AF527481

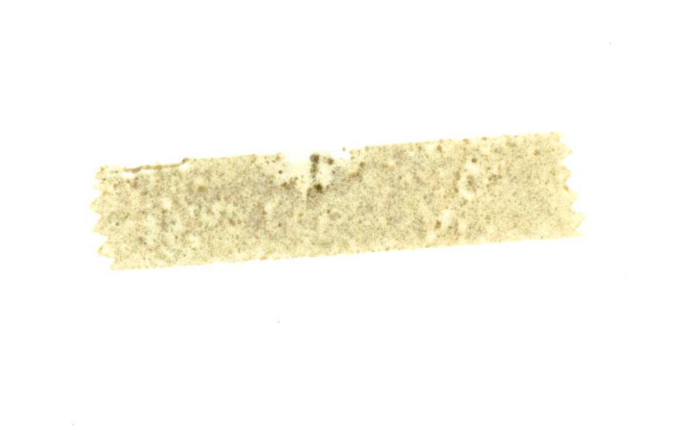

TEXTBOOK OF
SURGICAL GASTROENTEROLOGY

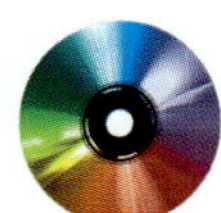

System requirements:

- Operating System—Windows Vista or above
- Web Browser—Internet Explorer 8 or above, Google Chrome and Mozilla Firefox
- Essential plugins—Java and PDF Reader
  - Facing problems in viewing content—it may be, your system does not have java enabled
  - You can test Java and download PDF reader by using the links from the help section of the **CD/DVD**

Accompanying **DVD-ROMs** is playable only in Computer and not in DVD player. CD/DVD has autorun function—it may take few seconds to load on your computer. If it does not work for you, then follow the steps below to access the contents manually:

- Click on my computer
- Select the CD/DVD drive and click open/explore—this will show list of files in the CD/DVD
- Find and double click file—"launch.html"

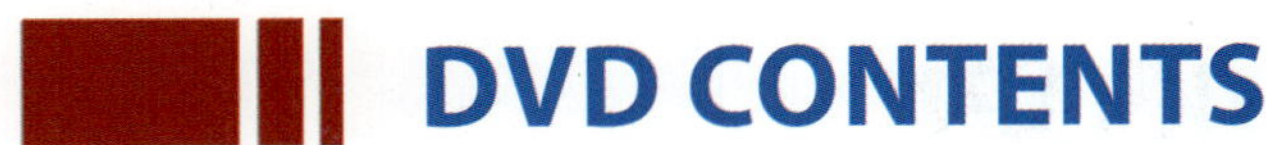

DVD CONTENTS

(Videos have no voice over)

TEXTBOOK OF
SURGICAL GASTROENTEROLOGY

VOLUME 1

Editor

PK Mishra

MS PhD
Professor
Govind Ballabh Pant Institute of
Postgraduate Medical Education and
Research
New Delhi, India

Foreword

Samiran Nundy

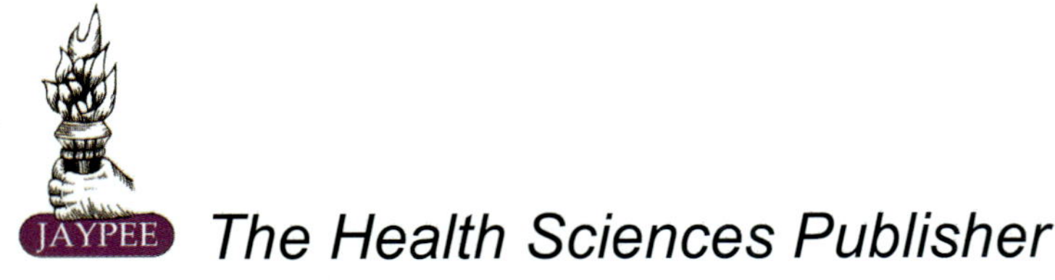

New Delhi | London | Philadelphia | Panama

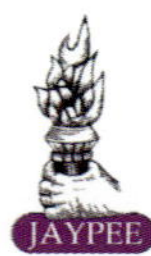

Jaypee Brothers Medical Publishers (P) Ltd.

Headquarters
Jaypee Brothers Medical Publishers (P) Ltd.
4838/24, Ansari Road, Daryaganj
New Delhi 110 002, India
Phone: +91-11-43574357
Fax: +91-11-43574314
E-mail: jaypee@jaypeebrothers.com

Overseas Offices
J.P. Medical Ltd.
83, Victoria Street, London
SW1H 0HW (UK)
Phone: +44-20 3170 8910
Fax: +44(0) 20 3008 6180
E-mail: info@jpmedpub.com

JP Medical Inc.
325, Chestnut Street
Suite 412
Philadelphia, PA 19106, USA
Phone: +1 267-519-9789
E-mail: support@jpmedus.com

Jaypee Brothers Medical Publishers (P) Ltd.
Bhotahity, Kathmandu, Nepal
Phone: +977-9741283608
E-mail: kathmandu@jaypeebrothers.com

Jaypee-Highlights Medical Publishers Inc.
City of Knowledge, Bld. 237, Clayton
Panama City, Panama
Phone: +1 507-301-0496
Fax: +1 507-301-0499
E-mail: cservice@jphmedical.com

Jaypee Brothers Medical Publishers (P) Ltd.
17/1-B, Babar Road, Block-B, Shaymali
Mohammadpur, Dhaka-1207
Bangladesh
Mobile: +08801912003485
E-mail: jaypeedhaka@gmail.com

Website: www.jaypeebrothers.com
Website: www.jaypeedigital.com

Inquiries for bulk sales may be solicited at: jaypee@jaypeebrothers.com

Textbook of Surgical Gastroenterology (2 Volumes)

First Edition: **2016**

ISBN: 978-93-5152-998-9

Printed at Replika Press Pvt. Ltd.

Dedicated to

My Parents

Contributors

Abhijit Chandra MS MCh
Professor and Head
Department of Surgical Gastroenterology
King George's Medical University
Lucknow, Uttar Pradesh, India

Adarsh Chaudhary MS
Chairman
Department of Gastrointestinal Surgery
Gastrointestinal Oncology and
Bariatric Surgery
Medanta Institute of Digestive and
Hepatobiliary Sciences
Medanta—The Medicity
Gurgaon, Haryana, India

Ahmad Jan MRCS(Ed) ChM (Ed)
Asian Bariatrics
Ahmedabad, Gujarat, India

Ajit Sewkani MS DNB
Associate Professor
Department of Surgical Gastroenterology
and Clinical Nutrition
Bhopal Memorial Hospital and Research Centre
Bhopal, Madhya Pradesh, India

AK Sarada MS FACS FICS FAIS
Director Professor (Surgery)
Lok Nayak Jai Prakash Narayan Hospital and
Maulana Azad Medical College
New Delhi, India

AK Singh MS DNB
Senior Advisor
Gastrointestinal Surgery
Army Hospital (R and R)
New Delhi, India

Amar Mukund
Associate Professor
Interventional Radiology
Institute of Liver and Biliary Sciences (ILBS)
New Delhi, India

Ankur Arora MD DNB FRCR EDiR
Associate Professor (Radiology)
Institute of Liver and Biliary Sciences
New Delhi, India

Ankur Garg MS MCh HPB
Surgery and Liver Transplantation
Institute of Liver and Biliary Sciences
New Delhi, India

Ankur Goyal MD
Assistant Professor
Department of Radiology
All India Institute of Medical Sciences (AIIMS)
New Delhi, India

Anshuman Ray MD (Anatomy)
Associate Professor
Department of Anatomy
RG Kar Medical College and Hospital
Kolkata, West Bengal, India

Anubhav Vindal MS
Professor
Department of Surgery
Lok Nayak Jai Prakash Narayan Hospital and
Maulana Azad Medical College
New Delhi, India

Anuj Sharma (VSM)
MS DNB MNAMS DNB (GI Surg) FAIS FICS
Liver and Pancreas Transplant Fellowship
(UCLA)
R and R Hospital
Armed Forces, New Delhi, India

Anurag Mishra MS DNB MNAMS
Asistant Professor
Lok Nayak Jai Prakash Narayan Hospital and
Maulana Azad Medical College
New Delhi, India

Archana Thakur MD
Director Professor
Department of Microbiology
Govind Ballabh Pant Institute of Postgraduate
Medical Education and Research
New Delhi, India

Arun Kumar Rathi MDRT
Director Professor
Department of Radiotherapy and Oncology
Lok Nayak Jai Prakash Narayan Hospital and
Maulana Azad Medical College
New Delhi, India

Arvind Kumar MS
Director
Institute of Robotic Surgery
Sir Ganga Ram Hospital
New Delhi, India

AS Soin MS FRCS(Glos) FRCS (Edin)
Chief
Medanta Institute of Liver Transplant and
Regenerative Medicine
Medanta—The Medicity
Gurgaon, Haryana, India

Ashok Kumar MS MCh FRCS FACS FAMS
Professor
Departments of Surgical Gastroenterology
Sanjay Gandhi Postgraduate Institute of
Medical Sciences (SGPGIMS)
Lucknow, Uttar Pradesh, India

Ashwin Rammohan MS FRCS MCh
Surgical Gastroenterolgy
Surgical Fellow in Liver Transplantation
Institute of Liver Surgery and Transplantation
National Foundation for Liver Research
Global Hospital, Chennai, Tamil Nadu, India

Asit Arora MS MCh
Assistent Professor
Institute of Liver and Biliary Sciences (ILBS)
New Delhi, India

Atul K Sharma (AVSM) MS DNB
Senior Consultant (Gastrointestinal)
Laparoscopic and Bariatric Surgery
Chairman
Institute of Gastrointestinal Sciences
Alchemist Hospitals
Panchkula, Chandigarh Tricity, India

Atul Sharma MD DM FRCPC
Department of Internal Medicine
Section of Hematology/Oncology
University of Manitoba and Professor of
Medical Oncology
Dr BR Ambedkar, Institute—Rotary Cancer
Hospital (Dr BRA-IRCH)
All India Institute of Medical Sciences (AIIMS)
New Delhi, India

Avinash Supe MS FICS DNBE FCPS DHA PGDME
MHPE (UIC) FIAGES FMAS FAIS Dean
Professor (GI Surgery)
GS Medical College
KEM Hospital
Mumbai, Maharashtra, India

Baljit Singh MD FICA
Director Professor
Department of Anesthesiology and
Intensive Care
Govind Ballabh Pant Institute of Postgraduate
Medical Education and Research
New Delhi, India

Belal Bin Asaf MS
Consultant
Institute of Robotic Surgery
Sir Ganga Ram Hospital
New Delhi, India

Benjamin Perakath MS FRCS (G)
Consultant
Dr Grays's Hospital
Elgin, Scotland, UK

Bhawna Sirohi
Consultant Medical Oncologist-GI and Breast Cancers
Head of Medical Oncology
Mazumdar Shaw Cancer Centre
Narayana Health
Bengaluru, Karnataka, India

Biju Pottakat MS MCh
Professor of Surgical Gastroenterology
Jawaharlal Institute of Postgraduate Medical Education and Research (JIPMER)
Puducherry, India

BK Jain MS FICS MNAMS
Professor of Surgery and Medical Superintendent
Guru Teg Bahadur (GTB) Hospital
New Delhi, India

Brundavan Nahak MS Mch
Consultant Surgical Gastroenterologist
Kalinga Hospital
Bhubaneshwar, Odisha, India

C Palanivelu
MS MCh DNB DSc PhD FACS FRCS (Hon) Ed
Director
Gem Institute of Gastroenterology and Laparoscopy
Chairman
Gem Hospital and Research Centre
Coimbatore, Tamil Nadu, India

Chintamani Godbole
Senior Resident
Department of Surgical Gastroenterology
Jaslok Hospital and Research Centre
Mumbai, Maharashtra, India

Chirag Shah
Department of Gastroenterology
Seth GS Medical College and King Edward Memorial (KEM) Hospital
Mumbai, Maharashtra, India

CS Naidu
Professor and Head
Department of Surgery
AFMC, Pune, Maharashtra, India

CS Pramesh MS FRCS
Chief, Division of Thoracic Surgery
Tata Memorial Hospital
Mumbai, Maharashtra, India

Cyriac Abby Philips MD DM Fellow Hepatology
Institute of Liver and Biliary Sciences (ILBS)
New Delhi, India

D Nageshwar Reddy
MD DM DSc FAMS FRCP FASGE FACG MWGO
Chairman
Asian Institute of Gastroenterology
Hyderabad, Telangana, India

Debasis Mishra MBBS MD DM
Department of Gatroenterology
IMS and SUM Hospital
Bhubaneswar, Odisha, India

Deborshi Sharma MS MRCS Edin
Department of Surgery
Lady Hardinge Medical College and Associated
Ram Manohar Lohia Hospital
New Delhi, India

Deepak Govil MS PhD
Senior Consultant (GI Surgery and Oncology)
Indraprastha Appollo Hospital
New Delhi, India

DK Sharma MS MCh
Head
Department of Surgery
Udaipur, Rajasthan, India

Dronacharya Routh
Consultant GI Surgeon
Command Hospital
West Bengal, India

Durgatosh Pandey MS MCh
Consultant
Thoracic and Surgical Oncology
Max Superspecialty Hospital
New Delhi, India

George Karimunadackal MCh MRCS
Professor
Tata Memorial Hospital
Mumbai, Maharashtra, India

Girish K Pande
MBBS MS PhD FRCS Eng FRCS Edin FRACS
Specialist HPB and Upper GI Surgery
Launceston General Hospital
Charles Street, Launceston, Tasmania 7250, Australia

Gomathy Narasimhan MS ASTS Fellowship
Senior Consultant
Transplant Surgeon Institute of Liver Disease and Transplantation
Global Hospital and Health City
India and National Foundation for Liver Research, India

Gourdas Choudhuri
MD DM FAMS FICP FACG FRCPI
Director and Head
Department of Gastroenterology and Hepatobiliary Sciences
Fortis Memorial Research Institute
Gurgaon, Haryana, India

Govind K Makharia
MD DM DNB (Gastroenterology)
Additional Professor
All India Institute of Medical Sciences (AIIMS)
New Delhi, India

Harpal S Dhaliwal MD DM
Department of Gastroenterology
Postgraduate Institute of Medical Education and Research
Chandigarh, India

Harsh Shah MS MCh
Consultant Gastrointestinal Surgery and Liver Transplant
Gangaram Institute of Postgraduate Medical Education and Research (GRIPMER)
New Delhi, India

Himanshu Yadav
Department of Surgical Gastronterology
Sanjay Gandhi Postgraduate Institute of Medical Sciences (SGPGIMS)
Lucknow, Uttar Pradesh, India

Hirdaya H Nag MS
Professor of Surgical Gastroenterology
Govind Ballabh Pant Institute of Postgraduate Medical Education and Research
New Delhi, India

Ho-Seong Han MD
Department of Surgery
Seoul National University
Bundang Hospital
Seongnam, Korea

Indira Malik MD
Assistant Professor
Department of Anesthesiology and Intensive Care
Govind Ballabh Pant Institute of Postgraduate Medical Education and Research
New Delhi, India

Jagdish Chander MS FICLS FICS
Director
Institute of Minimal Access Surgery
Jaypee Hospital
Noida, Uttar Pradesh, India

Jayanth Reddy MCh MRCS
Associate Consultant of Surgical Gastroenterology
Minimal Access and Bariatric Surgery (BGS)
Global Hospital
Bengaluru, Karnataka, India

JK Banerjee MBBS MS DNB
Post Doctoral Training in GI Surgery
Command Hospital
Pune, Maharashtra, India

John Joseph MD DM
Center for Liver and Biliary Sciences
Indraprastha Apollo Hospital
New Delhi, India

Joseph George MS Mch
Rajagiri Hospital
Kerala, India

Kamal Kataria
Assistant Professor
Department of Surgery
Guru Teg Bahadur Hospital (GTB) and
University College of Medical Sciences (UCMS)
New Delhi, India

Kamal Yadav MS FMAS
Lady Hardinge Medical College and
Associated
Ram Manohar Lohia Hospital
New Delhi, India

Kamlesh Kumar MS
Senior Resident
Department of Surgery
All India Institute of Medical Sciences (AIIMS)
New Delhi, India

Kapileshwar Vijay MS DNB GI Surgery
Santokba Durlabhji Memorial Hospital
Jaipur, Rajasthan, India

Kaushal Madan MD DM
Consultant, Director
Gastroenterology Services
Artemis Hospital
Gurgaon, Haryana, India

Kishore GS Bharathy
Additional Professor
Surgical Gastroenterolgy
Institute of Liver and Biliary Sciences (ILBS)
New Delhi, India

Kishore Singh MDRT MNAMS
Director Professor
Department of Radiotherapy and Oncology
Lok Nayak Jai Prakash Narayan Hospital and
Maulana Azad Medical College
New Delhi, India

KJ Singh
Professor and Head
Department of Gastrointestinal Surgery
Command Hospital
Lucknow, Uttar Pradesh, India

Kunal Parasar MS MCh
Senior Resident
Department of Surgical Gastroenterology
Govind Ballabh Pant Institute of
Postgraduate Medical Education and
Research (GIPMER)
New Delhi, India

Kuriko Kudo PhD
Telemedicine Development Center of Asia
Kyushu Hospital, Fukoka, Japan

Mahendra Narwaria MS FICS FIAGES FALS
Director
Asian Bariatrics
Ahmedabad, Gujarat, India

Mahesh Goel MS
Associate Professor
Gastrointestinal and Hepato-Pancreato-
Biliary Service
Department of Surgical Oncology
Tata Memorial Centre
Mumbai, Maharashtra, India

Manav Wadhawan MD DM
Center for Liver and Biliary Sciences
Indraprastha Apollo Hospital
New Delhi, India

Manish Suresh Bhandare
MCh (Surgical Oncology)
Fellow in Gastrointestinal and Hepato-
Pancreato-Biliary Oncology
Tata Memorial Hospital
Mumbai, Maharashtra, India

Manoj Gupta MS
Associate Consultant
Jaypee Hospital
Noida, Uttar Pradesh, India

Manoj Kumar Sharma MD DM
Associate Professor
Department of Hepatology
Institute of Liver and Biliary Sciences
New Delhi, India

Masao Tanaka MD PhD FACS
Chief Director
Shimonoseki City Hospital
President Emeritus, Japan Pancreas Society
President, Asian-Oceanic Pancreatic
Association
Professor Emeritus
Kyushu University
Fukuoka 812-8582, Japan

Mihir K Mohapatra
Professor
Department of Surgical Gastroenterology
SCB Medical College
Cuttack, Odisha, India

Mohamed Rela MS FRCS
Director
Institute of Liver Disease and Transplantation
Global Hospital and Health City
National Foundation for Liver Research, India

Mohammad Ibrarullah MCh FACS
Senior Consultant
Surgical Gastroenterology
Apollo Hospitals
Bhubaneswar, Odisha, India

Mohammed A Nayeem MS MCH
Consultant Liver Transplant Surgeon
Indraprastha Apollo Hospital
New Delhi, India

Mohan N MS DNB
Consultant Surgeon
Department of Surgical Gastroenterology
Meenakshi Mission Hospital and
Research Centre
Madurai, Tamil Nadu, India

Mohd Qaleem Fellow DNB
Department of GI Surgery
Indraprastha Apollo Hospital
New Delhi, India

Monika Gupta MS MCh
Consultant
Surgical Gastroenterology and Minimally
Invasive Surgery
Soni Hospital
Jaipur, Rajasthan, India

MS Ansari MS Mch DNB
Additional Professor
Department of Urology
Sanjay Gandhi Postgraduate Institute of
Medical Sciences (SGPGIMS)
Lucknow, Uttar Pradesh, India

N Ananthakrishnan MS FRCS (Eng.) FRCS (Ed.)
FRCS (Glasg.) MNAMS FIMSA FAMS FICS FACS FACG
Professor of Surgery
Mahatma Gandhi Medical College and
Research Institute
Puducherry, India

Namrata Singh
Chief Dietician
Department of Gastroenterology and
Nutrition
All India Institute of Medical Sciences (AIIMS)
New Delhi, India

Naoki Nakashima MD PhD
Telemedicine Development Center of Asia
and Medical Information Center
Kyushu University Hospital, Fukuoka, Japan

Naresh Jangir MS
Senior Resident
Department of GI Surgery
Fortis Hospital
New Delhi, India

Neeraj Bhateja MS DNB GI Surg
Department of GI Surgery
Fortis Hospital
Jaipur, Rajasthan, India

Neeraj Goel MS MCh
Consultant
Max Hospital
New Delhi, India

Neerav Goyal
DNB (Gen Surgery) DNB (GI Surgery) MNAMS
Senior Consultant
Centre for Liver and Biliary Sciences
Indraprastha Apollo Hospital
New Delhi, India

Nikhil Aggarwal MS MCh
Assistant Professor
Institute of Liver and Biliary Sciences (ILBS)
New Delhi, India

Nikhil Gupta MS MCh
Consultant
Rajiv Gandhi Cancer Institute
New Delhi, India

Nilesh Doctor MS DNB FRCS
Consultant Surgeon
Department of Surgical Gastroenterology
Jaslok Hospital and Research Centre
Mumbai, Maharashtra, India

Nilesh Patil MS MCh
Fellow, HPB Surgery
Department of HPB Surgery and
Liver Transplant
Indraprastha Apollo Hospital
New Delhi, India

Nitesh Patidar MS MCh
Senior Resident
Department of Urology
Sanjay Gandhi Postgraduate Institute of
Medical Sciences (SGPGIMS)
Lucknow, Uttar Pradesh, India

Noushif M MCh
Department of Surgical Gastroenterology
King George's Medical University
Lucknow, Uttar Pradesh, India

NS Balaji
Consultant Surgeon
Esophagogastric and Bariatric Surgery
University Hospitals North Midlands
Stoke on Trent, UK

P Senthilnathan MS DNB MRCS (Ed) DNB (GI Surgery) FMAS FACS
Consultant Surgical Gastroenterologist
Division of Minimally invasive and
HPB Surgery
Gem Hospital and Research Centre
Coimbatore, Tamil Nadu, India

Paari Vijayraghavan MS DNB MCh
Consultant
Miot International Hospital
Chennai, Tamil Nadu, India

Palanippan Ramanathan MS MCh
Surgical Oncology
All India Institute of Medical Sciences (AIIMS)
New Delhi, India

Pankaj Agarwal MBBS DNB
Consultant
Max Hospital, New Delhi, India

Pankaj Kumar Garg MS
Department of Surgery
University College of Medical Sciences
(UCMS) and Guru Teg Bahadur (GTB) Hospital
New Delhi, India

Pankaj Sharma MS
Senior Consultant
Laparoscopic, Bariatric and GI Surgery
Sri Balaji Action Hospital
New Delhi, India

Pankaj Tyagi MD DM
Consultant
Jaypee Hospital
Noida, Uttar Pradesh, India

Patta Radhakrishna MS MCh
Chief Surgical Gastroenterologist
SRM Institute for Medical Sciences (SIMS)
Chennai, Tamil Nadu, India

Pavan Addala MS
Senior Registrar
Department of Surgical GE
Apollo Hospitals
Chennai, Tamil Nadu, India

Pawan Rawal MD DM
Senior Consultant
Fortis hospital
Gurgaon, Haryana, India

Peush Sahni MS Phd
Professor and Head
Department of Surgical Gastroenterology
All India Institute of Medical Sciences (AIIMS)
New Delhi, India

PK Garg
Department of Surgery
Guru Teg Bahadur (GTB) Hospital and
University College of Medical Sciences
(UCMS), New Delhi, India

PK Mishra MS PhD
Professor
Govind Ballabh Pant Institute of
Postgraduate Medical Education and
Research
New Delhi, India

Poonam Narang MD
Director Professor
Department of Radiology
GB Pant Institute of Medical Education
and Research
New Delhi, India

Pradeep Jain MS MCh
Director
Gastrointestinal Surgery,
Laparoscopy and Oncology
Sri Balaji Action Hospital
New Delhi, India

Prakash Jain MS
Consultant Surgeon
Mercy Hospital
Kolkata, West Bengal, India

Pramod Kumar Garg MD DM
Professor
Department of Gastroenterology
All India Institute of Medical Sciences (AIIMS)
New Delhi, India

Praneeth Moka MD DM
Department of Gastroenterology
All India Institute of Medical Sciences (AIIMS)
New Delhi, India

Prasad Thotton Veedu MD
Department of Radiology
All India Institute of Medical Sciences (AIIMS)
New Delhi, India

Priya Ranjan
Classified Specialist
GI Surgery
Command Hospital
Kolkata, West Bengal, India

Puneet Puri MS Mch
Department of Surgical Gastroenterology
Sanjay Gandhi Postgraduate Institute of
Medical Sciences (SGPGIMS)
Lucknow, Uttar Pradesh, India

Punit Singla MS DNB (GI Surgery)
Liver Transplant Surgeon
Fortis Hospital
Gurgaon, Haryana, India

Purak Mishra MS
Department of GI Surgery
Indraprastha Apollo Hospital
New Delhi, India

R Kalayarasan MS DNB MCh
Assistant Professor
Department of Surgical Gastroenterology
Jawaharlal Institute of Postgraduate
Medical Education and Research (JIPMER)
Puducherry, India

R Surendran MS MCh DSc
Director
HPB Surgery and Transplant
Miot International Hospital
Chennai, Tamil Nadu, India

RA Sastry MS FRCS (Glasg)
Professor of Surgical Gastroenterology
Krishna Institute of Medical Sciences
Hyderabad, Telangana, India

Raghavendra Raja
Kokilaben Dhirubhai Ambani Hospital
Mumbai, Maharashtra, India

Rajan Chaudhry AVSM VSM PHS
Air Marshal, Director General
Medical Service (Air)

Rajan Saxena
Professor and Head
Department of Surgical Gastroenterology and Liver Transplant
Sanjay Gandhi Postgraduate Institute of Medical Sciences (SGPGIMS)
Lucknow, Uttar Pradesh, India

Rajesh Bhojwani MS MCh
Consultant
Surgical Gastroenterolgist, Laparoscopic and Bariatric Surgeon
Santokba Durlabhji Memorial Hospital
Jaipur, Rajasthan, India

Rajesh Panwar MS Mch
Assistant Professor
Department of GI Surgery
All India Institute of Medical Sciences (AIIMS)
New Delhi, India

Rajesh Rajalingam MS MCh
Transplant Fellowship, HPB and Transplant Surgeon Global Hospital
Chennai, Tamil Nadu, India

Rajinder Parshad
Professor
Department of Surgical Disciplines
All India Institute of Medical Sciences (AIIMS)
New Delhi, India

Rajneesh Kumar Singh MS MCh
Additional Professor
Department of Surgical Gastroenterology
Sanjay Gandhi Postgraduate Institute of Medical Sciences (SGPGIMS)
Lucknow, Uttar Pradesh, India

Raju Sharma MD
Professor
Department of Radiology
All India Institute of Medical Sciences (AIIMS)
New Delhi, India

Rakesh Kochhar MD DM
Professor
Department of Gastroenterology
Postgraduate Institute of Medical Education and Research
Chandigarh, India

Rakesh Kumar Singh MS Mch
Department of Surgical Gastroenterology
Sanjay Gandhi Postgraduate Institute of Medical Sciences (SGPGIMS)
Lucknow, Uttar Pradesh, India

Rakesh Kumar MD PhD
Professor
Department of Nuclear Medicine
All India Institute of Medical Sciences (AIIMS)
New Delhi, India

Rakesh Rai MS FRCS (UK) MD (Newcastle) CCST (UK) ASTS Fellow
Senior Consultant Transplant Surgeon
Fortis Hospital
Mumbai, Maharashtra, India

Rakhi Maiwall MD DM
Associate Professor
Institute of Liver and Biliary Science (ILBS)
New Delhi, India

Rambha Pandey MD
Assistant Professor
Dr BR Ambedkar Institute—Rotary Cancer Hospital (Dr BRA-IRCH)
All India Institute of Medical Sciences (AIIMS)
New Delhi, India

Ramesh Ardhnari MS MCh FRCS
Senior Consultant
Meenakshi Mission Hospital and Research Centre
Madurai, Tamil Nadu, India

Ramkrishna Prabhu MS
Department of Surgical Gastroenterology
Seth GS Medical College
Mumbai, Maharashtra, India

RK Saran MD
Department of Pathology
Govind Ballabh Pant Institute of Postgraduate Medical Education and Research (GIPMER), New Delhi, India

Rohin Mittal MS
Consultant
Surgical Gastroenterology
Christian Medical College
Vellore, Tamil Nadu, India

S Rajesh MD PDCC
Assistant Professor
Department of Radiology
Institute of Liver and Biliary Sciences (ILBS)
New Delhi, India

S Sudhindran MS FRCS
Consultant Surgeon
HPB and Transplant
Amrita Institute, Kochi, Kerala, India

Sabita Jiwnani MS MRCS
Tata Memorial Hospital
Mumbai, Maharashtra, India

Saket Kumar MS
Department of Surgical Gastroenterology
King George's Medical University
Lucknow, Uttar Pradesh, India

Sanjay Govil MS FRCS
Senior Consultant
HPB Surgery and Liver Transplantation
Institute of Liver Surgery and Transplantation
National Foundation for Liver Research
Global Hospital, Chennai, Tamil Nadu, India

Sanjay Gupta MS
Head
Department of Surgery
University College of Medical Sciences
New Delhi, India

Sanjay Nagral MS
Consultant Hepatobiliary Surgeon
Department of Surgical Gastroenterology
Jaslok Fortis and Shushrusha Hospital
Mumbai Honorary Surgeon
KB Bhabha Municipal General Hospital

Sanjay Singh Negi MS MCh FEBS
Director
HPB Surgery and Liver Transplantation
BLK Superspecialty Hospital
New Delhi, India

Sanjoy Mandal MS DNB MRCS MCh
Director and Senior Consultant
Department of GI Surgery
Medica Superspecialty Hospital
Kolkata, West Bengal, India

Saroj K Sinha MD DM
Department of Gastroenterology
Postgraduate Institute of Medical Education and Research (PGIMER)
Chandigarh, India

Satish B Dharap
Professor
LTM Medical College and LTM General Hospital
Mumbai, Maharashtra, India

Satya Prasad Samantaray
Assistant Professor
Department of Surgical Gastroenterology
SCB Medical College
Cuttack, Odisha, India

Satyajit Godhi MS MCh
Senior Resident
Surgical Gastroenterology
Govind Ballabh Pant Institute of Postgraduate Medical Education and Research
New Delhi, India

Saurabh Kedia MD DM
All India Institute of Medical Sciences (AIIMS)
New Delhi, India

Saurabh Singhal
Junior Resident
Department of Surgical Disciplines
All India Institute of Medical Sciences (AIIMS)
New Delhi, India

Savio George Barreto
Consultant
Department of Gastrointestinal Surgery
Gastrointestinal Oncology and Bariatric Surgery
Medanta Institute of Digestive and
Hepatobiliary Sciences
Medanta—The Medicity
Gurgaon, Haryana, India

Sellam Karunanithi MD
Department of Nuclear Medicine
All India Institute of Medical Sciences (AIIMS)
New Delhi, India

Shagun Misra MD
Lecturer
Department of Radiation Oncology
Tata Memorial Hospital
Parel, Mumbai, Maharashtra, India

Shailesh V Shrikhande MS MD FRCS
Chief Gastrointestinal and Hepato-Pancreato-Biliary Service
Department of Surgical Oncology
Tata Memorial Centre
Mumbai, Maharashtra, India

Shaleen Agarwal MS Mch
Senior Consultant
Centre for Liver and Biliary Sciences
Indraprastha Apollo Hospital
New Delhi, India

Shaleen Kumar MD
Professor
Department of Radiotherapy
Sanjay Gandhi Postgraduate Institute of
Medical Sciences (SGPGIMS)
Lucknow, Uttar Pradesh, India

Shalimar MD DM
Associate Professor (Gastroenterology)
All India Institute of Medical Sciences (AIIMS)
New Delhi, India

Shivanand Gamanagatti MD
Additional Professor of Radiology
All India Institute of Medical Sciences (AIIMS)
New Delhi, India

Shivaram Prasad Singh MD DM
(Past President), ISG
Secretary General SAASL
Head, Department of Gastroenterology
SCB Medical College
Cuttack, Odisha, India

Shivendra Singh MS MCh
Head (Gastrointestinal Oncology)
Rajiv Gandhi Cancer Institute
New Delhi, India
Director Professor
Department of Radiology
Govind Ballabh Pant Institute of
Postgraduate Medical Education and Research
New Delhi, India

Shivendra Singh MS MCh
Head (Gastrointestinal Oncology)
Rajiv Gandhi Cancer Institute
New Delhi, India

Shivraj Bahadur Singh DM
HPB and Transplant Fellow
Department of Surgical Gastroenterology
and Liver Transplantation
Sir Ganga Ram Hospital
New Delhi, India

Shobna J Bhatia
Head
Department of Gastroenterology
Seth GS Medical College and King Edward
Memorial (KEM) Hospital
Mumbai, Maharashtra, India

Shuzi Shimizu MD PhD
Department Endoscopic Diagnostics and
Therapeutics and Telemedicine Development
Center of Asia
Kyushu University Hospital, 3-1-1 Maidashi,
Higashi-ku,
Fukuoka 812-8582, Japan

Shyamkumar N Keshava
Department of Radiology
Christian Medical College
Vellore, Tamil Nadu, India

Siddharth Srivastava MD DM
Professor
Department of Gastroenterology
Govind Ballabh Pant Institute of
Postgraduate Medical Education and
Research
New Delhi, India

SK Acharya MD DM
Head
Department of Gastroenterology
All India Institute of Medical Sciences (AIIMS)
New Delhi, India

SK Sarin MD DM
Senior Professor and Head
Department of Hepatology
Director
Institute of Liver and Biliary Science (ILBS)
Adjunct Professor
Molecular Medicine
Jawahar Lal Nehru University, New Delhi
Honorary Professor
Jawaharlal Nehru Center for Advanced
Scientific Research
New Delhi, India

Sreenivas
Additional Professor of Biostatistics
All India Institute of Medical Sciences (AIIMS)
New Delhi, India

Subhash Gupta MS FRCS
Chief Liver Transplant and HPB Surgery
Director Centre for Liver and Biliary Sciences
Indraprastha Apollo Hospital
New Delhi, India

Subhash Mishra DNB
Indraprastha Appollo Hospital
New Delhi, India

Subodh Varshney MS DNB MNAMS FRCS
Professor and Head
Department of Surgical Gastroenterology
and Clinical Nutrition
Bhopal Memorial Hospital and Research Centre
Bhopal, Madhya Pradesh, India

Sudeep R Shah MS DNB FRCS (Edin)
Consultant GI HPB and Liver Transplant Surgeon
PD Hinduja Hospital
Mumbai, Maharashtra, India

S Sudhindran MS FRCS
Consultant Surgeon (HPB and Transplant)
Amrita Institute
Kochi, Kerala, India

Suhar Kumar MS DNB
Resident
Rajiv Gandhi Cancer Institute
New Delhi, India

Sujoy Pal MS DNB MCh
Professor
Department of GI Surgery and Liver
Transplantation
All India Institute of Medical Sciences (AIIMS)
New Delhi, India

Sukanta Ray MS MCh
Professor of Surgical Gastroenterology
School of Digestive and Liver Disease
Institute of Postgraduate Medical Education
and Research
Kolkata, West Bengal, India

Sundeep Jain MS MCh
Senior Consultant
Gastrointestinal, HPB, Laparoscopic and
Bariatric Surgery
Fortis-Escorts Hospital
Jaipur, Rajasthan, India

Sundeep Singh Saluja MS MCh
Professor of Surgical Gastroenterology
Govind Ballabh Pant Institute of Postgraduate
Medical Education and Research
New Delhi, India

Sunil Kumar Gupta MD DM
Oncology Senior Consultant and
Chief of Head and Neck Medical Services
Rajiv Gandhi Cancer Institute and Research Centre
New Delhi, India

Sunil Kumar Puri MD FICRI
Director-Professor and Head (Radiology)
Govind Ballabh Pant Institute of Postgraduate Medical Education and Research
New Delhi, India

Sunil T MS Mch
Assistant Professor
Department of Surgical Gastroenterology
Sanjay Gandhi Postgraduate Institute of Medical Sciences (SGPGIMS)
Lucknow, Uttar Pradesh, India

Supriyo Ghatak MS MCh
Consultant HPB and GI Surgeon
Calcutta Medical Research Institute
Kolkata, West Bengal, India

Sushmita Nitin Bhatnagar MS MCh
Professor, Unit Head
Department of Pediatric Surgery
Baijerbai Hospital for Children
Mumbai, Maharashtra, India

Swarupa Mitra MD
Senior Consultant, Radiation Oncologist
Rajiv Gandhi Cancer Institute
New Delhi, India

TK Chattopadhyay ???
Senior Professor and Head
Department of Surgical Gastroenterolgy
Institute of Liver and Biliary Sciences (ILBS)
New Delhi, India

TP Elamurugan D Ortho MS DNB MNAMS
Assistant Professor
Jawaharlal Institute of Postgraduate Medical Education and Research (JIPMER)
Puducherry, India

Uday Somashekar MS DNB
Assistant Professor
Jabalpur Medical College
Jabalpur, Madhya Pradesh, India

Umesh Kapil
Professor
Public Health Nutrition
Human Nutrition Unit
All India Institute of Medical Sciences (AIIMS)
New Delhi, India

V Baskaran MS PhD FACS
Department of Surgical Gastroenterology
Minimal Access and Bariatric Surgery
Madras Institute of Orthopedics and Traumatology (MIOT) International Hospital
Chennai, Tamil Nadu, India

Vaageesh BG MS MCh
Senior Resident
Govind Ballabh Pant Institute of Postgraduate Medical Education and Research
New Delhi, India

Vaibhav Varshney MS MCh
Senior Resident
Department of Surgical Gastroenterology
Govind Ballabh Pant Institute of Postgraduate Medical Education and Research
New Delhi, India

Vedavyas Mohapatra MS
Senior Resident
Department of Surgery
SCB Medical College
Cuttack, Odisha, India

Venkatramani Sitaram MS DNB FRCS
Professor and Head
Department of HPB Surgery
Christian Medical College
Vellore, Tamil Nadu, India

Venu Madhav Thumma
MS MRCSEd DNB (Surg Gastro)
Reader
Department of Surgical Gastroenterology
Nizams Institute of Medical Sciences
Hyderabad, Telangana, India

Vibha Verma
MS DNB (General Surgry) DNB (GI surgery) MRCS (Edn)
Consultant Liver Transplant and HPB Surgery
Kokilaben Dhirubhai Ambani Hospital
Mumbai, Maharashtra, India

Vijay Vohra MD
Chairman
Liver Transplant Gastrointestinal Anaesthesia and Critical Care
Medanta—The Medicity
Gurgaon, Haryana, India

Vikas Gupta MS MCh
Department of Surgery
Postgraduate Institute of Medical Education and Research
Chandigarh, India

Vikram Chaudhary MS
Gastrointestinal and Hepato-Pancreato-Biliary Service
Department of Surgical Oncology
Tata Memorial Centre
Mumbai, Maharashtra, India

Vikram Kate MS FRCS (Eng.) FRCS (Ed.) FRCS (Glasg.) PhD (SGE) MAMS FIMSA FACS FACG MFST (Ed.)
Professor
Department of General Surgery and Surgical Gastroenterology
Jawaharlal Institute of Postgraduate Medical Education and Research
Puducherry, India

Eppa Vimlakar Reddy
Consultant Surgeon
Department of Surgical Gastroenterology
Meenakshi Mission Hospital and Research Centre
Madurai, Tamil Nadu, India

Vinay Gaikwad MS
Consultant
GI and HPB Surgical Oncologist
Artemis Health Institute
Gurgaon, Haryana, India

Vinay Kapoor FRCS FACS
Professor of Surgical Gastroenterology
Sanjay Gandhi Postgraduate Institute of Medical Sciences (SGPGIMS)
Lucknow, Uttar Pradesh, India

Vinay Kumaran MS Mch
Consultant and Head
Liver Transplant and HPB Surgery
Kokilaben Dhirubhai Ambani Hospital
Mumbai, Maharashtra, India

Vineet Ahuja MD DM
Addditional Professor
Department of Gastroenterology
All India Institute of Medical Sciences (AIIMS)
New Delhi, India

Vineeta Goel MBBS DNB
Consultant Radiation Oncologist
Max Superspecialty Hospital
New Delhi, India

Vinu Moses
Department of Radiology
Christian Medical College
Vellore, Tamil Nadu, India

Vishal Gupta MS MCh
Associate Professor
Department of Surgical Gastroenterology
King George's Medical University
Lucknow, Uttar Pradesh, India

Vivek Goel MS
Consultant
Department of Laparoscopy and GI Surgery
Sri Balaji Action Hospital
New Delhi, India

Vivek Mangla MS MCh
Consultant
Gastroenterology and Liver Transplantation
Sir Ganga Ram Hospital
New Delhi, India

Yasuaki Antoku PhD
Telemedicine Development Center of Asia and Medical Information Center
Kyushu University Hospital
Fukuoka, Japan

Yogesh Kumar Sarin MS MCh
Director Professor and Medical Superintendent
Lok Nayak Jai Prakash Narayan Hospital and Maulana Azad Medical College
New Delhi, India

Yoshiko Houkabe MD PhD
Kyushu University
Fukuoka, Japan

Zaheer MD DNB Gastroenterology
Consultant Gastroenterologist
Asian Institute of Gastroenterology
Hyderabad, Telangana, India

Editorial Board

Foreword

Thirty years ago, general surgeons did almost all abdominal operations including those for hernia, hydrocele, as well as for diseases of the stomach and intestines. At this time, medical gastroenterology was making rapid strides by using diagnostic and therapeutic techniques driven by the advent of fiberoptic endoscopy and advances in imaging modalities. This opened up whole new challenges such as the management of massive variceal bleeding and obstructive jaundice, but there was no complementary specialty of surgical gastroenterology. This meant that the more complex procedures like portosystemic shunts and liver and pancreatic resections received little attention because they were done infrequently, demanded a lot of extra time and effort and, unfortunately, were consequently accompanied by high morbidity and mortality rates. In the late 1980s, after a rather hesitant and uncertain beginning, a few stalwarts set up separate departments of surgical gastroenterology in Trivandrum, Chennai, Lucknow and Delhi, which confined themselves to dealing with complex gastrointestinal problems, which were neglected by general surgeons, and these have since spawned over thirty others all over the country. With the advent of liver transplantation, this specialty has now acquired a certain glamour as well as extensive coverage in the media. Consequently, in 2015, surgical gastroenterology has now become the most sought after subspecialty for doctors who have just completed their Master of Surgery qualification and is, fortunately, attracting the brightest and best.

Unfortunately, there are very few textbooks which can guide the neophyte trainees in this field. Professor PK Mishra, who is a member of one of the elite and pioneering departments in the specialty, and who, incidentally, did a good PhD at All India Institute of Medical Sciences (AIIMS) under my guidance, has gathered together nearly all of India's luminaries in this comparatively new specialty and succeeded in producing a reference book which will be a sine qua non for all who venture into this exciting field.

There are introductory chapters on the approach to patients, imaging and chemoradiotherapy, followed by detailed descriptions of the management of disorders of different organs from the esophagus to the anal canal, and a section on liver transplantation. I particularly enjoyed the last 'Miscellaneous' section which deals with upper GI bleeding, robotics, tumor markers and finally ethics in surgery.

The choice of topics has been imaginative and the writing simple, informative and helpful.

I have little doubt that the book will be a success and go into many subsequent editions.

Samiran Nundy
Dean
Ganga Ram Institute for
Postgraduate Education and Research
New Delhi, India

Preface

I feel so relieved to be writing this preface, now that this massive project is near completion. Serendipity is sometimes more important than the noble motivation later ascribed to an act. The origin of the book had a bit of both. When I was approached by M/s Jaypee Brothers Medical Publishers (P) Ltd, for this book, I was in a frame of mind to strive to return to the profession a bit of what I gained from it. Fortunately or otherwise, I had no idea as to what it actually involved.

Surgical gastroenterology is relatively a new superspecialization which has established itself in the last three decades. Most of the work in surgical gastroenterology was done by general surgeons with various other responsibilities. Evolution in gastroenterology pushed the requirement of specialized care for this group of patients. Resection of liver, surgery for portal hypertension, surgery of pancreas and esophagus, for example, required specialized training and dedicated care. The challenge was taken up by a few stalwarts like Professors Samiran Nundy, Aranya, Kaushik, Wig and Chatterjee in the North and Professors Rangabashyam, Khanduri and Anantkrishnan in the South. Thanks to their efforts, surgical gastroenterology has not only become an established specialty but also, it is the most wanted one for the residents completing their MS (General Surgery). I was fortunate to train under Professor Nundy, All India Institute of Medical Sciences (AIIMS), and have been at Govind Ballabh Pant Postgraduate Institute of Medical Education and Research for last many years. GB Pant is an established pioneering superspecialty academic institute for training MCh and DM residents.

In the last many years, enormous experience has been gathered in various institutes working in this field in India. However, we are still dependent mainly on textbooks from the West. The available textbooks in surgical gastroenterology are not comprehensive, do not adequately discuss some of the diseases which are specifically relevant in the Asian context and do not have Indian protocols for therapy and follow-up even for diseases which are commonly seen by us. I, therefore, worked to compile a book, which could serve as a textbook for the students of surgical gastroenterology and could also be of help to the practicing surgeons and the gastroenterologists.

With this in mind, I got together a team of editors. We chose the authors and chapters to be covered with lots of deliberation. Most authors of the chapters are surgeons with vast experience and are well known in their field of expertise. Eminent gastroenterologists have also written some chapters, as required. All the chapters have been reviewed to add some balance in the coverage. We have also included several chapters with clinical approach which are not usually covered in other textbooks. A chapter on statistics was especially included as this knowledge is now essential for interpreting or publishing research articles. We also incorporated some chapters on robotics and telemedicine to acquaint our readers with critical knowledge in these important areas. An entire section on liver transplantation was envisaged which has now become an important and established specialization by itself. Knowledge about radiology and antibiotics relevant to our practice has been included. The last chapter in the book had to be on ethics. While teaching ethics may not by itself be a remedy for all ills, it certainly promotes responsibility, integrity and accountability in medical practice. I wish that the students undertake medical learning and research guided by ethical principles. Ethics is the essence of being human and I believe that every human effort is wasted, if it is ethically incorrect.

The idea of the book was to be a comprehensive textbook of surgical gastroenterology. When we had started, I wished to bring together a complete volume that had all the essential knowledge for a person being initiated into surgical gastroenterology. I did not realize initially that it was such a colossal project. With the full load of clinical and teaching duties, editing such a volume was really a tough task. Time delays took such a toll that at times I felt like shelving the project. We had to reject or redo many chapters. Many other chapters had to be left out. It was the effort of the editorial team, residents, and colleagues and of several authors of the book that kept me on course. I sincerely trust that the book would be a single point reference book, to the residents, gastroenterologists and surgeons.

No textbook in the present day can have all the information a person seeks. In the fast-changing medical world, readers should treat this compilation as a starter pack. Authors have worked hard on these chapters and the chapters have also been reviewed by peers. Still, there may be many shortcomings and there may be many aspects that are not up to the desirable level of discussion. I fully realize that some of the pronouncements in the ensuing chapters may already be getting modified or even outdated. A textbook takes almost two years to come to the print. I offer this to you with no apologies. I request all the readers to mail me their opinions so that the shortcomings may be corrected in the subsequent editions. It is my sincere hope that with your help the work will raise its level even further in the subsequent editions. Thank you readers for choosing the book.

PK Mishra
surgeonmishra@yahoo.com

Acknowledgments

It is a privilege to thank all those who helped me complete this work. First of all, I thank my publishers M/s Jaypee Brothers Medical Publishers (P) Ltd, New Delhi, India, for choosing me to do this work. On behalf of Jaypee, Shri Jitendar P Vij (Group Chairman), Mr Ankit Vij (Group President), Mr Tarun Duneja (Director-Publishing), Mr KK Raman (Production Manager), Mr Subrata Adhikary (Commissioning Editor) and Mr Mohit Bhargava (Production Coordinator) kept goading me to get this textbook into shape. They were liaising with designers, language editors, designers, artists, management and all other people who worked hard to put the book in your hand. I thank all the members of the Jaypee team for their effort. I wish that we continue to collaborate in the same spirit in future as well.

I wish to thank all the members of the editorial board Dr Baskaran, Dr Sujoy, Dr Rajnish, Dr Shivendra, Dr Uday Somashekhar, Dr Sundeep Singh Saluja and Dr Nayeem for reviewing and editing various chapters and sections of the book. The book was impossible without their efforts and constant support. Being at Govind Ballabh Pant and always available, Dr Saluja was a sounding board for all my decisions. He deserves my special thank.

I wish to thank all the authors who have contributed their chapters in this book. Two DVD-ROMs set with videos of the procedures to accompany the book, was a last-minute decision. I especially thank all the contributors who provided the videos of the various procedures at the very last moment. This book is shaped by the immense experience put forth in these chapters by the authors. The book actually belongs to them. On their behalf, as well as mine, I wish to also thank all our patients who gave us this experience. I wish to thank all my teachers under whom I learned to treat these patients. I was privileged to have Dr Samiran Nundy, a pioneer surgeon in the field of surgical gastroenterology, as my teacher and guide at All India Institute of Medical Sciences (AIIMS). He is one of the most admired doctors in the country today and a guiding star for all of us in this field. I profusely thank him for all he has done for me and also for writing the foreword of the book.

Being in an MCh, teaching institutes gave me the opportunity to interact with some of the sharpest minds in the profession. Our residents come through a grueling selection process and are extremely hard-working. Some of our fellows have become consultants in prestigious hospitals and have also contributed in the chapters of the book. They have helped me in several ways from the intellectual inputs to proofreading. I wish to immensely thank our present and past residents for all their help. I need to especially mention, Drs Vaibhav, Kunal and Vaageesh amongst the present ones, and Drs Rajesh, Kalay, Asit, Nilesh, John, Neeraj, Dinesh, Satyajit and Harsh amongst the earlier ones.

Over the last two years, I have had extra-long hours and my contribution at home in my absence was borne by my family. I wish to thank my wife Yuthika and daughters Pragya and Bhavya for their constant support and encouragement. Above all, they make this effort worthwhile.

In the end, the book represents desire of my parents for my learning and higher education. My late mother with her simplicity and affection nurtured me. My father has always strived for excellence and discipline. His generosity and deep love for all of us is exceeded only by his desire for us to be useful to the society. My gratitude for them is more than I can ever express. I dedicate this book to them and seek their blessing for me, my patients and for all my future endeavors.

Contents

VOLUME 1

SECTION 1 General

SECTION 2 Esophagus

SECTION 3 Stomach, Duodenum, Small Intestine and Retroperitoneum

SECTION 4 Pancreas

SECTION 5 Gallbladder and Bile Ducts

VOLUME 2

SECTION 6 Liver

SECTION 7 Spleen

SECTION 8 Colon, Rectum and Anal Canal

SECTION 9 Liver Transplantation

SECTION 10 Miscellaneous

SECTION 1

General

CHAPTER 1

Approach to a Patient of Digestive Disease

PK Mishra

INTRODUCTION

Practicing medicine is both an art as well as science. Medical science has made giant strides, especially in diagnostic modalities. Sometimes, in the scientific pursuit of medicine, the art of healing and touch of empathy is ignored. History and examination greatly emphasized hitherto have been overtaken by glamorous diagnostic investigations. Many of these diagnostic tests are both costly and hazardous, and offer little advantage over precise history taking and examination. Needless to say, that a thorough history and good bedside examination bring us closer to diagnosis as well as to the patient, and reduces unnecessary investigations. It is also the first contact between the patient and doctor. It enables the doctor to evaluate the patient and his disease while the patient also judges the doctor and his competence. A humane and competent doctor can evoke a unique feeling in his patients which goes a long way in their treatment.

While the medical science is a logical, analytical left brain activity, importance of the right brain virtues like comprehension of the larger picture, empathy and understanding cannot be overemphasized. Many medical boards make communicating empathically and effectively an essential factor in a student doctors evaluation. Emotionally intelligent care makes a vast difference in a patient's healing.[1] Nowhere else is the integration of left and right brain activity more important, than during the history taking and examination of a patient. No set of rigid rules can be made for all patients in the vast variety of different situations. It is not the purpose of this monograph to go into the nitty gritty of history taking. Readers of this text, who have been brought up on a staple of books, like Hutchison and Das[2,3] which have molded our thinking over the years, already understand the value of history. Disease specific history would be covered with the specific chapters in different sections of this textbook. Some broad general aspects are mentioned briefly to sensitize the beginner in this exercise. It is also to remind the rest of us, lest we trip on some fundamental aspect after conquering the bastions of knowledge.

HISTORY AND EXAMINATION

The purpose of history is to move closer to the diagnosis of the ailment with which the patient has presented. This may not always be possible or precise. By history taking we try and arrive at diagnostic possibilities and conduct examinations with these possibilities in mind. History and examination begin with the way the patient enters the clinic or presents to the surgeon. A person breathless on walking a few steps may not be a suitable surgical candidate, although his cancer may be resectable. Observation and nonverbal communication are important in the assessment, diagnosis and assurance of the patient. Age old sequence of presenting complaints, history of present illness, history of past illness, treatment, family, gynecological and menstrual history and, social and occupational history is important to be recorded though may not be obtained from the patient in the same sequence. On this basis, a focused examination followed by a plan for further investigation or treatment is made. In fact, history and examination may go hand in hand with a lag phase determined by the patient and the situation. In a sick and serious patient, these may be simultaneous and examination and resuscitative measures may often precede any history taking.

Another purpose of history taking is to evaluate the stage and severity of the disease and complications, if present. Comorbid illness which may affect the treatment outcome and survival of the patient should also be determined along with treatments received or ongoing. Familial and genetic aspects of the disease are important for the patient as well as other family members. Social and preventive aspects of the disease should also not be ignored. A patient who has an infective disorder should be advised on the precautions to prevent its spread. Many times unnecessary fears on this account may also need to be allayed.

Social and financial aspect of the patient to undergo specific treatment modality should also be assessed. Often, the history taking may begin with these aspects of the patient. It establishes a contact and familiarity with the patient and his social situation. Ailment of the patient can then be evaluated within this perspective. A patient of extrahepatic portal vein obstruction and portal hypertension coming from a remote area with no access to blood or gastroenterology services may be helped better by one time surgery. A daily laborer may be admitted nearer his surgery date so that he does not lose his wages.

While writing, history should be recorded systematically and sequentially. On one side, time should be put and then event, complaint, intervention or investigation recorded. Timeline of the events is important determinant for any diagnosis. A history of off and on pain for the last 4 or 5 years is unlikely to be due to malignant etiology unless a change in the course or severity of pain has occurred recently. Treatment of the patient done before his arrival is very important. Thus endoscopic retrograde cholangiopancreatography (ERCP) may alter the jaundice or palpable gall bladder on examination. Pain and fever starting from the time of endoscopy and dilatation may hint at perforation or pancreatitis.

History and examination should be conducted in an unhurried and relaxed manner as far as possible. It should be done with due privacy. Whenever a male doctor is examining a female, a female attendant should always be close-by. While recording the examination, it should be written system wise. A diagram of lump, mass or organomegaly may convey important and easily understandable information. Important negative history as well as examination findings should also be recorded. A family tree may be made wherever necessary. At the end of this record, the most likely diagnosis and plan of action should be recorded. Wherever required, your thoughts may be put down for future reference. When recording history and examination, three benchmarks are to be cleared. First, it should be understandable and helpful during next consultation. Second, it should withstand in a court of law. Lastly, it should be satisfactory to the patient, if read out to him. Completely avoid any disparaging comments regarding the patient or the treatment received previously.

Once the history and examination have been done, the plan of investigation and likely course should be explained to the patient. When the diagnosis has been confirmed, different alternative choices for treatment, their advantages and problems should also be discussed with the patient. It is duty of the surgeon to discuss the details of the operation, likely problems and the outcome with the patients and family. An ileostomy or colostomy may be an everyday affair for the surgeons but they are a matter of great consequence for the patient. The need for permanent stoma should always be thoroughly explained. It must be ensured that the person has completely understood this. It is also required to assure the patient that he will be given the best services and, such skill and infrastructure is available. Alternatively, it is our responsibility to guide him or her to be able to obtain the same.

COMMON PITFALLS

Language is one of the common problems in accurate assessment of a patient's problem. It may be wiser to get a person who understands the language than to depend on an inaccurate history. Sometimes, within the same language patient's choice of words may not depict the situation properly. Communication skills of patients differ widely. Elderly patients may not remember events sequentially and assistance may be required from other family members. Children may not be forthcoming due to fear or shyness. These factors have to be kept in mind while interpreting history.

History and examination require both time and patience. In many observations, it has been seen that doctors interrupt the patients describing their ailments invariably by 20 seconds. Partly, it is lack of time, but more often it is lack of patience. It is true that some patients may take long before they come to the reason for which they require to be treated. However, small circumambulation should be allowed to extract the story in patient's own way. Although remaining focused is also important, frequent interruption and leading questions may actually lead them astray. Questions suggested for keeping them on track should be open-ended. Obtaining a history and evaluating and interpreting them are both logical as well as intuitive at most times. Which symptom of the patient is more important and how it fits in the diagnostic puzzle are matters of skill to be learnt over years. It needs to be remembered that the patient may have more than one ailment which may be responsible for his condition.

Another aspect during interaction with the patient is to refrain from critically commenting on the treatment received by the patient from his previous doctors. Often a bile duct injury may present to us and critical comments by the examining doctor may further stoke the anguish and dissatisfaction of the patient. Errors of judgment do not constitute negligence (Suggestion: Let us not be judges, unless specifically called upon to be so!). Simultaneously, it would be necessary to accurately assess and record the complication suspected and the treatment required for correction of the same.

WRITING A PRESCRIPTION

It is said that best prescription is without any drugs. Any pharmacological intervention has its own problems. Universally prescribed proton pump inhibitors are beneficial only when indicated. Otherwise they may only serve to reduce a patient's acid output which is a desirable body function. It is also our first line of defense against organisms entering through the gastrointestinal tract. Problems associated with excessive and unnecessary use of analgesics and antibiotics are also well known. All interventions should be carefully weighed in terms of side effects and benefits. Simple steam inhalation and breathing exercises may work better than fancy cough suppressants and mucolytics. For poor patients cost is another important consideration. Patient may exhaust his limited money on drugs peripheral to his disease. Prescription of multiple drugs has further problems. Drug compatibility and interaction with each other are not always known. Further, one medicine may be required to be taken 6 hourly, another 8 hourly and, yet another on twice daily basis. Coupled with his other diabetic or cardiac medicines, it may be enough to tax an elderly patient.

Latest drugs should not be prescribed just on the basis of coaching of the medical representatives. They are prone to hide certain problems which the drugs may have caused during trials. Fortunately for us, the competitor brands readily supply this information. Since the doctor is ultimately responsible for his prescription, he should well acquaint himself with all the potential effects of the drugs before prescribing any medicine. In short, prescriptions should be kept simple and clearly worded in a manner understandable to the dispenser and the patient. It should have only minimum essential number of drugs and should be cost-effective.

ANGRY AND VIOLENT PATIENTS

A dissatisfied patient or relative may sometimes turn violent. This may arise because of some misunderstanding, having to wait too long or due to guilt or grief. It may arise out of perceived medical failing. Patients and relatives may crack under the stress of the disease and the long process of investigation and treatment. In such situation, it is important to remain composed. It may be required to take the help of other patients or relatives. Try to explore the reason for the anger by listening to the person attentively and addressing the main issues. Sometimes the security is required to be called in before the situation turns ugly. Before pressing the panic button it is still necessary to ensure that the person is not critically ill.

PROGNOSIS AND END STAGE CARE

Frequently, surgeons in outpatients encounter diseases which are advanced and incurable. Prognosticating them is a delicate exercise. Whether this information should be conveyed to the relatives only and they be allowed to handle the situation or the patient be also involved differs in different cultural setups. If directly revealed to the patient there is a slim, but usually exaggerated, chance/perception that he may become depressed and deteriorate on getting this news. On the other hand, the patient remains in dark and cannot plan his life. Decision to convey the news has to be taken in consultation with the relatives and taking consideration of patient's age, maturity and education. Kind of social and family support available to the patient is also important. It should also be remembered that we are responsible to the patient and at times the agenda of the carers, relatives or friends may be different from that of the patient. In the absence of exceptional circumstances, the patient should be informed of his state of illness without taking away all hopes.

Similarly, breaking the news of death of patients to the relatives may bring out untoward and occasionally, extreme reactions. No set of rules can govern the diverse situations with variables of patient's age, maturity, type and knowledge of illness and preparedness of the relatives for this eventuality. A situation of accident or sudden emergency which is a catastrophe imposed on the family with little preparedness for the event may thus be more shocking than, if such a situation was expected to occur. Hence, when the relatives are kept briefed periodically about the state of illness and the efforts of the medical team, the relatives are better prepared to handle the eventuality. Senior most available member of the team should break the news of death to the relatives. The occasion of the loss of life in any family deserves to be handled with due sensitivity. This unfortunately is not taught in medical colleges and needs to be learnt diligently. Surgeons should learn to handle this delicate situation at any cost. The major reason for complaints and litigations is the absence of regular honest communications between doctors and their patients, and more importantly, with the relatives of patients.

GI SURGERY AS SUPER SPECIALTY

It is not possible for any surgeon to master diverse areas. With expanding horizons of investigations and treatments, need for specialization has increased. It takes many years of education and apprenticeship for learning the nuances which makes a difference in the life of a patient. While its medical counterpart gastroenterology, had long established itself, gastrointestinal (GI) surgery or surgical gastroenterology as a super specialty in this country has come up only in the last thirty years. In the last two or three decades, it has made giant strides in specialized, high level of care. It is one of the more direct extensions of general surgery and hence most popular for the general surgeons. Entry into this super specialty is fiercely contested and only the brightest make it into this branch. It is both challenging as well as satisfying. Already, areas like colorectal surgery, hepatobiliary surgery, upper GI surgery and liver transplant are recognized as further subspecialty within this broad realm. Laparoscopy and robotic skills have already made their mark as important tools. The debate about specialization versus generalization is endless. These are not exclusive or at the cost of one or the other. Better coordination and definitions of functioning is required. How many general surgeons, GI surgeons or liver transplant surgeons are required is a matter to be defined by the health policy makers. Requirement for each is established and beyond any doubt.

Gastrointestinal surgeon is required to deal with difficult patients. Often, intensive care unit (ICU) care is part of their management. Issues of ventilation, nutrition, fluid, electrolytes are important in their management. Care of a patient who has had operations, like esophagectomy, pancreatic necrosectomy, a Whipple's operation or transplant is indeed a difficult affair. Often these patients have many other comorbidities. No doubt, many specialists contribute to this care; however the GI surgeon has to integrate the final management. Thus, training of a GI surgeon has to include advanced level of supportive care besides the primary surgical management.

Integral to medical advancements are analysis of results and comparison with different modalities of treatment. A GI surgeon has to be able to sieve the evidence amongst the plethora of literature flooding the internet.

LIVER TRANSPLANT

Liver transplantation is one of the greatest strides in modern medicine. Thanks to the contributions of Thomas Starzl and Sir Roy Calne, liver transplant has become an undisputed standard of care for end stage liver disease and many other ailments. Liver transplantation is an example of teamwork and dedication. Organ donation from brain dead and living donors brings forth ethical issues. Setting of priorities for organ distribution, counseling for donations, cost to the individuals and societies are issues which require transparent and professional handling.

FOLLOW-UP OF PATIENTS

While treating the patients, it is also important to know how the patient has fared after our intervention. We may be repeating the same mistake again and again and call this as experience. Unless we assiduously follow our patients and document their results we would not be any wiser about the validity of our treatment. We would also not be able to compare our results with alternative forms of interventions. Whenever a patient is seen, his complete address and phone number should be recorded. A periodic review of follow-up should be done and those patients who have not reported on their due dates should be contacted for their condition and well-being.

RESEARCH

Research is important for advancement in any specialty. Periodic analysis of results, innovations, applications of newer drugs and technology should be done within the ambit of ethical propriety. Analysis and comparisons of data has a strong statistical component. To understand any data we require some background of statistical method. A primer on statistics is therefore included in this textbook. Readers are strongly advised to build a solid foundation taking the help of this primer and to go further ahead to advance their knowledge.

ETHICS

This book ends with a chapter on ethics. Ethical practice and research should remain at the heart of any medical practitioner. Medical practice is not about earning money, and more and more money. Some recent developments have lacerated the heart of this profession. Taking money for the services not rendered, taking cuts for referrals, performing unnecessary tests and procedures, helping predatory pharmaceutical companies instead of the patients and unethical research have brought disrepute to this noble profession. Insider accounts have narrated harrowing tales of "a collective malaise".[4] I implore the young minds to be ever watchful and take this profession forward in the most ethical manner. No amount of money can substitute for the joy of really helping a patient in his time of need.

REFERENCES

1. Pink DH. A whole New Mind. UK: Publisher Marshall Cavendish; 2008.
2. Glynn M, Drake WM (Ed). Hutchison's Clinical Method: An integrated approach to clinical practice. 23rd edition. W B Saunders Ltd; 2012.
3. Das S. A Manual on Clinical Surgery. 10th edition. S Das's publications; 2008.
4. Rajghatta C. A Heartless Profession? Times of India; 2014.

CHAPTER 2

Gastrointestinal Imaging

Raju Sharma, Ankur Goyal

INTRODUCTION

Imaging plays an important role in visualizing the anatomy and detecting the diseases of the gastrointestinal tract (GIT). The imaging armamentarium comprises of abdominal radiographs, barium studies, ultrasonography (USG), computed tomography (CT), magnetic resonance imaging (MRI) and positron emission tomography (PET). Imaging advancements like contrast-enhanced ultrasound (CEUS), USG elastography, multidetector CT (MDCT), CT enterography, dual-energy CT (DECT), diffusion and perfusion imaging and magnetic resonance (MR) spectroscopy have revolutionized the study of GIT.[1] Co-registration techniques allow fusion of multimodality data (USG-CT, PET-CT, PET-MR, etc.) with improved characterization of lesions. Each modality has its unique profile of indications, advantages and limitations (Table 1). The technique employed depends upon availability, usefulness, safety and costs.

PLAIN RADIOGRAPHS

Plain abdominal radiographs are frequently performed in the setting of acute abdomen and demonstrate normal and abnormal gas accumulations, bowel pathologies, air-fluid levels and calcifications. It is essential that all clinical details are conveyed to the radiologist so that relevant information is not overlooked. Supine abdomen and erect chest radiographs are must in case of acute bowel obstruction.[2,3] The supine radiograph should be taken with empty bladder and include the hernial orifices. Upright chest radiograph is better than upright abdominal projection for detection of pneumoperitoneum, because X-ray beam strikes the diaphragm tangentially at highest point and thus even 1 mL of free air can be demonstrated. Erect radiographs are taken only after patient remains erect for 10 minutes so that free air gets time to ascend to the highest point. Erect chest radiograph including the diaphragm not only detects bowel perforation but also rules out any chest disease that may present with abdominal symptoms. In sick patients unable to move, lateral decubitus view can be obtained with horizontal X-ray beam. Supine abdominal radiographs may show air in the right upper quadrant, hepatorenal fossa, along the falciform or umbilical ligaments and in the fissure for ligamentum teres. Rigler's (double wall) sign, football sign and scrotal air in chidren are other signs of pneumoperitoneum. Erect abdominal radiograph can depict the number and size of air-fluid levels but is not reliable in diagnosing obstruction or ileus[2,3] and is, therefore, no longer employed. More than two fluid levels, greater than 2.5 cm, in the dilated small bowel, are said to be abnormal.[4] Differential vertical height of more than 2 cm between air-fluid levels in the same bowel loop and small bowel to colon diameter ratio of greater than 0.5 also indicates distal small bowel obstruction. Colonic diameter can normally reach up to 5.5 cm. Commensurate dilatation of both small and large bowel suggests the diagnosis of paralytic ileus. Obliteration of the border of psoas, kidney, bladder, liver or spleen can give important information about respective pathologies. In evaluation of bowel obstruction, abdominal radiographs are diagnostic in 50–60% of cases, equivocal in about 20–30%, and normal or misleading in 10–20%.[5]

When dilated bowel loops are detected on radiograph, next step is to determine whether it is small or large bowel. Dilated small bowel loops are usually arranged centrally in the abdomen, are more numerous, show a small radius of curvature and never exceed 5 cm in diameter. The small bowel valvulae conniventes form thin, complete rings, which are closer together and are prominent in jejunum but less marked in ileum. Dilated colon is peripherally located, greater than 5 cms, haustrae form thick incomplete bands and are absent in descending and sigmoid colon. The presence of mottled air lucencies suggestive of fecal

Table 1: Overview of imaging modalities with their advantages and limitations			
Modality	*Best suited for*	*Advantages*	*Shortcomings*
Radiograph	Acute bowel obstruction, suspected perforation	Quick	Limited or equivocal information
USG	• First investigation in acute abdomen especially for GB, appendix, liver abscesss • Ideal for repeated examinations and in pregnant patients • Resolving solid vs cystic lesions	Inexpensive, Dynamic & Real-time, Bedside, no radiation, high soft tissue resolution	Operator dependent, not comprehensive, obscured by bowel gas and body habitus
Barium studies	Subacute bowel obstruction	Motility and function can be studied Mucosal details	Radiation, only luminal information
MDCT	Modality of choice for evaluating acute and chronic abdominal conditions	Comprehensive, High temporal and spatial resolution, Fast image acquisition	Radiation, contrast issues
MRI	Hepato-biliary and pancreas imaging	No radiation	Cost, availability, artifacts, long acquisition time

contents is the most reliable sign that the loop is large bowel. In addition to localizing the site of obstruction, radiographs may give information about complications like mesenteric ischemia by depicting thumbprinting, thickened valvulae conniventes and air in the bowel wall (pneumatosis intestinalis) or portal vein.

The diagnosis of sigmoid volvulus may be clinched on the radiograph in the presence of massively distended inverted U-shaped ahaustral bowel loop with apex under the diaphragm. Coffee-bean sign and inferior convergence in left pelvis further lend support to the diagnosis. In comparison, cecal volvulus occupies left upper or right lower abdominal quadrant and haustral markings can be usually made out.

One must also look for air in the gall bladder (emphysematous cholecystitis) or in abdominal abscesses. Pancreatic calcifications, calcified gall stones, calcified liver lesions, hydatid cysts and calcified granulomatous lesions may be evident on abdominal radiographs

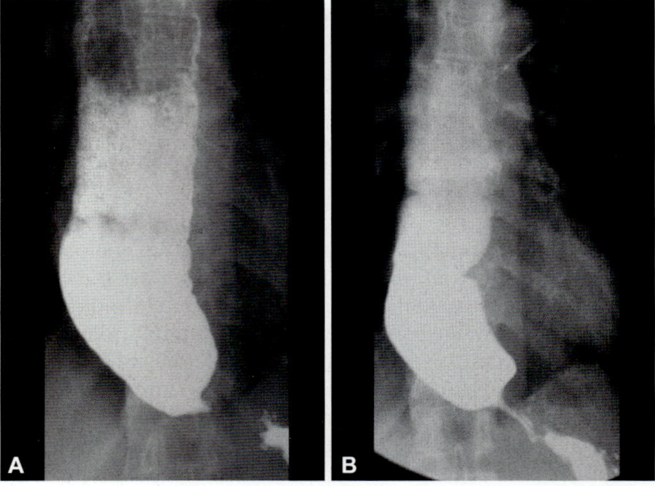

Figures 1A and B Barium swallow study (A and B) of a 36-year-old female patient shows massively dilated esophagus with smooth "beak-like" narrowing involving the gastroesophageal junction and proximal hold-up of barium. Note is made of multiple tertiary contractions in the thoracic esophagus in the absence of primary peristalsis. Findings are diagnostic of primary achalasia

BARIUM STUDIES AND FLUOROSCOPY

The role of barium studies has declined after the advent of endoscopy. Mucosal disease is much better evaluated by the latter, coupled with its ability to obtain biopsies. There are only certain niche indications for barium studies which are discussed below.

Motility of air-distended bowel can be visualized in real time under fluoroscopy. In single contrast examinations, the GIT lumen is filled with a positive contrast material to visualize peristalsis, emptying, anatomical disposition, calibre, outline, stenosis, dilatation, luminal-filling defects and extrinsic compression. In double contrast examinations, the inner surface is coated with contrast and lumen is distended with air. This allows detailed mucosal evaluation, especially useful in the detection of subtle pathologies.[6] Limitations of barium studies include inability to diagnose mural and extra-luminal pathologies.

Barium swallow is commonly requested for evaluation of dysphagia. It provides information regarding strictures, motility disorders, gastroesophageal reflux and malignancies (Figs 1 and 2). Main advantage over endoscopy is delineation of the GIT beyond the site of narrowing and functional information. Double contrast upper GI study demonstrates ulcerations and mucosal involvement in esophagitis/gastritis. Small bowel follow-through examination is indicated in cases of suspected inflammatory or obstructive small-bowel disease, including subacute bowel obstruction, malabsorption and jejunal diverticulosis (Figs 3 and 4). After preliminary fluoroscopy, patient drinks 300–500 mL of 50–70% barium suspension. Then various views are taken for stomach, duodenum, duodenojejunal flexure, small bowel and cecum. Prone view is must for small bowel evaluation and serves to spread out the bowel loops. Filled and mucosal relief views of the ileocecal junction are necessary to rule out any pathology. In cases, where ileocecal distension is equivocal, peroral pneumocolon using room air can be employed to identify abnormality. Problems with follow-through examination include lengthy examination time and false negative rate due to overlapping of bowel loops and their suboptimal distension. Barium enteroclysis used to be modality of choice for evaluation of small bowel, because of optimal bowel distension and opacification, however, has now

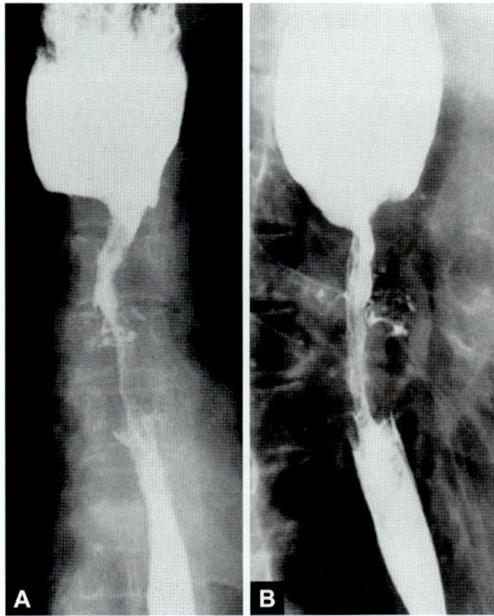

Figures 2A and B Barium swallow study (A and B) of a 50-year-old male patient shows a stricture in mid-thoracic esophagus with shelf-like margins, suggestive of malignant etiology. The narrowing appears to be circumferential with mucosal irregularity, ulceration and proximal holdup of barium. Endoscopic biopsy revealed squamous cell carcinoma

been replaced largely by CT. 600–1,200 mL of 20–40% w/v barium at the rate of 75 mL/minute is instilled through nasojejunal tube. Advantages over follow-through examination include bypassing of pylorus, better luminal distensibility, improved depiction of mucosal folds, ulceration, polyps, constrictions, simultaneous display of all bowel loops in the end and shorter examination time. Barium enema is done in cases of presumed large bowel involvement by strictures, inflammatory diseases or malignancy. Dye studies using water-soluble iodinated contrast media are very useful in detecting postoperative leaks, evaluating bowel continuity and motility.

ULTRASONOGRAPHY, CONTRAST-ENHANCED ULTRASOUND AND ULTRASOUND ELASTOGRAPHY

Transabdominal USG is an easy procedure without radiation exposure and allows quick assessment of the solid organs (including liver, biliary tree, pancreas and spleen) and bowel (especially in acute appendicitis). USG has excellent soft tissue imaging capabilities which make it ideal for evaluation of hepato-pancreato-biliary system and bowel loops. Problems with sonography include operator dependency, limited evaluation in the presence of bowel gas and obesity.

Ultrasonography permits accurate diagnosis of liver abscess, cholelithiasis, cholecystistis, pancreatitis, hepatosplenomegaly and free fluid. Differentiation of solid or cystic nature is the most useful application of USG in characterization of visceral mass lesions. Graded compression USG is a well-documented technique for evaluation of appendix.[7] USG signs of acute appendicitis include visualization of a blind-ending noncompressible, aperistaltic

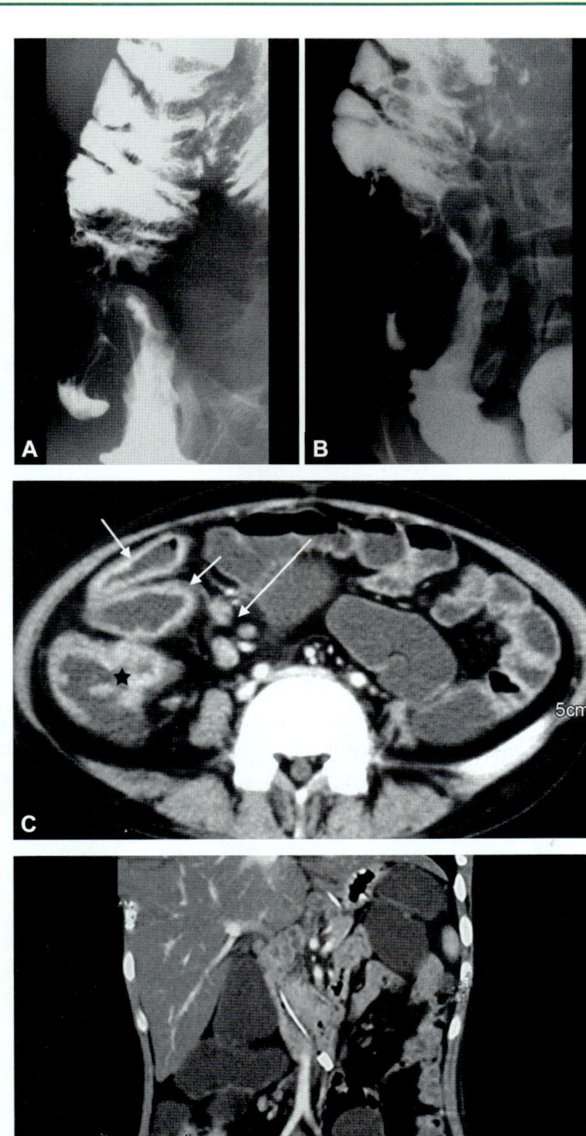

Figures 3A to D Barium meal follow-through study (A and B) of a 30-year-old male patient showing ileocecal Koch's. There is narrowing and mucosal irregularity of the terminal ileum with thin stream of barium seen in its lumen and resultant proximal dilatation. Cecum is contracted, irregular and shrunken. The normal acute angle of ileocecal junction is distorted (C and D) Computed tomography enteroclysis axial (C) and coronal (D) images of a 19-year-female patient (different patient) showing findings of tuberculous enteritis. There is wall thickening involving the distal (short arrows) and terminal ileum along with contiguous involvement of cecum (asterisk). Multiple enlarged regional lymph nodes are seen (long arrow). Note made of hepatomegaly in coronal image (D). There was near-complete resolution of the clinical and imaging findings post 9 months of antitubercular therapy

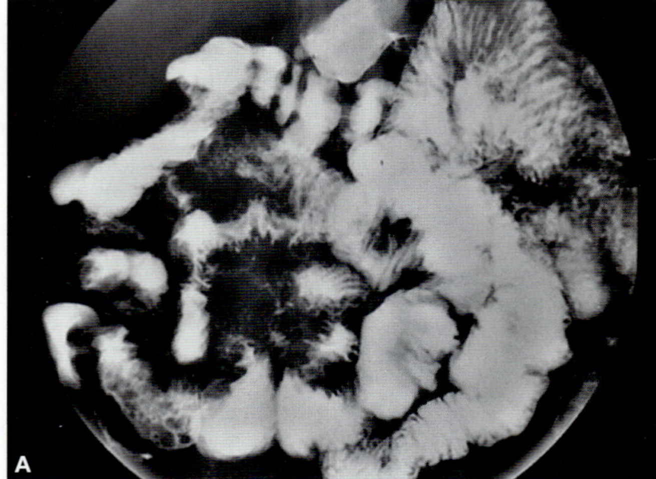

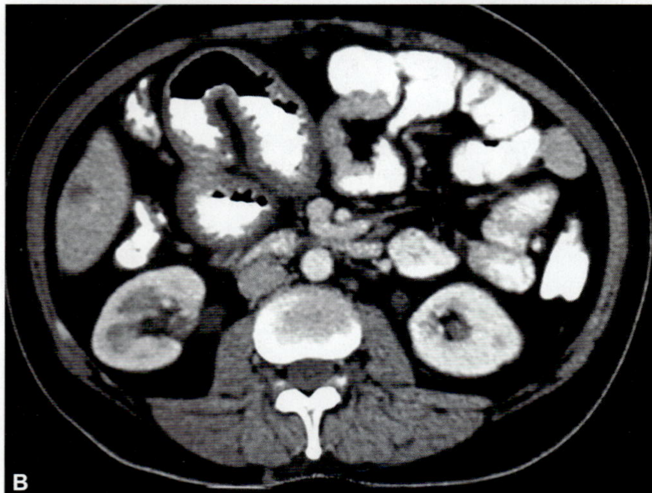

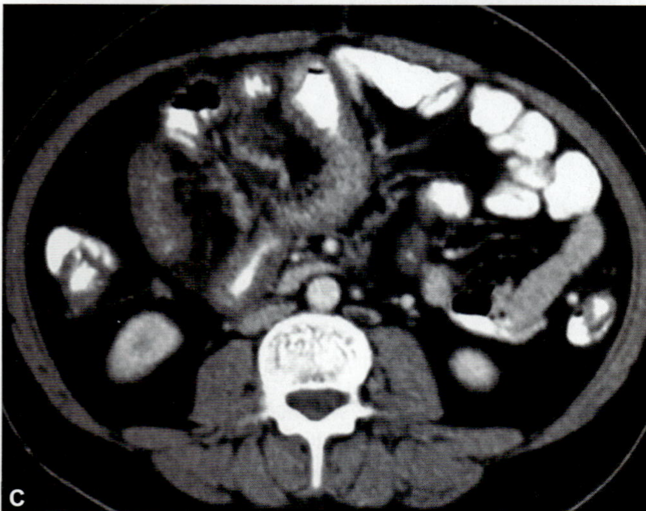

Figures 4A to C Non-Hodgkin lymphoma. (A) Barium meal follow-through study shows nodular mucosal fold thickening involving the small bowel. Axial contrast-enhanced computed tomography images of the same patient (B and C) show irregular wall thickening involving jejunal loops with alternating areas of dilatation and narrowing of the involved loops. The patient also had multiple heterogeneously enhancing liver lesions, one of them is seen in (B). Histology revealed B-cell non-Hodgkin lymphoma

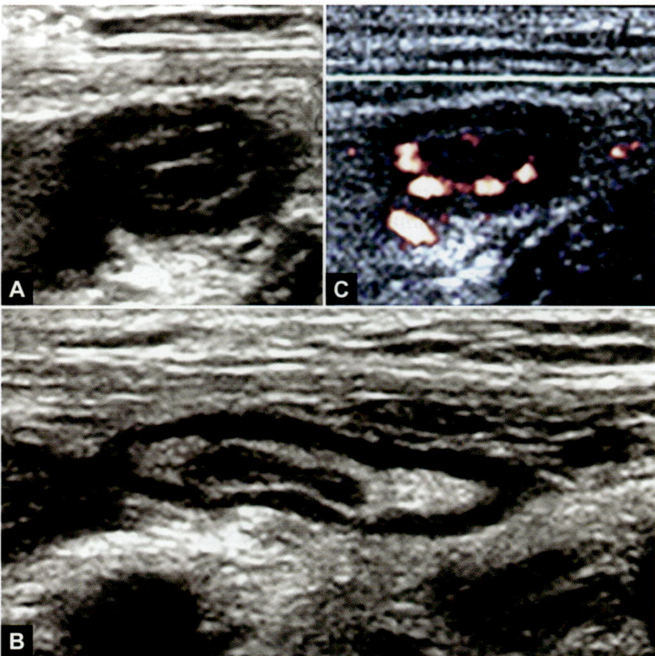

Figures 5A to C Ultrasound in acute appendicitis. Gray-scale sonography images (A and B) show thick-walled blind-ending structure in right iliac fossa which was aperistaltic and noncompressible in real time. Color doppler imaging (C) depicts increased vascularity in the bowel wall, further supportive of appendiceal inflammation. No surrounding collection was seen. Surgery confirmed inflamed appendix

tubular structure in right iliac fossa with more than 7 mm diameter and tender on compression (Fig. 5). An appendicolith may be seen and there may be regional inflammation or abscess formation. Intussusception and hypertrophic pyloric stenosis are other indications in children where USG is helpful.

Doppler examination enables noninvasive diagnosis of portal hypertension and hepatic venous outflow tract obstruction (HVOTO). The size and patency of vessels, direction and velocity of flow and presence of collaterals can be assessed. Sonography is used to diagnose extrahepatic portal venous obstruction and for evaluating the feasibility of surgery. It can also be used to assess the patency of lienorenal and transjugular intrahepatic portosystemic shunts (TIPS). Shrunken liver may however, limit the information gained through Doppler. Multiphasic CT or MRI is useful when sonography is equivocal.

In bowel diseases, USG may reveal bowel wall thickening and mesenteric lymphadenopathy in inflammatory diseases. In cases of fluid collections and abscesses, USG enables detection as well as provides guidance for percutaneous drainage. Doppler imaging allows assessment of perfusion of bowel wall. In bowel obstruction, proximally dilated bowel loops may be seen, showing increased or absent peristalsis. It may demonstrate abnormal bowel loops in obstructed hernias and may demonstrate zone of transition however, the negative predictive value is low.

Endoscopic USG (EUS) uses high frequency radial scanner mounted on the endoscope and enables sonographic evaluation of the upper GIT, especially valuable in evaluation of periampullary region and taking EUS-guided biopsies. EUS helps in evaluation of many diseases like depth of mural invasion of esophageal cancers, mediastinal adenopathy in esophageal and lung malignancies, evaluating hepatobiliary system and pancreas.[8]

Endosonography using intraluminal probes allows high-resolution imaging of the wall layers of the GIT.[9] Transrectal USG can be used for evaluating the mural invasion of rectal cancers while anal endosonography is useful for mapping traumatic defects of the external anal sphincter in patients with fecal incontinence and evaluating mural inflammation in Crohn's disease.[8] Intraoperative USG using high frequency transducers provides high resolution imaging for accurate detection of small lesions like neuroendocrine tumors of the pancreas. It is also used to localize deep-seated liver lesions that cannot be palpated by the surgeon.

Recently, use of intravenous microbubble contrast agents has enabled evaluation of vascularity of focal liver lesions and bowel wall without any radiation or risk of nephrotoxicity. This is helpful in characterizing liver lesions, assessing tumor response to ablative therapy or chemotherapy and evaluation of disease activity in inflammatory bowel diseases.[10-12] Elastography is a new method which permits assessment of tissue stiffness. The tissues are compressed manually or by shear waves and the deformation pattern is visualized as colors (from soft to stiff) on the image. The stiffness depends on the biomechanical properties, allowing differentiation between normal and abnormal tissues.[13] The indications include assessment of liver fibrosis, cirrhosis, characterizing liver lesions and measuring splenic stiffness as an indicator of portal hypertension.[14]

MULTIDETECTOR COMPUTED TOMOGRAPHY

Multidetector computed tomography with 16 or more rows of detectors allows fast acquisition of thin slices and permits isotropic multiplanar reformations (MPRs) in coronal, sagittal or oblique planes. Single breath-hold acquisition reduces peristaltic and breathing artifacts. With the advent of MDCT, multiphasic multiplanar information can be obtained during defined circulatory phases. Curved reformatting is employed for delineating pancreatic ductal anatomy, blood vessels and showing entire length of a bowel segment. Maximum intensity projections (MIP) accentuate high attenuating structures, like enhancing vessels and bones; prove beneficial in depicting pseudoaneurysms and active bleed. Volume rendering (VR) gives volumetric three-dimensional overview, displaying the CT numbers with varying colors and opacity levels. In shaded surface display (SSD), voxels located on the edges of a structure are selectively displayed by intensity thresholding. This technology is used in the evaluation of tubular structures like bowel (virtual colonoscopy), bronchi (virtual bronchoscopy) and blood vessels.

A typical abdominal CT protocol employs 0.6–1.2 mm collimation, 120–140 kV, 70–90 effective mAs. 100 mL of nonionic iodinated contrast media (iodine 300 mg/mL) is injected through an intravenous cannula and single phase acquisition is done at 60–70 seconds from the start of injection. In case of CT angiography, higher concentration of the contrast is used (350–400 mg/mL) and pressure injector (at rate of 4 mL/second) is employed. A noncontrast scan helps in demonstrating calcifications, calculi and hemorrhage. Multiphasic imaging protocol comprises of various combinations of unenhanced, early arterial at 15–25 seconds (for arterial anatomy and pathologies), late arterial at 25–35 seconds (for detecting hypervascular lesions), pancreatic phase at 35–45 seconds, portal venous phase at 55–70 seconds (parenchymal enhancement) and equilibrium phase at 3 minutes. Further delayed phases at 5 or 10 minutes may be acquired, as and when required (example in cholangiocarcinomas, adrenal lesions). One set of axial images are reconstructed at 5 mm thickness and 5 mm reconstruction interval for routine viewing and filming, while another set is reconstructed at thinner collimation for postprocessing and generation of MPRs, MIP and VR technique.

Contrast-enhanced CT is the investigation of choice for evaluation of acute abdomen including acute intestinal obstruction and abdominal trauma. It not only diagnoses obstruction but also demonstrates the transition zone, cause of obstruction and associated complications like strangulation and bowel ischemia. In the absence of acute obstruction, water or positive contrast agents are used to opacify bowel lumen. Neutral contrast (water) is used in case of CT angiograms and to depict bowel wall enhancement while 2% water-soluble iodinated contrast or barium sulfate is used in other scenarios. Latter is especially helpful in demonstrating bowel perforations, leaks or fistulas while drawback is obscuration of mucosal enhancement and blood vessels. The problem with water is that it gets absorbed early and this results in under-distention. Hence additives like mannitol, methyl cellulose, polyethylene glycol, low-density barium or milk are used to increase the osmolarity of water.

Multiphasic MDCT is the investigation of choice in the evaluation of focal hepatobiliary and pancreatic lesions, evaluating bowel ischemia and gastrointestinal (GI) bleeding (Figs 6 to 10). Widespread availability, low cost, shorter acquisition time and excellent spatial resolution make CT a very useful modality. The effective radiation dose in a single abdominopelvic CT acquisition is 5–7 millisievert, which is approximately equivalent to 300 digital chest radiographs.

Computed tomography enterography or enteroclysis have now replaced barium enteroclysis since CT gives wealth of extraluminal

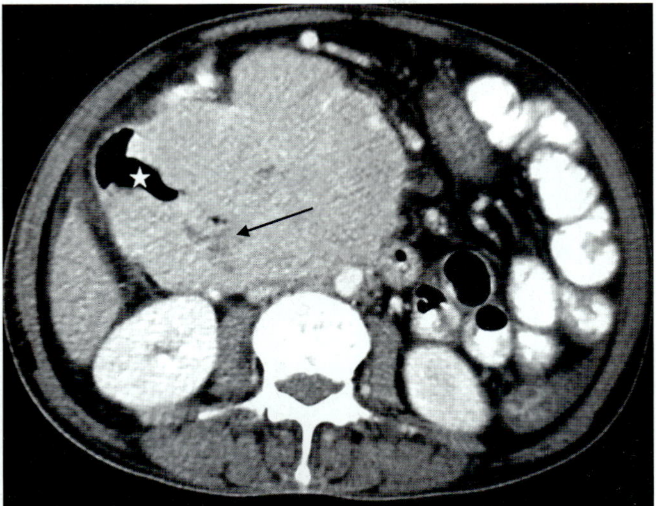

Figure 6 Computed tomography imaging of duodenal gastrointestinal stromal tumor (GIST). Axial contrast-enhanced computed tomography image shows lobulated enhancing soft tissue mass lesion eccentrically located along the medial wall of duodenum with large exophytic component. Presence of ulcer (asterisk) and areas of necrosis (arrow) further suggest the diagnosis of gastrointestinal stromal tumors. Endoscopic biopsy confirmed the diagnosis

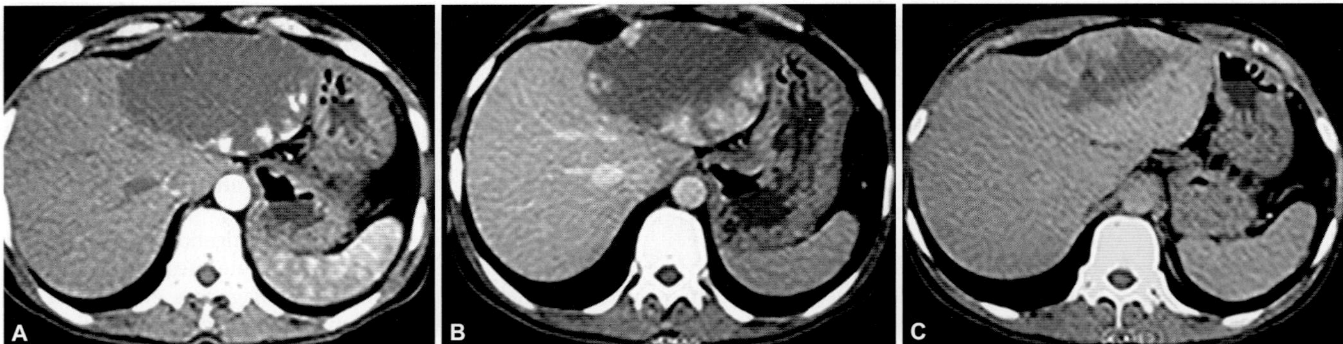

Figures 7A to C Axial multiphasic computed tomography images show a large liver lesion in left lobe showing peripheral discontinuous nodular enhancement in arterial phase (A) and progressive filling-in on venous and delayed phases (B and C), diagnostic of cavernous hemangioma. The enhancement follows the attenuation of aorta in all phases

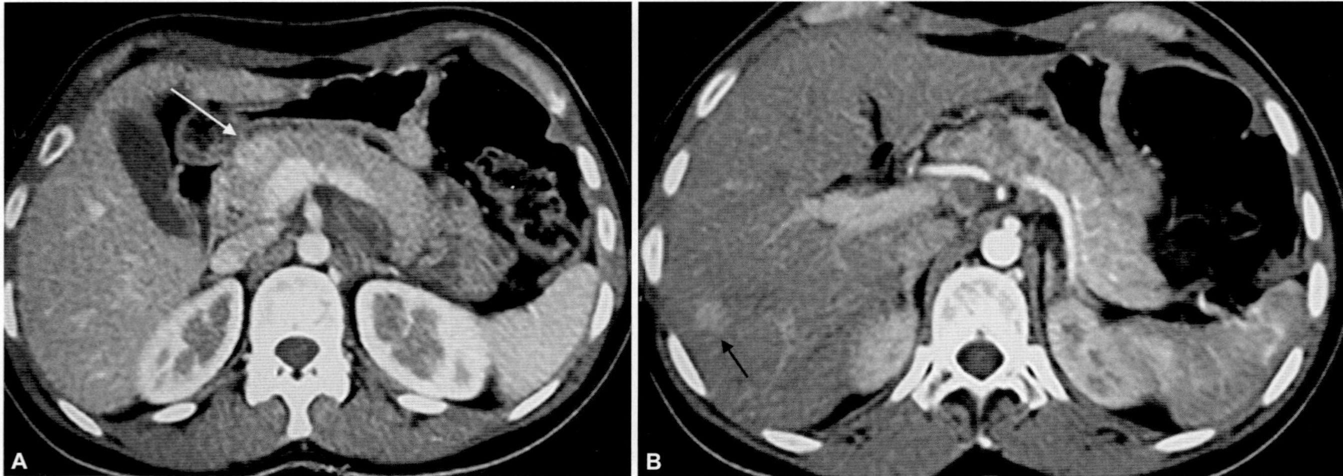

Figures 8A and B Axial contrast-enhanced computed tomography images (A and B) arterial phase show an intensely enhancing well-defined lesion in the pancreatic head (arrow in A) along with similar arterial enhancing lesion in liver (arrowhead in B). Multiple necrotic peripancreatic lymph nodes are also seen. Possibility of neuroendocrine pancreatic tumor with liver and nodal metastases was kept and the lesion proved to be insulinoma

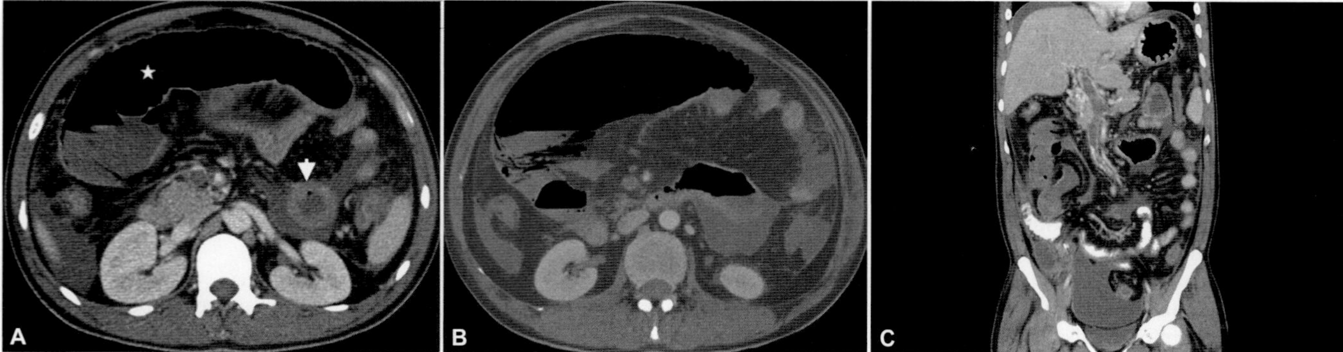

Figures 9A to C Mesenteric ischemia. Venous phase axial contrast-enhanced computed tomography image (A) shows hypodense filling defect in the superior mesenteric vein suggestive of thrombosis. One of the small bowel loops (asterisk) is massively distended and shows papery thin walls (suggestive of impending rupture). Another small bowel loop shows wall thickening (arrowhead). Free fluid is present. Use of wider window settings (B) enables clear demonstration of air in the mesenteric vessels (mesenteric vein tributaries) Coronal computed tomography image (C) venous phase permits excellent depiction of entire extent of thrombus in the superior mesenteric vein, extending into portal vein. There is free fluid in the abdomen-pelvis and in the root of mesentery

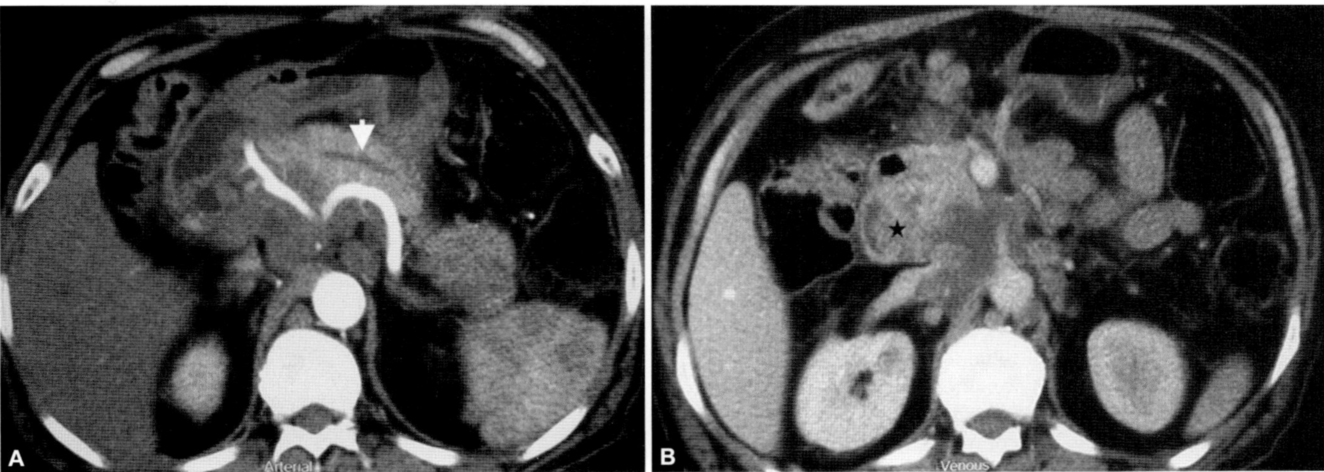

Figures 10A and B Pancreatic carcinoma with vascular involvement. Arterial (A) and venous phase (B) axial contrast-enhanced computed tomography images show an ill-defined heterogeneously enhancing mass lesion in the head of pancreas (asterisk) with multiple enlarged necrotic retropancreatic lymph nodes encasing the celiac trunk and superior mesenteric artery. Pancreatic duct is dilated in the body region (arrowhead)

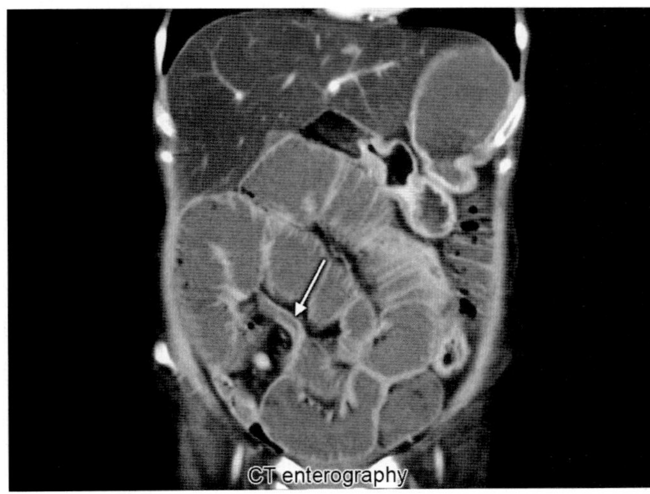

Figure 11 Computed tomography enterography study coronal image shows short segment narrowing in the distal small bowel with proximal dilatation. This was later proved to be a tubercular stricture. Note is made of fatty liver

information in addition to optimal bowel evaluation (Fig. 11). Enteroclysis involves small bowel distention by administration of high volume of contrast medium (1.5 L of water at 100 mL/minute) via a nasojejunal catheter (with tip beyond the duodenojejunal flexure) followed by CT acquisition. Enterography is more comfortable for the patient, since it does not involve inserting nasojejunal tube; rather patient is given fluids in fixed amounts at regular intervals to achieve optimal bowel distension. Enterography has been found to be almost equally reliable as enteroclysis in evaluation of bowel pathology and thus has replaced the latter.[15,16] Enteroclysis provides slightly better mucosal evaluation and specificity because it achieves better luminal distension.[17] Capsule endoscopy has higher sensitivity for mucosal evaluation but lower specificity and no extraluminal information.[16,18] Moreover, capsule endoscopy cannot be performed when the presence of a stricture is suspected because the capsule may become lodged at the diseased segment and cause obstruction.

Virtual colonography is a noninvasive way of studying the large bowel. After proper bowel preparation, the large intestine is distended with air or carbon dioxide and the patient is scanned in the prone and supine positions.[19] The examination is reviewed in multiple planes and as virtual endoscopy, allowing fly-through visualization of the colon in antegrade and retrograde directions. Colonic polyps more than 6 mm can be detected with high accuracy similar to that of conventional colonoscopy, while the accuracy for smaller polyps (those less than 6 mm) is less.[19,20] Newer softwares along with computer-aided detection (CAD) may further improve the diagnostic accuracy and reduce the imaging and interpretation time.[1] Moreover, CT enables detection of any extracolonic pathology as well. Virtual CT colonography may serve as a noninvasive screening alternative to colonoscopy and may replace the conventional barium enema studies in case of incomplete colonoscopy.

Software applications like CT volumetry help in planning the extent and nature of hepatic resection and evaluation of donor liver prior to transplant. In addition, it enables estimation of residual organ volume after surgical resection of the neoplastic lesions, especially useful in patients with cirrhosis.

Dual-energy CT is based on differential behaviour of tissues at different energies, which provides information about tissue composition.[21] GI applications of DECT include generation of virtual unenhanced scans, increased conspicuity of hypervascular liver lesions (on low energy images), quantifying iron deposition, characterizing adrenal nodules, differentiating normal and abnormal parenchyma in the pancreas, improved evaluation of calcified vessels and better bone removal softwares.[21] CT perfusion is a functional modality which provides quantitative assessment of tissue perfusion via various parameters, such as blood flow, blood volume, mean transit time, and permeability surface area product.[22] It is gaining value in evaluation and therapeutic response assessment of tumors of liver, pancreas and colon and to predict pancreatic necrosis in acute pancreatitis.[22,23]

Thus CT has almost replaced barium studies in bowel evaluation, provides a noninvasive alternative to colonoscopy and has replaced diagnostic angiography for mesenteric ischemia and GI bleed.

MAGNETIC RESONANCE IMAGING

Magnetic resonance imaging offers a radiation-free modality with better soft-tissue contrast and superior demonstration of contrast enhancement as compared to CT. Recent developments in MRI techniques and improved sequences allow faster and higher quality image acquisition.

The usual protocol for evaluation of hepato-biliary and pancreatic lesions involves T1-weighted gradient-echo sequence (to detect hemorrhage, fat), T2-weighted spin-echo (to identify abnormality) and dynamic postcontrast imaging. Fat suppression is frequently used with T2-weighted and postcontrast acquisition. In phase and opposed phase T1-weighted imaging serves to detect intracellular fat which is useful in evaluation of hepatic steatosis. Magnetic resonance cholangio-pancreaticography (MRCP) employs heavily T2-weighted sequences to image fluid-containing biliary tree with background suppression. Half-fourier acquisition single-shot turbo spin-echo (HASTE) sequence is acquired in axial and coronal planes along with thick slab images. Three-dimensional restore fast spin-echo sequence provides volumetric acquisition with isotropic resolution in all the directions. MRCP serves as a noninvasive alternative to endoscopic retrograde cholangio-pancreaticography (ERCP) for acquiring diagnostic information (Figs 12 and 13) and the latter is reserved for equivocal results and interventions. MRCP does not involve radiation, proves useful in case of incomplete or failed ERCP, and gives information about the ducts proximal to the site of obstruction.

Routinely used MR contrast media include extracellular agents like gadopentetate dimeglumine (Gd-DTPA), gadolinium-tetraazacyclododecanetetraacetic acid (Gd-DOTA) and gado-diamide. In evaluation of liver lesions, hepatobiliary agents like gadobenate dimeglumine (Gd BOPTA) and gadolinium ethoxybenzyl diethylenetriamine pentaacetic acid (Gd-EOB-DTPA) are employed. These contrast media actually serve as extracellular as well as hepatobiliary and even blood-pool agents. Hepatobiliary agents permit distinction between hepatocellular lesions and metastases. Also focal nodular hyperplasia (FNH) retains contrast on delayed phase and thus can be differentiated from liver adenomas. Superparamagnetic iron oxide (SPIO) is a reticuloendothelial system (RES) targeted contrast media which produces signal loss on T2-weighted MR images. Malignant lesions do not contain Kupffer cells and thus appear bright against background of hypointense liver parenchyma. Due to the associated risk of nephrogenic systemic fibrosis, gadolinium-based contrast agents should not be used, if glomerular filtration rate (GFR) is less than 30 mL/minute and reduced dose is to be used, if GFR is 30–60 mL/minute.

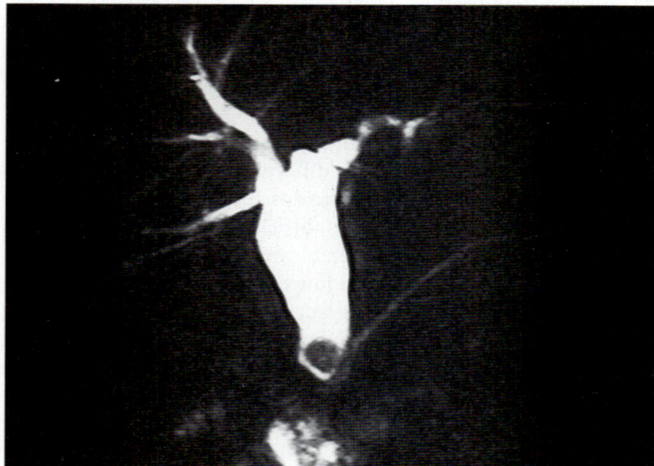

Figure 12 Type 1 choledochal cyst with choledocholithiasis. Projectional magnetic resonance cholangio-pancreaticography image shows fusiform dilatation of common bile duct with a rounded hypointense calculus in its lower end. There is mild dilatation of bilateral intrahepatic biliary radicals (stasis-related). Pancreatic duct is normal

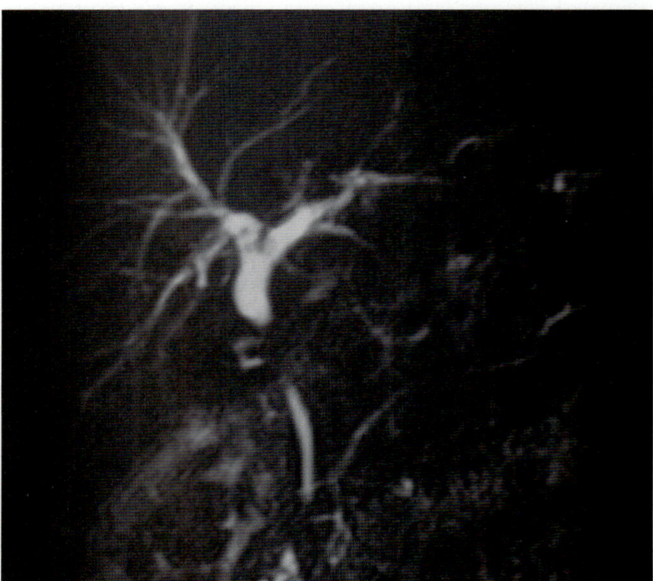

Figure 13 Postcholecystectomy benign biliary stricture. Projectional magnetic resonance cholangio-pancreaticography image shows non-visualization of mid portion of common bile duct, greater than 2 cm from the hilum suggesting type I benign biliary stricture. There is upstream dilatation of biliary radicals. Gall bladder and cystic duct are not seen (postoperative)

Magnetic resonance imaging facilitates superior detection and characterization of liver diseases, compared to CT. MRCP is the modality of choice for imaging of biliary and pancreatic ducts. MRI is the investigation of choice in the staging of rectal cancers.[24] MR enterography provides a radiation-free alternative, suited for repeated examinations especially in young patients with established inflammatory bowel disease (Fig. 14), and has equivalent sensitivity.[25] It is even superior in evaluation of anorectal fistulas (Fig. 15).[26] However, CT scores with respect to higher spatial resolution, better image quality and better interobserver agreement.[16,25] Fast sequences like true fast imaging and steady precession (FISP) and HASTE provide excellent image quality. HASTE thick slab generates conventional enteroclysis-like images.[27] T1-weighted images can depict fatty proliferation while post-gad fat-suppressed 3D volume interpolated breath-hold examination (VIBE) sequence shows disease activity. Functional cine-MRI can allow evaluation of intestinal motility along with detection of intra-

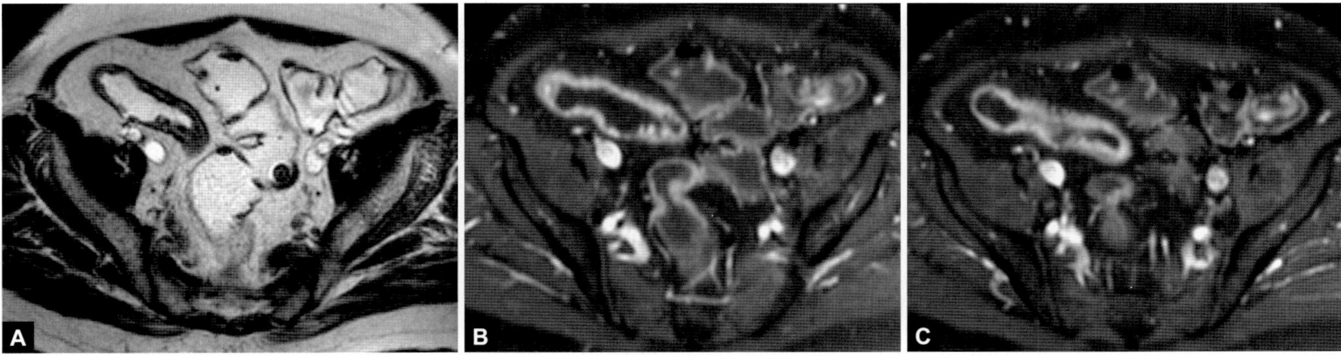

Figures 14A to C Magnetic resonance enterography in Crohn's disease. Axial true fast imaging and steady precession imaging (A) shows wall thickening involving distal ileum in the right iliac fossa. Axial contrast-enhanced fat suppressed volume interpolated breath-hold examination images (B and C) show abnormal wall thickening and enhancement in the distal small bowel loop with prominent vasa recta along it, suggesting inflammatory bowel disease. Multiple such segments were found on magnetic resonance imaging involving distal small bowel

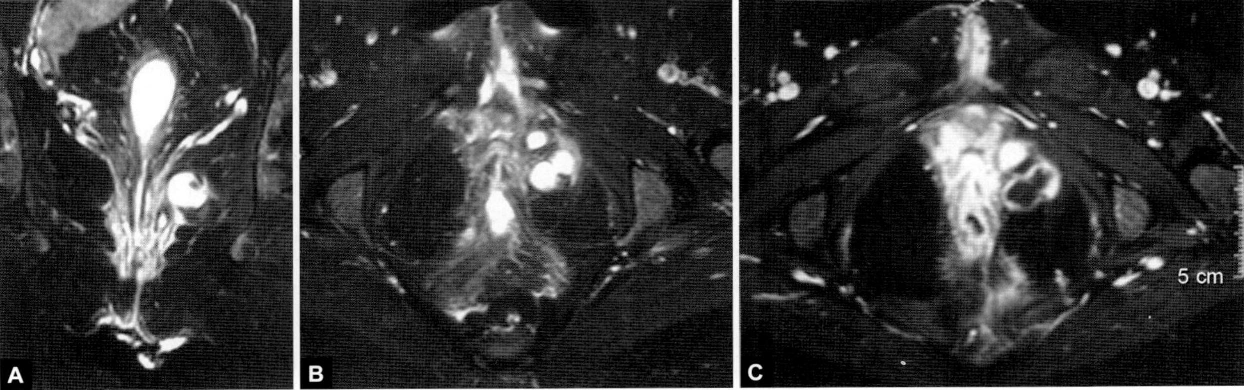

Figures 15A to C T2-weighted fat suppressed coronal image (A) shows multiple fluid collections in the left ischioanal fossa along with perianal fistula with multiple ramifications. T2 axial (B) and postgadolinium axial images (C) show that collections are located at 1-2 o' clock position, show rim enhancement with inflammatory changes also seen at 5 o' clock

abdominal adhesions.[28] The technique of MRI colonography is still evolving and may provide a radiation-free alternative to CT.[29]

Diffusion-weighted MRI is a relatively new technique in abdomen which can be incorporated into the existing protocols without any additional cost and minimal time penalty. It provides an additional paradigm for lesion characterization based on cellularity. Apparent diffusion coefficient (ADC) measurements may have a role in predicting response to chemotherapy in colorectal malignancies.[30] Low baseline ADC is associated with better response to chemotherapy. Also diffusion weighted imaging (DWI) is very sensitive in detecting liver metastases (Fig. 16). ADC values may aid to distinguish focal pancreatitis from adenocarcinoma.[31] Characterization of neoplastic lesions and infiltrative diseases is another application of DWI.[32] Hemangiomas and liver cysts show high ADC values while hepatocellular carcinoma and metastases depict lower values. DWI has a role in early evaluation of tumor response and identifying residual or recurrent lesions. Decreasing ADC values after chemoradiotherapy can be used as a marker of response before there is any appreciable change in the size of tumors. DWI also helps in the evaluation of patients with inflammatory bowel disease and can detect inflammation, abscesses and fistulas.[33]

Magnetic resonance spectroscopy provides information regarding relative tissue metabolite concentrations. Proton magnetic resonance spectroscopy (MRS) is used for noninvasive

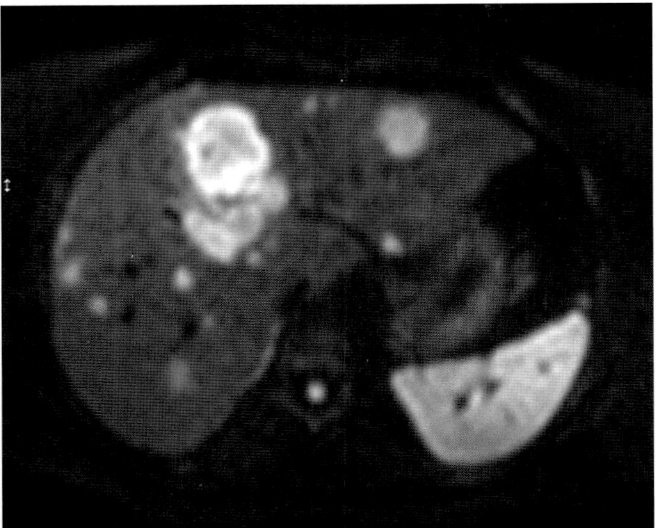

Figure 16 Axial diffusion weighted image at b-value of 800 second/mm^2 shows multiple hyperintense liver lesions, suggesting restricted diffusion. This was a case of colorectal malignancy where diffusion-weighted imaging (DWI) detected multiple liver metastases. DWI offers high lesion-to-background parenchyma contrast and is superior to T2W sequence for lesion detection

quantification of liver fat, diagnose malignancy based on elevated choline and identify inflamed bowel.[34,35] The advantages of higher field strength (3 Tesla) MR systems include improved detection of lesions on postcontrast scans, better image quality of MRCP and MR angiography, higher strength diffusion-weighted imaging with preserved image quality and improved spectral resolution in MRS.[36] Magnetic field homogeneities, chemical shift and susceptibility artifacts and increased acquisition time are the potential limitations.

DIGITAL SUBTRACTION ANGIOGRAPHY

Digital subtraction angiography (DSA) is the gold standard for the evaluation of arterial diseases. These days, diagnostic information is acquired through CT and MR angiograms while DSA is reserved for interventions. Transarterial embolizations in case of active bleeding or pseudoaneurysm, chemo-embolizations, angioplasty and stenting in mesenteric ischemia offer minimally invasive methods to manage many complex clinical problems.

RADIONUCLIDE STUDIES

Positron emission tomography provides functional metabolic information using various radiotracers. 18F-fluorodeoxyglucose (FDG) PET has demonstrated high accuracy in the detection and follow-up of cancers of esophagus and colon.[37] A combination of PET-CT is a potent tool in the primary staging and evaluation of any recurrent disease. PET-CT is superior in detecting hepatic and extrahepatic metastases in colorectal carcinomas. However, mucinous adenocarcinomas are less FDG avid and can produce false-negative results. PET-CT is a sensitive though nonspecific technique. Tuberculosis is an important confounding factor in our country and cannot be reliably differentiated from malignancy even on PET-CT.

Gallium-68 DOTA-NOC PET-CT has high sensitivity and specificity for the detection of neuroendocrine tumors. Technetium (Tc)-99m sulfur colloid and Tc-99m-labelled red blood cell (RBC) scan are used to detect obscure GI bleed. Tc-99m pertechnetate scan helps in detecting ectopic gastric mucosa in cases of Meckel's diverticulum. Tc-99m hexamethylpropyleneamine oxime (HMPAO) leukocyte scintigraphy is used in evaluation of inflammatory bowel diseases.

CONCLUSION

Imaging plays a vital role in the evaluation of virtually all GI and hepatobiliary diseases. A judicious use of the vast array of modalities available requires a close cooperation between the radiologist, gastroenterologist and GI surgeon. Indiscriminate use of ionizing radiation-based techniques must be avoided and repeat studies should be asked for only, if they significantly alter the course of management.

For evaluation of esophagus, endoscopy is the first-line study with barium swallow being complimentary and CT is used mainly for staging the malignancies. For stomach and duodenum, endoscopy is the modality of choice with barium meal helpful in evaluation of reflux, submucosal masses and infiltrative diseases. Small bowel evaluation is best achieved by enterography or enteroclysis and CT scores over barium giving mural and extraluminal information with short acquisition time. A follow-through or enterography study is required prior to capsule endoscopy to rule out small bowel obstruction. Latter is more sensitive in mucosal evaluation but is limited by long hours of patient preparation, small bowel transit and subsequent image analysis. Colonoscopy is the investigation of choice for evaluation of colorectal diseases with barium enema being reserved in cases of incomplete colonoscopy. Gastrograffin contrast studies are frequently used for evaluation of postoperative GIT. Radiographs and USG are the first-line investigations in acute abdomen and acute bowel obstruction, followed by CT for definitive diagnosis. Multiphasic MDCT and MRI are the modality of choice for evaluation of focal liver and pancreatic lesions. USG and MRCP are complementary for evaluation of the biliary tree. Side-viewing endoscopy and EUS are confirmatory to the findings of MRCP and CT in periampullary lesions. Newer techniques like DWI and perfusion CT are being explored for improving the accuracy of CT and MRI. Rational use of available modalities can enable prompt and accurate diagnosis of various GIT problems.

REFERENCES

1. Frokjaer JB, Drewes AM, Gregersen H. Imaging of the gastrointestinal tract-novel technologies. World J Gastroenterol WJG. 2009;15(2):160-8.
2. Field S, Guy PJ, Upsdell SM, Scourfield AE. The erect abdominal radiograph in the acute abdomen: should its routine use be abandoned? Br Med J Clin Res Ed. 1985;290(6486):1934-6.
3. Mirvis SE, Young JW, Keramati B, McCrea ES, Tarr R. Plain film evaluation of patients with abdominal pain: are three radiographs necessary? AJR Am J Roentgenol. 1986;147(3):501-3.
4. Gammill SL, Nice CM Jr. Air fluid levels: their occurrence in normal patients and their role in the analysis of ileus. Surgery. 1972;71(5):771-80.
5. Silva AC, Pimenta M, Guimaraes LS. Small Bowel Obstruction: What to look for. Radiographics. 2009;29(2):423-39.
6. Adam A, Dixon AK, Grainger RG, Allison DJ. Grainger and Allison's Diagnostic Radiology, 5th edition. Churchill Livingstone/Elsevier; 2008.
7. Puylaert JB. Acute appendicitis: US evaluation using graded compression. Radiology. 1986;158(2):355-60.
8. Schwartz DA, Wiersema MJ. The role of endoscopic ultrasound in hepatobiliary disease. Curr Gastroenterol Rep. 2002;4(1):72-8.
9. Wiersema MJ, Wiersema LM. High-resolution 25-megahertz ultrasonography of the gastrointestinal wall: histologic correlates. Gastrointest Endosc. 1993;39(4):499-504.
10. Serra C, Menozzi G, Labate AMM, Giangregorio F, Gionchetti P, Beltrami M, et al. Ultrasound assessment of vascularization of the thickened terminal ileum wall in Crohn's disease patients using a low-mechanical index real-time scanning technique with a second generation ultrasound contrast agent. Eur J Radiol. 2007;62(1):114-21.
11. Schlottmann K, Kratzer W, Scholmerich J. Doppler ultrasound and intravenous contrast agents in gastrointestinal tract disorders: current role and future implications. Eur J Gastroenterol Hepatol. 2005;17(3):263-75.
12. Nicolau C, Ripolles T. Contrast-enhanced ultrasound in abdominal imaging. Abdom Imaging. 2012;37(1):1-19.
13. Gilja OH, Hatlebakk JG, Odegaard S, Berstad A, Viola I, Giertsen C, et al. Advanced imaging and visualization in gastrointestinal disorders. World J Gastroenterol WJG. 2007;13(9):1408-21.
14. Frulio N, Trillaud H. Ultrasound elastography in liver. Diagn Interv Imaging. 2013;94(5):515-34.
15. Bruining DH. CT Enterography: is it the current state-of-the-art for small bowel diagnostics? Dig Dis. 2010;28(3):429-32.

16. Elsayes KM, Al-Hawary MM, Jagdish J, Ganesh HS, Platt JF. CT enterography: principles, trends, and interpretation of findings. Radiographics. 2010;30(7):1955-70.
17. Fisher LR. Invited commentary. Radiographics. 2010;30(7):1971-3.
18. Solem CA, Loftus EV Jr, Fletcher JG, Baron TH, Gostout CJ, Petersen BT, et al. Small-bowel imaging in Crohn's disease: a prospective, blinded, 4-way comparison trial. Gastrointest Endosc. 2008;68(2):255-66.
19. Blachar A, Sosna J. CT colonography (virtual colonoscopy): technique, indications and performance. Digestion. 2007;76(1):34-41.
20. Aschoff AJ, Ernst AS, Brambs H-J, Juchems MS. CT colonography: an update. Eur Radiol. 2008;18(3):429-37.
21. Coursey CA, Nelson RC, Boll DT, Paulson EK, Ho LM, Neville AM, et al. Dual-energy multidetector CT: how does it work, what can it tell us, and when can we use it in abdominopelvic imaging? Radiographics. 2010;30(4):1037-55.
22. Hansen M, Norling R, Lauridsen C, Fallentin E, Bæksgaard L, Kofoed K, et al. Computed tomography (CT) perfusion in abdominal cancer: technical aspects. Diagnostics. 2013;3(2):261-70.
23. Tsuji Y, Takahashi N, Tsutomu C. Pancreatic perfusion CT in early stage of severe acute pancreatitis. Int J Inflam. 2012;2012:497386.
24. Klessen C, Rogalla P, Taupitz M. Local staging of rectal cancer: the current role of MRI. Eur Radiol. 2007;17(2):379-89.
25. Siddiki HA, Fidler JL, Fletcher JG, Burton SS, Huprich JE, Hough DM, et al. Prospective comparison of state-of-the-art MR enterography and CT enterography in small-bowel Crohn's disease. AJR Am J Roentgenol. 2009;193(1):113-21.
26. Berman L, Israel GM, McCarthy SM, Weinreb JC, Longo WE. Utility of magnetic resonance imaging in anorectal disease. World J Gastroenterol WJG. 2007;13(23):3153-8.
27. Masselli G, Casciani E, Polettini E, Gualdi G. Comparison of MR enteroclysis with MR enterography and conventional enteroclysis in patients with Crohn's disease. Eur Radiol. 2008;18(3):438-47.
28. Buhmann-Kirchhoff S, Lang R, Kirchhoff C, Steitz HO, Jauch KW, Reiser M, et al. Functional cine MR imaging for the detection and mapping of intraabdominal adhesions: method and surgical correlation. Eur Radiol. 2008;18(6):1215-23.
29. Lauenstein TC. MR colonography: current status. Eur Radiol. 2006;16(7):1519-26.
30. Qayyum A. Diffusion-weighted imaging in the abdomen and pelvis: Concepts and applications. Radiographics. 2009;29(6):1797-810.
31. Fattahi R, Balci NC, Perman WH, Hsueh EC, Alkaade S, Havlioglu N, et al. Pancreatic diffusion-weighted imaging (DWI): comparison between mass-forming focal pancreatitis (FP), pancreatic cancer (PC), and normal pancreas. J Magn Reson Imaging JMRI. 2009;29(2):350-6.
32. Keogan MT, Edelman RR. Technologic advances in abdominal MR Imaging. Radiology. 2001;220(2):310-20.
33. Sinha R, Rajiah P, Ramachandran I, Sanders S, Murphy PD. Diffusion-weighted MR imaging of the gastrointestinal tract: technique, indications, and imaging findings. Radiographics. 2013;33(3):655-76.
34. Qayyum A. MR spectroscopy of the liver: principles and clinical applications. Radiographics. 2009;29(6):1653-64.
35. Varma S, Bird R, Eskin M, Dolenko B, Raju J, Bezabeh T. Detection of inflammatory bowel disease by proton magnetic resonance spectroscopy (1H MRS) using an animal model. J Inflamm Lond Engl. 2007;4:24.
36. Chang KJ, Kamel IR, Macura KJ, Bluemke DA. 3.0-T MR imaging of the abdomen: comparison with 1.5 T1. Radiographics. 2008;28(7):1983-98.
37. Esteves FP, Schuster DM, Halkar RK. Gastrointestinal tract malignancies and positron emission tomography: an overview. Semin Nucl Med. 2006;36(2):169-81.

CHAPTER 3

Infections and Antibiotics in Gastrointestinal Surgery

Archana Thakur

INTRODUCTION

Postoperative infections increase mortality, morbidity and prolong hospitalization leading to increase in cost of treatment. Many of these infections are believed to result from contamination of the operative site during the surgical procedure. Such contamination is unavoidable when the procedure involves a nonsterile area, such as the gastrointestinal tract (GIT), hence postoperative infections are common in gastrointestinal (GI) surgery. Incidence is higher in emergency surgery (16%) than in elective surgery (6%).[1,2] The operations which are complicated and of longer duration like colorectal and small intestine procedure, are more strongly associated with complications as compared to smaller operations. The incidence of infection is higher in lower gastrointestinal surgeries than in upper gastrointestinal surgeries as the bacterial load is higher in lower GIT.

COMMON INFECTIONS ENCOUNTERED IN GI SURGERY[1,3,4]

- Postoperative wound and tissue complications
  - Surgical-site infections: Which can be superficial or deep wound infection, wound abscess
  - Intra-abdominal infection: Abdominal abscess or peritonitis
  - Disruption of tissue, e.g. wound, fascia or leakage from anastomosis site
- Pulmonary complications and infections: Hypoxemia, collapse of alveoli (atelectasis), respiratory failure leading to endotracheal intubation and mechanical ventilation, ventilator-associated pneumonia, aspiration pneumonia, etc.
- Urinary tract infection
- Septicemia.

Wound and Tissue Infections

Wound and tissue infections after surgery occur in 2–30% cases depending upon risk factors[5] which are:

- Degree/density of bacterial contamination at the surgical site
- Duration of the operation
- Host susceptibility.

Density of Bacterial Contamination

Number and type of organisms present at the surgical site is the major factor influencing the risk of postoperative infection. This was recognized several decades ago in the wound classification system that divides all wounds into the four categories.[5-7]

Class I: Clean

Elective procedure, clean nontraumatic, not infected/inflamed wound, no break in technique, respiratory, gastrointestinal and genitourinary tracts not entered. Examples: elective inguinal hernia repair, splenectomy, exploratory laparotomy (no bowel involvement), *Staphylococcus aureus* is the most common pathogen and infection rate is 2% or less, depending on presence of other risk factors.

Class II: Clean contaminated

Emergency case, nontraumatic, clean wound, no unusual contamination, minor break in technique, controlled opening of gastrointestinal, respiratory or genitourinary tract with no or minor spillage. Examples: elective intestinal resection and other gastrointestinal procedures (including laparoscopy, colonoscopy, gastroscopy, vagotomy and pyloroplasty).

Contaminants are endogenous bacteria. For example, *Escherichia coli* and *Bacteroides fragilis* are common pathogens encountered in sigmoid colectomy wounds. Infection rate varies from of 4% to 10%.

Class III: Contaminated

Emergency procedures. Wound Created without normal antisepsis and sterile technique, operative wound contaminated, gross spillage from the GIT, nonpurulent inflammation.

Examples: Elective intestinal procedures with gross contamination of surgical site, intestinal spillage during laparotomy for penetrating injury, acute nonperforated, nongangrenous appendicitis.

Large spillage of intestinal bacteria in surgical field increases infection rate, which can be greater than 10–20% even with preventive antibiotics. Contaminants are the intestinal bacteria introduced by gross spillage in the surgical field.

Class IV: Dirty infected

Operative wound dirty and contaminated, acute bacterial inflammation of operative wound, traumatic wound from dirty source, presence of foreign body or devitalized tissue, fecal contamination, operative wound where clean tissue is transected to gain access to a collection of pus. Examples: abdominal exploration for acute peritonitis and intra-abdominal abscess, perforated appendicitis with abscess, wound debridement.

Unusual pathogens are often encountered and infection rate can be up to 30–40%.

Duration of the Operation

For duration of the operation, based on national nosocomial infections surveillance (NNIS) database, a standard T point was determined, which is the length of time in hours that represents the 75th percentile of procedures reported in the NNIS survey. It is different for different type of surgery. Longer the duration, higher the risk of infection. Depending on the duration of surgery risk category 0, 1, 2 or 3 is identified.[5,7-11]

Host Susceptibility

American Society of Anesthesiologists (ASA) has defined preoperative assessment score of 3, 4 or 5:[5,7]

- Class I: A patient in normal health
- Class II: A patient with mild systemic disease resulting in no functional limitations
- Class III: A patient with severe systemic disease that limits activity, but is not incapacitating
- Class IV: A patient with severe systemic disease that is a constant threat to life
- Class V: A moribund patient not likely to survive 24 hours.

Considering above variables a risk index has been developed. This has a range from 0 to 3 points. A point is added to the patient's risk index for each of the following three variables:[5,9,11]

- 1 point: The patient has a contaminated or dirty operation.
- 1 point: The duration of the operation exceeds the 75th percentile
- 1 point: The patient has an ASA preoperative assessment score of 3, 4 or 5.

The risk of postoperative wound infections increases with increase in risk index. The infection rate with risk point 0, 1, 2 or 3 being 1.5%, 2.9%, 6.8% and 13%, respectively. This risk can be used to decide preoperative prophylactic antibiotics administration.[5,6,9,11]

Other variables associated with increased risk of tissue and wound complications are smoking, comorbidity like diabetes, cardiovascular disease, lung disease, malnutrition, obesity, etc., perioperative blood loss and, type and site of surgery following elective operations.

Following emergency operations, gender (males more at risk), peritonitis (with localized or generalized pus more at risk), type of operation, (gastroduodenal, small bowel and colorectal surgery more risk) and if multiple operations are done, are some of the variables associated with wound infections.[1,3,7]

Diagnosis of Wound Infections

Diagnosis of postoperative wound is obvious when the wound opens and discharges pus. It is evident only after the fourth or fifth postoperative day except infections caused by beta-hemolytic Streptococci and by Clostridium species, which are evident within 24 hours. The classic signs of infection include localized erythema, localized pain, localized heat, cellulitis, edema, abscess, discharge, discoloration of tissues, friable and bleeding granulation tissue, abnormal smell, etc. Because most of the patients have some fever in the first several days after major operative procedure, fever is not a specific sign of postoperative infection.[5] Microbiological diagnosis can be made after culture of sample from local site. Common organisms causing infection will depend on the type of bacteria contaminating surgical site and that would be the flora of the viscera entered during surgical procedure. GIT is colonized by large number of aerobic and anaerobic bacteria. The number and type of organisms are different at different levels of GIT. The number of microorganisms varies from 10^4 organisms/g to 10^{11} organisms/g, increases at the distal portions of the GIT. Streptococci, Lactobacillus, Diphtheroids and few Peptostreptococcus usually colonize the stomach. Jejunum harbors Streptococci, Enterococci, aerobic Gram-negative bacteria and Bacteroides, whereas colon has predominantly *E. coli* and *B. fragilis*, concentration of anaerobes being many thousands times greater than aerobes.[12] Hence, the predominant bacteria causing infection are *E. coli,* Klebsiella spp., *Enterococcus faecalis*, Enterobacter spp. and anaerobic bacteria, like *B. fragilis*, Prevotella, Peptostreptococcus and Clostridium spp.

Hospital acquired abdominal infections, especially in the intensive care unit (ICU), are more likely to be caused by Pseudomonas species, Enterococcus species, *S. aureus* and fungi.[6,7,13]

Treatment of Wound Infections

In the event of infection, bacteriological identification and sensitivity of pathogen may not be available for more than 48–72 hours. Hence, empirical therapy by antibiotics has to be started as soon as possible along with other recommended procedures. Empirical therapy should be based on likely pathogen to be encountered and the local antibiogram of the hospital.

Mixed infections, aerobic and anaerobic are expected in gastrointestinal surgeries, so antimicrobials effective against both aerobic and anaerobic infection should be administered. Infection by *Pseudomonas aeruginosa* and Enterococcal species may also be considered when starting the treatment in patients in ICUs.

Single-agent or combination regimens can be considered.

Antimicrobials used as single agents are second generation cephalosporins (cefoxitin and cefotetan), carbapenems or combination of ticarcillin/clavulanic acid, piperacillin/tazobactam or ampicillin/sulbactam.[5,13]

The advantage of single-agent therapy is that aminoglycosides which are used in combination therapy and cause ototoxicity and nephrotoxicity are avoided. Single-agent therapy may also be less expensive. But single agent may not always be effective in hospital-acquired wound infection because they are mostly caused by multidrug resistant (MDR) bacteria.

If *S. aureus* is suspected, antistaphylococcal antimicrobials should be used. If methicillin-resistant *Staphylococcus aureus* (MRSA) is present or suspected, cefazolin, sulfamethoxazole/trimethroprim or vancomycin should be given.[5,13]

Combination regimens generally include two agents, one with activity against aerobic Gram-negative bacilli and the other against anaerobic bacteria.

Antimicrobials effective against the Enterobacteriaceae but not Bacteroides group are aminoglycosides (gentamicin, tobramycin, amikacin and netilmicin), third generation cephalosporins (cefotaxime, ceftriaxone, ceftazidime, cephoperazone and ceftizoxime), fourth generation cephalosporins (cefepime and cefpirome), quinolones and aztreonam. Antibiotics effective against *B. fragilis* group are metronidazole, cefoxitin, a combination of penicillin and beta-lactamase inhibitor (ticarcillin/clavulanic acid, piperacillin/tazobactam), newer quinolones (moxifloxacin) and carbapenems.[13-17]

Ampicillin/sulbactam combination is not effective in cases of infection with Pseudomonas species, hence it should be avoided for hospital-acquired infections (HAIs).

To cover infection with Enterococcus spp., ampicillin may be added as third agent.

Along with antibiotics, other recommended supportive treatment, e.g. opening of wound, surgical drainage, etc. should also be carried out for better outcome.

Perioperative Antimicrobial Prophylaxis

Perioperative antimicrobial prophylaxis is widely used to reduce the risk of postoperative wound infection. It can decrease morbidity, shorten hospital stay and contribute to reduce the overall cost of treatment. There is wide consensus and statements by various societies on specific procedures that warrant antimicrobial prophylaxis[5] and which do not need administration of prophylactic antibiotic. Recommendations are based on studies on animal models, randomized clinical trials and observational clinical data[6] and the principals of antimicrobial prophylaxis are well-defined.

Definition of Antimicrobial Prophylaxis

Prophylactic antibiotics are those antibiotics, which are given to the patients before contamination, or infection has occurred. They are recommended when the risk of postoperative infection is high or the expected consequence of infection is extreme morbidity or death.

Guidelines for Antimicrobial Prophylaxis in Surgery

The principles of antimicrobial prophylaxis in surgery involve the following considerations:[12]

- Surgical procedures for which prophylactic antimicrobials is to be used
- Selection of antimicrobial agent
- Timing of antimicrobial administration
- Route of antimicrobial administration
- Duration for which antimicrobial is to be given

Surgical procedures: Antimicrobial prophylaxis is beneficial in surgical procedures associated with a high risk of infection (clean contaminated, contaminated or dirty procedures), procedure in which the postoperative infection, however unlikely, may be severe or fatal, surgical procedures that enter the GIT (colorectal operations and high risk gastro duodenal and biliary-tract operations) and pose the risk of bacterial contamination or if the patient is immunocompromised (e.g. receiving immunosuppressive agents or neutropenic).

The number of organism is low in the stomach, duodenum and proximal small bowel, reducing the risk of infection associated with procedure entering these sites. For these procedures routine prophylaxis is not mandatory. However, number of bacteria increase with decrease in gastric acidity. So, the use of agents like antacids, histamine blocker or proton pump inhibitors or conditions, such as upper gastrointestinal bleeding or gastrointestinal stasis which reduce gastric acidity, increase the risk of wound infection.[18] Prophylactic antibiotics are indicated in such cases. Colorectal procedures have a high risk of infection, prophylaxis is strongly recommended for these procedures. Antibiotic prophylaxis for biliary tract procedure is recommended, if risk factors, like elderly patient (60 years or above), presence of jaundice, biliary obstruction, disease of the common duct, cholecystitis, etc. are associated.

Timing of antimicrobial administration: The timing of antimicrobial administration is important as antimicrobials given at inappropriate times can be ineffective for surgical prophylaxis. To be most effective in preventing postoperative infections an antimicrobial must be present in the contaminated tissues before bacteria enter the site (i.e. before the surgical incision) and must persist in tissues throughout the period of potential contamination.[19,20]

When antimicrobials are given after bacterial contamination, their ability to prevent infection is reduced. All the guidelines recommend that prophylaxis should be given, at induction of anesthesia or 30–60 minutes before incision.[21]

If an operation is expected to last more than 6–8 hours, an antimicrobial with a longer half-life and duration of action should be used. If short-acting agents are used, they should be readministered at intervals of twice the half-life of the agent. Increasing the dose of an agent provides less benefit than shortening the dosing interval because of drug clearance.[19,20]

Duration of antimicrobial prophylaxis: The shortest duration of antimicrobial administration that is effective in preventing postoperative operation is not known; however, recent studies document that postoperative antimicrobial administration is not necessary for many operations.[21,22]

Route of antimicrobial administration: Antimicrobials used for surgical prophylaxis may be administrated intravenously, intramuscularly, orally, rectally and topically (into the surgical wound). Most often intravenous and intramuscular routes are used. Oral antimicrobials are often used for gut decontamination in elective colorectal operations.[12]

Selection of antimicrobial agents: The antibiotic selected should be based on the site-specific flora, its spectrum of activity, its toxicity and pharmacokinetic properties. The agent selected should have antibacterial activity against the expected most common wound pathogens. In clean operations, Gram-positive cocci like staphylococci predominate, penicillinase-resistant penicillins (oxacillin and nafcillin) are suitable antibiotic. If methicillin-resistant staphylococci are suspected vancomycin or cephalosporins may be required.

For clean contaminated operations, the expected pathogen is bacteria found in the GIT. For these, first generation cephalosporin, such as cephazolin is the agent of choice due to its low cost, long duration of action and because it is effective against most of the pathogens commonly associated with clean and clean contaminated operations. The use of other first generation cephalosporins, such as cephalothin which although have a shorter duration of action, are more resistant to staphylococcal beta-lactamases, should be evaluated. First generation cephalosporins are as effective as second or third generation agents and a single preoperative dose is as effective as multiple dose.[12,23]

Pharmacological Considerations

Dosages of antimicrobial should be adjusted according to the minimum inhibitory concentration (MIC) against bacteria causing infection. Tissue concentrations at the operative site should be maintained higher than the MIC. Antimicrobial with short half-life have to be repeated if procedure is long.[7,21]

Antimicrobial should have bactericidal effect. Bactericidal effect of some antibiotics such as beta-lactams is not dose-dependent, rather it increases with contact time. Whereas bactericidal effect of aminoglycosides and quinolones depends on the concentration used rather than the contact time. They are called dose-dependent antibiotics.

Inoculum Effect

The MIC increases with the density of bacterial inoculums.[21]

Postantibiotic Effect

Some antibiotics show a persistent inhibitory effect on bacterial growth after elimination from tissue. Aminoglycosides have a postantibiotic effect (PAE) on Gram-negative bacteria and beta-lactam antibiotics on Gram-positive bacteria that persist for several hours. Fluroquinolones have PAE on both.[21]

Specific Recommendations for the Selection of Prophylactic Antimicrobials for Various Surgical Procedures (American Society of Health-System Pharmacists)

Biliary-Tract Surgery

Explorations of the common bile duct and choledochoenterostomies are among the most commonly performed abdominal procedures on biliary tract. In the majority of patients, the biliary tract is sterile and the risk of infection is no higher than that of other clean operation. If bacterial count increases in the biliary tract, the rate of infection may reach as high as 36%. Elderly patients above 70 years of age, patients of acute cholecystitis or with obstruction in biliary tract are at a higher risk of acquiring infection. The organisms most likely to be associated with wound infection are *E. coli*, Klebsiella and Enterococci.[5,23-25]

Recommendations: Antimicrobial prophylaxis is recommended for patients undergoing cholecystectomy. Single 1 g cefazolin should be given intravenously before or within 30 minutes of the start of the operation.

Gastroduodenal Surgery

Gastric operation for which antimicrobial prophylaxis is considered are resection with or without vagotomy for gastric or duodenal ulcers, resection for gastric carcinoma, and gastroplasty or gastric bypass for morbid obesity.[26] The risk of postoperative infection after gastroduodenal surgery varies markedly, depending on the type of operation performed and the patient's clinical condition. The wound infection rate was 4% after operation for duodenal ulcer, 29% for gastric ulcer and 33% for gastric resection for cancer. With gastric bypass operation a wound infection rate of 21% has been reported.[27-29] Other important factors associated with infection risk are the use of histamine H2 receptor blocker or the presence of achlorhydria, gastric obstruction or bleeding. They can increase bacterial concentration in stomach and may increase the risk of postoperative infection.[30,31] Wound infections after gastroduodenal surgery are polymicrobial and involve *E. coli* and Enterococci.

Recommendations: Prophylactic antimicrobials are not needed when the lumen of the intestinal tract is not entered. They should be used when the stomach or duodenum is entered surgically. Although some authors believe that antimicrobial are not necessary for patient undergoing gastric resection for non-obstructing ulcer, the widespread use of H2 receptor blockers make it likely that these patient will have high intraluminal bacterial concentration making antimicrobial prophylaxis advisable.

Cefazolin is preferred as a single preoperative dose.[12]

Colorectal Surgery

Surgical-site infection is the most common complication following colorectal surgery. It was believed to be because of large numbers of aerobic and anaerobic organisms are present in colon which causes bacterial contamination of surgical wound. Most frequently isolated organisms are *E. coli* and *B. fragilis*.

To reduce the risk of contamination of the surgical wound, it was considered necessary that resident bacterial concentration is reduced at site. It can be achieved by use of mechanical bowel preparation which decreases the total number of bacteria. Recently single day (12 hours or less) orthograde lavage techniques using an iso-osmotic nonabsorbable electrolyte solution or mannitol solution have been used.[32-34] Two liters of a polyethylene glycol-electrolyte lavage solution is given over 3 hours starting the morning of the day before surgery. It is used in conjunction with three doses of 1 g neomycin sulphate and 1 g erythromycin given orally at 19, 18 and 9 hours before surgery.

Antimicrobial agents combined with mechanical cleansing of the colonic lumen in some studies have significantly reduced postoperative wound infection rates from 30-60% to less than 10% in clean contaminated procedures.[35,36] However, level I evidence has now accumulated to omit mechanical preparation from the preoperative regimens. Several systematic reviews and meta-analysis have indicated that mechanical bowel preparation does not improve outcomes in terms of anastomotic leaks or surgical-site infections.

Recommendations:
Mechanical bowel preparation: Mechanical bowel preparation for surgery remains controversial, although frequently practiced. Bowel preparation is required for colonoscopy and can be omitted for bowel surgery.

A single intravenous dose of a 2 g cephalosporin that is effective against both aerobic and anaerobic bacteria and has a half-life of 60 minutes or longer (cefotetan, cefmetazole, cefotaxime or ceftizoxime) should be administered at induction of anesthesia.

If a cephalosporin with a half-life of 60 minutes or less is used (cefoxitin), and surgery lasts longer than 3 hours, a second dose of the intravenous antimicrobial should be given.

If the patient is to undergo a colostomy closure or rectal procedure, a combination of oral and intravenous agents should be given.[12]

Appendectomy

The incidence of infections depends on the condition of the appendix at the time of surgery. In uncomplicated appendectomy, the postoperative infection rate is reported to be between 0% and 30%.[37-39] However, if the appendix is gangrenous, perforated or abscessed (complicated appendicitis), wound infection rates approach 80% without antimicrobial prophylaxis.[40] Appropriate antimicrobial prophylaxis has reduced surgical wound infection rates to as low as 1% in both uncomplicated and certain complicated appendectomies. The majority of studies have shown that even when appropriate antimicrobials are used, infections will occur in 10–25% of patients with a gangrenous or perforated appendix.[40-42]

Microorganisms commonly isolated from wound infections after appendectomy are *E. coli* and *B. fragilis*. Streptococci, *S. aureus* and Enterococcus species have also been isolated frequently. Pseudomonas species has also been reported.[43,44]

Recommendations:
Uncomplicated appendicitis: Cephalosporin effective against both aerobic and anaerobic bacteria, i.e. cefoxitin, cefotetan, cefmetazole, cefotaxime or ceftizoxime. Dosage is 1–2 g intravenous at induction of anesthesia, to be repeated if surgery lasts longer than 3 hours.

Complicated appendicitis: Same regimen but to be continued for 3 to 5 days.

Alternatives are aminoglycosides or aztreonam plus metronidazole.[12]

Common Errors in Antibiotic Prophylaxis

Common errors in antibiotic prophylaxis include choosing the wrong antimicrobial, administering the prophylactic dose too early, omitting second dose in long operations or continuing the prophylactic antibiotic longer than required. The worst error is inappropriate use of valuable therapeutic agents with expanded spectrum and excessively long-term administration. Indiscriminate antibiotic use is costly and exposes the patients to adverse effects, and promotes resistance to the drugs.

Although prophylactic antimicrobials reduce the incidence of postoperative wound infections, but number of other factors, such as any underlying comorbid medical condition in the patient, break in sterile technique at any stage during operation, environment of operating-room, duration of procedure and the expertise of the surgeon also have a strong impact on wound infection rates. The drug-resistant organisms are selected as a result of inappropriate and indiscriminate use of prophylactic antibiotic and necessitate more expensive infection control measures and antibiotics. Along with antibiotic prophylaxis good infection control practices, good technique and good patient care is essential in reducing postoperative infections.[6]

Pulmonary Complications

Postoperative pulmonary complications can be atelectasis, endotracheal intubation and ventilation, aspiration pneumonia, ventilator-associated pneumonia (VAP), pleural effusion, respiratory failure, bronchospasm and exacerbation of chronic obstructive pulmonary disease.[45]

Pulmonary complications remain an important cause of mortality and morbidity in spite of many advances in anesthetic and surgical techniques.[46-48]

Most important risk factor of postoperative pulmonary complications is the site of incision; thoracic or upper abdominal procedure (e.g. cholecystectomy), in which the incision has to be near the diaphragm, carry higher risk than the procedures on lower abdomen or gynecology surgeries.[49-52] Other factors associated with higher probability of postoperative pulmonary complications include chronic respiratory disease, increasing age, obesity, history of smoking, malnutrition, long lasting anesthesia and a longer stay in hospital before operation. Men have two to three times higher incidences than women.[46]

Ventilator-Associated Pneumonia

Ventilator-associated pneumonia (VAP) is the pneumonia that develops 48 hours after mechanical ventilation by means of an endotracheal tube or tracheostomy is given. During intubation, the integrity of the oropharynx and trachea is compromised and microorganisms enter the lower respiratory tract and lung parenchyma leading to infection. Eight to twenty-eight percent of patients receiving mechanical ventilation develop ventilator-associated pneumonia. The mortality rate for VAP is very high varying from 24% to 50% and if the infection is caused by high-risk pathogens like *P. aeruginosa* and Acinetobacter, it can go up to 76%.[53-55]

Diagnosis of VAP

Ventilator-associated pneumonia is identified by using a combination of clinical, radiological and bacteriological criteria.

Clinically: Signs and symptoms of fever, purulent sputum, cough, dyspnea and raised total lung capacity (TLC) count or worsening gas exchange.

Radiologically: Persistent infiltration, consolidation and cavitation.

Bacteriologically: Positive culture growth in blood/pleural fluid/ quantitative culture of bronchoalveolar lavage (BAL).

By using a combination of presence of positive radiological findings and two of the clinical signs 69% cases of VAP can be diagnosed with specificity of 75%.[56]

Bacteriological Diagnosis

Appropriate antimicrobial treatment of patients with VAP significantly improves outcome, the goal should be rapid identification and accurate selection of antimicrobial agents.

Variety of samples and techniques has been used for culture to diagnose bacterial pneumonia.

For clinical diagnosis of VAP, nonquantitative or semiquantitative cultures of airway samples, e.g. endotracheal aspirate (ETA) can be done but it has less sensitivity and specificity (sensitivity of 82% but a specificity of only 27%)[57] as compared to quantitative cultures of airway specimens, such as quantitative endotracheal aspirate (QEA), blind bronchial sampling (BBS), bronchoscopic protected specimen brush (PSB) and BAL culture, etc. Specificity of this technique is more but it needs technical expertise and advance equipment.

Frequent method followed in labs is nonquantitative or semiquantitative cultures of endotracheal aspirate and BAL.[56]

Blood and Pleural Fluid Cultures

Although infection to the blood or pleural space spreads in less than 10% cases of VAP, it is recommended that two sets of blood cultures and a pleural fluid, if effusions is present should be part of investigation.[58] Blood culture is positive in less than 25% patients of VAP and in most of these positive cultures the organisms may originate from an extrapulmonary site of infection.[59,64]

Etiological Agents

The etiological agents responsible for infection differ according to the prevalent infections present in an ICU, prior antibiotic therapy and length of stay in the hospital. Prior antimicrobial therapy in the preceding 90 days, hospitalization of more than 5 days, prevalence of resistance in the community or local hospital, and immunosuppressive disease and/or therapy increases the risk of infection by MDR organisms.

Common causative organisms are *S. aureus*, *P. aeruginosa*, Acinetobacter spp. and Enterobacteriaceae group (Klebsiella, *E. coli*, proteus, Enterobacter, Citrobacter). *Streptococcus pneumoniae*, Haemophilus spp. and *Stenotrophomonas maltophilia* are also isolated from few patients. Candida spp. rarely causes invasive pulmonary disease. But if isolated in culture it indicates *P. aeruginosa* may be the cause of VAP in that patient.[48]

The prognosis of VAP is worse in patients having infection with aerobic Gram-negative bacilli as compared to infection with Gram-positive pathogens. Death rates are maximum in infections caused by *P. aeruginosa*, ranging from 70% to more than 80% in several studies[60,61] compared with 55% for pneumonias due to other organisms.[60]

Treatment of VAP

Selection of antibiotics: Patients with early-onset VAP and not likely to have infection with MDR organism, empirical therapy may be started with one of the following antibiotics:[56]

- Fluoroquinolones
- Ceftrioxone
- Ampicillin and sulbactum or
- Ertapenem.

In patients of VAP with late-onset or likely to have infection with MDR pathogens, initial single agents effective against Pseudomonas like:

- Cephalosporins (cefepime and ceftazidime)
- Carbapenems (imipenem and meropenem).

or

- Combination of beta-lactam/beta-lactamase inhibitors (piperacillin/tazobactam) and an antipseudomonal fluoroquinolone (ciprofloxacin and levofloxacin).

or

- Aminoglycoside (amikacin, gentamycin and tobramycin) and vancomycin or linezolid (if MRSA are suspected) may be considered for empirical treatment
- Telavancin is indicated in infections caused by methicillin-susceptible and resistant isolates, if the alternative treatments are not suitable.[56,62]

Probability of infection with MDR organisms increases if stay of the patient is prolonged (more than 5 days), patient is immunocompromised on immunosuppressive therapy, or had received antibiotics in last 90 days. The risk of infection with MDR organisms further increases if the incidence of resistant organism is more in the hospital or community.[56,63]

Development of resistance can be prevented by prescribing combination therapy. Combination therapy provides synergy and sufficient coverage also if the pathogen is resistant to the agent chosen as a single therapy, leading to improved outcome.[20]

Antibiotics should be changed on the basis of culture results.

Factors which Influence the Outcome of VAP

Early administration of antibiotics, choosing antibiotics based on the patient's risk for having MDR pathogens and local antibiogram, using combination therapy, using antibiotic of different class than received in the recent past and shortening the duration of antibiotic therapy if initial antibiotic was appropriate can influence the outcome of VAP.

Prevention

To reduce the incidence of postoperative pulmonary complications, supportive treatment for preoperative and postoperative chronic respiratory disease, such as breathing exercises, postural drainage, physiotherapy with or without intermittent positive-pressure breathing and incentive spirometry has been recommended.

Intra-abdominal Infections

Intra-abdominal infections (IAIs) include a variety of pathological conditions and can be categorized as being either uncomplicated or complicated.[63]

In uncomplicated case of IAI, the infection involves only a single organ and does not extend to the peritoneum.

In complicated IAI, the infectious process extends beyond the organ, causing either localized or diffuse peritonitis.

Many regimens have been recommended to treat IAI, e.g. guidelines by Surgical Infection Society and Infectious Diseases Society of America. The World Society of Emergency Surgery in consensus with surgeons, infectious disease specialists, pharmacologists, radiologists and intensivists defined following recommendations for early treatment of IAIs.[63]

Recommendations by the World Society of Emergency Surgery (WSES) for Management of Intra-Abdominal Infections (Table 1)

Community-acquired Extra-Biliary Intra-abdominal Infections (Table 2)

Empirical antibiotic treatment of community-acquired IAIs should be according to the most frequently isolated bacteria and the local trends of antibiotic resistance. The major pathogens involved in community-acquired IAIs are enterobacteriaceae, streptococci and anaerobes.

Treatment may be with either single or multiple antimicrobial regimens depending on the patient's condition as well as the specific microorganisms and resistance patterns.

For stable, non-critical patients presenting with no extended-spectrum β-lactamase (ESBL)-associated risk factors, amoxicillin/clavulanate and ciprofloxacin plus metronidazole regimens are recommended. For critically ill patients presenting with no ESBL-associated risk factors, treatments of piperacillin/tazobactam are recommended.

For stable, non-critical patients presenting with ESBL-associated risk factors, ertapenem or tigecycline are recommended. For critically ill patients presenting with ESBL-associated risk factors, meropenem or imipenem plus fluconazole regimens (the latter in the event of risk factors for *Candida*) are recommended.

Biliary Intra-abdominal Infections

The microorganisms, most often isolated in biliary infections are the Gram-negative aerobes; *E. coli* and *K. pneumoniae* and several anaerobes, especially *B. fragilis*.

The antimicrobial drug selection in biliary infections depends on antimicrobial activity against causative bacteria, the clinical condition of the patient, and the biliary levels of the antimicrobial agents and the manner in which it is secreted into the bile.

For stable, non-critical patients presenting with no ESBL-associated risk factors, amoxicillin/clavulanate or ciprofloxacin plus metronidazole is recommended.

For stable, non-critical patients presenting with ESBL-associated risk factors, tigecycline is recommended.

For critically ill patients presenting with no ESBL-associated risk factors, piperacillin/tazobactam is recommended.

For critically ill patients presenting with ESBL-associated risk factors, tigecycline plus piperacillin (plus fluconazole in the event of risk factors for *Candida*) is the recommended drug regimen.

Antimicrobial Regimens Recommended by WSES for Hospital-Acquired IAIs (Table 3)

The incidence of HAIs caused by resistant microorganisms has risen significantly because of higher levels of antibiotic exposure. The other factors, such as advanced age, comorbidity, degree of organ dysfunction, low albumin level, poor nutritional status, severity of illness and the presence of malignancy also contribute to acquiring HAIs due to resistant organisms. Common pathogens are MRSA, vancomycin-resistant *Enterococcus* species, carbapenem-resistant *P. aeruginosa*, ESBL producing *E. coli* and *Klebsiella* species and MDR *Acinetobacter* species. These infections have higher risks of complication and mortality than community-acquired disease. Hence, for these infections, complex multi-drug regimens are usually recommended.

For stable, non-critical patients presenting with risk factors for MDR pathogens, fluconazole and tigecycline plus piperacillin are recommended.

Table 1: Antimicrobial regime recommended by the World Society of Emergency Surgery (WSES) for treating community-acquired extrabiliary intra-abdominal infections

Condition of patient		*Antimicrobial agents*	*Dosage*
Stable patients	With no ESBL-associated risk factor	Amoxicillin/clavulanate Ciprofloxacin plus Metronidazole	2.2 g every 6 hours 400 mg every 8 hours 500 mg every 6 hours
	With ESBL-associated risk factor	Ertapenem or Tigecycline	1 g every 24 hours 100 mg LD than 50 mg 12 hours
Critically ill patients	With no ESBL-associated risk factor	Piperacillin/tazobactam	9 g LD then 18 g per day (continuous infusion) or 4.5 g every 6 hours
	With ESBL-associated risk factor	Meropenem or Imipenem plus Fluconazole	500 mg every 6 hours 500 mg every 6 hours 600 mg LD then 400 mg every 24 hours

Abbreviations: ESBL, extended-spectrum β-lactamase; LD, loading dose.

Table 2: Antimicrobial regime recommended by WSES for treating community-acquired biliary intra-abdominal infections

Condition of patient		*Antimicrobial agents*	*Dosage*
Stable patients	With no ESBL-associated risk factor	Amoxicillin/clavulanate Ciprofloxacin plus Metronidazole	2.2 g every 6 hours 400 mg every 8 hours 500 mg every 6 hours
	With ESBL-associated risk factor	Tigecycline	100 mg LD than 50 mg every 12 hours
Critically ill patients	With no ESBL-associated risk factor	Piperacillin/tazobactam	9 g LD then 18 g per day (continuous infusion) or 4.5 g every 6 hours
	With ESBL-associated risk factor	Piperacillin Plus Tigecycline plus/minus Fluconazole	9 g LD then 18 g per day (continuous infusion) or 4.5 g every 6 hours 100 mg LD than 50 mg every 12 hours 600 mg LD then 400 mg every 24 hours

Abbreviations: ESBL, extended-spectrum β-lactamase; LD, loading dose.

Table 3: Antimicrobial regimens recommended by WSES for hospital-acquired IAIs

Condition of patient	*Antimicrobial agents*	*Dosage*
Stable patients	Piperacillin plus Tigecycline plus Fluconazole	8 g LD then 16 g per day (continuous infusion) or 4 g every 6 hours 100 mg LD than 50 mg every 12 hours 600 mg LD then 400 mg every 24 hours
Critically ill patients	Piperacillin plus Tigecycline plus Echinocandin (capsofungin and micafungin) or Meropenem or Imipenem or Doripenem plus Teicoplanin Plus Echinocandin	8 g LD then 16 g per day (continuous infusion or 4 g every 6 hours 100 mg LD than 50 mg every 12 hours 500 mg every 6 hours 500 mg every 6 hours 500 mg every 8 hours 1.6 g via continuous infusion or 400 mg 6 hours

Abbreviation: LD, loading dose.

In critically ill patients presenting with risk factors for MDR pathogens, meropenem, imipenem/cilastatin and doripenem (plus an echinocandin and teicoplanin) or tigecycline (plus an echinocandin and piperacillin) are recommended.

Prevalence and Antimicrobial Profile of Pathogens Isolated from Patients having Postoperative Infections in GI Surgery in Govind Ballabh Pant Institute of Post Graduate Medical Education and Research

In our facility, which is a super specialty hospital, large number of gastrointestinal surgeries is done, and being a government organization, patients with various risk factors associated with infections are encountered.

Over a period of one year, 6517 culture positive samples, received from patients undergone gastrointestinal surgery, were evaluated in regards to type of organism isolated and antimicrobial sensitivity of these organisms. Only aerobic culture was done.

Type of samples received were wound swab, pus, discharge from surgical site, bile and drain fluids from various sites.

From 42.8% samples (2789), more than one type of organisms were isolated. Gram-negative bacteria (*Klebsiella pneumoniae, E. coli, Acinetobacter* and *Pseudomonas*) were predominant pathogens as shown in the Table 4.

Table 4: Predominant pathogens isolated

Organisms	*Number (%)*
Klebsiella pneumoniae	792 (12.15%)
Escherichia coli	739 (11.3%)
Acinetobacter spp.	505 (7.7%)
Pseudomonas spp.	399 (6.1%)
Enterococcus spp.	280 (4.2%)
Staphylococcus aureus	172 (2.6%)
Proteus mirabilis	162 (2.4%)
Enterobacter spp.	48 (0.7%)
Citrobacter spp.	37 (0.56%)
Providencia stuartii	34 (0.52%)

Other organisms isolated were *Burkholderia cepacia*, coagulase negative staphylococcus and *Morganella morganii.*

Antibiotics Susceptibility (Tables 5 and 6)

- For the Enterobacteriaceae group, tigecycline was the most effective antibiotic followed by amikacin, imipenem, ertapenem and piperacillin/tazobactam.

Table 5: Antibiotic (%) susceptibility pattern for Gram-negative bacteria						
Antibiotics	*Klebsiella species*	*E. coli*	*Acinetobacter species*	*Pseudomonas species*	*Proteus*	*Enterobacter spp.*
Ampicillin	0	0	0	0	0	20
Ampicillin-sulbactam	22.2	12.2	4.7	-	100	20
Piperacilli-tazobactum	59.6	43.3	28.5	62.5	100	40
Cefazolin	18.5	10.3	0	-	0	20
Ceftriaxone	22.2	16	19	36.8	0	20
Cefotaxime	0	20	0	-		
Cefepime	22.2	18.8	19	52	0	40
Aztreonam	18.5	9.4	0	14.5	0	20
Imipenem	62.9	34.5	57.1	58.4	100	60
Meropenem	54.9	33.5	57.1	33.5	100	60
Etrapenem	60.5	75	56.4	67.6	100	60
Amikacin	77.7	74.5	52.3	78.8	100	60
Gentamicin	44.4	30.1	23.8	36.2	0	60
Tobramycin	33.3	17.9	33.3	48	0	40
Ciprofloxacin	22.2	16	19	18.4	0	20
Ofloxcin	15	8.0	0	0		
Netilmicin	28.7	10.5	14	50.0		
Levofloxacin	37.2	43.7	17.6	53.7		
Moxifloxacin	22.2	13	14.2	-	0	20
Cotrimoxazole	18.5	9.4	4.7	-	0	20
Tigecycline	100	95.2	95.2	-	0	100
Ticarcillin-clavulanic acid	28.5	33.7	23.5	46.8		

- Isolates of *Pseudomonas spp.* were most sensitive to amikacin followed by ertapenem, imipenem, pipercillin/tazobactam, cefepime and netilmycin.
- Isolates of *Acinetobacter* spp. were most sensitive to tigecycline followed by carbapenems and amikacin.
- Linezolid was the most effective antibiotic for *S. aureus* and *Enterococcus* spp. followed by teicoplanin, cefuroxime, cefadroxyl and amoxy-clav.

Table 6: Antibiotic (%) susceptibility pattern for Gram-positive bacteria		
Antibiotics	*Enterococcus spp.*	*S. aureus*
Amoxy-clav	33.3	25.6
Ofloxacin	27.7	15.1
Netilmicin	14.8	63.6
Gantamicin	46.5	0
Amikacin	24.6	58
Roxithromycin	38.2	22.2
Teicoplanin	94.4	86.5
Linezolid	100	100
Cefuroxime	52.5	48.6
Cefadroxyl	42.8	55.3

Commonly used Antibiotics in Clinical Practice (Table 7)

Five functional groups cover most antibiotics are:

- Inhibitors of cell wall synthesis
- Inhibitors of protein synthesis
- Inhibitors of membrane function
- Inhibitors of nucleic acid synthesis
- Antimetabolites

Table 7: Commonly used antibiotics[65-71]

Class	*Drugs*	*Indications*	*Side effects*
Inhibitors of cell wall synthesis			
Penicillins (Bactericidal)			
Natural penicillins	Penicillin G Aqueous penicillin G Procaine penicillin G Benzathine penicillin G Penicillin V	• Drug of choice for infections due to: *S. pneumoniae* and other Streptococci, pharyngitis, bacteremia, endocarditis • *Neisseria meningitidis*-meningitis, meningococcemia • *Treponema pallidum*-syphilis • Actinomycosis other uses • Endocarditis prophylaxis in patients with valvular heart disease undergoing dental procedures at high risk for bacteremia. Prevention of rheumatic fever • Very little activity against *Staphylococcus* spp. due to penicillinase production • Anaerobes: good activity against Gram-positive mouth anaerobes such as *Peptococcus* spp., *Peptostreptococcus, Clostridium* spp. except *Clostridium difficile*	• Hypersensitivity reaction with serious anaphylactic reaction. Cross-allergenicity is observed among penicillins • Irritability, jerking, confusion, generalized seizures • Leukopenia, neutropenia or thrombocytopenia • Gastrointestinal upset and diarrhea • Brain and kidney damage (rare)
Penicillinase-resistant penicillins	Methicillin Nafcillin Oxacillin Cloxacillin Dicloxacillin	• Infections due to MSSA such as skin and soft tissue infections, septic arthritis, osteomyelitis, bacteremia, endocarditis, etc. • Not active against MRSA • No activity against Enterococcus spp. or *S. pneumoniae* • Gram-negative: No activity • Anaerobes: Limited	Above + transient increases in liver enzymes Interstitial nephritis
Aminopenicillins	Ampicillin Amoxicillin	• Because of activity against respiratory tract pathogens, useful for the treatment of mild to moderate pharyngitis, sinusitis, bronchitis and otitis media • Useful for uncomplicated urinary tract infections, Enterococcal infections and *Listeria monocytogenes* meningitis • Endocarditis prophylaxis in patients with valvular heart disease. Treatment of *Salmonella* (amoxicillin) and *Shigella* (ampicillin) • Ineffective against *S. aureus* • Gram-negative: Better activity than natural penicillins • Anaerobes: Activity similar to penicillin G	As natural penicillin
Carboxypenicillins	Carbenicillin Ticarcillin	• Due to enhanced activity against Gram-negative bacteria, including *P. aeruginosa*, useful for the treatment of serious infections such as bacteremia, pneumonia, complicated urinary tract infection, peritonitis, intra-abdominal infections, skin and soft tissue infections, bone and joint infections, and meningitis caused by Gram-negative bacteria (hospital-acquired infections) • May be used as empiric therapy in immunocompromised patients • Not active against *Klebsiella* spp. or *Serratia* • Not active against Enterococcus or *Staphylococcus* spp.	• As above + • Hypokalemia + • Sodium overload and fluid retention

Contd...

Contd...

Class	*Drugs*	*Indications*	*Side effects*
Ureidopenicillins	Piperacillin	• Same as above + active against *Klebsiella* spp. and *Serratia marcescens* • Piperacillin is the most active penicillin for infections due to *P. aeruginosa* • Anaerobes: Activity similar to penicillin G against *Clostridium* and *Peptostreptococcus* Some activity against *B. fragilis*	As above
Amidinopenicillins	Mecillinam	• Restricted use to urinary infection with *E. coli* • Active against penicillinase and low-level cephalosporinase producing organism	Gastrointestinal upset and diarrhea Hypersensitivity reaction
Combination-β-lactams and β-lactamase inhibitor			
With clavulanic acid	Amoxicillin-clavulanate	• Due to expanded activity against Gram-positive and Gram-negative bacteria (including anaerobes), often used in the treatment of polymicrobial infections, such as intra-abdominal infections, gynecological infections, diabetic foot infections, etc. • Useful for the treatment of otitis media, sinusitis, bronchitis, lower respiratory tract infections and human or animal bites	• Hypersensitivity reaction • Hemolytic anemia
	Ticarcillin/clavulanic acid	• Indicated for septicemia, lower respiratory infections, skin and skin structure infections and bone and joint infections, for UTIs, peritonitis caused by beta-lactamase-producing isolates of *S. aureus*, *Haemophilus influenzae*, *Klebsiella* spp., *E. coli*, *P. aeruginosa* and other Gram-negatives.	• Rash • Nausea • Diarrhea • Phlebitis at injection site • Increased eosinophils • Increased AST • Increased ALT
With sulbactam	Ampicillin-sulbactam	• Same activity of the parent penicillin against non β-lactamase producing organisms, and will have enhanced activity against beta-lactamase producing bacteria, e.g. *E. coli*, Proteus spp., Klebsiella spp., *H. influenza*, etc. • Not very active against beta-lactamase enzymes produced by *Serratia marcescens*, *P. aeruginosa*, *Proteus* spp., *Citrobacter* spp. and *Enterobacter* spp. • Useful for the treatment of mixed aerobic/anaerobic infections by susceptible bacteria	• Gastrointestinal upset and diarrhea, stomach pain, blood in stool • Hypersensitivity reaction • Painful urination • Vaginal yeast infection • Chest pain, dizziness
With tazobactam	Piperacillin/tazobactam	• Useful for the treatment of polymicrobial infections or other infections involving Gram-negative bacteria including hospital-acquired pneumonia, bacteremia, complicated urinary tract infections, complicated skin and soft tissue infections, intra-abdominal infections • And empiric therapy for febrile neutropenia	• Gastrointestinal upset and diarrhea • Hypersensitivity reaction
Cephalosporins (Bactericidal)			
First generation cephalosporins	Cefazolin Cephalothin Cephradine Cephapirin Cephalexin Cefadroxil	• Excellent activity against Gram-positive aerobes • Used for the treatment of mild to moderate infections of skin and soft tissue, septic arthritis, osteomyelitis and endocarditis due to MSSA and streptococci • Treatment of uncomplicated urinary tract infections. • Cefazolin is the drug of choice for surgical prophylaxis against surgical-site infection. • Also have activity against a limited number of Gram-negative aerobes • *P. mirabilis*, *E. coli*, *K. pneumoniae*	• Hypersensitivity reactions in patients with a history of penicillin allergy • Stevens-Johnson syndrome • Erythema multiforme • Exfoliative dermatitis • Gastrointestinal upset, diarrhea, nausea (if alcohol taken concurrently)

Contd...

Contd...

Class	*Drugs*	*Indications*	*Side effects*
Second generation cephalosporins	Cefamandole Cefonicid Cefaclor Cefprozil Cefuroxime Loracarbef Cefoxitin Cefotetan Cefmetazole	• Slightly less active than first generation agents against Gram-positive aerobes, such as Staphylococci and Streptococci, cefprozil and cefuroxime have the best Gram-positive coverage; cefoxitin and cefotetan have the worst but More active against Gram-negative aerobes and anaerobes • Cefuroxime is useful for the treatment of pharyngitis, tonsillitis, sinusitis, otitis media, bronchitis and mild to moderate community-acquired pneumonia. • Treatment of mild to moderate skin and soft tissue infections, and uncomplicated urinary tract infections due to susceptible bacteria. • Cefoxitin, cefotetan and cefmetazole have activity against Gram-negative aerobes and anaerobes, including *B. fragilis* • So they are useful for prophylaxis in abdominal surgical procedures and • For the treatment of polymicrobial infections such as intra-abdominal infections (diverticulitis, appendicitis, bowel perforation), pelvic infections (pelvic inflammatory disease), and skin and soft tissue infections in patients with diabetes	• Above + • Hypoprothrombinemia • Allergic reactions • Ethanol disulfiram reaction • Pseudomembranous colitis • Phlebitis • Drug fever • Interstitial nephritis (rare);
Third generation cephalosporins	Cefotaxime Ceftriaxone Ceftazidime Cefoperazone Ceftizoxime Moxalactam Cefixime Cefpodoxime Ceftibuten Cefdinir	• More activity than the second generation agents against Gram-negative aerobes (even beta-lactamase producing strains) • Are used for the treatment of bacteremia, pneumonia, complicated urinary tract infection, peritonitis, intra-abdominal infections, skin and soft tissue infections, bone and joint infections, and meningitis caused by Gram-negative bacteria (nosocomial infections) • If *P. aeruginosa* is known or suspected, ceftazidime or cefoperazone should be used • If anaerobes are known or suspected, metronidazole or clindamycin should be added • Ceftriaxone is used as a single intramuscular (dose for uncomplicated gonorrhea) • Cefotaxime and ceftriaxone have good activity against Gram-positive aerobes, and may be used for the treatment of infections due to PRSP (meningitis and pneumonia) • Ceftriaxone can be used for the treatment of endocarditis caused by *Streptococcus viridans*	• As above + • Biliary sludging (ceftazidime)
Fourth generation cephalosporins	Cefepime Cefpirome	• Cefepime is used for the treatment of community-and hospital-acquired pneumonia, bacteremia, uncomplicated and complicated urinary tract infections, skin and soft tissue infections, intra-abdominal infections • Empiric therapy for febrile neutropenia • Cefepime also has anti pseudomonal activity • If anaerobes are known or suspected, metronidazole or clindamycin should be added	Nonconvulsive status epilepticus (cefepime)
Fifth generation	Ceftraoline fosamil	• Broad spectrum, active against Gram-positive drug resistant bacteria (*S. pneumoniae*, MRSA, VRSA) • Also effective against *H. influenzae*, *M. catarrhalis* and some common Gram-negative bacteria	Gastrointestinal upset and diarrhea Allergic reaction *C. difficile*-associated diarrhea Direct Coombs test seroconversion

Contd...

Contd...

Class	*Drugs*	*Indications*	*Side effects*
Sixth generation	Ceftobiprole	• Broad spectrum, active against MRSA, methicillin-resistant *Staphylococcus epidermidis*, *E. faecalis* • Common Gram-negative bacteria *E. coli* and also *Pseudomonas*	• Nausea, diarrhea, vomiting • Infusion-site reaction • Headache • Dysgeusia (caramel-like taste)
Carbapenems	Imipenem (+ Cilastatin) Meropenem Doripenem Ertapenem	• Currently the most broad-spectrum antibiotics, with good activity against many Gram-positive and Gram-negative aerobes and anaerobes • Used for polymicrobial infections such as intra-abdominal infections or skin and skin structure infections in diabetic patients • Empiric therapy for nosocomial infections, such as serious lower respiratory tract infections, septicemia and complicated urinary tract infections, while waiting for the results susceptibility data • Ertapenem does not have activity against *P. aeruginosa* • Febrile neutropenia: imipenem or meropenem • Meningitis (children): meropenem • Carbapenems do not have activity against MRSA	• Hypersensitivity reactions in patients with a history of penicillin allergy. (5–15%) • Gastrointestinal upset, diarrhea, nausea • Insomnia, agitation, confusion, dizziness, hallucinations, and depression • Seizure • Antibiotic-associated pseudomembranous colitis (*C. difficile*)
Monobactams	Aztreonam	• Same as carbapenems + • Used for the treatment of infections caused by Gram-negative aerobes such as complicated and uncomplicated urinary tract infections, lower respiratory tract infections, meningitis, bacteremia, skin and skin structure infections, intra-abdominal infections and gynecologic infections caused by susceptible Gram-negative aerobes • Combination therapy is recommended to ensure coverage of Gram-positive and anaerobic bacteria • Aztreonam is especially useful for the treatment of Gram-negative infections in patients with a history of a severe penicillin allergy • If anaerobes are known or suspected, metronidazole or clindamycin should be added	• Hypersensitivity rash, pruritus, urticaria, angioedema, anaphylaxis (rare) • Negligible cross-reactivity with penicillin • Diarrhea, nausea, vomiting • Neutropenia, thrombocytopenia, eosinophilia, • Transient LFT increases • Phlebitis • Drug fever
Glycopeptides	Vancomycin Teicoplanin	• Infections due to methicillin-resistant staphylococci including bacteremia, pneumonia, empyema, endocarditis, peritonitis, osteomyelitis and skin and soft tissue infections • Intraventricular vancomycin is used for the treatment of meningitis • Serious Gram-positive infections in patients allergic to beta-lactam antibiotics • Infections caused by multidrug resistant Gram-positive organisms, such as *Corynebacterium*, *S. pneumoniae* • Perioperative prophylaxis to reduce the risk of infection in patients undergoing cardiac, neurosurgical, orthopedic, or vascular surgical procedures where the incidence of MRSA is high • Oral vancomycin. for the treatment of choice for moderate to severe *C. difficile* colitis • Vancomycin is not active against Gram-negative aerobes or anaerobes	Red-man syndrome characterized by flushing, pruritus, and a maculopapular or erythematous rash on the face, neck, chest, and upper extremities, may also be accompanied by hypotension. Resolves spontaneously after the discontinuation of the infusion Nephrotoxicity and Ototoxicity Neutropenia, thrombocytopenia

Contd...

Contd...

Class	*Drugs*	*Indications*	*Side effects*
Inhibitors of membrane function (Bactericidal)			
Lipopeptides (previously polypeptides)	Polymyxin B Polymyxin E Bacitracin Colistin	• Gram-negative MDR infections • Polymyxin can be used in combination against very resistant *Pseudomonas* • Used in Gram-negative infection of eye and ear usually applied directly to the eye • Bacitracin for topical Gram-positive infections • The use of polymyxin and colistin is experiencing a resurgence due to the emergence of multidrug resistant *Acinetobacter*, *Pseudomonas* and *Klebsiella* infections • Colistin is ineffective for *Proteus* and *Burkholderia* • Polymixin not effective against Gram-positives and anaerobes	• Kidney and nerve damage • Pruritis, rash
	Daptomycin	• Gram-positive organisms: Excellent activity • Reserved for the management of serious or complicated infections caused by resistant Gram-positive organisms where vancomycin and/or linezolid cannot be used • Daptomycin should not be used for the treatment of pneumonia since the compound is inactivated by pulmonary surfactant	• Nausea, diarrhea, headache • Injection site reactions • Rash • Myopathy and • CPK elevation
Inhibitors of protein synthesis			
Aminoglycosides (Bactericidal)	Gentamicin Neomycin Kanamycin Amikacin Tobramycin Netilmicin Streptomycin Paromomycin Spectinomycin	• Aminoglycosides are rarely used alone • Amikacin, gentamicin and tobramycin are used for the treatment of serious infections due to Gram-negative bacteria such as septicemia, bone and joint infections, skin and soft tissue infections, respiratory tract infections, intra-abdominal infections, and complicated urinary tract infections • Gentamicin or streptomycin may be used (with ampicillin, vancomycin, etc.) for the treatment of serious infections (endocarditis) due to enterococci, viridans streptococci or staphylococci • Streptomycin or amikacin is used in conjunction with other antituberculous medications in the treatment of non tuberculous infections • Anaerobes-aminoglycosides are inactive	• Nephrotoxicity • Ototoxicity auditory and vestibular • Vertigo • Kidney damage • Neuromuscular blockade (neomycin), • Hypersensitivity • Sterile abscess formation at intramuscular site
Tetracyclines Bacteriostatic	Tetracycline Doxycycline Minocycline Demeclocycline Oxytetracycline	• Tetracyclines display activity against Gram-positive and Gram-negative aerobic bacteria, as well as unusual bacteria • The emergence of bacterial resistance and the availability of more potent and useful antibiotics have limited the therapeutic usefulness of the tetracyclines • Can be used in community-acquired pneumonia due to penicillin susceptible *S. pneumoniae*, *Mycoplasma* spp. • Treatment of rickettsial infections • Chlamydial infections • Nongonococcal urethritis • Brucellosis, bartonellosis • Acne (minocycline)	• Gastrointestinal upset, nausea • Sensitivity to sunlight • Potential toxicity to mother and fetus during pregnancy • Impaired growth • Enamel hypoplasia • Permanent tooth discoloration • Transient depression of bone growth • Hepatotoxicity • Avoid in children less than 8 years of age • Rash, pruritus, urticaria, angioedema, anaphylaxis, serum sickness, • Stevens-Johnson syndrome • Lightheadedness, dizziness, vertigo, ataxia, headache

Contd...

Contd...

Class	*Drugs*	*Indications*	*Side effects*
		• Useful as either primary or alternative therapy for the treatment of plague,tularemia, chancroid, pertussis, Clostridial infections, anthrax, listeria, syphilis, Lyme disease, *Helicobacter pylori*, Cholera • Prevention of malaria (doxycycline) • Chronic SIADH (demeclocycline)	
Glycylcyclines	Tigecycline	• Active against a broad range of Gram-positive and Gram-negative aerobic and anaerobic bacteria • Tigecycline is approved for the treatment of polymicrobial infections • Complicated skin and skin structure infections • Complicated intra-abdominal infections • Tigecycline is not active against *Proteus mirabilis* or *P. aeruginosa*	Same as above
Macrolides Bacteriostatic	Erythromycin Azithromycin Clarithromycin Roxithromycin	• Useful alternative in penicillin-allergic patients • Respiratory tract infections, pharyngitis, tonsillitis, otitis media, sinusitis, acute exacerbations of chronic bronchitis • Azithromycin and clarithromycin are best if *H. influenzae* is suspected • Community-acquired pneumonia especially for atypical coverage, pertussis, *C. diphtheria* • Uncomplicated skin and soft tissue Infections. • Sexually-transmitted diseases: Azithromycin is effective for the treatment of nongonococcal urethritis or cervicitis due to *Chlamydia trachomatis* • Prophylaxis of bacterial endocarditis syphilis and gonorrhea. • *Mycobacterium avium* complex infections • *Campylobacter jejuni* infections, *H. pylori*	• Epigastric distress, abdominal pain, nausea, vomiting, diarrhea • Cholestatic hepatitis seen in adult patients • Allergic reactions • QT prolongation • Visual disturbance • Liver toxicity
Ketollides	Telithromycin Spiramycin	• The spectrum of activity of telithromycin is similar to that of azithro and clarithro with additional activity against macrolide-resistant *S. pneumoniae* • Currently approved only for the treatment of mild-moderate community-acquired pneumonia due to adverse effect. (risk outweighs benefit in treatment of sinusitis or bronchitis) • Acute bacterial sinusitis • Acute exacerbations of chronic bronchitis	• Diarrhea, nausea, vomiting, • Hepatotoxicity QT interval prolongation • Decreased visual acuity and blurred vision
Chloramphenicol Bacteriostatic		• Active against Gram-positives and Gram-negatives but not indicated as first line therapy for treatment of infections • Due to the low cost of this continues to be used for bacterial meningitis, pneumonia and typhoid fever • Not active against *P. aeruginosa*	• Aplastic anemia • Gray Baby Syndrome • Optic neuritis • Hypersensitivity reactions, anaphylaxis (rare) • Herxheimer-like responses • Nausea, vomiting diarrhea • Stomatitis • Acute attacks of porphyria • Interference during development of immunity and should not be given during active immunization

Contd...

Contd...

Class	*Drugs*	*Indications*	*Side effects*
Lincosamides Bacteriostatic	Clindamycin Lincomycin	• Primarily useful for infections due to anaerobes (including *B. fragilis*), pulmonary infections, pelvic infections, diabetic foot infections, decubitus ulcers • Alternative to penicillin in the treatment of infections due to *C. perfringens* • Treatment of skin and soft tissue infections due to *Staphylococcus* and Streptococci including MRSA • Alternative agent for the treatment of infections due to Gram-positive aerobes in patients allergic to penicillin (cellulitis, septic arthritis, osteomyelitis) • Alternative for the treatment of encephalitis due to *Toxoplasmosis gondii* in AIDS patients • Alternative for the treatment of *Pneumocystis carinii* pneumonia in AIDS patients allergic to sulfonamides • Treatment of bacterial vaginosis (vaginal cream)	• Nausea, vomiting, diarrhea • Pseudomembranous colitis • Antibiotic-associated diarrhea (*C. difficile*) • Hepatotoxicity Hypersensitivity
Oxazolinidinones	Linezolid	• Reserved for management of serious or complicated infections caused by resistant organisms, especially for infections where vancomycin cannot be used • Treatment of infections (bacteremia) due to vancomycin-resistant *Enterococcus* spp. • Complicated skin infections caused by MSSA or *S. pyogenes* • Community-acquired pneumonia due to PSSP, penicillinase producing Streptococci (MSSA) • Nosocomial pneumonia due to MSSA, MRSA and PSSP • Serious infections due to MRSA or VRE including endocarditis, meningitis and osteomyelitis	• Gastrointestinal nausea, diarrhea lactic acidosis • Headache • Peripheralneuropathy • Thrombocytopenia and anemia
Streptogramins	Quinupristin: Dalfopristin	• Dalfopristin is used for the treatment of vancomycin-resistant *Enterococcus faecium* bacteremia • Complicated skin and skin structure infections caused by MSSA or *S. pyogenes*; catheter-related bacteremia • Infections due to MRSA and community-acquired pneumonia (when vancomycin, linezolid and daptomycin cannot be used)	• Venous site irritation • Nausea, vomiting diarrhea • Myalgias • Arthralgias • Rash
DNA synthesis inhibitors (Quinolone/fluoroquinolones)			
First generation	Nalidixic acid	Only for Gram-negatives, used to treat urinary tract infections	• Stomach upset • Loss of appetite • Headache • Dizziness
Second generation	Ciprofloxacin Norfloxacin Enoxacin Ofloxacin Levofloxacin	• Gram-negative and Gram-positive coverage including anaerobes • More widespread tissue distribution • Used in UTI, bacterial prostatitis, osteomyelitis, community-acquired pneumonia, bacterial diarrhea, mycoplasma infections and gonorrhea • Effective against *Pseudomonas* also	• As above + • Phototoxicity • Tendinosis • Achilles tendon rupture • Impaired fracture healing • CNS damage

Contd...

Contd...

Class	*Drugs*	*Indications*	*Side effects*
Third generation	Gatifloxacin Sparfloxacin	• As above + expanded activity against Gram-positive organisms, particularly penicillin-sensitive and PRSP, and atypical pathogens such as *Mycoplasma pneumoniae* and *Chlamydia pneumoniae* • Acute sinus infections, skin infections, pneumonia, complications of chronic bronchitis, kidney and urinary tract infections, and gonorrhea • Less active than ciprofloxacin against Pseudomonas species • Used in ophthalmic infections	• Diarrhea, nausea stomach pain, vomiting • Dizziness, headache • Heart palpitations, high blood pressure • Labored breathing • Vaginal inflammation
Fourth generation	Moxifloxacin Gemifloxacin	• As above + anaerobes • Acute exacerbations of chronic bronchitis • Acute bacterial sinusitis • Community-acquired pneumonia • Uncomplicated skin and skin structure infections community-acquired pneumonia caused by multidrug resistant *S. pneumoniae* • Complicated skin and skin structure infections • Complicated intra-abdominal infections • In ophthalmology in conjuctival infections	• Diarrhea, nausea stomach pain, vomiting dizziness, headache • Reversible peripheral neuropathy • Spontaneous tendon rupture tendonitis • Acute liver failure or serious liver injury • QT prolongation, • *C. difficile* associated colitis
Other DNA inhibitors			
Metronidazole	Metronidazole (Flagyl®)	• Gram-positive and Gram-negative anaerobic bacterial • Protozoal infections	• Nausea, loss of appetite, headache, seizures • Cerebellar dysfunction • Ethanol disulfram reaction
Antimetabolites **Folic acid synthesis inhibitors**			
Sulfonamides	Trimethoprim/ sulfamethoxazole Sulfisoxazole Sulfadiazine	• Acute, chronic or recurrent infections of the urinary tract • Acute or chronic bacterial prostatitis • Acute bacterial exacerbations of chronic bronchitis • *P. carinii* pneumonia: The drug of choice for both treatment and prophylaxis • Skin and soft tissue infections due to MRSA • Acute otitis media, sinusitis • Nocardia infections • *Stenotrophomonas maltophilia* infections • Listeria meningitis if patient is allergic to penicillins • Toxoplasmosis • Not active against *P. aeruginosa*	• Thrombocytopenia Avoid in third trimester of pregnancy • Nausea, vomiting, diarrhea, anorexia, glossitis, abdominal pain • Hypersensitivity reactions, Stevens Johnson syndrome, exfoliative dermatitis, headache, insomnia, depression

Abbreviations: MSSA, methicillin-susceptible *Staphylococcus aureus*; MRSA, methicillin-resistant *Staphylococcus aureus*; AST, aspartate aminotransferase; ALT, alanine transaminase; VRSA, vancomycin-resistant *Staphylococcus aureus*; QT, Q wave and T wave; LFT, liver function test; PSSP, penicillin-susceptible *Streptococcus pneumoniae*; PRSP, penicillin-resistant *Streptococcus pneumoniae*; MDR, multidrug resistant; CPK, creatine phosphokinase; VRE, vancomycin-resistant enterococci; UTI, urinary tract infection; CNS, central nervous system; SIADH, syndrome of inappropriate antidiuretic hormone secretion.

REFERENCES

1. Sorensen LT, Hemmingsen U, Kallehave F, Wille-Jørgensen P, Kjaergaard J, Møller LN, et al. Risk factors for tissue and wound complications in gastrointestinal surgery. Ann Surg. 2005;241(4):654-8.
2. Medina M, Sillero M, Martinez-Gallego G, Delgado-Rodríguez M. Risk factors of surgical wound infection in patients undergoing herniorrhaphy. Eur J Surg. 1997;163(3):191-8.
3. Paunovic M. Predictors of postoperative complications in gastrointestinal surgery. Acta Medica Medianae. 2008. pp. 15-9.
4. Clarke JS, Condon RE, Bartlet JG, Gorbach SL, Nichols RL, Ochi S. Preoperative oral antibiotics reduce septic complications of colon operations: results of prospective, randomized, double-blind clinical study. Ann Surg. 1977;186(3):251-9.
5. Husted TL, Solomkin JS. Surgical Prophylaxis. In: Schlossberg D editor, Clinical infectious Disease. Cambridge University Press; 2008. pp. 797-806.

6. Page CP, Bohnen JM, Fletcher JR, McManus AT, Solomkin JS, Wittmann DH. Antimicrobial prophylaxis for surgical wounds. Guideline for clinical care. In: Arutyn, Goldmann, Schecker editors, Saunders Infection Control reference services, 1st edition, Philadelphia, Pennsylvania USA: W.B. Saunders Company; 1998; pp. 235-42.
7. Talbot TR. Surgical site infection and antimicrobial prophylaxis. Mandell, Douglas, and Bennett's Principles and practice of infectious diseases, 7th edition, Philadelphia Churchill Livingstone: Elsevier; 2010. pp. 3891-904.
8. Haley RW, Culver DH, Morgan WM, White JW, Emori TG, Hooton TM. Identifying patients at high risk of surgical wound infection: a simple multivariate index of patient susceptibility and wound contamination. Am J Epidemiol. 1985;121(2):206-15.
9. Culver DH, Horan TC, Gayens RP, Martone WJ, Jarvis WR, Emori TJ, et al. Surgical wound infection rates by wound class, operative procedure, and patient risk index. National Nosocomial Infections Surveillance System. Am J Med. 1991;91(3B):152S-157S.
10. National Nosocomial Infections Surveillance (NNIS) System Report, data summary from January 1992 to June 2002, issued August 2002. Centers for Disease Control, Atlanta, Georgia. http://www.cdc.gov/ncidod/hip/NNIS/2002NNISReport_AJIC.PDF
11. Owens WD, Felts JA, Spitznagel EL. ASA physical status classifications: a study of consistency of ratings. Anesthesiology. 1978;49(4):239-43.
12. ASHP guidelines on antimicrobial prophylaxis in surgery. Saunders Infection Control reference service Philadelphia, Pennsylvania USA: WB Saunders Company; 1998. pp. 244-6.
13. Bohnen JM. Antibiotic therapy for abdominal infection. World J Surg. 1998;22(2):152-7.
14. Dougherty SH, Sirinek KR, Schauer PR, Fink MP, Fabian TC, Martin DH, et al. Ticarcillin/clavulanate compared with clindamycin/gentamicin (with or without ampicillin) for the treatment of intra-abdominal infections in pediatric and adult patients. Am Surg. 1995;61(4):297-303.
15. Walker AP, Nichols RL, Wilson RF, Bivens BA, Trunkey DD, Edmiston CE, et al. Efficacy of a beta-lactamase inhibitor combination for serious intra-abdominal infections. Ann Surg. 1993;217(2):115-21.
16. Polk HC, Fink MP, Laverdiere M, Wilson SE, Garber GE, Barie PS, et al. Prospective randomized study of piperacillin/tazobactam therapy of surgically treated intra-abdominal infection. Am Surg. 1993;59(9):598-605.
17. Yellin AE, Heseltine PNR, Berne TV, Appleman MD, Gill MA, Riggio CE, et al. The role of Pseudomonas species in patients treated with ampicillin and sulbactam for gangrenous and perforated appendicitis. Surg Gynecol Obstet. 1985;161:303-7.
18. Gatehouse D, Dimock F, Burdon DW Alexander-Williams J, Keighley MR. Prediction of wound sepsis following gastric operations. Br J Surg. 1978;65(8):551-4.
19. Galanduik S, Polk HC, Jagelman DG, Fazio VW. Re-emphasis of priorities in surgical antibiotic prophylaxis. Surg Gynecol Obstet. 1989;169(3):219-22.
20. Bergamini TM, Polk HC. Pharmacodynamics of antibiotic penetration of tissue and surgical prophylaxis. Surg Gynecol Obstet. 1989;168(3):283-9.
21. Martin C. Antimicrobial prophylaxis in surgery: General concepts and clinical guidelines. Saunders Infection Control reference service Philadelphia, Pennsylvania USA: WB Saunders Company; 1998. pp. 267-73.
22. DiPiro JT, Cheung RP, Bowden TA, Mansberg JA. Single dose systemic antibiotic prophylaxis of surgical wound infections. Am J Surg. 1986;152:552-9.
23. Cainzos M, Potel J, Puente JL. Prospective randomized controlled study of prophylaxis with cefamandole in high risk patient undergoing operations upon the biliary tract. Surg Gynecol Obstet. 1985;160(1):27-32.
24. Lewis RT, Goodall RG, Marien B, Park M, Lloyd-Smith W, Wiegand FM. Biliary bacteria, antibiotic use and, wound infection in surgery of the gall bladder and common bile duct. Arch Surg. 1987:122(1):44-7.
25. Wells GR, Taylor EW, Lindsay G, Morton L. Relationship between bile colonization, high-risk factor and postoperative sepsis in patients undergoing biliary tract operation while receiving a prophylactic antibiotic: West of Scotland surgical infection study Group. Br J Surg. 1989;76:374-7.
26. Nichols RL, Webb WR, Jones JW, Smith JW, LoCicero J 3rd. Efficacy of antibiotic prophylaxis in high-risk gastroduodenal operation. AM J Surg. 1982;143(1):94-8.
27. Stone HH. Gastric Surgery. South Med J. 1977;70(Suppl 1):35-7.
28. Morris DL, Young D, Burdon DW, Keighley MR. Prospective randomized trial of single dose cefuroxime against mezlocilin in elective gastric surgery. J Hosp Infect. 1984;5(2):200-4.
29. Lewis RT, Allan CM, Goodal RG, Lloyd-Smith WC, Marien B, Wiegand FM. Discriminate use of antibiotics prophylaxis in gastroduodenal surgery. AM J Sur. 1979;138(5):640-3.
30. Rudell WS, Axon AT, Findley JM, Bartholomew BA, Hill MJ. Effect of Cimetidine on the gastric bacterial flora. Lancet. 1980;1:672-4.
31. LoCiero J 3rd, Nichols RL. Sepsis after gastroduodenal operations; relationship to gastric acid, motility, and endogenous microflora. South Med J. 1980;73(7):878-80.
32. Bartlett JG, Condon RE, Gorbach SL, Clarke JS, Nichols RL, Ochi S. Veterans Administration Cooperative study on bowel preparation for elective colorectal operations: Impact of oral antibiotics regimen on colonic flora, wound irrigation cultures and bacteriology of septic complication. Ann Surg. 1978;188(2):249-54.
33. Clarke JS, Condon R, Bartlett JG, Gorbach SL, Nichols RL, Ochi S. Preoperative oral antibiotics reduce septic complication of colon operations: result of a prospective randomized, double-blind clinical study. Ann Surg. 1977;186(3):251-9.
34. Nichols RL. Prophylaxis for elective bowel surgery. In: Wilson SE, Williams RA, Finegold S (Eds). Intra-abdominal infections. New York: McGraw Hill; 1982. pp. 267-85.
35. Baum ML, Anish DS, Chalmers TC, Sacks HS, Smith H, Fagerstrom RM. A survey of clinical trials of antibiotic prophylaxis in colon surgery: evidence against further use of no treatment controls. N Engl J Med. 1981;305(14):795-9.
36. Washington J, Dearing W, Judd E, et al. Effect of preoperative antibiotic regimen on development of infection after intestinal surgery. Ann Surg. 1974;180:567-72.
37. Gilmore OJ, Martin TD. Aetiology and prevention of wound infection in appendicetomy. Br J Surg. 1974;61(4):281-7.
38. Pinto DJ, Sanderson PJ. Rational use of antibiotic therapy after appendectomy. Br Med J. 1980;280:275-7.
39. Keighley MR. Infection: prophylaxis. Br Med Bull. 1988;44:374-402.
40. Donovan IA, Ellis D, Gatehouse D, Little G, Grimley R, Armistead S. One-dose antibiotic prophylaxis against wound infection after appendicectomy: a randomized trial of clindamycin, cefazolin sodium and a placebo. Br J Surg. 1979;66(3):193-6.
41. Jenson NG, Bach-Nilsen P, Damgaard B, et al. A Danish multicenter study; cefoxitin versus ampicillin versus metronidazole in perforated appendicitis. Br J Surg. 1984;71(2):144-6.
42. Stone HH. Bacterial flora of appendicitis in children. J Pediatr Surg. 1976;11(1):37-42.
43. Berne TV, Yellin AE, Appleman MD, Chenella FC, Gill MA, Heseltine PN. Surgically treated gangrenous or perforated appendicitis. A comparison of aztreonam and clindamycin versus gentamicin and clindamycin. Ann Surg. 1987;205(2):133-7.
44. Berne TV, Yellin AW, Appleman MD, Heseltine PN. Antibiotic management of surgically treated gangrenous or perforated appendicitis. Comparison of gentamicin and clilndamycin versus cefamandole versus cefoperazone. Am J Surg. 1982;144(1):8-13.

45. Windsor JA, Hill GL. Risk factor for postoperative pneumonia. The importance of protein depletion. Ann Surg. 1988;208(2):209-14.
46. Garibaldi RA, Britt MR, Coleman ML, Reading JC, Pace NL. Risk factors for postoperative pneumonia. Am J Med. 1981;70(3):677-80.
47. Bartlett RH, Gazzaniga AB, Geraghty TR. Respiratory maneuvers to prevent postoperative pulmonary complications. A critical review. JAMA. 1973 14;224(7):1017-21.
48. Chastre J, Fagon JY. Ventilator associated pneumonia. Am J Respir Crit Care Med. 2002;Vol 165(7):867-903.
49. Wightman JA. A prospective survey of the incidence of postoperative pulmonary complications. Br J Surg. 1968;55(2):85-91.
50. Williams CD, Brenowitz JB. "Prohibitive" lung function and major surgical procedures. Am J Surg. 1976;132(6):763-6.
51. Palmer KN. Post-operative pulmonary complications. Postgrad Med J. 1955;31(351):25-9.
52. Tisi GM. Preoperative identification and evaluation of the patient with lung disease. Med Clin North Am. 1987;71(3):399-412.
53. Pennington JE. Nosocomial respiratory infection. In: Mandell GL, Douglas RG, Bennet JE (Eds). Principles and practice of infectious diseases. St. Louis, MO: Churchill Livingstone; 1990. pp. 2199-2205.
54. Celis R, Torres A, Gatell JM, Almela M, Rodriguez-Roisin R, Agusti-Vidal A. Nosocomial pneumonia. A multivariate analysis of risk and prognosis. Chest 1988;93(2):318-24.
55. Rello J, Rue M, Jubert P, Muses G, Sonora R, Valles J, et al. Survival in patients with nosocomial pneumonia: impact of the severity of illness and the etiologic agent. Crit Care Med. 1997;25(11): 1862-7.
56. Koenig SM, Truwit JD. Ventilator-associated pneumonia: diagnosis, treatment, and prevention. Clin Microbiol Rev. 2006;19(4):637-57.
57. Marquette CH, Georges H, Wallet F, Ramon P, Saulnier F, Neviere R, et al. Diagnostic efficiency of endotracheal aspirates with quantitative bacterial cultures in intubated patients with suspected pneumonia. Comparison with the protected specimen brush. Am Rev Respir Dis. 1993;148(1):138-44.
58. Chastre J and Fagon JY. Ventilator-associated pneumonia. Am. J. Respir. Crit. Care Med. 2002;165:867-903.
59. Bryan CS. Nosocomial pneumonia: blood cultures remain useful. Chest. 1999;116(4):859-60.
60. Fagon JY, Chastre J, Domart Y, Trouillet JL, Pierre J, Darne C, et al. Nosocomial pneumonia in patients receiving continuous mechanical ventilation. Prospective analysis of 52 episodes with use of a protected specimen brush and quantitative culture techniques. Am Rev Respir Dis. 1989;139:877-84.
61. Stevens RM, Teres D, Skillman JJ, Feingold DS. Pneumonia in an ICU. A 30-month experience. Arch Intern Med. 1974;134(1):106-11.
62. American Thoracic Society. Infectious Diseases Society of America. Guidelines for the management of adults with hospital-acquired, ventilator-associated, and healthcare-associated pneumonia. Am J Respir Crit Care Med. 2005;171(4):388-416.
63. Sartelli M, Catena F, Coccolini F, Pinna AD. Antimicrobial management of intra-abdominal infections: Literature's guidelines. World J Gastroenterol. 2012;18(9):865-871.
64. Luna CM, Videla A, Mattera J, Vay C, Famiglietti A, Vujacich P, et al. Blood cultures have limited value in predicting severity of illness and as a diagnostic tool in ventilator-associated pneumonia. Chest. 1999;116(4):1075-84.
65. John H. Powers, Janet A Phoenix, Diana M. Zuckerman. Antibiotics usage and challenges - A comprehensive Review. NRCWF. Medscape. June 16, 2010.
66. Pelczar M.J., Chan, E.C.S. and Krieg, N.R. (1999) "Host-Parasite Interaction; Nonspecific Host Resistance", In: Microbiology Conceptsand Applications, 6th ed., McGraw-Hill Inc., New York, U.S.A. pp. 478-479.
67. Robert Berkow (ed.) Common Uses and possible side effects. The Merck manual of medical Information Sept 1999, ISBN 0-671-02727-1.
68. Casellas J.M Jr, Israele V, Martin M., Ishida M.T., Heguilen R, Soutric J, Arenoso H, Sibbald A, Stamboulian D. -Amoxicillin-sulbactam versus amoxicillin-clavulanic acid for the treatment of non-recurrent-acute otitis media in Argentinean children. Int J Pediatr Otorhinolaryngol 2005 Sep; 69(9):1225-33.
69. Derek Moore, Antibiotic classification and Mechanism. Retrieved on 25.10.13 from http://www.orthobullets.com/basic science/9059. Topic updated on 10.2.13.
70. List of Antibiotics. Retrieved on 26.10.13 from http://www.emedexpert.com/lists/antibiotics.shtml. Topic reviewed on 4.10.13.
71. Antibiotic classification and Mode of action. Retrieved on 25.10.13 from http://www.biomerieux-usa.com. Uploaded on March 2008.

CHAPTER 4

Nuclear Medicine Imaging in Gastrointestinal Diseases

Rakesh Kumar, Sellam Karunanithi

INTRODUCTION

Gastrointestinal (GI) imaging with radionuclide agents renders quantitative diagnostic information and noninvasive functional information which could not be obtained from anatomical imaging. GI imaging for various indications with positron emission tomography or computed tomography (PET/CT) and gamma camera scintigraphy including single-photon emission computed tomography (SPECT) and hybrid single photon emission tomography or computed tomography (SPECT/CT) are discussed below.

^{99m}TC-PERTECHNETATE MECKEL'S SCAN

Ectopic gastric mucosa in a Meckel's diverticulum can be a source of unexplained GI bleeding in pediatric patients. The indication for Meckel's scan is to localize the ectopic gastric mucosa. In the intestinal tract, gastric mucosa and the ectopic gastric mucosa shows ^{99m}Tc (Technetium-99m, $T_{1/2}$ = 6 hours)—pertechnetate uptake as the uptake is mainly localized to the mucin cell. Intravenous dose of 3.7 MBq/kg of body weight is usually given. Appearance of radioactivity in the ectopic gastric mucosa which appears at the same time as activity in the normal gastric mucosa is considered as positive study. Typical positive study occurs in gastric duplication and ectopic gastric mucosa which demonstrate simultaneous visualization with the stomach. Dynamic studies with intestinal duplication cysts show positive uptake even before the stomach is seen. Whereas delayed imaging is required in thoracic duplication cysts, as intrathoracic foregut duplication cysts show uptake on 24 hours delayed images after the gastric visualization.

^{99m}Tc-pertechnetate Meckel's scan has sensitivity and specificity of approximately 85% and 95%, respectively.[1] Priming with pentagastrin, H_2 blocker, and glucagon improves the detection rate. A subcutaneous dose of 6 mg/kg pentagastrin just before the imaging increases the metabolism of mucus producing cells. Glucagon is given at a dose of 50 mg/kg intravenously, 10 minutes after the ^{99m}Tc-pertechnetate administration. It inhibits the peristaltic dilution and washout of the radionuclide. Cimetidine is given orally for 2 days before imaging. It decreases the peptic secretion, thereby retarding the release of ^{99m}Tc-pertechnetate from the mucoid cells into the diverticulum lumen.[2,3] Intussusception, inflammatory lesions, obstructed loops of bowel, ulcers, arteriovenous malformations, and certain bowel tumors show false positive results.[4,5]

GASTROINTESTINAL BLEEDING

Nuclear medicine plays an important role in acute GI bleeding. Conventional endoscopy like gastroscopy, colonoscopy, and push-enteroscopy were used to confirm and localize hemorrhage from upper GI tract and colon. Conventional endoscopy has limited value in bleeding from the small intestine. ^{99m}Tc-labeled erythrocytes or radiolabeled sulfur colloid particles are the radionuclide agents used most commonly to detect active GI bleeding.

^{99m}Tc-labeled Autologous Erythrocyte (RBC) Scintigraphy

Red blood cells (RBCs) labeled by means of ^{99m}Tc can help to detect the source of GI bleeding in the small intestine in patients with bleeding in the lower GI tract from an uncertain source. It improves the disease management in patients presenting with obscure-overt bleeding, melena and hematochezia. Ready availability of good quality commercial kits enables rapid and reliable erythrocyte labeling. This technique is currently the most popular method as it provides dynamic early-phase imaging followed by extended equilibrium-phase. In vitro method has superior RBC labeling efficiency (98%) as compared with the in vivo (70%) and modified in vivo (90–95%) methods. Superior labeling efficiency makes the in vitro method preferable, yet on the contrary the in vivo method is simple.

Studies demonstrating radiotracer activity outside the region of normal vascular structures with retrograde or antegrade motion of radiotracer through bowel is considered positive. Bleeding from small intestine usually demonstrates a rapid distal progression through a series of multiple small, centrally located, curvilinear segments on cinematic display of the abdomen. On the contrary, large intestine bleeding demonstrates a more elongated pattern with peripheral location within the abdomen. Steady scintigraphic activity should not be diagnosed as an active bleeding site and usually results from a fixed vascular structure like hemangioma, accessory spleen, and ectopic kidney.[6]

Detecting intermittent bleeding is the main advantage of using ^{99m}Tc-RBCs as it permits visualization of GI bleeding over the course of several hours. Importantly bleeding rates as low as 0.1–0.4 mL/min can be detected by ^{99m}Tc-RBC scintigraphy. Also, entire GI tract can be visualized in ^{99m}Tc-RBC scintigraphy. It is an effective imaging modality in localizing lower GI bleeding especially in patients for whom all other diagnostic evaluation have failed to locate the site of bleeding.

^{99m}Tc-labeled Sulfur Colloid Scintigraphy

^{99m}Tc sulfur colloid is another radiotracer used in the evaluation of GI bleeding. It acts as an early phase vascular imaging agent. ^{99m}Tc sulfur colloid is extracted to liver, spleen and bone marrow and it get rapidly cleared from the vascular space. Extravasation from a vascular source, such as that which occurs during active GI bleeding, lacks rapid clearance and is easily detected ^{99m}Tc-labeled sulfur colloid scan.[7] Active bleeding occurring within a time-window of several minutes after radiotracer administration is the main dependent factor. It yields high target to background count ratio thereby has the advantage of detecting bleeding rates as low as 0.05–0.1 mL/min. As the liver and spleen show physiological ^{99m}Tc sulfur colloid accumulation those bleeding sites in close proximity to liver and spleen can show false negative results.

Scintigraphy with ^{99m}Tc-labeled RBC and ^{99m}Tc sulfur colloid has certain advantages over contrast angiography. Scintigraphy detects sources of venous and arterial GI bleeding, whereas angiography only detects arterial sources. Also, ^{99m}Tc RBC scintigraphy for GI bleeding has the ability to predict transfusion requirements and the need for angiography and surgery.[8-10] ^{99m}Tc RBC scintigraphy has prognostic importance as a negative study is predictive of good outcome in patients presenting with acute GI bleeding who are stabilized by transfusion and supportive care. Scintigraphy study with ^{99m}Tc-labeled RBC or ^{99m}Tc sulfur colloid is highly recommended before angiography as it plays an important role in assisting both radiological and surgical interventions.[11]

Other Techniques

^{99m}Tc-labeled albumin was the earliest intravascular agent used to detect GI bleeding.[12] ^{99m}Tc-labeled heat-damaged erythrocytes also have been used. These technique showed promising results but was soon surpassed by techniques using more reliable labeling techniques. ^{111}Indium-labeled erythrocytes also have been used with the aim of using the longer ($T_{1/2}$ = 2.80 days) of ^{111}In to facilitate prolonged imaging to detect intermittent GI bleeding. The increased radiation burden and, increased cost limit the potential clinical utility of this technique.[13]

GASTROESOPHAGEAL REFLUX SCINTIGRAPHY

^{99m}Tc sulfur colloid in water or milk/formula milk is often used for the assessment of gastroesophageal reflux (GER) in children. 0.2–1 mCi of ^{99m}Tc sulfur colloid is given orally in two thirds of the expected feeding volume. In order to clear any residual activity within the oropharynx and esophagus, the remaining unlabeled one third of the feeding volume is then swallowed. The patient is burped before imaging. Acquisition for 60 minutes with short-lasting 5-s anterior images is the usual protocol (Fig. 1). In order to look for evidence of aspiration, after the dynamic imaging at the end of 60 minutes, anterior and posterior static images of the thorax will be acquired.

Detection of GER on scintigraphy was found to be useful in the assessment of the outcome of antireflux surgery and in children presenting with caustic esophageal injury.[14,15] GER scan provides additional information such as aspiration, gastric emptying data, and abnormal esophageal contraction. In order to identify pulmonary aspiration, salivagram and milk scan are the two available scintigraphic studies. Aspiration during swallowing (antegrade events) is detected by salivagram while the milk scan detects the events related to GER (retrograde events). With patient in supine position, a small drop of liquid containing ^{99m}Tc-sulfur colloid is placed on the patient's tongue for salivagram and posterior images are obtained for 1 hour although the study often ends at 10–15 minutes. Demonstration of tracheobronchial activity and/or lung activity is considered positive. The salivagram is more frequently positive than the milk scan or videofluoroscopy in the detection of pulmonary aspiration.

ESOPHAGEAL TRANSIT SCINTIGRAPHY

Down syndrome, achalasia, systemic sclerosis, diffuse esophageal spasm, esophagitis, nutcracker esophagus, tracheoesophageal fistula, and diabetes mellitus are the usual esophageal motility disorders evaluated with esophageal transit scintigraphy. The major current indication is in patients with esophageal dysmotility to evaluate esophageal emptying and reflux. At least a 3-hour overnight fasting is required for the scan. The test is performed with the patient in the supine position and having him or her swallow a 10 mL bolus of water or milk labeled with 5.55 MBq of ^{99m}Tc sulfur colloid, followed by repetitive swallows of the bolus (dry swallows may also be obtained), and images are obtained via a gamma camera while the patient is in a supine or upright position. Images are analyzed and time-activity curves (TAC) are obtained from the regions of interest (ROI) drawn around the upper, middle, and lower thirds of the esophagus and the stomach. The normal transit time through the esophagus is typically less than 10 seconds which ranges from 3.4 ± 1 s for infants to 4.6 ± 1.9 s for patients 8–16 years of age.

Noninvasive nature, low radiation burden and its ability to quantify are major advantages of esophageal scintigraphy.

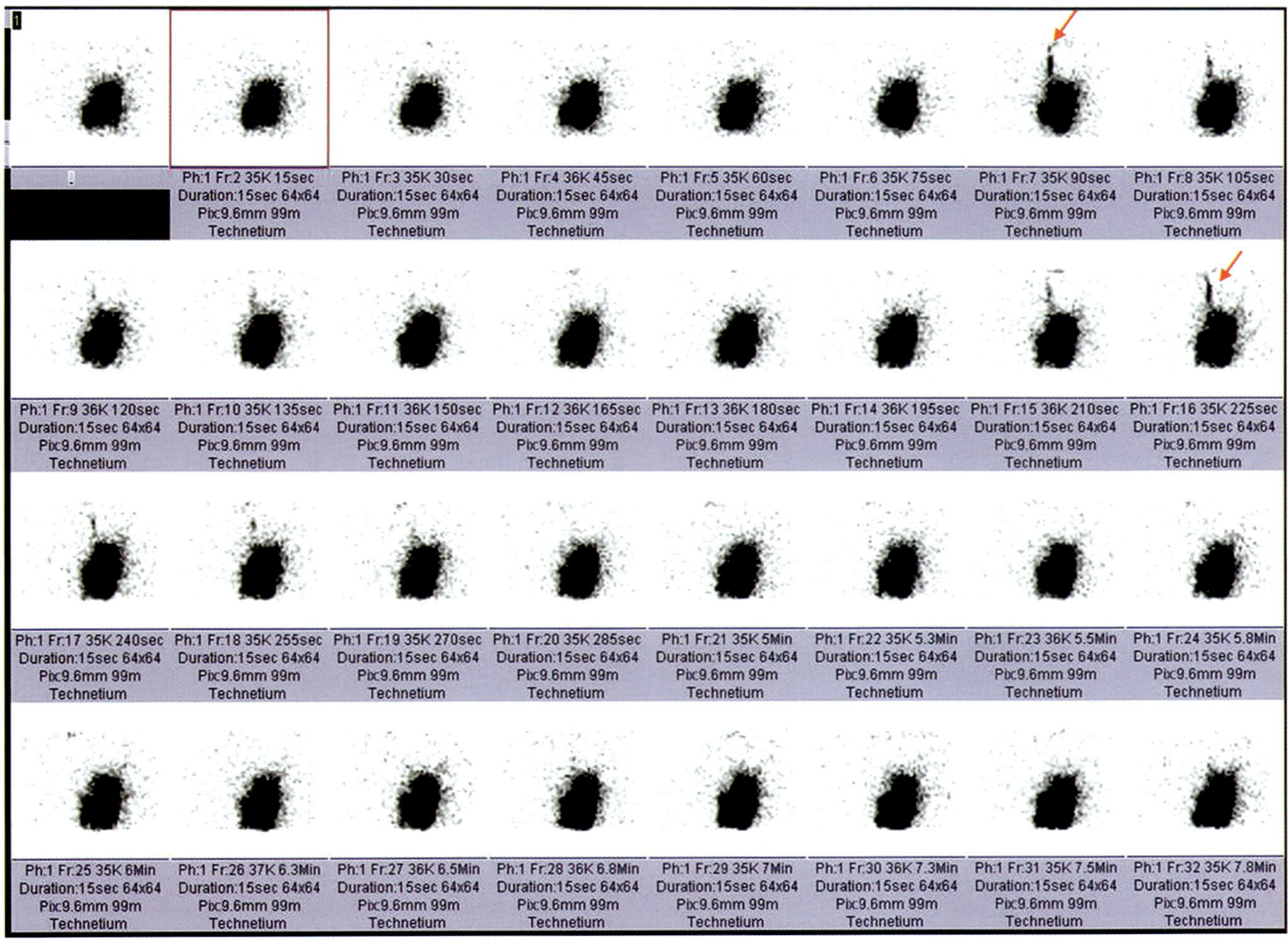

Figure 1 *Gastroesophageal reflux scintigraphic test*: Frequent reflux events are evident in this sequence (arrows), with retrograde extension of radiotracer up to the entire esophagus

Unavailability of esophageal manometry, equivocal manometry results, and negative manometry with high clinical suspicion of esophageal dysmotility are certain important indications for esophageal scintigraphy. It is also useful to monitor disease and its response to therapy.[16-18]

GASTRIC EMPTYING

Scintigraphy is the gold standard measurement of gastric emptying. It provides an objective assessment of the gastric transit abnormality preoperatively and postoperatively which guides treatment decisions.[19] Indications for scintigraphic gastric emptying include: (1) Diagnosis of dyspepsia with a normal endoscopic examination; (2) recalcitrant GER; (3) diabetics with symptoms of gastroparesis or erratic glycemic control and (4) suspected generalized motility disorders, postsurgical nausea, or vomiting.

The rate of scintigraphic gastric emptying is dependent on the nature of test meal used. Exponential clearance of activity will be noted with liquids. Solids generally demonstrate a lag period which is followed by near linear disappearance. In infants, milk or formula milk is used in assessment of gastric emptying. In older children, solid or combined solid and liquid emptying can be assessed. Idli or egg sandwich containing ^{99m}Tc-sulfur colloid is used for performing solid gastric emptying. ROI is drawn around the stomach region. Anterior images for 30 seconds are acquired for every 10 minutes. Images are acquired until 2 hours. Between image acquisitions the patient is allowed to sit upright. Simultaneous IV infusion of a prokinetic drug during gastric emptying study by scintigraphy has been used in a few nuclear medicine departments to identify patients ("responders" who have normalized gastric emptying) who are more likely to respond to chronic treatment with prokinetics.

Although scintigraphy is the accepted gold standard for diagnosis of gastroparesis[20] it has limited validation for detection of rapid gastric emptying, which has been observed in functional dyspepsia, cyclical vomiting, postgastric surgery symptoms, and diabetics with early stages of autonomic dysfunction. These patients cannot be distinguished from gastroparetics by symptoms alone. Patients should be off prokinetic or antikinetic medications for at least 48 hours before testing, and fasting blood glucose should be less than 180 mg/dL on the day of testing.

COLON TRANSIT

Indications for colon transit include evaluation of patients in whom surgery is considered for slow transit constipation; unexplained constipation or diarrhea; and constipated patients with upper GI symptoms.[21] A methacrylate-coated capsule containing ^{111}In-labeled activated charcoal particles is ingested. The coated capsule usually dissolves in the alkaline pH of the distal ileum and releases into the colon.[22] External markers are placed over the iliac crests to localize the position of the capsule in the small bowel. At the same time, a ^{99m}Tc-labeled egg meal is used to assess gastric and small bowel transit. Anterior and posterior images are obtained at specified times (e.g., 4, 24, and 48 hours) while the patient stands erect and an area of interest is drawn around the images of the regions of the colon. Radionuclide colon transit scintigraphy, a safe and noninvasive method, has been shown to correlate with radiopaque markers. Colon transit scintigraphy provides information on regional and overall colon transit.

The use of scintigraphy to measure GI transit is an important tool for the clinician in the diagnosis and treatment of common GI diseases. Studies such as colonic transit and SPECT for measuring gastric accommodation are gaining wider acceptance and availability; however, others such as rectoanal angle, and emptying, and esophageal scintigraphy are not widely available or lack standardization of the techniques and/or interpretation of the results. Gastric emptying scintigraphy still remains the most widely used GI scintigraphic test and has been established as the gold standard for measuring gastric emptying. Scintigraphy studies are easy to perform and usually well tolerated.

BILIARY ATRESIA VERSUS NEONATAL HEPATITIS

Biliary atresia and neonatal hepatitis share similar clinical features. In order to prevent complete deterioration of the extrahepatic biliary tree and irreversible liver damage, early detection of biliary atresia before 2–3 months of age is very important. ^{99m}Tc-hepatobiliary iminodiacetic acid (HIDA) derivatives like ^{99m}Tc-diisopropyl iminodiacetic acid (DISIDA) or ^{99m}Tc-mebrofenin are used in hepatobiliary scintigraphy. Priming the neonate with phenobarbital (5 mg/kg/d divided BID for 3–5 days before scintigraphy) is important. Phenobarbital increases the bile secretion and improves the sensitivity of the scan. Rarely, ursodeoxycholic acid has also been included in the bile secretion stimulation priming regimen.

Dynamic abdominal images are acquired for 1 hour (at some centers, only 15 minutes is acquired). Visualization of bowel excludes the presence of extra hepatic biliary atresia. Non-visualization of bowel activity till 24 hours delayed images is considered positive for biliary atresia. False positive results (normal liver uptake of tracer with no excretion up to 24 hours) can occur in severe cases of neonatal hepatitis, dehydration, total parenteral nutrition (TPN) cholestasis, Alagille syndrome, sepsis, and bile plug syndrome in cystic fibrosis. Poor liver uptake and poor hepatobiliary transit with passage of tracer into the bowel occurs typically in neonatal hepatitis. Severely impaired hepatocyte radiotracer uptake with non-visualization of bowel activity is considered as indeterminate and a repeat scintigraphy after priming with phenobarbital (if previously not performed) may prove useful in these cases. With the introduction of hybrid SPECT/CT accurate anatomical localization of questionable activity to bowel lumen versus genitourinary tract, liver, spleen, or elsewhere in equivocal cases can be performed.[23]

CHOLEDOCHAL CYST

A choledochal cyst is a congenital focal cystic or fusiform dilatation of the common bile duct (CBD) with or without associated proximal intrahepatic ductal dilatation. Patients with choledochal cysts usually present prior to the age of 10 years and females are affected more than males (4:1). Symptoms include pain (90%), intermittent jaundice (33%), right upper quadrant (RUQ) mass (25%), choledocholithiasis (50%), pancreatitis (33%), and cholangitis. Affected patients are at an increased risk of developing cholangiocarcinoma (10% of patients). Treatment consists of early surgical excision or anastomosis to the intestine in order to prevent biliary cirrhosis. Complications include: Cholangitis, pancreatitis, stone formation, and cholangiocarcinoma (20x's general population risk). Choledochal cysts may be sub-classified into five types (Type I–V).

HIDA scintigraphy with ^{99m}Tc-mebrofenin: A variety of appearances can be seen on the scintigraphic exam. Uptake of the radiotracer by the liver is usually normal. Initially the bile filled cyst may appear as a photopenic area, but on delayed images the cyst will fill with tracer and appear as a hot spot (Figs 2A to H). If the cyst is obstructive, there may be non-visualization of the CBD and bowel activity may not be identified.

BILIARY OBSTRUCTION AND CHOLECYSTITIS

Hepatobiliary scintigraphy is useful in the assessment of patients with right upper quadrant pain. Acute cholecystitis is associated with nonvisualization of the gallbladder on HIDA scintigraphy with ^{99m}Tc mebrofenin. A specificity of 100% and a diagnostic accuracy of 98% are documented in adult population.[24] However, in children, gallbladder visualization, though infrequent, is possible in acalculous cholecystitis. So visualization of the gallbladder in children does not exclude cholecystitis. Further assessment with 0.02 mg/kg sincalide infusion is advised if the gallbladder is visualized. Partial cystic duct obstruction, acalculous cholecystitis or chronic cholecystitis can cause poor contraction of the gallbladder following sincalide administration. A gallbladder ejection fraction (EF) of approximately less than 35% can be noted in patients with chronic cholecystitis. Also, chronic cholecystitis shows a delay in gallbladder filling in the absence of hepatic dysfunction. In scintigraphic evaluation for acute cholecystitis, morphine augmentation may help to reduce the number of false positive studies and decrease scanning time.[25]

BILIARY LEAK

Trauma and surgery are the common causes for biliary leak. In surgical cases, bile leaks occur most commonly at the cystic duct (70–75%). Intervention is required in large biliary leaks whereas small biliary leaks are allowed to heal spontaneously. Hepatobiliary scintigraphy is usually performed in such cases to identify biliary leak and to localize the site of leak. Also, scintigraphy provides a qualitative assessment of the severity of the leak. Hepatobiliary

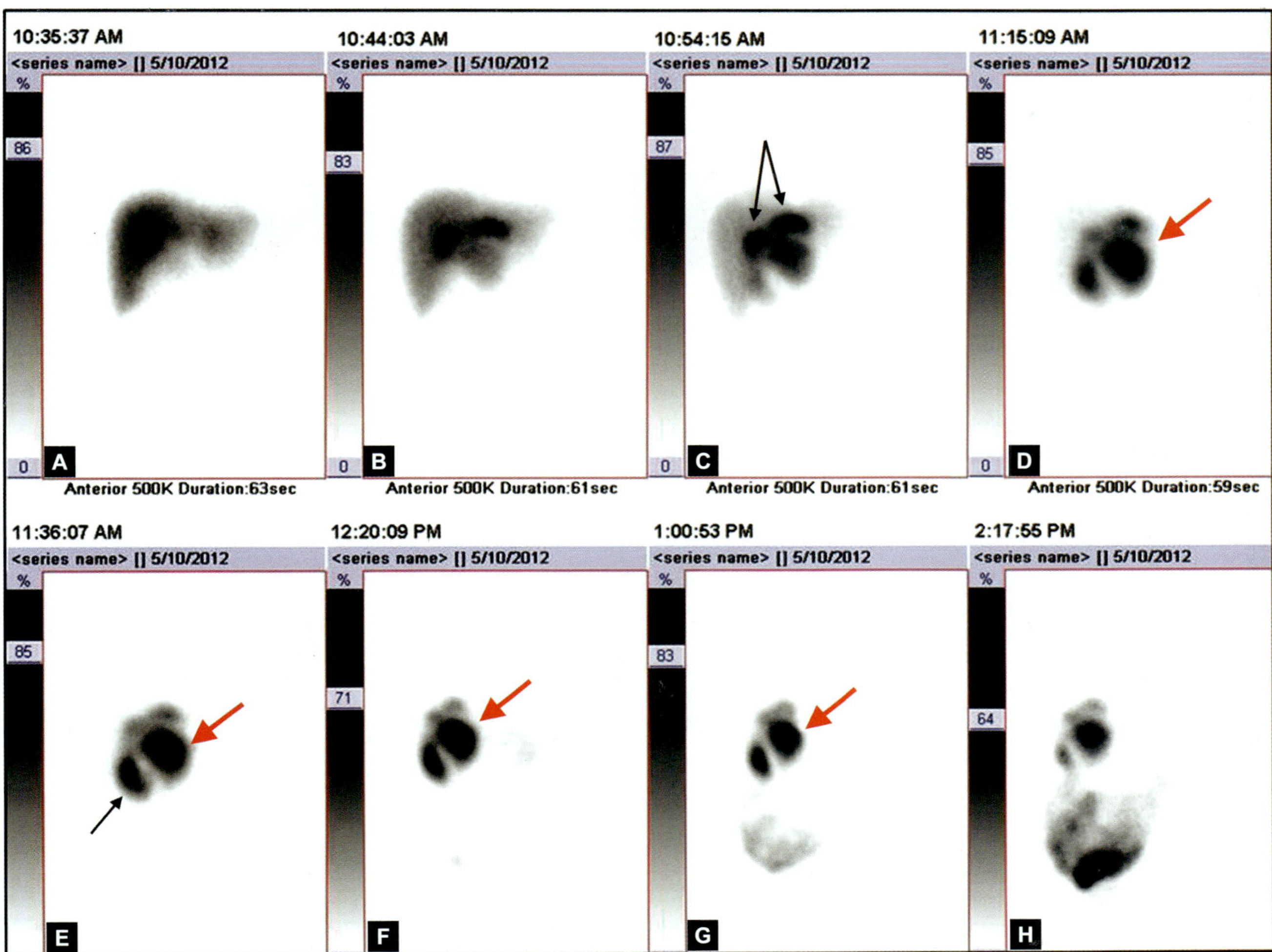

Figures 2A to H Hepatobiliary iminodiacetic acid (HIDA) scan with ^{99m}Tc-mebrofenin. Serial images reveal an initial photopenic area which as time progresses shows progressive accumulation of radiotracer (thick arrows). Also, appreciated are the right and left hepatic ducts (C; thin arrows) and gallbladder (E; thin arrows) with abdomen showing bowel activity in delayed images. These features are suggestive of non-obstructive choledochal cyst

scintigraphy is a sensitive, noninvasive and inexpensive test in this clinical setting. Positive scan reveal the presence of radiotracer within the peritoneal cavity (either adjacent to the liver or within the hepatic capsule) (Fig. 3). Infrequently, free bile ascites can be noted. Scintigraphy has better sensitivity and specificity in biliary leak detection as it can establish an active hepatobiliary component in fluid collection, whereas CT or ultrasonography (USG) can demonstrate only the presence of a fluid collection.[26] With the introduction of hybrid SPECT/CT accurate anatomical localization of bile leak can be documented which improves the patient management.

SPLENIC SCINTIGRAPHY

^{99m}Tc-denatured RBC is the ideal tracer for splenic scintigraphy. Denaturation of RBC improves the localization of spleen. Images are acquired at least 15 minutes after intravenous injection of ^{99m}Tc-labeled, denatured RBCs. Splenic scintigraphy alternatively can be performed by using ^{99m}Tc sulfur colloid. The tracer usually clears with a half-time of 2.5 minutes. Anatomic imaging may give the spleen a false appearance of abdominal tumor in patients with increased ligamentous laxity as they allow the spleen to become mobile within the abdomen. ^{99m}Tc-sulfur colloid or denatured RBC scan can distinguish the "wandering spleen" from abdominal tumor in these cases.[27]

Failure of early embryologic fusion of multiple buds of splenic tissue can result in accessory spleens or splenules which occurs in 40% of patients. Splenic hilum is the most common site. In patients with accessory spleens or splenules, after splenectomy hypertrophy of these residual buds occurs and can create an appearance of hypersplenism. Splenic scintigraphy with ^{99m}Tc-sulfur colloid or denatured RBC is helpful for establishing the presence of splenic tissue versus neoplastic proliferation. It is also useful in patients with splenic trauma where splenosis can occur with fragmentation of the spleen with subsequent auto-transplantation of splenic tissue. Associated rupture of diaphragm can result in thoracic splenosis. Splenic scintigraphy with ^{99m}Tc sulfur colloid or ^{99m}Tc denatured RBCs can be utilized in distincting thoracic splenosis from thoracic neoplasm in patient presenting with thoracic mass and a previous history of splenic trauma.[28] SPECT imaging gives a

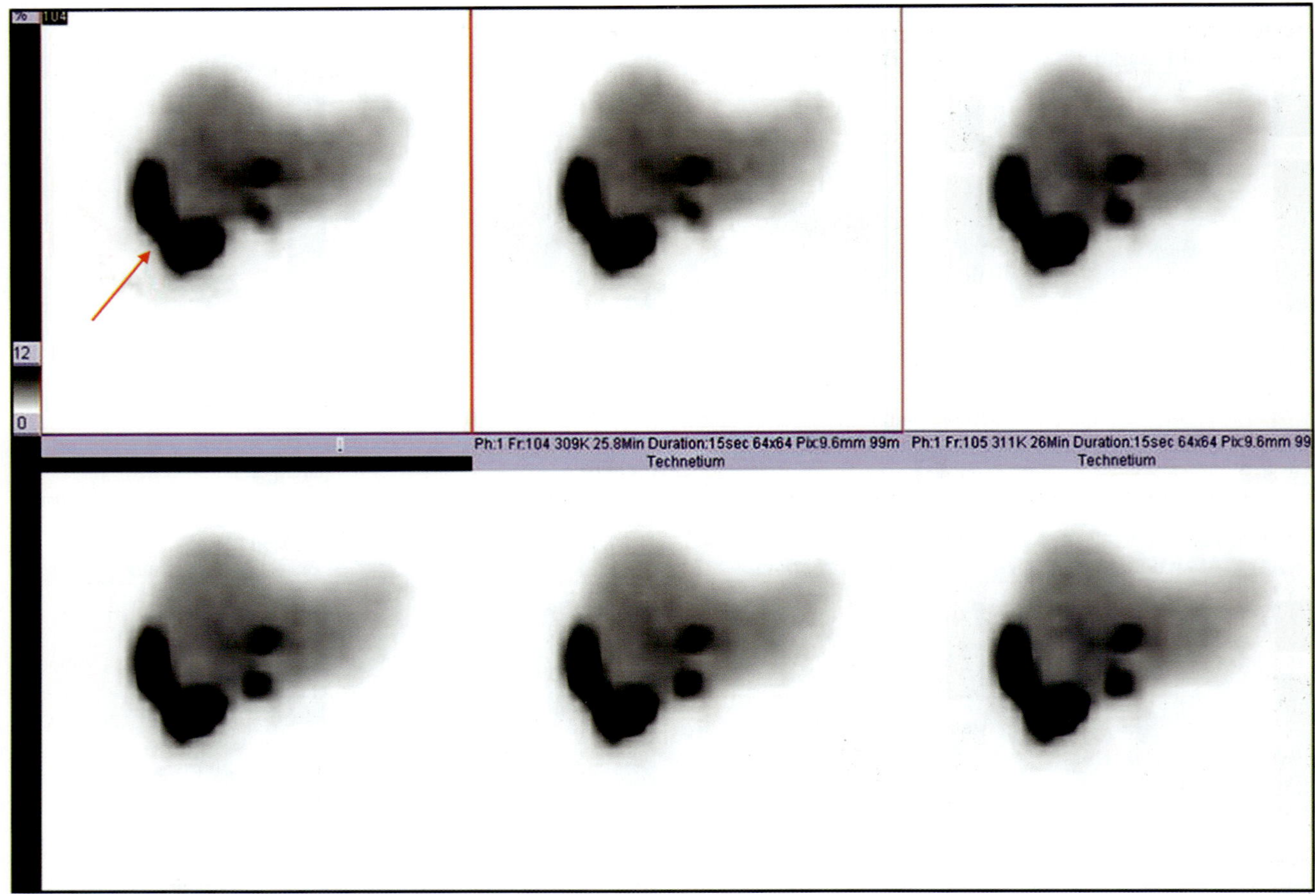

Figure 3 Hepatobiliary iminodiacetic acid (HIDA) scan with ^{99m}Tc-mebrofenin. Serial images reveal progressive accumulation of radiotracer in gallbladder fossa suggestive of bile leak (arrows) consequent to blunt injury to abdomen in a road traffic accident

three dimensional view which gives a better information regarding distribution and presence of splenic tissue. Hybrid SPECT/CT imaging provides precise anatomical correlation of splenic scintigraphic foci with its corresponding anatomical region.

PROTEIN-LOSING ENTEROPATHY

Protein-losing enteropathy refers to GI disorders associated with excessive plasma protein loss into the lumen of the gut. It is caused by loss of integrity of the cell membranes of enterocytes mucosal erosion or ulceration.[29,30] Patients can become edematous due to albumin loss and decreased plasma oncotic pressure. Scintigraphy for diagnosing protein losing enteropathy was initially performed using ^{131}I-polyvinylpyrrolidone, ^{131}I-albumin,[31] ^{51}Cr-albumin[29] and ^{99m}Tc-albumin. Imaging with ^{99m}Tc-albumin allows imaging of the GI tract thereby localizing the site of protein loss. It is useful in directing resection for surgically correctable causes. ^{99m}Tc-HSA (human serum albumin) scans were more likely positive in patients with higher rates of protein loss.[32,33] ^{99m}Tc-dextran and ^{111}In-transferrin are the other radiotracer available for diagnosing protein losing enteropathy. ^{99m}Tc-dextran when compared to ^{99m}Tc-HSA has faster background clearance and better in vivo stability. ^{111}In-transferrin has the ability to identify and quantify the protein loss in single examination.[34]

INFLAMMATORY BOWEL DISEASES

Localizing and quantifying the inflammation in inflammatory bowel diseases (IBDs) are very crucial in determining the diagnosis, prognosis, and optimal therapy. Evaluation with endoscopy is invasive and usually requires sedation. Limited segment of colon and the small intestine are particularly the sites that are inaccessible to evaluation. ^{99m}Tc-WBC imaging is noninvasive and has demonstrated less perceived discomfort and embarrassment when compared with barium enema and colonoscopy.[35]

Evaluation with ^{99m}Tc-WBC

The labeling of leukocytes with ^{99m}Tc with 20–45 mL of venous blood is done. Imaging is performed with a large field of view gamma camera and images are obtained at 0.5 hour and 2–3 hours after the injection of ^{99m}Tc-WBC. The patient voids before each imaging. Additional anterior chest images may be acquired in patients with suspicion of Crohn's disease (CD), to evaluate for esophageal and gastric activity. Static anterior supine view of the abdomen and pelvis are obtained followed by SPECT imaging.

Scintigraphy with ^{99m}Tc-WBC has been reported to be sensitive for the detection of inflammation in adults.[36] The agreement between colonoscopy and ^{99m}Tc-WBC imaging for the localization and evaluation of the extent of inflammation is excellent. Noninvasiveness, evaluation of the entire bowel in single study, and less radiation exposure compared with barium radiograph are the merits of ^{99m}Tc-WBC scan.[37] The ^{99m}Tc-WBC scan plays important role in the initial evaluation, and follow-up of patients with IBD.

^{99m}Tc-WBC scan has limitations in defining anatomic details such as prestenotic dilations, fistulas, or strictures which are best identifies with barium radiographic scans. The ^{99m}Tc-WBC scan is safe even in acutely ill patients who may not tolerate an endoscopic or radiological study. ^{99m}Tc-WBC scan is complementary to endoscopic or radiological studies in most patients.

Evaluation with Fluorodeoxyglucose (FDG) PET/CT

Positron emission tomography enabled researchers to correctly identify active IBD in 80% of children with IBD and showed no evidence of inflammation in children without IBD but present with recurrent abdominal pain.[38] Recently we evaluated the role of PET/CT enteroclysis and PET/CT colonography in IBDs. PET/CT enteroclysis in a single investigation detects a significantly higher number of lesions both in the small and large intestine in comparison to that detected by conventional barium and colonoscopy combined together.[39] PET/CT colonography is a novel noninvasive technique for the assessment of extent and activity of the disease in patients with ulcerative colitis (UC).[40]

FDG PET/CT IN GI MALIGNANCY

^{18}F-Fluorodeoxyglucose PET imaging has been used in clinical oncology since late 1980s. Large scientific data from 1990s consolidated the utility of PET in clinical oncology especially in lung malignancy, colorectal malignancy, lymphoma, and melanoma. FDG uptake is considered as a surrogate for the metabolic activity of a malignancy, specifically linked to glucose metabolism in malignant cells. The role of FDG-PET imaging, in fact, may be related to the Warburg effect-the observation made by Otto Warburg in 1924 that suggested that cancer cells metabolize glucose differently from normal nonmalignant cells. Glucose uptake by malignant cells is largely mediated by the glucose transporter 1 (GLUT-1) transporter. It has been correlated that the standardized uptake value (SUV) in FDG-PET correlate with the expression of GLUT-1 and the Ki-67 proliferative marker, indicating an association with tumor aggressiveness. PET combined with CT in the form of hybrid PET/CT allows accurate localization of lesions with improved spatial resolution.

Certain basic principles to be noted before advising FDG PET/CT:

- FDG-PET should be performed only after 4–6 weeks post-chemotherapy, 6–8 weeks post-radiotherapy and 8–12 weeks post-surgery as there are possibilities for false positive uptake during or early after therapy due to inflammation.
- Metabolic information is especially advantageous in detection of recurrent disease when sensitive serum markers such as carcinoembryonic antigen (CEA) are abnormal and anatomic imaging is unrevealing.

Colorectal Cancer

The primary indications for FDG-PET in colorectal carcinoma are for staging, restaging and detection of recurrence. Elevated serum CEA levels with unrevealing conventional diagnostic imaging findings is the scenario where FDG-PET is especially useful in the evaluation of recurrent colorectal cancer. FDG-PET is well established as the most accurate imaging modality for staging, restaging and evaluation of colorectal recurrence (Figs 4A to E).

FDG-PET imaging is useful in the detection of primary and premalignant lesions of the colon.[41-44] Size of the lesion and grade of dysplasia are the dependent factors that affect the sensitivity. Tumor larger than 1 cm has higher sensitivity (72%), FDG-PET has a sensitivity ranging from 33% in low-grade lesions up to 76% in high-grade lesions.[44] False positive uptake can be noted in IBDs and diverticulitis. Also, physiologic uptake in colonic mucosa, lymphoid tissue, and smooth muscle should be carefully analyzed which usually shows diffuse uptake. So the focal nature of hypermetabolism is important to differentiate between benign and malignant lesions. IBDs and physiologic uptake tend to be diffuse or segmental, whereas the accumulations of FDG in premalignant and malignant lesions are focal and intense. Focal uptake in the colon should lead to further invasive investigation.

In patients with rectal carcinoma main indications for FDG-PET are therapy monitoring and diagnosis of relapses, especially the differentiation between tumor and scar and also the localization of tumor manifestations in cases with increasing tumor markers. FDG-PET is very efficient in the imaging of pulmonic and hepatic metastases of colorectal cancer but not in lymph node staging. For patients who present with advanced stage disease FDG-PET imaging can serve as a baseline scan before the start of chemotherapy. Because the degree of FDG uptake before starting with assessment of the overall tumor burden can serve as a powerful tool to determine appropriate response to treatment on follow-up scans. Most recurrences after surgical resection for colorectal cancer occur within the first 4 years for which FDG-PET is very useful. FDG-PET imaging can be particularly useful in monitoring response to therapy with neoadjuvant chemoradiotherapy. FDG-PET can differentiate benign from malignant lesions based on their metabolic activity and its biological aggressiveness can be assessed which allows early assessment of response to treatment. Metabolically active tumors can be detected even before a morphologic change is noted on anatomical imaging. Meta-analysis studies[45] showed an overall sensitivity of 97% and specificity of 76% for FDG-PET in detecting recurrent colorectal cancer. FDG PET/CT is also found to be useful in malignant melanoma of anal canal, rectum and colon.

Minimally Invasive Radionuclide Interventional Therapies

In patients with unresectable liver metastases radiofrequency (RF) ablation and Yttrium-90 (^{90}Y) microspheres radioembolization are increasingly becoming the interventional techniques of choice. FDG-PET appears to have great potential in identifying residual tumor soon after RF ablation. Liver metastases depend primarily on the hepatic arteries for their nutrition and growth. The principle of radioembolization is similar to chemoembolization. Patients with liver-lung shunt fractions greater than 20% is a contraindication for radioembolization with ^{90}Y microspheres.

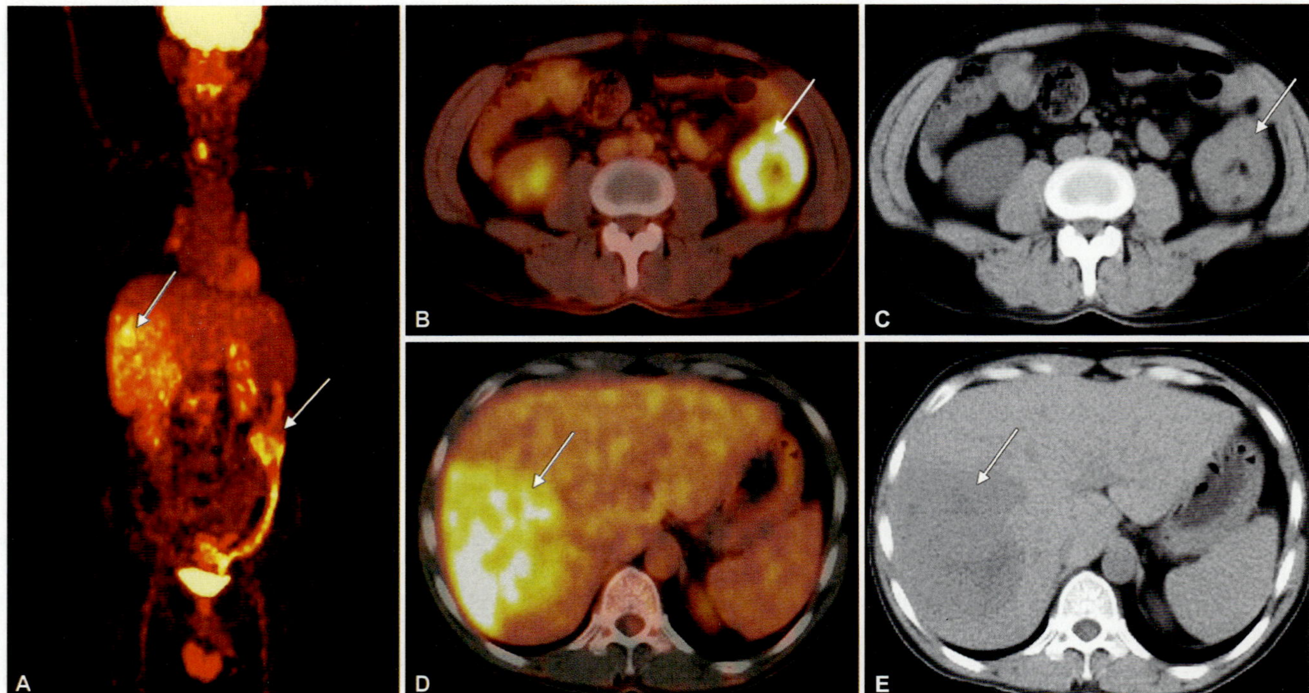

Figures 4A to E A 37-year-old male with colon carcinoma who underwent right hemicolectomy 8 years ago now presented with raising carcinoembryonic antigen (CEA) levels. He underwent ^{18}F-FDG PET/CT. Maximum intensity projection positron emission tomography (PET) image (A) and trans-axial PET/CT images (B to D) revealed recurrence in descending colon with hepatic metastatic lesions (arrows)

Esophageal Cancer

The sensitivity of detecting primary esophageal cancer with FDG-PET is high (90–100%).[46,47] It has superior sensitivity compared to CT alone. Esophagitis or other inflammation involving the esophagus can cause false positive uptake, which usually show mild linear diffuse uptake. Small or flat mucosal lesions and adenocarcinoma at or near the gastroesophageal junction can show false negative results with FDG-PET. Also, diffuse growth pattern and/or mucinous histopathology may show false negative results.[48,49]

Staging PET is limited in its ability to determine depth of tumor invasion. PET is complementary to CT for initial locoregional staging. The accuracy for distant metastasis was much higher than for CT-endoscopic ultrasound (CT-EUS). However, FDG-PET has lower accuracy for N staging when compared to CT-EUS. The lymph nodes adjacent to primary tumor usually show poor conspicuity due to intense primary tumor uptake. PET is also used in restaging, recurrence detection and in response evaluation to therapy (Figs 5A to D). FDG-PET is established as modality of highest sensitivity and accuracy for identifying distant metastatic disease in esophageal carcinoma. Also, response assessment to neoadjuvant therapy can be best performed with FDG PET/CT.

Gastric Carcinomas

The sensitivity of FDG-PET to detect locally advanced gastric carcinomas is dependent on the microscopic growth type of the tumor. Due to variable intense physiologic uptake of FDG within the gastric wall primary tumor of the stomach is difficult to identify with usual protocol FDG PET/CT. Distending the stomach with water improves the accuracy of detection of gastric lesions both preoperatively and in the postoperative remnant stomach. False positive FDG uptake can occur in acute inflammatory conditions such as superficial or erosive gastritis. The sensitivity of PET is low for the detection of metastatic lymph nodes, if size of the node is less than 6 mm as the spatial resolution is low for less than 6mm lesions.

Histologic subtype of the tumor is a strong dependent factor for FDG uptake and inversely correlates with the content of mucus.[50-52] The nonintestinal cell type, in the signet ring or mucinous cell types show low FDG uptake. If the primary tumor show FDG uptake, preliminary studies show a change in post-therapy uptake can serve as a good predictor of response to therapy and survival.

In response evaluation, the FDG-PET has advantage over CT. FDG-PET can demonstrate a decrease in FDG uptake at an earlier stage than could be demonstrated by CT and other conventional imaging methods. Also, CT response by RECIST (Response Evaluation Criteria in Solid Tumors) is measured by the change in size which may be a late manifestation of a response. FDG-PET has higher specificity (70–100%) for the detection of recurrent disease.

Gastrointestinal Stromal Tumors

Gastrointestinal stromal tumors (GIST) are considered as uncommon tumors of the GI tract and are now believed to be not sarcomas and to be arising from interstitial cells of Cajal or primitive

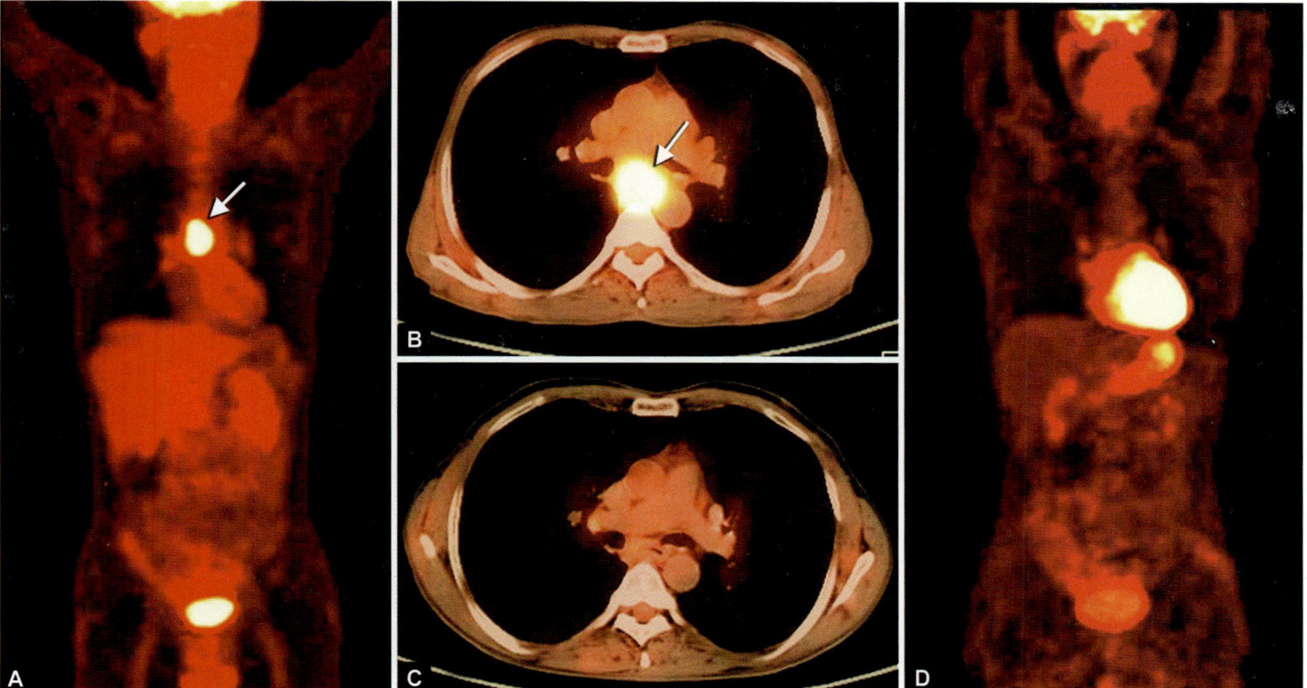

Figures 5A to D A 55-year-old male with esophageal carcinoma underwent ^{18}F-FDG PET/CT as a baseline study and as a response evaluation study. His baseline staging study revealed a mass lesion in lower esophagus (A, B; arrows) with no distant metastasis. His response evaluation study after three cycles of neoadjuvant chemotherapy (C and D) revealed complete resolution of the disease implying significant response to chemotherapy

cells in the GI tract. The prognostic information was better seen in FDG-PET images than in CT findings.[53] FDG-PET is useful for the recurrence detection (Figs 6A to G), monitoring of therapy and also in initial staging. GIST show highly variable uptake on FDG-PET. FDG-PET appears to be useful in assessing response to imatinib mesylate (Gleevec) therapy and prognosis if the tumor lesion show high uptake on the initial FDG scan.[54,55]

Hepatocellular Carcinoma

Hepatocellular carcinoma (HCC) is potentially curable by surgical resection, but surgery is the treatment of choice for only a small fraction of patients with localized disease. HCC has lower FDG accumulation in well-differentiated and low-grade tumors than in high-grade tumors (Figs 7A to F), as the much needed GLUT-1 concentration which is necessary for FDG uptake is low in well differentiated HCC.[56] Recently ^{11}C-acetate PET showed a good sensitivity of 87% compared with that of 47% with FDG-PET in HCC detection.[57] Hence the importance of ^{18}F-FDG-PET in the management of HCC is mainly in detecting extrahepatic spread. FDG-PET/CT may be helpful in surveillance after therapy and detection of local recurrence or occult metastatic disease in patients with unexplained serum alpha fetoprotein (AFP) elevation after interventional treatment (e.g., transarterial chemoembolization or RF ablation) and negative conventional imaging.[58] FDG-PET/CT sensitivity for detection of HCC depends on the underlying tumor grade. However, when assessed from the point of view of tumor characterization and prognosis, HCCs with low FDG uptake tend to be low grade and associated with improved patient outcome. High tumor FDG uptake in patients who are candidates for liver transplantation is associated with higher risk of tumor recurrence postoperatively (Figs 7A to F). Radiotracers of lipogenesis appear to be complementary to FDG. In particular, radiolabeled acetate and choline are useful in the imaging evaluation of well-differentiated tumors that do not sufficiently accumulate FDG.

Cholangiocarcinoma and Gallbladder Cancer

Limited data regarding use of FDG-PET, but evidence supports good sensitivity with potential false negative results in mucinous adenocarcinomas. Also, granulomatous disease, sclerosing cholangitis and stents can show FDG uptake and mimic malignancy.[59] Currently FDG PET/CT is used to detect distant metastasis, recurrence detection and in response evaluation (Figs 8A to H). Recently we evaluated the role of FDG PET/CT in recurrent gallbladder cancer (GBC).We found that FDG PET/CT can detect recurrence in GBC with high sensitivity and specificity and its routine use in these patients will detect recurrence early and change the subsequent management.[60]

Pancreatic Cancer

In diagnostic procedures for pancreatic carcinoma, FDG-PET can be recommended to explore the dignity of pancreatic lesions and in the imaging of tumor relapses. In order to stage the depth of invasion or to determine the invasion of local-regional structures

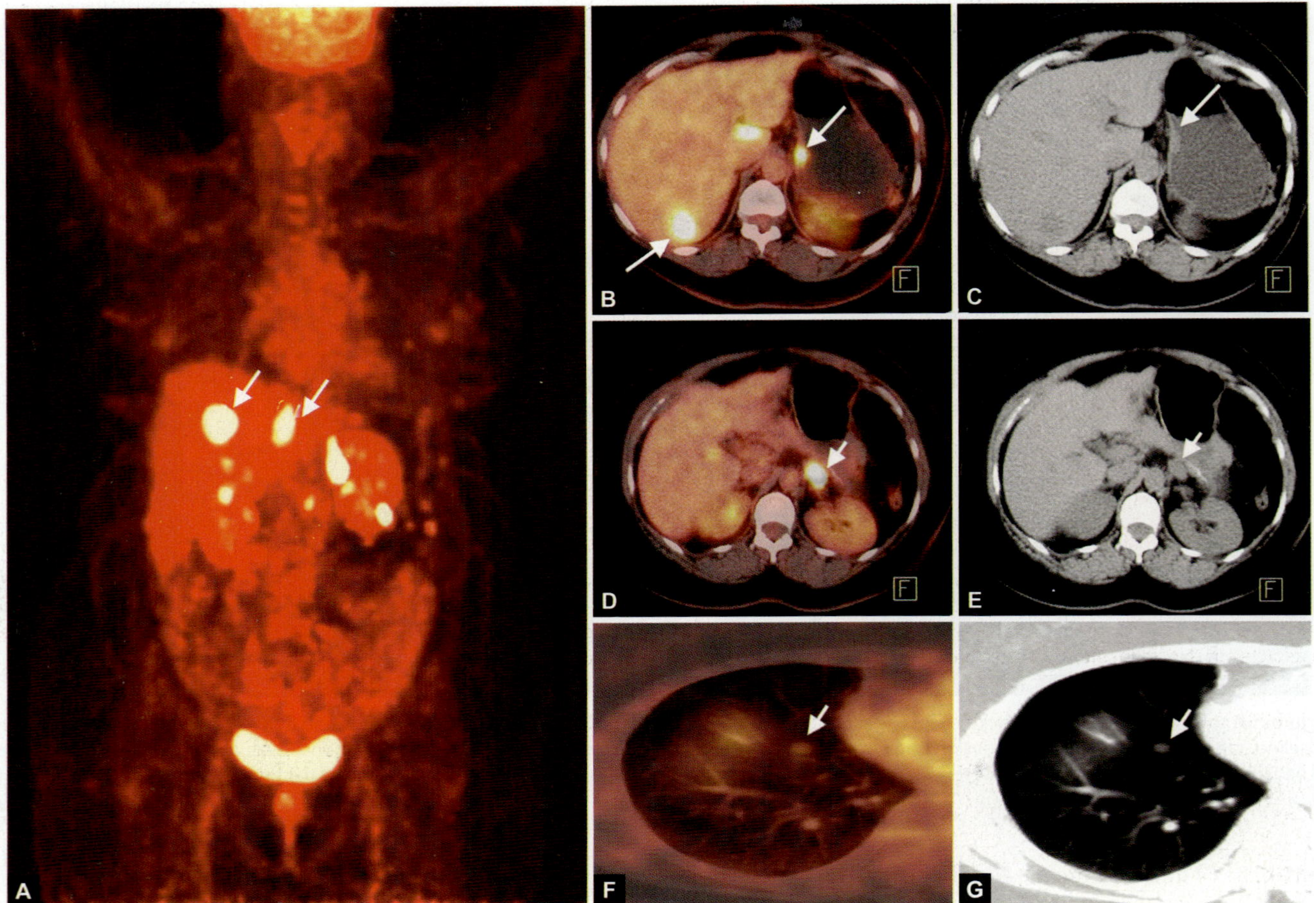

Figures 6A to G A 45-year-old female who was a known case of gastric gastrointestinal stromal tumor (GIST) underwent surgical resection now referred for PET/CT to rule out recurrence. She underwent ^{18}F-FDG PET/CT. Maximum intensity projection PET image (A) and transaxial PET/CT images (B to G) revealed recurrence in stomach with hepatic, perigastric lymph node and lung metastatic lesions (arrows)

by the primary tumor, thin slice CT or EUS are generally preferred. FDG-PET has limited role in delineating the anatomical boundaries of the primary tumor for respectability decision. Also, FDG-PET is poorly sensitive for the locoregional lymph node metastases detection, which may be due to their proximity to the primary lesion. FDG-PET is sensitive for the detection of metastatic disease to the liver and bone (Figs 9A to E).

The sensitivity of PET in detecting pancreatic cancer is similar to that of CT, but PET seems to be more specific. Sperti et al. found a sensitivity of 94% for both modalities, but PET was significantly more accurate in identifying malignancy.[61] FDG-PET is superior for detection of a treatment response to chemoradiotherapy. PET was superior to the combination of CT and MRI in the detection of recurrence (96% versus 39%). PET may be superior in the detection of recurrence within the tumor bed, but CT/MRI may have better discriminatory power within the hepatic parenchyma. PET may also complement the use of tumor markers or CT for the detection of recurrent disease when CT findings are equivocal. FDG-PET certainly plays a role in the detection of nonlocoregional and extra-abdominal metastases, but the role of FDG-PET in the initial diagnosis is questionable.

Carcinoma of Unknown Primary

For carcinoma of unknown primary (CUP), FDG-PET has shown overall modest sensitivity. The majority of these tumors prove to be from head and neck and lung carcinomas, but occult GI tumors are sometimes detected (< 10% incidence).[62,63]

In short, ^{18}F-FDG PET/CT imaging is highly accurate in restaging colorectal cancer, esophageal cancer and GISTs. Also, it has great potential in predicting treatment response early in the course of therapy. Initial staging with FDG-PET is usually restricted to patients with locally advanced disease who may benefit from curative resection if distant metastases are not found. For each GI malignancy, depth of invasion and nodal status are not well evaluated by FDG-PET scans. However, for locally-advanced malignancies, an FDG-PET scan may be used to identify occult metastatic disease which may then significantly change the treatment plan.

NEUROENDOCRINE TUMORS

Fluorodeoxyglucose PET/CT has revolutionized the imaging evaluation of patients with cancer. However, some cancers

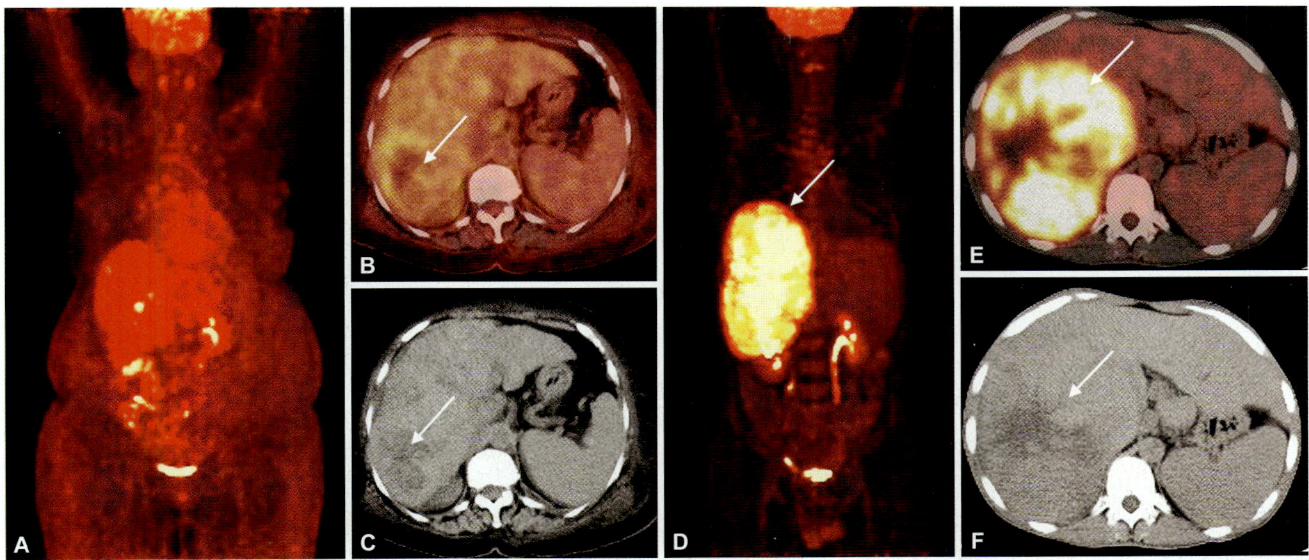

Figures 7A to F ^{18}F-FDG PET/CT studies in hepatocellular carcinoma (HCC) in two different scenarios. Well differentiated low grade HCC are often less fluorodeoxyglucose (FDG) avid lesions as depicted in maximum intensity projection positron emission tomography (PET) image (A) and trans-axial PET/CT images (B, C; arrows) where there is a hypodense lesion with less FDG avidity. High grade and poorly differentiated HCC are intense FDG avid lesions as depicted in maximum intensity projection PET image (D; arrows) and transaxial PET/CT images (E, F; arrows)

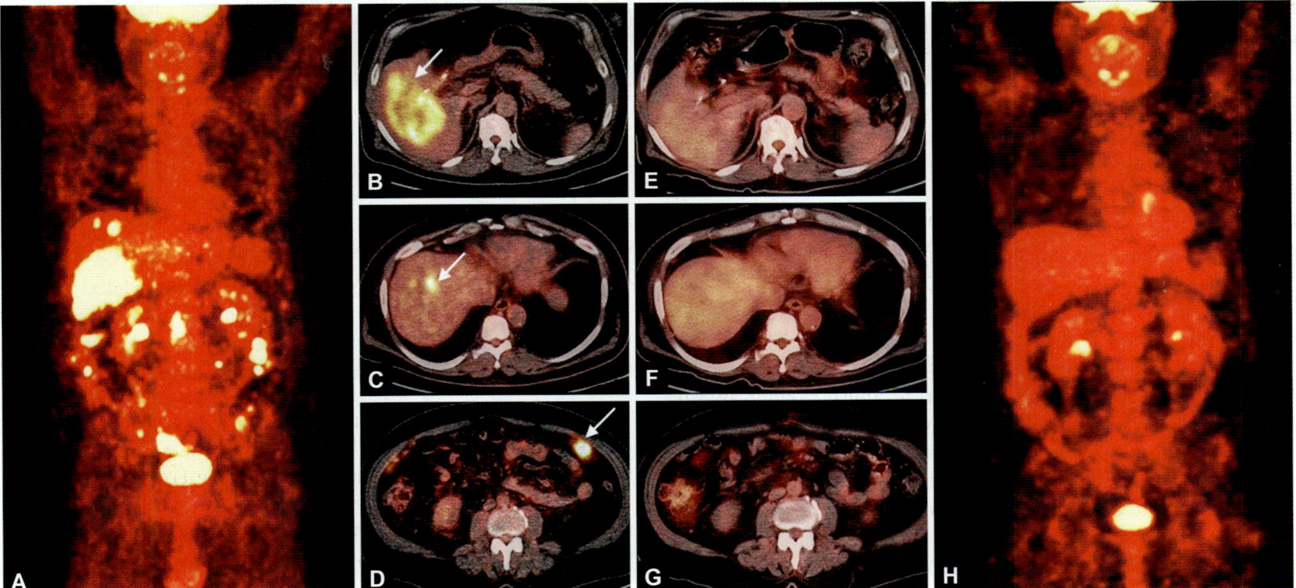

Figures 8A to H A 56-year-old male with gallbladder carcinoma underwent ^{18}F-Fluorodeoxyglucose positron emission tomography/computed tomography (^{18}F-FDG PET/CT) as a baseline study and as a response evaluation study. His baseline staging study revealed a mass lesion in gallbladder with adjacent hepatic involvement with hepatic and mesenteric lymph node metastasis (A to D; arrows). His response evaluation study after chemotherapy (E to H) revealed complete resolution of the disease implying significant response to chemotherapy

demonstrate low FDG avidity. It has been argued that although a negative FDG-PET scan may be interpreted as false-negative in terms of detectability of a tumor of sufficient size above the spatial resolution of PET, it should be considered true-negative with regard to tumor aggressiveness.[64] Other potentially useful PET radiotracers have been developed for tumors of hepatic, pancreatic, and GI origin, which may demonstrate low FDG uptake.

Neuroendocrine tumors (NETs) are a heterogeneous, generally indolent group of tumors that stem from the neural crest with main localization in the gastroenteropancreatic tract (e.g. carcinoids, insulinoma, glucagonoma, VIPoma, gastrinoma, somatostatinoma). A functioning NET, for instance in the pancreas, may be very small and yet give rise to severe endocrine symptoms whereas a patient with a small bowel tumor may present with diffuse symptoms and

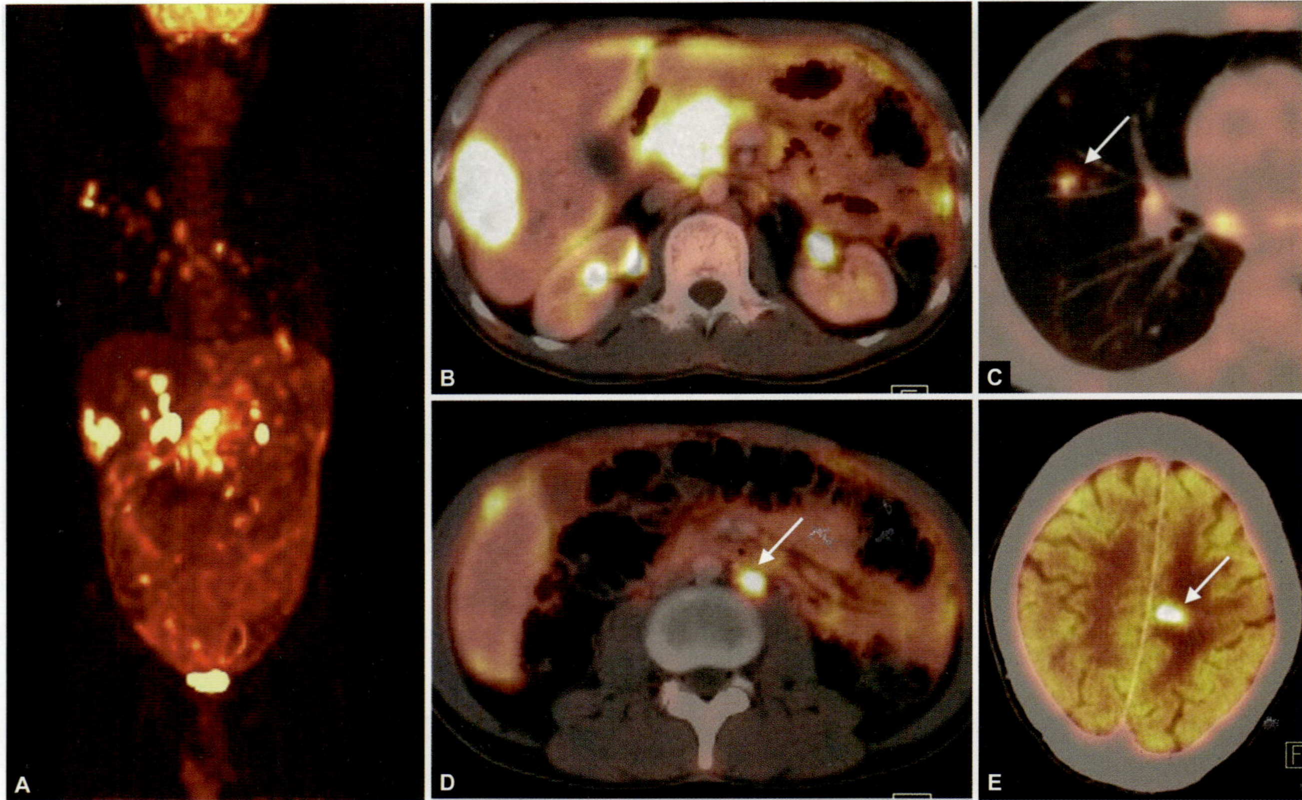

Figures 9A to E ^{18}F-Fluorodeoxyglucose positron emission tomography/computed tomography (^{18}F-FDG PET/CT) baseline staging study in a 57-year-old male with pancreatic cancer with raised cancer antigen (CA) 19.9 levels. Maximum intensity projection PET image (A) and trans-axial PET/CT images (B to E) revealed primary mass in pancreatic head with lung, para-aortic lymph node and brain metastatic lesions (arrows)

disseminated disease with a palpable bulky liver. The liver is a major site for metastases.

Imaging of NETs is therefore challenging and the imaging needs in the various patients are diverse. Imaging evaluation of NETs with PET has evolved rapidly in the recent years. The basic modalities for NET imaging are CT or MRI in combination with somatostatin receptor scintigraphy (SRS) with ^{111}In-labeled octreotide (OctreoScan) or more recently by PET with ^{68}Ga-labeled somatostatin analogues. Most of the NETs are well differentiated and low grade tumors which are less likely to be positive with FDG-PET. NETs express somatostatin tumor receptor (SSTR) which forms the basis for imaging with SRS. For SSTR imaging of the NET and its metastases, previously scintigraphy with somatostatin analogue pentetreotide radiolabeled SPECT agents by means of ^{111}In ($T_{1/2}$ = 2.8 days) or ^{99m}Tc-hydrazinonicotinyl (HYNIC)-Tyr3-octreotide were used.

Presently, PET tracer with somatostatin analogues as *68Ga-DOTA-NOC* ($T_{1/2}$= 68 min; ^{68}Ga-DOTA-1-NaI3-octreotide) that bind to the SSTR using the chelator 1,4,7,10-tetraazacyclododecane-*N,N=,N_,N_=*-tetraacetic acid (DOTA) is widely used and commonly performed (Figs 10A to F). ^{68}Ga-DOTA-peptides are generator produced unlike ^{18}F-FDG which is cyclotron produced. ^{68}Ga-DOTA-NOC uptake in gastroenteropancreatic NET correlates strongly with the tumor-associated overexpression of SSRT (subtypes 2A and 5).[65] Other current relevant tracers include the ^{68}Ga-DOTA-peptides (^{68}Ga-DOTAd- Phe1-Tyr3-octreotide, abbreviated as ^{68}Ga-DOTATOC; and ^{68}Ga-DOTA-DPhe1, Tyr3-octreotate, abbreviated as ^{68}Ga-DOTA-TATE).[65,66] First introduced in clinical application in 2005, ^{68}Ga-DOTATOC was reported to present a high tumor to non-tumor contrast and a higher sensitivity compared to SRS.[67,68] ^{68}Ga-DOTANOC has revealed promising results in preliminary studies for the main clinical indications: staging NET; suspected NET of unknown primary; follow-up, restaging and, finally for pre- and post-treatment evaluation of receptor radionuclide therapies.

In patients with inoperable or metastasized NETs, radiolabeled somatostatin analogues is a promising new tool in the treatment management. ^{111}In, ^{90}Y and ^{177}Lu labeled somatostatin analogues have been used for peptide receptor radionuclide therapy (PRRT). Symptomatic relief and tumor regression has been documented with [^{90}Y-DOTA0, Tyr3] octreotide and ^{177}Lu-DOTA-TATE therapy. Kidney protective agents are used to neutralize the side effects of this therapy. The patients' self-assessed quality of life increases significantly after ^{177}Lu-DOTA-TATE therapy. In our department we use ^{177}Lu-DOTA-TATE routinely for inoperable or metastasized NETs.

^{18}F-FDOPA ($T_{1/2}$ = 109 minutes; fluoro-3,4-dihydroxyphenylalanine)[69] is an another promising PET tracer recently being evaluated for NETs. ^{18}F-FDOPA uptake mechanism is different from SRS and ^{68}Ga-DOTA-NOC uptake mechanism.

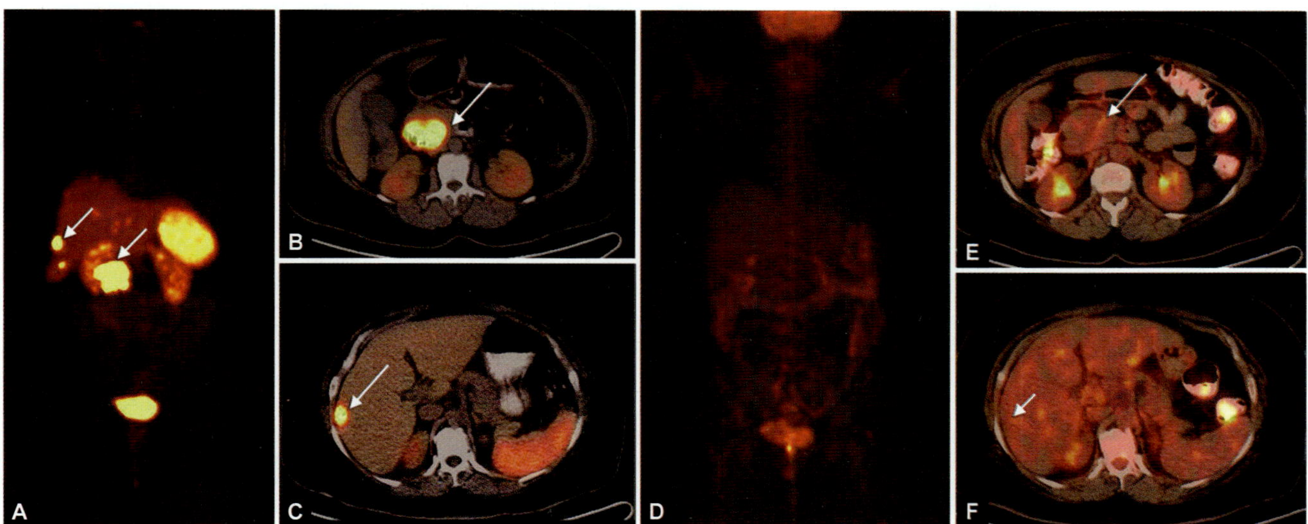

Figures 10A to F ^{68}Ga-DOTONOC positron emission tomography/computed tomography (PET/CT) and ^{18}F-FDG PET/CT studies in a case of pancreatic neuroendocrine tumor (NET). ^{68}Ga-DOTONOC PET/CT maximum intensity projection PET image (A) and trans-axial PET/CT images (B and C) revealed a DOTONOC avid primary pancreatic NET with hepatic metastasis (arrows). The same patient was false negative on ^{18}F-FDG PET/CT study as the corresponding lesions revealed no abnormal uptake (D to F; arrows)

^{18}F-FDOPA is concentrated by NETs through a large neutral amino acid transporter (LAT1)[70] that are upregulated and highly active in the cells of these tumors. Hybrid PET/CT allows for three-dimensional (3D) image acquisition and display as well as improved image interpretation.

In a recent investigation from our institution, we compared ^{68}Ga-DOTA-TOC PET/CT with FDG-PET/CT and contrast-enhanced CT to assess 20 patients with clinically suspected or known pancreatic NET.[71] The primary tumor was correctly localized in all 20 patients using ^{68}Ga-DOTA-TOC PET/CT, whereas contrast-enhanced CT correctly identified the tumors in 15 patients, and FDG-PET/CT, performing poorly with correct detection, identified the tumors in only two patients. Similar comparative findings were also noted for detection of metastatic disease.

Also, in another single-center study from our institution, 109 patients with gastroenteropancreatic NETs were evaluated with ^{68}Ga-DOTA-NOC PET/CT.[72] It performed significantly better than conventional imaging, with sensitivity and specificity of 78.3% and 92.5%, respectively, for detection of primary tumor and 97.4% and 100%, respectively, for identification of metastases. ^{68}Ga-DOTA-NOC PET/CT impacted the clinical management in 19% of patients. A potential confounding factor for PET tracer avidity to the somatostatin receptor may be competition with therapeutic unlabeled somatostatin analogs, such as octreotide or drug induced internalization of the somatostatin subtype 2 receptors. In summary, the experience with non-FDG tracers in NET is evolving and expanding rapidly. Recently, simultaneous ^{68}Ga-DOTATOC PET/MRI acquisition was shown to have special advantages in the characterization of abdominal lesions. Thus, hybrid imaging such as PET/CT or PET/MRI will play an important role in the future. Additional studies will be expected to define the exact role of these novel tracers in the imaging evaluation of patients with NET in the next several years.

Poorly differentiated neuroendocrine carcinomas (PDNEC) are rare tumors that can originate from any site of the GI tract. They usually exhibit an overall aggressive behavior which may vary between tumors according to the degree of cellular proliferation. Locally advanced nature and/or initial metastatic presentation are common. High mitotic rate, high Ki-67 labeling index and presence of necrosis can be noted on histology signifying aggressiveness. Somatostatin receptors expression is less in PDNEC and SRS is usually negative, whereas ^{18}F-FDG PET appears to be the best method of evaluating PDNEC.

Hyperinsulinism of Infancy

Congenital hyperinsulinism induces hypoglycemia in infants and treatment is required to prevent possible neurologic complications. Focal hyperinsulinism is cured by resection of the adenoma, whereas diffuse pancreatic involvement may be treated with subtotal pancreatectomy.[73] ^{18}F-FDOPA PET/CT has been used to preoperatively classify the form of infantile hyperinsulinism.[69,73]

REFERENCES

1. Treves ST, Grand RJ. Gastrointestinal bleeding. In: Treves ST (Ed). Pediatric Nuclear Medicine, 2nd edition. New York: Springer-Verlag; 1995. pp. 453-65.
2. Rossi P, Gourtsoyiannis N, Bezzi M. "Meckel's diverticulum: imaging diagnosis," American Journal of Roentgenology; 1996. pp. 567-73.
3. Yahchouchy EK, Marano AF, Etienne JF, Fingerhut AL. "Meckel's diverticulum," Journal of the American College of Surgeons; 2001. pp. 658-62.
4. Maurer AH. Gastrointestinal bleeding. In: Ell PJ, Gambhir GG (Eds). Nuclear Medicine in Clinical Diagnosis and Treatment, 3rd edition. Sydney: Churchill Livingstone; 2004. pp. 911-17.

5. Kumar R, Tripathi M, Chandrashekar N, Agarwala S, Kumar A, Dasan JB, et al. Diagnosis of ectopic gastric mucosa using ^{99m}Tc-pertechnetate: ^{99m}Tc-pertechnetate: spectrum of scintigraphic findings. Br J Radiol. 2005;78(932):714-20.
6. Ziessman HA, O'Malley JP, Thrall JH. Nuclear medicine. The Requisites in Radiology. Philadelphia: Elsevier, Mosby; 2006.
7. Alavi A, Ring EJ. Localization of gastrointestinal bleeding: superiority of ^{99m}Tc sulfur colloid compared with angiography. AJR Am J Roentgenol. 1981;137(4):741-8.
8. Alavi A, Worsley D, Zhuang H. Scintigraphic detection and localization of gastrointestinal bleeding sites. In: Sandler MP, Coleman RE, Patton JA (Eds). Diagnostic Nuclear Medicine, 4th edition. Philadelphia: Lippincott Williams and Wilkins; 2003. pp. 531-51.
9. Zuckier LS. Acute gastrointestinal bleeding. Semin Nucl Med. 2003;33:297-311.
10. Zettinig G, Staudenherz A, Leitha T. The importance of delayed images in gastrointestinal bleeding scintigraphy. Nuc Med Commun. 2002;23:803-8.
11. Ford PV, Bartold SP, Fink-Bennett DM, Jolles PR, Lull RJ, Maurer AH, et al. Procedure guidelines for gastrointestinal bleeding and Meckel's diverticulum scintigraphy. Society of Nuclear Medicine. J Nucl Med. 1999;40(7):1226-32.
12. Miskowiak J, Nielsen SL, Munck O, Andersen B. Abdominal scintiphotography with Tc99m technetium labelled albumin in acute gastrointestinal bleeding. Lancet. 1977;2:852-4.
13. Ferrant A, Dehasque N, Leners N, Meunier H. Scintigraphy with In-111- labeled red cells in intermittent gastrointestinal bleeding. J Nucl Med. 1980;21:844-5.
14. Ozcan Z, Ozcan C, Erinc R, Dirlik A, Mutaf O. Scintigraphy in the detection of gastro-oesophageal reflux in children with caustic oesophageal burns: a comparative study with radiography and 24-h pH monitoring. Pediatr Radiol. 2001;31:737-41.
15. Aktas A, Ciftci I, Caner B. The relationship between the degree of gasto-oesophageal reflux and the rate of gastric emptying. Nucl Med Commun. 1999;20:907-10.
16. Gainey MA. Radionuclide diagnosis. In: Walker WA, Durie PR, Hamilton JR (Eds). Pediatric Gastrointestinal Disease, 3rd edition. Canada: Decker CB; 2000. pp. 1655-75.
17. Mann MD, Wynchank S. Esophageal function (transport and motility). In: Ell PJ, Gambhir SS (Eds). Nuclear Medicine in Clinical Diagnosis and Treatment, 3rd edition. Edinburgh: Churchill Livingstone; 2004. pp. 789-803.
18. Da-Costa-Pinto EA, Dorsa TK, Altimani A, Andreollo NA, Cardoso SR, Morais DJ, et al. A functional study of caustic strictures of the esophagus in children. Braz J Med Biol Res. 2004;37:1623-30.
19. Chatterton BE. Gastric motility. In: Ell PJ, Gambhir SS (Eds). Nuclear Medicine in Clinical Diagnosis and Treatment, 3rd edition. Edinburgh: Churchill Livingstone; 2004. pp. 805-18.
20. Parkman HP, Hasler WL, Fisher RS. American Gastroenterological Association technical review on the diagnosis and treatment of gastroparesis. Gastroenterology. 2004;127:1592-1622.
21. Cook BJ, Lim E, Cook D, Hughes J, Chow CW, Stanton MP, et al. Radionuclear transit to assess sites of delay in large bowel transit in children with chronic idiopathic constipation. J Pediatr Surg. 2005;40:478-83.
22. Burton DD, Camilleri M, Mullan BP, Forstrom LA, Hung JC. Colonic transit scintigraphy labeled activated charcoal compared with ion exchange pellets. J Nucl Med. 1997;38:1807-10.
23. Kim CK, Norton KI, Shneider BL. Neonatal hyperbilirubinemia. In: Ell PJ, Gambhir SS (Eds). Nuclear Medicine in Clinical Diagnosis and Treatment, 3rd edition. Edinburgh: Churchill Livingstone; 2004. pp. 927-34.
24. Wessmann HS, Frank MS, Bernstein LH, Freeman LM. Rapid and accurate diagnosis of acute cholecystitis with ^{99m}Tc-HIDA cholescintigraphy. Am J Roentgenol. 1979;132:523-8.
25. Freitas JE. Cholescintigraphy. In: Ell PJ, Gambhir SS (Eds). Nuclear Medicine in Clinical Diagnosis and Treatment, 3rd edition. Edinburgh: Churchill Livingstone; 2004. pp. 919-26.
26. Ziessman HA, Zeman RK, Akin EA. Cholescintigraphy: correlation with other hepatobiliary imaging modalities. In: Sandler MP, Coleman RE, Patton JA (Eds). Diagnostic Nuclear Medicine, 4th edition. Philadelphia: Lippincott Williams and Wilkins; 2003. pp. 503-29.
27. Shuckett B. Cross-sectional imaging: ultrasonography, computed tomography, magnetic resonance imaging. In: Walker WA, Durie PR, Hamilton JR (Eds). Pediatric Gastrointestinal Disease, 3rd edition. Canada: Decker BC; 2000. pp. 1591-660.
28. Nadel HR. Hepatobiliary scintigraphy in children. Semin Nucl Med. 1996;26:25-42.
29. Gleason WA. Protein-losing enteropathy. In: Wyllie R, Hyams JS (Eds). Pediatric Gastrointestinal Disease, 2nd edition. Philadelphia: Saunders; 1999. Pp. 298-305.
30. Proujansky R. Protein-losing enteropathy. In: Walker WA, Durie PR, Hamilton JR (Eds). Pediatric Gastrointestinal Disease, 3rd edition. Canada: Decker CB; 2000. pp. 89-102.
31. Freeman T, Gordon AH. Measurement of albumin leak into the gastrointestinal tract using 131-I-albumin and ion exchange resins by mouth. Gut. 1964;6:155-7.
32. Shah ND, Chitkara DK, Locke GR, Meek PD, Talley NJ. Ambulatory care for constipation in the United States, 1993-2004. Am J Gastroenterol. 2008;103:1746-53.
33. Choung RS, Locke GR 3rd, Schleck CD, Zinsmeister AR, Talley NJ. Cumulative incidence of chronic constipation: a population-based study 1988-2003. Aliment Pharmacol Ther. 2007;26: 1521-8.
34. Burton DD, Camilleri M, Mullan BP, Forstrom LA, Hung JC. Colonic transit scintigraphy labeled activated charcoal compared with ion exchange pellets. J Nucl Med. 1997;38:1807-10.
35. Nelson RL, Schwartz A, Pavel D. Assessment of the usefulness of a diagnostic test: A survey of patient preference for diagnostic techniques in the evaluation of intestinal inflammation. BMC Med Res Methodol. 2001;1:5.
36. Charron M, Fernando del Rosario J, Kocoshis S. Distribution of acute bowel inflammation determined by technetium-labeled white blood cells in children with inflammatory bowel disease. Inflamm Bowel Dis. 1998;4:84-8.
37. Shields RA, Lawson RS. Effective dose equivalent. Nucl Med Commun. 1987;8:851-5.
38. Lemberg DA, Issenman RM, Cawdron R, Green T, Mernagh J, Skehan SJ, et al. Positron emission tomography in the investigation of pediatric inflammatory bowel disease. Inflamm Bowel Dis. 2005;11:733-8.
39. Das CJ, Makharia G, Kumar R, Chawla M, Goswami P, Sharma R, et al. PET-CT enteroclysis: a new technique for evaluation of inflammatory diseases of the intestine. Eur J Nucl Med Mol Imaging. 2007;34:2106-14.
40. Das CJ, Makharia GK, Kumar R, Kumar R, Tiwari RP, Sharma R, et al. PET/CT colonography: a novel non-invasive technique for assessment of extent and activity of ulcerative colitis. Eur J Nucl Med Mol Imaging. 2010;37:714-21.
41. Friedland S, Soetikno R, Carlisle M, Taur A, Kaltenbach T, Segall G, 18-Fluorodeoxyglucose positron emission tomography has limited sensitivity for colonic adenoma and early stage colon cancer. Gastrointest Endosc. 2005;61:395-400.
42. Gutman F, Alberini JL, Wartski M, Vilain D, Le Stanc E, Sarandi F, et al. Incidental colonic focal lesions detected by FDG PET/CT. AJR Am J Roentgenol. 2005;185:495-500.
43. Kamel EM, Thumshirn M, Truninger K, Schiesser M, Fried M, Padberg B, et al. Significance of incidental 18F-FDG accumulations in the gastrointestinal tract in PET/CT: correlation with endoscopic and histopathologic results. J Nucl Med. 2004;45:1804-10.

44. Van Kouwen MC, Nagengast FM, Jansen JB, Oyen WJ, Drenth JP. 2-(18F)-fluoro-2- deoxy-D-glucose positron emission tomography detects clinical relevant adenomas of the colon: a prospective study. J Clin Oncol. 2005;23:3713-7.
45. Huebner RH, Park KC, Shepherd JE, Schwimmer J, Czernin J, Phelps ME, et al. A meta-analysis of the literature for whole-body FDG PET detection of recurrent colorectal cancer. J Nucl Med. 2000;41:1177-89.
46. Yoon YC, Lee KS, Shim YM, Kim BT, Kim K, Kim TS. Metastasis to regional lymph nodes in patients with esophageal squamous cell carcinoma: CT versus FDG PET for presurgical detection prospective study. Radiology. 2003;227:764-70.
47. Heeren PA, Jager PL, Bongaerts F, van Dullemen H, Sluiter W, Plukker JT. Detection of distant metastases in esophageal cancer with (18)F-FDG PET. J Nucl Med. 2004;45:980-7.
48. Sihvo EI, Rasanen JV, Knuuti MJ, Minn HR, Luostarinen ME, Viljanen T, et al. Adenocarcinoma of the esophagus and the esophagogastric junction: Positron emission tomography improves staging and prediction of survival in distant but not in locoregional disease. J Gastrointest Surg. 2004;8:988-96.
49. Flamen P, Lerut T, Haustermans K, Van Cutsem E, Mortelmans L. Position of positron emission tomography and other imaging diagnostic modalities in esophageal cancer. Q J Nucl Med Mol Imaging. 2004;48:96-108.
50. Ott K, Weber WA, Fink U, Helmberger H, Becker K, Stein HJ, et al. Fluorodeoxy glucose positron emission tomography in adenocarcinomas of the distal esophagus and cardia. World J Surg. 2003;27:1035-9.
51. Stahl A, Ott K, Weber WA, Becker K, Link T, Siewert JR, et al. FDG PET imaging of locally advanced gastric carcinomas: correlation with endoscopic and histopathological findings. Eur J Nucl Med Mol Imaging. 2003;30:288-95.
52. Yoshioka T, Yamaguchi K, Kubota K, Saginoya T, Yamazaki T, Ido T, et al. Evaluation of 18F-FDG PET in patients with a, metastatic, or recurrent gastric cancer. J Nucl Med. 2003;44:690-9.
53. Goerres GW, Stupp R, Barghouth G, Hany TF, Pestalozzi B, Dizendorf E, et al. The value of PET, CT and in-line PET/CT in patients with gastrointestinal stromal tumors: Long-term outcome of treatment with imatinib mesylate. Eur J Nucl Med Mol Imaging. 2005;32:153-62.
54. Goerres GW, Stupp R, Barghouth G, Hany TF, Pestalozzi B, Dizendorf E, et al. The value of PET, CT and in-line PET/CT in patients with gastrointestinal stromal tumors: long-term outcome of treatment with imatinibmesylate. Eur J Nucl Med Mol Imaging. 2005;32:153-62.
55. Antoch G, Kanja J, Bauer S, Kuehl H, Renzing-Koehler K, Schuette J, et al. Comparison of PET, CT, and dual-modality PET/CT imaging for monitoring of imatinib (STI571) therapy in patients with gastrointestinal stromal tumors. J Nucl Med 2004;45:357-65.
56. Lee JD, Yang WI, Park YN, Kim KS, Choi JS, Yun M, et al. Different glucose uptake and glycolytic mechanisms between hepatocellular carcinoma and intrahepatic mass-forming cholangiocarcinoma with increased (18)F-FDG uptake. J Nucl Med. 2005;46:1753-9.
57. Ho CL, Yu SC, Yeung DW. 11C-acetate PET imaging in hepatocellular carcinoma and other liver masses. J Nucl Med. 2003;44:213-21.
58. Shiomi S, Nishiguchi S, Ishizu H, Iwata Y, Sasaki N, Tamori A, et al. Usefulness of positron emission tomography with fluorine-18-fluorodeoxyglucose for predicting outcome in patients with hepatocellular carcinoma. Am J Gastroenterol. 2001;96: 1877-80.
59. Anderson CD, Rice MH, Pinson CW, Chapman WC, Chari RS, Delbeke D, et al. Fluorodeoxyglucose PET imaging in the evaluation of gallbladder carcinoma and cholangiocarcinoma. J Gastrointest Surg. 2004;8:90-7.
60. Kumar R, Sharma P, Kumari A, Halanaik D, Malhotra A. Role of 18F-FDG PET/CT in detecting recurrent gallbladder carcinoma. Clin Nucl Med. 2012;37:431-5.
61. Sperti C, Pasquali C, Decet G, Chierichetti F, Liessi G, Pedrazzoli S. F-18-fluorodeoxyglucose positron emission tomography in differentiating malignant from benign pancreatic cysts: a prospective study. J Gastrointest Surg. 2005;9:22-9.
62. Delgado-Bolton RC, Fernandez-Perez C, Gonzalez-Mate A, Carreras JL. Meta-analysis of the performance of 18F-FDG PET in primary tumor detection in unknown primary tumors. J Nucl Med. 2003;44:1301-14.
63. Gutzeit A, Antoch G, Kuhl H, Egelhof T, Fischer M, Hauth E, et al. Unknown primary tumors: detection with dual-modality PET/CT—initial experience. Radiology. 2005;234:227-34.
64. Kwee TC, Basu S, Saboury B, Ambrosini V, Torigian DA, Alavi A. A new dimension of FDG-PET interpretation: Assessment of tumor biology. Eur J Nucl Med Mol Imaging. 2011;38:1158-70.
65. Wild D, Mäcke HR, Waser B, Reubi JC, Ginj M, Rasch H, et al. 68Ga-DOTANOC: a first compound for PET imaging with high affinity for somatostatin receptor subtypes 2 and 5. Eur J Nucl Med Mol Imaging. 2005;32:724.
66. Bushnell DL, Baum RP. Standard imaging techniques for neuroendocrine tumors. Endocrinol Metab Clin North Am. 2011;40:153-62.
67. Hofmann M, Maecke H, Borner R, Weckesser E, Schöffski P, Oei L, et al. Biokinetics and imaging with the somatostatin receptor PET radioligand (68)Ga-DOTATOC: preliminary data. Eur J Nucl Med. 2001;28:1751-7.
68. Kowalski J, Henze M, Schuhmacher J, Mäcke HR, Hofmann M, Haberkorn U. Evaluation of positron emission tomography imaging using [68Ga]-DOTA-D Phe (1)-Tyr (3)-Octreotide in comparison to [111In]-DTPAOC SPECT. First results in patients with neuroendocrine tumors. Mol Imaging Biol. 2003;5:42-8.
69. Balogova S, Talbot JN, Nataf V, Michaud L, Huchet V, Kerrou K, et al. (18)F-Fluorodihydroxyphenylalaninevs other radiopharmaceuticals for imaging neuroendocrine tumors according to their type. Eur J Nucl Med Mol Imaging. 2013;40: 943-66.
70. Jager PL, Chirakal R, Marriott CJ, Brouwers AH, Koopmans KP, Gulenchyn KY. 6-L-18F-fluorodihydroxyphenylalanine PET in neuroendocrine tumors: basic aspects and emerging clinical applications. J Nucl Med. 2008;49:573-86.
71. Kumar R, Sharma P, Garg P, Karunanithi S, Naswa N, Sharma R, et al. Role of (68)Ga-DOTATOC PET-CT in the diagnosis and staging of pancreatic neuroendocrine tumors. Eur Radiol. 2011;21:2408-16.
72. Naswa N, Sharma P, Kumar A, Nazar AH, Kumar R, Chumber S, et al. Gallium-68-DOTA-NOC PET/CT of patients with gastroenteropancreatic neuroendocrine tumors: a prospective single-center study. AJR Am J Roentgenol. 2011;197:1221-8.
73. Barthlen W, Blankenstein O, Mau H, Koch M, Höhne C, Mohnike W, et al. Evaluation of [18F]fluoro-L-DOPA positron emission tomography-computed tomography for surgery in focal congenital hyperinsulinism. J Clin Endocrinol Metab. 2008;93:869-75.

CHAPTER 5

Radiation Therapy

Kishore Singh, Arun Kumar Rathi

BASIC ASPECTS OF RADIATION THERAPY

Radiation therapy is a century old treatment method. It is defined as "treatment of diseases by ionizing radiation". About 60% of patients require radiation therapy, either alone or in combination with surgery. It is often combined with chemotherapy to improve results. The aim of this chapter is to give an idea of basic and overall aspects of radiotherapy; site-specific chapters will deal with organ-specific description of radiotherapy.

Advantage of radiotherapy over surgery in treatment of malignancy is:

- Control of cancer with organ-function preservation
- Wider area can be treated with radiation therapy.

On the other hand disadvantage of radiation therapy over surgery is:

- Prolonged period of treatment, often 6–7 weeks
- Radiation hazards to both patient and personnel.

Conventionally radiotherapy is mainly employed to improve local control and cure or relief of symptoms. When cure is not possible it is very useful for improving quality of life. New indications of radiation therapy are evolving in the form of stereotactic radiosurgery (SRS) or stereotactic radiotherapy (SRT) for ablation of small residual or metastatic tumors.

HISTORY

Radiation was discovered by Wilhelm Konrad von Rontgen in December 1895. Within few months, a person was treated with it. Soon after this Henri Becquerel discovered natural radioactivity in uranium (1896) and Madame Marie Curie isolated "radium" in 1898.

The initial period of radiotherapy (1900–1940) was "kilovoltage era", when radiotherapy was given with the help of "X-ray" machines. Since they have limited penetration capability, attempt has been made to develop beams with higher energy. First linear accelerator (LINAC) was started in 1948 and telecobalt machine (Fig. 1) went into use in 1951. This heralded the beginning of "megavoltage era" (1946–1996). Gradually high-energy equipment have taken over and replaced X-ray machines for treatment of cancer. With the development in electronics and computers; they have been extensively utilized for delivery of radiation. This has led to modern era of radiotherapy. Techniques like 3D conformal radiotherapy (3D CRT), intensity-modulated radiotherapy (IMRT), image-guided radiotherapy (IGRT), SRT, etc. have revolutionized the treatment of tumor by radiation therapy. Aptly, it is called "computer-assisted high precision radiotherapy era" (1996 onward). Now a day's modern radiotherapy extensively use imaging, computers and patient-positioning devices to accurately track tumor and precisely deliver radiation to the target.

TYPES OF RADIOTHERAPY

- *Radical or curative radiotherapy:* Here high doses of radiation are given, often till tolerance level of normal tissues, with the hope to achieve maximum probability of tumor control.
- *Adjuvant or neoadjuvant radiotherapy:* In this, surgery is followed by radiation therapy and/or chemotherapy as supplementary treatment. Moderate doses of radiation therapy are used to control microscopic disease only, whereas bulky tumor is removed by surgery. When administered preoperatively it is called as neoadjuvant.
- *Palliative radiotherapy:* It is utilized in hopeless cases where cure is not possible, mainly to relieve symptoms like pain, obstruction, bleeding, compression, etc. Usually short course, hypofractionated treatment with doses of 30 Gray (Gy) or 10 fractions is used.

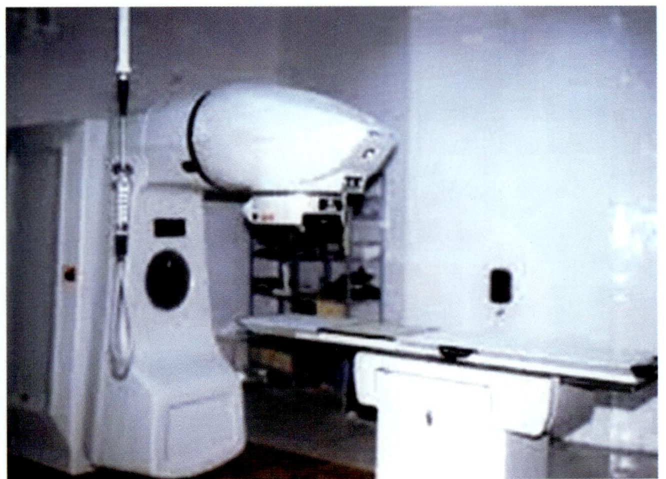

Figure 1 Telecobalt therapy machine

COMBINATION OF RADIATION THERAPY WITH SURGERY

Radiotherapy sometimes can be used before surgery (preoperative) to shrink the tumor to facilitate surgery or it may be used after radical or conservative surgery (postoperatively) to control the microscopic residual tumor left in the surgical bed. In the organ preservation setting (e.g. anal carcinoma), surgery is kept in reserve after completion of radical radiation therapy for salvage of residual or recurrent disease.

COMBINATION OF RADIATION THERAPY WITH CHEMOTHERAPY

Combination of chemotherapy-radiotherapy with concurrent delivery of both has become a popular strategy in therapy of locally advanced carcinoma. Improved local control and survival has been achieved with traditional chemotherapy agents, such as 5-fluorouracil and cisplatin. Clinical experience in tumors of anus, esophagus and rectum has established it, as useful modality.[1,2] Interactions of chemoradiotherapy are listed in Tables 1 and 2.

MODES OF RADIOTHERAPY

There are three main ways of irradiation:

1. Teletherapy

Here radiation source is away from body like telecobalt therapy or LINAC.

X-rays

X-rays are of two types: superficial (50–150 kVp) and deep X-rays (150–500 kVp). These are historical method to treat cancer. X-rays are produced by X-ray tubes. In which fast electrons are suddenly decelerated on special targets, kinetic energy is transformed in target into heat, and a small proportion is emitted in the form of X-rays.

Therapeutic X-ray machines consist of X-ray tube, target cooling system and power generator. The electrons are generated by heating the cathode and accelerated in vacuum toward anode (target) by applying a potential difference, created by X-ray generator. Efficiency of X-ray production is low; 99% of kinetic energy is converted into heat and only 1% is transmitted as X-ray.

Gamma Ray Units

The kilovoltage units were replaced by megavoltage beams like cobalt teletherapy and LINAC (6–15 MV). Megavoltage beams are superior in terms of skin sparing, deeper penetration, use of wedge filters, etc. over kilovoltage rays.

Telecobalt unit contains ^{60}Co isotope, it has high γ-ray energy (1.37 and 1.18), high-specific activity (small source size) and long half-life (5.3 years). Because of these properties it is an ideal isotope for teletherapy. They are the work horse for most of the developing and low resource countries and limited access to trained resources. These are isocentrically mounted units, having source to surface distance (SSD) of 80 cm. Machine is composed of head, which house source, collimator and source moving mechanism, a gantry and shaft to move machine isocentrically, treatment couch and machine console. These are very simple machines with high γ-ray energy, long half-life of radioisotope, high-specific activity and low maintenance requirement. However, LINAC is increasingly used world over as teletherapy machine for its superior beam over cobalt teletherapy.

Table 1: Chemotherapy and irradiation interactions

Strategy	*Advantages*	*Disadvantages*
Sequential	Least toxic, optimal systemic treatment.	Increase treatment time.
Concurrent	Short treatment time, radiation enhancement.	Compromised systemic toxicity, higher local toxicity.
Concurrent chemotherapy-radiotherapy and adjuvant chemotherapy	Maximize systemic therapy, radiation enhancement, both local and systemic therapy delivered up front.	Higher toxicity, increase treatment time, difficult to complete chemotherapy after chemotherapy-radiotherapy.
Induction chemotherapy and concurrent chemotherapy-radiotherapy	Maximum systemic therapy, radiation effect enhancement.	Higher toxicity, increase treatment time, difficult to complete radiotherapy after chemotherapy.

Table 2: Disease sites for which newer cytotoxic chemotherapy or targeted agents are under investigation for concurrent use with radiation

S.No.	Agent	Site
Cytotoxic chemotherapies		
1.	Oxaliplatin	Rectal cancer
2.	5-fluorouracil or capecitabine	Rectal cancer, pancreatic cancer
3.	Gemcitabine	Pancreatic cancer
Targeted therapies		
4.	Cetuximab	Pancreatic cancer
5.	Erlotinib	Rectal cancer
6.	Bevacizumab	Rectal cancer

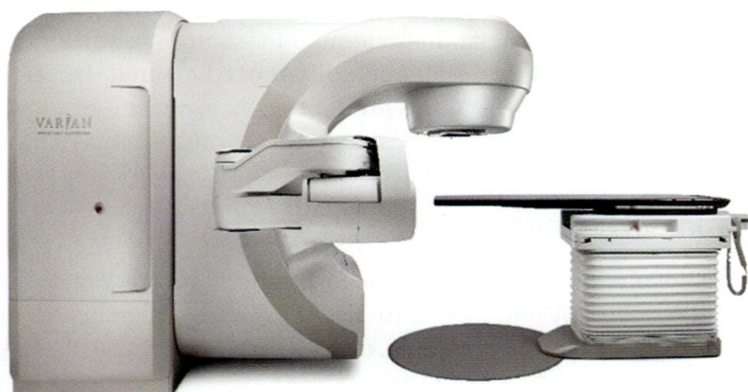

Figure 2 Modern linear accelerator

Linear Accelerators (Fig. 2)

These are the device used to accelerate particles to high energy through electromagnetic wave in a linear tube. In this machine electrons are accelerated in vacuumed waveguides using electromagnetic field (microwave) from 0.6 c to 0.99 c (the speed of light) before they hit target to produce high energy X-rays of megavoltage range. The energy achieved range from 4 MeV to 25 MeV. In LINAC very high electric or magnetic field is produced by injecting radiofrequency energy into confined cavity bounded by conducting material. The particle to be accelerated is injected into the electron gun. High-power radiofrequency fields (operating in S band of 2,856 MHz) generated by magnetron or klystron. Components of LINAC are:

- Power supply
- Modulator
- Magnetron or klystron
- Electron gun
- Waveguide
- Accelerator tube
- Bending magnet
- Treatment head

The various categories of LINAC developed over a period of time are:

- Low energy photons: 4 and 6 MeV
- Medium energy photons and electrons: 10–15 MeV

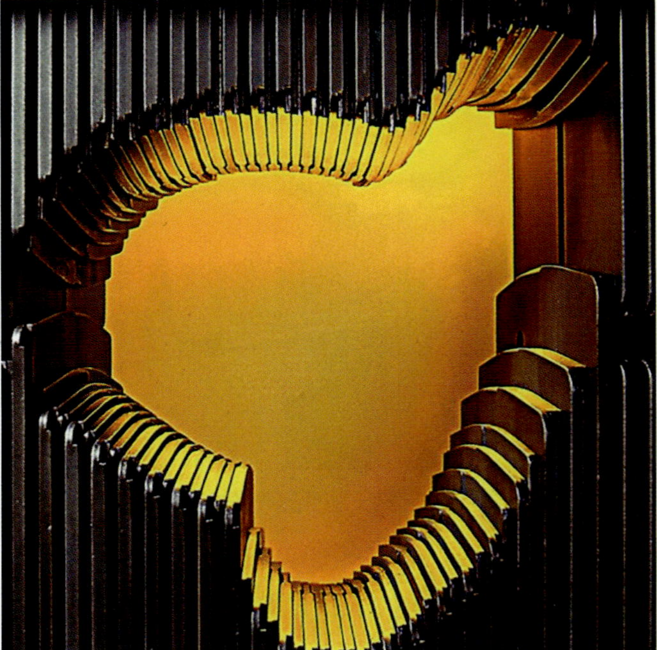

Figure 3 High definition multileaf collimator

- High energy photons and electrons: 18–25 MeV
- High energy photons and electrons with multileaf collimator (MLC) (Fig. 3) for IMRT.
- High energy photons and electrons with IGRT.

With this advancement of technology various technique of radiation therapy possible through LINAC like:

- 3D conformal radiotherapy
- Intensity-modulated radiotherapy
- Stereotactic radiotherapy
- Stereotactic radiosurgery
- Dynamic adaptive radiotherapy (DART)
- Image-guided radiotherapy.

Besides this simulators are extensively used in treatment of patients for acquisition of data, localization of target and critical structures, delineation and marking of treatment fields, transfer of data to treatment planning system and verification of plan.

2. Brachytherapy

Here small, sealed radiation source is kept close to target. Therefore it delivers very high doses only to local area in a short period of time and spares adjacent normal tissues (inverse square law). Early period of brachytherapy was done by low-dose rate (0.4–2 Gy or hour) or medium-dose rate (2–12 Gy or hour), replaced by high-dose rate (HDR) brachytherapy (>12 Gy or hour) in recent times.

Various method of placing the radiation sources are:

- Intracavitary (Source is kept in body cavity close to tumor)
- Interstitial (Source is implanted within the tumor)
- Intraluminal (Source is placed in the lumen close to tumor)
- Intraoperative brachytherapy is mainly used for esophagus, gall bladder, bile-ducts and anorectal tumors.

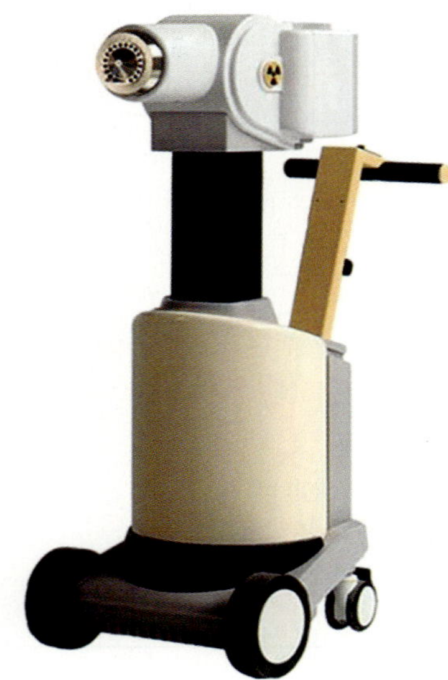

Figure 4 High-dose rate brachytherapy machine

Iridium 192 is the most commonly used radioisotope for the purpose of brachytherapy, have typical activity of 10 Curie (370 GBq).

Process of brachytherapy is clinical evaluation, decision about aim (curative or palliative), applicator insertion, image acquisition [magnetic resonance imaging (MRI) or computed tomography (CT) scan], treatment planning, treatment delivery, treatment summary and follow up. For specific site:

Esophagus: High-dose rate brachytherapy (Fig. 4) is used for boost following external beam radiation therapy or palliation of advanced disease.

Bile duct: Tumor bed is boosted with implant in tumor positive area, if positive margin or nodes. This is an effective palliation for advanced disease. Intraluminal HDR brachytherapy alone is used to relieve biliary duct obstruction along with percutaneous drainage.

Anorectal: Lesions are treated with interstitial, intraluminal or intraoperative HDR brachytherapy. Selected anal lesions can be treated radically by HDR brachytherapy alone or by boost after external beam radiation therapy.

Equipment: This is a small machine housing radioactive source inside safe box. A computer operated through remote control to place radioactive source inside applicator for a predefined dwell position (with accuracy of 1 mm or less) and time to impart irradiation. Various applicators for interstitial, intraluminal, contact or intracavitary are available.

3. Internal Therapy

Here radioisotope gets incorporated into body tissue and deposit radiation into cells, e.g. radioimmunothearapy.

RADIOBIOLOGY

The radiation used for treatment of cancer is electromagnetic radiations (Photons). The high energy X-rays or γ-rays form bottom part of spectrum of electromagnetic radiation, which range from very low energy radio waves to cosmic rays.

Main sources of high energy X-rays or γ-rays are radioactive decay of material like in nuclear reactor and machines such as X-ray machines, cyclotron, etc. Division of radioactive nuclei produces γ-rays, along with α and β particles.

Radiation produces their effect by ionization. This can be "direct" or "indirect". Most of particulate radiation like neutron, heavy ions, etc. directly ionize the atom and damage molecular structure of cell by this mechanism.

On the contrary photons (X-ray and γ-rays) are indirectly ionizing. When a photon passes through matter, energy is imparted in a random and discrete manner to it. The first step is deposition of energy. This extra energy leads to ejection of orbital electron out of its orbit (called secondary electrons). These secondary electrons then produce ionization by interacting with orbital electrons. This two-step process is called indirect method of ionization. Since water is most abundant material in cell (about 80–90%), ionization of water predominates the interaction of photon with matter.

The type of interaction depends upon energy of photons. In kilovoltage range, "photoelectric effect" is predominantly observed, whereas "Compton effect" dominates at the megavoltage range and pair production takes over at energy above 10 MV. Photoelectric effect is interaction of photon with tightly bound orbital electrons. In contrast Compton effect is interaction of loosely bound outer orbital electrons. Third type of interaction is pair production, here photon disappears and combined pair of electron and positron of 1.02 MeV is produced.

Linear energy transfer (LET) is measure of energy deposited per unit length of track. It is expressed as keV or µm. It indicates quality of radiation and is related with biological effect. LET is low for photons (sparsely ionizing) and high for particulate radiations (densely ionizing).

Table 3 showing the LET value of ionizing radiations.

Relative biological effectiveness (RBE) is measure of effectiveness of radiation beam. It is ratio of doses of test radiation and X-rays (standard radiation) required to produce the particular biological effect. Now X-rays are replaced by γ-rays of cobalt-60. RBE increases with increasing LET, till 100 keV or µm. After that it starts decreasing, because of "overkill" effect.

Radiation-induced Cell Kill

Deoxyribonucleic acid (DNA) is the main target of radiation-induced damage. Any dysfunction of it leads to cell death. Besides this cell membrane damage is also considered important. Ionization of water leads to production of free radical (•OH) which interact with DNA and breaks chemical bonds of molecule. This

Table 3: Linear energy transfer value of ionizing radiations

S.No.	*Type of radiation*	*Value of linear energy transfer*
1.	X-rays (250 kVp)	2.0
2.	^{60}Co γ-rays	0.3
3.	3 MeV X-rays	0.3
4.	10 MeV protons	0.5
5.	2 GeV Fe ions	1,000

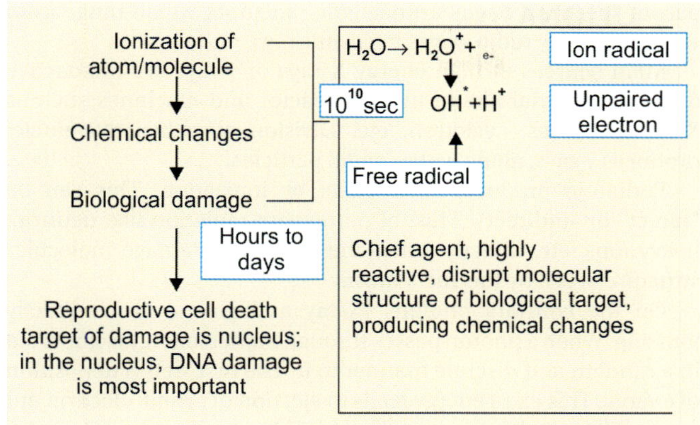

Figure 5 Biological basis of cell kill
Abbreviation: DNA, deoxyribonucleic acid.

disrupts intracellular mechanisms, resulting in loss of the capacity to divide (reproductive death). This is "indirect method of radiation damage" (Fig. 5).

Time Frame of Reaction

Time for transfer of energy to tissue is approximately 10^{-18} sec, 1 Gy produces approximately 10^5 ionizations, primarily H_2O^+ and e^-, shortly followed by excitation ($H_2O^{\bullet}$) and ionization of water into H and $OH^{\bullet}$ (Free radical), in about 10^{-14} sec. They produce radiochemical in approximately 10^{-12} sec. Per 1 Gy leads to approximately 25 DNA double-strand breaks (DSBs), approximately 900 single-strand breaks (SSBs), the range of free radical is approximately 4 nm.

Repair of Deoxyribonucleic Acid Damage

Deoxyribonucleic acid consists of double helix, linked by strands. The hydroxyl radical ($OH^{\bullet}$) being highly reactive (availability of an unpaired electron in outer orbit), take out hydrogen atoms from other molecules and damages the structure of DNA. This is expressed as damage to base, SSB or DSB. Radiation-induced damage to bases is repaired by base excision repair, SSB repair and DSB repair (homologous recombination and nonhomologous end joining).

CELL SURVIVAL CURVE

Radiation-induced cell kill is expressed in terms of loss of reproductive integrity. This is best measured by semi log plotting of cell survival against radiation dose (Fig. 6). Linear-quadratic model is the most common model used to do this. This uses two constants α and β to show relation between dose (D) and survival (S).

$$S = e - (\alpha D + \alpha D^2)$$

CELL CYCLE EFFECT

All dividing cells participate in cell cycle (except resting G_0 phase). Average cell cycle time is 10–40 hours. During cell cycle it passes through G1 to S, then to G2 and finally M followed by G1 again. Among these most sensitive phase of cell cycle is G2 or M phase (mitosis) and most resistant is S phase (synthesis). G2 or M phase takes about 20% time of cell cycle. The poor repair capacity during G2 or M phase is due to decrease access to repair enzyme and chromatin compaction, possibly results in reduced capacity to recovery from radiation damage. On the other side converse is true for radioresistance of S phase, which has higher capacity of repairing radiation-induced damage.

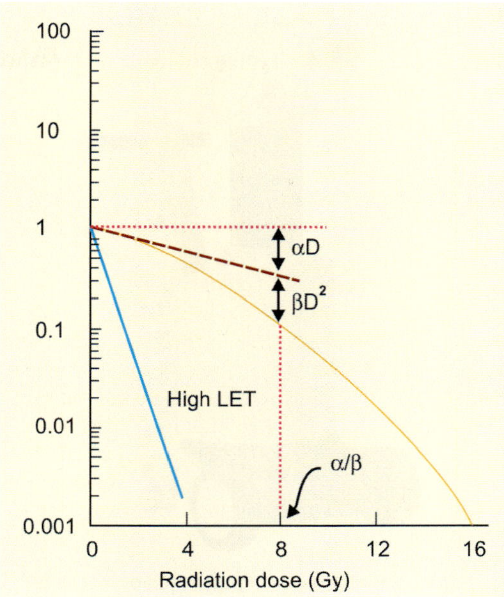

Figure 6 Cell survival curve

Oxygen Effect

It is most potent radio sensitizer. The PO2 level between 0 mmHg and 20 mmHg are associated with maximum modulation in effect. At level below 10 mmHg cells are considered hypoxic and becoming relatively resistant to radiation. Oxygen enhancement ratio (OER) is ratio of dose required to produce cell kill in hypoxic and fully oxic condition. An OER of 3 is seen between anoxic and fully oxic condition. As LET increases OER decreases. Differential sensitivity between hypoxic and well oxic cells is also reduced with high LET radiations. Recently it was seen that increased expression of hypoxia-induced factor is considered to be a factor in higher radioresistance of these cells. During fractionated radiotherapy this effect plays only a minor role on outcome but is considered to be an important cause of radiation therapy failure.

REPAIR OF RADIATION DAMAGE

Cells attempt to repair radiation-induced DNA damage between two fractions. The sublethal damage (SLD) is repairable injury, which occur between two fractions. This is also known as "Elkind repair", named after discoverer of phenomenon. This takes about 6–8 hours in most tissues to fully repair the SLD. SLD repair is nonexistent in malignant tissues. With increase in LET or RBE, there is increase in nonrepairable lesions. Also repair predominates in low dose-rate range and nonexistent at HDR range.

Another type of injury is potentially lethal damage (PLD). PLD recovery happens in malignant cells under hypoxic conditions. This mechanism enables them to attain radioresistant.

RADIATION RESPONSE MODIFIERS

There are three types of modifiers: Radiosensitizers, radioprotectors and bioreductive drugs.

1. Radiosensitizers

These are the agents associated with increase in cell killing by radiation. An ideal radiosensitizer has to be devoid of toxicity and associated purely with enhancement of lethal action of radiation. Whereas apparent radiosensitizers produce higher radiosensitization and cell killing but neither synergistic nor devoid of toxicity. Typically they should sensitize the tumor tissue only, but it is not seen in practice. In fact there is little therapeutic window between action on normal and tumor tissue by a radiosensitizer.

- *Hypoxic cell radiosensitizer:* It has been studied extensively. These are nitroimidazole group of drugs, having property of electron affinity. With this property they tend to mimic the oxygen effect at the time of free radical production. By this they fix the radiation-induced damage, leading to greater cell kill. Nimorazole has been successfully used to treat head and neck cancer.
- *Proliferating cell radiosensitizers:* These cells divide so fast that cell loss by radiation-induced cell killing is neutralized by new cell production and net result is tumor proliferation. Halogenated pyrimidines like bromodeoxyuridine and iododeoxyuridine are under study.

2. Bioreductive Drug

They are relatively less toxic to normal cells. But once they get inside hypoxic cells they got metabolize to produce active toxic molecules. Thus they preferentially kill relatively radioresistant tumor cell. Typical drug of this type is mitomycin C. It gets activated inside the cell to damage DNA of hypoxic cells in tumor only. Another drug under active study is tirapazamine.

3. Radioprotectors

Certain sulfhydryl compounds like cysteine and cysteamine are free radical scavengers. By virtue of this they remove free radical before it breaks bonds, thus preventing the cell damage. A dose reduction factor (DRF) of 1.8 was seen in whole body radiation of mice. Amifostine or phosphorothioate (WR-2721) is converted into active thiol compound inside the cell by alkaline phosphatase. Since tumor has poor vasculature, not much of drug gets infused inside it. Thereby amifostine give selective normal tissue radioprotection. Trial has shown successful xerostomia reduction in patients of head and neck cancer treated by radiotherapy. Pentoxifylline and vitamin E have shown reduction in radiation-induced morbidity like mucositis, enteritis, proctitis, fibrosis, etc.

RADIATION DOSE AND UNITS

Amount of radiation absorbed per unit mass is defined as "radiation dose". In SI system one Gy is amount of radiation required for imparting of 1 Joule of energy to 1 kg of material. The older unit of radiation measurement was "rad", one Gy is equivalent to 100 rad (1 cGy = 1 rad).

FRACTIONATION

Practice of using multiple exposures for completing total radiation dose is termed as fractionation. This is done to enhance the tolerance of normal tissues. The division of total dose into multiple fractions permits normal tissue to recover from radiation-induced damage by repair of radiation damage and proliferation of remaining cells. This repair mechanism is deficient in tumor tissue (abnormal cells); therefore they get eliminated by accumulated damage, whereas normal tissue survives.

Total number of fractions vary from one to thirty five, usually given daily from Monday to Friday, i.e. five days a week, dose per fraction range from 180–200 cGy or fraction. There are four R's behind the practice dividing dose into multiple smaller increments:

1. *Redistribution:* Since fractionated radiotherapy is given over a period of five days in a week, allowing cells to go through cell cycle. Thereby increasing the chances of exposure of cells to radiation, in their most sensitive phase of cycle, i.e. G2 or M phase. Thereby maximizing the chances of cell kill by radiation therapy.
2. *Reoxygenation:* During the fractions tumor cells get killed, allowing redistribution of oxygen in remaining fewer cells. Thereby improving the availability of oxygen to them. Better oxygenation gets translated into higher radio sensitivity.
3. *Repair:* There are minimum numbers of target in each cell required to be hit before the target get inactivated, consequently killing the cell. Between the two fractions gap few hours is given. In this period cells attempt to repair SLD produced by radiation. The repair mechanism is intact in normal cells, allowing them to recover from damage to a great extent. But it is not true for tumor, leading to accumulation of SLD in these cells. Once this crosses the threshold limit, cell loses its reproductive capacity.
4. *Repopulation:* Since radiotherapy course is generally given over a period of weeks, cells try to make up for the lost number by increasing the pace of multiplication. This phenomenon is good for recovery of normal tissue damage, but may become detrimental, if fractionation is too prolonged to permit regrowth of tumor.

Recruitment of G_0 cell into active cell cycle is also seen, in response to cell killing.

Therapeutic Ratio (Fig. 7)

It is defined as percentage of tumor control with acceptable level of normal tissue complication rates (usually 5%). The shape of curve is "sigmoid". Among "radiocurable" tumors gap between two curves is large, with tumor control curve is on left of normal tissue complication curve. In the radioresistant tumors the gap between two is narrower.

Effect of Tumor Volume

Tumor control probability (TCP) is directly proportional to tumor volume (Fig. 8). Therefore smaller tumors are controlled easily, whereas bigger tumor requires additional efforts to achieve local control. This difference is attributed to presence of higher amount of cancer stem cells. Further larger tumors have chronically hypoxic areas, related with deficient blood supply. Since these areas are relatively radioresistant, they often lead to failure with the use of standard doses of radiotherapy.

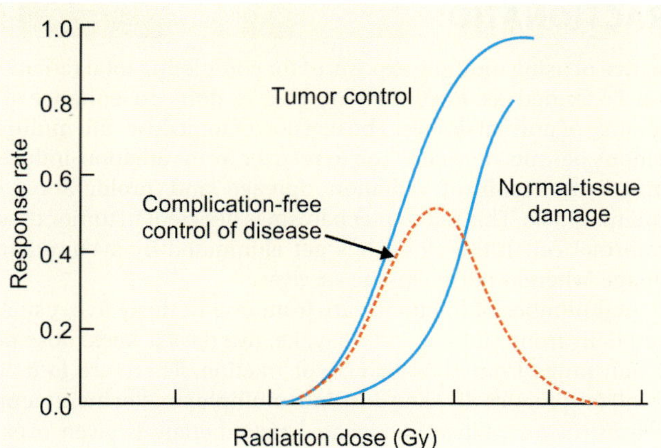

Figure 7 Therapeutic ratio

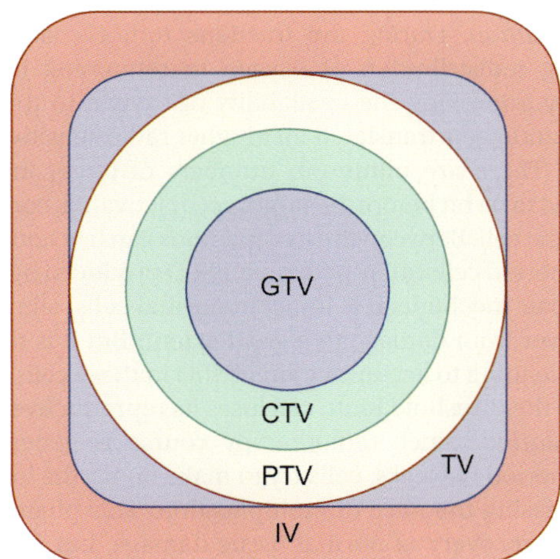

Figure 8 Tumor volume

Abbreviations: GTV, Gross tumor volume; CTV, GTV + subclinical disease; PTV, CTV + safe margin; TV, Treatment volume; IV, Irradiated volume.

Effect of Fractionation

- Conventional fractionation utilize daily dose of 180–200 cGy given for five days a week to a total dose of 60–70 Gy for gross disease and 45 Gy for preoperative and 50 Gy postoperatively.
- Radiosensitive tumor requires lesser doses of 35–45 Gy like in lymphoma, seminoma, etc. In contrast radioresistant tumors like osteosarcoma, glioblastoma, etc. will require doses in excess of 70 Gy, which is beyond tolerance limit of normal tissues. On the other hand most of the carcinomas (squamous or adeno) are moderately sensitive and usually controlled with doses of 60–70 Gy.

  Hyperfractionation is the use of doses less than 180–200 cGy per fraction. Therefore total numbers of fractions are higher than conventional fractionation. Most commonly two fractions are given per day, with a gap of six hours between them. Since the dose per fraction is smaller than conventional, it allows sparing of late-reacting tissues like nerves, bone and muscle, etc. damage in these late-reacting tissues, are dependent upon amount of dose given in each fraction. Lower dose per fraction means lower damage. The total dose given with this type of fractionation is higher, to compensate for decrease in efficacy with increased number of fractions. The delivery of higher dose may be associated with better tumor control and lesser late toxicity. This is found to be better for rapidly dividing tumor like head and neck, glioblastoma, etc.
- Hypofractionation involves delivery of dose of more than 200 cGy per fraction. Therefore total numbers of fractions are reduced and whole treatment is completed in lesser period of time. This is proven to be beneficial in tumor behaving more like late-reacting tissues like prostate. Also hypofractionation is frequently applied for palliation of symptoms. Usual doses are 30 Gy in 10 fractions.

Time Factor

The tumor cells start dividing rapidly after radiation-induced cell kill, to compensate for radiation-induced cell loss. However, it becomes clinically apparent after fourth week of radiotherapy. This accelerated repopulation of tumor cells may compromise tumor control, if treatment is prolonged beyond a reasonable period. Also to compensate for spurt in tumor growth higher doses of radiation are required. Withers (1988) found that for treatment time longer than four weeks additional dose of 0.6 Gy per day is needed to negate effect of proliferation.[3]

DELINEATION OF TUMOR

This is the most important step in treatment. Conventionally 2D planning is done with the help of bony landmarks. Here X-rays are taken on dedicated treatment planning machine known as simulators. This has now improved upon by 3D planning with the help of CT simulators and positron emission tomography (PET)-CT simulators.

With the help of imaging, tumor is identified and gross tumor volume (GTV), i.e. gross disease (palpable or visible), clinical target volume (CTV), i.e. microscopic disease are marked. CTV is addition of margin to cover subclinical disease and GTV, projected target volume (PTV) is marked to account for day to day variation in setup of treatment and tumor position, by putting margin of approximately 5 mm around CTV. Finally treatment volume is defined as one, enveloped by 100% isodose line. Organ at risk and irradiated volume are also documented to avoid damage by radiation.

Conventional or 2D image uses simple two, three or four-field planning on same isocenter. In contrast to this 3D radiotherapy contour is taken with CT scan to get dose volume histograms. Thereby, shapes of the beam constructed from each side conforming to the target volume. Newer method of doing this is by asymmetrical jaws and noncoplanar beams known as IMRT. Here intensity of beams changes in each field and even inside the field, thus maximizing radiation to tumor and sparing of normal organs. Latest in the technique of teletherapy is IGRT[4]. This involves real-time tracking of tumor before, during and after treatment to ensure coverage tumor by radiation beams all the times. Usually CT scan is employed for this purpose.

Dose is usually calculated at isocenter. It consists of total dose, number of fractions, dose per fraction and duration of treatment. Usual prescription for a radical radiotherapy is 70 Gy or 35 fractions over 7 weeks, consisting of 1.8 Gy per fraction.

Table 4: Grades of mucositis (oral)

Grade	*Changes*	*RTOG/EORTC*	*CTCAEv3*	*WHO*
0	No change	No change	No change	No change
1	Mild	Erythema, painless	Erythema, normal diet	Soreness, erythema
2	Moderate	Painful erythema, edema or ulcers, can eat	Patchy ulceration, modified diet	Erythema, ulcer, can eat
3	Severe	Painful erythema, edema or ulcers, unable to eat	Confluent ulceration, bleeding, unable to eat	ulcers, liquid diet only
4	Life threatening	Need of parenteral or enteral support	Significant bleeding, necrosis	Parenteral alimentation
5	Death	Death owing to side effects	Death owing to side effects	Death owing to side effects

Abbreviations: RTOG, radiation therapy and oncology group; EORTC, European Organization for Research and Treatment of Cancer; CTCAEv3, common terminology criteria for adverse events version 3; WHO, World Health Organization.

Adjuvant preoperative dose is limited to 45 Gy or 25 Fr or 5 Wks and postoperative doses are 50.4 Gy or 30 Fr or 6 Wks.

CARE DURING RADIOTHERAPY

All patients need to be monitored during and after radiotherapy for sequelae. Acute effects appear within three months of radiotherapy and late effects are seen after six months of completion of radiation therapy.

Acute effects like anorexia, fatigue, nausea, vomiting, mucositis (Table 4), erythema, alopecia and myelosuppression are seen in almost all patients. These are self-limiting and recovery takes place completely in most cases. These effects are severe with concomitant administration of chemotherapy, especially with 5-fluorouracil. Antiemetic is routinely given before abdominal irradiation.

Early radiation damage starts with vascular changes, expressed as erythema, followed by development of inflammatory changes. With continued radiation there is depletion of basal cells by disruption of vascular supply and resultant nonreplacement of continued cell loss. This leads to breakage in covering, manifest as ulceration and secondary infection. After completion of radiation healing occur by surviving stem cells or migration of these cells from nearby nonirradiated area.

Measurement of early changes is done on weekly basis, especially in latter half of treatment. Various systems for recording early sequelae are:

Subacute effects occur 4–8 weeks after completion of radiotherapy. Loss of appetite usually seen after abdominal irradiation, radiation hepatopathy occur 1–3 months following liver irradiation, lung exposure leads to mild radiation pneumonitis in 2–3 months.

Late Effects

All cancer treatments are associated with late effects which generally occur from 90 days to many years after therapy. Severity is related to total dose and fraction size. Bone growth stunning after 30 Gy is common in children. Radio necrosis of gut is now a thing of past, was reported at doses of more than 45 Gy. Stricture may be seen when radiation therapy is given in postoperative cases, where intestine get fixed. Rarely late subacute intestinal obstruction or ulceration is recorded.

Chronic radiation-induced changes are result of complex pathophysiological changes. These are expressed as loss of parenchymal cell, fibrosis and reduced vascularity. Radiation-induced damage releases inflammatory cytokines and growth factors. Progression of changes leads to loss of function by parenchymal damage. Producing symptoms of variable degree, dependent upon chronic radiation changes and volume treated.

Monitoring of late effects initially done at six monthly interval thereafter annually for lifelong period. Certain long-term effects, especially after low dose exposure takes decades to manifest, hence need long term plan. Late effects in normal tissue (LENT) or subjective objective management analytic (SOMA) system is used for scoring late sequelae arising from radiation therapy (Table 5).

Secondary Neoplasm

Cumulative incidence 1% at 10 years and 1.6% at 15 years. Almost 90% of cured patients suffer from late sequelae of irradiation. The age, radiation and concomitant chemotherapy are independent risk factors. Flank or abdominal irradiations are important risk factors for radiation-related sequelae. Females are at higher risk of development of grade 3–5 event. However, majority of incidents were mild to moderate. Current protocol with use of IMRT results in reduction in severity and number of event due to better sparing of normal tissues and organs.

CONCLUSION

Radiation therapy remains an essential component of the multidisciplinary management of many gastrointestinal tract (GIT) cancers undergoing curative therapy or organ function conservation. Use of ionizing radiation demands balance between efficacy and potential long-term toxicity (which are more pronounced in abdomen). Second malignant neoplasm is always an issue with an overall risk of 510% over 3 decades of 5-fluorouracil. Modern techniques should continue to improve cure rates and reduce both acute and late effects.

FUTURE

Hadron therapy (particulate beam irradiation) using proton, carbon ions, etc. are under development and presently available at selected places only.

Table 5: Late sequelae of radiotherapy

Target organ	*Symptom/Lesion*	*Period of manifestation*	*Tolerance dose for total volume*	*Remarks*
Esophagus	Dysphagia, ulcer, fistula, stenosis	0–24 months	~ 45 Gy	Mucositis as early symptom and pre-existing stricture
Stomach	Atony Ulcer	0 month 624 months	20 Gy ~ 50 Gy	Nausea, vomiting after radiation therapy
Small intestine	Malabsorption ulceration, obstruction	0 month 624 months	30 Gy 40 Gy	Greater frequency in postoperative radiation therapy (Fixation of loops)
Large intestine	Diarrhea/Pain, obstruction/Ulcer	0 month 624 months	10 Gy 45 Gy	Symptoms of ileus
Rectum	Proctitis Ulcer	0 month 624 months	~ 55Gy 60 Gy	Related to volume receiving high dose
Liver	Veno-occlusive disease (VOD) Fibrosis	3 weeks 612 months	30 Gy	Whole liver radiation, Late manifestation, if partial organ radiation therapy
Biliary tract	Stenosis/stricture	624 months	~ 55Gy	—
Pancreas	Fibrosis	624 months	~ 50 Gy	Part of radiation sickness syndrome

Protons, unlike photon beams generated on traditional treatment units, protons are produced by cyclotrons and have an advantage in the characteristic of the beam such that there is a sharp fall off between high- and low-dose areas, due to phenomenon termed the Bragg peak.[5] Unlike photons protons deposit their energy at a predetermine depth, which can be regulated. Thus all of energy deposited at one place with no radiation beyond that depth. This allows increase in dose (1520%) at local site with precision. High-dose irradiation with protons could lead to improved local control and long-term survival without excessive risk to normal tissues injury in patients with esophageal cancer.

REFERENCES

1. Mierzwa ML, Nyati MK, Morgan MA, Lawrence TS. Recent advances in combined modality therapy. The Oncologist. 2010;15:372-81.
2. Lawrence TS, Haffty BG, Harris JR. Milestones in the use of combined-modality radiation therapy and chemotherapy. J Clin Oncol. 2014;32:1173-9.
3. Withers HR, Taylor JM, Maciejewski B. The hazard of accelerated tumor clonogen repopulation during radiotherapy. Acta Oncol. 1988;27:131-46.
4. Jaffray DA. Image-guided radiation therapy: from concept to practice. Semin Radiat Oncol. 2007;17(4):243-4.
5. Brada M, Pijls-Johannesma M, De Ruysscher D. Proton therapy in clinical practice: current clinical evidence. J Clin Oncol. 2007;25(8):965-70.

BIBLIOGRAPHY

1. Hall EJ, Giaccia AJ. Radiobiology for the radiologist. Philadelphia: Lippincott Williams and Wilkins; 2006.
2. Halperin EC, Brady LW, Perez AC, Wazer DE. Perez and Brady's Principle and Practice of Radiation Oncology, 6th edition. Philadelphia: Lippincott Williams and Wilkins; 2013.
3. Podgorsak EB. Radiation oncology physics: A Handbook for Teachers and Students. Vienna: International Atomic Energy Agency; 2005.

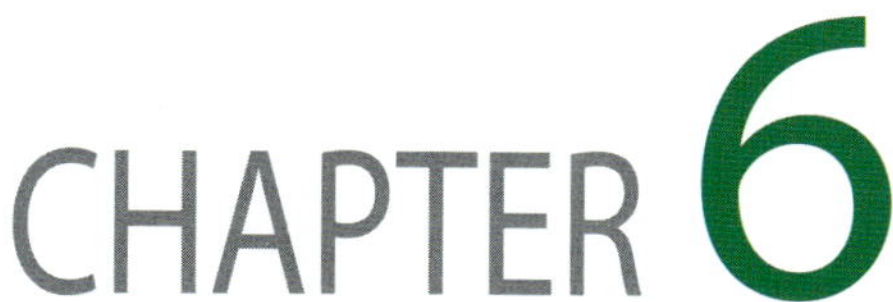

Chemotherapy Principles and Techniques for GI Cancers

Atul Sharma

INTRODUCTION

Identification of chemotherapeutic drugs and successful use of this new modality resulted in cure of many hematological and solid tumors in middle of last century, and prolongation of life in many other cancers.[1] This led to the idea that chemotherapy may be used in several ways as a therapeutic tool for treatment of cancers.

Adjuvant Therapy

After the successful local therapy in early stage disease, i.e. surgery or local radiotherapy to control micrometastases. Best examples among the GI cancers are stomach, colon, pancreas, etc.

Neoadjuvant Therapy

To reduce the size and bulk of tumor so as to facilitate surgery with clear margins or delivery of radiation to reduced tumor volume. Examples are: esophagus, stomach, sometimes pancreaticobiliary tract and colorectal cancers.

Concurrent Chemoradiation

This means when chemotherapy and radiotherapy are used simultaneously or concurrently. This may be used as in three ways: (i) only modality for treatment: as sometime used in esophageal cancer anal canal cancers, (ii) as adjuvant therapy: gastric cancer, rectal cancer or (iii) neoadjuvant therapy: rectal cancer, pancreatic cancer.

Palliative Therapy

To control the symptoms of unresectable/metastatic or recurrent disease and, if possible, prolongs the life and improves quality of life. Palliative chemotherapies have role in most of GI cancers but role is very well defined in gastric, pancreatic, gallbladder (including cholangiocarcinoma), hepatocellular carcinoma (HCC) and colorectal cancers.

Since chemotherapy drugs do not differentiate between normal cells and tumor cells most of growing cells are affected that may result into side effects and this is one of the main concern when using these drugs. The knowledge and application of molecular techniques to analyze gene expression of normal and malignant cells at the level of DNA, RNA and/or protein has helped to identify some of the important mechanisms by which chemotherapy exerts its effect and activate the program of cell death.[1]

The doses of most of chemotherapy drugs are calculated taking body surface area (BSA) into account and expressed as per meter square ($/m^2$). An antiemetic is used most of the time along with chemotherapy drugs. In cases of deranged organ function particularly bone marrow, hepatic and renal the doses need to be modified and used with extreme caution or particular cytotoxic drugs may be avoided.

DRUGS USED IN GI CANCERS

Disclaimer: The following listed drugs may not have been approved by the FDA for the indication listed below or perhaps have been used as offlabel drugs.

Chemotherapy Drugs: Largely in the Order of Alphabets

Capecitabine

This is an oral antimetabolite and a form of fluoropyrimidine. This is converted into active form 5-fluorouracil (5-FU) by the enzyme thymidine phosphorylase. Higher concentration of this enzyme is expressed in tumor tissues than normal tissue. This may also be considered as a form of continuous infusion of 5-FU.[2]

The usual dosage is 1,250 mg/m^2 PO bid for days 1–14 to be repeated every 3 weeks, when used as a single agent. However, for combination therapy, the dose may be reduced to 825–1,000 mg/m^2 PO bid for days 1–14 to be repeated every 3 weeks.

It should preferably been taken before meals with water. It may require dose adjustment in severe liver and renal dysfunctions.

The common side effects include but not limited to: diarrhea, mucositis, hand-foot syndrome (also known as plantar-palmar erythrodysesthesia), nausea and vomiting, myelosuppression, cardiac symptoms, etc.

The drug is used in Gastric or gastroesophageal cancer (adjuvant, neoadjuvant or palliative setting), colorectal cancer (single agent or along with oxaliplatin in adjuvant with oxaliplatin in recurrent or metastatic disease and along with radiotherapy in concurrent chemoradiation schedule for rectal cancer.[3]

Carboplatin

Carboplatin is a platinum compound which forms DNA adducts resulting into inhibition of DNA synthesis and function. Unlike the other drugs, the dose of carboplatin is calculated as a target area under the curve (AUC) which is usually 4–6 mg/mL/minute. In esophageal cancer this is used along with paclitaxel and radiation as a definitive concurrent chemoradiotherapy.[4,5]

Cisplatin

This is also known as cisdiamminedichloroplatinum (CDDP) or diaminodichloroplatinum (DDP). This is a platinum compound and one of the most commonly and efficacious drugs used in oncology. It forms DNA adducts which result in inhibition of DNA synthesis and function.

The dosage may vary 50–100 mg/m^2 each cycle depending upon the indication. Cisplatin should be used very cautiously particularly in patients with impaired renal function. Creatinine clearance needs to be calculated at baseline and before each cycle. Also it is very important to monitor electrolytes (Na, K, Mg) once a patient is on cisplatin. It is mandatory to hydrate patient before, during and after cisplatin infusion. The preferred way will be to give a liter before and a liter of 0.9% NaCl (normal saline) with 20 mEq of KCl after the cisplatin infusion. Idea is to keep urine output equal or greater to 100 mL/hour. If needed furosemide or mannitol may be used. Since this is a highly emetogenic agent it is required to use strong antiemetic agents (dexamethasone and 5HT-3 antagonists) along with cisplatin.

The common side effects include but not limited to: nephrotoxicity, nausea and vomiting, neurotoxicity, ototoxicity, vascular events, alopecia, etc.

It is used in esophagus, gastroesopahgeal, gastric, pancreatic, gallbladder and anal canal cancers.[4]

Epirubicin

This is an anticancer antibiotic which acts by intercalating into DNA and inhibiting topoisomerage II enzyme. Epirubicin is a component of a common regimen, ECF, used in gastric cancer (early or advanced stage). It is used in the dose of 50 mg/m^2 every 3 weeks as intravenous (IV) infusion. The common side effects associated with its use are myelosuppression, mild nausea, vomiting and diarrhea. It may also cause cardiotoxicity.[6]

5-Fluorouracil

5-Fluorouracil as commonly this is known as is by far one of the earliest and most extensively used drugs in GI cancers. 5-FU is an antimetabolite fluoropyrimidine derivative. It inhibits the enzyme thymidylate synthase and inhibits DNA synthesis and also affects RNA. It is available both for oral or parenteral use but parenteral use is much more common than oral. It is used as intravenous bolus, continuous intravenous infusion or some times intraperitoneally. Efficacy and toxicity is dependent upon duration of infusion; bolus or continuously. It is used in almost every part of GI tract malignancy.

It is or has been used in the neoadjuvant, adjuvant or palliative therapy of esophagus, gastric, pancreaticobiliary, colorectal, or anal canal cancers. Various dosing schedule are practiced: (a) 425 mg/m^2 bolus IV days 1–5 every 4 weeks, (b) 2,400–2,600 mg/m^2 46 hours infusion every 2 weeks, (c) 800–1,000 mg/m^2/day continuous infusion for 96 hours, or (d) 200 mg/m^2/day protracted infusion for 3 weeks.

Toxicity: Myelosuppression is more severe and common when used as bolus; whereas mucositis and diarrhea are common and severe were continuous infusion. This may lead to dehydration and other complications. Other side effects are hand-foot syndrome, changes in nails, lacrimal duct stenosis, increased lacrimation. Cardiac symptoms in the form of chest pain, ECG changes are not very uncommon and it should be used very cautiously or should be avoided in a patient with known history of cardiac disorders.[7]

Gemcitabine

This again is an antimetabolite which is used in the treatment of pancreaticobiliary cancer as single agent or in combination with other drugs. It is administered by intravenous route. With longer infusion the drug is widely distributed into body tissues. Gemcitabine is used as 1000 mg/m2 30 minutes IV infusion weekly for 7 week followed by 1 week rest. Subsequent infusions are days 1, 8, 15 every 4 weeks. It is also used as a radiosensitizer. The common indications are: neoadjuvant, adjuvant or palliative therapy for pancreatic adenocarcinoma or palliative treatment of biliary tract cancers along with cisplatin or oxaliplatin. The toxicity includes: myelosuppression, nausea and vomiting, flu-like symptoms. Rarely pulmonary toxicity has also been reported.[8,9]

Irinotecan

This is a semi-synthetic derivative of camptothecin and a topoisomerase I inhibitor. After IV infusion this is converted to its active form SN-38. Irinotecan is among the first new drugs in the treatment of colorectal cancers since 5-FU. It is used along with 5-FU and folinic acid in the treatment of metastatic colorectal cancer. It also can be combined with antibodies in the treatment of metastatic colorectal cancer. The common schedules followed are either 180 mg/m^2 every 2 weeks or less commonly 250–350 mg/m^2 every 3 weeks. Activity of irinotecan in other GI cancers is being explored.

The side effects are myelosuppression and more commonly early or late diarrhea which may be very severe in some cases.[10,11]

Mitomycin-C

Mitomycin-C belongs to the group of anticancer antibiotic. This is available for IV use and used in the treatment of gastric and anal canal cancer. It is used in the dose of 10 mg/m^2 on day 1 and 29 in the treatment of anal canal cancer where this is combined with 5-FU and radiation. In the treatment of gastric cancer this is used in the same dose but repeated after 8 weeks. Side effects other than nausea and vomiting are myelosuppression and typically this is delayed.[12]

Oxaliplatin

Oxaliplatin a new platinum analog is a drug which is being increasingly used in the GI cancers because of its efficacy and safety profile. It forms DNA adducts either interstand or intrastand and causes inhibition of DNA synthesis. It is extensively used in GI cancers; advanced or metastatic gastroesophageal and gastric cancer, adjuvant therapy in gastric cancer, pancreatic and biliary tract cancer, and most importantly adjuvant and advanced colorectal cancer in combination with 5-FU/LV. The usual doses are 80–85 mg/m^2 IV infusion day 1 and 8 every 3 weeks or 130 mg/m^2 IV infusion every 3 weeks. Unlike most other drugs oxaliplatin is given in dextrose 5%.

One of the most common and important toxicity of oxaliplatin is neurotoxicity which is both acute and chronic. It is peripheral sensory and might manifest as paraesthesia on exposure to cold, numbness, burning sensation in palms/soles, changes in voice, laryngopharyngeal dysesthesia, or difficulty in swallowing or breathing. Chronic neurotoxicity is usually dose dependent and reversible. Nausea, vomiting and mild to moderate myelosuppression are other side effects.[4,13]

Taxanes

The three drugs which come under this category are: (1) docetaxel, (2) paclitaxel and (3) Nab paclitaxel (nano albumin bound paclitaxel). They act by acting against microtubule.

Docetaxel is used as an intravenous infusion agent in advanced and unresectable gastric cancer in the dose of 75 mg/m^2 every 3 weeks. Docetaxel is known to causes fluid retention and dexamethasone in the dose of 8 mg orally for 3 days starting a day prior to infusion is prescribed with this.[14]

The main side effects are myelosuppression, hypersensitivity reactions, fluid retention, skin rashes, GI disturbances, deranged liver function tests, fatigue and asthenia.

Paclitaxel is the first drug from this group to be used and approved in clinical setting. It causes stabilization of microtubule. Paclitaxel in the weekly dose of 60 mg/m^2 and carboplatin along with radiation are used as definitive or neoadjuvant therapy in esophageal cancer. Paclitaxel is also used in unresectable gastric cancer along with platinum compound. In one of the regimen low doses of paclitaxel, DDP and etoposide are used in a twice a week schedule. Otherwise the usual dosing is 175–200 mg/m^2 in a 3 weekly schedule and 60–80 mg/m^2 in weekly schedule.

The main adverse effect is hypersensitivity reactions which usually occur in first few minutes. It is recommended to use premedication a night before and in the morning of paclitaxel infusion to reduce and minimize these reactions. Other side effects are myelosuppression, neurotoxicity (sensory), alopecia and myalgias which may require use of analgesics.[15]

Nano albumin bound or Nab Paclitaxel is used and found to be effective in combination with gemcitabine for treatment of unresectable pancreatic cancer. The dose is 125 mg/m^2 day 1, 8 and 15 every 4 weeks (weekly × 3 in a 4 week cycle). Myelosuppression and neuropathy are main side effects.

Targeted Agents

Recent knowledge in understanding of various molecular and cellular pathways has helped the scientific community to identify various targets for therapeutic interventions. Targeted therapy has made a significant impact in many cancers (solids and hematological). Among various cancers colorectal cancer is a leading cause of morbidity and mortality. Epidermal growth factor receptor (EGFR) is overexpressed in these and some gastric cancers making it an obvious choice for therapeutic target. Angiogenesis and binding of vascular endothelial growth factor (VEGF) to its receptors is known to start activation of series of intracellular signaling pathways in endothelial cells leading to formation of neovascularization and tumor cell spread.[16,17]

Antibodies against EGFR and VEGF have been developed and are being used successfully in some GI cancers to improve survival especially in advanced or metastatic cancers. Antibodies act by inhibition of signaling pathways. The drugs which have been approved or are used in clinical practice are:

a. *Bevacizumab (Avastin)*: It is a humanized antibody against VEGF for use in metastatic colorectal cancer in combination with IV 5-FU/LV or oral capecitabine. The recommended dose is 5–10 mg/kg every 2–3 weeks IV infusion. A patient on bevacizumab should be regularly monitored for any bleeding or hypertension. Administration of bevacizumab has been associated with encounter of bleeding disorders, would dehiscence, GI perforation, infusion related reactions, arterial thromboembolic phenomenon, etc.[18]
b. *Cetuximab (Erbitux)*: It is a chimeric IgG1 antibody against EGFR. The important thing to remember about cetuximab is that this is ineffective in patients who have KRAS mutation. Hence, it is mandatory to do KRAS mutation analysis before recommending cetuximab, and if KRAS is wild type only then this drug should be used. This is approved for use with infusional 5-FU/LV and irinotecan or other cytotoxic therapy as a first line or subsequent therapy in KRAS wild type tumor. The recommended dose is 400 mg/m^2 as loading dose followed by 250 mg/m^2 weekly till intolerance or disease progression. Of late a new schedule is practiced where 500 mg/m^2 of cetuximab is given every 2 weeks. It is advisable to use antihistaminic before infusing cetuximab. Since hypomagnesemia and hypocalcemia are observed after infusion a blood tests to check their values before infusion should be done. The adverse events include mainly skin toxicity (this is considered a surrogate marker of response) in the form of dryness, acneiform rashes, and pustules, peeling of skin, nail changes and hypomagnesemia.[19]

c. *Panitumumab*: Similar to cetuximab this is an antibody against EGFR the difference being that this is fully humanized. Used either as monotherapy in patients who have become refractory to other agents or as an initial therapy with other chemotherapy drugs. Currently this is not available in India. This is not used in the patients with KRAS mutation. The prescribed dose is 6 mg/kg infusion every 2 weeks. Infusion related reactions, skin toxicity and hypomagnesemia are main adverse reactions.
d. *Aflibercept*: This prevents the activation of VEGFR-1 and VEGFR-2. Recently this drug in combination with FOLFIRI improved survival in patients with metastatic colorectal cancer who were previously treated with oxaliplatin containing regimens. The dose is 4 mg/kg every 2 weeks. The infusion related reactions are main adverse reactions observed.[20]
e. *Regorafenib (Stivarga)*: This is an oral small molecule which is multikinase inhibitor of VEGFR, PDGFR, c-KIT, FGFR, etc. Recently regorafenib has been approved for use in metastatic colorectal cancer patients who have failed all other options. The dose is 160 mg orally for days 1–21 in a 28 days cycle. Hypertension and skin toxicity are the important side effects.[21]
f. *Sorafenib (Nexavar)*: Sorafenib is a multikinase inhibitor that is somewhat structurally similar to regorafenib. In the dose of 400 mg BD this is approved for the treatment of unresectable HCC with Child-Pugh score of A and possible B. GI disturbances in the form of diarrhea, hypertension and skin reactions are main side effects.[22]
g. *Trastuzumab (Herceptin)*: Trastuzumab is a humanized antibody against human epidermal growth receptor 2. This is one of the common antibodies mostly used in Her-2neu (HER-2) positive breast cancer. A subset of advanced gastric cancer patients (10–20%) also over expresses Her-2neu and get benefit in the form of increased survival when given trastuzumab in combination with chemotherapy (DDP and 5-FU or capecitabine). The dose is loading dose of 4 mg/kg IV infusion followed by 2 mg/kg weekly. The main adverse reactions are: infusion related and cardiotoxicity.[23]
h. *Erlotinib (Tarceva)*: Erlotinib is selective inhibitor of EGFR tyrosine kinase. This is used in the dose of 100 mg daily orally in combination with gemcitabine in the treatment of unresectable adenocarcinoma of pancreas where this was found to marginally improve survival. Diarrhea and skin reactions are commonly encountered toxicities.[24]

COMMON PROTOCOLS USED IN GI CANCERS[25]

Anal Canal

- Concurrent chemoradiation is preferred for localized disease
- 5-FU 1000 mg/m^2/day continuous infusion days 1–4 and days 29–32
- Mitomycin-C 10 mg/m^2 IV on days 1 and 29
- Concurrent radiotherapy 45 Gy/25#/5 weeks (25 fractions in 5 week).[12]

Biliary Tract Cancers (for Unresectable Tumors)

Gem-Cis:
- Cisplatin 25 mg/m^2 IV infusion day 1 and 8
- Gemcitabine 1000 mg/m^2 IV infusion on day 1 and 8 every 3 weeks up to eight cycles.[26]

mGEMOX:
- Gemcitabine 900 mg/m^2 IV infusion on day 1 and 8
- Oxaliplatin 80 mg/m^2 IV infusion day 1 and 8 every 3 weeks up to six cycles.[27]

At our center we prefer to use mGEMOX and for adjuvant therapy we use McDonalds Protocol which is as follows.[28]

Cycle 1 will be chemotherapy alone:
- 5-FU: 425 mg/m^2 IV bolus on days 1–5
- Leucovorin: 20 mg/m^2 IV on days 1–5.

28 days later this will be followed by chemoradiotherapy as:
- 5-FU: 400 mg/m^2 IV on days 1–4 and days 23–25 of radiation therapy
- Leucovorin: 20 mg/m^2 IV on days 1–4 and days 23–25 of radiation therapy.

Chemoradiotherapy is followed by two cycles of chemotherapy that are given 28 days apart and include:
- 5-FU: 425 mg/m^2 IV bolus on days 1–5
- Leucovorin: 20 mg/m^2 IV on days 1–5.

Colon-Rectal

The treatment of metastatic disease is same whether colon or rectum. The main difference in early stage/operable is that in rectal cancer it is preferred to give neoadjuvant chemoradiation before surgical resection except in very early disease. This is followed by adjuvant therapy for about 4 months.

Adjuvant Therapy

Mayo Clinic regimen: 5-FU + Leucovorin
- 5-FU: 425 mg/m^2 IV on days 1–5
- Leucovorin: 20 mg/m^2 IV on days 1–5, administered before 5-FU
- Cycles are repeated every 4–5 weeks for a total of six cycles.[29]

FOLFOX 4 protocol: Oxaliplatin + 5-FU + Leucovorin
- Oxaliplatin: 85 mg/m^2 IV on day 1
- 5-FU: 400 mg/m^2 IV bolus, followed by 600 mg/m^2 IV continuous infusion for 22 hours on days 1 and 2
- Leucovorin: 200 mg/m^2 IV on days 1 and 2 as a 2-hour infusion before 5-FU
- Cycles are repeated every 2 weeks for a total of twelve cycles (6 months total).[30]

Oxaliplatin + Capecitabine (XELOX)
- Oxaliplatin: 130 mg/m^2 IV on day 1
- Capecitabine: 1,000 mg/m^2 PO bid on days 1–14
- Repeat cycle every 3 weeks for a total of eight cycles (6 months total)
- Dose of capecitabine may be decreased to 850 mg/m^2 PO bid days 1–14 to reduce risk of toxicity without compromising efficacy.[31]

Capecitabine:
- Capecitabine 1,250 mg/m^2 PO bid on days 1–14
- Cycles are repeated every 21 days for a total of eight cycles
- Dose may be decreased to 850–1,000 mg/m^2 PO bid on days 1–14 to reduce risk of toxicity without compromising clinical efficacy.[32]

Metastatic Disease

FOLFIRI regimen:
- Irinotecan + 5-FU + Leucovorin
- Irinotecan: 180 mg/m^2 IV on day 1
- 5-FU: 400 mg/m^2 IV bolus on day 1, followed by 2,400 mg/m^2 IV continuous infusion for 46 hours
- Leucovorin: 200 mg/m^2 IV on day 1 as a 2-hour infusion prior to 5-FU
- Cycles are repeated every every 2 weeks until unacceptable toxicity or disease progression.[33,34]

Oxaliplatin + 5-FU + Leucovorin (FOLFOX4)
- Oxaliplatin: 85 mg/m^2 IV on day 1
- 5-FU: 400 mg/m^2 IV bolus, followed by 600 mg/m^2 IV over 22 hours on days 1 and 2
- Leucovorin: 200 mg/m^2 IV on days 1 and 2 as a 2-hour infusion before 5-FU
- Cycles are repeated every every 2 weeks until unacceptable toxicity or disease progression.[30,35]

Oxaliplatin + 5-FU + Leucovorin (FOLFOX6)
- Oxaliplatin: 100 mg/m^2 IV on day 1
- 5-FU: 400 mg/m^2 IV bolus on day 1, followed by 2,400 mg/m^2 IV continuous infusion for 46 hours
- Leucovorin: 400 mg/m^2 IV on day 1 as a 2-hour infusion before 5-FU
- Cycles are repeated every 2 weeks until unacceptable toxicity or disease progression.[36]

Oxaliplatin + Capecitabine (XELOX)
- Oxaliplatin: 130 mg/m^2 IV on day 1
- Capecitabine: 1,000 mg/m^2 PO bid on days 1–14
- Cycle are repeated every 3 weeks until disease progression or unacceptable toxicity
- Dose of capecitabine may be decreased to 850 mg/m^2 PO bid days 1–14 to reduce risk of toxicity without compromising.[18,37]

Capecitabine + Irinotecan (XELIRI):
- Capecitabine: 1,000 mg/m^2 PO bid on days 1–14
- Irinotecan: 250 mg/m^2 IV on day 1
- Cycle are repeated every 3 weeks until disease progression or unacceptable toxicity.
- May decrease dose of capecitabine to 850 mg/m^2 PO bid and dose of irinotecan to 200 mg/m^2 IV to reduce risk of toxicity without compromising clinical efficacy.[38]

FOLFOX4 + Bevacizumab:
- Oxaliplatin: 85 mg/m^2 IV on day 1
- 5-FU: 400 mg/m^2 IV bolus, followed by 600 mg/m^2 IV continuous infusion on days 1 and 2
- Leucovorin: 200 mg/m^2 IV on days 1 and 2 as a 2-hour infusion before 5-FU
- Bevacizumab: 10 mg/kg IV every 2 weeks
- Repeat cycle every 2 week until disease progression or unacceptable toxicity.[39]

Capecitabine + Oxaliplatin (XELOX) + Bevacizumab:
- Capecitabine: 850 mg/m2 PO bid on days 1–14
- Oxaliplatin: 130 mg/m^2 IV on day 1
- Bevacizumab: 7.5 mg/kg every 3 weeks
- Cycle are repeated every 3 weeks until disease progression or unacceptable toxicity.[18,40]

FOLFIRI + Cetuximab:
- Irinotecan: 180 mg/m^2 IV on day 1
- 5-FU: 400 mg/m^2 IV bolus followed by 2,400 mg/m^2 IV continuous infusion for 46 hours on days 1 and 2
- Leucovorin: 400 mg/m^2 IV on day 1 as a 2-hour infusion prior to 5-FU
- Cetuximab: 400 mg/m^2 IV loading dose, then 250 mg/m^2 IV weekly
- Cycle are repeated every 2 weeks until disease progression or unacceptable toxicity.[19]

FOLFOX4 + Cetuximab:
- Oxaliplatin: 85 mg/m^2 IV on day 1
- 5-FU: 400 mg/m^2 IV bolus followed by 600 mg/m^2 IV continuous infusion for 6 hours on days 1 and 2
- Leucovorin: 200 mg/m^2 IV on days 1 and 2 as a 2-hour infusion prior to 5-FU
- Cetuximab: 400 mg/m^2 IV loading dose, then 250 mg/m^2 IV weekly
- Cycle are repeated every 2 weeks until disease progression or unacceptable toxicity.[41]

For rectal cancer requiring neoadjuvant therapy

PreOp CT +RT (5-FU/capecitabine)[42]

This is followed by adjuvant chemotherapy for about 4 months (same protocols as in colon cancer).

Gastric Cancer and Gastroesophageal

Neoadjuvant

ECF:
- Epirubicin: 50 mg/m^2 IV on day 1
- Cisplatin: 60 mg/m^2 IV on day 1
- 5-FU: 200 mg/m^2 IV infusion continuously
- Repeat cycle every 21 days x three cycles[43]

Adjuvant

Start with cycle 1 as:
- 5-FU: 425 mg/m^2 IV bolus on days 1–5
- Leucovorin: 20 mg/m^2 IV on days 1–5

28 days later this will be followed by chemoradiotherapy as:
- 5-FU: 400 mg/m^2 IV on days 1-4 and days 23–25 of radiation therapy
- Leucovorin: 20 mg/m^2 IV on days 1-4 and days 23–25 of radiation therapy.

Concurrent chemoradiation is followed by two cycles of chemotherapy that are given 28 days apart as:
- 5-FU: 425 mg/m^2 IV bolus on days 1–5
- Leucovorin: 20 mg/m^2 IV on days 1–5.[28]

Capecitabine + Oxaliplatin
- Capecitabine: 1,000 mg/m^2 PO bid on days 1–14
- Oxaliplatin: 130 mg/m^2 IV on day 1
- Repeat cycle every 21 days for 6 months.[44]

Unresectable/Metastatic

DCF:
- Docetaxel: 75 mg/m^2 IV on day 1
- Cisplatin: 75 mg/m^2 IV on day 1
- 5-FU: 750 mg/m^2/day IV continuous infusion on days 1–5
- Repeat cycle every 21 days.[45]

PF:
- Cisplatin: 100 mg/m^2 IV on day 1
- 5-FU: 1,000 mg/m^2/day IV continuous infusion on days 1–5
- Repeat cycle every 28 days.

ECX:
- Epirubicin: 50 mg/m^2 IV on day 1
- Cisplatin: 60 mg/m^2 IV on day 1
- Capecitabine: 625 mg/m^2 PO bid continuously
- Repeat cycle every 21 days.[43]

EOX:
- Epirubicin: 50 mg/m^2 IV infusion on day 1
- Oxaliplatin: 130 mg/m^2 IV infusion on day 1 (2 hours)
- Capecitabine: 625 mg/m^2 PO bid daily
- Cycles to be repeated every 21 days.[44]

CPE:
- Cisplatin 15 mg/m^2
- Etoposide 40 mg/m^2
- Paclitaxel 50 mg/m^2, all given on day 1 and 4 every week for 3 weeks in a 28-day cycle.[45]

Esophagus

Chemotherapy Protocols

5-FU + Cisplatin (PF) + RT
- 5-FU: 800 mg/m^2/day IV continuous infusion on days 1–4 of week 1, 5, 8, and 11, nowadays this may be given via infusor pump
- Cisplatin: 100 mg/m^2 IV on day 1[46]
- We prefer to use low dose (5-FU: 750 mg/m^2/day IV continuous infusion on days 2–5 over 6 hours cisplatin: 75 mg/m^2 IV on day 1 and 2—divided doses).

ECX:
- Epirubicin: 50 mg/m^2 IV infusion on day 1
- Cisplatin: 60 mg/m^2 IV infusion on day 1 along with hydration
- Capecitabine: 625 mg/m^2 PO bid daily from days 1 through 21
- Cycles to be repeated every 21 days.[42]

EOX:
- Epirubicin: 50 mg/m^2 IV infusion day 1
- Oxaliplatin: 130 mg/m^2 IV infusion day 1
- Capecitabine: 625 mg/m^2 PO bid daily from days 1 through 21
- Cycles to be repeated every 21 days.[47]

Paclitaxel + Carboplatin
Paclitaxel: 200 mg/m^2 IV infusion over 24 hours on day 1
Carboplatin: dose calculated asAUC of 5 IV infusions on day 2
Cycles to be repeated every 21 days

OR
Paclitaxel + Carboplatin
Paclitaxel: 200 mg/m^2 IV over 24 hours on day 1
Cisplatin 75 mg/m^2 IV on day 2
Cycles to be repeated every 21 days[48]

Paclitaxel + Carboplatin
Paclitaxel: 50 mg/m^2 IV infusion
Carboplatin: calculated as with AUC 2 IV infusion weekly for 5 weeks
Radiation: 41.3 Gy in 23[49]

Pancreas

Adjuvant

- Gemcitabine 1,000 mg/m^2 IV infusion on day 1, 8 and 15 every 4 weeks for six cycles.[50,51]

Unresectable/Metastatic

- Gemcitabine 1,000 mg/m^2 IV infusion qw × 7 weeks followed by 1 week rest, and then on day 1, 8 and 15 every 4 weeks [52,53]
- Gemcitabine 1,000 mg/m^2 IV infusion on day 1 and 15 every 4 weeks
- Cisplatin 50 mg/m^2 IV infusion on day 1 and 15 every 4 weeks[54]
- Gemcitabine 1,000 mg/m^2 IV infusion on day 1, 8 and 15 every 4 weeks.[54]

FOLFIRINOX

All given day 1
- Oxaliplatin, 85 mg/m^2
- Irinotecan, 180 mg/m^2
- Leucovorin, 400 mg/m^2
- 5-FU 400 mg/m^2 given as a bolus followed by 2,400 mg/m^2 given as a 46-hour continuous infusion, every 2 weeks for 6 months[55]

Gemcitabine + Abraxane
- Gemcitabine 1,000 mg/m^2 IV infusion day 1, 8 and 15 every 4 weeks
- Abraxane 125 mg/m^2 infusion day 1, 8 and 15 every 4 weeks.[56]

REFERENCES

1. DeVita Vincent T, Chu E. Principles of medical oncology. Devita, Hellman & Rosenberg's Cancer: Principles & Practice of Oncology, 8th edition. Phidelphia: Lipponcott William & Wilkins; 2008.
2. Shimma N, Umeda I, Arasaki M, Murasaki C, Masubuchi K, Kohchi Y, et al. The design and synthesis of a new tumor-selective fluoropyrimidine carbamate, capecitabine. Bioorg Med Chem. 2000;8:1697-906.
3. Chu E. Efficacy and safety of capecitabine therapy for colorectal cancer. Am J Oncol Rev. 2003;2(Suppl 3):4-28.
4. Reed E. Cisplatin, caboplatin and oxaliplatin. Devita, Hellman & Rosenberg's Cancer: Principles & Practice of Oncology, 8th edition. Phidelphia: Lipponcott William & Wilkins; 2008. pp. 420-6.
5. Calvert AH, Newell DR, Gumbrell LA, O'Reilly S, Burnell M, Boxall FE, et al. Carboplatin dosage: prospective evaluation of a simple formula based on renal function. J Clin Oncol. 1989;7:1748-56.
6. Rasheed ZA, Rubin EH. Devita, Hellman & Rosenberg's Cancer: Principles & Practice of Oncology, 8th edition. Phidelphia: Lipponcott William & Wilkins; 2008. p. 444.
7. Grem JL. 5-Fluorouracil: forty-plus and still ticking. A review of its preclinical and clinical development. Invest New Drugs. 2000;18(4):299-313.
8. Ryan DP, Garcia-Carbonero R, Chabner BA. Cytidine analogs. In: Chabner BA, Longo DL (Eds). Cancer Chemotherapy and Biotherapy: Principles and Practice, 4th edition. Philadelphia: Lippincottâ€"Raven, 2006. p. 183.
9. Mini E, Nobili S, Caciagli B, Landini I, Mazzei T. Cellular pharmacology of gemcitabine. Ann Oncol. 2006;17(Suppl 5):v7-12.
10. Douillard JY, Cunningham D, Roth AD, Navarro M, James RD, Karasek P, et al. Irinotecan combined with fluorouracil compared with fluorouracil alone as first-line treatment for metastatic

colorectal cancer: a multicentre randomised trial. Lancet. 2000;355(9209):1041-7.

11. Saltz LB, Cox JV, Blanke C, Rosen LS, Fehrenbacher L, Moore MJ, et al. Irinotecan plus fluorouracil and leucovorin for metastatic colorectal cancer. Irinotecan Study Group. N Engl J Med. 2000;343(13):905-14.
12. Ajani JA, Winter KA, Gunderson LL, Pedersen J, Benson AB 3rd, et al. Fluorouracil, mitomycin, and radiotherapy vs fluorouracil, cisplatin, and radiotherapy for carcinoma of the anal canal: a randomized controlled trial. JAMA. 2008;299(16):1914-21.
13. Chaney SG, Vaisman A. Specificity of platinum-DNA adduct repair. J Inorg Biochem. 1999;77:71-81.
14. Lee JJ, Harris LN. Devita, Hellman & Rosenberg's Cancer: Principles & Practice of Oncology, Principles of Oncology—Pharmacology of Cancer Chemotherapy: Antimicrotubule Agents 8th edition. Phidelphia: Lipponcott William & Wilkins; 2008. pp. 450-6.
15. Van Cutsem E, Moiseyenko VM, Tjulandin S, Majlis A, Constenla M, Boni C, et al. Phase III study of docetaxel and cisplatin plus fluorouracil compared with cisplatin and fluorouracil as first-line therapy for advanced gastric cancer: a report of the V325 Study Group. J Clin Oncol. 2006;24(31):4991-7.
16. Sun W. Angiogenesis in metastatic colorectal cancer and the benefits of targeted therapy. J Hematol Oncol. 2012;5:63.
17. Dvorak HF. Vascular permeability factor/vascular endothelial growth factor: a critical cytokine in tumor angiogenesis and a potential target for diagnosis and therapy. J Clin Oncol. 2002;20:4368-80.
18. Cassidy J, Clarke S, Diaz-Rubio E, Scheithauer W, Figer A, Wong R, et al. Randomized phase iii study of capecitabine plus oxaliplatin compared with fluorouracil/folinic acid plus oxaliplatin as first-line therapy for metastatic colorectal cancer. J CLin Oncol. 2008;26:2006-12.
19. Van Cutsen E, Kohne C S, Hitre E, Zaluski J, Chang Chien CR, Makhson A, et al. Cetuximab and chemotherapy as initial management of metastatic colorectal cancer. N Eng J Med. 2009;360:1408-17.
20. Van Cutsem E, Tabernero J, Lakomy R, Prenen H, Prausová J, Macarulla T, et al. Addition of aflibercept to fluorouracil, leucovorin, and irinotecan improves survival in a phase III randomized trial in patients with metastatic colorectal cancer previously treated with an oxaliplatin-based regimen. J Clin Oncol. 2012;30:3499-506.
21. Grothey A, Van Cutsem E, Sobrero A, Siena S, Falcone A, Ychou M, et al. Regorafenib monotherapy for previously treated metastatic colorectal cancer (CORRECT): an international, multicentre, randomised, placebo-controlled, phase 3 trial. Lancet. 2013; 381:303-12.
22. Llovet JM, Ricc S, Mazzafero V, et al. Sorafenib in advanced hepatocellular carcinoma. N Eng J Med. 2008;359:378-90.
23. Bang YJ, Cutsem EV, Feverreisolva A, Chung HC, Shen L, Sawaki A, et al. Trastuzumab in combination with chemotherapy versus chemotherapy alone for treatment of HER2-positive advanced gastric or gastro-oesophageal junction cancer (ToGA): a phase 3, open-label, randomised controlled trial. The Lancet. 2010;376:687-97.
24. Moore MJ, Goldstein D, Hamm J, Figer A, Hecht JR, Gallinger S, et al. Erlotinib plus gemcitabine compared with gemcitabine alone in patients with advanced pancreatic cancer: a phase III trial of the National Cancer Institute of Canada Clinical Trials Group. J Clin Oncol. 2007;25:1960-6.
25. Chu E, DeVita TV (Eds). Physician's Cancer Chemotherapy Drug Manual, 2008. Jones and Bartlet Publishers. http://johnjhaddad.weebly.com/uploads/2/5/2/0/2520519/physician's cancer chemotherapy drug manual 2008 (pdf accessesd 24.9.14).
26. Valle JW, Wasan HS, Palmer DD, Cunningham D, Anthoney A, Maraveyas A, et al. Cisplatin plus gemcitabine versus gemcitabine for biliary tract cancer. N Engl J Med. 2010;362:1273-81.
27. Sharma A, Dwary AD, Mohanti BK, Deo SV, Pal S, Sreenivas S, et al. Best supportive care compared with chemotherapy for unresectable gallbladder cancer: a randomized controlled study. J Clin Oncol. 2010;28:4581-6.
28. Macdonald JS, Smalley SR, Benedetti J, Hundahl SA, Estes NC, Stemmermann GN, et al. Chemoradiotherapy after surgery compared with surgery alone for adenocarcinoma of the stomach or gastroesophageal junction. N Engl J Med. 2001;345:725-30.
29. O'Connell MJ, Malliard JA, Kahn MJ, Macdonald JS, Haller DG, Mayer RJ, et al. Controlled trial of fluorouracil and low-dose leucovorin given for 6 months as postoperative adjuvant therapy for colon cancer. J Clin Oncol. 1997;15:246-50.
30. Andre T, Boni C, Mounedji-Boudiaf L, et al. Oxaliplatin, fluorouracil, and leucovorin as adjuvant treatment for colon cancer. N Eng J Med. 2004;350:2343-51.
31. Schmoll H, Cartwright T, Tabernero J, Nowacki MP, Figer A, Maroun J, et al. Phase III trial of capecitabine plus oxaliplatin as adjuvant adjuvant therapy for stage III colon cancer: a planned safety analysis in 1,864 patients. J Clin Oncol. 2007;25:102-9.
32. Twelves C, Wong A, Nowacki NP, Abt M, Burris H 3rd, Carrato A, et al. Capecitabine as adjuvant treatment of stage III colon cancer. N Eng J Med. 2005;352:2696-704.
33. Andre T, Louvet C, Maindrault-Goebel F, Couteau C, Mabro M, Lotz JP, et al. CPT-11 (irinotecan) addition to bimonthly, high-dose leucovorin and bolus and continuous-infusion 5-fluorouracil (FOLFIRI) for pretreated metastatic colorectal cancer. GERCOR. Eur J Cancer. 1999;35:1343-7.
34. Fuchs CS, Marshall J, Mitchell E, Wierzbicki R, Ganju V, Jeffery M, et al. Randomized, controlled trial of irinotecan plus infusional, bolus, or oral fluoropyrimidines in first-line treatment of metastatic colorectal cancer: results from the BICC-C Study. J Clin Oncol. 2007;25:4779-86.
35. Goldberg RM, Tabah-Fisch I, Bleiberg H, de Gramont A, Tournigand C, Andre T, et al. Pooled analysis of safety and efficacy of oxaliplatin plus fluorouracil/leucovorin administered bimonthly in elderly patients with colorectal cancer. J Clin Oncol. 2006;24:4085-91.
36. Tournigard C, Andre T, Achille E, Lledo G, Flesh M, Mery-Mignard D, et al. FOLFIRI followed by FOLFOX6 or the reverse sequence in advanced colorectal cancer: a randomized GERCOR study. J Clin Oncol. 2004;22:229-37.
37. Diaz-Rubio E, Tabernero J, Gomez-Espana A, Massutí B, Sastre J, Chaves M, et al. Phase III study of capecitabine plus oxaliplatin compared with continuous-infusion fluorouracil plus oxaliplatin as first-line therapy in metastatic colorectal cancer: final report of the Spanish Cooperative Group for the Treatment of Digestive Tumors Trial. J Clin Oncol. 2007;25:4224-30.
38. Patt YZ, Lee FC, Liebmann JE, Diamandidis D, Eckhardt SG, Javle M, et al. Capecitabine plus 3-weekly irinotecan (XELIRI regimen) as first-line chemotherapy for metastatic colorectal cancer: phase II trial results. Am J CLin Oncol. 2007;30:350-7.
39. Giantonio BJ, Catalano PJ, Meropol NJ, O'Dwyer PJ, Mitchell EP, Alberts SR, et al. Bevacizumab in combination with oxaliplatin, fluorouracil, and leucovorin (FOLFOX4) for previously treated metastatic colorectal cancer: results from the Eastern Cooperative Oncology Group Study E3200. J Clin Oncol. 2007;25:1539-44.
40. Saltz LB, Clarke S, Diaz-Rubio E, Scheithauer W, Figer A, Wong R, et al. Bevacizumab in combination with oxaliplatin-based chemotherapy as first-line therapy in metastatic colorectal cancer: a randomized phase III study. J CLin Oncol. 2008;26:2013-9.
41. Tabernero J, Van Cutsem E, Diaz-Rubio E, Cervantes A, Humblet Y, André T, et al. Phase II trial of cetuximab in combination with fluorouracil, leucovorin, and oxaliplatin in the first-line treatment of metastatic colorectal cancer. J Clin Oncol. 2007;25:5225-32.
42. De Paoli A, Chiarra S, Luppi G, Friso ML, Beretta GD, Del Prete S, et al. Capecitabine in combination with preoperative

radiation therapy in locally advanced, resectable, rectal cancer: a multicentric phase II study. Ann Oncol. 2006:17:246-51.
43. Cunningham D, Allum WH, Stenning SP, Thompson JN, Van de Velde CJ, Nicolson M, et al. Perioperative chemotherapy versus surgery alone for resectable gastroesophageal cancer. N Eng J Med. 2006;355:11-20.
44. Bang YJ, Kim YW, yang HK, Chung HC, Park YK, Lee KH, et al. Adjuvant capecitabine and oxaliplatin for gastric cancer after D2 gastrectomy (CLASSIC): a phase 3 open-label, randomised controlled trial. Lancet. 2012;379:315-21.
45. Sharma A, Raina V, Lokeshwar N, Deo SV, Shukla NK, Mohanti BK. Phase II study of cisplatin, etoposide and paclitaxel in locally advanced or metastatic adenocarcinoma of gastric/ gastroesophageal junction. Indian J Cancer. 2006;43:16-9.
46. Herskovic A, Martz K, al-Sarraf M, Leichman L, Brindle J, Vaitkevicius V, et al. Combined chemotherapy and radiotherapy compared with radiotherapy alone in patients with cancer of the esophagus. N Eng J Med. 1992;326:1593-8.
47. Bölke E, Peiper M, Budach W. Capecitabine and oxaliplatin for advanced esophagogastric cancer. N Eng J Med. 2008;358:1965.
48. Ilson DH, Forastiere A, Aequette M, Costa F, Heelan R, Huang Y, et al. A phase II trial of paclitaxel and cisplatin in patients with advanced carcinoma of the esophagus. Cancer J. 2000;6:316-23.
49. Meerten E, Muller K, Tilanus HW, Siersema PD, Eijkenboom WM, van Dekken H, et al. Neoadjuvant concurrent chemoradiation with weekly paclitaxel and carboplatin for patients with oesophageal cancer: a phase II study. Br J Cancer. 2006;94:1389-94.
50. Oettle H, Post S, Neuhaus P, Gellert K, Langrehr J, Ridwelski K, et al. Adjuvant chemotherapy with gemcitabine vs observation in patients undergoing curative-intent resection of pancreatic cancer: a randomized controlled trial. JAMA. 2007;297:267-77.
51. Neoptolemos JP, Stocken DD, Bassi C, Ghaneh P, Cunningham D, Goldstein D, et al. Adjuvant chemotherapy with fluorouracil plus folinic acid vs gemcitabine following pancreatic cancer resection: a randomized controlled trial. JAMA. 2010;304:1073-81.
52. Neoptolemos JP, Stocken DD, Friess H, Bassi C, Dunn JA, Hickey H, et al. A randomized trial of chemoradiotherapy and chemotherapy after resection of pancreatic cancer. N Eng J Med. 2004;350:1200-10.
53. Burris HA 3rd, Moore MJ, Andersen J, Green MR, Rothenberg ML, Modiano MR, et al. Improvements in survival and clinical benefit with gemcitabine as first-line therapy for patients with advanced pancreas cancer: a randomized trial. J Clin Oncol. 1997;15:2403-13.
54. Heinemann V, Quietzsch D, Gieseler F, Gonnermann M, Schönekäs H, Rost A, et al. Randomized phase III trial of gemcitabine plus cisplatin compared with gemcitabine alone in advanced pancreatic cancer. J Clin Oncol. 2006;24:3946-52.
55. Conroy T, Desseigne F, Ychou M, Bouché O, Guimbaud R, Bécouarn Y, et al. FOLFIRINOX versus gemcitabine for metastatic pancreatic cancer. N Engl J Med. 2011;364:1817-25.
56. Von Hoff DD, Ervin T, Arena FP, Chiorean G, Infante J, Moore M, et al. Increased survival in pancreatic cancer with nab-paclitaxel plus gemcitabine. N Eng J Med 2013; 369: 1691-1703.

CHAPTER 7

Nutritional Support to Hospitalized Patients

Umesh Kapil, Namrata Singh

Malnutrition in hospitalized patients is associated with higher infection and complication rate,[1-4] increased muscle loss,[4-6] delayed wound healing,[2,7] longer hospital stay[8-10] with increased morbidity and mortality.[11-15] The nutrition support to a hospitalized patient is an area about which all physicians should have an adequate knowledge. This chapter focuses on: (1) basic concepts in nutrition, (2) assessment of nutritional status of hospitalized patients, (3) nutritional requirements of the hospitalized patients and (4) nutritional support to be provided to the hospitalized patients.

The guidelines mentioned in this chapter are essentially aimed for "Adult patients who are ambulatory, not critically ill and are not suffering from any specific major disease" which could lead to adverse outcome.

BASIC CONCEPTS IN NUTRITION

Nutrition is the study of assimilation of food by living organism and its utilization for growth and maintenance of the tissues. It is also defined as the science of food where action, interaction and balance of food, nutrients and other substances are studied in relation to health and disease. In general, it is the study of the processes by which an organism ingests, digests, absorbs, transports and utilizes nutrients and disposes the end products.[16] Food consists of the nutrients which are utilized by the body for various biological functions. Nutrients are chemical substances found in the food which nourishes the body. Nutrients can be classified as macronutrients and micronutrients (MN).

Macronutrients

Macronutrients are the nutrients that provide energy to the body. These are needed in relatively larger amount on a daily basis ("Macro" means large). They are essential for maintenance of nutritional health and well-being of an individual. The key macronutrients are described hereunder.

Carbohydrate

Carbohydrates (CHOs) are sugars or polymers of sugars such as starch. These are hydrolyzed to simple sugars in the body by the action of digestive enzymes.[16] Food like glucose and canesugar are simple carbohydrates. Starch is a complex carbohydrate made up of glucose units. Glucose is the main source of energy for the body. This is derived from starch and other sugars in the diet.

Role of carbohydrates: (1) Carbohydrates are the most cost-effective sources of energy, (2) carbohydrates have a protein sparing action, i.e. they serve as a primary source of energy and thus spare utilization of protein for energy, (3) when there is an excess of carbohydrates in diet, additional energy gets stored as fat in the adipose tissues, which is utilized later, when the body needs energy, (4) glucose is the principal source of energy for the central nervous system (CNS) and heart muscle. *Sources of carbohydrates*: Cereals (wheat, rice, maize, *jowar*), pulses (Bengal gram, green gram, *rajmah*, peas), roots (carrot, radish, beet root), tubers (potato, onion, colocasia) and sugar are the common sources of carbohydrate. One gram of carbohydrate yields 4 kcal of energy.

Dietary Fiber

Dietary fiber (DF) is defined as indigestible carbohydrates present in the plant foods. It plays an important role in nutrition along with macronutrient and micronutrient. The DF is the sum of the polysaccharides and lignins which are not digested by the endogenous secretions (enzymes) of the human gastrointestinal tract (GIT). Depending upon its solubility in the water, DF is further divided into two categories: (1) insoluble dietary fiber (IDF) and (2) soluble dietary fiber (SDF). The sum of these two categories is known as total dietary fiber (TDF).[17]

Role of dietary fiber: (1) Foods with high DF, because of their consistency, encourage mastication of food and stimulate the secretion of digestive juices and improves digestion,[18] (2) DF lowers serum LDL cholesterol level,[19] (3) DF increases fecal bulk in the colon due to increased water retention property. DF also reduces transit time decreasing the contact time between carcinogen and intestinal mucosa. The conversion of sterols to carcinogenic polycyclic aromatic hydrocarbons occurs in colon. DF binds toxins, bile acids and carcinogens.[20] All these processes lead to reduced risk of bowel cancer. (4) DF has a beneficial role in weight reduction. It adds bulk to the diet. It leads to delay in emptying of the stomach which in turn stimulates the satiety center and thereby reduces the desire to have more food by the subject,[21,22] (5) DF reduces the rate of absorption of CHO and leads to slow increase in blood glucose levels.

Sources of dietary fiber: The common sources of DF are whole grain cereals (wheat, *bajra*, maize, *ragi*, brown rice), whole pulses and legumes (Bengal gram, green gram, green peas, black gram, lentil, *rajmah*), whole fruits (apple, guava, pomegranate, pear, dates, *amla*), vegetables (brinjal, cucumber, green peas, mustard leaves, spinach), nuts and oilseeds (almonds, sesame seeds) and fenugreek seeds (Appendix III).

Fat

Fat is composed of three elements: (1) carbon, (2) hydrogen and (3) oxygen (fat in liquid state at room temperature is known as oil). Dietary fat is of two types: (1) visible fat and (2) invisible fat. The visible fats are derived from animal fats (butter, ghee) and from vegetable oils (groundnut, mustard, coconut, safflower and *til* oil). Invisible fat are present in food but are not visible to naked eyes. The common food items containing invisible fats are nuts, oil seeds, cereals and pulses.

Role of fat: (1) Fat is a concentrated source of energy and consists of essential fatty acids. It is also required for the absorption of fat soluble vitamins (like A, D and E) and is an essential component of cell membranes, (2) Fat contributes to energy density of the diet, (3) fat deposited beneath the skin acts as an insulator and prevents the heat loss from the body, (4) fat enhances taste and flavor of the food, thereby increases the food intake by the subject.

Sources of fats: The common sources of fat are butter, ghee, vegetable oils, *vanaspathi*, groundnut etc. A small amount of fat is usually present as invisible fat in majority of foods. The visible fat and invisible fat contribute to the total fat intake in the diet. One gram of fat yields 9 kcal of energy.

Protein

Proteins are complex organic nitrogenous compound composed of carbon, hydrogen, oxygen, nitrogen and sulfur in varying amounts.[23] Proteins are essential constituent of tissues and cells of the body. Dietary protein is vital during growth when new tissues are being developed. Foods rich in protein are often called "body building foods". Protein derived from cereals is deficient in lysine but rich in methionine while the protein derived from pulses is deficient in methionine but rich in lysine. When rice and pulses are eaten together in a proportion of 5:1 (Rice:Pulses), they make a complete protein. The mix vegetable protein has a net protein utilization (NPU) of 65% relative to egg protein. NPU indicates the proportion of ingested protein that is retained in the body under specified conditions for the maintenance and/or growth of the tissues.[23]

Role of protein: (1) Proteins are the body building material and compensate the loss which occurs due to tissue breakdown, (2) proteins are required as antibodies which defend against infections and (3) proteins form an important constituent of muscles, connective tissue, immune bodies, blood-clotting factors, lipoproteins, visual pigments and other body tissues.

Sources of protein: The common plant sources are: wheat, soyabean, pulses, legumes, groundnut etc. The common animal sources are: chicken, meat, fish, egg, milk, cheese, curd, *paneer*, etc. On an average, cereals contain 7–13% of protein. Pulses contain 22–25% of protein. Dry fruits like almonds, cashew nut and pistachio contain 20–30% of protein. One gram of protein yields 4 kcal of energy.

Water

Water is a chemical compound consisting of two hydrogen and one oxygen atom. It is the main constituent of the human body. The total body water accounts for about 70% of the body mass in human adults.

Role of water: (1) Water helps in maintenance of body temperature. (2) Water is a source of dietary minerals such as calcium, magnesium, sodium, zinc, copper, iodide and fluoride. (iii) It is an important vehicle for excretion of metabolic products from the body.

Sources of water: Ground well, ponds, spring, tube well, rivers and other water bodies. Water is also present in many food items.

Micronutrients

Micronutrients (MN) are nutrients which are required in smaller amounts by the body. MN are needed to be supplied through the diet. MN participate in many vital body functions and metabolic processes. MN include: vitamins and minerals.

Vitamins

Vitamins can be defined as organic substances necessary to carry out many vital functions in the body. Vitamins are utilized by the body to regulate various chemical processes. They participate in the utilization of the major nutrients like carbohydrates, fats and proteins. Vitamins do not directly yield energy but they act as energy-yielding catalysts. On the basis of their solubility, vitamins can be classified as: (1) fat soluble vitamins: vitamin-A (retinol), vitamin-D (cholecalciferol), vitamin-E (tocopherol) and vitamin-K (phylloquinone) and (2) water soluble vitamins: vitamin-B1 (thiamine), vitamin-B2 (riboflavin), vitamin B3 (niacin), biotin, vitamin-B5 (pantothenic acid), vitamin-B6 (pyridoxine), vitamin-B12 (cyanocobalamine), folate and vitamin-C (ascorbic acid).

Minerals

Minerals are chemical elements necessary for the maintenance of essential functions of the body. Minerals form an integral part of structural components of the body and also act as catalytic agents in many metabolic processes. The common minerals of human importance are calcium, iron, iodine, phosphorus, magnesium, sodium, potassium, zinc, fluorine, copper, chromium and selenium.

POINTS TO REMEMBER

- Nutrition is a prerequisite to sustain life
- 1 g of CHO yields 4 kcal of energy:
  - 1 g of protein yields 4 kcal of energy
  - 1 g of fat yields 9 kcal of energy
- Fats and oils are concentrated source of energy
- 100 g of cereals provides 330–360 kcal of energy
- 100 g of pulses provides 320–370 kcal of energy.

Balanced Diet

Balanced diet contains different types of foods in such quantities and proportions so that the need for energy, proteins, vitamins, minerals and other nutrients is adequately fulfilled and a small provision is made for extra nutrients to withstand short duration of leanness.[16] A balanced diet should comprise foods from all the five food groups namely: (1) cereals and their products, (2) pulses and legumes, (3) milk and meat products, (4) fruits and vegetables and (5) fats and sugar. In a balanced diet, the energy should be derived in the following proportion: (1) carbohydrates—50-60%, (2) protein—10-15% and (3) fats—20-30% (half from visible and the other half from invisible fat).[24] A balanced diet should be planned in such a manner that recommended dietary allowances (RDAs) for specific age and gender are fulfilled. Indian traditional diet consisting of cereals, pulses, seasonal vegetables and fruits consumed in adequate quantity provides all the essential nutrients including CHO, protein, fat, minerals and vitamins.

Recommended Dietary Allowance

The recommended dietary allowance (RDA) is an average daily intake level of dietary nutrients, which meets the nutrient requirements of nearly all healthy individuals commensurate with their life stage and gender group in a given population. The RDA for energy is calculated by estimating basal metabolic rate (BMR). BMR is the amount of energy required to carry out the involuntary work of the body. It includes functional activities of the various organs such as brain, liver, lungs, heart and kidney, and the secretory activities of glands, peristaltic movement of GIT, oxidation occurring in tissue, maintenance of muscle tone and body temperature.[16] The total energy requirement (TER) is calculated by multiplying the BMR with the physical activity level (PAL) factor. RDA includes a safety margin to cover differences between individuals, dietary traditions and practices. The RDAs for adult Indian population is given in Appendix I.

For hospitalized patients, it is necessary to assess TER based on age and gender so that the nutrition support can be provided accordingly.[25]

NUTRITIONAL SUPPORT FOR PATIENT ADMITTED IN A HOSPITAL

Hospital Malnutrition is associated with increased morbidity and mortality; prolonged hospital stay and hospital costs; and increased risk of infections, delayed wound healing, impaired respiratory function, electrolyte disturbances and postoperative complications. Nutritional status can decline significantly during the course of a patient's stay in the hospital, due to a combination of reduced nutrition intake by the patient and/or increased requirements secondary to the impact of the disease process. The concept of nutritional support services was initiated in 1970. Since then, a large body of evidence has been collected to establish the benefits of nutritional support to the hospitalized patients in outcome of the disease process. The following three steps are recommended to establish nutritional support for each patient admitted to the hospital:

1. Assessment of nutritional status
2. Assessment of the energy requirements
3. Determining the type of diets/nutrition support to be given and mode of its administration.

Assessment of Nutritional Status

The assessment of nutritional status of the subject should be undertaken by utilizing simple indicators. These can be assessed as a part of routine clinical care after the patient is admitted to the hospital. The objectives of nutritional assessment are: (1) to assess the energy requirements, (2) To decide the type of nutrition support to be provided, (3) to quantify the malnutrition, (4) to determine the type of diets/nutrition support to be given and mode of its administration and (5) to monitor the efficacy of the nutritional support.[26] The following parameters may be used for assessment of nutritional status.

Body Weight

It is the best indicator of the nutritional assessment as it is sensitive to changes in the nutritional status. It indicates the body mass and is a composite index of all body nutrients like water, minerals, fat, protein, CHO, etc. It is essential to remember that body weight include both fat mass and fat free mass. The fat free mass (cell mass) represents the active metabolizing tissue and therefore a better measure of depletion than whole body weight. It reflects both past (chronic) and/or present (acute) undernutrition. Short-term changes reflect changes in fluid balance while long-term changes reflect in tissue mass provided no edema or fluid shifts are present. Weight in relation to height, i.e. weight for height provides a simple indicator of nutritional status. For the hospitalized patients who are bedridden and unable to stand, the bed scales are available incorporating a weighing sling to determine the weight. The individual is positioned comfortably in the weighing sling, and the sling is raised slowly until the individual is fully suspended.[27] The sequential measurement of bodyweight during the course of hospitalization is an indicator of change in the nutritional status. Hence, it should be undertaken during the course of the patient's stay in the hospital. The change in body weight can be calculated by comparing the present weight with the pre-illness weight.

a. The standard weight of the patient in kilogram can be calculated using Broca's index which is as follows: Height of the subject in centimeters minus 100.

   For example a subject with height of 176 cm, using Broca's index. The standard weight of the subject should be 76 kg.

$$176 - 100 = 76$$

b. The percent ideal body weight (IBW) can be calculated by the following formula:

$$\frac{\text{Actual body weight} \times 100}{\text{Standard body weight}}$$

Interpretation of IBW can be done with following cutoffs: (1) mild malnutrition—80-90%, (2) moderate malnutrition—70-79%, (3) severe malnutrition—less than 69%, (4) overweight—110-120%, (5) obese—more than or equal to 130% and (6) morbidly obese—more than or equal to 200%.

c. During the course of hospital stay, the patient's body weight should be sequentially monitored. The percent body weight change can be calculated by following formulas:

$$\text{Percent body change weight} = \frac{\text{Usual body weight} - \text{Actual current body weight}}{\text{Usual body weight}} \times 100$$

The degree of loss of weight with respect to duration of hospital stay can be interpreted as per the Table 1:[28]

The body weight before the onset of the illness should be recorded by the recall of the body weight by the patient or this can be obtained from the records of the outpatient department. The pre-illness body weight is recorded and compared with the present weight of the hospitalized patient. This would reflect the current nutritional status of the patient.

Height

The height of an individual is influenced both by the genetic and environmental factors. It is a measure of achieved linear growth which indicates the past nutritional status. When a patient is unable to stand due to any disease condition, the knee height method is an appropriate method to calculate the height of the subject. It is measured with a sliding broad-blade caliper. In this method, the "bed fast patients" should lie supine (lying on the back), with the knee and ankle each bend at 90°. For this measurement, observer stands on the left side. Fixed blade of the caliper is placed under the heel of the foot and the movable blade lies snugly over the thigh about 4 cm proximal to patella. The shaft of the caliper passes over the lateral malleolus posterior to the head of the fibula and is parallel to the shaft of Tibia. Measurements are recorded to the nearest 0.1 cm, and two measurements taken in immediate succession should not vary more than 0.5 cm from each other.[27] The average of the two measurements provides height of the subject using the following equations (Fig. 1).[28]

Male: 64.19 – (0.04 × age of the patient) + (0.02 + knee height)
Females: 84.88 – (0.24 × age of the patient) + (1.83 + knee height)

Table 1: Impact of weight loss on nutritional risk

Duration of stay in hospital	*Significant weight loss (%)*	*Severe weight loss (%)*
1 week	1–2	>2
1 month	5	>5
3 months	7.5	>7.5
6 months	10	>10

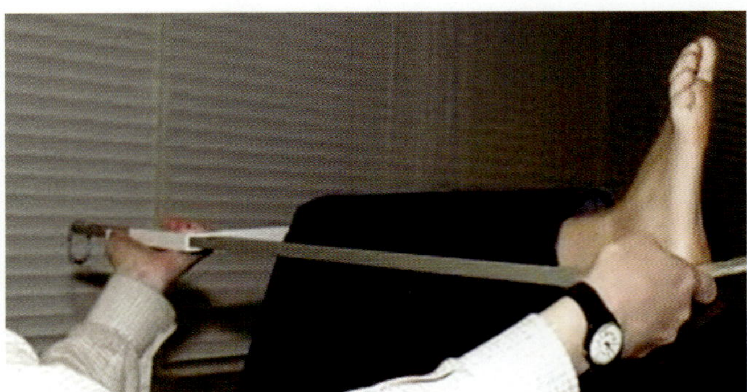

Figure 1 Knee height method

Body Mass Index (BMI) of the Patient

It is a simple indicator for estimation of nutritional status. The BMI is calculated by the following formula:

$$\text{BMI} = \frac{\text{Weight in kilograms}}{\text{Height in meters}^2}$$

The BMI cut-offs indicate nutritional status as follows: (1) severely malnourished—less than 16, (2) moderately malnourished—16.0-16.9, (3) mildly malnourished—17.0-18.4, (4) normal—18.5-24.9, (5) overweight—25.0-29.9, (6) obese (class I)—30.0-34.9, (7) obese (class II)—35.0-39.9 and (8) obese (class III)—≥40.[28] Although it is a valuable screening tool but may not be reliable especially when fat free mass is depleted while overall weight is normal due to increased fat mass.

Mid Upper Arm Circumference

The arm includes subcutaneous fat and muscle. A reduction in mid upper arm circumference (MUAC) reflects either a decrease in muscle mass or subcutaneous tissue, or both. Changes in MUAC measurements during the course of hospitalization are used to monitor progress of nutritional support,[29-31] correlating positively with changes in weight. MUAC measurements should be undertaken using a flexible, non-stretch tape made up of fiberglass. The measurement is taken to the nearest millimeter with a tape wrapped at the midpoint of the upper left arm, between the acromion process and the tip of olecranon.[32] It is a simpler measure than BMI, requiring minimum equipment and has been demonstrated to predict morbidity and mortality as accurately as underweight.[33] Measurements of MUAC are known to reflect changes in adult body weight.[34] MUAC is less affected than BMI by the localized accumulation (or removal) of excess fluid (pedal edema, periorbital edema, ascites). Thus, it is a more sensitive index of tissue atrophy than decrease in body weight. It is also relatively independent of height.[35] The standard reference values of MUAC for males and females are 27.7 mm and 21.1 mm, respectively.[36]

Skin-fold Thickness

The triceps skin-fold thickness (TSKFT) indicates subcutaneous fatness and thereby energy reserves of an individual. The depletion in subcutaneous fat indicates that the body is utilizing its reserve for meeting its energy requirements, which is not being met through the diet. The skin fold thickness can be measured by Harpendens skin fold calipers. Skin fold thickness is measured at several sites, and the assumption is made that the amount of fat stored subcutaneously at these sites (as measured by the skin fold thickness) will be representative of the total amount of body fat. Typically, skin fold thickness is determined at four sites: over the triceps muscle, over the biceps, in the subscapular region; and in the supra-iliac region. However, the TSKFT is the single best indicator of status of subcutaneous fat. The serial monitoring of TSKFT provides data on nutritional status of the subject over a period of time. The TSKFT values obtained are expressed as percentage of the reference standards and then compared with the standard values. The standard values of TSKFT for males and females are 12.5 mm and 16.5 mm[37] respectively. Based on the percentage of standard obtained of the TSKFT, the subject is categorized in following grades of malnutrition: (1) mild deficit—more than 90%, (2) moderate deficit—60–90% and (3) severe deficit—less than 60%.[38]

The percent of standard of TSKFT can be calculated by the following formula:

$$\frac{\text{Measurement obtained}}{\text{Standard}} \times 100$$

Clinical Nutritional Examination

The subject is examined from head to toe for the presence of clinical signs of nutritional deficiencies. The following signs may be assessed routinely in adults:

- Conjuctival pallor, pallor of palm/sole and spoon shaped nails: Indicative of anemia.
- Pale skin: Indicative of biotin, folic acid, vitamin B6 and iron deficiencies.
- Glossitis, angular stomatitis, cheilosis (cracked lips and corners of the mouth), fissured tongue: Indicative of vitamin B-complex deficiencies.
- Gingivitis (bleeding gums): Indicative of vitamin C deficiency.
- Magenta color tongue: Indicative of Vitamin B2 deficiency.
- Edema: Indicative of vitamin B6 and zinc deficiency, severe undernutrition.

Current Dietary Intake of the Nutrients

The routine dietary intake of a subject reflects the adequacy of nutrients consumed by the subject. Most common method utilized to assess the intake of nutrients is 24 hour-dietary recall method. Under this method the subject is inquired about raw and cooked foods consumed during the last 24-hours since the time of interview. The amount of cooked food consumed by the subject is converted to the raw amount. The nutritive value of the raw foods is calculated with the help of data published by ICMR on nutritive value of Indian foods and nutrient intake in last 24-hours is calculated. The data on intake of nutrients helps in advising the subject to consume a balanced diet. It also helps in predicting whether the nutritional status of patients is likely to improve or deteriorate. This method is useful in managing patients who are at risk to develop malnutrition.

Laboratory Investigations

The laboratory tests are undertaken to determine the status of individual nutrients in a subject. These can be measured by their individual or metabolite concentration in blood or urine. The common laboratory examinations for hospitalized patients which can be done are:

Hemoglobin: Hemoglobin is the iron containing oxygen transport metalloprotein in the red blood cells.[37] Hemoglobin estimation is an important test and useful index of the overall nutritional status. Besides anemia, it also determines status of protein and trace element in the body. A subject whose hemoglobin level is below 12 g/dL of blood is considered anemic. Deficiency of nutrients like iron, folate and vitamin B12 is a common cause of Anemia.[39]

Serum prealbumin: It is synthesized in the liver and partially catabolized in the kidneys. Its concentration decreases in protein-energy malnutrition and is restored to normal levels upon nutritional repletion. The half-life of the prealbumin is 2–3 days. Hence it responds rapidly to protein deprivation and also responds quickly with nutrition support. It is a sensitive indicator of nutritional status. Its normal values range 15.7–29.6 mg/dL. Serum values between 10–15 mg/dL show mild visceral depletion, between 5–10 mg/dL moderate visceral depletion and values less than 5 mg/dL show severe depletion. The serum albumin concentration does not reflect acute changes in food intake over a short period of time as it has a long half-life of 18–21 days. Moreover, it is a marker of inflammation.

Transferrin: Although transferrin has shorter half-life (7 days), it again reflects inflammation. It decreases during inflammation while rises in patients with iron deficiency anemia. Level less than 200 mg/mL indicate malnutrition.

Plasma creatinine: It reflects hydration status and muscle mass. It is low in patients with low muscle mass. Urinary excretion of creatinine is measure of muscle mass in patients with stable renal function.

Nitrogen balance: It is a precise measure whether the organism is anabolic or catabolic. In severely ill patients it is difficult to measure a reliable balance because various factors interplay like unaccounted loss from wound and use of blood and its product. It is predominantly used as research tool.

Delayed hypersensitivity skin test: It reflects cell mediated immunity. The response to intradermal injection with various antigens is mainly used in research setting. Lymphocyte counts less than 1,500 cell/mm^3 are considered to indicate undernutrition.

Functional Test

Hand dynamometry measures the voluntary hand strength which corresponds to the nutritional status and surgical outcome. It can be measured at the bedside and reflect the changes in muscle strength due to refeeding. It requires patient's cooperation. Direct muscle stimulation can be performed by electrical stimulation of adductor pollicis muscle in a non-cooperative patient.

Direct subjective global assessment (SGA) tool by Jeejeebhoy and Graham Hill classifies patients into three categories using a standardized questionnaire that incorporate the patient's history (food intake, complaints like vomiting, diarrhea and weight loss), physical examination and the clinician's overall judgment of the patient's nutritional status. It has great validity in elective situation but not in elderly patients.

Five features of patient's history are discussed here.

1. Weight loss in 6 months: Less than 5% small; 5–10% potentially significant; more than 10% definitely significant. The rate and pattern of patient's weight loss are considered.
2. Food consumption compared to a patient's usual pattern: Abnormal or normal. Duration and degree of abnormality.
3. Presence of abnormal gastrointestinal symptoms (anorexia, nausea, vomiting and diarrhea) persisting on daily basis for a period more than 2 weeks.
4. Functional capacity or energy level (bedridden to full energy).
5. Metabolic demands of the underlying disease state (low to high stress).

Four features of a physical examination are noted as normal, mild, moderate or severe:

1. Loss of subcutaneous fat in triceps region and at the level of lower ribs in mid-axillary line.
2. Muscle wasting in the deltoids and quadriceps.
3. Presence of edema in the ankles and sacral region.
4. Presence of ascites.

On the basis of these features of history and physical examination, the clinician subjectively identifies a rank to indicate a patient's nutritional status as—

SGA A: Well nourished; SGA B: Moderate or suspected malnutrition and SGA C: Severe malnutrition.

Malnutrition universal screening tool (MUST) established at consensus conferences of European Society of Enteral and Parenteral Nutrition is a tool adapted for special circumstances (when weight and height cannot be measured or there are fluid disturbances).

Calculation of the Energy Requirements

The nutrient requirements of the subject depend upon its TER. If adequate food is provided through the diet which can meet TER, generally the protein, carbohydrate, fat, vitamins and minerals requirements of a subject are met. The energy requirements of a subject can be assessed by the following two methods:

Calculation of TER (Method I)

Step I (Calculate the BMR): Based on the age, gender and weight of the subject, the BMR of the subject is calculated with help of the equations given in the Table 2.[25]

Step II (Assess the type of physical activities undertaken by the subject): The type of physical activity determines the energy requirements. The physical activities undertaken by an adult subject has been divided into three categories namely: (1) sedentary, (2) moderate and (3) heavy level of physical activity. The constant factor for each level of physical activity is: (1) sedentary—1.53, (2) moderate—1.8 and (3) heavy—2.3. Please see Appendix II for the detailed classification.

Step III (Assess the stress factors to which patient is exposed): Depending upon the medical condition of the patient, the stress factor of the subjects[40] should be determined based on the values given in the Table 3.

The TER of a subject can be calculated by utilizing the following formula:

TER = BMR × PAL value × Stress factor

Table 2: Equation for calculation of BMR (kcal expenditure/24 hour)

Gender	*Age (years)*	*Prediction equation*
Male	18–30	14.5 × Body weight (kg) + 645
	30–60	10.9 × Body weight (kg) + 833
	>60	12.6 × Body weight (kg) + 463
Female	18–30	14.0 × Body weight (kg) + 471
	30–60	8.1 × Body weight (kg) + 788
	>60	9.1 × Body weight (kg) + 565

Table 3: Stress factor to which patient is exposed

Patient condition		*Stress factor*
	Hospitalized patients without any stress	1.1
Infection	Fever	1.0 For 1°C increase in body temperature, add stress factor of 0.13
	Peritonitis	1.2–1.37
	Sepsis	1.4–1.8
Trauma	Soft tissue trauma	1.14–1.37
	Closed head injury	1.4–1.6
	Skeletal trauma	1.2–1.37
Burns	<20% total body surface area	1.0–1.5
	40% total body surface area	1.5–1.85
	100% total body surface area	1.5–2.05

Example: The TER of a 35-year-old male subject with a body weight of 60 kg and height of 172 cm with a sedentary level of physical activity and without any stress, admitted to the hospital can be calculated as follows:

Age = 35 years
Body weight = 60 kg
Height = 172 cm
PAL value = 1.53
Stress factor =1.1
BMR = 10.9 × Body weight (kg) + 833 (Take BMR values of male between 30–60 years as given in Table 2)
= 10.9 × 60 + 833
= 1,487 kcal
TER = BMR × PAL value × Stress factor
= 1,487 × 1.53 × 1.1
= 2,503 kcal (total energy requirement)

Calculation of TER (Method II)

Step I (Calculate the BMR of the subject): The BMR of the subject can be calculated by Harris and Benedict formula which is as follows:

Male BMR = 66.5 + 13.7 × weight (kg) + 5.0 × height (cm) - 6.75 × age (year)

$$\text{Female BMR} = 655.1 + 9.5 \times \text{weight (kg)} + 1.85 \times \text{height (cm)} - 4.67 \times \text{age (year)}$$

Step II [Assess the activity factor (AF)]: The AF determines the energy requirement of the subject. The type of activity undertaken by a subject is divided into three categories with a constant activity factor: (1) in bed—1.2, (2) in bed but mobile—1.25 and (3) mobile—1.3.

Step III [Asses the injury factor (IF)]: Depending upon the medical condition of the patient, the injury factor of the subject should be determined based on the values given in the Table 4.[28]

Step IV [Calculate the thermal factor (TF)]: The TF is for body temperature. It is determined by assessing the body temperature of the subject. The TF for various body temperatures is given in Table 5.

Based on the above steps, the TER of a subject can be calculated by utilizing the following formula:

$$\text{TER} = \text{BMR} \times \text{AF} \times \text{IF} \times \text{TF}$$ [28]

Example: The TER of a 35-year-old male subject with a body weight of 60 kg and height of 172 cm with a sedentary level of physical activity and without any stress, admitted to the hospital can be calculated as follows:

$$\begin{aligned} \text{Male BMR} &= 66.5 + 13.7 \times \text{weight (kg)} + 5.0 \times \text{height (cm)} - 6.75 \times \text{age (year)} \\ &= 66.5 + 13.7 \times 60 + 5.0 \times 172 - 6.75 \times 35 \\ &= 1{,}513 \text{ kcal} \\ \text{TER} &= \text{BMR} \times \text{AF} \times \text{IF} \times \text{TF} \\ &= 1{,}513 \times 1.25 \times 1.0 \times 1.1 \\ &= 2{,}080 \text{ kcal (total energy requirement)} \end{aligned}$$

The sources and proportions from which TER should be derived are as follows: (1) carbohydrates—50-60%, (2) protein—10-15% and (3) fats—20-30% (half from visible and other half from invisible fat).[24]

Table 4: Injury factor of the patient

Patient condition	*Injury factor (IF)*
Uncomplicated patients	1.0
Postoperative or cancer	1.1
Fracture	1.2
Sepsis	1.3
Polytrauma	1.6
Burns:	
30–50%	1.7
50–70%	1.8
70–90%	2.0

Table 5: Thermal factor for body temperature of the subject

Body temperature (oC)	*Thermal factor (TF)*
38	1.1
39	1.2
40	1.3
41	1.4

Type of Diets and Mode of their Administration

The type of diets and mode of their administration primarily depend upon the physical conditions and the type of disease from which a patient is suffering. As a golden rule, all patients should be given diets or nutritional support orally as it has limited side effects and toxicity. When the food is eaten orally, the body physiology regulates the absorption of the nutrients from GIT according to its requirements unlike when the nutrition support is given through parenteral route, in which the body physiology has limited role to play.

Oral Nutrition

The diet given to the hospitalized patients through mouth is called oral nutrition. Oral route is the best method for delivering diet or nutrition support to a hospitalized patient with a functional GIT.[41] This method can meet the energy requirements of the patient with fewer modifications in routine diet and is psychologically more acceptable by the patients. Majority of the patients can tolerate normal diet but few subjects require modifications in the consistency and texture of the diet.

Based upon the consistency, oral diet can be classified into three categories: (1) liquid diet, (2) semisolid diet and (3) soft diet.

Liquid diet can be further classified into: (1) clear liquid diet and (2) full fluid diet. A clear liquid diet is one which provides nutrients through an oral route in the form of a clear fluid. It leaves minimal residue in the GIT. It is used as an initial diet following surgery, or during acute gastrointestinal dysfunction. It is usually given for 3–4 days. A clear liquid diet is nutritionally adequate after addition of nutritional supplements.

A full fluid diet is given to patients with chewing difficulties. It is an intermediate diet before starting a solid diet after surgery or intravenous feeding. It is nutritionally adequate after addition of nutritional supplements. Once a patient starts tolerating liquid diet, he/she is progressed to semi-solid diet. A semi-solid diet is also known as pureed foods diet. It is given to patients in postoperative period. It includes foods which are high in protein but low in fat, fiber and energy. Scrambled egg, low-fat cottage cheese or lean meats can be blenderized and used for preparing semi-solid diet.

A soft diet is defined as a diet that consists of tender and soft foods that can be chewed more easily than those in a regular diet. The raw fruits, vegetables, whole grain cereals and pulses are not utilized for preparing soft diet. Soft diets are nutritionally adequate when a sufficient quantity and a variety of the nutrients are added. Main issues in developing oral nutrition support are given in the guidelines below which can be taken into account for planning the diet for a hospitalized patient:

- To increase the energy density of the diet, its fat content can be increased. The common Indian foods which have high content of fat are given in Appendix IV.
- The patients requiring tissue growth or suffering from burns and cancer are ones requiring high protein diet. They should be given foods with high protein content. The common Indian foods with high protein content are given in Appendix IV.
- The patients suffering from hypertension require diets with low sodium and high potassium. The sodium and potassium content of common Indian foods is given in Appendix V.
- The diabetic patients should be given diet made from foods with low glycemic index. The common Indian foods with low glycemic index are given in Appendix VI.

Enteral Nutrition

Definition: Enteral nutrition (EN) is the delivery of nutrition in the liquid form directly into the stomach/duodenum/jejunum. Nutrients are given through a tube or stoma directly into the stomach or small intestine, thus by passing the upper digestive tract. The nutritionally adequate feed containing protein, carbohydrate, fat, water, minerals and vitamins is administered.[42]

The GIT is the most effective method to feed a patient. If the patient has a functioning GIT with sufficient length and absorptive capacity, but is unable to meet his nutritional needs through oral route, then enteral nutrition therapy is the best mode to feed the patient.[43]

Routes of Administration

Short-term enteral nutrition which is administered to a patient for a period of less than 4 weeks is called a short-term enteral nutrition. It can be given through the following routes.

Nasogastric route: The site of administration is stomach. Feeding tubes which are inserted in the stomach are called "nasogastric" tubes (Fig. 2).[44]

Indications: Patients who are unable to consume adequate nutrition through oral route, e.g. patient intubated, sedated and patients in hypercatabolism state with partially functional GIT.[43]

Type of diet: The blenderized diet made from locally available food items like cereals, pulses, milk, egg, sugar, salt, oil, curd should be administered. The commercial preparations are also available; however, they are not cost effective as compared to blenderized diet made from locally available foods. Both the diets are equally effective.

Nasojejunal route and nasoduodenal route: In nasojejunal route, the site of administration is jejunum. A tube is inserted into the jejunum. It is called jejunal tube. In nasoduodenal route, duodenum is the site of administration (Figs 3 and 4).[44]

Indications: Functional GI tract with a proximal obstruction of upper GIT, inadequate gastric motility, esophageal reflux, upper GI surgery.[43]

Type of Diet: Same as for Nasogastric Route

Long term enteral nutrition: Enteral nutrition support which is administered for a longer duration, i.e. more than 4 weeks is called long-term enteral nutrition. This can be given through:

Gastrostomy: It is a surgical procedure for inserting a feeding tube into the stomach through the abdomen wall. The diet goes directly into the stomach (Fig. 5).

Indications: Head and neck cancers, malignant bowel obstruction including esophageal cancer, head injury, mechanical obstruction to swallowing, e.g. esophageal strictures, long-term intestinal malfunction requiring supplementary intake, e.g. cystic fibrosis, neurological disorders of swallowing (cerebral palsy, multiple sclerosis, parkinson's diseases, brain tumors, neonatal encephalopathy), Crohn's disease and burn patients.

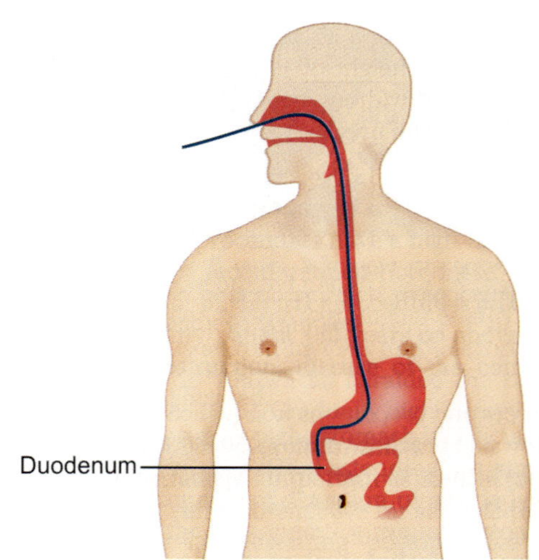

Figure 3 Nasoduodenal route

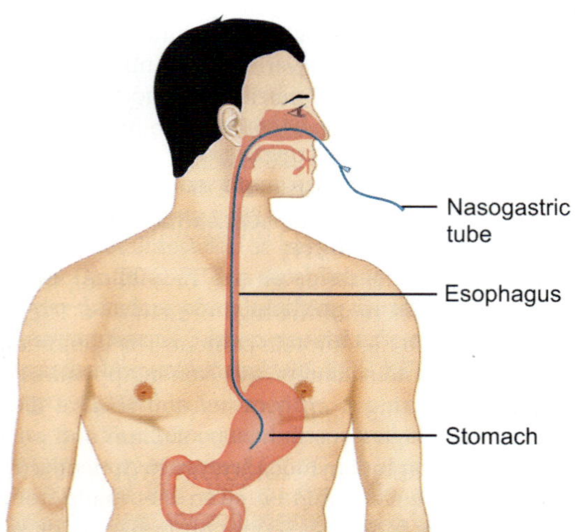

Figure 2 Nasogastric route

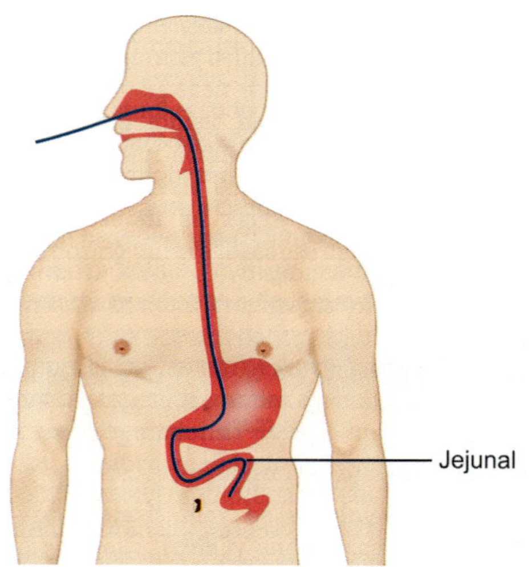

Figure 4 Nasojejunal route

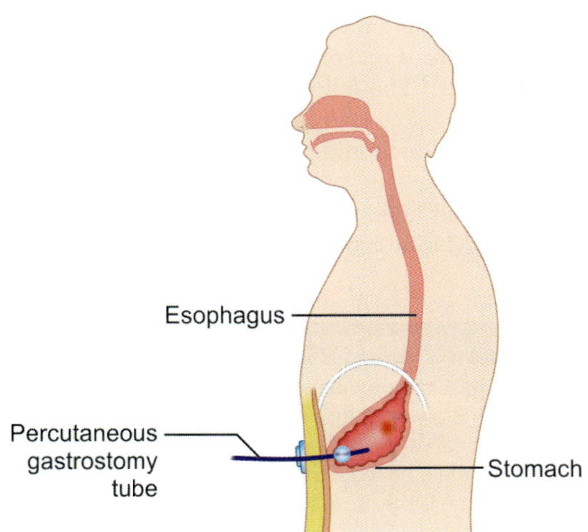

Figure 5 Gastrostomy

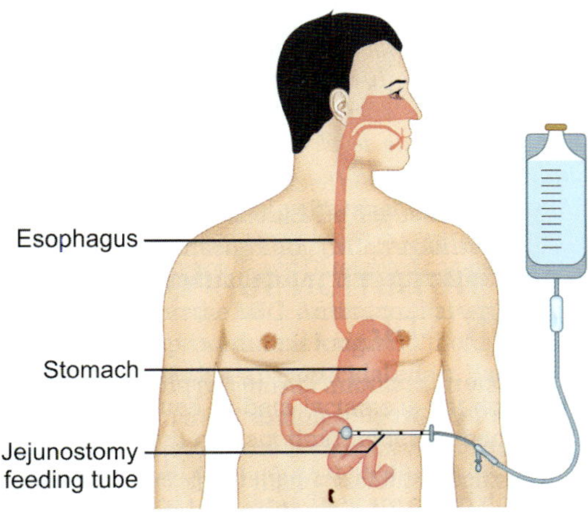

Figure 6 Jejunostomy

Type of Diet: Same as for Nasogastric Route

Jejunostomy: It is an artificial opening made by surgical procedure to the jejunum through the abdominal wall for feeding a patient. The feed goes directly into the jejunum (Fig. 6).

Indications: Functioning GI tract with an obstruction in the proximal jejunum (long term), upper GI stricture or fistula, inadequate gastric motility and long-term transpyloric feeding.[43]

Type of Diet: Same as for Nasogastric Route

Complications of enteral feeding: Many complications can be observed during enteral feeding. These may be tube related or due to feeding itself. *Tube related: insertion complications*: Failure of insertion and misplacement. Other common complications of insertion include peristomal infection, hemorrhage, peritonitis, colonic perforation and necrotizing fasciitis. *Accidental removal*: Nasoenteral feeding tubes are usually secured with adhesive tape to the patient's cheek. Still they are often removed accidentally either by patients or by staff. Gastrostomy and jejunostomy tubes, which are secured with sutures, are less often removed accidentally unless the sutures have cut through. *Tube blockage and damage*: Food precipitation leads to blockage especially in fine bore tubes. After every feed they should be flushed with saline. In case of blockage, they should be flushed with carbonated drinks. *Miscellaneous complications*: Feeding tubes may slip into the bowel lumen with peristalsis. They can also cause erosions and ulcers. *Gastrointestinal Complications: Gastrointestinal symptoms*: Nausea, abdominal bloating constipation or diarrhea are commonly seen. Diarrhea may be related to change of flora due to use of antibiotics. *Infection*: Milk and commercial feeds are an excellent growth medium for pathogenic organisms. Long time taken for these feeds to be delivered may lead to their contamination.[41] *Metabolic symptoms*: Hypertonic feed or rapid delivery may also lead to problems. Overhydration, hyperglycemia, hypertonic dehydration and electrolyte imbalance may occur. Vitamin and trace element deficiency and refeeding syndromes are also seen. *Aspiration*: The delivery of a large volume of feed into the stomach through a nasogastric tube or gastrostomy may result in reflux of feed into the esophagus and trachea and can lead to pulmonary aspiration.

Parenteral Nutrition

Definition: Parenteral nutrition (PN) refers to the administration of nutrients through intravenous route. This method of feeding may be required when the GIT is not functional, cannot be accessed, or the patient cannot be adequately nourished by oral or enteral route.[45] PN support is a relatively expensive treatment and is recommended which can only be justified for patients with specific diseases and indications.[45]

Indications: (1) Loss of functional bowel (massive small-bowel resection/short bowel syndrome, Crohn's disease, radiation enteritis, severe diarrhea, steatorrhea/malabsorption), (2) intestinal obstruction, paralytic ileus or intestinal pseudo-obstruction, (3) catabolic state when GIT is not usable or inability to obtain enteral access, (4) inability to provide sufficient nutrients/fluids enterally, (5) persistent GI hemorrhage, (6) prolonged fasting due to lengthy GI work-up, (7) enterocutaneous fistula, (8) trauma requiring repeat surgical procedures.[43]

Routes of Administration

Peripheral parenteral nutrition (PPN): This type of PN is administered through the small superficial veins of the extremities. The veins accessed to administer PPN are smaller in diameter therefore a lower concentration of nutrients (isotonic or slightly hypertonic solutions) solution is administered (Fig. 7).

Indications: (1) Patients requiring short-term (period <2 weeks) nutrition support, (2) patients who do not suffer from any fluid restrictions and (3) patients with increased nutritional requirements because of stress or malnutrition.

Type of diet: The type of nutritional support/diet to be given through PN cannot be prepared in the hospital. The nutrition support has to be procured from commercially available preparations, which consists dextrose, amino acids, fats, electrolytes, vitamins, trace elements, etc.

Central parenteral nutrition (CPN): CPN is the delivery of nutrients via central venous access.[46] CPN allows administration of nutrients in higher concentrations (hypertonic solutions) and in smaller fluid volumes as compared to PPN. CPN is administered into a vein with a large diameter such as superior vena cava. Dilution of hypertonic parenteral feeding formulation due to high

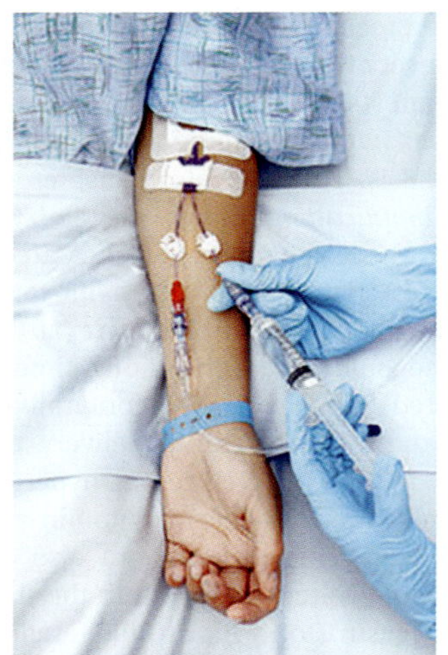

Figure 7 Peripheral parenteral nutrition

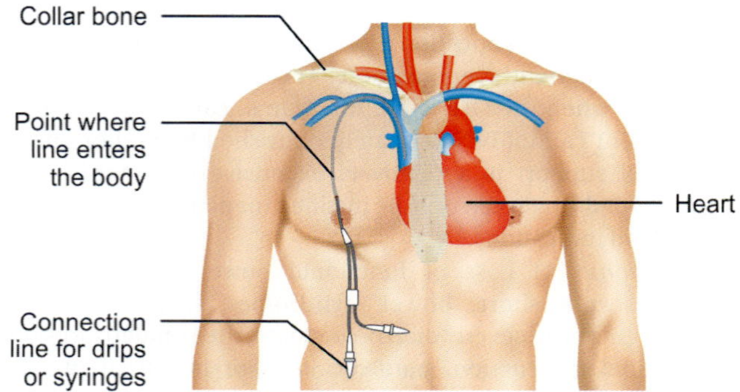

Figure 8 Central parenteral nutrition

blood flow minimizes the risk of complications associated with intravenous infusion of hypertonic solutions (Fig. 8).

Indications: (1) Patients requiring intravenous nutrition for period longer than 14 days, (2) patients with poor peripheral venous access and (3) patients who cannot be given large amounts of fluid due to primary condition such as congestive heart failure, chronic renal failure and hepatic failure. The type of diet in CPN is same as for PPN route.

Complications associated with parenteral nutrition: Potential complications of PN are metabolic complications (hyperglycemia), gastrointestinal complications (steatohepatitis, cholestasis), manganese toxicity, refeeding syndrome, infection/sepsis, metabolic bone disease.[43]

Monitoring nutritional support of hospitalized patients: enteral and parenteral nutrition: Patients receiving nutritional support need to be closely monitored. Metabolic parameters prior to the initiation of nutritional intervention should be done subsequently and periodically metabolic indicators should be monitored during nutritional therapy. Monitoring of daily nutrition helps in maintaining adequate calorie intake, detection of deficiencies, complications and nutrition losses. Vigilant fluid balance records are essential. Patients, who are at high risk for refeeding syndrome (acute intracellular shift of electrolytes as cell anabolism is stimulated) and other metabolic complications, should be monitored vigilantly. Prevention of refeeding syndrome is of utmost importance.[42] The following parameters should be given due consideration:

- The position and functioning of NG/NJ tubes should be checked before feeding.
- Gastrostomy and jejunostomy exit sites and erosions on the routes of NG/NJ tubes should be checked and care given each day.[47]

POINTS TO REMEMBER

- Oral feeding is best and provides complete nutrition.
- Enteral nutrition is given when a patient is unable to take food orally but has a functional GIT.
- Feeding tubes should be regularly cleaned to avoid tube blockage.
- Parenteral nutrition is the intravenous infusion of specialized nutrition solution.
- Regular monitoring is necessary to assess the success of the nutrition support.

Bluzby and the Veteran Affairs Total Parental Nutrition Cooperative study group found that 7–10 days of preoperative parental nutritional support followed by postoperative support could restore nutritional status to a intermediate level between severe malnutrition and normal individual. It might reduce the complication rate (Source: N Engl J Medicine. 1991;325:525).

STATUS OF NUTRITION SUPPORT SERVICES IN INDIA

Nutritional support services (NSS) in hospital settings should be a part of comprehensive and holistic patient management of the patient to ensure recovery and health outcomes. In India nutritional assessment of the hospitalized patients is not a routine practice and often malnutrition goes undiagnosed amongst patients. The critical issues in providing adequate nutritional support services to hospitalized patients are: (1) lack of education, training and awareness about benefits of nutrition support to physician, dietician, nurses and pharmacist, (2) inappropriate allocation of funds, (3) reluctance on the part of physicians to take advice from dieticians, (4) inappropriate quality of hospital food served to the patient's pilferage.[48] There is limited scientific evidence on status of nutritional support services in India. A study conducted on status of hospital malnutrition: a prospective evaluation of patients during hospitalization found that mean daily intake of energy amongst hospital patients was 819 kcal and that of protein was 22 g. During the course of hospitalization, 74% patients lost body weight. The mean weight loss was 2.13 kg. The timings at which the hospital food was served were not suitable to the patients. The patients often shared the served food with their attendants in the hospital.[49] Another study conducted to assess the nutrition support services in 50 hospitals attached medical colleges in different regions of the country documented that the dietician-to-patient ratio was 0.28 dieticians per 100 hospital beds. About 12% hospitals did not have any dietician. Only 64% of the hospitals had a dietetics department and 5% of the hospitals prepared disease specific therapeutic diets for the patients. The nursing staff did not participate in nutrition support services.[50]

Appendix I

Recommended Dietary Allowances for Indians

Group	Particulars	Body weight (kg)	Net Energy (kcal/d)	Protein (g/d)	Visible fat (g/d)	Calcium (mg/d)	Iron (mg/d)	Vitamin A (mg/d)		Thiamin (mg/d)	Riboflavin (mg/d)	Niacin (mg/d)	Pyridoxin (mg/d)	Ascorbic acid (mg/d)	Folate (mg/d)	Vit. B_{12} (mg/d)	Magnesium (mg/d)	Zinc (mg/d)
								Retinol	B-carotene									
Men	Sedentary work	60	2,320	60	25					1.2	1.4	16						
	Moderate work		2,730		30	600	17	600	4,800	1.4	1.6	18	2.0	40	200	1	340	12
	Heavy work		3,490		40					1.7	2.1	21						
Women	Sedentary work	55	1,900	55	20					1	1.1	12						
	Moderate work		2,230		25	600	21	600	4,800	1.1	1.3	14	2.0	40	200	1		10
	Heavy work		2,850		30					1.4	1.7	16						
	Pregnant woman		+350	82.2	30	1,200	35	800	6,400	+0.2	+0.3	+2	2.5	60	500	1.2	310	
	Lactation 0-6 months		+600	77.9	30	1,200	25	950	7,600	+0.3	+0.4	+4	2.5	80	300	1.5		12
	6-12 months		+520	70.2	30					+0.2	+0.3	+3	2.5					

Source: Dietary Guidelines for Indians, ICMR.

Appendix II

Classification of Physical Activities (Nutritive Value of Indian Foods, 2007)

Sedentary Activities of PAL Value of 1.53

Male: Teacher, tailor, doctor, driver, barber, executives, shoemaker, priest, retired personnel, landlord, postman, peon, etc.

Female: Teacher, tailor, executives, housewife, nurses, etc.

Moderate Activities of PAL Value of 1.8

Male: Fisherman, basket-maker, potter, goldsmith, agricultural labor, carpenter, mason, driver rickshaw-puller, electrician, fitter, turner, welder, industrial laborer, *cooli*, weaver, etc.

Female: Servant/maid, basket-maker, weaver, agricultural laborer, *beedi* maker, etc.

Heavy Activities of PAL Value of 2.3

Male: Intense manual work, stone-cutter, blacksmith, mine worker, woodcutter, gangman, etc.

Female: Stone cutter.

Appendix III

Approximate Range of Nutrient Contents of Various Food Groups (All values are per 100 g of edible portion)

S. no.	*Food groups*	*Energy (kcal)*	*Carbohydrates (g)*	*Protein (g)*	*Fat (g)*
1.	Cereal grains and products	245–352	52–79	6–12	0.4–2
2.	Pulses and legumes	323–432	16–61	7–43	0.1–20
3.	Vegetables				
	Leafy vegetables	26–49	2–6	2–5	0.1–1
	Roots and tubers	43–120	3–83	0.2–3	0.1–0.3
	Other vegetables	10–51	2–30	0.2–7	0.1–1
4.	Nuts and oil seeds	570–687	11–27	7–26	40–65
5.	Fruits	32–74	3–76	0.2–2	0.1–1
6.	Egg	173	-	13.3	13.3
7.	Milk and milk products	60–292	3–7.9	3.1–13.4	4–23
8.	Fats and edible oils	729–900	-	-	81–100
9.	Sugars	319–398	80–99	0.1–0.4	-

Source: Nutritive Value of Indian Foods, 2007.

Dietary Fiber Common Indian Foods (All values are per 100 g of edible portion)

S. No.	*Name of the foodstuff*	*TDF (g)*	*IDF (g)*	*SDF (g)*
Cereal grains and products:				
1.	Wheat (*Gehu*)	12.5	9.6	2.9
2.	Ragi	11.5	9.9	1.6
3.	*Bajra*	11.3	9.1	2.2
4.	Jowar	9.7	8.0	1.7
5.	Rice (*Chawal*)	4.1	3.2	0.9
Pulses and legumes:				
6.	Bengal gram (whole) (*Chola*)	28.3	25.2	3.1
7.	Red gram (whole)	22.6	19.8	2.8
8.	Black gram (whole)	20.3	15.4	4.9
9.	Bengal gram (*Chane-ki-daal*)	15.3	12.7	2.6
10.	Lentil (*Masoor daal*)	10.3	8.3	2.0
11.	Green gram (*Mung daal*)	8.2	6.5	1.7
Other vegetables:				
12.	Broad bean	8.9	6.7	2.1
13.	Peas, green	8.6	7.2	1.4
Fruits:				
14.	Guava (*Amrud*)	8.5	7.1	1.4
15.	Apple (*Sev*)	3.2	2.3	0.9
16.	Pomegranate (*Anar*)	2.8	2.3	0.5

Source: Nutritive Value of Indian Foods, 2007.

Abbreviations: TDF, total dietary fiber; IDF, insoluble dietary fiber; SDF, soluble dietary fiber

Note: Indian names in Hindi of the foodstuff are given in parentheses in italics.

Appendix IV

Common Indian Foods with High Calorie, Low Calorie, High Fat (≥25 g/100 g of edible portion) and High Protein (All values are per 100 g of edible portion)

Common Indian Foods with High Calorie Content		
S. No.	*Common Indian foods*	*Caloric content (kcal)/100g of edible portion*
1.	Ghee	900
2.	Butter (*Makhan*)	729
3.	Almond (*Badam*)	655
4.	Groundnut (*Moongphali*)	567
5.	Soyabean	432
6.	*Khoya*	421
7.	Sugar (*Chini*)	398
8.	Bengal gram daal (*Chane-ki-daal*)	372
9.	Milk buffalo's	117
10.	Banana (*Kela*)	116
11.	Mango (*Aam*)	74
Common Indian Foods with Low Calorie Content		
S. No.	*Common Indian foods*	*Caloric content (kcal)/100 g of edible portion*
1.	Butter milk (*Chach*)	15
2.	Skimmed milk	29
3.	Fruits	16–71
4.	Coconut water (*Nariyalpanni*)	24
5.	Other vegetables (*Sabjiyan*)	12–158
6.	Green leafy vegetables (*Haripattedar sabjiyan*)	30–97
7.	Peas green (*Matar*)	93
Common Indian Foods with High Fat Content (≥25 g/100 g of edible portion)		
S. No	*Common Indian foods*	*Fat content (g)/100 g of edible portion*
1.	Ghee	100
2.	Vanaspati	100
3.	Butter (*Makhan*)	81.0
4.	Walnut (*Akhrot*)	64.5
5.	Coconut dry (*Nariyal*)	62.3
6.	Almond (*Badam*)	58.9
7.	Pistachio nut (*Pista*)	53.5
8.	Cashewnut (*Kaju*)	46.9
9.	Groundnut (*Moongphali*)	40.1
10.	*Khoya*	31.2
11.	Cheese	25.1
Common Indian Foods with High Protein Content		
S. No.	*Common Indian foods*	*Protein content (g)/100 g of edible portion*
1.	Soyabean	43.2
2.	Chicken	25.9
3.	Groundnut (*Moongphali*)	25.3
4.	Lentil (*Masoor daal*)	25.1

Contd...

Contd...

Common Indian Foods with High Protein Content		
S. No.	*Common Indian foods*	*Protein content (g)/100 g of edible portion*
5.	Green gram daal (*moong daal*)	24.5
6.	Cheese	24.1
7.	Black gram daal (*urad daal*)	24.0
8.	Rajmah	22.9
9.	Bengal gram daal (*chane-ki-daal*)	20.8
10.	Almond (*badam*)	20.8
11.	Egg	13.3
12.	Milk	3.2

Source: Nutritive value of Indian foods, 2007.
(Indian names in Hindi of the foodstuff are given in parentheses)
Note: All the fries and processed foods like *samosa, mathri*, pastries, cakes, potato chips, etc. are rich in energy and should be avoided by people aiming for weight reduction and management.

Appendix V

Sodium and Potassium Content of Common Indian Foods (All values are per 100 g of edible portion)

Sodium Content of Common Indian Foods		
S. No.	*Common Indian foods*	*Sodium content (mg)/100 g of edible portion*
1.	Musk melon (*Kharbooza*)	104.6
2.	Fenugreek leaves (*Methi sag*)	76.1
3.	Milk cow's (*Doodh*)	73.0
4.	Spinach (*Palak*)	58.5
5.	Cauliflower (*Phulgobhi*)	53.0
6.	Banana (*Kela*)	36.6
7.	Carrot (*Gajar*)	35.6
8.	Pineapple (*Ananas*)	34.7
9.	Mutton	33.0
10.	Curd (*Dahi*)	32.0
11.	Redgram daal (*Arhar daal*)	28.5
12.	Apple (*Sev*)	28.0
13.	Watermelon (*Tarbuz*)	27.3
14.	Mango (*Aam*)	26.0
15.	Wheat flour (Whole) (*Gehu ka atta*)	20.0
16.	Rice flakes (*Poha*)	10.9
17.	Cucumber (*Kheera*)	10.2
18.	Pear (*Nashpati*)	6.1
19.	Papaya (*Papita*)	6.0
Potassium Content of Common Indian Foods		
S. No.	*Common Indian foods*	*Potassium content (mg)/100 g of edible portion*
1.	Green gram daal (*Mung daal*)	1,150
2.	Black gram daal (*Udad daal*)	800
3.	Lime sweet (*Mausambi*)	490

Contd...

Contd...

Potassium Content of Common Indian Foods		
S. No.	*Common Indian foods*	*Potassium content (mg)/100 g of edible portion*
4.	Amaranthus (*Chaulai sag*)	341
5.	Melon, musk (*Kharbooza*)	341
6.	Wheat, flour (Whole) (*Gehu ka atta*)	315
7.	Spinach (*Palak*)	206
8.	Brinjal (*Baingan*)	200
9.	Curd (cow's milk) (*Dahi*)	130
10.	French beans (*Gawar falli*)	120
11.	Carrot (*Gajar*)	108
12.	Milk, cow's (*Doodh*)	73

Source: Nutritive Value of Indian Foods, 2007.
(Indian names in Hindi of the foodstuff are given in parentheses)
Note: All the processed foods like pickles, sauces, cheese, salted butter, *namkeens, papads*, potato chips, etc. are rich in sodium and should be avoided by a person suffering from hypertension.
1 Teaspoon salt = 5 g of NaCl = 2 g.

Appendix VI
Glycemic Index of Common Indian Foods

S. No.	*Common Indian foods*	*Glycemic index*
1.	*Jowar*	110
2.	Semolina (*Suji*)	94
3.	Potato (*Aloo*)	85
4.	White rice (*Chawal*)	73
5.	White bread	70
6.	Brown rice (*Chawal*)	68
7.	Sugar (*Cheeni*)	65
8.	Whole wheat flour (*Chapatti*)	62
9.	Black gram (*Urad daal*)	61
10.	Rice (*Chawal*)	58
11.	Honey (*Shahad*)	58
12.	Banana (*Kela*)	55
13.	Green gram daal (*Moong daal*)	54
14.	Multigrain bread	53
15.	Curd (*Dahi*)	44
16.	Apple (*Sev*)	36
17.	Milk (*Doodh*)	27
18.	Rajmah	27
19.	Peanuts (*Moongfali*)	18
20.	Carrot (*Gajar*)	16

Appendix VII
Hospital Diet—Few Important Issues

The following points should be considered while planning diets for hospitalized patients:

i. Restrict food products prepared with processed grain (*maida* and *maida* products)
ii. Limit consumption of red meat and processed meat
iii. Avoid consumption of preserved foods high in salt and sugar
iv. Salt consumption should be restricted to less than 5 g/day
v Avoid intake of saturated fat
vi The subject should consume 5-6 meals/day. Small frequent meals should be provided
vii Promote consumption of fermented and germinated foods like sprouts as they are easy to digest and has an enhanced nutrient content.

In general, Hospitalized patients could consume the following foods liberally:

i Salads (uncooked vegetables)
ii Sprouts (whole pulses)
iii Roasted *channa*
iv Fruits
v Drinking water.

Some points to remember:

i. An attempt should be made to give dietary advice similar to routine diet consumed by patient before illness. Also, the dietary advice should be to eat the foods routinely prepared in the subject family
ii. Proper washing of fruits and vegetables before consuming
iii. Boiling, steaming and pressure-cooking should be preferred as a method of cooking over frying
iv. Eat food in a relaxed manner
v. Wash hands before eating.

ABBREVIATIONS

BMI—Body mass index
BMR—Basal metabolic rate
BW—Body weight
CPN—Central parenteral nutrition
CHO—Carbohydrates
Cm—Centimeter
CNS—Central nervous system
DF—Dietary fiber
EN—Enteral nutrition
FAO—Food and agricultural organization
GI—Gastrointestinal
GIT—Gastrointestinal tract
IBW—Ideal body weight
ICMR—Indian Council of Medical Research
IDF—Insoluble dietary fiber
kcal—Kilocalories
kg—Kilogram
LDL—Low density lipoprotein
MN—Micronutrients
NPU—Net protein utilization
NSS—Nutrition support services
PAL—Physical activity level
PN—Parenteral nutrition
PPN—Peripheral parenteral nutrition
RDA—Recommended dietary allowances
SDF—Soluble dietary fiber
TBSA—Total body surface area
TDF—Total dietary fiber
UNU—United Nations University
WHO—World Health Organization

GLOSSARY OF DEFINITIONS

Food: Anything which goes below our glottis. Food consists of nutrients.
Diet: The sum of food consumed by a person or other organism.
Catalyst: A substance, usually used in small amounts relative to the reactants, that modifies and increases the rate of a reaction without being consumed in the process.
Patient: A person who is under medical care or treatment.
Stress: It is the body's reaction to a change that requires a physical, mental or emotional adjustment or response.
Intravenous: Within or administered into a vein.
Anorexia: the symptom of poor appetite whatever the cause is.
Esophageal reflux: Chronic symptom of mucosal damage caused by stomach acid coming up from the stomach into the esophagus.
Fistula: It is an abnormal connection or track between two epithelium-lined organs or vessels that normally do not connect.
Necrosis: It is a form of cell injury that results in the premature death of cells in living tissue.
Enteritis: Enteritis is inflammation of the small intestine.
Cholestasis: It is a condition where bile cannot flow from the liver to the duodenum.
Malnutrition: It is a condition that occurs when a person's diet does not contain the right amount of nutrients.

REFERENCES

1. DiMaria-Ghalili RA. Changes in nutritional status and postoperative outcomes in elderly CABG patients. Biol Res Nurs. 2002;4:73-84.
2. Baldwin C, Parson TJ. Dietary advice and nutrition supplements in the management of illness-related malnutrition: a systematic review. Clin Nutr. 2004;23:1267-79.
3. Hoffer LJ. Clinical nutrition: 1. Protein-energy malnutrition in the inpatient. Can Med Assoc J. 2001;165:1345-9.
4. Chandra RK. Nutrition and the immune system: an introduction. Am J Clin Nutr. 1997;66:460S-3S.
5. Hill GL. Body composition research: implications for the practice of clinical nutrition. J Parenter Enteral Nutr. 1992;16:197-218.
6. Winter TA, Lemmer E, O'Keefe SDJ, Ogden JM. The effect of severe undernutrition, and subsequent refeeding on digestive function in human patients. Eur J Gastroenterol Hepatol. 2000;12:191-6.
7. Mechanick JI. Practical aspects of nutrition support for wound healing patients. Am J Surg. 2004;188:52-6.
8. Braunschweig C, Gomez S, Sheean PM. Impact of declines in nutritional status on outcomes in adult patients hospitalized for more than 7 days. J Am Diet Assoc. 2000;100:1316-22.
9. Gout BS, Barker LA, Crowe TC. Malnutrition identification, diagnosis and dietetic referrals: are we doing a good enough job. Nutr Diet. 2009;66:206-11.
10. Neumayer LA, Smout RJ, Horn HG, Horn SD. Early and sufficient feeding reduces length of stay and charges in surgical patients. J Surg Res. 2001;95:73-7.
11. Allison SP. The uses and limitations of nutritional support. Clin Nutr. 1992;11:319-30.
12. Holmes S. The effects of undernutrition in hospitalised patients. Nurs Stand. 2007;22:35-8.
13. Kubrack C, Jensen L. Malnutrition in acute care patients. Int J Nurs Stud. 2007;44:1036-54.
14. Allison SP. Malnutrition, disease and outcome. Nutrition. 2000;16:590-3.
15. Middleton MH, Nazarenko G, Nivison-Smith I, Smerdely P. Prevalence of malnutrition and 12-month incidence of mortality in two Sydney teaching hospitals. Int Med J. 2001;31:455-61.
16. Srilakshmi B. Dietetics, 6th edition. New Delhi: New Age International Publishers; 2011. pp. 189-90.
17. Gopalan C, Ramashahtri BV, Balasubramanian SC, Narasinga Rao BS, Deosthale YG, Pnat KC, et al. Nutritive Value of Indian Foods. New Delhi: Indian Council of Medical Research; 2007.
18. Leclere CL, Champ M, Boillot J, Guille G, Lecannu G, Molis C, et al. Role of viscous guar guam in lowering the glycemic response after a solid meal. Am J Nutr. 1994;59:914-21.
19. Glore SR, van Treeck D, Knehans AW, Guild M. Soluble fiber and serum lipids: a literature review. J Am Diet Assoc. 1994;94:425-36.
20. Reddy BS, Watanabe K, Sheinfil A. Effect of dietary wheat bran, alfalfa, pectin and carrageenan on plasma cholesterol and fecal bile acid and neutral sterol excretion in rats. J Nutr. 1980;110:1247-54.
21. Anderson JW, Tietyen-ClarkJ. Dietary fiber: hyperlipidemia, hypertension, and coronary heart disease. Am J Gasteroenterol. 1986;81:907-19.
22. WHO/FAO. Diet, nutrition and prevention of chronic diseases. WHO Technical Report Series 916; 2003. pp. 1-148.
23. Park K. Park's Textbook of Preventive and Social Medicine, 16th edition. Delhi: M/s Banarsidas Bhanot Publishers; 2000.
24. ICMR. Dietary guidelines for Indians. National Institute of Nutrition, Hyderabad, 2010.

25. ICMR. Nutrient Requirement and Recommended dietary allowances for Indians. A report to the expert group of the Indian Council of Medical Research, 2010.
26. Payne-James J. Artificial Nutrition Support in Clinical Practices, 1st edition. Edward Arnold, A division of Hodder Headline PLC; 1995. p. 128.
27. WHO Expert Committee Report. Physical Status: The Use and Interpretation of Anthropometry Physical Status. WHO Technical Report Series-854; 1995. pp. 396-7.
28. Joshi YK. Basics of Clinical Nutrition, 2nd edition. New Delhi: Jaypee Brothers Medical Publishers (P) Ltd.; 2008. pp. 36-56.
29. Hofvander Y, Eksmyr R. Changes in upper arm circumference and body weight in a 2-year follow-up of children in an applied nutrition programme in a representative Ethiopian highland village. Journal of Tropical Pediatrics. 1969;15:251-2.
30. Bray GA, Greenway FL, Molitch ME, Dahms WT, Atkinson RL, Hamilton K. Use of anthropometric measures to assess weight loss. American Journal of Clinical Nutrition. 1978;31:769-73.
31. Harries AD, Jones LA, Heatley RV, Newcombe RG, Rhodes J. Precision of anthropometric measurements: the value of midarm circumference. Clinical Nutrition. 1984;2:193-6.
32. Gibson RS. Principles of Nutritional Assessment, 1st edition. Oxford University Press; 1990.
33. Briend A, Garenne M, Maire B, Fontaine O, Dieng K. Nutritional status, age and survival: the muscle mass hypothesis. European Journal of Clinical Nutrition. 1989;43:715-6.
34. Ohlson MA, Biester A, Brewer WD, Hawthorne BE, Hutchinson MB. Anthropometry and nutritional status of adult women. Annals of Human Biology. 1956;28:89-202.
35. Olukoya AA. Identification of underweight women by measurement of arm circumference. International Journal of Gynecology and Obstetrics. 1990;31:231-5.
36. Frisancho AR. New norms of upper limbs fat and muscle area for assessment of nutritional status. Am J Clin Nutr. 1981;34:2540-5.
37. Jellife DB. The Assessment of the Nutritional Status of the Community, Geneva, World Health Organisation Monograph No. 53, 1966.
38. Maton, Anthea, Hopkins J, McLaughlin C, Johnson S, Warner M, et al. Englewood cliffs. New Jersey, USA: Prentice Hall. Human Biology and Health; 1993. ISBN O-13-981176.
39. Anjankar SP. Comparision of Haemoglobin Percentage and Nutritional Status of Post Graduate Girl Students Residing In Hostel, Rented Rooms and Home. Bioscience Discovery. 2012;3(2);243-50.
40. Slone DS. Nutritional support of the critically ill and injured patient. Critical Care Clinics. 2004;20:135-57.
41. Lloyd DAJ, Powell-Tuck J. Artificial nutrition: principles and practice of enteral feeding. Clinics in Colon and Rectal Surgery. 2004;17(2):107-18.
42. Bankhead R, Boullata J, Brantley S, Corkins M, Guenter, Krenitsky L. A.S.P.E.N. Enteral nutrition practice recommendations. Journal of Parenteral and Enteral Nutrition. 2009;33:122-67.
43. Department of nutrition services. Adult Enteral and Parenteral Nutrition Handbook, 5th edition. 2011. pp. 16-9.
44. Nilesh MR, Vilas PA, Ambadas JS, Sharadchandra MN. Formulation development of enteral nutrition products. International Research Journal of Pharmacy. 2011;2(3):19-28.
45. NSW Agency for Clinical Innovation. Parenteral Nutrition Pocketbook: For Adults. 2011, Accessed on www.health.nsw.gov.au/gmct.
46. Madsen H, Frankel EH. The Hitchhiker's guide to parenteral nutrition management for adult patients. Nutrition issues in Gastroenterology. 2006;40:46-68.
47. Enteral feeding. Accessed on www.patient.co.uk/doctor/Enteral-Feeding.html.
48. Sriram K. Suboptimal use of nutrition support services and products in India. Gastroenterology Today. 1998;2(4):249-50.
49. Kaul S, Kapil U, Joshi YK, Gupta MC, Acharya SK, Tandon BN. Hospital malnutrition: a prospective evaluation of patients during hospitalisation. Trop Gastroenterol. 1991;12(2):101-3.
50. Kapil U, Singh P, Singh, N. Status of nutrition support services in selected hospitals in India. Trop Gatroenterol. 2003;24(2):66-9.

CHAPTER 8

Statistics for Surgeons

Sreenivas

NUMBERS, DATA, INFORMATION AND VARIABLES

Numbers are pure numerical entities. They do not convey any meaning unless some units are attached to them. For example, 140 is pure number that does not convey anything to us on its own. But if we add some units, such as mm Hg or g/dL, they convey some idea about what we are talking about. If we say 140 mm Hg, one can guess that we are talking about the systolic blood pressure.

Data is a collection of raw, unorganized facts. Depending on the context, it could be simple or very complex. For example, the data on how many patients admitted in a trauma center undergo neurosurgery (yes or no) during a month is simple. On the other hand, if we collect some facts, such as gestation, birth weight, maternal and perinatal aspects, etc. associated with neonatal sepsis on daily basis among the neonates admitted in a neonatal intensive care unit (ICU) of large children's hospital, it could be complex. It is extremely difficult, if not impossible, to delineate meaningful interpretations from the data in its original form. We need to reorganize this "raw data" so that meaningful interpretations could be made. In addition, we may need to apply some analytical principles to make some conclusions about the meaningful interpretations that can be made after the reorganization of the data. When data is processed, organized, structured or presented in a given context so as to make it useful, it is called information. Intraocular pressure (IOP) of 34 mm is one piece of "data" from a patient of glaucoma. If we collect similar data from a set of patients, "process" that data and summarize that the average IOP among the glaucoma patients attending the clinic is 36 mm, it is information.

In any scientific research, we want to investigate phenomena that are not uniform across all subjects or situations. If the phenomenon of study is constant throughout without any change with respect to person to person, time to time or place to place, there is no need to "investigate". A mere observation of one subject will tell us what we want to know. Such phenomena are common in exact or pure sciences, such as physics, chemistry, etc. For example, Boyle's law stating that the product of pressure and volume of a gas at given temperature is constant is universally true whether we test it in India or Brazil. Entities that do not vary are called constants. We can find such many constants in physics, chemistry or mathematics. π is a constant indicating a relation between the circumference and diameter of a circle, earth's gravitational pull is a constant at a given altitude, etc. are examples of constants. Unfortunately, in biology or medicine, we rarely find such constants. We come across phenomena that are not fixed. Because there is variation, we need to study them empirically and come to an understanding about them. In this process, we deal with entities or characteristics that are not same for all subjects/patients. These entities or characteristics are called variables. Any given study can have one or more number of variables depending upon the type of investigation and objectives.

Variables that convey only a trait or an attribute are generally labeled as qualitative variables. They do not have any units of measurement. Blood group of patients, sex of the newborns and histological picture of a tumor are some such variables. These variables can further be categorized as nominal and ordinal. Nominal variables only convey the trait and there is no inherent grading or order. For example, blood group of patients can be of A, B, AB or O and there is no inherent hierarchy or order in these categories. So, it is a nominal variable. Other examples of nominal variables in clinical medicine could be etiology of the disease—infectious/alcoholic/idiopathic; histology of a tumor—squamous/adeno/other; smoking status of a patient—yes/no, etc. The other type of qualitative variables, the ordinal variable has some inherent hierarchy involved. Examples of such variables are stage of the disease—mild/moderate/severe; socioeconomic status—low/middle/high; educational achievement—illiterate/primary/middle/high school and above, etc. It can be noted there is an order in these categories as they convey some sense of increase or decrease in the phenomena being studied as the response category changes from one to another.

The other major type of variables is the quantitative variables. As the name suggests, they convey some quantity that is measureable and so they have some units of measurement. Systolic blood pressure (mm Hg), total serum albumin (mg/dL), glomerular filtration rate (mL/minutes), vitamin D (ng/dL), etc. are some examples of quantitative variables. Differences between values of a quantitative variable have numerical meaning. Like qualitative variables, quantitative variables are also of two types. Variables that can take any specific value within a given range are called continuous variables. For example, diastolic blood pressure can be any specific value, may be between 60 mm and 130 mm. It is for our convenience and practical purposes we measure it up to millimeters. In fact, the markings on a sphygmomanometer are of 2 mm that does not mean a subject's diastolic blood pressure can be 84 mm or 86 mm and no in between values possible. By the same token, if the reading shows as 88 mm, the exact pressure could be 87.9453 or 88.1423 or some such value close to 88. The phenomenon can take any value, but for practical convenience we measure it up to some convenient units. In the case of blood pressure, we take it up to millimeters. In case of serum vitamin D estimation, it could be nano grams. Because they can take any value in a continuous range, they are referred to as continuous variables.

The other type of quantitative variables is the countable variable. These variables convey the number of events, entities or persons of specific type. Examples of countable variables can be the cluster of differentiation 4 (CD4) count of a human immunodeficiency virus (HIV) patient, thin-layer chromatography (TLC) or platelets in a patient, number of days a patient stayed in the hospital after surgery, etc. As can be noted, these variables can take fixed values within a range but they cannot take any value between two consecutive integers. The CD4 count of a HIV patient can be either 254 or 255 but can never be 254.6 or 155.3, etc.

Generally, quantitative variables are more informative and amenable for in depth analyses than qualitative variables. Further, a quantitative variable can always be converted in to a qualitative variable, but vice versa is not possible. For example, birth weight of a newborn collected as exact weight in grams can be converted into a qualitative variable, low birth weight (yes/no) depending on the weight being less than 2500 g or not, at the time of analysis. If at the collection stage itself, it is recorded as normal/low birth weight, there is no way of knowing how many are with birth weight more than 2,000 g or 3,000 g or the average birth weight, etc. Further, the type of variables determines the type of analysis to be performed after the data collection. So it is important to decide at the planning stage itself what variables to collect and in what form.

Data is also referred to as primary and secondary. Data collected from the source by the investigators themselves is called primary data. Secondary data refers to the data collected by investigators other than the study investigators. Most of the clinical studies are based on primary data involving the investigators collecting the data on the patients attending their clinics. Data from large surveys such as national family health survey (NFHS), district level health survey (DLHS) and population census are good examples of secondary data which many investigators use for different purposes, once the official reports of these surveys are published.

TABULATION

As mentioned earlier, the raw data, as it is collected, is not useful to understand the messages that the data convey. We need to reorganize the raw data into form that is helpful to understand about the data itself. The first step in this process is tabulation of data. Tabulation of qualitative data is relatively simpler as involves only counting the number of observations of each type and expressing the frequency of each type in terms of percentages, etc. Tabulation of quantitative variables involves categorizing the study variable in to convenient ranges and then counting the number of observations within each range. The ranges are called the class intervals and the number of observations falling within each class interval is called the frequency of observations in that interval.

Tabulating the etiology of cirrhosis cases is an example of tabulation of a qualitative data. We simply count how many are of alcoholic etiology, viral etiology and cryptogenic and express these as proportions(%). Tabulating the age of these patients is an example of tabulating the quantitative data, as age is a quantitative variable. We divide the age into suitable ranges, such as above 20 years, 20–29 years, 30–39 years and above or equal to 40 years and within each of these intervals, count the number of cases whose age falls in the specific interval.

Once the tabulation is done, we are better placed to understand how many are of each type or where the maximum/minimum number lies, how many are above a specified limit, etc. These days personal computers and statistical software make the task of all statistical computing, including the tabulation quite easy.

AVERAGES

Tabulation, no doubt helps one to get some preliminary answers to our questions for which we collected the data. If we have two or more data sets, such as details of cirrhosis patients from two liver clinics, tabulation does not lead to good understanding with respect to the differences between the two data sets. This is more so when we deal with quantitative variables. In the example of age of cirrhosis cases, we may find high frequency of observations in one interval in the first data set, while high frequency may be observed in another interval in the second data set. Sometimes, the differences in the frequencies may not be so marked for any given interval, but small differences for each interval, with the direction of the differences changing interval to interval. The scenario becomes more complex, if we have more than two data sets. In view of these, comparison of the pattern or distribution of the study characteristic among the two data sets becomes difficult. Therefore, we need one index that tells about the characteristic we are interested in. These indices are called measures of "central tendency", as we wish to know about the core nature or the central value or the typical value of the whole data that can be considered as a representative of the total data.

The most common measure of central tendency is the average, also called as the arithmetic mean. It is calculated as the sum of all observations divided by the number of observations. For example, if the dual energy ratio of three cysteine stones in the urinary bladder were 1.2, 1.1 and 1.3, the average dual energy ratio would be $(1.2 + 1.1 + 1.3)/3 = 1.2$. Now, that we have only one index that is representative of the total data set, it is easy to compare such indices from different data sets to understand the similarities/dissimilarities among them.

The arithmetic mean or simply called mean is a good measure to indicate the typical value of the total data, more so if the number of observations is large (at least 30). Also, it is a good measure when the data distribution is symmetric. Data is said to have a symmetric distribution when the maximum frequency of observations is at a particular level and the frequencies of observations above and below that level gradually taper off as the difference from the maximum frequency level increases in either direction; and the frequencies away from the maximum frequency level are similar in either direction, for given difference from the maximum frequency level. If we erect bars, whose height is proportional to the frequencies at each level, the shape of the diagram looks like a bell. Much of the statistical theory is based on a bell-shaped distribution called normal distribution.

A variant of the arithmetic mean is the geometric mean. To put it simply, it is the arithmetic mean of the log values of individual observations in the original scale. After calculating the arithmetic mean on log values, we take the antilog so that the index calculated can have the original units of the variable. Geometric mean can be viewed in another perspective. If we have n observations in the sample, take the product of all n observations and the nth root of this product would be the geometric mean. It is often used in laboratory measurements, such as hepatitis B virus (HBV), viral load, etc. Taking the log transformation of individual values has another advantage as the distance between two specific values will be reduced and consequently the shape of the distribution will tend to be closer to then distribution. All results obtained on such transformed data are interpreted as though they are with the original scale.

Another measure of central tendency is the median. It is the middle most value, when the data is arranged in ascending or descending order. This measure is particularly useful to convey the typical value of the data set when the data shape is not symmetrical or skewed. If the distribution is skewed, there will be a few observations with very high value (positively skewed) or with very low values of the variable (negatively skewed). In such situations, arithmetic mean may be misleading. To convey this point let us consider the CD4 counts in HIV+ patients. Most of the HIV+ cases will have low CD4 counts, but there can be a few patients with high CD4 counts as well. The arithmetic average calculated from such data will be pulled towards the few high values, thereby making the representativeness questionable. But the median is not affected by these extreme values and so it would be a more reliable estimate of the central tendency. Therefore, it is important to understand the nature of the variable(s) that we deal with and also the nature of the data, before we start a formal analysis.

Another common measure of central tendency is the most frequent value observed in the data set. It is called mode. For example, if the ages of five colorectal cancer patients undergoing surgery were 65, 74, 59, 74 and 81, the modal age of such patients is 74 years as 74 occurred maximum number of times in the sample data. Sometimes, the dataset may not have any mode at all, as no repetition of any value of the variable could take place. Similarly, a dataset can have more than one mode as two or more specific values of the variable could occur with equal frequency. Because of its simplicity, mode can be easily understood. However, this measure is rarely used in clinical/medical applications.

MEASURES OF DISPERSION

Measures of central tendency help us to compare two or more data sets with respect to the typical value of the respective datasets. But to know completely about the dataset, a measure of central tendency alone is not enough. For example, consider the ages of five patients each undergoing gastrointestinal surgery and neurosurgery. Suppose the ages of five gastrointestinal surgery cases were 53, 58, 63, 68 and 73 and that of neurosurgery were 59, 61, 63, 65 and 67. If we calculate the average age of these two types of cases, it is the same 63 years. But looking at the raw data, we do understand that the ages of patients undergoing neurosurgery were closer to each other as compared to the ages of patients undergoing gastrointestinal surgery. In other words, the dispersion or the scatter of the values in one data set is different from the scatter in the other. When we want to know about a data, we cannot ignore this concept of variability or dispersion. Therefore, we need measures that can quantify the variation in any characteristic that we are interested in. These are called measures of variation or measures of dispersion and one measure called the standard deviation, is the most popular one. It quantifies the average distance (in either direction, positive or negative) of each observation for the arithmetic mean. A small value of standard deviation for a data set implies that each observation is close to the arithmetic mean or the values are close to each other. On the other hand, a large value of standard deviation implies there is greater scatter or dispersion in the data. Standard deviation also has the same units that the variable has. For example, if we say that birth weight of 16 newborns born on a particular day is 2250 g on the average with a standard deviation of 100 g, it implies that on the average, each of the 16 observations in the sample is 100 g away from the average birth weight of 2250 g. Naturally, the more the standard deviation, the more is the spread of values in the sample. So, a measure of central tendency (usually the arithmetic mean) and a measure of the variation (usually the standard deviation) are essential to convey about the behavior or nature of the variable under study. Generally, in medical literature, it is presented as mean ± standard deviation, 2250 ± 100 g in the birth weight example. Summary measures such mean, standard deviation and proportion are called parameters of the distribution of the variable.

STANDARD ERROR AND CONFIDENCE INTERVAL

We discussed how to summarize a variable in terms of its central tendency along with its measure of dispersion. Because of the variation in the phenomena, we want to know how likely we can get a similar summary measure if we repeat the study with similar sample size, type of subjects and evaluation methods. By repeated studies also, if we get similar summary measure, we can be confident of the result that we obtained. In the birth weights example, if we obtained the average birth weight of 16 newborns was 2250 g, we need to ascertain how this average would change if we repeat the study with another set of 16 newborns on another day in the same clinic. If the average value obtained on the second occasion is widely different from the one obtained on the first, the result that we obtained is of doubtful validity. Conceptually, we can extend this repeated studying to third time, fourth time or innumerable number of times and then ascertain how the summary measure obtained from each occasion is spread or varying. There are two possibilities for such repeated experimentation. First one is carrying out the same study empirically, number of times. But this is impractical in view of the time, resources, etc.

Alternatively, using the underlying statistical theory, we estimate the standard deviation associated with the sample estimates that would have been obtained, if we repeated the study. Here, we need to make a distinction between the standard deviation of the sample values and standard deviation of the summary measures that we obtain if we repeat the study number of times. The distribution of the parameter, such as mean or proportion that we get for each repetition is called the sampling distribution of the parameter and the standard deviation associated with the sampling distribution is referred to as standard error. Both standard error and standard deviation are standard deviation only, but standard error refers to the variation in the sample estimates that we would obtain by repeated studies, while standard deviation refers to the variation in the sample data that we collected. The interpretation of standard error is exactly same as that of standard deviation. To get back to the example of birth weight data, standard deviation of 100 g refers to the dispersion in the data set of 16 observations. From this we can obtain (through the statistical theory) the standard error associated with this mean based on a sample size of 16. It is obtained as the ratio of standard deviation to the square root of the sample size. In this example, the standard error is 100 ÷ square root (16) = 100 ÷ 4 = 25 g. It means that if we repeat the study number of times, every time with a sample size of 16 from the same clinic, using the same instrument for weight measurement, the average birth weight that we obtain from each such repeated study would on the average be 25 g away from the mean of 2250 g that we obtained. So, based on the variation observed in the sampled values, we are in a position to understand how our result is likely to vary in repeated studies.

As we have seen when we estimate the mean of a characteristic, we can estimate the standard error of a proportion also. Suppose, from a series of 100 patients of patients undergoing a surgical procedure, we observe that 20% are children. The proportion p is 0.2 or 20% that we estimated from a sample of size 100. The standard error of this proportion would be square root of [proportion × (1-proportion)] ÷ sample size. If terms of notations standard error of a proportion is square root ($p \times q \div n$), where q is the complement of p and n is the size of the sample. In our example, the standard error of the proportion of children would be square root of 0.2 × 0.8/100 = 0.04 or 4%. So, we can expect that the proportion of children undergoing the specific surgery would be 4% away from the estimated 20%, if we repeat the study from the same population with same sample size.

The real benefit of calculating the standard error is in identifying the probable range of values of the parameter, such that any estimated value with the specific sample size from similar population will lie in that identified range with 95% probability. The range of values or interval is called the confidence interval (CI). Our real intention of calculating this confidence interval is to alert a reader how fluctuating our result could be over repeated studies. If the fluctuations are minimal, our result is robust and likely to remain same in repeated studies. On the other hand, if the fluctuations are wide, indicating estimates that have significant clinical/practical implications on one side and estimates of little practical value on the other side, one would not like to take our estimated value of the parameter seriously. We will elaborate this concept further after we discuss the calculation of the confidence interval for a given study parameter.

A distribution of a variable is the description of how frequently a particular value that the variable can take. For example, if 90% of the communities in a country are Rh+ and the remaining 10% are Rh–, the variable Rh factor is distributed with 90% being Rh+ and 10% being Rh-. Another variable, say smoking among HIV+ cases can be distributed with different proportions of smokers and nonsmokers. Variables that can take only two values such as yes/no are called binary variables and they follow a distribution called binomial distribution.

Variables of quantitative nature, as described already in the section on averages, often take values that are close to the central tendency and as we go away from the central tendency in either direction, fewer and fewer values of the variable occur. In addition, the frequencies of the variable in either direction from the center, tend to be similar, thereby making a bell shaped symmetric curve. Such a distribution is called normal distribution. It has the mean, median and mode, all close to each other at the center of the distribution. This occurrence of different values of the variable can be expressed in a mathematical form, which is called the distribution function.

Every distribution is characterized by certain quantities called the parameters of that distribution. Binomial distribution has two parameters p and n. p is the proportion of one of the two outcomes and n the sample size. Similarly, normal distribution has two parameters μ and σ, where μ is the mean and σ is the standard deviation. Normal distribution is the backbone of much of the statistical theory. It is such a versatile distribution that even if the variable does not follow a symmetric distribution, its arithmetic mean follows a distribution close to the normal distribution. Likewise, other distributions like the binomial follow a normal distribution when the sample size increases or the probability of one of the two outcomes is closer to 50% and so on.

Once we know the pattern or distribution of the estimates that we obtain, we can use the properties of such distribution to guess about the range of values that can happen with 95% or 99% probability. Normal distribution has the property that mean – standard deviation to mean+ standard deviation covers 68% of the observations or data. Similarly, mean – 2 standard deviation to mean + 2 standard deviation covers 95% of the data and mean – 2.58 standard deviation to mean + 2.58 standard deviation includes 99% of the data. If our estimate based on sample also follows this distribution, the same logic should apply for the estimates derived from repeated studies. The calculation of the standard deviation of the estimate, i.e. the standard error has already been described earlier and so we can easily obtain the possible range that we are interested in.

Suppose, the bone mineral density (BMD) of L1 vertebra in 100 elderly women (60+ years) was observed to have a mean of 0.611 g/cm^2 with a standard deviation of 0.11 g/cm^2. We know that mean BMD over repeated studies also follows a normal distribution with mean as the obtained mean and standard deviation as sample standard deviation ÷ square root (sample size). Accordingly, the standard error of the mean BMD from this sample would be [0.11/square root (100)] = 0.011 g/cm^2.

Now using the property of normal distribution, we know that mean – SE to mean + SE = [0.611 – 0.011 to 0.611 + 0.011] = [0.60 to 0.622] includes 68% of the data. In other words, if we repeat the study 100 times from the same population, with the same sample size and using the same techniques of measuring bone density, there 68% chance that our obtained mean bone density would be in these two limits. This interval is called confidence interval and the associated probability is called the confidence coefficient. We can also describe it as 68% confidence interval. Similarly, the 95% confidence interval can be calculated as:

$$\begin{aligned}95\%\ \text{CI} &= [\text{mean} - 2\text{SE to mean} + 2\text{SE}]\\ &= [0.611 - (2 \times 0.011) \text{ to } 0.611 + (2 \times 0.011)]\\ &= [0.589 \text{ to } 0.633].\end{aligned}$$

So, we are 95% certain that over repeated study, the estimated BMD can be at the worst 0.589 g/cm^2 and at the best could be 0.633 g/cm^2. There is still a 5% chance that it can be either lower than 0.589 or more than 0.633 g. Naturally, the narrower this band is, the more precise is our result. Now a reader can understand the fluctuations associated with the estimated mean from our study and decide whether it is precise enough for him/her. This is the main purpose of calculating the confidence interval. Another useful interpretation of confidence interval is like saying; we do not know the true mean BMD. But we are 95% certain that it is somewhere between 0.589 g and 0.633 g. When we say this, be aware that we are not implying that the true value of BMD varies between the limits. True value is unknown but fixed. The probability is for the limits that we are trying to put around the true fixed value.

Same approach can also be used to construct a confidence interval for a proportion.

Generally, descriptive studies end with quoting the estimated parameter value and its 95% or 99% confidence interval.

STATISTICAL TESTING OF HYPOTHESIS, NULL HYPOTHESIS, ALTERNATIVE HYPOTHESIS, TYPES OF ERRORS AND POWER OF A TEST

As mentioned earlier, because of the variation in the phenomena, we need to base our conclusions empirically by observing a series of subjects/patients. In this process, we may need to compare two or more data sets with respect to the same phenomena. We compare the summary measures, such as mean and standard deviation in each category or strata of the variable. For example, one might be interested in know whether the neurocognitive functioning is similar among cases of idiopathic hypoparathyroidism with and without calcification in the basal ganglia region of the brain. Whatever the difference among the data sets, we are never sure it occurred because of the intrinsic differences between the groups or just due to chance. What all we can do is to assess this chance happening of the observed difference in terms of probability and then conclude whether chance play is substantial or minimal. If the chance play is substantial, we tend to say that whatever difference observed is just because of chance and conclude that there is no difference between the groups. On the other hand, if the chance play is minimal, we tend to say, that the difference observed is beyond chance and conclude that there is a significant difference between the groups. Because we are inferring about the population, based on a sample, this branch of statistics is called statistical inference. Further, the branch of statistical inference that deals with the issues of comparing groups, etc. is called testing of hypotheses. The other branch of statistical inference is estimation which involves estimating the parameter of interest and calculating the confidence interval that we have discussed earlier.

In testing of hypotheses, we proceed in a very logical manner in a step by step approach. We can describe these steps easily by considering a situation involving comparison of mean of a characteristic between two groups. So, we will have mean1 of sample1 and mean2 of sample2 with the respective standard deviations and sample sizes at hand. First, we propose a neutral or null stance stating that there is no difference between the two groups and state that both means are equal. This statement is called the 'null hypothesis' and we want to accept or reject this "null hypothesis". As against this null hypothesis, we can have an "alternative hypothesis", stating that both means are unequal or mean1 is more/less than mean2. If we accept the null hypothesis, we conclude that there is no significant difference between the two means and the difference that is observed is just a play of chance (chance probability is considerable). On the other hand, if we reject the null hypothesis, it implies we are ready to accept the alternative hypothesis and conclude that there is significant difference between the two means or one is more than the other etc. When we propose these null and alternative hypotheses, we must be sure that the null hypothesis is testable with the type of the design that we adopted and the data that was collected.

Once we are ready with the two hypotheses, we need to calculate an index based on the data that we have. This index is called the test statistic and is in the form of a ratio, the numerator being the difference of the two estimates of the parameter and the denominator being the standard error of the numerator. So, if we are comparing two means, the numerator is the absolute value of mean1 – mean2 and the denominator is the standard error of difference of means. Calculation of standard error involves the standard deviations of the two samples along with the respective sample sizes, etc. and it varies from situation to situation, depending on the type of variables that we are comparing, their distributional properties, etc. The details of calculation of the test statistic for various situations are beyond the scope of this book, but the concept of standard error, the key component in calculating the test statistic value has already been described earlier.

The test statistic that we calculate as difference of the two estimates divided by the standard error of the difference follows certain distributional patterns such as a normal distribution, *t* distribution, chi-square distribution, etc. for a given scenario. This has been already proven by the statistical theory. We need only to ensure that the underlying assumptions, such as the sample size, type of variable (qualitative, quantitative, etc.) and the distribution of the variable are met at least reasonably well.

We have an index calculated from the collected data and we also know that this ratio follows certain distributional patterns. These distributions have been well studied and their properties have been well documented in the statistical theory. Recall that while calculating the confidence interval, we already used certain properties of the normal distribution. Using the properties of the specific distribution that is applicable for our ratio, we can know the chance or probability of obtaining the test statistic value as much as we observed if the null hypothesis is correct.

Now, we have our null hypothesis, alternative hypothesis, the value of the test statistic based on our data, the distribution of the test statistic and the probability of observing the value of the test statistic that that has been observed, if the null hypothesis is correct. We have to probe on the probability of observing the test statistic value that has been observed to make a meaning out of it. If the null hypothesis is true, then whatever the magnitude of the ratio that we calculated, the chance of such magnitude should be high. It is for us to decide when to say the probability is considerable or cannot be dismissed as of little practical consequence. Suppose, we say that a probability of observed statistic is 2%, and if we are ready to accept that 2% is a very small chance that can be ignored, then we imply that chance play is very minimal and the statistic value that we have has happened because of the intrinsic differences between the two groups that are being compared. So we "reject" the null hypothesis, because if it is correct, the value that has been observed should have happened more by chance alone. On the other hand, if the probability of observing the statistic value under the null hypothesis is 20%, we can infer that there is a 20% chance that the observed difference could have arisen due to chance play only. This prompts us to go with the null hypothesis saying that the null hypothesis is accepted and the conclusion is no significant difference between the two groups.

It is debatable when to say that the probability of observed result under the null hypothesis is small or high. Without getting into the details, enough to know that less than a 5% chance is generally considered to be small enough to rule out chance as an explanation for the observed results. Beyond that it considered that observed results are due to chance. If one wants to be strict, 1% can be taken as an upper limit for ruling out chance as an explanation. In statistical terminology, this probability of 5% or 1% is called level of significance and is fixed at the time of designing the study. At the end of the data collection and analysis, the actual probability of obtaining the test statistic ratio that has been obtained is called the "p value". If the p value obtained is smaller than the level of confidence that was fixed initially at the designing stage, we reject the null hypothesis. Otherwise, we accept the null hypothesis.

Another way of viewing the p value is alerting the reader about the result that we obtained. If we conclude that response (60%) to treatment A is significantly more than the response (50%) to treatment B, and the obtained p value is 0.01, it implies that there is a 1% probability that the 10% excess response observed with treatment A can happen by chance alone. It also implies that we can be wrong in concluding that response to treatment is better 1% of times or 1 in 100 times. It will help any reader for better understanding of the results. This error that we are willing to accept is analogs to the false positivity of a diagnostic test and is called type I error in statistical testing. Similarly, we can have another error, there could be significant difference in reality between the groups being compared, but we fail to detect it. This is analogs to a false negativity of a diagnostic test and is called type II error in statistical testing of hypothesis.

We need to consider these two errors and their consequences at the design stage and appropriately fix them in advance. The maximum allowable type I error fixed at the planning stage is called the level of significance (also called α error) and the complement of the maximum type II error (also called β error) allowable is called the power of the test. Usually, we limit type I error at 5% and type II error at 20% (power = 100 – 20% = 80%). Accordingly, the sample size required will be calculated. After completing the study, we can calculate the actual type I and type II errors committed. The actual type I error committed is the p value, which is relevant if we are saying that groups are significantly different, etc. Statistical power of the test is important when one reports a nonsignificant finding.

Just as we alert the reader by quoting the p value in a significant finding, we need to alert if there is a negative or nonsignificant finding. This we convey through the power of the test. Statistical power of the test is the complement of type II error and it is analogs to the sensitivity of a diagnostic test. So if we report a negative result by a diagnostic test, one would like to know the sensitivity of the diagnostic test first. If the sensitivity is high, yet the result is negative, one tends to believe that the negative result is perhaps a truly negative result. On the other hand, if the sensitivity of the diagnostic test is poor and a negative result is reported by that test, one would suspect that the negative result declared could be a false negative. Applying the same analogy, if the statistical power ($1-\beta$) of test is low, we need to be circumspect about the negative result being reported. So, if the statistical testing indicates a nonsignificant finding, it is imperative on the part of the investigator to indicate the power of the test, so that a reader can have a better idea about the genuineness of the result. The calculation of power of the test is beyond the scope of this book.

Types of Statistical Tests

By this time, you should have a fair idea that when you want to statistically test a hypothesis, typically we have two entities—the exposure on one side and the outcome on the other. For example, in testing the association of breast cancer among women and the history of the same among their mothers, the maternal history is the exposure and the presence of breast cancer among women is the outcome. Again, both the exposure and outcome can be of different types of variables. In the above example, the exposure, maternal history of breast cancer is either yes or no, a binary variable and so is also the breast cancer status of a woman. Likewise, in a study of the association between the levels of alpha-fetoprotein (AFP) and presence of liver cancer, the exposure variable AFP level is quantitative and the outcome variable presence of the diseases is binary. We can extend the groups being compared (disease present and absent in this example) to more than two groups such as normal, benign and malignant tumors, etc.

Depending on the combination of the types of exposure and outcome variables, the test statistic varies from situation to situation. But the basic philosophy and the principles of obtaining the p value and the interpretation, etc. remain same. The details of deriving the test statistic for every situation are beyond the scope of this book and we will describe the test procedure for common situations.

COMPARISON OF MEAN BETWEEN TWO INDEPENDENT GROUPS

When you have a quantitative characteristic to be studied, it can be summarized as a mean along with the standard deviation from the sampled observations. To compare this summarized value of the characteristic between two groups that are independent, we use a statistical test called student's *t* test or simply *t* test. The test statistic is:

$$t_{(n_1+n_2-2)} = \frac{|\bar{x}_1 - \bar{x}_2|}{S\sqrt{\left(\frac{1}{n_1}+\frac{1}{n_2}\right)}} \quad ...(1)$$

Where $\bar{x}_1$ and $\bar{x}_2$ are means calculated from sample 1 and 2; n_1 and n_2 are the sample sizes. S is the pooled standard deviation of the two samples and is calculated as:

$$S = \frac{(n_1 \times s_1^2) + (n_2 \times s_2^2)}{(n_1 + n_2 - 2)} \quad ...(2)$$

in which s_1^2 and s_2^2 are the variances of sample 1 and 2, respectively. The index $n_1 + n_2 - 2$ associated with the test statistic t is called the degrees of freedom of t, which characterizes the distribution with our study sample sizes in each group.

After collecting the data and calculating the index (1) above, we look into the statistical tables of t distribution with $n_1 + n_2 - 2$ degrees of freedom at the level of confidence fixed at the planning stage (usually 5%) and note the t value that could happen with a probability of 5% or more when the null hypothesis is correct. If our observed t value is more than this theoretical limit, we conclude that our obtained statistic value has happened with a chance of less than 5% and so it is statistically significant. On the other hand, if our t value is less than the theoretical threshold value, we say that our result could be a chance observation and this chance is greater than 5%.

Nowadays with the advent of personal computers and statistical software implemented on them, we can calculate the exact probability of observing the obtained test statistic value under the experimental conditions. The conclusion depends on this probability (p value), whose upper limit is the confidence level that we fixed at planning stage, to declare a significant finding. We will explain the test procedure through an example.

Example: In a study to assess the impact of antenatal care visits by pregnant women on the birth weight of their newborns, an investigator collected the birth weight of newborns of 100 pregnant women who had at least three antenatal clinic (ANC) visits and 80 women who had less than three ANC visits. The mean birth weights were 2875 g and 2450 g; and the standard deviation were 225 g and 210 g respectively in samples with and without at least three ANC visits.

The question to be answered is: is the difference in the birth weights between the two groups statistically significant? The data that we have can be arranged as:

	Sample 1 (≥ 3 ANC)	Sample 2 (< 3 ANC)
Sample size:	$n_1 = 100$	$n_2 = 80$
Mean:	$\bar{x}_1 = 2875$ grams	$\bar{x}_2 = 2450$ grams
Standard deviation:	$S_1 = 225$ grams	$S_2 = 210$ grams

The null hypothesis H_0: The difference between the two means is by chance and there is no real difference between the two. In other words H_0: $\bar{x}_1 = \bar{x}_2$. Against this null hypothesis we have an alternative hypothesis H_1: $\bar{x}_1 \neq \bar{x}_2$. That is, both the estimates of mean are different from each other.

To test the null hypothesis, we use the student's t test as (1) we have two groups at hand; (2) the two groups are independent of each other (there is no overlap); and (3) the parameter that we are interested (birth weight) in comparing is of quantitative nature.

After plugging in the respective value in the test statistic (1) above, we get the t statistic value of 13.0, which has 100 + 80 – 2 = 178 degrees of freedom. Using the properties of the theoretical t distribution with 178 degrees of freedom, we know that a t value of 13.0 or more can occur with a probability of 0.000001. Since the chance of observing a t value of 13 with the sample sizes that we studied is so low, we tend to believe that perhaps the null hypothesis was not correct. So we reject the null hypothesis and conclude that the average birth weights in the two groups are statistically different. In other words, the birth weight in the group with a minimum of three ANC visits is significantly more than that in the group with fewer ANC visits. One should remember here that our conclusion that the ANC group had more birth weight can be wrong in 1/0.000001 = 1 million times.

Assumptions for a Student's *t* Test

Before we apply a statistical test, we should ensure that the data satisfies the assumptions needed to apply such a test. It should not be confused with the conditions for which the test is indicated. The three conditions mentioned above are indicated for the application of a student's t test. Student's t test requires two assumptions to be met. First, the two groups being compared have similar variances. So, we should have more or less similar standard deviations in the both samples. Most often a cursory look at the values of the standard deviation in the two groups is enough to guess about the similarity/dissimilarity. In case of doubt, formal statistical tests are available to know about the similarity of the two standard deviations. In the example above, the standard deviations are 225 g and 210 g, which appear to be similar.

The second assumption is that the quantitative characteristic that we are comparing should have a normal distribution. Tabulating data into some grouped frequencies or a diagrammatic presentation of the data as a histogram or a stem and leaf plot would help us to have quick idea about this. The shape of the plot should appear as a symmetric bell. Again there are formal statistical tests to see whether the data confirms to normal distribution or not. But most often, if the sample size in each group is at least 30 and the standard deviations are not large (relative to mean), it can be safely taken that the data confirms to normal distribution.

Tests that have this type of restrictive assumptions to be satisfied are called parametric tests of significance, while tests that do not require any assumptions to be met are called distribution free tests or nonparametric tests.

We can extend comparison of mean between two groups to among more than two groups. The statistical test that is useful for this is the analysis of variance (ANOVA) technique.

COMPARISON OF MEAN BETWEEN TWO DEPENDENT OR PAIRED GROUPS

To compare the mean of a characteristic from two groups that are not independent of each other, we use a statistical test called paired t test, another version of the t test. The test statistic is:

$$t_{(n-1)} = \frac{\bar{d}}{S/\sqrt{n}} \quad ...(3)$$

where, $\bar{d}$ is the average difference in the paired observations; n is the sample size; and S is the standard deviation of differences of the paired measurements. The statistic t has n-1 degrees of freedom here.

Table 1: Systolic blood pressure measurements of 10 women before and after using oral contraceptive pills

No.	Systolic blood pressure (mm Hg)		Difference (di)
	Before OCP usage	After OCP usage	
1	115	128	13
2	112	115	3
3	107	106	−1
4	119	128	9
5	115	122	7
6	138	145	7
7	126	132	6
8	105	109	4
9	104	102	−2
10	115	117	2
$\bar{x}$	115.6	120.4	4.8
SD	10.31	13.23	4.57

Abbreviations: OCP, oral contraceptive pill; SD, standard deviation.

Example: An investigator wanted to assess the impact of the usage of oral contraceptive pills (OCPs) on the blood pressure among women and collected systolic blood pressure before they started using OCPs and after 3 months of OCPs consumption. The data is shown in the Table 1.

Looking at the data, we understand that the average systolic blood pressure was 115.6 mm before the OCPs usage, which increased to 120.4 mm after 3 months usage of OCPs. The increase in each woman is on the average 4.8 mm with a standard deviation of 4.57 mm. We want to assess this 4.8 mm average increase is statistically significant or not. Recall that in the earlier example we dealt with two groups that have no overlap or interrelationship. In contrast, here we have only one group, but studied twice with some intervening period. So the student's *t* test is not appropriate here. We use paired *t* test whose form is shown in (3) above.

Plugging in the values of $\bar{d}$ (= 4.8), S (= 4.57) and n (= 10) in the formula (3), we obtain a *t* value of 3.38 which will have nine degrees of freedom. Once we have the test statistic calculated, the same procedure that we did in the two-sample *t* test will be followed. In fact, it is same for all statistical tests. So, we look at the theoretical *t* distribution with nine degrees of freedom and obtain the probability that a *t* value with nine degrees of freedom can happen by chance. In the present example, we realize it is 0.009. So, if there is no association between the usage of OCPs and systolic blood pressure (when the null hypothesis is true), a *t* value of 3.38 with nine degrees of freedom can arise only in nine out of 1,000 times. This chance being very small, we interpret that the role of chance in the observed result is minimal and there is a significant increase in the systolic blood pressure after the usage of OCPs. Again we can be wrong in concluding so in nine out of 1,000 times.

The assumption required for this paired *t* test is only one that the variable under consideration should be distributed as normal, at least approximately.

Comparison of a Proportion in Two Independent Samples

Just as we need to compare two estimates of a mean, we may need to compare two or more estimates of a proportion. To begin with we consider only two samples that are independent. Consider for example, the proportion of low birth weight babies (< 2500 g) among babies born to mothers on nutritional supplements and the same proportion in another group of mothers without any supplementation. We have the two sample sizes n_1 and n_2. Let p_1 and p_2 be the proportions in the respective groups. If the sample sizes in both the groups are large, the test statistic to assess the significance of the difference between the two proportions is:

$$Z = \frac{|p_1 - p_2|}{\sqrt{p \times q\left(\frac{1}{n_1} + \frac{1}{n_2}\right)}} \quad \text{...(4)}$$

Where p is the overall proportion estimates as

$$p = \frac{(n_1 \times p_1) + (n_2 \times p_2)}{(n_1 + n_2)} \quad \text{...(5)}$$

This statistic Z is expected to follow a Normal distribution and after calculating the Z value from our data, we can assess how likely our observed Z value can occur by chance alone, by looking at the theoretical normal distribution probability tables.

Comparison of Two proportions from Independent Samples: Contingency Table Method

Another way of comparing two independent proportions is by a test called chi-square test. To apply this test, we need to arrange the data in the form of a contingency table. Let us consider the same example as we discussed above. Further, let us suppose that among 100 babies born to mothers on supplements, 25 are of low birth weight while 35 out of 100 babies born to mothers without supplements are of low birth weight.

The data in a tabular form would appear as shown in Table 2.

We have n_1 = 100 and n_2 = 100 subjects in sample 1 and 2 respectively, making the total sample N = 200. Within the 100 of group 1, we have 25 as of low birth weight (a) and so the remaining 75 are of normal birth weight (b). Similarly, out of the 100 in group 2, 35 were of low birth weight (c) and so the remaining 65 were of normal birth weight (d). We have the two column totals ($a + c$) indicated as n_3 (= 60) and ($b + d$) indicated as n_4 (= 140) respectively.

The key to all chi-square tests is the calculation of expected values under the null hypothesis. Here we have a null hypothesis saying that the proportion of low birth weights is similar in the two

Table 2: Birth weight categories according the maternal groups

Group	Birth weight		Total
	Low	Normal	
With supplements	25 (a)	75 (b)	100 (n_1)
Without supplements	35 (c)	65 (d)	100 (n_2)
Total	60 (n_3)	140 (n_4)	200 (N)

groups or there is no association between maternal supplements and newborns birth weight.

We observed 25 babies of low birth weight in the first group. If the null hypothesis is correct, the expected number babies with low birth weight is similar to that we observed, then we tend to go with the null hypothesis and conclude that the differences are a play of chance only and no significant difference in the proportions between the two groups. We use this logic in developing the test statistic and use the differences between the observed and expected frequencies in the 4 cells of the table.

Calculation of Expected Frequency for the Cell (*a*)

Out of the 200 babies, 100 are with mothers on supplementations. So chance of mother being on supplements is 100/200.

Out of the 200 babies, 60 are of low birth weight. So chance of a baby having low birth weight is 60/200.

If the null hypothesis of no association is correct, the probability of the joint occurrence of these two events should be equal to the product of the two individual probabilities. So the joint probability of a mother on supplements and a newborn be of low birth weight would be (if the null hypothesis is correct): 100/200 × 60/200. So, with this probability, out of 200 total newborns, we expect (100/200) × (60/200) × 200 babies to be the expected frequency for the 25 that we observed as (*a*) in the Table 2. Simplifying the product terms we the expected frequency = (100 × 60)/200 or the corresponding row total x the corresponding column total divided by the grand total. So as against the 25 observed low birth weight babies belonging to the mothers on supplements, we expect 30 babies, if the null hypothesis is correct.

Similarly, we can calculate for the remaining 3 cells also. Because we have only 2 rows and 2 columns in our table, the expected frequencies for the other cells can easily be obtained (without calculating the frequencies) by subtracting the expected frequency one cell that we already obtained from the respective row and column totals. Therefore, the expected values for *b*, *c* and *d* are: 100 – 30 = 70; 60 – 30 = 30 and 140 – 70 = 70, respectively.

So for the four cells we have the observed frequencies and the expected frequencies. If the null hypothesis is correct, the difference between these two types of frequencies should be small in all the four cells. We denote the observed frequencies as O_i and expected frequencies as E_i. The subscript *i* stands for the cell number. In our example we have 4 cells, so, *i* ranges from 1 to 4. The test statistic is:

$$\chi_1^2 = \sum_{i=1}^{4} \frac{(O_i - E_i)^2}{E_i} \quad \text{...(6)}$$

The statistic is called chi-square and the subscript indicates the degrees of freedom associated with it. In our example the chi-square has 1 degree of freedom. As for the *t* distribution, the degrees of freedom characterize the chi-square distribution.

The chi-square statistic has a value of $(25 - 30)^2/30 + (75 - 70)^2/70 + (35 - 30)^2/30 + (65 - 70)^2/70 = 2.38$. Looking at the theoretical chi-square distribution tables, we understand that a chi-square with 1 degree of freedom can take a value of 2.38 or more extreme in 12.3% times. This chance of 12.3% being considerable, we conclude that the observed result is consistent with the null hypothesis and we accept it. In other words there is no significant association between maternal supplements and the birth weight.

The same test statistic can be calculated without resorting to the calculation of expected frequencies. The formula is:

$$\chi_1^2 = \frac{\text{N}\times(|a\times d - b\times c|)^2}{(n_1\times n_2\times n_3\times n_4)} \quad \text{...(6)}$$

Where *a*, *b*, *c* and *d* are the frequencies of the 4 cells in the contingency table shown above and n_1, n_2, n_3 and n_4 are the marginal totals, and N is the grand total. The symbol '| |' in the numerator indicates the absolute value ignore the sign.

Going back to the numerical example that we discussed above:

$$\chi_1^2 = \frac{200\times(|25\times65 - 75\times35|)^2}{(100\times100\times60\times140)} = \frac{200\times(1000)^2}{(100\times100\times60\times140)}$$

$$= \frac{200\times1000\times1000}{100\times100\times60\times140} = \frac{200}{84} = 2.38$$

which is exactly same as we got earlier with the calculation of expected values.

The chi-square test can be extended to more than two groups among which the proportion of particular characteristic is to be compared. For example, the proportion of low birth weight babies can be compared between low, middle and high socioeconomic group of mothers. The principle remains the same, that is calculation of expected frequencies and obtaining an index based on the differences between observed and expected frequencies. Formula based directly on the cell frequencies that avoid the calculation of expected frequencies is also available. In general if there are *r* rows and *c* columns in a contingency table, the chi-square calculated from such table will have $(r - 1) \times (c - 1)$ degrees of freedom.

Chi-square distribution is a distribution applicable for a quantitative variable and when there are only two rows and two columns (when the degrees of freedom is one), the continuous nature of the distribution is broken. To make it a continuous one, a correction called "Yates continuity correction" is applied in the calculation of the test statistic value. This is nothing but a subtraction of N/2 from the $|a \times d - b \times c|$ in the numerator of 6 above. Continuity correction makes the test more conservative, leading to the acceptance of the null hypothesis more often.

It should be noted that chi-square test uses only the absolute frequencies and not percentages or relative frequencies. Further, it does not require any assumptions to be met, unlike the *t* test. If the variable under consideration is binary or categorical, we can safely apply the test. So, chi-square test is a distribution free or nonparametric test.

If the expected frequencies in some cells are very small or zeros, chi-square test is not appropriate. A technique called Fisher's exact test is useful in such situations. This test is numerically very intensive and is usually applied with the help of computer software.

There are a number of statistical tests of hypothesis. Discussion of all tests is beyond the scope of this book. Interested readers might refer to books dealing with detailed statistical presentations.

STUDY DESIGNS

In epidemiological work, we are interested to seek answers for some prestated questions. These questions can be simple queries or postulated relations between two or more characteristics. The type of questions determines the approach that one needs to adopt in his/her work to find the answers. Also some times, same question can be answered by more than one approach. The approach that one adopts to find answers to his/her questions is broadly referred to as study designs. Here we discuss some commonly used designs in epidemiological work.

There are two broad types of studies, namely observational and experimental. Observational studies involve just measuring or observing certain characteristics of the study subjects at one or more points of time, but the study has nothing to do in determining the way that the patients are managed or the subjects are exposed to the study factor. In contrast, in experimental studies, the investigator determines which subject/patient should receive which treatment or exposure. Thus, there is greater control on the exposure/treatment allocation to the subjects in experimental studies.

For example, if we want to know the role of smoking in the causation of coronary artery disease (CAD), we can take a group of subjects who are currently smoking and free of the disease and follow them up to see who, when and how many develop the disease. Simultaneously, we can have another group who are not smokers and follow them to see the incidence of the condition and compare it with that in the exposed group. Alternatively, we can study simultaneously a group of CAD cases and a group free of CAD and ascertain how many smokers in each group. Yet another way is assemble two groups of subjects, one with and another without the disease, and ascertain about their past history of smoking habits. By comparing their past exposures in the two groups, we can have an idea about the role of the smoking in the causation of CAD. Even further, one can think of a homogenous group of nonsmoking individuals free of CAD now and then randomly put some of them on smoking (if the participating subjects consent and ethics committee permits) while remaining continue as nonsmokers, follow both the groups for considerable time to see the incidence of the condition in each group. Thus for a given question, we have different ways to find answers and these approaches are called the study designs. Needless to say that each approach/design has certain advantages and disadvantages associated with it. We need to be aware of these and plan any study that is best suitable taking into consideration of the feasibility in terms of number of cases/subjects, time, money, scientific validity and the ethics concerned etc. Each type of approach has been labeled as a specific design in scientific/research methodology parlance. We will discuss these commonly encountered designs briefly here.

Cross-sectional Design

The main characteristic of this approach is that the exposure and outcome variables are assessed simultaneously at the same time. For example, in studying the association between alcohol consumption and presence of liver disease, we can collect the present alcohol consumption status and the diagnosis of liver disease among persons attending a hospital. This design provides us a one-time snap-shot of the association between the two. Studies with this type of design can be quickly initiated and often provide a quick idea of the association of the exposure with the outcome. They may not involve huge expenditure also. The major limitation of this design is that the exposure might have been changed after the onset of the symptoms or before the diagnosis of the condition. Thus assessing the present status of the exposure may not reflect the true picture of its association with the outcome. To continue with our example of association between alcohol consumption and liver disease, a patient presenting today at a liver clinic might be suffering from the disease or symptoms related to it for some time before arriving at this liver clinic and his habit of alcohol consumption might have changed during this time. So the present status of alcohol consumption will not reflect the true picture. We can think of many such examples such as physical activity with diabetes, CAD; smoking with chronic obstructive pulmonary disease (COPD) or asthma, etc. Therefore, a cross-sectional design would be suitable when the exposure under consideration is likely to unaffected by the presence of the condition. This is generally true with some genetic mutations, etc. In general, cross-sectional studies form the first line of investigations in establishing an association between an exposure and an outcome. Because the participating subjects are observed only for different aspects, not involving any maneuvering of their management, cross-sectional studies are observational studies.

Prospective Study or Cohort Design

As the name suggests studies with this design involve a "cohort" that is observed prospectively over time. A cohort is defined as a group of persons similar on some respect. For example, primary school children, persons employed in an industry or profession, such as police, army, etc. In this approach, we enroll a group of similar persons (called a cohort) and measure their exposure and observe them over a certain length of time beginning from the enrolment. We must note that all the enrolled persons are free from the outcome at enrollment. During the follow-up, we observe who, when and how many develop the outcome of interest and at the end of the study we compare the proportions developing the outcome among the exposed and unexposed. Using these numbers we arrive at a summary measure of the association between the exposure and outcome. This design has a desirable feature of avoiding the biased assessment of exposure as the exposure status of each subject is assessed well before the occurrence of the outcome. Because the outcome has not yet happened at the initiation of the study, the temporality between the exposure and outcome provides a better basis for the causality of the association.

Cohort studies generally involve large number of subjects to be followed periodically for long time. In view of this, the expenditure involved tends to be high. Further, the longer the follow-up, the more likely for subjects to get dropped out and also more likely that the exposure initially measured might change. Cohort studies are suitable to study the different outcomes associated with a single exposure, such as methyl isocyanate (MIC) gas leakage, atomic radiation and natural calamities such as the recent floods in the state of Uttarakhand.

The third common type of an observational study design is the case-control. In this design, we enroll two groups of subjects, namely, one with the disease already diagnosed (called cases) and the other that the disease under investigation is absent (called controls). We then try to ascertain the status of past exposure among the two groups and compare the proportion of exposed in each group to know the magnitude of association between the exposure and the disease. This type of design is very easy and quick to mount. The answers to the research questions can be found quickly and because of this, the budget requirements are also likely to be lesser.

Case-control design is very useful to study rare diseases as against rare exposures suitable for cohort studies. Again, as many outcomes can be studied with the same exposure in cohort design, case-control design provides clues on the role many exposures on the same condition/disease.

Though the case-control design appears to be simple, it is prone for serious biases. The single most important bias that can creep in is due to the differential ability to recall the exposure details by patients and controls. Because of this it is not uncommon to find conflicting results with the same case series, but different series of controls. This is analogs to the riddle of making a drawn line shorter or longer, without touching the drawn line. One can make the drawn line longer or shorter by simply drawing another line shorter or longer, adjacent to the first one. Just as the first line drawn is well defined, so is our cases group. But this group can be declared more exposed by taking a control group which is less exposed. Alternatively, the case group can be declared less exposed, by comparing it with a control group that is more exposed. Therefore, the case and control groups should ideally be exactly similar with respect to their background characteristics and proneness for the exposure, etc. But it is often very difficult to find an ideal group of controls.

Case-control studies often provide the first line of evidence of association between an exposure and a disease.

Another type of study design is the experimental design. Randomized clinical trials, animal experiments, bioassays, etc. fall under this category. The major difference between these studies and the observational studies is the manipulation of the exposure/intervention. As mentioned before, in observational studies we only observe and no manipulation of the exposures/interventions is involved. In experimental studies, the investigator allots the type of exposure/intervention to different participants and then assesses the outcome with different exposure categories. Because of this the investigator has a lot of control over the study. Because of the manipulation of the interventions/exposures and the possible adverse effects associated with the allotted exposure, these studies should be carried out with a great deal of planning, care and ethical considerations. Since majority of experimental studies in medicine are clinical trials, we briefly describe the important features of clinical trials.

Trials can be therapeutic or prophylactic, each of which is carried out in a phased manner before a new drug/vaccine is introduced. In phase one, the pharmacokinetics of the drug is studies in terms of the maximum tolerable dose, half-life, time to reach maximum concentration, etc. Usually phase-I studies on health volunteers or volunteers with the disease. Sample size is not a consideration. In phase-II, the first attempt to see the efficacy of the drug is made. The focus is on safety. A concurrent comparison group may also be present some times. Issues such as randomization, blinding (if comparison group is present), and sample size are not given prominence. Based on the results of the phase-II, the next phase (phase-III) is initiated which is a full scale evaluation of the new drug with the existing standard.

The issues specific to a phase-III trial are sample size, randomization, blinding, inclusion/exclusion criteria. Blinding, also called as masking, assumes great relevance when the outcome of interest is subjective and is likely to get influenced by the knowledge about the intervention received by a specific patient/subject. It can occur from the patient him/her self or from the treating/assessing physician. In studies with hard outcomes such as death or relapse of the condition or estimation of a biochemical parameter, etc. the issue of blinding may not be very important.

Though there are common issues for any trial, it should be remembered that every trial is unique in its own as the type of interventions, durations, adverse events, type of population involved, etc.

We discussed the broad types of study designs. One should not jump to a conclusion that always one particular design is the best. Every study design has its advantages and disadvantages. One should assess the best suitable design with the resources available. In general in any disease control activities, a hypothesis is generated though a cross-sectional study, which is assessed through case-control studies. Further, the generated hypothesis established through a cohort study and randomized control studies before launching an intervention.

SAMPLE SIZE

Sample size is the most important hurdle for any clinician which makes them think that statistician is helpful for this only. In reality, a statistician can contribute a lot to the success of a study if involved right from the very beginning. Sample size is important for any study because of various reasons. All investigators want their study result to be not just a chance occurrence. By studying appropriate number of subjects, the chance occurrence is minimized as much as desired, so that the hypothesized relation only can be an explanation for the observed results. Thus ruling out chance play is the primary aim of studying a statistically required number. Similarly, no one wants to waste resources by studying more than the necessary number of subjects. One important reason that is often not realized is that we tend to get spurious or clinically unimportant results to be statistically significant by studying excessively large number of subjects. For example, by studying thousands of subjects, we can declare a reduction of 1 mm Hg in systolic blood pressure as statistically significant, but it may have very little practical implications or meaning. Another important reason to have appropriate sample size for any study is to be ethically correct, more applicable in clinical trials. When we study large numbers in a trial and our trial resulted in showing significantly better response in one arm, we have put some patients unnecessarily on an inferior treatment. By the same token, if our trial size is small, our efforts do not help to arrive at any conclusion. But the experimentation with humans cannot or should not be permitted for such futile research.

The sample size calculation involves a dialogue between the investigator and the statistician. The investigator should have a thorough knowledge about the topic that he/she plan to work on. When we say this, the investigator should have a fair idea about the earlier works on similar topic and what type of results that one can expect. The magnitude of the excess or decrease in the event/outcome is called the effect size and the investigator should be clear about the effect size that he/she considers practically/clinically important. He/she can get this information from the literature, experience, medical records or by talking to experts. If nothing is available, one may try a pilot work to have some idea and based on that one can plan larger investigation. For example, if one is trying to study the success rates of two treatments, the investigator should know the success with the standard available treatment and what he/she expects from the new treatment that he/she wants to study. If the objective is to estimate a single characteristic, such as hemoglobin, he/she should provide to the statistician that what is the average value that one expects along with the standard deviation of the characteristic.

The actual calculation of the sample size involves a mathematical formula, which depends on the type of variables and the type of study design, etc. Nevertheless, without going into the theory of sample size calculation, we present here the calculation method for some common study problems. Each is explained through a practical example.

Estimating the Sample Size for the Presence of a Condition or Prevalence of a Condition

Suppose, the prevalence of the condition that we want to estimate is expected to be P%, then the proportion of subjects without the condition would be 100 – P%. The investigator should have a fair idea about this P. We should also be ready to accept some error in this estimate that we want to make. This is expressed as the magnitude that we are prepared to be away from the assumed value of true, unknown P. Obviously, the farther from the truth we are ready to accept, the smaller would be the sample size and the closer we want to be to the assumed true value of P, the larger would be the sample size needed. So, before deciding on the allowable error margin, the investigator should ponder over the practical consequences of the error margin that he/she can be prepared to accept and accordingly decide how much error can be allowable. Another consideration is the number of times that the investigator wants to be certain that his/her estimated value of the P lies within the allowable error margin from the true P value. This is most often taken as 95% times and rarely taken as 99%. Once these are decided, the values are put in a formula shown below to arrive at the desired sample size with the desired features.

$$n = \frac{4 \times P \times (100 - P)}{d^2} \quad ...(7)$$

Where, n is the sample size required, P is the assumed prevalence of the condition and d ids the allowable margin that we are ready to accept. The constant 4 is for the number of times that we want to be certain that our estimated P is within a range from the true unknown P value. Here, it is for 95% times. If one is interested to be certain 99% times, the multiplier would be 7 (6.7 to be more accurate) instead of 4 in the above formula.

Example: We wish to estimate prevalence of smoking habit among the adolescent school going children in Delhi. Literature search indicated that the prevalence is of the order of 10% and would like to be within ± 2% of the assumed true prevalence, 95% times. In this example, our $P = 10$, $d = 2$ and the constant is 4 as we are interested to be certain at least 95% times.

Using the formula (7) above, $n = \frac{4 \times 10 \times (100 - 10)}{2^2} = \frac{4 \times 10 \times 90}{4}$

$$= 900$$

Therefore, we need to study 900 adolescent school children to estimate the prevalence of smoking habit among them, assuming that the true prevalence is 10%. This number would enable us to be within 2% of the truth in either direction, 95% of the times. This explanation of the sample size calculation needs to be documented in a study protocol.

Estimating the Sample Size for a Diagnostic Study

Most often diagnostic studies involve estimating the sensitivity and specificity of new diagnostic procedure taking an established diagnostic procedure as the reference or gold standard. Sensitivity, specificity and predictive values being proportions, the sample size calculation procedure for estimating prevalence can also be used for diagnostic studies. After the number is obtained it needs to be adjusted for the required number of suspected cases to be studied.

Example: Suppose a neonatologist wants to assess the role of preductal perfusion index (PI) in detecting the patent ductus arteriosus (PDA). She supposes (based on her experience and discussions with her mentors) that an elevated (≥1.1) preductal perfusion index will have about 60% sensitivity in picking up hemodynamically significant PDA (hsPDA) diagnosed by echocardiography. If she wants to plan a study to estimate the sensitivity of perfusion index in diagnosing hsPDA and an absolute error margin of 10% is allowable in a two-sided 95% confidence interval, she should study:

$$n = \frac{4 \times 60 \times (100 - 60)}{10^2} = \frac{4 \times 60 \times 40}{100} = 96$$

Since we are talking about sensitivity, the estimated number is the number of confirmed cases of hsPDA by the echocardiography. If the experience indicates that about 15% of preterm infants undergoing echocardiography have hsPDA, we need to study 96/0.15 = 640 preterm infants. This sample of 640 neonates would give us 96 cases of hsPDA as diagnosed by echo so that our estimated sensitivity of perfusion index will have a ± 10% absolute error, 95% times.

Similarly, one can calculate sample size required for specificity, positive predictive value or negative predictive value. If more than one index is to be studied, calculate the sample size required for all and take the sample size as the number that is the largest.

Estimating the Sample Size for Estimating the Mean of a Characteristic

The method of calculating the sample size to estimate the mean of a quantitative trait, such as hemoglobin, serum bilirubin or creatinine, etc. is similar to the calculation to estimate a proportion or prevalence. The only difference is that instead of P × (100 – P), we replace with the variance S^2 associated with the characteristic. The denominator is the absolute amount of allowable error in the estimate that we want to make. So, the sample size required is given by the formula:

$$n = \frac{4 \times s^2}{d^2} \quad ...(8)$$

This formula gives a sample size required so that, our sample estimate of the quantitative trait is within an absolute error margin of d in either direction, 95% of times. As in the case of calculating sample size to estimate prevalence, we need to use the constant 7 in place of 4, if we want to be 99% certain.

Example: We want to estimate the hemoglobin level (Hg%) among pregnant women attending a clinic and we expect that the average hemoglobin among them would be 10.5% with a standard deviation of 2.3%. If we are prepared to accept a relative error of 10%, 95% of times, the required number would be:

Error that can be allowable is 10% relative. It implies the absolute error margin d is 10% of 10.5 = 1.05.

$$n = \frac{4 \times s^2}{d^2} = \frac{4 \times 2.3 \times 2.3}{(1.05)^2} = 19.2 = 20$$

So if we presume that the true hemoglobin level is about 10.5% with a standard deviation of 2.3%, to estimate such hemoglobin with an absolute error margin of 1.05% (10% relative error) in a two-sided 95% confidence interval, we require 20 pregnant women to be studied.

Estimation of Sample Size for Studies Involving Testing of Hypothesis

In the previous 3 situations, we only estimated a parameter (either a proportion or a mean). Sometimes, we need to estimate the mean in 2 or more groups and then test whether these estimates are similar or significantly different. We will describe the methods for such cases now.

Estimation of Sample Size for Testing Hypothesis Involving Two Paired Means

When we want to test whether there is a significant change (increase or decrease) in a quantitative characteristic, we measure the variable initially and after some intervention or exposure. So we have two measurements of the same variable from each patient or participant. The research question would be whether the change from preintervention to post intervention is significant or not.

In this type of investigations, the investigator should propose a realistic amount of change in the quantitative characteristic that he/she wants to study. In addition, the investigator should also provide the statistician the value of the standard deviation of the change. Then the allowable errors of type I and type II are to be specified. It may be recalled that generally we allow a type I error of 5% (rarely 1%) and 20% of type II error.

With this combination of type I and type II allowable errors, the required sample size would be given by the formula:

$$n = \frac{8 \times s^2}{d^2}$$

Where S is the standard deviation of the expected difference and d is the expected difference. The constant 8 is for a maximum of 5% type I error and 20% type II error. If one is interested in different combination of type I and type II errors, the Table 3 below shows the value of the constant in the formula (9) above. As can be seen if we want to be accurate in the calculated number, we need to take 7.84 in the numerator. But for easy remembrance and quick calculation, we take it as 8. Similarly, for the constants for other combinations of the two types of errors can be taken from the table. The same constants can also be used for sample size calculations for other situations involving a testing of hypothesis.

Table 3: Constant values for the sample size calculations involving testing of hypothesis

Type I error (α)	*Type II error (β)*	*Constant*	
		Exact value	*Approximate value*
5%	20%	7.84	8
5%	10%	10.50	10
1%	20%	11.70	12
1%	10%	14.90	15

For the calculation of sample size in different scenarios described below we take the constant as 8 that correspond to a 5% alpha error and 20% beta error (80% power), which is the most commonly used combination of alpha and beta errors.

Example: Suppose a cardiologist wants assess the efficacy of an antihypertensive and by experience he knows that patients coming to his clinic have on the average a systolic blood pressure of 160 mm Hg. He expects that the antihypertensive can reduce the systolic blood pressure by about 5 mm Hg after a specified time with a standard deviation (S) of 12 mm Hg. If he wants to estimate the reduction in systolic blood pressure after using the antihypertensive and he is prepared to accept an alpha error of 5% and β error of 20%, the required sample size would be:

$$n = \frac{8 \times s^2}{d^2} = \frac{8 \times 12 \times 12}{(5)^2} = \frac{1152}{25} = 46.08 \text{ or } 47$$

So 47 subjects are needed to have 80% power (equivalent to say that 20% type II error) to detect a difference of 5.0 mm in means, assuming a standard deviation of differences is 12 mm and using a large sample Z test with a 5% (type I error) two-sided significance level.

The sample size calculation formula has been derived assuming that a large sample Z test will be used after the data collection is over. Instead, one wants to use a paired t test, the formula will slightly vary and hence the calculated sample size.

Estimation of Sample Size for Testing Hypothesis Involving Two Independent Means

In the previous example, we considered two paired or correlated means as we measured the variable (systolic blood pressure) in the same subject, but twice.

Another variant of the same objective could be to have two independent groups but similar with respect to the baseline value of the parameter (systolic blood pressure in this example) and put them on two antihypertensives and observe the change in the systolic blood pressure after some time in both groups and test for their equality.

In this type of situations, the method of calculating the sample size is same as in the previous example. The formula (9) will be slightly changed. If both groups have similar standard deviation value S, then the formula would be:

$$n = \frac{8 \times 2 \times s^2}{d^2} = \frac{16 \times s^2}{d^2} \quad ...(10)$$

If both groups have more or less similar standard deviation values, we can take the average as S. If they are expected to be different as S_1 and S_2, the sum of the squares of these two replaces $2S^2$ in the formula (10), which then becomes:

$$n = \frac{8 \times (s_1^2 + s_2^2)}{d^2} \quad ...(11)$$

Example: If the hemoglobin in pregnant women without supplements is on the average 10.5 grams with a standard deviation of 2.3, and supposing pregnant women with iron supplements would have average 2 g more with a standard deviation of 3.2, how many women per group need to be studied?

In this example difference $d = 2$ g, $S_1 = 2.3$, $S_2 = 3.2$

With 1% alpha error and 80% power, the constant term is 12. Therefore, the required sample size would be:

$$n = \frac{12 \times (s_1^2 + s_2^2)}{d^2} = 12 \times (2.3^2 + 3.2^2)/(2 \times 2) = 12 \times (5.29 + 10.24)/4$$

$= 46.6$ or 47 cases per group.

So, we require 47 pregnant women each with and without supplements (total 94 women) so that our study will have at most 1% alpha error and 80% power.

Estimation of Sample Size for Testing Hypothesis Involving Two Independent Proportions

In this situation, the sample size calculation formula is similar to the situation of comparing two means arising from two independent samples (formula 11 above) with minor modifications.

We have two proportions expected to be P_1 and P_2. The sample size required to test the hypothesis that the difference between them is not statistically significant is given by:

$$n = \frac{8 \times [(P_1 \times (100 - P_1) + P_2 \times (100 - P_2)]}{d^2} \qquad ...(12)$$

Example: Sample size required to compare the medical and surgical treatments for children with excessive number of episodes of otitis media (OTM) during the first 3 years of life, assuming the success rate is 50% in medical and 70% in surgical treatment, with 5% two sided level of significance and with 80% power.

We have $P_1 = 50$, $P_2 = 70$, $d = 20$

$$n = \frac{8 \times [(P_1 \times (100 - P_1) + P_2 \times (100 - P_2)]}{d^2} = \frac{8 \times [(50 \times 50) + (70 \times 30)]}{20^2}$$

$= 8 \times (2500 + 2100)/400 = 92$

Therefore, we need to study 92 children on medical management another 92 on surgical management, so that our comparison will have at most 5% type I error and 20% type II error.

Likewise, the sample size calculation is specific for each type of study design and the variables involved. Whatever the situation and the method of calculating the sample size, it should be understood clearly that the computed sample size gives only an idea of required number and the calculated number is not very sacrosanct. It only gives us an idea so that we can decide about the feasibility, budget, etc. The calculated number is rounded upwards to the nearest multiple of 5 or 10. Also, it is prudent to calculate for 3 or 4 possible scenarios with the assumed parameter values and combinations of the two errors and then choosing the best suitable number under the circumstances.

For any study there are bound to be some losses in the follow-up etc. so due allowance for this needs to be made in the calculated sample size. For example if the calculated sample size in the OTM example is 92 per arm and if we expect 20% losses in the follow-up, we need to enhance the sample size from 92 to 92/0.8 = 115 per arm so that at the end of the study we have 92 per arm.

There are free softwares available for sample size calculations on the internet. Not all can be vouched for correctness. One such free software which is useful for most frequent usage is power and sample size software from the Vanderbilt University, which can be downloaded from biostat.mc.vanderbilt.edu/twiki/bin/view/Main/PowerSampleSize. Another one is the Epicalc, which can be downloaded from www.brixtonhealth.com/epicalc.html.

If the study design is complex, expert help in sample size determination is strongly advised.

MEASURES OF ASSOCIATION

Comparison is extremely important in epidemiology. When we interpret measures of occurrence in two or more groups, we use some comparison either explicit or implicit. For example, a cardiologist trying to persuade a patient to quit smoking tells the patient that he had a 30% risk of developing CAD over the next 15 years, if he continued to smoke. Though the cardiologist did not mention the patient's risk of having CAD if he stopped smoking, he implied that if the patient stopped smoking, the risk of CAD would be reduced. Thus, it is an implicit comparison. According to sample registration system bulletin October 2012, the birth rate in the state of Kerala was 15.2 while that in the state of Uttar Pradesh was 27.8/1000. Here, we have an explicit comparison, so that one can more easily understand the difference.

In epidemiology, we are interested to know the possible cause(s) of an outcome. This branch of epidemiology is referred to as analytical epidemiology and it is based on explicit comparisons. If we suspect that a particular factor may be causing a specific outcome, we first look for an association between the factor and the outcome. Towards this aim, we compare the occurrence of outcome in a group of people exposed to the suspected factor to the occurrence of the outcome in a group of people unexposed to the same factor. The suspected factor is called as the "exposure", which can be a harmful substance or a specific behavior or personal characteristic.

In a study of association between an exposure and an outcome, the first requirement is have a clear definition of "case" and "population at risk". Once we have the definition of these, we observe the number of cases that occurred in the population at risk during the specified period. The number of observed events/cases linked to the denominator number of subjects at risk can give us an estimate of the risk of being a case in the population at risk.

Let us consider an example of the association between presence of cerebral edema and hospital mortality among patients of acute liver failure (ALF) admitted in a liver clinic. If we examine, say 100 admitted cases and note that 60 died during the hospital stay, it gives us an idea that 60% of ALF patients admitted are dead in the hospital. At this stage, this information does not tell us about the association of cerebral edema with mortality in the hospital. If we had also collected the status of each subject attending the clinic with respect to their cerebral edema status at admission, we can relate the mortality to the edema status. Suppose, out of the 100 we studied, 55 patients had cerebral edema and the rest 45 did not have cerebral edema. Further, out of 55 with edema 42 died during the hospital stay and out of 45 without cerebral edema 18 died during the hospital stay, we can use this information to quantify the association between the outcome mortality and the exposure of cerebral edema.

Risk of death in the hospital among all ALF patients admitted = 60/100 = 60.0%

Risk among those admitted with cerebral edema: 42/55 = 76.4%

Risk among those admitted without cerebral edema: 18/45 = 40.0%

Armed with these details, we now know that the risk of hospital mortality among patients of ALF is higher with cerebral edema than without cerebral edema. But we are not sure how much higher. Now to quantify the difference between the risks of mortality in those with and without cerebral edema, we have two ways of comparing the measures of occurrence.

The first one is by calculating the ratio of the two measures of occurrence and the second one is calculate the absolute difference of the two measures. Thus, we have two ways of calculating the excess risk of mortality.

$$\text{Ratio} = \frac{\text{Risk of mortality among those with cerebral edema}}{\text{Risk of mortality among those without cerebral edema}}$$

$$= \frac{76.4}{40.0} = 1.9$$

The ratio of risks or risk ratio measures how much more likely subjects of one group are to have the event of interest than subjects of the other group. In our example, ALF patients admitted with cerebral edema are nearly two times more likely to die before discharge than those cases admitted without cerebral edema.

In the difference measure, we calculate the difference in the risks by subtracting the risk of mortality without cerebral edema from the risk with cerebral edema.

Risk difference = (incidence risk in the exposed group) – (incidence risk in the unexposed group)

Risk difference = 76.4 – 40.0 = 26.4/100 or 264/1,000. Risk difference is also called attributable risk (AR).

Risk difference is an absolute measure of the excess risk of mortality with cerebral edema compared to the risk of mortality without cerebral edema. In our example, it shows that there were about 26 deaths excess due to cerebral edema per 100 ALF cases admitted.

Using either of these 2 measures, we are in a position to quantify the association between the exposure (cerebral edema at admission) and the outcome (mortality during the hospital stay).

Ratio measures are useful to compare any type of measure of occurrence—incidence risks, incidence rates, prevalence, odds, etc. These measures measure the strength of the association between the exposure and the outcome. The ratio measures are generally called relative risk (RR). But this term relative risk does not convey whether the ratio being referred to is based on risks or rates. A risk ratio is useful to assess the causative role of a suspected factor/exposure on a certain outcome while the rate ratio is useful to compare the incidence rate of an outcome in exposed and unexposed groups. Rate ratio takes into account the person-time at risk in each exposure group while other ratio measures do not. Rate ratio is a suitable measure in cohort studies involving patients/subjects entering or leaving the study at different time points. Because of the differences in rate ratio and a risk ratio, it would be more informative to use these terms instead of a generic term relative risk.

In analytical epidemiology, the measure odds ratio (OR) is used often as it has some desirable statistical properties than the risk ratio. We will briefly describe the calculation of odds ratio through an example.

Suppose 6 out of 10 ALF patients were found to be alcoholics, the probability of a patient being alcoholic = 6/10 = 0.6. Odds of a patient being alcoholic = 6/(10-6) = 1.5. The ratio of two odds (e.g. with and without exposure) is an odds ratio. Table 4 makes the calculation clear.

Table 4: Calculation of odds ratio

Exposure	*Cesarian delivery*		*Total*
	Yes	*No*	
Private Hospital	180 (*a*)	60 (*b*)	240
Government Hospital	200 (*c*)	400 (*d*)	600
Total	380	460	840 (*N*)

Odds of exposure among the diseased = a/c
Similarly, odds of exposure among nondiseased = b/d
Odds ratio = (a/c) ÷ (b/d) = (a × d)/(b × c)

Example: We have the details of type of delivery in 240 deliveries from private institutes and 600 from the government run institutions. Out of the 240 deliveries in the private institutes, 180 (75%) were cesarian deliveries as compared to 200 of the 600 (33%) deliveries in the government institutes. Thus, there is an apparent increase in the proportion of cesarian deliveries among the private institutes. We will quantify this association in terms of odds ratio.

Odds of cesarian delivery among private hospitals = a/b = 180/60
Odds of cesarian delivery among government hospitals = c/d = 200/400
Odds ratio = (180/60) ÷ (200/400) = 3 ÷ 1/2 = 6, which can also be obtained as $(a \times d) \div (b \times c)$
Odds ratio = $(a \times d)/(b \times c)$ = (180 × 400) ÷ (60 × 200) = 6

It should be noted that odds ratio based on odds of exposure among two outcome categories is same as odds ratio based on odds of outcome in the two exposure categories. The interpretation of odds ratio is on similar lines as any ratio measure. In our example, OR = 6 implies the odds of a delivery being cesarian is 6 times more in private hospital compared to a government hospital. If there is no association between the type of delivery and the type of the institute, we would expect the odds should be similar, so the odds ratio should be one. On the other hand, if the odds of the event/exposure are less in private hospitals, it will lead to a OR less than one. Accordingly, if the event under consideration is harmful or undesirable, a OR of more than one will imply that the exposure is a risk factor for the outcome and if the OR is less than one, it implies the exposure is a protective factor. The interpretation is vice versa if we are dealing with a desirable outcome.

Another ratio measure is hazards ratio (HR). This measure is specific to studies involving outcome as time to an event. Survival of cancer patients after therapy is one example where we use this measure. We calculate the survival probability at each time point in the follow-up and then plot in a diagram called Kaplan-Meir survival curves. The analysis itself is called survival analysis and it is a distinct branch of statistical analytical procedures. The main aim of this analysis is to describe the survival experience of the whole group over the length of follow-up time. This may involve one group or more than one group depending on the status of different exposures such as stage, etiology of disease and type of treatment, etc.

A hazard is defined as the slope of the survival curve— a measure of how rapidly the event is happening. Hazard itself may increase or decrease for a group over time but the ratio of hazards between two groups may be constant over time. Under this assumption, the HR is computed from all the data in the survival curve and not computed at any one time point. If the hazard ratio is 2.0, then the rate of the event in group is twice the rate in the other group.

NUMBER NEEDED TO TREAT

Risk difference can also be used as an indicator of effectiveness of different types of treatments/interventions in a trial set up. The index called number needed to treat (NNT) is defined as the inverse of the risk difference.

$$\text{NNT} = \frac{1}{RD}$$

Number needed to treat conveys the number of patients who would need to receive specific type of treatment in order for one additional patient to benefit from the treatment. Obviously, smaller the NNT, more the benefit of a treatment.

Example: Let us consider mortality rate from diarrhea in infants. Suppose, it is 49.6/1,000 infants per year among those who are not breastfed. Let us suppose further that the mortality is 7.4/1,000 infants per year in infants who were breastfed. Rate difference for mortality from diarrhea = 42.2/1,000 infants per year.

$$\text{NNT} = 1{,}000/42.2 = 23.7$$

It implies, to save one additional death, 24 babies have to be put on breast feeding. The index NNT has very useful interpretation in therapeutic trials.

Whatever the measure of association, we can calculate the 95% or 99% confidence interval for it and assess its statistical significance by appropriate tests of significance.

UNIVARIATE AND MULTIVARIABLE ANALYSES

By this time it should be clear that most often we have an outcome phenomenon on one side and one or more factors that may be associated with the outcome. Our aim is to find out how each of the many exposure factors is related to the outcome. Our main goal is if some exposures are significantly associated with the outcome and if these significantly associated factors are amenable for modification, we can modulate the outcome by manipulating these factors, so that it will lead to better health outcomes or quality of life for the patients.

In this process of quantifying the association between an outcome and each of the study factors; and identifying the significantly associated factors, we begin with studying the association one factor at a time. This type of analysis, though includes two variables—the outcome variable and the exposure variable, is often called univariate analysis because outcome is common and only one exposure is examined at a time. Some authors prefer to call it bivariate analysis as there are two variables involved—the outcome and the exposure.

The main aim of univariate analysis is to pick up those factors that have some bearing on the outcome. This forms the bedrock of any analysis as it explains how each study variable is associated with the outcome. The investigators should prod over these results as to the consistency or inconsistency of the observed association with the literature and possible reasons there of etc. The real understanding of the results comes from this stage of analysis and hence forms a crucial factor in writing the report or preparing a manuscript based on the study. An investigator who fails to understand and comprehend the results of univariate analysis cannot do proper justice to the whole work when he/she prepares the report/manuscript.

What we do in univariate analysis is describe how frequent or what is the magnitude of the outcome in the exposure categories along with 95% confidence intervals. In addition, the statistical significance of the difference in outcome between the categories of the exposure is also assessed, using the appropriate tests of hypothesis. Important findings that need to be highlighted are also shown diagrammatically to emphasize these aspects.

Multivariable Analysis

Most often, as we all know, any biological phenomenon depends on many factors. For example, a newborn's birth weight may depend on the gestation, maternal nutritional status, antenatal care received and pregnancy complications, etc. Each of these might show a significant association with the outcome, birth weight. But these exposure variables themselves may be related to each other. For example, a mother's nutritional status may be better if her antenatal care was good. Because these two exposures among themselves are related or associated, the association that has been observed between birth weight and mother's nutritional status includes in part at least, some association due to her antenatal care. Similarly, the association of antenatal care with newborn's birth weight might also include some part due to maternal nutritional status. Therefore, we need to disentangle the effect of each with the outcome, removing the overlap, if any. We attempt this through multivariable analysis, after developing a full understanding of the role of each of the study factor, one at a time in the univariate analysis.

Again, some authors make a distinction between multivariate and multivariable analysis. A multivariate analysis generally has more than one dependent variable or outcome variable where as a multivariable analysis involves a well defined single outcome but many independent or exposure factors. Most often we deal with single outcome in clinical medicine, so we deal with multivariable analysis.

There are many multivariable analysis techniques and most of them are regression procedures. Briefly, these procedures involve fitting a mathematical relation between the outcome (in its original form or a transformed form) on one side and the different exposure variables on the other side. Statistical methods help us to get the parameters estimates of the mathematical relation between the outcome and exposures, that best describe the presumed type of relation. So it is for the investigator and the statistician to postulate a type of relation between the outcome and the exposures. The relation could be like a line (linear relation) or nonlinear. The preliminary descriptions and univariate analyses help us to know the type of relation between the outcome and each exposure variable. Accordingly, we decide whether a linear model should be tried or a nonlinear model. Many of the nonlinear relations can be made linear by working with appropriate transformed data and such models are called log-linear models.

Whatever the type of the model is, all give us some parameter estimates called regression coefficients, which convey the average change in the dependent variable per unit change in the independent variable. For example, if we want to fit a linear relation (regression) between the birth weight of newborns and gestation, birth weight is our outcome variable or dependent variable and gestation is the independent or exposure variable. The regression analysis gives the regression coefficient that is interpreted as the average change (increase) in the newborn's birth weight for every one week increase in the gestation. Like for any estimate that we make, the regression coefficient also can have the standard error associated with it and we can assess the statistical significance of the obtained regression coefficient.

If we include only one exposure variable in our regression, it is called univariate regression. If we add more exposure variables such as maternal age, hemoglobin, etc. the regression is called multiple regression or multivariable regression. By studying exposure variables simultaneously, the statistical calculations give us the regression coefficient associated with a particular exposure, after other exposure variables have been held at constant level. In other words we get the effect of one exposure variable on the outcome after adjusting for the effect of other exposures. If gestation (weeks) and maternal hemoglobin (g%) are two exposures that we consider to be related with newborn's birth weight (g), a multiple regression would give us the average increase in the birth weight for every one week increase in the gestation, after adjusting for the maternal hemoglobin and; average increase in birth weight for every one g% increase in hemoglobin after adjusting for the gestation. It is also possible that both or only one of the two is statistically significant. This can be extended to more number of exposure variables. Thus, many exposures may be related with the outcome (as can be noted from a univariate analysis), but in reality only a few are independently associated with the outcome, which is known with the help of multivariable analysis. So, multivariable analysis is a very powerful and important analysis technique to identify significant and independently associated factors/exposures with the outcome.

The actual calculations, method of fitting the regression models and assessment of the models etc. are beyond the scope of this book. Interested readers should see books on detailed statistical models.

COMMON PITFALLS IN STATISTICAL CALCULATIONS AND INTERPRETATIONS

Benjamin Disraeli, a British politician of the nineteenth century said "There are three types of lies: lies, damn lies and statistics". It is not uncommon to hear the same quoted or some similar disdainful comments made on the subject statistics and its applications. In medical science and research, we keep reading conflicting views on the same topic from time to time. We get confused with these statements and wonder which one to be believed. For example, one scientific report in 1991 quoted significant positive association between coffee drinking and the risk of bladder cancer, while another in the year 2001 stated that coffee reduces risk of bladder cancer. Again in June 2006, another report quoted increased risk of bladder cancer with coffee consumption. Though the reasons for such conflicting and confusing statements are many, invariably the blame is put on statistics.

The basic truth that all must remember is that there is no way of knowing the truth and one has to depend on the results obtained by studying the sampled patients/data. As the results based only on a sample vary from sample to sample, there is always a possibility that our conclusions made on one sample can be wrong. In addition, various biases that can creep in due to the method of selecting/ including subjects for research and the method of ascertaining the exposures and the outcomes, lead to conclusions which may prove to be fallacious later. Generating evidence for or against a postulated relation is a process. We become wiser and wiser with every day and with every study leading to improved understanding of the issue.

Another contributing factor for the deriding views on statistics is the lack of full understanding the statistical principles. All statistical analytical techniques can never prove anything for certain and there is always a probability that our observed results could have arisen purely by chance. Unethical practices to promote vested or commercial interests are other contributing factor. This is more common in clinical trials as the results could have huge financial implications.

Some of the issues like chance, statistical errors and biases, etc. have been briefly described in the previous sections. We discuss briefly some common malpractices and misinterpretations of statistical analyses.

WRONG ANALYSIS TECHNIQUES

One of the common mistakes leading to inappropriate conclusions is incomplete or inappropriate analysis. Unfortunately, with the advent of desktop computers with sophisticated statistical software, these days anybody can do the statistical analyses, irrespective of their training and competence. Because of these facilities, naïve analysts tend to jump to more formal or advanced analyses without preliminary analyses that enhance the understanding of the phenomenon being investigated. Analysis should proceed in a logical manner. A preliminary descriptive analysis is a must before one goes further for more formal procedures. Otherwise the conclusion drawn from the advanced analysis could be misleading. Anscombe FJ described this pitfall very clearly taking four data sets on two variables. Each data set having distinctly different relation between the two variables show similar indices of association between the two variables. This illustration underlines the importance of understanding the data before applying advanced statistical techniques (graphs in statistical analysis, American statistician. 1973;27(1):17-21).

Another inappropriate application of statistical techniques is ignoring the paired nature of data and analyze as though the groups were independent. When the groups on which the data is collected are related such as preintervention and postintervention, the two groups of observations are not independent from each other. Essentially they belong to the same patient/subject, but measured twice and hence it is logical to expect that they are correlated. Analysis ignoring this aspect is flawed and so the conclusions may not be valid.

In situations where one intends to assess the agreement between measurements made by different methods, instruments or professionals, using the Pearson correlation coefficient as an index of agreement is inappropriate. It stems from lack of complete understanding of the concepts of agreement and correlation. For example, in assessing the agreement of blood pressure measurements made by a cardiologist and a trained nurse, we can have the measurements of the trained nurse consistently more (or less) by specified units (say 10 mm Hg) than those of the cardiologist. Common sense tells that there is poor agreement between the two if such a difference exists. But if we were to go by the correlation coefficient, we will conclude there is perfect agreement since the correlation between the two would be perfectly positive (+1). It should be remembered that correlation does not mean agreement, but agreement implies high positive correlation. The methods specific for agreement assessment such as paired *t* test, linear regression, Altman-Bland plots, etc. should be the basis for assessing the agreement.

Another inappropriate usage of statistical techniques is the application of the chi-square test on percentages. All chi-square tests should be applied on absolute frequencies and not relative frequencies. By taking the percentage of subjects with an attribute/trait, one tends to take the denominator as 100 in each of groups being compared. If the actual sample size in each group is less than 100, one would tend to get a statistically significant result, as the sample size has been enhanced. Similarly, one would tend to get a nonsignificant difference among groups, if the actual sample sizes are more than 100 in each group. Therefore, application of chi-square test with relative frequencies instead of absolute frequencies can lead to wrong conclusions.

MISLEADING PRESENTATION OF DATA THROUGH DIAGRAMS AND FIGURES

Frequency tables and numerical presentation of data undoubtedly provide a concise or compact view of the data and its principal characteristics. Diagrams on the other hand provide a visual method of examining the data as they make a lasting impression than numbers, convey the idea more forcefully and help us get a real grasp of the overall picture quickly. Though there are many types of diagrams and graphs to depict different types of data, the main purpose of any diagrammatic presentation is to convey information quickly. This very purpose is defeated, if the diagrammatic presentation is poor or not clear in conveying the intended message(s).

Graphs with Y-axis values starting from nonzero should be viewed with caution as they depict artificial steep increase or decrease in the frequencies, compared to the gradual rise or decrease in the data over different groups or time points. If X-axis is also starts with a nonzero value, the effect of this phenomenon is more dramatic.

Diagrams with equal intervals on the horizontal axis for unequal data intervals are not appropriate. Similarly, for unequal data intervals showing total frequency in that interval on the vertical axis is also not appropriate. We need to convert the frequency of the interval of unequal width as a frequency for standard width and then plot the converted frequency on the vertical axis.

Decoration of diagrams such as adding three-dimensional appearance to make them more exciting should be avoided as the accuracy of the diagram may be compromised. Pictograms that replace bars by columns of pictures to make the diagram more appealing can be misleading as we see the volume representing the frequency when in fact the height of the bar of pictures represents the frequency.

STATISTICAL SIGNIFICANCE VERSUS CLINICAL OR PUBLIC HEALTH SIGNIFICANCE

Many investigators with an intention to hit headlines in newspapers or scientific magazines/journals report results based only on statistical significance without proper consideration or explanation on clinical implications of such significance. For example, a report saying that a particular exposure increases the risk of a disease 10 times is very provoking and will attract attention of any reader. But what it really implies is that the risk of disease is 10 times more if the exposure is present as compared to when exposure is absent. So, when we really want to know the effect of the exposure, we need to consider the risk of the disease without the exposure or background risk. Suppose, it is 1 in a million. It then implies that exposure made the risk increase from 1 in a million to 10 in a million. In other words, the association between the exposure and disease is highly significant statistically but the public health impact of such exposure is at best very limited. This scenario is entirely different when the background risk is 1 in say 100, which increases to 10 in 100 with the presence of the exposure under consideration. Without explaining this, simply quoting that risk increases by 10 times, etc. makes a sensational reading and lay public might view the message in literal sense.

DATA MANIPULATION/FUDGING

The most glaring misuse of statistics is data manipulation and fudging. When an investigator deliberately wants to show a result of specific connotation, these types of malpractices take place. The values in the sample data are changed as it suits to the investigator's intentions or a data is fabricated without really studying any subjects. This artificial "creation" could be complete or partial, depending upon the proportion of cases/subjects actually studied and the number claimed to have been studied. Changing or discarding the values of extreme observations, outliers or unfavorable observations also falls in this category. Results generated from such data are likely to be proven wrong later.

DATA DREDGING

This is also commonly known as fishing expedition. Usually any study is planned with some specific primary objectives and a few more secondary objectives. The sample size and power calculations generally are to suit for the primary objectives. When the data is analyzed at the end of the study, it might be possible that the study might throw up a negative or uninterested finding for the primary objectives. Over enthusiastic investigators might overemphasize the results of the secondary objectives or some aspect that was not even planned initially, but turned out to be statistically significant. It should be remembered that when a large numbers of tests are performed in a data set, there is a chance that some tests produce positive results by chance alone. There are statistical procedures to overcome these problems. Without such corrective measures, the reported significant results that are mere artifacts of random variation can easily mislead the readers. Therefore, one should not over analyze any data and the analysis should be limited to the stated objectives only.

CHAPTER 9

Interventional Radiology of the Gastrointestinal Tract and Hepatobiliary System

Amar Mukund, S Rajesh

INTRODUCTION

The subspecialty of *Interventional Radiology* (IR) includes minimally invasive diagnostic and therapeutic procedures performed under imaging guidance. The emergence of this field over the past three to four decades has been made possible by the tremendous advancements in catheter and instrument design, imaging technology and radiological expertise. Many conditions that once required surgery can now be treated non-surgically by radiological interventions while other interventional techniques offer completely new therapeutic options. It also offers a less invasive alternative to surgical management of postoperative complications. By minimizing the physical trauma to the patient, radiological interventions can decrease the rates of infection and hasten recovery time resulting in shorter hospital stay. In addition, diagnostic procedures, such as percutaneous biopsies and fluid aspiration have obviated the need for diagnostic laparoscopy in majority of the patients, and play an important role in the management algorithm. Another area of application of IR is in patients who need to be stabilized before any surgical intervention (e.g. cholecystostomy and percutaneous drainage of infected pancreatic necrosis) or in patients who need down-staging of tumors before they can be taken for surgical resection or transplant like in cases of primary or metastatic liver tumors. Moreover, procedures such as transjugular intrahepatic portosystemic shunt and hepatic vein angioplasty or stenting can act as a bridge to liver transplant in patients who cannot immediately undergo surgery due to non-availability of donors or financial issues. The vast majority of IR procedures are performed under conscious sedation using local anesthesia. This chapter appraises the role of various radiological interventions in the management of pathologies affecting the gastrointestinal tract and hepatobiliary system. The emphasis is on the indications, contraindications, and likely outcomes, rather than on detailed technical descriptions.

GENERAL INTERVENTIONS

Fine Needle Aspiration/Biopsy

Image-guided percutaneous fine needle aspiration and biopsy is the most commonly performed radiological intervention in the abdomen.[1,2] It is widely accepted for its excellent efficacy and safety and has largely replaced the more invasive diagnostic laparoscopy and exploratory laparotomy.[2] The vast majority of biopsies are performed to confirm suspected malignancy, particularly in a patient with a known primary tumor. In addition, many biopsies are performed in oncologic patients with residual masses after therapy to determine whether such a mass represents residual viable tumor or necrotic tissue.[3] Depending on the operator preference, imaging guidance in the form of ultrasound or CT can be used.[4] Although magnetic resonance interventional systems are used in clinical practice, their role in performing routine biopsies is limited by cost and lack of widespread availability. Fine needle biopsies are obtained with 20- to 25-gauge needles. Large-gauge needle biopsies (14- to 18-gauge) are almost universally performed with an automated, spring-activated, Tru-Cut system. Many such systems of variable gauge, throw length and design are available. Endobiliary brush biopsies are also increasingly being performed for periductal infiltrating variety of cholangiocarcinomas. All abdominal biopsies can be performed on outpatient basis using no more than local anaesthesia. Preprocedural preparation involves assessment of coagulation studies (international normalized ratio or prothrombin time) and platelet count. Any derangements in these can be corrected by administration of vitamin K, fresh frozen plasma or platelet concentrates, as the need may be.[5]

Drainage of Abdominal Abscesses and Fluid Collections

Advances in imaging technology and improvements in the methods of percutaneous drainage have revolutionized the way abdominal abscesses and complex fluid collections are treated in the modern era. When compared with surgical exploration, especially in critically ill or postoperative patients, the rapid imaging localization and percutaneous treatment of abdominal collections have significantly less morbidity and mortality rates, and are now the accepted techniques for draining abscesses in abdomen, including the ones in difficult anatomical locations like subphrenic space or deep pelvis.[6,7]

Indications

Diagnostic

Mostly for the assessment of nature of fluid, i.e. whether the fluid is transudative or exudative, infected or sterile, for malignant cytology or to ascertain the organ of origin like bile, urine, lymph and pancreatic secretions.[8]

Therapeutic

- Treatment of sepsis.
- Alleviate pressure symptoms and pain due to a large cystic lesion (like simple hepatic cyst or pancreatic pseudocyst).
- Obliterating recurring cysts or collections using sclerosing agents.[9]

Image guidance: Most of the drainage procedures are performed under ultrasound or CT with or without fluoroscopy. Ultrasound is widely available, portable and enables real-time visualization of anatomy and the needle during the procedure, and hence is the most desirable in ICU setting. Sometimes ultrasound visualization may not be optimal especially in deep seated lesion or may be degraded by body habitus in obese patients or interference with bowel gases. CT overcomes these limitations, but does not allow real time imaging making the procedure lengthy. Moreover, patient needs to be shifted to CT suite and radiation dose imparted to the patient and operator may be of concern. Fluoroscopy is usually used to guide catheter exchange and upsizing.

Types of Drainage

Needle aspiration: One-time needle aspiration is usually used for diagnostic purposes or in cases of small abscesses or complex collections which do not require continuous drainage.

Catheter drainage: Continuous catheter drainage is performed for large abscesses or collections. Percutaneous catheters are placed using modified Seldinger or trocar technique. Generally, large superficial collections are drained using trocar technique while Seldinger technique is preferred for deep seated collections or potentially difficult drainages having limited access. In Seldinger technique, the collection is accessed using a thin 18–20 G Chiba or ring needle and a guidewire is passed through the needle into the collection. The tract is then serially dilated till insertion of a large bore catheter is possible.

Catheter Care

The catheter should be routinely inspected and drain volume and nature should be monitored. Special care should be taken to keep the catheter free of kinks. Any significant change in the nature/color/consistency of the drain fluid should warrant an evaluation to look for catheter retraction/migration. Pericatheter leak may suggest catheter block and requires either clearance of block or replacement of catheter. Drainage catheter placed within abscess or infected collections having thick collection should also be flushed with 5–10 mL of saline every 8–12 hours both towards the collection and towards the bag to prevent occlusion.

Catheter Removal

Catheter can be removed when the drainage is less than 10–20 mL/day and vital signs have returned to normal with no significant residual collection. Repeat cross-sectional imaging may be required if the patient's condition is not improving, there is less than expected drainage or when there is sudden reduction in the drainage of the catheter. If the catheter output remains unusually high even after 4–5 days of insertion, possibility of fistula to the bowel or pancreatic or biliary duct should be suspected.

SPECIAL CONSIDERATIONS

Enteric Abscesses

Enteric abscesses can arise as a result of appendicitis, diverticulitis or Crohn's disease. A complicating abscess in these conditions makes immediate surgery extremely difficult. In these circumstances, percutaneous drainage, in combination with appropriate antibiotic therapy, can be used to effectively drain the abscess. Elective surgery can then be performed at an appropriate interval after resolution of sepsis. These abscesses occur in close proximity to bowel loops, and CT guidance may be necessary to ensure that small or large bowel is not traversed by the catheter during drainage. Success rates between 80–100% can be achieved in percutaneous drainage of enteric abscesses, permitting single-stage surgery.[10-14]

Abscess-Fistula Complex

Fistulization to collections can occur from various structures including the biliary system, pancreatic duct and bowel. Persistent high outputs (>50–100 mL/day) or an increase in output after 4–5 days of drainage should alert the treating physician to the possibility of a probable fistula.[15,16] Management principles include draining the abscess and proximal diversion of bowel contents or biliary/pancreatic ductal stenting. The catheter placed in the fistulous track is left in situ for approximately 2 weeks to allow a mature fibrous track to form. When catheter output recedes to less than 20 mL/day the catheter can be withdrawn. Fistulas are designated as high-output when drainage is greater than 200 mL/day.[15,16] With high-output fistulas it is important to monitor and correct electrolyte and fluid losses to expedite fistula healing.

Subphrenic Abscess

Majority of subphrenic abscesses are postoperative, often resulting from pancreatic, gastric or biliary surgery. Anatomically, they are

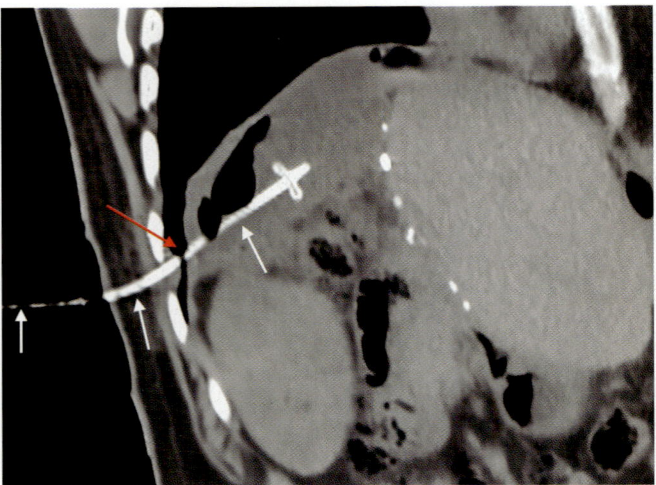

Figure 1 Coronal-oblique CT image demonstrating a drainage catheter (white arrows) being placed in the right subphrenic collection through transpleural route (red arrow)

located in a difficult position making an extrapleural access route a technical challenge. Traditionally, these abscesses were drained using a subpleural or extrapleural approach.[17] However, it has become apparent that an intercostal approach can be used to good effect in these patients without any significant increase in the rate of major complications including pneumothorax and empyema (Fig. 1). It is still important, however, to go through the lowest intercostal space possible that gives access to the abscess.

Hepatic Abscess

Percutaneous drainage of hepatic abscess is very successful and should be curative in more than 90% of cases even when the abscess appears loculated with multiple septations or has solid portions on imaging.[18,19] Access can be intercostal or subcostal depending on the location of the abscess. Catheter drainage is preferred in large abscesses while needle aspiration may suffice for the smaller ones.

Pancreatic Collections

Pancreatic Pseudocyst

Not all pancreatic pseudocysts require drainage. The most common reasons for drainage include pain, pressure symptoms or infection. The access route is usually transperitoneal. CT guidance is preferred because the precise relationship of the pseudocyst with surrounding organs can be seen clearly. Usually an 8–10 French catheter suffices for drainage.

The relationship of the pseudocyst with the pancreatic duct determines the length of drainage. If there is communication with the pancreatic duct, the duration of drainage is prolonged for 1–2 months or longer. The duration of drainage can be decreased by the use of antisecretory agents like somatostatin or its analog octreotide. If there is communication and the downstream pancreatic duct is obstructed by a stricture or stone, pseudocyst drainage will not be successful unless the downstream obstruction is relieved. Percutaneous drainage is successful in up to 90% of pancreatic pseudocysts.[20-23]

Pancreatic Abscess

Pancreatic abscess is mostly seen in patients having acute severe pancreatitis and usually have a severe systemic illness. In addition, pancreatic abscesses are often multilocular and the contents are usually very viscous, requiring large bore catheters (14–26 French) for drainage.

CT is the preferred guidance modality, as these patients have an associated ileus, making ultrasound guidance difficult. In majority of the cases, more than one catheter will be required due to the viscous nature, associated necrotic debris and/or multiloculation. Vigorous irrigation and careful monitoring of the patient are important for favorable outcomes. Success rates for drainage of pancreatic abscess vary from 32% to 80%.[22-24] Percutaneous drainage may not always be an ultimate cure; however, it may delay the surgery till the acute episode is over with relatively better patient condition and improved surgical outcomes.

Pancreatic Necrosis

As opposed to pancreatic abscess, pancreatic necrosis occurs early in the course (<2 weeks) of severe acute pancreatitis. The principal role of IR in patients with pancreatic necrosis is to differentiate sterile from infected necrosis. This differentiation cannot be made clinically, because sepsis indicators can be raised in patients with both sterile and infected necrosis. Percutaneous sampling of the necrotic area with a 20-gauge needle under ultrasound or CT guidance can help determine the nature of the fluid. Pancreatic necrosis is generally not suitable for percutaneous drainage because of its viscous contents. Occasionally, if the necrotic contents have liquefied, percutaneous drainage may be attempted (Figs 2 to 4). Large-bore 24–26 French catheters will be required for effective drainage.[24] Once an image-guided percutaneous tract is established by a retroperitoneal route, a wide array of minimally invasive techniques are now available as an alternative to open surgical necrosectomy. Minimally invasive necrosectomy via a flank tract has evolved from an adjunct to open debridement through lumbar incision to a primarily endoscopic technique. The procedure is now known as video-assisted retroperitoneal debridement (VARD). VARD involves intraoperative dilatation of the percutaneous drain tract followed by irrigation, lavage and suction using a nephroscope or flexible endoscope. A large bore catheter is then left in place, so that more treatments can be performed if required.[24-26]

Retroperitoneal Abscess

Retroperitoneal abscesses are usually located in the iliopsoas compartment and can have varied etiologies ranging from spinal osteomyelitis to Crohn's disease or hematogenous spread. These abscesses usually require CT guidance for drainage because of their deep location. Between 80% and 90% success rates have been reported for percutaneous catheter drainage (PCD) of iliopsoas abscesses.[27]

Splenic Abscess

Because the spleen is a highly vascular organ and there is a propensity of hemorrhage, splenic abscesses were traditionally managed with conservative measures. However, catheter drainage

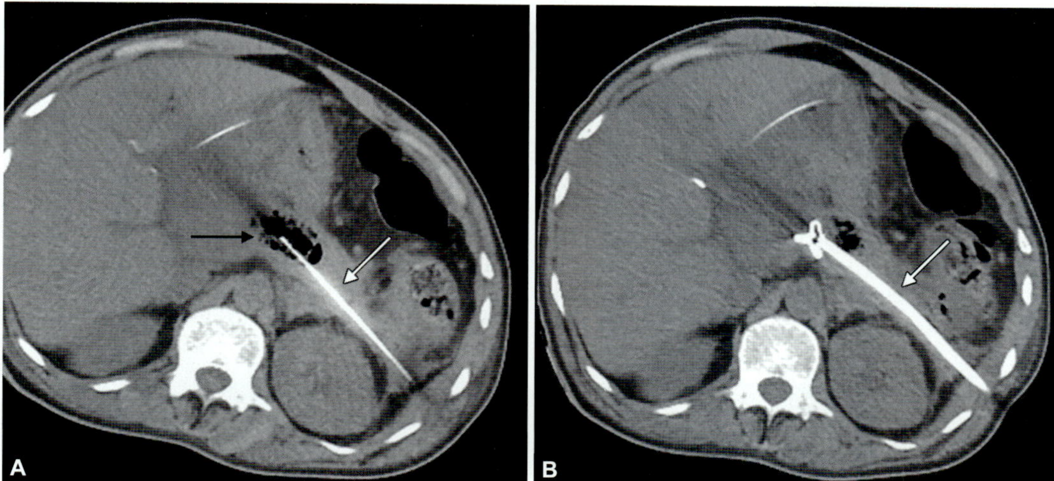

Figures 2A and B Axial-oblique CT images demonstrating a Chiba needle (white arrow in A) being used to access the infected necrotic collection (black arrow in A) in the peripancreatic region. This was followed by placement of a drainage catheter (white arrow in B) after serially dilating the tract over a guidewire

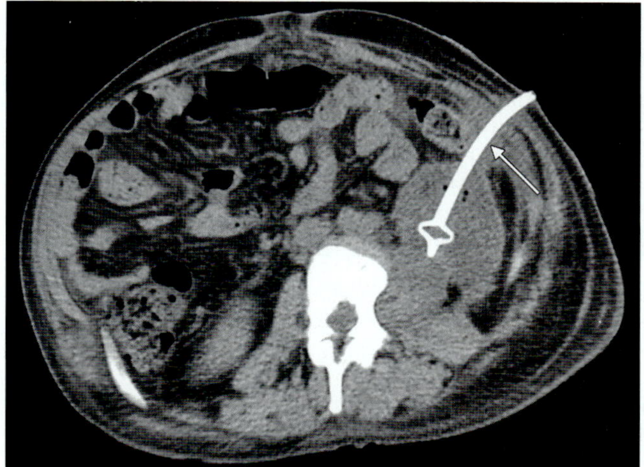

Figure 3 Axial-oblique CT image demonstrating a drainage catheter (arrow) in the left flank collection in a patient with acute pancreatitis

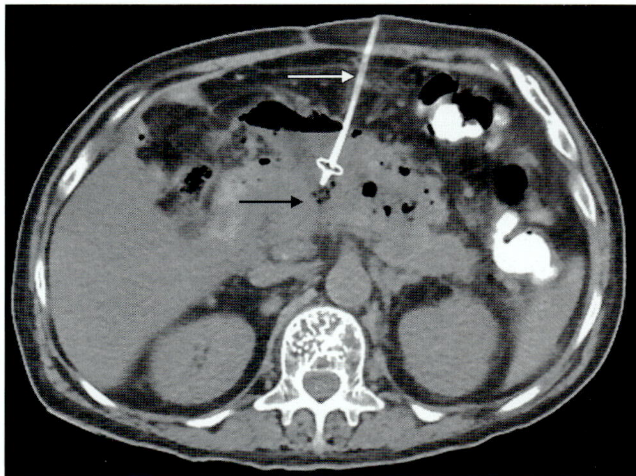

Figure 4 Another example of a drainage catheter (white arrow) being placed in the infected necrotic peripancreatic collection (black arrow)

is now increasingly being used for these patients without any significant increase in the rate of major complications.[28-30] Catheter should traverse minimal amount of normal splenic parenchyma while draining the abscess. Both ultrasonographic and CT guidance can be used for this purpose. Small 8–10 French catheters are preferred because of the vascular nature of the spleen.

Transvaginal and Transrectal Access

Transvaginal and transrectal routes have been gaining in popularity for draining abscesses in the rectouterine or rectovesical pouches because they are the most direct routes to abscesses in the deep pelvis and permit truly dependent drainage.[31,32]

ORGAN OR DISEASE SPECIFIC INTERVENTIONS

Vascular Diseases of Liver

Budd-Chiari Syndrome/Hepatic Venous Outflow Tract Obstruction

Budd-Chiari syndrome (BCS) refers to a group of disorders resulting from hepatic venous outflow tract obstruction which may be present in the hepatic veins or in the inferior vena cava (IVC) just above where hepatic veins drain into IVC. Depending on the rapidity of venous obstruction and the development of venous collaterals to decompress the liver sinusoids, it may have a fulminant, acute, subacute or chronic presentation.[33-35] Patients with acute thrombosis of hepatic veins present with severe ascites and acute hepatic failure, and those with the more common subacute or chronic presentation due to segmental/membranous occlusion of hepatic veins, IVC or both present with multiple intrahepatic venovenous collateral formation with minimal ascites, abdominal discomfort, upper gastrointestinal bleed and progress to end stage liver disease and its related complications.[36-38]

The treatment of BCS is complex depending on the presentation and must follow a step by step strategy. Acute thrombosis of hepatic veins is managed medically with anticoagulation and symptomatic therapy of ascites, portal hypertension and its complications. In chronic BCS, management depends on the length of venous obstruction, available hepatic reserve and severity of hepatic parenchymal fibrosis. While surgical creation of portosystemic shunt used to be the preferred therapeutic option for patients refractory to medical treatment in the past, with the advent of interventional radiological techniques, nonoperative endovascular management with angioplasty and stenting has become the standard practice at most centers (Figs 5A and B), liver transplant being reserved as a salvage procedure.[39-42] The protocol followed for endovascular management of BCS has been summarized in Flow chart 1.

Acute Portal and Mesenteric Vein Thrombosis

Traditional treatment of acute portomesenteric vein thrombosis includes conservative medical therapy and/or surgical treatment. Medical treatment mainly includes thrombolysis and anticoagulation. However, efficacy of the conservative treatment is limited and it cannot directly remove the obstruction due to the thrombosis. High mortality due to bleeding also needs to be considered. Surgical approach is invasive with its own complications. Therefore, it is seldom used as a standard treatment unless intestinal necrosis occurs. As radiological techniques have matured, catheter-directed thrombolysis has become the

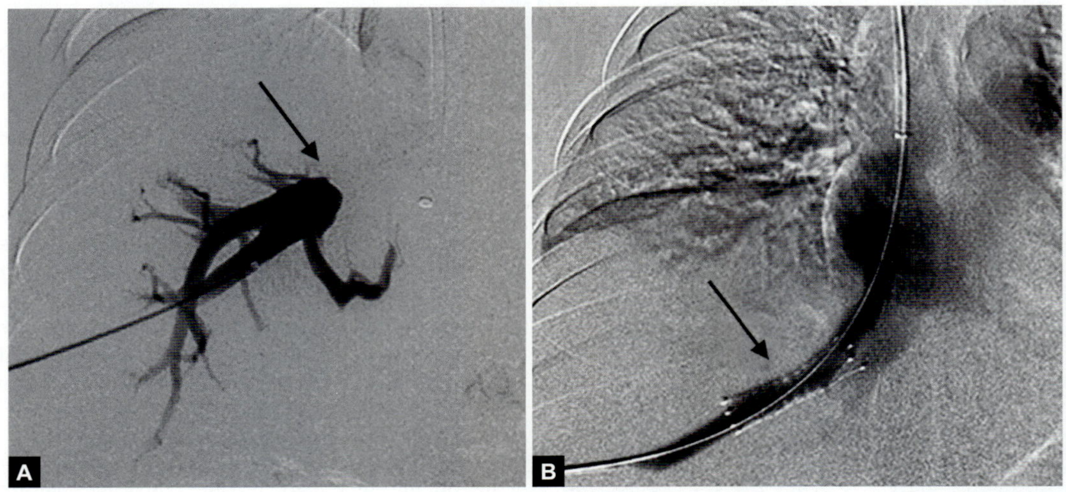

Figures 5A and B Angiographic images demonstrating obstruction of the right hepatic vein (arrow in A) which gets relieved after stenting (arrow in B)

Flow chart 1 Protocol followed for endovascular management of BCS

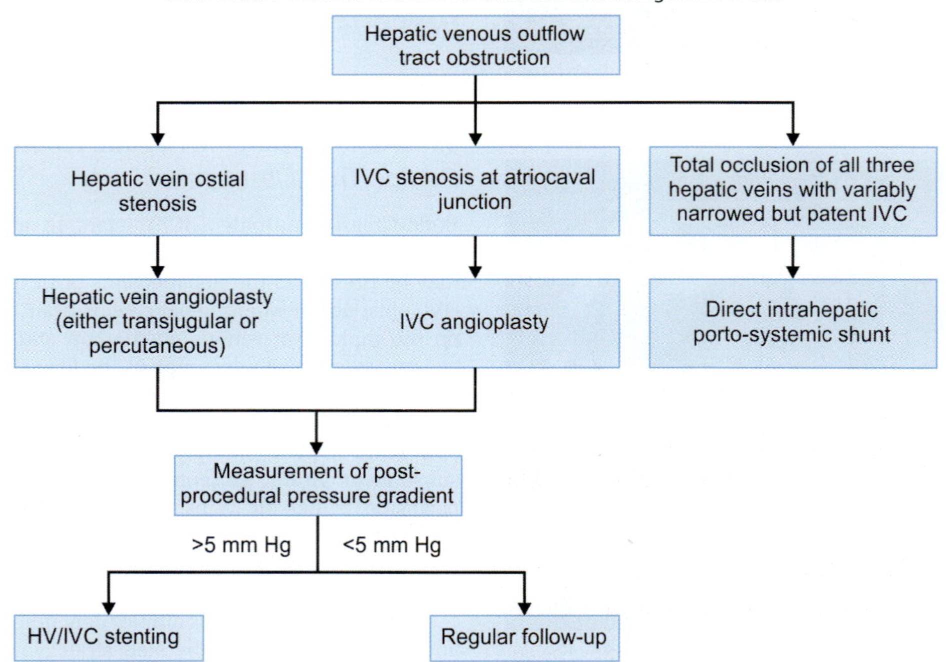

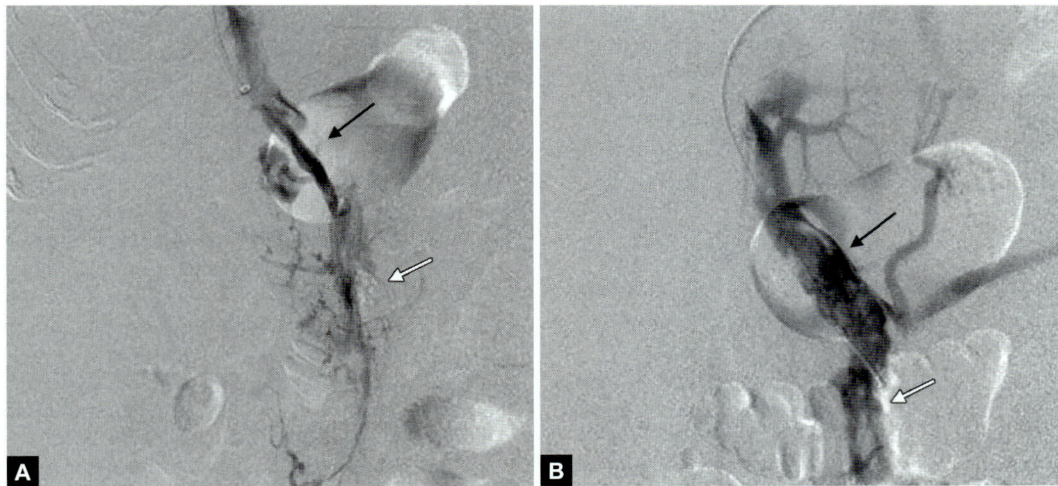

Figures 6A and B Angiographic image demonstrating partially thrombosed portal and superior mesenteric vein (black and white arrows in A, respectively). This was thrombolysed using a catheter inserted through the transjugular route. Post-thrombolysis image (B) demonstrating significant resolution of thrombus (arrows)

preferred means of treating acute-subacute portomesenteric vein thrombosis.[43,44] Image-guided thrombolysis can be performed by two approaches (Flow chart 2):

1. *Direct approach:* This involves placement of a catheter directly into the portal or mesenteric vein thrombus either via transjugular route (through transjugular intrahepatic portosystemic shunt) or direct percutaneous transhepatic route. Through this approach, both mechanical thrombectomy and pharmacological thrombolysis can be performed. It is preferred in patients with existing ascites and coagulative dysfunction because the way does not pass through the intraperitoneal route and there are less chances of bleeding and hepatic surface injury (Figs 6A and B). Transjugular intrahepatic portosystemic shunt (TIPS) diverts portal blood flow and reduces portal pressure effectively. It is thus suitable for patients with gastro-oesophageal varices requiring a portosystemic shunt. TIPS is however a technically complex procedure with attendant complications. In patients without ascites or coagulative dysfunction percutaneous transhepatic portal vein cannulation in comparison is simpler and cheaper than TIPS.
2. *Indirect approach:* When direct approach is not feasible, catheter can be placed in the superior mesenteric artery and thrombolytic agent can be infused.

Direct thrombolysis has been shown to be better than indirect treatment. Directly injected thrombolytic agents enhance thrombolysis, reduce the dose of thrombolytic agent and reduce the bleeding complication. Mechanical aspiration and mashing, stenting and balloon expanding can quickly restore perfusion and establish blood circulation in a short time. Results of thrombolysis are poor in patients when the disease duration is more than 2 weeks or lateral branch angiogenesis is seen on angiography around the main vessels.[44]

Chronic Portal Vein Thrombosis

When acute portal vein thrombosis (PVT) is asymptomatic and goes undetected, patients present later in life and are diagnosed

Flow chart 2 Protocol followed for endovascular management of acute portomesenteric vein thrombosis

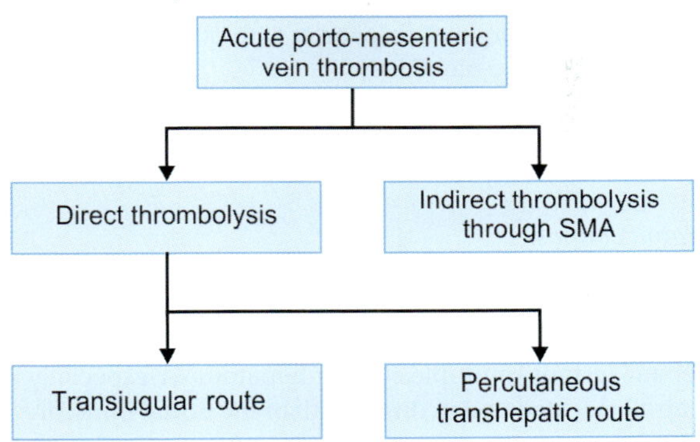

either incidentally on imaging done for unrelated issues or when investigations for portal hypertension related complications are carried out. The development of gastro-oesophageal varices and its propensity for massive hemorrhage is the most dangerous manifestation of chronic PVT. It is an important cause of portal hypertension in developing countries, where it is the most common cause of upper gastrointestinal bleeding in children (up to 70% in some series).[45]

Complications of chronic PVT:

- Variceal bleeding
- Biliary dilatation due to extrinsic compression caused by port-portal paracholedochal collaterals with associated sludge and/or stone formation (called as portal biliopathy)
- Splenomegaly and resultant hypersplenism.

The role of interventional radiology depends on the clinical presentation and includes:

- Patients with massive acute variceal bleeding refractory to medical and/or endoscopic therapy can be considered for an emergency TIPS or B-RTO. Recanalization of the portal vein remnant may also be possible in a selected cohort of cases.[46]

- Patients with intrahepatic biliary radical dilatation due to portal biliopathy might benefit from placement of an internal-external biliary drain, until the portal venous system is decompressed by surgical shunt creation.
- Pharmacological thrombolysis and/or mechanical thrombectomy can be used in patients with thrombosed portosystemic surgical shunts to prevent redo surgery.

Complications of Chronic Liver Disease and Portal Hypertension

Transjugular Intrahepatic Portosystemic Shunt

Transjugular intrahepatic portosystemic shunt refers to creation of a portosystemic shunt by transjugular placement of a metal stent between the hepatic and portal veins. Its primary goal is to decrease portal pressure and associated complications.

Indications:

- Acute variceal bleeding not responding to medical or endoscopic therapy
- Secondary prevention of variceal bleed
- Refractory ascites and hepatic hydrothorax
- Hepatorenal syndrome
- Budd-Chiari syndrome
- Before a major surgery in a patient with portal hypertension to decrease operative blood loss.

Since TIPS is associated with a high risk of hepatic encephalopathy, it is not recommended as a primary therapy for variceal bleed.

Contraindications:

- Severe pulmonary hypertension or congestive heart failure
- Uncontrolled hepatic encephalopathy
- Uncontrolled systemic infection
- Hepatic lesions (multiple cysts or hepatomas), especially when centrally located and in direct path of the portal puncture.

Procedure: The procedure can be performed under conscious sedation and analgesia. Hepatic vein is first cannulated through transjugular approach and portal puncture is done using a long needle passed through the metallic cannula. The tract is then dilated using a balloon and after calibration, metallic stent is deployed. Portal pressures are measured before and after the procedure. A technically successful outcome is defined as a decrease in portosystemic gradient to less than 12 mm Hg or more than 20% decrease in the portal pressures from baseline.[47,48] If the portosystemic gradient remains elevated despite dilatation of the stent or, if the varices continue to fill, embolization of the varices can be performed (Figs 7A to D).

Results: Technical success rates of the procedure are more than 95%.[49] With the use of covered stents, patency rates have also improved significantly.[50]

Partial Splenic Artery Embolization

Splenectomy and splenic artery ligation have been used for the treatment of hypersplenism caused by chronic liver disease. However, splenectomy is associated with high morbidity and significant mortality rate due to the high rates of postsplenectomy sepsis. Splenic artery ligation is not very effective in relieving hypersplenism due to the development of collaterals. Partial splenic artery embolization (PSE) is an alternative to surgical splenectomy and splenic artery ligation. In PSE, the vascular supply to spleen is occluded distally so that collateralization does not take place. Moreover, since only partial embolization is carried out, chances of sepsis and length of hospital stay is less compared to surgical splenectomy.[51,52] The procedure can be done even in patients who are poor candidates for surgery. It has also been used in patients who cannot undergo interferon therapy for treatment of hepatitis-C infection due to thrombocytopenia.[53] PSE increases platelet counts via two mechanisms: (1) by reducing the splenic size, thereby reducing the trapping of thrombocytes in the embolized spleen and (2) decreasing levels of platelet-associated immunoglobulin G (IgG). Reduction of platelet-associated IgG leads to decreased immunologic induction of thrombocytopenia. The increase in leukocytes after PSE can be attributed to the activation of body defense mechanisms against infarcted splenic tissues.[54-56] More recently, total splenic artery embolization has been used in liver transplant recipients with splenohepatic steal syndrome because it decreases the portal blood flow.[57]

Procedure: Splenic artery is selectively cannulated through femoral route. The catheter is placed distal to the origin of last pancreatic artery and embolizing agents such as polyvinyl alcohol particles or gelfoam soaked in antibiotic solution are injected.

Balloon-occluded Retrograde Transvenous Obliteration (B-RTO)

Gastric varices bleed less frequently than esophageal varices but their different hemodynamics including presence of large portocaval shunts and high blood flow volume, predisposes them to more severe hemorrhage with higher rebleeding rates and high mortality rates.[58-60]

Shunt surgery is usually contraindicated in these patients as they have poor liver function. Although endoscopic sclerotherapy and glue injection is the most frequently used treatment modality with high success rates approaching 100% in treating the initial episode of acute bleeding from gastric varices, the rebleeding rates are high, approaching almost 25%.[61,62] The rates of bleeding as well as rebleeding post endoscopic sclerotherapy treatment are especially higher in the isolated gastric varices (IGV) (78% and 53% respectively) due to their unique hemodynamic characteristics and associated large draining shunts.[63,64] TIPS also has decreased success rate for IGV with hepatic encephalopathy and shunt obstruction being other problems.

B-RTO of gastric varices is a novel interventional radiological procedure which has been shown to have very high success rates in treating gastric varices, including isolated gastric varices with large shunts, with very low recurrence and rebleeding rates.[63-65]

More recently, B-RTO has also been used effectively for the management of refractory hepatic encephalopathy secondary to large spontaneous portosystemic shunts (Fig. 8).[66]

Procedure: The procedure is performed under conscious sedation. A right IJV or right femoral vein approach is used to selectively cannulate the left renal vein and then subsequently the gastrorenal, lienorenal or gastrocaval shunt. A balloon catheter is then placed proximally into the shunt and complete occlusion of the shunt is confirmed by injecting contrast. The sclerosing agent is infused with the goal of filling the full extent of varices. After infusion of

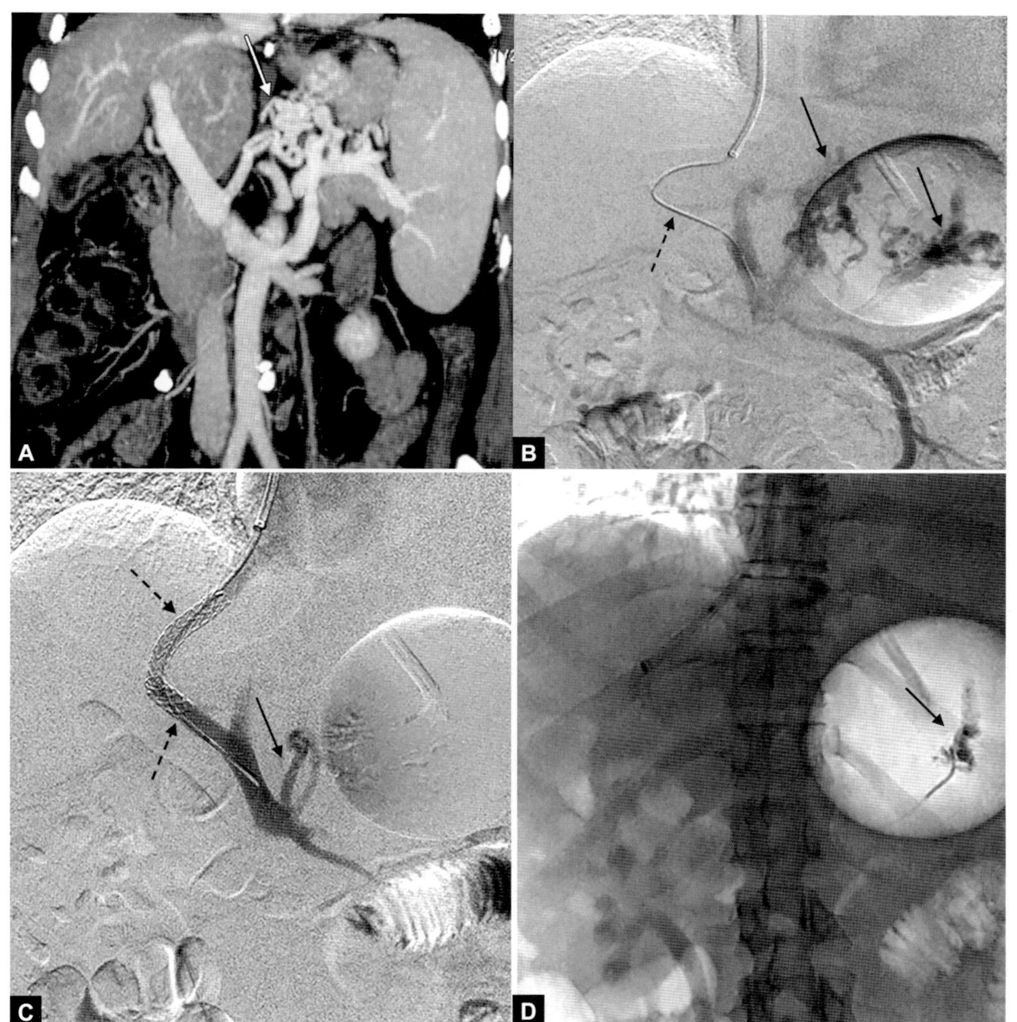

Figures 7A to D Coronal CT image (A) showing gastroesophageal collaterals (arrow) in a patient with chronic liver disease. Angiographic images demonstrating an angiogram obtained through a catheter placed in the portal vein (interrupted arrow in B) through transjugular route with opacification of the collaterals (black arrows in B). TIPS stent being deployed (interrupted arrows in C) with persistence of opacification of the left gastric vein (solid arrow in C). Thus, glue (arrow in D) was injected in these collaterals to occlude them and prevent any further episodes of variceal bleeding

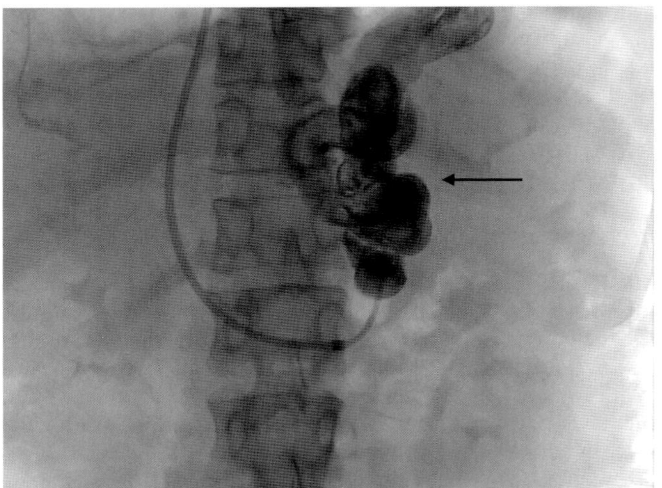

Figure 8 Angiographic image demonstrating stasis of the sclerosing agent in the large lienorenal shunt (arrow). B-RTO in this patient was performed to relieve symptoms of hepatic encephalopathy

the sclerosing agent, the balloon is kept inflated for 4–6 hours and removed after thrombotic occlusion of shunt and varices. Worsening of gastroesophageal varices and ascites formation are few complications which may be seen secondary to B-RTO, hence regular endoscopic follow-up should be done to monitor development of esophageal varices.

Interventional Radiology in the Management of Hepatocellular Carcinoma

The management of hepatocellular carcinoma (HCC) involves a multidisciplinary approach depending on the disease status and extent including the patient's performance status. Curative treatments of HCC include surgical resection or liver transplantation if it is diagnosed at an early stage. Only 15% of patients are diagnosed at an early stage and are eligible for curative treatments as others present with advanced disease.[67] This is mostly because most of the patients have no symptoms other than that of cirrhosis. Even if HCC is diagnosed at an early stage; all patients may not be fit to undergo liver resection, also liver transplantation may not be possible due to organ unavailability. In such a scenario interventional therapies for HCC remain a minimally invasive and most promising alternative to surgical therapies. Most of these therapies are planned as per Barcelona Clinic Liver Cancer (BCLC) classification, which helps in prognosticating as well as guiding the treatment strategies.

According to BCLC classification, patients with early stage HCC, who have been excluded from surgery, are best suited for image guided tumor ablation. Whereas patients with large or multinodular HCC but preserved liver function, no major vascular invasion or extrahepatic spread, good performance status should be considered for transarterial therapies such as transarterial chemoembolization (TACE). Current literature also suggests that newer therapies such as transarterial radioembolization (TARE) may be offered to selected group of patients. Similarly few patients may be best treated with multimodal therapies. Interventional treatment not only offers a palliative cure but may be used as neoadjuvant treatment in the setting of liver transplantation. It may be used to prevent dropout of patients waiting for organ and defined as a bridging procedure. Moreover it may be used to treat patients who are initially out of transplant criteria with intent to decrease the tumor burden so that they can fit into the transplantation criteria; hence these therapies are labeled as downstaging procedures.

Image-guided Tumor Ablation

Image guided tumor ablation is direct application ablative therapies and include percutaneous injection therapies consisting of ethanol or acetic acid and percutaneous application of energy mostly thermal such as radiofrequency ablation (RFA), microwave ablation (MWA), cryoablation and laser ablation. Newer non-thermal ablation techniques include irreversible ablation (IRE) and light activated drug therapy. However, amongst all, RFA has shown to be superior to ethanol injection in effectiveness and survival in various randomized control trial and is considered as standard treatment for local control of tumor.[68,69] Contraindications for percutaneous ablative therapy are ascites, uncorrectable coagulopathy, and lack of a safe pathway to localize the lesion, large lesion and lesions adjacent vascular structure due to risk of incomplete ablation. Post ablation follow-up is done with imaging to assess treatment response based on modified RECIST criteria. Complications of percutaneous ablative techniques range from immediate/periprocedural hemorrhage and self-limiting post ablation syndrome comprising of systemic inflammatory response that is managed conservatively.

Chemical Ablation

Ethanol (95%) and acetic acid (50%) have been used to treat small HCC by direct injection into the liver tumor from center to periphery using a thin 22G or 21G needle under ultrasound or CT guidance. This causes tumor necrosis by inducing intense cell dehydration, protein denaturation and small vessel thrombosis leading to coagulative necrosis and fibrosis of the tumor. This technique is ideally suited for small HCC (<3 cm in diameter) but not for larger lesions. Multiple sessions may be required for complete response. This technique is contraindicated in presence of ascites or coagulopathy.

Radiofrequency Ablation

Radiofrequency ablation induces thermal injury by depositing electromagnetic energy within the tumor. An alternating current of high oscillating frequency (200–1200 kHz and 200–250 watts) is produced from an RF generator and passed into tumoral tissue through a 14–17 guage electrode probe which causes ionic agitation with frictional heat production and cell death. Ideally a rim of 0.5–1.0 cm normal tissue should be ablated along with the tumor to achieve complete ablation. Presently RFA is considered to be the best treatment option for the treatment of early stage HCC (Figs 9 and 10).

Microwave Ablation

Involves application of electromagnetic radiation generated from a microwave generator that leads to oscillation of dipole water molecules with alternating field, increasing the kinetic energy and direct radiant heating of the tissue around the antenna. MWA is emerging as an alternative to RFA having advantages of consistent high temperature, large tumor volume, and fast ablation time. Charred tissue does not limit the heat propagation and is less susceptible to heat sink effect offering better results than radio frequency ablation.

Laser Ablation

In laser ablation light energy is applied via fibers directly inserted into the tissue to cause tissue necrosis. Single bare 400-lm laser fiber is capable of ablating spherical volume of up to 2 cm in diameter. Fewer data is available regarding the clinical efficacy of laser treatment.

Cryoablation

Single needle design cryoprobe has a closed loop circulation of specialized gases like argon, nitrogen and helium which creates a high pressure zone at the tip of the probe creating a freezing and thawing cycle. This leads to formation of both intra and extra cellular ice crystals (ice ball) with osmotic imbalance, cell membrane damage and cell death. At present there are no major literature supporting the use of cryoablation for treatment of HCC.

New Nonchemical Nonthermal Ablation Techniques

Irrerversible Electroporation

This is a novel technique wherein electrical field is used to produce focused apoptotic cell death by creating permanent pores in the cell membrane while preserving adjacent extracellular matrix and vessels. In contrast to thermal ablation, IRE leads to complete cell death without any residual tumor pertaining to heat sink effect, moreover there is no inflammation or necrosis. This produces a precise zone of ablation without affecting the adjacent tissues like blood vessels, bile duct, urethra and nerves. This technique however requires the patient to be in general anesthesia due to the risk of inducing muscle twitching or contractions during the procedure. Although IRE appears to be a promising tool, human

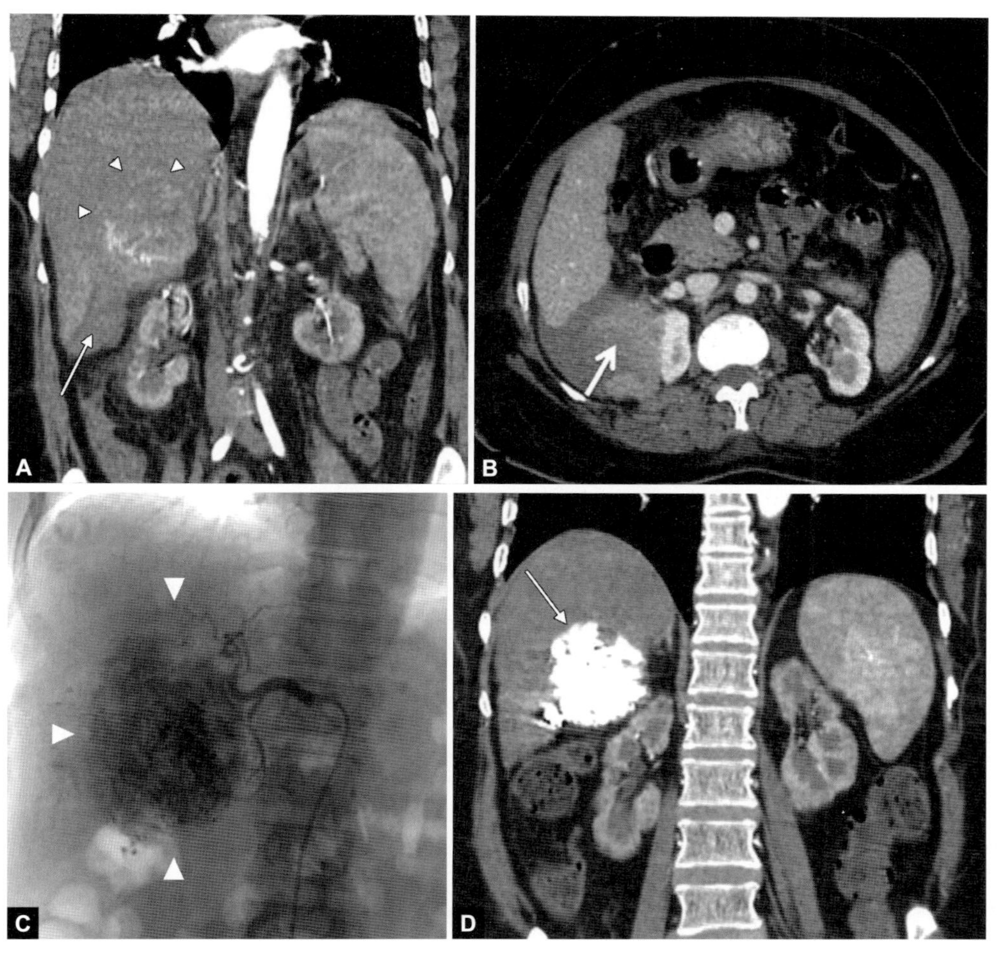

Figures 9A to D Coronal (A) and axial (B) CT images demonstrating a ruptured hepatocellular carcinoma (arrowheads in A) with hemorrhagic collection in the subhepatic region (arrows in A and B). Angiographic (C) and CT image (D) showing deposition of chemoembolic agent in the tumor (arrowheads in C and arrow in D)

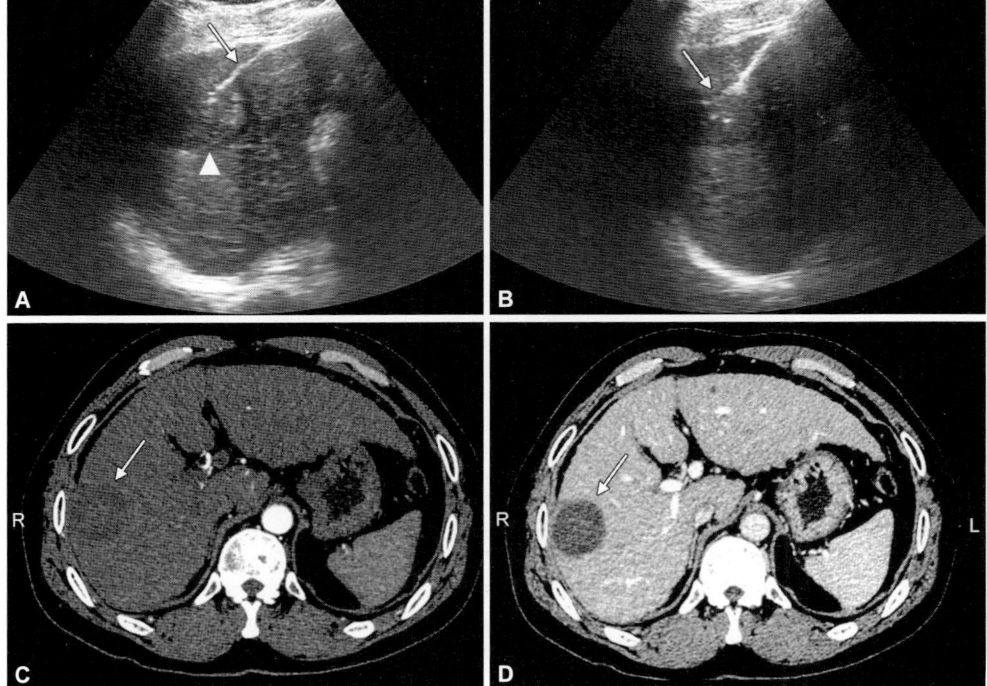

Figures 10A to D Gray-scale ultrasound images (A and B) demonstrating the RFA probe (arrow in A) being positioned within the HCC (arrowhead in A) and opening up of its prongs (arrow in B). Post-ablation CT images (C and D) showing complete ablation of the tumor as evidenced by lack of any enhancement within the tumor in the arterial (C) or venous phase (D) images

experience with IRE is limited and further comparative studies are needed to validate the results.

Light Activated Drug Therapy

Light activated drug therapy utilizes long wavelength light to activate drug which has been administered intravenously. The drug molecule developed for this treatment is talaporfin sodium (Aptocine; Light Sciences Oncology, Bellevue, WA), which is synthesized from a chlorophyll derivative. After IV administration, talaporfin sodium concentrates within the tumors. Drug is then activated by a light emitting activator which is inserted percutaneously within the tumor under imaging guidance. Activated drug produces singlet oxygen which causes apoptotic cell death through oxidation.[70]

Transarterial Embolization Therapies

Transarterial Chemoembolization

Transarterial chemoembolization is a form of palliative therapy that combines transarterial embolization and regional chemotherapy. The embolotherapy selectively interrupts the arterial blood flow to the tumor while maintaining the dominant portal vein blood flow and prevents washout of the injected chemotherapeutic agents from tumor having a synergistic antitumor effect with limited or low systemic drug levels and hence toxicity. TACE is mostly performed for patients having intermediate stage HCC.

Best candidates for TACE are those with unresectable HCC (stage A-C), Child Pugh's class A/B, liver dominant disease with no extrahepatic spread, preserved portal vein flow and liver function with performance status 0-2. Presence of extrahepatic disease with portal vein invasion, intractable systemic infection, hepatic encephalopathy, biliary obstruction, renal insufficiency and uncorrectable coagulopathy are contraindications for the procedure.

In TACE procedure, selective catheterization of the artery supplying the tumor is performed and an emulsion of lipiodol with the chemotherapeutic agent (doxorubicin, mitomycin or cisplatin ranging 50–100 mg) is injected selectively into the artery feeding the tumor followed by embolization with gelfoam or polyvinyl alcohol particles (Figs 11A to F). Currently, specialized particles (drug eluting beads) are available that can be preloaded with the chemotherapeutic agents like doxorubicin that releases the drug in a slow and sustained manner offering better results.

Post TACE, about 60–80% patients have post-embolization syndrome constituting non-specific symptoms of fatigue, fever, nausea and anorexia secondary to ischemia of liver parenchyma and elevated transaminases. This condition is self-limiting and requires no specific treatment except for symptomatic management. Other not so common complications like bile duct ischemia with stricture formation, cholecystitis, and pancreatitis do occur in 10% of patients due to non-targeted embolization.

Follow-up post TACE is done with imaging to look for amount of tumor necrosis and reduction in size. The treatment response is assessed employing the modified RECIST (response evaluation criteria in solid tumors) criteria.

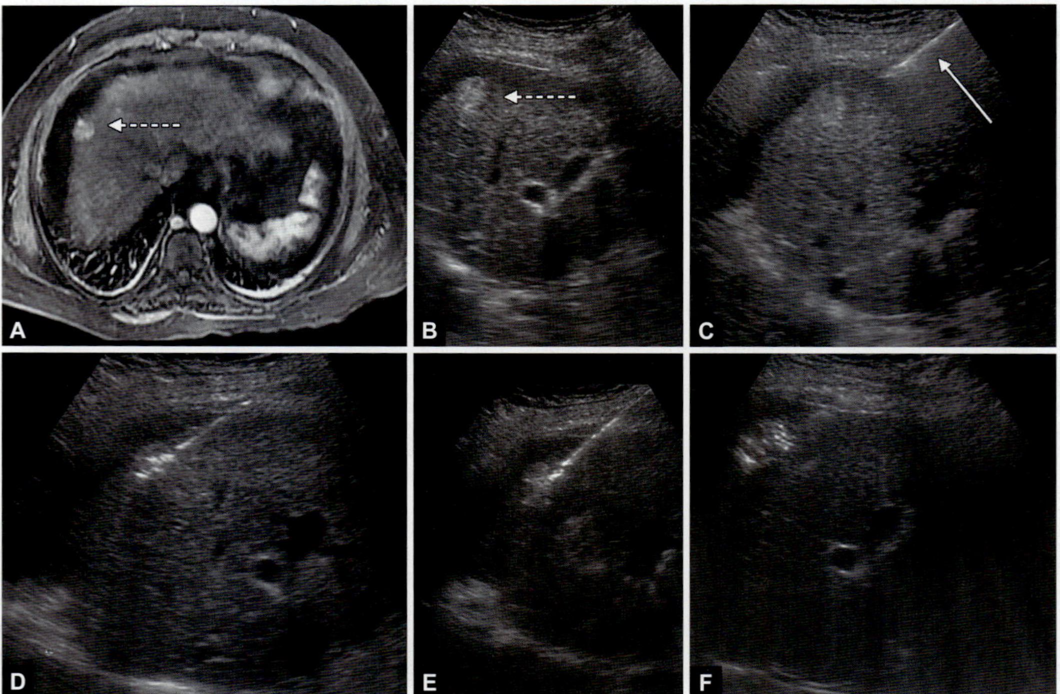

Figures 11A to F Axial contrast-enhanced T1-weighted MR image showing a tiny subcapsular enhancing HCC (arrow in A) in the right lobe of liver. Gray-scale ultrasound image (B to F) showing the echogenic tumor (arrow in B) targeted using the RFA probe (arrow in C) and ablated

Transarterial Radioembolization

Transarterial radioembolization or selective internal radiation therapy (SIRT) is a form of intra-arterial brachytherapy that involves injection of isotopes directly into the arteries supplying the tumor. This technique is ideally indicated in patients with unresectable HCC with or without portal vein thrombosis or as a bridge to liver transplantation. Yttrium-90 is a high energy beta emitting radioisotope that can be incorporated into glass or resin microspheres. Microspheres are selectively injected into the hepatic arteries supplying the tumor, where they emit their beta energy and irradiate the tumor. Most feared complication of this procedure is non-target embolization of Yttrium-90 microspheres which can cause radiation gastritis, cholecystitis, pneumonitis and hepatitis with progressive hepatopulmonary insufficiency. Compared to TACE, TARE is safe in treatment of patients with unresectable HCC with coexisting portal vein invasion, with a median survival of 8–14 months.

RADIOLOGICAL INTERVENTIONS FOR POST-LIVER TRANSPLANT COMPLICATIONS

Interventional radiology plays an important role in the management of complications after liver transplant.

Vascular

1. *Hepatic artery interventions:* Hepatic arterial complications include stenosis, thrombosis, trauma, arterioportal fistula and steal syndrome.[71-76] Since biliary tree is almost entirely supplied by the hepatic artery, diminished arterial flow to liver can result in ischemic biliary strictures.
   Indications:
   - *Diagnostic angiography:* When noninvasive tests like ultrasound Doppler, CT or MR angiography are inconclusive, catheter angiography can be performed. However, with the advancements in imaging technology, this indication is rarely, if ever used nowadays.
   - *Angioplasty and/or stenting for hepatic arterial stenosis or thrombosis:* The entire hepatic artery should be first assessed for the length of stenosis and presence of any tandem lesions.[71] Angioplasty is preferred with stenting reserved for cases with refractory lesions or when there are complications like traumatic injury to the vessel with bleeding (Figs. 12A to D).
   - *Embolization for hepatic arterial pseudoaneurysms and arterioportal fistulas:*[76] Spontaneous extrahepatic pseudoaneurysms due to contained rupture of mycotic aneurysms usually require surgical management, while

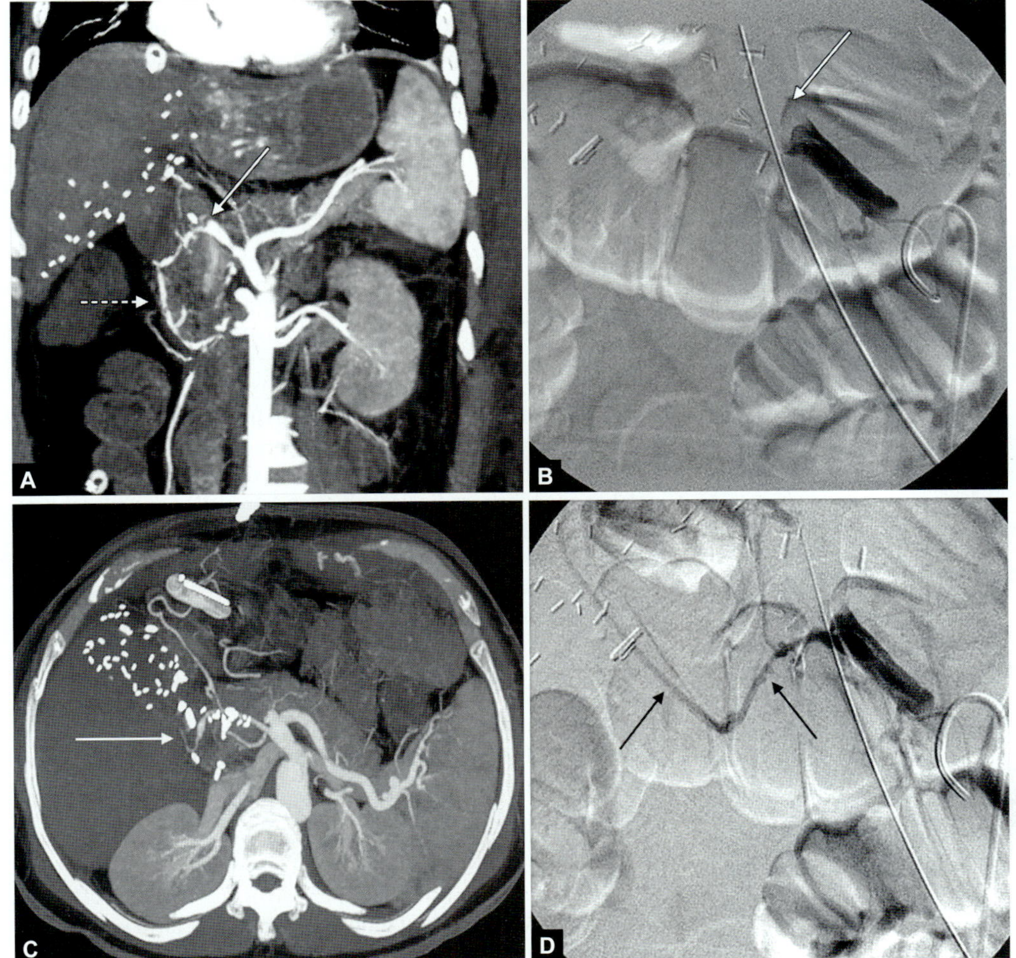

Figures 12A to D Coronal CT (A) and angiographic image (B) demonstrating abrupt cut-off of the hepatic artery (solid arrows) in a post-liver transplant patient. Axial CT (C) and angiographic image (D) after thrombolysis showing restoration of the patency of intrahepatic arterial branches (arrows in C and D)

iatrogenic extrahepatic pseudoaneurysms can be treated with stent grafts or balloon tamponade. Intrahepatic pseudoaneurysms should be treated with superselective coil embolization.[74] If endovascular access is not technically feasible, percutaneous embolization with glue, thrombin and/or microcoils can be attempted. Arterioportal fistulas are assessed using selective hepatic arteriography.[76] However, visualization of the actual fistulous tract is rare. Therefore, microcoils are deployed superselectively into the involved hepatic arterial branch. Complete obliteration is usually not possible and the aim of the procedure is to reduce the flow in the portal vein as much as possible. Additional fistulous communications may be unmasked once the dominant fistula is closed-off; therefore, hepatic arteriogram should be repeated after the deployment of coils.

- *Arterial steal syndromes:* It can of two types—(1) splenohepatic (more common; 85% of cases) and (2) gastroduodenal hepatic (15%). A celiac artery angiogram is essential for diagnosis. Splenic steal syndrome can be treated by reduction of the splenic blood flow by placing coils or hour-glass shaped stent-graft in the proximal splenic artery (Fig. 13). Gastroduodenal hepatic steal syndrome can be managed by coil embolization of the gastroduodenal artery after confirming the patency of superior mesenteric artery, so that collateral circulation to gut is maintained post embolization.[72]

2. *Portal venous interventions:* Portal vein can be accessed using either transjugular or percutaneous approach. Transjugular approach is preferred when patient's coagulation parameters are deranged or when portal vein thrombolysis is contemplated. Direct percutaneous transhepatic approach is the more commonly used route because it is in-line with the long axis of the portal vein and allows easy manipulation of the devices across the lesion.[77] The principal disadvantage is the increased risk of bleeding and the need to close the percutaneous tract after the procedure.[77]
   Indications:
   - *Portal vein stenosis:* Hemodynamic significance of stenosis is confirmed first by taking pressure gradients across the suspected area of narrowing. A gradient of more than 5 mm Hg is generally considered to be an indication for active intervention. Balloon dilatation is performed initially and if the residual stenosis on the post-dilatation venogram is more than 30%, a balloon-expandable or self-expandable stent is deployed.
   - *Portal vein thrombus:* The full-extent of thrombus is evaluated on venogram. Mechanical thrombectomy can then be performed followed by thrombolytic infusion using urokinase or tPA. Infusion can be continued for a maximum of 48 hours and the results are intermittently assessed by venography at intervals of 12–24 hours.
3. *Hepatic venous outflow interventions:* Occlusive disease can either involve the hepatic veins or the IVC.
   - *Occlusive disease of the hepatic veins:* Hepatic veins can be accessed from either transjugular (preferred route) or percutaneous transhepatic approach. The stenosed segment is traversed with guidewire and pressure gradients are measured. In case of significant stenosis (gradient >5 mm Hg) balloon dilatation with or without stenting is performed. In case there is significant thrombus, mechanical and pharmacological thrombolysis can be performed before proceeding to balloon dilatation.
   - *IVC occlusion:* If the occlusion is near the cavoatrial junction, right common femoral route is preferred over transjugular route. Rest of the procedure is same as that for hepatic vein occlusion.

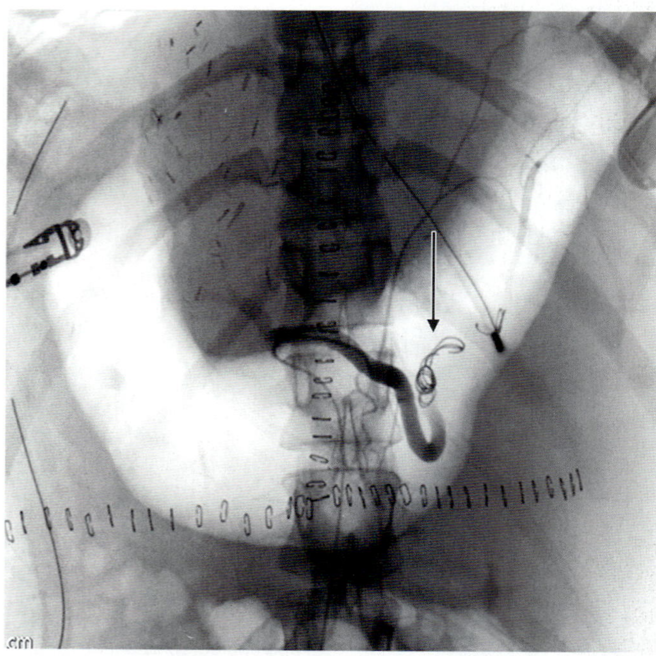

Figure 13 Angiographic image demonstrating coils (arrow) being placed to occlude the splenic artery in liver transplant recipient with splenohepatic steal syndrome

Nonvascular

Biliary Interventions

In up to 40% of transplant recipients with biliary obstruction, biliary tree is not significantly dilated. Therefore, percutaneous drainage is technically difficult and often requires puncture of central/hilar intrahepatic biliary radicals with attendant risk of vascular injury. Moreover, biliary disease in this setting is usually chronic and requires multiple sessions of dilatation (Figs 14A and B).[78] Rest of the procedural details are same as described below in the section on percutaneous transhepatic biliary drainage (PTBD).

Percutaneous Liver Biopsy

Ultrasound guided percutaneous liver biopsy is preferred at many centers over fluoroscopic approach for the evaluation of patients with suspected graft dysfunction due to its excellent efficacy and safety profile.

Drainage of Abdominal Collections

Abdominopelvic or pleural fluid collections that form in the post-transplant period may need to be aspirated for diagnostic purposes

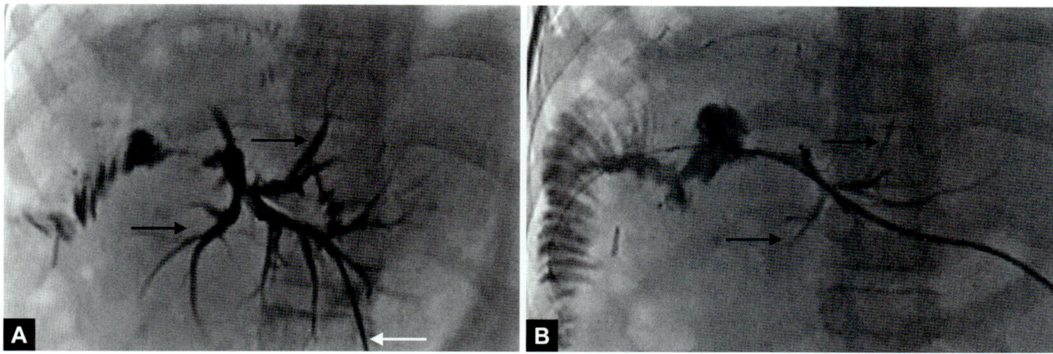

Figures 14A and B Angiographic image (A) demonstrating hepaticojejunostomy stricture with intrahepatic biliary radical dilatation (black arrows in A). This was relieved after stricture dilatation with decompression of the biliary radicals (black arrows in B)

to assess the nature of fluid and rule out infection. Drainage procedures may be planned accordingly.

Percutaneous Biliary Interventions

Percutaneous Transhepatic Biliary Drainage

Malignant bile duct obstruction can result in significant deterioration of patient's quality of life. In addition, obstructive jaundice precludes the use of certain chemotherapeutic agents. Similarly, biliary drainage and stricture dilatation is an integral part of management of benign biliary strictures.[79-83] For lesions involving the mid or distal common bile duct, endoscopic approach is usually preferred. However, for hilar lesions, percutaneous approach is associated with a higher success rate. In addition, when ERCP is not possible due to anatomy altering surgery like biliary-enterostomy, or when it fails, PTBD is the only option.

Indications:

In malignancy,

- Cholangitis
- Pruritus
- To lower the bilirubin for chemotherapy

In benign disease,

- Evaluation and treatment of biliary obstruction at biliary-enteric anastomoses
- Evaluation and/or treatment of biliary obstruction/leak following surgical procedures with suspected ductal transection or ligation
- Percutaneous treatment of biliary stone disease.

Procedure: The procedure consists of sterile puncture of a peripheral biliary radical under image guidance followed by placement of a catheter or stent for internal or external drainage of bile. Biliary puncture can be done either under ultrasonography or fluorosopic guidance. Internal drainage should ideally be attempted a few days after the initial PTBD to allow decompression of the biliary system and the inflammatory edema to subside. The external drainage catheter is replaced with an internal external drainage catheter over a stiff guidewire. This catheter should be left to external drainage initially. The external end of the catheter can be capped once the bile is clear of clots or debris and the patient is afebrile. Close monitoring and regular follow-up of the catheter is necessary to detect catheter migration, pericatheter leak or obstruction at an early stage. Bile output, color and vital signs should be recorded daily along with regular sonographic examination. Catheter should be exchanged every 4-6 weeks to prevent blockage.

Biliary Stent Insertion

Biliary endoprosthesis can be either plastic or metallic. An internal stent is more comfortable and acceptable to the patient because there is no drainage bag to carry around. An internal stent also prevents the complications of pericatheter leak or slippage. Metallic stents have been traditionally used for malignant obstruction, as they could not be retrieved later; however, retrievable metallic stents are now available and being used in the management of benign biliary strictures as well.[78,79,84] The major advantage of metallic stents is that they can be inserted in a contracted state and expand on their own after positioning. Also, they are less prone to migration and show a better patency rate than plastic stents (Fig. 15). However, up to 50% of these stents lose their patency in

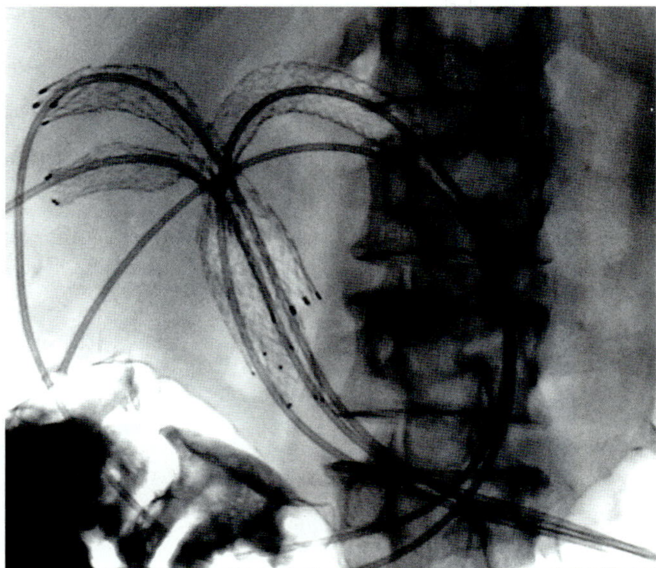

Figure 15 Radiographic image demonstrating hilar reconstruction using multiple metallic stents in a patient with malignant hilar obstruction

their first 6–8 months due to progressive tumor ingrowth through the openings between the struts of the stent, leading to recurrent episodes of jaundice and cholangitis.[85,86] The optimal strategy for the management of patients with malignant biliary obstruction who present with occluded SEMS is still controversial. Standard techniques used to tackle this problem include mechanical cleaning of the existing stent, use of covered stents, and repeat stenting using plastic stent or SEMS. Covered stents have shown better clinical patency rates compared to the standard bare metal stents for malignant obstruction.[85] These stents can be deployed across the cystic duct, pancreatic duct, and biliary duct origin with acceptable complication rates. Recently, endobiliary RFA has also been used to good effect for reopening of occluded metallic biliary stents.[87,88]

Biliary-enteric Anastomotic Strictures

Most of the benign biliary strictures are treated surgically with creation of biliary-enteric anastomosis. However, despite the refinements in surgical techniques, biliary-enteric anastomotic strictures following surgical repair of iatrogenic bile duct injuries and liver transplantation continue to be a significant cause of morbidity and mortality in this group of patients.[89-91] These strictures can occur following 28–32% of live donor liver transplantations and 10–30% of surgeries on native livers.[89,90] With the advances in interventional radiological and endoscopic procedures, the primary management of these patients over the years has shifted from a predominantly surgical approach to these less invasive methods.[90,91] Since endoscopic approach is technically difficult in patients with biliary-enteric anastomoses, percutaneous serial balloon dilatation and catheter maintenance over an extended period has become common at most centers[89,91,92] (Figs. 14A and B). However, due to the fibrotic nature of these strictures, failure rates are high with the reported long-term success rates after percutaneous management ranging from 55% to 83%.[92,93] Recently, cutting balloons, which were originally introduced to treat fibrosis and intimal hyperplasia in coronary vessels, have been utilized to good effect in the management of resistant biliary-enteric anastomotic strictures[94] (Fig. 16).

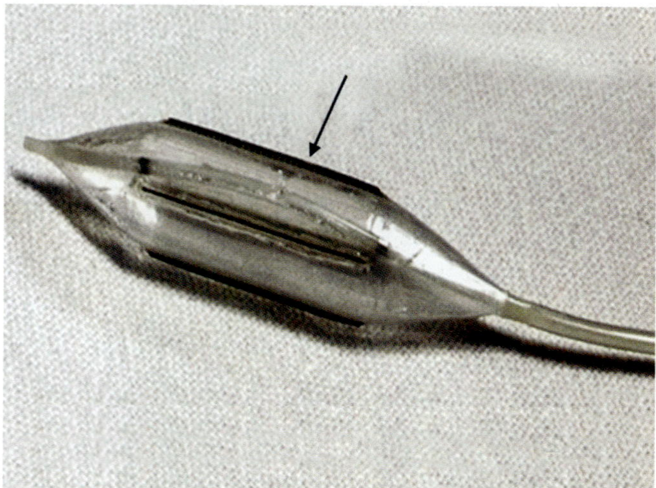

Figure 16 Photograph of a cutting balloon with the arrow pointing to one of its microtomes

Management of Hepaticolithiasis

Biliary stone removal can be performed in the same sitting as dilatation. In case of a well-developed percutaneous or T-tube tract, stones can be fragmented using a balloon, laser or intracorporeal lithotripsy and either flushed internally or removed via the tract with the help of a basket. A flexible endoscope can also be used for this purpose. Alternatively, ampulla can be over dilated to flush the stones into the bowel.[95,96]

Intraluminal Brachytherapy with PTBD

Through PTBD, high dose rate intraluminal brachytherapy using Iridium-192 can be delivered selectively to the tumor while avoiding the risks of external radiotherapy. It can be offered to patients with stricture length less than 6 cm with absence of distant disease. The brachytherapy catheter can be passed through the biliary drainage catheter and positioned with its tip 1 cm beyond the distal end of the stricture.[97,98]

Percutaneous Cholecystostomy

Cholecystostomy may be used as a temporary measure in patients of acute cholecystitis who are critically ill and cannot undergo surgery.[99,100] It can also be used as an access route to biliary tree when all other measures have failed.[101] Gall bladder is punctured under ultrasound guidance. Both transhepatic and transperitoneal approaches have been used. Transhepatic route is usually preferred as the transperitoneal approach carries a greater risk of bile leak and resultant peritonitis. After dilating the tract, an 8 French pigtail catheter is placed with its tip within the gall bladder and sutured to skin. If surgery is not considered as in cases of acalculus cholecystitis, the catheter can be removed once the patient's symptoms have resolved and a sufficient time has elapsed for the tract to mature.[102]

Preoperative Portal Vein Embolization

Surgical resection with complete removal of all cancerous tissue is the only way to provide patients with primary and metastatic liver disease a chance of cure or long-term survival. This radical treatment often requires extended hepatectomy. However, patients with limited liver remnant volumes may not be eligible for this surgery because of the increased risk of postsurgical liver failure. To reduce the risk of postoperative liver failure in such patients, portal vein embolization (PVE) has been effectively used.[103-105] PVE induces hypertrophy of the non-embolized future liver remnant (FLR) (expressed as a percentage of total liver volume) while causing the atrophy of tumor bearing hepatic lobe. PVE enables resection of livers previously considered unresectable due to borderline FLR. It decreases postoperative liver insufficiency. An FLR volume larger than 25–30% with normal liver parenchyma and more than 40% in diseased parenchyma (as in post-chemotherapy hepatic damage, liver cirrhosis/fibrosis and long-lasting cholestasis) is considered mandatory.

Although intraoperative portal branch ligation and transileocolic PVE (minilaparotomy technique) has been described, percutaneous transhepatic embolization using fluoroscopic guidance by an interventional radiologist is the preferred technique.[104]

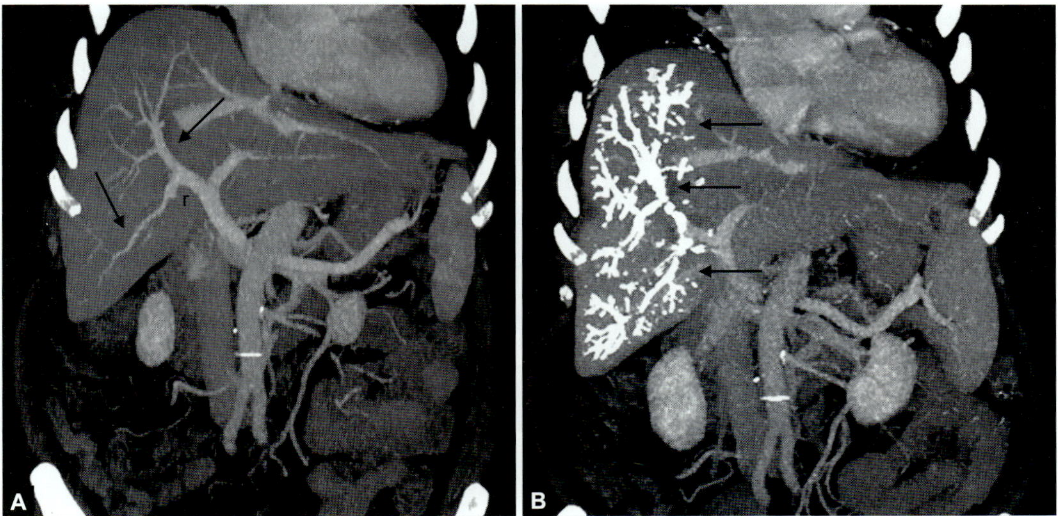

Figures 17A and B Preoperative portal vein embolization. Preprocedural coronal CT image (A) demonstrating the portal venous radicals (arrows in A) which were embolized using glue. Glue has formed a cast in the portal venous branches (arrows in B)

Procedure

Portal vein can be accessed percutaneously through ipsilateral or contralateral approach.

- *Ipsilateral approach* punctures the side which is planned to be removed. Thus complications in the FLR like hemorrhage, portal vein thrombosis or dissection are avoided. Also, ipsilateral approach facilitates embolization of segment 4 branch. However, depending on the material used for embolization, reverse-curved catheters or multiple lumen balloon occlusion catheters are usually necessary.
- *Contralateral approach* is easier in catheterization of the right portal branches and delivering the embolization material in the direction of the portal flow (Figs 17A and B). This reduces the chance of migration of embolization material in the portal branches of the FLR.

Postprocedural Management

Optimal waiting time between PVE and liver resection is still contentious.[105] The possible risk of tumor growth demands a waiting time as short as possible while a longer time interval allows extra growth of the FLR. Unresectable disease ranging from 6.4% to 33% has been described after PVE. The interval is mainly determined by the time required to attain sufficient FLR volume or function which was the primary aim of the PVE. In most cases surgery is performed after a period of 3–4 weeks of PVE.[105]

Visceral Arterial Interventions

Visceral Artery Aneurysms

Visceral artery aneurysms (VAAs) include aneurysms of the splanchnic circulation and those of the renal artery. VAAs are rare in comparison to aortic and iliac, femoral, and popliteal artery aneurysms. The most commonly affected arteries are the splenic, hepatic and celiac; multiple aneurysms have been found in one-third of patients in some series.[106-109] The etiology of the aneurysm has a great influence on whether it will be a true or pseudoaneurysm. Pseudoaneurysm is defined as dilatation of the artery with focal disruption of the arterial wall while true aneurysms are defined as dilatation of all wall layers. Aneurysms related to degenerative processes, fibromuscular dysplasia, inherited disorders of the vascular wall, segmental arterial mediolysis and vasculitis are true aneurysms unless they have ruptured. Aneurysms related to pancreatitis, infection, trauma or surgery are always pseudoaneurysms. All pseodoaneurysms require treatment as there is a high risk of rupture (up to 25%) with high mortality rates of up to 50%.[106-109] True aneurysms have a lower risk of rupture and the decision to treat is based on the size of the aneurysm, symptoms, interval growth and the vessel involved. Intervention is probably warranted in any pregnant patient with a splenic artery aneurysm, or any symptomatic aneurysm. There are no firmly defined size criteria for intervention in asymptomatic non-pregnant patients, but 2 cm in diameter has been recommended as the threshold for intervention, especially in young women.[106-109]

Endoluminal management serves to exclude a pseudoaneurysm from the circulation. It can either be done by embolization or placement of a stent graft across the parent artery (Flow chart 3).[106-113]

Selecting the optimal method depends on the:

- Size of the pseudoaneurysm
- Diameter of the neck
- Expendability of the donor artery.

A. Embolization

1. Endoluminally accessible:
    - Transcatheter embolization:
        - Embolization of pseudoaneurysm itself
        - Proximal coil embolization of donor artery
        - Proximal and distal coil embolization of donor artery (Figs 18A to F).

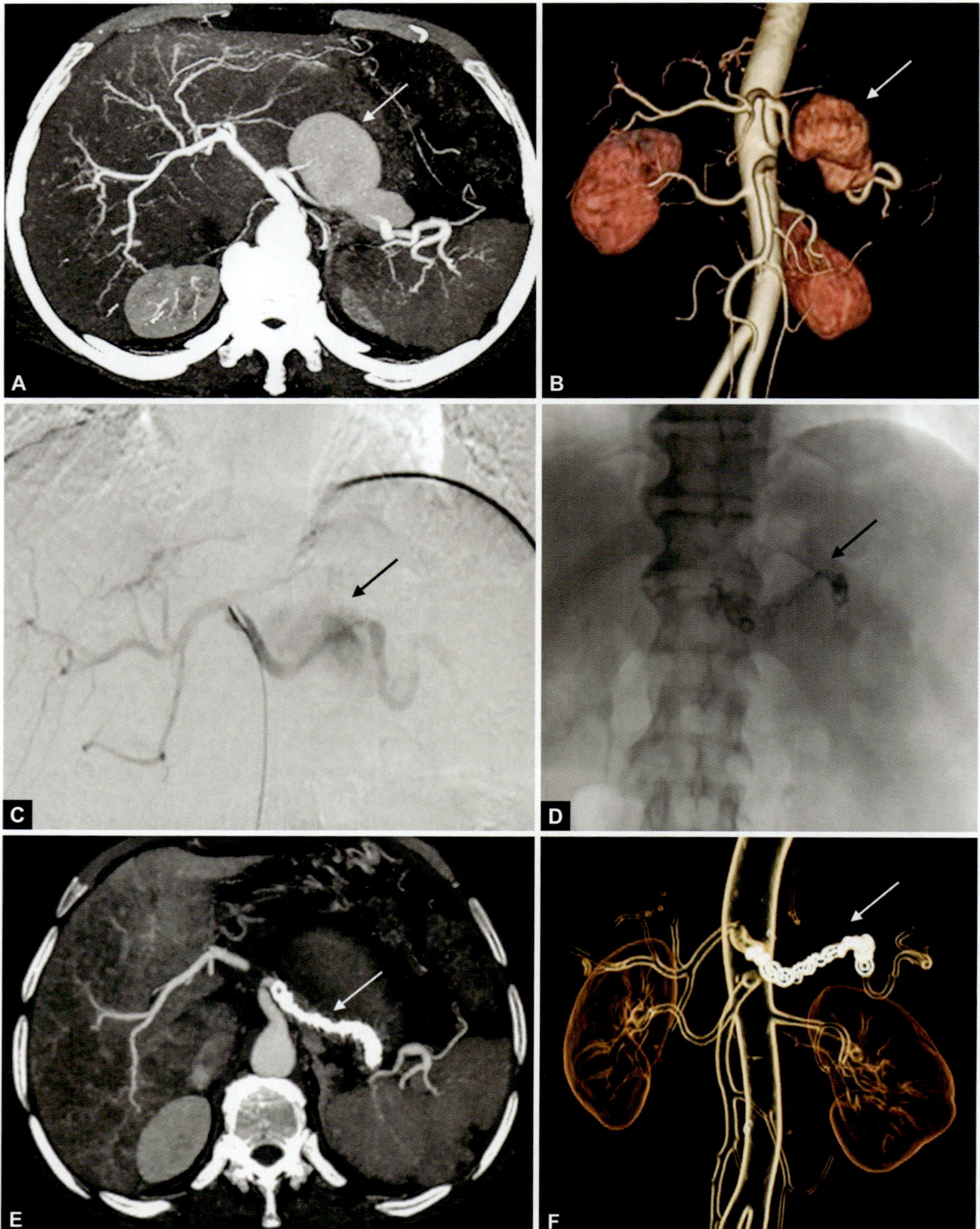

Figures 18A to F Axial MIP (A) and 3D volume-rendered image (B) demonstrating a large pseudoaneurysm (arrow) in a patient with acute necrotizing pancreatitis. Angiographic image (C) showing active leak of contrast in the pseudoaneurysm (arrow). This was embolized with coils (arrow in D to F) using the sandwich technique (front and back door embolization)

2. Endoluminally inaccessible:
   - Percutaneous interventional techniques:
     - Direct coil embolization
     - Direct glue embolization (Figs. 19A to D)
     - Direct thrombin embolization.

B. Stent placement: Patients who have undergone Whipple procedure can develop a characteristic type of delayed postoperative bleeding from gastroduodenal or pancreatic artery pseudoaneurysms. It usually presents after the fifth postoperative day with a "sentinel bleed" from a drain, the

Flow chart 3 Proposed algorithm[113] for the management of visceral artery pseudoaneurysms

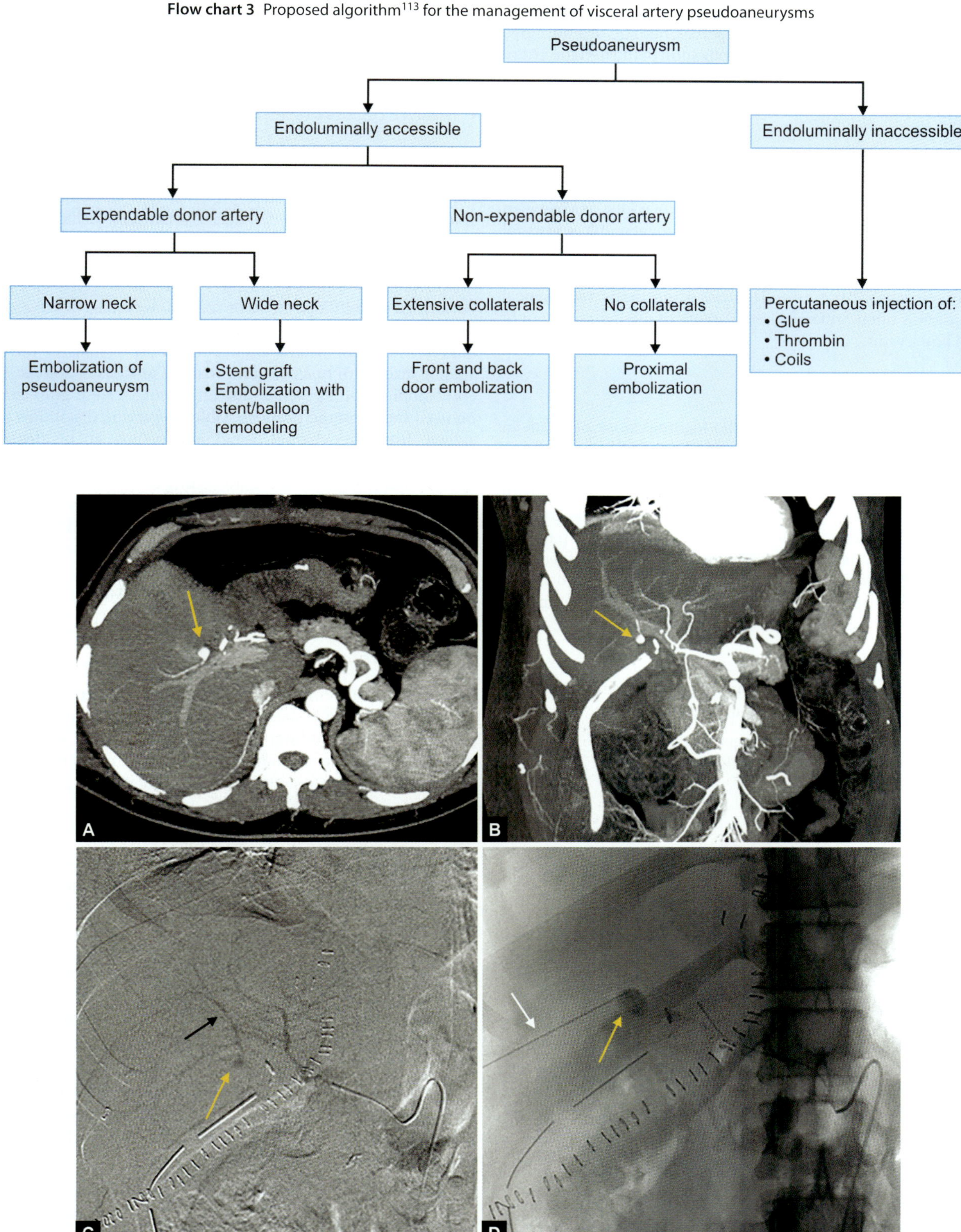

Figures 19A to D Axial (A) and coronal MIP (B) images and angiographic image (C) demonstrating a hepatic artery pseudoaneurysm (yellow arrows) in a patient with blunt abdominal trauma. This was not accessible through endovascular route and had to be embolized with glue injected through a needle (white arrow in D) percutaneously (yellow arrow in D)

gastrointestinal tract, or both. When the origin is the GDA stump, stent-graft placement preserves hepatic arterial flow. When this is not feasible, coil embolization of the hepatic artery across the GDA stump is usually well tolerated if the portal vein is patent. Pancreaticoduodenal artery pseudoaneurysms can usually be coil embolized.

Results

Overall technical success rate of the procedure is between 90–100%.[106,108,109] Data on endovascular management of visceral aneurysm repair is limited and there are no trials comparing endovascular management with surgical repair. However, due to its minimally invasive nature and low risk of morbidity, radiological intervention is often preferred over surgery in the management of visceral aneurysms.

Abdominal Trauma

Traumatic injury continues to be the leading cause of death in patients under the age of 45 years.[114] Blunt abdominal trauma in isolation represents 5% of trauma mortality.[115] Excessive bleeding accounts for 80–90% of these deaths.[114] Patients with trauma can be broadly divided into two groups on the basis of hemodynamic stability. In hemodynamically unstable patients, surgical exploration is often urgently required to control bleeding. The non-surgical group is more stable on presentation and can be managed with conservative measures or endovascular therapy.

Hepatic Injury

Clinically significant traumatic hemorrhage from the liver most commonly arises from the hepatic arterial system.

Indications for endovascular management:

- Recurrent hemodynamic instability despite resuscitation and CT findings of hepatic injury.
- Persistent hemobilia.
- Repeat hemorrhage after initial surgical management.

Procedure

In case of single point of extravasation, subselective catheterization of the involved artery can be done using a microcatheter and embolization can be performed using gelfoam, PVA particles or coils (Figs. 20A to D). When there are multiple points of extravasation non-selective embolization can be done using gelfoam pledgets. In cases of fistulas between hepatic artery and portal vein, hepatic vein or bile ducts, the parent artery can be isolated with the help of microcoils. Stent grafts can also be used for main hepatic artery fistulas. Technical success rates for hepatic artery embolization ranges from 85% to 100%.[116,117] Complications include liver infarct, gall bladder necrosis and hepatic abscess formation.

Splenic Injury

Once treated solely with splenectomy, hemodynamically stable patients of splenic trauma can now be nonoperatively managed with splenic artery embolization.[118-120] It is minimally invasive and allows preservation of splenic function.

Indications

- Hemodynamically unstable patients with imaging findings of splenic injury or active extravasation.
- Intrasplenic pseudoaneurysm or arteriovenous fistula.
- Delayed rupture of spleen.

Procedure

For intrasplenic hemorrhage proximal coil embolization of the splenic artery is performed. It decreases the splenic flow to control the bleeding and at the same time has a low risk of splenic infarction because the collateral circulation is preserved. For extrasplenic hemorrhage subselective distal splenic artery embolization is performed with PVA particles or coils. However, it carries a greater risk of splenic infarction and requires more time than proximal embolization. For pseudoaneurysms or AV fistulas of the main splenic artery are treated with proximal and distal splenic artery coil embolization to exclude the aneurysm. A stent graft can also be used for the same purpose while preserving distal flow to the spleen. Intraparenchymal pseudoaneurysms can be treated by knocking off the conduit artery by coils. Success rates of proximal splenic artery embolization in the setting of trauma have a technical success rate of 90–95% with low risk of complications.[118-120] Distal embolization has a similar success rate but a higher risk of splenic infarction.

Percutaneous Vascular Gastrointestinal Tract Interventions

Acute Gastrointestinal Tract Bleeding

With the advancements in noninvasive imaging techniques, angiography is rarely used nowadays for the diagnosis of acute gastrointestinal bleeding. However, transarterial embolization plays a critical role in management of gastrointestinal bleeding and many a times may act as a lifesaving therapy.

Upper Gastrointestinal Bleeding

Upper gastrointestinal bleeding is generally defined as bleeding that occurs in the digestive tract proximal to the ligament of Treitz; in practice from the esophagus, stomach and duodenum, followed by hepatic and pancreatic bleeding.

It can be due to:

- Direct bleeding into the stomach usually due to primary gastric pathology
- Transpapillary hemorrhage (hemobilia, pancreatic duct hemorrhage) or
- Variceal bleeding.

Endoscopy is the diagnostic and therapeutic mainstay in the management of acute upper gastrointestinal bleeding since a diagnosis can be made in the majority of cases and the bleeding can be controlled at the same time.

Indications for radiologic intervention:

- Failure of endoscopy
- Significant rebleeding after 1st–2nd endoscopy
- Ongoing transfusion requirement
- Need for more than 5 units over 24 hours
- Earlier for elderly, multiple comorbidities.

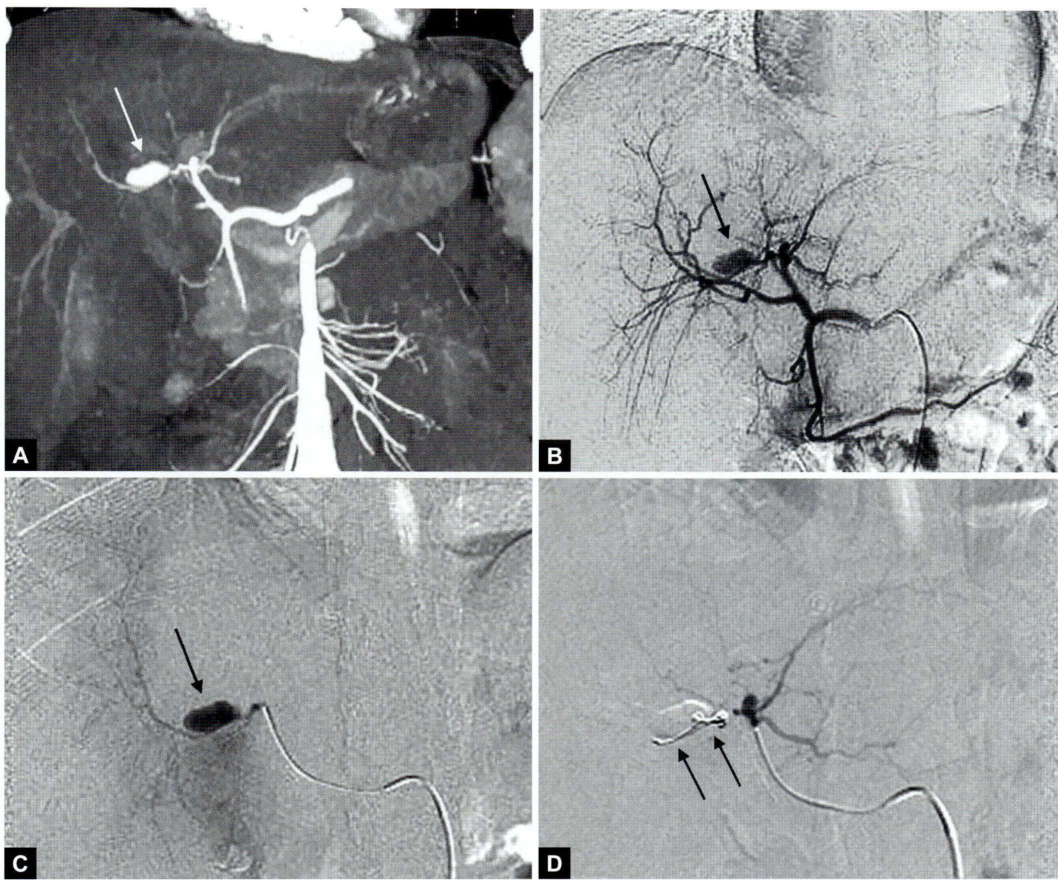

Figures 20A to D Coronal MIP image (A) and angiographic images (B and C) demonstrating a hepatic artery pseudoaneurysm (arrows) in a patient with liver laceration secondary to road-traffic accident. This was embolized with coils (arrows in D)

Procedure

Based on the preprocedural imaging, the site of bleeding is localized and selectively accessed. The vessel supplying the bleed (usually gastroduodenal or left gastric artery) is then subselectively catheterized. A variety of embolizing agents can be used. For left gastric artery, a common technique is embolization with gelfoam particles allowing blood flow to the carry particles to peripheral branches. For GDA bleeding, either coils or gelfoam can be used. Coils must be deposited both proximal and distal to the origin of the bleed to avoid reconstitution of flow to the bleeding site by collaterals. Variceal bleeding not responding to medical or endoscopic management can be treated with TIPS (discussed previously).

Lower Gastrointestinal Bleeding

In practice, lower gastrointestinal bleeding is defined as bleeding occurring from jejunum, ileum and colon. It is much less common than upper gastrointestinal bleeding and seen in a more elder population. Endoscopy plays a more limited role and is less often used as the initial approach than in upper gastrointestinal bleed.

Etiology

- Diverticulosis
- Angiodysplasia
- Neoplasia
- Inflammatory conditions
- Radiation
- Hemorrhoids

Since collateral circulation is less extensively developed in the hindgut, superselective catheterization is more important while managing lower gastrointestinal bleeds to avoid ischemic complications to the bowel. For colonic bleeds, it is often possible to advance all the way into the vasa recta in the bowel wall. If the catheter can be advanced right up to the site of bleeding, microcoils can be used for embolization. However, if the bleeding site is more diffuse or if the microcatheter cannot be advanced up to the exact site of bleeding, then polyvinyl alcohol particles are commonly injected as embolizing agents.

Results

Upper gastrointestinal embolization: Clinical success is considerably lower than technical success because of multitude of collaterals in the celiac arterial system and because upper gastrointestinal bleed often arises from more diffuses processes such as gastritis. Control of bleeding without any further interventions can be achieved in up to 56–88% of cases.[121-123] Studies comparing embolization with surgery in the management of upper gastrointestinal bleed refractory to endoscopic therapy have yielded comparable results in terms of hemostasis and mortality rates.[124,125]

Lower gastrointestinal embolization: Clinical success for lower gastrointestinal embolization is high at 84–92% because microcatheters can usually be advanced close to the site of bleed and collateral supply is less extensive.[126-129] Rebleeding is more common in small bowel than colon because of more collateral vessels in the small bowel mesentery.

Mesenteric Ischemia

Acute Mesenteric Ischemia

Acute mesenteric ischemia is a potentially life-threatening abdominal emergency. It can be due to occlusive and non-occlusive etiologies affecting the arterial or venous system. Occlusive causes include embolic or thrombotic occlusion of superior or inferior mesenteric artery or less commonly mesenteric venous thrombosis. Non-occlusive ischemia is due to mesenteric arterial vasoconstriction secondary to hypotension or use of vasopressors [non-occlusive mesenteric ischemia (NOMI)]. Patients usually present with abdominal pain out of proportion to the physical findings, nausea, vomiting, and constipation, with or without bloody diarrhea. Abdominal symptoms may then gradually worsen with the development of peritonitis, which indicates intestinal infarction. In most series, the mortality rate exceeds 60% without early and aggressive intervention.[130,131]

A pre-procedural contrast enhanced computed tomography combined with angiography of the abdomen is done to look for signs of bowel wall ischemia or necrosis with associated emboli or thrombus in the major arteries perfusing the bowel or the presence of mesenteric vein thrombosis.

Endovascular techniques are indicated when there is early (<12 hours) or minimal bowel ischemia without evidence of bowel wall necrosis or peritonitis clinically or on imaging, while urgent exploratory laparotomy with bowel resection is indicated when there are signs of impending bowel infarction and bowel necrosis. The various endovascular options include vasodilator administration, pharmacological/mechanical thrombolysis and angioplasty/stenting.

Occlusive acute mesenteric ischemia:

1. *Catheter suction embolectomy:* After retrograde puncture of the femoral artery, a selective catheter is placed in the affected mesenteric artery adjacent to the embolus, then the embolus is aspirated using a large caliber sheath (8 French) advanced over the wire placed adjacent to the embolus.
2. *Catheter directed thrombolysis:* After placing the catheter in the thrombosed artery, the thrombus or embolus is crossed with a hydrophilic guidewire. The catheter is then replaced with a coaxial infusion catheter with multiple side-holes. After an initial bolus dose, continuous infusion of the thrombolytic agent is done. The fibrinolytic or thrombolytic medications used are tissue plasminogen activator or recombinant tPA that include alteplase, reteplase or tenecteplase. Concomitant adjuvant heparinization may be done. The patient is then closely monitored with fibrinogen level and activated plasma thromboplastin time in an intensive care unit. Periodic assessment of the thrombolysis progress is done with angiograms performed through the guiding sheath. If thrombolysis is successful and an underlying stenosis is identified, then angioplasty with stenting is performed. The patient is taken for surgery if there is no improvement with development of peritoneal signs. Management of mesenteric vein thrombosis has already been explained previously.

Non occlusive acute mesenteric ischemia: Direct intra-arterial continuous infusion of papaverine can be done via catheter placed in the affected artery. The infusion rate is based on the clinical response typically requiring at least 24 hours and can be continued if vasospasm persists on serial angiograms performed via the infusion catheter. There is little role for surgical intervention in these patients.

Chronic Mesenteric Ischemia

Chronic mesenteric ischemia is caused by chronic stenotic or occlusive disease of the bowel's arterial supply usually secondary to atherosclerosis. Median arcuate ligament syndrome attributed to compression of celiac artery ostium by median arcuate ligament is another variant causing chronic low perfusion. Patients with chronic mesenteric venous ischemia are often asymptomatic due to extensive venous collateralization and are unlikely to develop intestinal infarction Postprandial pain is the defining symptom.

The traditional therapy for chronic mesenteric ischemia is surgery. Transaortic endarterectomy and aorta-visceral artery bypass are common operations for atherosclerotic lesions. However, these approaches are now used more often for occlusions and for symptomatic atherosclerotic ostial and proximal visceral artery stenosis. Percutaneous therapy with stents are now usually considered the first treatment option. Once the flow limiting stenosis or occlusion is confirmed on pre-procedural CT angiography, selective catheterization of the SMA is performed via the transfemoral route. The stenosis is crossed with a hydrophilic guidewire. Initially angioplasty is performed with an appropriately oversized balloon of the stenosis followed by deployment of a balloon mounted stent bridging the stenosis. The position of the stent is confirmed with contrast injection via the guiding sheath. Stenting offers better outcomes in cases of near total occlusion rather than angioplasty alone. Post stenting, the patients are put on antiplatelets lifelong and followed up with CT angiography to detect in stent occlusion secondary to intimal hyperplasia.[132-134]

Outcome and complications: The immediate periprocedural complication of revascularization procedure is development of reperfusion syndrome due to generation of oxygen free radical that leads to bowel inflammation. This condition is managed conservatively. The most feared complication is development of ischemic bowel infarction which requires surgery and bowel resection. Hemorrhagic episodes secondary to thrombolysis can be avoided with close monitoring of the coagulation status.

Percutaneous Nonvascular Interventions in Gastrointestinal Tract

For patients who require long-term nutrition, percutaneously placed tubes offer the best option. Enteral tubes can be placed through either natural orifices or percutaneous routes. They are simpler, associated with low morbidity and mortality and considered to be safer than endoscopic and surgical placement.[135-137]

Types of Tubes

- Single lumen tubes are used for a single dedicated function of either feeding or decompression. They are technically easy to place requiring minimal manipulation.
- Split lumen gastrojejunostomy tube has a separate gastric lumen and a one or more jejunal lumens. Gastric lumen is used either for decompression in patients with gastroparesis or gastric outlet obstruction or administering medications that are absorbed only by stomach while jejunal lumen can be used for feeding.

Percutaneous Gastrostomy

Indications

- Nutritional support for patients with inadequate oral intake due to dysphagia caused by esophageal obstruction or neurological disorders.
- Diversion of feed from esophageal leaks caused by recent surgery or trauma.
- Gastric decompression.

Procedure

Air is insufflated into the gastric lumen till adequate distension is achieved and the anterior gastric wall is opposed against the anterior abdominal wall. Site of puncture is usually the distal body of stomach equidistant from the lesser and greater curvatures to minimize the risk of arterial injury. Gastric puncture is performed with the kit needle pre-loaded with an anchor system. Stomach is gently approximated to the anterior abdominal wall by gentle traction. After serial dilatation of the tract, desired pigtail-retained gastrostomy catheter is placed. Contrast is injected to confirm the position.[138-140]

Percutaneous Gastrojejunostomy

In patients with history of gastroesophageal reflux disease or aspiration, percutaneous transgastric jejunostomy is considered. It can be performed as an initial feeding tube placement or by converting a prior gastrostomy tube to a gastrojejunostomy tube.[139,140]

Percutaneous Jejunostomy

It is indicated for patients with a history of chronic aspiration or gastric surgery. Because jejunum is highly mobile and easily collapsible, jejunostomy is technically more demanding. Dilatation of jejunal loops is achieved by slow saline injection through nasojejunostomy tube. On frontal and lateral fluoroscopy, the catheter tip is located in an air-filled proximal jejunal loop located close to the anterior abdominal wall and used as a target for puncture.

Percutaneous Cecostomy

Cecostomy is indicated for decompression or diversion in the setting of fecal incontinence, colonic pseudo-obstruction, or cecal volvulus.[141-143] It can also be used to deliver laxatives for antegrade irrigation for patients who have chronic constipation. An anterior intraperitoneal approach is used for cecostomy. Cecum can be distended using a foley's catheter placed through the rectum. Single wall puncture is made under fluoroscopic guidance and the catheter placed using the technique described previously for gastrostomy.[143]

REFERENCES

1. Mueller PR, vanSonnenberg E. Interventional radiology in the chest and abdomen. N Engl J Med. 1990;322(19):1364-74.
2. Silverman SG, Deuson TE, Kane N, Adams DF, Seltzer SE, Phillips MD, et al. Percutaneous abdominal biopsy: cost-identification analysis. Radiology. 1998;206(2):429-35.
3. Gupta S. Role of image-guided percutaneous needle biopsy in cancer staging. Semin Roentgenol. 2006;41(2):78-90.
4. Silverman SG, Mueller PR, Pinkney LP, Koenker RM, Seltzer SE. Predictive value of image-guided biopsy: analysis of results of 101 biopsies. Radiology. 1993;187:715-8.
5. Silverman SG, Mueller PR, Pfister RC. Hemostatic evaluation before abdominal interventions: an overview and proposal. Am J Roentgenol. 1990;154(2):233-8.
6. vanSonnenberg E, Mueller PR, Ferrucci JT Jr. Percutaneous drainage of 250 abdominal abscesses and fluid collections. Part I: Results, failures, and complications. Radiology. 1984;151(2):337-41.
7. Mueller PR, vanSonnenberg E, Ferrucci JT Jr. Percutaneous drainage of 250 abdominal abscesses and fluid collections. Part II: Current procedural concepts. Radiology. 1984;151(2):343-7.
8. Bakal CW, Sacks D, Burke DR, Cardella JF, Chopra PS, Dawson SL, et al. Society of Interventional Radiology Standards of Practice Committee. Quality improvement guidelines for adult percutaneous abscess and fluid drainage. J Vasc Interv Radiol. 2003;14(9 Pt 2):S223-5.
9. vanSonnenberg E, Wroblicka JT, D'Agostina HB, Mathieson JR, Casola G, O'Laoide R, et al. Symptomatic hepatic cysts: percutaneous drainage and sclerosis. Radiology. 1994;190:387-92.
10. Mueller PR, Saini S, Wittenbeurg J, Simeone J, Hahn PF, Steiner E, et al. Sigmoid diverticular abscesses: percutaneous drainage as an adjunct to surgical resection in 24 cases. Radiology. 1987;164:321-5.
11. Stabile BE, Puccio E, vanSonnenberg E, Neff CC. Preoperative percutaneous drainage of diverticular abscesses. Am J Surg. 1990;159(1):99-104.
12. Lasson A, Lundagårds J, Lorén I, Nilsson PE. Appendiceal abscesses: primary percutaneous drainage and selective interval appendicectomy. Eur J Surg. 2002;168(5):264-9.
13. Casola G, vanSonnenberg E, Neff CC. Abscesses in Crohn disease: percutaneous drainage. Radiology. 1987;163:19-22.
14. Neff CC, vanSonnenberg E, Casola G, Wittich GR, Hoyt DB, Halasz NA, et al. Diverticular abscesses: percutaneous drainage. Radiology. 1987;163:15-8.
15. Lambiase RE, Cronan JJ, Dorfman GS, Paolella LP, Haas RA. Post-operative abscesses with enteric communication: percutaneous treatment. Radiology. 1989;171:497-500.

16. Kerlan RK, Jeffrey RB, Pogany AC, Ring EI. Abdominal abscess with low-output fistula: successful percutaneous drainage. Radiology. 1985;155:73-5.
17. Eisenberg PJ, Lee MJ, Boland GW, Mueller PR. Percutaneous drainage of a subphrenic abscess with gastric fistula. Am J Roentgenol. 1994;162:1233-7.
18. Cai YL, Xiong XZ, Lu J, Cheng Y, Yang C, Lin YX, et al. Percutaneous needle aspiration versus catheter drainage in the management of liver abscess: a systematic review and meta-analysis. HPB (Oxford). 2015;17(3):195-201.
19. Slaughter MR. Use of percutaneous drainage for treatment of pyogenic liver abscess. JAAPA. 2013;26(1):43-6.
20. Loveday BP, Mittal A, Phillips A, Windsor JA. Minimally invasive management of pancreatic abscess, pseudocyst, and necrosis: a systematic review of current guidelines. World J Surg. 2008;32(11):2383-94.
21. Lee MJ, Wittich GR, Mueller PR. Percutaneous intervention in acute pancreatitis. RadioGraphics. 1998;18:711-24.
22. Lee MJ, Rattner DW, Legemate DA, Saini S, Dawson SL, Hahn PF, et al. Acute complicated pancreatitis: redefining the role of interventional radiology. Radiology. 1992;183:171-4.
23. Balthazar EJ, Freeny PC, vanSonnenberg E. Imaging and intervention in acute pancreatitis. Radiology. 1994;193:297-306.
24. Bucher P, Pugin F, Morel P. Minimally invasive necrosectomy for infected necrotizing pancreatitis. Pancreas. 2008;36(2):113-9.
25. Rosenberg A, Steensma EA, Napolitano LM. Necrotizing pancreatitis: new definitions and a new era in surgical management. Surg Infect (Larchmt). 2015;16(1):1-13.
26. Hollemans RA, van Brunschot S, Bakker OJ, Bollen TL, Timmer R, Besselink MG, et al. Dutch Pancreatitis Study Group. Minimally invasive intervention for infected necrosis in acute pancreatitis. Expert Rev Med Devices. 2014;11(6):637-48.
27. Maher MM, Gervais DA, Kalra MK, Lucey B, Sahani DV, Arellano R, et al. The inaccessible or undrainable abscess: how to drain it. Radiographics. 2004;24(3):717-35.
28. Yeom JS, Park JS, Seo JH, Park ES, Lim JY, Park CH, et al. Multiple large splenic abscesses managed with computed tomography-guided percutaneous catheter drainage in children. Pediatr Neonatol. 2013;54(6):409-12.
29. Conzo G, Docimo G, Palazzo A, Della Pietra C, Stanzione F, Sciascia V, et al. The role of percutaneous US-guided drainage in the treatment of Splenic abscess. Case report and review of the literature. Ann Ital Chir. 2012;83(5):433-6.
30. Lee WS, Choi ST, Kim KK. Splenic abscess: a single institution study and review of the literature. Yonsei Med J. 2011;52(2):288-92.
31. Saokar A, Arellano RS, Gervais DA, Mueller PR, Hahn PF, Lee SI. Transvaginal drainage of pelvic fluid collections: results, expectations, and experience. AJR Am J Roentgenol. 2008;191(5): 1352-8.
32. Sudakoff GS, Lundeen SJ, Otterson MF. Transrectal and transvaginal sonographic intervention of infected pelvic fluid collections: a complete approach. Ultrasound Q. 2005;21(3):175-85.
33. Menon KV, Shah V, Kamath PS. The Budd-Chiari syndrome. N Engl J Med. 2004;350:578-85.
34. Gandini R, Konda D, Simonetti G. Transjugular intrahepatic portosystemic shunt patency and clinical outcome in patients with Budd-Chiari syndrome: covered versus uncovered stents. Radiology. 2006;241(1):298-305.
35. Patil P, Deshmukh H, Popat B, Rathod K. Spectrum of imaging in Budd-Chiari syndrome. Journal of Medical Imaging and Radiation Oncology. 2012;56:75-83.
36. Amarapurkar DN, Punamiya SJ, Patel ND. Changing spectrum of Budd-Chiari syndrome in India with special reference to non-surgical treatment. World Journal of Gastroenterology. 2008;14(2):278-85.
37. Datta DV, Saha S, Singh SA, Gupta BB, Aikat BK, Chugh KS, et al. Chronic Budd-Chiari syndrome due to obstruction of the intrahepatic portion of the inferior vena cava. Gut. 1972;13:372-8.
38. Alam S, Khanna R, Mukund A. Clinical and prothrombotic profile of hepatic vein outflow tract obstruction. Indian J Pediatr. 2014;81(5):434-40.
39. Dhiman RK, Saraswat VA, Radhakrishnan S, Parashar A, Agarwal DK, Naik SR. Multiple venous thromboses and membranous obstruction of inferior vena cava in association with hereditary protein C deficiency: a case report. Journal of Gastroenterology and Hepatology. 1992;7:434-8.
40. Mukund A, Gamanagatti S. Imaging and interventions in Budd-Chiari syndrome. World J Radiol. 2011;3(7):169-77.
41. Mukund A, Gamanagatti S, Acharya SK. Radiological interventions in HVOTO—practical tips. Trop Gastroenterol. 2011;32(1):4-14.
42. Mancuso A. Budd-Chiari syndrome management: lights and shadows. World Journal of Hepatology. 2011;3(10):262-4.
43. Hollingshead M, Burke CT, Mauro MA, Weeks SM, DixonRG, Jaques PF. Transcatheter thrombolytic therapy for acute mesenteric and portal vein thrombosis. J Vasc Interv Radiol. 2005;16:651-61.
44. Liu FY, Wang MQ, Fan QS, Duan F, Wang ZJ, Song P. Interventional treatment for symptomatic acute-subacute portal and superior mesenteric vein thrombosis. World J Gastroenterol. 2009;15(40):5028-34.
45. Khanna R, Sarin SK. Non-cirrhotic portal hypertension—diagnosis and management. J Hepatol. 2014;60(2):421-41.
46. Alberti D, Colusso M, Cheli M, Ravelli P, Indriolo A, Signorelli S, et al. Results of a stepwise approach to extrahepatic portal vein obstruction in children. J Pediatr Gastroenterol Nutr. 2013;57(5):619-26.
47. Boyer TD, Haskal ZJ, American Association for the Study of Liver Diseases. The Role of transjugular intrahepatic portosystemic shunt (TIPS) in the management of portal hypertension: update 2009. Hepatology. 2010;51(1):306.
48. Haskal ZJ, Radhakrishnan J. Transjugular intrahepatic portosystemic shunts in hemodialysis-dependent patients and patients with advanced renal insufficiency: safety, caution, and encephalopathy. J Vasc Interv Radiol. 2008;19(4):516-20.
49. Haskal ZJ, Martin L, Cardella JF, Cole PE, Drooz A, Grassi CJ, et al. Quality improvement guidelines for transjugular intrahepatic portosystemic shunts. J Vasc Interv Radiol. 2003;14 (9 Pt 2):S265-70.
50. Bureau C, Garcia-Pagan JC, Otal P, Pomier-Layrargues G, Chabbert V, Cortez C, et al. Improved clinical outcome using polytetrafluoroethylene-coated stents for TIPS: results of a randomized study. Gastroenterology. 2004;126(2):469-75.
51. Koconis KG, Singh H, Soares G. Partial splenic embolisation in the treatment of patients with portal hypertension: a review of the english language literature. J Vasc Interv Radiol. 2007;18(4):463-81.
52. Xu ZJ, Zheng LQ, Pan XN. Partial embolisation as re-treatment of hypersplenism after unsuccessful splenic artery ligation. World J Gastroenterol. 2015;21(4):1365-70.
53. Takahara M, Miyake Y, Miyatake H, Imagawa A, Nakatsu M, Ando M, et al. Partial splenic embolization facilitates the adherence to peginterferon in chronic hepatitis C with thrombocytopenia. Intern Med. 2011;50(22):2731-6.
54. Wang HY, Shih SC, Lin SC, Chang WS, Wang TE, Lin FJ, et al. Partial splenic embolisation: 12-month hematological effects and complications. Hepatogastroenterology. 2008;55(86-87):1838-42.
55. Guan YS, Hu Y. Clinical application of partial splenic embolisation. ScientificWorldJournal. 2014;2014:961345.
56. Gu JJ, He XH, Li WT, Ji J, Peng WJ, Li GD, et al. Safety and efficacy of splenic artery coil embolization for hypersplenism in liver cirrhosis. Acta Radiol. 2012;53(8):862-7.

57. Bárcena R, Moreno A, Foruny JR, Moreno A, Sánchez J, Gil-Grande L, et al. Improved graft function in liver-transplanted patients after partial splenic embolisation: reversal of splenic artery steal syndrome? Clin Transplant. 2006;20(4):517-23.
58. De Franchis R, Primignani M. Natural history of portal hypertension in patients with cirrhosis. Clin Liver Dis. 2001;5:645-63.
59. Trudeau W, Prindiville T. Endoscopic injection sclerosis in bleeding gastric varices. Gastrointest Endosc. 1986;32:264-8.
60. Sarin SK, Lahoti D, Saxena SP, Murthy NS, Makwana UK. Prevalence, classification and natural history of gastric varices: a long-term follow-up study in 568 portal hypertension patients. Hepatology. 1992;16:1343-9.
61. Sarin SK. Long-term follow-up of gastric variceal sclerotherapy: an eleven year experience. Gastrointest Endosc. 1997;46:8-14.
62. Rajoriya N, Forrest EH, Gray J, Stuart RC, Carter RC, McKay CJ, et al. Long-term follow-up of endoscopic histoacryl glue injection for the management of gastric variceal bleeding. QJM. 2011;104:41-7.
63. Fukuda T, Hirota S, Sugimura K. Long-term results of balloon-occluded retrograde transvenous obliteration for the treatment of gastric varices and hepatic encephalopathy. J Vasc Interv Radiol. 2001;12:327-36.
64. Hiraga N, Aikata H, Takaki S, Kodama H, Shirakawa H, Imamura M, et al. The long-term outcome of patients with bleeding gastric varices after balloon-occluded retrograde transvenous obliteration. J Gastroenterol. 2007;42:663-72.
65. Ninoi T, Nishida N, Kaminou T, Sakai Y, Kitayama T, Hamuro M, et al. Balloon occluded retrograde transvenous obliteration of gastric varices with gastrorenal shunt: long-term follow-up in 78 patients. AJR. 2005;184:1340-6.
66. Mukund A, Rajesh S, Arora A, Patidar Y, Jain D, Sarin SK. Efficacy of balloon-occluded retrograde transvenous obliteration of large spontaneous lienorenal shunt in patients with severe recurrent hepatic encephalopathy with foam sclerotherapy: initial experience. J Vasc Interv Radiol. 2012;23(9):1200-6.
67. Roxburgh P, Evans TR. Systemic therapy of hepatocellular carcinoma: are we making progress? Adv Ther. 2008;25(11): 1089-104.
68. Orlando A, Leandro G, Olivo M, Andriulli A, Cottone M. Radiofrequency thermal ablation vs. percutaneous ethanol injection for small hepatocellular carcinoma in cirrhosis: meta-analysis of randomized controlled trials. Am J Gastroenterol. 2009;104(2):514-24.
69. Germani G, Pleguezuelo M, Gurusamy K, Meyer T, Isgrò G, Burroughs AK. Clinical outcomes of radiofrequency ablation, percutaneous alcohol and acetic acid injection for hepatocelullar carcinoma: a meta-analysis. J Hepatol. 2010;52(3):380-8.
70. Lencioni R, Cioni D, Della Pina C, Crocetti L. Hepatocellular carcinoma: new options for image-guided ablation. J Hepatobiliary Pancreat Sci. 2010;17(4):399-403.
71. Saad WE, Davies MG, Sahler L, et al. Hepatic artery stenosis in liver transplant recipients: primary treatment with percutaneous transluminal angioplasty. J Vasc Interv Radiol. 2005 Jun;16(6):795-805.
72. Saad WE. Management of nonocclusive hepatic artery complications after liver transplantation. Tech Vasc Interv Radiol. 2007;10(3):221-32.
73. Saad WE. Management of hepatic artery steno-occlusive complications after liver transplantation. Tech Vasc Interv Radiol. 2007;10(3):207-20.
74. Saad WE, Dasgupta N, Lippert AJ, Turba UC, Davies MG, Kumer S, et al. Extrahepatic pseudoaneurysms and ruptures of the hepatic artery in liver transplant recipients: endovascular management and a new iatrogenic etiology. Cardiovasc Intervent Radiol. 2013;36(1):118-27.
75. Saad WE, Davies MG, Saad NE, Westesson KE, Patel NC, Sahler LG, et al. Catheter thrombolysis of thrombosed hepatic arteries in liver transplant recipients: predictors of success and role of thrombolysis. Vasc Endovascular Surg. 2007;41(1):19-26.
76. Saad WE, Davies MG, Rubens DJ, Sahler LG, Patel NC, Lee DE, et al. Endoluminal management of arterioportal fistulae in liver transplant recipients: a single-center experience. Vasc Endovascular Surg. 2006 Dec-2007 Jan;40(6):451-9.
77. Saad WE. Portal interventions in liver transplant recipients. Semin Intervent Radiol. 2012;29(2):99-104.
78. Saad WE, Saad NE, Davies MG, Lee DE, Patel NC, Sahler LG, et al. Transhepatic balloon dilation of anastomotic biliary strictures in liver transplant recipients: the significance of a patent hepatic artery. J Vasc Interv Radiol. 2005;16(9):1221-8.
79. Lee MJ, Dawson SL, Mueller PR, Krebs TL, Saini S, Hahn PF. Palliation of malignant bile duct obstruction with metallic biliary endoprostheses: technique, results, and complications. J Vasc Interv Radiol. 1992;3:665-71.
80. Mauri G, Mattiuz C, Sconfienza LM, Pedicini V, Poretti D, Melchiorre F, et al. Role of interventional radiology in the management of complications after pancreatic surgery: a pictorial review. Insights Imaging. 2015;6(2):231-9.
81. Xu C, Lv PH, Huang XE, Sun L, Wang SX, Wang FA. Internal-external percutaneous transhepatic biliary drainage for patients with malignant obstructive jaundice. Asian Pac J Cancer Prev. 2014;15(21):9391-4.
82. Zhao XQ, Dong JH, Jiang K, Huang XQ, Zhang WZ. Comparison of percutaneous transhepatic biliary drainage and endoscopic biliary drainage in the management of malignant biliary tract obstruction: a meta-analysis. Dig Endosc. 2015;27(1):137-45.
83. Bezzi M, Bonomo G, Salvatori FM, et al. Ten years follow-up percutaneous management if benign biliary strictures: how successful are we? RSNA 1995. Radiol Suppl. 1995;197:241.
84. Hausegger KA, Kugler C, Uggowitzer M, Lammer J, Karaic R, Klein GE, et al. Benign biliary obstruction: is treatment with the Wallstent advisable? Radiology. 1996;200:437-41.
85. Loew BJ, Howell DA, Sanders MK, Desilets DJ, Kortan PP, May GR, et al. Comparative performance of uncoated, self-expanding metal biliary stents of different designs in 2 diameters: final results of an international multicenter, randomized, controlled trial. Gastrointest Endosc. 2009;70(3):445-53.
86. Das A, Sivak MV Jr. Endoscopic palliation for inoperable pancreatic cancer. Cancer Control. 2000;7(5):452-7.
87. Steel AW, Postgate AJ, Khorsandi S, Nicholls J, Jiao L, Vlavianos P, et al. Endoscopically applied radiofrequency ablation appears to be safe in the treatment of malignant biliary obstruction. Gastrointest Endosc. 2011;73(1):149-53.
88. Mukund A, Arora A, Rajesh S, Bothra P, Patidar Y. Endobiliary radiofrequency ablation for reopening of occluded biliary stents: a promising technique. J Vasc Interv Radiol. 2013;24(1):142-4.
89. Laštovi-ková J, Peregrin J. Biliary strictures after orthotopic liver transplantation: long-term results of percutaneous treatment in patients with nonfeasible endoscopic therapy. Transplant Proc. 2012;44(5):1379-84.
90. Ryu CH, Lee SK. Biliary strictures after liver transplantation. Gut Liver. 2011;5(2):133-42.
91. Choo SW, Shin SW, Do YS, Liu WC, Park KB, Sung YM, et al. The balloon dilatation and large profile catheter maintenance method for the management of the bile duct stricture following liver transplantation. Korean J Radiol. 2006;7(1):41-9.
92. Glas L, Courbière M, Ficarelli S, Milot L, Mennesson N, Pilleul F. Long-term outcome of percutaneous transhepatic therapy for benign biliaryenteric anastomotic strictures. J Vasc Interv Radiol. 2008;19(9):1336-43.

93. Tocchi A, Costa G, Lepre L, Liotta G, Mazzoni G, Sita A. The long-term outcome of hepaticojejunostomy in the treatment of benign bile duct strictures. Ann Surg.1996;224(2):162-7.
94. Mukund A, Rajesh S, Agrawal N, Arora A, Arora A. Percutaneous management of resistant biliary-enteric anastomotic strictures with the use of a combined cutting and conventional balloon cholangioplasty protocol: a single-center experience. J Vasc Interv Radiol. 2015;26:560-5.
95. Ozcan N, Kahriman G, Mavili E. Percutaneous transhepatic removal of bile duct stones: results of 261 patients. Cardiovasc Intervent Radiol. 2012;35(3):621-7.
96. Tsuyuguchi T, Miyakawa K, Sugiyama H, Sakai Y, Nishikawa T, Sakamoto D, et al. Ten-year long-term results after non-surgical management of hepatolithiasis, including cases with choledochoenterostomy. J Hepatobiliary Pancreat Sci. 2014; 21(11):795-800.
97. Mattiucci GC, Autorino R, Tringali A, , Perri V, Balducci M, Deodato F, et al. A Phase I study of high-dose-rate intraluminal brachytherapy as palliative treatment in extrahepatic biliary tract cancer. Brachytherapy. 2015;14(3):401-4.
98. Yoshioka Y, Ogawa K, Oikawa H, Onishi H, Kanesaka N, Tamamoto T, et al. Impact of intraluminal brachytherapy on survival outcome for radiation therapy for unresectable biliary tract cancer: a propensity-score matched-pair analysis. Int J Radiat Oncol Biol Phys. 2014;89(4):822-9.
99. Peters R, Kolderman S, Peters B, Simoens M, Braak S. Percutaneous cholecystostomy: single centre experience in 111 patients with an acute cholecystitis. JBR-BTR. 2014;97(4):197-201.
100. Viste A, Jensen D, Angelsen JH, Hoem D. Percutaneous cholecystostomy in acute cholecystitis; a retrospective analysis of a large series of 104 patients. BMC Surg. 2015;15:17.
101. Hatzidakis A, Venetucci P, Krokidis M, Iaccarino V. Percutaneous biliary interventions through the gall bladder and the cystic duct: what radiologists need to know. Clin Radiol. 2014;69(12):1304-11.
102. Khasawneh MA, Shamp A, Heller S, Zielinski MD, Jenkins DH, Osborn JB, et al. Successful laparoscopic cholecystectomy after percutaneous cholecystostomy tube placement. J Trauma Acute Care Surg. 2015;78(1):100-4.
103. Barbaro B, Caputo F, Tebala C, Di Stasi C, Vellone M, Giuliante F, et al. Preoperative right portal vein embolisation: indications and results. Radiol Med. 2009;114(4):553-70.
104. Fischman AM, Ward TJ, Horn JC, Kim E, Patel RS, Nowakowski FS, et al. Portal vein embolisation before right hepatectomy or extended right hepatectomy using sodium tetradecyl sulfate foam: technique and initial results. J Vasc Interv Radiol. 2014;25(7):1045-53.
105. van Gulik TM, van den Esschert JW, de Graaf W, van Lienden KP, Busch OR, Heger M, et al. Controversies in the use of portal vein embolisation. Dig Surg. 2008;25(6):436-44.
106. Spiliopoulos S, Sabharwal T, Karnabatidis D, Brountzos E, Katsanos K, Krokidis M, et al. Endovascular treatment of visceral aneurysms and pseudoaneurysms: long-term outcomes from a multicenter European study. Cardiovasc Intervent Radiol. 2012;35(6):1315-25.
107. Jana M, Gamanagatti S, Mukund A, Paul S, Gupta P, Garg P, et al. Endovascular management in abdominal visceral arterial aneurysms: a pictorial essay. World J Radiol. 2011;3(7):182-7.
108. Etezadi V, Gandhi RT, Benenati JF, Rochon P, Gordon M, Benenati MJ, et al. Endovascular treatment of visceral and renal artery aneurysms. J Vasc Interv Radiol. 2011;22(9):1246-53.
109. Ferrero E, Ferri M, Viazzo A, Robaldo A, Carbonatto P, Pecchio A, et al. Visceral artery aneurysms, an experience on 32 cases in a single center: treatment from surgery to multilayer stent. Ann Vasc Surg. 2011;25(7):923-35.
110. Amesur NB, Zajko AB, Costa G, Abu-Elmagd KM. Combined surgical and interventional radiologic management strategies in patients with arterial pseudo-aneurysms after multivisceral transplantation. Transplantation. 2014;97(2):235-44.
111. Sfyroeras GS, Liapis CD. Endovascular management of visceral artery aneurysms with flow-diverting stents. Ann Vasc Surg. 2014;28(4):1080.
112. Vaquero C, San Norberto E, Martin-Pedrosa M, Del Río L, Cenizo N, Taylor J, et al. Endovascular management of splenic artery aneurysms. Rev Port Cir Cardiotorac Vasc. 2013;20(2):97-101.
113. Saad NE, Saad WE, Davies MG, Waldman DL, Fultz PJ, Rubens DJ. Pseudoaneurysms and the role of minimally invasive techniques in their management. Radiographics. 2005;25(Suppl 1):S173-89.
114. Parks SN. Initial assessment In: Trauma, 5th edition. New York: McGraw- Hill Publishers; 2004. pp. 159-75.
115. Stanescu AL, Gross JA, Bittle M, Mann FA. Imaging of blunt abdominal trauma. Semin Roentgenol. 2006;41(3):196-208.
116. Hagiwara A, Yukioka T, Ohta S, Tokunaga T, Ohta S, Matsuda H, et al. Nonsurgical management of patients with blunt hepatic injury: efficacy of transcatheter arterial embolisation. AJR Am J Roentgenol. 1997;169(4):1151-6.
117. Monnin V, Sengel C, Thony F, Bricault I, Voirin D, Letoublon C, et al. Place of arterial embolisation in severe blunt hepatic trauma: a multidisciplinary approach. Cardiovasc Intervent Radiol. 2008;31(5):875-82.
118. Raikhlin A, Baerlocher MO, Asch MR, Myers A. Imaging and transcatheter arterial embolisation for traumatic splenic injuries: review of the literature. Can J Surg. 2008;51(6):464-72.
119. Hagiwara A, Yukioka T, Ohta S, Nitatori T, Matsuda H, Shimazaki S. Nonsurgical management of patients with blunt splenic injury: efficacy of transcatheter arterial embolisation. AJR Am J Roentgenol. 1996;167(1):159-66.
120. Sclafani SJ, Shaftan GW, Scalea TM, Patterson LA, Kohl L, Kantor A, et al. Nonoperative salvage of computed tomography-diagnosed splenic injuries: utilization of angiography for triage and embolisation for hemostasis. J Trauma. 1995;39(5):818-25.
121. Larssen L, Moger T, Bjørnbeth BA, Lygren I, Kløw NE. Transcatheter arterial embolisation in the management of bleeding duodenal ulcers: a 5.5-year retrospective study of treatment and outcome. Scand J Gastroenterol. 2008;43(2):217-22.
122. Padia SA, Geisinger MA, Newman JS, Pierce G, Obuchowski NA, Sands MJ. Effectiveness of coil embolisation in angiographically detectable versus non-detectable sources of upper gastrointestinal hemorrhage. J Vasc Interv Radiol. 2009;20(4):461-6.
123. Poultsides GA, Kim CJ, Orlando R 3rd, Peros G, Hallisey MJ, Vignati PV. Angiographic embolisation for gastroduodenal hemorrhage: safety, efficacy, and predictors of outcome. Arch Surg. 2008;143(5):457-61.
124. Defreyne L, De Schrijver I, Decruyenaere J, Van Maele G, Ceelen W, De Looze D, et al. Therapeutic decision-making in endoscopically unmanageable nonvariceal upper gastrointestinal hemorrhage. Cardiovasc Intervent Radiol. 2008;31(5):897-905.
125. Eriksson LG, Ljungdahl M, Sundbom M, Nyman R. Transcatheter arterial embolisation versus surgery in the treatment of upper gastrointestinal bleeding after therapeutic endoscopy failure. J Vasc Interv Radiol. 2008;19(10):1413-8.
126. Funaki B. Superselective embolisation of colonic bleeding. Semin Intervent Radiol. 2005;22(2):139-40.
127. Kickuth R, Rattunde H, Gschossmann J, Inderbitzin D, Ludwig K, Triller J. Acute lower gastrointestinal hemorrhage: minimally invasive management with microcatheter embolisation. J Vasc Interv Radiol. 2008;19(9):1289-96.
128. Lipof T, Sardella WV, Bartus CM, Johnson KH, Vignati PV, Cohen JL. The efficacy and durability of super-selective embolisation in the treatment of lower gastrointestinal bleeding. Dis Colon Rectum. 2008;51(3):301-5.

129. Koh DC, Luchtefeld MA, Kim DG, Knox MF, Fedeson BC, Vanerp JS, et al. Efficacy of transarterial embolisation as definitive treatment in lower gastrointestinal bleeding. Colorectal Dis. 2009;11(1):53-9.
130. Sachs SM, Morton JH, Schwartz SI. Acute mesenteric ischemia. Surgery. 1982;92:646-53.
131. Mamode N, Pickford I, Leiberman P. Failure to improve outcome in acute mesenteric ischemia: seven year review. Eur J Surg. 1999;165:203-8.
132. Park WM, Gloviczki P, Cherry KJ Jr, Hallett JW Jr, Bower TC, Panneton JM, et al. Contemporary management of acute mesenteric ischemia: factors associated with survival. J Vasc Surg. 2002;35:445-52.
133. Turba UC, Saad WE, Arslan B, Sabri SS, Trotter S, Angle JF, et al. Chronic mesenteric ischaemia: 28-year experience of endovascular treatment. Eur Radiol. 2012;22:1372-84.
134. Zeller T, Rastan A, Sixt S. Chronic atherosclerotic mesenteric ischemia (CMI). Vasc Med. 2010;15:333-8.
135. Perona F, Castellazzi G, De Iuliis A, Rizzo L. Percutaneous radiologic gastrostomy: a 12-year series. Gut Liver. 2010;4(Suppl 1):S44-9.
136. Leeds JS, McAlindon ME, Grant J, Robson HE, Lee FK, Sanders DS. Survival analysis after gastrostomy: a single-centre, observational study comparing radiological and endoscopic insertion. Eur J Gastroenterol Hepatol. 2010;22(5):591-6.
137. Rossi UG, Petrocelli F, Seitun S, Patrone L, Ferro C. Percutaneous radiological gastrostomy: single-puncture double-anchor technique. Radiol Med. 2013;118(3):356-65.
138. Ho SG, Marchinkow LO, Legiehn GM, Munk PL, Lee MJ. Radiological percutaneous gastrostomy. Clin Radiol. 2001;56(11):902-10.
139. Bazarah SM, Al-Rawas M, Akbar H, Qari Y. Percutaneous gastrostomy and gastrojejunostomy: radiological and endoscopic approach. Ann Saudi Med. 2002;22(1-2):38-42.
140. Lyon SM, Pascoe DM. Percutaneous gastrostomy and gastrojejunostomy. Semin Intervent Radiol. 2004;21(3):181-9.
141. Tewari SO, Getrajdman GI, Petre EN, Sofocleous CT, Siegelbaum RH, Erinjeri JP, et al. Safety and efficacy of percutaneous cecostomy/colostomy for treatment of large bowel obstruction in adults with cancer. J Vasc Interv Radiol. 2015;26(2):182-8.
142. Khan WU, Satkunasingham J, Moineddin R, Jamal I, Afzal S, Chait P, et al. The percutaneous cecostomy tube in the management of fecal incontinence in children. J Vasc Interv Radiol. 2015;26(2):189-95.
143. Chait PG, Shlomovitz E, Connolly BL, Temple MJ, Restrepo R, Amaral JG, et al. Percutaneous cecostomy: updates in technique and patient care. Radiology. 2003;227(1):246-50.

SECTION 2

Esophagus

CHAPTER 10

Anatomy and Physiology of the Esophagus

Nikhil Aggarwal

ANATOMY

Esophagus serves as a one way tube for food transport from pharynx to stomach. It starts at the level of C6 at the base of pharynx and ends at the cardia of stomach at T11. It spans across three body cavities: (1) neck, (2) chest and (3) abdomen and is correspondingly divided into cervical, thoracic and abdominal esophagus (Fig. 1). It is flanked by two high pressure zones: (1) upper esophageal sphincter (UES) and (2) lower esophageal sphincter (LES).

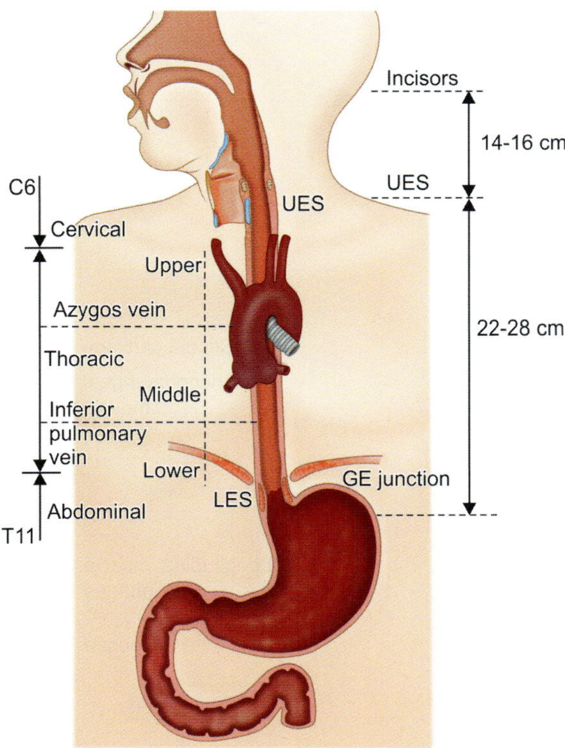

Figure 1 Topography and divisions of esophagus

It lies in front of the vertebral column and is anteriorly related to larynx, trachea, right pulmonary artery, left main bronchus, pericardium and diaphragm from above downward. In the chest it lies in the posterior mediastinum with mediastinal pleura, lungs and their hila on both sides. On the right lie the subclavian artery and the azygous vein. The thoracic duct ascends in groove between aorta and azygous vein and crosses behind the esophagus to the left side at the level of T4-T5. On the left are situated aortic arch and aorta (Fig. 2). The esophagus moves anterior to aorta at the level of eighth thoracic vertebra and exits the diaphragm through the esophageal hiatus at T10 level accompanied by both the vagus nerves. The esophageal hiatus is formed by the right and left crura of the diaphragm and the median arcuate ligament.

The American Joint Committee on Cancer (AJCC, 2010) divides esophagus into cervical, thoracic and abdominal esophagus for the location of the primary tumor.[1] The thoracic esophagus is further subdivided into upper, middle and lower thoracic esophagus. The cervical esophagus is superiorly bordered by the hypopharynx and inferiorly by the thoracic inlet at the level of the sternal notch. The thoracic inlet marks the superior border of upper thoracic esophagus which is inferiorly demarcated by the lower border of the azygous vein. The middle thoracic esophagus starts from the lower border of the azygous vein to end at the inferior pulmonary veins. The lower thoracic esophagus extends from the inferior pulmonary veins to the esophageal hiatus (Fig. 1).

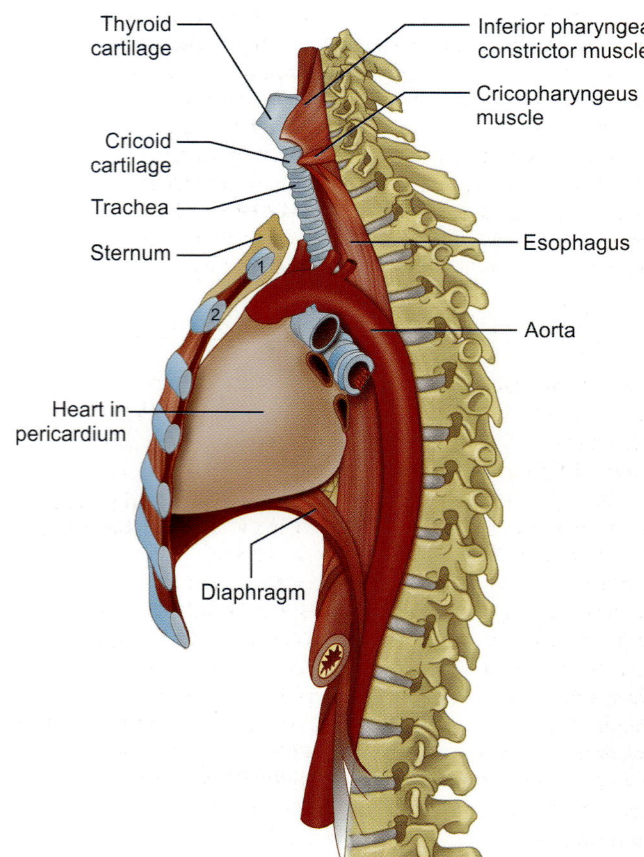

Figure 2 Course of the esophagus

The esophageal length varies from 22 to 28 cm (24 ± 5 SD).[2] Endoscopically, incisors are used as the landmark for measuring the length. UES lies at 14–16 cm and LES 40–45 cm from incisors (Fig. 1). The esophagus starts as a midline structure and has three deviations in its course. It deviates slightly to the left at thoracic inlet, to the right at carina to accommodate arch of aorta and to the left as it enters esophageal hiatus. It also bends in an anteroposterior plane to follow the cervicothoracic curvatures of vertebral column. The diameter of the esophagus varies from 1.6 to 2.5 cm. There are three narrowing: (1) cricopharyngeus—14 mm, (2) bronchoaortic constriction just below carina—15–17 mm and (3) diaphragmatic constriction—16–19 mm.[3]

The inferior pharyngeal constrictor bridges the pharyngeal and esophageal musculature. It is composed of thyropharyngeus and cricopharyngeus which originate from lateral processes of thyroid and cricoid cartilages respectively (Fig. 3). The fibers of thyropharyngeus are oblique and that of cricopharyngeus are horizontal. The area of weakness between these two muscle bundles is known as Killian's triangle, which is the site of Zenker's diverticulum. The UES is a musculocartilaginous structure. The high pressure at the UES is due to cricopharyngeus muscle. The cricopharyngeus is attached to the cricoid cartilage forming a C-shaped muscular band. The pressure profile at UES is asymmetric as the semicircular cricopharyngeus exerts pressure toward posterior plane of cricoid. The UES pressure is 100 mm Hg in the anteroposterior plane and 50 mm Hg laterally.[4]

The esophagus is anchored in its upper end by insertion of its longitudinal muscles at the posterior ridge of cricoid cartilage via the cricoesophageal tendon (Fig. 4). Numerous delicate undulated membranes composed of collagen and elastic fibers connect the esophagus with the trachea, bronchi, pleura and prevertebral fascia.[2] The distal end of the esophagus and the gastroesophageal junction is anchored by phrenoesophageal membrane, also known as Laimer ligament or Allison membrane. It splits into two sheets,

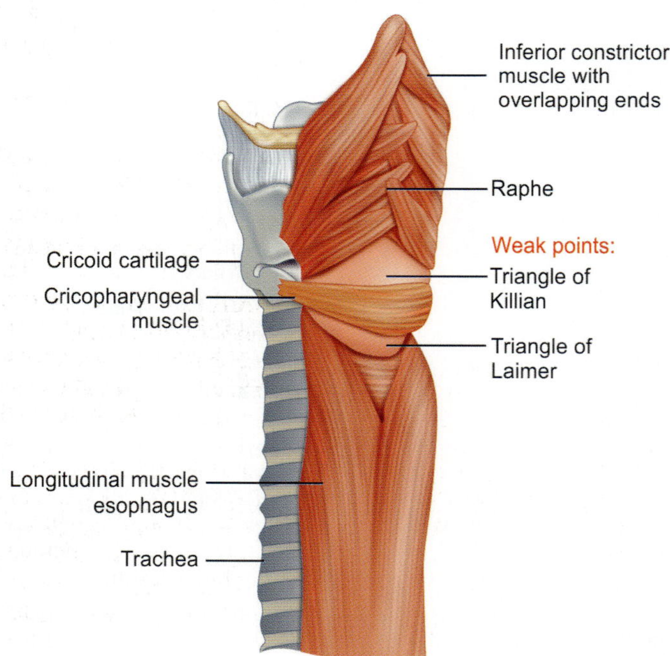

Figure 3 The pharyngoesophageal junction

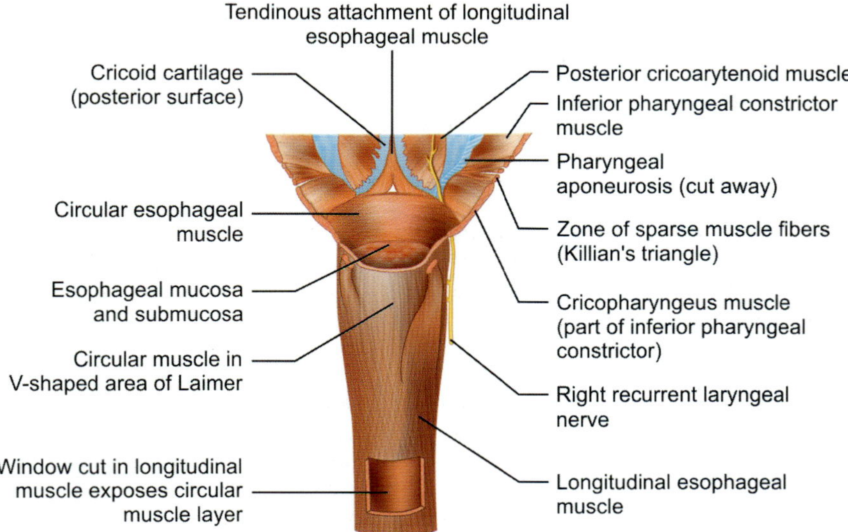

Figure 4 The pharyngoesophageal junction (posterior view with pharynx opened)

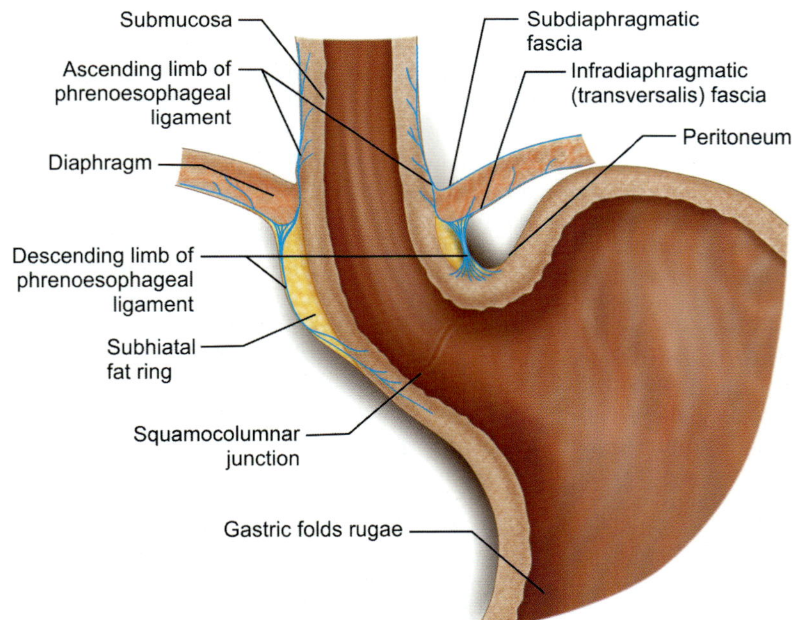

Figure 5 The gastroesophageal junction

one passing upward for 2–4 cm inserting on submucosa of the esophagus and the other passing down and blending into gastric serosa at fundus, gastrohepatic ligament and the dorsal gastric mesentery (Fig. 5).

The esophagus is composed of mucosa, submucosa and muscularis propria (Fig. 6). It lacks serosa and mesentery unlike other parts of gastrointestinal tract. It is enveloped by an adventitia; thin loose connective tissue containing small vessels, nerves and lymphatic channels. The mucosal layer consists of epithelium, basement membrane, lamina propria and muscularis mucosa. The epithelium is non-keratinized, stratified squamous epithelium along the whole length and its distal 1–2 cm transitions to cardiac mucosa or junctional columnar epithelium at Z line. The muscularis mucosa forms the long mucosal folds that run in the longitudinal axis of the esophagus. The submucosa has a network of lymphatic and vascular structures, mucous glands and Meissner's neural plexus. The muscular layer is composed of two layers of muscles: (1) inner layer is circular and (2) outer layer is

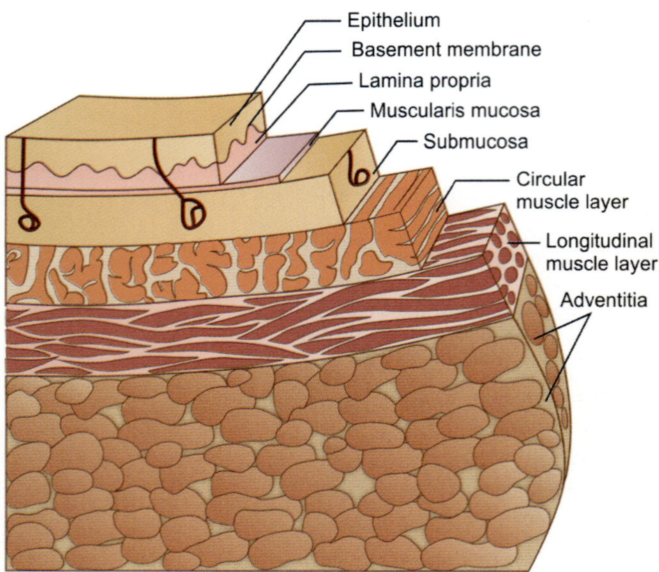

Figure 6 Layers of the esophagus

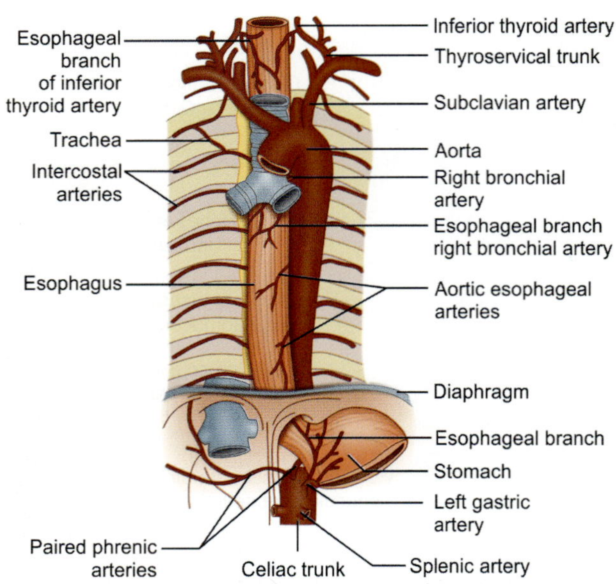

Figure 7 The arterial supply of the esophagus

longitudinal. The longitudinal muscles attach to posterior surface of cricoid and in the process leave an area devoid of musculature—Laimer triangle (Fig. 4). The circular muscle layer is an extension of cricopharyngeus. While both the muscle layers of upper third of the esophagus are striated, that of the middle third is mixed and lower one-third is smooth muscle. The transition from striated to smooth muscle is gradual.

The esophagus joins the stomach at gastroesophageal junction. Various definitions have been used to identify the gastroesophageal junction. Some of them include: (a) the location of the peritoneal reflection onto the stomach, (b) the location of the junction between the tubular esophagus and the saccular stomach, (c) the region adjacent to the acute angle of His, (d) the distal extent of the white esophageal squamous epithelium, (e) the proximal extent of gastric oxyntic mucosa, (f) the proximal limit of the gastric rugal folds, (g) the manometric distal end of the LES, (h) the point beyond which no submucosal esophageal glands are found and (i) the change in the muscularis propria from a circular and longitudinal layer in the esophagus to a less defined muscularis propria of the stomach with a third oblique layer.[5]

Lower esophageal sphincter is not a true sphincter anatomically. However, a distinct high pressure zone can be identified during manometry. It spans across the esophageal hiatus being 1–2 cm intra-abdominally. Three to four centimeter cranial to junction with stomach, the circular muscle layer increases in number and produces a stepwise thickening of terminal esophageal musculature.[6] Radial and axial thickness is variable and asymmetric at gastroesophageal junction which corresponds with the manometric pressure profile.[7] At the gastroesophageal junction circular muscle fiber bundles on lesser curvature side form short muscle clasps while those on greater curvature change direction to oblique gastric sling fibers.[2] Upper and lower halves of the LES show reversed variations in respiratory phases. Inspiration causes an increase in pressure in the lower half whereas in the upper half inspiration causes a drop in pressure. The point at which they reverse is called respiratory inversion point.

Arterial Supply

The cervical esophagus receives blood from superior and inferior thyroid arteries. The cricopharyngeus is supplied by superior thyroid artery. The thoracic esophagus is supplied by esophageal arteries coming off aorta, esophageal branches off the right and left bronchial arteries, descending braches off the inferior thyroid arteries, intercostal arteries and ascending branches of the paired inferior phrenic arteries. The lower thoracic and abdominal esophagus are supplied by left gastric artery, paired inferior phrenic arteries and branches of the splenic artery (Fig. 7). Studies of Liebermann-Meffert D et al. could not confirm the supply from intercostal, phrenic or direct branches off the aorta.[8] All the major arterial vessels arborize into minute branches before entering the esophageal wall and form a fine capillary network. They go on to form dense submucosal interconnected network.[8]

Venous Drainage

Butler classified esophageal veins into intrinsic and extrinsic veins.[9] The intrinsic veins include a subepithelial plexus in lamina propria, a submucous plexus and perforating veins. There are no valves in the esophageal venous circulatory system. The extrinsic veins drain into the inferior and superior thyroid veins, into the azygous and hemiazygous veins and into the gastric and splenic veins (Fig. 8). Vianna et al. showed presence of palisade zone at gastroesophageal junction. Venous flow is bidirectional at the palisade zone, which acts as a intercommunication between the portal and azygous systems.[10]

Lymphatic Drainage

The lymph capillaries unite to form blind endothelial sacculations. These initial lymphatics form a network within the submucosa that runs longitudinally. It gives off branches that pass the muscle

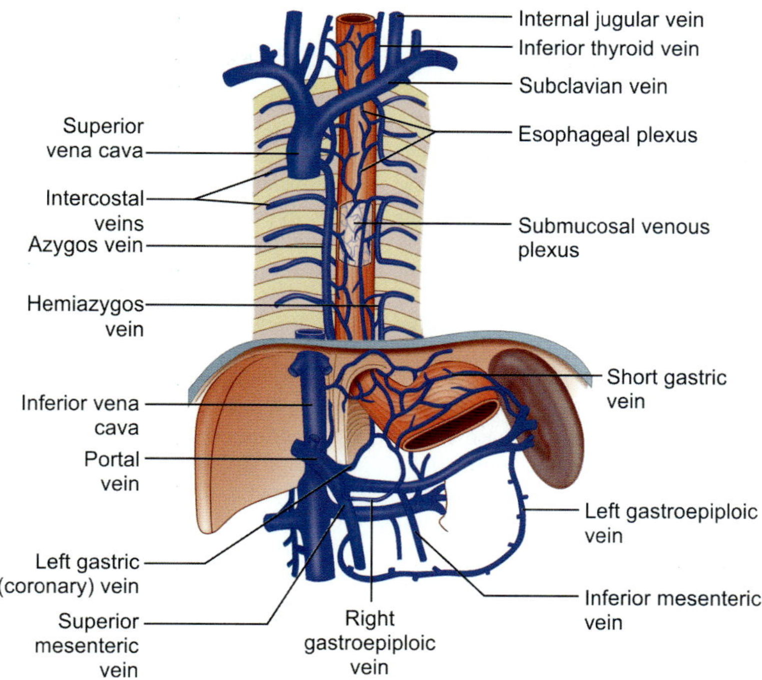

Figure 8 The venous drainage of the esophagus

layers and empty into the collecting subadventitial and surface trunks and then drain into regional lymph node beds. These entire lymphatic channels possess valves. The lymphatic flow is upward for upper two-thirds of the esophagus and downward for the distal third. In the neck drainage occurs to paratracheal, deep lateral cervical and internal jugular nodes. In the thorax it drains into mediastinal nodes, thoracic ducts, paratracheal, subcarinal, paraesophageal, retrocardiac and infracardiac nodes. It also drains posteriorly in the nodes along the esophagus and azygos vein. Lymphatics of the lower esophagus drain into the celiac nodes via left gastric lymphatics. This rich network of lymphatics makes esophageal cancers prone to early spread.

Innervation

The esophagus is innervated through the sympathetic and the parasympathetic nervous system.

Superior cervical ganglion in the neck gives rise to cervical sympathetic truck which terminates in cervicothoracic (stellate ganglion). The thoracic sympathetic trunk continues from here giving off branches to the esophageal plexus which envelops the thoracic esophagus. Inferiorly, the greater and lesser splanchnic nerves innervate the distal esophagus.

The parasympathetic supply is through the vagus nerve. The vagus nerve gives rise to superior and recurrent laryngeal nerve. The superior laryngeal nerve branches into external and internal laryngeal nerves, which provide motor innervation to the cricothyroid muscle and inferior pharyngeal constrictor muscle and sensory innervation to the larynx, respectively. The recurrent laryngeal nerves both right and left, loop underneath right subclavian artery and aortic arch respectively and travel back upward in the tracheoesophageal groove, the left being closer to the groove. Both give off branches to the esophagus and the trachea and enter the pharynx and innervate all muscles of the laryngopharynx except cricothyroid. Distally the vagal trunk forms esophageal plexus which join again to become left (anterior) and right (posterior) vagal trunk before exiting the diaphragm.

In the esophagus dense network of nerves and ganglia are situated in the muscular layer (Auerbach's plexus) and in the submucosa (Meissner's plexus).

PHYSIOLOGY

The function of the esophagus is to actively transport ingested food to stomach. It also prevents reflux while permitting occasional retrograde movement for evacuation of gas (belching) and gastric contents (vomiting). During these retrograde movements the esophagus itself remains a passive conduit.

Swallowing

The act of swallowing occurs in three stages: (1) oral stage, (2) pharyngeal stage and (3) esophageal stage. These stages are a continuous process closely coordinated through the medullary swallowing centers.[11] It takes approximately 8-10 seconds for food bolus to reach the stomach from initiation of swallow.

The UES is 4-5 cm in length with mean resting pressure of 60 mm Hg and a short relaxation time of 0.58 seconds. It prevents steady flow of air into the esophagus. The LES is 3-5 cm in length with mean resting pressure of 24 mm Hg and relaxation time of 8.4 sec. It prevents excessive material from refluxing back into the esophagus.[3]

The oral phase is voluntary. The swallowing is initiated when it is sensed that the food particles have been reduced sufficiently in size. The tongue lubricates and moves the bolus backward. The tongue with hard palate and closed glossopalatal gate forms an expulsion chamber. The bolus is loaded and pushed through the glossopalatal opening and it enters the pharynx.

The pharyngeal phase is involuntary. The receptors at the base of the tongue, anterior and posterior pillars, posterior pharyngeal wall, soft palates, tonsils, epiglottis and larynx initiate swallowing reflex.[12] The sensory input is integrated with cortical input in swallowing center in the brainstem, and efferent information is sent to oropharyngeal musculature. A rapid series of pharyngeal effects occurs almost simultaneously. The pharynx is transformed from a respiratory to a swallowing conduit by shutting of openings of the pharynx to the nasal passages, oral cavity and laryngeal vestibule.[13] UES is opened, aided by forward displacement of pharynx and relaxation of cricopharyngeus muscle. Longitudinal contraction of the pharynx brings UES close to the base of the tongue. The posterior pharyngeal wall contracts and sequentially comes in contact with the posterior surface of the tongue, the epiglottis, the laryngeal, arytenoid and interarytenoid muscles and the cricoid cartilage.[14] The UES, which remains in a constant state of tone, relaxes and the bolus passes from the pharynx, across the UES into the proximal esophagus, while preventing the food from entering the airways. The UES shows postrelaxation contraction, close to 90 mm Hg and then returns to resting pressure.

Movement of bolus along the length of the esophagus is caused by propulsive motility pattern known as peristalsis. The esophageal peristalsis is the result of coordinated contractions of the circular and longitudinal esophageal muscles. Contraction of the more distal segments occurs at longer latencies following the swallow than those in the proximal segments. Sequential contraction of circular muscle in a proximal to distal direction propels the food bolus toward the stomach (Fig. 9). The esophageal peristalsis is controlled by the medullary swallowing center via the vagus nerve. Nucleus ambiguous provides motor innervation to striated muscle of the proximal esophagus. Dorsal motor nucleus of the vagus provides innervations to the distal smooth muscle of the esophagus. The myenteric (Auerbach) plexus mediates the vagal innervation and coordinates peristalsis in the smooth muscle portion of the esophagus. Three types of contractions have been described: (1) primary, (2) secondary and (3) tertiary.

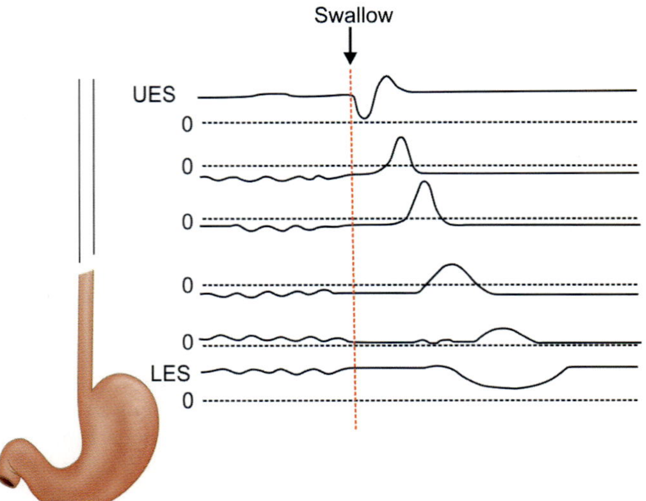

Figure 9 Relaxation of the UES, LES and progressive peristalsis in the esophagus

When swallows are very closely spaced, contraction of the distal esophagus is inhibited (deglutitive inhibition). If a series of rapid swallows are taken, peristalsis is inhibited till the last swallow and a single peristaltic contraction at the end allows proper clearance.[15]

Primary peristalsis is progressive and follows the act of swallowing. They travel at 2–4 cm/sec and generate pressure of 40–80 mm Hg. During primary peristalsis LES relaxation starts at the initiation of the swallow and lasts till the peristalsis reaches the LES. The secondary peristalsis is also progressive but occurs in response to distension or irritation and is without UES relaxation or pharyngeal contraction. It clears the esophagus of residual ingested material and refluxed content. The tertiary contractions are nonprogressive and nonperistaltic contraction waves. They are primarily identified on barium X-ray studies. Their physiologic role is uncertain.

Factors influencing peristalsis include esophageal site, posture, consistency and resistance to movement of the bolus, size of bolus, temperature of bolus. The amplitude of contraction is higher in the proximal and distal esophagus with a low pressure zone at the junction of striated and smooth muscle. The strength of the propulsive force decreases in upright compared to the supine position. A larger bolus leads to stronger contractions. Warmth increases the strength of contraction while cold decreases it. Osmolality and age has no effect on contractions.

In addition to peristaltic contractions, Winship et al.[16] have shown existence of esophageal propulsive force, generated by the muscles above the bolus, when passage of a bolus is obstructed. This increases with increase in the diameter of the bolus and is greatest in the distal end of the esophagus.

The LES prevents gastroesophageal reflux and relaxes with swallowing to allow passage of food bolus into the stomach. The pressure is maintained by intrinsic muscle activity of circular muscle layer and augmented by phasic diaphragmatic pressure. LES relaxation starts less than 2 seconds after the initiation of a swallow. The relaxation is for 8–10 seconds and is followed by an after contraction. LES tone is modulated by many hormones and neurotransmitters. These include relaxants such as nitrates and nitric oxide, nicotine, dopamine, vasoactive intestinal peptide, adenosine, β-adrenergic agonists, secretin-cholecystokinin, calcitonin gene-related peptide and prostaglandin E. Muscarinic M2 and M3 receptor agonists, substance P, gastrin and α-adrenergic agonists increase LES tone.[17] The function of LES depends upon its overall length, the abdominal length and pressure of the sphincter.[18] The shorter length requires higher pressure to remain competent.

Lower esophageal sphincter relaxation also occurs without a swallow which is called transient lower esophageal sphincter relaxation (tLESR). They are defined as periods (lasting 10–60 sec) of spontaneous (not preceded by a swallow), simultaneous relaxation of the LES and crural diaphragm.[19] tLESRs are vagally mediated and occur in response to proximal gastric fundus distension and permit gastroesophageal reflux, belching, retching and vomiting. The proportion of tLESRs associated with reflux varies from 10% to 93%.[20]

REFERENCES

1. Edge SB, Byrd DR, Compton CC, Fritz AG, Greene FL, Trotti A. AJCC Cancer Staging Manual, 7th edition. Springer; 2010.
2. Liebermann-Meffert D. Human foregut anatomy, adjacent structures, and their relation to surgical approaches. In: Yeo CJ, Matthews JB, McFadden DW, Pemberton JH, Peters JH (Eds). Shackelford's Surgery of the Alimentary Tract, 7th edition. Philadelphia: Elsevier; 2013. pp. 9-31.
3. Maish MS. Esophagus. In: Courtney M. Townsend J, Beauchamp RD, Evers BM, Kenneth L. Mattox (Eds). Sabiston Textbook of Surgery, 19th edition. Elsevier; 2012. pp. 1012-66.
4. Tutuian R, Castell DO. Physiology of the Esophagus and Its Sphincters. In: Yeo CJ, Matthews JB, McFadden DW, Pemberton JH, Peters JH (Eds). Shackelford's Surgery of the Alimentary Tract, 7th edition. Philadelphia: Elsevier; 2013. pp. 50-7.
5. Oezcelik A, DeMeester SR. General anatomy of the esophagus. Thoracic Surgery Clinics. 2011;21(2):289-97.
6. Liebermann-Meffert D, Allgower M, Schmid P, Blum AL. Muscular equivalent of the lower esophageal sphincter. Gastroenterology. 1979;76(1):31-8.
7. Stein HJ, Liebermann-Meffert D, DeMeester TR, Siewert JR. Three-dimensional pressure image and muscular structure of the human lower esophageal sphincter. Surgery. 1995;117(6):692-8.
8. Liebermann-Meffert DM, Luescher U, Neff U, Ruedi TP, Allgower M. Esophagectomy without thoracotomy: is there a risk of intramediastinal bleeding? A study on blood supply of the esophagus. Annals of Surgery. 1987;206(2):184-92.
9. Butler H. The veins of the oesophagus. Thorax. 1951;6(3):276-96.
10. Vianna A, Hayes PC, Moscoso G, Driver M, Portmann B, Westaby D, et al. Normal venous circulation of the gastroesophageal junction. A route to understanding varices. Gastroenterology. 1987;93(4):876-89.
11. Weisbrodt NW. Neuromuscular organization of esophageal and pharyngeal motility. Archives of Internal Medicine. 1976;136(5):524-31.
12. Jean A, Car A. Inputs to the swallowing medullary neurons from the peripheral afferent fibers and the swallowing cortical area. Brain Research. 1979;178(2-3):567-72.
13. Dua KS, Ren J, Bardan E, Xie P, Shaker R. Coordination of deglutitive glottal function and pharyngeal bolus transit during normal eating. Gastroenterology. 1997;112(1):73-83.
14. Kahrilas PJ, Logemann JA, Lin S, Ergun GA. Pharyngeal clearance during swallowing: a combined manometric and videofluoroscopic study. Gastroenterology. 1992;103(1):128-36.
15. Tutuian R, Jalil S, Katz PO, Castell DO. Effect of interval between swallows on oesophageal pressures and bolus movement in normal subjects—Studies with combined multichannel intraluminal impedance and oesophageal manometry. Neurogastroenterol Motil. 2004;16(1):23-9.
16. Winship DH, Zboralske FF. The esophageal propulsive force: esophageal response to acute obstruction. J Clin Invest. 1967;46(9):1391-401.
17. Hershcovici T, Mashimo H, Fass R. The lower esophageal sphincter. Neurogastroenterol Motil. 2011;23(9):819-30.
18. Bonavina L, Evander A, DeMeester TR, Walther B, Cheng SC, Palazzo L, et al. Length of the distal esophageal sphincter and competency of the cardia. Am J Surg. 1986;151(1):25-34.
19. Dodds WJ, Dent J, Hogan WJ, Helm JF, Hauser R, Patel GK, et al. Mechanisms of gastroesophageal reflux in patients with reflux esophagitis. N Engl J Med. 1982;307(25):1547-52.
20. Mittal RK, McCallum RW. Characteristics of transient lower esophageal sphincter relaxation in humans. Am J Physiol. 1987;252(5 Pt 1):G636-41.

CHAPTER 11

Diagnostic Tests in Esophageal Diseases

Shobna J Bhatia, Chirag Shah

INTRODUCTION

The esophagus is a muscular tube extending from the upper to the lower esophageal sphincters (LES). Its function is to transport food by peristalsis from the pharynx to the stomach. The two sphincters are necessary to prevent proximal reflux of contents. Diseases of the esophagus occur frequently, the presenting symptoms in most cases being heartburn, sour regurgitation, dysphagia, odynophagia, chest pain, globus sensation or hiccups.

Differentiating various disorders only on clinical grounds is sometimes difficult. Hence, we need to use investigations like endoscopy, imaging studies and manometry. The choice of investigation depends on the symptom complex that the patient presents with. For instance, endoscopy is the investigation of choice for mucosal diseases, whereas manometry is useful when a motor disorder is suspected. Barium swallow is useful in patients with dysphagia to locate the site and length of stricture and in assessment of motor disorders. Investigations, like computed tomography (CT) scan and endoscopic ultrasound, are useful in cases where depth of lesions is to be assessed or extra-esophageal pathologies are suspected (mediastinal lymph nodes, depth of tumors and invasion of tumors into aorta).

ENDOSCOPY

Basics

There are many flexible endoscopes available for various applications, but they all have similar features. Basically, an endoscope has a head with controlling valves (buttons) for air insufflations and suction, a flexible shaft (insertion tube) housing the light (and image) transmitting fiber optic bundles and one or more service channels, and ending distally with a maneuverable bending tip. An umbilical or universal cord (also called "light guide connecting tube") connects the endoscope to the light source and processor, air supply and suction. Like in all electronic image processing systems, the image is captured using a charge-coupled device (CCD) chip, after processed electronically, and the video image is displayed on a monitor. Illumination is provided from an external high-intensity light source which provides required illumination at the tip transmitted through light-carrying fiber bundles passing through the umbilical cord and the shaft of the endoscope.[1] In recent years, high definition endoscopes with special imaging techniques, such as Narrow-Band Imaging (NBI), Fujinon Intelligent Chromoendoscopy (FICE) and i-SCAN, are being used to identify early malignant lesions.

Image Enhancement Techniques

Staining of esophageal mucosa with iodine-based and other stains has been used to pick up and report Barrett's esophagus and early malignancy. Recently, NBI (Olympus) and post-acquisition image processing [i-SCAN (Pentax) and FICE (Fujinon)] have been used for image enhancement to pick up early malignancy and Barrett's esophagus.[2] The principle employed here is enhancement of vascular pattern and mucosal pattern with a particular bandwidth of visible light waves.[3]

Indications

Dysphagia

The first step in assessing dysphagia is to determine whether it is oropharyngeal or esophageal in origin. Based on the likely site and causes, subsequent investigation and management can differ greatly. This can usually be achieved through a carefully-taken history, which has been shown to differentiate between oropharyngeal, esophageal and neuromuscular causes of dysphagia accurately in up to 85% of patients.[4] Symptoms, such as difficulty in initiation of swallow, nasal regurgitation, cough immediately after swallow, associated neurological disease, history of neck surgery, stroke, suggest possibility of oropharyngeal dysphagia.[5] Feeling of something stuck in the throat even when a person is not swallowing suggests potential sensory dysfunction, and most common such a disorder is globus hystericus. It is clinically important to distinguish between mechanical and motor dysphagia before planning investigation; this helps in directing investigations well and minimizes costs. Mechanical lesions cause dysphagia which is more for solids than liquids, may be intermittent (web, Schatzki's ring) or progressive (benign or malignant stricture), and weight loss can occur (prominent with malignant obstruction). Motor dysphagia is usually for both solids and liquids, nonprogressive or slowly progressive; weight loss may be prominent with severe dysmotility, e. g. achalasia cardia.

After a detailed history, a barium radiograph, including a solid bolus challenge, is often advocated as the first test. This is particularly so when oropharyngeal or motor dysphagia is suspected. Alternatively, many experts have advocated endoscopy as the first test. The choice of the initial test should be based on available expertise and preference of the individual physician. If the barium examination shows a mechanical obstruction, endoscopy should be done for confirmation, and obtaining a biopsy. Gastroscopy is preferred first-line investigation in patients with mechanical dysphagia. In patients with motor dysphagia, manometry can be considered as the next investigation after a negative endoscopy. In elderly patients with dysphagia, it is better to do barium swallow even before endoscopy to rule out compression due to osteophytes and Zenker's diverticulum (Fig. 1). Barium swallow is also useful when endoscopy shows a tight stricture which cannot be negotiated by the endoscope; in these cases, the status of the esophagus beyond the stricture can be assessed.

Peptic Stricture

There is usually a history of gastroesophageal reflux disease (GERD) or dyspeptic symptoms. These strictures are short, and usually located in lower esophagus (Figs 2 and 3). Endoscopy can be used to diagnose and treat these strictures using controlled radial expansion balloon dilators or bougie dilators. These balloons are available in various sizes. In resistant cases, options include removable metal stents and surgery.[6] Patients require long-term proton pump inhibitor (PPI) therapy to prevent frequent recurrence[7] or anti-reflux surgery.

Schatzki's ring is a partial or complete mucosal ring (Fig. 4). Patients present with intermittent dysphagia and sometimes with food impaction. The ring is seen at the level of the gastroesophageal mucosal junction in association with GERD and hiatus hernia; Schatzki's ring is sometimes considered a forme fruste of an early peptic stricture. Endoscopic dilatation is not difficult; the strictures are easy to dilate endoscopically as there is no muscle involvement. Most can be treated with single time dilatation with Savary type dilators.[8]

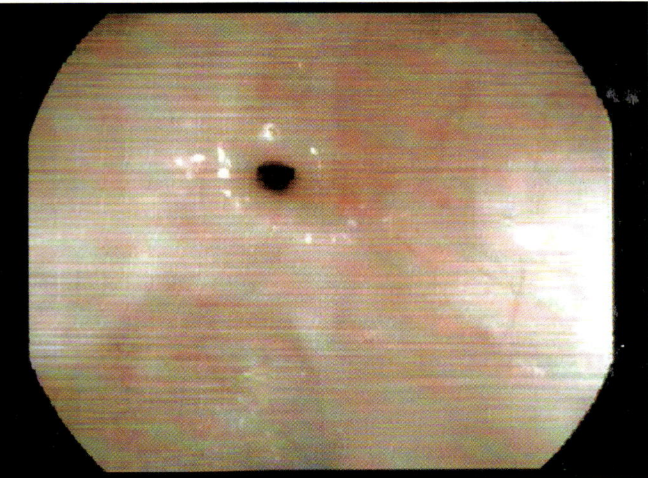

Figure 2 Endoscopic view of a peptic stricture; there is a narrowing in the distal esophagus. These strictures are often associated with a hiatal hernia

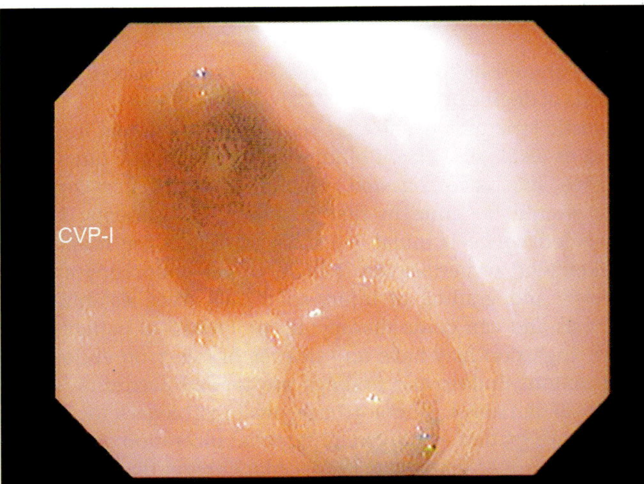

Figure 1 Endoscopic view of Zenker's diverticulum. The lumen of the esophagus may be confused with the lumen of the diverticulum

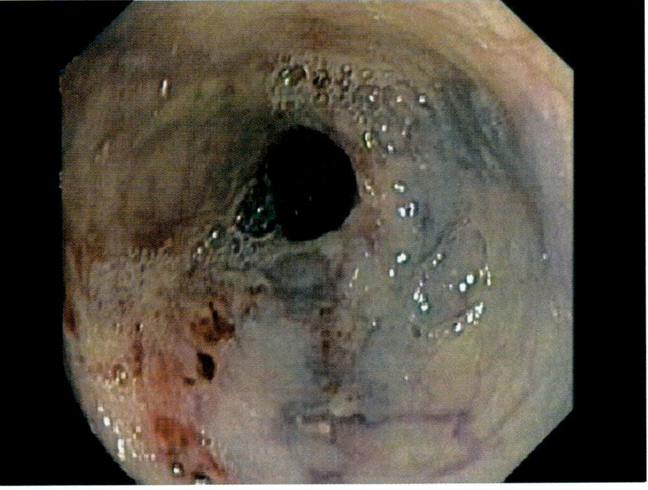

Figure 3 Peptic stricture in the distal esophagus along with circumferential esophagitis

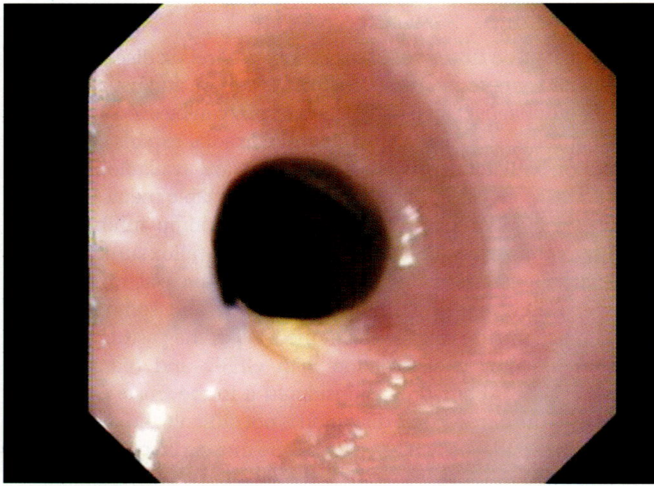

Figure 4 Endoscopy shows a ring in the lower esophagus

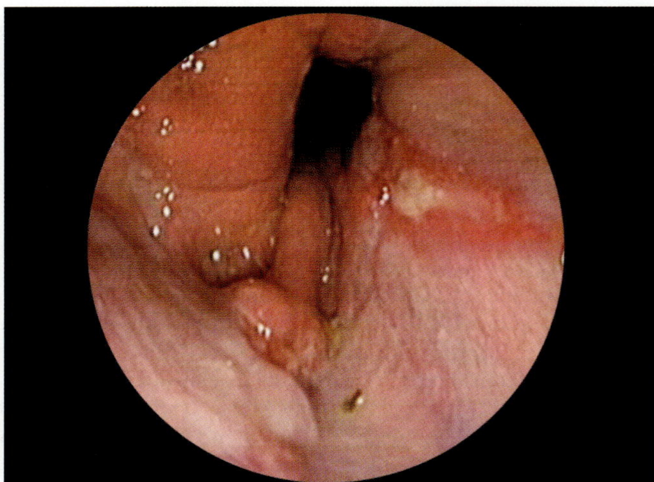

Figure 6 Circumferential esophageal ulceration after corrosive injury

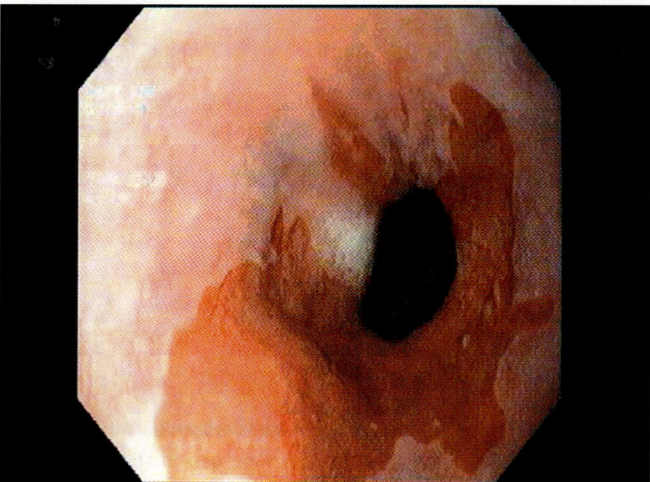

Figure 5 *Barrett's esophagus*: Endoscopy shows reddish, velvet-like gastric mucosa extending into the esophagus. The esophageal mucosa is pink and has a glossy appearance

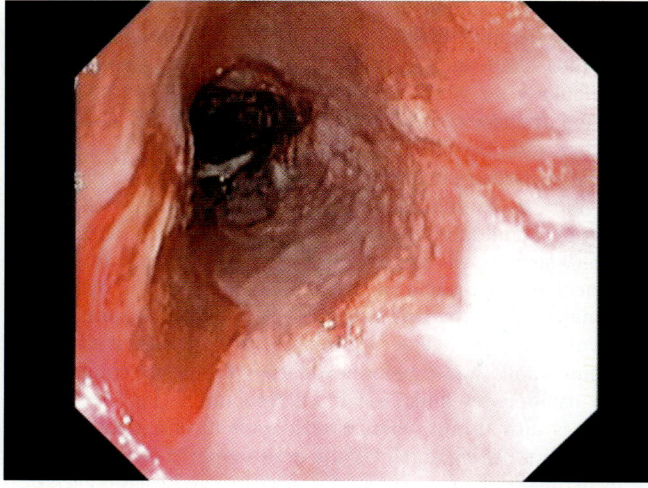

Figure 7 Endoscopy shows a narrowing in distal esophagus with proximal ulceration, following corrosive ingestion

Esophageal webs present as intermittent dysphagia or food impaction. They are most commonly seen in the upper esophagus as a part of Plummer-Vinson syndrome; the syndrome is more common in women. Patients have dysphagia, esophageal webs and iron-deficiency anemia. One-time endoscopic dilatation is usually sufficient; the web may be missed at endoscopy if it is ruptured during the initial passage of the endoscope. Recurrence is reduced with treatment of iron deficiency anemia. Some patients require repeat dilatations.

Barrett's esophagus is a complication of severe GERD in which the normal squamous mucosa of the esophagus is replaced by potentially precancerous columnar mucosa with goblet cells. Endoscopy is important for diagnosis and measuring extent of Barrett's esophagus (Fig. 5). Endoscopy shows velvety mucosa extending into the esophagus. It is reported as per Prague classification.[9] Barrett's esophagus should be confirmed by histological diagnosis; biopsies should be examined for dysplasia. Patients should be followed-up with endoscopic surveillance on the basis of degree of dysplasia.[10]

Caustic strictures occur after suicidal or accidental ingestion of acid or alkali. The extent of injury depends on the quantity of corrosive substance ingested. First endoscopy after corrosive injury should be done in first 36 hours.[11] Endoscopy should be avoided between initial 3–5 days as tissues are friable and the likelihood of perforation is high. Upper endoscopy enables diagnosis and grading of injury to the GI tract, establishes a prognosis and can guide therapy; up to 40–80% of patients with caustic ingestion may have no evidence of injury on endoscopic examination. Endoscopic findings are graded according to the severity of damage, e.g. hemorrhage, erosions, blisters, ulcers with exudate are graded as IIa, circumferential ulceration as grade III and multiple deep ulcers with brown, black or gray discoloration as grade IV (Fig. 6). Once a stricture (Fig. 7) has occurred, the extent of stricture should be assessed on barium swallow with concentration on degree of narrowing, length, tortuosity and gastric involvement. Further endoscopic treatment can be done with gradual sequential dilatations with Savary type dilators. Injection therapy with steroids,[12] needle-knife technique,[13] esophageal stent, retrograde dilatation help in difficult patients. Patients who have co-morbidities, refractory strictures or complications of endoscopic therapy require surgical management.

Radiation Injury

Radiation injury usually occurs in patients with head and neck malignancies who have received radiotherapy. These strictures are usually located in upper esophagus and the length of the strictures range from 0.5 cm to 13.5 cm (median, 5 cm) and the luminal diameter from 1 mm to 11 mm (median, 6 mm).[14] The treatment is endoscopic dilatation with Savary-Gillard type bougies. More than two-thirds patients respond well to dilatations.[14]

Eosinophilic Esophagitis

Eosinophilic esophagitis (EE) is a disorder histologically characterized by presence of greater than 15 eosinophils/HPF in a mid-esophageal biopsy. Endoscopically, it presents as web, furrows, fissures, rings, stricture, mucosal avulsions, erosions and even normal endoscopy. Diagnosis is always on histology. At least four mid-esophageal biopsies should be taken to reliably diagnose EE. It is preferable to take biopsies after a 6 weeks trial of PPI to avoid confusion with GERD-related infiltration of eosinophils. Treatment is food elimination diets, and drug therapy with budesonide viscous or spray. Stricture can be managed with endotherapy and recurrence can be reduced with proper medical management.[15]

Extrinsic Compression

- Benign inflammatory mediastinal lymph node usually causes compression in midesophagus. Endoscopically mucosa may be normal or show a bulge, erosions or ulceration. Endoscopic biopsies should be taken; however, diagnostic yield may be low.
- Spine osteophytes usually do not cause dysphagia, except in old patients. They are usually detected on barium or lateral X-ray. The endoscopist should be careful doing endoscopy in these patients as forceful insertion of the endoscope could lead to perforation.
- Vascular compression: Abnormal vasculature can cause dysphagia, i.e. dysphagia lusoria. Most common vascular abnormalities are double aortic arch and right aortic arch, others being abnormal innominate artery. On endoscopy, this may be seen as indentation in midesophagus with transmitted pulsations. Treatment will be surgical in symptomatic patients.
- Large Zenker's diverticulum can cause compression of the upper esophagus; therefore, care should be taken during endoscopy to look for esophageal opening, and not to enter the diverticulum forcefully. Endoscopic treatment of Zenker's diverticulum is being accepted rapidly.
- External compression by pulmonary or cardiac mass is usually present in midesophagus and can lead to severe obstruction occasionally. Endoscopy shows an extrinsic compression with normal mucosa.
- Post-fundoplication dysphagia can be due to mechanical or motor cause. A tight wrap is the most common cause of mechanical dysphagia. On endoscopy, there may be resistance at gastroesophageal junction. Manometry can guide treatment decisions.[16]

Malignant Strictures

Esophageal cancer can appear as a growth, ulceration or stricture with varying degree of luminal occlusion (Figs 8 to 10). Tumor tissue is usually friable. In some patients with a tight stricture, mucosal irregularity is not apparent and the lesion can be seen after dilatation. At least six biopsies with standard forceps, or four biopsies with jumbo biopsy forceps should be taken to avoid the need for repeated sampling; brush cytology can be done after obtaining biopsy. The extent of growth should be mentioned in relation to upper esophageal sphincter (UES) and

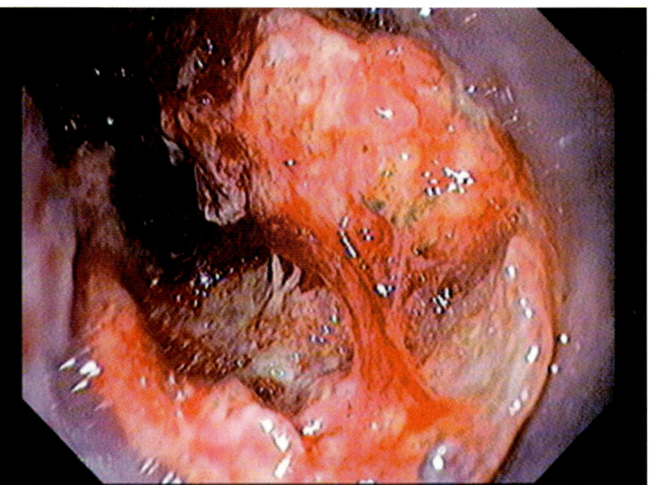

Figure 8 Endoscopy shows an ulcerated lumen-occluding growth in the midesophagus. Biopsy showed squamous cell carcinoma

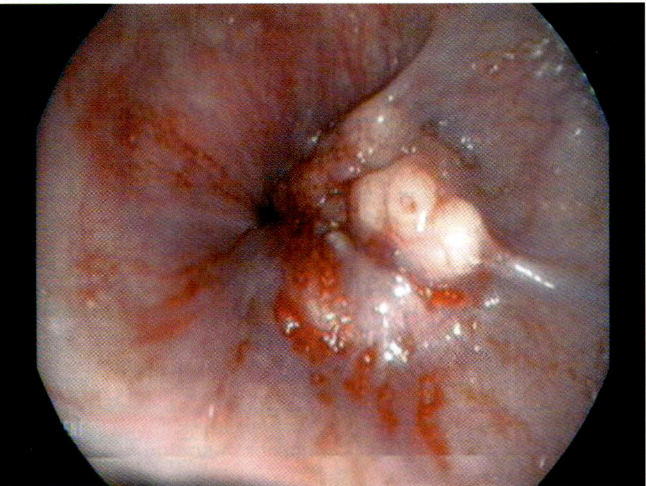

Figure 9 A nodular lesion is seen in the distal esophagus. Biopsy showed adenocarcinoma

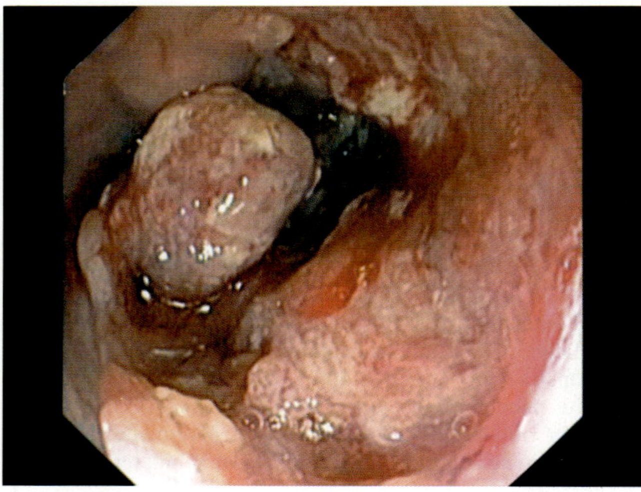

Figure 10 Endoscopy shows an ulcerated and nodular, circumferential lesion

gastroesophageal junction. Extent of the tumor in stomach should be mentioned in case of growth at gastroesophageal junction. In squamous cell carcinoma, palliation can be achieved with both radiation and esophageal stent. The former has the advantage of sustained effect,[17] and the latter has the advantage of immediate effect. Malignant fistula can also be managed with esophageal stenting. Adenocarcinomas do not respond well to radiation.

Role of Endoscopy in Evaluation of Heartburn, Odynophagia, Chest Pain, Hiccups

Gastroesophageal reflux disease is the most common cause of heartburn and sour regurgitation. On endoscopy, it is seen as erythema, erosions and ulceration. The severity of esophageal lesions is graded using Los Angeles classification (Table 1, Figs 11 and 12).[18] Approximately 50% of patients with symptoms of GERD do not have obvious esophagitis and are labeled as nonerosive reflux disease; these patients require further work up with pH-metry if they do not respond to acid suppression using PPI.

A patient, who has symptoms of uncomplicated typical heartburn, may be given an initial trial of therapy without endoscopic evaluation. When there are alarm symptoms that suggest that the reflux may be severe or that complications have occurred, endoscopy is the procedure of choice. Such symptoms include dysphagia or odynophagia, persistent or progressive symptoms despite therapy and extra-esophageal symptoms. Endoscopy should also be considered in immunosuppressed patients, suspected mass, stricture or ulcer on imaging, gastrointestinal bleeding or iron deficiency anemia and in an elderly patient with recent onset symptoms and weight loss. The sole finding of a hiatus hernia on barium studies is not an indication for endoscopy. Also, routine follow-up endoscopy is not necessary unless there is a change in pattern or severe symptoms, or alarm symptoms as above. Endoscopy should always be done prior to surgery for GERD, and is part of the surgical preoperative workup.

Table 1: Los Angeles' grading of esophagitis[19]

Grade of esophagitis	*Description*
Grade A	One (or more) mucosal break no longer than 5 mm, that does not extend between the tops of two mucosal folds
Grade B	One (or more) mucosal break more than 5 mm long that does not extend between the tops of two mucosal folds
Grade C	One (or more) mucosal break that is continuous between the tops of two or more mucosal folds but which involves less than 75% of the circumference
Grade D	One (or more) mucosal break which involves at least 75% of the esophageal circumference

Source: Adapted from reference 19.

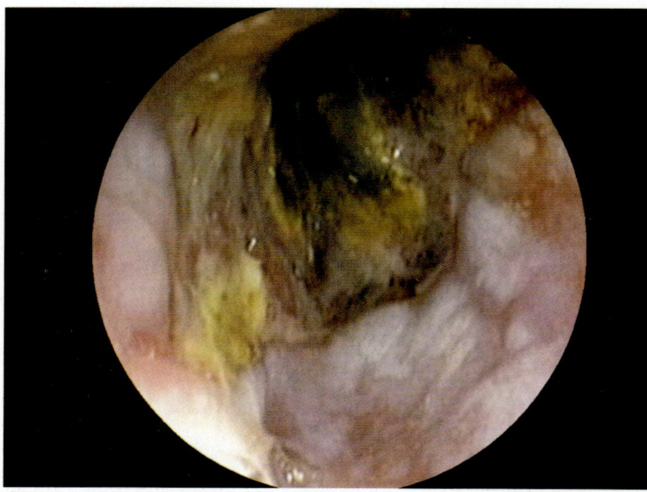

Figure 11 Endoscopy shows mucosal break more than 5 mm long that does not extend between the tops of two mucosal folds, suggestive of grade B esophagitis

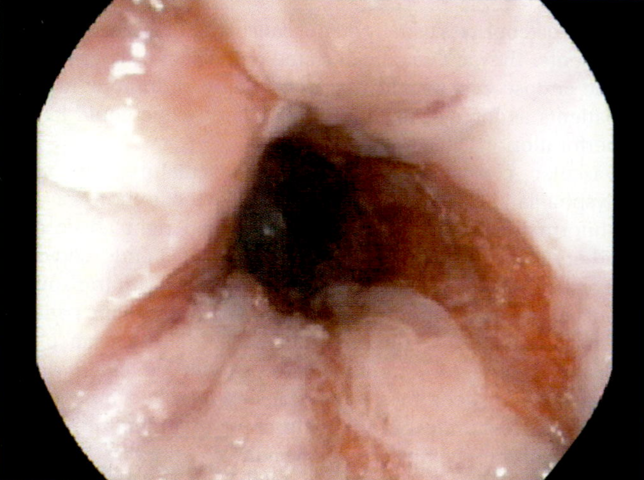

Figure 12 The distal esophagus shows large mucosal break, which occupies less than 75% of the circumference

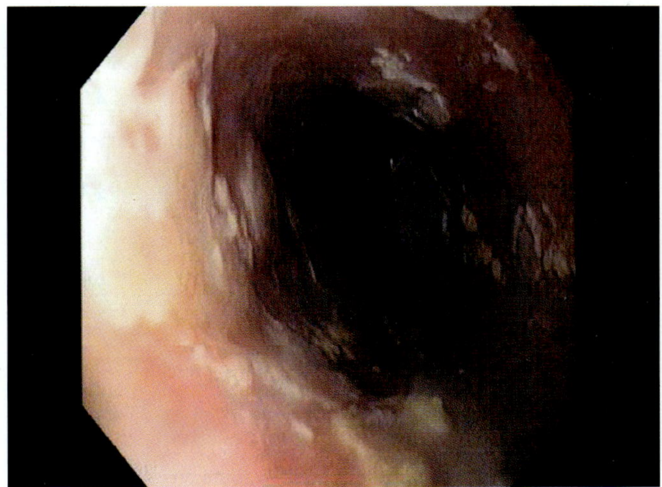

Figure 13 Endoscopy shows multiple white flakes in esophagus, suggestive of candidiasis

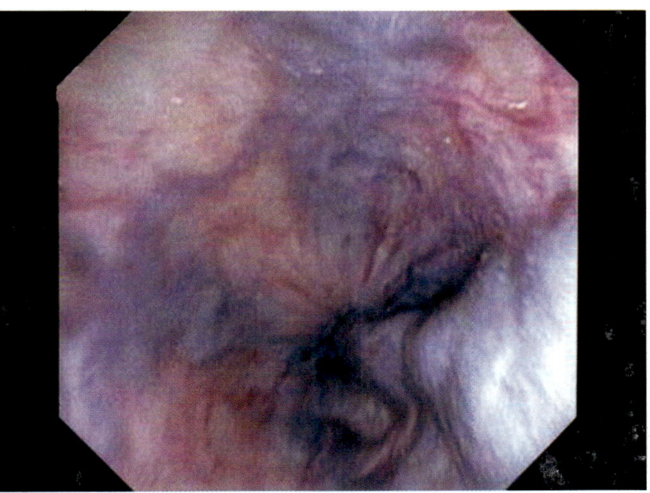

Figure 15 Endoscopy shows linear dilated submucosal veins in the distal esophagus

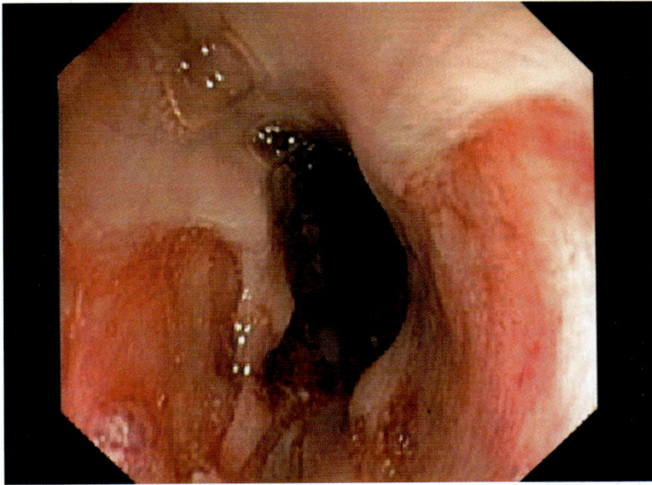

Figure 14 Endoscopy shows solitary, large ulcer in midesophagus. Biopsy from the center of the ulcer confirmed cytomegalovirus infection

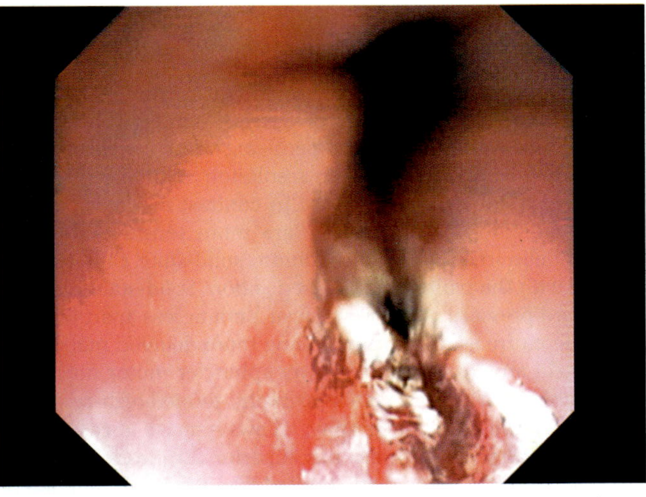

Figure 16 A longitudinal mucosal tear with overlying fibrinous exudate is seen in the distal esophagus, suggestive of Mallory-Weiss tear

Candidal esophagitis is usually associated with mild odynophagia. Biopsy for candidiasis is to be taken from white flakes (Fig. 13) visible on endoscopy. Cytomegalovirus (CMV) esophagitis is associated with significant odynophagia. Herpes simplex virus (HSV) esophagitis is associated with superficial ulcers, which coalesce with each other. When CMV infection (Fig. 14) is suspected, biopsy should be taken from the center of the ulcer, and for herpes from the periphery of the ulcer.[20]

ESOPHAGEAL CAUSES OF GI BLEED

In patients presenting with upper GI bleeding, endoscopy is usually the first investigation, and should be done once the patient is hemodynamically stable. Endoscopy helps to identify the bleeding site and allows therapeutic hemostasis in most patients.

The most common cause of esophageal bleeding is esophageal varices due to cirrhotic or noncirrhotic portal hypertension. Varices appear as bluish linear columns starting at the esophagogastric (EG) junction (Fig. 15) or in continuation with a gastric varix.

Mallory-Weiss tears are gastroesophageal junction mucosal or submucosal lacerations (Fig. 16) and usually present with hematemesis or coffee-ground emesis, typically after single or multiple episodes of vomiting without blood or retching. Endoscopy commonly reveals a solitary gastroesophageal junction tear. Bleeding is self-limited; occasionally, it can be severe. In such cases, endoscopic hemoclip application is used to close the tear and arrest the bleeding.

Patients with severe erosive esophagitis can present with bleeding; this bleeding is usually mild and history of heartburn is obtained in less than half of the patients. Severe bleeding is treated medically with a PPI. Endoscopy is useful in diagnosis, but endoscopic therapy has very little role, except in cases where an ulcer is found (Fig. 17). Occasionally, patients with candida, HSV, CMV or pill-induced esophagitis may present with GI bleed.

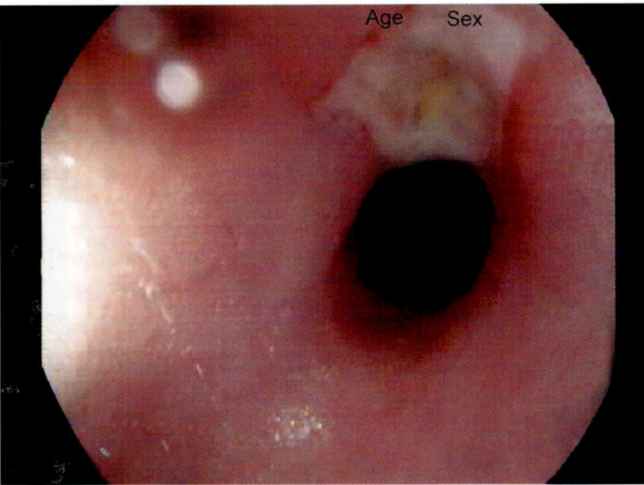

Figure 17 A large ulcer irregular edge is seen in the distal esophagus

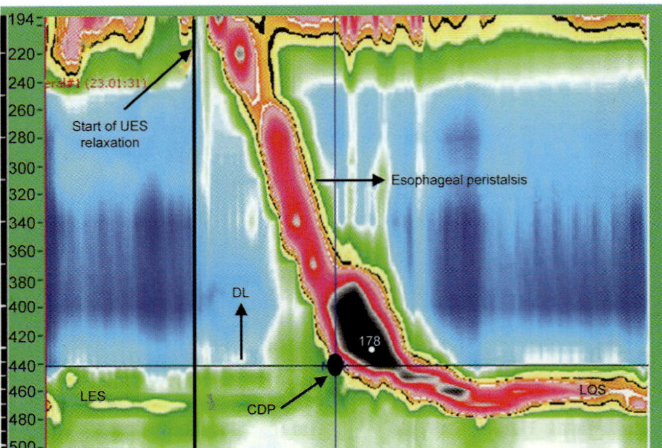

Figure 18 Clouse plots of a normal swallow. Data are acquired using a water perfusion system. The pressure signals are converted into color and pressure topography plot is obtained; the X-axis indicates time, Y-axis indicates the position of the catheter along the esophagus. The anatomic high-pressure zones of upper (UES) and lower (LES/esophagogastric junction) are seen. The start of the swallow is highlighted by the thick black line at the start of UES relaxation. The CDP is highlighted as a black dot and should reside within 3 cm of the LES. DL is the time between onset of swallow and CDP.

Abbreviations: UES, upper esophageal sphincter; LES, lower esophageal sphincter; CDP, contractile deceleration point; DL, distal latency; DCI, distal contractile integral

ESOPHAGEAL MANOMETRY

Manometry is the most sensitive and accurate technique to diagnose esophageal motility disorders. Standard manometry is performed with a number of perfusing catheters with 8 or 16 recording points, whereas high-resolution manometry (HRM) utilizes up to 36 recording points. In contrast to water perfused catheters, solid state transducers are more sensitive and have higher fidelity recordings. In addition, solid-state catheters can be used with the patient in upright position. Solid-state catheters can record pressure measurements at 1 cm or less apart intervals along the entire esophagus, providing more detailed mapping of esophageal and its upper and lower sphincter motor function.[21] The combination of HRM with topography, termed high-resolution esophageal pressure topography, allows precise measurement of esophageal pressures, and has superior diagnostic sensitivity for achalasia compared with limited conventional manometry (72% vs 56%).[22]

By convention, an esophageal pressure topography study comprises a series of ten test swallows of 5 mL water each, swallowed in a supine posture. The analysis is done using dedicated software. The normal values and analysis as per the Chicago classification are currently based on this convention.[23] In special situations, studies are done with patients in upright position, or swallowing boluses with varying consistencies (solid, semisolid food).

Important parameters that are measured during manometry (Fig. 18) are:

- Integrated relaxation pressure (mm Hg): This parameter indicates lower esophageal sphincter (LES) relaxation, and is measured for four contiguous or noncontiguous seconds of relaxation in the ten-second window following deglutition and UES relaxation. It is the most important parameter as it is used to define diagnostic categories.
- Distal contractile integral (mm Hg-s-cm) indicates the strength of contraction and is the composite of amplitude × duration × length (mm Hg-s-cm) of the distal esophageal contraction.
- Contractile deceleration point (CDP) is the inflection point along the 30 mm Hg isobaric contour where propagation velocity slows demarcating the tubular esophagus from the phrenic ampulla.
- Contractile front velocity (cm/s) is the slope of the tangent approximating the 30 mm Hg isobaric contour in the distal esophagus.
- Distal latency (DL) (s) is the time interval between UES relaxation and the CDP. A short DL indicates a spastic contraction.
- Peristaltic breaks (cm) are gaps in the 20 mm Hg isobaric contour of the peristaltic contraction between the UES and esophagogastric junction (EGJ).
- Motility disorders are classified as per Chicago classification (Table 2).[23]

It is important to know that this classification is of primary esophageal motility disorders and is not to be used in patients who have mechanical stricture (peptic stricture) or have undergone esophageal surgery (fundoplication, laparoscopic gastric banding or Heller myotomy).

A hierarchical analysis approach to the analysis during HRM was suggested in the Chicago classification.[23] The classification is valid only for swallow in supine position, and most studies have been done using solid state manometry. The earlier Chicago classification had defined three types of achalasia of which type II responded best to treatment and type III worst.[24]

Indications for Manometry

Manometry is useful in patients with motor dysphagia in whom no mechanical cause for dysphagia (stricture, ulcer) is identified. In

Table 2: Chicago classification of motility disorders of esophagus

Diagnosis	*Diagnostic criteria*
Achalasia (Figs 19A to C)	
Type I achalasia: classic achalasia	Mean IRP > upper limit of normal, 100% failed peristalsis
Type II achalasia	Achalasia with esophageal compression: mean IRP > upper limit of normal, no normal peristalsis, panesophageal pressurization with >20% of swallows
Type III achalasia	Mean IRP > upper limit of normal, no normal peristalsis, preserved fragments of distal peristalsis or premature (spastic) contractions with >20% of swallows
EGJ outflow obstruction	Mean IRP > upper limit of normal, some instances of intact peristalsis or weak peristalsis with small breaks such that the criteria for achalasia are not met
Motility disorders	Patterns not observed in normal individuals
Distal esophageal spasm (Fig. 20)	Normal mean IRP >20% premature contractions
Hypercontractile esophagus (Jackhammer esophagus) (Fig. 21)	At least one swallow DCI > 8,000 mm Hg-s-cm with single peaked or multipeaked contraction
Absent peristalsis	Normal mean IRP, 100% of swallows with failed peristalsis
Weak peristalsis with large peristaltic defects (Fig. 22)	Mean IRP < 15 mm Hg and >20% swallows with large breaks in the 20 mm Hg isobaric contour (>5 cm in length)
Weak peristalsis with small peristaltic defects	Mean IRP < 15 mm Hg and >30% swallows with small breaks in the 20 mm Hg isobaric contour (2–5 cm in length)
Frequent failed peristalsis	>30%, but <100% of swallows with failed peristalsis
Rapid contractions with normal latency	Rapid contraction with >20% of swallows, DL > 4.5 sec
Hypertensive peristalsis (nutcracker esophagus)	Mean DCI > 5,000 mm Hg-s-cm, but not meeting criteria for hypercontractile esophagus
Normal	Not meeting any of the above diagnostic criteria

Abbreviations: IRP, integrated relaxation pressure; EGJ, esophagogastric junction; DCI, distal contractile integral.

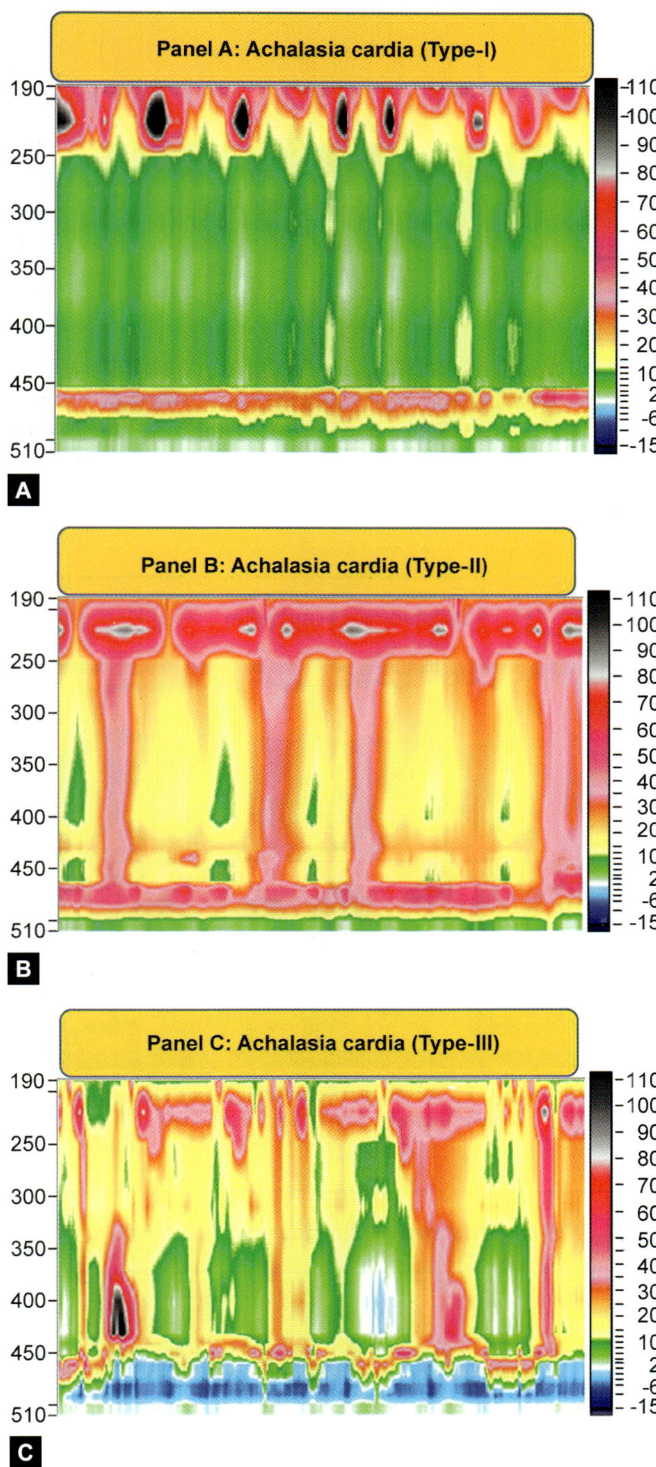

Figures 19A to C *Achalasia cardia*: The three panels show achalasia types I–III as defined in the Chicago classification

patients with GERD, it is used to localize the LES prior to pH-metry; it is useful to perform manometry prior to fundoplication to rule out other motor disorders like achalasia as also to assess degree of dysmotility.

ESOPHAGEAL pH-METRY

Esophageal pH-metry is a method to detect reflux of acidic gastric contents in esophagus. Ambulatory reflux monitoring measures intraesophageal acidity by placing a pH-sensitive electrode placed in a predetermined site of the esophagus. By convention, reflux is defined as a drop in esophageal pH to below four. The number of reflux episodes, as well as the acid exposure time (percentage time with pH < 4), are measured over 24–48 hours. The correlation between symptoms and reflux episodes as per occurrence is expressed using the symptom index (SI)

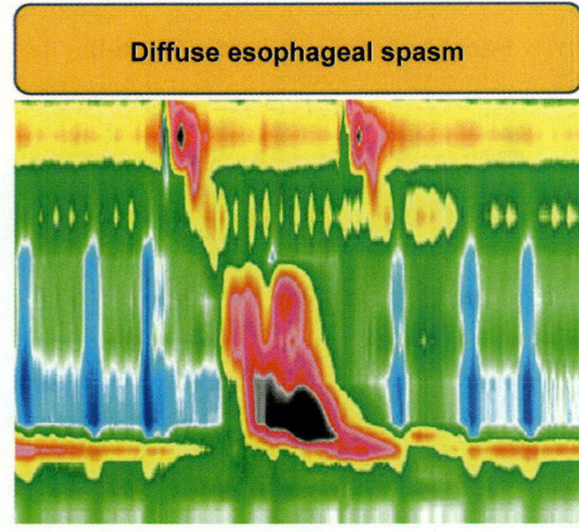

Figure 20 Manometry shows diffuse esophageal spasm. The LES is relaxing, the contraction is premature in onset (DL<4.5 sec)
Abbreviations: LES, lower esophageal sphincter; DL, distal latency.

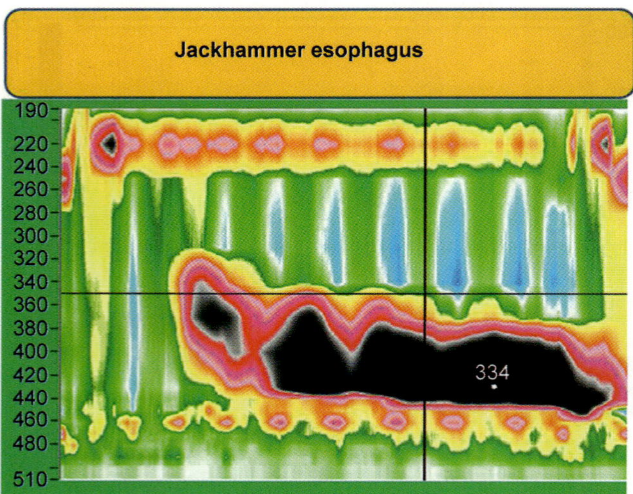

Figure 21 *Jackhammer esophagus*: Plot shows repetitive contractions after a swallow

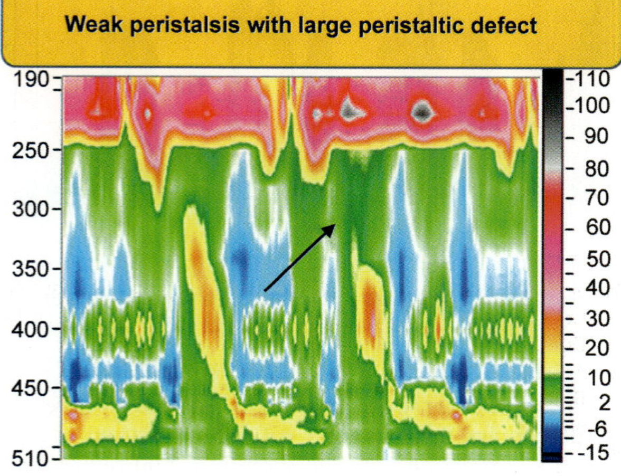

Figure 22 Weak peristalsis with large peristaltic defect

or symptom association probability (SAP). A positive SI and/or SAP statistically, suggests a high probability that the relationship between reflux and symptoms which was recorded, did not occur by chance and thereby suggests a causal relationship.[25]

Procedure

There are two types of pH systems: (i) catheter and (ii) capsule based. For catheter-based systems, antimony or glass electrode probes are placed with the recording sensor at 5 cm proximal to EG junction. The catheter is attached to a portable recorder, which remains with patient throughout 24 hours. The Bravo capsule is placed at 5 cm proximal to EG junction by an endoscopic clipping device, and connects to the recorder using telemetry.

The patient is asked to discontinue antacids for 12 hours, prokinetics for 24 hours, H2 blockers for 48 hours and PPI for at least 1 week before the procedure. The patient is advised to consume normal diet, and stick to his daily activity level if possible; events, like food, sleep, supine or sitting position, are recorded using predesigned buttons on the recorder. The data are downloaded to a computer and analyzed using a dedicated software. Data are reported as esophageal acid exposure time, acid clearance time, number of reflux episodes and longest duration of reflux episode and area under pH 4; the Johnson and Demeester score is calculated based on these parameters.

Indications of pH-Metry

Ambulatory pH-metry is useful in the following groups of patients with GERD: those presenting with atypical symptoms, treatment failures, for step-up treatment, documented Barrett's esophagus for monitoring therapy, to confirm or exclude GERD as a cause of noncardiac chest pain, before anti-reflux surgery in the absence of endoscopic evidence of esophagitis, post anti-reflux surgery if suspected to have ongoing reflux, suspected reflux related asthma or upper respiratory tract symptoms.

It is unrewarding if there is endoscopic esophagitis, symptoms have responded to empirical PPI, for suspicion of Barrett's metaplasia, nonnuclear dyspepsia, *H. pylori*-related ulcer disease or malignant ulcer.

IMPEDANCE pH MONITORING

Ambulatory pH-metry, a method based on detection of changes in acid content, was considered gold standard for detection of GERD until recently. GER-type symptoms often persist in many patients despite adequate acid reducing medications. It has been suggested that these symptoms may be due to reflux of gastric contents having pH greater than 4 (i.e. nonacid reflux).[26]

Multichannel intraluminal impedance (MII) is a novel technique for detecting esophageal gastroesophageal reflux, the nature of reflux as well as the presence of refluxate presence, its distribution and its clearing by esophageal motility. MII can thus detect presence of reflux, identify its pH and as to whether the refluxate is liquid or gas as well as the refluxate clearance time while pH measurement component can only measure the acid clearance time.

Multichannel intraluminal impedance works on the principle of impedance. The presence of bolus inside the esophageal lumen with variable density, ionic contents and conductivity offers resistance to alternating current between two metal electrodes, which work as impedance measuring segment. Electric conductivity (the opposite of resistance or impedance) is directly related to the ionic concentration of the intraluminal content; content with high ionic concentrations (i.e. refluxate, food) have low resistance (high conductivity) compared to the esophageal lining or air.[27]

Impedance systems are also available in combination with pH-metry and manometry. Currently, combined pH-impedance is more commonly used.

Combined impedance-pH monitoring is useful to assess gastroesophageal reflux in the postprandial period, and in patients with persistent symptoms on therapy and those with atypical symptoms.[28] It also has been used in pediatric patients and infants with GER[29] and apnea in infants and premature babies.[30]

Ambulatory combined-pH monitoring and bilirubin monitoring (Bilitec®) require the presence of bilirubin and therefore is not useful in bile-free nonacid reflux, which accounts for 90% of nonacid reflux.[31]

ENDOSCOPIC ULTRASOUND FOR ESOPHAGEAL DISORDERS

Endoscopic ultrasound (EUS) is an important investigation to aid diagnosis in esophageal disorders. There are two basic echoendoscope designs: (i) A radial array system where the scanning is done using circumferential views that range from 270° to 360°, (ii) A curvilinear array system where the view is linear mainly, and high-frequency catheter-based miniprobes. The curvilinear array design permits direct needle aspiration, biopsies and fine needle injection (FNI) under ultrasonographic guidance. Catheter-based miniprobes are used in mechanical echoendoscopes. These oblique-viewing optical systems scan at frequencies from 5.0 MHz to 20 MHz and permit diagnostic procedures. Some even possess Doppler capabilities. Therapeutic echoendoscopes with larger 3.8 mm channels permit large-diameter devices such as large-bore (10F) stents.[32]

Endoscopic ultrasound has excellent highly accuracy in evaluating intramural lesions in terms of spread, depth, possible causes as well as evaluating extraluminal lesions (lymph nodes) in the gastrointestinal tract. With surgery or clinical follow-up as gold standard, the accuracy is 96%.[33]

Endoscopic ultrasound-guided fine-needle aspiration cytology (EUS-FNAC) most useful in individuals with esophageal subepithelial lesions and with EUS characteristics suggestive of malignancy. Endoscopic features of subepithelial lesions that correlate with malignancy include irregular extraluminal border, echogenic foci larger than 3 mm, cystic spaces larger than 4 mm and size on EUS greater than 4 cm. Each of these features when present increases the risk of malignancy incrementally by 30%.[34]

The sensitivity of EUS-FNAC TNM staging of esophageal cancer is greater than 85%. Ultrasonography with fine-needle aspiration cytology (EUS FNAC) is more accurate than CT for local staging of mediastinal lymph nodes. EUS helps to identify the subset most likely to benefit from endoscopic mucosal resection and neoadjuvant chemotherapy. Dilation of malignant esophageal strictures enables completion of EUS examination, aiding treatment planning in up to 20% of patients.[33] The risk of malignant cell seeding of the needle track following EUS- and CT-guided percutaneous biopsy is very low (only case reports). EUS has limitation in detecting postoperative or postradiation recurrence as accuracy deceases due to inflammation and fibrosis and should not be used for this purpose unless tissue sampling is required.

REFERENCES

1. Cotton PB, Williams CB, Saunders BP, Hawes RH. Endoscopic equipment. Practical Gastrointestinal Endoscopy: The Fundamentals, 6th edition. West Sussex, Wiley: Oxford University Press; 2008. pp. 7-21.
2. Yoshida T, Inoue H, Usui S, Satodate H, Fukami N, Kudo SE. Narrow-band imaging system with magnifying endoscopy for superficial esophageal lesions. Gastrointest Endosc. 2004;59(2):288-95.
3. ASGE Technology Committee, Adler DG, Conway JD, Diehl DL, Farraye FA, Kantsevoy SV, et al. Narrow band imaging and multiband imaging. Gastrointest Endosc. 2008;67(4):581-9.
4. Spieker MR. Evaluating dysphagia. Am Fam Physician. 2000;61(12): 3639-48.
5. Cook IJ. Oropharyngeal dysphagia. Gastroenterol Clin North Am. 2009;38(3):411-31.
6. Bansal A, Kahrilas PJ. Treatment of GERD complications (Barrett's, peptic stricture) and etra-esophageal syndromes. Best Pract Res Clin Gastroenterol. 2010;24(6):961-8.
7. Pregun I, Hritz I, Tulassay Z, Herszényi L. Peptic esophageal stricture: medical treatment. Dig Dis. 2009;27(1):31-7.
8. Smith MS. Diagnosis and management of esophageal rings and webs. Gastroenterol Hepatol (N Y). 2010;6(11):701-4.
9. Sharma P, Dent J, Armstrong D, Bergman JJ, Gossner L, Hoshihara Y, et al. The development and validation of an endoscopic grading system for Barrett's esophagus: the Prague C and M criteria. Gastroenterology. 2006;131(5):1392-9.
10. Fitzgerald RC, di Pietro M, Ragunath K, Watson P, Trudgill N, Patel P, et al. British Society of gastroenterology guidelines on the diagnosis and management of Barrett's esophagus. Gut. 2014;63(1):7-42.
11. Zargar SA, Kochhar R, Nagi B, Mehta S, Mehta SK. Ingestion of corrosive acids. Spectrum of injury to upper gastrointestinal tract and natural history. Gastroenterology. 1989;97(3):702-7.
12. Kochhar R, Ray JD, Sriram PV, Kumar S, Singh K. Intralesional steroids augment the effects of endoscopic dilation in corrosive esophageal strictures. Gastrointest Endosc. 1999;49(4 Pt 1):509-13.
13. Hordijk ML, Siersema PD, Tilanus HW, Kuipers EJ. Electrocautery therapy for refractory anastomotic strictures of the esophagus. Gastrointest Endosc. 2006;63(1):157-63.
14. Swaroop VS, Desai DC, Mohandas KM, Dave UR, Gulla RI, Dinshaw KA, et al. Dilation of esophageal strictures induced by radiation therapy for cancer of the esophagus. Gastrointest Endosc. 1994;40(3):311-5.
15. Papadopoulou A, Koletzko S, Heuschkel R, Dias JA, Allen KJ, Murch SH, et al. Management guidelines of eosinophilic esophagitis in childhood. J Pediatr Gastroenterol Nutr. 2014;58(1):107-18.
16. Wilshire CL, Niebisch S, Watson TJ, Litle VR, Peyre CG, Jones CE, et al. Dysphagia postfundoplication: more commonly hiatal outflow resistance than poor esophageal body motility. Surgery. 2012;152(2):584-92.
17. Shridhar R, Almhanna K, Meredith KL, Biagioli MC, Chuong MD, Cruz A, et al. Radiation therapy and esophageal cancer. Cancer Control. 2013;20(2):97-110.
18. Armstrong D, Bennett JR, Blum AL, Dent J, De Dombal FT, Galmiche JP, et al. The endoscopic assessment of esophagitis: a progress report on observer agreement. Gastroenterology. 1996;111(1):85-92.
19. Lundell LR, Dent J, Bennett JR, Blum AL, Armstrong D, Galmiche JP, et al. Endoscopic assessment of oesophagitis:

clinical and functional correlates and further validation of the Los Angeles classification. Gut. 1999;45:172-80.
20. Mel Wilcox C. Gastrointestinal consequences of infection with human immunodeficiency virus. In: Feldman M, Friedman LS, Brandt LJ (Eds). Sleisenger and Fordtran's Gastrointestinal and Liver Disease: Pathophysiology, Diagnosis, Management, 10th edition. Philadelphia: Saunders; 2010. pp. 524-36.
21. Bogte A, Bredenoord AJ, Oors J, Siersema PD, Smout AJ. Reproducibility of esophageal high-resolution manometry. Neurogastroenterol Motil. 2011;23(7):e271-6.
22. Clouse RE, Staiano A, Alrakawi A, Haroian L. Application of topographical methods to clinical esophageal manometery. Am J Gastroenterol. 2000;95(10):2720-30.
23. Bredenoord AJ, Fox M, Kahrilas PJ, Pandolfino JE, Schwizer W, Smout AJ, et al. Chicago classification criteria of esophageal motility disorders defined in high resolution esophageal pressure topography. Neurogastroenterol Motil. 2012;24 Suppl 1:57-65.
24. Gyawali CP, Bredenoord AJ, Conklin JL, Fox M, Pandolfino JE, Peters J, et al. Evaluation of esophageal motor function in clinical practice. Neurogastroenterol Motil. 2013;25(2):99-133.
25. Bredenoord AJ. Impedance-pH monitoring: new standard for measuring gastro-esophageal reflux. Neurogastroenterol Motil. 2008;20(5):434-9.
26. Stein HJ, Feussner H, Kauer W, DeMeester TR, Siewert JR. Alkaline gastroesophageal reflux: assessment by ambulatory esophageal aspiration and pH monitoring. Am J Surg. 1994;167(1):163-8.
27. Silny J. Intraluminal multiple electric impedance procedure for measurement of gastrointetinal motility. J Gastrointest Motil. 1991;3:151-62.
28. Castell DO, Mainie I, Tutuian R. Non-acid gastroesophageal reflux: documenting its relationship to symptoms using multichannel intraluminal impedance (MII). Trans Am Clin Climatol Assoc. 2005;116:321-34.
29. Skopnik H, Silny J, Heiber O, Schulz J, Rau G, Heimann G. Gastroesophageal reflux in infants: evaluation of a new intraluminal impedance technique. J Pediatr Gastroenterol Nutr. 1996;23(5):591-8.
30. Wenzl TG, Schenke S, Peschgens T, Silny J, Heimann G, Skopnik H. Association of apnea and nonacid gastroesophageal reflux in infants: investigations with the intraluminal impedance technique. Pediatr Pulmonol. 2001;31(2):144-9.
31. Sifrim D, Holloway RH, Silny J, Dent J. Non-acid gastroesophageal reflux. Gastroenterology. 2001;120:A436.
32. ASGE Standards of Practice Committee, Gan SI, Rajan E, Alder DG. Role of EUS. Gastrointest Endosc. 2007;66:425-34.
33. Maluf-Filho F, Dotti CM, Halwan B, Queiros AF, Kupski C, Chaves DM, et al. An evidence-based consensus statement on the role and application of endosonography in clinical practice. Endoscopy. 2009;41(11):979-87.
34. Chak A, Canto MI, Rösch T, Dittler HJ, Hawes RH, Tio T, et al. Endosonographic differentiation of benign and malignant stromal cell tumors. Gastrointest Endosc. 1997;45(6):468-73.

CHAPTER 12

Approach to a Patient with Dysphagia

Vishal Gupta

INTRODUCTION

Dysphagia (Greek: *dys-* difficulty; *phagia-* to eat) refers to the abnormal sensations associated with disordered bolus transit from mouth to stomach. Patient can have the sensation of food being held up somewhere in the passage after ingestion so they complain that food bolus sticks, holds up or just complain that they need to ingest more water to push the food down in the stomach. Dysphagia is a common symptom, is reported to affect 5–8% of general population[1] and becomes more common with aging affecting up to 16% elderly population.[2]

It is important to remember that dysphagia *always* indicates problem in the oropharynx or esophagus, and *always* needs further evaluation.

PHYSIOLOGY OF SWALLOWING

To understand the problem of dysphagia it is important to review the physiology of swallowing which is a complex but highly coordinated neuromuscular activity. Briefly, process of normal swallowing can be divided into oral, pharyngeal and esophageal phases.

During *oral phase* (lasting < 1 second) food bolus passes rapidly posteriorly toward the posterior tonsil pillars by the elevation of the tongue in anterior to posterior direction. This phase is voluntary and is under the control of peripheral nervous system.

The *pharyngeal phase*, which also lasts for less than 1 second, begins when the food bolus passes the anterior tonsil pillars. Soft palate elevates and retracts to close the nasopharynx thus preventing food regurgitation into the nasopharynx. At the same time the laryngeal valves close and the larynx is elevated under the base of the tongue by the contraction of the pharyngeal constrictor muscles. This prevents laryngeal aspiration during the passage of the food which is propelled across the pharynx toward the cricopharynx by the posterior movement of the base of the tongue. This phase is involuntary and is under the control of peripheral nervous system.

The *esophageal phase* begins with the entry of food bolus in the esophagus across the upper esophageal sphincter (UES) and ends when it passes into the stomach through the lower esophageal sphincter. This phase lasts about 8–20 seconds. Food bolus passes through the esophagus with the help of sequential peristaltic waves (primary and secondary) which are under the control of autonomic nervous system thus this phase is involuntary. It is important to know that the composition of esophageal muscle changes proximal to distal: striated muscles only in proximal 5% length, mixed striated and smooth muscles in next 40% and only smooth muscle in distal 55–60%.

PATHOPHYSIOLOGY OF DYSPHAGIA

The normal transport of the food bolus from the oral cavity to stomach through pharynx and esophagus depends on many factors like size of the food bolus, diameter of the lumen, peristaltic force, and normal coordinated relaxation of the upper and lower esophageal sphincters. Thus dysphagia can be classified as *mechanical* or *motor* depending on the underlying mechanism, and also as *oropharyngeal* or *esophageal* depending on the site of problem. So both oropharyngeal and esophageal dysphagia can have motor or mechanical etiologies (Tables 1 and 2).

Oropharyngeal dysphagia results from disordered oral and pharyngeal phases of swallowing. Usually both the phases are affected by the same underlying problem thus they are usually grouped together. Oropharyngeal dysphagia is usually motor type as it is usually associated with neuromuscular disorders while esophageal dysphagia is usually mechanical in nature.

Table 1: Causes of oropharyngeal dysphagia

Neuromuscular diseases
1. Neurogenic: • Cerebrovascular accidents/stroke • Polio • Parkinson disease • Dementia • Tabes dorsalis • Brainstem tumor • Other congenital or degenerative disorders • Diabetes mellitus • Recurrent laryngeal nerve injury • Paraneoplastic syndromes • Diphtheria • Rabies 2. Myogenic disorders: • Polymyositis, dermatomyositis • Scleroderma • Mixed connective tissue disorder • Dystrophies • Hyperthyroidism • Hypothyroidism • Amyloidosis
Structural lesions
1. Intrinsic: • Oropharyngeal carcinoma • Cervical esophageal carcinoma • Esophageal web • Benign cervical esophageal stricture, e.g. corrosive stricture • Inflammatory disorder (tonsillar abscess) • Postsurgical • Postradiation • Foreign body 2. Extrinsic: • Thyroid enlargement • Cervical lymphadenopathy • Vertebral osteophytes

Table 2: Causes of esophageal dysphagia

Motility (neuromuscular) disorder
• Idiopathic hypomotility disorder • Motility disorder secondary to systemic disorders (hypothyroidism, scleroderma, diabetes mellitus, amyloidosis) • Reflux induced dysmotility • Achalasia and achalasia variants • Diffuse esophageal spasm • Nutcracker esophagus • Hypertensive lower esophageal sphincter
Mechanical (structural) lesions
1. Intrinsic: • Benign esophageal tumors • Esophageal carcinoma • Peptic stricture • Reflux esophagitis • Corrosive stricture • Rings and webs (e.g. Schatzki's ring, Plummer-Vinson/Patterson-Kelley Syndrome) • Foreign body, e.g. impacted denture • Postsurgical, e.g. fundoplication, esophagectomy, myotomy • Postradiation • Diverticulum • Eosinophilic esophagitis • Pill esophagitis 2. Extrinsic: • Vascular abnormalities (e.g. dysphagia lusoria) • Mediastinal tumors and lymphadenopathy • Osteophytes • Gastric volvulus

Mechanical dysphagia can result from ingestion of a very large bolus (intraluminal cause), intrinsic narrowing of the lumen (intrinsic cause) or external compression (extraluminal cause). Like any other part of the gastrointestinal tract, esophagus can distend during the passage of the bolus. Normally it can distend up to 4 cm in diameter. Patient becomes symptomatic for dysphagia when lumen cannot distend beyond 2.5 cm, but dysphagia is always present when lumen cannot distend beyond 13 mm.[3]

Motor dysphagia results from difficulty in initiating a swallow, abnormal peristalsis or abnormal relaxation of upper or lower esophageal sphincters or combination of these factors. It may be neurogenic or myogenic in origin. Diseases affecting skeletal muscles (e.g. myasthenia gravis) may cause dysphagia by involving the pharynx, UES or cervical esophagus. So oropharyngeal motor dysphagia may result from neuromuscular disorders causing muscle paralysis, simultaneous non-peristaltic contractions or non-relaxation of UES.

As thoracic esophagus, including LES, is predominantly a smooth muscle segment, this part is mainly affected in smooth muscle disorders, e.g. scleroderma. This segment is under the control of autonomic nervous system (parasympathetic through vagus nerve). It controls the peristaltic contraction of the esophageal body and swallows induced relaxation of LES, thus allowing the bolus to pass smoothly across the esophagus and LES into the stomach. Any interference with this coordinated process due to defect in vagal innervation (as in achalasia) or muscle disorders can lead to weak contraction, non-peristaltic contractions, aperistalsis or non-relaxation of LES leading to dysphagia.

It is important to know that mechanical and motor causes are not mutually exclusive and they may coexist in same patient, e.g. gastroesophageal reflux disease (causing peptic stricture and esophageal dysmotility), scleroderma or Zenker's diverticulum (dysphagia due to UES dysmotility and by the compression by distended diverticulum).[4]

APPROACH TO A PATIENT WITH DYSPHAGIA (FLOW CHART 1)

History

Importance of a careful history in the evaluation of a patient with dysphagia cannot be overemphasized. It needs a patient and careful listening to the patient as many factors may act as barriers during history taking, e.g. language, literacy, sociocultural factors (females may be reluctant to provide greater details of their problem), etc. For patients, depending upon their understanding of the perception, dysphagia can mean anything from a common oral pathology (causing odynophagia actually) to esophageal cancer (causing true dysphagia).

Flow chart 1 Algorithm of approach to a patient with dysphagia

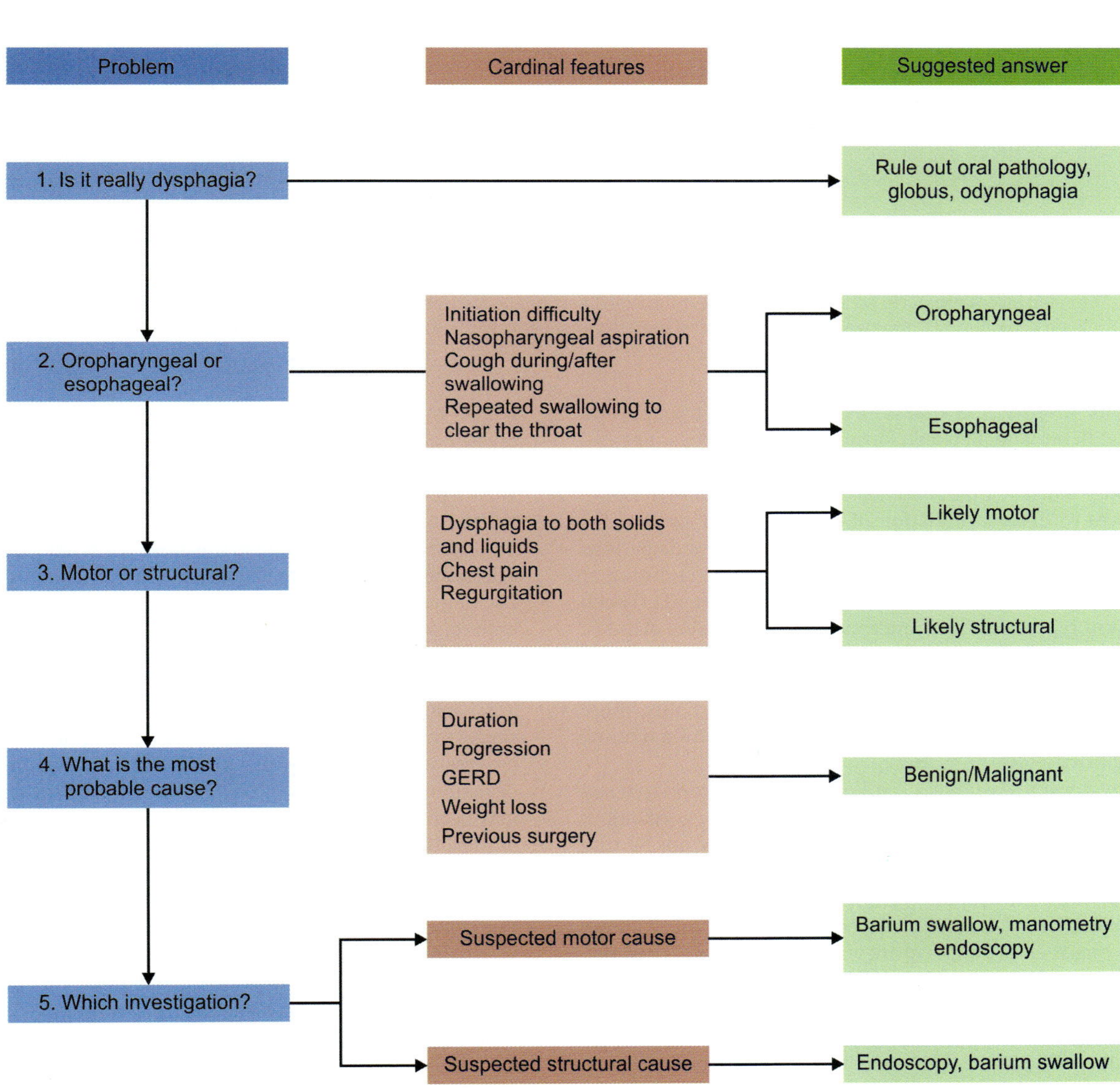

Careful history can provide a presumptive diagnosis in terms of anatomical site and likely cause in up to 80% of cases[5] thus accurate history facilitates further workup.

Art of history taking in dysphagic patient include a targeted approach with four basic aims to be kept in mind. *First* to establish whether patient is actually having dysphagia; *second* to determine the site of the problem (i.e. to differentiate between oropharyngeal and esophageal dysphagia), *third* to differentiate between motor and mechanical dysphagia, and *lastly* to elaborate associate symptoms that can help to ascertain the underlying cause.

1. It is important to ascertain the presence of true dysphagia, and to differentiate it from common oral pathology, odynophagia and globus sensation. Patient with common oral pathology (e.g. oral ulcers, pharyngitis, tonsillitis, carries tooth, etc.) may have difficulty in chewing or have odynophagia.

Odynophagia is pain during swallowing. It is generally more transient and persists only for the duration that the bolus takes to pass through the esophagus. Odynophagia can occur with or shortly after the start of the swallow, and may reflect different underlying problem.

Globus sensation refers to the sensation that something is continuously lodged in the throat giving a sensation of lump, fullness or tightness. There is no structural or motor abnormality in the transport of the bolus. It is more common in females, has psychological component, and most importantly it is present in between the swallows and rather alleviated by eating. Nasopharyngeal and tracheobronchial aspirations are always absent.

2. Once the presence of true dysphagia is confirmed, it becomes important to (1) grade the dysphagia (Table 3) to

Table 3: Dysphagia grading

Grade	Mellow & Pinkas[1]	Ogilvie et al.[2]	Sugahara et al.[3]
0	Able to eat normal diet	Able to eat normal diet	
1	Able to eat some solid food	Able to eat some solid food	Normal eating
2	Able to eat semisolids only	Able to eat semisolids only	Requires liquids with meals
3	Able to swallow liquids only	Able to swallow liquids only	Can take semisolids only
4	Unable to swallow anything, including saliva	Complete dysphagia even for liquids	Can take liquids only
5			Unable to take liquids, can swallow saliva only
6			Absolute dysphagia

[1] Mellow MH, Pinkas H. Endoscopic laser therapy for malignancies affecting the esophagus and gastroesophageal junction: analysis of technical and functional efficacy. Arch Intern Med. 1985;145:1443-6.
[2] Ogilvie AL, Dronfield MW, Ferguson R, Atkinson M. Palliative intubation of esophagogastric neoplasms at fibreoptic endoscopy. Gut. 1982;23(12):1060-7.
[3] Sugahara S, Ohara K, Yoshioka H. Improvement of swallowing function in patients with esophageal cancer treated by radiology. J Jpn Soc Cancer Ther. 1996;31:1124-30.

assess its severity and assess response to the therapy and (2) to differentiate between oropharyngeal and esophageal dysphagia. There are four cardinal symptoms of high specificity indicating the presence of *oropharyngeal dysphagia*[6]: (1) absent or delayed initiation of oropharyngeal swallow (or dysphagia within 1 second of swallowing); (2) postdeglutitive nasopharyngeal regurgitation; (3) cough or choking during or after swallow (due to tracheobronchial aspiration) and (4) need to swallow repetitively in an attempt to clear the throat of bolus. Supportive, though less specific, symptoms are oral drooling, hoarseness of voice, bolus hold up in the neck, garbled voice and expectoration rather than regurgitation of the bolus. There may be history of recurrent bolus impaction requiring manual dislodgment.

Esophageal dysphagia differs from oropharyngeal dysphagia by the absence of nasopharyngeal regurgitation, absence of tracheobronchial aspiration [this may not be true in case of carcinoma esophagus with tracheoesophageal fistula or corrosive esophageal stricture with tracheo (brocho)-esophageal fistula], by the fact that it is not immediate, it allows further ingestion of liquids to alleviate dysphagia and presence of regurgitation of retained secretions or food itself. Site of food hold up can give some clue to underlying site of obstruction. Patient may have a sensation of retrosternal food hold up in esophageal dysphagia. However, 30% of cases can perceive hold up of bolus in suprasternal or cervical region when the actual problem lies within the esophageal body.[6] Thus based on the site of dysphagia perceived it can be difficult to differentiate between the oropharyngeal and esophageal dysphagia.

3. Once the site of problem causing dysphagia is ascertained, it becomes important to ascertain the type of dysphagia: motor or structural. Duration and nature of dysphagia may help in such differentiation.

In *motor* disorder, dysphagia is for both liquids and solids because of inherent problem with peristaltic and/or sphincteric mechanisms. In structural lesions, dysphagia is initially for solids. This aggravates to dysphagia for liquids and dysphagia for a smaller bolus as the disease progresses compromising the lumen.[7]

Dysphagia, chest pain and regurgitation are three cardinal symptoms of esophageal motility disorder.[8] Chest pain, especially retrosternal chest pain, occur in achalasia or diffuse esophageal spam. It may mimic heartburn of gastroesophageal reflux, may occur during meals, and may be sporadic or nocturnal. Spontaneous regurgitation in between meals, during meals or at night strongly suggests motility disorder.[8] This regurgitation is to be differentiated from regurgitation in gastroesophageal reflux disease in which regurgitated food/fluid is noxious in taste due to the presence of acid and/or bile, thus patient is not able to reswallow it due to its nature.

4. Eliciting associated symptoms and nature of dysphagia are important in narrowing down the differential diagnosis (Tables 1 and 2) and ascertaining the underlying cause of dysphagia.

A short history of progressive dysphagia with weight loss suggests malignancy especially if there are other suggestive symptoms like hoarseness. A long history of slowly progressing dysphagia with a history of heartburn may suggest development of peptic stricture, though at a later stage patient may become less symptomatic for reflux either due to stricture or development of Barrett's esophagus. A long history of intermittent, non-progressive dysphagia for solid food may suggest the presence of a fixed structural lesion, e.g. Schaztki ring (*Steakhouse syndrome*) or motor disorder.

History of recent intake of oral medications (to rule out pill esophagitis), corrosive ingestion, viral infection, pulmonary tuberculosis, neck surgery (thyroid), gastroesophageal surgery (e.g. fundoplication) are also important in addition to eliciting the history of gastroesophageal reflux, stroke and other neuromuscular disorder, and history suggestive of connective tissue disorder as esophagus may be involved in scleroderma (CREST syndrome: calcinosis, Raynaud's phenomenon, esophageal dysmotility, sclerodactyly, telangiectasia).

A very useful way to elicit above mentioned points during history taking is to let the patient describe what happens when he/she eats or take liquids.

Examination

Physical examination is important for the assessment of the general condition of the patient that can guide whether patient can tolerate the invasive procedures that may be required to investigate and treat the cause of dysphagia. Occasionally, it can provide the clues to the specific cause of dysphagia, e.g. presence of left supraclavicular lymphadenopathy may suggest the presence of esophageal malignancy as a cause of dysphagia.

Anemia may be present due chronic blood loss (ulcer/esophagitis/tumor) or poor oral intake. Patient may be dehydrated due to poor oral intake especially in case of absolute dysphagia. Abdomen examination should focus on the presence of hepatomegaly, ascites and any epigastric lump may raise the suspicion of gastric malignancy or liver metastases. Chest should be assessed for aspiration. Assessment for neuromuscular disorder (e.g. Parkinson's disease) is important in oropharyngeal dysphagia as it is usually motor in type. However, absence of neurological signs does not preclude the presence of neuromuscular etiology of oropharyngeal dysphagia. Patient can have features of connective tissue disorder like calcinosis, sclerodactyly, telengiectasia, rashes or joint abnormalities, muscle wasting or weakness due to neuromuscular disorders.

Investigations

Oropharyngeal dysphagia is usually investigated with indirect laryngoscopy, barium swallow and videofluoroscopy. Generally evaluation of oropharyngeal dysphagia come under the purview of ENT surgeons, thus only the evaluation of esophageal dysphagia will be discussed in detail.

Most important investigations in the evaluation of esophageal dysphagia are endoscopy, barium swallow and esophageal manometry.

Endoscopy

It is the initial investigation of choice because of its high diagnostic yield, provision of mucosal biopsy and therapeutic potential. Presently, wide availability of this facility and expertise has also made it the first line investigation for esophageal dysphagia. So endoscopy is recommended to establish the diagnosis, look for associated problem, e.g. esophagitis, exclude malignancy and implement therapy, if required. A normal endoscopy, however, does not rule the presence of esophageal pathology as a cause of dysphagia. In such case other investigations, e.g. barium swallow or manometry, can be helpful as discussed later. Esophageal biopsies should be taken to exclude eosinophilic esophagitis.

Barium Swallow

Safety, wider availability and accuracy have made endoscopy the preferred investigation over barium studies. Barium studies can, however, be useful in certain situations for the assessment of esophageal anatomy as well as esophageal function especially the emptying. Barium study has been found to be more sensitive than endoscopy for strictures having a luminal diameter more than 10 mm, distal rings, and for achalasia and other motility disorders. For the diagnosis of achalasia, it is considered to be more sensitive than endoscopy which is mainly performed to exclude malignancy. Classical signs of achalasia are dilated esophagus with air fluid level and bird beak appearance representing tapered contracted LES. In addition, fluoroscopic examination can detect abnormalities of esophageal motility (e.g. corkscrew esophagus in diffuse esophageal spasm). For esophageal stricture additional information, like length and tightness of stricture, can be useful for therapy planning and also for post-therapy comparison. In addition, it can identify lesions that can be difficult to assess or create diagnostic problem during endoscopy, e.g. Zenker's or epiphrenic diverticulum, and paraesophageal hernia. Its importance in defining gastroesophageal anatomy in postsurgical dysphagia cases cannot be underestimated. Cause of post-fundoplication dysphagia (tight wrap, slipped wrap, herniated wrap, etc.) or post-myotomy dysphagia can be very well ascertained on barium studies. Similar information can be provided on barium studies for dysphagia after bariatric surgery (sleeve gastrectomy, Roux-en gastric bypass, gastric banding), after gastric or colonic transposition for various indications and recurrence of dysphagia after esophageal stenting.

Another recently described technique of barium study is *timed barium esophagogram.*[9] It objectively assesses the esophageal emptying. Multiple sequential films at pre-decided time interval are taken after a single swallow of a fixed volume of a specific density barium solution. Height and width of the barium column is used to assess the esophageal emptying. This test is being used in patients with achalasia, especially in long standing cases, to assess its severity and to follow-up after treatment.

Manometry

Esophageal manometry remains the gold standard test for assessment of esophageal motility disorders. It is also advised in patients with normal endoscopy. However, this test is not commonly used because of limited availability at a few centers. When available it is used in cases where endoscopy and barium studies remain non-diagnostic or when motor dysphagia is strongly suspected based on clinical evaluation. Based on the manometric findings, specific motility disorder can be diagnosed[10] as per classification given by *Spechler and Castell.* Classic manometric findings of *achalasia* are aperistaltic esophagus and non-relaxing LES. LES pressure may be low (32%), normal (25%) or high (43%).[11] *Esophageal spasm* is diagnosed by synchronous peristaltic waves (>20% of wet swallows), intermittent but normally progressive esophageal peristalsis, and normally relaxing LES. In *scleroderma*, LES is hypotonic or atonic with aperistaltic esophageal body leading to severe reflux. Dysphagia generally develops due to reflux peptic stricture.

In conventional manometry esophageal pressure is measured using a catheter with several water-perfused sideholes and with or without the addition of a sleeve sensor or solid state pressure transducers. Conventional manometry catheters are limited by gaps between the pressure sensors. In contrast in *high resolution manometry* (HRM) catheters are placed with smaller spacing between sideholes making it more accurate in pressure measurement as compared to conventional manometry. With HRM, the clinician can simultaneously measure pressures from hypopharynx to stomach as compared to time-consuming pull through techniques which are no longer used. With the introduction of HRM, esophageal motor disorders have been classified with refinement (*Chicago classification*).[12] Achalasia has been classified into three types based on HRM: type I is classical achalasia with minimal esophageal pressurization; type II is achalasia with compression and type III is achalasia with body spasm. This classification has prognostic importance and may help choosing the correct treatment modality. Patients with type II achalasia respond better to myotomy or dilatation while type I achalasia respond better to myotomy than to dilatation, and type III remains most difficult to treat with poor response to either myotomy or dilatation.[13]

Recently, impedance manometry catheters which have additional sensors for liquid and viscous bolus transit have been developed allowing further assessment of esophageal function especially in cases with non-obstructing dysphagia.[14]

Further Evaluation

There remain a small group of patients in which endoscopy, barium studies and manometry do not yield any specific diagnosis. Further evaluation requires reviewing the patient's history to ascertain the cause: motor or structural. Next step is to repeat the endoscopy with careful examination with sufficient insufflation that can detect small (large diameter) ring and specifically examine blind areas, e.g. gastroesophageal junction by retroflexion of the endoscope to rule out gastroesophageal junction malignancy presenting as pseudoachalasia. Esophageal mucosal biopsies should be taken at this time if already not taken during previous endoscopy, to rule out eosinophilic esophagitis. Barium examination may be repeated with proper views and videofluoroscopic sequences. Empiric esophageal dilation has been advocated by some authors.[6]

SPECIAL SITUATION: POSTOPERATIVE DYSPHAGIA

Post-reflux Surgery Dysphagia

Transient dysphagia occurs in 40–70% of patients after Nissen's fundoplication most probably secondary to edema at the gastroesophageal junction. Dysphagia usually resolves spontaneously within 2–3 months in most of the cases. Persistent dysphagia, however, is reported by 3–24% of patients. The risk factors and causes include presence of preoperative dysphagia, presence of preoperative esophageal dysmotility, laparoscopic approach, Nissen-Rosetti fundoplication (as compared to floppy Nissen's), recurrence of hiatal hernia and consequent wrap herniation above the diaphragm, twisted fundoplication, slippage of fundoplication and tight diaphragmatic hiatus.[15-17]

These patients require extensive evaluation to identify the exact cause of persistent dysphagia for correct management. Review of original symptoms, workup before the previous surgery, operative records, immediate outcomes after primary surgery, and timing of symptom occurrence are important aspect of evaluation. A routine preoperative workup includes endoscopy preferably by the operating surgeon, manometry, barium esophagogram, and a gastric emptying study, if possible.[16]

Post-esophagectomy Dysphagia

Development of dysphagia after esophagectomy can result from benign causes like anastomotic stricture (at esophagoenteric anastomotic site), narrow gastric tube, tight hiatus, or oropharyngeal dysfunction due to recurrent laryngeal nerve injury. Tumor recurrence can also be a cause of anastomotic narrowing.

Benign anastomotic stricture after esophagectomy is quite common (incidence 26–42%).[18] Symptomatic strictures have been defined as presence of dysphagia along with endoscopic or radiographic (on esophagogram) evidence of stricture.[19] Dysphagia after esophagectomy can compromise early outcome and quality of life. Most of these patients present within 2–3 months. Well defined risk factors include use of gastric tube (vs colonic conduit), anastomotic leak, and associated cardiovascular comorbidities. However, site of anastomosis (chest vs neck), method of anastomosis[20,21] (hand sewn vs stapled; though side to side semi-mechanical method is associated with lower rates of leak and stricture[22,23]), and neoadjuvant treatment have not been found to be risk factors. While most of these anastomotic strictures are minimal or mild (>9 mm), some may develop refractory strictures requiring multiple sessions of dilations. Risk factors for such refractory strictures include anastomotic leak, development of stricture within 3 months of surgery, and neoadjuvant chemoradiotherapy.[18] In case of colonic transposition, anastomotic stricture can develop due to acid reflux and these peptic strictures mainly involve cologastric anastomosis.[24]

Post-esophagectomy dysphagia requires evaluation with barium esophagogram revealing the presence of stricture or any other anatomical abnormality. This may be followed by endoscopy that can confirm the diagnosis and exclude tumor recurrence. Dilatation which can be performed at the same time remains the primary treatment modality for benign anastomotic strictures.

Dysphagia after Achalasia Treatment

Recurrent dysphagia after myotomy is seen in ~10% cases on long-term follow-up.[25] Causes of treatment failure are incomplete myotomy (especially on gastric site), healing with fibrosis of myotomy edges, tight fundoplication, gastroesophageal reflux, type III/IV megaesophagus/sigmoid esophagus, and late occurrence of carcinoma.

Persistent dysphagia after treatment for achalasia should be evaluated with a combination of endoscopy, barium swallow and manometry. Endoscopy can detect esophagitis due to reflux, esophageal narrowing due to tight wrap or incomplete myotomy, or paraesophageal hernia. Barium swallow similarly can detect anatomic abnormality in addition to providing emptying function (especially with timed barium examination as discussed earlier). Manometry is useful in quantifying LES pressure and helps predict the success of further therapy.

REFERENCES

1. Lindgren S, Janzon L. Prevalence of swallowing complaints and clinical findings among 50-79-year-old men and women in an urban population. Dysphagia. 1991;6(4):187-92.
2. Bloem BR, Lagaay AM, van Beek W, Haan J, Roos RA, Wintzen AR. Prevalence of subjective dysphagia in community residents aged over 87. BMJ. 1990;300(6726):721-2.
3. Goyal RK. Dysphagia. In: Longo DL, Fauci AS (Eds). Harrison's Gastroenterology and Hepatology, 1st edition. McGraw Hills; 2010.
4. Arora AS, Conklin JL. Practical approaches to dysphagia caused by esophageal motor disorders. Curr Gastroenterol Rep. 2001;3(3):191-9.
5. Edwards DA. Discriminative information in the diagnosis of dysphagia. J R Coll Physicians Lond. 1975;9(3):257-63.
6. Cook IJ. Diagnostic evaluation of dysphagia. Nat Clin Pract Gastroenterol Hepatol. 2008;5(7):393-403.
7. Gyawali CP, Clouse RE. Approach to the patient with dysphagia, odynophagia, or noncardiac chest pain. In: Yamada T, Aplers DH, Kalloo AN, Kapolwitz N, Owyang C, Powell AW (Eds). Principles of Clinical Gastroenterology, 1st edition. Blackwell Publishing; 2008.

8. Howard PJ, Maher L, Pryde A, Cameron EW, Heading RC. Five year prospective study of the incidence, clinical features, and diagnosis of achalasia in Edinburgh. Gut. 1992;33(8):1011-5.
9. Neyaz Z, Gupta M, Ghoshal UC. How to perform and interpret timed barium esophagogram. J Neurogastroenterol Motil. 2013;19(2):251-6.
10. Spechler SJ, Castell DO. Classification of oesophageal motility abnormalities. Gut. 2001;49(1):145-51.
11. Langerman A, Patti MG. Epidemiology, pathophysiology and clinical features of achalasia. In: Yeo CJ (Ed). Shackelford's Surgery of the Alimentary Tract, 7th edition. Elseviers Saunders; 2013.
12. Pandolfino JE, Ghosh SK, Rice J, Clarke JO, Kwiatek MA, Kahrilas PJ. Classifying esophageal motility by pressure topography characteristics: a study of 400 patients and 75 controls. Am J Gastroenterol. 2008;103(1):27-37.
13. Pandolfino JE, Kwiatek MA, Nealis T, Bulsiewicz W, Post J, Kahrilas PJ. Achalasia: a new clinically relevant classification by high-resolution manometry. Gastroenterology. 2008;135(5):1526-33.
14. Kessing BF, Smout AJ, Bredenoord AJ. Clinical applications of esophageal impedance monitoring and high-resolution manometry. Curr Gastroenterol Rep. 2012;14(3):197-205.
15. Herron DM, Swanström LL, Ramzi N, Hansen PD. Factors predictive of dysphagia after laparoscopic Nissen fundoplication. Surg Endosc. 1999;13(12):1180-3.
16. Légner A, Tsuboi K, Bathla L, Lee T, Morrow LE, Mittal SK. Reoperative antireflux surgery for dysphagia. Surg Endosc. 2011;25(4):1160-7.
17. Sato K, Awad ZT, Filipi CJ, Selima MA, Cummings JE, Fenton SJ, et al. Causes of long-term dysphagia after laparoscopic Nissen fundoplication. JSLS. 2002;6(1):35-40.
18. van Heijl M, Gooszen JA, Fockens P, Busch OR, van Lanschot JJ, van Berge Henegouwen MI. Risk factors for development of benign cervical strictures after esophagectomy. Ann Surg. 2010;251(6):1064-9.
19. Williams VA, Watson TJ, Zhovtis S, Gellersen O, Raymond D, Jones C, et al. Endoscopic and symptomatic assessment of anastomotic strictures following esophagectomy and cervical esophagogastrostomy. Surg Endosc. 2008;22(6):1470-6.
20. Hsu HH, Chen JS, Huang PM, Lee JM, Lee YC. Comparison of manual and mechanical cervical esophagogastric anastomosis after esophageal resection for squamous cell carcinoma: a prospective randomized controlled trial. Eur J Cardiothorac Surg. 2004;25(6):1097-101.
21. Laterza E, de' Manzoni G, Veraldi GF, Guglielmi A, Tedesco P, Cordiano C. Manual compared with mechanical cervical oesophagogastric anastomosis: a randomised trial. Eur J Surg. 1999;165(11):1051-4.
22. Orringer MB, Marshall B, Iannettoni MD. Eliminating the cervical esophagogastric anastomotic leak with a side-to-side stapled anastomosis. J Thorac Cardiovasc Surg. 2000;119(2):277-88.
23. Collard JM, Romagnoli R, Goncette L, Otte JB, Kestens PJ. Terminalized semimechanical side-to-side suture technique for cervical esophagogastrostomy. Ann Thorac Surg. 1998;65(3):814-7.
24. Cassivi SD. Leaks, strictures, and necrosis: a review of anastomotic complications following esophagectomy. Semin Thorac Cardiovasc Surg. 2004;16(2):124-32.
25. Zaninotto G, Costantini M, Rizzetto C, Zanatta L, Guirroli E, Portale G, et al. Four hundred laparoscopic myotomies for esophageal achalasia: a single centre experience. Ann Surg. 2008;248(6):986-93.

CHAPTER 13

Gastroesophageal Reflux Disease

V Baskaran

INTRODUCTION

The "Montreal Global Definition of gastroesophageal reflux disease (GERD)" worked out by a global panel of experts is "a condition which develops when the reflux of stomach contents causes troublesome symptoms, characteristically retrosternal burning (often labeled as heartburn) and regurgitation."[1] The definition is dependent upon subjective symptoms as perceived by an individual rather than on an objective or measurable criterion.

Gastroesophageal reflux disease is common in the Western hemisphere and the wide variation in its reported prevalence going up to 42%[2,3] is more due to inclusion criteria for diagnosis, than to difference in true prevalence. GERD grabs attention, as the quality of life in those with GERD is significantly lower than that of the general population.[2-4]

Deemed infrequent in developing countries a decade ago, GERD is now increasingly seen in India with a prevalence as high as 16% in the urban population[5,6] and with similar rates in the rest of Asia.[7,8] Ethnic differences exist even among Asians, with Indians having higher incidence of GERD compared to the Chinese and Malays.[8] GERD afflicts all age groups starting from infancy with a high prevalence in childhood and reduced prevalence in teens and young adults. This chapter, however, will focus on GERD in the adult population only.

PATHOPHYSIOLOGY

Under normal conditions, food passes along the esophagus into the stomach in a prograde manner aided by esophageal body peristalsis with choreographed relaxation of the gastroesophageal junction. What causes continence of the gastroesophageal junction in the absence of a recognizable anatomical sphincter has been the subject of major studies. However, in reality the lower esophageal sphincter (LES) is a physiological sphincter of about 2.5–4 cm length with a complex structure ending about 4 mm above the endoscopic squamocolumnar line.[9] This is recognizable on manometry as a high-pressure zone (HPZ). The LES can also be determined by anatomic, pharmacologic dissection, as well as by high definition CT scan. Under resting conditions, this zone maintains a pressure of 15–30 mm Hg above gastric pressure. It should be remembered that intragastric pressure is normally higher than esophageal pressure and hence, in the absence of or the impaired function of this sphincter, reflux would be the rule rather than the exception.

Morphologically, the LES is composed of (a) one striated muscle, *i.e.* the diaphragmatic crura constituting the hiatus, and (b) two smooth muscles, one proximal and the other distal. The proximal smooth muscle is the more pronounced part of the distal circular muscles of the esophagus (Figs 1 and 2). The distal smooth muscles are located in the cardia and are specialized fibers of the intermediate layer of proximal stomach muscles.[10] These are generally referred to as sling and clasp fibers of cardia (Fig. 1). Contraction of these muscles narrows and closes the cardia and increases the length of the abdominal esophagus. The state of tonic contraction of the sling muscles contributes to the angle of His. These muscles are said to be the first line of defense against reflux.[11,12]

The crural mechanism by a strong and oblique pinchcock type constriction of the distal esophagus offers a good antireflux protection.[9] This pinchcock effect is more during coughing, sneezing, etc. However, during inspiration, the esophagus ascends and reduces the compactness of the HPZ by moving the smooth muscle components away from the diaphragmatic skeletal muscle environment.[9,13] Hence, during inspiration the protective effect is reduced.

Gastroesophageal reflux disease occurs due to a failure of a complex set of protective barriers as well as due to alterations in the way the refluxed material is dealt with. While the first set causes reflux across the gastroesophageal junction, the second

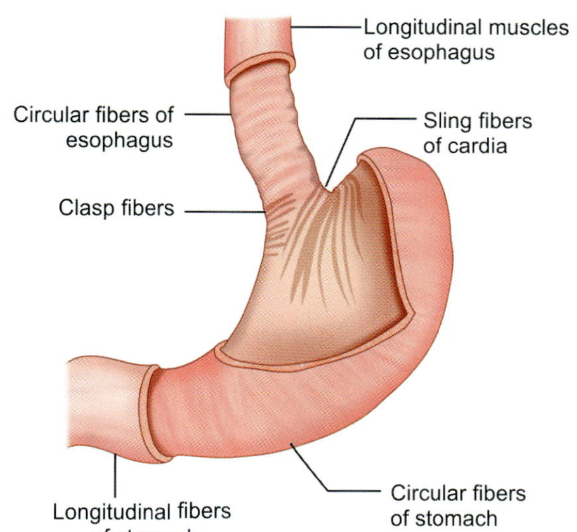

Figure 1 Anatomy of "sling and clasp" fibers of the LES and cardia. It is easy to comprehend how the contraction of these fibers would strengthen the competence of LES

Table 1: Various factors that lead to GERD	
Factors encouraging reflux across gastroesophageal junction	*Factors encouraging prolonged acid stasis in esophagus*
• Failure of the sphincter • Hiatus hernia • Transient LES relaxation • Change in the angle of His • Delayed gastric emptying	• Impaired esophageal motility • Decreased salivary secretion • Change in salivary composition • Supine posture

set of factors encourages stasis of acid in the esophagus leading to mucosal injury. The various factors that may lead to GERD are shown in Table 1 (Figs 3 and 4).

It is necessary to understand various mechanisms that cause reflux, so that therapy, especially surgical therapy, can be meticulously planned to address each of these issues.

If the LES pressure drops to less than 6 mm Hg, the gastric contents tend to reflux into the esophagus. Aberrations in the LES in patients with GERD have been documented in the form of abnormalities in the contractility and density of muscarinic receptors which appear to be the cause for GERD.[11,12] Certain drugs, such as calcium channel blockers, theophylline, nitrates, diazepam, morphine, meperidine and barbiturates are known to lower LES pressures. Similarly, fat, chocolate, ethanol and peppermint lower LES pressure, possibly by causing gastric stasis. The angle of His has a great role in preventing reflux. Various studies have shown that the narrower the angle, the better is the continence (Fig. 4). It has been mentioned earlier in this chapter that the sling fibers of cardia also contribute to the acuity of the angle of His and to the integrity of the LES. This geometry also causes the gastroesophageal flap valve, which is the sharp fold between the distal esophagus and the fundus seen on J maneuver view of the gastroesophageal junction. This valve is essential for continence of the LES. Various authors classify this valve for objectivity to delineate its relationship to reflux. The commonly used system is that of Hill which classifies the flap valve into four grades: Grade I being the best flap valve and Grades II to IV with correspondingly worsening reflux.[14] Others simplify the flap valve into intact (corresponding to Hill Type I) and impaired (corresponding to Hill types II to IV) with impaired valves associated with reflux.[15]

A major cause for reflux is the transient LES relaxation (TLESR). Normally, the LES relaxes following an act of swallowing, whether it is wet or dry or subsequent to peristalsis. When there is brief relaxation of the LES without any such trigger, it is called TLESR. This is a common occurrence seen in response to gastric

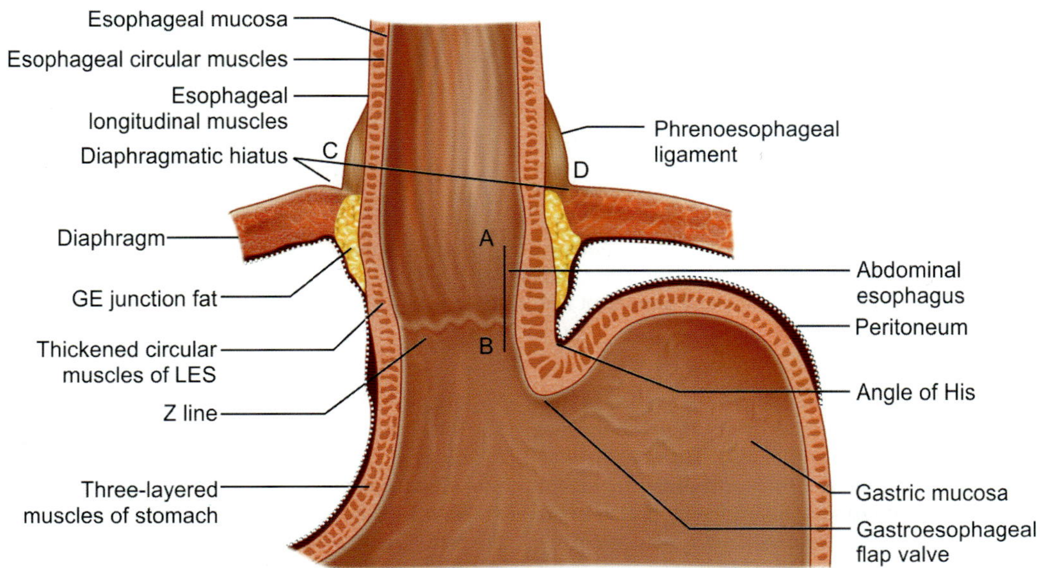

Figure 2 Anatomy of GE junction. Note two layered muscles of the esophagus changes to 3 layers of stomach at GE junction. The acute angle of His is discernable. The point A shows proximal aspect of abdominal esophagus and the line AB denotes the length of abdominal esophagus. The distance between points C and D is the width of the esophageal hiatus. The figure explains various aspects of GE junction that help in preventing reflux

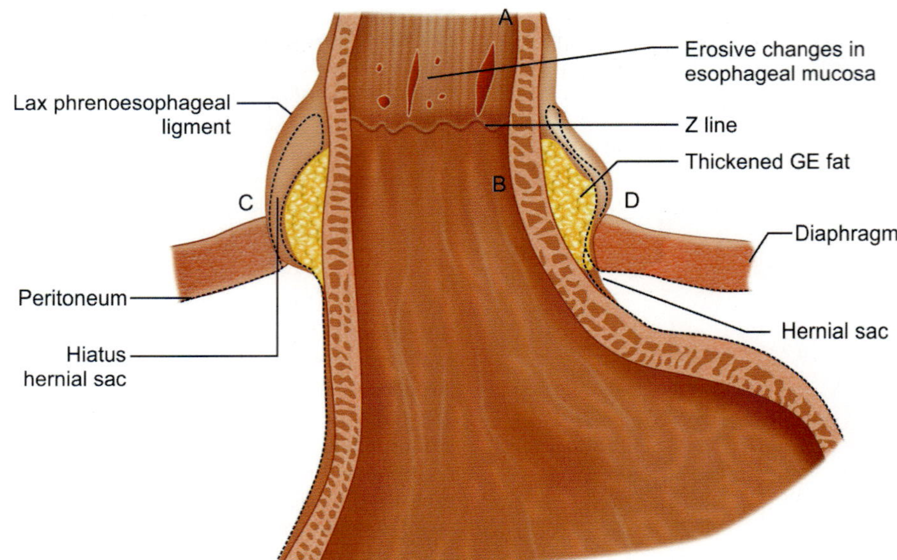

Figure 3 Anatomy of GE junction in a patient with sliding hiatus hernia. Please compare with Figure 2 and note the significant increase in the size of the esophageal hiatus (distance between points C and D), upward displacement of both points A and B as well as Z line. Complete absence of abdominal esophagus, ineffective LES, nonexistent angle of His and obliteration of GE junction flap valve facilitate reflux. In addition, the proximal migration of GE junction with other structures result in lax phrenoesophageal ligament, increase in GE junction fat pads and peritoneal hiatal hernial sac

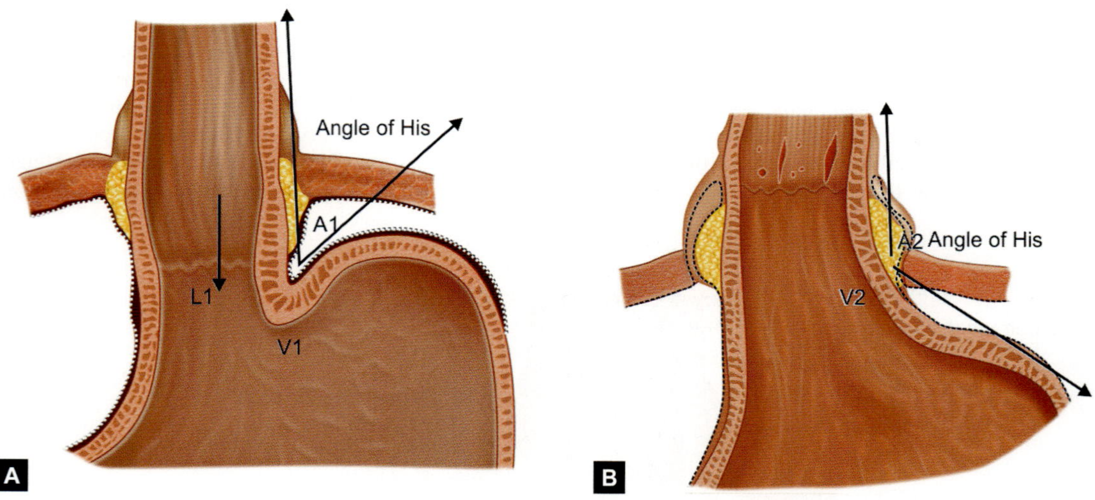

Figures 4A and B Correlation between the angle of His and continence of LES is related to the length of abdominal esophagus. The acute angle of His in Figure A is related to the length of abdominal esophagus L1. Compare these with A2 which is wider and L2 which is nonexistent in Figure B. Also note that GE flap valve V1 in Figure A is likely to more competent than V2 in Figure B

distension and is the cause for physiologic reflux in the normal population. The refluxed acid is cleared by normal esophageal clearance mechanism. In patients with GERD, the occurrence of TLESR is not increased, but the quantity and proximal extent of reflux is increased or its subsequent clearance by peristalsis is impaired. This leads to increased or prolonged acid exposure of the esophagus in these patients.[16] Even though TLESR is a major cause for reflux in the normal population, in patients with GERD, the actual reflux occurs because of LES hypotonia or hiatus hernia.[17]

Whenever intra-abdominal pressure increases during episodes like coughing or sneezing, the abdominal pressure is transmitted to the stomach. The elevated intragastric pressure then tends to propel gastric contents into the esophagus. Intrinsic LES pressure, the length of the abdominal esophagus, acuity of Angle of His and the hiatus are responsible for preventing this reflux. As LES pressure cannot rise simultaneously with the sudden explosive increase in abdominal pressure, it has a limited role in preventing reflux. However, a normal hiatus contracting vigorously during coughing, sneezing, *etc.* can prevent reflux by pinching and closing the lower esophagus. Similarly, the longer the length of the abdominal esophagus, the more is the closing pressure exerted on it by the suddenly raised intra-abdominal pressure. So the very pressure that can push gastric contents into the esophagus can also exert an extrinsic occluding pressure on the distal esophagus at the hiatus. An acute angle of His works better against reflux by enabling the fundus with higher pressure to compress the distal esophagus. Thus it is obvious that hiatus hernia is a major structural cause for GERD.

In the absence of raised intra-abdominal pressure, intragastric pressure can go up by simple distension. Whenever gastric distension occurs irrespective of the cause, the LES gets effaced by the distending the stomach leading to reflux. Gastric stasis seen in more than 10% of patients with GERD, may cause reflux by similar effacement of the LES.

The basic factor for esophageal injury in GERD is prolonged contact between esophageal mucosa and gastric acid. When acid reaches the esophagus, its contact time with its mucosa is reduced by two factors: (1) the neutralization of the acid by saliva and (2) esophageal clearance achieved by its contractions. The buffering activity of saliva which has a pH of 7.8–8.0 is due to bicarbonates and proteins. The buffering may fail if the bicarbonate concentration is low or if the volume of saliva is inadequate. The reduced salivary secretion during sleep is an important cause for severe forms of GERD. In many patients with GERD, motility of esophagus is impaired and the more the severity, the more is the impairment. Gravity also plays a major role in GERD as the acid contact time in supine refluxers is more than double the normal people.[18]

PATHOGENESIS

The basic abnormality in GERD is the injury to esophageal mucosa caused by the reflux. Both acidic and nonacidic refluxate can induce erosive changes in the esophageal mucosa, especially in the lower esophagus. However, up to 70% of patients with GERD do not exhibit mucosal erosions. It was believed that acid exposure causes direct mucosal injury. It is proved now that the injury is caused by cytokines released by esophageal mucosal cells.[19] One mechanism for cytokine release and development of reflux esophagitis and Barrett's esophagus is the change in the bacterial flora in the distal esophagus following GERD. The type I microbiome, seen in normal esophagus, is dominated by Gram-positive bacteria, while the type II microbiome, mainly associated with abnormal esophagus, including reflux esophagitis and Barrett's esophagus, contains a larger proportion of Gram-negative bacteria.[20] The Gram-positive bacterial wall components, such as lipopolysaccharides (LPS), can up-regulate gene expression of proinflammatory cytokines *via* activation of the TLR4 and NF-kB pathway.[20]

Three forms of GERD are recognized based on the presence of erosions and other morphological features: erosive reflux disease (ERD), non-erosive reflux disease (NERD) and Barrett's esophagus. The three groups differ not only in their morphology, but also in their prognosis. There are arguments as to whether these three entities are three different segments in the spectrum of reflux disease or three different diseases or categories. Many patients shift from one entity to another over time with or without treatment and it appears that these are manifestation of the same disease, the difference lying in the severity of the reflux.[21]

Prolonged or chronic reflux leads to further complications. Erosions may involve larger areas of the esophagus and may lead to ulcers. Ulcers may heal with cicatrization leading to strictures, which are classically in the distal esophagus, though they may occur proximally as well. Other important sequelae of submucosal inflammation are shortening of the LES.

Pathogenesis of Columnar Lined Epithelium

A serious complication of GERD is the development of columnar lined epithelium (CLE) in the esophagus, and subsequently a particular type of CLE better known as Barrett's esophagus. Classically, tongues of columnar lined mucosa creep upward into the esophagus replacing the normal squamous lined mucosa. CLE is of three kinds: cardiac mucosa and oxyntic cardiac mucosa are the common types seen in GERD. The third type of columnar cells is different from gastric type cells and is composed of cells normally seen in the distal intestine. This is referred to as intestinal type metaplasia and is integral to the definition and diagnosis of Barrett's esophagus. These specialized columnar epithelial cells are now postulated to originate from the esophageal stem cells located in the basal layers of the epithelium or submucosal glands. This differentiation is induced by bile salt and acid and invokes the transcription factor CDX2 and many cellular signaling pathways which are usually involved in intestinal differentiation.[22] Aberrations—actual or relative—in Wnt, Notch, BMP, Sonic HH and TGFB signaling pathways have been identified in this process.[22] Increased acid and bile exposure leads to esophagitis with the widening of tight junctions in the superficial layers of epithelium and the action of acid and bile possibly induces esophageal stem cells to express CDX1 and CDX2 genes and the basal cells to express BMP-4 and other morphogenetic factors. This combination promotes the change from squamous to intestinal type mucosa which is an adaptive change, as this mucosa tolerates onslaught by gastric reflux.[23] BMP pathway promotes intestinal metaplasia and Wnt pathway is incriminated in the development of dysplasia.[24] There is more than enough evidence to suggest that alkaline reflux is associated with higher grades of esophagitis and Barrett's esophagus.[25]

Two new histological concepts contribute to the understanding of Barrett's esophagus. One of them is the squamo-oxyntic gap (SOG) and the other is the dilated distal esophagus.[26,27] The gap between squamous cell lined esophageal mucosa proximally and proper oxyntic cell lined mucosa in the cardia distally, traditionally marked as Z-line, is almost zero in normal people. However, when GERD occurs, CLE replaces squamous epithelium starting from the Z-line, thus increasing the SOG. While the SOG is the histological evidence of GERD, the length of SOG is a reflection of its severity.[26] The importance of Barrett's esophagus lies in the fact that intestinal metaplasia is a premalignant condition and dysplasia and subsequent transformation into adenocarcinoma can occur with time.[27,28] Its seriousness lies in the recognition that Barrett's esophagus is seen in up to 25% of patients with GERD,[28,29] even if endoscopy appears normal.[27]

The dilated distal esophagus is reflux-damaged and it possesses gastric type folds, and is indistinguishable from the proximal stomach on endoscopy. This occurs due to shortening of the LES and destruction of the abdominal esophagus.[27] The usual practice of endoscopists is to biopsy only those areas of the esophagus which show erosive disease and not to take any biopsy in those with no mucosal changes. Chandrasoma et al. have biopsied areas below the Z-line and histologically showed that what appeared to be rugae bearing proximal stomach was actually the distal esophagus which was damaged and dilated because of reflux and more than 20% of these biopsies showed Barrett's esophagus.[27] Hence they recommend that biopsy of normal appearing rugae bearing mucosa up to 1 cm below Z-line should also be done.[27] If not done, there is a risk of missing the diagnosis of GERD and even Barrett's esophagus.[27] Diagnosis of CLE in these specimen should be taken as proof of GERD and dilated distal esophagus.[27]

Pathological Basis of Symptoms

The pathogenesis of heartburn is not fully understood. It is reasonable to conclude that acid causes heartburn by injuring the mucosa or by permeation through esophageal mucosa. However, patients with NERD have fewer and less acidic reflux episodes, but have similar symptoms. Hence, there possibly are other mechanisms for pain. These include distension of the esophagus caused by refluxate and exaggerated pain sensitivity.[30] Acid sensitive TRPV1 receptors have been identified in sensory nerve fibers and in epithelial cells of the esophageal mucosa, which have a specific role in pain perception.[31]

The symptomatology of reflux disease is variable and has no correlation with esophageal morphology as seen on endoscopy. It is now well recognized that differential esophageal hypersensitivity to acid exposure occurs in patients.[32,33] This phenomenon is due to a malfunction of the brain-gut system, where the aberration may be at the gut level in the spinal cord or at the brain.[32] Various regions of the brain, on fMRI, show differential activity to acid exposure in the esophagus. The activity patterns are very different in patients with different types of reflux disease.[34] In addition, an abnormality in the brain system which monitors the visceral neuronal activity has been shown in patients with reflux disease.[35] All these factors prove that the esophageal symptomatology in patients with GERD is due to a complex interaction between esophageal mucosa and various regions of the brain, forming a neurological background for differential pain perception and psychological anticipation of pain.

The association between *Helicobacter pylori* infection and GERD has been a subject of much speculation and research. Many reports have documented that *H. pylori* infection has a moderating influence on the severity of erosive esophagitis associated with GERD.[36] This has been attributed to reduced gastric acid secretion in patients with *H. pylori* infection. High gastric acid secretion as documented by low serum gastrin-17 levels, higher age, hiatus hernia and the absence of *H. pylori* appear to be the best predictors of erosive esophagitis development.[36]

CLINICAL FEATURES

The classic or diagnostic symptoms of GERD are heartburn and acid regurgitation. About 60–70% of people with these symptoms actually have GERD. These symptoms are often seen in other gastrointestinal diseases such as peptic ulcers, achalasia, esophageal cancers, gastric stasis, etc.

The atypical symptoms of GERD include epigastric pain or burning, vomiting, nausea, chest pain, choking sensation, post-prandial discomfort and fullness. GERD is a chronic and often persistent problem. The symptoms persist even after years and the need for medication increases with age, thereby increasing the cost of treatment.[37]

The common extra esophageal presentations of GERD are chronic cough, laryngitis and asthma. However, as these diseases are common problems in the population, it may be erroneous to attribute them to GERD readily. In such cases, local causes are to be excluded and coexistence of GERD should be proven. However, GERD can be considered as a potential cofactor.[38] Patients with symptoms of laryngeal reflux in the absence of local causes often have GERD and Barrett's esophagus as well. Hence such patients should be screened by upper GI endoscopy when no local pathology is found. Cherry Donner Syndrome (reflux laryngitis in the elderly) and Sandifer syndrome (Torticollis and abnormal neck movements and spasms in neonates and infants due to GERD) are named syndromes of extra esophageal presentations.

The association between bronchial asthma and GERD has been investigated extensively. A report from India stated that GERD was associated in the majority (57.14%) of patients with bronchial asthma as documented by history, Bernstein test, bronchial hyper responsiveness to acid instillation into the esophagus and response to PPI therapy.[39] In fact, the authors recommend that bronchial asthma patients with history suggestive of GERD are likely to improve with acid suppression. Recurrent chest infections may be secondary to GERD, silent or otherwise.

Risk factors for reflux diseases are many. Some patients are genetically predisposed to develop GERD.[40] Obesity, sedentary life style, smoking, dietary predilection and reduced sleep all seem to have a role to play and contribute to the increasing trend of GERD in most populations.[41,42] Obesity contributes to the development of GERD while physical activity reduces it.

The association between obesity and GERD needs further discussion. As obesity is increasing worldwide, including in India, the incidence of GERD is also increasing correspondingly. There may be many compounding factors in the obese, such as genetic and dietary factors, reduced physical activity, sleep disorders, etc. which make them more susceptible to developing GERD. However, there appears to be a definite correlation between high BMI and GERD which is independent of dietary factors, physical activity, etc.[42,43] The mechanism that causes GERD in the obese is identified as the increased pressure exerted on the viscera by the weight of the anterior abdominal wall and excess intra-abdominal fat. In addition, adipocytokines including interleukin-6 and tumor necrosis factor α produced by the metabolically active adipose tissue are believed to contribute to GERD development.[44]

DIAGNOSIS

The presence of reflux is detectable by (a) symptoms, (b) endoscopic findings, (c) 24-hour pHmetry and (d) radiological/radioisotope studies. In a number of patients the symptoms are so classical and specific, that a diagnosis of GERD can be made relatively easily. However, in patients with atypical presentation, diagnosis would be difficult and even impossible at times. On the other hand, a number of patients with functional disorders of the esophagus may mimic symptoms of GERD, resulting in a false diagnosis of GERD in them. Endoscopic findings when present definitely suggest GERD, but absence of such findings does not exclude GERD, a fact often dismissed by clinicians.

Endoscopy

An upper GI endoscopy is the initial test for assessing patients with GERD, as in most esophageal and gastric symptoms. In the presence of typical GERD symptoms, endoscopy is not warranted (ACG guidelines). However, endoscopic assessment of the esophagus may be needed for the detection of (a) the presence and extent of esophagitis and its complications, (b) presence and size of hiatus hernia and (c) for other esophageal diseases such as malignant strictures, achalasia, etc. Endoscopy can also detect gastric and duodenal pathologies such as ulcers, gastric stasis, gastric malignancy, etc. that may actually be responsible for the symptoms.

However, less than half of the patients with GERD exhibit endoscopic evidence of esophageal injury due to acid reflux. Explaining the association between reflux symptoms and endoscopic findings is a major problem for the physician. Patients with erosive esophagitis in the absence of gastric stasis do not need any further test for diagnosing GERD, whereas patients with a normal esophagus would pose problems and often need additional investigations for diagnosis. When GERD is proved in these patients by further investigations such as 24-hour pHmetry (see below), such patients will be deemed to have non-erosive esophagitis (NERD). It is worth remembering that erosive esophageal signs may vanish with PPI therapy and hence endoscopy may be normal in patients who have been on PPIs. Therefore, it is advisable to ask for endoscopy in patients with suspected GERD at least 10 days after cessation of PPI therapy for better endoscopic yield rate.

Detection of abnormalities in the esophagus consequent to GERD has increased with the advent of additional light waves, and narrow band imaging which pick up subtle changes and aid in early detection of lesions.[45]

Many classifications exist for categorizing erosive esophageal injuries with a view to assessing and comparing response to therapies. The following are some of the classification systems used: (a) Savary-Miller, (b) Hetzel-Dent, (c) MUSE (M-metaplasia, U-ulcer, S-stricture and E-erosions) and (d) Los Angeles classification.[46]

Most of these classifications use early or subtle changes to detect esophagitis and employ many features, which are often prone to subjective interpretations, for staging of severity. Since reproducibility is an issue with these systems, the Los Angeles (LA) system of classification, which uses objective features for assessing the severity of disease, has become the preferred classification for assessing response to therapy and for ease of comparison. The LA classification of esophagitis[47] is reproduced in the Table 2.

Table 2: The LA classification of esophagitis

Grade A	One (or more) mucosal break no longer than 5 mm that does not extend between the tops of two mucosal folds
Grade B	One (or more) mucosal break more than 5 mm long that does not extend between the tops of two mucosal folds
Grade C	One (or more) mucosal break that is continuous between the tops of two or more mucosal folds but which involve less than 75% of the circumference
Grade D	One (or more) mucosal break which involves at least 75% of the esophageal circumference

The criticism against LA classification is that it does not recognize early or subtle changes in the mucosa, thereby excluding those with early disease. Similarly by not including ulcers and strictures it eliminates those with complicated GERD. By including these features, the MUSE classification may have a wider application, but is prone to a high level of subjective notation by endoscopists. Due to the very nature of the difference in classification of changes in esophageal mucosa between various systems, the response to therapy is also differently assessed. For example, if there is an improvement by two stages in one classification, the improvement may be only by one stage in another classification. Hence, comparison of benefit using different classification systems would be unreliable.[48]

Another major advantage of endoscopy is its ability to detect Barrett's esophagus. It is cautioned that endoscopic diagnosis of columnar cell lined mucosa may be seen in high proportion of patients with GERD, but documentation of metaplasia on biopsy is essential for diagnosis of Barrett's esophagus and this may bring down its actual prevalence rates.[29] It is well known that Barrett's esophagus is a major and sinister complication of reflux disease and the rate of progression of esophagitis to Barrett's esophagus is related to its severity. For example, patients with LA grade D esophagitis are at a higher risk of developing Barrett's esophagus as compared to those with less severe grades. Interestingly, the presence of erosive esophagitis can also be detected non-invasively using PET scans with SUV correlating with the severity score of LA system.[49]

pHmetry

Twenty-four-hour pHmetry that records the measurements of pH at selected locations in the esophagus over a 24-hour period has come to stay as the "gold standard" for determining GERD. This involves the placement of a flexible wire at the tip of which is a pH sensor. The pH probe is passed transnasally and stationed proximal to the gastroesophageal junction as determined by esophageal manometry. The pH probe continuously records the pH and stores the data in a portable recorder, which the patient wears usually for 24 hours. By convention, the probe is placed 5 cm proximal to the gastroesophageal junction as determined on manometry. An acid reflux is defined as a recording of esophageal pH of 4 or less and alkaline reflux as a recording of 7 or above. In order to distinguish patients with GERD from those with normal levels of reflux, Johnson and DeMeester[50] devised a composite score taking into consideration the following six parameters:

1. Percent total time pH < 4
2. Percent upright time pH < 4
3. Percent supine time pH < 4
4. Number of reflux episodes
5. Number of reflux episodes ≥5 min
6. Longest reflux episode (minutes)

A composite score (also known as JD score and DeMeester score) above 14.72 is diagnostic of acid reflux[50] (Table 3). The score is different for alkaline reflux.[51] A pH value above 7 is usually due to alkaline gastric reflux, which is secondary to duodenogastric reflux. At present, 24-hour esophageal pH monitoring can be done with a single channel single probe wire, single channel dual probe wire or wireless systems. The most popular wireless system (Bravo)

Table 3 24-hour impedence-pHmetry report of a 21-year-old woman with significant GERD. Note the predominantly upright reflux with a very high DeMeester score. Her endoscopy showed no esophagitis, no Barrett's esophagus, no hiatus hernia, but a lax sphincter

Impedance-pH monitoring Details

Reflux Study

Acid Exposure (pH)

	Upright	*Upright Normal*	*Recumbent*	*Recumbent Normal*	*Total*	*Total Normal*
Clearance pH: Channel 7						
Number of Acid Episodes	16		3		19	
Time	646.2 min		35.7 min		681.8 min	
Percent Time	**64.7%**	(< 6.3%)	**9.7%**	(< 1.2%)	**49.9%**	(< 4.2%)
Mean Acid Clearance Time	2423 sec		714 sec		2153 sec	
Longest Episode	357.7 min		34.4 min		357.7 min	

Acid Exposure normal values in parentheses are valid for un-medicated 95th percentile adult.

Statistics (pH)

	Upright	*Upright Normal*	*Recumbent*	*Recumbent Normal*	*Total*	*Total Normal*
Clearance pH: Channel 7						
Minimum	0.00		0.02		0.00	
Maximum	7.47		7.20		7.47	
Mean	2.78		1..50		2.16	
Median	2.10		1.48		1.65	
Standard Deviation	1.56		0.63		1.37	
Variance	2.44		0.40		1.87	

Acid Reflux Composite Score Analysis (DeMeester) (pH)

	Patient Value	*Patient Score*	*Normal Threshold*
Upright Time in Reflux	64.7%	27.6	< 8.4
Recumbent Time in Reflux	9.7%	10.1	< 3.5
Total Time in Reflux	49.9%	36.6	< 4.5
Episodes over 5 min.	8.4	7.4	< 3.5
Longest Episode	357.7 min	45.7	< 19.8
Total Episodes	20.0	1.1	< 46.9
Composite Score		**128.6**	**< 14.7**

Note: Composite Score patient values are normalized for 24 hours.

uses a capsule which is placed at a specific place (usually 6 cm above endoscopically identified Z-line) and offers the advantage of comfort to the patient, enhanced study time up to 48 hours as well as improved yields.[52]

The new kid on the block is the multi-channel impedancemetry in combination with pHmetry. This technique addresses the major drawback of 24-hour esophageal pH monitoring namely, the inability to detect weak acid or non-acid reflux. Impedancemetry employs a multichannel probe with a pH sensor at the tip and ring electrodes along the esophageal length. The ring electrodes lying at various levels detect the appearance of a bolus of fluid irrespective of volume and pH by impedance changes. Thus when there is reflux of gastric fluid in the pH range of 4–7 which is not recognized as abnormal by conventional 24-hour esophageal pH monitoring, impedancemetry detects it. Thus, when the symptomatology is suggestive of GERD, but endoscopy and 24 hour esophageal pH monitoring are not supportive, a positive multichannel impedance recording, would clinch the diagnosis of GERD. In addition, the height of reflux as measured by this technique, throws light on the reflux of gastric contents into the mouth or respiratory tree, thereby aiding in the diagnosis of extra esophageal reflux.[53] Impedancemetry, however, cannot distinguish between small and large volumes and hence is unable to distinguish large volume refluxers. In combination with pHmetry, impedance study can assess response to PPI therapy.[54]

Based on the pattern of abnormal recording of reflux on 24-hour pHmetry, patients with GERD can be divided into three distinct groups: upright refluxers who show abnormal reflux only in upright posture, supine refluxers who show reflux activity only in the supine position and combined refluxers who have reflux in both positions. It appears that these three groups form a spectrum with upright refluxers having a milder disease while supine refluxers have a more severe and combined refluxers having the most severe disease.[55]

The supine and combined refluxers have more severe disease as they reflux more while sleeping and their esophageal clearance is impaired during sleep. Gravity also plays an important role in aiding faster esophageal clearance and hence, in the supine position esophageal acid clearance is delayed. Ambulatory pH monitoring is unnecessary in patients who have Barrett's esophagus.[38]

Manometry

Whenever a diagnostic confusion exists, manometry is required to exclude other esophageal diseases such as achalasia. It is useful, if not mandatory[38] before a patient is planned for surgery. Manometry is done using saline infusing catheters or high precision transducer mounted catheters, which are passed through the nostrils into the stomach. The catheter is gradually withdrawn and the pressure recordings are analyzed. The most common pressure recordings in GERD is hypotensive LES (Fig. 5). A mechanically defective LES is characterized by three parameters: (1) total length shorter than 2 cm, (2) abdominal length shorter than 1 cm and (3) a resting pressure less than 6 mm Hg.[56] Manometry will also throw light on the nature of esophageal contractions and the presence of hiatus hernia, if any (Fig. 5). One major reason for mandating manometry before surgery is to exclude achalasia or diffuse esophageal spasm (DES), as these conditions would preclude antireflux surgery or precipitate dysphagia after surgery. Another manometry finding which is important is the esophageal contraction amplitude. Amplitude more than 30 mm Hg is required for propulsion of food across a 360 degree fundoplication.[56] The nature of esophageal contractions thus helps the surgeon to determine the type of surgery that would benefit the patient most (see below).

Radiological Imaging

In the past, detection of reflux of radio opaque material proximal to diaphragmatic hiatus was deemed to suggest GERD. The quantity and proximal extent of reflux in the supine position or Trendelenburg position were assessed to determine the degree or severity of the reflux. Imaging studies do accurately identify the presence of hiatus hernia, but currently reliance on imaging

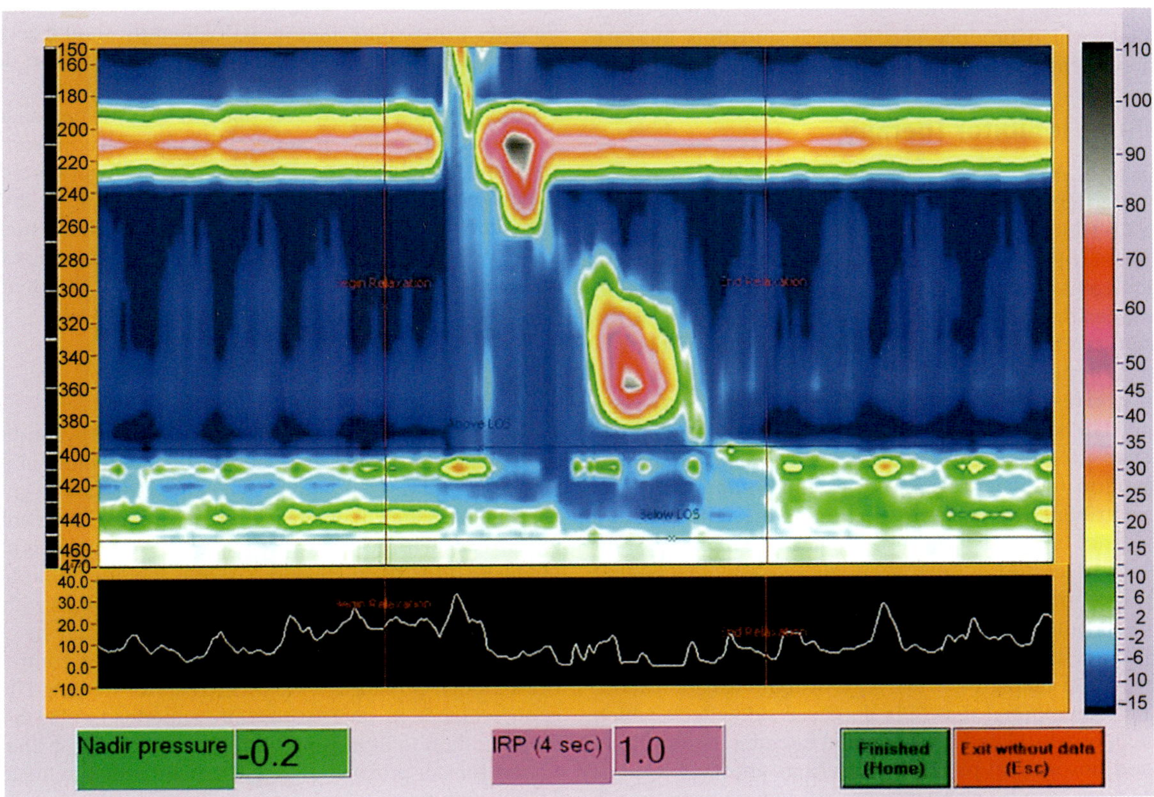

Figure 5 Manometry recording of a male with GERD associated with hiatus hernia. Note: (a) hypotensive LES-pressures lower than 6 mm Hg; (b) two strata of high-pressure zones corresponding to LES location-LES proper as the upper one and hiatus as the lower one; (c) normal propulsion along the length of the esophagus and (d) relaxation of LES with wet swallow thus excluding achalasia

techniques has decreased. Hiatus hernia is often incidentally detected on CT images of thoracoabdominal area done for other purposes. The actual size of the hiatus hernia can be easily determined by CT. The current recommendation is that barium radiographs should not be performed for diagnosing GERD.[38]

Nuclear Imaging

Radionuclear scintigraphy using radioactive nucleotide such as ^{99m}Tc may be used to assess the presence and extent of gastroesophageal reflux and to evaluate gastric paresis. This study is often used in children and in adults only for the evaluation of gastric stasis.

MEDICAL MANAGEMENT

Lifestyle Changes

Medical management of GERD starts with non-medical life style changes. As obesity is one of the most common risk factors, patients who are above the permissible BMI (22.9 for Indians and other Asians and 24.9 for others) should be encouraged to reduce weight. As reflux is more common after heavy meals, patients with GERD should refrain from going to sleep or lying down flat for 2–3 hours after meals. This is especially so for patients with nocturnal GERD.[38] Head end elevation by 15–20 degrees is recommended for supine position and mixed type refluxers.

Dietary restriction of fats and other substances such as coffee and chocolate which produce gastric stasis and thus increase reflux is routinely advocated.

Proton Pump Inhibitor Therapy

The mainstay of medical therapy now revolves around proton pump inhibitors (PPIs). PPIs can be started in those with typical symptoms of GERD even without waiting for endoscopy. An 8-week course of PPIs is indicated. Despite enormous literature favoring one agent over another, there are no major differences in efficacy between the different PPIs.[57] For efficient acid control, the drug is taken once a day in the proper dose on an empty stomach and at least 30 minutes before the first meal of the day.

Patients who respond to 8 weeks of therapy should ideally stop PPIs and need to be followed up for return of symptoms. Patients who have had no relief to PPI therapy need to be evaluated in detail to confirm the diagnosis and to exclude other conditions that may contribute to symptoms. If reflux is present, it gives a positive evidence of GERD. If the tests are negative after cessation of PPI therapy at least for a week, then it is safe to conclude that the patient's symptoms are not due to GERD. They do not need PPIs anymore, but may need to be investigated for non-GERD causes. This issue is particularly important in this country where people have been taking PPIs for years without an indication. It should be remembered that PPIs do cause side effects which include osteoporosis-related hip and spine fractures, community-acquired and nosocomial pneumonia, various enteric and non-enteric infections, fundic gland polyps and hypomagnesemia.[58] Evidence indicates that earlier referral for pHmetry can save on the cost of unnecessary PPI administration.[59] This author has stopped PPIs in many patients including some doctors who have been taking PPIs for many years when investigations showed no evidence of reflux. If tests are to be performed while the patient is on PPIs, the investigation of choice is pH monitoring combined with impedance monitoring. The tests would identify the subset of non-responders whose symptoms are caused by weak or non-acid reflux and also those who have no reflux at all.[60]

Patients who have had only partial response may be considered for increasing the dose to twice daily therapy or switching to a different PPI. Additional night dosing may be beneficial to patients who are night time refluxers.[38]

Patients with typical symptoms of GERD with associated extraesophageal symptoms can be given PPIs without endoscopy, as mentioned earlier. Relief in extra esophageal symptoms following PPI therapy may be indicative of GERD as a cofactor in the laryngeal and pulmonary disease. However, tests for confirmation of reflux are mandatory in those with extraesophageal symptoms without typical GERD symptoms. Interestingly, there is a new twist in the association between reflux and chronic cough. New technology has enabled us to distinguish between reflux-induced cough and cough-induced reflux.[61] Understandably, treating of some patients would remain complicated.

Maintenance PPI therapy should be administered for two groups of patients: (1) GERD patients who have recurrence of symptoms after PPI is discontinued and (2) patients with complications including erosive esophagitis and Barrett's esophagus. Patients with Barrett's esophagus seem to get chemoprophylaxis from developing adenocarcinoma while on PPIs.[62] Most surgeons, however, recommend surgery for the same goal[54,63] (see below). Patients, who require long-term PPI therapy, should get the lowest effective dose of the chosen drug or get the drug on demand or intermittent therapy.[38]

There is dichotomy of opinion in the management of complications such as strictures. Physicians recommend dilatation with long-term PPI therapy. At times intralesional steroid injection is practiced by them to delay fibrosis and to defer the need for subsequent dilatation.[38,64] Most surgeons believe that patients with strictures would be best served by a good antireflux surgery for better control of reflux—both acid and non acid—after adequate dilatation.[56,63]

Other Drugs

There appears to be very little role for other drugs in the current therapy of GERD. Sucralfate has no role, excepting in pregnancy where it can be given empirically while PPIs can be given only if clinically indicated. Raft forming alginate preparations are safer and effective in all trimesters of pregnancy.[65] When relief is inadequate following PPI alone, bedtime H2RA therapy is added to PPI therapy administered in the day in selected patients with objective evidence of night-time reflux. At times, H2RA may be considered as a maintenance option, especially if PPIs are contraindicated. Even though prokinetics are prescribed for treating GERD, there is no evidence to say that they are superior to placebo[66] or that their addition to PPIs improve efficacy of therapy.[67] There may be a small role for prokinetics in the management of refractory GERD. TLESR inhibitors like baclofen may also be tried in this situation.

The reasons for non-response or partial response to PPIs are many. As mentioned earlier, many non-responders may have other coexisting diseases and their symptoms may be secondary to them. There is evidence that some non-responders may have very high proximal extent of reflux and may have a hypersensitive esophagus.[68]

Therapy of Barrett's Esophagus

Barrett's esophagus *per se* produces no specific symptom in a patient with GERD. On the other hand, because of its resistance to erosive action of reflux, heartburn may reduce. Barrett's esophagus requires treatment solely due to its neoplastic potential with an annual incidence of 0.5–1.0% of developing esophageal adenocarcinoma.[69] Hence, endoscopic screening is recommended for patients with Barrett's esophagus. Endoscopic surveillance at intervals of 3–5 years is recommended for patients without dysplasia.[69,70]

Treatment of Barrett's esophagus is that of underlying GERD, *i.e.* similar to those without Barrett's esophagus. This would be PPIs according to physicians.[38,61,68] However, surgeons strongly favor antireflux surgery[56,63,70] for Barrett's esophagus for two reasons: (1) the presence of Barrett's esophagus suggests long standing and/or severe disease and hence is better treated by surgery; and (2) surgery reduces not only the acid reflux, but also biliopancreatic reflux which is deemed to be the sinister agent in the pathophysiology of Barrett's esophagus. Metaplastic changes of Barrett's esophagus are reported to regress to a greater degree following surgery than after PPI therapy. However, there is no demonstrable improvement in esophageal adenocarcinoma rates.[56,71]

Conventionally Barrett's esophagus with high-grade dysplasia and cancers were treated by esophagectomy. In view of morbidity and mortality associated with esophagectomy, attention was diverted toward endoscopic ablation of Barrett's mucosa. Experience has shown that endotherapy is effective and at par with surgery in reducing progression to neoplasia, though a small subset of patients who undergo endotherapy may have cancer recurrence and will need surgery.[72,73] Options for endoscopic ablation of the involved mucosa include photodynamic therapy, radio frequency ablation, argon beam coagulation and cryotherapy, of which RFA has proven to be the most effective.[74] This procedure is also an option for Barrett's esophagus with low grade dysplasia but is not recommended for patients with nondysplastic Barrett's esophagus.[70] With the increasing skill levels and the availability of better instruments, endoscopic mucosal resection has become the most efficient technique of endoablation for managing Barrett's esophagus with high grade dysplasia and mucosal Barrett's cancer.[75,76] Current recommendations endorse endotherapy for Barrett's esophagus with high-grade dysplasia as well as for mucosal Barrett's cancer.[38,70] More advanced cancers and recurrences are managed by surgery.

SURGICAL MANAGEMENT

The aim of surgical intervention is to enhance the sphincteric action of the LES without making it unduly hypertensive or less yielding, conditions, which may predispose patients to dysphagia. Any surgical procedure aimed at treating GERD should fulfill the following criteria: (a) at least 2 cm of the abdominal esophagus should be present, as the best protection against reflux comes from the length of abdominal esophagus. (b) Wide hiatal opening should be reduced to a level of 60Fr bougie size. Further tightening of the hiatus is likely to lead to dysphagia. (c) The wrap around the esophagus should be constituted by the fundus alone and never by the body of the stomach. This is because of the fact that the fundus, unlike gastric body, exhibits relaxation similar to the distal esophagus when food induced peristalsis occurs, thereby offering no obstruction to the passage of the bolus of food across the LES. (d) The length of wrap should not be more than 2 cm, as this may cause dysphagia (e) The angle of His should be restored or augmented, as far as possible.

Initially, TLESR was deemed to be an intrinsic failure of the LES and was not expected to reduce following antireflux procedures. However, evidence points to its amelioration after antireflux surgery.[77]

Indications for Surgery

There is discordance between physicians and surgeons regarding indications for surgery in patients with GERD. This is evident when guidelines issued by professional societies such as American College of Gastroenterology[38] and SAGES (Society of American Gastrointestinal and Endoscopic Surgeons)[63] are compared. Universally accepted indications for antireflux surgery in patients with GERD are the following:

- Patients with documented reflux who have failed medical management (inadequate symptom control, severe regurgitation not controlled with acid suppression, or medication side effects)
- Patients who opt for surgery despite successful medical management (due to quality of life considerations and lifelong need for medication)
- Patients with GERD due to hiatus hernia
- Selected patients with extra-esophageal manifestations with classical symptoms of GERD or positive test evidence of GERD.

The best treatment options for complications of GERD (e.g. Barrett's esophagus, peptic stricture) again differ between physicians and surgeons.[38,64] These are discussed in detail subsequently.

When PPI therapy and surgery are two options for the same problem, it is inevitable that comparisons would be made to assess the superiority of one over the other. The oft-quoted LOTUS trial showed that the results of antireflux surgery and therapy with esomeprazole were similar at 3 and 5 years.[78] The Cochrane review on the efficacy of antireflux surgery stated that laparoscopic fundoplication surgery is more effective than medical management for the treatment of GERD at least in the short to medium term.[79] The reviewers felt that treatment decisions for GERD should be based on patient and surgeon preference.[79]

The REFLUX Trial that was done in 21 UK hospitals has come out with its findings recently. The trial found that after 5 years, laparoscopic fundoplication continued to provide better relief than medical management.[80] Contrary to earlier reports of side effects of surgery, the study found no evidence of long-term adverse symptoms.[80,81] Antireflux surgery offers excellent relief of symptoms and increases the quality of life, much more than achievable with medical therapy.[80,81] Even though, the cure rates declined from 98% at 3 years to 73% after 10 years, most patients were happy with surgery and their quality of life scores were the same as the general population.[81,82]

Surgical Options

Surgical options were many in the past: some needed thoracic approach, while most could be done by abdominal approach. Abdominal operations differed mainly on the type of wrap—whether complete or partial. Nissen's 360 degree fundoplication is the only operation that involves a complete wrap and also happens to be the most tested of the antireflux operations.

A number of surgical procedures such as Belsey's Mark IV, Hill's repair and Colle's gastroplasty are described routinely in standard textbooks of surgery. However, these operations are seldom performed now as laparoscopic Nissen's fundoplication and its modifications have established themselves as reliable and effective at par with the open operations and without the disadvantages of open surgery. Colle's gastroplasty at times will be required when short esophagus is encountered. Surgeons have started doing this procedure also through minimal access, often through thoracoscopy.

The original operation described by Nissen in 1956 involved a tight wrap of the anterior and posterior walls of the gastric fundus of about 5 cm length.[83] The procedure did not involve division of the short gastric vessels. Even though the control of reflux was excellent, some patients had troublesome dysphagia. One of Nissen's students, Dr Mario Rossetti, modified the Nissen's procedure by having a floppy wrap using only the anterior wall of the fundus. So, when a short floppy complete wrap is done without dividing the short gastric vessels, this procedure is often referred to as Nissen-Rossetti procedure. Some authors believe that by retaining short gastric connections between the spleen and the fundus, the fundus remains in its location which prevents the proximal migration of the wrap.[83] The most common mechanical failure after surgery is the proximal migration of the wrap in to the chest. There lies the importance of adequate mobilization of the esophagus and any other technique that would help in preventing proximal migration of the wrap.

There were other modifications to Nissen's fundoplication. Those suggested by Donohue and De Meester involve division of the short gastric vessels and the formation of a floppy, but short (not exceeding 2 cm) wrap. De Meester also suggested the usage of Teflon strips on the wrap to prevent breakdown. There are many procedures, which use only a partial wrap. The most popular of these are anterior wrap (Dor's) and posterior wrap (Toupet's).

Nissen Fundoplication

The gold standard of antireflux surgery is the 360 degree floppy Nissen fundoplication performed laparoscopically. This chapter will not go into the details of the operative steps, but merely highlight the essential steps. The camera port is usually placed well above the umbilicus and to the left of midline with 3–4 additional 5 mm ports. A liver retractor which can be fixed such as Nathanson's retractor makes the procedure easier and eliminates the need for an assistant. The key components of a good fundoplication are shown below (Figs 6A to F).

a. Dissection of hiatus safeguarding the hepatic branches of vagus, esophagus and anterior and posterior vagii. Though many surgeons do not spare the hepatic branches, there is a possibility of antral denervation in an occasional patient when these fibers are divided (Fig. 6A).
b. Mobilization of about 6–8 cm of esophagus and even more if there is a bigger hiatus hernia. Mobilization of this extent will ensure 2–4 cm of intra-abdominal esophagus. Unless there is adequate mobilization of esophagus, there is a high risk of failure of antireflux mechanism and even cephalad displacement of wrap into the chest (Figs 6B and C).
c. Mobilization of the fundus completely from lateral aspect, from the diaphragm and posteriorly. The retroesophageal opening should not extend onto the stomach and when done with complete mobilization of esophagus would be wide enough to take the fundus freely (Fig. 6D).
d. The crura should be appropriately tightened with nonabsorbable sutures, ideally over a bougie, to ensure that the hiatus opening is not less than 60Fr.
e. The wrap should be made only from the fundus and identification of the left and right anchor points of the wrap should be done diligently. The so-called "drop test" and "shoeshine maneuver" help in ensuring a proper untwisted wrap. Floppiness of the wrap should be ensured. Anchoring of the wrap through bites through anterior wall of esophagus and to the right crus helps in prevention of its migration (Figs 6E and F).

Complete or Partial Fundoplication

Detailed analysis of the outcome of various procedures shows that the initial response after all types of operations tends to be similar in preventing reflux.[84] Collective experience highlights that a complete wrap tends to produce more side effects—dysphagia being the prime one. Hence, in early to mid-term follow-up, patients with a complete wrap tend to have lower satisfaction scores compared to those with partial wraps. However, on long-term follow-up, patients who have had partial wraps are prone to develop recurrence of reflux, whereas those who have had complete wraps have less treatment failure and many of them show improvement in their dysphagia. Hence, overall satisfaction scores tend to be equal in all groups in the long-term follow-up. Thus, the outcome after surgical procedures forms a spectrum, with Nissen's at one end with low recurrence, but higher side effects and anterior wrap at the other end with higher recurrence, but lower side effects and with the posterior wrap occupying the middle position. In the end, it boils down to a tradeoff between recurrence and side effects when one chooses a particular procedure over another.[85]

Engstrom et al. compared anterior and posterior partial wraps and found that the posterior wrap was very good in controlling reflux with practically no side effects, whereas the anterior 180 degree wrap was inadequate in controlling reflux.[86] The authors felt that anterior fundoplication should not be recommended for control of GERD.

Generally it is believed that GERD often coexists with esophageal motility disorders such as DES, hypomotility or hypertensive LES. Hence, most authors recommend that a partial fundoplication is preferable to a 360 degree Nissen's fundoplication in patients with esophageal motility disorders. Hitherto the teaching has been that the type of surgery should be tailored according to the esophageal manometry report. If the esophageal peristalsis is good, the 360 degree Nissen's fundoplication is the most appropriate option and if the peristalsis is suboptimal (pressure amplitude <30 mm Hg), the partial wrap should be preferred. However, some surgeons believe that Nissen's fundoplication is an adequate procedure

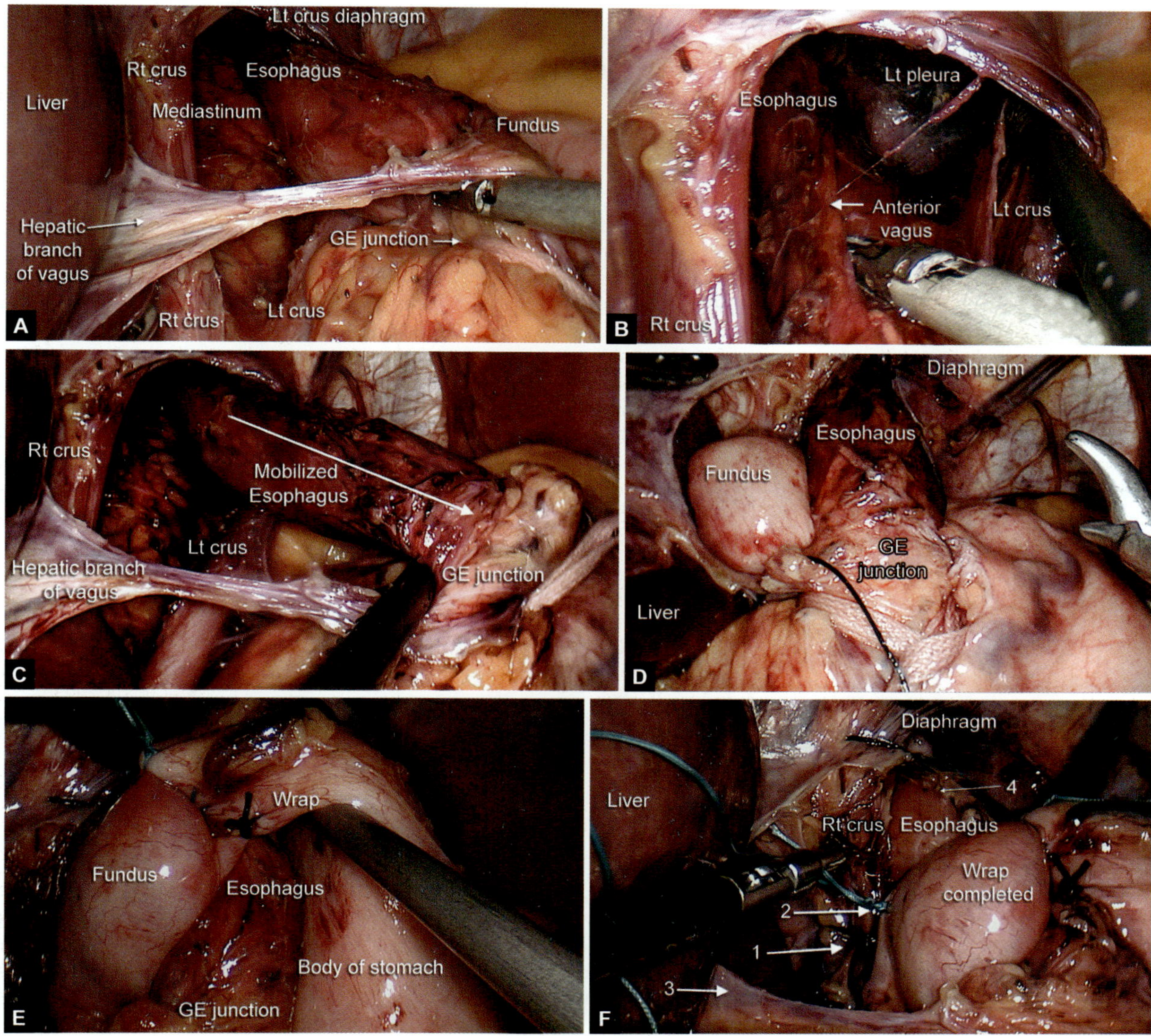

Figures 6A to F Operative pictures of laparoscopic 360 degree floppy fundoplication. (A) Please see clear dissection of the hiatus retaining the hepatic branch of the vagus. The esophagus is mobilized on the posterior and right sides; (B) Anterior and left dissection of the esophagus, safeguarding anterior vagus. Left pleura is seen and attempt would be made not to open the pleura while dividing adhesions. Note the wide hiatus; (C) Extent of dissection of the esophagus. When 8–10 cm of the esophagus is mobilized about 3–4 cm of the esophagus can be brought into abdomen (white arrow); (D) Complete mobilization of the fundus ensures that the fundus brought to the right of the esophagus remains there only (the 'drop test'). Retraction of the fundus back to left side suggests that mobilization of the fundus and/or the retroesophageal space is inadequate. Please note adequate length of intra-abdominal esophagus and snug hiatus, after hiatal closure; (E) Floppiness of wrap and its correct positioning just above GE junction; (F) Completed 360 degree floppy fundoplication.

Note: (1) Hiatus closure with nonabsorbable suture making it snug. (2) Suturing of wrap onto right crus. (3) Intact hepatic branch of vagus. (4) Adequate intra-abdominal length of the esophagus

even when GERD is associated with dysmotility.[56,87] According to them, the dysphagia is transient and dysmotility improves after surgery.[56,87]

Complications of Antireflux Surgery

Specific surgical complications of fundoplication (Figs 7A to F) can be grouped as follows:

1. Dysphagia:
   a. Overzealous tightening of the wrap or the hiatus that may lead to dysphagia
   b. Fibrosis around esophagus at the site of wrap, usually due to microabscesses along the suture.
2. Recurrence of symptoms:
   a. Slipped wrap, which can be perigastric or migration of the wrap into the chest.

      Herniation of antireflux fundoplication into chest is due to a short esophagus or inadequate mobilization of thoracic esophagus. Reflux symptoms tend to remain controlled reasonably as fundoplication continues to work like transthoracic fundoplication performed for short esophagus.[88] Perigastric slippage results in wrap coming

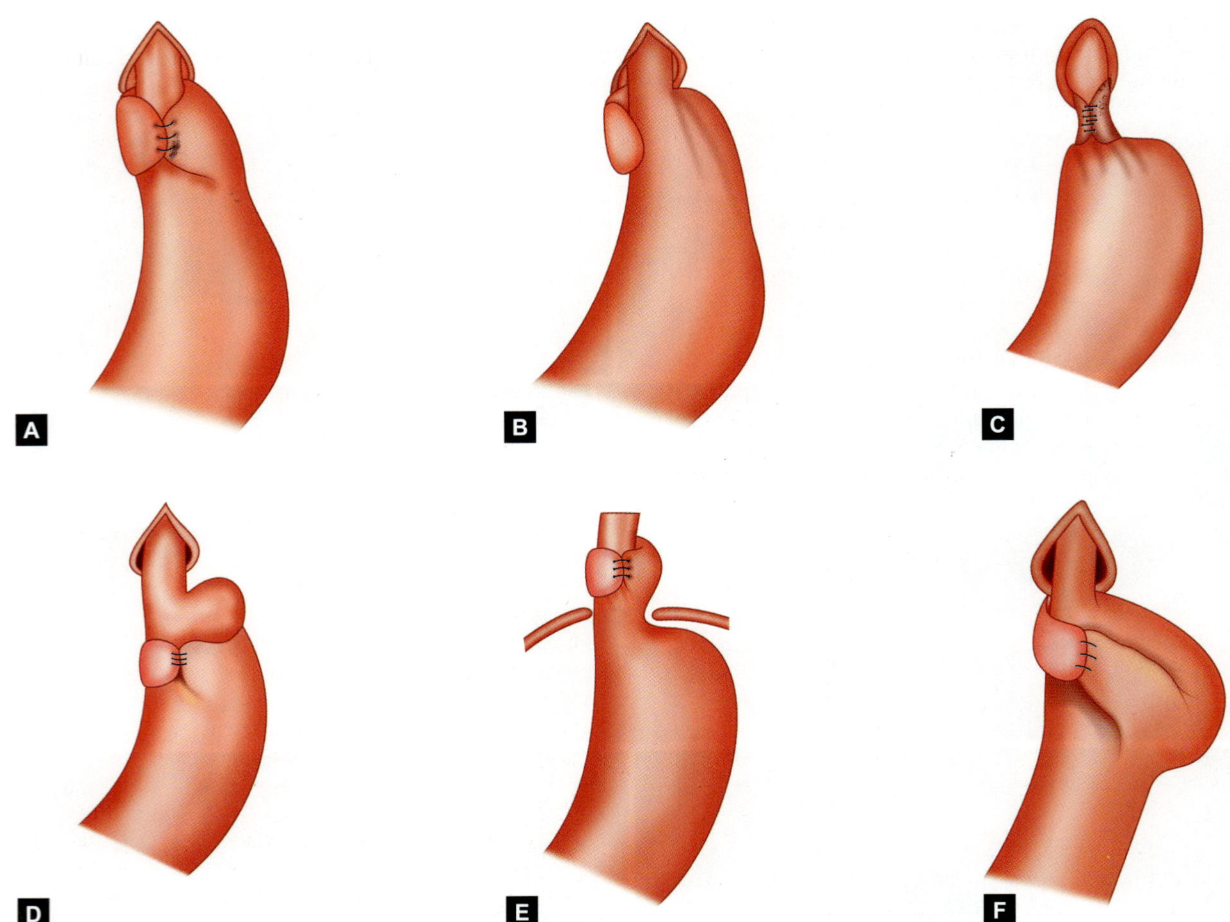

Figures 7A to F Complications of 360 degree fundoplication. (A) Normal and well executed 360 degree fundoplication. (B) Disrupted or dehisced wrap. (C) Overzealous tightening of the wrap. Sometimes, the wrap may appear not too tight, but the hiatus may be very tight beneath the wrap. Both the situations lead to dysphagia. (D) Slipped wrap, which is perigastric in location. With time, due to obstruction caused by the wrap, more and more of the body of stomach slips proximally under the wrap leading to double stomach or hour glass stomach. (E) Transdiaphragmatic migration of the wrap. (F) Faulty construction of the wrap with body of stomach rather than with fundus only

over the body of the stomach which results in inadequate reflux control and may cause dysphagia.

b. Dismantled or loosened wrap and/or hiatal widening due to dehiscence may occur when the sutures cut through or dissolve. This will result in undoing of the wrap or loosening of the hiatus resulting in recurrence of symptoms.
c. Faulty wrap constructed with body of stomach.

3. Bloating and vomiting:
   a. Inability to belch is common after a nonfloppy fundoplication in the short term.
   b. Injury to vagii may result in gastric stasis.

The largest reported series on 285 redo fundoplications (including 54 out of 1892), Smith et al. from Emory found transdiaphragmatic herniation to be the commonest cause of failure.[89] Possible reasons are short esophagus, inadequate mobilization of esophagus or disruption of hiatal closure or a combination of these three. Experience of these authors with Collis gastroplasty for lengthening esophagus has shown acid exposure in 80% of these patients.[90] In order to diminish the risk of hiatal repair disruption, many suggest use of mesh for crural repair.

Based on a study of 208 patients who underwent revision surgery for failed fundoplication, it was reported that the pattern of failure was 61 disrupted fundoplications, 52 slipped fundoplications, 30 intrathoracic fundoplications, 25 twisted fundoplications and 14 two-compartment stomachs.[90] Redo fundoplication is the procedure of choice, but in subgroups of patients with morbid obesity, significant comorbidities or esophageal dysmotility, Roux-en-Y gastric bypass is preferable.[91]

Total disruption of wrap is often due to technical failures such as use of absorbable suture material when creating the wrap, inadequate suturing of tissues, incomplete bites and tension on the suture line due to insufficient mobilization of the fundus. Hence many surgeons recommend division of short gastric vessels on a routine basis. Another factor that needs emphasis is the fixation of the wrap onto the right crus which helps in retaining the wrap in place. Should gastrogastric sutures completing the wrap anteriorly come off, the wrap sutured over right crus would still work as 270 degree posterior wrap. Slipping of the wrap can rarely be acute in onset due to violent retching or vomiting in the immediate post op period and may present as acute retrosternal discomfort and severe dysphagia. Usually it occurs gradually during the postoperative period if the sutures are not passed through the esophageal wall or cardia or the sutures have cut through due to any reason. These patients usually complain of heartburn and dysphagia occurring after a symptom free postoperative interval. The other patterns of failure such as twisted or slipped fundoplications often are due to incorrect techniques used in creation of the wrap, especially suturing too distal area along the greater curvature to the fundus.

Gastric denervation symptoms (i.e. abdominal fullness, delayed emptying and/or diarrhea) may occur when the vagii are injured during antireflux surgery. With meticulous surgical technique, vagal injury should be avoided.

Apart from the above mentioned complications, there may be failure of fundoplication in terms of relief from symptoms, or in terms of restoration of physiological functions. Table 4 lists some of the predictors, which are defined as failure of physiologic improvement on tests, patient dissatisfaction, or the need for reoperation.[92]

Table 4: Lists of some predictors

Strong predictors	*Weak predictors*
• Hiatus hernia >3 cm	• Poor motility of esophagus
• Preoperative atypical symptoms	• BMI >30 kg/m^2
• Poor response to preoperative antacids	
• Postoperative vomiting	

Surgery of Hiatus Hernia

There is some debate as to how to manage hiatus hernia. Surgery for hiatus hernia needs to be decided on the following criteria:

- Paraesophageal hiatus hernia producing symptoms (both GERD and non-GERD) needs surgery.
- Asymptomatic hiatus hernia does not need intervention. Decision on asymptomatic or minimally symptomatic paraesophageal hernia should be made taking the age and other risk factors of the patient into consideration.
- GERD associated with hiatus hernia is best treated with an antireflux surgery.
- Hiatal repair along with mobilization of the distal esophagus may be undertaken, if any surgery is contemplated for the stomach such as partial gastrectomy or sleeve gastrectomy for any reason. Troublesome reflux may be avoided by this approach.
- Though commonly mesh reinforcement of large hiatal defect (>5 square cm) is recommended to prevent failure of the repair in the short and medium terms, complications of the mesh have seriously raised a question mark over its usefulness on a long-term basis.

Prosthesis-based Antireflux Surgery

A new addition to the surgical techniques is an implantable antireflux valve. The LINX™ Reflux Management System is a flexible band that is placed laparoscopically around the distal esophagus. This band comprises of interlinked titanium beads with magnetic activity. The beads can slide over a wire like pearls on a string. The magnetic attraction keeps the beads together making the band short thus compressing and occluding the esophagus. When a bolus of food reaches the LES, the peristaltic pressure opens the band. The size of the band and the magnetic force are so designed that they prevent reflux, but not produce complications. Current data on this implant with 4 years of follow-up shows that it offers consistent symptom relief and pH control with markedly fewer side effects than traditional laparoscopic fundoplication and no adverse effects in well-selected patients.[93] The limitations of its use include inability to subject these patients to MRI examination, implantation of pace makers and the high cost.

GERD and Bariatric Surgery

Bariatric surgery is a better therapeutic option than a fundoplication for obese patients with high BMI, whenever surgical therapy for GERD is considered for them.[38,63] Of course the qualifying BMI range for bariatric surgery should be respected. Gastric bypass would be the preferred operation in these patients.[38,63]

Gastroesophageal reflux disease is more prevalent in the morbidly obese than in the normal population. Some of these patients may also have hiatus hernia. The presence of GERD seems to dictate the bariatric procedure to be chosen till now. Commonly, it is believed that patients with reflux should be offered Roux-en-Y-gastric bypass rather than sleeve gastrectomy.[30] Controversy exists as to whether sleeve gastrectomy actually increases reflux symptoms. According to a recent review, 8 papers suggested an increase in GERD symptoms, while 5 papers showed an actual decrease.[94] Evidence suggests that following sleeve gastrectomy, GERD symptoms reduce in many mainly due to reduction in weight and intra-abdominal fat. In addition, as a major portion of the parietal cell bearing stomach is excised, acid secretion is also reduced, thereby reducing refluxable acid. Usually, gastric emptying is enhanced after sleeve gastrectomy, which also helps in reducing reflux. Lozoura et al. showed that heartburn reduced after sleeve gastrectomy, whereas regurgitation and vomiting increased after surgery.[95] They attributed the increase in vomiting to a tubular stomach without any fundal or antral pouch.[95] It should be remembered in this context that vomiting is not infrequent after any type of bariatric surgery.

Daes et al. from Columbia reported a remarkable improvement of 94% in symptoms of GERD with or without hiatus hernia. In 382 patients who underwent sleeve gastrectomy[96] the authors performed standardized technique that included mobilization of distal esophagus to ensure adequate intra-abdominal esophagus and crural repair in all. Others also have reported similar excellent clearance of GERD following sleeve gastrectomy combined with crural repair in morbidly obese patients.[97]

ENDOTHERAPY OF GERD

A number of endoscopic procedures caught the fancy of the scientific community because of their ingenuity and projected ability to augment the LES pressure and to be nearly as effective as fundoplication. These procedures can be classified to include: (1) radiofrequency based LES stimulation techniques, (2) bulking agents to increase bulk of the LES and (3) endoscopic suturing/buttressing techniques.

One of the foremost forms of endoscopic therapy was the Stretta procedure which involved applying controlled radio frequency to the tissues of the LES and the gastric cardia. The intended goals were increasing LES muscle mass and decreasing the LES compliance and possibly reducing TLESR. This procedure seemed to enjoy initial enthusiasm, but did not provide durable long-term relief from GERD. Only a small percentage of patients actually benefit and complications in the form of dysphagia and gastroparesis are troublesome enough in the others requiring further treatment.[98] SAGES guidelines recommend this procedure for selected adult patients who are unwilling for surgery.[99]

Endoscopic injection of inert bulking agents can be given into the LES either in the muscles under endoscopic and fluoroscopic guidance (Enteryx, a biopolymer) or into the submucosa [Durasphere, pyrolytic carbon-coated zirconium oxide spheres and the Plexiglas, polymethylmethacrylate (PMMA)]. The underlying principle is the premise that increasing the bulk of the LES would improve its continence, by decreasing its compliance. In practice, however, it produced mixed results.[100,101] The procedure performed with Enteryx was associated with severe complications, including pneumomediastinum, embolization of the polymer, leading to renal failure and esophageal stenosis. Following a death due to intra-aortic injection of the polymer Enteryx was withdrawn from the market.[100] The Gatekeeper Reflux Repair System utilizes a soft, pliable, expandable prosthesis made of a polyacrylonitrile-based hydrogel. The prosthesis is implanted into the esophageal submucosa, and with time, the prosthesis absorbs water and expands, creating bulk in the region of implantation.

Currently, three FDA approved endoscopic suturing devices (EndoCinch™, NDO Plicator™, and EsophyX®) are available for the treatment of GERD. These vary in technology, but achieve plication of tissues in the lower esophageal region with sutures, transmural fasteners, or staples, which can be placed during endoscopy. These help create a gastroesophageal valve of full thickness from inside the stomach.

EsophyX™ System with SerosaFuse™ Fastener creates transoral incisionless fundoplication. Present data suggests that the majority of patients require additional medical therapy or a revisional fundoplication at mid- to long-term follow-up. Currently existing endoscopic therapy or transoral incisionless fundoplication cannot be commended as an alternative to medical or traditional surgical therapy.[64,99,102]

CONCLUSION

Gastroesophageal reflux disease is a common disorder of the upper digestive tract and its prevalence in India and other Asian countries is on the rise. Diagnosis of GERD may be possible in many patients on their symptomatology alone, but investigations are often required for definite diagnosis in the rest. Some of the most researched aspects of GERD include erosive esophagitis and the premalignant potential of Barrett's esophagus. Medical management including life style modifications remains the mainstay of therapy for uncomplicated GERD. Accumulated evidence shows better results following surgery, compared to PPI therapy. Antireflux surgery should ideally be offered to patients who have chronic or severe disease that is poorly controlled as well as to those with Barrett's esophagus and other complications of reflux. Laparoscopic floppy 360-degree fundoplication appears to be the choice of procedure, unless the patient has poor or low amplitude peristaltic contractions, in which case a partial wrap may be offered. Management guidelines for hiatus hernia exist. Barrett's esophagus with high-grade dysplasia or intramucosal cancers is better managed by endoscopic mucosal ablation, failing which esophagectomy should be considered. Obesity and GERD are interlinked and when they coexist, bariatric surgery is preferable to pure antireflux procedures provided existing criteria for bariatric surgery are met with.

Acknowledgment

The author wishes to thank Lt Col R Saranga Bharathi for valuable inputs in the preparation of the manuscript and wife Sujayalakshmi Baskaran for editing the manuscript.

REFERENCES

1. Vakil N, van Zanten SV, Kahrilas P, Dent J, Jones R. Global Consensus Group. The Montreal definition and classification of gastroesophageal reflux disease: a global evidence-based consensus. Am J Gastroenterol. 2006;101:1900-20.
2. Hansen JM, Wildner-Christensen M, Schaffalitzky de Muckadell OB. Gastroesophageal reflux symptoms in a Danish population: a prospective follow-up analysis of symptoms, quality of life, and health-care use. Am J Gastroenterol. 2009;104:2394-403.
3. Delaney BC. Review article: prevalence and epidemiology of gastro-oesophageal reflux disease. Aliment Pharmacol Ther. 2004;20(Suppl 8):2-4.
4. Hwang H. Quality of life and surgical outcomes following laparoscopic surgery for refractory gastroesophageal reflux disease in a regional hospital. Can J Surg. 2012;55:41-5.
5. Bhatia SJ, Reddy DN, Ghoshal UC, Jayanthi V, Abraham P, Choudhuri G, et al. Epidemiology and symptom profile of gastroesophageal reflux in the Indian population: report of the Indian Society of Gastroenterology Task Force. Indian J Gastroenterol. 2011;30:118-27.
6. Sharma PK, Ahuja V, Madan K, Gupta S, Raizada A, Sharma MP. Prevalence, severity, and risk factors of symptomatic gastroesophageal reflux disease among employees of a large hospital in northern India. Indian J Gastroenterol. 2011;30:128-34.
7. Hye-Kyung Jung. Epidemiology of gastroesophageal reflux disease in Asia: a systematic review. J Neurogastroenterol Motil. 2011;17:14-27.
8. Rajendra S, Kutty K, Karim N. Ethnic differences in the prevalence of endoscopic esophagitis and Barrett's esophagus: the long and short of it all. Dig Dis Sci. 2004;49:237-42.
9. Kwiatek MA, Pandolfino JE, Kahrilas PJ. 3D-high resolution manometry of the esophagogastric junction. Neurogastroenterol Motil. 2011;23:e461-9.
10. Brasseur JG, Ulerich R, Dai Q, Patel DK, Soliman AMS, Miller LS. Pharmacological dissection of the human gastro-oesophageal segment into three sphincteric components. J Physiol. 2007;580 (Pt 3):961-75.
11. Miller LS, Dai Q, Vegesna AK, Korimilli A, Ulerich R, Schiffner B, et al. A missing sphincteric component of the gastro-esophageal junction in patients with GERD. Neurogastroenterol Motil. 2009;21:813-e52.
12. Miller LS, Vegesna AK, Brasseur JG, Braverman AS, Ruggieri MR. The osophagogastric junction. Ann N Y Acad Sci. 2011;1232:323-30.
13. Delattre JF, Avisse C, Marcus C, Flament JB. Functional anatomy of the gastroesophageal junction. Surg Clin North Am. 2000;80: 241-60.
14. Koch OO, Spaun G, Antoniou SA, Rabl C, Köhler G, Emmanuel K, et al. Endoscopic grading of the gastroesophageal flap valve is

correlated with reflux activity and can predict the size of the esophageal hiatus in patients with gastroesophageal reflux disease. Surg Endosc. 2013;27:4590-5.
15. Kaneyama H, Kaise M, Arakawa H, Arai Y, Kanazawa K, Tajiri H. Gastroesophageal flap valve status distinguishes clinical phenotypes of large hiatal hernia. World J Gastroenterol. 2010;16:6010-5.
16. Iwakiri K, Hayashi Y, Kotoyori M, Tanaka Y, Kawakami A, Sakamoto C, et al. Transient lower esophageal sphincter relaxations (TLESRs) are the major mechanism of gastroesophageal reflux but are not the cause of reflux disease. Dig Dis Sci. 2005;50:1072-7.
17. Van Herwaarden MA, Samsom M, Smout AJ. Excess gastroesophageal reflux in patients with hiatus hernia is caused by mechanisms other than transient LES relaxations. Gastroenterology. 2000;119:1439-46.
18. Kahrilas PJ. GERD pathogenesis, pathophysiology, and clinical manifestations GERD pathogenesis, pathophysiology, and clinical manifestations. Cleveland Cli J Med. 2003;70:S4-19.
19. Altomare A, Guarino MP, Cocca S, Emerenziani S, Cicala M. Gastroesophageal reflux disease: update on inflammation and symptom perception. World J Gastroenterol. 2013;19:6523-8.
20. Yang L, Francois F, Pe Z. Molecular pathways: pathogenesis and clinical implications of microbiome alteration in esophagitis and Barrett esophagus. Clin Cancer Res. 2012;18:2138-4.
21. Labenz J. Prospective follow-up data from the ProGERD study suggest that GERD is not a categorial disease. Am J Gastroenterol. 2006;101:2457-62.
22. Peters JH, Avisar N. The molecular pathogenesis of Barrett's esophagus: common signaling pathways in embryogenesis metaplasia and neoplasia. J Gastrointest Surg. 2010;14(Suppl 1): S81-7.
23. Souza RF, Krishnan K, Spechler SJ. Acid, Bile, and CDX: the ABCs of making Barrett's metaplasia. Am J Physiol. 2008;295:G211-8.
24. Moyes LH, McEwan H, Radulescu S, Pawlikowski J, Lamm CG, Nixon C, et al. Activation of Wnt signalling promotes development of dysplasia in Barrett's oesophagus. J Pathol. 2012;228:99-112.
25. Attwood EA, DeMeester TR, Bremner CG, Barlow AP, Hinder RA. Alkaline gastroesophageal reflux: implications in the development of complications in Barrett's columnar-lined lower esophagus. Surgery. 1989;106:764-70.
26. Chandrasoma PT. Histologic definition of gastro-esophageal reflux disease.1. Curr Opin Gastroenterol. 2013;29:460-7.
27. Chandrasoma P, Wijetunge S, Ma Y, Demeester S, Hagen J, Demeester T. The dilated distal esophagus: a new entity that is the pathologic basis of early gastroesophageal reflux disease. Am J Surg Pathol. 2011;35:1873-81.
28. Chandra S, Gorospe EC, Leggett CL, Wang KK. Barrett's esophagus in 2012: updates in pathogenesis, treatment, and surveillance. Curr Gastroenterol Rep. 2013;15:322.
29. Balasubramanian G, Singh M, Gupta N, Gaddam S, Giacchino M, Wani SB, et al. Prevalence and predictors of columnar lined esophagus in gastroesophageal reflux disease (GERD) patients undergoing upper endoscopy. Am J Gastroenterol. 2012;107: 1655-61.
30. Bredenoord AJ. Mechanisms of reflux perception in gastroesophageal reflux disease: a review. Am J Gastroenterol. 2012;107:8-15.
31. Matthews PJ, Aziz Q, Facer P, Davis JB, Thompson DG, Anand P. Increased capsaicin receptor TRPV1 nerve fibres in the inflamed human oesophagus. Eur J Gastroenterol Hepatol. 2004;16:897-902.
32. Yang M, Li ZS, Chen DF, Zou DW, Xu XR, Fang DC, et al. Quantitative assessment and characterization of visceral hyperalgesia evoked by esophageal balloon distention and acid perfusion in patients with functional heartburn, nonerosive reflux disease, and erosive esophagitis. Clin J Pain. 2010;26:326-31.
33. Hunt RH. Precise role of acid in non-erosive reflux disease. Digestion. 2008;78(Suppl 1):31-41.
34. Wang K, Duan LP, Zeng XZ, Liu JY, Xu-Chu W. Differences in cerebral response to esophageal acid stimuli and psychological anticipation in GERD subtypes—an fMRI study. BMC Gastroenterol. 2011;26:11-28.
35. Sun H, Chen Y, Zhao X, Wang X, Jiang Y, Wu P, et al. Abnormal activity of default mode network in GERD patients. BMC Neurosci. 2013;14:69.
36. Chourasia D, Misra A, Tripathi S, Krishnani N, Ghoshal UC. Patients with helicobacter pylori infection have less severe gastroesophageal reflux disease: a study using endoscopy, 24-hour gastric and esophageal pH metry. Indian J Gastroenterol. 2011;30:12-21.
37. Van Meer S, Bogte A, Siersema PD. Long-term follow up in patients with gastroesophageal reflux disease with specific emphasis on reflux symptoms, use of anti-reflux medication and anti-reflux surgery outcome: a retrospective study. Scand J Gastroenterol. 2013;48:1242-8.
38. Katz PO, Gerson LB, Vela MF. Guidelines for the diagnosis and management of gastroesophageal reflux disease. Am J Gastroenterol. 2013;108:308-28.
39. Gopal B, Singhal P, Gaur SN. Gastroesophageal reflux disease in bronchial asthma and the response to omeprazole. Asian Pac J Allergy Immunol. 2005;23:29-34.
40. Cameron AJ, Lagergren J, Henriksson C, Nyren O, Locke GR 3rd, Pedersen NL. Gastroesophageal reflux disease in monozygotic and dizygotic twins. Gastroenterology. 2002;122:55-9.
41. Djärv T, Wikman A, Nordenstedt H, Johar A, Lagergren J, Lagergren P. Physical activity, obesity and gastroesophageal reflux disease in the general population. World J Gastroenterol. 2012;18:3710-4.
42. Lindam A, Jansson C, Nordenstedt H, Pedersen NL, Lagergren J. A population-based study of gastroesophageal reflux disease and sleep problems in elderly twins. PLoS One. 2012;7(10):e48602.
43. Nandurkar S, Locke GR 3rd, Fett S, Zinsmeister AR, Cameron AJ, Talley NJ. Relationship between body mass index, diet, exercise and gastro-oesophageal reflux symptoms in a community. Aliment Pharmacol Ther. 2004;20:497-505.
44. Emerenziani S, Rescio MP, Guarino MP, Cicala M. Gastro-esophageal reflux disease and obesity, where is the link? J Gastroenterol. 2013;19:6536-9.
45. Banerjee R, Reddy DN. Enhanced endoscopic imaging and gastroesophageal reflux disease. Indian J Gastroenterol. 2011;30: 193-200.
46. Armstrong D. Endoscopic evaluation of gastro-esophageal reflux disease. Yale J Biol Med. 1999;72:93-100.
47. Lundell LR, Dent J, Bennett JR, Blum AL, Armstrong D, Galmiche JP, et al. Endoscopic assessment of oesophagitis: clinical and functional correlates and further validation of the Los Angeles classification. Gut. 1999;45:172-80.
48. Yaghoobi M. Impact of oesophagitis classification in evaluating healing of erosive oesophagitis after therapy with proton pump inhibitors: a pooled analysis. Eur J Gastroenterol Hepatol. 2010;22:583-90.
49. Tsai MK, Ding HJ, Lai HC, Yen KY, Li CI, Lin YY, et al. Detection of gastroesophageal reflux esophagitis using 2-fluoro-2-deoxy-d-glucose positron emission tomography. ScientificWorld Journal. 2012;2012:702803.
50. Johnson LF, DeMeester TR. Twenty-four hour pH monitoring of the distal esophagus, a quantitative measure of gastroesophageal reflux. Am J Gastroenterol. 1974:62:325-32.
51. DeMeester TR, Wang Ching-I, Wernly JA, Pellegrini CA, Little AG, Klementschitsch P, et al. Technique, indications, and clinical use of 24 hour esophageal pH monitoring. J Thoracic Cardiovasc Surg. 1980;79:656-67.

52. Seren S, Bayraktar UB, Ehrinpreis MN. Esophageal pH monitoring with Bravo™ capsule in patients with suspected gastroesophageal reflux disease. Am J Gastroenterol. 2007;102:S119-56.
53. Zentilin P, Dulbecco P, Savarino E, Giannini E, Savarino V. Combined multichannel intraluminal impedance and pH-metry: a novel technique to improve detection of gastro-oesophageal reflux literature review. Dig Liver Dis. 2004;36:565-9.
54. Hong SK, Vaezi MF. Gastroesophageal reflux monitoring: pH (catheter and capsule) and impedance. Gastrointest Endosc Clin N Am. 2009;19:1-22.
55. Saraswat VA, Dhiman RK, Mishra A, Naik SR. Correlation of 24-hr esophageal pH patterns with clinical features and endoscopy in gastroesophageal reflux disease. Dig Dis Sci. 1994;39:199-205.
56. Minjarez RC, Jobe BA. Surgical therapy for gastroesophageal reflux disease. GI Motility Online. 2006 May16; doi:10.1038/gimo56.
57. Gralnek IM, Dulai GS, Fennerty MB, Spiegel BM. Esomeprazole versus other proton pump inhibitors in erosive esophagitis: a meta-analysis of randomized clinical trials. Clin Gastroenterol Hepatol. 2006;4:1452-8.
58. Florentin M, Elisaf MS. Proton pump inhibitor-induced hypomagnesemia: A new challenge. World J Nephrol. 2012;1:151-4.
59. Kleiman DA, Beninato T, Bosworth BP, Brunaud L, Ciecierega T, Crawford CV Jr, et al. Early referral for esophageal pH monitoring is more cost-effective than prolonged empiric trials of proton-pump inhibitors for suspected gastroesophageal reflux disease. J Gastrointest Surg. 2014;18:26-33.
60. Roman S, Bruley des Varannes S, Pouderoux P, Chaput U, Mion F, Galmiche JP, et al. Ambulatory 24-h oesophageal impedance-pH recordings: reliability of automatic analysis for gastro-oesophageal reflux assessment. Neurogastroenterol Motil. 2006;18:978-86.
61. Smith JA, Decalmer S, Kelsall A, McGuinness K, Jones H, Galloway S, et al. Acoustic cough-reflux associations in chronic cough: potential triggers and mechanisms. Gastroenterology. 2010;139:754-62.
62. Singh S, Garg SK, Singh PP, Iyer PG, El-Serag HB. Acid-suppressive medications and risk of oesophageal adenocarcinoma in patients with Barrett's oesophagus: a systematic review and meta-analysis. Gut. 2014;63(8):1229-37.
63. The Society of American Gastrointestinal and Endoscopic Surgeons. [Internetß Guidelines for the Surgical Treatment of Gastroesophageal Reflux Disease (GERD) Feb2010. Available from http://www.sages.org/publications/guidelines/guidelines-for-surgical-treatment-of-gastroesophageal-reflux-disease-gerd/
64. Vakil N. Review article: the role of surgery in gastro-oesophageal reflux disease. Aliment Pharmacol Ther. 2007;25:1365-72.
65. Quartarone G. Gastroesophageal reflux in pregnancy: a systematic review on the benefit of raft forming agents. Minerva Ginecol. 2013;65:541-9.
66. Khan M, Santana J, Donnellan C, Preston C, Moayyedi P. Medical treatments in the short term management of reflux oesophagitis. Cochrane Database Syst Rev. 2007;(2):CD003244.
67. Miwa H, Inoue K, Ashida K, Kogawa T, Nagahara A, Yoshida S, et al. Randomised clinical trial: efficacy of the addition of a prokinetic, mosapride citrate, to omeprazole in the treatment of patients with non-erosive reflux disease—a double-blind, placebo-controlled study. Aliment Pharmacol Ther. 2011;33:323-32.
68. Rohof WO, Bennink RJ, de Jonge H, Boeckxstaens GE. Increased proximal reflux in a hypersensitive esophagus might explain symptoms resistant to proton pump inhibitors in patients with gastroesophageal reflux disease. Clin Gastroenterol Hepatol. 2014;12(10):1647-55.
69. Armstrong D. Should patients with Barrett's oesophagus be kept under surveillance? The case for. Best Pract Res Clin Gastroenterol. 2008;22:721-39.
70. Spechler SJ. Barrett esophagus and risk of esophageal cancer: a clinical review. JAMA. 2013;310:627-36.
71. Rossi M, Barreca M, de Bortoli N, Renzi C, Santi S, Gennai A, et al. Efficacy of Nissen fundoplication versus medical therapy in the regression of low-grade dysplasia in patients with Barrett esophagus: a prospective study. Ann Surg. 2006;243:58-63.
72. Perry KA, Walker JP, Salazar M, Suzo A, Hazey JW, Melvin WS. Endoscopic management of high-grade dysplasia and intramucosal carcinoma: experience in a large academic medical center. Surg Endosc. 2014;28:777-82.
73. Wu J, Pan YM, Wang TT, Gao DJ, Hu B. Endotherapy versus surgery for early neoplasia in Barrett's esophagus: a meta-analysis. Gastrointest Endosc. 2014;79:233-41.
74. Ertan A, Zaheer I, Correa AM, Thosani N, Blackmon SH. Photodynamic therapy vs radiofrequency ablation for Barrett's dysplasia: efficacy, safety and cost-comparison. World J Gastroenterol. 2013;19:7106-13.
75. Mori H, Kobara H, Rafiq K, Nishiyama N, Fujihara S, Ayagi M, et al. Radical excision of Barrett's esophagus and complete recovery of normal squamous epithelium. World J Gastroenterol. 2013;19:5195-8.
76. Spechler SJ, Sharma P, Shaheen NJ. American Gastroenterological Association technical review on the management of Barrett's esophagus. Gatroenterology. 2011;140(3):e18-52.
77. Bahmeriz F, Dutta S, Allen CJ, Pottruff CG, Anvari M. Does laparoscopic antireflux surgery prevent the occurrence of transient lower esophageal sphincter relaxation? Surg Endosc. 2003;17:1050-4.
78. Galmiche JP, Hatlebakk J, Attwood S, Ell C, Fiocca R, Eklund S, et al. Laparoscopic antireflux surgery vs esomeprazole treatment for chronic GERD: the LOTUS randomized clinical trial. JAMA. 2011;305:1969-77.
79. Khan M, Santana J, Donnellan C, Preston C, Moayyedi P. Medical treatments in the short term management of reflux oesophagitis. Cochrane Database Syst Rev. 2007 Apr 18;(2):CD003244.
80. Grant AM, Cotton SC, Boachie C, Ramsay CR, Krukowski ZH, Heading RC, et al. Minimal access surgery compared with medical management for gastro-oesophageal reflux disease: five year follow-up of a randomised controlled trial (REFLUX). BMJ. 2013;346:f1908.
81. Kellokumpu I, Voutilainen M, Haglund C, Färkkilä M, Roberts PJ, Kautiainen H. Quality of life following laparoscopic Nissen fundoplication: assessing short-term and long-term outcomes. World J Gastroenterol. 2013;19:3810-8.
82. The TEF VATER International Support Group. [Internet] c1990. The history of the Nissen fundoplication [Internet] Available from http://www.tefvater.org/esophageal/fundoplications.htm
83. Del Genio G, Rossetti G, Brusciano L, Maffettone V, Napolitano V, Pizza F, et al. Laparoscopic Nissen-Rossetti fundoplication is effective to control gastro-oesophageal and pharyngeal reflux detected using 24-hour oesophageal impedance and pH monitoring (MII-pH). Acta Otorhinolaryngol Ital. 2006;26:287-92.
84. Watson DI, Jamieson GG, Pike GK, Davies N, Richardson M, Devitt PG. Prospective randomized double-blind trial between laparoscopic Nissen fundoplication and anterior partial fundoplication. Br J Surg. 1999;86:123-30.
85. Woodcock SA, Watson DI, Lally C, Archer S, Bessell JR, Booth M, et al. Quality of life following laparoscopic anterior 90 degrees versus Nissen fundoplication: results from a multicenter randomized trial. World J Surg. 2006;30:1856-63.
86. Engström C, Lönroth H, Mardani J, Lundell L. An anterior or posterior approach to partial fundoplication? Long-term results of a randomized trial. World J Surg. 2007;31:1221-5.
87. Dell'Acqua-Cassão B, Mardiros-Herbella FA, Farah JF, Bonadiman A, Silva LC, Patti MG. Outcomes of laparoscopic Nissen

fundoplication in patients with manometric patterns of esophageal motility disorders. Am Surg. 2013;79:361-5.
88. Deswysen Y, Volonté F, Gutschow C, Romagnoli R, Strignano P, Ouazzani A, et al. Herniation of an abdominal antireflux fundoplication into the chest: what does it mean? Eur J Cardiothorac Surg. 2014;46(1):121-6.
89. Smith CD, McClusky DA, Rajad MA, Lederman AB, Hunter JG. When fundoplication fails redo? Ann Surg. 2005;241:861-71.
90. Juhasz A, Sundaram A, Hoshino M, Lee TH, Filipi CJ, Mittal SK. Endoscopic assessment of failed fundoplication: a case for standardization. Surg Endosc. 2011;25:3761-6.
91. Yamamoto SR, Hoshino M, Nandipati KC, Lee TH, Mittal SK. Long-term outcomes of reintervention for failed fundoplication: redo fundoplication versus Roux-en-Y reconstruction. Surg Endosc. 2014;28:42-8.
92. Davis CS, Baldea A, Johns JR, Joehl RJ, Fisichella PM. The evolution and long-term results of laparoscopic antireflux surgery for the treatment of gastroesophageal reflux disease. JSLS. 2010;14:332-41.
93. Lipham JC, DeMeester TR, Ganz RA, Bonavina L, Saino G, Dunn DH, et al. The LINX® reflux management system: confirmed safety and efficacy now at 4 years. Surg Endosc. 2012;26:2944-9.
94. Laffin M, Chau J, Gill RS, Birch DW, Karmali S. Sleeve gastrectomy and gastroesophageal reflux disease. J Obes. 2013;2013:741097. doi:10.1155/2013/741097.
95. Lazoura O, Zacharoulis D, Triantafyllidis G, Fanariotis M, Sioka E, Papamargaritis D, et al. Symptoms of gastroesophageal reflux following laparoscopic sleeve gastrectomy are related to the final shape of the sleeve as depicted by radiology. Obes Surg. 2011; 21:295-9.
96. Daes J, Jimenez ME, Said N, Dennis R. Improvement of gastroesophageal reflux symptoms after standardized laparoscopic sleeve gastrectomy. Obes Surg. 2014;24(4):536-40.
97. Soliman AM, Maged H, Awad AM, El-Sheikh O. Laparoscopic crural repair with simultaneous sleeve gastrectomy: a way in gastroesophageal reflux disease treatment associated with morbid obesity. J Minim Invasive Surg Sci. 2012;1:67-73.
98. Yatto RP, Russell G, Hargis D, Gunter N. Long term follow up of patients treated with stretta. Am J Gastroenterol. 2007;102:S119-56.
99. Auyang ED, Rauth T, Fannel RD, SAGES Guidelines Committee. [Internet] Endoluminal Treatments for Gastroesophageal Reflux. 2013 Feb. Available from http://www.sages.org/publications/guidelines/endoluminal-treatments-for-gastroesophageal-reflux-disease-gerd/
100. Ganz RA, Fallon E, Wittchow T, Klein D. A new injectable agent for the treatment of GERD: results of the durasphere pilot trial. Gastrointest Endosc. 2009;69:318-23.
101. Watson TJ, Peters JH. Lower esophageal sphincter injections for the treatment of gastroesophageal reflux disease. Thorac Surg Clin. 2005;15:405-15.
102. Frazzoni M, Conigliaro R, Manta R, Melotti G. Reflux parameters as modified by EsophyX or laparoscopic fundoplication in refractory GERD. Aliment Pharmacol Ther. 2011;34:67-75.

CHAPTER 14

Motility Disorders of the Esophagus

NS Balaji

INTRODUCTION

Motility disorders of the gastrointestinal (GI) tract in general are relatively poorly understood and their diagnosis and management hence, unsurprisingly challenging. Esophageal motility disorders are probably the better understood entities. Improving knowledge of the pathophysiology and availability of investigations has helped us with the treatment of this rather unusual spectrum of conditions.

This unique group of disorders is increasingly recognized as a cause for varied and subtle symptoms which make these patients see different specialists, such as ear, nose and throat (ENT) surgeons, cardiologists, physicians and predominantly medical gastroenterologists. Rarely do they come to a surgical consultant's room until surgical option is in the picture either as a treatment of choice or occasionally desperation. However, it is at this point the surgeon has to understand and be wary to what the scalpel can offer and what it may not. Appropriate selection of patients based on a good history taking and thorough investigation using the available methods of evaluation would benefit the patient and the surgeon equally.

Achalasia is undoubtedly the best understood esophageal motility disorder despite ongoing debates of their etiology. Nutcracker esophagus (NE), diffuse esophageal spasm (DES), hypertensive esophageal sphincter and ineffective esophageal motility (IEM) form the majority of other esophageal motility disorders. With better understanding of the varied clinical presentation and the aid of esophageal physiology studies diagnosis has become easier to plan appropriate treatment and prognosticate treatment outcomes.

Esophageal motility disorders are either classified broadly from a clinical perspective as achalasia and non-achalasia motility disorders or primary and secondary motility disorders. Definition of motility disorders were initially based on Castell's conventional manometric criteria that are increasingly being replaced by the Chicago classification system based on high-resolution manometry (HRM).

CLASSIFICATION OF MOTILITY DISORDERS: WHY?

Primary versus Secondary

Primary motility disorders of the esophagus are those that have no other identifiable cause (Table 1). The most commonly identifiable "other" primary cause is gastroesophageal reflux disease (GERD) that is known to contribute to a spectrum of esophageal dysmotility patterns secondary to varied degrees of injury to the esophageal mucosa and the body. It is hence imperative that GERD is ruled out as a causative factor in all non-achalasia motility disorders. Other known causative factors are generalized connective tissue disorders, such as scleroderma, malignant diseases (pseudoachalasia), postoperative states, etc. (Table 2). The importance of diagnosing secondary motility disorders is for the treatment to be aimed primarily at the causative factor, such as GERD, malignancy, etc.

Achalasia versus Non-achalasia Disorders

A primary reason for segregating achalasia from the rest of the disorders is the availability of a reasonable consensus on the diagnosis and management of achalasia with resultant good clinical outcomes and the absence of the same for the rest. Hence, a diagnosis of achalasia is seen upon as a light bulb in the bigger spectrum of motility disorders of the esophagus. Similarly, the

Table 1: Classification of primary esophageal motility disorders

Category	*Disorder*
Inadequate LOS relaxation	Classic achalasia Atypical disorders of LOS relaxation
Uncoordinated contraction	Diffuse esophageal spasm
Hypercontraction	Nutcracker esophagus Isolated hypertensive LOS
Hypocontraction	Ineffective esophageal motility

Abbreviation: LOS, lower esophageal sphincter

Table 2: Causes of secondary esophageal motility disorders

Primary disease	*Motility disturbances*
Systemic sclerosis Connective tissue disorders	Loss of distal (smooth muscle) peristalsis Weak lower esophageal sphincter pressure (<10 mm Hg); Normal proximal esophagus and UES (striated muscle)
Gastroesophageal reflux disease	IEM Hypotensive lower esophageal sphincter
Chagas disease	Similar to achalasia
Diabetes mellitus	Combination of motility abnormalities
Tumors	Achalasia (pseudo)
Postoperative states (antireflux surgery, bariatric surgery)	Achalasia (pseudo) Ineffective motility Hypertensive LOS

Abbreviations: LOS, lower esophageal sphincter; UES, upper esophageal sphincter; IEM, ineffective esophageal motility.

diagnosis of a non-achalasia disorder forewarns the treating physician on the rather not so predictable positive outcome upon treatment, and helps to appropriately counsel the patient.

DEFINITION OF VARIOUS ESOPHAGEAL MOTILITY DISORDERS

Esophageal manometric criteria have always stood as the gold standard for defining esophageal motility disorders. The various pressure profiles (dynamic and static) of the lower esophageal sphincter (LES) and the esophageal body formed the basis of the criteria developed by Castell et al. on conventional manometric studies (Table 3). However, the emergence of HRM and the establishment of criteria based on both dynamic and static profiles have led to the more recent Chicago classification and a later modification (Table 4).

CLINICAL DIAGNOSIS

The classical/typical symptoms of an esophageal disease dysphagia, heartburn and regurgitation can happen in varying combinations in different motility disorders in spite of a preponderance of dysphagia being the principal symptom in most of the patients. Typically dysphagia to liquid and solids from the onset or to liquids alone without any alarm symptoms are more favoring an underlying motility disorder. Atypical symptoms such as chest pain tend to be more common in the nonmotility disorders and this must be ascertained in the not so infrequent patient who has been extensively investigated by the cardiologist to rule out a cardiac source. Suggestive features of a potential esophageal source of chest pain would be pain in association with food, relief with antacids or proton pump inhibitors (PPIs), non-association with exercise and presence of additional symptoms, such as heartburn and regurgitation.

Table 3: Manometric (conventional) features of primary esophageal motility disorders

Disorder	*Manometric features*
Achalasia	Absent, incomplete LOS relaxation Absent peristalsis
Diffuse esophageal spasm	More than 20% of swallows result in simultaneous contractions May have multipeaked and/or prolonged contractions
Nutcracker esophagus	Peristaltic contractions of increased amplitude (>180 mm Hg)
Hypertensive LOS	Increased resting LOS pressure (> 40 mm Hg)
IEM	Decreased amplitude (<30 mm Hg) peristaltic or nonperistaltic contractions in distal esophagus with more than or equal to 30% of wet swallows

Abbreviations: LOS, lower esophageal sphincter; IEM, ineffective esophageal motility.

Hence, it is always imperative to rule out a malignancy in anyone with dysphagia and a cardiac source in anyone with chest pain.

However, symptoms on their own are not reliable for the diagnosis of motility disorders including the patient who may present with a combination of heartburn, regurgitation and dysphagia. Regurgitation of static food material from the esophagus and secondary heartburn due to fermentation can confuse the diagnosis with GERD and lead to an erroneous labeling of GERD. Progressive dysphagia can also happen in benign strictures and worsening scleroderma.

Patti et al. reported that dysphagia was the most common symptom and was present in 94% of 145 patients with untreated achalasia. Regurgitation was present in 76%, heartburn in 52%, and chest pain in 41% of these patients. It was also noted that at the time of referral, 45% of patients were on acid reducing medications on the presumed diagnosis of GERD.

When dealing with patients with esophageal diseases, significant weight loss should alert the clinician of an underlying malignancy or a recent surgery for GERD. The latter suggests the possibility of a secondary achalasia due to a tight wrap or an undiagnosed achalasia in the first place prior to anti-reflux surgery. Clinical examination may reveal stigmata of a systemic disease that may contribute to a secondary motility disorder. No significant findings are seen in any primary motility disorder of the esophagus.

Table 4: Chicago classification of motility disorders of the esophagus

Diagnosis	*Diagnostic criteria*
Achalasia	
Type I achalasia	Classic achalasia: mean IRP more than upper limit of normal, 100% failed peristalsis
Type II achalasia	Achalasia with esophageal compression: mean IRP more than upper limit of normal, no normal peristalsis, pan esophageal pressurization with more than or equal to 20% of swallows
Type III achalasia	Mean IRP more than upper limit of normal, no normal peristalsis, preserved fragments of distal peristalsis or premature (spastic) contractions with more than or equal to 20% of swallows
EGJ outflow obstruction	Mean IRP more than upper limit of normal, some instances of intact peristalsis or weak peristalsis with small breaks such that the criteria for achalasia are not met.
Other motility disorders	(Patterns not observed in normal individuals)
Distal esophageal spasm	Normal mean IRP, more than or equal to 20% premature contractions
Hypercontractile esophagus (Jackhammer esophagus)	At least one swallow DCI more than 8,000 mm Hg-s-cm with single peaked or multipeaked contraction
Absent peristalsis	Normal mean IRP, 100% of swallows with failed peristalsis
Other peristaltic abnormalities	(Defined by exceeding statistical limits of normal)
Weak peristalsis with large peristaltic defects	Mean IRP less than 15 mm Hg and more than 20% swallows with large breaks in the 20 mm Hg isobaric contour (more than 5 cm in length)
Weak peristalsis with small peristaltic defects	Mean IRP less than 15 mm Hg and more than 30% swallows with small breaks in the 20 mm Hg isobaric contour (2–5 cm in length)
Frequent failed peristalsis	More than 30%, but less than 100% of swallows with failed peristalsis
Rapid contractions with normal latency	Rapid contraction with more than or equal to 20% of swallows, DL more than 4.5 s
Hypertensive peristalsis (nutcracker esophagus)	Mean DCI more than 5,000 mm Hg-s-cm, but not meeting criteria for hypercontractile esophagus
Normal	Not achieving any of the above diagnostic criteria

Abbreviations: IRP, integrated relaxation pressure; DCI, distal contractile integral; EGJ, esophagogastric junction.

Symptoms should be used as an initial screening tool to localize the probable site of disease in the esophagus and not as a diagnostic method to base treatment.

INVESTIGATIONS

A thorough history taking and clinical examination for stigmata of systemic disease is of paramount importance in directing further investigative modalities. After this the journey to localize the cause, begins.

Upper GI Endoscopy and Biopsy

An endoscopic evaluation of the esophagus is mandatory and is usually the initial investigation in a patient with suspected motility disorders. It can detect structural lesions and simultaneously combine multiple biopsies even in the absence of structural lesions with the increasing awareness of eosinophilic esophagitis as a cause for dysphagia. The endoscopist should have a low threshold for obtaining biopsies in the above clinical context of dysphagia without an obviously identifiable lesion. However, it is not uncommon to find a normal upper gastrointestinal endoscopy finding in a background of motility disturbances within the esophagus.

In the absence of a structural mucosal abnormality to account for the patient's symptoms, indirect evidences for a potentially underlying motility issue are a dilated esophagus, food stasis, presence of a diverticulum, a difficult entry into the stomach past the area of the LES zone. Active peristalsis that is unusual during the course of a normal upper gastrointestinal endoscopy should be noted. The presence of an extrinsic compression may guide the clinician to pursue further investigations, if felt appropriate.

Identifiable causative factors directing a diagnosis toward a secondary motility disorder include GERD (evidence of esophagitis, peptic strictures and large hiatal hernias), strictures and malignancy.

Radiology Studies

Contrast studies have always been an important tool in the investigation of disorders of the esophagus. These have remained as a "road map" to esophageal anatomy. Barium swallow examinations in these disorders are done either to assess static or dynamic function.

Cineradiography with concomitant fluoroscopic monitoring of bolus passage, esophageal structure and contractility would be the ideal investigation of choice over static films, if facilities permit the same. The need of an experienced radiologist with a special interest in performing dynamic esophageal barium examinations cannot be overemphasized. Timed barium examination in the prone oblique, supine and upright positions with concentrating on various phases and segments of esophageal function can be of immense use in the interpretation of even subtle abnormalities that may guide decision making.

The identification of structural problems, such as a web, stricture, diverticula, corkscrew esophagus and hiatal hernia are easily observed on static films to the mindful eyes of an experienced radiologist. Dynamic imaging identifies swallowing problems at the level of the thoracic inlet, peristaltic activity in the body, bolus passage, anatomy of the hiatus and region of the LES, reflux into the esophagus and emptying into the stomach.

There may be a few instances that may warrant a contrast swallow examination prior to an upper gastrointestinal endoscopy in situations such as a suspected Zenker's diverticulum or high esophageal/pharyngeal lesions that may have a potential to cause iatrogenic injuries during endoscopic intubation. Computed tomography (CT) scans with oral contrast can also be useful in specific clinical circumstances where extraluminal pathology should be excluded such as instances when a pseudoachalasia is considered secondary to an obstructing lesion from without.

Esophageal Physiology Studies

Esophageal manometry is the gold standard investigation for assessment of esophageal body function, competence and relaxation of the lower and upper esophageal sphincters and the finally to derive at a clinically appropriate correlation of symptoms and esophageal dysfunction.

High-Resolution Manometry

The emergence of HRM and esophageal pressure topography has widened the understanding of esophageal function and has led to the recent Chicago classification of esophageal motility disorders based on HRM criteria. The subclassification of types of achalasia to predict the treatment outcomes based on body peristaltic characteristics is a welcome addition to prognosticate success in selective subtypes.

Ambulatory pH Studies

Ambulatory pH and impedance studies are to be used more liberally to rule out a secondary esophageal motility disorder resulting from GERD. It is to be noted that a significant proportion of non-achalasia primary esophageal motility disorders are secondary to GERD and it is imperative that it is to be ruled out. It is a wrong notion that pH studies would not be indicated in motility disorders of the esophagus.

MANAGEMENT OF ESOPHAGEAL MOTILITY DISORDERS

Achalasia

"Cure of achalasia is impossible. Any treatment is palliative."

All treatment modalities are aimed at reducing outflow resistance and improving dysphagia. This has to be borne in mind when counseling the patient and care taken not to offer cure of disease. It is disturbing and inappropriate to guarantee cure in achalasia although it is seen in medical practice. Moreover, there always remains a chance of symptom recurrence or even progression of the disease in the long-term and alternate methods of treatment must have to be considered at every step in the history of the disease. It is widely accepted that medical management without any endoscopic or surgical intervention has little role in the treatment of achalasia (Table 5).

Table 5: Management of achalasia

Surgical management	Laparoscopic Heller's myotomy and partial fundoplication Esophagectomy (end stage disease)
Endoscopic management	Pneumatic dilatation Botulinum toxin injection Per oral endoscopic myotomy (POEM)
Medical management (Ineffective)	Nitrates, calcium channel blockers Tricyclics

The standard endoscopic methods have been pneumatic dilatation, injection of botulinum toxin and more recently the availability and emerging acceptance of per oral endoscopic myotomy (POEM). Surgical therapies that have stood the test of time are Heller's myotomy with or without an anti-reflux procedure and esophagectomy for end-stage achalasia or failed other methods of surgery.

Surgical versus Nonsurgical Methods

The controversies surrounding the effectiveness of surgical and nonsurgical management still continue although the verdict clearly favors the surgical management groups. Recent meta-analysis have demonstrated an obvious superiority in the surgical arms both in the effectiveness of symptom relief and continued long-term success rates. However, in patients who may not be candidates for a surgical procedure are best offered nonsurgical methods accepting a relatively less favorable long-term outcome. The superiority of surgery has been questioned in a recent publication comparing surgery versus pneumatic dilatation, which had similar outcomes at 2 years. The nonsurgical fraternity has welcomed this but in depth analysis expose a number of caveats in the conclusion. It is the efficacy and longevity of sustained symptom relief, which makes surgery a more attractive alternative to nonsurgical treatment.

Surgical Management of Achalasia Cardia

Heller's myotomy with anti-reflux surgery is the current gold standard surgical procedure for the treatment of achalasia.

We have moved beyond the controversies of open versus laparoscopic repair and questioning the need for an additional fundoplication. Current debates revolve around the type of partial fundoplication (anterior versus posterior) and the benefit of an extended myotomy onto up to 3–4 cm the stomach versus the traditional 1–2 cm.

Current evidence points to equivalent efficacy of both the anterior and posterior partial fundoplications with no established superiority of one over the other. The benefit of an extended myotomy over the standard myotomy has been proposed predominantly by the Seattle group and has not been reproduced by others.

It is hence justifiable to accept that a standard laparoscopic Heller's myotomy with a partial fundoplication based on surgeon's preference is the preferred surgical procedure for achalasia.

The details of the surgical technique are beyond the realms of this chapter but the principles of surgery are to be strictly adhered to:

- Thorough physiological preoperative evaluation
- Patient counseling (symptom control, not cure)
- Optimal port positioning (Fig. 1)
- Adequate esophageal mobilization (Fig. 2)
- Adequate length of myotomy (esophagus) (Fig. 3)
- Adequate extended length of myotomy (stomach)
- Appropriately done sound partial (anterior or posterior) fundoplication (Fig. 4).
- Optimal follow-up

Surgery performed with above-mentioned principles is associated with a good intraoperative, short-term and long-term outcomes. Complications such as bleeding and perforation intraoperatively are relatively low and controllable as it is within the surgeon's reach all the time unlike nonsurgical methods.

Pneumatic Dilatation

Controlled pneumatic dilation of the LES aims at disrupting the integrity of the sphincter radially and hence decreasing outflow resistance. The efficiency of this technique in terms of postprocedural symptom relief, which is usually an outpatient procedure, or with an overnight stay in hospital is reported to be up to 90%. The procedure can be repeated based on symptomatic need or radiologic evidence of outflow obstruction. Over a follow-up period of 10 years the need for repeat dilatation has been reported to be between 25% and 65%. It is the relative lapse in durability of the procedure that makes it inferior to surgical myotomy in the long-term data.

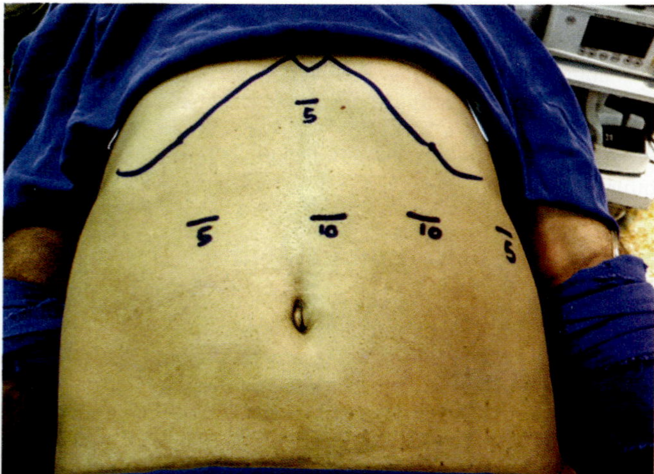

Figure 1 Port positions

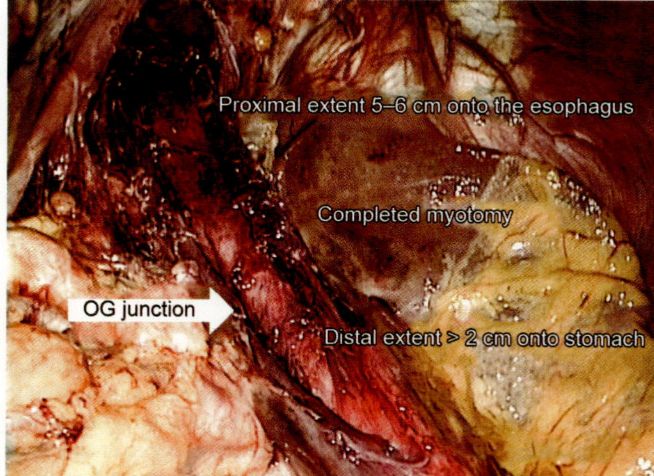

Figure 3 Completed myotomy

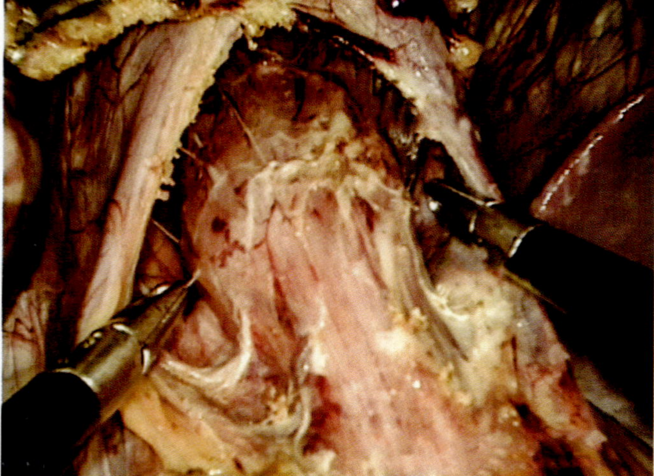

Figure 2 Proximally dilated esophagus with a waistline at the OG junction

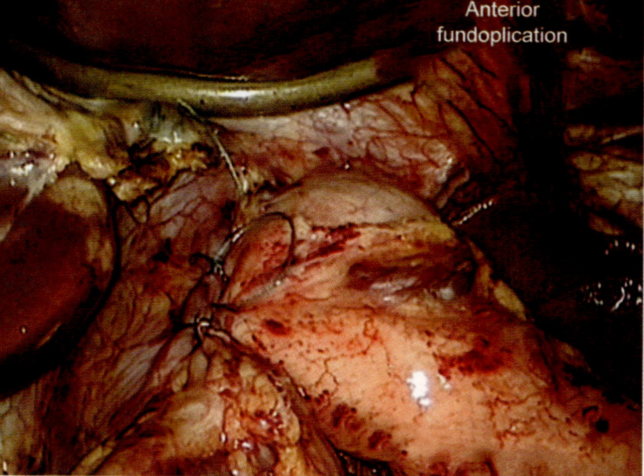

Figure 4 Anterior fundoplication

Pneumatic balloon dilatation is undoubtedly one of the few alternates in patients who are either unfit for surgery or unwilling for surgery. It is our normal practice to offer surgery as the first option in patients except for the above-mentioned circumstances.

Based on available evidence the efficacy of pneumatic dilatation in relieving symptoms in the short-term may be equivalent or slightly inferior to surgery, but it scores lower in long-term symptom control. The need for repeated dilatations over the years after the initial procedure can be high and has to be informed to the patient when options are discussed. Complications associated with the procedure especially perforation up to 5% based on the technique and pressures used, can be quite challenging to manage. Surgery, drainage and more recently stenting are options in the setting of perforations.

Botox Injection

Injection of botulinum toxin derivatives for smooth muscle relaxation is widely applied in many fields of medicine. The application in achieving relaxation of the smooth muscle of the LES is also aimed at relief of outflow resistance. It mainly acts at the terminal nerve endings of the monaural junction by preventing the release of acetylcholine from vesicles, causing chemical denervation and paralysis of the muscles.

It is a much safer procedure compared to the surgical option or pneumatic dilatation as it involves purely an endoscopic injection. Equally the symptom control after the procedure is also acceptable and probably comparable to pneumatic dilatation. However, the durability of action of botox injection is short-lived in the region of 6–8 months and a repeat session becomes nearly inevitable.

POEM for Achalasia

Per oral endoscopic myotomy (POEM) is the new kid on the block with considerable attention and interest on the future of this novel technique. This ingenious endoscopic esophagomyotomy first reported by Pasricha et al. in porcine models was performed by Inoue et al. in humans. Endoscopic dissection and division of the inner circular muscular layer of the esophagus by way of a small proximal opening of the esophageal mucosa and a submucosal tunnel is achieved by this novel procedure.

Initial series have strongly established the efficacy and safety profile of this technique that has taken the endoscopic world into a different realm of innovation after natural orifice transluminal endoscopic surgery (NOTES). However, the issues that have been thrown for discussion are twofold. Firstly, the critics cite that the absence of an inherent anti-reflux procedure may predispose the patient to pathological reflux after the procedure. However, the proponents of the procedure argue that there may not be the need to perform an additional anti-reflux procedure as it is only the circular muscle fibers that are divided and the esophageal hiatus and outer longitudinal fibers remain undisturbed. The initial reports suggest that there can be postoperative reflux of up to 50% reported by Swanstrom et al.

In one series of 16 patients treated with POEM, symptom relief at 3 months was achieved in 15 patients (94%) and mean LES pressure decreased from a pretreatment value of 27 mm Hg to a post-treatment value of 12 mm Hg. No patient developed symptoms of gastroesophageal reflux, but one patient had mild esophagitis on follow-up upper endoscopy. Second issue is of the long term results and their comparison with other modalities of treatment. Long-term data from randomized trials are necessary to compare POEM with laparoscopic surgical myotomy and pneumatic dilation before POEM can be recommended.

NUTCRACKER ESOPHAGUS

Nutcracker esophagus (NE) is a primary motility disorder of the esophagus characterized by a hypercontractile distal esophageal body. It is hence sometimes referred to as a "super squeeze" esophagus. It was traditionally defined manometrically with distal esophageal body amplitudes of greater than 180 mm hg in the background of normal peristaltic function and a manometrically normal LES. The HRM criteria for the diagnosis of nutcracker esophagus necessitates the distal contractile integral (DCI) of greater than 5,000 mm Hg*sec*cm. Another variant called as the "Jackhammer esophagus" is said to exists, if there is more than one peristalsis with a DCI of greater than 8,000 mm Hg*sec*cm.

The clinical presentation of hypertensive esophageal body disorders is predominantly characterized by chest pain. Dysphagia is the next common symptom and may be mixed with symptoms of GERD, such as heartburn, regurgitation, etc. The more common picture is a patient presenting to the cardiologist with chest pain and after all cardiac investigations negating a cardiac source referred to an esophagologist. It is a rarity for a patient with nutcracker esophagus to reach a surgeon's consulting room per se.

The treatment of nutcracker esophagus is primarily medical aimed at reducing the peristaltic vigor. The main agents used in this are nitrates and calcium channel blockers with or without acid suppression. The results are very variable and predominantly not very satisfactory to the surgeon and the patient. The usual therapy recommended is diltiazem 180–240 mg per day or a tricyclic antidepressant at bedtime. Isosorbide 10 mg as an "on need" protocol can also be used. It is also unclear if the contractile amplitude in these patients has any bearing to symptoms control that makes treatment prognostication difficult.

The role of surgery in nutcracker esophagus according to Patti et al. who have amongst the highest experience is limited only to patients who have a predominant symptom of dysphagia. They claim up to an 80% symptom relief if dysphagia is the predominant symptom and only a 50% relief when chest pain is the predominant symptom. Other groups have reported a recurrence rate of up to 75%. Hence, the role of surgery in nutcracker esophagus is to be taken with a nihilistic approach, limiting the same to patients with failed all other methods and a predominant symptom of dysphagia plus a hypertensive LES. The patient has to be counseled appropriately on the same lines.

DIFFUSE ESOPHAGEAL SPASM

Diffuse esophageal spasm (DES) is defined manometrically by the presence of normal peristalsis intermittently interrupted by simultaneous contractions in 20–60% of all swallows. The main prerequisite is the presence of normal intervening peristalsis that would differentiate DES from achalasia, which is characterized by 100% of simultaneous contractions. The HRM criteria for DES is the presence of premature contractions characterized with a distal latency (DL) less than 4.5 seconds in more than 20% of contractions.

The predominant clinical symptoms are chest pain and dysphagia. DES is variably viewed as within the spectrum of progression to achalasia at a later stage in the course of disease as evidenced by a few follow-up studies when repeat manometry in some of these patients revealed progression to achalasia. LES abnormalities are seen to coexist in up to 50% of patients with either a hypertensive sphincter or partial relaxation further supporting the achalasia correlation.

Treatment options remain limited to the use of medications as mentioned in nutcracker esophagus with similar results. However, surgery seems to be more favorable in comparison to nutcracker esophagus. The standard surgical option that is described is a long myotomy either using the thoracoscopic or laparoscopic route. The proximal extent of the myotomy should be guided by manometric findings.

Following myotomy, dysphagia is said to be relieved in 80–86% of patients and chest pain in 75–80% of the patients. Relief is more after laparoscopic approach than thoracoscopic approach. Regurgitation and heartburn scores were also significantly improved after operation. Similar reports on significant improvement in symptoms score regarding chest pain, dysphagia, regurgitation and heartburn have been published.

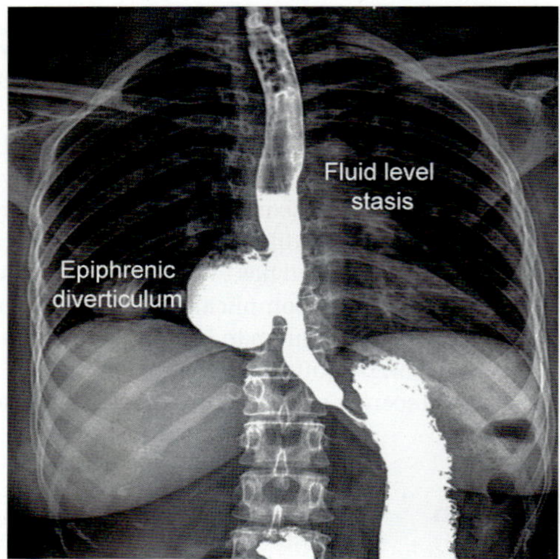

Figure 5 Preoperative esophagogram-epiphrenic diverticulum

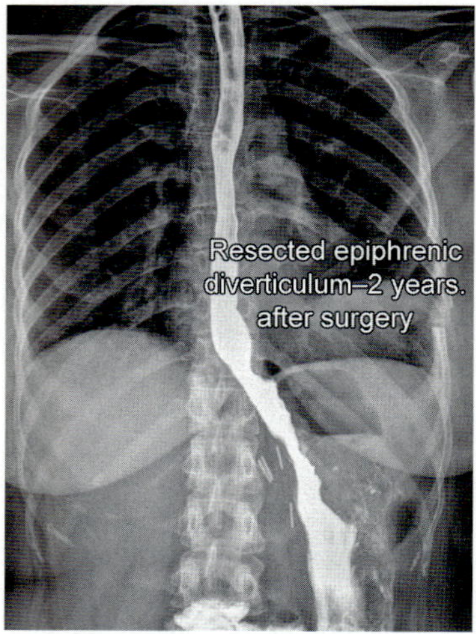

Figure 6 Postoperative esophagogram after excision of diverticulum, myotomy and fundoplication

HYPERTENSIVE ESOPHAGEAL SPHINCTER

The finding of an isolated hypertensive esophageal sphincter is uncommon but has been reported and is classified as a distinct motility disorder. The presenting symptom is usually dysphagia secondary to the functional outflow obstruction at the level of the gastroesophageal junction. It may associate with other motility abnormalities such as mentioned above with a DES pattern.

In a patient with dysphagia as the predominant symptom and a manometric evidence of a hypertensive LES, a surgical myotomy combined with a partial fundoplication gives good symptomatic relief and is accepted. However, a trial of pneumatic dilatation prior to offering a surgical correction in this uncommon entity is an acceptable alternative to predict the outcome of surgical correction.

EPIPHRENIC ESOPHAGEAL DIVERTICULUM

An epiphrenic diverticulum is a pulsion diverticulum, usually located in the distal esophagus. It is due to herniation of the mucosa and submucosa through the muscle layers of the esophageal wall. Most patients complain of dysphagia and respiratory symptoms that are often present due to aspiration. An endoscopy as the initial investigation usually gives a hint to the abnormality depending on the size and position. A barium swallow is the investigation of choice as it shows the position of the diverticulum (more frequently on the right side), the width of the diverticular neck and its distance from the gastroesophageal junction (Fig. 5).

It is more commonly accepted and proven that an epiphrenic diverticulum is always caused by an underlying esophageal motility disorder. Conventional manometry demonstrates a motility disorder in about 70% of patients. These findings support the rationale for performing a myotomy in all patients with an epiphrenic diverticulum. Therefore, the operation of choice is resection of the diverticulum, esophageal myotomy and partial fundoplication (Fig. 6). Traditionally, the operation was performed through a left thoracotomy. The development of minimally invasive surgery has brought a drastic change, as today most of these diverticula are resected through a laparoscopic approach.

CONCLUSION

Motility disorders of the esophagus are increasingly recognized but relatively poorly understood conditions. Achalasia remains the best-understood disorder with predictable prognostication of treatment outcomes.

The appropriate use of good history taking, esophageal physiology studies, upper gastrointestinal contrast studies and consultation and counseling with a physician/surgeon with the best understanding of the disease would direct the patient toward best treatment. Both medical and surgical treatment has predictable outcomes in achalasia with a better long-term success with surgical myotomy in achalasia. On the contrary, both medical and surgical treatments are less predictable and less rewarding in non-achalasia motility disorders and this has to be borne in mind when offering surgical treatment.

BIBLIOGRAPHY

1. Achem SR. Noncardiac chest pain-treatment approaches. Gastroenterol Clin North Am. 2008;37(4):859-78.
2. Achem SR. Treatment of non-cardiac chest pain. Dis Mon. 2008;54(9):642-70.
3. Allaix ME, Patti MG. What is the best primary therapy for achalasia: medical or surgical treatment? Who owns achalasia? J Gastroint Surg. 2013;17(9):1547-9.
4. Almansa C, Heckman MG, DeVault KR, Bouras E, Achem SR. Esophageal spasm: demographic, clinical, radiographic, and manometric features in 108 patients. Dis Esophagus. 2012;25(3): 214-21.
5. Bredenoord AJ, Fox M, Kahrilas PJ, Pandolfino JE, Schwizer W, Smout AJ: Chicago classification criteria of esophageal motility disorders defined in high resolution esophageal pressure topography. Neurogastroenterol Motil. 2012;Suppl 1:57-65.
6. Campos GM, Vittinghoff E, Rabl C, Takata M, Gadenstatter M, Lin F, et al. Endoscopic and surgical treatments for achalasia: a systematic review and meta-analysis. Ann Surg. 2009;249(1):45-57.
7. Carlson DA, Pandolfino JE. High-resolution manometry and esophageal pressure topography: filling the gaps of convention manometry. Gastroenterol Clin North Am. 2013;42(1):1-15.
8. Carlson DA, Pandolfino JE. The Chicago criteria for esophageal motility disorders: What has changed in the past 5 years? Curr Opin Gastroenterol. 2012;28(4):395-402.
9. Chuah SK, Chiu CH, Tai WC, Lee JH, Lu HI, Changchien CS, et al. Current status in the treatment options for esophageal achalasia. World J Gastroenterol. 2013;19(33):5421-9.
10. Da Silveira EB, Rogers AI. Treatment of achalasia with botulinum A toxin. Am J Ther. 2002;9(2):157-61.
11. Eypasch EP, DeMeester TR, Klingman RR, Stein HJ. Physiologic assessment and surgical management of diffuse esophageal spasm. J Thorac Cardiovasc Surg. 1992;104(4):859-68.
12. Fass R, Achem SR. Noncardiac chest pain: diagnostic evaluation. Diseases of the esophagus: official journal of the International Society for Diseases of the Esophagus. 2012;25(2):89-101.
13. Fisichella PM, Patti MG. From Heller to POEM (1914-2014): A 100-Year History of Surgery for Achalasia. J Gastrointestinal Surgery. 2014;18:1870-1875.
14. Fisichella PM, Raz D, Palazzo F, Niponmick I, Patti MG. Clinical, radiological, and manometric profile in 145 patients with untreated achalasia. World J Surg. 2008;32(9):1974-9.
15. Herbella FA, Raz DJ, Nipomnick I, Patti MG. Primary versus secondary esophageal motility disorders: diagnosis and implications for treatment. J Laparoendosc Adv Surg Tech A. 2009;19(2):195-8.
16. Herbella FA, Tineli AC, Wilson JL, Del Grande JC. Surgical treatment of primary esophageal motility disorders. Journal of gastrointestinal surgery: official journal of the Society for Surgery of the Alimentary Tract. 2008. pp. 604-8.
17. Hirano I, Pandolfino J. New technologies for the evaluation of esophageal motility disorders: impedance, high-resolution manometry, and intraluminal ultrasound. Gastroenterol Clin North Am. 2007;36(3):531-51.
18. Inoue H, Tianle KM, Ikeda H, Hosoya T, Onimaru M, Yoshida A, et al. Peroral endoscopic myotomy for esophageal achalasia: technique, indication, and outcomes. Thorac Surg Clin. 2011; 21(4):519-25.
19. Lamb PJ, Myers JC, Thompson SK, Jamieson GG. Laparoscopic fundoplication in patients with a hypertensive lower esophageal sphincter. J Gastrointest Surg. 2009;13(1):61-5.
20. Leconte M, Douard R, Gaudric M, Dumontier I, Chaussade S, Dousset B. Functional results after extended myotomy for diffuse oesophageal spasm. Br J Surg. 2007;94(9):1113-8.
21. Patti MG, Fisichella PM. Laparoscopic Heller myotomy and Dor fundoplication for esophageal achalasia. How I do it. J Gastrointest Surg. 2008;12(4):764-6.
22. Patti MG, Gasper WJ, Fisichella PM, Nipomnick I, Palazzo F. Gastroesophageal reflux disease and connective tissue disorders: pathophysiology and implications for treatment. J Gastrointest Surg. 2008;12(11):1900-6.
23. Patti MG, Gorodner MV, Galvani C, Tedesco P, Fisichella PM, Ostroff JW, et al. Spectrum of esophageal motility disorders: implications for diagnosis and treatment. Arch Surg. 2005;140(5):442-8.
24. Patti MG, Herbella FA. Achalasia and other esophageal motility disorders. J Gastrointest Surg. 2011;15(5):703-7.
25. Richter JE, Boeckxstaens GE: Management of achalasia: surgery or pneumatic dilation. Gut. 2011;60(6):869-76.
26. Roll GR, Rabl C, Ciovica R, Peeva S, Campos GM. A controversy that has been tough to swallow: is the treatment of achalasia now digested? J Gastrointest Surg. 2010;4(Suppl 1):S33-45.
27. Salvador R, Costantini M, Rizzetto C, Zaninotto G. Diffuse esophageal spasm: the surgical approach. Diseases of the esophagus: official journal of the International Society for Diseases of the Esophagus. 2012. pp. 311-8.
28. Sharata A, Kurian AA, Dunst CM, Bhayani NH, Reavis KM, Swanstrom LL. Peroral endoscopic myotomy (POEM) is safe and effective in the setting of prior endoscopic intervention. Journal of gastrointestinal surgery: official journal of the Society for Surgery of the Alimentary Tract. 2013. pp. 1188-92.
29. Sifrim D, Fornari F. Non-achalasic motor disorders of the oesophagus. Best practice & research. Clinical gastroenterology. 2007. pp. 575-93.
30. Soares R, Herbella FA, Prachand VN, Ferguson MK, Patti MG. Epiphrenic diverticulum of the esophagus. From pathophysiology to treatment. Journal of gastrointestinal surgery: official journal of the Society for Surgery of the Alimentary Tract. 2010;14(12): 2009-15.
31. Spechler SJ, Castell DO. Classification of oesophageal motility abnormalities. Gut. 2001;49(1):145-51.
32. Stavropoulos SN, Modayil RJ, Friedel D, Savides T. The International Per Oral Endoscopic Myotomy Survey (IPOEMS): a snapshot of the global POEM experience. Surg Endosc. 2013;27(9):3322-38.
33. Tamhankar AP, Almogy G, Arain MA, Portale G, Hagen JA, Peters JH, et al. Surgical management of hypertensive lower esophageal sphincter with dysphagia or chest pain. J Gastrointest Surg. 2003;7(8):990-6.
34. Tutuian R, Castell DO. Esophageal motility disorders (distal esophageal spasm, nutcracker esophagus, and hypertensive lower esophageal sphincter): modern management. Curr Treat Options Gastroenterol. 2006;9(4):283-94.
35. Vanuytsel T, Bisschops R, Farre R, Pauwels A, Holvoet L, Arts J, et al. Botulinum toxin reduces Dysphagia in patients with nonachalasia primary esophageal motility disorders. Clin Gastroenterol Hepatol. 2013;11(9):1115-21.
36. Yaghoobi M, Mayrand S, Martel M, Roshan-Afshar I, Bijarchi R, Barkun A. Laparoscopic Heller's myotomy versus pneumatic dilation in the treatment of idiopathic achalasia: a meta-analysis of randomized, controlled trials. Gastrointest Endosc. 2013;78(3): 468-75.
37. Zhao X, Pasricha PJ. Botulinum toxin for spastic GI disorders: a systematic review. Gastrointest Endosc. 2003;57(2):219-35.

CHAPTER 15

Esophageal Perforation: Diagnosis and Management

Rajneesh Kumar Singh, Puneet Puri

INTRODUCTION

Esophageal perforation is a rare condition. As a result, the diagnosis is difficult to make and management protocols are not standardized. It has a high morbidity and mortality that may be reduced by quick and appropriate decision making with regard to the management of such patients. The diverse etiology and presentation of esophageal perforation make it a challenge to tailor the management to the needs of the given patient. A number of factors influence the outcome and impact the management of such patients. This chapter is an attempt to review the often confusing literature on the subject and outline the salient points that the reader would wish to be acquainted with in managing patients with an esophageal perforation.

EPIDEMIOLOGY

Esophageal perforation is an uncommon problem. The worldwide incidence is not known. However, a population based study from Iceland put the age-standardized incidence as 3.1/1,000,000/year.[1] In a recent large review, the mean frequency of esophageal perforation in 37 studies was 3.9±2.3 cases per year (range 1.1–11.9).[2] It seems to occur slightly more commonly in males.[3]

ETIOLOGY

With the increasing number of endoscopic procedures in the modern era, iatrogenic perforation is an important cause of esophageal perforation. The etiology of esophageal perforation can be divided into several subsets for purpose of understanding this diverse condition. These can be iatrogenic versus non-iatrogenic perforation, previously diseased versus healthy esophagus, spontaneous versus nonspontaneous perforation, traumatic versus nontraumatic perforation, etc. The list of various causes, by no means exhaustive, is as follows:

- Trauma
  - Iatrogenic trauma: During diagnostic or therapeutic endoscopic procedures; during various surgical procedures in the neck, thorax or abdomen like thyroidectomy, fundoplication; transesophageal echocardiography; etc.
  - Non-iatrogenic trauma: Penetrating trauma in the neck, thorax and abdomen. Foreign body ingestions like fish bone perforation, swallowed denture, corrosive perforation of esophagus, barotrauma, etc.
- Spontaneous perforation: Boerhaave's syndrome.

Iatrogenic trauma during endoscopy is the most common cause of esophageal perforation.[4,5] The posterior wall of the pharynx is the most unsupported by muscle coat and is the most common site of perforation during diagnostic endoscopy by aggressive attempts to cross the cricopharyngeal sphincter without proper vision. The other causes of perforation during endoscopy are during dilatation of benign and malignant strictures. These perforations usually occur either just proximal to or at the stricture. External trauma mostly leads to cervical esophageal injury followed by thoracic and abdominal esophagus respectively.[6] The incidence of cervical esophageal injury in penetrating neck trauma is 5–6%.[7,8] The thoracic esophagus is less vulnerable to external trauma due to its location in protective thoracic cage. The important mechanisms of injury include gunshot wounds and stab wounds. Spontaneous esophageal rupture (Boerhaave's syndrome) is caused by sudden rise in intraluminal pressure of esophagus through patent lower esophageal sphincter during vomiting. The possible cause for sudden rise in intraluminal pressure is failure of relaxation of upper esophageal sphincter. The brunt of this sudden rise in pressure falls on the weak area of left wall of lower esophagus.[9] Most of the spontaneous perforations occur on the left side and lead to massive contamination of the mediastinum and pleural cavities with food and secretions from the esophagus and stomach.

PATHOPHYSIOLOGY

Perforation of the esophagus leads to contamination of the surrounding tissues with food, secretions and the accompanying bacteria. The significance of this depends on the site and the severity of the perforation. In intramural and some transmural perforations, the contamination remains limited and only a local abscess may form that can resolve with antibiotics. In most other patients, there is significant contamination of the mediastinum and pleural spaces. In the thorax, the result is often mediastinitis, sepsis and multiorgan dysfunction, if not treated in time. In the cervical region, this mostly leads to formation of an abscess that may resolve after drainage. In the abdomen due to poor supporting tissues, there is usually peritoneal contamination and peritonitis.

CLINICAL FEATURES

As may be clear from the pathophysiology, esophageal perforation can have varied presentations ranging from self-limiting condition to florid sepsis involving multiorgan failure leading to death. The clinical features of esophageal perforation depend on site of injury, degree of contamination and length of time elapsed after injury. The cervical esophageal perforation often present with neck pain, stiffness and surgical emphysema. The surgical emphysema may be detected in 60% of cases on clinical examination.[10] Other features can be hoarseness of voice and dysphagia. The systemic symptoms occur less commonly as mediastinal contamination is limited by attachment of the prevertebral fascia.[11]

With regard to the thoracic esophageal perforations, the symptoms may be nonspecific. Due to close proximity of thoracic esophagus to heart, symptoms may be attributed to that of coronary artery disease. Patients usually present with severe chest pain, retrosternal discomfort that are common presentation of coronary artery disease or aortic dissection. Hence, diagnosis may be delayed unless high index of suspicion is kept while interpreting history of such patients. A missed esophageal perforation can have more severe consequences than that of well-diagnosed coronary event. The constellation of chest pain, vomiting and surgical emphysema described as Mackler's triad is found in less than 50% of patients.[9] The breach of adjacent pleurae lead to hydropneumothorax resulting in respiratory distress. The left pleural cavity is usually involved in lower thoracic esophageal perforations and right is more often contaminated in upper thoracic esophageal perforations. Hematemesis or melena is an uncommon presentation. The pleural and mediastinal contamination lead to bacterial proliferation and systemic inflammatory response syndrome (SIRS) due to release of cytokines leading to fluid sequestration, hypotension and eventually septic shock and multiorgan failure.

Abdominal esophageal perforation leads to generalized peritoneal contamination and development of peritonitis. Patients present with sharp epigastric pain usually with rapid development of signs of peritonitis.

DIAGNOSIS AND WORK UP

After perforation, there occurs a systemic inflammatory response in the next 24–48 hours. The inflammatory phase is soon followed by infection. The mediastinal infection can lead to development of multiorgan dysfunction syndrome (MODS) and may prove fatal. Hence, once suspected the diagnosis must be established at the earliest and appropriate management should be initiated. A delay of more than 24 hours in the diagnosis and treatment is consistently associated with poor outcome of these patients. The clinical features may not be suggestive during the first contact with the patient, so frequent repeat examinations are warranted. The diagnostic modalities aim to establish the diagnosis of esophageal perforation as well as to delineate collections and abscesses secondary to perforations.

IMAGING MODALITIES

Plain X-ray neck and chest (posteroanterior and lateral view) can demonstrate pleural effusion, hydropneumothorax, lung collapse, pneumomediastinum, subcutaneous emphysema and free gas under diaphragm.

Water-soluble contrast study is conventionally the first confirmatory investigation undertaken and can demonstrate the site and severity of leak (Fig. 1). While this is possible in a stable patient, it is difficult to execute in a sick patient in the intensive care unit, often with multiorgan dysfunction. In addition, false negative water-soluble contrast study is not uncommon due to the poor mucosal coating property of the water-soluble contrast and rapid passage of contrast in certain parts of the esophagus, e.g. cervical esophagus. In case of a negative study, a repeat study may be done after few hours if the index of suspicion remains high. Alternatively, a dilute barium study may be undertaken, albeit at the risk of barium leakage into the mediastinum and perpetuating an inflammatory response.[12]

Contrast enhanced computerized tomography, in addition to demonstrating the leak from the esophagus, helps to delineate collections in mediastinum, pleural cavity and peritoneal cavity (Figs 2A and B). A recent study showed that CT scan may in fact render the contrast esophagography unnecessary thereafter. In their study on patients with pneumomediastinum, Wu et al. found that the negative predictive value of CT scan was 100%.[13] Hence, in a patient with a negative CT scan, no further investigation is

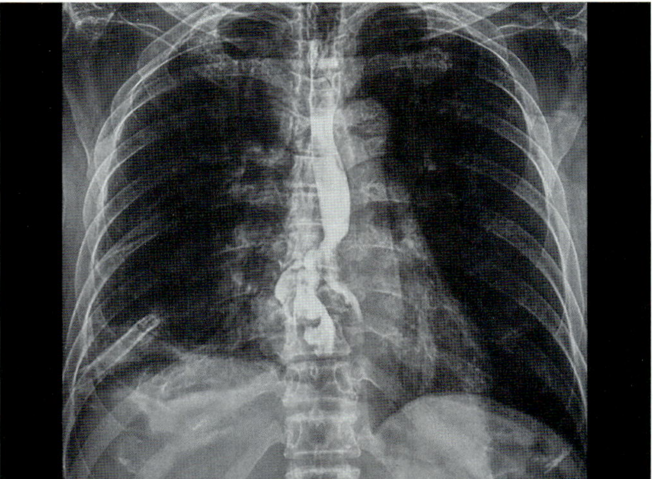

Figure 1 Water-soluble contrast study of patient following dilatation for corrosive stricture of midesophagus (shows contrast spill into the mediastinum and right pleural cavity)

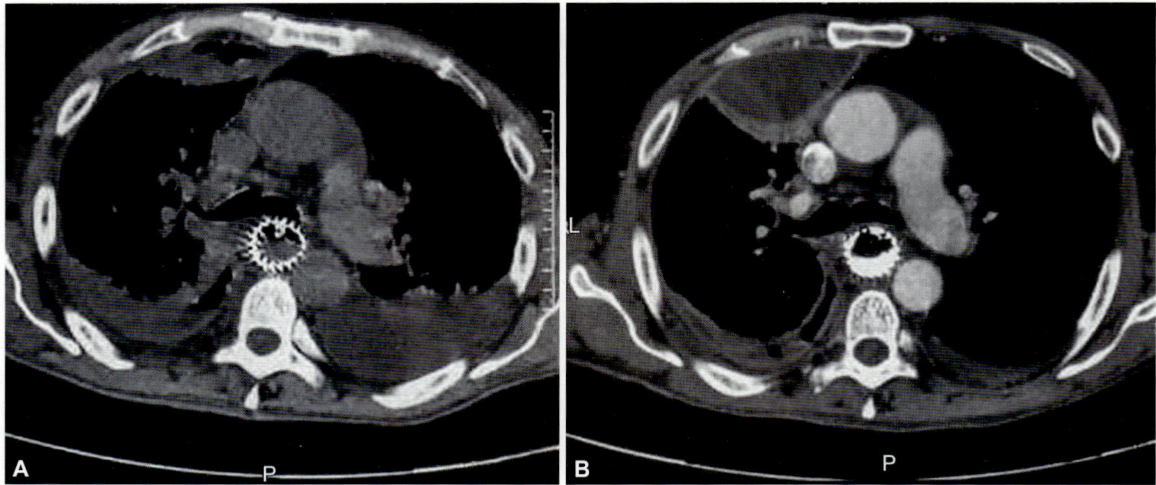

Figures 2A and B CT scan following SEMS inserted for the same perforation as Figure 1. It shows SEMS without and with oral/IV contrast showing complete sealing of the perforation (no leakage of oral contrast). Multiple collections in both pleural cavities are also seen
Abbreviations: CT, computed tomography; SEMS, self-expanding metallic stent.

necessary. However, the positive predictive value of CT scan was 62%, meaning thereby that there were quite a few false positive tests. They concluded that if the CT scan was positive then a contrast esophagography should be done.

Conventionally, endoscopy was thought to be contraindicated in patients with suspected esophageal perforation.[14] However, there is some information to suggest that endoscopy done by an experienced operator with minimal insufflation is quite safe in these patients. Endoscopy has been shown to be quite effective in diagnosis of esophageal injuries in patients with penetrating trauma and also in patients with anastomotic leaks following a mediastinal esophagogastric anastomosis.[15,16] The role of endoscopy is presently considered to be limited to a subset of patients in whom there is high index of suspicion, but radiography is negative and secondly those who can't swallow contrast due to technical reasons. However, Kuppusamy et al. objectively assessed the usefulness of endoscopy in series of 52 patients and concluded the benefit of endoscopy as follows: detection of additional secondary pathology (perforation, stricture, cancer) (n = 10), treatment of secondary pathology (ballooning, stenting) (n = 6), stent and drain management (nasomediastinal drain, etc.) (n = 6), changes in initial planned treatment approach (no repair, resection, diversion) (n = 5).[17]

MANAGEMENT

Early confirmation of diagnosis and institution of appropriate therapy is crucial in avoiding the high morbidity and mortality associated with this feared problem. The delay in treatment is one of the most important factors determining mortality. A systematic review of several studies found that for patients treated within 24 hours of perforation, the pooled morality was 7.4% and this was 20.3% in patients with a delay in treatment greater than 24 hours.[17] Having said this, the treatment of esophageal perforation is mostly based on retrospective studies because of rarity of this condition. However, no uniform management protocol has been universally agreed upon, there are some facts that should be taken into account while managing these patients.[18]

General measures like intravenous fluid resuscitation, nil per-orally, proton pump inhibitors, broad spectrum antibiotics, intravenous and/or enteral nutrition and organ specific support, where needed, and monitoring are as important as making specific decisions with regard to management of the perforation. Antibiotics should also cover anaerobes found in the upper GI tract. Patients, who are quite sick with impending organ failure, should be managed in the intensive care. As the pleural cavities are frequently contaminated therefore pulmonary care should be instituted early, including oxygen supplementation, physiotherapy and incentive spirometry. Early institution of antifungal therapy is now recognized as an important measure to reduce mortality in sick patients. Hoffmann et al. isolated candida in 30% of the patients with esophageal perforations and showed that the mortality was 41% in Candida-positive patients versus 23% in Candida-negative patients.[19] While prophylactic fluconazole has become a norm for these patients, this study recommended echinocandins (e.g. caspofungin) in the sickest of patients due to the fear of growing resistance to fluconazole.[19] Early institution of parenteral and thereafter enteral nutrition is of utmost importance if other measures are to be effective. Often these patients are septic as well as malnourished because of the delay in diagnosis or referral for appropriate therapy. In our published series, we found that a low serum albumin (<3 g/dL) after resuscitation is an important predictor of high mortality.[20]

The factors that need to be taken into account while deciding specific management of the esophageal perforation include etiology, time from perforation, site of perforation, intramural or transmural perforation, preexisting pathology, degree of contamination, severity of sepsis, hemodynamics, general physical condition of the patient and comorbid conditions. This list, while detailed, is not exhaustive. Hence, the experience of the center or surgeon and the general outlook of the patient plays a major role in choosing a given treatment strategy. There are several treatment strategies for the perforation. However, it is not uncommon to see various individualized modifications and hybrid approaches. The aims of choosing a specific strategy are as follows:

- To control the sepsis by draining the collections and abscesses supplemented with antimicrobial or antifungal cover
- To prevent the ongoing contamination
- To augment the healing of damaged tissue.

The various treatment strategies may be grouped as follows:

- Nonoperative treatment
- Surgical treatment
  - Primary repair
  - Drainage
  - Esophageal exclusion and diversion
  - Esophagectomy
- Endoscopic treatment
  - Endoscopic stents
  - Endoscopic closure techniques
  - Endoscopic drainage or vacuum therapy.

NONOPERATIVE TREATMENT

The interpretation of the term is quite varied across publications. In the strictest sense, it meant treatment only with antibiotics, nil by mouth and parenteral nutrition along with other general measures. Some authors have also included percutaneous drainage and provision for a feeding jejunostomy in nonoperative treatment.[21] Therefore, there is a frequent overlap with so-called "conservative treatment". Frequent monitoring of the clinical condition of the patient and frequent use of radiology (esophagography or CT scan) to follow-up the perforation to closure are important aspects of nonoperative treatment. Cameron[22] defined the criteria for applying nonoperative treatment in a small series of eight patients as follows: (a) The esophageal disruption should be well contained within the mediastinum or between the mediastinum and visceral lung pleura. (b) The cavity should be well-drained back into the esophagus (c) Minimal symptoms should be present. (d) There should be minimal evidence of clinical sepsis. Cameron did acknowledge the difficulty in interpreting the "severity" of clinical sepsis.

From old literature, the following groups of patients seem suitable for nonoperative treatment: (a) instrumental perforations, particularly in the cervical region, (b) small perforations occurring during dilatation of corrosive or peptic strictures, or associated with endoscopic sclerotherapy of varices, (c) late presentation of perforation with minimal symptoms. For the large part, the patient may select himself/herself for nonoperative treatment if he/she presents late and appears to tolerate the perforation well with minimal sepsis.[23]

Alorjay et al. recognized the challenge of choice of nonoperative treatment in patients who present early following the perforation.[24] Therefore, nonoperative treatment comes with rider of frequent monitoring with esophagography or CT scan along with monitoring the clinical condition of the patient. If, for any reason, the patient seems to be deteriorating then an alternative treatment plan is chosen. Altorjay et al. proposed extended criteria for nonoperative treatment as follows:[24]

- Intramural perforation (all)
- Transmural perforation
  - Perforation detected early or when detected late, circumscribed (contained) one
  - The lesion in the mediastinum or in the space between the mediastinum and visceral pleura causes well encapsulated extravasation
  - From the cavity surrounding the esophagus, the contrast medium flows adequately back into the esophageal lumen.
  - The tissue defect is not in neoplastic tissue, not in the abdominal cavity and is not accompanied by simultaneous obstructive esophageal disease.
  - Symptoms are minimal.
  - Symptoms and signs of septicemia are absent.
  - Availability of adequate radiology support such as contrast swallow study, CT scan, etc.
  - Adequate thoracic surgical experience and skills.

SURGICAL TREATMENT

This can be discussed in individual heads with the caveat that there is a frequent overlap and not all procedures conform to strict definitions.

Primary Repair

The patients, who present early (within 24 hours), have an otherwise healthy esophagus (good local tissues) and are acceptable risk for general anesthesia, primary repair of the perforation is the best option. It must be remembered that the mucosal tear is often longer than the muscular tear. Hence, a myotomy is required at the corners to define the full limits of the perforation. The mucosa and muscle layers should be carefully sutured in two layers with interrupted absorbable sutures. Stapled closure is an alternative if the local tissues permit. Reinforcement of the repair may be done with vascularized flaps of pleura, pericardium, intercostal muscle, diaphragm, omentum or fundus of stomach. Some authors have reported the use of extraneous materials, like absorbable mesh and fibrin glue, to reinforce the repair.[25] While some authors[26] have shown that the leak rates are lower for reinforced repairs than otherwise, others have reported similar results for reinforced and nonreinforced repair.[27] Regardless of the controversy, it is clear that the most important steps are diligent identification of the margins of the perforation and careful suture placement. In some cases, like achalasia cardia, where perforation occurs after pneumatic dilatation, it is common sense to protect the mucosal repair with an anterior fundoplication. In other cases, it may be decided on case per case basis. Two additional steps should always be carried out with primary repair: (i) the first is adequate local drainage, and (ii) the second is a provision for enteral feeding by a feeding jejunostomy.

There are several modifications reported for primary repair. Conventionally, primary repair had been reserved for patients presenting within 24 hours. Primary repair even beyond 24 hours delay is now considered acceptable by most centers.[26-28] Several authors have presented acceptable results with primary repair even beyond 24 hours. Bhatia et al. presented a mortality rate of 8%, 6% and 8% respectively in patients undergoing primary repair within 24 hours, between 24–72 hours and beyond 72 hours, in a series of 119 patients with esophageal perforation.[3] For the most part, the time limit on primary repair is now not considered important. The condition of the patient, sepsis and condition of the local tissues are considered more important in taking this decision. Most surgeons would reinforce or buttress the primary repair in this situation, despite the controversy surrounding reinforcement of primary repair. Another interesting modification is primary repair over a T-tube. In patients undergoing primary repair for late perforations, the repair is done over a T-tube placed in the esophagus and the long limb is brought out through the chest wall. Linden et al. carried out primary repair over either a 16 Fr T-tube or a trimmed percutaneous gastrostomy tube in patients with severely inflamed local tissues that were not able to hold sutures.[29] In their series, out of 36 patients, 11 had a leak demonstrated on postoperative barium swallow. However, in the presence of adequately placed drains, most of these leaks did not need any more intervention. In the absence of prospective controlled trials, the benefit of T-tube is difficult to judge but it seems to appeal to common sense when the tissues seem not to be able to hold sutures very well.

Drainage

Drainage procedures, as a group, include a variety of surgical and percutaneous drainage procedures. In late presentation of cervical perforations, surgical drainage of the abscess is adequate treatment.[30] The subsequent salivary fistula gradually heals satisfactorily with good nutrition. Placement of radiology-guided drains is needed for abscesses within the pleural cavity or mediastinum. Drainage is also an adjunct to other surgical procedures such as primary repair, decortication, esophagectomy, etc. Indeed good drainage is the most important step in the source control of septic focus. Often no other intervention is needed for patients who undergo adequate drainage of collections. Hence, good round the clock intervention-radiology support is very important for surgical units dealing for esophageal perforation. Vogel et al. managed 28 patients with thoracic perforations with percutaneous drainage of collections and no mortality.[21] Of these patients, only 3 subsequently needed thoracotomy for persisting sepsis and underwent debridement and drainage.

Conservative Treatment

Conservative treatment is often confused with "nonoperative" treatment that was defined earlier by Cameron et al. Most authors include percutaneous drainage as a part of conservative treatment. Martinez et al. described successful conservative management of thoracic perforation in 17 children with success all but one.[31] Vogel managed 32 patients with "aggressive conservative" management in their series of 47 patients.[21] Of these 4 patients with cervical perforations underwent purely "nonoperative" treatment and 28 patients with thoracic perforation underwent "nonoperative" or "conservative" treatment. These authors seem to use the two terms interchangeably and add percutaneous drainage when needed. The results of their series were quite remarkable in that there was no mortality in this subgroup, albeit at the cost of prolonged intensive care and hospital stay (mean 25 days). Therefore, conservative (nonsurgical) treatment with drainage, as needed, seems to have a definite role in some patients. The problem seems to be one of patient selection and there are still no clearly defined criteria that help in this matter. Some patient can clearly be selected for conservative treatment (± drainage) as follows: cervical perforation, thoracic perforation with localized collection or abscess and mild sepsis or severe comorbidities.

Esophageal Exclusion and Diversion

The "bipolar" exclusion of the esophagus bearing the perforated segment is a last ditch effort in trying to control ongoing contamination in very sick patients with severe sepsis and multiorgan dysfunction. As is apparent, it is a salvage procedure and is usually reserved for septic patients with late presentation in whom esophagectomy is considered unsafe and too high risk. It usually implies stapling or division of the esophagus in the neck and the abdomen, cervical loop or end esophagostomy, tube gastrostomy, feeding jejunostomy and wide drainage. If the esophagus is only stapled across in the neck (and not divided), the stapled segment usually recanalizes in 2–4 weeks. If a longer period of exclusion is required then the esophagus needs to be divided in the neck with an end esophagostomy. It must be noted that Urschel had originally described the procedure as "esophageal diversion in continuity" and the esophagus was tied off in the neck and the abdomen using umbilical tapes ligatures.[32]

A modification of the exclusion procedure consists of primary repair of the perforation in the thoracic esophagus and temporary esophageal exclusion using absorbable staples. The absorbable staples in the cervical esophagus lead to recanalization of esophageal lumen much earlier (1–2 weeks) than that reported for nonabsorbable staples (2–4 weeks).[33,34] Others have tried to circumferentially tie off the esophagus at both ends with heavy (absorbable) suture in the hope that it will recanalize later.

Most of the experiences quoted here have been of small numbers of patients and individualized treatment of the severely septic patient. We managed 52 patients of esophageal perforation at the All India Institute of Medical Sciences, New Delhi.[20] Of these, 32 patients presented beyond 2 days of perforation (late presentation). Twenty-two patients (42%), who were severely septic, underwent esophageal exclusion procedure including division of the esophagus in the neck and end esophagostomy. In this subgroup, 6 patients died, 2 were lost to follow-up and 14 underwent staged reconstruction. There was one postoperative mortality following reconstructive surgery. All the remaining patients were dysphagia free on follow-up. The high mortality must be seen in light of the fact that these were very sick patients with late presentation of esophageal perforation and severe sepsis.

Esophagectomy

Esophagectomy eliminates the source of sepsis in one stroke and prevents further contamination of the mediastinum. While that may be true, it remains a major surgical undertaking in very sick and septic patients. The risk of resection in a sick patient should be weighed against the risk of sepsis due to mediastinal contamination and this decision is usually not an easy one. A recent review of seven studies including 147 patients with delayed presentation of esophageal perforation compared esophagectomy (n = 86) to conservative procedures (n = 57) and found that the mortality was the lowest in the esophagectomy arm (0–18%) than exclusion (50%) or primary repair (68%). However, the bias toward esophagectomy cannot be disregarded in these retrospective studies, particularly as others have reported much better results with conservative procedures (as primary repair) even beyond 24 hours. The key seems to be proper patient selection for esophagectomy and

Altorjay defined the following criteria for selecting patients for esophagectomy:[35]

- Concomitant obstructive esophageal disease is present
- There is an extensive injury, even one treated within 24 hours, associated with serious mediastinal or intrapleural contamination
- Primary repair would cause a 50% narrowing of the esophageal lumen
- There is a spontaneous perforation associated with substantial sepsis
- There is circumscribed extravasation caused by a neglected impacted foreign body.

Gupta et al. described a series of 57 patients of esophageal perforation from Post Graduate Institute of Medical Education and Research (PGIMER), Chandigarh.[36] Of these 33 patients (58%) underwent esophagectomy and the mortality of esophagectomy was an acceptable 9%. Their criteria of esophagectomy included patients with distal obstructive pathology (such as malignancy, corrosive stricture and achalasia with megaesophagus). The good results of their series may be seen in light of the fact that the current therapy of choice for perforated esophageal malignancy is a self-expanding metallic stent (SEMS) and quite a few patients with perforation during dilatation of corrosive stricture can be managed with less aggressive surgery or drainage. In fact, some patients with previously healthy esophagus may require an esophagectomy when the esophagus is considered too badly damaged to be salvageable.

While the criteria for patient selection are not very clearly defined, esophagectomy is chosen as surgical therapy of choice when the esophagus is deemed unsalvageable (previously healthy or diseased) and the patient is considered at reasonable risk for esophagectomy. Sometimes this decision may be needed to be taken during surgery when attempting a primary repair and the esophagus is found to be too badly damaged for repair. If the patient is considered at high risk then a lesser procedure such as exclusion and diversion may be a better choice.

Functional Outcome of Esophageal Perforation

There is very little data on the follow-up of patients with esophageal perforation who have undergone successful management of their acute problem. Orringer's group has published one such uncommon series.[37] In their series of 42 patients, 25 underwent primary repair, 15 underwent esophagectomy and 2 underwent drainage as the first modality of treatment. Of those (n = 25) who underwent primary repair, 10 (40%) required dilatations and 5 of these later needed esophagectomy for tight peptic strictures. Of those (n = 15) who underwent esophagectomy, 8 (53%) required dilatations and none required reoperation. Of those (n = 2) who initially underwent drainage only one required primary repair and one required esophagectomy. Mortality (including follow-up) related to esophageal perforation was 12%. At a mean follow-up of 3.7 years, 55.8% patients reported a better quality of swallowing than before perforation, 33.3% patients same as before and 11.1% patients worse than before.

While it is difficult to interpret the results of a single retrospective series, there are a few learning points. The first point is that while the indications of primary repair have expanded in the recent years, careful patient selection is needed as some of these patients need esophagectomy for continuing dysphagia on follow-up. Another learning point relates to the need for long-term follow-up before any particular therapy is concluded as being successful in the treatment of esophageal perforation.

ENDOSCOPIC TREATMENT

Endoscopic Stent Therapy

Endoscopic treatment of esophageal perforation has certainly crossed the threshold of vain attempts of the endoscopist to contain morbidity of the perforation caused by him/her, to being successful treatment in some situations. SEMS are the most promising of all endoscopic therapies. Properly positioned covered self-expanding stents can seal off the perforation site and maintain luminal patency. Such stents are deployed endoscopically and a follow-up contrast study within 24 hours is mandatory to document complete sealing. Incompletely sealed perforations require early surgical treatment. After successful deployment of stent, oral feeding can be resumed after 3–5 days. The stent can be left in position for 6–8 weeks and can then be removed endoscopically.[38-40]

A recent review of 25 studies of esophageal stenting for perforation or anastomotic leaks, included 267 patients with complete follow-up.[41] The stents used could be grouped as self-expanding plastic stents (SEPS), fully covered self-expanding metallic stents (FSEMS) and partially covered self-expanding metallic stents (PSEMS). Clinical success (successful deployment and removal) was achieved in 85% of patients and was not different between stent types. Sixty-five (34%) patients had a stent-related complication. Stent migration occurred more often with SEPS (31%) and FSEMS (26%) than with PSEMS (12%), whereas the tissue in- and overgrowth was slightly more with PSEMS (12%) than with FSEMS (7%) and SEPS (3%). A large proportion (59%) of patients needed radiology-guided drainage of associated abscesses or collections. The overall mortality was 13% and the cause of death was mostly an abscess outside the esophagus. An endoscopic reintervention was performed in 53 (25%) patients; however, more with SEPS or FSEMS (both 26% respectively) than with PSEMS (13%). A surgical intervention for incomplete sealing, a procedure-related or stent-related complication, was performed in 13% of patients and was not different between stent designs. The time to stent removal was 6–8 weeks.

The data with regard to stent placement is quite heterogeneous and difficult to interpret. In summary, these series demonstrate the urgent need to drain abscesses and collections along with stent deployment as integral to the treatment. Stent migration is a problem that may be overcome with use of partially covered stents, albeit at the cost of more tissue ingrowth that may hamper successful removal. In effect, covered stents deployed for 6–8 weeks are effective in treating majority of patients with perforation that have been reported in these series.

Patient selection has been the bugbear of stent treatment. An analysis of unsuccessful stent placement was done by Freeman et al. to find out the predictive factors for failure of stent therapy.[42] Over a 7-year period, 187 patients were treated with esophageal stents and 15 patients (8%) required surgical intervention for inadequate sealing of perforation.[42] Stent failure was significantly more frequent in patients who had an esophageal leak of the proximal cervical esophagus, that traversed the gastroesophageal junction, an esophageal injury longer than 6 cm or an anastomotic leak associated with a more distal conduit leak. Malignancy or previous radiation therapy was not associated with treatment failure.

Endoscopic Endoluminal Vacuum Therapy

The initial drawback of endoscopic therapy was the inability to deal with collections or abscesses in the mediastinum and pleural cavities and the subsequent need for percutaneous or surgical drainage. The first attempts were to place transnasal drainage tubes endoscopically through the perforation into periesophageal collections. However, these were not very successful. The concept of vacuum-assisted wound closure for postsurgical wounds has been extended, innovatively, to treat esophageal perforation as well. A recent paper described the endoluminal vacuum therapy in 10 patients with esophageal perforation.[43] A small polyurethane sponge is endoscopically inserted through the perforation into the adjacent abscess cavity and connected by a naso-esophageal tube to a vacuum device. As the cavity collapses over the next few days, the sponge needs to be changed about twice a week until the cavity is small enough to be left alone. If the perforation persists then a stent can be deployed at this time. This series reported sponge changes over mean of 5.4 sessions.[43] One patient died during treatment, one needed surgical resection and one needed stent therapy. However, it is quite early, but it seems that the therapy may serve as a bridge for sick patients prior to more aggressive surgical therapy.

Other Endoscopic Therapies

Endoscopic clips have been used by endoscopists for some time.[44] Initially, the through-the-scope (TTS) clips were used. These were small in size and could only be used for closing small defects. The over-the-scope (OTS) clips are larger and have been FDA approved for closing mucosal defects up to 20 mm in size, although closure of defects up to 30 mm is feasible. However, the scope needs to be withdrawn every time to load a new OTS clip.

PREDICTIVE FACTORS AND PATIENT SELECTION FOR MANAGEMENT

Several factors have been found to be related to increased mortality of esophageal perforation. These include advanced age, comorbid diseases, late presentation beyond 24 hours, severe sepsis, etc. However due to the retrospective nature of all studies and small number of patients, there is significant heterogeneity in the predictive factors of mortality.

A recent large review collated the results of 75 studies (total 2,971 patients).[2] The pooled overall morality was 11.9% and the mean hospital stay was 32.9 days. Studies with a mean age greater than 60 years had a mortality of 14.8% as compared to those with a mean age of less than 60 years (10.5%). Gender did not seem to make a difference in the pooled morality. With regard to the site of perforation the pooled mortality for cervical, thoracic and abdominal perforations were 5.9%, 10.9% and 13.2% respectively. With regard to the cause, the pooled morality was 13.2% for iatrogenic perforations and 14.8% for spontaneous perforation. The delay in starting treatment more than 24 hours was associated with a pooled morality of 20.3% as compared to those with treatment started within 24 hours (7.4%). With regard to the type of treatment, the pooled mortality was 9.5% for primary repair, 13.8% for esophagectomy, 20% for T-tube and other repairs and 7.3% for stent therapy. While this review obviously suffers from severe limitations due to the heterogeneous nature of included studies, it is nevertheless a good source of a large volume of collated literature on esophageal perforations.

Abbas et al. in a series of 119 patients with esophageal perforation proposed a severity score to sum up factors affecting outcome and mortality.[45] In this score, the individual factors were given separate weightage as follows (Table 1):

Table 1: Esophageal perforation severity score

Variable	*Score*
Age >75 years	1
Tachycardia >100 beats/min	1
Leukocytosis >10,000 WBC/mL	1
Pleural effusion (on CXR or CT)	1
Fever >38.5 degree C	2
Non-contained leak (on CT or barium swallow)	2
Respiratory compromise (respiratory rate >30, mechanical ventilation)	2
Time to diagnosis >24 h	2
Cancer	3
Hypotension	3
Total potential score	18

Abbreviations: CXR, chest X-ray; CT, computed tomography.

In this study, for scores of less than 2, 2–5 and greater than 5, the complication rate was 53%, 65% and 81% respectively; the length of hospital stay was 10, 16 and 28 days respectively and the mortality was 2%, 6% and 27% respectively.[45] In their series, the presence of non-contained (free) perforation and respiratory compromise or failure were independently associated with operative treatment as opposed to nonoperative treatment. The authors proposed that patients with low scores (e.g. contained perforations and no respiratory compromise) were suitable for nonoperative management. The severity score proposed by them seems quite reasonable but has not been validated by any other study for the purpose of selection of treatment.

Maier et al. managed 14 patients with spontaneous esophageal perforation with primary repair or esophagectomy.[46] The choice of surgical procedure was made based on the duration of leak, patients overall status and extent of mediastinal and pleural contamination. The problem lies with the subjective nature of criteria used for patient selection. Furugaki et al. used the presence of SIRS for choosing patients for surgical treatment.[47] They carefully monitored patients for SIRS and converted conservative treatment to surgery if SIRS developed during monitoring.

In a recent multicenter study, the factors predictive of mortality were advanced age, preexisting coronary artery disease and esophageal malignancy.[48] In a large single center Canadian series, the predictors of mortality on multivariate logistic regression analysis were preoperative respiratory failure, malignant perfora-

Flow chart 1 Algorithm for management of esophageal perforation
Abbreviation: SEMS, self-expandable metal stents.

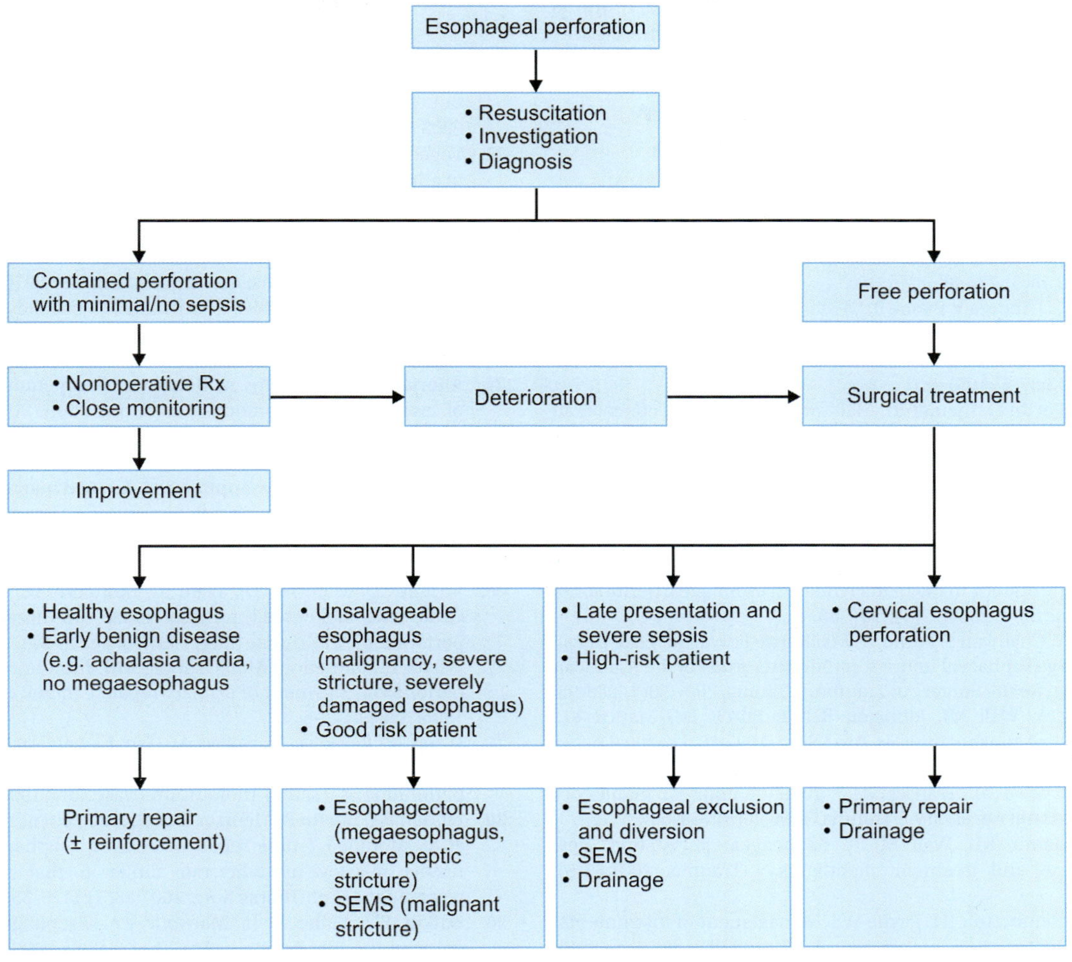

tions, high Charlton comorbidity index, pulmonary comorbidity and sepsis.[3] In our series from New Delhi, the factors predictive of mortality were delayed presentation, low serum albumin and perioperative ventilation.[20]

The various treatment options may be tailored to the patients' clinical presentation as follows (Flow chart 1):

- Nonoperative management
  - Contained perforation
  - No significant sepsis
- Primary repair (± reinforcement)
  - Usually early presentation (<24) or late presentation (good risk patients) also included
  - Healthy local tissues
- Drainage
  - Delayed presentation (mostly cervical and thoracic perforations)
  - No mediastinitis or sever systemic sepsis
- Esophagectomy
  - Unsalvageable esophagus (malignancy, severe peptic or corrosive stricture)
  - Good risk patient (can withstand major resection)
- Esophageal exclusion
  - Delayed presentation
  - With mediastinitis and severe sepsis
- Endoscopic stenting
  - Malignant structure
  - High-risk patient (sepsis and/or comorbid conditions).

SUMMARY

Esophageal perforation is an uncommon problem that is often iatrogenic. The presentation can vary from an asymptomatic extraluminal air to free leakage of the esophageal contents into the surrounding tissues leading a severe inflammatory reaction, sepsis and sometimes multiorgan failure. A high index of suspicion for any out of the ordinary symptoms after an endoscopic procedure can help in early diagnosis and treatment. Early institution of appropriate treatment is a very important determinant of good outcome in esophageal perforation. Most of the mortality due to esophageal perforation is related to delayed diagnosis, severe sepsis and resultant multiorgan failure. Surgery has been the standard of care for most patients with esophageal perforation and primary repair of the perforation is the procedure of choice. Intervention radiology support is crucial in obtaining good drainage and control of sepsis. Endoscopic interventions are making rapid advances and their role will become clearer in the near future, with more patients undergoing endoscopic procedures for esophageal perforations.

REFERENCES

1. Vidarsdottir H, Blondal S, Alfredsson H, Geirsson A, Gudbjartsson T. Oesophageal perforations in Iceland: a whole population study on incidence, aetiology and surgical outcome. Thorac Cardiovasc Surg. 2010;58(8):476-80.
2. Biancari F, D'Andrea V, Paone R, Di Marco C, Savino G, Koivukangas V, et al. Current treatment and outcome of esophageal perforations in adults: systematic review and meta-analysis of 75 studies. World J Surg. 2013;37(5):1051-9.
3. Bhatia P, Fortin D, Inculet RI, Malthaner RA. Current concepts in the management of esophageal perforations: a twenty-seven year Canadian experience. Ann Thorac Surg. 2011;92(1):209-15.
4. Younes Z, Johnson DA. The spectrum of spontaneous and iatrogenic esophageal injury: perforations, Mallory-Weiss tears, and hematomas. J Clin Gastroenterol. 1999;29:306-17.
5. Brinster CJ, Singhal S, Lee L, Marshall MB, Kaiser LR, Kucharczuk JC. Evolving options in the management of esophageal perforation. Ann Thorac Surg. 2004;77(4):1475-83.
6. Asensio JA, Chahwan S, Forno W, MacKersie R, Wall M, Lake J, et al. Penetrating esophageal injuries: multicenter study of the American Association for the Surgery of Trauma. J Trauma. 2001;50(2):289-96.
7. Hirshberg A, Wall MJ, Johnston RH Jr, Burch JM, Mattox KL. Transcervical gunshot injuries. Am J Surg. 1994;167(3):309-12.
8. Demetriades D, Theodorou D, Cornwell E, Asensio J, Belzberg H, Velmahos G, et al. Transcervical gunshot injuries: mandatory operation is not necessary. J Trauma. 1996;40(5):758-60.
9. Wu JT, Mattox KL, Wall MJ Jr. Esophageal perforation: new perspectives and treatment paradigms. J Trauma. 2007;63(5): 1173-84.
10. Sarr MD, Pemberton JH, Payne WS. Management of instrumental perforations of the esophagus. J Thorac Cardiovasc Surg. 1982;84(2):211-8.
11. Jones WG II, Ginsberg RJ. Esophageal perforation: a continuing challenge. Ann Thorac Surg. 1992;53(3):534-54.
12. Buecker A, Wein BB, Neuerburg JM, Guenther RW. Esophageal perforation: comparison of use of aqueous and barium-containing contrast media. Radiology. 1997;202(3):683-6.
13. Wu CH, Chen CM, Chen CC, Wong YC, Wang CJ, Lo WC, et al. Esophagography after pneumomediastinum without CT findings of esophageal perforation: is it necessary? AJR Am J Roentgenol. 2013;201(5):977-84.
14. Pasricha PJ, Fleischer DE, Kalloo AN. Endoscopic perforations of the upper digestive tract: a review of their pathogenesis, prevention, and management. Gastroenterology. 1994;106(3):787-802.
15. Arantes V, Campolina C, Valerio SH, de Sa RN, Toledo C, Ferrari TA, et al. Flexible esophagoscopy as a diagnostic tool for traumatic esophageal injuries. J Trauma. 2009;66(6):1677-82.
16. Griffin SM, Lamb PJ, Dresner SM, Richardson DL, Hayes N. Diagnosis and management of a mediastinal leak following radical oesophagectomy. Br J Surg. 2001;88(10):1346-51.
17. Kuppusamy MK, Felisky C, Kozarek RA, Schembre D, Ross A, Gan I, et al. Impact of endoscopic assessment and treatment on operative and non-operative management of acute oesophageal perforation. Br J Surg. 2011;98(6):818-24.
18. Biancari F, D'Andrea V, Paone R, Di Marco C, Savino G, Koivukangas V, et al. Current treatment and outcome of esophageal perforations in adults: systematic review and meta-analysis of 75 studies. World J Surg. 2013;37(5):1051-9.
19. Hoffmann M, Kujath P, Vogt FM, Laubert T, Limmer S, Mulrooney T, et al. Outcome and management of invasive candidiasis following oesophageal perforation. Mycoses. 2013;56(2):173-8.
20. Singh RK, Sahni P, Chattopadhyay TK. Esophageal perforation– the problems of late presentation. Hepatogastroenterology. 2008;55(88):2103-7.
21. Vogel SB, Rout WR, Martin TD, Abbitt PL. Esophageal perforation in adults: aggressive, conservative treatment lowers morbidity and mortality. Ann Surg. 2005;241(6):1016-21
22. Cameron JL, Kieffer RF, Hendrix TR, Mehigan DG, Baker RR. Selective nonoperative management of contained intrathoracic esophageal disruptions. Ann Thorac Surg. 1979;27(5):404-8.
23. Lyons WS, Seremetis MG, deGuzman VC, Peabody JW Jr. Ruptures and perforations of the esophagus: the case for conservative supportive management. Ann Thorac Surg. 1978;25(4):346-50.
24. Altorjay A, Kiss J, Vörös A, Bohák A. Nonoperative management of esophageal perforations. Is it justified? Ann Surg. 1997; 225(4):415-21.
25. Bardaxoglou E, Manganas D, Meunier B, Landen S, Maddern GJ, Campion JP, et al. New approach to surgical management of early esophageal thoracic perforation: primary suture repair reinforced with absorbable mesh and fibrin glue. World J Surg. 1997;21(6): 618-21.
26. Wright CD, Mathisen DJ, Wain JC, Moncure AC, Hilgenberg AD, Grillo HC. Reinforced primary repair of thoracic esophageal perforation. Ann Thorac Surg. 1995;60(2):245-8.
27. Whyte RI, Iannettoni MD, Orringer MB. Intrathoracic esophageal perforation. The merit of primary repair. J Thorac Cardiovasc Surg. 1995;109(1):140-6.
28. Wang N, Razzouk AJ, Safavi A, Gan K, Van Arsdell GS, Burton PM, et al. Delayed primary repair of intrathoracic esophageal perforation: is it safe? J Thorac Cardiovasc Surg. 1996;111(1):114-21.
29. Linden PA, Bueno R, Mentzer SJ, Zellos L, Lebenthal A, Colson YL, et al. Modified T-tube repair of delayed esophageal perforation results in a low mortality rate similar to that seen with acute perforations. Ann Thorac Surg. 2007;83(3):1129-33.
30. Bufkin BL, Miller JI Jr, Mansour KA. Esophageal perforation: emphasis on management. Ann Thorac Surg. 1996;61(5):1447-51.
31. Martinez L, Rivas S, Hernández F, Avila LF, Lassaletta L, Murcia J, et al. Aggressive conservative treatment of esophageal perforations in children. J Pediatr Surg. 2003;38(5):685-9.
32. Urschel HC, Razzuk MA, Wood RE, Galbraith N, Pockey M, Paulson DL. Improved management of esophageal perforation: exclusion and diversion in continuity. Ann Surg. 1974;179(5):587-91.
33. Chang CH, Lin PJ, Chang JP, Hsieh MJ, Lee MC, Chu JJ. One-stage operation for treatment after delayed diagnosis of thoracic esophageal perforation. Ann Thorac Surg. 1992;53(4):617-20.
34. Bardini R, Bonavina L, Pavanello M, Asolati M, Peracchia A. Temporary double exclusion of the perforated esophagus using absorbable staples. Ann Thorac Surg. 1992;54(6):1165-7.
35. Altorjay A, Kiss J, Vörös A, Szirányi E. The role of esophagectomy in the management of esophageal perforations. Ann Thorac Surg. 1998;65(5):1433-6.
36. Gupta NM, Kaman L. Personal management of 57 consecutive patients with esophageal perforation. Am J Surg. 2004;187(1):58-63.
37. Iannettoni MD, Vlessis AA, Whyte RI, Orringer MB. Functional outcome after surgical treatment of esophageal perforation. Ann Thorac Surg. 1997;64(6):1606-9.
38. Dai Y, Chopra SS, Kneif S, Hünerbein M. Management of esophageal anastomotic leaks, perforations, and fistulae with self-expanding plastic stents. J Thorac Cardiovasc Surg. 2011;141(5):1213-7.
39. Ben-David K, Lopes J, Hochwald S, Draganov P, Forsmark C, Collins D, et al. Minimally invasive treatment of esophageal

perforation using a multidisciplinary treatment algorithm: a case series. Endoscopy. 2011;43(2):160-2.
40. Ben-David K, Behrns K, Hochwald S, Rossidis G, Caban A, Crippen C, et al. Esophageal perforation management using a multidisciplinary minimally invasive treatment algorithm. J Am Coll Surg. 2014;218(4):768-74.
41. van Boeckel PG, Sijbring A, Vleggaar FP, Siersema PD. Systematic review: temporary stent placement for benign rupture or anastomotic leak of the oesophagus. Aliment Pharmacol Ther. 2011;33(12):1292-301.
42. Freeman RK, Ascioti AJ, Giannini T, Mahidhara RJ. Analysis of unsuccessful esophageal stent placements for esophageal perforation, fistula, or anastomotic leak. Ann Thorac Surg. 2012;94(3):959-64.
43. Heits N, Stapel L, Reichert B, Schafmayer C, Schniewind B, Becker T, et al. Endoscopic endoluminal vacuum therapy in esophageal perforation. Ann Thorac Surg. 2014;97(3):1029-35.
44. Jay Yuan, Baichoo E, Wong Kee Song LM. Endoscopic therapies for acute esophageal perforations and leaks. Techniques in Gastrointestinal Endoscopy. 2014;16(1):53-61. Available on Science direct - Not quoted in Pubmed.
45. Abbas G, Schuchert MJ, Pettiford BL, Pennathur A, Landreneau J, Landreneau J, et al. Contemporaneous management of esophageal perforation. Surgery. 2009;146(4):749-55.
46. Maier A, Pinter H, Anegg U, Fell B, Tomaselli F, Sankin O, et al. Boerhaave's syndrome: a continuing challenge in thoracic surgery. Hepatogastroenterology. 2001;48(41):1368-71.
47. Furugaki K, Yoshida J, Hokazono K, Emoto T, Nakashima J, Ohyama M, et al. Esophageal ruptures: triage using the systemic inflammatory response syndrome score. Gen Thorac Cardiovasc Surg. 2011;59(3):220-4.
48. Biancari F, Saarnio J, Mennander A, Hypén L, Salminen P, Kuttila K, et al. Outcome of patients with esophageal perforations: a multicenter study. World J Surg. 2014;38(4):902-9.

CHAPTER 16

Corrosive Injury of Esophagus and Stomach

N Ananthakrishnan, R Kalayarasan, Vikram Kate

INTRODUCTION

Corrosive injuries of the esophagus, while less frequent in developed countries are by far the most common cause of benign esophageal obstruction in India.[1] The devastating effect of corrosive ingestion on the upper gastrointestinal tract can pose a significant management challenge. Treatment of these patients can consume considerable health resources since management is long drawn and punctuated by fresh complaints that appear from time to time. Every management decision taken right from the occurrence of the corrosive incident has a bearing on the outcome of these patients. In view of the relative low incidence of corrosive ingestion, individual physicians have little clinical experience with management of these patients. An incorrect management decision or an inappropriate surgical procedure by the clinician can delay or adversely affect the outcome of these patients or make future surgery impossible. Hence, a good understanding of the clinical manifestation and management of corrosive injuries of the esophagus and stomach is essential to avoid such pitfalls. This chapter aims to provide an outline of the diagnosis and management of a patient with corrosive injury of the esophagus and stomach.

EPIDEMIOLOGY

A corrosive substance can cause destruction or damage to living tissue on contact. The word "corrosion" is derived from the Latin verb *corrodere* which means "to gnaw". This term signifies how the corrosive substances "gnaw" their way through the flesh. Corrosives are broadly classified into acids and alkali. The commonly used term "lye" refers to a strong alkali.[2] The alkalis commonly implicated in corrosive poisoning include sodium hydroxide containing bathroom cleaners and dish washing agents. The usual acid containing substances incriminated in corrosive poisoning are toilet cleaning agents which contain Nitric or hydrochloric acid and antirust compound with hydrochloric, oxalic and hydrofluoric acid as constituent.

The chemical agents responsible for corrosive poisoning are not uniform worldwide. In the annual report of the American Association of Poison Control Centers (AAPCC) in 2008, sodium hypochlorite, a usual alkali constituent in various cleaning agents was the most commonly implicated corrosive agent.[2] Reports from other countries in the West also showed that ingestion of alkalis was the most common cause of corrosive poisoning.[3-6] In contrast to the Western data, the majority of corrosive ingestions in India are due to acids as these are most commonly used in toilet cleaners compared to a more expensive caustic soda. In a study from a center in South India, the predominant acid containing substances implicated in corrosive poisoning were hydrochloric acid containing toilet cleaners and aqua regia or goldsmith's solvent which contains hydrochloric and nitric acid in 3:1 proportion.[7]

Accidental corrosive ingestion is common in children especially male child due to their curious nature and tendency to scan household goods and ingest corrosive containing products. According to the 2008 AAPCC annual report, ingestion of corrosives was an important cause of poisonings in children after cosmetics and analgesics.[2] A study from India reported that consumption of corrosives was responsible for approximately 8% of acute poisoning cases among children admitted to a referral center.[8] A multicenter study of poisoning among Indian children revealed that corrosive ingestion was an important cause of poisoning ranking behind kerosene, drugs and pesticide poisonings.[9]

Corrosive ingestion in adults could be suicidal or accidental. In a Singaporean study published in 1950s corrosive poisoning accounted for approximately 30% of all suicidal deaths.[10] After the introduction of the law to ban over-the-counter sale of caustic soda the proportion of suicidal deaths secondary to corrosive ingestion showed a steady decline. In addition, there is a steady increase in the suicide rate worldwide and non-corrosive methods were often used by people who intend to commit suicide. The reflection of this trend is the recent data from USA where only 4.5% of all corrosive ingestions were with suicidal intent.[2] The major problem with Indian data on suicides is attempted cases of suicides are grossly under-reported. According to 2005 data the national suicide rate was 10.3/100,000 population and Puducherry with the suicide rate of 52.1/100,000 population topped the list.[11,12] In this data corrosive ingestion was clubbed with other poisons and hence the data on the frequency of suicidal deaths secondary to corrosive ingestion could not be ascertained. As a result, in India hospital admission data of poisoning due to corrosives in referral centers is an important source of data, which suggest that one in two corrosive ingestion are with suicidal intent.[1] Some authors have suggested that suicidal ingestion tends to be associated with higher grades of tissue injury.[13] Since patients who consume corrosive with suicidal intent tend to ingest it with some hesitancy oral cavity, oropharynx and proximal esophagus are severely injured. On the other hand, accidental intake is often associated with rapid consumption of corrosives in larger amount without knowing that they are corrosives and are frequently associated with gastric injuries.

Data from the USA have shown that the poisonings related to corrosive intake has remained unchanged at approximately 9% over the years.[2] However, the introduction of strict safety laws like use of child-proof safety caps on toilet cleaners bottles reduced the incidence of corrosive poisoning in children. However, such safety laws to limit accidental corrosive ingestion among children are not there in many developing countries including India.

PATHOPHYSIOLOGY

The extent of injury following corrosive ingestion is determined by the nature and amount of corrosive ingested. Since Alkaline agents are usually colorless and relatively tasteless with less marked odor, they are often consumed in larger quantity. Alkalis produce liquefaction necrosis that often results in deep tissue injury. Caustic soda (sodium hydroxide), a common constituent in cleaning agents, is very dangerous, particularly in liquid form. It has been found in experimental animals that a 30% solution of caustic soda can cause full-thickness esophageal necrosis with just 1-second exposure. The combination of the viscous nature of alkali with tendency to adhere to the esophageal mucosa and the process of liquefaction necrosis increase the likelihood of transmural injuries. In addition, alkalis are more likely to produce periesophageal injury with damage to adjacent organs like the respiratory tract. Tissue injury following alkali ingestion can be classified into an acute necrotic phase (phase 1) which lasts for 24–72 hours after injury followed by an ulceration and granulation phase (phase 2) which lasts approximately for 3–12 days.[14] The esophagus is at its weakest point during this second phase. Cicatrization and scarring (phase 3) begins approximately 3 weeks after the initial injury resulting in stricture formation.

Acids usually cause coagulation necrosis as opposed to alkalis. The coagulum formed in response to acid ingestion prevents the transmural spread of corrosive agent thereby reducing the likelihood of full thickness injury. Hydrofluoric acid is an exception as it produces liquefactive necrosis. In addition, severe transmural injury with or without perforation may occur if acids in concentrated form are consumed in larger quantity. Usually, acids with a pH < 2 are corrosive, but pH alone does not determine the severity of injury, other parameters of acid like molarity and complexing capacity play an important role in determining the extent of injury. Due to their strong odor and obnoxious taste, acids are usually taken in a little amount, are consumed quickly and tend to cause more damage to the stomach compared to esophagus. While there is a dictum that "Acid licks the esophagus and bites the stomach" a few authors have questioned the dictum and shown that damage to esophagus is common even after acid ingestion.[15] It is also proposed that injuries of the gastric antrum is more common in fasting state, and the body of the stomach is more commonly affected if the ingestion occurs in the postprandial state.[1] In the largest Indian experience, reported from author's center, 82.6% of 109 gastric injuries were secondary to acid ingestion.[7] The majority of the patients had strictures in the prepyloric region (83.5%), and others had strictures in the region of antrum, body, pyloroduodenal area or diffuse gastric stricture.

Small bowel injuries are uncommon with corrosive ingestion since experimental studies have shown that soon after ingested corrosives enter the stomach there is a reflex pyloric spasm which limits the passage of the corrosive into the duodenum. However, following gastric surgeries involving pyloric ablation or bypass, ingested acid can enter the small intestine rapidly and can cause significant injury. In addition, in rare circumstances when corrosives are taken in considerable amount especially when mixed with other fluids which can dilute the acids, it can enter the small bowel in significant amount causing full thickness necrosis with relative sparing of the proximal gastrointestinal tract (Fig. 1).[16]

Sequelae of corrosive ingestions depend upon the extent of the initial injury. Mild injuries involving only the mucosa usually heal without any complications. While moderate injuries extending beyond mucosa heal with esophageal stricture severe transmural injuries results in perforation in the acute phase, or dense, undilatable stricture in the recovery phase.

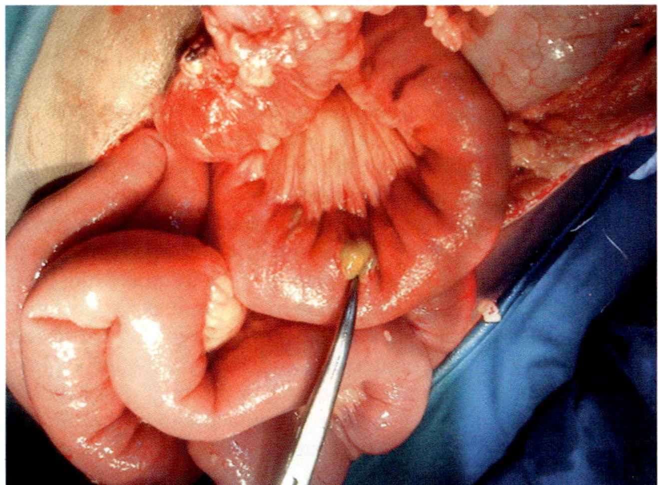

Figure 1 Isolated jejunal necrosis in a patient sparing the esophagus and the stomach

CLINICAL FEATURES

Clinical presentation depends upon the extent of injury which is determined by the amount of corrosive ingested, nature of the substance (strong or weak corrosive) and physical form of the corrosive (solid or liquid). In the mildest form, the patient may be asymptomatic or presents with mild symptoms like throat pain without any voice change or dysphagia. On examination of the oral cavity, there may be normal mucosa or mild erythema in the oropharynx. In moderate to severe injuries, the patient presents with significant symptoms. Odynophagia and dysphagia indicate extensive esophageal involvement.[17] Presence of stridor or hoarseness suggests upper airway involvement. Epigastric pain and hematemesis suggest involvement of the stomach; although significant overlap of symptoms can occur.[18] On examination of patients with severe injuries there may be respiratory distress with tachycardia and drooling saliva. The oropharyngeal mucosa and lips may show ulceration or adherent slough. Presence of abdominal tenderness and peritoneal signs is an ominous sign suggesting gastric necrosis. Gastric or esophageal perforation can occur at any time during the first 2 weeks, although the incidence is maximum between day 3 and 12 following ingestion.[2] Therefore, any alteration in the patient's clinical course in the form of worsening abdominal pain (indicating gastric perforation) or development of chest pain (indicating esophageal perforation) requires immediate radiological evaluation. Clinical manifestation of late sequelae depends upon the location and extent of stricture. While dysphagia is the typical symptom of patients with esophageal stricture patients with isolated gastric stricture present with symptoms of gastric outlet obstruction.

INVESTIGATIONS

In corrosive ingestion, diagnosis can be established in the majority of the patients by history and clinical examination and investigations are required only to document the extent of injury. Upper gastrointestinal endoscopy is a valuable investigation for planning management of caustic ingestion. However, there is some controversy regarding the timing of endoscopy. Some authors recommend early endoscopy within 24 hours after ingestion, while others recommend between 48 and 72 hours after ingestion. Proponents of early endoscopy suggest that early endoscopic grading of injury permits early discharge of patients with no evidence of gastrointestinal injury and facilitates appropriate management of patients with severe injury.[19] Authors recommend between 48-72 hours after ingestion since early endoscopy carries the risk of misdiagnosing the extent of transmural damage in the presence of extensive hyperemia; in addition endoscopic procedure related risk does not increase until 96 hours post-ingestion.[20] However, due to increased risk of iatrogenic perforation, upper gastrointestinal endoscopy is better avoided between 5 and 15 days after ingestion. A thorough but cautious examination of the esophagus and stomach should be tried in contrast to the earlier recommendation that the endoscopy should not be advanced past the first sign of injury. The modern, flexible narrow-caliber endoscopes passed with minimal insufflation by a skilled operator do not increase the risk of perforation, and the initial recommendation stemmed from rigid scopes used in the past. The findings on endoscopy are usually graded using the classification proposed by Zargar et al.

- Grade 1—only erythema and edema.
- Grade 2a—hemorrhage, erosions, blisters and ulcers with exudate.
- Grade 2b—circumferential esophageal ulceration.
- Grade 3a—scattered deep ulcers with brown, black and gray discoloration.
- Grade 3b—extensive deep ulcers with brown, black and gray discoloration.
- Grade 4—esophageal perforation.

Patients with Grade 1 and 2a injury usually recover without any sequelae, whereas a significant proportion of patients with Grade 2b injury and almost all patients with Grade 3 injury will develop stricture of the esophagus or stomach, or both, which will require therapeutic intervention.[20]

The role of radiographic examination in the acute phase is limited to plain X-rays. Serial chest and abdominal radiographs are indicated in patients with doubtful chest and abdominal examination findings to diagnose perforation. Barium or water soluble contrast study is contraindicated in the acute phase since in patients with perforation extravasated barium can induce severe inflammatory reaction. While water soluble contrast study is relatively safe in patients with perforation, aspiration of these agents (common in the acute phase) can result in severe pulmonary complications. However, contrast study of upper digestive tract is an essential investigation in the late phase to diagnose the location and extent of stricture. A computed tomography (CT) scan is indicated for a patient with equivocal findings on endoscopic examination, and there is a strong index of suspicion for a perforation. Millar et al. reported that technetium labeled sucralfate swallow is an accurate investigation to assess the extent of esophageal injury. Since sucralfate adheres to the ulcerated mucosa, it can be used as an alternative to endoscopy especially in children who require general anesthesia for endoscopy.[21] Some authors advocate diagnostic laparoscopy in patients with higher grades of injury on endoscopic examination to rule out full thickness injury to stomach.[22]

MANAGEMENT: ACUTE PHASE

Nonoperative Treatment

Acute phase management follows basic principles of resuscitation with maintenance of airway and circulation. Both gastric lavage and induced emesis are contraindicated as this result in additional esophageal injury secondary to re-exposure of the esophagus to the corrosive agent.[22] Similarly, neutralization of acids with alkali and vice versa is contraindicated as heat generated by the exothermic chemical reaction might aggravate the tissue injury. Similarly, there is very little role for measures to dilute the corrosive with milk or water, as the extent of the injury is usually determined within minutes after ingestion of corrosive agent. Broad-spectrum antibiotics are recommended in patients with second or greater degree injuries, although no controlled data are available. Some advocate antibiotics only in patients receiving steroids. Since the oropharynx and upper esophagus are home to many virulent bacteria, there is potential for systemic sepsis in higher grade injuries. Hence, broad-spectrum intravenous antibiotics active against oral and intestinal flora should be administered. Intravenous proton pump inhibitors should be given in patients with higher grade injuries to minimize the insult to the injured gastric mucosa and avoid exacerbation of the esophageal injury by superimposed gastroesophageal reflux.[23] The debate on the use of corticosteroids in patients with corrosive injury to avert stricture formation has been laid to rest with the conclusion of two recent meta-analyses that the corticosteroids do not prevent the development of strictures following corrosive ingestion and their use may lead to the development of serious adverse effects.[24,25] Some advocate nasogastric tube insertion in the acute phase of corrosive injury.[26] The advantages of early nasogastric tube placement are it facilitates enteral feeding and can provide a lumen for dilatation if a tight stricture develops. This is particularly important in high esophageal or pharyngoesophageal strictures to avoid complete closure of the pharyngoesophageal junction. However, placement of a nasogastric tube itself can facilitate the development of long strictures.[26] Hence nasogastric tube placement is not routinely advocated, and the decision has to be taken on a case to case basis. Few authors have advocated early placement of stents to prevent stricture formation.[27] Specially, designed silicone rubber or polyflex stents are used for this purpose. However, drawbacks associated with stent placement are limited success rate (< 50%), a high incidence of migration (up to 25%) and the potential for hyperplastic response to placed stents. Recently biodegradable stents made of poly-*L*-lactide or polydioxanone have been introduced. Theoretically prolonged dilatory effect before progressive degradation of biodegradable stents makes them ideal for prevention and treatment of benign esophageal strictures.[28] However, in limited clinical experience the success rate is only 45% and is associated with 10% migration rate.[29] Considering the cost, limited success rate and association with potential complications like migration, stents are not routinely recommended in the acute management of corrosive injuries. Early dilatation starting after injury as advocated by few authors is not recommended as it is associated with increased risk of perforation.[26] Many pharmacological agents including mitomycin C, 5-fluorouracil, vitamin E, octreotide and interferon-alfa-2b have been tried in experimental and clinical setting to prevent stricture formation; however, none of them have been proven to be of significant benefit.[29]

Surgical Management

Indications for surgical intervention in the acute phase include:

- Esophageal perforation
- Peritonitis
- Uncontrolled massive hematemesis.

Since the interval between ingestion and time of surgery in the acute phase is an important determinant of outcome following surgery, there should be a low threshold for consideration of laparotomy at the earliest clinical suspicion. Presence of hemodynamic instability and extensive injury on endoscopy is a strong indication for emergency surgical intervention even in the absence of obvious peritoneal signs or mediastinitis. Cheng et al. have shown that the presence of metabolic acidosis predicts transmural necrosis in these patients and can guide the decision for operative intervention.[30] Some advocate laparoscopy before formal laparotomy in these patients to avoid non-therapeutic laparotomy. The concern with this approach is that diagnostic laparoscopy is not a substitute for a thorough abdominal exploration, especially of the posterior aspects of the stomach and duodenum which are the usual locations for more severe injuries. In addition, laparoscopy should not overly extend the duration of surgery as time is a major determinant of outcome in this situation.

Surgical options depend upon the extent of injury, and radical removal of all necrotic tissue is recommended to improve outcome in these patients. In patients with isolated extensive gastric necrosis, a total or partial gastrectomy is performed depending upon the extent of involvement.[31] In the presence of equivocal findings, before planning a resection, an anterior gastrotomy is made to assess the extent of transmural and mucosal necrosis, since mucosal necrosis is more extensive than what is apparent from the serosal side. After total gastrectomy, decision for reconstruction depends upon the general condition of the patient. Critically ill patients do not withstand lengthy reconstructive procedures, hence it is appropriate to perform only drainage of the esophageal, and duodenal stump, with a feeding jejunostomy, leaving reconstruction (using a jejunal loop) for a more opportune moment should the patient comes out of the acute phase. There is no role for procedures such as direct closure of a perforation since the stomach is like wet blotting paper around the site of perforation.

In the more common scenario of associated esophageal injury with gastric injury, subtotal esophagectomy with gastrectomy is recommended. A significantly higher mortality (66%) has been reported in patients in whom a thoracoabdominal approach was used for esophageal resection. Brun et al. reported that blunt esophageal stripping avoids thoracotomy and reduces mortality in these critically ill patients.[32] The thrombosis of perivisceral vessels, corrosive induced periesophageal edema and the lack of mediastinal adhesions in the acute phase facilitates blunt esophageal stripping. It is preferable to avoid reconstruction in the acute phase. The proximal esophagus is brought out as an esophagostomy, and a feeding jejunostomy is done. In some patients, corrosive injury can extend beyond the stomach and the esophagus to the adjacent organs like pancreas, colon and small bowel. These patients require the additional visceral resection such as pancreatoduodenectomy, colonic or small bowel resection in addition to esophagogastrectomy. Morbidity and mortality is high after extensive surgical resection.[33]

MANAGEMENT: CHRONIC PHASE

Endoscopic Dilatation of Stricture

Stricture is an important late sequel following corrosive ingestion. It begins within the first 2–3 weeks and may progress rapidly. Endoscopic dilatation can be done by using either bougie (like Savary-Gilliard dilators) or balloon dilators. Savary bougie dilators offer the operator the advantage of feeling the dilatation occurring under his hands whereas balloon dilators allow the dilatation to be performed under vision.[29] The accepted endoscopic dilatation procedure for esophageal stricture is frequent dilatation at appropriate intervals to achieve an esophageal lumen size of 15 mm with complete relief of dysphagia.[1] Afterwards, repeat dilatation is performed whenever dysphagia recurs. The data from various Indian centers show encouraging results with endoscopic dilatation in those selected group of patients where the type of stricture permits endoscopic therapy.[1] Only a limited number of studies have assessed the long-term outcomes and

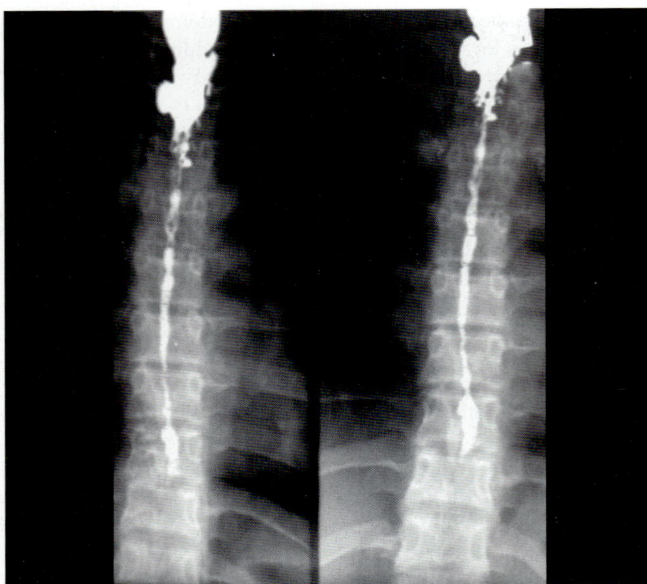

Figure 2 Upper gastrointestinal contrast study of a patient with long esophageal stricture

stricture recurrence rate with endoscopic therapy in patients with the corrosive stricture.[1,34] Recurrence rate following endoscopic dilatation is more in corrosive stricture compared to benign peptic stricture in one study.[34] But, there is a progressive decrease in the recurrence rate with time and the difference between corrosive and peptic stricture groups becomes insignificant after 36 months. However, not all strictures are amenable for endoscopic dilatation and surgery is indicated in following circumstances:

- Long esophageal strictures (>10 cm) as dilatation of these strictures are associated with a high incidence of perforation (Fig. 2).
- Multiple esophageal strictures defined as more than three in one study.[35]
- Irregular narrowing with sacculations of the esophageal lumen which is prone for dilatation induced perforation.
- Failed dilatation that is defined as the requirement of more than five sessions of endoscopic dilatation in one study.[35]
- Need for frequent dilatation to maintain satisfactory swallowing.
- Previous dilatation related complications like perforation.

SURGICAL MANAGEMENT OF STRICTURE

Optimum Time for Reconstruction

Waiting for the scarring process to end before undertaking reconstruction for caustic injury is imperative to avoid anastomotic stricture formation. However, the optimum time for reconstruction after corrosive ingestion has not been clearly defined in the literature, with the reported period for reconstruction ranging from 2 months to several years in different series.[36] Demirbilek et al. in an experimental study on rats found that although collagen deposition peaked during the second week it continued for a long time post-corrosive induced esophageal injury.[37] The fact that fibrosis continued for about 6–12 months following corrosive injury suggests that the edge of the esophageal stricture might not be defined until then. Better results are achieved in the series where the reconstruction has been delayed for 6–12 months. Longer waiting time is preferred especially in patients with associated pharyngeal strictures. Another factor which determines the optimum time of reconstruction is the nutritional status of these patients, since the majority are malnourished secondary to dysphagia. If nasogastric tube was placed in the acute phase it can be used for feeding. However, long-term tolerance is poor with nasogastric tube feeding. Hence, a feeding jejunostomy or gastrostomy is required. Since stomach will also be frequently affected in corrosive injury and gastrostomy precludes stomach as an option for esophageal replacement, feeding jejunostomy is the preferred method for enteral nutrition in patients with corrosive stricture of the esophagus and stomach.

ESOPHAGEAL RESECTION VERSUS ESOPHAGEAL BYPASS WITHOUT RESECTION

A major controversy in surgical management of esophageal stricture is whether to resect the damaged esophagus. Many authors advocate esophageal resection for all corrosive esophageal strictures for fear of complications such as malignancy, mucoceles, abscess formation or rupture of esophagus left insitu.[38,39] However, the risk of malignancy, the most feared complication of leaving esophagus in situ has been over emphasized, and the true incidence of malignancy remains uncertain. Several facts need to be considered in assessing the risk of malignancy. Some series report a 2–13% incidence of malignancy after corrosive esophageal injury while others report a very low incidence ranging from 0–2%.[40-43] It is not clear whether any of this data is based on long-term prospective follow-up or pertains only to extrapolated data from a few index cases. In nearly 100 years from 1904–2003, only about 118 cases of post-corrosive carcinoma had been reported worldwide.[44,45] Of 650 patients treated by Kocchar et al. for carcinoma of the esophagus, there were only 2 patients with the history of corrosive ingestion and of 156 patients with corrosive ingestion only 2 patients developed carcinoma.[45] In the authors experience of over 500 corrosive injuries managed over a 30-year period, a single case of a cricopharyngeal cancer occurred in a smoker following caustic esophageal injury and a solitary case of peri-gastroenterostomy stomal cancer 17 years post-acid ingestion.[46] In the latter, the malignancy could be either secondary to corrosive ingestion or chronic bile reflux gastritis.

The next issue regards the relationship of the incidence of carcinoma to the nature of corrosive ingested. Almost all described cases of post-corrosive malignancy in literature had occurred following ingestion of alkali.[43,47] In the highest reported incidence of 13% of malignancy after corrosive ingestion by Kim et al. every one of which was following lye ingestion.[43] The third issue is the risk of carcinoma in a scarred esophagus left after bypass surgery. It has been mentioned in one report that the risk of malignancy decreases after surgery.[47] It has also been mentioned that the possibility of malignant change in strictured esophagus left in situ is negligible as there is no continued mechanical, chemical or thermal irritation of the scarred esophagus.[43,48,49] In addition many of the published reports do not distinguish between cancer in the bypassed segment and cancer in the portion of the esophagus in the food stream. In fact, it has been stated that there is only one reported carcinoma arising in a post-cricoid strictured esophagus that has been excluded from the transit of food.[50]

The fourth issue is whether less serious injuries that are managed by dilatation or no treatment have less risk of malignancy. Published reports state that patients with mild esophageal injury not requiring major reconstructive surgery are also at risk of malignancy.[51] Also, patients requiring frequent endoscopic dilatation could be at a higher risk of carcinoma due to repeated trauma and irritation.[45] If the risk of malignant change were significant, one would find it unethical to offer any non-resectional treatment like the dilatation to a patient who has corrosive induced esophageal injury. Acceptance of endoscopic dilatation as the primary therapeutic modality in patients whose stricture allows endoscopic therapy and the fact that majority of these patients do not develop esophageal malignancy indicates that the fear of malignant change in corrosive injury of the esophagus is overestimated.

The final issue on this subject is the risk of resection versus bypass. Gerzic et al. stated that the routine resection of the esophagus is unnecessary in most patients and can be hazardous.[48] The mortality rate for esophageal resection with reconstruction in their hands was 11.11% versus only 5.68% for bypass alone. Others also advocate bypass over resection since esophagectomy is difficult in these patients and may be associated with injury to adjacent structures due to periesophageal fibrosis and may require a thoracotomy thus adding to the morbidity.[49] To summarize, bypass is preferred over resection in patients with corrosive esophageal stricture in view of:

- The low incidence of malignancy that may approach zero in acid burns which form the predominant cause in Indian scenario.
- The fact that this very low risk is accepted in the vast majority of patients subjected to dilatation,
- The absence of any evidence to suggest that there is an increased risk of malignancy in patients requiring surgery and
- The poor general condition of patients in whom resection with bypass is likely to be associated with a higher mortality and morbidity.

CHOICE OF ESOPHAGEAL REPLACEMENT

The strictured esophagus may be replaced using the stomach, colon or the jejunum.[52] The jejunum is not a preferred conduit because of its limited length. However, supercharged jejunal grafts can be used in the absence of another alternative conduit. Free jejunal grafts may be used to bridge short defects after excision of a localized esophageal stricture. Advantages of the stomach as an esophageal substitute include the relative ease of mobilization and the need for only a single anastomosis. However, frequent involvement of the stomach in the scarring process particularly after acid ingestion makes it a less suitable alternative in patients with corrosive esophageal stricture compared to esophageal cancer.[46] In addition, functional results of gastric conduit tend to deteriorate with time, with the development of symptomatic reflux, stricture and columnar metaplasia of the residual squamous epithelium above the anastomosis in the proximal esophageal remnant.

While colon interposition is a more extensive procedure requiring three anastomoses, the functional results remain stable or improve with time. In addition, colon has a good vascularity and long vascular arcades allow for the transfer without tension and a better luminal match. The choice between right and left colon for esophagocoloplasty is still debated, and results are difficult to compare due to inconsistencies in patient selection and surgical technique used in the reported series. In conventional right colon conduit ileum, ascending colon and the proximal portion of the transverse colon based on middle colic artery and vein is used as conduit and ileum is anastomosed to cervical esophagus (Fig. 3A). The proposed advantages of right colon esophagocoloplasty are prevention of pharyngeal reflux by the preservation of the ileocecal valve, ease of the ileocolic anastomosis compared to a colocolic anastomosis which is required during conventional left coloplasty and, possibility of using the left colon as a rescue conduit in case of postoperative right colon conduit necrosis.[35] The drawback of right colon esophagocoloplasty is vascular anatomy of the right colon is highly variable which predispose to conduit ischemia.

In the conventional left colon esophagocoloplasty transverse colon distal to the hepatic flexure and the proximal portion of descending colon based on ascending branch of left colic artery is used as the conduit (Fig. 3B). The proposed advantages of left colon esophagocoloplasty are reliable vascular supply, and the wall thickness and caliber of the lumen of the left colon make it more suitable for esophageal replacement than the right colon.[52] Drawback of left colon esophagocoloplasty is that the left colon is not infrequently involved by diverticulosis, although it is uncommon in Indian population. Authors proposed a modified technique termed as mid-colon esophagocoloplasty (modified left colon coloplasty) utilizing the benefits of both right colon and left colon (Figs 3C and 4).[53] In this technique, the colon is mobilized

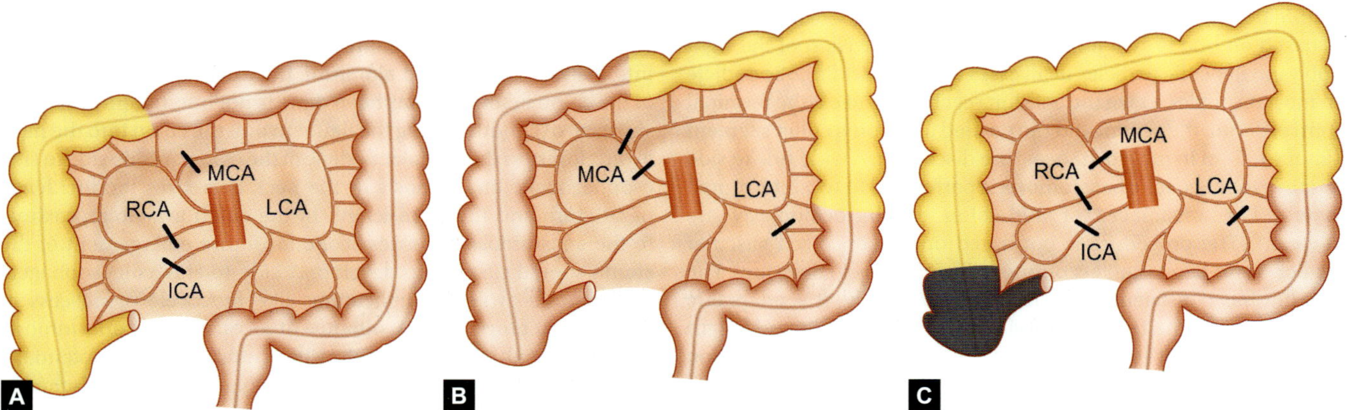

Figures 3A to C Segment of colon used in: (A) right colon esophagocoloplasty; (B) left colon esophagocoloplasty; (C) mid colon esophagocoloplasty.
Abbreviations: ICA, Ileocolic artery; RCA, Right colic artery; MCA, Middle colic artery; LCA, Left colic artery.

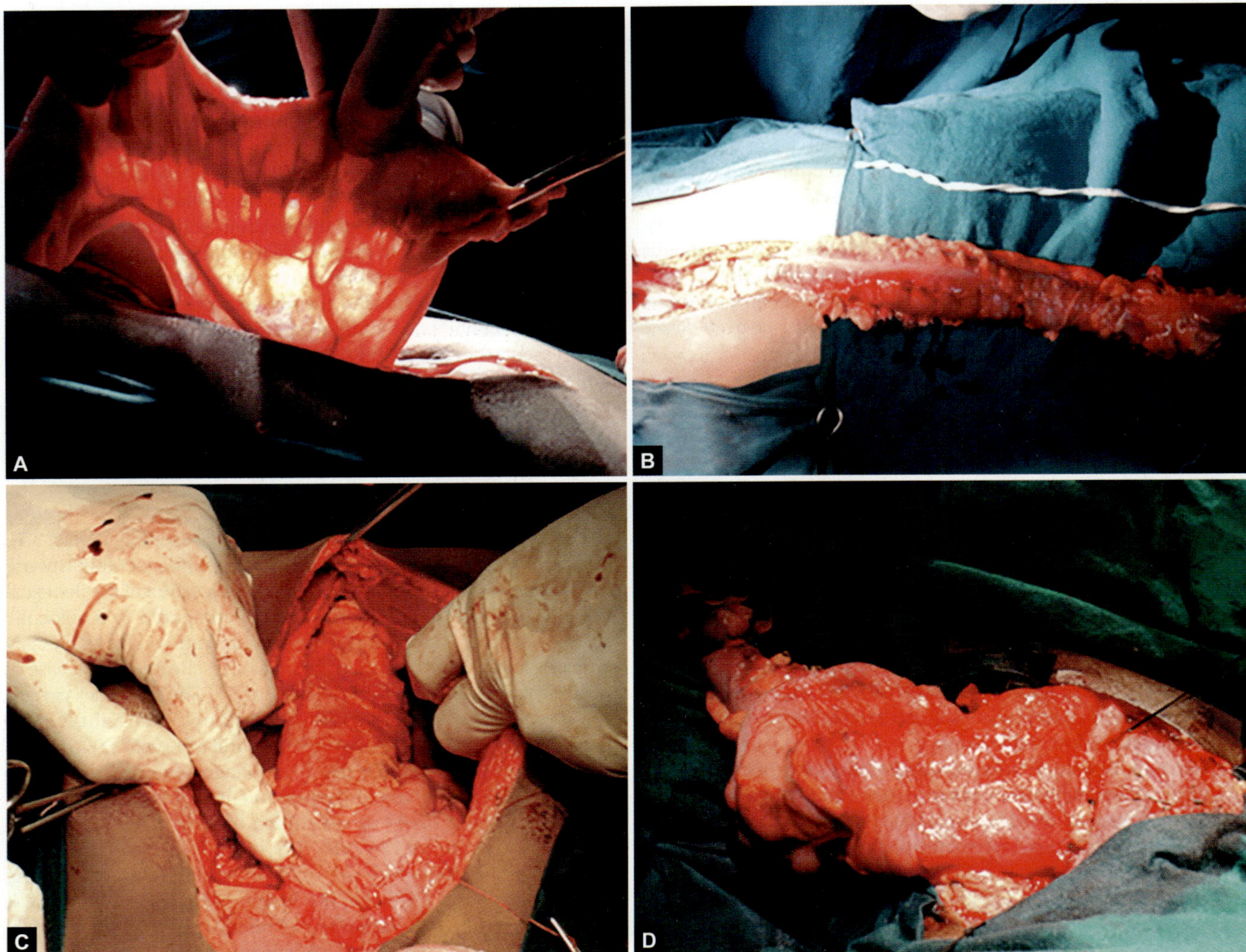

Figures 4A to D Mid-colon esophagocoloplasty: (A) transillumination to demonstrate vascular arcade (conduit based on ascending branch of left colic artery); (B) testing for adequacy of the colonic length by placing it on the chest before drawing it through retrosternal tunnel; (C) conduit placed in the retrosternal tunnel; (D) completed esophagocolic anastomosis. Note the extra length of colon available after anastomosis which can be excised

from the terminal ileum to the mid descending colon. The descending colon is divided beyond the left colic vessels and the terminal ileum about 2 cm from the ileocecal valve. Colonic conduit is based on one or two left colic vessels with division of the right colic and ileocolic pedicles in all cases and the middle colic pedicle in most instances. Once the conduit reaches the neck, the terminal 2 cm of ileum, the cecum and the unused ascending colon segment (about 4–5 cm in most instances) are discarded. A wide side to side (5 cm) esophagocolic anastomosis is performed in two interrupted layers. The advantages of mid-colon esophagocoloplasty are several.[46] The procedure is not based on preconceived vascular pedicles and hence can accommodate variations in anatomy. The conduit has consistent and good vascular supply. It is adaptable with respect to the feeding vessels. There is no problem of length since the segment to be used is not divided until after the colon is drawn into the neck without tension. The main problems with conventional right and left esophagocoloplasty are shortage of colonic length leading to tension at the end to side anastomotic site which contributes to both a fistula and a cervical anastomotic stenosis and necrosis of the colon due to poor vascularity. Authors have consistently found that the correct length of the colon required can be accurately assessed only when it has been mobilized, pulled into the neck and placed alongside the esophagus. Prior division of the colon before this has been done is not infrequently met with shortage of conduit. Using the ileum to pull the colon into the neck avoids injury to the vascular pedicle of the colon. A wide side to side esophagocolic anastomosis in the neck decreases the incidence of stricture and the extra length of the colon available proximal to the anastomosis provides scope for future enlargement of the stoma should a stricture develop. A side to side coloesophageal anastomosis avoids complications like mucocele or abscess in the residual esophagus. Avoidance of an end to side anastomosis ensures that the terminal end of the colon, which is potentially ischemic, does not form part of the anastomosis. An ischemic colon is the most frequent cause of a cervical salivary fistula. Authors had only one instance of colonic necrosis in 105 instances.

A mid colon conduit is possible irrespective of gastric involvement and previous gastroenterostomy also does not preclude its use. In the author's experience of modified left colon esophagocoloplasty in 105 patients over a period of 30 years 72 (68.6%) patients had normal swallowing and 33 (31.4%) had only occasional minor difficulty with solid food on long-term follow-up.

ROUTES FOR ESOPHAGEAL BYPASS

The routes available for the conduit transfer are the posterior mediastinum, the anterior mediastinum (retrosternal route) or the subcutaneous route. Unlike esophageal cancer where graft is positioned in the posterior mediastinum in the bed of the excised esophagus, the retrosternal route is commonly used in surgery for corrosive stricture as the native esophagus is left in situ in the majority of the patients. When the conduit is placed substernally few authors recommend an enlargement of the thoracic inlet by removing the medial aspect of the left clavicle, the left half of the manubrium, and the medial portions of the first and second ribs.[52] However, in the authors experience, it is not required in the vast majority of the patients.[46] Excision of xiphoid process is recommended to avoid sharp pressure on the colon at the junction of the retrosternal tunnel and peritoneal cavity. The subcutaneous route is generally not recommended as it results in poor cosmetic outcome. However, it may be required in following scenarios:

- Previous esophageal perforation with mediastinitis.
- Inadequate space in the anterior mediastinum especially in children.
- Gross posterior protrusion of sternoclavicular joints.
- Presence of coexistent conditions like heart disease that may require thoracotomy later.

Questionable viability of the conduit is not a reason to place it subcutaneously since such a conduit should not be used for bypass.

MANAGEMENT OF PHARYNGEAL STRICTURES

Before embarking on a procedure to bypass, the thoracic esophageal stricture one must be sure that there is a patent cervical esophageal segment of adequate length to make the proximal anastomosis of the conduit. Any attempt to go proximal to the cervical stricture and construct a pharyngocolic anastomosis is ill advised and is associated with serious risks of aspiration due to the difficulty in learning to swallow. Hence in high strictures every attempt should be made to do anastomosis below the level of cricopharyngeal sphincter. For the purpose of management, pharyngeal strictures are classified into five types and treatment option depend on the type of stricture.[54]

Type I—Pharyngeal stricture with residual lumen that can permit a guide wire. In these patients, endoscopic dilatation should be considered the first line of therapy. Esophageal bypass should be considered only if multiple endoscopic dilatation is required or strictures rapidly restenosed or if they had an associated esophageal stricture which is not feasible for endoscopic dilatation.

Type II—Pharyngeal stricture with no demonstrable residual lumen or pharyngeal stricture in proximity to the laryngeal inlet. In these patients, endoscopic dilatation is either not possible or it can result in respiratory embarrassment secondary to the occlusion of the glottic inlet by the inflated balloon. These patients should undergo an initial right neck exploration. After identification and opening of the cervical esophagus, a passage to the hypopharynx is established by retrograde dilatation. The esophageal opening is then converted into an esophagostomy and a nasogastric tube inserted through the nose is brought out through the esophagostomy. This tract can be used for repeated dilation of the pharyngoesophageal stricture using over the wire Savary-Gilliard dilators. After each session of dilatation, the nasogastric tube should be reinserted and brought out through the esophagostomy to keep the tract open. Frequent dilatations are performed to achieve adequate lumen. Subsequently an esophagocoloplasty will be done distal to the dilated stricture through a left neck approach along the anterior border of the left sternocleidomastoid. The right cervical esophagostomy usually undergoes spontaneous closure in majority of the patients. In rare patients in whom spontaneous closure is delayed, sutured closure of the esophagostomy can be performed after separation from the skin.

Type III—Short segment pharyngoesophageal obstruction due to granulation tissue or synechiae. These patients are managed by excision of granulation tissue and adhesiolysis under the guidance of a direct laryngoscope. To achieve a satisfactory lumen size these patients might require multiple sessions.

Type IV—Tight stricture of the pharyngoesophageal junction refractory to endoscopic dilatation with a normal esophagus of at least 5 cm length distal to the pharyngoesophageal stricture. Use of spiral CT neck after the air swallow with sagittal neck reconstruction is a good technique for identification of distal residual esophageal lumen.[55] In these patients stricture can be repaired using an island pectoralis major myocutaneous flap or sternomastoid muscle myocutaneous inlay flap.[56,57] Since the pectoralis major myocutaneous flap leaves an unsightly chest wall scar the authors prefer sternomastoid muscle myocutaneous inlay flap over the pectoralis major flap. In patients in whom there is no distal obstruction these flaps can be a definitive treatment. However, in patients with additional distal obstruction either endoscopic dilatation or esophageal bypass will be required.

Type V—Pharyngeal stricture with no demonstrable lumen in the cervical esophageal segment. In these patients if there is an associated laryngeal involvement requiring tracheostomy, mid colon esophagocoloplasty with pharyngocolic anastomosis above the level of pharyngeal stricture can be performed. However, in patients with the patent airway this procedure is associated with high incidence of aspiration and should not be performed. While a tracheostomy can be added to avoid aspiration there is a risk that these patients might end up with a permanent tracheostomy and inability to swallow since many patients may not learn to swallow normally in the presence of high anastomosis. A simple feeding gastrostomy or jejunostomy results in a better quality of life compared to an ill fashioned high pharyngeal anastomosis in these patients.

MANAGEMENT OF CORROSIVE GASTRIC STRICTURE

Gastric strictures can be isolated or more commonly associated with esophageal stricture.[58] Hence, it is imperative to rule out an associated gastric stricture in all patients with corrosive injury, as it can have a significant impact on the management of stricture in the esophagus. The magnitude of the gastric involvement can be usually assessed with an endoscopic evaluation and a barium study. However, in patients with absolute dysphagia, both these techniques cannot be used to evaluate the type of gastric injury. In that scenario, a cheaper alternative to CT scan is a plain abdominal radiograph done after overnight fasting, and if it shows a gastric air fluid level, gastric outlet obstruction can be diagnosed.[59] As is the case for esophageal strictures, the need for gastrectomy to prevent malignant change has been overrated. Authors have not encountered any instance of malignancy in the scarred stomach.[7] For the purpose of management gastric strictures are classified into five types:

- Type I: Short pre-pyloric stricture.
- Type II: Stricture extending proximally up to the antrum.
- Type III: Mid gastric stricture involving the body and sparing the proximal and distal portion of the stomach.
- Type IV: Diffuse gastric involvement producing a linitis plastica like appearance (Figs 5 and 6).
- Type V: Gastric stricture associated with a stricture of the first part of the duodenum.

In patients with isolated Type I gastric stricture, a limited resection with a gastroduodenal reconstruction is the treatment of choice (Figs 7 and 8). Loop gastrojejunostomy should be performed only in patients in whom an esophageal stricture can be confidently ruled out as it can preclude the use of stomach as a conduit. Isolated Types II and III strictures are best treated by distal gastrectomy with polya reconstruction. In patients with poor general condition a loop gastrojejunostomy can be used in Type II strictures; however, a retrocolic gastrojejunostomy should be avoided as it increases the technical difficulty or sometimes preclude future colonic bypass by interfering with the middle colic vascular arcade. Gastrojejunostomy should be avoided in Type III structure as the anastomosis is usually non-dependent. A non-dependent gastrojejunostomy significantly affects the patient's quality of life as it produces refractory bile reflux in addition to inadequate gastric drainage. Isolated Type IV gastric stricture is

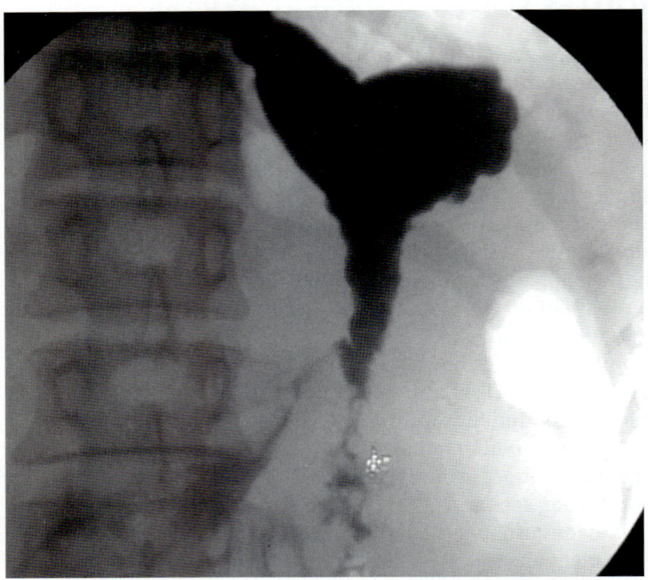

Figure 6 Upper gastrointestinal contrast study of a patient with Type IV gastric stricture

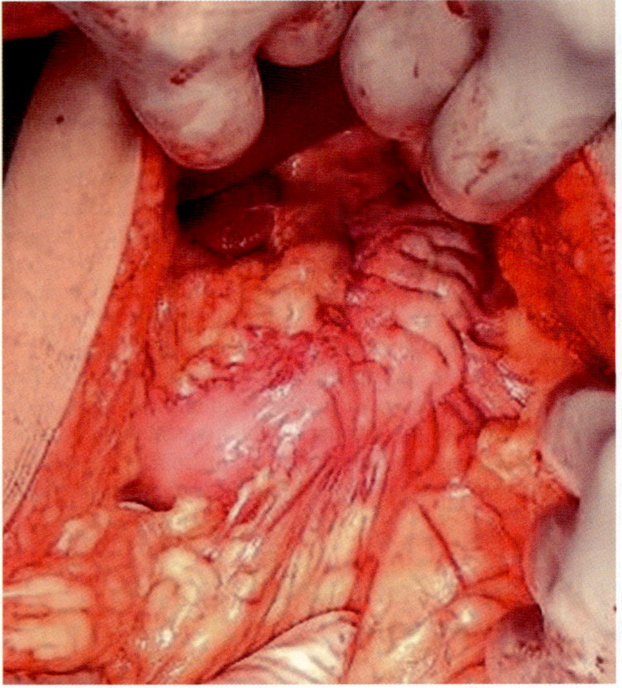

Figure 5 Intraoperative view of a Type IV gastric stricture

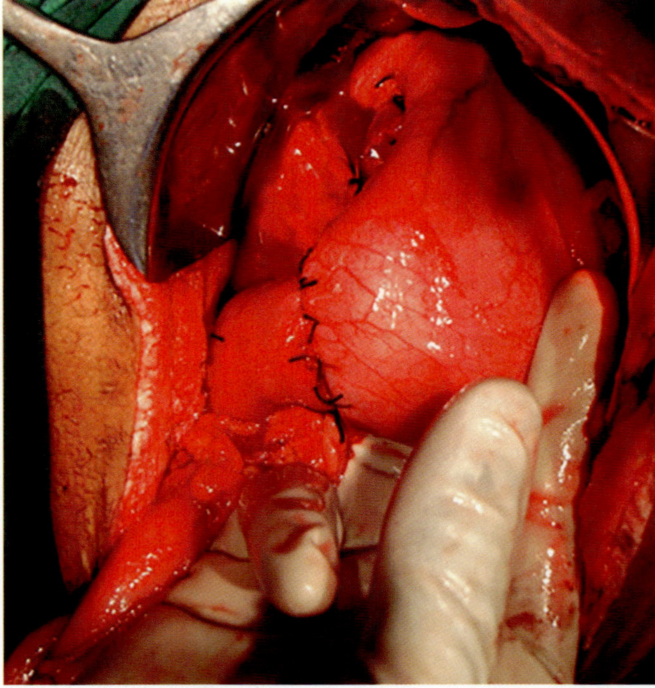

Figure 7 Limited gastric resection with gastroduodenal reconstruction for isolated Type I gastric stricture

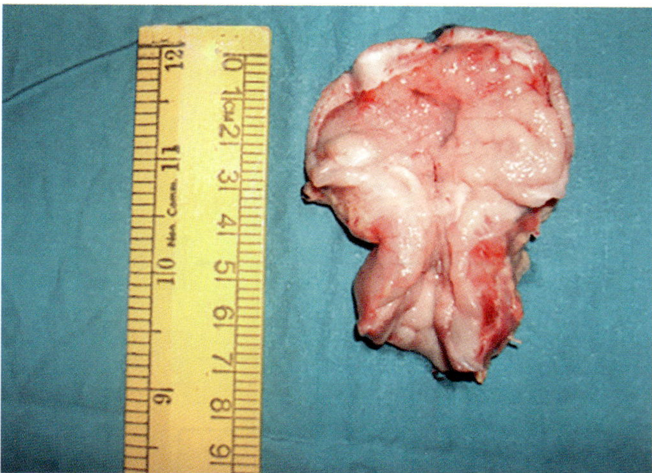

Figure 8 Specimen of prepyloric stricture—limited resection

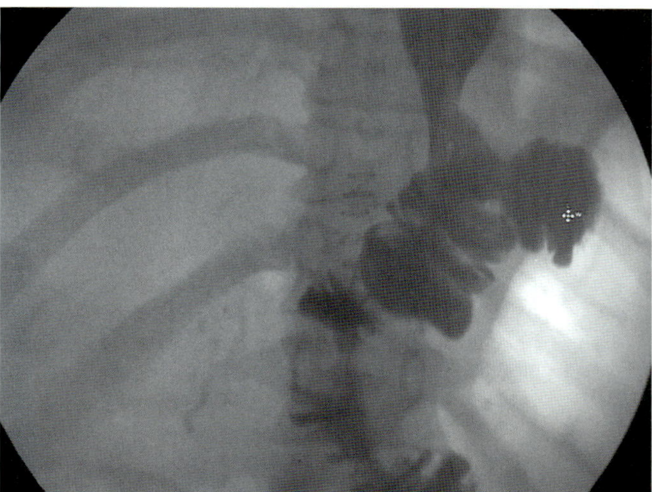

Figure 9 Esophagojejunostomy reconstruction following total gastrectomy for Type IV gastric stricture

best treated by total gastrectomy in fit patients. Reconstruction is carried out with esophagojejunostomy with feeding jejunostomy (Fig. 9). Type V gastric stricture presents a management challenge. Since any major resective procedure is associated with significant complications in these poor risk patients an antecolic dependent gastrojejunostomy is a safer option.

SIMULTANEOUS ESOPHAGEAL AND GASTRIC STRICTURES

Management of these patients depends upon the presentation time of the gastric and esophageal stricture. If the stricture in the stomach manifests before the stricture in the esophagus, a limited distal gastrectomy with gastroduodenal reconstruction can be performed, leaving esophageal bypass to a later date, should it become necessary. However, gastric strictures can present in a delayed fashion sometimes weeks to several months after the appearance of stricture in the esophagus. The delayed presentation of a gastric stricture can be a consequence of overlooked mild narrowing in the pylorus at the time of endoscopic dilatation of esophageal stricture that had progressed, over months, to total obstruction. An alternate possibility is the presence of subclinical gastric outlet obstruction that remained asymptomatic in the presence of the dysphagia secondary to stricture in the esophagus; subsequently when the patient resumes oral diet after esophageal bypass the gastric outlet obstruction becomes overt. These delayed gastric strictures have significant implications when one contemplates gastric conduit for esophageal replacement.

In patients who present with simultaneous esophageal and gastric stricture, it is recommended to combine esophagocoloplasty with a gastrojejunostomy distal to the cologastric anastomosis. In patients with combined esophageal and Type IV gastric stricture it is preferable to do colonic bypass for the esophagus and anastomosing the distal end of the colon to the proximal jejunum, leaving the stomach in situ, as addition of total gastrectomy with esophageal bypass significantly increase the morbidity in these frail patients. Delayed gastric outlet obstruction after esophageal bypass is a significant problem as it often manifests as dilatation of the conduit.[58] This condition should not be misdiagnosed as stenosis of the cologastric anastomosis. The distinction can be easily done by endoscopy, and gastric stricture can be managed either a limited gastrectomy or a gastrojejunostomy distal to the cologastric anastomosis. Delayed gastric outlet obstruction can pose a complex management challenge if it occurs in patients in whom esophageal replacement was done using a gastric conduit. In this scenario, a limited gastrectomy or gastrojejunostomy is rarely feasible, and a jejunal interposition might be the only available option. In a rare scenario, a pyloroplasty might be feasible. Algorithmic approach for the management of a corrosive stricture of the esophagus and stomach is illustrated in Flow chart 1.

LAPAROSCOPIC ESOPHAGEAL BYPASS

Technical feasibility of laparoscopic retrosternal gastric bypass has been recently reported in a single small series of 4 patients.[60] Whole stomach instead of the gastric tube was used as a conduit in that series. Similarly, technical feasibility of laparoscopic colonic bypass has been reported in one series of four patients.[61] However, long-term follow-up data is not available in these series. Since esophageal bypass is a technically challenging procedure requiring an utmost care in handling of the conduit, these procedures should be attempted laparoscopically only in high volume centers with significant experience in advanced laparoscopic procedures.

SOCIOECONOMIC IMPACT OF CORROSIVE INGESTION

The social and economic impact of severe corrosive injuries is very significant. Protracted treatment requiring numerous diagnostic and interventional procedures puts a significant burden on the health care system. Economic productivity of the family is also affected since the family members have to shift closer to a major referral center, where these complicated interventions are performed. In addition to the economic

Flow chart 1 Algorithmic approach for the management of corrosive stricture of the esophagus and stomach

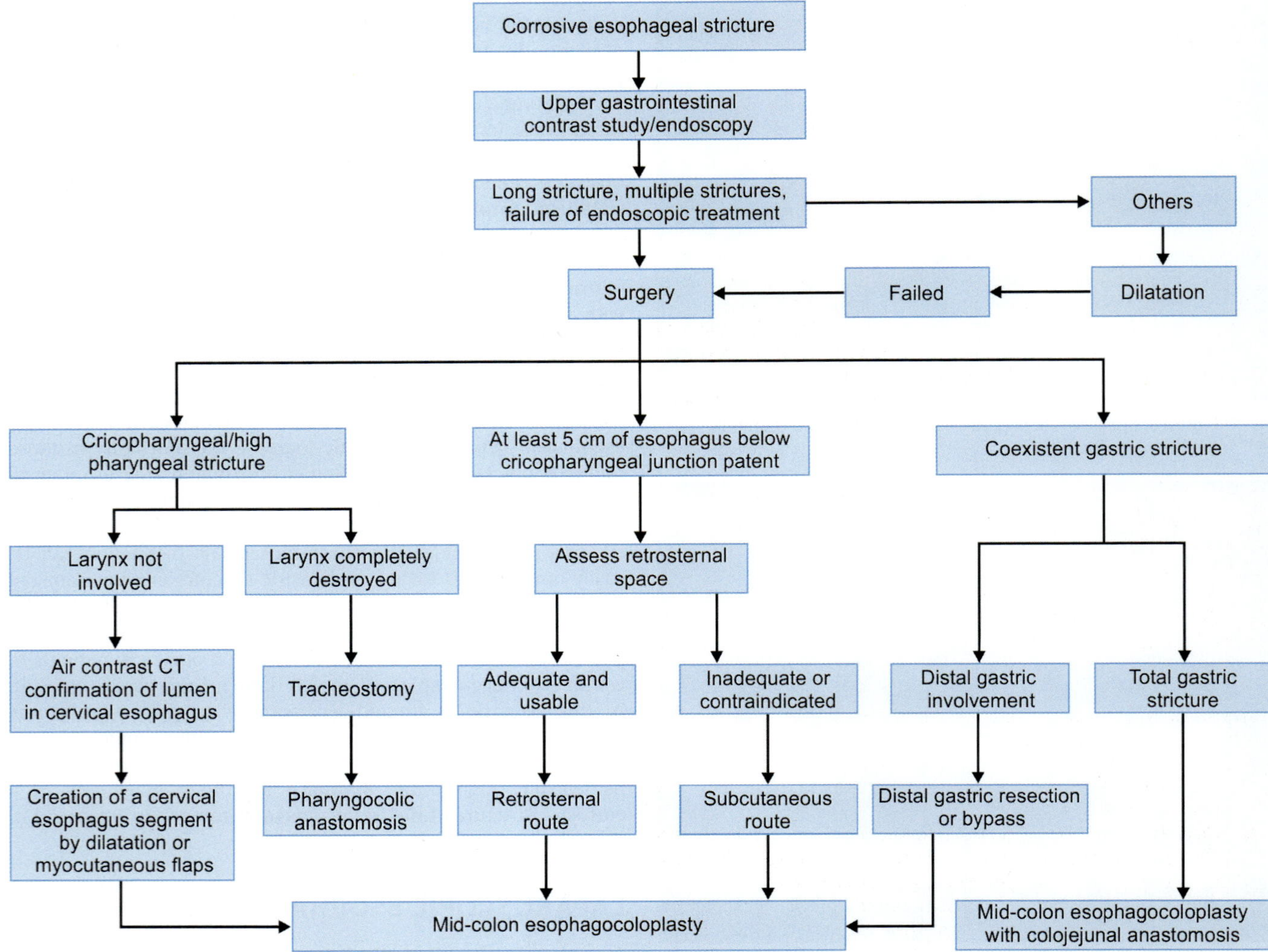

consequences, there is significant social impact as the stress of protracted treatment results in the breakup within the family and recurrence of psychiatric symptoms in these patients with risk of repeat suicidal attempts. Hence, active measures should be taken to reduce the incidence of corrosive ingestion and its consequences.

REFERENCES

1. Lakshmi CP, Vijayahari R, Kate V, Ananthakrishnan N. A hospital-based epidemiological study of corrosive alimentary injuries with particular reference to the Indian experience. Natl Med J India. 2013;26:31-6.
2. Bronstein AC, Spyker DA, Cantilena LR Jr, Green JL, Rumack BH, Giffin SL. 2008 Annual Report of the American Association of Poison Control Centers' National Poison Data System (NPDS): 26th Annual Report. ClinToxicol (Phila). 2009;47:911-1084.
3. Arévalo-Silva C, Eliashar R, Wohlgelernter J, Elidan J, Gross M. Ingestion of caustic substances: a 15-year experience. Laryngoscope. 2006;116:1422-6.
4. Stiff G, Alwafi A, Rees BI, Lari J. Corrosive injuries of the oesophagus and stomach: experience in management at a regional paediatric centre. Ann R Coll Surg Engl. 1996;78:119-23.
5. Rodríguez MA, Meza Flores JL. Clinical-epidemiological characteristics in caustic ingestion patients in the Hipólito Unanue National Hospital. Rev Gastroenterol Peru. 2003;23:115-25.
6. Bautista Casasnovas A, Estevez Martinez E, Varela Cives R, Villanueva Jeremias A, Tojo Sierra R, Cadranel S. A retrospective analysis of ingestion of caustic substances by children: ten-year statistics in Galicia. Eur J Pediatr. 1997;156:410-4.
7. Ananthakrishnan N, Parthasarathy G, Kate V. Chronic corrosive injuries of the stomach—a single unit experience of 109 patients over thirty years. World J Surg. 2010;34:758-64.
8. Jayashree M, Singhi S. Changing trends and predictors of outcome in patients with acute poisoning admitted to the intensive care. J Trop Pediatr. 2011;57:340-6.
9. Dutta AK, Seth A, Goyal PK, Aggarwal V, Mittal SK, Sharma R, et al. Poisoning in children: Indian scenario. Indian J Pediatr. 1998;65:365-70.
10. Ting SK, Tan KK. Post mortem survey of suicides in Singapore. Singapore Med J. 1969;10:248-58.

11. Soman CR, Safraj S, Kutty VR, Vijayakumar K, Ajayan K. Suicide in South India: a community-based study in Kerala. Indian J Psychiatry. 2009;51:261-4.
12. Gajalakshmi V, Peto R. Verbal autopsy of 80,000 adult deaths in Tamil Nadu, South India. BMC Public Health. 2004;4:47.
13. Gumaste VV, Dave PB. Ingestion of corrosive substances by adults. Am J Gastroenterol. 1992;87:1-5.
14. Osman M, Russell J, Shukla D, Moghadamfalahi M, Granger DN. Responses of the murine esophageal microcirculation to acute exposure to alkali, acid, or hypochlorite. J Pediatr Surg. 2008;43:1672-8.
15. Zargar SA, Kochhar R, Nagi B, Mehta S, Mehta SK. Ingestion of corrosive acids: spectrum of injury to upper gastrointestinal tract and natural history. Gastroenterology. 1989;97:702-7.
16. Pankaja S, Valooran G, Das S, Suvasini L, Aravind R, Kate V, et al. Isolated full thickness jejunal necrosis following sulphuric acid cocktail ingestion—a clinical case report—isolated corrosive jejunal necrosis. Surgical Science. 2011;2:338-40.
17. Gorman RL, Khin-Maung-Gyi MT, Klein-Schwartz W, Oderda GM, Benson B, Litovitz T, et al. Initial symptoms aspredictors of esophageal injury in alkaline corrosive ingestion. Am J Emerg Med. 1992;10:189-94.
18. Gupta SK, Croffie JM, Fitzgerald JF. Is esophagogastroduodenoscopy necessary in all caustic ingestions? J Pediatr Gastroenterol Nutr. 2001;32:50-3.
19. Lahoti D, Broor SL. Corrosive injury to the upper gastrointestinal tract. Indian J Gastroenterol. 1993;12:135-41.
20. Zargar SA, Kochhar R, Mehta S, Mehta SK. The role of fiberoptic endoscopy in the management of corrosive ingestion and modified endoscopic classification of burns. Gastrointest Endosc. 1991;37:165-9.
21. Millar AJ, Numanoglu A, Mann M, Marven S, Rode H. Detection of caustic oesophageal injury with technetium 99m-labelled sucralfate. J Pediatr Surg. 2001;36:262-5.
22. Hugh TB, Kelly MD. Corrosive ingestion and the surgeon. J Am Coll Surg. 1999;189:508-22.
23. Cakal B, Akbal E, Köklü S, Babalı A, Koçak E, Taş A. Acute therapy with intravenous omeprazole on caustic esophageal injury: a prospective case series. Dis Esophagus. 2013;26:22-6.
24. Pelclová D, Navrátil T. Do corticosteroids prevent oesophageal stricture after corrosive ingestion? Toxicol Rev. 2005;24:125-9.
25. Howell JM, Dalsey WC, Hartsell FW, Butzin CA. Steroids for the treatment of corrosive esophageal injury: a statistical analysis of past studies. Am J Emerg Med. 1992;10:421-5.
26. Ramasamy K, Gumaste VV. Corrosive ingestion in adults. J Clin Gastroenterol. 2003;37:119-24.
27. De Peppo F, Zaccara A, Dall'Oglio L, Federici di Abriola G, Ponticelli A, Marchetti P, et al. Stenting for caustic strictures: esophageal replacement replaced. J Pediatr Surg. 1998;33:54-7.
28. Repici A, Vleggaar FP, Hassan C, van Boeckel PG, Romeo F, Pagano N, et al. Efficacy and safety of biodegradable stents for refractory benign esophageal strictures: the BEST (Biodegradable Esophageal Stent) study. Gastrointest Endosc. 2010;72:927-34.
29. Contini S, Scarpignato C. Caustic injury of the upper gastrointestinal tract: a comprehensive review. World J Gastroenterol. 2013;19: 3918-30.
30. Cheng YJ, Kao EL. Arterial blood gas analysis in caustic ingestion injuries. Surg Today. 2003;33:483-5.
31. Ananthakrishnan N, Parthasarathy G, Kate V. Acute corrosive injuries of the stomach: a single unit experience of thirty years. ISRN Gastroenterol. 2011;2011:914013.
32. Brun JG, Celerier M, Koskas F, Dubost C. Blunt thorax oesophageal stripping: an emergency procedure for caustic ingestion. Br J Surg. 1984;71:698-700.
33. Javed A, Pal S, Krishnan EK, Sahni P, Chattopadhyay TK. Surgical management and outcomes of severe gastrointestinal injuries due to corrosive ingestion. World J Gastrointest Surg. 2012;4:121-5.
34. Broor SL, Raju GS, Bose PP, Lahoti D, Ramesh GN, Kumar A, et al. Long term results of endoscopic dilatation for corrosive oesophageal strictures. Gut. 1993;34:1498-501.
35. Bothereau H, Munoz-Bongrand N, Lambert B, et al. Esophageal reconstruction after caustic injury: is there still a place for right coloplasty? Am J Surg. 2007;193:660-4.
36. Chirica M, Veyrie N, Munoz-Bongrand N, Zohar S, HalimiB, Celerier M, et al. Late morbidity after coloninterposition for corrosive esophageal injury: risk factors, management, and outcome. A 20-years experience. Ann Surg. 2010;252:271-80.
37. Demirbilek S, Aydin G, Yucesan S, Vural H, Bitiren M. Polyunsaturated phosphatidylcholine lowers collagen deposition in a rat model of corrosive esophageal burn. Eur J Pediatr Surg. 2002;12:8-12.
38. Mannell A, Epstein B. Exclusion of the esophagus—is this a dangerous maneuver? Br J Surg. 1984;71:442-5.
39. Ribet M, Chambon JP, Pruvot FR. Oesophagectomy for severe corrosive injuries: is it always legitimate? Eur J Cardiothorac Surg. 1990;4:347-50.
40. Marchand P. Caustic strictures of the oesophagus. Thorax. 1955;10: 171-81.
41. Carver CM Jr, Sealy WC, Dillon ML Jr. Management of alkali burns of the esophagus. J Am Med Assoc. 1956;160:1447-50.
42. Mamede RC, de Mello Fillo FV. Ingestion of caustic substances and its complications. Sao Paolo Med J. 2001;119:10-5.
43. Kim YT, Sung SW, Kim JH. Is it necessary to resect the diseased esophagus in performing reconstruction for corrosive esophageal stricture? Eur J Cardiothorac Surg. 2001;20:1-6.
44. Agarwal R, Kocchar R, Nagi B, Mehta SK. Carcinoma developing in a patient long standing lye stricture of the esophagus. J Assoc Physicians India. 1989;37:233-4.
45. Kocchar R, Sethy PK, Kocchar S, Nagi B, Gupta NM. Corrosive induced carcinoma of the esophagus: report of three patients and review of literature. J Gastroenterol Hepatol. 2006;21:777-80.
46. Ananthakrishnan N, Subbarao KSVK, Parthasarathy G, Kate V, Kalayarasan R. Long term results of esophageal bypass for corrosive strictures without esophageal resection using a modified left colon esophagocoloplasty—a report of 105 consecutive patients from a single unit over thirty years. Hepatogastroenterology. 2014;61: 1033-1041. doi 10.5754/he 12872.
47. Hopkins RA, Postlethwait RW. Caustic burns and carcinoma of the esophagus. Ann Surg. 1981;194:146-8.
48. Gerzic BZ, Knezevic JB, Milicevic MN, Jovanovic BK. Esophagocoloplasty in the management of postcorrosive stricture of the esophagus. Ann Surg. 1990;211:329-36.
49. Ogura JH, Roper CL, Burford TH. Complete functional restitution of the food passage in extensive stenosing burns of the esophagus. J Thorac Cardiovasc Surg. 1961;42:340-5.
50. Fekete F. Cancer of the esophagus; indications for resection and for by-pass. Serono Symposia, Proceedings. 1981;43:300-3.
51. Bigelow NH. Carcinoma of the esophagus developing at the site of lye stricture. Cancer. 1953;6:1159-64.
52. DeMeester SR. Colon interposition following esophagectomy. Dis Esophagus. 2001;14:169-72.
53. Ananthakrishnan N, Subba Rao KSVK, Radjendirin P. Mid-colon esophagocoloplasty for corrosive esophageal strictures. Aust N Z J Surg. 1993;63:389-95.
54. Ananthakrishnan N, Kate V, Parthasarathy G. Therapeutic options for management of pharyngoesophageal corrosive strictures. J Gastrointest Surg. 2011;15:566-75.

55. Ananthakrishnan N, Parthasarathy G, Kate V. Use of spiral CT to demonstrate esophageal lumen in corrosive strictures. Indian J Gastroenterol. 2007;26:101.
56. Ananthakrishnan N, Nachiappan M, Subba Rao KSVK. Island pectoralis major myocutaneous flap for pharyngo-oesophageal strictures prior to esophagocoloplasty. J R Coll Surg Edinb. 2001;46:202-4.
57. Ananthakrishnan N, Parthasarathy G, Maroju NK, Kate V. Sternocleidomastoid muscle myocutaneous flap for corrosive Pharyngo-esophageal strictures. World J Surg. 2007;31:1592-6.
58. Ananthakrishnan N, Subba Rao KSVK, Rajendran P. Delayed gastric outlet obstruction after esophagocoloplasty: clinical presentation with massive megacolon. Indian J Thorac Cardiovasc Surg. 1991;7:99-10.
59. Ananthakrishnan N, Parthasarathy G, Kate V. Gastric fluid level after overnight fast: test to diagnose gastric outlet obstruction in corrosive esophageal stricture. Indian J Gastroenterol. 2006;25: 269-70.
60. Javed A, Agarwal AK. Laparoscopic retrosternal bypass for corrosive stricture of the esophagus. Surg Endosc. 2012;26:3344-9.
61. Javed A, Agarwal AK. Total laparoscopic esophageal bypass using a colonic conduit for corrosive-induced esophageal stricture. Surg Endosc. 2013;27:3726-32.

CHAPTER 17

Benign Tumors of the Esophagus

Vivek Mangla, Manoj Gupta

INTRODUCTION

Benign esophageal tumors are rare and often asymptomatic. They constitute less than 1% of all esophageal neoplasms as malignant tumors far outnumber benign esophageal tumors.[1]
Nevertheless, they pose a challenge in establishing a definitive diagnosis and deciding management.

The exact incidence is difficult to determine as most benign esophageal tumors are asymptomatic and detected incidentally. Incidental detection is becoming more common with the increasing use of upper gastrointestinal endoscopy. In one series of nearly 20,000 autopsies over a 50-year period, there were only 90 cases of benign esophageal tumors.[2] Recent advancements have resulted in better understanding of diagnosis, classification and minimally invasive methods for treatment of these tumors.

EPIDEMIOLOGY

Two separate series by Moersch and Harrington[3] and Plachta[4] have reported a prevalence of benign esophageal tumors and cysts of 0.59% (44 out of 7459) and 0.45% (90 out of 19982), respectively. In a review by Plachta, out of 504 esophageal tumors identified at autopsy, 82% were malignant and 18% benign. Benign tumors were more common in males than females. The mean age of patients was 45 years for symptomatic and 68 years for asymptomatic patients, respectively. The most common tumors were leiomyomas in 49 (54%), polyps in 23 (26%), cysts in 3 (3%), hemangioma in 3 (3%) and papillomas in 2 (2%). There was a slight predilection for the lower third of the esophagus.[4]

CLASSIFICATION

Various systems have been used to classify benign esophageal tumors. Classification systems, by Sweet et al. as well as Moersch and Harrington, were based on both clinical and gross pathologic findings.[3,5] Tumors have been classified according to the esophageal layer (mucosa, submucosa or muscularis) from which they originate. Another classification system has been proposed by Nemir et al. in which esophageal tumors are organized by cell of origin into epithelial, non-epithelial and heterotopic tumors.[6] Another classification system which is commonly used because of its clarity has classified these tumors into three groups, intramural–extramucosal, mucosal–intraluminal and cysts and duplications.[7-9]

INTRAMURAL/EXTRAMUCOSAL TUMORS

Mesenchymal Tumors

Leiomyoma

Leiomyoma is a rare benign tumor and comprises 0.4%–1% of all esophageal tumors.[10] It is the most common benign tumor (67%–80%) of the esophagus.[11] Leiomyoma usually presents as a solitary intramural, oval-shaped mass which originates in the muscularis propria or the muscularis mucosae.[11] Multiple leiomyomas (leiomyomatosis) may be seen in about 5% of cases. Leiomyomas are seen most commonly in the distal third of esophagus followed by mid- and proximal third of the esophagus.[12]

Clinical features: With increasing use of endoscopy, leiomyomas are frequently detected in asymptomatic patients. Esophageal leiomyomas are mostly asymptomatic, especially when they are smaller than 5 cm in diameter. Large tumors can cause dysphagia (most common symptom), vague retrosternal discomfort, chest pain, esophageal obstruction and regurgitation. Rarely, patients may present with gastrointestinal bleeding, with erosion through the mucosa. In extremely rare cases, large lesions may cause severe esophageal obstruction and weight loss and muscle wasting may be observed.[13]

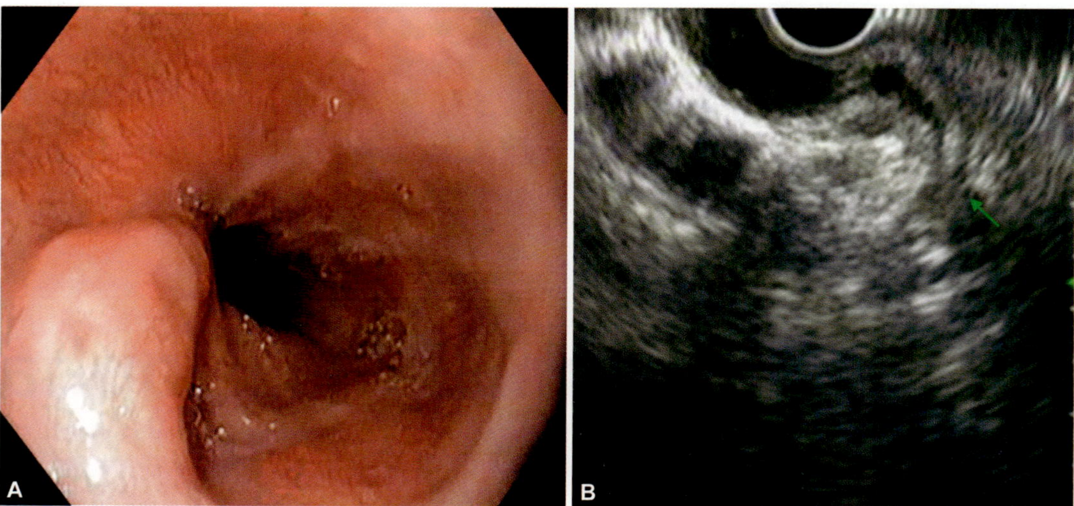

Figures 1A and B Esophageal leiomyoma. (A) Endoscopy showing a lesion causing a bulge in distal esophageal lumen just above the gastroesophageal junction covered by intact mucosa endoscopic ultrasound; (B) Showing a hypoechoic mural lesion likely arising from the 4th sonographic layer (muscularis propria). In this location, the likely possibility would be a leiomyoma. GIST has an identical appearance but is rare in the esophagus
Source: Dr Mandhir Kumar, Sir Ganga Ram Hospital, New Delhi.

Diagnosis: It is based on characteristic findings on oral contrast studies, endoscopy and endoscopic ultrasound (EUS). On oral contrast study with barium, leiomyoma appears as a focal smooth bulge impinging on the esophageal lumen without any obstruction to the flow of contrast. Endoscopically, leiomyoma is seen as a bulge into the esophageal lumen covered in most cases, by an intact normal esophageal mucosa (Fig. 1A). Mucosal erosion is rare.[14] On EUS, leiomyomas appear as oval shaped, smooth hypoechoic lesions usually arising from the second (muscularis mucosa) or the fourth endoscopic layer, i.e. muscularis propria[15] (Fig. 1B). One large study has reported that leiomyomas more often arise from muscularis mucosae rather than muscularis propria as was previously thought.[16] EUS-guided needle biopsy is generally not recommended as it can result in adhesions between the mucosa and the tumor and subsequently complicate extramucosal enucleation during surgical procedure.[17,18] In cases of ulcerated mucosa and suspicion of cancer, endoscopic biopsy should be considered.[17]

Histology: Histologically, leiomyoma comprises of bundles of interlacing smooth muscle cells, well-demarcated from adjacent tissue by a definitive connective tissue capsule (Figs 2A and B). The tumor cells have blunt-ended elongated nuclei with minimal atypia and few mitotic figures.[19]

Asymptomatic or smaller leiomyomas may be followed-up with barium swallow and endoscopy as they have slow growth rate, a characteristic radiographic appearance and minimal risk of malignant transformation.[11]

Treatment: Surgical excision is considered for symptomatic leiomyomas and for tumors greater than 5 cm. Leiomyomas involving the mid-third esophagus have conventionally been approached using a right thoracotomy. Tumors in the distal third of the esophagus may be resected through a left thoracoabdominal approach or a transhiatal approach. The outer esophageal muscle is incised longitudinally for extramucosal excision or enucleation. Careful dissection is done to separate and remove the leiomyoma from the underlying submucosa. If the mucosa is inadvertently opened during dissection, the underlying mucosa is re-approximated, followed by closure of the longitudinal muscle. Segmental esophageal resection (esophagogastrectomy) may be indicated for giant leiomyomas of the cardia. Total esophagectomy is needed rarely for very large leiomyomas involving long segment of the esophagus (Figs 3A and B) or for patients with leiomyomatosis.

Videothoracoscopic enucleation was reported for the first time in 1992[20,21] and is now, considered the surgical treatment of choice for esophageal leiomyomas. For leiomyomas of the distal third of esophagus, especially those of the intra-abdominal esophagus, enucleation by laparoscopy is a good option.[22] Minimally invasive approaches are associated with less pain, and pulmonary complications and hence faster recovery.[23] Intraoperative endoscopy can be useful for localizing the lesion in small leiomyomas, for identifying the border between esophageal mucosa and leiomyoma during dissection, and for confirming the integrity of the esophageal mucosa after enucleation.[23] There are some recent reports describing endoscopic removal of leiomyoma.[24] However, experience with this technique is limited and hence endoscopic resection for leiomyoma is not commonly done.[25]

Gastrointestinal Stromal Tumors

Gastrointestinal stromal tumors (GIST) are a heterogeneous group of mesenchymal tumors of the gastrointestinal tract (GIT). They are the most common sarcomas of the GIT and are commonly seen in stomach and small bowel. In contrast, esophageal GISTs are rare, accounting for 12.7–28% of mesenchymal esophageal tumors or 2% of all GISTs.[26-28] Esophageal GISTs are difficult to differentiate preoperatively from leiomyomas as their clinical presentation, endoscopy, EUS or computed tomography (CT) scan findings are almost similar.[26,29,30] On EUS, both GISTs and leiomyomas are

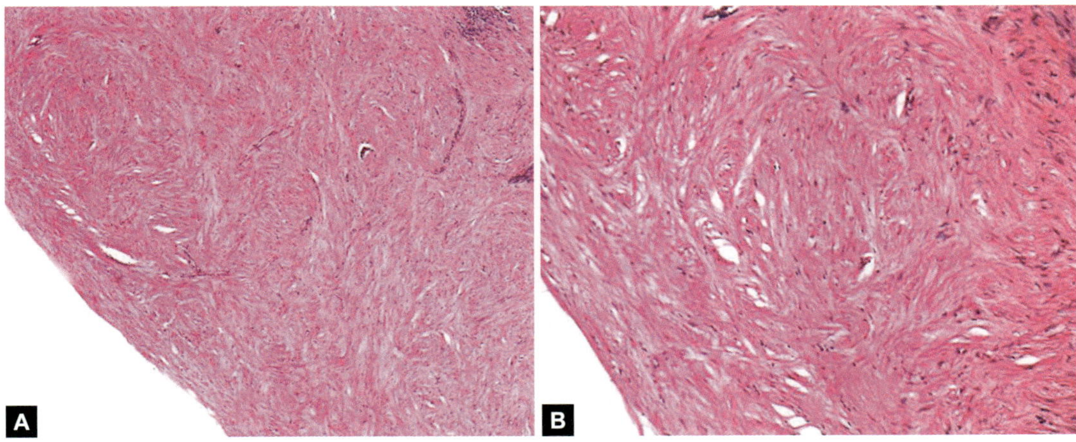

Figures 2A and B Photomicrograph showing esophageal leiomyoma, showing well circumscribed benign tumor comprising of fascicles of smooth muscles. No mitosis or necrosis is seen
Source: Dr Prasenjit Das, AIIMS, New Delhi.

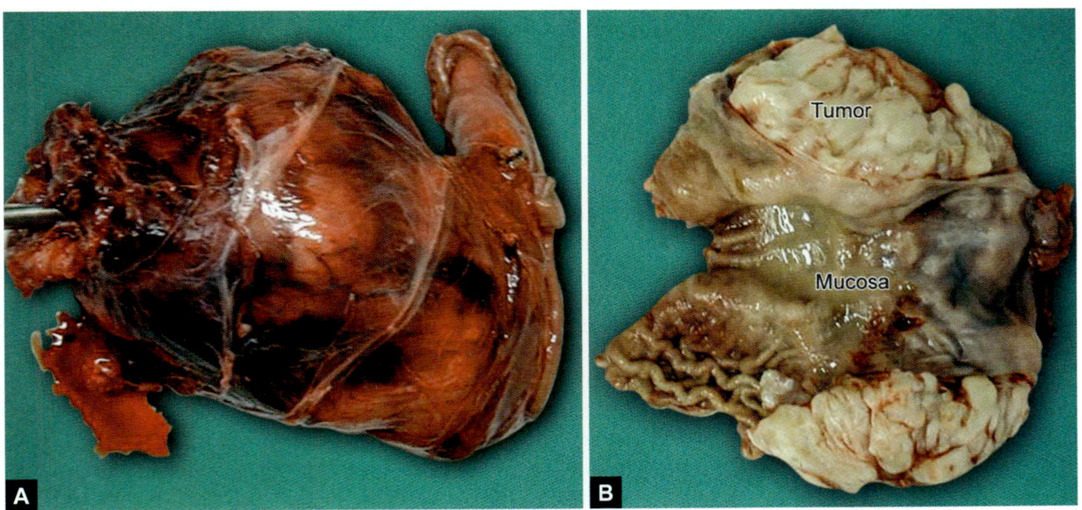

Figures 3A and B Large esophageal leiomyoma. (A) Requiring esophagectomy with gastric pull up; (B) Operative specimen showing intact mucosa over the tumor
Source: Prof TK Chattopadhyay, ILBS, New Delhi.

hypoechoic lesions and may originate from the muscularis propria or muscularis mucosa.

Fine-needle aspiration is usually avoided in case of esophageal submucosal lesions, as it may induce scarring that might make safe enucleation difficult. Blum et al. recommended biopsy for tumors larger than 2 cm, enlarging tumors or tumors positive on positron emission tomography (PET) scan.[29]

Immunohistochemical staining can differentiate GISTs, which have c-kit mutations and are positive for cluster of differentiation CD117 and CD34 from leiomyomas, which are CD34 and CD117 negative, with no c-kit mutations. Leiomyomas are also positive for desmin and smooth muscle actin (SMA), while GISTs are usually (but not always) negative.[30]

Benign and malignant tumors are differentiated on the basis of size of tumor and number of mitotic figures per high-power field (HPF). Tumors with size greater than 10 cm in diameter and presence of greater than or equal to 5 mitotic figures per HPF have higher malignant potential. However, metastatic disease may occur even with small tumors and tumors with low mitotic figures. Symptoms, diagnostic methods and treatment options are as for leiomyoma.[31] GISTs often attain large size and mucosal ulceration may occur. These lesions, therefore, are more often symptomatic with dysphagia and bleeding. CT is used to assess extent of lesion and relationship to surrounding structures. Small lesions may be treated with enucleation. However, large lesions usually require esophagectomy.

Generally, adjuvant therapy has been shown to result in increased recurrence-free survival in patients with GISTs at high risk of recurrence.[32] Imatinib is effective as an adjuvant therapy in GISTs. However, there is no study which has specifically looked at role of adjuvant or neoadjuvant therapy with imatinib in patients with esophageal GIST. Extrapolating from GISTs at other sites, adjuvant treatment with imatinib is usually recommended for patients with esophageal GISTs at high risk of recurrence.

Schwannoma

Schwannoma (synonym, neurilemmoma) is the least common esophageal mesenchymal tumor. The age at presentation ranges from 47–62 years with no gender predilection. These usually arise from the muscularis propria.[15] Histologically, these lesions have moderate cellularity comprising of spindle cells and a characteristic peripheral rim of lymphoid cells. These tumors are positive for S-100 and glial fibrillary acidic protein (GFAP) and negative for CD34 and SMA. Clinical presentation and diagnostic work up is similar to leiomyoma. Symptoms depend on the size and location of the tumor, and even airway compression and esophageal obstruction have been reported.[33,34] Treatment options are similar to those described for leiomyoma. Treatment with modalities ranging from endoscopic resection to minimally invasive methods has been reported.[35,36] Larger tumors tend to be malignant. Complete resection and benign histology are associated with better prognosis.

Other Intramural/Extramucosal Tumors

Granular Cell Tumors

Granular cell tumors (GCTs) were first described by Abrikossoff. These tumors usually occur in the skin, tongue, breast and GIT but rarely involve the esophagus. Approximately 10% percent arise in the GIT, most commonly in the distal esophagus.[37] The mean age at diagnosis for these tumors is 45 years with male preponderance.[37] Most patients are asymptomatic, up to one-third of patients have dysphagia.[37] On endoscopy, GCTs are typically small, sessile, yellowish-white, and covered by normal-appearing translucent mucosa.[38] Most patients have solitary lesions but up to 10% patients may have two or more lesions at diagnosis.[37]

Histologically, the tumor is composed of sheets or nests of plump, round or polygonal cells having abundant light amphophilic but strikingly granular cytoplasm with small, round, pyknotic central uniform nuclei.[38] Under electron microscopy, they resemble Schwann cells and stain positive for S-100 protein and neuron-specific enolase, suggesting that they originate from cells of neural origin.[8]

Superficial biopsies may be normal and may miss the diagnosis, showing only fragments of normal squamous mucosa or revealing hyperplastic changes that can be misdiagnosed as squamous cell carcinoma.[38] In this regard, a Lugol staining technique, suggested for use by Tada et al. can help differentiate GCT from squamous cell carcinoma endoscopically.[39]

Granular cell tumors may be malignant, especially larger lesions and those that exhibit growth.[40] Fanburg-Smith JC have assessed six histological criteria: necrosis, spindling, vesicular nuclei with large nucleoli, increased mitotic activity, high nuclear to cytoplasmic (N:C) ratio and pleomorphism.[41] Neoplasms that meet three or more of these criteria have been classified as histologically malignant; those that meet one or two criteria have been classified as atypical; and those that display only focal pleomorphism but fulfill none of the other criteria have been classified as benign.

Management of patients with GCT still remains controversial due to paucity of literature. Some authors have suggested aggressive treatment with surgical removal on diagnosis as it is difficult to distinguish between benign and malignant tumors on preoperative evaluation.[42] Other authors have suggested endoscopic follow-up for small and symptomatic lesions. Successful endoscopic mucosal resection has been reported using laser, banding, standard endoscopic mucosal resection methods and alcohol injection.[43] Tumors with size less than 20 mm which are not attached to the muscularis propria are best suited for endoscopic resection.[44]

Transthoracic excision of GCTs is the most definitive treatment and is indicated for tumors not amenable to endoscopic resection. Recent advances in minimally invasive surgery may allow for decreased perioperative morbidity and hospital stay.

Hemangioma

Esophageal hemangioma is rare. A literature review by Govoni in 1982, analyzed 56 cases with esophageal hemangioma, mostly single case reports or studies of 2 or 3 cases.[45] Their prevalence in the general population was 0.04% based upon an autopsy series.[3] Hemangioma occurs more often in mid or distal esophagus. The majority are cavernous (i.e. have cavernous vascular spaces seen histologically), although capillary lesions have also been described. Although, usually hemangiomas are solitary, multiple lesions may be seen in patients with Osler-Weber-Rendu disease, Klippel-Trénaunay syndrome or congenital blue rubber bleb nevus syndrome.[46]

Hemorrhage and dysphagia are the most common symptoms. Hemorrhage from an esophageal vascular tumor can be massive or even fatal. Dysphagia is usually mild due to esophageal elasticity and usually seen with larger lesions. Death has been reported from obstruction and subsequent aspiration pneumonitis.[47]

On endoscopy, hemangiomas appear as nodular, soft, bluish-red and typically blanch when pressed with biopsy forceps. They must be differentiated from Kaposi's sarcoma, which may have a similar endoscopic appearance. Hemangioma appears as well-defined hypoechoic mass arising from the second or third endosonographic layer on EUS.[48,49] CT findings of an intramural mass; with marked enhancement, following intravenous contrast enables the diagnosis to be established preoperatively.[50]

For mucosal or submucosal hemangioma, endoscopic resection should be considered.[51] Superficial tumors with size less than 2.5 cm in diameter and those with a thin pedicle are better suited for endoscopic resection. If endoscopic resection is deemed difficult, either endoscopic injection sclerotherapy (EIS) or a surgical resection should be considered.[52,53] Recently developed techniques include fulguration using potassium titanyl phosphate/yttrium aluminium garnet laser.[54]

Rhabdomyoma

Rhabdomyomas are rare, striated skeletal muscle tumors. They occur most often in the upper-third of the esophagus as a submucosal mass.

Lipoma

Lipoma appears as a soft, pale yellow submucosal tumor with intact overlying mucosa. These are usually found incidentally. On

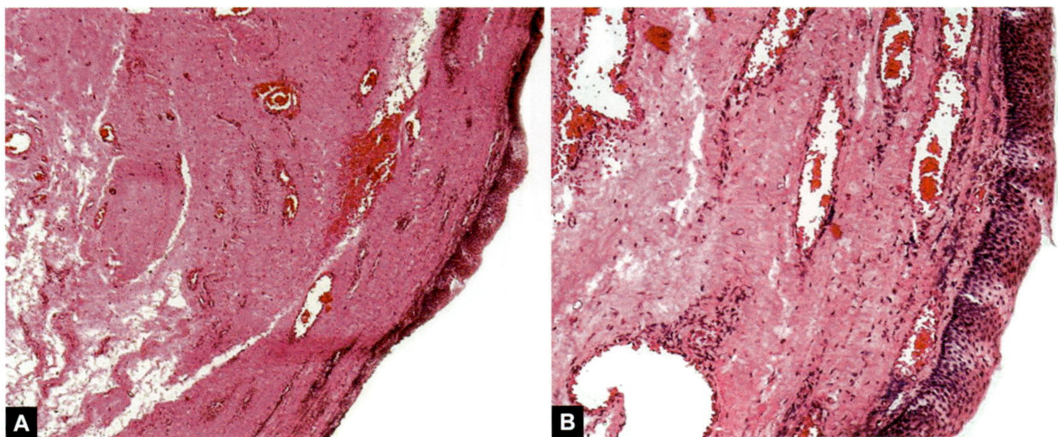

Figures 4A and B Photomicrograph showing features of benign fibrovascular polyp, covered by stratified squamous epithelium. The subepithelium shows hypocellular fibrocollagenous stroma with congested blood vessels (magnifications of both 40x)
Source: Dr Prasenjit Das, AIIMS, New Delhi.

EUS, they are hyperechoic, homogeneous lesions. Biopsy samples are difficult to obtain as lipomas do not involve the mucosa. As they have no malignant potential, most do not require treatment or further follow-up unless symptomatic.[14] Symptomatic lesions may be treated with enucleation.

INTRALUMINAL/MUCOSAL TUMORS

Fibrovascular Polyps

Fibrovascular polyps (FVPs) are the second most common benign esophageal tumor after leiomyoma. They contain a mixture of fibrous, vascular and adipose tissue covered by squamous epithelium (Figs 4A and B). They are most commonly encountered in the upper-third of the esophagus and typically attach directly to the inferior aspect of the cricopharyngeus. FVPs are mostly reported in men, in their 6th or 7th decade.[7]

It has been hypothesized that FVPs arise from a nodular thickening of a redundant mucosal fold. As a result of propulsive forces during repeated swallowing, these areas can enlarge in size so much so as to even reach the stomach.[7,55]

Most FVPs are asymptomatic. Some case reports have described dramatic presentations with prolapse of large lesions into the larynx causing asphyxiation; lesions as large as 20 cm have been reported. Lesions that protrude into the proximal stomach are exposed to an acidic environment, which can lead to ulceration and bleeding.[7]

On barium swallow study, FVP appears as a large intraluminal mass within the esophagus (Figs 5A and B). Endoscopy shows a fleshy polypoid lesion usually arising from the cricopharynx (Figs 6A and B). On sagittal and coronal T2-weighted magnetic resonance imaging (MRI), FVP appear as a large well marginated intraluminal polyp within the thoracic esophagus extending for a variable length depending on the size (Figs 7A and B). On axial T1-weighted and T2-weighted images, the lesion displays hypointense and hyperintense signal respectively (Figs 8A and B).[56]

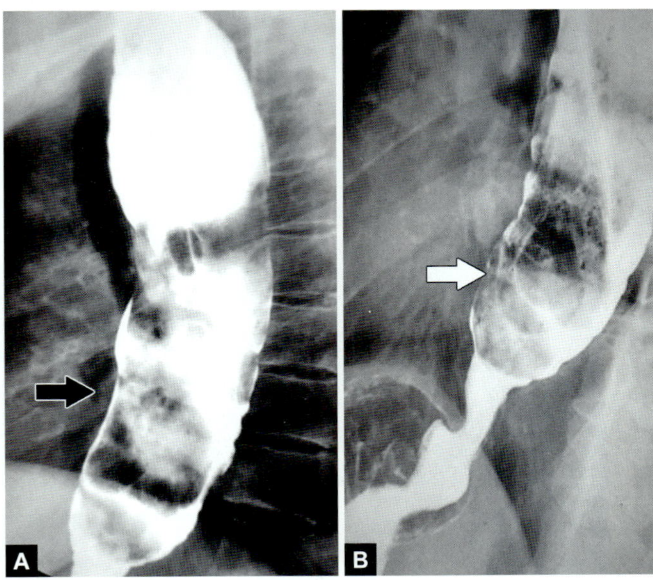

Figures 5A and B Barium swallow showing a large intraluminal filling defect (black arrow) within mid and distal thoracic esophagus with normal esophageal mucosa (white arrow)
Source: Dr Vijay Ramachandran.

Considering its progressive nature and the risk of asphyxiation and sudden death, surgical removal of the polyp is usually recommended. Local excision of the polyp is curative and recurrence is rare.[57] Traditionally, the most common approach has been through a cervical esophagotomy (since most lesions arise from the region of cricopharyngeus) with complete excision of the polyp. Endoscopic removal of symptomatic polyps may be done using a snare, as these polyps often have a stalk. EUS should be performed before endoscopic excision to rule out the presence of a large vessel feeding the stalk of the lesion. Surgical resection still may be required, if the base of the

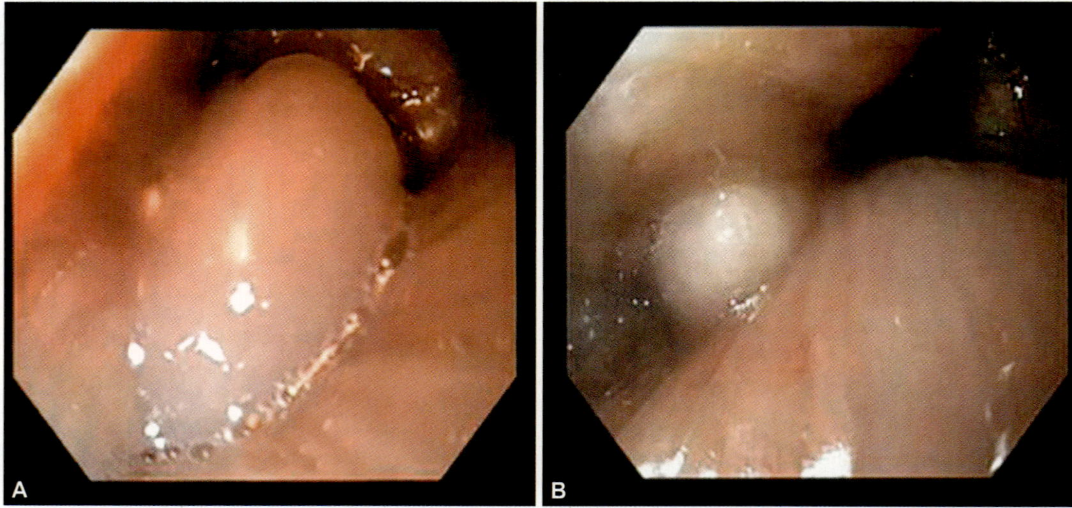

Figures 6A and B Fibrovascular polyp in a middle aged male patient. (A) Endoscopy showing fleshy polypoid lesion arising at 20 cm from incisors (B) Prolapsing into hypopharynx
Source: Dr Vikram Bhatia, New Delhi.

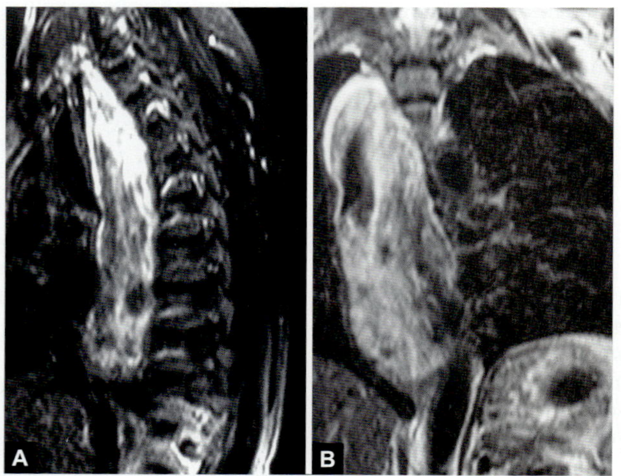

Figures 7A and B Sagittal and coronal T2-weighted MRI showing a large well marginated intraluminal polyp within the thoracic esophagus extending from the thoracic inlet level to just above the level of the diaphragm
Source: Dr Vijay Ramachandran.

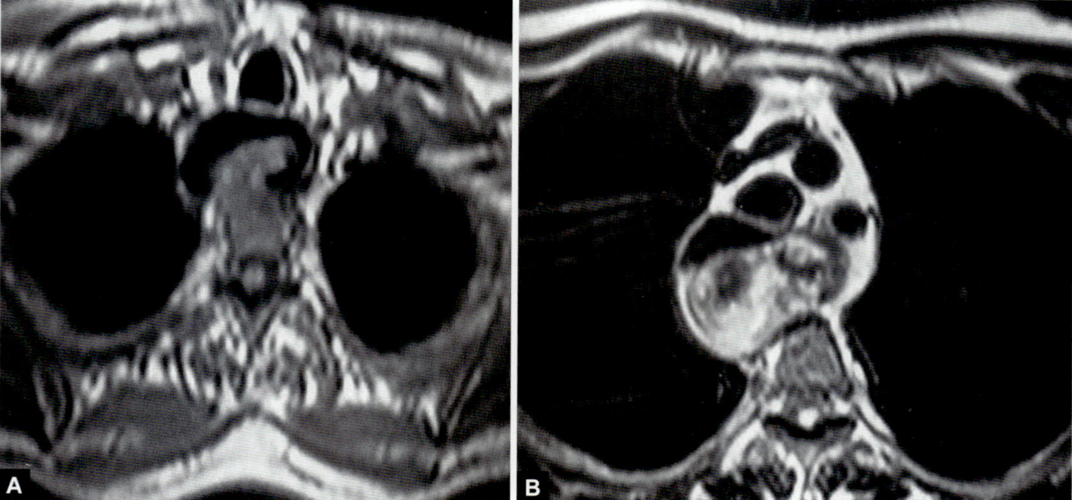

Figures 8A and B (A) Axial T1-weighted and; (B) T2-weighted images show that the lesion displays hypointense signal on T1-weighted and hyperintense signal on T2-weighted images
Source: Dr Vijay Ramachandran.

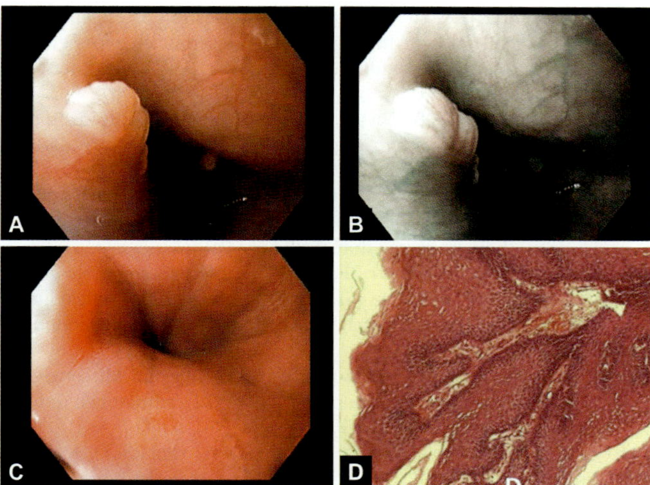

Figures 9A to D Esophageal squamous papilloma in a 45-year-old male patient. (A) Endoscopy showing a fleshy pink lesion in esophagus; (B) Narrow band imaging showing a small, sessile lesion in the upper third of esophagus. No tumor neovascularization is seen on the surface. The adjacent mucosa is normal; (C) Lesion was completely removed endoscopically by snaring; (D) Biopsy showing squamous papilloma composed of multilobulated hyperplastic benign stratified squamous epithelium lined papillae with fibrovascular cores (HE, x40)
Source: Dr Vikram Bhatia and Dr Archana Rastogi, ILBS, New Delhi.

stalk is endoscopically inaccessible or if a large feeding vessel is present.

Papilloma

Esophageal papillomas are rare benign epithelial lesions, mostly diagnosed in patients who are in their 50s.[58-60] They are more common in men.[58-60] Majority of the papillomas present as a solitary lesion, although patients with over 10 lesions have been reported.[59] Approximately, 70% of papillomas occur in the distal one-third of the esophagus,[58] and have been associated with documented reflux and esophagitis.[59]

On endoscopy, they appear as small, fleshy pink lesions, either sessile or pedunculated lesions (Figs 9A and B). Papillomas may be associated with tylosis and acanthosis nigricans.[61] The association of human papilloma virus (HPV) with esophageal papillomas has been described.[62,63] Rarely, malignant degeneration of papilloma has been reported.[64]

Histologically, papillomas are characterized by finger-like projections of tissue lined by squamous cells and a core of connective tissue that contains small blood vessels (Fig. 9C).[58] Most lesions are asymptomatic, but large lesions can cause dysphagia.[59]

Papillomas are usually amenable to endoscopic resection (Fig. 9D). Lesions smaller than 1 cm can usually be removed with a cold-forceps biopsy, but larger lesions require endoscopic mucosal resection. Recurrence after resection is rare.[59]

Adenomas

Esophageal adenomas are mostly associated with Barrett's esophagus. They present as a polypoid or nodular lesion[65] and lesions as large as 1.5 cm have been reported.[66] Enhanced endoscopic techniques such as narrow band imaging or chromoendoscopy can be used to evaluate the adjacent Barrett's mucosa.

There is limited literature available regarding management of esophageal adenomas. If adenoma is not associated with Barrett's esophagitis, lesions smaller than 1 cm should be resected endoscopically using a biopsy forceps or snare. More than 1 cm lesions and those containing high-grade dysplasia can be removed using endoscopic mucosal resection. Advanced lesions may require surgery.

REFERENCES

1. Seremetis MG, Lyons WS, deGuzman VC, Peabody JW. Leiomyomata of the esophagus. An analysis of 838 cases. Cancer. 1976;38:2166-77.
2. Coutinho DS, Soga J, Yoshikawa T, Miyashita K, Tanaka O, Sasaki K, et al. Granular cell tumours of the esophagus: a report of two cases and review of the literature. Am J Gastroenterol. 1985;80:758-62.
3. Moersch HJ, Harrington SW. Benign tumor of the esophagus. Ann Otl Rhnol Laryngol. 1944;53:800.
4. Plachta A. Benign tumours of the esophagus. Review of literature and report of 99 cases. Am J Gastroenterol. 1962;38:639-52.
5. Sweet RH, Soutter L, Valenzuela CT. Muscle wall tumors of the esophagus. J Thorac Surg. 1954;27:13-31.
6. Nemir P, Wallace HW, Fallahnejad M. Diagnosis and surgical management of benign diseases of the esophagus. Curr Probl Surg. 1976;13:1-74.
7. Avezzano EA, Fleischer DE, Merida MA, Anderson DL. Giant fibrovascular polyps of the esophagus. Am J Gastroenterol. 1990;85:299-302.
8. Reed CE. Benign tumors of the esophagus. Chest Surg Clin N Am. 1994;4:769-83.
9. Herrera JL. Benign and metastatic tumors of the esophagus. Gastroenterol Clin North Am. 1991;20:775-89.
10. Shamji F, Todd TR. Benign Tumors. In: Pearson FG, Hiebert CA, Deslauries J (Eds). Esophageal surgery. New York: Churchill Livingstone; 1995. pp. 519-53.
11. Mutrie CJ, Donahue DM, Wain JC, Wright CD, Gaissert HA, Grillo HC, et al. Esophageal leiomyoma: a 40-year experience. Ann Thorac Surg. 2005;79:1122-5.
12. Hatch GF, Wertheimer-Hatch L, Hatch KF, Davis GB, Blanchard DK, Foster RS, et al. Tumors of the esophagus. World J Surg. 2000;24:401-11.
13. Rendina EA, Venuta F, Pescarmona EO, Facciolo F, Francioni F, Di Tolla R, et al. Leiomyoma of the esophagus. Scand J Thorac Cardiovasc Surg. 1990;24:79-82.
14. Rice TW. Benign esophageal tumours: esophagoscopy and endoscopic esophageal ultrasound. Semin Thorac Cardiovasc Surg. 2003;15:20-6.
15. Bhatia V, Tajika M, Rastogi A. Upper gastrointestinal submucosal lesions--clinical and endosonographic evaluation and management. Trop Gastroenterol. 2010;31:5-29.
16. Yasuda K, Cho E, Nakajima M, Kawai K. Diagnosis of submucosal lesions of the upper gastrointestinal tract by endoscopic ultrasonography. Gastrointest Endosc. 1990;36(2 Suppl):S17-20.
17. Punpale A, Rangole A, Bhambhani N, Karimundackal G, Desai N, de Souza A, et al. Leiomyoma of esophagus. Ann Thorac Cardiovasc Surg. 2007;13(2):78-81.
18. Xu GQ, Zhang BL, Li YM, Chen LH, Ji F, Chen WX, et al. Diagnostic value of endoscopic ultrasonography for gastrointestinal leiomyoma. World J Gastroenterol. 2003;9(9):2088-91.

19. Evans HL. Smooth muscle tumours of the gastrointestinal tract. A study of 56 cases followed for a minimum of 10 years. Cancer. 1985;56(9):2242-50.
20. Bardini R, Segalin A, Ruol A, Pavanello M, Peracchia A. Videothoracoscopic enucleation of esophageal leiomyoma. Ann Thorac Surg. 1992;54(3):576-7.
21. Everitt NJ, Glinatsis M, McMahon MJ. Thoracoscopic enucleation of leiomyoma of the oesophagus. Br J Surg. 1992;79(7):643.
22. Marmuse JP, Johanet H, Louvent F, Benhamou G. [Leiomyomas of the lower third of the esophagus. Value of transhiatal enucleation]. Ann Chir. 1994;48:446-51.
23. Zaninotto G, Portale G, Costantini M, et al. Minimally invasive enucleation of esophageal leiomyoma. Surg Endosc. 2006;20: 1904-8.
24. Kinney T, Waxman I. Treatment of benign esophageal tumours by endoscopic techniques. Semin Thorac Cardiovasc Surg. 2003;15:27-34.
25. Lee LS, Singhal S, Brinster CJ, Marshall B, Kochman ML, Kaiser LR, et al. Current management of esophageal leiomyoma. J Am Coll Surg. 2004;198:136-46.
26. Lee HJ, Park SI, Kim DK, Kim YH. Surgical resection of esophageal gastrointestinal stromal tumours. Ann Thorac Surg. 2009;87(5):1569-71.
27. von Rahden BH, Stein HJ, Feussner H, Siewert JR. Enucleation of submucosal tumours of the esophagus: minimally invasive versus open approach. Surg Endosc. 2004;18:924-30.
28. Jiang P, Jiao Z, Han B, Zhang X, Sun X, Su J, et al. Clinical characteristics and surgical treatment of oesophageal gastrointestinal stromal tumours. Eur J Cardiothorac Surg. 2010;38:223-7.
29. Blum MG, Bilimoria KY, Wayne JD, de Hoyos AL, Talamonti MS, Adley B. Surgical considerations for the management and resection of esophageal gastrointestinal stromal tumors. Ann Thorac Surg. 2007;84:1717-23.
30. Miettinen M, Sarlomo-Rikala M, Sobin LH, Lasota J. Esophageal stromal tumours: a clinicopathologic, immunohistochemical, and molecular genetic study of 17 cases and comparison with esophageal leiomyomas and leiomyosarcomas. Am J Surg Pathol. 2000;24:211-22.
31. Horton KM, Juluru K, Montogomery E, Fishman EK. Computed tomography imaging of gastrointestinal stromal tumours with pathology correlation. J Comput Assist Tomogr. 2004;28:811-7.
32. Dematteo RP, Ballman KV, Antonescu CR, Maki RG, Pisters PW, Demetri GD, et al. Adjuvant imatinib mesylate after resection of localised, primary gastrointestinal stromal tumour: a randomised, double-blind, placebo-controlled trial. Lancet. 2009;373:1097-104.
33. Chen HC, Huang HJ, Wu CY, Lin TS, Fang HY. Esophageal schwannoma with tracheal compression. Thorac Cardiovasc Surg. 2006;54:555-8.
34. Mizuguchi S, Inoue K, Imagawa A, Kitano Y, Kameyama M, Ueda H, et al. Benign esophageal schwannoma compressing the trachea in pregnancy. Ann Thorac Surg. 2008;85:660-2.
35. Kent M, d'Amato T, Nordman C, Schuchert M, Landreneau R, Alvelo-Rivera M, et al. Minimally invasive resection of benign esophageal tumors. J Thorac Cardiovasc Surg. 2007;134:176-81.
36. Naus PJ, Tio FO, Gross GW. Esophageal schwannoma: first report of successful management by endoscopic removal. Gastrointest Endosc. 2001;54:520-2.
37. Orlowska J, Pachlewski J, Gugulski A, Butruk E. A conservative approach to granular cell tumours of the esophagus: four case reports and literature review. Am J Gastroenterol. 1993;88:311-5.
38. Ordonez NG, Mackay B. Granular cell tumor: a review of the pathology and histogenesis. Ultrastruct Pathol. 1999;23(4): 207-22.
39. Tada S, Iida M, Yao T, Miyagahara T, Hasuda S, Fujishima M. Granular cell tumor of the esophagus: endoscopic ultrasonographic demonstration and endoscopic removal. Am J Gastroenterol. 1990;85(11):1507-11.
40. Vuyk HD, Snow GB, Tiwari RM, van Velzen D, Veldhuizen RW. Granular cell tumor of the proximal esophagus. A rare disease. Cancer. 1985;55:445-9.
41. Fanburg-Smith JC, Meis-Kindblom JM, Fante R, Kindblom LG. Malignant granular cell tumor of soft tissue: diagnostic criteria and clinicopathologic correlation. Am J Surg Pathol. 1998;22:779-94.
42. Postlethwaite RW, Lowe JE: Benign tumours and cysts of the esophagus. In: Zuidema GD, Orringer MB (Eds). Shackelford's surgery of the alimentary tract, 4th edition. Philadelphia: Saunders; 1996.
43. Catalano F, Kind R, Rodella L, Lombardo F, Festini M, Tomezzoli A, et al. Endoscopic treatment of esophageal granular cell tumors. Endoscopy. 2002;34(7):582-4.
44. Yasuda I, Tomita E, Nagura K, Nishigaki Y, Yamada O, Kachi H. Endoscopic removal of granular cell tumors. Gastrointest Endosc. 1995;41:163-7.
45. Govoni AF. Hemangiomas of the esophagus. Gastrointest Radiol. 1982;7(2):113-7.
46. Rasalkar DD, Chiu PW, Teoh AY, Chu WC. Oesophageal haemangioma: imaging characteristics of this rare condition. Hong Kong Med J. 2010;16(3):230-1.
47. Hanel K, Talley NA, Hunt DR. Hemangioma of the esophagus: an unusual cause of upper gastrointestinal bleeding. Dig Dis Sci. 1981;26:257-63.
48. Oda, Kondo H, Yamao T, Saito D, Ono H, Gotoda T, et al. Metastatic tumors to the stomach: analysis of 54 patients diagnosed at endoscopy and 347 autopsy cases. Endoscopy. 2001;33:507-10.
49. Yoshikane H, Suzuki T, Yoshioka N, Ogawa Y, Ochi T, Hasegawa N. Hemangioma of the esophagus: endosonographic imaging and endoscopic resection. Endoscopy. 1995;27(3):267-9.
50. Dumbleton SA, Warshauer DM, Koruda MJ, Woosley JT. Haemangioma of the oesophagus: CT demonstration. Australas Radiol. 1997;41:65-6.
51. Araki K, Ohno S, Egashira A, Saeki H, Kawaguchi H, Ikeda Y, et al. Esophageal hemangioma: a case report and review of the literature. Hepatogastroenterology. 1999;46:3148-54.
52. Folia M, Naiman N, Dubois R, Ayari S, Froehlich P. Management of postcricoid and upper esophageal hemangioma. Int J Pediatr Otorhinolaryngol. 2007;71:147-51.
53. Wu YC, Liu HP, Liu YH, Hsieh MJ, Lin PJ. Minimal access thoracic surgery for esophageal hemangioma. Ann Thorac Surg. 2001;72(5):1754-5.
54. Shigemitsu K, Naomoto Y, Yamatsuji T, Ono K, Aoki H, Haisa M, et al. Esophageal hemangioma successfully treated by fulguration using potassium titanyl phosphate/yttrium aluminum garnet (KTP/YAG) laser: a case report. Dis Esophagus. 2000;13(2):161-4.
55. Owens JJ, Donovan DT, Alford EL, McKechnie JC, Franklin DJ, Stewart MG, et al. Life-threatening presentations of fibrovascular esophageal and hypopharyngeal polyps. Ann Otol Rhinol Laryngol. 1994;103:838-42.
56. Goenka AH, Sharma S, Ramachandran V, Chattopadhyay TK, Ray R. Giant fibrovascular polyp of the esophagus: report of a case. Surg Today. 2011;41:120-4.
57. Rice TW, Murthy SC. Surgical treatment of benign esophageal diseases. In: Sellke FW, Del Nido PJ, Swanson SJ (Eds). Sabiston & Spencer Surgery of the Chest. 7th edition. Philadelphia: Elsevier Saunders; 2005. pp. 583-609.
58. Quitadamo M, Benson J. Squamous papilloma of the esophagus: a case report and review of the literature. Am J Gastroenterol. 1988;83:194-201.

59. Carr NJ, Monihan JM, Sobin LH. Squamous cell papilloma of the esophagus: a clinicopathologic and follow-up study of 25 cases. Am J Gastroenterol. 1994;89(2):245-8.
60. Odze R, Antonioli D, Shocket D, Noble-Topham S, Goldman H, Upton M. Esophageal squamous papillomas. A clinicopathologic study of 38 lesions and analysis for human papillomavirus by the polymerase chain reaction. Am J Surg Pathol. 1993;17:803-12.
61. Brinson RR, Schuman BM, Mills LR, Thigpen S, Freedman S. Multiple squamous papillomas of the esophagus associated with Goltz syndrome. Am J Gastroenterol. 1987;82:1177-9.
62. Szanto I, Szentirmay Z, Banai J, Nagy P, Gonda G, Vörös A, et al. [Squamous papilloma of the esophagus. Clinical and pathological observations based on 172 papillomas in 155 patients]. Orv Hetil. 2005;146(12):547-52.
63. Syrjanen KJ. HPV infections and oesophageal cancer. J Clin Pathol. 2002;55:721-8.
64. Mourra N, Flejou JF, Arrive L. Clinical challenges and images in GI. Extrahepatic biliary cystadenoma with mesenchymal stroma. Gastroenterology. 2008;134:1295-637.
65. Lee RG. Adenomas arising in Barrett's esophagus. Am J Clin Pathol. 1986;85:629-32.
66. Keeffe EB, Hisken EC, Schubert F. Adenomatous polyp arising in Barrett's esophagus. J Clin Gastroenterol. 1986;8:271-4.

CHAPTER 18

Carcinoma Esophagus

Kishore GS Bharathy, TK Chattopadhyay

INTRODUCTION

Carcinoma of the esophagus is the eighth most common cancer worldwide[1] and is still associated with high mortality rates. Accurate diagnosis and staging permits appropriate prognostication and management. Surgery is the mainstay of curative treatment and multidisciplinary approach to care ensures that patients with this disease derive the best chance of survival and good quality of life.

EPIDEMIOLOGY AND RISK FACTORS

There is a striking geographic variation in the distribution of esophageal cancer worldwide. Esophageal adenocarcinoma (EAC) is common in Western Europe, North America, Australia whereas squamous cell carcinoma (SCC) is the predominant variety in India, eastern countries and an area that extends from the border of the Caspian Sea, Turkey through Russia and Northern China, called the "esophageal cancer belt".[2] Each of these types has characteristic epidemiological profiles and risk factors.

Esophageal Adenocarcinoma

The incidence of EAC has shown the fastest rise in the last three decades among any solid malignancy in the western world.[3] It is a dramatic and starkly visible epidemic related to many interrelated risk factors. Barrett's esophagus (BE), which is a columnar metaplasia of the distal esophagus generally containing intestinal differentiation, is considered to be the most important of these. Endoscopic studies have shown that BE develops in 6% to 14% of individuals with GERD, and approximately 0.5% to 1% of patients with BE develop adenocarcinoma.[4,5] Relative to the general population, BE increases adenocarcinoma risk 30-fold, and the presence of BE is associated with a 0.12% annual risk of developing adenocarcinoma.[6] Age (>50 years), male sex, white race, hiatal hernia, chronic gastroesophageal reflux disease (GERD), increased body mass index (BMI), and intra-abdominal body fat distribution constitute established risk factors.[7] Inherited polymorphisms of the epidermal growth factor (EGF) gene causing increased serum EGF have been associated with increased adenocarcinoma risk, especially in patients with BE.[8] BE also aggregates in families. Familial BE can be confirmed in 7.3% of persons presenting with BE or adenocarcinoma of the distal esophagus or gastroesophageal junction (GEJ).[9] The role of endoscopic screening and surveillance for BE is out of scope of discussion of this chapter.

Many pre-existing conditions may increase the risk of developing EAC secondary to increasing gastric acid production or increasing esophageal exposure to refluxed gastric acid or bile. These include myotomy or dilation of the lower esophageal sphincter (LES), scleroderma, Zollinger-Ellison syndrome and any condition requiring medications known to relax the LES.[10] There is data to indicate that bile salt exposure to the distal esophagus likely induces intestinal differentiation and this process is mediated through the transcription factor CDX-2 through the epidermal growth factor receptor. Progression of BE to adenocarcinoma is associated with inflammation, cyclooxygenase 2 activation, and epigenetic modifications.[10] Obesity and metabolic syndrome are important risk factors associated with BE and adenocarcinoma. Metabolic syndrome is more prevalent in people with BE than in the general population and is positively associated with the length of specialized intestinal metaplasia (SIM). Sixty percent of patients with long-segment BE had metabolic syndrome, and 92% were centrally obese compared with 23.8% and 62%, respectively (p=0.007 and 0.005) in short-segment BE.[11] A large observational study found that the use of NSAIDs, proton pump inhibitors, and statins in patients with BE was associated with a reduced progression to adenocarcinoma.[12] Smoking is associated with an increased risk of

Table 1: Risk factors for the development of esophageal adenocarcinoma

Reference	*Risk factor studied*	*Main findings*	*Type of study*
Rubenstein JH[18]	GERD	At least weekly symptoms of GERD increased the odds of EAC fivefold (OR=4.92; 95% CI=3.90–6.22), and daily symptoms increased the odds sevenfold (random effects summary OR=7.40, 95% CI=4.94–11.1)	Meta-analysis
Hvid Jensen F[8]	Barrett's esophagus	As compared with the risk in the general population, the RR of adenocarcinoma among patients with BE was 11.3 (95% CI, 8.8–14.4)	Population based cohort study
Turati F[19]	Obesity	The overall RR of esophageal cancer was 1.71 (95% CI 1.50–1.96) for BMI between 25 and 30, and was 2.34 (95% CI 1.95–2.81) for BMI ≥30 kg/m^2. The association was stronger for adenocarcinoma (RR for BMI ≥30 kg/m^2=2.73, 95% CI 2.16–3.46)	Meta-analysis
Cook MB[20]	Smoking	The summary ORs demonstrated strong associations between cigarette smoking and EAC (OR=1.96, 95% CI=1.64–2.34), AEJ (OR=2.18, 95% CI=1.84–2.58). There was a strong dose-response association between pack-years of cigarette smoking and incidence (p <0.001). Smoking cessation was associated with reduced risks	Meta-analysis
Bhat S[21]	Gender	The risk of cancer was statistically significantly elevated in men compared with women (0.28% per year vs. 0.13% per year; HR=2.11, 95% CI=1.41–3.16, p <.001)	Population based study
Islami F[22]	*H.pylori* infection	EAC is inversely associated with *H.pylori* infection. The summary OR (95% CI) was 0.56 (0.46–0.68). Further analysis showed that colonization with CagA-positive strains was inversely associated with EAC risk (OR, 0.41; 95% CI, 0.28–0.62) but colonization with CagA-negative strains was not (OR, 1.08; 95% CI, 0.76–1.53)	Meta-analysis

Abbreviations: GERD, gastroesophageal reflux disease; EAC, esophageal adenocarcinoma; OR, odds ratio; CI, confidence interval; RR, relative risk; BE, Barrett's esophagus; BMI, body mass idex; AEJ, adenocarcinoma of the esophagogastric junction.

developing esophageal carcinoma (squamous>junctional>adenocarcinoma).[13] Alcohol consumption is associated with an increased risk of SCC whereas it has not implicated in the development of EAC.[14,15] While H.pylori infection is associated with an increased risk of gastric carcinoma, meta-analyses indicate that that H.pylori infection is inversely associated with EAC risk. Treatment of H.pylori infection is thought to be linked to the epidemiological increase in the incidence of EAC.[16] Male sex is associated with more than 8 fold risk of developing EAC.[17] The evidence for risk factors in development of EAC is summarized in Table 1.

Squamous Cell Carcinoma

SCC has well established risk factors some of which are exclusive to certain geographic areas and are closely linked to dietary habits, lifestyle and low socio-economic status.[23] Poor oral hygiene has been shown to be associated with the development of esophageal SCC.[24] Smoking is perhaps one of the most important of the risk factors. The major carcinogenic activity of tobacco smoke is contained in the tar fraction. The volatile nitrosamines and polynuclear aromatic hydrocarbons are the primary initiators.[2] Snuff (smokeless tobacco) is the most powerful risk factor of esophageal cancer in Jammu region, followed by the salt tea, smoking and the sundried food.[25]. Hookah smoking and nass chewing are associated with SCC risk.[26] Alcohol has a synergistic effect with smoking on risk. Both intensity and duration of alcohol use affects risk, but unlike smoking, intensity is more important. The relative risk for SCC increases with the amount of alcohol consumed, being approximately 1.8 for 5 to 11 drinks per week and increasing to 7.4 for more than 30 drinks per week.[2] Tylosis is a rare disorder associated with hyperkeratosis of the palms of the hands and soles of the feet and a high rate of SCC. The inherited type of tylosis (Howell-Evans syndrome) is an autosomal dominant disease with a gene locus mapped to 17q 25. There are several preexisting conditions that increase the risk of developing SCC. These include caustic injury, achalasia, current or past history of SCC of the head and neck, Plummer Vinson syndrome and Zenker diverticulum.[2] The deficiency of Zinc and Molybdenum can be correlated to the development of SCC.[27] Infection with human papilloma virus (HPV) type 52 has been correlated with the development of SCC.[28] Out of a total of 101 biopsy specimens of carcinoma esophagus analyzed, the frequency of HPV was found to be the highest 14/32 (44%) in Dibrugarh followed by 33% (11/33) in Kashmir, but, interestingly, no high-risk HPV could be detected in New Delhi patients who showed the highest frequency (30.6%) of p53 mutation as against only 12.5% in Dibrugarh and 6.1% in Kashmir.[29] Smoking is strongly associated with viral infection. Tumor suppressor genes, genetic polymorphisms have been studied as risk factors for the development of esophageal cancer in many excellent Indian studies.[30-34] p53 expression was threefold higher than normal in dysplasias of squamous epithelium and adenocarcinoma, while it was eightfold higher in SCC.[35] In an Indian study, the p53 exon 7 appeared to be the 'hot-spot' for esophageal cancer as it alone was responsible for more than 76% (13/17) of mutations and more than 95% (20/21) of the patients with p53 mutation were smokers.[29] SCC with DNA replication errors are associated with p16/pRb loss and wild-type p53.[36]

CLINICAL PRESENTATION

More often than not, esophageal cancer presents at an advanced stage in our country. The most common symptom is progressive dysphagia (74%-83%).[37] At times the dysphagia is of a sudden onset which results from impaction of food at the site of the tumor and aggravated by the local spasm of the esophagus. Similarly, the dysphagia can be suddenly relieved following necrosis and sloughing of the tumor. Other important symptoms include loss of weight (58%), appetite in a patient with a fitting epidemiological profile. Symptoms and signs of locally advanced disease include hoarseness of voice due to recurrent laryngeal nerve involvement, cough during eating or drinking indicating a malignant tracheo-esophageal fistula, a deep boring pain in the chest and back due to infiltration of the tumor into the mediastinum and regional adenopathy. Features of metastatic disease reflect the organ system involved and may include jaundice, ascites, dyspnea, pleural effusion, signs of an intracranial space occupying lesion or a bony swelling. In patients diagnosed with recent esophageal cancer, metastases were seen in the liver in 35%, lung in 20%, bone in 9%, adrenal gland and brain in 2% each, and 1% each in the pericardium, pleura, soft tissues, stomach, pancreas, and spleen.[38] At the other end of the spectrum is a cancer detected incidentally on endoscopy performed as a part of screening for BE or in patients with GERD. These patients may have non-specific symptoms, reflux, or a sensation of food occasionally getting stuck in the chest. A high index of suspicion helps in detecting these tumors early.

STAGING

The 7th UICC-AJCC staging system for esophageal cancer is summarized in Table 2.[39]

The application of the 7th edition staging system results in a better prognostic stratification of overall survival for EAC compared to the 6th edition.[41] Improvements include new definitions of Tis, T4, regional lymph node, N classification, and M classification, and addition of nonanatomic cancer characteristics: histopathologic cell type, histologic grade, and cancer location. Indeed, the latest 7th edition has acknowledged the importance of the number of involved nodes by revising the N category from site-dependent staging to a numerically based classification into N0 to N3.[42]

Summary of Stage Grouping

Stage 0 is high grade dysplasia without the presence of invasive carcinoma. Stages I and II comprise of node negative T1-T3 tumors and are staged separately for EAC and SCC. Adenosquamous carcinomas are staged as SCC. For EAC, histological grading

Table 2: The AJCC-TNM staging for esophageal cancer
T: Primary Tumor
T0 No evidence of tumor Tis High-grade dysplasia T1 Tumor invades the lamina propria, muscularis mucosa (T1a), or submucosa (T1b). T2 Tumor invades into but not beyond the muscularis propria T3 Tumor invades the paraesophageal tissue, but does not invade adjacent structures T4a Resectable tumor invades adjacent structures, such as pleura, pericardium, diaphragm T4b Unresectable tumor invades other adjacent structures, such as aorta, vertebral body, trachea
N: Regional Lymph Nodes Any paraesophageal lymph node from cervical lymph nodes to celiac nodes
N0 No regional lymph node metastases N1 1 to 2 positive regional lymph nodes N2 3 to 6 positive regional lymph nodes N3 7 or more positive regional lymph nodes
M: Distant Metastasis
M0 No distant metastases M1 Distant metastases
Non-anatomic Cancer Characteristics
Histopathologic cell type Adenocarcinoma Squamous cell carcinoma
Histologic grade G1 Well differentiated G2 Moderately differentiated G3 Poorly differentiated G4 Undifferentiated
Tumor location
Upper thoracic 20–25 cm from incisors (sternal notch to azygous vein) Middle thoracic greater than 25–30 cm from incisors (azygous vein to inferior pulmonary vein) Lower thoracic greater than 30–40 cm from incisors (inferior pulmonary vein to esophagogastric junction)
Adenocarcinoma of the esophagogastric junction (AEG) is classified according to its topographic location into three types as per the well-known Siewert system.[40] Type I AEG occurs between 1 and 5 cm proximal to the cardia; type II tumors occur 1 cm proximal and 2 cm distal to the cardia; type III tumors occur between 2 and 5 cm distal to the cardia. Typing of tumors that show infiltration across these arbitrary anatomical boundaries is dictated by the epicenter of the tumor. AEGs are stage grouped similar to adenocarcinoma of the esophagus.

is incorporated into the staging system; for SCC in addition to grade, location of the tumor is important. Lower thoracic SCC has a better survival than middle/upper thoracic tumors. Stage III disease comprises of various combinations of node positive resectable tumors (T1 through T4a). Stage IV is presence of unresectable disease/distant metastases.

INVESTIGATIONS

Investigations are directed towards diagnosis, staging evaluation, assessment of fitness to undergo major surgery/multimodality therapy. Blood investigations (hemogram, liver, kidney function tests, blood grouping), chest radiography and ECG are mandatory. Cardiopulmonary evaluation (echocardiogram, pulmonary function test) is routinely done as the population is often elderly, nutritionally depleted, with comorbidities. The following paragraphs summarize the role of specific investigative modalities in carcinoma esophagus in the light of available evidence.

Barium Esophagography

The principal finding on a barium esophagogram is a stricture. The radiographic appearance is an asymmetric, abrupt, irregular narrowing with shelf like margins and a nodular or ulcerated surface within the stricture. Other useful information available on barium study includes the site and length of the stricture, relationship to the GEJ, evidence of tracheoesophageal fistula and status of the stomach. In most centers, endoscopy has replaced barium esophagography as the initial investigation of choice.

Endoscopy

Endoscopy and biopsy is the first investigation in the evaluation of dysphagia and forms the mainstay of the diagnosis of esophageal carcinoma.[42] Endoscopy detects the location of the tumor (distance from the incisor teeth/GEJ), its extent (longitudinal as well as circumferential) and morphology (flat/ulcerated/nodular, described in standard terminology[43]) and provides an opportunity for biopsy for tissue diagnosis. Careful endoscopy detects Barrett's epithelium, dysplasia, and carcinoma. A cancer length greater than 5 cm is predictive of T3 cancer, with 89% sensitivity, 92% specificity, 89% positive predictive value, and 92% negative predictive value.[44] Endoscopy and biopsy is mandatory in all patients being evaluated for BE/dysplasia/invasive cancer. Chromoendoscopy, narrow band imaging, confocal fluorescence microscopy, elastic scattering spectroscopy and optical coherence tomography are some of the techniques available to detect early lesions in the setting of BE, dysplasia.

Endoscopic Ultrasonography (EUS)

EUS gives a stratified view of the wall of the esophagus and helps in accurate T staging. It also helps in evaluating regional nodes and permits sampling by a guided fine needle aspiration. Reported pooled sensitivity and specificity are 81.6% and 99.4%, respectively, for T1 classification; 81.4% and 96.3% for T2; 91.4% and 94.4% for T3; and 92.4% and 97.4% for T4[45] Conventional EUS tends to overstage early esophageal cancers, a phenomenon that occurs in 10% to 28% of the patients with T1, T2 lesions[46,47] EUS is not accurate in distinguishing Tis from T1 cancers, and other examinations such as pathologic examination of endoscopic mucosal resection (EMR) specimens are necessary for this distinction. A meta-analysis of 49 publications[45] reported pooled sensitivity of 84% and specificity of 85%, for EUS determination of N classification. Overall, sensitivity, specificity, and positive and negative predictive values of EUS evaluation without performance of the fine needle aspiration (FNA) for lymph node staging were 75%, 97%, 75%, and 98%, respectively[46] Round well demarcated hypoechoic nodes are considered malignant. EUS-FNA may not be feasible if the biopsy tract has to traverse the primary tumor. If the EUS probe is not negotiable across a circumferential lesion, it is indicative of advanced disease.

Computed Tomography (CT)

CT is essential to rule out distant metastases. Despite improved technology, CT is only 37% to 66% sensitive in screening for distant metastases in patients with esophageal cancer.[42] The preservation of fat planes between an esophageal cancer and adjacent structures at CT excludes T4 cancers and is the only T determination provided by this examination. A recent meta-analysis of 20 publications[48] reported a pooled sensitivity and specificity for CT determination of N stage to be 59% and 81%, respectively. If the short axis of intrathoracic or abdominal lymph nodes is greater than 1 cm on CT, they are likely to be metastatic. Supraclavicular lymph nodes with a short axis greater than 0.5 cm and retrocrural lymph nodes greater than 0.6 cm are radiographically pathologic.[42]

Positron Emission Tomography (PET)

Many authors also advocate PET along with CT prior to planning operative intervention and to assess response to neoadjuvant therapy. A meta-analysis of 12 publications reported a pooled sensitivity and specificity for flurodeoxy glucose (FDG) PET in determination of N stage to be 59% and 81%, respectively.[48] PET/CT is reported to detect distant metastases in 25% of patients that was missed by CT.[49] The combination of FDG PET and CT has a diagnostic accuracy of 80% to 92% and avoids unnecessary surgery in 90%.[42]

Staging Laparoscopy

Laparoscopy was reported to change therapy in 10% of patients, allowing resection in 2% who are over-staged and avoiding resection in 8% with newly detected M1 cancer.[50] The sensitivities of laparoscopy in detecting peritoneal and liver metastases are 71% and 86%, respectively.[50] Staging laparoscopy is routinely done at the time of undertaking curative resection.

Bronchoscopy

Bronchoscopy is necessary part of the staging work of tumors of the upper and middle third of the esophagus. It helps in ruling out infiltration if the trachea and bronchus which may contraindicate surgical resection or radical radiotherapy. During the procedure either mucosal infiltration or a bulge may be visualized.

MANAGEMENT

Management options should be tailored to suit the type, location and stage of the tumor, performance status of the patient and expertise of the treating team for optimal results.

SURGERY

The fundamental aim of surgical management of esophageal carcinoma is to achieve R0 resection at acceptable morbidity and minimal mortality rates. Surgery still remains the cornerstone of curative management. Several studies have shown that both perioperative mortality and morbidity are lower for esophageal resection when the procedure is performed in high-volume centers.[51,52] The following section provides an overview of various operative approaches and evidence for them. Operative techniques and complications of surgery are covered elsewhere in this book.

Types of Surgery

It depends on the experience, philosophy of the treating center, surgeon; the location of the tumor, its stage and patient profile. The largest randomized trial comparing transhiatal esophagectomy (THE) vs. transthoracic esophagectomy (TTE)[53] included a total of 220 patients with adenocarcinoma who were assigned to THE or TTE with 2-field lymphadenectomy. The transhiatal group had shorter duration of surgery, less blood loss, and less overall morbidity. By contrast, significantly more lymph nodes were retrieved in the TTE group. Nevertheless, there was no significant difference in perioperative mortality. In addition, the R0 resection rate was similar for both groups. There was no statistically significant difference between the two groups in terms of survival. Other trials, including meta-analyses, have confirmed a lack of survival difference between the two techniques.[54] Minimally invasive esophagectomy (MIE) is a viable alternative to open techniques. Meta-analytic evidence finds equivalent oncologic outcomes to conventional open esophagectomy.[55] In a review of an experience of more than 1000 MIEs performed over a 15-year period, modified McKeown MIE was performed in 481 patients and Ivor Lewis MIE in 530. The median length of stay (8 days) and ICU stay (2 days) were similar between the two approaches. The median number of lymph nodes resected was 21. The overall operative mortality was 1.7%. The Ivor Lewis MIE group had both a significantly lower incidence of recurrent nerve injury (1%) and a significantly lower operative mortality rate (0.9% at 30 days) than the modified-McKeown MIE group.[56] In the recently published TIME trial,[57] fifty six patients were assigned to the open esophagectomy group and 59 to the MIE group after randomization. There was significantly less blood loss, significantly fewer pulmonary infections during MIE than during open esophagectomy (9% vs. 29%), shorter hospital stay (11 days vs 14 days) and better short-term quality of life, assessed 6 weeks after surgery. R0 resection, lymph node yield and perioperative mortality were similar between the two approaches. Totally laparoscopic esophagectomy with thoracoscopic part performed in prone position has been demonstrated to be technically feasible, with a low incidence of respiratory complications.[58]

Extent of Lymphadenctomy

A RCT comparing 2-field and 3-field lymphadenectomy in SCC failed to demonstrate any survival advantage for extended lymph node dissection. Five year survival rates were 48% with 2-field and 66% with 3-field lymphadenectomy (not significant).[59] The 3-field approach has been associated with higher operative morbidity including higher recurrent laryngeal nerve paralysis and pulmonary complications.[60] In a retrospective review of stage matched patients treated with either a transhiatal or an en bloc resection, it was shown that with extensive nodal disease (>9) the type of resection did not impact survival because there was nearly universal systemic disease in this group of patients.[61] In contrast, for those with limited nodal disease (1–8 nodes) the type of resection significantly impacted survival in favor of the en bloc resection.[61] In the RCT comparing THE vs. TTE alluded to earlier, in a subgroup analysis, a survival advantage was demonstrated in patients with 1–8 positive lymph nodes among those undergoing the TTE (64% vs. 23%, p=0.02).[62] The relative advantages and disadvantages of various surgical approaches are compared in Table 3.

Surgical considerations for AEG are summarized in Table 4.

The salient surgical principles of performing a successful esophagectomy (irrespective of the approach used) are essentially (i) careful dissection of the esophagus from the surrounding structures, (ii) adequate lymphadenectomy (iii) gentle handling, preparation of the gastric conduit (iv) tension free esophago-gastric anastomosis. These are illustrated in Figures 1A through F.

Table 3: Comparison of various surgical approaches to esophageal resection

Surgical approach	*Advantages*	*Disadvantages*
THE	Commonly performed in training institutes in the country. Lesser morbidity as the thorax is not opened. Equal survival benefit as compared to TTE.	Does not permit extended lymphadenectomy in the middle/ upper mediastinum.
TTE	Permits dissection of mid-thoracic and upper thoracic tumors under vision. Permits performance of extended mediastinal lymphadenectomy.	Reported higher pulmonary morbidity.
MIE	Advantages of the minimally invasive approach. Magnified dissection under vision. Similar oncological clearance, better lymph node yield in some studies.	Steep learning curve.
ELD	Occult lymph node metastases are detected in distant nodes even in T1/T2 tumors. These are cleared with ELD. Survival advantage has been reported in pN1 disease.	Higher morbidity due to recurrent laryngeal nerve injuries, tracheal ischemia. Learning curve involved. May result in stage migration rather than true survival benefit.

Abbreviations: THE, transhiatal esophagectomy; TTE, transthoracic esophagectomy; MIE, minimally invasive esophagectomy; ELD, extended lymphadenectomy

Table 4: Surgery for adenocarcinoma of the esophagogastric junction

Siewert type	*Visceral resection*	*Lymph node clearance*	*Approach*
I	Subtotal esophagectomy, sleeve gastric resection	Posterior mediastinal, paracardial, lesser curve, left gastric	Right posterolateral thoracotomy in early tumors for two field lymph node clearance; alternatively a transhiatal approach may be used
II	Distal esophagectomy, proximal/total gastrectomy	Paracardiac, lesser curve, left gastric, celiac, common hepatic/formal D2, posterior mediastinal	Transhiatal is the preferred approach; thoracotomy if esophageal invasion is more than 1.5–2 cm
III	Distal esophagectomy, total gastrectomy	D2, posterior mediastinal	Same as above

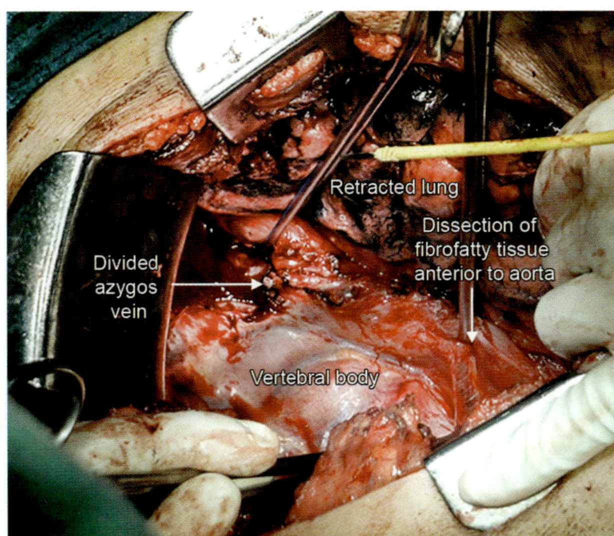

Figure 1A Transthoracic esophagectomy; esophagus looped with a plastic sling

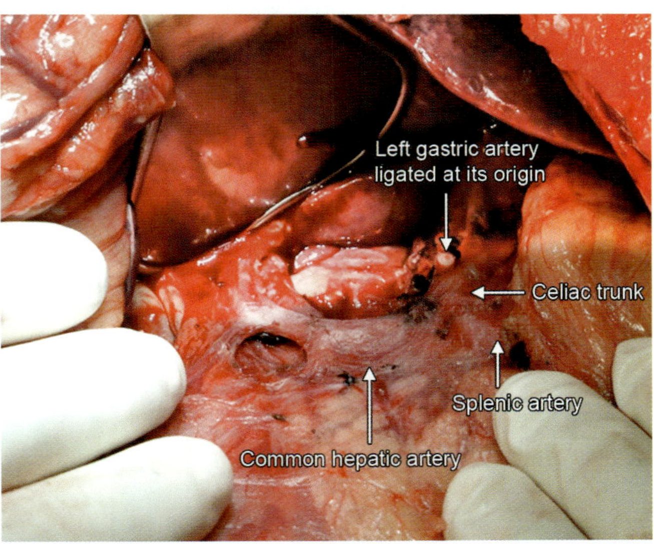

Figure 1C Completed abdominal lymphadenectomy

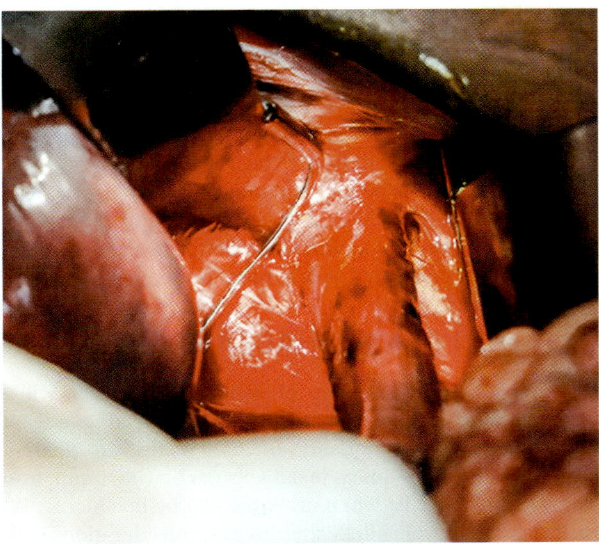

Figure 1B Lower mediastinal dissection under vision during transhiatal esophagectomy

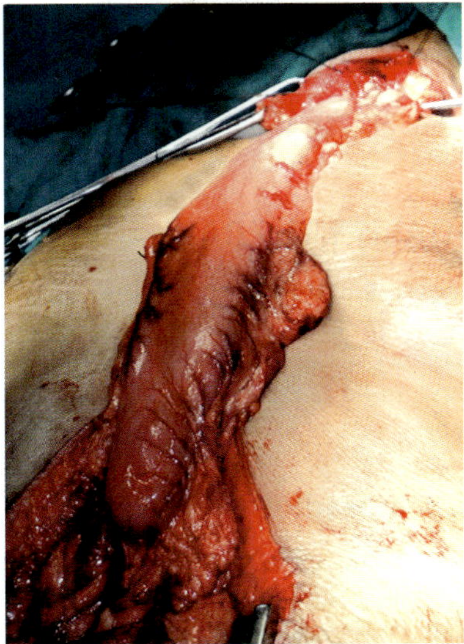

Figure 1D Stomach conduit based on the right gastroepiploic arcade; reaches the neck without tension

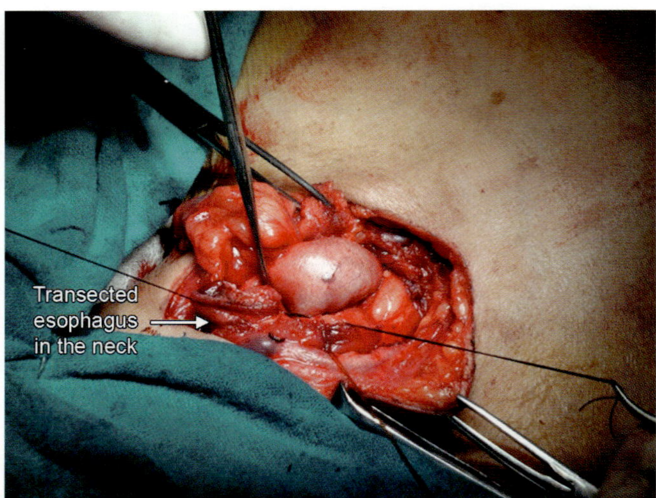

Figure 1E Stomach conduit 'pink' in the neck

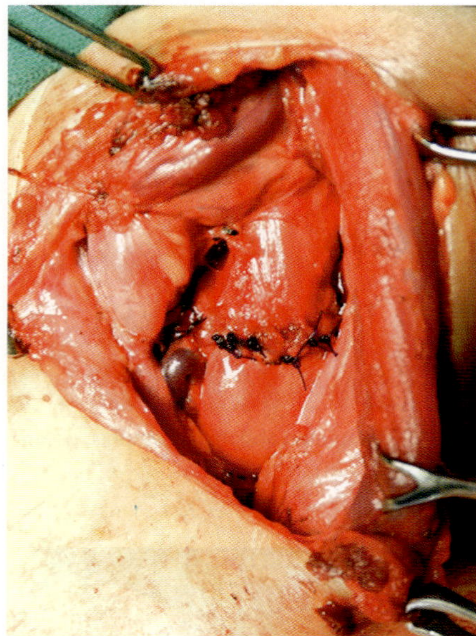

Figure 1F Completed esophagogastric anastomosis

MULTIMODALITY THERAPY

Stage of disease, type and location of tumor determine the type of multimodality approach one might adopt. Standard treatment options and evidence is discussed in the following section. Details of chemotherapy, radiotherapy regimens and adverse effects are not covered here.

Definitive Chemoradiotherapy (CRT)

This is an alternative to surgery for SCC, especially located in the upper third of the esophagus. In a randomized control trial (RCT) comparing surgery vs. definitive CRT for resectable SCC of the mid/lower thoracic esophagus, 5 year overall survival (OS) was similar and there was a trend to improved OS with CRT in node positive disease, trend to better disease free survival (DFS).[63] Though there is no survival benefit, treatment related morbidity is lower with CRT.[64]

Neoadjuvant Therapy

While surgery is alone sufficient in T1 and most T2 tumors, neoadjuvant therapy is the standard of care in T3 and T4a tumors. There is level 1 evidence to support the use of neoadjuvant therapy in carcinoma esophagus. While there is no clear evidence of advantage of neoadjuvant CRT over chemotherapy,[65] most centers prefer the former, especially when SCC is the histological type.

Neoadjuvant CRT

In a meta-analysis of 9 RCTs, the hazard ratio (HR) for OS favored neoadjuvant CRT over surgery alone 0·81 (95% CI 0·70-0·95; P=0·008).[64] In another meta-analysis of 12 RCTs of neoadjuvant CRT vs. surgery alone (n=1854), the HR for all-cause mortality strongly favored the former (0.78; 95% CI 0.70-0.88; p<0.0001).[65] In a recent RCT[66] of 366 patients (75% EAC, 23% SCC and 2% large-cell undifferentiated carcinoma), the R0 resection rate (92% vs. 69%; p<0.001) and median OS (49.4 months vs. 24 months; HR, 0.657; 95% CI, 0.495 to 0.871; p=0.003) favored neoadjuvant CRT over surgery alone. The in hospital mortality rates were similar in both groups (4% each). The authors concluded that neoadjuvant CRT improves survival among patients with potentially curable esophageal or esophagogastric-junction cancer with acceptable adverse-event rates.

Neoadjuvant Chemotherapy

In an updated meta-analysis[65] involving 9 RCTs of neoadjuvant chemotherapy vs. surgery alone (n=1981) in resectable esophageal carcinoma, the HR for all-cause mortality favored the former (0.87; 0.79-0.96; p=0.005), providing strong evidence for a survival benefit. This effect was statistically significant for EAC (HR 0.83; 0.71-0.95; p=0.01) as opposed to SCC (HR0.92; 0.81-1.04; p=0.18).[65]

Perioperative Chemotherapy

Perioperative chemotherapy is the standard of care in resectable adenocarcinoma of the lower esophagus, GEJ, or stomach. In a recent multicenter phase III RCT,[67] the 5 year OS (38% vs. 24%; HR: 0.69; 95% CI, 0.50–0.95; p=.02), 5 year DFS (34% vs. 19%; HR, 0.65; 95% CI, 0.48–0.89; p=.003) and curative resection rates (84% vs. 73%; p=0.04) were all significantly better with perioperative chemotherapy as compared with surgery alone.

PALLIATION OF ESOPHAGEAL CANCER

Majority (~80%) of the cases of esophageal cancer will not be amenable to curative treatment. While treating advanced esophageal carcinoma, quality of life issues are extremely important. Multidisciplinary team approach with input from a palliative care specialist when available can be invaluable. While choosing a modality to palliate this disease, considerations include the predominant symptom, morphology and location of the tumor, life expectancy of the patient, expertise of the treating team, expectations, wishes of the patient and costs. The indications, relative advantages and disadvantages of various modalities available are summarized in the following paragraphs.

Esophageal Stenting

This is the most widespread modality for palliation of dysphagia in advanced tumors and can be use even in patients with poor performance status or recurrent tumors. Covered stents resist tumor ingrowth, but are associated with a high rate of stent migration. Uncovered stents migrate less, but are prone to tumor ingrowth. Partially covered stents are uncovered at their ends. Initial stricture dilation is generally recommended, and the diameter of the stent to be deployed should not be greater than 2 mm of the estimated stricture diameter. The length of the stenosis must be accurately measured and a stent chosen is at least 4 cm longer than the stricture.[68] Patients with bulky, proximal tumors can develop tracheal compression after stent deployment; hence the treating team should be prepared for endotracheal intubation/airway stenting. For stent placement in the very distal esophagus, it is important to avoid leaving an excessive length of stent within the stomach to prevent contact with the opposite gastric wall, which could result in obstruction and/or ulceration. Greater than 95% of patients undergoing stent placement for malignant esophageal obstruction are able to tolerate a liquid diet.[69] In patients with malignant dysphagia in the presence of a tracheoesophageal fistula, SEMS restored luminal patency in about 98% and sealed the fistula in 70–100% of patients.[70] Serious complications after stent placement are low. They can occur during the procedure, or be delayed, important of which are migration (6.8%), bleeding (3.9%).[68] Perforation and mortality occur in less than 1% of the cases. Rare cases of delayed aorto-esophageal fistula have been reported prompting caution while considering stenting for tumors abutting the thoracic aorta. There is level 1 evidence to suggest that SEMS insertion is safer and more effective than rigid plastic tube insertion. In a recent meta-analysis of 1027 patients from 16 RCTs, stenting resulted in lesser re-intervention while locoregional therapy resulted in slightly better one year survival.[71]

Surgery

With the availability of endoscopic techniques and stenting, there is seldom a role for palliative esophagectomy even in the presence of a bleeding or a perforated tumor. A feeding jejunostomy is an excellent option for providing nutritional support in patients with advanced tumors discovered at surgery/staging laparoscopy.

External Beam Radiotherapy

It is useful for the palliation of dysphagia if the life expectancy is low (~3–6 months). If patients are expected to live longer and are reasonable fit, combination chemotherapy may be added. The risks associated with treatment include development of post radiotherapy strictures, tracheo-esophageal fistula. Also it takes around 4–6 weeks for therapy to become effective; time spent in visiting treatment facilities also consumes a significant amount of quality time of patients. In a recent RCT from India,[72] comparing esophageal stenting with SEMS alone (Group I), vs. a combination of stenting followed by EBRT (Group II), better dysphagia relief and median survival were noted in Group II. Conventional SEMS and anti-reflux stents were equally effective. Previous CRT had no impact on complications, procedural deaths, and overall patient survival.

Endoluminal Brachytherapy

It is not used routinely due to a short dysphagia free interval (~2.5 months), significant complication rates including severe esophagitis, stricture formation (25%), fistulization (10%) and requirement of multiple endoscopies for catheter placement.[73]

Photodynamic Therapy

It provides good palliation of dysphagia in patients, with improvement in 85% and a dysphagia free interval of 66 days.[74] It also provided control of bleeding in over 90% of the cases. Additional sessions/stent placement can be done in patients who develop recurrent dysphagia. Photodynamic therapy is extremely useful in patients with cervical esophageal malignancies, long segment strictures. Disadvantages include high cost of equipment, risk of developing photosensitivity (~10%), need to remain indoors for 6 weeks post procedure, risk of esophageal perforation (~1–2%) especially in patients who have undergone prior chemoradiation.[73]

Laser Therapy

Treatment with the Nd:YAG laser can provide short term relief of dysphagia in up to 90% of the patients. High costs, requirement of multiple treatment sessions and a high perforation rate (up to 5%) are disadvantages.[73]

Other methods available for palliation include endoscopic ethanol injection, local injection of chemotherapy, cryoablation, argon plasma coagulation and esophageal dilatation. These have short term benefits, need repeated sessions, are associated with complications and are selectively used if at all and usually in combination with other modalities of palliation.

A management algorithm for esophageal cancer is depicted in Flow chart 1.

PROGNOSIS AND SURVIVAL

The 7th edition of the AJCC-TNM staging manual is data-driven and advanced stage correlates with poorer survival. The N stage perhaps is the best prognostic marker and patients with N3 disease (≥7 lymph nodes) have poor survival.[61] Various immunophenotypic and genetic markers have been demonstrated to affect survival. Vascular epidermal growth factor immunopositivity has been shown to be associated with lymph node metastasis.[75] In a study elucidating molecular markers of tumor aggressiveness, multiple logistic regression analysis revealed that loss of p16 immunoreactivity was a significant risk factor for tumor stage (OR=3.3), whereas the loss of pRb was a significant risk factor for nodal metastasis (OR=8.8). MDM2 (an E3 ubiquitin ligase) over-expression emerged as the most significant risk factor for distant organ metastasis (OR=4.6).[76] Results also suggest that stromelysin-3 positive and tissue inhibitor of matrix metalloproteinase-2 negative phenotype is an adverse prognosticator in esophageal cancer patients.[77] Estrogen receptor beta is believed to be a marker

Flow chart 1 Algorithm depicting management strategies for esophageal carcinoma stratified by T, N stage

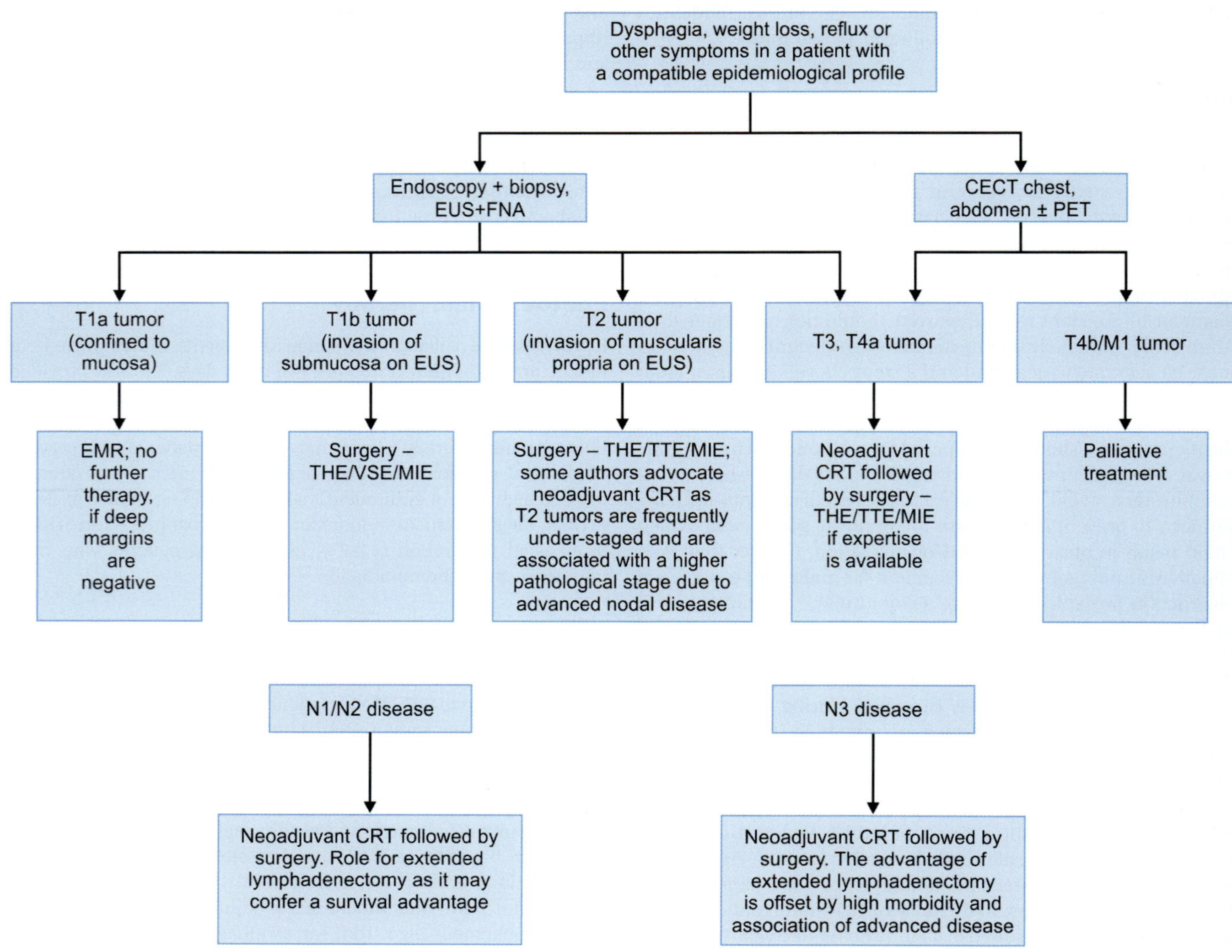

Abbreviations: EUS, endoscopic ultrasound; FNA, fine needle aspiration; CECT, contrast enhanced computed tomogram; PET, positron emission tomography; EMR, endoscopic mucosal resection; THE, transhiatal esophagectomy; VSE, vagal sparing esophagectomy; MIE, minimally invasive esophagectomy; TTE, transthoracic esophagectomy; CRT, chemoradiotherapy.

for poor biological behavior, that is dedifferentiation or higher stage of disease.[78] In a study evaluating genetic polymorphism of epidermal growth factor receptors, patients with EGF +61AG genotype had median survival of 25.5 months (95% CI=5.2–45.5), whereas those with EGF +61GG genotype had survival of only 3.7 months (95% CI=0.0–9.8, p=0.006).[79] HER2neu positive tumors (around 25% of AEG) are responsive to trastuzumab. This drug has demonstrated a survival advantage for patients with advanced AEG.[80] Other novel molecular targets are being explored. Personalized medicine, evaluation of proteomic profile might be used to prognosticate patients and direct therapy in the future.

Despite advances in surgical technique, multi-modality therapy and molecular diagnostics, survival rates for esophageal cancer remain modest at best. The poor survival rates of EAC are mostly related to the fact that symptomatic disease correlates with advanced stage (T3N1), whereby only 1 in 7 patients is predicted to be alive at 5 years, despite all the therapeutic efforts to achieve a cure.[81] In the senior author's experience, the overall actuarial survival rates at 2, 5, and 10 years for esophageal carcinoma patients were 54%, 38%, and 18% respectively.[82]_The 5-year survival rate for EAC and AEG was 21.27% with a median survival of 13.48 months.[83] The resectability rate of the SCC group has been reported to be significantly higher (76%) than in the EAC group (55%). In this series, the 5-year survival achieved in SCC was higher than in the EAC group (11.6% vs. 7.2%) but the difference was not statistically significant.[17] Survival data from select Indian and international series is summarized in Table 5.

SUMMARY

Carcinoma of the esophagus has well defined epidemiological risk factors. EAC is associated with GERD, BE, obesity while SCC is associated with smoking, snuff, alcohol consumption, low socio-economic status. Symptomatic clinical presentation usually

Table 5: Overall survival of esophageal and gastroesophageal junctional tumors after surgery

Author	*Year of publication*	*Total number of patients*	*Type of tumor*	*Overall survival**
Prashad[83]	1999	78	EAC, AEG	21.27%
Siewert JR[40]	2000	1002	AEG	32.3%, 24.3% (10YSR)
Gupta NM[17]	2001	169	SCC, EAC	11.6%, 7.2% respectively for SCC, EAC
Rao YG[82]	2002	367	SCC, EAC	54%,(2YSR) 38%, and 18% (10YSR)
Omloo JM[62]	2007	220	EAC	35%
Palanivelu C[84]	2007	32	AEG	62%, 42%, 46%, 15% (3YSR) for stages I, IIA, IIB & III respectively
Orringer MB[85]	2007	1482	EAC, SCC	65%, 28.5%, 11%, 10% for Stages I, II, III and IV A respectively
Hasegawa S[86]	2010	147	AEG	44.2%, 31% for types II,III respectively
van Hagen P[66]	2012	366	EAC, SCC	Median OS 49.4 months with NACRT
Blom RL[87]	2013	165	EAC, SCC	3YSR 57–61% with NACRT

*Numbers indicate 5-year survival rates in percentages unless indicated otherwise in parenthesis.

Abbreviations: EAC, esophageal adenocarcinoma; AEG, adenocarcinoma of the esophago-gastric junction; YSR, year survival rate; SCC, squamous cell carcinoma; NACRT, neoadjuvant chemoradiotherapy

correlates with advanced disease. Early cancers may be detected while screening for BE. Endoscopy with biopsy, EUS with FNA and CECT±PET are considered mandatory for diagnosis and staging. Endoscopy provides an assessment of the morphology and extent of the tumor with an opportunity for biopsy. EUS clearly defines the depth of infiltration of the esophageal wall, detects regional nodes and is able to sample them. CT detects T4 or M1 disease, the efficacy of the latter being increased by PET. The 7th edition of the AJCC-TNM classification has made improvements over the previous version. Nodal disease is stratified based on the number of involved nodes. EAC, SCC are staged similarly for stages 0, III, IV, while grading and location of the tumor is taken into account while stratifying stage I, II tumors. Surgery remains the cornerstone for the curative treatment of esophageal cancer, except in two instances: T1a tumors confined to the mucosa while EMR with negative deep margins is considered an alternative, in SCC of the upper thoracic esophagus where definitive CRT has shown to have equal survival. The type of surgical approach employed depends on the experience and comfort level of the treating team and been shown to have equal survival benefit. THE is believed to have less morbidity while TTE provides the opportunity for extended mediastinal lymphadenectomy which may have a survival advantage in limited nodal disease. MIE improves short term quality of life and has comparable oncological outcome to open approaches; however it has a learning curve. Neoadjuvant CRT is becoming the standard of care in T3/N1 disease. Neoadjuvant chemotherapy is an acceptable alternative, especially in EAC. Perioperative chemotherapy is beneficial in type III AEG which is treated like gastric cancers. Palliative therapy with stenting and external beam radiotherapy can prolong survival in advanced disease. Apart from conventional prognostic indicators like R0 resection, N staging, reponse to neoadjuvant CRT, there are numerous studies on genetic polymorphism, immunophenotypic markers which are making inroads into clinical practice. All in all, esophageal cancer remains a challenging disease to treat and the astute surgeon should select therapeutic options that entail the least morbidity while guaranteeing best possible survival and quality of life to patients.

REFERENCES

1. Cancer Statistics, World Cancer Research Fund International. Available at: www.wcrf.org/int/cancer-facts-figures/worldwide-data.
2. Wheeler JB, Reed CE. Epidemiology of esophageal cancer. Surg Clin North Am. 2012;92:1077-87.
3. Edgren G, Adami HO, Weiderpass E, Nyrén O. A global assessment of the oesophageal adenocarcinoma epidemic. Gut. 2013;62: 1406-14.
4. Connor MJ, Weston AP, Mayo MS, Sharma P. The prevalence of Barrett's esophagus and erosive esophagitis in patients undergoing upper endoscopy for dyspepsia in a VA population. Dig Dis Sci. 2004;49:920-4.
5. Reynolds JC, Waronker M, Pacquing MS, Yassin RR. Barrett's esophagus. reducing the risk of progression to adenocarcinoma. Gastroenterol Clin North Am. 1999;28:917-45.
6. Hvid-Jensen F, Pedersen L, Drewes AM, Sorensen HT, Funch-Jensen P. Incidence of adenocarcinoma among patients with Barrett's esophagus. N Engl J Med. 2011;365:1375-83.
7. American Gastroenterological Association, Spechler SJ, Sharma P, Souza RF, Inadomi JM, Shaheen NJ. American Gastroenterological Association medical position statement on the management of Barrett's esophagus. Gastroenterology. 2011;140:1084-91.
8. Lanuti M, Liu G, Goodwin JM, Zhai R, Fuchs BC, Asomaning K, et al. A functional epidermal growth factor (EGF) polymorphism, EGF serum levels, and esophageal adenocarcinoma risk and outcome. Clin Cancer Res. 2008;14:3216-22.
9. Chak A, Ochs-Balcom H, Falk G, Grady WM, Kinnard M, Willis JE, et al. Familiality in Barrett's esophagus, adenocarcinoma of the esophagus, and adenocarcinoma of the gastroesophageal junction. Cancer Epidemiol Biomarkers Prev. 2006;15:1668-73.
10. Denlinger CE, Thompson RK. Molecular basis of esophageal cancer development and progression. Surg Clin North Am. 2012; 92:1089-103.
11. Ryan AM, Healy LA, Power DG, Byrne M, Murphy S, Byrne PJ, et al. Barrett esophagus: prevalence of central adiposity, metabolic syndrome, and a proinflammatory state. Ann Surg. 2008;247:909-15.
12. Nguyen DM, Richardson P, El-Serag HB. Medications (NSAIDs, statins, proton pump inhibitors) and the risk of esophageal adenocarcinoma in patients with Barrett's esophagus. Gastroenterologist. 2010;138:2260-6.

13. Pandeya N, Williams GM, Sadhegi S, Green AC, Webb PM, Whiteman DC. Associations of duration, intensity, and quantity of smoking with adenocarcinoma and squamous cell carcinoma of the esophagus. Am J Epidemiol. 2008;168:105-14.
14. Toh Y, Oki E, Ohgaki K, Sakamoto Y, Ito S, Egashira A, et al. Alcohol drinking, cigarette smoking, and the development of squamous cell carcinoma of the esophagus: molecular mechanisms of carcinogenesis. Int J Clin Oncol. 2010;15:135-44.
15. Tramacere I, Pelucchi C, Bagnardi V, Rota M, Scotti L, Islami F, et al. A meta-analysis on alcohol drinking and esophageal and gastric cardia adenocarcinoma risk. Ann Oncol. 2012;23:287-97.
16. Polk DB, Peek RM Jr. Helicobacter pylori: gastric cancer and beyond. Nat Rev Cancer. 2010;10:403-14.
17. Gupta NM, Jindal R, Prakash O, Gupta R, Bhasin DK. Comparison of the clinical profile and outcome for squamous cell carcinoma and adenocarcinoma of the distal esophagus and cardia in India. Surg Today. 2001;31:400-4.
18. Rubenstein JH, Taylor JB. Meta-analysis: the association of oesophageal adenocarcinoma with symptoms of gastro-oesophageal reflux. Aliment Pharmacol Ther. 2010;32:1222-7.
19. Turati F, Tramacere I, La Vecchia C, Negri E. A meta-analysis of body mass index and esophageal and gastric cardia adenocarcinoma. Ann Oncol. 2013;24:609-17.
20. Cook MB, Kamangar F, Whiteman DC, Freedman ND, Gammon MD, Bernstein L, et al. Cigarette smoking and adenocarcinomas of the esophagus and esophagogastric junction: a pooled analysis from the international BEACON consortium. J Natl Cancer Inst. 2010;102:1344-53.
21. Bhat S, Coleman HG, Yousef F, Johnston BT, McManus DT, Gavin AT, et al. Risk of malignant progression in Barrett's esophagus patients: results from a large population-based study. J Natl Cancer Inst. 2011;103:1049-57
22. Islami F, Kamangar F. Helicobacter pylori and esophageal cancer risk: a meta-analysis. Cancer Prev Res (Phila). 2008;1:329–38.
23. Dar NA, Shah IA, Bhat GA, Makhdoomi MA, Iqbal B, Rafiq R, et al. Socioeconomic status and esophageal squamous cell carcinoma risk in Kashmir, India. Cancer Sci. 2013;104:1231-6.
24. Dar NA, Islami F, Bhat GA, Shah IA, Makhdoomi MA, Iqbal B, et al. Poor oral hygiene and risk of esophageal squamous cell carcinoma in Kashmir. Br J Cancer. 2013;109:1367-72.
25. Sehgal S, Kaul S, Gupta BB, Dhar MK. Risk factors and survival analysis of the esophageal cancer in the population of Jammu, India. Indian J Cancer. 2012;49:245-50.
26. Dar NA, Bhat GA, Shah IA, Iqbal B, Makhdoomi MA, Nisar I, et al. Hookah smoking, nass chewing, and oesophageal squamous cell carcinoma in Kashmir, India. Br J Cancer. 2012;107:1618-23.
27. Ray SS, Das D, Ghosh T, Ghosh AK. The levels of zinc and molybdenum in hair and food grain in areas of high and low incidence of esophageal cancer: a comparative study. Glob J Health Sci. 2012;4:168-75.
28. Vaiphei K, Kochhar R, Bhardawaj S, Dutta U, Singh K. High prevalence of human papillomavirus in esophageal squamous cell carcinoma: a study in paired samples. Dis Esophagus. 2013;26:282-7.
29. Katiyar S, Hedau S, Jain N, Kar P, Khuroo MS, Mohanta J, et al. p53 gene mutation and human papillomavirus (HPV) infection in esophageal carcinoma from three different endemic geographic regions of India. Cancer Lett. 2005;218:69-79.
30. Sharma A, Das BC, Sehgal A, Mehrotra R, Kar P, Sardana S, et al. GSTM1 and GSTT1 polymorphism and susceptibility to esophageal cancer in high- and low-risk regions of India. Tumour Biol. 2013;34:3249-57.
31. Jain M, Kumar S, Rastogi N, Lal P, Ghoshal UC, Tiwari A, et al. GSTT1, GSTM1 and GSTP1 genetic polymorphisms and interaction with tobacco, alcohol and occupational exposure in esophageal cancer patients from North India. Cancer Lett. 2006;242:60-7.
32. Rasool S, Khan T, Qazi F, Ganai BA. ECRG1 and its relationship with esophageal cancer: a brief review. Onkologie. 2013;36:213-6.
33. Rai AK, Freddy AJ, Banerjee A, Kurkalang S, Rangad GM, Islam M, et al. Distinct involvement of 9p21-24 and 13q14.1-14.3 chromosomal regions in raw betel-nut induced esophageal cancers in the state of Meghalaya, India. Asian Pac J Cancer Prev. 2012;13:2629-33.
34. Chava S, Mohan V, Pasupuleti N, Latha MM, Khan IA, Upendram P, et al. Evaluation of Aurora-A gene polymorphism and esophageal cancer risk in a South Indian population. Genet Test Mol Biomarkers. 2011;15:185-9.
35. Chava S, Mohan V, Shetty PJ, Manolla ML, Vaidya S, Khan IA, et al. Immunohistochemical evaluation of p53, FHIT, and IGF2 gene expression in esophageal cancer. Dis Esophagus. 2012;25:81-7.
36. Mathew R, Arora S, Mathur M, Chattopadhyay TK, Ralhan R. Esophageal squamous cell carcinomas with DNA replication errors (RER+) are associated with p16/pRb loss and wild-type p53. J CancerRes Clin Oncol. 2001;127:603-12.
37. Bharat A, Crabtree T. Management of advanced-stage operable esophageal cancer. Surg Clin North Am. 2012;92:1179-97.
38. Quint LE, Hepburn LM, Francis IR, Whyte RI, Orringer MB. Incidence and distribution of distant metastases from newly diagnosed esophageal carcinoma. Cancer. 1995;76:1120-5.
39. Edge S, Byrd DR, Compton CC, Fritz AG, Greene FL, Trotti A. eds. Esophagus and esophagogastric junction. In: AJCC cancer staging manual. 7th ed. New York, NY: Springer, 2009;103-115.
40. Rüdiger Siewert J, Feith M, Werner M, Stein HJ: Adenocarcinoma of the esophagogastric junction: Results of surgical therapy based on anatomical/topographic classification in 1,002 consecutive patients. Ann Surg. 2000;232:353-61.
41. Talsma K, van Hagen P, Grotenhuis BA, Steyerberg EW, Tilanus HW, van Lanschot JJ, et al. Comparison of the 6th and 7th Editions of the UICC-AJCC TNM Classification for Esophageal Cancer. Ann Surg Oncol. 2012;19:2142-8.
42. Li Z, Rice TW. Diagnosis and staging of cancer of the esophagus and esophagogastric junction. Surg Clin North Am. 2012;92:1105-26.
43. Pech O, Gossner L, Manner H, May A, Rabenstein T, Behrens A, et al. Prospective evaluation of the macroscopic types and location of early Barrett's neoplasia in 380 lesions. Endoscopy. 2007;39:588-93.
44. Bhutani MS, Barde CJ, Markert RJ, Gopalswamy N. Length of esophageal cancer and degree of luminal stenosis during upper endoscopy predict T stage by endoscopic ultrasound. Endoscopy. 2002;34:461-3.
45. Puli SR, Reddy JB, Bechtold ML, Antillon D, Ibdah JA, Antillon MR. Staging accuracy of esophageal cancer by endoscopic ultrasound: a meta-analysis and systematic review. World J Gastroenterol. 2008;14:1479-90.
46. Pech O, Günter E, Dusemund F, Origer J, Lorenz D, Ell C. Accuracy of endoscopic ultrasound in preoperative staging of esophageal cancer: results from a referral center for early esophageal cancer. Endoscopy. 2010;42:456-61.
47. Fernández-Sordo JO, Konda VJ, Chennat J, Madrigal-Hoyos E, Posner MC, Ferguson MK, et al. Is Endoscopic Ultrasound (EUS) necessary in the pre-therapeutic assessment of Barrett's esophagus with early neoplasia? J Gastrointest Oncol. 2012;3:314-21.
48. Sgourakis G, Gockel I, Lyros O, Hansen T, Mildenberger P, Lang H. Detection of lymph node metastases in esophageal cancer. Expert Rev Anticancer Ther. 2011;11:601-12.
49. Kumar P, Damle NA, Bal C. Role of F18-FDG PET/CT in the Staging and Restaging of Esophageal Cancer: A Comparison with CECT. Indian J Surg Oncol. 2011;2:343-50.

50. Bonavina L, Incarbone R, Lattuada E, Segalin A, Cesana B, Peracchia A. Preoperative laparoscopy in management of patients with carcinoma of the esophagus and of the esophagogastric junction. J Surg Oncol. 1997;65:171-4.
51. van Lanschot JJ, Hulscher JB, Buskens CJ, Tilanus HW, ten Kate FJ, Obertop H. Hospital volume and hospital mortality for esophagectomy. Cancer. 2001;91:1574-8.
52. Wouters MW, Wijnhoven BP, Karim-Kos HE, Blaauwgeers HG, Stassen LP, Steup WH, et al. High volume versus low volume for esophageal resection for cancer: the essential role of case-mix adjustments based on clinical data. Ann Surg Oncol. 2008;15:80-7.
53. Hulscher JB, van Sandick JW, de Boer AG, Wijnhoven BP, Tijssen JG, Fockens P, et al. Extended transthoracic resection compared with limited transhiatal resection for adenocarcinoma of the esophagus. N Engl J Med. 2002;347:1662-9.
54. Pennathur A, Zhang J, Chen H, Luketich JD. The "best operation" for esophageal cancer? Ann Thorac Surg. 2010;89:S2163-7.
55. Dantoc M, Cox MR, Eslick GD. Evidence to support the use of minimally invasive esophagectomy for esophageal cancer: a meta-analysis. Arch Surg. 2012;147:768-76.
56. Luketich JD, Pennathur A, Awais O, Levy RM, Keeley S, Shende M, et al. Outcomes after minimally invasive esophagectomy: review of over 1000 patients. Ann Surg. 2012;256:95-103.
57. Biere SS, van Berge Henegouwen MI, Maas KW, Bonavina L, Rosman C, Garcia JR, et al. Minimally invasive versus open oesophagectomy for patients with oesophageal cancer: a multicentre, open-label, randomized controlled trial. Lancet. 2012;379:1887-92.
58. Palanivelu C, Prakash A, Senthilkumar R, Senthilnathan P, Parthasarathi R, Rajan PS, et al. Minimally invasive esophagectomy: thoracoscopic mobilization of the esophagus and mediastinal lymphadenectomy in prone position--experience of 130 patients. J Am Coll Surg. 2006;203:7-16.
59. Nishihira T, Hirayama K, Mori S. A prospective randomized trial of extended cervical and superior mediastinal lymphadenectomy for carcinoma of the thoracic esophagus. Am J Surg. 1998;175:47-51.
60. Hermansson M, DeMeester SR. Management of stage 1 esophageal cancer. Surg Clin North Am. 2012;92:1155-67.
61. Johansson J, DeMeester TR, Hagen JA, DeMeester SR, Peters JH, Oberg S, et al. En bloc vs transhiatal esophagectomy for stage T3 N1 adenocarcinoma of the distal esophagus. Arch Surg. 2004;139: 627-31.
62. Omloo JM, Lagarde SM, Hulscher JB, Reitsma JB, Fockens P, van Dekken H, et al. Extended transthoracic resection compared with limited transhiatal resection for adenocarcinoma of the mid/distal esophagus: five-year survival of a randomized clinical trial. Ann Surg. 2007;246:992-1000.
63. Teoh AY, Chiu PW, Yeung WK, Liu SY, Wong SK, et al. Long-term survival outcomes after definitive chemoradiation versus surgery in patients with resectable squamous carcinoma of the esophagus: results from a randomized controlled trial. Ann Oncol. 2013;24: 165-71.
64. Kranzfelder M, Schuster T, Geinitz H, Friess H, Büchler P. Meta-analysis of neoadjuvant treatment modalities and definitive non-surgical therapy for oesophageal squamous cell cancer. Br J Surg. 2011;98:768-83.
65. Sjoquist KM, Burmeister BH, Smithers BM, Zalcberg JR, Simes RJ, Barbour A, et al; Australasian Gastro-Intestinal Trials Group. Survival after neoadjuvant chemotherapy or chemoradiotherapy for resectable oesophageal carcinoma: an updated meta-analysis. Lancet Oncol. 2011;12:681-92.
66. van Hagen P, Hulshof MC, van Lanschot JJ, Steyerberg EW, van Berge Henegouwen MI, Wijnhoven BP, et al; CROSS Group. Preoperative chemoradiotherapy for esophageal or junctional cancer. N Engl J Med. 2012;366:2074-84.
67. Ychou M, Boige V, Pignon JP, Conroy T, Bouché O, Lebreton G, et al. Perioperative chemotherapy compared with surgery alone for resectable gastroesophageal adenocarcinoma: an FNCLCC and FFCD multicenter phase III trial. J Clin Oncol. 2011;29:1715-21.
68. Vignesh S, Hoffe SE, Meredith KL, Shridhar R, Almhanna K, Gupta AK. Endoscopic therapy of neoplasia related to Barrett's esophagus and endoscopic palliation of esophageal cancer. Cancer Control. 2013;20:117-29.
69. Rozanes I, Poyanli A, Acunas B. Palliative treatment of inoperable malignant esophageal strictures with metal stents: one center's experience with four different stents. Eur J Radiol. 2002;43:196-203.
70. Verschuur EM, Kuipers EJ, Siersema PD. Esophageal stents for malignant strictures close to the upper esophageal sphincter. Gastrointest Endosc. 2007;66:1082-90.
71. Sgourakis G, Gockel I, Radtke A, Dedemadi G, Goumas K, Mylona S, et al. The use of self-expanding stents in esophageal and gastroesophageal junction cancer palliation: a meta-analysis and meta-regression analysis of outcomes. Dig Dis Sci. 2010;55: 3018-30.
72. Javed A, Pal S, Dash NR, Ahuja V, Mohanti BK, Vishnubhatla S, et al. Palliative stenting with or without radiotherapy for inoperable esophageal carcinoma: a randomized trial. J Gastrointest Cancer. 2012;43:63-9.
73. Freeman RK, Ascioti AJ, Mahidhara RJ. Palliative therapy for patients with unresectable esophageal carcinoma. Surg Clin North Am. 2012;92:1337-51.
74. Little VR, Luketich JD, Christie NA, Buenaventura PO, Alvelo-Rivera M, McCaughan JS, et al. Photodynamic therapy as palliation for esophageal cancer: experience in 215 patients. Ann Thorac Surg. 2003;76:1687-92.
75. Mukherjee T, Kumar A, Mathur M, Chattopadhyay TK, Ralhan R. Ets-1 and VEGF expression correlates with tumor angiogenesis, lymph node metastasis, and patient survival in esophageal squamous cell carcinoma. J Cancer Res Clin Oncol. 2003;129:430-6.
76. Mathew R, Arora S, Khanna R, Mathur M, Shukla NK, Ralhan R. Alterations in p53 and pRb pathways and their prognostic significance in oesophageal cancer. Eur J Cancer. 2002;38:832-41.
77. Sharma R, Chattopadhyay TK, Mathur M, Ralhan R. Prognostic significance of stromelysin-3 and tissue inhibitor of matrix metalloproteinase-2 in esophageal cancer. Oncology. 2004;67: 300-9.
78. Kalayarasan R, Ananthakrishnan N, Kate V, Basu D. Estrogen and progesterone receptors in esophageal carcinoma. Dis Esophagus. 2008;21:298-303.
79. Jain M, Kumar S, Upadhyay R, Lal P, Tiwari A, Ghoshal UC, et al. Influence of apoptosis (BCL2, FAS), cell cycle (CCND1) and growth factor (EGF, EGFR) genetic polymorphisms on survival outcome: an exploratory study in squamous cell esophageal cancer. Cancer Biol Ther. 2007;6:1553-8.
80. Bang YJ, Van Cutsem E, Feyereislova A; ToGA Trial Investigators. Trastuzumab in combination with chemotherapy versus chemotherapy alone for treatment of HER2-positive advanced gastric or gastro-oesophageal junction cancer (ToGA): a Phase 3, open-label, randomized controlled trial. Lancet. 2010;376:687-97.
81. Cancer Research UK. 2012. Available at: http://www.cancerresearchuk.org/about-cancer/type/oesophageal-cancer/treatment/statistics-and-outlook-for-oesophageal-cancer.
82. Rao YG, Pal S, Pande GK, Sahni P, Chattopadhyay TK. Transhiatal esophagectomy for benign and malignant conditions. Am J Surg. 2002;184:136-42.
83. Parshad R, Singh RK, Kumar A, Gupta SD, Chattopadhyay TK. Adenocarcinoma of distal esophagus and gastroesophageal junction: long-term results of surgical treatment in a North Indian Center. World J Surg. 1999;23:277-83.

84. Palanivelu C, Prakash A, Parthasarathi R, Senthilkumar R, Senthilnathan PR, Rajapandian S. Laparoscopic esophagogastrectomy without thoracic or cervical access for adenocarcinoma of the gastroesophageal junction: an Indian experience from a tertiary center. Surg Endosc. 2007;21:16-20.
85. Orringer MB, Marshall B, Chang AC, Lee J, Pickens A, Lau CL. Two thousand transhiatal esophagectomies: changing trends, lessons learned. Ann Surg. 2007;246:363-72.
86. Hasegawa S, Yoshikawa T. Adenocarcinoma of the esophagogastric junction: incidence, characteristics, and treatment strategies. Gastric Cancer. 2010;13:63-73.
87. Blom RL, Sosef MN, Nap M, Lammering G, van den Berkmortel F, Hulshof MC, et al. Comparison of two neoadjuvant chemoradiotherapy regimens in patients with potentially curable esophageal carcinoma. Dis Esophagus. 2014;27:380-7.

CHAPTER 19

Esophageal Cancer: Operative Strategies and Lymphadenectomy

C S Pramesh, George Karimundackal, Sabita Jiwnani

SURGICAL TREATMENT OF ESOPHAGEAL CANCER

Esophageal cancer is a morbid disease and globally, is a common cause of cancer-related death.[1] Worldwide, squamous cell carcinoma remains the major type of esophageal cancer in spite of a virtual epidemic of adenocarcinomas in the western world over the past three decades.[2-4] The spectrum of disease is widely variant with squamous cancers being common in Asia (China, Iran, India, Japan and Korea) in contrast to North America and Europe where adenocarcinomas of the gastroesophageal junction and lower esophagus are more common.[5] Several large randomized trials and meta-analysis[6] addressing various aspects of treatment have been performed in the past few years, resulting in considerable improvement in survival; yet, the overall prognosis of the disease remains grim.

A number of recent randomized trials have firmly established that patients treated with neoadjuvant chemotherapy or chemoradiotherapy have superior survival over surgery alone. However, currently there is no evidence to suggest that surgery can be avoided even in carefully selected subgroups and it remains the mainstay of treatment for localized, nonmetastatic esophageal cancer. Recent progress in nonsurgical treatment have included endoscopic mucosal resection (EMR) showing promising results for very early mucosal lesions and definitive concurrent chemoradiation being advocated for more advanced squamous esophageal cancer. Nevertheless, in most experienced centers, esophagectomy after neoadjuvant therapy remains the standard of care, primarily because the volume of evidence is much higher for surgery than nonsurgical treatment.[4,7] However, concerns remain that it is a major surgical procedure with considerable morbidity and mortality, even in experienced centers.[8] Even in highly developed healthcare systems like the United States, postoperative mortality rates range from 8% in high-volume centers to 23% in low-volume centers.[9] Although there is relatively low volume and quality of evidence supporting it, the high postoperative morbidity and mortality have been used as arguments to promote nonsurgical therapy in the form of definitive chemoradiation as an alternative. The National Comprehensive Cancer Network (NCCN) treatment guidelines[10] now offer definitive chemoradiation as an "acceptable alternative" to esophagectomy. Esophageal surgeons are now making concerted efforts to reduce the morbidity and mortality of esophageal resectional surgery by careful patient selection, concentration of surgery in high volume, experienced centers, adopting different, potentially less morbid surgical approaches and by enhanced recovery programs.[11-14] In this chapter, we enumerate and discuss the different issues and controversies related to surgery for esophageal cancer, including patient selection and preoperative preparation, principles of surgical therapy, different surgical procedures for esophageal cancer and some points of surgical technique and postoperative care.

PATIENT SELECTION AND PREOPERATIVE PREPARATION

Esophagectomy is a formidable operation and careful patient selection and optimization of comorbid conditions is the key to good perioperative outcomes. Nutritional status and cardiorespiratory function are specific parameters to be evaluated while considering patients for surgical resection.[15] Many patients with squamous esophageal cancer are malnourished and are likely to benefit from supplemental enteral feeding, especially those with more than 10% weight loss and/or grade III or more dysphagia. Though some units advocate a feeding jejunostomy, we prefer to avoid an additional surgical procedure by using an endoscopically-guided nasogastric tube bypassing the malignant growth for preoperative feeding. As most patients get neoadjuvant therapy, this permits 6–8 weeks of enteral nutrition before surgery. Pulmonary complications are the most common morbidity after esophagectomy and chronic obstructive pulmonary disease, bronchial asthma and a low forced expiratory volume in 1 second (FEV1) and diffusion capacity to carbon monoxide (DLCO) are important predictive factors. We prefer a transhiatal approach to reduce pulmonary complications in such patients and in those with extensive pulmonary fibrosis. Patients with a history of myocardial infarction and ischemic heart disease with a low ejection fraction are at high risk for perioperative cardiac complications. Our preference is to evaluate these patients with a stress two-dimensional (2D) echocardiography to accurately estimate perioperative cardiac risk. Although chronological age alone is not a risk factor, some studies have shown increased morbidity with advancing age.[16,17] Correctable preoperative risk factors include smoking cessation, correction of malnutrition (by enteral feeding) and optimizing pre-existing pulmonary dysfunction (by pulmonary rehabilitation including chest physiotherapy, incentive spirometry and judicious use of bronchodilators). A dedicated multidisciplinary team including surgeons, anesthesiologists, intensivists, pulmonary physicians, physiotherapists and nutritionists is invaluable both in patient selection and preoperative optimization. In addition to the involvement of these specialists in the routine workup of patients, our unit also has a weekly multidisciplinary meeting to aid decision making and optimization of high-risk patients planned for esophagectomy.

TECHNIQUES IN SURGICAL MANAGEMENT

This section of the chapter will discuss the principles and techniques of esophageal resection, some specific issues and the evidence related to it.

Principles of Esophageal Resection

The basic principles of radical esophagectomy for cancer include:

- A complete (R-0) resection of the tumor with adequate proximal, distal and circumferential margins
- Dissection of the associated lymph node drainage area
- Reconstruction of the esophagus with a substitute organ, most commonly the tubularized stomach.

Types of Esophageal Resection

Esophageal resection may be performed by various techniques as follows:

- Transthoracic esophagectomy
  - Modified McKeown's three stage esophagectomy
  - Ivor-Lewis esophagectomy
- Transhiatal esophagectomy
- Minimally invasive esophagectomy (MIE)
  - Complete MIE
  - Hybrid MIE
  - Robotic esophagectomy
- Left thoracoabdominal partial esophagogastrectomy.

The extent of lymphadenectomy varies from single-field (abdominal), two-field standard, extended and total (abdominal and mediastinal) and three-field (abdominal, mediastinal and cervical) lymphadenectomy. The variability of adoption of different techniques of esophagectomy and lymphadenectomy by different surgeons is a direct reflection of the lack of high quality evidence favoring a particular technique. A good esophageal surgeon should be versatile and have expertise with most of these approaches to enable individualized decision making according to the specific characteristics of the disease and the patient. Our personal preference is to perform a three stage modified McKeown's transthoracic esophagectomy (open and MIE); we reserve the transhiatal esophagectomy only for patients with extensive emphysema or pulmonary fibrosis.

Operative Technique

Transthoracic esophagectomy (modified McKeown's): The procedure is performed under general anesthesia with epidural analgesia as an important adjunct for pain relief. While some surgeons prefer single-lung ventilation for the thoracic part of the procedure, we find it necessary only when we do a thoracoscopic esophageal mobilization. We position the patient at the near end of the operating table in a left lateral position; we enter the thoracic cavity through a fifth interspace posterolateral thoracotomy, dividing the lattissimus dorsi and sparing the serratus anterior muscle. A preliminary assessment of the thoracic cavity is made to rule out obviously advanced disease and pleuropulmonary metastases. We start the procedure by making two parallel incisions in the mediastinal pleura (anterior and posterior to the esophagus) at the level of the tumor. We initially dissect the esophagus immediately above and below the level of the growth and confirm operability. We then proceed to mobilize the esophagus circumferentially throughout its intrathoracic course along with the adjacent draining lymph nodes. In an en bloc esophagectomy, the azygos vein and thoracic duct are also included in the resected specimen; this has the advantage of giving a wider circumferential resection margin. We prefer to preserve the horizontal part of the azygos vein along with the bronchial artery (except in growths around that area), as we believe that it reduces postoperative pulmonary complications.[18] Complete esophageal dissection along with appropriate mediastinal lymphadenectomy (Figs 1 to 3) is performed and the thorax is closed with an (no. 24) intercostal drainage tube.

The patient is then positioned supine and the abdomen is opened with a vertical midline incision starting at the xiphisternum and ending just above the umbilicus. The abdominal cavity is inspected for unsuspected hepatic or peritoneal metastatic disease, which has become increasingly uncommon with technological advances in preoperative imaging techniques. We then proceed with the mobilization of the stomach, which is performed by serial ligation of the vessels of the gastrocolic omentum, taking care to maintain a safe distance from the right gastroepiploic vascular arcade. Mobilization of the stomach is continued by ligation of the left gastroepiploic vessels and the short gastric vessels. Extreme care is necessary while ligating the terminal short gastric vessels, especially in obese patients to avoid inadvertent bleeding which might necessitate a splenectomy. Once the mobilization of the greater curvature is complete, we mobilize the gastrohepatic omentum, taking care to identify and preserve aberrant replaced hepatic arteries, which may be present occasionally. We then take a transverse skin crease incision parallel to, and one finger breadth above the medial third of the left clavicle for esophageal dissection at the neck. The sternomastoid is retracted laterally, the medial fibers of the strap muscles divided (or retracted medially)

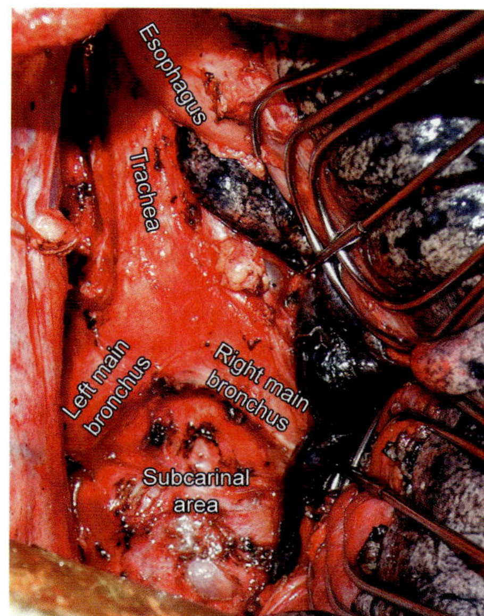

Figure 1 Standard mediastinal lymphadenectomy—clearance of the subcarinal lymph nodes

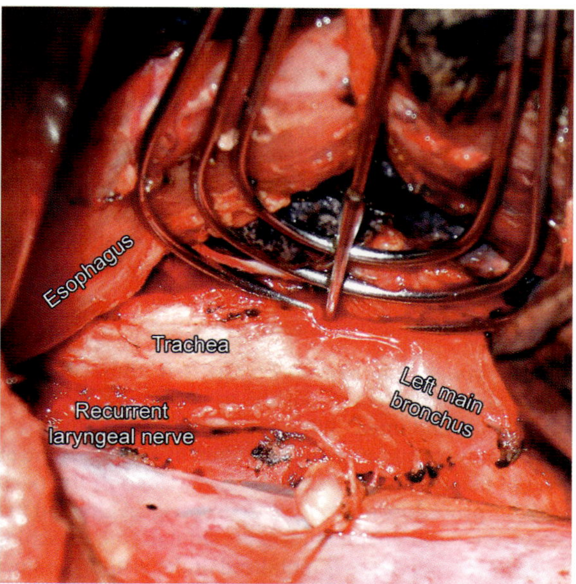

Figure 3 Total mediastinal lymphadenectomy—clearance of the left recurrent laryngeal nerve group of lymph nodes

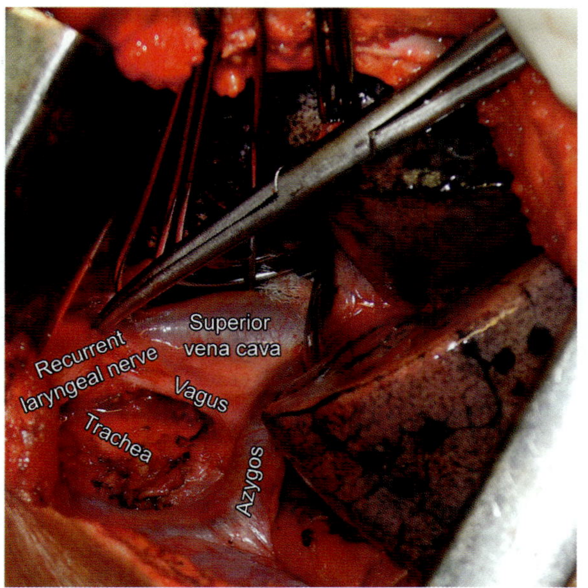

Figure 2 Extended mediastinal lymphadenectomy—clearance of the right recurrent laryngeal nerve group of lymph nodes

and the carotid sheath (with the carotid artery and internal jugular vein within) retracted laterally. The cervical esophagus is then carefully dissected, taking care not to injure the left recurrent laryngeal nerve. The esophagus is encircled using a tape and then divided at the neck (taking care that the mucosa does not retract), and stay sutures are taken on the proximal esophageal stump. The distal esophageal stump is closed and sutured to a Penrose drain or tape and the specimen is delivered into the abdominal wound. The stomach tube is formed using a linear stapler, simultaneously clearing the lymph nodes along the lesser curvature. We perform a D2 lymph node dissection including the splenic, left gastric, hepatic, and coeliac groups of lymph nodes. We suture the tip of the gastric tube to the Penrose drain and carefully guide the stomach tube through the posterior mediastinum to the cervical incision, taking care to maintain the correct orientation (this can be confirmed by the staple line being seen on the right of the stomach tube when it is delivered in the neck). We perform a stapled (triangulated linear staple technique) anastomosis at the neck. Alternative anastomotic techniques include a single layer, interrupted or continuous hand-sewn technique. Our current preference is to place a nasojejunal tube (for postoperative enteral feeding) after the posterior layer of the anastomosis is complete; other authors favor a formal feeding jejunostomy. We also place a nasogastric tube for decompression of the stomach tube. The abdominal and neck wounds are closed without drains to complete the procedure.

Ivor Lewis esophagectomy: The Ivor Lewis operation starts with the abdominal part of the procedure almost identical to the gastric mobilization described above. The abdomen is closed after the D2 lymphadenectomy and a feeding jejunostomy. The thorax is then opened through the fifth interspace (as described above) and the infra azygos part of the esophagus is mobilized. The dissected esophagus along with the stomach is delivered into the chest and the specimen removed and stomach tube completed. The esophagogastric anastomosis is performed in the mediastinum at the level of the azygos vein, usually using a circular end to end anastomosis (EEA) stapler.

Transhiatal esophagectomy: The procedure for a transhiatal esophagectomy is similar to the modified McKeown operation described above, except that the mediastinal dissection is performed from the abdominal and neck incisions without a thoracotomy. After complete gastric mobilization through a midline laparotomy and cervical esophageal mobilization through the neck incision, the transhiatal part of the dissection is begun. The lower esophageal mobilization can be performed almost always under vision from the abdomen by wide retraction of the esophageal diaphragmatic hiatus. The upper and middle esophageal mobilization is performed by blunt dissection using the fingers of either hand introduced through the diaphragmatic hiatus and the cervical incision respectively, maintaining traction on the thoracic esophagus. The dissection is carried out sequentially: anterior, posterior and the lateral attachments from above and below. It is important to stay on the esophageal wall to avoid injury to adjoining structures, viz the tracheobronchial tree, azygos vein and the bronchial artery. Once the thoracic esophagus is mobilized completely, the rest of the procedure is similar to that described in the modified McKeown procedure.

Left thoracoabdominal approach: The left thoracoabdominal approach gives excellent exposure to the lower mediastinum and the upper abdomen. While other authors perform a total esophagectomy (combining this with blunt dissection at and above the level of the aortic arch) with an anastomosis in the neck, we perform this procedure only for gastroesophageal junction tumors with gastric involvement precluding the stomach tube reaching the neck. The lower esophagus is mobilized under vision, the stomach mobilization done as described above, the tumor resected with adequate proximal and distal margins and a stapled anastomosis done in the lower mediastinum using an EEA stapler.

Minimally invasive esophagectomy: Esophagectomy is ideally suited for a minimally invasive approach and can be performed with the same radicality as open surgery. Details of MIE are discussed in another chapter of the book.

Postoperative Care

Most experienced high-volume centers including ours adopt an enhanced recovery program after esophagectomy. Key principles include early (usually on-table) extubation, postoperatively shifting to high dependency units or even the wards [rather than intensive care units (ICUs)], early mobilization with initiation of chest physiotherapy (often on the day of surgery), early enteral (jejunal) feeding starting the morning after surgery and early removal of the nasogastric tube[19] (typically on the second postoperative day in our unit, if there is no gastric tube dilatation on the chest X-ray), urinary catheters and intercostal drains. While many centers start oral feeding after a contrast swallow between the sixth and tenth postoperative days, we do not perform a contrast swallow before initiating oral feeding. Typically, we start water orally on the fourth postoperative day, gradually increasing to full liquid feeds by the sixth–seventh postoperative day and solid feeds by the seventh-eighth day. A crucial aspect of good outcomes after esophagectomy is an aggressive postoperative rehabilitation program with a dedicated multidisciplinary team consisting of surgeons, anesthesiologists, intensivists, nurses, physiotherapists and nutritionists.

ISSUES IN SURGICAL TREATMENT OF ESOPHAGEAL CANCER

There are several controversial issues in the surgical management of esophageal cancer. These include:

- Surgical approach: Transthoracic versus transhiatal versus MIE
- Extent of lymphadenectomy
- Anastomotic technique: Stapled versus hand-sewn
- Route of reconstruction: Posterior mediastinal versus retrosternal
- Need for pyloric drainage.

Surgical Approach

The debate between a transthoracic and a transhiatal approach has been longstanding with equally strong proponents for both. This controversy has now been further compounded by the growing popularity of MIE.[20] There has been a low volume and quality of evidence to conclusively answer the question of the optimal operative approach. Theoretical advantages of the transthoracic approach include operating under direct vision, more radical surgery including more extensive lymph node dissection and possibly lower chance of injury to vital structures including the aorta, tracheobronchial tree and the thoracic duct. The disadvantages of this approach include the need for thoracotomy and resultant postoperative pain, which can at least theoretically translate into a higher incidence of pulmonary complications. Proponents of the transhiatal approach claim equivalent survival with lower morbidity while opponents criticize the lack of radical circumferential clearance and mediastinal lymphadenectomy. Theoretical advantages of MIE include: smaller incisions, avoiding prolonged, forcible retraction of the thoracic cage, less trauma to the intercostal nerves, better visualization at surgery, less postoperative pain, fewer pulmonary complications and reduced hospital stay. Limited availability of expertise and need for specialized equipment are deterrents for more universal adoption of the minimally invasive approach, which otherwise has the potential to combine the advantages of the transthoracic and transhiatal approaches.

There have been five randomized trials[21-26] and three meta-analyses[27-29] comparing transthoracic with transhiatal esophagectomy. The meta-analyses concluded that survival rates were similar with the two approaches with reduced morbidity with transhiatal esophagectomy. However, the meta-analyses had several flaws, primarily the inclusion of a large number of non-randomized and non-comparative studies which lacked scientific rigor. An interesting feature of the meta-analysis was that when only randomized and comparative studies were included in the analysis, strong trends toward superior survival and better postoperative outcomes were seen with the transthoracic approach. The largest randomized trial,[24] which included 220 patients of only adenocarcinoma of the esophagus, showed no statistically significant differences between the transhiatal and transthoracic approaches. The absolute survival figures in the intention to treat analysis however, showed 39% 5-year survival with the transthoracic approach compared to 29% with the transhiatal approach. Clearly, the study was underpowered to detect a clinically important difference in survival between the two groups. A subsequent updated publication of the same trial[25] giving longer term results showed no difference in outcomes between the two groups. In the absence of high quality evidence, the controversy continues with no clear superiority being demonstrated by either approach.

In a recent systematic review[30] which analyzed the oncological outcomes after minimally invasive surgery (MIS) esophagectomy, 17 case-control studies were included; surgeries were classified into open (718 patients), MIE (494 patients) and hybrid (386 patients). Though these were non-randomized studies, it appeared that MIS esophagectomy had similar lymph nodal yield and survival compared to open surgery. Previous systematic reviews[31,32] had demonstrated superior results with MIS esophagectomy in the following parameters: blood loss (312 mL vs 577 mL), ICU (4.5 days vs 7.6 days) and hospital (14.9 days vs 19.6 days) stay, lymph node yield (23.8 nodes vs 20.2 nodes), pulmonary morbidity (15.1% vs 22.9%), overall morbidity (43.8% vs 60.4%) and mortality (1.9% vs 4.5%). A recently published randomized trial[33] showed a significantly lower incidence of pulmonary complications with MIS esophagectomy (9%) compared to open esophagectomy (29%).

There have been some recent reports of successful robotic esophagectomy for cancer.[34-36] Most of these report initial experiences of few patients with limited data on long-term results. In a comparative study[34] of 11 patients who underwent robotic-assisted MIE and 26 patients who underwent conventional MIE, no differences were found in the immediate postoperative results. A recent study[35] evaluated the results of 21 patients undergoing robot-assisted MIE, while it was feasible and operative time reduced with increasing experience, three of the 21 patients had airway fistulae. Currently, it appears that more data from other centers is required about robotic esophagectomy, and definite superiority needs to be demonstrated before it is adopted for the routine management of esophageal cancer.[37]

From the above discussion, it is clear that the optimum approach for esophageal resection is still not clear and is heavily dependent on individual surgeons' biases. In an international survey of surgical technique involving 269 surgeons from 41 countries in six continents, 52% responders favored an open transthoracic esophagectomy, 26% favored a transhiatal esophagectomy and 14% preferred a minimally invasive approach.[38] As mentioned earlier, the versatile esophageal surgeon should be equally comfortable with all these surgical techniques to be able to choose the best approach for an individual patient.

Extent of Lymphadenectomy

The optimum extent of lymphadenectomy during esophageal resections is a controversial issue, with two widely divergent views: one which considers lymph node metastases as only indicators and not governors of prognosis, implying that lymph node dissection will therefore not improve survival[39] and the opposite view that radical lymphadenectomy not only impacts on locoregional recurrence but also on survival.[40,41] Radical lymphadenectomy including three-field lymph node dissection is widely practiced in Japan[42-44] and some parts of the western world[45,46] while in most parts of the United States and Europe, a less radical lymphadenectomy is performed. While there are undoubted benefits with superior staging and possibly better locoregional control when a three-field esophagectomy is performed, questions remain about a survival benefit.[47] The increased morbidity and mortality associated with three-field lymphadenectomy, combined with the need for highly expert surgical skills have deterred most surgeons from performing this procedure. In most series, three-field lymphadenectomy has been associated with a higher incidence of recurrent laryngeal nerve paresis, pulmonary complications and ischemic tracheabronchitis.

A stage by stage comparison by Akiyama[42] and colleagues suggested that survival was superior with three-field lymphadenectomy compared to two-field lymphadenectomy. However, such comparisons are prone to be biased by stage migration as the three-field lymphadenectomy group is more likely to have more accurate staging compared to the two-field group. Other Japanese authors[42-44] have also shown clearly superior survival with radical three-field lymphadenectomy. Two small randomized studies[48,49] (one of which was a quasi-randomized study) again showed improved survival with three-field lymphadenectomy, Kato and colleagues[48] showing a 48.7% vs 33.7% 5-year survival and Nishihara and colleagues[49] showing a 66.2% vs 48% 5-year survival. In two separate surgical series from the western world, Altorki[45] and Lerut[46] showed a 51% and 41.9% 5-year survival with radical three-field lymphadenectomy. A large nation-wide study[50] of nearly 5600 patients undergoing esophageal resection in 96 institutions in Japan showed a 5-year survival of 34% with 1800 three-field (1800 patients) and 27% with two-field (2800 patients) lymphadenectomy. Most of the evidence supporting extensive lymphadenectomy has originated from Japan where the predominant histology is squamous carcinoma. As seen from the above discussion, it is obvious that there is a lack of high quality evidence to conclusively answer this question. We are currently accruing patients in a large randomized trial comparing radical three-field lymphadenectomy with standard lymphadenectomy in operable esophageal cancer (NCT 00193817).

Several large studies in the last decade have demonstrated improved outcomes with extended lymphadenectomy for esophageal cancer. Two large studies[51,52] analyzing data from the surveillance epidemiology and end results (SEER) database and two large multicentric studies looked at the impact of extended lymphadenectomy on overall survival after esophagectomy regardless of the operative approach. In a study[51] of approximately 2600 patients undergoing esophagectomy who had complete nodal staging information, the total number of lymph nodes dissected was an independent prognostic factor, with an almost linear improvement in survival with the number of lymph nodes dissected, regardless of nodal status (positive or negative). On linear regression modeling, there was a 10% and 3% improvement in overall survival for every 10 extra lymph nodes dissected in N0 and N+ patients respectively; the best overall survival was seen when more than 30 lymph nodes were dissected. In another study[52] of the SEER database involving 4882 patients, recursive partitioning analysis was used to stratify patients based on the total number of lymph nodes dissected at surgery. Similar to the previous study, a lymph node yield of 30 nodes was associated with the maximum all cause and cancer-specific survival.

Two large multi-institutional studies[53,54] were also published confirming the effect of dissecting more lymph nodes on survival after esophagectomy. In a study[53] of a cumulative database of over 2300 patients from nine high-volume centers worldwide, Cox regression analysis showed the total number of lymph nodes examined as an independent predictor of survival; the optimum threshold defined by this analysis was 23 lymph nodes. The Worldwide Esophageal Cancer Collaboration (WECC) database [on which the seventh tumor, nodes, metastases (TNM) staging system for esophageal cancers was based] analyzed data of over 4600 patients who underwent esophagectomy from 13 different centers from across the world.[54] Optimum lymphadenectomy was defined as approximately 10, 15 and 30 lymph nodes for pT1, pT2 and pT3/4 esophageal cancers respectively. All the above studies provide strong evidence for the added value of extended lymph node dissection during esophageal cancer surgery.

Anastomotic Technique

Anastomotic leaks and strictures are dreaded early and late complications after esophageal resection respectively and several studies have been done to evaluate the optimal anastomotic technique. There have been several non-randomized, 10 randomized studies and three reviews[55-57] comparing hand-sewn with stapled esophagogastric anastomosis. Most of these studies were heterogeneous with the location and type of anastomotic techniques compared and had few patients. The meta-analysis[56] published in 2001 combined data from five randomized trials and concluded that hand-sewn and stapled anastomotic techniques had similar leak rates and that stapled anastomoses had a higher incidence of postoperative stricture formation. However, most of the studies on stapled anastomoses used an end to end anastomotic technique which is prone for stricture formation. Most recent studies have described a linear stapling technique[58] using an end to side or a triangulating technique.[59,60] These techniques have a far lower rate of anastomotic strictures as the technique involves creating a voluminous anastomosis.

Route of Reconstruction

There are three available routes to reconstruct the esophagus, they include the posterior mediastinal, retrosternal and the subcutaneous. The subcutaneous route is almost never used and the commonly used routes are the former two. A meta-analysis of six randomized trials[61] compared the posterior mediastinal with the retrosternal routes of reconstruction and concluded that outcomes were similar between the two routes with respect to mortality, anastomotic leaks and cardiac and pulmonary complications. There were however, some trends toward lower mortality and cardiopulmonary morbidity with the posterior mediastinal route which failed to reach statistical significance. The total number of patients in the six randomized controlled trials (RCTs) constituting the meta-analysis was only 342, strongly raising the possibility that an inadequate sample size could be the reason for not finding real differences in outcomes between the two groups. This is clearly one of the areas in esophageal surgery where further research is mandated.

Pyloric Drainage

The need for pyloric drainage after esophageal resection has been studied in retrospective as well as randomized trials. In a meta-analysis of nine randomized trials with a total of 553 patients,[62] a statistically significant difference was found only for immediate postoperative gastric outlet obstruction favoring the pyloric drainage group with the scintigraphic gastric emptying time ratio (drainage vs no drainage) of 0.53; there were no differences in other early outcomes including mortality, anastomotic leaks, cardiac complications, pulmonary morbidity or fatal aspiration though some trends were in favor of the pyloroplasty arm. Late outcomes also showed a nonsignificant trend toward improved outcomes with pyloroplasty with respect to delayed outcomes including nutritional status, gastric emptying and obstructive foregut symptoms. A more recent systematic review[63] of recent retrospective studies (668 patients) also concluded that there were no differences in postoperative mortality, anastomotic leaks and cardiopulmonary complications between the pyloric drainage and no drainage groups.

SUMMARY

Esophagectomy offers the best chance at long-term cure for localized esophageal cancer with neoadjuvant chemotherapy or chemoradiation proven to improve overall survival. Controversy exists over the ideal surgical approach and the extent of lymphadenectomy to be performed. While esophagectomy is a formidable surgery, it can be performed safely and with relatively low morbidity and mortality by experienced surgeons in high-volume centers. A multidisciplinary team comprising surgeons, anesthesiologists, intensivists, nurses, nutritionists and physiotherapists is crucial for favorable perioperative outcomes.

REFERENCES

1. Siegel R, Naishadham D, Jemal A. Cancer statisics, 2012. CA Cancer J Clin. 2012;62:10-29.
2. Vaughan TL, Davis S, Kristal A, Thomas DB. Obesity, alcohol and tobacco as risk factors for cancer of the esophagus and gastric cardia: adenocarcinoma versus squamous cell carcinoma. Cancer Epidemiol Biomarkers Prev. 1995;4(2):85-92.
3. Devesa SS, Blot WJ, Fraumeni JF. Changing patterns in the incidence of esophageal and gastric carcinoma in the United States. Cancer. 1998;83:2049-53.
4. DeMeester SR. Adenocarcinoma of the esophagus and cardia: a review of the disease and its treatment. Ann Surg Oncol. 2006;13: 12-30.
5. Kamangar F, Dores GM, Anderson WF. Patterns of cancer incidence, mortality and prevalence across five continents: defining priorities to reduce cancer disparities in different geographic regions of the world. J Clin Oncol. 2006;24(14):2137-50.
6. Sjoquist KM, Burmeister BH, Smithers BM Zalcberg JR, Simes RJ, Barbour A, et al. Survival after neoadjuvant chemotherapy or chemoradiotherapy for resectable oesophageal carcinoma: an updated meta-analysis. Lancet Oncol. 2011;12:681-92.
7. Blom D, Peters JH, DeMeester TR. Controversies in the current management of carcinoma of the esophagus. J Am Coll Surg. 2002;195:241-50.
8. Kelsen DP, Ginsberg R, Pajak TF, Sheahan DG, Gunderson L, Mortimer J, et al. Chemotherapy followed by surgery compared with surgery alone for localized esophageal cancer. N Engl J Med. 1998;339:1979-84.
9. Birkmeyer JD, Siewers AE, Finlayson EVA, Stukel TA, Lucas FL, Batista I, et al. Hospital volume and surgical mortality in the United States. N Engl J Med. 2002;346:1128-37.
10. National Comprehensive Cancer Network. NCCN guidelines version 1.2013. Esophageal and esophagogastric junction cancers. [Online] Available from www.nccn.org/professionals/physician_gls/pdf/esophageal.pdf [Accessed March, 2013].
11. Dimick JB, Goodney PP, Orringer MB, Birkmeyer JD. Specialty training and mortality after esophageal cancer resection. Ann Thorac Surg. 2005;80:282-6.
12. Dimick JB, Pronovost PJ, Heitmiller RE, Lipsett PA. Intensive care unit staffing is associated with decreased length of stay, hospital cost, and complications after esophageal resection. Crit Care Med. 2001;29:904-5.

13. Luketich JD, Pennathur A, Awais O, Levy RM, Keeley S, Shende M, et al. Outcomes after minimally invasive esophagectomy. Review of over 1000 patients. Ann Surg. 2012;256:95-103.
14. Stein HJ, Brucher BLDM, Sendler A, Siewert JR. Esophageal cancer: patient evaluation and pre-treatment staging. Surg Oncol. 2001;10:103-11.
15. Reed CE. Surgical management of esophageal carcinoma. Oncologist. 1999;4:95-105.
16. Alexiou C, Beggs D, Salama FD, Brackenbury ET, Morgan WE, et al. Surgery for esophageal cancer in elderly patients: the view from Nottingham. J Thorac Cardiovasc Surg. 1998;116:545-53.
17. Tsutsui S, Moriguchi S, Morita M Kuwano H, Matsuda H, Mori M, et al. Multivariate analysis of postoperative complications after esophageal resection. Ann Thorac Surg. 1992;53:1052-6.
18. Pramesh CS, Mistry RC, Sharma S, Pantvaidya GH, Raina S. Bronchial artery preservation during transthoracic esophagectomy. J Surg Oncol. 2004;85:202-3.
19. Mistry RC, Vijayabhaskar R, Karimundackal G, Jiwnani S, Pramesh CS. Effect of short-term vs prolonged nasogastric decompression on major postesophagectomy complications: a parallel-group, randomized trial. Arch Surg. 2012;147:747-51.
20. Lazzarino AI, Nagpal K, Bottle A, Faiz O, Moorthy K, Aylin P. Open versus minimally invasiveesophagectomy: trends of utilization and associated outcomes in England. Ann Surg. 2010;252:292-8.
21. Fok M, Siu KF, Wong J. A comparison of transhiatal and transthoracic resection for carcinoma of the thoracic esophagus. Am J Surg. 1989;158:414-9.
22. Goldminc M, Maddern G, Le Prise E, Meunier B, Campion JP, Launois B. Oesophagectomy by a transhiatal approach or thoracotomy: a prospective randomized trial. Br J Surg. 1993;80:367-70.
23. Chu KM, Law SY, Fok M, Wong J. A prospective randomized comparison of transhiatal and transthoracic resection for lower-third esophageal carcinoma. Am J Surg. 1997;174:320-4.
24. Hulscher JBF, van Sandick JW, de Boer AG, Wijnhoven BP, Tijssen JG, Fockens P, et al. Extended transthoracic resection compared with limited transhiatal resection for adenocarcinoma of the esophagus. N Eng J Med. 2002;347:1662-9.
25. Omloo JMT, Lagarde SM, Hulscher JB, Reitsma JB, Fockens P, van Dekken H, et al. Extended transthoracic resection compared with limited transhiatal resection for adenocarcinoma of the mid/distal esophagus. Five-year survival of a randomized clinical trial. Ann Surg. 2007;246:992-1000.
26. Areja D, SubhanA, Mirza MR, Anis N. Transhiatal versus Ivor-Lewis procedure for the treatment of Carcinoma esophagus. Pak J Surg. 2006;22:126-9.
27. Rindani R, Martin CJ, Cox MR. Transhiatal versus Ivor-Lewis oesophagectomy: is there a difference? Aust N Z J Surg. 1999;69: 187-94.
28. Hulscher JBF, Tijssen JJP, Obertop H, van Lanschot JJB. Transthoracic versus transhiatal resection for carcinoma of the esophagus: a meta-analysis. Ann Thorac Surg. 2001;72:306-13.
29. Boshier PR, Anderson O, Hanna GB. Transthoracic versus transhiatal esophagectomy for the treatment of esophageal cancer. A meta-analysis. Ann Surg. 2011;254:894-906.
30. Dantoc MM, Cox MR, Eslick GD. Does minimally invasive esophagectomy (MIE) provide for comparable oncologic outcomes to open techniques? A systematic review. J Gastrointest Surg. 2012;16:486-94.
31. Verhage RJ, Hazebroek EJ, Boone J, Van Hillegersberg R. Minimally invasive surgery compared to open procedures in esophagectomy for cancer: a systematic review of the literature. Minerva Chir. 2009;64:135-46.
32. Nagpal K, Ahmed K, Vats A, Yakoub D, James D, Ashrafian H, et al. Is minimally invasive surgery beneficial in the management of esophageal cancer? A meta-analysis. Surg Endosc. 2010;24:1621-9.
33. Biere SS, van Berge Henegouwen MI, Maas KW, Bonavina L, Rosman C, Garcia JR, et al. Minimally invasive versus open oesophagectomy for patients with oesophageal cancer: a multicenter, open-label randomized controlled trial. Lancet. 2012;379:1887-92.
34. Weksler B, Sharma P, Moudgill N, Chojnacki KA, Rosato EL. Robot-assisted minimally invasive esophagectomy is equivalent to thoracoscopic minimally invasive esophagectomy. Dis Esophagus. 2012;25:403-9.
35. Sarkaria IS, Rizk NP, Finley DJ, Bains MS, Adusumilli PS, Huang J, et al. Combined thoracoscopic and laparoscopic robotic-assisted minimally invasive esophagectomy using a four-arm platform: experience, technique and cautions during early procedure development. Eur J Cardiothorac Surg. 2013;43(5):e107-15.
36. Cerfolio RJ, Bryant AS, Hawn MT. Technical aspects and early results of robotic esophagectomy with chest anastomosis. J Thorac Cardiovasc Surg. 2013;145:90-6.
37. Clark J, Sodergren MH, Purkayastha S, Mayer EK, James D, Athanasiou T, et al. The role of robotic assisted laparoscopy for oesophagogastric oncological resection: an appraisal of the literature. Dis Esophagus. 2011;24:240-50.
38. Boone J, Livestro DP, Elias SG, Borel Rinkes IH, van Hillegersberg R. International survey on esophageal cancer: part I surgical techniques, Dis Esophagus. 2009;22:195-202.
39. Orringer MB, Marshall B, Stirling MC. Transhiatal esophagectomy for benign and malignant disease. J Thorac Cardiovasc Surg. 1993;105:265-77.
40. Skinner DB. En bloc resection for neoplasms of the esophagus and cardia. J Thorac Cardiovasc Surg. 1983;85:59-71.
41. Akiyama H, TsurumaruM, Udagawa H, Kajiyama Y. Systemic lymph node dissection for cancer—effective or not? Dis Esophagus. 1994;7:1-12.
42. Akiyama H, Tsurumaru M, Udagawa H, Kajiyama Y. Radical lymph node dissection for cancer of the thoracic esophagus. Ann Surg. 1994;220:364-73.
43. Ando N, Ozawa S, Kitagawa Y, Shinozawa Y, Kitajima M. Improvement in the results of surgical treatment of advanced squamous esophageal carcinoma during 15 consecutive years. Ann Surg. 2000;232:225-32.
44. Fujita H, Kakegawa T, Yamana H, Shima I, Toh Y, Tomita Y, et al. Mortality and morbidity rates, postoperative course, quality of life, and prognosis after extended radical lymphadenectomy for esophageal cancer: comparison of three-field lymphadenectomy with two-field lymphadenectomy. Ann Surg. 1995;222:654-62.
45. Altorki N, Kent M, Ferrara C, Port J. Three-field lymph node dissection for squamous cell and adenocarcinoma of the esophagus. Ann Surg. 2002;236:177-83.
46. Lerutm T, Nafteux P, Moons J, Coosemans W, Decker G, De Ley P, et al. Three-Field Lymphadenectomy for carcinoma of the esophagus and gastroesophageal junction in 174 R0 resections: Impact on staging, disease-free survival, and outcome. A plea for adaptation of TNM Classification in upper-half esophageal carcinoma. Ann Surg. 2004;240:962-74.
47. Lerut T, Coosemans W, de Leyn P, Decker G, Deneffe G, Van Raemdonck D. Is there a role for radical esophagectomy? Eur J Cardiothorac Surg. 1999;16 Suppl 1:S44-7.
48. Kato H, Watanabe H, Tachimori Y, lizuka T. Evaluation of neck lymph node dissection for thoracic esophageal carcinoma. Ann Thorac Surg. 1991;51:931-5.
49. Nishihara T, Hirayama K, Mori S. A prospective randomized trial of extended cervical and superior mediastinal lymphadenectomy for carcinoma of the thoracic esophagus. Am J Surg. 1998;175:47-51.
50. Isono K, Sato H, Nakayama K. Result of nationwide study on the three field lymph dissection of esophageal cancer. Oncology. 1991;48:411-20.

51. Schwarz RE, Smith DD. Clinical impact of lymphadenectomy extent in resectable esophageal cancer. J Gastrointest Surg. 2007; 11:1384-93.
52. Groth SS, Virnig BA, Whitson BA, DeFor TE, Li ZZ, Tuttle TM, et al. Determination of the minimum number of lymph nodes to examine to maximize survival in patients with esophageal carcinoma: data from the Surveillance Epidemiology and End Results database. J Thorac Cardiovasc Surg. 2010;139:612-20.
53. Peyre CG, Hagen JA, DeMeester SR, Altorki NK, Ancona E, Griffin SM, et al. The number of lymph nodes removed predicts survival in esophageal cancer: an international study on the impact of extent of surgical resection. Ann Surg. 2008;248:549-56.
54. Rizk NP, Ishwaran H, Rice TW, Chen LQ, Schipper PH, Kesler KA, et al. Optimum lymphadencectomy for esophageal cancer. Ann Surg. 2010;251:46-50.
55. Beitler AL, Urschel JD. Comparison of stapled and hand-sewn esophagogastric anastomosis. Am J Surg. 1998;175:337-40.
56. Urschel JD, Blewett CJ, Bennett WF, Miller JD, Young JE. Handsewn or stapled esophagogastric anastomoses after esophagectomy for cancer: Meta-analysis of randomized controlled trials. Dis Esophagus. 2001;14:212-7.
57. Kim RH, Takabe K. Methods of esophagogastric anastomosis following esophagectomy for cancer: a systematic review. J Surg Oncol. 2010;101:527-33.
58. Orringer MB, Marshall B, Lannettoni MD. Eliminating the cervical esophagogastric anastomotic leak with a side-to-side stapled anastomosis. J Thorac Cardiovasc Surg. 2000;119:277-88.
59. Toh Y, Sakaguchi Y, Ikeda O, Adachi E, Ohgaki K, Yamashita Y, et al. The triangulating stapling technique for cervical esophagogastric anastomosis after esophagectomy. Surg Today. 2009;39:201-6.
60. Takemura M, Yoshida K, Fujiwara Y. Modified triangulating stapling technique for esophagogastrostomy after esophagectomy for esophageal cancer. Surg Endosc. 2013;27:1249-53.
61. Urschel JD, Urschel DM, Miller JD, Bennett WF, Young JE. A meta-analysis of randomized controlled trials of route of reconstruction after esophagectomy for cancer. Am J Surg. 2001;182:470-5.
62. Urschel JD, Blewett CJ, Young JE, Miller JD, Bennett WF. Pyloric drainage (pyloroplasty) or no drainage in gastric reconstruction after esophagectomy: a meta-analysis of randomized controlled trials. Dig Surg. 2002;19:160-4.
63. Gaur P, Swanson SJ. Should we continue to drain the pylorus in patients undergoing an esophagectomy? Dis Esophagus. 2014;27(6):568-73.

CHAPTER 20

Multimodality Treatment in Carcinoma of the Esophagus

Shaleen Kumar, Shagun Misra, Rajneesh Kumar Singh

INTRODUCTION

This chapter is an attempt to present multimodality treatment in carcinoma of the esophagus from the perspective of a surgeon who must decide whether a patient is a surgical candidate or not? If so, can the patient be offered potentially curative surgery as sole treatment? Surgery alone is considered appropriate if the tumor is confined to the mucosa, and often such disease would have been detected incidentally or in a screening program. By the time a patient presents with dysphagia, which is the most common reason for patients to seek medical attention, tumors would have spread around the circumference and laterally and such muscle invasive or transmural disease also frequently present with regional nodal spread or distant metastasis. Following surgery for patients with muscle invasive disease, local or systemic failures are common, shortening survival and have been the reason to use adjuvant therapies. In the Indian subcontinent, probably fewer than 10% of patients with cancer esophagus would be candidates for resection (i.e. disease in the middle or lower third, with regional spread alone) and after excluding those with medical or other reasons for inoperability, even fewer would go on to receive surgery. Almost all resected patients would be candidates for adjuvant treatments given the high rates of local and distant failures.

So what adjuvant therapies can be offered? Radiotherapy (RT) and chemotherapy (CT) have been combined with surgery, given singly or in combination, upfront to surgery (also called preoperative, neoadjuvant or anterior) and/or following surgery (also called postoperative, adjuvant or posterior). For a review of all possible surgical adjuvant approaches, the interested reader is referred to an easily accessible review on the web, permitting in this chapter a critique of the most successful and controversial approaches that include neoadjuvant chemoradiotherapy (NACRT) and perioperative CT (i.e. neoadjuvant alone or also as adjuvant) to be presented in some detail.[1]

If the patient for medical or other reasons is not undergoing surgery, or there is likely to be gross or microscopic residual disease following surgery due to periesophageal spread for example, what are the most important considerations that help to decide whether the patient be offered RT alone or concurrently with CT (CRT)? Should a patient with non-regional nodal metastasis AJCC M1a or other oligometastasis be offered a standard course of CRT or an abbreviated course of RT alone? What are the priorities for management of patients with advanced disease in poor general condition and how are they best palliated? And finally, what does the published Indian experience offer by way of practical guidance.

SHOULD PATIENTS WITH RESECTABLE CANCER OF THE ESOPHAGUS BE OFFERED PREOPERATIVE OR POSTOPERATIVE THERAPY TOGETHER WITH SURGERY?

Surgical esophagectomy remains the treatment of choice for localized thoracic esophageal carcinoma as twice the proportion of patients remain dysphagia free compared to radiotherapy.[2] Patterns of failure, reported following surgery will depend upon selection criteria (e.g. length of primary tumor), preoperative staging procedures used and the vigour of post-treatment follow-up. A perusal of randomized trials of cancer esophagus published in the past decade, that used CT scans of the thorax, abdomen and pelvis but not 18F-Fluorodeoxyglucose positron emission tomography (FDG-PET) scans for preoperative staging, reported local failures of the order of 40% and distant metastases ranging between 30–60% for their exclusive surgery arms.[3-5] In similarly staged patients, the additional use of FDG-PET scans would identify up to 20% patients with distant nodal or organ metastases, excluding these from surgery, with an apparent improvement in surgical results.[6]

Addition of radiotherapy or systemic CT to surgical resection by targeting micrometastases can prolong survival for resectable esophageal cancer. An updated clinical practice guideline by Cancer Care Ontario,[1] has exhaustively reviewed published literature on the adjuvant use of RT or CT and have concluded as follows: there is no incremental benefit of the following strategies when added to surgery; (1) preoperative RT compared to surgery alone: endpoint, mortality at 1 year; (2) postoperative CT versus surgery alone: endpoint, mortality at 5 years; (3) postoperative CT versus postoperative chemoradiotherapy; (4) Surgery and postoperative RT versus surgery alone: endpoint, mortality at 3–5 years; (5) preoperative RT versus postoperative RT: endpoint, survival at 5 years; (6) preoperative and postoperative RT versus postoperative RT; (7) preoperative CT plus postoperative CT versus surgery alone: endpoint, survival at 3–5 years; (8) postoperative CT versus postoperative RT; (9) preoperative CT versus preoperative RT; (10) preoperative chemoradiotherapy versus preoperative RT; and (11) immunotherapy or hyperthermia combined with CT and/or RT and surgery.

Patients after esophagectomy are debilitated making the administration of CT difficult and in addition have the remodeled stomach or colon lying in proximity to the tumor bed, anastomosed with the proximal cut end of the esophagus, which limit the dose of RT that can be safely delivered to the tumor bed, in the postoperative setting. The volumes of RT are usually larger than those used in the preoperative setting and the absence of a gross disease does not permit an assessment of response to CT or RT.[7] The focus therefore has been on adjuvant treatments delivered before surgical resection as being the more doable option.

NEOADJUVANT CHEMORADIOTHERAPY FOLLOWED BY SURGERY: EVIDENCE BASE AND CRITIQUE

The Australasian Gastro-Intestinal Trials Group published a meta-analysis which included 13 studies for the comparison of NACRT followed by surgery with surgery alone in patients with resectable esophageal cancer with a sample size of 1,932 patients.[8] CT preceded RT in three trials and was given concurrently in the remaining 10. There was variability in RT doses, individual fractions sizes, number of fractions a week and total treatment duration. Most commonly two cycles of cisplatin [cis-dichlorodiammineplatinum (CDDP)] and 5-fluorouracil (5-FU) have been given spaced 3 weeks apart during RT. The hazard of death from all causes was lower for NACRT followed by surgery compared to surgery alone [hazard ratio, HR 0.78 (95% confidence interval, CI 0.70–0.88; p<0.0001)]. The absolute survival benefit at 2 years was 8.7% and the number needed to treat (NNT) of 11, i.e. this corresponds to treating 11 patients with NACRT with the expectation of 1 patient living longer. NACRT improved outcomes both in patients with squamous cell carcinoma (SCC) (HR 0.80, 95% CI 0.68–0.93; p=0.004) and adenocarcinoma (AC) (HR 0.75, 95% CI 0.59–0.95; p=0.02).

The current interest in NACRT has been fuelled by the multicenter phase III trial from the Netherlands.[9] In a rigorous quality assured trial setting, preoperative RT (41.4 Gy, 1.8 Gy per fraction, treated 5 days a week) was delivered with once-a-week CT [paclitaxel 50 mg/m^2 of body surface area (BSA) and carboplatin area-under-the-curve, AUC 2, for 5 cycles] followed at a median interval of 6.6 weeks by surgery and compared to surgery alone for middle third, lower third and esophagogastric junction tumors (AC, 75% and SCC, 23%); median age 60 years; a median length of 4 cm; resectable [i.e. cT2 and cT3, i.e. transmural spread but not invading adjacent structures as determined by endoscopic ultrasound (EUS) and with regional nodal spread in 65%]; in patients who were fully active (84%), or at worst not able to carry out heavy physical work; and with adequate nutritional intake, having lost no more than 10% of the usual body weight and good pulmonary function, i.e. forced expiratory volume in 1 sec, FEV1 more than 1.5 liter. The complication rates for NACRT + surgery versus surgery alone were—pulmonary, 46% versus 44%, anastomotic leaks, 22% versus 30%; deaths in hospital or after 30 days, 6% versus 7% and grade 3 leucopenia of 6%. In the NACRT arm, 94% went on to receive surgery (due to patient refusal, disease progression or death) and achieved an R0 resection rate of 92% (vs 69% for surgery alone), and a pathologically complete response (pCR) rate of 29% (AC, 23% and SCC, 49%). At a median follow-up of 45 months for survivors, the median, 1, 2 and 5 year survival for NACRT plus surgery versus surgery alone arms were 49.4 mo, 82%, 67% and 47% versus 24 mo, 70%, 50% and 34%, log rank p<0.001, HR 0.498, 95% CI 0.357–0.693.

What are the Realistic Risks of NACRT in the Western Literature?

In order to decide whether a given patient should be offered NACRT, it is worth while to review the risks associated with this strategy to justify its use. A reading of a comprehensive review on this subject of fairly contemporary publications (2000–2008, 38 retrospective and prospective trials including randomized comparisons, comprising 3,640 patients) would provide useful insights as the inclusion of observational studies can provide important additional information and suggest what might be encountered in practice as opposed to a closely monitored environment of a randomized clinical trial.[10] The RT doses most commonly used were of the order of 45 Gy, in 1.8–2.0 Gy per fraction, 5 days a week. CDDP + 5-FU were the most commonly used combinations.

What Proportions of Patients Who Start a Course of NACRT Go on to Surgery?

This data is difficult to glean from most papers as most retrospective studies report on patients completing all assigned treatment. In 12 of the 38 studies reviewed comprising 1,333 patients, 83.6% patients underwent esophagectomy. Reasons for exclusion of nearly 1 out of every 5 patients that were started on NACRT included: disease progression (5.9%); unfit for surgery (4.5%); refusal following NACRT (4.1%); poor tolerance and persistent toxicity (0.2% each); died during or following NACRT (1.5%). Excluding disease progression, it would not be unreasonable to attribute the figures (*vide supra*) of poor motivation, being unfit for surgery, refusal, poor tolerance, toxicity and death (a total of ≈ 10.5%, or 1 in 10 patients) to the effects of combined CT and RT. Data on toxicity were provided in 10 papers out of 38 reviewed. Grade 3 or 4 toxicity was as follows: neutropenia, 1–60%; neutropenic fever, 1–23%; nausea and vomiting, 0–16%; esophagitis, 0–43%; dehydration, 17%; fever, 10%; thrombosis, 8%; pneumonia, 2% and fistula, 2%.

Enteral or parenteral nutritional support was required in 6–35% and in 9 of these 10 studies, a mortality of 2.3% was reported after start of NACRT but before surgery.

What Proportion of Patients Achieved a Complete Resection, i.e. an R0 Resection Both in Longitudinal and Circumferential Resections Margins (CRMs)?

Data was reported on 23 of the 38 trials reviewed and this varied from 56% to 100%, with a weighted mean of 88.4% (slightly lower at 85.9% for CRMs). The vast majority used CDDP/5-FU combinations and very few, a platinum plus taxane.

What Proportions of Operated Specimens had a Pathologically Complete Response?

Data was reported in 32 of 38 trials reviewed and this ranged from 13% to 49%, with a mean of 25.8% or 1 in 4 patients. An important observation was that the pCR rates were independent of histology (i.e. identical for SCC, mean 25.9% and AC, mean 21.2%), CT agent (i.e. CDDP + 5-FU compared to other platinum/taxane combinations were equivalent), timing of or percentage of patients proceeding for surgery and radiation dose. In another report, pCRs were associated with clinically and significantly higher survival rates than those without pCRs.[11] There are refinements to tumor response seen on histological assessment, categorizing tumor response grade, TRG into no residual tumor, TRG 1; rare residual cancer cells, TRG 2; predominant fibrosis with residual cancer cells, TRG 3; residual cancer cells outgrowing fibrosis, TRG 4 and complete absence of regression change, TRG 5.[12] Responders (TRG 1 to 3) had a longer disease free survival than non-responders (TRG 4 and 5), but there are other prognostic indices such as pathological nodal status that are also predictive of outcome.

Postoperative Morbidity?

This may be influenced by the time interval between completion of NACRT and surgery. Anastomotic leakage varied between 1% and 44%, pulmonary complications, 5–57% and cardiac complications between 2–25% for an overall complication rate of 47.6% in patients who underwent resections.[10] Postoperative mortality was reported in 22/38 studies, and was variously recorded as 0–11%, with a weighted mean of 5.2%.

Indian Experience

Several groups in India practice NACRT preceding surgery for operable cancer esophagus, but a PubMed search on 9 February 2014 using the search strings, '((“carcinoma” [MeSH Terms] OR “carcinoma” [All Fields]) AND (“esophagus” [All Fields] OR “esophagus” [MeSH Terms] OR “esophagus” [All Fields])) AND (“India” [MeSH Terms] OR “India” [All Fields])' returned 244 articles, none of which dealt with this topic.

The authors would therefore like to share their modest experience in a tertiary care academic university hospital.[13] Thirty-six non-metastatic patients of SCC (July 2005 to October 2010) staged with CT scans of the thorax/abdomen and Tc99MDP bone scan if indicated but without EUS, bronchoscopy or FDG-PET received ether short-course RT, 20 Gy/5fx/1 week (n=13) and 1-cycle of concurrent cisplatin (CDDP) 75 mg/m^2 (n=10), or long-course RT 45 Gy/25fx/5 weeks (n=23), and concurrent weekly CDDP 35 mg/m^2 (n=10) or with 5-FU 325 or 500 mg/m^2 (n=13) followed 2–4 weeks later by surgery (n=25) (short-course, n=11 and long-course, n=14) of whom 23 were resected. The median age (range) was 55.5 years (30–68); 81% males; 81% Karnofsky performance score of 80 or better; median weight loss of 8.5% (0–40%); 97% with mid/lower third locations and a median length of 7 cm (1–15); 50%-stage II and 47%-stage III (clinical staging 1992 TNM system). RT was completed without interruptions with median number of cycles in short-course RT + CDDP – 1, long-course RT + CDDP/5-FU – 4 and long-course RT + CDDP – 5. Worst hematological toxicity was grade 2 white cell count and emesis in 6% each. Reasons for not undergoing surgery in about one-third, 31% (2/13-short-course, 9/23-long-course) included refusal-7, disease progression-2, worsening general condition-1 and administrative error-1. Esophagectomy-92% (23/25) was carried out via transhiatal-44%, transthoracic-36% or thoracoscopic-12% routes, using the stomach as conduit, with pulmonary complications in 43%, anastomotic leak in 17% and operative deaths in 8% (2/23). Complete responders-ypT0 + ypN0 were 12.5% (1/8-short-course RT + CDDP) and 25% (3/12-long course RT, 2 with CDDP and 1 with CDDP/5-FU). Of the 23 resected, with 9 (40%) dead, 8 [34% lost to follow-up (LFU)] and 6 (26%) alive at a median follow-up of 27.5 mo (4.4–56.4), the median and 2-year survival was likely to range between 34.3 mo and 76% (best case scenario where those LFU were censored) versus 13.9 mo and 40% (worst case scenario were those LFU were treated as events). Of the 11 not operated, with a median follow-up of 6 mo (4.3–43.9 mo), the median and 2-year survival was 7 mo and 21% (worst case scenario, the 3 patients LFU considered events). Local failures were documented in 17% (resected) versus 72% (not operated), while distant failures were 40% and 18% respectively. The interpretation is that 45 Gy RT and weekly CDDP 35 mg/m^2 +/- 5-FU 325–500 mg/m^2 results in pCRs in about 25% of patients and is doable in the context of resource constrained environments, and it is likely that this patient population is more representative of the clinical practice in university hospitals in India.

To place this patient profile in perspective, the Dutch multicenter study[9] recruited patients with smaller tumors (median 4 cm), fitter patients, none with weight loss more than 10%, histology being AC in 75%, a drop-out of only 6% following NACRT, pCR rates of 29% similar to the long course RT + CDDP +/- 5-FU regimen, similar operative mortality and no patient lost to follow-up.

NEOADJUVANT CHEMOTHERAPY FOLLOWED BY SURGERY: EVIDENCE BASE AND CRITIQUE

The Australasian Gastro-Intestinal Trials Group, also included 10 studies for the comparison of neoadjuvant chemotherapy (NACT) followed by surgery compared with surgery in patients with resectable esophageal cancer with a sample size of 2,062 patients.[8] Most commonly two or three cycles of cisplatin (CDDP) and 5-FU were given spaced 3 weeks apart before undertaking surgical resection. The hazard of death from all causes was lower for NACT followed by surgery compared to surgery alone (hazard ratio, HR 0.87 (95% CI 0.79–0.96; p=0.005). The absolute survival benefit at 2 years was 5.1% and the number needed to treat, NNT of 19, i.e. this corresponds to treating 19 patients with NACT with the expectation of 1 patient living longer. Survival following NACT in patients with SCC gave an HR of 0.92, 95% CI 0.81–1.04; p=0.18 and for AC an HR 0.83, 95% CI 0.71–0.95; p=0.01. However, the two largest RCTs in this meta-analysis reached opposite conclusions, which are elaborated next.

Comparison of the Medical Research Council (UK) and the Radiation Therapy Oncology Group (USA) Trials

The Medical Research Council (MRC) trial (OEO2 trial) randomized 802 patients to either two 4 day cycles 3 weeks apart, of CDDP 80 mg/m^2 plus 5-FU 1,000 mg/m^2 daily by continuous infusion, CI for 4 days followed by surgery (CS group, n=400) or surgery alone (S group, 402).[14] The median age was 63 years; mid or lower third location in 89%, cardia in 10%; AC 66% and SCC 31%; normal activity possible (66%) or could do light household work (31%). CT compliance was 96% (94% had both cycles and 6% had one cycle—reasons, intercurrent disease 0.02%, refusal 0.02%, death 0.02% or progressive disease 0.01%); 3% in CS and 1% in S died before surgery; postoperative deaths were 10% in each arm; R0 resection was observed in 60% (CS) and 54% (S), p<0.0001 and postoperative complications in 41% (CS) and 42% (S). At a median follow-up of 6 years, the OS was better for the CS group, HR 0.84, 95% CI, 0.72–0.98; p<0.03, and the 5-year OS was 23.0% for CS compared with 17.1% for S. The first disease-free survival event was macroscopic residual disease from incomplete resection (R2) or no resection in 26.4% of the S group versus 14.3% of the CS p<0.001. Three-year survival by type of resection was R0 42.4%, R1 was 18.0%, and R2 was 8.6%. In absolute terms, the 5-year survival for AC was 22.6% (CS) and 17.6% (S) and for SCC was 25.5% (CS) and 17.0% (S).[14,15]

The Radiation Therapy Oncology Group (RTOG) trial 8,911 used similar drugs, CDDP 100 mg/m^2 plus 5-FU 1,000 mg/m^2 for 5 days every 28 days for 3 cycles preceding surgery and 2 cycles following surgery with CDDP 75 mg/m^2 and same 5-FU doses (CS group, n=213) and compared outcomes with surgery alone (S group, n=227).[16] The median age was 62 years and the histology, AC, 54% and SCC 46%. The CT compliance was 70.5% (3 cycles), 13% (2 cycles) and 16% (1 cycle). In the postoperative phase 52% received one and 38% received two cycles of CT. The usual reasons for non compliance were cited as patient or physician choice, disease progression, death, toxicity or others. Grade 3 or higher toxicity was seen in 29% (neutropenia) and 25% (mucositis). Mortality attributed to CT was recorded in 2%. The median time from registration to surgery was 9 days (S group) and 93 days (CS group). Surgical mortality was 6% in each arm. R0 resections were 59% (S group) and 62% (CS group). At a median FU of 8.8 years, the median survival was identical at 15.6 months.[16,17]

There are several reasons that have been offered to explain why the MRC trial reported positive results and the RTOG trial was a negative one. In the RTOG trial, 93 (40%) of 234 patients registered in the preoperative CT group could not undergo surgery or had no tumor resection, compared with only 34 (15%) of 227 in the surgery-alone group. In the MRC trial, the corresponding numbers were 52 (13%) of 400 and 67 (17%) of 402. A possible explanation is that the three CT courses used in the RTOG trial were too toxic, induced a detrimental delay for surgery in non-responders' tumors, or both. In the RTOG study, a 12-week duration of the CT compared to 6 weeks in the MRC study meant that failure to respond to preoperative CT would delay definitive treatment twice as much in the RTOG compared to the MRC study which may have allowed disease progression and therefore obscured benefits of NACT preceding surgery.

Indian Experience

There has been at least one observational study (n=50) published on the role of preoperative CT in operable SCC of esophagus in Kashmir, where patients received NACT with CDDP + 5-FU followed by surgery and compared with another group that received only surgery and demonstrated a pCR of 12% and an R0 resection rate of 80%.[18] The thoracic disease management group at the Tata Memorial Hospital in Mumbai has easily the largest Indian experience of NACT and attest to its doability in a review article.[19]

THE CHOICE BETWEEN NEOADJUVANT CHEMOTHERAPY COMPARED WITH NEOADJUVANT CHEMORADIOTHERAPY, BOTH TO BE FOLLOWED BY SURGERY: EVIDENCE BASE AND CRITIQUE

The Australasian Gastro-Intestinal Trials Group, also included two studies to address this issue.[8] In the German study that was prematurely closed due to poor accrual, patients with locally advanced AC of the lower esophagus or esophagogastric junction received either 15 weeks of NACT followed by surgery (arm A) or 12 weeks of NACT plus 3 weeks of NACRT followed by surgery (arm B).[20] NACT consisted of weekly fluorouracil (2 g/m^2, 24-hour infusion) and leucovorin (500 mg/m^2, 2-hour infusion) as well as biweekly cisplatin (50 mg/m^2), while the NACRT consisted of CDDP, etoposide and 30 Gy of RT in 2 Gy per fraction. The pCR was significantly increased in arm B (2.0% vs 15.6%; p<0.03), but at the expense of greater operative mortality 3.8% vs 10.2%.

In the Australian randomized phase II trial, patients received preoperative CT with CDDP 80 mg/m^2, day 1 and 5-FU 1,000 mg/m^2/day CI for 4 days, repeated 3 weeks later.[21] In the CRT arm the second cycle began concurrently with 35 Gy in 15 fractions of RT (and a reduced dose of 5-FU, 800 mg/m^2/day). The pCR for CRT was 13% versus 0% for CT, p=0.02 and R1 resection rate for CRT 0% versus CT 11%, p=0.04 favored those receiving CRT with no treatment related deaths in either arm.

Neither trial showed any advantage for NACRT compared to NACT, as both were underpowered. The HR was 0.77, 95% CI 0.53–1.12, p=0.17 in favor of NACRT.

There is an RCT underway at the Tata Memorial Hospital, Mumbai, testing the relative merits of these alternate approaches to adjuvant therapy in operable esophageal cancer.[19]

Recommendations

So although the recommendations are to use platinum based NACRT or cisplatin based NACT as the "preferred" modality in the management of surgically resectable patients with esophageal cancers, these come with some caveats.[1] The survival advantages are minimal (NNT of 11 for NACRT and 19 for NACT, *vide supra*), come at a price of enhanced morbidity and so should be based on patient preferences, comorbidities and suitability for trimodality treatment, besides available expertise and motivation of the multidisciplinary group of surgeons, oncologists and skills of perioperative teams involved.

Further, and this needs emphasis, that these therapies are for operable patients and should not be used to downstage incurable disease.

There is a proportionately larger benefit for the use of NACRT to NACT but many argue that the favorable results of the UK MAGIC trial (perioperative epirubicin, CDDP and 5-FU in resectable lower esophagus, GEJ and gastric ACs),[22] the MRC trial[15] and the French multicenter trial[23] with an identical design to the UK MAGIC trial justify exclusion of preoperative RT for this group of patients.[8] But these trials were mainly of ACs and there is a lot of overlap with gastric, GEJ and lower esophageal tumors. Besides, there is no good direct evidence to support the use of NACRT to NACT (or perioperative CT), *vide supra* and therefore concerns remain. In the USA, NACRT is favored over perioperative CT given the "negative" RTOG trial 8911[17] while in the UK the latter is the favored approach. NACRT also has a profound, but temporary negative effect on most aspects of health related quality of life.[10] Clearly, it is only the fittest amongst the operable esophageal cancer patients who may be able to tolerate NACRT, and the rest could possibly be offered NACT (or perioperative CT) as an alternative.

POSTOPERATIVE THERAPY FOR NODE POSITIVE (N+), MICROSCOPIC (R1), OR GROSS RESIDUAL (R2) DISEASE

In contemporary RCTs, 5-year survival in the surgery alone arms has varied between 17% and 20%,[14,17] but they can hardly be characterized as a medical success story, especially when we keep in mind that much of this improvement is the result of better clinical staging and better patient selection.

Surgery remains the mainstay of treatment for operable mid and lower third esophageal cancers, as not all surgeons remain convinced about the use of neoadjuvant treatments and prefer to offer postoperative RT (PORT) when indicated, for example in node positive, R1 or R2 disease.[7] Although the pooled randomized evidence[1] indicates no survival benefit for PORT, a perusal of some of the randomized trials suggest that in the specific subgroup of N+ or residual disease, patients will experience significantly fewer local recurrences with its use.[24] In retrospective analysis of patients with 3 or more positive nodes in the mediastinum, a survival advantage has also been observed.[25] Further intensification of treatment in the form of postoperative chemoradiotherapy (POCRT) in N+ cancers of the esophagus, have suggested a survival advantage over and above RT alone, but once again, at the expense of significantly more neutropenia, esophagitis and gastrointestinal reactions of all grades.[26]

For patients who have received NACRT followed by surgery, and have R2 disease, there is retrospective data to suggest that giving further CT (mainly single agent taxane) in the postoperative phase may result in better disease free survival, DFS and overall survival, OS. This benefit was however not conferred in those with R0 or R1 resections.[27]

Indian Experience

A policy of offering PORT to all patients with resected cancers of the esophagus was followed at a university hospital setting between the years 1990–2002 as the surgeons believed that in the absence of a systematic lymph node dissection in the mediastinum, they would prefer to label the procedure as "non-curative".[28] The audit revealed that a third of the 139 operated patients could not comply with the advice of PORT and it was reflective of poor motivation after stressful interventions in a group of patients already debilitated by their disease. The postsurgical convalescence period was prolonged in some patients; nearly half of the patients could not start PORT by 6 weeks, 79% commenced within 2 months and 96% within 3 months. A 5-year survival of 17% was observed after accounting for 13% of patients lost to follow-up, who were considered as dead for computation of the survival curve assuming the worst case scenario. One cannot draw inferences on efficacy of PORT from such audits, and given the rationale and interest in preoperative approaches, this strategy was abandoned. However, possibly a case for POCRT or PORT can be made in postoperative patients with residual disease or N+, which hopefully should be as few as possible in surgical practice by careful patient selection or by accepting the philosophy of greater feasibility of NACRT/ NACT/perioperative CT *vide supra*.

COMBINED MODALITY TREATMENT IN THE NON-SURGICAL MANAGEMENT OF CANCER ESOPHAGUS

Radiotherapy is applicable to a diverse patient population and most series comprise patients with disease too advanced for surgery.[29] RT treats the primary tumor, surrounding tissues and lymphatics and the doses are limited by tolerances of the surrounding lung, heart and spinal cord. Historically there was a lot of interest in NACT followed by RT as the tumors responses are very gratifying, with responders to NACT having better OS compared to non-responders, but a meta-analysis of three randomized trials has shown no survival benefit of sequential chemoradiotherapy in patients with SCC with an HR for mortality 0·90, 95% CI 0·72–1·03; p=0·18.[30]

The current interest in RT and CT delivered concurrently, i.e. CRT stems from the Radiation Therapy Oncology Group (RTOG 85-01) trial where RT to a dose of 50 Gy in 25 fractions, 2 Gy per fraction, spread over 5 weeks was delivered concurrently on weeks 1 and 5 (CDDP 75 mg/m^2 day 1 and 5-FU 1,000 mg/m^2 CI for days 1-4) and as adjuvant on weeks 8 and 11 (CRT arm, n=61), and compared with 64 Gy (RT arm, n=60).[31] At long-term follow-up, the median OS was 14.1 mo versus 9.3 mo and the 5-year OS 26% versus 0%, p<0.001 favoring the CRT arm.[32] On the Karnofsky scale, 93% of patients had a score of 70 or higher (i.e. patient at least cares for self); 88% were SCC; 80% had disease in mid or lower third; weight loss as a percentage of usual body weight was not mentioned, not were the median length of the tumors. By 1 year, the rates of persistence or recurrence of tumor were 44% versus 62% (p=0.01) and distant metastasis were 22% versus 38%, p=0.005 favoring the CRT arm. Side effects were severe in 44% and life threatening in 20% in the CRT arm compared to 25% and 3% for the RT arm. The CT compliance for all four cycles was 54%.

With the RTOG 85-01 trial as a new bench mark, three routes of dose intensification were pursued:

1. Intergroup Trial 0122 (RTOG 90-12), a phase II trial, that incorporated the following modifications to the CRT arm of the RTOG 85-01, *vide supra*.[33] (a) The 5-FU continuous infusion was increased from 4 to 5 days; (b) the total number of cycles of CT was increased from 4 to 5 cycles; (c) three cycles of full dose neoadjuvant 5-FU/cisplatin were delivered prior to the start of combined modality therapy and (d) the radiation dose was increased from 50 Gy to 64.8 Gy but at 1.8 Gy per fraction. Forty-five were enrolled, 31% did not complete the neoadjuvant CT (reasons, death, toxicity, progression or refusal), grade 3 or higher toxicity was witnessed in 72% and a treatment mortality of 11% (6/45). The median OS was 20 mo and at 5-years, 20%. This strategy was not pursued further.
2. RTOG 92-07, a phase I/II trial similar to CRT arm of RTOG 85-01 with the addition of esophageal brachytherapy, EB, three sittings of 5 Gy each (high dose rate, HDR) in weeks 8, 9 and 10 or one sitting of 20 Gy low-dose-rate, LDR in week 8.[34] Fifty were enrolled; the overall compliance to external RT, CT and EB was 50%; severe toxicity, mainly hematologic and gastrointestinal was observed in 58%, life threatening in another 26% and fatal toxicity in 8% with 12% patients developing fistulae. The median OS was 11 mo and by 1-year, 48% were alive. This strategy was not pursued further.
3. Intergroup 0123 (RTOG 94-05), a phase III trial with the control arm being the CRT arm of RTOG 85-01 versus the higher dose arm delivering 64.8 Gy, but CT dose and schedules remained quite similar.[35] Two hundred and eighteen eligible patients were randomized equally. About 60% had a Karnofsky score of 90 or 100 (at worst with minor signs/symptoms, essentially normal); median tumor length 5 cm; about 60% having lost less than 10% of usual body weight and 86% SCC. Grade 3 or higher toxicities were seen in two-thirds of patients; 10% (11/109) died in the high dose arm but of note, 6% (7/11) deaths occurred in patients who had received 50.5 Gy or less. The median OS was 13 mo versus 18.1 mo and 2-year survival 31% versus 40% in the high dose arm and control arms respectively, both differences non significant. This finding is widely misunderstood to suggest a detrimental effect of dose escalation beyond 50 Gy, but most deaths occurred by 50.4 Gy.

With modern RT planning, which may include the use of FDG-PET scans for tumor delineation, 4D CT planning (which means factoring physiological motion such as breathing) to reduce doses to lung, heart or spinal cord, patterns of failure following the CRT protocol as in the current standard of care in the US (RTOG 85-01) result in local failures within the gross tumor in about 50% of patients and the same number have distant failures and some have both.[36]

Other treatment intensive approaches include a Phase II RCT (RTOG 0113) of induction taxane-platin-5-FU followed by taxane-platin concurrent with 50.4 Gy (n=41) versus induction with taxane-platin and similar CRT (n=43). Two-thirds of the patients had a weight loss of less than 10%, tumor size less than 5 cm and histology AC. Both arms had over 80% grade III/IV toxicities with 3% and 6% deaths respectively and 2-year OS of 56% and 37% respectively and neither have been pursued further.[37]

In the UK, a phase II/III RCT randomized patients to receive CRT, CDDP 60 mg/m^2 day 1 and capecitabine 1,250 mg/m^2 day 1–21 for four cycles with cycle 3 and 4 given along with 50 Gy/25fx RT (n=129) or similar CRT plus cetuximab 400 mg/m^2 day 1 followed by 250 mg/m^2 weekly (n=129). All patients were fit, at best restricted in strenuous physical activity (ECOG 0 or 1), over 70% has SCC histology while over 85% had a mid/lower third location and were FDG-PET staged. Overall compliance to CT as planned was close to 55% and grade III/IV non-hematologic toxicities were 80%, and those in the CRT + cetuximab experienced shorter median survival 22·1 mo versus 25·4 mo HR 1·53, 95% CI 1·03–2·27, p=0·035. These median survivals are better than other series in part due to FDG-PET used to exclude AJCC M1a (non-regional nodes) and AJCC M1b disease. Cetuximab is not recommended along with CDDP-capecitabine combination.[38]

The RTOG 1010 trial is currently evaluating the addition of trastuzumab to chemoradiation with the RT doses of 50.4 Gy plus weekly carboplatin AUC 2 and paclitaxel 50 mg/m^2 in AC of the esophagus.

Indian Data

Currently there is at least one published Indian trial on the subject of definitive CRT in esophageal cancer that is searchable on PubMed. Following a phase II experience,[39] an RCT of unresectable patients with SCC evaluated a doable regimen of once-a-week CDDP 35 mg/m^2 delivered concurrently with RT to doses of 66 Gy/33fx/6.5 weeks (or 50 Gy/25Fx/5wks plus two fractions of 6 Gy HDR brachytherapy), CRT arm (n=65) versus RT alone (n=60). Patients ranged in Karnofsky scale from 50 (requires considerable assistance and frequent medical care) to 90 (normal activity, minor signs of disease), median weight loss about 10%, over 80% in upper/mid esophagus locations, all SCC and a median length of 7.5 cm. Compliance to RT was 78% (47/60) in RT group and 89% (58/65) of the CRT group p=0.10; more than or equal to six cycles of CDDP could be delivered in 63% (41/65), with grade 3 neutropenia of 3%. Eighteen percent (23/125) patients were lost to follow-up and considered as events in the survival analysis, i.e. worst case scenario. At a median (range) follow-up of 113 months (65–135) of all patients alive and with 120/125 events, the median, 1, 2 and 5 year survival was 6.5 months, 30%, 21.6% and 11.7% versus 14.5 months, 58.5%, 38.5% and 18.5% for the RT and CRT groups respectively, HR 1.55, 95% CI 1.08–2.22, p=0.016, with a greater hazard of dying in the RT arm.[40,41] One may infer that the addition of concurrent CDDP to RT results in a modest improvement in survival and is associated with manageable additional acute morbidity.

Recommendations

A meta-analysis of seven RCTs suggests a 1-year survival benefit in favor of CRT compared to RT alone, OR 0.61, 95% CI 0.44–0.84, p<0.00001. When expressed as an absolute mortality rate, the survival by 1 year for CRT versus RT alone was 44% versus 33%. This is an absolute difference of 11% and an NNT of 9, at the expense of significant increase in adverse effects, including life threatening toxicities, compared to RT alone.[42] This practice guideline states that CDDP based CT is reasonable to use, but patients must be made aware of the increased acute toxicity, balancing risks and benefits.

On a practical note, if a patient can manage an intake of at least 1,000 kcal/m^2 BSA/day; has lost not more than 10% of usual body weight in the preceding 6 months; is at least able to care for self although unable to carry on normal activity or do active work, i.e. Karnofsky score of more than or equal to 70; has no major comorbidities; and is not aspirating his saliva due to an absolute block in the food passage that puts at risk for pneumonia, a platinum based weekly CRT regimen that permit closer monitoring of toxicity can be offered, always under close supervision. For the rest, RT as sole treatment is safer, with the caveat, that maintaining calorie intake and recognizing and managing aspiration early (such as seeking and investigating any fever or cough or worsening motivation/general condition of the patient) is *sine qua non* for steering a patient safely through a course of RT. The experienced clinical oncologist needs to discuss with the patient and decides rather than a one-size-fits-all prescription of "concurrent chemoradiotherapy" for all not-for-surgery patients.

CHEMORADIOTHERAPY OR NACRT FOLLOWED BY SURGERY FOR OPERABLE PATIENTS?

In the meta-analysis comparing preoperative CT plus surgery to surgery alone the 5-year survival expectation of patients randomized to surgery was 16%.[1] In the RTOG 85-01 trial, the OS by 5 years of patients randomized to the CRT arm (*vide supra*) was 26%, 95% CI, 15–37%, while the non-randomized CRT cohort that followed the main trial reported a figure of 14%, 95% CI 6–23%.[32] It appears that CRT, even in not-for-surgery patients can approximate the survival expectations of patients undergoing surgery alone. Further, given the encouraging data of CRT preceding surgery, it would seem logical to determine to what extent surgery can add to the prognosis of patients treated with CRT.

A German study randomized surgically eligible patients to NACT (three cycles of 5-FU, folinic acid, etoposide and CDDP every 3 weeks) followed by 40 Gy RT and concurrent CDDP plus etoposide on days 2–8 of RT followed by surgery (surgery arm, n=86) versus same NACT and either 65 Gy by external RT or 60 Gy plus esophageal brachytherapy and concurrent CDDP plus etoposide on days 2–8 of RT (RT arm, n=86). Importantly 34% patients in the surgery arm did not proceed to surgery which is not surprising.[10] Overall treatment mortality was 12.8% versus 3.5%, median survival 16.4 mo versus 14.9 mo and 2-year survival 39.9% versus 35.4% in the surgery and RT arms respectively. The outcomes were deemed equivalent, p=0.007.[43]

The French, in a more pragmatic design asked the same question. They carried out an RCT in responders to CRT by randomizing to either further CRT or to surgery. Two cycles of CDDP 15 mg/m^2 plus 5-FU 800 mg/m^2 over 5 days were delivered on days 1 and 22 with 46 Gy/23 fx or 15 Gy/5fx-gap-15 Gy/5fx (n=444). Those who responded by way of improvement in dysphagia or shrinkage in tumor and provided they were fit to proceed were then randomized to surgery (Arm A, n=129) or further CRT (Arm B, n=130) to either 20 Gy/10 fx (total 66 Gy) or 15 Gy/5x (total 45 Gy) as per initial RT plan plus three more cycles of identical CT on days 43, 64 and 92. Deaths in the first 3 months were 9% versus 1% for arms A and B, p=0.002, while median survival were 17.7 mo versus 19.3 mo and 2-year survivals 33.6% versus 39.8% respectively, p=0.44. Stents were required for 5% versus 32%, p<0.001, while any intervention to correct for dysphagia was required in 24% versus 46%, p<0.001 for arms A and B respectively. The interpretation is that in responders to CRT, survivals are unchanged by the addition of surgery, although additional procedures to alleviate dysphagia are required twice as often with CRT alone.[44]

Identifying Responders to NACRT Using FDG-PET

If an FDG-PET study were done after completion of a course of CRT, the resulting esophagitis and ulceration would result in a high false positive rate, and will therefore not reliably differentiate between responders and non-responders to decide whether to continue with CRT or suggest surgery respectively. Hence, it has been suggested that if PET were to be performed for this purpose, it should be done about 2 weeks into CRT as inflammation just about starts to set in around that time resulting in low false positive rates, sensitivity 93% and specificity 95%. In a meta-analysis of twenty reports comprising 849 patients, sensitivity of PET for this specific objective ranged between 33% and 100% (pooled estimate 67%) and specificity also from 30% to 100% (pooled estimate 68%), with significant heterogeneity and a recommendation of not using PET to guide decisions in respect of neoadjuvant therapy.[45]

MANAGEMENT OF PATIENTS WITH NON-REGIONAL NODAL METASTASIS AJCC M1A OR OTHER SMALL VOLUME OLIGOMETASTASIS IN GOOD GENERAL CONDITION

For a primary tumor located in the upper third (i.e. at 18–24 cm), AJCC staging assigns spread to the supraclavicular node (surgical neck node level IV) as a "non-regional node" categorizing it as M1a. If the primary was located in the mid third (i.e. 24–32 cm), this node would represent distant spread and be categorized M1b. A similar situation exists with celiac lymphnode metastases from lower third locations (i.e. 32–40 cm), i.e. M1a, and if spread from a mid-third location, M1b. The category M1a is distinct from M1b as the latter includes lung, liver, suprarenal, bone or other metastases.

Radiation morbidity is volume dependent. If these nodes (M1a) can be encompassed in a reasonable volume after factoring: (i) the primary disease (the so-called gross tumor volume, GTV); (ii) with a margin of 3 cm along the esophagus, and sometimes 1 cm radially for mucosal spread [the so-called clinical target volume (CTV)]; and then factoring in known and measured uncertainties in the treatment planning and execution chain, currently about 1.5 cm in three dimensions in the authors institution [the so-called planning target volume (PTV)], then if other factors are favorable (*vide supra*), such patients may be included in a course of CRT with an intent to effect growth restraint for as long as possible. This philosophy is also extended to subpleural or small pulmonary parenchymal metastases seen currently with high resolution CT imaging or PET-CT scans with the argument that before these higher resolution scanners became available, a fit patient would have invariably undergone CRT. The aim, once again is to sustain local control and dysphagia relief for as long as possible. CRT then, is appropriate not only for appropriately selected non-surgical candidates (*vide supra*), but also for selected M1a and M1b patients, providing always, that it can be delivered in doable strategies safely. As a matter in fact, the stage migration afforded by PET-CT scans and patient selection is one of the main reasons for apparently better outcomes of modern treatments in both early and advanced stages, the well-known Will-Rogers phenomenon.[46]

The counter argument is that with M1b disease, the metastases would be the Achilles heel (i.e. responsible for the patients demise), but then, responses to CT are not as durable as those with RT, and therefore some rational combination of both CT and RT may be appropriate for sustained dysphagia relief and local control in addition to growth restraint of the metastases in selected patients. The treatments offered will be often timed and tailored to the individual requirements.

PRIORITIZING MANAGEMENT OF PATIENTS WITH ADVANCED DISEASE, M1B IN POOR GENERAL CONDITION

On occasion, patients are brought to the clinic exceedingly debilitated. The cause of debilitation is often a combination of: (i) starvation, severe weight loss and cachexia due to dysphagia; (ii) dehydration, especially in summer months in most of India, due to dysphagia; (iii) aspiration pneumonia/septicemia due to regurgitation of pooled saliva and attempts at swallowing food or water, again consequent to dysphagia; (iv) constipation due to use of narcotic analgesia (codeine, tramadol, pentazocine, buprenorphine or morphine) consequent to severe chest/back pain due to periesophageal spread in the mediastinum, epigastric pain referred to the back due to celiac nodes encasing nerves, low back ache due to para-aortic lymphnodes, capsule stretch of the liver with metastases or bone metastases; (v) other symptoms due to a respiratory fistula, hoarseness from recurrent laryngeal nerve invasion, hiccups from phrenic nerve invasion or symptoms specific to metastatic disease to the lungs, liver and central nervous system, and sometimes hypercalcemia. A patient and careful history and brief physical examination will often identify easily remediable causes of debility which are best managed as an in-patient, e.g. correct dehydration, antibiotics for lung infection, institute pain control according to the WHO ladder, enemas for constipation and a Ryles tube (often helped by the radiologist or gastroenterologist) to feed safely as a better option than parenteral nutrition (expensive, allergic reactions and not sustainable). With these correctable causes of debility rectified in the short term, a better assessment of the impact of locoregional and metastatic disease is possible and permits calm and rational decision-making to institute further palliative procedures as follows.

If there is no active infection, CDDP 75 mg/m^2 day 1 and 5-FU 600 mg/m^2 days 1-4 would be a good starting point to address most metastasis, and the primary tumor. Fitter patients can receive any one of the doable combinations of an anthracycline-platin-fluoropyrimidine combination with response rates of over 40%.[47]

A passage through the esophageal stricture can be addressed by a variety of approaches that include stents, argon plasma coagulation (APC), photodynamic therapy (PDT), esophageal brachytherapy, CT, radiotherapy and chemoradiotherapy.

Short course RT would be appropriate for brain and bone metastases.

CONCLUSION

Safe and rational decision-making in what serves the best interest of a patient afflicted with esophageal cancer, involves the combined skills of a surgeon with interest in esophageal malignancies, a clinical oncologist (or alternatively a radiation and medical oncologist) evaluating a patient in real time and sharing the pros and cons of alternate strategies with both patient and family as the treatments can be onerous, disease debilitating, outcomes uncertain, significant toxicity, costs containments are always welcome, and trust building between treating team and family, which comes to the rescue of all concerned in a disease where at best 1 person in 5 would survive 5 years even in the controlled and highly quality assured environment of clinical trials, which are quite removed from clinical practice.

REFERENCES

1. Malthaner RA, Wong RKS, Spithoff K, Rumble RB, Zuraw L, Gastrointestinal Cancer Disease Site Group. Preoperative or postoperative therapy for resectable esophageal cancer. Toronto (ON): Cancer Care Ontario; 2008 May 21 [Endorsed 2013 Apr 02]. Program in Evidence-based Care Evidence-based Series No.: 2-11 Version 3. Available from https://www.cancercare.on.ca/common/pages/UserFile.aspx?serverId=6&path=/File%20Database/CCO%20Files/PEBC/pebc2-11f.pdf [accessed 26 January 2014].
2. Badwe RA, Sharma V, Bhansali MS, Dinshaw KA, Patil PK, Dalvi N, et al. The quality of swallowing for patients with operable esophageal carcinoma: a randomized trial comparing surgery with radiotherapy. Cancer. 1999;85:763-8.
3. Urba SG, Orringer MB, Turrisi A, Iannettoni M, Forastiere A, Strawderman M. Randomized trial of preoperative chemoradiation versus surgery alone in patients with locoregional esophageal carcinoma. J Clin Oncol. 2001;19:305-13.
4. Burmeister BH, Smithers BM, Gebski V, Fitzgerald L, Simes RJ, Devitt P, et al. Surgery alone versus chemoradiotherapy followed by surgery for resectable cancer of the oesophagus: a randomised controlled phase III trial. Lancet Oncol. 2005;6:659-68.
5. Lv J, Cao XF, Zhu B, Ji L, Tao L, Wang DD. Long-term efficacy of perioperative chemoradiotherapy on esophageal squamous cell carcinoma. World J Gastroenterol. 2010;16:1649-54.
6. Heeren PA, Jager PL, Bongaerts F, van Dullemen H, Sluiter W, Plukker JT. Detection of distant metastases in esophageal cancer with (18)F-FDG PET. J Nucl Med. 2004;45:980-7.
7. Jabbour SK, Thomas CR Jr. Radiation therapy in the postoperative management of esophageal cancer. J Gastrointest Oncol. 2010;1:102-11.
8. Sjoquist KM, Burmeister BH, Smithers BM, Zalcberg JR, Simes RJ, Barbour A, et al. Survival after neoadjuvant chemotherapy or chemoradiotherapy for resectable oesophageal carcinoma: an updated meta-analysis. Lancet Oncol. 2011;12:681-92.
9. van Hagen P, Hulshof MC, van Lanschot JJ, Steyerberg EW, van Berge Henegouwen MI, Wijnhoven BP, et al. Preoperative chemoradiotherapy for esophageal or junctional cancer. N Engl J Med. 2012;366:2074-84.
10. Courrech Staal EF, Aleman BM, Boot H, van Velthuysen ML, van Tinteren H, van Sandick JW. Systematic review of the benefits and risks of neoadjuvant chemoradiation for oesophageal cancer. Br J Surg. 2010;97:1482-96.
11. van Hagen P, Wijnhoven BP, Nafteux P, Moons J, Haustermans K, De Hertogh G, et al. Recurrence pattern in patients with a pathologically complete response after neoadjuvant chemoradiotherapy and surgery for oesophageal cancer. Br J Surg. 2013;100:267-73.
12. Mandard AM, Dalibard F, Mandard JC, Marnay J, Henry-Amar M, Petiot JF, et al. Pathologic assessment of tumor regression after preoperative chemoradiotherapy of esophageal carcinoma. Clinicopathologic correlations. Cancer. 1994;73:2680-86.
13. Misra S, Lokesha HM, Chaudhuri T, Khurana R, Tewari A, Singh RK, et al. P-0020 Preoperative cisplatin with/without 5-FU

concurrent with short or long course radiotherapy preceding surgery for operable squamous cell cancer of esophagus. Ann Oncol. 2011;22(Suppl 5):v31.
14. Medical Research Council Oesophageal Cancer Working Group. Surgical resection with or without preoperative chemotherapy in oesophageal cancer: a randomised controlled trial. Lancet. 2002;359:1727-33.
15. Allum WH, Stenning SP, Bancewicz J, Clark PI, Langley RE. Long-term results of a randomized trial of surgery with or without preoperative chemotherapy in esophageal cancer. J Clin Oncol. 2009;27:5062-7.
16. Kelsen DP, Ginsberg R, Pajak TF, Sheahan DG, Gunderson L, Mortimer J, et al. Chemotherapy followed by surgery compared with surgery alone for localized esophageal cancer. N Engl J Med. 1998;339:1979-84.
17. Kelsen DP, Winter KA, Gunderson LL, Mortimer J, Estes NC, Haller DG, et al. Long-term results of RTOG trial 8911 (USA Intergroup 113): a random assignment trial comparison of chemotherapy followed by surgery compared with surgery alone for esophageal cancer. J Clin Oncol. 2007;25:3719-25.
18. Lone GN, Sheikh AA, Sheikh ZA, Baba KM, Qurieshi MA, Mufti GN, et al. Role of preoperative chemotherapy in squamous cell carcinoma of esophagus in Kashmir, a cancer belt—a pilot study. Asian Pac J Cancer Prev. 2011;12:465-70.
19. Keditsu KK, Jiwnani S, Karimundackal G, Pramesh CS. Multimodality management of esophageal cancer. Indian J Surg Oncol. 2013;4:96-104.
20. Stahl M, Walz MK, Stuschke M, Lehmann N, Meyer HJ, Riera-Knorrenschild J, et al. Phase III comparison of preoperative chemotherapy compared with chemoradiotherapy in patients with locally advanced adenocarcinoma of the esophagogastric junction. J Clin Oncol. 2009;27:851-6.
21. Burmeister BH, Thomas JM, Burmeister EA, Walpole ET, Harvey JA, Thomson DB, et al. Is concurrent radiation therapy required in patients receiving preoperative chemotherapy for adenocarcinoma of the oesophagus? A randomised phase II trial. Eur J Cancer. 2011;47:354-60.
22. Cunningham D, Allum WH, Stenning SP, Thompson JN, Van de Velde CJ, Nicolson M, et al. Perioperative chemotherapy versus surgery alone for resectable gastroesophageal cancer. N Engl J Med. 2006;355:11-20.
23. Ychou M, Boige V, Pignon JP, Conroy T, Bouché O, Lebreton G, et al. Perioperative chemotherapy compared with surgery alone for resectable gastroesophageal adenocarcinoma: an FNCLCC and FFCD multicenter phase III trial. J Clin Oncol. 2011;29:1715-21.
24. Ténière P, Hay JM, Fingerhut A, Fagniez PL. Postoperative radiation therapy does not increase survival after curative resection for squamous cell carcinoma of the middle and lower esophagus as shown by a multicenter controlled trial. French University Association for Surgical Research. Surg Gynecol Obstet. 1991;173:123-30.
25. Chen J, Pan J, Zheng X, Zhu K, Li J, Chen M, et al. Number and location of positive nodes, postoperative radiotherapy, and survival after esophagectomy with three-field lymph node dissection for thoracic esophageal squamous cell carcinoma. Int J Radiat Oncol Biol Phys. 2012;82:475-82.
26. Chen J, Pan J, Liu J, Li J, Zhu K, Zheng X, et al. Postoperative radiation therapy with or without concurrent chemotherapy for node-positive thoracic esophageal squamous cell carcinoma. Int J Radiat Oncol Biol Phys. 2013;86:671-7.
27. Kim GJ, Koshy M, Hanlon AL, Horiba MN, Edelman MJ, Burrows WM, et al. The benefit of chemotherapy in esophageal cancer patients with residual disease after trimodality therapy. Am J Clin Oncol. 2014 Jan 30.
28. Kumar S, Dimri K, Balachandran P, Kumar A, Lal P, Sikora SS, et al. An audit of postoperative radiotherapy after non-curative resection for cancer of the oesophagus. Clin Oncol (R Coll Radiol). 2005;17:352-7.
29. Suntharalingam M. Definitive chemoradiation in the management of locally advanced esophageal cancer. Semin Radiat Oncol. 2007;17:22-8.
30. Gebski V, Burmeister B, Smithers BM, Foo K, Zalcberg J, Simes J, et al. Survival benefits from neoadjuvant chemoradiotherapy or chemotherapy in oesophageal carcinoma: a meta-analysis. Lancet Oncol. 2007;8:226-34.
31. Herskovic A, Martz K, al-Sarraf M, Leichman L, Brindle J, Vaitkevicius V, et al. Combined chemotherapy and radiotherapy compared with radiotherapy alone in patients with cancer of the esophagus. N Engl J Med. 1992;326:1593-8.
32. Cooper JS, Guo MD, Herskovic A, Macdonald JS, Martenson JA Jr, Al-Sarraf M, et al. Chemoradiotherapy of locally advanced esophageal cancer: long-term follow-up of a prospective randomized trial (RTOG 85-01). Radiation Therapy Oncology Group. JAMA. 1999;281:1623-7.
33. Minsky BD, Neuberg D, Kelsen DP, Pisansky TM, Ginsberg RJ, Pajak T, et al. Final report of Intergroup Trial 0122 (ECOG PE-289, RTOG 90-12): Phase II trial of neoadjuvant chemotherapy plus concurrent chemotherapy and high-dose radiation for squamous cell carcinoma of the esophagus. Int J Radiat Oncol Biol Phys. 1999;43:517-23.
34. Gaspar LE, Qian C, Kocha WI, Coia LR, Herskovic A, Graham M. A phase I/II study of external beam radiation, brachytherapy and concurrent chemotherapy in localized cancer of the esophagus (RTOG 92-07): preliminary toxicity report. Int J Radiat Oncol Biol Phys. 1997;37:593-9.
35. Minsky BD, Pajak TF, Ginsberg RJ, Pisansky TM, Martenson J, Komaki R, et al. INT 0123 (Radiation Therapy Oncology Group 94-05) phase III trial of combined-modality therapy for esophageal cancer: high-dose versus standard-dose radiation therapy. J Clin Oncol. 2002;20:1167-74.
36. Welsh J, Settle SH, Amini A, Xiao L, Suzuki A, Hayashi Y, et al. Failure patterns in patients with esophageal cancer treated with definitive chemoradiation. Cancer. 2012;118:2632-40.
37. Ajani JA, Winter K, Komaki R, Kelsen DP, Minsky BD, Liao Z, et al. Phase II randomized trial of two nonoperative regimens of induction chemotherapy followed by chemoradiation in patients with localized carcinoma of the esophagus: RTOG 0113. J Clin Oncol. 2008;26:4551-6.
38. Crosby T, Hurt CN, Falk S, Gollins S, Mukherjee S, Staffurth J, et al. Chemoradiotherapy with or without cetuximab in patients with oesophageal cancer (SCOPE1): a multicentre, phase 2/3 randomised trial. Lancet Oncol. 2013;14(7):627-37.
39. Kumar S, Dimri K, Datta NR, Rastogi N, Lal P, Das KJ, et al. Safety and efficacy of concurrent cisplatin and radiotherapy in inoperable or metastatic squamous cell esophageal cancer. Acta Oncol. 2002;41:457-62.
40. Kumar S, Dimri K, Khurana R, Rastogi N, Das KJ, Lal P. A randomised trial of radiotherapy compared with cisplatin chemo-radiotherapy in patients with unresectable squamous cell cancer of the esophagus. Radiother Oncol. 2007;83:139-47.
41. Pandey A, Misra S, Choudhuri T, Dimri K, Khurana R, Lal P, et al. PD-0001 mature results of a randomised trial of radiotherapy compared with cisplatin chemoradiotherapy in patients with unresectable squamous cell cancer of the esophagus. Annals of Oncology. 2011;22(Supplement 5):v19-26.
42. Members of the Gastrointestinal Cancer Disease Site Group. Combined modality radiotherapy and chemotherapy in the non-surgical management of localized carcinoma of the esophagus. In: Wong R, Tey R (reviewers). Toronto (ON): Cancer Care Ontario; 2011 Sep 15 [Endorsed 2010 Sep 29]. Program in Evidence-based Care Evidence-Based Series No.: 2-12 Version 2.

43. Stahl M, Stuschke M, Lehmann N, Meyer HJ, Walz MK, Seeber S, et al. Chemoradiation with and without surgery in patients with locally advanced squamous cell carcinoma of the esophagus. J Clin Oncol. 2005;23:2310-7. Erratum in: J Clin Oncol. 2006;24(3):531.
44. Bedenne L, Michel P, Bouché O, Milan C, Mariette C, Conroy T, et al. Chemoradiation followed by surgery compared with chemoradiation alone in squamous cancer of the esophagus: FFCD 9102. J Clin Oncol. 2007;25:1160-8.
45. Kwee RM. Prediction of tumor response to neoadjuvant therapy in patients with esophageal cancer with use of 18F FDG PET: a systematic review. Radiology. 2010;254:707-17.
46. Feinstein AR, Sosin DM, Wells CK. The Will Rogers phenomenon. Stage migration and new diagnostic techniques as a source of misleading statistics for survival in cancer. N Engl J Med. 1985;312:1604-8.
47. Cunningham D, Starling N, Rao S, Iveson T, Nicolson M, Coxon F, et al. Capecitabine and oxaliplatin for advanced esophagogastric cancer. N Engl J Med. 2008;358:36-46.

CHAPTER 21

Minimal Invasive Esophagectomy

Rajesh Bhojwani, Kapileshwar Vijay

INTRODUCTION

Esophageal carcinoma is a lethal disease, if left untreated. Surgery has remained the mainstay of treatment. Esophagectomy is a highly invasive surgery, and thus is associated with significant morbidity and mortality. Minimal invasive approaches have also been incorporated into esophageal cancer surgery in an attempt to improve postoperative outcomes of esophagectomy. Various modifications of minimal invasive esophagectomy have been developed; however, the safety, efficacy, advantages and disadvantages are still under debate. In general, the surgical community has been hesitant to use minimally invasive techniques as part of cancer treatment, because of concerns that a minimally invasive surgical approach will compromise the oncologic principles of treatment.

Over the last decade, many centers and surgeons have taken up minimal invasive oesophagectomy as the preferred modality for esophageal resection. However, there exist regional differences on local, national and international level that make it difficult to generalize the available data. Recently, there has been evidence for improved short-term outcome and many studies have shown equivalence with open esophagectomy in terms of oncological issues. More studies and prospective data will be required to prove the superiority of minimal invasive oesophagectomy, and standardize various techniques of the procedure.

HISTORY

The first report for minimally invasive application to esophageal resection came from Cuschieri et al. who reported 5 patients that underwent thoracoscopic mobilization of the esophagus in 1992.[1] Mediastinoscopic assisted transhiatal esophagectomy was first reported in 1993 by Bumm R et al. A total laparoscopic approach was then described by DePaula and colleagues in 1995,[2] and then by Swanstrom and Hansen in1997.[3] During the same time, Akaishi and colleagues from Japan described the thoracoscopic en bloc esophagectomy with radical mediastinal lymphadenectomy in 1996.[4]

In 1999, Watson et al. described the total endoscopic Ivor-Lewis esophagectomy.[5] The first report of a combined thoracoscopic and laparoscopic approach was described by Nguyen et al. in the same year.[6] In 2003, the robot assisted thoracolaparoscopic approach was developed at UCMU, Netherlands.[7] However, the first report of robot assisted thoracoscopic esophagectomy came in 2004 from Kernstein and colleagues.[8]

CLASSIFICATION OF MINIMAL INVASIVE ESOPHAGECTOMY

Minimal invasive esophagectomy has been performed with many different approaches toward the three cavities involved namely abdomen, chest and the cervical region. The chest has been approached in many positions by the surgeons. Based on these approaches toward specific cavities involved the MIE can be classified as mentioned below.

Variations of minimally invasive esophagectomy (MIE):[9]

- Total MIE (thoracoscopic and laparoscopic esophagectomy)
- Hybrid MIE (either thoracoscopic or laparoscopic approach)
- Laparoscopic-assisted transhiatal esophagectomy
- Video-assisted mediastinoscopic transhiatal esophagectomy
- Robot assisted MIE.

Based on the position of the patient for thoracoscopic part of the procedure, MIE may be classified as:

- Left lateral decubitus position
- Prone position
- Semiprone position.

Based on the site of gastroesophageal anastomosis after resection, the MIE can be classified into:

- Modified McKeown MIE (anastomosis in the neck)
- Ivor Lewis MIE (intrathoracic anastomosis).

Anesthetic Considerations

An invasive arterial blood pressure monitoring is advisable. Subclavian route is preferred for central venous catheterization, or instead, a brachial line may be used. A jugular central venous access is avoided to minimize interference with the surgical procedure on the neck. A double lumen endotracheal tube would be required when performing the thoracoscopic part in the left lateral decubitus position. However, the esophageal and mediastinal dissection in the prone position can be performed comfortably over a single lumen endotracheal tube.

Appropriate fluid administration is important for optimum outcome as inadequate intravascular volume cause inadequate tissue perfusion and oxygenation which can leads to anastomotic failure and leak. On the other hand, excessive fluid may lead to pulmonary complications. Significant volume loading is required during the laparoscopic phase, secondary to the pneumoperitoneum and steep reverse Trendelenburg position. Hypercarbia and acidosis need to be monitored, given the high flow of CO_2 during the procedure. Vasopressors need to be administered with caution, as they may compromise the viability of the newly created gastric conduit. Hypercarbia may be reversed by deflating the pneumoperitoneum or pneumothorax if created, allowing the patient time to compensate and clear the excess carbon dioxide. The preload may be increased by volume loading, lowering the insufflation pressure and limiting the duration and angle of reverse Trendelenburg position. Prolonged nature of surgery and involvement of three body compartments leads to loss of substantial amount of temperature leading to hypothermia which has been associated with decreased oxygen delivery, increased stress response and myocardial work and postoperative infection. Normothermia should be aggressively maintained with proper patient covering, application of Bair Hugger (body warmer) and warm fluids.

Thoracic Epidural

Thoracic epidural not only decreases postoperative pain and related pulmonary complications but also improves microcirculation of gastric conduit by improving local gastric vasomotor tone. However, aggressive epidural bolus should be avoided to avoid reduction in flow at the end of gastric tube.

SURGICAL TECHNIQUE

Thoracoscopic Esophageal Mobilization and Mediastinal Dissection in the Left Lateral Decubitus Position

These techniques have been described by various authors including Maloney and colleagues[10] and Luketich et al. The thoracoscopic technique as described by Luketich et al.[11] is briefly described here. Their technique involves a total laparoscopic and thoracoscopic approach and currently involves an intrathoracic anastomosis and has been featured as Ivor-Lewis MIE. This has been an improvisation by the authors over their previous experience of modified McKeown MIE wherein a cervical anastomosis was being performed.

Thoracoscopic Phase (As Described by Luketich et al.)[11]

Positioning and Port Placement

The patient is kept in the left lateral decubitus position. A double lumen endotracheal tube is required and the right lung is kept deflated while the surgical procedure goes on. Correct placement of double lumen endotracheal tube is essential. The surgeon operates from the right side of the patient (i.e. near the patient's back) while the assistant stands on the left side. Five thoracoscopic ports are inserted.

A 10 mm camera port is inserted in the eighth or ninth intercostal space (ICS) in the midaxillary line. The surgeon uses two ports, a 10mm port placed in the eighth or ninth ICS in the posterior axillary line for the right hand, and another 5 mm just inferior to the angle of scapula for the left hand. Two ports are inserted for the assistant—a 10 mm port in the anterior axillary line in the fourth ICS to insert the retractor to retract the lungs and another 5 mm in the sixth ICS at the anterior axillary line to utilize the suction.

The diaphragm is retracted down with the help of a retraction stitch taken through the central tendon and brought out through the lateral chest wall at the level of the insertion of the diaphragm through a small stab incision. This retraction helps in exposing the distal thoracic esophagus.

Mobilization of the esophagus begins by dividing the inferior pulmonary ligament. It is then taken up exposing the right pulmonary vein and further up along the pericardium to the level of subcarinal lymph nodes (level-VII nodes are dissected en bloc with the esophagus). The pleura overlying the esophagus is then divided and then, the azygos vein is transected with the help of endo GIA staplers. The vagus nerve is transacted to prevent any traction injuries to the recurrent nerve during the mobilization. Above the azygos, the dissection is performed close to the esophagus. The pleura is then divided along the posterior groove between the aorta and the esophagus. Care is taken to avoid injury to the thoracic duct. Lymphatics and the aortoesophageal vessels are controlled with endoclips or an energy source. The dissection is carried deep and likewise, the esophagus is circumferentially mobilized from the hiatus to the thoracic inlet.

Thoracoscopic Phase in Prone Position

Cuschieri[12] performed the first prone position thoracoscopic esophageal mobilization in 1994. Jarrral et al. published a review of thoracoscopic esophagectomy in prone position and identified 20 articles published in 20 years (1990–2010) on a series of patients operated by this technique.[13]

Author of this chapter has also used the prone position for thoracoscopic esophageal mobilization in 104 cases since 2008 and the technique that is currently being used at Santokba Institute of Digestive Surgical Science (SIDSS) is described here. Several modifications have been done over the learning curve, and the technique has remained standardized in the last 5 years.

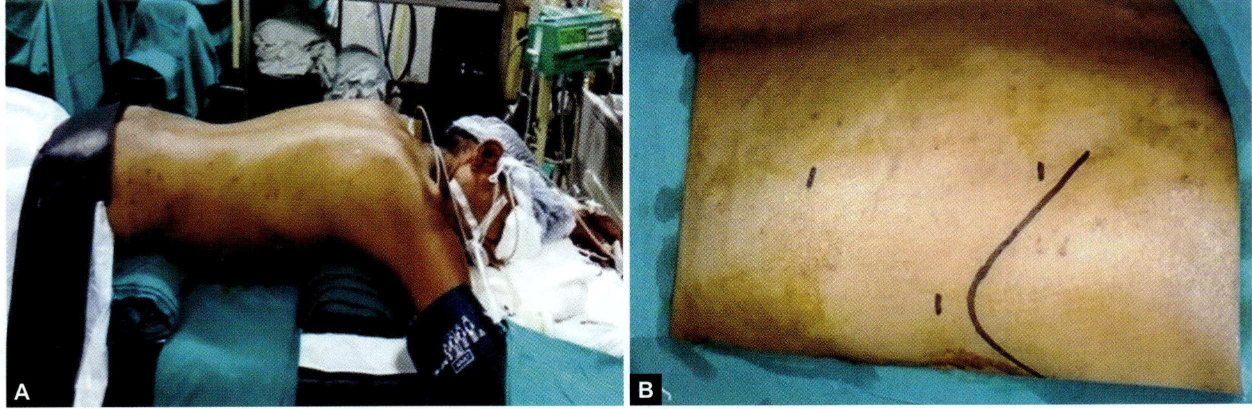

Figures 1A and B (A) Patient position and (B) port placement

After general anesthesia on a trolley adjacent to the operating table the patient is rolled over, on to the operative table and put in a prone position with the right shoulder abducted to 90° and the forearm fixed so as to rotate the scapula. A soft cushion is placed under the chest and the pelvis so as to keep a potential space for the abdomen to expand during inspiration. The monitor is kept to the left side of the patient, while the surgeon and assistant on the right side of the patient (Figs 1A and B).

A three port technique is utilized in most of the cases. The camera is inserted through a 10 mm port which is inserted just inferior to the angle of scapula usually in the sixth or seventh ICS in the midaxillary line. Another 10 mm port is inserted posterior to the posterior axillary line along the border of scapula in the fourth or fifth ICS. A 5 mm port is inserted in the posterior axillary line in the ninth ICS. The three port positions form a triangle and provide good ergonomics for the procedure.

A 30° 10 mm telescope is utilized for the entire dissection. A pneumothorax is created with CO_2 insufflation and the pressure kept at 10 mm Hg. This pressure and the effect of gravity help the right lung stay deflated and out of the field of esophageal and mediastinal dissection.

The procedure is done with the help of a Harmonic Scalpel (Ethicon, Somerville, NJ, USA) for the dissection and Force-Triad (Covidien, Norwalk, CT, USA) for coagulating the aortoesophageal vessels the dissection begins near the lower end by incising the inferior pulmonary ligament deep up to the pericardium and is carried upward over the right pulmonary vein. The incised pleura, fat and the lymph nodal tissue are all taken en bloc with the esophagus. The azygos vein is then divided between clips and sutures. The dissection then goes along the margin of the right bronchus, the carina and then to the left bronchus. At this point the pleura over the posterior groove (aortoesophageal groove) is incised, and with the blunt dissection the aortoesophageal vessels and lymphatics are identified, clipped and divided. At this point the thoracic duct if encountered or any tubular structure running along the aorta is clipped to prevent postoperative chylous leak. An umbilical tape is then passed over the pericardium and the esophagus is then retracted with a loop of umbilical tape around. The traction on this tape allows circumferential dissection as well as the dissection of the left bronchial nodes. The vagus nerve is divided at this point and the supra-azygos dissection is carried out close to the esophageal wall. Extent of dissection ranges from the hiatus inferiorly to the thoracic inlet superiorly, and the paraesophageal, subcarinal, paratracheal, bilateral tracheobronchial and right pulmonary nodes are dissected en bloc with the specimen. The important steps have been depicted underneath with the help of intraoperative photographs and the schematic diagrams depicting the anatomy (Figs 2 to 5).

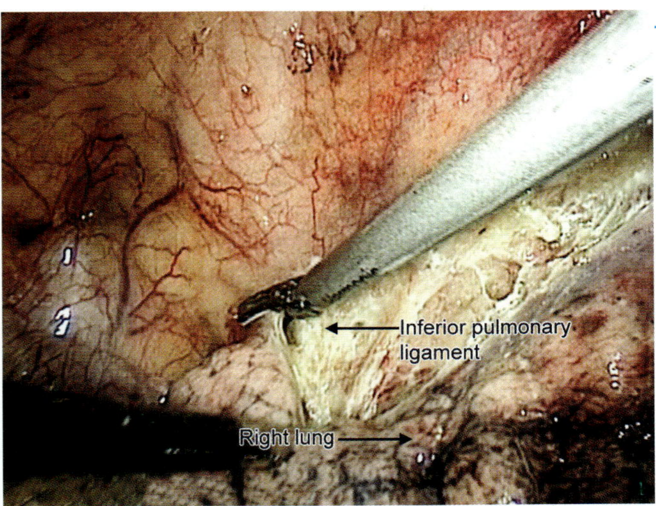

Figure 2 Division of inferior pulmonary ligament

VISUALIZATION OF THE OPERATIVE FIELD DURING THORACOSOPY

Esophageal dissection during thoracoscopy requires optimal visualization of the mediastinal field wherein the right lung has been retracted away. Apart from the prone and the semiprone position as has been described earlier, where the position of the patient itself, partly retracts the lung away from the field, various makeovers have been described. The lung can be retracted with a lung retractor[14] or a retracting suture[4] in the left lateral decubitus position.

In the prone position, the gravity, helps the lung to fall anteriorly and gives good exposure of the mediastinum. This can

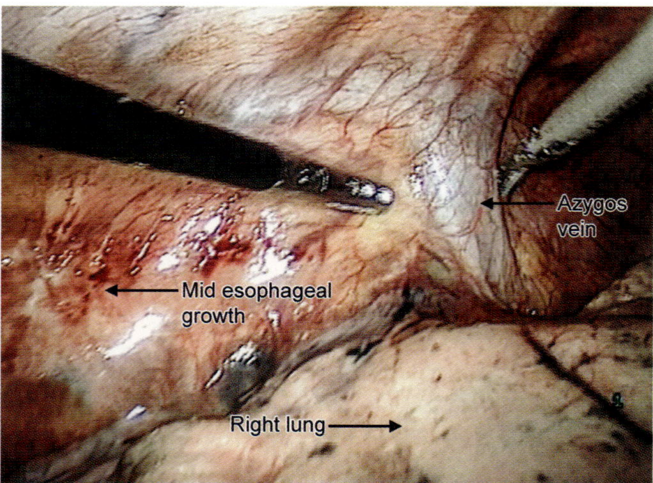

Figure 3 Division of azygos vein

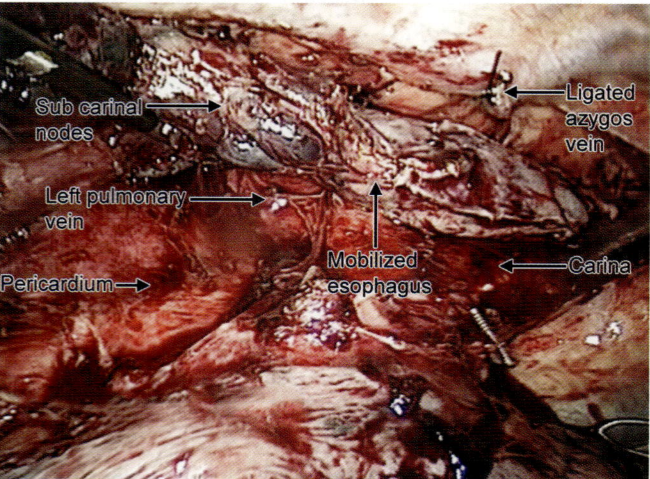

Figure 4 Completed thoracic esophageal mobilization with en bloc lymph nodes

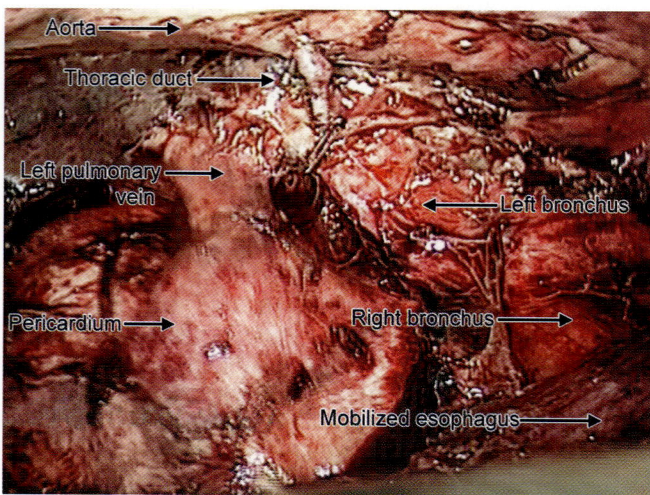

Figure 5 Completed thoracic esophageal mobilization depicting mediastinal anatomy

be further aided by a low pressure carbon dioxide insufflation up to 8–10 mm Hg which maximizes the exposure of the intrathoracic esophagus.[15] A hand assisted technique has been described wherein a small upper abdominal incision has been used to insert the hand through the anterior phrenomediastinal route into the right thoracic cavity.[16]

TECHNICAL ADVANTAGES OF THE PRONE POSITION TECHNIQUE

The prone position technique appears to be associated with a less steep learning curve.[13] Lungs do not obscure the field because they fall away with the gravity and also with the pneumothorax. The blood also gets pooled in the dependent portion, and does not obscure the esophagus and mediastinum which always remain visible. This is further aided by a 30° telescope which can be rotated at different angles to visualize the crevices and the depth of dissection. The surgeon operates in a plane parallel to the camera, much similar to conventional laparoscopy that makes it easier for a surgeon who is used to laparoscopic procedures.[13] It is advisable to keep the height of the table at the elbow position, so as to facilitate the movements at the elbow of the surgeon, parallel to the field of operation, making the operation easier. The esophagus with its long axis adherent to the aorta and a self-retracted state makes it easier to make an incision on the pleura over the esophagopulmonary groove and complete the nodal dissection of the aortopulmonary window and the carinal area en bloc with the esophagus. This dissection does not require any retraction but just a gentle push by the left hand of the surgeon himself. An assistant surgeon is not required in most of the cases. The prone position also allows good dissection around the left recurrent laryngeal nerve nodes which may have a proposed oncological significance.[17] The prone position also provides a good view of the carina and the left bronchus and may help in reducing the incidence of tracheobronchial compilations.[18] Diaphragmatic retraction is not required since the hiatus is adequately visible in all the cases in the prone position.

BENEFITS AND LIMITATIONS OF PRONE ESOPHAGEAL SURGERY[13]

Potential Advantages

- Shortened learning curve
- Ergonomic position of hands
- Fewer thoracoscopic ports required
- Only one assistant required for the camera
- Theoretically improved oxygenation in prone position
- One lung ventilation not necessarily required
- Lungs and blood do not obscure operative field due to the effects of gravity.

Potential Disadvantages

- Longer setup time to position
- Unfamiliar anatomical orientation to surgeons

- Difficult airway management if the endotracheal tube gets displaced
- Emergency conversion to open procedure difficult in prone position
- Limited clinical data.

Minimally Invasive Esophagectomy in Semiprone Position

Thoracoscopic mobilization usually has been performed in left lateral decubitus or in prone position. All comparative studies are retrospective analysis and have failed to prove significant difference in clinical outcome.[15,17,19] Prone position has been shown to be associated with better surgical exposure and ergonomics which minimize operative time and surgical fatigue. However, in case of conversion, especially in case of bleeding, changing posture is troublesome. To overcome this problem and to retain the advantage of prone position, semiprone position has been described for MIE.

After double lumen endotracheal intubation, the patient at the outset is placed in the LLP and inclined forward 45°, with the arm placed on an arm rest. Four thoracoscopic ports are used: camera port (Port I) in the seventh ICS in posterior axillary line, and the remaining three ports are placed at the fourth ICS (Port II) in the mid-axillary line, and the seventh (Port III) and ninth ICS (Port IV) inferior to the scapular tip.[20]

In the semiprone approach, the surgeon and the camera are aligned in the same plane and the esophageal mobilization is done with a "rolling type" of motion.

Both the lateral decubitus position and semiprone position have benefits and limitations. Semiprone position gives better exposure of the posterior mediastinum, subcarinal and paratracheal spaces as lung retraction is partly aided by gravity. Cephalad and caudal extremes of the esophagus are approached better. This position minimizes fatigue and maximizes ergonomic function at the level of the wrist. Compared with the full-prone position, the port incisions are sited more anterior and thus safer positions. Subsequent chest tube placement is also better in semiprone position.[21]

ROLE OF AZYGUS VEIN PRESERVATION

Traditionally, an en bloc esophagectomy involved resection of azygos vein from diaphragm to its insertion at superior vena cava along with ligation of multiple intercostal veins. Purported advantage was of proper lymphadenectomy. Disadvantage of the azygos vein resection with intercostal branches is the difficult, time consuming and may cause ischemic spinal cord injury with severe neurologic deficits.[22] In addition, severe bleeding from hemiazygos and intercostal veins is also possible. En bloc esophagectomy has therefore been modified and the azygos vein is divided just over the esophagus. However, the azygos vein may become a restrictive band, reducing blood flow to the tip of the conduit, causing venous congestion, or potentially narrowing the conduit.[23] Extent of mediastinal lymph node dissection is not substantially affected by preserving the azygos vein.[24] Many practitioners are preserving the azygos vein with the notion that it helps to maintain the orientation of the conduit in the mediastinum without any adverse effect on extent of lymphadenectomy or conduit necrosis. Although no definite evidence is available, presently azygos preserving MIE is considered safe and feasible.

LAPAROSCOPIC PHASE (TECHNIQUE AS FOLLOWED AT SIDSS)

Position

The patient is placed in the supine position with legs apart, with arms abducted out and a foot support in place. The surgeon operates from between the legs and the monitor is placed on the head end of the patient. The camera assistant is on the right side of the patient while the surgical assistant stands on the left.

Five abdominal ports are utilized for the gastric mobilization, conduit creation, pyloroplasty and feeding jejunostomy (Figs. 6 to 9). When bulky tumors are involved in non-obese patients, a 5 cm epigastric vertical incision is used to deliver the specimen out and fashion a gastric conduit. The feeding jejunostomy and pyloroplasty are also performed through the same incision.

The abdomen is mapped and the camera port is created in the midline approximately 18–20 cm below the xiphisternum. Nathanson's liver retractor is used to retract the left lobe of liver and it is inserted through a small hole (approximately 4 mm) just

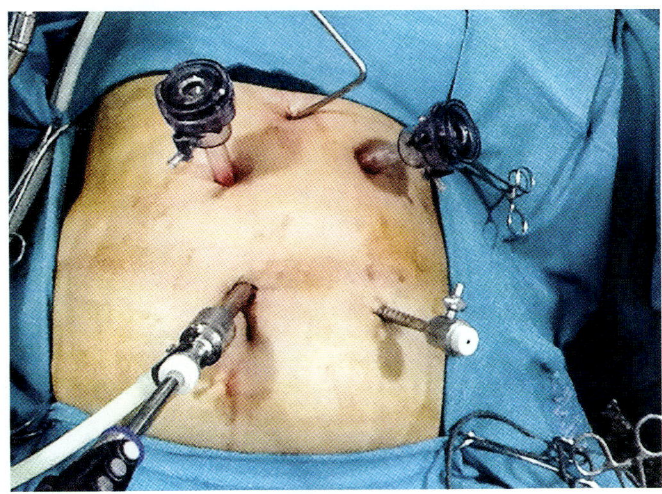

Figure 6 Port position

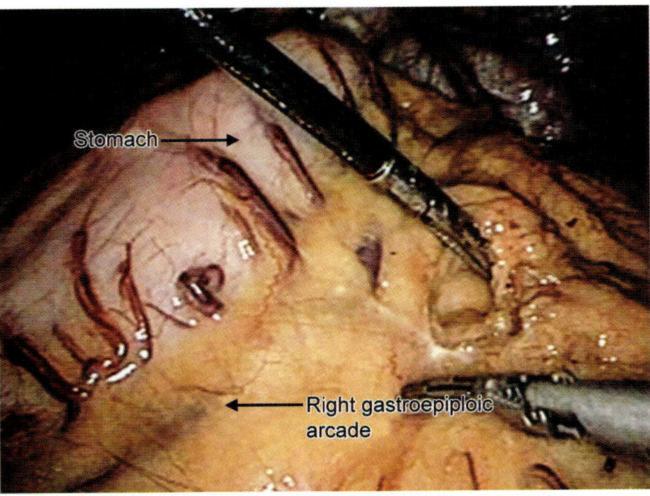

Figure 7 Gastric mobilization with preservation of right gastroepiploic arcade

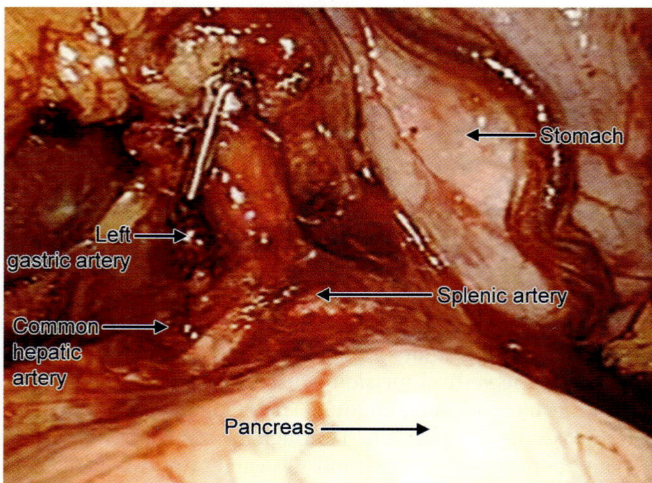

Figure 8 Left gastric lymphadenectomy

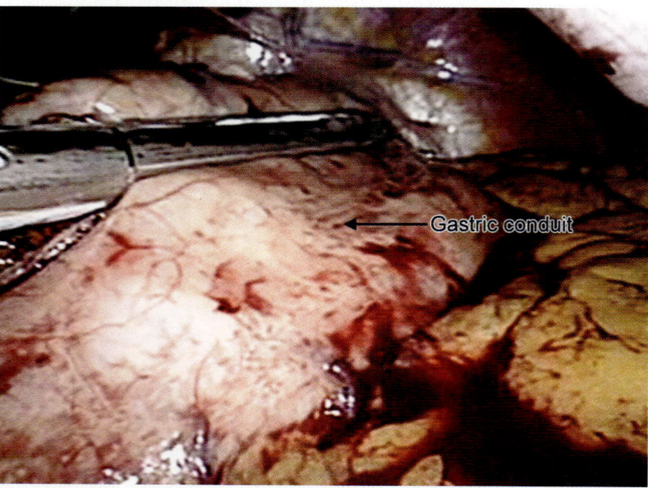

Figure 9 Gastric conduit fashioning

below the xiphisternum in the midline. A 5 mm working port is used parallel to the camera port in the left mid clavicular line. A 10 mm assisting port is created in the mid clavicular line in the left subcostal region 1 cm below the costal line. Another working port (12 mm) is created in the right mid clavicular line at a level midway between the xiphisternum and the camera port. The camera port is inserted by an open method and all other ports are created under direct vision.

The abdomen is inspected over both the lobes of liver, peritoneum and the omentum to rule out a metastatic disease. The gastrocolic omentum is opened away from the right gastroepiploic arcade. The arcade is identified clearly and protected throughout the procedure. The short gastric vessels are divided with ultrasonic shears (Harmonic scalpel; Ethicon, Somerville, NJ, USA). The greater curve is mobilized from the level of the pylorus up to the left crus.

The stomach is then flipped over to the right of the patient and all the retrogastric attachments are dissected off. The left gastric pedicle is then dissected, and the left gastric vein and the artery serially clipped at the base, and all the nodal and adjacent tissue is swept up with the specimen. The dissection is then carried forward cranially along the crura up till the hiatus. The anterior peritoneum over the esophagus is divided, and the dissection is carried out circumferentially all around through the hiatus till it becomes contiguous with the thoracic dissection and the entire esophagus is found free from all attachments. The dissection then concentrates on mobilizing the antropyloric part, dividing all the posterior gastric taking care of the right gastroepiploic arcade. Partial or complete kocherization of the duodenum may be required to ensure that the pylorus reaches the hiatus. The state is now ready for fashioning the gastric conduit. The stapler is then introduced through the right mid clavicular port. The first stapler fire is done with the vascular load to divide the lesser omentum above the level of right gastric artery. Subsequently, purple loads on stapler (Endo GIA Reloads with Tristaple technology, Covidien) are used to create a 4–5 cm, wide gastric conduit parallel to the greater curve. Three to four fires may be required. The last portion of 2–4 cm of attached fundus to the esophagus is not stapled divided to enable pulling the specimen and the conduit up the chest and the final division is done in the neck to resect the specimen out.

At this point, before pulling the specimen up through the chest, a pyloroplasty is performed with 4-0 PDS interrupted suture. A feeding jejunostomy is also performed at this point. The esophagus and the conduit are then pulled up in the neck, the specimen resected off and a gastroesophageal anastomosis performed.

In patients with bulky esophageal tumors which cannot be delivered through the neck, a small (5 cm) incision is created in the epigastrium as mentioned earlier. The esophagus is divided in the neck and the specimen with the tumor is delivered out through the incision under the wound cover. The gastric conduit is then fashioned outside with the help of a linear stapler. Specimen is resected and the gastric conduit pulled up through the posterior mediastinum over a tube inserted from the neck and a gastroesophageal anastomosis is performed.

Ivor Lewis Minimally Invasive Esophagectomy

The approach for MIE depends on the preference of the surgeon; however, fear of recurrent laryngeal nerve injury, vocal cord paralysis, conduit necrosis and anastomotic leak have led to popularization of minimally invasive Ivor Lewis technique especially in the western hemisphere where GE junction adenocarcinoma, premalignant Barrett esophagus are more common than esophageal squamous cell carcinoma. For laparoscopic portion of the MIE, the patient is positioned supine in steep reverse-Trendelenburg with a footboard in place. The surgeon stands on the patient's right, and the assistant stands on the patient's left. For the thoracoscopic portion of the procedure, the patient is repositioned to the left lateral decubitus position. The surgeon remains to the right of the patient, and the first assistant remains to the left of the patient and the esophagogastric anastomosis is done with circular stapler. Most dreaded complication of Ivor Lewis is anastomotic leak which can cause severe mediastinitis and is associated with high mortality.

Results

Kunisaki[25] and colleagues reported the first series of Ivor Lewis MIE in 2004. There was no operative mortality in this 15-patient series, but the rate of anastomotic leak was high (13%), and the average hospital stay was lengthy (30 days). In 2008, Nguyen[26] and colleagues reported an updated series of 104 MIEs; 51 were performed using an Ivor Lewis approach. Anastomotic leak occurred in 10% of the patients who underwent Ivor Lewis MIE, and major postoperative complications occurred in 12%. The average hospital stay was 10 days, with an average of 3 days in the ICU. Recently, Luketich[27] et al. have published a retrospective analysis of over 1,000 patients with MIE. The MIE-neck was performed in 481 (48%) and MIE-Ivor Lewis in 530 (52%). Patients undergoing MIE-Ivor Lewis were operated in the current era. The median number of lymph nodes resected was 21. The operative mortality was 1.68%. Median length of stay (8 days) and ICU stay (2 days) were similar between the two approaches. Mortality rate was 0.9%, and recurrent nerve injury was less frequent in the Ivor Lewis MIE group ($p < 0.001$).

ROBOT-ASSISTED MINIMALLY INVASIVE ESOPHAGECTOMY

Robot-assisted minimally invasive esophagectomy is a technological advancement over current thoracoscopic and laparoscopic techniques. Robotic surgery offers high-definition with increased magnification and three-dimensional vision. The use of its surgical wrists, motion scaling, and tremor filtration, allows the surgeon to perform precise esophageal en bloc surgery.

Robotic MIE was first reported in 2002 by Melvin which was a brief report without technical details.[28] In 2003, Kernstine K reported first oncological robotic MIE. Kim et al.[29] published a series of 21 patients who underwent a three stage esophagectomy. It was shown that the docking time of robot reduces significantly with learning curve. None of the patients developed pneumonia, respiratory failure or 90 days mortality. These were done by single surgeon with no previous experience of MIE. It is possible that robotic prone esophagectomy may shorten the learning curve.

Since then many authors have reported their experience with robotic MIE but all are retrospective analysis and the perioperative parameters and postoperative outcome like intraoperative blood loss, duration, postoperative complication are not different from MIE. Although robotic MIE has several advantages, there are many disadvantages like getting accustomed to the space and setup requirements. The fixed cost of the system and the maintenance costs are also a huge concern.

OUTCOME OF MINIMALLY INVASIVE ESOPHAGECTOMY

Adaptation of MIE has been slow and has not surpassed open esophagectomy as the operation of choice, possibly due to the complexity of anatomy, technical difficulties and a very steep learning curve. Very few centers have mastered the technique and reported the results.

Learning Curve

Esophagectomy in considered as one of the most challenging procedure to perform minimally invasively. Extensive mediastinal nodal dissection requires even more experience. The normal learning curve in thoracoscopic esophagectomy has been shown to be in excess of 30 cases to achieve a standardized techniques and plateau.

Osugi et al.[30] reported that basic skills could be learned during the first 17 cases. Ninomiya et al.[31] thought that this could be reduced to only 10 cases when performed under the direction of an experienced surgeon and with a regular surgical team. A fully trained surgeon can thus facilitate a new surgeon to safely perform minimally invasive esophagectomy during the induction period. The primary education of the regular surgical team by post-accreditation supervision is essential for safe and rapid start to minimally invasive esophagectomy.

SURGICAL OUTCOME

Minimally invasive esophagectomy has shown several advantages over open esophagectomy including better cosmesis, less tissue trauma, lesser pain, reduced postoperative inflammatory response and lesser morbidity. The results of MIE have been compared to open esophagectomy in multiple series in the literature. In a meta-analysis[32] of 672 patients, including open esophagectomy, MIE and hybrid MIE, it was found that patients with MIE had better operative and postoperative outcome in terms of less blood loss, shorter ICU stay and hospital stay and significant reduction in respiratory complications. However, there was no significant difference in anastomotic leak rates, stricture rates, incidence of conduit ischemia, chyle leak, vocal cord palsy or 30 days mortality. Moreover in subgroup analysis it was found that patients who underwent hybrid MIE had better outcome as compared to open esophagectomy. A multicenter, open label randomized controlled trial (TIME)[33] has shown better short come outcomes with MIE in terms of hospital stay (11 days in MIE vs 14 days in open), incidence of pulmonary infection at 2 weeks (9% vs 29%) and pulmonary infection during hospital stay, pain scores and intraoperative blood loss. Duration of hospitalization and quality of life 6 weeks after surgery was significantly better in MIE group.[33] TIME trial and a report by Schoppmann et al.[34] showed a significantly less incidence of recurrent laryngeal nerve palsy in MIE. It was hypothesized that the pneumatic dissection by CO_2 from thoracic cavity to the neck can open the planes and simplify neck dissection. In a sub-group analysis of the same RCT based on the immunological markers, it was shown that level of leukocyte count, IL-8 and prolactin levels (inflammatory markers) after 168 hours of surgery were significantly less in MIE group.[35] Another study by Parameswaran et al.[36] showed better physical recovery in the first 6 months in MIE group with low level of fatigue and higher activity patterns (Table 1).

ONCOLOGICAL OUTCOME

Since the adaptation of MIE, the adequacy of oncological resection in terms of long-term survival, adequacy of margins and lymph node yield compared to that of open esophagectomy has been questioned. A first determinant of oncologic safety is the proportion of microscopically radical (R0) resections. Remarkably, comparisons of R0 resection rates between open and minimally invasive esophagectomy have rarely been reported. In three recent comparative studies R0 resection rates were reported. In the TIME trial a non-significant difference of 8% (92% vs 84%) in favor of minimally invasive esophagectomy was observed.[33] A similar non-significant difference was shown by Sihag et al.[37]

Table 1: Comparison of complications and mortality between minimally invasive and open esophagectomy

Parameters	*Schoppmann et al.*			*TIME trial*			*Parameswaran et al.*		
	Open (30)	*MIE (50)*	*P value*	*Open (56)*	*MIE 59)*	*P value*	*Open (30)*	*MIE (50)*	*P value*
Blood loss	4 (12.9%)	13 (41.9%)	0.011	475 (50–3000)	200 (20–1200)	< 0.001	9 (30%)	7 (14%)	0.09
Hospital stay	15 (8.46)	29 (6–79)	0.001	14 (1–120)	11 (7–80)	0.044	10 (6–56)	12 (8–86)	0.01
ICU stay	3 (0–45)	10 (1–40)	0.001	1 (0–106)	1 (0–50)	0.706	5 (2–16)	11 (2–38)	0.27
Operative time	411 (270–600)	400 240–550)	NS	299 (66–570)	329 (90–559)	0.002	266 (209–390)	442 (305–580)	< 0.01
Respiratory complication	3 (9.7%)	12 (38.7%)	0.008	19 (34%)	7 (12%)	0.005	7 (23%)	4 (8%)	0.05
Anastomotic leak rate	1 (3.2%)	2 (6.4%)	0.24	4 (70%)	7 (12%)	0.390	1 (3%)	4 (8%)	0.52
Vocal cord palsy	4 (12.9%)	12 (38.7%)	0.005				0	6 (12%)	0.07
30 days mortality	0	0	0	0 (0%)	1 (2%)	0.590	1 (3%)	1 (2%)	NS

Table 2: Comparison of minimally invasive and open esophagectomy for R0 resection and lymph node harvest

Parameter	*Time Trial*			*Sihag et al.*			*Sundarm et al.*			*Dantoc et al.*		
	Open (56)	*MIE (59)*	*P value*	*Open (76)*	*MIE (38)*	*P value*	*Open (26)*	*MIE (47)*	*P value*	*Open (718)*	*MIE (494)*	*P value*
R0 resection rate	47 (84%)	54 (92%)	0.080	71 (93.4%)	38 (100%)	0.163	24 (92.3%)	45 (93.61%)	0.318	–	–	–
Total number of nodes (median)	21 (7–47)	20 (3–44)	0.852	21 (16–27)	19 (15–28)	0.740	19 (17.75–24.75)	20 (14–27)	NS	10 (3–32.8)	16 (5.7–33.9)	0.04

(100% vs 93.4%) and to a lesser extent by Sundaram et al.[38] (93.6% vs 92.3%). Contrary to R0 resection rates, the total number of retrieved lymph nodes is a very commonly reported outcome measure. One of the three meta-analyses on this topic resulted in a significant difference in median number of nodes,16 versus 10, in favor of minimally invasive esophagectomy. In the same review the described increase in lymph node retrieval did not seem to translate to a survival benefit as no significant differences were found in 1-, 2-, 3- and 5-year survival.[39] Another multicenter trial ECOG 2202 showed similar lymph node yield in both the groups.[40] Smithers et al.[41] reported 5-year stage-specific survival rates after MIE as follows: 85% in stage I, 33% in stage IIA, 37% in stage IIB and 16% in stage III (TNM classification, 6th edition). Osugi et al.[42] compared long-term survival of patients undergoing VATS esophagectomy with those undergoing OE as historical controls, as stratified by the oncological background. There were no marked differences in 3- and 5-year survival between the two groups Other studies also showed statistical equivalency in long-term survival between MIE and OE (Table 2).[43]

A meta-analysis by Sgourakis et al.[44] showed that there were no significant differences in survival within each time interval (30 days, 1, 2, 3 and 5 years), although the difference favored the MIE. However, the oncological benefits to patients undergoing MIE have not been scientifically proven because there have been no RCTs comparing long-term survival of patients undergoing MIE with patients undergoing OE.

QUALITY OF LIFE

Although oncological superiority of MIE has not yet been proven, MIE shows significant improvement in quality of life when compared with open esophagectomy. A multicenter RCT (TIME trail) has shown MIE has been associated with significant improvement of quality of life as measured by the short form -36 and the European Organization for Research and Treatment of Cancer (EORTC).[33]

AUTHOR'S EXPERIENCE

The first thoracolaparoscopic esophageal resection was performed at Santokba Institute of Digestive Surgical Sciences (SIDSS) in March 2005. A total of 114 minimal invasive esophageal resections have been attempted since. The learning curve has been steep, and the procedure has been standardized to its current form for the last 5 years. There have been ten cases where the procedure was abandoned for various reasons like detection of unresectability or metastases on the operation table. There were six conversions of thoracoscopy to thoracotomy, two for complications of bleeding not controlled with laparoscopy, and four for non-progression of dissection.

Another 3 patients were converted from thoracoscopic to open transhiatal esophageal resection for inability to sustain adequate oxygenation in prone position with pneumothorax.

A total of 104 MIEs have been performed till August 2013. First two procedures were performed in left lateral decubitus position, out of which one was converted to open thoracotomy, due to inability to retract the lung adequately, and the resultant suboptimal exposure of tissues. The remaining cases have been performed in the prone position.

There were 58 squamous cell carcinomas and 41 adenocarcinomas, 3 leiomyomas of the middle third, 1 GIST of middle third and 1 benign stricture not amenable to dilatation and 1 malignant stricture of middle third form a breast primary 17 years after breast resection. Nineteen tumors were classified as GE junction tumors, 27 were lower third lesions and the rest were middle third lesions. Only 9 patients were classified as non-bulky lesions, and in these cases, specimen was withdrawn from the neck, and a total thoracolaparoscopic esophageal resection was performed. The other lesions were deemed bulky, and in all of these cases, either a hybrid MIE was performed with a laparotomy or a small 5 cm incision in the epigastrium was used to extract the specimen out, and fashion the gastric conduit.

A neck anastomosis was performed in all cases, and there have been no intrathoracic anastomosis, in cases operated upon with a minimal invasive intent. However, there have been 11 other cases during the same time interval, which have undergone an open esophageal resection, with a primarily open approach, and an intrathoracic anastomosis has been performed in three of these patients.

A hybrid approach with a laparotomy has been performed in 27 cases, primarily because of cost constraints in these patients, and 9 of them with other indications like previous abdominal operations, adhesions, etc. Major morbidity was seen in 9/104 (9.3%) patients and the mortality was 5/104 (5.2%). However, a significant improvement in results was observed in the last 73 cases over the last 3 years with major morbidity of 6/73 (4.3%) and mortality of 2/73 (1.4%).

The major intraoperative complications encountered during the learning curve included a port insertion induced diaphragmatic and liver injury, and this patient required a conversion. Another patient developed a dissection induced small 3 mm rent in the membranous part of carina. This was repaired thoracoscopically with interrupted vicryl, and the patient made an uneventful recovery. One patient had bleed from the aortoesophageal perforator which required a thoracotomy and bleeder control. Another patient had major bleed from the bronchial artery while the conduit was being pulled up, and required and required a thoracotomy for control.

REFERENCES

1. Cuschieri A, Shimi S, Banting S. Endoscopic oesophagectomy through a right thoracoscopic approach. J R Coll Surg Edinb. 1992;37:7-11.
2. Depaula AL, Hashiba K, Ferreira EA, de Paula RA, Grecco E. Laparoscopic transhiatal esophagectomy with esophagogastroplasty. Surg Laparosc Endosc. 1995;5:1-5.
3. Swanstrom LL, Hansen P. Laparoscopic total esophagectomy. Arch Surg. 1997;132:943-7.
4. Akaishi T, Kaneda I, Higuchi N, Kuriya Y, Kuramoto J, Toyoda T, et al. Thoracoscopic en bloc esophagectomy with radial mediastinal lymphadenectomy. J Thorac Cardiovasc Surg. 1996;112:1533-40.
5. Watson DI, Davies N, Jamieson GG. Totally endoscopic Ivor Lewis esophagectomy. Surg Endosc. 1999;13;293-7.
6. Nguyen NT, Schauer PR, Luketich JD. Combined laparoscopic and thoracoscopic approach to esophagectomy. J Am Coll Surg. 1999;188:328-32.
7. Van Hillegersberg R, Boone J, Draaisma WA, Broeders IA, Giezeman MU, Borel Rinkes IH. First experience with robot-assisted thoracoscopic esophagolymphadenectomy for esophageal cancer. Surg Endosc. 2006;20:1435-9.
8. Kernstein KH, DeArmond DT, Karimi M, Van Natta TL, Campos JC, Yoder MR, et al. The robotic, 2-stage, 3 field esophago-lymphadenectomy. J Thorac Cardiovas Surg. 2004;127:1847-9.
9. Watanabe M, Baba Y, Nagai Y, Baba H. Minimally invasive esophagectomy for esophageal cancer: an updated review. Surg Today. 2013;43(3):237-44.
10. Maloney JD, Weigel TL. Minimally invasive esophagectomy for malignant and premalignant diseases of the esophagus. Surg Clin North Am. 2008;88(5):979-90.
11. Levy RM, Trivedi D, Luketich JD. Minimally invasive esophagectomy. Surg Clin North Am. 2012;92(5):1265-85.
12. Cuschieri A. Thoracoscopic subtotal oesophagectomy. Endosc Surg Allied Technol. 1994;2:21-5.
13. Jarral OA, Purkayastha S, Athanasiou T, Darzi A, Hanna GB, Zacharakis E. Thoracoscopic esophagectomy in the prone position. Surg Endosc. 2012;26(8):2095-103.
14. Osugi H, Takemura M, Higashino M, Takada N, Lee S, Ueno M, et al. Video-assisted thoracoscopic esophagectomy and radical lymph node dissection for esophageal cancer. A series of 75 cases. Surg Endosc. 2002;16:1588-93.
15. Fabian T, Martin J, Katigbak M, McKelvey AA, Federico JA. Thoracoscopic esophageal mobilization during minimally invasive esophagectomy: a head-to-head comparison of prone versus decubitus positions. Surg Endosc. 2008;22:2485-91.
16. Kawano T, Iwai T. Hand-assisted thoracoscopic esophagectomy using a new supportive approach. Surg Endosc. 2001;15:330.
17. Noshiro H, Iwasaki H, Kobayashi K, Uchiyama A, Miyasaka Y, Masatsugu T, et al. Lymphadenectomy along the left recurrent laryngeal nerve by a minimally invasive esophagectomy in the prone position for thoracic esophageal cancer. Surg Endosc. 2010;24:2965-73.
18. Dexter SP, Martin IG, McMahon MJ. Radical thoracoscopic esophagectomy for cancer. Surg Endosc. 1996;10:147-51.
19. Kuwabara S, Katayanagi N. Comparison of three different operative methods of video-assisted thoracoscopic esophagectomy. Esophagus. 2010;7:23-9.
20. Lin J, Kang M, Chen C, Lin R. Thoracoscopic oesophageal mobilization during thoracolaparoscopy three-stage oesophagectomy: a comparison of lateral decubitus versus semiprone positions. Interact Cardiovasc Thorac Surg. 2013;17(5):829-34.
21. Agasthian T. Revisiting the prone position in video-assisted thoracoscopic surgery. Asian Cardiovasc Thorac Ann. 2010;18: 364-7.
22. Zantl N, Stein HJ, Brücher BL, Bartels H, Siewert JR. Ischemic spinal cord syndrome after transthoracic esophagectomy: two cases of a rare neurologic complication. Dis Esophagus. 2000;13:328-32.
23. Lin FCF, Russel H, Ferguson MK. Strangulation of reconstructive gastric tube by the azygos vein. Ann Thorac Surg. 2006;82:8-10.
24. Boone J, Schipper ME, Bleys RL, Borel Rinkes IH, van Hillegersberg R. The effect of azygos vein preservation on mediastinal lymph

node harvesting in thoracic esophagolymphadenectomy. Dis Esophagus. 2008;21(3):226-9.
25. Kunisaki C, Hatori S, Imada T, Akiyama H, Ono H, Otsuka Y, et al. Video-assisted thoracoscopic esophagectomy with a voice-controlled robot: the AESOP system. Surg Laparosc Endosc Percutan Tech. 2004;14(6):323-7.
26. Nguyen NT, Hinojosa MW, Smith BR, Chang KJ, Gray J, Hoyt D. Minimally invasive esophagectomy: lessons learned from 104 operations. Ann Surg. 2008;248(6):1081-91.
27. Luketich JD, Pennathur A, Awais O, Levy RM, Keeley S, Shende M, et al. Outcomes after minimally invasive esophagectomy: review of over 1000 patients. Ann Surg. 2012;256(1):95-103.
28. Melvin WS, Needleman BJ, Krause KR, Schneider C, Wolf RK, Michler RE, et al. Computer enhanced robotic telesurgery. Initial experience in foregut surgery. Surg Endosc. 2002;16:1790-2.
29. Kim DJ, Hyung WJ, Lee CY, Lee JG, Haam SJ, Park IK, et al. Thoracoscopic esophagectomy for esophageal cancer: feasibility and safety of robotic assistance in the prone position. J Thorac Cardiovasc Surg. 2010;139:53-9.
30. Osugi H, Takemura M, Higashino M, Takada N, Lee S, Ueno M, et al. Learning curve of video-assisted thoracoscopic esophagectomy and extensive lymphadenectomy for squamous cell cancer of the thoracic esophagus and results. Surg Endosc. 2003;17:515-9.
31. Ninomiya I, Osugi H, Fujimura T, Kayahara M, Takamura H, Takemura M, et al. Results of video-assisted thoracoscopic surgery for esophageal cancer during the induction period. Gen Thorac Cardiovasc Surg. 2008;56:119-25.
32. Nagpal K, Ahmed K, Vats A, Yakoub D, James D, Ashrafian H, et al. Is minimally invasive surgery beneficial in the management of esophageal cancer? A meta-analysis. Surg Endosc. 2010;24:1621-9.
33. Biere SS, van Berge Henegouwen MI, Maas KW, Bonavina L, Rosman C, Garcia JR, et al. Minimally invasive versus open oesophagectomy for patients with oesophageal cancer: a multicentre, open-label, randomised controlled trial. Lancet. 2012;379(9829):1887-92.
34. Schoppmann SF, Prager G, Langer FB, Riegler FM, Kabon B, Fleischmann E, et al. Open versus minimally invasive esophagectomy: a single-center case controlled study. Surg Endosc. 2010;24(12):3044-53.
35. Maas KW, Biere SS, van Hoogstraten IM, van der Peet DL, Cuesta MA. Immunological changes after minimally invasive or conventional esophageal resection for cancer: a randomized trial. World J Surg. 2013;38:131-7.
36. Parameswaran R, Titcomb DR, Blencowe NS, Berrisford RG, Wajed SA, Streets CG, et al. Assessment and comparison of recovery after open and minimally invasive esophagectomy for cancer: an exploratory study in two centers. Ann Surg Oncol. 2013;20(6):1970-7.
37. Sihag S, Wright CD, Wain JC, Gaissert HA, Lanuti M, Allan JS, et al. Comparison of perioperative outcomes following open versus minimally invasive Ivor Lewis oesophagectomy at a single, high-volume centre. Eur J Cardiothorac Surg. 2012;42(3):430-7.
38. Sundaram A, Geronimo JC, Willer BL, Hoshino M, Torgersen Z, Juhasz A, et al. Survival and quality of life after minimally invasive esophagectomy: a single-surgeon experience. Surg Endosc 2012;26(1):168-76.
39. Dantoc M, Cox MR, Eslick GD. Evidence to support the use of minimally invasive esophagectomy for esophageal cancer: a meta-analysis. Arch Surg. 2012;147:768-76.
40. Luketich JD, Pennathur A, Catalano PJ, et al. Results of a phase II multicenter study of MIE (Eastern Cooperative Oncology Group Study E2202). J Clin Oncol. 2009;27:15S.
41. Smithers BM, Gotley DC, Martin I, Thomas JM. Comparison of the outcomes between open and minimally invasive esophagectomy. Ann Surg. 2007;245:232-40.
42. Osugi H, Takemura M, Higashino M, Takada N, Lee S, Kinoshita H. A comparison of video-assisted thoracoscopic oesophagectomy and radical lymph node dissection for squamous cell cancer of the oesophagus with open operation. Br J Surg. 2003;90:108-13.
43. Takeuchi H, Kawakubo H, Kitagawa Y. Current status of minimally invasive esophagectomy for patients with esophageal cancer. Gen Thorac Cardiovasc Surg. 2013;61(9):513-21.
44. Sgourakis G, Gockel I, Radtke A, Musholt TJ, Timm S, Rink A, et al. Minimally invasive versus open esophagectomy: metaanalysis of outcomes. Dig Dis Sci. 2010;55:3031-40.

CHAPTER 22

Esophageal Replacement Procedures

Sundeep Jain, Neeraj Bhateja

INTRODUCTION AND HISTORY

Esophageal resection and its replacement has always been a challenge for surgeons. There are few peculiarities with its replacement like long length and thoracic location, which has made it technically difficult. Broadly it is done for malignant lesions and corrosive injury to the esophagus. Historically the operations for esophageal replacements were done extrapleurally as there were problems due to wound infections, esophageal anastomotic leaks, severe cardiorespiratory instability and high risk of operative mortality. Subsequent successes in this field were only possible due to the development of anesthesia techniques like ways of tracheal intubation and positive pressure ventilation.

Skin flaps were initially tried for esophageal replacement[1-4] followed by use of stomach,[5,6] jejunum[7] and colon[8] in that order. Torek[9] in 1913, after successful esophagectomy, placed an external tube between cervical esophagus and stomach. That patient survived for 11 years. Skin flaps continued to be used as the main means of reconstruction though those were possible only in staged operation.[10,11] They were marked by need of staged procedures, high fistula rates and overall poor results. Thus these are largely obsolete.

Stomach: Kirschner[6] first successfully used stomach as esophageal replacement. The safety of cervical esophagogastrostomy was shortly established[12] and now this is the standard organ especially for patients of esophageal cancers.[13]

Jejunum: First successful intrathoracic esophagojejunostomy was done by Reinhoff in 1942.[14] This was later advanced to free pedicled grafts.[15]

Colon: It was the last organ used successfully for esophageal replacement and this was started in 1950s. Orsoni and Lemaire described the routine use of transverse and descending colon for reconstruction along with its placement through posterior mediastinum and retrosternal routes.[16] Goligher & Robin concluded that the left colon was best suited for reconstruction of pharynx and esophagus.[17] Finally Belsey proposed that left colon is best choice for its smaller diameter and more reliable blood supply.[18]

PLANNING OF ESOPHAGEAL REPLACEMENT

Esophageal replacement can be planned in either single stage with resection or in two staged procedure after resection in first stage. In case of staged operation things which need to be thought of are: choice of access incisions, length of esophagus and stomach to be resected, placements of drainage tubes in stomach and enteral feeding tubes.

Indications of One Stage Operation

- Planned esophagectomy (most commonly for cancer)
- Esophageal perforation with minimal soilage (posterior mediastinal route)
- Perforation with moderate soilage (nonanatomic route like retrosternal route).

Contraindications for One Stage Operation

- Perforation or necrosis with severe mediastinitis
- Cardiorespiratory instability during esophagectomy
- Failed initial attempt at reconstruction with unprepared remaining organs.

Timing of Second Stage Operation

- Second operation must be planned only after there is no sign of ongoing local inflammation and infection and when patient is nutritionally fit with good to fair performance status.

SELECTION OF ESOPHAGEAL SUBSTITUTE

Stomach, colon and jejunum (free or pedicled) are the organs used for esophageal replacements in that order of preference.

Contraindications for the Use of Stomach as Esophageal Substitute

- Partial gastrectomy
- Loss of right gastroepiploic vessels (due to omentectomy, inflammation)
- Prior procedure on stomach like gastrojejunostomy, cysto-gastrostomy or gastrostomy

Contraindications for the Use of Colon as Esophageal Substitute

- Partial/total colectomy
- Abdominal aortic surgery with loss of inferior mesenteric or left colic arteries
- Atherosclerosis affecting left, right or middle colic arteries
- Diverticulosis
- Multiple polyps
- Ulcerative colitis
- Dense fibrous adhesions
- Radiation enteritis.

Contraindications for the Use of Jejunum as Esophageal Substitute

- Crohn's disease
- Short bowel syndrome
- Radiation enteritis
- Superior mesenteric artery syndrome.

Factors Affecting the Choice of Replacement Organ

- Anatomy:
  - Vascular supply
  - Available length
  - Diameter match
  - Tissue strength
- Technique:
  - Technical ease of operation
  - Operative morbidity and mortality
  - Duration of operation
  - Number of anastomoses
  - Risk of vascular insufficiency
- Others:
  - Patient age
  - Type of disease (benign or malignant)
  - Surgeons experience in any particular technique.

ROUTES FOR ESPOPHAGEAL REPLACEMENTS

Posterior Mediastinal Route (Orthotopic)

This is the most commonly used route after esophagectomy. Its advantages are that it needs no specific preparation and gives straightest and shortest connection between cervical esophagus and abdomen. This is 1.9 cm shorter than the substernal route and 3.7 cm shorter than the subcutaneous route as found in cadavers.[19] Posterior mediastinum is wide to accommodate the replaced organ and it minimizes the cardiorespiratory compromise which can be seen more often during substernal route. It has better long-term swallowing function,[20] and it permits the possibility of anastomosis at any level in the chest or neck.

Contraindications of this Route

- Esophageal replacement without resection
- Severe mediastinal inflammation after prior urgent esophagectomy for acute corrosive injury (i.e. in cases of staged reconstruction).

Technique

After esophagectomy no further procedure is needed to prepare the posterior mediastinum to accommodate the organ. Preservation of the azygos vein can help in preventing the migration of the replaced organ.

Substernal/Retrosternal Space (Heterotopic)

The next most common space used is this route. The main indication is when esophageal replacement is done without esophagectomy or when replacement is done as a second stage operation after prior esophagectomy for acute injuries like corrosive or perforation. Figure 1 shows the barium swallow after retrosternal colon transposition.

Disadvantages

Only cervical anastomosis is possible thus needing a longer organ, associated with higher incidence of anastomotic leaks and operative mortality than orthotopic route.[21,22] Also it is associated with higher incidence of dysphagia possibly due to angulation of the conduit as it passes from posterior cervical space to retrosternal space and due to narrow thoracic inlet.[23] In some patients clavicular head and part of manubrium needs to be removed to accommodate the organ through the narrow inlet. Usage of this route is associated with more frequent compromise of cardiopulmonary function during early postoperative period. The blood flow to the retrosternally placed organ may be decreased by positive pressure ventilation if needed in the postoperative period.[22,24]

Technique

With patient in supine position, fascia underlying the xiphoid process is divided and the substernal space is widened by surgeon's fingers so as to permit the entire hand of surgeon into that space. It is important to stay in the middle as laterally there is risk of bleeding from internal thoracic vessels. Cervical incision is then given (along left sternocleidomastoid muscle or transversely) and at least three fingers of the surgeon should come out into the cervical wound. If the inlet is narrow the head of left clavicle and portion of manubrium needs to the resected preserving the subclavian vessels.

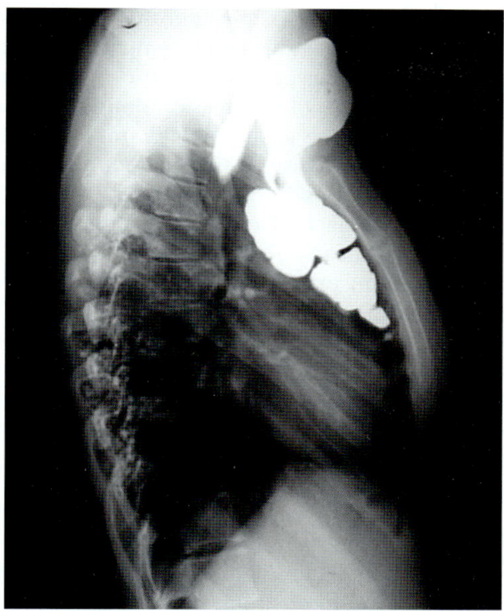

Figure 1 Barium after colon transposition showing the esophagocolonic anastomosis in the neck and the retrosternal position of the colonic graft

Subcutaneous Route/Antesternal (Heterotopic)

Historically this was quite frequent route of replacement but it has got very few indications these days. Its advantages include no or less incidence of cardiopulmonary compromise, lower incidence of postoperative ventilation.[25] This is the only option in certain situations like fibrosed posterior mediastinum, history of transsternal thoracic surgery in the past.

Drawbacks

This is the longest route thus needs greater length of the organ, thus more chance of anastomosis under tension with higher leak rates, more possibility of dysphagia due to more acute angulation, more chance of delayed passage of food into abdomen due to acute angulation at the level of abdomen. Lastly cosmetically it is most undesirable route.

Technique

This tunnel starts at the level of xiphoid process, and the space is widened enough to accommodate surgeon's entire hand. Again it is important to stay in the middle as there is risk of injury to the perforating vessels from the pectoralis muscles. Sometimes sternocleidomastoid muscle needs to be divided to provide adequate space.

STOMACH AS THE ESOPHAGEAL REPLACEMENT

Stomach is the most commonly used organ as the esophageal replacement due to various advantages like technical ease to use, less number of anastomoses, reliable blood supply and good function.

Stomach is used in two forms most commonly, i.e. gastric tube (Figs 2 to 5) constructed from the greater curvature or the whole stomach.

Operative Technique

The anatomic preparation of the stomach as the replacement needs to be done in such a way that it has an adequate length along with good vascularity in terms of both the arterial supply and venous drainage and its safe transposition in to the chest or neck.

Stomach is mobilized by dividing the greater omentum preserving the right gastroepiploic artery along with the arcade

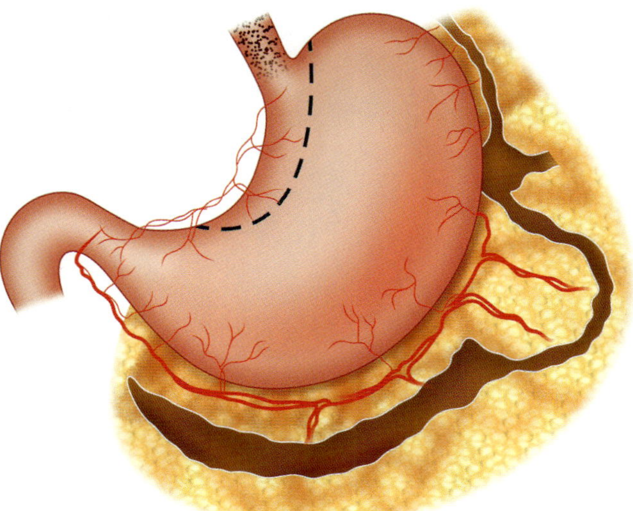

Figure 2 Line of transection to create tubularized gastric conduit

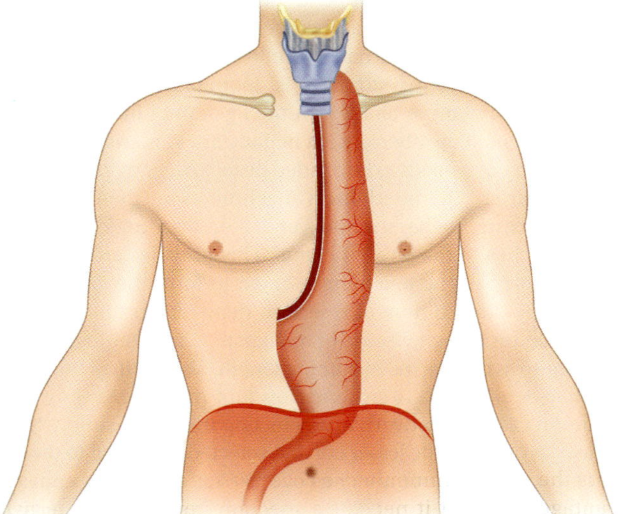

Figure 3 Tubularized gastric conduit replacing esophagus

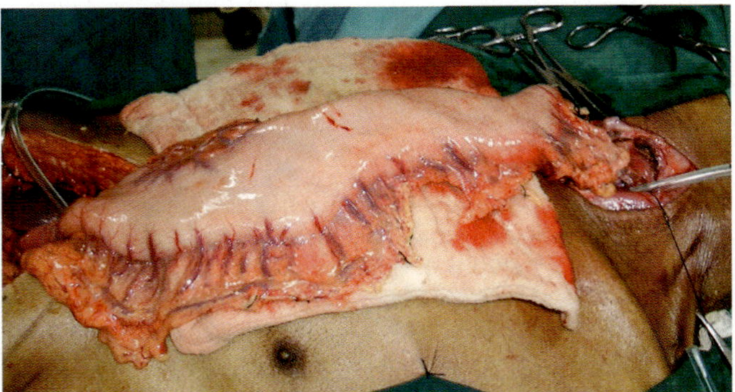

Figure 4 Gastric tubularized conduit after esophagectomy for cancer esophagus

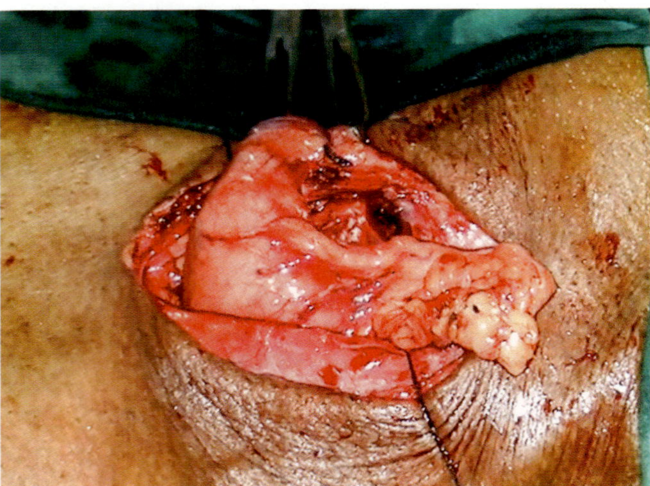

Figure 5 Gastric conduit in the neck for esophagogastric anastomosis (coming through the posterior mediastinum after esophagectomy)

along the greater curve followed by the division of the short gastric vessels, left gastroepiploic and left gastric vessels. In some cases if the blood supply needs to be augmented the length of one or two short gastric vessels may be preserved so that they can be anastomosed with the internal mammary vessels or neck vessels.[26]

The lesser curve of stomach is mobilized by dividing the gastrohepatic omentum along with the ligation of inferior phrenic artery if present. If the aberrant left hepatic artery is arising from the left gastric artery, it needs to be divided distal to the origin of aberrant left hepatic artery. Retroperitoneal attachments are then divided till the level of cruri. Kocher's maneuver is then performed so that the pylorus reaches to the level of hiatus. This provides an extra 5 cm length. The lesser curve is then resected to form the gastric tube. The proximal limit of line of resection depends on the indication whether it is for benign disease or malignancy. The fundus is mostly preserved so as to have the maximum length. The width of the gastric tube must be around 8–10 cm as narrow tube may cause injury to the intramural vascular network thus affecting the blood supply to the fundus.[27] A point on the lesser curve is selected just distal to the fifth branch of the left gastric artery as over 90% of the lymph nodes on lesser curve will be resected.[28] The resection line can be created with staplers or suturing.

In cases of benign diseases and mid thoracic tumors whole stomach can be used as the replacement. The important difference here is the preparation of the lesser curve. The terminal branches of the gastric vessels along the lesser curve are divided flush with the gastric serosa from fifth branch of left gastric artery proximally till the level of cardia removing all the fat, lymph nodes and nerve branches. This helps in the lengthening of the stomach. If additional length is still required the seromuscular layer can be incised transversely from lesser to greater curve providing extra 1–2 cm of length.[29] The stomach is divided at the cardia.

Transposition of the stomach is easy when done during transthoracic surgery. After transhiatal or thoraco-laparoscopic surgery it needs to be pushed or pulled into the space. It is important to do it with minimal trauma and torsion to the stomach.

Complications after Gastric Pull-up

- Anastomotic leak—most common complication. The cervical anastomoses are three times more prone to leak than thoracic anastomoses.[30] Oral feeds are most often allowed along with jejunal feeds if needed.
- Anastomotic stricture—mostly related to leaks. Mostly treated with endoscopic dilatations.
- Gastric necrosis—rare complication. Only treatment is immediate removal of stomach and adequate drainage of the route with esophageal exteriorization. If the necrosis is partial and if there is adequate length, reanastomosis can be performed. If the initial anastomoses is in chest replace the stomach in abdomen after closing its end along with decompressive gastrostomy and cervical esophagostomy. Reconstruction then has to be planned as the second stage procedure.
- Gastric torsion—it leads to necrosis if the torsion is more than 90–180 degrees. It is a totally preventable complication by careful transpositioning of the stomach.

Postoperative Function of Gastric Conduit

Long-term quality of life with gastric replacement of esophagus is reported to be good with 86% patients reported very good functional results, with 90% having stable weight, 5% dumping and 10% diarrhea, 15–20% had dysphagia and heartburn or regurgitation.[31]

COLON AS THE REPLACEMENT

This is the second most common organ used for esophageal replacement. Colon transposition is technically a bigger challenge than the gastric pull up and most commonly done for corrosive injury of esophagus (Fig. 6).

Special Anatomic Considerations

The blood supply of the colon is from the superior and inferior mesenteric vessels. Its blood supply is variable thus making it a very important consideration for colonic replacement. The classic vascular pattern of colon is seen in only 25% of patients with middle, right and left colonic arteries forming the marginal artery of Drummond.[32] In 5–10% patients there is no right colic artery and in 5–15% the middle colic artery is absent.[32-34] The blood supply of left

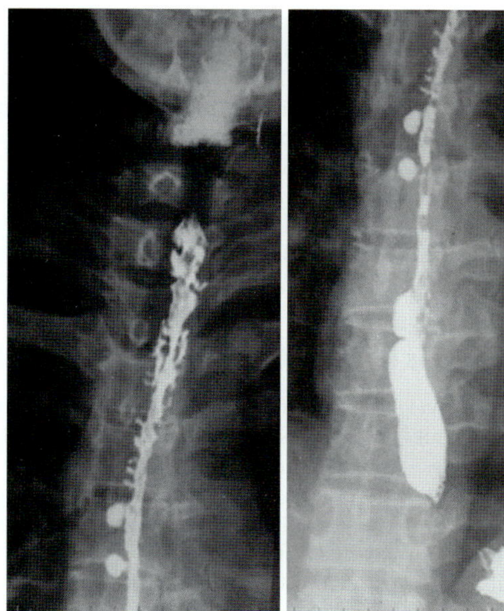

Figure 6 Patient with corrosive injury of esophagus below the hypopharynx level. She was treated with pharyngocoloplasty

colon from inferior mesenteric artery (IMA) is more constant. The first branch of IMA is left colic artery dividing further into ascending and descending branches. The ascending branch is present in 95% patients.[34] The marginal artery of Drummond is the communication between the superior and the inferior mesenteric arterial supply to the colon and is vital to the successful colonic transposition.

Types of Colonic Conduits for Replacements

Two main options include use of right or the left colon for replacement. The left colon is preferred as it has consistent blood supply, thick wall and smaller diameter giving a better size match for end to end anastomosis. These are pedicled grafts based on one of the main vessels like right, middle or left colonic artery. The ascending branch of left colonic artery is most often used for long or short segment transpositions using descending and transverse colon in isoperistaltic manner. The middle and right colonic artery based grafts are used less often. Sometimes free colonic grafts can be used along with microvascular anastomoses. Most often the proximal anastomosis is in the neck and if stomach is intact the distal anastomoses are with the body of stomach. When the stomach is not available then the colon is anastomosed with the Roux loop of jejunum. The orientation of the colon transposition is not a major determinant of postoperative function.

Operative Technique

The operative technique described here is the most commonly performed type that is isoperistaltic left colon transposition based on ascending branch of left colic artery (Figs 7 to 11). This can be done both by open and minimal access methods. The omentum is separated from colon in the avascular plane. Entire colon is mobilized with its mobilization from the retroperitoneal structures. The length of the graft is measured using a tape placed on the mesenteric border and it is divided at some extra length so as to allow contraction after division. Then the two branches of left colonic, middle colonic and ileocolic arteries are dissected and bulldog clamps are applied on them (except the ascending branch) along with the clamp on the distal colon to check for the adequacy of the blood supply to the proposed

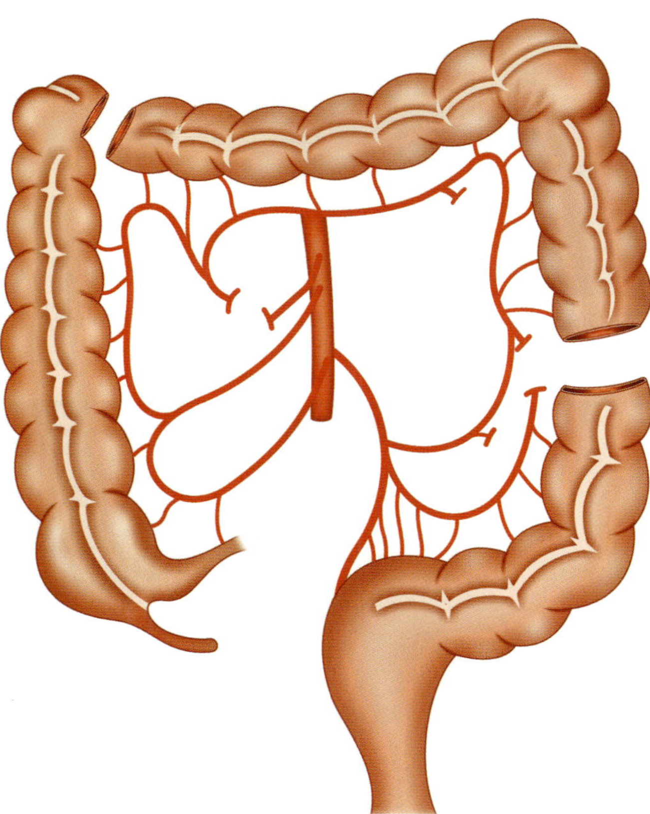

Figure 7 Showing line of division of colon with division of descending branch of left colonic and middle colonic artery to create left sided colonic graft based on ascending branch of left colonic artery

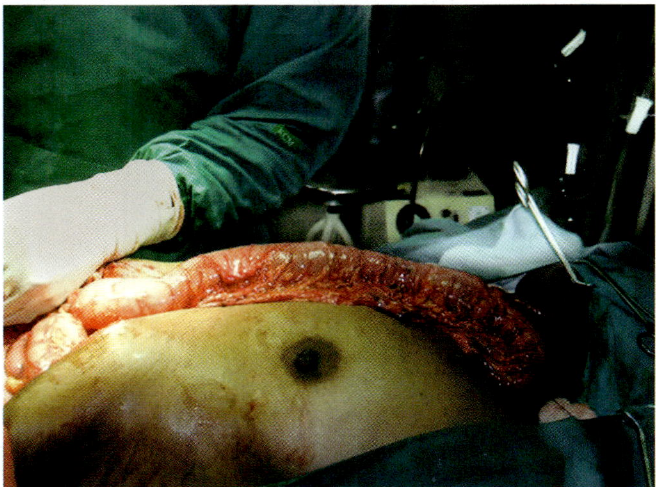

Figure 8 Colonic conduit in a patient undergoing pharyngocoloplasty for corrosive injury esophagus

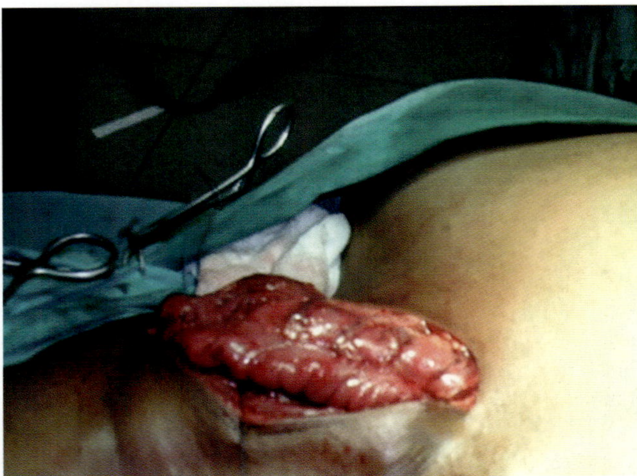

Figure 9 Colonic end in the neck for pharyngocolonic anastomosis (coming through the retrosternal space)

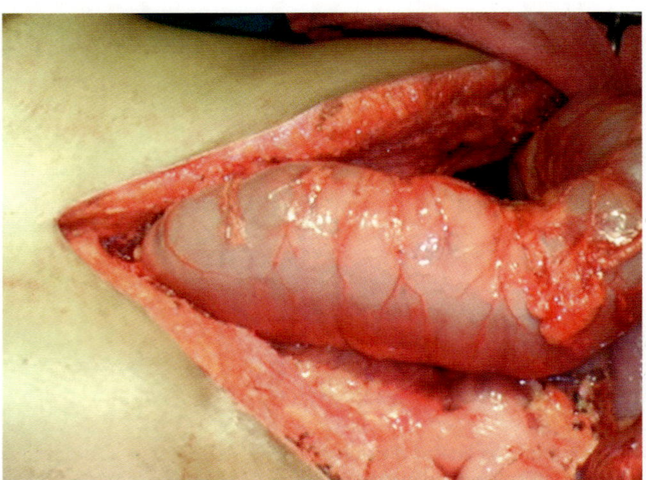

Figure 10 Colonic end in the abdomen ready for anastomosis with the stomach

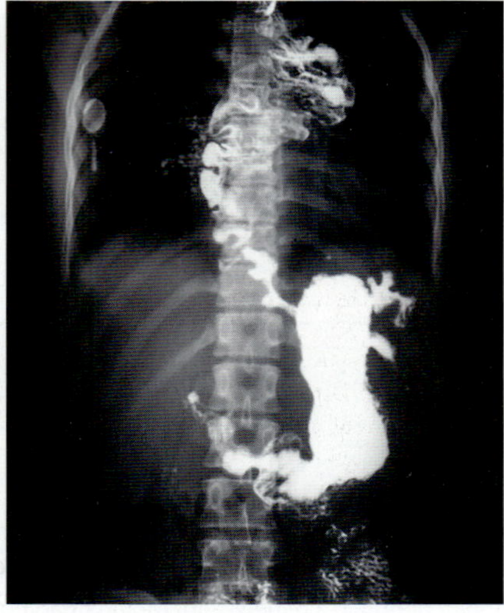

Figure 11 Barium study showing colonic conduit after colon transposition

graft from the single vessel that is ascending branch of left colic artery. After this neck dissection is done and finally the colon is divided at the desired level. This is followed by the creation of the retrosternal route and various anastomoses. The proximal anastomosis is done first followed by distal anastomosis so that the redundant portion can be resected if there is any. As final position of the cecum and appendix is on the middle or the left side of the abdomen appendicectomy is added to prevent any future diagnostic dilemmas. On the same principles right colonic and ileocolic transpositions can be done.

Complications Related to Colonic Transpositions

- Graft necrosis—it is seen in up to 5% patients.[35,36] This is the result of inadequate perfusion. It can be prevented by doing the microvascular anastomosis in the neck or with the internal mammary artery to supercharge the colon thus reducing the risk of ischemia.[37,38] This complication is difficult to diagnose early, and endoscopy showing mucosal ischemia is one such method. Once it remove the necrosed organ is removed with drainage of the route and esophagostomy and closure of the distal anastomotic site followed by second stage reconstruction.
- Anastomotic leak and stricture—the incidence is around 10% and is lower than the gastric pull up.[34,39] The strictures are the results of subclinical leaks. Treatment is the endoscopic dilatation.
- Graft redundancy—this can cause dysphagia, obstruction, regurgitation and bacterial overgrowth.[40] Surgical corrections may be needed in severe cases and it is easier with subcutaneous route than with posterior and retrosternal routes.[41]
- Chronic ischemia—this occurs due to inadequate venous drainage and treated by endoscopic dilatations.[42]
- Development of cancer or diverticulitis in the transpositioned colon.[43,44]

Postoperative Function of the Transpositioned Colon

The transit time of transpositioned colon is short so there is no absorption. The macroscopic and histological changes in the colon are almost nil.[45] There is only rare inflammation or fibrosis. Nutritionally there is no advantage of colon over stomach. Quality of life after colonic transposition is good with 75–90% patients having good to excellent level of satisfaction.[46,47] Gastrointestinal symptoms are common like early satiety in 20–75%, regurgitation in 10–40%, eructations in 50% and postprandial abdominal pain in 40% and diarrhea in 10%.[47,48]

JEJUNAL GRAFTS

Jejunum is another organ used for esophageal replacement. It is not a popular choice as its blood supply is segmental thus making it prone to ischemia. It can be used in two ways—as pedicled graft (Figs 12 and 13) and as free jejunal grafts.

Pedicled Jejunal Grafts

These are suitable mainly for short segment esophageal replacements in an isoperistaltic fashion for the distal esophagus. Though, long segment replacements are also reported.

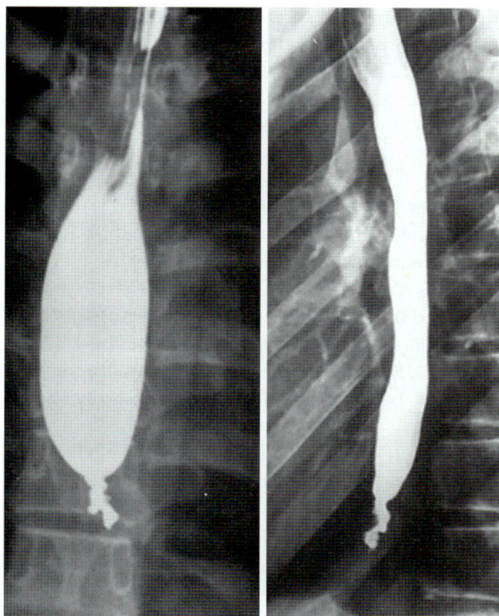

Figure 12 Patient with lower end esophageal corrosive stricture treated with pedicled jejunal graft

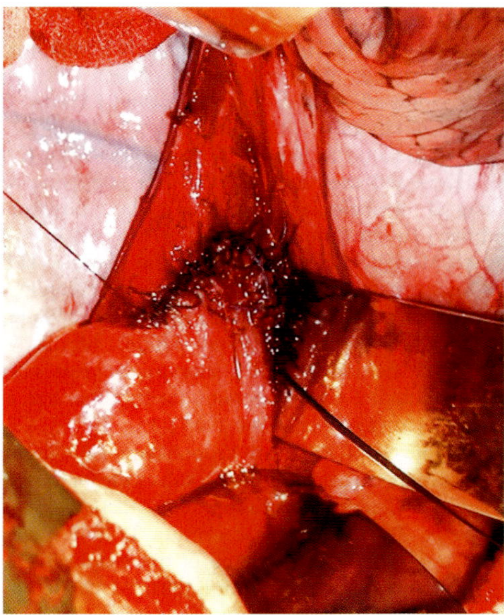

Figure 13 Completed pedicled jejunal graft between esophagus and stomach

These procedures require much greater skill and experience and we recommend that these should only be considered if stomach or colonic replacement is not feasible. In practice this is of utmost rarity.

Complications after Jejunal Interposition

- Graft ischemia/necrosis, anastomotic dehiscence, chronic ischemia and graft redundancy.

Postoperative Function after Jejunal Interposition

The patients after jejunal interposition have less incidence of dysphagia, regurgitation and heartburn with being able to take a normal diet.[49,50] Though, diarrhea occurs in around 20% patients.[51]

Free Jejunal Grafts

This is the most common method used for cervical esophageal replacement. With the help of microvascular anastomoses a short jejunal segment is used to replace cervical esophagus.

Its proximal end is anastomosed to the hypopharynx and distal end either to the remaining esophagus or to another organ (stomach or colon) forming a composite graft.

Complications

Graft necrosis with its loss in 8%, fistula rate of 20%, strictures in 20% (mostly distal) and graft redundancy.[52]

Postoperative Function after Free Jejunal Grafts

The functional status after free jejunal grafts for cervical esophageal replacement is good. Most are able to take oral feeds with 15-20% patients requiring additional supplements by gastrostomy or jejunostomy feeds.[53] Regurgitation and heartburn are rare.

ARTIFICIAL TUBES FOR ESOPHAGEAL REPLACEMENTS

The use of artificial tube dates back to 1913 when Torek[9] for the first time used an external tube to connect cervical esophagus with gastrostomy. Subsequently rubber and silastic tubes were used for the same purpose. From 1950s onward efforts are on to create an artificial internal esophageal tube using materials like autologous tissues, homologous tissues, wire mesh, plastics, rubber, silicone and polymers like Teflon and Dacron.[54-58]

Need of Artificial Esophagus

The use of autologous organs for esophageal replacement involves one or more complicated surgeries with their attendant morbidity, risk of loss of primary function of the harvested organ, and it may sometimes not be feasible due to previous disease or surgery. Thus the need of an artificial substitute was felt.

Regenerative medicine is being used to try various kinds of acellular synthetic or biologic scaffoldings alone or with seeding of epithelial and muscle cells on to the scaffolds. They can be used without any need of immunosuppression. Acellular scaffolds are populated with silicone, vicryl or polyvinyllidene fluoride (PDFE) and the biologic scaffolds are populated with epithelial or muscular seeds.[59,60] Recently decellularized matrices are used as scaffolds made from the human and animal tissues.[61]

OUR EXPERIENCE

From August 2005 till June 2014, we have operated on 56 cases of cancer esophagus, initial 26 by open method (TTE/THE) and the later 30 by thoraco-laparoscopic (TLE) approach. In all but one, a tubularised gastric conduit placed in the posterior mediastinum was used as the esophageal replacement. In one case the colon was used as the stomach was short of length for a cervical anastomosis. Complications in the form of anastomotic leak occurred in 2/56 cases, which were managed conservatively.

During the similar period we have operated upon 13 patients of corrosive injury esophagus. Two of them presented with acute injury with profuse bleeding and perforations. These two patients were managed with initial esophagogastrectomy with cervical esophagostomy, gastrostomy and feeding jejunostomy, followed by second stage colon transposition. In one of them clavicular head needed to be removed due to narrow thoracic inlet. One of these patients is well on follow-up. The other patient who had initially failed suicidal corrosive ingestion, finally committed suicide 1½ years after his surgery. Remaining 11 patients presented to us in chronic stage with feeding jejunostomy tube in situ. Among them 3/11 had complete cervical esophageal cicatrization so pharyngocoloplasty was done with proximal anastomosis with hypopharynx and distal with stomach in two and Roux loop of jejunum in one. Six of eleven patients had colon transposition with proximal anastomosis with cervical esophagus and distal with stomach in four and Roux loop of jejunum in two of them. One of eleven patients had non-passable stricture in the distal esophagus which was treated with segmental pedicled jejunal graft anastomosed proximally to the thoracic esophagus and distally to the stomach after resection of the strictured esophageal segment, through the right abdominothoracic incision. One of eleven patients had the history of transsternal resection of benign esophageal tumor with cervical esophagostomy and feeding jejunostomy done elsewhere in cardiothoracic department. In this patient colon transposition was done through the subcutaneous route from the left of the sternal scar. In all but one patient colon was placed through retrosternal route. All had uneventful recovery and are doing fine as of now.

REFERENCES

1. Mikulicz J. Ein Fall von resection des carcinomatosen oesophagus mit plastischen ersatz des excirdirten stuckes. Prager Med Wschr. 1886;11:93-4.
2. Bircher E. Ein Beitrag zur plastischen bildung eines neuen oesophagus. Zbl Chir. 1907;34:1479-82.
3. Garre C. Ueber oesophagus—resection und oesophagoplastik. Langenbeck's Arch Klin Chir. 1898;57:719-22.
4. Payr. Antethorakaler oesophagusplastik. Munchen Med Wschr. 1917;64:783.
5. Beck C, Carrell A. Demonstration of specimens illustrating a method of formation of a prethoracic esophagus. Ill Med J. 1905;7:463-4.
6. Kirschner. Ein neues Verfahren der Oesophagoplastik. Arch Klin Chir. 1920;114:606-63.
7. Roux. L'oesophago-jejuno-gastrostomose, nouvelle operation pour retrecissement infranchissable de l'oesophage. Semaine Med. 1907;27:37-40.
8. Kelling G. Oesophagoplastik mit hilfe des querkolon. Zbl Chir. 1911;36:1209-12.
9. Torek F. First successful case of resection of the thoracic portion of the oesophagus for carcinoma. Surg Gynecol Obstet. 1913;16:614-7.
10. Wookey H. The surgical treatment of cancer of the pharynx and upper esophagus. Surg Gynecol Obstet. 1942;75:499-506.
11. Bricker EM, Burford TH. Experiences with tubed pedicle grafts in esophageal reconstruction following resection for cancer. Ann Surg. 1957;145:979-92.
12. Rapant V, Hromada J. Surgical treatment of corrosive stenoses of the thoracic part of the esophagus by a single stage palliative anastomosis. J Thorac Surg. 1950;20:454-73.
13. Le Roux BT. An analysis of 700 cases of carcinoma of the hypopharynx, the esophagus, and the proximal stomach. Thorax. 1961;16:226-55.
14. Reinhoff WF Jr. Intrathoracic esophagojejunostomy for lesions of the upper third of the esophagus. South Med J. 1946;39:928-40.
15. Kasai M, Abo S, Makino K, Yoshida S, Taguchi Y. Reconstruction of the cervical esophagus with a pedicled jejuna graft. Surg Gynecol Obstet. 1965;121:102-6.
16. Orsoni P, Lemaire M. Technique des oesophagoplasties par le colon transverse et descendant. J Chirurgie. 1951;67:491-505.
17. Goligher JC, Robin IG. Use of left colon for reconstruction of pharynx and oesophagus after pharyngectomy. Br J Surg. 1954; 42:283-90.
18. Belsey R. Reconstruction of the esophagus with left colon. J Thorac Cardiovasc Surg. 1965;49:3-55.
19. Ngan SY, Wong J. Lengths of different routes for esophageal replacement. J Thorac Cardiovasc Surg. 1986;91:790-2.
20. Kuwano H, Ikebe M, Baba K, Kitamura K, Toh Y, Matsuda H, et al. Operative procedures of reconstruction with resection of esophageal cancer and the postoperative quality of life. World J Surg. 1993;17:773-6.
21. Hirai T, Iwata T, Yamashita Y, Mukaida H, Saeki S, Toge T. Investigation of suitability of devascularized upper half of the whole stomach as replacement for the esophagus. Hiroshima J Med Sci. 1992;41:25-30.
22. Bartels H, Thorban S, Siewert JR. Anterior versus posterior reconstruction after transhiatal esophagectomy: a randomized controlled trial. Br J Surg. 1993;80:1141-4.
23. Shiraha S, Matsumoto H, Terada M, Noguchi J, Sankouji T, Hayashi M. Motility studies of the cervical esophagus with intrathoracic gastric conduit after esophagectomy. Scand J Thorac Cardiovasc Surg. 1992;26:119-23.
24. Jacob L, Boudaoud S, Rabary O, Payen D, Sarfati E, Gossot D, et al. Decreased mesenteric blood flow supplying retrosternal esophageal ileocoloplastic grafts during positive pressure breathing. J Thorac Cardiovasc Surg. 1994;107:68-73.
25. Tsutsui S, Moriguchi S, Morita M, Kuwano H, Matsuda H, Mori M, et al. Multivariate analysis of postoperative complications after esophageal resection. Ann Thorac Surg. 1992;53:1052-6.
26. Murakami M, Sugiyama A, Ikegami T, Ishida K, Maruta F, Shimizu F, et al. Revascularization using the short gastric vessels of the gastric tube after subtotal esophagectomy for intrathoracic esophageal carcinoma. J Am Coll Surg. 2000;190:71-7.
27. Pierie JP, de Graaf PW, van Vroonhoven TJ, Obertop H. The vascularisation of a gastric tube as a substitute for the esophagus is affected by its diameter. Dis Esoph. 1998;11:231-5.
28. Akiyama H, Tsurumaru M, Kawamura T, Ono Y. Principles of surgical treatment for carcinoma of the esophagus: analysis of lymphnode involvement. Ann Surg. 1981;194:438-46.
29. Perrachia A, Bardini R, Narne S. Resections for pharyngo-oesophageal cancer. In: Jamieson GG (Ed). Surgery of the Oesophagus. Edinburgh: Churchill Livingstone; 1988. pp. 689-99.
30. McManus K, Anikin V, McGuigan J. Total thoracic oesophagectomy for oesophageal carcinoma: has it been worth it? Eur J Cardio-Thorac Surg. 1999;16:261-5.
31. De Leyn P, Coosemans W, Lerut T. Early and late functional results in patients with intrathoracic gastric replacement after oesophagectomy for carcinoma. Eur J Cardio-Thorac Surg. 1992;6:79-85.
32. Sonneland J, Anson BJ, Beaton LE. Surgical anatomy of the arterial supply to the colon from the superior mesenteric artery based upon a study of 600 specimens. Surg Gynecol Obstet. 1958;106: 385-98.
33. Sage M, Calmat A, Leguerrier A, Honnart F, Cabrol C, Guerin-Surville H. Vascularization du colon transverse. Bull Assoc Anat. 1977;61:397-406.

34. Peters JH, Kronson JW, Katz M, DeMeester TR. Arterial anatomic considerations in colon interposition for esophageal replacement. Arch Surg. 1995;130:858-63.
35. Khan AR, Stiff G, Mohammed AR, Alwafi A, Ress BI, Lari J. Esophageal replacement with colon in children. Pediatr Surg Int. 1998;13:79-83.
36. Thomas P, Fuentes P, Giudicelli R, Reboud E. Colon interposition for esophageal replacement: current and long term function. Ann Thorac Surg. 1997;64:757-64.
37. O'Rourke IC, Threlfall GN. Colonic interposition for esophageal reconstruction with special reference to microvascular reinforcement of graft circulation. Aust N Z J Surg. 1986;56:767-71.
38. Golshani SD, Lee C, Cass D, Thomas A, Mandpe AH. Microvascular "supercharged" cervical colon: minimizing ischemia in esophageal reconstruction. Ann Plast Surg. 1999;43:533-8.
39. Cheng B-C, Lu S-Q, Gao S-Z, Tu ZF, Lin DM, Wang TS. Colon replacement from espophagus. Clinical experience from 240 cases. Chin Med J. 1994;107:216-8.
40. Schien M, Conlan AA, Hatchuel MD. Surgical management of the redundant transposed colon. Am J Surg. 1990;160:529-30.
41. Bonavina L, Chella B, Segalin A, Luzzani S. Surgical treatment of the redundant interposed colon after retrosternal esophagoplasty. Ann Thorac Surg. 1998;65:1446-8.
42. Cheng W, Heitmiller RF, Jones B. Subacute ischemia of the colon esophageal interposition. Ann Thorac Surg. 1994;57:899-903.
43. Lee SJ, Koay CD, Thompson H, Nicolaides AR, Das Gupta AR. Adenocarcinoma arising in an esophageal colonic interposition graft. J Laryngol Otol. 1994;108:80-3.
44. Isolauri J, Markkula H. Recurrent ulceration and colopericardial fistula as late complications of colon interposition. Ann Thorac Surg. 1987;44:84-5.
45. Isolauri J, Helin H, Markkula H. Colon interposition for esophageal disease: histologic findings of colonic mucosa after a follow up of 5 months to 15 years. Am J Gastroenterol. 1991;86:277-80.
46. Curet-Scott MJ, Ferguson MK, Little AG, Skinner DB. Colon interposition for benign esophageal disease. Surgery. 1987;102: 568-74.
47. Cerfolio RJ, Allen MS, Deschamps C, Trastek VF, Pairolero PC. Esophageal replacement by colon interposition. Ann Thorac Surg. 1995;59:1382-4.
48. Collard J-M, Otte J-B, Reynaert M, et al. Quality of life three years or more after esophagectomy for cancer. J Thorac Cardiovasc Surg. 1992;104:391-4.
49. Gaissert HA, Mathisen DJ, Grillo HC, et al. Short segment intestinal interposition of the distal esophagus. J Thorac Cardiovasc Surg. 1993;106:860-7.
50. Watson TJ, Demeester TR, Kauer WKH, et al. Esophageal replacement for end stage benign esophageal disease. J Thorac Cardiovasc Surg. 1998;115:1241-9.
51. Nishihira T, Oe H, Sugawara K, et al. Reconstruction of the thoracic esophagus with jejuna pedicled segments for cancer of the thoracic esophagus. Dis Esoph. 1995;8:30-9.
52. Kato H, Watanabe H, Iizuka T, et al. Primary esophageal reconstruction after resection of the cancer in the hypopharynx or cervical esophagus: comparison of free forearm skin tube flap, free jejuna transplantation, and pull through esophagectomy. Jpn J Clin Oncol. 1987;17:255-61.
53. Fisher SR, Cameron R, Hoyt DJ, Cole TB, Seigler HF, Meyers WC. Free jejunal interposition graft for reconstruction of the esophagus. Head Neck. 1990;12:126-30.
54. Neuhof H, Ziegler JM. Experimental reconstruction of the esophagus by granulations tubes. Surg Gynecol Obstet. 1922; 34:767-75.
55. Rob CG, Bateman GH. Reconstruction of the trachea and cervical esophagus. Br J Surg. 1949;37:202-5.
56. Edgerton MT. One stage reconstruction of the cervical esophagus or trachea. Surgery. 1952;31:239-50.
57. Fryfogle JD, Cyrowski GA, Rothwell D, Rheault G, Clark T. Replacement of the middle third of the esophagus with a silicone rubber prosthesis. Dis Chest. 1963;43:464-75.
58. Fukushima M, Kako N, Chiba K, Kawaguchi T, Kimura Y, Sato M, et al. Seven year follow up study after the replacement of the esophagus with an artificial esophagus in the dog. Surgery. 1983;93:70-7.
59. Lynen JP, Klinge U, Anurov M, Titkova S, Mertens PR, Jansen M. Surgical mesh as a scaffold for tissue regeneration in the esophagus. Eur Surg Res. 2004;36:104-11.
60. Takimoto Y, Nakamura T, Yamamoto Y, Kiyotani T, Teramachi M, Shimizu Y. The experimental replacement of a cervical esophagus segment with an artificial prosthesis with the use of collagen matrix and a silicone stent. J Thorac Cardiovasc Surg. 1998;116: 98-106.
61. Badylak SF, Hoppo T, Nieponice A, Gilbert TW, Davison JM, Jobe BA. Esophageal preservation in five male patients after endoscopic inner layer circumferential resection in the setting of superficial cancer: a regenerative medicine approach with a biologic scaffold. Tissue Eng Part A. 2011;17:1643-50.

SECTION 3

Stomach, Duodenum, Small Intestine and Retroperitoneum

CHAPTER 23

Stomach and Duodenum

Neeraj Goel, PK Mishra

Anatomy of Stomach

STOMACH

Stomach is the most dilated part of the gastrointestinal tract (GIT). It is the first intra-abdominal part of the GIT interposed between the esophagus and the first part of the duodenum. Stomach occupies the left hypochondrium, the epigastrium and the umbilical region with majority of it being under the left rib cage. It is a highly vascular muscular bag which is fixed at its proximal and distal ends. It is a distensible organ which is highly variable in its size according the contents present inside the lumen. The two fixed points are:

1. Gastroesophageal junction (GEJ) (cardia) is the most fixed part located 2.5 cm to left of midline at the level of tenth thoracic (T10) vertebra and is approximately 40 cm from the incisor teeth.
2. Gastroduodenal junction (pylorus) is located to the right of the midline at the level of first lumbar (L1) vertebra but can be located at lower levels also.

Gross Anatomy

The stomach has three main parts, namely: fundus, body and the pyloric part; two borders, namely: lesser curvature (the right border) and the greater curvature (the left border) and two surfaces, namely: anterior and posterior surface (Fig. 1).

Peritoneal Arrangement

The stomach is completely intraperitoneal with peritoneum except at two fixed points near GE junction and pylorus. It forms a double layered lesser omentum from lesser curvature to the liver and greater omentum which hangs from the greater curvature. The omentum contains variable amount of fat and carry the important vessels to supply the stomach.

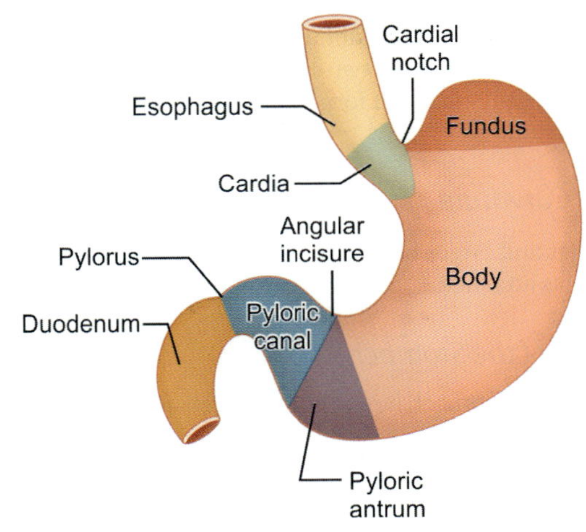

Figure 1 Parts of stomach

Cardia

It is the part of the stomach at the GEJ. It ends at the cardial notch from where the fundus starts.

Fundus

It is the part of the stomach which projects above the cardia and appear as a hump. It usually is in contact with the left hemidiaphragm. Due to its position this part of the stomach is usually filled with air. Fundus when stretched gives extra length which is important during the formation of the gastric tube.

Endoscopically the fundus is not seen until retroflex maneuver is performed.

Body

Body is the largest part of the stomach. It starts from the funds and reaches up to the incisura angularis, a notch which is present on the lesser curvature of the stomach. A variable part of the body may be above and below the costal margin depending upon the amount of distension of the abdomen. In cases of massive dilatation the body part can reach even up to umbilical or hypogastric region.

Pyloric Part

This is the distal most part of the stomach. It starts from the incisura angularis to the duodenopyloric junction. It has a wide part which is called the antrum and a narrow canal-like part which is called the pyloric canal which continues with the duodenal lumen. The circular muscle at the distal end of the pylorus is thick and forms a sphincter which is known as the pyloric sphincter. On the surface the pyloroduodenal area is identified by the presence of the prepyloric vein of Mayo. The pyloric canal is situated at the head and the neck of the pancreas.

Lesser Curvature

It is the right border of the stomach. It has a notch approximately at the junction of proximal two-thirds and distal one-third, known as incisura angularis and it forms the junction of the body and the pyloric antrum.

Greater Curvature

It is the left and larger border of the stomach to which the greater omentum is attached.

Relations of the Stomach

Posterior to the stomach lie structures which are collectively known as the stomach bed. Posterior to the stomach and anterior to the stomach bed structures lays the lesser sac. It constitutes left crus and dome of the diaphragm, splenic artery, body of pancreas, transverse mesocolon and upper part of left kidney, left suprarenal gland, spleen and left colic flexure. Right sided relations of the lesser curvature in the midline are formed by the aorta with the coeliac trunk, the coeliac plexus and ganglia and coeliac lymph nodes.

Greater and Lesser Omentum

The stomach is attached to lesser omentum on the lesser curvature and to the greater omentum onto the greater curvature.

Lesser Omentum

It is formed by turning of the peritoneum at the lesser curvature and contains variable amount of fat. It has one free border toward the right side which is called as the hepatoduodenal ligament and contains the hepatic artery, bile duct and the portal vein. Along the lesser curvature the right gastric and the left gastric arteries run between the two layers of the lesser omentum.

Greater Omentum

It is the policeman of the abdomen as its free floating part reaches anywhere in the abdomen where there is inflammatory process going on. It is four layered peritoneal fold with variable amount of the fat. It has a very rich vasculature formed by multiple anastomosing vessels arising from the right gastroepiploic, left gastroepiploic and the short gastric arteries. It has a very formidable capacity of regeneration. It has very rich lymphatic supply. Recent studies have shown that the greater omentum is a storehouse for the oval cells which are the progenitor cells and can be utilized for regeneration (Fig. 2).

BLOOD SUPPLY

Stomach has a very robust blood supply such that it can survive even on a single blood vessel.

The main arteries supplying the stomach are (Fig. 3):

- Right gastric artery (RGA)
- Left gastric artery (LGA)
- Right gastroepiploic artery (RGEA)
- Left gastroepiploic artery (LGEA) and the
- Short gastric arteries

Left Gastric Artery

In more than 90% of the individuals, it is a branch of the celiac axis and in rest may arise as a branch of common hepatic, splenic, superior mesenteric artery and sometimes even directly from aorta. After arising from the celiac axis it ascends toward the GEJ and gives cardioesophageal branch and then descends along the lesser curvature giving anterior and posterior branches. In 24% of cases it may give rise to aberrant left hepatic artery which should be positively sought for and LGA should be ligated beyond its branching to prevent liver vascularity.

Right Gastric Artery

It is usually a small branch from the proper hepatic artery. It remains suprapyloric giving few pyloric branches before anastomosing to the LGA along the lesser curvature.

Left Gastroepiploic Artery

In most cases it originates from the distal splenic artery. With the RGEA it forms the arc of Barkow in the greater omentum.

Right Gastroepiploic Artery

It may be a continuation of gastrodudoenal artery or a direct branch of it. It travels toward the pylorus and gives infrapyloric branches before it travels along the greater curvature. At the greater curvature, it anastomosis to the LGEA to complete the arc of Barkow.

Short Gastric Arteries

Approximately 5–7 branches arise from the terminal branch of the splenic artery and travel toward the stomach fundus to supply

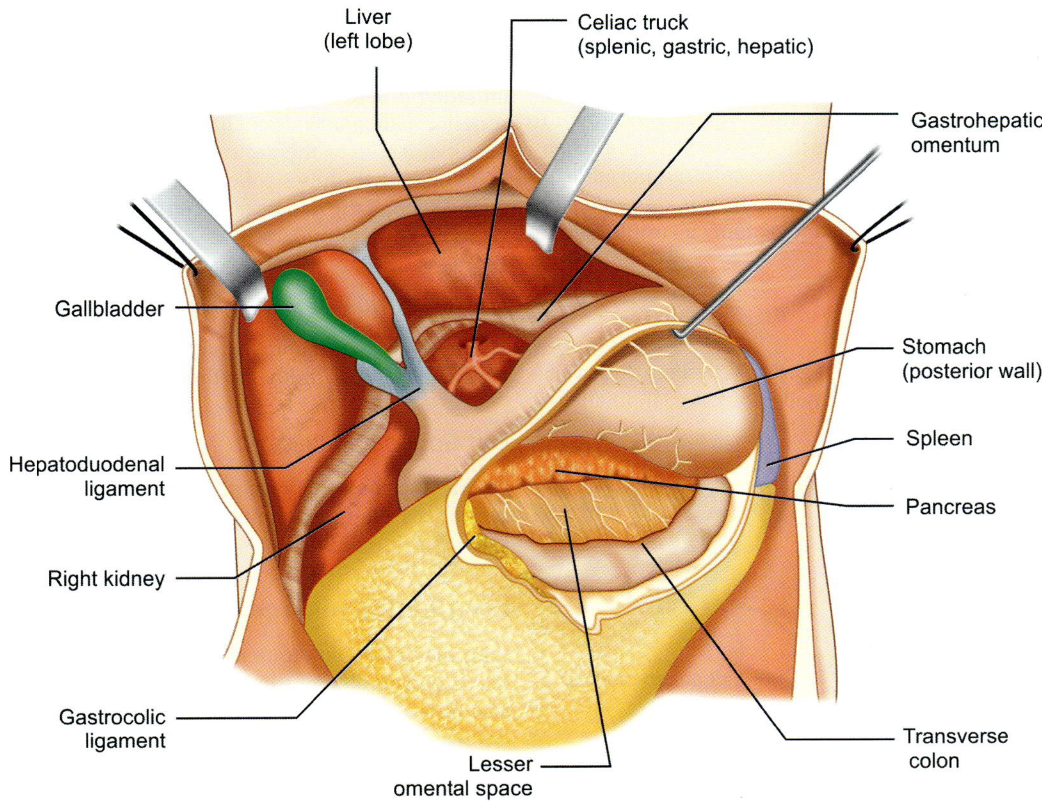

Figure 2 Relations of stomach

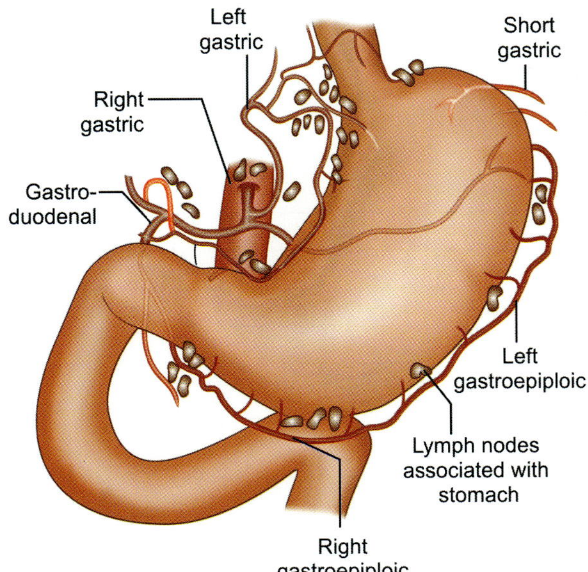

Figure 3 Arterial supply of stomach

this area. While performing splenectomy the short gastric arteries should be ligated carefully so as to avoid the injury to stomach.

Arterial Circulation of the Gastric Wall

Stomach can survive on a single vessel. The smaller branches of these arteries penetrate muscularis and anastomose with the submucosal plexus. This submucosal plexus allows stomach to survive on single vessel even when the three others are ligated.

Thus,

- Stomach remains viable when gastric tube is made based on RGA and RGEA
- With 90–95% gastrectomy remnant remains viable due to supply from esophageal arteries.

But this not absolute as:

- Ligation of all extrinsic arteries may sometimes not stop gastric ulcer bleed
- Necrosis of the lesser curvature is known during selective vagotomy.

A special note is made here about the inferior phrenic arteries which supply the GEJ (left in ~50% of cases and right in 3% of cases).

Veins of the Stomach (Fig. 4)

Left Gastric (Coronary) Vein

It starts at the middle of the lesser curvature, travels upward and then at the hiatus turns down along the lesser curvature to go behind the common hepatic artery to enter into the portal vein (73%). It can also drain into the splenic vein. It is important to recognize this vein during the lymphadenectomy as troublesome bleeding can occur.

Right Gastric Vein

This is a small vein which joins the left gastric vein. Prepyloric vein of Mayo is its tributary which as explained earlier is a landmark for gastroduodenal junction.

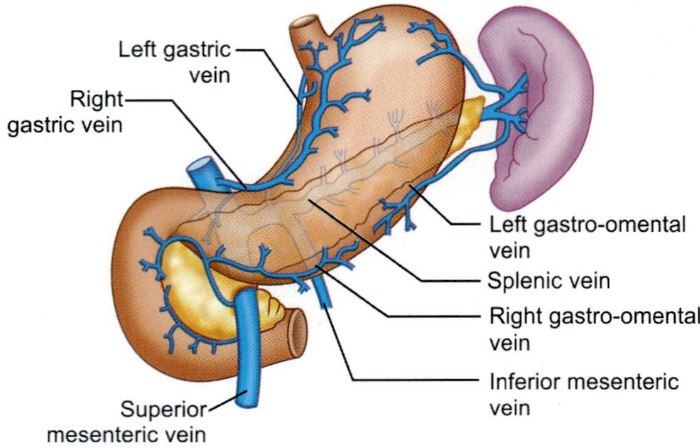

Figure 4 Venous drainage of stomach

Right Gastroepiploic Vein

It accompanies the RGEA before draining into the superior mesenteric vein posterior to the neck of pancreas, it receives superior pancreaticoduodenal vein and the middle colic vein. Trunk of Henle or the gastrocolic trunk is formed by the joining RGEV and right upper colic vein. It is a short vein which travels on the head of the pancreas. It can give rise to bleeding during the Whipple's operation.

Short Gastric Veins

These veins travel along the named arties and drain the fundus of the stomach. They drain into the splenic vein.

Left Gastroepiploic Vein

Drains into the splenic vein. Due to this rich venous networking the varices can occur in the case of occlusion of the splenoportal axis.

Lymphatic Drainage of the Stomach

With the developing understanding of the cancer of the stomach the understanding of the lymphatic drainage of the stomach has also improved drastically. The following discussion on lymphatic drainage is in accordance with the latest guidelines for radical lymph node dissection for the gastric cancer (Table 1 and Fig. 5).

- Total gastrectomy
  - D0: Lymphadenectomy less than D1
  - D1: Nos. 1–7
  - D1+: D1+ Nos. 8a, 9, 11p
  - D2: D1 + Nos. 8a, 9, 10, 11p, 11d, 12a.

Table 1: Anatomical definition of lymph node status (Japanese classification of gastric cancer: 3rd edition. 2011)

Station number	*Location*	*Description (lymph nodes along)*
1	Right paracardial	First branch of ascending limb of LGA
2	Left paracardial	Esophagogatstric branch of left subphrenic artery
3a		Branches of LGA
3b		Second branch and distal part of RGA
4sa	Left greater curvature	SGA
4sb	Left greater curvature	LGEA
4d	Right greater curvature	Second branch and distal part of RGEA
5	Suprapyloric	First branch and proximal part of RGA
6	Infrapyloric	First branch and proximal part of RGEA to the confluence of RGEA and ASPDV
7		Trunk of LGA from its origin to ascending branch
8a	Common hepatic	Anterosuperior to CHA
8p	Common hepatic	Posterior to CHA
9	Celiac	Celiac
10	Splenic hilar	Splenic artery at hilum of spleen
11p	Proximal splenic	Origin of splenic artery to halfway of the pancreatic tail end
11d	Distal splenic	From halfway point (above) to end of pancreatic tail

Contd...

Contd...

Station number	*Location*	*Description (lymph nodes along)*
12a	Hepatoduodenal ligament	Proper hepatic artery in caudal half from confluence of RHD and LHD to superior border of pancreas
12b	Hepatoduodenal ligament	Bile duct in caudal half from confluence of RHD and LHD to superior border of pancreas
12p	Hepatoduodenal ligament	Portal vein in caudal half from confluence of RHD and LHD to superior border of pancreas
13		Posterior surface of pancreas cranial to papilla
14v		SMV
15		Middle colic vessels
16a1	Para-aortic	Aortic hiatus
16a2	Para-aortic	Between upper margin of origin of celiac axis and lower border of LRV
16b1	Para-aortic	Between lower border of LRV and upper border of origin of IMA
16b2	Para-aortic	Between upper border of origin of IMA and aortic bifurcation
17		Anterior surface of pancreas beneath sheath
18		Along inferior border of pancreatic body
19	Infradiaphragmatic	Subphrenic artery
20	Paraesophageal	Esophageal hiatus
110	Paraesophageal	Lower thorax
111	Subdiaphragmatic	Separate from esophagus
112	Posterior mediastinal	Separate from esophagus and esophageal hiatus

Abbreviations: LGA, left gastric artery; RGA, right gastric artery; SGA, short gastric artery; LGEA, left gastroepiploic artery; RGEA, right gastroepiploic artery; CHA, common hepatic artery; ASPDV, anterior superior pancreatoduodenal vein; RHD, right hepatic duct; LHD, left hepatic duct; SMV, superior mesenteric vessels; IMV, inferior mesenteric vein; LRV, left renal vein.

- Distal gastrectomy
  - D0: Lymphadenectomy less than D1
  - D1: Nos. 1, 3, 4sb, 4d, 5, 6, 7
  - D1+: D1+ Nos. 8a, 9
  - D2: D1 + Nos. 8a, 9, 11p, 12a.
- Pylorus-preserving gastrectomy
  - D0: Lymphadenectomy less than D1
  - D1: Nos. 1, 3, 4sb, 4d, 6, 7
  - D1+: D1+ Nos. 8a, 9.
- Proximal gastrectomy
  - D0: Lymphadenectomy less than D1
  - D1: Nos. 1, 2, 3a, 4sa, 4sb, 7
  - D1+: D1+ Nos. 8a, 9, 11p.

NERVE SUPPLY

The left and the right vagus nerves accompany the esophagus through the esophageal hiatus in anterior and posterior position respectively. Each trunk then divides into the two divisions. Anterior vagus divides into the hepatic branch which goes toward the liver and another branch which descends along the lesser curvature to go toward the pylorus (the so called anterior nerve of Latarjet). The anterior nerve of Latarjet divides into multiple branches, 10–12 in number in the formation of the Crow's foot.

Posterior vagus gives rise to celiac branch which goes to celiac plexus and posterior branch which supplies the posterior wall of stomach (posterior nerve of Latarjet).

The above presented pattern is the most common at the hiatus but variations do occur which may involve presence of more than two structures at the hiatus. It is important to recognize these patterns during the vagotomy. It should be remembered that during the vagotomy posterior vagus will be seen slightly away from the GEJ but the anterior vagus will be seen onto the wall of the GEJ, sometimes inseparable from the musculature.

During the selective vagotomy one should be vigilant in identifying the criminal nerve of Grassi which is the early posterior branch of the vagus nerve. Failure to divide this nerve leads to incomplete cessation of acid and ulcer recurrence (Fig. 6).

Anatomy of Duodenum

Duodenum is the first, shortest and the widest portion of the small intestine. It is approximately 10–12 inches in length and is subjected to very few variations. It starts at the pyloroduodenal junction and ends at the duodenojejunal flexure. It is mainly a retroperitoneal structure. It is a C shaped structure in the loop of which is located to the head of the pancreas.

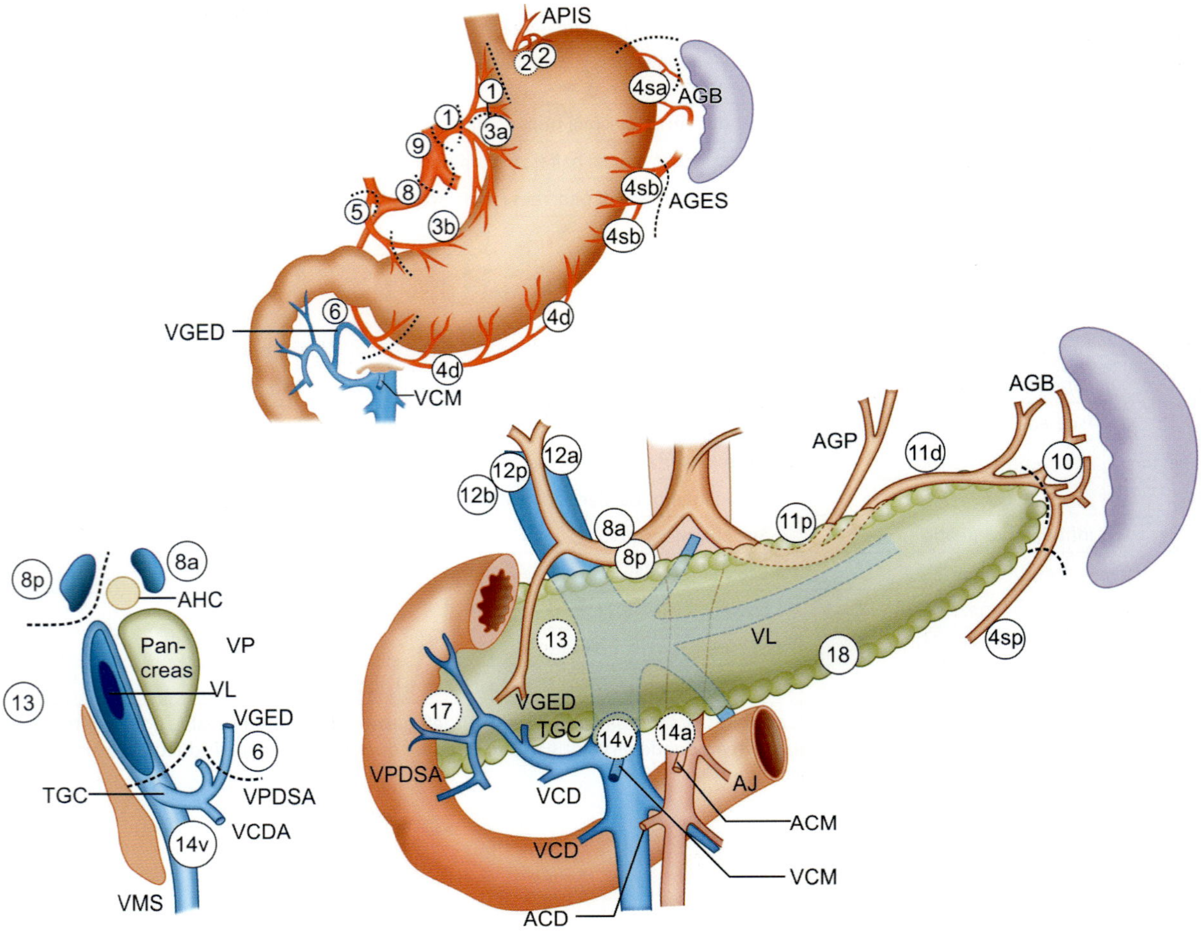

Figure 5 Extent of lymph node dissection required for gastric cancer (Japanese gastric cancer treatment guidelines 2010)

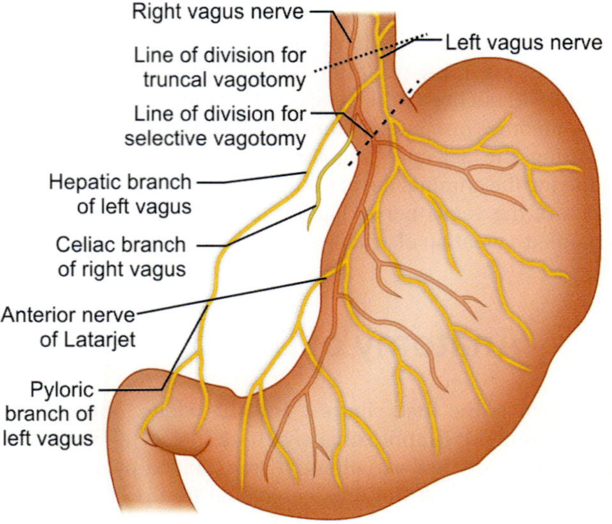

Figure 6 Nerve supply of stomach

Parts of Duodenum

It is divided into four parts (Fig. 7):

First ascending part: It is nearly horizontal and measures approximately 2 inches (~5 cm) and begins at the gastroduodenal junction. It is a relatively mobile portion than any other portion of the duodenum. From the pylorus it ascends upward, laterally and posteriorly to reach the neck of the gall bladder. This portion is completely intraperitoneal. Relations (Fig. 8);

Superiorly: Lesser omentum and the foramen of Winslow
Inferiorly: Head of the pancreas
Anterosuperiorly: Liver, gall bladder
Posterosuperiorly: Common bile duct (CBD), hepatic artery, portal vein and gastroduodenal artery.

Second descending part: It descends almost vertically from the D1 and is approximately 3 inches (~7.5 cm) in length. It reaches up to L3 vertebral level. It is totally retroperitoneal covered anteriorly by the anterior layer of mesocolic peritoneum.

Medially, it is fixed to the head of pancreas by connective tissue. Relations;

Anterior: Transverse colon

Posterior: Common bile duct, right kidney, renal vessels and vena cava

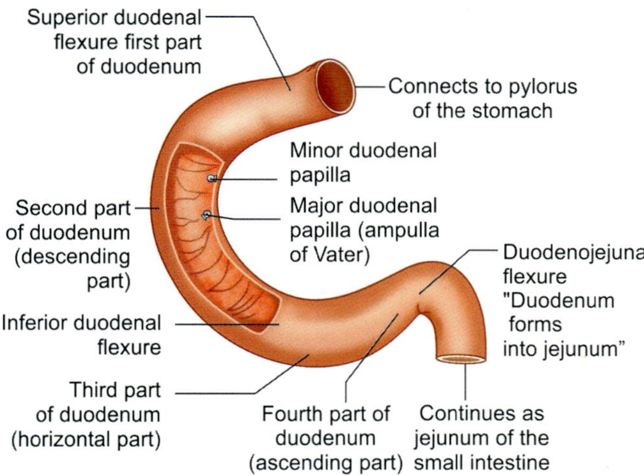

Figure 7 Parts of duodenum

Left: Common bile duct, pancreatic duct, head of the pancreas and superior and inferior pancreaticoduodenal arteries. The CBD and the pancreatic duct travel into the posteromedial wall of the duodenum obliquely and open into the lower portion of D2 at the papilla.

Third part: It the longest, narrowest portion approximately 5 inches (~13 cm) in length. It crosses the midline over the L3 vertebral level from right to left side to end at the level of L2 vertebra. It is also totally retroperitoneal and is covered by descending layer of transverse mesocolon. Relations;

Anterior: Superior mesenteric vessels, jejunum and transverse mesocolon

Posterior: Diaphragmatic crura, vena cava and abdominal aorta

Superior: Superior mesenteric vessels, pancreas and inferior pancreaticoduodenal arteries

Inferior: Mesentery.

Fourth part: It is the shortest part approximately 1 inch (2.5 cm) in length. It ascends from the level of L2 vertebra to the point where the mesentery begins, i.e. at the beginning of the jejunum. It is fixed to the left crus of diaphragm by a connective tissue called as suspensory ligament of Treitz which at times also contain some vessels. This junction of duodenum and jejunum is called as duodenojejunal flexure.

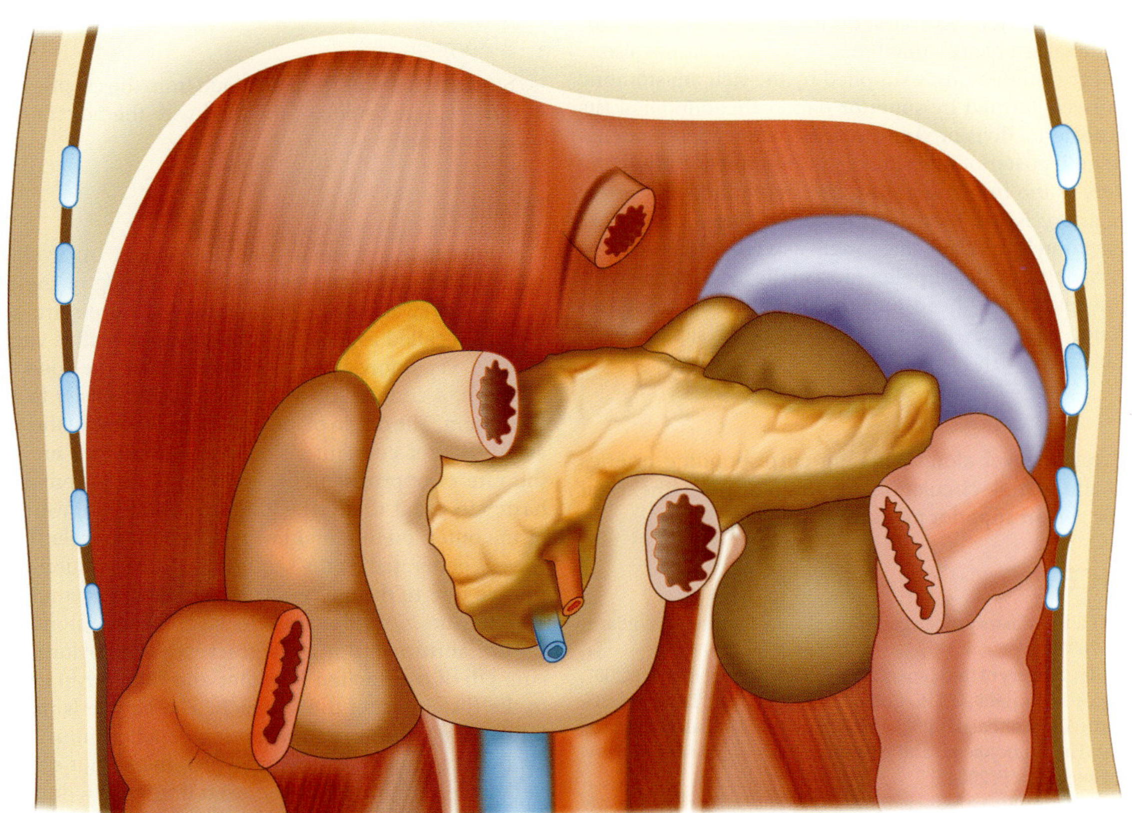

Figure 8 Relations of duodenum

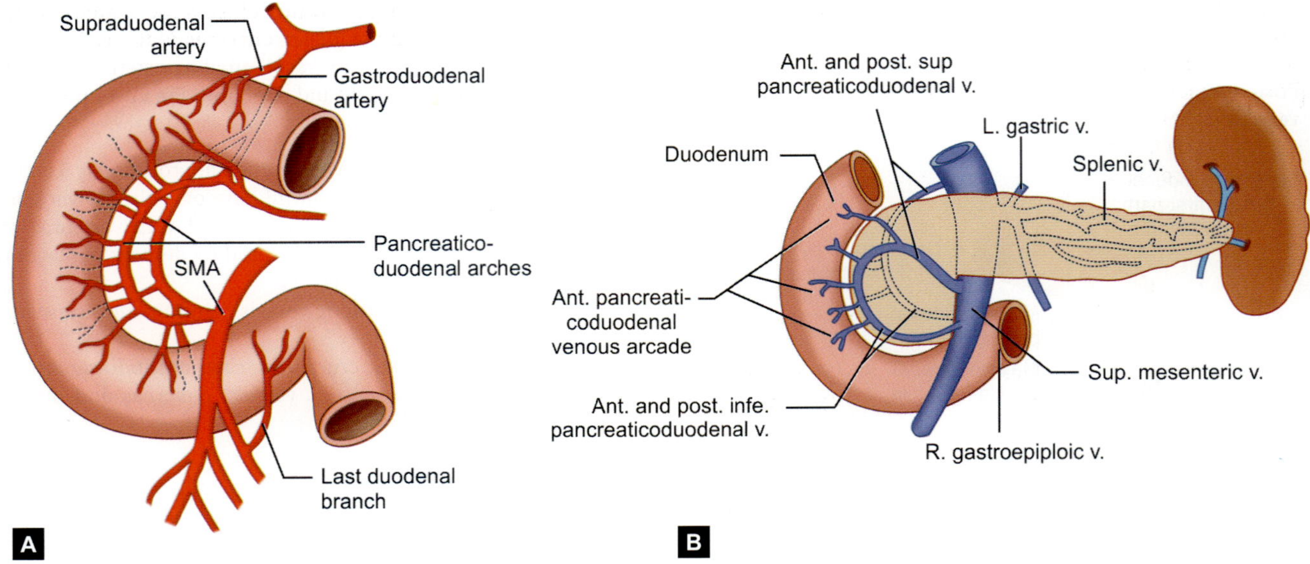

Figures 9A and B Arterial supply and venous drainage of duodenum
Abbreviation: SMA, superior mesenteric artery.

Blood Supply

Arteries

Superior pancreaticoduodenal artery branch of gastroduodenal artery supplies the first part. This artery may arise variably from superior mesenteric artery also. Other arteries supplying this part are supraduodenal artery and sometimes right gastric artery also.

The rest of the duodenum is supplied by the rich anastomotic network of vessels formed by superior pancreaticoduodenal (its anterior and posterior divisions) and inferior pancreaticoduodenal (its anterior and posterior divisions). As described earlier, the superior artery is the branching from the gastroduodenal artery and inferior artery is the branch of superior mesenteric artery either arise separately or divide after origin as a common trunk.

This arterial network also supplies most of the head of pancreas. Therefore, the pancreatic head and duodenum are resected in unison and not separately and resection of either separately is challenging task (Fig. 9A).

Veins

The named veins travel along with the corresponding arteries to end into the portal circulation by draining into the right gastroepiploic vein or superior mesenteric vein (Fig. 9B).

REFERENCES

1. Bland KI (Eds). Mastery of Surgery, 5th edition. Lippincott William-Wilkins; 2007.
2. Yeo CJ (Eds). Surgery of the alimentary tract, 6th edition. Elsevier; 2007.
3. Skandalakis LJ, Skandalakis JE, Colborn GL, Weidman TA, Foster RS, Kingsnorth AN, Skandalakis PN, Mirilas PS (Eds). Skandalakis Surgical Anatomy: The Embryologic and Anatomic Basis of Modern Surgery. Athens, Greece: PMP; 2004.
4. Japanese Gastric Cancer Association. Japanese classification of gastric carcinoma: 3rd English edition. Gastric Cancer. 2011;14:101-12.
5. Japanese Gastric Cancer Association. Japanese gastric cancer treatment guidelines 2010 (ver. 3). Gastric Cancer. 2011;4:113-23.

Physiology of Stomach

All the organs of the gastrointestinal tract (GIT) serve one or more of the following functions:

- Motility
- Secretion
- Absorption

Stomach receives the eaten food from the esophagus and stores it. It helps in digestion of the food with the help of its motor and secretory functions.

Motility

The muscular system of the stomach is involved in storage, mixing, trituration and controlled emptying of the food. At the start of the swallowing stomach musculature starts to relax with a process called as receptive relaxation (which is vagal mediated as after vagotomy it is abolished). After the food reaches the stomach, a contraction wave (called peristalsis) is set in by the distension. The origin of the peristaltic wave is in the fundal region at the greater curvature. The electrical signals are generated at the rate of approximately 3/minutes (the pacemaker potential, basic electrical rhythm).[1] It travels aborally toward the pylorus in the outer longitudinal layer of smooth muscle. The peristaltic wave is generated by the sequential depolarization of the circular muscle due to the successively migrating pacemaker potentials. The thickness of the muscle layer of the stomach increases toward antrum and it is the thickest at the pylorus, likewise the strength of contraction is higher and they travel at higher speed in the distal part of the stomach. The chyme is pushed into the funnel shaped antrum for getting expelled into the duodenum via pylorus (gastric emptying) which relaxes for a very short time to deliver 5–15 mL of chyme each time to the duodenum. Thus, most of the chyme is pushed back to the body of the stomach. This sequential contraction of the stomach leads to breaking down of the food particles into smaller and smaller size. Interstitial cell of

Cajal, located in the muscularis propria are also important for the gastric motility.

The gastric motility is influenced by a variety of stimuli.[2] Vagal reflexes are facilitatory for the peristalsis of the stomach. Gastrin released by the G cells has an inhibitory effect on the gastric emptying. Intrinsic nervous system of the stomach releases a variety of neurotransmitters of which the important inhibitory ones are vasoactive intestinal peptide (VIP) and nitric oxide (NO) and excitatory are neurokinin A, acetylcholine, substance P and tachykinins. Smaller particles are emptied faster, as do the lower osmolar foods.[3] The osmolarity of the gastric contents is sensed by the duodenum which inhibits the emptying (enterogastric reflex), if the osmolarity is higher than 200 mOsm/L.

The volume of the empty stomach is only 50 mL which can go up to 1,000 mL with the coordinated neuromuscular system of the stomach.

Secretion

The structure of a gastric gland should be understood before going on to secretory functions (Fig. 10).

Isthmus is the opening of the gland, lining epithelium is made by the parietal cells and the surface mucus cells. Mucus cells are located at the neck and the parietal and the chief cells are located lower down. Oxyntic glands (acid secreting) are more numerous in the fundus and body region. These glands also contain D cells which secrete somatostatin and enterochromaffin-like cells (ECL cells) which secrete histamine. Mucus-secreting cells are more numerous in the pyloric (antral) glands but also present in sufficient numbers in oxyntic glands. Gastrin is secreted by the pyloric gland G cells. Endocrine cells are scattered throughout the stomach and located at the bases of the glands (Table 2).

Exocrine

It is involved mainly the acid secretion and its control and the mucosal barrier.

Approximately 500 mL-1,000 mL of gastric juice is secreted in the fasting state. After each meal, around 1,000 mL of juices are secreted. The main constituents of the gastric juice are:

Mucus: It is the product of mucus cells of oxyntic and pyloric glands. It is a mixture of glycoproteins and provides a weak barrier from acids to gastric mucosa.

Pepsinogen: It is stored in the chief cells in vesicles in the oxyntic glands. Under the influences of vagal, gastrin and secretin stimuli they are secreted. At a pH less than 5, the precursor molecule gets cleaved and forms the pepsin which cleaves the peptide bonds. It is amongst the three most potent enzymes of the GIT (pepsin, chymotrypsin and trypsin). It is functioning at highest level at pH of 2 and gets denatured at a pH of more than 8.

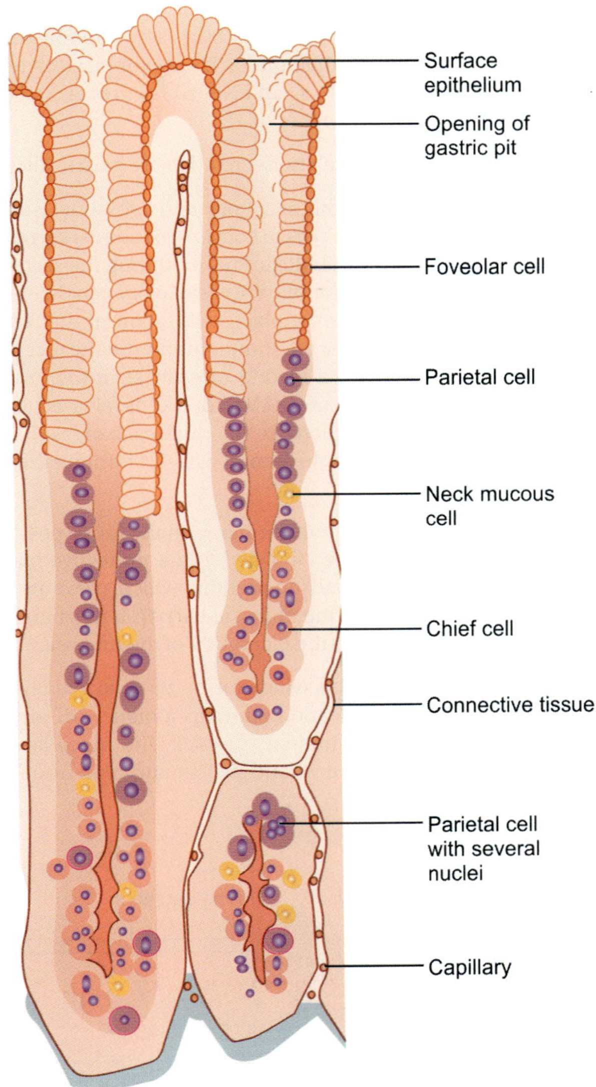

Figure 10 Gastric gland showing the location of various secretory cells

Table 2: Various cells and their location in gastric glands and stomach

Gastric gland	*Cell(s)*	*Location*	*Secretory product*
Isthmus	Mucous cells	Body, pyloric	Mucus gel layer
Body	Parietal (oxyntic) cells	Only body	Intrinsic factor, gastric acid
Base	Chief (zymogenic) cells	Only body	Gastric lipase, pepsinogen
Base	Enteroendocrine (APUD) cells	Body, pyloric	Hormones of GIT(see later)

Abbreviations: APUD, amine precursor uptake and decarboxylation; GIT, gastrointestinal tract.

Intrinsic factor: It is a mucoprotein which helps in absorption of vitamin B_{12} and is secreted by the parietal cells. Its deficiency can lead to pernicious anemia. After gastrectomy due to nonsecretion of it, patient develops vitamin B_{12} deficiency anemia.

Electrolytes: The secretion of the electrolytes is the function of parietal cells which are the major cells which secrete H^+ ions into the gastric lumen. The interplay of the various secretory and inhibitory stimuli on the parietal cells leads to secretion of the hydrochloric acid (HCl) into the lumen. The major electrolytes in the gastric secretion are H^+, Cl^-, K^+ and Na^+ which are regulated by the H^+ K^+ ATPase pump.

Blood group antigens: They are also secreted in the gastric juice.

The gastric acid secretion: Both secretory and inhibitory stimuli interact and signal the parietal cells to control gastric acid secretion. The parietal cells show a morphologic change during the secretion of the acid. After a secretory stimulus, the secretory canaliculus of the parietal cells expand, it is the place of location of the proton pumps which secrete acid. After the stimulants bind at the receptors at the basolateral membrane a second messenger in the form of cyclic adenosine monophosphate (cAMP) or Ca^{2+} is released which binds to the proton pump and activates it, which exchanges H^+ with K^+ with H^+ being secreted into the lumen with Cl^- forming the HCl (Fig. 11).[4]

The mucosal barrier: The pH in the lumen is in the range of 1-2, at this pH the mucosa should be damaged, but a protective barrier is present in the stomach and duodenum which prevents this from occurring, it is called as the mucosal barrier. If this barrier is somehow disturbed it leads to the ulceration of the mucosa.

Mucus: It is gel of glycoproteins which forms an unstirred layer at the surface of gastric mucosa and maintains a higher pH around the mucosal cells than the luminal pH of 2. The outer layer is persistently degraded by the acid and pepsin and replenished by the mucus cells. The mucus secretion is enhanced by the acid in the lumen, cholinergic stimuli and prostaglandin E_2.

Figure 11 Acid secretion
Abbreviations: PGE_2, prostaglandin E_2; ATP, adenosine triphosphate; AMP, adenosine monophosphate.

Bicarbonate: In addition to the mucus, the secretion of HCO_3^- probably mediated by the prostaglandins; also plays a part in the mucosal barrier. It is stimulated by glucagon, cholecystokinin (CCK) and prostaglandins. It is inhibited by nonsteroidal anti-inflammatory drugs (NSAIDs), alcohol and bile acids.

Restitution is the process by which the adjacent cells migrate and rapidly replace the sloughed or denuded surface epithelial cells.

Oxygen and nutrients for cellular functions, involved in protection of cell, are provided by the mucosal blood flow.

Bombesin, a neurohormonal peptide is also involved in mucosal protection. It is secreted from noncholinergic afferents in response to stimuli like capscacin and increases the prostaglandin levels.[5]

The duodenal mucosa has a similar protective mechanism. It also receives highly alkaline secretion from the pancreas which also helps neutralize the acidic contents received (Fig. 12).

The regulation of the acid secretion:[6,7,8] Gastric acid has certain important functions to perform as activation of pepsinogen to facilitate protein digestion, facilitating vitamin B_{12} absorption. It also helps killing harmful bacteria. But how is it controlled? It is

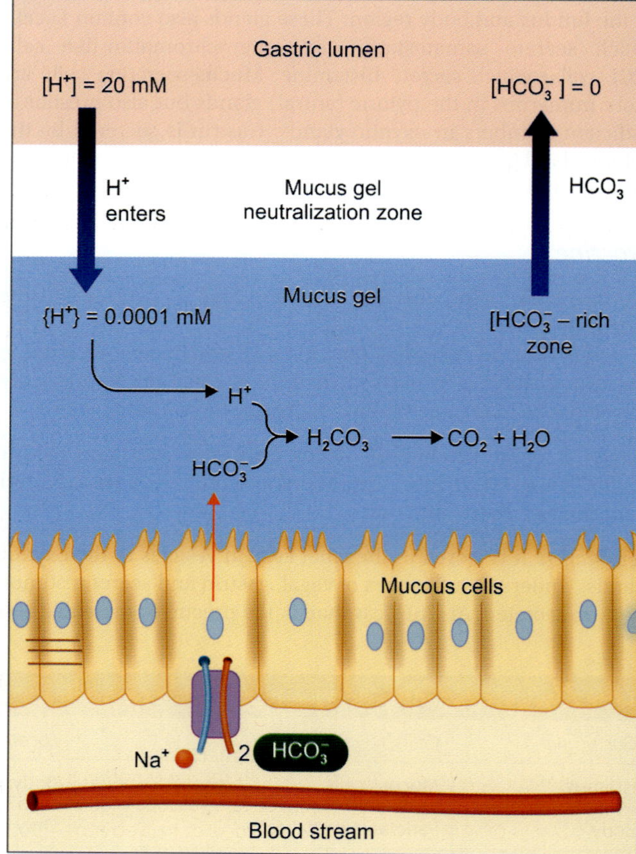

Figure 12 Pathway for mucosal barrier

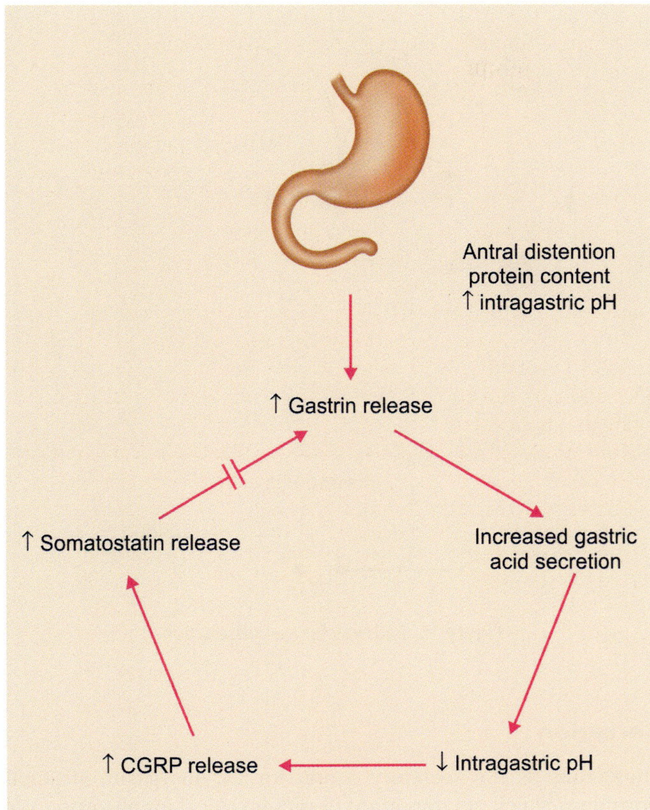

Figure 13 Negative feedback loop for acid control
Abbreviation: CGRP, calcitonin gene-related peptide.

the interplay of the various stimulating and inhibiting pathways (Fig. 13).

Interprandial basal acid secretion is 2 to 5 mEq of HCl per hour. It makes about 10% of total maximal acid output. It is more at nighttime. Low bacterial count of stomach is due to basal acid secretion. There is up to 90% decrease in secretion after vagotomy or H2 receptor blockade.

Stimulation of gastric secretion (three phases)	*Inhibition of gastric secretion*
Cephalic phase: This phase is initiated at the cranial level with the sight, smell or even thought of food. It is mediated by vagus as after vagotomy it is abolished. *Gastric phase:* Food in the stomach causes gastrin release from antrum. Distension also gets gastrin released (via intramural cholinergics). Histamine mediates majority of acid stimulatory effects of gastrin and acetylcholine. ECL cells release histamine. *Intestinal phase:* Food in the intestinal lumen releases entero-oxyntin which stimulates the acid secretion.	*Antral inhibition:* Gastrin secretion starts getting inhibited with a pH of less than 2.5 in the antrum and completely inhibited at a pH of 1.2 with any stimulus. Somatostatin in the antral cells (D cells) is the physiologic inhibitor of gastrin release. *Intestinal inhibition:* After the acidic food reaches the intestine, it inhibits gastrin secretion by release of hormones now labelled as enterogastrone. Secretin does not block acid secretion in physiologic conditions.

Endocrine

Gastrin: Antral G cells produce gastrin. It is the major stimulant of gastric acid secretion. G17 is the major form of gastrin (others are G34 and G71). Its secretion is stimulated by luminal peptides and amino acids. Its most potent inhibitor is luminal acid (which acts in paracrine manner through somatostatin). Gastrin is trophic factor for parietal cells and enterochromaffin cells.

Somatostatin: D cells of antral mucosa secrete somatostatin. Inhibited secretions are histamine release, acid secretion and gastrin. It controls acid secretion in a paracrine manner. Gastrin releasing peptide (GRP) stimulates its release in feedback manner.[9]

Ghrelin: It is a potent secretagogue of pituitary growth hormone. It is orexigenic hormone, i.e. it increases appetite when at high levels. It increases gastric motility and shows resemblance to motilin. It is thought to be secreted from the endocrine cells in the fundus and body, particularly oxyntic glands and its levels are suppressed after sleeve gastrectomies and gastric bypass.[10]

Absorption

Main absorptive functions are done by the small intestine, certain products are absorbed in the stomach, such as drugs, like aspirin, alcohol (a part of it) and few amino acids. The acidic environment provided by the stomach aids in the absorption of calcium and iron. The intrinsic factor secreted by stomach aids in absorption of the vitamin B_{12}.

How do all these physiologic processes integrate?

In the mouth during chewing the food is mixed with salivary amylase and reaches stomach. The stimulation of gastric acid is initiated. Gastrin levels increase and peak at 30 minutes after meal. Acidity cleaves the pepsinogen to active pepsin which initiates the protein digestion. The food is broken down into smaller particles and mixes thoroughly by the coordinated motility of the stomach. In the stomach protein digestion is only ~10% complete but carbohydrate digestion is ~40% complete. Fat digestion is almost minimal. Volume, texture, acidity and osmolality of the meal determine the rate at which gastric contents are sent to the duodenum.

PHYSIOLOGY OF DUODENUM

Absorption

The duodenum is the major site for absorption of Calcium (Ca) and Iron (Fe). It also furthers the breakdown of the food products.

Calcium Absorption

The Ca absorption is influenced by the renal, cutaneous and bony systems. The duodenum is the major site of absorption which can actively absorb 80–100% of the Ca intake. Some Ca is also passively absorbed by the jejunum. Vitamin D is the major controller of the Ca absorption. Through the receptors it can change Ca levels within minutes. As said earlier that there is passive absortpiton in the small intestine which occurs through the paracellular pathway which is concentration gradient dependent and ensures absorption in the absence of vitamin D (Fig. 14).

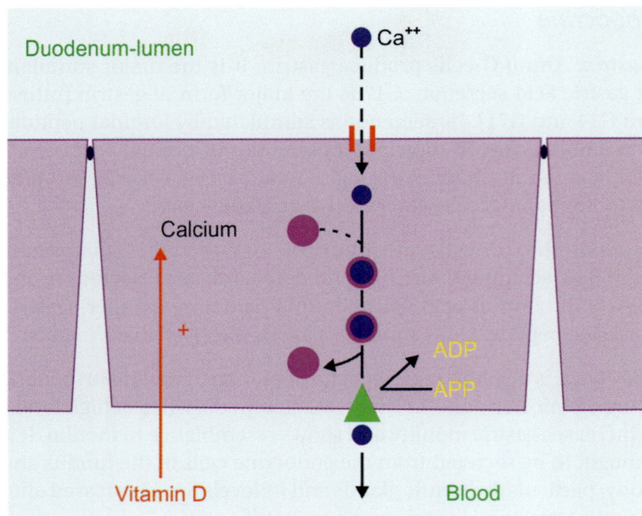

Figure 14 Pathway for calcium absorption

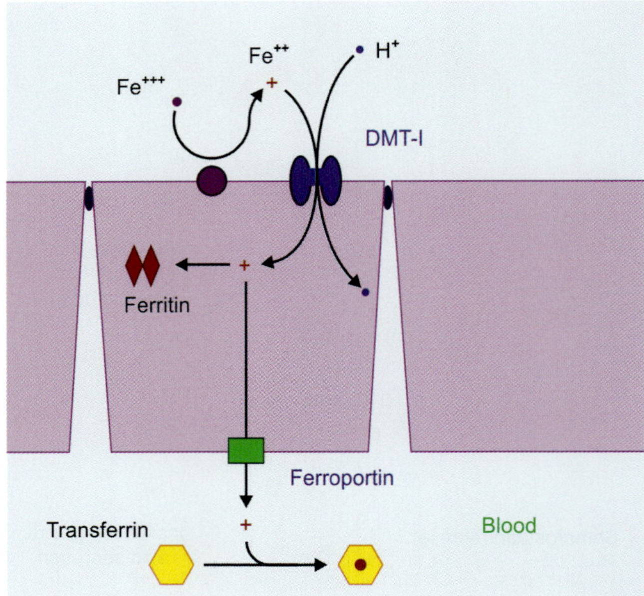

Figure 15 Pathway for iron absorption

Iron Absorption

Nearly all of the dietary iron is absorbed by the duodenum. This includes absorption from heme (10%) and nonheme (90%) dietary sources. Heme iron which is the most bioavailable form is absorbed with the help of a membrane bound protein. It can be directly available as heme or can be successively processed intracellularly before being released into blood stream as reduced form. The absorption of iron is directly reduced by the increases in gastric acidity, high fiber diet and caffeine consumption. *Helicobacter pylori* can produce atrophic gastritis and hence to iron deficiency anemia (Fig. 15).

Carbohydrate Absorption

Once in duodenum, chyme mixes with pancreatic enzyme alpha amylase which cleaves carbohydrates into maltose, maltotriose and alpha limit dextrins. These sugar forms are further broken down at brush border of jejunum into glucose, fructose and galactose for absorption by different glucose transporters.

Protein Absorption

Protein cleavage starts in the stomach. Trypsin (activated trypsinogen) activates pancreatic enzymes in duodenum which further cleaves the protein in dipeptide or tripeptide forms which are absorbed in duodenum and upper jejunum. Up to 50% of protein is absorbed in the duodenum.

Fat Absorption

Pancreatic lipase (activated by CCK) leads to hydrolysis of lipids in the duodenum. Biliary phospholipids are hydrolyzed by phospholipase A_2. Bile emulsifies the fat and forms micelles and liposomes which when come in contact with brush border get absorbed. Most fat is absorbed in duodenum and upper jejunum.

Secretion

Duodenum is the secretory center for various gastrointestinal hormones which are important or rather critical for absorption of nutrients and motility.

The major gastrointestinal hormones secreted by the duodenum are as follows (Figs 16A to C):

- Gastrin: Secreted from G cells of duodenum and antrum. It is stimulated by GRP, distension of antrum, vagal and adrenergic stimulation, amino acids and proteins. It stimulates secretion of acid and pepsinogen in stomach.
- Cholecystokinin: Secreted from I cells of jejunum and duodenum. Its secretion is stimulated by amino acids, peptides and fats. It stimulates contraction of gall bladder and relaxes sphincter of Oddi. It stimulates pancreatic enzyme secretion. It is one of potent inhibitors of gastric emptying.
- Secretin: Secreted by S cells of duodenum and jejunum. It is stimulated by bile salts and fatty acids. Acidity of the lumen also stimulates its secretion. It causes release of water and bicarbonate from pancreas. It increases the flow of bile. It inhibits gastric acid secretion and gastrin. Motility is also inhibited.
- Somatostatin: Secreted by D cells of duodenum, antrum and pancreatic islets. In the gut, fats, acid and protein stimulate its secretion. Other hormones also stimulate it. In pancreas glucose, CCK and amino acids stimulate its secretion. It is universal off switch inhibiting release of hormones, gastric acid, pancreatic hormones secretion and water and electrolytes from small bowel.
- Gastric inhibitory peptide: Secreted by K cells of duodenum and jejunum. It is stimulated by adrenergic stimulation, fats, protein and glucose. It inhibits gastric acid and pepsin secretion. It stimulates insulin secretion.

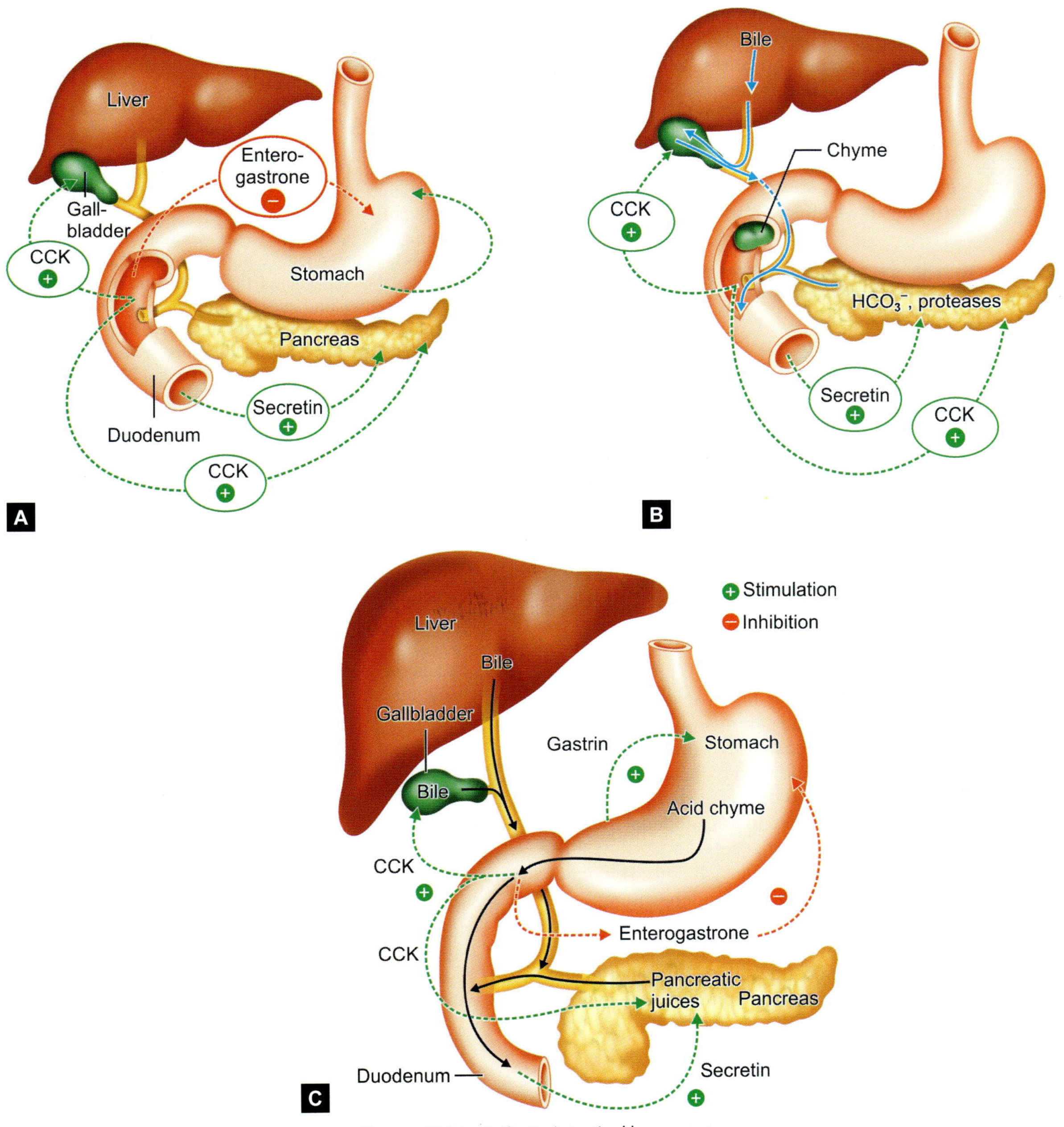

Figures 16A to C Gastrointestinal hormones
Abbreviations: cholecystokinin; HCO_3^-, bicarbonate.

- Motilin: Secreted by duodenum and jejunum. It is stimulated by fat and distension of stomach. It initiates migrating motor complex. Stimulates upper GIT motility. Erythromycin exerts its prokinetic effects through motilin receptors.
- Vasoactive intestinal peptide: It is secreted throughout the GIT in response to vagal stimulation. It is a neuropeptide. It is a potent vasodilator and stimulates pancreatic and intestinal secretions. It inhibits gastric acid secretion.

Other important neurotransmitters that are secreted by the duodenum are serotonin and NO. Serotonin relaxes stomach and enhances intestinal motility. Nitric oxide relaxes the smooth muscles of stomach and small intestine. It also actively regulates the tone of lower esophageal sphincter.

Motility

As with other parts of the GIT, the duodenal motility is regulated by the neural system (both intrinsic and extrinsic) and, endocrine and paracrine mechanisms.

The intrinsic neural system of duodenum has autonomous electric pacemaker which generates signal such as to provide propagation velocity of ~15 cm/minutes which is higher than the jejuna speed hence resulting in net propulsion to the jejunum.

The extrinsic nervous system comprises of sympathetic innervations from the celiac and superior mesenteric ganglia. This innervation is mainly inhibitory. Because of both excitatory and inhibitory neuronal connections vagus nerve exhibits a variety of responses. Such as in stomach it stimulates acid secretion and in duodenum it inhibits motility.

Various neurohormones have effect on the motility as follows (Table 3):

Table 3: Neurohormones and their effects on intestinal motility

	Stimulatory	*Inhibitory*
Neurohormones	Acetylcholine	Calcitonin gene regulated peptide
	Bombesin	Peptide YY
	Cholecystokinin	Neurotensin
	Motilin	Vasoactive intestinal peptide
	Serotonin	Secretin
	Substance P	Somatostatin
	Gastrin-releasing peptide	

Mucosal Defense

The chime received from the stomach is highly acidic which can damage the duodenal mucosa. Alkalinization is one of the major functions of the duodenum. Various mechanisms are involved in this. The foremost is the bicarbonate secretion. With the acidic contents in the duodenal lumen, a number of products are activated which in turn increase the secretion of bicarbonate in the duodenal mucosa, pancreas and liver. These compounds are secretin, vasoactive VIP, melatonin, motilin and vagally produced acetylcholine. The major component is bicarbonate secretion from the duodenal bulb.

Certain other mechanisms are also present like mucus secretion and increased blood flow. Enteroglucagon, calcitonin gene-related peptide and NO increase the blood flow. With interplay of the cyclooxygenase activity mucus production is increased by goblet and Brunner's glands. The thickened mucosal coat buffers the duodenum helping small amount of bicarbonate neutralize a large amount of gastric acid.

REFERENCES

1. van Halden DF, Layer Dr, Holdsworth J et al. Generation and propagation of gastric slow waves. Clin Exp Pharmacol Physiol 37:516,2010.
2. Henning JW, Brookes SJ, Costa M: Excitatory and inhibitory motor reflexes in isolated guinea pig stomach. J Physiol 501:197,1996.
3. Camilleri M, Malagelada JR, Brown ML et al. Relation between antral motility and gastric emptying of solids and liquids in humans. Am J Physiol Gastrointest Liver Physiol 249:G580,1985.
4. Athmann C, Zeng N, Scott DR, Sachs G: Regulation of parietal cell calcium signaling in gastric glands. Am J Physiol 279:G1048,2000.
5. Gyries K. Neuropeptides and gastric mucosal homeostasis. Curr Top Med Chem 4:63,2004.
6. Schubert ML, Peura Da: Control of gastric acid secretion in health and disease. Gastroenterology 134:1842,2008.
7. Katschinski M: Nutritional implications of cephalic phase gastrointestinal responses. Appetite 34:189,2000.
8. Schiller LR, Walsh Jh, Feldman M: Distention induced gastrin release: effects of luminal acidification and intravenous atropine. Gastroenterology 78:912,1980.
9. Makhlouf GM, Schubert ML: Gastric somatostatin: A paracrine regulator of gastric acid secretion. Metabolism 39:138,1990.
10. Ariyasu H, Takaya K, Tagami T et al: Stomach is a major source of circulating ghrelin, and feeding state determines plasma ghrelin like immunoreactivity levels in humans. J Clin Endocrinol Metab 86:4753,2001.

BIBLIOGRAPHY

1. Barrett KE, Susan MB et al Eds. Ganong's Review of Medical Physiology, 24th e. McGrawHill, 2012.
2. Doherty G. CURRENT Diagnosis and Treatment Surgery, 13th e. McGrawHill, 2009.
3. Townsend CM, Beauchamp RD Eds. Sabiston Textbook of Surgery. The biological basis of modern surgical practice. 19th e. Elseivier, 2012.
4. Yeo CJ, Matthews JB et al Eds. Shackelford's Surgery of the Alimentary Tract, 6th e. Saunders, 2006.

CHAPTER 24

Surgery for Peptic Ulcer Disease

Vikram Kate, R Kalayarasan, TP Elamurugan, N Ananthakrishnan

INTRODUCTION

Peptic ulcer disease (PUD) is one of the common gastrointestinal disorders which shows striking geographical variations in incidence and prevalence. The understanding of its pathogenesis and treatment changed significantly with the discovery of *Helicobacter pylori (H. pylori)* by Warren and Marshall in 1982.[1] While the incidence of PUD has decreased in the developed countries, it remains a problem in developing countries primarily due to the differences in the prevalence of *H. pylori* infection.[2] In a recent Indian study a reduction in the overall frequency of PUD was noted in the last two decades, the decline more marked in duodenal ulcer compared to gastric ulcer.[3] However, worldwide, complications related to PUD still remain high possibly related to wide use of ulcerogenic drugs such as non-steroidal anti-inflammatory drugs (NSAIDs) and selective serotonin reuptake inhibitors.[4] With the advent of effective medical treatment there has been a marked decrease in the rate of elective surgery for PUD; however, its effect on emergency surgery has been less dramatic.[5] Even in the authors' experience, the frequency of elective surgery for peptic ulcer declined over a three decade period (1970-2000) by nearly 90%, whereas surgery for peptic ulcer perforation increased by about 20%. Patients with past history of surgery for PUD can present with long-term complications like anastomotic ulcer perforation, gastrojejunocolic fistula or rarely retrograde jejunogastric intussusception. Hence, knowledge of the surgical management for PUD is important for all gastrointestinal surgeons. In this chapter we describe the surgical options for management of PUD with an emphasis on emergency surgery for the management of PUD complications.

HISTORY AND EVOLUTION OF PEPTIC ULCER SURGERY

"Those who don't know history are destined to repeat it"

— Edmund Burke (1729-1797)

The first operative treatment for PUD was performed in 1881 by Rydygier who resected the pylorus in a patient with gastric outlet obstruction (GOO).[6,7] In 1882, Kriege performed suture closure of a perforated duodenal ulcer. Gastric resection for ulcer was popularized by Billroth who initially described the reconstruction by gastroduodenostomy in 1881 (Billroth I) and subsequently the antecolic gastrojejunostomy (Billroth II).[8,9] Gastroenterostomy for an uncomplicated gastric ulcer was first introduced in 1893 by Codivilla.[10] Loop gastrojejunostomy was a popular procedure in the late 19th century and early 20th century since it was associated with less morbidity. However, in the 1920s surgeons realized that 50% of patients who underwent isolated gastrojejunostomy developed marginal ulceration secondary to hypergastrinemia which occurs as a result of antral alkalinization (from enterogastric reflux).[6,7,10] In 1918, Phemister introduced subtotal gastrectomy (two-thirds distal gastrectomy) for the management of PUD and suggested that this decreased marginal ulceration by reducing acid.[10] This surgery was popular till mid 1900s when it was realized that the problems created by the gastric resection were greater than the PUD for which the operation had been originally done. In 1943, Dragstedt and colleagues proposed truncal vagotomy (TV) for PUD which had lower morbidity than distal gastrectomy and lower recurrence rate compared to gastrojejunostomy.[11,12] Vagotomy caused an 85% decrease in basal acid output and a 50% decrease in maximal acid output. Initially TV was performed through the transthoracic route. However, as one-third of patients developed gastric stasis secondary to antral denervation, the transabdominal route with an added drainage procedure (gastrojejunostomy or pyloroplasty) was adopted. Heineke-Mikulicz pyloroplasty was first described by Heineke (1881) and Mikulicz (1888) as a procedure in which the pylorus was opened longitudinally and closed transversely in two layers.[6,7] Later in 1951, Weinberg and associates modified two layers closure to a single layer suturing. This was done to reduce in folding of excessive tissue and thus to decrease postoperative gastric stasis.[13] While vagotomy and drainage was a safe alternative it was associated with an ulcer recurrence rate of 10% and various long-term postoperative complications like dumping and diarrhea. In 1957 Griffith and Harkins introduced selective vagotomy in which vagal fibers are divided from the anterior vagus distal to the origin of the hepatic and from the posterior vagus distal to the celiac branches.[14] This operation was done to avoid the side effects due to denervation of the extra gastric viscera. Since antral fibers are denervated in selective vagotomy a drainage procedure was still obligatory. Soon it was recognized that drainage procedure rather than the vagotomy was the cause of most of the difficulties following vagotomy and drainage. Since selective vagotomy was technically demanding it soon went out of favor.

To avoid a drainage procedure, proximal gastric vagotomy or highly selective vagotomy (HSV) was introduced in 1957.[15] Vagal fibers to the portion of stomach that controlled gastric emptying was preserved whereas the nerves that controlled acid secretion are divided. Preganglionic efferent vagal fibers reach the parietal cell mass in stomach in seven different surgical sites (Fig. 1). In the extended HSV described by Donahue and colleagues all seven sites except site 5 are routinely divided since nerves at site 5 cannot be divided without sacrificing blood supply to the proximal stomach.[16] Routine intraoperative testing for the completeness of vagotomy was also performed. However, in the more commonly performed HSV, described by two separate groups, Johnston and Wilkinson and Amdrup and Jensen in 1970, only areas 1–4 are routinely divided.[7] Although HSV avoided a drainage procedure it had a higher rate of recurrent ulcer than the other procedures and was surgeon dependent. In the 1970s, TV and antrectomy became the procedure of choice as it abolished both cephalic and gastric phase of acid secretion and had the least ulcer recurrence rate. It was labeled as the gold standard surgical procedure for ulcer disease.[17] However, antrectomy was technically difficult in patients with excessive scarring of the duodenum and these patients experienced both vagotomy and gastrectomy related complications. Efforts were made to simplify the complex procedure of HSV while maintaining its benefits. Taylor described a modified HSV in which anterior seromyotomy was combined with posterior TV.[18]

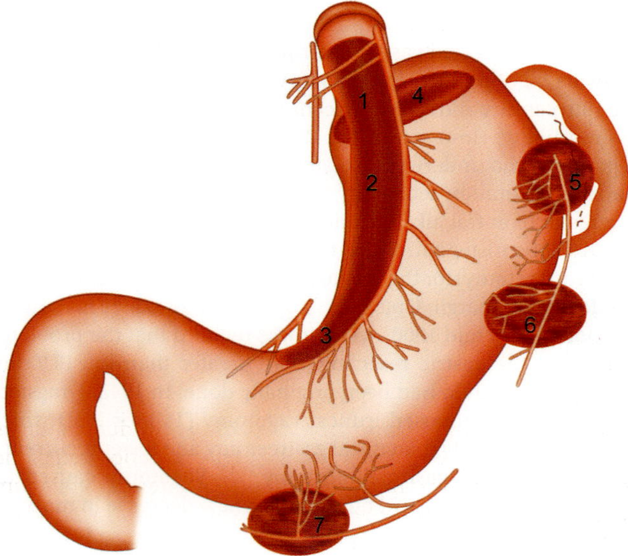

Figure 1 Seven surgical sites where preganglionic efferent vagal nerves enter the parietal cell mass

In the late 20th century with the advent of laparoscopic surgery and a description of modified HSV (Taylor's procedure) which was ideally suited for laparoscopic surgery there was a renewed interest in HSV. Soon minimally invasive surgery was used for the management of PUD complications like perforation and GOO. Current indications for elective surgery in PUD are restricted to ulcers where malignancy cannot be ruled out with certainty and PUD refractory to medical therapy. In the present era majority of the surgeries are performed for the management of complications of PUD which include bleeding, perforation and GOO.

ELECTIVE SURGERY FOR PEPTIC ULCER DISEASE

The choice of surgical procedure depends upon the location (gastric or duodenal) and type of ulcer. An ideal surgery for PUD should permit ulcer healing, prevent ulcer related complications and correct the underlying etiology with minimal postoperative complications. However, none of the surgery described for PUD fulfills all the criteria and the decision making depends upon the type of the ulcer and patient related factors.

Surgery for Intractable Duodenal Ulcer

Intractable duodenal ulcer is defined as an ulcer which does not heal after *H. pylori* eradication and complete course of PPI for a period of 8–12 weeks.[6] This also includes patients who are *H. pylori* negative and have not responded to the conventional antisecretory therapy. However, before contemplating surgery it is necessary that in patients with *H. pylori* infection, *H. pylori* eradication is conclusively achieved. Temporary suppression of the organism following first line therapy for *H. pylori* can result into a negative test which may later become positive due to recrudescence of *H. pylori* infection.[19,20] In these patients the appropriate rescue therapy for *H. pylori* should be used to achieve eradication.[19] Since gastric acid hypersecretion plays an important role in the pathogenesis of duodenal ulcer, an acid reduction procedure is recommended for the treatment. Surgical options include:

- TV with drainage procedure
- HSV
- TV with antrectomy

Of these, TV with antrectomy is associated with the least ulcer recurrence rate of 0–2%, and HSV has the maximum ulcer recurrence rate of 10–15%.[6] The ulcer recurrence rate with TV and drainage is approximately 10%; moreover in 10–15% it is associated with significant complications secondary to drainage procedure.

Table 1: Randomized controlled trials comparing surgical procedures for the management of PUD

Surgical procedures compared	*Author*	*Year*	*Number of patients*	*Duration of follow-up (years)*	*Results (p value)*	*Conclusion*
HSV with TV and antrectomy	Dorricott et al.[21]	1978	116 vs. 106	1	Ulcer recurrence rate 4.3% vs 1% (NS) Good functional outcome (Visick grades I and II) 82% vs 56% (<0.05)	HSV produced good functional outcome in spite of high recurrence rate
	De Vries et al.[22]	1983	71 vs 74	7	Ulcer recurrence rate 9.9% vs 1.4% (<0.05) Excellent functional outcome (Visick grade I) 33% vs 17% (<0.05)	HSV is associated with high recurrence rate; however, it is associated with excellent functional outcome
HSV with Taylor procedure	Oostvogel et al.[23]	1988	43 vs 48	2	Ulcer recurrence rate 9.3% vs 8.7% (NS) Good functional outcome (Visick grades I and II) 84% vs 89% (NS)	Taylor procedure is as good as HSV for the treatment of refractory duodenal ulcer
	Wallia et al.[24]	1994	50 vs 50	3–8	Ulcer recurrence rate 14% vs 12% (NS) Good functional outcome (Visick grades I and II) 76% vs 76% (NS)	Taylor procedure is as good as HSV for the treatment of refractory duodenal ulcer
HSV with Billroth I gastrectomy	Reid et al.[31]	1982	26 vs 30	8	Ulcer recurrence rate 23.1% vs 16.7% (NS) Symptomatic result (Visick grading III or more) 0 vs. 26.67% (<0.05)	No difference in ulcer recurrence rate; however, symptomatic result better with HSV
	Emås et al.[32]	1994	16 vs 14	10	Ulcer recurrence rate 18.8% vs 14.3% (NS) Symptomatic result (Visick grading III or more) 25% vs 28.6% (NS)	No difference in ulcer recurrence rate, or symptomatic results

Abbreviations: HSV, highly selective vagotomy; TV, truncal vagotomy; NS, not significant.

Therefore TV with drainage procedure is no longer recommended for the management of intractable duodenal ulcer.

Two RCTs comparing HSV with TV and antrectomy reported that while HSV is associated with a higher recurrence rate, it is associated with less long-term complications (Table 1).[21,22] Functional outcomes were assessed using Visick grading which includes 5 grades: grade 1—no gastric symptoms, grade 2—mild symptoms easily controlled by adjustment of diet or way of life, grade 3—mild symptoms not controlled by care, but not interfering with life or work, grade 4—symptoms as bad as before operation and interfering with life or work and grade 5—symptoms worse than before operation and incapacitating. Good functional outcome (Visick Grade I & II) was reported in these trials with both HSV and TV with antrectomy.[21,22] However, as these trials were carried out in the pre *H. pylori* era, the effect of *H. pylori* eradication on the surgical outcome (ulcer recurrence) of these procedures is not known. One practical consideration is that in the present era, experience with HSV is limited. Taylor's procedure could overcome this potential limitation. The two RCTs which compared HSV with Taylor's procedure showed equivalent results in terms of ulcer recurrence and functional outcome (Table 1).[23,24] Hence the recommended surgical procedure for patients with intractable duodenal ulcer is HSV or the Taylor procedure. If experience with these is a limiting factor, TV with antrectomy can be done.

Management of Difficult Duodenal Stump

Closure of the duodenal stump may be difficult in patients with refractory large duodenal ulcer undergoing a Billroth II reconstruction and there is a possibility of duodenal stump blowout. Since duodenal stump blowout is associated with high morbidity and mortality, a few techniques have been described for the management of difficult duodenal stump:

- Nissen's closure
- Bancroft's closure
- Tube duodenostomy
- Roux-en-Y limb closure.

Nissen's closure is used in patients with large, penetrating, posterior duodenal ulcers.[25,26] The posterior duodenal wall is separated sharply from the proximal two-thirds of the ulcer and no attempt is made to excise the ulcer. Following transection of anterior duodenum, the anterior wall of the duodenum is sutured to the distal edge of the ulcer and the posterior wall of the duodenum. Then a seromuscular fold of the anterior duodenum was sutured to the proximal edge of ulcer crater. To minimize the tension along suture line a Kocher maneuver is carried out (Figs 2A to C).

Bancroft's closure is used when surgeon is committed to antrectomy but scarring prevents mobilization of the pylorus and

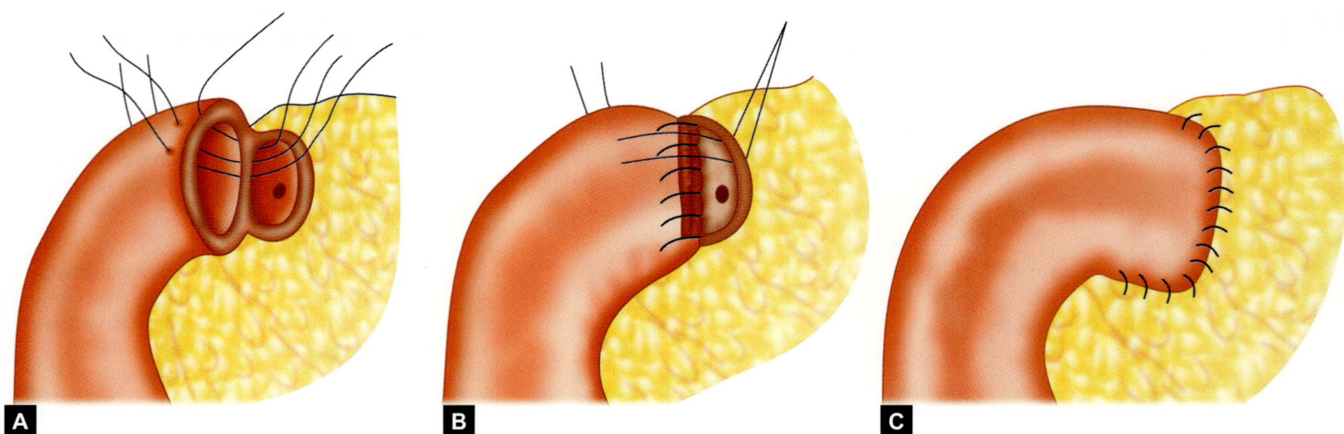

Figures 2A to C Technique of Nissen's closure for management of difficult duodenal stump: (A) anterior wall of the duodenum is sutured to the distal edge of the ulcer and the posterior wall of the duodenum; (B) seromuscular fold of the anterior duodenum sutured to the proximal edge of ulcer crater; (C) completed seromuscular sutures

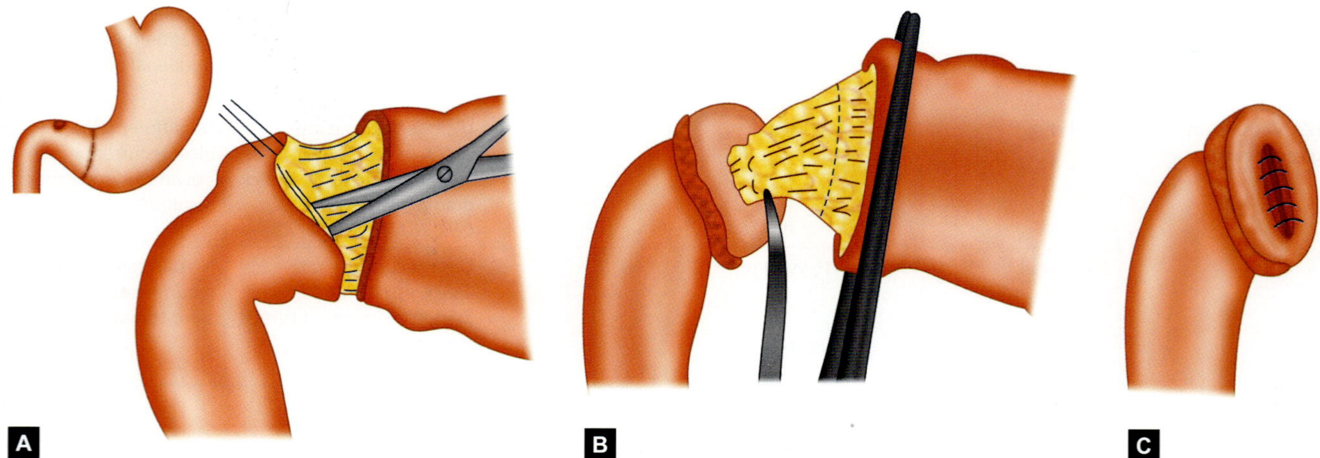

Figures 3A to C Technique of Bancroft's closure for management of difficult duodenal stump: (A) plane is created between the submucosa and muscular layer at the level of distal antrum; (B) dissection of the entire pylorus completed and the entire dissected gastric mucosa is excised; (C) duodenal mucosa and submucosa closed with a running absorbable suture and then closure of the duodenum is completed with a non-absorbable suture of the trimmed antral muscle

duodenal bulb.[25,27] The decision for Bancroft's closure should be taken before ligating the right gastric and right gastroepiploic arteries as they provide blood supply to the preserved distal antrum. In this technique a plane is created between the submucosa and muscular layer at the level of distal antrum and the dissection is carried toward the pylorus till the duodenum is reached. The entire dissected gastric mucosa is excised and the frozen section of distal margin done to confirm duodenal mucosa. The mucosa and submucosa of duodenum is then secured with continuous absorbable suture. The excess antral muscle is trimmed and the closure completed with a non-absorbable suture (Figs 3A to C).

For tube duodenostomy a 16/18 F Foley's catheter is placed in the cut end of duodenum and fixed using purse string suture.[28] The junction of tube and the duodenum is buttressed with a viable omental pedicle. An alternative to tube duodenostomy is to use two nasogastric tubes, one placed in the stomach proximal to the gastrojejunal anastomosis.[29] The duodenal stump is decompressed by placing a second nasogastric tube across the anastomosis, through the afferent jejunal loop with its tip in the second part of the duodenum (Figs 4A to C).

In Roux-en-Y limb closure the jejunum is anastomosed to the duodenum in an end to side or side-to-side fashion.[25] Side-to-side duodenojejunostomy is used in patients with a giant duodenal ulcer penetrating into pancreas head. In a recent study the Roux-en-Y limb closure was found to be superior to the Nissen's closure.[30]

Surgery for Intractable Gastric Ulcer

Surgery for intractable gastric ulcer depends upon the type of gastric ulcer. Johnson originally classified gastric ulcers into three types based on the location, gastric acid hypersecretion and association with duodenal ulcers. Csendes et al. added a fourth type for ulcers located high along lesser curve. Subsequently NSAID related ulcers were classified as Type V gastric ulcers. The modified Johnson classification is summarized in Table 2.[6]

Table 2: Modified Johnson classification of gastric ulcers

Type	*Location*	*Gastric acid secretion*	*Complications*		
			Bleeding	*Perforation*	*Obstruction*
I	Body, along lesser curve in the region of incisura angularis	Normal or low	+	+++	-
II	Body, associated with duodenal ulcer	High	+++	+++	+++
III	Prepyloric	High	+++	+++	+
IV	High on lesser curve near gastroesophageal junction	Low	++	+++	-
V	Anywhere induced by ulcerogenic drugs	Normal	++	++	+

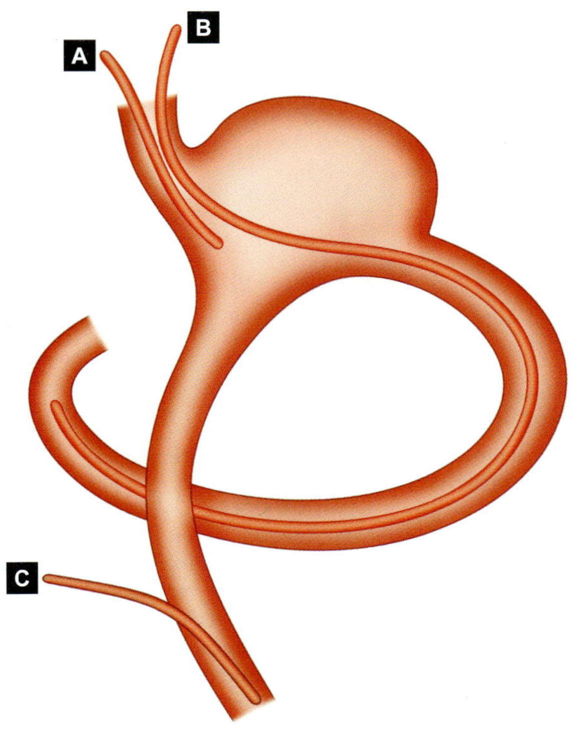

Figures 4A to C Technique of using two nasogastric tubes to prevent duodenal stump blowout: (A) one nasogastric tube placed in the stomach; (B) second nasogastric tube advanced into afferent jejunal loop with its tip in the second part of the duodenum; (C) feeding jejunostomy

Surgical options for Type I gastric ulcer include distal gastrectomy with Billroth I or II reconstruction and HSV with ulcer excision. While distal gastrectomy removes the ulcer and the diseased antrum it may be associated with postgastrectomy complications. HSV with ulcer excision is a less morbid procedure compared to distal gastrectomy. Two RCTs compared distal gastrectomy with Billroth I reconstruction to HSV with ulcer excision and concluded that ulcer recurrence rate is comparable between two procedures (Table 1).[31,32] While the follow-up is adequate the numbers of patients included in these RCTs are small. Hence the choice depends upon expertise with the procedure and the ulcer size and location as HSV with ulcer excision may not be possible in large ulcers with excessive scarring extending on to the incisura as it may damage antral innervation.

Types II and III gastric ulcers are associated with gastric acid hypersecretion and hence their treatment is similar to duodenal ulcers. Surgical options include HSV, TV with antrectomy, and TV with drainage.[6] However, HSV is associated with high incidence of ulcer recurrence rate especially in Type III ulcers where the recurrence rate can be up to 44%. Antral stasis secondary to relative GOO in addition to gastric acid hypersecretion could explain the high recurrence rate with HSV in these ulcers. Hence TV with antrectomy is the recommended surgical procedure for Types II and III gastric ulcers. In Type II gastric ulcer when associated with an active ulcer in the duodenum and GOO, TV with drainage is the recommended procedure due to the difficulties in duodenal closure (hot duodenum) following antrectomy.

Type IV ulcers are pathophysiologically similar to Type I ulcers and the proximal location might be due to proximal migration of antral mucosa since these ulcers usually occur at the junction of the antral and parietal cell mucosa. Surgical resection is difficult because of their location and to avoid total gastrectomy various procedures have been described including Csendes operation, Pauchet gastrectomy, the Schoemaker procedure and the Kelling-Madlener procedure (Figs 5A to D).[33,34] In the Csendes operation a subtotal gastrectomy including the ulcer is performed and reconstruction is by Roux-en-Y esophagogastrojejunostomy. In the Pauchet procedure a distal gastrectomy is performed with tongue shaped excision along lesser curve to include the proximal gastric ulcer. Reconstruction is by Billroth II gastrojejunostomy. Schoemaker procedure is a modification of Billroth I resection, while the resection is similar to Pauchet procedure reconstruction is by anastomosing the duodenum to the greater curvature of the stomach. In Kelling-Madlener procedure a distal gastrectomy is performed along with biopsy of ulcer (ulcer is not excised) to rule out malignancy.

Management of Type V gastric ulcer is focused on stopping ulcerogenic medications, adding prostaglandin analogs or PPI. If the ulcerogenic drugs cannot be stopped vagotomy is indicated to reduce acid secretion.

Gastric Ulcer: Benign or Malignant

The main diagnostic dilemma in patients with gastric ulcer is to differentiate benign from a malignant gastric ulcer. The incidence of malignancy in gastric ulcer ranges from 6% to 30%, the incidence increases with the ulcer size.[35] Clinical symptoms are unreliable in making the distinction. Endoscopic findings suggestive of a malignant ulcer are giant gastric ulcer (>3 cm), irregular ulcer edge, mucosal folds stopping short of ulcer edge and ulcer associated

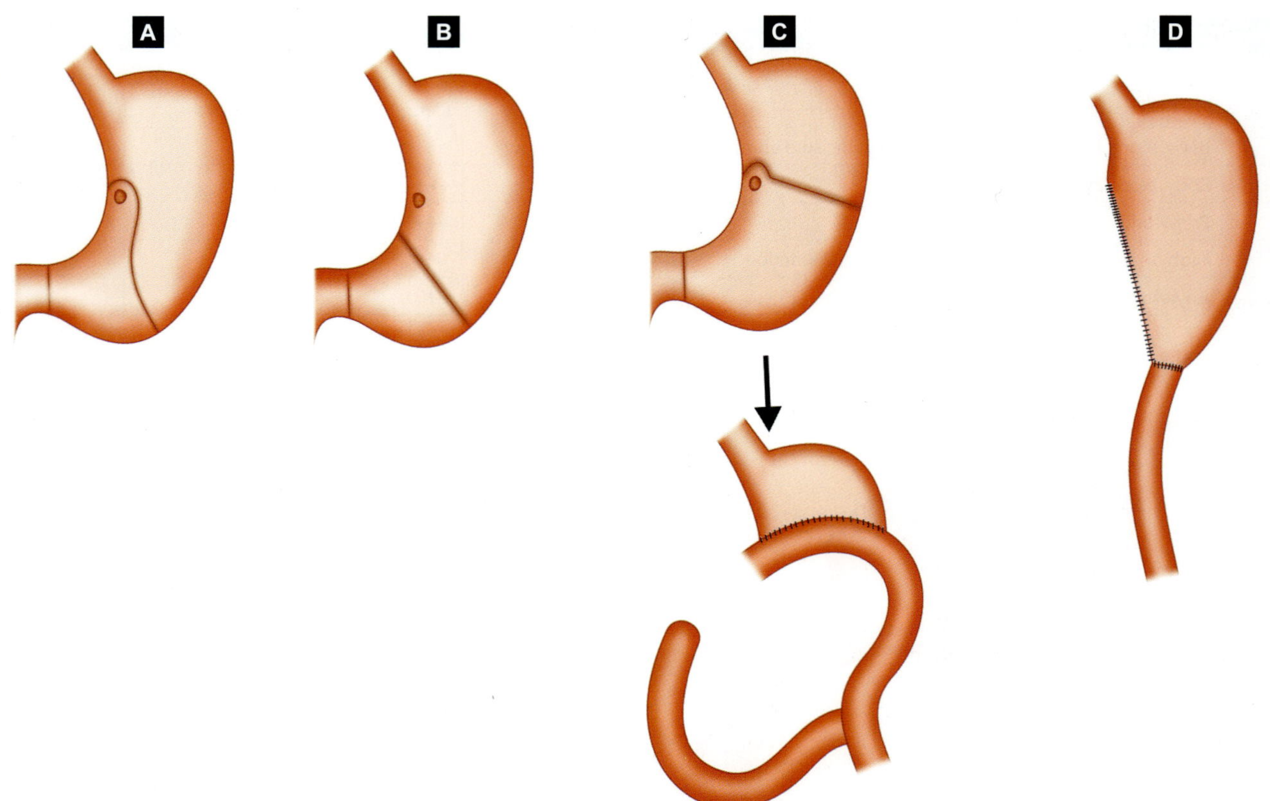

Figures 5A to D Surgical procedures for Type IV gastric ulcer: (A) Pauchet procedure; (B) Kelling-Madlener procedure; (C) Csendes procedure; (D) Schoemaker procedure

with a growth.[36] Sometimes these findings can be deceiving and gastrectomy rather than vagotomy may be a safer option if the patient is considered for surgery (Fig. 6). Multiple biopsies should be taken from the ulcer edge to rule out malignancy. If the biopsy is not suggestive of malignancy, further management depends upon the degree of suspicion. If the degree of suspicion based on endoscopic appearance is high, gastrectomy is recommended; if the degree of suspicion is low a course of PPI can be tried for 4–8 weeks. If the ulcer does not heal with PPI, gastrectomy is recommended, the extent of which depends upon the location of ulcer. Vagotomy can be added for Types II and III gastric ulcers.

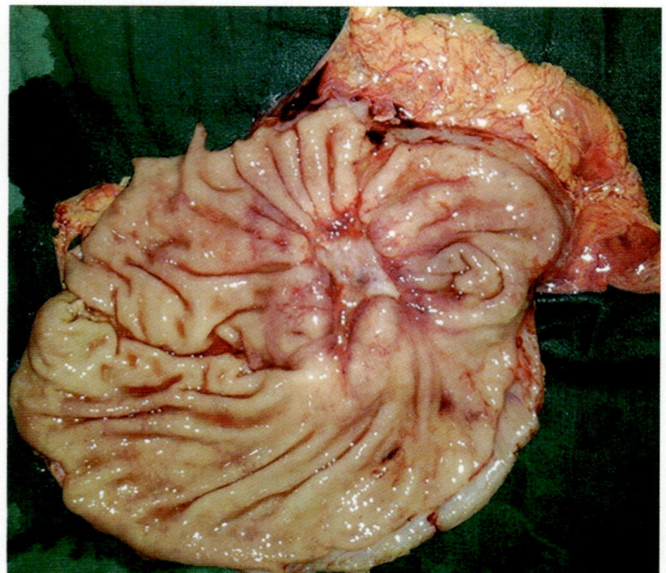

Figure 6 Malignant ulcer masquerading as benign ulcer with gastric mucosal folds radiating up to the ulcer edge

EMERGENCY SURGERY FOR PEPTIC ULCER DISEASE

Perforation

Peptic ulcer perforation occurs in 2–10% of patients with PUD and is a common surgical emergency in India. It is associated with high incidence of morbidity and mortality.[37] Perforation is more common in males; however, perforation in females is associated with higher mortality. Seasonal variation has been noted in one Indian study with the peak incidence of perforation between November and January and lowest incidence in the months of April and May.[38] Anterior wall of the first part of duodenum is the most common site of perforation followed by perforation of prepyloric and lesser curve gastric ulcers. However, gastric ulcer perforations are associated with higher incidence of morbidity and mortality. Factors associated with poor prognosis in patients with perforated peptic ulcer are old age, comorbid conditions, shock at presentation, large size of perforation and delay in presentation.[39] While non-operative therapy has been suggested in a select group of patients, surgery remains the mainstay of therapy.[40] Since the management of perforated duodenal and gastric ulcers is different it will be discussed separately.

Simple Perforated Duodenal Ulcer

Conservative or operative therapy: Conservative therapy is reserved for a small group of patients with perforation of less than 24 hours duration, hemodynamically stable, with minimal peritoneal signs, and no evidence of extravasation of oral water soluble contrast.[41,42] However, these patients, especially if elderly, should be closely followed up since the risk of failure with conservative treatment is more with advancing age.

Need for omentoplasty: The most common surgical procedure performed in patients with perforated duodenal ulcer is pedicled omental patch closure. While this technique was first described by Cellan-Jones in 1929 it is attributed to Grahams who had actually described a free-omental patch.[43,44] In pedicled omental patch closure, no attempt is made to close the perforation but it is plugged with omentum (Figs 7A to C). Sutures used to fix the omentum should not be too tight as it may strangulate the pedicled omental patch. Another important step is copious irrigation of peritoneal cavity with at least 6–10 L of warm saline. There is limited role for adding vagotomy to omentoplasty since postoperative *H. pylori* eradication prevents ulcer recurrence in these patients.[45] However, in patients with reperforation and perforation associated with GOO, a concomitant acid reducing procedure can be added if the patient does not have adverse risk factors. While drains are commonly placed there is no strong evidence to support routine drainage of peritoneal cavity.[46] In fact, drains can be a source of infection and are not always helpful in detecting a leak.

Large Perforated Duodenal Ulcer

Duodenal ulcer perforations measuring more than 2 cm are described as giant duodenal ulcer perforation. These perforations are associated with a high incidence of post-surgical leakage following simple omental patch closure. Various surgical options described are partial gastrectomy, jejunal serosal patch, jejunal pedicle graft, gastric disconnection, pyloric exclusion and controlled tube duodenostomy.[28,47-50] Since these patients are often very sick, an ideal procedure should be less complex and associated with less incidence of releak.

The two common recommended procedures are pyloric exclusion and controlled tube duodenostomy.[28,50,51] In pyloric exclusion; the duodenal perforation is closed with an omental plug or primary repair. The pylorus is occluded with a nonabsorbable suture material placed through a gastrotomy in the distal stomach, a side-to-side gastrojejunostomy is carried out at the site of gastrotomy (Figs 8A to E).[50] Vagotomy is not added. In very sick patients not fit to undergo pyloric exclusion, controlled tube duodenostomy can be performed.[50,51] In this procedure of triple-tube-ostomy, a primary repair of duodenal perforation is carried out. The duodenum is decompressed by a retrograde tube duodenostomy performed by retrograde passage of a tube through an enterotomy in jejunum 15 cm distal to duodenojejunal flexure. The tip of the tube is positioned at the junction of second and third part of duodenum (Figs 9A to D). Stomach is decompressed by a nasogastric tube or by a tube gastrostomy. An antegrade feeding jejunostomy is added. A lateral duodenostomy through the perforation should be avoided as lateral duodenal fistulas do not heal well and presence of a catheter through the perforation precludes healing. A partial gastrectomy if feasible with an end tube-duodenostomy is a safer option in these patients.

Laparoscopic or Open Repair

While laparoscopy has been used commonly in elective surgery for PUD it is less frequently used in patients with perforation peritonitis. A few RCTs have shown the feasibility of the laparoscopic repair of duodenal ulcer perforation (Table 3).[52-54] Both suture (omental patch closure) and suture less repair were used in these trials. In the latter group fibrin glue with or without gelatin sponge was used. Operative time in the laparoscopic group was more in two of the three trials and the principal reason was the time taken for laparoscopic peritoneal lavage. However, use of high-volume irrigation systems can shorten this duration. While the laparoscopy group had less morbidity, this was not statistically significant in any of the trials. A significant decrease in hospital stay was demonstrated in only one trial. Reperforation was more common in patients in whom the suture less technique was used. Conversion was reported in all three trials, common reasons being large perforation (>10 mm), inability to localize the perforation and difficulties in placing reliable sutures due to friable ulcer

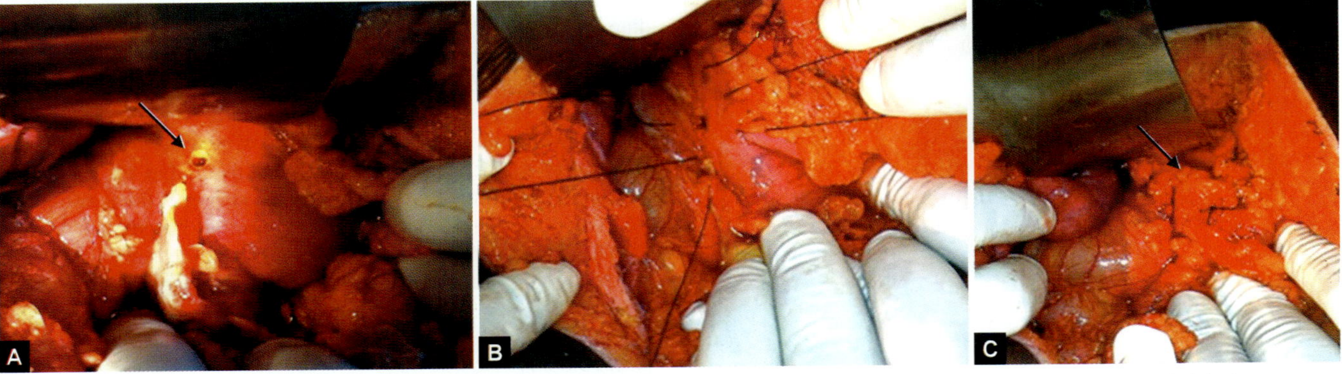

Figures 7A to C Pedicled omental patch closure of duodenal perforation: (A) perforation in the first part of duodenum (arrow); (B) full thickness stay sutures used to plug the omentum are placed across the perforation; (C) sutures tied to close the perforation with pedicled ometum (arrow)

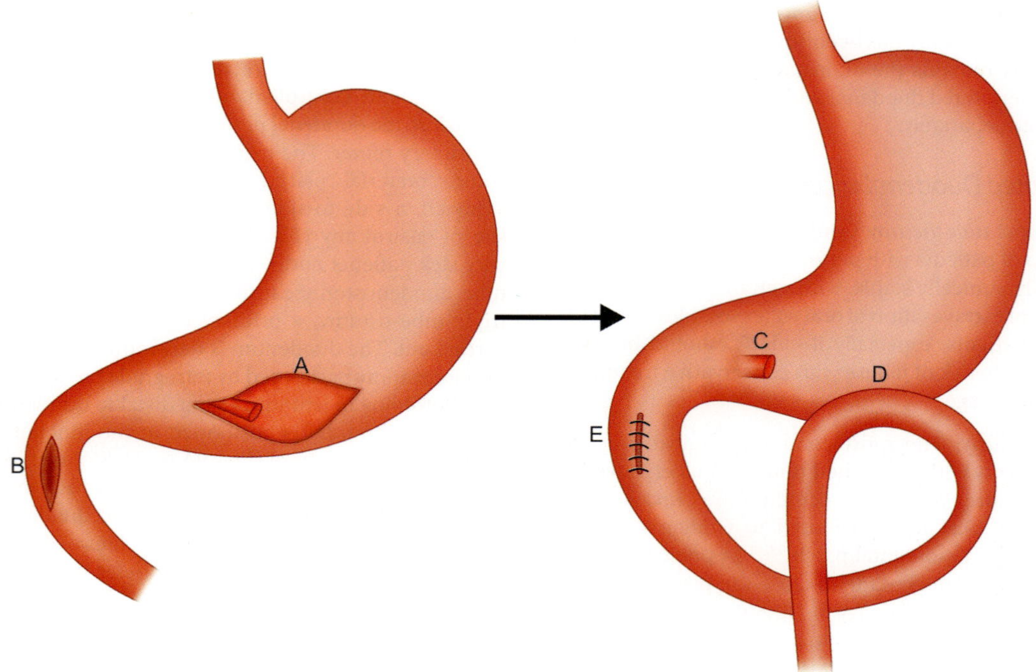

Figures 8A to E Technique of pyloric exclusion: (A) gastrotomy to occlude pylorus; (B) large duodenal ulcer perforation; (C) pylorus occluded with non-absorbable suture; (D) gastrotomy used for gastrojunostomy; (E) closed duodenal perforation

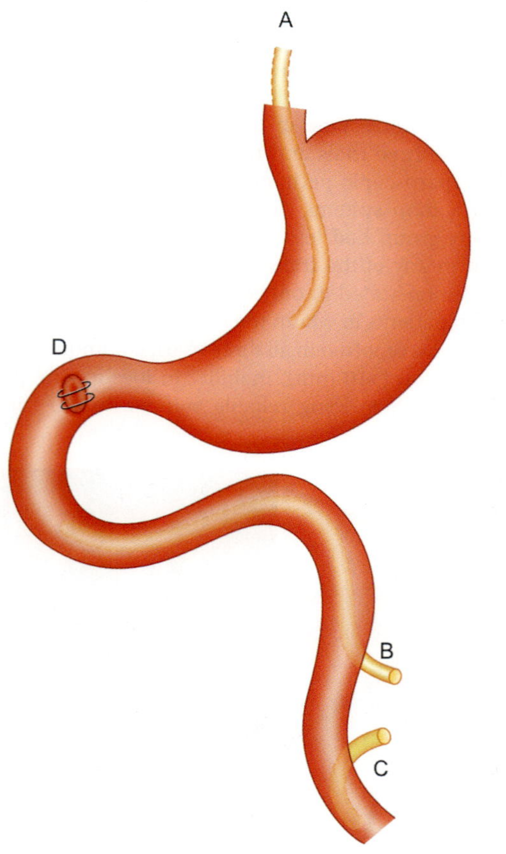

Figures 9A to D Technique of controlled tube duodenostomy: (A) nasogastric tube to decompress stomach; (B) retrograde duodenostomy; (C) feeding jejunostomy; (D) closed duodenal perforation

edge.[52-54] While mortality was less in the laparoscopic group in all three trials, the difference was not statistically significant. The limitations of these RCTs are that comparative data of laparoscopic and open repair in patients stratified according to the risk factors (like ASA score) are not available. Two of the three RCTs were published more than 10 years back and since laparoscopic skills have improved with time, further trials are required to demonstrate its superiority over the open approach.

Role of Natural Orifice Transluminal Endoscopic Surgery

Natural orifice transluminal endoscopic surgery (NOTES) repair of perforated peptic ulcers was proposed to be less invasive than laparoscopy. The feasibility of NOTES repair of perforated peptic ulcer was first demonstrated in animal studies and subsequently Bingener et al. reported its feasibility in humans.[55] Since it was the first human study, laparoscopy was used for confirmation of diagnosis and for surveillance of the procedure. The endoscope was advanced through the perforation into the peritoneal cavity, irrigation was performed and a viable mobile segment of omentum was pulled intraluminally through the site of perforation. The omentum was then fixed to the mucosa of the wall with endoscopic clips. After repair, the duodenum was insufflated to test for air leakage. The authors had done an earlier survey of the feasibility of NOTES and could select patients appropriately based on it.[56] While NOTES is feasible, further studies with a larger sample size are required to demonstrate its superiority over open or laparoscopic approach.

Perforated Gastric Ulcer

Gastric ulcer perforation though less common is associated with a greater morbidity and mortality compared to duodenal

Table 3: Randomized controlled trials comparing laparoscopic and open repair of perforated peptic ulcer

Author	*Year of publication*	*No. of patients Total (Lap/open)*	*Mean operative time (minute) Lap/open (p value)*	*Median hospital stay (days) Lap/open (p value)*	*Morbidity Lap/open (p value)*	*Reoperation rate Lap/open (p value)*	*Mortality Lap/open (p value)*
Lau et al.[52]	1996	93 (48/45)	94.3/53.7 (<0.001)	5/5 (NS)	11/10 (NS)	1/2 (NS)	0/1 (NS)
Siu et al.[53]	2002	121 (63/58)	42.0/52.3 (0.025)	6/7 (0.004)	15/25 (NS)	3/1 (NS)	1/3 (NS)
Bertleff et al.[54]	2009	101 (52/49)	75/50	6.5/8 (NS)	9/15 (NS)	NR	2/4 (NS)

ulcer perforation since it is common in elderly with history of intake of ulcerogenic drugs.[57] However, in one Indian study, a preponderance in young male patients with previous history of peptic ulcer has been reported.[58] Management of perforated gastric ulcers depends upon the type of gastric ulcer perforation, condition of the patient and presence of peptic ulcer symptoms. There is no role for conservative management of a perforated gastric ulcer since it is not possible to rule out malignancy in this situation as prior endoscopic biopsy would not have been done. Surgical options for perforated gastric ulcer include omental patch closure with ulcer biopsy, local excision of the ulcer with primary repair and gastric resection with reconstruction.[59]

Definitive surgery with gastric resection is preferred in stable patients with long history of peptic ulcer symptoms. The arguments in favor of resection procedure are: (a) that 6–14% of perforated gastric ulcers will have a malignant etiology, (b) the outcome of patients with gastric perforation depends on their preoperative condition and not on the type of surgery and (c) a low association of gastric ulcer with *H. pylori* when compared to duodenal ulcer.[58-61] Arguments against resection procedures are that even if the histopathology confirms gastric cancer, survival following resection for a perforated gastric cancer is dismal. While the outcome of patients with gastric perforation is determined by their preoperative condition, gastric resection requires more operative time and requires more postoperative blood transfusions, increased requirement of postoperative ventilation and has other morbidity. Also, performing a simple patch repair in the emergency setting, compared to a gastrectomy, is within the competence of the non-specialist emergency general surgeon.[58-61]

For patients with Type I gastric ulcer perforation distal gastrectomy is preferred in stable patients. In unstable patients omental patch closure with biopsy of the ulcer is recommended. Primary repair of gastric perforation is not recommended as it is associated with a high incidence of postoperative leak.[59,61] Type II gastric ulcer perforation is managed similar to duodenal ulcer perforation with an omental patch closure and biopsy from the ulcer edge to rule out malignancy. In stable patients and patients with chronic symptoms of PUD a vagotomy can be added. If vagotomy is not carried out and the patients are positive for *H. pylori*, eradication therapy can be administered postoperatively. Diagnosis of *H. pylori* in the postoperative setting can be carried out by noninvasive tests such as urea breath test or a stool antigen test since endoscopy with gastric insufflation may not be safe for few weeks following gastroduodenal surgery. Patients with Type III gastric perforation have a high incidence of GOO following omental patch closure; hence in a stable patient antrectomy with vagotomy is recommended. Type IV gastric ulcers present a management dilemma since resection requires total gastrectomy which is considered a morbid procedure in a critically ill patient. Hence an omental patch closure with biopsy from ulcer edge may be preferred over resection.

Bleeding

Bleeding from peptic ulcer is the most common cause for nonvariceal upper gastrointestinal bleeding in India.[62] Similar to other PUD related complications the incidence of bleeding peptic ulcer has also decreased due to widespread use of PPIs and *H. pylori* eradication.[63] This trend has been documented in a recent Indian study, with the decrease in incidence being more pronounced for duodenal ulcer bleeding compared to gastric ulcer bleeding.[62] While endoscopic therapy is the first line treatment, it fails in 5–20% of patients and these require emergency surgical intervention.[63]

Chronic blood loss in patients with peptic ulcer is due to erosion of mucosal vessels whereas significant bleeding results from erosion of an underlying major vessel which is usually gastroduodenal artery in case of duodenal ulcer and left gastric artery in gastric ulcers along the lesser curve.[63] Various risk scores have been proposed to determine the need for hospitalization and intervention in these patients (Table 4).[64,65] In general presence of tachycardia, hypotension, nasogastric aspiration of fresh blood and a hemoglobin concentration less than 8 g/dL predict severe bleed and a need for urgent evaluation. Initial management includes volume resuscitation with crystalloids. Blood transfusion is recommended for a hemoglobin concentration of less than or equal to 7 g/dL as studies have shown that restrictive transfusion compared to liberal transfusion is associated with less incidence of rebleeding by decreasing splanchnic blood flow and coagulopathy.[66] Early administration of intravenous PPI is recommended as it has been shown to decrease the number of patients requiring endoscopic therapy.

Upper gastrointestinal endoscopy plays an important role in the management of peptic ulcer bleeding as it allows both diagnosis and treatment. The timing of endoscopy depends upon the patient's general condition. Patients with active hematemesis should be offered urgent endoscopy whereas patients who are hemodynamically stable after initial resuscitation can undergo endoscopy the next morning.[63,67] The Forrest classification is commonly used to categorize endoscopic appearances of bleeding ulcers (Ia—active pulsatile bleeding, Ib—active non-pulsatile bleeding, IIa—non-bleeding visible vessel, IIb—an adherent clot, IIc—a flat pigmented spot and III—an ulcer with a clean base) and patients with Forrest I and IIa ulcers have high incidence

Table 4: Risk scores used for classification of patients with bleeding peptic ulcer

Rockall score[64]

Variable	*Clinical score*			
	0	*1*	*2*	*3*
Age (years)	<60	60–79	≥80	
Shock	"No shock" Systolic BP ≥100, Pulse <100	"Tachycardia", Systolic BP ≥100, Pulse ≥100	"Hypotension", Systolic BP <100	
Comorbidity			Cardiac failure, ischemic heart disease, any major comorbidity	Renal failure, liver failure, disseminated malignancy
Diagnosis	Mallory-Weiss tear, no lesion identified and no stigmata of recent hemorrhage	All other diagnoses	Malignancy of upper GI tract	
Major stigmata of recent hemorrhage	None or dark spot only		Blood in upper GI tract, adherent clot, visible or spurting vessel	
Low risk ≤3, Moderate risk 4–7, High risk ≥8.				

AIMS65 score[65]

Variable	*Clinical score*	
	0	*1*
Serum albumin	<60	60–79
International normalized ratio (INR)	<1.5	>1.5
Mental status	Normal	Altered
Systolic BP	>90	≤90
Age	≤65	>65
Low risk <2, High risk ≥2.		

of recurrent bleeding.[67] Endoscopic treatment is indicated in patients with Forrest I, IIa and IIb ulcers. In patients with IIB, the ulcer clot should be washed since presence of clot is contiguous with a breach in an artery and, when it is present, endoscopic treatment is mandatory. Endoscopic treatment options include adrenaline injection, electrocautery and mechanical methods like hemoclips. Studies have shown that a combination treatment yields better results compared to monotherapy. Routine second look endoscopy after initial successful endoscopic hemostasis is not recommended.[68] Failure of endoscopic therapy occurs in 8–15% of patients. This is defined either as continued massive bleeding in patients in whom initial endoscopic control fails or those with recurrent bleeding after initial successful endoscopic hemostasis. The options for managing such patients includes: repeat endoscopic therapy (successful in 75% cases),[69] angiographic embolisation[70] and surgical intervention. A large ulcer in the posterior bulbar duodenum and lesser curvature which erodes into major underlying vessels, a high Rockall score, Forrest Types I and II ulcers are predictive of failure of endoscopic treatment. Relative indications for surgery or angiography include: exsanguinating hemorrhage, resuscitation with more than 6U blood, continued bleeding at more than 1 unit/8hour, persistent hypotension, rebleed uncontrolled by a second therapeutic endoscopy. The thresholds are lower in elderly or with lesions at high risk of rebleeding (as above); and with complex patients (such as rare blood group, multiple anti-red cell antibodies, or those refusing blood transfusion) in whom bleeding is not readily controlled.

Surgery for Bleeding Duodenal Ulcer

The common surgical procedure performed for bleeding duodenal ulcer is under running of the ulcer with pyloroplasty and TV.[6] A wide Kocher maneuver is performed. A longitudinal pyloroduodenotomy is made to expose the bleeding ulcer which is usually located in the posterior wall of first part of duodenum. If active bleeding is encountered usually from the gastroduodenal artery, it is initially controlled by digital pressure and subsequently ligated using a U stitch. If no bleeding is encountered the ulcer base should be cleaned to identify an underlying visible vessel which should be ligated. The pyloroduodenotomy is closed transversely as a Heineke-Mikulicz pyloroplasty.

Role of adding an acid-reduction procedure in emergency surgery has been questioned in the era of effective anti *H. pylori* medical treatment. The arguments in favor of adding acid reduction procedure are only that 40–70% of patients with a bleeding duodenal ulcer are positive for *H. pylori, and H. pylori* testing in the presence of hemorrhage is unreliable. On the contrary there is evidence that eradication of *H. pylori* reduces the risk of rebleed and is recommended in patients with *H. pylori* infection.[71]

Bleeding Gastric Ulcer

For Types I, II and III bleeding gastric ulcer gastric resection with reconstruction is preferred, whereas for Type IV gastric ulcer especially in an unstable patient wedge resection of the ulcer bearing segment and primary closure is a good alternative to total gastrectomy.[6]

Gastric Outlet Obstruction

There has been a steady decline in the incidence of GOO with the advent of effective medical therapy. In a recent Indian study, GOO was reported as the least common complication of PUD.[72] GOO can occur with both acute and chronic peptic ulcers. While spasm and edema secondary to inflammation play an important role in the former, fibrosis and scarring contributes in the chronic stages. Typical symptoms of GOO include gastric retention, vomiting, epigastric pain and weight loss. Recurrent vomiting also results in electrolyte and acid-base imbalance characterized by hyponatremic, hypokalemic metabolic alkalosis with paradoxical aciduria. A saline load test can confirm GOO and determine the need for intervention in these patients.[73] A 16 F nasogastric tube is placed in the stomach and the stomach contents are emptied. Around 750 mL of normal saline is instilled over 3–5 minutes. The tube is blocked for 30 minutes and then aspirated to measure the gastric residual volume. A gastric residual volume more than 400 mL is suggestive of definite GOO, 300–400 mL is suggestive of probable GOO, 200–300 mL is indeterminate and less than 200 mL rules out GOO. Upper GI endoscopy with biopsy should be performed in all patients with clinical GOO to rule out malignancy.

Initial management includes fluid resuscitation with normal saline and correction of hypokalemia till adequate urine output is established. Nasogastric decompression and parenteral PPI should be initiated. Patients with acute GOO usually respond to these conservative measures. In patients with chronic GOO not responding to conservative measures intervention is required. Endoscopic balloon dilatation (EBD) and surgery are the two options. Benjamin et al. first reported the use of EBD of the pylorus as a treatment for peptic ulcer induced GOO.[74,75] Success rates range from 45.4–100%.[75-79] The reason for these variable results includes simultaneous use of PPIs, *H. pylori* eradication and duration of follow-up. While immediate relief has been noted in majority of patients, long-term success is better in patients who had received *H. pylori* eradication therapy (Table 5). While EBD can be associated with serious complications like bleeding and perforation, they are uncommon with dilatation less than 15 mm. The present evidence suggests that balloon dilatation can be a reasonable option especially in patients not fit for surgery although more studies with long duration of follow-up are required to make a definite recommendation.

Surgery remains the treatment of choice especially in patients presenting with refractory GOO and patients with chronically scarred and occluded pylorus or post-bulbar region. Surgical options include vagotomy and antrectomy, TV and gastrojejunostomy or HSV and gastrojejunostomy.[6] While TV and antrectomy is an ideal procedure, inflammation and scarring at the duodenal bulb may preclude a safe antrectomy (Figs 10A to D). TV and gastrojejunostomy is a commonly preferred procedure. In a small subset of patients with long standing obstruction and a hugely dilated stomach, it may be advisable to add a feeding jejunostomy to the procedure as chronically dilated stomach might take time to regain its tone. Patients in this group may have a high nasogastric tube aspirate for a prolonged time. Although the need for bypass would theoretically negate the advantages of HSV, few studies have shown that preservation of the antropyloric innervation may preserve controlled gastric emptying and minimize bile reflux.[16] Laparoscopic gastrojejunostomy for the relief of GOO has emerged as a procedure with a more rapid postoperative recovery and shorter hospital stay compared with open surgery.[80] In time laparoscopic TV with gastrojejunostomy may become the new gold standard.

COMPLICATIONS FOLLOWING PEPTIC ULCER SURGERY

Complications following surgery for PUD can be divided into postoperative complications and postgastrectomy syndromes. Postgastrectomy syndromes can be further divided into complications secondary to gastric resection, secondary to vagotomy, and related to reconstruction.

Postoperative Complications

Immediate postoperative complications include bleeding, anastomotic leak, infection and a duodenal stump blowout. Significant bleeding through abdominal drain or main wound is usually secondary due to slippage of ligatures and requires prompt re-exploration for hemostasis. Anastomotic line bleeding following gastrectomy with gastroenterostomy usually manifests as bleeding through the nasogastric tube. Initial management is conservative: gastric lavage, blood transfusion if required, and close monitoring. If bleeding is persistent surgical exploration is required, the anterior layer of the gastroenterostomy is opened and bleeding which

Table 5: Results of endoscopic balloon dilatation for gastric outlet obstruction

Author	*Year of publication*	*Number of patients*	*Response rate with H. pylori eradication*	*Response rate without H. pylori eradication*	*Duration of follow-up (months), median (range)*
Benjamin et al.[75]	1984	6	83.33%	—	5–14
Cherian et al.[76]	2007	23	100%	—	43 (5–90)
Boylan et al.[77]	1999	40	88.8%	64.5%	24
Kochhar et al.[78]	2004	11	100%	—	12–30
Lam et al.[79]	2004	25	78.6%	45.4%	24 (16–40)

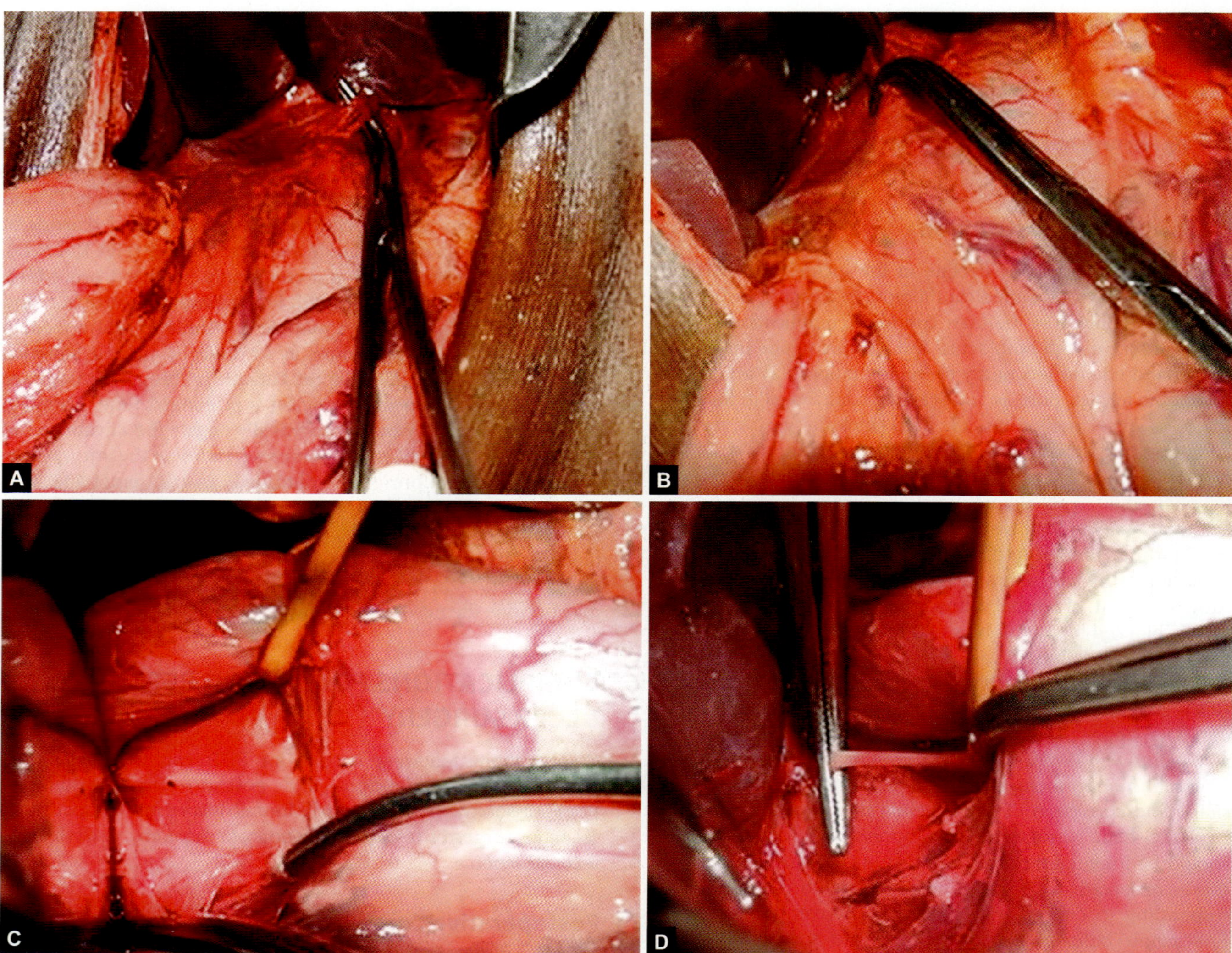

Figures 10A to D Technique of truncal vagotomy: (A and B) dissection of anterior vagus; (C and D) dissection of posterior vagus

usually occurs from the posterior anastomotic line is controlled by hemostatic sutures. Anterior layer of gastroenterostomy is then resutured.

Anastomotic leak usually occurs around the fourth to seventh postoperative day. It is associated with high morbidity and mortality and requires re-exploration with peritoneal lavage, drainage and a feeding jejunostomy. Duodenal stump blowout is the most feared complication following Billroth II gastrectomy.[81] It usually occurs around fifth postoperative day and presents as increased bilious output from drains in patients who have a drain in situ. If the drain is not placed or has been removed it can manifest as a localized intra-abdominal collection or diffuse peritonitis. The management depends upon the clinical presentation. In patients with a drain in situ, if the duodenal contents are draining well without any signs of peritonitis a trial of conservative treatment with nil per oral, total parenteral nutrition or jejunostomy (if present) feeds may allow resolution of fistula. Signs of peritonitis necessitate prompt re-exploration, lavage and drainage and feeding jejunostomy. Definitive repair of the duodenum with omental patch reinforcement, if feasible, can be done. If the duodenum is friable and edematous, a tube duodenostomy is preferable.

Postgastrectomy Syndromes

H. pylori therapy and potent antisecretary drugs have reduced the overall need for gastric acid-reducing surgery; hence it is rare to come across patients with postgastrectomy syndromes. However, one needs to be familiar with these disorders as a late presentation decades following the index operation is well known.

Secondary to Gastric Resection

Dumping syndrome: Dumping syndrome is the most common and often disabling syndrome after gastrectomy with gastroenterostomy.[82,83] Clinically significant symptoms with characteristic alimentary and cardiovascular manifestations occur in approximately 10–20% of patients and are more common with Billroth II reconstruction compared to Billroth I reconstruction. Based on the time interval between intake of meal and appearance of symptoms, dumping syndrome is classified into early and late dumping syndrome.

Early dumping syndrome occurs within 30 minutes of eating.[82,83] The rapid emptying of hyperosmolar gastric contents into the duodenum results in fluid shift from the intravascular compartment into the bowel lumen, leading to distension of small bowel associated with increased amplitude and frequency of bowel contractions. This manifest clinically as crampy abdominal pain, bloating, diarrhea (secondary to bowel distension), palpitations and lightheadedness (secondary to intravascular volume contraction). Symptoms of early dumping syndrome can be prevented by intake of smaller but more frequent meals, limiting the amount of liquids ingested during meals and avoiding hyperosmolar fluids. Exercise must be avoided soon after meal. Lying down in a supine position produces symptomatic relief when symptoms develop. In the majority of patients early dumping syndrome can be managed by these dietary modifications and surgical management is required in less than 1% of patients. Surgical options include conversion of Billroth II to Billroth I reconstruction, interposition of iso/anti peristaltic 10–20 cm jejunal loop to delay gastric emptying or creation of long limb (60–70 cm) Roux-en-Y gastrojejunostomy.[82,84]

"Late dumping syndrome", a less common syndrome compared to early dumping occurs 2–3 hours after a meal and usually causes milder and shorter lasting symptoms. It is attributed to the functional hyperinsulinism that occurs in response to the postprandial hyperglycemia caused by two factors: (1) rapid gastric emptying due to gastrectomy and (2) loss of parasympathetic innervation of the pancreas due to the vagotomy. Symptoms are alleviated by glucose administration. Along with dietary measures described for early dumping syndrome, pectin (carbohydrate gelling agent) or acarbose (α glucosidase inhibitor) may be prescribed as they prevent postprandial hyperglycemia. Octreotide has been found to be useful in both early and late dumping syndrome as it inhibits insulin and other gut hormone release, restores fasting migratory motor complex and inhibits food induced circulatory changes. Recent studies have shown that long acting somatostatin analogs provide better quality of life compared to thrice a day octreotide.[85] However, in a long-term study it was found that somatostatin analogs tend to lose their efficacy for the treatment of dumping syndrome over a period of time.[86] For refractory symptoms an antiperistaltic jejunal loop interposition or Roux-en-Y gastrojejunostomy can be performed.

Metabolic disturbances: It includes iron and vitamin B_{12} deficiency anemia, calcium deficiency and steatorrhea.[87,88] Iron deficiency anemia is secondary to impaired gastric acid secretion which interferes with iron absorption in the proximal small bowel.[82,87] Vitamin B_{12} deficiency is secondary to deficiency of the intrinsic factor produced by parietal cells. Iron deficiency can be corrected by oral iron supplements, whereas B_{12} deficiency requires intramuscular injection of cyanocobalamin every 3 months. Inefficient mixing of food, bile and pancreatic enzymes results in fat malabsorption and steatorrhea which may require restriction of fat intake in some patients. Osteoporosis and osteomalacia occur secondary to impaired calcium and vitamin D absorption.[88] These changes can occur within two years after gastrectomy; hence supplementation should be started immediately after surgery. Severe copper deficiency with clinical features mimicking vitamin B_{12} deficiency (ataxia, myelopathy and peripheral neuropathy) can occur following gastrectomy since copper is absorbed in the proximal duodenum.[89]

Weight loss: Weight loss is common after gastrectomy.[82] It is multifactorial and the patient enters a stage of negative nitrogen balance during which the weight loss is proportional to the amount of stomach resected. Usually it is temporary and with appropriate dietary modifications weight gain can be achieved.

Secondary to Gastric Reconstruction

Afferent loop syndrome: It is due to complete or partial mechanical obstruction of the afferent loop at the site of gastrojejunostomy or at a point along the afferent loop leading to its distension with bile and other enteric secretions.[6,82] The syndrome is common in patients with a long afferent loop and can present in an acute or a chronic (more common) form. The typical presentation is with nausea and colicky abdominal pain within 10 minutes of a meal which progressively increases in severity and is followed by bilious vomiting and resolution of clinical symptoms. Stasis secondary to afferent loop obstruction facilitates bacterial overgrowth which predisposes the patient to steatorrhea, malnutrition and vitamin B_{12} deficiency. In patients with these symptoms diagnosis can be confirmed by non-filling of the afferent loop on a barium study. However, even a non-obstructed afferent loop may not show filling in 20% of patients.[90] Recent studies have shown that dilated, fluid filled, C loop appearance of the afferent loop on CT abdomen is more sensitive for the diagnosis of afferent loop syndrome.[91] Since medical treatment is ineffective reoperation is usually required. Surgical options include conversion of the Billroth II to a Billroth I or Roux-en-Y anastomosis or creating a Braun enteroenterostomy between afferent and efferent limb. While Roux-en-Y anastomosis is used for the treatment, afferent loop obstruction can occur following Roux-en-Y reconstruction as well.[92] The afferent loop, in this scenario the biliopancreatic limb, can get obstructed by internal herniation which occurs in one of the following three points: (a) the mesenteric defect of the transverse mesocolon; (b) the jejunal mesenteric gap at the jejunojejunostomy and (c) Petersen's space, which is the space between the mesentery of the alimentary limb and the transverse mesocolon. Hence, these mesenteric gaps should be closed while performing Roux-en-Y anastomosis.

Efferent loop syndrome: It mimics small bowel obstruction and is caused by obstruction of the efferent loop secondary to intra-abdominal adhesions or by herniation of the efferent limb behind the anastomosis in a right to left manner.[6,82] Surgical option depending upon the cause could be intra-abdominal adhesiolysis or reduction of the hernia with obliteration of the hernial space. Braun enteroenterostomy between afferent and efferent limb can also prevent retroanastomotic herniation.

Retained antrum syndrome: It occurs following Billroth II gastrectomy when the gastrin producing cells of antral mucosa are present in the duodenal stump.[93] These gastrin secreting cells are over stimulated due to repeated exposure to alkaline intestinal content. This in turn leads to increased acid secretion which may result in recurrent ulceration. Serum gastrin levels, radionuclide scan or endoscopic biopsies of the duodenal stump to document gastric antral mucosa can be done for confirming the diagnosis.

It may be medically treated with PPIs. Refractory cases require excision of the duodenal cuff or revision of Billroth II to Billroth I anastomosis.

Alkaline reflux gastritis: It is secondary to reflux of bile into the stomach and is more common following Billroth II reconstruction.[6,82] Bile acids permit hydrogen ions to diffuse from the lumen into the submucosa by disrupting the gastric mucosal barrier.[94] While endoscopic evidence of bile reflux gastritis is present in significant number of patients, only a small proportion have symptoms attributable to bile reflux which underscores the need for careful evaluation. Symptomatic patients with bile reflux have a higher concentration of deoxycholic acid in their gastric remnant compared with asymptomatic patients.[95] Clinical symptoms include nausea, bilious vomiting and epigastric pain. Pain is aggravated by ingestion of food and is not relieved by ingestion of alkali or with vomiting. Medical treatment is usually ineffective and patients with refractory symptoms require reoperation with Roux-en-Y revision, interposition jejunal loop or Braun enteroenterostomy. In a recent study both Roux-en-Y anastomosis and jejunal loop interposition was found to be equally effective in the management of alkaline reflux gastritis.[96]

Roux limb stasis syndrome: It is characterized by nausea and non-bilious vomiting of food.[97] However, patients do not have postprandial pain. On endoscopy, the gastric remnant and the Roux limb is dilated, without evidence of mechanical obstruction on oral contrast examination. The length of the Roux limb and amount of remnant stomach were identified as the major risk factor for this condition. A trial of conservative treatment with promotility agents can be attempted. Since an ectopic pacemaker with retrograde peristalsis was considered as one mechanism for stasis, endoscopic placement of temporary electrodes near the gastrojejunostomy with gastric electrical stimulation was used in few studies with variable success.[98] If conservative measures fail, surgical options include near total gastrectomy in patients with significant gastric remnant, excision of Roux limb and reconstruction by Billroth II anastomosis with a Braun's enteroenterostomy between the afferent and efferent limb.

Gastrojejunocolic fistula: Gastrojejunocolic fistula is a rare late complication of gastrojejunostomy. It is common after gastrojejunostomy without acid reduction procedures or gastrojejunostomy with an incomplete vagotomy, which results in formation of stomal (anastomotic) ulcer. The ulcer progressively erodes into the transverse colon resulting in a gastrojejunocolic fistula. It is more common following a retrocolic gastrojejunostomy compared to antecolic gastrojejunostomy.[99,100] The patient usually presents with feculent vomiting, diarrhea and weight loss. Feculent vomiting and diarrhea are secondary to bacterial overgrowth in the small bowel. Barium enema is the investigation of choice to demonstrate the fistula. Endoscopy or colonoscopy or both should be performed to rule out malignancy and contrast enhanced computed tomography to rule out extraluminal causes for the fistula. Traditionally these are managed with a three-staged procedure when the patients are severely malnourished: an initial diversion colostomy, followed by resection of the fistula, and stoma closure in the third stage. Later a two stage procedure (Lahey's procedure) was described. However, currently a single stage procedure is preferred with adequate perioperative nutritional support using parenteral or enteral nutrition.[100]

Jejunogastric intussusception: It is common after simple gastrojejunostomy or Billroth II gastrectomy. Three anatomical types of jejunogastric intussusception have been described: Type I is herniation of the afferent loop into stomach, Type II is the herniation of the efferent loop into stomach and Type III represents a combined form. Type II accounts for 80% of all jejunogastric intussusception.[101] Clinical features include abdominal pain and vomiting with a palpable mass in the upper abdomen. It is a surgical emergency since delay can result in gangrene of the intussuscepted segment. If the intussusceptum is viable, it is reduced and the afferent and efferent limbs of jejunum are fixed to adjacent tissue (mesocolon, colon or stomach) to prevent recurrence. An alternative operative approach is to convert the Billroth II anastomosis to a Billroth I. If there is any doubt regarding strangulation, resection of the intussuscepted small bowel is preferred. In situ resection has also been reported without dismantling the existing gastrojejunostomy.[102]

Secondary to Vagotomy

Gastric stasis: Gastric stasis is a common complication following TV or selective vagotomy and hence these are always combined with a drainage procedure.[103] Despite a drainage procedure some patients develop epigastric fullness and vomiting secondary to gastric atony. While the diagnosis of gastroparesis can be confirmed by scintigraphic assessment of gastric emptying, other causes of gastroparesis like diabetes mellitus, electrolyte imbalance and mechanical causes of GOO should be excluded before attributing the cause to vagotomy. First line of management is with prokinetic agents such as metoclopramide (dopamine antagonist), erythromycin (motilin receptor agonist) or one of the newer agents like levosulpiride.[104] Supplemental nutrition (enteral or parenteral) should be given till the stomach regains its tone. Majority of patients improve with conservative treatment and surgery in the form of near total or total gastrectomy is reserved for rare patients who do not respond to a conservative trial of at least 3 months.[105]

Diarrhea: Distinct from other causes of diarrhea (like dumping syndrome), vagotomy itself can cause diarrhea in approximately 10% of patients. While vagal denervation of small bowel was initially thought to be the main cause, other causes like bacterial growth (secondary to impaired gastric emptying and decreased gastric acid secretion) and bile acid malabsorption also play an important role.[106] Most patients improve with medical treatment in the form of antimotility agents (loperamide) or bile acid binding resins (cholestyramine).[107] Interposition of a 10 cm reversed jejunal loop (Henle's loop), 60–70 cm distal to ligament of Treitz is required in rare patients' refractory to medical therapy.[6]

REFERENCES

1. Warren JR, Marshall B. Unidentified curved bacilli on gastric epithelium in active chronic gastritis. Lancet. 1983;321:1273-5.
2. Lam SK. Differences in peptic ulcer between East and West. Baillieres Best Pract Res Clin Gastroenterol. 2000;14:41-52.
3. Dutta AK, Chacko A, Balekuduru A, Sahu MK, Gangadharan SK. Time trends in epidemiology of peptic ulcer disease in India over two decades. Indian J Gastroenterol. 2012;31:111-5.
4. Garcia Rodriguez LA, Barreales TL. Risk of upper gastrointestinal complications among users of traditional NSAIDs and COXIBs in the general population. Gastroenterology. 2007;132:498-506.

5. Wang YR, Richter JE, Dempsey DT. Trends and outcomes of hospitalizations for peptic ulcer disease in the United States, 1993 to 2006. Ann Surg. 2010;251:51-8.
6. Harbison SP, Dempsey DT. Peptic ulcer disease. Curr Probl Surg. 2005;42:346-454.
7. Blalock JB Jr. History and evolution of peptic ulcer surgery. Am J Surg. 1981;141:317-22.
8. Newton SE 3rd, Judd ES. Long term follow-up proves Billroth I gastric resection inadequate for permanent control of duodenal ulcer. Surg Gynecol Obstet. 1963;116:170-4.
9. Rhea WG Jr, Killen DA, Scott HW Jr. Long term results of partial gastric resection without vagotomy in duodenal ulcer disease. Surg Gynecol Obstet. 1965;120:970-4.
10. Harkins HN. The surgical treatment of duodenal ulcer 1884 to 1965. J Natl Med Assoc. 1965;57:365-73.
11. Dragstedt LF, Harper PV, Tovee FR, Woodward ER. Section of the vagus nerves to the stomach in the treatment of peptic ulcer. Ann Surg. 1947;126:687-92.
12. Dragstedt LR. Vagotomy for gastroduodenal ulcer. Ann Surg. 1945;122:973-89.
13. Weinberg JA. Vagotomy and pyloroplasty in the treatment of duodenal ulcer. Am J Surg. 1963;105:347-51.
14. Griffith CA, Harkins HN. Selective gastric vagotomy: physiologic basis and technique. Surg Clin North Am. 1962;42:1431-41.
15. Griffith CA, Harkins HN. Partial gastric vagotomy: an experimental study. Gastroenterology. 1957;32:96-102.
16. Donahue PE, Griffith C, Richter HM. A 50-year perspective upon selective gastric vagotomy. Am J Surg. 1996;172:9-12.
17. Herrington JL Jr. Gastroduodenal ulcer: overview of 150 papers presented before the Southern Surgical Association 1888-1986. Ann Surg. 1988;207:754-69.
18. Taylor TV, Lythgoe JP, McFarland JB, Gilmore IT, Thomas PE, Ferguson GH. Anterior lesser curve seromyotomy and posterior truncal vagotomy versus truncal vagotomy and pyloroplasty in the treatment of chronic duodenal ulcer. Br J Surg. 1990;77:1007-9.
19. Kate V, Ananthakrishnan N, Tovey FI. Is Helicobacter pylori infection the primary cause of duodenal ulceration or a secondary factor? A review of the evidence. Gastroenterol Res Pract. 2013;2013:425840.
20. Kate V, Maroju NK, Ananthakrishnan N. Helicobacter pylori infection and upper gastrointestinal disorders. Gastroenterol Res Pract. 2013;2013:896209.
21. Dorricott NJ, Mcneish AR, Alexander-Williams J, Royston CM, Cooke WM, Spencer CJ, et al. Prospective randomized multicentre trial of proximal gastric vagotomy or truncal vagotomy and antrectomy for chronic duodenal ulcer: interim results. Br J Surg. 1978;65:152-4.
22. De Vries BC, Schattenkerk ME, Smith EE, Spencer J, Jackson DS, Alexander-Williams J, et al. Prospective randomized multicentre trial of proximal gastric vagotomy or truncal vagotomy and antrectomy for chronic duodenal ulcer: results after 5-7 years. Br J Surg. 1983;70:701-3.
23. Oostvogel HJ, van Vroonhoven TJ. Anterior lesser curve seromyotomy with posterior truncal vagotomy versus proximal gastric vagotomy. Br J Surg. 1988;75:121-4.
24. Walia HS, Abd el-Karim HA. Anterior lesser curve seromyotomy with posterior truncal vagotomy versus proximal gastric vagotomy: results of a prospective randomized trial 3-8 years after surgery. World J Surg. 1994;18:758-63.
25. Burch JM, Cox CL, Feliciano DV, Richardson RJ, Martin RR. Management of the difficult duodenal stump. Am J Surg. 1991;162:522-6.
26. Nissen R. ZurResektion da tietsitzenden duodenal Geschwurs. ZentralblChir. 1933;60:483-5.
27. Bancroft FW. A modification of the devine operation of pyloric exclusion for duodenal ulcer. Am J Surg. 1931;16:223-30.
28. Lal P, Vindal A, Hadke NS. Controlled tube duodenostomy in the management of giant duodenal ulcer perforation: a new technique for a surgically challenging condition. Am J Surg. 2009;198:319-23.
29. Raman RS, Kate V, Ananthakrishnan N. A technique to prevent duodenal blowout after difficult gastrectomies. Indian J Gastroenterol. 2013;32:60-1.
30. Vashist YK, Yekebas EF, Gebauer F, Tachezy M, Bachmann K, König A, et al. Management of the difficult duodenal stump in penetrating duodenal ulcer disease: a comparative analysis of duodenojejunostomy with "classical" stump closure (Nissen-Bsteh). Langenbecks Arch Surg. 2012;397:1243-9.
31. Reid DA, Duthie HL, Bransom CJ, Johnson AG. Late follow-up of highly selective vagotomy with excision of the ulcer compared with Billroth I gastrectomy for treatment of benign gastric ulcer. Br J Surg. 1982;69:605-7.
32. Emås S, Grupcev G, Eriksson B. Ten-year follow-up of a prospective, randomized trial of selective proximal vagotomy with ulcer excision and partial gastrectomy with gastroduodenostomy for treating corporeal gastric ulcer. Am J Surg. 1994;167:596-600.
33. Lewis A, Qvist G. Operative treatment of high gastric ulcer with special reference to Pauchet's method. Br J Surg. 1972;59:1-4.
34. Csendes A, Braghetto I, Calvo F, De la Cuadra R, Velasco N, Schutte H, et al. Surgical treatment of high gastric ulcer. Am J Surg. 1985;149:765-70.
35. Cohn I, Sartin J. Giant gastric ulcers. Ann Surg. 1958;147:749-59.
36. Barragry TP, Blatchford JW 3rd, Allen MO. Giant gastric ulcers. A review of 49 cases. Ann Surg. 1986;203:255-9.
37. Jhobta RS, Attri AK, Kaushik R, Sharma R, Jhobta A. Spectrum of perforation peritonitis in India—review of 504 consecutive cases. World J Emerg Surg. 2006;1:26.
38. Arveen S, Jagdish S, Kadambari D. Perforated peptic ulcer in South India: an institutional perspective. World J Surg. 2009;33:1600-4.
39. Buck DL, Vester-Andersen M, Møller MH; Danish Clinical Register of Emergency Surgery. Surgical delay is a critical determinant of survival in perforated peptic ulcer. Br J Surg. 2013;100:1045-9.
40. Møller MH, Adamsen S, Wøjdemann M, Møller AM. Perforated peptic ulcer: how to improve outcome? Scand J Gastroenterol. 2009;44:15-22.
41. Songne B, Jean F, Foulatier O, Khalil H, Scotté M. Non operative treatment for perforated peptic ulcer: results of a prospective study. Ann Chir. 2004;129:578-82.
42. Crofts TJ, Park KG, Steele RJ, Chung SS, Li AK. A randomized trial of nonoperative treatment for perforated peptic ulcer. N Engl J Med. 1989;320:970-3.
43. Cellan-Jones CJ. A rapid method of treatment perforated duodenal ulcer. Br Med J. 1929;1:1076-7.
44. Graham RR. The treatment of perforated duodenal ulcers. Surg Gynecol Obstet. 1937;64:235-8.
45. Bose AC, Kate V, Ananthakrishnan N, Parija SC. Helicobacter pylori eradication prevents recurrence after simple closure of perforated duodenal ulcer. J Gastroenterol Hepatol. 2007;22:345-8.
46. Pai D, Sharma A, Kanungo R, Jagdish S, Gupta A. Role of abdominal drains in perforated duodenal ulcer patients: a prospective controlled study. Aust N Z J Surg. 1999;69:210-3.
47. Sharma D, Saxena A, Rahman H, Raina VK, Kapoor JP. Free omental plug: a nostalgic look at an old and dependable technique for giant peptic perforations. Digest Surg. 2000;17:216-8.
48. McIlrath DC, Larson RH. Surgical management of large perforations of the duodenum. Surg Clin North Am. 1971;51:857-61.
49. Cranford CA Jr, Olson R, Bradley EL III. Gastric disconnection in the management of perforated giant duodenal ulcer. Am J Surg. 1988;155:439-42.

50. Vaughn G, Frazier O, Graham D, Mattox KL, Petmecky FF, Jordan GL. The use of pyloric exclusion in the management of severe duodenal injuries. Am J Surg. 1977;134:785-90.
51. Fujikuni N, Tanabe K, Yamamoto H, Suzuki T, Tokumoto N, Ohdan H. Triple-tube-ostomy: a novel technique for the surgical treatment of iatrogenic duodenal perforation. Case Rep Gastroenterol. 2011;5:672-9.
52. Lau WY, Leung KL, Kwong KH, Davey IC, Robertson C, Dawson JJ, et al. A randomized study comparing laparoscopic versus open repair of perforated peptic ulcer using suture or sutureless technique. Ann Surg. 1996;224:131-8.
53. Siu WT, Leong HT, Law BK, Chau CH, Li AC, Fung KH, et al. Laparoscopic repair for perforated peptic ulcer: a randomized controlled trial. Ann Surg. 2002;235:313-9.
54. Bertleff MJ, Halm JA, Bemelman WA, van der Ham AC, van der Harst E, Oei HI, et al. Randomized clinical trial of laparoscopic versus open repair of the perforated peptic ulcer: the LAMA trial. World J Surg. 2009;33:1368-73.
55. Bingener J, Loomis EA, Gostout CJ, Zielinski MD, Buttar NS, Song LM, et al. Feasibility of NOTES omental plug repair of perforated peptic ulcers: results from a clinical pilot trial. Surg Endosc. 2013;27:2201-8.
56. Bonin EA, Moran E, Gostout CJ, McConico AL, Zielinski M, Bingener J. Natural orifice transluminal endoscopic surgery for patients with perforated peptic ulcer. Surg Endosc. 2012;26:1534-8.
57. Svanes C, Lie RT, Svanes K, Lie SA, Soreide O. Adverse effects of delayed treatment for perforated peptic ulcer. Ann Surg. 1994;220:168-75.
58. Sarath Chandra S, Kumar SS. Definitive or conservative surgery for perforated gastric ulcer?—An unresolved problem. Int J Surg. 2009;7:136-9.
59. Madiba TE, Nair R, Mulaudzi TV, Thomson SR. Perforated gastric ulcer—reappraisal of surgical options. S Afr J Surg. 2005;43:58-60.
60. Kuwabara K, Matsuda S, Fushimi K, Ishikawa KB, Horiguchi H, Fujimori K. Reappraising the surgical approach on the perforated gastroduodenal ulcer: should gastric resection be abandoned? J Clin Med Res. 2011;3:213-22.
61. Leeman MF, Skouras C, Paterson-Brown S. The management of perforated gastric ulcers. Int J Surg. 2013;11:322-4.
62. Simon EG, Chacko A, Dutta AK, Joseph AJ, George B. Acute nonvariceal upper gastrointestinal bleeding—experience of a tertiary care center in southern India. Indian J Gastroenterol. 2013;32:236-41.
63. Lau JY, Barkun A, Fan DM, Kuipers EJ, Yang YS, Chan FK. Challenges in the management of acute peptic ulcer bleeding. Lancet. 2013;381:2033-43.
64. Rockall TA, Logan RF, Devlin HB, Northfield TC. Risk assessment after acute upper gastrointestinal hemorrhage. Gut. 1996;38: 316-21.
65. Saltzman JR, Tabak YP, Hyett BH, Sun X, Travis AC, Johannes RS. Simple risk score accurately predicts in-hospital mortality, length of stay, and cost in acute upper GI bleeding. Gastrointest Endosc. 2011;74:1215-24.
66. Villanueva C, Colomo A, Bosch A, Concepción M, Hernandez-Gea V, Aracil C, et al. Transfusion strategies for acute upper gastrointestinal bleeding. N Engl J Med. 2013;368:11-21.
67. Laine L, McQuaid KR. Endoscopic therapy for bleeding ulcers: an evidence based approach based on meta-analyses of randomized controlled trials. Clin Gastroenterol Hepatol. 2009;1:33-47.
68. Marmo R, Rotondano G, Piscopo R, Bianco MA, D'Angella R, Cipolletta L. Dual therapy versus monotherapy in the endoscopic treatment of high-risk bleeding ulcers: a meta-analysis of controlled trials. Am J Gastroenterol. 2007;102:279-89.
69. Lau JY, Sung JJ, Lam YH, Chan AC, Ng EK, Lee DW, et al. Endoscopic re-treatment compared with surgery in patients with recurrent bleeding after initial endoscopic control of bleeding ulcers. N Engl J Med. 1999;340:751-6.
70. Loffroy R, Guiu B. Role of transcatheter arterial embolization for massive bleeding from gastroduodenal ulcers. World J Gastroenterol. 2009;21:5889-97.
71. Kate V, Ananthakrishnan N, Badrinath S, Amarnath SK, Ratnakar C. Bleeding duodenal ulcer: is Helicobacter pylori a risk factor? Indian J Gastroenterol. 1998;17:34-5.
72. Appasani S, Kochhar S, Nagi B, Gupta V, Kochhar R. Benign gastric outlet obstruction—spectrum and management. Trop Gastroenterol. 2011;32:259-66.
73. Soll AH, Graham DY. Peptic ulcer disease. In: Yamada T (Ed). Yamada Textbook of Gastroenterology, 5th edition. Oxford, UK: Wiley-Blackwell Publishing Ltd; 2009. pp. 936-81.
74. Benjamin SB, Cattau EL, Glass RL. Balloon dilation of the pylorus: therapy for gastric outlet obstruction. Gastrointest Endosc. 1982;28:253-4.
75. Benjamin SB, Glass RL, Cattau EL Jr, Miller WBl. Preliminary experience with balloon dilation of the pylorus. Gastrointest Endosc. 1984;30:93-5.
76. Cherian PT, Cherian S, Singh P. Long-term follow-up of patients with gastric outlet obstruction related to peptic ulcer disease treated with endoscopic balloon dilatation and drug therapy. Gastrointest Endosc. 2007;66:491-7.
77. Boylan JJ, Gradzka MI. Long-term results of endoscopic balloon dilatation for gastric outlet obstruction. Dig Dis Sci. 1999;44:1883-6.
78. Kochhar R, Sethy PK, Nagi B, Wig JD. Endoscopic balloon dilatation of benign gastric outlet obstruction. J Gastroenterol Hepatol. 2004;19:418-22.
79. Lam YH, Lau JY, Fung TM, Ng EK, Wong SK, Sung JJ, et al. Endoscopic balloon dilation for benign gastric outlet obstruction with or without Helicobacter pylori infection. Gastrointest Endosc. 2004;60:229-33.
80. Zhang LP, Tabrizian P, Nguyen S, Telem D, Divino C. Laparoscopic gastrojejunostomy for the treatment of gastric outlet obstruction. JSLS. 2011;15:169-73.
81. Zivic EJ. Duodenal stump blow-out in the Billroth II gastric resection. J Natl Med Assoc. 1969;61:17-9.
82. Bolton JS, Conway WC 2nd. Postgastrectomy syndromes. Surg Clin North Am. 2011;91:1105-22.
83. Le Blanc-Louvry I, Savoye G, Maillot C, Denis P, Ducrotté P. An impaired accommodation of the proximal stomach to a meal is associated with symptoms after distal gastrectomy. Am J Gastroenterol. 2003;98:2642-7.
84. Richards WO, Golzarian J, Wasudev N, Sawyers JL. Reverse phasic contractions are present in antiperistaltic jejunal limbs up to twenty-one years postoperatively. J Am Coll Surg. 1994;178:557-63.
85. Arts J, Caenepeel P, Bisschops R, Dewulf D, Holvoet L, Piessevaux H, et al. Efficacy of the long-acting repeatable formulation of the somatostatin analogue octreotide in postoperative dumping. Clin Gastroenterol Hepatol. 2009;7:432-7.
86. Penning C, Vecht J, Masclee AA. Efficacy of depot long-acting release octreotide therapy in severe dumping syndrome. Aliment Pharmacol Ther. 2005;22:963-9.
87. Beyan C, Beyan E, Kaptan K, Ifran A, Uzar AI. Post-gastrectomy anemia: evaluation of 72 cases with post-gastrectomy anemia. Hematology. 2007;12:81-4.
88. Sipponen P, Häkönen M. Hypochlorhydric stomach: a risk condition for calcium malabsorption and osteoporosis? Scand J Gastroenterol. 2010;45:133-8.
89. Tan JC, Burns DL, Jones HR. Severe ataxia, myelopathy, and peripheral neuropathy due to acquired copper deficiency in a patient with history of gastrectomy. J Parenter Enteral Nutr. 2006;30:446-50.
90. Gayer G, Barsuk D, Hertz M, Apter S, Zissin R. CT diagnosis of afferent loop syndrome. Clin Radiol. 2002;57:835-9.

91. Juan YH, Yu CY, Hsu HH, Huang GS, Chan DC, Liu CH, et al. Multidetector-row CT for the diagnosis of afferent loop syndrome following gastroenterostomy reconstruction. Yonsei Med J. 2011;52:574-80.
92. Aoki M, Saka M, Morita S, Fukagawa T, Katai H. Afferent loop obstruction after distal gastrectomy with Roux-en-Y reconstruction. World J Surg. 2010;34:2389-92.
93. Gibril F, Lindeman RJ, Abou-Saif A, Shojamanesh H, Roy PK, PeghiniPL, et al. Retained gastric antrum syndrome: a forgotten, treatable cause of refractory peptic ulcer disease. Dig Dis Sci. 2001;46:610-7.
94. Ivey KJ, Den Beston I, Clifton JA. Effect of bile salts on ionic movement across the lumen gastric mucosa. Gastroenterology. 1970;59:683-7.
95. Gadacz TR, Zuidema GD. Bile acid composition in patients with and without symptoms of postoperative reflux gastritis. Am J Surg. 1978;135:48-52.
96. Tireli M. The results of the surgical treatment of alkaline reflux gastritis. Hepatogastroenterology. 2012;59:2352-6.
97. Britton JP, Johnston D, Ward DC, Axon AT, Barker MC. Gastric emptying and clinical outcome after Roux-en-Y diversion. Br J Surg. 1987;74:900-4.
98. Daram SR, Tang SJ, Vick K, Aru G, Lahr C, Amin O, et al. Novel application of GI electrical stimulation in Roux stasis syndrome (with video). Gastrointest Endosc. 2011;74:683-6.
99. Umasankar A, Kate V, Ananthakrishnan N, Smile SR, Jagdish S, Srinivasan K. Anterior or posterior gastro-jejunostomy with truncal vagotomy for duodenal ulcer—are they functionally different? Trop Gastroenterol. 2003;24:202-4.
100. Subramaniasivam N, Ananthakrishnan N, Kate V, Smile SR, Jagdish S, Srinivasan K. Gastrojejunocolic fistula following surgery for peptic ulcer. Trop Gastroenterol. 1997;18:183-7.
101. Shackman R. Jejunogastric intussusception. Br J Surg. 1940;27: 475-80.
102. Jain BK, Lodh U, Chandra SS, Hadke NS, Ananthakrishnan N, Mehta RB, et al. Jejunogastric intussusception: therapeutic options. Aust N Z J Surg. 1989;59:865-8.
103. Srinivasan K, Ananthakrishnan N, Chezian C, Sahai A. Truncal vagotomy and gastrojejunostomy for chronic duodenal ulcer in India. Natl Med J India. 1996;9:57-60.
104. McClelland RN, Horton JW. Relief of acute, persistent postvagotomy atony by metoclopramide. Ann Surg. 1978;188:439-47.
105. Speicher JE, Thirlby RC, Burggraaf J, Kelly C, Levasseur S. Results of completion gastrectomies in 44 patients with postsurgical gastric atony. J Gastrointest Surg. 2009;13:874-80.
106. Duncombe VM, Bolin TD, Davis AE. Double-blind trial of cholestyramine in post-vagotomy diarrhoea. Gut. 1977;18:531-5.
107. Cuschieri A. Postvagotomy diarrhoea: is there a place for surgical management? Gut. 1990;31:245-6.

CHAPTER 25

Carcinoma Stomach

Durgatosh Pandey, Palaniappan Ramanathan, Pankaj Kumar Garg, Rambha Pandey

EPIDEMIOLOGY

The first anatomic description and natural history of gastric cancer was made by Cruveilhier in 1835.[1] An estimated 952,000 patients were diagnosed of gastric cancer worldwide in 2012, accounting for 6.8% of the total cancer incidence. According to worldwide statistics, its incidence is after cancers of the lung, breast, colorectum and prostate, making it the fifth most common malignancy in the world today. More than 70% of cases of gastric cancer occur in the developing countries, and 50% the world's gastric cancer load is from Eastern Asia. Gastric cancer is more common in men than in women (rate ratio 2.2:1). The countries with highest incidence rates of gastric cancer in 2008 were Republic of Korea (62 per 100,000) for males and Guatemala (26 per 100,000) for females. In Japan, approximately 50% of gastric tumors are diagnosed early; by contrast, only 5–10% of cases in the United States are diagnosed early.[2] Stomach cancer is the third leading cause of cancer death in both sexes worldwide, and is responsible for about 723,000 deaths (8.8% of the total cancer deaths) with a high fatality to case ratio of 70%.[3,4]

ETIOPATHOGENESIS

Helicobacter pylori

H. pylori is a WHO class I carcinogen related to the development of antral and body gastric cancers but indirectly protective in proximal gastric cancers.[5] Chronic *H. pylori* infection causes severe atrophic gastritis associated with reduced acid production, thereby reducing the risk of gastroesophageal reflux disease (GERD) significantly. This reduces the risk of gastroesophageal adenocarcinoma related to GERD.[6,7] There is a twofold increased risk in gastric cancer development in patients with previous *H. pylori* infection.[8] The presence of the cytoxan-associated gene A (*cagA*) is associated with increased virulence and risk of gastric cancer. Ebstein Barr virus was found to be associated with gastric cancer but the exact mechanism of action is not known.[9]

Dietary Factors

Increased dietary intake of high salt foods, such as miso soup of Japan, pickled vegetables, dried and salted fish, have been associated with increased incidence and mortality of gastric cancer.[10,11] The incidence increases significantly when salt intake exceeds 10 g/day.[12] Increased fruit and vegetable consumption reduces the incidence of gastric cancer by 44%. Vitamin C also reduces the incidence.[13,14] Alcohol consumption more than 60 g/day and more than 4 drinks/day is also associated with increased risk of gastric cancer.[15,16] Smoking is an independent risk factor.[17]

Hereditary and Genetic Factors

Majority of gastric cancers are sporadic but 1–3% are hereditary. The most common familial gastric cancer is hereditary diffuse gastric cancer (HDGC). HDGC is an autosomal dominant disease characterized by early onset of diffuse gastric adenocarcinoma associated with a higher risk for lobular breast cancer and signet ring cell colon cancer. It is caused by a germ line mutation in CDH1 gene. This gene that encodes for E-cadherin, a calcium dependent cell adhesion protein is located on chromosome 16q22 and is responsible for cell-cell interaction and cell polarity. According to International Gastric Cancer Linkage Consortium, a family is diagnosed with HDGC if they meet the following criteria:

- Two or more documented cases of diffuse gastric cancer in first-degree or second-degree relatives, with at least one diagnosed before the age of 50 years, or

- Three or more cases of documented diffuse gastric cancer in first-degree or second-degree relatives, independent of age of onset.[18,19]

Family members of HDGC should undergo testing for CDH 1 mutations after genetic counseling. There is no absolute age at which patients positive for the CDH1 mutant should undergo surgery; however, total gastrectomy is recommended in any CDH1-positive patient with a positive biopsy and/or age greater than 20 years. Annual surveillance endoscopy should be performed in patients who deny prophylactic gastrectomy and until the patient is ready to proceed based on genetic risk alone.[20] So far, over 80 prophylactic gastrectomies have been reported. In most of these specimen, occult signet ring cell carcinoma was identified in the submucosa. This implies that these patients have occult carcinoma within their gastric wall for much of their adult life, and that invasive malignancy awaits an unidentified trigger.[18]

Gastric cancer is also identified in other hereditary diseases like Lynch syndrome, Li Fraumeni syndrome and familial adenomatous polyposis (FAP). In Lynch syndrome, MLH1 and MSH2 carriers had increased risk whereas none of the MSH6 carriers developed gastric cancer.[21] Polyps greater than 2 cm in size and sessile polyps are more prone to for malignancy.

Other Risk Factors

Family history of gastric cancer, presence of chronic atrophic gastritis, pernicious anemia, gastric adenomatous polyps, Menetrier disease, obesity, and occupational exposure to coal, metal and rubber industries are some of the documented risk factors associated with gastric cancers.

CLINICAL FEATURES

The most common symptoms at presentation are anorexia induced weight loss (40%) and vague abdominal pain (58%). Dysphagia is common in proximal tumors and nausea, vomiting and gastric outlet obstruction are the presenting features in distal tumors. Early satiety is seen in linitis plastica the diffuse infiltrative form of disease. Chronic anemia seen in 40% of patients often manifests as iron deficiency anemia in patients with heme-positive stool; frank gastrointestinal bleeding with hematemesis is rare (5%).[22] Metastases can be clinically detected. Jaundice, ascites or hepatomegaly suggests hematogenous metastases to liver. Palpable left supraclavicular (Virchow node), periumbilical lymph node (Sister Mary Joseph nodule), palpable ovarian mass (Krukenberg tumor) on pelvic examination, or an extraluminal mass on rectal examination (Blumer shelf), ascites are indicative of disseminated disease. Nonspecific cutaneous findings include acanthosis nigricans and eruption of multiple seborrheic keratoses (sign of Leser-Trélat).[23]

CLASSIFICATION

Majority (95%) of stomach cancers are adenocarcinomas, with the remaining 5% being a mix of lymphoma, carcinoid, leiomyosarcoma, gastrointestinal stromal tumors, adenosquamous, and squamous cell carcinomas. In 1963, Laurens classified gastric cancer into diffuse and intestinal types after reviewing 1,344 cases of gastric cancer.[24] On endoscopy, diffuse gastric cancer appears as ulcers whereas intestinal variety is bulky and exophytic. On pathologic examination, diffuse type microscopically appears as a mass of mucocellular cells with poor glandular differentiation, whereas the intestinal types have well-formed glands or branching tubular structures.[25,26] Submucosal infiltrative growth is characteristic of diffuse type. Peritoneal metastasis is common in diffuse type and liver metastases in intestinal type. E-cadherin loss is observed in diffuse type. Disease progression through chronic gastritis-intestinal metaplasia-dysplasia- then malignancy is observed in intestinal type.[27,28]

STAGING

According to American Joint Committee on Cancer (7th edition), 2010, the TNM staging[29] is described in Box 1.

For an adequate sampling, 15 lymph nodes need to be removed to accurately differentiate between pN2 and pN3 disease. Different staging has been discussed in Table 1.

BOX 1 The TNM staging

Primary Tumor (T)

Tx—Primary tumor cannot be assessed
T0—No evidence of primary tumor
Tis—Carcinoma in situ: intraepithelial tumor without invasion of the lamina propria
T1—Tumor invades lamina propria, muscularis mucosae, or submucosa
T1a—Tumor invades lamina propria or muscularis mucosae
T1b—Tumor invades submucosa
T2—Tumor invades muscularis propria
T3—Tumor penetrates subserosal connective tissue without invasion of visceral peritoneum or adjacent structures*,**,***
T4—Tumor invades serosa (visceral peritoneum) or adjacent structures**,***
T4a—Tumor invades serosa (visceral peritoneum)
T4b—Tumor invades adjacent structures

Regional Lymph Nodes (N)

Nx—Regional lymph node (s) cannot be assessed
N0—No regional lymph node metastasis#
N1—Metastasis in 1–2 regional lymph nodes
N2—Metastasis in 3–6 regional lymph nodes
N3—Metastasis in 7 or more regional lymph nodes
N3a—Metastasis in 7–15 regional lymph nodes
N3b—Metastasis in 16 or more regional lymph nodes

Distant Metastases (M)

M0—No distant metastasis (no pathologic M0; use clinical M to complete stage group)
M1—Distant metastasis

*A tumor may penetrate the muscularis propria with extension into the gastrocolic or gastrohepatic ligaments, or into the greater or lesser omentum, without perforation of the visceral peritoneum covering these structures. In this case, the tumor is classified T3. If there is perforation of the visceral peritoneum covering the gastric ligaments or the omentum, the tumor should be classified T4.
**The adjacent structures of the stomach include the spleen, transverse colon, liver, diaphragm, pancreas, abdominal wall, adrenal gland, kidney, small intestine and retroperitoneum.
***Intramural extension to the duodenum or esophagus is classified by the depth of the greatest invasion in any of these sites, including the stomach.
#A designation of pN0 should be used, if all examined lymph nodes are negative, regardless of the total number removed and examined.

Table 1: Staging	
Stage 0	Tis N0 M0
Stage IA	T1 N0 M0
Stage IB	T2 N0 M0 T1 N1 M0
Stage IIA	T3 N0 M0 T2 N1 M0 T1 N2 M0
Stage IIB	T4a N0 M0 T3 N1 M0 T2 N2 M0 T1 N3 M0
Stage IIIA	T4a N1 M0 T3 N2 M0 T2 N3 M0
Stage IIIB	T4b N0 M0 T4b N1 M0 T4a N2 M0 T3 N3 M0
Stage IIIC	T4b N2 M0 T4b N3 M0 T4a N3 M0
Stage IV	Any T Any N M1

Table 2: Depth of tumor invasion using T classification	
T1	Tumor invasion of mucosa and/or muscularis mucosa (M) or submucosa (SM)
T2	Tumor invasion of muscularis propria (MP) or subserosa (SS)
T3	Tumor penetration of serosa (SE)
T4	Tumor invasion of adjacent structures (SI)
TX	Unknown

Japanese Gastric Cancer Association (1998) described a new classification. Depth of tumor invasion is recorded using T classification. Anatomical levels of invasion of the gastric wall are also recorded in Table 2.

The depth of invasion (M, SM1, SM2) are determined and recorded only when the vertical margin (VM) is negative (SM1; submucosal invasion <0.5 mm, SM2; invasion >0.5 mm).

Macroscopic appearance of the tumor during endoscopy was included (adapted from Borrmann classification) (Table 3).[30]

The Japanese Research Society for Gastric Cancer (JRSGC) established a different classification system for nodal metastasis based on anatomic location of the nodes and designated by stations (Fig. 1) and (Table 4).

Extent of Node Metastasis

- N0: No evidence of LN metastasis
- N1: Metastasis to Group 1 LNs, but no metastasis to Groups 2 or 3 LNs
- N2: Metastasis to Group 2 LNs, but no metastasis to Group 3 LNs
- N3: Metastasis to Group 3 LNs
- NX: Unknown

Table 3: Macroscopic appearance of the tumor	
Type 0	Superficial, flat tumors with or without minimal elevation or depression
Type 0 I	Protruded type
Type 0 IIa	Superficial elevated type
Type 0 IIb	Flat type
Type 0 IIc	Superficial depressed type
Type 0 III	Excavated type
Type 1	Polypoid tumors, sharply demarcated from the surrounding mucosa, usually attached on a wide base
Type 2	Ulcerated carcinomas with sharply demarcated and raised margins
Type 3	Ulcerated carcinomas without definite limits, infiltrating into the surrounding wall
Type 4	Diffusely infiltrating carcinomas in which ulceration is usually not a marked feature
Type 5	Non-classifiable carcinomas that cannot be classified into any of the above types

Patients with peritoneal cytology that is positive for malignant cells (up to 60% of patients with locally advanced disease on imaging) should be treated as having metastatic disease because their survival following resection is similar to those with overt metastases.[31]

INVESTIGATIONS

Routine blood investigations including complete blood count, liver function test, random blood sugar and renal function test are done. Chest X-ray and ECG are basic preoperative requirements.

Conventional endoscopy is the standard investigation for gastric cancer. For assessing depth of invasion, endoscopic ultrasonography (EUS) remains the primary choice for determining T staging. EUS has a T-stage accuracy of 60–80% and a lymph node accuracy of 50–65%. Additionally, EUS allows for fine-needle aspiration of suspicious lymph nodes and can detect liver metastases missed by conventional imaging studies.[32-34]

To detect early gastric cancers (EGCs) chromoendoscopy is more sensitive than conventional endoscopy. Magnification endoscopy is also useful. Lateral extent of the tumor must be identified for endoscopic resection and this is well seen by chromoendoscopy. Dyes used in chromoendoscopy are indigocarmine with or without acetic acid, congo red, methylene blue. During chromoendoscopy, the mucus adhering to the mucosa is washed away as thoroughly as possible before the examination of the lesion; then 10–20 mL of 1.5% acetic acid is sprinkled evenly over and around the lesion followed by 10–20 mL of 0.2% indigocarmine dye sprinkled 30–60 seconds later and finally the area is washed with clean water 20–30 seconds later for the final view. Gastric cancers appear unstained on final examination. Lesions with flat/elevated morphology show clear images. Tumor size, location and depth of tumor do not affect the clarity of the images. Lee et al. showed that the borders of the lesions were distinct in 66.9% with conventional endoscopy and in 84.1% with acetic acid-indigocarmine (AI) chromoendoscopy ($P < 0.001$).[35]

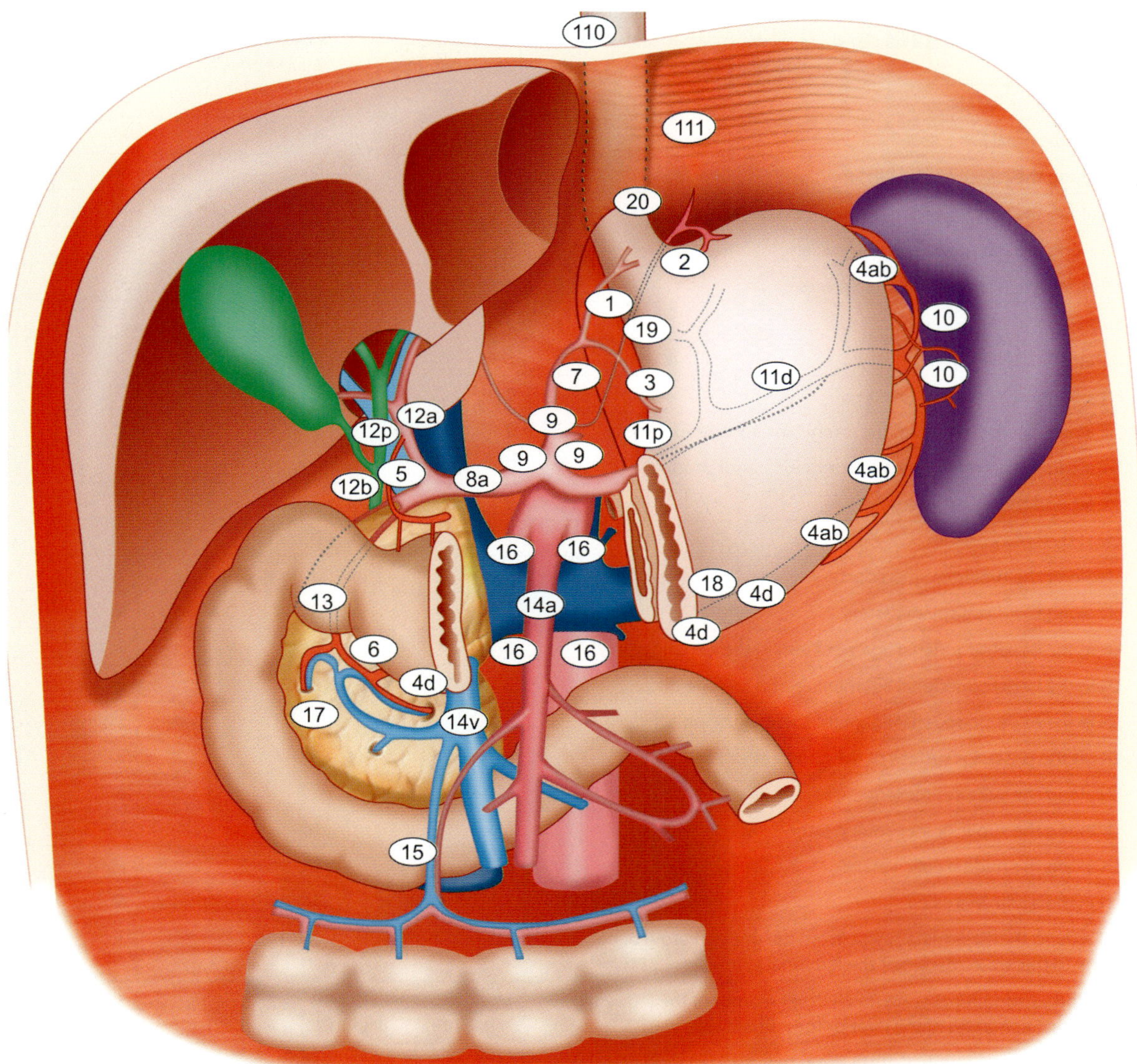

Figure 1 Location of nodal stations based on the JRSGC
Source: Japanese Gastric Cancer Association. Japanese Classification of Gastric Carcinoma, 2nd english edition. Gastric Cancer. 1998;1:16

A system consisting of a magnification endoscope combined with narrow-band imaging (NBI), with the spectral bandwidth narrowed by optical filters, has been developed to enhance visualization of mucosal surface structure and vascular architecture. This differentiates cancerous from non-cancerous lesions and also undifferentiated tumor from differentiated tumor with an accuracy of 90%.[36]

Computed tomography (CT) remains the best investigation for staging gastric cancer. The sensitivity of a CT scan to determine nodal status ranges from 50% to 95% and specificity from 40% to 99%. PET is not currently a primary staging modality for gastric cancer. It may have a role in assessing the response to neoadjuvant chemotherapy in locally advanced disease.[37,38] At laparoscopy, radiologically occult metastases are documented in up to 40% of patients with gastric cancer and a negative CT, who would have been considered potentially resectable. Laparoscopic ultrasound is a valuable adjunct to detect and evaluate liver metastases that are not visualized from the surface.[39]

Higher levels of serum tumor markers, such as carcinoembryonic antigen (CEA), carbohydrate antigen (CA 19-9), and α-fetoprotein (AFP), correlate with depth of tumor invasion, pathologic stage, presence of vascular invasion, and liver and lymph node metastases.[40,41]

MANAGEMENT

Gastric cancer management is based on staging. Gastric cancer is broadly classified into EGC (involvement of mucosa and submucosa), locally advanced (other than early and metastatic) and advanced disease (metastatic). Early stage is managed

Table 4: Lymph node groups based on the JRSGC (1 = D1, 2 = D2, 3 = D3, M = distant metastasis)

Station No.	*Description*	*Upper one-third*	*Middle one-third*	*Lower one-third*
1	Right paracardial LN	1	1	2
2	Left paracardial LN	1	3	M
3	LN along the lesser curvature	1	1	1
4sa	LN along the short gastric vessels	1	3	M
4sb	LN along the left gastroepiploic vessels	1	1	3
4d	LN along the right gastroepiploic vessels	2	1	1
5	Suprapyloric LN	3	1	1
6	Infrapyloric LN	3	1	1
7	LN along the left gastric artery	2	2	2
8a	LN along the common hepatic artery (anterosuperior group)	2	2	2
8p	LN along the common hepatic artery (posterior group)	3	3	3
9	LN around the celiac artery	2	2	2
10	LN at the splenic hilum	2	3	M
11p	LN along the proximal splenic artery	2	2	2
11d	LN along the distal splenic artery	2	3	M
12a	LN in the hepatoduodenal ligament (along the hepatic artery)	3	2	2
12b	LN in the hepatoduodenal ligament (along the bile duct)	3	3	3
12p	LN in the hepatoduodenal ligament (behind the portal vein)	3	3	3
13	LN on the posterior surface of the pancreatic head	M	3	3
14v	LN along the superior mesenteric vein	M	3	2
14a	LN along the superior mesenteric artery	M	M	M
15	LN along the middle colic vessels	M	M	M
16a1	LN in the aortic hiatus	3	M	M
16a2	LN around the abdominal aorta (from the upper margin of celiac trunk to the lower margin of the left renal vein)	M	3	3
16b1	LN around abdominal aorta (from lower margin of the left renal vein to the upper margin of the inferior mesenteric artery)	M	3	3
16b2	LN around the abdominal aorta (from the upper margin of inferior mesenteric artery to the aortic bifurcation)	M	M	M
17	LN on the anterior surface of the pancreatic head	M	M	M
18	LN along the inferior margin of the pancreas	M	M	M
19	Infradiaphragmatic LN	3	M	M
20	LN in the esophageal hiatus of the diaphragm	3	M	M
110	Paraesophageal LN in the lower thorax	M	M	M
111	Supradiaphragmatic LN	M	M	M
112	Posterior mediastinal LN	M	M	M

by endoscopic surgeries, locally advanced by multimodality treatment with surgery as primary modality and advanced disease by palliative management. Management also differs based on whether the tumor is proximal or distal in location. The three modalities of management are surgery, radiotherapy and chemotherapy. Multimodality management is essential for optimal results.

SURGERY

Early gastric cancer is defined as being confined to the mucosa or the submucosa, regardless of the presence or absence of regional lymph node metastasis. Eastern countries have intense screening programs that detect up to 70% of cancers at an early stage. EGC can be treated either with simple gastrectomy or selected cases by endoscopic intervention. Two types of endoscopic interventions have been described: (1) endoscopic mucosal resection and (2) endoscopic submucosal dissection.

Endoscopic Mucosal Resection

Endoscopic mucosal resection (EMR) was first introduced in 1984, and is also known as "Strip biopsy". EMR are indicated in well differentiated adenocarcinoma, tumors less than or equal to 20 mm in elevated type, less than or equal to 10 mm in depressed type, not associated with peptic ulcer and invasion limited to the mucosa.[42,43]

Advantages: Minimal invasion, low cost, better patient tolerance, and better postoperative quality of life.

Disadvantages: Larger-sized lesions cannot be resected completely by EMR at one time. Thus, the entire pathologic specimen cannot be submitted for proper analysis.

Techniques: EMR-precut, EMR-cap and EMR-ligation.

Endoscopic Submucosal Dissection

Endoscopic submucosal dissection (ESD) was developed for en bloc resection of large superficial lesions. ESD uses the needle-knife to strip the tumors from the submucosal layer. ESD has a relatively higher incidence rate of complications such as bleeding and perforation.[44] A comparison between ESD and EMR has shown that ESD has:

- a longer operation time
- a higher en bloc resection rate and higher histologically complete resection rate (even for tumors >20 mm)
- a lower recurrence rate
- a higher chance of perforation, but bleeding is similar in both procedures.

It has been noted that tumor location in the upper and middle portions of the gastric body, ulceration, unskillful operation and blind hemostasis, and lesions more than 3 cm are risk factors of perforation. The perforation can be repaired by metal clips and the majority does not require surgical operations.[45-52]

GASTRECTOMY

It is essential to have a good knowledge of the anatomy and the lymphatic drainage of the stomach (Fig. 1).

Staging laparoscopy should precede laparotomy during the same anesthesia in a patient with gastric cancer. This would help in identifying small liver metastases or peritoneal deposits in a substantial proportion of patients, thereby avoiding many unnecessary laparotomies. Staging laparoscopy is indicated before any neoadjuvant therapy, not only to know the status of the disease also to collect peritoneal fluid or wash for cytology. Staging laparoscopy is indicated in T3 or N1 disease before upfront surgery in the same sitting as locally advanced disease has high chances of occult metastases. Staging laparoscopy detects 40% of radiologically occult metastases, thereby reducing unnecessary laparotomies.

Gastrectomy can be classified into the following types:

- Total gastrectomy
- Distal gastrectomy
- Pylorus preserving gastrectomy (PPG)
- Proximal gastrectomy
- Segmental gastrectomy
- Local resection

Gastrectomy is indicated for locoregional gastric cancers (Stages I–III). The standard surgical procedure for clinically node-positive or T2 to T4a tumors is either distal or total gastrectomy. Distal gastrectomy is performed when a satisfactory proximal margin can be achieved. Depending on the extent of stomach resected, distal gastrectomy can be further classified into partial, subtotal or near total gastrectomy. If a satisfactory proximal margin cannot be achieved, total gastrectomy should be performed. Total gastrectomy is also considered for proximal tumors and gastroesophageal junction cancers. Such tumors may also be considered for proximal gastrectomy, although the popularity of this procedure has declined. In selected patients in whom the tumor invades distal pancreas/spleen, addition of distal pancreatectomy-splenectomy may enhance the ability to achieve R0 resection.

For cT1 cN0 tumors, gastric resections can be modified according to tumor location. For proximal tumors where more than 50% of the distal stomach can be preserved, proximal gastrectomy can be performed. For tumors in the mid-body of stomach with distal border at least 4 cm proximal to pylorus, PPG may be performed. Segmental gastrectomy and local resection are investigational for superficial gastric cancers.

Reconstruction after gastrectomy can be done by several means:

- Following total gastrectomy:
  - Roux-en-Y esophagojejunostomy
  - Jejunal interposition
- Following distal gastrectomy:
  - Billroth I gastroduodenostomy
  - Billroth II gastrojejunostomy
  - Roux-en-Y gastrojejunostomy
- Following pylorus-preserving gastrectomy:
  - Gastrogastrostomy
- Following proximal gastrectomy:
  - Esophagogastrostomy
  - Jejunal interposition.

The most common reconstruction done after total gastrectomy is the Roux-en-Y esophagojejunostomy. Gertler et al. conducted a meta-analysis on numerous reconstructive options after total gastrectomy. Roux-en-Y bypass, jejunal interposition and jejunal pouch were compared and concluded that jejunal pouch reconstruction has improved quality of life when compared to others. Jejunal pouch can be done without significant increase in operative time, length of hospital stay, increased morbidity or mortality.[53] Distal radical gastrectomy with Billroth I or Billroth II anastomosis is done for distal gastric cancers. Both the lesser curvature and greater curvature of the stomach need to be cleared of nodal tissue for transection.

Frequent meals in small quantities are advised after total gastrectomy. Nutritional deficiency results in anemia due to impaired iron absorption or due to lack of intrinsic factor results in megaloblastic anemia. Calcium deficiency results in osteoporosis and even fat malabsorption have been reported. It is necessary that on follow-up, nutritional deficiency surveillance is kept and supplemented by iron, vitamins and calcium.

SENTINEL LYMPH NODE BIOPSY

This is under investigation for clinically node-negative gastric cancers. Two percent patent blue dye, 1% isosulfan blue, technetium-99m(Sn) colloid, or a combination is injected in submucosa or subserosa, endoscopically or during open procedure. Sentinel lymph nodes are identified by direct visualization of the node or by using gamma probe. Average yield of 1.5–4 sentinel lymph nodes were identified with sensitivity, specificity, accuracy and negative predictive of 72.7–93%, 75%, 74–100% and 50% respectively. High false-negative rates were observed as the tumor cause lymphatic obstruction resulting in tracer flowing to secondary negative nodes. Skip metastasis and surgeon experience are the other factors affecting sentinel lymph node identification.[54-57]

SYSTEMATIC LYMPH NODE DISSECTION

The degree of lymph node dissection was traditionally based on the Japanese staging system in which nodal stations were assigned into groups N1, N2 or N3. A rough conceptualization of the types of lymph node dissection can be understood as:

- D1 dissection—If a dissection removes N1 nodes (perigastric nodes along the left and right pericardial nodes, lesser and greater curvature, suprapyloric and infrapyloric)
- D0 dissection—anything less than a D1
- D2 dissection—D1 plus removal of nodes along the left gastric artery, common hepatic artery, celiac trunk and splenic artery
- D3 dissection—D2 plus removal of nodes along the hepatoduodenal ligament and root of the mesentery
- D4 dissection—D3 plus removal of para-aortic and paracolic lymph nodes.

A more accurate description of different types of lymph node dissection is based on the nodal stations to be dissected based on the location of the tumor (proximal, body, distal stomach) as given in Table 5.

In 1942, Tamaki Kajitani, a Japanese surgeon first proposed D2 nodal dissection for the treatment of a gastric cancer.[58] D2 nodal dissection is recommended for gastric adenocarcinoma of Stage Ib or higher (higher than cT2 or cN1). Modifications of nodal dissection by T stages and procedures is described in Table 5.

Figure 2 shows the operative field after the completion of total gastrectomy with D2 lymph node dissection, with preservation of pancreas and spleen. An omentectomy and bursectomy is an integral part of the D2 nodal dissection. Some important steps are highlighted for proper D2 dissection.

- A distinctive plane between the nodal tissue and the pancreas parenchyma should be recognized and the dissection should be maintained in this plane to avoid injury to the pancreas.
- Injury to coronary vein results in profuse bleeding and is difficult to control. Careful dissection and vessel control before division is recommended.

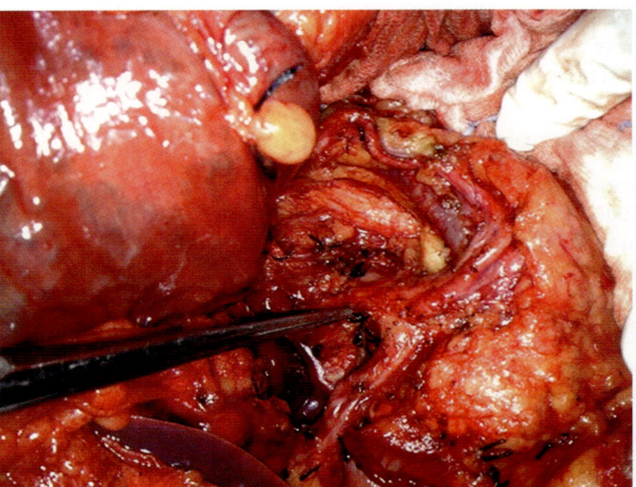

Figure 2 Operative photograph showing the field after D2 dissection in a patients undergoing total gastrectomy. The common hepatic artery, splenic artery and vein up to splenic hilum and celiac axis have been cleared. The forceps points to the stump of left gastric artery. Spleen and pancreas have been preserved

- The right accessory colic vein is located in the right side of the transverse colon mesentery, this joins with the right gastroepiploic vein, and the venous drainage from the pancreatic head then forms a gastrocolic trunk. Nodal station 6 is located proximal to the junction of the right accessory colic vein and the right gastroepiploic vein. For complete dissection of station 6, the right gastroepiploic vein should be ligated at this junction.
- For complete clearance of the left greater curvature nodal tissue (station 4sb), ligation of left gastroepiploic artery and vein should be done at its origin at the level of lower pole of the spleen and the tail of the pancreas.[58]

A summary of prospective randomized trials on the extent of lymphadenectomy is described in Table 6.

Initial studies in the West showed higher morbidity and mortality with no survival benefit in D2 dissection versus D1 dissection. But recent trials and long follow-up are in favor of modified D2 dissection (pancreas and spleen preserving) having a survival benefit in D2 arm with acceptable increased morbidity. This is true for western patients also. Studies in favor of D2 dissection are as follows:

- In an update of Dutch D1 vs D2 trial patients randomly assigned to the D1 group (n=380) and to the D2 group (n=331) were followed up for a median time of 15.2 years. Overall 15-year survival of the total of 711 patients was 21% (82 patients) for the D1 group and 29% (92 patients) for the D2 group (p=0.34). Gastric-cancer-related death rate was significantly higher in the D1 group (48%, 182 patients) compared with the D2 group

Table 5: Modifications of nodal dissection by T stages and procedures

	Total gastrectomy	*Distal gastrectomy*	*Proximal gastrectomy*
cTis (mucosal)	D1 (1–7)	D1 (1, 3, 4sb, 4d, 5, 6, 7)	D1 (1, 2, 3a, 4sa, 4sb, 7)
cT1 (submucosal), cN0	D1 plus (D1 and 8a, 9, 11p)	D1 plus (D1 and 8a, 9)	D1 plus (D1 and 8a, 9, 11p)
cT2 or deeper or cN1	D2 (D1 plus and 10, 11d, 12a)	D2 (D1 plus and 11p, 12a)	Should be treated with total with D2

Table 6: Summary of prospective randomized trials addressing extent of lymphadenectomy

Author	*Stages*	*LND (n)*	*5-year survival (%)*	*Morbidity n (%)*	*Mortality n (%)*
Cape Town trial,[59] 1988	I–IIIA	D1 (22) D2 (21)	78 (3-y) 76 (3-y)	3 (4) 7 (9)	0 (0) 0 (0)
Hong Kong trial,[60] 1994	I–IV	D1 (25) D3 (30)	45 35	0 (0) 24 (57)*	0 (0) 1 (3)
Dutch trial,[61] 1995	I–IV	D1 (380) D2 (331)	45 47	94 (25) 142 (43)*	15 (4) 32 (10)*
UK MRC trial,[62,63] 1996 and 1999	I–IIIB	D1 (200) D2 (200)	35 33	55 (28) 92 (46)*	13 (7) 26 (13)*
Italian trial[64] (IGCSG) 2004	I–IIB	D1 (76) D2 (86)	— —	8 (11) 14 (16)	1 (1.3) 0 (0)
Taiwanese trial,[65,66] 2004, 2006	I–IV	D1 (110) D3 (111)	54 60*	8 (7) 19 (17)*	0 (0) 0 (0)

*$p < 0.05$

Abbreviations: IGCSG, Italian Gastric Cancer Study Group; LND, lymph node dissection; MRC, Medical Research Council.

(37%, 123 patients), whereas death due to other diseases was similar in both groups. Local recurrence was 22% (82 patients) in the D1 group versus 12% (40 patients) in D2, and regional recurrence was 19% (73 patients) in D1 versus 13% (43 patients) in D2. Patients who had the D2 procedure had a significantly higher operative mortality rate than D1 [n=32 (10%) vs n=15 (4%); p=0.004], higher complication rate [n=142 (43%) vs n=94 (25%); p <0.0001], and higher reoperation rate [n=59 (18%) vs n=30 (8%); p=0.00016].[67]

- Austrian study in favor of radical lymph node dissection for gastric cancer yielded survival rates similar to those in Japanese investigations without sacrificing low postoperative mortality.[68]
- Spanish study showed no significant difference in the length of hospital stay, overall morbidity, or operative mortality between D1 and D2. Five-year survival in the D2 group was longer (50.6%) than in the D1 group (41.4%) for tumor stages (tumor-node-metastasis) more than I.[69]
- Italian Gastric Cancer Study Group showed that the rate of complications following D2 dissection is less than in published randomized Western trials.[70]
- Earlier trials show that D2 dissections had higher operative mortality, while recent trials have lower rates. A trend of improved survival exists among D2 patients who did not undergo resection of the spleen or pancreas, as well as for patients with T3/T4 cancers.[71]
- Taiwanese trial showed a survival advantage of extended lymphadenectomy (5-year survival being 60% in D3 dissection arm versus 54% in D1 dissection arm, p< 0.05).

In a Japanese trial comparing D2 dissection and D2 plus para-aortic dissection, there was no improvement in survival when para-aortic dissection was added to the procedure.[72]

Metastatic Lymph Node Ratio

Metastatic lymph node ratio (MLR; the ratio between metastatic lymph nodes and total evaluated lymph nodes) as opposed to the total number of positive nodes may be more valuable in cases in which inadequate node evaluation has been performed. Several groups have found MLR to be one of the strongest negative prognostic factors for survival on multivariate analyses.[73]

MARUYAMA INDEX (MI)

This was used to analyze the completeness of a nodal dissection based on data from 4,302 patients treated at the National Canter Hospital in Japan between 1968 and 1989. A computer software was used to predict the possibility of each nodal station involvement based on several clinical (preoperative) data points like histology type, gross appearance of the tumor, size and tumor depth. A calculated value (MI) was used to estimate the sum of the percentages of undissected nodal stations that reflect potentially untreated disease left behind. A low MI is associated with better overall survival and an MI of more than 5 is an indicator of inadequate nodal dissection. As it is based on preoperative data, marginal error in estimation might lead to over or under treatment. High value of MI may be due to inadequate nodal dissection or advanced disease beyond surgical treatment. So, high MI values have to be interpreted cautiously.[74,75]

LAPAROSCOPIC GASTRECTOMY

The first laparoscopic-assisted distal gastrectomy with lymph node dissection for gastric cancer was performed by Kitano and colleagues in 1994.[76] Numerous retrospective analyses and prospective trial by Huscher et al. and Hayashi et al. have shown that laparoscopic gastric resection for malignancy is both feasible and safe, with no increased morbidity when compared with open resection. Mean number of lymph nodes harvested was similar to open surgery. Advantage of laparoscopy is decreased blood loss, earlier postoperative flatus passage and shorter hospital stay. Operative time is longer than open procedure.[77-82] The conversion rate to open is around 2.3–25% and majority are due to extensive disease rather than intraoperative complications.[83] At least 60–90 cases are required for complete learning of the technique.[84] Long-term outcome for Stages I and II is comparable with open procedure.[85] Multiple severe comorbidities, high BMI, those who have received neoadjuvant therapy, or those who have undergone previous laparotomy may not be good candidates for laparoscopic surgery. Poor cardiopulmonary reserve is an absolute contraindication. Decreased surgical visibility, dissection plane hindered by adipose tissue and difficulty with anastomoses have been reported in obese patients. Higher BMI has also been reported as an independent risk factor for increased risk of pancreatic fistula following laparoscopic distal gastrectomy.[86,87] Tumor dissemination and trocar-site metastasis are most likely related to poor technique or advanced disease. Precautions to prevent trocar site metastasis include minimal handling of tumor, securing trocars to skin with suture to prevent dislodgment, irrigation of trocar sites with tumoricidal agent, and the use of wound protector at the tumor extraction site.[88]

ROBOTIC SURGERY

Song et al.[89] demonstrated that robotic gastrectomy with lymphadenectomy could be done safely and effectively for patients with gastric cancer. Out of 100 cases, 33 underwent total gastrectomy and 67 had subtotal gastrectomy with D1 or D2 lymphadenectomy. The mean total operation time and console time were 231 and 150 minutes, respectively. The first flatus was noted on postoperative day 2.9, soft diet was started on postoperative day 4.2, and the mean postoperative hospital stay was 7.8 days. The mean number of retrieved lymph nodes was 36.7 (range, 11–83). There were 13 postoperative complications and one postoperative death.

NEOADJUVANT TREATMENT

Even after potentially curative surgery, overall survival at 5 years remains as low as 20–30% in gastric adenocarcinoma. Theoretically, administration of chemotherapy before surgical resection can address micrometastatic lesions, downstage disease and allow an in vivo assessment of chemotherapeutic efficacy in those patients with measurable disease (primary or perigastric nodal disease) on imaging. Progression of disease before resection and the potential for surgery-preventing toxicity are the main concerns with preoperative therapy. Progressive disease on preoperative therapy may be spared unnecessary laparotomy as disease is likely to be beyond surgical therapy at presentation. Toxicity remains an issue, because the platinum-based regimens that are often used can be difficult to tolerate.[90,91] A recent meta-analysis of trials by Li and colleagues assessed survival following surgery for locally advanced gastric cancer with either neoadjuvant chemotherapy or surgery alone, with a median follow-up time of 3 years. The neoadjuvant group had a marginal improvement in overall survival compared with the control group (48.1% vs 46.9%), significant downstaging and higher complete resection (R0) rate. Later stages of disease (pT3-4) benefited more from neoadjuvant therapy than those at earlier stages (pT1-2). Combination therapy and intravenous administration were more effective than monotherapy, oral administration, or intra-arterial administration.[92]

A landmark study on the role of chemotherapy for resectable gastric cancer was the Medical Research Council Adjuvant Gastric Cancer Infusional Chemotherapy (MAGIC) trial. Patients with Stages II to IVA gastric cancer (74%), distal esophageal (11%), and gastroesophageal junction (15%) cancers were randomized to receive perioperative chemotherapy (n=250) or surgery alone (n=253). The chemotherapy regimen consisted of three cycles of epirubicin, cisplatin and 5-FU (ECF) before and after surgery. Data indicated that 5-year survival was better (36% vs 23%, HR 0.75, 95% CI 0.60–0.93, p<0.009), progression-free survival was longer (HR for progression 0.66, 95% CI 0.53–0.81, p<0.001), and local recurrence rates were lower (14.4% perioperative chemotherapy group; 20.6% surgery group) in the ECF arm. Tumor downstaging was also seen for both T and N stage. Limitations of the trial include inability to determine the contribution of preoperative versus postoperative chemotherapy on survival because of the trial design, and the differential impact on distal esophageal and gastroesophageal junction tumors could not be assessed because they were both included in the study.[93,94]

In a European study, 102 patients were randomized to either preoperative radiation or surgery alone. In a 20-year follow-up period, no significant improvement in survival was seen.[95] The Radiation Therapy Oncology Group trial (RTOG 9904) similarly examined neoadjuvant chemoradiation therapy in patients with resectable gastric cancer; a pathologic complete response was seen in 26% and R0 resection completed in 77%. In spite of favorable results, large prospective randomized trials are lacking. Thus neoadjuvant therapy can be administered in carefully selected patients, with radiotherapy alone having limited benefit.[96,97]

ADJUVANT THERAPY

The benefit of adjuvant radiotherapy alone has not been validated. Modest improvement in overall survival has been described in patients receiving adjuvant chemotherapy especially in Asian population and in node positive cancers. In Japanese patients receiving adjuvant S-1, an oral fluoropyrimidine after surgery have shown significant better survival than surgery alone.[98]

The Southwest Oncology Group Intergroup trial (SWOG 9008/ INT-0116) by Macdonald and colleagues randomized 556 patients who underwent complete resection for Stages IB to IVA gastric or gastroesophageal junction cancer to surgery alone (n=275) or surgery with postoperative chemoradiotherapy (n=281). The regimen consisted of 425 mg/m^2 of 5-FU with leucovorin 20 mg/m^2/day for 5 days followed by 45 Gy of radiation at 180 cGy per day for 5 weeks with modified doses of 5-FU/leucovorin. One month after completion of the radiotherapy, two additional 5-day cycles of 5-FU/leucovorin were administered. Median follow-up period was 6 years. They found that the surgery plus adjuvant chemoradiotherapy resulted in improved overall survival (35 vs 26 months, p<0.006) and disease-free survival (30 vs 19 months, p<0.001) compared with surgery only. One of the strongest criticisms of the study concerned the inadequate extent of lymph node dissection.[99,100]

Yan et al.[101] conducted a meta-analysis on intraperitoneal chemotherapy and concluded that there was a significant survival benefit with hyperthermic intraoperative intraperitoneal chemotherapy (HIIC) and HIIC combined with early postoperative intraperitoneal chemotherapy (EPIC) but no comments on locoregional control. No survival benefit was observed in normothermic intraoperative intraperitoneal chemotherapy (NIIC), delayed postoperative intraperitoneal chemotherapy (DPIC) and early postoperative intraperitoneal chemotherapy (EPIC) alone. Complications were neutropenia and higher rate of intra-abdominal abscesses.

PALLIATIVE THERAPY

In metastatic disease, performance status plays an important role in modality of treatment or best supportive care. Wagner et al. showed benefit (including improvement in quality of life) following palliative chemotherapy over best supportive care.[102] A prognostic model of Royal Marsden remained effective for discriminating different survival groups and includes four major factors—(1) performance status, (2) liver metastases, (3) peritoneal metastases and (4) alkaline phosphatase more than 100 UI/L.[103] Several drugs can be used either singly or in combination: cisplatin, capecitabine, oxaliplatin, docetaxel, irinotecan, etc. Palliative surgeries—gastrectomy in bleeding and gastrojejunostomy in obstruction can be done if a long survival is expected. Otherwise percutaneous endoscopic gastrostomy (PEG), open gastrostomy or stenting (SEMS) is recommended.

Majority of patients with advanced disease die of organ failure due to metastases.

TARGETED THERAPY

HER2 is a key driver of tumorigenesis in gastric cancer. Amplification of HER2 amplification or over expression is seen in 7–34% of gastric cancer. The first clinical evidence of efficacy of an anti-HER2 treatment (trastuzumab) was demonstrated by the ToGA trial.[104] Median overall survival was 13.8 months in those assigned to trastuzumab plus chemotherapy compared with 11.1 months in those treated with chemotherapy alone (HR 0.74; 95% CI 0.60–0.91; p=0.0046).

TREATMENT SUMMARY

Medically fit patients undergo standard treatment as per NCCN 2013 guidelines:[105]

1. Endoscopic treatment is an option for Tis and T1a tumors in experienced centers.
2. Surgery with lymph node dissection for medically fit patients with resectable disease. Laparotomy should be preceded by staging laparoscopy.
3. Gastric resection should include at least D1 and preferably D2 lymphadenectomy with a goal of examining at least 15 lymph nodes. Routine or prophylactic splenectomy is not indicated.
4. Patients with resectable disease (clinically T2 or more) have an option of preoperative chemotherapy followed by surgery. In such patients, postoperative chemotherapy should be considered if R0 resection is achieved. In case of R1 or R2 resection, postoperative chemoradiation is preferred.
5. In patients who have undergone upfront surgery without receiving preoperative treatment, postoperative chemoradiation is recommended following R0 resection in all patients with T3-T4 or node positive tumors. Postoperative chemoradiation may also be considered for selected patients with T2 N0 tumors with high risk features.

Patients with gastric cancer, who are not fit for standard treatment, should undergo chemoradiation, palliative chemotherapy or best supportive care depending on the stage of the disease.

SURVEILLANCE

Follow-up should include a complete history and physical examination every 3-6 months for 1–2 years, then every 6–12 months for 3–5 years, and annually thereafter. Laboratory tests, including complete blood counts and liver function tests, should be performed as clinically indicated. Radiologic imaging and endoscopic examination is done as clinically indicated. Patients should be monitored for nutritional deficiencies (e.g. vitamin B_{12} and iron) in surgically resected patients and treated accordingly.

REFERENCES

1. Santoro E. The history of gastric cancer: legends and chronicles. Gastric Cancer. 2005;8:71-4.
2. Altekruse SF, Kosary CL, Krapcho M, Neyman N, Aminou R, Waldron W, et al. (Eds). Surveillance, Epidemiology, and End Results (SEER) Cancer Statistics Review, 1975-2007. National Cancer Institute; 2010. Available at: http://seer.cancer.gov/statfacts/html/stomach.html. Accessed on January, 2014.
3. Jemal A, Bray F, Center MM, Ferlay J, Ward E, Forman D. Global cancer statistics. CA Cancer J Clin. 2011;61:69-90.
4. http://globocan.iarc.fr/Pages/fact_sheets_cancer.aspx[GLOBOCAN 2012] Accessed on January, 2014.
5. Pounder RE, Ng D. The prevalence of Helicobacter pylori infection in different countries. Aliment Pharmacol Ther. 1995;9:33-9.
6. Raghunath A, Hungin AP, Wooff D, Childs S. Prevalence of Helicobacter pylori in patients with gastro-esophageal reflux disease: systemic review. BMJ. 2003;326:737-44.
7. Warburton-Timms VJ, Charlett A, Valori RM, Uff JS, Shepherd NA, Barr H, et al. The significance of cag A(+) Helicobacter pylori in reflux esophagitis. Gut. 2001;49:341-6.
8. Eslick GD, Lim LL, Byles JE, Xia HH, Talley NJ. Association of Helicobacter pylori infection with gastric carcinoma: a meta-analysis. Am J Gastroenterol. 1999;94:2373-9.
9. Murphy G, Pfeiffer R, Camargo MC, Rabkin CS. Meta-analysis shows that prevalence of Epstein-Barr virus-positive gastric cancer differs based on sex and anatomic location. Gastroenterology. 2009;137:824-33.
10. Joossens JV, Hill MJ, Elliott P, Stamler R, Lesaffre E, Dyer A, et al. Dietary salt, nitrate and stomach cancer mortality in 24 countries. European Cancer Prevention (ECP) and the INTERSALT Cooperative Research Group. Int J Epidemiol. 1996;25:494-504.
11. Guggenheim DE, Shah MA. Gastric cancer epidemiology and risk factors. J Surg Oncol. 2013;107:230-6.
12. Shikata K, Kiyohara Y, Kubo M, Yonemoto K, Ninomiya T, Shirota T, et al. A prospective study of dietary salt intake and gastric cancer incidence in a defined Japanese population: The Hisayama study. Int J Cancer. 2006;119:196-201.
13. Larsson SC, Bergkvist L, Wolk A. Fruit and vegetable consumption and incidence of gastric cancer: a prospective study. Cancer Epidemiol Biomarkers Prev. 2006;15:1998-2001.
14. Ma JL, Zhang L, Brown LM, Li JY, Shen L, Pan KF, et al. Fifteeen-year effects of Helicobacter pylori, garlic, and vitamin treatments on gastric cancer incidence and mortality. J Natl Cancer Inst. 2012;104:488-92.
15. Tramacere I, Negri E, Pelucchi C, Bagnardi V, Rota M, Scotti L, et al. A meta-analysis on alcohol drinking and gastric cancer risk. Ann Oncol. 2012;23:28-36.
16. Duell EJ, Travier N, Lujan-Barroso L, Clavel-Chapelon F, Boutron-Ruault MC, Morois S, et al. Alcohol consumption and gastric cancer risk in the European prospective investigation into cancer and nutrition (EPIC) cohort. Am J Clin Nutr. 2011;94:1266-75.
17. Smyth EC, Capanu M, Janjigian YY, Kelsen DK, Coit D, Strong VE, et al. Tobacco use is associated with increased recurrence and death from gastric cancer. Ann Surg Oncol. 2012;19:2088-94.
18. Fitzgerald RC, Hardwick R, Huntsman D, Carneiro F, Guilford P, Blair V, et al. Hereditary diffuse gastric cancer: updated consensus guidelines for clinical management and directions for future research. J Med Genet. 2010;47:436-44.

19. Carneiro F, Oliveira C, Seruca R. Pathology and genetics of familial gastric cancer. Int J Surg Pathol. 2010;18(Suppl 3):33S-6S.
20. Patel SH, Kooby DA. Gastric adenocarcinoma surgery and adjuvant therapy. Surg Clin N Am. 2011;91:1039-77.
21. Capelle LG, Van Grieken NC, Lingsma HF, Steyerberg EW, Klokman WJ, Bruno MJ, et al. Risk and epidemiological time trends of gastric cancer in lynch syndrome carriers in The Netherlands. Gastroenterology. 2010;138:487-92.
22. Yao JC, Schnirer II, Reddy S, Chiang S, Najam A, Yu C, et al. Effects of sex and racial/ethnic group on the pattern of gastric cancer localization. Gastric Cancer. 2002;5:208-12.
23. Yeh JS, Munn SE, Plunkett TA, Harper PG, Hopster DJ, du Vivier AW. Coexistence of acanthosis nigricans and the sign of Leser-Trelat in a patient with gastric adenocarcinoma: a case report and literature review. J Am Acad Dermatol. 2000;42:357-62.
24. Lauren P. The two histological main types of gastric carcinoma: diffuse and so-called intestinal-type carcinoma. An attempt at the histoclinical classification. Acta Pathol Microbiol Scand. 1965;64:31-49.
25. Vauhkonen M, Vauhkonen H, Sipponen P. Pathology and molecular biology of gastric cancer. Best Pract Res Clin Gastroenterol. 2006;20:651-74.
26. Munson JL, O'Mahony R. Radical gastrectomy for cancer of the stomach. Surg Clin North Am. 2005;85:1021-32.
27. Correa P, Shiao YH. Phenotypic and genotypic events in gastric carcinogenesis. Cancer Res. 1994;54:1941s-3s.
28. Mahvi DM, Krantz SB. Stomach. ln: Townsend CM Jr, Beauchamp RD, Evers BM, Mattox KL (Eds). Sabiston Textbook of Surgery, 19th edition. Philadelphia, PA: Saunders Elsevier; 2012.
29. Edge SB, Byrd DR, Compton CC, Fritz AG, Greene FL, Trotti A (Eds). AJCC Cancer Staging Manual, 7th edition. New York: Springer Science and Business Media LLC (SBM); 2010.
30. JGCA. Japanese classification of gastric carcinoma-2nd English edition. Gastric Cancer. 1998;1:10-24.
31. Bentrem D, Wilton A, Mazumdar M, Brennan M, Coit D. The value of peritoneal cytology as a preoperative predictor in patients with gastric carcinoma undergoing a curative resection. Ann Surg Oncol. 2005;12:347-53.
32. Goldfarb M, Brower S, Schwaitzberg SD. Minimally invasive surgery and cancer: controversies part 1. Surg Endosc. 2010;24:304-34.
33. Bentrem D, Gerdes H, Tang L, Brennan M, Coit D. Clinical correlation of endoscopic ultrasonography with pathologic stage and outcome in patients undergoing curative resection for gastric cancer. Ann Surg Oncol. 2007;14:1853-9.
34. Jones DB. Role of endoscopic ultrasound in staging upper gastrointestinal cancers. ANZ J Surg. 2007;77:166-72.
35. Lee BE, Kim GH, Park do Y, Kim DH, Jeon TY, Park SB, et al. Acetic acid-indigo carmine chromoendoscopy for delineating early gastric cancers: its usefulness according to histological type. BMC Gastroenterology. 2010;10:97.
36. Li HY, Dai J, Xue HB, Zhao YJ, Chen XY, Gao YJ, et al. Application of magnifying endoscopy with narrow-band imaging in diagnosing gastric lesions: a prospective study. Gastrointest Endosc. 2012;76:1124-32.
37. Bhandari S, Shim CS, Kim JH, Jung IS, Cho JY, Lee JS, et al. Usefulness of three-dimensional, multidetector row CT (virtual gastroscopy and multiplanar reconstruction) in the evaluation of gastric cancer: a comparison with conventional endoscopy, EUS, and histopathology. Gastrointest Endosc. 2004;59:619-26.
38. Chen J, Cheong JH, Yun MJ, Kim J, Lim JS, Hyung WJ, et al. Improvement in preoperative staging of gastric adenocarcinoma with positron emission tomography. Cancer. 2005;103:2383-90.
39. Samee A, Moorthy K, Jaipersad T, Crisp W, Cheruvu C, Elder J, et al. Evaluation of the role of laparoscopic ultrasonography in the staging of oesophagogastric cancers. Surg Endosc. 2009;23:2061-5.
40. Mihmanli M, Dilege E, Demir U, Coskun H, Eroglu T, Uysalol MD. The use of tumor markers as predictors of prognosis in gastric cancer. Hepatogastroenterology. 2004;51:1544-7.
41. Liu X, Cheng Y, Sheng W, Lu H, Xu Y, Long Z, et al. Clinicopathologic features and prognostic factors in alpha-fetoprotein-producing gastric cancers: analysis of 104 cases. J Surg Oncol. 2010;102:249-55.
42. Wang KK, Prasad G, Tian J. Endoscopic mucosal resection and endoscopic submucosal dissection in esophageal and gastric cancers. Curr Opin Gastroenterol. 2010;26:453-8.
43. Eguchi T, Gotoda T, Oda I, Hamanaka H, Hasuike N, Saito D. Is endoscopic one-piece mucosal resection essential for early gastric cancer? Dig Endosc. 2003;15:113-6.
44. Lian J, Chen S, Zhang Y, Qiu F. A meta-analysis of endoscopic submucosal dissection and EMR for early gastric cancer. Gastrointest Endosc. 2012;76:763-70.
45. Oka S, Tanaka S, Kaneko I, Mouri R, Hirata M, Kawamura T, et al. Advantage of endoscopic submucosal dissection compared with EMR for early gastric cancer. Gastrointest Endosc. 2006;64:877-83.
46. Min BH, Lee JH, Kim JJ, Shim SG, Chang DK, Kim YH, et al. Clinical outcomes of endoscopic submucosal dissection (ESD) for treating early gastric cancer: comparison with endoscopic mucosal resection after circumferential precutting (EMR-P). Dig Liver Dis. 2009;41:201-9.
47. Nakamoto S, Sakai Y, Kasanuki J, Kondo F, Ooka Y, Kato K, et al. Indications for the use of endoscopic mucosal resection for early gastric cancer in Japan: a comparative study with endoscopic submucosal dissection. Endoscopy. 2009;41:746-50.
48. Oda I, Saito D, Tada M, Iishi H, Tanabe S, Oyama T, et al. A multicenter retrospective study of endoscopic resection for early gastric cancer. Gastric Cancer. 2006;9:262-70.
49. Catalano F, Trecca A, Rodella L, Lombardo F, Tomezzoli A, Battista S, et al. The modern treatment of early gastric cancer: our experience in an Italian cohort. Surg Endosc. 2009;23:1581-6.
50. Hoteya S, Iizuka T, Kikuchi D, Yahagi N. Benefits of endoscopic submucosal dissection according to size and location of gastric neoplasm, compared with conventional mucosal resection. J Gastroenterol Hepatol. 2009;24:1102-6.
51. Hoteya S, Iizuka T, Kikuchi D, Yahagi N. Clinical advantages of endoscopic submucosal dissection for gastric cancers in remnant stomach surpass conventional endoscopic mucosal resection. Dig Endosc. 2010;22:17-20.
52. Watanabe T, Kume K, Taip M, Shibata M, Kubo H, Ejiri Y, et al. Gastric mucosal cancer smaller than 7 mm can be treated with conventional endoscopic mucosal resection as effectively as with endoscopic submucosal dissection. Hepatogastroenterology. 2010;57:668-73.
53. Gertler R, Rosenberg R, Feith M, Schuster T, Friess H. Pouch vs. no pouch following total gastrectomy: meta-analysis and systematic review. Am J Gastroenterol. 2009;104:2838-51.
54. Coburn NG. Lymph nodes and gastric cancer. J Surg Oncol. 2009;99:199-206.
55. Kitagawa Y, Fujii H, Mukai M, Kubota T, Ando N, Watanabe M, et al. The role of the sentinel lymph node in gastrointestinal cancer. Surg Clin North Am. 2000;80:1799-809.
56. Cozzaglio L, Bottura R, Di Rocco M, Gennari L, Doci R. Sentinel lymph node biopsy in gastric cancer: possible applications and limits. Eur J Surg Oncol. 2011;37:55-9.
57. Lee JH, Ryu KW, Nam BH, Kook MC, Cho SJ, Lee JY, et al. Factors associated with detection failure and false-negative sentinel node biopsy findings in gastric cancer: results of prospective single center trials. J Surg Oncol. 2009;99:137-42.
58. Hoshi H. Standard D2 and modified nodal dissection for gastric adenocarcinoma. Surg Oncol Clin N Am. 2012;21:57-70.
59. Dent DM, Madden MV, Price SK. Randomized comparison of R1 and R2 gastrectomy for gastric carcinoma. Br J Surg. 1988;75:110-2.

60. Robertson CS, Chung SC, Woods SD, Griffin SM, Raimes SA, Lau JT, et al. A prospective randomized trial comparing R1 subtotal gastrectomy with R3 total gastrectomy for antral cancer. Ann Surg. 1994;220:176-82.
61. Bonenkamp JJ, Songun I, Hermans J, Sasako M, Welvaart K, Plukker JT, et al. Randomised comparison of morbidity after D1 and D2 dissection for gastric cancer in 996 Dutch patients. Lancet. 1995;345:745-8.
62. Cuschieri A, Fayers P, Fielding J, Craven J, Bancewicz J, Joypaul V, et al. Postoperative morbidity and mortality after D1 and D2 resections for gastric cancer: preliminary results of the MRC randomised controlled surgical trial. The Surgical Cooperative Group. Lancet. 1996;347:995-9.
63. Cuschieri A, Weeden S, Fielding J, Bancewicz J, Craven J, Joypaul V, et al. Patient survival after D1 and D2 resections for gastric cancer: long-term results of the MRC randomized surgical trial. Surgical Co-operative Group. Br J Cancer. 1999;79:1522-30.
64. Degiuli M, Sasako M, Calgaro M, Garino M, Rebecchi F, Mineccia M, et al. Morbidity and mortality after D1 and D2 gastrectomy for cancer: interim analysis of the Italian Gastric Cancer Study Group (IGCSG) randomised surgical trial. Eur J Surg Oncol. 2004; 30:303-8.
65. Wu CW, Hsiung CA, Lo SS, Hsieh MC, Chen JH, Li AF, et al. Nodal dissection for patients with gastric cancer: a randomised controlled trial. Lancet Oncol. 2006;7:309-15.
66. Wu CW, Hsiung CA, Lo SS, Hsieh MC, Shia LT, Whang-Peng J. Randomized clinical trial of morbidity after D1 and D3 surgery for gastric cancer. Br J Surg. 2004;91:283-7.
67. Songun I, Putter H, Kranenbarg EM, Sasako M, van de Velde CJ. Surgical treatment of gastric cancer: 15-year follow-up results of the randomised nationwide Dutch D1D2 trial. Lancet Oncol. 2010;11:439-49.
68. Jatzko GR, Lisborg PH, Denk H, Klimpfinger M, Stettner HM. A 10-year experience with Japanese-type radical lymph node dissection for gastric cancer outside of Japan. Cancer. 1995;76:1302-12.
69. Sierra A, Regueira FM, Hernández-Lizoáin JL, Pardo F, Martínez-Gonzalez MA, A-Cienfuegos J. Role of the extended lymphadenectomy in gastric cancer surgery: experience in a single institution. Ann Surg Oncol. 2003;10:219-26.
70. Degiuli M, Sasako M, Ponti A, Italian Gastric Cancer Study Group. Morbidity and mortality in the Italian Gastric Cancer Study Group randomized clinical trial of D1 versus D2 resection for gastric cancer. Br J Surg. 2010;97:643-9.
71. Seevaratnam R, Bocicariu A, Cardoso R, Mahar A, Kiss A, Helyer L, et al. A meta-analysis of D1 versus D2 lymph node dissection. Gastric Cancer. 2012;15(Suppl 1):S60-9.
72. Sasako M, Sano T, Yamamoto S, Kurokawa Y, Nashimoto A, Kurita A, et al. D2 lymphadenectomy alone or with para-aortic nodal dissection for gastric cancer. N Engl J Med. 2008;359:453-62.
73. Lee SY, Hwang I, Park YS, Gardner J, Ro JY. Metastatic lymph node ratio in advanced gastric carcinoma: a better prognostic factor than number of metastatic lymph nodes? Int J Oncol. 2010;36:1461-7.
74. Hundahl SA, Macdonald JS, Benedetti J, Fitzsimmons T; Southwest Oncology Group and the Gastric Intergroup. Surgical treatment variation in a prospective, randomized trial of chemoradiotherapy in gastric cancer: the effect of undertreatment. Ann Surg Oncol. 2002;9:278-86.
75. Bollschweiler E, Boettcher K, Hoelscher AH, Sasako M, Kinoshita T, Maruyama K, et al. Preoperative assessment of lymph node metastases in patients with gastric cancer: evaluation of the Maruyama computer program. Br J Surg. 1992;79:156-60.
76. Kitano S, Iso Y, Moriyama M, Sugimachi K. Laparoscopy-assisted Billroth I gastrectomy. Surg Laparosc Endosc. 1994;4:146-8.
77. Huscher CG, Mingoli A, Sgarzini G, Sansonetti A, Di Paola M, Recher A, et al. Laparoscopic versus open subtotal gastrectomy for distal gastric cancer: five-year results of a randomized prospective trial. Ann Surg. 2005;241:232-7.
78. Lee JH, Han HS. A prospective randomized study comparing open vs laparoscopy-assisted distal gastrectomy in early gastric cancer: early results. Surg Endosc. 2005;19:168-73.
79. Kim YW, Baik YH, Yun YH, Nam BH, Kim DH, Choi IJ, et al. Improved quality of life outcomes after laparoscopy-assisted distal gastrectomy for early gastric cancer: results of a prospective randomized clinical trial. Ann Surg. 2008;248:721-7.
80. Kim HH, Hyung WJ, Cho GS, Kim MC, Han SU, Kim W, et al. Morbidity and mortality of laparoscopic gastrectomy versus open gastrectomy for gastric cancer: an interim report—a phase III multicenter, prospective, randomized trial (KLASS Trial). Ann Surg. 2010;251:417-20.
81. Hayashi H, Ochiai T, Shimada H, Gunji Y. Prospective randomized study of open versus laparoscopy-assisted distal gastrectomy with extraperigastric lymph node dissection for early gastric cancer. Surg Endosc. 2005;19:1172-6.
82. Memon MA, Khan S, Yunus RM, Barr R, Memon B. Meta-analysis of laparoscopic and open distal gastrectomy for gastric carcinoma. Surg Endosc. 2008;22:1781-9.
83. Shiraishi N, Yasuda K, Kitano S. Laparoscopic gastrectomy with lymph node dissection for gastric cancer. Gastric Cancer. 2006;9:167-76.
84. Zhang X, Tanigawa N. Learning curve of laparoscopic surgery for gastric cancer, a laparoscopic distal gastrectomy-based analysis. Surg Endosc. 2009;23:1259-64.
85. Lee SW, Nomura E, Bouras G, Tokuhara T, Tsunemi S, Tanigawa N. Long-term oncologic outcomes from laparoscopic gastrectomy for gastric cancer: a single-center experience of 601 consecutive resections. J Am Coll Surg. 2010;211:33-40.
86. Jiang X, Hiki N, Nunobe S, Kumagai K, Nohara K, Sano T, et al. Postoperative pancreatic fistula and the risk factors of laparoscopy-assisted distal gastrectomy for early gastric cancer. Ann Surg Oncol. 2012;19:115-21.
87. Strong VE. Laparoscopic resection for gastric carcinoma: Western experience. Surg Onc Clin N Am. 2012;21:141-58.
88. Phillips JD, Nagle AP, Soper NJ. Laparoscopic gastrectomy for cancer. Surg Oncol Clin N Am. 2013;22:39-57.
89. Song J, Oh SJ, Kang WH, Hyung WJ, Choi SH, Noh SH. Robot-assisted gastrectomy with lymph node dissection for gastric cancer: lessons learned from an initial 100 consecutive procedures. Ann Surg. 2009;249:927-32.
90. Sano T, Sasako M, Yamamoto S, Nashimoto A, Kurita A, Hiratsuka M, et al. Gastric cancer surgery: morbidity and mortality results from a prospective randomized controlled trial comparing D2 and extended para-aortic lymphadenectomy—Japan Clinical Oncology Group Study 9501. J Clin Oncol. 2004;22:2767-73.
91. Rajdev L. Treatment options for surgically resectable gastric cancer. Curr Treat Options Oncol. 2010;11:14-23.
92. Li W, Qin J, Sun YH, Liu TS. Neoadjuvant chemotherapy for advanced gastric cancer: a meta-analysis. World J Gastroenterol. 2010;16:5621-8.
93. Cunningham D, Allum WH, Stenning SP, Thompson JN, Van de Velde CJ, Nicolson M, et al. Perioperative chemotherapy versus surgery alone for resectable gastroesophageal cancer. N Engl J Med. 2006;355:11-20.
94. Ng K, Meyerhardt JA, Fuchs CS. Adjuvant and neoadjuvant approaches in gastric cancer. Cancer J. 2007;13:168-74.
95. Skoropad VY, Berdov BA, Mardynski YS, Titova LN. A prospective, randomized trial of pre-operative and intraoperative radiotherapy versus surgery alone in resectable gastric cancer. Eur J Surg Oncol. 2000;26:773-9.
96. Ajani JA, Mansfield PF, Janjan N, Morris J, Pisters PW, Lynch PM, et al. Multi-institutional trial of preoperative chemoradiotherapy in

patients with potentially resectable gastric carcinoma. J Clin Oncol. 2004;22:2774-80.
97. Ajani JA, Winter K, Okawara GS, Donohue JH, Pisters PW, Crane CH, et al. Phase II trial of preoperative chemoradiation in patients with localized gastric adenocarcinoma (RTOG 9904): quality of combined modality therapy and pathologic response. J Clin Oncol. 2006;24:3953-8.
98. Sakuramoto S, Sasako M, Yamaguchi T, Kinoshita T, Fujii M, Nashimoto A, et al. Adjuvant chemotherapy for gastric cancer with S-1, an oral fluoropyrimidine. N Engl J Med. 2007;357:1810-20.
99. Macdonald JS, Smalley SR, Benedetti J, Hundahl SA, Estes NC, Stemmermann GN, et al. Chemoradiotherapy after surgery compared with surgery alone for adenocarcinoma of the stomach or gastroesophageal junction. N Engl J Med. 2001;345:725-30.
100. Macdonald J, Smalley S, Benedetti J. Postoperative combined radiation and chemotherapy improves disease-free survival and overall survival in resected adenocarcinoma of the stomach and gastroesophageal junction: update of the results of Intergroup Study INT- 0116 (SWOG 9008). Presented at the Am Soc Clin Oncol Gastrointestinal Cancers Symposium [abstract 6]. San Francisco, January 22–24, 2004.
101. Yan TD, Black D, Sugarbaker PH, Zhu J, Yonemura Y, Petrou G, et al. A systematic review and meta-analysis of the randomized controlled trials on adjuvant intraperitoneal chemotherapy for resectable gastric cancer. Ann Surg Oncol. 2007;14:2702-13.
102. Wagner AD, Unverzagt S, Grothe W, Kleber G, Grothey A, Haerting J, et al. Chemotherapy for advanced gastric cancer. Cochrane Database of Systematic Reviews 2010, Mar 17;(3):CD004064.
103. Chau I, Ashley S, Cunningham D. Validation of the royal marsden hospital prognostic index in advanced esophagogastric cancer using individual patient data from the REAL 2 study. J Clin Oncol. 2009;27:e3–4.
104. Bang YJ, Van Cutsem E, Feyereislova A, Chung HC, Shen L, Sawaki A, et al. Trastuzmab in combination with chemotherapy versus chemotherapy alone for treatment of HER2-positive advanced gastric or gastro-oesophageal junction cancer (ToGA): a phase 3, open-label, randomized controlled trial. Lancet. 2010;376:687-97.
105. NCCN guidelines version 2.2013 gastric cancer (accessed on 8.9.2013) [http://www.nccn.org/professionals/physician_gls/pdf/gastric.pdf].

CHAPTER 26

Duodenal and Small Intestinal Tumors

Monika Gupta

Duodenal Tumors

INTRODUCTION

Duodenal tumors in the periampullary region are treated like periampullary tumors which are dealt with elsewhere. An overview of duodenal tumors is presented briefly. A special category of duodenal tumors is near the duodenojejunal flexure where proximity of superior mesenteric artery and veins may present special issues in resection. Tumors arising from third part of duodenum may be resected without concomitant pancreatic resection, if they do not involve the inner medial aspect.

PATHOLOGY AND CLINICAL FEATURES

Benign Tumors

Duodenal Adenomas

After leiomyomas, adenomas are the second most common benign tumors of the small intestine. The duodenum is the most common site of involvement, and the lesion most commonly is a villous adenoma. Villous adenomas constitute 45% of all benign lesions of the duodenum. Common presentation of villous adenomas is with jaundice (69%), abdominal pain (40%) anemia or melena (19%), weight loss (18%) and fever (18%). The passing of mucous with dyselectrolytemia, described with colorectal villous adenomas is rarely seen with duodenal adenomas.[1]

Duodenal adenomas can be part of various syndromes, like familial adenomatous polyposis (FAP), Gardner's syndrome, Peutz-Jeghers syndrome, etc. In patients of FAP who have previously undergone total proctocolectomy, periampullary carcinomas arising in duodenal polyps are the most common cause of mortality.

Duodenal villous adenomas can coexist with invasive tumors of the duodenum. A villous adenoma more than 4 cm is suggestive of malignancy. Duodenal polyps with malignant potential especially villous adenomas need to be screened as they may need radical resection. Histologically, carcinoma in situ (CIS) and invasive carcinoma (INV) are considered as malignant while an adenoma with or without cellular atypia is considered as benign (Komorowski and Cohen).[2]

Brunner's Gland Adenomas

These are extremely rare, comprising 10.6% of benign duodenal tumors. The literature contains predominantly case reports, with only one large case series. Brunner's gland adenomas (BGAs) are usually benign and primary carcinomas arising in Brunner's glands are extremely rare. Only one case of atypical BGA and two cases of definite primary malignancy arising in a BGA have been reported in the literature till date.[3] Brunner's gland hyperplasia is asymptomatic or may present with abdominal pain, upper gastrointestinal bleeding and may be associated with chronic pancreatitis. Careful evaluation for differentiation from duodenal malignancy with contrast-enhanced computed tomography (CECT), endoscopic ultrasound (EUS) and biopsy; along with prolonged follow-up confirms the diagnosis.

Other Benign Tumors

Lipomas, hyperplastic polyps, lymphangiomas and hemangiomas can occur in the duodenum. A specific preoperative diagnosis is very difficult to establish. Pathological diagnosis can be established after resection of symptomatic tumors.

Malignant Tumors

Duodenal adenocarcinomas are rare, comprising 0.5% of all gastrointestinal malignancies. Amongst these about 45% of all adenocarcinomas arise within the duodenum and 55% in the jejunum and ileum.[4] Periampullary carcinoma constitute a different entity in terms of both presentation and management and are hence not included within small intestinal tumors. In FAP, the relative risk of developing proximal small bowel malignancy increases 50- to 300-fold.

DIAGNOSIS AND TREATMENT

Endoscopy is best to diagnose suspected adenomas. Adenomas are resected and biopsied. False negative biopsy rate can be high (25–56%) in villous adenomas so care must be taken to perform a wide excision. Nowadays, even large lateral adenomas can be resected endoscopically. If endoscopic excision fails, surgical excision in the form of transduodenal excision, sleeve duodenectomy or segmental duodenectomy can be done. In tumors which are invasive on imaging, large (>4 cm), recurrent, associated with lymph nodes (LNs), or when the ampulla is involved a more radical excision (pancreaticoduodenectomy) should be preferred.[1,5]

In biopsy proven resectable duodenal carcinomas pancreaticoduodenectomy with peripancreatic nodes excision is the radical treatment. Some centers perform this laparoscopically but long-term survival data is still awaited. Carcinomas of the distal third portion and fourth portion of the duodenum are often amenable to segmental duodenectomy with lymphadenectomy.[6] Tumors in third part of duodenum or at duodenojejunal flexure (Figs 1 to 5) are to be assessed closely. Proximity to superior mesenteric artery (SMA) and superior mesenteric vein (SMV) presents difficulty in radical resection. Adequate mobilization of the flexure is helpful. Advanced-stage small bowel tumors causing substantial hemorrhage or obstruction should be resected, if the patient's performance status and clinical circumstances permit.

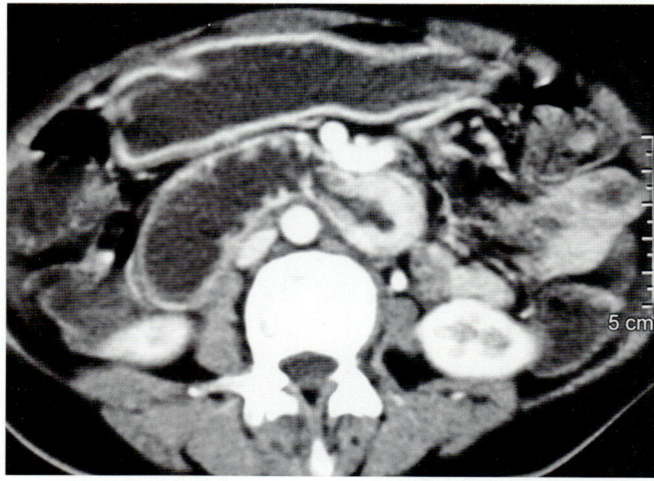

Figure 2 Contrast-enhanced computed tomography showing irregular thickening at D4 suggestive of malignancy

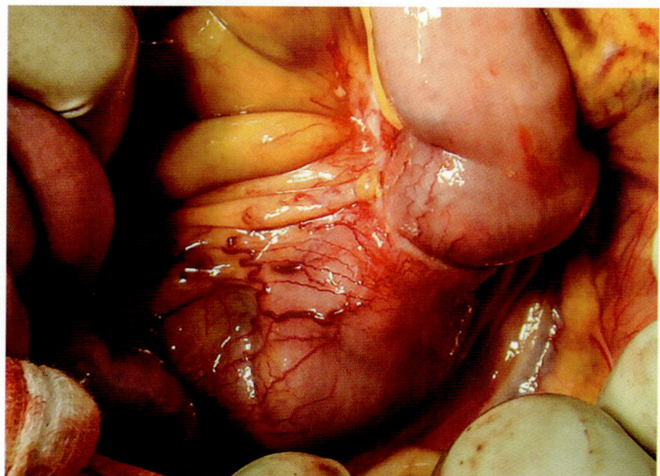

Figure 3 Same patient as in Figure 2. Operative picture showing D4 mass reaching DJ flexure

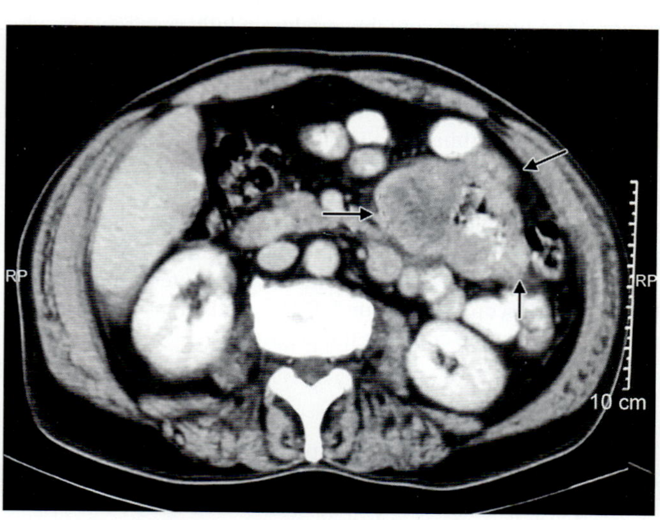

Figure 1 Carcinoma duodenojejunal flexure

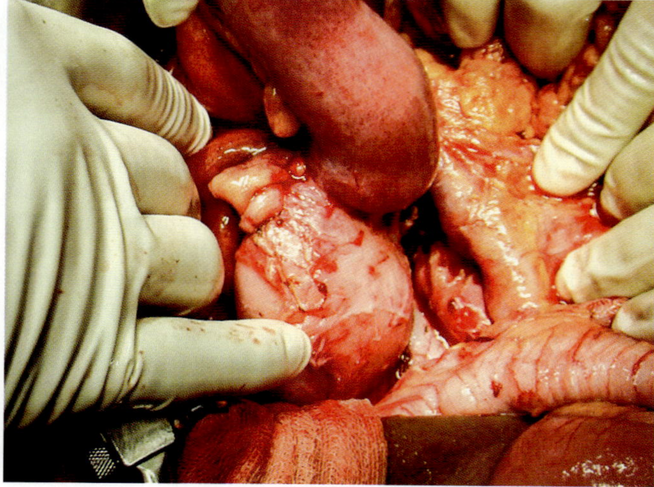

Figure 4 D4 mass being mobilized from retro-peritoneal structures

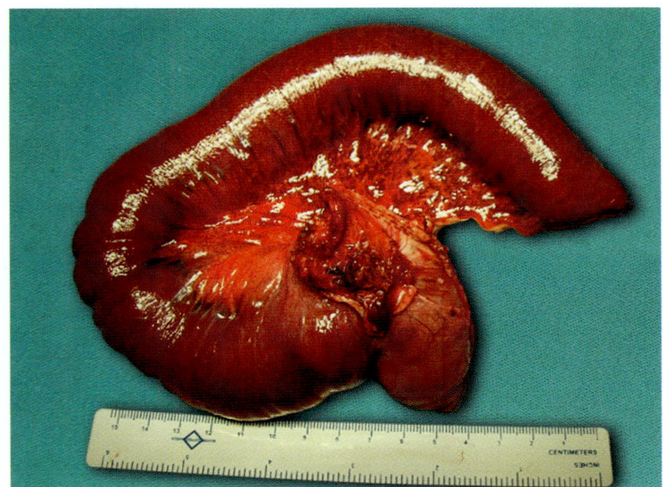

Figure 5 Radically resected specimen of D4 mass with mesentric nodes

PROGNOSIS

While benign polyps have very good prognosis, patients with syndromic polyps should be followed lifelong. After radical resection, malignant lesions of duodenum can have a 5-year survival of 50% which is better than other periampullary tumors.

REFERENCES

1. Chappuis CW, Divincenti FC, Cohn I. Villous tumors of the duodenum. Ann Surg. 1989;209:593-8.
2. Komorowski RA and Cohen EB. Villous tumors of the duodenum. A clinicopathologic study. Cancer. 1981;47:1377-86.
3. Tripathi M, Walsh J, Grin A, Karamchandani J, Lategan B, Sapp H, et al. Brunner's gland adenoma with typical and atypical features. Gastrointest Endosc. 2013;77(5S):1647.
4. Singhal N, Singhal D. Adjuvant chemotherapy for small intestine adenocarcinoma. Cochrane Database Syst Rev. 2007;18;(3): CD005202.
5. Catania G, Cardi F, Migliore M, Romeo G. Villous adenocarcinoma of the duodenum invading the ampulla of Vater. Case Report and Review of Literature. HPB Surg. 1996;10:105-9.
6. Kaklamanos IG, Bathe OF, Franceschi D, Camarda C, Levi J, Livingstone AS. Extent of resection in the management of duodenal adenocarcinoma. Am J Surg. 2000;179:37-41.

Tumors of the Small Intestine

INTRODUCTION

Small intestinal tumors both benign and malignant are rare considering that the small intestine constitutes 75% of the total gastrointestinal tract. Less than 2% of gastrointestinal malignancies originate from small intestines.[1-3] Malignant small intestinal tumors account for 0.1% to 0.3% of all malignancies. Benign tumors seen usually are leiomyoma, lymphangioma, lipoma, desmoid tumors and hamartomas. They are generally asymptomatic but may present with complications. On the other hand, malignant lesions of the small intestine are usually symptomatic. These include adenocarcinoma, lymphoma, leiomyosarcoma and carcinoids. The presenting signs and symptoms are nonspecific.[1] The most common symptoms include abdominal pain, nausea and vomiting, bleeding and weight loss. These are often ignored until severe symptoms develop and present as surgical emergencies. The small intestine may also be the site of metastasis, the spread being contiguous, hematogenous or by peritoneal metastases.[4]

One of the reasons for the delayed diagnosis is the relative inaccessibility of the small intestine to the endoscope. Several diagnostic tools have now been developed for earlier diagnosis. Small bowel enteroscopy can access large parts of small intestine. Operative resection is the main stay of the treatment in most lesions and prognosis is determined by stage and aggressiveness of the disease.

ADENOCARCINOMA

Small bowel adenocarcinoma is an uncommon disease that can be difficult to diagnose. There is usually delay in diagnosis due to inaccessibility of small intestine.

Clinical Presentation

The most common symptom at diagnosis is abdominal pain (43%), followed by nausea and vomiting (16%), fatigue and anemia (15%), upper or lower gastrointestinal tract bleeding (7%) and jaundice (6%). The histologic diagnosis is most often obtained at laparotomy (56%), followed by upper endoscopy (41%). Overall 15% patients may have history of other diseases like colorectal cancer (5%), Crohn's disease (5%), celiac disease (3%) and FAP (2%). Before 1990, patients with small bowel adenocarcinoma were more likely to have the diagnosis established with laparotomy, than patients diagnosed thereafter. Every attempt to diagnose the cause of symptoms should be made in elderly patients with suggestive sign and symptoms.

Pathology and Risk Factors

The low incidence of small bowel malignancies is attributed to certain protective factors. A rapid transit time reduces mucosal contact with potential carcinogens. Production of potential carcinogens from degradation products of bile acids and other substrates is reduced by alkaline pH and lower bacterial counts in the small intestines. Fluidity of the contents makes it less irritating. Abundant digestive enzymes and benzopyrene hydroxylase detoxify carcinogens. Besides these there is a high concentration of lymphoid tissue and thus immunoglobulin A for an early immune response.[1,5]

Small intestinal adenocarcinomas are mostly located proximally, nearly 80% are found in the duodenum or jejunum. Approximately 45% arise in the duodenum, while 55% arise in the jejunum and ileum.[6]

The etiopathogenesis of small bowel adenocarcinoma is similar to the adenoma-carcinoma sequence seen in colon. A pre-existing adenoma, either single or in association with one of the multiple polyposis syndromes[7-9] and Crohn's disease are important risk factors for small bowel adenocarcinoma. Other risk factors are coeliac sprue, cystic fibrosis, peptic ulcer and dietary risk factors like smoked and salt-cured foods and red meat.

Small intestine is well endowed with lymphatics. Invasion of the lymphatics by the cancer leads to early dissemination. Thus most small bowel carcinomas are already advanced when diagnosed.[10] Early diagnosis and surgical treatment before dissemination is the most important positive predictor of survival. Advanced stage, high-grade, incomplete resection and greater lymph node ratio are markers of poor prognosis.[11-15]

Diagnosis

Unlike conventional enteroclysis, cross-sectional imaging studies have the potential to simultaneously demonstrate intraluminal, mural and metastatic lesions. Contrast-enhanced and water-enhanced multidetector computed tomographic (CT) enteroclysis has an overall accuracy of 84.7% for detecting small bowel neoplasms.

However, conventional CECT cannot diagnose small mucosal or bleeding lesions or polyps causing obscure gastrointestinal bleed. For such lesions capsule endoscopy (CE) has high sensitivity compared to small bowel follow-through, push enteroscopy and CT, but it is time consuming and expensive with no therapeutic or biopsy potential. In stricturing or malignant disease capsule retention rate is 1.5–5% so CT enteroclysis/magnetic resonance (MR) enteroclysis is the initial investigation of choice.[16]

In contrast, double-balloon enteroscopy (DBE) has advantage of being able to perform biopsy or therapeutic intervention. DBE could also serve as a complementary approach after an initial diagnostic imaging using capsule endoscopy.[17]

Endoscopic or percutaneous biopsy for diagnosis is not necessary as resection is the better option for all patients who can safely undergo an operation. Besides, percutaneous biopsy of palpable small bowel tumors can be harmful as it can cause bile leak, bleed and metastatic spread in the peritoneal cavity. In case of failure of or unavailability of advanced investigating techniques, intraoperative endoscopy is the last resort (Flow chart 1).

Flow chart 1 Diagnostic workup of suspected small bowel neoplasm

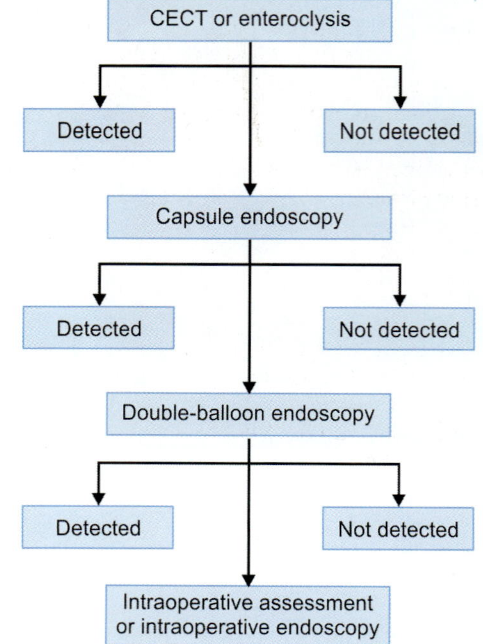

Abbreviation: CECT, contrast-enhanced computed tomography.

Treatment

Surgical Management

The optimal treatment of small bowel adenocarcinoma continues to be a complete radical resection. Curative resection is feasible in 40% to 65% of patients, with 5-year survival rates of 40%–60% for resected tumors versus 15%–30% for non-resected tumors.[12]

Carcinomas of the distal third portion and fourth portion of the duodenum are often amenable to segmental duodenectomy with or without distal pancreatectomy.[18] Jejunal and ileal carcinomas should be resected with at least 10 cm of normal bowel proximally and distally and with sufficient mesentery to include any involved lymph nodes. Distal ileal cancers generally are resected with at least part of the right colon, if not a formal right colectomy.[1] Both laparoscopic and open resections are feasible for most jejunal or ileal carcinomas. Most pancreaticoduodenectomies for cancer of D2 are still performed as open procedures, although laparoscopic resection is feasible.

Advanced-stage small bowel tumors causing substantial hemorrhage or obstruction should be resected when the patient's performance status and clinical circumstances allow.

In cases of resected small bowel tumors with an uncertain lymph nodes status, further re-resection or the use of adjuvant treatment is not substantiated by literature. Similarly, there is inadequate evidence to support the use of postoperative adjuvant therapy to improve survival rates.[6,11,13,15]

Treatment of Locally Advanced Disease

Endoscopic placement of self-expandable metallic stents under fluoroscopy is a safe and effective treatment for the palliation of patients with inoperable malignant duodenal obstruction. The median stent patency is about 100 days.[19]

Treatment of Metastatic Disease

Resectable hepatic metastases should be considered for resection, especially for jejunal and ileal adenocarcinomas, although no data exists to prove that this aggressive therapy is as effective as colorectal hepatic metastasectomy.

Chemotherapy prolongs survival for patients with either unresectable or metastatic disease. The median OS was significantly better for patients who had undergone a Whipple procedure compared with any other type of resection (82 months vs. 29 months; P 0.0001). Adjuvant chemotherapy after a Whipple procedure or resection did not appear to significantly affect the survival curve (P 0.49) (Table 1). Conversely, chemotherapy, in a subset analysis, improved OS when given to patients who did not undergo surgery or who had Stage IV disease compared with patients who received no treatment (12 months vs. 2 months; P 0.02).[15]

Radiotherapy is difficult for small bowel malignancies because of its mobility as well as radiation enteritis. Radiation alone or with 5-fluorouracil (5FU), is reserved for duodenal cancers with a positive resection margin. In advanced unresectable duodenal carcinoma, palliative radiotherapy may help control chronic blood loss.[20]

LYMPHOMA

About 5-10% of gastrointestinal tumors are lymphomas of which 20-30% are located in small intestines. Primary gastrointestinal lymphoma is the second most common tumor of the small intestine. Lymphomas may be sporadic or be associated with autoimmune and immunodeficiency syndromes, inflammatory bowel disease and posttransplant status. The various aspects of gastrointestinal lymphomas are dealt with in another chapter of this section.

CARCINOIDS

The term Karzinoide (carcinoma like), was introduced by Oberndorfer in 1907. The incidence of carcinoid tumors is about 1 to 2 per 100,000 population. The gastrointestinal tract (64%) and lungs and bronchi (28%) are the organs most commonly involved. Within the gastrointestinal tract, carcinoids are most frequently found in the small intestine (41.8%), rectum (27.4%), stomach (8.7%) and appendix (5%).[21] The previously reported highest incidence in the appendix was due to higher rates of incidental appendectomies, and is not supported by current data.

Classification

Embryologically carcinoids are classified as: foregut (bronchus, thymus, stomach, duodenum, pancreas); midgut (small bowel, appendix, right colon); and hindgut (transverse and descending colon, rectum). Midgut carcinoids are argentaffin-positive and have high 5-hydroxytryptamine (5-HT) content. They also secrete tachykinins, prostaglandins and bradykinins into the circulation.

Clinical Features

Small bowel carcinoids usually present in sixth or seventh decade with pain and small bowel obstruction. Symptoms of carcinoid syndrome like flushing (90%), diarrhea (80%), wheezing or carcinoid heart disease (40-50%) may be the presenting feature in 20-30% patients. The liver deactivates biogenic amines secreted by carcinoid tumors. Therefore, carcinoid syndrome is seen in patients with hepatic metastasis, or with retroperitoneal disease, liver dysfunction or significant tumor burden. Due to its indolent nature, patients usually have symptoms for 4-5 years before being diagnosed.

Table 1: WHO classification of neuroendocrine tumors (2010)[22]
NET G1 (carcinoid)
NET G2 (If Ki67 index >20%, this may be labeled G3)
NEC G3 (large cell or small cell type)
Mixed adenoneuroendocrine carcinoma (MANEC)
Hyperplastic and preneoplastic lesions

Abbreviations: NET, neuroendocrine tumor–well-differentiated; NEC, neuroendocrine carcinoma–poorly differentiated; G, grade.

Pathology

Unlike adenocarcinomas which affect the proximal small bowel, carcinoid tumors usually involve the terminal ileum. They are often small (1-2 cm) and arise in the submucosa. These tumors are advanced at the time of diagnosis with 70% having lymph nodal metastases and 50% having liver metastases. Thirty percent may have multiple small bowel tumors.

Treatment

Surgery

Radical resection of involved small gut with lymphadenectomy and wide excision of the mesentery (fibrosed part) is curative in localized disease with 5-year and 10-year survival rates of 73% and 65% respectively. A wide side to side anastomosis may be preferred to prevent leaks or strictures due to suboptimal mesenteric flow at the ends. Surgical resections palliate the symptoms and improve survival even in metastatic disease.[23,24] Resecting the primary may reduce the supply of hormones which induce the growth of secondaries in liver.

Cytoreductive surgery for liver metastases can be undertaken along with resection of primary tumor or may be done later. This may be in the form of anatomical/nonanatomical liver resections or liver transplant. Other forms of therapy used for liver metastases are hepatic artery embolization, radiofrequency ablation (RFA) and cryoablation. None has been proven to be superior to the others.

Medical Therapies

Long acting analogs of octreotide, like lanreotide, sandostatin or somatuline depot have been used for control of carcinoid syndrome. They effectively control symptoms in 50-75% of somatostatin receptor containing tumor metastasis, but true tumor response (size reduction) is rare. Interferon alpha has also been used for symptomatic relief in carcinoid syndrome but it is associated with myelosuppression.

Cytotoxic chemotherapy is effective in poorly differentiated carcinoids. An etoposide cisplatin combination shows response rates of up to 60%. There are two randomized controlled trials (RCTs) using combination of 5FU and streptozocin showing 22-33% response rates but with no survival advantage.

Radioactive agents like Lutetium (^{177}Lu) and Yttrium (^{90}Y) have been combined with long acting somatostatin analogs and used as adjuvant therapies.

In a multivariate analysis of patients with well to moderately differentiated neuroendocrine tumors (NETs), disease stage, primary tumor site, histologic grade, sex and age were predictors of outcome.[25]

In summary, resectable disease has a good prognosis with reasonable survival in surgically resected metastatic disease. Novel therapies have an increasing role in the management of carcinoid syndrome.

BENIGN TUMORS AND POLYPS

Other tumors which can occur in the duodenum and small bowel are lipomas, hyperplastic polyps, lymphangiomas and hemangiomas. Specific preoperative diagnosis is very difficult to establish. Pathological diagnosis can be established after resecting the tumor in symptomatic patients.

Small Bowel Polyposis

Small bowel polyps can be sporadic or associated with various polyposis syndromes. The hamartomatous polyposis syndromes are a heterogenous group of autosomal dominant disorders. These include familial juvenile polyposis syndrome, Peutz-Jeghers syndrome, phosphatase and tensin homolog gene hamartoma (Cowden's and Bannayan-Riley-Ruvalcaba syndromes), MEN syndrome type 2B, hereditary mixed polyposis syndrome, Cronkhite-Canada syndrome, basal cell nevus syndrome, and neurofibromatosis type 1. These comprise less than 1% of inherited gastrointestinal cancer predisposition syndromes.[26]

Juvenile polyposis can be diagnosed when any one of the following conditions is fulfilled: (1) 5 juvenile polyps in the colorectum; (2) juvenile polyps throughout the gastrointestinal tract; or (3) any number of juvenile polyps with a family history of juvenile polyposis.

Classification

Juvenile polyposis can be classified according to clinical presentation and location of polyps: (1) juvenile polyposis coli; (2) juvenile polyposis of infancy with a very early age of onset, severe hypoalbuminemia and failure to thrive; (3) generalized juvenile polyps of both the upper and lower gastrointestinal tract.

Presentation

The polyposis usually present as intestinal obstruction, intussusception and rectal bleeding. Patients with multiple juvenile polyps have considerable mucus secretion with hypokalemia and protein-losing enteropathy, leading to hypoalbuminemia and hypoproteinemia. Solitary juvenile polyps [as opposed to juvenile polyposis syndrome (JPS)] usually present at 4–5 years of age with rectal bleed and are mainly located in the colon or rectum. These have a propensity to autoamputate or prolapse.

Patients with hamartomatous polyposis have an increased lifetime risk of gastrointestinal and extraintestinal malignancies. Juvenile polyposis coli is associated with increased risk for colorectal, gastric and pancreatic malignancy. In a meta-analysis of Peutz-Jeghers syndrome patients the cumulative risk of developing any cancer was 93%.[9,26]

Treatment and Prevention

Small bowel hamartomas can be diagnosed and treated with double balloon enteroscopy. In patients with genetically proven syndromes the screening should begin soon after birth. It is necessary to clear all small intestinal polyps (>5 mm) as far as possible. Timely clearance of all small intestinal polyps and careful screening is the gold standard of management.

In patients undergoing surgery or when DBE is not available, intraoperative endoscopy with polypectomy helps in diagnosis and excision without multiple enterotomies. In patients with diagnosis of malignancy of small bowel, radical resection with intraoperative endoscopic excision of polyps is indicated. Massive resections of small bowel should be avoided to prevent short bowel syndrome.

Chemoprevention for intestinal polyposis with sirolimus (rapamycin) and cyclooxygenase-2 (COX-2) inhibitors is under investigation.

REFERENCES

1. Ashley SW, Wells SA. Tumors of the small intestine. Semin Oncol. 1988;15:116-28.
2. Zollinger RM. Primary neoplasms of the small intestine. Am J Surg. 1986;151:654-8.
3. Frost DB, Mercado PD, Tyrell JS. Small bowel cancer: A 30-year review. Ann Surg Oncol. 1994:1:290-5.
4. Coco C, Rizzo G, Manno A, Mattana C, Verbo A. Surgical treatment of small bowel neoplasms. Eur Rev Med Pharmacol Sci. 2010;14:327-33.
5. Turan M, Karadayi K, Duman M, Ozer H, Arici S, Yildirir C, et al. Small bowel tumors in emergency surgery. Ulus Travma Acil Cerrahi Derg. 2010;16:327-33.
6. Singhal N. Singhal D. Adjuvant chemotherapy for small intestine adenocarcinoma. Cochrane Database Syst Rev. 2007;18(3):CD005202.
7. Sellner F. Investigations on the significance of the adenoma-carcinoma sequence in the small bowel. Cancer. 1990;66:702-15.
8. Kurtz RC, Sternberg SS, Miller HH, Decosse JJ. Upper gastrointestinal neoplasia in familial polyposis. Dig Dis Sci. 1987;32:459-65.
9. Giardiello FM, Brensinger JD, Tersmette AC, Goodman SN, Petersen GM, Booker SV, et al. Very high risk of cancer in familial Peutz-Jeghers syndrome. Gastroenterology. 2000;119:1447-53.
10. Schottenfeld D, Beebe-Dimmer JL, Vigneau FD. The epidemiology and pathogenesis of neoplasia in the small intestine. Ann Epidemiol. 2009;19:58-69.
11. Halfdanarson TR, McWilliams RR, Donohue JH, Quevedo JF. A single-institution experience with 491 cases of small bowel adenocarcinoma. Am J Surg. 2010;199:797-803.
12. Ouriel K, Adams JT. Adenocarcinoma of the small intestine. Am J Surg. 1984;147:66-71.
13. Zhou Z, Wan D, Shi M. [Diagnosis and treatment of primary malignant tumors of the small bowel]. Zhonghua Zhong Liu Za Zhi. 1997;19:297-9.
14. Talamonti MS, Goetz LH, Rao S, Joehl RJ. Primary cancers of the small bowel: analysis of prognostic factors and results of surgical management. Arch Surg. 2002;137:564-70.
15. Dabaja BS, Suki D, Pro B, Bonnen M, Ajani J. Adenocarcinoma of the small bowel: presentation, prognostic factors, and outcome of 217 patients. Cancer. 2004;101:518-26.
16. Dye CE, Gaffney RR, Dykes TM, Moyer MT. Endoscopic and radiographic evaluation of the small bowel in 2012. Am J Med. 2012;125:1228.e1-1228.e12.
17. Li XB, Ge ZZ, Dai J, Gao YJ, Liu WZ, Hu YB, et al. The role of capsule endoscopy combined with double-balloon enteroscopy in diagnosis of small bowel diseases. Chin Med J (Engl). 2007;120:30-5.
18. Kaklamanos IG, Bathe OF, Franceschi D, Camarda C, Levi J, Livingstone AS. Extent of resection in the management of duodenal adenocarcinoma. Am J Surg. 2000;179:37-41.
19. Caglar E, Dobrucali A. Self-expandable metallic stent placement in the palliative treatment of malignant obstruction of gastric outlet and duodenum. Clin Endosc. 2013;46:59-64.
20. Brennan MF. Duodenal cancer. Asian J Surg. 1990;13:204.
21. Modlin IM, Lye KD, Kidd M. A 5-decade analysis of 13,715 carcinoid tumors. Cancer. 2003;97:934-59.
22. Bosman F, Carneiro F, Hruban R, Theise N (Eds). WHO Classification of tumors of the digestive system. Lyon, France: IARC Press; 2010.

23. Hellman P, Lundstrom T, Ohrvall U, Eriksson B, Skogseid B, Oberg K, et al. Effect of surgery on the outcome of midgut carcinoid disease with lymph node and liver metastases. World J Surg. 2002;26: -991-7.
24. Givi B, Pommier SJ, Thompson AK, Diggs BS, Pommier RF. Operative resection of primary carcinoid neoplasms in patients with liver metastases yields significantly better survival. Surgery. 2006;140:891-7.
25. Yao JC, Hassan M, Phan A, Dagohoy C, Leary C, Mares JE, et al. One hundred years after "carcinoid": epidemiology of and prognostic factors for neuroendocrine tumors in 35,825 cases in the United States. J Clin Oncol. 2008;26:3063-72.
26. Kopacova M, Tacheci I, Rejchrt S, Bures J. Peutz-Jeghers syndrome: diagnostic and therapeutic approach. World J Gastroenterol. 2009;15:5397-408.

CHAPTER 27

Gastric Bezoar and Gastric Volvulus

KJ Singh

Gastric Bezoar

INTRODUCTION

Bezoars are conglomerate masses of foreign material that are retained in the GIT. This happens commonly in the stomach but has also been seen in the esophagus and rectum. Most commonly the foreign material is the residue of plants and vegetables (phytobezoar) while less commonly it may be hair (trichobezoars), medication (pharmacobezoar) and persimmons (disopyrobezoar). This article focuses on gastric bezoars.

The word "bezoar" comes from the Persian word *pād-zahr*, meaning "antidote"[1] as it was believed that a drinking glass containing a bezoar would neutralize any poison poured into it.

INCIDENCE

The true incidence is uncertain because many patients may be asymptomatic. However, the reported prevalence is 0.4%. Asymptomatic bezoars are more common in patients who have undergone an antrectomy.

ETIOLOGY

While the formation of bezoars is multifactorial and not well understood, some factors are:

- Altered gastric motility and emptying due to disorders like diabetes mellitus,[2] non-diabetic neuropathies, hypothyroidism, amyloidosis, myotonic dystrophy, progressive systemic sclerosis, Guillain-Barre syndrome, gastric carcinoma and gastric ulcer can all predispose to bezoar formation. Medications impairing gastric emptying include anticholinergics, phenothiazines, tricyclic antidepressants, levodopa and ethanol.
- Size and digestibility of swallowed food material.
- Missing teeth, poor mastication, xerostomia, poorly fitting or painful dentures.
- Prior gastric surgery, like antrectomy, pyloroplasty, Roux-en-Y gastric bypass, partial gastrectomy and gastric stapling procedures. The rise in bariatric surgery procedures have led to a significant rise in bezoar formation.[3-5] It has also been reported after surgery for gastric carcinoma.[6,7]

TYPES

Depending on the content, bezoars can be classified as:

a. *Lactobezoar* is a type of food bezoar, usually seen in premature infants receiving formula foods and comprising of inspissated milk.
b. *Pharmacobezoar* (or medication bezoars) is made up of tablets or a semiliquid mass of drugs, normally found following overdose of sustained-release medication.[8]
c. *Phytobezoar* is composed of undigestible plant material mainly cellulose, frequently reported in patients with impaired digestion and decreased gastric motility.
d. *Disopyrobezoar* is type of phytobezoar formed from unripe persimmons.
e. *Trichobezoar* (Figs. 1 to 4) consists of large quantities of hair that have been ingested (trichophagia). Around 80% patients are less than 30 years of age and more than 90% are women. The incidence is highest in childhood and adolescence. Occasionally the individual may have psychiatric disorder or the hair-pulling disorder trichotillomania. It may be the manifestation of a personality maladjustment or frank psychosis. Human hair is resistant to digestion. Also, its smooth surface prevents peristaltic propulsion and thus remains between the gastric mucosal folds. Progressive hair ingestion leads to the conglomerate of hair with food and mucus, forming

a trichobezoar. Acid induced denaturation of hair protein gives a black color to the bezoar while entrapment of undigested fat and bacterial colonization in the interstices leads to a foul smelling mass with a slimy mucoid coat. While usually the trichobezoar remains within the stomach, it may sometimes extend distally into the jejunum, ileum or even colon. This has been called as Rapunzel syndrome[9] (Fig. 3), by Vaughan et al. in 1968[10] after the long-haired girl in the fairy tale by the Brothers Grimm named Rapunzel.

PRESENTATION

In the early stages, patients may be asymptomatic or have nonspecific symptoms. Gastric bezoar patients commonly present with pain abdomen (70%), nausea and vomiting suggestive of gastric outlet obstruction (64%). Obstructive features may also be because of a ball-valve type of mechanism. In patients with trichobezoars, denaturation of hair protein may result in foul odor. However, foul breath can persist after trichobezoar removal suggesting an underlying motility disorder.[11] Patients often complain of early satiety and weight loss. In Rapunzel syndrome, intestinal obstruction may arise by part of the tail breaking off and migrating to the small intestine. Post-antrectomy, the incidence of bezoars is higher. Ulceration may occur (10–24%) with hematemesis or malena but massive GI bleed is rare. Patients may have low BMI and may have a palpable abdominal mass (57–88%) on physical examination. Patients may present with iron deficiency anemia. Concomitant gastric cancer has been reported although the causal relation has not been established.[12]

The large size of the trichobezoar hinders the blood supply to the mucosa of the stomach or part of the intestine leading to ulceration and eventually perforation. Perforation is the most common complication. In addition, complications of trichobezoar include intussusception, protein-losing enteropathy, obstructive jaundice, pancreatitis and even death.

DIAGNOSIS

A high degree of suspicion is required since presenting symptoms may be indistinguishable from other common GI illnesses. A careful history including psychiatric illnesses, previous surgeries and medication needs to be taken. A history of unusual eating habits or alopecia due to trichotillomania may suggest ingestion of oral hair and may point to the diagnosis. Other psychiatric disorders including obsessive compulsive disorder, pica, depression and anorexia nervosa may also be present with trichobezoar. Occupational history related to ingestion of furniture polish or shellac (because of high alcohol content), etc. may be a pointer.

Endoscopy is the investigation of choice for gastric bezoars. It also offers therapeutic possibilities for smaller bezoars that can be endoscopically fragmented and removed. It determines the extent and nature of the gastric mass and enables the distinction between trichobezoars and other foreign bodies. The phytobezoar is seen in the stomach as a dark greenish-blackish ball of amorphous material.[13] Plain X-ray of abdomen may demonstrate features of intestinal obstruction. In the area of stomach a filling defect outlined by gas may be seen.

Barium studies may show a characteristic mottled or streaked appearance or an outline of stomach with the filling defect inside.[14]

On contrast-enhanced computed tomography (CECT) a bezoar appears as a well-circumscribed ovoid intraluminal lesion, with concentric whorls of different densities and air pockets enmeshed within. Oral contrast fills the more peripheral interstices, and a thin band of contrast circumscribes it. Non-enhancement after intravenous contrast excludes neoplasms. CECT also reliably demonstrates complications such as obstruction or perforation.

TREATMENT

The ultimate goal of treatment is to remove the bezoar and prevent its recurrence. DeBakey and Oschsner did a review of the condition in 1938 and at that time mentioned that the only viable treatment was surgical removal. However, since then, various medical and surgical therapies have been devised the most significant being newer endoscopic approaches. The appropriate therapy depends upon the location, size and composition of the bezoar.

Surgery

Surgery remains the mainstay in the management of bezoars. Surgery may be performed by open method (Figs 1 to 4) or laparoscopically.[15,16] For gastric bezoars, an anterior gastrotomy is made between stay sutures and the bezoar retrieved. Any distal obstruction is ruled out and the gastrotomy closed in one or two layers or with stapler. Laparoscopic removal could be piecemeal or in toto depending on the size and weight of the bezoar. However, an impervious endobag is a must to prevent spillage and infection.[17] Careful examination of the entire intestine and stomach is somewhat more difficult laparoscopically. However, this is necessary to prevent intestinal obstruction due to satellite fragments from the bezoars.

Endoscopic Therapy

If feasible, endotherapy is the ideal treatment for bezoars. It is minimally invasive with low morbidity as compared to surgery. Endotherapy has been classified into three broad categories: (1) direct endoscopic retrieval, (2) retrieval following mechanical fragmentation and (3) retrieval following chemical fragmentation.

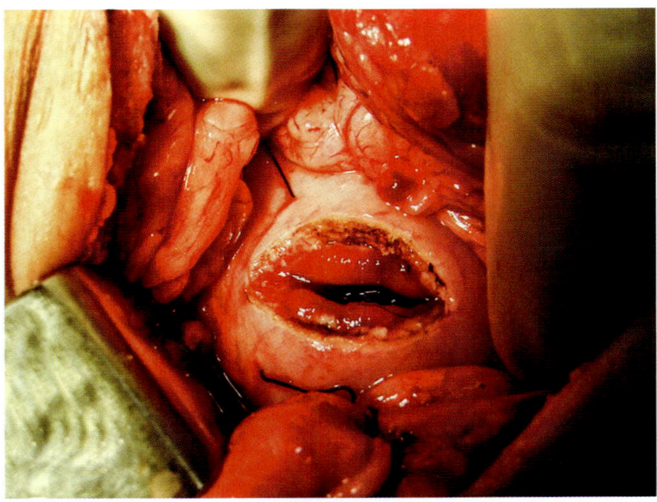

Figure 1 Trichobezoar in a 6-year-old girl. Stomach opened by a small gastrotomy

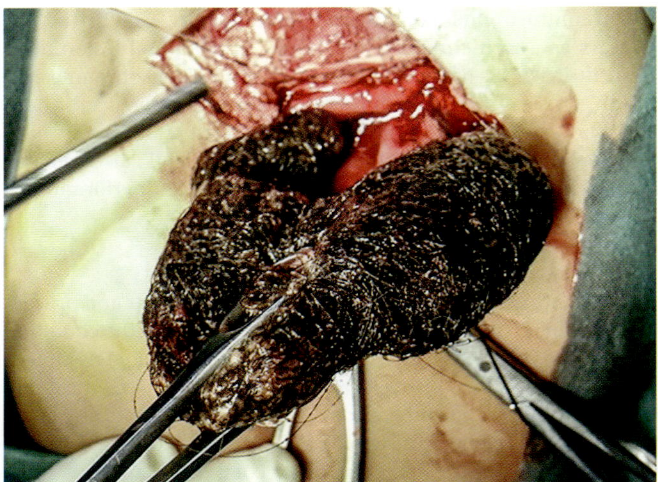

Figure 2 Organized tuft of hair being gently eased out

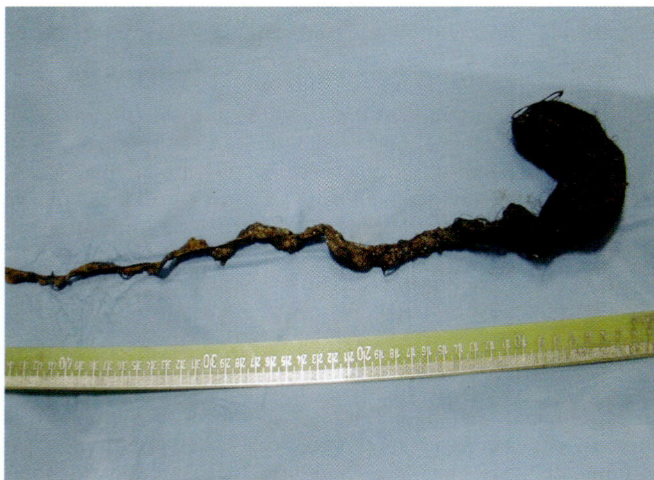

Figure 3 Trichobezoar taken out intact. Showing a long wavy continuation into duodenum and jejunum—"Rapunzel"

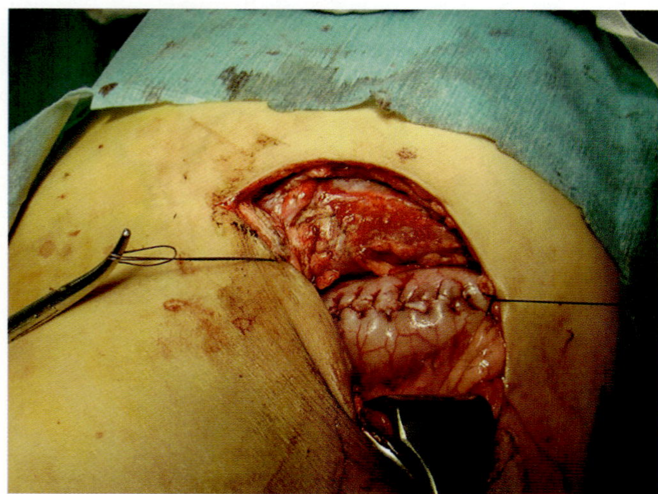

Figure 4 Gastrotomy was closed in two layers. First layer being completed

Equipment like dormia basket, suction through large channel endoscopes, snares and adjuncts like electrohydraulic lithotripsy, laser therapy and enzymatic preparations have been used.[18] Having said that, the reports in literature are single case reports or short series and endoscopic option may be possible in small bezoars only.

Currently endoscopic therapy is limited by the difficulty of fragmentation because of density, large size and hardness. As repeated passage of the endoscope is needed to remove all the fragments complications like esophagitis, ulceration and esophageal perforation can occur. Fragments of gastric bezoar can also migrate distally causing intestinal obstruction.

Medical Therapy

In early cases, medical therapy includes observation with correction of dehydration. Gastric lavage tube with saline lavage or 0.1N HCl, $NaHCO_3$ for about 2 weeks has been advocated with variable success. Enzymatic dissolution directed against specific components of a bezoar includes mucolytics, proteolytics and cellulose. Phytobezoars are most amenable while disopyrobezoar and trichobezoars are resistant. Sodium carbonate or N-acetylcysteine helps to dissolve the proteinaceous component of the bezoar. The most successful agent has been cellulose with successful dissolution rates reported from 83% to 100%.[19] The use of promotility agents is mainly of historical interest. Occasionally they may precipitate an obstruction. Psychiatric counseling and support is essential for many of these patients.

PREVENTION

After the successful management of gastric bezoars recurrence is reported in almost 13% cases.[20] Prevention is directed toward the underlying pathology. To prevent phytobezoars patients should avoid raw citrus fruits, persimmons and high-fiber food. If gastric stasis is a component, prokinetics may be helpful. For underlying psychiatric disorders specific therapy is required.

REFERENCES

1. DeBakey M, Ochsner A. Bezoars and concretions. Surgery. 1938;4:934-63.
2. Ahn Y-H, Maturu P, Steinheber FU, Goldman JM. Association of diabetes mellitus with gastric bezoar formation. Arch Intern Med. 1987;147:527-8.
3. Deitel M, Bendago M. Endoscopy of vertical banded gastroplasty. Am Surg. 1989;55:287-90.
4. White NB, Gibbs KE, Goodwin A, Teixeira J. Gastric bezoar complicating laparoscopic adjustable gastric banding, and review of literature. Obes Surg. 2003;13:948-50.
5. Veronelli A, Ranieri R, Laneri M, Montorsi M, Bianchi P, Cosentino F, et al. Gastric bezoars after adjustable gastric banding. Obes Surg. 2004;14:796-7.
6. Diettrich NA, Gau FC. Postgastrectomy phytobezoars—endoscopic diagnosis and treatment. Arch Surg. 1985;120:432-5.
7. Van Thiel DH, DeBelle RC, Painter TD, McMillan WB, Haradin AR. Phytobezoar occurring as a complication of gastric carcinoma. Gastroenterology. 1975;68:1292-6.
8. Buckley NA, Dawson AH, Reith DA. Controlled release drugs in overdose. Clinical considerations. Drug Safe. 1995;12:73-84.
9. Rabie ME, Arishi AR, Khan A, Ageely H, Seif El-Nasr GA, Fagihi M. Rapunzel syndrome: the unsuspected culprit. World J Gastroenterol. 2008;14:1141-3.

10. Vaughan ED Jr, Sawyers JL, Scott HW Jr. The Rapunzel syndrome. An unusual complication of intestinal bezoar. Surgery. 1968;63:339-43.
11. Hayes PG, Rotstein OD. Gastrointestinal phytobezoars: presentation and management. Can J Surg. 1986;29:419-20.
12. Scwab KS, Cheng EH. Postgastrectomy bezoar secondary to gastric cancer. J Clin Gastroenterol. 1993;16:45-7.
13. Eisenberg RL. Gastrointestinal Radiology: A Pattern Approach, 4th edition. Philadelphia, USA: Lippincott Williams and Wilkins; 2003. pp. 262-3, 274-5.
14. Halpert RD. Gastrointestinal Imaging: The Requisites, 3rd edition. Philadelphia, USA: Mosby Elsevier; 2006. pp. 52-3.
15. Palanivelu C, Rangarajan M, Senthilkumar R, Madankumar MV. Trichobezoars in the stomach and ileum and their laparoscopy-assisted removal: a bizarre case. Singapore Med J. 2007;48:e37-9.
16. Shami SB, Jararaa AA, Hamade A, Ammori BJ. Laparoscopic removal of a huge gastric trichobezoar in a patient with trichotillomania. Surg Laparosc Endosc Percutan Tech. 2007;17:197-200.
17. Sharma D, Manish S, Raghavendra B, Rama A, Anurag R, Shaji T. Laparoscopic treatment of gastric bezoar.JSLS. 2010;14:263-7.
18. Blam ME, Lichtenstein GR. A new endoscopic technique for the removal of gastric phytobezoars. Gastrointest Endosc. 2000;52:404-8.
19. Andrus CH, Ponsky JL. Bezoars: classification, pathophysiology and treatment. Am J Gastroenterol. 1988;83:476-8.
20. Williams RS. The fascinating history of bezoars. Med J Aust. 1986;145:613-4.

Gastric Volvulus

INTRODUCTION AND HISTORY

Gastric volvulus is an uncommon clinical entity in which the stomach abnormally rotates by at least 180°. Berti was the first person to describe gastric volvulus in a female autopsy patient in 1866.[1] Berg, in 1896 is credited with performing the first successful operation for this condition.[2] The classic triad associated with gastric volvulus is of severe epigastric pain, retching without vomiting, and inability to pass a nasogastric tube. The same was described by Borchardt in 1904.[3]

The actual incidence and prevalence of gastric volvulus is unknown since many cases of chronic volvulus do not become acute and are not diagnosed. Males and females are equally affected. About 10–20% of cases occur in children.[4]

CLASSIFICATION

Gastric volvulus can be classified according to anatomy, etiology and onset.

Anatomical Classification

This is the most frequently used classification system of gastric volvulus and was proposed by Singleton.[5] It relates to the axis around which the stomach rotates. There are the following three types.

Organoaxial Type

The transverse line connecting the gastroesophageal junction and the pylorus forms an axis around which the stomach rotates. This is the most common type of gastric volvulus, occurring in about two-thirds of cases.[6] Strangulation and necrosis have been reported in 5–28% of cases.[7]

Mesenteroaxial Type

Here, the stomach rotates about a longitudinal axis parallel to gastrohepatic omentum. Typically, the antrum rotates anteriorly and superiorly causing the posterior surface of the stomach to come anteriorly. This comprises approximately one-third of cases.[6] The rotation is usually intermittent and incomplete. Vascular compromise is uncommon.

Combined Type

This is a rare variety and usually observed in patients with chronic volvulus.[8]

Etiological Classification

According to etiology, gastric volvulus is classified as Type 1 (primary or idiopathic) and Type 2 (secondary—congenital or acquired).

Type 1

Primary gastric volvulus accounts for about one-third of cases and is supposedly due to abnormal laxity of the ligaments attaching the stomach namely gastrosplenic, gastroduodenal, gastrophrenic and gastrohepatic. It has been seen in association with congenital asplenia and with "wandering spleen".[9]

Primary gastric volvulus is usually mesenteroaxial. It is consequent to approximation of the cardia and pylorus on a full stomach. The pylorus rotates anteriorly (more commonly) or posteriorly from right to left.[9] This type of volvulus is usually incomplete (<180°) and is accompanied by chronic or intermittent symptoms.[8]

Type 2

Secondary gastric volvulus is found in two-thirds patients. It is related to congenital or acquired defects of diaphragm that cause uncharacteristic mobility of the stomach. It is usually organoaxial and results in an intrathoracic stomach lying upside down. Invariably the greater curve rotates up into the chest either anteriorly (more common) or posterior with respect to the fixed duodenum and esophagus.[8] Despite the rich blood supply of the stomach, strangulation can occur with torsion greater than 180°.[7]

Both in adults and children, paraesophageal hiatal hernia is the most common cause.[10] In children, congenital diaphragmatic hernia (Bochdalek on the left side) is another common cause.[11] Sometimes it occurs after traumatic hernia; diaphragmatic eventration;[12] Morgagni's hernia and surgical procedures like fundoplication. It has also been reported as a complication of liver transplantation and may be caused by the ligation of the gastrohepatic ligament during hepatectomy.[13] In patients with severe postural deformities like kyphoscoliosis, there is a potential for volvulus.[14]

CLASSIFICATION ACCORDING TO ONSET

It may be an acute or chronic gastric volvulus. The difference in presentation depends on the extent of twisting and the speed of onset, manifesting as an acute abdomen or as a chronic intermittent problem.

Acute Gastric Volvulus (Usually Organoaxial Type)

The classical clinical triad diagnostic of acute volvulus occurs in about 70% cases.[15] Carter et al. observed three additional findings that may be very indicative of gastric volvulus: negligible abdominal findings when the stomach is in the thorax; Radiograph showing a viscus filled with gas in the lower chest or upper abdomen, especially when associated with a paraesophageal hernia; and upper gastrointestinal series showing obstruction at the site of the gastric volvulus.[7,16]

Intrathoracic gastric volvulus causes chest pain mimicking an acute myocardial infarction due to gastric distention. Abdominal findings may be minimal. Hiccups may be a subtle sign in the clinical diagnosis.[17]

Intra-abdominal gastric volvulus usually manifests as sudden onset of severe epigastric or left upper abdominal pain. Patients may have upper abdominal distention and tenderness. If gastrointestinal bleed or sepsis sets in, gastric strangulation or perforation has invariably occurred.

Chronic Gastric Volvulus (Usually Mesenteroaxial Type)

The signs and symptoms are vague and intermittent or it may be an incidental finding. Patients present with intermittent epigastric pain, early satiety, chest discomfort, dyspnea and abdominal fullness after a meal. Dysphagia occurs when the gastroesophageal junction is distorted. In view of the vague and nonspecific nature of the symptoms, however, patients are often investigated for other common conditions such as peptic ulcer disease and cholelithiasis.

DIAGNOSIS AND DIFFERENTIAL DIAGNOSIS

Physical examination findings can often be misleading and nonspecific. A differential diagnosis of cholecystitis, pancreatitis, hiatal hernia, myocardial infarction or peptic ulcer disease may be considered depending on the severity and type of volvulus and the location of the stomach.

Biochemistry

In case of ischemia or perforation, leucocytosis and neutrophilia may be present. Hyperamylasemia may lead to a misdiagnosis of pancreatitis.[18,19]

Imaging

In view of the intermittent nature of the volvulus, on radiology, the diagnosis of primary gastric volvulus may be difficult to establish. Imaging is often only diagnostic at the time when patients have symptoms.[14]

1. *Chest and abdominal radiography:* On chest radiography, the diagnosis is confirmed by a retrocardiac, gas-filled viscus seen in cases of intrathoracic stomach (Figs 5A and B).

In organoaxial volvulus, abdominal films may show a horizontally oriented stomach with a single air-fluid level,[11] a downward pointing stomach and a lack of distal gas.[20]

In mesenteroaxial volvulus, a spherical stomach is seen on supine films and two air-fluid levels on erect films, with the antrum positioned superior to the fundus.[8]

2. *Upper gastrointestinal contrast studies:* Barium or gastrografin contrast studies may show an upside-down stomach above a normally located GEJ. Contrast studies have a diagnostic yield of 81–84%.[10,21,22]

3. *CT Scanning:* CECT is the best imaging modality with numerous benefits. It can quickly diagnose the condition based on a few coronal reconstructed images; the presence or absence of free air or gastric pneumatosis can be made; predisposing factors like diaphragmatic or hiatal hernias can be picked up and other abdominal pathology excluded (Figs 6A and B).[18,23]

Endoscopy

Upper gastrointestinal endoscopy may be helpful in the diagnosis of gastric volvulus. Usually the endoscopist has difficulty in intubating the stomach or pylorus. Depending on the degree of torsion, there is significant distortion of the gastric anatomy.[23]

MANAGEMENT

The management mainly depends upon whether the condition is acute or chronic. However, for both varieties the principles are same, namely: decompression, reduction and prevention of recurrence. In case of established vascular compromise, a major resection may be required. The morbidity and mortality may be significant in such cases.

The standard treatment of an acute gastric volvulus is emergency laparotomy. The favored procedure is the one in which the greater curve of the stomach is fixed to the anterior abdominal wall or the anterior gastropexy. This can also be achieved laparoscopically as shown in recent series.[24,25] In patients unfit for surgery (secondary to comorbidities or an inability to tolerate anesthesia), endoscopic reduction may be attempted which may convert an emergency operation to an urgent one.

With chronic gastric volvulus, surgery is performed on a planned basis to prevent complications and recurrent symptoms. Recently endoscopic treatment with or without laparoscopic approach has also been adopted.

OPEN SURGICAL APPROACH

Preoperative Management

Upon confirmation of the diagnosis of gastric volvulus, the patient is resuscitated, and medically optimized. In adults, early gastric decompression with a nasogastric tube should be done although

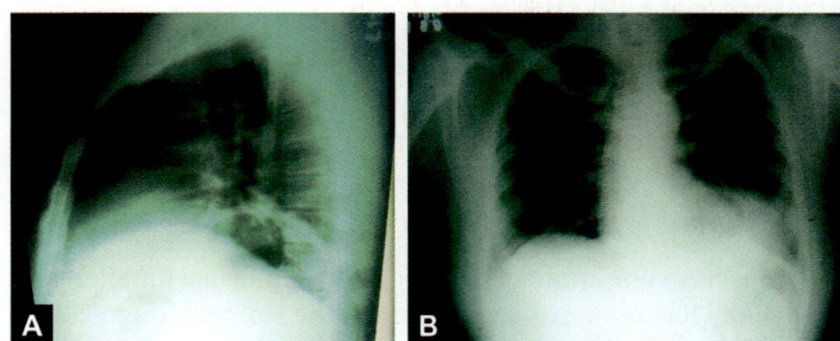

Figures 5A and B Plain X-ray demonstrating retrocardiac gas-filled viscus in a 56-year-old male who presented with acute upper abdominal and lower chest pain mimicking acute myocardial infarction

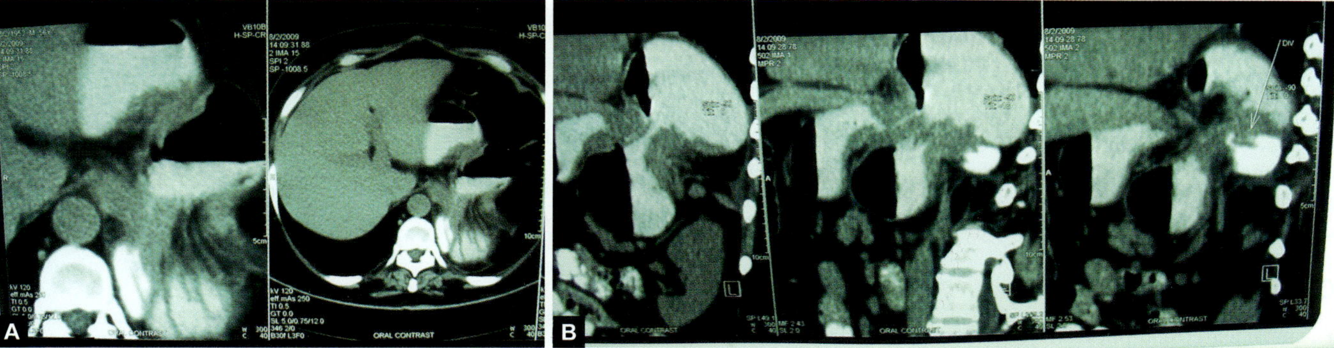

Figures 6A and B Coronal reconstructed CECT showing secondary acute gastric volvulus associated with paraesophageal hernia and partially intrathoracic stomach. Acute inflammation and fat stranding are seen in the region of the volvulus

this may not be easy if the gastroesophageal junction is obstructed. Aggressive placement of the nasogastric tube may cause perforation, hence due care should be taken especially in the pediatric population. For the same reason, it is not advocated in children.[9]

Surgical Approach

The surgical approach is usually through an upper midline incision. The condition of the stomach is assessed. In case of gangrene, a major resection—segmental, subtotal or total gastrectomy—is needed. If a diaphragmatic hernia is present the gastric herniation is reduced and the hernial sac excised. The crural defect is repaired. The use of mesh to reinforce the crural defect is controversial. Additionally a gastropexy is done to the anterior abdominal wall with a gastrostomy tube or suture to prevent recurrence. Fundoplication is occasionally done. In patients who are medically high risk, septic, or with a limited life expectancy, gastropexy alone is safer and sufficient (Figs 7 and 8).

Laparoscopic repair should be performed by experts. Owing to the distorted anatomy the risk of gastric and esophageal perforation is high. It is preferable to keep the insufflation pressure low and to use an ultrasonic dissector to remove the hernia sac. The dissection is usually begun in the left crural region, dividing the short gastric vessels and starting excision of the sac along the inner border of the left crus. Excessive traction on the stomach should be avoided as it may cause gastric injury. The pleural interface with the sac is low on both left and right sides above the crura and may accidently get opened; hence, a rim of sac is left on the pleura. Extra caution is required in dissecting near the base of the right crus, because of likely injury to the left gastric vessels which may have herniated into the chest across the edge of the crus.

Endoscopic Reduction

In very high-risk patients, endoscopic reduction may be attempted.[22,26-32] A significant number of patients of chronic gastric volvulus are being managed endoscopically.[22,27,31,32] Various studies have reported a high recurrence rate but very few serious complications.[33]

Endoscopic treatment is done by advancing the scope beyond the point of torsion and then untwisting the stomach by rotating it. In view of the high risk of gastric perforation, endoscopic reduction should not be attempted in patients who are found to have vascular compromise during the procedure. Surgery is indicated if there is failure to untwist the volvulus or evidence of strangulation.

Following endoscopic reduction, a percutaneous endoscopic gastrostomy tube is placed to decrease the incidence of recurrence.[27,32]

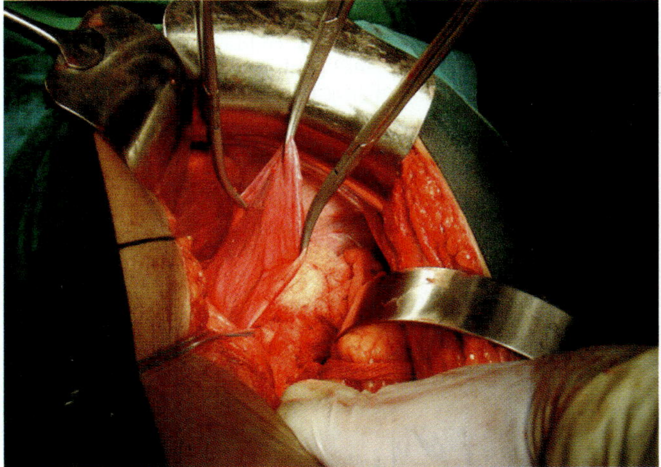

Figure 7 Reduction and excision of sac

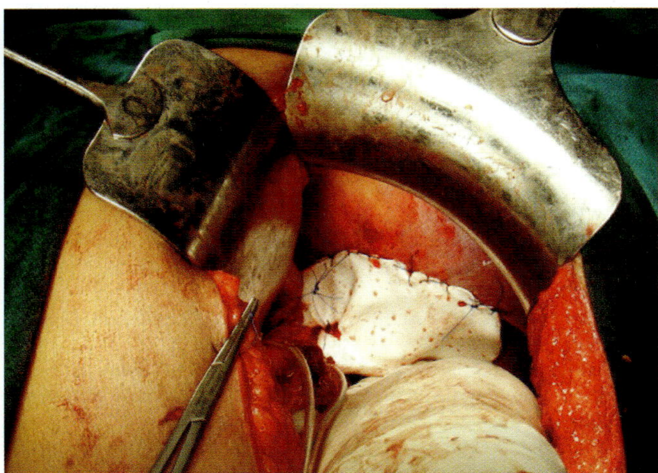

Figure 8 Repair of large diaphragmatic defect with "Goretex" mesh

Future Trends

There are increasing reports of laparoscopic and endoscopic procedures in the treatment of gastric volvulus.[24,25,34-37] Purely endoscopic technique is best reserved for high risk patients because it does not address the underlying defect. In contrast, laparoscopy with or without endoscopy has the potential to combine minimal invasive approach with repair of diaphragmatic defect.

Complications

The most feared complications of gastric volvulus are strangulation and necrosis. They can be a life threatening and occur most commonly with organoaxial gastric volvulus (5–28% of cases).[7] Gastric perforation is a result of ischemia and necrosis and can result in sepsis and cardiovascular collapse. As brought out, perforation can also be a complication of endoscopic reduction. Operative complications are akin to those seen in other conditions requiring major abdominal surgery.

Prognosis

If not surgically intervened, mortality rate for acute gastric volvulus is reportedly as high as 80%.[24] Historically, mortality rates of 30–50% have been reported for acute gastric volvulus, with the major cause of death being strangulation leading to necrosis and perforation.[7,8,25] Currently, with advances in diagnosis, management and supportive care, the mortality rate from acute gastric volvulus is 15–20% and that for chronic gastric volvulus is 0–13%.[35]

REFERENCES

1. Berti A. Singulare attortigliamento dele' esofago col duodeno seguita da rapida morte. *Gazz Med Ital.* 1866;9:139.
2. Berg J. Zwei Falle von axendrehung des magens operation; heilung. *Nord Med Arkiv.* 1897;30:1.
3. Borchardt M. Aus pathologie und therapie des magenvolvulus. *Arch Klin Chir.* 1904;74:243.
4. Harford WV, McArthur KE. Diverticula, hernias, volvulus, and rupture. In: Sleisenger MH, Fordtran JS (Eds). *Gastrointestinal Disease: Pathophysiology, Diagnosis, Management,* 5th edition. Philadelphia, PA: Saunders; 1993. pp. 481-3.
5. Singleton AC. Chronic gastric volvulus. *Radiology.* 1940;34:53-61.
6. Milne LW, Hunter JJ, Anshus JS, Rosen P. Gastric volvulus: two cases and a review of the literature. *J Emerg Med.* 1994;12:299-306.
7. Carter R, Brewer LA 3rd, Hinshaw DB. Acute gastric volvulus. A study of 25 cases. *Am J Surg.* 1980;140:99-106.
8. Wasselle JA, Norman J. Acute gastric volvulus: pathogenesis, diagnosis, and treatment. *Am J Gastroenterol.* 1993;88:1780-4.
9. UC A, Kao SC, Sanders KD, Lawrence J. Gastric volvulus and wandering spleen. Am J Gastroenterol. 1998;93:1146-8.
10. Gourgiotis S, Vougas V, Germanos S, Baratsis S. Acute gastric volvulus: diagnosis and management over 10 years. *Dig Surg.* 2006;23:169-72.
11. Cameron AE, Howard ER. Gastric volvulus in childhood. *J Pediatr Surg.* 1987;22:944-7.
12. Oh A, Gulati G, Sherman ML, Golub R, Kutin N. Bilateral eventration of the diaphragm and perforated gastric volvulus in an adolescent. J Pediatr Surg. 2000; 35:1824-7.
13. Franco A, Vaughan KG, Vukcevic Z, Thomas S, Mazariegos GV. Gastric volvulus as a complication of liver transplant. *Pediatr Radiol.* 2005;35:327-9.
14. Rashid F, Thangarajah T, Mulvey D, Larvin M, Iftikhar SY. A review article on gastric volvulus: a challenge to diagnosis and management. Int J Surg. 2010;8:18-22.
15. Miller DL, Pasquale MD, Seneca RP, Hodin E. Gastric volvulus in the pediatric population. *Arch Surg.* 1991;126:1146-9.
16. Ayala JA, Naik MB, Olutoye OO. Delayed presentation of congenital diaphragmatic hernia manifesting as combined-type acute gastric volvulus: a case report and review of literature. J Pediatr Surg. 2008;43:E35-9.
17. McElreath DP, Olden KW, Aduli F. Hiccups: a subtle sign in the clinical diagnosis of gastric volvulus and a review of the literature. Dig Dis Sci. 2008;53:3033-6.
18. Godshall D, Mossallam U, Rosenbaum R. Gastric volvulus: case report and review of the literature. *J Emerg Med.* 1999;17:837-40.
19. Williams L, Lansdown MR, Larvin M, Ward DC. Gastric volvulus: a rare cause of hyperamylasaemia. *Br J Clin Pract.* 1990;44:708-9.
20. Sevcik WE, Steiner IP. Acute gastric volvulus: case report and review of the literature. *CJEM.* 1999;1:200-3.
21. Cozart JC, Clouse RE. Gastric volvulus as a cause of intermittent dysphagia. *Dig Dis Sci.* 1998;43:1057-60.
22. Tsang TK, Walker R, Yu DJ. Endoscopic reduction of gastric volvulus: the alpha-loop maneuver. *Gastrointest Endosc.* 1995;42:244-8.
23. Woon CY, Chung AY, Low AS, Wong WK. Delayed diagnosis of intermittent mesenteroaxial volvulus of the stomach by computed tomography: a case report. *J Med Case Reports.* 2008;2:343.
24. Palanivelu C, Rangarajan M, Shetty AR, Senthilkumar R. Laparoscopic suture gastropexy for gastric volvulus: a report of 14 cases. *Surg Endosc.* 2007;21:863-6.
25. Teague WJ, Ackroyd R, Watson DI, Devitt PG. Changing patterns in the management of gastric volvulus over 14 years. *Br J Surg.* 2000;87:358-61.
26. Kulkarni K, Nagler J. Emergency endoscopic reduction of a gastric volvulus. *Endoscopy.* 2007;39(Suppl 1):E173.
27. Ghosh S, Palmer KR. Double percutaneous endoscopic gastrostomy fixation: an effective treatment for recurrent gastric volvulus. *Am J Gastroenterol.* 1993;88:1271-2.
28. Wolfgang R, Lee JG. Endoscopic treatment of acute gastric volvulus causing cardiac tamponade. *J Clin Gastroenterol.* 2001;32:336-9.
29. Kodali VP, Maas LC. Endoscopic reduction of acute gastric volvulus. *J Clin Gastroenterol.* 1995;21:331-2.
30. Lowenthal MN, Odes HS, Fritsch E. Endoscopic reduction of acute gastric volvulus complicating motor neuron disease. *Isr J Med Sci.* 1985;21:552-3.
31. Bhasin DK, Nagi B, Kochhar R, Singh K, Gupta NM, Mehta SK. Endoscopic management of chronic organoaxial volvulus of the stomach. *Am J Gastroenterol.* 1990;85:1486-8.
32. Baudet JS, Armengol-Miró JR, Medina C, Accarino AM, Vilaseca J, Malagelada JR. Percutaneous endoscopic gastrostomy as a treatment for chronic gastric volvulus. *Endoscopy.* 1997;29:147-8.
33. Hsu YC, Perng CL, Chen CK, Tsai JJ, Lin HJ. Conservative management of chronic gastric volvulus: 44 cases over 5 years. *World J Gastroenterol.* 2010;16:4200-5.
34. Hani MB. A combined laparoscopic and endoscopic approach to acute gastric volvulus associated with traumatic diaphragmatic hernia. *Surg Laparosc Endosc Percutan Tech.* 2008;18:151-4.
35. Katkhouda N, Mavor E, Achanta K, Friedlander MH, Grant SW, Essani R, et al. Laparoscopic repair of chronic intrathoracic gastric volvulus. Surgery. 2000;128:784-90.
36. Beqiri A, VanderKolk WE, Scheeres D. Combined endoscopic and laparoscopic management of chronic gastric volvulus. Gastrointest Endosc. 1997;46:450-2.
37. Newman RM, Newman E, Kogan Z, Stien D, Falkenstien D, Gouge TH. A combined laparoscopic and endoscopic approach to acute primary gastric volvulus. J Laparoendosc Adv Surg Tech A. 1997;7:177-81.

CHAPTER 28

Intestinal Obstruction

Sanjoy Mandal

Intestinal obstruction (IO) is an entity, which is very commonly encountered by general surgeons and gastrointestinal surgeons alike.[1,2] It has been observed that IO accounts for 1% of all hospital admissions and 7-8% of emergency surgeries.[3] IO is defined as absence of normal propulsion of enteric contents. A female preponderance is seen due to the fact that women have higher incidence of pelvic surgeries and endometriosis. IO can occur because of an organic lesion or due to inadequate peristalsis of the intestinal wall, in which case it is referred to as paralytic ileus and/or pseudo-obstruction. IO can be broadly classified as obstruction in the small (Box 1) and large bowel (Box 2).

While in the west the common causes of obstruction are postoperative adhesions and malignancy,[4] in India hernias still are the predominant cause[5] with malignancy, adhesions, tuberculosis and volvulus being the other important entities.[2] However, with the changing health scenario especially in tertiary care hospitals, the patient spectrum increasingly resembles that of the west.[5] Whereas in the past Crohn's disease was considered a rarity in India, its prevalence has increased.[6]

BOX 1 Etiology of small bowel obstruction

A. Lesion in the lumen
   a. Gallstone ileus
   b. Impacted fecal matter
   c. Bezoars
   d. Worms
   e. Foreign body
B. Lesion in the wall of the bowel
   a. Inflammatory stricture
      i. TB
      ii. Crohn's disease
      iii. Ulcerative colitis
   b. Malignant stricture
      i. GIST
      ii. Adenocarcinoma
      iii. Carcinoid tumors
      iv. Lymphoma
   c. Ischemic stricture
   d. Drug induced strictures, e.g. NSAIDs
   e. Intramural hematoma
   f. Intussusception
   g. Radiation strictures
   h. Paralytic ileus
C. Lesion outside the wall
   a. Adhesion and band
   b. Hernias
   c. Metastatic tumors
   d. Intra-abdominal abscess
   e. Intra-abdominal hematoma
   f. Pancreatic pseudocyst
   g. Intra-abdominal drains
   h. Tight fascial opening at stoma

BOX 2 Etiology of colonic obstruction

Common causes

- Malignancy-adenocarcinoma (primary, anastomotic, metastatic)
- Volvulus
- Obstructed hernia
- Anastomotic stricture

Unusual causes

- Intussusceptions
- Fecal impaction
- Strictures (Tubercular, inflammatory bowel disease, endometriosis, radiation therapy, ischemia)
- Foreign body
- Extrinsic compression by a mass (e.g. pancreatic pseudocyst)
- Hematoma
- Metastasis
- Diverticulitis
- Pseudo-obstruction

PATHOPHYSIOLOGY

Obstruction can be classified into dynamic and adynamic varieties. Dynamic obstruction occurs when a physical obstruction prevents the bowel contents from being propelled forward. As a result, more and more contents accumulate in the lumen with a resultant stretching of the bowel wall. This results in vigorous contraction of the intestinal muscle in an effort to overcome the obstruction which translates into the colicky pain experienced by patients. The presentation and subsequent progress depends on the level and type of obstruction, and whether the obstruction is complete or partial. The presence of bowel ischemia complicates the situation. If the obstruction is at a single point then the bowel proximal to it dilates. But if the obstruction is at two points then it forms a closed loop obstruction with high possibility of bowel ischemia and perforation. This situation is likely to happen in colonic obstruction with a competent IC valve or a strangulated hernia. Distention in bowel obstruction is essentially due to secreted fluid and swallowed air. Increasing fluid and gas in the bowel leads to increased intraluminal pressures. This can cause compression of mucosal lymphatics, leading to bowel wall edema hampering the venous return causing further congestion in the bowel wall, with ensuing translocation of bacteria and their exotoxins. Ultimately there is compromise of the arterial inflow, and terminating in infarction of the bowel wall and perforation. As the duration of obstruction progresses there is progressive loss of fluids and electrolytes leading to hyponatremia, hypokalemia and metabolic acidosis. In cases of bowel strangulation and gangrene there is increased risk of bacteremia and endotoxemia with associated hypotension, acidosis and septic shock. The possibility of bowel perforation is also higher.

Adynamic obstruction occurs when there is no physical obstruction but inability of the musculature of the bowel wall to contract with the consequence that bowel contents keep collecting. The whole bowel tends to be dilated in contrast to mechanical obstruction where the bowel is dilated proximal to the point of obstruction.[7]

In obstruction there is a marked change in the flora of the small bowel with E. coli, S. faecalis and Klebsiella species predominating. Currently with the increased incidence of ESBL producing species, even in community acquired infection, the situation has become alarming.[8]

Clinical Features

Most patients present with sudden or gradual onset colicky pain abdomen, which is generalized in nature. In proximal small bowel obstruction, bilious vomiting is a pronounced and early feature while abdominal distention may not be prominent. The onset of obstipation is also delayed. Distal small bowel obstruction on the other hand is associated with central abdominal distention, colicky pain, bilious vomiting and obstipation.

Large bowel obstruction tends to be associated with distention, pain, and pronounced early obstipation. The course tends to be different in patients who have a competent ileal valve where a blind loop tends to get formed with extensive dilatation of the colon and increased chances of cecal perforation.

On examination patients may have dehydration, with a rapid and thready pulse. There may be associated drowsiness due to dyselectrolytemia. Abdominal examination may reveal visible peristalsis (Fig. 1), distention, and tenderness. Guarding and rigidity may be present if there is associated peritonism due to bowel gangrene or perforation. A detailed examination of all the hernial sites should be made which includes the inguinal, femoral and obturator areas. Howship-Romberg sign, which is pain along the medial aspect of the thigh and knee, is due to compression of the anterior branch of the obturator nerve by the hernia sac. This is seen in almost half of patients of obturator hernia. Hannington-Kiff sign is also seen in obturator hernias, in which the adductor reflex is absent in the thigh.[9] Note should also be made of scars of previous abdominal surgery and any evidence of herniation through those scars. A per-rectal examination should always be done to assess for rectal neoplasia or stricture.

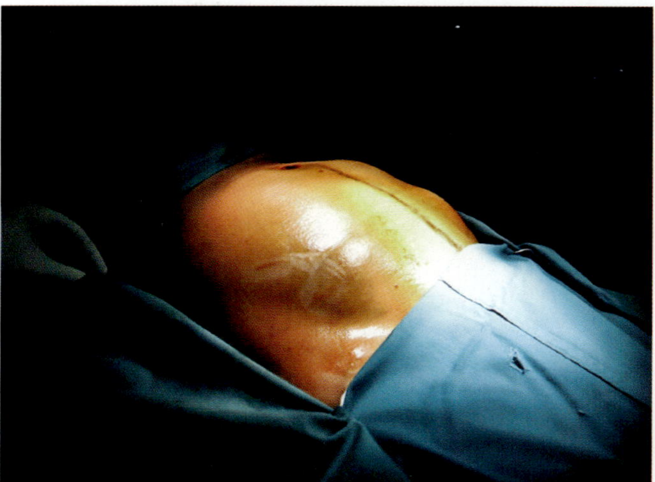

Figure 1 Visible peristalsis and distended bowel loops seen on abdominal wall

Investigation

The preliminary investigations done in these patients are a complete blood count, which would show relative hemoconcentration and raised total count with an increased neutrophil count. Dehydration may be associated with raised urea and creatinine and dyselectrolytemia.

An erect and supine x-ray of the abdomen with a chest x-ray should be performed. The erect films show air fluid levels, which is ideal for diagnosing obstruction. Other than the gastric fluid level, up to two other air fluid levels may be normal—one near the duodenal bulb and the other near the terminal ileum. Presence of more than this is considered abnormal (Fig. 2). The erect film is also important as a perforation can be detected by free air under the diaphragm. In patients who are unable to stand, a sitting film or a left lateral decubitus film may be taken. In a patient who has had prior surgery adhesions may hinder appearance of free gas under the diaphragm. The supine film is important in assessing the level of the obstruction by seeing the character of the bowel loops. Jejunal loops appear as concertina pattern, ileal loops are characterless while colonic loops have haustrations (Fig. 3). Dilatation of small bowel more than 3 cm, right colon more than 9 cm and sigmoid more than 5 cm is considered significant but not diagnostic. Serial x-rays which show fixed dilated loops are likely to

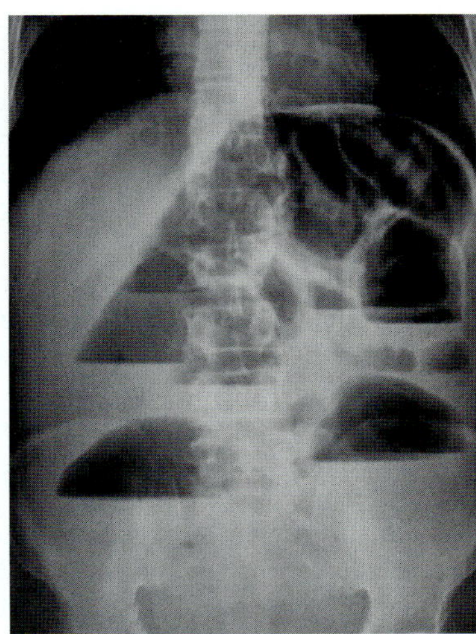

Figure 2 Multiple air fluid level on erect plain X-ray film of the abdomen

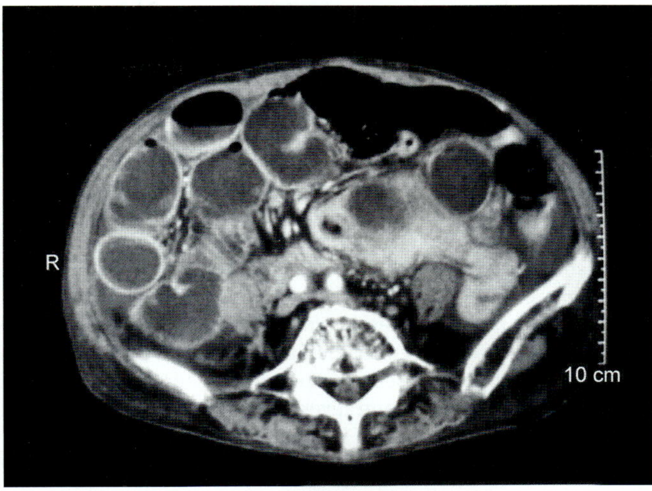

Figure 4 CT scan of the abdomen showing dilated small bowel loops

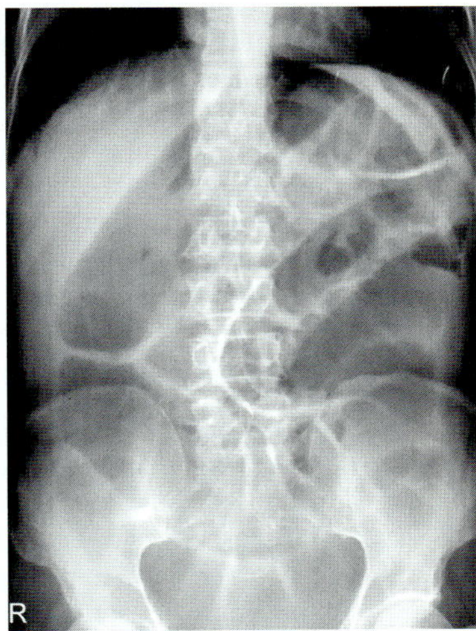

Figure 3 Dilated ileal loops seen on a supine plain X-ray film. Ileal loops are identified as 'characterless'

indicate an obstruction which is unlikely to get relieved by medical management. An X-ray which shows dilated small bowel loops with absence of air in the large bowel is highly suggestive of small bowel obstruction but the presence of gas in the large bowel does not rule out small bowel obstruction.

Ultrasound of the abdomen can identify dilated bowel loops and at times help in identifying the cause of the obstruction but is very operator dependent and its resolution is limited by gas filled bowel loops.[10,11]

Use of barium is not recommended in bowel obstruction as it may precipitate a complete obstruction. Barium is very thick and tenacious and impacted barium in the bowel is very difficult to handle during surgery. In the presence of perforation, barium spill will cause very severe peritonitis.

Contrast Enhanced Computed Tomography (CECT) abdomen is an important investigation modality. It can be done fairly rapidly, and with the current multi-slice technology, high definition 3D reconstruction imaging can be obtained. Characteristic features of small bowel obstruction on CT are dilated bowel caliber, specific transition point, distal collapsed bowel loops and fecal matter in the small bowel (Fig. 4).[12]

It is sensitive and specific in defining the site and cause of obstruction. It has a sensitivity of 93%, specificity of close to 100% and a positive predictive value of 94% in small bowel obstruction.[13] Hence it has become the investigation of choice in most centers. CT is also very accurate in identifying whether there is strangulation or volvulus. Oral contrast with hyperosmolar agents has been found to be safe though not absolutely necessary for assessing intestinal obstruction. The advantage of the hyperosmolar oral contrast is that it draws out fluid from the bowel wall into the lumen, which can be therapeutic in case of adhesive bowel obstruction where it decreases the time to spontaneous relief of obstruction but it does not alter the need for surgical treatment.[14,15]

MRI abdomen has been found to give good results for assessing obstruction on T1 weighted images[16] but has limited ability in assessing the cause of obstruction.[17,18] The long scan time is a major drawback. In our experience, patients with pain, distention and vomiting, find it difficult to undergo a prolonged investigation in a deep claustrophobic tunnel!

Conventional X-rays have a sensitivity of 69% and a specificity of 57%.[19] CT on the other hand has a sensitivity of 94–100% and an accuracy of 90–95%.[20] Thus though conventional radiology remains the initial investigation for IO, but due to its ability to determine the site, level, cause, and severity of obstruction CT has become the investigation of choice.[21]

Management

One of the most important decisions that must be taken by the surgeon in a patient of IO is whether to operate or to manage conservatively. If conservative management is pursued, what should be its duration? Hence treatment for each and every patient has to be individualized.

Patients who are present with symptoms suggestive of obstruction should undergo resuscitation and evaluation hand in hand. Patients should be started on IV fluids for resuscitation. IV Fluids of choice are Ringer's lactate and 0.9% normal saline with or without potassium supplementation. These should be given in such a volume so as to ensure urine output of at least 0.5 ml/kg/hr. The patients should be catheterized to ensure hourly urine output measurement. A large bore 16 or 18 F nasogastric tube should be placed and put on continuous drainage and 2 hourly aspirations for gastrointestinal decompression. Broad-spectrum IV antibiotics preferably a combination of 2nd or 3rd generation cephalosporin's with metronidazole should be started. Patients who have co-morbidities like age, uncontrolled diabetes, patients with features of sepsis, should be started on antibiotics like piperacillin-tazobactam, or cefoperazone-sulbactam or even carbapenems. However, antibiotics are not a replacement for surgical intervention. If there is organ failure or overt sepsis the patients should be managed in the ICU and proper resuscitation performed. Intra-arterial blood pressure monitoring and central venous catheters may be placed if required. An arterial blood gas should be performed and necessary optimization of the patient should be done. All patients with overt mechanical obstruction should undergo surgery at the earliest after necessary work up and resuscitation. The old dictum that 'the sun should never rise and set' in a patient of intestinal obstruction still holds true in most cases, but in cases of adhesive obstruction a longer period of watchful expectancy can be done.

Barring patients with partial obstruction or adhesive obstruction all other patients in whom the obstruction gets relieved with initial conservative management for e.g., hernias getting reduced or volvulus getting derotated, early elective surgery must be performed in the same admission as the problem is likely to recur. Patients who have obvious evidence of bowel ischemia should be operated on an urgent basis as soon as the initial resuscitation and evaluation has been performed. No attempt should be made to treat these patients conservatively.

Surgery for any patient of obstruction should be well planned. This can be performed by open or laparoscopic methods. Laparoscopy is contraindicated in patients with excessive bowel dilation where lack of working space may prove technically difficult in performing the procedure. Laparoscopy would also be contraindicated if there is coagulopathy, hemodynamic instability and marked cardiopulmonary problems. Laparoscopy, when feasible, results in earlier return of bowel function and a shorter hospital stay.

When open surgery is contemplated midline exploratory laparotomy is preferred as it provides rapid access to all quadrants of the abdomen enabling the surgeon to deal with any eventuality. Possible measures needed to relieve the obstruction include—adhesiolysis, band release, bowel resection and anastomosis, stricturoplasty, bypass, and stoma formation. As a number of patients undergoing surgery for IO may require a stoma, a preoperative informed consent for the same must be obtained from all patients. Due risk should also be explained to the patient and relatives. In today's era of litigation, a well-informed and well-counseled patient and relatives translates into peace of mind for the surgeon. Stoma should be marked preoperatively.

SPECIAL PROBLEMS AND THEIR MANAGEMENT

Obstructed Hernia

The probability of a hernia getting obstructed or strangulated varies from 0.29% up to 2.9%.[22] The most common obstructed hernias are inguinal hernias in male and incisional hernias in female. But the hernia most likely to get obstructed is the obturator hernia followed by the femoral. Though these hernias are rare and are almost exclusively seen in elderly females, due to the very narrow and tight neck they have a very high likelihood of getting obstructed. Obturator hernia represents less than 1% of all hernias[23] and is often referred to as "little old lady's hernia".[24]

Since these hernias are rare and easily missed, they are like to get detected late and hence the prognosis is worse. Preoperative diagnosis is made in only 10–30%.[25] More than 90% of patients of obturator hernia present with obstruction.[26]

Obstructed hernias, whether strangulated or not should be operated on an emergency basis. In case the hernia does get reduced spontaneously one should keep a close watch as the hernia may still remain obstructed and strangulated due to existing internal adhesions and being reduced en-masse. When operating on an obstructed inguinal hernia the incision is given along the groin crease extending down toward the scrotum. The hernia sac should be opened at the fundus and not at the neck as adhesion are less likely. Also, since there is a possibility of strangulation, the infected contents can be drained out without the peritoneal cavity being contaminated. After inspection of the contents the neck is dissected and opened. The bowel is thoroughly inspected for any ischemia, gangrene or perforation. The constriction ring should be carefully divided. If required, the viability of the bowel is assessed after covering it with warm mops and 100% oxygen. In case of any doubt the concerned bowel should be resected. For repairing the hernia a polypropylene mesh is used if there has been no infection or contamination otherwise an anatomical repair is performed.

Obstruction Due to Adhesions or Bands

This is the most common form of obstruction seen in the west accounting for up to 75% cases.[27] Incidence of adhesion after any surgery is about 67%. After multiple surgeries it may reach 93%. The incidence is less after laparoscopic surgery. It has been seen that 71% of all adhesions after surgery form in the laparotomy scar, hence reducing the size of this scar will decrease the incidence of adhesions. Also given the fact that laparoscopy is associated with less bowel handling, less bowel abrasion by gauze or mops and less bowel desiccation all lead to decreased adhesion formation.[28] Even in patients who have not undergone any surgery the incidence may be up to 28%.[29,30] Most of these are innocuous and do not cause significant problem. It is only in14.3% patients who have undergone open surgery that obstruction is seen and 2.6% require adhesiolysis.[31] In the absence of peritonitis all cases should initially be managed conservatively with nasogastric aspiration and IV fluids.[32,33] A period of at least 48 hours should be given for the obstruction to resolve spontaneously. In 65–90% cases the non-operative approach will lead to relief of obstruction, especially in cases where the obstruction is partial. In 85–95% cases the relief occurs in the first 48 hours. In situations with a complete obstruction the chances of failure of non-operative management is higher.[34,35,36] Small bowel obstruction in the scenario of a recent surgery in the past 4–6 weeks should preferably be managed non-operatively. An exception to this is when the obstruction follows laparoscopic surgery where the threshold for operative intervention should be higher as there might be the possibility of bowel incarceration in a port site or internal hernial defect.[27] Surgery should be carried out in all cases where the obstruction

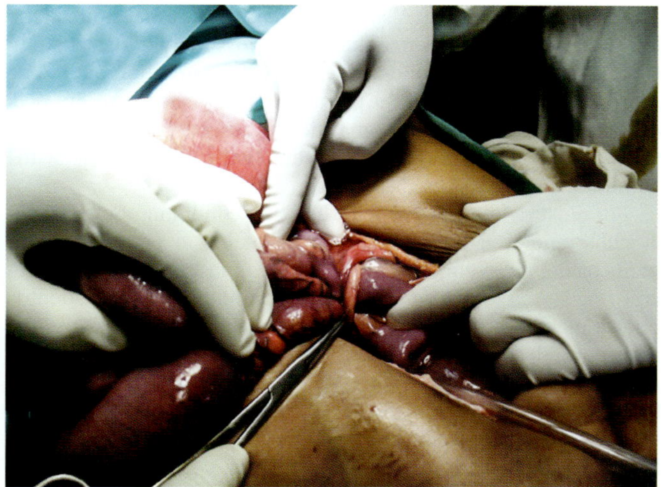

Figure 5 Small bowel obstruction due band

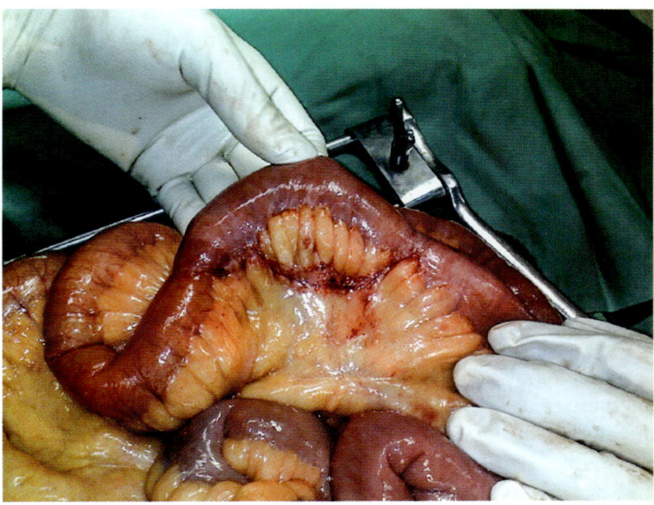

Figure 6 Constriction ring after relief of band obstruction

does not resolve with conservative management (Figs 5 and 6). Adhesiolysis should be carried out and any ischemic bowel resected. It cannot be emphasized that minimizing bleeding, tissue handling, infection and contamination risk, drying of tissues, use of cautery, use of sutures, foreign bodies and using starch free gloves is important in preventing further adhesions.[37] Various compounds like Seprafilm, Prevadh etc, have been developed which claim to reduce the incidence of adhesions but none have been proven in clinical trials.[38,39] An adhesion barrier may be used in high risk patients (myomectomy, endometriosis or pelvic inflammatory disease). Also, oxidized regenerated cellulose (Interceed, surgicel) should not be used as it may increase the risk of adhesions in this situation.[40] In cases where the bowel distention is not extreme and some working space can be created after pneumoperitoneum, the adhesiolysis should be performed by laparoscopy. Not only is recovery quicker, the chance of further bowel adhesions is also less.[41,42]

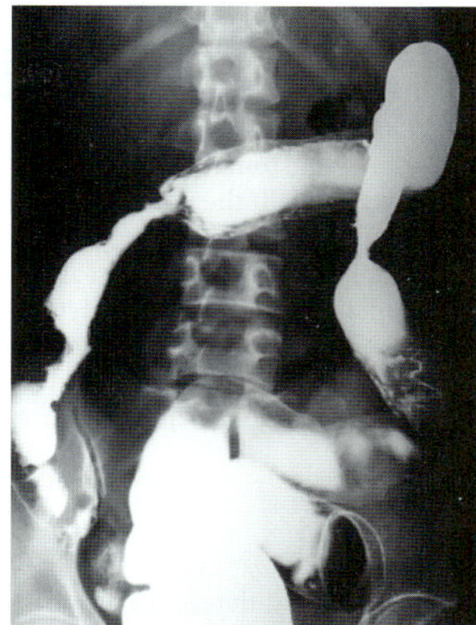

Figure 7 Barium enema showing multiple benign strictures of the colon (at the descending colon and transverse colon), these as smooth taperings unlike those with shouldering seen in malignancy. These strictures turned out to tubercular in etiology.

TUBERCULAR OBSTRUCTION

Abdominal TB constitutes almost 11% of all cases of extra-pulmonary tubercular patients. It can involve any part of the GI tract. In Indians, the spread to the GI tract is hematogenous and not by the oral route. This is mainly because of the fact that in India milk is boiled before consumption. Due to its high prevalence in India, TB of the GI tract should be kept as a differential in most cases of obstruction.[43,44] Tubercular strictures mainly involve the small bowel and most commonly the distal ileum and the ileo-colic region. This is followed by the jejunum. Rarely is the large bowel involved (Fig. 7).[45-48] The high propensity for affecting the ileal and ileocecal region is the physiological stasis and rich lymphoid tissue of this area.

Tubercular ulcers are single or multiple with normal mucosa in between. They are generally superficial and do not penetrate beyond the muscularis.[49] They are transversely oriented in contrast to typhoid ulcers and Crohn's disease which are longitudinal or serpiginous respectively.[50] Healing of the ulcers by arterial occlusion and subsequent ischemia can lead to stricture formation.[51] Also ATT may lead to healing of ulcers with fibrosis and subsequent stricture formation. GI tuberculosis has been described as ulcerative and hypertrophic forms.[52] Ulcerative form is seen more often in malnourished adults. Hypertrophic form on the other hand is more usual in the well-nourished adults.

Patients who present with subacute obstruction which gets relieved with initial conservative management can be followed up with ATT. Addition of steroids may decrease the adhesive complication.[53] Some of these patients may not require surgery, as some studies have shown strictures disappearing after ATT being started.[54,55] But patients who develop repeated episodes of obstruction should undergo surgery. Tubercular strictures can be managed either by stricturoplasty or by resection. Radical resections are not recommended.[56,57] If stricturoplasty is performed a biopsy of the margin should always be taken.[56,58] In up to 60% of case the strictures can be multiple.[59] In these situations it is prudent to resect them in continuity to avoid having multiple anastomosis or stricturoplasty sites. In some cases due to the distribution of the strictures, multiple anastomosis and/or stricturoplasties may be unavoidable. In cases where the general condition of the patient is very poor and where there is high probability of non healing and subsequent anastomotic leak it may be preferable to perform a stoma, especially if the concerned area is distally in the ileum. Lesion located very close to or involving the ileocecal junction should undergo a limited ileo-colectomy[60] unlike radical resections for malignancies. In addition to strictures, other causes of intestinal obstruction in TB are adhesions to abdominal lymph nodes, compression or kinking caused by nodes—e.g. affecting 3rd part of duodenum and duodeno-jejunal flexure, and intestinal cocoon.

CROHN'S' STRICTURE

Crohn's strictures need to be differentiated from TB strictures as the approach is somewhat different. These are initially managed conservatively with medications. Crohn's strictures are known to recur and surgery in these cases was thought to be associated with leaks and fistula formation. However the incidence of such complications has been overstated. A number of studies have reported the safety of surgery in patients of CD. It is to be emphasized that those patients who are otherwise not responding to medical management should not be denied surgery solely out fear of fistula formation. Some preoperative clues to the diagnosis of Crohn's disease are foreshortening of the mesentery with the mesenteric fat creeping on to the bowel. Surgical management involves stricturoplasty with biopsy of the margin or resection. Longer strictures can be managed by the Finley type stricturoplasty. For obstructing lesions close to or involving the IC junction a limited ileo-colectomy should be performed. Any bowel resection in CD needs to be conservative as there are high chances of recurrence which may need further resections leading to short bowel syndrome.

GALLSTONE ILEUS

This is seen almost exclusively in the elderly age group with long standing gallstone disease. These patients develop a fistula between the gall bladder and the duodenum through which a large gall bladder stone passes into the intestine. Since the distal ileum is the narrowest part of the small bowel, such stones would get stuck there and lead to small bowel obstruction. X-rays would show small bowel obstruction. If the stone is radio-opaque it may be seen on plain X-ray. Pneumobilia may also be apparent (Rigler's Triad). Since these patients are usually sick and in a compromised condition, surgery should involve enterotomy and removal of the stone or stones. This can be performed laparoscopically also.[61,62] The cholecystoduodenal fistula should not be disturbed as it would prolong the surgery which would be detrimental for the patient. This fistula should be tackled later in an elective setting after the patient's condition is optimized.

COLONIC MALIGNANCY

Colonic malignancies present with obstruction very late in the course of the disease. It has been classically found that left sided tumors tend to be stricturing growths hence are more likely to present with obstruction. Also important is the fact that stool on the left side is more solid hence the higher possibility of obstruction. Colonic tumors which tend to present with obstruction tend to be more advanced and hence the prognosis tends to be worse. Surgical options include: diverting stoma without resection, resection with stoma without anastomosis, resection with anastomosis with/without a diverting stoma.

For most right sided growth where the condition of the patient is stable and well preserved, it is acceptable to perform a right hemicolectomy with an ileotransverse anastomosis without a covering stoma.[63-68] Where the general condition of the patient is poor it may be prudent to perform a resection and exteriorize the ends as an ileostomy and mucus fistula or even in extremely poor risk cases performing only a diverting stoma so as to provide for time for the patient to recover before performing a definitive surgery.

For obstructing lesion in the transverse colon extended right hemicolectomy with an ileo-descending colon anastomosisit may be preferred over a transverse colectomy with colo-colic anastomosis.

For obstructing lesions in the left colon, surgical options include Hartmann's Procedure (Resection with end colostomy with closure of the distal end),[69-74] resection with primary anastomosis, with/without a proximal diverting stoma and Subtotal colectomy with an ileorectal anastomosis.

For obstructing growths of the rectum and anal canal, a lower anterior resection or an abdominoperineal resection in the emergency setting is not recommended. These patients should preferably undergo a diverting stoma or placement of a SEMS as a bridge to surgery. This may be followed by neoadjuvantchemo radiotherapy,[75] with definitive surgery being performed 6-12 weeks after completion of chemo radiation.[76]

DIVERTICULITIS

Diverticular disease is seen commonly in the west, but is very uncommon in Asia and Africa. This has been mainly attributed to the high fiber diet in these parts of the world. It most commonly affects the sigmoid colon. Though most cases of diverticular disease are uncomplicated, up to 25% of cases are associated with features of obstruction, perforation and fistula formation.[77] Recurrent episodes of inflammation can lead to stricturing and obstruction. This occurs most commonly in the sigmoid colon.[78] Differentiating a diverticular obstruction form a malignant one is very difficult considering the similar age of presentation and the radiological findings. Moreover the two entities can co-exist. A sigmoidoscopy should be performed to get a biopsy. It may also be used to provide temporary relief by dilatation and stenting so that an elective surgery may be performed, though the role of stenting is debatable.[79,80] These patients should undergo a sigmoid colectomy with colostomy (Hartmann's procedure). Only performing a diverting colostomy is generally not justified as the diseased sigmoid, even if there is no malignancy, if left in-situ can continue to create problems.[81]

VOLVULUS

Volvulus is an entity when the small or large intestine twists around itself leading to intestinal obstruction and can compromise in its blood supply leading to gangrene. Volvulus is one of the causes of intestinal obstruction which leads to massive abdominal distention. It is seen very commonly in the 'volvulus belt' involving countries such as India, the Middle East and Africa. The most common site of volvulus is the sigmoid (60%), followed by cecum (20–40%).[82,83] Less common causes include ileosigmoid knotting and small bowel volvulus as a result of adhesions. Cecal bascule is another entity in which there is upward and anterior folding of the cecum. It also has the potential to form obstruction and strangulation. The age of presentation tends to vary from region to region. In India the age of presentation is in 3rd or 4th decade whereas in the west it is in the 6th decade with multiple co-morbidities.[84] In the 'volvulus belt', it is seen in those consuming high volumes of roughage, while in the west it seen among those consuming processed food.[85]

The risk factors for developing a volvulus are a very loaded and bulky intestine, long mesentery with a narrow base and fixation at the apex on the antimesenteric side. Clinically the patients present with symptoms of large bowel obstruction with massive abdominal distention.

Plain X-ray films in sigmoid volvulus classically reveal a 'coffee bean sign' or a 'bent inner tube sign' as a result of a dilated bowel loop extending from the left iliac fossa into the right upper quadrant. Similar findings can be seen in cecal volvulus but the bowel distention is less and the bowel loops are diametrically opposite placed.[86] Instillation of rectal contrast shows a 'bird's beak' sign at the site of obstruction. In case of doubt a CT scan should be done which is very accurate at identifying the volvulus which shows up as a 'whirl sign'.[87]

When patients present with a suspected sigmoid volvulus, an attempt may be made to pass a flatus tube or colonoscope per rectally to derotate the sigmoid. This should be carried out only if there are no signs of peritonitis or gangrene. Derotation leads to immediate passage of large amounts of flatus and stools and relief of distention. Patient should then be planned for surgery on a semi-urgent basis in the same admission. Resection of the involved bowel is the optimal procedure but is associated with increased operative time. Primary anastomosis can be performed if the patient is stable and the bowel is healthy. If the bowel is gangrenous, resection with a diverting stoma may be preferable. The bowel continuity is restored after 8–12 weeks. For selected high risk patients sigmoidopexy with broadening of the base of the sigmoid mesentery can be performed. However there is a high rate of recurrence of the volvulus in this situation.

INTUSSUSCEPTION

This is usually seen in children in the age group of 6–12 months as a result of hypertrophy of the Peyer's patches and presents with the classic triad of colicky abdominal pain, bloody diarrhea and a sausage shaped periumblical mass. In adults it is rare and can be attributed to about 1–5% of all causes of obstruction.[88] This occurs invariably due a protruding intraluminal lesion, e.g. polyp in atleast 80% of cases. In 10–20% cases it is idiopathic. As a result of intestinal peristalsis the lesion with the bowel wall gets telescoped into the bowel lumen. Intussusceptions can be classified into 4 different types depending upon the location, entero-enteric (small bowel telescoping into small bowel), enterocolic (small bowel telescoping into large bowel), colocolic (large bowel telescoping into large bowel) and ileocecal (where IC valve is the lead point of intussusceptions). This last type is difficult to differentiate from the enterocolic type.[89,90,91] On plain X-rays multiple air fluid levels are seen and barium or gastrograffin series may show a 'stacked coin' or 'coiled spring' appearance.[92,93,94] Intussusceptions are well seen on ultrasonography as a 'target sign' or 'doughnut sign' ('bowel in bowel' appearance) on transverse imaging while on longitudinal sections it is seen as a 'pseudo-kidney sign' or 'hay fork sign' (Fig. 8). Contrast CT scan is considered one of the best diagnostic tools with a diagnostic accuracy of 58–100%. In adults there is no role of conservative treatment as there is always an underlying lesion, which will lead to recurrence unless the offending lesion is removed.[95] Surgeries involves reducing the intussusception and resecting the offending segment of bowel. Intussusceptions should be reduced carefully and gently by pushing and not by pulling (Fig. 9). Adhesions between the intussusception and the intussuscepiens are gently dissected if required. Intussusceptions

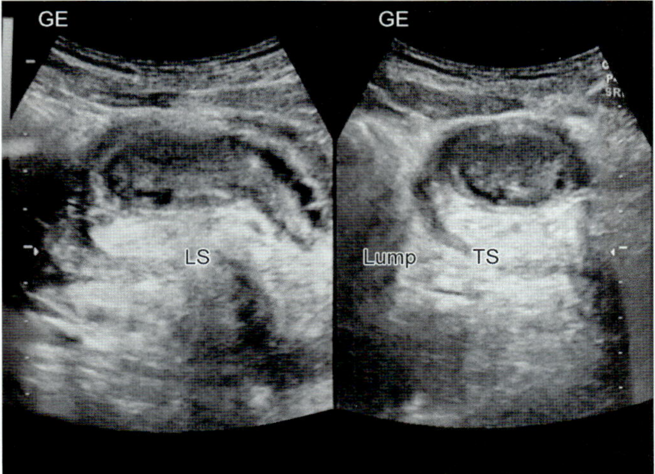

Figure 8 Ultrasound of the abdomen showing typical bowel-in-bowel appearance, 'pseudo kidney' sign on longitudinal imaging while on transverse scans it is the 'Target' sign which is suggestive of intussusception

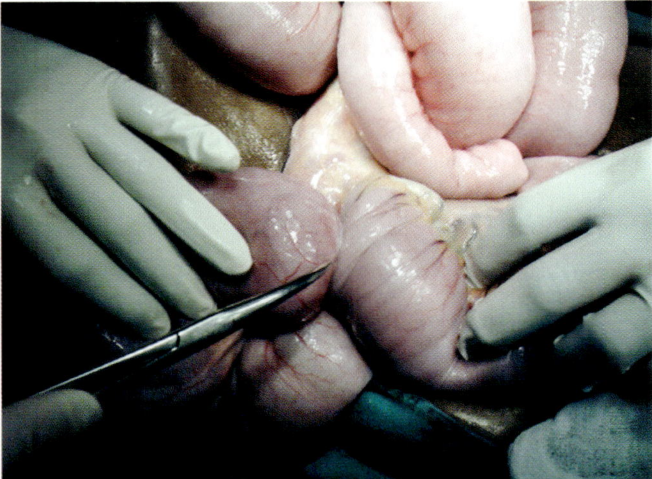

Figure 9 Small bowel intussusception due to small bowel polyp. This patient had multiple polyps. The oral mucosa had pigmentation (below). Diagnosed as a case of Peutz-Jegher's syndrome

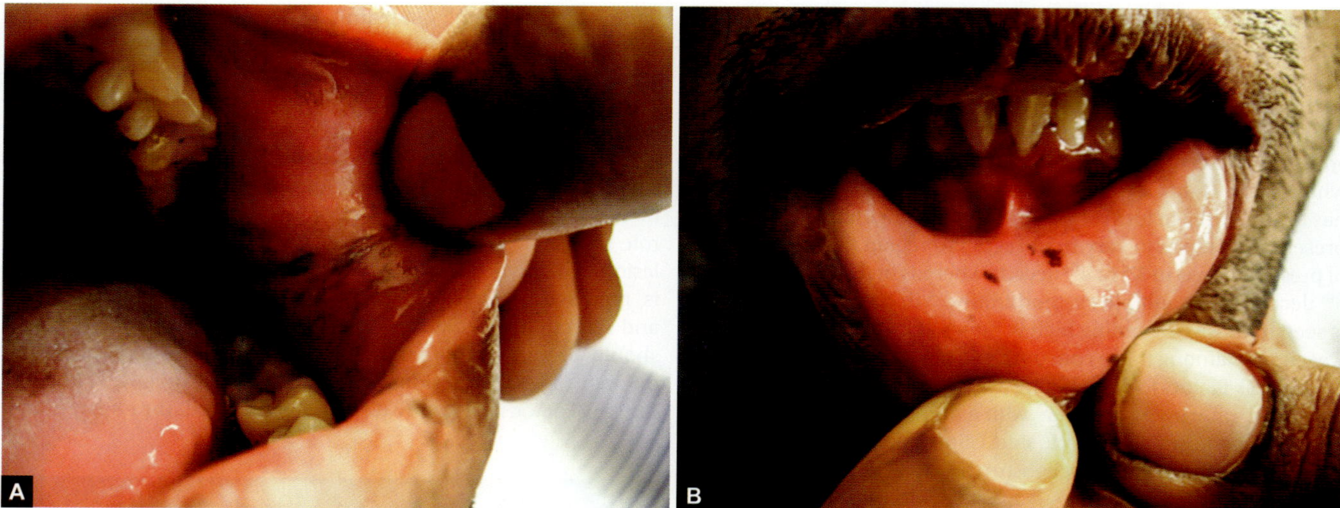

Figures 10A and B A & B showing pigmentation of the oral mucosa

in the elderly are known to harbor underlying malignancy and hence reduction should be avoided as there is a possibility of tumor cell dissemination. Reduction of the lesion should also be avoided if there is doubt of bowel viability. In these situations it is always better to directly resect the concerned segment. The rest of the bowel should be inspected for any other lesion as there is a possibility of multiple lesions in some cases (Figs 10A and B).

POSTOPERATIVE ILEUS (POI)

Postoperative bowel function should resume by 72 hours unless there has been history of prolonged preoperative intestinal obstruction, sepsis, or dyselectrolytemia. Preventive measures include keep operating times short, reducing opioid use by alternative techniques like epidural analgesia, minimal bowel handling and by adopting laparoscopic surgery. Studies have shown laparoscopic surgery to be associated with much less trauma and a less inflammatory state with a resultant early return of bowel motility. Other measures include avoiding nasogastric tubes, early resumption of oral feeds, and early ambulation. Prokinetic medications like levosulpiride and metoclopramide have been recommended to treat POI. Any abnormality of serum sodium, potassium and magnesium should be corrected.[96]

CONCLUSION

Intestinal obstruction continues to be a challenge for surgeons. In the foreseeable future it is expected that surgical technique will get more refined and better intensive care will help manage critically ill patient better.

BIBLIOGRAPHY

1. Irvin TT. Abdominal pain: a surgical audit of 1190 emergency admissions. Br J Surg. 1989;76:1121-5.
2. Adhikari S, Hossein MZ, Das A, Mitra N, Ray U. Etiology and Outcome of Acute Intestinal Obstruction: A Review of 367 Patients in Eastern India. Saudi J Gastroenterol. 2010;16:285-7.
3. Miller G, Boman J, Shrier I, Gordon PH. Natural history of patients with adhesive small bowel obstruction. Br J Surg. 2000;87:1240-7.
4. van der Wal JB, Lordens GI, Vrijland WW, van Veen RN, Lange J, Jeekel J. Adhesion prevention during laparotomy: long-term follow-up of a randomized clinical trial. Ann Surg. 2011;253:1118-21.
5. Tamijmarane A, Chandra S, Smile SR. Clinical aspects of adhesive intestinal obstruction. TropGastroenterol. 2000;21:141-3.
6. Pai CG, Khandige GK. Is Crohn's disease rare in India? Indian J Gastroenterol. 2000;19:17-20.
7. Luckey A, Livingston E, Tache Y. Mechanisms and treatment of postoperative ileus. Arch Surg. 2003;138:206-14.
8. Chaudhuri BN, Rodrigues C, Balaji V, Iyer R, Sekar U, Wattal C, et al. Incidence of ESBL producers amongst Gram-negative bacilli isolated from intra-abdominal infections across India (based on SMART study, 2007 data). J Assoc Physicians India. 2011;59: 287-92.
9. Kammori M, Mafune K, Hirashima T, Kawahara M, Hashimoto M, Ogawa T, et al. Forty-three cases of obturator hernia. Am J Surg. 2004;187:549-52.
10. Cappell MS, Batke M. Mechanical obstruction of the small bowel and colon. Med Clin North Am. 2008;92:575-97.
11. Suri S, Gupta S, Sudhakar PJ, Venkataramu NK, Sood B, Wig JD. Comparative evaluation of plain films, ultrasound and CT in the diagnosis of intestinal obstruction. Acta Radiol. 1999;40:422-8.
12. Maglinte DD, Reyes BL, Harmon BH, Kelvin FM, Turner WW Jr, Hage JE, et al. Reliability and role of plain radiography and CT in the diagnosis of small bowel obstruction. Am J Roentgenol. 1996;167:1451-5.
13. Muchha P Jr. Small intestinal obstruction. SurgClin N Am. 1987;67:597-620.
14. Abbas SM, Bissett IP, Parry BR. Meta-analysis of oral water-soluble contrast agent in the management of adhesive small bowel obstruction. Br J Surg. 2007;94:404-11.
15. Abbas SM, Bissett IP, Parry BR. Oral water soluble contrast for the management of adhesive small bowel obstruction. Cochrane Database Syst Rev. 2007;18(3):CD004651.
16. Umschaden HW, Szolar D, Gasser J, Umschaden M, Haselbach H. Small bowel disease: comparison of MR enteroclysis images with conventional enteroclysis and surgical findings. Radiology. 2000;215:717-25.

17. Diaz JJ Jr, Bokhari F, Mowery NT, Acosta JA, Block EF, Bromberg WJ, et al. Guidelines for management of small bowel obstruction. J Trauma. 2008;64:1651-64.
18. Maglinte DD, Heitkamp DE, Howard TJ, Kelvin FM, Lappas JC. Current concepts in imaging of small bowel obstruction. Radiol Clin North Am. 2003;41:263-83.
19. Maglinte DD, Gage SN, Harmon BH, Kelvin FM, Hage JP, Chua GT, et al. Obstruction of the small intestine: accuracy and role of CT in diagnosis. Radiology. 1993;188:61-4.
20. Frager D, Medwid SW, Baer JW, Mollinelli B, Friedman M. CT of small-bowel obstruction: value in establishing the diagnosis and determining the degree and cause. Am J Roentgenol. 1994;162:37-41.
21. Boudiaf M, Soyer P, Terem C, Pelage JP, Maissiat E, Rymer R. CT evaluation of small bowel obstruction. Radiographics. 2001;21: 613-24.
22. Gallegos NC, Dawson J, Jarvis M, Hobsley M. Risk of strangulation in groin hernias. Br J Surg. 1991;78:1171-3.
23. Chang SS, Shan YS, Lin YJ, Tai YS, Lin PW. A review of obturator hernia and a proposed algorithm for its diagnosis and treatment. World J Surg. 2005;29:450-4.
24. Dundamadappa SK, Tsou IY, Goh JS. Clinics in diagnostic imaging (107). Singapore Med J. 2006;47:89-94.
25. Gray SW, Skandalakis JE, Soria RE, Rowe JS Jr. Strangulated obturator hernia. Surgery. 1974;75:20-7.
26. Lo CY, Lorentz TG, Lau PW. Obturator hernia presenting as small bowel obstruction. Am J Surg. 1994;167:396-8.
27. Sarraf-Yazdi S, Shapiro ML. Small bowel obstruction: The eternal dilemma of when to intervene. Scand J Surg. 2010;99:78-80.
28. Lundorff P, Hahlin M, Kallfelt B, Thorburn J, Lindblom B. Adhesion formation after laparoscopic surgery in tubal pregnancy: a randomized trial versus laparotomy. Fertil Steril. 1991;55:911-5.
29. Weibel MA, Majno G. Peritoneal adhesions and their relation to abdominal surgery. A postmortem study. Am J Surg. 1973;126:345-53.
30. Yesildaglar N, Koninckx PR. Adhesion formation in intubated rabbits increases with high insufflation pressure during endoscopic surgery. Hum Reprod. 2000;15:687-91.
31. Beck DE, Opelka FG, Bailey HR, Rauh SM, Pashos CL. Incidence of small-bowel obstruction and adhesiolysis after open colorectal and general surgery. Dis Colon Rectum. 1999;42:241-8.
32. Diaz JJ Jr, Bokhari F, Mowery NT, Acosta JA, Block EF, Bromberg WJ, et al. Guidelines for management of small bowel obstruction. J Trauma. 2008;64:1651-64.
33. Rocha FG, Theman TA, Matros E, Ledbetter SM, Zinner MJ, Ferzoco SJ. Nonoperative management of patients with a diagnosis of high-grade small bowel obstruction by computed tomography. Arch Surg. 2009;144:1000-04.
34. Cappell MS, Batke M: Mechanical obstruction of the small bowel and colon. Med Clin North Am. 2008;92:575-97.
35. Hayanga AJ, Bass-Wilkins K, Bulkley GB: Current management of small-bowel obstruction. Adv Surg. 2005;39:1-33.
36. Fevang BT, Jensen D, Svanes K, Viste A. Early operation or conservative management of patients with small bowel obstruction. Eur J Surg. 2002;168:475-81.
37. Diamond MP, Wexner SD, diZereg GS, Korell M, Zmora O, Van Goor H, et al. Adhesion prevention and reduction: current status and future recommendations of a multinational-interdisciplinary consensus conference. Surg Innov. 2010;17:183-8.
38. Mabrut JY, Favre JP, Desrousseaux B, Chipponi J, Arnaud JP, Domergue J, et al. Safety and long-term outcome of a new concept for surgical adhesion-reduction strategies (Prevadh): a prospective, multicenter study. Hepatogastroenterology. 2008;55:517-21.
39. Zeng Q, Yu Z, You J, Zhang Q. Efficacy and safety of Seprafilm for preventing postoperative abdominal adhesion: systematic review and meta-analysis. World J Surg. 2007;31:2125-31.
40. Robertson D, Lefebvre G, Leyland N, Wolfman W, Allaire C, Awadalla A, et al. Adhesion prevention in gynaecological surgery. J Obstet Gynaecol Can. 2010;32:598-608.
41. Schuster KM, Davis KA, Rosenbaum SH: Emergency and urgent surgery. Med Clin North Am. 2009;93:1131-48.
42. Szomstein S, Lo Menzo E, Simpfendorfer C, Zundel N, Rosenthal RJ. Laparoscopic lysis of adhesions. World J Surg. 2006;30:535-40.
43. Wig KL, Chitkara NK, Gupta SP, Kishore K, Manchanda RL. Ileocecal tuberculosis with particular reference to isolation of *Mycobacterium tuberculosis*. With a note on its relation to regional ileitis (Crohn's disease). Am Rev Respir Dis. 1961;84:169-78.
44. Vij JC, Malhotra V, Choudhary V, Jain NK, Prasad G, Choudhary A, et al. A clinicopathological study of abdominal tuberculosis. Indian J Tuberc. 1992;39:213-20.
45. Bhansali SK. Abdominal tuberculosis. Experiences with 300 cases. Am J Gastroenterol. 1977;67:324-37.
46. Tandon RK, Sarin SK, Bose SL, Berry M, Tandon BN. A clinico-radiological reappraisal of intestinal tuberculosis – changing profile? Gastroenterol Jpn. 1986;21:17-22.
47. Palmer KR, Patil DH, Basran S, Riordan JF, Silk DBA. Abdominal tuberculosis in urban Britain: a common disease. Gut. 1985;26: 1296-305.
48. Joshi MJ. The surgical management of intestinal tuberculosis a conservative approach. Indian J Surg. 1978;40:79-83.
49. Tandon HD, Prakash A. Pathology of intestinal tuberculosis and its distinction from Crohn's disease. Gut. 1972;13:260-9.
50. Anand BS. Distinguishing Crohn's disease from intestinal tuberculosis. Natl Med J India. 1989;2:170-5.
51. Kapoor VK. Abdominal tuberculosis. Postgrad Med J. 1998;74: 459-67.
52. Tandon HD, Prakash A. Pathology of intestinal tuberculosis and its distinction from Crohn's disease. Gut. 1972;13:260-9.
53. Singh MM, Bhargava AN, Jain KP. Tuberculous peritonitis. An evaluation of pathogenetic mechanisms, diagnostic procedures and therapeutic measures. N Engl J Med. 1969;281:1091-4.
54. Anand BS, Nanda R, Sachdev K. Response of tuberculous stricture to antituberculous treatment. Gut. 1988;29:62-9.
55. Balasubramanian R, Ramachandran R, Joseph P, et al. Interim results of a clinical study of abdominal tuberculosis. Indian J Tubercul. 1989;36:117-21.
56. Pujari BD. Modified surgical procedures in intestinal tuberculosis. Br J Surg. 1979;66:180-1.
57. Joshi MJ. The surgical management of intestinal tuberculosis-a conservative approach. Indian J Surg. 1978;40:79-83.
58. Parikh AJ. Conservative approach in management of intestinal tuberculosis. Indian J Surg. 1978;40:85-90.
59. Bhansali SK. Abdominal tuberculosis. Experiences with 300 cases. Am J Gastroenterol. 1977;67:324-37.
60. Prakash A. Ulceroconstrictive tuberculosis of the bowel. Int Surg. 1978;63:23-9.
61. Yakan S, Engin O, Tekeli T, Calik B, Deneçli AG, Coker A, et al. Gallstone ileus as an unexpected complication of cholelithiasis: diagnostic difficulties and treatment. Ulus Travma Acil Cerrahi Derg. 2010;16:344-8.
62. Shiwani MH, Ullah Q. Laparoscopic enterolithotomy is a valid option to treat gallstone ileus. JSLS. 2010;14:282-5.
63. Welch JP, Donaldson GA. Management of severe obstruction of the large bowel due to malignant disease. Am J Surg. 1974;127:492-9.
64. Phillips RK, Hittinger R, Fry JS, Fielding LP. Malignant large bowel obstruction. Br J Surg. 1985;72:296-302.
65. Jiang JK, Lan YT, Lin TC, Chen WS, Yang SH, Wang HS, et al. Primary vs. delayed resection for obstructive left-sided colorectal cancer: impact of surgery on patient outcome. Dis Colon Rectum. 2008;51:306-11.

66. Runkel NS, Schlag P, Schwarz V, Herfarth C. Outcome after emergency surgery for cancer of the large intestine. Br J Surg. 1991;78:183-8.
67. De Salvo GL, Gava C, Pucciarelli S, Lise M. Curative surgery for obstruction from primary left colorectal carcinoma: primary or staged resection? Cochrane Database Syst Rev. 2004;(2): CD002101.
68. Carty NJ, Corder AP. Which surgeons avoid a stoma in treating left-sided colonic obstruction? Results of a postal questionnaire. Ann R Coll Surg Engl. 1992;74:391-4.
69. Lee YM, Law WL, Chu KW, Poon RT. Emergency surgery for obstructing colorectal cancers: a comparison between right-sided and left-sided lesions. J Am Coll Surg. 2001;192:719-25.
70. Caiazzo P, Di Palma R, Pesce G, Pede A. Obstructing colon cancer–what's the surgical strategy? Ann Ital Chir. 2004;75:455-60.
71. Isbister WH, Prasad J. Emergency large bowel surgery: a 15-year audit. Int J Colorectal Dis. 1997;12:285-90.
72. Parc R, Bouteloup PY, Kartheuser A. Must we reject primary colostomy in left colonic obstruction caused by cancer? Chirurgie. 1989;115 Suppl 2:112-6.
73. Cugnenc PH, Berger A, Zinzindohoue F, Quinaux D, Wind P, Chevallier JM. 2-stage surgery of neoplastic left colonic obstruction remains the safest procedure. J Chir (Paris) 1997;134:275-8.
74. Finan PJ, Campbell S, Verma R, MacFie J, Gatt M, Parker MC, et al. The management of malignant large bowel obstruction: ACPGBI position statement. Colorectal Dis. 2007;9 Suppl 4:1-17.
75. Liu Y, Li DC, Feng HY, Zhu Y, Liu LY. Effects of enterostomy in treating locally advanced rectal cancer with combined chemoradiotherapy and operation. Zhonghua Wai Ke Za Zhi. 2007;45:455-8.
76. Sebag-Montefiore D, Stephens RJ, Steele R, Monson J, Grieve R, Khanna S, et al. Preoperative radiotherapy versus selective postoperative chemoradiotherapy in patients with rectal cancer (MRC CR07 and NCIC-CTG C016): a multicentre, randomised trial. Lancet. 2009;373:811-20.
77. Kang JY, Hoare J, Tinto A, Subramanian S, Ellis C, Majeed A, et al. Diverticular disease of the colon–on the rise: A study of hospital admissions in England between 1989/1990 and 1999/2000. Aliment Pharmacol Ther. 2003;17:1189-95.
78. Stollman N, Raskin JB. Diverticular disease of the colon. Lancet. 2004;363:631-9.
79. Small AJ, Young-Fadok TM, Baron TH. Expandable metal stent placement for benign colorectal obstruction: outcomes for 23 cases. Surg Endosc. 2008;22:454-62.
80. Keränen I, Lepistö A, Udd M, Halttunen J, Kylänpää L. Outcome of patients after endoluminal stent placement for benign colorectal obstruction. Scand J Gastroenterol. 2010;45:725-31.
81. Constantinides VA, Tekkis PP, Athanasiou T, Aziz O, Purkayastha S, Remzi FH, et al. Primary resection with anastomosis vs. Hartmann's procedure in nonelective surgery for acute colonic diverticulitis: A systematic review. Dis Colon Rectum. 2006;49:966-81.
82. Lal SK, Morgenstern R, Vinjirayer EP, Matin A. Sigmoid volvulus an update. Gastrointest Endosc Clin N Am. 2006;16:175-87.
83. Pirró N, Corroller LE, Solari C, Merad A, Sielezneff I, Sastre B, et al. Cecal volvulus: anatomical bases and physiopathology. Morphologie. 2006;90:197-202.
84. Rabinovici R, Simansky DA, Kaplan O, Mavor E, Manny J. Cecal volvulus. Dis Colon Rectum. 1990;33:765-9.
85. Northeast AD, Dennison AR, Lee EG. Sigmoid volvulus: New thoughts on epidemiology. Dis Colon Rectum. 1984;27:260-1.
86. Moore CJ, Corl FM, Fishman EK. CT of cecal volvulus: unraveling the image. AJR Am J Roentgenol. 2001;177:95-8.
87. Rappaport A, Roland T, Pringot J, Billemont MF, Ghijselings L, Van Campenhoudt M. The whirl sign in caecal volvulus: a decisive diagnostic clue. JBR-BTR. 2007;90:532-4.
88. Azar T, Berger DL. Adult intussusception. Ann Surg. 1997;226:134-8.
89. Weilbaecher D, Bolin JA, Hearn D, Ogden W 2nd. Intussusception in adults. Review of 160 cases. Am J Surg. 1971;121:531-5.
90. Nagorney DM, Sarr MG, McIlrath DC. Surgical management of intussusception in the adult. Ann Surg. 1981;193:230-6.
91. Cotlar AM, Cohn I Jr. Intussusception in adults. Am J Surg. 1961;101:114-20.
92. Eisen LK, Cunningham JD, Aufses AH Jr. Intussusception in adults: institutional review. J Am Coll Surg. 1999;188:390-5.
93. Zubaidi A, Al-Saif F, Silverman R. Adult intussusception: a retrospective review. Dis Colon Rectum. 2006;49:1546-51.
94. Wiot JF, Spitz HB. Small bowel intussusception demonstrated by oral barium. Radiology. 1970;97:361-6.
95. Begos DG, Sandor A, Modlin IM. The diagnosis and management of adult intussusception. Am J Surg. 1997;173:88-94.
96. Zeinali F, Stulberg JJ, Delaney CP. Pharmacological management of postoperative ileus. Can J Surg. 2009;52:153-7.

CHAPTER 29

Abdominal Tuberculosis

Nilesh Patil, RK Saran, Uday Somashekar

INTRODUCTION

Tuberculosis (TB) has infected nearly one-third of the world's population.[1] It continues to be prevalent in developing countries like India due to low socioeconomic status, malnutrition, overcrowding, poor education and limited access to the healthcare facilities. In developed countries, the incidence is rising due to increasing incidence of human immunodeficiency virus (HIV) infection, use of immunosuppressants and emergence of multidrug-resistant strains of *Mycobacterium tuberculosis*. In 2010, approximately two million cases in the world were estimated to be from India.[2] Extrapulmonary tuberculosis is present in 15–20% of patients while in HIV positive patients, the incidence of extrapulmonary tuberculosis is reported up to 50%.[3,4,5] It can coexist with pulmonary tuberculosis in around 5–36% of patients.[6] Abdominal tuberculosis is the sixth most common form of extrapulmonary tuberculosis,[7] constituting 11–16% of it and overall 1–3% of the total load.[8,9] It mainly includes involvement of gastrointestinal tract, peritoneum and lymph nodes; although solid organs can also be rarely involved. It often presents with nonspecific clinical features, mimicking many clinical conditions, such as inflammatory bowel disease, malignancy and other infectious diseases. Because of the limited accuracy of laboratory tests and imaging techniques in diagnosing abdominal tuberculosis, it is a formidable challenge for treating physicians. A high index of suspicion is needed as delay in diagnosis and improper management can lead to considerable morbidity and mortality due to complications.

ETIOPATHOGENESIS AND PATHOLOGY

Abdominal tuberculosis has been attributed to hematogenous spread from primary pulmonary focus acquired during childhood with later reactivation of latent infection, swallowing of infected bacilli from active pulmonary tuberculosis, local spread from adjacent viscera and ingestion of infected food or milk.[10,11] Almost all cases of abdominal tuberculosis are caused by *M. tuberculosis* and infection due to *M. bovis* is now rare because of its eradication due to public health measures, such as use of pasteurized milk products. Atypical mycobacteria like *M. avium* intracellular have become a major pathogen in HIV positive patients.[12] In gastrointestinal tuberculosis, M (microfold) cells associated with Peyer's patches phagocytose tubercle bacilli and then they are transported to mesenteric lymph nodes. Mesenteric lymph nodes may get matted and also may caseate. Inflammatory cellular infiltration, lymph node enlargement and local edema can lead to the formation of inflammatory masses.[5] Endarteritis and caseating necrosis cause transverse mucosal ulceration. Increased fibroblastic activity results in local bowel wall thickening and intestinal narrowing which leads to multiple bowel strictures (Figs 1 and 2).[10] The histological picture includes epitheloid cell granulomata with a peripheral rim of lymphocytes and plasma cells, Langhans' giant cells and central caseating necrosis. In addition, fibrosis and calcification (commonly occurs in lymph nodes) are seen in healing lesions. Granulomas are of various sizes, confluent and are mainly seen in the submucosal layer (Fig. 3). Sometimes characteristic granulomas are seen only in the mesenteric lymph nodes, especially in the patient who has received antitubercular treatment (ATT) for some time. On colonoscopic biopsies granulomas have been visualized in 8–48% of the patients with caseation being seen only in one-third of them.[13] The ileocecal region is the most commonly affected due to high density of lymphoid tissue, physiological stasis, increased fluid and electrolyte absorption and minimal digestive activity. However, tuberculosis can have a focus at any site in the abdomen with associated lymph node and peritoneal involvement. The peritoneum and mesenteric lymph nodes are usually infected by hematogenous spread from

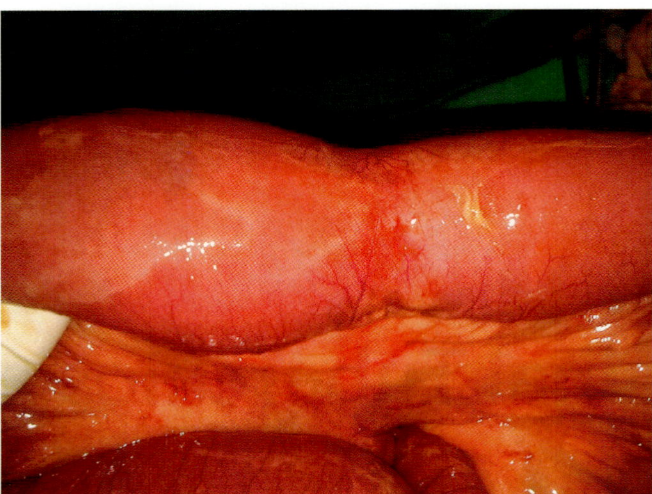

Figure 1 Small bowel stricture

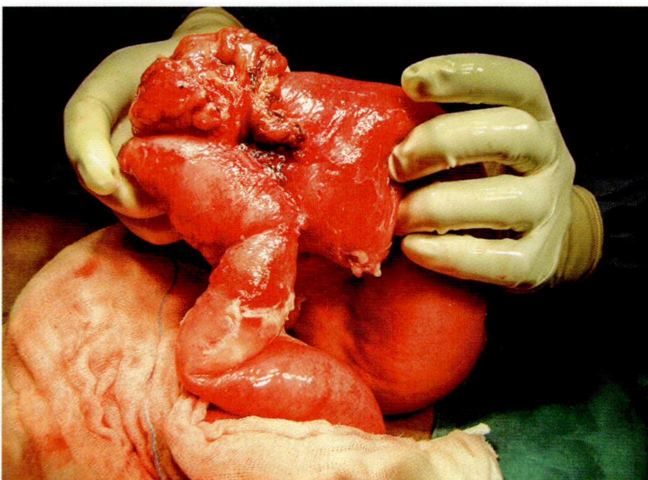

Figure 2 Tubercular abdomen with stricture ileum

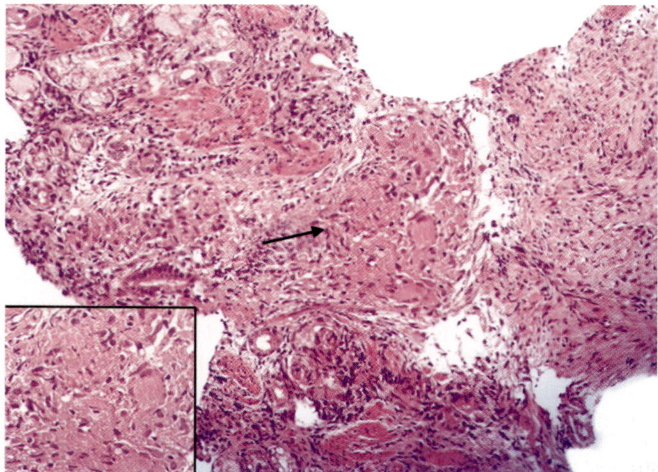

Figure 3 Duodenal biopsy. Hematoxylin and eosin stain (H&E) x 10 granuloma in submucosa. Arrow and inset x 20 granuloma. Mucosal glands were seen in photograph

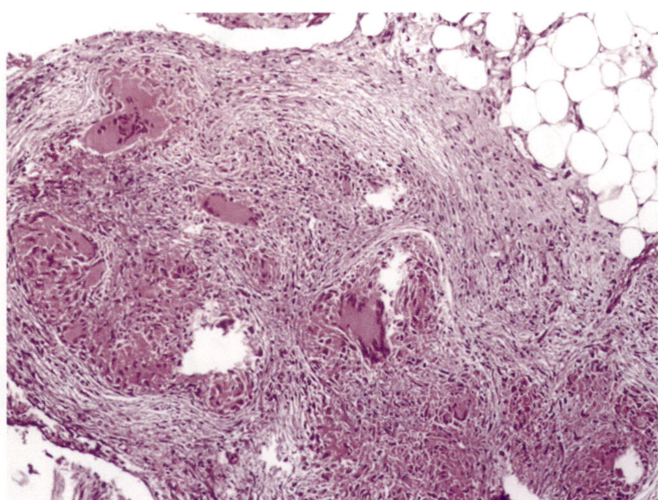

Figure 4 Peritoneal tubercular nodule. Hematoxylin and eosin stain (H&E) x 4 a tubercle is seen in peritoneal fatty tissue. Langerhans type giant cells and epithelioid cells. Necrosis not seen

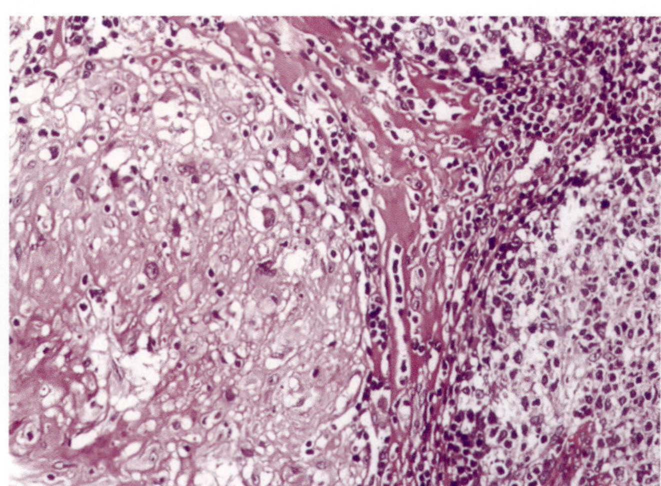

Figure 5 Healing phase of epithelioid granuloma in lymph node. Hematoxylin and eosin stain (H&E) X 20. Peripheral sclerosis and presence of foamy histiocytes is predominant population. No frank epithelioid cells, Langerhans cells or necrosis noted. Acid-fast bacillus stain was negative

pulmonary tuberculosis.[14] Reactivation of this dormant infection produces clinical manifestations, often without any associated active lung focus. Infection can also reach the peritoneum (Fig. 4) by direct spread from lymph nodes, from affected regions of gastrointestinal tract, tubercular salpingitis in women or by direct contamination during peritoneal dialysis. Abdominal lymph nodal (Fig. 5) and peritoneal tuberculosis (Fig. 6) may be seen in one-third of cases without associated involvement of gastrointestinal tract.[15]

In 1950, Hoon et al.[15] categorized the intestinal lesions into ulcerative, ulcerohyperplastic and hyperplastic varieties. Ulcerative form has been more commonly seen in malnourished patients, while hypertrophic form in relatively well nourished cases

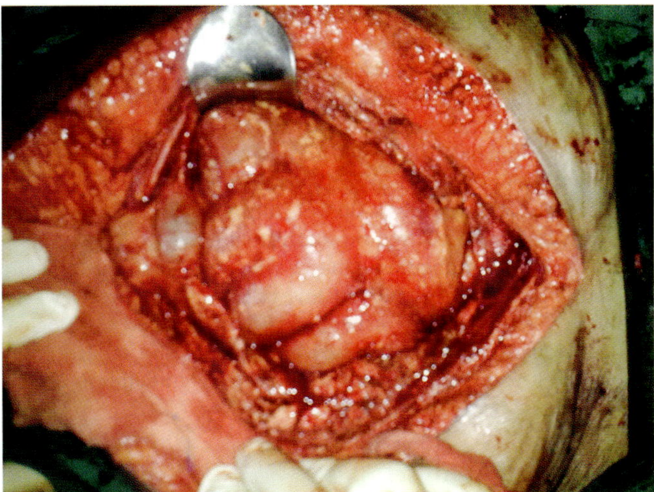

Figure 6 Koch's abdomen showing peritoneal tubercles

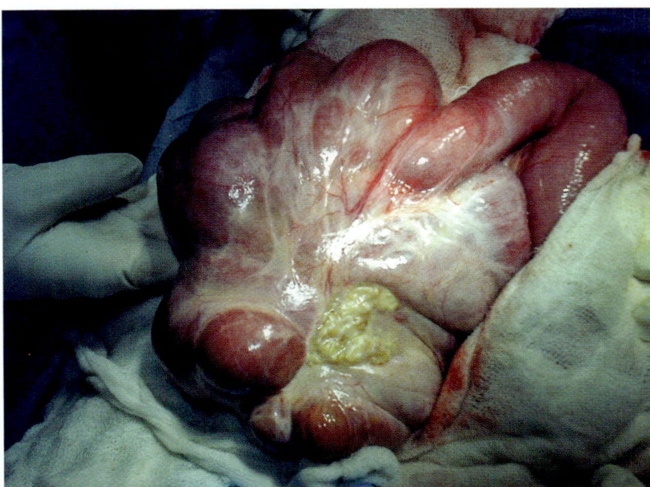

Figure 7 Fibroadhesive tuberculosis with matted bowel loops

with strong host resistance. Ulcerative and stricturous lesions are frequently seen in the small bowel. Colonic and ileocecal lesions are usually ulcerohypertrophic. Peritoneal tuberculosis can be of (i) wet type with ascites which may be generalized or encysted; (ii) fibroadhesive type composed of matted bowel loops (Fig. 7) with thickened mesentery and rolled up omentum. A combination of these forms may also be seen.

CLINICAL FEATURES

It is commonly seen in young adults between the age group 20–40 years. Although some studies[5,16] from India reported a female preponderance, the sex incidence is equal. It also affects children with more common involvement of peritoneum and lymph nodes as compared to intestines (90% vs <10%).[5,17] In immunocompromised patients, abdominal tuberculosis occurs in the disseminated form usually with lymph nodal and solid organ involvement. Abdominal tuberculosis is generally a chronic illness, having insidious onset, with intermittent acute attacks. Sometimes peritoneal and lymph nodal disease is found incidentally during laparotomy for other disease. Constitutional symptoms such as low-grade fever with evening rise, lethargy, malaise, night sweats and anorexia and weight loss are more frequently seen in patients with either ulcerative intestinal tuberculosis or ascitic type of peritoneal tuberculosis. Other clinical features depend upon the site and type of the involvement. In general abdominal distension (82%), ascites (79%), weight loss (62%), pain abdomen (58%) (either colicky or dull and continuous), bowel disturbances such gurgling, diarrhea (16%), alternating constipation and diarrhea and abdominal mass (20%) are common presenting complaints of abdominal tuberculosis.[18] In one-third of patients there may be associated other organ involvement[19] with lung and pleura being common sites of involvement. Few studies reported active pulmonary disease in 15–20% of patients with abdominal tuberculosis.[20,21] Ten percent of women with abdominal tuberculosis may have concomitant genital tract involvement.[22] Cervical or axillary lymph nodes involvement may be seen in 3–10% of patients.[23] Rarely acute abdomen may be the initial presentation in patients of abdominal tuberculosis[20,24] with intestinal obstruction being the most common followed by perforation. Other rare acute modes of presentation of abdominal tuberculosis are pancolitis, massive lower gastrointestinal bleed and acute peritonitis without bowel perforation or acute mesenteric lymphadenitis. Sometimes patients with peritoneal tuberculosis or miliary tuberculosis with multisystem involvement may present with toxemia.

INVESTIGATIONS

As the correct diagnosis is made only in 35–50% of patients on the basis of clinical manifestations,[25] a variety of investigative methods have been used to diagnose abdominal tuberculosis. Anemia and hypoalbuminemia are frequently seen in these patients due to chronicity and malnutrition. Other nonspecific findings include leukocytosis with relative lymphocytosis, raised erythrocyte sedimentation rate (ESR) and elevated C-reactive protein (CRP) levels, but they may be useful in assessing the response to the ATT. Serum CA125 level may be raised in tuberculosis, however CA19.9 and carcinoembryonic antigen (CEA) are normal. Tuberculin skin test is of limited value as it cannot differentiate between active disease and previous sensitization by contact or Bacillus Calmette-Guérin (BCG) vaccination. Also, it may be negative in patients with malnutrition, concurrent HIV infection, lymphomas, chronic renal failure and fulminant tuberculosis and in patients on steroids. Radiological imaging has important role in the diagnosis of abdominal tuberculosis. Chest X-ray reveals abnormalities (either active focus or healed lesion) in 15–50% of patients with abdominal tuberculosis.[26-28] A positive findings on chest X-ray supports the diagnosis of abdominal tuberculosis, however normal chest radiograph does not rule it out. Plain X-ray abdomen may show features of intestinal obstruction (dilated bowel loops with multiple air fluid levels) and perforation (free air) or ground glass appearance due to ascites. Also calcified lymph nodes, enteroliths and calcified granulomas in the solid viscera may be found. Barium studies are helpful but cannot differentiate tuberculosis from Crohn's disease and malignancy and it does not show peritoneal lesions. In addition, Tandon et al.[29] reported false-negative barium studies in 25% of patients. Small bowel barium meal study may reveal increased intestinal transit, hypersegmentation of the barium column, precipitation and flocculation of barium, thickened mucosal folds and hour glass strictures. Multiple strictures with segmental dilatation and fixed and matted bowel loops may also be seen. Kapoor VK et al.[30] reported following features on barium enema: thickened ileocecal valve and/or incompetent valve with narrowing of the terminal ileum ("Fleischner" or "inverted umbrella sign"), thickened mucosal folds and contour irregularity of the terminal ileum, pulled up contracted and deformed cecum (conical cecum), straightening of ileocecal valve and "gooseneck deformity" (dilated terminal ileum, appearing suspended from a retracted deformed cecum). Both "Stierlin" sign (absence of barium retention in the inflamed segments of the ileum, caecum and ascending colon, with a normal column of barium on either side) and "String" sign (persistent narrow stream of barium suggestive of stenosis) seen on barium enema are not specific for tuberculosis as they can also be seen in Crohn's disease. Ultrasonography (USG) is a cheap and easily available modality for imaging peritoneal tuberculosis. It may reveal free or loculated intraperitoneal fluid with debris or septae inside, interbowel loop ascites ("sliced bread" sign), uniform and concentric bowel wall thickening in the ileocecal region and pulled up ileocecal mass in subhepatic space giving "pseudokidney" appearance.[30] However, complex inflammatory tuberculosis masses may be difficult to differentiate from malignancy and lymphomas while septations within ascites may also develop in peritoneal carcinomatosis and nontubercular pyogenic peritonitis.[31] On USG, lymph nodes in tuberculosis may be either discrete or matted with heterogenous echotexture, while homogeneously hypoechoic nodes are suggestive of lymphomas. Calcifications within tubercular granulomas may produce discrete posterior acoustic shadows. Computed tomography (CT) is better than USG in detecting abdominal lymphadenopathy and high density ascites.[32] In addition, it helps to differentiate abdominal tuberculosis from peritoneal carcinomatosis. Uniform circumferential thickening of bowel wall, thickened nodular mesentery and abdominal lymphadenopathy with low attenuation centers and peripheral rim enhancement and diffuse regular thickening of the peritoneum are highly suggestive of abdominal tuberculosis. Computed tomography with enteroclysis allows better visualization of transmural abnormalities and helps to differentiate tuberculosis from Crohn's disease.[33] Complications, such as obstruction, perforation and fistulisation are also seen on computed tomography. Computed tomography is preferred over magnetic resonance imaging (MRI) as it is a quick, cheap investigation with better spatial resolution and lesser artefacts. It can also simultaneously evaluate chest and abdomen with pelvis in a single examination. MRI is useful in patients with contraindication for intravenous contrast media and for evaluation of anorectal tuberculosis.

Microscopy and Culture

Demonstration of acid-fast bacilli on microscopy or culture is considered as the gold standard for diagnosis of tuberculosis anywhere in the body. In 1964, Paustian[34] reported that one or more of the following four criteria must be fulfilled to diagnose abdominal tuberculosis: (i) histological evidence of tubercles with caseation necrosis; (ii) typical operative findings with biopsy of mesenteric nodes showing histologic evidence of tuberculosis; (iii) animal inoculation or culture of suspected tissue resulting in growth of *M. tuberculosis*; and (iv) histological demonstration of acid-fast bacilli in a lesion. But yield of acid-fast bacilli in abdominal tuberculosis is low. Tubercular bacilli can be detected on smear or histology by Zeihl-Nielsen and auramine-rhodamine fluorescent stain. In addition, they can be cultured in Lowenstein-Jenesen medium or BACTEC 460 liquid medium with yield of latter being better. Sinkala E et al.[35] reported very low sensitivity with microscopy (yielding only 10–30% of culture positive samples). But yield can be increased by immunohistochemical (IHC) staining with monoclonal antibodies to the *M. tuberculosis* complex specific antigen.[36,37] Culture is highly sensitive but it may require 6–8 weeks to obtain positive result. Tissues for microscopic and histological examination may be obtained by endoscopic and laparoscopic biopsy or ultrasound (US)/endoscopic US/CT-guided fine-needle aspiration and cytology (FNAC).

Ascitic Fluid Analysis

The ascitic fluid in tuberculosis is usually straw colored with protein greater than 3 g/dL, cell count greater than 1,000/mL, consisting predominantly of lymphocytes (>70%) and serum ascites albumin gradient is less than 1.1 g/dL. Adenosine deaminase activity (ADA) in ascitic fluid is helpful in differentiating tuberculosis from other causes of ascites. Various studies reported sensitivities and specificities of 93–100% and 92–98% respectively with cut-off values of between 30 and 32 U/L.[38-41] Sensitivity of the ADA may be lower in patients of HIV and concomitant cirrhosis whereas ADA level may be elevated in patients with malignant ascites. Recently, Bandyopadhyay R et al.,[42] with an aim to differentiate between tubercular and malignant ascites reported that ascitic fluid lactate dehydrogenase (LDH) less than 110 U/L and ADA greateer than 33 U/L has a sensitivity of 97% and specificity of 100% for tuberculosis. Ascitic fluid interferon-γ may also be raised in tubercular peritonitis.[40] Diagnosis of tuberculosis can also be done by Ziehl-Neelsen (ZN) staining or culture of ascitic fluid, but they are associated with limitation of low yield of 3% and 20% respectively.[43] However, centrifugation of large amount of ascitic fluid may increase their yield.[44]

Endoscopy

Upper gastrointestinal endoscopy can easily access the lesions in esophagus, stomach and duodenum. Colonic or ileocecal disease is well seen in lower gastrointestinal endoscopy. Double-balloon enteroscopy or push enteroscopy are helpful in visualizing lesion in the proximal jejunum while capsule endoscopy should be used with caution in patients with suspected intestinal obstruction.

Colonoscopy with retrograde ileoscopy is a useful diagnostic modality in 60–80% of patients with combination of histology and culture.[13,43,45,46] Involvement may be focal or multifocal. Ulcers in tuberculosis are usually superficial, transversely oriented with sharp irregular margins and undermined edges with normal or hyperemic intervening mucosa. Mucosal nodules are of variable size (2–6 mm) and friable and may be confluent or scattered. In addition, pseudopolyps, cobblestoning and strictures are seen. Alvares et al.[47] reported ulcers (70%), nodules (56%), a deformed ileocecal valve (40%), strictures (23%), and polypoid lesions (14%) on colonoscopy. In addition, more than one site was involved in 50% of patients. Pancolitis is less common and seen in 4–8% of patients.[13,45] Sometimes tubercular lesions may mimic inflammatory bowel disease or malignancy.[13,46] Bhargava et al.[48] suggested obtaining 8 to 10 biopsies for histology and 3 to 4 specimens for culture. Biopsies should be taken from the edge of ulcer. Yield is low due to predominant involvement of submucosa.

Laparoscopy

Laparoscopy has been considered as an important modality for early detection in suspected tubercular peritonitis[49-51] with a positive diagnostic yield of up to 85%.[26,49] Bhargava et al.[52] reported intraoperative findings during laparoscopy being more helpful (95% accurate) than either histology or culture in diagnosing tubercular peritonitis. It should be used with caution in patients of fibroadhesive peritoneal tuberculosis due to the risk of perforation. Biopsy should be taken from suspicious areas and adequacy of the biopsy is assessed with frozen section. Caseating granulomas may be seen on biopsy in 85–90% of patients. In a study by Krishnan P et al.,[53] laparoscopic biopsy established diagnosis in 80% of patients suspected to have abdominal tuberculosis without evidence of extra-abdominal disease. The laparoscopic findings in peritoneal tuberculosis include thickened, hyperemic, inflamed peritoneum, multiple yellowish uniform (3–5 mm) tubercles over peritoneum, omentum and viscera, omental caking, adhesion between organs and peritoneum. The laparoscopic features may mimic disseminated abdominal malignancies, especially ovarian cancer, therefore histological confirmation is mandatory.

Serological Tests

In a review on commercially available serological tests [including enzyme-linked immunosorbent assay (ELISA)], Steingart KR et al.[54] reported variable sensitivity and specificity for extrapulmonary tuberculosis. Most of these tests remain positive even after antitubercular therapy and also their results are not reproducible. Their role in diagnosing abdominal tuberculosis is not yet defined. Makharia GK et al.[55] reported no significant difference in positivity of anti-saccharomyces cerevisiae antibodies (ASCA) in patients with Crohn's disease versus intestinal tuberculosis. ASCA immunoglobulin A (IgA) and ASCA IgG, either alone or in combination cannot differentiate between Crohn's disease and intestinal tuberculosis.

Amplification Methods

They directly detect *M. tuberculosis* deoxyribonucleic acid (DNA) in clinical samples using *M. tuberculosis* complex specific primers. Moatter et al.[56] reported use of polymerase chain reaction (PCR) in abdominal tuberculosis. PCR is a noninvasive method and can provide rapid diagnosis with very high specificity up to 100%.[57] It can differentiate intestinal tuberculosis from Crohn's disease (discussed in detail in the chapter on Crohn's Disease). Limitations of PCR are high cost and low sensitivity reported in some studies.[58,59] In addition, it cannot assess bacterial sensitivity to antitubercular drugs.

Intestinal Tuberculosis

The hypertrophic form is the most common type and presents with colicky abdominal pain, vomiting and borborygmi, palpable mass in the right iliac fossa. Ulcerative variant is less frequently seen and patients with this type of tuberculosis may manifest with diarrhea and melena. Isolated colonic tuberculosis without ileocecal involvement can be seen 9% patients of abdominal tuberculosis.[60] Sigmoid, ascending and transverse colon are commonly affected and multifocal involvement has been reported in 28–44% of cases with colonic tuberculosis.[48,61] Abdominal pain is the common presenting complaint in these patients while hematochezia is noted in less than one-third of cases.[61,62] It should be differentiated from inflammatory bowel disease and malignancy.

Complications

Most frequent complications are intestinal obstruction (acute or subacute), perforation, abscess formation and gastrointestinal bleeding. Obstruction is caused due to narrowing of lumen in hypertrophic type of tuberculosis, small bowel strictures, and fixity of bowel loops by adhesions and extrinsic compression by enlarged lymph nodes or omental mass. Its incidence ranges from 12% to 30% and in India, tuberculosis accounts for 3% to 25% cases of intestinal obstruction.[63] Tubercular perforations occur proximal to stricture and are usually single.[5] It may be generalized or localized and pneumoperitoneum is found in 50% of patients.[43] The reported incidence of free intestinal perforation in abdominal tuberculosis varies from 1% to 15% and in India, it is second most common cause after typhoid.[64,65] Tuberculosis accounts for nearly 4% cases of lower gastrointestinal bleed.[66] Gastrointestinal bleeding is frequently minor and life threatening massive bleed is uncommon. Bhargava et al.[46] reported bleeding in 70% of patients with colonic tuberculosis while Singh et al.[13] found bleeding in 31% cases and it was massive in 13% of patients. Many studies in India reported tuberculosis as second most common cause of malabsorption after tropical sprue.[64,67,68] It was commonly seen in patients with intestinal strictures as compared to non-stricturing form. Malabsorption has been attributed to the various factors such as decreased absorption due to ulcers, involvement of lymphatics and lymph nodes and bacterial overgrowth with secondary deconjugation of bile salts. Internal fistulas such as enteroenteric, enterocolic or coloduodenal may complicate intestinal tuberculosis. External fistulas are rare but may occur following surgical intervention.

Intestinal tuberculosis can be differentiated from Crohn's disease based on combination of clinical, radiological and histological findings. Male preponderance, prolonged illness, chronic diarrhea, blood in stool, perianal disease, extraintestinal manifestations, involvement of left colon, skip lesions, aphthous ulcers, cobblestoning, longitudinal ulcers and microgranulomas are more common in Crohn's disease.[69] On the other hand, equal sex distribution, fever, weight loss, constipation partial intestinal obstruction, transversely oriented ulcers with surrounding hyperemic mucosa, nodular lesions and large caseating granulomas are highly suggestive of tuberculosis.[69,70] On barium study, strictures in Crohn's disease are long and often multiple, while in tuberculosis they are short and usually single. Also, configuration of ileocecal valve is usually preserved in Crohn's disease. Abdominal computed tomography in Crohn's disease shows symmetric bowel wall thickening and creeping mesenteric fat. Asymmetric mural thickening thickened nodular mesentery, omental caking, caseating lymphnodes and ascites on computed tomography point toward tuberculosis.

Tubercular Peritonitis

It accounts for 31–58% cases of abdominal tuberculosis[71] and commonly present as a subacute illness with slow development over weeks to months. Ascitic form (either generalised or localized) is the most common type, seen in 97% of cases.[11,20] In a review on tubercular peritonitis, Sanai FM et al.[72] reported abdominal pain as the most common presenting complaint (65%), frequently associated with abdominal distension. Pain abdomen is usually generalized and nonspecific in nature. Other clinical symptoms include diarrhea (61%), fever (59%), weight loss (21%) and constipation (11%).[72] Ascites (73%), abdominal tenderness (48%), hepatomegaly (28%) and splenomegaly (14%) may be detected on clinical examination while a doughy abdomen is rarely found.[72] Tubercular ascites should be differentiated from ascites due to cirrhosis as most of the antitubercular drugs are hepatotoxic. In addition, encysted tubercular ascites may mimic pancreatic pseudocyst, mesenteric cyst or ovarian cyst. Other less common form, i.e. fibroadhesive type is seen in 3% of cases. In this type bowel loops get stuck to the peritoneum and mesentery by adhesions. Sometimes peritoneal space gets obliterated due to encasement of small bowel loops by a fibrocollagenous membrane giving appearance like a cocoon. It may present with intestinal obstruction (either acute or subacute), abdominal distension, weight loss or palpable abdominal lump[73] while ascites is uncommon. Barium studies show slow transit of barium or classic "cauliflower sign". Computed tomography abdomen reveals matted small bowel loops with surrounding soft tissue density membrane.

Lymph Nodal Disease

Tuberculosis commonly involves mesenteric, celiac, periportal and peripancreatic group of lymph nodes with sparing of retroperitoneal lymph nodes.[74] They get matted and may form large conglomerate masses. In addition, dystrophic calcification can occur in these lymph nodes, which is unusual in malignancy.[75] Concomitant bowel involvement may be absent.[76] Tuberculosis lymph node involvement can lead to bowel obstruction due to narrowing, traction and fixity of bowel loops while rupture of caseous lymph nodes may cause acute tubercular peritonitis. Enlarged periportal and pericholedochal lymph nodes can cause obstructive jaundice or portal hypertension. Also, patients with tubercular lymphadenitis may present with pyrexia of unknown origin, dull aching pain abdomen or abdominal mass (mobile or fixed).

Esophageal Tuberculosis

It has been reported in 0.2–1% of all gastrointestinal tuberculosis cases[77] and usually affects mid-esophagus. Esophageal tuberculosis is usually secondary, due to spread from adjacent organs, such as lymph nodes, the lungs, spine and rarely the blood.[78] The most common presenting feature is dysphagia, while odynophagia, retrosternal pain and hematemesis are associated other clinical symptoms. In addition, weight loss and other systemic symptoms has been reported.[79,80] Pulmonary symptoms become predominant when fistulisation occurs into tracheobronchial tree. Endoscopy reveals either ulcerative, hyperplastic or granular type lesions.[81] Also, it can present as a tumorlike growth with a stricture.[82,83] Computed tomography thorax reveals mid esophageal thickening with mediastinal lymphadenopathy and it may help in identifying concomitant lung lesions and complications such as a bronchoesophageal fistula. Differentiation of esophageal tuberculosis from malignancy based on endoscopic and radiological findings may be difficult.

Gastroduodenal Tuberculosis

Involvement of stomach (Figs 8 and 9) and duodenum is rare with incidence of around 0.5%.[84] It has been reported that ingestion of histamine 2 (H2) blockers over long-term increases the incidence of gastroduodenal tuberculosis.[85] It is usually attributed to either hematogenous spread from pulmonary lesions or local spread from adjacent lymph nodes. In stomach, it commonly involves antrum and prepyloric region while duodenal involvement is rare. Gastric outlet obstruction occur either in hypertrophic type of gastric tuberculosis or due to extrinsic compression by tubercular lymph nodes in duodenal tuberculosis.[86] Diagnosis of gastroduodenal tuberculosis should be kept in mind in young patients particularly

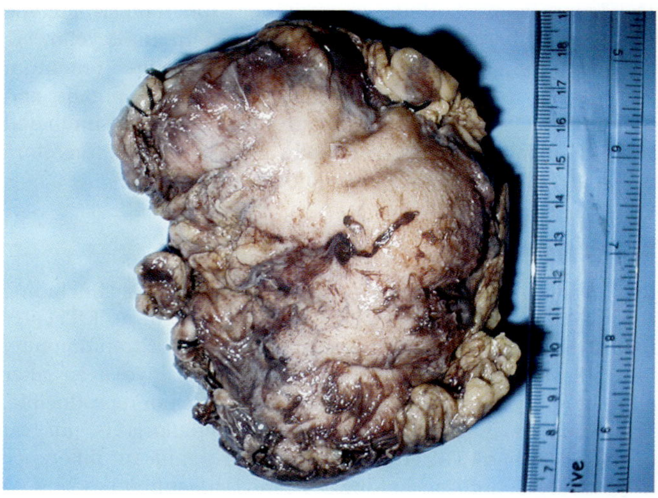

Figure 8 Tuberculosis of stomach

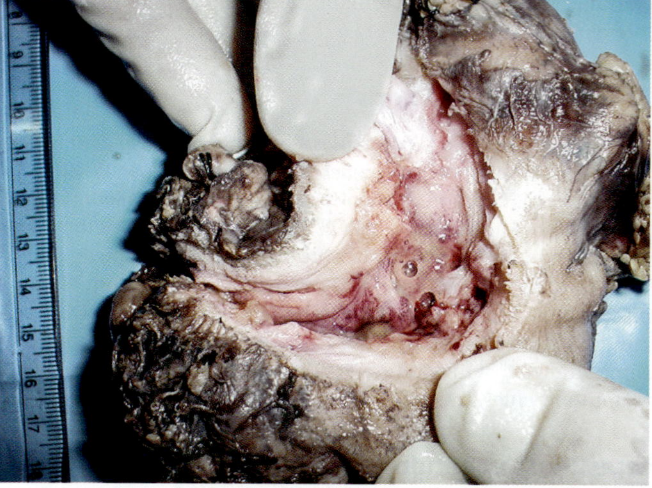

Figure 9 Opened specimen of stomach showing hypertrophied fibrous wall with thickened irregular mucosa

from endemic areas, presenting with gastric outlet obstruction and those with non-response to antisecretory therapy. The clinical features are often vague, mimicking peptic ulcer disease or malignancy. Rao YG et al.[87] reported vomiting (61%), epigastric pain (56%) and weight loss (30%) as common presenting complaints. Upper gastrointestinal bleeding and jaundice was noted in 26% and 9% of patients respectively. Bleeding is usually mild and intermittent.[87] Endoscopic and radiological findings are frequently nonspecific while intraoperatively it may masquerade as malignancy. Rarely complications such as perforation and fistulisation into adjacent structures may occur.

Anorectal Disease

Involvement of rectum due to tuberculosis is less common. Puri AS et al.[88] reported hematochezia and constipation in 88% and 37% of patients respectively, while constitutional symptoms were seen in 75% of patients. Lower third of rectum is commonly affected[13] and perrectal and proctoscopic examinations reveals annular stricture or areas of ulceration with nodularity. It is very rare to see perianal disease concomitant with rectal tuberculosis.[43] Development of rectovesical or rectourethral fistulae may complicate rectal tuberculosis. Anal tuberculosis commonly presents with multiple fistulae in ano with anal discharge, however perianal abscesses, ulcers or nodules are also seen.[89-91] There may be associated inguinal lymphadenopathy. Shukla et al.[89] reported tuberculosis as an etiology in 14% of patients with fistula in ano. Perianal swelling was present in one-third of cases while none of the patients had systemic symptoms.

Pancreatic Tuberculosis

Isolated pancreatic involvement by tuberculosis is uncommon, with incidence of 2–5% in autopsy series of military tuberculosis.[92,93] It has higher incidence in endemic areas and in the immunocompromised patients. Chaudhary et al.[94] reported incidence of 23% in HIV positive patients. Pancreas is involved in tuberculosis due to spread from the peripancreatic lymph nodes or hematogenous spread. It presents with diverse clinical features, such as abdominal pain (75%), weight loss (69%), generalized weakness (64%), fever (50%) and jaundice (31%).[95] In addition, pancreatic tuberculosis has also been reported to cause acute[96] or chronic[97] pancreatitis, portal hypertension,[98] gastrointestinal bleed,[99] pancreatic cyst or abscess[100] and pancreatic mass mimicking malignancy.[101] Radiological findings are usually nonconclusive. USG shows bulky, heteroechoic pancreas and hypoechoic intrapancreatic collections.[102] Computed tomography findings include hypodense lesions with irregular borders (commonly in the head of the pancreas), enlarged peripancreatic necrotic lymph nodes or diffuse enlargement of the pancreas.[102] Also, there may be associated mural thickening of ileocecal region. Recently, endoscopic ultrasound (EUS) has evolved as an important diagnostic tool for pancreatic lesions. In a series of Song et al.,[103] EUS-FNA diagnosed pancreatic/peripancreatic tuberculosis in 76.2% of patients.

Hepatobiliary Tuberculosis

Involvement of liver in tuberculosis is uncommon with reported incidence of only 1.2% in a study from South Africa.[104] It has been attributed most commonly to hematogenous spread in military tuberculosis[105] while rarely liver can be affected due to spread through lymphatics or portal vein from a tubercular focus in gastrointestinal tract.[106] The clinical course is usually protracted with nonspecific symptoms, like abdominal pain, vomiting, fever, anorexia and weight loss. Jaundice may be seen in 28% of patients with isolated hepatic tuberculosis.[107] Clinical examination reveals hepatomegaly in 95% of patients and splenomegaly is found in 18–55% of cases.[106] Laboratory investigations show mild elevation of liver enzymes. Pathologically, it can occur in miliary, nodular and focal tuberculoma or abscess form.[108,109] Radiological findings are usually nonspecific mimicking abscess or tumor. Therefore, FNAC or trucut biopsy is needed to confirm the diagnosis. Isolated biliary tuberculosis is rare with reported incidence of 3% in autopsy series.[110] Biliary tract tuberculosis occurs secondary to liver (tubercle bacilli excreted into bile), direct spread from periportal lymph nodes or infection through the papilla. Symptoms develop due to strictures (including post ATT strictures) or extrinsic compression by lymph nodes. In addition, cholangitis may develop following rupture of caseating granuloma within the biliary tree. Saluja et al.,[111] Chong et al.[112] and Govindasamy M et al.[113] reported abdominal pain and jaundice as the most common presenting complaints in patients of biliary tuberculosis while in a study of Amarapurkar et al.,[114] fever and weight loss were the most commonly presenting symptoms. Serum bilirubin level is usually lower than that found in malignant biliary stricture.[113] Radiological investigations including cholangiography [magnetic resonance cholangiopancreatography/endoscopic retrograde cholangiopancreatography (MRCP/ERCP)] help to identify any mass lesion and level and extent of biliary obstruction. Clinical features and cholangiographic findings cannot differentiate biliary tuberculosis from carcinoma gall bladder or cholangiocarcinoma. Also, the yield of tubercular bacilli in the bile aspirated during ERCP is very low (0–10%).[111,115] USG/EUS/CT-guided FNAC of the periportal or pericholedochal lymph nodes may be helpful in diagnosis. In most of the patients the diagnosis is made either intraoperatively or postoperatively.

Medical Management

Radiological and endoscopic findings cannot diagnose abdominal tuberculosis conclusively while the yield of acid-fast bacilli is low with microscopy or culture. Most physicians recommend ATT after demonstration of caseating granulomas on histopathology. A therapeutic trial based on clinical or radiological findings may simply delay the treatment in many clinical conditions such as inflammatory bowel disease, lymphomas and malignancy. In addition, it may alter histological picture of tuberculosis, which makes later confirmation of diagnosis more difficult. Antitubercular therapy is highly effective in peritoneal, lymph nodal and solid organ tuberculosis. Many patients with gestrointestinal tuberculosis also respond well to it. Commonly used drugs are isoniazid, rifampicin, pyrazinamide, ethambutol and streptomycin. Usually, these drugs are used in various combinations to prevent emergence of drug-resistant strains. The frequently used protocol is four drugs (isoniazid, rifampicin, pyrazinamide and ethambutol) given daily for 2 months followed by 4 months combination of isoniazid and rifampicin. There is no evidence in the literature to continue ATT beyond 6 months in abdominal tuberculosis. In a randomized controlled trial, Balasubramanian R et al.[116] reported equivalent cure rates (99% vs 94%) with 6 months short course ATT and 12 months standard chemotherapy. Compliance to ATT is must as incomplete treatment leads to multidrug-resistant tuberculosis. Directly observed therapy is highly effective modality to facilitate curative treatment and curative rate of 85% to 90% with relapse rate of only 5% has been reported with it.[117,118] The important adverse effect of ATT is hepatotoxicity and its risk increases with underlying liver disease, particularly cirrhosis. Liver function tests should be monitored routinely during treatment. Besides dug toxicity, complications such as intestinal obstruction,[119] perforation and biliary strictures may occur during treatment. Coinfection with HIV may complicate ATT due to altered drug absorption, unfavorable drug interactions and increased risk of relapse. The use of corticosteroids is still uncertain, although some studies reported decreased risk of stricture or adhesion formation following use of steroids during initial 2 months of ATT.[120,121]

Emergence of multidrug-resistant strains in some endemic areas poses a challenge for clinicians. Second-line drugs are used for their treatment. These include fluoroquinolones, ethinamide, cycloserine and para-aminosalicylic acid (PAS). Consideration should be given to four drugs (include a parenteral drug) in intensive phase and three drugs in later phase. Bedaquiline fumarate has been used recently in some trials where other drugs have failed.

SURGICAL TREATMENT

Surgery is usually indicated for complications such as intestinal obstruction not responding to conservative treatment, perforation, fistulisation, massive hemorrhage or when malignancy cannot be ruled out. As these patients are chronically malnourished and poor surgical candidates with increased risk of postoperative complications, conservative surgical procedures are preferred to radical ones. Vigorous resuscitation is must before any surgical intervention. Strictureplasty is useful for small bowel strictures, but segmental surgical resection is preferred for tight strictures with complete obliteration of the lumen and for multiple strictures over a short segment. Some studies reported resolution of stricturous intestinal lesion with ATT alone even in patients with subacute intestinal obstruction.[122,123] In one study obstructive symptoms resolved after mean duration of 6 months.[123] Limited ileocecal resection is commonly done for hypertrophic ileocecal lesions causing intestinal obstruction. Nowadays, bypass procedures are rarely performed because of risk of malabsorption due to blind loop formation and progression of residual disease. Excessive adhesiolysis should be resisted in patients with fibroadhesive type peritoneal tuberculosis to avoid iatrogenic enterotomies. In patients with tubercular intestinal perforations, resection of affected segment of bowel is preferred over primary closure due to increased risk of leak associated with primary closure.[124] If the general condition of the patient is very poor, it is wiser to exteriorize the bowel loop as a stoma at the site of perforation. Surgery for persistent bleeding from ulcerative intestinal tuberculosis usually requires resection. Esophageal tuberculosis responds well to ATT. Surgery may be indicated for perforation and fistulisation into tracheobronchial tree. However, endoscopic stenting may be considered in selected patients. In patients of gastroduodenal tuberculosis presenting with gastric outlet obstruction, gastrojejunostomy (GJ) is preferred over pyloroplasty as fibrosis around pyloroduodenal area makes the pyloroplasty technically difficult.[125] Feeding jejunostomy is always performed along with gastrojejunostomy as gastric atony secondary to prolonged stasis may affect the nutrition of patient in the postoperative period. Some authors reported good outcome following endoscopic balloon dilatation of duodenal strictures along with ATT.[126] Tubercular gastric ulcer with a persistent bleed can be treated with vagotomy and antrectomy.[87] ATT can cure hepatobiliary and pancreatic tuberculosis, but surgery may be required sometimes when malignancy cannot be ruled out pre operatively[127] or in persistent biliary obstruction despite ATT.

REFERENCES

1. World Health Organization. (2010). Global tuberculosis control. [Online] Available from http://www.who.int/tb/publications/global_report/2010/en/index.html. [Accessed April, 2015].
2. TB India 2010, RNTCP status report.
3. Aston NO. Abdominal tuberculosis. World J Surg. 1997;21:492-9.
4. Singhal A, Gulati A, Frizell R, Manning AP. Abdominal tuberculosis in Bradford, UK: 1992-2002. Eur J Gastroenterol Hepatol. 2005;17:967-71.
5. Kapoor VK. Abdominal tuberculosis. Postgrad Med J. 1998;74:459-67.
6. Bolukbas C, Bolukbas FF, Kendir T, Dalay RA, Akbayir N, Sokmen MH, et al. Clinical presentation of abdominal tuberculosis in HIV seronegative adults. Boston Medical Centre Gastroenterology. 2005;5:21.
7. Donoghue HD, Holton J. Intestinal tuberculosis. Curr Opin Infect Dis. 2009;22:490-6.
8. Farer LS, Lowell AM, Meador MP. Extrapulmonary tuberculosis in the United States. Am J Epidemiol. 1979;109:5-15.
9. Sheer TA, Coyle WJ. Gastrointestinal tuberculosis. Curr Gastroenterol Rep. 2003;5:273-78.
10. Horvath KD, Whelan RL. Intestinal tuberculosis: return of an old disease. Am J Gastroenterol. 1998;93:692-6.
11. Singh MM, Bhargava AN, Jain KP. Tuberculous peritonitis. An evaluation of pathogenetic mechanisms, diagnostic procedures and therapeutic measures. N Engl J Med. 1969;281:1091-4.
12. Diagnosis and management of mycobacterial infection and disease in persons with human immunodeficiency virus infection. Centers for Disease Control. Ann Intern Med. 1987;106:254-6.
13. Singh V, Kumar P, Kamal J, Prakash V, Vaiphei K, Singh K. Clinicocolonoscopic profile of colonic tuberculosis. Am J Gastroenterol. 1996;91:565-8.
14. Rangabashyam N. Abdominal tuberculosis. In: Oxford Textbook of Surgery, Morris PJ, Malt RA (Eds). New York: Oxford University Press; 1994. pp. 2484-92.
15. Hoon JR, Dockerty MB, Pemberton Jde J. Ileocaecal tuberculosis including a comparison of this disease with non-specific regional enterocolitis and noncaseous tuberculated enterocolitis. Int Abstr Surg. 1950;91:417-40.
16. Wig KL, Chitkara NK, Gupta SP, Kishore K, Manchanda RL. Ileocecal tuberculosis with particular reference to isolation of Mycobacterium tuberculosis. Am Rev Respir Dis. 1961;84:169-78.
17. Sharma AK, Aggarwal LD, Sharma CS, Sarin YK. Abdominal tuberculosis in children: experience over a decade. Indian Pediatr. 1993;30:1149-53.
18. Marshall JB. Tuberculosis of the gastrointestinal tract and peritoneum. Am J Gastroentero. 1993;88:989-99.
19. Vij JC, Malhotra V, Choudhary V, Jain NK, Prasaed G, Choudhary A, et al. A clinicopathological study of abdominal tuberculosis. Indian J Tuberc. 1992;39:213-20.
20. Manohar A, Simjee AE, Haffejee AA, Pettengell KE. Symptoms and investigative findings in 145 patients with tuberculous peritonitis

diagnosed by peritoneoscopy and biopsy over a five year period. Gut. 1990;31:1130-2.
21. al Karawi MA, Mohamed AE, Yasawy MI, Graham DY, Shariq S, Ahmed AM, et al. Protean manifestation of gastrointestinal tuberculosis: report on 130 patients. J Clin Gastroenterol. 1995; 20:225-32.
22. Klimach OE, Ormerod LP. Gastrointestinal tuberculosis: a retrospective review of 109 cases in a district general hospital. Q J Med. 1985;56:569-78.
23. Innes JA. Non-respiratory tuberculosis. J R Coll Physicians Lond. 1981;15:227-31.
24. Kapoor VK, Gupta S, Sikora SS, et al. Acute tubercular abdomen. Indian J Surg. 1991;53:71-5.
25. al-Hadeedi S, Walia HS, al-Sayer HM. Abdominal tuberculosis. Can J Surg. 1990;33:233-7.
26. Marshall JB. Tuberculosis of the gastrointestinal tract and peritoneum. Am J Gastroenterol. 1993;88:989-99.
27. Lingenfelser T, Zak J, Marks IN, Steyn E, Halkett J, Price SK. Abdominal tuberculosis: still a potentially lethal disease. Am J Gastroenterol. 1993;88:744-50.
28. Balthazar EJ, Gordon R, Hulnick D. Ileocecal tuberculosis: CT and radiologic evaluation. AJR Am J Roentgenol. 1990;154:499-503.
29. Tandon RK, Sarin SK, Bose SL, Berry M, Tandon BN. A clinico-radiological reappraisal of intestinal tuberculosis changing profile? Gastroenterol Jpn. 1986;21:17-22.
30. Kapoor VK, Chattopadhyay TK, Sharma LK. Radiology of abdominal tuberculosis. Australas Radiol. 1988;32:365-7.
31. Sheikh A. TB or not TB. BMJ. 1999;318:979.
32. Denton T, Hossain J. A radiological study of abdominal tuberculosis in a Saudi population, with special reference to ultrasound and computed tomography. Clin Radiol. 1993;47:409-14.
33. Dave-Verma H, Moore S, Singh A, Martins N, Zawacki J. Computed tomographic enterography and enterolysis: pearls and pitfalls. Curr Probl Diagn Radiol. 2008;37:279-87.
34. Paustian FF. Tuberculosis of the intestine. In: Bockus HL, (Ed). Gastroenterology, 2nd edition. Philadelphia: WB Saunders Co; 1964. p. 311.
35. Sinkala E, Gray S, Zulu I, Mudenda V, Zimba L, Vermund SH, et al. Clinical and ultrasonographic features of abdominal tuberculosis in HIV positive adults in Zambia. BMC Infect Dis. 2009;9:44.
36. Purohit MR, Mustafa T, Wiker HG, Mørkve O, Sviland L. Immunohistochemical diagnosis of abdominal and lymph node tuberculosis by detecting Mycobacterium tuberculosis complex specific antigen MPT64. Diagn Pathol. 2007;2:36.
37. Goel MM, Budhwar P. Species-specific immunohistochemical localization of Mycobacterium tuberculosis complex in fine needle aspirates of tuberculous lymphadenitis using antibody to 38 kDa immunodominant protein antigen. Acta Cytol. 2008;52: 424-33.
38. Voigt MD, Kalvaria I, Trey C, Berman P, Lombard C, Kirsch RE. Diagnostic value of ascites adenosine deaminase in tuberculous peritonitis. Lancet. 1989;1:751-4.
39. Burgess LJ, Swanepoel CG, Taljaard JJ. The use of adenosine deaminase as a diagnostic tool for peritoneal tuberculosis. Tuberculosis (Edinb). 2001;81:243-8.
40. Sathar MA, Simjee AE, Coovadia YM, Soni PN, Moola SA, Insam B, et al. Ascitic fluid gamma interferon concentrations and adenosine deaminase activity in tuberculous peritonitis. Gut. 1995;36:419-21.
41. Dwivedi M, Misra SP, Misra V, Kumar R. Value of adenosine deaminase estimation in the diagnosis of tuberculous ascites. Am J Gastroenterol. 1990;85:1123-5.
42. Bandyopadhyay R, Bandyopadhyay S, Ghoshal J, Kumar U, Dutta A. Study of biochemical parameters of ascitic fluid in exudative ascites with special reference to tuberculous peritonitis. J Indian Med Assoc. 2006;104:174, 176-7,185.
43. Sharma MP, Bhatia V. Abdominal tuberculosis. Indian J Med Res. 2004;120:305-15.
44. Selvakumar N, Vanajakumar, Thilothammal N, Paramasivan CN. Isolation of Mycobacterium tuberculosis from cerebrospinal fluid by the centrifugation & filtration methods. Indian J Med Res. 1996;103:250-2.
45. Shah S, Thomas V, Mathan M, Chacko A, Chandy G, Ramakrishna BS, et al. Colonoscopic study of 50 patients with colonic tuberculosis. Gut. 1992;33:347-51.
46. Bhargava DK, Kushwaha AK, Dasarathy S, Shriniwas, Chopra P. Endoscopic diagnosis of segmental colonic tuberculosis. Gastrointest Endosc. 1992;38:571-4.
47. Alvares JF, Devarbhavi H, Makhija P, Rao S, Kottoor R. Clinical, colonoscopic, and histologic profile of colonic tuberculosis in a tertiary hospital. Endoscopy. 2005;37:351-6.
48. Bhargawa DK, Tandon HD, Chawla TC, Shriniwas S, Tandon BN, Kapur BM. Diagnosis of ileocecal and colonic tuberculosis by colonoscopy. Gastrointest Endosc. 1985;31:68-70.
49. Wolfe JH, Behn AR, Jackson BT. Tuberculous peritonitis and role of diagnostic laparoscopy. Lancet. 1979;1:852-3.
50. Jorge AD. Peritoneal tuberculosis. Endoscopy. 1984;16:10-2.
51. Sandikci MU, Colakoglu S, Ergun Y, Unal S, Akkiz H, Sandikçi S, et al. Presentation and role of peritoneoscopy in the diagnosis of tuberculous peritonitis. J Gastroenterol Hepatol. 1992;7:298-301.
52. Bhargava DK, Shriniwas, Chopra P, Nijhawan S, Dasarathy S, Kushwaha AK. Peritoneal tuberculosis: laparoscopic patterns and its diagnostic accuracy. Am J Gastroenterol. 1992;87:109-12.
53. Krishnan P, Vayoth O, Dhar P, Surendran S, Ponnambathayil S. Laparoscopy in suspected abdominal tuberculosis is useful as an early diagnostic method. ANZ J Surg. 2008;78:987-9.
54. Steingart KR, Henry M, Laal S, Hopewell PC, Ramsay A, Menzies D, et al. A systematic review of commercial serological antibody detection tests for the diagnosis of extrapulmonary tuberculosis. Thorax. 2007;62:911-8.
55. Makharia GK, Sachdev V, Gupta R, Lal S, Pandey RM. Anti-Saccharomyces cerivisiae antibody does not differentiate between Crohn's disease and intestinal tuberculosis. Dig Dis Sci. 2007;52: 33-9.
56. Moatter T, Mirza S, Siddiqui MS, Soomro IN. Detection of Mycobacterium tuberculosis in paraffin embedded intestinal tissue specimens by polymerase chain reaction: characterization of IS6110 element negative strains. J Pak Med Assoc. 1998;48:174-8.
57. Wiener RS, Della-Latta P, Schluger NW. Effect of nucleic acid amplification for Mycobacterium tuberculosis on clinical decision making in suspected extrapulmonary tuberculosis. Chest. 2005;128:102-7.
58. Pulimood AB, Peter S, Rook GW, Donoghue HD. In situ PCR for Mycobacterium tuberculosis in mucosal biopsy specimens of intestinal tuberculosis and Crohn disease. Am J Clin Pathol. 2008;129:846-51.
59. Pai M, Minion J, Steingart K, Ramsay A. New and improved tuberculosis diagnostics: evidence, policy, practice, and impact. Curr Opin Pulm Med. 2010;16:271-84.
60. Chawla S, Mukerjee P, Bery K. Segmental tuberculosis of the colon (a report of ten cases). Clin Radiol. 1971;22:104-9.
61. Arya TVS, Jain AK, Kumar M, Agarwal AK, Gupta JP. Colonic tuberculosis: a clinical and colonoscopic profile. Indian J Gastroenterol. 1994;13(Suppl) A 116.
62. Puri AS, Vij JC, Chaudhary A, Kumar N, Sachdev A, Malhotra V, et al. Diagnosis and outcome of isolated rectal tuberculosis. Dis Colon Rectum. 1996;39:1126-9.
63. Gill SS, Eggleston FC. Acute intestinal obstruction. Arch Surg. 1965;91:589-91.
64. Bhansali SK. Abdominal tuberculosis. Experiences with 300 cases. Am J Gastroenterol. 1977;67:324-37.

65. Bhansali SK, Desai AN, Dhaboowala CB. Tuberculous perforation of the small intestine. A clinical analysis of 19 cases. J Assoc Physicians India. 1968;16:351-5.
66. Kapoor VK. Abdominal tuberculosis: the Indian contribution. Indian J Gastroenterol. 1998;17:141-7.
67. Ranjan P, Ghoshal UC, Aggarwal R, Pandey R, Misra A, Naik S, et al. Etiological spectrum spsoradic malabsorption syndrome in Northern Indian adults at a tertiary hospital. Indian J Gastreoenterol. 2004;23:94-8.
68. Tandon RK, Bansal R, Kapur BML, Shriniwas. A study of malabsorption in intestinal tuberculosis: stagnant loop syndrome. Am J Clin Nutr. 1980;33:244-50.
69. Makharia GK, Srivastava S, Das P, Goswami P, Singh U, Tripathi M, et al. Clinical, endoscopic, and histological differentiations between Crohn's disease and intestinal tuberculosis. Am J Gastroenterol. 2010;105:642-51.
70. Amarapurkar DN, Patel ND, Rane PS. Diagnosis of Crohn's disease in India where tuberculosis is widely prevalent. World J Gastroenterol. 2008;14:741-6.
71. Dorairajan LN, Gupta S, Deo SV, Chumber S, Sharma L. Peritonitis in India–a decade's experience. Trop Gastroenterol. 1995;16:33-8.
72. Sanai FM, Bzeizi KI. Systematic review: tuberculous peritonitis-presenting features, diagnostic strategies and treatment. Aliment Pharmacol Ther. 2005;22:685-700.
73. Mohanty D, Jain BK, Agrawal J, Gupta A, Agrawal V. Abdominal Cocoon: clinical presentation, diagnosis, and management. J Gastrointest Surg. 2009;13:1160-2.
74. Gulati MS, Sarma D, Paul SB. CT appearances in abdominal tuberculosis. A pictorial assay. Clin Imaging. 1999;23:51-9.
75. Kedar RP, Shah PP, Shivde RS, Malde HM. Sonographic findings in gastrointestinal and peritoneal tuberculosis. Clin Radiol. 1994;49:24-9.
76. Jakubowski A, Elwood RK, Enarson DA. Clinical features and abdominal tuberculosis. J Infect Dis. 1988;158:687-92.
77. Welzel TM, K awan T, Bohle W, Richter GM, Bosse A, Zoller WG. An unusual cause of dysphagia: esophageal tuberculosis. J Gastrointestin Liver Dis. 2010;19:321-4.
78. Peixoto PC, Ministro PS, Sadio AD, Cancela EM, Araújo RN, Machado JL, et al. Esophageal tuberculosis: an unusual cause of dysphagia. Gastrointest Endosc. 2009;69:1173-6.
79. Leung VK, Chan WH, Chow TL, Luk IS, Chau TN, Loke TK. Oesophageal tuberculosis mimicking oesophageal carcinoma. Hong Kong Med J. 2006;12:473-6.
80. Mokoena T, Shama DM, Ngakane H, Bryer JV. Oesophageal tuberculosis: a review of eleven cases. Postgrad Med J. 1992;68: 110-5.
81. Jain SK, Jain S, Jain M, Yaduvanshi A. Esophageal tuberculosis: is it so rare? Report of 12 cases and review of the literature. Am J Gastroenterol. 2002;97:293-6.
82. Patnayak R, Reddy MK, Parthasarathy S, Yootla M, Reddy V, Jena A. Unusual presentation of esophageal tuberculosis mimicking malignancy. Saudi J Gastroenterol. 2008;14:103-4.
83. Fujiwara Y, Osugi H, Takada N, Takemura M, Lee S, Ueno M, et al. Esophageal tuberculosis presenting with an appearance similar to that of carcinoma of the esophagus. J Gastroenterol. 2003;38: 477-81.
84. Palmer ED. Tuberculosis of the stomach and the stomach in tuberculosis: a review with particular reference to gross pathology and gastroscopic diagnosis. Am Rev Tuberc. 1950;61:116-30.
85. Di Placido R, Pietroletti R, Leardi S, Simi M. Primary gastroduodenal tuberculosis infection presenting as pyloric outlet obstruction. Am J Gastroenterol. 1996;91:807-8.
86. Gupta SK, Jain AK, Gupta JP, Agrawal AK, Berry K. Duodenal tuberculosis. Clin Radiol. 1988;39:159-61.
87. Rao YG, Pande GK, Sahni P, Chattopadhyay TK. Gastroduodenal tuberculosis management guidelines, based on a large experience and a review of the literature. Can J Surg. 2004;47:364-8.
88. Puri AS, Vij JC, Chaudhary A, Kumar N, Sachdev A, Malhotra V, et al. Diagnosis and outcome of isolated rectal tuberculosis. Dis Colon Rectum. 1996;39:1126-9.
89. Shukla HS, Gupta SC, Singh G, Singh PA. Tubercular fistula in ano. Br J Surg. 1988;75:38-9.
90. Sultan S, Azria F, Bauer P, Abdelnour M, Atienza P. Anoperineal tuberculosis: diagnostic and management considerations in seven cases. Dis Colon Rectum. 2002;45:407-10.
91. Ani AN, Solanke TF. Anal fistula: a review of 82 cases. Dis Colon Rectum. 1976;19:51-5.
92. Auerbach O. Acute generalized miliary tuberculosis. Am J Pathol. 1944;20:121-36.
93. Paraf A, Menager C, Texier J. [Tuberculosis of the pancreas and tuberculosis of the lymph nodes of the upper region of the abdomen]. Rev Med Chir Mal Foie. 1966;41:101-26.
94. Chaudhary A, Negi SS, Sachdev AK, Gondal R. Pancreatic tuberculosis: still a histopathological diagnosis. Dig Surg. 2002;19:389-92.
95. Xia F, Poon RT, Wang SG, Bie P, Huang XQ, Dong JH. Tuberculosis of pancreas and peripancreatic lymph node in immunocompetent patients: experience from China. World J Gastroenterol. 2003;9:1361-4.
96. Rushing JL, Hanna CJ, Selecky PA. Pancreatitis as the presenting manifestation of military tuberculosis. West J Med. 1978;129:432-6.
97. Patankar T, Prasad S, Laxminarayan R. Diabetes mellitus: an uncommon manifestation of pancreatic tuberculosis. J Assoc Physicians India. 1999;47:938-9.
98. Ruttenberg D, Graham S, Burns D, Solomon D, Bornman P. Abdominal tuberculosis: a cause of portal vein thrombosis and portal hypertension. Dig Dis Sci. 1991;36:112-5.
99. Fan ST, Yan KW, Lau WY, Wong KK. Tuberculosis of the pancreas: a rare cause of massive gastrointestinal bleeding. Br J Surg.1986;73:373.
100. Kouraklis G, Glinavou A, Karayiannakis A, Karatzas G. Primary tuberculosis of the pancreas mimicking a pancreatic tumour. Int J Pancreatol. 2001;29:151-3.
101. Tan KK, Chen K, Liau KH, Ho CK. Pancreatic tuberculosis mimicking pancreatic carcinoma: series of three cases. Eur J Gastroenterol Hepatol. 2009;21:1317-9.
102. Nagar AM, Raut AA, Morani AC, Sanghvi DA, Desai CS, Thapar VB. Pancreatic tuberculosis: a clinical and imaging review of 32 cases. J Comput Assist Tomogr. 2009;33(1):136-41.
103. Song TJ, Lee SS, Park do H, Lee TY, Lee SO, Seo DW, et al. Yield of EUS-guided FNA on the diagnosis of pancreatic/peripancreatic tuberculosis. Gastrointest Endosc. 2009;69:484-91.
104. Essop AR, Posen JA, Hodkinson JH, Segal I. Tuberculosis hepatitis: a clinical review of 96 cases. Q J Med. 1984;53:465-77.
105. Terry RB, Gunnar RM. Primary miliary tuberculosis of the liver. J Am Med Assoc. 1957;164(2):150-7.
106. Hersch C. Tuberculosis of the liver. A study of 200 cases. S Afr Med J. 1964;38:857-63.
107. Desai CS, Joshi AG, Abraham P, Desai DC, Deshpande RB, Bhaduri A, et al. Hepatic tuberculosis in absence of disseminated abdominal tuberculosis. Ann Hepatol. 2006;5(1):41-3.
108. Chien RN, Lin PY, Liaw YF. Hepatic tuberculosis comparison of miliary and local form. Infection. 1995;23:5-8.
109. Achem SR, Kolts BE, Grisnik J, MacMath T, Monteiro CB, Goldstein J: Pseudotumoral hepatic tuberculosis: atypical presentation and comprehensive review of literature. J Clin Gastroenterol. 1992;14:72-7.
110. Stemmerman M. Bile duct tuberculosis. Q Bull Sea View Hosp. 1941;6:316-24.

111. Saluja SS, Ray S, Pal S, Kukeraja M, Srivastava DN, Sahni P, et al. Hepatobiliary and pancreatic tuberculosis: a two decade experience. BMC Surg. 2007;7:10.
112. Chong VH, Lim KS. Hepatobiliary tuberculosis. Singapore Med J. 2010;51(9):744-51.
113. Govindasamy M, Srinivasan T, Varma V, Mehta N, Yadav A, Kumaran V, et al. Biliary Tract Tuberculosis-a diagnostic dilemma. J Gastrointest Surg. 2011;15(12):2172-7.
114. Amarapurkar DN, Patel ND, Amarapurkar AD. Hepatobiliary tuberculosis in western India. Indian J Pathol Microbiol. 2008;51: 175-81.
115. Bearer EA, Savides TJ, McCutchan JA. Endoscopic diagnosis and management of hepatobiliary tuberculosis. Am J Gastroenterol. 1996;91:2602-4.
116. Balasubramanian R, Nagarajan M, Balambal R, Tripathy SP, Sundararaman R, Venkatesan P, et al. Randomised controlled clinical trial of short course chemotherapy in abdominal tuberculosis: a five-year report. Int J Tuberc Lung Dis. 1997;1:44-51.
117. Tuberculosis control and research strategies for the 1990s: memorandum from a WHO meeting. Bull World Health Organ. 1992;70:17-21.
118. Morse DI. Directly observed therapy for tuberculosis. BMJ. 1996;312: 719-20.
119. Seabra J, Coelho H, Barros, H, Alves JO, Goncalves V, Rocha-Marques A. Acute tuberculous perforation of the small bowel during antituberculous therapy. J Clin Gastroenterol. 1993;16: 320-2.
120. Alrajhi AA, Halim MA, al-Hokail A, Alrabiah F, al-Omran K. Corticosteroid treatment of peritoneal tuberculosis. Clin Infect Dis. 1998;27:52-6.
121. Findlay JM. Medical management of gastrointestinal tuberculosis. J R Soc Med. 1982;75:583-4.
122. Anand BS, Nanda R, Sachdev GK. Response of tuberculous stricture to antituberculous treatment. Gut. 1988;29:62-9.
123. Balasubramanian R, Ramachandran R, Joseph PE, Nagarajan M, Thiruvengadam KV, Tripathy SP, et al. Interim results of a clinical study of abdominal tuberculosis. Indian J Tuberc. 1989;36:117-21.
124. Ara C, Sogutlu GK, Yildiz R, Kocak O, Isik B, Yilmaz S, et al. Spontaneous small bowel perforations due to intestinal tuberculosis should not be repaired by simple closure. J Gastrointest Surg. 2005;9(4)514-7.
125. Thompson JN, Keshavarzian A, Rees HC. Duodenal tuberculosis. J R Coll Surg Edinb. 1984;29:292-5.
126. Vij JC, Ramesh GN, Choudhary V, Malhotra V. Endoscopic balloon dilation of tuberculous duodenal strictures. Gastrointest Endosc. 1992;38:510-1.
127. Singh DK, Haider A, Tatke M, Kumar P, Mishra PK. Primary pancreatic tuberculosis masquerading as pancreatic tumour leading to Whipple's pancreaticoduodenectomy. A case report and review of literature. JOP. 2009;10(4):451-6.

CHAPTER 30

Gastrointestinal Lymphomas

Anurag Mishra, AK Sarda

INTRODUCTION

Lymphoma is the third most common neoplasm arising in the small intestine, and it accounts for 15–20% of all malignant small bowel tumors. The incidence of intestinal lymphoma has doubled between 1985 and 1990 which was attributed to an upsurge in the lymphoma among immunocompromised patients. However, the incidence stabilized in the 1990s, predominantly due to decline in acquired immunodeficiency syndrome-related malignancy.[1]

Lymphoma may involve any part of the GI tract, and GI tract in turn is the most common site of extra nodal disease.[2,3] The incidence appears to depend on geographic location. In Western and Middle Eastern regions, gastric lymphoma is the most common followed by the small intestine, colon, pancreas and all other sites; however, in other regions like India, Africa, and the South Pacific, intestinal lymphoma is the predominant form, followed by the stomach, colon and other organs (Table 1).[2,4]

Criteria for primary GI lymphoma,[5] (Dawson et al.):

- Absence of palpable lymphadenopathy
- Normal peripheral blood smear and bone marrow biopsy
- Absence of mediastinal lymphadenopathy on chest X-ray
- Disease grossly confined to the affected small bowel segment as confirmed by diagnostic imaging, endoscopy or laparotomy

Table 1: Frequency and sites of extranodal lymphomas in series from different countries

	USA (1972)	*The Netherlands (1989)*	*Denmark (1991)*	*Canada (1992)*	*Hong Kong (1984)*	*Pakistan (1992)*	*Egypt (1994)*	*Switzerland (1997)*
Stomach	24	23	19		39	10	10	36
Small intestine	8	5	9	24	24	17	5	11
Colon and rectum	5	7	2		—	10	6	4
Head and neck	21	23	8	34	22	18	23	19
Orbit	2	3	1	4	1	<1	<1	5
Central nervous system	2	6	7	10	—	2	1	1
Lung, pleura	4	5	5	1	—	—	—	1
Bone	5	3	9	4	4	2	11	3
Soft tissue	9	2	3	5	3	—	—	1
Breast	2	2	1	2	—	—	—	3
Skin	8	2	11	4	3	8	4	6
Genitourinary tract	3	4	6	5	8	12	6	5

Table 2: Symptoms at diagnosis in primary NHL of the GI tract[8]

Symptoms	*Stomach*	*Small bowel*	*Ileocecal region*	*Multiple GI sites*
Pain	78.0	75.0	76.9	58.3
Loss of appetite	47.3	40.6	23.1	58.3
Loss of weight	24.5	34.4	15.4	25.0
Bleeding	18.8	6.3	11.5	8.3
Vomiting	18.1	31.3	7.7	20.8
Night sweats	11.2	12.5	19.2	45.8
Bone	3.6	—	—	—
Diarrhea	3.6	12.5	19.2	29.2
Constipation	3.2	25.0	23.1	12.5
Fever	2.2	6.3	7.7	4.2
Perforation	1.8	9.4	—	—
Ileus	—	37.5	19.2	4.2
B symptoms (fever, night sweats)	11.9	15.6	11.5	25.0
Median time to diagnosis (days)	93	135	76	142

- Regional lymphadenopathy only
- Absence of hepatic or splenic tumor involvement except via direct extension from the primary bowel involvement.

Gastric lymphoma is a disease of elderly, with a peak incidence in the 6th and 7th decades and has a male preponderance of 2–3:1.[4,6] However, recent studies have demonstrated an increasing incidence in younger patients, predominantly because of increased incidence in HIV-infected patients.[4] Antrum and distal body is the most common site of gastric lymphomas; however, the involvement of other parts of stomach is not infrequent.[6] Primary gastric lymphoma is typically unifocal whereas secondary lymphoma shows a multifocal gastric and duodenal involvement. Small intestinal lymphomas, like gastric lymphomas, tend to occur in patients older than 50 years; however, it is the most common intestinal neoplasm in children younger than 10 years, thus resulting in a bimodal distribution.[6,7] Small bowel lymphoma is most commonly located in the ileum, the site of the highest concentration of gut-associated lymphoid tissue.[6]

SYMPTOMS

Symptoms depend on the site of involvement. Presentation is usually late as the early is marked by non-specific symptoms (Table 2).

STAGING

A variety of staging systems exist for primary intestinal lymphoma all based on the classic Ann Arbor staging system (Tables 3 and 4). All of these systems have a similar plan, in which stage I is local disease, stage II is regional involvement, and stages III and IV are for advanced disease stage. More recently, a TNM (tumor, node, metastasis)-like staging system has been proposed by the European Gastrointestinal Lymphoma Study Group. This classification system is believed to be suited for the unique aspects of primary GI lymphomas in being able to predict the response to therapy, as well as the clinical staging of the disease (Table 5).

Table 3: Ann Arbor staging for lymphoma[2]

Stage I	Involvement of a single lymph node region; or localized involvement of a single extralymphatic organ or site in the absence of any lymph node involvement
Stage II	Involvement of two or more lymph node regions on the same side of the diaphragm; or localized involvement of a single extralymphatic organ or site in association with regional lymph node involvement, with or without involvement of other lymph node regions on the same side of the diaphragm
Stage III	Involvement of lymph node regions on both sides of the diaphragm, which also may be accompanied by extra-lymphatic extension in association with adjacent lymph node involvement, or by involvement of the spleen, or both
Stage IV	Diffuse or disseminated involvement of one or more extralymphatic organs, with or without associated lymph node involvement; or isolated extralymphatic organ involvement in the absence of adjacent regional lymph node involvement, but in conjunction with disease in distant site(s); any involvement of the liver or bone marrow, or nodular involvement of the lungs

Table 4: Musshoff's criteria for staging of gastric lymphomas[3]

Stage	*Definition*
IE	Lymphoma restricted to the GI tract on one side of the diaphragm
IE_1	Infiltration limited to the mucosa and submucosa
IE_2	Lymphoma extending beyond the submucosa
IIE	Lymphoma additionally infiltrating lymph nodes on the same side of the diaphragm
IIE_1	Infiltration of regional lymph nodes
IIE_2	Infiltration of lymph nodes beyond the regional nodes
IIIE	Lymphoma infiltrating the GI tract and/or the lymph nodes on both sides of the diaphragm
IVE	Localized infiltration of associated lymph nodes together with diffuse or disseminated involvement of extra-GI organs

Table 5: TNM classification of gastric lymphoma[9]	
Primary tumor (T):	
TX	Primary tumor cannot be assessed
T0	No evidence of primary tumor
Tis	Carcinoma in situ
T1	Tumor invades the lamina propria or submucosa
T2	Tumor invades the muscularis propria or subserosa
T3	Tumor penetrates the serosa (visceral peritoneum) without invasion of adjacent structures
T4	Tumor invades adjacent structures
Lymph node (N):	
NX	Regional lymph node(s) cannot be assessed
N0	No regional lymph node metastasis
N1	Metastasis in perigastric lymph node(s) within 3 cm of the edge of primary tumors
N2	Metastasis in perigastric lymph node(s) more than 3 cm from the edge of the primary tumor or in lymph nodes along the left gastric, common hepatic, splenic, or celiac arteries
Distant metastasis:	
MX	Presence of distant metastasis cannot be assessed
M0	No distant metastasis
M1	Distant metastasis

DIAGNOSIS

A high index of suspicion is required to make the diagnosis of GI lymphoma because the clinical and radiologic features are often vague. A careful physical examination should include palpation of all lymph node regions and evaluation of the abdomen for palpable masses or hepatosplenomegaly.[10] Laboratory evaluation should include a complete and differential blood count, routine biochemical assays, lactate dehydrogenase level, and serum protein electrophoresis.[10] Once the diagnosis of GI lymphoma is established, evidence of metastatic disease should be sought by performing an upper airway examination, bone marrow biopsy, and CT of the chest and abdomen to evaluate for lymphadenopathy; any enlarged lymph nodes should be biopsied.[6]

Gastric Lymphoma

Gastric lymphoma is usually diagnosed on the basis of upper GI endoscopy and biopsy, with a diagnostic yield of approximately 90%.[11] The most frequent endoscopic finding is ulceration in both low-grade and high-grade lesions. Diffuse infiltration and polypoid masses are also common findings.[11] Such appearances are mistaken for benign conditions such as gastritis or peptic ulcer disease in up to 25–50% of patients, thus reinforcing the importance of biopsy.[11,12] Endoscopic ultrasound is an important adjunct for detecting intramural tumor infiltration and determining tumor stage and is more reliable than routine CT scanning. The sensitivity of lymph node detection is more variable, with 45–90% accuracy.[11] Like Gastric adenocarcinomas, gastric lymphoma also has perigastric lymphadenopathy but is only more pronounced and reaching as far as beyond renal hilum and this finding is more suggestive of lymphoma. On CECT gastric lymphoma appears as thickened gastric folds with preserved perigastric fat planes, a picture distinct from adenocarcinoma but at the same time various other etiologies like hypertrophic gastritis or Ménétrier disease which also gives similar radiologic picture needs to be ruled out. It is also advisable to perform *Helicobacter pylori* testing on biopsy.[6]

Gastric lymphomas may present as infiltrating type which can be either focal or diffuse but unlike gastric adenocarcinoma it rarely ever causes gastric outlet obstruction. Other presentation of gastric lymphoma is ulcerative type which may have single or multiple ulcers, are usually irregular and at times mimic benign ulcers. Gastric lymphoma can also present like polypoidal intraluminal growths with appearance very similar to carcinoma. Another very characteristic feature of gastric lymphoma is multiple submucosal nodules with central ulceration which gives a peculiar bull's eye appearance on barium study.

Intestinal Lymphoma

As many as 90% of small bowel lymphomas are diagnosed intraoperatively either as part of a treatment plan or to establish a diagnosis.[13] Commonly used preoperative imaging modalities include CT of the abdomen and pelvis (Figs 1 and 2), lymphangiography, gallium scanning, upper GI series, barium enema, upper GI endoscopy and colonoscopy; the appropriate work-up depends on the suspected location of the tumor, and decisions should be made on an individual basis.[13]

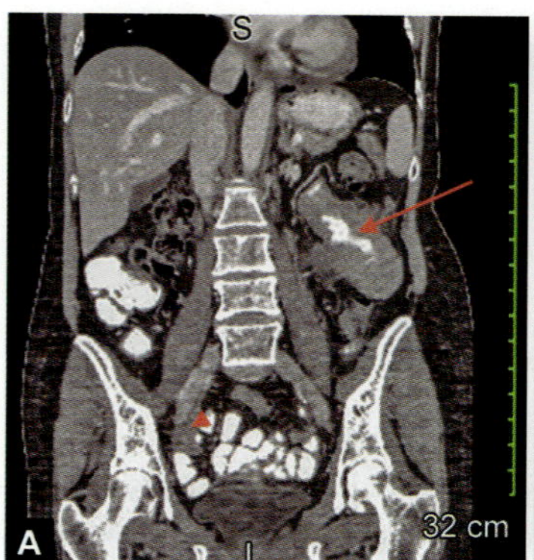

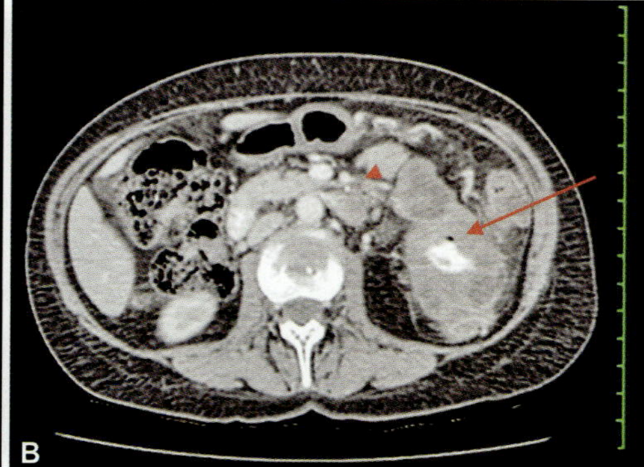

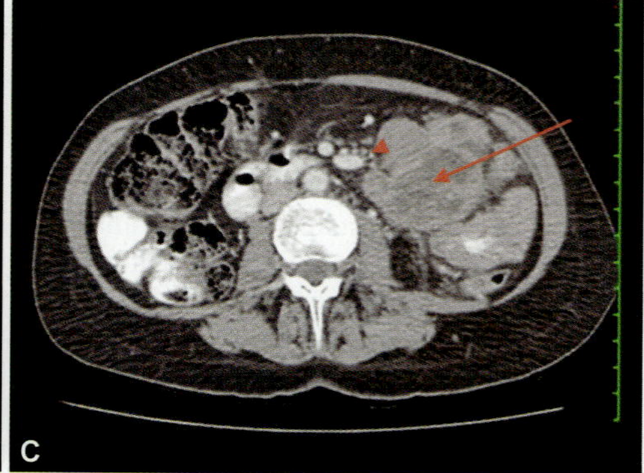

Figures 1A to C CT scans showing circumferential thickening of jejunum (arrow) with lymph node enlargement in mesentery and right iliac region (arrowhead)

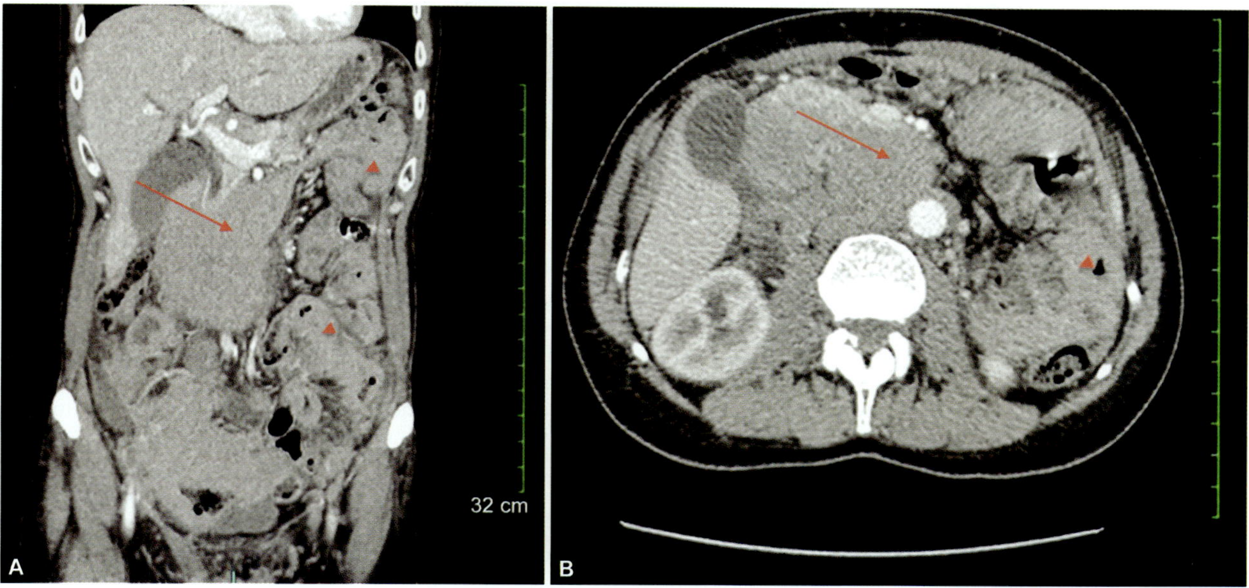

Figures 2A and B CT scans showing large retroperitoneal lymph node mass pushing aorta to left (arrow)and thickening of jejunum and ileum (arrowhead)

Table 6: *H. pylori* treatment[15]

Regimen 1 (Treatment of choice)	*Regimen 2 (Penicillin sensitive patient)*	*Regimen 3*
Omeprazole (20 mg, twice a day)	Omeprazole (20 mg, twice a day)	Omeprazole (20 mg, twice a day)
Amoxicillin (1 g, twice a day)	Metronidazole (500 mg, twice a day)	Tetracycline (500 mg, 4 times a day)
Clarithromycin (500 mg, twice a day)	Clarithromycin (500 mg, twice a day)	Metronidazole (500 mg, 4 times a day)
		Bismuth (525 mg, 4 times a day)

Four distinct radiographic features of small bowel lymphoma have been described:

1. Multiple luminal filling defects signifying lesions in the small bowel wall.
2. Discrete mass that forms the lead point for an intussusception that can be identified as a target lesion on the CT scan, usually longer segments of the small bowel that are involved, as opposed to the adenocarcinoma.
3. Aneurysmal dilatation of the small bowel with intermittent obstruction.
4. Findings of cavitary masses that appears arising from the mesentery with aggressive large cell lymphomas.

TREATMENT

Initial treatment of both gastric and intestinal lymphomas should take into account *H. pylori* status because approximately 70–80% of mucosal-associated lymphoid tissue (MALT) lymphomas and a variable number of diffuse large B cell lymphomas (DLBCL) regress after *H. pylori* eradication in patients harboring the bacterium.[14]

Currently, management of gastric lymphoma takes a predominantly conservative, nonsurgical approach, whereas treatment of many intestinal lymphomas involves a multidisciplinary approach with surgical management being a key component of therapy.

Gastric Lymphoma

The indolent nature of low-grade MALT lymphomas lends itself to conservative treatment, with antibiotic therapy being the sole initial agent, given that the patient can be monitored closely.[16] A significant proportion of these patients (up to 77%) will have complete remission within 12 months of after *H. pylori* eradication.[17] Current *H. pylori* eradication therapy should include a 2-week regimen of either (1) omeprazole or lansoprazole, clarithromycin, and amoxicillin; (2) omeprazole or lansoprazole, metronidazole, and clarithromycin; or (3) omeprazole or lansoprazole, bismuth, metronidazole, and tetracycline (Table 6). Strict endoscopic surveillance with biopsy is recommended 2 months after treatment and at least 6 monthly for 2 years to monitor response to treatment regression.[16] Indicators of possible failure of *H. pylori* eradication include lymphomas of stage IIE and above, stage IE_2 cases that involve the muscularis propria or serosa, lymphomas demonstrating t(11;18) (q21;q21) or t(1;14) (p22;q32) translocations or nuclear expression of Bcl-10, or lymphomas associated with underlying autoimmune disorders.[17] However, eradication should still be pursued in these patients.

Management of patients demonstrating antibiotic failure is still not clear. Surgical therapy is highly curative for localized tumors, but many gastric lymphomas disseminate widely within the mucosa, with frequent tumor relapse in the gastric stump and eventual need for total gastrectomy, which has a significant impact on quality of life.[17] Thus, a multimodal approach consisting of any combination of chemotherapy, radiation therapy and surgery is common.[3] Chemotherapy with an alkylating agent, like cyclophosphamide or chlorambucil, is useful either alone or as an adjunct to surgical resection for *H. pylori* eradication-resistant MALT lymphomas.[16,17] Combination chemotherapy with CHOP [cyclophosphamide, hydroxydaunomycin, Oncovin (vincristine), and prednisone], with the possible addition of rituximab (a chimeric monoclonal antibody against the CD20 B-cell antigen), is preferred for the treatment of high-grade MALT lymphoma or DLBCL.[16,18,19] MALT lymphomas are also highly radiosensitive, and the use of low-dose localized radiation alone is highly effective in the management of lymphomas unresponsive to *H. pylori* eradication, with a 5-year survival in excess of 90%.[17] The combination of surgery and radiotherapy has been advocated for management of low-grade disease, whereas high-grade disease also requires additional chemotherapy, but no consensus has been reached[3,19] (Flow charts 1 and 2).

Intestinal Lymphoma

Patients with *H. pylori* positive intestinal lymphomas also benefit from eradication therapy, as with gastric lymphoma.[7] Initial management of stage I or II small bowel lymphoma should otherwise include segmental surgical resection with regional lymph node excision, regardless of patient age or lymphoma type, given the increased risk for perforation and obstruction associated with these tumors.[2] An aggressive multimodal

Flow chart 1 Treatment algorithm for low grade gastric lymphoma

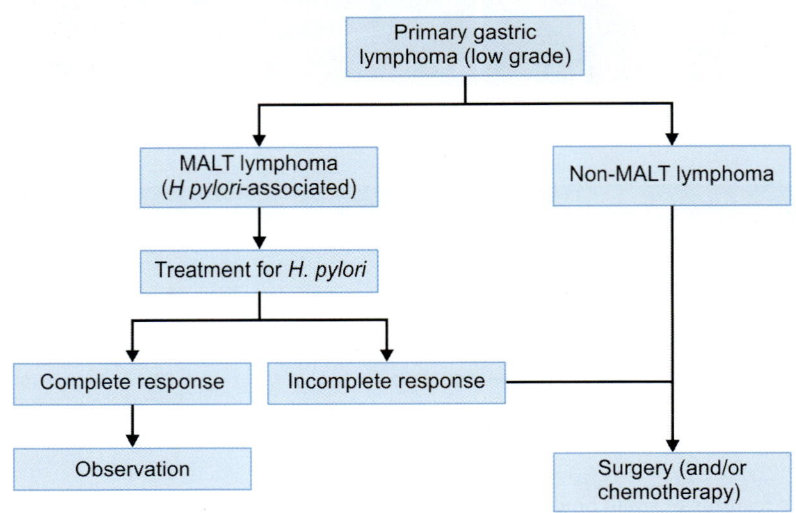

Flow chart 2 Management of high grade gastric lymphomas

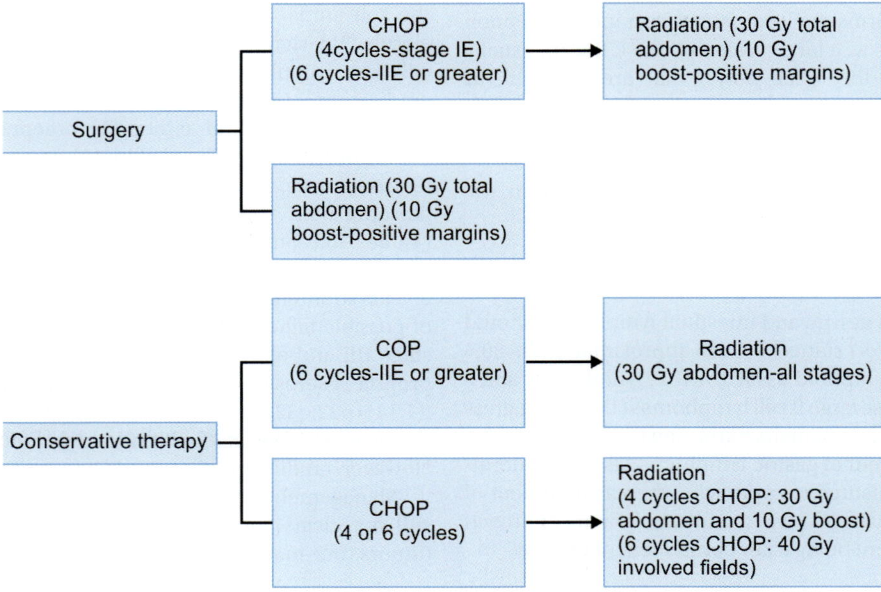

therapeutic approach combining both surgical resection and poly chemotherapy can improve the outcome in patients with all intestinal lymphoma variants, but decisions on the appropriate course of therapy must be made on an individual basis.[7,20] The most commonly applied chemotherapy regimen for patients with intestinal DLBCL or MALT lymphoma is CHOP, with the addition of rituximab in those with mantle cell or follicular variants.[2,7] Treatment of Burkitt's lymphoma is similar to CHOP, with the substitution of methotrexate for prednisone.[2] T-cell lymphomas are notoriously chemotherapy resistant; the best chance for cure in this patient population is achieved by enrollment in clinical trials.[2] Radiotherapy is infrequently used in the treatment of intestinal lymphomas because of a high risk of late complications.[20]

PROGNOSIS

Factors affecting prognosis in patients with GI lymphoma include:

- Lymphoma type,
- Grade,
- Stage,
- Location,
- Molecular markers,
- Genetic rearrangements, and
- Age of the patient.

Mucosal-associated lymphoid tissue and MALT-derived lymphomas have the best overall prognosis, regardless of location.[2,7] Gastric lymphomas have a better overall prognosis than intestinal lymphomas do; 5-year survival rates for tumors localized to the stomach are approximately 91% for low-grade, 73% for secondary high-grade and 56% for primary high-grade tumors, whereas the 5-year survival rate for aggressive small intestinal lymphomas is approximately 25–30%.[4,21,22] Intestinal B-cell lymphomas are associated with a better prognosis than those of T-cell origin, with average 5-year survival rates of 75% and 25%, respectively.[21,23]

Subtypes of Lymphoma Arising in the Small Intestine

Numerous classification schemes exist for non-Hodgkin's lymphomas, including the Kiel-Rappaport, Lukes-Collins, Revised European-American Lymphoma (REAL), Working Formulation, and World Health Organization classifications. Lymphomas arising in the GI tract generally fall into one of four categories from these classification schemas:

1. Diffuse large cell lymphoma,
2. MALT associated lymphomas,
3. Peripheral T-cell lymphoma, and
4. Burkitt's lymphomas.

Diffuse Large B-cell Lymphoma

It is the most common non-Hodgkin's lymphoma occurring in the small bowel, with ileocecal region being the most common affected site. It has a male preponderance with peak incidence in 6th decade of life. They usually present as focal or segmental lesions in the distal small intestine. As the names suggest these tumors are made of diffuse large B cell with large nuclei which are double the size of a lymphocyte. These tumor cells are CD19, CD20+, CD22+, CD79a+ and a large proportion of them demonstrate BCL2 gene mutations.

HIV and other general immunodepressed states are established risk factors. Surgery with adjuvant chemoradiotherapy is the mainstay of treatment for localized disease. In a prospective trial surgery was confirmed as an effective treatment of this disease.[24] Treatment with CHOP (cyclophosphamide, doxorubicin, vincristine and prednisone) or CHOP and radiation appeared equivalent to surgery in gastric disease.[8] The multimodality treatment has been reported to yield an overall 5-year survival rate of 50–70%.[2]

Mucosal-associated Lymphoid Tissue Lymphoma

Mucosal-associated lymphoid tissue also known as marginal zone B-cell lymphoma and in small intestine are of two different histological sub types:

1. Western type MALT lymphoma or
2. Immunoproliferative small intestine disease.

These lymphomas are characterized by cellular heterogeneity, bearing close resemblance to normal gut-associated lymphoid tissue (Peyer's patch and mesenteric nodal tissue). There is a dominant expression of immunoglobulin M as compared to immunoglobulin G or immunoglobulin A on these tumor cells. They also express B-cell associated antigens, including CD19, CD20, CD22 and CD79a. They are usually CD5, CD10, CD23 and CD43 variable. Unlike the large diffuse B cells, they are not associated with BCL2 or BCL1 rearrangements. Studies suggest that MALT tumors may be antigen driven, especially Campylobacter jejuni, *H. pylori*.[25] Patients mostly present with localized stage I or II disease involving the small intestine. Treatment is multimodal, including surgical resection and/or chemoradiation therapy. In early stages of immunoproliferative small intestine disease treatment may consist of antibiotics, usually tetracycline.[25]

Burkitt's Lymphoma

Burkitt's lymphoma accounts for a meager 5% of all small intestinal lymphomas and may present as an endemic, sporadic type or immunodeficiency associated type. It demonstrates a rapid growth with short doubling time. Cell of Burkitt's lymphoma are monomorphic having around nuclei and abundant basophilic cytoplasm. Most striking feature of Burkitt's lymphoma is a starry-eyed pattern, imparted by the numerous benign macrophages that have ingested apoptotic tumor cells. In the National Cancer Institute series of sporadic Burkitt's lymphoma, one-fourth of the patients presented with a mass in the right lower quadrant, mimicking appendicitis. Treatment consists primarily of chemotherapy, usually vincristine, cyclophosphamide, doxorubicin and methotrexate.[26]

T-cell Lymphomas of the Small Intestine

Initially designated as malignant histiocytosis of the intestine, nomenclature has lately been changed to T-cell lymphoma of the small intestine. It constitutes as little as 15% of all lymphomas arising in the small intestine. Tumor is characterized by presence of small, medium and large cells along with high content of intraepithelial T cells in the adjacent mucosa. The tumor cells are CD3+, CD7+,

CD8+, CD4- and CD103+. Many of these lymphomas are associated with celiac disease and malabsorption, commonly known as Enteropathy Associated T cell Lymphoma (EATL). It is believed that the relative risk of developing a lymphoma in the setting of celiac disease is 25- to 100-fold higher than in normal patients. The link between refractory sprue disease, which is not responsive to a gluten-free diet, and the development of lymphoma is controversial.[27] Several authors have suggested that development of a lymphoma may be simply a monoclonal outgrowth of reactive T cells.

SUMMARY

Gastrointestinal lymphomas are a diverse group of neoplasms that are often associated with vague symptoms that imitate common intra-abdominal pathologies; a high degree of suspicion is frequently required to make the diagnosis. Many advances have been made in the diagnosis and management of GI lymphomas over the past decade. The importance of *H. pylori* infection to the development of lymphomas has only recently been realized, and this realization has revolutionized treatment of the disease. Gastric lymphoma, once a surgical disease, is now managed conservatively, with *H. pylori* eradication being central to treatment. Although surgery remains the mainstay of treatment of small intestinal lymphoma, *H. pylori* eradication has proved to be a useful adjunct in its management as well.

REFERENCES

1. Cancer Facts and Figures 2005. American Cancer Society, Atlanta.
2. Koniaris LG, Drugas G, Katzman PJ, Salloum R. Management of gastrointestinal lymphoma. J Am Coll Surg. 2003;197:127-41.
3. Ahmad A, Govil Y, Frank BB. Gastric mucosa-associated lymphoid tissue lymphoma. Am J Gastroenterol. 2003;98:975-86.
4. Al-Akwaa AM, Siddiqui N, Al-Mofleh IA. Primary gastric lymphoma. World J Gastroenterol. 2004;10:5-11.
5. Dawson IMP, Cornes JS, Morrison BC. Primary malignant lymphoid tumours of the intestinal tract. Br J Surg. 1961;49:80-9.
6. Mercer DW, Robinson EK. Stomach. In: Townsend CM (Ed). Sabiston's Textbook of Surgery: The Biological Basis of Modern Surgical Practice. Philadelphia: Elsevier; 2004. pp. 1265-321.
7. Nakamura S, Matsumoto T, Takeshita M, Kurahara K, Yao T, Tsuneyoshi M, et al. A clinicopathologic study of primary small intestine lymphoma: prognostic significance of mucosa-associated lymphoid tissue-derived lymphoma. Cancer. 2000;88:286-94.
8. Koch P, del Valle F, Berdel WE, Willich NA, Reers B, Hiddemann W, et al. Primary gastrointestinal non-Hodgkin's lymphoma: I. Anatomic and histologic distribution, clinical features, and survival data of 371 patients registered in the German Multicenter Study GIT NHL 01/92. J ClinOncol. 2001;19:3861-73.
9. Green FL, Page DL, Fleming ID, et al. AJCC Cancer Staging Manual, 6th edition. New York: Springer-Verlag; 2001.
10. Yoon SS, Coit DG, Portlock CS, Karpeh MS. The diminishing role of surgery in the treatment of gastric lymphoma. Ann Surg. 2004;240:28-37.
11. Boot H, de Jong D. Gastric lymphoma: the revolution of the past decade. Scand J Gastroenterol Suppl. 2002;236:27-36.
12. Ernst M, Stein H, Ludwig D, Boese-Landgraf J, Ritz J, Häring R. Surgical therapy of gastrointestinal non-Hodgkin's lymphomas. Eur J Surg Oncol. 1996;22:177-81.
13. Ha CS, Cho MJ, Allen PK, Fuller LM, Cabanillas F, Cox JD. Primary non-Hodgkin lymphoma of the small bowel. Radiology. 1999;211:183-7.
14. Sepulveda AR, Coelho LG. Helicobacter pylori and gastric malignancies. Helicobacter. 2002;7(Suppl 1):37-42.
15. Kahl BS. Update: Gastric MALT lymphoma. Curr Opin Oncol. 2003;15:347-52.
16. Zucca E, Conconi A, Cavalli F. Treatment of extranodal lymphomas. Best Pract Res Clin Haematol. 2002;15:533-47.
17. Du MQ, Isaccson PG. Gastric MALT lymphoma: from aetiology to treatment. Lancet Oncol. 2002;3:97-104.
18. Couderc B, Dujols JP, Mokhtari F, Norkowski JL, Slawinski JC, Schlaifer D. The management of adult aggressive non-Hodgkin's lymphomas. Crit Rev Oncol Hematol. 2000;35:33-48.
19. Coiffier B, Lepage E, Briere J, Herbrecht R, Tilly H, Bouabdallah R, et al. CHOP chemotherapy plus rituximab compared with CHOP alone in elderly patients with diffuse large-B-cell lymphoma. N Engl J Med. 2002;346:235-42.
20. Geara F. Radiotherapy for gastrointestinal lymphomas: indications and techniques. Cancer Radiother. 1999;3:141-8.
21. Gill SS, Heuman DM, Mihas AA. Small intestinal neoplasms. J Clin Gastroenterol. 2001;33:267-82.
22. Kocher M, Muller RP, Ross D, Hoederath A, Sack H. Radiotherapy for treatment of localized gastrointestinal non-Hodgkin's lymphoma. Radiother Oncol. 1997;42:37-41.
23. Rodriguez J, Munsell M, Yazji S, Hagemeister FB, Younes A, Andersson B, et al. Impact of high-dose chemotherapy on peripheral T-cell lymphomas. J Clin Oncol. 2001;19:3766-70.
24. Fischbach W, Dragosics B, Kolve-Goebeler ME, Ohmann C, Greiner A, Yang Q, et al. Primary gastric B-cell lymphoma: results of a prospective multicenter study. The German-Austrian Gastrointestinal Lymphoma Study Group. Gastroenterology. 2000;119:1191-202.
25. Suarez F, Lortholary O, Hermine O, Lecuit M. Infection-associated lymphomas derived from marginal zone B cells: a model of antigen-driven lymphoproliferation. Blood. 2006;107:3034-44.
26. Blum KA, Lozanski G, Byrd JC. Adult Burkitt leukemia and lymphoma. Blood. 2004;104:3009-20.
27. Al-Toma A, Verbeek WH, Hadithi M, von Blomberg BM, Mulder CJ. Survival in refractory coeliac disease and enteropathy associated T cell lymphoma: retrospective evaluation of single centre experience. Gut. 2007;56:1373-8.

CHAPTER 31

Visceral Artery Aneurysms

RA Sastry, Venu Madhav Thumma

INTRODUCTION

Visceral artery aneurysms (VAA) are rare entities and are increasingly being diagnosed thanks to the advances in imaging techniques. Increased manipulations of biliary tract by both percutaneous and endoscopic techniques, intravascular chemoembolization catheters and increasing radical resections with inadvertent arterial trauma and subadventitial dissections have perhaps contributed to the increased incidence. VAA are important to recognize because they are potentially lethal as 25% may rupture with the resultant mortality of 25–70%.

Visceral aneurysms may be recognized in three types of clinical settings: (1) incidental discovery, (2) a false aneurysm as a consequence of neighboring GI pathology, e.g. following pancreatitis etc. and (3) as a complication of a visceral abdominal aneurysm, e.g. gastrointestinal bleeding. Large published series are sparse and there are only a few case series published with more than 30 cases. The natural history of VAA is still largely unknown. With the increasing utilization of endovascular techniques for management of VAA, the role of surgery is decreasing.

EPIDEMIOLOGY

Visceral artery aneurysms have an incidence of 1% in the general population[1-3] and between 0.1–10% in autopsy series.[2] Majority of VAA originate in either splenic or hepatic artery with a frequency of 60% and 20% respectively. Though rarely, aneurysms have been reported in virtually all visceral arteries including SMA, celiac, gastric, gastroepiploic, jejunal, ileal, colic, pancreatic, gastroduodenal and IMA in the decreasing order, incidence ranging from 5.5% to less than 1%.[4,5] Aneurysms of the hepatic arteries were the most frequently reported VAA in some of the recent series. This increase in frequency is attributed not only to increasing numbers of percutaneous biliary interventions but also to increasing conservative management of blunt liver trauma.[5,6]

ETIOLOGY

Visceral artery aneurysms can be both true and pseudoaneurysms. A true aneurysm is composed of all three layers of vessel wall, i.e. tunica intima, media and externa, whereas in pseudoaneurysm wall is deficient of one or more layers. Atherosclerosis, fibromuscular dysplasia, medial degeneration and portal hypertension are the predominant causes of true aneurysms. Patients with fibromuscular dysplasia are 6 times more likely to have visceral aneurysms than normal population whereas 10–30% of patients with portal hypertension and massive splenomegly have splenic artery aneurysms (SAAs) often multiple. Multiple pregnancies is considered another risk factor and the pathogenesis is attributed to hormonal effects and increased AV shunting that occurs during pregnancy. In the pre-antibiotic era mycotic pseudoaneurysm secondary to endocarditis were the most frequent.[7] Abdominal and surgical traumas along with infectious or inflammatory diseases are other important causes of pseudoaneurysms. The causes of VAA are summarized in Table 1.[8] Forty cases of visceral aneurysms were seen at Nizam's Institute of Medical Sciences, Hyderabad, between 2000 and 2010. A break-up of the aneurysms and the etiology are described in Tables 2 and 3.

DIAGNOSIS

Most visceral aneurysms do not produce any symptoms. This is particularly true for aneurysms of hepatic, gastroepiploic and pancreatoduodenal arteries whose first presentation itself is often after rupture. Symptoms of the primary inflammatory pathology such as pancreatitis may mask the initial subtle

Table 1: Etiology of visceral artery aneurysm

True aneurysms
Common causes: • Arteriosclerosis • Fibromuscular dysplasia • Cystic medial necrosis • Portal hypertension
Uncommon causes: • Autoimmune/collagen vascular diseases • Polyarteritis nodosa • Systemic lupus erythematosus • Takayasu arteritis • Ehlers-Danlos syndrome • Marfan syndrome • Neurofibromatosis • Hypertension • Congenital • α1-Antitrypsin deficiency
Pseudoaneurysms
Common causes: • Inflammatory conditions • Pancreatitis • Blunt or penetrating abdominal trauma • Anastomotic pseudoaneurysm (after orthotopic liver transplantation) • Percutaneous intervention of biliary tract • Arterial dissection
Uncommon causes: • Infectious diseases • Mycotic aneurysms • Syphilis • Infective endocarditis • Tuberculosis

symptoms of aneurysm. A sentinel bleeding during the course of acute necrotizing pancreatitis or in a back ground of chronic pancreatitis should warn a clinician of an impending major bleed and should prompt him to a definitive action. The "double rupture phenomenon" is the result of initial tamponade of the bleeding within the confines of lesser sac followed by an intraperitoneal rupture.[9]

Table 2: Location and nature of visceral aneurysms seen at NIMS between 2000 and 2010 (n=40)

	Total number (40)	*True (8)*	*False (32)*
Splenic artery A	20	5	15
HAA	8	-	8
GDAA	4	-	4
SMAA	2	1	1
Celiac AA	2	2	-
Lt. Gastric AA	1	-	1
PDAA	1	-	1
Jejunal AA	1	-	1
Lt. Colic A	1	-	1

Table 3: Etiology of visceral aneurysms seen at NIMS (n=40)

Etiology	*Number*
Acute pancreatitis	9
Chronic pancreatitis	8
Trauma	6
Postoperative	4
Infective	2
Polyarteritis nodosa	1
Idiopathic	10 (True aneurysms: 8)

In the past, invasive intra-arterial angiography used to be the gold standard for detecting aneurysms, but nowadays CT angiography and 3D contrast-enhanced MR angiography (CE-MRA) have replaced conventional angiography for diagnostic purposes.[10] CT and MR angiography can not only diagnose aneurysms with great accuracy but can also provide information about regional anatomy and its variations, feeder vessels and collateral blood supply (Figs 1A and B). In addition, 3D anatomic information can be acquired which is helpful for surgical or endovascular intervention planning. Furthermore, they also provide information regarding the severity of the underlying disease.

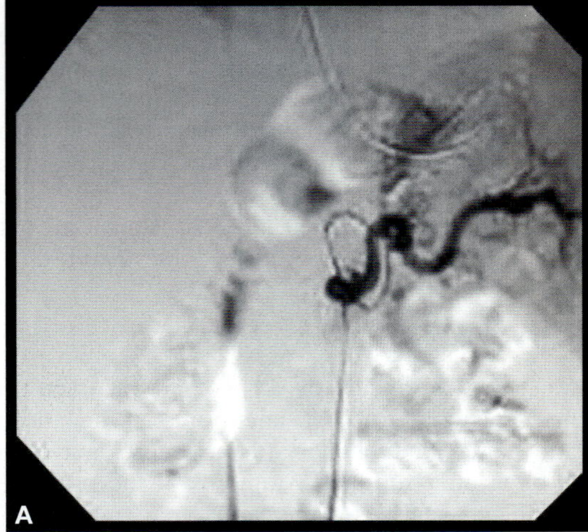

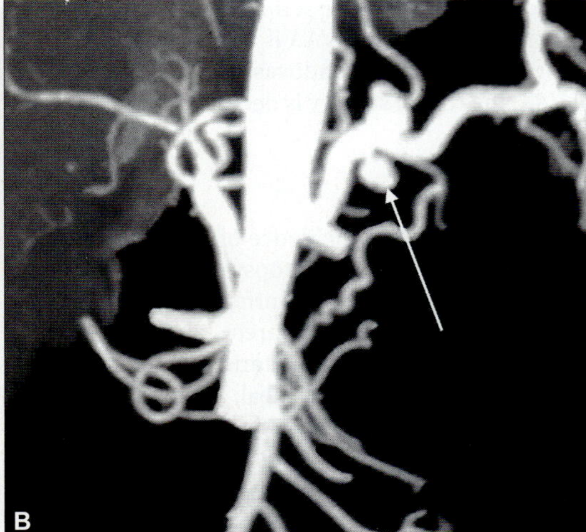

Figures 1A and B (A and B) Aneurysm missed on conventional angiogram; demonstrated on CT angiogram

TREATMENT

In the years gone by close observation or surgery used to be the treatment options for VAA. Surgically, aneurysm resections with revascularization, aneurysm ligation, or end-organ resection (i.e. splenectomy) are the available options. However, they suffer from the disadvantages of being technically difficult procedures and having a hostile environment due to coexisting pancreatitis, hepatobiliary disease, portal hypertension, pregnancy, etc.

Ligating an aneurysm without reconstruction can be resorted to in an emergency situation especially if collateral circulation is adequate (Fig. 2). Simple ligation is a reasonable option for ruptured aneurysm of small visceral arteries also as there is very low risk of resulting ischemia and there is associated technical difficulty of reconstruction. For large arteries like celiac trunk and common hepatic artery, ligation can be thought of as an emergency option without inciting liver ischemia if ligation can be performed proximal to a functional gastroduodenal artery.[10] Though splenectomy was most commonly resorted to for SAA, with increasing awareness of post-splenectomy septic complications splenic preservation is attempted wherever possible. It is also made possible by the fact that SAAs are saccular and located proximally making aneurysectomy and anastomosis safe and feasible. Endovascular approaches to managing VAA score over conventional open surgery due to less procedure related complications and have now become the first line of management in most centers (Figs 3A and B). Endovascular management of VAA utilizing either coil embolization or covered stent placement is feasible in almost all clinical and anatomical scenario, emergency and elective alike. There are some perceived limitations of endovascular techniques in emergency settings like risk of failure[11] and availability of expertise and facilities during odd hours but these can be easily overcome in dedicated centers with expert operators. Different techniques are utilized for true and pseudoaneurysms. True aneurysms are dealt with by coil packing of the aneurysm while pseudoaneurysms require isolation with distal and proximal coiling.[12] Even though the data for endovascular management of VAA is still evolving, impressive results with low morbidity and mortality with good success rates are already evident.

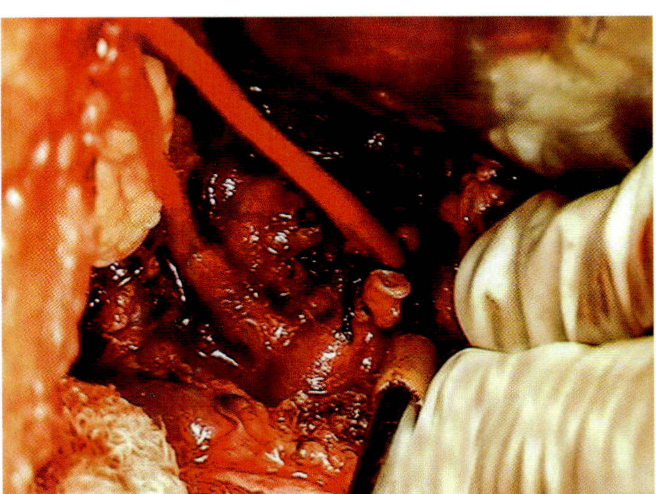

Figure 2 Ligation of splenic artery

SPLENIC ARTERY ANEURYSM (SAA)

True aneurysms are predominantly seen in females and affect population in their fifth to sixth decade of life.[11] These aneurysms are usually saccular in shape and the most common site is the distal third of the splenic artery (75%) followed by the middle third (20%).[12,13] Association of SAA has been described with conditions like pregnancy, systemic hypertension and cirrhosis[14-18] and less commonly with, arteritis, collagen vascular disease, and inflammatory and infectious disorders.[15] Histopathological examination of SAA specimens reveal atherosclerotic changes in as much as 80–90% of cases, but these are secondary changes occurring due to degeneration of tunica media rather than a cause of aneurysm.[19-21] Concomitant splanchnic aneurysms are found in 3% of patients and non-splanchnic aneurysms have been documented in up to 14% of cases, most of which occur in the renal artery.[19]

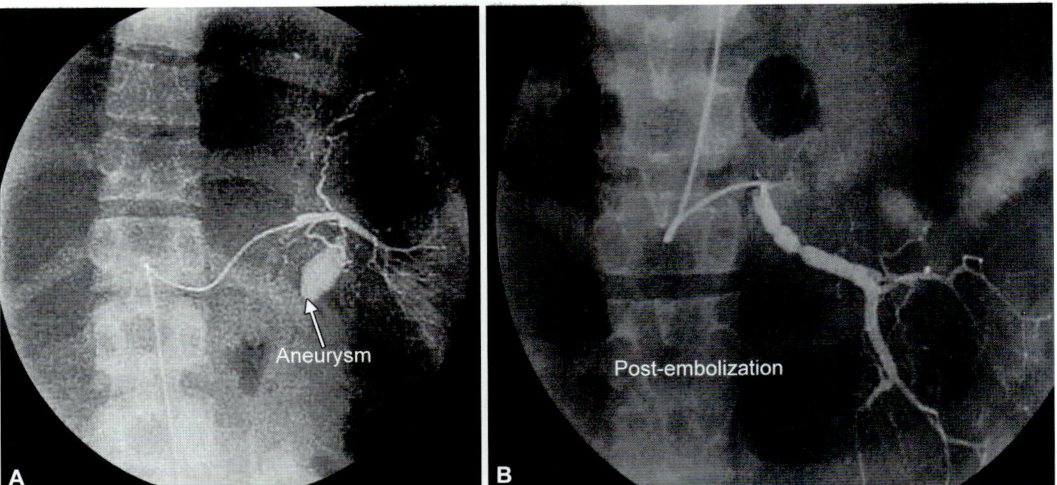

Figures 3A and B (A and B) Embolization of splenic artery aneurysm

Splenic Artery Aneurysm and Pregnancy

Splenic artery aneurysms have a female preponderance. They have a tendency to rupture during third trimester of pregnancy and this risk is highest during last 2 weeks of gestation.[21,22] Increased levels of circulating estrogen and progesterone during pregnancy leads to medial degeneration resulting in aneurysmal dilation.[13,17] Another hormone relaxin enhances the effect of estrogen and progesterone by increasing the elasticity of splenic artery.[23] Multiparous women have increased incidence of SAA rupture due to repeated exposure of high circulating hormones. Another factor which facilitates formation of SAA during pregnancy is the hyperdynamic state of increased cardiac output and circulating blood volume. Enlarged uterus compresses on aorta and IVC thereby further increases the splenic artery blood flow and portal congestion and contributes to the formation of SAA.[18,24,25] Though very rare, spontaneous rupture of SAA has also been reported during 1st trimester.[26]

Splenic Artery Aneurysm and Portal Hypertension

Patients suffering from portal hypertension are particularly at risk with an incidence of 7.1–13.0%.[17,18] In one of the series of cirrhotic patients incidence of SAA was found to be 8.8%.[27] Increased blood flow is thought to be the causative factor for SAA in cases of portal hypertension of liver transplant recipient. Conversely SAA may lead to EHPVO and resulting portal hypertension.[28-32] SAA can compress the adjoining splenic vein leading to thrombosis and thus sinistral portal hypertension. The authors had one such patient in their series (Fig. 4). Splenectomy with excision of aneurysm is curative for these cases.

False Aneurysm

False or pseudoaneurysms of the splenic artery are less prevalent than true SAA. However, they are increasingly being reported in recent literature. Unlike true SAA, these have a male predominance. The underlying causes in most of the cases are pancreatitis, postoperative (usually associated with pancreatic fistula), trauma or infection. There have been 160 reported cases of splenic artery pseudoaneurysm in last four decades, with the size ranging from 0.3 to 17 cm, and 11% of them being giant pseudoaneurysms.[19] A giant pseudoaneurysm is defined as a pseudoaneurysm equal to or greater than 5 cm in size. In the literature, size has ranged from 5 to 18 cm.[20,31] Erosion of the splenic artery by an enlarging pseudocyst due to enzymatic digestion and, thus, conversion of the pseudocyst into a pseudoaneurysm can explain the formation of a giant pseudoaneurysm (Figs 5A and B).

Pancreatitis and Pseudoaneurysm

Pseudoaneurysms are more common after chronic pancreatitis than after acute pancreatitis.[21] The incidence has been reported

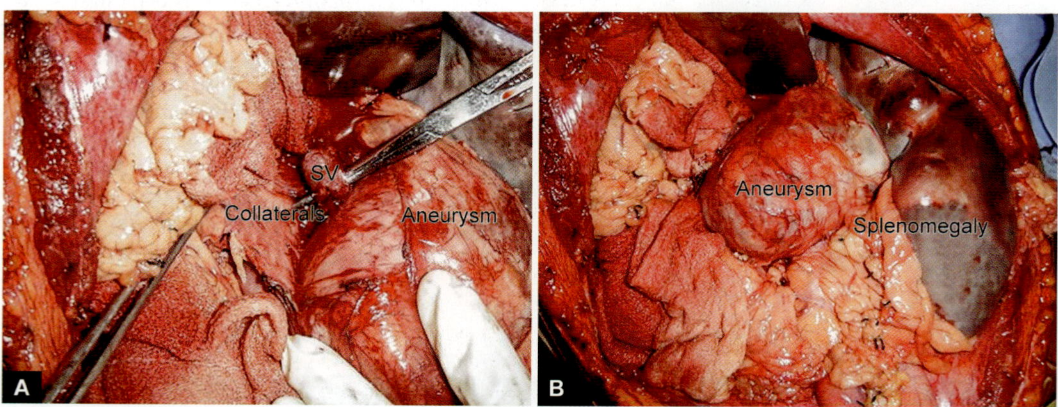

Figure 4 True aneurysm compressing SV causing portal hypertension

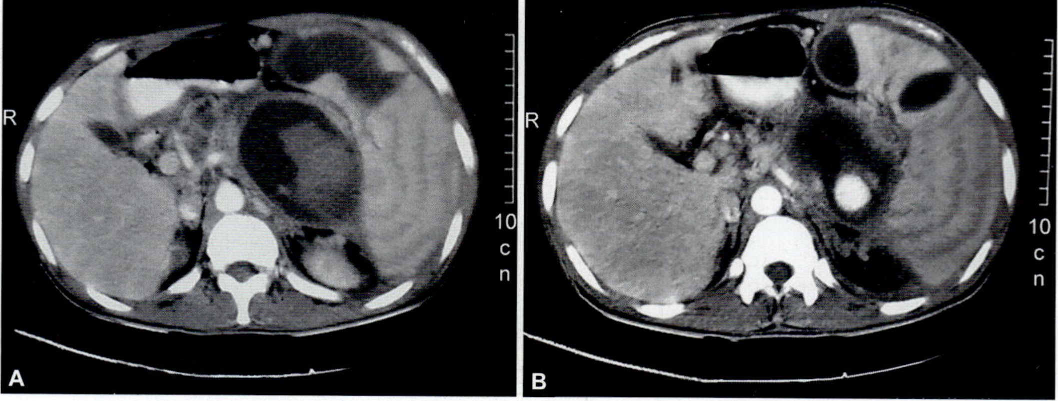

Figures 5A and B (A and B) Massive pseudoaneurysm after bleed into pseudocyst

as 10–17% in chronic pancreatitis[22,23] whereas for acute pancreatitis it is not well defined.

The splenic artery is the most common artery involved followed by pancreaticoduodenal artery and gastroduodenal artery.[33] In some series the gastroduodenal artery was the most common followed by the splenic artery.[24] Even though rare pseudoaneurysms of superior and inferior posterior pancreaticoduodenal arteries, the splenic vein and the superior mesenteric artery (SMA) have also been reported.[34]

A ruptured pseudoaneurysm in pancreatitis can be fatal in 20% of cases.[25]

Natural History and Clinical Symptoms

Splenic Artery Aneurysms are associated with progressive increase in size leading ultimately to rupture. Symptomatic SAA may present with abdominal pain in the epigastrium or left upper quadrant. In some nonspecific symptoms may be present which lead to the final diagnosis by abdominal imaging. With increasing availability of modern imaging up to 80% aneurysms are discovered incidentally in one series.[26] Rarely a mass, pulsatile or otherwise, may be detected on clinical examination.

Rupture of Splenic Artery Aneurysm

Spontaneous rupture of the aneurysm is reported to occur in 2–10% of patients as the initial presentation.[13] Risk factors for rupture of the aneurysms include pregnancy, development of symptoms, expanding aneurysms, a diameter greater than 2 cm, portal hypertension, portocaval shunt and liver transplantation.[13,33]

False aneurysms have a significantly higher risk of rupture compared to true aneurysms. A rupture presents with sudden onset severe pain in the epigastrium or more often left upper quadrant, left shoulder tip pain (Kehr's sign) and hemodynamic instability. Occasionally they may present with the double rupture phenomena within 48 hours. In this scenario the first hemorrhage occurs in to the lesser sac leading to temporary tamponade. This is followed by flooding through the epiploic foramen into the peritoneal cavity with resultant severe shock. The double rupture phenomenon was first described by Bockerman in 1930.[22,27]

Apart from intra-peritoneal bleeding, secondary erosion of the aneurysm into an adjacent viscous may lead to gastrointestinal hemorrhage. This has been described in up to 13% of patients with rupture of the aneurysm into the stomach, colon or the pancreatic duct (hemosuccus pancreaticus) in the pancreas.[5,28] Erosion in to the splenic vein may result in an arteriovenous fistula and portal hypertension.

Although relatively rare, false aneurysm of the splenic artery may be the cause of necrosis of the walls of the organs adhering to the aneurysm, and the cause of bleeding to both the lower and upper parts of the gastrointestinal tract. Aneurysm rupture to the stomach and colon have been reported.[29,30]

A large pseudoaneurysm may also result from a direct splenic artery rupture into a pseudocyst cavity.[33]

Spontaneous rupture is the most serious complication of SAA with an overall mortality rate of 25%. This is particularly high when it occurs in pregnancy where it has been found to be as high as 75%.

Postoperative

Pseudoaneurysms that develop in the presence of pancreatic fistula resulting from surgery or severe pancreatitis often present with a small sentinel bleed that precedes the major hemorrhage. In the postoperative situation a third of such patients would suffer from intraluminal hemorrhage while the majority will bleed intra-abdominally which will be detected in the abdominal drains if present.

Diagnosis

Multidetector computed tomography (MDCT) scan with three-dimensional rendering would be the initial investigation of choice to diagnose suspected VAA. SAA gives a well-defined and uniform appearance on contrast-enhanced CT, but may also show mural thrombus and peripheral calcification.

Visceral angiography is gold standard for diagnosing VAA. It can be therapeutic also. However, even visceral angiography can be false negative. In one series 11% had false negative rate and 6% needed repeat angiographic intervention for localizing the aneurysm.[31] Vasoconstriction in response to acute hemorrhage is the cause of many of these false negative results especially in postoperative settings.

Angiography has been reported to be 94–100% accurate in identifying the source of hemorrhage, its efficacy in arresting hemorrhage by embolization ranges from 64–78%.[32]

Management

True SAAs with features suggestive of low risk for rupture may be successfully managed without intervention. Radiological follow-up with 6 monthly ultrasound or CT scan should be mandatory to assess progression of the aneurysm. Active intervention should be considered if the aneurysm is symptomatic, enlarging, more than 2 cm in diameter or if found in pregnancy or childbearing age.[33] All false aneurysms of the splenic artery should be treated as soon as possible. Trastek et al. suggest that all incidental asymptomatic aneurysms detected during or before planned pregnancy should be treated before term.[20] In addition all asymptomatic aneurysms greater than 2 cm in diameter and those increasing in size during surveillance regardless of size should also be treated.[20] It is generally accepted that any SAAs detected in patients undergoing liver transplantation should also be treated.

Endovascular

It is now considered by many to be the first line of treatment in most patients with SAAs. Complications of this technique include migration of the coil and distal infarction, abscess formation and rarely aneurysm rupture. Recanalization may occur in up to 12.5% of patients after successful embolization.[34] This can be treated by either a repeat embolization or surgery.

Recent innovations in the management of SAAs include the use of endovascular stent grafts. This is a minimally invasive technique that excludes the aneurismal dilatation of the artery while preserving normal blood flow. The size and tortuosity of the splenic artery as well as the position of the aneurysm may have limitations in the deployment of the stent graft. They are more suitable for proximal aneurysms.[35] There are two major varieties of stent grafts. One is a self-expanding stent graft which has the advantage of being very flexible. The other is a balloon-expanding stent graft which has a capacity for more accurate deployment.

Stent grafts have a significantly lower risk of splenic infarction compared to embolization.

Staged combination therapy has been advocated for specific situations, especially in the management of giant aneurysms and in patients with significant comorbidities. Embolization of the aneurysm is followed by surgical excision.[36]

Patients with false SAA are usually unwell due to the underlying disease, usually pancreatitis or pancreatic fistulae. Mortality rate after open surgical intervention of false aneurysms near the head of the pancreas is reported to be around 16% and may reach up to 50% for those near the body and tail.

Combination of coils and Gelfoam gelatin can be used in case of voluminous false SAA.

Percutaneous injection of thrombin is another option in the treatment of false aneurysms in selected patients especially where catheterization may prove impractical.

Pseudoaneurysm in presence of pancreatic pseudocyst poses some special challenges. Operation and embolization play complementary management roles. Embolization is the preferred initial therapy.[36] Surgery should be reserved for failure of endovascular therapy or in an actively bleeding and hemodynamically unstable patient or for the patients who have secondary complications of pseudocyst like infection or compression.[36]

Surgery

Emergency Indications

- Failure of endovascular therapy
- Facilities for endovascular therapy not available
- Rupture into stomach or colon
- Hemodynamically unstable patients.

Elective

- Giant aneurysm not amenable to endovascular therapy
- Pseudoaneurysm associated with a pseudocyst—initially treated with endovascular therapy. However, transcatheter embolization has a higher failure rate (20%) as a primary treatment in these patients than in those without pseudocysts (13%)[32]
- Secondary complications such as infection and extrinsic compression.

Open surgery is associated with a morbidity and mortality rates of 9% and 1.3% respectively.

Splenic artery aneurysms may be approached anteriorly or laterally. The anterior approach tends to disrupt the short gastric and left gastroepiploic vessels and may increase the risk of splenic infarction. The lateral retroperitoneal approach preserves the collateral perfusion to spleen.

Laparoscopic excision of SAA has been considered by a number of authors as a less invasive alternative to open surgery at the expense of increased technical challenge.

HEPATIC ARTERY ANEURYSM (HAA)

For extrahepatic arteries true aneurysms used to be the most common, but due to ever increasing use of interventional procedures and also more prevalent use of CT scan post liver trauma pseudoaneurysms now account for 50% of all aneurysms of hepatic artery.[8]

Clinical Presentation

Hepatic artery aneurysm is predominantly seen in males (male/female ratio 3:2) and mostly during sixth and seventh decade of life. More than half of the patients present with pain in the right hypochondrium radiating to back. Free peritoneal rupture leading to severe abdominal pain along with hypovolemic shock may be seen in 20–30% cases. Relatively uncommon but intraluminal rupture into stomach or duodenum may also occur. Of all the aneurysms presenting with rupture, 50% do so by rupturing into biliary tree and of them one-third present with triad of hemobilia-biliary colic, obstructive jaundice and melena.[37] Hemobilia was found after a mean interval of 2 months secondary to rupture intrahepatic pseudoaneurysm after conservative management of blunt trauma liver.[38] Even rarer is the presentation in the form of obstructive jaundice by aneurysm causing compression on biliary tree or liver abscess. The author had a patient who developed pseudoaneurysm of right hepatic artery following Whipple's resection for periampullary carcinoma that was initially embolized had recurred due to collateral vascularization and had to be operated (Figs 6A and B).

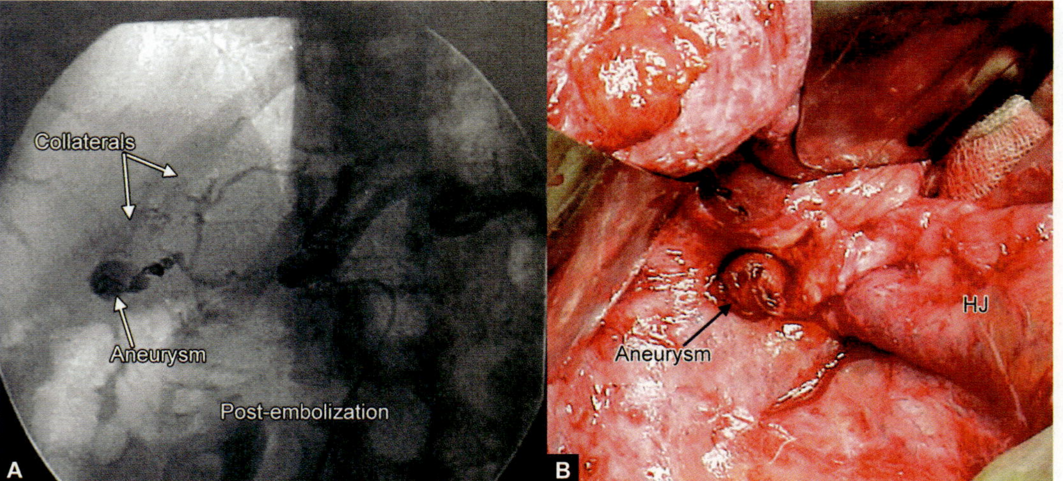

Figures 6A and B (A and B) Post whipple right hepatic artery pseudoaneurysm refilling after embolization requiring surgery

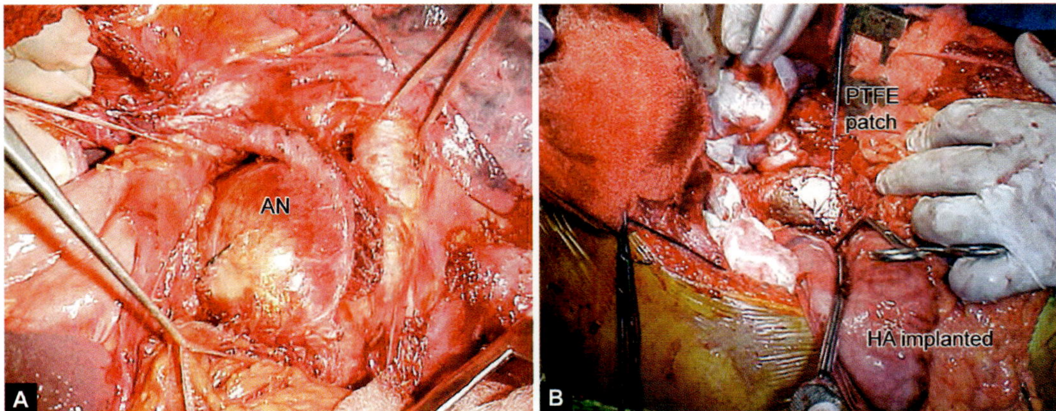

Figures 7A and B (A and B) Celiac A aneurysm excised and hepatic artery reimplanted into the PTFE patch graft

Management

Association of size and its risk of rupture for HAAs are as yet undefined. On the basis of a report of 22 patients who were followed for mean duration of 68.4 months with no reported complications, authors recommended interventions for symptomatic and high risk group (multiple aneurysms and a non-atherosclerotic etiology) patients. Ligation or embolization of hepatic artery should only be done if the portal vein patency is assured. Otherwise there is risk of hepatic infarction.

It is prudent to ensure portal vein patency prior to attempting ligation or embolization of aneurysm or affected artery. On one hand aneurysms arising from common hepatic artery or distal to that can be embolized or ligated without need for reconstruction, on the other hand aneurysms of hepatic artery proper demands vascular reconstruction to prevent hepatic ischemia as in this scenario collaterals from gastroduodenal and right gastric arteries are also disrupted. Stent graft by the virtue of their ability to maintain prograde flow is the desired technique for patients of hepatic artery proper aneurysms and for patients with hepatic insufficiency.

CELIAC ARTERY ANEURYSM

True celiac arterial aneurysms comprise of 5.9% of all VAA with male preponderance (M:F = 2:1) and a mean age of 64.2 years. Majority of them are detected incidentally, but when symptomatic may mimic pancreatitis.[39] Risk for rupture also depends on etiology. In the historic era of 1950s infectious symptomatic aneurysms were high and 87% ruptured. Etiologically, 40% were infectious (usually luetic), 7% were traumatic, and 52% were of undetermined cause.[40] However, infectious cause is uncommon in recent series where most are atherosclerotic origin with very low incidence of rupture.[41] Non-visceral arterial aneurysms are frequently associated.

Management

Intervention is indicated in aneurysms more than 2 cm size in an otherwise fit patient. In a series of 18 patients, none with size less than 2 cm in diameter had rupture. Aneurysms of the celiac artery can be treated with celiac ligation, followed by aortohepatic bypass or direct aortic reimplantation (Figs 7A and B). For patients requiring revascularization, prosthetic grafts offer better patency than saphenous vein grafts. Emergency intervention may include ligation or percutaneous transcatheter embolization in case the aneurysm ruptures.

SUPERIOR MESENTERIC ARTERY ANEURYSM (FIG. 8)

Up to a third of superior mesenteric artery aneurysms result from septic emboli. Non-hemolytic streptococci, staphylococci, and Gram-negative bacteria are the most commonly implicated organisms. Other etiologies like atherosclerosis, cystic medial dysplasia and collagen vascular disorders and polyarteritis nodosa have also been reported.[42] Mean size of the aneurysms in patients who did not rupture was 2.2 cm. Of the 13 patients who did not rupture, 10 were asymptomatic. Superior mesenteric artery is the most common site for the aneurysms arising out of arterial dissection.[43] More than 90% of superior mesenteric artery aneurysms are symptomatic, with associated abdominal pain and gastrointestinal bleeding. Acute mesenteric ischemia may result from thromboembolism of the artery.

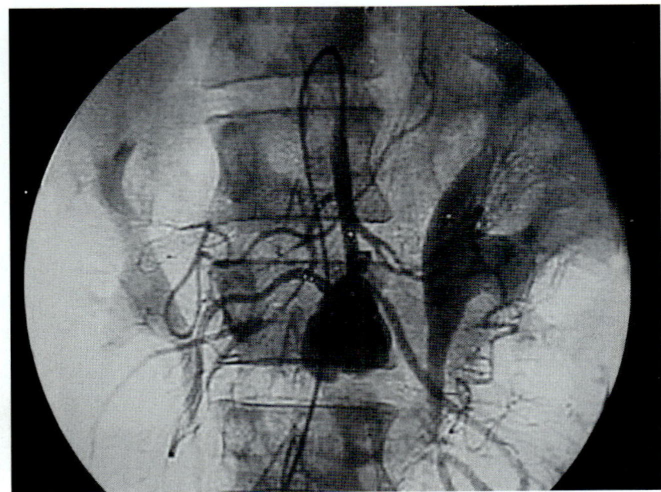

Figure 8 Mycotic aneurysm of SMA

Management

Indications for elective repair are size more than 2 cm in a good-risk patient, growth, and symptoms. Proximal and distal ligation of aneurysm bearing vessel is one of the more popular methods to treat SMA aneurysms. Trial occlusion can be performed with peroperative assessment for bowel ischemia. Usually collaterals from inferior mesenteric arteries and celiac artery provide adequate circulation to prevent ischemia. Endoaneurysmorraphy and arterial reconstruction with bypass after ligation using either vein or prosthetic graft can also be done. Venous graft is preferred for reconstruction in infected aneurysm. Proximal SMA is exposed with medial visceral rotation while distal SMA aneurysms may be approached transmesenterically.

GASTRODUODENAL ARTERY (GDA) ANEURYSM AND PANCREATICODUODENAL ARTERY (PDA) ANEURYSM

Pseudoaneurysms of pancreaticoduodenal and gastroduodenal arteries are more common than true aneurysms which account for only 3.5% of all VAA. Pancreatitis and pancreatoduodenectomy are two most usual causes for formation of pseudoaneurysm in this location.[44] In a review of 74 cases, only 7.5% of GDA aneurysms remained asymptomatic while acute presentation with rupture was seen in 52%.[45] Ruptured aneurysms usually manifest with hematemesis, melena, and hemodynamic shock. Though less frequent GDA aneurysms may present with retroperitoneal or intraperitoneal bleeds. Bleeding into the pancreatic duct (hemosuccus pancreaticus) or bleeding into the common bile duct (hemobilia) are also seen.[46] After pancreatoduodenectomy, "herald" or "sentinel" bleeding from a drain may indicate a pseudoaneurysm. A ruptured aneurysm is managed by ligation or resection, with or without vascular reconstruction, or preferably by transcatheter embolization or stenting. Although transcatheter embolization is preferred in elective and emergency settings there are limitations for it. Because of the rich collateral circulation, it is necessary to confirm that retrograde filling of the aneurysm does not occur from collateral vessels (e.g. inferior pancreaticoduodenal artery). Therefore, treatment of these aneurysms may involve embolization of both the afferent and efferent arteries (Figs 9A and B). When performing embolization in saccular aneurysms of the GDAs, either isolation of the aneurysm neck or both proximal and distal embolization should be performed rather than proximal embolization alone as the aneurysm may recruit a new vascular supply in a retrograde manner.

Complications of embolization are usually limited because of well-formed collateral circulation. However, this may be jeopardized by previous radiation or surgery. If the origin of either the CAA or SMA is occluded, embolization of GDA and PDA becomes much more complex. In this situation, maintaining patency of the parent artery is essential to prevent bowel ischemia.[47]

Others

Other rare aneurysms include inferior mesenteric artery aneurysm, aneurysm arising from branches of superior mesenteric artery, branches of inferior mesenteric artery[48] (Fig. 10) and gastroepiploic arteries.

CONCLUSION

Visceral artery aneurysms are rare. Rupture occurs in up to 25% cases and is associated with high mortality. They are detected more frequently due to widespread use of CT scans. Treatment is usually dictated by the presentation, location and the associated risk factors. Various options for treating VAA include endovascular treatment, open surgical repair and laparoscopic surgery. Treatment is recommended for all VAA larger than 2 cm and aneurysms in women of childbearing age.

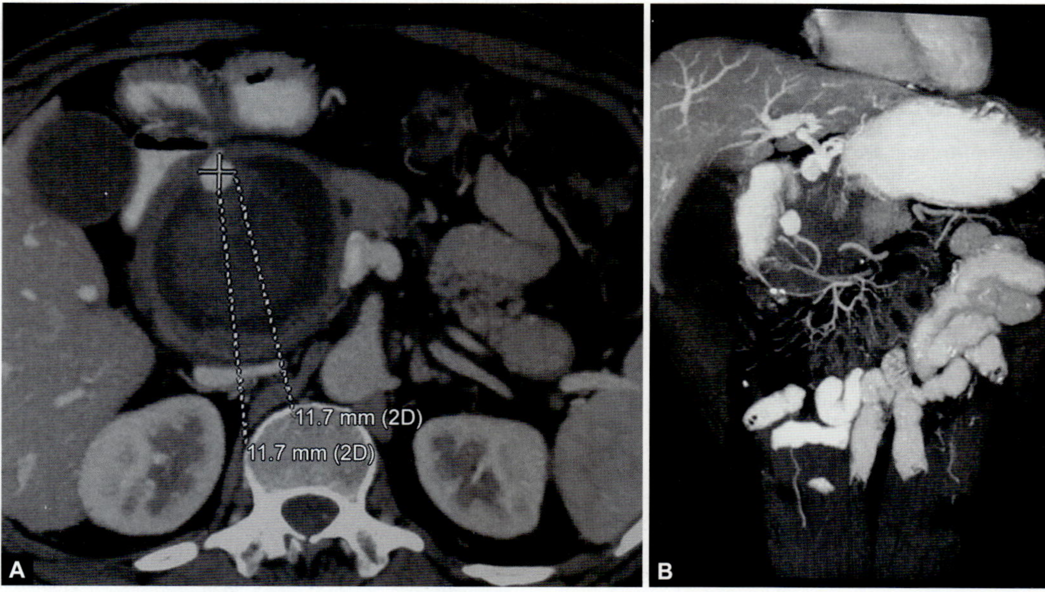

Figures 9A and B (A and B) PDA arch aneurysm

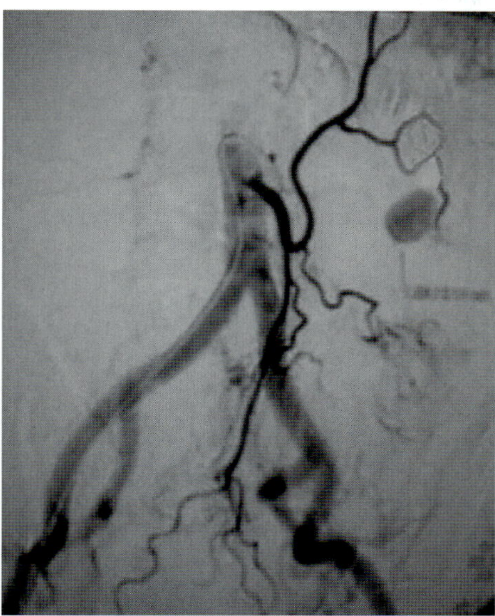

Figure 10 Pseudoaneurysm of left colic artery after Tenckhoff catheter removal

REFERENCES

1. Carmeci C, McClenathan J. Visceral artery aneurysms as seen in a community hospital. Am J Surg. 2000;179:486-9.
2. Hossain A, Reis ED, Dave SP, Kerstein MD, Hollier LH. Visceral artery aneurysms: experience in a tertiary-care center. Am Surg. 2001;67:432-7.
3. Panayiotopoulos YP, Assadourian R, Taylor PR. Aneurysms of the visceral and renal arteries. Ann R Coll Surg Engl. 1996;78:412-9.
4. Stanley JC, Thompson NW, Fry WJ. Splanchnic artery aneurysms. Arch Surg. 1970;101:689-97.
5. Messina LM, Shanley CJ. Visceral artery aneurysms. Surg Clin North Am. 1997;77:425-42.
6. Shanley CJ, Shah NL, Messina LM. Common splanchnic artery aneurysms: splenic, hepatic, and celiac. Ann Vasc Surg. 1996;10:315-22.
7. Wig JD, Khanna SK, Nair PM, Suri S, Dutta BN, Talwar BL. Unusual mycotic aneurysms. J Indian Med Assoc. 1980;75(7):143-5.
8. Pasha SF, Gloviczki P, Stanson AW, Kamath PS. Splanchnic artery aneurysms. Mayo Clin Proc. 2007;82:472-9.
9. de Vries JE, Schattenkerk ME, Malt RA. Complications of splenic artery aneurysm other than intraperitoneal rupture. Surgery. 1982;91:200-4.
10. Pilleul F, Beuf O. Diagnosis of splanchnic artery aneurysms and pseudoaneurysms, with special reference to contrast enhanced 3D MR angiography: a review. Acta Radiol. 2004;45:702-8.
11. Kenningham R, Hershman MJ, McWilliams RG, Campbell F. Incidental splenic artery aneurysm. J R Soc Med. 2002;95:460-1.
12. Mattar SG, Lumsden AB. The management of splenic artery aneurysms: experience with 23 cases. Am J Surg. 1995;169:580-4.
13. Siablis D, Papathanassiou ZG, Karnabatidis D, Christeas N, Katsanos K, Vagianos C. Splenic arteriovenous fistula and sudden onset of portal hypertension as complications of a ruptured splenic artery aneurysm: successful treatment with transcatheter arterial embolization. A case study and review of the literature. World J Gastroenterol. 2006;12:4264-6.
14. Abbas MA, Stone WM, Fowl RJ, Gloviczki P, Oldenburg WA, Pairolero PC, et al. Splenic artery aneurysms: two decades experience at Mayo clinic. Ann Vasc Surg. 2002;16:442-9.
15. Lee PC, Rhee RY, Gordon RY, Fung JJ, Webster MW. Management of splenic artery aneurysms: the significance of portal and essential hypertension. J Am Coll Surg. 1999;189:483-90.
16. Selo-Ojeme DO, Welch CC. Review: spontaneous rupture of splenic artery aneurysm in pregnancy. Eur J Obstet Gynecol Reprod Biol. 2003;109:124-7.
17. Garbagna G, Cornalba G, Rota L. Splenic artery aneurysms in patients with portal hypertension (author's transl). Radiol Med. 1980;66:239-42.
18. Puttini M, Aseni P, Brambilla G, Belli L. Splenic artery aneurysms in portal hypertension. J Cardiovasc Surg (Torino). 1982;23:490-3.
19. Goldberg RF, Maley W, Kennedy EP, Yeo CJ, Lavu H. Giant splenic artery pseudoaneurysm. J Gastrointest Surg. 2011;15:1063-6.
20. Tessier DJ, Stone WM, Fowl RJ, Abbas MA, Andrews JC, Bower TC, et al. Clinical features and management of splenic artery pseudoaneurysm: case series and cumulative review of literature. J Vasc Surg. 2003;38:969-74.
21. de PM, Berney T, Buhler L, Delgadillo X, Mentha G, Morel P. Management of bleeding pseudoaneurysms in patients with pancreatitis. Br J Surg. 1999;86:29-32.
22. White AF, Baum S, Buranasiri S. Aneurysms secondary to pancreatitis. AJR Am J Roentgenol. 1976;127:393-6.
23. Kiviluoto T, Kivisaari L, Kivilaakso E, Lempinen M. Pseudocysts in chronic pancreatitis. Surgical results in 102 consecutive patients. Arch Surg. 1989;124:240-3.
24. Carr JA, Cho JS, Shepard AD, Nypaver TJ, Reddy DJ. Visceral pseudoaneurysms due to pancreatic pseudocysts: rare but lethal complications of pancreatitis. J Vasc Surg. 2000;32:722-30.
25. Balachandra S, Siriwardena AK. Systematic appraisal of the management of the major vascular complications of pancreatitis. Am J Surg. 2005;190:489-95.
26. de CJ, Quinn T, Gagner M. Laparoscopic exclusion of a splenic artery aneurysm using a lateral approach permits preservation of the spleen. Surg Laparosc Endosc Percutan Tech. 2001;11:221-4.
27. O'Grady JP, Day EJ, Toole AL, Paust JC. Splenic artery aneurysm rupture in pregnancy. A review and case report. Obstet Gynecol. 1977;50:627-30.
28. Harper PC, Gamelli RL, Kaye MD. Recurrent hemorrhage into the pancreatic duct from a splenic artery aneurysm. Gastroenterology. 1984;87:417-20.
29. Rosales-Zabal JM, Navarro-Jarabo JM, Rivera-Irigoin R, et al. Rupture of a splenic pseudoaneurysm in the colon as an unusual cause of rectal bleeding. Colorectal Dis. 2012;14:e425-6.
30. Wierzbicki T, Szmeja J, Borejsza-Wysocki M, Męczyński M, Smuszkiewicz P, Katulska K, et al. Massive bleeding from upper gastrointestinal tract as a symptom of rupture of splenic artery aneurysm to stomach. Med Sci Monit. 2012;18:CS8-11.
31. Zyromski NJ, Vieira C, Stecker M, Nakeeb A, Pitt HA, Lillemoe KD, et al. Improved outcomes in postoperative and pancreatitis-related visceral pseudoaneurysms. J Gastrointest Surg. 2007;11:50-5.
32. Belli AM, Markose G, Morgan R. The role of interventional radiology in the management of abdominal visceral artery aneurysms. Cardiovasc Intervent Radiol. 2012;35:234-43.
33. Al-Habbal Y, Christophi C, Muralidharan V. Aneurysms of the splenic artery—a review. Surgeon. 2010;8:223-31.
34. Carr SC, Pearce WH, Vogelzang RL, McCarthy WJ, Nemcek AA Jr, Yao JS. Current management of visceral artery aneurysms. Surgery. 1996;120:627-33.
35. Karaman K, Onat L, Sirvanci M, Olga R. Endovascular stent graft treatment in a patient with splenic artery aneurysm. Diagn Interv Radiol. 2005;11:119-21.
36. Bakhos CT, McIntosh BC, Nukta FA, Fiedler PN, Denatale RW, Sweeney TF, et al. Staged arterial embolization and surgical resection of a giant splenic artery aneurysm. Ann Vasc Surg. 2007;21:208-10.

37. Zachary K, Geier S, Pellecchia C, et al. Jaundice secondary to hepatic artery aneurysm: radiological appearance and clinical features. Am J Gastroenterol. 1986;81:295-8.
38. Thumma VM, Bheerappa N, Sastry RA. Has incidence of haemobilia increased with increasing conservative management of blunt liver injuries? HPB. 2008;10:31.
39. Sachdev-Ost U. Visceral artery aneurysms: review of current management options. Mt Sinai J Med. 2010;77:296-303.
40. Graham LM, Stanley JC, Whitehouse WM, Jr., Zelenock GB, Wakefield TW, Cronenwett JL, et al. Celiac artery aneurysms: historic (1745-1949) versus contemporary (1950-1984) differences in etiology and clinical importance. J Vasc Surg. 1985;2:757-64.
41. Stone WM, Abbas MA, Gloviczki P, Fowl RJ, Cherry KJ. Celiac arterial aneurysms: a critical reappraisal of a rare entity. Arch Surg. 2002;137:670-4.
42. Stone WM, Abbas M, Cherry KJ, Fowl RJ, Gloviczki P. Superior mesenteric artery aneurysms: is presence an indication for intervention? J Vasc Surg. 2002;36:234-7.
43. Cormier F, Ferry J, Artru B, Wechsler B, Cormier JM. Dissecting aneurysms of the main trunk of the superior mesenteric artery. J Vasc Surg. 1992;15:424-30.
44. Otah E, Cushin BJ, Rozenblit GN, Neff R, Otah KE, Cooperman AM. Visceral artery pseudoaneurysms following pancreatoduodenectomy. Arch Surg. 2002;137:55-9.
45. Habib N, Hassan S, Abdou R, Torbey E, Alkaied H, Maniatis T, et al. Gastroduodenal artery aneurysm, diagnosis, clinical presentation and management: a concise review. Ann Surg Innov Res. 2013;7:4.
46. Fodor M, Fodor L, Ciuce C. Gastroduodenal artery pseudoaneurysm ruptured in the common bile duct. Acta Chir Belg. 2010;110:103-5.
47. Belli AM, Markose G, Morgan R. The role of interventional radiology in the management of abdominal visceral artery aneurysms. Cardiovasc Intervent Radiol. 2012;35:234-43.
48. Ram R, Swarnalatha G, Varma V, Desai M, Prasad N, Sastry RA, et al. Pseudoaneurysm of left colic artery after Tenckhoff catheter removal, with unrecognized fungal peritonitis. J Nephrol. 2008;21:962-4.

CHAPTER 32

Mesenteric Ischemia

D K Sharma

INTRODUCTION

Gastrointestinal blood flow is termed as splanchnic circulation and includes circulation to pancreas, liver, spleen and omentum apart from the stomach, small bowel and colorectum. Mesenteric circulation refers to blood supply to the latter group of gastrointestinal organs. Since most of the vascular disorders of splanchnic circulation affect the intestines, mesenteric ischemia is the more important entity and focus of this chapter.

Mesenteric ischemia is a challenging disease process with difficulties involved in its diagnosis, the limited time window it offers for carrying out a potentially effective management, its complex pathophysiology, its associations with other highly morbid diseases and the high morbidity and mortality associated with it. Early diagnosis and appropriate, timely treatment are essential if the patient is to survive. At the same time, clinical signs and symptoms are hardly specific, investigations are difficult to choose, perform and interpret and both these factors impact prompt treatment also. Moreover, the treatment modalities require highly specialized services ranging from gastrointestinal surgery, intensive care medicine to vascular surgery. Even when optimally managed, the mortality rate is nearly 40% overall.[1,2]

There is a wide range of etiologic processes leading to mesenteric ischemia. Moreover, pathophysiology of these etiologies differs enough to lead to a significant difference in their management. The clinical course also varies depending on the site as well as type (i.e., arteries or veins) of vascular involvement. The clinician, therefore, has to be able to recognize subtle differences in presentations of different etiologies as well as different vessels involved.

Nevertheless, even with this gloomy background, there is hope for the patient afflicted with this dreadful condition if high index of suspicion is maintained, appropriate investigations are chosen and prompt and suitable treatment is instituted. To this end, a thorough understanding of all aspects of the disease is necessary.

ANATOMIC CONSIDERATIONS

Arterial Supply

There are four major areas of the gastrointestinal tract (GIT) based on the primary arterial source. The primary arteries of the GIT are—celiac artery/axis (CA), superior mesenteric artery (SMA) and inferior mesenteric artery (IMA). Apart from the origin, course and distribution of these major GI vessels, it is of crucial importance to understand the intercommunications and collateral circulation among them. The ensuing text is an attempt at description of these two aspects of intestinal arterial supply.

The celiac axis (CA) is the largest branch of the abdominal aorta and arises at the level of lower portion of T12 or upper portion of L1 vertebra, projecting at a right angle to the anterior surface of aorta (Fig. 1).[3] The CA gives rise to splenic artery, common hepatic artery and left gastric artery in its most common (93%) presentation.[4]

The SMA arises approximately 1–1.5 cm distal to the origin of CA, at an angle of 20–30 degrees from anterior surface of the aorta, at the level of upper portion of L1 (Fig. 1). It is approximately 1 cm in diameter at its origin and passes behind the body and then anterior to uncinate process of the pancreas, to finally emerge under lower pancreatic border, anterior to third part of duodenum. Named branches of SMA are—inferior pancreaticoduodenal artery, middle colic artery (MCA), right colic artery (RCA) and ileocolic artery (Fig. 2). Inferior pancreaticoduodenal artery is the first branch of SMA and communicates with pancreaticoduodenal branches of the gastroduodenal artery which in turn is a branch of the hepatic artery. This is the most important communication between the CA and SMA arterial system and provides a collateral route in vascular occlusive pathologic states. The MCA is the second branch of SMA, arising just caudal to the inferior pancreaticoduodenal artery, in proximity to the inferior border

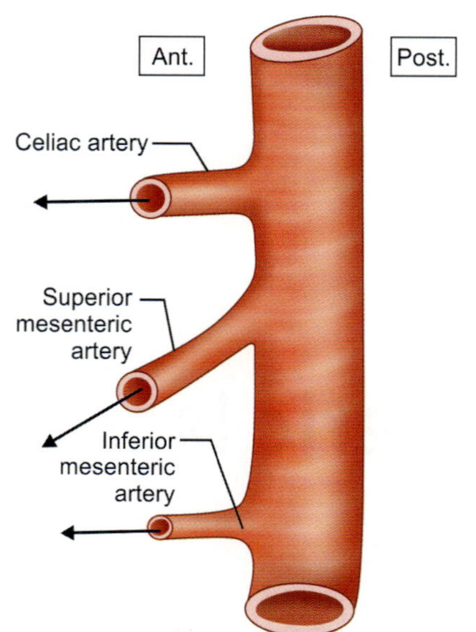

Figure 1 Schematic representation of the three mesenteric branches of aorta, illustrating their angles and levels of origin. The superior mesenteric artery (SMA) arises at an acute angle, making it the most susceptible to thromboembolism

of pancreas. Its right branch communicates with ascending limb of RCA while the left branch communicates with ascending limb of the left colic artery (LCA). The latter is a branch of the IMA and constitutes an important communication between SMA and IMA. The RCA may arise separately from SMA (40%) or as a common trunk with MCA (50%), or may have a common trunk with ileocolic artery. The latter may arise separately from SMA and from its left aspect gives off branches (12–20) to the small bowel, after entering the mesentery. Importantly, in about 20% individuals MCA may be absent wherein the RCA and hypogastric artery become important sources of supply to the colon if IMA is blocked or sacrificed.

The IMA arises from aorta at the level of L3 (Fig. 1) and divides into LCA, multiple sigmoid arteries (usually 3–4 in number) and superior rectal artery. The LCA divides into an ascending and a descending branch. The sigmoid arteries may also arise from distal portion of the descending branch of LCA (Fig. 3).

These three arterial systems intercommunicate. For the sake of understanding, these intercommunications can be categorized in eight regions: (1) among CA branches; (2) CA and SMA; (3) among SMA branches; (4) SMA and IMA; (5) among IMA branches; (6) IMA and internal iliac arteries; (7) CA and IMA and (8) parietal and gastrointestinal branches (parietovisceral communications) of aorta.

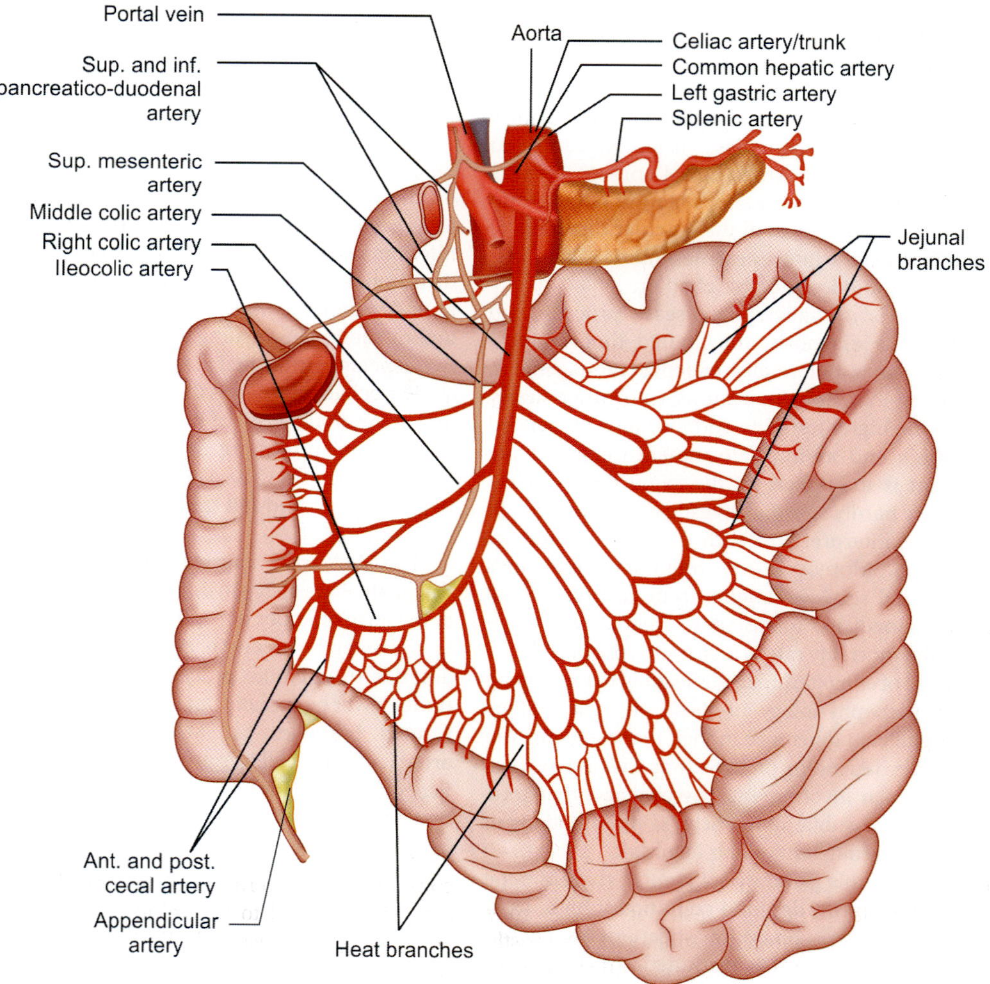

Figure 2 Branches and distribution of the superior mesenteric artery (SMA)

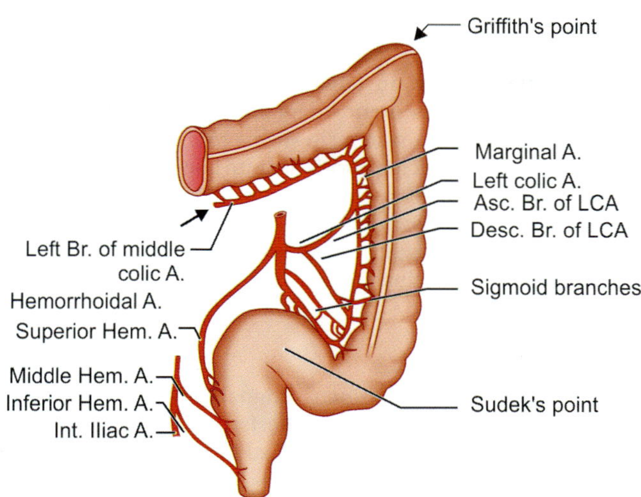

Figure 3 Representation of branches and distribution of inferior mesenteric artery (IMA). Marginal artery, Arch of Riolan and critical points (of Griffith & Sudek) are also shown

Left gastroepiploic artery, a branch of splenic artery communicates with right gastroepiploic artery arising from gastroduodenal branch of the common hepatic artery. Right gastric artery, also arising from the hepatic artery communicates with the left gastric artery along the lesser curvature of the stomach. The large size of CA, multiple blood supply, profuse extramural and intramural communications among the supplying vessels ensure that stomach is mostly immune to ischemia (Fig. 4).

Celiac artery and SMA can communicate through various channels—a common origin of SMA and CA (rare, 1% incidence); an embryologic remnant channel directly communicating these two (Arch of Buhler) (Fig. 5); dorsal pancreatic artery arising from splenic artery and communicating with branches of MCA; etc. Thus, if the CA is blocked, gastrohepatic circulation is maintained through these channels from the SMA system.

Main communication between SMA and IMA systems are through meandering mesenteric artery and the marginal artery of Drummond. Meandering mesenteric artery[5] joins the ascending limb of LCA to SMA just proximal to origin of MCA. It is often long, follows an inconstant course and is present in approximately 2/3 of individuals.

There has been a lot of confusion regarding this often vitally important communicating vessel which explains the profusion of names that have been given to it—meso-mesenteric artery, arch of Riolan, marginal artery of Drummond, arch of Treves, central anastomotic artery of the colon, middle-left colic collateral, accessory MCA, etc. One of the important clarifications in this regard is that the marginal artery of Drummond is distinct from meandering mesenteric artery. This vessel connects ascending branch of LCA to left branch of MCA and is quite constant in position along the transverse and descending portions of colon (Fig. 6).

The marginal artery of Drummond extends in region of transverse, descending, sigmoid colon and across the rectosigmoid junction. Griffith point is the area where left branch of MCA and ascending branch of LCA anastomose in region of splenic flexure of colon to provide continuity to the marginal artery and this anastomosis can be functionally lacking or inadequate in approximately 5% cases, hence the term "Critical Point of Griffith".[6] Continuity of the marginal artery may be lacking in relation to descending colon (5%), sigmoid colon (20%) and rectosigmoid region (most often).[7]

Superior rectal artery—the terminal branch of IMA—communicates with middle and inferior rectal arteries arising from hypogastric vessels, thus enabling a major potential collateral circulation to the rectum and sigmoid colon. Although Sudek had postulated a critical point in blood supply to the sigmoid colon in the region between the last sigmoid branch of LCA and the superior rectal artery, this has later been shown to be incorrect.[6] As can be discerned, these communications are also systemic-visceral communications.

Other systemic visceral communications of note are—iliolumbar arteries and superior and inferior epigastric arteries through circumflex iliac and femoral arteries.

Branches from splenic artery may communicate with the LCA branches, often in the region of splenic flexure.

The following scenarios illustrate the importance of these communications/collateral systems in pathologic states as well as

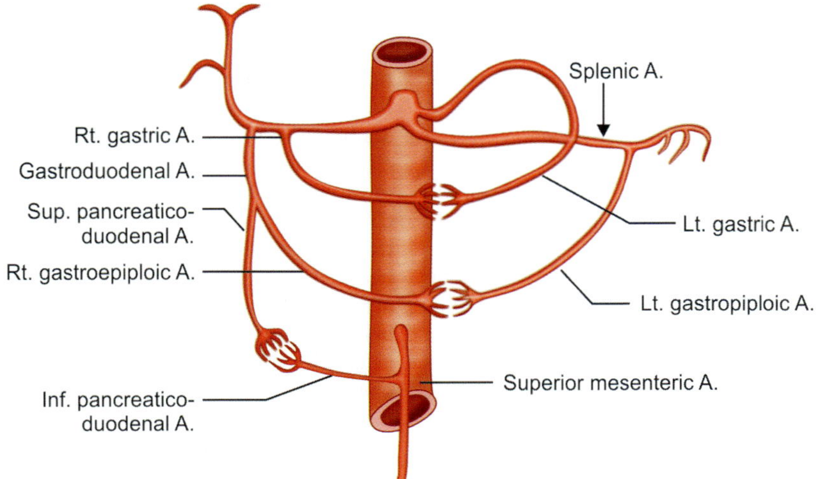

Figure 4 Schematic representations of main celiac axis (CA) and superior mesenteric artery (SMA) communications

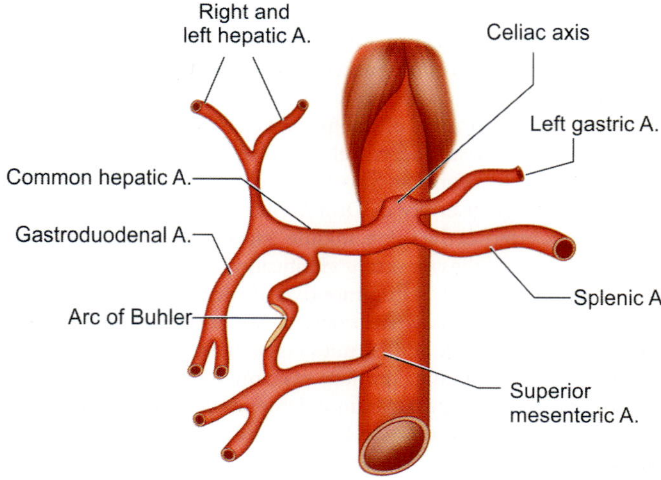

Figure 5 The Arch of Buhler

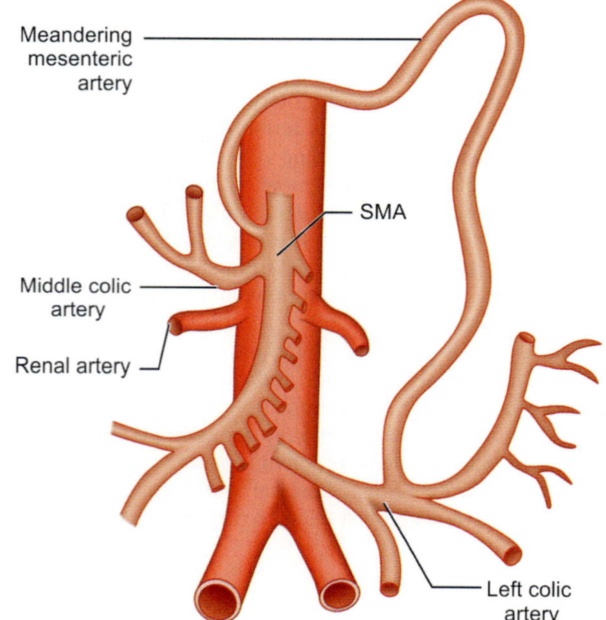

Figure 6 Meandering mesenteric artery in one of its described positions. The blood flow can be in either direction, depending upon the site of blockage. Exact points of the SMA-IMA it connects are variable.

practical implications when dealing with possibility of mesenteric ischemia.

Superior mesenteric artery occlusion is often compensated by collateralization from CA through the pancreaticoduodenal loop described above, and from IMA through the meandering mesenteric artery. It is especially important to recognize contribution of the latter to an occluded SMA during aortic reconstruction surgery, because if it is sacrificed, the whole of midgut might become gangrenous.[8,9] In chronic arteriosclerosis, IMA is the most commonly occluded vessel (of the three mesenteric vessels), and it is involved in almost all abdominal aortic aneurysms.[10] Therefore if an occluded IMA system is being maintained by collaterals from SMA or is involved in an aortic aneurysm, it is important to preserve these collaterals while performing surgery for arteriosclerosis or aortic aneurysm. Again an important aspect is the recognition of the meandering mesenteric artery and whether blood flow in this is from SMA to IMA system; in such a case, if it is damaged or sacrificed, bowel in IMA territory is likely to become gangrenous.[10] In chronic obstruction of the IMA, compensatory blood flow also comes from hypogastric circulation. It must however be remembered that hypogastric collaterals have practically no part to play in acute IMA occlusion.[8]

Venous Drainage

By and large, mesenteric venous drainage follows the arterial supply. The superior mesenteric vein formed by veins draining regions corresponding to those supplied by the SMA merges with the splenic vein posterior to the pancreas to form the portal vein. The splenic vein receives tributaries from fundus and left portion of the greater curvature of the stomach (short gastric veins), left gastroepiploic vein, pancreatic veins draining body and tail of the pancreas and the inferior mesenteric vein. The superior mesenteric vein receives right gastroepiploic vein, anterior and posterior inferior pancreaticoduodenal veins (anterior and posterior superior pancreaticoduodenal veins usually drain into right gastroepiploic and portal veins, respectively), apart from venous drainage of small bowel and large bowel up to the transverse colon. The inferior mesenteric vein begins as superior rectal vein and ascends, receiving tributaries from sigmoid and left colic veins, thus draining the rectum, sigmoid colon, descending colon and the splenic flexure. The portocaval anastomoses and potential collaterals between these two systems become important in mesenteric venous occlusion.

PHYSIOLOGY

In terms of the proportion of blood received, mesenteric circulation is one of the largest regional circulations in the body, receiving approximately 25% of the cardiac output under resting conditions.[11] The SMA supplies the maximum blood flow to the splanchnic circulation among the three main arteries. After penetrating the bowel wall, arteries divide and successively become smaller, finally becoming arterioles when the diameter reaches approximately 25 μm. Arterioles are the resistance vessels of splanchnic circulation because a small change in their internal diameter has a highly disproportionate effect on splanchnic circulation resistance.[12] Their thick muscle coat is highly responsive to various stimuli and they modulate and determine the intestinal circulation to a large extent.[13,14] Further division of arterioles transforms them into capillaries, termed the exchange vessels because nutrients, oxygen, electrolytes and fluid are exchanged across their thin walls. The junctions of arterioles and capillaries bear precapillary sphincters which control entry of blood into capillaries. Only a small number of precapillary sphincters are open at any time, hence ensuring that only a small part of the total nutrient bed is perfused at any given time. These sphincters therefore are the principal determinants of quantum and place of exchange of various substances as well as redistribution of blood from one nutrient bed to another, leading to what is referred to as physiologic shunting.[15]

Distal to the capillary bed, the venules join successively to form veins and these vessels serve as capacitance vessels in that they contain a large amount of blood at any time. Veins are thinner, but contain proportionately more smooth muscle. When the smooth muscle in their walls contracts there is shifting of a large amount of blood into the general circulation. Moreover, the raised venous pressure is conducted to the capillaries, leading to increased efflux of fluid across their walls with resultant edema and luminal fluid accumulation.

Regulation of Mesenteric Blood Flow

The basal vascular smooth muscle tone is modulated by various contractile and dilatory forces, in turn changing the intestinal blood flow. These forces can be either extrinsic or intrinsic.

Extrinsic Control

Hemodynamic factors (systemic arterial blood pressure, cardiac output and blood volume), autonomic nervous system (mainly sympathetic neural system) and neurohormonal substances contribute to extrinsic control of the mesenteric blood flow. Parasympathetic nerve supply, essentially from the vagi, can indirectly affect intestinal blood flow through mechanical (by altering intestinal motility) and metabolic (by influencing gastrointestinal secretions) effects, but there is no appreciable direct vascular effects. Main effect of sympathetic stimulation is mesenteric arteriolar constriction leading to reduction of intestinal blood flow and is mediated mainly by α-adrenergic receptors. This leads to redistribution of blood within the mesenteric circulation. Moreover, constriction of venous smooth muscle causes blood volume shift to the systemic circulation.[16] Overall, the main physiologic effect of sympathetic stimulation is decrease of mesenteric blood flow, during conditions that require increase of blood flow to systemic circulation, e.g. during physical stress or activity. When sympathetic discharge becomes excessive or continued, it can cause mesenteric hypoperfusion and resultant ischemia.[17-19]

Sympathetic stimulation also causes redistribution of blood flow away from intestinal mucosa, making it more vulnerable to ischemic damage.

Some substances cause dilatation of mesenteric arterial bed by increasing levels of cyclic AMP (cAMP), either by stimulating adenylate cyclase, or by inhibiting phosphodiesterase. It is by the latter mechanism that papaverine exerts its action (Flow chart 1).

Various circulating neurohormonal substances cause changes in mesenteric circulation. However, the exact effect of each of these is not yet known. The effects of some of these substances have been summarized in Table 1. Similarly, drugs can have profound effects on mesenteric circulation (Table 1). Their impact is important from both etiologic as well as therapeutic point of view.

Flow chart 1 Role of cyclic AMP in mesenteric arterial vasodilatation

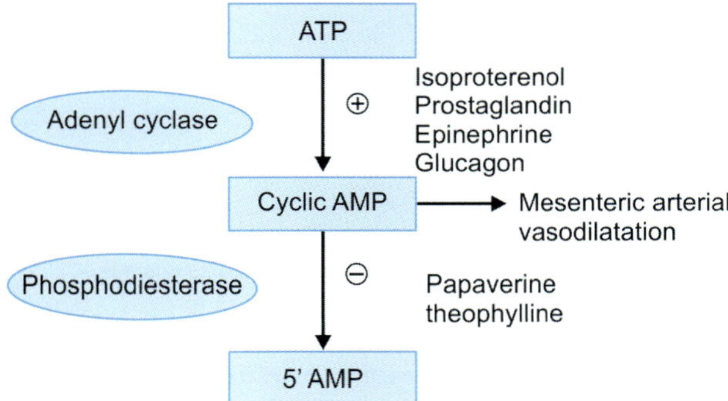

Table 1: Effects of various pharmacologic agents/substances on mesenteric circulation

Agent/Drug	*Mechanism*	*Effect*	*Comment*
Norepinephrine Methoxamine, Metaraminol, Phenylephrine	α-adrenoreceptor stimulation	Constriction of mesenteric vasculature	
Phentolamine	α-adrenoreceptor blockage	Dilatation of mesenteric vasculature	Causes decreased systemic arterial pressure, therefore may decrease intestinal blood even while dilating local mesenteric vasculature
Isoproterenol	β-adrenoreceptor stimulant	Mesenteric vasodilatation	Increases intestinal blood flow unless SAP falls significantly enough to cause reduced regional blood flow
Propranolol	β-adrenoreceptor antagonist	Blocks intestinal vasodilatation	
Epinephrine	α- and β-adrenoreceptor agonist at low and high levels respectively	Various effects: low concentration—intestinal vasodilatation; high concentration—vasoconstriction	
Dopamine	Low concentration—agonist action on dopaminergic receptors in mesenteric vessels; high concentration (>10 μg/kg/min)—α-adrenoreceptor stimulation	Low concentration—vasodilatation; high concentration—vasoconstriction	

Contd...

Contd...

Agent/Drug	*Mechanism*	*Effect*	*Comment*
Histamine		Dilation of mesenteric blood vessels; constriction of non-vascular intestinal smooth muscle	Increase in intestinal blood flow due to vasodilation limited by non-vascular smooth muscle contraction
Serotonin	?Physiologic role	Variable responses	High concentration required for any potentially therapeutic use
Bradykinin		Vasodilation	
Vasopressin		Vasoconstriction of intestinal circulation; release triggered by systemic hypotension; may exacerbate mesenteric ischemia if systemic hypotension is due to mesenteric ischemia	Selective effect on splanchnic resistance vessels, more than systemic circulation; clinically used in GI bleed. Can precipitate occlusive intestinal ischemia
Angiotensin II		Vasoconstriction of intestinal circulation	Systemic hypotension causes release
Gastrointestinal and pancreatic hormones			Administration in physiologic doses shows no appreciable effect on GI blood flow
Pentagastric, ?Gastrin		Decrease mesenteric vascular resistance	Increase in intestinal blood flow
Secretin		Vasodilatation	
Glucagon			Variable responses
Cholecystokinin		Vasoconstriction/vasodilatation under different conditions	
Tolazoline	Direct smooth muscle relaxation		More rapid onset of action; preferred for intra-arterial injection
Papaverine	Phosphodiesterase inactivation→Direct smooth muscle relaxation		More effective for infusing in mesenteric arterial circulation since it is almost completely inactivated by single passage through liver
Sodium nitroprusside	Direct smooth muscle relaxation		Used for acute systemic arterial hypertension; extremely short duration of action
Caffeine		Vasodilator; may be modulated due to associated sympathomimetic action	
Sodium nitrite, aminophylline	Direct smooth muscle action	Vasodilatation	
Digoxin		Intestinal vasoconstriction	Predisposing factor in nonocclusive mesenteric ischemia
Ergotamine		Vasoconstriction	Used for migraine; Predisposing factor for mesenteric ischemia
PG E1	Increased cAMP	Vasodilatation	Used for diagnostic and therapeutic purpose

Intrinsic Regulation

Mesenteric circulation is also intrinsically controlled by local mechanisms that include instantaneously effective myogenic and metabolic controls, along with other regulatory mechanisms. Myogenic mechanisms involve arteriolar constriction or relaxation in response to increased or decreased arterial transmural pressures, resulting in maintenance of a constant capillary pressure and thereby transcapillary fluid exchange. This process of maintenance of a uniform total intestinal blood supply despite wide variations in systemic blood pressures is referred to as auto-regulation.[20] Even when pressures drop from 100 mm Hg to 30 mm Hg, intestinal villus blood flow has been shown to remain constant.[21]

Metabolic regulatory mechanism comes into play when there is tissue hypoxia and is mediated by both reduced oxygen level and accumulation of metabolites, leading to arteriolar smooth muscle relaxation. Indirectly, hypoxia may affect the circulation by causing changes in intestinal tone and motility.

Mesenteric ischemia can be of two types: (1) acute and (2) chronic. Acute mesenteric ischemia (AMI) refers to a sudden occlusion of intestinal blood supply, sufficient to affect its metabolic activity as well as threaten its viability. Chronic mesenteric ischemia, as the name suggests, is an insidious process of intestinal blood flow, allowing development of collaterals and thereby leading to less dramatic consequences.

ACUTE MESENTERIC ISCHEMIA

There is high morbidity and mortality associated with AMI. This is possibly due to three factors—its occurrence in a relatively elderly age group, having associated comorbid conditions which may also be causally related; a delay in diagnosing the condition due to low index of suspicion; and difficulty in optimizing the patient before interventions. A confusion regarding who would best manage such a patient as well as an imperative need for an often unattainable interdisciplinary coordination also contribute to the dismal prognosis.

Etiopathogenesis

Most of the blood reaching the intestine supplies the mucosa, it being the most metabolically active among the three intestinal layers. Consequently, when there is sudden compromise of the intestinal blood supply, mucosa is the worst affected. Most of the pathologic consequences of acute intestinal ischemia also arise from mucosal injury. Capillary integrity is compromised, leading to exudation and thereby bowel wall edema. The concomitant loss of barrier function allows bacterial translocation and endotoxemia. There is also efflux of fluid into the bowel lumen, leading to its distension, which may further worsen the mucosal blood supply. The mucosa may then slough, leading to formation of mucosal ulcers. If blood supply is further compromised, muscular and serosal layers also will get ischemic and later on gangrenous. In addition, if the intestinal blood supply is restored, further insult may occur due to "reperfusion injury", ensuing due to free oxygen radicals,[22] vasopressin and rennin-angiotensin system,[23-25] among others.

An additional important mechanism is mesenteric vasoconstriction that ensues in response to arterial occlusion, which further worsens the ischemia.

Acute mesenteric ischemia is caused by one of four precipitating causes—(1) acute embolism, (2) acute thrombosis, (3) nonocclusive mesenteric ischemia (NOMI) and (4) mesenteric venous thrombosis (MVT). It is important to recognize differences among clinical syndromes caused by each of these mechanisms since there are marked differences in their managements and early institution of correct management is so crucial in determining successful outcomes.

Acute Arterial Embolism

It is the most common cause of AMI, being reported to cause 25–50% of all cases of AMI.[26] The affected patient is usually elderly with risk factors like recent myocardial infarction, congestive heart failure, arrhythmias or rheumatic heart disease. There are usually no preceding/chronic symptoms of abdominal pain which might suggest long standing vascular occlusion, as is the case with thrombotic occlusion.

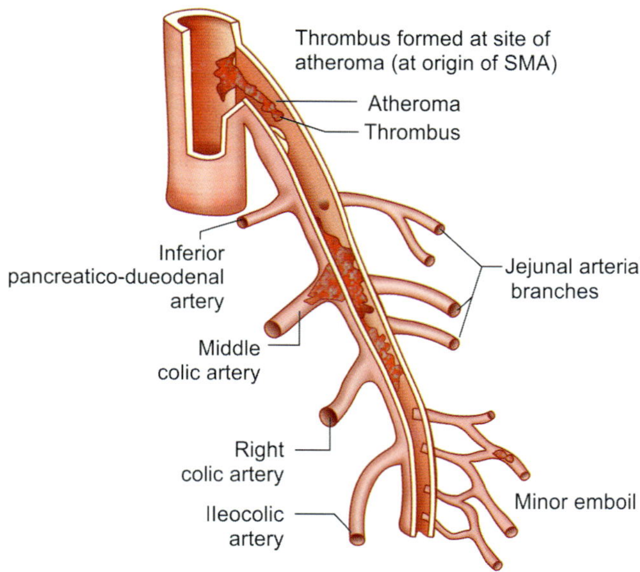

Figure 7 Common sites of superior artery thrombosis and embolism

Emboli can originate from left ventricle (after myocardial infarction, from a hypokinetic segment or ventricular aneurysm), left atrium (atrial fibrillation), proximal aorta (atheroemboli), systemic venous system [venous thrombus from extremities, as in deep venous thrombosis (DVT), gaining access to left heart through an intracardiac shunt—the so-called paradoxical embolus], or during endovascular procedures, due to manipulations. Many times, the source of embolus remains unrecognized.

Among the major mesenteric arteries, SMA is the one most frequently affected. Classically, the embolus tends to lodge somewhat beyond its origin, where it starts to taper (Fig. 7). Classically, this is just beyond the origin of MCA, although it can be more distal also. The extent of intestinal involvement depends upon the site of occlusion. Due to the classic site of occlusion, first part of jejunum is usually spared. However, if the occlusion is at origin of the SMA, as occurs in some cases, whole of small intestine, starting at the ligament of Treitz will be compromised. In case emboli lodge more distally, the corresponding bowel portion will be affected. In this scenario, since usually multiple emboli become impacted at various sites, there is patchy involvement of the bowel.

In addition to the SMA, in many instances, other mesenteric arterial systems[27] and/or multiple systems may be involved leading to corresponding consequences.

As mentioned above, acute mesenteric arterial occlusion also leads to further mesenteric vasoconstriction, thus worsening the ischemia.

Mesenteric Artery Thrombosis

Acute mesenteric arterial thrombosis affects up to 25% cases of AMI[26] and most commonly occurs over pre-existing chronic arteriosclerotic or atherosclerotic arterial occlusive disease. Other etiologies include aortic dissection extending to mesenteric vessel ostia, mesenteric arterial dissection—spontaneous or consequent on diagnostic or therapeutic arterial catheter manipulations, Takayasu arteritis and fibromuscular dysplasia. Infrequently, thrombosis may occur spontaneously, without any pre-existing arterial disease, usually in the setting of a hypercoagulable state.

Atherosclerosis of mesenteric arteries usually occurs at the ostia of these vessels. Therefore, when thrombosis supervenes over a pre-existing atherosclerosis, as is usually the case, occlusion occurs at these sites, rendering almost the whole of the region of supply of the particular vessel ischemic. This is in contrast to embolism, which tends to spare the most proximal segment of SMA and the corresponding segment of intestine as well (Fig. 7).

Since atherosclerosis is a slowly progressive pathology, it entails development of collaterals which prevent symptoms of arterial ischemia from developing for a long time. In fact, most of the patients with atherosclerotic occlusion are practically free of clinical manifestations of intestinal ischemia before an acute thrombotic episode supervenes. On the other hand, some patients do have postprandial abdominal symptoms—referred to as "intestinal angina" prior to the acute event. Presumably, in this latter group of patients, the collateral circulation is not able to cope with increased demand in the postprandial period. These pre-existing symptoms are again in contrast to acute mesenteric arterial embolism, in which almost invariably there are no pre-existing symptoms.

Apart from the etiologic factors leading to thrombosis, there are certain precipitating factors which contribute to occurrence of thrombosis. Most of these pertain to a state of relative hypotension and dehydration. Hemorrhage in an already critically occlusive atheromatous lesion may lead to complete occlusion and thereby ischemia.

Nonocclusive Mesenteric Ischemia

As the name suggests, in this condition mesenteric ischemia occurs in absence of physical occlusion of mesenteric arteries. Instead, the diminution of blood supply is caused by vasoconstriction of mesenteric arteries in response to various stimuli and conditions (Fig. 8).

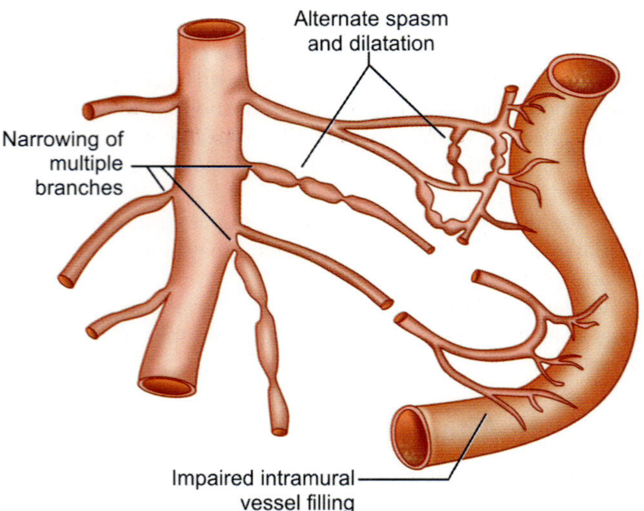

Figure 8 Various patterns of mesenteric vascular involvement in NOMI. These are reflected in angiographic findings in NOMI. Alternate spasm and dilatation leads to "String of sausages" sign, whereas the overall peripheral attenuation of mesenteric circulation is seen as "prune tree" appearance

Pathogenesis of NOMI involves release of neurohormonal substances such as angiotensin II, vasopressin or catecholamines in response to a shock state. The shock state may be consequent to sepsis, myocardial infarction, severe hemorrhage, etc. This leads to widespread vasoconstriction in the mesenteric arterial system and overwhelms the autoregulatory mechanisms described above.[28] Secondly, even after the precipitating cause has been dealt with and the systemic circulation is restored, the mesenteric vasoconstriction persists, thus perpetuating the mesenteric ischemia. Thirdly, after restoration of circulation, the element of reperfusion injury comes into play, as mentioned above, further worsening the insult. Finally, due to the often repetitive nature of precipitating conditions, ischemic intestinal injury in NOMI is also repetitive, which is cumulatively far worse than the single time insult encountered in occlusive pathologies like embolism or thrombosis.[29]

Prognosis of NOMI is much worse than occlusive ischemic pathologies and this is because of three reasons. First is the inherently worse injury suffered due to the reasons enumerated above in pathogenesis of the condition. Secondly, general condition of these patients is already compromised because of the shock state and its precipitating causes which comprise the etiology of NOMI. Finally and probably most significantly, is the likelihood of not suspecting or completely missing the occurrence of NOMI in these patients due to the general unawareness of this condition. Mortality rate among the most severely affected patients has been reported to be in excess of 90%.[28] A high index of suspicion, early diagnosis and appropriate timely institution of treatment are crucial to decrease the mortality.

NOMI is not uncommon, comprising approximately 20% of all cases of AMI,[28] although some studies report it to be less common[30]—most likely due to its going unrecognized. A lookout for risk factors and precipitating causes is essential to recognize and treat the condition. Various risk factors that ought to be kept in mind and recognized are summarized in Table 2.

Mesenteric Venous Thrombosis

Mesenteric venous occlusion, usually consequent upon its thrombosis leads to three sequential and concomitant pathogenetic mechanisms. Venous occlusion leads to rise in hydrostatic pressure within the mesenteric venous system. This causes bowel wall edema as well as intraluminal sequestration of fluid which compromise the mural circulation. The resultant hypovolemia may then lead to vasoconstriction, with its consequences. If perpetuated, there is loss of mucosal barrier function which allows endotoxemia and bacteremia, further worsening the condition.

Mesenteric venous thrombosis as cause of AMI has been reported to be much less common than other causes, comprising approximately 6% of all cases.[32] It also differs from other causes of AMI in that the patients affected are much younger (usually in fourth to seventh decade of life), are more likely to be females, and have much better prognosis in terms of mortality.

Mesenteric venous thrombosis has been classified in two ways. It has been referred to as acute or chronic according to whether the symptom duration is less than or more than 4 weeks. If, as may happen, there are no symptoms, it is still considered chronic MVT.[32] The second method of classification depends upon the etiology. If there is no identifiable cause of MVT, it is termed

Table 2: Risk factors and precipitating causes of NOMI

Risk factor/Precipitating factor	*Examples*	*Mechanism*
Age		Associated low cardiac output states
Shock	Septicemia, hemorrhage, MI	Hypoperfusion
Dehydration	Severe diarrhea	Hypovolemia and hypoperfusion
Conditions of high third space losses	Burns, acute pancreatitis	Low intravascular volume, low cardiac output
Drugs administered to combat shock	Epinephrine, phenylephrine, high dose dopamine, norepinephrine	Vasoconstriction
Other drugs	Ergot alkaloids (for migraine); beta blockers; digitalis; cocaine (substance abuse)	Vasoconstriction
	Diuretics	Hypovolemia, ADH release, renin-angiotensin system stimulation
	Somatostatin	Specific reduction of mesenteric blood flow
Cardiac surgical procedure[31]	Intra-aortic balloon pump use, prolonged pump time, coronary angioplasty (esp. if failed), emergency cardiac procedures	Hemodynamic disturbance

primary and if a cause is identifiable, it is called secondary MVT. Most cases belong to the secondary MVT group. Causes of MVT include hypercoagulable states (most commonly polycythemia vera), trauma, intra-abdominal infections, obstruction of venous flow with resultant stasis, etc. Tobacco use and previous MVT have been recognized as further risk factors for developing MVT.[32]

Usually the clinically important MVT involves portal venous and superior mesenteric venous systems. Thrombosis of the inferior mesenteric venous system is not often clinically significant due to the abundant collateral circulation pathways available.

Clinical Features

Symptoms

The most important clinical feature of AMI, especially due to embolism or thrombosis is abdominal pain, usually severe, out of proportion of corresponding abdominal signs. Unfortunately, it is this absence of abdominal signs that contributes significantly to the dismal prognosis associated with AMI, since it leads to a crucial delay in diagnosing an emergent condition unless a high index of suspicion and general awareness of the condition is present.

The abdominal pain is severe, usually anterior, colicky—at least in early stages, and may be diffuse or localize in any of the abdominal quadrants.

The abdominal pain may be less acute and severe in some patients of mesenteric arterial thrombosis who have had progressive occlusion of arterial lumen over a period of time, usually due to atherosclerosis, with accompanying development of collateral circulation. These patients often give a preceding history of postprandial abdominal pain, anorexia, aversion to food—often due to fear of precipitating the pain, weight loss, or recent illness. These symptoms are useful indicators of thrombosis as underlying pathology and should be actively sought when evaluating a patient with AMI. Of course, as noted earlier, many of the patients with atheromatous or arteriosclerotic obstruction do not have any preceding symptoms at all and these patients are difficult to distinguish from embolic AMI patients on the basis of history. In some of the patients with thrombotic AMI, due to the presence of collaterals, onset of symptoms is less acute and may evolve over a period of days instead of hours and severity of pain may also be less. In other aspects, pain of thrombotic AMI is similar to that of embolic AMI.

The critical condition of patients who are usually afflicted with NOMI makes it difficult to assess the symptoms. Most of these patients are mentally obtunded so that a meaningful history pertaining to abdominal pain is usually not forthcoming. In conscious patients, however, the pain is similar to embolic or thrombotic pain. The important thing in evaluating a suspected NOMI patient is recognition of risk and precipitating factors detailed above and keeping a high index of suspicion.

In MVT, the pain is less acute—often developing over several days instead of hours,[33] less severe and more diffuse. The pain is often accompanied by anorexia, abdominal distension, diarrhea, nausea and vomiting.

Vomiting often accompanies abdominal pain. Other less common symptoms include abdominal distension and diarrhea. There may be occult blood in stools or frank hematochezia, especially in late cases.

Signs

Physical examination in patients with AMI, in the early stages, is unrewarding in that there are few, if any, signs. The general condition of the patient depends upon the underlying etiologic or associated condition, as well as whether ischemia has or has not progressed to bowel infarction. General physical examination findings like condition of mucous membranes, pallor, temperature of extremities, pulse rate, blood pressure, respiratory status, etc. also depend upon these two factors.

In contrast to symptoms, abdominal signs in patients with AMI are minimal or absent in the early stages. When signs develop, they are due to an irreversible ischemic injury to the bowel wall leading to peritonism or peritonitis. Continuous pain, guarding, rebound tenderness or rigidity of abdomen, absent bowel sounds, etc. develop late and indicate bowel necrosis or perforations.

Abdominal fullness can be due to bowel distension or peritoneal fluid consequent upon bowel perforation or ascites. The latter is often an accompaniment of MVT.

Whereas symptoms of the various causes of AMI show subtle differences, abdominal signs, once they develop are almost the same, since they usually result when bowel vitality is compromised.

MANAGEMENT

Investigations

Laboratory Investigations

Like the clinical features of AMI, laboratory investigations do not contribute much to diagnosis of AMI. They are primarily useful in excluding other causes of acute abdomen, like acute pancreatitis or hollow viscus perforation. Also, they may indicate presence of or impending irreversible bowel injury. Common laboratory investigations performed in a patient with AMI include complete blood counts, coagulation profile, serum amylase and lipase, liver function tests, renal function tests and arterial blood gas analysis. Leukocytosis, acidosis and hyperamylasemia may indicate advanced ischemic bowel injury and are important in this regard, but their normal levels do not exclude bowel ischemia. Other enzyme levels like those of alkaline phosphatase, lactate dehydrogenase, creatinine phosphokinase, mucosal diamine oxidase have been evaluated as early markers of bowel ischemia, but have not shown any practical utility.[34] Hypercoagulable state might indicate MVT and hemoconcentration on CBC may be a pointer toward NOMI, being almost always present in this condition.[35]

Laboratory investigations are also necessary for optimizing the patient should any surgical procedure be required.

Radiological Investigations

Abdominal X-ray: Since the presentation of AMI is usually of acute abdominal pain, abdominal X-ray is often the first investigation advised or available. The main role of this investigation is to rule out other pathologies presenting with acute abdominal pain, like intestinal obstruction or hollow viscus perforation. In AMI, certain findings can be demonstrated—a fixed, dilated intestinal loop, dilated bowel loops of paralytic ileus,[36] "thumbprinting", etc. However, these findings are non-specific, and often detected in retrospect or if high index of suspicion is maintained. Moreover, in about a fourth of patients with AMI, they are not present.[37] Other findings like pneumatosis intestinales[38] and air in the portal circulation or biliary tree can be seen in late cases. However, pneumatosis intestinalis can be seen in other conditions like COPD and inflammatory bowel disease. It must be kept in mind that free peritoneal air can also be seen in late cases of AMI, at a stage when bowel perforation has occurred.

Barium studies: Barium studies are considered inappropriate in patients suspected of AMI since intraluminal barium can precipitate bowel perforation and also spill into the peritoneal cavity if bowel is perforated, as occurs in late cases; or the presence of barium will interfere with angiography if and when it is required. Moreover, these do not contribute much to diagnosis and management of this condition.

Ultrasound: Duplex ultrasound is an attractive option in these patients since it may potentially demonstrate blood flow in the mesenteric circulation. However, it is hampered by presence of bowel gas, requirement of high technical expertise, and the presence of proximal blood flow in mesenteric vessels in embolic AMI, which can therefore not be excluded. The main utility of this investigation is in excluding MVT, by demonstrating normal flow in portal vein and SMA. Absence of blood flow in portal venous system or presence of ascites in appropriate clinical setting is highly suggestive of MVT,[39] though these cannot be considered as confirmatory of this condition at present. Overall, the role of duplex scanning in AMI is useful but not fully established.

Transgastric ultrasonography: It has been suggested as means to visualize and assess abdominal aorta, and thereby at least proximal parts of mesenteric arterial system, but its utility is unknown at present.

Abdominal CT scan: It is considered investigation of choice in MVT.[40] Enlargement of and presence of intraluminal hypodense lesion (filling defect) in portal vein or superior mesenteric vein and "bull's eye" appearance (due to peripheral rim enhancement of vein wall along with the luminal filling defect)[41] are important and diagnostic findings. Bowel wall thickening and ascites are other significant corroborative findings.

Much like abdominal X-ray, CECT of abdomen is considered an important tool in assessing a patient presenting with acute abdomen. In the setting of suspected AMI its utility lies in excluding other abdominal pathologies apart from diagnosing MVT. Demonstration of findings like contrast distribution within the bowel, presence of intra-abdominal masses, bowel wall thickening, status of fat planes around bowel loops is useful. Intramural gas, air in portal system or biliary tract, lack of bowel wall enhancement, or liver and splenic infarcts have been shown as important findings in AMI.[42]

It can demonstrate presence of calcified plaque in abdominal aorta at the origin of mesenteric vessels or in the SMA (Fig. 9) which might be an important corroborative finding along with bowel changes for thrombotic AMI. However, differentiation of acute

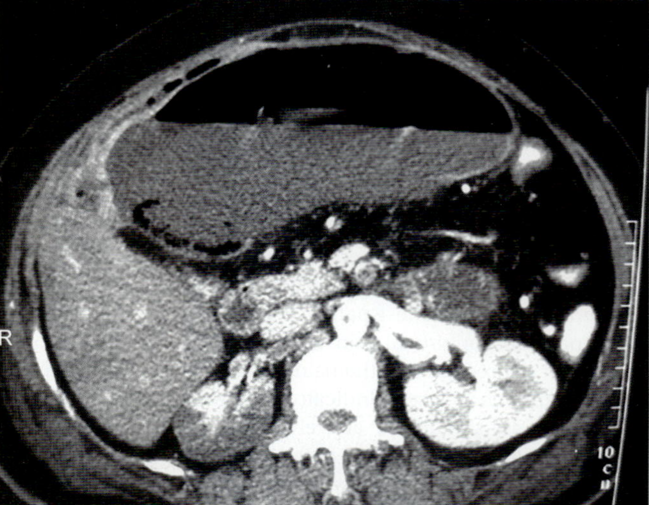

Figure 9 Thrombosed SMA and right renal artery with small thrombus also seen in aorta; A grossly dilated bowel loop is seen anteriorly.

from chronic occlusion of mesenteric arteries may not always be possible and it can be normal in embolic or thrombotic AMI, thus limiting its usefulness in these conditions.

Magnetic resonance imaging (MRI): This investigation has been reported to offer a high level of accuracy in MVT, but its utility in this condition is yet to be established fully.

Arteriography: Arteriography is undoubtedly the gold standard investigation in AMI. It can confirm the diagnosis, show the level of occlusion and can also be used as therapeutic tool in selected patients. The information obtained can be useful in deciding the surgical approach when operative intervention is required. Or, it can identify patients in whom surgical intervention is not required, e.g., NOMI.

However, it is not feasible as well as desirable to be performed in every patient. A stable patient with suspicion of AMI, seen early in the course of the disease, is perhaps the best candidate. Arteriography is not without complications, morbidity and mortality, requires high degree of expertise as well advanced equipment, and takes time to perform if meaningful results are to be expected. Therefore, it is very important to select patients for this study with the prime question being whether the risks, effort, expertise and delay in surgical intervention consequent on performing this investigation is going to benefit the patient.

When performed, arteriography gives information regarding three important aspects of AMI. First, it helps in differentiating between embolic and thrombotic AMI, which is important from management point of view in that the surgical approaches of these two conditions are different. The differences in arteriographic findings amongst the various causes of AMI have been summarized in Table 3. Second, and perhaps even more importantly, it can demonstrate NOMI as being the cause of AMI, the treatment of this condition being altogether different from AMI due to thromboembolic causes. Finally, it can establish the diagnosis of MVT, largely by exclusion of other causes but also by certain findings (Table 3).

Additionally, the catheter placed at the origin of a mesenteric vessel can be used to infuse drugs—vasodilators or thrombolytics, and can thus be therapeutic as well.

Infusion of papaverine (or other agents like tolazoline or nitroglycerin) and observation of reversal of constriction of mesenteric vessels is an important diagnostic maneuver in differentiating NOMI from patients with hypovolemia or those on high dose vasopressors. Among these patients, it is important to correct hypovolemia and reduce dose of vasopressors before concluding presence of NOMI on arteriography. Other false interpretations can also occur. In a patient with embolic occlusion, with passage of time there may be deposition of secondary thrombus on top of the embolus, with disappearance of meniscus sign. The embolus may lodge more proximally, giving rise to appearance similar to thrombosis or there may be some flow around the embolus in the early stages leading to unusual appearances.

TREATMENT

Medical

Volume Resuscitation

Patients with AMI have significant third space fluid losses resulting from loss of protein rich fluid within the gut lumen. The resultant hypovolemia and consequent hypoperfusion lead to mesenteric vasoconstriction, thus perpetuating the ischemic process. It is important to emphasize that mesenteric vasoconstriction is an important pathophysiologic phenomenon in both occlusive as well as nonocclusive etiologies. In addition, the vasospasm confuses the picture on diagnostic imaging, especially arteriography, as alluded to earlier. Moreover, the resultant hypotension requires administration of vasopressors, which again are detrimental to mesenteric circulation.

Volume resuscitation is therefore the first step in managing patients with AMI. Since many of these patients have additional

Table 3: Arteriographic findings of various causes of acute mesenteric ischemia

	Opacification of proximal segments of mesenteric arteries	*Collaterals*	*Appearance*	*Other findings*
Thrombosis	Usually absent, or only the proximal-most portion is opacified	Usual; demonstrable in delayed films due to retrograde filling		Diffuse atheromatous disease in abdominal aorta in supraceliac or suprarenal segments
Embolism	Proximal few centimeters are opacified; proximal jejunal branches are also opacified[43]	Unusual	Inverted meniscus sign; may be obscured if secondary thrombus deposition in relatively chronic cases	Relatively undiseased abdominal aorta and mesenteric vessels
NOMI	Patent mesenteric vessels; narrowing at origins of these vessels or at intermittent levels	Unusual	"String of sausages" or "string of lakes"[28] (Fig. 9)	Abdominal aorta and mesenteric vessels may or may not be diseased; reflux of contrast from a selectively injected SMA
MVT	Arterial vasospasm may be present; reflux of contrast into aorta; prolonged arterial phase; more intense opacification of mesenteric capillaries	Not relevant; venous collaterals not usually seen		Diagnosis of exclusion; prolonged venous phase—inadequate filling of major veins; thrombus may sometimes be demonstrated

comorbidities, volume resuscitation has to be well monitored. The patient must have a central venous line and Foley's catheter in place; CVP measurements and urine output acting as guides to volume resuscitation. In selected patients, placement of Swan-Ganz catheter is also required. An arterial line is placed if significant hemodynamic instability is present.

The volume resuscitation is aggressively performed, especially in patients who have hemodynamic compromise. The goal in the latter group of patients is to taper off the vasopressors since these have especially deleterious effect on mesenteric circulation.

Choice of Vasopressors and Other Drugs

Although no vasopressor is safe in AMI, certain agents have relatively more deleterious effect on mesenteric circulation. Noradrenaline and phenylephrine are especially notorious in this regard. Dopamine in low doses acts as mesenteric vasodilator, and might be preferred to the other two. Other "bad" drug in this regard includes digitalis which also causes mesenteric ischemia.

Intestinal Decompression

Early placement of nasogastric tube serves to decompress the distended, fluid and gas filled bowel loops. Decrease in intraluminal pressure can decrease ischemic mucosal injury. Moreover, the resultant decrease in abdominal distension is helpful in improving respiratory effort. It also lessens the probability of intestinal perforation and risk of aspiration.[44]

Antibiotics

Prophylactic broad spectrum antibiotics, including anaerobic coverage are indicated because loss of mucosal barrier, translocation of bacteria and endotoxemia are important accompaniments of mesenteric ischemia as described earlier.

Anticoagulation

Since thromboembolism is a predominant cause in AMI, it is pertinent to consider anticoagulation in its management. However, the decision is not straightforward, and depends upon the etiology.

In patients with acute thrombotic or embolic occlusions, anticoagulation may help in controlling the progression of thrombus. However, many of these patients may have to undergo operative intervention, in which case anticoagulation is contraindicated. Moreover, anticoagulation may increase chances of gastrointestinal bleeding; the intestinal mucosa being ischemic is more prone to hemorrhage. Also, most of these patients already have a degree of hypocoagulability consequent on systemic effects of mesenteric ischemia. Overall, formal anticoagulation does not play a significant role in the majority of these patients.

However, in MVT, anticoagulation is indicated and forms the cornerstone of management. In the acute stage, anticoagulation is required to limit the progression of thrombus. And in chronic cases, long-term anticoagulation with oral agents is required to prevent recurrences.

In the postoperative period, embolic AMI patients require anticoagulation in order to diminish chances of further embolization. On the other hand, patients with thrombotic AMI do not require anticoagulation postoperatively.

Interventional (Nonsurgical)

Selective Vasodilator Infusion

Since mesenteric vasoconstriction is the primary pathology in NOMI and a very important constituent of pathophysiology in thromboembolic AMI, including MVT, it follows that attempt at mesenteric vasodilatation holds a very important place in management of AMI. It also implies that while mesenteric vasodilatation is the primary therapy in NOMI, it also has significant adjunctive role in the treatment of other causes of AMI.

Mesenteric vasodilatation is achieved by selective catheterization of the concerned mesenteric vessel and infusing a vasodilator, most commonly papaverine.[45] Since arteriography is performed in a setting of an unestablished diagnosis, the first step is infusion of a test dose (60 mg) of papaverine, which is followed by a repeat contrast injection. If a reversal of vasoconstriction is noted, along with other suggestive findings, NOMI is diagnosed and an infusion of papaverine at a rate of 30–60 mL/hour is continued. On the other hand, if thromboembolic etiology is diagnosed but with vasoconstriction and reversal as described above, the infusion is still continued while an appropriate surgical intervention is planned, since vasoconstriction has been shown to play an important pathogenic role in even these conditions.[45]

Papaverine is useful in this setting because of its high first pass metabolism (it is inactivated to the tune of >90% on its first pass through the liver), thus making its side effects like cardiac dysrhythmias, etc. much less when administered selectively. Angiographic evaluation is repeated after 8–24 hours in order to assess effects of vasodilation. The catheter is flushed with saline for a period of approximately 30 minutes before repeating the contrast injection, so that this assessment is in absence of continuing vasodilatation and presumably gives better idea of how patient will fare after vasodilatation is stopped. At this time it may be decided to stop the infusion, or continue it for further 24 hours, depending upon angiographic findings and patient's condition. It is not clear as to how long the infusion can continue, but periods of as long as 4–5 days have been reported.

More important in taking the decision to continue the infusion is the patient's condition and laboratory parameters. Repeated abdominal examinations, assessment of general condition of patient and appropriate laboratory investigations are mandatory and give indication whether the infusion is succeeding or not. Appearance of abdominal signs and deterioration of patient—clinically or biochemically—are indications for surgical intervention.

It is important to note that even after it has been decided to intervene surgically, the catheter is left in place. After surgical exploration and possible resection of non-viable parts of gut, it may be helpful to continue the infusion postoperatively so as to support intestinal segments with marginal circulation.

Tolazoline 25 mg bolus followed by 25–50 mg/hour infusion has also been used.

Selective catheter vasodilator therapy is usually accompanied by administration of heparin in order to reduce chances of thrombus formation at catheter site or thrombus propagation.

Thrombolysis

Unlike coronary artery thrombosis, lysis of mesenteric vascular thrombosis has not been conclusively proven to be useful. The main reasons are the risk of intestinal hemorrhage that lysis can precipitate and the time taken for the thrombus to lyse sufficiently. However, successful thrombolysis using streptokinase[46,47] and urokinase[48] for AMI due to thrombosis/thromboembolism and for MVT[49,50] has been reported. For the latter, access is achieved in a transjugular or selective arterial manner.

Bowel viability can be ascertained laparoscopically, if required. There is no consensus or even a guideline regarding the use of this modality in AMI but some authors have recommended its use in elderly patients with significant morbidities, picked up in sufficiently early course of the disease and in whom bowel viability can be laparoscopically confirmed.[48,51]

Angioplasty

Again, in contrast to coronary occlusion, experience in use of angioplasty for mesenteric arterial occlusion is very limited. Initial technical success (86%) with low complication rate (6%) among patients with chronic visceral ischemia has been reported.[52] It can also be used in thrombotic occlusion following lysis of the thrombus, to deal with the underlying narrowing.

Other Interventions

Transluminal endovascular fenestration of false lumen of aortic aneurysm causing AMI has been reported to lead to relief of the ischemia.[53]

Surgery

Surgical intervention is the cornerstone of management of AMI. It cannot be emphasized enough that the dismal prognosis is contributed to in no small proportion by the delay in operating upon the patient, for various reasons. As mentioned in the earlier sections, nonoperative and medical therapies are applicable in selected subgroup of patients with this condition and that too, often as preoperative measures. Although in NOMI surgery does not play any part in dealing with the primary pathology, it is diagnostically important in patients who either cannot undergo arteriography or if the diagnosis of NOMI is not sufficiently certain. Moreover, even in NOMI, exploration is essential if there is compromise of bowel viability.

The goals of surgery in AMI are twofold. Firstly, exploration of a patient with suspected AMI serves to confirm the diagnosis, determine the etiology, and perform definitive procedure according to the etiology. It is reiterated here that although preoperative studies, especially arteriography, are useful in elucidating the etiology, their universal application is hampered by the delay they entail. Secondly, an equally importantly, bowel viability is assessed and resection of non-viable gut is carried out (Fig. 10).

Operating Room Set-up and Requirements

Overall setup of the operating room is essentially that for any major abdominal surgery. Since many of these patients are hemodynamically compromised or have significant cardiorespiratory comorbidities, the OT should be equipped to deal with these conditions as well. The special requirements include equipment to assess mesenteric blood flow and bowel viability. Wood's lamp, fluorescein and Doppler ultrasound with intraoperatively usable probes should be available.

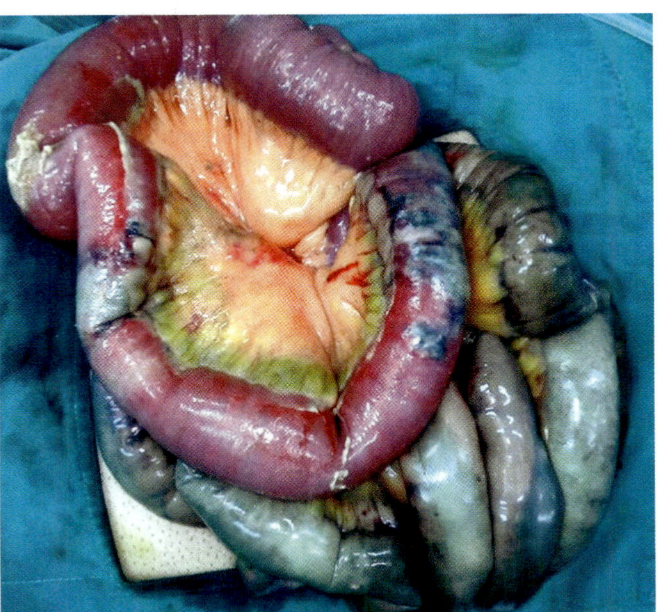

Figure 10 Operative photograph of gangrenous bowel loops

Incision and Exposure

The patient is placed supine and prepared from clavicles to the knees. The draping is done so as to keep the area from nipples to thighs exposed. Exposure of thighs can come in handy in case harvesting of great saphenous vein for grafting is required.

A long midline incision is made. Whole of the bowel from stomach to the deepest portion of rectum is inspected and evaluated. The pattern of involvement often gives clues to the etiology. Thrombotic occlusion of SMA usually involves whole of the small bowel up to the right third of transverse colon in contrast to an embolic occlusion which spares proximal most portion of the jejunum, due to the site of occlusion as described earlier. In NOMI, the involvement is more unpredictable and pulsations can often be felt in mesentery of affected intestine. In MVT, the bowel and mesentery are congested and edematous, often with cyanotic discoloration, affecting almost whole of the bowel extent along with presence of mesenteric pulsations.

Pulsations in mesentery are assessed both manually and with Doppler ultrasound. However, presence of pulsations does not rule out occlusion, since these may be due to collateral circulation as well. Absence of pulsations is important and can indicate site as well etiology of AMI. However, final determination of bowel viability as well as interpretation of pulsations is done at the end of procedure when revascularization has already been performed.

The next step is exposure and assessment of the relevant mesenteric artery. SMA can be exposed dividing the ligament of Treitz and exposing it where it exits from the pancreas. Celiac artery exposure is achieved either through gastrohepatic ligament or by medial visceral rotation, as described later. In the case of SMA, proximal few centimeters are exposed and pulsations evaluated. Presence or otherwise of pulsations at the origin can indicate embolism or thrombosis, respectively. Celiac artery branches are similarly evaluated for pulsations. If MVT is suspected, SMV is exposed inferior to pancreas and assessed for presence of a thrombus. Thrombectomy can then be performed if indicated.

Nonocclusive mesenteric ischemia is suspected during exploration if mesenteric pulsations are present throughout, with distal attenuation. In such a scenario, handling of bowel is reduced to a minimum, so as to reduce further mesenteric vasoconstriction. Evaluation of bowel viability is carried out, any necessary resections done and abdomen is closed. Patient is then taken for arterial vasodilator therapy.

Revascularization

Embolism: Superior mesenteric artery is mobilized and taken control of, proximally and distally. If diagnosis of embolus is certain, a transverse arteriotomy is performed some centimeters distal to the SMA origin. Usually the embolus can be localized at this site. Alternatively, if the diagnosis is not certain or if the vessel is especially narrow, a longitudinal arteriotomy is performed at a similar site. A number 3 embolectomy catheter followed by a number 4 catheter is passed successively proximally and into the aorta to confirm brisk inflow. A number 3 embolectomy catheter is then passed distally to dredge out the embolus. A smaller number 2 catheter is passed subsequently to clear out smaller, more distal portion of the vessel. Sometimes parts of the embolus can be milked out. At this stage dilute heparin is infused distally. Short infusion of thrombolytic agent has also been recommended at this stage. Infusion of a bolus of papaverine before closing the arteriotomy is also considered appropriate considering the significant role coexistent vasoconstriction plays in pathogenesis of AMI (Fig. 11).

Transverse arteriotomy can be closed primarily, with fine (6-O or 7-O) interrupted monofilament sutures. A longitudinal arteriotomy, or transverse arteriotomy in a narrow vessel usually requires patch angioplasty.

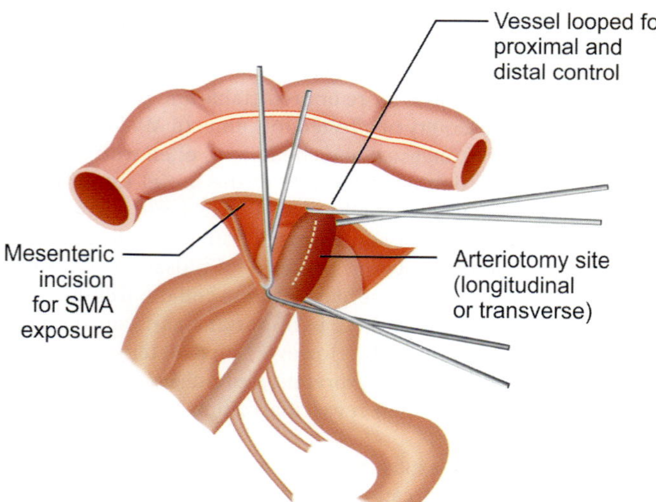

Figure 11 Superior mesenteric artery embolectomy. The vessel has been exposed through incision in mesentery and taken control of proximally and distally, including any proximal branches if required. Following arteriotomy, Fogarty catheter is passed to clear out the embolus/debris. Arteriotomy is closed primarily, or with a vein patch.

Thrombosis: Revascularization is more complex in thrombotic AMI. The occlusion is proximal, at the origin of the vessel and is usually associated with diseased aorta as well as the mesenteric vessel. Revascularization can be carried out by either bypass grafting or by thomoarterectomy, the former being the preferred method.

Bypass grafting: The most common procedure performed is bypass of thrombosed portion of the mesenteric vessel using a conduit from aorta. Major variables deciding the procedure used are: bowel viability and need or otherwise of resection, status of aorta to be used for proximal anastomosis, the conduit used and the extent of revascularization required.

Either supraceliac or infrarenal aorta can be used for inflow. Infrarenal aorta is easy to approach and expose, but is more often diseased and likely to be less appropriate for inflow, usually requires proximal and distal clamping in order to perform the proximal anastomosis (with ensuing increase in afterload while the anastomosis is being performed), and the graft assumes an inverted U configuration, more prone to kinking. While the supraceliac aorta is more difficult to expose, the extra time taken to do so is offset by having a less diseased inflow channel, by using side clamping instead of proximal and distal clamping, and the straighter, shorter course of the graft.

Possibilities of bowel compromise, bacterial transmigration or frank devitalization with peritoneal contamination limit the utility of synthetic grafts in this scenario. Great saphenous grafts have therefore been preferred as conduits. However, if the bowel is not compromised and if native venous graft is not available, synthetic conduits like PTFE or Dacron can be used.

Proximal anastomosis: A 1–1.5 cm arteriotomy is made on the aorta, in a longitudinal fashion. The graft is anastomosed in an end to side fashion using monofilament synthetic sutures (usually 3-O polypropylene).

Distal anastomosis: In the case of SMA, the distal anastomosis is performed just proximal or distal to origin of the MCA in an end to side fashion, using fine (6-O or 7-O) monofilament synthetic sutures.

Route of the conduit: When supraceliac aorta is used as the inflow channel and is approached through the lesser sac, the conduit has to be placed posterior to pancreas after creating a tunnel. When medial visceral rotation is used, the graft is more easily placed, and since origins of both CA and SMA are exposed, either or both can be bypassed. It must be mentioned here that usually a single vessel is bypassed in this situation.

When infrarenal aorta is used, the graft has to take a longer route and takes an inverted U configuration, as mentioned earlier. This configuration, especially when saphenous vein graft is used, is more prone to kinking and thereby obstruction.

Thromboendarterectomy: Alternatively, especially if saphenous venous graft is not available in presence of contamination, thromboarterectomy can be performed. Retrograde thromboarterectomy performed through a distal arteriotomy has been shown to lead to poor results. The procedure of choice, although more technically demanding, is to perform an antegrade thromboarterectomy by exposing the origin of the involved mesenteric vessel as well as the supraceliac aorta. This exposure can be done through either the lesser sac or by medial visceral rotation.

Mesenteric venous thrombosis: The primary treatment of MVT is anticoagulation. However, during exploration, if MVT is found, or if exploration is carried out to deal with compromised bowel, mesenteric venous exploration can be attempted. SMV is exposed inferior to the pancreas and a transverse venotomy is performed somewhat distal to where it appears. Thrombus from portal vein is extracted using a thrombectomy catheter. Distal thrombi can be milked out. It must be remembered that in MVT thrombotic process is more generalized than it appears and results of thrombectomy may not be gratifying.

Resection

As mentioned earlier, one of the goals of surgical intervention in AMI is to assess bowel viability or otherwise and to deal with it accordingly. Also, the final assessment of bowel viability should be made only after revascularization has been performed. In fact it is recommended to wait for at least 30–45 minutes before such assessment is made. Subjective assessment by evaluation of bowel and mesenteric color, bowel wall edema, mucosal hemorrhages, peristalsis, bleeding from cut edges and even mesenteric pulsations has been found to be inaccurate. It is important to make an accurate assessment so as to avoid resecting too much of the intestine on one hand and leaving behind non-viable intestine on the other as both are equally detrimental to the patient. Objective assessment using fluorescein and Wood's lamp or the Doppler ultrasound should be considered an essential part of assessment of bowel viability.

In the fluorescein test, Sodium Fluorescein (1,000 mg over 30 seconds) is administered intravenously. A hand held Wood's lamp (it emits ultraviolet light) is then used to illuminate the bowel with OT lights dimmed. The intensity as well as pattern of fluorescence is assessed. This test has been reported to be more accurate than Doppler and clinical assessment.[54] Some workers have not reproduced the same results, however.[55] Although cited as an objective test, assessment of intensity and pattern of fluorescence is subjective to some extent, explaining the conflicting results regarding its accuracy. Once injected, fluorescein remains in circulation for up to 24 hours, so that it is a one-time test, making it mandatory that revascularization and hemodynamic stabilization must be fully done before performing it.

Continuous wave Doppler ultrasound intraoperative probe can be used to assess for pulsations in the mesentery as well as bowel wall. The problem with this method is that it is operator dependent and also small patchy areas of non-viability are likely to be missed. The main utility of this investigation is in assessing clinically doubtful areas for presence of pulsations. The ease and rapidity with which it can be performed are its advantages.

All bowels judged to be non-viable (*see* Fig. 10) should be resected. The decision to reconstruct or anastomose after resection depends upon the patient's condition, condition of remaining bowel, etiology of AMI and the part of bowel involved. If the patient is in extremis, or is hemodynamically unstable especially if vasopressors are required, it is better to staple or over sew the ends or bring out as multiple ostomies with the plan for reconstruction at a later stage. If the remaining bowel has healthy, briskly bleeding edges, anastomosis can be performed; otherwise it is best avoided. In cases of MVT, the extent of bowel involvement is wider than is obvious; hence the need to resect more than what is obviously non-viable and also to be circumspect in reconstruction. Additionally, thrombotic process in MVT has a potential to further extend. If part of colon is resected, standard practice is to bring out the ends as ostomies.

It is imperative that decision regarding second look operation and its timing (often 18–24 hours later) is decided at the time of first laparotomy. The "second look" operation is then performed, regardless of the patient's condition. This is because postoperatively, patient's vital signs, abdominal signs, general condition and results of laboratory investigations are poor indicators of bowel viability.

PROGNOSIS

Acute mesenteric ischemia is associated with considerable mortality. It is still in the range of 60% despite improvements in diagnostic as well as therapeutic modalities. The main reasons for this are the patient's comorbidities and delay in institution of appropriate treatment.

Among the main etiologies of AMI, MVT has the best prognosis and NOMI the worst.[56] Acute arterial thromboembolism has intermediate result. Between the two, patients with embolic AMI fare better, presumably because of the less extensive bowel involvement (due to more distal occlusion) and association with less comorbidities and relatively less diseased vessels.

REFERENCES

1. Schoots IG, Koffeman GI, Legemate DA. Systematic review of survival after acute mesenteric ischemia according to disease aetiology. Br J Surg. 2004;91:17-27.
2. Edwards MS, Cherr GS, Craven TE, Olsen AW, Plonk GW, Geary RL, et al. Acute occlusive mesenteric ischemia: surgical management and outcomes. Ann Vasc Surg. 2003. Epub 2003;17:72-9.
3. Feller I, Woodburne RT. Surgical anatomy of the abdominal aorta. Ann Surg. 1966;154(Suppl):239-52.
4. Ruzicka FF, Rossi P. Normal celiac and hepatic arteriogram. NY State J Med. 1968;68:3032-4.
5. Muscowitz M, Zimmerman H, Felson B. The meandering mesenteric artery of the colon. Am J Roentgenol. 1964;92:1088-99.
6. Griffiths JD. Surgical anatomy of the blood supply of the distal colon. Ann R Coll Surg Engl. 1956;19:241-56.
7. Steward JA, Rankin FW. Blood supply of large intestine: its surgical considerations. Arch Surg. 1933;26:843.
8. Iliopoulos JI, Pierce GE, Hermreck AS, Haller CC, Thomas JH. Hemodynamics of the inferior mesenteric arterial circulation. J Vasc Surg. 1990;11:120-4.
9. Connolly JE, Kwaan JHA. Prophylactic revascularization of the gut. Ann Surg. 1979;190:514-22.
10. Ernst CB, Hagihara PF, Daughtery ME, Sachatello CR, Griffen WO Jr. Ischemic colitis incidence following abdominal aortic reconstruction: a prospective study. Surgery. 1976;80:417-21.
11. Bond JH, Prentiss RA, Levitt MD. The effects of feeding on blood flow to the stomach, small bowel and colon of the conscious dog. J Lab Clin Med. 1979;93:594-9.
12. Folkow B, Neil E. Circulation. London: Oxford University Press; 1971.
13. Eade MN. Gut circulation and absorption: a review, part 1. N Z Med J. 1976;84:10-4.
14. Eade MN. Gut circulation and absorption: a review, part 2. N Z Med J. 1976;84:58-62.
15. Sernka T, Jacobson E. Gastrointestinal Physiology: The Essentials. Baltimore: Williams & Wilkins; 1979.

16. Rothe CF. Reflex control of veins and vascular capacitance. Physiol Rev. 1983;63:1281-342.
17. Boley SJ, Regan JA, Tunick PA. Persistent vasoconstriction: a major factor in nonocclusive mesenteric ischemia. Curr Top Surg Res. 1971;3:425.
18. Folkow B, Lewis DH, Lundgren O, Mellander S, Wallentin I. The effect of graded vasoconstrictor fiber stimulation on the intestinal resistance and capacitance vessels. Acta Physiol Scand. 1964;61:445-57.
19. Folkow B, Lewis D, Lundgren O, Mellander S, Wallentin I. The effect of the sympathetic vasoconstrictor fibers on the distribution of the capillary blood flow in the intestine. Acta Physiol Scand. 1964;61:458-66.
20. Johnson PC. Origin, localization and homeostatic significance of autoregulation in the intestine. Circ Res. 1964;14(Suppl):225-33.
21. Lundgren O, Svanvik J. Mucosal hemodynamics in the small intestine of the cat during reduced perfusion pressure. Acta Physiol Scand. 1973;88:551-63.
22. Hoang MP, Lee EL, Anand A. Histologic spectrum of arterial and arteriolar lesions in acute and chronic cocaine-induced mesenteric ischemia: report of three cases and literature review. Am J Surg Pathol. 1998;22(11):1404-10.
23. Kauraluoma MI, Karkola P, Heikinnen E. Mesenteric infarction. Am J Surg. 1977;133:188-93.
24. Rosenblum JD, Boyle CM, Schwartz LB. The mesenteric circulation: anatomy and physiology. Surg Clin North Am. 1997;77(2): 289-306.
25. Heys SD, Brittenden J, Crofts TJ. Acute mesenteric ischemia: the continuing difficulty in early diagnosis. Postgrad Med J. 1993;69: 48-51.
26. Stoney RJ, Cunninham CG. Acute mesenteric ischemia. Surgery. 1993;114:489-90.
27. Kaleya RN, Summartano RJ, Boley SJ. Aggressive approach to acute mesenteric ischemia. Surg Clin North Am. 1992;72(1):157-82.
28. Boley SJ, Brandt LJ, Veith FJ. Ischemic disorders of the intestine. Curr Probl Surg. 1978;15:1-85.
29. Clark ET, Gewerz BI. Intermittent ischemia potentiates intestinal reperfusion injury. J Vasc Surg. 1991;13:606-61.
30. Howard TJ, Plaskon LA, Wiebke EA. Nonocclusive mesenteric ischemia remains a diagnostic dilemma. Am J Surg. 1996;171(4): 405-8.
31. Klempnauer J, Grothues F, Bektas TH. Acute mesenteric ischemia following cardiac surgery. J Cardiovasc Surg. 1997;38:639-43.
32. Rhee RY, Gloviczki P, Medonca CT. Mesenteric venous thrombosis: still a lethal disease in the 1990s. J Vasc Surg. 1994;20:688-97.
33. Rhee RY, Gloviczki P. Mesenteric venous thrombosis. Surg Clin North Am. 1997;77(2):327-38.
34. Thompson JS, Bragg LE, West WW. Serum enzyme levels during intestinal ischemia. Ann Surg. 1990;211:369-73.
35. Britt LG, Cheek RC. Non-occlusive mesenteric vascular disease: clinical and experimental observations. Ann Surg. 1969;169:704-11.
36. Gennaro M, Ascer E, Matano R. Acute mesenteric ischemia after cardiopulmonary bypass. Am J Surg. 1993;166:231-6.
37. Smerud MJ, Johnson CD, Stephens DH. Diagnosis of bowel infarction: a comparison of plain films and CT scans in 23 cases. Am J Roentgenol. 1990;154:99-103.
38. Wolfe EL, Sprayregen S, Bakal CW. Radiology in intestinal ischemia. Surg Clin North Am. 1992;72:107-24.
39. Miller VE, Beland LL. Pulsed Doppler duplex sonography and CT of portal vein thrombosis. Am J Roentgenol. 1985;145:73-6.
40. Vogelzang RL, Gore RM, Anschnetz SL. Thrombosis of the splanchnic veins: CT diagnoses. Am J Roentgenol. 1988;150:93-6.
41. Boley SJ, Kaleya RN, Brandt LJ. Mesenteric venous thrombosis. Surg Clin North Am. 1992;72:183-201.
42. Taourel PG, Deneuville M, Pradel JA. Acute mesenteric ischemia: diagnosis with contrast enhanced CT. Radiology. 1996;199(3):632-6.
43. Eldrup-Jorgensen J, Hawkins RE, Bredenberg CE. Abdominal vascular catastrophies. Surg Clin North Am. 1997;77:1305-20.
44. McKinsey JF, Gewertz BL. Acute mesenteric ischemia. Surg Clin North Am. 1997;77(2):307-18.
45. Boley SJ, Feinstein FR, Sammartano R. New concepts in the management of superior mesenteric artery embolus. Surg Gynecol Obstet. 1981;153:561-6.
46. Jamieson AC, Thomas RJF, Cade JF. Lysis of a superior mesenteric artery embolus following local infusion of streptokinase and heparin. Aust N Z J Surg. 1979;49:355-6.
47. Flickinger EJ, Johsrude IS, Ogburn NL. Local streptokinase infusion for superior mesenteric artery thromboembolism. Am J Roentgenol. 1983;140:771-3.
48. Regan F, Karlstad RR, Magnuson TH. Minimally invasive management of acute superior mesenteric artery occlusion: combined urokinase and laparoscopic therapy. Am J Gastroenterol. 1996;91(5):1019-21.
49. Rivitz SM, Geller SC, Hahn C, Waltman AC. Treatment of acute mesenteric venous thrombosis with transjugular intramesenteric urokinase infusion. J Vasc Interv Radiol. 1995;6(2):219-23.
50. Rijs J, Depreitere B, Beckers A. Mesenteric venous thrombosis: diagnostic and therapeutic approach. Acta Chir Belg. 1997;97(5):247-9.
51. Walsh RM, Popovich MJ, Hoadley J. Bedside diagnostic laparoscopy and peritoneal lavage in the intensive care unit. Surg Endosc. 1998;12(12):1405-9.
52. Matsumoto AH, Angle JF, Tegtmeyer CJ. Mesenteric angioplasty and stenting for chronic mesenteric ischemia. In: Perler BA, Becker GJ (Eds). Vascular Intervention: A Clinical Approach. New York: Thieme; 1998.
53. Williams DM, Brothers TE, Messina LE. Relief of mesenteric ischemia in type III aortic dissection with percutaneous fenestration of the aortic septum. Radiology. 1990;174:450-2.
54. Bulkley GB, Zuidema GD, Hamilton SR. Intraoperative determination of small intestinal viability following ischemic injury. Ann Surg. 1981;193:628-37.
55. Ballard JL, Stone WM, Hallett JW. A critical analysis of adjuvant techniques used to assess bowel viability in acute mesenteric ischemia. Ann Surg. 1993;59(5):309-11.
56. Bassiouny HS. Nonocclusive mesenteric ischemia. Surg Clin North Am. 1997;77:319-26.

CHAPTER 33

Radiation Enteritis: Pathophysiology, Prevention and Management

Vineeta Goel, Pankaj Agarwal

INTRODUCTION

Radiation enteritis is defined as a clinical syndrome resulting from radiation exposure to the small and large intestines. While giving radiotherapy to various abdominal and pelvic tumors, the small and large intestine often act as dose limiting structures as they lie within the radiation treatment portals. In the last decade with rapid evolution of highly conformal/focused radiation techniques, e.g. Intensity modulated radiation therapy (IMRT), 3 dimensional conformal radiation therapy (3DCRT) and stereotactic body radiation therapy (SBRT); the incidence of radiation enteritis has declined.[1,2] With present day radiation techniques, incidence of severe chronic radiation enteritis has come down to less than 5%.[3] Chen et al. have shown in a study that early radiation therapy techniques were associated with higher rate of complications that required corrective surgery. With newer precise radiation techniques, the incidence of severe radiation enteritis has significantly reduced.[4]

Decline in the incidence of radiation enteritis is also reflected in the present day management of gastrointestinal and genitourinary cancers, with radiation therapy being integrated as a multimodality component of neoadjuvant or adjuvant therapy. Earlier radiation for abdominopelvic malignancies was often avoided because of fear of radiation enteritis. But now radiation therapy is routinely added in the management of gastric, pancreatic, hepatobiliary, rectal, prostatic, cervical and uterine cancers.[5]

PATHOPHYSIOLOGY

Acute injury to small and large intestine starts in the mucosal lining. Moreover radiation has a cytotoxic effect on rapidly proliferating mucosal epithelial cells. Crypt cell wall necrosis occurs within 12–24 hours after a dose of 1.5–3 Gy. In following days and weeks, there is more progressive loss of cells, villous atrophy and cystic crypt dilation. Signs and symptoms of acute enteritis usually settle in 2–3 weeks after completion of radiation and mucosa gradually gets normal.[3,6]

In contrast to acute radiation injury (which affects only mucosal lining), chronic radiation enteritis manifests in the whole thickness of bowel wall causing fibrosis and adhesions with areas of stenosis or ulceration. Chronically injured intestinal mucosa often becomes pale and telangiectatic. Fistula formation is an extreme form of chronic enteritis and can be life threatening.[3]

On microscopic examination, chronic radiation enteritis changes are seen in the submucosa in the form of atypical fibroblasts and collagen proliferation. However, these changes are not limited to submucosa and can be seen in the lamina propria and muscularis propria too. Vessel wall becomes thickened with proliferation of intimal foam cell and formation of recanalized fibrin thrombi within the lumen. This obliterative endarteritis leads to tissue ischemia, necrosis and subsequent transmural fibrosis results in mucosal ulceration, intestinal wall necrosis and serosal adhesions.[3]

5-FU based chemotherapy is often added with radiation therapy. Chemotherapy agent 5-FU does not affect mucosal stem cells but acts on rapidly proliferating transit cell population.[7] Vascular toxicity due to radiation may also add to the toxic effects of 5-FU on bowel mucosa.[8]

Various factors which affect the incidence of radiation enteritis are:

- Presence of comorbidities such as diabetes mellitus and hypertension. These are associated with chronic vasculitis and are generally associated with a higher incidence of acute and chronic enteritis.
- Previous abdominal surgery leads to intestinal adhesions and fibrosis leading to an increase in incidence of radiation enteritis.

- Inflammatory bowel disease is a relative contraindication to radiation therapy due to high risk of both acute and late radiation enteritis.
- The concurrent use of chemotherapy increases the incidence of radiation induced enteritis. In a study on gynecologic malignancies, the incidence of grade 3–4 GI toxicity was 14% in patients treated with radiation therapy as compared to 55% in patients treated with concurrent chemoradiotherapy.[9]

CLINICAL MANIFESTATIONS

Radiation enteritis can be acute or chronic. It is the chronic effects which are of more concern to both patients and the radiation oncologist. The sections most frequently affected are the lower ileum, cecum, and rectosigmoid. The midgut and transverse colon are usually free of radiation effects.[10] Severe acute effects may also manifest as consequential chronic injury to the bowel.

Patients of acute radiation enteritis may present with nausea, vomiting, abdominal pain or cramps and diarrhea. This may result in malabsorption of fat, lactose, bile salts and vitamins (B_{12}). Nausea and vomiting may occur immediately or within hours after radiation. Abdominal cramping and diarrhea usually develops 1–2 weeks after start of radiation therapy. Acute radiation injury to rectum may lead to mucoid rectal discharge, pain, tenesmus or rectal bleeding resulting into weight loss. Acute radiation enteritis generally resolves 2–3 weeks after completion of radiation therapy.[3,11]

Late chronic small bowel injury usually manifest after 3 months post radiation up to 3 years. The most common symptoms of chronic radiation enteritis are abdominal cramping, persistent diarrhea and bloody or mucus discharge per rectum. Chronic small bowel enteritis leads to thickened intestinal folds leading to malabsorption of bile salts and consequently osmotic diarrhea. Such diarrhea responds to bile salt sequestering agents as discussed later.[12]

Chronic radiation proctitis is associated with decreased rectal compliance and patients present with symptoms of frequent diarrhea along with tenesmus and bloody or mucus discharge. Rectal pain may be present if proctitis extends into the anal canal.

The above presentation is indicative of mild chronic enteritis and can be managed by dietary modifications and symptomatic treatment. Severe chronic enteritis manifests as intestinal obstruction, severe bleeding, ulceration, perforation, fistula formation or intractable diarrhea and requires surgical and medical intervention.

GRADING

The Radiation Therapy Oncology Group (RTOG) grades numerous types of GI toxicity.[13]

Acute Enteritis

Grade 1: Increased frequency or change in quality of bowel habits not requiring medication/rectal discomfort not requiring analgesics.

Grade 2: Diarrhea requiring parasympatholytic drugs (e.g. Lomotil)/mucous discharge not necessitating sanitary pads/rectal or abdominal pain requiring analgesics.

Grade 3: Diarrhea requiring parenteral support/severe mucous or blood discharge necessitating sanitary pads/abdominal distention.

Grade 4: Acute or subacute obstruction, fistula or perforation; GI bleeding requiring transfusion; abdominal pain or tenesmus requiring tube decompression or bowel diversion.

Chronic Enteritis

Grade 1: Mild diarrhea; mild cramping; bowel movement 5 times daily; slight rectal discharge or bleeding.

Grade 2: Moderate diarrhea and colic; bowel movement more than 5 times daily; excessive rectal mucus or intermittent bleeding.

Grade 3: Obstruction or bleeding, requiring surgery.

Grade 4: Necrosis/perforation fistula.

DIAGNOSIS AND MANAGEMENT

Various imaging and endoscopic modalities can aid in diagnosis of radiation enteritis. Acute radiation enteritis is usually a clinical diagnosis in a patient presenting with abdominal pain, nausea, vomiting, diarrhea and abdominal distension within 3 months of radiation to abdomen or pelvis.

Chronic radiation enteritis needs high index of suspicion, investigations and early intervention. Contrast enhanced CT scan is very helpful, as it delineates the diseased intestine segment with thickened wall. CT scan may also show intestinal strictures and exclude other bowel pathologies. Occult mucosal bleeding, erosions, ulcerations, etc. can be seen by appropriate endoscopies. While radiation proctitis can be easily diagnosed with proctosigmoidoscopy, diagnosis of small bowel enteritis is often difficult.[14]

The diagnosis of radiation induced enteritis or proctitis is difficult to confirm without biopsy as it may clinically appear similar to postoperative adhesive bowel obstruction, which may also be an incidental finding.[15]

Radiation enteritis can cause mucosal ulcerations in the small bowel which may not be detected by traditional endoscopy and imaging. In such cases capsule endoscopy allows for direct and minimally invasive visualization of small bowel mucosa.[14] The main limitation of capsule endoscopy is its inability to get tissue for histopathological confirmation. Another limitation of capsule endoscopy is a risk for capsule retention due to underlying intestinal strictures. Incidence of capsule retention is around 2%.[16]

Conservative Management

Acute enteritis is managed with symptomatic treatment of diarrhea and resultant dehydration and malabsorption. Symptoms usually resolve with medications, dietary changes and treatment break for severe symptoms. Dietary changes include lactose free, low fat and low residue diet. Diarrhea due to small bowel injury often responds to bile salt sequestering agents like cholestyramine.[12] Short-chain fatty acids (SCFAs) are useful in the management of radiation proctitis.[17] Some patients may benefit with replacement of pancreatic enzymes, anti-motility agents and probiotics.

Chronic radiation enteritis and proctitis have different clinical presentation and management.

Mild cases of chronic enteritis can be managed with low fiber diet and stool softeners and sometimes with anticholinergics and opioid agonists such as diphenoxylate although, no standard recommendations are available. Fiber laxatives add form and consistency to stools and help in management of patients with reduced rectal compliance. Severe cases require surgical intervention. Initial attempt is always toward conservative management with bowel decompression and bowel rest.[3,6]

Persistent chronic radiation proctitis is initially managed with hydrocortisone enemas. Sucralfate enemas have also been reported with mixed results. Chronic proctitis not responding to symptomatic treatment with hydrocortisone and sucralfate enemas will require endoscopic treatment with argon plasma coagulation (APC).[18] APC reduces rectal bleeding in 80–90% patients and even reduces diarrhea and urgency.[19] Role of hyperbaric oxygen is discussed later.

Chemical cauterization by formalin application for chronic radiation induced rectal bleed has been established in many studies and case reports. In a retrospective study by Parikh et al., rectal instillation of 4% formalin resulted in cessation of symptoms in 88% patients.[20] Sharma et al. in a similar study treated radiation proctitis with instillation of 50 mL of 4% formalin for 3 minutes with 100% overall response and complete cessation of bleeding in 60% patients.[21]

Surgical Management

Surgical intervention is indicated in cases presenting with features of intestinal obstruction, strictures or intestinal fistula. Intestinal obstruction is initially managed conservatively by bowel rest and total parenteral nutrition. However, if obstruction is not relieved by conservative measures, surgical exploration is mandatory. Type and extent of surgery will depend on location, single or multiple affected segments and length of affected bowel segment. Goal of surgery is relief of obstruction with preservation of maximum bowel length. Surgery would include adhesiolysis, release of obstructing bands, strictureplasty or internal by pass of obstructed segment. Strictureplasty is effective and useful means of conserving intestinal length in selected patients. Dietz et al. in their study showed that strictureplasty is effective in selected patients with chronic radiation enteritis resulting into small intestine strictures with limited intestinal reserve. Strictureplasty is however not indicated in the presence of perforation, hemorrhage or fistula.[22]

If the affected bowel is too unhealthy because of radiation injury or edema then ileostomy or colostomy is preferred. Radical resection of involved segment with primary anastomosis is usually done as a last resort and in highly selected patients with localized involvement, healthy proximal and distal bowel.

For patients presenting with intestinal fistulae and/or peritonitis, surgical intervention is required. Spontaneous healing of small intestinal fistulae usually does not occur due to poor healing capacity of irradiated tissue resulting from stromal fibrosis and vascular ischemia. Patients with radiation related intestinal fistulae sometimes require resection, diversion procedure or creation of stoma. There is no consensus regarding choice of surgery with intestinal bypass and resection of diseased bowel having comparable results. Other surgical options may include small intestine bypass or resection and primary anastomosis.[3,4]

Rectourethral, rectovaginal and rectovesicular fistulae may occur as delayed complication of pelvic radiation. Patients mostly present with infection, intractable pain and/or incontinence. Due to poorly vascularized, unhealthy previously irradiated tissue, local debridement, excision of fistulae and repair are not helpful. Additional options include improving success of fistula repair using interposition of pedunculated flaps from neighboring non-irradiated areas such as Gracilis or Martius muscle flap. If flap interposition is not feasible, urinary or fecal diversion is a good option for palliation of symptoms. Pelvic exenteration is best avoided due to significant morbidity and perineal wound complications.[23-25]

MEDICAL MANAGEMENT OF RADIATION ENTERITIS

Hyperbaric Oxygen Therapy

Hyperbaric oxygen therapy is also effective for delayed refractory hemorrhagic proctitis and necrosis. Hyperbaric therapy is postulated to act by improving angiogenesis and also by reversing the fibro-atrophic effect associated with radiation injury of bowel. Fibro-atrophic effect refers to fibrosis and depletion in stem cells seen with chronic proctitis and enteritis. Neovascularization increases the blood supply and reduces incidence of ischemic necrosis responsible for severe complications. Hyperbaric therapy is believed to mobilize stem cells from bone marrow and also reduce fibrosis. There are also few clinical reports on the preoperative use of hyperbaric oxygen, to possibly allow for conservative management with avoidance of surgery.[26] Marshall et al. reported the use of hyperbaric oxygen for chronic radiation enteritis with overall response rate of 68% (43% complete and 25% partial).[27]

Role of Sulfasalazine

Eicosanoids and free radical release is one of the pathways in the pathogenesis of acute radiation enteritis. Mesalazine (5-ASA), a potent inhibitor of free radical release in mucosa could therefore be useful in preventing acute radiation injury. However, a randomized double blind study of mesalazine for acute enteritis by Resbeut et al. did not show benefit of sulfasalazine.[28] Yeoh et al. reported expression of NFkappaB (NF-kB) and COX-2 expression in radiated bowel. Such expression suggests similar pathways for both radiation enteritis and inflammatory bowel disease and possible benefit with 5-ASA and tumor-necrosis factor alpha blocker for treatment of radiation enteritis.[29]

There are contradictory reports in literature regarding effectiveness of sulfasalazine in prevention of acute radiation enteritis. Sulfasalazine tried for prophylactic use for prevention of radiation enteritis was found to be effective in reducing incidence of diarrhea by 30% at doses of 2 g/day.[30] However, in a similar study by Baughan et al., sulfasalazine was not found to be effective.[31]

PREVENTION OF RADIATION-INDUCED INTESTINAL INJURY

Over the years our understanding of radiation Dose-Volume and consequential enteritis has improved. Incidence of radiation enteritis is related to the volume of bowel exposed to radiation and total dose received. Various treatment approaches that can minimize the risk of severe radiation enteritis include the following.

Radiation Delivery Techniques

Radiation fields were earlier based on clinical and anatomical bony landmarks. But in the present times radiation fields are guided by 3 dimension volumetric imaging like CT, MRI and PET scans. This has helped radiation oncologists to identify and focus radiation to desirable targets and minimize unwarranted radiation to small and large bowel.

At the same time radiation therapy machines have evolved with new sophisticated hardware and software. Earlier the radiation to abdomen and pelvis was generally with anteriorly and posteriorly directed beams called AP-PA beams. AP-PA beams deliver radiation dose to a large volume of bowel. These are now often replaced by newer techniques like 3DCRT, IMRT and SBRT which help to generate concave shaped dose distributions and limit both dose and volume of bowel irradiation (Figs 1 and 2). Image guided radiation therapy (IGRT) further helps in reducing daily set up variations and thereby minimizes bowel dose uncertainty.

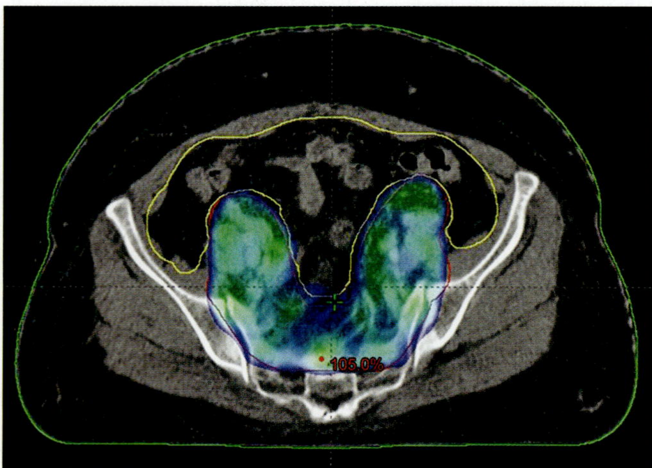

Figure 1 Dose distribution by IMRT showing treatment of pelvic lymph node area with sparing of adjacent organs

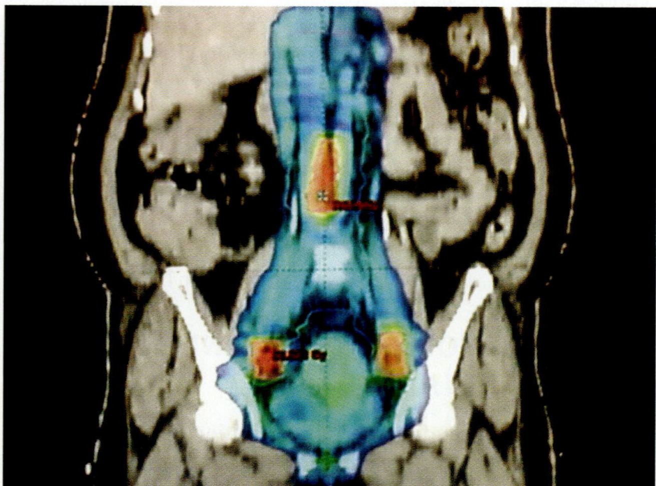

Figure 2 Coronal view of radiation dose distribution of pelvic and para-aortic radiation with sparing of adjacent bowel and kidneys with IMRT technique

With the use of these precision radiation techniques the incidence of both acute and chronic radiation enteritis has come down significantly. These also facilitate combining radiation therapy with chemotherapy as the overall toxicity is reduced.

Patient Positioning Techniques

Appropriate positioning of the patient also helps in removing as much small bowel from the treatment field as possible. For rectal cancers, as reported by Gallagher et al., radiation therapy with patient in prone position with full urinary bladder can reduce volume of small bowel from 600–1,000 cc to 145–385 cc.[32] The benefits of treating in prone position have also been reported by Martin et al. He observed that relative to supine, prone position with a belly board significantly reduced the volume of small bowel receiving 80–100% of the prescribed dose during pelvic treatment for gynecologic cancers.[33,34]

Defining Bowel Loops in Simulation and Image Segmentation

It is sometimes challenging to differentiate small bowel from vessels, nodes and large bowel on planning CT images. Herbert et al. showed that use of small bowel contrast and bowel shielding reduced the incidence of small bowel complications.[35]

Preoperative Radiation Therapy

Postoperative radiation therapy of pelvic malignancies, like cervical, uterine, rectal and urinary bladder, is associated with increased incidence of radiation enteritis. In postoperative setting a larger volume of small bowel falls into the pelvis and is often immobile due to postoperative adhesions. Consequently there is more bowel in the radiation fields and increased incidence of enteritis.

In the Phase III German Rectal Cancer Study Group, preoperative versus postoperative pelvic radiation were associated with a 9% versus 15% rate of long-term incidence of chronic diarrhea respectively (p=0.07).[36] Green et al. reported that 65% patients referred for postoperative radiation had fixed loops of small bowel within the pelvis; and only 18% in patients with no prior surgery.[37] Due to lack of normal bowel movement, the radiation dose gets deposited at a particular segment of bowel leading to increased risk of bowel wall damage in postoperative cases.

Because of above mentioned reasons we generally try to avoid surgery in bulky carcinoma cervix (which are likely to require postoperative radiation) and manage it with equally effective combination of concurrent chemoradiotherapy. In locally advanced carcinoma rectum preoperative chemoradiotherapy is preferred over postoperative treatment. Additionally, in patients planned for postoperative radiotherapy, surgical clips placed at high-risk areas during surgery helps to better define the location of tumor bed during radiation treatment planning.

Role of Surgical Bowel Displacement before Radiation

If radiation therapy is planned after surgery, an attempt should be made during surgery to displace as much bowel outside the radiation field as possible. Use of polyglycolic, biodegradable mesh helps in keeping the intestine loops out of the pelvis. This procedure is simple and does not add to morbidity or operative time. The mesh usually gets absorbed 3–4 months postoperatively. Placement of a mesh during surgery decreases the small intestine exposure by 50%.[38-41] However, this technique is not popular nowadays.

Other surgical techniques which can be used to exclude bowel in the pelvis include cystopexy, omentopexy, transposition of large bowel and synthetic pelvic sling placement. These surgical techniques reduce the volume of bowel at risk of high for radiation exposure by 50–60%.[42]

These techniques stand outdated and are of historical importance. Non-surgical techniques of bowel displacement such as bladder distention, abdominal compression and pretreatment positioning are easier and preferred in current era of conformal radiation therapy.

PHARMACOLOGICAL PREVENTION OF RADIATION ENTERITIS

Role of Sulfasalazine in preventing acute radiation enteritis has been briefed above.

COX-2 inhibitors have also been shown to suppress cytokine expression and to reduce acute bowel damage in animal experiments following abdominal radiation.[43]

Various studies have reported involvement of Rho/Rho kinase pathway in radiation fibrosis and intestinal smooth muscle cell fibrogenic differentiation via NF-kB inhibition, suggesting potential role of Rho kinase inhibitors in decreasing radiation induced bowel damage.[44]

Role of Amifostine in preventing radiation proctitis could not be reproduced in studies, despite it being labeled as a radiation protector.

Dietary supplementation of selenium and zinc may reduce anorectal sequelae of abdominopelvic radiotherapy. Zinc supplementation in diet induces heat shock proteins which help by preserving the structure of normal proteins and repairing or removing damaged ones.[45]

Prostaglandins (PGs) have also been investigated for their role as radioprotectors. Misoprostol suppositories reduce symptoms of acute radiation colitis by pro-proliferative and anti-apoptotic effects on epithelial cells in gastrointestinal injury. PGE2 decreases radiation induced apoptosis and increases crypt survival. Many other compounds have been described in the pathogenesis of radiation injury and cytoprotection such as glutamine, insulin like growth factors-1 (IGF-1), glucagon like peptide-2 (GLP-2). Presently no clinical benefit has been established of these compounds and future studies are awaited.[46]

Radiation therapy induces NF-kB overexpression, and octreotide treatment decreases the end organ damage and inflammation of the small intestine. Therefore use of octreotide has beneficial effects on intestinal damage in abdominal irradiation through the inflammatory process.[17]

CONCLUSION

Radiation enteritis is a well-known complication of abdominal and pelvic radiation therapy. With the availability of high precision radiation therapy techniques the incidence of late radiation enteritis has reduced significantly.

REFERENCES

1. Nutting CM, Convery DJ, Cosgrove VP, Rowbottom C, Padhani AR, Webb S, et al. Reduction of small and large bowel irradiation using an optimized intensity-modulated pelvic radiotherapy technique in patients with prostate cancer. Int J Radiat Oncol Biol Phys. 2000;48:649-56.
2. Portelance L, Chao KS, Grigsby PW, Bennet H, Low D. Intensity modulated radiation therapy (IMRT) reduces small bowel, rectum, and bladder doses in patients with cervical cancer receiving pelvic and para-aortic irradiation. Int J Radiat Oncol Biol Phys. 2001;51:261-6.
3. Coia LR, Myerson RJ, Tepper JE. Late effects of radiation therapy on the gastrointestinal tract. Int J Radiat Oncol Biol Phys. 1995;31: 1213-36.
4. Chen MC, Chiang FF, Hsu TW, Chen JB, Chao TH, Ma HF, et al. Clinical experience in 89 consecutive cases of chronic radiation enterocolitis. J Chin Med Assoc. 2011;74:69-74.
5. NCCN Guidelines(R) Updates. J Natl Compr Canc Netw. 2013;11(8):xxix-xxxiv.
6. Hauer-Jensen M, Wang J, Denham JW. Bowel injury: current and evolving management strategies. Semin Radiat Oncol. 2003;13: 357-71.
7. Pritchard DM, Watson AJ, Potten CS, et al. Inhibition by uridine but not thymidine of p53-dependent intestinal apoptosis initiated by 5-fluorouracil: evidence for the involvement of RNA perturbation. Proc Natl Acad Sci USA. 1997;94:1795-9.
8. Kakinuma S, Ohwada S. Gastric mucosal blood flow and gastric secretion following intravenous administration of 5-fluorouracil in anesthetized rats. Cancer Chemother Pharmacol. 1997;39: 357-60.
9. Keys HM, Bundy BN, Stehman FB, Muderspach LI, Chafe WE, Suggs CL 3rd, et al. Cisplatin, radiation and adjuvant hysterectomy compared with radiation and hysterectomy for bulky stage IB cervical carcinoma. N Eng J Med. 2001;340:725-30.
10. Meissner K. Late radiogenic small bowel damage: guidelines for the general surgeon. Dig Surg. 1999;16:169-74.
11. Miller AR, Martenson JA, Nelson H, Schleck CD, Ilstrup DM, Gunderson LL, et al. The incidence and clinical consequences of treatment—related bowel injury. Int J Radiat Oncol Biol Phys. 1999;43:817-25.
12. Heusinkveld RS, Manning MR, Aristizabal SA. Control of radiation-induced diarrhea with cholestyramine. Int J Radiat Oncol Biol Phys. 1978;4:687-90.
13. Cox JD, Stetz J, Pajak TF. Toxicity criteria of the Radiation Therapy Oncology Group (RTOG) and the European Organization for Research and Treatment of Cancer (EORTC). Int J Radiat Oncol Biol Phys. 1995;31(5):1341-6.
14. Hussain A, Mahmood H, Thomas A, Frazer C, Hasani SE. Does chronic radiation enteritis pose a diagnostic challenge? A report of three cases. Hong Kong Med J. 2008;14:327-30.
15. Nussbaum ML, Compana TJ, Weese JL. Radiation-induced intestinal injury. Clin Plast Surg. 1993;20:573-80.
16. Ho KK, Joyce AM. Gastrointest Endosc Clin N Am. 2007;17(1): 169-78, viii-ix.
17. Kountouras J, Zavos C. Recent advances in the management of radiation colitis. World J Gastroenterol. 2008;14(48):7289-301.
18. Hanson B, MacDonald R, Shaukat A. Endoscopic and medical therapy for chronic radiation proctopathy: a systematic review. Dis Colon Rectum. 2012;55:1081-95.
19. Postgate A, Saunders B, Tjandra J, Vargo J. Argon plasma coagulation in chronic radiation proctitis. Endoscopy. 2007;39:361-5.

20. Parikh S, Hughes C, Salvati EP, Eisenstat T, Oliver G, Chinn B, et al. Treatment of hemorrhagic radiation proctitis with 4 percent formalin. Dis Colon Rectum. 2003;46:596-600.
21. Sharma B, Kumar R, Singh KK, Chauhan V. Intrarectal application of formalin for chronic radiation proctitis: a simple, cheap and effective treatment. Tropical Gastroenterology. 2010;31(1):37-40.
22. Dietz DW, Remzi FH, Fazio VW. Strictureplasty for obstructing small-bowel lesions in diffuse radiation enteritis—successful outcome in five patients. Dis Colon Rectum. 2001;44:1772-7.
23. Pricolo VE, Shellito PC. Surgery for radiation injury to the large intestine: variables influencing outcome. Diseases of the Colon and Rectum. 1994;37(7):675-84.
24. Anseline PF, Lavery IC, Fazio VW. Radiation injury of the rectum. Evaluation of surgical treatment. Annals of Surgery. 1981;194(6):716-24.
25. Lucarotti ME, Mountford RA, Bartolo DCC. Surgical management of intestinal radiation injury. Diseases of the Colon and Rectum. 1991;34(10):865-9.
26. Feldmeier JJ, Hampson NB. A systematic review of the literature reporting the application of hyperbaric oxygen prevention and treatment of delayed radiation injuries: an evidence based approach. Undersea Hyperb Med. 2002;29:4-30.
27. Marshall GT, Thirlby RC, Bredfeldt JE, Hampson NB. Treatment of gastrointestinal radiation injury with hyperbaric oxygen. Undersea Hyperb Med. 2007;34:35-42.
28. Resbeut M, Marteau P, Cowen D, Richaud P, Bourdin S, Dubois, et al. A randomized double blind placebo controlled multicenter study of mesalazine for the prevention of acute radiation enteritis. Radiother Oncol. 1997;44:59-63.
29. Yeoh AS, Bowen JM, Gibson RJ, Keefe DM. Nuclear factor kappaB (NFkappaB) and cyclooxygenase-2 (Cox-2) expression in the irradiated colorectum is associated with subsequent histopathological changes. Int J Radiat Oncol Biol Phys. 2005;63:1295-303.
30. Kiliç D, Egehan I, Ozenirler S, Dursun A. Double-blinded, randomized, placebo-controlled study to evaluate the effectiveness of sulphasalazine in preventing acute gastrointestinal complications due to radiotherapy. Radiother Oncol. 2000;57:125-9.
31. Baughan CA, Canney PA, Buchanan RB, Pickering RM. A randomized trial to assess the efficacy of 5-aminosalicylic acid for the prevention of radiation enteritis. Clin Oncol (R Coll Radiol). 1993;5:19-24.
32. Gallagher MJ, Brereton HD, Rostock RA, Zero JM, Zekoski DA, Poyss LF, et al. A prospective study of treatment techniques to minimize the volume of pelvic small bowel with reduction of acute and late effects associated with pelvic irradiation. Int J Radiat Oncol Biol Phys. 1986;12:1565-73.
33. Martin J, Fitzpatrick K, Horan G, McCloy R, Buckney S, O'Neill L, et al. Treatment with a belly-board device significantly reduces the volume of small bowel irradiated and results in low acute toxicity in adjuvant radiotherapy for gynecologic cancer: results of a prospective study. Radiother Oncol. 2005;74:267-74.
34. Ghosh K, Padilla LA, Murray KP, Downs LS, Carson LF, Dusenbery KE. Using a belly board device to reduce the small bowel volume within pelvic radiation fields in women with postoperatively treated cervical carcinoma. Gynecol Oncol. 2001;83:271-5.
35. Herbert SH, Curran WJ, Solin LJ, Stafford PM, Lanciano RM, Hanks GE. Decreasing gastrointestinal morbidity with the use of small bowel contrast during treatment planning for pelvic irradiation. Int J Radiat Oncol Biol Phys. 1991;20:835-42.
36. Sauer R, Becker H, Hohenberger W, Rödel C, Wittekind C, Fietkau R et al. Preoperative versus postoperative chemoradiotherapy for rectal cancer. N Engl J Med. 2004;351:1731-40.
37. Green N. The avoidance of small intestine injury in gynecologic cancer. Int J Radiat Oncol Biol Phys. 1991;9:1385-90.
38. Waddell BE, Rodriguez-Bigas MA, Lee RJ, Weber TK, Petrelli NJ. Prevention of chronic radiation enteritis. J Am Coll Surg. 1999;189:611-24.
39. Rodier JF, Janser JC, Rodier D, Dauplat J, Kauffmann P, Le Bouedec G, et al. Prevention of radiation enteritis by an absorbable polyglycolic acid mesh sling. A 60-case multicentric study. Cancer. 1991;68:2545-9.
40. Logmans A, van Lent M, van Geel AN, Olofsen-Van Acht M, Koper PC, Wiggers T, et al. The pedicled omentoplasty, a simple and effective surgical technique to acquire a safe pelvic radiation field; theoretical and practical aspects. Radiother Oncol. 1994;33:269-71.
41. Chen JS, ChangChien CR, Wang JY, Fan HA. Pelvic peritoneal reconstruction to prevent radiation enteritis in rectal carcinoma. Dis Colon Rectum. 1992;35:897-901.
42. Van Garderen JA, Wiggers TH, Van Geel AN. Complications of the pedicled omentoplasty. Neth J Surg. 119;43:171-4.
43. Keskek M, Gocmen E, Kilic M, Gencturk S, Can B, Cengiz M, et al. Increased expression of cyclooxygenase-2 (COX-2) in radiation-induced small bowel injury in rats. J Surg Res. 2006;135:76-84.
44. Bourgier C, Haydont V, Milliat F, Francois A, Holler V, Lasser P, et al. Inhibition of Rho kinase modulates radiation induced fibrogenic phenotype in intestinal smooth muscle cells through alteration of the cytoskeleton and connective tissue growth factor expression. Gut. 2005;54:336-43.
45. Tytell M, Hooper PL. Heat shock proteins: new keys to the development of cytoprotective therapies. Expert Opin Ther Targets. 2001;5:267-87.
46. Khan AM, Birk JW, Anderson JC, Georgsson M, Park TL, Smith CJ, et al. A prospective randomized placebocontrolled double-blinded pilot study of misoprostol rectal suppositories in the prevention of acute and chronic radiation proctitis symptoms in prostate cancer patients. Am J Gastroenterol. 2000;95:1961-6.

CHAPTER 34

Gastrointestinal Stromal Tumor

Subodh Varshney, Ajit Sewkani

INTRODUCTION AND HISTORICAL ASPECT

The term gastrointestinal stromal tumor (GIST) came into existence in late 1980s and early 1990s. The term stromal tumor was coined by Mazur and Clark in 1983.[1] Earlier, from 1930s to 1950s, these stromal tumors were considered as part of group of smooth muscle tumor which were categorized as leiomyoma, leiomyoblastoma or leiomyosarcoma depending on their degree of differentiation. Subsequently with advent of electron microscopy in late 1960s and 1970s, it was observed that there is differentiation among the smooth muscles. This concept was further supported by advent of immunohistochemistry in 1980. Since then tumors, which were CD34 positive, were considered stromal tumor. Later, CD117 became more specific marker for the GIST.

These tumors have a variable expression for smooth muscle markers such as desmins and actins. Other markers, specific for neural crest origin, neuron specific enolase and S-100, were positive in subgroup of patients with stromal tumors while they were absent in the smooth muscle tumors. This raised a debate whether these tumors show a significant neural differentiation and should be classified as gastrointestinal autonomic nerve tumor. Now it is well accepted that gastrointestinal autonomic nerve tumor is a morphologic variant of GIST.

Gastrointestinal stromal tumors (GIST) are the most common types of mesenchymal tumors of GI tract. Improved diagnostic modalities have led to an increase in incidence of these tumors.

The genetic and immunophenotypic profiling allow to differentiate these tumors from other mesenchymal tumors of GI tract.[2] These tumors are CD 34 positive and express c-KIT oncoprotein. The specific feature of GIST is mutation of c-KIT oncoprotein that results in activation KIT kinase enzyme.[3] The development of tyrosine-kinase inhibitor (TKI) imatinib (STI571) has led a major change in treatment of GIST.[3,4] A mutation in the gene encoding KIT receptor tyrosine kinase has been identified in about 80% of patients, while platelet-derived growth factor receptor alpha (PDGFRA) mutations are found in another 5–10% of patients. Although 10–15% of patients do not have detectable KIT or PDGFRA mutations (wild type GISTs), but the lack of mutation does not rule out the possibility of GIST. In addition, the strong correlation between the presence and type of KIT and PDGFRA mutations and the prognosis has not been fouind. Most of the KIT mutations occur in exon 11 and some are identified in the exon 9. In addition, very rarely they can affect exon 13 and 17. Majority of the PDGFRA mutations affect exon 18. Mutations involving KIT exon 11 are most commonly found in GISTs of all sites, whereas those affecting exon 9 are specific for intestinal GISTs and PDGFRA exon 18 mutations are frequently detected in gastric GISTs. Although the deficiencies in succinate dehydrogenase (SDH) are asscociated with majority of wild type GISTs, other mutations such as alterations in the neurofibromatosis-1 (NF1) gene, activational mutations in BRAF oncogene and RAS-family mutations are also reported. In addition, developments of GISTs have been aasscociated with certain familial syndromes, e.g. Carney-Stratkis, Carney's triad and Familial GIST.

At laparotomy, GISTs are often cystic and hemorrhagic. Morphologically GIST is categorized into three types; (1) spindle cell (70%), (2) epitheloid (20%) or (3) mixed (10%). The epitheloid variety is more frequently detected in the stomach, omentum and disseminated intra-abdominal tumors of undefined origin; while Spindle cell type are more often seen in the intestinal GISTs. The prediction of biological behavior both clinicaly and pathologically is difficult, as it is decided by tumor site, size and mitotic activity.[5]

A stem cell of Cajal is believed to be the principle cell of origin. The comlex network formed by interstitial cells of Cajal (ICCs) within the muscle wall of the gut generally controls gut motility through a muscular pacemaker system.[6] Developmemt of ICC system needs expression of the c-KIT proto-oncogenes. The expression of c-KIT has been broadly accepted as a molecular marker of ICCs, although its expression is not limited to this cell type.[7] Constitutive activation of mutant c-KIT tyrosine kinase receptors in the absence of its ligand in the stem cell result in malignant transformation of cells.[6,7]

EPIDEMIOLOGY

The annual incidence of GIST is estimated to be 10–20 per million people. However, because of the incomplete definition and classification, the precise incidence is not known. Adults over 40 years constitute over 90% cases of GIST. However, GISTs can develop in all age groups including children.[8] They occur with equal frequency in both males and females (Fig. 1).

It can arise in any part of GI tract, most common being stomach (60%) and small intestine (30%). The remaining sites include esophagus, large intestine (colon and rectum), and anus. Rarely, they can develop in the gallbladder, pancreas, liver and urinary bladder. In addition, they may arise in extra-gastroinetsinal sites such as mesentery, retroperitoneum and omentum, called as extra-gastrointestinal stromal tumor (EGIST).[9]

The risk of malignancy vary from 20% to 30% depending up on site, size and mitotic activity of the tumor. Majority of the GISTs are sporadic (not inherited) and have no clear cause. Their incidence is not affected by geographic location, ethnicity, race or occupation. At present, very few risk factors are known for GISTs.

FAMILIAL GASTROINTESTINAL STROMAL TUMOR SYNDROMES

There is an increased risk of development of stromal tumors in this inherited condition. This is a rare syndrome and tumors develop at a younger age and are multiple in many occasions. In this syndrome abnormal copy of c-KIT genes are transmitted from parents to child and are found in all the cells. In sporadic GIST, the same gene is mutated but found only in cancer cells.[10] Recently, germ line mutations encoding SDH subunits have been detected in familial GISTs in addition to germ line KIT mutations. Rarely, GISTs can develop in association with NF type 1. They are often multiple in number and arise in small intestine. Further, Carney's triad constitutes the association of gastric GIST, extra-adrenal paraganglioma and pulmonary chondroma, while Carney-Stratakis syndrome comprises GIST and paragangliomas.

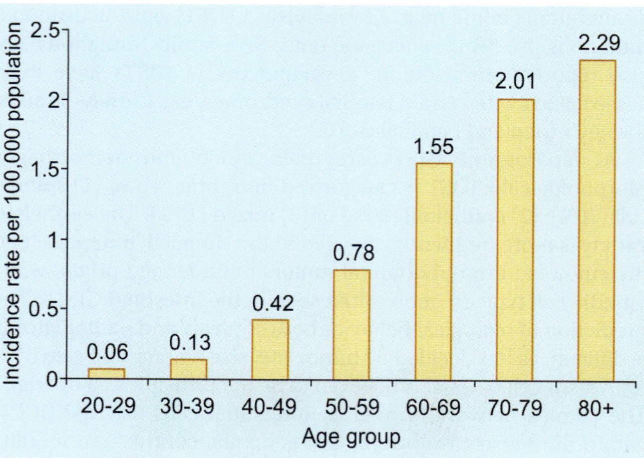

Figure 1 Age-adjusted incidence rates of GIST

ANATOMICAL LOCATION OF TUMOR

Anatomical distribution of GIST has been shown in Figure 2.

Esophagus

Very rarely GIST can arise in the esophagus. Majority of the esophageal GISTs are large in size: more than 5 cm, localized in the lower 3rd part and show more than 5 mitoses/50 HPF. Sometimes large ulcerated masses may involve the proximal part of the stomach and adjacent structures. As only few cases with long-term follow-up have been reported in the literature, the conclusive risk categorization of the esophageal GISTs has not been defined yet. As in other locations, esophageal GISTs have mutations in exon 11 of c-KIT.[7]

Stomach

Stomach is the most common site for GIST. Fundus and body of stomach are most frequent site of GIST (55%), followed by antrum (20–25%) and pylorus (20%). Mostly GIST are submucosal (60%) or subserosal (30%) and rarely intramural (10%).

Most common symptoms of gastric GIST are bleeding, abdominal pain, malaise or fatigue. Overall, majority of the gastric GISTs behave in an indolent manner. But there some which have poor outcome. The poor prognostic factors are large size (>8 cm), more mitoses (≥ 3/HPF), higher histologic grade more than or equal to 2 or R_1/R_2 resection. Debulking surgery for palliation prolongs survival in various instances[11] but still R_0 resection has best chance of cure and prolonged survival (Fig. 3).

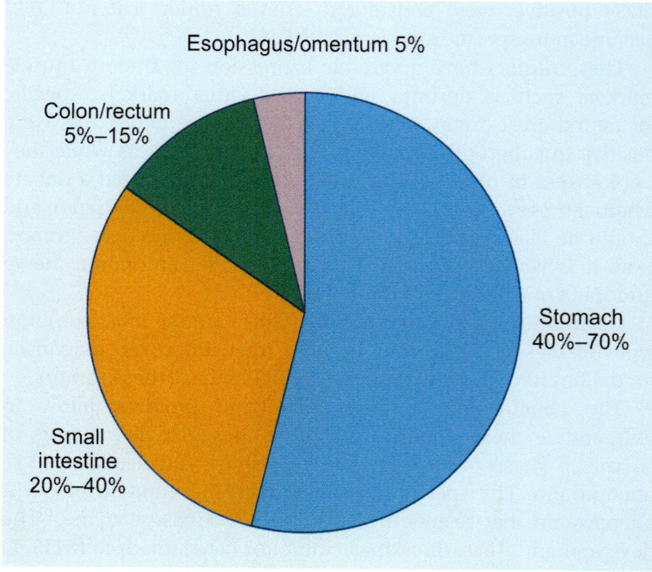

Figure 2 Anatomical distribution of GIST

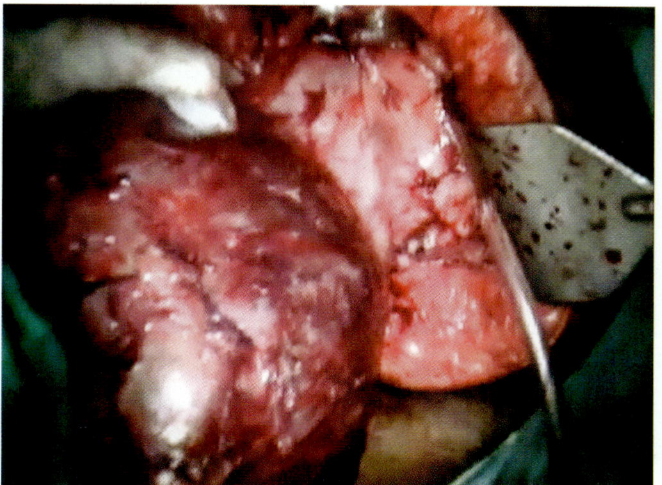

Figure 3 Operative picture of gastric GIST

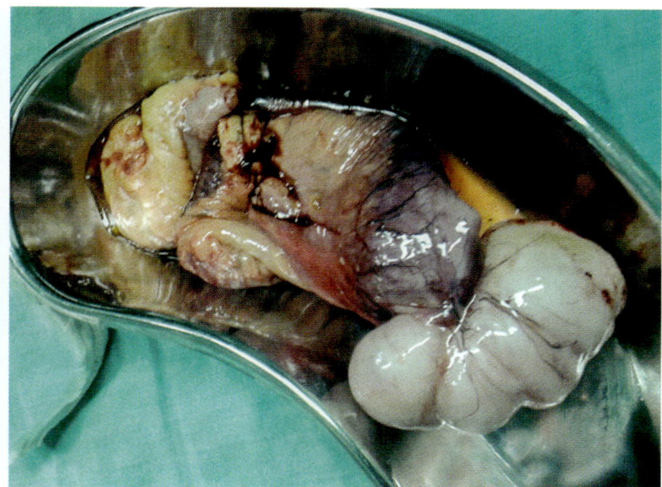

Figure 4 Specimen of small bowel (jejunal) GIST

Small Bowel

Small intestinal GIST have vague and nonspecific symptoms, making an early diagnosis difficult. As compared to gastric GISTs, small intestinal GISTs tend to be more aggressive outcome with a tumor related mortality up to 50%.

Duodenal GIST can be benign when they are small in size (<5 cm), have fewer mitoses less than 2/50 HPF and are paucicellular spindle cells type. Those with larger size (>5 cm) epitheliod cells with hypercellularity and have mitosis more than 2/50 HPF are malignant. There is an increased risk of distal ileal GIST in patients with Crohn's disease (Fig. 4).[12]

Colon and Rectum

It is very rare to find GIST arising from colon, with incidence of 1–2%. GISTs of the colon most commonly arise in anorectal region. Their presentation varies from incidental small tumors to large masses, occupying entire pelvis. The prognosis is again determined by mitotic rate and tumor size. Size less than 2 cm and mitotic rate less than 1 mitosis/50 HPF are suggestive of benign lesion, while size more than 5 cm and mitotic more than 5/10 HPF are generally accepted as predictors of malignancy (Figs 5A and B).

PRESENTATION

Signs and Symptoms of Gastrointestinal Stromal Tumors

The most common presentation of GIST is an asymptomatic mass. The symptoms depend up on the tumor size and location, the most common being abdominal pain. Few patients may present as acute abdomen due to tumor rupture, gastrointestinal obstruction or acute appendicitis.

The common symptoms related to GISTs include:

- Abdominal discomfort or pain
- A mass or swelling in the abdomen
- Nausea, vomiting
- Early satiety
- Loss of appetite
- Weight loss
- Dysphagia (for tumors in the esophagus)
- GI bleed (small bowel GIST)
- Altered bowel habits (rectal GIST)
- Anemic symptoms.

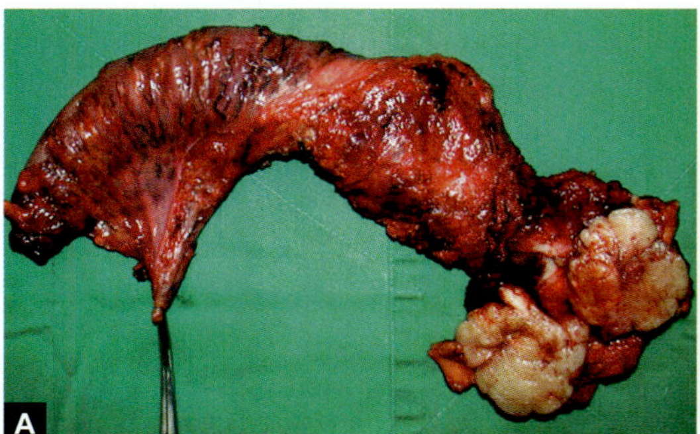

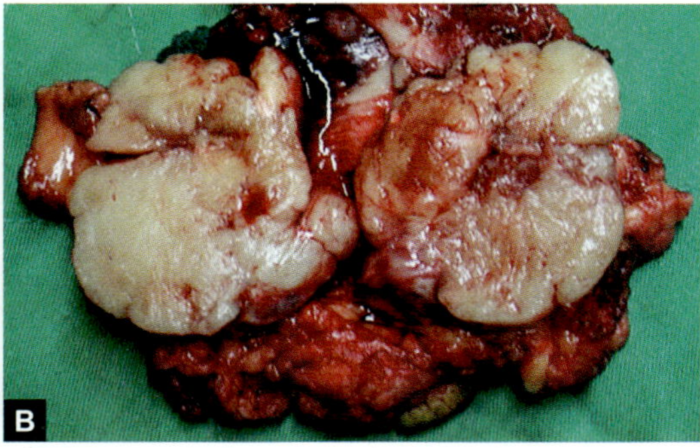

Figures 5A and B Specimen of rectal GIST (APR Specimen)

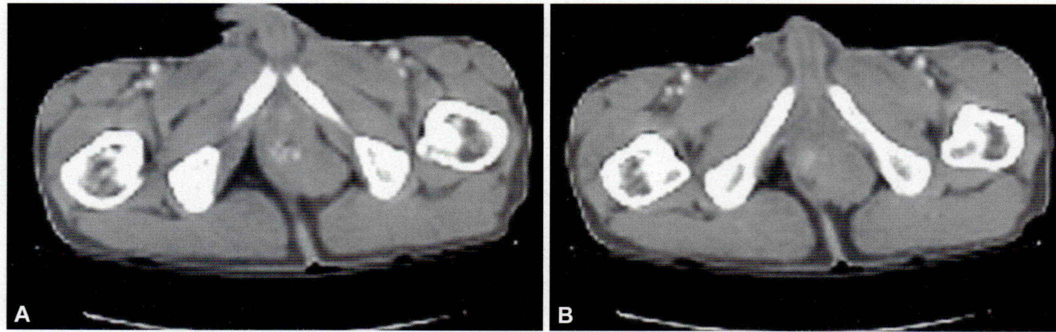

Figures 6A and B CECT showing rectal GIST

Generally, benign behavior has been reported with the tumors which are confined locally at diagnosis and detected incidentally during surgery. However, as their behavior is uncertain and they need to be examined pathologically, resection of these tumors is considered. The most common site for metastasis are liver and/or dissemination within the abdominal cavity. Metastasis to lymph nodes is very rare, while that to the lungs and other extra-abdominal sites can occur in advanced cases.

EVALUATION

Routine screeing is not recommended, as there are no effective screening tests for diagnosing GISTs. Rarely, a GIST may detected incidentally during endoscopy, CT scan, barium study or abdominal surgery performed for another reason. Further evaluation may be required to confirm the diagnosis, if the GIST is suspected.

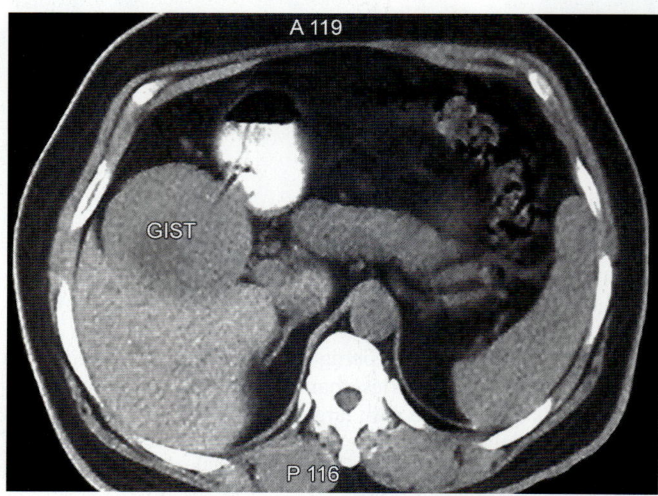

Figure 7 CT scan showing colonic GIST

IMAGING TESTS

Reasons for performing imaging test include:
- To find out whether tumor is malignant
- To assess tumor extent
- To assess efficacy of treatment
- To look for tumor recurrence.

BARIUM X-RAYS

Depending on the location of tumor, a barium swallow, follow through, enteroclysis or enema may be chosen. Although these tests can suggest the diagnosis of GI tumors, small intestine tumors may be missed. In most cases they have been supplanted by endoscopy which has the advantage of taking biopsy from suspicious area.

COMPUTED TOMOGRAPHY (CT) SCAN

Contrast-enhanced computed tomography (CECT) abdomen is the preferred imaging modality to characterize an abdominal mass, to define its extent and to look for metastases. It is a good tool to guide a percutaneous biopsy and to assess tumor response to targeted therapy. A decrease in tumor size or tumor density on CT indicate positive reponse to therapy. Sometimes the decrease in tumor density may be the only sign (even with increasing tumor size) and may precede tumor shrinkage. In addition, in neoadjuvant settings, the decline in tumor density can predict response to therapy early. Similarly, the increase in intra tumoral density (giving a "nodule within the nodule" appearance) despite similar size may suggest disease progression (Figs 6A and B).

MAGNETIC RESONANCE IMAGING SCANS

Magnetic resonance imaging (MRI) is equivalent to CT in evaluating the primary tumor; however, it provides better anatomical definition of liver secondaries and rectal GIST. Similar to CT, it also helps in evalution of tumor reponse to TKIs therapy. In addition, it is an excellent modality to evaluate secondaries to other distant organs, particularly the brain or spine (Fig. 7).

POSITRON EMISSION TOMOGRAPHY (PET) SCAN

Positron emission tomography (PET) scan cannot show accurate anatomical details like CT or MRI images, but it can detect the possible areas of tumor spread. It can also help in clarifying the doubtful findings on CT or MRI. In addition, PET has ability to differentiate necrotic tissue from an active tumor and non-descript benign changes from recurrent tumor. It adds important value to standard CT images because anatomical changes on CT often lag behind the changes in the metabolic activity of tumors. The PET scan can be useful to assess response to the imatinib at 2–4 weeks after initiation of therapy.[13] Recently, many imaging centers can provide both anatomical and functional evaluation of tumors in one step as they are equipped with combined PET-CT scanners (Figs 8 and 9).

ENDOSCOPY

Most of the GISTs are submucosal; this makes them difficult to diagnose with endoscopy. Tumor breaks through the mucosa is easily seen on endoscopy, and these have a greater chance of malignancy (Figs 10 and 11).

Capsule endoscopy can evaluate whole of the small intestine. However, it can not show the exact anatomical location of the lesion and also biopsy of the abnormal areas cannot be done during the test. But, while performing double balloon enteroscopy, it is possible to define the site of lesion and also to conduct the biopsy (Fig. 12).

Figures 8A and B FDG-PET scans of a patient with metastatic GIST (A) prior to and (B) show no 18FDG uptake in all prevoius tumor sites following response to 1 month Imatinib therapy

ENDOSCOPIC ULTRASOUND

Endoscopic ultrasound has an additional diagnostic value especially in gastric and rectal GISTs because of its ability to differentiate the various layers of intestinal wall which confirms the origin of lesion from muscle layer. It may be used as guide for endoscopic biopsy.

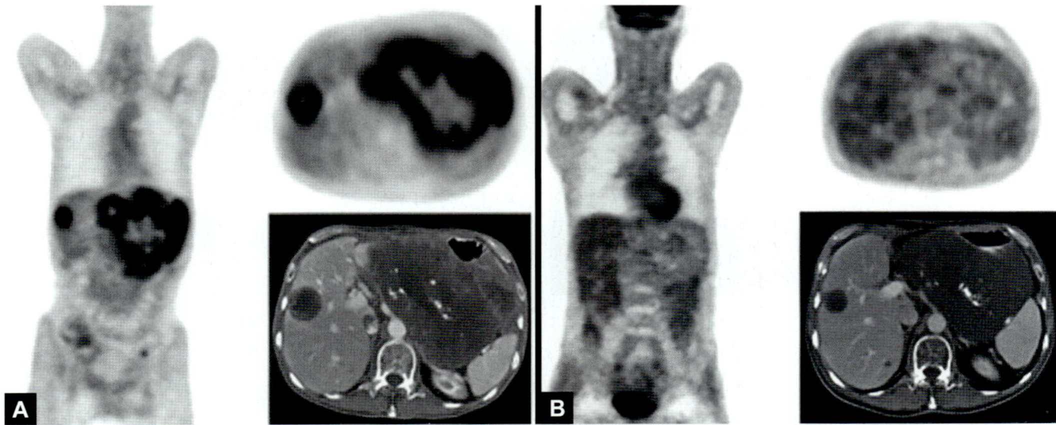

Figures 9A and B FDG-PET and correlating CT scans of a patient prior to and 1 month after imatinib therapy (consistent with response to imatinib therapy despite the fact that the gastric and hepatic lesions are stable; however, that the densities of the gastric mass and the hepatic lesion have significantly decreased on CT)

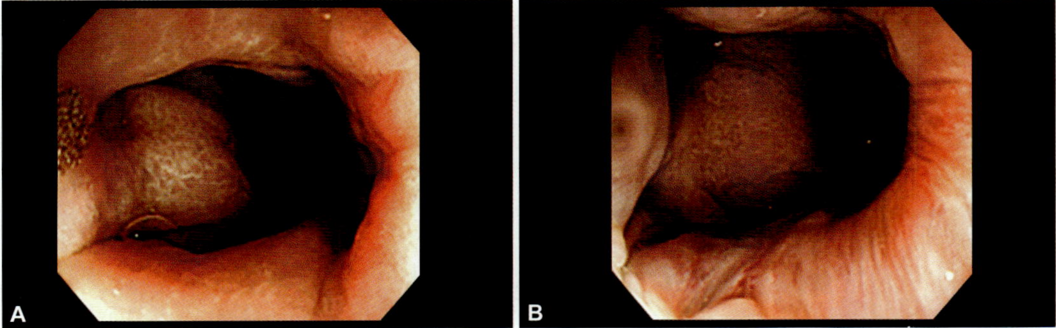

Figures 10A and B Endoscopic pictures of rectal GIST

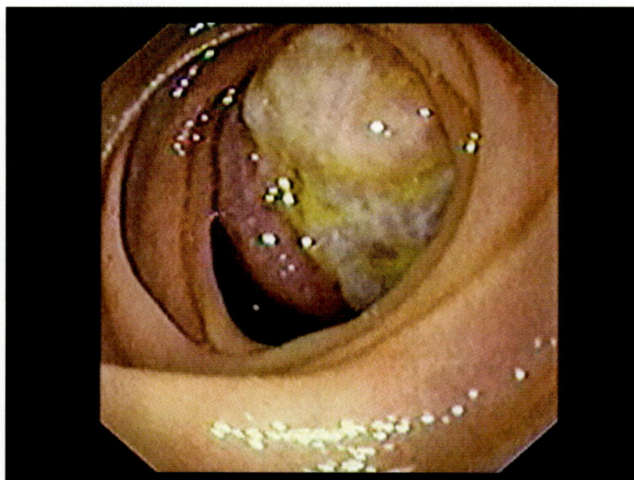

Figure 11 Stromal tumor of the jejunum (GIST). Large polypoid tumor with a deep central ulceration

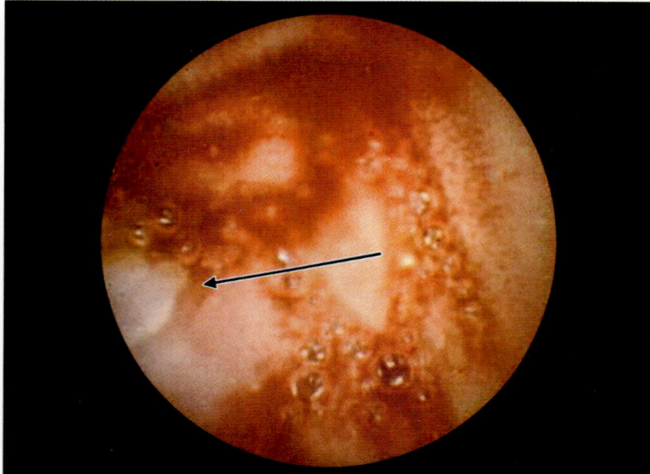

Figure 12 GIST of the jejunum. Large polypoid tumor in jejunum with a deep central ulceration (arrow) with oozing bleeding

Presence of two or three of the endosonographic features such as tumor size of more than 4 cm, irregular extraluminal border, echogenic foci and cystic spaces suggest malignancy with 80–100% confidence (Figs 13A and B).[14]

BIOPSY AND IMMUNOHISTOCHEMISTRY

There are several ways to take a sample from a GI tract tumor:

- Endoscopic biopsy
- Image guided fine needle biopsy
- Surgical biopsy.

Biopsy is usually required to confirm the diagnosis of primary GIST before initiation of preoperative TKI therapy. Due to risk of tumor hemorrhage and intra-abdominal dissemination, EUS guided biopsy is preferred over percutaneous biopsy. Percutaneous biopsy under image guidance may be used for the confirmation of metastatic disease.

The diagnosis of GIST on biopsy tissue sample is usually achieved with the help of immunohistochemical staining for CD117 and molecular genetic testing for KIT and PDGFRA mutations. If GIST is diagnosed, the *mitotic rate* needs to be assessed to grade the tumor as it has a prognostic value. It is expressed as number of mitosis per 50 HPF.

Other IHC markers in GIST are CD 34 (70%), SMA—smooth muscle actin (20–30%), S 100 protein (10%) and desmin (<5%). The expression of CD34 and SMA is often reciprocal. Colorectal and esophageal GISTs consistently show CD 34 positivity while small bowel lesions are more often SMA positive.

DOG1 is chloride dependent protein activated by calcium dependent receptor. It is expressed by GISTs irrespective of mutation type. Its immunostaining may be helpful for cases that cannot be diagnosed as GIST on the basis of CD 117 immunostaining and KIT and PDGFRA mutation testing (Figs 14 to 16).

STAGING

Staging for tumors is an important factor in selecting treatment options and in predicting the patient's prognosis.

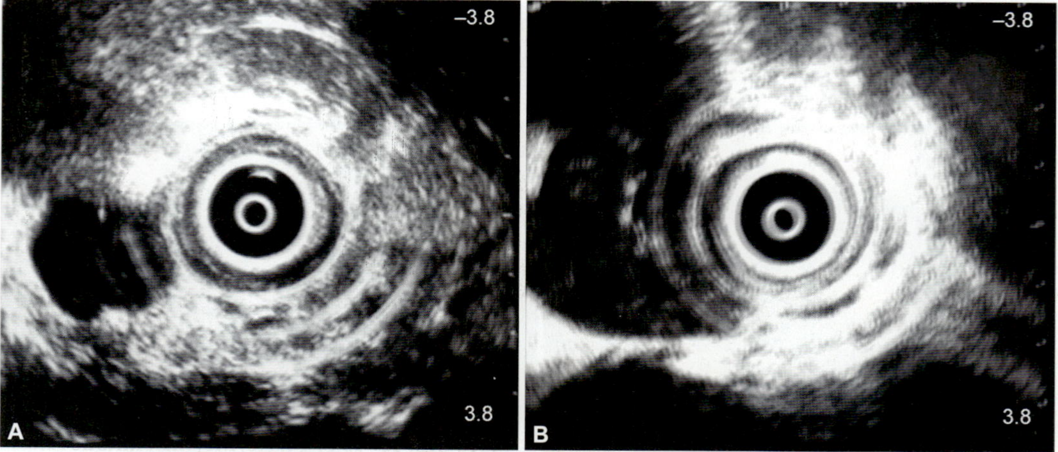

Figures 13A and B Endoeono (TRUS) picture showing rectal GIST

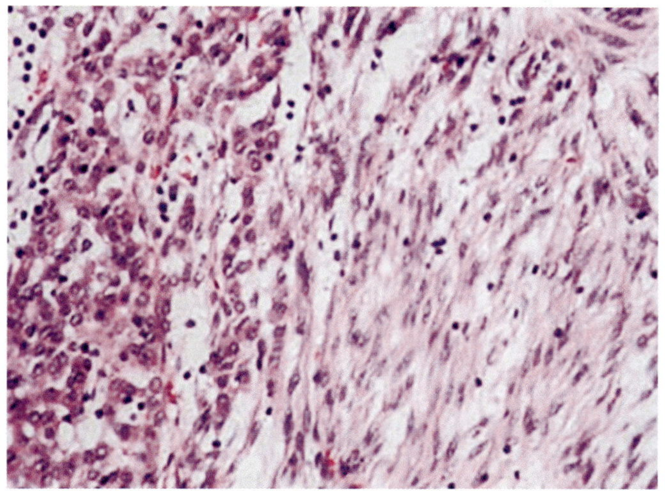

Figure 14 GIST-high power maginification. Tumor shows plasmacytoid (left hand side), as well as spindle-cell (right hand side) growth pattern

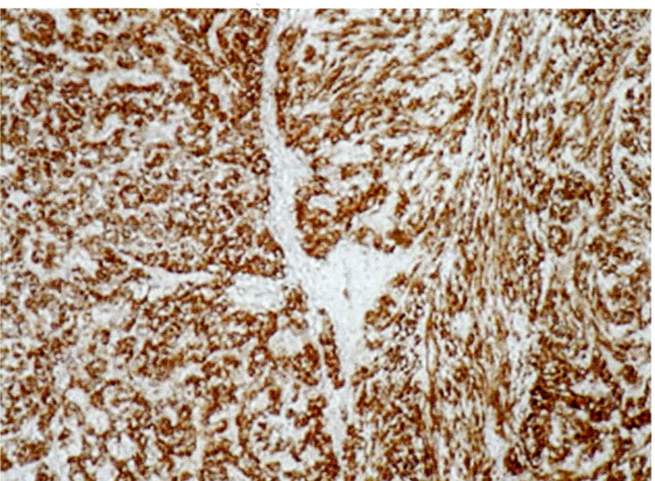

Figure 15 The same picture. All tumor cells show strong expression of c-KIT (CD117)

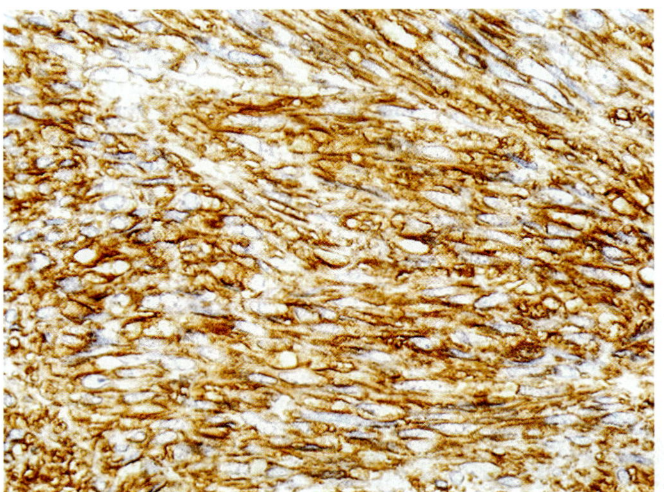

Figure 16 Histopathologic image of GIST arising in the stomach. CD34 immunostain

AJCC TNM Staging System

The AJCC recently developed a TNM staging system for GISTs.

T Categories for Gastrointestinal Stromal Tumor

TX: The primary (main) tumor cannot be assessed
T0: No signs of a primary tumor
T1: The tumor is ≤2 cm across
T2: The tumor is >2 cm but ≤5 cm across
T3: The tumor >5 cm across but ≤10 cm across
T4: The tumor is >10 cm across

N Categories for Gastrointestinal Stromal Tumor

NX: Assessment of regional lymph node not done
N0: Regional lymph nodes free of cancer
N1: Regional lymph nodes involved by cancer

M Categories for Gastrointestinal Stromal Tumor

M0: Cancer is localized to site, not metastasized
M1: Cancer has metastasized to distant organs or sites.

Histological Grade

GX: Grade cannot be assessed
G1: Low grade; mitotic rate ≤5/50 HPF
G2: High grade; mitotic rrate >5/50 HPF

Stage Grouping

The T, N and M categories are combined, with the mitotic rate, in a process called stage grouping. The stage grouping depends on the organ of origin.

Gastric Gastrointestinal Stromal Tumor

Stage IA: T1 or T2, N0, M0, low mitotic rate
Stage IB: T3, N0, M0, low mitotic rate
Stage II: T1 or T2, N0, M0, high mitotic rate or T4, N0, M0, low mitotic rate
Stage IIIA: T3, N0, M0, high mitotic rate
Stage IIIB: T4, N0, M0, high mitotic rate
Stage IV: Any T, N1, M0, any mitotic rate or any T, any N, M1, any mitotic rate.

Small Intestinal Gastrointestinal Stromal Tumor

Stage IA: T1 or T2, N0, M0, low mitotic rate
Stage II: T3, N0, M0, low mitotic rate
Stage IIIA: T1, N0, M0, high mitotic rate or T4, N0, M0, low mitotic rate
Stage IIIB: T2, T3 or T4, N0, M0, high mitotic rate
Stage IV: Any T, N1, M0, any mitotic rate or any T, any N, M1, any mitotic rate.

PROGNOSTIC FACTORS

The clinical behavior of GISTs can be benign to very malignant. The outcome can be very unpredictable. There is no accepted single staging system of a GIST. Several prognostic factors have been studied like size, molecular studies, histology and immunohistochemistry. Most useful predictors for malignancy are large size and high mitotic counts.[15]

Histopathology	*Size (cm)*	*Mitosis (HPF)*
Benign	<5	<1/10
Borderline	>5	<1/10
Malignant	>10	>1/10

Grading of Gastrointestinal Stromal Tumors

Grade	*Mitoses (HPF)*	*Cellularity*	*Atypia*	*Necrosis*
I	<3/10	Mild-Moderate	Absent	Absent
II	<6/10	Moderate	Mild	Absent
III	>6/10	Marked	Moderate	Focal
IV	>6/10	Marked	Marked	Prominent

Larger GIST (>5 cm) has a higher malignant potential than smaller GIST (<5 cm). Similarly, mitoses more than 5/50 HPF has a higher malignant potential unless if it is duodenal GIST where more than 2/50 HPF mitoses have a higher malignant potential. Gastric GIST (5–10 cm) with low mitotic or Ki 67 count have a good prognosis while small bowel GIST more than 5 cm are aggressive tumors, irrespective of mitotic count. Any GIST which is more than 10 cm behave in a malignant way.

Sclerosis is a favorable prognostic feature while hypercellular sarcomatous feature predicts malignant behavior.[5]

KIT exon 11 mutation is a bad prognostic marker and is generally seen in larger tumors. In Gastric GIST, deletion in exon 11 has a worse prognosis than point mutation.[3-5]

In 2002, Fletcher et al.[16] estimated the risk of progression in GISTs based upon tumor size and mitotic rate, while Miettinen et al.[17] extended this risk stratification by adding tumor site. The clinical utility of the Miettinen-Lasota classification has been proven in large dataset. The Modified NIH Joensuu Criteria[18] has included the presence of tumor rupture in addition to tumor size, mitotic rate and site of tumor. Recently, a nomogram has been developed by Gold and colleagues[19] to predict recurrence-free survival after resection of localized primary GIST. It takes into account tumor size, site and mitotic index.

Resectable versus Unresectable Tumors

Resectability depends upon various factors such as tumor size, its location and presence of spread to other parts of body. Resectable tumors can be removed certainly without significant risk of morbidity, while unserectable tumors cannot be removed completely because of their spread and other reasons. Targeted therapy may be a viable option to downsize the tumor, if the tumor is found to be unresectable or marginally resectable.

Survival Rates for Gastrointestinal Stromal Tumors

The survival rates of GISTs are difficult to determine because these tumors are uncommon. Moreover in past many of these tumors were classified in other types of tumors. Finally because after the invention of targeted therapy, the treatment of GISTs has changed substantially over last few years.

The overall 5-year survival rate of patients with malignant GIST has been found to be about 45% based on the historical data of the patients treated between 1990 and 2010. However, the 5-year relative survival of about 64% has been reported for the tumors that were confined to the organ of origin.

TREATMENT OPTIONS AND ALGORITHM

The tumor characteristics (such as size, location, growth rate, and whether it has spread) and overall general condition of the patient are taken into consideration while deciding the treatement.

Surgery and targeted drug therapy are two important reasonable therapeutic options for GISTs, while other options, such as chemotherapy and radiation therapy are useful only in palliative settings. All therapeutic choices along with their potential adverse effects should be discussed with the patient.

Surgery for Gastrointestinal Stromal Tumors

Surgical resection is the ideal treatment for localized and potentially resectable GISTs. Rupture of the pseudocapsule should be avoided while handling of the tumor, as spillage might increase the risk of local recurrence and spread. The primary aim should be to achieve R0 resection as 5-year survival of patients with complete gross resection is better than that of patient with incomplete excision (45% vs 9%).[20,21] In addition, surgical resection may be needed in case of advanced or recurrent disease following a favorable response or a stable diasease after TKI therapy and for limited disease progression on systemic therapy. However, upfront surgery may be needed for complications such as perforation, hemorrhage or obstruction. Even in patients presenting with tumor rupture, every effort should be made to remove all visible tumor as recurrence free survival of such patients (with microscopic positive margin) at a median of 4 years is similar to that of patients who have undergone R0 resection. Large GISTs with invasion into surrounding structures may require en bloc resection of infiltrated organs. Wedge resection (for stomach), sphincter sparing resection (rectum) or organ sparing resection (for esophagus and duodenum) to obtain negative resection margin should be considered whenever possible. Preoperative TKI therapy can enble such resections and improve the outcome.[22] As GIST metastasize seldom to lymph nodes, lymphadenectomy is warrented only for enlarged suspicious lymph nodes. The role of laparoscopic approach in resection of GISTs is continuously expanding. Although there are no prospective studies in the literature, the retrospective analyses have reported low morbidity, short hospital stay and low recurrence rate with laparoscopic or laparoscopic assisted resections. Laparoscopic approach may be amenable for selected patients having GISTs in favorable anatomical sites such as gastric anterior wall, jejunum and ileum. In addition, small rectal GISTs can also be considered for laparoscopic resection.[21]

The liver secondaries from GISTs are usually multifocal, so they may not suitable for hepatic resection, However, they can be tackled with cryosurgery, radiofrequency ablation, embolization, or ethanol ablation. The value of these treatments in patients with a GIST is not fully known as there are not enough studies.

TARGETED THERAPY FOR GASTROINTESTINAL STROMAL TUMOR

Tyrosine-kinase inhibitors inhibit activation of enzyme tyrosine kinase by occupying its active site and subsequently stop the cell division.[23] Besides imatinib, many other TKIs such as sunitinib,[24] nilotinib, masatinib, mosetanib, sorafenib, regorafenib, and dasatinib are available. Ability to inhibit one or several tyrosine kinases differ among these drugs. The impact of imatinib therapy is decided by the primary KIT and PDGFRA mutation status. GISTs with exon 11 KIT mutations show the substantial response, while those with exon 9 mutations usually benefit from higher imatinib dosage (800 mg/day). Patients with wild type GIST do not benefit from imatinib. In addition, among the GISTs with PDGFRA mutations, exon 18 mutated GISTs generally show the response with exception of GIST with exon 18 D842V mutation.

Imatinib is generally well tolerated and safe. Edema (mostly periorbital), muscle cramps and gastrointestinal disturbances are commonly encountered clinical side effects of this drug. These side effects do not require interruption of therapy, and can be managed symptomatically. Sometimes they may subside with prolonged therapy. Rarely serious side effects such as low blood count, LFT abnormalities, lung toxicity and GI bleeding can occur. However, these side effects usually improve with interruption of therapy.

Sunitinib inhibits multiple tyrosine kinases. It can produce objective response and control the disease progression in imatinib resistant GISTs. Sunitinib is a reasonable alternative TKI for the patients intolerant to imatinib. The commonly reported adverse effecs of sunitinib in clinical trials are nausea, fatigue and vomitting. Other side effects comprise of anorexia, abdominal pain, diarrhea, hematological toxicities and skin discoloration. In addition, a remarkable risk of hand foot skin reaction (HFSR) is associated with sunitinib. Regular application of emollient lotion can prevent it. If the above side effects are severe, dose reduction or interruption of sunitinib should be considered. Recent reports have revealed the association of hypertension, cardiotoxicity and hypothyroidism with the use of sunitinib. Thus, patients with cardiac risk factors or a history of heart disease should be closely monitored for hypertension and left ventricular ejection fraction. In addition, serum TSH levels are measured every 3–6 months.

Resistance to Imatinib

Although patients with advanced GISTs benefit from imatinib, resistance to the drug can develop in some patients. The clinical progression occurring during initial 6 months of therapy constitutes primary resistance. It is frequently seen in wild type GISTs, GISTs with PDGFRA exon 18 D284V mutations or GISTs carrying exon 9 mutation treated with 400 mg of imatinib daily. Secondary resistance is defined as disease progression after initial reponse or stabilization on imatinib for more than 6 months. Outgrowth of tumor clones with secondary mutations in KIT is the most common cause of secondary imatinib resistance. Increasing the dose to 800 mg/day or shfting to sunitinib is a sensible alternative for patients with disease progression on 400 mg/day of imatinib.

Assessment of Response

The response to systemic treatment in solid tumors is traditionally assessed with RECIST criteria. However, these criteria are not sensitive in GISTs.[25] Choi et al.[26,27] developed criteria (including tumor size and density) based on CT to assess response. Although these criteria correlate with PET and are superior to RECIST criteria, they lack universal acceptance, validation in cases treated previously with various targeted therapies and simplicity for use outside the specialized centers. Metabolic response criteria based on PET have been proposed by EORTC[28] and they define complete reponse, partial reponse, stable disease and disease progression. However, as the information provided by CECT correlates with that from PET-CT in up to 95% cases, contrast enchanced CT scan is the preferred imaging modality for the assessment of the treatment reponse in patients with GIST on preoperative TKI therapy.

Adjuvant Therapy

Surgery alone does not provide long-term survival for majority of the GIST patients due to increased risk of postoperative recurrence, especially in those with high risk features. Depending upon the results of phase III ACOSOG Z9001 and SSG XVIII/AIO trials, postoperative imatinib (400 mg/day) therapy is recommended following complete resection of primary GIST in patients with high risk recurrence potential such as size of tumor more than 10 cm and any no. of mitoses, no. of mitoses more than 10 and any tumor size, mitotic index more than 5 and tumor size more than 5 cm, tumor size less than 5 cm and no. of mitoses more than 5 (non-gastric GIST), tumor size 5–10 cm and no. of mitoses less than 5 (non-gastric GIST) and those with no preoperative imatinib therapy.[29,30] This treatment must be continued for at least 36 months. Athough 3 years of adjuvant imatinib in high risk patients reduces the risk of recurrence, it does not prolong the overall survival. The continuation of imatinib therapy is also warranted for patients with complete resection following preoperative imatinib therapy. In addition, imatinib needs be continued, if the persistent metastatic or residual tumor remains following surgical resection.

Preoperative Therapy

By causing tumor shrinkage, preoperative TKI facilitates R0 resection, allows function or organ sparing resection and also mutilating surgeries can be avoided. In addition, the risk of intraoperative tumor rupture and peritoneal seeding is reduced secondary to decreased tumor size and vascularity.

There is lack of evidence in the literature regarding the role preoperative TKI therapy, especially in neoadjuvant setting. Only observational studies and few phase II trials constitute the available data in the literature. Even in the prospective BFR 14 phase III study, the preoperative therapy data was solely acquired by a retrospective subgroup analysis of only 9 patients.[31] Most of the series involved only cases with unresectable or metastatic GISTs, focusing on the downsizing therapy. Although these prospective studies have revealed safety and beneficial effect of preoperative therapy, the survival benefit could not be evaluated because of the lack of control arm and the potential confounding effect of administration of adjuvant imatinib therapy. Thus, at present, the use of preoperative TKI therapy in locally advanced/unresectable or resectable primary or recurrent GIST should be decided on individual basis.

Before the initiation of preoperative imatinib, baseline CECT is obtained. Imatinib needs to be continued until maximal reponse (two successive CT scans showing no further improvement or lesion becomes surgically resectable on scan) is seen and 6–12 months may be required to achieve this reponse. But, it is not always needed to delay the surgery until a maximal response is seen and presence of symptoms or complications may require early surgical intervention. Careful evaluation of the response is undertaken to avoid missing of the best window for surgical intervention. CT scan is performed every 8–12 weeks. If it shows no progression, the same dose of imatinib is continued and surgical resection must be considered if possible. But if the CT scan reveals progression of the disease, surgery is advocated after stoppage of imatinib therapy.

Palliative Therapy

At present the standard of care for patients with metastatic or recurrent GISTs which are c-KIT positive is imatinib. In these

Flow chart 1 Algorithm for management of GIST

Evidence of intra-abdominal tumor, differential diagnosis GIST
→ Staging biopsys if needed for therapeutical concept
→ Histological evidence of GIST[1]

- Metastatic: imatinib 400 mg/d or 600 mg/d
  - Progression → Evaluate → Dose escalation to 800 mg/d
  - Stable disease response → Continue imatinib 400 mg/d or 600 mg/d → (back to Stable disease response)
- Inoperable[2] imatinib 400 mg/d or 600 mg/d
  - Progression → Evaluate → Dose escalation to 800 mg/d
  - Stable disease response → Secondary operable: resection[3]
- Secondary operable: resection[3] → Continue imatinib 400 mg/d or 600 mg/d
- Primary operable: resection
  - Incomplete resection: imatinib 400 mg/d or 600 mg/d
  - Complete resection: adjuvant therapy with imatinib in clinical trials

Dose escalation to 800 mg/d
- Progression
  - Local progression → 800 mg/d[4] + Local treatment (surgery, RFA, LITT[5])
  - Systemic progression → Clinical trials: imatinib + RAD001, imatinib + PKC412, imatinib + AMN107, sunitinib
- Stable disease response → Continue imatinib 800 mg/d → (back to Stable disease response)

patients, imatinib needs to be continued until progression. Interruption of therapy leads to either increased risk of relapse (patients with no residual disease on imaging) or flare up of the disease (patients with stable or responsive disease). Also, patients should be evaluated at 3 monthly intervals for assessement of tumor reponse. Patients with progressive disease requires escalation of dose of imatinib up to 800 mg/day as tolerated or switching to sunitinib. The role of surgery is very limited in this group of patients. Although benefit of surgery is not proven in clinical trials, selected patients with limited progression or stable/responsive disease on imatinib, which is resectable, may get maximum benefit from the surgery. If the patient is not a surgical candidate, other options such as RFA, chemoembolization or palliative RT (in case of boney metastases) may be considered.

Follow-up Care

Follow-up is required to detect the tumor recurrence early and also the potential adverse effects of treatment. Generally relapse occurs within 2–3 years in patients with high risk GISTs, while patients with low risk disease can relapse later. Thus, risk stratification can help in selecting individualized surveillance program. There is no published data regarding the optimal follow-up strategy for the patients with localized disease treated surgically. The National Comprehensive Cancer Network (NCCN) consensus panel suggests a thorough history and physical examination and CECT abdomen along with pelvis at the interval of 3–6 months during the first 5 years, followed by annual CT scan thereafter.[32] More frequent follow-up is advocated by ESMO guidelines[33] for the patients with intermediate-risk and high-risk GISTs (CT at the interval of 3–4 months for the first 3 years, then every 6 months through 5 years, then yearly thereafter) as compared to those with low-risk tumors (CT every 6 months for 5 years) (Flow chart 1).

REFERENCES

1. Mazur MT, Clark HB. Gastric stromal tumors. Reappraisal of histogenesis. Am J Surg Pathol. 1983;7(6):507-19.
2. El-Rifai W, Sarlomo-Rikala M, Andersson LC, et al. DNA sequence copy number changes in gastrointestinal stromal tumors: tumor progression and prognostic significance. Cancer Res. 2000;60: 3899-903.
3. de Silva CM, Reid R. Gastrointestinal stromal tumors (GIST): C-kit mutations, CD117 expression, differential diagnosis and targeted cancer therapy with imatinib. Pathology Oncology Research. 2003;9(1):13-9.
4. Din OS, Woll PJ. Treatment of gastrointestinal stromal tumor: focus on imatinib mesylate. Ther Clin Risk Manag. 2008;4(1):149-62.
5. Miettinen M, El-Rifai W, HL Sobin L, Lasota J, et al. Evaluation of malignancy and prognosis of gastrointestinal stromal tumors: a review. Hum Pathol. 2002;33:478-83.
6. Min KW, Leabu M. Interstitial cells of Cajal (ICC) and Gastrointestinal stromal tumors (GIST): facts, speculations and myths. J Cell Mol Med. 2006;10(4):995-1013.
7. Rubin BP, Singer S, Tsao C, Duensing A, Lux ML, Ruiz R, et al. KIT activation is a ubiquitous feature of gastrointestinal stromal tumors. Cancer Res. 2001;61:8118-21.
8. Kaemmer DA, Otto J, Lassay L, Steinau G, Klink C, Junge K, et al. The Gist of literature on paediatric GIST: review of clinical presentation. J Pediatr Hematol Oncol. 2009;31(2):108-12.
9. Col C, Yilmaz F. A case report of an extraintestinal GIST presenting as a giant abdominopelvic tumors. Gastrointest Cancer Res. 2013;6(4):120-2.
10. Postow MA, Robson ME. Inherited gastrointestinal stromal tumor syndrome: mutation clinical features and therapeutic implications. Clin Sarcoma Res. 2012;2:16.
11. El-Hanafy E, El-Hemaly M, Hamdy E, El-Raouf AA, El-Hak NG, Atif E. Surgical management of gastric gastrointestinal stromal tumor: a single centre esperience. Saudi J Gastroenterol. 2011;17(3): 189-93.
12. Pfeffel F, Stiglbauer W, Depisch D, Oberhuber G, Raderer M, Scheithauer W. Coincidence of Crohn's disease and a high-risk gastrointestinal stromal tumor of the terminal ileum. Digestion. 1999;60:363-6.
13. Basu S, Mohadas KM, Peshwe H, Asopa R, Vyawahare M. FDG-PET and PET/CT in the clinical management of gastrointestinal stromal tumor. Nuclear Medicine Communications. 2008;29:1026-39.
14. Chak A, Canto MI, Rosch T, Dittler HJ, Hawes RH, Tio TL, et al. Endosonographic differentiation of benign and malignant stromal cell tumors. Gastrointest Endosc. 1997;45:468-73.
15. Amin MB, Ma CK, Linden MD, Kubus JJ, Zarbo RJ. Prognostic value of proliferating cell nuclear antigen index in gastric stromal tumors. Correlation with mitotic count and clinical outcome. Am J Clin Pathol. 1993;100:428-32.
16. Fletcher CD, Berman JJ, Corless C, Gorstein F, Lasota J, Longley BJ, et al. Diagnosis of gastrointestinal stromal tumors: a consensus approach. Int J Surg Pathol. 2002;10(2):81-9.
17. Miettinen M, Lasota J. Gastrointestinal stromal tumors: pathology and prognosis at different sites. Semin Diagn Pathol. 2006;23(2): 70-83.
18. Joensuu H. Risk stratification of patients diagnosed with gastrointestinal stromal tumor. Hum Pathol. 2008;39:1411-9.
19. Gold JS, Gönen M, Gutiérrez A, Broto JM, García-del-Muro X, Smyrk TC, et al. Development and validation of a prognostic nomogram for recurrence-free survival after complete surgical resection of localised primary gastrointestinal stromal tumour: a retrospective analysis. Lancet Oncol. 2009;10(11):1045-52.
20. Pierie JP, Choudry U, Muzikansky A, Yeap BY, Souba WW, Ott MJ, et al. The effect of surgery and grade on outcome of gastrointestinal stromal tumors. Arch Surg. 2001;136(4):383-9.
21. Otani Y, Furukawa T, Yoshida M, Saikawa Y, Wada N, Ueda M, et al. Operative indications for relatively small (2–5 cm) gastrointestinal stromal tumor of the stomach based on analysis of 60 operated cases. Surgery. 2006;139:484-92.
22. Joensuu H, Roberts PJ, Sarlomo-Rikala M, Andersson LC, Tervahartiala P, Tuveson D, et al. Effect of the tyrosine kinase inhibitor STI571 in a patient with a metastatic gastrointestinal stromal tumor. N Engl J Med. 2001;344:1052-6.
23. Heinrich MC, Griffith DJ, Druker BJ, Wait CL, Ott KA, Zigler AJ. Inhibition of c-kit receptor tyrosine kinase activity by STI 571, a selective tyrosine kinase inhibitor. Blood. 2000;96:925-32.
24. Demetri GD, van Oosterom AT, Garrett CR, Blackstein ME, Shah MH, Verweij J, et al. Efficacy and safety of sunitinib in patients with advanced gastrointestinal stromal tumour after failure of imatinib: a randomised controlled trial. Lancet. 2006;368:1329-38.
25. Benjamin RS, Choi H, Macapinlac HA, Burgess MA, Patel SR, Chen LL, et al. We should desist using RECIST, at least in GIST. J Clin Oncol. 2007;25:1760-4.
26. Choi H. Critical issues in response evaluation on computed tomography: lessons from the gastrointestinal stromal tumor model. Curr Oncol Rep. 2005;7:307-11.
27. Choi H, Charnsangavej C, Faria SC, Macapinlac HA, Burgess MA, Patel SR, et al. Correlation of computed tomography and positron emission tomography in patients with metastatic gastrointestinal

stromal tumor treated at a single institution with imatinib mesylate: proposal of new computed tomography response criteria. J Clin Oncol. 2007;25:1753-9.
28. Young H, Baum R, Cremerius U, et al. Measurement of clinical and subclinical tumour response using [18F]-fluorodeoxyglucose and positron emission tomography: review and 1999 EORTC recommendations. European Organization for Research and Treatment of Cancer (EORTC) PET Study Group. Eur J Cancer. 1999;35(13):1773-82.
29. Dematteo RP, Ballman KV, Antonescu CR, Maki RG, Pisters PW, Demetri GD, et al. Adjuvant imatinib mesylate after resection of localised, primary gastrointestinal stromal tumour: a randomised, double-blind, placebo-controlled trial. Lancet. 2009;373(9669):1097-104.
30. Joensuu H, Eriksson M, Sundby Hall K, Hartmann JT, Pink D, Schütte J, et al. One vs three years of adjuvant imatinib for operable gastrointestinal stromal tumor: a randomized trial. JAMA. 2012;307(12):1265-72.
31. Blesius A, Cassier PA, Bertucci F, Fayette J, Ray-Coquard I, Bui B, et al. Neoadjuvant imatinib in patients with locally advanced non metastatic GIST in the prospective BFR14 trial. BMC Cancer. 2011;11:72.
32. Demetri GD, Delaney T. NCCN: sarcoma. Cancer Control. 2001;8:94-101.
33. Casali PG, Blay JY. Gastrointestinal stromal tumours: ESMO Clinical Practice Guidelines for diagnosis, treatment and follow-up. Ann Oncol. 2010;21(Suppl 5):v98-102.

CHAPTER 35

Retroperitoneal Tumors

Sanjay Gupta

INTRODUCTION

Retroperitoneal tumors are a heterogeneous group of lesions, discussed together because of their anatomical location in the retroperitoneum. Traditionally, tumors of kidney, colon, adrenal and pancreas are not included in this group, though these structures are located in the retroperitoneum. Late presentation, large size and difficult surgical resection are some of the challenges which make prognosis of many of these lesions poor. Primary retroperitoneal tumors are distinct from tumors arising from named retroperitoneal organs and metastases to retroperitoneal lymph nodes.

ANATOMY OF RETROPERITONEAL SPACE

Retroperitoneum is the space behind the abdominal cavity and extends from the posterior peritoneum in the front to the transversalis fascia covering spine and the muscles of the posterior abdominal wall at the back. It is limited by the diaphragm above and the pelvic floor muscles below. The anterior and posterior layers of Gerota's fascia subdivide the retroperitoneal space into anterior and posterior pararenal spaces and the perirenal space (Fig. 1). The anterior pararenal space contains pancreas, duodenum, ascending and descending colon. The perirenal space contains kidney, ureter, adrenal and perinephric fat on either side. The posterior pararenal space contains fatty and areolar tissue traversed by an extensive network of vessels, neural structures and lymphatics. These spaces are separated superiorly but they communicate with the extraperitoneal space of the pelvis inferiorly and the two compartments become continuous. Due to a large potential space and loose connective tissue in the retroperitoneum, tumors can become large with widespread extension before clinical presentation.[1,2,3]

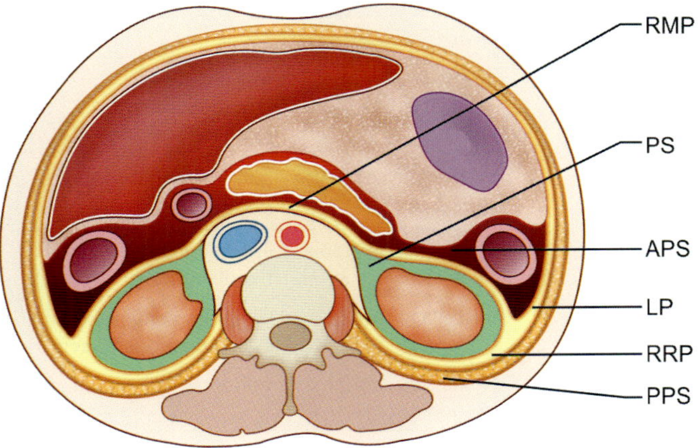

Figure 1 The retroperitoneal space

Abbreviations: RMP, Retromesenteric plane; PS, Para renal space; APS, Anterior para renal space; LP, Lateral conal planes; RRP, Retro renal plane; PPS, Posterior pararenal space

PATHOLOGY OF RETROPERITONEAL TUMORS

Primary retroperitoneal masses can broadly be divided into two groups: solid and cystic. These could be neoplastic or non-neoplastic and further divided on the basis of predominant cell type. Tables 1 and 2 give a broad pathological classification of these lesions.[2] Use of immune markers provides important additional information for classification of these tumors.

In adult patients, liposarcoma, leiomyosarcoma and undifferentiated pleomorphic sarcoma are the commonest malignant retroperitoneal tumors. The most common retroperitoneal sarcoma in the pediatric age is rhabdomyosarcoma, followed by fibrosarcoma and liposarcoma.[4] A retrospective analysis of 69 retroperitoneal

Table 1: Classification of solid retroperitoneal masses

Type of mass	*Germ layer*	*Tissue of origin*	*Benign*	*Malignant*
Neoplastic	Mesodermal	Adipose tissue	Lipoma	Liposarcoma
		Smooth muscle	Leiomyoma	Leiomyosarcoma
		Connective tissue	Fibroma	Fibrosarcoma, malignant fibrous histiocytoma
		Miscellaneous from striated muscle, blood vessels, primitive mesenchyme, remnant of notochord		
	Neurogenic	Nerve sheath	Neurofibroma, schwannoma	Neurofibrosarcoma, malignant schwannoma
		Sympathetic nerves	Ganglioneuroma	Neuroblastoma
		Chromaffin tissue	Paraganglioma, pheochromocytoma	Malignant paraganglioma and pheochromocytoma
	Germ cell, sex cord and stromal cell	Germ cell	Teratoma	Malignant teratoma
		Sex cord stromal cell	Granulosa cell tumor, thecoma, Sertoli-Leydig cell tumor	
	Lymphoid or hematologic origin			Lymphoma, extramedullary plasmacytoma
Non-neoplastic	Pseudotumoral lipomatosis, retroperitoneal fibrosis, Erdheim-Chester disease, and extramedullary hematopoiesis.			

Table 2: Classification of cystic retroperitoneal masses

Type of mass	*Germ layer*	*Lesion*
Neoplastic	Epithelial	Mucinous/serous cystadenoma and cystadenocarcinoma
	Mesothelial	Mesothelioma
	Germ cell	Cystic teratoma
	Cystic change in solid neoplasm	Paraganglioma, neurilemmoma, sarcoma
	Miscellaneous	Lymphangioma, epidermal cyst, bronchogenic cyst
Non-neoplastic	Hematoma, urinoma, lymphocele, non-pancreatic pseudocyst	

Table 3: Symptomatology of retroperitoneal tumors

Symptoms and signs	*Characteristics*
Palpable mass	Large, firm and irregular, usually fixed. May be confined to one half of the abdomen initially. Areas of resonance on percussion suggest retroperitoneal location.
Pain	Vague, mostly in the flanks
Urological	Colic, hematuria, Lower urinary tract symptoms (LUTS)
Gastrointestinal	Dyspepsia, post-prandial fullness, constipation, melena/hematemesis
Neurological	Neuralgic pain, motor or sensory deficit
Vascular	Lower limb edema, varicocele, features of vena cava obstruction with abdominal wall collateral veins
Paraneoplastic	Hypoglycemia, hypertension
Fever	Due to tumor necrosis

tumors in a report from Italy showed 70% malignant, 25% benign and 5% uncertain histology. Of the malignant lesions, leiomyosarcoma (25%), liposarcoma (18%) and malignant fibrous histiocytoma (10%) were the three commonest histological diagnoses. Benign schwannoma (29%), cysts of uncertain origin (23%), lipoma (11%) and cystic teratoma (11%) were the most frequent benign lesions.[5]

CLINICAL FEATURES OF RETROPERITONEAL TUMORS

Due to their location in retroperitoneum, which is a large space with loose areolar tissue, lesions can grow to a large size before they become symptomatic. Patients often present with a large (17–18 cm) asymptomatic lump (Figs. 4 and 5) or the mass is incidentally detected on imaging. In one series of 500 patients, 80% of patients presented with an abdominal mass, 42% with lower extremity neurologic symptoms, and 37% with pain.[6] Table 3 lists the symptoms which could occur in a patient with retroperitoneal mass.[7] Lymph node bearing areas should be examined in all patients to detect enlarged lymph nodes of lymphoma. Testes should always be examined in males as some patients with testicular neoplasm may initially present with abdominal mass.

Most of the patients with retroperitoneal sarcoma do not have identifiable risk factors, but a meticulous history should be elicited. Incidence of radiation related sarcomas have increased with increasing dose and duration of radiation. Genetic disorders such as neurofibromatosis 1 (NF1)[9] is another risk factor.

INVESTIGATION OF A RETROPERITONEAL MASS

Investigations are done in a retroperitoneal mass for precise localization of the lesion, determining the extent of local and systemic spread and characterizing the specific pathological type.

Imaging

Imaging forms the mainstay of detection, characterization, staging, grading, treatment planning and follow up of retroperitoneal masses.[8] For this CT scan and MRI are the most important imaging modalities. Conventional radiological investigations like plain X-rays, barium studies, intravenous urogram (IVU) and angiography are of historical interest and have been replaced by CT and MRI.

If a retroperitoneal tumor is clinically suspected, thin slice multi-detector CT scan with gastrointestinal and intravenous contrast is the investigation of choice. MRI gives improved soft tissue resolution and is useful for assessment of encasement or invasion of blood vessels. MRI gives a better assessment of malignant potential and resectability and is of help when CT scan is either not possible or its findings are uncertain. Although ultrasound can detect larger retroperitoneal masses, presence of overlying bowel gas interferes with detection of fat and calcification, both of which are essential in characterization of the lesion. The relationship of the mass to the adjacent structures cannot be clearly defined by an ultrasound. For this reason, if the mass is initially detected on ultrasound examination, a CT scan should follow. Clear delineation of adjoining structures alerts the surgeon and helps in planning the operation accordingly (Figs 2 and 3).

Tumor Detection and Characterization

A lesion which displaces retroperitoneal organs anteriorly (e.g., kidneys, adrenals, ureter, colon, pancreas and duodenum) and is not arising from them is likely to be a primary retroperitoneal tumor.[9]

Some retroperitoneal masses tend to extend between retroperitoneal organs without compressing them. Lymphangioma and lymphoma typically show this pattern of spread. Tumors arising from sympathetic ganglia tend to grow in the direction of sympathetic chain and characteristically assume an elongated shape.

Some tumor contents on imaging provide good characterization of the tissues and help in differentiating the tumor. Fat is detected on CT by its low attenuation value while on T1 weighted MRI images it shows strong signals which disappear in fat suppressed images. Presence of fat is typical of lipoma, liposarcoma and teratoma.

Presence of myxoid stroma, which gives strong signal intensity on T2 weighted MRI images and shows delayed contrast enhancement, is typical of neurogenic tumors. Necrosis within tumors is seen as low attenuation on CT and does not enhance with contrast. It is hyper intense on T2-weighted MR imaging. Necrosis is typically present in tumors of high-grade malignancy like leiomyosarcoma.

Occurrence of cystic areas is characteristic of tumors such as lymphangioma and mucinous cystic tumors. Neurogenic tumors may show partly solid and partly cystic areas.

Another important consideration at imaging is the vascularity of these tumors. Paraganglioma and hemangiopericytoma are extremely hypervascular. Moderately hypervascular tumors include myxoid malignant fibrous histiocytoma and leiomyosarcoma while hypovascular tumors include low grade liposarcoma, lymphoma, and many other benign tumors. Table 4 lists some specific diagnostic imaging features of retroperitoneal masses.[2]

Tumor Staging

10–20% of retroperitoneal tumors present with metastatic disease, commonly to lung and liver. For a high grade tumor, CT scan of chest and abdomen are done to rule out metastatic disease. Chest x-ray is sufficient in cases of low grade retroperitoneal tumors. The role of PET or PET-CT is not yet clearly defined. However, many tumors show increased uptake and this investigation can be used to assess treatment response and follow up the patients.[6]

Imaging Follow Up

Imaging forms an important tool for following up the patients subsequent to surgical excision of the primary tumor. Recurrence in these cases is local and initially asymptomatic. Both CT and MRI can be used for imaging in the follow up. Follow up is done every three months for first two years then every six months for five years and yearly thereafter. Frequency of imaging depends on the type

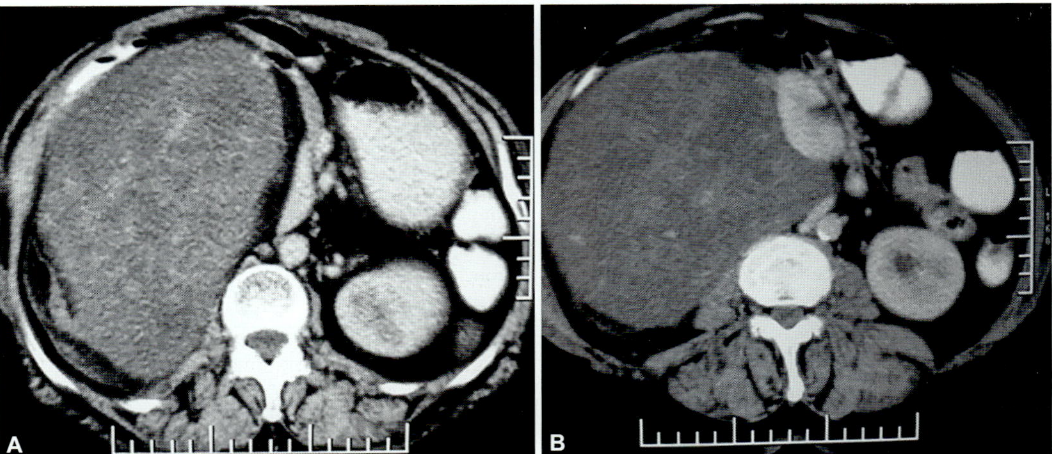

Figures 2A and B Large retroperitoneal mass pushing IVC (A) and right kidney medially (B)

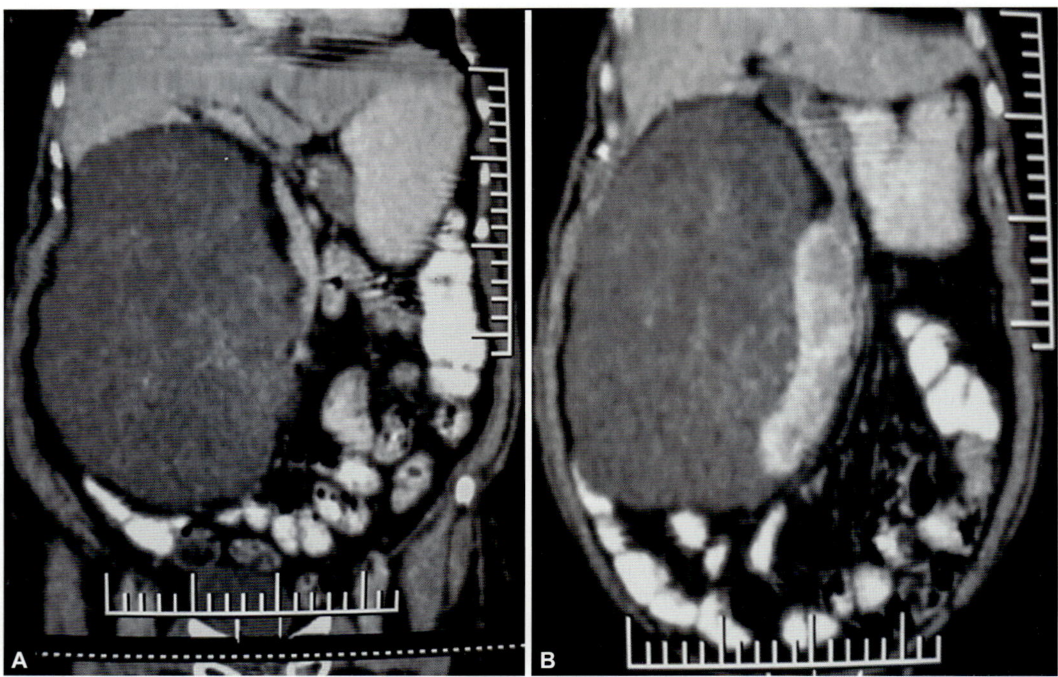

Figures 3A and B Showing Coronal reconstruction. IVC and Right kidney seen toward medial aspect

Table 4: Imaging features suggestive of a specific diagnosis for retroperitoneal masses[2]

Imaging feature	*Diagnosis*
Pure fat containing mass	Lipoma, well-differentiated liposarcoma
Heterogeneous mass with fat	Dedifferentiated liposarcoma, myelolipoma
Fat-fluid level, calcification, teeth	Teratoma
Myxoid stroma	Neurogenic tumor, myxoid liposarcoma
Large mass, extensive necrosis, invasion of IVC	Leiomyosarcoma
Extremely hypervascular	Paraganglioma, hemangiopericytoma
Hypovascular	Lymphoma, low-grade liposarcoma, benign tumor
T2 hypointensity	Lymphoma, desmoid tumor, small round cell tumor, retroperitoneal fibrosis
Paravertebral mass	Neurogenic tumor
Extension between normal structures, encasement without luminal compression	Lymphangioma, ganglioneuroma, lymphoma (floating aorta or CT angiogram sign)
Extension along normal structures	Paraganglioma, ganglioneuroma
Soft-tissue mass with calcification	Malignant fibrous histiocytoma, teratoma, extraosseous chondrosarcoma Ewing sarcoma, synovial sarcoma, dedifferentiated liposarcoma
Cystic mass with solid tumor enhancement	Myxoid liposarcoma, schwannoma, neurofibroma
Cystic mass with slow, progressive enhancement	Lymphangioleiomyoma, urinoma
Multilocular cystic mass, calcification, elongated shape, crossing retroperitoneal compartments	Lymphangioma
Unilocular cyst in subdiaphragmatic space	Bronchogenic cyst
Presacral unilocular cyst	Epidermoid cyst
Presacral multilocular cyst	Tailgut cyst

and aggressiveness of the tumor, completeness of the operative resection, grade of the tumor, clinical examination and probability of re-resection. Postoperative scarring may make the interpretation of images difficult.[8] For this reason an early postoperative CT scan with oral and intravenous contrast is done, which forms the baseline for future follow up scans.[10] As mentioned earlier, PET scan may become a tool for following up patients treated for primary retroperitoneal tumors.

Biopsy

The role of biopsy in management of retroperitoneal tumors is not clearly defined. Image guided core biopsy is accurate in 90% of the cases, though it may not define the histological subtype and nuclear grade in many cases. It is preferred over FNAC.[1] The advantage of the accurate pretreatment diagnosis is obvious. Appropriate treatment can be instituted in diseases such as lymphoma, where chemotherapy or radiotherapy is indicated and unnecessary surgery is avoided. Preoperative biopsy carries the risk of tumor seeding, bleeding, injury to adjacent structures and sampling a non-representative area of the tumor. Using image guidance and coaxial core biopsy technique avoids some of these problems.[6] Open biopsy of retroperitoneal tumors is discouraged as it violates virgin planes. It is indicated only if repeated core needle biopsies are inconclusive and it is felt that correct histopathological diagnosis may substantially change the management.[10]

Tumor Markers

Metastases from testicular tumors may mimic primary retroperitoneal tumors. Elevated levels of Alpha-fetoprotein (AFP) may suggest a diagnosis of metastases from nonseminomatous testicular tumor. Elevated levels of CEA and CA 19-9 have also been reported in patients with primary retroperitoneal sarcoma, though these are not specific.[11]

PROGNOSTIC FACTORS

The grade of tumor and completeness of resection are two most important prognostic factors in primary retroperitoneal tumors. Unifocal lesions carry a better prognosis than multifocal lesions.[6] While the 5-year disease specific survival after R0/R1 resection for primary retroperitoneal sarcoma is 69%, a similar resection for recurrent disease is much lower at 30%.[10]

TREATMENT

Surgical resection forms the cornerstone of treatment of retroperitoneal tumors. Studies from the USA have shown an 80% resectability rate from specialized centres.[10] While chemotherapy and radiotherapy are given both in neoadjuvant and in adjuvant settings, their role is not clearly defined.

Surgery for Retroperitoneal Tumors

Excision of the primary retroperitoneal tumor with microscopically negative margins is most likely to give a long tumor-free survival. The ability to achieve an R0/R1 resection can be enhanced by better patient selection, critical analysis of preoperative imaging, potential tumor downsizing with neoadjuvant therapy, and an improved intraoperative approach to resection. The surgeon should be prepared to resect and reconstruct any organ that composes the margin of the tumor, including viscera, musculoskeletal and major neurovascular structures. This resection might require participation by surgeons from other subspecialties. Based on review of the imaging, the primary surgeon should plan for these possibilities, rather than compromising the resection because of a lack of available subspecialty expertise at the time of surgery.[10]

Since important structures such as pancreas, kidney and ureter, colon, aorta, vena cava and iliac vessels are in close proximity to the tumor (Figs 2 and 3), wide excision in the usual sense with 2 cm margin of normal tissue all around the tumor is often not possible, unless the adjacent organ is removed, especially in high grade tumors. European surgeons have tried the concept of 'compartment excision' where both involved and uninvolved organs of the compartment are removed along with the primary tumor. Such an extensive excision has been shown to reduce the rate of local recurrence, though it is associated with increased postoperative morbidity and mortality. Reconstruction following such extensive resection may be quite challenging. Though this concept is more in tune with 'wide local excision', it is still not widely accepted.[12]

The standard surgical approach is through a long midline incision (Fig. 6). Often these tumors are pushing in nature. Even large masses can be successfully removed with due diligence (Figs 4 and 5). Tumors may share their blood supply with adjoining structure. Attempt should be to preserve the structures unless

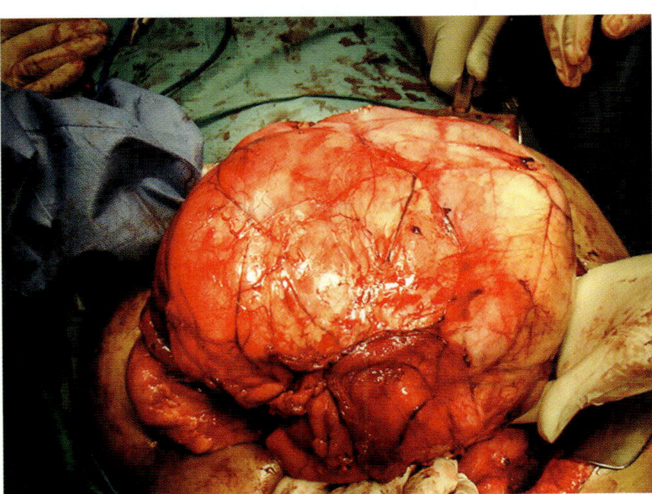

Figure 4 Same patient as in Figures 1 & 2 showing mobilized retroperitoneal mass being lifted out of abdomen

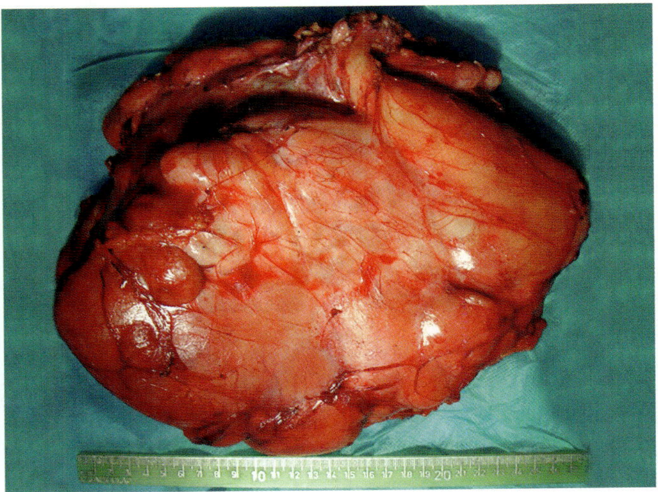

Figure 5 Resected tumor

they come in the way of R0 resection. It is suggested that areas of the tumor which are easier to dissect should be tackled before concentrating on more difficult areas.[13] Tumors located under the diaphragm and in the pelvis, especially the latter, pose additional difficulty in surgical resection. Proximity to rib cage or pelvis prevents exposure for the tumor for safe resection. This problem can partly be overcome by converting the abdominal incision to abdominothoracic or abdominoinguinal incision (Fig. 7).[14]

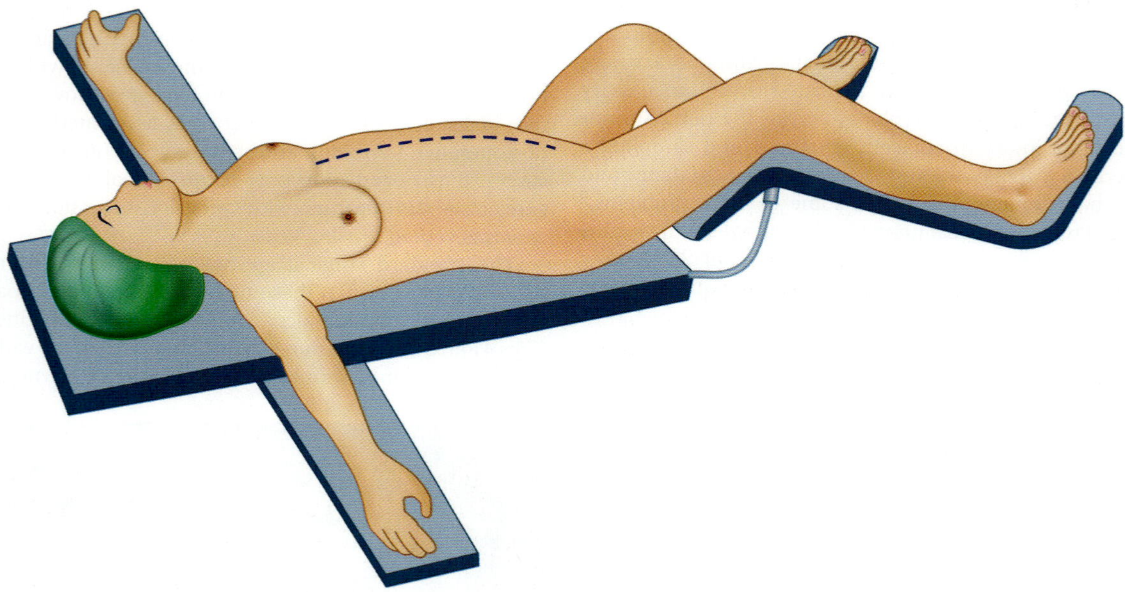

Figure 6 Lithotomy position with dorsolumbar hyperextension for retroperitoneal exposure and to allow perineal access

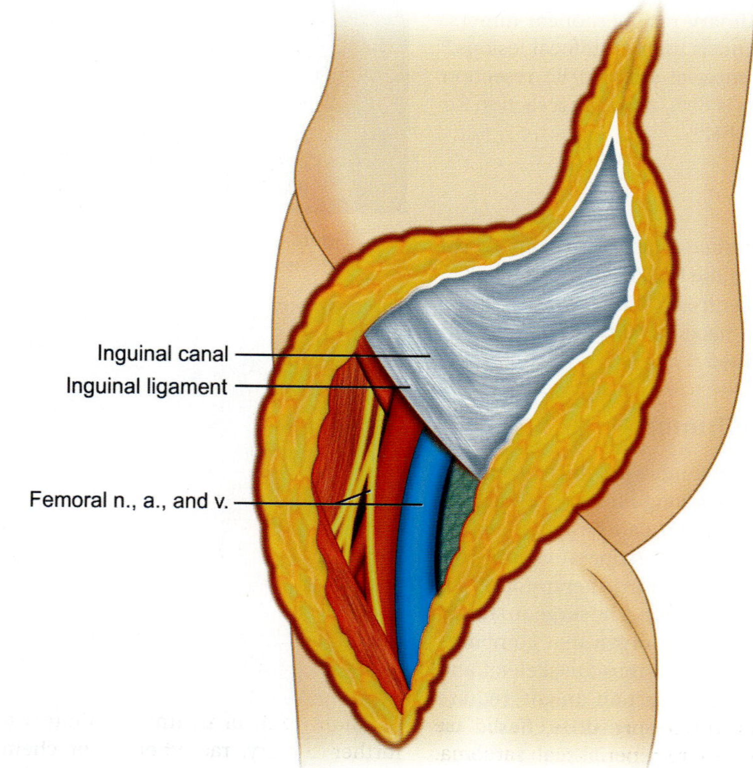

Figure 7 Showing abdominoinguinal incision

Inoperability of a retroperitoneal tumor is often due to extensive peritoneal or vascular involvement.[15]

Radiation Therapy

Radiotherapy has been used both in preoperative and postoperative settings in retroperitoneal tumors, though there is no strong evidence to support its use. Radiotherapy in postoperative setting is associated with significant wound and bowel complications.

Preoperative radiotherapy is less likely to cause injury to surrounding organs as these are displaced by the tumor. Additionally, the tumor is more vascular and its extent is more clearly defined. Additional boost radiation is given to areas which are expected to have positive margins (e.g., adjacent to surrounding viscera or vascular structure). Advances in radiotherapy including Intensity Modulated RT (IMRT) and Image Guided RT (IGRT) have significantly reduced post-RT complications. Brachytherapy and intraoperative radiotherapy has also been given to improve the outcome, though the numbers are not sufficient to draw any definite conclusion.[12]

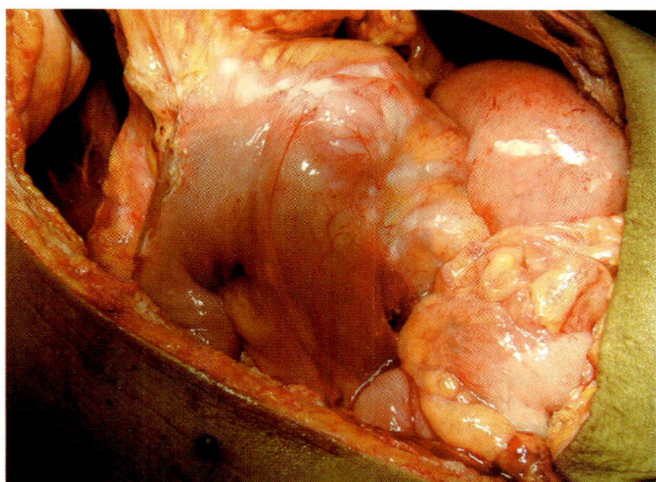

Figure 8 Recurrent lipsarcoma lifting the DJ flexure. Clear planes with surrounding structures were lost with extensive peritoneal disease

Chemotherapy

Systemic chemotherapy has been given as neoadjuvant cytoreductive therapy to improve R0 resectability for locally advanced disease, as a radiation sensitizer, or as definitive therapy for unresectable tumors. Commonly used drugs with known activity against retroperitoneal sarcomas include doxorubicin, ifosfamide, dacarbazine, gemcitabine, and docetaxel. The front-line regimen includes the combination of doxorubicin and ifosfamide.[4]

Neoadjuvant chemotherapy has been tried in intermediate or high grade tumors with the goal to reduce the extent of surgery and get improved tumor-free and overall survival. Another argument in favor of neoadjuvant chemotherapy is the better tolerance of potentially nephrotoxic chemotherapy in those patients who are likely to require nephrectomy due to renal involvement.

A recent Cochrane review has determined that while adjuvant chemotherapy reduces tumor recurrence and improves disease-free survival, overall survival cannot be commented upon.[12] Chemotherapy has also been used in the setting of bulky recurrent peritoneal disease. After surgical debulking, Hyperthermic Intraperitoneal Chemotherapy (HIPEC) is given in the intraoperative setting. The chemotherapy is typically platinum based. While the therapy is safe, conclusive data based on large studies is lacking.[12]

Recurrent Disease

50–80% of retroperitoneal sarcomas, undergoing complete resection with curative intent, show loco-regional recurrence at five years. Recurrences continue to rise with time and may occur as late as 20 years after the primary surgery.[10]

Local Recurrence

A large number of patients present with locally recurrent disease (Fig. 8) after the initial treatment of retroperitoneal sarcoma. A re-surgery may be attempted with curative intent if the recurrence is limited. However, this is complicated by the distorted anatomy and any reconstruction done at the time of initial surgery. Palliative resection may be done for relief of specific symptoms. Systemic therapy may be attempted for intermediate or high grade malignancies.[12]

Metastatic Disease

Multiple metastases, which present early after the primary surgery in a patient with poor performance status, are best treated by systemic therapy. Attempts have been made to excise the metastases from lung or liver if they are solitary or few, with long disease-free interval and good performance status of the patient. Because of the limited number of patients, no definite conclusion can be drawn regarding the appropriateness of metastatectomy.[12]

Palliative Procedures

Palliative treatment in the form of bypass or ostomy may be done for intestinal obstruction due to recurrent or advanced retroperitoneal sarcoma.

SUMMARY

Primary retroperitoneal sarcomas continue to pose diagnostic and therapeutic challenge. While CT forms the cornerstone for diagnosis, MRI adds to the details about local invasion, especially vascular involvement. While localized tumors can be excised without tissue diagnosis, core needle biopsy should be done if a disease such as lymphoma is suspected. Surgical excision is the primary treatment modality. The success of surgical treatment depends on the preparedness of the surgeon to resect and reconstruct adjacent structures. Local recurrence is the most common form of treatment failure which may be managed by further surgery, radiotherapy or chemotherapy. The treatment of primary retroperitoneal sarcoma is still evolving with further progress likely in the fields of radiotherapy and chemotherapy.

REFERENCES

1. Larson SD, Evers BM. Diseases of peritoneum, retroperitoneum, mesentery and omentum. In: Yamada T (ed). Textbook of Gastroenterology. 5th edition. Sussex: Blackwell Publishing; 2009. p. 2516.
2. Rajiah P, Sinha R, Cuevas C, Dubinsky TJ, Bush WH Jr, Kolokythas O. Imaging of uncommon retroperitoneal masses. Radiographics. 2011;31:949-76.
3. Pavlica P, Valentino M, Barozzi L. Retroperitoneal masses. In Morcos SK, Thomsen HS (eds). Urogenital Imaging: A problem Oriented Approach. Sussex: Wiley Blackwell; 2009. pp. 21–41.
4. Raval B, Pollock RE, Guadagnolo A, Patel SK. In Silverman PM (ed). Oncologic Imaging: A Multidisciplinary Approach. Philadelphia: Elsevier Saunders; 2012. pp. 403-21.
5. Serio G, Tenchini P, Nifosi F, Iacono C. Surgical strategy in primary retroperitoneal tumours. Br J Surg. 1989;76:385-9.
6. Bartlett E, Yoon SS. Current treatment for the local control of retroperitoneal sarcomas. J Am Coll Surg. 2011;213:436-46.
7. Bratu O, Mischianu D, Spanu D, Barla R, Hoara P, Constantinoiu S. Paraneoplastic syndrome in primitive retroperitoneal tumours. Chirurgia (Bucur). 2013;108:26-31.
8. Francis IR, Cohan RH, Varma DG, Sondak VK. Retroperitoneal sarcomas. Cancer Imaging. 2005;5:89-94.
9. Nishino M, Hayakawa K, Minami M, Yamamoto A, Ueda H, Takasu K. Primary retroperitoneal neoplasms: CT and MR imaging findings with anatomic and pathologic diagnostic clues. Radiographics. 2003;23:45-57.
10. Swallow CJ, Catton CN. Improving outcomes for retroperitoneal sarcomas: a work in progress. Surg Oncol Clin N Am. 2012;21: 317-31.
11. Gatcombe HG, Assikis V, Kooby D, Johnstone PA. Primary retroperitoneal teratomas: a review of the literature. J Surg Oncol. 2004;86:107-13.
12. Mullinax JE, Zager JS, Gonzalez RJ. Current diagnosis and management of retroperitoneal sarcoma. Cancer Control. 2011;18:177-87.
13. Malkowicz SB. Retroperitoneal tumors. In: Wein AJ, Kavoussi LR, Novick AC, Partin AW, Peters CA (Eds). Campbell- Walsh Urology, 10th edition. Philadelphia: Elsevier; 2012. pp. 1506-15.
14. Behranwala KA, A'Hern R, Thomas JM. Primary malignant tumors of the iliopsoas compartment. J Surg Oncol. 2004;86:78-83.
15. Dalal KM, Antonescu CR, Singer S. Diagnosis and management of lipomatous tumors. J Surg Oncol. 2008;97:298-313.

SECTION 4

Pancreas

CHAPTER 36

Pancreas: Embryology, Anatomy and Physiology

Harsh Shah, Sundeep Singh Saluja

INTRODUCTION

The pancreas (Greek word, *pancreas* means all flesh) is a soft, elongated, lobulated organ that extends from the splenic hilum to the C loop of the duodenum. Galen named it pancreas thinking that it protected and supported the blood vessels. Vesalius thought that pancreas was a cushion for the stomach. Wirsung was the one who described about the pancreatic ducts in the humans way back in 1642. In 1664, de Graaf described about the nature of pancreatic secretion from the pancreatic fistula in dogs. The pancreas is located in the retroperitoneum. It is an area replete with major blood vessels, nerves and lymphatics. This makes pancreatic access and surgery difficult. The knowledge of anatomy would be helpful while managing problems related to pancreas.

EMBRYOLOGY

The pancreas develops from the endoderm of the primitive duodenum in early fourth week of embryonic life. The endoderm gives rise to a dorsal pancreatic bud (DPB) and a ventral pancreatic bud (VPB), which fuse to form a single organ. The ventral bud arises from the hepatic diverticulum while dorsal bud grows out from the foregut endoderm into dorsal mesoduodenum.

The ventral bud forms the whole of uncinate process along with posterior portion of pancreatic head while dorsal bud forms the remaining portion of pancreatic head, body and tail of pancreas. The distribution of pancreatic polypeptide (PP) cells, fat infiltration and shape of islets cells helps in differentiating the pancreatic tissue that arises from VPB from DPB. The ventral pancreas has abundance of PP cells. The ventral pancreas has less fatty infiltration compared to dorsal pancreas.[1] The pancreatic tissue arising from ventral bud has islets cells which are irregular in shape while those from dorsal bud have round or oval-shape.

The growth of the dorsal bud surpasses ventral bud by fifth week. Due to differential growth of the wall of the duodenum, there is an anticlockwise movement of the ventral bud and it moves behind the bile duct to a dorsal position compared to dorsal bud. Failure of migration of ventral bud results in an anomaly called **annular pancreas**.

Both ventral and dorsal buds fuse by the sixth week. The main pancreatic duct (MPD) also known as duct of Wirsung is formed from union of distal part of dorsal pancreatic duct with ventral pancreatic duct. The remaining part of dorsal pancreatic duct is patent in about 60% of population and is known as duct of Santorini.[2] In the remaining 40% population, it may just be obliterated. The MPD opens into the medial wall of second part of duodenum at major papilla. Fusion of ducts may not occur in 10% of individuals, in which case drainage of pancreatic secretion mainly occurs through duct of Santorini into the duodenum at minor papilla while the uncinate process and posterior portion of head drain through the opening of main duct at major papilla. This anomaly is known as **pancreatic divisum**.

The MPD formed from secondary ducts which further receive the terminal ductules. The exocrine component of pancreas consists of pancreatic acini that arise from the cell clusters around the terminal ducts. The endocrine component of the pancreas known as islets of Langerhans arises from the epithelial cells along the pancreatic acini. They constitute 1–2% of the adult gland. It has four types of cells. The beta cells constitute majority of pancreatic endocrine cells. It produces insulin and amylin (an insulin antagonist). Insulin secretion begins around fifth month of embryonic life. The other types of cells include alpha cells, delta cells and PP cells. Alpha cells secrete glucagon, delta cells secrete somatostatin and cells secrete pancreatic polypeptide. These PP cells do not arise from a single progenitor PP cells. There is a variable distribution of these cells within the pancreas. Alpha cells are located mainly in the body and tail while PP cells are mainly located in the head of pancreas. Delta and beta cells are present throughout the pancreas.[3] Blood vessels, lymphatics and connective tissue, are formed from the mesodermal tissue. Nerves supplying the pancreas develop from the ectoderm.

DEVELOPMENTAL ANOMALIES

Aplasia is defined as complete agenesis of pancreas. Complete pancreatic aplasia is usually fatal in the newborn. Aplasia is associated with mutation of the pancreatic and duodenal homeobox 1 (Pdx-1) gene. Mature-onset diabetes of the young (MODY) is associated with heterozygous mutation of the Pdx-1 gene. Partial pancreatic agenesis is defined as absence of a portion of pancreas while rest of the pancreas is normal. It is not associated with any endocrine or exocrine insufficiency. Dorsal pancreas is most often affected part in partial agensis of pancreas.

Hypoplasia or lipomatous pseudohypertrophy of the pancreas is defined as congenital absence of secondary exocrine structure. In such a pancreas, the ductal structures are replaced by fat while the islets cells are normal.

Pancreas divisum (PD) occurs when the dorsal and ventral pancreatic ducts fail to join. It is the most common variation of pancreatic duct anatomy. When the ducts fail to join completely, it is known as classic pancreas divisum. When this occurs partially, it is known as partial pancreas divisum. In this abnormality, most of the pancreatic secretions are drained via the duct of Santorini through minor papilla. Larger studies on pancreas divisum have shown that the occurrence of idiopathic pancreatitis was similar to that in the general population.[4]

Annular pancreas occurs due to incomplete migration of VPB during embryogenesis, where in a band of pancreatic tissue encircles the second portion of the duodenum. It is the most common pancreatic anomaly reported in children.[5] Duodenal obstruction is the most common presentation with more than 50% patients are symptomatic at birth or become during the first year of life. It is frequently associated with trisomy of twenty first chromosome and duodenal atresia. There are several theories for its development. The role of mutation in hedgehog signaling pathway and familial inheritance in the development of annular pancreas are still under investigation. Lecco et al.[6] (1910) suggested that free end of the ventral bud gets fixed to the duodenal wall. As the duodenal rotation occurs, the base moves along with it and forms a band of pancreatic tissue around the duodenum. According to Baldwin's theory[7] (1910), persistence of the left portion of the ventral bud growing in opposition to the right portion of the ventral bud forms a compressing ring circumferentially around the duodenum. Tieken[8] (1901) postulated that hypertrophy of the ventral and dorsal buds which eventually fused resulted in an annular structure. However, no consensus has been reached and none of the theory explains the ductal anatomy in the annular pancreas.

Ectopic pancreas is the presence of pancreatic tissue outside pancreas. It is usually found with in the gastrointestinal tract. Ectopic pancreatic tissue results from migration of the embryonic remnant that gives rise to pancreatic tissue along the gastrointestinal tract during the development. Second theory suggests that pancreatic metaplasia of the endodermal tissues located in the submucosa may occur during embryogenesis and result in ectopic pancreatic rest. The most common location is in the stomach (27%). The other common sites include duodenum (25%), jejunum (15%)[9] or within a Meckel's diverticulum.[5]

It is usually asymptomatic, however it can cause ulcerations and bleeding within the gastrointestinal tract. According to Modified Heinrich Classification,[10] Type 1 heterotopia consists of pancreatic tissue similar to those seen in normal pancreas. It has acini, ducts and islets cells. In Type 2, the ectopic tissue is referred as canalicular variety as it has only pancreatic ducts. Type 3 heterotropia is known as exocrine pancreas as it is characterized by acinar tissue only. Type 4 is known as endocrine pancreas as it is made up of islet cells only. Malignant transformation is extremely rare in the ectopic pancreatic tissue. Around 30 cases of malignant transformation of ectopic pancreatic tissue have been reported in literature.[11] Most of them occur in stomach and are adenocarcinoma on histology. The prognosis seems to be better than malignancy that arising from pancreas itself, probably due to earlier presentation.[12]

ANATOMY

Pancreas measures 12–20 cm in length and weighs around 70–110 g. It is located in retroperitoneum. It is divided into head, uncinate, neck, body and tail (Fig. 1). The pancreas is covered with a fine connective tissue but does not have a true capsule.

The head lies to the right of lumbar 2 (L2) vertebra in apposition with the duodenum. It has three borders (superior, duodenal and inferior) and two surfaces (anterior and posterior). The pancreatic head lies in front of the inferior vena cava (IVC), right renal artery, both renal veins, and the superior mesenteric vessels. The boundary between head and neck is often marked anteriorly by a groove for the gastroduodenal artery (GDA) and posteriorly by a similar but deeper groove that contains the union of the superior mesenteric vein and splenic vein (SPV) as they form the portal vein.

The neck is a narrow (2.0 cm) portion of the gland behind which lies the portal vein. The vertebral bodies of L1 and L2 are in posterior relation while the first portion of the duodenum is superior. It is important to remember that the plane between neck and superior mesenteric vein (SMV) is avascular. This information is useful while making plane between SMV and pancreas which is one of the critical steps during Whipple's pancreaticoduodenectomy.

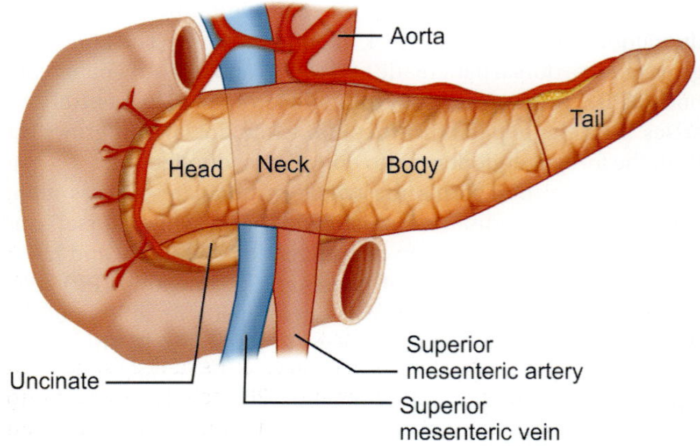

Figure 1 Divisions of pancreas

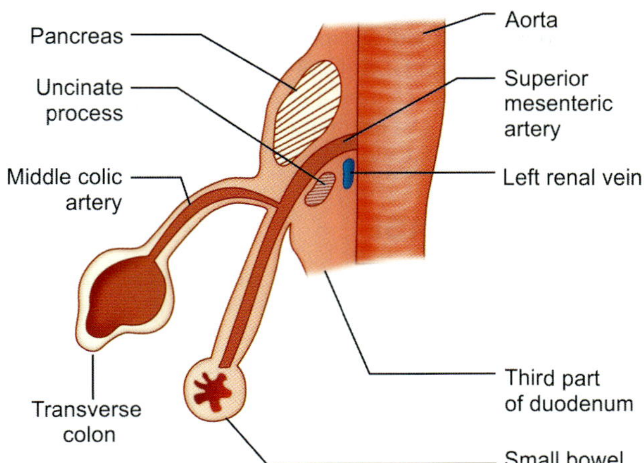

Figure 2 Sagittal section through neck of pancreas

The pancreatic body is triangular in cross section. The three borders (superior, anterior and inferior) divide it into three surfaces—anterosuperior, anteroinferior and posterior. The stomach lies anterior to the body and tail of the pancreas, whereas the aorta, left adrenal gland and left kidney are in posterior relation to the body of the pancreas. The SPV lies on posterior surface of the pancreas. Occasionally, it is embedded within the pancreatic tissue. The splenic artery lies at the superior edge of the gland and runs a tortuous course.

Pancreatic tail is the narrowest portion of the gland, measuring 1.5-3.5 cm in length. It lies between the two layers of splenorenal ligament. Therefore, it is prone to injury while performing splenectomy.

The uncinate process which is located posterior to the head extends variably between the IVC and the superior mesenteric vessels. Posteriorly, it is in close relation to vena cava and aorta (Fig. 2) and inferiorly, it lies on the upper surface of the third part of the duodenum.

Tumors of the uncinate process do not usually present with jaundice as they lie away from common bile duct (CBD) however present with gastric outlet obstruction as they compress the third part of the duodenum.

PANCREATIC DUCTS

The pancreatic ductal system consists of duct of Santorini and duct of Wirsung. The MPD (Wirsung) is usually located midway between the superior and inferior margins in a slightly posterior plane. It is formed by union of duct draining ventral bud and the distal part of the duct draining dorsal bud. It terminates at the second part of duodenum at major papilla. The proximal part of duct of dorsal bud continues as a duct of Santorini opening into minor papilla. In 10% of patients ductal system from the two buds fails to fuse. This variation is known as pancreatic divisum as described above. The secondary ductules usually arise at right angles to the main duct. Approximately, 20 such ducts drain into MPD. The various intercalated ducts in a lobule join to form an interlobular duct which then join to form a secondary duct.

MAJOR PAPILLA

Major papilla is a hoodlike elevation of duodenal mucosa at the point where MPD and CBD enter into duodenum. It is also known as the papilla of Vater. It is located on the medial wall of second part of duodenum 7-10 cm distal to the pylorus. The CBD and MPD come together to constitute a common channel of variable length. Three types of configurations are described as follow:

Type 1: It is the most common type and constitutes 85% of cases. In this type, the MPD opens into the CBD to form a common channel at a variable distance from the papilla.

Type 2: In type 2, the MPD and CBD lie close to each other but open separately at the papilla. It is the least common variety and constitutes approximately 5%.

Type 3: Where the MPD and CBD open separately into the duodenum. Seen in about 10%.

MINOR PAPILLA

The minor papilla is located 2 cm anterior and proximal to the major papilla and is seen in approximately 70% of patients. Minor papilla drains the accessory pancreatic duct of Santorini. The GDA is a useful landmark to identify the location of minor papilla. The duct of Santorini and the minor papilla lie in front of the vessel. Therefore, one should not go beyond the GDA while transecting the duodenum during gastrectomy.

There is no sphincter around the minor papilla. When present, it is known as sphincter of Helly. In around 10% of population, most of the pancreatic secretion may be drained by the duct of Santorini. Inadvertent ligation of this dominant duct along with the GDA could be disastrous.

SPHINCTER OF ODDI

Sphincter of Oddi consists of annular fibers that surround the intramural portion of pancreatic and bile ducts. Francis Glisson described it in 1654. It has three components sphincter choledochus (around CBD), sphincter pancreaticus (around pancreatic duct) and sphincter papillae. The sphincter lies within the ampulla and works in response to hormonal and neural signals to control biliary and pancreatic secretions. The length of the sphincter varies between 4 mm and 10 mm.

ARTERIAL SUPPLY

The pancreas receives an opulent blood supply from the branches of coeliac artery and superior mesenteric artery (SMA).

The head of the pancreas and duodenum are supplied mainly from the two arcades that run along the pancreaticoduodenal groove. The anterior pancreaticoduodenal arcade is formed by union of anterior superior pancreaticoduodenal artery (ASPDA) and anterior inferior pancreaticoduodenal artery (AIPDA). The ASPDA is the onward continuation of the GDA. It descends between duodenum and pancreas to anastomose with the AIPDA along the medial surface of the duodenum. The posterior pancreaticoduodenal arcade is formed by union of posterior superior pancreaticoduodenal artery (PSPDA) and

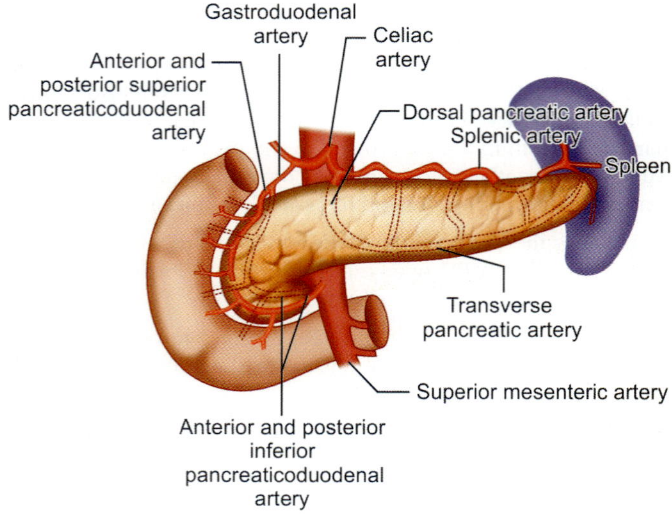

Figure 3 Arterial supply of pancreas

posterior inferior pancreaticoduodenal artery (PIPDA). The PSPDA is a branch of GDA that arises near the superior border of pancreas and runs behind the pancreas into pancreaticoduodenal groove to anastomose with the PIPDA coming from below. AIPDA and PIPDA may arise together from SMA as the inferior pancreaticoduodenal artery (IPDA) or separately. The IPDA may itself arise from the right side of the SMA directly or from the left side together with the first jejunal artery (J1A) (Fig. 3).

Body and tail of pancreas are supplied by inferoanterior and inferoposterior pancreatoduodenal vessels. They arise from the SMA or one of its branches. Together they form an arcade and supply body and tail of pancreas along with duodenojejunal junction and neck of pancreas.

The dorsal pancreatic artery (DPA) arises from either celiac or splenic artery. It is an inconsistent vessel. It courses along the superior border of the body and the tail of the pancreas. The branch from the GDA (the superior pancreatic branch) and the branch from the DPA (the suprapancreatic branch) form an arcade along the superior margin of the pancreas. The transverse pancreatic artery (TPA) courses along the inferior margin of pancreas and arises from SMA, ASPDA or the posterosuperior pancreatic artery.

The splenic artery, as it runs along the superior border of pancreas, give rise to numerous branches that provide blood supply to the body and tail of pancreas. The great pancreatic artery (GPA) is the largest branch of splenic artery. It originate near the junction of body and tail pancreas and divide into left and right branches to provide blood supply to the body and tail of the pancreas. The smaller branches from the splenic artery that provide blood to body and tail of pancreas are known as the caudal pancreatic arteries (CPAs).

One of the most common anatomical variations among arterial supply to liver is origin of the right hepatic artery from SMA. Right hepatic artery may then course either through or posterior to pancreatic head and then passing posterolateral to the CBD. Rarely, the common hepatic artery (CHA) may arise from SMA and have such a course. While performing Whipple's procedure, the reconstruction of artery is important in either situation to avoid postoperative complications related to it.

The GDA is important to any discussion in relation to arterial supply of pancreas. Due to extensive collateral network, hepatic artery may remain well perfused in severe atherosclerotic narrowing of celiac artery through GDA. GDA should be test clamped with non-crushing vascular clamps, prior to ligation. Checking the pulsation of CHA after test clamping of GDA is an essential step in Whipple's procedure to avoid ischemic complication to liver.

VENOUS DRAINAGE

It is important to have a complete knowledge of the variations in the inferior mesenteric vein (IMV), SPV and SMV in relation to venous drainage of the pancreas. The SMV, SPV and the portal vein are closely related to the pancreas. The SMV passes posterior to the neck of the pancreas and rarely receives any branch from it. The numerous tributaries from the body tail pancreas drain into the SPV along its course. It joins the SMV to form portal vein behind the neck of pancreas. The IMV is variable in its drainage into either the SPV or the SMV. In an autopsy study of 38 patients, Kimura et al. reported that the IMV drain into the SMV in 42% cases, SPV in 34% cases, and the confluence of the SPV and the SMV in 24%.[13]

The left gastric vein runs along the lesser curve of the stomach. It is constant in its course but terminates either into the portal vein few cm above the spleno-portal junction or directly at the spleno-portal junction.

The head of the pancreas is drained by several pancreaticoduodenal veins forming an arcade which ultimately drains into portal or SMV. The venous drainage of superior part of the body and tail of the pancreas is via multiple small veins that drain into the SPV. While the remaining inferior part of the body and tail is drained by inferior pancreatic vein coursing along the inferior border of pancreas to join SMV.

Care must be taken while dissecting neck of the pancreas from the vein, when small venous channels are encountered, draining the neck into the portal vein. Small tributaries are often present draining the uncinate process into SMV, which must be ligated with care to avoid bleeding from the SMV.

LYMPHATIC DRAINAGE

Multiple groups of nodes may receive drainage from each region of the gland. Pancreatic cancer often presents with positive lymph nodal disease and a high incidence of local recurrence after resection due to this well-endowed lymphatic drainage. Lymph capillaries commence around the pancreatic acini. The larger lymph vessels follow the arterial supply and drain into the lymph nodes around the pancreas. Lymphatics from the tail and the body drain mostly into the pancreaticosplenic nodes, although some drain directly to preaortic nodes. Lymphatics from the neck and the head drain more widely into nodes along the pancreaticoduodenal, superior mesenteric and hepatic arteries, and some also drain to the preaortic nodes and coeliac axis nodes. There is no evidence of lymphatic channels within the pancreatic islets.

NERVE SUPPLY

Pancreatic innervation mostly accompanies the vascular structures. Sympathetic fibers arising from the thoracic spinal nerve 6–10 (T6–T10), travel via celiac ganglion to reach the pancreas.

The parasympathetic fibers have their cell bodies in the brain. The postganglionic fibers innervate the pancreas via branches from the vagus nerve. Pancreatic parenchyma is supplied by both sympathetic and parasympathetic nerve fibers while vasomotor supply consists of sympathetic fibers only. The parasympathetic system stimulates both endocrine and exocrine secretion and the sympathetic system inhibits exocrine secretion.

Both the sympathetic and parasympathetic systems mediate the pain and other sensory information from the pancreatic tissue. Pain arising from the pancreas can present as referred pain to both epigastrium and the retroperitoneum. Inflammatory or infiltrative processes arising from the gland can involves the tissues of the retroperitoneum that are innervated by somatic nerves supplying the posterior paravertebral region. This can result in referred pain to the posterior paravertebral region around the lower thoracic spine. Clinical implication of thermal or chemical ablation of the nerve plexus can be used as therapeutic option to control pain in chronic pancreatitis or inoperable pancreatic tumors.

PHYSIOLOGY

Pancreas has both exocrine and endocrine component. The exocrine pancreas constitutes 85% of the pancreatic mass while endocrine tissue comprises of only 1–2% mass. The extracellular matrix (10%) and blood vessels and ducts (4%) constitute the remaining part. The physical approximation of endocrine and endocrine components, presence of islets cell receptor on the acinar cells and the presence of portal blood system between acinar and islet cells allow close co-ordination between exocrine and endocrine function.

Even 20% of the normally functioning pancreatic gland can prevent exocrine/endocrine insufficiency. However, in many patients undergoing pancreatic resection where the remaining pancreas is not normal, pancreatic endocrine and exocrine insufficiency can develop with removal of smaller portions of the gland.

Exocrine Pancreas

Around 500–800 mL of pancreatic juice is secreted per day. It is colorless, odorless, isoosmotic and alkaline in nature. Both acinar and duct cells secretion constitute the pancreatic juice. An acinus consists of around 40 cells arranged in a spherical unit. The acinar cell secretion is enzyme rich containing proteases, lipases and amylases that help in digestion of all three kinds of food. Each of the acinar cells can secrete all three types of enzymes. The type and amount of enzymes released are adjusted according the composition of digested food through nonparallel regulation of secretion.

Centroacinar cells are located centrally within the acinus. They along with cells of intercalated duct maintain fluid and electrolyte secretion within the pancreatic juice. These cells are rich in carbonic anhydrase, enzyme needed for bicarbonate secretion. The quantity of bicarbonate secreted varies according to the rate of its secretion. Bicarbonate secretion increases as the amount of pancreatic secretion increases. Chloride secretion varies inversely with bicarbonate levels such that the sum of two remains constant. On a contrary, sodium ion (Na^+) and potassium ion (K^+) concentrations remain constant throughout all the phases of secretion.[14]

The acidic chyme is the main stimulant for bicarbonate release in pancreatic juice. It is mediated through release of the secretin hormone from duodenal cells. Cholecystokinin (CCK) also stimulates the bicarbonate secretion, but to a lesser extent than secretin. CCK potentiates the secretin stimulated bicarbonate secretion. Somatostatin, pancreatic polypeptide and glucagon inhibit the exocrine secretion. The truncal vagotomy reduces the bicarbonate and the fluid secretion from the pancreas.[15]

The pancreatic enzymes are released from the zymogen granules in the acinar cells into the acinar lumen. These proteins combine with the water and bicarbonate secretions of the centroacinar cells to form pancreatic juice. There is a continuous exchange of anions and cations during the passage of juice through the ductal system. In patients with chronic pancreatitis repeated inflammation, scarring and stone deposition result in damage of both islet cells and acinar tissue. This eventually results in exocrine and endocrine insufficiency.

The nature of pancreatic secretion varies in fasting and fed state. The amount and composition of the secretion is influenced by dietary composition of food. The presence of food in the duodenum is the most important stimulus for the enzyme release. Nutrient load of about 1 kcal/minutes in the duodenum is required to convert the fasting pattern of secretion to the fed pattern.

The most potent stimulant for enzyme secretion in pancreatic juice is lipid. Free fatty acids stimulate the release of CCK from the duodenum which then causes enzyme rich release of pancreatic juice. Chronic ingestion of a high-fat diet is associated with higher enzyme output in fasting and postprandial state, while acute changes increases the postprandial output only.

Digested protein rather than whole protein stimulate pancreatic secretion with essential amino acids such as tryptophan, valine and phenylalanine being the most important ones. Hydrolysis of protein in the stomach yields peptides. These substances on reaching duodenum, stimulate the release of hormones such as secretin and CCK. They stimulate the enzyme and bicarbonate secretion in the pancreatic juice.

Amylase is the only enzyme that is released in its active form. The carbohydrates ingested in the form of starch and glycogen are hydrolyzed into dextrins, isodextrins, maltose and glucose by pancreatic amylase. These are then transported across the intestinal cells by an active mechanism.

The various enzymes that help in the digestion of proteins are secreted as proenzymes. Enterokinase released in succus entericus convert trypsinogen into its active form trypsin. Trypsin activates other proteolytic enzymes. Protease inhibitors stored in acinar cells prevent enzyme activation within the cell. A failure to express a normal trypsinogen inhibitor, pancreatic secretory trypsin inhibitor (PSTI) or serine protease inhibitor Kazal type 1 (SPINK1), is the cause of familial pancreatitis. Trypsinogen is expressed in several isoforms and a missense mutation on the cationic trypsinogen, or protease, serine, 1 (PRSS1), results in premature, intrapancreatic activation of trypsinogen. This accounts for about two-thirds of cases of hereditary pancreatitis.

Trypsin converts chymotrypsinogen into chymotrypsin. It also activates the other enzymes such as carboxypeptidase A and B, elastase and phospholipase. Carboxypeptidase cleaves the amino acid at the end of peptide chain. The elastase, chymotrpsin and trypsin cleave the bonds between amino acids within the peptide chain. Smaller fragment like dipeptides and amino acids are absorbed in the small intestine via active transport mechanism.

Triglycerides are hydrolyzed to 2-monoglyceride and fatty acid through pancreatic lipase. Co-lipase increases the activity level of lipase after binding thereby changing its molecular configuration. It is also secreted by pancreas. Phospholipase A2 hydrolyzes phospholipids. It is also activated by trypsin. Bile salts are required for fat absorption. They along with hydrolyzed fat form micelles which are transported across the intestinal cells. Here, they are reassembled and packaged inside the chylomicrons for transport into the bloodstream through lymphatics.

Endocrine Pancreas

Typical adult pancreas contains approximately 1 million islets of Langerhans. The size of the islets varies from 50 to 900 μm. Islets located closer to the major arterioles are large in size while those located deep in the pancreatic tissue are small in size. Most islets contain around 3,000–4,000 cells. There are five types of cells. These include beta cells that produce insulin, alpha cells that secrete glucagon, delta cells which secrete somatostatin, epsilon cells that produce ghrelin, and PP cells that secrete pancreatic polypeptide.

Insulin is a 56-amino acid peptide. It has two chains, alpha and beta, joined by two disulfide bridges and a connecting peptide known as C-peptide. Insulin is secreted in two phases. In the first phase, stored insulin is released. This phase lasts for about 5 minutes after a glucose challenge. The second phase of secretion is a longer and sustained release. It is due to ongoing production of new insulin. Beta cell synthesis of insulin is regulated by three main factors: (i) plasma glucose level; (ii) neural signals and (iii) the paracrine influence of other islet cells.

Oral glucose not only enters the bloodstream but also stimulates the release of enteric hormones such as glucagon-like peptide-1 (GLP-1), gastric inhibitory peptide (GIP) also known as glucose-dependent insulinotropic polypeptide and CCK. These hormones augment the secretion of insulin, and are therefore referred to as incretins. Therefore, oral glucose is a more vigorous stimulus to insulin secretion than intravenous glucose. Plasma levels of amino acids such as leucine, lysine, arginine and free fatty acids also influence insulin secretion. The neural control of insulin secretion is through both sympathetic and parasympathetic fibers. The insulin release is stimulated by beta sympathetic and cholinergic fibers and inhibited by alpha sympathetic fibers. The paracrine control means control of secretion of cells by secretion from the adjacent cells. Insulin secretion is inhibited by somatostatin, amylin, and pancreastatin.[16]

Insulin lowers plasma glucose levels by inhibiting hepatic glucose production and facilitating glucose transport into cells. It inhibits glycogenolysis. It also decreases fatty acid breakdown and ketone production. Insulin stimulates the protein synthesis and thus has anabolic properties. Body has sufficient functional reserve in insulin secretory capacity. Patient do not develop diabetes even after resection of 80% of the pancreas, if the remaining pancreas is healthy.[17]

Glucagon is a single-chain peptide with 29 amino acids. It increases plasma glucose level by stimulating hepatic glycogenolysis and gluconeogenesis. Glucagon secretion is inhibited by glucose. GIP stimulates its secretion while GLP-1 inhibits its secretion. Somatostatin and insulin have paracrine action and exert negative influence on glucagon secretion. Glucagon secretion is stimulated by both beta adrenergic and cholinergic fibers. Alpha sympathetic fibers inhibit the release of glucagon.[18]

Somatostatin is a peptide hormone, which inhibits both endocrine and exocrine secretion. It also inhibits both gastrointestinal and biliary motility. Intestinal absorption is also decreased. Five different somatostatin receptors (SSTRs) have been cloned.[19] The hexapeptide and octapeptide analogues such as octreotide bind only to SSTR2, SSTR3 and SSTR5. These analogs have a longer serum half-life, and their potent inhibitory effect has been used clinically. For example, octreotide has been shown to decrease fistula output and speed the time it takes for enteric and pancreatic fistulas to close.[20] The major stimulant is food probably intraluminal fat. Cholinergic nerves also inhibit the somatostatin release.

Pancreatic polypeptide is produced by the PP cells. The most potent stimulus for release of PP is protein, followed by fat.[21,22] PP secretion is increased through cholinergic stimulation by hypoglycemia.[23] Vagus plays an important role in stimulation of the pancreas. In fact, vagotomy eliminates the rise in PP level usually seen after a meal. This can be used as a test for the completeness of a surgical vagotomy or for the presence of diabetic autonomic neuropathy. PP is known to inhibit gallbladder contraction, bile as well as exocrine pancreatic secretion. Deficiencies in PP secretion due to severe chronic pancreatitis or proximal resections are accompanied by reduced hepatic insulin sensitivity due to decreased hepatic insulin receptors.[24] These effects are reversed by PP administration.

A fifth islet peptide, ghrelin, is secreted from a distinct population of islet cells, called epsilon cells.[25,26] Ghrelin is also present in the gastric fundus in large amounts and stimulates growth hormone secretion via growth hormone releasing hormone released from the pituitary. It is an orexigenic, or appetite-stimulating, peptide the plasma levels of which are increased in obesity. Ghrelin has also been shown to block insulin effects on the liver, and inhibits the beta cell response to incretin hormones and glucose.[27] Therefore, ghrelin secretion from and within the islet may modulate the responses of other islet cells to nutrient and hormonal stimuli.

The other peptides produced by pancreas include neuropeptides such as serotonin, vasoactive intestinal polypeptide (VIP) and galanin. It also produces amylin and pancreastatin. Amylin, also known as islet amyloid polypeptide is stored in the beta cells along with insulin.[28] The proposed function of amylin is modulation of insulin secretion. Pancreastatin augments glucagon while inhibiting somatostatin and insulin release.[29,30] Pancreatic exocrine secretion is also inhibited by pancreastatin.[31]

Intra-Islet Regulation

The beta cells constitute about 70% of the total islet cell mass. They are situated in the central portion of each islet while the other cell types are largely peripheral in location. The delta cells make only 5% while the alpha cells make up 10%, and the PP cells make up 15% of the total islet cell mass.[32] Individual islet cells can secrete multiple hormones. For example, the beta cells secrete both insulin and amylin, which counter-regulates the actions of insulin. Actually, more than 20 different hormones are secreted by the islets, and the exact functions of this milieu are very complex. There is diversity among the islets depending on their location within the pancreas. In general, islets located closer to major arterioles are larger than islets located more deeply in the parenchyma of the pancreas. The beta and delta cells are evenly distributed throughout the pancreas, while PP cells are predominantly located in the head and uncinate process while alpha cells are predominant in the body and tail. This is clinically significant because pancreatoduodenectomy removes 95% of the PP cells in the pancreas. This may partially explain the higher incidence of glucose intolerance after the Whipple procedure than after distal pancreatectomy. In addition, chronic pancreatitis, which disproportionately affects the pancreatic head, is associated with PP deficiency and pancreatogenic diabetes.[33]

The islets receive about 20–30% of the pancreatic blood flow although it forms only 2% of total pancreatic mass. The manner in which the blood flows through an individual islet can affect the islet function because the four types of cells have a different location. Blood flow within islet can vary from the center of the islet to the periphery, from the periphery to the center, or from one pole of the islet to the other. The predominant pattern of blood flow through the islets in the human pancreas is still conjectural. However, there is a strong component of paracrine regulation. Secretions from one islet cells influence the secretions from neighboring islet cells. Somatostatin inhibits the secretions of insulin, glucagon and PP from their respective cells. Therefore, somatostatin may have an important role in intra islet control of islet cell secretions.[34] Islet hormone secretions are also regulated by the feedback mechanisms. For example, small rise in arterial levels of insulin secretion inhibits further secretion from beta cells.

Although most of the blood supply to the acinar cells comes directly from the pancreatic arterioles, small quantity of blood comes from the islet capillaries. Perfusion of acinar cells with this venous blood has some kind of influence on exocrine secretion as well from these acini. Thus, insulin release, increased by high carbohydrate content of the meal, also promotes an amylase-rich exocrine secretion.

REFERENCES

1. Suda K, Mizuguchi K, Hoshino A. Differences of the ventral and dorsal anlagen of pancreas after fusion. Acta Pathol Jpn. 1981;31: 583-9.
2. Skandalakis JE, Gray SW. Embryology for surgeons: the embryological basis for the treatment of congenital anomalies, 2nd edition. Baltimore: Williams & Wilkins; 1994.
3. Beger HG. The pancreas. Oxford; Malden, MA: Blackwell Science; 1998.
4. Kamisawa T, Egawa N, Tsuruta K, Okamoto A, Mtsukawa M. Pancreatitis associated with congenital abnormalities of the pancreaticobiliary system. Hepatogastroenterology. 2005;52:223-9.
5. Kiernan PD, ReMine SG, Kierman PC, ReMine WH. Annular pancreas: May Clinic experience from 1957 to 1976 with review of the literature. Arch Surg. 1980;115(1);46-50.
6. Lecco TM Zur Morphologie des Pankreas annulare. Sitzungsb. Akad. Wissensch. Math Naturw. CL. 1910;119:391-406.
7. Baldwin W. A specimen of annular pancreas. Anat Rec. 1910;4: 299-304.
8. Tieken. Annular pancreas [transl.]. Chicago Pathol Soc. 1901; 4:180.
9. Dolan RV, ReMine WH, Dockerty MB. The fate of heterotopic pancreatic tissue. A study of 212 cases. Arch Surg. 1974;109: 762-5.
10. Gaspar Fuentes A, Campos Tarrech JM, Fernandez Burgui JL, Castells Tejon E, Ruiz Rossello J, Gomez Perez J, et al. Pancreatic ectopias. Rev Esp Enferm Apar Dig. 1973;39:255-68.
11. Goodarzi M, Rashid A, Maru D. Invasive ductal adenocarcinoma arising from pancreatic heterotopia in rectum: case report and review of literature. Hum Pathol. 2010;41:1809-13.
12. Eisenberger CF, Gocht A, Knoefel WT, Busch CB, Peiper M, Kutup A, et al. Heterotopic pancreas--clinical presentation and pathology with review of the literature. Hepatogastroenterology. 2004;51: 854-8.
13. Kimura W. Surgical anatomy of the pancreas for limited resection. J Hepatobiliary Pancreat Surg. 2000;7:473-9.
14. Davenport HW. Pancreatic secretion. In: Davenport HN (Ed). Physiology of the Digestive Tract, 5th edition. Chicago: Year Book Medical Publishers; 1982. p. 143.
15. Konturek SJ, Becker HD, Thompson JC. Effect of vagotomy on hormones stimulating pancreatic secretion. Arch Surg. 1974;108:704.
16. Ebert R, Creutzfeldt W. Gastrointestinal peptides and insulin secretion. Diabetes Metab Rev. 1987;3:1-26.
17. Leahy JL, Bonner-Weir S, Weir GC. Abnormal glucose regulation of insulin secretion in models of reduced B-cell mass. Diabetes. 1984;33:667-73.
18. Brunicardi FC, Sun YS, Druck P, Goulet RJ, Elahi D, Andersen DK. Splanchnic neural regulation of insulin and glucagon secretion in the isolated perfused human pancreas. Am J Surg. 1987; 153:34.
19. Yamada Y, Post SR, Wang K, Tager HS, Bell GI, Seino S. Cloning and functional characterization of a family of human and mouse somatostatin receptors expressed in brain, gastrointestinal tract, and kidney. Proc Natl Acad Sci U S A. 1992;89:251-5.
20. Voss M, Pappas T. Pancreatic fistula. Curr Treat Options Gastroenterol. 2002;5:345.
21. Feldman M, Richardson CT, Taylor IL, Walsh JH. Effect of atropine on vagal release of gastrin and pancreatic polypeptide. J Clin Invest. 1979;63:294-8.
22. Floyd JC, Fajans SS, Pek S. Regulation in healthy subjects of thesecretion of human pancreatic polypeptide, a newly recognized pancreaticislet polypeptide. Trans Assoc Am Physicians. 1976;89:146-58.
23. Adrian TE, Bloom SR, Besterman HS, Cooke TJ, Barnes AJ, Russell RC. Mechanism of pancreatic polypeptide release in man. Lancet. 1977;1:161-3.
24. Seymour NE, Andersen DK. Pancreatic polypeptide and glucosemetabolism, In: Greenly GH (Ed). Gastrointestinal Endocrinology. Totowa NJ. Humana Press; 1999. p. 321.
25. Wierup N, Svensson H, Mulder H, Sundler F. The ghrelin cell: a novel developmentally regulated islet cell in the human pancreas. Regul Pept. 2002;107:63.
26. Prado CL, Pugh-Bernard AE, Elghazi L, Sosa-Pineda B, Sussel L. Ghrelin cells replace insulin-producing beta cells in two mouse models of pancreas development. Proc Natl Acad Sci U S A. 2004;101:2924-9.
27. Sun Y, Asnicar M, Saha PK, Chan L, Smith RG. Ablation of ghrelin improves the diabetic but not obese phenotype of ob/ob mice. Cell Metab. 2006;3:379-86.
28. Westermark P, Wilander E, Westermark GT, Johnson KH. Islet amyloid polypeptide-like-immunoreactivity in the islet B-cells of type II (non-insulin-dependent) diabetic and non-diabetic individuals. Diabetologia. 1987;30:887-92.

29. Tatemoto K, Efendic S, Mutt V, Makk G, Feistner GJ, Barchas JD. Pancreastatin, a novel pancreatic peptide that inhibits insulin secretion. Nature. 1986;324:476-8.
30. Efendic S, Tatemoto K, Mutt V, Quan C, Chang D, Ostenson CG. Pancreastatin and islet hormone release. Proc Natl Acad Sci. U S A. 1987;84:7257-60.
31. Funakoshi A, Miyasaka K, Nakamura R, Kitani K, Tatemoto K. Inhibitory effect of pancreastatin on pancreatic exocrine secretion in the conscious rat. Regul Pept. 1989;25:157-66.
32. Gorelick FS, Jamieson JD. Structure-function relationship of the pancreas, In Johnson LR (Ed). Physiology of the Gastrointestinal Tract. New York: Raven Press; 1981. p. 773.
33. Kennedy FP. Pathophysiology of pancreatic polypeptide secretion in human diabetes mellitus. Diabetes Nutr Metab. 1990;2:155.
34. Kleinman R, Ohning G, Wong H, Watt P, Walsh J, Brunicardi FC. Regulatory role of intra islet somatostatin on insulin secretion in the isolated perfused human pancreas. Pancreas. 1994;9: 172-8.

CHAPTER 37

Acute Pancreatitis

Pramod Kumar Garg

INTRODUCTION

Acute pancreatitis is a common gastrointestinal emergency.[1] Abdominal pain is its predominant presenting symptom. The severity of acute pancreatitis varies from mild interstitial pancreatitis to severe necrotizing pancreatitis.[2] Severe acute pancreatitis is associated with a significant mortality of 10–40%.[3]

DEFINITION

Acute pancreatitis can be defined as an acute inflammatory disease of the pancreas resulting from a variety of insults and characterized clinically by a sudden onset of upper abdominal pain and biochemically by an increase of pancreatic enzymes in the blood.[4]

MAGNITUDE

The exact magnitude of acute pancreatitis is not well known. The incidence of acute pancreatitis varies from 30–80/100,000 population in different countries and has been increasing over the past 2 decades.[5,6] Acute pancreatitis ranked first among all gastrointestinal related hospitalization in the United States in 2009 and accounted for 274,119 admissions annually with more than $2.5 billion cost of treatment.[7]

CLINICAL PRESENTATION

The most common symptom is a sudden onset of severe abdominal pain. Like any other visceral pain, the pain in acute pancreatitis is ill defined and poorly localized. It usually starts in the upper abdomen and often radiates to the back. It persists for several hours to a few days. Associated features may include vomiting, abdominal fullness, and low grade fever. Fever beyond the first week usually suggests super-added infection. Paralytic ileus may complicate severe pancreatitis. Acute pancreatitis may also present without pain. Painless acute pancreatitis may occur due to: (1) upper abdominal surgery with handling of the pancreas, (2) dialysis and (3) certain drugs. The diagnosis of painless acute pancreatitis is challenging but should be suspected if there is unexplained deterioration in a patient's condition in such a setting.

On physical examination, there is mild tenderness in the upper abdomen particularly in the epigastrium. The abdomen may be slightly distended and the bowel sounds sluggish. Unlike other acute abdominal emergencies, the signs are subtle while the pain is quite severe in acute pancreatitis. In patients with severe pancreatitis however, there may be generalized abdominal distension with some rigidity and guarding. In a minority of patients, there may be intra-abdominal hypertension with markedly tense abdomen. Unlike peritonitis, rebound tenderness is not a feature of acute pancreatitis. Periumbilical reddish discoloration known as Cullen's sign and/or flank discoloration known as the Grey Turner's sign are rarely seen. Subcutaneous fat necrosis may also be rarely seen. Systemic examination may show presence of systemic inflammatory response syndrome (SIRS) and organ dysfunction. Tachycardia, tachypnea, dyspnea, hypotension, and oliguria indicate impending or established organ dysfunction. Persistent SIRS indicates likelihood of a severe pancreatitis.

ETIOLOGY

The common causes of acute pancreatitis include gallstones, alcohol abuse, trauma, post-endoscopic retrograde cholangio-pancreatography (ERCP) and miscellaneous. The miscellaneous causes include drugs, trauma, viral infections, small periampullary tumors (especially in elderly), biliary ascariasis and microlithiasis (<3 mm gallstones). No cause is discernible in about 10–25% of patients and these cases are labeled as idiopathic pancreatitis.

Table 1: Common causes of acute pancreatitis	
Gallstones	40–45%
Alcohol	25–30%
Post-ERCP	5%
Post-trauma	1%
Idiopathic	10–25%
Miscellaneous	5%

Table 1 shows the various causes of pancreatitis and their relative frequencies.[1,3]

Mechanism of Pancreatic Injury and Inflammation

The mechanism of pancreatitis varies depending on the etiology. A gallstone may cause pancreatitis when it obstructs the common channel at the papilla and consequently the pancreatic duct as demonstrated elegantly by Opie[8] way back in 1901. Another remarkable study showed recovery of small stones in the stool samples of patients within 2–3 days of the onset of acute pancreatitis supporting this hypothesis.[9] The events subsequent to obstruction are not well understood—either there is increased pressure within the pancreatic duct which is transmitted to the acinar cells leading to disruption of the cellular secretory processes or there is reflux of bile from the bile duct into the pancreatic duct causing toxic injury.

The mechanism of injury due to alcohol is most likely related to its toxic effects. Chronic consumption of alcohol is required to cause pancreatitis. At least more than 60 grams of alcohol for more than 5 years is required to cause alcohol related pancreatitis and less than 10% of alcoholics develop alcoholic pancreatitis. Alcohol abuse is generally associated with the risk of chronic pancreatitis but it can also cause acute pancreatitis.[10] A binge of alcohol may at times precipitate an acute attack but only in those abusing alcohol. Pancreatic injury and inflammation are related to the toxic effects of alcohol metabolites such as acetaldehyde and fatty acid ethyl esters, and also to oxidative stress induced by the alcohol metabolism.

Abdominal trauma is another common cause of pancreatitis in both children and adults. Trauma may lead to fracture of the pancreas usually at the level of genu where it lies over the spine causing pancreatic duct disruption. Pancreatic trauma is usually associated with injury to other intra-abdominal organs such as liver and intestine, which lead to more obvious clinical manifestations and govern the prognosis. However, it is essential to recognize pancreatic injury as it often requires early surgical intervention.

Endoscopic retrograde cholangiopancreatography may cause acute pancreatitis in 5–7% of patients.[11] The mechanism of injury is related to microtrauma of the papilla induced by the procedure leading to edema, obstruction to the pancreatic duct outflow and increased intraductal pressure. Another cause of increased intraductal pressure is injection of contrast dye into the pancreatic duct during ERCP. The major risk factors of post-ERCP pancreatitis are difficult cannulation, repeated cannulation of the pancreatic duct, and injection of contrast into the pancreatic duct especially under pressure.

Many drugs have been implicated to cause acute pancreatitis but the causality has not been fully established in most cases. The drugs may cause acute pancreatitis by hypersensitivity/idiosyncratic reaction, or due to their toxic metabolites. The drugs most likely to be associated with acute pancreatitis include: Azathioprine, angiotensin-converting-enzyme (ACE) inhibitors, Mesalazine, Simvastatin, Fenofibrate, Thiazides and Valproic acid.

Common viral infections that may cause acute pancreatitis are Coxsackie, EB virus, mumps virus, hepatitis A, E and B viruses, and HIV.[12] Presence of fever preceding the onset of acute pancreatitis may be a clue to infectious etiology of acute pancreatitis. Ascaris induced acute pancreatitis has been commonly reported from India particularly Kashmir.[13]

Small periampullary tumors may cause acute pancreatitis and must be ruled out in elderly patients with unexplained acute pancreatitis.

Pathophysiological Perturbations in the Initiation and Progression of Acute Pancreatitis

The sequence of events in the development of acute pancreatitis can be divided into three major phases: (1) initiation phase, (2) perpetuation phase, and (3) secondary escalation phase. The initiating phase starts in the pancreatic acinar cells and involves premature and unphysiological activation of pancreatic digestive enzymes mainly trypsin. Intracellular activation of enzymes leads to cellular injury through apoptosis and/or necrosis. The mechanism of cellular injury is not well understood and is an area of ongoing research. Cellular injury particularly the necrotic form leads to activation of the central inflammatory mediator NF-kappaB (NFkB) in the acinar cells. NFkB activation is the major inflammation initiating factor by upregulating the transcription of various proinflammatory cytokines. It is pertinent to note that acinar cell itself acts as an inflammatory cell in the beginning by generating cytokines and chemokines such as TNF-α, IL-8, etc.[14]

Following the initiation of the inflammation, perpetuation of inflammation occurs due to recruitment of effector cells mainly leukocytes of the innate and adaptive immune systems. The migration of leukocytes is an orderly process that requires upregulation of vascular endothelial adhesion molecules and interaction of activated leukocytes with these adhesion molecules via their ligands namely selectins and integrins. Neutrophils, monocytes, lymphocytes play important role in escalating the local inflammation as well as the systemic inflammatory response leading to distant organ injury. The other important event in this phase is microcirculatory disturbances in the pancreas which contribute to pancreatic necrosis. Microcirculatory changes include reduced pancreatic blood flow leading to pancreatic ischemia and increased capillary permeability. The reduction in blood flow is multifactorial. Leukocyte adhesion, platelet aggregation, hemoconcentration secondary to fluid loss, vasoconstriction and reduced capillary perfusion have all been shown to contribute to pancreatic ischemia. Coagulation disturbances may also cause microthrombi in the pancreatic vasculature.

In the escalation phase, superadded infection of the necrotic pancreatic and peripancreatic tissue, and fluid collections is the culprit. The necrotic pancreatic tissue, and peripancreatic fluid collections are susceptible to infection. Infected pancreatic necrosis (IPN) usually occurs after the first week of illness, results in secondary escalation of local and systemic inflammation, and carries a high mortality. The route of infection is most likely transmigration of gut bacteria secondary to increased intestinal permeability. The deleterious effects of the superadded infection are similar to any septic process but the outcome of pancreatic infection is more sinister due to its deep location and spread of infection within the abdomen particularly in the retroperitoneum leading to difficulty in controlling the infection. The septic process further leads to exacerbation of SIRS with release of cytokines and chemokines thus aggravating the process set in motion by the underlying pancreatitis.

DIAGNOSIS AND DIFFERENTIAL DIAGNOSIS

The diagnosis of acute pancreatitis can be made if two out of the following three criteria are present:[15]

1. Abdominal pain suggestive of acute pancreatitis (acute onset of a persistent, constant upper abdominal pain often radiating to the back).
2. Serum amylase and/or lipase activity at least more than or equal to three times the upper limit of normal.
3. Characteristic findings of acute pancreatitis on imaging, e.g. on transabdominal ultrasonography (USG), or contrast enhanced computed tomography (CECT) or magnetic resonance imaging (MRI) scan of the abdomen.

Differential Diagnosis

In patients presenting with acute upper abdominal pain, the important differential diagnoses include acute cholecystitis, intestinal obstruction, intestinal perforation, peritonitis, acute appendicitis and peptic ulcer disease. Other uncommon differential diagnoses include mesenteric ischemia, myocardial infarction, dissection of aorta, etc. Plain X-ray of the abdomen in erect and supine position, USG of the abdomen, serum amylase and an electrocardiogram (ECG) are important investigations which should always be done in a patient presenting with acute abdomen. A computed tomography scan of the abdomen may be required in problematic cases where the diagnosis is in doubt even after these tests. Table 2 shows the main differential diagnoses and their differentiating features from acute pancreatitis.

Investigations

As mentioned above, the basic investigations which should be done in the emergency room itself include a plain X-ray of the abdomen in erect and supine position, USG of the abdomen, serum amylase and an ECG. Serum amylase is elevated to more than 3 times the upper normal in most patients with acute pancreatitis. It falls rapidly over the first 3 days and thus loses its diagnostic value thereafter. The level of serum amylase has no correlation with the severity of acute pancreatitis. Repeated measurement of serum amylase as a guide to improvement in acute pancreatitis is not recommended as either the fall or rise in levels has no correlation with the clinical course. Serum amylase may be elevated in some other conditions such as parotitis, acute cholecystitis, intestinal obstruction, renal failure, etc. and may thus lead to a diagnostic dilemma. Lipase is more specific than amylase and may remain elevated for a few more days after serum amylase level comes down. Asymptomatic elevation of serum amylase has no clinical significance and may be due to macroamylasemia.

Hematocrit is a maker of fluid balance and should be monitored especially in the first 24–48 hours. The fluid requirement is high in the initial period. Hematocrit has been used as a guide to optimize fluid administration as a part of goal directed therapy. Total leucocyte count is a marker of SIRS in the initial period and of infection later. Serum electrolytes and serum pH should be monitored periodically in patients with severe pancreatitis. Blood urea (or blood urea nitrogen) has been shown to be a good prognostic marker. Liver function tests during the first 48 hours indicate biliary etiology of acute pancreatitis. It has been shown that serum alanine transferase (ALT) more than 150 IU/L and bilirubin more than 3 mg/dL predict biliary pancreatitis with a 84–96% sensitivity.[16,17] Serum calcium may fall during the acute phase and may have prognostic significance. Hypercalcemia may be a cause of acute pancreatitis in patients with hyperparathyroidism. It may, however, be normal during the acute phase and should be repeated after recovery. Lipid profile should be done to rule out hypertriglyceridemia as a cause of pancreatitis

Imaging Investigations

A plain X-ray of the abdomen may show a dilated transverse colon with abrupt cut off near the splenic flexure, known as the "colon cut-off sign". An isolated loop of dilated jejunum, known as the "sentinel loop" may be present. These dilated segments are due

Table 2: Differential diagnosis of acute pancreatitis

S. No.	*Diagnosis*	*Differentiating clinical features*	*Investigative findings*
1.	Acute cholecystitis	Tender gallbladder lump (Murphy's sign)	Distended and thickened GB with stone on USG of the abdomen
2.	Acute intestinal obstruction	Abdominal distension, constipation, recurrent vomiting, exaggerated bowel sounds	Air-fluid levels on a plain X-ray of the abdomen in erect posture
3.	Intestinal perforation with peritonitis	Abdominal distension, rebound tenderness, guarding, absent bowel sounds	Free air under diaphragm on an erect plain X-ray of the abdomen
4.	Acute appendicitis	Tenderness in the right iliac fossa	USG and/or CECT scan of the abdomen showing inflamed appendix
5.	Ureteric colic	Pain radiating from loin to groin	USG may show hydronephrosis/hydroureter and a stone; urine shows RBCs
6.	Liver abscess	History of fever, tender hepatomegaly	USG shows liver abscess
7.	Acute myocardial infarction	Upper abdominal or chest pain, radiation to left upper limb, dyspnea, sweating	ECG showing typical changes, elevated cardiac enzymes

to inflammation induced localized ileus. In patients with chronic pancreatitis presenting with an acute exacerbation, pancreatic calculi may be seen on the plain film.

Ultrasonography is an important investigation. It may show features of acute pancreatitis in the form of bulky, enlarged and hypoechoic pancreas, and blurring of peripancreatic margins. There may be fluid collections in and around the pancreas. It may also show gallstones as the cause of acute pancreatitis and a dilated bile duct with or without bile duct stone. The limitations of USG are that it cannot diagnose pancreatic necrosis and it may not visualize the pancreas well due to the presence of fat and bowel gas.

A CECT scan of the abdomen is an important imaging test for acute pancreatitis. However, all patients do not require a CECT scan. The indications for a CECT scan are: (1) if the diagnosis is in doubt at the time of presentation, (2) to look for the presence of pancreatic and peripancreatic necrosis between day 4 and 7 (Figs 1 to 5) in severe pancreatitis and (3) for complications such as IPN and pseudocyst before planning intervention,

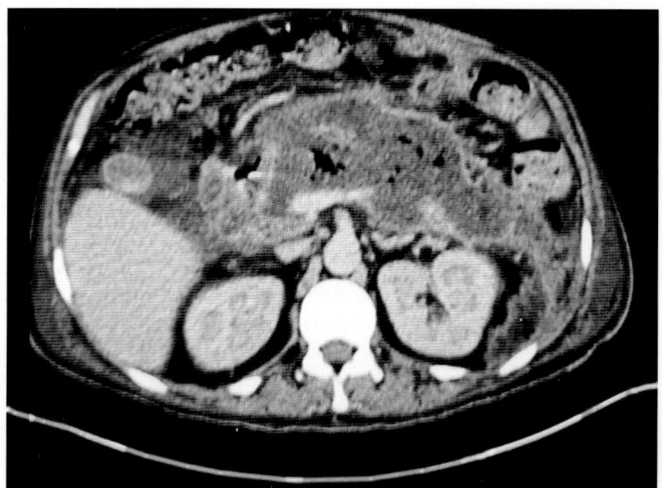

Figure 3 Contrast enhanced CT scan showing infected pancreatic necrosis with extra intestinal air within the collection

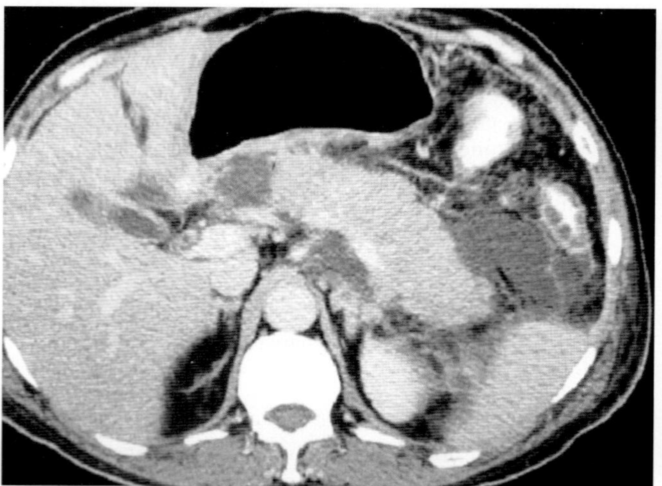

Figure 1 Contrast enhanced CT scan showing minimal necrosis of the pancreas in the head region and an acute fluid collection in the tail region

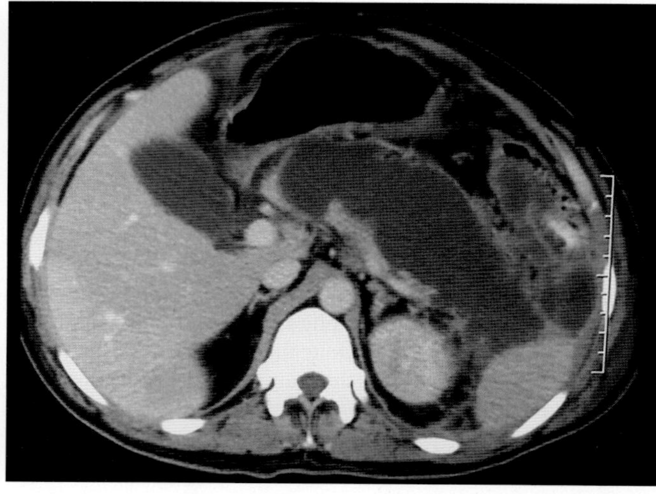

Figure 4 Contrast enhanced CT scan showing a sterile walled off pancreatic necrosis

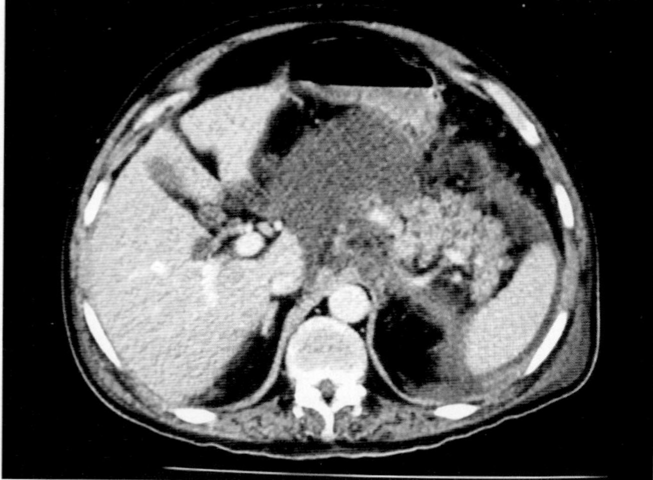

Figure 2 Contrast enhanced CT scan showing more than 50% necrosis involving the head and body of the pancreas

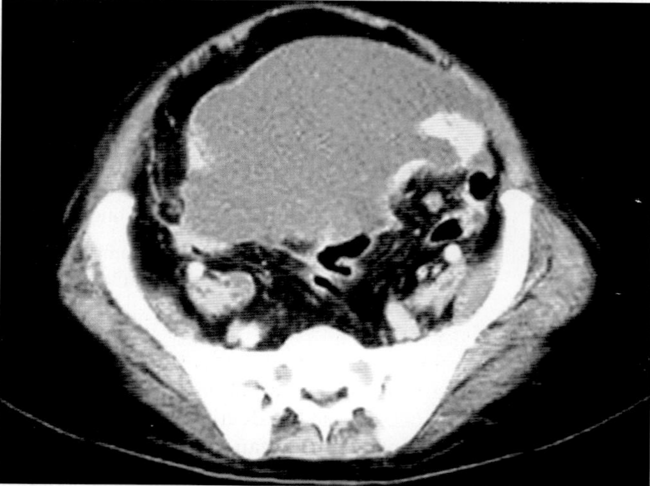

Figure 5 Contrast enhanced CT scan showing a large pseudocyst

Table 3: Balthazar's scoring for CT severity index

CT finding	*Score*
CT Grade:	
A. Normal pancreas	0
B. Pancreatic enlargement	1
C. B + Peripancreatic inflammation	2
D. 1 peripancreatic fluid collection	3
E. >1 peripancreatic fluid collections	4
Pancreatic necrosis:	
No necrosis	0
1/3rd necrosis	2
1/2 necrosis	4
>1/2 necrosis	6

e.g. percutaneous/endoscopic drainage or surgery. A CECT is not required in patients with clinically mild pancreatitis who improve with conservative treatment. Pancreatic necrosis is diagnosed as non-enhancing (non-viable) areas of pancreas on a CECT scan. The amount of pancreatic necrosis should be graded as less than 30%, 30–50% and more than 50%. It is also important to look for peripancreatic necrosis. A CT severity index should be calculated according to Balthazar et al. (Table 3).[18]

Microbiological Investigations

Development of infection further complicates the course of the illness. The most important cause of worry is infection of the pancreatic and peripancreatic necrosis, and fluid collections. The diagnosis of infected necrosis can be confirmed by culture of the necrotic material and/or fluid. Other sources of infection like central line, cholangitis, urinary and chest infection should also be looked for. Appropriate cultures of sputum, central line, intravenous catheter and urine should be done periodically.

CLINICAL COURSE AND COMPLICATIONS

The clinical course of acute pancreatitis depends on the severity of illness which is governed by local and systemic complications. Pathologically, pancreatic inflammation may or may not be associated with necrosis of the gland. Acute edematous (or interstitial) pancreatitis is seen in 70–80% of patients and runs a mild course. Most patients with acute interstitial pancreatitis do not develop significant local or systemic complications. On the other hand, acute necrotizing pancreatitis is present in 20–30% of patients and usually has a severe course. The severity classification of acute pancreatitis takes into account the local and systemic complications and thus will be discussed after the description of the various complications. There are two phases of mortality in patients with acute pancreatitis—early and late. Early mortality is defined as death within 1–2 weeks of admission. It occurs mainly due to organ failure in patients with severe necrotizing pancreatitis.[2,19] Late mortality is due to sepsis related to IPN and persistence or development of new organ failure.[20]

Local Complications

The local complications of acute pancreatitis include inflammation, fluid collections and pancreatic necrosis. In addition, adjacent organ involvement may lead to bowel, biliary and/or vascular complications.

Fluid Collections

Acute fluid collections develop in approximately 50% of all acute pancreatitis as a consequence of inflammation, exudation and pancreatic ductal leakage.[21]

Definitions of fluid collections according to the revised Atlanta classification: Recently, the revised Atlanta classification[22] has defined the various fluid collections according to the time of their development and associated necrosis. The new classification divides fluid collections into two broad categories—early, i.e. less than 4 weeks and late, i.e. more than 4 weeks:

Early collections (<4 weeks) are of two types:

- *Type 1*: Acute peripancreatic fluid collection (APFC) is defined as a collection of fluid associated with interstitial edematous pancreatitis (IEP) without pancreatic or peripancreatic necrosis.
- *Type 2*: Acute necrotic collection (ANC) is a collection of fluid containing variable amounts of both fluid and necrotic material following acute necrotizing pancreatitis.

Late collections (≥4 weeks) are also of two types:

- *Pancreatic pseudocyst*: It is defined as a collection of fluid outside the pancreas with minimal or no necrosis with a defined inflammatory wall. Pseudocysts by definition contain no or minimal necrotic debris.
- *Walled-off necrosis*: It is defined as an organized collection of fluid and pancreatic and/or peripancreatic necrosis following acute necrotizing pancreatitis with a defined inflammatory wall. It has been shown that pancreatic necrosis liquefies gradually over a period of time. Coupled with a variable degree of peripancreatic fluid collections, liquefying pancreatic necrosis becomes organized and walled off over a period of 4–8 weeks. In other words, acute necrotic collections become organized and well defined over time to evolve into what has been termed as "Walled Off Necrosis" (WON). A T2 weighted MRI scan is very useful to differentiate a WON from a pseudocyst (Figs 6A and B).

Natural course of fluid collections: The fluid collections may either resolve or persist. The extent of pancreatic necrosis, and size and duration of fluid collections determine their outcome.[23] In general, acute fluid collections after acute interstitial pancreatitis usually resolve. Acute necrotic collections are more likely to persist and may become infected. True pseudocysts are very uncommon following acute pancreatitis because APFC usually resolve. On the other hand, acute necrotic collections evolve into WON which are more likely to persist. It has now been recognized that most patients with acute pancreatitis have WON rather than true pseudocysts because of the presence of necrotic debris. The differentiation between a pseudocyst and WON is best made on an MRI scan although a USG can also show presence of necrotic debris within the collection. CT scan is not a good modality for this purpose.

Complications of pancreatic fluid collections: The common complications of fluid collections include infection, hemorrhage, compression, rupture and pancreatic ascites. Infection is the most common complication.

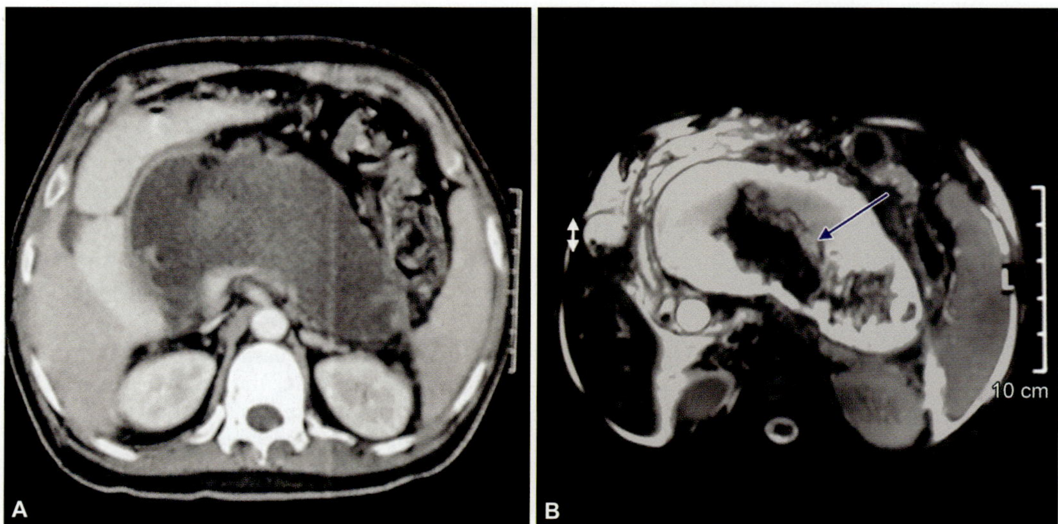

Figures 6A and B (A) An MRI scan showing a large collection on T1 weighted sequence. (B) T2 weighted sequence of the collection showed necrotic debris (arrow) within the collection suggesting walled off necrosis

Necrosis

Pancreatic necrosis is a critical and ominous development during the course of acute pancreatitis. It may lead to a mortality of up to 40%.[24] In addition to pancreatic necrosis, necrosis of peripancreatic fat may also occur. In fact, it has now been recognized that peripancreatic necrosis may occur alone without pancreatic necrosis with similar risk of infection. For this reason, peripancreatic necrosis alone has also been included in the revised Atlanta classification to define necrotizing pancreatitis. Pancreatic necrosis may be limited or extensive. More extensive the pancreatic necrosis, more are the chances of local and systemic complications. Necrosis may either remain sterile or become infected. IPN is the cause of severe sepsis and further complicates the course of acute pancreatitis with worsening of clinical condition of the patient. It has been shown that the extent and infection of the pancreatic necrosis correlate with organ failure and mortality.[3] The diagnosis of IPN is suspected in the presence of fever, raised leukocyte count and worsening clinical course. It can be confirmed by demonstrating the presence of bacteria in the pancreatic necrotic tissue or fluid collection either on Gram's stain or on culture. Pancreatic tissue/fluid can be obtained by a fine needle aspiration (FNA) under either CT or USG guidance using a 20–22 G needle. The FNA is usually performed in the second or third week of the illness when there are maximum chances of infection. The issue of FNA, however, is debatable. Most experts recommend that the management of suspected infected necrosis should be guided by the clinical condition of the patient rather than the results of FNA and hence routine FNA is no more advisable to confirm infected necrosis.[15] Fluid from the percutaneous drainage or that obtained during surgery should be cultured to diagnose infected necrosis. Presence of extra-intestinal air in the pancreatic bed or within the collection is another sign of IPN.

Other Non-pancreatic Local Complications

Peripancreatic inflammation may involve adjacent bowel. Involvement of the antroduodenal area may lead to gastric outlet obstruction (GOO). Rarely, colonic necrosis may occur in severe necrotizing pancreatitis which may prove to be catastrophic. Fluid collection in the head of pancreas may cause biliary obstruction. Vascular complications may also complicate the course of acute pancreatitis and may involve both arteries and veins. Venous thrombosis of the splenic and portal veins occurs in up to 10% of patients. Fortunately, vascular thrombosis does not lead to significant problems in the majority of patients. On the other hand, arterial involvement leads to the formation of a pseudoaneurysm, which may cause massive bleeding and further compromise a patient's condition.

Systemic Complications

Systemic complications manifest in the form of systemic inflammatory response syndrome (SIRS) and organ failure. Organ failure usually involves respiratory and renal systems but may also involve cardiovascular system. Three important characteristics of organ failure should be taken into account, i.e. the timing, grade and the dynamics. Transient organ failure does not adversely affect the outcome. Persistent organ failure for more than 48 hours is considered as suggestive of severe acute pancreatitis. With regard to the timing, early organ failure within the first 7 days has a worse prognosis compared with late organ failure. Patients with early onset organ failure are termed as having early severe acute pancreatitis (ESAP).[2] Organ failure should be graded preferably according to modified Marshall's grading system (Table 4). Understandably, patients with more severe grade of organ failure have a worse outcome.

Prediction of Severity of Acute Pancreatitis

Predicting the severity is important for prognostication and referral of a patient to a higher center. The methods for predicting severity of acute pancreatitis include: (1) Scoring systems based on clinical and laboratory parameters, (2) single prognostic markers and (3) imaging criteria based on CECT scan findings.

Table 4: Severity of acute pancreatitis according to the revised Atlanta classification

- Severe acute pancreatitis: Persistent organ failure of at least grade 2 >48 hours
- Moderate acute pancreatitis: At least one of the following should be present:
  - transient organ failure
  - exacerbation of existing organ dysfunction
  - local complications requiring prolonged hospital stay or intervention
- Mild acute pancreatitis: Absence of systemic or local complication

Scoring Systems

Ranson's, Imirie's, BISAP and APACHE II are common scoring systems to prognosticate the disease. Of these, the first two are generally not used nowadays because they require multiple parameters and take at least 48 hours to obtain all the parameters to calculate the score. *B*edside *I*ndex of *S*everity in *A*cute *P*ancreatitis (BISAP) score takes into account the following parameters—*B*lood urea, *I*mpaired mental status, *S*IRS, *A*ge, and *P*leural effusion.[25] It is a relatively new scoring system which has been shown to predict severe acute pancreatitis fairly accurately and has been validated. APACHE II is the most commonly used scoring system to assess and predict the severity of acute pancreatitis. It is not specific for acute pancreatitis and has been used for other acute illnesses. An APACHE II score of more than 8 suggests severe pancreatitis. However, it is somewhat cumbersome to calculate as it requires multiple parameters (the software can be downloaded at *http://apache-ii-score-calculator.soft112.com/*).

Single Prognostic Markers

In addition to the multiple scoring systems which are often considered complex, many single prognostic markers have been proposed to simplify the prognostication. Such markers include: c-reactive protein (CRP), trypsinogen activated peptide, granulocytic elastase, α-2 macroglobulin, IL-6, etc.[26] Among these markers, CRP is the most commonly used. Serum procalcitonin may be used as an indirect marker of infection particularly in suspected cases of infected necrosis. Obesity has been found to be an independent prognostic marker. However, the overall clinical utility of these single prognostic markers is limited.

Imaging-based Assessment of Severity

Contrast enhanced computed tomography scan of the abdomen is considered an important investigation not only for the diagnosis but also for assessing the severity of pancreatitis. The extent of inflammation, fluid collections and necrosis have been shown to have a prognostic value. Balthazar et al.[18] have devised a score based on these findings and correlated that with the outcome of acute pancreatitis (Table 3; Figs 1 to 5). A CT severity index of more than 7 is suggestive of severe pancreatitis.

Classification of the Severity of Acute Pancreatitis

In order to classify the disease into different categories of severity, the most widely used classification has been the Atlanta classification of 1992.[21] This classification divided severity into two categories, i.e. mild and severe pancreatitis based on the local and systemic complications. The defining features of severe acute pancreatitis were presence of organ failure, an APACHE II score more than 8, and/or local complications, i.e. necrosis, pseudocyst, and abscess. Atlanta classification defined organ failure as follows: Respiratory failure—paO_2 less than 60 mm, acute renal failure—serum creatinine more than 2.0 mg/dL, cardiovascular failure—systolic blood pressure less than 90 mm Hg and/or severe gastrointestinal bleeding of more than 500 mL/24 hours.

While the original classification served its purpose and helped crystallize the prevalent concepts about acute pancreatitis, there were some important shortcomings as follows:

- The definition of organ failure did not take into account the timing, grade or the dynamics of organ failure. For example, it is well known that transient organ failure does not significantly affect the outcome. Early organ failure has a worse prognosis compared with late organ failure.
- All local complications were included in the list of criteria for severe pancreatitis regardless of their severity although different local complications have variable significance.

In addition to these concerns about the original classification, our understanding of acute pancreatitis has undergone a sea change over the past 20 years. Thus, the Atlanta classification was revised and published in 2012.[21] The revised classification has divided severity of acute pancreatitis in to three categories: mild, moderate and severe (Table 4). The criteria of different severity grades are as follows:

- *Severe acute pancreatitis*: The only defining criterion for severe acute pancreatitis is persistent organ failure of at least grade 2 severity according to the Modified Marshall's grading system persisting for more than 48 hours (Table 5).
- *Moderate acute pancreatitis*: It is defined as presence of transient organ failure, exacerbation of existing organ dysfunction and/or presence of local complications requiring prolonged hospital stay or intervention.

Table 5: Modified Marshall's scoring system for grading organ failure

Organ system	*Grade*				
	0	*1*	*2*	*3*	*4*
Respiratory (PO_2/FIO_2)	>400	301–400	201–300	101–200	≤101
Renal (serum creatinine) (mg/dL)	<1.5	1.5–1.9	1.9–3.5	3.5–4.9	≥5
Cardiovascular (systolic blood pressure) (mm Hg)	>90	<90 Fluid responsive	<90 Not fluid responsive	<90 (pH<7.3)	<90 (pH<7.2)

- *Mild acute pancreatitis*: Absence of systemic or local complication defines mild acute pancreatitis.

Although the revised classification has made significant changes, a few limitations must be appreciated. There are two phases of mortality in patients with acute pancreatitis—early and late. Early mortality, defined as death within 1-2 weeks of admission, is because of organ failure in severe pancreatitis.[27] Sixty per cent of patients developed organ failure at admission and those with persistent organ failure had a worst outcome according to one study.[28] Late mortality is sepsis related. This occurs due to IPN and persistence or development of new organ failure.[29] It has been shown that only a small subset of patients with early severe acute pancreatitis account for almost half of the deaths, e.g. in a study, 11% of patients with fulminant/subfulminant pancreatitis accounted for 47% of all deaths.[2] The revised Atlanta classification has not clearly defined the early severe group for much better prognostication and early aggressive treatment. Another limitation of the new classification is that it did not assign adequate prognostic significance to IPN, which is the cause of most of the late mortality in acute pancreatitis.

Treatment

The treatment of acute pancreatitis comprises of the following:

- Initial stabilization and resuscitation
- Nutritional support
- Prevention and treatment of infection
- Management of organ failure
- Management of fluid collections and necrosis
- Management of complications
- Prevention of recurrence

INITIAL STABILIZATION AND RESUSCITATION

The initial management consists of analgesics for relief of pain. Usually parenteral diclofenac is given for pain relief. Opioid analgesic may be required if there is unsatisfactory response. The most important goal in the first 48 hours is replacement of fluid. There is significant amount of fluid loss in acute pancreatitis due to inflammation, exudation and capillary leak. The fluid losses may be in excess of 3-4 L/day for the first 2-3 days hence that much of intravenous fluid should be given per day for the first 24-48 hours.[30] However, one should be cautious and avoid a fluid overload situation especially in the elderly, in patients with cardiovascular disease, and in patients with acute renal failure. Central venous pressure (CVP) monitoring is not a good guide for fluid therapy especially in ventilated patients. Crystalloids are preferred for fluid therapy.[31] Early goal directed therapy may be used with monitoring of mean arterial pressure and mixed venous oxygen saturation as recommended in patients with severe sepsis.[32] The goal for fluid resuscitation could be maintenance of hematocrit, blood urea nitrogen (BUN) or clinical parameter of urine output. Ringer lactate has been shown to be better than normal saline in a randomized controlled trial as the latter may cause acidosis.[33] Although there are still controversy about the optimal fluid therapy in acute pancreatitis, maintenance of fluid and electrolyte balance is the key to initial resuscitation and must be pursued with care.[34] H_2 blockers are generally advised to prevent stress induced gastrointestinal bleeding. A nasogastric tube for aspiration should not be placed unless there is paralytic ileus or recurrent vomiting. Interventions to decrease pancreatic enzymes secretion have proved to be futile because by the time clinical manifestations of acute pancreatitis set in, the intracellular activation of enzymes has no more role to play. Hence, drugs such as glucagon, somatostatin, atropine, etc. have not been found to be useful in clinical trials. Similarly, interventions to inhibit pancreatic enzymes have not been successful, e.g. antiproteases aprotinin and gabexate maleate are not useful; the reason being that the process of acute pancreatitis is driven mainly by the activation of the inflammatory cascade after the initial intracellular events in the pancreatic acinar cells and not by the proteolytic action of these enzymes.

Nutritional Support

Nutrition should be started as soon as the patient is pain free and is able to tolerate oral feeds. The concept of giving rest to the pancreas by keeping the patient fasting has been discarded. In fact, early enteral nutrition has been shown to reduce complications including infection of the necrotic tissue by maintaining gut mucosal integrity and preventing transmigration of bacteria. In patients with mild pancreatitis, oral feeding should be resumed soon after abdominal pain subsides. Feeding may be started with clear liquids and then soft semisolid diet may be introduced followed by almost a normal diet as per patient's tolerance. A recent randomized trial has shown that early nasogastric tube feeding might be better than keeping the patient fasting in patients with mild to moderate acute pancreatitis with less pain and oral feed intolerance.[35] In patients with severe pancreatitis too, attempts should be made to start enteral nutrition early by nasogastric or nasojejunal tube feeding. A recent meta-analysis has shown that nasogastric and nasojejunal tube feeding are equally well tolerated.[36] Nasojejunal tube feeding might be required if a patient does not tolerate nasogastric feeding. The liquid enteral feeds should be isotonic and contain standard recommended combination of carbohydrates, proteins and fats. There is no restriction in giving fats to such patients. The calorie intake should be increased gradually to about 2,000 kcal/day over a few days depending on the tolerability. Refeeding pain may be an issue in some patients that might delay institution of oral feeding. Parenteral nutrition is required only if a patient has severe ileus, is not able to tolerate even the nasojejunal feeding due to pain or distension, and if there is active gastrointestinal bleeding. Intravenous parenteral nutrition is generally given using a commercial preparation. The risks of parenteral nutrition are sepsis, electrolyte imbalance and increased gut permeability. Thus, it should be changed to enteral feeding as soon as possible.

Prevention and Treatment of Infection

Infection of the fluid collections and necrotic tissue is a major concern in patients with acute pancreatitis. IPN is a dreaded complication of acute pancreatitis. Prophylactic antibiotics showed some benefits in earlier trials but have failed to show any benefit in many recent randomized trials and meta-analyses.[37] In fact, the use of prophylactic antibiotics may lead to more resistant bacterial and fungal infections. However, despite no clear evidence of their benefit, antibiotics are often used by most practitioners but their use must be restricted. It is generally advisable to use antibiotics only if there is demonstrable pancreatic or extrapancreatic infection such as cholangitis, chest infection, etc. The choice of antibiotics should be guided by the antibiotic sensitivity pattern in a hospital and the ability of antibiotics to penetrate the blood pancreatic barrier such as third generation cephalosporins, ureidopenicillins, carbapenem, quinolones and metronidazole.

Management of Organ Failure

Organ failure is the most important complication that requires management in an intensive care unit (ICU). Any patient showing signs of organ dysfunction must be immediately transferred to a secondary/tertiary care center where ICU facilities are available. Patients with respiratory failure may require ventilator support, those with renal failure may require dialysis and fluid non-responsive hypotension requires vasopressors such as noradrenaline. A good ICU care is the key to a successful outcome. Organ failure may also develop later during the course of the illness secondary to sepsis and similar care must be provided at that stage as well.

MANAGEMENT OF FLUID COLLECTIONS AND NECROSIS

Acute fluid collections usually do not require any intervention and should be managed conservatively. The indications for drainage include: (1) if the collections are large and causing significant pressure symptoms, (2) contributing to increased intra-abdominal pressure and (3) get infected. If drainage is indicated, percutaneous drainage is preferred. Acute fluid collections without necrosis usually resolve spontaneously. Acute necrotic fluid collections generally persist and may require intervention.

Patients with sterile necrosis should be managed conservatively. Pancreatic necrosis is almost always accompanied by some fluid collections. Most patients with sterile necrosis and fluid collections do not require drainage or necrosectomy. The emphasis in such patients should be on nutrition, organ support if required, and prevention of infection. Nasojejeunal feeding may be preferred if there is intolerance to oral feeding due to pressure symptoms over the stomach. Over a period of time, the sterile necrosis and associated fluid collections evolve into "WON". Drainage of WON is indicated only if the patient is symptomatic. Symptoms include pain, early satiety, vomiting due to GOO, and jaundice due to biliary obstruction by a collection in the head of the pancreas. If required, drainage may be done either percutaneously or endoscopically. Percutaneous drainage may lead to a persistent fistula. Thus, internal drainage is preferred either surgically or endoscopically. In addition to drainage, necrosectomy may also be required.

Infected pancreatic necrosis is the most sinister complication in patients with acute pancreatitis and may develop in the second to third week of illness or later. While conservative treatment is recommended for sterile necrosis, surgical necrosectomy has generally been considered the standard of care for IPN. It is recommended that surgery should be performed after 3–4 weeks of the onset of pancreatitis so that the necrosis becomes organized and surgical planes are well-defined. Early surgery results in a high mortality in patients with IPN. Most surgeons thus prefer to operate on patients with IPN beyond fourth week of the illness.[38] Many recent studies and a meta-analysis have shown that conservative treatment might be successful in a substantial percentage of patients with infected necrosis.[39] Conservative therapy for IPN includes intensive care, combination antibiotics, and nutritional support, with or without drainage of the infected fluid collections. Drainage should be performed usually at the stage of "WON". In patients with infected WON, percutaneous drainage is generally preferred as the first line of treatment. If a patient is not improving even after PCD, then necrosectomy is required. This treatment strategy is referred to as "Step-up" therapy, i.e. starting with conservative treatment then performing percutaneous drainage and finally scaling up to necrosectomy.[40]

Pancreatic Necrosectomy

Necrosectomy has traditionally been performed by open surgery. However, open surgery is associated with many problems such as intraoperative collateral tissue damage, bleeding, worsening organ failure due to surgical trauma, multiple operations, stormy postoperative course, lengthy stay in ICU, and a high mortality. For this reason, minimally invasive necrosectomy techniques have evolved mainly through the retroperitoneal route using the percutaneously placed catheter as a guide. Minimally invasive necrosectomy is much safer and effective. Video-assisted retroperitoneal debridement (VARD) has been shown to be a safe and effective minimally invasive technique.[40] Among other minimally invasive procedures for treating IPN, per-oral direct endoscopic necrosectomy (DEN) has been shown to be quite effective in many case series and studies (Figs. 7A to D). A multicenter study from Germany reported results of DEN in 93 patients with WON showed a success rate of 80% and a complication rate of 26%.[41] A multicenter study from the United States reported results of DEN in 104 patients with WON with success was 91% and 14% complications.[42] However, endoscopic necrosectomy should be done in relatively stable patients with WON by expert endoscopists.

Management of Complications

Biliary obstruction may occur due either to a bile duct stone in patients with gallstone pancreatitis or due to collection in the head of the pancreas. It may manifest in the form of jaundice or abnormal liver function tests. Biliary obstruction may be complicated by the development of acute cholangitis. USG of the abdomen is diagnostic for biliary obstruction. The treatment consists of ERCP and providing biliary drainage by removal of a stone if present and placing a plastic biliary stent in the bile duct. ERCP may also be required very early, i.e. within the first 24–48 hours of the onset of pancreatitis if a CBD stone is still causing obstruction (although the stone passes out on its own in most cases). Routine ERCP within the first 48 hours in patients with acute gallstone pancreatitis is not recommended in the absence of biliary obstruction or cholangitis.[43]

Gastric outlet obstruction might develop but usually does not require any intervention except that a nasojejunal tube may be placed under endoscopic guidance for feeding. The collection causing GOO may need to be drained.

Portal/splenic vein thrombosis may occur in up to 10% of patients with consequent development of esophagogastric varices. If a patient presents with gastrointestinal bleeding due to variceal bleeding, endoscopic hemostasis may be achieved by sclerotherapy/band ligation. Another important cause of

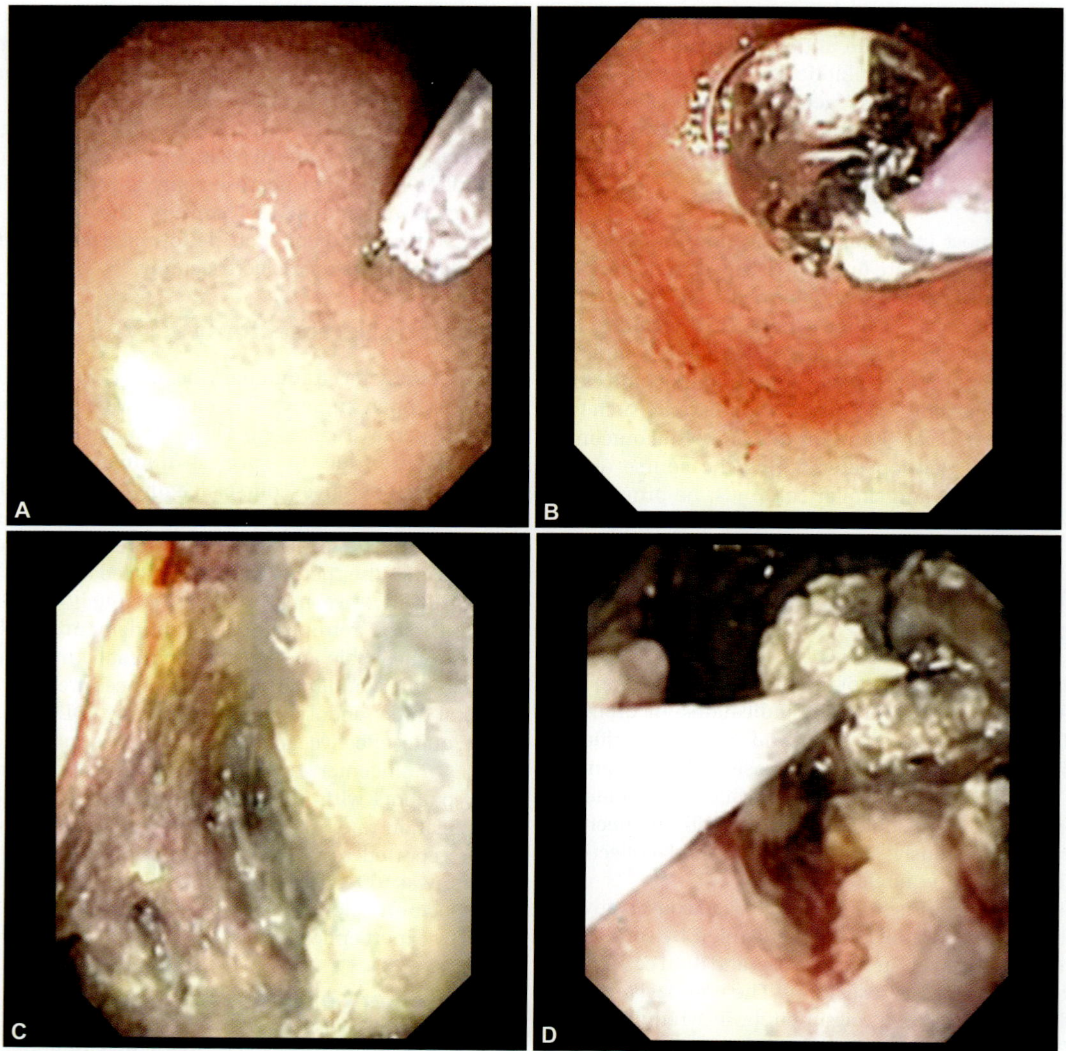

Figures 7A to D (A) Endoscopic view of needle puncture being made over the bulge in the stomach due to a large collection; (B) Endoscopic view of balloon dilation of the cystogastrostomy tract; (C) Endoscopic view necrotic debris inside the collection; (D) Endoscopic view of necrotic debris being removed by a snare

bleeding could be a pseudoaneurysm that may bleed either directly into the gut lumen or into a collection. The diagnosis of pseudoaneurysm can be made by CT angiography and confirmed by digital substraction angiography. The treatment of choice for pseudoaneurysmal bleeding is angiographic embolization.[44]

Pleural effusion is commonly seen in severe acute pancreatitis and requires drainage only if it causes respiratory compromise.

Colonic necrosis is a rare but catastrophic complication and may remain unnoticed until late. The best option is surgical exploration, peritoneal lavage and ileostomy.

PSEUDOCYST

Pseudocyst is a relatively late complication. Most pseudocysts resolve spontaneously. Asymptomatic pseudocysts are best treated expectantly, i.e. a wait and watch policy should be adopted. The indications for draining a pseudocyst are pain, obstructive symptoms, infection and an enlarging cyst. Pseudocyst can be drained by three methods: (1) percutaneous, (2) surgical and (3) endoscopic.[45] Percutaneous drainage is effective but may lead to a fistula formation if the pseudocyst is communicating with the main pancreatic duct. Surgical drainage has been the standard treatment for pseudocyst. It provides internal drainage in the form of cystoenterostomy (either cystogastrostomy or cystoduodenostomy) (Figs 7A and D). Endoscopic drainage of pseudocyst has been shown to be comparable to surgery. A randomized trial has recently shown that the efficacy of surgical and endoscopic cystogastrosotmy is similar but endoscopic drainage is associated with shorter hospital stay and lesser cost.[46] Because of its minimally invasive nature, endoscopic cystoenterostomy is preferred over surgical cystoenterostomy if the expertise is available. "WON" should be treated endoscopically with caution. Endoscopic drainage alone may not be sufficient if significant debris is present and there is a risk of it getting secondarily infected. Thus, in addition to drainage, WON may require endoscopic necrosectomy as mentioned above. Endoscopic drainage of pseudocyst under endosonography (EUS) guidance may be safer as demonstrated by a randomized study especially in non-bulging cysts.[47]

Prognosis

Two most important determinants of mortality are IPN and organ failure. There is almost no mortality in patients with acute interstitial pancreatitis. In patients with severe acute pancreatitis defined by the presence of organ failure, the mortality is high in those with early organ failure within the first week (i.e. early severe acute pancreatitis).[2] In patients with IPN also, the mortality is high and varies from 15% to 40%. The significant predictors of mortality are older age, comorbid conditions, obesity, early onset organ failure, extensive necrosis and infected necrosis. Patients with both infected necrosis and organ failure have the highest risk of mortality.[3,48]

Prevention of Recurrence

Most patients, who have had an attack of acute pancreatitis, are at risk of having a recurrence of pancreatitis if the offending cause/agent is not eliminated. Fortunately, most causes of pancreatitis can be removed/treated, e.g. gallstones, alcohol, drugs, trauma, ERCP, etc. In patients with gallstone pancreatitis, cholecystectomy should be done within the same admission in patients with mild pancreatitis and after about 6–8 weeks in those with severe pancreatitis to prevent recurrence.[49] Patients with alcohol related pancreatitis must be counseled during hospitalization and after discharge for abstinence.

However, the risk of recurrence in patients with idiopathic pancreatitis is difficult to predict. After an index episode of pancreatitis, the cause is not apparent in up to 25% of patients. Determining the cause in such patients is important to prevent recurrence. The causes can be grouped into mechanical, toxic-metabolic, anatomic and miscellaneous (Table 6).[50] Work-up for patients with idiopathic acute pancreatitis should be done after recovery from the acute episode. The work-up should include a metabolic profile to rule out hypercalcemia and hypertriglyceridemia, and a repeat USG abdomen. Special investigations such as magnetic resonance cholangiopancreaticography (MRCP) and EUS are often required for a complete work-up.

Table 6: Causes of idiopathic acute pancreatitis

Mechanical	*Toxic-metabolic*
• Microlithiasis • Sphincter of Oddi dysfunction • Pancreas divisum • Other congenital anomalies • Pancreaticobiliary tumors • Trauma • Parasitic infestations	• Hypertriglyceridemia • Hypercalcemia • Medications
	Miscellaneous • Vascular • Hereditary pancreatitis
	Chronic pancreatitis: presenting as recurrent acute pancreatitis

REFERENCES

1. Banks PA. Practice guidelines in acute pancreatitis. Am J Gastroenterol. 1997;92:377-86.
2. Sharma M, Banerjee D, Garg PK. Characterization of newer subgroups of fulminant and subfulminant pancreatitis associated with a high early mortality. Am J Gastroenterol. 2007;102:2688-95.
3. Garg PK, Madan K, Pande GK, Khanna S, Sathyanarayan G, Bohidar NP, et al. Association of extent and infection of pancreatic necrosis with organ failure and death in acute necrotizing pancreatitis. Clin Gastroenterol Hepatol. 2005;3:159-66.
4. Isenmann R, Beger HG. Natural history of acute pancreatitis and the role of infection. Best Pract Res Clin Gastroenterol. 1999;13: 291-301.
5. Spanier BW, Dijkgraaf MG, Bruno MJ. Epidemiology, aetiology and outcome of acute and chronic pancreatitis: an update. Best Pract Res Clin Gastroenterol. 2008;22:45-63.
6. Lowenfels AB, Maisonneuve P, Sullivan T. The changing character of acute pancreatitis: epidenmiology, etiology, and prognosis. Curr Gastroenterol Rep. 2009;1:97-103.
7. Peery AF, Dellon ES, Lund J, Crockett SD, McGowan CE, Bulsiewicz WJ, et al. Burden of gastrointestinal disease in the United States: 2012 Update. Gastroenterology. 2012;143(5):1179-87.
8. Opie EL. The etiology of acute hemorrhagic pancreatitis. John Hopkins Med Bull. 1901;12:182-8.
9. Acosta JM, Ledesma CL. Gallstone migration as a cause of acute pancreatitis. N Engl J Med. 1974;290:484-7.
10. Sarles H, Sarles JC, Camatte R, Muratore R, Gaini M, Guien C, et al. Observations on 205 confirmed cases of acute pancreatitis, recurring pancreatitis and chronic pancreatitis. Gut. 1965;6: 545-59.
11. Bhatia V, Garg PK, Tandon RK, Madan K. Endoscopic retrograde cholangio-pancreatography induced acute pancreatitis often has a benign outcome. J Clin Gastroenterol. 2006;40;726-31.
12. Makharia GK, Garg PK, Tandon RK. Acute pancreatitis associated with acute hepatitis E infection. Trop Gastroenterol. 2003;24:200-1.
13. Khuroo MS, Zargar SA, Mahajan R. Hepatobiliary and pancreatic ascariasis in India. Lancet. 1990;335(8704):1503-6.
14. Sah RP, Garg P, Saluja AK. Pathogenic mechanisms of acute pancreatitis. Curr Opin Gastroenterol. 2012;28:507-15.
15. Working Group IAP/APA Acute Pancreatitis Guidelines. IAP/APA evidence-based guidelines for the management of acute pancreatitis. Pancreatology. 2013;13(4 Suppl 2):e1-15.
16. Tenner S, Dubner H, Steinberg W. Predicting gallstone pancreatitis with laboratory parameters: a meta-analysis. Am J Gastroenterol. 1994;89(10):1863-6.
17. Grau F, Almela P, Aparisi L, Bautista D, Pascual I, Pena A, et al. Usefulness of alanine and aspartate aminotransferases in the diagnosis of microlithiasis in idiopathic acute pancreatitis. Int J Pancreatol. 1999;25:107-11.
18. Balthazar EJ, Robinson DL, Megibow AJ, Ranson JH. Acute pancreatitis: value of CT in establishing prognosis. Radiology. 1990;174:331-6.
19. Isenmann R, Rau B, Beger HG. Early severe acute pancreatitis: characteristics of a new sub group. Pancreas. 2001;22:274-8.
20. Gloor B, Muller CA, Worni M, Martignoni ME, Uhl W, Buchler MW. Late mortality in patients with severe acute pancreatitis. Br J Surg. 2001;88:975-9.
21. Bradley EL 3rd. A clinically based classification system for acute pancreatitis: summary of the International Symposium on Acute Pancreatitis, Atlanta, GA, September 11 through 13, 1992. Arch Surg. 1993;128:586-90.
22. Banks PA, Bollen TL, Dervenis C, Gooszen HG, Johnson CD, Sarr MG, et al. Classification of acute pancreatitis—2012: revision of the

Atlanta classification and definitions by international consensus. Gut. 2013;62:102-11.
23. Brun A, Agarwal N, Pitchumoni CS. Fluid collections in and around the pancreas in acute pancreatitis. J Clin Gastroenterol. 2011;45:614-25.
24. Forsmark CE, Baillie J. AGA Institute technical review on acute pancreatitis. Gastroenterology. 2007;132:2022-44.
25. Singh VK, Wu BU, Bollen TL, Repas K, Maurer R, Johannes RS, et al. A prospective evaluation of the bedside index for severity in acute pancreatitis score in assessing mortality and intermediate markers of severity in acute pancreatitis. Am J Gastroenterol. 2009;104: 966-71.
26. Sathyanarayan G, Garg PK, Prasad H, Tandon RK. Elevated level of interleukin-6 predicts organ failure and severe disease in patients with acute pancreatitis. J Gastroenterol Hepatol. 2007;4:550-4.
27. Renner IG, Savage WT 3rd, Pantoja JL, Renner VJ. Death due to acute pancreatitis. A retrospective analysis of 405 autopsy cases. Dig Dis Sci. 1985;30:1005-18.
28. Johnson CD, Abu-Hilal M, Members of the British Acute Pancreatitis Study Group. Persistent organ failure during the first week as a marker of fatal outcome in acute pancreatitis. Gut. 2004;53:1340-4.
29. Lowham A, Lavelle J, Leese T. Mortality from acute pancreatitis: late septic deaths can be avoided but some early deaths still occur. Int J Pancreatol. 1999;25:103-6.
30. de-Madaria E, Banks PA, Moya-Hoyo N, Wu BU, Rey-Riveiro M, Acevedo-Piedra NG, et al. Early factors associated with fluid sequestration and outcomes of patients with acute pancreatitis. Clin Gastroenterol Hepatol. 2014;12(6):997-1002.
31. Trikudanathan G, Navaneethan U, Vege SS. Current controversies in fluid resuscitation in acute pancreatitis: a systematic review. Pancreas. 2012;41:827-34.
32. Rivers E, Nguyen B, Havstad S, Ressler J, Muzzin A, Knoblich B, et al. Early goal-directed therapy in the treatment of severe sepsis and septic shock. N Engl J Med. 2001;9:1368-77.
33. Wu BU, Hwang JQ, Gardner TH, Repas K, Delee R, Yu S, et al. Lactated Ringer's solution reduces systemic inflammation compared with saline in patients with acute pancreatitis. Clin Gastroenterol Hepatol. 2011;9:710-7.
34. Haydock MD, Mittal A, Wilms HR, Phillips A, Petrov MS, Windsor JA. Fluid therapy in acute pancreatitis: anybody's guess. Ann Surg. 2013;257:182-8.
35. Petrov MS, McIlroy K, Grayson L, Phillips AR, Windsor JA. Early nasogastric tube feeding versus nil per os in mild to moderate acute pancreatitis: a randomized controlled trial. Clin Nutr. 2013;32: 697-703.
36. Chang YS, Fu HQ, Xiao YM, Liu JC. Nasogastric or nasojejunal feeding in predicted severe acute pancreatitis: a meta-analysis. Crit Care. 2013;17(3):R118.
37. Villatoro E, Mulla M, Larvin M. Antibiotic therapy for prophylaxis against infection of pancreatic necrosis in acute pancreatitis. Cochrane Database Syst Rev. 2010;(5):CD002941.
38. Besselink MG, Verwer TJ, Schoenmaeckers EJ, Buskens E, Ridwan BU, Visser MR, et al. Timing of surgical intervention in necrotizing pancreatitis. Arch Surg. 2007;142:1194-201.
39. Mouli VP, Sreenivas V, Garg PK. Efficacy of conservative treatment, without necrosectomy, for infected pancreatic necrosis: a systematic review and meta-analysis. Gastroenterology. 2013;144:333-40.
40. van Santvoort HC, Besselink MG, Bakker OJ, Hofker HS, Boermeester MA, Dejong CH, et al. A step-up approach or open necrosectomy for necrotizing pancreatitis. N Engl J Med. 2010;362:1491-502.
41. Seifert H, Biermer M, Schmitt W, Jürgensen C, Will U, Gerlach R, et al. Transluminal endoscopic necrosectomy after acute pancreatitis: a multicenter study with long-term follow-up (the GEPARD Study). Gut. 2009;58:1260-6.
42. Gardner TB, Coelho-Prabhu N, Gordon SR, Gelrud A, Maple JT, Papachristou GI, et al. Direct endoscopic necrosectomy for the treatment of walled-off pancreatic necrosis: results from a multicenter U.S. series. Gastrointest Endosc. 2011;73:718-26.
43. van Geenen EJ, van Santvoort HC, Besselink MG, van der Peet DL, van Erpecum KJ, Fockens P, et al. Lack of consensus on the role of endoscopic retrograde cholangiography in acute biliary pancreatitis in published meta-analyses and guidelines: a systematic review. Pancreas. 2013;42:774-80.
44. Sharma PK, Madan K, Garg PK. Hemorrhage in acute pancreatitis: should gastrointestinal bleeding be considered an organ failure? Pancreas. 2008;36:141-5.
45. Fisher JM, Gardner TB. Endoscopic therapy of necrotizing pancreatitis and pseudocysts. Gastrointest Endosc Clin N Am. 2013;23:787-802.
46. Varadarajulu S, Bang JY, Sutton BS, Trevino JM, Christein JD, Wilcox CM. Equal efficacy of endoscopic and surgical cystogastrostomy for pancreatic pseudocyst drainage in a randomized trial. Gastroenterology. 2013;145:583-90.
47. Varadarajulu S, Christein JD, Tamhane A, Drelichman ER, Wilcox CM. Prospective randomized trial comparing EUS and EGD for transmural drainage of pancreatic pseudocysts (with videos). Gastrointest Endosc. 2008;68:1102-11.
48. Petrov MS, Shanbhag S, Chakraborty M, Phillips AR, Windsor JA. Organ failure and infection of pancreatic necrosis as determinants of mortality in patients with acute pancreatitis. Gastroenterology. 2010;139:813-20.
49. Gurusamy KS, Nagendran M, Davidson BR. Early versus delayed laparoscopic cholecystectomy for acute gallstone pancreatitis. Cochrane Database Syst Rev. 2013;9:CD010326.
50. Kedia S, Dhingra R, Garg PK. Recurrent acute pancreatitis: an approach to diagnosis and management. Trop Gastroenterol. 2013;34:123-35.

CHAPTER 38

Surgery in Acute Pancreatitis

Mohammad Ibrarullah, Jayanth Reddy, V K Kapoor

Management of acute pancreatitis has undergone considerable evolution in the last two decades. Better understanding of the pathophysiology, availability of excellent imaging modalities, improved intensive care facilities and non-surgical treatment options have changed the treatment paradigm so that surgical intervention is required only in a limited number of patients.

NATURAL HISTORY OF ACUTE PANCREATITIS

Acute pancreatitis is classified into acute interstitial edematous pancreatitis and necrotizing pancreatitis. Fortunately, more than 80% of patients suffer from acute interstitial edematous pancreatitis, a milder form of the disease where spontaneous recovery is expected in a few days without any major sequel. Approximately 20% of patients develop necrotizing pancreatitis that involves either pancreas or peripancreatic tissue or both.[1,2] Impairment of pancreatic perfusion, resulting in necrosis of the inflamed tissue, takes few days to evolve.[3,4] Imaging studies to assess the extent of tissue necrosis should, therefore, be performed toward the end of the first week after the onset of pancreatitis.[5]

The natural history of inflamed pancreatic and peripancreatic tissue is unpredictable. It may remain solid or liquefy over a period of time. Similarly, the necrotic tissue may remain sterile or get infected. The generally reported incidence of infection is approximately 60–70%, though it has dropped to 20–40% in some recent studies.[6] Earlier studies indicated that the risk of infection increases with the extent of necrosis[7,8] and duration of symptoms.[9] But, some recent studies contradict this view.[10,11] Infection, however, is rare in the first week of the attack.[10,12] Clinically, acute pancreatitis is classified as mild, moderately severe and severe. Severe pancreatitis has a bimodal presentation; in the first week, the systemic involvement is due to the activation of cytokine cascades by the pancreatic inflammation, manifesting clinically as the systemic inflammatory response syndrome (SIRS).[9] Persistence of SIRS may lead to organ failure, which may be transient and resolve within 48 hours or persistent. This phase usually lasts for 1 week or may spill over to the second week. Deterioration in the second or third week of the attack is usually due to infection of the pancreatic and peripancreatic necrosis. Persistent infection is considered the major risk factor resulting in nearly fivefold increase in organ failure[8] and threefold increase in death.[13] There is no conclusive evidence that infected necrosis can be prevented by antibiotics.[14] The only viable treatment option is its removal by various available techniques.

DIAGNOSIS OF INFECTED PANCREATIC NECROSIS

Clinically, infected pancreatic necrosis should be suspected when patients having necrotizing pancreatitis continue or present with signs of sepsis like fever, leukocytosis, or organ failure beyond 7–10 days. On CT scan, presence of gas bubble in the necrotic tissue (Fig. 1) is a pointer toward infection.[15] Serum procalcitonin level of 1.8 ng/mL or more on two consecutive days has also been used to predict infected necrosis with a sensitivity of 75–95% and specificity of 83-91%.[16-18] CT scan guided fine needle aspiration (FNA) of the necrotic tissue was recommended as a routine to establish infection.[2,5] Gram stain or culture positive aspirate is considered the conclusive evidence of infected necrosis. Positive FNA is an indication for early surgical intervention to salvage a deteriorating patient. This practice, in the recent times, has become questionable on several accounts.[6,12,19] It has now been well established that early surgery in acute pancreatitis is counterproductive and associated with a very high morbidity and mortality.[1] The surgical intervention, therefore, should be delayed at least by 4-6 weeks.

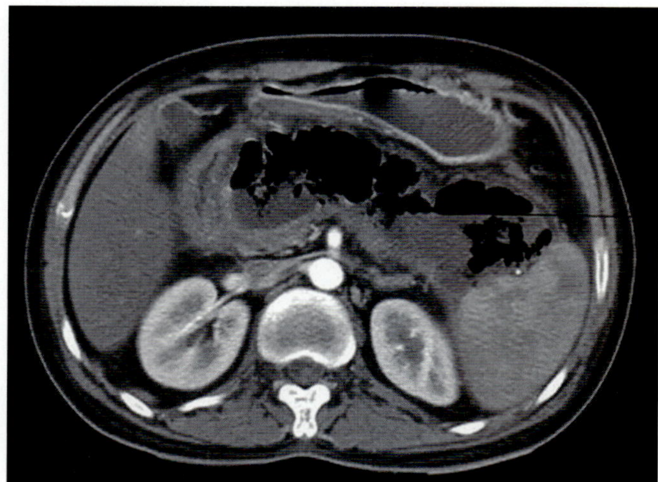

Figure 1 Peripancreatic necrosis with air—infected

In the interim period, the patient should receive supportive care in the ICU. Any need for intervention during this period can be non-surgical, in the form of CT guided or endoscopic drainage. Only those patients who continue to be in sepsis or multiorgan failure despite adequate conservative and non-surgical management are candidates for surgical necrosectomy. It has also been reported that in a sub-group of clinically stable patients, infected necrosis can be managed conservatively.[20-24] On the contrary, necrosectomy is seldom required in patients with sterile necrosis. It should be performed only if the patient fails to show clinical improvement. Hence at present, there are very few indications for diagnostic FNA; these would be suspicion of superimposed fungal infection and clinical deterioration especially in patients who are presumed to have IPN and are on long-term broad spectrum antibiotics.[25] The recently published IAP/APA guidelines on acute pancreatitis also state that routine FNA to diagnose IPN is not indicated, because clinical signs [i.e. persistent fever, increasing total leukocyte count (TLC)] and imaging signs (i.e. presence of gas in the areas of necrosis or peripancreatic collections) are accurate predictors of IPN in majority of the patients.[26] Routine FNA may produce false negative results in 12–25% of patients, it does not shorten the time to diagnose IPN or help in tailoring antibiotic treatment.[27] Therefore, it is apparent that necrosectomy is more often decided on clinical grounds like persistent sepsis and multiorgan failure rather than presence or absence of infection alone, thereby making the role of FNA rather redundant.

TIMING OF INTERVENTION

In the past, surgical intervention was decided on the basis of clinical deterioration and presence of infection detected on FNA performed early in the course of an attack. However, a very high mortality rate (up to 65%) questioned the rationale of such an approach.[28] A prospective randomized trial comparing early (within 72 hours) with late (at least 12 days after the onset) intervention had to be terminated because of high mortality associated with the former—56% versus 27% with the latter approach.[29] In 2002, the International Association of Pancreatology (IAP) recommended that surgery in necrotizing pancreatitis should not be performed within 2 weeks of the onset of an attack.[2] Subsequent studies have provided evidence that the mortality remains high when necrosectomy is performed within the first 2–3 weeks. This can be reduced to less than 8% when the surgery is delayed beyond 4 weeks.[30,31] Delayed surgical intervention, i.e. after at least 3–4 weeks is now the accepted practice[1] because of several reasons: (1) it is now reasonably established that early deterioration in acute pancreatitis is due to systemic inflammatory response and surgical intervention at this stage may further aggravate it, (2) infection of the necrotic tissue is rare in the first week, (3) sterile necrosis rarely requires debridement, (4) delay beyond 4 weeks helps in demarcation and loosening of the necrotic tissue which can be removed with relative ease, less complications and better long-term endocrine and exocrine function.

CURRENT MANAGEMENT GUIDELINES

In the modified Atlanta Classification,[32] the morphological abnormalities of the pancreatic and peripancreatic region based on contrast enhanced CT scan serve as a guide to decide on a specific modality of treatment. Management of acute pancreatitis is essentially conservative in the first 2 weeks. It has been reported that at least 50% of the patients recover with initial intensive care management.[33,34] Therapeutic interventions—radiological, endoscopic or surgical—are indicated to treat local complications. Unlike the practice in 1980s, in the present day scenario, most of the centers practice a "step-up" approach, i.e. starting with least invasive approach like percutaneous catheter drainage (PCD) (Fig. 2) and upgrading to most invasive approach like open necrosectomy.[12,35-38] Acute necrotic collection (ANC) can be drained by CT guided percutaneous catheter. Walled-off necrotic collection (WNC) is amenable to treatment by the same technique or by endoscopy through transgastric approach. When these modalities fail, necrosectomy should be attempted by minimally invasive approach. Open necrosectomy, in the current scenario, is reserved for the sub-group of patients in whom the preceding modalities fail or not feasible. In a prospective randomized study (PANTER trial), 35% of the patients assigned for the "step-up" approach could be salvaged only by percutaneous drainage.

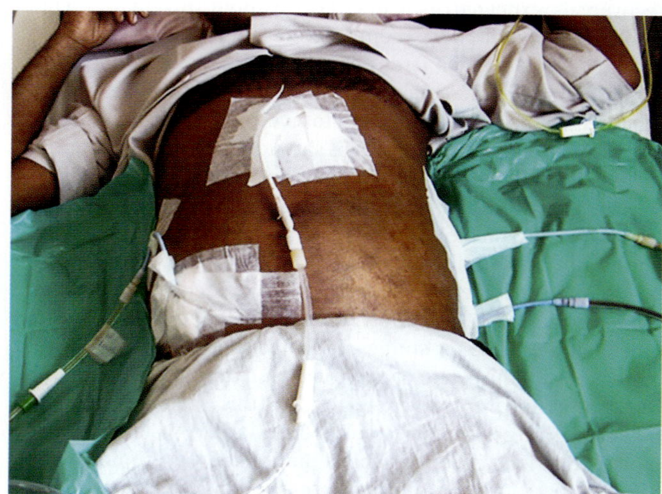

Figure 2 Multiple PCDs

Table 1: Summary of minimally invasive techniques for pancreatic necrosectomy

Technique	*Selection criteria*	*Advantages*	*Limitations*
Percutaneous	Mainly for collections in body and tail of pancreas	Early use for control of sepsis. Avoids surgery in >1/3 of patients	Dedicated team for multiple procedures and catheter upsizing. High rate of EPF
Laparoscopic	Collections must be organized	Complete removal possible in single stage. Simultaneous cholecystectomy, if needed and access to extrapancreatic collections (pericolic and perinephric space). Lower morbidity over open surgery	Peritoneal contamination. Adverse effects of pneumoperitoneum in critically-ill patients
Retroperitoneal	Mainly for collections in body and tail of pancreas	Limits peritoneal contamination and has favorable outcome over open surgery	Limited access to extrapancreatic collections. Need for multiple procedures and inability to perform simultaneous procedures

The morbidity in this group with respect to new-onset multiorgan failure, postoperative diabetes mellitus and incisional hernia was significantly less compared to open surgical necrosectomy group.[12] Another publication on the step-up approach was a US-Canadian multicenter prospective study[38] using the videoscopic assisted retroperitoneal debridement (VARD) technique in 40 patients. One quarter of patients could be treated by PCD only and the overall mortality was 0%. The PGIMER Chandigarh group[39] recently published their experience of managing patients with severe acute pancreatitis using the step-up approach. Of the 70 consecutive patients with SAP in this series, 14 were managed medically and 29 managed with PCD alone, whereas 27 required surgery after initial PCD. Sepsis reversal was achieved with PCD alone in 63%. PCD alone was curative in 27 patients (48%). Overall mortality in the whole group was 24%. These studies support the current evidence on merits of the step-up approach in infected pancreatic necrosis. As it stands today, the step-up approach may be considered as the reference standard intervention. As suggested by the Dutch Pancreatitis Study Group, although the individual components of the step-up approach may be subject to improvement, the concept of the step-up approach, i.e. delay, drain and debride, seems to be here to stay.[40]

ROLE OF PERCUTANEOUS CATHETER DRAINAGE IN PANCREATIC NECROSIS

With the ever increasing use of step-up approach in the management of severe acute pancreatitis, use of PCD has become an important and integral part of the same. The rationale of using PCD in the initial stage of the treatment of patients with SAP is to improve the clinical condition of these seriously ill patients by drainage of the infected fluid under pressure. This is done with an intention, either to postpone the surgical intervention or even to obviate the need for surgical necrosectomy, thereby allowing the target necrosis to mature and also for secondary treatment of residual collection and necrosis after surgery. A recent systematic review on PCD placement by the Dutch Pancreatitis Study Group, included 11 studies, predominantly retrospective, with 384 patients, of whom two-thirds had infected necrosis and organ failure.[40] PCD size ranged from 8 F to 22 F with two or more catheters used per patient. In four series, the drains were placed early in the course of the disease, within 2 weeks of admission. The drains were flushed with saline every 8 hours and were replaced when occluded. The success rate (no further need of surgical necrosectomy) was 56%. The complication rate was 21% and majority of the complications were EPFs and pancreaticoenteric fistulas. The overall mortality rate was 17%. As illustrated in the study by the PGIMER Chandigarh group,[39] the number and size of the initial catheters is determined by the size and location of collection/necrosis, by the viscosity of the initially aspirated fluid, and by the amount of the aspirated particulate debris. In their study, total number of catheters used in 56 patients was 94 and the total number of interventional procedures (repositioning, replacement, flushing, upsizing and additional catheter placement under image guidance) was 292. The diameter of PCD catheters varied from 8 F to 14 F. A 10 F diameter was the most common size used in this study. The success of PCD placement in SAP depends thereby largely on the diligent catheter care, need for repeated sessions of catheter repositioning, replacement or upsizing by a dedicated team of interventional radiologists. Many patients with infected and/or suspected infected necrotizing pancreatitis can recover with PCD as the first and only intervention (Table 1).

INDICATIONS FOR SURGERY

- Infected necrosis with ongoing sepsis and organ dysfunction which is not amenable to treatment with lesser invasive measures.
- Symptomatic walled off necrosis late in the course (>4–8 weeks after onset).
- Sterile necrosis with persistent organ dysfunction or patients who remain persistently unwell beyond 4 weeks with fever, anorexia, vomiting and/or unable to resume oral intake; such situations are, however, uncommon.
- Complications:
  - Perforated/Obstructed viscus
  - Acute bleeding (Fig. 3)
  - Abdominal compartment syndrome
  - Bowel ischemia

The various surgical options available for necrotizing pancreatitis are:

- Minimally invasive necrosectomy (MIN):
  - Transperitoneal/Laparoscopic approach
  - Retroperitoneal approach

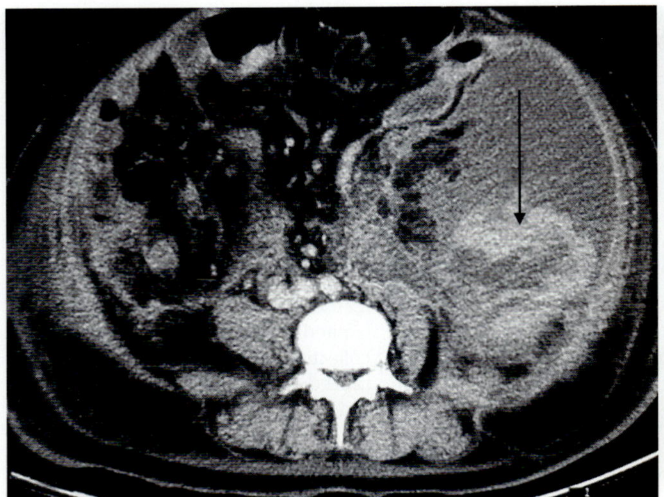

Figure 3 Acute necrotizing pancreatitis with bleed (hyperdense on CECT) in necrosis

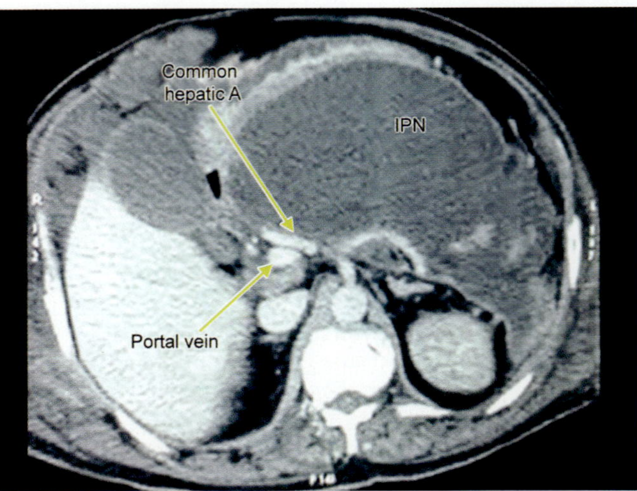

Figure 4 Large collection suitable for lap drainage

- Open necrosectomy:
  - Closed continuous lavage
  - Planned staged relaparotomies with repeated lavage
  - Ventral open packing
  - Closed packing

Loveday et al.[41] recently provided a comprehensive classification of interventional procedures for treating the local complications of acute pancreatitis based on visualization, route and purpose. The purpose of this classification system was to introduce uniformity into the documentation of interventions worldwide thereby allowing effective comparison between studies.

MINIMALLY INVASIVE APPROACHES TO NECROSECTOMY (TABLE 1)

The gold standard of treatment for patients with infected pancreatic necrosis remains open pancreatic necrosectomy. Open necrosectomy for infected necrosis carries substantial risks, however, with mortality rates of up to 20–40% reported even from specialist centers.[39,42,43] The physiological stress to the patient of severe acute pancreatitis with infected necrosis is further exacerbated by the "second hit" of a laparotomy and open necrosectomy. A number of less invasive surgical techniques have therefore been developed in an attempt to minimize the excess disturbance of necrosectomy. The two most commonly used techniques of MIN are the laparoscopic and the retroperitoneal approaches.

Laparoscopic Transperitoneal Necrosectomy

Laparoscopic transperitoneal necrosectomy (Figs 4 and 5) has been reported to be feasible,[44,45] though not widely practiced. The procedure essentially follows the principles of open surgery. The necrotic cavity is usually approached from the infracolic compartment. Distended bowel can cause impediment to adequate vision and access. Hand-ports have also been used to facilitate necrosectomy.[44] Drainage catheters are left behind in the debrided cavity like in open necrosectomy. The procedure can be repeated if required. Laparoscopic techniques can largely be categorized into three different approaches: (1) hand-assisted, (2) conventional laparoscopic approach and (3) robotic approach. Potential advantages of the laparoscopic approach include access to areas inaccessible by an endoscope, e.g. right and left paracolic gutters, perinephric space, retroduodenal space and root of the mesentery, and the ability to perform simultaneous cholecystectomy and less wound infections and pulmonary adverse events compared to open necrosectomy. The limitations of laparoscopic approach include risk of dissemination of retroperitoneal infection into the peritoneum and also the need for inducing pneumoperitoneum, which may adversely affect the already critically ill and hemodynamically unstable patients. In a limited review, the conversion rate and mortality following this procedure have been reported to be 11% and 7%, respectively.[45] A retrospective study from China has the largest number of patients managed with laparoscopic pancreatic necrosectomy till date.[46] In this study, traditional open necrosectomy (n=51) was compared with laparoscopic necrosectomy (n=25). The technique utilized pneumoperitoneum, four to five trocar, laparoscopic debridement of necrotic collections and use of postoperative catheters for continued lavage. The laparoscopic necrosectomy group showed a significant decrease in estimated intraoperative blood loss, incidence of postoperative pancreatic fistula (32% vs 55%), incision infection (0% vs 18%) and length of stay (34 vs 43 days); mortality was similar in the two groups.

Minimally Invasive Retroperitoneal Necrosectomy

Retroperitoneal approach to the necrotic tissue by an incision in the left flank (Fig. 6) was first described by Fagniez in 1989 and subsequently by other authors.[47-49] The procedure, though considered less morbid, failed to gain wide acceptance because the results were no different from that of conventional (transperitoneal) approach. Major morbidity like hemorrhage and fistulae formation were reported in 25–68% of patients. Relatively blind dissection of the necrotic tissue was considered the major drawback of this

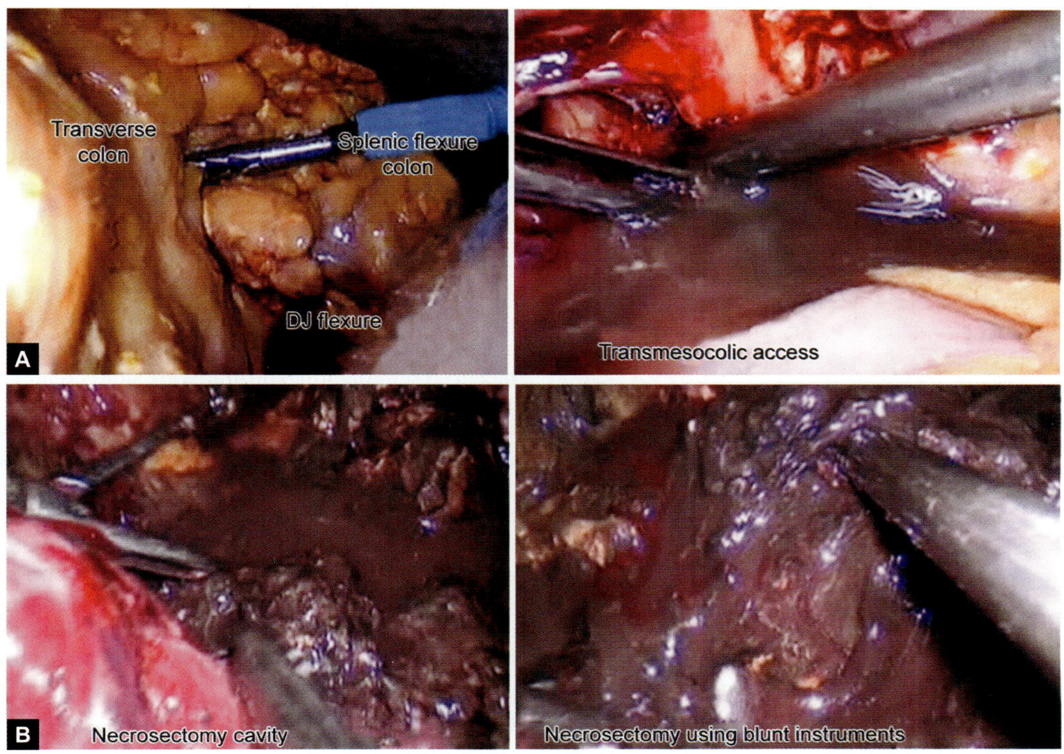

Figures 5A and B Lap necrosectomy

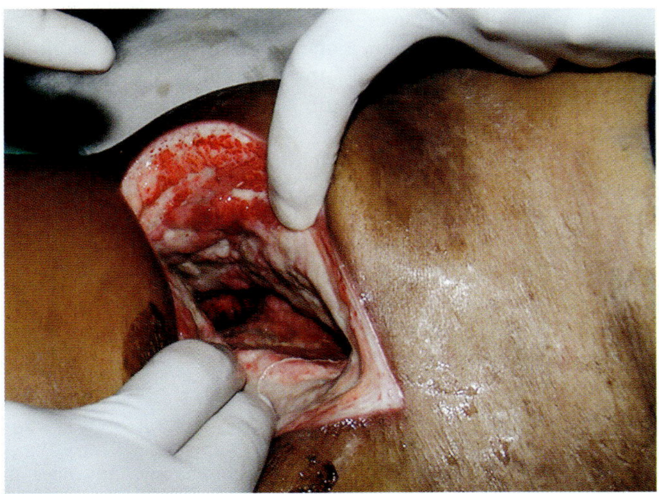

Figure 6 Flank incision for drainage of collection near tail of pancreas

procedure. In a major development, with the use of videoscope, the retroperitoneal approach has re-emerged in a big way and is poised to become the "standard of care" replacing the conventional necrosectomy.[45,50] The various types of videoscopes used for this purpose are: nephroscope, mediastinoscope, bronchoscope or laparoscope. In this technique, a 12–14 F percutaneous drainage catheter is first placed into the necrotic cavity under CT guidance. The catheter tract is subsequently dilated under fluoroscopy to 30 F to allow passage of a rigid scope. Necrosectomy is carried out under direct vision using long grasping forceps and continuous irrigation. At the end of the procedure, two tube drains are left in the cavity for irrigation and drainage. Complete necrosectomy often requires multiple sittings. This technique has been variously called sinus tract endoscopy,[51] minimally invasive retroperitoneal necrosectomy (MIRPN)[52] or minimal access retroperitoneal pancreatic necrosectomy (MARPN).[53] Alternatively, the procedure can be performed by making a small incision close to the exit point of the percutaneous drainage catheter. The necrotic cavity is accessed by using the catheter as the guide. The loose necrotic tissues are removed during the procedure by grasping forceps and later using frequent irrigation. Subsequently, an extra-long laparoscopic port is placed through which videoscope is introduced and CO_2 insufflation of the cavity is performed. Using laparoscopic forceps, further debridement of the cavity is carried out under direct vision. After removing most of the loose necrotic tissue, the percutaneous catheter is replaced by two wide bore tube drains for the purpose of irrigation and drainage. This technique of video assisted retroperitoneal debridement (VARD) has been claimed to be more effective and less time consuming than the "sinus tract endoscopy" since the approach is through a mini incision that permits removal of larger chunks of the necrotic tissue.[54]

With increasing experience, the minimally invasive approach can be applied to a large proportion of patients with pancreatic necrosis. The expected advantages of the procedure over the conventional approach are: (1) minimal surgical trauma, i.e. tissue damage and systemic proinflammatory response in an otherwise septic patient, (2) no contamination of peritoneal cavity, (3) better preservation of the healthy pancreatic parenchyma thereby minimizing long-term endocrine and exocrine deficiency.[45,50] In a series of 137 patients, up to 85% of patients were found suitable for MARPN.[53] The only limitation of the procedure is inability to find a safe track for the initial guidewire placement and its inability to remove necrosis present in relation to head and uncinate process. In a systematic review of five studies comprising of 197 patients, the procedure was successful in 88% of patients with a mortality rate of 17%. Complications were reported in 46% of patients, the major ones being bowel fistula, gastric and duodenal perforation, colonic necrosis, bleeding and pancreatic fistula.[50] A recent metanalysis including a total of 336 patients across four studies comparing MIN (n=215) to open necrosectomy (ON) (n=121) demonstrated significant advantages of MIN in terms of postoperative incidence of multiorgan failure, incisional hernias, new-onset diabetes mellitus and use of pancreatic enzyme supplements.[55] There were no differences in terms of mortality, need for surgical reintervention, intra-abdominal bleeding, enterocutaneous fistulas and pancreatic fistulas.

Open Necrosectomy

In the 1980s, open necrosectomy was introduced as a salvage procedure for pancreatic necrosis. Aggressive removal of the necrotic tissue and wide drainage helped in bringing down the mortality figures significantly to less than 20% in most of the centers.[1] Pancreatic necrosis involving more than 30% of the parenchyma along with peripancreatic necrosis, sterile or infected was considered the indication for open necrosectomy. The current trend, however, relegates open necrosectomy to a procedure of last resort for a symptomatic patient in whom all other lesser invasive modalities have failed.

Depending on the extent of necrosis, as assessed on preoperative CT scan, the abdomen is opened by a long midline or bilateral subcostal incision. The duodenum is Kocherized and the colonic flexures are brought down for wide exposure. The necrotic cavity is approached from the retrocolic or retrogastric area after dividing the gastrocolic and duodenocolic ligaments. Loose necrotic tissues are removed by gentle finger dissection or by using sponge holder. Healthy looking pancreas or tissues of doubtful viability should be left behind for a reassessment at a later date. The procedure is completed in one of the following ways.

Closed Continuous Lavage

After necrosectomy two double lumen Salem type sump drains (20–24 F) and two single lumen tube drains (28–32 F) are placed, two from each side directed to the opposite side in relation to the head and tail of the pancreas. The gastrocolic and duodenocolic ligaments are sutured back to create a closed cavity. The smaller lumen tubes are used for inflow of the irrigation fluid. Initially a large volume, approximately 35–40 liters, of lavage fluid peritoneal dialysis fluid is used. Postoperative lavage is continued till the effluent appears clear and free from any solid material. Drains are subsequently removed when the output is less than 10 mL and its amylase content is within normal limits.[56]

Planned Staged Relaparotomies with Repeated Lavage

After necrosectomy the abdomen is closed with a zipper sewn to the fasciae. This is done to facilitate relaparotomy every 48 hours to carry out further debridement. After complete necrosectomy is achieved the zipper is removed and abdomen is closed over drains.[57]

Ventral Open Packing

After necrosectomy, the cavity is packed and left open. Planned re-exploration and necrosectomy is carried out every 48–72 hours. Once complete necrosectomy is achieved and healthy granulation tissues appear in the debrided cavity, it is closed with drainage tubes.[58]

Closed Packing

After necrosectomy, the residual cavity is packed with multiple gauze filled penrose drains and closed-suction catheters. Irrigation and drainage are performed using peritoneal dialysis fluid or balanced salt solution. The drains are slowly removed after at least 1 week allowing the cavity to gradually collapse.[59]

The mortality following open necrosectomy ranges from 8% to 47%, with most centers reporting a figure of less than 20%. The most common procedure related complications are bowel fistula in 1–52%, pancreatic fistula in 13–53% and hemorrhage in 2–50%. Complications are more common with open packing and planned relaparotomy procedures.[60] Heinrich et al.[61] in an evidence based review suggested that careful single necrosectomy and postoperative lavage without planned relaparotomies are less harmful and should be preferred for surgical treatment of IPN.

CONCLUSION

Necrotizing pancreatitis should be initially managed conservatively in the high dependency unit/intensive care unit. Morbidity in the first 2 weeks is a consequence of systemic inflammatory response caused by the inflamed pancreas. Infected necrosis is an indication for therapeutic intervention, not necessarily surgical. Modified Atlanta classification based on morphological delineation of pancreatic and peripancreatic tissue serves as a guide to therapeutic intervention in the second week. Current wisdom recommends a "step-up" approach to treat pancreatic necrosis. Open surgical necrosectomy is required in a small sub-group of patients in whom alternative lesser invasive modalities are either not feasible or have failed. Necrosectomy followed by closed cavity drainage appears to be better than planned relaparotomies or ventral open packing. A planned and systematic approach has brought down the mortality of necrotizing pancreatitis to less than 20% in most centers.

REFERENCES

1. Stern J, Matthews JB. Pancreatic necrosectomy. Advances in Surgery. 2011;45:155-76.
2. Andrew WU, Warshaw C, Imrie C, Bassi C, McKay CJ, Lankisch PG, et al. IAP guidelines for the surgical management of acute pancreatitis. Pancreatology. 2002;2:565-73.
3. Spanier BWM, Nio Y, van der Hulst RWN, Tuynman HA, Dijkgraaf MG, Bruno MJ. Practice and yield of early CT scan in acute pancreatitis: a Dutch observational multicenter study. Pancreatology. 2010;10:222-8.
4. Bollen TL, Singh VK, Maurer R, Repas K, van Es HW, Banks PA, et al. A comparative evaluation of radiologic and clinical scoring systems in the early prediction of severity of acute pancreatitis. Am J Gastroenterol. 2012;107:612-9.
5. UK Working Party on Acute Pancreatitis. UK guidelines for the management of acute pancreatitis. Gut. 2005;54(Suppl III):iii1-9.

6. Haney JC, Papas TN. Necrotizing pancreatitis: diagnosis and management. Surg Clin North Am. 2007;87:1431-46.
7. Hughes SJ, Papachristou GI, Federle MP, Lee KK. Necrotizing pancreatitis. Gastroenterol Clin North Am. 2007;36:313-23.
8. Buchler MW, Gloor B, Muller CA, Fries H, Seiler CA, Uhl W. Acute necrotizing pancreatitis: treatment strategy according to the status of infection. Ann Surg. 2000;232:619-26.
9. Beger HG, Rau BN, New advances in pancreatic surgery. Curr Opin Gastroenterol. 2007;23:522-34.
10. Besselink MG, van Santvoort HC, Boermeester MA, Nieuwenhuijs VB, van Goor H, Dejong CH, et al. Timing and impact of infections in acute pancreatitis. Br J Surg. 2009;96:267-73.
11. van Santvoort HC, Bakker OJ, Bollen TL, Besselink MG, Ahmed Ali U, Schrijver AM, et al. A conservative and minimally invasive approach to necrotizing pancreatitis improves outcome. Gastroenterology. 2011;141:1254-63.
12. van Santvoort HC, Besselink MG, Bakker OJ, Hofker HS, Boermeester MA, Dejong CH, et al. A step-up approach or open necrosectomy for necrotizing pancreatitis (PANTER trial). N Engl J Med. 2010;362:1491-502.
13. Frossard J, Steer ML, Pastor CM. Acute pancreatitis. Lancet. 2008;371:143-52.
14. Villatoro E, Mulla M, Larvin M. Antibiotic therapy for prophylaxis against infection of pancreatic necrosis in acute pancreatitis. Cochrane Database Syst Rev. 2010;5:CD002941.
15. Casas JD, Diaz R, Valderas G, Mariscal A, Cuadras P. Prognostic value of CT in the early assessment of patients with acute pancreatitis. Am J Roengtenol. 2004;182:569-74.
16. Rau B, Steinbach G, Gansauge F, Mayer JM, Grunert A, Beger HG. The potential role of procalcitonin and IL-8 in the prediction of infected necrosis in acute pancreatitis. Gut. 1997;41:832-40.
17. Rau BM, Kemppainen EA, Gumbs AA, Buchler MW, Wegscheider K, Bassi C, et al. Early assessment of pancreatic infections and overall prognosis in severe acute pancreatitis by procalcitonin: a prospective international multicenter study. Ann Surg. 2007;245:745-54.
18. Toh SK, Phillips S, Johnson CD. A prospective audit against national standards of the presentation and management of acute pancreatitis in the South of England. Gut. 2000;46:239-43.
19. Sakorafas GH, Lappas C, Mastoraki A, Delis SG, Safioleas M. Current trends in the management of infected necrotizing pancreatitis. Infect Disord Drug Targets. 2010;10:9-14.
20. Rau BM, Bothe A, Beger HG. Surgical treatment of necrotizing pancreatitis by necrosectomy and closed lavage: changing patient characteristics and outcome in a 19 year, single-centre series. Surgery. 2005;138:28-39.
21. Runzi M, Niebel W, Goebell H, Gerken G, Layer P. Severe acute pancreatitis: nonsurgical treatment of infected necrosis. Pancreas. 2005;30:195-9.
22. Ramesh H, Prakash K, Lekha V, Jacob G, Venugopal A. Are some cases of infected pancreatic necrosis treatable without intervention? Dig Surg. 2003;20:296-9.
23. Lee J, Kwak KK, Park JK, Yoon WJ, Lee SH, Ryu JK, et al. The efficacy of non-surgical treatment of infected pancreatic necrosis. Pancreas. 2007;34:399-404.
24. Sivsankar A, Kannan DG, Ravichandran P, Jeswanth S, Balachandar TG, Surendran R. Outcome of severe acute pancreatitis: is there a role of conservative management of infected necrosis? Hepatobiliary Pancreat Dis Int. 2006;5:599-604.
25. Freeman ML, Werner J, van Santvoort HC, Baron TH, Besselink MG, Windsor JA, et al. Interventions for necrotizing pancreatitis: summary of a multidisciplinary consensus conference. Pancreas. 2012;41(8):1176-94.
26. Working Group IAP/APA Acute Pancreatitis Guidelines. IAP/APA evidence-based guidelines for the management of acute pancreatitis. Pancreatology. 2013;13(4 Suppl 2):e1-15.
27. Rau B, Pralle U, Mayer JM, Beger HG. Role of ultrasonographically guided fine needle aspiration cytology in the diagnosis of infected pancreatic necrosis. Br J Surg. 1998;85:179-84.
28. Werner J, Feuerbach S, Uhl W, Buchle MW. Management of acute pancreatitis: from surgery to interventional intensive care. Gut. 2005;54:426-36.
29. Mier J, Leon EL, Castillo A, Robledo F, Blanco R. Early versus late necrosectomy in severe necrotizing pancreatitis. Am J Surg. 1997;173:71-5.
30. Hartwig W, Maksan FM, Foitzik T, Schmidt J, Herfarth C, Klar E. Reduction in mortality with delayed surgical therapy of severe pancreatitis. J Gastrointest Surg. 2002;6:481-7.
31. Basselink M, Verwer TJ. Schoenmaeckers EJ, Buskens E, Ridwan BU, Visser MR, et al. Timing of surgical intervention in necrotizing pancreatitis. Arch Surg. 2007;142:1194-201.
32. Banks PA, Bollen TL, Dervenis C, Gooszen HG, Johnson CD, Sarr MG, et al. Classification of acute pancreatitis—2012: revision of the Atlanta classification and definitions by international consensus. Gut. 2013;62:102-11.
33. Le Mée J, Paye F, Sauvanet A, O'Toole D, Hammel P, Marty J, et al. Incidence and reversibility of organ failure in the course of Sterile or infected necrotizing pancreatitis. Arch Surg. 2001;136:1386-90.
34. Flint R, Windsor JA. Early physiological response to intensive care as a clinically relevant approach to predicting the outcome in severe acute pancreatitis. Arch Surg. 2004;139:438-43.
35. Pascual I, Sabater L, Añón R, Calvete J, Pacheco G, Muñoz E, et al. Surgical versus nonsurgical treatment of infected pancreatic necrosis: more arguments to change the paradigm. J Gastrointest Surg. 2013;17:1627-33.
36. Windsor JA. Infected pancreatic necrosis: drain first, but do it better. HPB. 2011;13:367-8.
37. Parekh D. Laparoscopic-assisted pancreatic necrosectomy: a new surgical option for treatment of severe necrotizing pancreatitis. Arch Surg. 2006;141:895-902.
38. Horvath K, Freeny P, Escallon J, Heagerty P, Comstock B, Glickerman DJ, et al. Safety and efficacy of video-assisted retroperitoneal debridement for infected pancreatic collections: a multicenter, prospective, single-arm phase 2 study. Arch Surg. 2010;145(9):817-25.
39. Babu RY, Gupta R, Kang M, Bhasin DK, Rana SS, Singh R. Predictors of surgery in patients with severe acute pancreatitis managed by the step-up approach. Ann Surg. 2013;257(4):737-50.
40. Besselink MG. The "step-up approach" to infected necrotizing pancreatitis: delay, drain, debride. Dig Liver Dis. 2011;43(6):421-2.
40a. van Baal MC, van Santvoort HC, Bollen TL, Bakker OJ, Besselink MG, Gooszen HG, et al. Systematic review of percutaneous catheter drainage as primary treatment for necrotizing pancreatitis. Br J Surg. 2011;98(1):18-27.
41. Loveday BP, Petrov MS, Connor S, Rossaak JI, Mittal A, Phillips AR, et al. A comprehensive classification of invasive procedures for treating the local complications of acute pancreatitis based on visualization, route, and purpose. Pancreatology. 2011;11(4):406-13.
42. Beger HG, Büchler M, Bittner R, Oettinger W, Block S, Nevalainen T. Necrosectomy and postoperative local lavage in patients with necrotizing pancreatitis: results of a prospective clinical trial. World J Surg. 1988;12(2):255-62.
43. Babu BI, Sheen AJ, Lee SH, O'Shea S, Eddleston JM, Siriwardena AK. Open pancreatic necrosectomy in the multidisciplinary management of postinflammatory necrosis. Ann Surg. 2010; 251(5):783-6.
44. Zhu JF, Fan XH, Zhang XH. Laparoscopic treatment of severe acute pancreatitis. Surg Endosc. 2001;15:146-8.
45. Babu BI, Siriwardena AK. Current status of minimally invasive necrosectomy for post-inflammatory pancreatic necrosis. HPB. 2009;11:96-102.

46. Tan J, Tan H, Hu B, Ke C, Ding X, Chen F, et al. Short-term outcomes from a multicenter retrospective study in China comparing laparoscopic and open surgery for the treatment of infected pancreatic necrosis. J Laparoendosc Adv Surg Tech A. 2012;22(1):27-33.
47. Fagniez PL, Rotman N, Kracht M. Direct retroperitoneal approach to necrosis in severe acute pancreatitis. Br J Surg. 1989;76:264-7.
48. Nakasaki H, Tajima T, Fujii K, Makuuchi H. A surgical treatment of infected pancreatic necrosis: retroperitoneal laparotomy. Dig Surg. 1999;16:506-11.
49. Villazon A. Retroperitoneal drainage in the management of the septic phase of severe acute pancreatitis. World J Surg. 1991;15: 408-9.
50. Bello B, Matthews JB. Minimally invasive treatment of pancreatic necrosis. World J Gastroenterol. 2012;18:6829-35.
51. Carter CR, McKay CJ, Imrie CW. Percutaneous necrosectomy and sinus tract endoscopy in the management of infected pancreatic necrosis: an initial experience. Ann Surg. 2000;232:175-80.
52. Connor S, Ghaneh P, Raraty M, Sutton R, Rosso E, Garvey CJ, et al. Minimally invasive retroperitoneal pancreatic necrosectomy. Dig Surg. 2003;20:270-7.
53. Raraty MGT, Halloran CM, Dodd S, Ghaneh P, Connor S, Evans J, et al. Minimal access retroperitoneal pancreatic necrosectomy-improvement in morbidity and mortality with a less invasive approach. Ann Surg. 2010;251:787-93.
54. Santvoort HCV, Besselink MGH, Horvath KD, Sinanan MN, Bollen TL, van Ramshorst B, et al. Videoscopic assisted retroperitoneal debridement in infected necrotizing pancreatitis. HPB. 2007;9:156-9.
55. Cirocchi R, Trastulli S, Desiderio J, Boselli C, Parisi A, Noya G, et al. Minimally invasive necrosectomy versus conventional surgery in the treatment of infected pancreatic necrosis: a systematic review and a meta-analysis of comparative studies. Surg Laparosc Endosc Percutan Tech. 2013;23(1):8-20.
56. Rau BM, Beger HG. Necrosectomy and closed lavage. In: Beger HG, Matsuno S, Cameron JL, Rau BM, Sunamura M, Schulick RD (Eds). Diseases of the Pancreas Current Surgical Therapy. Berlin, Germany: Springer; 2008. pp. 231-40.
57. Sarr MG, Nagorney DM, Mucha P Jr., Farnell MB, Johnson CD. Acute necrotizing pancreatitis: management by planned, staged pancreatic necrosectomy/debridement and delayed primary wound closure over drains. Br J Surg. 1991;78:576-81.
58. Bradley EL. Management of infected pancreatitis necrosis by open drainage. Ann Surg. 1987;206:542-50.
59. Castillo CF, Rattner DW, Makary MA, Mostafav A, McGrath D, Warshaw AL. Debridement and closed packing for the treatment of necrotizing pancreatitis. Annals of Surgery. 1998;228:676-84.
60. Vasiliadis K, Papavasiliou C, Nimer AA, Lamprou N, Makridis C. The role of open necrosectomy in the current management of acute necrotizing pancreatitis: a review article. ISRN Surgery, Volume 2013, Article ID 579435.http://dx.doi.org/10.1155/2013/579435.
61. Heinrich S, Schäfer M, Rousson V, Clavien PA. Evidence-based treatment of acute pancreatitis: a look at established paradigms. Ann Surg. 2006;243(2):154-68.

CHAPTER 39

Pseudocyst and Other Complications of Pancreatitis

Chintamani Godbole, Nilesh Doctor

INTRODUCTION

Acute pancreatitis is often followed by a variety of sequelae with distinct morphological and clinical manifestations. All these are direct effects of the inflammatory process, necrosis and the physiological capacity of body to localize the inflammation. Most of these are the different points in the temporal sequence of events that occur following acute pancreatitis and are just known to us by different names. Modern imaging techniques have enabled their accurate diagnosis and distinction from one another. As clear is their diagnosis, the treatment guidelines still are being debated with a lack of consensus on when, how and in whom to intervene.

DEFINITION AND NOMENCLATURE

Acute pancreatitis has been one of the diseases marked by a considerable amount of confusion in nomenclature and definition of various disease stages. Lack of access to biopsy of this retroperitoneal and vascular organ is the prime reason for the same. Over five consensus conferences have attempted to "define" various stages of the disease. Following is a synopsis of the various consensus meetings[1] (Table 1).

The revised Atlanta Classification was published in March 2013 by the same working group that gave the Atlanta Classification. The authors accepted that the terms formulated in the Atlanta Classification led to considerable amount of confusion and a lot of patients did not fit into any of the categories of the classification. The revised Atlanta Classification aimed at resolving these confusions and provided objective definition of acute pancreatitis and its local complications based on cross sectional imaging. It indeed comprehensively covers and defines all the local complications following acute pancreatitis and has provided clarity which no prior classification system ever did.

Table 1: Synopsis of various classification systems for acute pancreatitis[1]

Classification	*Consensus*
Marseille (1965)	Pure histology based and hence of no practical benefit. Only defined acute and chronic pancreatitis and no other complications
Cambridge (1984)	First time gave names—necrosis, pseudocyst, phlegmon, pancreatic abscess based on morphological characters on imaging
Marseille-Rome (1988)	Definitions of various sequelae of pancreatitis same as before Main feature was the statement made about the reversibility of sequelae like necrosis, pseudocyst following acute pancreatitis Etiologies of acute pancreatitis were addressed
Atlanta (1992)	Defined entities—acute pancreatitis, pancreatic necrosis, post-acute collections, pseudocyst and pancreatic abscess based on their morphology and content

Following is a detail account of various definitions as per the revised Atlanta Classification:

The *revised Atlanta Classification* divides acute pancreatitis into two broad types—(1) interstitial edematous pancreatitis and (2) necrotizing pancreatitis.

Interstitial edematous pancreatitis is characterized on a contrast-enhanced computed tomography (CECT) with a diffuse or localized swelling and edema of the pancreas with a relatively homogenous enhancement. There may be presence of peripancreatic fat stranding and peripancreatic fluid. The symptoms and signs of this pancreatitis usually resolve within a week (Fig. 1A).

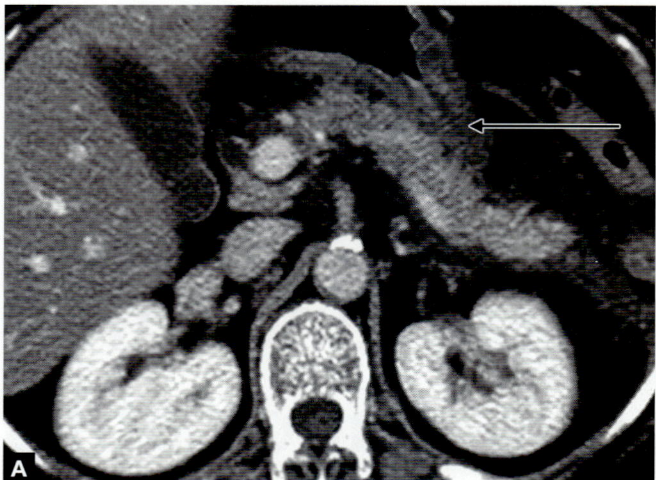

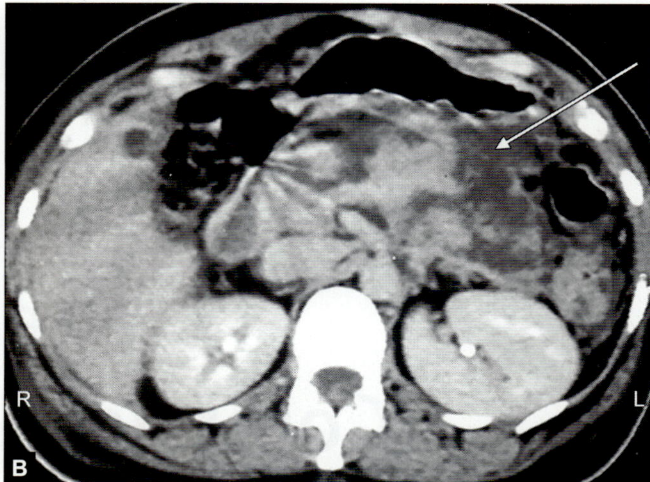

Figures 1A and B (A) Axial section of CECT image showing an acute peripancreatic fluid collection in the setting of acute edematous pancreatitis; (B) Axial section of CECT image showing acute necrotic collection characterized by non-enhancing areas both within and around the pancreas with lack of a well-defined wall suggestive of acute necrotizing pancreatitis

Necrotizing pancreatitis is characterized by presence of pancreatic and/or peripancreatic non-enhancing areas suggestive of necrosis. Most commonly there is necrosis of pancreatic parenchyma along with part of surrounding fat. Rarely pancreatic necrosis and peripancreatic fat necrosis are seen alone (Fig. 1B).

Both types of pancreatitis mentioned above lead to a variety of sequelae which have been defined as below:

- Acute peripancreatic fluid collection (APFC): It is defined as presence of fluid collection around pancreas seen within 4 weeks after onset of pancreatitis without any defined wall. It is usually associated with interstitial edematous pancreatitis.
- Pancreatic pseudocyst: Pseudocyst is defined as presence of fluid collection around pancreas with minimal or no necrosis and has a well-defined wall. It occurs more than 4 weeks after onset of pancreatitis and is usually associated with interstitial pancreatitis.
- Acute necrotic collection (ANC): Any collection containing both fluid and necrosis in variable amount seen within 4 weeks of onset on pancreatitis is defined as acute necrotic collection. It is usually associated with necrotizing pancreatitis.
- Walled-off necrosis (WON): A mature, encapsulated collection of pancreatic and/or peripancreatic necrosis with a well-defined inflammatory wall. It usually occurs more than 4 weeks after onset of necrotizing pancreatitis.

CLINICAL FEATURES

A pseudocyst or a walled off necrosis may present as persistent abdominal pain following episode of acute pancreatitis. A new onset of pain after the initial pain of acute pancreatitis has subsided indicates infection, bleeding or just mere increase in size of the collection. New onset systemic inflammatory response syndrome (SIRS) or organ failure more than 1 week after the onset of pancreatitis indicates infection of the existing acute necrotic collection, pseudocyst or walled-off pancreatic necrosis (WOPN). Other symptoms may include early satiety, nausea and vomiting or low grade fever. A subset of patients may just have anorexia, weight loss and failure to thrive. Pseudocyst or WOPN in the region of head of pancreas can present with obstructive jaundice due to compression of the common bile duct. Splenic vein thrombosis can result in isolated left sided portal hypertension. These patients can develop fundal varices which may be either asymptomatic or present as upper gastrointestinal (UGI) bleed. Clinical examination may reveal fullness or a lump palpable in the epigastric or right or left hypochondrium. Disease involving the tail of pancreas with extension along the left paracolic gutter may result in palpable fullness along the left flank.

DIAGNOSIS

The diagnosis of the various complications following acute pancreatitis is based essentially on their morphological characteristics on CECT scan. Following are the diagnostic features of each on CECT as per the revised Atlanta Classification:

- Acute peripancreatic fluid collection (Fig. 1A):
  - Homogeneous collection with fluid density
  - Confined by normal peripancreatic fascial planes
  - No definable wall encapsulating the collection
  - Adjacent to pancreas (no intra-pancreatic extension)
- Pancreatic pseudocyst (Fig. 2):
  - Well circumscribed, usually round or oval
  - Homogeneous fluid density with no solid component
  - Well defined wall
  - More than 4 weeks after onset of acute pancreatitis
- Acute necrotic collection (Fig. 3):
  - CECT criteria
  - Occurs only in the setting of acute necrotizing pancreatitis
  - Heterogeneous density (liquid and non-liquid component) of varying degrees in different locations (some appear homogeneous early in their course)
  - No definable wall encapsulating the collection
  - Location—intrapancreatic and/or extrapancreatic

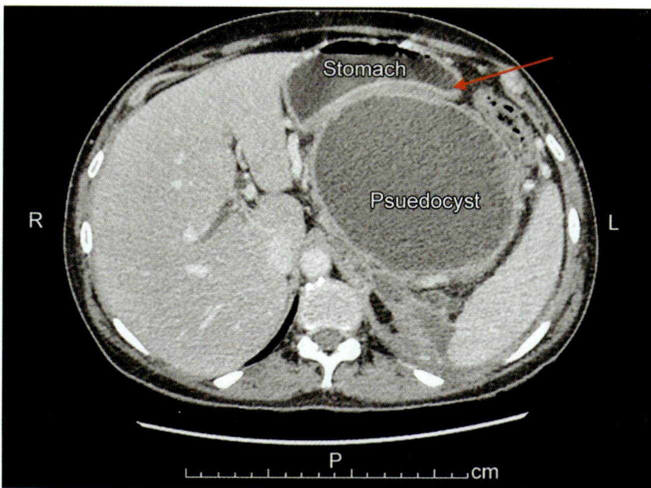

Figure 2 Axial section of contrast enhanced CT scan abdomen showing a large fluid collection in region of body and tail pancreas with a well-defined wall suggestive of a pseudocyst. It is abutting the posterior wall of the stomach

- Walled off pancreatic necrosis (WON) (Fig. 4):
  - Intrapancreatic and/or extrapancreatic collection
  - Heterogeneous density (both liquid and non-liquid density) with varying degrees of loculations
  - Well defined wall
  - More than 4 weeks after onset of acute pancreatitis.

ROLE OF OTHER IMAGING MODALITIES

Magnetic resonance imaging (MRI) abdomen can provide details and information as much as a CT scan for diagnosis of acute pancreatitis and its complications. Miller et al. have described the MRI imaging characteristics of acute pancreatitis and its complications. MRI takes longer scan time and lacks the anatomical details provided by CT scan. Different settings of the MRI need to be interpreted by a trained radiologist. Surgeons are usually more comfortable with CT scan. However, MRI can be repeated without fear of radiation. MRI scores over a CT scan in providing following additional information:

- A cystic lesion of the pancreas seen on a CT scan may be a pseudocyst, walled off pancreatic necrosis or a cystic neoplasm.

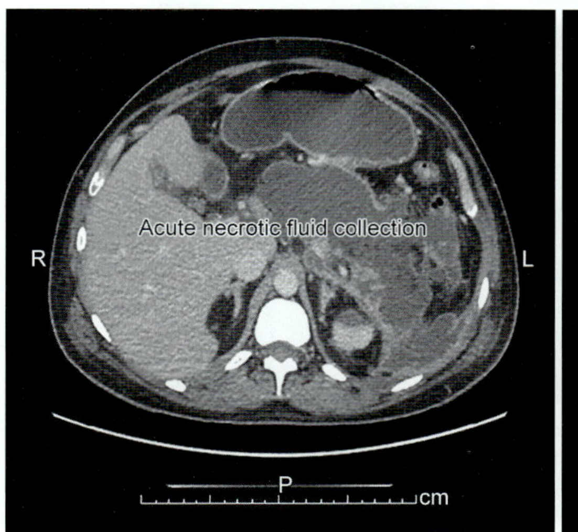

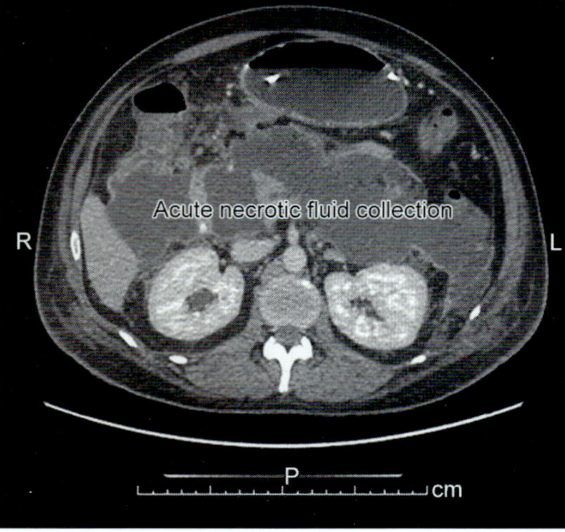

Figure 3 Axial sections of contrast enhanced CT scan abdomen showing a heterogeneous collection in and around pancreas with no well-defined wall suggestive of acute necrotic fluid collection (ANFC)

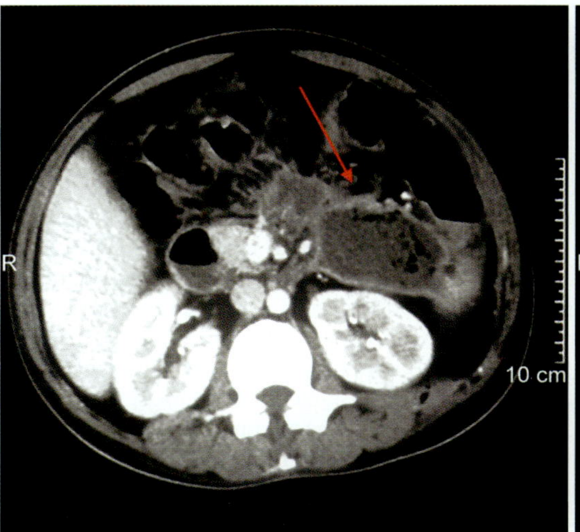

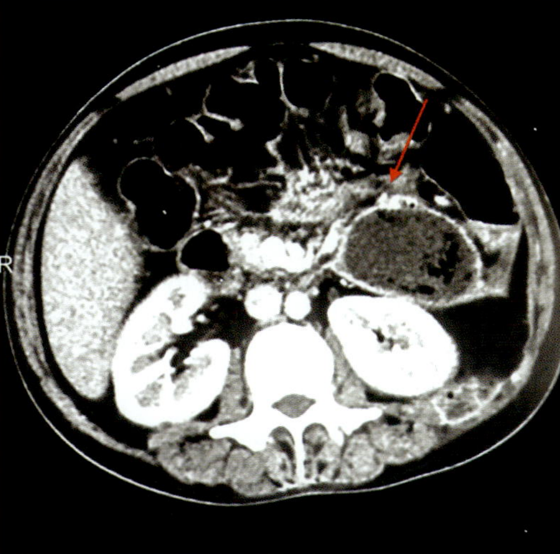

Figure 4 Axial section of contrast enhanced CT scan abdomen showing an encapsulated collection with necrosis located near tail region of pancreas with a well-defined inflammatory wall suggestive of a walled of necrosis (WON)

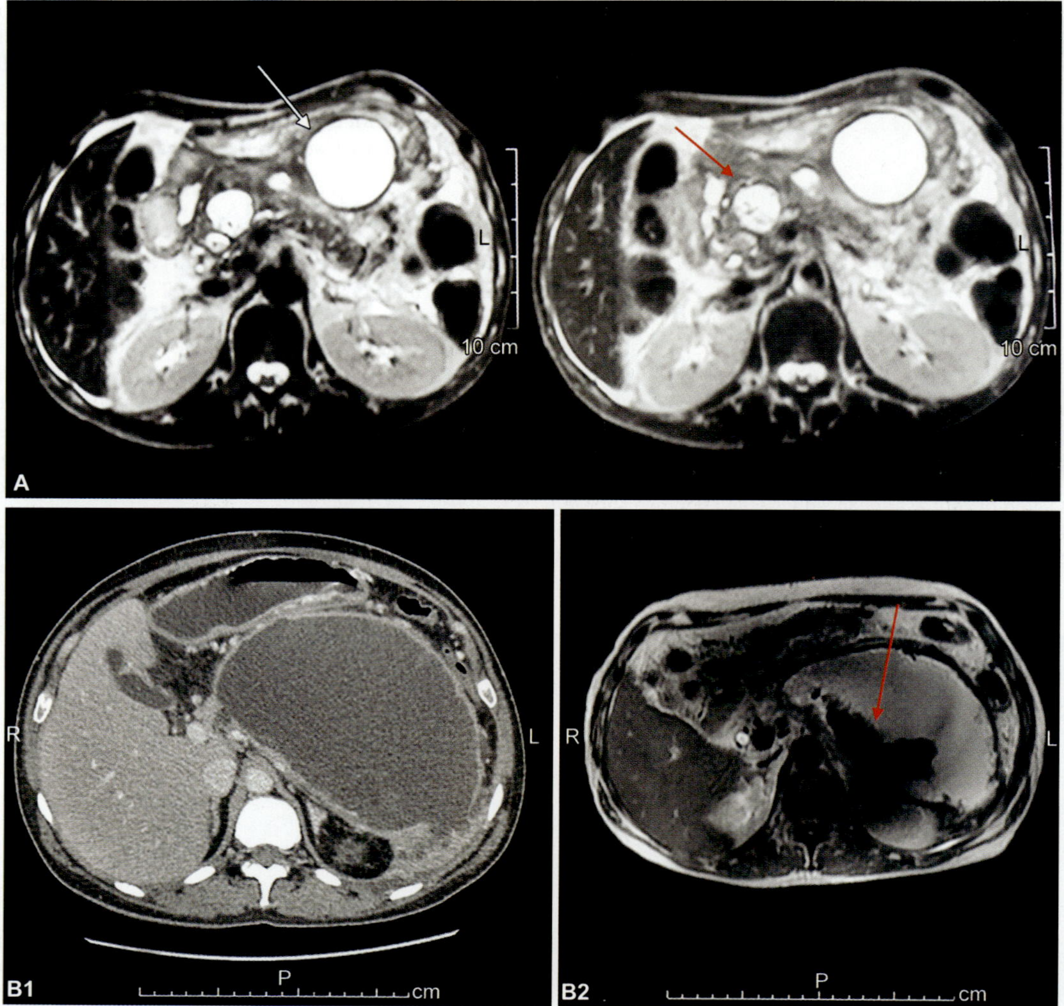

Figures 5A and B (A) Axial section of T2-weighted MRI shows a pseudocyst in the tail of pancreas containing fluid (white arrow) and another small cyst in head region containing both fluid and some necrotic component (red arrow); (B) (5B1) Axial section of CECT scan abdomen showing a homogenous density of fluid collection in region of body and tail pancreas showing a pseudocyst without any necrotic component. (5B2) Axial section of T2-weighted MRI of the same lesion shows that pseudocyst contains both fluid (white) and necrotic component (red arrow)

An MRI especially the T2-weighted images may show the content, whether it is completely cystic or has some solid tissue or necrotic debris within and can aid in the diagnosis (Figs 5A and B).

- Hemorrhage into a collection of pancreatitis is better diagnosed on MRI as a result of high signal intensity on T1-weighted images by methemoglobin and presence of low-signal-intensity hemosiderin rim on T2-weighted images.
- Addition of a magnetic resonance cholangiopancreatography (MRCP) enables visualization of the bile duct in detail.

TREATMENT

We would like to reiterate that the various complications following acute pancreatitis discussed above are different points along the natural history of this continuous evolving process. Therefore the principles behind their management are essentially the same and are discussed under one heading.

Before discussing management options we would like to brief on the *current status of CT guided fine needle aspiration (FNA)* for diagnosis of infected pancreatic necrosis. In order to determine whether pancreatic necrosis is infected in a clinical setting of a patient with necrotizing pancreatitis who is showing features of sepsis and organ failure, a CT guided aspiration of the pancreatic necrosis for culture has been advised in literature.[2] Clancy et al. have discussed role of CT guided FNA with Gram stain and culture as a deciding factor to perform surgical necrosectomy in patients who deteriorate clinically with sepsis and organ failure.[2]

Freeman et al. in multidisciplinary consensus conference have discussed the role of FNA to establish infection in necrotizing pancreatitis. They have made following arguments against an FNA:[3]

- Nowadays most interventions done for necrotizing pancreatitis are minimally invasive like an image guided percutaneous drainage. In a patient in whom infected pancreatic necrosis is expected an image guided pigtail catheter drainage can

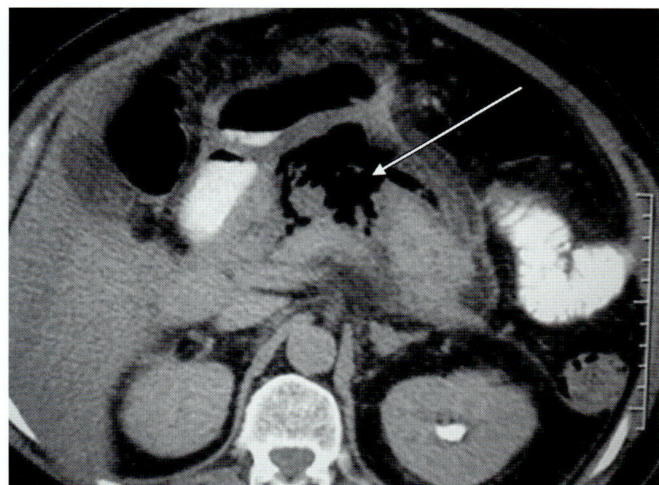

Figure 6 Axial section of CECT scan showing air within acute necrotic collection, diagnostic of infected pancreatic necrosis

achieve two tasks—getting tissue or pus for culture as well as drainage of the liquid component of the collection. Therefore an additional FNA is often not required as the risks associated with an image guided catheter insertion are the same and it serves both purposes of diagnosis and drainage.

- A number of studies have shown that infected pancreatic necrosis can be successfully treated conservatively with antibiotics. Mouli et al. in their meta-analysis evaluating conservative management of infected pancreatic necrosis have shown that successful medical management is possible in 64% of cases and that surgical necrosectomy may be avoided.[4]
- Whenever there is presence of air in the necrosis, it is diagnostic of infected pancreatic necrosis (Fig. 6). In all other cases a diagnosis of infected pancreatic necrosis should be made on presence of clinical evidence like the presence of SIRS and organ failure at 2 weeks or more after the onset of acute pancreatitis. A new onset of SIRS and organ failure especially after the second week of the attack, in a patient who had recovered from the acute phase also points toward infection of the necrosis.

Freeman et al. have thus not recommended an FNA for diagnosis of infected pancreatic necrosis. The only clinical setting in which an FNA would be accepted is that of a patient of necrotizing pancreatitis who deteriorates clinically on antibiotics and a fungal super infection of the necrosis is suspected.

The main questions regarding intervention in acute pancreatitis are—when, in whom and how to intervene?

When to Intervene?

A number of studies have shown that more the delay for any intervention for necrotizing pancreatitis, better is the outcome and lesser are the complications. The later the intervention the better is the demarcation of necrotic tissue and fluid from the surrounding vital tissue enabling its easier separation and lesser bleeding. Moreover, the systemic inflammatory response and organ failure seen after a necrosectomy is also less if intervention is delayed.

Mier et al. in their study comparing early versus late necrosectomy showed that necrosectomy done within 5 days of onset of acute necrotizing pancreatitis had higher APACHE II scores, organ failure and mortality compared to the ones performed at least 12 days after onset.[5] Large single center retrospective studies[6-8] have shown that a change in approach in performing more and more delayed interventions for necrotizing pancreatitis resulted in a statistically significant lesser morbidity and mortality.

In our own published study, we analyzed 61 patients of necrotizing pancreatitis who underwent open necrosectomy from 1998 to 2009. The mean duration from the onset of pancreatitis to the intervention was 29 days. We could achieve single stage necrosectomy in 90% of the patients with a reoperation rate of only 8%. The overall mortality was 9.5%. We could clearly experience benefits of a delayed necrosectomy in the form of easy separation of the necrosum from vital tissue with less bleeding and local complications. The patients were in a more hemodynamically stable state compared to what they were in earlier phase of acute pancreatitis and could tolerate surgery much better.[9]

Whom to Intervene?

The complications following pancreatitis that may require any intervention include infected pancreatic necrosis, acute necrotic collection, pseudocyst and WOPN. The indications of intervention are essentially the same in all, only the type of intervention varies.

We would like to classify *indications of intervention* in acute pancreatitis into early and late phase.

- Early phase:
  - Acute peripancreatic fluid collections never require and acute necrotic collections seldom require intervention.
  - Absolute indications of early intervention include acute pancreatitis with bowel perforation and abdominal compartment syndrome. However, in both these scenarios, pancreatic debridement is not indicated.[3]
  - Other indications would be an infected acute necrotic collection evident by presence of systemic sepsis or organ failure. As previously discussed, even in this scenario first a trial of conservative treatment has to be given with hydration, antibiotics, nutrition and intensive care. If there is no clinical improvement despite above, only then any intervention should be considered.
- Late phase:
  - The main indication still remains infected necrosis or collection with systemic sepsis and organ failure as mentioned above and underlying principle remains the same of waiting as much as possible.
  - Mechanical gastric outlet obstruction or biliary obstruction due to mass effect of a large WOPN or a pseudocyst remains an indication of intervention.
  - Persistent pain causing poor appetite, weight loss and failure to thrive should also be considered as an indication for intervention.

How to Intervene?

A number of modalities have been described for intervention in acute pancreatitis. They can be classified into the following types:

- Open surgical
- Minimally invasive surgical
- Image guided percutaneous
- Endoscopic
- Hybrid.

Loveday et al. have proposed a nomenclature and classification system of various interventions for pancreatitis based on method of visualization, the route of entry into the collection and the purpose of drainage.[10] The details of this system are given in Table 2. This taxonomy has been shown to have excellent inter-observer agreement. Although this system may be cumbersome to use in day to day practice, it allows standardization for nomenclature for use in audit, analysis and data publication.[10]

Following is a detail account of the various types of interventions:

- **Open procedures:** Open procedures can be classified into two types:
  - Internal drainage: Open cystogastrostomy; Open cystojejunostomy.
  - External drainage: Open necrosectomy followed by:
    - Open packing
    - Closed packing
    - Continuous postoperative lavage
- **Internal drainage:** These are done for pseudocyst and WOPNs with a well formed wall usually done after 4 weeks of the onset of pancreatitis. If the collection is abutting the posterior wall of the stomach, an open transgastric cystogastrostomy can be done. If the collection is abutting into the transverse mesocolon, then an open cystojejunostomy can be done. The essential requirement for these procedures is a well formed cyst wall that can hold sutures and can be anastomosed with the gut.
- **External drainage:** An open necrosectomy essentially involves a wide laparotomy. Entry into the cavity with necrosis may be through the gastrocolic omentum or through the transmesocolic window. Removal of necrosum is done with a combination of blunt dissection, irrigation and suction. Following the necrosectomy, there are three approaches described to deal with the cavity.
  - Open packing: This involves putting packs and keeping the abdomen open. The patient is taken back to the operation

Table 2: Classification of interventions for pancreatic necrosis based on route, visualization, purpose (Loveday et al.)[10]

		Route	
Type	*Name*	*Entry point*	*Internal route*
R1	Per os transpapillary	External orifice	Duodenal papilla to enter pancreatic duct
R2	Per os transmural	External orifice	Traversing gastrointestinal wall
R3	Percutaneous retroperitoneal	Skin	Traversing retroperitoneum
R4	Percutaneous transperitoneal	Skin	Traversing peritoneum
R5	Percutaneous transmural	Skin	Traversing gastrointestinal wall
Rx		Insufficient information	
Rz		Other route	
		Visualization	
V1	Radiological	Using only radiological modalities (e.g. fluoroscopy, CT, ultrasound, MR) to visualize and assist entering the target lesion	
V2	Endoscopic	Using any white light endoscopic instrument (e.g. flexible, or rigid endoscope, urological endoscope) to visualize the target lesion	
V3	Hybrid	Using an endoscopic technique as the primary mode of visualization, assisted by a real time radiological modality (e.g. EUS)	
V4	Open	Using any method where skin and any other body layers are cut to expose the site of the procedure	
Vx		Insufficient information	
Vz		Other visualization technique	
		Purpose	
P1	Drainage	Fluid and/or solid material are removed either externally or internally into the GI tract	
P2	Lavage	Facilitate external or internal drainage by flushing away solid matter using fluid	
P3	Fragmentation	Facilitate external or internal drainage by breaking down solid matter by instrumental or mechanical disruption	
P4	Debridement	Taking or cutting out solid matter with either sharp or blunt dissection	
P5	Excision	Remove necrotic tissue by cutting out the damaged pancreas	
Px		Insufficient information	
Pz		Other purpose	

theatre on one or more occasions and further debridement is done if required.
  - Closed packing: The cavity is packed after necrosectomy, multiple drains are placed and the abdomen is closed. A relaparotomy is planned after 24–48 hours to remove the packs and do further debridement if necessary.
  - Continuous lavage: Two or more drains are placed into the cavity, the abdomen is closed and postoperatively the cavity is continuously irrigated with warm saline. Continuous irrigation loosens the necrosum which allows its separation and helps in its drainage.
- As per various series of publications on open necrosectomy, it is associated with a relatively high morbidity (34% to 95%) and mortality ranging from 6% to 25%.[3]

Among the three types mentioned above, Continuous postoperative lavage has been shown to be superior to the other two in terms of lesser morbidity whereas the mortality is more or less the same. A relaparotomy significantly increases the morbidity of the patient by increasing the systemic inflammatory response as well as the chances of local complications like bleeding or bowel perforation.[3]

IMAGE-GUIDED PERCUTANEOUS APPROACHES

- Usually these procedures are done under guidance of a contrast enhanced CT scan. The collection is accessed from the percutaneous approach after identifying a window on imaging that is avoids injury to the colon, stomach, spleen and major blood vessels. A USG guided approach may also be done in selected cased with large collections reaching the abdominal wall. Aspiration alone without drainage of pseudocysts or any acute collections is no longer recommended due to high failure rates.[11]
- For drainage, usually pigtail catheters of size varying from 12 Fr to 24 Fr can be inserted under CT guidance. Often multiple catheters may be required for complete drainage of collections.[12]
- Percutaneous catheter drainage may be done as:
  - A primary modality for treatment
  - As a part of the "step-up approach", details of which we shall be described below
  - As a salvage modality to drain undrained collections following a surgical necrosectomy.
- Van Baal MC et al. in a review article have evaluated 11 studies with 384 patients in whom image guided catheter drainage was used as a primary modality for the treatment of infected or symptomatic pancreatic necrosis. They have shown that in 55.7% patients no further necrosectomy was required and they could be successfully managed with drainage alone. The overall mortality in this series was 17.4%.[12]

A brief word on the *"step-up" approach*:

- Van Santvoort HC et al. in the Dutch PANTER trial randomized patients of infected pancreatic necrosis into two groups—one underwent open necrosectomy and the other was subjected to a "step approach".[13]

As per the step-up approach:

Patients were subjected to percutaneous CT-guided drainage of the pancreatic collections (Fig. 7). Pigtail catheters of median size 14 Fr were used for drainage. Multiple catheters were used in some patients. Following drainage, catheters were continuously irrigated with warm saline for 72 hours and patients were assessed for clinical improvement. If there was no improvement then a CT scan was repeated and any undrained foci of collection were looked for. If undrained collections were seen, they were drained by percutaneous catheters. If there were no collections seen or if they were not amenable for drainage, then the patients were subjected to minimally invasive surgical necrosectomy. The necrosectomy in most patients was done by the video-assisted retroperitoneal debridement technique. Important to note is that 35% patients in the step-up group did not require a necrosectomy indicating that percutaneous drainage was sufficient for adequate source control.

Van Santvoort showed that in the "step-up approach" group there was a statistically significant lower incidence of major

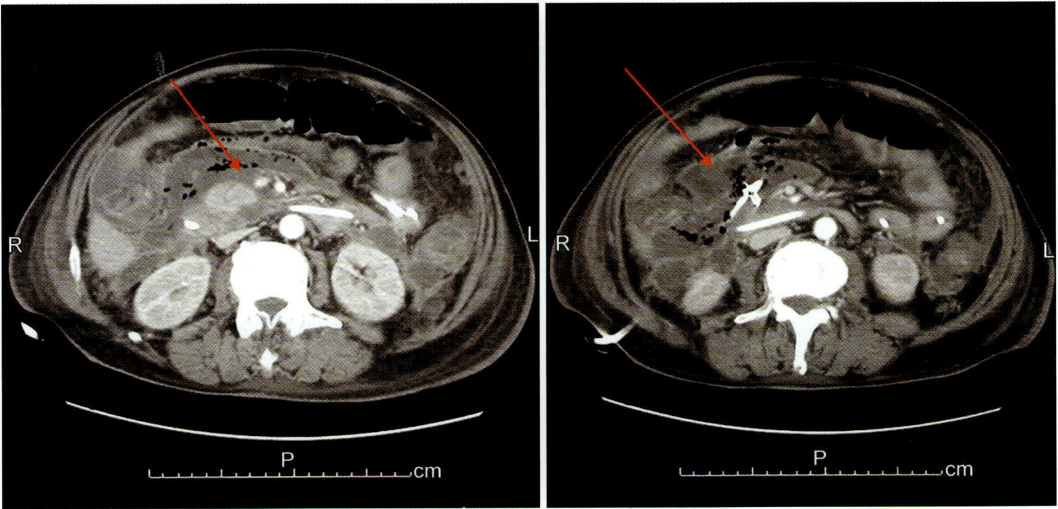

Figure 7 Axial section of contrast enhanced CT scan abdomen showing a walled of necrotic collection containing air around head of pancreas. Pig tail in place (red arrow) shows that WON is being managed via step up approach

postoperative complications like organ failure and lesser long-term complications like new onset diabetes and incisional hernia compared to the "open necrosectomy group".[13] The step-up approach benefits by delaying surgical necrosectomy as much as possible and avoiding surgery in a significant number of patients who improve following percutaneous drainage alone.

Minimally invasive approaches for pancreatic necrosectomy can be classified as:

- Transperitoneal approach
- Retroperitoneal approach

Transperitoneal Approach

- A laparoscopic transperitoneal approach involves opening of the necrosum cavity, removal of the necrosum by irrigation, suction and use of blunt tissue holding forceps. The laparoscope can be used to visualize the cavity internally and remove any remaining necrosis which is easily separable. The cavity then can be left open with drains in situ. In case of a well formed pseudocyst or WOPN in the retrogastric region, the cavity may be opened through a transgastric approach and a laparoscopic cystogastrostomy can be done using an endostapler.
- The advantages of the transperitoneal approach include ability to visualize and drain the entire necrosis containing cavity, smaller wound with lesser infection and that a cholecystectomy may be added if the pancreatitis is of biliary etiology. The main disadvantage is that a retroperitoneal infective focus may get disseminated into the peritoneum.
- As shown in the Table 3 are major studies showing that a laparoscopic approach may be used in acute necrotizing pancreatitis with reasonable success rates and mortality.[14-16]

Retroperitoneal Approach

The minimally invasive retroperitoneal approach is known by many names—*"sinus tract endoscopy"* and *"video assisted retroperitoneal debridement"*.

The principles are the following:

- A percutaneous drain is inserted into the retroperitoneum through the left lumbar region for drainage of the pancreatic collection. The drain track is dilated or a small incision is used to guide a laparoscope, a rigid nephroscope or a flexible endoscope into the collection. Necrosectomy is done with a combination of irrigation, suction and use of blunt grasping forceps along the side of the telescope.
- A number of studies have shown that this approach can be used to achieve success rates about 70–80% with low reoperation rates (Table 4).
- Retrospective studies comparing minimally invasive retroperitoneal approach with open necrosectomy have shown lesser organ failure, major complications and ICU stay in the minimally invasive approach group.[17]

ENDOSCOPIC TREATMENT TECHNIQUES

Endoscopic transmural necrosectomy through the posterior gastric wall was first reported in 1996 by T. Baron et al. This procedure involves accessing the pancreatic collection through the posterior gastric wall. Removal of necrosis is by irrigation, aspiration, use of endoscopic baskets and other instruments. Following the debridement multiple large bore double pigtail stents can be placed into the cavity to facilitate drainage. Often multiple sessions are required for adequate drainage. Use of endoscopic ultrasound (EUS) can help in guiding the direction of the transgastric needle puncture. Advantages of EUS include ability to visualize precise depth and direction of the collection, avoiding major vessel and viscus injury and to assess the contents of the collection.

Haghshenasskashani A, in a systematic review of studies of endoscopic necrosectomies comprising of 260 total patients with over a thousand endoscopic procedures have shown that endoscopic necrosectomy alone resulted in resolution of necrosis in 70% of cases. The overall morbidity and mortality rate in this series was 27% and 5% respectively.[18]

Bakker et al. from the Dutch pancreatitis study group have published results of an on-going trial comparing endoscopic necrosectomy to surgical necrosectomy (VARD). They have shown that the endoscopy group has significantly lower post-procedure inflammatory response, organ failure and pancreatic fistulae.[19]

Table 3: Studies showing results of laparoscopic transperitoneal necrosectomy

Study	*Patients*	*Success rate (%)*	*Reoperation rate (%)*	*Mortality (%)*
Gagner (1996)	8	75	38	-
Zhu (2001)	10	70	-	10
Zhou (2003)	13	92	0	15
Parekh (2006)	19	84	11	11

Table 4: Studies showing results of video-assisted retroperitoneal debridement

Study	*No. of patients*	*Timing of intervention (mean)*	*Success rate (%)*	*Reoperation rate (%)*	*Mortality (%)*
Connor (2005)	47	28	75	5	19
Horvath (2010)	25	80	60	8	0
Van Santvoort (2010)	24	30	63	NA	17
Raraty (2010)	137	32	84	33	19

Hybrid Approaches

Often more than one type approach may be required in a patient for adequate drainage of the pancreatic collection or necrosis. The "step-up" approach is a good example of a hybrid approach wherein lesser invasive approaches are used first and more invasive interventions are done only if required. Ross et al. have reported combined use of endoscopic with percutaneous drainage for the management of symptomatic pancreatic necrosis. They have shown that this approach results in low procedure related morbidity, avoidance of surgical necrosectomy and minimizes chances of post-intervention pancreatic fistula.[20]

Pseudocyst

Pseudocyst is defined as the presence of fluid collection around the pancreas with minimal or no necrosis and has a well-defined wall. It occurs more than 4 weeks after the onset of pancreatitis and is usually associated with interstitial pancreatitis. It accounts for more than 75% of cystic lesions of pancreas.

The incidence of pseudocyst following acute pancreatitis reported in various series varies from 5% to 15%. It occurs more frequently in patients with alcohol related pancreatitis (50–60%) than gall stone (15%). Trauma is another important cause for occurrence of pseudocyst especially in children and young adults. The incidence of pseudocyst is also higher in the setting of acute on chronic pancreatitis (20–40%). Around 50% of cysts are located near head of pancreas, while remaining are distributed evenly in body and tail region. Around 10% of patients have multiple pseudocysts.

CLASSIFICATION

In 1991, D'Egidio and Schein classified pseudocyst into three types based on type of pancreatitis (acute or chronic), pancreatic ductal anatomy and communication of cyst with the pancreatic duct.[21] Type I or Post-necrotic pseudocysts occur usually after an episode of acute pancreatitis, are associated with normal pancreatic duct anatomy and rarely have any cyst duct communication. Type II pseudocysts occur in a setting of acute on chronic pancreatitis, have diseased pancreatic duct without any stricture and usually have a duct cyst communication. Both Types I and II are cysts are large in size and extra-pancreatic in location. Type III pseudocysts, also known as retention cysts occur in patients with chronic pancreatitis, have dilated main pancreatic duct (MPD) with stricture and have ductal communication with the cyst. Chronic pseudocysts are usually small in size (<4 cm), intrapancreatic in location, occur in setting of chronic pancreatitis and have a communication with pancreatic duct. It is important to differentiate chronic pseudocyst from Types I and II because these patients require management of chronic pancreatitis in addition to drainage of pseudocyst. Pseudocyst in these cases may not require separate drainage procedure since most of them are drained in the procedure performed for chronic pancreatitis.

Another classification proposed by Nealon and Walser in 2002[22] became popular since many pseudocyst are now treated with endoscopic method. They classified them into seven types:

Type I have normal MPD without any communication with cyst

Type II have normal MPD with a duct-cyst communication

Type III have otherwise normal duct with a stricture and no cyst- duct communication

Type IV have normal duct with a stricture and also a cyst-duct communication

Type V have normal duct with a complete cut-off

Type VI have chronic pancreatitis with no cyst-duct communication

Type VII have chronic pancreatitis with a cyst-duct communication

CLINICAL FEATURES

Abdominal pain is the most common symptom of pseudocyst. It is seen in more than 90% of cases. The presentation of pseudocyst can vary from asymptomatic pseudocyst to acute abdomen secondary to complications related to cyst. Persistence or recurrence of abdominal pain following the episode of acute pancreatitis suggests that patient may be developing a pseudocyst. It is important to differentiate this from other causes like infection or bleeding that may result in new onset pain after the initial pain of acute pancreatitis has subsided. Other symptoms of pseudocysts are related to pressure symptoms secondary to a large collection. These vary according to the size and location of the pseudocyst. These include early satiety, nausea and vomiting (50–60%), weight loss (20–50%), jaundice (10%) and low grade fever (10%). Symptoms may also be secondary to complication occurring in the pseudocyst like bleeding, infection and rupture.

Clinical examination may reveal fullness or a palpable lump in the epigastric or right or left hypochondrium. Pseudocyst involving the tail of pancreas with extension along the left paracolic gutter may result in palpable fullness along the left flank. Peritoneal sign suggest cyst rupture or infection in the cyst.

Traumatic pseudocysts have similar clinical features but the symptoms may occur at a time remote from trauma.

The *acute complications* include bleed/hemorrhage in the cyst, cyst rupture or infection. While *chronic complications* are gastric outlet obstruction, obstructive jaundice secondary to pressure effects and portal hypertension secondary to splenic vein thrombosis.

DIAGNOSIS

Laboratory Parameters

Although serum amylase and lipase are elevated in approximately 50% of patients with pseudocyst, but these tests have limited utility in diagnosis. Imaging remains the cornerstone for diagnosis as described above.

Ultrasonography has certain limitations in initial diagnosis of pseudocyst due to presence of bowel gases. However, presence of echoic structure with distal acoustic enhancement is suggestive of pseudocyst. It appears complex especially when there is hemorrhage, infection or necrotic debris within the cyst. It has value in follow-up of pseudocyst planned for conservative management as it is cheap, easily available and does cause any radiation injury.

CECT Scan

The imaging findings are described above. The imaging findings on CT scan are diagnostic of pseudocyst. In addition it provides information regarding surrounding anatomy and underlying pancreatic pathology to formulate management. CT angiography is useful in delineating pseudoaneurysm. CECT scan may not be able to differentiate debris with fluid component which may be useful when contemplating endoscopic treatment. Another limitation of CT is in differentiating a pseudocyst from cystic neoplasm especially mucinous cystadenoma and intraductal papillary mucinous neoplasms (IPMN).

MRI/MRCP

Magnetic resonance imaging scores over a CT scan (Figs. 5B1 and B2) in providing following additional information:

a. An MRI especially the T2-weighted images may show the content, whether it is completely cystic or has some solid tissue or necrotic debris within and can aid in the diagnosis.
b. Hemorrhage into a collection of pancreatitis is better diagnosed on MRI as a result of high signal intensity on T1-weighted images produced by methaemoglobin and by presence of low-signal-intensity hemosiderin rim on T2-weighted images.
c. Addition of an MRCP enables visualization of the bile duct and pancreatic duct in detail.

Therefore MRI is useful when contemplating endoscopic treatment for pseudocyst drainage, a situation where one has difficulty in differentiating bleeding from complex fluid collection on CECT.

Endoscopic Ultrasound

The main indications for Endoscopic Ultrasound (EUS) in patients with pseudocyst are:

a. To differentiate from cystic neoplasm of pancreas. Presence of cyst wall thickness more than 3 mm, macro septation, presence of a mass or nodule or cystic dilatation of main pancreatic duct suggest cystic neoplasm. EUS-guided fluid aspiration further helps in differentiating from cystic neoplasm. Cyst fluid CEA levels more than 400 ng/mL and low amylase levels support mucinous cystic neoplasm while both levels being low support serous cyst adenoma. A high amylase and low CEA levels support a diagnosis of pseudocyst.[23]

   Sperti et al.[24] found that high serum CA 19-9 and high fluid CA 72-4 levels to have 95% specificity and 80% sensitivity for detecting mucinous and malignant cyst.
b. EUS helps in guiding therapeutic endoscopic drainage.

MANAGEMENT

Expectant Treatment

Many cysts can resolve with conservative expectant treatment therefore this is the first line of management for these patients. This includes intravenous fluid, analgesics and antiemetics. Oral feeding is started once the pain subsides with low fat diet. Vitas et al.[25] followed 114 patients with pseudocyst for 5 years. They had 68 patients in expectant group; of which only 6 patients required emergency treatment of life threatening complication and 19 patients required elective operation. Other studies suggest that size and duration of cyst is poor predictor for resolution or complication of the cyst.

The main indications for intervention are presence of symptoms or presence of complications.

The various modalities include surgical, endoscopic and radiological drainage of cyst. They are complementary and their use depends upon the expertise available.

Percutaneous drainage is done using ultrasound or CT scan. The prerequisite include the cyst should not have associated strictured pancreatic duct, any visible cyst to duct communication and/or blood or necrosis in the cyst cavity. The long-term success rate is reported to be around 50–60%. The major complications include pancreatic fistula, infection in the cyst cavity and injury to adjacent structures.

Internal Drainage

These are done for pseudocysts with a well formed wall and usually done after 4 weeks of the onset of pancreatitis. If the collection is abutting the posterior wall of the stomach, an open transgastric cystogastrostomy can be done. If the collection is abutting into the transverse mesocolon, then an open cystojejunostomy can be done. The essential requirement for these procedures is a well formed cyst wall that can hold sutures and can be anastomosed with the gut. These operations are now being performed laparoscopically as well.

Endoscopic Drainage

It can be done either through transpapillary approach or direct drainage across stomach or duodenum. The transpapillary route is preferred when cyst is communicating with MPD. This is usually observed at the level of genu. The prerequisite for direct drainage include cyst wall thickness less than 1 cm, absence of varices or large intervening vessel. It is either under fluoroscopy or using EUS. Presence of necrosis has become only a relative contraindication with advent of removable stents, although presence of necrosis results in higher rate of complication.

Other complications following acute pancreatitis:

1. Pancreatic fistula and disconnected duct syndrome: Necrosis of pancreatic parenchyma involving a portion of the duct may lead to leakage of pancreatic secretions into the peripancreatic space resulting in a pancreatic fistula. Such leakage can have a variety of clinical manifestations such as—recurrent peripancreatic collections, pancreatic ascites, pancreatic pleural effusion or persistence of amylase rich fluid in a previously placed drain. Such pancreatic fistulae are often seen after a necrosectomy.

As per the International Study Group on Pancreatic Fistula criteria a pancreatic fistula is defined as output via a previously placed catheter of any measurable volume of fluid with amylase content greater than 3 times the serum amylase activity.[26]

In a study and literature review done by the Dutch pancreatitis study group, Bakker et al. have shown that in patients of acute necrotizing pancreatitis who underwent any intervention like percutaneous catheter drainage or a necrosectomy, the incidence of pancreatic fistulae was about 30%. The authors also compared subgroups of patients who underwent endoscopic transpapillary stenting versus subgroup of patients treated conservatively. They found that patients treated with stenting had fistula closure rates about 84% whereas in the ones treated conservatively it was 75%. They concluded that endoscopic therapy is a safe alternative which may hasten closure rates of pancreatic fistulae following acute pancreatitis. However, the study being retrospective, no treatment recommendations were made.[27]

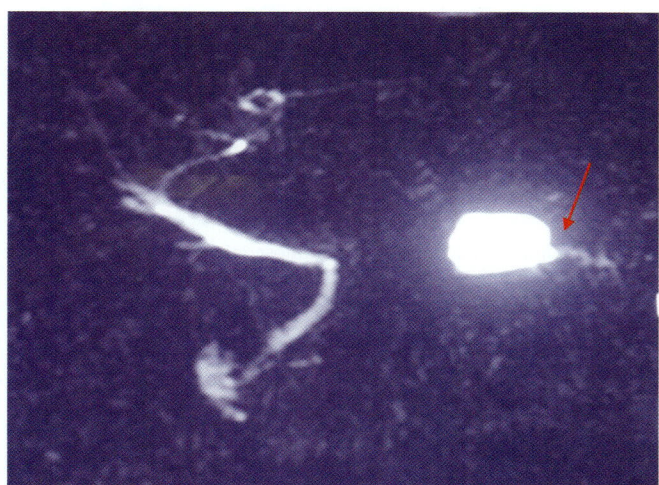

Figure 8 MRCP of a patient undergone necrosectomy shows a fluid collection in region of tail of pancreas with upstream dilatation of main pancreatic duct and normal proximal MPD suggestive of disconnected duct syndrome

Howard et al. classified pancreatic fistulae following necrotizing pancreatitis into side fistulae and end fistulae based on findings on endoscopic pancreatography. They showed that side fistulae have a high incidence of spontaneous closure (>80%) whereas all the patients with end fistulae did not close spontaneously and required surgery.[28] This entity was further defined as the "disconnected duct syndrome" which has the following diagnostic criteria[29] (Fig. 8):

- Evidence of main pancreatic duct cut-off or discontinuity with the inability of accessing or cannulating the upstream pancreatic duct on endoscopic retrograde pancreatography.
- Necrosis of at least 2 cm of pancreas with evidence of viable pancreatic tissue distal to the disruption on CT scan.
- Demonstrable pancreatic fistula in the form of drainage, pancreatic ascites, effusion or recurrent collections in proximity to the site of disruption.

Many endoscopic and surgical treatment modalities have been described for treatment of disconnected duct syndrome. Surgical treatment modalities include fistula-jejunostomy, cystogastrostomy and distal pancreatectomy. Solanky et al. in their review article on surgical procedures for disconnected duct syndrome have shown that both resection as well as roux en Y pancreaticojejunostomy have comparable success rate in fistula closure and that resectional procedures have a slight higher incidence of postoperative complications. They recommend that endoscopic treatment can be used temporarily till pancreatic inflammation reduces, but almost all patients invariably require a surgical procedure.[30] However, if one sees data from high volume endoscopy centers, a predominance of endoscopic treatment approaches successfully managing patients of disconnected duct is seen.

Pelaez-Luna M et al. from the Mayo Clinic retrospectively analyzed 31 patients of disconnected duct syndrome. Twenty-six patients were treated with transpapillary endoscopic drainage of the pancreatic collection. Nineteen patients had long-term improvement and did not require further surgery. Rest 7 patients failed treatment and required operation.[31]

Varadarajulu S et al. retrospectively analyzed 97 patients of ductal disruption following pancreatitis. Endoscopic transpapillary stenting was successful in 92 patients. Overall success rate of stenting was 55%. On univariate and multivariate analysis of factors predicting success of endotherapy, a partially disrupted pancreatic duct, successful bridging of gap between two duct ends by the stent and longer duration of stent placement were the factors significantly associated with success of endotherapy.[32]

2. Splenic vein thrombosis: Splanchnic venous thrombosis is not an uncommon complication following acute pancreatitis. It is usually seen in severe acute pancreatitis with local complications like necrosis. The pathophysiology is said to be perivascular inflammation and thrombosis due to proximity of splenic and portal vein with the inflamed pancreas.

In a retrospective study by Gonzalez et al.,[33] the incidence of splanchnic venous thrombosis was found to be about 15% among patients admitted with acute pancreatitis. The most common vessel involved was splenic vein followed by portal vein. All the patients who developed venous thrombosis had severe pancreatitis as per the Atlanta Classification. Laboratory investigations for hypercoagulable states were negative in all patients suggesting that they were due to the pancreatitis itself. None of the patients developed significant clinical features as a result of the thrombosis except 1 patient who developed colonic ischemia as he had extensive thrombosis of portal, splenic and superior mesenteric vein.[33]

On follow-up recanalization was seen in 30% of patients. Anticoagulation was used only in 4 out of 20 patients. There was no obvious benefit of anticoagulation seen. Left sided portal hypertension leading to gastric fundal varices with bleeding following acute pancreatitis related splenic vein thrombosis has been reported but is rare. The treatment involves doing a splenectomy or splenic artery embolization.

3. Hemorrhage following acute pancreatitis: Inflammation and necrosis associated with acute pancreatitis results in erosion into vessel wall and may result in hemorrhage (1–3%) by direct vessel damage or commonly is preceded by formation of pseudoaneurysms. Splenic artery is the most common vessel involved followed by unnamed pancreatic vessels, portal vein or rarely the spleen itself due to parenchymal involvement. The bleeding may occur in the gastrointestinal tract causing melena, within the pancreatic collection presenting as sudden onset pain and increase in size of abdominal lump or rarely into free peritoneal cavity causing hemoperitoneum. Interventional radiological techniques involving angiography and coiling of the pseudoaneurysm are able to control bleeding in most of the scenarios. In cases not controlled with radiological techniques, exploration with ligation, salvage emergency pancreatectomy or open packing may be deployed.[34]

CONCLUSION

An array of complications with a wide range of clinical features can be seen after acute pancreatitis. Cross section imaging like a CT scan or an MRI is essential to morphologically characterize these complications for their correct diagnosis. Various types of interventions done for acute pancreatitis have come a long way from the traditional open necrosectomies to minimally invasive approaches at present. The principle of delaying and possibly avoiding any intervention is now the validated approach of treatment. Decision to intervene is best made on clinical parameters and not on radiological or microbiological criteria. Uses of minimally invasive surgical approaches clearly offer advantages over conventional surgical methods. Endoscopic approaches of intervention are the upcoming modalities whose results look promising. Acute pancreatitis still however is a disease with considerable mortality, morbidity and often a prolonged hospital stay. Complications like pseudocyst, hemorrhage, splenic vein thrombosis, pancreatic fistula and disconnected duct syndromes need careful management. Further research in the form of randomized trials comparing various treatment modalities are required to establish treatment guidelines to give the best possible outcome to our patients.

REFERENCES

1. Jarnagin WR. Blumgart's Surgery of the Liver, Biliary tract and Pancreas, 5th edition. Elsevier Saunders.
2. Clancy TE, Benoit EP, Asley SW. Current management of acute pancreatitis. J Gastrointest Surg. 2005;9:440-52.
3. Freeman ML, Werner J, van Santvoort HC, Baron TH, Besselink MG, Windsor JA, et al. Interventions for necrotizing pancreatitis. Summary of a multidisciplinary consensus conference. Pancreas. 2012;41(8):1176-94.
4. Mouli VP, Sreenivas V, Garg PK. Efficacy of conservative treatment, without necrosectomy, for infected pancreatic necrosis: a systematic review and meta-analysis. Gastroenterology. 2013;144(2):333-40.
5. Mier J, Leon EL, Castillo A, Robledo F, Blanco R. Early versus late necrosectomy in severe necrotizing pancreatitis. Am J Surg. 1997;173:71-5.
6. Wittau M, Scheele J, Gölz I, Henne-Bruns D, Isenmann R. Changing role of surgery in necrotizing pancreatitis: a single-center experience. Hepatogastroenterology. 2010;57:1300-4.
7. Besselink MG, Verwer TJ, Schoenmaeckers EJ, Buskens E, Ridwan BU, Visser MR, et al. Timing of surgical intervention in necrotizing pancreatitis. Arch Surg. 2007;142:1194-201.
8. Hartwig W, Maksan SM, Foitzik T, Schmidt J, Herfarth C, Klar E. Reduction in mortality with delayed surgical therapy of severe pancreatitis. J Gastrointest Surg. 2002;6:481-7.
9. Doctor N, Philip S, Gandhi V, Hussain M, Barreto SG. Analysis of the delayed approach to the management of infected pancreatic necrosis. World J Gastroenterol. 2011;17(3):366-71.
10. Loveday BP, Petrov MS, Connor S, Rossaak JI, Mittal A, Phillips AR, et al. A comprehensive classification of invasive procedures for treating the local complications of acute pancreatitis based on visualization, route, and purpose. Pancreatology. 2011;11:406-13.
11. Heider R, Meyer AA, Galanko JA, Behrns KE. Percutaneous drainage of pancreatic pseudocysts is associated with a higher failure rate than surgical treatment in unselected patients. Ann Surg. 1999;229:781-7.
12. Van Baal MC, van Santvoort HC, Bollen TL, Bakker OJ, Besselink MG, Gooszen HG, et al. Systematic review of percutaneous catheter drainage as primary treatment for necrotizing pancreatitis. Br J Surg. 2011;98:18-27.
13. Van Santvoort HC, Besselink MG, Bakker OJ, Hofker HS, Boermeester MA, Dejong CH, et al. A step-up approach or open necrosectomy for necrotizing pancreatitis. N Engl J Med. 2010;362: 1491-502.
14. Parekh D. Laparoscopic-assisted pancreatic necrosectomy: a new surgical option for treatment of severe necrotizing pancreatitis. Arch Surg. 2006;141(9):895-902.
15. Zhu JF, Fan XH, Zhang XH. Laparoscopic treatment of severe acute pancreatitis. Surg Endosc. 2001;15:146-8.
16. Zhou ZG, Zheng YC, Shu Y, Hu WM, Tian BL, Li QS, et al. Laparoscopic management of severe acute pancreatitis. Pancreas. 2003;27:e46-50.
17. Raraty MG, Halloran CM, Dodd S, Ghaneh P, Connor S, Evans J, et al. Minimal access retroperitoneal pancreatic necrosectomy: improvement in morbidity and mortality with a less invasive approach. Ann Surg. 2010;251:787-93.
18. Haghshenasskashani A, Laurence JM, Kwan V, Johnston E, Hollands MJ, Richardson AJ, et al. Endoscopic necrosectomy of pancreatic necrosis: a systematic review. Surg Endosc. 2011; 25:3724-30.
19. Bakker OJ, van Santvoort HC, van Brunschot S, Geskus RB, Besselink MG, Bollen TL, et al. Endoscopic transgastric vs surgical necrosectomy for infected necrotizing pancreatitis: a randomized trial. JAMA. 2012;307:1053-61.
20. Ross A, Gluck M, Irani S, Hauptmann E, Fotoohi M, Siegal J, et al. Combined endoscopic and percutaneous drainage of organized pancreatic necrosis. Gastrointest Endosc. 2010;71:79-84.
21. D'Egidio A, Schein M. Pancreatic pseudocysts: a proposed classification and its management implications. Br J Surg. 1991;78:981-4.
22. Nealon WH, Walser E. Main pancreatic ductal anatomy can direct choice of modality for treating pancreatic pseudocysts (surgery versus percutaneous drainage). Ann Surg. 2002;235:751-8.
23. Hammel P, Levy P, Voitot H, Levy M, Vilgrain V, Zins M, et al. Preoperative cyst fluid analysis is useful for the differential diagnosis of cystic lesions of the pancreas. Gastroenterology. 1995;108:1230-5.
24. Sperti C, Pasquali C, Guolo P, Polverosi R, Liessi G, Pedrazzoli S. Serum tumor markers and cyst fluid analysis are useful for the diagnosis of pancreatic cystic tumors. Cancer. 1996;78:237-43.
25. Vitas GJ, Sarr MG. Selected management of pancreatic pseudocysts: operative versus expectant management. Surgery. 1992;111: 123-30.
26. Bassi C, Dervenis C, Butturini G, Fingerhut A, Yeo C, Izbicki J, et al. Postoperative pancreatic fistula: an international study group (ISGPF) definition. Surgery. 2005;138:8-13.
27. Bakker OJ, van Baal MC, van Santvoort HC, Besselink MG, Dutch Pancreatitis Study Group. Endoscopic transpapillary stenting or conservative treatment for pancreatic fistulas in necrotizing pancreatitis: multicenter series and literature review. Ann Surg. 2011;253(5):961-7.
28. Howard TJ, Stonerock CE, Sarkar J, Lehman GA, Sherman S, Wiebke EA, et al. Contemporary treatment strategies for external pancreatic fistulas. Surgery. 1998;124:627-32.
29. Sandrasegaran K, Tann M, Jennings SG, Maglinte DD, Peter SD, Sherman S, et al. Disconnection of the pancreatic duct: an important but overlooked complication of severe acute pancreatitis. Radiographics. 2007;27:1389-400.
30. Solanki R, Koganti SB, Bheerappa N, Sastry RA. Disconnected duct syndrome: refractory inflammatory external pancreatic fistula following percutaneous drainage of an infected peripancreatic fluid collection. A case report and review of the literature. JOP. 2011;12(2):177-80.
31. Pelaez-Luna M, Vege SS, Petersen BT, Chari ST, Clain JE, Levy MJ, et.al. Disconnected pancreatic duct syndrome in severe acute pancreatitis: clinical and imaging characteristics and outcomes in a cohort of 31 cases. Gastrointest Endosc. 2008;68:91-7.
32. Varadarajulu S, Noone TC, Tutuian R, Hawes RH, Cotton PB. Predictors of outcome in pancreatic duct disruption managed by endoscopic transpapillary stent placement. Gastrointest Endosc. 2005;61:568-75.
33. Gonzelez HJ, Sahay SJ, Samadi B, Davidson BR, Rahman SH. Splanchnic vein thrombosis in severe acute pancreatitis: a 2-year, single-institution experience. HPB (Oxford). 2011;13(12):860-4.
34. Flati G, Andrén-Sandberg A, La Pinta M, Porowska B, Carboni M. Potentially fatal bleeding in acute pancreatitis: pathophysiology, prevention, and treatment. Pancreas. 2003;26(1):8-14.

CHAPTER 40

Medical Management of Chronic Pancreatitis

Harpal S Dhaliwal, Saroj K Sinha, Rakesh Kochhar

INTRODUCTION

Chronic pancreatitis (CP), traditionally, has been defined as progressive, permanent and irreversible damage to the pancreas with histological evidence of chronic inflammation, fibrosis and destruction of exocrine (acinar cells) and endocrine (islets of Langerhans) tissue.[1] But this definition based on histology as the reference standard, is imperfect for more than one reason. First, because of its deep retroperitoneal location, pancreatic tissue is difficult and morbid to obtain. Second, the histologic changes of chronic pancreatitis are often patchy and a small biopsy, even if procured, might lead to sampling error. Third, individuals may harbor the histologic features of chronic pancreatitis in the absence of symptoms or complications from the disease. And fourth, the histologic abnormalities of chronic pancreatitis are not pathognomonic and may occur in other conditions as well (such as diabetes, renal failure and aging). Thus, chronic pancreatitis is diagnosed based upon clinical features (pain, exocrine and endocrine insufficiency) combined with radiological abnormalities on plain abdominal radiographs, cross-sectional imaging, endoscopic ultrasonography (EUS) or pancreatography. Chronic pancreatitis is distinguished from acute pancreatitis by the complete recovery of the gland after acute episode in the latter.[1]

EPIDEMIOLOGY

The incidence and prevalence of chronic pancreatitis may vary depending upon the differences in the availability and sophistication of the imaging techniques used, as also the magnitude of risk factors such as alcohol abuse in a particular community. Estimates of annual incidence in western series vary from 3 to 9 cases per 100,000 individuals.[1-3] In a recent nationwide survey in Japan,[4] the annual incidence was 14.4 per 100,000 population which is much higher than the incidence estimated in that country in 1994; and the prevalence also increased from 28.5 per 100,000 to 32.9 in 1999. Epidemiological data from India are scarce. One study from south India found the prevalence of chronic pancreatitis as 126 per 100,000 individuals.[5]

In contrast to this, two prominent autopsy studies have reported chronic pancreatitis in 5.3% and 13% out of 394 and 3821 unselected autopsies, respectively.[6,7] The clinical diagnosis of chronic pancreatitis was made in only 0.5% of those patients and the prevalence of chronic pancreatitis was much higher (11.2–19%) in patients with diabetes mellitus compared to patients without the diagnosis of diabetes (5.3–7%).

ETIOLOGICAL CLASSIFICATION OF CHRONIC PANCREATITIS

Chronic pancreatitis can be due to a number of etiologies. An etiological classification, toxic idiopathic genetic autoimmune recurrent obstructive (TIGAR-O) classification, was proposed by Etemad and Whitcomb in 2001[8] and is summarized in Table 1. The common causes of chronic pancreatitis in India are idiopathic, alcohol, pancreas divisum alone, pancreas divisum along with excessive alcohol consumption, and hyperparathyroidism.[9] Whereas idiopathic chronic pancreatitis is the predominant form reported in most Indian studies, alcohol-related chronic pancreatitis and idiopathic chronic pancreatitis are equally common in north India.[9]

At the molecular level, idiopathic chronic pancreatitis has been linked to a number of genetic mutations. The common genetic mutations found in idiopathic chronic pancreatitis in India[10] are serine protease inhibitor kazal type 1 (SPINK1) mutation (42%), cystic fibrosis transmembrane conductance regulator (CFTR) gene mutation (9%) and CFTR gene polymorphisms

Table 1: Diverse etiologies of chronic pancreatitis (TIGAR-O classification)[8]

1. Toxic/metabolic: 1. Alcohol 2. Tobacco smoking 3. Hypercalcemia 4. Hyperparathyroidism 5. Chronic renal failure 6. Medications 7. Organotin compounds, e.g. dibutyltin dichloride (DBTC).
2. Idiopathic: 1. Early onset 2. Late onset 3. Tropical calcific pancreatitis (TCP) 4. Fibrocalculous pancreatic diabetes (FCPD).
3. Genetic: 1. Autosomal dominant: cationic trypsinogen (codon 29 and 122 mutations in PRSS1) 2. Autosomal recessive/modifier genes: CFTR mutations, SPINK1 mutations, cationic trypsinogen (codon 16, 22, 23 mutations), antitrypsin deficiency.
4. Autoimmune: 1. Isolated autoimmune chronic pancreatitis 2. Syndromic autoimmune chronic pancreatitis: Sjogren syndrome associated chronic pancreatitis, inflammatory bowel disease associated chronic pancreatitis, and primary biliary cirrhosis associated chronic pancreatitis.
5. Recurrent and severe acute pancreatitis: 1. Postnecrotic (severe acute pancreatitis) 2. Recurrent acute pancreatitis 3. Vascular diseases/ischemic pancreatitis 4. Post-irradiation pancreatitis.
6. Obstructive pancreatitis: 1. Pancreas divisum 2. Sphincter of Oddi disorders (controversial) 3. Duct obstruction (e.g. tumor) 4. Periampullary duodenal wall cysts 5. Post-traumatic pancreatic duct scar.

Abbreviations: CFTR, cystic fibrosis transmembrane conductance regulator; SPINK1, serine protease inhibitor kazal type 1.

(41%). Chymotrypsinogen C (CTRC) degrades trypsinogen, and its loss-of-function variants also predispose to idiopathic chronic pancreatitis.[9]

CLINICAL FEATURES

Alcoholic chronic pancreatitis mainly affects men in fourth or fifth decade of life.[11] Idiopathic chronic pancreatitis has early onset (second decade) and late onset (sixth decade) forms, with equal gender distribution.[11] Hereditary disease manifests at around 10 years[12] and tropical pancreatitis at 20–30 years of age.[13] The more common type 1 form of autoimmune disease afflicts males in their sixth decade.[14] The three main clinical manifestations of chronic pancreatitis are abdominal pain, exocrine insufficiency and endocrine insufficiency and these will be discussed in detail subsequently.

Tropical pancreatitis is a type of idiopathic pancreatitis which is diagnosed, if there are following features: onset of disease before 30 years, malnutrition (BMI<18.5 kg/m^2), evidence of large pancreatic calculi and grossly dilated main pancreatic duct (MPD) on imaging, diabetes and absence of other known causes of chronic pancreatitis.[10] It shares similar features with other forms of chronic pancreatitis for pain. But diabetes due to tropical pancreatitis is more ketoacidosis resistant and gross steatorrhea is uncommon, possibly due to the low fat diet consumed by Asians. The disease was reported to have an aggressive course with patients dying in the prime of their lives because of complications related to chronic pancreatitis including pancreatic carcinoma.

In the early years, patients of tropical pancreatitis were very poorly nourished with bilateral parotid gland enlargement. However, with improvement in global nutritional status and enzyme replacement therapy, these features are rarely seen. A recent study has confirmed the significant increase in body mass index and other anthropometric parameters of patients with modern tropical pancreatitis.[15]

Pancreatic calcification is a marker of more advanced pancreatic disease with more extensive gland fibrosis and destruction. Hence, most studies have shown a higher prevalence of endocrine and exocrine insufficiency in calcific pancreatitis compared to non-calcific pancreatitis. But pseudocysts and portal hypertension appear to be more common in non-calcific pancreatitis. It is speculated that in the absence of calcifications, the relatively preserved parenchymal functions lead to more severe and widespread peripancreatic inflammation and a higher frequency of these complications.

DIAGNOSIS

A number of tests are available for the diagnosis of chronic pancreatitis.[1] This bewildering array is not only confusing but also attests to the fact that no individual test is reliable enough to replace the others. In general, the diagnostic tests are divided into two groups, depending upon whether they detect abnormalities of pancreatic function or its structure (Table 2). All of them are more accurate in advanced disease, when gross functional and structural abnormalities have set in. The various tests used are:

Tests of Function

Direct Hormonal Stimulation Test (With Secretin or Cholecystokinin)

They are believed to be the most sensitive tests for the diagnosis of chronic pancreatitis.[16,17] A double-lumen nasoduodenal tube is placed: the gastric lumen is used to aspirate gastric secretions so that they do not dilute the pancreatic secretions after entering the duodenum. The duodenal lumen is used to aspirate the pancreatic juice after intravenous injection of secretin (1 U/kg). Secretin stimulates bicarbonate secretion; maximal bicarbonate concentration less than 80 mEq/L is considered to indicate functional insufficiency. Similarly, the maximal concentration of pancreatic enzymes can be estimated after injecting cholecystokinin (but this is not as commonly used as secretin stimulation).

Direct hormonal stimulation tests have a number of drawbacks: first, being cumbersome, time-consuming and expensive, they are available at only very few referral centers. Second, the institutions offering these tests use their own protocols and there

Table 2: Various tests used to diagnose pancreatic diseases

Tests of function
• Direct hormonal stimulation tests (with secretin or cholecystokinin or both) for bicarbonate and/or enzyme concentration/output in pancreatic juice • Magnetic resonance cholangiopancreatography (MRCP) with secretin stimulation • Fecal elastase • Fecal chymotrypsin • Serum trypsinogen • ^{13}C-mixed triglyceride (^{13}C-MTG) test • Fecal fat estimation (quantitative, semiquantitative, qualitative) • Blood glucose level.
Tests of structure
• Plain abdominal radiograph • Abdominal ultrasonography • Computed tomography • MRI with MRCP • Endoscopic retrograde cholangiopancreaticography (ERCP) • Endoscopic ultrasonography.

Abbreviations: MRI, magnetic resonance imaging; MRCP, magnetic resonance cholangiopancreatography.

is no standardization. Third, they are difficult for the patient to tolerate because of their inherent invasiveness. Fourth, accurate estimation of bicarbonate concentration or enzyme output may be challenging. And fifth, exocrine pancreatic function is frequently disturbed in diseases other than chronic pancreatitis including pancreatic diseases (pancreatic tumors, acute necrotizing pancreatitis, cystic fibrosis, diabetes mellitus), extrapancreatic disorders (celiac disease, Crohn's disease, Zollinger-Ellison syndrome) and postoperative states (gastrectomy and pancreatico-duodenectomy). So, they are not highly specific for the diagnosis of chronic pancreatitis and have to be interpreted in the overall context of patient's symptomatology.

Magnetic Resonance Cholangiopancreatography with Secretin Stimulation (sMRCP)

It provides dynamic information about both ductal morphology and pancreatic function, after secretin injection (0.5 IU/kg). Secretin stimulates fluid and bicarbonate secretion from the ductal cells (and enzymes from acinar cells to a lesser extent) leading to distension of pancreatic ducts and hence their better visualization on magnetic resonance cholangiopancreatography (MRCP).

The subsequent filling of the duodenum with pancreatic secretions (as assessed by the duodenal diameter during MRCP) can be used to evaluate the pancreatic exocrine function semiquantitatively. The mean duodenal diameter on MRCP after secretin injection in mild chronic pancreatitis, severe chronic pancreatitis and healthy controls is 4.12 ± 1.33 mm, 1.70 ± 0.77 mm and 15.38 ± 1.73 mm respectively ($p<0.05$).[18]

With secretin stimulation, the sensitivity of MRCP for detecting chronic pancreatitis changes increases from 77% to 89%, and the negative predictive value from 84% to 98%.[19] The main advantage of sMRCP over direct functional tests is its noninvasiveness and to provide the morphological information of the MPD as well.

Fecal Elastase Levels

Elastase is highly stable along the gastrointestinal transit and hence its fecal levels correlate significantly with the amount produced by the pancreas (i.e. with pancreatic exocrine functions). The methodology for fecal elastase quantification is based upon human-specific monoclonal antibodies; the oral pancreatic enzyme replacement therapy (PERT) which contains porcine enzymes (including proteases), does not interfere with its estimation and need not to be stopped before such estimation.

Fecal elastase concentration more than 200 mcg/grams of stool is considered normal and value less than 50 mcg/grams signifies exocrine dysfunction. Although this test is relatively insensitive to detect mild chronic pancreatitis, its sensitivity for moderate-to-severe chronic pancreatitis is very high, close to 100%.

Fecal Chymotrypsin Activity

Chymotrypsin is variably inactivated during intestinal passage so that its fecal activity does not precisely estimate the pancreatic exocrine functions. Hence, this test is less sensitive than fecal elastase in diagnosing chronic pancreatitis. It is universally normal in mild chronic pancreatitis and in 50% of patients with moderate-to-severe chronic pancreatitis. A low value (<3 U/gm) is taken as cut-off defining the exocrine insufficiency to improve its performance. As PERT interacts with fecal chymotrypsin activity estimation (by the colorimetry-based assay used for this purpose), it should be stopped at least 48 hours preceding the stool sample collection.

For these reasons, the main role of fecal chymotrypsin estimation is not to diagnose pancreatic exocrine dysfunction or chronic pancreatitis but to check the patient's compliance to PERT. The colorimetry-based assay will detect the combined activity of both endogenous and exogenous enzymes. In this context, the fecal chymotrypsin activity should increase substantially, if enzyme supplements are correctly administered.

^{13}C-Mixed Triglyceride Breath Test

In the ^{13}C-mixed triglyceride (^{13}C-MTG) test, patient ingests a small amount of ^{13}C-marked triglycerides along with butter on a piece of toasted bread, after an overnight fast. In the presence of normal lipase activity, ^{13}C-triglycerides will be degraded in the intestinal lumen and ^{13}C-marked fatty acids so released, will be absorbed into circulation. These fatty acids will, in turn, be metabolized in the liver, and $^{13}CO_2$ so produced, can finally be measured in exhaled air. Values below 58% are considered as pathological, and the test has got a sensitivity and specificity of more than 90% for fat maldigestion.[20]

^{13}C-mixed triglyceride is a simple, noninvasive and reasonably accurate test for not only diagnosing chronic pancreatitis but also monitoring the efficacy of PERT in these patients. It is easily performed in routine practice and can be safely repeated as per requirement.

Fecal Fat Estimation

The gold standard for fecal fat quantification is 72-hour fecal collection and fat estimation by chemical titration, first described by van de Kamer. The patient should be on standard diet containing

100 g of daily fat for 5 consecutive days; the whole amount of feces produced over the last 3 days of this period are collected. This is done to minimize the variability that can occur, if the collection period is short. The collected feces are converted (saponified) to potassium salts of fatty acids or soaps by heating in ethanolic potassium hydroxide. The soaps are reacted with hydrochloric acid so that free fatty acids are released, which (after extraction into ether) are titrated against sodium hydroxide to derive the total fatty acid content. Fecal fat quantities more than or equal to 7 grams/day are considered abnormal. Coefficient of fat absorption (CFA) should be used to better quantify the steatorrhea; in healthy subjects, it is usually greater than 80%. CFA is calculated by the equation:

$$\text{CFA}(\%) = 100 \times (\text{mean fat intake} - \text{mean stool fat}) \div \text{mean fat intake}$$

The 72-hour fecal fat quantification has several disadvantages limiting its routine clinical applicability. First, the strict dietary instructions for 5 consecutive days may not be complied by the predominant alcoholic population afflicted by this disorder. Second, the collection and handling of the collected stools in laboratory is highly unpleasant and cumbersome: the stool sample must be first homogenized and then processed following a manual protocol. And third, fecal fat quantification is a nonspecific test, since maldigestion or malabsorption of any etiology could lead to falsely positive test results.

Steatocrit is a more convenient semiquantitative alternative to the 72-hour fecal fat test, as it requires only a single random homogenized stool sample. It has been widely used to assess steatorrhea due to pancreatic insufficiency in pediatric practice. It is akin to the determination of hematocrit of blood by centrifugation, except that the stool suspension separates into three layers (solid, aqueous and fatty layer) in steatocrit, compared to two layers [red blood cells (RBCs) and plasma] in hematocrit. Steatocrit is estimated by using the formula:

$$\text{Steatocrit}(\%) = 100 \times \text{height of fatty layer} \div \text{combined height of fatty and solid layer}$$

Acidification of stool markedly improves the performance of this test.[21] An acid steatocrit value of more than 10% has a high sensitivity (100%) and specificity (95%) for diagnosing steatorrhea when compared to 72-hour quantitative fat analysis.[22]

Sudan III staining on a random stool sample is a qualitative test to assess fecal fat loss. Greater than six droplets of fat per high power field suggest steatorrhea. This test is, however, insensitive and detects steatorrhea only if daily fecal fat loss is more than 25 g.

Although steatocrit and Sudan staining avoid the nuisance of prolonged fecal collection, they suffer many of the drawbacks of 72-hour fecal fat estimation including the need of consuming high fat diet for several days before the collection of stool samples, need to stop the oral enzyme supplements, patient embarrassment and the nonspecificity of test results.

Tests of Structure

Tests of structure are more important practically for making the diagnosis of chronic pancreatitis. Based upon these tests, chronic pancreatitis can be classified as either large duct disease or small duct disease and this classification has got diagnostic as well as therapeutic implications.[1] Large duct disease implies substantial abnormalities of the MPD (>5 mm dilatation on cross-sectional imaging or pancreatography) and small duct disease means lack of these findings (i.e. pancreatic duct less than or equal to 5 mm in diameter). The diagnosis of large duct disease is easy and straightforward, the disease is usually alcohol-related, exocrine and endocrine insufficiency is usually present and the treatment options focus on decompressing the dilated pancreatic duct endoscopically or surgically. On the contrary, small duct disease is more challenging to diagnose as the functional and morphological parameters of the gland can be minimally deranged or equivocal, the etiology is generally idiopathic and the management includes measures other than ductal decompression (Flow chart 1).

The various tests of structure are discussed below:

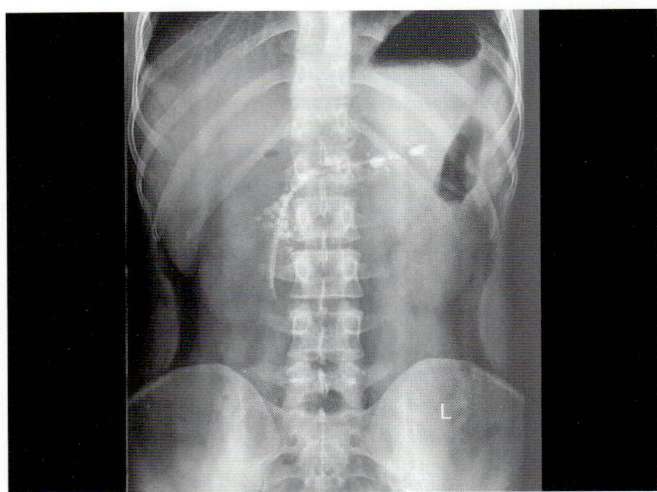

Figure 1 Plain abdominal radiograph showing diffuse, chunky calcification in the pancreatic parenchyma [at the level of lumbar 1 (L1) and L2 vertebrae]. A stent has been placed in the main pancreatic duct

Plain Abdominal Radiographs

Calcifications superimposed on lumbar 2 (L2) or L1 vertebrae, if diffuse, are quite specific for chronic pancreatitis (Fig. 1). However, focal calcification may occur in the tumors of pancreas (cystic and islet cell tumors) and in peripancreatic vessels. Pancreatic calcifications on plain radiographs can be seen in up to 30% of patients with chronic pancreatitis.

Ultrasound

Transabdominal ultrasound is often the first investigation while evaluating a patient presenting with acute or chronic abdominal pain. As such, it is often the first investigation giving a clue to the possibility of chronic pancreatitis by demonstrating dilated pancreatic duct, shadowing ductal stones, altered gland echotexture or by suggesting complications of chronic pancreatitis, e.g. pseudocyst or bile duct obstruction. Various studies have shown a sensitivity of 60–80% and specificity of 80–90% in diagnosing chronic pancreatitis. However, further evaluation is generally needed in the work-up of these patients including cross-sectional imaging or pancreatography.

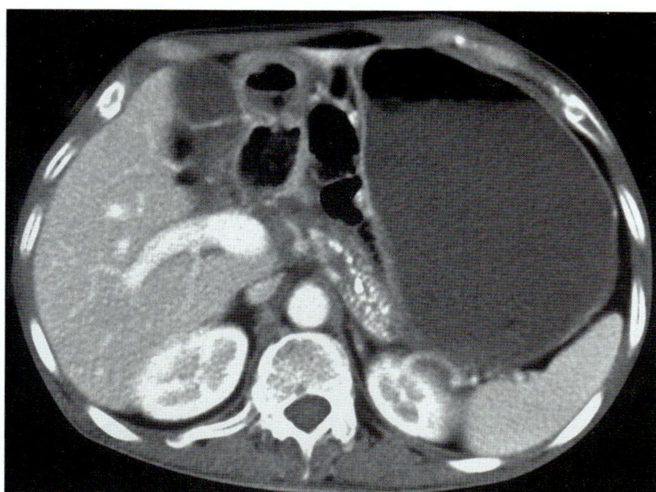

Figure 2 Contrast-enhanced computed tomography of abdomen showing calcification in the body of pancreas

CT or MRI

Both these cross-sectional imaging modalities are more sensitive and specific than ultrasound. Structural abnormalities that can be highly suggestive include changes in the MPD (dilatation, strictures, irregularity or intraductal stones), side branches of MPD (dilatation, irregularity) or pancreatic parenchyma (lobularity of the gland, cysts, enlargement or atrophy). Figure 2 is the CT of a patient with chronic pancreatitis showing calcification in the body of pancreas.

Endoscopic Retrograde Cholangiopancreatography

Endoscopic retrograde cholangiopancreatography (ERCP) can be used as a diagnostic as well as therapeutic tool in patients with chronic pancreatitis (Fig. 3). It can detect dilatations and stenoses of pancreatic duct, pancreatic stones or cysts.[23] Aberrations in the structure of the duct can also be staged by ERCP using the Cambridge classification[24] as detailed in Table 3. The disadvantages of ERCP are the risk of complications seen in around 5% of cases (in as many as 20% of certain high-risk subgroups) leading to a mortality rate of up to 0.5%.

Magnetic Resonance Cholangiopancreatography

Magnetic resonance cholangiopancreatography (MRCP) is fast replacing ERCP as a noninvasive diagnostic modality for chronic pancreatitis with MPD involvement (Fig. 4). It is especially preferred in cases at high risk of post-ERCP pancreatitis or in those with poorly accessible pancreatic duct as a result of gastric or pancreatic surgery.[25] It is superior to ERCP in demonstrating the pancreatic duct distal to an obstructing lesion.

Endoscopic Ultrasound

Endoscopic ultrasound is well-suited to the examination of the retroperitoneal organ pancreas because of the probe's proximity to the pancreatic parenchyma. As higher frequency means lower depth of penetration, transabdominal ultrasound is restricted to a lower frequency (along with associated lower resolution) to overcome the distance between the skin and retroperitoneum. Furthermore, EUS avoids the intervening fat and bowel air that degrade the quality of images of pancreas produced by transabdominal ultrasound.

Table 3: Cambridge grading of chronic pancreatitis[24]

Grade	*Main pancreatic duct*	*Side branches*
Normal	Normal	Normal
Equivocal	Normal	<3 Abnormal
Mild	Normal	≥3 Abnormal
Moderate	Abnormal	>3 Abnormal
Severe	Abnormal with (at least one): • Large cavity (>10 mm) • Obstruction • Filling defect • Severe dilatation or irregularity	>3 Abnormal

Endoscopic ultrasound is better than computed tomography (CT), magnetic resonance imaging (MRI), MRCP and ERCP for diagnosing chronic pancreatitis. Computed tomography and MRI rely on MPD dilatation, moderate-sized cysts and calcifications, all of which are markers of severe disease by the Cambridge criteria. MRCP is slightly better than CT/MRI for detecting MPD irregularity and dilated side branches; however its resolution is too poor to detect the wall irregularity when the ducts are not dilated or minimally dilated. ERCP permits only ductal imaging and not the parenchymal changes (other than the stones in the parenchyma large enough to be radiopaque on plain radiographs). Fibrotic or inflammatory parenchymal changes cannot be assessed with ERCP until they cause ductal irregularity or obstruction. ERCP also carries the risk of invoking pancreatitis.

Endoscopic ultrasound boasts of fine resolution of pancreatic parenchyma, MPD walls and side branches in real-time. It can more reliably identify smaller parenchymal cysts, more subtly dilated or clubbed side branches and a few millimeter specks of calcifications (as shadowing hyperechoic reflections) which can be missed even on computed tomography (Fig. 5). Hence, it is superior to all other modalities, including MRCP and ERCP in patients with early changes of chronic pancreatitis as well as small duct involvement.

Conventionally, EUS diagnosis of chronic pancreatitis relies on nine criteria (four parenchymal and five ductal), each criteria being given equal weightage (Table 4). The finding of only two or less criteria has a high negative predictive value while presence of five or more criteria or calcifications has a high positive predictive value. Fulfillment of 3–4 criteria is considered equivocal.

An expert-based consensus classification system (Rosemont classification)[26] was devised by 32 expert endosonographers in an American Society of Gastrointestinal Endoscopy (ASGE) endorsed international conference in 2007 at Rosemont, Illinois. In contrast to the conventional classification, relative weights to the individual criteria (major A, major B and minor) were given, depending upon its specificity for chronic pancreatitis. The five ductal criteria were the same as in conventional classification but parenchymal criteria were expanded to six from four by further qualifying two of these criteria: hyperechoic foci with or without shadowing, and hypoechoic lobules with or without honeycombing. The details of Rosemont's classification are provided in Table 4.

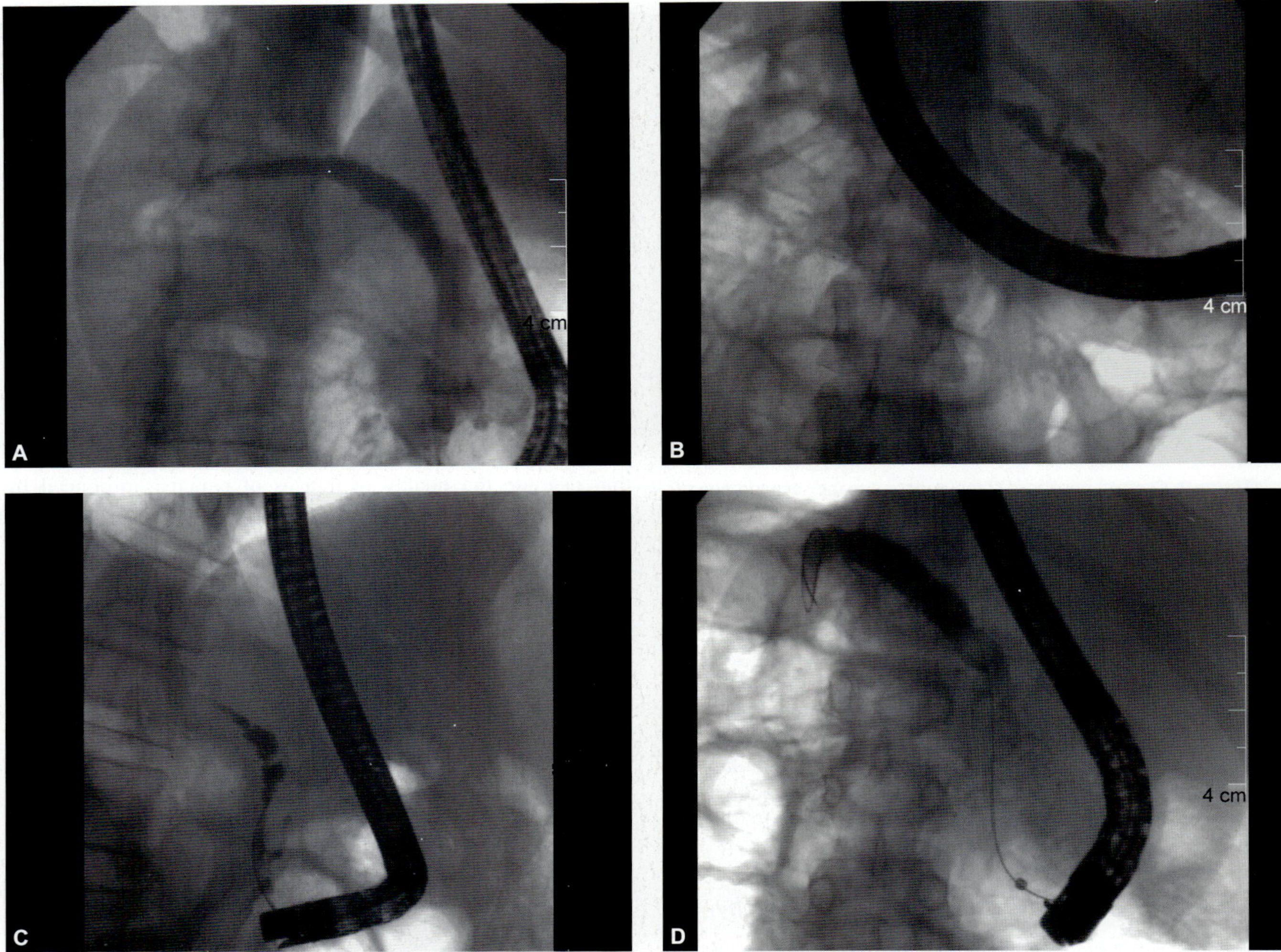

Figures 3A to D Endoscopic retrograde cholangiopancreatography films to show the typical findings on pancreatograms of chronic pancreatitis. (A) uniformly dilated main pancreatic duct with irregular margins; (B) dilated, irregular main pancreatic duct with clubbed side branches; (C) dilated main pancreatic duct with multiple strictures; (D) dilated main pancreatic duct with a proximal filling defect suggestive of intraductal calculus

Prospective studies are needed to establish that the Rosemont's criteria perform better than conventional criteria, have got better inter- and intra-observer agreement and have sufficient advantages justifying its complexity for being more widely used.

MEDICAL MANAGEMENT OF CHRONIC PANCREATITIS

Diet and Life-style Modifications

Historically, a low-fat diet has been recommended in pancreatic exocrine insufficiency (PEI) to reduce steatorrhea. This recommendation has been abandoned in modern dietary counseling due to the risk of aggravating PEI-related weight loss and deficiencies of lipid-soluble vitamins.[27] By optimization of the PERT dose, most patients with PEI will tolerate a normal-fat diet. A fiber-rich diet is to be avoided because the fibrous material interferes with the lipolytic enzyme activity; proteolytic and amylolytic activity is also affected to a lesser extent.

Medium-chain triglycerides (MCTs) have not been shown to be effective in alleviating maldigestion in patients with PEI. Evidence suggests that MCTs also require enzyme supplements for proper digestion and absorption. The energy content of MCTs is limited (8.3 kcal/g) and their poor palatability and high cost reduce patient compliance. They should be used only as a last resort in patients with persistence of symptoms or weight loss despite adequate enzyme supplementation.

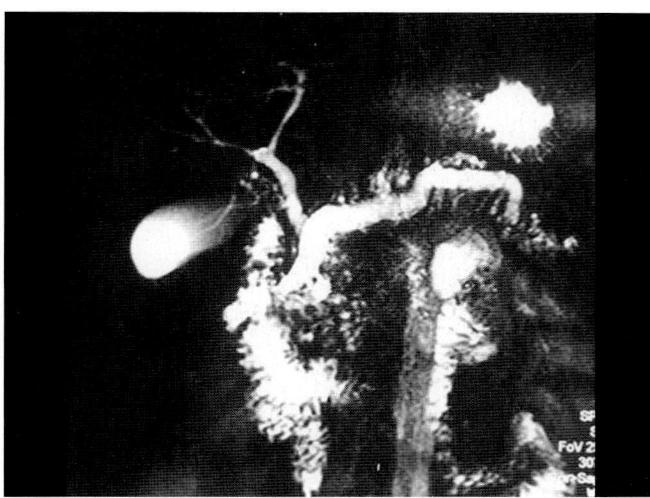

Figure 4 Magnetic resonance cholangiopancreatography showing grossly dilated dorsal pancreatic duct with clubbed side branches, in a patient with chronic pancreatitis due to pancreas divisum

In patients with an alcoholic etiology of chronic pancreatitis, cessation of alcohol beneficially effects the pain and disease progression.[28,29] Moreover, there is increasing data implicating smoking as an important and independent etiological factor for chronic pancreatitis. Cigarette smoking also accelerates the progression of alcohol-related pancreatitis.[30,31] Hence, complete abstinence of alcohol and tobacco consumption is highly recommended in these patients.

Abdominal Pain

Pain is the over-riding symptom in all but ~10% cases of chronic pancreatitis; painless disease is usually seen in elderly patients with idiopathic chronic pancreatitis or patients of autoimmune pancreatitis who might otherwise present with jaundice, steatorrhea or diabetes. Persistent, worsening or recurrent abdominal pain is the most compelling reason that drives patients to seek medical care.

The natural history of abdominal pain varies and its course is difficult to determine in an individual patient. Once it develops, pain generally fluctuates in severity, frequency and character in an unpredictable manner. Pain eventually vanishes in around half of the cases in the natural history of the disease. Few studies have shown the occurrence of pain relief near the time of disease burn-out (development of glandular calcifications and functional failure, i.e. steatorrhea and diabetes).

Chronic pancreatitis is a complex disease with significant heterogeneity in pain mechanisms. Traditionally, ductal hypertension has been held responsible for pain and patients are often subjected to endoscopic or surgical decompression of pancreatic duct. But, since the pain mechanisms are many and complex (Table 5), there might be partial or no response to single modality treatment in a significant proportion of patients. So, a holistic understanding of pathophysiology behind pain genesis is imperative and accordingly patients should be subjected to various medical, endoscopic and surgical modalities of pain relief, as outlined in Flowchart 1. Also, dietary (antioxidant rich diet) and lifestyle (absolute abstinence of alcohol and smoking) modifications need to be thoroughly stressed to all patients at all stages of the disease.

In routine pancreatology practice, after ruling out the causes of pain due to complications, treatment side-effects and unrelated problems, the pancreatic causes are considered (Flow chart 1). The medical therapy is tried first (as detailed below) and is successful in around one-third of all chronic pancreatitis patients. If medical therapy fails, the ductal morphology is reviewed. For the patients with large duct disease (MPD dilatation due to stones/strictures), ductal decompression (endoscopic or surgical) is offered. Those with only pancreatic parenchymal changes, without MPD dilatation, are considered to have small duct disease and are managed by ventral-plasty (V-plasty) or total pancreatectomy with islet cell transplantation. Celiac plexus block (EUS-guided) can be tried but generally, is not as successful as in patients with carcinoma pancreas and pain.

The medical treatment of pain mainly focuses on parenchymal and neural components of pain genesis mechanisms and the various medical options are discussed below:

Analgesics: They can be tried for short-term relief of worsening or recurrent pain. The World Health Organization pain ladder[32] is followed, starting with a nonsteroidal anti-inflammatory drug. Long-term administration of high potency opiates like morphine should be avoided due to the risk of dependence, narcotic bowel syndrome and the fact that they can lead to activation and degranulation of mast cells,[33] thereby worsening the inflammation and neuroimmune interactions. Tramadol, a low potency selective μ-receptor agonist, is as effective as higher potency narcotics, but with a significantly better safety profile.[34] Other options for severe unremitting pain include epidural buprenorphine and transdermal fentanyl patch. An open label randomized crossover trial compared transdermal fentanyl plaster with sustained-release morphine tablets in an equipotent dosage regimen.[35] Patients' preference, pain relief and quality of life were similar in both the groups, but 44% of patients using transdermal fentanyl developed dermatological side-effects. Considering the increased costs incurred by transdermal formulations, it was concluded that they cannot be recommended as first-line route for opioid therapy in chronic pancreatitis, but should be used selectively in patients having trouble with tablet ingestion.

Drugs for neuropathic pain: Tricyclic antidepressants (amitriptyline), serotonin-norepinephrine reuptake inhibitors (SNRIs, e.g. duloxetine) and anticonvulsants (gabapentin and pregabalin) are effective for neuropathic pain and have been used in chronic pancreatitis as well. Pregabalin is an $\alpha 2\delta$ receptor blocker that decreases presynaptic release of glutamate, noradrenaline and substance P; and has been shown to improve pain in chronic pancreatitis by inhibiting central sensitization.[36] A recent randomized controlled trial[37] evaluated the effect of increasing doses (150–600 mg/d) of pregabalin for 3 weeks on pain in 64 patients with chronic pancreatitis; and demonstrated significant pain relief in the pregabalin arm.

The various drugs used for pain relief in chronic pancreatitis along with their usual starting dose and maximum dose in adults are tabulated in Table 6.

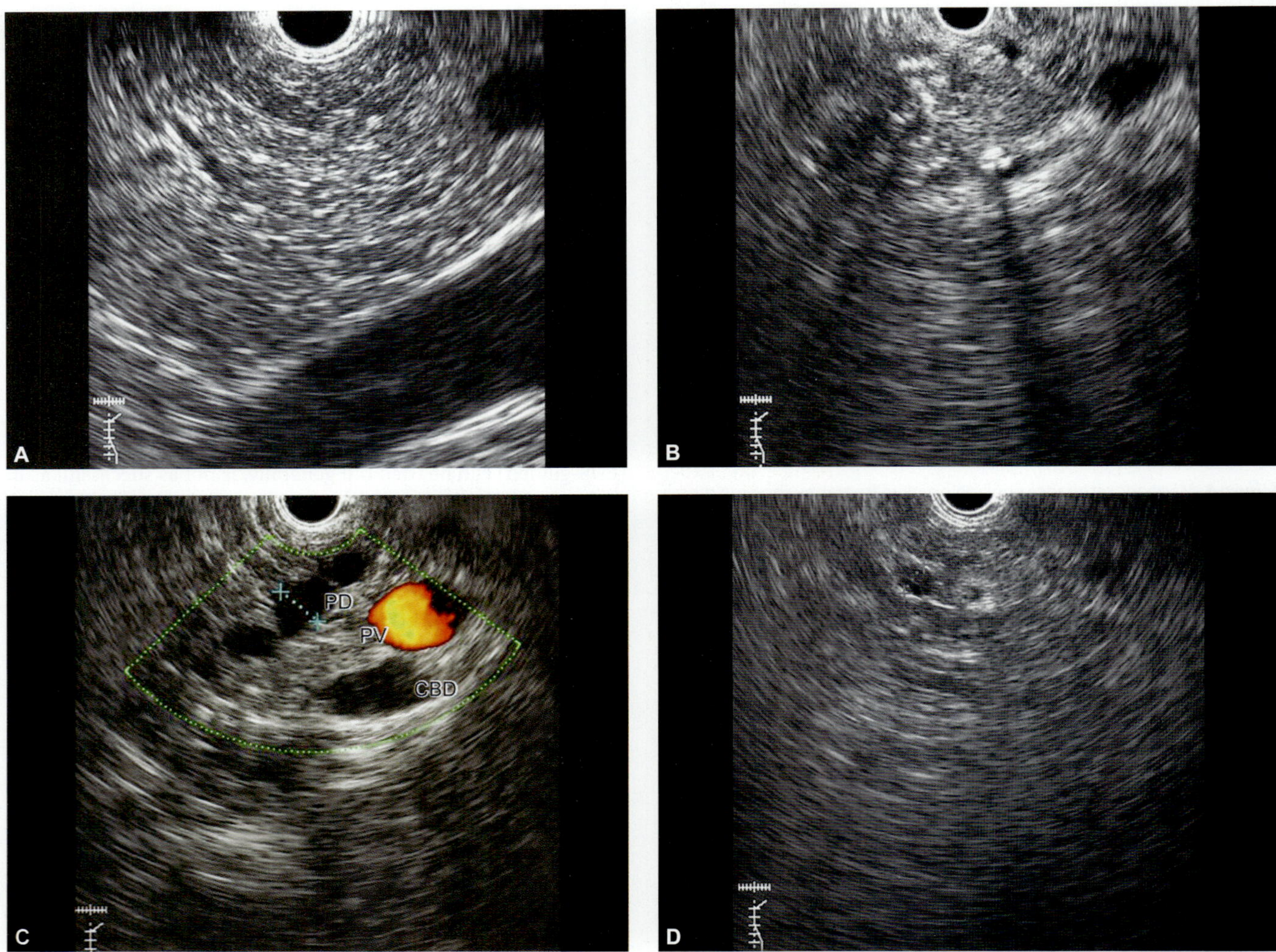

Figures 5A to D Typical linear array echoendoscopic findings in chronic pancreatitis. (A) hyperechoic strands and hyperechoic foci without shadowing in a patient with early chronic pancreatitis; (B) hyperechoic strands and hyperechoic foci with shadowing; (C) transgastric view showing dilated main pancreatic duct (8.8 mm) in the neck region of pancreas, without hyperechoic margins of main pancreatic duct; ((D) transgastric view showing dilated pancreatic duct (6.6 mm) in the body of pancreas, with hyperechoic margins of main pancreatic duct

Antioxidants: It is known that the increase in MPD pressure can activate pancreatic stellate cells (PSCs), which in turn can generate oxidative stress.[38] Also, ethanol and smoking can lead to oxidative stress within the PSCs.[39,40] Oxidative stress generates a pro-inflammatory state by activating immune cells, increasing expression of pro-inflammatory cytokines, and activating cytokine receptors and transcription factors [e.g. tumor necrosis factor alpha, nuclear factor-kappaB (NF-κB)]. Clinical studies have shown a significant reduction in antioxidant defenses in patients with chronic pancreatitis.

Antioxidant therapy in chronic pancreatitis supplies methyl and thiol moieties for the trans-sulfuration pathway, which is essential for protection against reactive oxygen species (ROS) mediated electrophilic stress.[41] Studies have used an antioxidant cocktail consisting of methionine, organic selenium, ascorbic acid, beta carotene, and alpha tocopherol. Methionine preserves the trans-sulfuration pathway in acinar cells and is believed to be the most important antioxidant in the setting of chronic pancreatitis.

Table 4: Endoscopic ultrasound criteria for the diagnosis of chronic pancreatitis

Conventional criteria		
Parenchymal abnormalities	*Ductal abnormalities*	
Hyperechoic foci Hyperechoic strands Hypoechoic lobules Cysts	Main duct dilatation Main duct irregularity Hyperechoic ductal walls Dilated side branches Calcification	
Diagnosis of chronic pancreatitis by the number of conventional criteria fulfilled:		
1–2 criteria: high negative predictive value 3–4 criteria: equivocal ≥5 criteria: high positive predictive value		
Rosemont's criteria[26]		
	Parenchymal abnormalities	*Ductal abnormalities*
Major A	Hyperechoic foci with shadowing	Calculi
Major B	Lobularity with honeycombing	—
Minor	Hyperechoic foci without shadowing	MPD dilatation
	Hyperechoic strands	Irregular MPD contour
	Lobularity without honeycombing	Hyperechoic MPD margins
	Cysts	Dilated side branches
Diagnosis of chronic pancreatitis by Rosemont's criteria:		
Consistent with chronic pancreatitis	1 major A + ≥3 minor features, or 1 major A + major B, or 2 major A features	
Suggestive of chronic pancreatitis	1 major A + <3 minor features, or 1 major B + ≥3 minor features, or ≥5 minor features	
Indeterminate for chronic pancreatitis	3 or 4 minor features, or major B feature alone, or with <3 minor features	
Normal	Two minor features, no major features	

Abbreviation: MPD, main pancreatic duct.

Antioxidants have been extensively used in pain management of chronic pancreatitis patients. A randomized Indian trial by Bhardwaj et al.[42] reported a significant beneficial effect on pain after antioxidant supplementation. This trial used a daily dose of 600 mcg organic selenium, 540 mg ascorbic acid, 9,000 IU beta carotene, 270 IU alpha tocopherol and 2 g methionine for 6 months.

However, these findings were negated by another randomized western trial by Siriwardena et al. (ANTICIPATE study)[43], which showed that antioxidants offered no beneficial effect on pain or quality of life at 6-month evaluation, although the blood levels of antioxidants were significantly raised after the therapy. An important difference between these 2 landmark but contradictory trials may be the different patient populations included in the two.[44] In the Bhardwaj study, most patients were young and undernourished non-alcoholics with idiopathic chronic pancreatitis while the ANTICIPATE study mainly enrolled adult patients with alcohol-related chronic pancreatitis without malnutrition. Similarly, the prevalence of smoking, which is likely an important factor in the pathogenesis of pancreatic pain, was also significantly different (28% vs 80%, respectively). Also, in the Bhardwaj study, a subgroup analysis of the patients with alcohol-related pancreatitis demonstrated no benefit of antioxidants.

Table 5: Causes of pain in chronic pancreatitis

• **Disease-related**
a. Ongoing inflammation leading to neuroimmune interactions between inflammatory cells and nociceptive neurons within the pancreas b. Altered nociception leading to hyperalgesia (exaggerated pain sensation from nociceptive stimuli) and allodynia (pain sensation triggered by a normal non-painful stimuli) due to neuropathic/neuroplastic mechanisms: – Neural edema and perineural disruption – Schwann cell proliferation – Neural hypertrophy and sprouting c. Self-perpetuating pain, in the absence of stimuli, due to: – Visceral nerve sensitization – Central nervous system sensitization d. Ductal hypertension e. Parenchymal hypertension f. Tissue ischemia g. Oxidative stress leading to the genesis of reactive oxygen species.
• **Complications-related**
a. Inflammatory mass in the head of pancreas b. Obstruction of the bile duct or duodenum c. Pseudocyst d. Carcinoma of pancreas.
• **Treatment-related**
Opiate gastroparesis or constipation.
• **Unrelated causes**
a. Peptic ulcer b. Gallstones c. Mesenteric ischemia d. Small bowel stricture e. Somatic (e.g. surgical scar).

Pancreatic enzymes: The proteases in pancreatic enzyme supplements degrade cholecystokinin (CCK) releasing factor (secreted from the duodenal mucosa) so that the plasma CCK levels are lowered. The elevated CCK stimulates exocrine pancreas and causes pain by increasing intraductal pressures (CCK-A receptors).[45] It also causes direct activation of nociceptive pathways in the central nervous system (CCK-B receptors).[46]

The duodenal protease activity is only seen with non-enteric coated formulations and studies using such formulations have documented improvement in pain.[47,48] Due to reduced bicarbonate secretion in chronic pancreatitis, release of the enzymes from enteric-coated preparations (which occurs at pH >5.5) in the duodenum is erratic and they are generally released more distally in the jejunum and ileum. In line with this, most studies using enteric-coated enzymes (which cannot degrade the

Flow chart 1 Management of pain in chronic pancreatitis

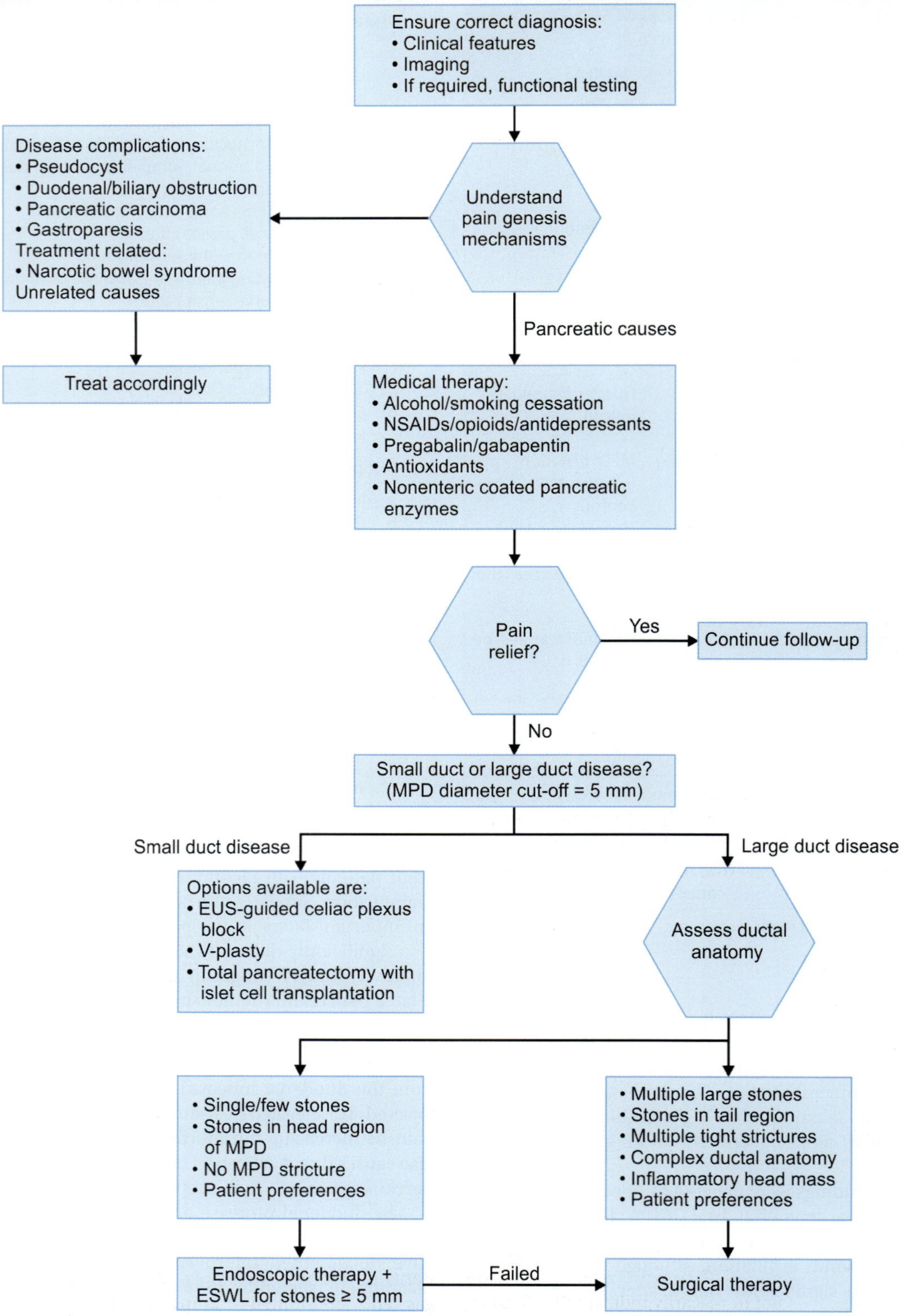

Ensure correct diagnosis:
- Clinical features
- Imaging
- If required, functional testing

Understand pain genesis mechanisms

Disease complications:
- Pseudocyst
- Duodenal/biliary obstruction
- Pancreatic carcinoma
- Gastroparesis

Treatment related:
- Narcotic bowel syndrome

Unrelated causes

Treat accordingly

Pancreatic causes

Medical therapy:
- Alcohol/smoking cessation
- NSAIDs/opioids/antidepressants
- Pregabalin/gabapentin
- Antioxidants
- Nonenteric coated pancreatic enzymes

Pain relief?

Yes

Continue follow-up

No

Small duct or large duct disease? (MPD diameter cut-off = 5 mm)

Small duct disease

Options available are:
- EUS-guided celiac plexus block
- V-plasty
- Total pancreatectomy with islet cell transplantation

Large duct disease

Assess ductal anatomy

- Single/few stones
- Stones in head region of MPD
- No MPD stricture
- Patient preferences

- Multiple large stones
- Stones in tail region
- Multiple tight strictures
- Complex ductal anatomy
- Inflammatory head mass
- Patient preferences

Endoscopic therapy + ESWL for stones ≥ 5 mm

Failed

Surgical therapy

Abbreviations: NSAIDs, nonsteroidal anti-inflammatory drugs; MPD, main pancreatic duct; EUS-guided, endoscopic ultrasonography-guided; V-plasty, ventral plasty; ESWL, extracorporeal shock wave lithotripsy.

Table 6: Drugs used in chronic pancreatitis for pain relief and their dosages for adults

Drug	*Starting dose*	*Maximum dose*	*Comment*
Acetaminophen	650 mg PO 4–6 hourly	4 grams/day	Side-effects uncommon
Ibuprofen	200–400 mg PO 4–6 hourly	3200 mg/day	More potent than acetaminophen
Ketorolac	15 mg IV/IM 6 hourly	120 mg/day	Available for parenteral use
Indomethacin	25 mg PO 8 hourly	200 mg/day	GI side-effects common
Tramadol	50 mg PO 6 hourly	400 mg/day	Mixed opioid/adrenergic action
Codeine sulphate	15–60 mg PO 4 hourly	360 mg/day	Nausea common
Morphine	4–15 mg IV 4 hourly 5–30 mg PO 4 hourly	1600 mg/day orally in opioid tolerant patients	High risk of opioid dependence
Levorphanol	1–2 mg IV 6–8 hourly 2–4 mg PO 6–8 hourly	16 mg/day	Longer acting than morphine
Amitryptyline	10–25 mg PO HS	150 mg/day	Variety of GI, neurological and cardiac side-effects at high dose
Fluoxetine	20 mg PO daily	80 mg/day	Fewer side-effects than tricyclic antidepressants; Also less effective in relieving pain
Duloxetine	20 mg PO daily	60 mg/day	May cause nausea, constipation
Pregabalin	75 mg PO 12 hourly	600 mg/day	Inhibits central sensitization
Gabapentin	900 mg PO daily	3600 mg/day	Less preferred than pregabalin

Abbreviations: GI, gastrointestinal; IV, intravenous; PO, per oral; IM, intramuscular; HS, hour of sleep.

CCK-releasing factor present in the duodenum) have not shown any improvement on pain measures.

In the 2 studies[47,48] which demonstrated pain relief with pancreatic enzymes, the predictors of response were early disease (small duct chronic pancreatitis), female sex and idiopathic chronic pancreatitis. On the other hand, patients with large-duct disease (mainly advanced alcoholic chronic pancreatitis) generally do not respond well. The usual dose of pancreatic enzymes for pain relief is 240,000 ubiquitin-specific proteases (USP) of protease (8 tablets of Viokase-8) with meals and at night. It is important to prescribe non-enteric preparations along with a proton pump inhibitor in order to protect the enzymes from gastric acid mediated inactivation in the stomach.

Pancreatic Exocrine Insufficiency

Pancreatic exocrine insufficiency (PEI) is a state of maldigestion as a result of reduced pancreatic enzyme activity in the intestinal lumen to a level below the threshold required to maintain normal digestion. This concept is crucial to understand two consequences important for diagnosing and treating PEI. First, pancreatic exocrine secretion can be significantly reduced without PEI being present. In a landmark paper, DiMagno et al.[49] demonstrated that steatorrhea only occurs when pancreatic lipase output is reduced to less than 10% of normal. Hence, the demonstration of moderately reduced bicarbonate or enzyme output in sensitive tests of pancreatic secretion, such as the secretin/cholecystokinin stimulation test or fecal elastase-1, although a reliable indicator of chronic pancreatitis, does not necessarily indicate PEI. Second, any pathology, including extrapancreatic conditions that interrupt the chain of events required for the normal digestion of ingested food by pancreatic enzymes, may cause PEI. Examples include Zollinger-Ellison syndrome (in which excess acid inactivates the pancreatic enzymes and precipitates the bile salts) and upper gastrointestinal surgery (which leads to impaired mixing of ingested food and the pancreatic enzymes).

The progression to exocrine burn-out of the gland depends on the etiology of chronic pancreatitis. Patients with alcohol-related pancreatitis develop exocrine failure as early as 10 years of disease onset, while this only occurs after 20 to 25 years in idiopathic chronic pancreatitis.[10] Furthermore, in autoimmune pancreatitis, PEI is one of the presenting feature in more than 75% of cases.[50,51]

In general, in PEI, fat maldigestion predates and is clinically more apparent than carbohydrate or protein maldigestion. Several factors are responsible for that. First, fat is primarily digested by lipase and co-lipase of pancreatic origin, whereas other digestive enzymes have extrapancreatic sources as well. Second, with the progression of functional failure in chronic pancreatitis, lipase output diminishes earlier and more rapidly compared with the production of other pancreatic enzymes. Third, pancreatic lipase is much more acid-labile than other enzymes. Low bicarbonate secretion in chronic pancreatitis predisposes to a fall in pH of duodenum and lipase in particular gets inactivated. And lastly, the acidic duodenal pH also precipitates bile salts; thus mixed micelles are not formed and lipid digestion and absorption is further impaired.[1]

Clinical features of PEI: Steatorrhea (loose, greasy, foul-smelling stools that are difficult to flush) is a feature of advanced chronic pancreatitis. Under such circumstances, patient may even pass frank oil-droplets in stools. Watery diarrhea, bloating, excess gas and abdominal cramps are rare and generally suggest malabsorption of small bowel origin. Even with substantial amount of fecal fat loss, most patients have only three or four motions per day and some may have only one.[1]

Fat malabsorption in chronic pancreatitis predisposes to deficiencies of fat-soluble vitamins (vitamin A, D, E and K).

Particularly common in this population is the vitamin D deficiency, which may lead to symptomatic metabolic bone disease with associated morbidity.

Diagnosis of PEI: Steatorrhea, weight loss and diarrhea are indicators of symptomatic severe PEI and are strong reasons to start PERT. However, many patients lack these overt features of PEI but still may be harboring subclinical malabsorption, which can only be identified by sensitive tests of pancreatic function.

The ^{13}C-mixed triglycerides (^{13}C-MTG) breath test is considered the most physiological test for diagnosing PEI, as it directly measures the clinically most relevant end-effect of pancreatic exocrine function: the degradation of triglycerides. This makes this test preferable to the tests that measure pancreatic secretion (such as the secretin/CCK test or fecal elastase-1 assay) which are more useful to diagnose chronic pancreatitis rather than PEI. ^{13}C-MTG breath test is, however, only sparsely done in few specialized centers across the globe and is not available ubiquitously. CFA calculation after 72-hour fecal collection and fat estimation can also be used to diagnose PEI, although this test has a number of limitations, as previously discussed.

PEI can be predicted with reasonable certainty by the number of EUS criteria for chronic pancreatitis fulfilled in an individual patient. Patients with more than or equal to 8 EUS criteria have a probability of more than 70% of having PEI.[52] Moreover, specific criteria are significantly associated with PEI. MPD calculi suggest PEI with a probability of 80% and this increases to 83%, if additionally, MPD dilatation is also present. On the other hand, the probability reduces to mere 12%, if both of these features are absent.[52]

Management of PEI: Cornerstones in the treatment of PEI are PERT, cessation of smoking and alcohol abuse, consultation with a dietician and a systematic follow-up to ensure optimal treatment effect. The goal of this treatment concept is to normalize digestion, alleviate PEI-related symptoms and prevent malnutrition-related morbidity and mortality.

Modern pancreatic enzyme preparations are extracts from the porcine pancreas that are administered as enteric-coated mini-microspheres. PERT is started at 50,000 lipase units per major meal and 25,000 lipase units per snack; these doses can be doubled if there is lack of response. PERT should be taken with meals and the dose should be adjusted to the fat content of the meal. If maldigestion persists, proton pump inhibitors can be added. If PERT is still ineffective, despite the optimization described above, alternative possibilities (small intestinal bacterial overgrowth and celiac disease) are considered, and the evidence for the diagnosis of PEI is revised (Flow chart 2).

In general, PERT is very well tolerated. Rare side-effects include flatulence, bloating, abdominal cramps, allergic reactions, hyperuricemia, hyperuricosuria, iron and folate deficiency, and Salmonella infections. The most feared but fortunately very rare complication is fibrosing colonopathy, which was only reported in children with cystic fibrosis given very high doses of PERT.

Monitoring of treatment response in PEI: Fecal fat quantification or ^{13}C-MTG breath test are the most appropriate methods for verifying elimination of fat maldigestion. However, this approach may not be feasible in clinical practice. Most guidelines recommend a re-evaluation of symptoms, weight and serum markers of malnutrition (hemoglobin, albumin, prealbumin and retinol-binding protein).

A recent randomized, double-blind, placebo-controlled trial in chronic pancreatitis patients has established the substantial therapeutic efficacy of modern enzyme preparations in decreasing stool frequency, improving its consistency and reducing the amount of fat excretion.[53] These findings have been confirmed by means of ^{13}C-MTG breath test, measurement of CFA and assessment of nutritional parameters in another prospective study on 49 patients of chronic pancreatitis with fat maldigestion.[20]

Flow chart 2 Management of pancreatic exocrine insufficiency

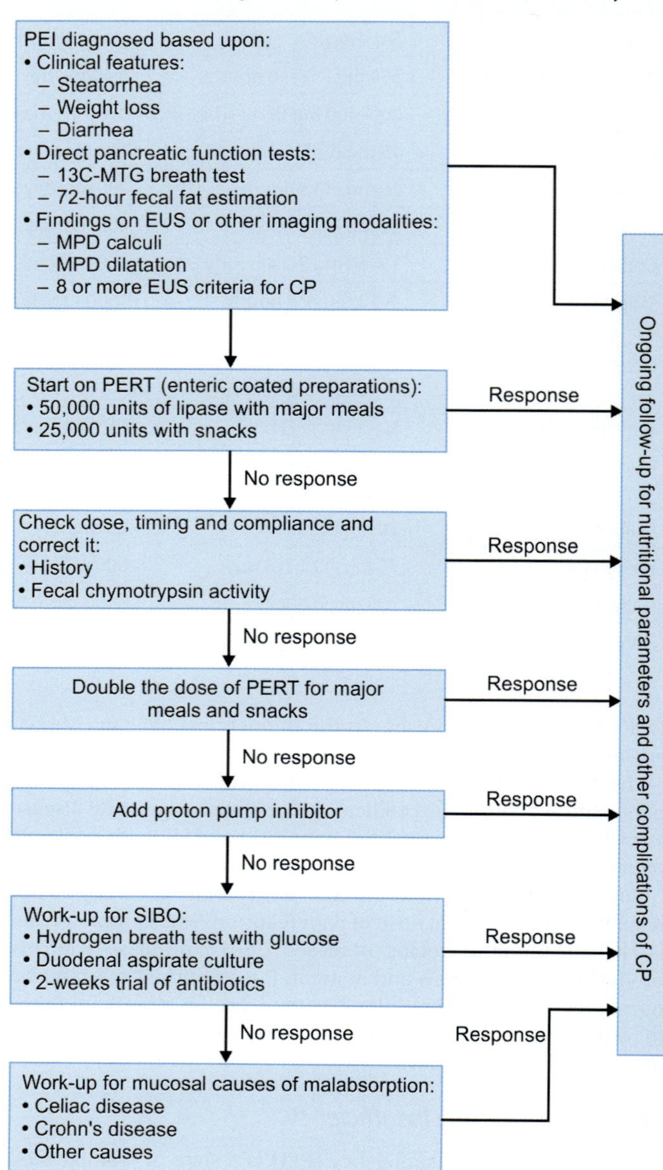

Abbreviations: PEI, pancreatic exocrine insufficiency; ^{13}C-MTG, ^{13}C-mixed triglyceride; EUS, endoscopic ultrasonography; CP, chronic pancreatitis; PERT, pancreatic enzyme replacement therapy; SIBO, small intestinal bacterial overgrowth.

PEI in cystic fibrosis: Cystic fibrosis is a rare autosomal recessive disease that affects the lung and pancreatic functions from birth. The thick mucus blocks the small airways and the pancreatic ducts leading to dyspnea and pancreatic dysfunction. Around 85% of patients with cystic fibrosis have some evidence of PEI, clinically or sub-clinically. Standard treatment of this disease comprises of chest physiotherapy, aerosolized antibiotics, mucolytics and pancreatic enzyme supplements.

Several randomized placebo-controlled trials have established that PERT ameliorates the symptoms and improves the coefficients of fat and nitrogen absorption in patients with cystic fibrosis, with favorable safety profiles. However, very high doses of PERT in pediatric cystic fibrosis have been associated with fibrosing colonopathy. Hence, maximum dose of PERT used in children should not exceed 10,000 IU lipase/kg/day.

Pancreatogenic Diabetes

Pancreatogenic or type 3c diabetes (T3cDM) occurs due to inherited or acquired diseases of the pancreas or its resection. T3cDM accounts for up to 10% of the western diabetic population; 75% of this burden is attributed to chronic pancreatitis. Depending upon the etiology, extent of calcification and duration of the disease, 40–80% of patients with chronic pancreatitis develop diabetes and its spectrum ranges from mild to severe disease. In its extreme form (brittle diabetes), the condition is difficult to manage because of a paradoxical combination of accentuated peripheral insulin sensitivity and attenuated hepatic insulin sensitivity. Without insulin replacement, progressive hyperglycemia sets in and the affected patients have the same long-term risk of microvascular complications as diabetes mellitus type 1 (T1DM) patients, owing to persistently high levels of glycosylated proteins. However, they quickly turn hypoglycemic when insulin therapy is barely excessive, as a consequence of the increased peripheral insulin sensitivity and low glucagon secretion from the diseased gland. Moreover, blood glucose control may be extremely labile because of carbohydrate malabsorption, variable alcohol intake and inconsistent eating patterns due to pain.

Ascribing diabetes mellitus to chronic pancreatitis (hence labeling it as T3cDM) can be challenging at times. Patients with long-standing T1DM or T2DM may develop features of pancreatic functional insufficiency and patients with diabetes mellitus are at higher risk of developing acute or chronic pancreatitis anyway. Moreover, patients with already diagnosed chronic pancreatitis may also develop T2DM or T1DM, independently of pancreatitis-related failure of the gland. In distinguishing between the different diabetes types, the presence of islet cell antibodies is consistent with T1DM, and the presence of clinical or biochemical evidence of insulin resistance is associated with T2DM. Specific diagnostic criteria for T3cDM have been proposed[54] and are tabulated in Table 7.

Table 7: Diagnostic criteria for T3cDM, as proposed by Evald et al.[54]

Major criteria (must be present):
• Presence of pancreatic exocrine insufficiency (as detected by fecal elastase-1 test or direct function tests) • Pathological pancreatic imaging (endoscopic ultrasound, MRI, CT) • Absence of type 1 diabetes mellitus associated autoimmune markers
Minor criteria:
• Absent pancreatic polypeptide secretion • Impaired incretin secretion (e.g., GLP-1) • No excessive insulin resistance (e.g., HOMA-IR) • Impaired beta cell function (e.g., HOMA-B, C-Peptide/glucose-ratio) • Low serum levels of lipid soluble vitamins (A, D, E and K)

Abbreviations: MRI, magnetic resonance imaging; CT, computed tomography; GLP-1, glucagon-like peptide-1; HOMA-IR, homeostasis model assessment of insulin resistance; HOMA-B, homeostasis model assessment of beta cell.

Pathophysiology of pancreatogenic diabetes: Although the predominant cause is relative insulin deficiency, T3cDM has a unique pattern of endocrine and metabolic disturbances, not shared by other forms of diabetes. Hepatic insulin resistance, characteristic of T3cDM, occurs due to deficient pancreatic polypeptide (PP) secretion from the diseased gland, while peripheral insulin sensitivity is increased because of relative hypoinsulinemia. The secretion of the enteric glucoregulatory hormones [incretins: glucose-dependent insulinotropic peptide (GIP) and glucagon-like peptide 1 (GLP-1)] is impaired because of protein and fat malabsorption.[55,56] The pancreatic alpha cells are also affected; as a result of depressed glucagon production, patients are at an increased risk of both spontaneous and treatment-related hypoglycemia. The combined multi-hormonal abnormalities of T3cDM due to chronic pancreatitis therefore result in a severely perturbed endocrine environment which is, however, different than the pattern of abnormalities seen in either T1DM or T2DM.

Complications of pancreatogenic diabetes: Diabetic ketoacidosis (DKA) is distinctly uncommon in pancreatogenic diabetes. There are several reasons for that: relatively preserved beta cell function (and hence insulin secretion) compared to patients with T1DM; diminished production of glucagon, an important ketogenic stimulus and depleted adipose tissue stock of triglycerides (because of malabsorption), a key substrate for ketogenesis. Nevertheless, rare case reports of ketoacidosis in chronic pancreatitis are available. Four important settings for the development of DKA in chronic pancreatitis are: infection coupled with non-compliance to antidiabetic medications, acute exacerbation of chronic pancreatitis, use of potent enzyme supplementations and after pancreatic duct decompression. The last two factors lead to correction of maldigestion, resulting in an increase in body fat stores, thereby increasing the predisposition to ketoacidosis. O'Keefe et al.[57] studied the effect of potent pancreatic enzyme supplements in patients with chronic pancreatitis, a significant number of whom were taking insulin for the control of diabetes. The enzyme supplements led to abnormally high blood glucose levels in most of the patients, one of whom developed DKA as well.

Until the 1980s, it was assumed that microvascular complications were rare in all secondary forms of diabetes including pancreatogenic diabetes. The basis of this belief might be the fact that patients succumb to the primary illness (responsible for diabetes) long before they could develop such complications, which typically evolve after 10–15 years duration of persistent hyperglycemia. Subsequent studies, therefore, clearly showed that if patients are followed-up long enough, microvascular complications in secondary diabetes do occur with the same frequency and severity as they are otherwise known in diabetes mellitus. For example, Barman et al.[58] in their study on 277 patients of fibrocalculus pancreatic diabetes (FCPD), matched with an equal number of controls with T2DM, showed that the retinopathy was as frequent in FCPD (36.1%) as it was in T2DM (37.2%). Mohan et al.[59] performed the fundoscopic evaluation of 40 patients with tropical pancreatic diabetes and diabetic retinopathy was diagnosed in 13 patients. Three patients had proliferative retinopathy which required laser photocoagulation and two more patients had diabetic maculopathy. So, even severe forms of retinopathy are known in pancreatogenic diabetes. Similarly, nephropathy and neuropathy are equally common in pancreatogenic diabetes compared to diabetes mellitus of similar duration.

Special considerations in pancreatogenic diabetes: There is a growing body of basic and clinical research which implies that special considerations are needed for the treatment of T3cDM, in the light of high risk of pancreatic malignancy and associated exocrine insufficiency (leading to metabolic complications). Epidemiologic studies suggest that several risk factors associated with pancreatic malignancy independently operate in these patients: chronic pancreatitis per se, diabetes per se, various antidiabetic drugs (insulin, insulin secretagogues, incretin analogs and dipeptidyl peptidase-4 inhibitors) and other factors like smoking, etc.

Chronic pancreatitis and diabetes are both risk factors which promote the development of pancreatic cancer, as shown in several epidemiologic studies.[60,61] The risk of pancreatic cancer is increased 10–20 fold in patients with chronic pancreatitis.[61] Jee et al. similarly found a positive linear relationship between fasting glucose and the risk of developing pancreatic cancer across all categories of obesity in a cohort analysis of 1,298,385 Korean patients.[62]

Recent cohort and population-based studies also propose that antidiabetic medications differentially alter the risk of developing pancreatic carcinoma; insulin and sulfonylureas clearly increase the risk.[63,64] Concerns have been raised over incretin-based antidiabetic therapies, in view of their trophic effects on the pancreas.[65] A recent analysis of adverse outcomes from the Food and Drug Administration database also revealed a 2.9-fold higher incidence of pancreatic cancer with exenatide and sitagliptin usage, in comparison with other antidiabetic medications.[66] On the contrary, metformin therapy reduces the risk of pancreatic carcinoma by as much as 60%.[64,67] Metformin should, therefore, be the first line of therapy in T3cDM and continued, if additional insulin needs to be started for achieving euglycemia.

Management of pancreatogenic diabetes: There are no specific recommendations for the treatment of T3cDM in the current standards of medical care in diabetes, published by the American Diabetes Association, nor are there any prospective randomized trials of therapy in T3cDM. This serves to perpetuate the widespread misconception that T3cDM is managed exactly on the lines of T1DM and T2DM.

The goal of therapy in T3cDM is reduction in hemoglobin A1c (HbA1c) levels below 7%. The treatment should probably always incorporate metformin, so as to exploit its beneficial effects on the risk of pancreatic carcinoma. The initial choice of insulin versus metformin therapy depends on the clinical presentation of the patient. For patients presenting with DKA or who are profoundly hyperglycemic (fasting glucose >180 mg/dL and/or HbA1c levels >8.5%) and catabolic with glycosuria and weight loss, insulin treatment is directly started. Metformin should be added as early as possible. For all other patients, metformin is the first line therapy and insulin is only added, if blood sugars are not controlled with maximal dose of metformin (2 grams/day). Due to the enhanced peripheral sensitivity to insulin, dose of insulin required to achieve and maintain glycemic control is significantly less than that used in other insulin-dependent patients.

The management of T3cDM should also incorporate concentrated efforts to correct lifestyle factors contributing to hyperglycemia and the risk of malignancy. Weight reduction in obese patients, physical activity, low carbohydrate diet, abstinence of alcohol and smoking are critical elements which should be reinforced at every visit.

In patients with T3cDM, PEI is nearly ubiquitous.[54] This not only contributes to nutritional deficiencies and the development of metabolic bone disease, but also to poor glycemic control due to defective release of incretins from the gut.[55,56] PERT is therefore required in virtually all patients with T3cDM.[54]

OTHER COMPLICATONS OF CHRONIC PANCREATITIS

Apart from pain, exocrine and endocrine insufficiency, chronic pancreatitis is associated with other complications like pseudocysts, gastrointestinal bleeding due to pseudoaneurysms, pancreatic fistulas (internal or external), bile duct obstruction, duodenal obstruction and malignancy. The management of these complications requires a multidisciplinary approach involving the endoscopists, interventional radiologists and surgeons and is beyond the scope of this review.

Studies on the natural history of chronic pancreatitis have indicated a higher mortality and significantly reduced life-span in these patients. In a nationwide retrospective cohort study, data of 11,972 patients of chronic pancreatitis were collected from Danish registries from 1995 through 2010 and compared with 119,720 age- and sex-matched controls.[68] Patients with chronic pancreatitis had a 5-fold increased risk of death and their life expectancy was approximately 8 years less compared with the controls. In this cohort, younger patients in particular had a higher risk of death. Pancreatic cancer was the most common cause of death among chronic pancreatitis patients.[68]

REFERENCES

1. Forsmark CE. Chronic pancreatitis. Sleisenger and Fordtran's Gastrointestinal and liver disease. 10th edition.
2. O'Aullivan JN, Norbrega FT, Morlock CG, Brown AL, Bartholomew LG. Acute and chronic pancreatitis in Rochester, Minnesota 1940-1969. Gastroenterology. 1973;62:373-9.
3. Anderson BN, Pedersen NT, Scheel J, Worning H. Incidence of alcoholic chronic pancreatitis in Copenhagen. Scand J Gastroenterol. 1982;17:247-52.
4. Otsuki M. Chronic pancreatitis in Japan: epidemiology, prognosis, diagnostic criteria and future problems. J Gastroenterol. 2003;38:315-26.
5. Balaji LN, Tandon RK, Tandon BN, Banks PA. Prevalence and clinical features of chronic pancreatitis in southern India. Int J Pancreatol. 1994;15:29-34.
6. Joshi RA, Probstein JG, Blumenthal HT. A survey of experiences with three hundred clinical and one hundred and eight autopsy cases of acute pancreatitis. Am Surg. 1957;23:34-42.
7. Olsen TS. The incidence and clinical relevance of chronic inflammation in the pancreas in autopsy material. Acta Pathol Microbiol Scand. 1978;86A:361-5.
8. Etemad B, Whitcomb DC. Chronic pancreatitis: diagnosis, classification and new genetic developments. Gastroenterology. 2001;120:682-707.
9. Sinha SK, Kochhar R. Is the profile of chronic pancreatitis in India changing? Indian J Gastroenterol. 2014;33:216-8.

10. Midha S, Khajuria R, Shastri S, Kabra M, Garg PK. Idiopathic chronic pancreatitis in India: phenotypic characterization and strong genetic susceptibility due to SPINK1 and CFTR gene mutations. Gut. 2010;59:800-7.
11. Layer P, Yamamoto H, Kalthoff L, Clain JE, Bakken LJ, DiMagno EP. The different courses of early and late onset idiopathic and alcoholic chronic pancreatitis. Gastroenterology. 1994;107:1481-87.
12. Rosendahl J, Bodeker H, Mossner J, Teich N. Hereditary chronic pancreatitis. Orphanet J Rare Dis. 2007;2:1.
13. Barman KK, Premalatha G, Mohan V. Tropical chronic pancreatitis. Postgrad Med J. 2003;79:606-15.
14. Park DH, Kim MH, Chiari S. Recent advances in autoimmune pancreatitis. Gut. 2009;58:1680-89.
15. Padmalayam I, John S, Mohan V, Ramchandran A, Viswanathan M. Anthropometric studies in diabetes in the tropics. Acta Diabetol Lat. 1991;28:55-60.
16. Chowdhury RS, Forsmark CE. Pancreatic function testing. Aliment Pharmacol Ther. 2003;17:733-50.
17. Niederau C, Grendell JH. Diagnosis of chronic pancreatitis. Gastroenterology. 1985;88:1973.
18. Czako L. Diagnosis of early-stage chronic pancreatitis by secretin-enhanced magnetic resonance cholangiopancreatography. J Gastroenterol. 2007;42:113-7.
19. Hellerhoff KJ, Helmberger H 3rd, Rosch T, Settles MR, Link TM, Rummeny EJ. Dynamic MR pancreatography after secretin administration: image quality and diagnostic accuracy. AJR Am J Roentgenol. 2002;179:121-9.
20. Dominguez-Munoz JE, Iglesias-Garcia J, Vilarino-Insua M, Iglesias-Rey M, Lourido V. 13C-mixed triglyceride breath test to assess the oral enzyme substitution therapy in patients with chronic pancreatitis. Clin Gastroenterol Hepatol. 2007;5:484-8.
21. Tran M, Forget P, Van den Neucker A, Strik J, van Kreel B, Kuijten R. The acid steatocrit: a much improved method. J Pediatr Gastroenterol Nutr. 1994;19:299-303.
22. Amann ST, Josephson SA, Toskes PP. Acid steatocrit: a simple, rapid gravimetric method to determine steatorrhea. Am J Gastroenterol. 1997;92:2280-4.
23. Witt H, Apte MV, Keim V, Wilson JS. Chronic pancreatitis: challenges and advances in pathogenesis, genetics, diagnosis and therapy. Gastroenterology. 2007;132:1557-73.
24. Sarner M, Cotton PB. Classification of pancreatitis. Gut. 1984;25: 756-9.
25. Calvo MM, Bujanda L, Calderon A, Heras I, Cabriada JL, Bernal A, et al. Comparison between MRCP and ERCP for evaluation of the pancreatic duct. Am J Gastroenterol. 2002;97:347-53.
26. Catalano MF, Sahai A, Levy M, Romagnuolo J, Wiersema M, Brugge W, et al. EUS-based criteria for the diagnosis of chronic pancreatitis: the Rosemont classification. Gastrointest Endosc. 2009;69:1251-61.
27. Domínguez-Muñoz JE. Pancreatic exocrine insufficiency: diagnosis and treatment. J Gastroenterol Hepatol. 2011;26:12-6.
28. Strum WB. Abstinence in alcoholic chronic pancreatitis. Effect on pain and outcome. J Clin Gastroenterol. 1995;20:37-41.
29. Coté GA, Yadav D, Slivka A, Hawes RH, Anderson MA, Burton FR, et al. Alcohol and smoking as risk factors in an epidemiology study of patients with chronic pancreatitis. Clin Gastroenterol Hepatol. 2011;9:266-73.
30. Maisonneuve P, Lowenfels AB, Müllhaupt B, Cavallini G, Lankisch PG, Andersen JR, et al. Cigarette smoking accelerates progression of alcoholic chronic pancreatitis. Gut. 2005;54:510-4.
31. Tolstrup JS, Kristiansen L, Becker U, Grønbaek M. Smoking and risk of acute and chronic pancreatitis among women and men: a population-based cohort study. Arch Intern Med. 2009;169:603-9.
32. World Health Organization. Cancer Pain Relief and Palliative Care: Report of a WHO Expert Committee. Geneva: World Health Organization, 1990.
33. Sheen CH, Schleimer RP, Kulka M. Codeine induces human mast cell chemokine and cytokine production: involvement of G-protein activation. Allergy. 2007;62:532-8.
34. Wilder-Smith CH, Hill L, Osler W, O'Keefe S. Effect of tramadol and morphine on pain and gastrointestinal motor function in patients with chronic pancreatitis. Dig Dis Sci. 1999;44:1107-16.
35. Niemann T, Madsen LG, Larsen S, Thorsgaard N. Opioid treatment of painful chronic pancreatitis. Int J Pancreatol. 2000;27:235-40.
36. Bouwense SA, Olesen SS, Drewes AM, Poley JW, van Goor H, Wilder-Smith OH. Effects of pregabalin on central sensitization in patients with chronic pancreatitis in a randomized, controlled trial. PLoS One. 2012;7:e42096.
37. Olesen SS, Bouwense SA, Wilder-Smith OH, van Goor H, Drewes AM. Pregabalin reduces pain in patients with chronic pancreatitis in a randomized, controlled trial. Gastroenterology. 2011;141:536-43.
38. Asaumi H, Watanabe S, Taguchi M, Tashiro M, Otsuki M. Externally applied pressure activates pancreatic stellate cells through the generation of intracellular reactive oxygen species. Am J Physiol Gastrointest Liver Physiol. 2007;293:G972-8.
39. Asaumi H, Watanabe S, Taguchi M, Tashiro M, Nagashio Y, Nomiyama Y, et al. Green tea polyphenol-epigallocatechin-3-gallate inhibits ethanol-induced activation of pancreatic stellate cells. Eur J Clin Invest. 2006;36:113-22.
40. Jianyu-Hao, Guang-Li, Baosen-pang. Evidence for cigarette smoke-induced oxidative stress in the rat pancreas. Inhal Toxicol. 2009;21: 1007-12.
41. Braganza JM, Dormandy TL. Micronutrient therapy for chronic pancreatitis: rationale and impact. JOP. 2010;11:99-112.
42. Bhardwaj P, Garg PK, Maulik SK, Saraya A, Tandon RK, Acharya SK. A randomized controlled trial of antioxidant supplementation for pain relief in patients with chronic pancreatitis. Gastroenterology. 2009;136:149-59.
43. Siriwardena AK, Mason JM, Sheen AJ, Makin AJ, Shah NS. Antioxidant therapy does not reduce pain in patients with chronic pancreatitis: the ANTICIPATE study. Gastroenterology. 2012;143:655-63.
44. Forsmark CE, Liddle RA. The challenging task of treating painful chronic pancreatitis. (Editorial) Gastroenterology. 2012;143:533-5.
45. Okazaki K, Yamamoto Y, Ito K. Endoscopic measurement of papillary sphincter zone and pancreatic main ductal pressure in patients with chronic pancreatitis. Gastroenterology. 1986;91:409-18.
46. Xie JY, Herman DS, Stiller CO, Gardell LR, Ossipov MH, Lai J, et al. Cholecystokinin in the rostral ventromedial medulla mediates opioid-induced hyperalgesia and anti-nociceptive tolerance. J Neurosci. 2005;25:409-16.
47. Isaksson G, Ihse I. Pain reduction by an oral pancreatic enzyme preparation in chronic pancreatitis. Dig Dis Sci. 1983;28:97-102.
48. Slaff J, Jacobson D, Tillman CR, Curington C, Toskes P. Protease-specific suppression of pancreatic exocrine secretion. Gastroenterology. 1984;87:44-52.
49. DiMagno EP, Go VL, Summerskill WH. Relations between pancreatic enzyme ouputs and malabsorption in severe pancreatic insufficiency. N Engl J Med. 1973;288:813-5.
50. Chari ST, Smyrk TC, Levy MJ, Topazian MD, Takahashi N, Zhang L, et al. Diagnosis of autoimmune pancreatitis: the Mayo Clinic experience. Clin Gastroenterol Hepatol. 2006;4:1010-6.
51. Finkelberg DL, Sahani D, Deshpande V, Brugge WR. Autoimmune pancreatitis. N Engl J Med. 2006;355:2670-6.
52. Dominguez-Munoz JE, Alvarez-Castro A, Larino-Noia J, Nieto L, Iglesias-Garcia J. Endoscopic ultrasonography of the pancreas as an indirect method to predict pancreatic exocrine insufficiency in patients with chronic pancreatitis. Pancreas. 2012;41:724-8.
53. Safdi M, Bekal PK, Martin S, Saeed ZA, Burton F, Toskes PP. The effects of oral pancreatic enzymes (Creon 10 capsule) on steatorrhea: a multicenter, placebo-controlled, parallel group trial in subjects with chronic pancreatitis. Pancreas. 2006;33:156-62.

54. Ewald N, Hardt PD. Diagnosis and treatment of diabetes mellitus in chronic pancreatitis. World J Gastroenterol. 2013;19:7276-81.
55. Ebert R, Creutzfeldt WO. Reversal of impaired GIP and insulin secretion in patients with pancreatogenic steatorrhea following enzyme substitution. Diabetologia. 1980;19:198-204.
56. Knop FK, Visboll T, Larsen S, Højberg PV, Vølund A, Madsbad S. Increased post-prandial responses of GLP-1 and GIP in patients with chronic pancreatitis and steatorrhea following pancreatic enzyme substitution. Am J Physiol Endocrinol Metab. 2007;292:E324-30.
57. O'Keefe SJ, Cariem AK, Lewy M. The exacerbation of pancreatic endocrine dysfunction by potent pancreatic exocrine pancreatic supplements in patients with chronic pancreatitis. J Clin Gastroenterol. 2001;32:319-23.
58. Barman KK, Padmanabhan M, Premalatha G, Deepa R, Mohan R, Mohan V. Prevalence of diabetic complications in fibrocalculous pancreatic diabetic patients and type 2 diabetic patients: A cross-sectional comparative study. J Diabetes complications. 2004;18:264-70.
59. Mohan R, Rajendran B, Mohan V, Ramachandran A, Viswanathan M, Kohner EM. Retinopathy in tropical pancreatic diabetes. Arch Ophthalmol. 1985;103:1487-89.
60. Lowenfels AB, Maisonneuve P, Cavallini G, Ammann RW, Lankisch PG, Andersen JR, et al. Pancreatitis and the risk of pancreatic cancer. N Engl J Med. 1993;328:1433-7.
61. Magruder JT, Elahi D, Andersen DK. Diabetes and pancreatic cancer: chicken or egg? Pancreas. 2011;40:339-51.
62. Jee SH, Ohrr H, Sull JW, Yun JE, Ji M, Samet JM. Fasting serum glucose level and cancer risk in Korean men and women. JAMA. 2005;293:194-202.
63. Bowker SL, Majumdar SR, Veugelers P, Johnson JA. Increased cancer-related mortality for patients with type 2 diabetes who use sulfonylureas or insulin. Diabetes Care. 2006;29:254-58.
64. Li D, Yeung SC, Hassan MM, Konopleva M, Abbruzzese JL. Antidiabetic therapies affect risk of pancreatic cancer. Gastroenterology. 2009;137:482-8.
65. Stoffers DA, Kieffer TJ, Hussain MA, Drucker DJ, Bonner-Weir S, Habener JF, et al. Insulinotropic glucagon-like peptide-1 agonists stimulate expression of homeodomain protein IDX-1 and increase islet size in mouse pancreas. Diabetes. 2000;49:741-8.
66. Elashoff M, Matveyenko AV, Gier B, Elashoff R, Butler PC. Pancreatitis, pancreatic and thyroid cancer with glucagon-like peptide-1-based therapies. Gastroenterology. 2011;141:150-6.
67. Libby G, Donnelly LA, Donnan PT, Alessi DR, Morris AD, Evans JM. New users of metformin are at low of incident cancer: a cohort study among people with type 2 diabetes. Diabetes Care. 2009;32:1620-5.
68. Bang UC, Benfield T, Hyldstrup L, Bendtsen F, Jensen JE. Mortality, cancer and comorbidities associated with chronic pancreatitis: a Danish nationwide matched-cohort study. Gastroenterology. 2014;146:989-94.

CHAPTER 41

Surgery for Chronic Pancreatitis

Vikas Gupta

INTRODUCTION

Chronic pancreatitis (CP) is a chronic debilitating, progressive inflammatory condition characterized by disabling pain and pancreatic insufficiency (includes both exocrine and endocrine). It usually involves a young population and has enormous socioeconomic burden to the patient and his family due to loss of working hours because of pain. Patients suffering from chronic pancreatitis usually have a poor quality of life and a shortened life expectancy.[1,2]

The disease has a latent period of about 5-10 years prior to the onset of clinically significant pancreatic insufficiency. During this period pain remains the predominant symptom. Primarily being a disease of exocrine pancreas, its dysfunction predates the onset of endocrine insufficiency. Continued alcohol consumption and smoking can accentuate the inflammatory process and rapid progression of pancreatitis.[1,3,4] In the normal course of the disease uninterrupted by surgical intervention, about 30-50% of patients will eventually become diabetic.[1,3,4]

Ongoing inflammation in the pancreas can lead to the formation of a mass in the head of pancreas. It is seen in about 30-50% of the patients.[5] This can be associated with the development of biliary (about 30%) or duodenal stenosis (5-7%),[5,6] portomesenteric compression (8-10%) and splenic vein thrombosis (3-5%).[7]

INDICATIONS FOR SURGERY

Pain is the most common indication of surgery. During the course of the disease, about three-fourths of the patients may require surgical intervention. Failure of medical and endoscopic management to provide adequate pain relief is the classical indication for surgery. Medical management should not be prolonged as much as to make the patient opioid dependent.[8] van der Gaag et al. have shown that preoperative use of opioids was associated with poor pain relief in the postoperative period.[9]

Other indications for surgery include:
- Development of inflammatory mass
- Presence of multiple narrowing of the pancreatic duct which makes it unsuitable for endotherapy
- Development of biliary or duodenal stenosis
- Compression of portal and/or superior mesenteric vein
- Inflammatory mass suspicious of malignancy.

Rationale of Surgery in Chronic Pancreatitis

Intraductal and interstitial hypertension have been the proposed as the mechanisms of pain in chronic pancreatitis. This situation is quite similar to the occurrence of compartment syndrome in pancreas. Both the etiologies can be very effectively addressed by the surgical decompression and adequate drainage of the pancreas.[8]

Pancreatic head has been found to be enlarged in about half of the patients with chronic pancreatitis. Radiological size more than 4 cm is considered as inflammatory head mass. Focal inflammation of the head has been found in almost all the patients with chronic pancreatitis.[5] Pancreatic head has been considered as a 'pacemaker of pain' in chronic pancreatitis. Head mass is often addressed with resectional procedures.

Surgery has been proved to be superior to endoscopic treatment of chronic pancreatitis. Dite et al. in a study of 72 patients randomized into surgery and endotherapy, found similar immediate success in both the groups. However, complete pain relief and increase in body weight at 5 years were significantly superior in patients undergoing surgical treatment. New onset of diabetes was similar in both the groups.[10] Another randomized trial comparing surgery and endotherapy showed a lower pain score, better physical health scores and better quality of life in patients undergoing surgical treatment for chronic pancreatitis at 24 months of follow up. More so, there was a significantly higher number of patients with complete and partial pain relief in the surgery group. The trial was terminated early after interim analysis on the basis of significant differences in the outcome favoring surgery.[11]

Timing of Surgery

Effect on pain relief: A recent study of 266 patients followed for a median of 62 months, showed pain relief in 58% of the patients. Surgery within three years of onset of symptoms was associated with more pain relief (OR 1.8, 95% CI, 1–3.4; p=0.03) on both multivariate and univariate analysis. In addition more pain relief was observed in patients not taking opioids preoperatively (OR, 2.1; 95% CI, 1.2–4.0; p=0.006) and those who had fewer than five endoscopic interventions (OR, 2.5; 95% CI, 1.1–6.3; p=0.04) prior to surgery.[12] A recent meta-analysis has shown that early surgery was associated with an increased likelihood of complete postoperative pain relief (RR=1.67, 95 % CI 1.09–2.56, p=0.02).[13]

Effect of pancreatic insufficiency: Ali et al in a study showed that early surgery (within three years of onset) lowered the odds of developing de novo pancreatic endocrine insufficiency (OR 0.57, 95% CI, 0.33–0.96), on multivariate analysis. However, it did not have any effect on the exocrine insufcifency.[12] A previous study has shown delayed surgery to be associated with higher possibility of developing postoperative exocrine pancreatic insufficiency (OR 2.47, p=0.002). Furthermore, they showed a trend towards a higher incidence of new onset diabetes (21 vs 30 %, p=0.12) after late surgery.[14]

Need for reintervention: It has consistently been seen over the years that the need for reintervention after surgical treatment has been lower after surgery than after endoscopic treatment[13]. A previous study has shown preoperative opioid usage was associated with three time's higher reoperation rates.[15]

Number of endoscopic interventions and use of opioid analgesics are indirectly related to the duration of symptoms. A study from UK has shown patients who used opioids prior to surgery had statistically longer duration of preoperative symptoms (mean, 2.0 vs. 5.9 years) and larger number of hospitalizations prior to surgery (mean, 3 vs. 10).[15]

Risk of malignancy: Chronic pancreatitis is an independent risk factor for malignancy. The risk of malignancy increases with the duration of disease. The cumulative risk of developing adenocarcinoma at 10 and 20 years is 1.8% and 4% respectively.[16] At times it can be difficult to establish the exact nature of pancreatic head mass. Another study has identified elevated Serum bilirubin and CA 19-9, and dilated MPD and CBD as predictors of malignancy in patients with CCP with head mass.[17]

Surgical intervention should be performed early in the course of the disease. Not only does it achieve a better pain relief but also it can delay the onset of insufficiency in these patients. It can slow down the ongoing inflammatory process by providing surgical decompression. It is imperative to have intervention before the changes become irreversible and cause permanent damage to the pancreas.[13]

Surgical Options

The main aim of the surgical procedure is to provide a lasting pain relief and at the same time preserve endocrine and exocrine functions. Despite so many innovations over the last century, still there is not a single ideal procedure.[18,19] This is probably due to variations in the pathomorphological features of the disease. Surgical procedures can be divided into drainage procedures, resectional procedures and combined procedures (Box 1).

BOX 1 Classification of surgical procedures for chronic pancreatitis

Resectional procedures

Major resection:
- Kausch-Whipple pancreaticoduodenectomy
- Total pancreatectomy with or without duodenum preservation
- Total pancreatectomy with islet cell autotransplantation

Organ preserving resection:
- Pylorus preserving pancreaticoduodenectomy
- Left sided resection

Drainage procedures
- Duval's procedure
- Puestow-Gillesby procedure
- Partington-Rochelle variant of the Puestow procedure

Hybrid procedures
- Head coring and drainage (Frey's procedure)
- Duodenum preserving pancreatic head resection (Beger's procedure)

Modifications:
- Izbicki (Hamburg) modification
- Berne modification
- Imiazumi modification

Denervation procedures

Preoperative Assessment

Surgical success mandates appropriate procedures for appropriate patients. So, a proper patient selection is essential to have good outcome. Components of assessment should achieve: (a) confirmation of the diagnosis of chronic pancreatitis and to ascertain the head mass if present to be benign in nature; (b) determine the anatomy of pancreas with special attention to duct, head mass and parenchyma; (c) evaluate the patency of spleno-porto-mesenteric axis; (d) assessment of exocrine and endocrine function; (e) evaluation of complications of pancreatitis such as biliary and duodenal obstruction; and (f) assessment of patient's nutritional, medical and psychosocial comorbidities with special attention to alcoholism and opioid dependence.

A contrast enhanced CT with pancreatic protocol can delineate the anatomy of pancreas and should be done in all the patients. The diagnosis of chronic pancreatitis can be very easily made with the presence of radio dense ductal calcifications, dilated pancreatic duct and atrophic pancreas (Figs 1A and B). However, in the presence of inflammatory head mass (Fig. 2), it can at times be difficult to distinguish it from pancreatic cancer.[16,17,20] Measurement of CA 19-9 and Carcinoembryonic antigen can be helpful in differentiating the two conditions. Though it is elevated in both the conditions, the degree of elevation will be higher in malignancy than in chronic pancreatitis. If CA 19-9 is elevated, it is imperative to rule out malignancy before accepting the diagnosis of chronic pancreatitis.[17,20,21] Endoscopic ultrasound can help to distinguish the two conditions and, if need be, a guided fine needle

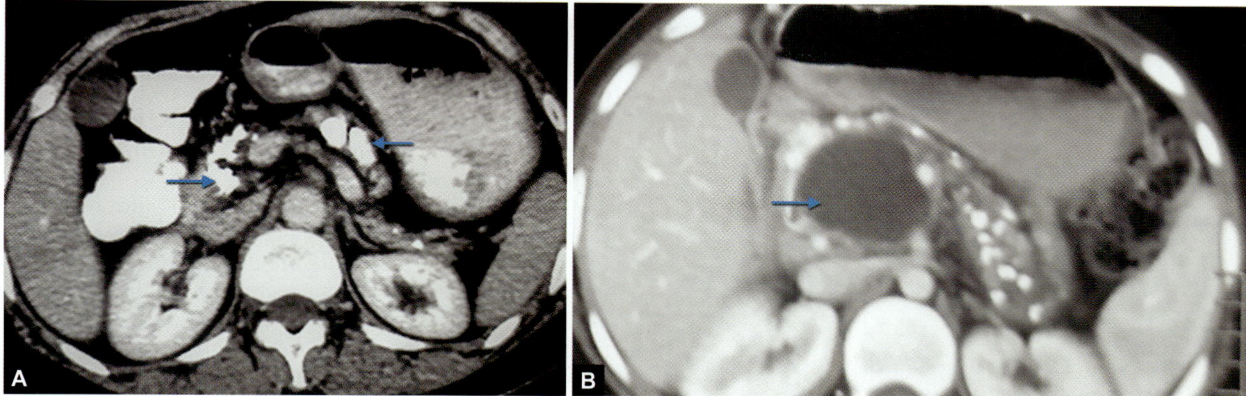

Figures 1A and B (A) Shows atrophic pancreas with ductal calcifications (arrows), suitable for lateral pancreaticojejunostomy. (B) Chronic pancreatitis with multiple calcifications and a large cyst (arrow) in the head region. The cyst can be incorporated into the pancreaticojejunal anastomosis

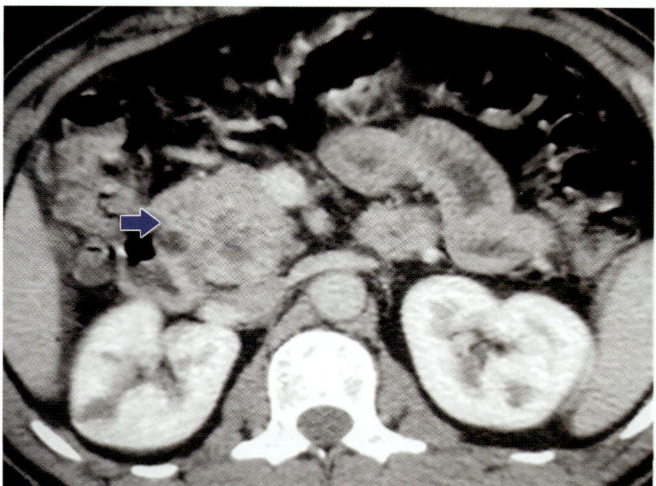

Figure 2 Contrast enhanced CT scan showing an inflammatory mass (arrow) in the head and uncinate of pancreas. CA 19-9 was normal and patient underwent Frey procedure

aspiration biopsy can be performed to ascertain the diagnosis of malignancy.[22] However, a negative biopsy does not rule out malignancy.

In addition CT can be helpful in detecting associated pseudocysts, biliary or duodenal obstruction and evaluation of splenoportal axis. Some of the patients might have undergone endoscopic intervention [Endoscopic retrograde cholangiopancreaticography (ERCP)] prior to surgical referral. Magnetic resonance cholangiopancreatography (MRCP) (Fig. 3) can be done to exactly delineate the anatomy of the duct so as to plan the extent of drainage in a given patient.[23] However, due to invasiveness, diagnostic ERCP should be avoided as far as possible.

Cross-sectional imaging and knowledge of ductal anatomy is helpful in decision making regarding the choice of procedure. A duct diameter of at least 5mm or more without a head mass is suitable for a drainage procedure. Presence of an inflammatory head mass on imaging needs resection (partial or total). Inability to conclusively exclude malignancy requires en bloc surgical resection.[18,19,21]

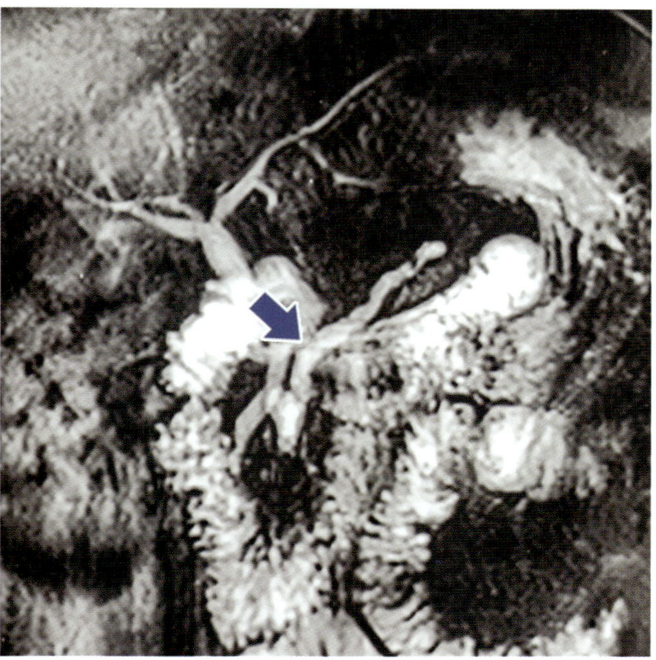

Figure 3 Magnetic resonance cholangiopancreatography showing dilated pancreatic duct (arrow) with a single dominant stricture in the head region. The bile duct is not dilated

All patients should undergo upper GI endoscopy for evaluation of varices, esophagogastric or fundal as an indirect evidence of chronic pancreatitis related portal hypertension.[7,24]

Preoperative assessment of severity of pain and degree of disability should be established in all the patients. Pain should be quantified as far as possible by analog scale or by Izbicki score.[25] Special attention should be given to the need for narcotics to control pain. Alcohol abuse is a common phenomenon in these patients. Continued alcohol consumption is associated with poor postoperative pain relief and recurrence of symptoms after surgery. It is imperative to reform before contemplating any surgical intervention.[21,24] At the same time other potential causes of pain such as peptic ulcer and biliary calculus should be excluded.

BOX 2 Preoperative evaluation for chronic pancreatitis

History and physical exam
- Etiologic evaluation: alcohol, smoking
- Symptom evaluation: pain, weight loss, endocrine and exocrine insufficiency
- Previous treatment: drug treatment (analgesics, enzymes), endoscopic interventions

Laboratory parameters
- Routine evaluation with liver function tests, blood sugar, blood urea and creatinine, hemogram, serum albumin and serum electrolytes
- Tumor markers like CA19-9, CEA

Not essential
- Endocrine function (glucose tolerance, insulin, C peptide, etc.
- Exocrine function test (fecal elastase, etc.)

Mandatory Imaging (cross-sectional)
- Computed tomography (CT) or magnetic resonance imaging (MRI)

Imaging for ductal anatomy
- Magnetic resonance cholangiopancreaticography [MRCP (preferable)]*
- Endoscopic retrograde cholangiopancreaticography (ERCP)*

Provided by physician prior to referral (*useful, but not essential*)
- Upper GI endoscopy
- Endoscopic retrograde cholangiopancreaticography (ERCP)*
- Endoscopic ultrasound (EUS)

Not required
- Preoperative tissue diagnosis

* Either ERCP or MRI with MRCP has to be performed for reliable evaluation of the pancreatic duct

In one study it was found that as many as 32% of the patients had a BMI less than 20 kg/m^2; 50% had hypoalbuminemia; 57% had chronic diarrhea and 24% had steatorrhea. Malnutrition is often multifactorial in these patients: depletion of nutrients due to alcohol consumption and pain; malabsorption due to exocrine insufficiency; increase metabolic activity due to chronic inflammatory component of the disease.[26] Generally, patients with poor nutrition status have more perioperative complications. Nutritional assessment should be done in all the patients and deficiencies should be corrected by dietary and enzyme supplements. Particularly patients with tropical pancreatitis have severe malnutrition due to nutritional metabolities.[27] The work up[28] of chronic pancreatitis is as listed in Box 2.

RESECTIONAL PROCEDURES

Partial or total resection of pancreas is an attractive and permanent solution for the recurrent problem of pain associated with CP. What so ever may be the etiology of pain, surgical extirpation of the affected part of pancreas would be curative. However, it is always associated with the risk of developing permanent pancreatic insufficiency; the greater the resection, the greater the risk.

Pancreaticoduodenectomy

Kausch-Whipple pancreaticoduodenectomy (PD) includes the resection of pancreatic head along with the entire duodenum, distal third of the stomach, bile duct, and proximal jejunum. PD was initially advocated for malignant lesions of head of pancreas as it was associated with high morbidity and mortality rates. Over a period of time the safety of the procedure has increased and this has led to the expansion of indications for benign lesions like chronic pancreatitis as well.[29] Pancreatic head acts as a pacemaker of pain and total resection of head in PD should be able to relieve pain.

However, classical PD is associated with nutritional sequelae, so it is not the preferred operation for chronic pancreatitis. Pylorus-preserving procedure (PPPD) on the other hand does not entail the removal of stomach (Figs 4A and B) and hence avoids the long term consequences of gastrectomy. It is the preferred procedure whenever resection is planned for chronic pancreatitis.[30] In patients with strictures in the distal remnant,

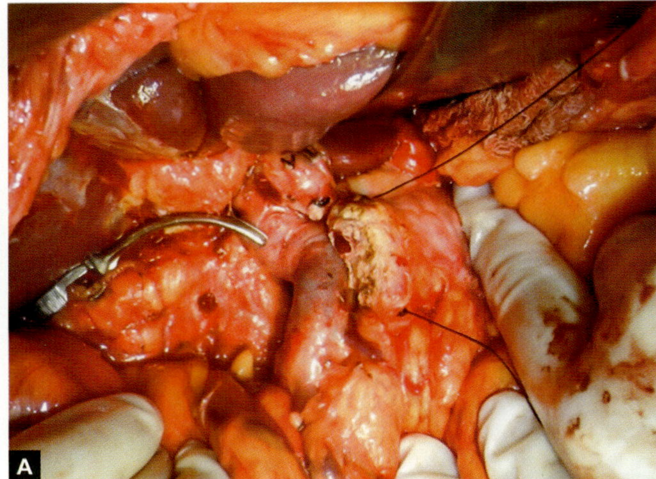

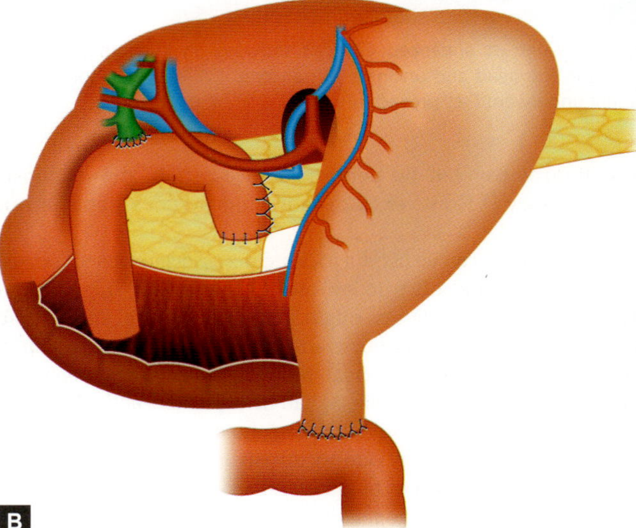

Figures 4A and B (A) Pancreaticoduodenal resection in a patient with head mass suspicious of malignancy. Note is made on the atrophic pancreas with dilated pancreatic duct and a un-dilated bile duct (clamped); (B) Schematic representation of reconstruction after pylorus preserving pancreaticoduodenectomy (PPPD)

Table 1: Outcome of PPPD for chronic pancreatitis

Author	*N*	*Operative morbidity (%)*	*Operative mortality (%)*	*Pain relief (%)*	*Diabetes (%)*	*Weight gain (%)*
McAfee et al.[31]	12	27	0	-	-	92
Morel et al.[32]	20	35	0	85	-	95
Martin et al.[33]	44	31	4	93	42	74
Stapleton and Williamson[34]	52	46	0	47	23	-
Traverso and Kozarek[29]	42	36	0	76	22	81

Traverso and Longmire had suggested decompression of the entire duct by adding longitudinal lateral pancreaticojejunostomy along the anterior aspect of the remnant.[29]

In most of the high volume centres, the mortality associated with PD has declined to below 2%, but the morbidity associated with the procedure remains as high as 20–30%. The major concern of performing a PD remains that of pancreatic anastomotic complications. In malignancy, the reported incidence of all anastomotic leaks is about 15–20%. However, in chronic pancreatitis, the firm texture of the gland and dilated main pancreatic duct help to make a secure anastomosis.[29-34]

The major advantage of PD is the resection of an unrecognized adenocarcinoma in a patient with head mass. The procedure in itself is sufficient to address the patients with duodenal and distal bile duct stricture. The procedure can also be curative in patients with groove pancreatitis.

With pancreaticoduodenectomy, the long term pain relief has been reported in 85% of the patients. However, it is associated with 50% incidence of new onset of diabetes and almost half of the patients developing exocrine insufficiency (Table 1) at a follow up of ten years.[29-34]

Distal Pancreatectomy

Majority of the patients with chronic pancreatitis have a dominant disease in the head region and the changes in the distal pancreas are secondary to changes in the head. Only small percentage of patients (5–15%) have disease confined to the body and tail of pancreas.[35,36] This happens in patients with isolated duct stricture, pseudocyst, or both at the neck of the pancreas. This is emerging as a special entity known as disconnected duct syndrome. These patients with focal disease confined to the body and tail, are suitable for distal partial (40–80%) pancreatectomy.[36,37] Distal pancreatectomy is a less morbid procedure than PD. It leaves major portion of the gland untreated. Therefore this procedure is associated with a significant incidence of recurrence. It is imperative to have a normal head before contemplating this procedure. Even in selected patients, the reported incidence of pain relief varies from 31–80%.[35-38]

Distal Pancreatectomy (95%)

Fry and Child in 1965 reported good outcome of 16 patients who had undergone near total pancreatectomy.[18,39] The procedure entails removal of almost entire pancreas leaving a very thin rim of tissue over the duodenum. This tissue accounts for only 5% of the pancreatic parenchymal tissue. This in turn helps in preserving the pancreaticoduodenal arcade and intrapancreatic portion of the bile duct. Child's rationale for performing this procedure was to avoid pancreaticoduodenectomy, which was associated with a high mortality and morbidity at that time. About 40% of the patients experienced perioperative complications like abscesses and fistulas. The procedure was able to achieve a pain relief of 80% at six years follow up.[40] The remnant pancreas was insufficient for glycemic control. The incidence of postoperative diabetes was 72%, which was unacceptably high. In the same report, patients undergoing PD had similar pain relief with a lower incidence of pancreas endocrine dysfunction. So the procedure of 95% distal pancreatectomy was put to disrepute.

Total Pancreatectomy

Total pancreatectomy is inherently associated with significant morbidity in terms of glycemic control and malabsorption and should not be performed as a first line treatment for chronic pancreatitis. Total pancreatectomy should be performed with islet cell transplantation as a salvage procedure in patients who continue to have severe pain with poor quality of life after simpler procedures (completion pancreatectomy).[21]

Linehan et al. in a study of 29 patients undergoing total pancreatectomy reported prolonged hospital stay mainly due to poor diabetes control.[41] About 25% patients experienced major hypoglycemic episodes. Another report of forty patients undergoing total or completion pancreatectomy demonstrated 5% postoperative mortality and 8% reoperation rate. Eighty per cent patients had complete or substantial pain relief.[42] Majority of late mortality was attributed to pancreatic insuficiency. Others have also demonstrated total pancreatectomy as an effective procedure in relieving pain but at the risk of severe hypoglycemic attacks.[43,44]

Total pancreatectomy can provide an excellent pain relief but at the cost of worsening of endocrine and exocrine insufficiency. Therefore this procedure may be offered with autologous pancreatic islet cell transplant to those patients who are not insulin dependent. Patients need to be counselled about this procedure and its consequences before offering this procedure.

Autologous Islet Transplantation

Without autologous islet transplantation (AIT), total pancreatectomy was fraught with the complication of brittle diabetes, and was not acceptable modality to get pain relief in CP.[41-44] AIT alleviates the problem of brittle diabetes associated with total or subtotal pancreatectomy. In addition benefits of preserving endocrine function are reduced risk of long term complications like neuropathy, nephropathy, retinopathy and other complications. Autologous islet cell transplantation (AIT) with total pancreatectomy has proved to be an effective method of pain relief in chronic pancreatitis (CP).[45-48]

In AIT the islets are carefully isolated from explanted pancreas in a laboratory and then transplanted back into the patient by infusion through the portal vein.[45-47] In successful cases, patients will be euglycemic. Majority of the cases may become independent of insulin or require only a small dose.[47,48]

Despite poor initial success rate of allogeneic pancreas transplantation, AIT has been effectively performed since the 1970s. Improvement in isolation techniques has increased success of the procedure.[45] Few authors recommend performing this procedure earlier in the course of the disease before irreversible damage occurs.[48]

DRAINAGE PROCEDURES

Gould in 1898 was first to successfully remove pancreatic calculi from Wirsung's duct.[49] Later, Moynihan removed pancreatic calculus through transpancreatic route while Mayo-Robson described transduodenal route through the papilla of Vater.[50] Goethe Link reported successful pain relief with external drainage of the pancreatic duct through the skin to decompress obstruction.[51] Safety of intestinal anastomosis with pancreas in experimental studies led to the evolution of pancreaticojejunostomy.

Duval and Zollinger et al. in separate studies in 1954 reported distal pancreatosplenectomy with caudal pancreaticojejunostomy (Fig. 5A) as a drainage procedure for chronic pancreatitis.[52,53] It mandated resection of distal pancreas and spleen. The procedure was effective if there was a dominant stricture between the ampulla and tail. However, it failed to provide a lasting pain in the presence of multiple stricture with classical 'Chain of lakes' appearance because of the ineffective drainage provided by the procedure.

The concept was later improvised by Puestow and Gillesby in 1958 by the addition of longitudinal pancreaticojejunostomy (Fig. 5B) with implantation of the divided tail into the Roux en Y limb of the jejunum.[54] This was done with an aim of providing adequate ductal drainage. This procedure could decompress a greater length of pancreatic duct but failed to do so in the head region as the jejunum limb was not brought beyond the superior mesenteric vessels. More over the procedure required splenectomy also.

In 1960, Partington and Rochelle modified the procedure performed by Puestow and Gillesby by creating a side to side anastomosis with jejunum after longitudinally incising the anterior surface of pancreas to identify the duct.[55] This procedure did not require mobilization of the pancreas from its posterior (retroperitoneal) attachments and had an advantage of avoiding distal pancreatectomy and splenectomy; and hence the consequences of the same. The procedure had a theoretical advantage of decompressing the pancreatic duct from head to the tail region of pancreas. This procedure has been widely performed over the years.

Technique of Lateral Pancreaticojejunostomy (LPJ)

A duct diameter of at least 7 mm (5 mm according to some authors) or more, with chain of lakes appearance and absence of a head mass is suitable for this procedure.

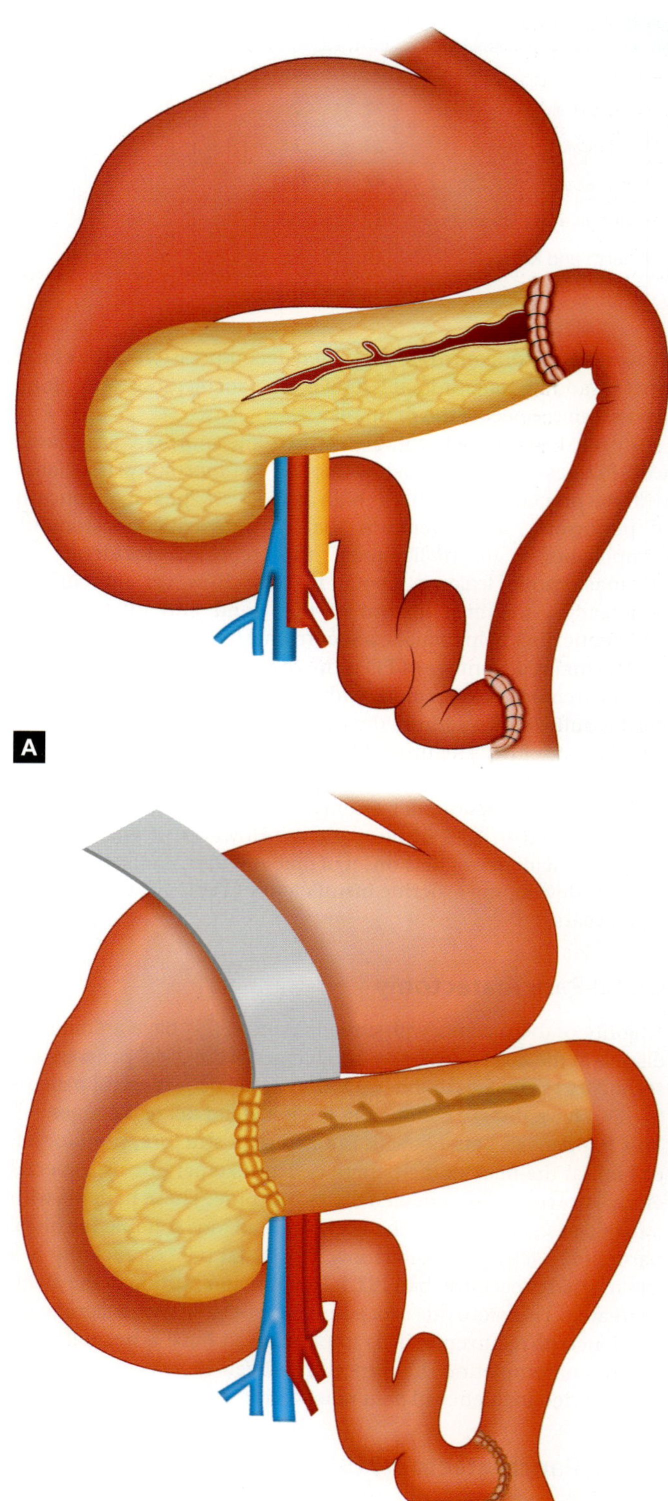

Figures 5A and B (A) Schematic representation of Duval's procedure; reconstruction after caudal pancreaticosplenectomy; (B) Schematic representation of Puestow's procedure; extended drainage of the duct after caudal pancreaticosplenectomy

Exposure: A midline or a bilateral subcostal incision is used to enter the abdomen depending upon the built of the patient. Gastrocolic omentum is divided so as to expose the pancreas right from the duodenum to the tail of the pancreas. Fibrous adhesions between the stomach and pancreas are divided. Hepatic flexure should be taken down completely so as to fully expose the head. Anterior pancreaticoduodenal and gastroduodenal veins are suture ligated and divided. Pylorus and the first part of the duodenum should be lifted off the pancreas head so as to have adequate delineation. Kocher's maneuver is performed so as to hold the pancreatic head while opening the duct in the head region. The head should be palpated for any suspicious mass and frozen biopsy should be sent if required. At this point of time, superior and inferior borders of pancreas should be defined and fibrofatty tissue along the anterior surface of pancreas should be removed, as it will subsequently facilitate the placement of sutures during anastomosis.

Duct management: Pancreatic duct can be identified easily by palpation in the neck or body region where it is superficial, as thin parenchyma overlies a dilated duct. In patient with duct packed with stones, the needle can be used to sound the stone for subsequent opening of the duct. Once the duct is located, it is confirmed by aspirating by using a thin needle (21G). Keeping the needle in position, small ductotomy is made using diathermy to gain sufficient access so as to place a fine instrument into the duct (Figs 6A and B). The ductotomy is extended towards the left using diathermy over the closed tip of a fine hemostat in the duct. It is extended till about 1 cm short of the tip of tail. The calculi in the pancreatic duct can be removed as and when they are encountered while opening the duct. Effort should be made to remove the calculi from the side branches whenever palpated. The gastroduodenal artery is often hidden in the inflammatory tissue and difficult to visualize. It should preferably be ligated before dividing whenever feasible. Towards, the right, the ductotomy is extended just short of duodenum. A small intraparenchymal cyst encountered during operation should be incorporated into the ductotomy and drained along with it into the jejunum. A small sliver of tissue should be taken for frozen biopsy to rule out cancer and IPMN. Bleeding from the pancreatic margin is usually controlled with diathermy or a fine monofilament non absorbable suture. Once the duct is completely opened, it is preferable to pack it with gauze till the time Roux limb is prepared. It serves as a tamponade for the small bleeding points and one gets a nearly clear field by the time pancreatic anastomosis is done.

Roux limb: About 15 cm from ligament of Treitz, jejunum is divided with a stapler cutter device (GIA, blue load). The point is chosen in order to have natural ligament attachment and avoid internal

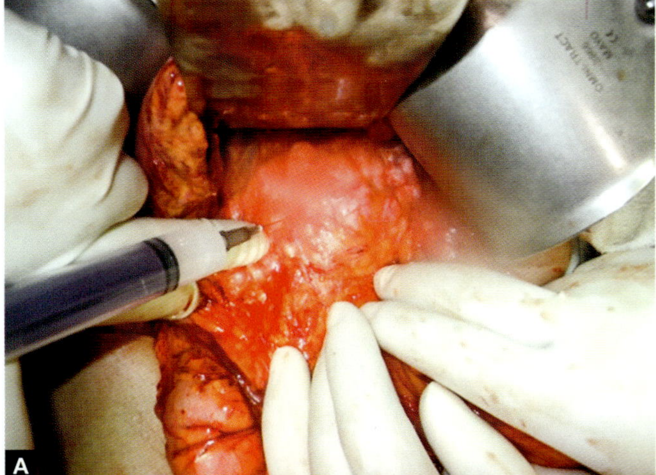

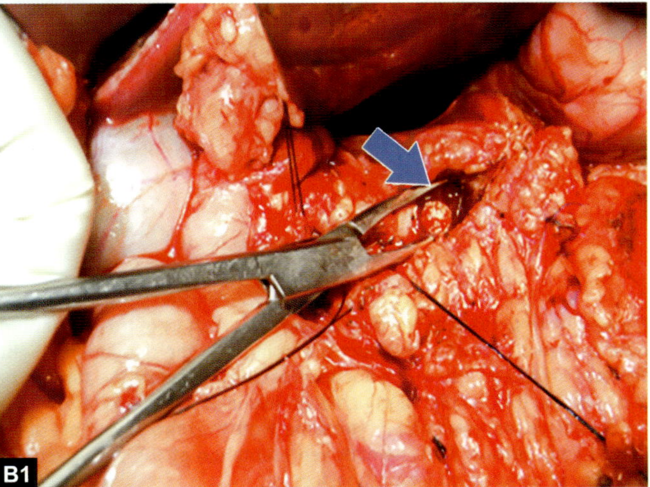

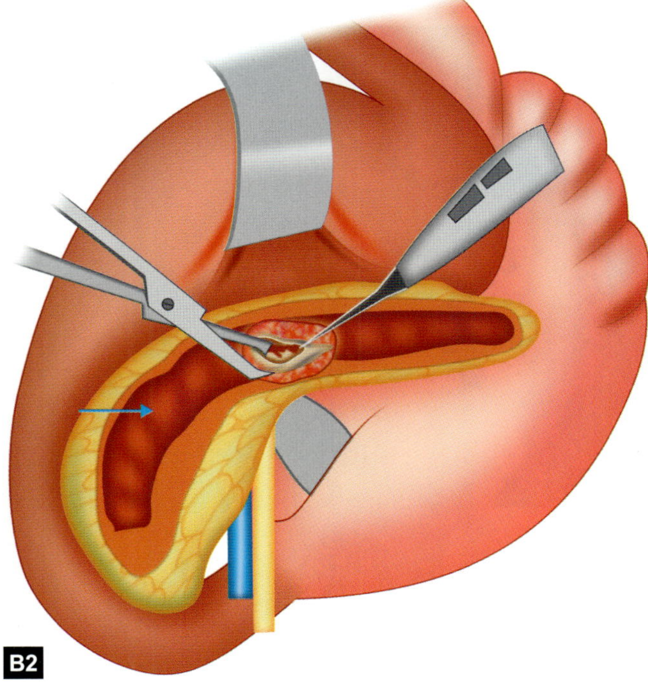

Figures 6A and B (A) Needle aspiration for identification of the pancreatic duct, once identified, the needle is kept in place and parenchyma is divided to access the duct; (B1) Left: The duct is opened over a hemostatic forceps, note the stone in the duct (arrow); (B2) Schematic representation of the same, pancreatic duct is marked with arrow

herniation. jejunojejunostomy is constructed about 45–50 cm downstream in a side to side fashion either using a stapler cutter or hand sewn. The mesenteric defect is closed with a fine suture. The Roux limb is brought up through retrocolic route via creating a defect in the avascular portion of transverse mesocolon usually to the left of middle colic artery.

Pancreaticojejunal anastomosis: Jejunum is placed over the pancreatic surface and opened longitudinally serially to match the length of ductotomy. It is important not to open the jejunum in its entire length initially as the eventration of the opened jejunum poses difficulties while suturing. Usually a single layer continuous anastomosis with a long lasting fine monofilament

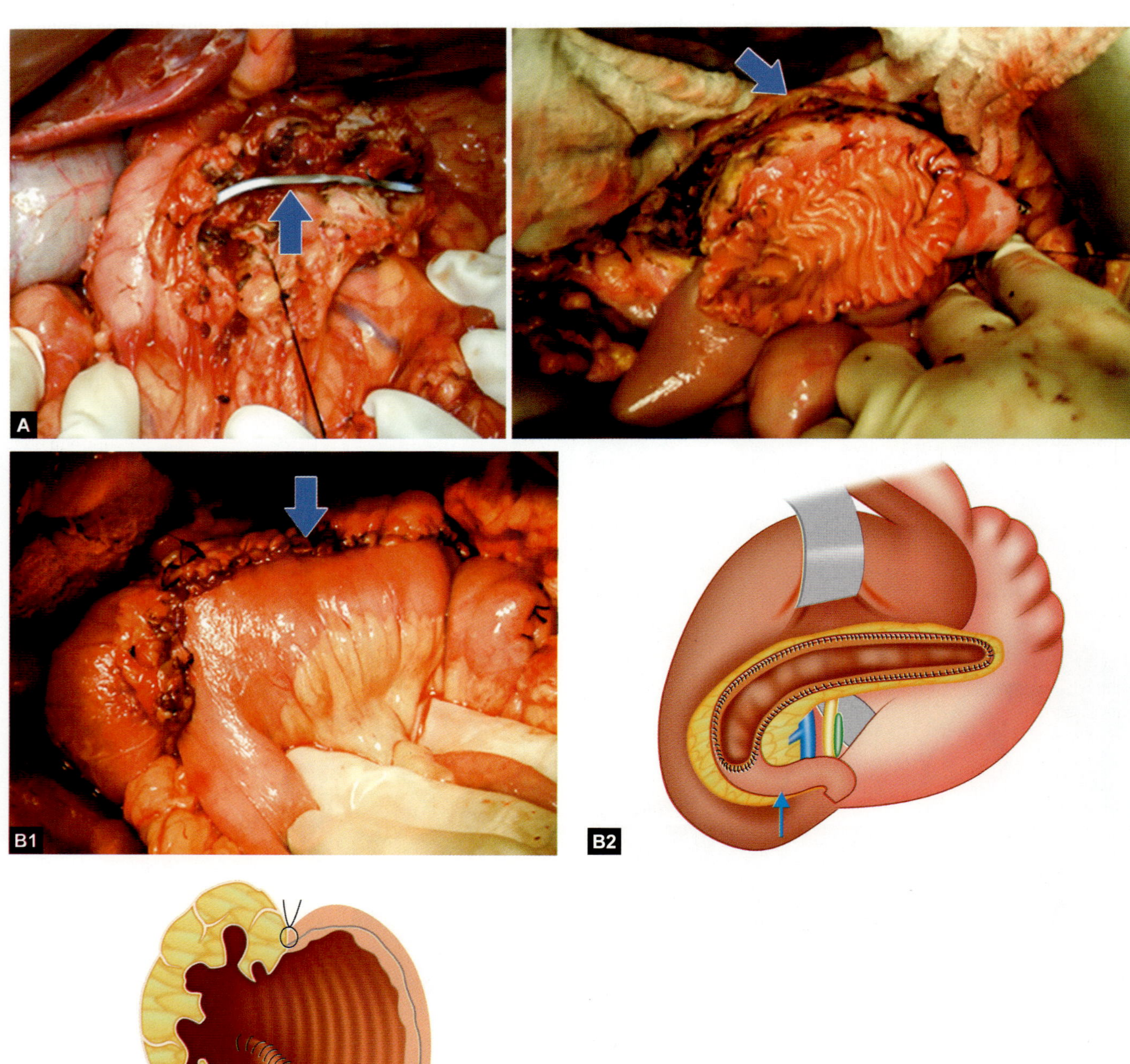

Figures 7A to C (A) Left: The duct is opened just short of the duodenum, note the stent (arrow) in the duct is dipping into the duodenum; Right: Jejunum is placed close to the opened duct (arrow) before the start of the anastomosis; (B) Completed pancreatico-jejunal anastomosis (arrow) and the schematic representation of the same. Note the retro-colic route of the jejunal limb (arrow); (C) Schematic representation of the cross-sectional anatomy of pancreatico-jejunal anastomosis

Table 2: Outcome of patients with lateral pancreaticojejunostomy

Author	*Year*	*N*	*Operative mortality (%)*	*Pain relief (%)*	*Follow up (years)*
Schnelldorfer et al.[56]	2007	170	-	48	5.5
Nealon et al.[58]	2001	124	0	86	6.5
Delcore et al.[59]	1994	28	-	86	3.5
Adams et al.[60]	1994	62	0	68	6.3
Greenlee et al.[61]	1990	50	4.2	82	7.9
Bradley et al.[57]	1987	48	0	66	5.8
Sato et al.[62]	1986	46	0	91	9.1
Holmberg et al.[63]	1985	51	0	72	8.2
Warshaw[64]	1985	36	3	83	3.6

suture is performed. Difficult part of the anastomosis should be performed first and we always prefer to start from the tail region and proceed towards the inferior and superior borders. Full thickness jejunal bites are sutured with pancreatic capsule taking partial thickness of parenchyma (Figs 7A to C). No attempt should be made to sew directly the mucosa of pancreatic duct except the tail region where the parenchyma is very thin. Deep bites into the parenchyma can occlude the side branches of the gland and may limit the drainage.

A 16 F closed suction drain is placed along the inferior border of anastomosis prior to closure.

Postoperatively, nasogastric decompression can be removed and orals can be resumed after 24 hours.

Results of LPJ: With the introduction of coring out (see below) of the head of pancreas, simple LPJ as a drainage procedure is being rarely performed. Even in patients without inflammatory head mass, some amount of the head is usually cored out in order to provide adequate decompression.

This procedure can be performed with a morbidity of 6-35% and mortality of less than 5%. Recent series have reported less than 1% mortality rates.[56-65] Relief of pain is the primary end point of the operation and has been reported from 48-91%[56-65] (Table 2). Bradley et al. have reported a good pain relief in all the patients with a duct diameter of 7 mm or more while those with a duct diameter of less than 6 mm had inadequate pain relief. Continued alcohol use is one of the reasons for development of recurrent pain.[57] Despite early pain relief in more than 80% of the patients, about 30-35% of patients develop pain at a follow up of 3-5 years.[18,56-66] There is no evidence to suggest that this procedure worsens the pancreatic insufficiency as it is associated with minimal loss of the functioning pancreatic parenchyma. Nealon & Thompson reported benefit from operation in patients with mild to moderate disease compared to their non operative counterparts as measured by weight loss and need for enzyme replacement.[65] Prinz and Greenlee reported less than half the patients became diabetic on long term follow-up.[66]

HYBRID PROCEDURES

Frey Procedure

With the variable results of Partigton and Rochelle procedure, and about a third of patients developing recurrence of pain, the need to develop a new procedure was realized.[56-66] It has been found that pancreatic head is a pacemaker for pain in chronic pancreatitis. Without excising the head, it is difficult to achieve pain relief in patients with inflammatory head mass.[5,8,12,13,14,18,19,21] In 1987 Frey and Smith described a procedure which entails partial excision of head with drainage of duct.[67]

Rationale of Frey's Procedure: About 30-50% patients have inflammatory head mass associated with dilated duct.[5,13,14,18,19,21,68] Partial excision of the head improves the drainage of Wirsung's and Santorini's ducts. It also helps to remove calculi from the ducts in the head and also partially removes the head which is thought to be an epicenter for pain.[18,19,21,68] Frey and Smith in their original article had described more posterior location of the main pancreatic duct in the head region and presence of thick pancreatic tissue between the posteriorly placed duct and medial duodenal wall (Figs 8A and B). Inability to excise this tissue will hamper the drainage of duct and incomplete relief.[67]

Surgical technique: The exposure of pancreas and opening of the pancreatic duct is performed as described above (Lateral pancreaticojejunostomy section). In patients with non dilated duct, there can be difficulty in locating the duct, intraoperative ultrasound can be a useful tool in such a situation.

Local excision of head: Attention should be given to the location of superior mesenteric vein and portal vein in relation to pancreas. This is important as pancreas at this point will not be divided and one should be careful while coring out in this area. After the duct is opened till the neck of pancreas, coring of pancreatic tissue is performed in the head region. Pancreaticoduodenal groove should be palpated if possible; however it is difficult in patients with a head mass. Absorbable sutures should be placed on to the pancreas, about 5 mm parallel and medial to the inner aspect of duodenum. These sutures are hemostatic and mark as a point for the medial most part of dissection. This helps to preserve the superior and inferior pancreaticoduodenal arcade. As most of the times, gastroduodenal artery is embedded in inflammatory fibrotic tissue and is difficult to preserve in most of the cases, so it is imperative to preserve the pancreato-duodenal arcade to avoid ischemic complications. The pancreatic tissue is removed in small bits, and one should secure hemostasis after removal of each and every bit. Use of bipolar cautery is very helpful in this sitation. Excised pancreatic tissue should always be sent for frozen biopsy to reconfirm the nature of head mass. While coring out the pancreatic tissue, care should be exercised to avoid injuring common bile duct. If need be the bile duct can be intubated with a

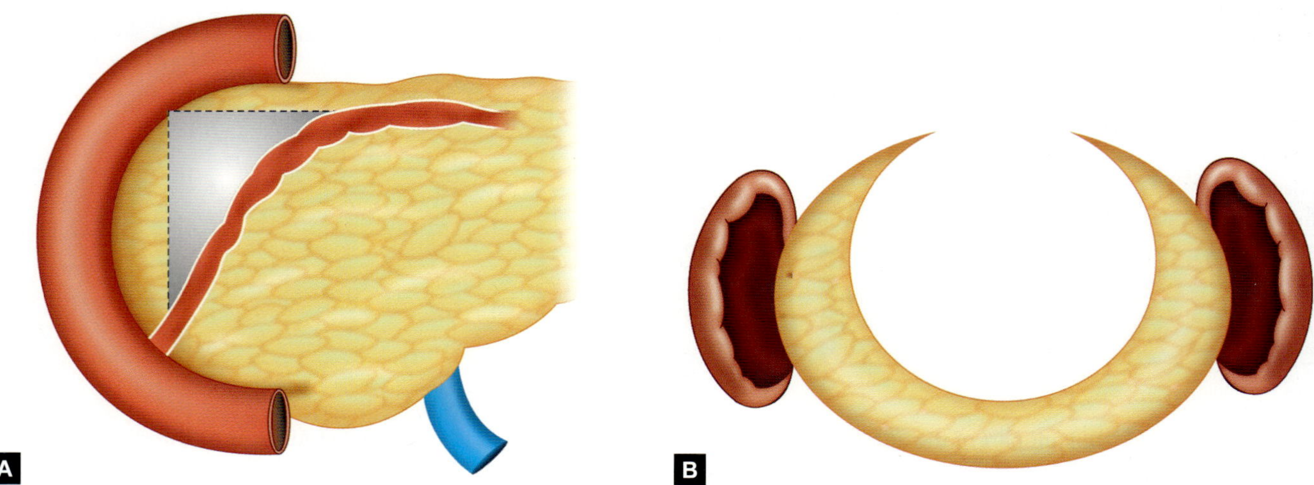

Figures 8A and B (A) Triangular area of the pancreatic head between posteriorly placed duct and medial wall of the duodenum, which needs to be cored out for the adequate ductal decompression in Frey procedure; (B) Schematic representation of the cross-sectional anatomy of pancreatic head at the end of Frey procedure

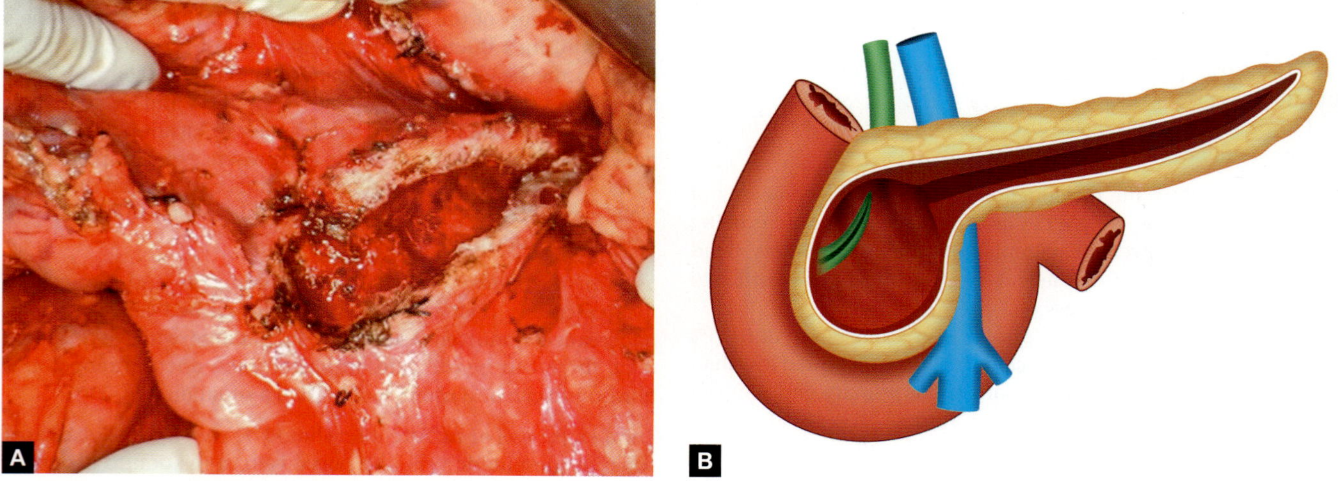

Figures 9A and B (A) Picture at the end of cored out pancreatic head in Frey procedure. Note the extent of ductal dilatation; (B) Schematic representation of the extent of resection at the end of Frey procedure. Note the bile duct is getting decompressed after the resection

metal dilator for ease in identification. The coring is carried on to the uncinate taking care to avoid complete transection of pancreas particularly in the region of SMV and PV. At the end of coring, a thin rim of pancreatic tissue should remain over the duodenum to preserve the superior and inferior arcade (Figs 9A and B). Only a short length of pancreatic duct (about 15 mm) should remain unopened from pancreatic parenchyma to duodenum. This should be probed for the presence of calculi and removed if any. Very little amount of pancreatic tissue should remain over the bile duct at the end of coring. In more than two-thirds of the patients, with biliary obstruction, this is sufficient to relieve the obstruction. During the process of coring, hand should always be kept behind the posterior pancreatic capsule, so that the surgeon is aware of the posterior limit of excision. Posteriorly, a thin rim of pancreatic tissue should remain between the cored out head, uncinate and vascular structures (vena cava, SMV, PV). It is imperative not to open the posterior pancreatic capsule, so as to avoid postoperative leak into the retroperitoneum.

The cored out head is in continuity with the main pancreatic duct and drained in a Roux en Y limb of the jejunum as described above. In the head region, the jejunum is sutured with the rim of pancreatic tissue left on the duodenal wall.

Complications: It can be performed with a mortality of about 2%. The incidence of complications like pancreatic fistula, intra-abdominal collection, hemorrhage, pulmonary complications, etc has been reported variably from 7–40% in various series.[68-71] Arterial bleed occurs due to formation of peripancreatic pseudoaneurysm secondary to anastomotic failure, occurs in 2–3% of patients.[70] However, contrary to pancreaticoduodenectomy for malignancy, anastomotic disruptions occurs less frequently in these patients, due to the presence of dilated duct and extensive fibrosis secondary to chronic pancreatitis.

Predictors of outcome: About 10–20% of patients have persistent symptoms after the surgery.[14,19,68-73] Frey and Amikura[72] found chronic narcotic use and multiple interventions prior to surgery were associated with poor outcome. Another series[14] had reported preoperative exocrine insufficiency and occurrence of surgical complications as the predictors of poor pain relief. Negi et al.[74] found use of preoperative opiates, continuous pattern of pain and postoperative complications to be associated with poor pain relief. Although, studies have shown poor pain relief in patients taking narcotics, but surgical intervention in these patients have been found to decrease pain scores and need for hospital readmissions. This can be extrapolated to the fact that preoperative narcotic use should not deter surgical intervention in these patients. These patients should be referred for surgery early in the course of disease before the development of drug addiction.

A recent small study has shown increasing pancreatic fibrosis to be associated with resolution of pain in patients treated with the Frey procedure.[75] They advocated major resectional procedures in patients with mild or minimal fibrosis.

The correlation between main pancreatic duct diameter and pain relief after the Frey procedure remains debated.[72,76] Few studies have shown a good association between ductal dilation beyond 4 mm and better pain relief.[75] In the absence of ductal dilatation, Frey's procedure in itself is insufficient to provide adequate decompression.

A few studies have found a `good correlation between weight of the cored out pancreas with pain relief. However, due to variability of head size, the amount of cored tissue will be variable.[72,77] Mean percent volume of excised head mass of about 60% has also been found to be associated with pain relief.

Outcome: The occurrence of de novo diabetes has been reported in 8–34% of the patients while exocrine insufficiency occurs in 60–80%, with a pain relief in 70–100% of the patients.[14,68-77] An Indian series has reported sustained complete and partial pain relief in 75% of the patients at a follow up of six years.[74] Keck et al. reported 62% complete pain relief at five years of follow up,[69] while Falconi et al. found complete or partial pain relief in 90% after Frey's procedure.[78] Hildebrand et al. showed improved quality of life after surgical intervention.[79] Comparison of Frey's procedures with other operations for chronic pancreatitis is discussed in subsequent section.

Duodenum Preserving Head Resection

Rationale: Inflammatory head mass (size ≥3 cm), which is considered as pacemaker of pain, is observed in 30–50% of the patients with chronic pancreatitis. The head enlargement leads on to obstruction of main pancreatic duct, common bile duct. In addition it can lead to formation of stones in pancreatic duct, bile duct, pseudocystic cavities, and portomesenteric compression.[5,8,12,13,14,18,19,21,80] Duct drainage procedures are useful only in patients with dilated duct. Those with non dilated ducts get little benefit from simple drainage procedures.[75,77] Presence of head mass is associated with a risk of malignancy also.[16,17]

The procedure entails 95% resection of pancreatic head, leaving a small rim of pancreatic tissue along the medial duodenal wall (Fig. 10). This allows the preservation of enteroduodenal axis which has the major advantage over pancreaticoduodenectomy, however this is associated with loss of pancreatic tissue leading on to the development of brittle diabetes.[18,21,40]

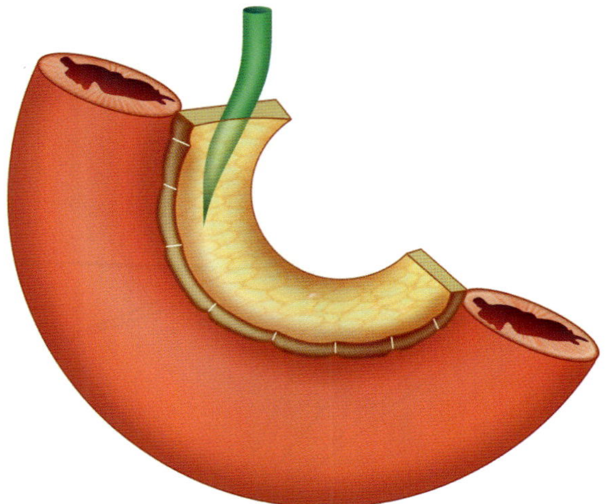

Figure 10 Schematic representation of the extent of resection of pancreatic head at the end of Beger procedure

Technique: This procedure entails the subtotal resection of head mass between PV and the intrapancreatic portion of bile duct.[80] The head of the pancreas is exposed by dividing gastrocolic ligament. After taking down the hepatic flexure, duodenocolic attachments are divided. Duodenum is Kocherized to expose the posterior part of head. Superior mesenteric vein (SMV) is identified below the pancreatic head. Common hepatic artery and the CBD are identified isolated and looped. Starting from SMV and tracing upwards, the tunnel between the pancreas and portal vein is completed. This can be a very difficult in the presence of lot of inflammation and adhesions. A step wise mobilization of vein from pancreas neck is desirable in this situation to avoid inadvertent injury to former. In difficult situations, it is better to loop and have control over the SMV and PV, so as to control any possible bleeding. A sling is passed anterior to PV to lift up the pancreas from it. Gastrodudenal artery is identified and ligated at its origin. Neck of pancreas is divided after placing hemostatic stay sutures at the superior and inferior border of pancreas. While dividing the pancreas, pancreatic duct is easily identified by the sudden release of gush of pancreatic juice. The bleeding points from the cut surface are ligated using a fine monofilament suture (5'O polypropylene). Pancreas is separated from the PV by ligating and dividing the small branches entering directly from the head. The pancreas near the medial transection plane is completely separated from the vascular structures (artery and vein) by anterior and posterior rotation of the pancreas (Figs 11A and B). The lateral limit (duodenal) of the transaction is marked about 5 mm medial to the inner duodenal. It is imperative to identify the wall of bile duct as it enters the pancreas and always remain medial to CBD. If required, a metal dilator can be placed from the supraduodenal part of CBD for ease of identification. The transection is completed by dividing the head mass along the wall of intrapancreatic bile duct towards the papilla. The parenchymal thickness of pancreas on the duodenal wall usually is 5mm anterior and 20–25 mm posterior to the pancreatic duct opening. Once the dissection at the level of papilla is accomplished, the pancreatic transection is completed leaving small amount of tissue along the medial wall of the duodenum till the place where uncinate has previously been separated from the mesenteric vasculature. At the end of

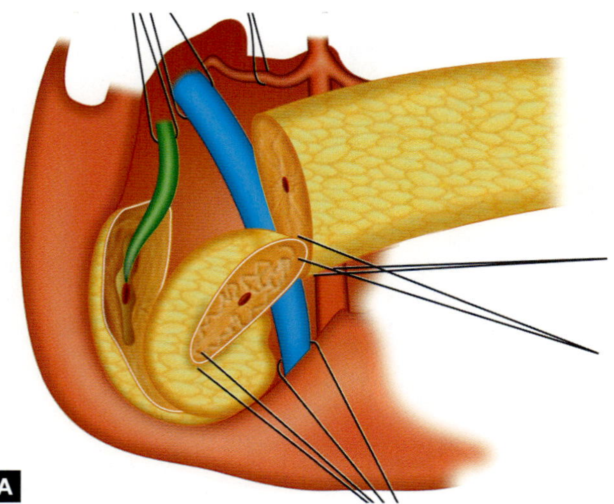

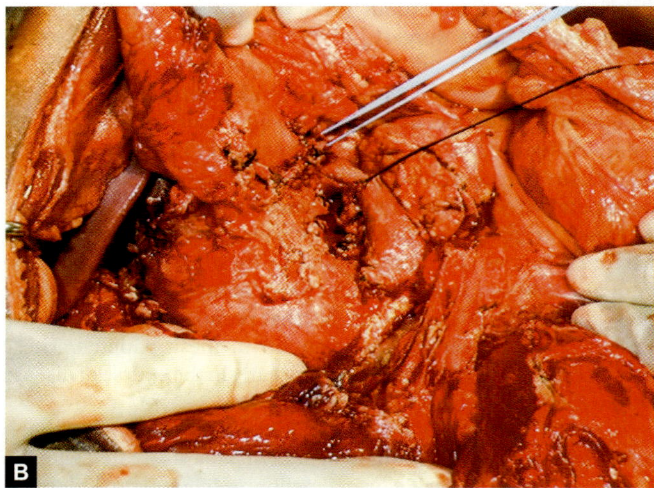

Figures 11A and B (A) Schematic representation of pancreatic head resection after separating pancreas from vascular structures; (B) Picture at the end of duodenum preserving pancreatic head resection (Beger procedure). Note the small diameter of the pancreatic duct at the cut end of pancreas

the procedure, a small rim of tissue remains between the CBD and duodenal wall. Mostly, removal of inflammatory head mass is sufficient to decompress bile duct, but in the presence of persistant stricture, prepapillary bile duct can be opened longitudinally for decompression into the jejunal loop.[80]

About 20-25 cm distal to the ligament of Treitz, a 40 cm Roux limb of jejunum is brought to the pancreas, through retrocolic route to the right of the middle colic artery. End to side anastomosis with mucosa to mucosa approximation is performed between the left pancreas (at the point of transection) and jejunum. About 5-8 cm distal of the left pancreatic anastomosis, jejunal loop is anastomosed to the rim of pancreatic tissue left in the head region in a side to side fashion using interrupted sutures. About 4-5 cm long jejunal incision is required for this anastomosis. Bowel continuity is restored about 40 cm distal to the right anastomosis (Fig. 12). In patients with persistent bile duct stricture, a longitudinal choledochotomy is given in the suprapapillary portion and included in the anastomosis.

In patients with a dilated main pancreatic duct with multiple strictures, the duct can be opened longitudinally on the ventral aspect towards the tail region and a side to side anastomosis is fashioned as done in the drainage procedure.[80]

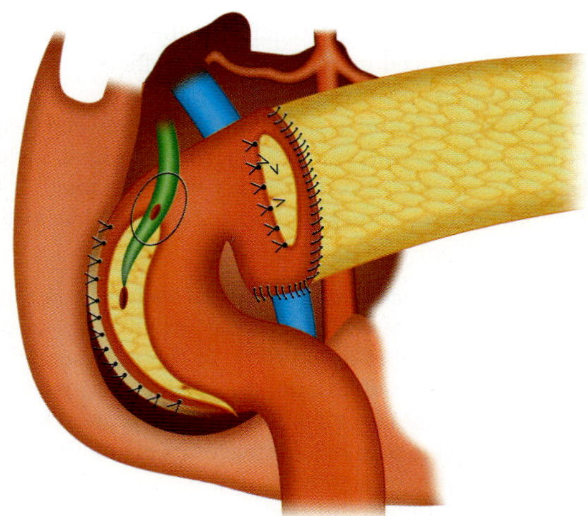

Figure 12 Schematic representation of reconstruction after DPPHR, note two anastomosis are made, one with the neck and another with rim of pancreatic tissue in the head. In the presence of bile duct stricture, the duct can be opened (marked by circle) and drained into the jejeunal loop

Complications: Major complications have been reported variably from 8-40%. These include anastomotic disruptions, arterial hemorrhage, abdominal abscess, surgical site infections and medical complications like pulmonary infections. Need for reoperation has been reported in 2-8% of the patients.[18,21,68,69,80-83]

Outcome: Preservation of enteroduodenal axis helps in better regulation of glucose metabolism because of the good endocrine capacity of the duodenum. Moreover, preservation of duodenum regulates gastric emptying and hence better glycemic control. Complete removal of pancreatic head reduces the circulating glucagon and somatostatin.[84] Decreasing levels of these hormones have been proposed to be responsible for improvement in the endocrine function. Aspelund et al. reported 8% incidence of new onset diabetes at a follow up of 36 months,[82] while Reidiger et al. reported 26% incidence at a median follow up of 44 months.[14] Keck et al. reported 17% incidence of development of de novo diabetes at a median follow up of 62 months.[69] Beger et al. reported 44% incidence of insulin dependent diabetes after a median follow up of 5.7 years.[80]

Exocrine insufficiency has been variably reported from 20-100% of patients in various controlled and uncontrolled studies.[14,80-86] Riediger et al. have reported 75% exocrine deficiency at follow up, however, only 12% had de novo insufficiency.[14]

Complete or partial pain relief is achieved in 70-100% of the patients in various randomized trials.[81,83,86] However, a study of 42 patients, 57% pain relief was observed at 62 months of follow up.[14] While Beger et al. observed 91% pain relief in 388 patients at 5.7 years of follow up.[80]

Modifications of Hybrid Procedures

Bern modification: This is a technical simplification of the Beger-procedure with equivalent outcome.[87-89] The excavation of the pancreatic head is performed identical to that of Beger-procedure. However, in contrast to the latter; there is no need to separate pancreas from the portomesenteric axis. Transaction of the pancreas at that level is not required. This makes the procedure technically easy and safer as it eliminates the difficult dissection of pancreas from the portomesenteric axis particularly in patients with dense inflammation and portal hypertension.[28] A continuous single anastomosis is performed with the pancreatic rim and jejunal Roux limb. The distal duct is probed with a soft feeding tube to ensure the patency. The procedure is ideal for patients with a dominant inflammatory head mass without left side stenosis.[18,28,87] In the event of distal stenosis, the duct should be longitudinally opened and drained towards the left as done in Frey procedure. In patients with concomitant stricture of the bile duct, it can be opened longitudinally and drained into the jejunum as is done in Frey or DPPHR.

Izbicki modification: It is also known as 'Hamburg Modification'. The procedure is most suitable for patients with small duct pancreatitis (SDP).[24,90] A duct diameter of less than 3 mm is classified as small duct disease. In a large series of 978 patients, the incidence of SDP was 5.2%.[91] After the exposure of pancreas, and Kocherization of the duodenum, intrapancreatic common bile duct is identified by placing a metal dilator in the duct. Starting from the upper and lower edges of the gland, the ventral pancreatic aspect is longitudinally excised.[90] This forms a longitudinal triangular cavity along the ventral aspect of pancreas. This V-shaped excision provides adequate drainage of secondary and tertiary order pancreatic ducts (Fig. 13). Subsequently, this V shaped cavity is anastomosed to a Roux-en-Y loop jejunum in a side-to-side manner using a single-layer monofilament running suture. Kutup et al. have reported 17% morbidity associated with the procedure, with complete pain relief in 75%, weight gain in 89%, improved quality of life and return to work. However, they didn't notice any significant change in pancreatic function from the preoperative levels.[92]

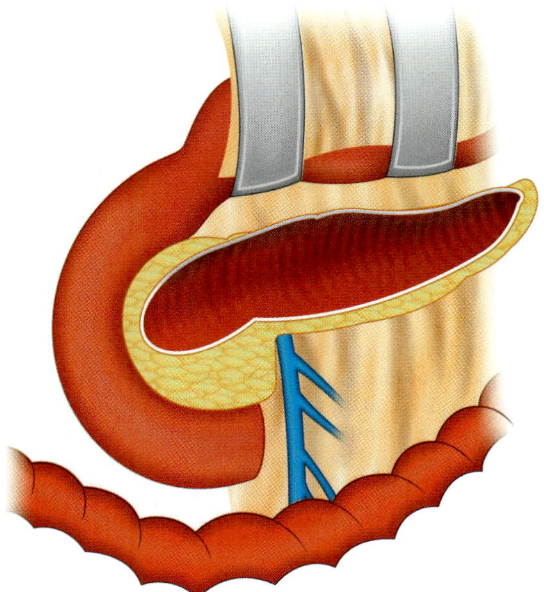

Figure 13 Schematic representation of Izbicki modification. The duct is opened in the shape of longitudinal 'V' shape

Imiazumi modification: Imiazumi modification entails removal of pancreatic head including intraparenchymal bile duct. This allows removal of more pancreatic head than Beger procedure. This procedure is particularly useful while treating patients of chronic pancreatitis bile duct stenosis.[93]

Comparison of Operative Procedures

There are predominantly three major operative procedures: Pancreaticoduodenectomy (PD), Local resection with LPJ (Frey's procedure) and duodenum preserving head resection (Beger's procedure) with or without some modifications, which are performed for chronic pancreatitis (Table 3).

Frey's versus Pancreaticoduodenectomy

A recent meta-analysis comparing the two procedure has shown a shorter operation time, lower intraoperative blood loss and less need for transfusion with the Frey procedure,[94] Chiang et al., in a prospective study comparing Frey with classical Whipple's procedure, found no difference in morbidity, mortality, pain relief and improvement in pancreatic exocrine and endocrine function at 3 and 6 months of follow up.[95] Aspelund et al. found a significantly lower incidence of de novo diabetes (8% vs 25%) after the Frey procedure when compared with pancreaticoduodenectomy.[82] There are two randomized control trials comparing the two procedures. Izbicki et al. in a randomized study found similar pain relief with Frey and PD, however the quality of life was better in patients undergoing the former operation.[86] Moreover, the incidence of complications was significantly lower (19% *vs* 53%) after the Frey procedure.[86] Another randomized control trial by Farkas et al. concluded lesser postoperative complications with similar pain relief and a better long-term quality of life with Frey procedure.[96] Strate et al. in a long term follow-up study (mean of 7 years) found no difference between Frey and pancreaticoduodenectomy in terms of exocrine and endocrine insufficiency, late mortality and survival rates.[97] On the contrary, a 15-year follow-up study of a randomized controlled trial reported poor outcome of pancreaticoduodenectomy in terms of long-term mortality rate.[98] Frey procedure showed better outcome with regards to return to work and weight gain (Tables 3 and 4).[79]

A recent meta-analysis has shown lower postoperative morbidity and mortality and similar pain relief with Frey procedure when compared to PD.[94]

Beger versus Pancreaticoduodenectomy

There are three randomized trial comparing the two procedures. Buchler et al. demonstrated better pain relief and pancreatic function in patients undergoing DPPHR when compared with PPPD.[81] Similar results in terms of pain relief and pancreatic function were reported by in a recent RCT by Keck et al.[99] Klempa et al. in a RCT comparing Beger's procedure with classical PD

Table 3: Randomized controlled trials comparing the three different procedures for chronic pancreatitis

Author	*Place*	*Procedure*	*N*	*Op morbidity (%)*	*Op mortality (%)*	*Pain relief (%)*	*New DM (%)*	*Exo insuf (%)*
Frey versus Pancreaticoduodenectomy								
Frakas et al.[96]	Hungary	Frey PPPD	20 20	0 40	0 0	100 100	0 15	- -
Izbicki et al.[86]	Germany	Frey PPPD	31 30	19 53	3 0	80 75	0 10	58 83
Duodenum preserving pancreatic head resection versus pancreaticoduodenectomy								
Klempa et al.[83]	Germany	DPPHR PD	22 21	54 51	1 0	100 70	12 38	20 100
Buchler et al.[81]	Germany	DPPHR PPPD	20 20	15 20	0 0	94 77	- -	100 100
Keck et al.*[99]	Germany	DPPHR PPPD	42 43	33 30	0 0	67 67	10 8	76 63
Frey versus duodenum preserving pancreatic head resection								
Izbicki et al.[100]	Germany	Frey DPPHR	22 20	9 20	0 0	70 70	0 0	50 50
Kroninger et al.[88]	Germany	OPPHR DPPHR	33 32	21 20	0 0	- -	- -	- -

*includes both Frey and Beger procedure;

Abbreviations: DM: diabetes mellitus; exo: exocrine; op: operative; PPPD: pylorus preserving pancreaticoduodenectomy; DPPHR: duodenum preserving pancreatic head resection; OPPHR: organ preserving pancreatic head resection.

Table 4: Long term outcome (beyond 7 years) of Randomized control trials comparing the three procedures

Author	*Procedure*	*N*	*Late mortality (%)*	*Pain relief (%)*	*New DM (%)*	*Exo insuf (%)*	*Change in QOL*
Klempa et al.[83]	DPPHR PD	22 21	5 5	100 70	25 20	20 100	- -
Izbicki et al.[86]	Frey PPPD	31 30	3 0	90 87	29 37	58 83	71 43
Strate et al.[97]	Frey PPPD	31 30	20 13	81 81	61 65	86 96	58 50
Bachmann et al. [98]	Frey PPPD	32 32	53 30	43 24	81 86	86 93	67 58

Abbreviations: DM: diabetes mellitus; exo: exocrine; PD: pancreaticoduodenectomy; PPPD: pylorus preserving pancreaticoduodenectomy; DPPHR: duodenum preserving pancreatic head resection.

found comparable pain relief with both the procedures.[83] A recent metaanalysis has shown, DPPHR and PD to be equally effective in achieving complete pain relief.[94]

Witzigmann et al. found a higher incidence of developing diabetes following the Whipple procedure.[101] Muller et al. at a follow up of 14-year found a higher incidence of insulin-dependent diabetes following PPPD when compared with Beger's procedure (50% vs 79%), however the need for pancreatic enzyme replacement was similar in both groups.[102] Klempa et al. in a long term study found a favorable outcome with DPPHR in terms of return to work and pain relief, however, the incidence of pancreatic insufficiency was similar.[83]

Frey versus Beger

Two randomized controlled trial have compared Frey procedure with Beger procedure. Kroninger et al. has reported similar perioperative morbidity and mortality with both the procedure.[88] They reported similar quality of life with both the procedures.[88] While another RCT by Izbicki et al. has shown increased morbidity (9% vs 20%) associated with duodenum preserving head resection.[86] They found comparable outcome in terms of pain relief, endocrine, exocrine function, weight gain, return to work and quality of life. The results of the study 8-year follow up study showed equivalent mortality, pain relief, exocrine/endocrine insufficiency, rate of reintervention and quality of life.[103] Keck et al. in a comparative study of 92 patients showed a trend toward better pain control but similar pancreatic insufficiency, weight gain after the Frey procedure when compared to the Beger procedure.[69]

Denervation Procedure

Whatever the mechanism of pain, afferent pain fibers traverse from the pancreas to the brain via the sympathetic nerves.[104]

Afferent fibers course via the celiac ganglion and some of them may travel across the midline. Afferent impulses (pain) travel to the sympathetic ganglia (T5 - T10) via the splanchnic nerves[21]. The greater splanchnic nerve descends on the ribs. The azygous and hemiazygous veins are the main anatomic landmark for identification of respectively the right and left greater splanchnic nerves.[105] The major nerve trunks pierce the ipsilateral diaphragmatic crura and reach the celiac ganglion. Several attempts to interrupt the neural pain pathway by non-surgical or surgical neurolysis (temporary or permanent), have been reported with varying success.[104] Celiac ganglia block can be used as a prognostic marker for pain relief after resection. Patient having a reduction in pain after celiac ganglion blockade are more likely to profit from splanchnicectomy. Those who improve with celiac ganglia neurolysis have a higher possibility of pain relief after pancreatic resection with or without islet cell transplantation.[21]

Neural ablation is an alternative method of pain palliation without resection and hence preservation of the function of residual organ.[104]

Besides radiological and endosonography guided neural blocks, surgical ablation of splanchnic nerves can be offered as a treatment modality in patients with intractable pain not suitable for pancreatic resection or drainage. With the advent of Video-assisted thoracoscopic surgery (VATS) the procedure can be performed with minimum morbidity.[106,107] *One* study of 14 patients undergoing VATS for chronic pancreatitis has reported complete resolution of pain in 25% of the patients, with a low morbidity and a short hospital stay.[24] However, pain relief is variable and over longer duration most develop recurrent pain within several months of their procedure.[106,107]

MANAGEMENT OF COMPLICATIONS OF CHRONIC PANCREATITIS

Biliary Obstruction

The incidence of biliary obstruction in chronic pancreatitis varies from 3–46% depending upon the methodology of evaluation. Majority of the patients don't develop jaundice secondary to obstruction.[6,21,24,108,109]

The stricture associated with CP is usually long segment. One study has reported a mean length of the stricture to be 40.7 mm (range 16–57 mm).[110] Based on the morphology of stricture, Caroli and Nora classified stricture into five types:[111] type I - long retropancreatic stenosis [commonest in CP, (Fig. 14)], type II dilatation of the main bile duct, stricture of the sphincter of oddi, type III: hourglass stricture, type IV: symptomatic of either a cyst or a malignancy and type V: cancer of the pancreas. The importance lies in planning the surgical strategy in these patients. Type IV (malignancy) and V strictures always require oncological resection, whereas type I to III does not always require intervention. The indications of biliary drainage are as listed[112] in Box 3.

Endoscopic management of biliary obstruction has high technical success rates but is associated with complications of stent clogging and septic complications on long term basis. It should be reserved only for emergency situations and in patients with severe comorbidities who are not suitable for surgical interventions.[6,108]

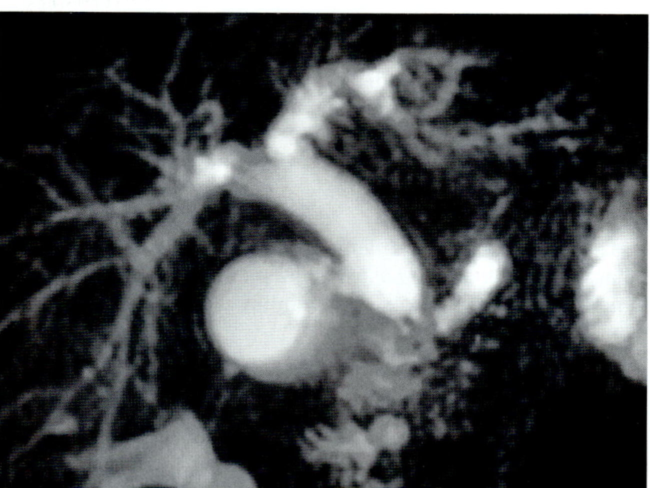

Figure 14 MRCP showing type I biliary stricture in association with chronic pancreatitis

BOX 3 Indications of surgery in biliary obstruction due to chronic pancreatitis[112]

- Symptomatic cholangitis or infected bile.
- Biliary cirrhosis (biopsy proven).
- CBD stones in association with common bile duct stricture.
- Inability to rule out cancer of the pancreas.
- Progression of the common bile duct structure based on radiological assessment of increased dilatation of the common and intrahepatic bile ducts.
- Persistent jaundice for over a month.
- Persistently elevated alkaline phosphatase (more than 3 times normal levels beyond 1 month).

In about two thirds of the patients, excision of the pancreas (Frey or DPPHR) head is sufficient to decompress the biliary obstruction. However, if the biliary dilatation persists even after head resection, it is advisable to add biliary decompression.[108,112,113] Bile duct can be decompressed by a lateral longitudinal choledochotomy in the intrapancreatic portion of the duct after completing the head excision.[18,19,80] The choledochotomy is drained in the same jejunal loop used for pancreatic anastomosis. Imiazumi modification of DPPHR can address the issue of biliary obstruction very effectively.[93] Alternatively, in patients with long stricture beyond pancreas, chledochoduodenostomy or choledochojejunostomy can be performed.[109] Cholecystojejunostomy, though easy to construct is associated with a failure rate of about 23%, and should be avoided.[108]

Duodenal Obstruction

Duodenal obstruction occurs less frequently in CP than biliary obstruction. The reported incidence is 1.2% with a range of 0.5–10%.[6,21,24] Two different types of obstruction have been defined—acute transient obstruction and persistent fibrous stenosis.[6] The former is more common during acute exacerbation as a result of mucosal edema, and does not need any intervention and usually resolves with supportive treatment.

Patients with complete duodenal obstruction, who have persistent symptoms beyond 4 weeks period, and who have recurrent episodes of duodenal obstruction should be suspected of having duodenal stenosis and considered for surgical intervention[6].

Gastrojejunostomy should be performed in these patients and vagotomy should preferably be added in view of benign condition.

Chronic pancreatitis patients with a head mass and combined biliary and duodenal obstruction should be considered for pancreaticoduodenectomy or a combined biliary and duodenal bypass.

Portal Hypertension

Extrahepatic portal hypertension is a well-known complication of CP. Total or subtotal occlusion of the spleno-porto-mesenteric axis may occur variably.[114,115,116] Splenic vein is the most common to be involved and has been reported variably from 2-45 %.[7,117,118] The incidence of portal and/or mesenteric vein obstruction has been described in about 5-10%.[7,114-118] The presence of spleno-porto-mesenteric occlusion per se is not an indication for surgery.[119] Occurrence of bleeding and esophageal, gastric varices has been reported respectively in 0.5% and 2% of the patients.[7,117] Compression of spleno-porto-mesenteric axis in the inflammatory process has been proposed to be the cause for non-occlusive portal hypertension.

Surgery is done for the pancreatic symptoms, not for portal hypertension. Presence of portal hypertension opens up portosystemic collaterals (Fig. 15) prolongs the surgery, increases blood loss, increases hospital stay. However, the long term outcome of these patients was similar to those without portal hypertension.[114,115,116] Bockhorn et al. has shown the similar outcomes in patients of portal hypertension with or without cavernomatous transformation of portal vein.[116] In the event of cavernomatous transformation of portal vein, procedure which entail separation of pancreas from portal vein (pancreaticoduodenectomy or Beger) should not be attempted.[116] In such a situation Frey or Hamburg procedure is more suitable. In patients with non occlusive portal hypertension, a prospective randomized trial has shown better restoration of splanchnic flow in patients undergoing resectional procedure (PPPD and DPHR) when compared to Frey procedure.[120] Dissection along the portomesenteric axis releases the vessels from the inflammatory and fibrous tissue and decompresses the vasculature. Resectional operations can prevent the late complications associated with extrahepatic portal hypertension.

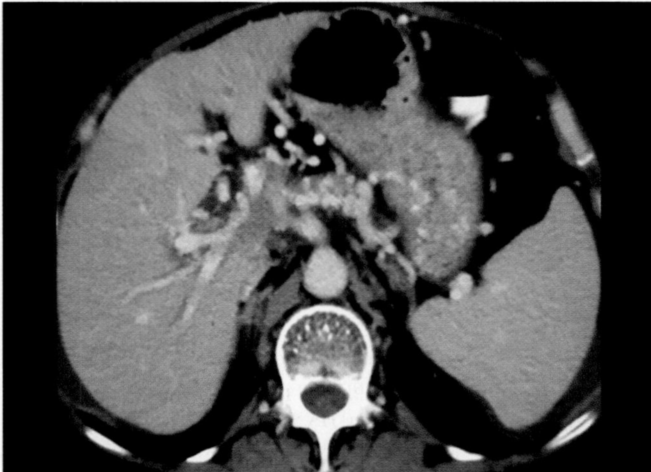

Figure 15 CECT showing cavernomatous transformation of the portal vein. Note is made on the presence of multiple collaterals in hepatoduodenal and peripancreatic area

Patients with extensive collaterals which could preclude a safe pancreatic drainage or resection should undergo a staged procedure—shunt surgery followed by a definitive pancreatic surgery.[114] Patients with isolated thrombosis of splenic vein can be treated by splenectomy as it eliminates all the venous outflow collaterals, thereby decompressing the varices.[7] Patients with bleeding or high risk varices should undergo splenectomy. The role of prophylactic splenectomy in the absence of bleed is debatable. This is because of the rarity of bleed and lack of progression of varices on follow-up endoscopy in patients with asymptomatic varices.[117] However, if laparotomy is performed for other purposes in a patient with known asymptomatic varices, a splenectomy should be performed. In patients with combined occlusion of splenic and portal vein, a gastric revascularization procedure or a meso caval shunt can give protection against variceal bleeding.

Table 5: Choice of surgical procedure in chronic pancreatitis

Procedure	*Pathomorphology*
Drainage procedures	
Caudal drainage (Duval) Puestow Procedure	Obsolete, replaced by newer procedures
Lateral pancreatico-jejunostomy	Dilated main pancreatic duct (>7mm) without presence of inflammatory head mass
Resection procedures	
PD/ PPPD	• Suspected neoplasia • Presence of fixed duodenal stenosis
Distal pancreatectomy	Focal disease localized to the body and tail region of pancreas
Total pancreatectomy	• Only as a salvage procedure • Caution of brittle diabetes
Total pancreatectomy with AIT	• Intractable pain, Preserves endocrine function • Caution severe exocrine insufficiency
Hybrid procedures	Exclude malignancy by frozen section
Frey procedure	• Ductal obstruction with a small inflammatory head mass • Technically easier
Beger procedure	• Large Inflammatory head mass without a distal stricture • Technically difficult, separation from portomesenteric axis
V shaped excision	Small duct pancreatitis (<3 mm)

CONCLUSION

Pain is the dominant symptom which dictates the need for surgical intervention. The therapy should be tailored to the symptoms of the patient, the stage of the disease and pathomorphology of the pancreas. Choice of surgical procedure is dictated by the status of the main pancreatic duct and inflammatory head mass (Table 5). Pain relief is similar for hybrid procedures and pancreaticoduodenectomy. Resectional procedures should be avoided as far as possible as it leads to the permanent extirpation of functioning parenchyma. Presence of biliary, duodenal and vascular compression needs to be addressed appropriately. Surgical intervention provides an effective long term pain relief and improved quality of life, but does not stop the progression of functional deterioration of pancreas. Development of endocrine or exocrine dysfunction after surgical intervention is not a failure of therapy but is the natural course of the disease. More research should be directed towards improvement of the pancreatic function.

REFERENCES

1. Layer P, Yamamoto H, Kalthoff L, Clain JE, Bakken LJ, DiMagno EP. The different courses of early- and late-onset idiopathic and alcoholic chronic pancreatitis. Gastroenterology. 1994;107:1481-7.
2. Di Sebastiano P. The quality of life in chronic pancreatitis: the role of surgery. JOP. 2006;7:120-1.
3. Lankisch PG, Lohr-Happe A, Otto J, Creutzfeldt W. Natural course in chronic pancreatitis: pain, exocrine and endocrine pancreatic insufficiency and prognosis of the disease. Digestion. 1993;54: 148-55.
4. Ammann RW, Muellhaupt B. The natural history of pain in alcoholic chronic pancreatitis. Gastroenterology. 1999;116:1132-40.
5. Beger HG, Buchler M, Bittner RR, Oettinger W, Roscher R. Duodenum-preserving resection of the head of the pancreas in severe chronic pancreatitis: early and late results. Ann Surg. 1989;209:273-8.
6. Vijungco JD, Prinz RA. Management of biliary and duodenal complications of chronic pancreatitis. World J Surg. 2003;27:1258-70.
7. Weber SM, Rikkers LF. Splenic vein thrombosis and gastrointestinal bleeding in chronic pancreatitits. World J Surg. 2003;27:1271-4.
8. D'Haese JG, Ceyhan GO, Demir IE, Tieftrunk E, Friess H. Treatment option in painful chronic pancreatitis: a systematic review. HPB (Oxford). 2014;16:512-21.
9. van der Gaag NA, van Gulik TM, Busch OR, Sprangers MA, Bruno MJ, Zevenbergen C, Gouma DJ, et al. Functional and medical outcomes after tailored surgery for pain due to chronic pancreatitis. Ann Surg. 2012;255:763-70.
10. Dite P, Ruzicka M, Zboril V, Novotny I. A prospective, randomized trial comparing endoscopic and surgical therapy for chronic pancreatitis. Endoscopy. 2003;35:553-8.
11. Cahen DL, Gauma DJ, Nio Y, Rauws EA, BoermeesterMA, Busch OR, et al. Endoscopic versus surgical drainage of the pancreatic duct in chronic pancreatitis. N Engl J Med. 2007:356:676-84.
12. Ahmed Ali U, Nieuwenhuijs VB, van Eijck Ch, Gooszen HG, van Dam RM, Busch OR, et al. Clinical outcome in relation to timing of surgery in chronic pancreatitis: a nomogram to predict pain relief. Arch Surg. 2012;147:925-32.
13. Yang CJ, Bliss LA, Schapira EF, Freedman SD, Ng SC, Windsor JA, Tseng JF. Systematic review of early surgery for chronic pancreatitis: impact on pain, pancreatic function and re-intervention. J Gastrointest Surg. 2014;18:1863-9.
14. Riediger H, Adam U, Fischer E, Keck T, Pfeffer F, Hopt UT, Makowiec F. Long-term outcome after resection for chronic pancreatitis in 224 patients. J Gastrointest Surg. 2007;11:949-59.
15. Alexakis N, Connor S, Ghaneh P, Raraty M, Lombard M, Smart H, et al. Influence of opioid use on surgical and long-term outcome after resection for chronic pancreatitis. Surgery. 2004;136:600-8.
16. Lowenfels AB, Maisonneuve P, Cavallini G, Ammann RW, Lankisch PG, Andersen JR, et al. Pancreatitis and the risk of pancreatic cancer. International Pancreatitis Study Group. N Engl J Med. 1993;328:1433-7.
17. Perumal S, Palaniappan R, Pillai SA, Velayutham V, Sathyanesan J. Predictors of malignancy in chronic calcific pancreatitis with head mass. World J Gastrointest Surg. 2013;5:97-103.
18. Andersen DK, Frey CF. Evolution of surgical treatment of chronic pancreatitis. Ann Surg. 2010;251:18-32.
19. Frey CF, Andersen DK. Surgery for chronic pancreatitis. Am J Surg. 2007;194(Suppl):S53-60.
20. Merdrignac A, Sulpice L, Rayar M, Rohou M, Quehen E, Zamreek A, et al. Pancreatic head cancer in patients with chronic pancreatitis. Hepatobiliary Pancreat Dis Int. 2014;13:192-7.
21. Ahmed SA, Wary C, Rilo HL, Choe KA, Gelrud A, Howington JA, et al. Chronic pancreatitis: recent advances and ongoing challenges. Curr Probl Surg. 2006;43:127-238.
22. Zhu M, Xu C, Wu Y, Li C, Zhang M, Li Z. Differentiation of pancreatic cancer and chronic pancreatitis using computer-aided diagnosis of endoscopic ultrasound (EUS) images: a diagnostic test. PLoS One. 2013;8:e63820.
23. Cote GA, Smith J, Sherman S, Kelly K. Technologies for imaging the normal and diseased pancreas. Gastroenterology 2013;144: 1262-71.
24. Bachmann K Izbicki JR, Yekebas EF. Chronic pancreatitis: modern surgical management. Langenbecks Arch Surg 2011;396:139-49.
25. Bloechle C, Izbicki JR, Knoefel WT, Keuchler T, Broelsch CE. Quality of life in chronic pancreatitis: results after duodenum-preserving resection of the head of the pancreas. Pancreas. 1995;11:77-85.
26. Rasmussen HH, Irtun O, Olesen SS, Drewes AM, Holst M. Nutrition in chronic pancreatitis. World J Gastroenterol. 2013;19:7267-75.
27. Pothula Rajendra VK, Sivanpillay Mahadevan S, Parvathareddy SR, Nara BK, Gorlagunta Ramachandra M, Tripuraneni Venkata AC. Frey's pancreaticojejunostomy in tropical pancreatitis: assessment of quality of life. A prospective study. World J Surg. 2014;13:3235-47.
28. Strobel O, Buchler MW, Werner J. Surgical therapy of chronic pancreatitis: indications, techniques and results. Int J Surg. 2009;7:305-12.
29. Traverso LW, Kozarek RA. The Whipple procedure for severe complications of chronic pancreatitis. Arch Surg. 1993;128:1047-50.
30. Jimenez RE, Fernandez-Del Castillo C, Rattner DW, Warshaw AL. Pylorus-preserving pancreaticoduodenectomy in the treatment of chronic pancreatitis. World J Surg. 2003;27:1211-6.
31. Martin RF, Rossi RL, Leslie KA. Long-term results of pylorus-preserving pancreatoduodenectomy for chronic pancreatitis. Arch. Surg. 1996;131:247-52.
32. McAfee MK, van Heerden JA, Adson MA. Is proximal pancreatoduodenectomy with pyloric preservation superior to total pancreatectomy? Surgery. 1989;105:347-51.
33. Morel P, Mathey P, Corboud H, Huber O, Egeli RA, Rohner A. Pylorus-preserving duodenopancreatectomy: long-term complications and comparison with the Whipple procedure. World J. Surg. 1990;14:642-6.
34. Stapleton GN, Williamson RC. Proximal pancreatoduodenectomy for chronic pancreatitis. Br. J. Surg. 1996;83:1433-40.
35. Duffy JP, Delano MJ, Reber HA Pancreatic surgery. Curr Opin Gastroenterol. 2002; 18:568-73.
36. Sawyer R, Frey CF. Is there still a role for distal pancreatectomy in surgery for chronic pancreatitis? Am J Surg. 1994;168:6-9.
37. Hutchins RR, Hart RS, Pacifico M, Bradley NJ, Williamson RC Long-term results of distal pancreatectomy for chronic pancreatitis in 90 patients. Ann Surg. 2002;236:612-8.

38. Schoenberg MH, Schlosser W, Ruck W, Beger HG Distal pancreatectomy in chronic pancreatitis. Dig Surg. 1999;16:130-6.
39. Fry WJ, Child CG III. Ninety-five per cent distal pancreatectomy for chronic pancreatitis. Ann Surg. 1965;162:543-9.
40. Frey CF, Child CG, Fry W. Pancreatectomy for chronic pancreatitis. Ann Surg. 1976;184:403-13.
41. Linehan IP, Lambert MA, Brown DC, Kutz AB, Cotton PB, Russell RC. Total pancreatectomy for chronic pancreatitis. Gut. 1988;29:358-65.
42. Fleming WR, Williamson RC. Role of total pancreatectomy in the treatment of patients with end-stage chronic pancreatitis. Br J Surg. 1995;82:1409-12.
43. Cooper MJ, Williamson RC, Benjamin IS, Carter DC, Cuschieri A, Linehan IP, et al. Total pancreatectomy for chronic pancreatitis. Br J Surg. 1987;74:912-5.
44. Stone WM, Sarr MG, Nagorney DM, Mcllrath DC. Chronic pancreatitis. Results of Whipple's resection and total pancreatectomy. Arch Surg. 1988;123:815-9.
45. White SA, Robertson GS, London NJ, Dennison AR. Human islet cell autotransplantation to prevent diabetes after pancreas resection. Dig Surg. 2000;17:439-50.
46. Farney AC, Najarian JS, Nakhleh RE Lioveras G, Field MJ, Gores PF, et al. Autotransplantation of dispersed pancreatic islet tissue combined with total or near-total pancreatectomy for treatment of chronic pancreatitis. Surgery. 1991;110:427-37; discussion 437-9.
47. Shapiro AM, Ricordi C, Hering BJ, Auchincloss H, lindblad R, Robertson RP, et al. International trial of the Edmonton protocol for islet transplantation. N Engl J Med. 2006;355:1318-30.
48. Rodriguez Rilo HL, Ahmad SA, D'Alessio D, Iwanaga Y, Kim J, Choe KA, et al. Total pancreatectomy and autologous islet cell transplantation as a means to treat severe chronic pancreatitis. J Gastrointest Surg. 2003;7:978-89.
49. Gould AP. Pancreatic calculi: transaction of the clinical Society of London. Lancet. 1898;2:1532.
50. Mayo-Robson AW. The pathology and surgery of certain diseases of the pancreas. Lancet. 1904:773.
51. Link G. Pancreatostomy for chronic pancreatitis with calculi in the duct of Wirsung and diffuse calcinosis of the pancreatic parenchyma. Ann Surg. 1953;138:287-8.
52. DuVal MK Jr. Caudal pancreatico-jejunostomy for chronic relapsing pancreatitis. Ann Surg. 1954;140:775-85.
53. Zollinger RM, Keith LM Jr, Ellison EH. Pancreatitis. N Engl J Med. 1954;251:497-502.
54. Puestow CB, Gillesby WJ. Retrograde surgical drainage of pancreas for chronic relapsing pancreatitis. AMA Arch Surg. 1958;76: 898-907.
55. Partington PF, Rochelle RE. Modified Puestow procedure for retrograde drainage of the pancreatic duct. Ann Surg. 1960;152: 1037-43.
56. Schnelldorfer T, Lewin DN, Adams DB. Operative management of chronic pancreatitis: longterm results in 372 patients. J Am Coll Surg. 2007 May;204(5):1039-45; discussion 1045-7.
57. Bradley EL. Long-term results of pancreaticojejunostomy in patients with chronic pancreatitis. Am J Surg. 1987;153:207-13.
58. Nealon WH, Matin S. Analysis of surgical success in preventing recurrent acute exacerbations in chronic pancreatitis. Ann Surg. 2001;233:793-800.
59. Delcore R, Rodriguez FJ, Thomas JH, Forster J, Hermreck AS. The role of pancreaticojejunostomy in patients without dilated pancreatic ducts. Am J Surg. 1994;168:598-601; discussion 601-2.
60. Adams DB, Ford MC, Anderson MC Outcome after lateral pancreaticojejunostomy for chronic pancreatitis. Ann Surg. 1994; 219:481-7.
61. Greenlee HB, Prinz RA, Aranha GV. Longterm results of side-to-side pancreaticojejunostomy. World J Surg. 1990;14:70-6.
62. Sato T, Miyashita E, Yamauchi H, Matsuno S. The role of surgical treatment for chronic pancreatitis. Ann Surg. 1986;203:266-71.
63. Holmberg JT, Isaksson G, Ihse I. Long-term results of pancreaticojejunostomy in chronic pancreatitis. Surg Gynecol Obstet. 1985;160:339-46.
64. Warshaw AL. Conservation of pancreatic tissue by combined gastric, biliary, and pancreatic duct drainage for pain from chronic pancreatitis. Am J Surg. 1985;149:563-9.
65. Nealon WH, Thompson JC Progressive loss of pancreatic function in chronic pancreatitis is delayed by main pancreatic duct decompression. A longitudinal prospective analysis of the modified puestow procedure. Ann Surg. 1993;217:458-68.
66. Prinz RA, Greenlee HB. Pancreatic duct drainage in 100 patients with chronic pancreatitis. Ann Surg. 1981;194:313-20.
67. Frey CF, Smith GJ. Description and rationale of a new operation for chronic pancreatitis. Pancreas. 1987;2:701-7.
68. Roch A, Teyssedou J, Mutter D, Marescaux J, Pessaux P. Chronic pancreatitis: a surgical disease? Role of Frey procedure. World J Gastrointest Surg. 2014;6:129-35.
69. Keck T, Wellner UF, Riediger H, Adam U, Sick O, Hopt UT, et al. Long-term outcome after 92 duodenum-preserving pancreatic head resections for chronic pancreatitis: comparison of Beger and Frey procedures. J Gastrointest Surg 2010;14:549-56.
70. Pessaux P, Kianmanesh R, Regimbeau JM, Sastre B, Delcenserie R, Sielezneff I, et al. Frey procedure in the treatment of chronic pancreatitis: short-term results. Pancreas. 2006;33:354-8.
71. Roch AM, Brachet D, Lermite E, Pessaux P, Arnaud JP. Frey procedure in patients with chronic pancreatitis: short and long-term outcome from a prospective study. J Gastrointest Surg 2012;16:1362-9.
72. Frey CF, Amikura K. Local resection of the head of the pancreas combined with longitudinal pancreaticojejunostomy in the management of patients with chronic pancreatitis. Ann Surg. 1994;220:492-504; discussion 504-7.
73. Ho HS, Frey CF. Frey procedure combined: local resection of pancreatic head combined with lateral pancreaticojejunostomy. Arch Surg. 2001;136:1353-8.
74. Negi S, Singh A, Chaudhary A. Pain relief after Frey's procedure for chronic pancreatitis. Br J Surg.2010;97:1087-95.
75. Cooper MA, Makary MA, Ng J, Cui Y, Singh VK, Matsukuma K, et al. Extent of pancreatic fibrosis as a determinant of symptom resolution after the Frey procedure: a clinico-pathologic analysis. J Gastrointest Surg. 2013;17:682-7.
76. Shrikhande SV, Kleeff J, Friess H, Büchler MW. Management of pain in small duct chronic pancreatitis. J Gastrointest Surg. 2006;10: 227-33.
77. Frey CF, Reber HA. Local resection of the head of the pancreas with pancreaticojejunostomy. J Gastrointest Surg. 2005;9:863-8.
78. Falconi M, Bassi C, Casetti L, Mantovani W, Mascetta G, Sartori N, et al. Long-term results of Frey's procedure for chronic pancreatitis: a longitudinal prospective study on 40 patients. J Gastrointest Surg. 2006;10:504-10.
79. Hildebrand P, Duderstadt S, Jungbluth T, Roblick UJ, Bruch HP, Czymek R. Evaluation of the quality of life after surgical treatment of chronic pancreatitis. JOP 2011;12:364-71.
80. Beger HG, Rau BM, Poch B. Duodenum-preserving pancreatic head resection. In Beger HG, Matsuno S, Cameron JL, editors, Diseases of the pancreas current surgical therapy; Springer, 1st edn. pp. 399-412.
81. Buchler MW, Friess H, Muller MW, Wheatley AM, Beger HG. Randomized trial of duodenum preserving pancreatic head resection versus pylorus-preserving Whipple in chronic pancreatitis. Am J Surg. 1995;169:65-9; discussion 69-70.

82. Aspelund G, Topazian MD, Lee JH, Andersen DK. Improved outcomes for benign disease with limited pancreatic head resection. J Gastrointest Surg. 2005;9:400-9.
83. Klempa I, Spatny M, Menzel J, Baca I, Nustede R, Stockmann F, et al. Pancreatic function and quality of life after resection of the head of the pancreas in chronic pancreatitis. A prospective, randomized comparative study after duodenum preserving resection of the head of the pancreas versus Whipple's operation. Chirurg. 1995;66:350-9.
84. Bittner R, Butters M, Buchler M, Nagele S, Roscher R, Beger HG. Glucose homeostasis and endocrine pancreatic function in patients with chronic pancreatitis before and after surgical therapy. Pancreas 1994;9:47-53.
85. McClaine RJ, Lowy AM, Matthews JB, Schmulewitz N, Sussman JJ, Ingraham Am, et al. A comparison of pancreaticoduodenectomy and duodenum-preserving head resection for the treatment of chronic pancreatitis. HPB (Oxford). 2009;11:677-83.
86. Izbicki JR, Bloechle C, Broering DC, Knoefel W, Kuechler T, Broelsch CE. Extended drainage versus resection in surgery for chronic pancreatitis: a prospective randomized trial comparing the longitudinal pancreaticojejunostomy combined with local pancreatic head excision with the pylorus-preserving pancreatoduodenectomy. Ann Surg. 1998;228:771-9.
87. Gloor B, Friess H, Uhl W, Buchler MW. A modified technique of the Beger and Frey procedure in patients with chronic pancreatitis. Dig Surg. 2001;18:21-5.
88. Koninger J, Seiler CM, Sauerland S, Wente MN, Reidel MA, Muller MW, et al. Duodenum-preserving pancreatic head resection–a randomized controlled trial comparing the original Beger procedure with the Berne modification (ISRCTN No. 50638764). Surgery. 2008;143:490-8.
89. Muller MW, Friess H, Leitzbach S, Michalski CW, Berberat P, Ceyhan GO, et al. Perioperative and follow-up results after central pancreatic head resection (Berne technique) in a consecutive series of patients with chronic pancreatitis. Am J Surg. 2008;196:364-72.
90. Izbicki JR, Bloechle C, Broering DC, Kuechler T, Broelsch CE. Longitudinal V-shaped excision of the ventral pancreas for small duct disease in severe chronic pancreatitis: prospective evaluation of a new surgical procedure. Ann Surg. 1998; 227: 213-9.
91. Yekebas EF, Bogoevski D, Honarpisheh H, Cataldegirmen G, Habermann CR, Seewald S, et al. Long-term follow up in small duct chronic pancreatits: A plea for extended drainage by "V-shaped excision" of the anterior aspect of the pancreas. Ann Surg. 2006; 244: 940-8.
92. Kutup A, Vashisht Y, Kaifi JT, Yekebas EF, Izbicki JR. For which type of chronic pancreatitis is the "Hamburg procedure" indicated? J Hepatobiliary Pancreat Sci. 2010;17: 758-62.
93. Hatori T, Imaizumi T, Harada N, Fukuda A, Suzuki M, Hanyu F, et al. Appraisal of Imaizumi modification of the Beger procedure: the TWMU experience. J Hepatobiliary Pancreat Sci. 2010;17: 752-7.
94. Yin Z, Sun J, Yin D, Wang J. Surgical treatment strategies in chronic pancreatitis: a meta-analysis. Arch Surg. 2012;147:961-8.
95. Chiang KC, Yeh CN, Hsu JT, Chen HM, Chen HY, Hwang TL, et al. Pancreaticoduodenectomy versus Frey's procedure for chronic pancreatitis: preliminary data on outcome and pancreatic function. Surg Today. 2007;37:961-6.
96. Farkas G, Leindler L, Daroczi M, Farkas G Jr. Prospective randomised comparison of organ-preserving pancreatic head resection with pylorus-preserving pancreaticoduodenectomy. Langenbecks Arch Surg. 2006;391:338-42.
97. Strate T, Bachmann K, Busch P, Mann O, Schneider C, Bruhn JP, et al. Resection vs drainage in treatment of chronic pancreatitis: long-term results of a randomized trial. Gastroenterology. 2008;134:1406-11.
98. Bachmann K, Tomkoetter L, Kutup A, Erbes J, Vashist Y, Mann O, et al. Is the Whipple procedure harmful for long-term outcome in treatment of chronic pancreatitis? 15-years follow-up comparing the outcome after pylorus-preserving pancreatoduodenectomy and Frey procedure in chronic pancreatitis. Ann Surg. 2013;258:815-20; discussion 820-1.
99. Keck T, Adam U, Makowiec F, Reidiger H, Wellner U, Tittelbach-Helmrich D, et al. Short and long-term results of duodenum preservation versus resection for the management of chronic pancreatitis: a prospective randomized study. Surgery. 2012;152: S95-102.
100. Izbicki JR, Bloechle C, Knoefel WT, Kuechler T, Binmoeller KF, Broelsch CE. Duodenum-preserving resection of the head of the pancreas in chronic pancreatitis: a prospective, randomized trial. Ann Surg. 1995;221:350-8.
101. Witzigmann H, Max D, Uhlmann D, Geissler F, Schwarz R, Ludwig S, et al. Outcome after duodenum-preserving pancreatic head resection is improved compared with classic Whipple procedure in the treatment of chronic pancreatitis. Surgery. 2003;134:53-62.
102. Muller MW, Friess H, Martin DJ, Hinz U, Dahmen R, Buchler MW. Long-term follow-up of a randomized clinical trial comparing Beger with pylorus-preserving Whipple procedure for chronic pancreatitis. Br J Surg. 2008;95:350-6.
103. Strate T, Taherpour Z, Bloechle C, Mann O, Bruhn JP, Schneider C, et al. Long-term follow-up of a randomized trial comparing the beger and frey procedures for patients suffering from chronic pancreatitis. Ann Surg. 2005;241:591-8.
104. Bradley EL, Bem J. Nerve blocks and neuroablative surgery for chronic pancreatitis. World J Surg. 2003;27:1241-8.
105. Noppen M, Meysman M, D'Haese J, Vincken W. Thoracoscopic splanchnicolysis for the relief of chronic pancreatitis pain: experience of a group of pneumologists. Chest. 1998;113:528-31.
106. Maher JW, Johlin FC, Heitshusen D. Long-term follow-up of thoracoscopic splanchnicectomy for chronic pancreatitis pain. Surg Endosc. 2001;15:706-9.
107. Hammond B, Vitale GC, Rangnekar N, Vitale EA, Binford JC. Bilateral thoracoscopic splanchnicectomy for pain control in chronic pancreatitis. Am Surg 2004;70:546-9.
108. Abdallah AA, Krige JEJ, Bornman PC. Biliary tract obstruction in chronic pancreatitis. HPB (Oxford). 2007;9:421-8.
109. Saluja SS, Kalayarasan R, Mishra PK, Srivastava S, Chandrasekar S, Godhi S. Chronic pancreatitis with benign biliary obstruction: management issues. World J Surg. 2014;38:2455-9.
110. Snape WJ, Long WB, Trotman BW, Marin GA, Czaja AJ. Marked alkaline phosphatase elevation with partial common bile duct obstruction due to calcific pancreatitis. Gastroenterology. 1976;70:70-3.
111. Caroli J, Nora J. L'hepato-choledoque dans les pancreatitis. Ille Congres Europeen des Societes Nationales de Gastroenterologie. Bologne 1952.
112. Frey C, Suzuki M, Isaji S. Treatment of chronic pancreatitis complicated by obstruction of the common bile duct or duodenum. World J Surg. 1990;14:59-69.
113. Rebibo L, Yzet T, Cosse C, Delcenserie R, Bartoli E, Regimbeau JM. Frey procedure for the treatment of chronic pancreatitis associated with common bile duct stricture. Hepatobiliary Pancreat Dis int. 2013;12: 637-44.
114. Ramesh H, Jacob G, Venugopal A, Lekha V, Jacob M. Surgical management of chronic pancreatitis with portal hypertension – a 19 year experience. Surgery. 2008,143:252-8.
115. Adam U, Makoweic F, Riediger H, Keck T, Kroger JC, Uhrmeister P, et al. Pancreas head resection for chronic pancreatitis in patients

with extrahepatic generalized portal hypertension. Surgery. 2004;135:411-8.

116. Bockhorn M, Gebauer F, Bogoevski D, Molmenti E, Cataldegirmen D, Vashisht YK, et al. Chronic pancreatitis complicated by cavernoustransformation of the portal vein: contraindication to surgery? Surgery. 2011;149:321-8.
117. Agarwal AK, Raj Kumar K, Agarwal S, Singh S. Significance of splenic vein thrombosis in chronic pancreatitis. Am J Surg. 2008;196:149-54.
118. Bernades P, Baetz A, Levy P, Belghiti J, Menu Y, Fekete F. Splenic and portal venous obstruction in chronic pancreatitis. A prospective longitudinal study of a medical-surgical series of 266 patients. Dig Dis Sci. 1992;37:340-6.
119. Izbicki JR, Yekebas EF, Strate T, Eisenberger CF, Hosch SB, Steffani K, et al. Extrahepatic portal hypertension in chronic pancreatitis: an old problem revisited. Ann Surg. 2002;236:82-9.
120. Beger HG, KrautzbergerW, Bittner R, Buchler M, Limmer J. Duodenum-preserving resection of the head of the pancreas in patients with severe chronic pancreatitis. Surgery. 1985;97:467-73.

CHAPTER 42

Pancreatic and Periampullary Cancer

Savio George Barreto, Adarsh Chaudhary

INTRODUCTION

Pancreatic and periampullary cancer affects individuals all over the world and is one of the leading causes of cancer-related deaths. It was recently estimated that 250,000 individuals are annually afflicted with this cancer.[1] While there was a slight decrease in pancreatic cancer a few years ago, it is now becoming more evident that the incidence of this malignancy is on the rise.[1,2] In India, too, the incidence of pancreatic and periampullary cancer was noted to be increasing.[3]

While surgery offers the best chance of long-term survival, only a small fraction (10–20%) of patients with pancreatic cancer will be amenable to a curative resection at presentation[4] owing to the insidious nature of the cancer with symptoms developing only once the tumor has invaded locally or metastasized. Patients with periampullary cancer, on the other hand, tend to present earlier and are more amenable to curative resection as the disease causes an obstructive jaundice early in the course of development of the tumor.

Recent efforts have thus focused on trying to improve survival further in patients amenable to resection by the addition of chemotherapy and radiotherapy in the adjuvant setting. In patients with locally advanced disease, attempts have been made to downstage the cancer by administering neoadjuvant chemotherapy alone or chemoradiotherapy and aggressive surgery, thereafter.[5]

This chapter provides a concise, evidence-based perspective on the management of pancreatic and periampullary cancer.

FACTORS IMPLICATED IN PATHOGENESIS

Less than 10% of pancreatic cancer patients have a hereditary predisposition.[6] This implies that environmental factors thus play a significantly role in the development of sporadic pancreatic cancer. Some of the more important factors linked to the development of pancreatic cancer include:

- Smoking—Individuals who smoke cigarettes have a 75% increased risk of developing pancreatic cancer compared to non-smokers[7] with the risk for developing the cancer reducing only after 10 years of cessation.[8]
- Alcohol—A study by the International Pancreatic Cancer Case-Control Consortium recently found a positive association between heavy alcohol consumption (≥9 drinks per day) and the risk of pancreatic cancer[9] which was independent of tobacco consumption or prior acute pancreatitis.
- Diabetes mellitus—Long-term diabetes mellitus has also been noted to be associated with a 1.5–2 fold increase in the risk of pancreatic cancer.[10,11]
- Obesity—An elevated body mass index has been shown to be an independent risk factor for the development of pancreatic cancer.[12]
- Chronic pancreatitis—Pre-existing chronic pancreatitis is also known to predispose to the development of pancreatic cancer accounting for up to 5% of cases.[13]
- Bacterial infections—Emerging evidence has implicated helicobacter pylori and a pathogen for periodontal disease, Porphyromonas gingivalis, as putative agents in the development of a host immune response mediated pathway in the development of the cancer.[14]
- Pancreatic cystic neoplasia—Intraductal papillary mucinous neoplasia (IPMN) and mucinous cystic neoplasia (MCN) are now widely accepted as preneoplastic conditions of the pancreas. The recent revised International Consensus Guidelines (2012) have provided objective features in these lesions focusing on the magnetic resonance imaging morphology of the main pancreatic duct (MPD) and the cyst to guide decision-making.[15]

Table 1: Seventh edition of American Joint Committee on cancer staging of exocrine pancreatic cancer[19]

Primary tumor (T)			
TX	Primary tumor cannot be assessed		
T0	No e/o primary tumor		
Tis	Carcinoma in situ		
T1	Tumor limited to the pancreas, 2 cm or less in greatest dimension		
T2	Tumor limited to the pancreas, more than 2 cm in greatest dimension		
T3	Tumor extends beyond the pancreas but without involvement of the celiac axis or the superior mesenteric artery		
T4	Tumor involves the celiac axis or the superior mesenteric artery (unresectable primary tumor)		
Regional lymph nodes (N)			
NX	Regional lymph node(s) cannot be assessed		
N0	No regional lymph nodal metastasis		
N1	Regional lymph node metastasis		
Distant metastases (M)			
M0	No distant metastases		
M1	Distant metastases		
Anatomic stage			
Stage 0	Tis	N0	M0
Stage IA	T1	N0	M0
Stage IB	T2	N0	M0
Stage IIA	T3	N0	M0
Stage IIB	T1-3	N1	M0
Stage III	T4	Any N	M0
Stage IV	Any T	Any N	M1

- Pancreatic Intraepithelial Neoplasia (PanIN)[16]—These premalignant pathological changes arise in the smaller ducts of the head of pancreas more frequently than in the tail region. They have been classified into three grades[16-18] ranging from less invasive to invasive nature and have been labeled, PanIN-1, 2 and 3.

TNM Classification of Pancreatic Cancer

The American Joint Committee on Cancer staging—7th edition recently provided an[19] updated tumor node metastasis (TNM) staging that has been highlighted in Table 1.

Signs and Symptoms of Pancreatic Cancer[20,21]

Patients with cancer of the pancreatic head generally present late when the tumor invades the retroperitoneum locally resulting in pain radiating to the back, impinges on the lower end of bile duct or duodenum resulting in painless progressive jaundice or features of gastric outlet obstruction, respectively or when it has metastasized resulting in features of asthenia, anorexia and weight loss. New onset diabetes mellitus or an episode of acute pancreatitis in an elderly patient should arouse the suspicion of an underlying neoplasm.

Cancers of the periampullary region generally present early as painless jaundice with or without cholangitis as these lesions obstruct the biliary passages early in the course of the disease. The classical reported pattern of "waxing and waning" of obstructive jaundice is encountered in only one-third patients.[22]

Unfortunately, patients with cancers in the body and tail of pancreas present even later as there is no scope for compression of surrounding organs to produce early symptoms. Thus, they normally present with a lump in the abdomen often at a stage when the tumor has already metastasized.[23]

In patients with chronic pancreatitis, a new symptom or change in the nature of pain should alert the clinician to investigate for an evolving neoplastic process.[24]

Icterus is the most common clinical sign in periampullary and pancreatic cancer. Given that the jaundice results from an obstructive process, features such as scratch marks on the trunk and extremities owing to the pruritus from the cuticular deposition of bile salts, high colored urine and pale stools are pathognomonic of these tumors in the absence of gallstones. A palpable globular mass in the right hypochondrium, consistent with an enlarged gallbladder is another sign of an underlying pancreatic cancer.

Clinical features in keeping with advanced cancer are the enlarged supraclavicular lymph node of Virchow, Blumer's shelf on digital rectal examination and ascites.

INVESTIGATIONS

A complete work-up of patients presenting with a periampullary or pancreatic cancer should include the following:

Blood/serum investigations:

- Serum carbohydrate antigen 19-9 (CA 19-9)
- Complete blood counts—especially in patients with suspected cholangitis
- Liver function tests—especially in patients with jaundice
- Renal function tests—especially in patients with jaundice and planned for any procedure under anesthesia
- Prothrombin time and international normalized ratio (INR)—especially in patients with jaundice.

Radiological investigations:[25]

- Multi-detector computed tomography (MDCT, Figs 1A and B) scan of the abdomen and pelvis with an associated angiography, if feasible (for delineating vascular anatomy)
- MRI and MR cholangiopancreatography (MRCP, Fig. 2)—may be an alternative to MDCT.

Endoscopy (ERCP and EUS):

- Endoscopic retrograde cholangiopancreatography (ERCP)—to obtain tissue for biopsy and to permit drainage of an obstructed biliary tree in patients with cholangitis resulting from the obstructing cancer with or without renal impairment, or in those unfit for surgery in whom optimization prior to surgery is essential.[26-28]
- Endoscopic ultrasonography (EUS)—
  - If accurate determination of T-stage is essential prior to surgery [e.g. in ampullary adenomas—to determine if ampullectomy or pancreatoduodenectomy is warranted]

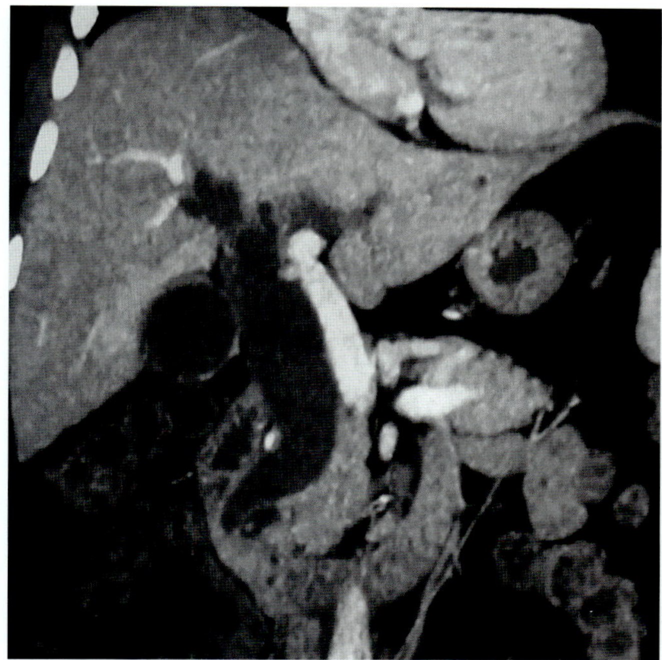

Figure 1A Periampullary carcinoma CECT coronal section showing dilated CBD and pancreatic duct (double duct). Portal vein and SMA are away from tumor and well delineated

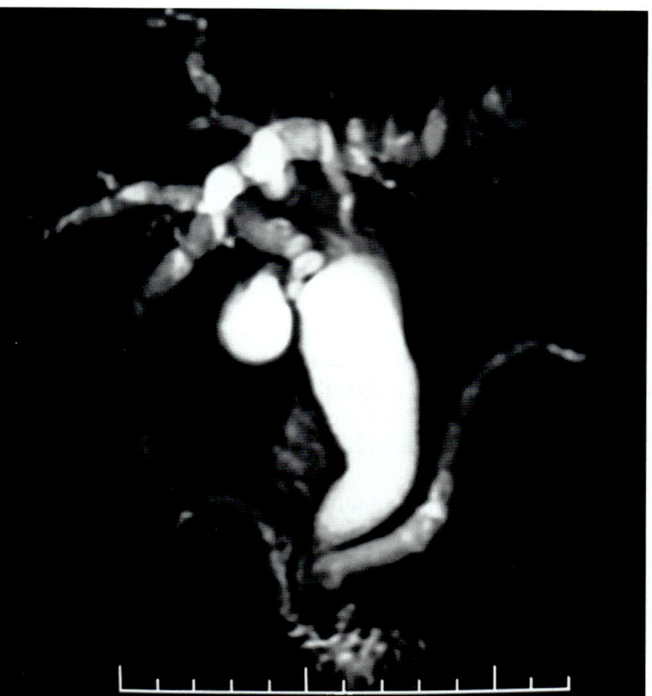

Figure 2 MRCP showing dilated pancreatic and bile ducts with periampullary mass projecting into lumen

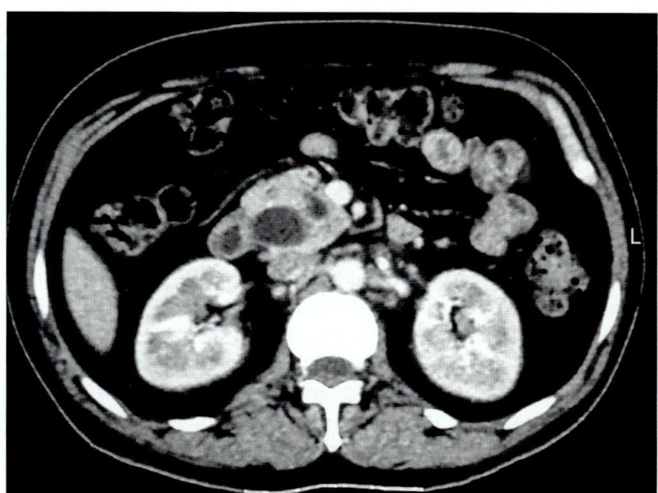

Figure 1B Periampullary Ca axial view—showing double duct

- In borderline resectable tumors to determine vascular involvement and/or to obtain tumor biopsies.[29]

Complementary Investigations

- Positron emission tomography-CT (PET-CT)—May play an adjunctive role to MDCT or MRCP in patients with locally advanced or borderline-resectable tumors to detect or rule out metastases outside the abdominal cavity.[30]
- Diagnostic laparoscopy and laparoscopic ultrasonography—May have a role in patients with unresectable disease on conventional imaging. Diagnostic laparoscopy shown to downstage these tumors rendering them amenable to curative resections.[31]

DIAGNOSIS OF IPMN/MCN

The International Consensus Guidelines 2012[15] for the management of pancreatic cystic neoplasms were recently published. Patients with cystic lesions of the pancreas more than or equal to 10 mm should preferably undergo a pancreatic protocol CT scan or gadolinium-enhanced MRI/MRCP.[32]

The subsequent algorithm for managing these cystic lesions takes into account the size of the lesion, the presence of solid components, the diameter of the MPD, and the presence of mural nodules.

Patients with cysts more than or equal to 10 mm in the head of pancreas causing obstructive jaundice and demonstrating features such as enhanced solid component and an MPD more than 10 mm should be advised a surgical resection.

Patients with cysts more than or equal to 30 mm and presenting with features described as "worrisome" such as, clinical history of pancreatitis, thickened enhanced cyst walls, MPD size of 5-9 mm, non-enhanced mural nodules, abrupt change in the MPD caliber with distal pancreatic atrophy, and lymphadenopathy,[33-39] an EUS would be the next choice of investigation. Surgical resection would be warranted in the case of lesions demonstrating the presence of mural nodules, intraductal mucin, thickening of any wall and/or cytological analysis indicative of malignant cells or high grade epithelial atypia.[15]

Patients with cysts less than 30 mm without the "worrisome features" described above or with "worrisome features" on imaging but not corroborated on EUS, should be offered surveillance with the regimen being determined by the size of the largest cyst:[15]

- <10 mm—Repeat CT/MRI in 2-3 years.
- 20-30 mm—Repeat EUS in 3-6 months. The subsequent interval for surveillance could be lengthened alternating between EUS and MRI.
- >30 mm—Close surveillance alternating MRI with EUS every 3-6 months. In these patients, surgery should be considered especially in younger fit patients.

Cystic lesions in the pancreas measuring less than 10 mm are of low malignant potential for which no immediate treatment is warranted.[33,34] However, patients with such lesions may be offered surveillance with CT or MRI every year for 2 years. Thereafter, the frequency of surveillance would depend on the interval change in the size of the lesion.

Endoscopic ultrasonography-guided fine needle aspiration (EUS FNA) is recommended only in the evaluation of small BD-IPMNs without "worrisome features".[15]

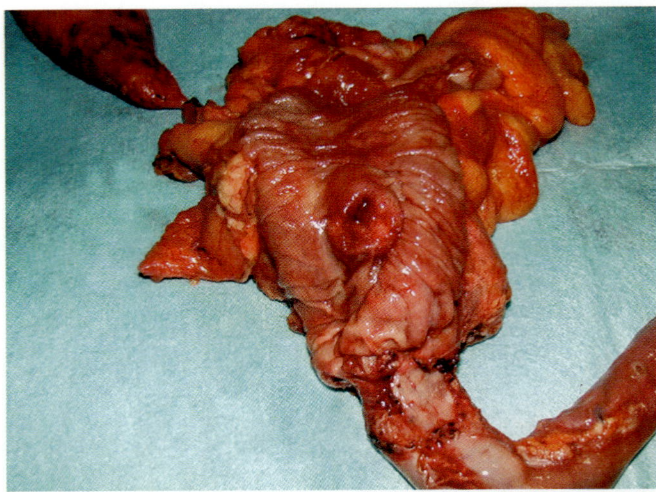

Figure 3 Resected specimen of WPD showing ampullary mass in opened duodenum

SURGICAL MANAGEMENT

Surgery offers the only chance of cure in patients with pancreatic and periampullary cancer. However, it should only be attempted in patients in whom a complete (R0) resection is deemed feasible. The available evidence does not support the role of a palliative pancreatoduodenectomy or pancreatic resection for pancreatic cancer. The operative treatment for pancreatic head and neck cancers is a pancreatoduodenectomy, a distal pancreatectomy for cancers of the body and tail and a subtotal pancreatectomy for tumors at the junction of the neck and body.

Resectable Pancreatic Cancer

Head, Uncinate Process and Proximal Neck of Pancreas (Including Periampullary Cancer)

Pancreatoduodenectomy (Fig. 3): The curative resection for pancreatic cancer involving the head, uncinate process and/or proximal neck of the pancreas as well as periampullary region is the pancreatoduodenectomy. This procedure involves removal of the duodenum and pancreatic head, uncinate process and neck along with the distal common bile duct (and gallbladder). Based on the location of transaction of the stomach/duodenum there are two named procedures, viz. the Classical Whipple's procedure (proximal transection at the junction of distal body and antrum of the stomach) and the pylorus-preserving pancreatoduodenectomy (PPPD). The reconstruction is then achieved by anastomosing the pancreatic remnant, the common hepatic duct and the stomach to the bowel. While the common hepatic duct and stomach are anastomosed with the jejunum, the choice of anastomosis of the pancreatic remnant is between the stomach (pancreaticogastrostomy) or the roux loop of jejunum (pancreaticojejunostomy). Similarly, the stomach may be joined to the jejunum in front of (ante-colic) or behind (retrocolic) the transverse colon.

Based on the existing evidence in literature, there is no oncological benefit of performing a PPPD as compared to a Classical Whipple's procedure.[40] However, specific indication in which only a Classical Whipple procedure should be performed includes large pancreatic head cancers invading stomach or duodenum and duodenal cancers.

Despite studies promulgating the benefits of a pancreatico-gastrostomy versus a pancreaticojejunostomy[41] or vice versa, the current literature has indicated that both anastomoses are equally efficacious.[42]

Performance of an antecolic duodenojejunostomy after PPPD leads to a reduction in the rate of delayed gastric emptying (DGE)[43] possibly by avoiding torsion or angulation that may result from a retrocolic anastomosis.

An important component of an oncological surgery is the performance of a lymphadenectomy as part of curative surgery. A standard lymphadenectomy involves removal of lymph nodes of the right side of the hepatoduodenal ligament (12b1 and 12c), posterior pancreaticoduodenal nodes (13a and 13b), nodes to the right side of the superior mesenteric artery from the origin of the superior mesenteric artery at the aorta to the inferior pancreaticoduodenal artery (14a and 14b) and anterior pancreaticoduodenal nodes (17a and 17b). Some authors have suggested that there may be a role for an extended lymphadenectomy. However, the current literature indicates that an extended lymphadenectomy confers no further oncological benefit over a standard lymphadenectomy[44-46] at the expense of an increased risk of intractable diarrhea in the early postoperative phase.

Distal Neck, Body and Tail of Pancreas

Distal/subtotal pancreatectomy:[23] Brennan et al. advocated an aggressive resection for tumors of the body and tail of the pancreas.[47] Current literature consistently reports the need for inclusion of a splenectomy as part of a distal/subtotal pancreatectomy to attain a complete en bloc resection for carcinomas.[48]

Staplers or suture closure of the pancreatic stump after a distal or subtotal pancreatectomy are equally efficacious.[49,50] Irrespective of the technique used to transect/close the pancreatic stump, attention needs to be paid to transfixing the pancreatic duct.

Middle or central pancreatectomy may be considered only in benign or borderline malignant lesions of the mid body of the pancreas and should not be performed for malignant tumors.

Resectable Locally Advanced Pancreatic Cancer

Up to one-third of patients with pancreatic body and tail cancers at the time of surgery have evidence of involvement of surrounding organs either as a result of direct tumor infiltration or inflammatory adhesions.[51] An en bloc resections in these patients should be attempted only if a complete (R0) resection can be achieved. If an R0 resection can be achieved in these patients, the long-term survival rates have been noted to be similar to patients undergoing standard resection for resectable tumors.[52-54] Moreover, the long-term survival rates in these patients are markedly improved as compared to patients with unresectable locally advanced disease.[53] These resections should preferably be undertaken in high volume centers with the necessary expertise.[55]

Borderline Resectable Tumors

"Borderline resectable pancreatic tumor or cancer (BRT)" of the head and body of pancreas has been defined by the National Comprehensive Cancer Network (NCCN) as tumor abutment of the superior mesenteric artery (SMA), encasement of gastroduodenal artery (GDA) up to its origin from the hepatic artery, severe unilateral superior mesenteric vein (SMV) or portal vein impingement, or colon and mesocolon involvement.[56] To date there is no consensus on the ideal management of these patients with the choice of management varying between neoadjuvant chemoradiotherapy[57] followed by surgery versus up front surgery and adjuvant chemoradiotherapy or chemoradiotherapy.[58,59]

Vascular Resections

There is increasing evidence that performing a venous resection (SMV/portal vein) could lead to improved outcomes (5-year survival rates of 23%) so long as an R0 resection can be obtained.[60]

However, certain factors that need to be taken into account when deciding on performing venous resections as part of pancreatic resections include[55] the depth[61] and length[60] of venous invasion. This is because even a complete resection with involvement of tunica media and intima is associated with poor outcomes. Similarly, length of involvement more than 3 cm is associated with poor outcomes.

There is no evidence to support the performance of arterial resections in pancreatic cancer[55] as such resections are associated with poor short-term outcomes as well as survival.[62]

PANCREATIC RESECTION IN METASTATIC DISEASE

Studies have demonstrated a feasibility of performing metastasectomy along with resection of the primary tumor in pancreatic cancer.[63] However, to date, there exists no clear evidence to demonstrate a survival benefit even in patients with resectable pancreatic cancer.[55,64]

LAPAROSCOPY AND ROBOTIC SURGERY FOR PANCREATIC AND PERIAMPULLARY CARCINOMA

Laparoscopic and robotic surgery have been demonstrated to be feasible for performing distal pancreatectomy with some series even demonstrating the feasibility of these procedures for pancreatoduodenectomy for benign lesions of the pancreas.[65-70] However, to date there exists no convincing high-level evidence to suggest that laparoscopic pancreatoduodenectomy or even distal pancreatectomy is equal to, or superior, to open surgery in terms of overall survival for pancreatic and periampullary cancer.[69] Another important factor which does not lend support to the role for laparoscopy or robotic surgery for pancreatic cancer surgery is the complexity of procedure in itself. Morbidity associated with the procedure (pancreatic leak, hemorrhage, DGE) is thus not related to the length of the abdominal incision but rather to the extensive nature of the surgical procedure on pancreas.[71] This has been better elucidated in a well conducted trial of accelerated recovery after laparoscopic distal pancreatectomy that indicated a high readmission rate.[72]

SURGICAL MANAGEMENT GUIDELINES FOR INVASIVE AND NON-INVASIVE IPMN AND MCN

Recommendations from the International Consensus Guidelines 2012[15]

- The standard treatment for invasive and noninvasive MCNs and IPMNs is a pancreatectomy with standard lymph node dissection.
- Laparoscopic surgery may be considered in patients with low-grade and possibly high-grade dysplasia of IPMN and MCN.
- In patients with a strong family history of PDAC and multifocal BD-IPMNs, the performance of a total pancreatectomy needs to be considered.

FAST-TRACK PROTOCOLS/ENHANCED RECOVERY[20]

An interesting innovative approach borrowed from other surgical specialties such as colorectal and vascular surgery are the evidence-based clinical pathways collectively termed as Enhanced recovery after surgery protocols. While these protocols have been tried by some centers for almost a decade, their general acceptance in pancreatic surgical units has not been very enthusiastic for fears of an increased morbidity rate.[73] However, level 1 evidence is now available to support the use of enhanced recovery protocols after pancreatic surgery given that they not only resulted in improved gastric emptying and reduced postoperative stay and hospital costs[74,75] but also contributed to significantly reduced morbidity, in general, as well as no increase in readmission rates.[76]

PALLIATIVE GASTROENTEROSTOMY AND/OR BILIODIGESTIVE BYPASS[77]

The available evidence strongly recommends the performance of a triple bypass, if feasible, in patients with unresectable periampullary[78] as well as pancreatic cancer[79] undergoing an exploratory laparotomy irrespective of the presence of features of gastric outlet obstruction. While these procedures do not appear to significantly impair short-term outcomes they have certainly contributed to avoiding long-term gastroduodenal obstruction.[79]

CHEMOTHERAPY AND CHEMORADIO-THERAPY FOR RESECTABLE PANCREATIC CANCER

Adjuvant Therapy

There have been seven randomized controlled trials that have examined the role of chemotherapy and chemoradiotherapy in patients with resectable pancreatic cancer.[80-86] While three trials demonstrated a benefit of adjuvant chemotherapy (5-fluorouracil or gemcitabine) in terms of overall survival,[82-84] two trials indicated a benefit of 5-fluorouracil-based chemoradiotherapy.[81,86] Single agent gemcitabine remains the preferred drug in the adjuvant setting while the role of combination therapies including targeted agents remains investigational.[87]

Neoadjuvant Therapy

Given the fact that up to 40% of patients with pancreatic cancer present in the locally advanced and borderline resectable category, there has been considerable interest in the use of chemotherapy and chemoradiation in the neoadjuvant setting with an aim to downsize the tumors rendering them amenable to a curative resection.[88] These strategies have been met with some success resulting in an ability to perform a resection (R0/R1) in up to 40% of patients with previous locally advanced, unresectable pancreatic cancer.[89,90] In one the largest series, Strobel et al.[89] noted that survival rates in these patients were similar to those observed for initially resectable pancreatic cancer. Katz et al.[90] noted a significantly longer survival in those patients who could complete the therapy and undergo a resection compared to those who could not.

Palliative Therapy

Gemcitabine was favored as a single agent monotherapy in advanced pancreatic cancer for a long time.[91] However, despite the lack of convincing benefit of gemcitabine-based combination therapies on overall survival, they are preferred over gemcitabine monotherapy on account of their effects on response rates and progression-free survival.[92]

SUMMARY

The overbearing nihilism in our perception of pancreatic cancer is preventing us from appreciating the small, but certain, advances in the management of this cancer. Periampullary cancer, on the other hand, remains a less investigated entity possibly due to its early presentation and hence relatively better outcomes as compared to pancreatic cancer. Scientifically-tempered surgical aggression aimed at complete surgical resection coupled with the use of adjuvant chemotherapy or chemoradiotherapy (when indicated) offer the best possible outcome in patients with resectable or locally advanced but resectable disease. Data on the role of neoadjuvant chemotherapy in borderline resectable is encouraging and this deserves further attention. Palliative surgery may yet possess a valuable role in pancreatic cancer in terms of improving quality of life coupled with gemcitabine-based mono- or combination therapies.

REFERENCES

1. Yeo TP, Lowenfels AB. Demographics and epidemiology of pancreatic cancer. Cancer J. 2012;18(6):477-84.
2. Bosetti C, Bertuccio P, Malvezzi M, Levi F, Chatenoud L, Negri E, et al. Cancer mortality in Europe, 2005-2009, and an overview of trends since 1980. Ann Oncol. 2013;24(10):2657-71.
3. Dhir V, Mohandas KM. Epidemiology of digestive tract cancers in India IV. Gallbladder and pancreas. Indian J Gastroenterol. 1999;18(1):24-8.
4. Krempien R, Muentier M, Harms W, Debus J. Neoadjuvant chemoradiation in patients with pancreatic adenocarcinoma. HPB (Oxford). 2006;8(1):22-8.
5. Gillen S, Schuster T, Buschenfelde CMZ, Friess H, Kleeff J. Preoperative/neoadjuvant therapy in pancreatic cancer: systematic review and meta-analysis of response and resectino percentages. PLOS Med. 2010;7(4):e1000267.
6. Segura PP, Ponce CG, Ramon YCT, Blanch RS, Aranda E. Hereditary pancreatic cancer: molecular bases and their application in diagnosis and clinical management: a guideline of the TTD group. Clin Transl Oncol. 2012;14(8):553-63.
7. Iodice S, Gandini S, Maisonneuve P, Lowenfels AB. Tobacco and the risk of pancreatic cancer: a review and metaanalysis. Langenbecks Arch Surg. 2008;393:535-45.
8. Duell EJ. Epidemiology and potential mechanisms of tobacco smoking and heavy alcohol consumption in pancreatic cancer. Mol Carcinog. 2012;51:40-52.
9. Lucenteforte E, La Vecchia C, Silverman D, Petersen GM, Bracci PM, Ji BT, et al. Alcohol consumption and pancreatic cancer: a pooled analysis in the International Pancreatic Cancer Case-Control Consortium (PanC4). Ann Oncol. 2012;23(2):374-82.
10. Ben Q, Xu M, Ning X, Liu J, Hong S, Huang W, et al. Diabetes mellitus and risk of pancreatic cancer: a meta-analysis of cohort studies. Eur J Cancer. 2011;47(13):1928-37.
11. Kasuga M, Ueki K, Tajima N, Noda M, Ohashi K, Noto H, et al. Report of the Japan Diabetes Society/Japanese Cancer Association joint committee on diabetes and cancer. Cancer Sci. 2013;104(7):965-76.
12. Jiao L, Berrington de Gonzalez A, Hartge P, Pfeiffer RM, Park Y, Freedman DM, et al. Body mass index, effect modifiers, and risk of pancreatic cancer: a pooled study of seven prospective cohorts. Cancer Causes Control. 2010;21(8):1305-14.
13. Zavoral M, Minarikova P, Zavada F, Salek C, Minarik M. Molecular biology of pancreatic cancer. World J Gastroenterol. 2011;17(24):2897-908.
14. Michaud DS. Role of bacterial infections in pancreatic cancer. Carcinogenesis. 2013;34(10):2193-7.
15. Tanaka M, Fernandez-Del Castillo C, Adsay V, Chari S, Falconi M, Jang JY, et al. International consensus guidelines 2012 for the management of IPMN and MCN of the pancreas. Pancreatology. 2012;12(3):183-97.
16. Hruban RH, Maitra A, Goggins M. Update on pancreatic intraepithelial neoplasia. Int J Clin Exp Pathol. 2008;1(4):306-16.

17. Hruban RH, Adsay NV, Albores-Saavedra J, Compton C, Garrett ES, Goodman SN, et al. Pancreatic intraepithelial neoplasia: a new nomenclature and classification system for pancreatic duct lesions. Am J Surg Pathol. 2001;25(5):579-86.
18. Hruban R, Pitman M, Klimstra D (Eds). Tumors of the Pancreas Atlas of Tumor Pathology, 4th series. Washington DC: American Registry of Pathology and Armed Forces Institute of Pathology; 2007.
19. Edge S, Byrd D, Compton C, et al. (Eds). AJCC Cancer Staging Manual, 7th edition. New York: Springer Verlag; 2009.
20. Shrikhande S, Barreto S. Surgery for pancreatic carcinoma: state of the art. Indian J Surg. 2012;74:79-86.
21. Barreto G, Shukla PJ, Ramadwar M, Arya S, Shrikhande SV. Cystic tumours of the pancreas. HPB (Oxford). 2007;9(4):259-66.
22. Barreto S, Shukla P, Shrikhande S. Periampullary carcinoma. In: Shrikhande S, Friess H, Buchler M (Eds). Surgery of Pancreatic Tumors. New Delhi: BI Publications; 2007. pp. 206-15.
23. Barreto S, Shukla P, Shrikhande S. Tumors of the pancreatic body and tail. World Journal of Oncology. 2010;1(2):52-65.
24. Shrikhande S, Barreto G, Koliopanos A. Pancreatic carcinogenesis: the impact of chronic pancreatitis and its clinical relevance. Indian J Cancer. 2009;46:288-96.
25. Shrikhande S, Barreto S, Goel M, Arya S. Multimodality Imaging of Pancreatic Ductal Adenocarcinoma: A Review of the Literature HPB (Oxford). 2012.
26. Jagannath P, Dhir V, Shrikhande S, Shah RC, Mullerpatan P, Mohandas KM. Effect of preoperative biliary stenting on immediate outcome after pancreaticoduodenectomy. Br J Surg. 2005;92(3):356-61.
27. Sewnath ME, Birjmohun RS, Rauws EA, Huibregtse K, Obertop H, Gouma DJ. The effect of preoperative biliary drainage on postoperative complications after pancreaticoduodenectomy. J Am Coll Surg. 2001;192(6):726-34.
28. Coates JM, Beal SH, Russo JE, Vanderveen KA, Chen SL, Bold RJ, et al. Negligible effect of selective preoperative biliary drainage on perioperative resuscitation, morbidity, and mortality in patients undergoing pancreaticoduodenectomy. Arch Surg. 2009;144(9):841-7.
29. Soriano A, Castells A, Ayuso C, Ayuso JR, de Caralt MT, Gines MA, et al. Preoperative staging and tumor resectability assessment of pancreatic cancer: prospective study comparing endoscopic ultrasonography, helical computed tomography, magnetic resonance imaging, and angiography. Am J Gastroenterol. 2004;99(3):492-501.
30. Farma JM, Santillan AA, Melis M, Walters J, Belinc D, Chen DT, et al. PET/CT fusion scan enhances CT staging in patients with pancreatic neoplasms. Ann Surg Oncol. 2008;15(9):2465-71.
31. Hariharan D, Constantinides VA, Froeling FE, Tekkis PP, Kocher HM. The role of laparoscopy and laparoscopic ultrasound in the preoperative staging of pancreatico-biliary cancers—a meta-analysis. Eur J Surg Oncol. 2010;36(10):941-8.
32. Berland L, Silverman S, Gore R, Mayo-Smith W, Megibow A, Yee J, et al. Managing incidental findings on abdominal CT: white paper of the ACR incidental findings committee. J Am Col Radiol. 2010;7:754-73.
33. Castillo CF-d, Targarona J, Thayer S, Rattner D, Brugge W, Warshaw A. Incidental pancreatic cysts: clinicopathologic characteristics and comparison with symptomatic patients. Arch Surg. 2003;138:427-34.
34. Das A, Wells C, Nguyen C. Incidental cystic neoplasms of pancreas: what is the optimal interval of imaging surveillance? Am J Gastroenterol. 2008;103:1657-62.
35. Bassi C, Crippa S, Salvia R. Intraductal papillary mucinous neoplasms (IPMNs): is it time to (sometimes) spare the knife? Gut. 2008;57:287-9.
36. Brounts L, Lehmann R, Causey M, Sebesta J, Brown T. Natural course and outcome of cystic lesions in the pancreas. Am J Surg. 2009;197:619-23.
37. Javle M, Shah P, Yu J, Bhagat V, Litwin A, Iyer R, et al. Cystic pancreatic tumors (CPT): predictors of malignant behavior. J Surg Oncol. 2007;95:221-8.
38. Lee S, Shin C, Park J, Woo S, Yoo J, Ryu J, et al. Outcomes of cystic lesions in the pancreas after extended follow-up. Dig Dis Sci. 2007;52:2653-9.
39. Salvia R, Crippa S, Falconi M, Bassi C, Guarise A, Scarpa A, et al. Branch-duct intraductal papillary mucinous neoplasms of the pancreas: to operate or not to operate? Gut. 2007;56:1086-90.
40. Diener MK, Fitzmaurice C, Schwarzer G, Seiler CM, Antes G, Knaebel HP, et al. Pylorus-preserving pancreaticoduodenectomy (pp Whipple) versus pancreaticoduodenectomy (classic Whipple) for surgical treatment of periampullary and pancreatic carcinoma. Cochrane Database Syst Rev. 2014;11:CD006053.
41. Topal B, Fieuws S, Aerts R, Weerts J, Feryn T, Roeyen G, et al. Pancreaticojejunostomy versus pancreaticogastrostomy reconstruction after pancreaticoduodenectomy for pancreatic or periampullary tumours: a multicentre randomised trial. Lancet Oncol. 2013;14(7):655-62.
42. He T, Zhao Y, Chen Q, Wang X, Lin H, Han W. Pancreaticojejunostomy versus pancreaticogastrostomy after pancreaticoduodenectomy: a systematic review and meta-analysis. Dig Surg. 2013;30(1):56-69.
43. Su AP, Cao SS, Zhang Y, Zhang ZD, Hu WM, Tian BL. Does antecolic reconstruction for duodenojejunostomy improve delayed gastric emptying after pylorus-preserving pancreaticoduodenectomy? A systematic review and meta-analysis. World J Gastroenterol. 2012;18(43):6315-23.
44. Iqbal N, Lovegrove RE, Tilney HS, Abraham AT, Bhattacharya S, Tekkis PP, et al. A comparison of pancreaticoduodenectomy with extended pancreaticoduodenectomy: a meta-analysis of 1909 patients. Eur J Surg Oncol. 2009;35(1):79-86.
45. Michalski CW, Kleeff J, Wente MN, Diener MK, Buchler MW, Friess H. Systematic review and meta-analysis of standard and extended lymphadenectomy in pancreaticoduodenectomy for pancreatic cancer. Br J Surg. 2007;94(3):265-73.
46. Sergeant G, Melloul E, Lesurtel M, Deoliveira ML, Clavien PA. Extended lymphadenectomy in patients with pancreatic cancer is debatable. World J Surg. 2013;37(8):1782-8.
47. Brennan MF, Moccia RD, Klimstra D. Management of adenocarcinoma of the body and tail of the pancreas. Ann Surg. 1996;223(5):506-11.
48. Shoup M, Brennan MF, McWhite K, Leung DH, Klimstra D, Conlon KC. The value of splenic preservation with distal pancreatectomy. Arch Surg. 2002;137(2):164-8.
49. Knaebel HP, Diener MK, Wente MN, Buchler MW, Seiler CM. Systematic review and meta-analysis of technique for closure of the pancreatic remnant after distal pancreatectomy. Br J Surg. 2005;92(5):539-46.
50. Diener MK, Seiler CM, Rossion I, Kleeff J, Glanemann M, Butturini G, et al. Efficacy of stapler versus hand-sewn closure after distal pancreatectomy (DISPACT): a randomised, controlled multicentre trial. Lancet. 2011;377(9776):1514-22.
51. Christein JD, Kendrick ML, Iqbal CW, Nagorney DM, Farnell MB. Distal pancreatectomy for resectable adenocarcinoma of the body and tail of the pancreas. J Gastrointest Surg. 2005;9(7):922-7.
52. Sasson AR, Hoffman JP, Ross EA, Kagan SA, Pingpank JF, Eisenberg BL. En bloc resection for locally advanced cancer of the pancreas: is it worthwhile? J Gastrointest Surg. 2002;6(2):147-57.
53. Shoup M, Conlon KC, Klimstra D, Brennan MF. Is extended resection for adenocarcinoma of the body or tail of the pancreas justified? J Gastrointest Surg. 2003;7(8):946-52.

54. Hartwig W, Hackert T, Hinz U, Hassenpflug M, Strobel O, Buchler MW, et al. Multivisceral resection for pancreatic malignancies: risk-analysis and long-term outcome. Ann Surg. 2009;250(1):81-7.
55. Shrikhande SV, Barreto SG. Extended pancreatic resections and lymphadenectomy: an appraisal of the current evidence. World J Gastrointest Surg. 2010;2(2):39-46.
56. Oberg K, Akerstrom G, Rindi G, Jelic S. Neuroendocrine gastroenteropancreatic tumours: ESMO Clinical Practice Guidelines for diagnosis, treatment and follow-up. Ann Oncol. 2010;21(Suppl 5):v223-7.
57. Varadhachary GR, Tamm EP, Abbruzzese JL, Xiong HQ, Crane CH, Wang H, et al. Borderline resectable pancreatic cancer: definitions, management, and role of preoperative therapy. Ann Surg Oncol. 2006;13(8):1035-46.
58. Tucker ON, Rela M. Controversies in the management of borderline resectable proximal pancreatic adenocarcinoma with vascular involvement. HPB Surg. 2008;2008:839503.
59. Shrikhande SV, Arya S, Barreto SG, Ingle S, D'Souza MA, Hawaldar R, et al. Borderline resectable pancreatic tumors: is there a need for further refinement of this stage? Hepatobiliary Pancreat Dis Int. 2011;10(3):319-24.
60. Kaneoka Y, Yamaguchi A, Isogai M. Portal or superior mesenteric vein resection for pancreatic head adenocarcinoma: prognostic value of the length of venous resection. Surgery. 2009;145(4):417-25.
61. Fukuda S, Oussoultzoglou E, Bachellier P, Rosso E, Nakano H, Audet M, et al. Significance of the depth of portal vein wall invasion after curative resection for pancreatic adenocarcinoma. Arch Surg. 2007;142(2):172-9.
62. Ravikumar R, Holroyd D, Fusai G. Is there a role for arterial reconstruction in surgery for pancreatic cancer? World J Gastrointest Surg. 2013;5(3):27-9.
63. Niess H, Conrad C, Kleespies A, Haas F, Bao Q, Jauch KW, et al. Surgery for metastasis to the pancreas: is it safe and effective? J Surg Oncol. 2013;107(8):859-64.
64. Michalski CW, Erkan M, Huser N, Muller MW, Hartel M, Friess H, et al. Resection of primary pancreatic cancer and liver metastasis: a systematic review. Dig Surg. 2008;25(6):473-80.
65. Kendrick ML, Cusati D. Total laparoscopic pancreaticoduodenectomy: feasibility and outcome in an early experience. Arch Surg. 2010;145(1):19-23.
66. Palanivelu C, Rajan PS, Rangarajan M, Vaithiswaran V, Senthilnathan P, Parthasarathi R, et al. Evolution in techniques of laparoscopic pancreaticoduodenectomy: a decade long experience from a tertiary center. J Hepatobiliary Pancreat Surg. 2009;16(6):731-40.
67. Ammori BJ. Laparoscopic hand-assisted pancreaticoduodenectomy: initial UK experience. Surg Endosc. 2004;18(4):717-8.
68. Staudacher C, Orsenigo E, Baccari P, Di Palo S, Crippa S. Laparoscopic assisted duodenopancreatectomy. Surg Endosc. 2005;19(3):352-6.
69. Kendrick ML. Laparoscopic and robotic resection for pancreatic cancer. Cancer J. 2012;18(6):571-6.
70. Boggi U, Signori S, De Lio N, Perrone VG, Vistoli F, Belluomini M, et al. Feasibility of robotic pancreaticoduodenectomy. Br J Surg. 2013;100(7):917-25.
71. Shrikhande SV, Barreto SG, Shukla PJ. Laparoscopy in pancreatic tumors. J Minim Access Surg. 2007;3(2):47-51.
72. Baker MS, Bentrem DJ, Ujiki MB, Stocker S, Talamonti MS. Adding days spent in readmission to the initial postoperative length of stay limits the perceived benefit of laparoscopic distal pancreatectomy when compared with open distal pancreatectomy. Am J Surg. 2011;201(3):295-9.
73. Ypsilantis E, Praseedom RK. Current status of fast-track recovery pathways in pancreatic surgery. JOP. 2009;10(6):646-50.
74. Balzano G, Zerbi A, Braga M, Rocchetti S, Beneduce AA, Di Carlo V. Fast-track recovery programme after pancreatico-duodenectomy reduces delayed gastric emptying. Br J Surg. 2008;95(11): 1387-93.
75. Kennedy EP, Rosato EL, Sauter PK, Rosenberg LM, Doria C, Marino IR, et al. Initiation of a critical pathway for pancreaticoduodenectomy at an academic institution—the first step in multidisciplinary team building. J Am Coll Surg. 2007;204(5):917-23.
76. Coolsen MM, van Dam RM, van der Wilt AA, Slim K, Lassen K, Dejong CH. Systematic review and meta-analysis of enhanced recovery after pancreatic surgery with particular emphasis on pancreaticoduodenectomies. World J Surg. 2013;37(8):1909-18.
77. Shrikhande S, Barreto S, Shrikhande V. Pancreatic cancer. In: Haribhakti S (Ed). Clinical GI Surgery; 2011.
78. Gurusamy K, Kumar S, Davidson B. Prophylactic gastrojejunostomy for unresectable periampullary carcinoma. Cochrane Database Syst Rev. 2010;10:CD008533.
79. Huser N, Michalski C, Schuster T, Friess H, Kleeff J. Systematic review and meta-analysis of prophylactic gastroenterstomy for unresectable advanced pancreatic cancer. Br J Surg. 2009;96(7): 711-9.
80. Ueno H, Kosuge T, Matsuyama Y, Yamamoto J, Nakao A, Egawa S, et al. A randomised phase III trial comparing gemcitabine with surgery-only in patients with resected pancreatic cancer: Japanese Study Group of Adjuvant Therapy for Pancreatic Cancer. Br J Cancer. 2009;101(6):908-15.
81. Regine WF, Winter KA, Abrams RA, Safran H, Hoffman JP, Konski A, et al. Fluorouracil vs gemcitabine chemotherapy before and after fluorouracil-based chemoradiation following resection of pancreatic adenocarcinoma: a randomized controlled trial. JAMA. 2008;299(9):1019-26.
82. Oettle H, Post S, Neuhaus P, Gellert K, Langrehr J, Ridwelski K, et al. Adjuvant chemotherapy with gemcitabine vs observation in patients undergoing curative-intent resection of pancreatic cancer: a randomized controlled trial. JAMA. 2007;297(3): 267-77.
83. Neoptolemos JP, Stocken DD, Friess H, Bassi C, Dunn JA, Hickey H, et al. A randomized trial of chemoradiotherapy and chemotherapy after resection of pancreatic cancer. N Engl J Med. 2004;350(12):1200-10.
84. Neoptolemos JP, Stocken DD, Bassi C, Ghaneh P, Cunningham D, Goldstein D, et al. Adjuvant chemotherapy with fluorouracil plus folinic acid vs gemcitabine following pancreatic cancer resection: a randomized controlled trial. JAMA. 2010;304(10): 1073-81.
85. Klinkenbijl JH, Jeekel J, Sahmoud T, van Pel R, Couvreur ML, Veenhof CH, et al. Adjuvant radiotherapy and 5-fluorouracil after curative resection of cancer of the pancreas and periampullary region: phase III trial of the EORTC gastrointestinal tract cancer cooperative group. Ann Surg. 1999;230(6):776-82.
86. Kalser MH, Ellenberg SS. Pancreatic cancer. Adjuvant combined radiation and chemotherapy following curative resection. Arch Surg. 1985;120(8):899-903.
87. Antoniou G, Kountourakis P, Papadimitriou K, Vassiliou V, Papamichael D. Adjuvant therapy for resectable pancreatic adenocarcinoma: review of the current treatment approaches and future directions. Cancer Treat Rev. 2014;40(1):78-85.
88. Papavasiliou P, Chun YS, Hoffman JP. How to define and manage borderline resectable pancreatic cancer. Surg Clin North Am. 2013;93(3):663-74.

89. Strobel O, Berens V, Hinz U, Hartwig W, Hackert T, Bergmann F, et al. Resection after neoadjuvant therapy for locally advanced, "unresectable" pancreatic cancer. Surgery. 2012;152(3 Suppl 1): S33-42.
90. Katz MH, Pisters PW, Evans DB, Sun CC, Lee JE, Fleming JB, et al. Borderline resectable pancreatic cancer: the importance of this emerging stage of disease. J Am Coll Surg. 2008;206(5):833-46.
91. Burris HA, 3rd, Moore MJ, Andersen J, Green MR, Rothenberg ML, Modiano MR, et al. Improvements in survival and clinical benefit with gemcitabine as first-line therapy for patients with advanced pancreas cancer: a randomized trial. J Clin Oncol. 1997;15(6): 2403-13.
92. Paulson AS, Tran Cao HS, Tempero MA, Lowy AM. Therapeutic advances in pancreatic cancer. Gastroenterology. 2013;144(6):1316-26.

CHAPTER 43

Pancreatic Surgery

Rajesh Rajalingam, PK Mishra

INTRODUCTION

Pancreas is a fleshy visceral organ of unique importance in the portomesenteric axis. In view of the anatomical proximity to various organs and vessels, especially at the head of pancreas, even small lesion of this location requires major resection and reconstruction. This makes pancreatic surgery one of the most demanding and technically difficult ones. In fact, there is no organ that has evoked such a curious attraction, both medically and surgically.

Traditionally, neoplasm involving the pancreas has poor prognosis, where its incidence almost equals the mortality rate.[1] Only 25–35% of the pancreatic neoplasm are operable with the rest ultimately going for palliative treatments. Their management evolved by better understanding the biological nature of each pathologic variant, and progress in their diagnosis, perioperative optimization and care. Despite all improvements 5-year survival has not improved, especially for adenocarcinoma of the pancreas, which is still around 10–20%. Perioperative outcomes have improved and currently the accepted pancreatic resection (pancreaticoduodenectomy) mortality is around 4%.[2-6] This relatively low perioperative mortality rate from over 15% in the 1970s, makes pancreaticoduodenectomy a much more attractive option now, than it has been at any time in its long history (Table 1).

Table 1: Tumor types and their overall survival figures from large series

Tumor		*5-year survival (%)*
Ductal adenocarcinoma head	Without resection Resection with N1[5] Resection with N0[5]	0 18 32
Ductal adenocarci-noma—body and tail	Standard resection[7] Radical resection RAMPS[8]	8 35.5
Other periampullary carcinoma	Ampullary carcinoma[9] Lower CBD carcinoma[9] Duodenal carcinoma[10]	51 26 74

Proximal Pancreatic Neoplasm (Head/Uncinate Process)

CEPHALIC PANCREATICODUODENECTOMY

Though scattered attempts were made since 1898 by Alessandro Codivilla, the first pancreaticoduodenectomy was successfully performed by Walther Carl Eduard Kausch in 1912, and later popularized by Allen Oldfather Whipple in 1940s.[11]

Pancreaticoduodenectomy, in addition to the primary malignancies of the head of pancreas and duodenum, is also indicated in chronic pancreatitis with suspicious head mass. It is also required in extended resections for locally advanced gallbladder, biliary and colorectalmalignancies. In grade IV/V pancreaticoduodenal injury, emergency pancreaticoduodenectomy is an effective option.

Preoperative Preparation

Diagnosis and Staging

The minimum required for a patient who undergoes pancreatico-duodenectomy is a pancreatic protocol multidetector computer tomography (MDCT) of 1–2 mm slice thickness.[12] The advantages of this MDCT is in assessing the vascularity of the lesion (hyperdense-NET, hypodense-adenocarcinoma), any field change [intraductal papillary mucinous neoplasm (IPMN)-multiple lesions], assessment of the vascular involvement and its extent, helping in defining borderline resectable lesions and additionally detecting aberrant vascular and biliary anatomy for technical considerations.[13] If the lesion is in doubt and does not warrant the risk of pancreaticoduodenectomy further imaging with magnetic resonance cholangiopancreatography (MRCP) or endoscopic ultrasound (EUS) guided biopsy should be performed.

Optimization of the Patient

General health and nutritional status: As these cancers tend to occur in older age group, optimizing cardiopulmonary and nutritional status is important. As such, old age is no more a contraindication.[14] Anorexia and weight loss are the most common presentations of pancreatic malignancy. When the serum albumin is less than 3 g/dL, or if surgery is delayed for more than 2 weeks, supplemental nutrition should be preferred. Nutrition can usually be provided enterally, but occasionally parenteral alimentation is indicated (gastric outlet obstruction).[15]

Preoperative biliary drainage (PBD): Since most of these patients present with progressive obstructive jaundice and itching, it is important to evaluate the effects of this hyperbilirubinemia like coagulopathy, acute kidney injury, cholangitis and indirectly malnutrition. As these complications increase the morbidity and mortality of the procedure, there are certain absolute indications for PBD.

- Cholangitis
- Intractable pruritus
- Coagulopathy
- Renal dysfunction.

Other indications for preoperative drainage are neoadjuvant treatment or any delay in surgery. Most surgeons would consider preoperative stenting in their patients if the bilirubin levels are above 15 mg/dL. These issues are further discussed in the chapter on perioperative management. If stenting is performed, a plastic biliary stent (at least 10 Fr) should be placed preferably endoscopically. Metal stents often incite a severe inflammatory reaction and may be incorporated into the bile duct wall, making it difficult to remove them at the time of surgery. However, metallic stenting is not a contraindication for resectable tumors.[16] Routine PBD is controversial as many randomized controlled trials have shown mixed results.[17] The largest and most recent randomized trial on PBD (10 Fr plastic stent) versus no drainage in 202 patients with pancreatic head malignancy showed a non-significant trend toward more surgery-related complications with PBD (47% vs 37%) including more readmissions for stent related complications with one postprocedural death.[18]

Deep venous thrombosis prophylaxis: All patients should receive 5,000 units aqueous low molecular weight heparin subcutaneous, preoperatively. Thigh-length sequential compression devices are applied preoperatively.

Operative Management

Patient Positioning and Incision

The patient is placed in supine position. Optionally, a logroll (at first lumbar vertebra level) can be used in obese patients to wide open the upper abdomen. The operation is performed either through a midline, a bilateral subcostal incision, a reverse L incision or a transverse incision with the curve facing downward for opening the lower flap. The latter is preferred in obese patients. Any self-retaining retractors, like Bookwalter, Thomson, Omni retractors, can be used and wide exposure of the operative field helps for further dissection.

Staging Laparoscopy

The role of staging laparoscopy in malignancy of the pancreas is justified in distal pancreatic adenocarcinoma and borderline pancreatic head tumors especially the large size lesions where the yield varies from 10% to 36%. The addition of CA 19-9 values, positive peritoneal cytology and laparoscopic ultrasound further improve the yield.[19-21] The most common reasons for unresectability are small hepatic or peritoneal metastases, which are not evident by preoperative imaging. The role of staging laparoscopy for periampullary cancer and cystic neoplasm of the head of pancreas is not proven and hence optional.

Initial Assessment for Metastatic Disease

Thorough exploration especially the subdiaphragmatic and inferior surface of the liver, root of the mesocolon and the pelvic cavity are evaluated. Occasionally an uncinate process mass mimics a nodal lesion at the root of the mesentry, hence this needs caution before deciding inoperability. A biopsy with frozen section should be taken of any suspicious lesion to rule out metastatic disease.

The following are the steps in pancreaticoduodenectomy (Fig. 1).

Mobilization of the duodenum and pancreatic head: The first step is to bring down the hepatic flexure from the liver—Cattell-Braasch maneuver mobilizing the right colon till the midline. Extensive Kocher's maneuver is performed to mobilize the "C" loop of the duodenum posteriorly till the aorta and left renal vein (LRV) are clearly visible. The vena cava and the aorta are cleaned off soft tissue exposing the LRV. Routine removal of the nodal tissue between the vena cava and aorta is not required. However, firm nodes or nodules in these areas need to be confirmed for metastasis by frozen biopsy (Fig. 2).[22]

Exposing the anterior surface of the pancreatic head and SMV: Attention is now turned to the anterior aspect of the head of the pancreas which is exposed by opening the lesser sac (gastrocolic ligament). Laterally, recognition of the avascular plane of dissection between the transverse mesocolon and the first part of duodenum is necessary for exposing the head of the pancreas. This step usually exposes the accessory middle colic vein (AMC), which joins the larger right gastroepiploic (RGE) vein to form the gastrocolic trunk before draining into superior mesenteric vein (SMV) (Fig. 3).

Careful exposure and ligation of these venous structures are required to expose the infra-pancreatic SMV, as any attempt to expose the anterior pancreas without tackling these veins result in significant bleeding and losing the advantage of having clear field. Usually middle colic vein is retracted medially after adequate exposure of the head of pancreas and its drainage does not interfere

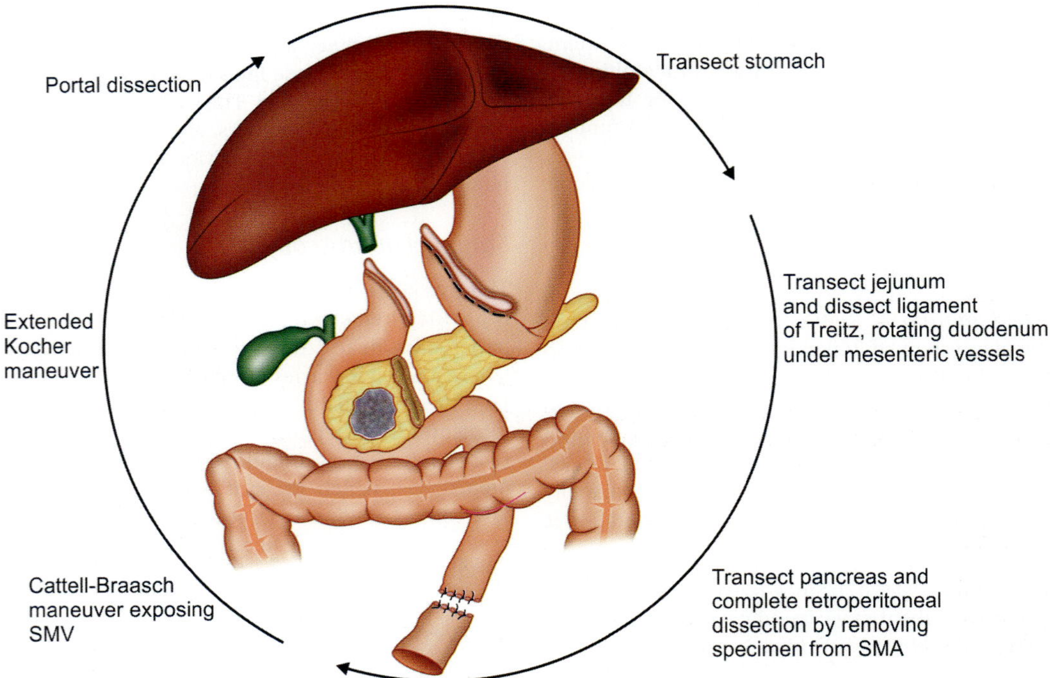

Figure 1 The surgical steps of pancreaticoduodenectomy (clockwise resection)

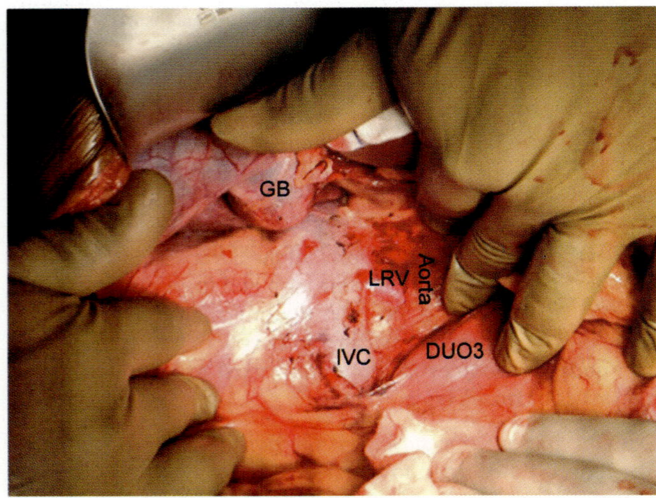

Figure 2 Post Cattell-Braasch/Kocherized intraoperative picture showing the mobilized "C" loop of duodenum exposing the LRV draining into the inferior vena cava (IVC) and the right side of abdominal aorta (AORTA). Gallbladder (GB), 3rd part of the duodenum (DUO 3)

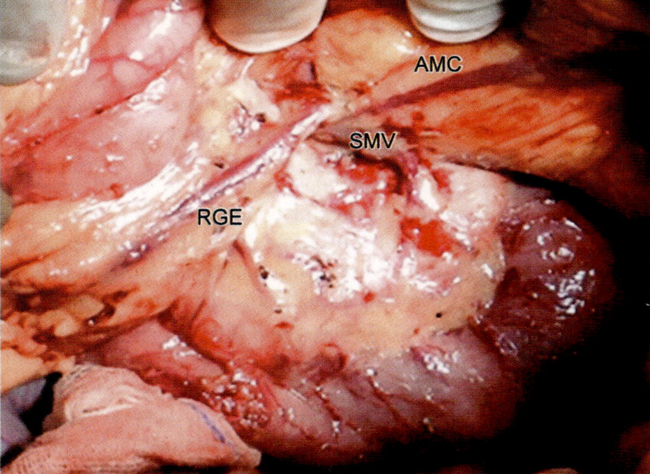

Figure 3 Intraoperative picture showing the anterior surface of the pancreas with accessory middle colic vein (AMC) joining the right gastroepiploic (RGE) vein to form the gastrocolic trunk and drain into superior mesenteric vein (SMV)

with creation of tunnel of love. Completion of the tunnel of love can be postponed till suprapancreatic dissections are completed.

Suprapancreatic dissection: Before starting this dissection, any aberrant hepatic arterial anatomy should be ruled out. Gallbladder is then mobilized after ligation of cystic artery and duct. The common hepatic duct is mobilized and looped after ensuring the location and safety of right hepatic artery. The replaced right hepatic artery runs along the lateral most margin of the hepatoduodenal ligament and is usually in posterior relation to the duct. Common hepatic duct is transected with scissors or cautery taking care of any biliary stent. The nature of the bile helps us in identifying patients who were in cholangitis and demand extra care. Bile and stent are sent for culture and sensitivity. The distal duct is suture ligated after sending the margin for histopathological examination. Bull dog clamp can be applied to the proximal duct or

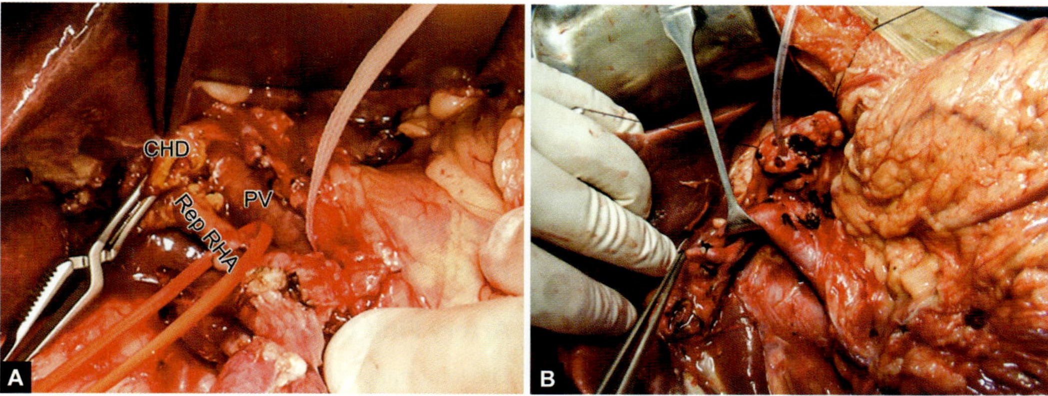

Figures 4A and B Intraoperative picture (A) showing the suprapancreatic dissection with common hepatic duct (CHD) cut after preserving the replaced right hepatic artery (Rep RHA) and exposing the right side of main portal vein (PV) (B) showing hepatic artery traversing posterior to portal vein

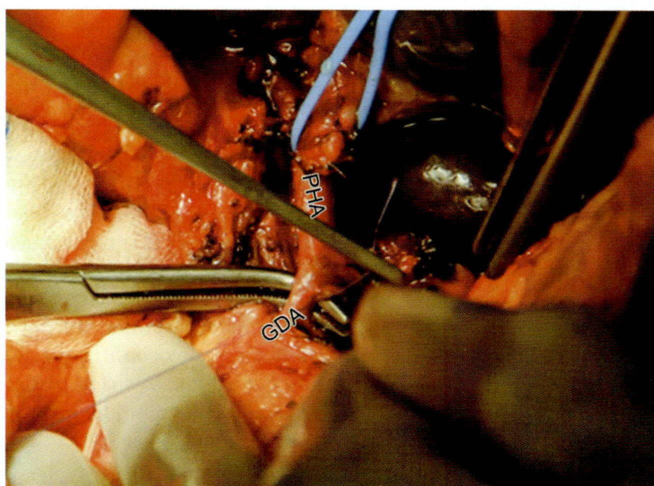

Figure 5 Intraoperative picture showing gastroduodenal artery (GDA) being tied and exposing the suprapancreatic part of the main portal vein

it can just be allowed to drain in the abdominal cavity. Preserving the right hepatic artery, the soft tissue and lymph nodes behind the bile duct are separated from the portal vein and allowed to remain in continuity with the pancreas (specimen). This step helps in exposing the RHA and the lateral border of the main portal vein (Figs 4A and B).

Tracing the RHA along the anterior surface of the portal vein helps in identifying the origin of Gastroduodenal artery (GDA). However, identification of the GDA can be done once the lesser omentum is opened and common hepatic artery is traced from the superior border of pancreas, laterally. Before ligation, clamp test [clamp the GDA and palpate hepatic artery at the hilum of liver to rule out hepatic supply from GDA as in celiac artery stenosis/median arcuate ligament (MAL) syndrome] is performed. After confirming, GDA is ligated and divided, leaving 1 cm stump which is secured with both prolene stitch and a metal clip. These steps help in exposing the suprapancreatic portal vein, the superior margin of tunnel of love (Fig. 5).

Finally the tunnel of love is carefully opened with blunt dissection, as much as possible under vision, taking care that there is no invasion. Usually, there are no anterior tributaries to the SMV at this location. Opening the tunnel of love only confirms that anterior surface of portal vein is free from tumor adherence. It does not mean that there is no vascular invasion as it is still possible that tumor is invading along the posterolateral border especially in cases where mass is arising from uncinate. Looping of the portal vein superiorly and SMV inferiorly is required in venous vascular resection and should be done whenever a tumor invasion is suspected.

Transection of the proximal duodenum or stomach and proximal jejunum: By this time, it is often evident whether the tumor is resectable. If this is the case, the distal stomach and proximal duodenum are mobilized and the right gastric vessels are divided. The arcade along the duodenal stump is maintained with the nerve of Latarjet preserved to the pylorus, the 1–2 cm duodenal stump is transected with a stapling device for a pylorus preserving technique. However, gastric antrum is transected when conventional pancreaticoduodenectomy is contemplated. Next the duodenojejunal flexure and the proximal jejunum are mobilized preserving the IMV. Dividing the jejunum about 5–8 cm from the duodenojejunal flexure, helps in further mobilization and ligation of the mesenteric vessels, releasing the duodenojejunal flexure. This step can be hastened with the use of the harmonic scalpel. The proximal jejunal segment, which is part of the specimen, is delivered to the right side.

Transection of the pancreatic neck and uncinate process dissection: In order to avoid bleeding and provide traction, two hemostatic polypropylene sutures are placed at both the inferior and superior margin of the pancreas, on either side of the proposed line of transection (i.e. four sutures total), which usually overlies the portal vein (Fig. 6). Caution is advised in taking the superior suture on the remnant side as main pancreatic duct is closer to this location. The pancreatic parenchyma is divided with scalpel and any bleeding is usually stopped with electrocoagulation or a fine suture. Good pancreatic stump helps in pancreatic reconstruction.

The principle of uncinate process dissection is the complete removal of the uncinate process with the so-called mesopancreas, baring the portal vein/SMV and right side of the superior mesenteric artery. Early ligation of the IPDA helps in avoiding excessive bleeding during this dissection as it prevents congestion of the specimen. This dissection can be done in two ways.

The classical technique involves retraction of the specimen to the right and careful identification and ligation of the vessels from superior mesenteric artery and vein, usually in a caudocranial direction. The surgeon's fingers guide the left extent of the dissection by the SMA pulsations (Figs 7A and B).

Artery first dissection follows the same steps as above helping in exposure of the origin of SMA from the aorta, thereby allowing further separation of SMA from the pancreatic mass. IPDA can be easily visualized as the first branch of SMA, whose early ligation has been advocated to significantly reduce the venous blood loss while doing further dissection.[23] Aberrant hepatic artery can mimic IPDA at this location, hence needs early recognition to avoid disaster.

In the posterior approach of SMA first technique, when there is possibilty of venous resection, uncinate dissection is done before the pancreatic transection. Uncinate is dissected craniocaudally with the assistant lifting and retracting the specimen to the left. This exposes the posterior surface of the pancreatic head and portal vein (Fig. 8). Technically the pancreatic transection with venous resection is easier once the uncinate dissection is done. Arterial stumps and portal axis venous tributaries are suture ligated with nonabsorbable sutures.

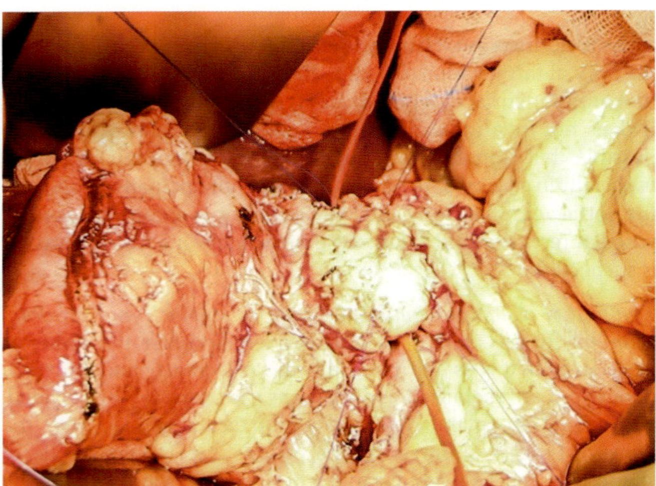

Figure 6 Intraoperative picture showing the four stitches on both sides of pancreatic transection

MODIFICATIONS OF PANCREATICODUODENECTOMY

Artery First Dissection

The importance of negative surgical margin along with the search for potential curative option for borderline pancreatic cancer has led to this approach. "Borderline resectable" disease has been defined as those tumors with:

- Venous involvement of SMV/PV without encasement of the nearby arteries
- Gastroduodenal artery and short-segment hepatic artery encasement without extension on to the celiac axis
- Tumor abutment of the SMA not exceeding 180° of the circumference of the vessel wall.[24,25]

The basis of this approach is to rule out arterial invasion rather than venous invasion as venous resection with R0 resection still has a comparable survival.[26] This technique was first described in 1993;[27] however, various approaches for artery first techniques have evolved over the last few years in view of the tumor location, specific artery involvement (SMA vs CHA) and technical expertise. Though six different approaches have been described till now, the "artery first" approach technically means to confirm the R0 resectability of the tumor and to rule out arterial invasion before proceeding to irreversible steps in pancreaticoduodenectomy rather than literally an initial artery first dissection[28] (Fig. 9).

The different approaches are:

- *Posterior approach (P):* Technically easy, especially for posteromedial tumors and helps in early identification of the

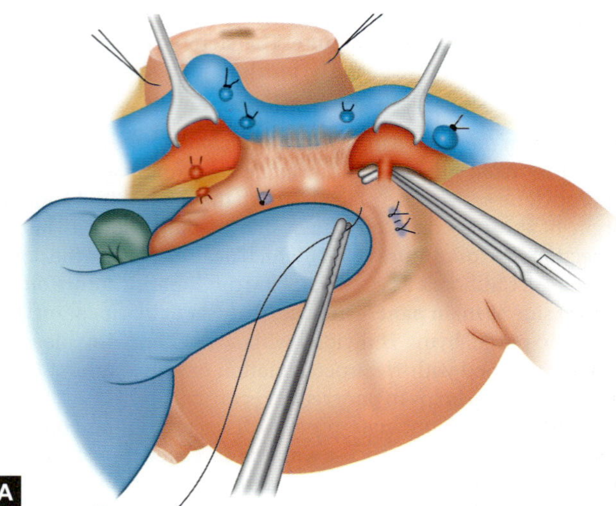

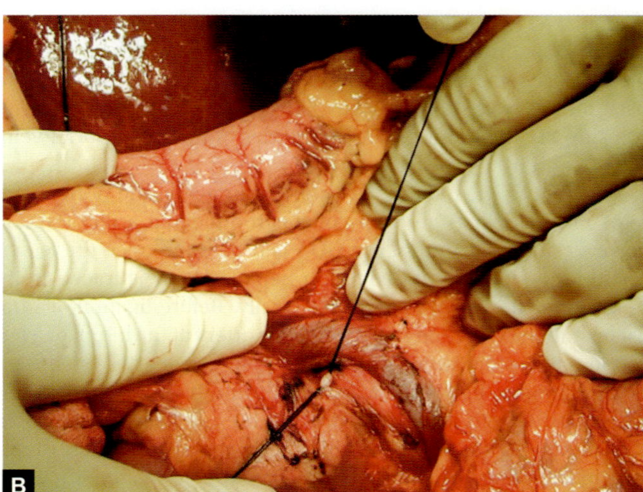

Figures 7A and B (A) Schematic diagram showing the uncinate dissection and (B) operative picture showing ligation of inferior pancreaticoduodenal artery (IPDA)

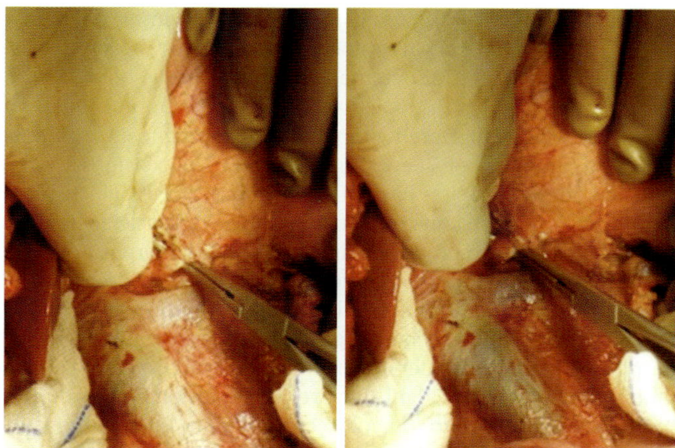

Figure 8 Intraoperative picture showing the posterior approach of artery first dissection with ligation of the IPDA after exposing the SMA first (*Abbreviation*: LRV, left renal vein)

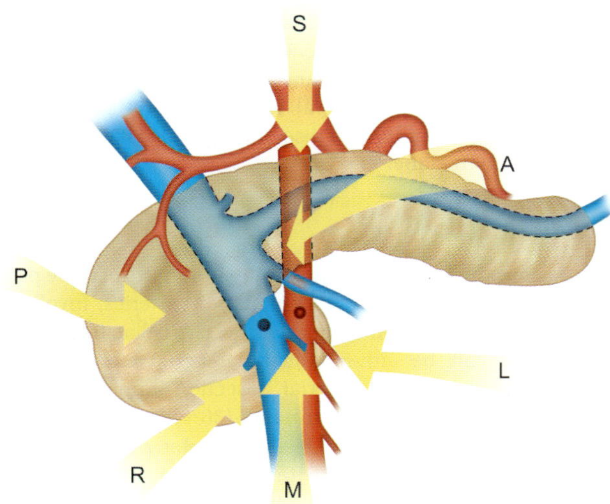

Figure 9 Schematic diagram for the different approaches to artery first dissection

aberrant vessels from SMA. Also helps in early identification of SMV involvement and facilitates en bloc resection (Fig. 9).

- *Medial uncinate approach:* Mainly for uncinate process lesions allowing early dissection and confirming the resectability, early ligation of IPDA reducing the blood loss and for patients requiring total pancreatectomy.
- *Inferior infracolic (mesenteric) approach:* Followed especially in locally advanced tumors allowing better exposure and dissection of region posterior to SMA.
- *Left posterior approach:* For tumors along uncinate and ventral pancreas, facilitates skeletonization of SMA in the retroperitoneum without Kocherization of the duodenum. So it helps in better SMA clearance at the cost of postoperative diarrhea requiring antidiarrheals.
- *Inferior supracolic approach:* For tumors along inferior border of the pancreas. Facilitates better retroperitoneal dissection, especially with locally advanced tumors with neoadjuvant treatment. "No-touch" technique with en bloc Kocherization theoretically prevents tumor cell dissemination.
- *Superior approach:* For tumors of the superior border of pancreas, helps in early identification of CHA, celiac and SMA involvement.

Though the results of artery first dissection have not shown clear advantage on survival, lymph node retrieval or R0 resection, they definitely improve the outlook of borderline resectable patients, reduce intraoperative blood loss with early ligation of IPDA and help to be better prepared for vascular resections. These approaches also help when extended pancreatic resection is required onto the body of pancreas.

Standard versus Pylorus Preserving (PPPD) versus Subtotal Stomach Preserving Pancreaticoduodenectomy (SSPPD)

Standard pancreaticoduodenectomy includes distal gastrectomy or antrectomy for better oncological clearance and to reduce the risk of marginal ulceration. However, it was found that these patients have more long-term GI morbidities in the form of dumping syndrome, postoperative alkaline reflux and weight loss. Pylorus preserving pancreaticoduodenectomy (PPPD) was initially described by Kenneth Watson in 1944 for "ensuring maximal protein and carbohydrate digestion in the stomach". However, it was William Traverso Longmire in 1977, who propagated this procedure extensively in patients with chronic pancreatitis initially with the specific intent of preserving the pylorus and first part of duodenum to make this procedure more physiological, hence called as "Longmire III operation".[29] He hypothesized that preserving the antrum, pylorus and first part of the duodenum with intact nerve supply (along with ligation of the right gastric and gastroepiploic vessels at the origin) helps in relieving the GI symptoms due to gastroenterostomy. This was confirmed in few retrospective studies. However, there was increased incidence of delayed gastric emptying (DGE) and increased hospital stay along with doubt about oncological clearance. Hence many randomized trials comparing PPPD with standard pancreaticoduodenectomy for pancreatic head neoplasm and periampullary lesions were conducted. The recent meta-analysis of these randomized trials suggest that, though these studies had some heterogenous data, PPPD was faster (around 1 hour quicker with less blood loss and significantly better quality of life in form of better appetite, less nausea and vomiting, lesser incidence of diarrhea and better weight gain.[30] Though incidence of DGE was initially high in patients undergoing PPPD, recent meta-analysis on DGE showed presence of preoperative diabetes, postoperative pancreatic fistulas, and postoperative complications were the clinical risk factors responsible for DGE. Antecolic duodenojejunal reconstruction and PBD resulted in a decrease in incidence of DGE and there was no difference in PPPD versus standard pancreaticoduodenectomy. Also there was no significant difference in lymph node yield, tumor recurrence and overall survival between these two procedures.[31] PPPD is avoided in locally advanced pancreatic malignancy involving or adjacent to the first part of duodenum and when the duodenal stump is ischemic.

Subtotal stomach-preserving pancreaticoduodenectomy was introduced with the aim to preserve as much stomach as possible, minimizing problems related to DGE that are associated with preserving the pyloric ring with lost vagal innervation. The duodenum, pylorus, and 1–2 cm of stomach are resected with the pancreatic specimen and the jejunal anastomosis fashioned to the distal antrum. However, studies have shown no significant difference in the DGE compared to standard or PPPD and the incidence of ulceration may be higher than that with conventional pancreaticoduodenectomy (due to retained antrum producing large amounts of gastrin). No improvements in median survival or disease-free survival have been demonstrated with this procedure.[32]

Vascular Resection

Fortner described extensive pancreatic surgery with vascular resection for advanced tumors over 30 years back, though he had dismal results.[33] Recent introduction of neoadjuvant therapy along with better imaging techniques, operative advancements and perioperative care have helped in increasing the borderline resectable patient pool. There is also improved ability to diagnose and execute vascular resection. Because of the anatomical proximity, venous involvement of pancreatic head malignancy is more common than arterial involvement and similarly prognosis differs between their involvements. There is no 5-year survival after arterial resections.[34] Presently contrast enhanced CT with EUS has the highest accuracy for detecting vascular involvement.[35]

Venous Resection

Currently there is no contraindication for venous resection unless R0 resection is not possible or reconstructable veins are absent, i.e. SMV is replaced by collaterals. Hence any surgeon contemplating pancreatic resection should be well versed with venous resection and reconstruction to avoid R1/R2 resection. Nakao and Ishikawa had classified venous involvement into two main groups where in bilateral involvement is associated with worse prognosis than unilateral involvement.[36,37] Bilateral involvement confirms the vascular, perineural invasion along with probable arterial involvement thereby implying an aggressive tumor. Similarly, the depth of portal vein invasion also influences the prognosis. The tumors involving tunica media or more are associated with large tumors (>4.5 cm), poor tumor differentiation and bilateral venous involvement thereby implying worse prognosis.[38] Venous resection can be either sleeve (Figs 10A and B) or excision

Theoretically excision has better clearance. If the defect is less than 3 cm, primary reconstruction is possible. Larger defect require interposition graft. Internal jugular vein is used as interposition graft when required as it has good size match and is easily retrievable. If inferior mesenteric venous drainage is compromised try to reimplant the splenic vein into the graft if possible, to avoid congestion in spleen and stomach after major surgery. Portal circulation clamp time should be short (<30 min) to avoid reperfusion syndrome and bowel edema leading to difficult reconstruction. Preparedness for these issues holds the key in the success of this operation.[22] Tumors of the uncinate process usually involve the distal SMV needing segmental resection without requiring portal clamping and splenic vein sacrifice[39] (Figs 11A and B).

Recent meta-analysis on studies with pancreaticoduodenectomy showed overall incidence of venous resection was 26% with 60% of them had histological invasion. Median morbidity and mortality rates were 42% and 5.9%, respectively which did not differ much from patients undergoing pancreaticoduodenectomy without venous resection. The survival rate of these tumors is more influenced by their grade, R0 resection and LN status rather than venous resection alone.[40]

Arterial Resection

After the introduction of neoadjuvant therapy, more of these patients are referred for vascular resections. Of the arteries, involvement of SMA is more common compared to CHA/celiac trunk. Arterial involvement can be either adherence (<180°) or encasement (>180°). The results of arterial resection are unsatisfactory, because of high in-hospital mortality (36%) and poor quality of life (intractable diarrhea and feeding intolerance). The survival rates are similar to patients without any resection.[41] However, there is a subgroup of patients where adherence is a possibility. In tumors with good prognosis like NET, arterial resection can be contemplated in selected cases. The selection criteria include

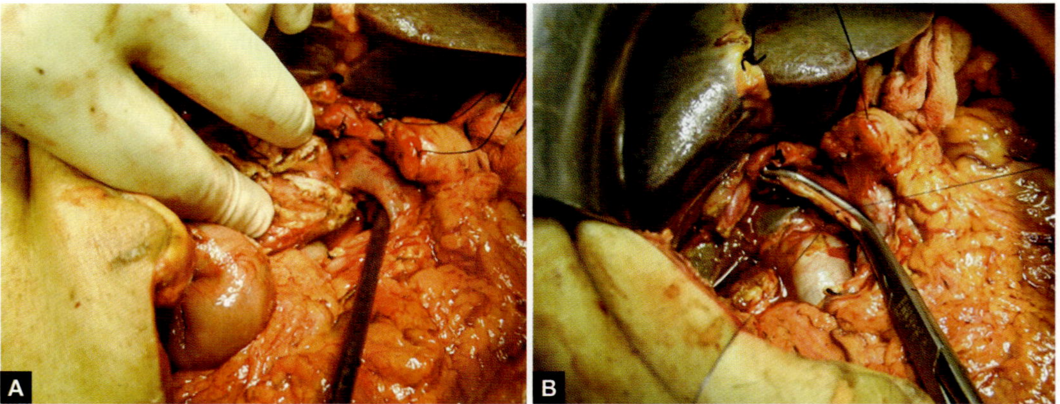

Figures 10A and B Operative picture showing (A) pancreatic tumor adherent to portal vein (B) sleeve resection with reconstruction with the help of Satinsky vascular clamp

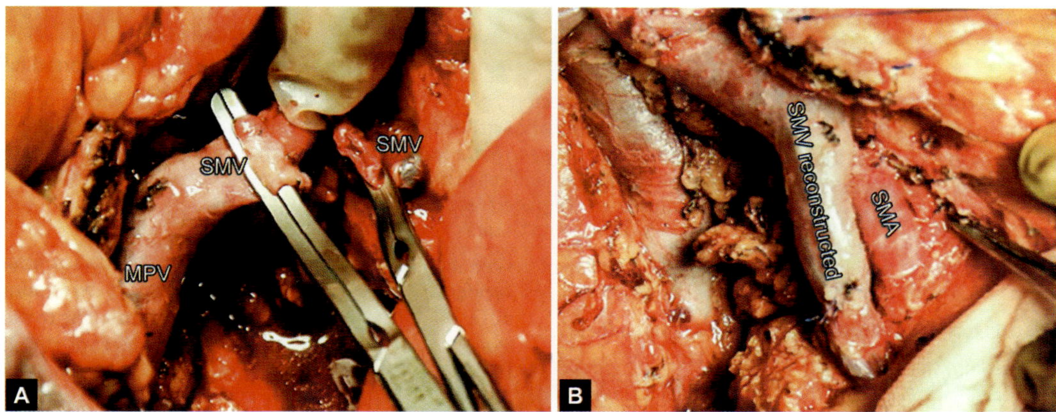

Figures 11A and B Intraoperative picture showing (A) distal SMV resection and (B) primary reconstruction for an uncinate mass
Abbreviations: PV, portal vein; SMA, superior mesenteric artery

patient's age less than 55 years, good performance status (ECOG score 0 or 1) and feasibility of the procedure (i.e. extent and location of the tumor, suitability of the artery proximal and distal to the tumor for reconstruction, adequate collateral blood supply via the SMA, pancreatoduodenal arcades and gastroduodenal artery for patients undergoing resection of the CA and common HA, respectively).[41] A rare technique of infrarenal aortic implantation of SMA might be useful in difficult cases of reconstruction.[42]

Multivisceral Resection

The efficacies of multivisceral resection for adjacent organ involvement in pancreatectomy have been studied in recent series.[43] More than 40% of pancreatic tumors are locally advanced with adjacent organ involvement at presentation. Though case series in the past have shown higher morbidity and inoperability, recent series have shown the feasibility of the extended resections along with equivalent survival if R0 resection is achieved. The most common adjacent structures resected are colon, stomach, liver, adrenal and kidney. Multivisceral resections are associated with higher morbidities (55.5% vs 42.8%) in the form of septic complications and re-explorations with longer ICU stay and higher intraoperative blood loss. The 30-day and hospital mortality rates were twice as high in multivisceral when compared with the standard resection group (3.0% and 6.9% vs 1.5% and 3.5% respectively), though this difference did not reach significance.[43] The risk for increased morbidity is associated with longer operating time more than 300 minutes and more than two organ resection. However, the overall survival and the long-term results are comparable to the standard resection, hence justifying the extended resection. Liver resection with pancreaticoduodenectomy is commonly performed in gallbladder malignancy and cholangiocarcinomas. They have acceptable inhospital mortality results if done with minor liver resection rather than major liver resection.

Role of Extended Lymphadenectomy

Fortner in 1973 proposed "extended radical lymphadenectomy (ERL)" along with vascular resection, as a method for more aggressive nodal and marginal clearance. As with any other GI malignancy, the rationale for extended lymphadenectomy in pancreatic adenocarcinoma was the high incidence of lymph nodal involvement (70%) and perineural invasion (67%) and preferential retroperitoneal lymphatics involvement (60%) of these tumors.[44] After the excellent result of extended lymphadenectomy by Ishikawa (1988) on the overall 3-year survival (38% vs 13%) and reduced local recurrence (67% vs 16%), ERL became the procedure of choice in Japan and few other centres.[45] However, these results were not reproduced in other centers and resulted in persistent, exhausting diarrhea for at least 6 months postoperatively. In 1998 Italy conference, the extent of lymphadenectomy for pancreatic head adenocarcinoma was classified as standard (SL), radical (RL) and extended (ERL) (Table 2, Fig. 12).

Recent meta-analysis of 4 RCTs and 11 non-RCTs on the role of lymphadenectomy in pancreatic head adenocarcinoma clearly showed universal increase in the yield of lymph nodes (6–17 vs 12–41), hence increased operating time in all the studies.[46] However, this was not reflected in the increased overall or disease free survival in all four randomized trials except for one study by Pedrazzoli showing a survival advantage in the subgroup of node positive patients. In addition, the quality of life is severely hampered by the persistent diarrhea (10.8–76%) for almost 6 months, leading to malnutrition which was proven in two of the four randomized trials. However, the results of the meta-analysis are hampered by the non-standardization of the surgical techniques and lymph nodal mapping which was identified by less than 15 LN retrieval in more than 50% of the patients in three out of four RCTs. Hence pancreaticoduodenectomy with SL with at least 15 LN retrievals is the procedure of choice.[46]

Ultraradical Surgery

Ultraradical surgery with portal vein resection, total pancreatectomy, and retroperitoneal lymphadenectomy has been performed, primarily in Japan, in an attempt to improve the outcomes from resection. Proponents argue that the more extensive resection allows removal of multifocal disease and additional potentially involved peripancreatic nodes.[33] It also eliminates the need for pancreaticoenteric anastomosis, thereby removing the risk of a postoperative leak or pancreatic fistula. However, several reports failed to demonstrate improved survival. Moreover diabetes developing after total pancreatectomy is often difficult to control.[47]

Table 2: Classification of the lymphadenectomy for pancreatic head malignancies		
Standard lymphadenectomy	*Radical pancreatoduodenectomy*	*Extended radical pancreatoduodenectomy*
En bloc resection of the following lymph node groups is performed	Regional lymphadenectomy plus skeletonization of hepatic arteries, superior mesenteric artery between aorta and inferior pancreaticoduodenal, and celiac trunk, dissection of the anterolateral aspect of aorta and vena cava including Gerota's fascia	Radical lymphadenectomy plus clearance of anterior aorta between the diaphragmatic hiatus (around the celiac trunk) and the origin of the common iliac arteries
12b1, 12b2, 12c (Lymph nodes of the right side of the hepatoduodenal ligament)	All 8-Skeletonization of the common and proper hepatic artery lymph nodes	All 16-clearance of all connective and lymphatic tissue, starting from 3 cm to the right of the duodenum, and extending to the mid-portion of the left kidney; and from the inferior margin of the liver across the diaphragmatic hiatus, well above the origin of the celiac trunk to the origin of the common iliac arteries. Clearance of the anterior aorta of all lymphatic and neurovascular tissue including the tissue around the celiac axis is performed. Left adrenalectomy is optional
13a, 13b (Posterior pancreaticoduodenal nodes)	9-Celiac axis nodes	
14a, 14b (Nodes to the right side of the SMA from the origin of the SMA at the aorta to the inferior pancreaticoduodenal artery)	All 12-lymph nodes of the left and right side of the hepatoduodenal ligament	
17a, 17b (Anterior pancreaticoduodenal nodes)	All 14-Circumferential skeletonization of SMA between the aorta and the inferior pancreaticoduodenal artery	
Lymph nodes of the anterior-superior region of the common hepatic artery (8a)	16a2, 16b1 All lymph nodes of the anterolateral aspect of the aorta and of the inferior vena cava, in continuity with Gerota's fascia, between the celiac axis and the inferior mesenteric artery	

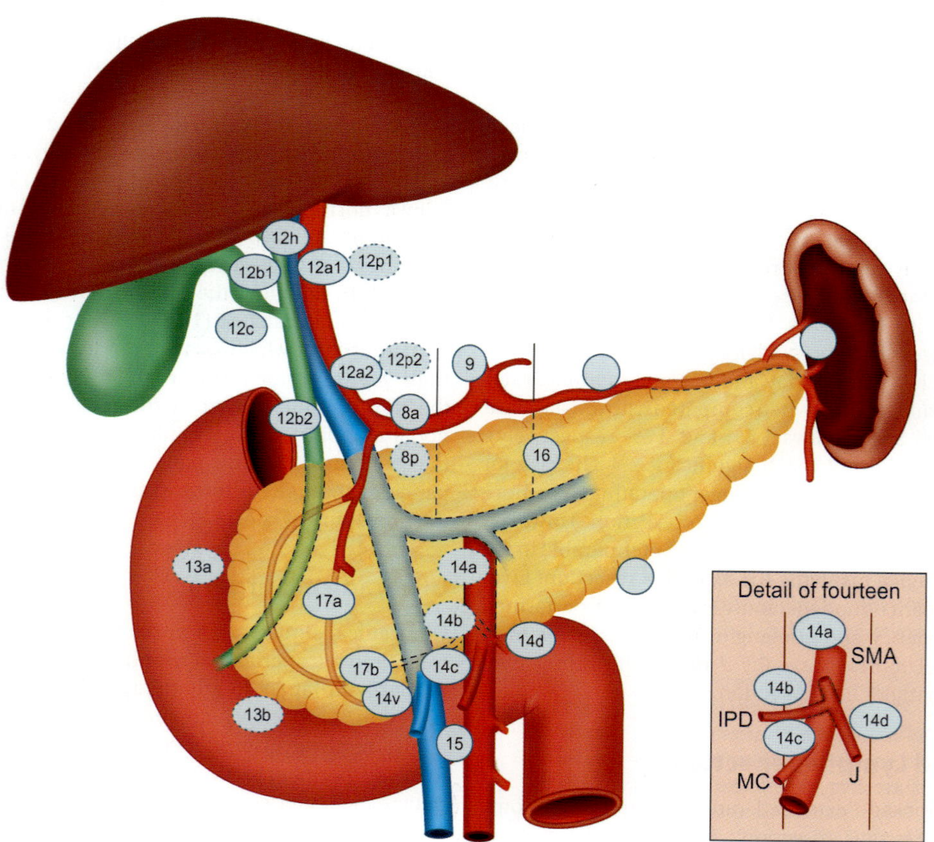

Figure 12 Schematic diagram of the extent of lymphadenectomy in pancreatic head malignancies

Minimally Invasive Pancreaticoduodenectomy

This has been covered in the chapter on Minimally invasive Pancreaticoduodenectomy.

RECONSTRUCTION OF GASTROINTESTINAL CONTINUITY

Pancreatic Reconstruction

Pancreatic reconstruction is the Achilles heel of pancreatico-duodenectomy and various technical modifications have been described. Initially, when pancreaticoduodenectomy was performed, pancreatic duct was ligated considering that pancreatic juice is not essential. However, Cattell, in 1943, stressed on the indispensible pancreaticojejunal anastomosis. It was also the cause for majority of the complications. He recommended a direct anastomosis of the pancreatic duct and the jejunum in patients in whom the main pancreatic duct had sufficient diameter. Coffey, in 1909, tried the technique of invaginating the pancreatic stump into jejunal limb in human cadavers, and Child, in 1941, attempted this technique in humans.[48,49] Whipple's introduced the technique of tube pancreaticojejunostomy in 1946, which we follow now as stented anastomosis.[50] Many types of operations have been devised since that time, although most of them are variations of the ideas of Cattell, Child and Whipple.[51]

We follow Blumgart's technique which is described here with our modifications to it.[52] Pancreaticojejunal anastomosis is constructed using 2–3 transpancreatic U sutures on either side of the main pancreatic duct (Fig. 13A). U sutures are placed 1 cm distal to the transected edge of the pancreas going from front to back. The seromuscular bite of the jejunum is taken, nearer the mesenteric edge, and the suture is reverted back to front through the pancreas completing the U. U sutures were taken 5 mm from each other. These sutures approximate the jejunum to dorsal surface of the pancreatic stump. Sutures with needles on them were kept separately and held with rubber shod clamps. A duct-to-mucosa anastomosis is then constructed after creating a small opening in the jejunum. Anastomosis was done using 6–8 interrupted 4-0/5-0 polyglactin sutures (Fig. 13B). A short internal stent using appropriate infant feeding tube is placed and fixed with ends of tied-up sutures of the posterior wall of duct-to-mucosa anastomosis. Previously held U sutures were then tied on the anterior surface of pancreas. Needles were then passed through seromuscular antimesenteric edge of jejunum bringing the jejunum toward and covering the front of pancreatic cut edge (Fig. 13C). Knots were tied again at the ventral part of the pancreas (Fig. 13D). The placement of sutures at two sites in the jejunal wall and the full thickness of the pancreas prevent them from cutting through. More recently, we have given up internal stenting almost entirely. In difficult cases an external stent may, however, be beneficial.

Biliary Anastomosis

The hepaticojejunostomy is performed at a distance from pancreatojejunostomy, which should be tension free as well as

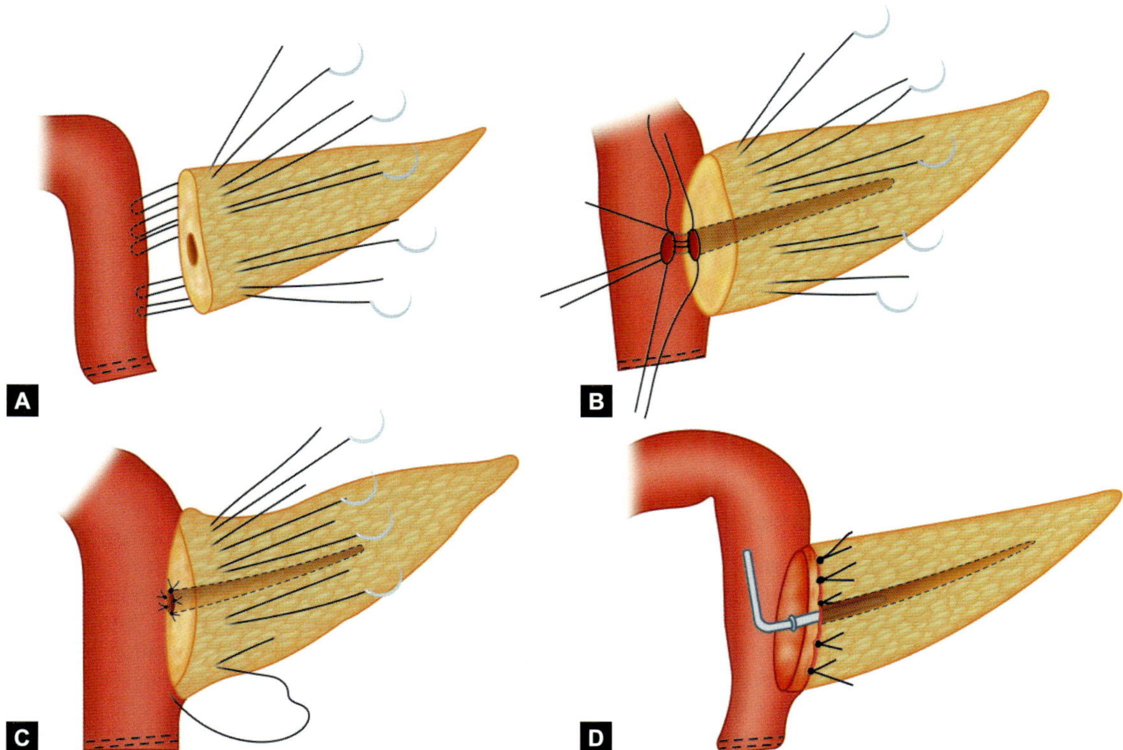

Figures 13A to D Schematic diagrams illustrating the modified Blumgart's technique for pancreaticojejunal anastomosis; internal stent has now been given up by us: (A) Transpancreatic U sutures; (B) Duct to mucosa anastomosis with 4-0 polygalactin; (C) Duct to mucosa completed; next the transpancreatic sutures are tied. Seromuscular sutures in progress; (D) Second layer of seromuscular sutures tied up with completed anastomosis kink free, arbitrarily 10 cm from pancreatojejunostomy. A single layer anastomosis using interrupted sutures of 5-0 polydioxanone (PDS) or 4-0 polyglactin is usually performed (continuous sutures are acceptable in a dilated duct). The bowel lumen is opened with electrocautery for a length equivalent or less than the bile duct diameter and the sutures are placed easily in a dilated duct. We do both corner sutures first followed by posterior sutures, placed equidistance (2 mm interval) at varying depths. Then the knots are thrown inside the lumen. Rarely, in a difficult anastomosis, the anterior rows of bile duct sutures are placed before doing the posterior wall anastomosis.

Duodenal Anastomosis

Finally, an antecolic/retrocolic gastro(duodeno) jejunostomy is constructed approximately 45 cm distal to the choledochojejunostomy in standard two-layer fashion.

Role of Drains

There has been controversy regarding whether drain placement after pancreatic resections including pancreaticoduodenectomy is useful or not. Earlier studies revealed that prophylactic drainage increases the risk of intra-abdominal abscess and infectious complications rather than reducing it. Moreover, the management of pancreatic fistula did not change significantly with prophylactic drainage. Recently, two large retrospective studies (2013) and a systematic review including these two studies also suggested that prophylactic drainage can be safely abandoned as it is associated with more complications.[53,54] However, if a drain is placed, prospective randomized studies demonstrate that early removal is safe in patients with postoperative day 1 drain amylase values less than 5,000 U/L and is associated with a lower rate of fistula than delayed removal.[55,56] These claims have been strongly refuted by a multicenter randomized controlled trial published recently (2014) and has provided level one evidence in favor of drainage. There was increased morbidity and mortality in the group where drainage was not used and the trial was stopped prematurely.[57] Thus it seems that drain may be omitted in some patients but this subgroup needs to be identified. We use drains in all our patients. Our practice of keeping the drains for 3–5 days has served well for our patients and has not caused any additional morbidity. Drain fluid amylase and amount of drainage are monitored daily. Drains are removed when both the amylase levels and the amount have reduced to acceptable levels.

Postoperative Management

Complications Related to Pancreaticoduodenectomy

Pancreatic fistula: Postoperative pancreatic fistula (POPF) is the most common procedure related complication after pancreaticoduodenectomy. It not only contributes to the morbidity but also the mortality in these patients. Hence it is called the Achilles heel of the pancreaticoduodenectomy reconstruction. The reported incidence of pancreatic fistula is not similar worldwide due to the different criteria defining pancreatic fistula are used. In 2005, the International Study Group on Pancreatic Fistula (ISGPF) defined pancreatic fistula as a level of amylase in a drain or an abdominal collection over three times the serum level starting on the third postoperative day, regardless of the flow.[58]

Table 3: ISGPF grading of postoperative pancreatic fistula[58]

Grade of PF	*Clinical condition*	*Specific treatment*	*US/CT (if obtained)*	*Reoperation*	*Signs of infection*	*Sepsis*
A	Well	No	Negative	No	No	No
B	Often well	Yes/No	Negative/ Positive	No	Yes	No
C	Ill appearing/Bad	Yes	Positive	Yes	Yes	Yes

In most studies, incidence of pancreatic fistula varies between 10% and 15% of patients undergoing pancreaticoduodenectomy. Though there is reduction in the mortality after pancreaticoduodenectomy, there is not much improvement in the incidence of pancreatic fistula, except in few series. Since pancreaticoduodenectomy is a multivisceral resection, the POPF after pancreaticoduodenectomy is more worrisome as the fistula content is mixed with digestive pancreaticobiliary secretion and has bacterial contamination (74%).[59] The diagnosis of pancreatic fistula after pancreaticoduodenectomy is typically made at the end of the first postoperative week. However, presently, evaluating drain fluid amylase early (3rd day) has helped in early identification of pancreatic fistula and cautious management of these patients. POPF has been classified into three grades according to the clinical manifestation and requirement of intervention (Table 3).

Various risk factors have been identified for pancreatic fistula; however, the texture of the pancreatic parenchyma (soft or firm) and size of the pancreatic duct are the most important ones along with volume of pancreatic work. This is further evident from the review of 2,664 patients, where reported incidence of pancreatic fistula after pancreaticoduodenectomy is 5% for chronic pancreatitis, 12% for adenocarcinomas of the pancreas, 15% for cancer of the ampulla of Vater and 33% for lower bile duct cholangiocarcinoma.[60] Pancreatic fistula is evaluated with contrast enhanced CT of the upper abdomen. In approximately half of the cases, pancreatic fistula is associated with a perianastomotic collection. Though these collections may be asymptomatic, they require adequate drainage due to their risk of abscess formation or vascular erosion. Routine CT on POD 7 has been studied and found to detect asymptomatic pancreatic fistula in 80% of patients who would have otherwise recovered normally. Currently there is no consensus on the prophylactic CT. It should be considered in patients who have undergone vascular reconstruction especially arterial (aberrant vessels or SMA/Celiac axis) even when the biochemical criteria are not met.

Treatment: Grades A and B pancreatic fistula can be managed conservatively. The principle is to ensure adequate drainage of the pancreatic fistula by abdominal drains or pigtail insertion under imaging guidance. Nutritional support is maintained through enteral route. Enteral nutrition is associated with significantly higher and early closure rates of pancreatic fistulas[61] contrary to the earlier belief. However, oral feeding is avoided in pancreaticogastrostomy anastomosis and the stomach is drained using a nasogastric tube with gentle aspiration. Inhibition of pancreatic secretions using somatostatin or its analogs may speed up healing of the pancreatic fistula.[62] The role of prophylactic antibiotic is not clear. The outcome of conservative management is successful in around 85% of patients. Most fistula close within an average duration of 1 month.[63] Re-exploration is required in cases where abdominal collection not amenable for drainage, or when clinical condition deteriorate or in cases of hemorrhage that are amenable to endovascular treatment. The mortality associated with these interventions is high. When the anastomotic disruption is large, the surgical procedure contemplated is based on the timing of reintervention, clinical status and viability of pancreatic stump. Early disruption requires evaluation of the pancreatojejunostomy jejunal limb to rule out obstruction/kinking. In this group of patients, excision of the edematous jejunal limb and redoing the anastomosis with external pancreatic drain should be considered. Another option is conversion to a pancreaticogastric anastomosis.[64] In late interventions, ligation or glue injection of the remnant ischemic stump or externalizing drain to the pancreaticoduodenectomy may be available options. Rarely completion pancreatectomy is the option, but is associated with high mortality (between 24% and 80%).[65]

Prevention: Various modifications have been tried to reduce the complications related pancreaticodigestive anastomotic leak. Interestingly apart from few exceptions, no single technique has been found to reduce this complication. Overall, it is the volume of pancreatic work and the surgeons' comfort that has most impact in reducing this complication. Thus tailoring your own technique from experience to the need of the hour is all that matters.[66] However, it is essential to understand the different modifications and the concepts favoring them.

The various anastomotic techniques tried are duct to mucosa, dunking (invagination) and binding anastomosis. Further external and internal stents have been used in these variations. The most common pancreaticodigestive anastomosis performed worldwide is pancreaticojejunostomy. Our method is Blumgart's duct to mucosa anastomosis that has been described above. A review revealed that binding pancreatojejunostomy, where the cut end of the pancreas is completely invaginated into a jejunal limb (end to end or end to side) seemed to be a safe and secure technique that reduces the rate of pancreatic fistula.[67] However, only one RCT supported this along with few observational studies. Experience of other surgeons with this anastomosis has not been so good. The uses of external and internal stents in pancreatojejunostomy anastomosis have also been analyzed. It was found that external stent (3 RCTs) reduced the incidence of POPF by diverting the pancreatic enzymes from the pancreatojejunostomy anastomosis thereby preventing the digestive action.[68-70] The use of an internal stent was not found to be helpful. There is no evidence to recommend biological wrap (omental or falciform ligament) or somatostatin analogs to prevent or reduce POPF.

Pancreaticogastrostomy vs pancreaticojejunostomy: Pancreaticogastrostomy was first described by Waugh and Clagett in 1944. It has several physiological and technical benefits like close proximity of the pancreatic remnant to the posterior wall of the stomach for a tension free anastomosis, thick well vascularized stomach for approximating, use of nasogastric tube to decompress stomach, absence of enterokinase, acidic pH in the stomach to neutralize and deactivate pancreatic enzymes and use of endoscopy for surveillance. However, its opponents argued for the difficulty in treating pancreatic fistula occurring in conjunction with gastric fistula and long-term effects of pancreatic enzymes deactivation. In view of the favorable results of pancreaticogastrostomy with respect to POPF formation in various observational studies, 4 RCTs were performed against pancreatojejunostomy including one performed on high risk soft pancreas alone to confirm this hypothesis. Except for the recent RCT by Fernández-Cruz (2008), all the other RCTs did not show any advantage of pancreaticogastrostomy over pancreatojejunostomy in the POPF formation. A recent meta-analysis revealed the heterogeneity involved in the study groups and difficulty in comparisons. They concluded that pancreaticogastrostomy has similar mortality compared to pancreatojejunostomy. Pancreaticogastrostomy may reduce the risk of biliary fistula, DGE and intra-abdominal collections but with increased risk for intraluminal hemorrhage.[71] Overall, there is not much advantage for either pancreaticogastrostomy or pancreatojejunostomy in terms of postoperative complications. Pancreatojejunostomy may be favored for the long-term benefits.

Isolated roux loop pancreaticojejunostomy: Machado in 1976, introduced the isolated pancreatojejunostomy, thereby avoiding intestinal and bile contents from activating the pancreatic juice and hence minimizing the incidence and severity of anastomotic erosion.[72] Potential disadvantages are increased operating time, the need for an additional anastomosis and additional loss of 45 cm of absorptive jejunum. Several earlier cohort studies reported decreased pancreatic fistula rate for duct to mucosa isolated pancreatojejunostomy.[73,74] However, recent prospective studies including an RCT does not support isolated pancreatojejunostomy compared to the conventional pancreatojejunostomy. It adds extra 70 minutes to the operating time besides making another 40 cm of bowel non-functional.[75-77] In the event of pancreatic fistula, it may reduce its severity and thereby the hospital stay.[78]

Delayed gastric emptying: Delayed gastric emptying is the second most common complication after pancreaticoduodenectomy. Although it is not life threatening, it significantly hampers nutrition and increases the hospital stay thereby delaying the convalescence and adjuvant treatment. Its incidence varies from 19% to 70% mainly because of the difference in definition. Hence in 2007 consensus, the International Study Group of Pancreatic Surgery (ISGPS) defined DGE as "any nasogastric tube intubation lasting more than three postoperative days (POD)" or "the inability to tolerate a solid diet by POD 7". They further stratified DGE into different grades of severity, A to C as stated in Table 4.

Table 4: Grading of delayed gastric emptying (DGE) in pancreatic surgeries

DGE grade	*Nasogastric tube required*	*Table of tolerate solid oral intake by POD*	*Vomiting/ Gastric distension*	*Use of prokinetics*
A	4–7 days or reinsertion >POD 3	7	±	±
B	8–14 days or reinsertion >POD 7	14	+	+
C	>14 days or reinsertion >POD 14	21	+	+

Various theories proposed for primary DGE include vagal denervation, ischemia of the pylorus, decreased serum motilin, angulation of the duodenojejunal anastomosis. More common is secondary DGE that is related to intra-abdominal complications like pancreatic fistula, intra-abdominal bleed and abscess.[79] Hence diagnosis of DGE is considered as an alarm and warrants detailed evaluation for these complications. The other reported risk factors are advanced age, male gender, preoperative cholangitis, long operating time, pancreatic fibrosis and prior abdominal surgery. Though PPPD was earlier considered a risk factor for DGE, recent meta-analyses has disproved this. Retrocolic reconstruction of duodenojejunal was considered to be associated with higher incidence of DGE compared to antecolic duodenojejunal[80] but this fact is not supported by a recent randomized trial. Prophylactic erythromycin which triggers phase 3 of the gastric migratory motor activity complex has been shown to reduce 53–75% incidence of DGE.[81] DGE is usually treated with nasogastric decompression along with nutritional support. Motility drugs like perinorm or lesuride are tried initially after ruling out any mechanical obstruction. If no response is there, Erythromycin 250 mg thrice daily for 1–3 weeks may resolve the problem.

Postoperative hemorrhage: The incidence of bleeding after pancreaticoduodenectomy varies from 4% to 16%. The ISGPS defined postpancreatectomy hemorrhage using three parameters: (1) onset, (2) location and (3) severity.[82] The onset is either early (≤24 hours after the end of the index operation) or late (>24 hours). The location is either intraluminal or extraluminal. The severity of bleeding may be either mild or severe.

Three different grades A, B and C are defined according to the time of onset, site of bleeding, severity and clinical impact (Table 5). Early hemorrhages are usually due to technical reasons and majority are from the intra-abdominal sites in 85% and rest from intra-luminal sites such as GI suture line and pancreatojejunostomy stump site. The main reasons for differentiating early from late hemorrhages are, early ones are easily detectable and early surgical intervention and control of the bleeding results in good outcome.[83] Late hemorrhages are usually associated with intra-abdominal septic complications like pancreatic fistula and biliary fistula. They are mostly arterial origin and intraluminal bleed.[84] The most common artery to be involved is the GDA stump followed by IPDA, CHA, splenic artery and, rarely, the aberrant arteries.[85] The hemorrhage may present initially as slow bleed that spontaneously stops (herald bleed) followed by significant bleed with shock.[86] In stable patients CT angiography is the investigation of choice to evaluate the site of extravasation and intra-abdominal collection. Usually this is best managed by angiographic embolization or endovascular stenting which has 80% success rate.[87] Recent availability of covered stents has helped in better management of the pseudoaneurysms. Endoscopy can be a useful adjunct in localizing intra-luminal bleeds. Patients with hemodynamic instability and intra-abdominal infections, require re-exploration and damage control surgery. Recurrent bleeds after re-exploration is still a possibility. Postoperative angiogram is done in such cases to avoid further catastrophe. Mortality after later hemorrhages is between 10% and 20% as the risk of ischemic complications increases with these interventions.

Ischemic complications: Ischemic complications of pancreatico-duodenectomy have been recognized recently and it attracts early attention in view of its one-third contribution to the perioperative mortality after pancreaticoduodenectomy. The incidence has been reported as 1–3% and has been attributed to arterial trauma while operating. The common presentations of these complications are hepatic ischemia, intrahepatic abscess, biliary complications and mesenteric ischemia.[79] A careful preoperative evaluation and good technique can completely avoid this catastrophe.

Preoperative CT angiography helps in evaluation of the etiology such as course of aberrant arteries or presence of celiac artery/SMA stenosis. Routine CT angiography reveals 11% celiac/SMA stenosis in patients undergoing pancreaticoduodenectomy of which 5% are hemodynamically significant. Celiac artery stenosis is either caused by MAL compression or intrinsic stenosis while isolated SMA stenosis is usually intrinsic. By identifying these etiology preoperatively, they can be managed before contemplating pancreaticoduodenectomy. The intrinsic stenoses are managed with preoperative endovascular stenting. Significant MAL compression diagnosed intraoperatively with GDA clamping test requires intervention. It should be borne in the mind that an equivocal GDA clamping test performed at the beginning of pancreaticoduodenectomy could be subsequently altered by interruption of other peripancreatic collateralls, including dorsal pancreatic artery and the arc of Bühler. Further, celiac axis compression varies during inspiratory and expiratory phases, including under intraoperative mechanical ventilation, thus impeding determination of a clear threshold. Division of MAL seems to be safe and effective if indications and technique are appropriate. By following this protocol, majority of unexpected ischemic complications are avoided.[88]

Table 5: Proposed classification of postpancreatectomy hemorrhage (PPH) by the International Study Group of Pancreatic Surgery (ISGPS) of onset, location

Grade	*Time of onset, location, severity and clinical impact of bleeding*		*Clinical condition*	*Therapeutic consequence*
A	Early, intraluminal or extraluminal, mild		Well	None
B	Early, intraluminal or extraluminal severe	Late, intraluminal or extraluminal, mild	Often well/intermediate, very rarely life-threatening	Transfusion of fluid/blood, intermediate care unit (or ICU), therapeutic endoscopy, embolization, relaparotomy for early PPH
C		Late, intraluminal or extraluminal, severe	Severely impaired, life-threatening	Localization of bleeding, angiography and embolization, endoscopy or relaparotomy, ICU

Biliary complications: The biliary complications can be either primary or secondary to pancreatic leaks, which need to be treated accordingly. Their incidence ranges from 2% to 5%. It is diagnosed by a bilirubin concentration in the drain fluid of at least three times the serum level on or after postoperative day 3. They are classified as grades A, B and C according to the need of intervention. The long-term implication of bile leak is that there is a chance of 8% stricture after 5 years and 13% stricture after 10 years follow-up.[89] Usually these complications are managed by converting it into a controlled fistula and tackling the stricture with delayed definitive surgery/PTBD dilatation. Most bile collections can be managed with radiologic interventions.

Other complications: Chylous leak has been reported as 1.3-16.3%.[90-92] Various definitions used account for the wide variation. A milky drain output with triglyceride level more than 110 mg/dL is the commonly accepted definition. Its implications are large fluid volume losses together with protein, electrolyte, immunoglobulin and lymphocytes. This takes heavy toll on already debilitated patients with prolonged abdominal drainage and hospital stay. Radical lymphadenectomy, concomitant vascular resection, early institution of enteral nutrition and portomesenteric thrombosis have been identified as the risk factors for chyle leak. However, managing these patients conservatively with fat restricted diet helps in complete resolution.[93]

Implication of acute pancreatitis, diagnosed incidentally (25%) on 1 week postoperative CT, on recovery is still not clear. Healthy pancreatic parenchyma (soft pancreas) is a risk factor.[94]

PERIOPERATIVE MORBIDITY AND MORTALITY

As noted earlier, the R0 conventional pancreaticoduodenectomy is associated with a 5-year survival of 20-30% and a perioperative mortality rate of less than 4%. Pancreatic anastomotic dehiscence, liver failure or bowel necrosis are the contributing factors for mortality. In a meta-analysis of 14 studies, there was a significant association between hospital volume and postoperative mortality as well as overall survival.[95]

The prognosis for pancreatic cancer remains poor and depends on:

T Stage[96]

Stage wise post-resection figures is given in Table 6.

Table 6: Stage-wise post-resection survival (%)

Stage	*Patients (%)*	*1-year (%)*	*5-year (%)*
IA	8.8	71.3	31.4
IB	11.0	67.3	27.2
IIA	17.9	60.7	15.7
IIB	36.4	52.7	7.7
III	13.2	44.5	6.8
IV	12.7	19.2	2.8

Nodal Status

Ten percent (10%) (node positive) versus 25–30% (node negative).

Margin Status

After a curative resection, margin status and nodal status determines the prognosis. The positive margin rate after a pancreaticoduodenectomy for pancreatic cancer was reported to range from 15% to 85%. Recent reports showed 25% margin positivity (R1 + R2) with 10–15% R2 resections.[97,98] However, R1/R2 pancreaticoduodenectomy have been shown to have a better role of palliation compared to bypass surgeries with relatively good overall survival.[99] The impact of these margin positivity resections is evaluated in a recent study of 388 pancreaticoduodenectomy patients with 207 bypass surgeries. When comparing periampullary cancers, the margin positivity is higher with pancreatic (51%) and distal cholangiocarcinoma (27%). However, there is an overall survival benefit after a pancreaticoduodenectomy regardless of the resection margin or primary origin of the periampullary adenocarcinoma, as compared with a bypass operation. R1 status has no influence on the survival. Although an R2 resection was associated with poorer outcome in periampullary adenocarcinomas, the resection status did not play a role in survival outcome in pancreatic head adenocarcinoma.

SPECIAL SITUATIONS

Aberrant Arteries

An aberrant arterial anomaly is a well-recognized risk factor for ischemic complications like hepatic ischemia, hepaticojejunostomy failure and hemorrhage in view of pseudoaneurysm. This is particularly avoided by preoperative multidetector CT, which increases the awareness of the vascular anomaly. Replaced or accessory RHA and replaced CHA from SMA are the anomalies of importance in pancreaticoduodenectomy, which are present in 11–21% of the pancreaticoduodenectomy. A surgeon is left with three options when he encounters intraoperatively—ligation, dissection and traction away from the site of dissection, or division and anastomosis. Ligation can be attempted if vessel caliber is small, as in accessory artery or the vessel is already involved and collaterals has developed, which can be tested with brisk backflow in the aberrant vessel. A replaced RHA or CHA should generally be recognized and preserved (Fig. 14). However, if oncological clearance is compromised, it is divided and reconstructed. Replaced RHA is usually reconstructed with the GDA stump. Routine postoperative CT at 2 weeks is recommended to rule out pseudoaneurysm.

Uncinate Process Tumors

They account for up to 10% of all pancreatic cancers, and presentation is usually delayed in view of late onset of jaundice (28%) which may account for lower resection rates (30%) and reduced overall survival. Understanding the anatomy of the uncinate process and its relationship to the mesenteric vessels

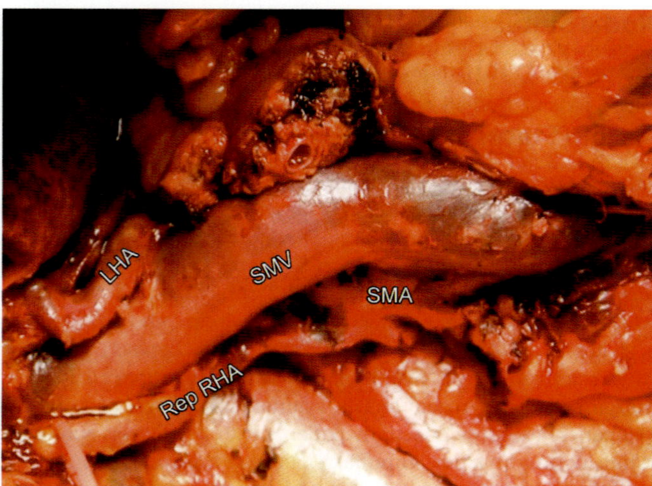

Figure 14 Intraoperative picture showing the replaced right hepatic artery (Rep RHA) from SMA preserved during pancreaticoduodenectomy

is the key. Synchronous venous resection will help in achieving negative resection margins. Artery first dissection should be performed to confirm its resectability.[39]

Pancreaticoduodenectomy in Non-pancreatic Neoplasm

Biliary cancers (cholangiocarcinoma and gallbladder cancer) are the main indications for adding pancreaticoduodenectomy and they usually involve liver resection (hepato-pancreaticoduodenectomy) to gain curative resection. Pancreaticoduodenectomy in non-pancreatic neoplasm is problematic as these patients have normal pancreas with non-dilated duct and usually require additional organ resection, thereby increasing the morbidity and mortality. The reported mortality is as high as 33% with major complications because of pancreatic fistula, hepatic failure and other infectious complications.[100,101] The reported incidence of pancreatic fistula can be as high as 95% in view of the above mentioned reasons and less chance of contained pancreatic leak in view of vast dead space.[102] Recently they found that prognosis is different for these two tumors undergoing pancreaticoduodenectomy. Bile duct cancers, even though they are invasive cancers, they tend to spread submucosally and involve hilum and intrapancreatic bile duct warranting HPD for R0 resection with good survival. Margin positivity with carcinoma in situ may not warrant pancreaticoduodenectomy as the results are same.[103]

The indications for gallbladder cancers requiring pancreaticoduodenectomy are:

- Cancers with direct infiltration which are almost always advanced with lymph node metastasis.
- Large nodes in the retropancreatic region, adherent to the pancreatic head warranting pancreaticoduodenectomy.

However, recent results are not in favor of HPD for gallbladder cancers when combined with major liver resection or with lymph nodal metastasis as long-term survivals are nil.[104] The reported long-term survivals for gallbladder cancer with pancreaticoduodenectomy has been in stage III or below tumors with pancreaticoduodenectomy added for adequate peripancreatic lymph nodal clearance.

Pancreaticoduodenectomy in Chronic Pancreatitis

This will be covered in chronic pancreatitis chapter.

Metastases to the Pancreas

Metastatic tumors of the pancreas are rare (<5%—living patients and up to 15% in autopsy of patients with malignancy).[105,106] A recent systematic review of 18 studies with 399 patients (minimum 10 patients) on curative pancreatectomy for metastatic disease has shown pancreatic metastasectomy confers a survival benefit in selected patients.[107] RCC is the most common primary (62.6%) followed by sarcoma (7.2%), ovarian carcinoma (4.7%) and melanoma (4%). Synchronous lesions are 10.1% and 14% have extra-pancreatic lesions. With median follow-up of 33 months, overall 5-year survival was 50.02%. However, survival outcome is better for RCC than for non-RCC related metastases (median survival 71.7 months vs 24.7 months, respectively). Patients with extra-pancreatic metastases have poor median survival of 26 months. Hence in selected patients pancreatectomy is justified, especially in metastatic RCC.

TRANSDUODENAL EXCISION OF PAPILLA OF VATER

Transduodenal excision (TDE) was first introduced by Sir William Halstead in 1899. However, currently its role is valid in a few and specific situations, in view of the advancement of endoscopic papillectomy and the superior results after pancreaticoduodenectomy. They are:[108]

- Large (≥2 cm) villous or tubulovillous adenomas of the papilla
- Adenomas of the papilla with high-grade dysplasia.

Its role in pT1/T2 is not justified in view of the high incidence of LN metastases in early tumor and the superior R0 resection rate along with better 5-year survival rates after pancreaticoduodenectomy for ampullary lesions. In patients unfit for pancreaticoduodenectomy, it may have a palliative role. The major advantages of TDE over endoscopic papillectomy are that specimen is obtained intact for pathological examination and with the advantage of conversion to pancreaticoduodenectomy in inadequate resection.

Technique

Abdomen is opened via a midline incision, in case a conversion to a more radical procedure is required. Adequate Kocherization is performed so that a long 6–8 cm duodenotomy is performed longitudinally in a lazy-S fashion along the antimesenteric border of 2nd part of the duodenum. Circumferential stay sutures are placed about 1 cm beyond the gross border of the lesion and it is resected allowing a full thickness excision including the biliopancreatic ductal junction. Once adequate resection is confirmed, pancreatic and bile ducts are reimplanted into the duodenum by creating a new common wall and further marsupialization with the duodenal mucosa after confirming the patency of the two openings. Drains are placed after closing the duodenum (Figs 15A and B).

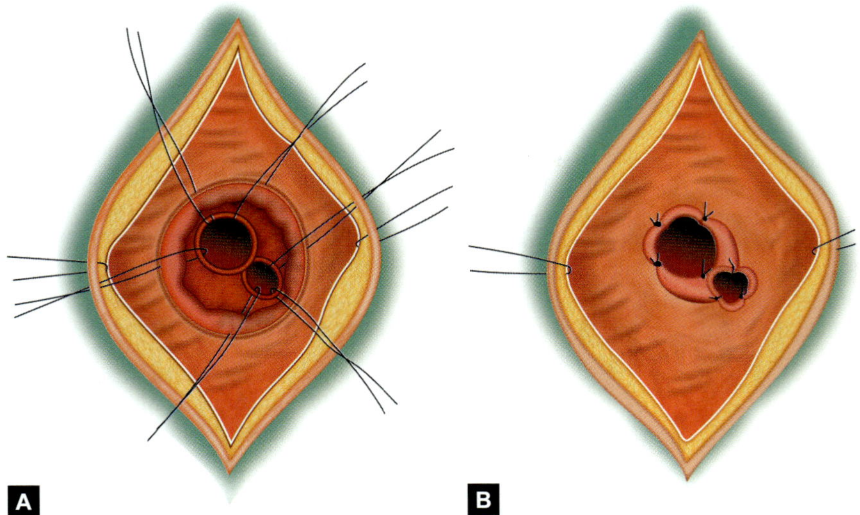

Figures 15A and B Schematic diagram of the intraoperative picture of TDE

Distal Pancreatic Neoplasm

INTRODUCTION

Lesion in these regions are both benign/low malignant like mucinous cystic neoplasm, NET, solid pseudopapillary lesions along with pseudocyst and malignant like ductal adenocarcinoma. Adenocarcinomas in these regions present in advanced stages as these are well away from digestive and biliary system to cause early symptoms. Hence their prognosis is poor though their biological behavior is same as the head of pancreas lesions.[109]

Usually distal pancreatic lesions were managed by distal pancreatectomy with splenectomy, because of the technical ease and shorter duration of operation. With better understanding of the tumor biology and oncological benefit of splenic preservation, various modifications have been introduced to reduce the amount of pancreatic resection and preserve spleen.

DISTAL PANCREATECTOMY

Billroth first described this procedure in 1884. Though distal pancreatectomy with splenectomy is the most common procedure performed in this region, various modifications were introduced to reduce the surgical trauma and preserve spleen when possible. Now distal pancreatectomy is commonly performed laparoscopically. The primary differences between the two procedures are the method of access (length and number of abdominal incisions), the method of exposure, and the extent of operative trauma.

STANDARD PROCEDURE: OPEN DISTAL PANCREATECTOMY WITH EN BLOC SPLENECTOMY

Staging laparoscopy has an important role in managing body/tail neoplasm as they have 44% yield of distant metastasis. A bilateral subcostal, straight transverse incision or midline incision can be used. Lesser sac is opened via the gastrocolic ligament and the greater curvature is fully mobilized till the short gastric vessels freeing the stomach from the upper pole of the spleen. The mobilized stomach is retracted superiorly after dividing the pancreaticogastric attachments. The body of the pancreas is mobilized superiorly and inferiorly at the probable level of transection, usually at the level of neck of pancreas (anterior to the portomesenteric axis). Dissection on the superior border of the pancreas helps in delineating the splenic artery from the celiac axis, lymphadenectomy and also in looping the neck of pancreas. The body of the pancreas is lifted from the retroperitoneum by working on the avascular plane till the splenic hilum. Splenic artery is ligated close to the origin. The spleen is completely mobilized from its diaphragmatic, colonic and renal attachments. Pancreatic transection is done after applying stay sutures exposing the splenic vein behind. Splenic vein is suture ligated and the distal pancreas is removed en bloc with the spleen. The remnant pancreatic stump is oversewn with 4 0 PDS, interrupted sutures after carefully closing the main pancreatic duct with finer prolene sutures. Drains are always placed after securing hemostasis. Arterial stumps are oversewn with 5 0 prolene sutures.

MODIFICATIONS OF DISTAL PANCREATECTOMY

Distal Pancreatectomy with Spleen Preservation

In view of the fear of overwhelming post-splenectomy infection (OPSI) and the oncological risk that splenectomy has in the development of lung and ovarian cancers, splenectomy is avoided in patients where distal pancreatectomy is indicated for benign or low malignant potential conditions.[110] This can be achieved with or without vessel preservation.

Warshaw, in 1988, performed open distal pancreatectomy with vessel ligation and transection.[111] The spleen survives on the short gastric vessels. This can be achieved by early transection of the splenic artery close to its origin, mobilization of the pancreas from the retroperitoneum, transection of the splenic hilum excluding the short gastric and left gastroepiploic vessels. These procedures are found to have less operating time and blood loss than vessel preserving technique. However, approximately 10% have splenic infarction with 3% undergoing splenectomy.[112]

Splenic vessel preservation (SVP) was initially practised by pediatric surgeons for nesidioblastosis. The small pancreatic vessel needs fine dissection and ligation and is better done laparoscopically. A recent systematic review of 23 studies comparing SVP with Warshaw technique (WT), revealed that the mean operating time (160 vs 215 min, $p<0.001$), mean estimated blood loss (301 vs 390 mL, $p<0.001$) and length of stay (8 vs 11 days, $p<0.001$) was significantly less in WT than SVP patients. Comparing complications, splenic infarction and splenectomy occurred more frequently in WT patients ($p<0.05$). Three risk factors for failure of WT include the size of the spleen, acute inflammation and variation in splenic vessel anatomy, such as paucity of short gastric vessels.[112]

Radical en bloc Distal Pancreatectomy

Radical Antegrade Modular Pancreaticosplenectomy (RAMPS)/Multivisceral Resection

Strasberg introduced this variant of radical distal pancreatectomy for invasive malignant tumors of the distal pancreas.[113] It aims at achieving negative margin and adequate regional lymphadenectomy as it may improve the survival. Here the dissection proceeds from right-to-left and the main difference from the conventional distal pancreatectomy is the posterior margin and targeted lymphadenectomy. There are two posterior plane of dissection described according to the involvement of left adrenal gland. However, the initial dissection is the same, transection of the pancreas at the neck and dissecting in sagittal plane down to reach the aorta exposing the left side of SMA and celiac artery along with lymphadenectomy. The anterior plane of posterior dissection (anterior RAMPS) follows on the LRV and on the surface of the left adrenal and kidney. However, when adrenal involvement is present, the posterior sagittal plane (posterior RAMPS) ends at the diaphragm and left renal artery forms the posterior plane of dissection with LRV, inferiorly. In a recent long-term analysis of 47 patients with RAMPS procedure (89% negative tangential margin with no perioperative mortality) showed 35.5% 5-year actuarial survival for adenocarcinoma pancreas.[114] However, in two retrospective studies which compared standard distal pancreatectomy versus RAMPS, there was no overall survival difference. One of the studies showed less tangential margin positivity for RAMPS.[8,115]

Modified Appleby's Procedure

Appleby initially described this technique for gastric cancers with celiac artery involvement for radical resection. It was modified (no gastrectomy) for malignant pancreatic body tumor with celiac axis involvement.[116] Technically celiac axis and the distal pancreas along with spleen are resected preserving the hepatic supply via SMA/GDA. This technique is feasible in rare patients where the malignant body tumors have:[117]

- Involved celiac axis/hepatic artery with no aortic involvement
- No distant metastasis
- Adequate hepatic perfusion through GDA
- No para-aortic lymphadenopathy along the transverse mesocolon
- R0 resection is possible.

These procedures have been attempted with multivisceral resection and portomesentric venous resection and reconstruction. However, this involves risking perfusion to the liver and higher complications. The reported complications are as high as 92%, along with hepatic ischemia and ischemic gastropathy which increases the mortality rate.[118]

Laparoscopic Distal Pancreatectomy

Laparoscopic resection results in improved operative and postoperative outcomes compared with open surgery according to the results of the present meta-analysis.[119] It may be a safe and feasible option for patients with lesions in the body and tail of the pancreas. Laparoscopic pancreatic resection is discussed in detail elsewhere.

COMPLICATIONS OF DISTAL PANCREATECTOMY

The operative mortality rate for distal pancreatectomy has been reduced to less than 1%. However, the morbidity still ranges from 30% to 50%.[79]

Pancreatic Fistula

The most frequent and worrying complication occurring after distal pancreatectomy is the formation of POPF leading to secondary complications in the form of intra-abdominal abscess, sepsis and rarely lethal hemorrhage. Its incidence ranges from 15–30%, slightly higher than pancreaticoduodenectomy. However, in contrast to pancreaticoduodenectomy, these fistulae are typically pure pancreatic juice rather than mixed digestive enzymes and have less frequent bacterial contamination (31%).[59] However, resolution takes longer, with less than half of pancreatic fistulas resolving during the first postoperative month. The risk factors for POPF are found to be soft pancreas and emergency distal pancreatectomy. POPF is regarded to have negative impact on patient's survival and is an independent risk factor for peritoneal recurrence. Various preventive measures are taken to reduce this complication. Although no technique is ideal, current evidence is as follows:[120]

- Stapler transection is not superior to handsewn anastomosis in reducing the POPF (DISPACT trial, 2011, 28% vs 32%, NS).[121] Stapling device with a mesh (SEAMGUARD) was found to reduce the POPF significantly in a RCT.[122]
- Various tissue coagulation techniques have been tried like harmonic scalpel, Tissue Link (radiofrequency device), CUSA, soft coagulation device (VIO) and LIGASURE. These show a trend toward reduced incidence of POPF. Here the concept is ligation of the main pancreatic duct followed by sealing by coagulation of the branch ducts with the stump left open without performing suture.[120]
- Seromuscular patches or anastomosis—Though found to have some role, it has not proven its efficacy for reducing Grade B/C POPF.[123]

- Fibrin sealants have been found to reduce the POPF but there is lack of high level evidence.[124]
- Pancreatic stenting—Prophylactic stenting has been of benefit in many recent studies though of small sample size.[125-128]
- Prophylactic somatostatin analogs do not reduce the clinically significant POPF.[129]

Endocrine and Exocrine Insufficiency

The incidence of diabetes after left pancreatectomy is very low when the resected volume of the gland amounts to no more than 70%. However, information from pancreas transplantation suggests that 25% of living pancreas donors who underwent left pancreatectomy had glucose intolerance after 1 year.[130] More recently the same group, despite using stringent criteria to select donors, reported that 43% of living organ donation between 1997 and 2003 were found to have abnormal fasting glucose levels, impaired glucose tolerance or diabetes at follow-up examination.

CENTRAL/MEDIAN PANCREATECTOMY OR REGIONAL PANCREATECTOMY

Central pancreatectomy otherwise called as "the *Dagradi-Serio-Iacono* procedure" is a parenchyma preserving surgery for the pancreatic neck and proximal body lesions.[131] In the past, though utilized as an alternative to distal pancreatectomy, its role has been clearly identified in benign and low malignant lesions with preservation of the pancreatic parenchyma and spleen. It is also useful in few malignant conditions like metastatic renal cell carcinoma and metastatic NET, where it serves for palliation.

Procedure

The initial steps are similar to distal pancreatectomy; however, it requires preservation of the spleen with reconstruction of the distal pancreatic stump. In a recent systematic review, 94% of central pancreatectomy patients have their proximal stump closed. For distal stump, pancreaticojejunostomy is the widely accepted mode of reconstruction (57.7%) compared to pancreaticogastrostomy (38.4%).[132] When they compared with distal pancreatectomy, central pancreatectomy is associated with long duration of surgery and hospital stay. In situations where distal pancreatectomy represents an alternative, central pancreatectomy is associated with a slightly higher risk of early complications like pancreatic fistula (40.9%), though most are clinically less significant, grade A/B fistula. However, they are not associated with other complications of distal pancreatectomy like DGE, bleeding, pancreatitis. They found that central pancreatectomy is a safe procedure with good long-term functional reserve. The difference between the two procedures on the cumulative incidence of diabetes (new-onset and worsening) is 4–5% after central pancreatectomy and 35–38% after distal pancreatectomy. Similarly exocrine insufficiency is slightly higher in distal pancreatectomy (19.1%) than central pancreatectomy (11.9%). The most important worry about this procedure is the recurrence which has been reported in 3.3% of the 559 central pancreatectomy patients. Most of them are in IPMN, hence intraoperative frozen section and probably pancreaticogastrostomy might help in direct endoscopic follow-up (Figs 16A to F).[131,133]

TOTAL PANCREATECTOMY

Total pancreatectomy, though tried earlier as a radical operation with no risk of pancreatic anastomosis, has shown poorer survival compared with its contemporary (7.9 vs 17.2 months).[134] Even worse, is the exocrine (persistent diarrhea, steatorrhea) and endocrine insufficiency (brittle diabetes, recurrent hypoglycemia in view of loss of glucagon). However, recent studies have proven its definite role with good survival in specific situations. With the advancement in imaging and better perioperative care, the indications for total pancreatectomy are:

- Main branch extensive IPMN especially with positive intraoperative frozen section. Margin positivity with carcinoma in situ or invasive lesion requires further resection.
- Pancreatic head tumors, in which the pancreatic anastomosis proves to be unsafe.
- Pancreatic head tumors, in which complete (R0) excision might be compromised. (Median survival—18 vs 10 months for conversion to total pancreatectomy and incomplete R1 resection, respectively).[135]
- Prophylactic total pancreatectomy because of the fear/risk of cancer in inherited cancer syndromes.

Technically, total pancreatectomy is essentially a combination of the above mentioned resection of the pancreatic head and a distal pancreatectomy. It is preferable, not to divide the neck of the pancreas but to remove the whole pancreas in toto. Usually distal pancreatomy steps are performed first, once the venous confluence of the portal vein has been dissected out and the remaining operation follows the steps of the pancreatic head resection. Duodenojejunostomy (pylorus preserving) is preferable in total pancreatectomy.

Recent series showed total pancreatectomy can be done safely and the postoperative mortality and morbidity range varies from 3% to 8.3% and from 24% to 55%, respectively.[134,136] Primary elective total pancreatectomy has been performed more frequently than completion total pancreatectomy.[137] IPMN and pancreatic metastases from renal cell carcinoma are the most common indications. The results are better along with good quality of life in total pancreatectomy done for non-ductal adenocarcinomas.[137]

ENUCLEATION

Enucleation, a parenchyma preserving procedure was first described by Ernesto Tricomi. Though superior in terms of preserving exocrine and endocrine functions, it still results in higher incidence of pancreatic fistula (27–50%) and oncologically inferior results.[138,139] Tumor pathology and the location of the lesion in the pancreas (depth) has been proven to be the risk factors for the inferior results.[139] With the advancement in imaging, incidental early lesions are diagnosed and their relationships with pancreatic duct are well delineated, thereby helping in proper selection of patients suitable for enucleation. Now, enucleation is an accepted procedure for lesions of less than 4 cm (2–3 mm away from the pancreatic duct) with benign or low malignant potential.[140,141] Endocrine tumors are the most common indication in most series. Among them most common ones are insulinomas and non-functioning tumors of less than 4 cm.[142] Gastrinomas, VIPomas and tumors with high malignant potential are avoided.[139] Serous or mucinous cystadenoma and benign lesion have favorable results.

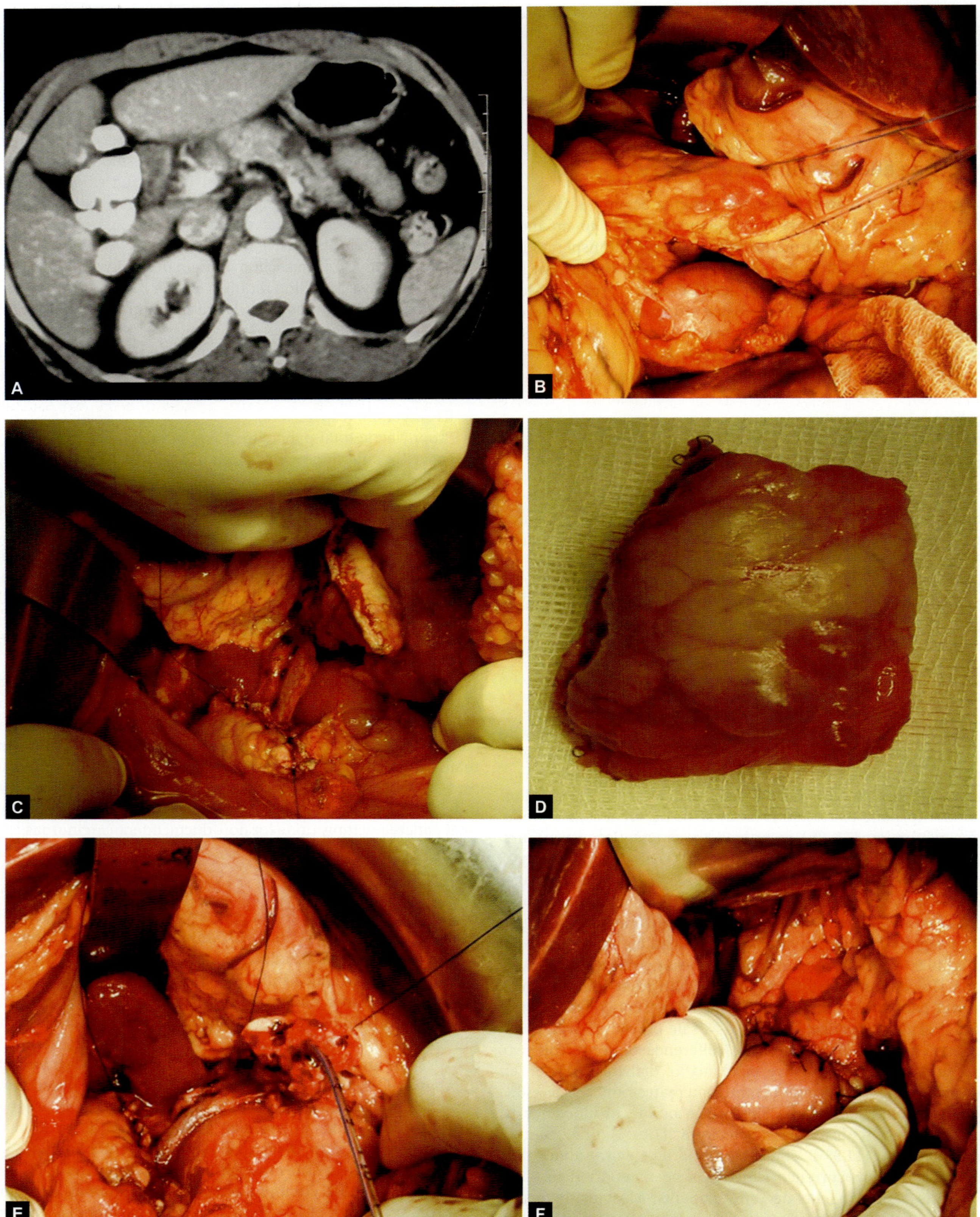

Figures 16A to F Median pancreatectomy: (A) CECT showing a suspected IPMN, (B) central pancreas mobilized, (C) proximal resection with stapler and oversewn with prolene sutures, (D) resected pancreas, (E) infant feeding tube in distal pancreas; splenic artery and vein seen, (F) distal pancreas joined to Roux loop with pancreatojejunostomy

Though branch duct IPMN has been enucleated accidentally, long-term results are still awaited. If final pathology suggests malignancy, reoperation for radical treatment is needed. Metastases should be ruled out with conventional/functional imaging. Intraoperative ultrasonography (IOUS) helps in confirming 2–3 mm margin free from the pancreatic lesion.[143] However, even with IOUS, the clinical pancreatic fistula rates are still around 23%, though most of them are managed conservatively.[139]

MIDDLE PRESERVING PANCREATECTOMY

Middle preserving pancreatectomy (MPP), though a new technique, is found to be a reasonable alternative to total pancreatectomy in multicenteric noninvasive lesions of the pancreas (head and tail lesion).[144-149] It can be done in single or two stage procedure. As almost 25% of the pancreatic tissue is preserved, exocrine and endocrine insufficiency is much better than total pancreatectomy.[150] This is also an option in metachronous metastatic lesion to the pancreas and invasive lesion.

REFERENCES

1. Parkin DM, Bray F, Ferlay J, Pisani P. Global cancer statistics, 2002. CA: A Cancer Journal for Clinicians. 2005;55(2):74-108.
2. Niederhuber JE, Brennan MF, Menck HR. The National Cancer Data Base report on pancreatic cancer. Cancer. 1995;76(9):1671-7.
3. Balcom JHt, Rattner DW, Warshaw AL, Chang Y, Fernandez-del Castillo C. Ten-year experience with 733 pancreatic resections: changing indications, older patients, and decreasing length of hospitalization. Archives of Surgery (Chicago, Ill: 1960). 2001;136(4):391-8.
4. Fong Y, Gonen M, Rubin D, Radzyner M, Brennan MF. Long-term survival is superior after resection for cancer in high-volume centers. Annals of Surgery. 2005;242(4):540-4.
5. Cameron JL, Riall TS, Coleman J, Belcher KA. One thousand consecutive pancreaticoduodenectomies. Annals of Surgery. 2006;244(1):10-5.
6. Kneuertz PJ, Pitt HA, Bilimoria KY, Smiley JP, Cohen ME, Ko CY, et al. Risk of morbidity and mortality following hepato-pancreato-biliary surgery. Journal of Gastrointestinal Surgery: Official Journal of the Society for Surgery of the Alimentary Tract. 2012;16(9): 1727-35.
7. Dalton RR, Sarr MG, van Heerden JA, Colby TV. Carcinoma of the body and tail of the pancreas: is curative resection justified? Surgery. 1992;111(5):489-94.
8. Mitchem JB, Hamilton N, Gao F, Hawkins WG, Linehan DC, Strasberg SM. Long-term results of resection of adenocarcinoma of the body and tail of the pancreas using radical antegrade modular pancreatosplenectomy procedure. Journal of the American College of Surgeons. 2012;214(1):46-52.
9. Nagakawa T, Kayahara M, Ikeda S, Futakawa S, Kakita A, Kawarada H, et al. Biliary tract cancer treatment: results from the Biliary Tract Cancer Statistics Registry in Japan. Journal of Hepato-Biliary-Pancreatic Surgery. 2002;9(5):569-75.
10. Sarela AI, Brennan MF, Karpeh MS, Klimstra D, Conlon KC. Adenocarcinoma of the duodenum: importance of accurate lymph node staging and similarity in outcome to gastric cancer. Annals of Surgical Oncology. 2004;11(4):380-6.
11. Whipple AO, Parsons WB, Mullins CR. Treatment of carcinoma of the ampulla of vater. Annals of Surgery. 1935;102(4):763-79.
12. Grenacher L, Klauss M. Computed tomography of pancreatic tumors. Der Radiologe. 2009;49(2):107-23.
13. Barabino M, Santambrogio R, Pisani Ceretti A, Scalzone R, Montorsi M, Opocher E. Is there still a role for laparoscopy combined with laparoscopic ultrasonography in the staging of pancreatic cancer? Surgical Endoscopy. 2011;25(1):160-5.
14. Oliveira-Cunha M, Malde DJ, Aldouri A, Morris-Stiff G, Menon KV, Smith AM. Results of pancreatic surgery in the elderly: is age a barrier? HPB: the Official Journal of the International Hepato Pancreato Biliary Association. 2013;15(1):24-30.
15. Braga M, Ljungqvist O, Soeters P, Fearon K, Weimann A, Bozzetti F. ESPEN Guidelines on parenteral nutrition: surgery. Clinical Nutrition (Edinburgh, Scotland). 2009;28(4):378-86.
16. Isayama H, Nakai Y, Kawakubo K, Kogure H, Togawa O, Hamada T, et al. Covered metallic stenting for malignant distal biliary obstruction: clinical results according to stent type. Journal of Hepato-Biliary-Pancreatic Sciences. 2011;18(5):673-7.
17. Mumtaz K, Hamid S, Jafri W. Endoscopic retrograde cholangiopancreaticography with or without stenting in patients with pancreaticobiliary malignancy, prior to surgery. The Cochrane Database of Systematic Reviews. 2007(3):Cd006001.
18. van der Gaag NA, van Gulik TM, Gouma DJ. Role of Preoperative biliary drainage in jaundiced patients who are candidates for pancreatoduodenectomy or hepatic resection. Ann Surg. 2014;259(4):e74-5.
19. Chang L, Stefanidis D, Richardson WS, Earle DB, Fanelli RD. The role of staging laparoscopy for intraabdominal cancers: an evidence-based review. Surgical Endoscopy. 2009;23(2):231-41.
20. Pietrabissa A, Caramella D, Di Candio G, Carobbi A, Boggi U, Rossi G, et al. Laparoscopy and laparoscopic ultrasonography for staging pancreatic cancer: critical appraisal. World Journal of Surgery. 1999;23(10):998-1002.
21. Hariharan D, Constantinides VA, Froeling FE, Tekkis PP, Kocher HM. The role of laparoscopy and laparoscopic ultrasound in the preoperative staging of pancreatico-biliary cancers—a meta-analysis. European Journal of Surgical Oncology: the Journal of the European Society of Surgical Oncology and the British Association of Surgical Oncology. 2010;36(10):941-8.
22. Masui T, Kubota T, Aoki K, Nakanishi Y, Miyamoto T, Nagata J, et al. Long-term survival after resection of pancreatic ductal adenocarcinoma with para-aortic lymph node metastasis: case report. World Journal of Surgical Oncology. 2013;11(1):195.
23. Ohigashi H, Ishikawa O, Eguchi H, Yamada T, Sasaki Y, Noura S, et al. Early ligation of the inferior pancreaticoduodenal artery to reduce blood loss during pancreaticoduodenectomy. Hepatogastroenterology. 2004;51(55):4-5.
24. Katz MH, Pisters PW, Evans DB, Sun CC, Lee JE, Fleming JB, et al. Borderline resectable pancreatic cancer: the importance of this emerging stage of disease. Journal of the American College of Surgeons. 2008;206(5):833-46.
25. Callery MP, Chang KJ, Fishman EK, Talamonti MS, William Traverso L, Linehan DC. Pretreatment assessment of resectable and borderline resectable pancreatic cancer: expert consensus statement. Annals of Surgical Oncology. 2009;16(7):1727-33.
26. Muller SA, Tarantino I, Martin DJ, Schmied BM. Pancreatic surgery: beyond the traditional limits. Recent results in cancer research Fortschritte der Krebsforschung Progres dans les Recherches sur le Cancer. 2012;196:53-64.
27. Nakao A, Takagi H. Isolated pancreatectomy for pancreatic head carcinoma using catheter bypass of the portal vein. Hepatogastroenterology. 1993;40(5):426-9.
28. Sanjay P, Takaori K, Govil S, Shrikhande SV, Windsor JA. 'Artery-first' approaches to pancreatoduodenectomy. The British Journal of Surgery. 2012;99(8):1027-35.
29. Traverso LW, Longmire WP Jr. Preservation of the pylorus in pancreaticoduodenectomy. Surgery, Gynecology & Obstetrics. 1978;146(6):959-62.

30. Iqbal N, Lovegrove RE, Tilney HS, Abraham AT, Bhattacharya S, Tekkis PP, et al. A comparison of pancreaticoduodenectomy with pylorus preserving pancreaticoduodenectomy: a meta-analysis of 2822 patients. European Journal of Surgical Oncology: the Journal of the European Society of Surgical Oncology and the British Association of Surgical Oncology. 2008;34(11):1237-45.
31. Diener MK, Rahbari NN, Fischer L, Antes G, Buchler MW, Seiler CM. Duodenum-preserving pancreatic head resection versus pancreatoduodenectomy for surgical treatment of chronic pancreatitis: a systematic review and meta-analysis. Annals of Surgery. 2008;247(6):950-61.
32. Fujii T, Kanda M, Kodera Y, Nagai S, Sahin TT, Hayashi M, et al. Preservation of the pyloric ring has little value in surgery for pancreatic head cancer: a comparative study comparing three surgical procedures. Annals of Surgical Oncology. 2012;19(1):176-83.
33. Fortner JG. Regional resection and pancreatic carcinoma. Surgery. 1973;73(5):799-800.
34. Marangoni G, O'Sullivan A, Faraj W, Heaton N, Rela M. Pancreatectomy with synchronous vascular resection—an argument in favour. The Surgeon: Journal of the Royal Colleges of Surgeons of Edinburgh and Ireland. 2012;10(2):102-6.
35. Andersson R, Vagianos CE, Williamson RC. Preoperative staging and evaluation of resectability in pancreatic ductal adenocarcinoma. HPB: the Official Journal of the International Hepato Pancreato Biliary Association. 2004;6(1):5-12.
36. Nakao A, Harada A, Nonami T, Kaneko T, Inoue S, Takagi H. Clinical significance of portal invasion by pancreatic head carcinoma. Surgery. 1995;117(1):50-5.
37. Ishikawa O, Ohigashi H, Imaoka S, Furukawa H, Sasaki Y, Fujita M, et al. Preoperative indications for extended pancreatectomy for locally advanced pancreas cancer involving the portal vein. Annals of Surgery. 1992;215(3):231-6.
38. Fukuda S, Oussoultzoglou E, Bachellier P, Rosso E, Nakano H, Audet M, et al. Significance of the depth of portal vein wall invasion after curative resection for pancreatic adenocarcinoma. Archives of Surgery (Chicago, Ill: 1960). 2007;142(2):172-9.
39. O'Sullivan AW, Heaton N, Rela M. Cancer of the uncinate process of the pancreas: surgical anatomy and clinicopathological features. Hepatobiliary & Pancreatic Diseases International: HBPD INT. 2009;8(6):569-74.
40. Siriwardana HP, Siriwardena AK. Systematic review of outcome of synchronous portal-superior mesenteric vein resection during pancreatectomy for cancer. The British Journal of Surgery. 2006;93(6):662-73.
41. Mollberg N, Rahbari NN, Koch M, Hartwig W, Hoeger Y, Buchler MW, et al. Arterial resection during pancreatectomy for pancreatic cancer: a systematic review and meta-analysis. Annals of Surgery. 2011;254(6):882-93.
42. Govil S. Is superior mesenteric artery reimplantation during surgery for pancreaticoduodenal tumors an underutilized procedure? Indian Journal of Gastroenterology: Official Journal of the Indian Society of Gastroenterology. 2013.
43. Hartwig W, Hackert T, Hinz U, Hassenpflug M, Strobel O, Buchler MW, et al. Multivisceral resection for pancreatic malignancies: risk-analysis and long-term outcome. Annals of Surgery. 2009;250(1):81-7.
44. Slidell MB, Chang DC, Cameron JL, Wolfgang C, Herman JM, Schulick RD, et al. Impact of total lymph node count and lymph node ratio on staging and survival after pancreatectomy for pancreatic adenocarcinoma: a large, population-based analysis. Annals of Surgical Oncology. 2008;15(1):165-74.
45. Ishikawa O, Ohhigashi H, Sasaki Y, Kabuto T, Fukuda I, Furukawa H, et al. Practical usefulness of lymphatic and connective tissue clearance for the carcinoma of the pancreas head. Annals of Surgery. 1988;208(2):215-20.
46. Svoronos C, Tsoulfas G, Katsourakis A, Noussios G, Chatzitheoklitos E, Marakis NG. Role of extended lymphadenectomy in the treatment of pancreatic head adenocarcinoma: review and meta-analysis. ANZ Journal of Surgery. 2013.
47. Yeo CJ, Cameron JL, Sohn TA, Lillemoe KD, Pitt HA, Talamini MA, et al. Six hundred fifty consecutive pancreaticoduodenectomies in the 1990s: pathology, complications, and outcomes. Annals of Surgery. 1997;226(3):248-57.
48. Coffey RC. XVII. Pancreato-enterostomy and pancreatectomy: a preliminary report. Annals of Surgery. 1909;50(6):1238-64.
49. Child CG. Carcinoma of the duodenum. Annals of Surgery. 1943;118(5):838-42.
50. Whipple AO. Observations on radical surgery for lesions of the pancreas. Surgery, Gynecology & Obstetrics. 1946;82:623-31.
51. Kakita A, Yoshida M, Takahashi T. History of pancreaticojejunostomy in pancreaticoduodenectomy: development of a more reliable anastomosis technique. Journal of Hepato-Biliary-Pancreatic Surgery. 2001;8(3):230-7.
52. Mishra PK, Saluja SS, Gupta M, Rajalingam R, Pattnaik P. Blumgart's technique of pancreaticojejunostomy: an appraisal. Digestive Surgery. 2011;28(4):281-7.
53. Correa-Gallego C, Brennan MF, D'Angelica M, Fong Y, Dematteo RP, Kingham TP, et al. Operative drainage following pancreatic resection: analysis of 1122 patients resected over 5 years at a single institution. Annals of Surgery. 2013;258(6):1051-8.
54. Mehta VV, Fisher SB, Maithel SK, Sarmiento JM, Staley CA, Kooby DA. Is it time to abandon routine operative drain use? A single institution assessment of 709 consecutive pancreaticoduodenectomies. Journal of the American College of Surgeons. 2013;216(4):635-42.
55. Kawai M, Tani M, Terasawa H, Ina S, Hirono S, Nishioka R, et al. Early removal of prophylactic drains reduces the risk of intra-abdominal infections in patients with pancreatic head resection: prospective study for 104 consecutive patients. Annals of Surgery. 2006;244(1):1-7.
56. Bassi C, Molinari E, Malleo G, Crippa S, Butturini G, Salvia R, et al. Early versus late drain removal after standard pancreatic resections: results of a prospective randomized trial. Annals of Surgery. 2010;252(2):207-14.
57. Buren GV, Bloomston M, Hughes SJ, Winter J,Behrman SW, Zyromski NJ, et al. A Randomized Prospective Multicenter Trial of Pancreaticoduodenectomy with and without routine Intraperitoneal Drainage. Annals of Surg. 2014;259:605-12.
58. Bassi C, Dervenis C, Butturini G, Fingerhut A, Yeo C, Izbicki J, et al. Postoperative pancreatic fistula: an international study group (ISGPF) definition. Surgery. 2005;138(1):8-13.
59. Vin Y, Sima CS, Getrajdman GI, Brown KT, Covey A, Brennan MF, et al. Management and outcomes of postpancreatectomy fistula, leak, and abscess: results of 908 patients resected at a single institution between 2000 and 2005. Journal of the American College of Surgeons. 2008;207(4):490-8.
60. Bartoli FG, Arnone GB, Ravera G, Bachi V. Pancreatic fistula and relative mortality in malignant disease after pancreaticoduodenectomy. Review and statistical meta-analysis regarding 15 years of literature. Anticancer Research. 1991;11(5):1831-48.
61. Klek S, Sierzega M, Turczynowski L, Szybinski P, Szczepanek K, Kulig J. Enteral and parenteral nutrition in the conservative treatment of pancreatic fistula: a randomized clinical trial. Gastroenterology. 2011;141(1):157-63, 63.e1.
62. Li-Ling J, Irving M. Somatostatin and octreotide in the prevention of postoperative pancreatic complications and the treatment of enterocutaneous pancreatic fistulas: a systematic review of randomized controlled trials. The British Journal of Surgery. 2001;88(2):190-9.

63. Munoz-Bongrand N, Sauvanet A, Denys A, Sibert A, Vilgrain V, Belghiti J. Conservative management of pancreatic fistula after pancreaticoduodenectomy with pancreaticogastrostomy. Journal of the American College of Surgeons. 2004;199(2):198-203.
64. Govil S. Salvage pancreaticogastrostomy for pancreatic fistulae after pancreaticoduodenectomy. Indian Journal of Gastroenterology: Official Journal of the Indian Society of Gastroenterology. 2012;31(5):263-6.
65. Gueroult S, Parc Y, Duron F, Paye F, Parc R. Completion pancreatectomy for postoperative peritonitis after pancreaticoduodenectomy: early and late outcome. Archives of Surgery (Chicago, Ill: 1960). 2004;139(1):16-9.
66. Trede M, Richter A, Wendl K. Personal observations, opinions, and approaches to cancer of the pancreas and the periampullary area. The Surgical Clinics of North America. 2001;81(3):595-610.
67. Hashimoto D, Chikamoto A, Ohmuraya M, Hirota M, Baba H. Pancreaticodigestive anastomosis and the postoperative management strategies to prevent postoperative pancreatic fistula formation after pancreaticoduodenectomy. Surg Today. 2014;44(7):1207-13.
68. Motoi F, Egawa S, Rikiyama T, Katayose Y, Unno M. Randomized clinical trial of external stent drainage of the pancreatic duct to reduce postoperative pancreatic fistula after pancreaticojejunostomy. The British Journal of Surgery. 2012;99(4):524-31.
69. Winter JM, Cameron JL, Campbell KA, Chang DC, Riall TS, Schulick RD, et al. Does pancreatic duct stenting decrease the rate of pancreatic fistula following pancreaticoduodenectomy? Results of a prospective randomized trial. Journal of Gastrointestinal Surgery: Official Journal of the Society for Surgery of the Alimentary Tract. 2006;10(9):1280-90.
70. Pessaux P, Sauvanet A, Mariette C, Paye F, Muscari F, Cunha AS, et al. External pancreatic duct stent decreases pancreatic fistula rate after pancreaticoduodenectomy: prospective multicenter randomized trial. Annals of surgery. 2011;253(5):879-85.
71. He T, Zhao Y, Chen Q, Wang X, Lin H, Han W. Pancreaticojejunostomy versus pancreaticogastrostomy after pancreaticoduodenectomy: a systematic review and meta-analysis. Digestive Surgery. 2013;30(1):56-69.
72. Machado MC, da Cunha JE, Bacchella T, Bove P. A modified technique for the reconstruction of the alimentary tract after pancreatoduodenectomy. Surgery, Gynecology & Obstetrics. 1976;143(2):271-2.
73. Kingsnorth AN. Duct to mucosa isolated Roux loop pancreaticojejunostomy as an improved anastomosis after resection of the pancreas. Surgery, Gynecology & Obstetrics. 1989;169(5):451-3.
74. Khan AW, Agarwal AK, Davidson BR. Isolated Roux loop duct-to-mucosa pancreaticojejunostomy avoids pancreatic leaks in pancreaticoduodenectomy. Digestive Surgery. 2002;19(3):199-204.
75. Ballas K, Symeonidis N, Rafailidis S, Pavlidis T, Marakis G, Mavroudis N, et al. Use of isolated Roux loop for pancreaticojejunostomy reconstruction after pancreaticoduodenectomy. World Journal of Gastroenterology: WJG. 2010;16(25):3178-82.
76. Kaman L, Sanyal S, Behera A, Singh R, Katariya RN. Isolated Roux loop pancreaticojejunostomy vs single loop pancreaticojejunostomy after pancreaticoduodenectomy. International Journal of Surgery (London, England). 2008;6(4):306-10.
77. Perwaiz A, Singhal D, Singh A, Chaudhary A. Is isolated Roux loop pancreaticojejunostomy superior to conventional reconstruction in pancreaticoduodenectomy? HPB: the official journal of the International Hepato Pancreato Biliary Association. 2009;11(4):326-31.
78. Ke S, Ding XM, Gao J, Zhao AM, Deng GY, Ma RL, et al. A prospective, randomized trial of Roux-en-Y reconstruction with isolated pancreatic drainage versus conventional loop reconstruction after pancreaticoduodenectomy. Surgery. 2013;153(6):743-52.
79. Lermite E, Sommacale D, Piardi T, Arnaud JP, Sauvanet A, Dejong CH, et al. Complications after pancreatic resection: diagnosis, prevention and management. Clinics and Research in Hepatology and Gastroenterology. 2013;37(3):230-9.
80. Tani M, Terasawa H, Kawai M, Ina S, Hirono S, Uchiyama K, et al. Improvement of delayed gastric emptying in pylorus-preserving pancreaticoduodenectomy: results of a prospective, randomized, controlled trial. Annals of Surgery. 2006;243(3):316-20.
81. Ohwada S, Satoh Y, Kawate S, Yamada T, Kawamura O, Koyama T, et al. Low-dose erythromycin reduces delayed gastric emptying and improves gastric motility after Billroth I pylorus-preserving pancreaticoduodenectomy. Annals of Surgery. 2001;234(5):668-74.
82. Wente MN, Veit JA, Bassi C, Dervenis C, Fingerhut A, Gouma DJ, et al. Postpancreatectomy hemorrhage (PPH): an International Study Group of Pancreatic Surgery (ISGPS) Definition. Surgery. 2007;142(1):20-5.
83. de Castro SM, Busch OR, Gouma DJ. Management of bleeding and leakage after pancreatic surgery. Best Practice & Research Clinical Gastroenterology. 2004;18(5):847-64.
84. Balachandran P, Sikora SS, Raghavendra Rao RV, Kumar A, Saxena R, Kapoor VK. Haemorrhagic complications of pancreaticoduodenectomy. ANZ Journal of Surgery. 2004;74(11): 945-50.
85. Otah E, Cushin BJ, Rozenblit GN, Neff R, Otah KE, Cooperman AM. Visceral artery pseudoaneurysms following pancreatoduodenectomy. Archives of Surgery (Chicago, Ill: 1960). 2002;137(1):55-9.
86. Yekebas EF, Wolfram L, Cataldegirmen G, Habermann CR, Bogoevski D, Koenig AM, et al. Postpancreatectomy hemorrhage: diagnosis and treatment: an analysis in 1669 consecutive pancreatic resections. Annals of Surgery. 2007;246(2):269-80.
87. Beyer L, Bonmardion R, Marciano S, Hartung O, Ramis O, Chabert L, et al. Results of non-operative therapy for delayed hemorrhage after pancreaticoduodenectomy. Journal of Gastrointestinal Surgery: Official Journal of the Society for Surgery of the Alimentary Tract. 2009;13(5):922-8.
88. Gaujoux S, Sauvanet A, Vullierme MP, Cortes A, Dokmak S, Sibert A, et al. Ischemic complications after pancreaticoduodenectomy: incidence, prevention, and management. Annals of Surgery. 2009;249(1):111-7.
89. Reid-Lombardo KM, Ramos-De la Medina A, Thomsen K, Harmsen WS, Farnell MB. Long-term anastomotic complications after pancreaticoduodenectomy for benign diseases. Journal of Gastrointestinal Surgery: Official Journal of the Society for Surgery of the Alimentary Tract. 2007;11(12):1704-11.
90. Assumpcao L, Cameron JL, Wolfgang CL, Edil B, Choti MA, Herman JM, et al. Incidence and management of chyle leaks following pancreatic resection: a high volume single-center institutional experience. Journal of Gastrointestinal Surgery: Official Journal of the Society for Surgery of the Alimentary Tract. 2008;12(11): 1915-23.
91. Malik HZ, Crozier J, Murray L, Carter R. Chyle leakage and early enteral feeding following pancreatico-duodenectomy: management options. Digestive Surgery. 2007;24(6):418-22.
92. van der Gaag NA, Verhaar AC, Haverkort EB, Busch OR, van Gulik TM, Gouma DJ. Chylous ascites after pancreaticoduodenectomy: introduction of a grading system. Journal of the American College of Surgeons. 2008;207(5):751-7.
93. Hilal MA, Layfield DM, Di Fabio F, Arregui-Fresneda I, Panagiotopoulou IG, Armstrong TH, et al. Postoperative chyle leak after major pancreatic resections in patients who receive enteral feed: risk factors and management options. World Journal of Surgery. 2013;37(12):2918-26.
94. Raty S, Sand J, Nordback I. Detection of postoperative pancreatitis after pancreatic surgery by urine trypsinogen strip test. The British Journal of Surgery. 2007;94(1):64-9.

95. Gooiker GA, van Gijn W, Wouters MW, Post PN, van de Velde CJ, Tollenaar RA. Systematic review and meta-analysis of the volume-outcome relationship in pancreatic surgery. The British Journal of Surgery. 2011;98(4):485-94.
96. Bilimoria KY, Bentrem DJ, Ko CY, Ritchey J, Stewart AK, Winchester DP, et al. Validation of the 6th edition AJCC Pancreatic Cancer Staging System: report from the National Cancer Database. Cancer. 2007;110(4):738-44.
97. Wang SE, Shyr YM, Su CH, Chen TH, Wu CW. Palliative pancreaticoduodenectomy in pancreatic and periampullary adenocarcinomas. Pancreas. 2012;41(6):882-7.
98. Raut CP, Tseng JF, Sun CC, Wang H, Wolff RA, Crane CH, et al. Impact of resection status on pattern of failure and survival after pancreaticoduodenectomy for pancreatic adenocarcinoma. Annals of Surgery. 2007;246(1):52-60.
99. Lillemoe KD, Cameron JL, Yeo CJ, Sohn TA, Nakeeb A, Sauter PK, et al. Pancreaticoduodenectomy. Does it have a role in the palliation of pancreatic cancer? Annals of Surgery. 1996;223(6):718-25.
100. Nimura Y, Hayakawa N, Kamiya J, Maeda S, Kondo S, Yasui A, et al. Hepatopancreatoduodenectomy for advanced carcinoma of the biliary tract. Hepato-gastroenterology. 1991;38(2):170-5.
101. Miyagawa S, Makuuchi M, Kawasaki S, Hayashi K, Harada H, Kitamura H, et al. Outcome of major hepatectomy with pancreatoduodenectomy for advanced biliary malignancies. World Journal of Surgery. 1996;20(1):77-80.
102. Sakamoto Y, Nara S, Kishi Y, Esaki M, Shimada K, Kokudo N, et al. Is extended hemihepatectomy plus pancreaticoduodenectomy justified for advanced bile duct cancer and gallbladder cancer? Surgery. 2013;153(6):794-800.
103. Igami T, Nagino M, Oda K, Nishio H, Ebata T, Yokoyama Y, et al. Clinicopathologic study of cholangiocarcinoma with superficial spread. Annals of Surgery. 2009;249(2):296-302.
104. Lim CS, Jang JY, Lee SE, Kang MJ, Kim SW. Reappraisal of hepatopancreatoduodenectomy as a treatment modality for bile duct and gallbladder cancer. Journal of Gastrointestinal Surgery: Official Journal of the Society for Surgery of the Alimentary Tract. 2012;16(5):1012-8.
105. Nakamura E, Shimizu M, Itoh T, Manabe T. Secondary tumors of the pancreas: clinicopathological study of 103 autopsy cases of Japanese patients. Pathology International. 2001;51(9):686-90.
106. Adsay NV, Andea A, Basturk O, Kilinc N, Nassar H, Cheng JD. Secondary tumors of the pancreas: an analysis of a surgical and autopsy database and review of the literature. Virchows Archiv: An International Journal of Pathology. 2004;444(6):527-35.
107. Adler H, Redmond CE, Heneghan HM, Swan N, Maguire D, Traynor O, et al. Pancreatectomy for metastatic disease: a systematic review. European Journal of Surgical Oncology: the Journal of the European Society of Surgical Oncology and the British Association of Surgical Oncology. 2014;40(4):379-86.
108. Paramythiotis D, Kleeff J, Wirtz M, Friess H, Buchler MW. Still any role for transduodenal local excision in tumors of the papilla of Vater? Journal of Hepato-Biliary-Pancreatic Surgery. 2004;11(4):239-44.
109. Kleeff J, Diener MK, Z'Graggen K, Hinz U, Wagner M, Bachmann J, et al. Distal pancreatectomy: risk factors for surgical failure in 302 consecutive cases. Annals of Surgery. 2007;245(4):573-82.
110. Linet MS, Nyren O, Gridley G, Mellemkjaer L, McLaughlin JK, Olsen JH, et al. Risk of cancer following splenectomy. International Journal of Cancer Journal International du Cancer. 1996;66(5): 611-6.
111. Warshaw AL. Conservation of the spleen with distal pancreatectomy. Archives of surgery (Chicago, Ill: 1960). 1988;123(5):550-3.
112. Jain G, Chakravartty S, Patel AG. Spleen-preserving distal pancreatectomy with and without splenic vessel ligation: a systematic review. HPB: the official journal of the International Hepato Pancreato Biliary Association. 2013;15(6):403-10.
113. Strasberg SM, Drebin JA, Linehan D. Radical antegrade modular pancreatosplenectomy. Surgery. 2003;133(5):521-7.
114. Strasberg SM, Fields R. Left-sided pancreatic cancer: distal pancreatectomy and its variants: radical antegrade modular pancreatosplenectomy and distal pancreatectomy with celiac axis resection. Cancer Journal (Sudbury, Mass). 2012;18(6):562-70.
115. Chang YR, Han SS, Park SJ, Lee SD, Yoo TS, Kim YK, et al. Surgical outcome of pancreatic cancer using radical antegrade modular pancreatosplenectomy procedure. World Journal of Gastroenterology: WJG. 2012;18(39):5595-600.
116. Liu B. Modified appleby operation in treatment of distal pancreatic cancer. Hepatobiliary & Pancreatic Diseases International: HBPD INT. 2003;2(4):622-5.
117. Bonnet S, Kohneh-Shahri N, Goere D, Deshayes I, Ayadi S, Elias D. Indications and surgical technique of Appleby's operation for tumor invasion of the celiac trunk and its branches. Journal de Chirurgie. 2009;146(1):6-14.
118. Smoot RL, Donohue JH. Modified Appleby procedure for resection of tumors of the pancreatic body and tail with celiac axis involvement. Journal of gastrointestinal surgery: official journal of the Society for Surgery of the Alimentary Tract. 2012;16(11):2167-9.
119. Iacobone M, Citton M, Nitti D. Laparoscopic distal pancreatectomy: up-to-date and literature review. World Journal of Gastroenterology: WJG. 2012;18(38):5329-37.
120. Makino I, Kitagawa H, Nakagawara H, Tajima H, Ninomiya I, Fushida S, et al. Management of remnant pancreatic stump fto prevent the development of postoperative pancreatic fistulas after distal pancreatectomy: current evidence and our strategy. Surgery Today. 2013;43(6):595-602.
121. Diener MK, Seiler CM, Rossion I, Kleeff J, Glanemann M, Butturini G, et al. Efficacy of stapler versus hand-sewn closure after distal pancreatectomy (DISPACT): a randomised, controlled multicentre trial. Lancet. 2011;377(9776):1514-22.
122. Hamilton NA, Porembka MR, Johnston FM, Gao F, Strasberg SM, Linehan DC, et al. Mesh reinforcement of pancreatic transection decreases incidence of pancreatic occlusion failure for left pancreatectomy: a single-blinded, randomized controlled trial. Annals of Surgery. 2012;255(6):1037-42.
123. Olah A, Issekutz A, Belagyi T, Hajdu N, Romics L, Jr. Randomized clinical trial of techniques for closure of the pancreatic remnant following distal pancreatectomy. The British Journal of Surgery. 2009;96(6):602-7.
124. Suzuki Y, Kuroda Y, Morita A, Fujino Y, Tanioka Y, Kawamura T, et al. Fibrin glue sealing for the prevention of pancreatic fistulas following distal pancreatectomy. Archives of Surgery (Chicago, Ill: 1960). 1995;130(9):952-5.
125. Abe N, Sugiyama M, Suzuki Y, Yamaguchi T, Mori T, Atomi Y. Preoperative endoscopic pancreatic stenting: a novel prophylactic measure against pancreatic fistula after distal pancreatectomy. Journal of Hepato-Biliary-Pancreatic Surgery. 2008;15(4):373-6.
126. Fischer CP, Bass B, Fahy B, Aloia T. Transampullary pancreatic duct stenting decreases pancreatic fistula rate following left pancreatectomy. Hepato-gastroenterology. 2008;55(81):244-8.
127. Rieder B, Krampulz D, Adolf J, Pfeiffer A. Endoscopic pancreatic sphincterotomy and stenting for preoperative prophylaxis of pancreatic fistula after distal pancreatectomy. Gastrointestinal Endoscopy. 2010;72(3):536-42.
128. Oida T, Mimatsu K, Kawasaki A, Kanou H, Kuboi Y, Kida K, et al. Transduodenal pancreatic juice drainage for preventing pancreatic fistula formation after distal pancreatectomy. Hepatogastroenterology. 2011;58(105):177-82.
129. Suc B, Msika S, Piccinini M, Fourtanier G, Hay JM, Flamant Y, et al. Octreotide in the prevention of intra-abdominal complications following elective pancreatic resection: a prospective, multicenter randomized controlled trial. Archives of Surgery (Chicago, Ill: 1960). 2004;139(3):288-94.

130. Kendall DM, Sutherland DE, Najarian JS, Goetz FC, Robertson RP. Effects of hemipancreatectomy on insulin secretion and glucose tolerance in healthy humans. The New England Journal of Medicine. 1990;322(13):898-903.
131. Iacono C, Verlato G, Ruzzenente A, Campagnaro T, Bacchelli C, Valdegamberi A, et al. Systematic review of central pancreatectomy and meta-analysis of central versus distal pancreatectomy. The British Journal of Surgery. 2013;100(7):873-85.
132. Knaebel HP, Diener MK, Wente MN, Buchler MW, Seiler CM. Systematic review and meta-analysis of technique for closure of the pancreatic remnant after distal pancreatectomy. The British Journal of Surgery. 2005;92(5):539-46.
133. Xu SB, Zhu YP, Zhou W, Xie K, Mou YP. Patients get more long-term benefit from central pancreatectomy than distal resection: a meta-analysis. European Journal of Surgical Oncology: the Journal of the European Society of Surgical Oncology and the British Association of Surgical Oncology. 2013;39(6):567-74.
134. Karpoff HM, Klimstra DS, Brennan MF, Conlon KC. Results of total pancreatectomy for adenocarcinoma of the pancreas. Archives of Surgery (Chicago, Ill: 1960). 2001;136(1):44-7.
135. Schmidt CM, Glant J, Winter JM, Kennard J, Dixon J, Zhao Q, et al. Total pancreatectomy (R0 resection) improves survival over subtotal pancreatectomy in isolated neck margin positive pancreatic adenocarcinoma. Surgery. 2007;142(4):572-8.
136. Muller MW, Friess H, Kleeff J, Dahmen R, Wagner M, Hinz U, et al. Is there still a role for total pancreatectomy? Annals of Surgery. 2007;246(6):966-74.
137. Casadei R, Monari F, Buscemi S, Laterza M, Ricci C, Rega D, et al. Total pancreatectomy: indications, operative technique, and results: a single centre experience and review of literature. Updates in Surgery. 2010;62(1):41-6.
138. Hackert T, Hinz U, Fritz S, Strobel O, Schneider L, Hartwig W, et al. Enucleation in pancreatic surgery: indications, technique, and outcome compared to standard pancreatic resections. Langenbeck's Archives of Surgery/Deutsche Gesellschaft fur Chirurgie. 2011;396(8):1197-203.
139. Crippa S, Bassi C, Salvia R, Falconi M, Butturini G, Pederzoli P. Enucleation of pancreatic neoplasms. Br J Sur. 2007;94(10):1254-9.
140. Norton JA. Surgery for primary pancreatic neuroendocrine tumors. Journal of Gastrointestinal Surgery: Official Journal of the Society for Surgery of the Alimentary Tract. 2006;10(3):327-31.
141. Tucker ON, Crotty PL, Conlon KC. The management of insulinoma. The British Journal of Surgery. 2006;93(3):264-75.
142. Zhang T, Xu J, Wang T, Liao Q, Dai M, Zhao Y. Enucleation of pancreatic lesions: indications, outcomes, and risk factors for clinical pancreatic fistula. J Gastrointest Surg. 2013;17(12): 2099-104.
143. Hiramoto JS, Feldstein VA, LaBerge JM, Norton JA. Intraoperative ultrasound and preoperative localization detects all occult insulinomas; discussion 1025-6. Archives of Surgery (Chicago, Ill: 1960). 2001;136(9):1020-5.
144. Aryal B, Komokata T, Kadono J, Motodaka H, Shimamoto Y, Kitazono I, et al. Middle-preserving pancreatectomy with reversed pancreaticogastrostomy: report of a case. Surg Today. 2014;44(8):1584-7.
145. Cheng K, Shen BY, Peng CH, Na LM, Cheng DF. Middle-preserving pancreatectomy: report of two cases and review of the literature. World J Surg Oncol. 2013;11:106.
146. Horiguchi A, Ishihara S, Ito M, Asano Y, Furusawa K, Yamamoto T, et al. Middle-segment-preserving pancreatectomy for biliary-pancreatic tumors. Hepatogastroenterology. 2011;58(107-8):1018-21.
147. Ohzato H, Yamamoto T, Fukunaga M, Imamura H, Furukawa H. Middle-preserving pancreatectomy for multifocal metastatic renal cell carcinoma located in the head, body and tail of the pancreas. A case report. JOP: Journal of the Pancreas. 2010;11(6):633-7.
148. Sperti C, Polizzi ML, Moro M, Beltrame V, Pedrazzoli S. Middle-preserving pancreatectomy: an interesting procedure for pancreas-sparing resection. JOP: Journal of the Pancreas. 2010;11(3):258-61.
149. Partelli S, Boninsegna L, Salvia R, Bassi C, Pederzoli P, Falconi M. Middle-preserving pancreatectomy for multicentric body-sparing lesions of the pancreas. American Journal of Surgery. 2009;198(3):e49-53.
150. Yasuda H, Takada T, Toyota N, Amano H, Yoshida M, Takada Y, et al. Limited pancreatectomy: significance of postoperative maintenance of pancreatic exocrine function. Journal of Hepato-Biliary-Pancreatic Surgery. 2000;7(5):466-72.

CHAPTER 44

Cystic Neoplasms of the Pancreas

Masao Tanaka

INTRODUCTION

Cystic neoplasms of the pancreas are not infrequently found as an incidental lesion when an imaging study, such as ultrasonography, computed tomography or magnetic resonance images (MRIs), is taken for diagnostic investigation of other diseases or just for a routine health check. Even when presenting with symptoms, most of the lesions only cause nonspecific abdominal symptoms like epigastric discomfort and/or fullness. It is rare for a cystic neoplasm to cause acute pancreatitis. However, if present, it is very specific and may be due to a mucin plug obstructing the ampulla of Vater in a patient with intraductal papillary mucinous neoplasm (IPMN) or compression to the main pancreatic duct (MPD) by any of the cystic neoplasms. In malignant cases, obstruction of the common bile duct may occur due to the same mechanisms, resulting in jaundice or cholangitis. However, most of the cystic neoplasms of the pancreas are usually asymptomatic.

The most frequent cystic neoplasm is IPMN, the incidence of which is reported to be 1/1,000 in individuals 60 years and older.[1] The second most frequent is mucinous cystic neoplasm (MCN) almost exclusively found in the body or tail of the pancreas in middle-aged women. Since both of IPMN and MCN have some common characteristics, including intratumoral mucin accumulation and malignant transformation following adenoma-carcinoma sequence, distinction between these two different pathological entities has been sometimes difficult, causing confusion of the differential diagnosis for a long time. However, the WHO classifications issued in 1996 and 2000[2,3] and subsequent publication of the international consensus guidelines for the management of IPMN and MCN in 2006[4] and their revision in 2012[5] have settled down the confused classification.

The other more infrequent entities of the cystic neoplasms of the pancreas include serous cystic neoplasm (SCN), solid pseudopapillary neoplasm, and dermoid cyst. Epidermoid cyst and lymphoepithelial cyst are also cystic lesions with enlarging tendency to be listed in the differential diagnoses of the cystic neoplasms of the pancreas, but these are non-neoplastic. This chapter of the text deals with these neoplastic and non-neoplastic cysts in this order. Neuroendocrine neoplasms and even adenocarcinomas and acinar cell carcinomas may sometimes show a cystic change due to central necrosis; however, these originally solid neoplasms are out of the scope of this chapter.

INTRADUCTAL PAPILLARY MUCINOUS NEOPLASM

General Aspects

Intraductal papillary mucinous neoplasms are characterized by intraductal papillary proliferation of mucinous cells. Due to abundant mucin production, IPMNs cause cystic, saccular or cylindrical dilation of the MPD, one or more of its branch ducts, or both, although the amount of mucin production is variable. When the mucin production is profuse, characteristic endoscopic features are noted at the ampulla of Vater, i.e., extrusion of mucin through the patulous orifice (Fig. 1). This finding drew attention and led to the epoch-making report of "mucin-secreting pancreatic cancer" published by Ohhashi et al.[6,7] in 1980 and 1982. When the duct of Santorini is involved, the characteristic dilation occurs at the minor papilla.

Intraductal papillary mucinous neoplasm is a rather uncommon type of pancreatic neoplasm, being 0.5% of all pancreatic neoplasms discovered at autopsy, 7.5% of clinically diagnosed pancreatic neoplasms, and 16.3% of pancreatic neoplasms resected.[8] Kimura et al.[9] reviewed 244 patients with duct-ectatic mucin-producing neoplasm of the pancreas, which corresponds to IPMN, from Japanese, European and American literature,

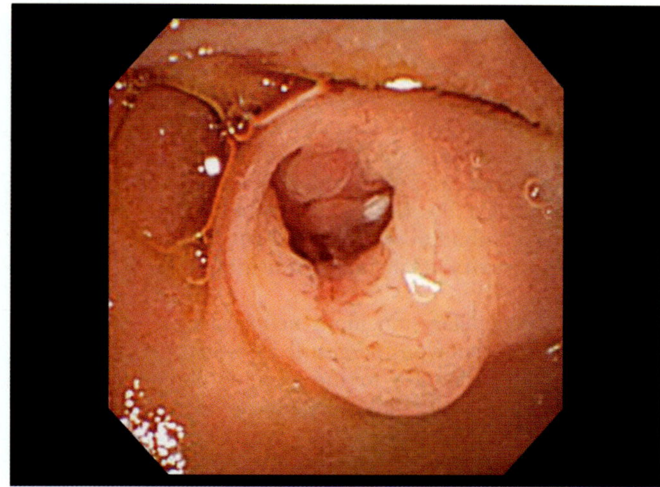

Figure 1 Dilated papilla

together with 15 patients of their own. The male to female ratio of the patients was 2.2, and the mean age 65.5 years. More than a half (62%) was found in the head of the pancreas. A history of pancreatitis, jaundice, and diabetes were noted in 15–19%. This neoplasm occurs in all races, but the largest number of patients have been reported from Japan.

Classification by Macroscopic Type

Clinical morphological forms of IPMNs are classified into three types, i.e. main duct type (MD-IPMN), branch duct type (BD-IPMN) and mixed or combined type (Figs 2A to D).[10] This classification is critically important in terms of malignant transformation closely associated with IPMNs. As summarized in the Sendai consensus guidelines, 70% on average of MD-IPMNs are malignant at the diagnosis, but the reverse is true in BD-IPMNs.[4] Mixed type IPMNs show clinicopathological characteristics similar to MD-IPMN. The classification may be changed by histological examination after resection, because

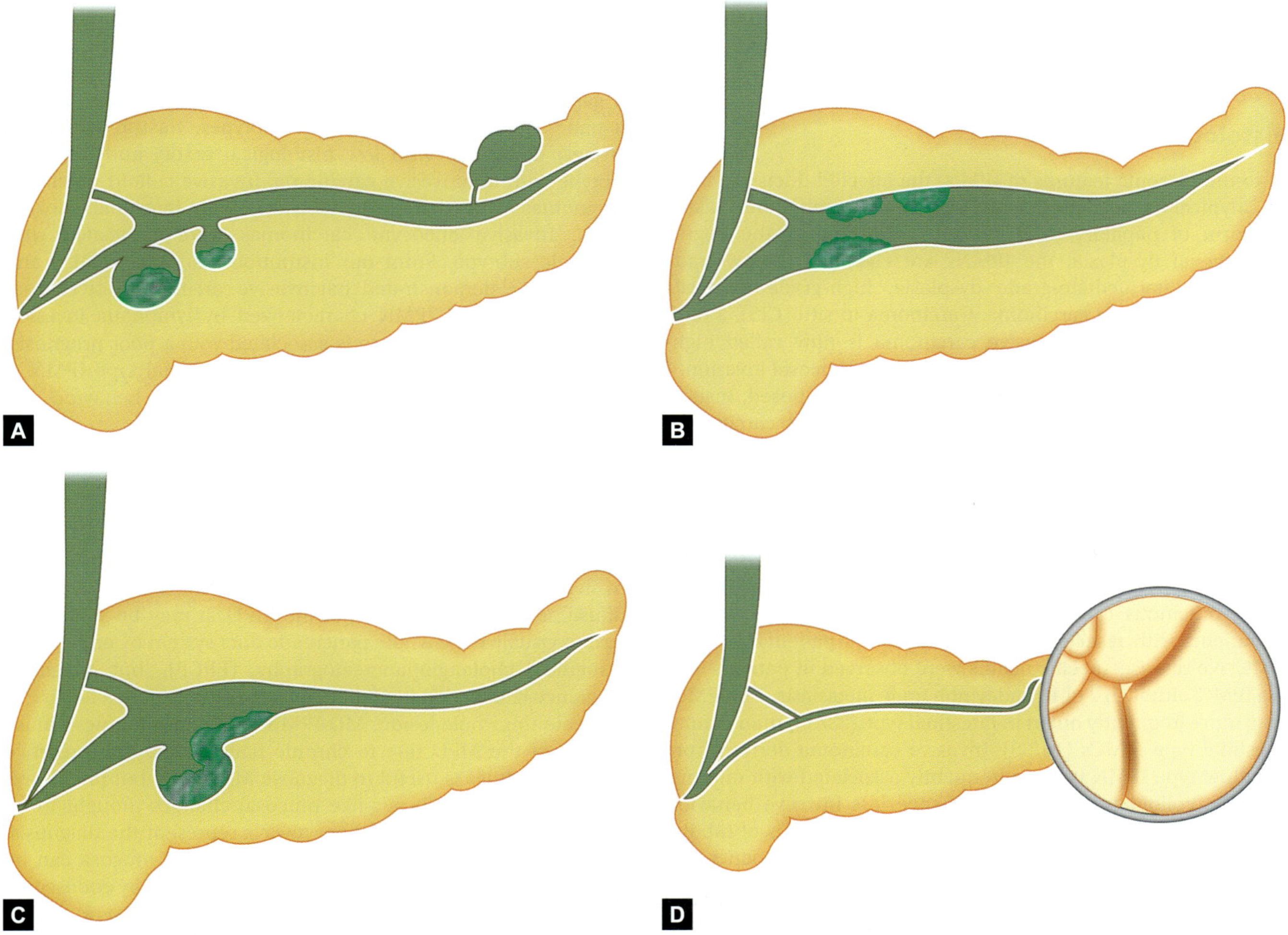

Figures 2A to D Schema of macroscopic types of IPMN (A: branch duct type, B: main duct type, C: mixed type) and characteristic features of MCN (D)

microscopic main duct involvement by IPMN is frequent even in BD-IPMNs. Therefore, every study must declare its standpoint of clinical morphological classification, either radiological or histological. Multiplicity is one of the unique features of IPMN, which is observed in 30% of all patients but not in other cystic neoplasms.[11]

Diagnosis

Among a variety of cystic neoplasms of the pancreas, IPMNs are most likely to present with some clinical symptoms. During the initial phase of the development of IPMNs, profuse mucin secreted by the IPMN may obliterate the orifice of the ampulla of Vater, precipitating an episode of epigastric discomfort or pain and hyperamylasemia consistent with acute pancreatitis. These symptoms are usually recurrent, but may become less severe or frequent with time due to dilation of the orifice caused by repeated passage of mucin (Fig. 1). However, severe pancreatitis is uncommon and some authors reported that 55–87% of the patients with IPMN are asymptomatic.[12-15] Patients with IPMN may develop insufficiency of pancreatic exocrine and endocrine functions in the long term, resulting in steatorrhea, diarrhea and diabetes mellitus secondary to persistent obliteration of the MPD in the head portion by mucin or papillary growth. By the similar mechanism, jaundice may occur when direct tumor invasion or viscid mucin obstructs the bile duct.

Histological Aspects

As to microscopic features of IPMN, the affected ducts are lined by atypical mucin-producing columnar epithelium taking the form of papillary proliferations. According to the degree of epithelial dysplasia, the IPMNs are classified as low-grade dysplasia, intermediate-grade dysplasia, high-grade dysplasia and further invasive carcinoma. Carcinoma in situ (CIS), a term formerly used for noninvasive carcinoma is now called high-grade dysplasia because of the absence of submucosal invasion.[16] Moreover, the Fukuoka consensus guidelines proposed, instead of the former description of "minimally invasive carcinoma" variably defined by the depth of invasion[17-19] or volume of the invasive part (<5%),[20] more clear definition of sub-staging the T1 category (those with invasive carcinoma <2 cm) into T1a for those that are ≤0.5 cm, T1b for those that are >0.5 cm and ≤1 cm, and T1c for those that are 1–2 cm employing standard TNM staging.[5] There have been few reports focusing on T1a intra ductal mucinous carcinoma (IPMC). Nakata et al.[21] evaluated 71 patients with resected IPMC, including 10 patients with T1a IPMC. No disease-specific deaths were observed in patients with T1a IPMC, although 2 of 10 had lymph node metastasis. T1a IPMCs were more frequently noted in intestinal type (23/33) than in non-intestinal type IPMCs (16/38). Invasive carcinoma derived from intestinal type IPMN is more frequently associated with minimal invasion, colloid carcinoma, and hence less invasive behavior. Invasive carcinoma derived from gastric type IPMN is of tubular carcinoma with aggressive behavior similar to usual pancreatic ductal adenocarcinoma (PDAC).

Grade of dysplasia of the neoplastic lining may vary from patient to patient, or even from area to area within one tumor. As there may be a tiny focal area of severe dysplasia within a vast majority of low grade to intermediate-grade dysplasia, extensive histological examination of the whole lesion is necessary in every patient with IPMN. The transition of different grades may be abrupt in some cases, or gradual or ill-defined in others. After the thorough examination of the whole sections, the classification of IPMN as low grade, intermediate-grade, high-grade dysplasia, or invasive carcinoma can be determined based on the most severe grade of epithelial dysplasia encountered in the neoplasm.[22] Macroscopic distribution of the dilated pancreatic ducts may not be always consistent with microscopic distribution of the dysplastic epithelium.

Intraductal papillary mucinous neoplasms are histologically classified into four subtypes, i.e. gastric, intestinal, pancreatobiliary and oncocytic, according to the histomorphological findings of papillae and immunohistochemical features of mucin glycoproteins.[23,24] The subtypes may vary within one lesion just as the histological grade of dysplasia; then the classification of the subtypes should depend on the most dominant component of the same histological grade or highest grade of dysplastic epithelium. This morphological variation of IPMNs is associated with sex, age, ductal dilation, histological grade, macroscopic type, invasiveness, stage, recurrence and prognosis of the patients with IPMNs.[25] Patients with pancreatobiliary subtype are more frequently female. Patients with oncocytic subtype IPMN are younger and those with pancreatobiliary subtype are older than those with other subtypes. Ductal dilation is more prominent in intestinal subtype than in gastric subtype. Mural nodules are more frequently present in pancreatobiliary and oncocytic subtypes. Gastric subtype is strongly associated with low histological grade, and intestinal subtype with noninvasive carcinoma. Invasive colloid mucinous carcinomas were definitely associated with intestinal subtype IPMN. Invasive oncocytic carcinomas were associated with oncocytic subtype. From our institution, Sadakari et al.[26] and Nakata et al.[21] demonstrated that invasive carcinoma derived from non-intestinal type IPMN characterized by lymphatic invasion and tubular invasive pattern is associated with a poor prognosis, while invasive carcinoma derived from intestinal type IPMN is associated with colloid carcinoma and less invasive behavior.

Characteristics of Each Macroscopic Type

MD-IPMN

Intraductal papillary mucinous neoplasm predominantly involving the MPD is classified as MD-IPMN with resultant diffuse or segmental dilation of the MPD. It may be sometimes hard to visualize the whole pancreatic duct system by endoscopic retrograde cholangiopancreatography (ERCP), but magnetic resonance cholangiopancreatography (MRCP) is quite effective to delineate the whole lesion. MD-IPMN sometimes mimics diffuse dilation of the MPD due to chronic pancreatitis. The presence of mural nodules is useful to diagnose MD-IPMN but not always present. Also, the fish egg-like mucosal changes thought to be characteristic of IPMNs may not always represent the diagnosis, as we previously reported that the fish egg-like mucosa can be present in patients with chronic pancreatitis treated by endoscopic stenting.[27] Demonstration of mucin extruding from a dilated duodenal papilla and/or mucin plugs in the MPD strongly suggest MD-IPMN, but may be present in those with BD-IPMN as well. The dilated papilla with mucin extrusion is more frequent in MD-IPMN than in BD-IPMN and correlated to malignant IPMN.[28]

Overall, 70% on average of MD-IPMNs were reported to be malignant.[4] The diagnosis of malignancy can be confirmed preoperatively by pancreatic juice cytology and/or transpapillary biopsy. However, the positive rate of transpapillary biopsy and cytology is relatively low, being around 50%[11,29] probably due to heterogeneity of dysplasia within a lesion and/or celluar atypia very well differentiated. The confirmative diagnosis must await the results of postoperative histological examinations of surgical specimens. Also, there may be a discrepancy between the localization of dysplastic neoplastic cells and the area of MPD dilation.

All fit patients are candidates for surgical resection. Only a part of dilated MPD with mural nodules may be resected while preserving the rest of the pancreas. However, total pancreatectomy may be performed in patients with diffuse MPD dilation with widespread mural nodules, but the indication for total pancreatectomy must be balanced against the age of the patient and resultant deficit of endocrine and exocrine pancreatic functions, because such a patient can survive even for several years without resection in case of minimally invasive carcinoma or high-grade dysplasia (formerly called CIS). Okada et al.[30] demonstrated that the mean tumor spread in the MPD was 41.6 ± 30.0 mm in 40 patients with resected MD or mixed type IPMN. One may be surprised by this long distance of the IPMN spread along the MPD; however, it should be recognized that they took all grades of dysplasia, even LGD, as positive.

BD-IPMN

Only IPMNs involving one or more branches of the pancreatic duct with the MPD ≤ 5 mm are now called BD-IPMN, because the revised international consensus guidelines defined MPD dilation of MD-IPMN to be more than 5 mm.[5] A BD-IPMN accompanying MPD dilation more than 5 mm should be classified as mixed type.

At the time of diagnosis only 30% on average of all BD-IPMNs are malignant.[4] Therefore, it is important to choose a possibly malignant BD-IPMN somehow. Carcinoma derived from BD-IPMN or intraductal papillary mucinous carcinoma (IPMC) of its invasive stage is rather easy to diagnose with recent imaging modalities. However, the preoperative and intraoperative diagnosis of high-grade dysplasia and "minimally invasive carcinoma" (<5 mm in depth of invasion) is still quite difficult, and has been the subject of many previous studies.[31-33]

In the preoperative diagnosis of malignancy in BD-IPMNs, the presence of mural nodules (>1 cm) and dilated MPD (>1 cm) have been reported to be most significant signs to suggest malignancy. Beside these, the international consensus (Sendai) guidelines included the presence of clinical symptoms such as acute pancreatitis and the size of the BD-IPMN (>3 cm) as malignant stigmata.[4] However, in view of the relatively low frequency of malignancy in flat-type (without mural nodules) BD-IPMNs, more than 3 cm in size, the cyst size has been excluded from the malignant stigmata and moved down to a category "worrisome features" (Flow chart 1).[5] Sadakari et al.[34] reported that the frequency of malignancy in flat BD-IPMNs more than or equal to 30 mm and MPD diameter less than 5 mm was only 3.6%, whereas it was 26.3% in those with MPD diameter more than or equal to 5 mm.

The presence of mural nodules is the most significant predictor of a malignant BD-IPMN. In particular, almost all BD-IPMNs are malignant when they have a large contrast-enhanced mural nodule. Tanaka[35] reviewed 246 patients reported in four series of BD-IPMN. All 15 patients with purely BD-IPMNs (i.e. without MPD dilation) less than 3 cm with mural nodules had carcinoma, but there was no single case of carcinoma in 124 patients with purely BD-IPMNs less than 3 cm without mural nodules. Shimizu et al.[36] reported that size of mural nodules, MPD diameter, and cyst size were independent predictors of malignancy in an analysis of 310 patients who underwent pancreatic resection for benign (n = 150) and malignant (n = 160; noninvasive 100, invasive 60) BD-IPMNs. With 7 mm as the cutoff value for the size of mural nodules, diagnostic sensitivity was 74.3% and specificity 72.7%. On the other hand, carcinoma without nodules accounted for only 9.4% of 160 patients with malignant BD-IPMNs.

Regarding the preoperative diagnosis of mural nodules, endosonography (EUS) gives superior images compared to other diagnostic methods, but the differentiation of a mucin plug from a mural nodule is still difficult. Ohno et al.[37] classified mural nodules into four types; low papillary nodule as type I, polypoid smooth-surfaced nodule as type II, papillary nodule with thickened wall or irregular structure as type III, and invasive nodule connected to an ill-defined hypoechoic area as type IV. Multivariable logistic regression analysis showed that types III and IV mural nodules and symptomatic IPMNs were significant for malignancy. For mural nodule diameter, invasive IPMNs were significantly larger, but types III and IV mural nodules were more frequently associated with malignancy, particularly invasive cancer, at 88.9% and 91.7%, respectively. The diagnosis of IPMNs with types III or IV mural nodule as malignant resulted in a sensitivity of 60%, specificity of 92.9%, and accuracy of 75.9%. Doppler and contrast-enhanced ultrasonography may be useful to detect blood supply to the solid component.[38]

When malignant BD-IPMN has been confirmed by pancreatic juice cytology or some other methods or is highly suspected, pancreatic resection with lymphadenectomy should be performed.[5] Lymphadenectomy must be extended to station two lymph nodes, i.e. D2 dissection, if the presence of invasive carcinoma is demonstrated by imagings. Only when the presence of invasive carcinoma can be negated, lymphadenectomy may be limited to some appropriate extent. A current problem is a difficulty in diagnosing "minimally invasive carcinoma", which is compatible with T1a (≤0.5 cm), by any currently available imaging modalities, while this subgroup of invasive carcinoma may be associated with lymph node metastasis.[21]

Whenever a BD-IPMN is resected, frozen section examination must be conducted intraoperatively. Resection can be completed only when no further spread of high-grade dysplasia of IPMN is demonstrated along the MPD beyond the resection line. In addition to the presence of continuous dysplastic epithelium, we repeatedly reported that we should pay more attention to the possible presence of concomitant but distinct invasive adenocarcinoma and/or CIS as mentioned later (not yet determined if this is PanIN 3 or high-grade dysplasia of IPMN).[31,39] Recently, we proposed the utilization of intraoperative irrigation cytology to examine the presence/absence of concomitant carcinoma in the pancreas to be left in situ when performing partial pancreatectomy for possibly malignant IPMN.[33] In 5 of 48 patients who underwent partial pancreatectomy, irrigation cytology was positive for malignant

Flow chart 1 Algorithm cited from pancreatology

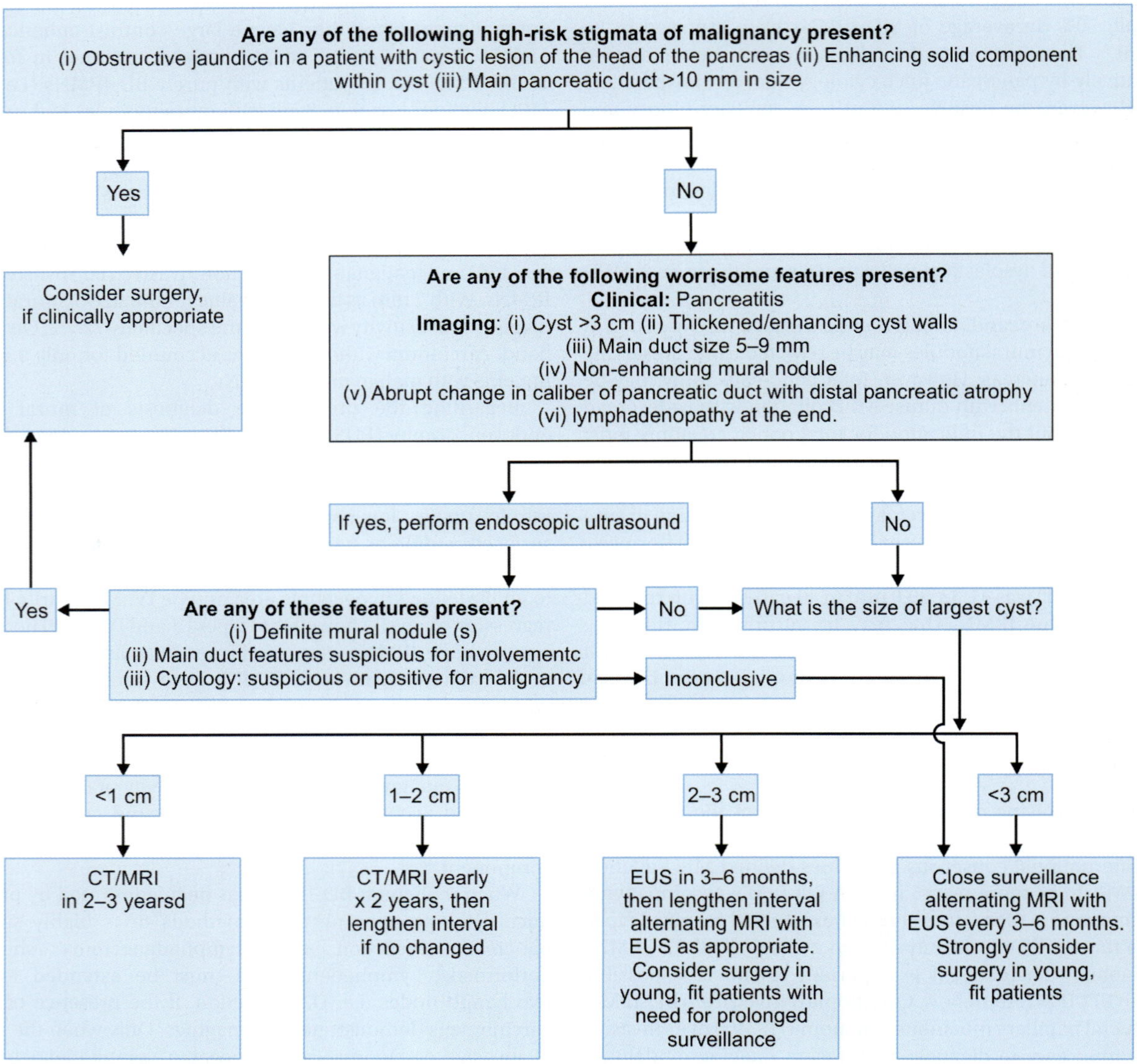

Are any of the following high-risk stigmata of malignancy present?
(i) Obstructive jaundice in a patient with cystic lesion of the head of the pancreas (ii) Enhancing solid component within cyst (iii) Main pancreatic duct >10 mm in size

Yes → Consider surgery, if clinically appropriate

No →

Are any of the following worrisome features present?
Clinical: Pancreatitis
Imaging: (i) Cyst >3 cm (ii) Thickened/enhancing cyst walls
(iii) Main duct size 5–9 mm
(iv) Non-enhancing mural nodule
(v) Abrupt change in caliber of pancreatic duct with distal pancreatic atrophy
(vi) lymphadenopathy at the end.

If yes, perform endoscopic ultrasound

No → What is the size of largest cyst?

Are any of these features present?
(i) Definite mural nodule (s)
(ii) Main duct features suspicious for involvementc
(iii) Cytology: suspicious or positive for malignancy

Yes → Consider surgery, if clinically appropriate

No → What is the size of largest cyst?

Inconclusive → Close surveillance

<1 cm → CT/MRI in 2–3 yearsd

1–2 cm → CT/MRI yearly x 2 years, then lengthen interval if no changed

2–3 cm → EUS in 3–6 months, then lengthen interval alternating MRI with EUS as appropriate. Consider surgery in young, fit patients with need for prolonged surveillance

<3 cm → Close surveillance alternating MRI with EUS every 3–6 months. Strongly consider surgery in young, fit patients

cells. In the additionally resected specimens, stage 0 distinct PDAC was found in four patients and stage 3 in one. Thus, every patient who undergoes pancreatectomy for IPMN should be informed with the possibility of total pancreatectomy as the Fukuoka consensus guidelines stated.[5]

Association of Pancreatic Ductal Adenocarcinoma with IPMN

Apart from malignant transformation of itself, IPMN may be associated with occurrence of distinct PDAC. Tanaka et al.[31] reported the first case of a BD-IPMN diagnosed as having a distinct CIS by preoperative pancreatic juice cytology. The site of origin of positive cytology was estimated by repeated segmental cytological examinations using a balloon catheter inserted by ERCP. Next, Yamaguchi et al.[39] claimed the role of IPMN as a sentinel to detect a CIS. Five years later, the same group reported 146 patients who underwent pancreatectomy for IPMN alone (69 patients), PDAC alone (70 patients), or both of IPMN and PDAC (7 patients).[40] The 7 patients with PDAC concomitant with IPMN were all male and corresponded to 9.2% of 76 patients with IPMN and 9.1% of 77 patients with PDAC. All IPMNs concomitant with PDAC are of branch duct type with a mean diameter of 3.0 cm and of low-grade dysplasia by histology. PDACs in 2 of the 7 patients were CIS, 1 minimally invasive carcinoma and the other 4 invasive carcinoma. Noteworthy was the fact that the presence of IPMN led to the diagnosis of PDAC in 4 of these patients. They further analyzed their consecutive 236 patients with IPMN on observation or resected to identify predictors of the presence of PDAC seen in 22 patients (9.3%).[41] Multivariate analysis revealed worsening diabetes mellitus and an abnormal serum level of carbohydrate antigen (CA) 19-9 as significant factors to predict the presence of PDAC.

Our Kyushu University experience with 405 patients with IPMN as of March 2013 includes 43 distinct PDACs concomitant with IPMN (Fig. 3). The overall frequency of concomitant PDAC is thus 11% (43/405) (Table 1). There were 38 distinct PDACs in 305 patients with BD-IPMN (12%), 2 in 55 patients with MD-IPMN (4%), and 3 in 45 patients with mixed type IPMN (7%). On the other hand, there were 106 patients who had a variety of cancers in the other organs in these 405 patients (26%).

After publication of many reports along the same line from Japan,[42-48] the Japan Pancreas Society reported a large-scale retrospective analysis and defined the clinicopathological features of IPMC and PDAC concomitant with IPMN.[49] Out of 765 patients with resected IPMNs, 122 were diagnosed as having IPMC, 31 (4.1% of all IPMNs) PDACs distinct from IPMN, and 30 PDACs with equivocal association with IPMN. When the clinicopathological data of these patients compared with that of 7,605 patients with usual PDAC registered in the Japan Pancreas Society pancreatic cancer registry, IPMC and PDAC concomitant with IPMN were significantly smaller, less invasive, and less extensive than usual PDAC. Hence the patients with the former two categories of carcinoma could survive significantly longer than those with usual PDAC, indicating that both of PDAC concomitant with IPMN and IPMC might have less aggressive biological behavior or be diagnosed earlier than usual PDAC. The group proposed histological continuity as a proof of carcinoma derived from IPMN or IPMC, but this study also revealed that there were the similar number of PDACs which were not clearly demonstrated as carcinoma derived from IPMN or carcinoma distinct from IPMN, as seen in 30 of 183 patients with PDAC associated with IPMN (16.4%).

Another large-scale retrospective analysis by the JPS[50] showed that only 62 (17.8%) of 349 patients with BD-IPMN observed

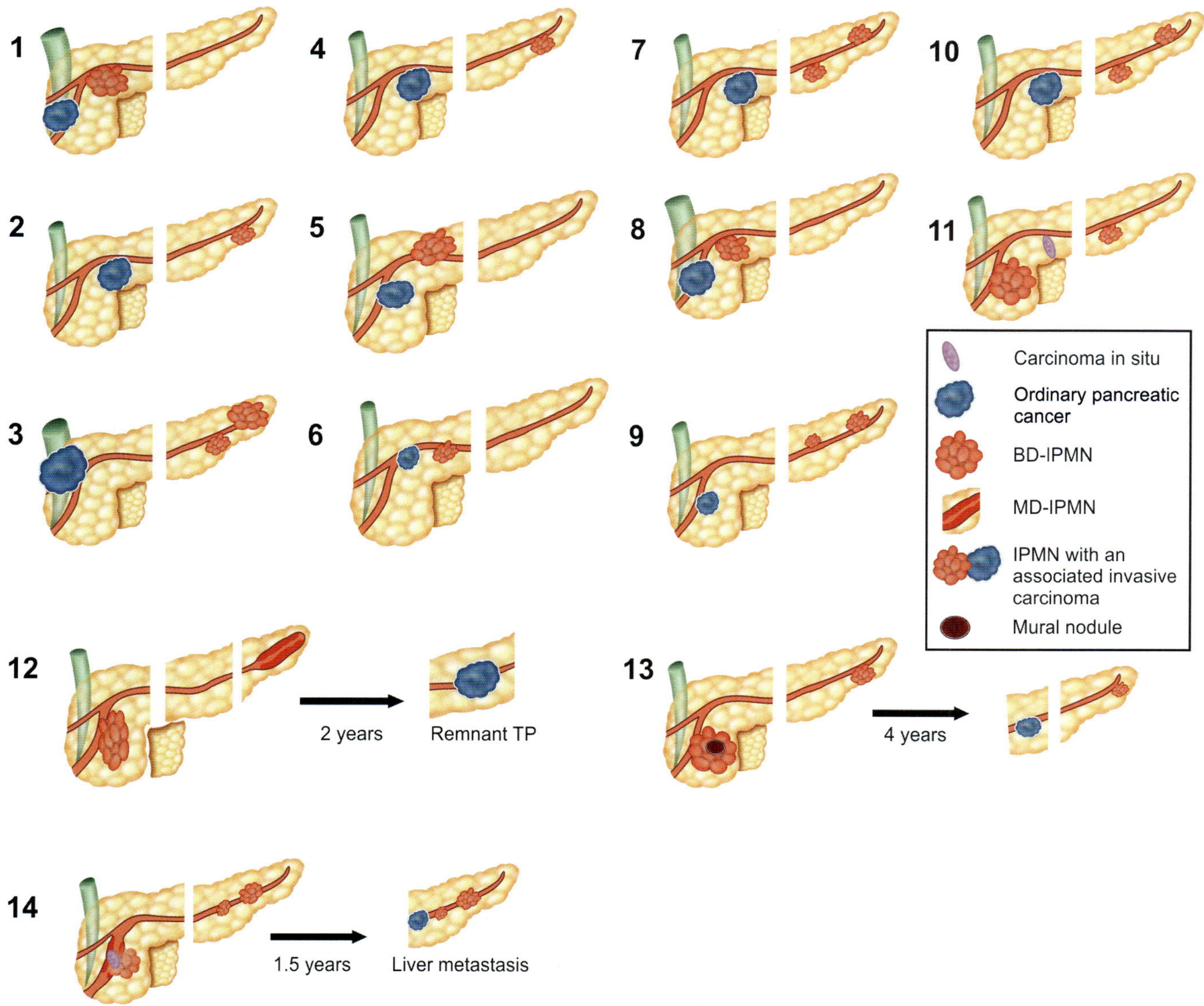

Figure 3A

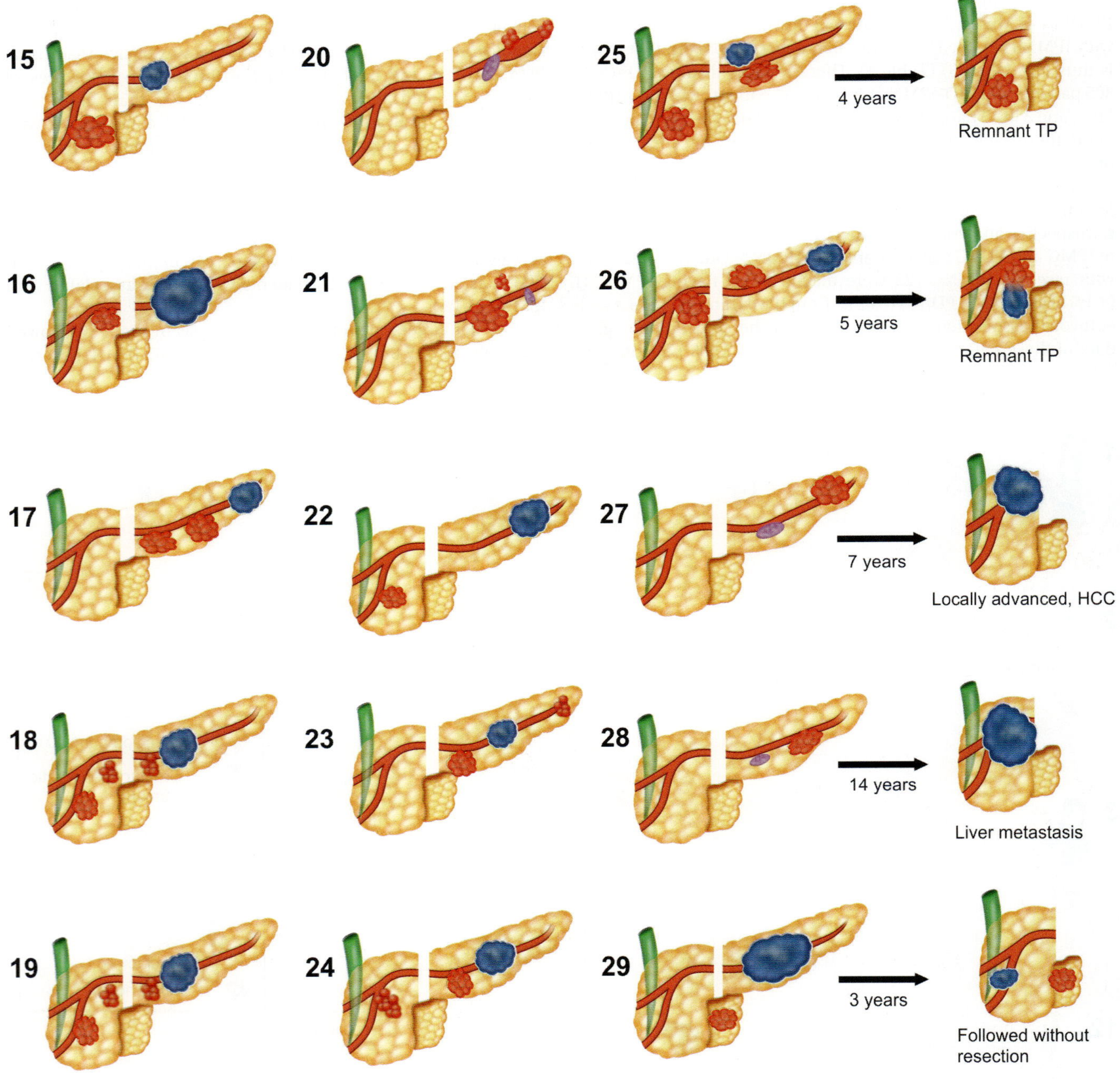
15
20
25
4 years
Remnant TP
16
21
26
5 years
Remnant TP
17
22
27
7 years
Locally advanced, HCC
18
23
28
14 years
Liver metastasis
19
24
29
3 years
Followed without resection

Figure 3B

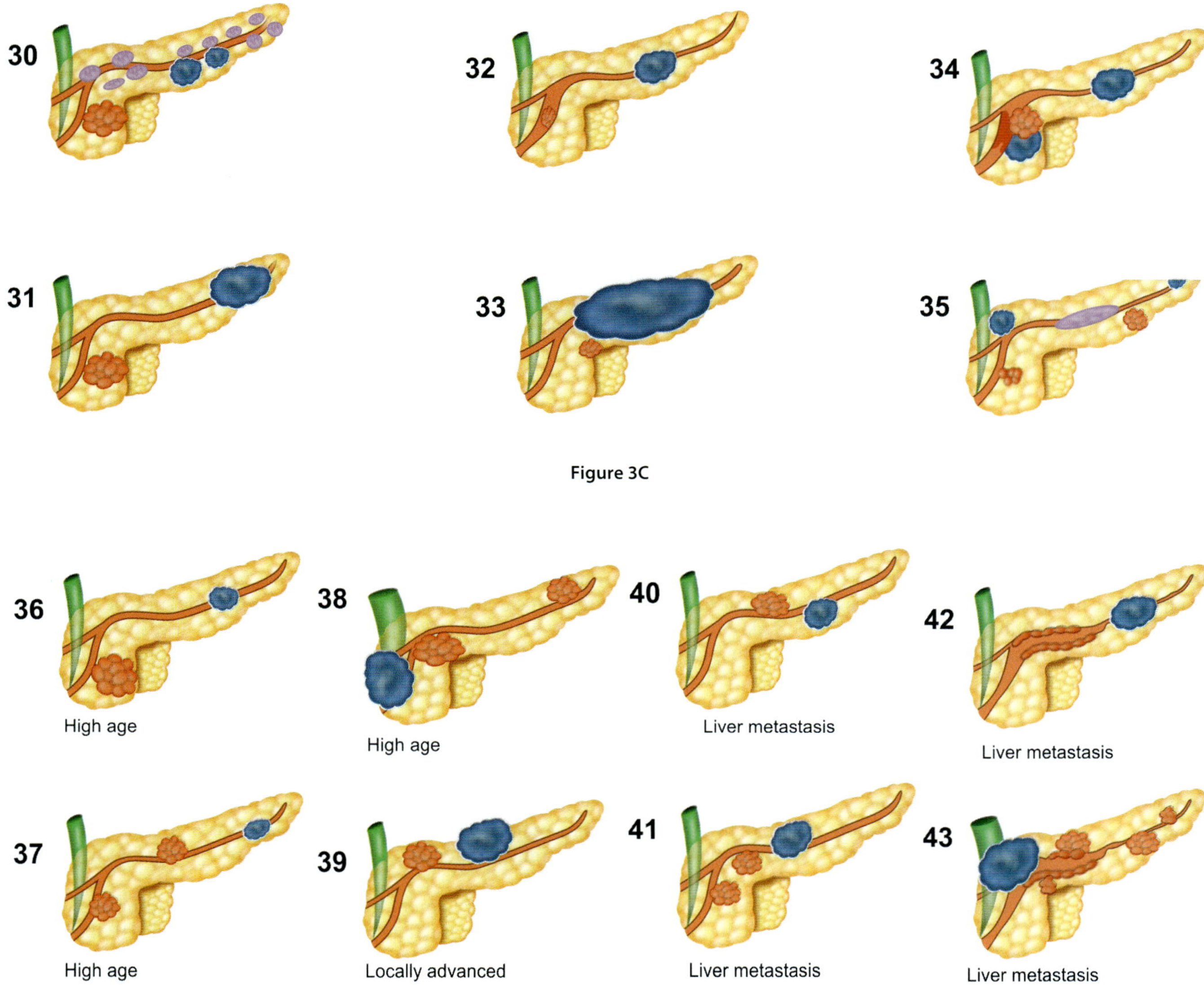

Figures 3A to D A: pancreatoduodenectomy, B: distal pancreatectomy, C: total pancreatectomy, D: unresctable.

Table 1: Carcinoma concomitant with IPMN

	Total	*Main duct type*	*Branch duct type*	*Mixed type*
Number of patients	405	55	305	45
Age, years (range)	69 (21-88)	70 (51–84)	68 (21–88)	71 (33–85)
Gender (M:F)	218:187	31:24	160:145	27:18
Size of BD, mm (range)	25 (5–2711)	-	25 (5–1218)	30 (7–2711)
Size of MPD, mm (range)	3.5 (2–40)	12 (6–40)	3 (2–5)	8 (6–13)
Mural nodule				
Present	100 (25%)	33 (60%)	50 (16%)	17 (38%)
Absent	305 (75%)	22 (40%)	255 (84%)	28 (62%)
Carcinoma				
Pancreas cancer	43 (11%)	2 (4%)	38 (12%)	3 (7%)
Other organs	106 (26%)	14 (25%)	82 (27%)	10 (22%)

for a median period of 3.7 years exhibited disease progression. However, distinct PDAC developed in 7 (2.0%) patients, thus the yearly incidence of distinct PDAC 0.41%. In all probability, IPMN of the pancreas seems to indicate the increased risk for developing PDAC of the entire pancreas. Considering IPMNs as a sentinel of subsequent development of PDAC, meticulous surveillance of the entire pancreas is mandatory to detect a PDAC derived from IPMN or arising in a distinct site of the pancreas. The intervals for surveillance of benign BD-IPMNs and the pancreatic remnant after resection of IPMNs should therefore not be lengthened to more than 6 months, although the best interval and modality for surveillance remain to be determined. Patients with a strong family history of PDAC are likely to have IPMNs before developing a PDAC during surveillance;[51,52] however, whether those with IPMN and a family history of PDAC should receive more frequent surveillance is unknown yet.

Prognosis of IPMN

When a benign IPMN causes acute pancreatitis, a complete removal can be obtained by limited non-anatomical pancreatectomy or even enucleation like ductal branch-oriented pancreatectomy.[53] Although the immediate postoperative course after non-anatomical pancreatectomy may be more frequently complicated by pancreatic fistula, the long-term outcome is always excellent.

The prognosis of noninvasive IPMN is favorable but invasive IPMN exhibits a spectrum of survival according to the proportion of the invasion in the whole lesion.[20] In addition, for patients with invasive IPMN, lymph node positivity was associated with poor outcome, the 5-year survival rate being 44.1% for node negatives versus 0% for node positives.[54] Stratification by nodal status demonstrated no difference in survival among lymph node-positive patients, but median survival of resected, lymph node-negative invasive IPMN was significantly better than that with lymph node-negative PDAC. Wasif et al.[55] reported that overall survival is better in invasive IPMN than PDAC, but the prognosis of lymph node-positive invasive IPMN mimicked that of lymph node-positive PDAC, and positive lymph nodes, high tumor grade, tumor size more than 2 cm, and age more than 66 years were adverse predictors of survival for patients with invasive IPMN. Partelli et al.[56] also emphasized that lymph node ratio (LNR) is a strong predictor of survival after resection of invasive IPMN, with 5-year disease-specific survival decreasing while the LNR increased (LNR=0, 86.5%; LNR >0 to 0.2, 34.4%; LNR >0.2, 11.1%; $p<0.05$).

Histological subtypes of IPMN consisting of gastric, intestinal, pancreatobiliary and oncocytic subtypes have been shown to be closely associated with the prognosis of invasive IPMN. Sadakari et al.[26] initiatively reviewed 30 patients with invasive IPMN and divided them into two pathologic subtypes, intestinal and non-intestinal. The prognosis of these patients was compared to that of 119 patients with conventional PDAC. The 5-year survival rate of patients with non-intestinal subtypes (0.0%) characterized by positive lymphatic invasion and tubular invasive pattern was as poor as that of patients with conventional PDAC (19.9%; $p=0.67$), whereas that of intestinal subtype (66.7%) was significantly better than that of conventional PDAC ($p<0.001$). In the next year, Furukawa et al.[25] also demonstrated that the subtypes of IPMN were associated with the histological types (tubular or colloid) of the invasive component and the prognosis of invasive IPMN. Nakata et al.[21] analyzed 71 patients with invasive IPMN and reported that there were no disease-specific deaths in 10 patients with minimally invasive (<5 mm, T1a) IPMN, although 2 of them had lymph node metastasis. T1a was more frequent in intestinal subtype (23/33 cases) than in non-intestinal subtype (16/38 cases; $p=0.019$). The prognosis of massively invasive intestinal subtype was significantly better than that of massively invasive non-intestinal subtype ($p=0.013$), being related to less frequent tubular invasion ($p<0.001$) and lymphatic ($p=0.001$) or serosal ($p=0.021$) invasion. Yopp et al.[57] also analyzed 59 patients resected for invasive IPMN. Tubular carcinoma subtype present in 59% of the patients and the presence of positive regional lymph nodes were predictive of decreased survival. The 5-year estimated survival rates for tubular carcinoma and colloid carcinoma were 55% and 87%, respectively ($p=0.01$). Survival of invasive tubular subtype was not different from that of matched patients with conventional PDAC. Within the same year, Kim et al.[58] reported 54, 56, 30 and 2 patients with gastric, intestinal, pancreatobiliary and oncocytic types of IPMNs, respectively, and reached the similar conclusion. Mino-Kenudson et al.[59] also studied 61 patients with invasive IPMN, including tubular in 38 (62%), colloid in 16 (26%), and oncocytic in seven (12%). Colloid and oncocytic carcinomas arose only from intestinal and oncocytic subtypes, respectively, mostly of MD type, while tubular carcinomas primarily grew from gastric subtype associated with BD-IPMN. Survival of patients with invasive carcinoma arising from gastric subtype was significantly worse than that of patients with non-gastric subtype ($p=0.016$), resembling PDAC. In 2013, Distler et al.[60] reported 103 resected IPMNs, including 45 intestinal subtype (44%), 41 pancreatobiliary subtype (40%), 13 gastric subtype (12%) and 4 oncocytic subtype (4%). The 5-year survival for intestinal IPMNs was significantly better than that for pancreatobiliary IPMNs (86.6% vs 35.6%; $p<0.001$). The pancreatobiliary subtype was strongly associated with malignancy, recurrence and short survival which are comparable with those of PDAC.

Adjuvant treatment for PDAC has proved to improve survival; however, adjuvant therapy after resection of invasive IPMN has not been fully investigated yet. Turrini et al.[61] reviewed 412 patients undergoing resection of IPMN, 98 of whom had invasive IPMN which recurred in 45 patients (46%). Adjuvant treatment did not affect median survival in node-positive or node-negative invasive IPMN; however, a subgroup of patients with resectable recurrence in the remnant pancreas appeared to have more favorable outcomes.

MUCINOUS CYSTIC NEOPLASM

Mucinous cystic neoplasm of the pancreas is a cystic tumor with the inner surface lined by columnar mucin-producing epithelium supported by ovarian-type stroma. Not only IPMNs but also MCNs produce an excessive amount of mucin. MCN occurs almost invariably in the body or tail of the pancreas of young to middle-aged women. This neoplasm was not thought to communicate with the pancreatic duct, but a recent study reported that ERCP or pancreatography of resected MCNs revealed a communication between the cyst and MPD in 18.1% of 156 MCNs.[62]

Mucinous cystic neoplasm is characterized by adenoma-carcinoma sequence, progressing from LGD to HGD and further to invasive carcinoma, just like IPMN. This is one of the most striking features of MCN that may make it difficult to distinguish this entity from IPMN. Conversely, the most prominent feature of MCN is the presence of ovarian-type stroma, which is defined as a prerequisite for MCN by WHO and AFIP classifications.[63,64] MCN can occur in male patients;[65] however, after the ovarian-type stroma was regarded as essential for the diagnosis, the proportion of male patients has become extremely lower than previously reported. Yamao et al.[62] reported only 3 male patients in their series of 156 patients with MCN proven by the presence of ovarian-type stroma. Likewise, MCNs are observed exclusively in the body or tail of the pancreas, but rarely in the head of the pancreas, as reported in only one of their series of 156 patients.[62]

Differentiation of IPMN and MCN is a matter of pathologic diagnosis, but their clinical management is quite similar.[66] Symptoms attributable to the presence of MCN were noted in about a half of the patients, depending on the size of the lesion and presence of communication with the MPD.[62] A large MCN may cause diabetes mellitus secondary to parenchymal replacement. In Yamao's series, 4.6% of the patients had diabetes, similar to the frequency of 3.8% previously reported by Thompson et al.[67] MCN of the pancreas very rarely contains gastrin-producing cells and produces Zollinger-Ellison syndrome as in the case of ovarian MCN.[68] Although relatively rare, some patients with MCN present with acute pancreatitis.[62] In that case, an MCN may possibly be misdiagnosed as a pseudocyst.[69]

Yamao et al.[62] reported that 82.7% of their 156 patients had adenoma, 13.4% noninvasive carcinoma, and 3.9% invasive carcinoma. The diameter of MCN and presence of mural nodule predict malignant MCN. Large MCNs and those with mural nodules must be treated as carcinoma by resection with lymph node dissection. On the other hand, small MCNs may be resected by laparoscopic pancreatectomy with preservation of the spleen and/or splenic vessels.[70-72] The Fukuoka consensus recommends surgical resection for all surgically fit patients with MCN, and laparoscopic resection as well as parenchyma-sparing resections and distal pancreatectomy with spleen preservation for MCNs less than 4 cm in size without mural nodules.[5]

The prognosis of patients with MCN depends on the grade of malignancy. According to Yamao et al.,[72] a significant difference in the survival rates was observed between adenomas and carcinomas and between minimally invasive carcinomas (T1a) and invasive carcinomas. The postoperative 3-, 5- and 10-year survival rates were 99.8%, 98.8% and 98.8% and 92.3%, 86.5% and 86.5% for patients with adenoma and carcinoma, respectively, and 100%, 100% and 100%, and 50.0%, 0% and 0% for patients with minimally invasive and invasive carcinomas, respectively.

Differentiation of IPMN and MCN

The differentiation of IPMN from MCN had been a major problem, but the international consensus Sendai guidelines contributed to better understanding of clinicopathological features for distinction of these two entities (Table 2). Using these features, it is possible to distinguish IPMN from MCN in most cases. However, if a BD-IPMN forms a multilocular spherical cyst in the tail of the pancreas, it may mimic an MCN (Figs 4A to C). When the tumor has high-risk stigmata like the presence of mural nodule, it should anyway be resected and subjected to histological examinations to determine the presence or absence of ovarian-type stroma. The Fukuoka consensus proposed that a mucinous neoplastic cyst which has imaging features of MCN but lacks ovarian-type stroma should be categorized as an "indeterminate" mucinous neoplasm.[5]

When the tumor does not exhibit any high-risk stigmata or worrisome features proposed in the Fukuoka guidelines,[5] the differentiation is more important to choose an appropriate surveillance protocol. An IPMN needs close observation at least every 6 months to check the emergence of mural nodules within the cyst and concomitant PDAC in other sites of the pancreas, while yearly ultrasonography or computed tomography is sufficient to check the growth and emergence of mural nodules within an MCN. In a case of benign, highly suspicious MCN, it may be judicious to subject the patient to laparoscopic distal pancreatectomy to confirm the histological diagnosis. If confirmed as an MCN, no postoperative surveillance is necessary; however, if confirmed as an IPMN, the remnant pancreas needs periodical life-long surveillance postoperatively.

SEROUS CYSTIC NEOPLASM

Serous cystic neoplasms are composed of true cystic structures lined by epithelial cells with the glycogen-rich cytoplasm and comprise 4–10% of all cystic lesions of the pancreas.[73,74] The lining

Table 2: Typical features of MCN and branch duct IPMN

Characteristic	*MCN*	*Branch duct IPMN*
Gender (female)	>95%	~30%
Age (decade)	4th and 5th	6th and 7th
Location (body/tail)	95%	~30%
Common capsule	Yes	No
Calcification	Rare, curvilinear, in the wall of cyst	No
Gross appearance	Orange-like	Grape-like
Internal structure	Cysts in cyst	Cyst by cyst
Pancreatic duct communication	Infrequent	Yes (though not always demonstrable)
Main pancreatic duct	Normal or deviated	Normal, or if dilated, suggests combined type

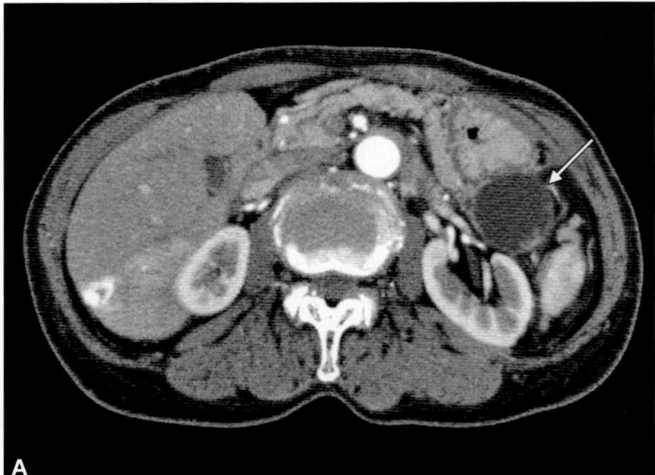

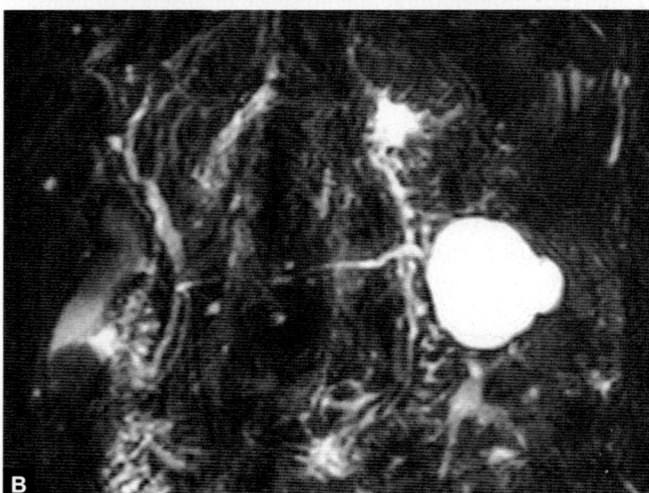

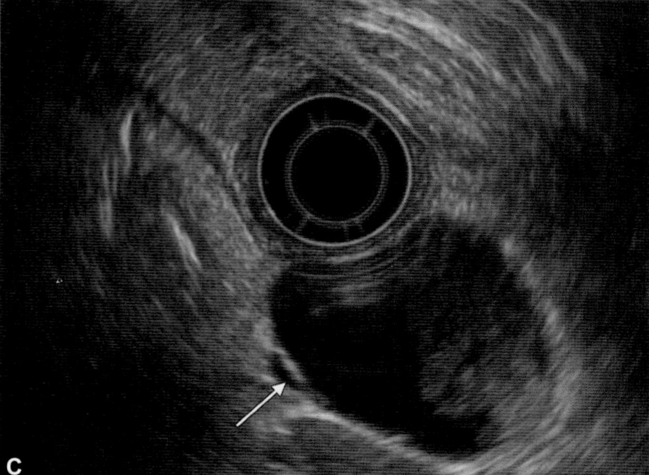

Figures 4A to C (A) CT, (B) MRCP and (C) EUS in a 73-year-old woman with an IPMN which mimics an MCN. A bilocular thick-walled cystic lesion, 39x27 mm in size, looks like an MCN with a mural nodule and cyst-in-cyst appearance (arrows), but actually was a noninvasive intraductal papillary mucinous carcinoma

of SCN is a single layer of simple cuboidal epithelium positive for periodic acid-Shiff staining of glycogen, which disappears after diastase digestion. This slowly growing neoplasm occurs more frequently in women (70%) with the mean age in the sixties,[75] and does not frequently cause clinical symptoms. A retrospective review of 172 patients with SCN, 90 surgical and 82 observed, showed some symptoms in only 20% of all patients.[76] The others were diagnosed just by incident. Clinical symptoms are mostly obscure and nonspecific, including abdominal discomfort, nausea, vomiting and weight loss caused by a mass or compression to the MPD. Obstructive pancreatitis or jaundice may occur according to the site (pancreatic body or head) of involvement by a hugely grown SCN. SCN is almost equally distributed in the whole pancreas, being in the head in 39%, the body in 35% and the tail in 22%.[76] Multifocal serous cystadenoma of the pancreas was reported in a 48-year-old Japanese woman.[77]

Serous cystic neoplasms take a variety of macroscopic forms, including most frequent microcystic type, oligocystic or macrocystic type, and solid type.[78-82] The most typical is the microcystic type, which demonstrates a clearly defined, multilocular cyst of "honeycomb appearance", occasionally with a "central stellate scar" composed of hyalinized tissue and a calcification of "sunburst type" on ultrasonography and computed tomography (Fig. 5).[83] Kimura et al.[76] reported that the honeycomb appearance was noted best by EUS (80.7%), compared to computed tomography (67.1%), ultrasonography (59.5%) and MRI (71.1%). The sunburst calcification was observed in 11.0% in their series. There is a tendency that larger cysts are located in the periphery and smaller cysts in the center.[84] SCNs are usually hypervascular and well enhanced by contrast. Therefore, this tumor must be distinguished from neuroendocrine neoplasms when it is small and appears as a solid mass. SCN does not usually communicate with the MPD and then ERP only shows a mass effect to or obstruction of the MPD. T2-weighted images of MRI reveal multilocular cysts with hyperintense contents, while T1-weighted images show a low intensity mass. Gadolinium study shows early and delayed enhancement.

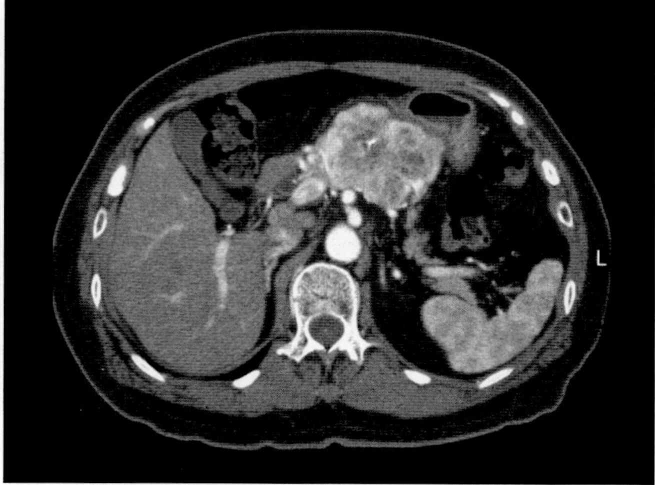

Figure 5 CT showing the honeycomb appearance and stellate scar of a well-enhanced microcystic SCN in a 64-year-old woman

The other forms of SCN, oligocystic/macrocystic and solid types, pose a difficulty in differentiating from other sorts of pancreatic neoplasms. Warshaw et al.[85] reported that 50% of SCNs showed the microcystic pattern, with the characteristic central scar or sunburst calcification observed in only 11%. A series of 172 patients with SCN reported by Kimura et al.[76] showed a microcystic (58.7%), macrocystic (19.8%), mixed (16.8%), solid (3.0%) or unclassified pattern (1.8%). A macrocystic SCN consisting of one or more large cysts with or without small cysts mimics an IPMN, an MCN, or a pseudocyst (Figs 6A to C). A careful inspection of the images of a macrocystic SCN may disclose some areas of the microcystic pattern.[86] If not, however, it is very difficult to distinguish macrocystic SCNs from IPMNs. EUS-guided fine needle aspiration (EUS-FNA) with determination of the carcinoembryonic antigen (CEA) level of the cyst fluid is helpful, demonstrating high levels in mucinous cysts like IPMN and MCN and low levels in SCN.[87] Immunohistochemical features are the same as those of microcystic SCN.[78,86,88,89]

It is well known that cystic neoplasms of the pancreas occur in 7–71% of patients with von Hippel-Lindau disease, most of them being SCNs.[90-92] Association of SCN and a variety of other diseases are also reported, including autoimmune hemolytic anemia and idiopathic thrombocytopenic purpura (Evan's syndrome).[93] SCNs are not infrequently associated with diabetes mellitus, cholelithiasis, pancreatic and extrapancreatic malignancies, but most of these associations may be coincidence related to the advanced age of the patients.[94]

The malignant change of SCNs is quite rare; indicating that SCN may be hamartomatous rather than neoplastic, but in adult patients differentiation of SCN from IPMN and MCN is of great importance, because these mucinous cysts would achieve malignant transformation.[95] The epithelial nature of SCN is indicated by the positivity of EMA, CEA and cytokeratin, and negativity of trypsin (acinar cell marker), insulin, glucagon, and somatostatin (endocrine markers), gastrin, chromogranin A, and synaptophysin (neuroendocrine markers), S-100 protein, actin, desmin, and vimentin (mesenchymal marker), and factor VIII-related antigen (endothelial marker). Immunohistochemical localization of CA19-9 was reported to be associated with clinical behavior of SCN, either benign (positive apical membrane and supranuclear cytoplasm) or malignant (positive entire surface and cytoplasm).[96]

Surgical intervention is needed only when SCNs are large and symptomatic, and/or when SCN is unequivocally malignant with the evidence such as liver metastasis or lymph node metastasis. Another not infrequent indication for surgery is the inability to clearly distinguish a macrocystic SCN from mucinous cysts like IPMN and MCN. The preoperative diagnosis did not correctly identify SCN in 57 (63%) of 90 patients with a resected SCN,[76] suggesting that macrocystic/oligocystic SCNs occupy a considerable proportion of resected SCNs. Of 80 SCNs treated at Massachusetts General Hospital over 15 years from 1976 through 1991, 5 (6.3%) were macrocystic SCN.[78] Laparoscopic resection would be a suitable option for the surgical treatment of SCNs.[97,98] As the risk of malignant transformation is minimal, the prognosis of SCNs is excellent.

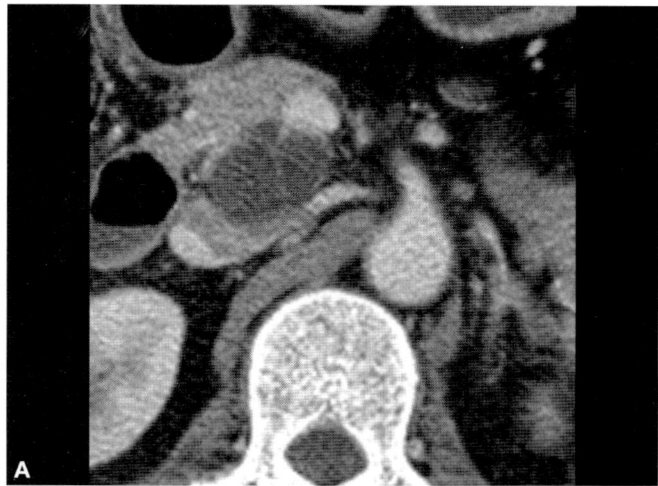

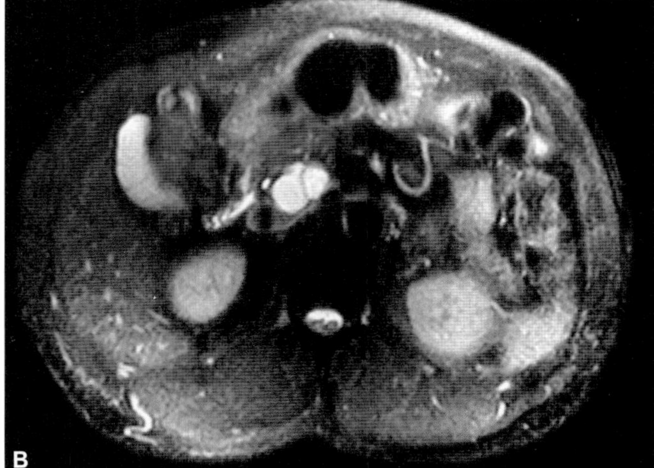

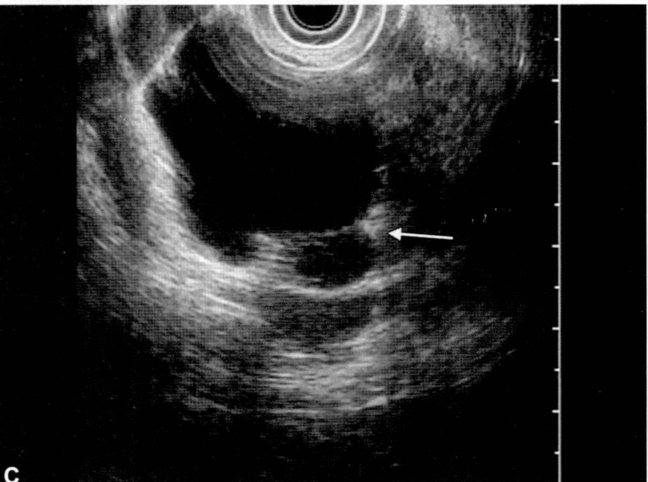

Figures 6A to C (A) CT, (B) T2-weighted MRI and (C) EUS demonstrating a macrocystic SCN mimicking an IPMN with cyst-by-cyst appearance in a 56-year-old man

SOLID-PSEUDOPAPILLARY TUMOR

Solid-pseudopapillary tumor (SPT) is a benign or low grade malignant neoplasm predominantly seen in young women and previously called a variety of names including solid cystic tumors, papillary cystic tumors, benign or malignant papillary neoplasms, solid and papillary epithelial neoplasms, and solid and cystic acinar cell tumors.[99-104] The name solid-cystic tumor was based on its macroscopic features, while papillary-cystic or solid and papillary tumor is related to the histologic features. The name SPT proposed by the WHO and AFIP classifications adequately represents the two most prominent histologic features, a mixture of solid and pseudopapillary regions.[63,105] The vast majority of SPTs are benign with a few exceptions.[102,106] The histological presence of vascular invasion, perineual invasion, and pancreatic parenchymal invasion shows the malignant potential, but even without these features of malignancy this tumor may behave as a malignancy. In reality, the malignant potential of SPT is neither fully understood nor predictable even with histologically benign tumors.[107]

Immunohistochemical demonstration of α1-antitrypsin in tumor cells indicates the possible acinar cell origin of SPTs, and neuron specific enolase and pancreatic hormones the endocrine cell origin. Also, electron microscopic demonstration of zymogen-like granules suggests the acinar cell origin, intercellular lumina with microvilli the ductular origin, and neurosecretory granules the endocrine cell origin.[100,103,104,108-113] Despite all these previous reports, the origin of SPT cells remains obscure. The expression of epithelial as well as mesenchymal markers, and the occasional presence of exocrine and endocrine features would suggest omnipotent stem cells as the origin of SPTs. In this context, Mao et al.[114] proposed a name of pancreatic embryonic tumor representing the omnipotent nature of ductular-centroacinar cell component during embryogenesis. However, the stem cell hypothesis does not explain the strong female preponderance (male <10%) of SPT. Increased levels of estrogen and/or progesterone receptors and enhanced growth of an SPT in a pregnant woman were reported,[115-120] whereas contradictory results were also described.[121,122] Abnormality in sex chromosomes may be important,[123] but further studies on the origin of this tumor are warranted.

Clinical symptoms of SPTs are nonspecific. Quite rarely, rupture of the capsule of SPT may result in hemoperitoneum as seen in 8 of 292 patients collected from the world literature.[114] Plain radiographs may show the tumor contour and/or calcification of the tumor. Cross section imagings (ultrasonography and computed tomography) demonstrate sharply demarcated solid and cystic masses without internal septa, which can be divided into three types, i.e. solid, mixed and cystic.[124] The completely solid type accounts for only 5.6% of 285 patients.[114] The others are at least partly cystic, and thus this tumor is always listed as one of cystic neoplasms of the pancreas. MRI depicts a multilocular tumor with high intensity areas on T2 images. MRCP shows a mass effect to cause deviation of the pancreatic ductal system.

The cells of SPT have two components, those with clear cytoplasm and eosinophilic cytoplasm. In both components, the uniform polygonal cells are arranged along delicate and often hyalinized fibrovascular stalks, resembling rosettes or ducts. The spaces between the pseudopapillary structures comprise red blood cells. Mitoses are rare, but in malignant SPT they may be prominent as well as vascular invasion. The tumor cells do not contain glycogen or mucin, but occasionally eosinophilic, diastase-resistant, PAS positive globes of varying size. Positive staining of immunohistochemical markers alpha-1-antitrypsin, alpha-1-antichymotrypsin, NSE, and vimentin is diagnostic of SPT. Alpha-1-antitrypsin also stains the aforementioned PAS positive globules. Some tumor cells of SPT may be stained by grimelius. DNA flow cytometry shows a diploid DNA pattern in benign SPTs but may show aneuploidy in metastasizing SPTs.[117,125] One study showed that in a malignant case the initial tumor and the first recurrent tumor showed a diploid result, but tumors in the second and third recurrences showed aneuploidy.[126] Positive synaptophysin stain may also be related to recurrence.[126]

Surgical resection is curative in 95% of patients with SPT.[121,127,128] Only a few patients suffer from recurrence and/or metastasis and a small proportion of them die of the disease.[100,101,129-134] Although the criteria of malignant SPT have not been established, unequivocal perineural invasion or angioinvasion, with or without deep invasion into the pancreatic parenchyma or peripancreatic tissue, and metastatic deposits indicate malignant behavior. Nishihara et al.[106] compared the histopathologic features of 3 metastasizing and 19 non-metastasizing SPTs and claimed that the degree of nuclear atypia, venous invasion, mitotic rate and prominence of necrobiotic cell nests (cells with pyknotic nuclei and eosinophilic cytoplasm) were useful indicators of malignancy. Thick capsules and aneuploidy of DNA histogram were also reported to be related to malignant potential.[135] The frequency of malignant SPT was 14.7% as suggested by 22 metastases (liver and/or peritoneal dissemination in 20, lymph node in 2) and 18 direct invasions (e.g. vessels, spleen, stomach, duodenum) in 292 patients collected from the world literature.[114] Even without all these findings a benign-appearing SPT may possibly show malignant behavior, thus featuring as a borderline malignancy.

DERMOID CYST

A dermoid cyst is an extremely rare cystic neoplasm of the pancreas, occurring at any age. This is a kind of teratoma taking a cystic form, i.e., "cystic teratoma" in other words,[136,137] one of the three entities included in "squamous-lined cysts of the pancreas", i.e. lymphoepithelial cyst, dermoid cyst, and epidermoid cyst in an intrapancreatic accessory spleen, proposed by Adsay et al.[138] The most recent review identified only 35 patients with a dermoid cyst in the world literature.[139] There is no preponderance in either gender. Most of the patients are asymptomatic, but this lesion may cause abdominal and/or back pain, nausea, vomiting, and palpable mass when it grows huge and causes a mass effect. It may arise from any part of the pancreas. Persistently high levels of serum CA19-9 has been reported in a patient with a dermoid cyst.[140] Cross section images show solid components in a cystic lesion often associated with calcification and adipose components. EUS and FNA cytology have recently been shown to be an effective adjunct for the preoperative diagnosis, yielding cyst fluid containing numerous benign, mature squamous cells, keratin debris and inflammatory cells.[141]

Surgical resection is the standard therapy to cure dermoid cyst and in order to exclude malignancy.[142] The presence of skin appendages (hair, sebaceous gland, etc.) or mesenchymal elements (bone, cartilage, nerve, etc.) in the cyst is characteristic of dermoid cyst.[137] Histologically, mucinous epithelium, respiratory-type mucosa and sebaceous units are identifiable in dermoid cysts.[138]

REFERENCES

1. Reid-Lombardo KM, St Sauver J, Li Z, Ahrens WA, Unni KK, Que FG. Incidence, prevalence, and management of intraductal papillary mucinous neoplasm in Olmsted County, Minnesota, 1984-2005: a population study. Pancreas. 2008;37:139-44.
2. Kloppel G, Solcia, E, Longnecker DS, Capella C, Sobin LH. World Health Organization International Histological Typing of Tumors of the Exocrine Pancreas. Berlin: Springer-Verlag; 1996. pp. 1-61.
3. Longnecker DS AG, Hruban RH, Kloppel G. Intraductal papillary-mucinous neoplasms of the pancreas. In: Hamilton SR, Aaltonen LA (Eds). World Health Organization Classification of Tumors. Pathology and Genetics of Tumors of the Digestive System. Lyon: IARC Press; 2000. pp. 237-41.
4. Tanaka M, Chari S, Adsay V, Fernández-del Castillo C, Falconi M, Shimizu M, et al. International consensus guidelines for management of intraductal papillary mucinous neoplasms and mucinous cystic neoplasms of the pancreas. Pancreatology. 2006;6:17-32.
5. Tanaka M, Fernández-del Castillo C, Adsay V, Chari S, Falconi M, Jang J-Y, et al. International consensus guidelines 2012 for the management of IPMN and MCN of the pancreas. Pancreatology. 2012:12:183-97.
6. Ohhashi K, Tajiri H, Gondo M, Yokoyama Y, Maruyama M, Takekoshi T, et al. A report of a resected case of pancreatic cystadenocarcinoma forming choledochopancreatic fistula. Prog Digest Endosc. 1980;17:261-4.
7. Ohhashi K, Murakami Y, Maruyama M, et al. Four cases of mucous secreting pancreatic cancer. Prog Digest Endosc. 1982;20:348-51 (in Japanese with English abstract).
8. Furuta K, Watanabe H, Ikeda S. Differences between solid and duct-ectatic types of pancreatic ductal carcinomas. Cancer. 1992;69:1327-33.
9. Kimura W, Sasahira N, Yoshikawa T, Muto T, Makuuchi M. Duct-ectatic type of mucin producing tumor of the pancreas—new concept of pancreatic neoplasia. Hepatogastroneterology. 1996;43:692-709.
10. Tanaka M. Intraductal papillary mucinous neoplasm of the pancreas: diagnosis and treatment. Pancreas. 2004;28:282-8. Tanaka M Pancreatology 2006;6:17-32.
11. Yamaguchi K, Chijiiwa K, Shimizu S, Yokohata K, Tanaka M. Intraductal papillary neoplasm of the pancreas: a clinical review of 13 benign and four malignant conditions. Eur J Surg. 1999;165: 223-9.
12. Obara T, Maguchi H, Saitoh Y, Ura H, Koike Y, Kitazawa S, et al. Mucin-producing tumor of the pancreas: a unique clinical entity. Am J Gastroenterol. 1991;86:1619-25.
13. Ringold DA, Shroff P, Sikka SK, Ylagan L, Jonnalagadda S, Early DS, et al. Pancreatitis is frequent among patients with side-branch intraductal papillary mucinous neoplasia diagnosed by EUS. Gastrointest Endosc. 2009;70:488-94.
14. Pelletier AL, Hammel P, Rebours V, Couvelard A, Vullierme MP, Maire F, et al. Acute pancreatitis in patients operated on for intraductal papillary mucinous neoplasms of the pancreas: frequency, severity, and clinicopathologic correlations. Pancreas. 2010;39:658-61.
15. Tsutsumi K, Ohtsuka T, Oda Y, Sadakari Y, Mori Y, Aishima S, et al. A history of acute pancreatitis in intraductal papillary mucinous neoplasms of the pancreas is a potential predictive factor for malignant papillary subtype. Pancreatology. 2012;10:707-12.
16. Adsay VN, et al. Intraductal neoplasm of the pancreas. In: Bosman FT, et al. (Eds). WHO Classification of Tumors of Digestive System. Lyon: WHO Press; 2010. pp. 304-13.
17. Nakagohri T, Asano T, Kenmochi T, Urashima T, Ochiai T. Long-term surgical outcome of noninvasive and minimally invasive intraductal papillary mucinous adenocarcinoma of the pancreas. World J Surg. 2002;26:1166-9.
18. Takahashi H, Nakamori S, Nakahira S, Tsujie M, Takahshi Y, Marubashi S, et al. Surgical outcomes of noninvasive and minimally invasive intraductal papillary-mucinous neoplasms of the pancreas. Ann Surg Oncol. 2006;13:955-60.
19. Nara S, Shimada K, Kosuge T, Kanai Y, Hiraoka N. Minimally invasive intraductal papillary-mucinous carcinoma of the pancreas: clinicopathologic study of 104 intraductal papillary-mucinous neoplasms. Am J Surg Pathol. 2008;32:243-55.
20. Kang MJ, Lee KB, Jang JY, Kwon W, Park JW, Chang YR, et al. Disease spectrum of intraductal papillary mucinous neoplasm with an associated invasive carcinoma: Invasive IPMN versus pancreatic ductal adenocarcinoma-associated IPMN. Pancreas. 2013;42(8):1267-74.
21. Nakata K, Ohuchida K, Aishima S, Sadakari Y, Kayashima T, Miyasaka Y, et al. Invasive carcinoma derived from intestinal-type intraductal papillary mucinous neoplasm is associated with minimal invasion, colloid carcinoma, and less invasive behavior, leading to a better prognosis. Pancreas. 2011;40:581-7.
22. Sessa F, Solcia E, Capella C, Bonato M, Scarpa A, Zamboni G, et al. Intraductal papillary-mucinous tumours represent a distinct group of pancreatic neoplasms: An investigation of tumour cell differentiation and K-ras, p53 and c-erbB2 abnormalities in 26 patients. Virchows Arch Pathol Anat. 1994;425:357-67.
23. Adsay NV, Merati K, Basturk O, Iacobuzio-Donahue C, Levi E, Cheng JD, et al. Pathologically and biologically distinct types of epithelium in intraductal papillary mucinous neoplasms: delineation of an "intestinal" pathway of carcinogenesis in the pancreas. Am J Surg Pathol. 2004;28:839-48.
24. Furukawa T, Klöppel G, Adsay NV, Albores-Saavedra J, Fukushima N, Horii A, et al. Classification of types of intraductal papillary-mucinous neoplasm of the pancreas: a consensus study. Virchows Arch. 2005;447:794-9.
25. Furukawa T, Hatori T, Fujita I, Yamamoto M, Kobayashi M, Ohike N, et al. Prognostic relevance of morphological types of intraductal papillary mucinous neoplasms of the pancreas. Gut. 2011;60:509-16.
26. Sadakari Y, Ohuchida K, Nakata K, Ohtsuka T, Aishima S, Takahata S, et al. Invasive carcinoma derived from the nonintestinal type intraductal papillary mucinous neoplasm of the pancreas has a poorer prognosis than that derived from the intestinal type. Surgery. 2010;147:812-7.
27. Nagayoshi Y, Aso T, Ohtsuka T, Kono H, Ideno N, Igarashi H, et al. Peroral pancreatoscopy using a SpyGlass system for the assessment of intraductal papillary mucinous neoplasms of the pancreas. J Hepatobiliary Pancreat Sci. 2014;21(6):410-7.
28. Aso T, Ohtsuka T, Ideno N, Kono H, Nagayoshi Y, Mori Y, et al. Diagnostic significance of a dilated orifice of the duodenal papilla in intraductal papillary mucinous neoplasm of the pancreas. Gastrointest Endosc. 2012;76:313-20.
29. Yamaguchi K, Ogawa Y, Chijiiwa K, Tanaka M. Mucin-hypersecreting tumors of the pancreas: assessing the grade of malignancy preoperatively. Am J Surg. 1996;171:427-31.
30. Okada K, Imaizumi T, Hirabayashi K, Matsuyama M, Yazawa N, Dowaki S, et al. The distance of tumor spread in the main pancreatic duct of an intraductal papillary-mucinous neoplasm: where to resect and how to predict it. J Hepatobiliary Pancreat Sci. 2010;17:516-22.
31. Tanaka M, Yokohata K, Konomi H, Yamaguchi K, Chijiiwa K, Ohta M. Segmental balloon cytology for preoperative localization of in situ pancreatic cancer. Gastrointest Endosc. 1997;46:447-9.
32. Eguchi H, Ishikawa O, Ohigashi H, Sasaki Y, Yamada T, Nakaizumi A, et al. Histology in detecting continuous and skip type intraductal cancer existence for intraductal papillary mucinous carcinoma of the pancreas. Cancer. 2006;107:2567-75.

33. Mori Y, Ohtsuka T, Tamura K, Ideno N, Aso T, Kono H, et al. Intraoperative irrigation cytology of the remnant pancreas to detect remnant distinct pancreatic ductal adenocarcinoma in patients with intraductal papillary mucinous neoplasm undergoing partial pancreatectomy. Surgery. 2014;155(1):67-73.
34. Sadakari Y, Ienaga J, Kobayashi K, Miyasaka Y, Takahata S, Nakamura M, et al. Cyst size indicates malignant transformation in branch duct intraductal papillary mucinous neoplasm of the pancreas without mural nodules. Pancreas. 2010;39:232-6.
35. Tanaka M. Controversies in the management of pancreatic IPMN. Nat Rev Gastroenterol Hepatol. 2011;8:56-60.
36. Shimizu Y, Yamaue H, Maguchi H, Yamao K, Hirono S, Osanai M, et al. Predictors of malignancy in intraductal papillary mucinous neoplasm of the pancreas: analysis of 310 pancreatic resection patients at multiple high-volume centers. Pancreas. 2013;42:883-8.
37. Ohno E, Hirooka Y, Itoh A, Ishigami M, Katano Y, Ohmiya N, et al. Intraductal papillary mucinous neoplasms of the pancreas. Differentiation of malignant and benign tumors by endoscopic ultrasound findings of mural nodules. Ann Surg. 2009;249:628-34.
38. Ohno E, Itoh A, Kawashima H, Ishikawa T, Matsubara H, Itoh Y, et al. Malignant transformation of branch duct type intraductal papillary mucinous neoplasms of the pancreas based on contrast-enhanced endoscopic ultrasonography morphological changes: focus on malignant transformation of intraductal papillary mucinous neoplasm itself. Pancreas. 2012;41:855-62.
39. Yamaguchi K, Nakamura K, Yokohata K, Shimizu S, Chijiiwa K, Tanaka M. Pancreatic cyst as a sentinel of in situ carcinoma of the pancreas. Report of two cases. Int J Pancreatol. 1997;22:227-31.
40. Yamaguchi K, Ohuchida J, Ohtsuka T, Nakano K, Tanaka M. Intraductal papillary-mucinous tumor of the pancreas concomitant with ductal carcinoma of the pancreas. Pancreatology. 2002;2: 484-90.
41. Ingkakul T, Sadakari Y, Ienaga J, Satoh N, Takahata S, Tanaka M. Predictors of the presence of concomitant invasive ductal carcinoma in intraductal papillary mucinous neoplasm of the pancreas. Ann Surg. 2010;251:70-5.
42. Tada M, Kawabe T, Arizumi M, Togawa O, Matsubara S, Yamamoto N, et al. Pancreatic cancer in patients with pancreatic cystic lesions: a prospective study in 197 patients. Clin Gastroenterol Hepatol. 2006;4:1265-70.
43. Uehara H, Nakaizumi A, Ishikawa O, Iishi H, Tatsumi K, Takakura R, et al. Development of ductal carcinoma of the pancreas during follow-up of branch duct intraductal papillary mucinous neoplasm of the pancreas. Gut. 2008;57:1561-5.
44. Kanno A, Satoh K, Hirota M, Hamada S, Umino J, Itoh H, et al. Prediction of invasive carcinoma in branch type intraductal papillary mucinous neoplasms of the pancreas. J Gastroenterol. 2010;45:952-9.
45. Tanno S, Nakano Y, Sugiyama Y, Nakamura K, Sasajima J, Koizumi K, et al. Incidence of synchronous and metachronous pancreatic carcinoma in 168 patients with branch duct intraductal papillary mucinous neoplasm. Pancreatology. 2010;10:173-8.
46. Tanno S, Nakano Y, Koizumi K, Sugiyama Y, Nakamura K, Sasajima J, et al. Pancreatic ductal adenocarcinomas in long-term follow-up patients with branch duct intraductal papillary mucinous neoplasms. Pancreas. 2010;39:36-40.
47. Ikeuchi N, Itoi T, Sofuni A, Itokawa F, Tsuchiya T, Kurihara T, et al. Prognosis of cancer with branch duct type IPMN of the pancreas. World J Gastroenterol. 2010;16:1890-5.
48. Sawai Y, Yamao K, Bhatia V, Chiba T, Mizuno N, Sawaki A, et al. Development of pancreatic cancers during long-term follow-up of side-branch intraductal papillary mucinous neoplasms. Endoscopy. 2010;42:1077-84.
49. Yamaguchi K, Kanemitsu S, Hatori T, Maguchi H, Shimizu Y, Tada M, et al. Pancreatic ductal adenocarcinoma derived from IPMN and pancreatic ductal adenocarcinoma concomitant with IPMN. Pancreas. 2011;40:571-80.
50. Maguchi H, Tanno S, Mizuno N, Hanada K, Kobayashi G, Hatori T, et al. Natural history of branch duct intraductal papillary mucinous neoplasms of the pancreas: a multicenter study in Japan. Pancreas. 2011;40:364-70.
51. Shi C, Klein AP, Goggins M, Maitra A, Canto M, Ali S, et al. Increased prevalence of precursor lesions in familial pancreatic cancer patients. Clin Cancer Res. 2009;15,7737-43.
52. Poley JW, Kluijt I, Gouma DJ, Harinck F, Wagner A, Aalfs C, et al. The yield of first-time endoscopic ultrasonography in screening individuals at a high risk of developing pancreatic cancer. Am J Gastroenterol. 2009;104,2175-81.
53. Yamaguchi K, Shimizu S, Yokohata K, Noshiro H, Chijiiwa K, Tanaka M. Ductal branch-oriented minimal pancreatectomy: two cases of successful treatment. J Hepatobiliary Pancreat Surg. 1999;6:69-73.
54. De Moor V, Arvanitakis M, Nagy N, Coppens E, Delhaye M, Closset J. Intraductal papillary mucinous neoplasms of the pancreas: clinicopathological features and long term outcome related to histopathological group. Hepatogastroenterology. 2012;59:565-9.
55. Wasif N, Bentrem DJ, Farrell JJ, Ko CY, Hines OJ, Reber HA, et al. Invasive intraductal papillary mucinous neoplasm versus sporadic pancreatic adenocarcinoma: a stage-matched comparison of outcomes. Cancer. 2010;116:3369-77.
56. Partelli S, Fernandez-Del Castillo C, Bassi C, Mantovani W, Thayer SP, Crippa S, et al. Invasive intraductal papillary mucinous carcinomas of the pancreas: predictors of survival and the role of lymph node ratio. Ann Surg. 2010;251:477-82.
57. Yopp AC, Katabi N, Janakos M, Klimstra DS, D'Angelica MI, DeMatteo RP, et al. Invasive carcinoma arising in intraductal papillary mucinous neoplasms of the pancreas: a matched control study with conventional pancreatic ductal adenocarcinoma. Ann Surg. 2011;253:968-74.
58. Kim J, Jang KT, Mo Park S, Lim SW, Kim JH, Lee KH, et al. Prognostic relevance of pathologic subtypes and minimal invasion in intraductal papillary mucinous neoplasms of the pancreas. Tumour Biol. 2011;32:535-42.
59. Mino-Kenudson M, Fernández-del Castillo C, Baba Y, Valsangkar NP, Liss AS, Hsu M, et al. Prognosis of invasive intraductal papillary mucinous neoplasm depends on histological and precursor epithelial subtypes. Gut. 2011;60:1712-20.
60. Distler M, Kersting S, Niedergethmann M, Aust DE, Franz M, Rückert F, et al. Pathohistological subtype predicts survival in patients with intraductal papillary mucinous neoplasm (IPMN) of the pancreas. Ann Surg. 2013;258:324-30.
61. Turrini O, Waters JA, Schnelldorfer T, Lillemoe KD, Yiannoutsos CT, Farnell MB, et al. Invasive intraductal papillary mucinous neoplasm: predictors of survival and role of adjuvant therapy. HPB (Oxford). 2010;12:447-55.
62. Yamao K, Yanagisawa A, Takahashi K, Kimura W, Doi R, Fukushima N, et al. Clinicopathological features and prognosis of mucinous cystic neoplasm with ovarian-type stroma: a multi-institutional study of the Japan pancreas society. Pancreas. 2011;40:67-71.
63. Kloeppel G, Solcia E, Longnecker DS, Capella C, Sobin LH. World Health Organization International Histological Classification of Tumours. Histological Typing of Tumours of the Exocrine Pancreas, 2nd edition. Berlin: Springer-Verlag; 1996. pp. 1-61.
64. Solcia E, Capella C, Kloeppel G. Tumors of the pancreas. In: Rosai J (Ed). Atlas of Tumor Pathology. Fascicle 20, 3rd Series. Washington DC: Armed Forces Institute of Pathology; 1997. pp. 1-262.
65. Wouters K, Ectors N, Van Steenbergen W, Aerts R, Driessen A, Van Hoe L, et al. A pancreatic mucinous cystadenoma in a man with mesenchymal stroma expressing oestrogen and progesterone receptors. Virchows Arch Pathol Anat. 1998;432:187-9.

66. Loftus ED Jr, Olivares-Pakad BA, Batts KP, Adkins MC, Stephens DH, Sarr MG, et al. Intraductal papillary-mucinous tumors of the pancreas: clinicopathologic features, outcome, and nomenclature. Gastroenterology. 1996;110:1909-18.
67. Thompson LDR, Becker RC, Przygodzki RM, Adair CF, Heffess CS. Mucinous cystic neoplasm (mucinous cystadenocarcinoma of low-grade malignant potential) of the pancreas. Am J Surg Pathol. 1999;23:1-16.
68. Margolis RM, Jang N. Zollinger-Ellison syndrome associated with pancreatic cystadenocarcinoma. N Engl J Med. 1984;311:1380-81, Baruch Y, Levy Y, Goldsher D, Munichor M, Eidelman S. Massive haematemesis—presenting symptoms of cystadenocarcinoma of the pancreas. Postgrad Med J. 1989;65:42-4.
69. Sperti C, Pasquali C, Davoli C, Polverosi R, Pedrazzoli S. Mucinous cystadenoma of the pancreas as a cause of acute pancreatitis. Hepatogastroenterology. 1998;45:2421-4.
70. Nakamura M, Nagayoshi Y, Kono H, Mori Y, Ohtsuka T, Takahata S, et al. Lateral approach for laparoscopic splenic vessel-preserving distal pancreatectomy. Surgery. 2011;150:326-31.
71. Song KB, Kim SC, Park JB, Kim YH, Jung YS, Kim MH, et al. Single-center experience of laparoscopic left pancreatic resection in 359 consecutive patients: changing the surgical paradigm of left pancreatic resection. Surg Endosc. 2011;25:3364-72.
72. Adam J-P, Jacquin A, Laurent C, Collet D, Masson B, Fernández-Cruz L, et al. Laparoscopic spleen-preserving distal pancreatectomy: splenic vessel preservation compared with the Warshaw technique. Arch Surg. 2012;19:1-7.
73. Didolkar MSD, Malhotra Y, Holyoke ED, Elias G. Cystadenoma of the pancreas. Surg Gynecol Obstet. 1975;140:925-8.
74. Nakamoto M, Minagawa N, Yamaguchi K. Serous cystadenoma of the pancreas showing enlargement on images: a case report. J UOEH. 2012;34:201-6.
75. Compagno J, Oertel JE. Microcystic adenomas of the pancreas (glycogen-rich cystadenomas). A clinicopathologic study of 34 cases. Am J Clin Pathol. 1978;69:289-98.
76. Kimura W, Moriya T, Hirai I, Hanada K, Abe H, Yanagisawa A, et al. Multicenter study of serous cystic neoplasm of the Japan pancreas society. Pancreas. 2012;41:380-7.
77. Tanno S, Obara T, Sohma M, Tanaka T, Izawa T, Fujii T, et al. Multifocal serous cystadenoma of the pancreas. A case report and review of the literature. Int J Pancreatol. 1998;24:129-2.
78. Lewandrowski K, Warshaw A, Compton C. Macrocystic serous cystadenoma of the pancreas: a morphologic variant differing from microcystic adenoma. Hum Pathol. 1992;23:871-5.
79. Huh JR, Chi JG, Jung KC, Choe KJ, Yoon YB. Macrocystic serous cystadenoma of pancreas: a case report. J Kor Med Sci. 1994;9:78-85. Gouhiri M, Soyer P, Barbagelatta M, Rymer R. Macrocystic serous cystadenoma of the pancreas: CT and endosonographic features. Abdom Imaging. 1999;24:72-4.
80. Egawa N, Maillet B, Schršder S, Mukai K, Klšppel G. Serous oligocystic and ill-demarcated adenoma of the pancreas: a variant of serous cystic adenoma of the pancreas. Virchows Arch Pathol Anat. 1994;424:13-7.
81. Inoue K, Yamaguchi K, Shimizu S, Yokohata K, Chijiiwa K, Tanaka M. Serous cystadenoma of the pancreas with atypical imaging features: a new variant of serous cystadenoma. Int J Pancreatol. 1997;16:102-6.
82. Perez-Ordonez B, Naseem A, Lieberman PH, Klimstra DS. Solid serous adenoma of the pancreas. The solid variant of serous cystadenoma? Am J Surg Pathol. 1996;20:1401-5.
83. Yamaguchi K, Hirakata R, Kitamura K. Serous cystadenoma of the pancreas: radiologic and clinicopathologic features in seven cases. Gastroenterol Jpn. 1990;25:607-12.
84. Fugazzola C, Procacci C, Bergano Andreis IA, Iacono C, Portuese A, Dompier P, et al. Cystic tumor of the pancreas: evaluation by ultrasonography and computed tomography. Gastrointest Radiol. 1991;16:53-61.
85. Warshaw AL, Compton CC, Lewandrowski K, Cardenosa G, Mueller PR. Cystic tumors of the pancreas: new clinical, pathologic, and pathologic observations in 67 patients. Ann Surg. 1990;212:432-45.
86. Inoue K, Yamaguchi K, Shimizu S, Yokohata K, Chijiiwa K, Tanaka M. Serous cystadenoma of the pancreas with atypical imaging features: a new variant of serous cystadenoma. Int J Pancreatol. 1997;16:102-6.
87. Pitman MB, Lewandrowski K, Shen J, Sahani D, Brugge W, Fernandez-del Castillo C. Pancreatic cysts: preoperative diagnosis and clinical management. Cancer Cytopathol. 2010;118:1-13.
88. Huh JR, Chi JG, Jung KC, Choe KJ, Yoon YB. Macrocystic serous cystadenoma of pancreas: a case report. J Kor Med Sci. 1994;9:78-85.
89. Egawa N, Maillet B, Schršder S, Mukai K, Klšppel G. Serous oligocystic and ill-demarcated adenoma of the pancreas: a variant of serous cystic adenoma of the pancreas. Virchows Arch Pathol Anat. 1994;424:13-7.
90. Neumann HP, Dinkel E, Brambs H, Wimmer B, Friedburg H, Volk B, et al. Pancreatic lesions in the von Hippel-Lindau syndrome. Gastroenterology. 1991;101:465-71.
91. Hough DM, Stephens DH, Johnson CD, Binkovitz LA. Pancreatic lesions in von Hippel-Lindau disease: prevalence, clinical significance, and CT findings. AJR Am J Roentgenol. 1994;162:1091-4.
92. Hammel PR, Vilgrain V, Terris B, Penfornis A, Sauvanet A, Correas JM, et al. Pancreatic involvement in von Hippel-Lindau disease. The Groupe Francophone d'Etude de la Maladie de von Hippel-Lindau. Gastroenterology. 2000;119:1087-95.
93. Doll DC, List AF, Yarbro JW. Evan's syndrome associated with microcystic adenoma of the pancreas. Cancer. 1987;59:1366-8.
94. Montag AG, Fossati N, Michelassi F. Pancreatic microcystic adenoma coexistent with pancreatic ductal carcinoma. A report of two cases. Am J Surg Pathol. 1990;14:352-5.
95. Lonser RR, Glenn GM, Walther M, Chew EY, Libutti SK, Linehan WM, et al. von Hippel-Lindau disease. Lancet. 2003;361:2059-67.
96. Ishikawa T, Nakao A, Nomoto S, Hosono J, Harada A, Nonami T, et al. Immunohistochemical and molecular biological studies of serous cystadenoma of the pancreas. Pancreas. 1998;16:40-4.
97. Weber AWS, Serrano FB, Cueto JG, Rodriguez GW. Laparoscopic treatment of pancreatic serous cystadenoma. Surg Laparosc Endosc. 1994;4:304-7.
98. Nakamura M, Nagayoshi Y, Kono H, Mori Y, Ohtsuka T, Takahata S, et al. Lateral approach for laparoscopic splenic vessel-preserving distal pancreatectomy. Surgery. 2011;150:326-31.
99. Kissane JM. Tumors of the exocrine pancreas in childhood. In: Humphrey GB, Grindey GB, Dehner LP, Acton RT, Pysher TJ (Eds). Cancer Treatment and Research. Hague/Boston/London: Martinus Nijhoff Publishers; 1982. pp. 99-129.
100. Oertel JE, Mendelsohn G, Compagno J. Solid and papillary epithelial neoplasms of the pancreas. In: Humphrey GB, Grindey GB, Dehner LP, Acton RT, Pysher TJ (Eds). Cancer Treatment and Research. Hague/Boston/London: Martinus Nijhoff Publishers; 1982. pp. 167-86.
101. Cubilla AL, Fitzgerald PJ. Tumors of the excorine pancreas. In: Hartmann WH (Eds). Atlas of Tumor Pathology. Washington, DC: Armed Forces Institute of Pathology; 1984. pp. 1-287.
102. Compagno J, Oertle JE, Kremzar M. Solid and papillary epithelial neoplasm of the pancreas. Lab Invest. 1979;40:248-9.
103. Lieber MR, Lack EE, Roberts JR, Merino MJ, Patterson K, Restrepo C, et al. Solid and papillary epithelial neoplasm of the pancreas. An ultrastructural and immunohistochemical study of six cases. Am J Surg Pathol. 1987;11:85-93.
104. Kloeppel G, Morohoshi T, John HD, Oehmichen W, Opitz K, Angekort A, et al. Solid and cystic acinar cell tumour of the

pancreas. A tumour in young women with favorable prognosis. Virchows Arch Pathol Anat. 1981;392:171-83.
105. Solcia E, Capella C, Klšppel G. Tumors of the pancreas. In: Rosai J (Ed). Atlas of Tumor Pathology. Washington DC: Armed Forces Institute of Pathology; 1997. pp. 1-262.
106. Nishihara K, Nagoshi M, Tsuneyoshi M, Yamaguchi K, Hayashi I. Papillary cystic tumors of the pancreas. Assessment of their grade of malignant potential. Cancer. 1993;71:82-92.
107. Park JK, Cho EJ, Ryu JK, Kim YT, Yoon YB. Natural history and malignant risk factors of solid pseudopapillary tumors of the pancreas. Postgrad Med. 2013;125:92-9.
108. Taxy JB. Adenocarcinoma of the pancreas in childhood. Report of a case and a review of the English literature. Cancer. 1976;37: 1508-18.
109. Boor PJ, Swanson MR. Papillary-cystic neoplasm of the pancreas. Am J Surg Pathol. 1979;3:69-75.
110. Benjamin E, Wright DH. Adenocarcinoma of the pancreas of childhood: a report of two cases. Histopathology. 1980;4:87-104.
111. Hamoudi AB, Misugi K, Grosfeld JL, Reiner CB. Papillary epithelial neoplasm of the pancreas in a child. Report of a case with electron microscopy. Cancer. 1970;26:1126-34.
112. Learmonth GM, Price SK, Visser AE, Emms M. Papillary and cystic neoplasm of the pancreas: an acinar cell tumour? Histopathology. 1985;9:63-79.
113. Schlosnagle DC, Campbell WG. The papillary and solid neoplasm of the pancreas: a report of two cases with electron microscopy, one containing neurosecretory granules. Cancer. 1981;47: 2603-10.
114. Mao C, Guvendi M, Domenico DR, Kim K, Thomford NR, Howard JM. Papillary cystic and solid tumors of the pancreas: a pancreatic embryonic tumor? Studies of three cases and cumulative review of the world's literature. Surgery. 1995;118:821-8.
115. Morales A, Ruiz Molina JM, Esteves HO, Robles-Diaz G, Diaz-Sanches V. Papillary-cystic neoplasm of the pancreas. A sex-steroid dependent tumor. Int J Pancreatol. 1998;24:219-25.
116. Ladanyi M, Mulay S, Arseneau J, Bettez P. Estrogen and progesterone receptor determination in the papillary cystic neoplasm of the pancreas. Cancer. 1987;60:1604-11.
117. Wrba F, Chott A, Ludvik B, Schratter M, Spona J, Reiner A, et al. Solid and cystic tumour of the pancreas: a hormonal-dependent neoplasm? Histopathology. 1988;12:338-40.
118. Stšmmer P, Kraus J, Stolte M, Giedl J. Solid and cystic pancreatic tumors. Clinical, histochemical and electron microscopic features in ten cases. Cancer. 1991;67:1635-41.
119. Carbone A, Ranelletti FO, Rinelli A, Vecchio FM, Lauriola L, Piantelli M, et al. Type II estrogen receptor in the papillary cystic tumor of the pancreas. Am J Clin Pathol. 1988;92:572-6.
120. Lee WY, Tzeng CC, Chen RM, Tsao CJ, Tseng JY, Jin YT. Papillary cystic tumors of the pancreas: assessment of malignant potential by analysis of progesterone receptor, flow cytometry, and ras oncogene mutation. Anticancer Res. 1997;17:2587-91.
121. Yamaguchi K, Miyagahara T, Tsuneyoshi M, Enjoji M, Horie A, Nakayama I, et al. Papillary cystic tumor of the pancreas: an immunohistochemical and ultrastructural study of 14 patients. Jpn J Clin Oncol. 1989;19:102-11.
122. Yamaguchi K, Miyagahara T, Tsuneyoshi M, Enjoji M, Horie A, Nakayama I, et al. Papillary cystic tumor of the pancreas. Is it a hormone-dependent neoplasm? Path Res Pract. 1993;189:521-6.
123. Matsubara K, Nigami H, Harigaya H, Baba K. Chromosome abnormality in solid and cystic tumor of the pancreas. Am J Gastroenterol. 1997;92:1219-21.
124. Friedman AC, Lichtenstein JE, Dachman AH. Cystic neoplasm of the pancreas. Radiological-pathological correlation. Radiology. 1983;149:45-50.
125. Cappellari JO, Geisinger KR, Albertson DA, Wolfman NT, Kute TE. Malignant papillary cystic tumor of the pancreas. Cancer. 1990;66:193-8.
126. Lai HW, Su CH, Li AF, Wu LH, Shyr YM, Chen TH, et al. Malignant solid and pseudopapillary tumor of the pancreas—clinicohistological, immunohistochemical, and flow cytometric evaluation. Hepatogastroenterology. 2006;53:291-5.
127. Yamaguchi K, Hirakata R, Kitamura K. Papillary cystic neoplasm of the pancreas: radiological and pathological characteristics in 11 cases. Br J Surg. 1990;77:1000-3.
128. Vassos N, Agaimy A, Klein P, Hohenberger W, Croner RS. Solid-pseudopapillary neoplasm (SPN) of the pancreas: case series and literature review on an enigmatic entity. Int J Clin Exp Pathol. 2013;6:1051-9.
129. Matsuda Y, Imai Y, Kawata S, Nishikawa M, Miyoshi S, Saito R, et al. Papillary-cystic neoplasm of the pancreas with multiple hepatic metastases: a case report. Gastroenterol Jpn. 1987;22:379-84.
130. Hernandez-Maldonado JJ, Rodriguez-Bigas MA, Gonzarez de Pesante A, Vazquez-Quintana E. Papillary cystic neoplasm of the pancreas: a report of a case presenting with carcinomatosis. Am Surg. 1989;55:552-9.
131. Matsunou H, Konishi F. Papillary-cystic neoplasm of the pancreas: a clinicopathologic study concerning the tumor aging and malignancy of nine cases. Cancer. 1990;65:283-91.
132. Sclafani LM, Reuter VE, Coit DG, Brennan MF. The malignant nature of papillary and cystic neoplasm of the pancreas. Cancer. 1991;68:153-8.
133. Jorgensen LJ, Hansen AB, Burcharth F, Philipsen E, Horn T. Solid and papillary neoplasm of the pancreas. Ultrastruct Pathol. 1992;16:659-66.
134. Horisawa M, Niinomi N, Sato T, Yokoi S, Oda K, Ichikawa M, et al. Frantz's tumor (solid and cystic tumor of the pancreas) with liver metastasis: successful treatment and long-term follow-up. J Ped Surg. 1995;30:724-6.
135. Cho NH, Go JH, Jung SH, Jung WH, Lee KK. Correlation between proliferating index and prognostic factors in papillary cystic tumors of the pancreas. J Kor Med Sci. 1995;10:342-51.
136. Mester M, Trajber HJ, Compton CC, de Camargo Júnior HS, de Almeida PC, Hoover HC Jr. Cystic teratomas of the pancreas. Arch Surg. 1990;125:1215-8.
137. Fernandez-Cebrian JM, Carda P, Morales V, Galindo J. Dermoid cyst of the pancreas: a rare cystic neoplasm. Hepatogastroenterology. 1998;45:1874-6.
138. Adsay NV, Hasteh F, Cheng JD, Klimstra DS. Squamous-lined cysts of the pancreas: lymphoepithelial cysts, dermoid cysts (teratomas), and accessory-splenic epidermoid cysts. Semin Diagn Pathol. 2000;17:56-65.
139. Lane J, Vance A, Finelli D, Williams G, Ravichandran P. Dermoid cyst of the pancreas: a case report with literature review. J Radiol Case Rep. 2012;6(12):17-25.
140. Micke O, Schafer U, Willich N. Persistent elevation of CA 19-9 levels in a patient with an extended retroperitoneal dermoid. Anticancer Res. 1999;19:2717-20.
141. Markovsky V, Russin VL. Fine-needle aspiration of dermoid cyst of the pancreas: a case report. Diagn Cytopathol. 1993;9:66-9.
142. Tucci G, Muzi MG, Nigro C, Cadeddu F, Amabile D, Servadei F, et al. Dermoid cyst of the pancreas: presentation and management. World J Surg Oncol. 2007;5:85.

CHAPTER 45

Neuroendocrine Tumors of the Pancreas

Vinay Gaikwad, Mahesh Goel, Bhawna Sirohi, Shailesh V Shrikhande

INTRODUCTION

After Oberndorfer coined the term "Karzinoide" which means "cancer-like" in 1907,[1] several advances have been made over the last century regarding the understanding and management of gastroenteropancreatic neuroendocrine tumors (GEP-NETs). Today, the term "neuroendocrine neoplasm" is considered appropriate since "carcinoid" does not account for the malignant potential of some of these tumors.[2] Pancreatic neuroendocrine tumors (pNETs), which are believed to arise from pancreatic islet cells, are low-grade to intermediate-grade neoplasms. These rare tumors account for less than 5% of pancreatic malignancies.[3]

Numerous classification systems have attempted to capture the diversity of these tumors. Recent large-scale collaborative trials have aided in enhancing our comprehension of the origin, molecular biology, and behavioral patterns of these tumors. Guidelines have been established and updated by various groups such as the European Neuroendocrine Tumour Society (ENETS),[4] the North American Neuroendocrine Tumor Society (NANETS)[5] and the United Kingdom Neuroendocrine Tumour Society (UKNETS),[6] some of which have been incorporated in different sections in this chapter. Detection or reporting of pNETs is rapidly increasing and therapeutic options are fast expanding, making this tumor type even more relevant for contemporary clinicians.[7]

EPIDEMIOLOGY

Early awareness regarding the diagnosis and reporting of neuroendocrine tumors (NETs) stemmed primarily from North America and Scandinavia. The reported incidence of primary pNETs according to the Surveillance, Epidemiology, and End Results (SEER) program, which spanned five decades, was 0.18–0.24 per 100,000 population. This was comparable to the 0.23 per 100,000 population incidence reported by the Norwegian Cancer Registry (NCR).[8] A study by the Mayo Clinic also found that the incidence of these tumors increase with age.[9] A similar annual incidence of 0.2 per 100,000 population has been reported from Hong Kong.[10] Data collection from India is currently ongoing, although available data indicate that this tumor type is not uncommon, and constitutes a significant entity among reported pancreatic neoplasms.[7,11-13]

PATHOLOGY

There exists heterogeneity in classification systems and pathological reporting, underscoring the ongoing evolution in the familiarity with these relatively rare tumors. Traditional classification based on differentiation divides pNETs into well-differentiated and poorly differentiated types, the latter being considered malignant. The well-differentiated tumors are further classified, based on the production of hormones (peptides/amines), into functional or nonfunctional tumors.[14] pNETs are usually solitary. Syndromes such as multiple endocrine neoplasia 1 (MEN 1) and von Hippel-Lindau syndrome should be suspected when multiple lesions are detected.[15]

Microscopically, well-differentiated tumors demonstrate organoid arrangements of uniform tumor cells. They display nesting, trabecular or gyriform patterns. These cells secrete profuse amounts of neurosecretory granules which cause strong and diffuse immunoexpression of chromogranin A and synaptophysin (Figs 1A to D). Poorly differentiated tumors have a more sheet-like or diffuse architecture with mitosis (Fig. 2). The cells have irregular nuclei with less cytoplasmic granularity which, in turn, demonstrate lesser immunoexpression of the neuroendocrine markers. Generally, infiltrating tumors more than 2 cm, the presence of angioinvasion, metastatic tumors and tumors with a high proliferative index portend a poorer prognosis.[2]

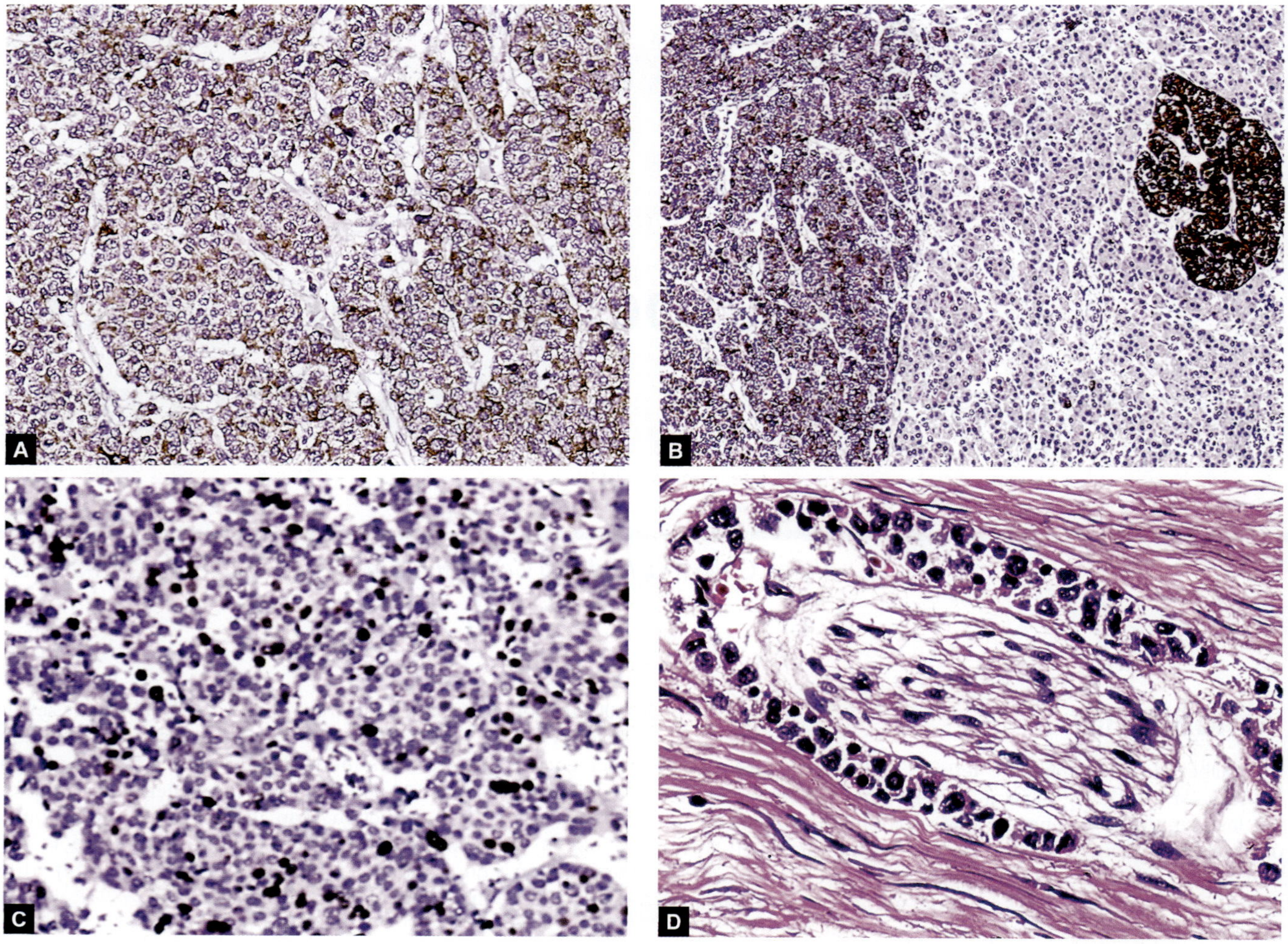

Figures 1A to D (A) Chromogranin staining, (B) Synaptophysin stain, (C) Showing high mib index, (D) Perineural infiltration

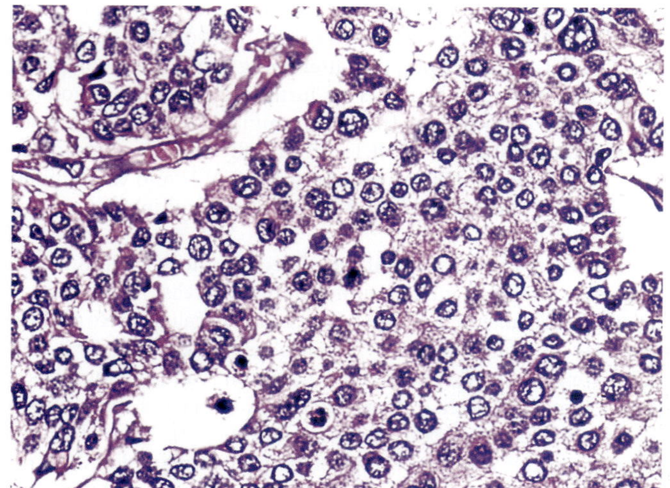

Figure 2 Showing sheet-like pattern with mitoses

In 2010, the World Health Organization (WHO) had updated its classification of GEP-NETs:[16]

I. Neuroendocrine tumor (NET)
   a. G1 (carcinoid)
   b. G2
II. Neuroendocrine carcinoma (NEC)
   a. G3 (large cell type)
   b. G3 (small cell type)
III. Mixed adenoneuroendocrine carcinoma (MANEC)
IV. Hyperplastic and preneoplastic lesions

Note: G indicates the grading which is provided in Table 1.

Table 1: Grading of pNETs

Grade	*Mitosis/10 HPF*	*Ki-67 labeling index (%)*
G1	<2	≤2
G2	2–20	3–20
G3	>20	>20

Other systems of classification include the ENETS classification,[17] the NANETS classification,[5] and a recently proposed classification by the Gastrointestinal Pathology Study Group of the Korean Society of Pathologists.[18]

STAGING

The two most widely used staging systems for pNETs are the American Joint Committee on Cancer (AJCC) staging and the ENETS staging.[19] The discrepancies between the two systems, especially of the T staging, may raise issues during evaluation of data using different systems. A simplified comparison of staging systems is provided in Table 2.

CLINICAL FEATURES

Nonfunctioning tumors, which are more common, are usually detected incidentally or found because of symptoms due to mass effect of the tumor. Tumors to the right of the superior mesenteric vessels produce symptoms of jaundice and gastric outlet obstruction while tumors to the left of the superior mesenteric vessels cause late onset of weight loss, cachexia and back pain. Pain is mainly due to invasion of the celiac axis or liver metastasis. Functioning tumors cause syndromes based on the hormones produced.[20] Table 3 summarizes the distribution, clinical presentations and survival of pNETs based on available epidemiological data.

SPECIFIC pNETs

The majority of pNETs are large, and around 50% are metastatic at presentation.[21] Forty percent of pNETs are nonfunctional, although with the increased understanding of this disease more nonfunctional tumors are being detected. Among functional tumors, insulinomas are the most common tumors, being typically hypervascular, small, solitary tumors. These tumors usually present with the well-known "Whipple's triad". Successful excision of these tumors leads to a normal life expectancy. Gastrinomas, which typically present within the gastrinoma triangle (bounded by the junction of common and cystic ducts superiorly, the second and third parts of duodenum inferiorly and head and neck of pancreas medially) (Fig. 3), are mostly highly malignant tumors.[20] They may present with the symptom-complex called Zollinger-Ellison syndrome. Between 70–80% of these tumors present with metastatic disease.[22] Glucagonomas are associated with the pathognomonic necrolytic migratory erythema. This is a red blistering rash which spreads over the lower abdomen, groin, buttocks and perineum. Blood sugar levels are hard to control and 50% mortality in these situations are due to thromboembolic

Table 2: Comparison of staging systems of pNETs

	AJCC	*ENETS*
T0	No evidence of primary tumor	
T1	Limited to the pancreas, ≤2 cm	Limited to the pancreas, <2 cm
T2	Limited to the pancreas, >2 cm	Limited to the pancreas, 2–4 cm
T3	Beyond the pancreas without involvement of celiac axis/SMA	Limited to the pancreas, >4 cm; invading duodenum or bile duct
T4	Celiac axis/SMA involvement	Involvement of other organs; celiac axis/SMA involvement
N0	No regional lymph node metastasis	
N1	Regional lymph node metastasis	
M0	No distant metastasis	
M1	Distant metastasis	

Table 3: Distribution, epidemiology, clinical characteristics and survival patterns of pNETs according to functionality

Tumor type	*%*	*Male:Female*	*Decade at diagnosis*	*Clinical features*	*Metastasis (%)*	*MEN-1 (%)*	*5-year survival rate (%)*
Nonfunctioning and PPoma	10–50	0.86:1	4th–5th	Mass effect	60	20–30	30–50
Insulinoma	20–30	0.7:1	5th	Neuroglucopenia, Whipple triad	10	5–10	80–95
Gastrinoma	15–20	1.5–2:1	6th	ZES (peptic ulcer, epigastric pain, diarrhea)	60–90	25	50–70
VIPoma	2–4	0.3:1	4th–5th	Watery diarrhea, hypokalemia, achlorhydria	80	10	40–50
Glucagonoma	1–3	1:1	5th	Necrolytic migratory erythema, diabetes mellitus, cachexia	80–90	5–17	50–60
Somatostatinoma	0–1	1:1	6th	Gallstones, diabetes mellitus, steatorrhea, achlorhydria	60–70	5–10	20–40

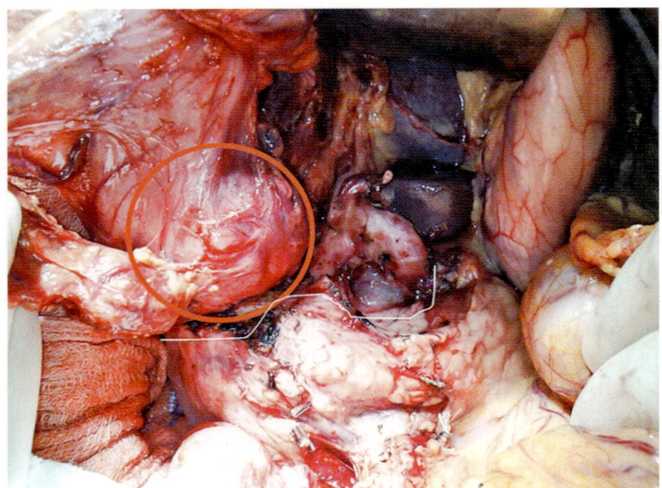

Figure 3 Intraoperative photograph of a G2 NET (encircled in orange) in the gastrinoma triangle bounded by the junction of common and cystic ducts superiorly, the second and third portions of duodenum inferiorly and head and neck of pancreas medially. The white line indicates the plane from where it was dissected away prior to resection

disease.[21] Reasonably good survival rates have been reported after surgery. VIPomas which are associated with Verner-Morrison syndrome, and somatostatinomas also have a good prognosis after surgery.

Investigations

Biochemical Tumor Markers

Serum Chromogranin A (Cg A) is a nonspecific but sensitive test. Cg A is an acidic glycoprotein expressed in the secretory granules of neuroendocrine cell types. Regarding measurement, enzyme-linked immunoadsorbent assay might be more sensitive than immunoradiometric assay.[23] The degree of elevation of this marker correlates well with the stage and extent of the disease, but not so well with the grade. Serum Cg A levels are found to elevate in 80–90% of pNETs, being elevated in 100% of gastrinomas and 70% of nonfunctioning tumors.[24] It has also been noted to be a good indicator for the response to treatment with somatostatin analogs and other therapeutic agents, a drop in the value indicating a better prognosis. Other conditions in which a raised serum Cg A level may be present include intake of proton-pump inhibitors, atrophic gastritis, acute pancreatitis, inflammatory bowel disease, renal failure, colon cancer, pancreatic cancer, hepatocellular carcinoma, and breast cancer.[25] These conditions should be taken into consideration, and proton-pump inhibitors should be stopped 2 weeks prior to sampling.

A 24-hour urinary 5-hydroxyindoleacetic acid (5-HIAA) which is a breakdown product of serotonin is also a helpful marker. Specific bioactive markers are also useful especially in functional tumors, usually suspected by relevant symptomatology.[26]

Immunohistochemical Markers

These markers aid in the diagnosis and prognostication of pNETs. Routine tissue staining with Ki-67 is recommended for all cases as this is essential for accurate classification.[14] Chromogranin and synaptophysin are recommended for diagnosis. Although not routinely recommended, other markers that can be used are chromogranin B, NCAM, CD57, CDX2, neuron-specific enolase and keratins.[27] These markers may help to identify tumor location and augment the diagnosis.

Imaging (Morphological)

A contrast-enhanced, multidetector computed tomography (MDCT) will display a heterogeneously or homogenously enhancing mass during the arterial and portal phases, without distortion of the contour of the pancreas, suggesting the presence of these highly vascular tumors.[28,29] A sensitivity of 94.4% has been reported by this modality[30] (Figs 4 and 5).

Magnetic resonance imaging (MRI) might be able to demonstrate lesions not detected on CT scan.[31] pNETs are usually seen as hypointense lesions in fat-suppressed T1-weighted images and hyperintense in T2-weighted images. Using gadolinium MRI scan a sensitivity of 91.6% has been reported. In contrast to cystic pancreatic neoplasms (when imaging findings are similar), a rim of enhancement with signal intensity different from the surrounding normal pancreatic parenchyma favors a pNET.[32,33] Either a CT scan or an MRI scan is a good initial imaging modality.

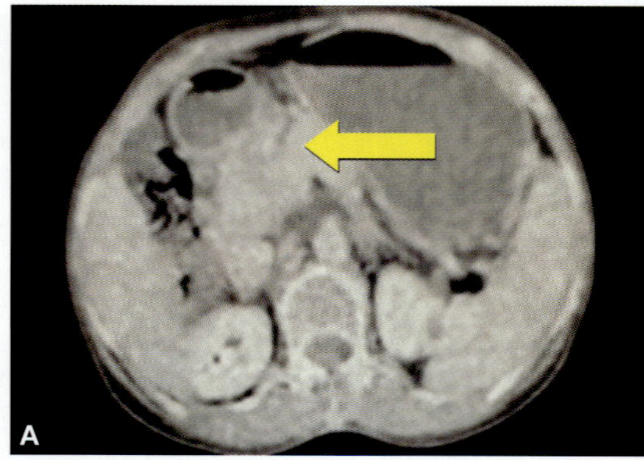

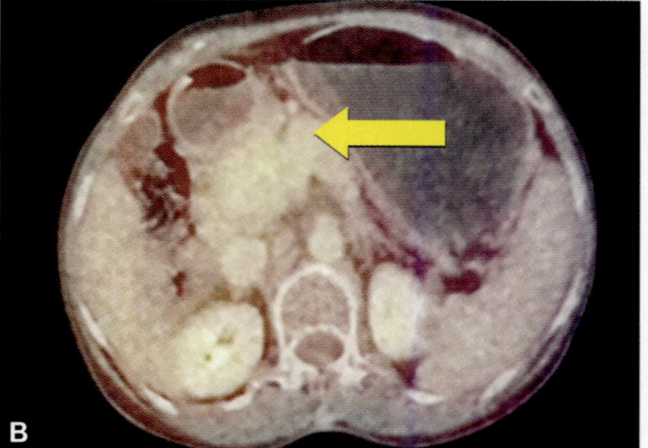

Figures 4A and B (A) Axial image of contrast enhanced CT scan showing a heterogeneous enhacing mass lesion in head of pancreas (yellow arrow). (B) The mass has DOTATEC uptake on DOTA PET scan suggestive of NET. Patient also had portal vein thrombosis

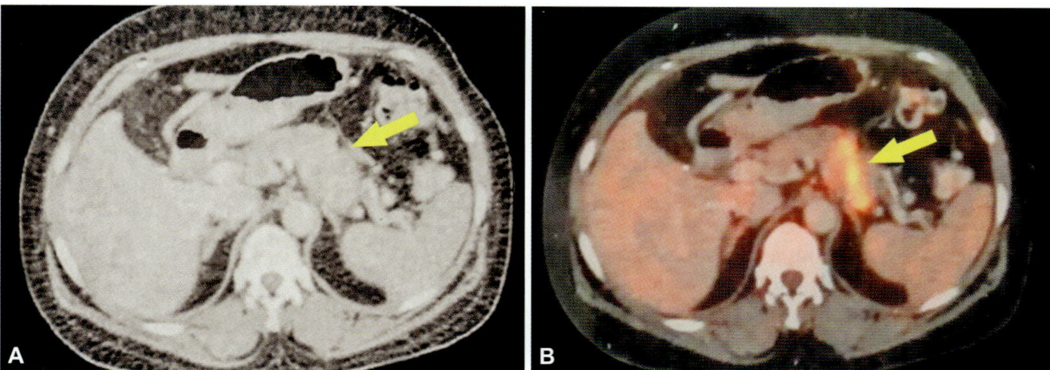

Figures 5A and B Axial section contrast enhanced CT scan showing a mass lesion in body and tail of pancreas. This patient had FDG avid tumor in body and tail of pancreas. The patient underwent radical distal pancreatectomy with splenectomy. The histopathology of tumor showed an NET with high Ki index (40–50%)

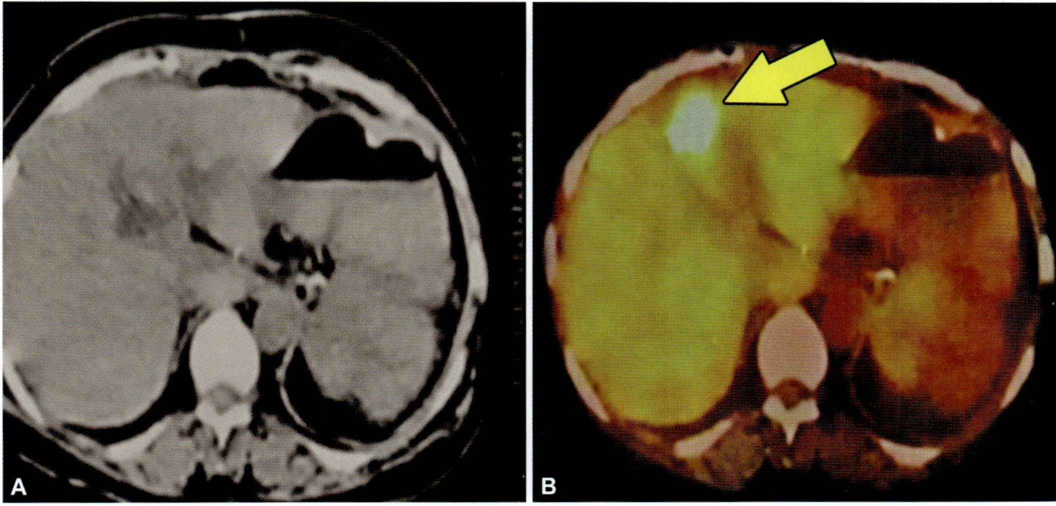

Figures 6A and B (A) Axial section of contrast enhanced CT scan done postoperatively did not show any local or systemic recurrence; (B) DOTATEC PET scan showed DOTATEC avid lesion in the liver suggestive of liver metastasis (yellow arrow) with no uptake in resection site. These lesions were not seen in preoperative FDG-PET scan

Endoscopic ultrasound (EUS) has been reported to have up to 95% sensitivity to pNETs.[34] A heterogenous echotexture is the feature most suggestive of tumors. This procedure is absolutely indicated in patients with MEN-1 because of the possibility of multifocality.[35] Fine needle aspiration via EUS has also been shown to have a sensitivity and diagnostic accuracy of up to 90%. Microscopic features showing a richly cellular aspirate with granular chromatin and plasmacytoid morphology aid in the diagnosis.[36,37] Contrast-enhanced sonography is superior to B-mode sonography for the detection of nonfunctioning pNETs.[38] There is also a correlation between the enhancement pattern and the Ki-67 index.

Imaging (Functional)

Somotostatin-receptor scintigraphy (SRS) using111-Indium-DTPA-octreotide is routinely recommended (along with CT scan or MRI) and is considered to be the gold standard in nuclear imaging of pNETs.[39] The sensitivity is between 60–90% but is lower for insulinomas. This scan should be used as the first staging modality, and can be used with therapeutic intent if uptake is present. A negative SRS indicates a worse prognosis. SRS is also the most sensitive modality for the detection of hepatic metastasis. Newer and perhaps better nuclear imaging modalities are up coming.

^{68}Ga-DOTA(0)-Phe(1)-Tyr(3)-octreotide positron emission tomography-computed tomography (68Ga-DOTATOC PET-CT) is a new modality about which evidence is generating.[40] (Figs 4B, 6A and B) One study even reports 100% sensitivity for detection of primary pNETs as well as metastatic disease.[41] Further evidence is required to substantiate this report, but this imaging modality is exciting also because it obviates the need for an in-house cyclotron. 6-[F]fluoro-3,4-dihydroxyphenylalanine (F-FDOPA) PET/CT is also showing promise.[42] The utility of these investigations, however, are presently limited due to the lack of widespread availability. The FDG-PET Scan is not routinely recommended for diagnosis of NET tumors, since it does not light up for NET tumors with a low proliferation index. Therefore it has a low sensitivity for diagnosis. But it may have a value in suggesting the grade of tumor without biopsy when combined with DOTA-PET scan. It has been seen that uptake on 18F-FDG PET occurs for tumors with a high proliferation index thereby suggesting presence of high grade tumor (Fig. 5B).

Treatment

A multidisciplinary approach cannot be overemphasized in the management of pNETs. It encompasses the diverse branches of surgical oncology, interventional radiology, radiation oncology, medical oncology, pathology and nuclear medicine. Thus treatment is tailored to suit the individual patient. Flow chart 1 outlines a proposed algorithm for treatment of patients with neuroendocrine liver metastasis (NELM).

Surgical Management

Surgery remains the modality of choice for cure in patients with limited disease. It has a role in cytoreduction and palliation as well.[43,44] Aggressive surgery, although universally thought to be the preferred approach for resectable disease,[45-47] has occasionally been questioned due to the lack of high-level evidence regarding its impact on local recurrence and metastasis.[48] Prospective studies, especially randomized ones, are sparse, primarily because of the relatively low patient numbers and lack of collaboration.

Although there is some conflicting evidence, surgery for localized disease seems not only justified, but only essential when a complete resection can be achieved with acceptable morbidity.[49-51] Based on the anatomical location in the pancreas and the tumor type, various resection procedures have been advocated. These include pancreatoduodenectomy with or without venous resection, distal pancreatectomy with or without splenectomy, median/central pancreatectomy and enucleation procedures. For pancreatic resection procedures, regional lymphadenectomy is recommended. Enucleation can be performed for benign lesions which are less than 2 cm and are away from the pancreatic duct (Fig. 7). Most of these tumors are insulinomas. Peripancreatic lymph node sampling is recommended. Intraoperative ultrasound is a useful tool especially for the detection of occult disease. An increasing number of reports of laparoscopic resection with acceptable results are now available.[52]

Flow chart 1 Suggested management algorithm for NELM

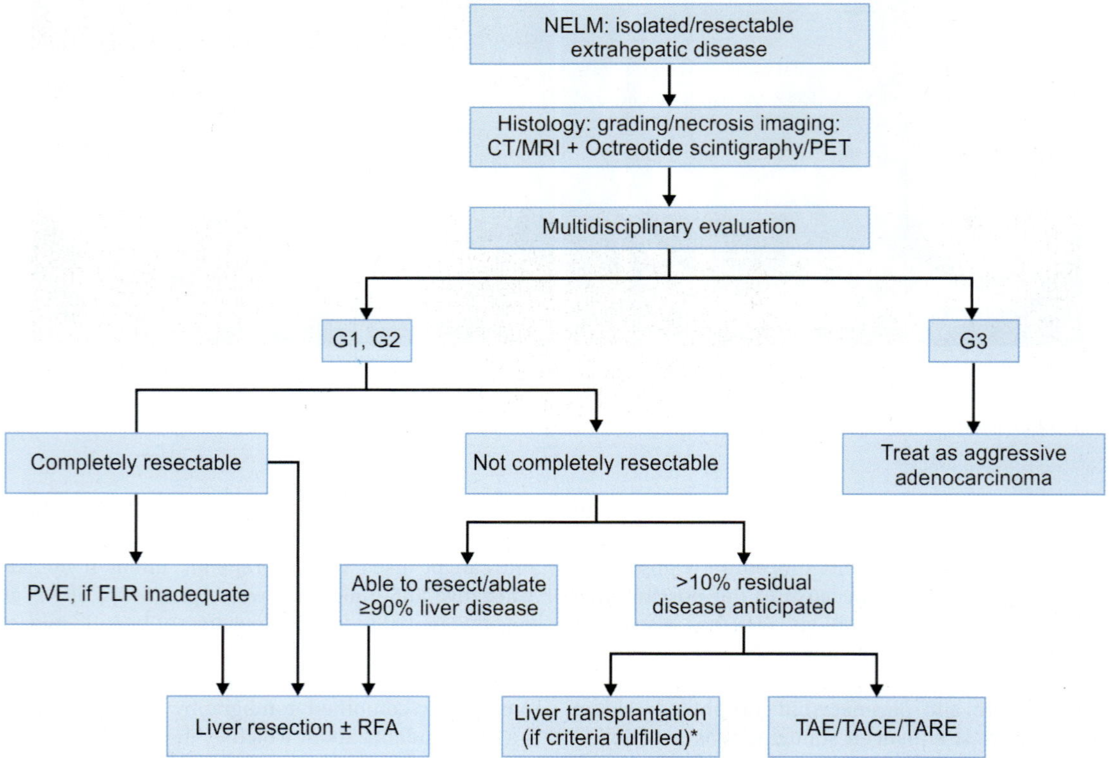

*Milan liver transplantation eligibility criteria for NELM:
Grade 1/2 NET
Primary tumor drained by portal system
>50% liver involvement by tumor
Good response/stable disease during pretransplantation period
Age ≤50 years
No medical/surgical contraindication, including previous tumors

More aggressive resections for pNETs have been performed involving vascular resection and involved contiguous organs (Figs 8A to D). Feasibility of these procedures with acceptable short-term and long-term outcomes has been reported.[53,54] Data on resection of the primary tumor in the presence of unresectable metastatic disease has been analyzed.[55,56] Although not without bias, studies indicate a possible benefit after these operations, stressing the need for randomized trials.

There is no doubt that liver metastasis from pNETs portends a worse prognosis; however, surgical resection has found a definite

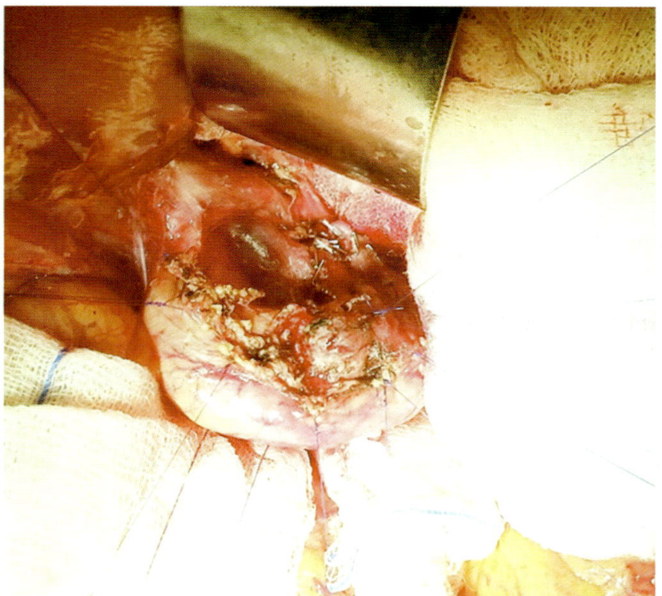

Figure 7 Intraoperative photograph of an enucleation of a G1 NET at the pancreatic neck-body junction at the superior border of the pancreas. The pancreatic neck has been dissected away from the common hepatic artery superiorly and the portal vein posteriorly

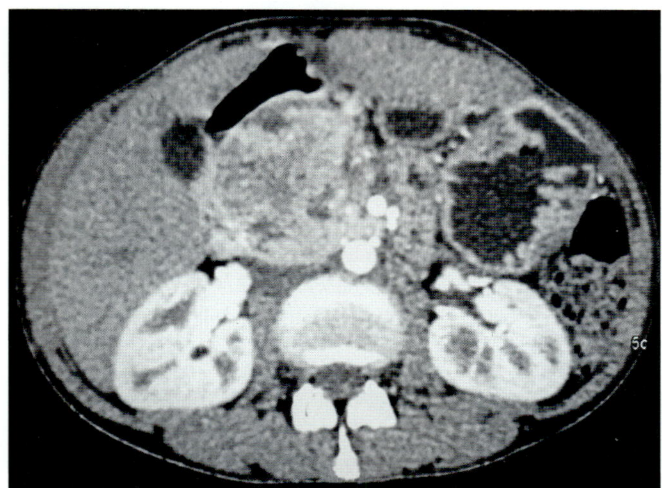

Figure 8A Showing large neuroendocrine tumor for which portal vein resection was required. MDCT axial view showing large pancreatic neuroendocrine tumor

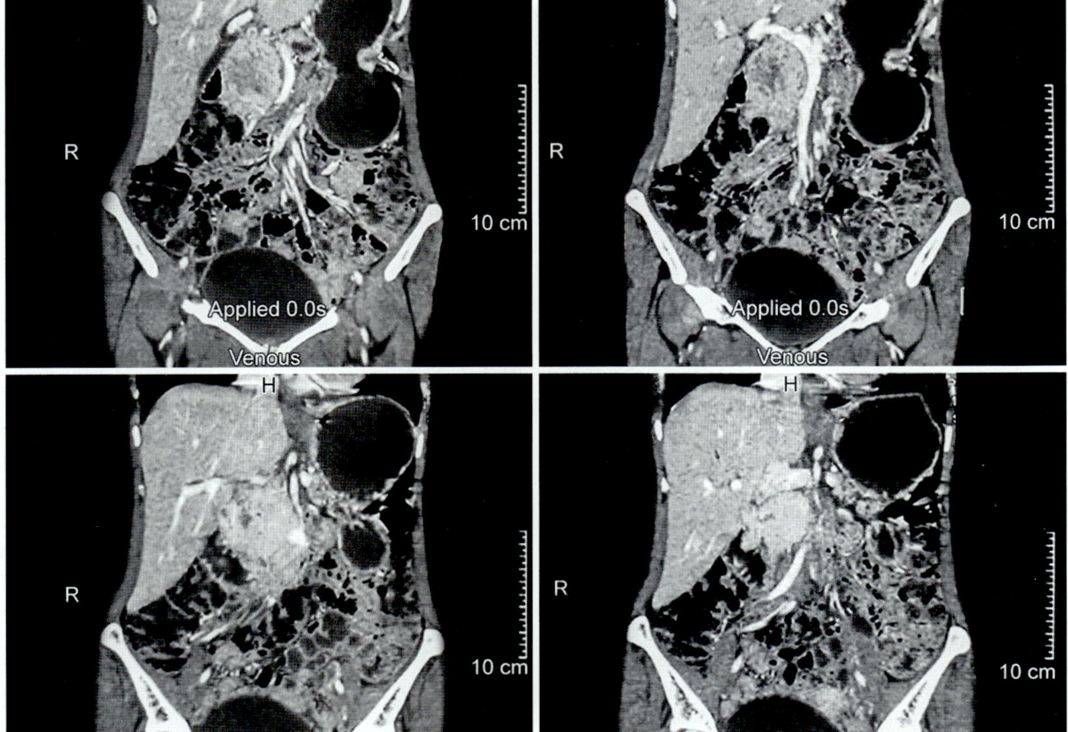

Figure 8B Showing large neuroendocrine tumor for which portal vein resection was required. MDCT axial view

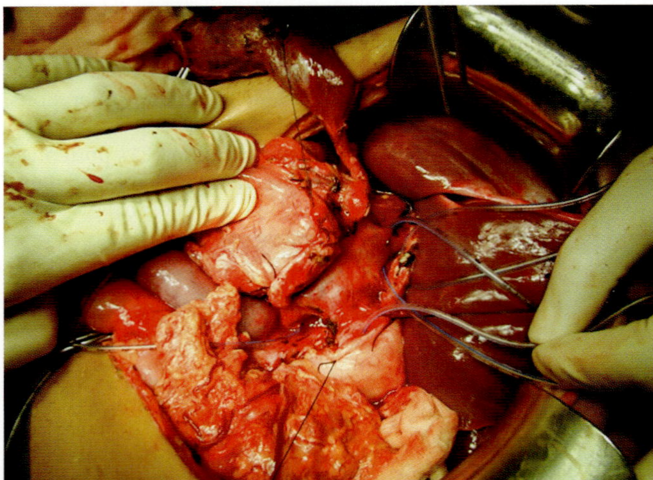

Figure 8C Showing large neuroendocrine tumor for which portal vein resection was required. Showing pancreatic transection above portal vein; sutures mark cut end of pancreas

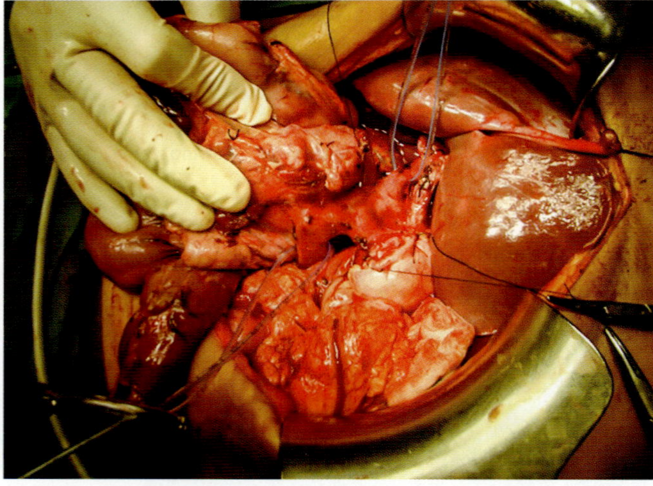

Figure 8D Showing large neuroendocrine tumor for which portal vein resection was required. Adherence to SMV. In preparation for transection, PV above and SMV below have been looped with infant feeding tubes

role in the management of this clinical scenario. Guidelines formulated by various groups support surgical therapy in specific situations.[5,57] The ENETS guidelines recommend surgery with curative intent in patients with resectable, well-differentiated liver-restricted metastatic disease, when the surgery can be performed with acceptable morbidity and less than 5% mortality. Debulking appears justified if more than 90% of the tumor mass can be removed.[58] Table 4 provides outcomes after liver resection.

More than 300 cases of orthotopic liver transplantation for NELM have been reported in literature.[66] Table 5 provides outcomes from available reports after liver transplantation. The United Network for Organ Sharing (UNOS) approves liver transplantation for metastatic NETs with metastasis restricted to the liver in patients with severe symptoms unresponsive to adjuvant treatment after aggressive surgical resection including

Table 4: Outcomes from selected studies following liver resection for NELM

Author	*Year*	*No. of patients*	*5-year survival (%)*
Ahlman[59]	1996	54	70
Sarmiento[60]	2003	170	61
Elias[61]	2003	47	71
Osborne[62]	2006	61	70
Ahmed[63]	2009	50	74.3
Glazer[64]	2010	172	77.4
Mayo[65]	2011	339	74

Table 5: Outcomes from selected studies following liver transplantation for NELM

Author	*Year*	*No. of patients*	*5-year survival (%)*
Rosenau[69]	2002	19	80
Le Treut[70]	2008	85	NA
Mathe[71]	2011	89	44
Gedaly[67]	2011	150	49

excision of the primary lesion and reduction of liver metastasis.[67] Young patients (<50 years) without extrahepatic metastatic disease with well-differentiated tumors are more likely to benefit from liver transplantation. A metaanalysis involving transplanted metastatic pancreatic NETs reported a 1-, 3- and 5-year survival rates of 71%, 55% and 41%, respectively.[68]

Liver-Directed Therapy

About 90% of the oxygenation and nutrition of these highly vascular tumors is derived from the hepatic artery. Several ablative techniques have been developed to exploit the dual blood supply of the liver, given that normal hepatocytes derive most of their blood supply from the portal vein.[72] Because of the high rates of recurrence, liver-directed therapies are essentially regarded as debulking modalities.

Thermal Ablation

These techniques employ focally induced non-physiologic temperatures produced by carefully placed probes into the liver to produce cytotoxic effects. The popular methods that utilize heat to induce cell death are Radio-frequency ablation (RFA) and microwave ablation (MWA).[73] RFA uses heat generated by the change in the direction of high-frequency alternating current, causing ionic vibration.[74] MWA induces coagulative necrosis using heat generated from friction of fluctuating intracellular water by non-ionizing radiation.[75] MWA is capable of generating higher temperatures when compared to RFA. It also allows for a decreased "heat sink" effect caused by nearby vasculature, so can be used more freely near major vessels.[76] There is a dearth of data comparing RFA with MWA.

Cryoablation, on the contrary, uses temperatures well below the freezing point of intracellular water. Cell death is determined by the lowest temperature attained.[77] Freezing does not seem be as effective as heating techniques and a higher complication and recurrence rate has been reported after cryoablation when compared to RFA or MWA.[78] Thermal ablative techniques can be used in inoperable disease or as an adjunct to resection. Table 6 provides outcomes after ablation therapy.

Transarterial Embolization (TAE) and Transarterial Chemoembolization (TACE)

Selective tumor ischemia by occlusion of the hepatic artery is an attractive option to improve the quality of life and reduce the metastatic burden for patients who are not surgical candidates. "Bland" embolization with polyvinyl alcohol particles or chemoembolization with agents such as doxorubicin or mitomycin is accomplished via a catheter selectively inserted into the hepatic artery under fluoroscopic guidance.[83,84] About 18 months is the median duration of response, with low and intermediate-grade NETs displaying more durable responses.[85] Postembolization syndrome which constitutes liver dysfunction, right upper abdominal pain, nausea/vomiting and fever can be reduced by highly selective cannulation of right or left hepatic artery.[86]

Selective Internal Radiation Therapy (SIRT)

This form of therapy, otherwise known as transarterial radioembolization (TARE), substitutes chemotherapeutic agents with radioactive microspheres of yttrium-90 (^{90}Y). Theraspheres (MDS Nordion, Ottawa, ON, Canada) and SIR-Spheres (SirtexMedical Limited, New South Wales, Australia) differ in the composition (glass vs resin) and diameter (20–30 µm vs 20–60 µm) of their microspheres.[87] TARE has been reported to manifest more tolerable postembolization sequelae. Preprocedural evaluation for hepatopulmonary shunts is mandatory to ensure less than 20% of blood flow is diverted to the lungs, avoiding radiation pneumonitis. Gastroduodenal artery reflux should also be ruled out to prevent GI toxicity. Pre-procedureTechnetium-99m-(99mTc-) labeled macroaggregated albumin (MAA) scans are able to rule out these conditions.[88,89]

Hepatic Artery Infusion

Hepatic artery infusion (HAI) involves direct delivery of chemotherapeutic agents into the hepatic artery via a pump. This technique is rarely used in NLM, mostly as an adjunct to TACE. No significant difference in outcome has been reported using HAI.[90,91] Table 7 provides outcomes after various intra-arterial therapies.

Percutaneous Alcohol Injection (PAI)

Ultrasound-guided injection of ethanol, a near-obsolete technique, is best used as an adjunct to other ablative techniques.[96] It is no more used as monotherapy and its use is limited to small lesions, especially near major vessels where the "heat sink" effect would make RFA less than ideal.[97]

Systemic Therapy

Somatostatin Analogs

Over 80% of NETs express a high density for somatostatin receptors.[98] Octreotide, a synthetic somatostatin analog, binds

Table 6: Outcomes from selected studies following ablation for NELM

Author	*Year*	*Modality*	*No. of patients*	*Median Overall Survival (months)*
Seifert[79]	1998	Cryoablation	13	NA
Mazzaglia[80]	2007	RFA	63	47
Martin[76]	2010	MWA	11	18
Akyildiz[81]	2010	RFA	89	72
Karabulut[82]	2011	RFA	68	73

Table 7: Outcomes from selected studies following intra-arterial therapy for NELM

Author	*Year*	*Modality*	*No. of patients*		*Median Overall Survival (months)*
Gupta[92]	2005	TAE TACE	74 49	123	28.5
Strosberg[86]	2006	TAE	84		36
Christante[91]	2008	HAI HAI+TACE	18 59	77	26 39
Kennedy[93]	2008	TARE	148		70
Dong[94]	2010	TACE	123		39.6
Paprottka[95]	2011	TARE	42		NA

with somatostatin receptors and inhibits the secretion of amines and peptides from neuroendocrine cells and has been used for symptomatic relief in "carcinoid" syndrome.[99] A long acting depot form of octreotide (octreotide LAR) which can be administered on a monthly basis is being increasingly used.[100]

PROMID[101] was the first prospective randomized trial regarding the antitumor effect of octreotide LAR. The study included well differentiated NETs of midgut origin. The results support the antiproliferative effects of octreotide with stabilization being the most frequent response. Octreotide LAR, however, did not decrease the time to progression when there was a large tumor burden. The authors concluded that octreotide LAR should be considered in newly diagnosed NETs with low liver tumor burden and resected primary tumor. National Comprehensive Cancer Network (NCCN) has included octreotide LAR as the management option in view of PROMID results. It can be used for tumor control in recurrent, unresectable metastatic NETs in asymptomatic patients as well as for tumor and symptom control in patients with functional NETs.

A phase III trial is ongoing regarding the antitumor effects of lanreotide autogel, another long acting monthly administered somatostatin analog. Another phase III study is recruiting patients with metastatic gastrointestinal NETs with disease-related symptoms inadequately controlled by somatostatin analogs. This study is comparing pasireotide LAR, a novel multireceptor targeted analog with octreotide LAR. The addition of interferon α has not shown a survival benefit when compared to octreotide monotherapy.[102]

Peptide Receptor Radionuclide Therapy

The high rate of somatostatin receptor expression in NETs has led to the interest in peptide receptor radionuclide therapy (PRRT) for metastatic or inoperable disease. The most frequently used radionuclides include yttrium (^{90}Y) and lutetium (^{177}Lu) linked with somatostatin analogs.[103] They differ from each other in terms of emitted particles, particle energy and tissue penetration. ^{177}Lu-DOTATATE and ^{90}Y-DOTATOC may be effective in smaller and larger tumors, respectively. An overall tumor response rate of up to 30% has been reported.[104] However, no prospective randomized trials are available. ^{111}Indium(^{111}In) and ^{131}I-MIBG have also been used with encouraging results.[105]

Systemic Chemotherapy

Cytotoxic chemotherapy is generally not considered as the first line, non-surgical treatment but rather can be used as a salvage therapy in advanced pancreatic NETs. Chemotherapeutic agents such as 5-flurouracil, streptozotocin, dacarbazine and doxorubicin have been studied alone or with combination therapies and have shown little benefit in symptom control or tumor shrinkage. In advanced pancreatic NETs, streptozotocin, in combination with other chemotherapeutic agents, has given encouraging response rates of about 40% and is regarded by many experts as the standard of treatment for this subset of tumors.[106] Temozolomide has also shown favorable antitumor effects in pancreatic NETs.[107] Platinum-based chemotherapy regimens may also be useful in high grade, poorly differentiated NETs. Systemic chemotherapy, with its limited benefits, remains the only therapeutic option for most patients with advanced poorly differentiated (WHO grade 3) NETs.[108]

Targeted Therapy

Studies regarding targeted therapy for pancreatic NETs have focused on inhibitors of vascular endothelial growth factor (VEGF) or mammalian target of rapamycin (mTOR). Bevacizumab and three tyrosine kinase inhibitors: (1) pazopanib, (2) sorafenib and (3) sunitinib have been evaluated for the treatment of advanced pancreatic NETs. Although all these targeted agents have shown promise, sunitinib in particular was associated with a remarkable median progression free survival (PFS) of 11.4 months as compared to 5.5 months for placebo.[109,110]

Everolimus is an mTOR inhibitor[111] which has also demonstrated significant improvement in PFS in progressive advanced pancreatic NETs in a phase III trial (RADIANT-3).[112,113] The PFS with everolimus was 11 months as compared to 4.6 months with placebo.

These benefits have, thus far, only been demonstrated in well to moderately differentiated pancreatic NETs. Combination therapy with a somatostatin analog has also shown promise in terms of clinical benefit and time to progression in advanced NETs. Studies regarding the combination of various targeted therapy molecules are also ongoing and have been demonstrated to be well tolerated.[114]

CONCLUSION

Worldwide, the awareness regarding the diagnosis and treatment of pNETs is increasing, including that in our country. Multi-institutional and multinational collaboration has greatly aided this progress. With the wide-acceptance of an aggressive surgical approach of these tumors, we can expect studies which will increase the body of evidence gathered. Newer non-surgical therapies are also encouraging, broadening the scope for the treatment of metastatic disease. Consensus guidelines are frequently updated due to the rapid evolution in the understanding of these tumors. One must keep abreast of recent developments which are anticipated in the near future to provide optimal care to this relatively rare group of patients, always keeping in mind the value of multidisciplinary management.

REFERENCES

1. Oberndorfer S. Karzinoide tumoren des dunndarms. Frankf Z Pathol. 1907;1:426-32.
2. Klimstra DS, Modlin IR, Coppola D, Lloyd RV, Suster S. The pathologic classification of neuroendocrine tumors: a review of nomenclature, grading, and staging systems. Pancreas. 2010;39(6): 707-12.
3. Davies K, Conlon KC. Neuroendocrine tumors of the pancreas. Curr Gastroenterol Rep. 2009;11(2):119-27.
4. Pavel M, Baudin E, Couvelard A, Krenning E, Oberg K, Steinmuller T, et al. ENETS Consensus Guidelines for the management of patients with liver and other distant metastases from neuroendocrine neoplasms of foregut, midgut, hindgut, and unknown primary. Neuroendocrinology. 2012;95(2):157-76.
5. Kunz PL, Reidy-Lagunes D, Anthony LB, Bertino EM, Brendtro K, Chan JA, et al. Consensus guidelines for the management and treatment of neuroendocrine tumors. Pancreas. 2013;42(4):557-77.
6. Ramage JK, Ahmed A, Ardill J, Bax N, Breen DJ, Caplin ME, et al. Guidelines for the management of gastroenteropancreatic neuroendocrine (including carcinoid) tumours (NETs). Gut. 2012;61(1):6-32.

7. Shrikhande SV, Sirohi B, Goel M, Barreto SG. Pancreatic neuroendocrine tumors. Indian J Gastroenterol. 2013;32(1):3-17.
8. Hauso O, Gustafsson BI, Kidd M, Waldum HL, Drozdov I, Chan AK, et al. Neuroendocrine tumor epidemiology: contrasting Norway and North America. Cancer. 2008;113(10):2655-64.
9. Halfdanarson TR, Rabe KG, Rubin J, Petersen GM. Pancreatic neuroendocrine tumors (PNETs): incidence, prognosis and recent trend toward improved survival. Ann Oncol. 2008;19(10):1727-33.
10. Lam KY, Lo CY. Pancreatic endocrine tumour: a 22-year clinico-pathological experience with morphological, immunohistochemical observation and a review of the literature. Eur J Surg Oncol. 1997;23(1):36-42.
11. Amarapurkar DN, Juneja MP, Patel ND, Amarapurkar AD, Amarapurkar PD. A retrospective clinico-pathological analysis of neuroendocrine tumors of the gastrointestinal tract. Trop Gastroenterol. 2010;31(2):101-4.
12. Bhatia P, Srinivasan R, Rajwanshi A, Nijhawan R, Khandelwal N, Wig J, et al. 5-year review and reappraisal of ultrasound-guided percutaneous transabdominal fine needle aspiration of pancreatic lesions. Acta Cytol. 2008;52(5):523-9.
13. Punpale AS, Shrikhande SV, Sumeet G, Shukla PJ. Primary neuroendocrine carcinoma presenting as mesenteric cyst. Indian J Gastroenterol. 2007;26(3):137-8.
14. Oberg K, Akerstrom G, Rindi G, Jelic S. Neuroendocrine gastroenteropancreatic tumours: ESMO Clinical Practice Guidelines for diagnosis, treatment and follow-up. Ann Oncol. 2010;21(Suppl 5):v223-7.
15. Kloppel G. Classification and pathology of gastroenteropancreatic neuroendocrine neoplasms. Endocr Relat Cancer. 2011;18 (Suppl 1):S1-16.
16. Rindi G, Klimstra DS, Arnold R, Bosman F, et al. Nomenclature and classification of neuroendocrine neoplasms of the digestive system. In: Bosman FCF, Hruban R, Theise N (Eds). WHO Classification of Tumors of the Digestive System. Lyon: IARC Press; 2010. pp. 13-4.
17. O'Toole D, Rindi G, Plockinger U, Wiedenmann B. ENETS consensus guidelines for the management of patients with rare metastases from digestive neuroendocrine tumors: rationale and working framework. Introduction. Neuroendocrinology. 2010;91(4):324-5.
18. Cho MY, Sohn JH, Jin SY, Kim H, Jung ES, Kim MJ, et al. Proposal for a standardized pathology report of gastroenteropancreatic neuroendocrine tumors: prognostic significance of pathological parameters. Korean J Pathol. 2013;47(3):227-37.
19. Rindi G, Kloppel G, Alhman H, Caplin M, Couvelard A, de Herder WW, et al. TNM staging of foregut (neuro)endocrine tumors: a consensus proposal including a grading system. Virchows Arch. 2006;449(4):395-401.
20. Turaga KK, Kvols LK. Recent progress in the understanding, diagnosis, and treatment of gastroenteropancreatic neuroendocrine tumors. CA Cancer J Clin. 2011;61(2):113-32.
21. Kaltsas GA, Besser GM, Grossman AB. The diagnosis and medical management of advanced neuroendocrine tumors. Endocr Rev. 2004;25(3):458-511.
22. Norton JA, Alexander HR, Fraker DL, Venzon DJ, Gibril F, Jensen RT. Possible primary lymph node gastrinoma: occurrence, natural history, and predictive factors: a prospective study. Ann Surg. 2003;237(5):650-7.
23. Zatelli MC, Torta M, Leon A, Ambrosio MR, Gion M, Tomassetti P, et al. Chromogranin A as a marker of neuroendocrine neoplasia: an Italian Multicenter Study. Endocr Relat Cancer. 2007;14(2): 473-82.
24. Nehar D, Lombard-Bohas C, Olivieri S, Claustrat B, Chayvialle JA, Penes MC, et al. Interest of chromogranin A for diagnosis and follow-up of endocrine tumours. Clin Endocrinol (Oxf). 2004;60(5):644-52.
25. Lawrence B, Gustafsson BI, Kidd M, Pavel M, Svejda B, Modlin IM. The clinical relevance of chromogranin A as a biomarker for gastroenteropancreatic neuroendocrine tumors. Endocrinol Metab Clin North Am. 2011;40(1):111-34, viii.
26. Eriksson B, Oberg K, Stridsberg M. Tumor markers in neuroendocrine tumors. Digestion. 2000;62(Suppl 1):33-8.
27. Lindholm DP, Oberg K. Biomarkers and molecular imaging in gastroenteropancreatic neuroendocrine tumors. Horm Metab Res. 2011;43(12):832-7.
28. Hayashi D, Tkacz JN, Hammond S, Devenney-Cakir BC, Zaim S, Bouzegaou N, et al. Gastroenteropancreatic neuroendocrine tumors: multimodality imaging features with pathological correlation. Jpn J Radiol. 2011;29(2):85-91.
29. Phan GQ, Yeo CJ, Hruban RH, Lillemoe KD, Pitt HA, Cameron JL. Surgical experience with pancreatic and peripancreatic neuroendocrine tumors: review of 125 patients. J Gastrointest Surg. 1998;2(5):472-82.
30. Gouya H, Vignaux O, Augui J, Dousset B, Palazzo L, Louvel A, et al. CT, endoscopic sonography, and a combined protocol for preoperative evaluation of pancreatic insulinomas. AJR Am J Roentgenol. 2003;181(4):987-92.
31. Ichikawa T, Peterson MS, Federle MP, Baron RL, Haradome H, Kawamori Y, et al. Islet cell tumor of the pancreas: biphasic CT versus MR imaging in tumor detection. Radiology. 2000;216(1): 163-71.
32. Owen NJ, Sohaib SA, Peppercorn PD, Monson JP, Grossman AB, Besser GM, et al. MRI of pancreatic neuroendocrine tumours. Br J Radiol. 2001;74(886):968-73.
33. Herwick S, Miller FH, Keppke AL. MRI of islet cell tumors of the pancreas. AJR Am J Roentgenol. 2006;187(5):W472-80.
34. Ishikawa T, Itoh A, Kawashima H, Ohno E, Matsubara H, Itoh Y, et al. Usefulness of EUS combined with contrast-enhancement in the differential diagnosis of malignant versus benign and preoperative localization of pancreatic endocrine tumors. Gastrointest Endosc. 2010;71(6):951-9.
35. Pais SA, Al-Haddad M, Mohamadnejad M, Leblanc JK, Sherman S, McHenry L, et al. EUS for pancreatic neuroendocrine tumors: a single-center, 11-year experience. Gastrointest Endosc. 2010;71(7):1185-93.
36. Figueiredo FA, Giovannini M, Monges G, Bories E, Pesenti C, Caillol F, et al. EUS-FNA predicts 5-year survival in pancreatic endocrine tumors. Gastrointest Endosc. 2009;70(5):907-14.
37. Atiq M, Bhutani MS, Bektas M, Lee JE, Gong Y, Tamm EP, et al. EUS-FNA for pancreatic neuroendocrine tumors: a tertiary cancer center experience. Dig Dis Sci. 2012;57(3):791-800.
38. Malago R, D'Onofrio M, Zamboni GA, Faccioli N, Falconi M, Boninsegna L, et al. Contrast-enhanced sonography of nonfunctioning pancreatic neuroendocrine tumors. AJR Am J Roentgenol. 2009;192(2):424-30.
39. Oberg KE, Reubi JC, Kwekkeboom DJ, Krenning EP. Role of somatostatins in gastroenteropancreatic neuroendocrine tumor development and therapy. Gastroenterology. 2010;139(3):742-53, 53 e1.
40. Versari A, Camellini L, Carlinfante G, Frasoldati A, Nicoli F, Grassi E, et al. Ga-68 DOTATOC PET, endoscopic ultrasonography, and multidetector CT in the diagnosis of duodenopancreatic neuroendocrine tumors: a single-centre retrospective study. Clin Nucl Med. 2010;35(5):321-8.
41. Kumar R, Sharma P, Garg P, Karunanithi S, Naswa N, Sharma R, et al. Role of (68)Ga-DOTATOC PET-CT in the diagnosis and staging of pancreatic neuroendocrine tumours. Eur Radiol. 2011;21(11):2408-16.
42. Yakemchuk VN, Jager PL, Chirakal R, Reid R, Major P, Gulenchyn KY. PET/CT using (1)(8)F-FDOPA provides improved staging of carcinoid tumor patients in a Canadian setting. Nucl Med Commun. 2012;33(3):322-30.

43. Bilimoria KY, Talamonti MS, Tomlinson JS, Stewart AK, Winchester DP, Ko CY, et al. Prognostic score predicting survival after resection of pancreatic neuroendocrine tumors: analysis of 3851 patients. Ann Surg. 2008;247(3):490-500.
44. Chen H, Hardacre JM, Uzar A, Cameron JL, Choti MA. Isolated liver metastases from neuroendocrine tumors: does resection prolong survival? J Am Coll Surg. 1998;187(1):88-92; discussion-3.
45. Nomura N, Fujii T, Kanazumi N, Takeda S, Nomoto S, Kasuya H, et al. Nonfunctioning neuroendocrine pancreatic tumors: our experience and management. J Hepatobiliary Pancreat Surg. 2009;16(5):639-47.
46. Schurr PG, Strate T, Rese K, Kaifi JT, Reichelt U, Petri S, et al. Aggressive surgery improves long-term survival in neuroendocrine pancreatic tumors: an institutional experience. Ann Surg. 2007;245(2):273-81.
47. Touzios JG, Kiely JM, Pitt SC, Rilling WS, Quebbeman EJ, Wilson SD, et al. Neuroendocrine hepatic metastases: does aggressive management improve survival? Ann Surg. 2005;241(5):776-83.
48. Hodul PJ, Strosberg JR, Kvols LK. Aggressive surgical resection in the management of pancreatic neuroendocrine tumors: when is it indicated? Cancer Control. 2008;15(4):314-21.
49. Hackert T, Hinz U, Fritz S, Strobel O, Schneider L, Hartwig W, et al. Enucleation in pancreatic surgery: indications, technique, and outcome compared to standard pancreatic resections. Langenbecks Arch Surg. 2011;396(8):1197-203.
50. Kimura W, Tezuka K, Hirai I. Surgical management of pancreatic neuroendocrine tumors. Surg Today. 2011;41(10):1332-43.
51. Falconi M, Zerbi A, Crippa S, Balzano G, Boninsegna L, Capitanio V, et al. Parenchyma-preserving resections for small nonfunctioning pancreatic endocrine tumors. Ann Surg Oncol. 2010;17(6):1621-7.
52. Fernandez-Cruz L, Blanco L, Cosa R, Rendon H. Is laparoscopic resection adequate in patients with neuroendocrine pancreatic tumors? World J Surg. 2008;32(5):904-17.
53. Norton JA, Alexander HR, Fraker DL, Venzon DJ, Gibril F, Jensen RT. Comparison of surgical results in patients with advanced and limited disease with multiple endocrine neoplasia type 1 and Zollinger-Ellison syndrome. Ann Surg. 2001;234(4):495-505.
54. Norton JA, Kivlen M, Li M, Schneider D, Chuter T, Jensen RT. Morbidity and mortality of aggressive resection in patients with advanced neuroendocrine tumors. Arch Surg. 2003;138(8):859-66.
55. Capurso G, Bettini R, Rinzivillo M, Boninsegna L, Delle Fave G, Falconi M. Role of resection of the primary pancreatic neuroendocrine tumour only in patients with unresectable metastatic liver disease: a systematic review. Neuroendocrinology. 2011;93(4):223-9.
56. Bettini R, Mantovani W, Boninsegna L, Crippa S, Capelli P, Bassi C, et al. Primary tumour resection in metastatic nonfunctioning pancreatic endocrine carcinomas. Dig Liver Dis. 2009;41(1):49-55.
57. Jagannath P, Chhabra D, Shrikhande S, Shah R. Surgical treatment of liver metastases in neuroendocrine neoplasms. Int J Hepatol. 2012;2012:782672.
58. Steinmuller T, Kianmanesh R, Falconi M, Scarpa A, Taal B, Kwekkeboom DJ, et al. Consensus guidelines for the management of patients with liver metastases from digestive (neuro)endocrine tumors: foregut, midgut, hindgut, and unknown primary. Neuroendocrinology. 2008;87(1):47-62.
59. Ahlman H, Westberg G, Wangberg B, Nilsson O, Tylen U, Schersten T, et al. Treatment of liver metastases of carcinoid tumors. World J Surg. 1996;20(2):196-202.
60. Sarmiento JM, Heywood G, Rubin J, Ilstrup DM, Nagorney DM, Que FG. Surgical treatment of neuroendocrine metastases to the liver: a plea for resection to increase survival. J Am Coll Surg. 2003;197(1):29-37.
61. Elias D, Lasser P, Ducreux M, Duvillard P, Ouellet JF, Dromain C, et al. Liver resection (and associated extrahepatic resections) for metastatic well-differentiated endocrine tumors: a 15-year single center prospective study. Surgery. 2003;133(4):375-82.
62. Osborne DA, Zervos EE, Strosberg J, Boe BA, Malafa M, Rosemurgy AS, et al. Improved outcome with cytoreduction versus embolization for symptomatic hepatic metastases of carcinoid and neuroendocrine tumors. Ann Surg Oncol. 2006;13(4):572-81.
63. Ahmed A, Turner G, King B, Jones L, Culliford D, McCance D, et al. Midgut neuroendocrine tumours with liver metastases: results of the UKINETS study. Endocr Relat Cancer. 2009;16(3):885-94.
64. Glazer ES, Tseng JF, Al-Refaie W, Solorzano CC, Liu P, Willborn KA, et al. Long-term survival after surgical management of neuroendocrine hepatic metastases. HPB (Oxford). 2010;12(6):427-33.
65. Mayo SC, Pawlik TM. Surgical management of neuroendocrine tumors: treatment of localized and metastatic disease. Oncology (Williston Park). 2011;25(9):806, 8, 10.
66. Fendrich V, Michl P, Habbe N, Bartsch DK. Liver-specific therapies for metastases of neuroendocrine pancreatic tumors. World J Hepatol. 2010;2(10):367-73.
67. Gedaly R, Daily MF, Davenport D, McHugh PP, Koch A, Angulo P, et al. Liver transplantation for the treatment of liver metastases from neuroendocrine tumors: an analysis of the UNOS database. Arch Surg. 2011;146(8):953-8.
68. Mathe Z, Tagkalos E, Paul A, Molmenti EP, Kobori L, Fouzas I, et al. Liver transplantation for hepatic metastases of neuroendocrine pancreatic tumors: a survival-based analysis. Transplantation. 2011;91(5):575-82.
69. Rosenau J, Bahr MJ, von Wasielewski R, Mengel M, Schmidt HH, Nashan B, et al. Ki67, E-cadherin, and p53 as prognostic indicators of long-term outcome after liver transplantation for metastatic neuroendocrine tumors. Transplantation. 2002;73(3):386-94.
70. Le Treut YP, Gregoire E, Belghiti J, Boillot O, Soubrane O, Mantion G, et al. Predictors of long-term survival after liver transplantation for metastatic endocrine tumors: an 85-case French multicentric report. Am J Transplant. 2008;8(6):1205-13.
71. Vernadakis S, Sotiropoulos GC, Brokalaki EI, Esser S, Kaiser GM, Cicinnati VR, et al. Long-term outcomes of liver transplant patients with human immunodeficiency virus infection and end-stage-liver-disease: single center experience. Eur J Med Res. 2011;16(8):342-8.
72. Diamandidou E, Ajani JA, Yang DJ, Chuang VP, Brown CA, Carrasco HC, et al. Two-phase study of hepatic artery vascular occlusion with microencapsulated cisplatin in patients with liver metastases from neuroendocrine tumors. AJR Am J Roentgenol. 1998;170(2):339-44.
73. Mayo SC, Pawlik TM. Thermal ablative therapies for secondary hepatic malignancies. Cancer J. 2010;16(2):111-7.
74. Curley SA. Radiofrequency ablation of malignant liver tumors. Oncologist. 2001;6(1):14-23.
75. Ong SL, Gravante G, Metcalfe MS, Strickland AD, Dennison AR, Lloyd DM. Efficacy and safety of microwave ablation for primary and secondary liver malignancies: a systematic review. Eur J Gastroenterol Hepatol. 2009;21(6):599-605.
76. Martin RC, Scoggins CR, McMasters KM. Safety and efficacy of microwave ablation of hepatic tumors: a prospective review of a 5-year experience. Ann Surg Oncol. 2010;17(1):171-8.
77. Bilchik AJ, Sarantou T, Foshag LJ, Giuliano AE, Ramming KP. Cryosurgical palliation of metastatic neuroendocrine tumors resistant to conventional therapy. Surgery. 1997;122(6):1040-7.
78. Shapiro RS, Shafir M, Sung M, Warner R, Glajchen N. Cryotherapy of metastatic carcinoid tumors. Abdom Imaging. 1998;23(3):314-7.
79. Seifert JK, Zhao J, Ahkter J, Bolton E, Junginger T, Morris DL. Cryoablation of human colorectal cancer in vivo in a nude mouse xenograft model. Cryobiology. 1998;37(1):30-7.
80. Mazzaglia PJ, Berber E, Siperstein AE. Radiofrequency thermal ablation of metastatic neuroendocrine tumors in the liver. Curr Treat Options Oncol. 2007;8(4):322-30.

81. Akyildiz HY, Mitchell J, Milas M, Siperstein A, Berber E. Laparoscopic radiofrequency thermal ablation of neuroendocrine hepatic metastases: long-term follow-up. Surgery. 2010;148(6):1288-93.
82. Karabulut K, Aucejo F, Akyildiz HY, Siperstein A, Berber E. Resection and radiofrequency ablation in the treatment of hepatocellular carcinoma: a single-center experience. Surg Endosc. 2012;26(4):990-7.
83. Proye C. Natural history of liver metastasis of gastroenteropancreatic neuroendocrine tumors: place for chemoembolization. World J Surg. 2001;25(6):685-8.
84. Clouse ME, Perry L, Stuart K, Stokes KR. Hepatic arterial chemoembolization for metastatic neuroendocrine tumors. Digestion. 1994;55(Suppl 3):92-7.
85. Gupta S, Yao JC, Ahrar K, Wallace MJ, Morello FA, Madoff DC, et al. Hepatic artery embolization and chemoembolization for treatment of patients with metastatic carcinoid tumors: the M.D. Anderson experience. Cancer J. 2003;9(4):261-7.
86. Strosberg JR, Choi J, Cantor AB, Kvols LK. Selective hepatic artery embolization for treatment of patients with metastatic carcinoid and pancreatic endocrine tumors. Cancer Control. 2006;13(1): 72-8.
87. King J, Quinn R, Glenn DM, Janssen J, Tong D, Liaw W, et al. Radioembolization with selective internal radiation microspheres for neuroendocrine liver metastases. Cancer. 2008;113(5):921-9.
88. Murthy R, Nunez R, Szklaruk J, Erwin W, Madoff DC, Gupta S, et al. Yttrium-90 microsphere therapy for hepatic malignancy: devices, indications, technical considerations, and potential complications. Radiographics. 2005;25(Suppl 1):S41-55.
89. Bester L, Salem R. Reduction of arteriohepatovenous shunting by temporary balloon occlusion in patients undergoing radioembolization. J Vasc Interv Radiol. 2007;18(10):1310-4.
90. Eadens MJ, Grothey A. Curable metastatic colorectal cancer. Curr Oncol Rep. 2011;13(3):168-76.
91. Christante D, Pommier S, Givi B, Pommier R. Hepatic artery chemoinfusion with chemoembolization for neuroendocrine cancer with progressive hepatic metastases despite octreotide therapy. Surgery. 2008;144(6):885-93.
92. Gupta S, Johnson MM, Murthy R, Ahrar K, Wallace MJ, Madoff DC, et al. Hepatic arterial embolization and chemoembolization for the treatment of patients with metastatic neuroendocrine tumors: variables affecting response rates and survival. Cancer. 2005;104(8):1590-602.
93. Kennedy AS, Dezarn WA, McNeillie P, Coldwell D, Nutting C, Carter D, et al. Radioembolization for unresectable neuroendocrine hepatic metastases using resin 90Y-microspheres: early results in 148 patients. Am J Clin Oncol. 2008;31(3):271-9.
94. Dong XD, Carr BI. Hepatic artery chemoembolization for the treatment of liver metastases from neuroendocrine tumors: a long-term follow-up in 123 patients. Med Oncol. 2011;28(Suppl 1): S286-90.
95. Paprottka PM, Hoffmann RT, Haug A, Sommer WH, Raessler F, Trumm CG, et al. radioembolization of symptomatic, unresectable neuroendocrine hepatic metastases using yttrium-90 microspheres. Cardiovasc Intervent Radiol. 2012;35(2):334-42.
96. Giovannini M, Seitz JF. Ultrasound-guided percutaneous alcohol injection of small liver metastases. Results in 40 patients. Cancer. 1994;73(2):294-7.
97. Giovannini M. Percutaneous alcohol ablation for liver metastasis. Semin Oncol. 2002;29(2):192-5.
98. Kvols LK, Moertel CG, O'Connell MJ, Schutt AJ, Rubin J, Hahn RG. Treatment of the malignant carcinoid syndrome. Evaluation of a long-acting somatostatin analogue. N Engl J Med. 1986;315(11): 663-6.
99. di Bartolomeo M, Bajetta E, Buzzoni R, Mariani L, Carnaghi C, Somma L, et al. Clinical efficacy of octreotide in the treatment of metastatic neuroendocrine tumors. A study by the Italian Trials in Medical Oncology Group. Cancer. 1996;77(2):402-8.
100. O'Toole D, Ducreux M, Bommelaer G, Wemeau JL, Bouche O, Catus F, et al. Treatment of carcinoid syndrome: a prospective crossover evaluation of lanreotide versus octreotide in terms of efficacy, patient acceptability, and tolerance. Cancer. 2000;88(4):770-6.
101. Rinke A, Muller HH, Schade-Brittinger C, Klose KJ, Barth P, Wied M, et al. Placebo-controlled, double-blind, prospective, randomized study on the effect of octreotide LAR in the control of tumor growth in patients with metastatic neuroendocrine midgut tumors: a report from the PROMID Study Group. J Clin Oncol. 2009;27(28):4656-63.
102. Modlin IM, Pavel M, Kidd M, Gustafsson BI. Review article: somatostatin analogues in the treatment of gastroenteropancreatic neuroendocrine (carcinoid) tumours. Aliment Pharmacol Ther. 2010;31(2):169-88.
103. Teunissen JJ, Kwekkeboom DJ, Kooij PP, Bakker WH, Krenning EP. Peptide receptor radionuclide therapy for non-radioiodine-avid differentiated thyroid carcinoma. J Nucl Med. 2005;46 (Suppl 1):107S-14S.
104. Bushnell DL, Jr., O'Dorisio TM, O'Dorisio MS, Menda Y, Hicks RJ, Van Cutsem E, et al. 90Y-edotreotide for metastatic carcinoid refractory to octreotide. J Clin Oncol. 2010;28(10):1652-9.
105. Kwekkeboom DJ, de Herder WW, Kam BL, van Eijck CH, van Essen M, Kooij PP, et al. Treatment with the radiolabeled somatostatin analog [177 Lu-DOTA 0,Tyr3]octreotate: toxicity, efficacy, and survival. J Clin Oncol. 2008;26(13):2124-30.
106. Sun W, Lipsitz S, Catalano P, Mailliard JA, Haller DG. Phase II/III study of doxorubicin with fluorouracil compared with streptozocin with fluorouracil or dacarbazine in the treatment of advanced carcinoid tumors: Eastern Cooperative Oncology Group Study E1281. J Clin Oncol. 2005;23(22):4897-904.
107. Kulke MH, Hornick JL, Frauenhoffer C, Hooshmand S, Ryan DP, Enzinger PC, et al. O6-methylguanine DNA methyltransferase deficiency and response to temozolomide-based therapy in patients with neuroendocrine tumors. Clin Cancer Res. 2009;15(1):338-45.
108. Strosberg JR, Fine RL, Choi J, Nasir A, Coppola D, Chen DT, et al. First-line chemotherapy with capecitabine and temozolomide in patients with metastatic pancreatic endocrine carcinomas. Cancer. 2011;117(2):268-75.
109. Raymond E, Dahan L, Raoul JL, Bang YJ, Borbath I, Lombard-Bohas C, et al. Sunitinib malate for the treatment of pancreatic neuroendocrine tumors. N Engl J Med. 2011;364(6):501-13.
110. Yao JC, Phan A, Hoff PM, Chen HX, Charnsangavej C, Yeung SC, et al. Targeting vascular endothelial growth factor in advanced carcinoid tumor: a random assignment phase II study of depot octreotide with bevacizumab and pegylated interferon alpha-2b. J Clin Oncol. 2008;26(8):1316-23.
111. Yao JC, Shah MH, Ito T, Bohas CL, Wolin EM, Van Cutsem E, et al. Everolimus for advanced pancreatic neuroendocrine tumors. N Engl J Med. 2011;364(6):514-23.
112. Yao JC, Lombard-Bohas C, Baudin E, Kvols LK, Rougier P, Ruszniewski P, et al. Daily oral everolimus activity in patients with metastatic pancreatic neuroendocrine tumors after failure of cytotoxic chemotherapy: a phase II trial. J Clin Oncol. 2010;28(1): 69-76.
113. Ito T, Okusaka T, Ikeda M, Igarashi H, Morizane C, Nakachi K, et al. Everolimus for advanced pancreatic neuroendocrine tumours: a subgroup analysis evaluating Japanese patients in the RADIANT-3 trial. Jpn J Clin Oncol. 2012;42(10):903-11.
114. Yao JC, Phan AT, Chang DZ, Wolff RA, Hess K, Gupta S, et al. Efficacy of RAD001 (everolimus) and octreotide LAR in advanced low- to intermediate-grade neuroendocrine tumors: results of a phase II study. J Clin Oncol. 2008;26(26):4311-8.

CHAPTER 46

Minimally Invasive Approach to Pancreatic Lesions

C Palanivelu, P Senthilnathan

INTRODUCTION

The introduction of laparoscopy to the surgical field has revolutionized several procedures including pancreatic surgery. But adaptation of laparoscopic pancreatic surgery has been relatively slow due to its proximity to the great vessels, retroperitoneal location and friability of pancreas. With enormous development in technology coupled with improved anatomical knowledge and refined skills, laparoscopic pancreatic surgery has grown out of its infancy and is an established speciality today. Although safety and outcomes are well-documented, the patient selection remains the key, especially during early experience. The criticism which led to delayed introduction of minimally invasive approach in pancreatic diseases during the last century were the technical complexity of these procedures demanding high expertise, associated high morbidity/mortality and concerns over oncologic adequacy of malignant lesions with long-term outcomes. With growing number of centers worldwide performing these procedures and availability of the research data, most of the concerns mentioned above have become irrelevant.

Initially, laparoscopic pancreatic surgeries focused mainly on diagnostic aspects like staging laparoscopy and biopsy. With increasing experience in laparoscopic techniques, advancements in hemostatic technology and better imaging systems, many centers across the globe started laparoscopic pancreatic work in high numbers. This has led to performance of surgeries, such as pancreaticoduodenectomy or segmental pancreatic resections which were once considered impossible by laparoscopy.

HISTORY

Bernheim in 1911 reported diagnostic laparoscopy in a patient with pancreatic mass. He stated that detection of liver metastasis saved a needless laparotomy. Cuschieri et al. in 1978 and Warshaw et al. in 1986 also performed diagnostic laparoscopy for the detection of liver metastasis and tumor resectability.

Pachter et al. in 1979 managed to transect pancreas during distal pancreatectomy using stapling device. Using this technology, Soper et al., established the safety and feasibility of laparoscopic distal pancreatectomy (LDP) in an animal model. Gagner and Pomp in 1994 reported the first successful laparoscopic pylorus preserving pancreaticoduodenectomy in a 30-year-old woman with chronic pancreatitis. Since then many laparoscopic pancreatic procedures including enucleation, distal pancreatectomy, necrosectomy and pancreaticoduodenectomy are being increasingly performed.

In 1996, Cuschieri et al. reported laparoscopic distal (70–80%) pancreatectomy with splenectomy in seven patients. During the same period, Gagner et al. attempted laparoscopic pancreatic distal resection with spleen preservation in seven patients with islet cell tumor. Warshaw et al. in 1988 were the first to describe the open technique of spleen preserving distal pancreatectomy. Their technique was adopted by Sussman and Vezakis et al. in 1996 for laparoscopic resections.

In 1993, Pietrabissa et al. was first to use laparoscopic ultrasonography for localization of insulinoma by laparoscopic infragastric inspection of the pancreas. In 1996, Gagner et al. did laparoscopic extirpation of insulinomas in four patients, followed by Bonjer et al. and Cuschieri et al. during 1998.

The authors have got two decades long experience in managing various pancreatic diseases by minimal access method. We started doing staging laparoscopy for staging pancreatic malignancy and tumor localization in pancreatic neuroendocrine tumors (PNET) as early as 1992. We started advanced pancreatic work like pancreaticoduodenectomy and distal pancreatectomy from 1998 onward.

TYPES OF RESECTION

Location, size, number and biological behavior of tumor decide the type of resection for any pancreatic lesion. Based on this, pancreatic resections are classified into:

- Pancreaticoduodenectomy
- Distal or left side pancreatectomy
- Distal or left side pancreatectomy with spleen preservation
- Central or median or middle pancreatectomy
- Duodenum preserving pancreatectomy
- Total pancreatectomy
- Enucleation.

Distal Pancreatectomy (Figs 1A to F)

In 1996, Sussman and colleagues described LDP in a patient of insulinoma involving tail of pancreas which was localized with intraoperative ultrasound. Since then it is the most commonly performed laparoscopic pancreatic resection. Initially, the procedure was combined with splenectomy mainly in view of technical reasons. With advent of growing expertise, coupled with the use of modern thermal devices, splenic preservation has become routine, unless indicated otherwise. Currently, laparoscopic distal pancreatic resection is an established procedure with large multicenter data available highlighting its feasibility and safety. Its efficacy compared with the open approach are also available in the literature.

Indications

Indications for LDP are similar to open distal pancreatectomy (ODP).

- Cystic tumors, like mucinous cystadenoma, serous cyst-adenoma, simple cysts, echinococcal cyst and unspecified cyst
- Neuroendocrine tumors, like insulinoma, gastrinoma and nonfunctioning tumors
- Isolated pseudocyst; isolated left-sided disease
- Chronic pancreatitis; isolated left-sided disease
- Small, incidentally detected carcinoma of pancreatic tail.

Contraindications

Laparoscopic distal pancreatectomy is an established procedure but still has some inherent limitations. Some of the relative contraindications for this procedure are:

- Previous pancreatic surgery
- Associated portal hypertension
- Tumor size of more than 8 cm
- Body mass index (BMI) more than 35.

Preoperative Preparation

Apart from routine work for fitness, some specific investigations needed are cross-sectional imaging either in the form of contrast-enhanced computed tomography (CECT) or magnetic resonance imaging (MRI) of abdomen, specific tumor markers and endoscopic ultrasound (US)-guided fine needle aspiration (FNA) in some patient to establish the diagnosis which alters the management. Bowel preparation will help in better handling of colon especially transverse colon, which is closely related to pancreas.

Operative Technique

Positioning and operative team: Patient is placed in supine position with leg split. Surgeon stands between the legs of the patient, camera surgeon stands on right and scrub nurse on left side of the patient. Monitor is placed at the head end of patient.

Exposure of the pancreas: Approach to pancreas starts with entry into the lesser sac by dividing the greater omentum below the gastroepiploic arcade starting half way along the greater curvature. The entire gastrocolic omentum from distal antrum up to the fundus of the stomach including the short gastric vessels is divided. Short gastric vessels should be preserved, if spleen preservation is planned. In case of associated chronic pancreatitis, the adhesions between the posterior wall of the stomach and anterior surface of the pancreas have to be released carefully.

Splenic artery ligation: The splenic artery is identified at the upper border of the body of the pancreas and dissected for an adequate distance proximal to the tumor. It is then ligated and divided to minimize the risk of major bleeding during later dissection. This step is omitted where splenic conservation is planned. In cases, where the splenic artery could not be identified due to bulky lesion in the body, it can be ligated posteriorly after complete mobilization of distal pancreas.

Mobilization of pancreas: Division of the splenocolic ligament gives way to the inferior border at the tail end of the pancreas. Division of anterior layer of the transverse mesocolon along the lower border of the pancreas opens the areolar tissue at the back of the pancreas. Dissection is pursued until the splenic vein is identified. The junction of the splenic and superior mesenteric vein is identified by opening the fascial layer in avascular plane. If the inferior mesenteric vein joins the splenic vein proximally to proposed transection, it is ligated and transected.

Division of the splenic vessels and pancreatic transection: If the splenic artery is not divided earlier, it can now be identified at the upper border of pancreas. It is clipped distal to the ligature and divided. Splenic vein is carefully separated from posterior aspect of pancreas after dividing direct draining vessels. Now splenic vein is doubly ligated with silk and divided. Alternatively, Endo GIA™ stapler can be used for transection, if adequate space can be created. After division of the splenic vessels, the body of the pancreas is transected with 1 cm tumor margin. We prefer gold/green cartridge for transection, advantage being approximation of both layers of pancreatic capsule with obliteration of duct. Alternately, white cartridge can also be used which seals the pancreatic duct but has the disadvantage of crushing the parenchyma. Harmonic shears can also be used for parenchymal division and the stump is overrun by 3-0 prolene sutures. Use of en-masse transection of pancreas along with splenic vein by using Endo GIA™ stapler can also be done in cases where separation of splenic vein from parenchyma is not possible.

Removal of specimen: Retraction of transected pancreas and the spleen facilitates the division of remaining attachments, generally being avascular. The short gastric vessels attached if any, are divided. The resected specimen of pancreas and spleen is placed in an endobag. A small suprapubic Pfannenstiel incision enables extraction of specimen, which provides better cosmesis and lesser pain.

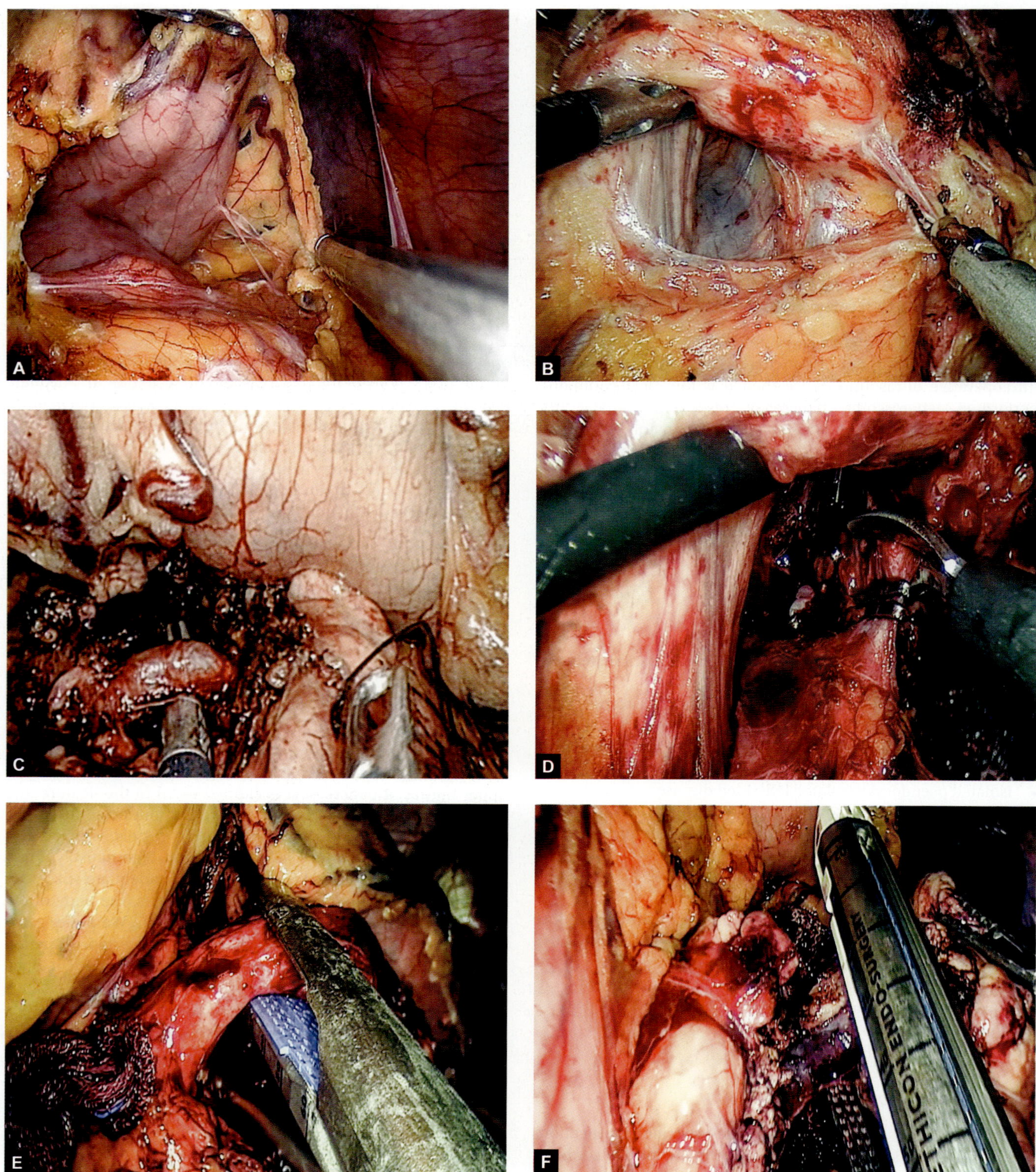

Figures 1A to F Distal pancreatectomy. (A) Division of gastrocolic omentum and exposure of pancreas; (B) Mobilization of inferior and posterior surface of pancreas. Splenic vein seen below; (C) Dissection of splenic artery proximal to the lesion; (D) Division of splenic artery between the clips; (E) Pancreatic parenchymal transection using endo GIA stapler (blue); (F) Splenic vein is transected using endo GIA stapler (white)

Table 1: Operative and postoperative results of laparoscopy and open distal pancreatectomy

Author	*No. of cases*		*Spleen preservation n (%)*		*Operation time (minutes)*		*Hospital stay days*		*Pancreatic fistula rate n (%)*	
	Lap.	*Open*	*Lap.*	*Open*	*Lap.*	*Open*	*Lap.*	*Open*	*Lap.*	*Open*
Kim et al. 11	93	35	38 (40.8)	2 (5.7)	195	190	10	16	8 (8.6)	5 (14.3)
Kooby et al. 12	23	189	43 (30)	24 (12)	230	216	5.9	9.0	37 (26)/16 (11)	64 (32)/36 (18)
Jayaraman et al. 13	100	100	14 (42.4)	33 (14.0)	195	160	5	6	8 (10.8)	13 (5.5)
DiNorcia et al.14	71	168	11 (15.5)	26 (15.8)	191	192	5	6	8 (11.3)	25 (14.9)
Casadei et al. 15	22	22	4 (18.2)	4 (18.2)	225	145	8.0	11.0	2 (9.1)	4 (18.2)
Waters et al. 16	18	22	5 (28)	3 (14)	224	234	6	8	2 (11.1)	4 (18.2)
Mehta et al. 17	30	30	21 (70)	9 (30)	188	226	8.7	12.6	5 (16.7)/5 (16.7)	4 (13.3)/4 (13.3)
Butturini et al. 18	43	73	19 (44.2)	8 (11)	180	180	8	9	12 (27.9)	10 (13.7)
Abu et al. 19	35	16	14 (40)	3 (19)	200	225	7	11	10 (29)	7 (44)
Fox et al. 20	42	76	15 (35.7)	17 (22.4)	304	281	5	7	12 (28.6)/0 (0)	10 (13.2)/4 (5.3)
Limongelli et al. 21	16	29	5 (31)	3 (14)	204	160	6.4	8.6	3 (18)/1 (6)	6 (20)/5 (17.2)

Abbreviation: Lap: laparoscopic.

Spleen preserving distal pancreatectomy: For known benign lesions of pancreas, spleen preserving distal pancreatectomy is the ideal procedure. Steps are similar till the exposure of pancreas. Splenic artery is to be carefully dissected away from superior border of pancreas. The separation of splenic vein from posterior surface of pancreas is achieved after carefully ligating small draining vessels. It is a technically challenging and rate limiting step of this operation and if damaged, may result in removal of the spleen. Alternatively, laparoscopic adaptation of Warren technique can be employed which involves division of splenic vessels with preservation of short gastric vessels.

Results and Review of Literature

In spite of early hesitation for laparoscopic pancreatic resections, LDP is now being performed world over with availability of sufficient literature support. Considering its advantages over open approach open pancreaticoduodenectomy (OPD), it can be considered the treatment of choice for benign and low-grade malignant lesions. We published our initial experience of LDP in 22 patients with excellent results. In this series, there were no conversions with good perioperative outcomes. We could preserve spleen in 32% of the cases with only one patient developing clinically significant pancreatic fistula [International Study Group of Pancreatic Fistula (ISGPF) grade B]. We could maintain the same outcomes after 75 cases with shortened operative time and less blood loss. Some authors have expressed concerns over its utilization for malignant lesions but multi-institutional trial by Kooby et al. comprising total of 212 patients demonstrated acceptable oncological safety. The study mentions margin positive rate, no of nodes retrieved, overall survival were same in LDP and ODP groups although had only 11% cases done by laparoscopic approach. Laparoscopic approach is associated with shorter operating times, lesser pain and early return of bowel function and of normal activities. Now, it is clear that in experienced hands, LDP is comparable with ODP in relation to complications and outcome, with added advantages of minimally invasive approach. It has been convincingly shown that LDP is feasible with short-term and long-term outcomes similar to ODP. The recent meta-analysis by Jin et al. showed advantages in laparoscopic arm like less intraoperative blood loss and transfusion requirements, early oral intake, fewer wound complications and shorter hospital stay. This meta-analysis included 15 studies that compared both laparoscopic pancreaticoduodenectomy (LPD) and OPD. The reported incidence of pancreatic fistula in the literature varies between 23% and 26% for open approach. In this meta-analysis, the pooled pancreatic fistula rates between laparoscopic (17%) and open (18%) group did not show any difference. The other advantage with laparoscopic approach is increased chances of spleen preservation that is reported to be around 40%. This figure is again statistically higher than open approach. Selected series comparing both open and laparoscopic approach with results are shown in Table 1. There were concerns about the use of laparoscopy for adenocarcinoma of body and tail pancreas for various reasons including port site metastasis, inadequate lymphadenectomy and margin status. Recent evidences suggest that even oncological procedures like radical antegrade modular pancreatosplenectomy (RAMPS) are possible by laparoscopy with comparable results (Table 1).

Parenchyma Preserving Pancreatectomy

Neoplastic lesions in the pancreatic head or tail are resected by pancreaticoduodenectomy or distal pancreatectomy but tumors in the body-neck of pancreas can be difficult for a surgeon. Extended right or left pancreatic resections can result in greater loss of glandular tissue increasing the risk of diabetes and impaired exocrine function.

Need for Parenchyma Preservation

Even in apparently normal pancreas, the incidence of postoperative exocrine and endocrine impairment is not predictable. Many factors, like duct obstruction, pre-existing chronic pancreatitis and diabetes, atrophy and fibrosis of the remnant may play a role.

After standard left-sided resection there is wide variation in the incidence of endocrine impairment and onset of diabetes from 17% to 85% of patients. It is reasonable that the extent of the resection be minimized to limit endocrine and exocrine insufficiency in long-term.

For these reasons, more conservative surgical techniques like enucleation has been advocated for small, benign tumors located in the neck of the gland. For benign and neoplastic lesions which are not small and superficial enough or otherwise fit to be simply enucleated, middle segment pancreatectomy should be considered.

Enucleation

Enucleation is the treatment option for small, benign and low-grade malignant tumors such as cystic neoplasms and endocrine tumors of the pancreas. Laparoscopic ultrasound helps in exact localization of the lesion and its relation to the main pancreatic duct. However, it should be remembered that enucleation cannot be always applicable. When the neoplastic lesion measures more than 2 cm or is encased within the pancreatic gland, enucleation is associated with a high risk of Wirsung's duct damage. In the case of tumors with uncertain biological behavior, this approach should be avoided because of the risk of tumor recurrence.

Median Pancreatectomy (Figs 2A to E)

Indications

- Tumor size 2–5 cm
- Small tumors deeply located in the gland, not eligible for enucleation
- Non-neoplastic cystic lesion such as lymphoepithelial, dermoid and hydatid cysts
- Solitary metastasis of pancreatic neck (renal metastasis), pancreatic endocrine tumor with metastases in a multimodal treatment
- Focal chronic pancreatitis with isolated and short stenosis of Wirsung's duct, cystic inflammatory lesion.

Contraindications

- Large lesions where it is not possible to preserve at least 5 cm distal to pancreatic stump
- Distal body-tail atrophy
- Malignant tumors (especially ductal carcinoma)
- Neoplastic involvement from other organs (stomach, transverse colon)
- Diffuse chronic pancreatitis
- Main duct intraductal papillary mucinous neoplasms (IPMN).

Our Operative Technique

Patient is placed in supine position with leg split; operating surgeon stands in between the legs.

Mobilization of pancreas: Pancreas is exposed by opening gastrocolic omentum and its inferior border is defined by dividing the transverse mesocolon attachment. Posterior mobilization of pancreas is done taking care to avoid injury to splenic vein and artery. Small pancreatic branches supplying the mobilized pancreas are clipped and divided.

Pancreatic division: Pancreas proximal to the tumor is divided with Endo GIA™ stapler and reinforced with 3-0 polydioxanone (PDS) sutures. Distally, pancreas is divided sharply and hemostasis achieved. Central portion with the tumor is removed.

Pancreatic anastomosis: Distal Pancreatic stump is anastomosed to Roux-en-y limb of jejunum intracorporeally in two layers. A drain is then placed near the site of anastomosis to complete the procedure.

Results and Review of Literature

Median pancreatectomy constitutes a small percentage of pancreatic resections and the literature is very much limited. Laparoscopic approach is even more restricted to few case reports and series. In a review of 51 patients who underwent laparoscopic median pancreatectomy, Machado et al. concluded that it is a feasible and useful technique for removal of tumors located in the neck of pancreas. The reported pancreatic fistula is about 46% and this relatively higher fistula rates when compared to both distal pancreatectomy and pancreaticoduodenectomy can be attributed to double pancreatic stump. Majority of the reconstruction is surprisingly pancreaticogastrostomy (67.7%). The hospital stay was 13.8 days which was not different from the published open series. However, there was no reported exocrine and endocrine insufficiency in this review.

Pancreaticoduodenectomy (Figs 3A to I)

First description of laparoscopic pancreatic head resection came in 1994 by Gagner and Pomp where they used a hybrid approach using right subcostal hand port for tumor assessment and anastomosis. In 2007, a large series of 45 patients was published showing excellent outcomes with regard to blood loss, length of hospital stay, with comparable morbidity and mortality to open approach. Recently, two large series reemphasized the feasibility and safety of this procedure and one of those studies compared its outcome with open surgery.

Indications

Selection of patient is extremely important for successful employment of laparoscopic approach. We stress on selecting early, small lesions for the beginners and later on larger tumors can be attempted. Moreover, associated conditions like obesity, previous upper abdominal surgeries and borderline resectable tumors are better avoided. The preferred indications include:

- Ampullary tumors
- Distal common bile duct (CBD) tumors
- Early carcinoma head of pancreas (less than 3 cm)
- Duodenal carcinoma.

Team Set-Up, Patient Positioning and Instrumentation

Patient is placed supine with leg split and reverse Trendelenburg position. Monitor lies at the head end of patient. Position of surgeon

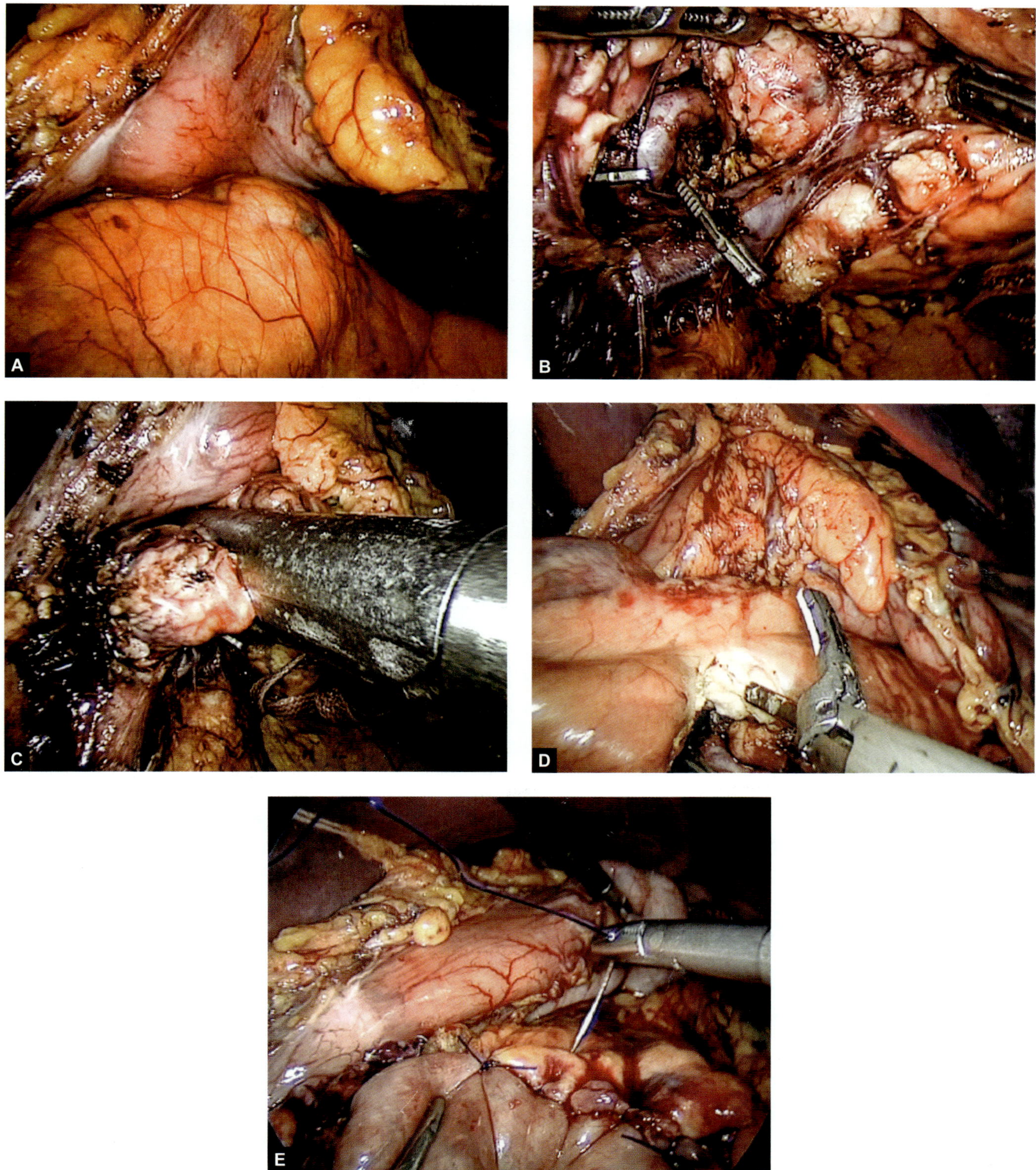

Figures 2A to E Median pancreatectomy. (A) Use of laparoscopic ultrasound to localize the lesion; (B) Separation of pancreas from the splenic vessels; (C) Proximal pancreatic division using linear cutter; (D) Distal pancreatic transection using ultrasonic energy source; (E) Completion of pancreato-jejunostomy

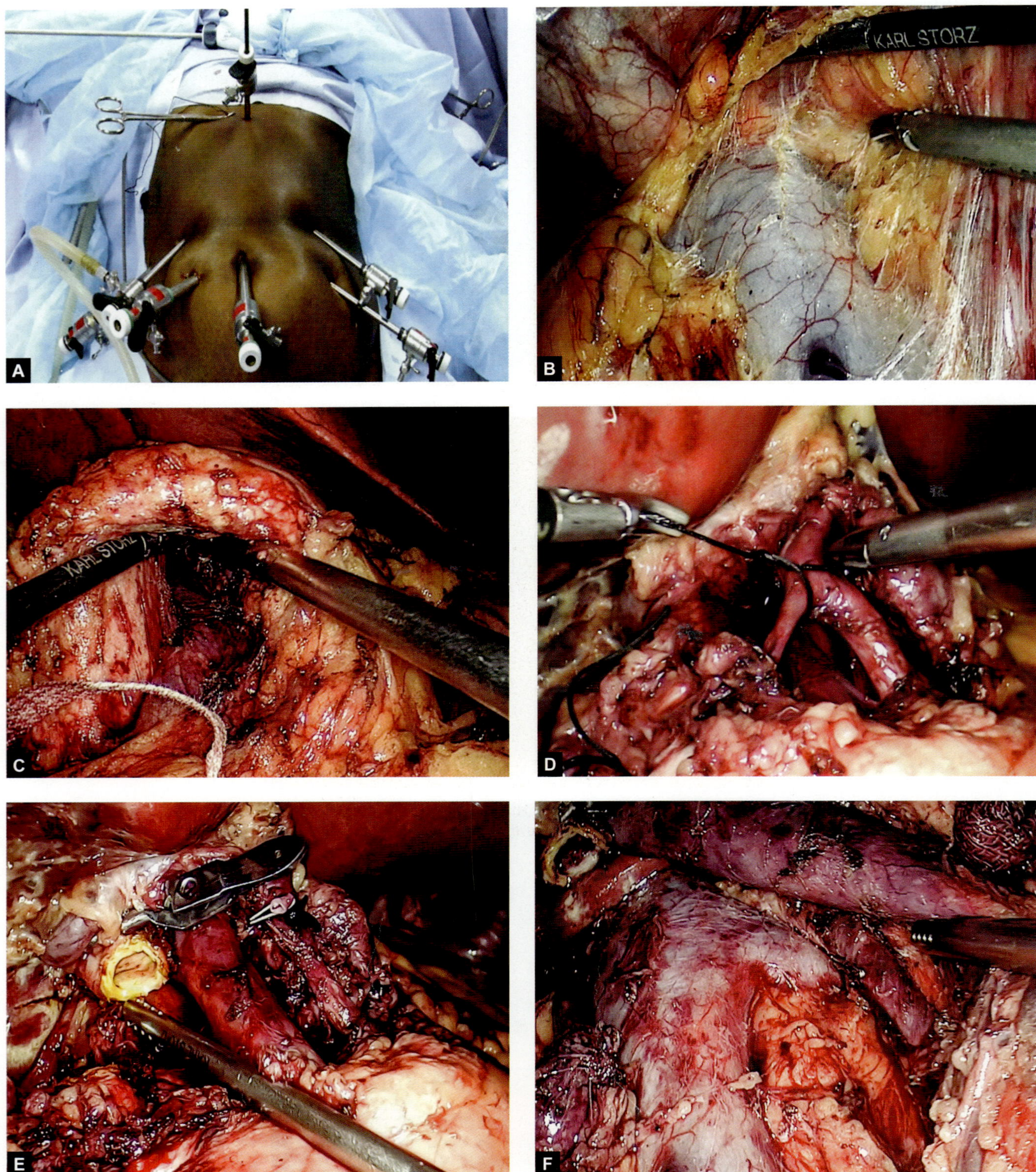

Figures 3A to F (A) Port placement for laparoscopic pancreaticoduodenectomy. Totally 7 ports are used. The camera alternates between midline and right pararectal ports; (B) Kocherisation of duodenum inferior vena cava is clearly seen along with the posterior surface of head of pancreas; (C) Dissection of neck of pancreas a way from the splenoportal confluence; (D) Ligation of gastroduodenal artery close to its origin from hepatic artery proper. Lymphadenectomy is carried out in the hepatoduodenal ligament; (E) Divided common hepatic duct with endo bulldog occluding the lumen to prevent bile spillage; (F) At the end of complete resection. IVC, left renal vein, superior mesenteric artery and cut surface of common hepatic duct clearly seen;

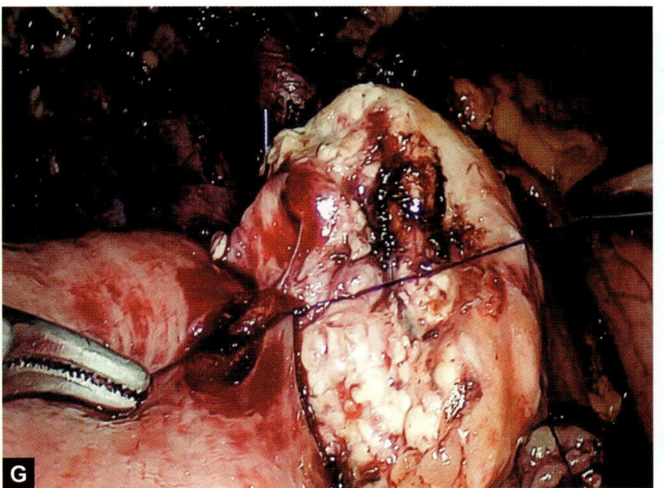

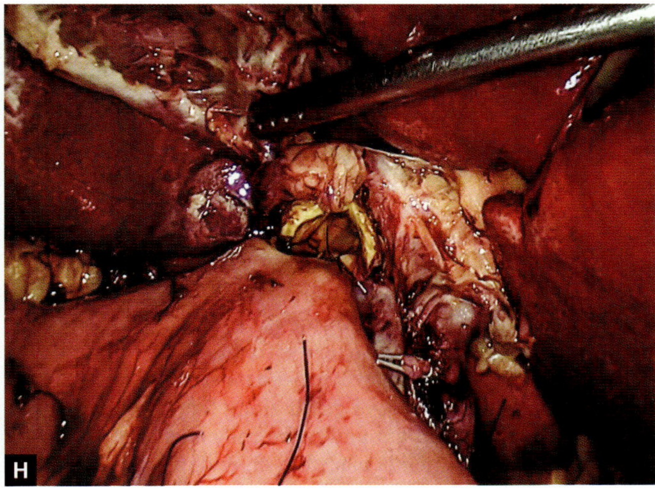

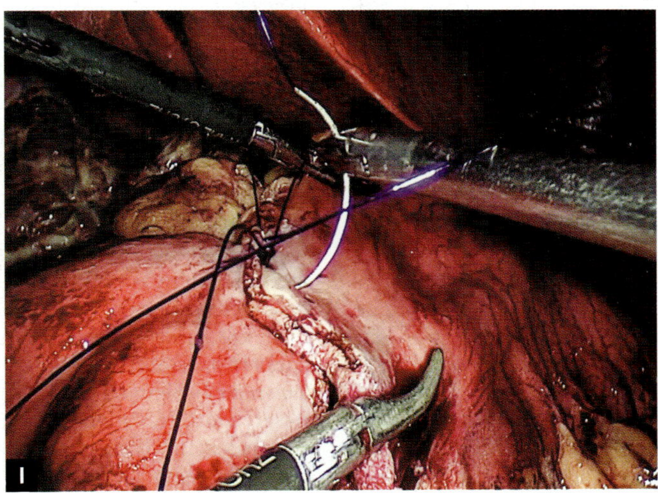

Figures 3G to I (G) Duct to mucosa pancreatojejunostomy is in progress; (H) posterior layer hepaticojejunostomy is completed; (I) Final reconstruction is duodenojejunostomy. Here anterior layer is being sutured.

varies depending on the area of dissection and reconstruction. The scheme of port placement is shown in the Fig. 3A.

Operative Details

For the purpose of description, the procedure can be divided into two phases; resection and reconstruction.

Phase 1: Resection

After staging laparoscopy to rule out any intra-abdominal distant metastasis, the resection is commenced by bringing down hepatic flexure colon and exposing the entire duodenum. The gastrocolic ligament is divided and lesser sac is entered. The head of pancreas is exposed completely by dividing right gastroepiploic vessels and gastrocolic trunk. The operability of the lesion is assessed by two important maneuvers. The first is the extended Kocherization which allows us to assess the superior mesenteric artery (SMA). The second one is tunneling behind the neck of pancreas to assess portal vein involvement. If both are free, irreversible steps are then commenced.

If decision is made to go ahead with resection, antrum or first part of duodenum is transected using Endo GIA™ stapler depending upon the type of resection (classical/pylorus preserving). This exposes the entire field of dissection. The dissection of portal structures begins with decompression of the gall bladder as it provides better visualization of the structures in porta. Calot's triangle is dissected, cystic artery and duct clipped and divided. Gall bladder is left attached to the liver until the reconstruction is over as it provides good retraction of liver. Common hepatic duct is transected above the level of cystic duct junction and the entire fibro-fatty and lymphatic tissues along the hepatoduodenal ligament is cleared exposing common hepatic artery and portal vein. Bile spillage from the opened hepatic duct is avoided by applying endo bulldog clamp. Hepatic artery traced down along superior border of pancreas in gastrohepatic omentum where the gastroduodenal artery is identified and ligated at its origin from common hepatic artery. Dissection continued toward common hepatic artery and celiac axis along the superior border of pancreas, taking down lymphatic tissue toward specimen.

The mobilization of duodenum continues toward third and fourth part including proximal 15 cm of jejunum after dividing jejunal mesentery. Care is taken to ligate the first jejunal branch followed by transection of jejunum with Endo GIA™ stapler (white cartridge). This facilitates delivery of transected jejunum toward the specimen side. Pancreatic transection at neck begins after placing stay sutures at superior and inferior border on either side of transection line which helps in retraction and hemostasis. It is done using harmonic shears while area of suspected duct is divided with scissors to avoid injury to ductal mucosa. The attachment of uncinate process with SMA is now visualized including inferior pancreaticoduodenal vessels which need to be clipped and divided ensuring complete removal of gland along right border of SMA. This is one of the important and technically challenging steps of this procedure. Specimen is placed in an endobag and delivered through Pfannenstiel incision at the end of procedure.

Phase 2: Reconstruction

The jejunum is brought to the supracolic compartment in retrocolic fashion. The pancreatic stump is mobilized for a length of 2–3 cm to facilitate the pancreatic anastomosis. We prefer pancreaticojejunal reconstruction which is done by end to side duct to mucosa technique using 4–0 PDS sutures. The mucosal anastomosis is reinforced using 3-0 polypropylene seromuscular to pancreatic capsule sutures all around where posterior layer is done prior to duct to mucosal anastomosis. If the pancreas is soft and duct is tiny, we prefer to do the dunking technique. Approximately, 7–8 cm distal to pancreaticojejunostomy anastomosis, hepaticojejunostomy is done by creating small opening in the jejunum and anastomosing it with cut end of hepatic duct. It is done in single layer with 4–0 PDS interrupted sutures and if the duct is dilated, the anterior layer can be completed using continuous sutures. Distal to hepaticojejunal anastomosis, duodenojejunostomy/gastrojejunostomy is performed in an antecolic fashion using 2–0 PDS, continuous, extramucosal sutures. In case of classical resection, gastrojejunostomy is done using Endo GIA™ linear stapler on the dependent posterior aspect of stomach. Nasojejunal and nasogastric tubes are used for feeding and decompression respectively. We routinely place tube drain at the pancreatic anastomotic site.

Results and Review of Literature

Gagner and Pomp reported the first laparoscopic pancreatoduodenectomy in 1994. They concluded laparoscopy is not worthwhile for such major resection and reconstruction. But their initial cases included chronic pancreatitis which is considered difficult to perform even now. Few other studies also concluded that there was no role for laparoscopy in pancreaticoduodenectomy at that time. In this background, we did not hurry up things in performing pancreaticoduodenectomy till we gained sufficient experience in other major laparoscopic procedures like colectomy, gastrectomy and choledochal cyst excision. During the initial phase of this series, we used to have stringent criteria for patient selection such as periampullary tumors or small pancreatic head mass. As we gained experience and confidence, we have successfully attempted a greater number of LPDs for carcinoma head of pancreas. In the latter part of our series, LPD for pancreatic head tumors were performed with almost the same frequency as periampullary tumors. We reported our early experience of 42 patients in the year 2006 which showed excellent perioperative outcomes reversing the initial trend. Few other studies confirmed the feasibility of this procedure. Over the years, we have made numerous technical modifications in terms of surgeon comfort, energy source, radicality of surgery, type of reconstruction and specimen extraction. These refinements in technique resulted in better outcomes as shown in our next publication in 2009 which included 75 patients. The mean operative time was 357 minutes, blood loss 74 mL, no conversions and overall postoperative morbidity was 26.7%. Pancreatic fistula developed in 5 patients which constitutes 6.67% which is very much acceptable and comparable to open approach. Oncologically, resection status and lymph nodal yield are comparable with open approach which translated into equal survival outcome. Recently, Asbun and colleagues compared their open and laparoscopic pancreatoduodenectomy and found to have better perioperative outcomes for laparoscopy in terms of blood loss, intensive care unit (ICU) stay and hospital stay.

CONCLUSION

Laparoscopic pancreatic resections were considered insurmountable till recently because of the intricacies involved in resection and reconstruction. But now the available evidence suggests that pancreatic resection by minimal access approach is here to stay. Among the resections done laparoscopically, distal pancreatectomy is now accepted as standard of care and should be offered as the preferred option for body and tail lesions. Though there are no well-designed randomized controlled studies to compare open and LDP, meta-analysis of case control studies have shown the benefits of laparoscopic approach like increased spleen preservation, less blood loss and shorter hospital stay. Radical pancreatectomy with adequate lymphadenectomy is also possible and evidence is accumulating for malignant lesions to be dealt with laparoscopy.

A retrospective review of a prospectively maintained database from March 1998 to April 2013 was done. A total of 130 patients were chosen for this study and patients who underwent LPD for benign diseases were excluded from the study (20 cases). We had one conversion to open in our series, overall postoperative morbidity being 29.7% and mortality rate was 1.53%. Pancreatic fistula rate was 8.46%. The mean operating time was 310±34 min, and the mean blood loss was 110±22 ml. The mean hospital stay was 8±2.6 days. Resected margins were positive in 9.23% of cases. The mean number of retrieved lymph nodes was 18.15±4.73. The overall 5 year actuarial survival (estimated from Kaplan Meir curve) is 29.42 % and the median survival is 33 months.

LPD had decreased transfusion requirements, shorter hospital stay, higher R0 margin status, increased lymph node retrieval. Well-controlled trials including case-control or prospective randomized studies should be performed in the future to explore the possible clinical advantages of LPD in terms of oncological radicality and overall outcomes.

Laparoscopic median pancreatectomy is technically feasible and safe surgical approach for removing pancreatic neck tumors in well-selected patients.[30] In experienced hands, it is associated with no mortality. Incidence of pancreatic fistula is although high. Most of the complications can be successfully managed conservatively.

It allows the surgeon to preserve pancreatic parenchyma and avoids long-term endocrine and exocrine pancreatic insufficiency especially in young patients.

Laparoscopic pancreaticoduodenectomy has thus crossed the feasibility stage and has come to be accepted as a viable alternative to open approach in selected centers across the world. From few case reports a decade ago, to large institutional trials currently, LPD has crossed the stage of infancy. The available evidence suggests comparable immediate postoperative and short-term outcomes to that of open surgery. However, certain issues like non-availability of randomized controlled trials (RCTs), oncological radicality, long-term survival and prolonged learning curve needs to be addressed in order to have a widespread acceptance and practice of LPD.

BIBLIOGRAPHY

1. Abu Hilal M, Hamdan M, Di Fabio F, Pearce NW, Johnson CD. Laparoscopic versus open distal pancreatectomy: a clinical and cost-effectiveness study. Surg Endosc. 2011;26:1670-4.
2. Asbun HJ, Stauffer JA. Laparoscopic vs open pancreaticoduodenectomy: overall outcomes and severity of complications using the Accordion Severity Grading System. J Am Coll Surg. 2012;215(6):810-9.
3. Butturini G, Inama M, Malleo G, Manfredi R, Melotti GL, Piccoli M, et al. Perioperative and longterm results of laparoscopic spleenpreserving distal pancreatectomy with or without splenic vessels conservation: a retrospective analysis. J Surg Oncol. 2012;105:387-92.
4. Casadei R, Ricci C, D'Ambra M, Marrano N, Alagna V, Rega D, et al. Laparoscopic versus open distal pancreatectomy in pancreatic tumours: a case-control study. Updates Surg. 2010;62:171-4.
5. Choi SH1, Kang CM, Lee WJ, Chi HS. Laparoscopic modified anterior RAMPS in well-selected left-sided pancreatic cancer: technical feasibility and interim results. Surg Endosc. 2011;25(7):2360-1.
6. DiNorcia J, Schrope BA, Lee MK, Reavey PL, Rosen SJ, Lee JA, et al. Laparoscopic distal pancreatectomy offers shorter hospital stays with fewer complications. J Gastrointest Surg. 2010;14:1804-12.
7. Fox AM, Pitzul K, Bhojani F, Kaplan M, Moulton CA, Wei AC, et al. Comparison of outcomes and costs between laparoscopic distal pancreatectomy and open resection at a single centre. Surg Endosc. 2012;26:1220-30.
8. Gagner M, Pomp A. Laparoscopic pylorus-preserving pancreatoduodenectomy, Surg Endosc. 1994;8(5):408-10.
9. Jayaraman S, Gonen M, Brennan MF, D'Angelica MI, DeMatteo RP, Fong Y, et al. Laparoscopic distal pancreatectomy: evolution of a technique at a single institution. J Am Coll Surg. 2010;211:503-9.
10. Jin T, Altaf K, Xiong JJ, Huang W, Javed MA, Mai G, et al. A systematic review and meta-analysis of studies comparing laparoscopic and open distal pancreatectomy. HPB (Oxford). 2012;14(11):711-24.
11. Kim SC, Park KT, Hwang JW, Shin HC, Lee SS, Seo DW et al. Comparative analysis of clinical outcomes for laparoscopic distal pancreatic resection and open distal pancreatic resection at a single institution. Surg Endosc. 2008;22:2261-8.
12. Kim SC, Song KB, Jung YS, Kim YH, Park DH, Lee SS, et al. Short-term clinical outcomes for 100 consecutive cases of laparoscopic pylorus-preserving pancreatoduodenectomy: improvement with surgical experience. Surg Endosc. 2013;27(1):95-103.
13. Kooby DA, Chu CK. Laparoscopic management of pancreatic malignancies. Surg Clin North Am. 2010;90(2):427-46.
14. Kooby DA, Gillespie T, Bentrem D, Nakeeb A, Schmidt MC, Merchant NB, et al. Left-sided pancreatectomy: a multicenter comparison of laparoscopic and open approaches. Ann Surg. 2008;248(3):438-46.
15. Kooby DA, Hawkins WG, Schmidt CM, Weber SM, Bentrem DJ, Gillespie TW, et al. A multicenter analysis of distal pancreatectomy for adenocarcinoma: is laparoscopic resection appropriate? J Am Coll Surg. 2010;210(5):779-85, 786-7.
16. Limongelli P, Belli A, Russo G, Cioffi L, D'Agostino A, Fantini C, et al. Laparoscopic and open surgical treatment of left-sided pancreatic lesions: clinical outcomes and cost-effectiveness analysis. Surg Endosc. 2012;26:1830-6.
17. Mabrut JY, Fernandez-Cruz L, Azagra JS, Bassi C, Delvaux G, Weerts J, et al. Laparoscopic pancreatic resection: results of a multicenter European study of 127 patients. Surgery. 2005;137(6):597-605.
18. Machado MA, Surjan RC, Epstein MG, Makdissi FF. Laparoscopic central pancreatectomy: a review of 51 cases. Surg Laparosc Endosc Percutan Tech. 2013;23(6):486-90.
19. Machado MA, Surjan RC, Goldman SM, Ardengh JC, Makdissi FF. Laparoscoic pancreatic resection. From enucleation to pancreatoduodenectomy. 11-year experience. Arq Gastroenterol. 2013;50(3):214-8.
20. Mehta SS, Doumane G, Mura T, Nocca D, Fabre JM. Laparoscopic versus open distal pancreatectomy: a single-institution case-control study. Surg Endosc. 2012;26:402-7.
21. Merchant NB, Parikh AA, Kooby DA. Should all distal pancreatectomies be performed laparoscopically? Adv Surg. 2009;43:283-300.
22. Palanivelu C, Jani K, Senthilnathan P, Parthasarathi R, Rajapandian S, Madhankumar MV. Laparoscopic pancreaticoduodenectomy: technique and outcomes. J Am Coll Surg. 2007;205(2):222-30.
23. Palanivelu C, Rajan PS, Rangarajan M, Vaithiswaran V, Senthilnathan P, Parthasarathi R, et al. Evolution in techniques of laparoscopic pancreaticoduodenectomy: a decade long experience from a tertiary center. J Hepatobiliary Pancreat Surg. 2009;16(6):731-40.
24. Palanivelu C, Shetty R, Jani K, Sendhilkumar K, Rajan PS, Maheshkumar GS. Laparoscopic distal pancreatectomy: results of a prospective non-randomized study from a tertiary center. Surg Endosc. 2007;21(3):373-7.
25. Røsok BI, Marangos IP, Kazaryan AM, Rosseland AR, Buanes T, Mathisen O, et al. Single-centre experience of laparoscopic pancreatic surgery. Br J Surg. 2010;97(6):902-9.
26. Sussman LA, Christie R, Whittle DE. Laparoscopic excision of distal pancreas including insulinoma. Aust N Z J Surg. 1996;66(6):414-6.
27. Ten years of experience with resection of left-sided pancreatic ductal adenocarcinoma: evolution and initial experience to a laparoscopic approach. Surg Endosc. 2010;24(7):1533-41.
28. Warshaw AL. Conservation of the spleen with distal pancreatectomy. Arch Surg. 1988;123(5):550-3.
29. Waters JA, Canal DF, Wiebke EA, Dumas RP, Beane JD, Aguilar-Saavedra JR, et al. Robotic distal pancreatectomy: cost-effective? Surgery. 2010;148:814-23.
30. Senthilnathan P, Gul SI, Gurumurthy SS, Palanivelu PR, Parthasarathi R, Palanisamy NV, Natesan VA, Palanivelu C. Laparoscopic central pancreatectomy: Our technique and long-term results in 14 patients. J Min Access Surg 2015;11:167-71.

CHAPTER 47

Pancreaticoduodenal Injuries

Satish B Dharap

INTRODUCTION

Duodenal and pancreatic injuries are relatively less common. However, they are often missed—not only while evaluating abdominal trauma but also during laparotomy. This leads to delayed recognition resulting in risk to life due to several complications particularly sepsis. Their management demands high degree of clinical acumen and surgical dexterity.

Asensio et al. have reported the incidence of pancreatic trauma in the range from 0.2% to 6% and that of duodenal injury from 3% to 5% of all patients with abdominal injury. Two-thirds of these occur due to penetrating injury.[1] While blunt injuries are usually isolated, penetrating injuries almost always have multiple associated intra-abdominal injuries.[1] Both are challenging with high mortality ranging 9–34% (mean 19%) in pancreatic injuries and 6–25% in duodenal injuries. Morbidity is reported in the range of 30–60%.[2]

CLINICAL PRESENTATIONS

The following four different settings can be considered:

1. Emergency setting, suspected abdominal trauma with unstable hemodynamics: The goal is to save life.
2. Emergency setting with stable hemodynamics: The goal is to achieve early diagnosis, plan appropriate definitive treatment in order to prevent morbidity and mortality
3. Elective setting: Delayed presentation with abdominal pain and lump or distension with past history of trauma with probable clinical diagnosis of pseudocyst or pancreatic ascites. Such patients merit elective evaluation and management by endotherapy or open surgery and will not be further discussed here.
4. Iatrogenic injuries: Duodenum in particular can be injured during operations in nearby vicinity and during procedures like endoscopic retrograde cholangio-pancreatography (ERCP). These have also been excluded.

Emergency Setting: Unstable Patient

While evaluating a trauma patient priority is always toward recognition and management of immediately life threatening conditions, i.e. relief of airway obstruction, relief of compromised breathing and rapid control of bleeding and fluid resuscitation.

In any patient with suspected abdominal injury in a state of shock, a surgeon has to swiftly decide about the need for a lifesaving laparotomy; which is indicated if ultrasound [focused assessment by sonography in trauma or (FAST)] reveals the presence of free fluid or if free flow of blood is obtained on the diagnostic peritoneal aspirate. In a patient with penetrating abdominal trauma immediate laparotomy is recommended in presence of shock, evisceration or high velocity weapon use. No further investigation is necessary.

Lifesaving Laparotomy for Abdominal Trauma[3]

Long midline incision is recommended as it gives adequate access to all parts of abdomen and can be easily extended from xiphisternum to pubis should the need arise. Hemorrhage control is the top priority and liver, splenic or retroperitoneal vascular injury which could be associated needs to be given an urgent attention. Entire bowel should be quickly taken out (eviscerated) and multiple large abdominal packs placed over the liver, spleen, paracolic gutters, on either side in the pelvis and over any bleeding area before proceeding with examination of supracolic and infracolic compartments. They are serially taken out taking care of any active bleeding appropriately. The diagnosis of injury to duodenum and pancreas is intraoperative and both being retroperitoneal organs, injuries can be missed on an exploratory laparotomy unless specifically looked for.

Exploration for Pancreatic or Duodenal Injury

Periduodenal hematoma, bile staining, bogginess or crepitus around the duodenum are suggestive of duodenal injury while a central hematoma should raise suspicion of pancreatic injury. Thorough exploration is necessary to assess retroperitoneal injury. This involves Kocher's maneuver (Kocherization of the duodenum) which exposes the second part of the duodenum and the pancreatic head; opening of lesser sac by laying open the gastrocolic omentum which exposes the body and the tail of the pancreas and Cattell-Braasch maneuver (dissection beginning around the cecum and the terminal ileum which lifts up the root of the mesentery) exposing the third part of the duodenum and duodenojejunal flexure. Further access to the body and the tail of the pancreas are provided by Mattox maneuver in which left colon and the spleen are rotated medially after a lateral peritoneal incision (left medial visceral rotation).

Extent and severity of injury should be assessed. The definitive treatment is planned as per the extent and severity of injury and patient's general condition.

Damage control approach should be adopted in a patient with persistent shock with metabolic failure, i.e. triad of hypothermia, coagulopathy and acidosis. Injuries involving distal pancreas with bleeding are best managed with expeditious splenectomy with distal pancreatectomy. If duodenum is also injured in such cases, reconstructive procedure should be deferred till a later date. Open bowel can be closed or stapled and duct can be drained or just tied. Temporary abdominal closure is carried out. Patient is shifted to intensive care for further resuscitation, metabolic correction and stabilization with a plan for re-laparotomy usually by 48–72 hours when definitive repair is carried out.

Main pancreatic duct injury appears to escalate pancreas specific morbidity and mortality[4] and all attempts should be made to recognize ductal injury in a stable patient. Direct visualization of ductal injury, more than 50% parenchymal laceration, central gland perforation, transection of pancreas, or severe contusion are strong indicators of ductal disruption.[4] Intraoperative pancreatic ductogram has been described—either by transduodenal cannulation through ampulla or by cannulation of the distal duct near the tail. Intraoperative cholangiogram has been used to diagnose bile duct injury. Intravenous secretin has been used to stimulate pancreatic secretion and the clear efflux of secretion from the severed pancreatic duct has been identified with the help of magnifying loupe.[5] Intraoperative ultrasound has also been used to identify pancreatic ductal injury.[5]

Emergency Setting: Stable Patient

When hemodynamically stable, the patient should undergo thorough clinical and radiological evaluation. In such cases, mechanism of injury often suggests pancreatico-duodenal injury.

Mechanism of Injury

Blunt pancreatico-duodenal injuries are often the result of a force which crushes these tissues against dorsolumbar spine. Bicycle handle bar injury is a common mechanism observed in children.[6] In a motor vehicle crash, a driver can sustain steering wheel injury leading to pancreatic or duodenal disruption. An inappropriately applied seat belt has also been implicated.[7] A severe forceful blow over the epigastrium could be responsible. It should also be suspected if there is any evidence of injury to dorsolumbar spine (Fig. 1). Duodenojejunal disruption can result from deceleration mechanism as it is a junction of the fixed and mobile part of intestine.

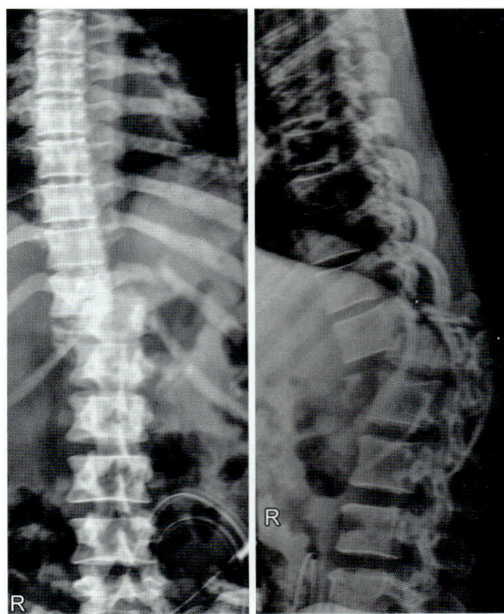

Figure 1 Dorsolumbar spine X-ray showing vertebral body fracture subluxation at dorsolumbar junction. CT scan abdomen revealed pneumoperitoneum. Laparotomy revealed D2 laceration. It was treated by pyloric exclusion with good recovery from duodenal injury

In patients with penetrating trauma, pancreatico-duodenal injuries should be suspected in all cases with high velocity weapon wounds.

Clinical Examination

Bruises, abrasions and entry or exit wounds may suggest internal injury. Tenderness, guarding and rigidity although expected may not be present in early stages due to retroperitoneal location of injury. Also these signs may be absent in patients with head injury and spinal injury with neurological deficit. Therefore further investigation to rule out internal injury is warranted in all patients with major trauma.

INVESTIGATIONS

Abdominal paracentesis: Although widely practiced in many places in India, this investigation is not recommended in view of high false negativity.[8]

Diagnostic peritoneal lavage: Diagnostic peritoneal lavage (DPL) is not reliable in the diagnosis of retroperitoneal injury.[7] A raised amylase level in lavage fluid indicates any bowel injury and is not specific for pancreatic injury.[1]

Ultrasonography: Presence of free fluid on FAST ultrasound scan suggests some abdominal injury and in stable patient indicates need to carry out further evaluation by CT scan. It is more often due to associated injuries rather than pancreatico-duodenal injuries. In emergency setting ultrasonographic evaluation of pancreas is not possible due to bowel gas. Like DPL, FAST is also not a reliable investigation to diagnose retroperitoneal injuries.[7]

Serum amylase and lipase levels may be elevated in case of pancreatic injury; but these tests are usually not asked for while evaluating a patient with acute trauma unless pancreatic injury is suspected. Although hyperamylasemia is encountered its sensitivity and specificity is not enough to consider it as diagnostic. Repeated amylase determination for 48 hours might be helpful in diagnosing major duct injury.[4]

Plain X rays: Free intraperitoneal air on chest X-ray suggests injury to hollow viscus and presence of retroperitoneal air outlining kidneys or psoas in abdominal films has been described to suggest retroperitoneal duodenal injury.[1] Spinal X-rays showing fracture of transverse process or vertebral body in L1, L2 region of dorsolumbar spine should raise suspicion of injury to the duodenum or pancreas.[1]

Contrast studies: Gastroduodenal series done after water soluble oral contrast was the investigation done in past to diagnose duodenal injuries. It is largely replaced by the CT scan.

CT scan: Contrast enhanced CT scan is the investigation of choice in diagnosing pancreatico-duodenal injuries. It may sometimes be precluded by raised creatinine. Duodenal injury should be suspected if there is evidence of retroperitoneal air or leak of contrast and duodenal wall thickening. Abdominal CT scan without oral contrast has been reported to pick about 75% of duodenal injuries.[9] Use of oral contrast enhances the diagnosis of retroperitoneal duodenal injury. Pancreatic transection appears as an area of hypodensity in the region of pancreas suggestive of disruption (Fig. 2). If disruption involves more than 50% of pancreatic tissue, ductal injury should be suspected. Unexplained thickening of the anterior renal fascia, pancreatic edema, gross enlargement of the gland, presence of fluid separating the splenic vein or pancreatic body are also considered consistent with pancreatic injury.[1] However, abdominal CT scan is only moderately sensitive in detecting severity of pancreatic injury. It may, both miss and underestimate the injuries.[4]

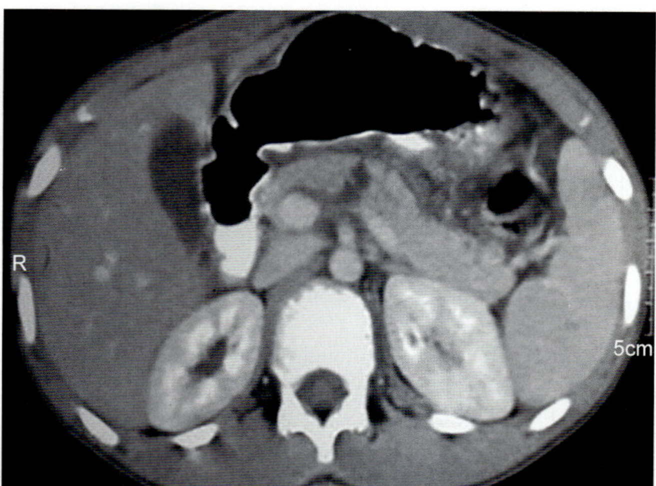

Figure 2 CT scan of abdomen showing hypodensity over the pancreatic neck, suggestive of pancreatic laceration

MR cholangiopancreatography (MRCP): If CT scan reveals pancreatic transection, ductal disruption should be evaluated by MRCP—particularly secretin stimulated MRCP.[10,11]

Endoscopic retrograde cholangio-pancreatography (ERCP): ERCP is usually not feasible in acute settings as it may be difficult to position the patient due to hemodynamic state or pain or associated injuries. Although invasive it has therapeutic benefit. When feasible it has been used for both the preoperative diagnosis of ductal disruption as well as endoscopic management including pancreatic sphincterotomy and pancreatic ductal stenting.[12]

GRADING OF INJURIES

Severity of organ injury guides the injury management. American Association of Surgery for Trauma (AAST) has adopted organ injury scale as shown in Tables 1 and 2.[13]

Table 1: Duodenum injury scale

Grade	*Type of injury*	*Description*
I	Hematoma	Involving single portion of duodenum
	Laceration	Partial thickness, no perforation
II	Hematoma	Involving more than one portion
	Laceration	Disruption <50% of circumference
III	Laceration	Disruption 50–75% of circumference of D2 Disruption 50–100% of circumference of D1, D3 or D4
IV	Laceration	Disruption >75% of circumference of D2 involving ampulla or distal common bile duct
V	Laceration	Massive disruption of duodeno-pancreatic complex
	Vascular	Devascularization of duodenum

Advance one grade for multiple injuries up to grade III

Table 2: Pancreatic injury scale

Grade	*Type of injury*	*Description*
I	Hematoma	Minor contusion without duct injury
	Laceration	Superficial laceration without duct injury
II	Hematoma	Major contusion without duct injury or tissue loss
	Laceration	Major laceration without duct injury or tissue loss
III	Laceration	Distal transection or parenchymal injury with duct injury
IV	Laceration	Proximal# transection or parenchymal injury involving ampulla
V	Laceration	Massive disruption of pancreatic head

#Proximal pancreas is to the right of the superior mesenteric vein.
Advance one grade for multiple injuries up to grade III.

DEFINITIVE TREATMENT

It must be remembered that it is rare to explore the patient with preoperative diagnosis of pancreatico-duodenal injuries. More often it is the diagnosis on table, and therefore, a thorough exploration of the retroperitoneum as described earlier is essential to detect the injuries. During any laparotomy for trauma, the priority is hemorrhage control and hemodynamic stabilization of the patient.

ISOLATED DUODENAL INJURIES

Second part of duodenum is the most frequently injured part (33%) followed by the third, fourth and first parts. In 14% patients multiple parts are injured.[1] Duodenal hematoma is the only injury which can be treated non operatively if diagnosed preoperatively or may be left alone if found on laparotomy.

Injuries to the second part of the duodenum are often diagnosed late, associated with contamination and friable edematous bowel, making primary closure technically difficult and anastomotic healing rare. A number of procedures have been described. The decision depends upon extent of tissue loss, involvement of the papilla, associated pancreatic injury and extent of contamination. If the duodenal wound allows primary closure, it should be carried out. In a clean cut stab injuries without contamination this alone may suffice. The serosal patch can be used to reinforce the suture line. Most injuries can be repaired by primary closure in one or two layers.[14] The closure should be oriented transversely if possible, to avoid luminal compromise. In case of complete duodenal transection, the preferred method of repair is primary anastomosis after appropriate debridement and mobilization. However, this is not possible in case of tissue loss. Such an injury involving duodenum above the papilla can be treated by antrectomy, closure of the duodenal stump and gastrojejunostomy. When it is distal to the ampulla, closure of the distal duodenum and Roux-en-Y duodenojejunal anastomosis is appropriate.[14] The decompression of the affected duodenum can be achieved by a duodenostomy which can be done either antegrade (transgastric), direct (transduodenal/lateral duodenostomy) or retrograde (transjejunal) (Fig. 3). Lateral duodenostomy is often complicated by leak as it is usually not possible to get the duodenum to the parietal wall.

Stone and Garoni have described "triple ostomy" comprising of a gastrostomy tube to decompress the stomach, a retrograde jejunostomy tube to decompress the duodenum and an antegrade feeding jejunostomy.[14] This technique involves making new openings in the uninjured bowel with the risk of leak. Also, the decompression is not as efficient as desired.[14]

In presence of delayed operation, edematous edges and contamination, the suture-line leak is a concern. In such cases, *pyloric exclusion* (Fig. 4) has been described consisting of closure of the duodenal wound, gastrotomy and suturing of the pylorus with absorbable sutures and gastrojejunostomy. Biliary drainage by T tube can also be added to facilitate diversion from the anastomotic site. Addition of vagotomy has been described to prevent the risk of marginal ulcers. This technique is usually used for wounds involving more than 50% of circumference of the duodenum or with associated pancreatic injury.[1] *Duodenal diverticulization* (Fig. 5) can also be attempted which consists of closure of the wound, vagotomy, antrectomy and gastrojejeunostomy. This technique is preferred when there is associated injury to gastric antrum and/or pylorus.[1]

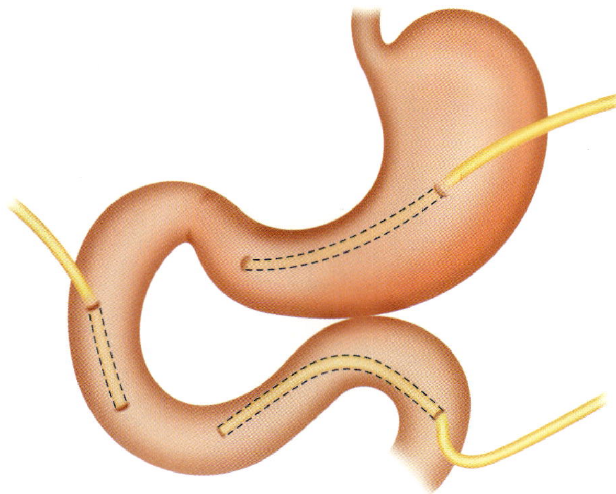

Figure 3 Techniques of duodenal decompression—transgastric (prograde), lateral duodenostomy, transjejunal (retrograde)

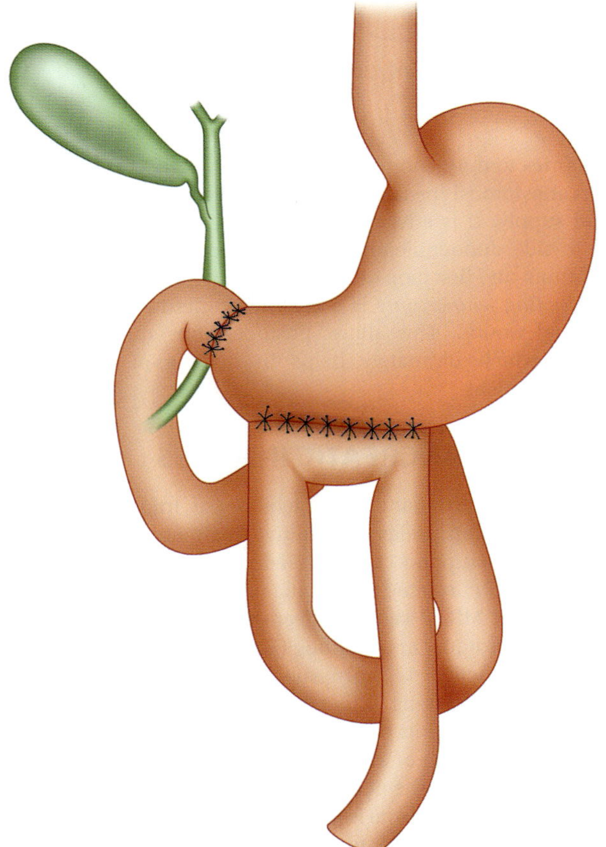

Figure 4 Pyloric exclusion: Pylorus is sutured with delayed absorbable sutures through a gastrotomy which is converted into a gastrojejunostomy

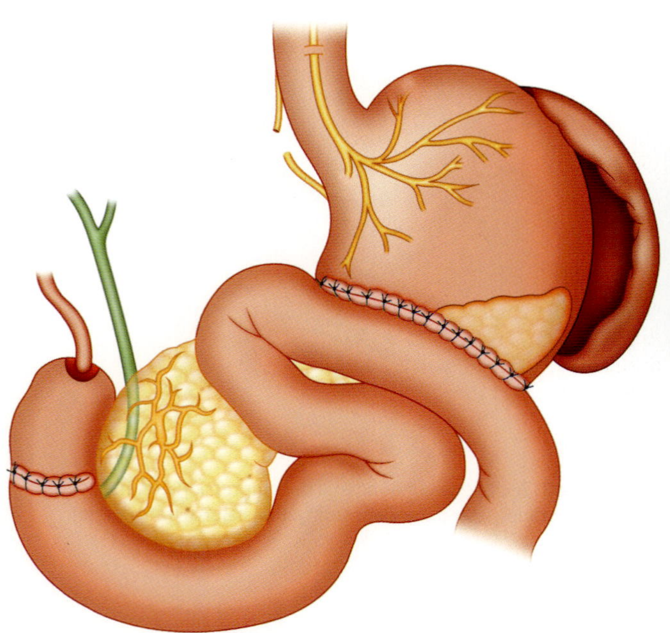

Figure 5 Duodenal diverticulization

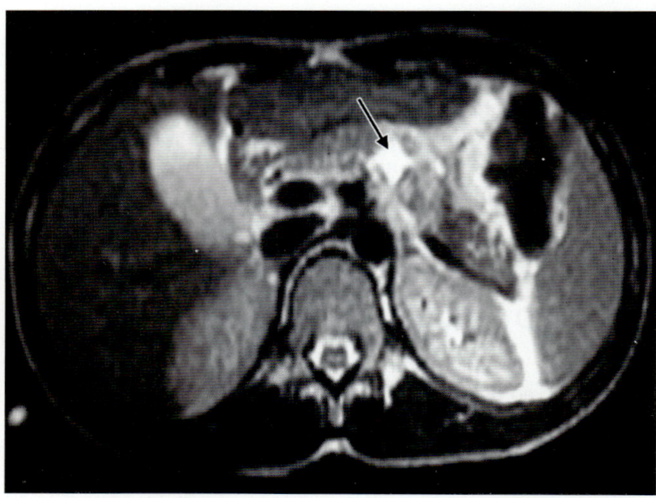

Figure 6 MRCP showing pancreatic duct transaction. ERCP revealed partial duct disruption. This 9-year-old child was successfully treated by pancreatic sphincterotomy. Stenting was not possible due to small size of the duct

Injuries to duodenojejunal junction are difficult to manage by direct anastomosis because of difficult access and have precarious blood supply. It is advisable to close the ends and to establish side to side duodenojejunostomy between the third part of the duodenum and first loop of the jejunum.

A feeding jejunostomy is a useful adjunct to management of duodenal wound. This allows postoperative enteral nutritional support which ultimately helps in healing of the probable anastomotic leak.

ISOLATED PANCREATIC INJURIES

Two major determinants of outcome are Injury to the main pancreatic duct and delay to definitive treatment.[2,4]

If ductal disruption can be ruled out, patient can be treated non-operatively. Isolated pancreatic injury with ductal disruption diagnosed on MRCP can be effectively managed by pancreatic duct sphincterotomy and stenting (Fig. 6). Proximal ductal injury without obstruction is more suitable for stenting than distal injury.[15] When stenting is not possible, surgical exploration is recommended. Patients treated non-operatively need to be closely observed. Worsening of abdominal signs and rising amylase and lipase levels indicate the need for surgical intervention.[5]

When there is no ductal injury (Grades I and II), drainage alone is sufficient.[4] Some are treated by pancreatorrhaphy, debridement of devitalized tissue and drainage.[1] In presence of ductal injury (Grade III and higher) resectional procedure and drainage of the stump should be undertaken to reduce morbidity.[4] Primary repair of ductal injury leads to postoperative complications and hence is not recommended.[4] Commonest site of injury is at the pancreatic neck followed by head, body and tail. In general, injuries to the left of the superior mesenteric vessels can be

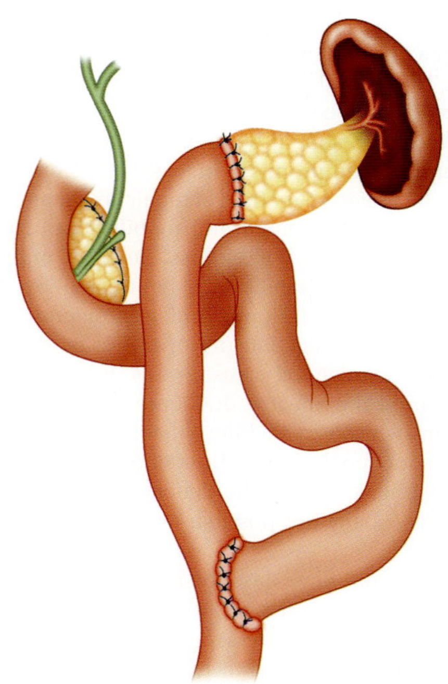

Figure 7 Roux-en-Y pancreaticojejunostomy to preserve distal pancreas after transaction

treated by distal pancreatectomy with or without splenectomy. Pancreatic tissue can be conserved by establishing an internal drainage of the injured pancreas into the roux-en-Y jejunal loop or pancreaticogastrostomy (Fig. 7).

Management of isolated pancreatic ductal disruption diagnosed early by imaging is often debated—whether to treat a stable patient by surgery or non-operatively? Sequelae of nonoperative treatment of pancreatic ductal injury could range from a more favorable pseudocyst formation (amenable to internal drainage at a later date), to morbid intra-abdominal infections (needing drainage leading to fistula) or multiple organ dysfunction syndrome (MODS) and death. Hamidian Jahromi et al. have reported similar rate of complications in two groups—(1) surgical and (2) nonsurgical; however, those treated non-operatively required significantly longer duration of parenteral nutrition and hospital stay.[16] In pediatric cases also operative treatment in cases of ductal injury has been found to reduce duration of hospital stay and complications when compared to nonoperative management.[4] Availability of facilities like ERCP for stenting and interventional radiology for guided drainage of intra-abdominal fluid collections and infections enhance the scope for nonoperative management. The management plan has to be individualized based on patient's condition and available resources.

COMBINED PANCREATICO-DUODENAL INJURY

These injuries have high mortality due to bleeding and sepsis. They are often due to penetrating trauma and are associated with multiple intra-abdominal injuries particularly major vascular injury. If the patient is unstable, biliary diversion, suture closure of the tear and drainage is all that is possible as a part of damage control surgery. If stable, biliary and pancreatic ductal integrity should be established if possible by an intraoperative ductography. If intact, the suture repair of the tear and drainage is all that is necessary.

Whipple's pancreatico-duodenectomy is rarely needed. It may be considered for uncontrollable bleeding from the head of the pancreas or neighboring vasculature or if there is irreparable injury to the duodenum or pancreatic head or ampulla or vascular compromise of the pancreatico-duodenal complex. Most such patients are hemodynamically unstable and therefore drainage may be a preferred option to pancreatico-duodenectomy.

Drainage

All pancreatic and duodenal injuries treated surgically should be drained with a closed system, avoiding juxtaposition to the suture line to avoid fistula formation.[1] Closed suction drain is better than sump drain which is better than penrose drain in reducing drain related complications like infection.[4]

Octreotide

Octreotide is often used by surgeons after pancreatic surgery and injury. But available evidence does not demonstrate any reduction in frequency and severity of complications after its usage.[4]

Outcome

Mortality for duodenal and pancreatic injury has been reported to range from 5-30% and 5-55% respectively.[1] Most early deaths are due to exsanguination while late deaths are due to complications of duodenal and pancreatic injury.

Complications

Anastomotic leak and intra-abdominal abscesses and duodenal fistula, pancreatic fistula, post-traumatic pancreatitis, pseudocyst and hemorrhage, sepsis, multiple organ dysfunction syndrome are frequently observed in pancreatico-duodenal injuries. [1]

AUTHOR'S VIEWS

High velocity penetrating trauma is uncommon in civilian practice. Most low velocity penetrating traumas undergo immediate laparotomy in view of peritoneal penetration. Such duodenal injuries are always clean cut without much contamination and respond well to primary suturing alone. Blunt duodenal injuries are often operated late due to delay in diagnosis. Because of contamination and tissue edema, primary repair is not sufficient. Author prefers pyloric exclusion because of its simplicity. Tube drainage of the area and feeding jejunostomy are a must. Suture-line leak is commonly observed, but if drain tube is functioning well, then a jejunostomy permits cost-effective enteral feeding with healing of the suture-line.

Most pancreatic injuries follow blunt trauma. When diagnosed preoperatively, in case of pancreatic ductal injury if stenting is not possible, author's preference is for surgical exploration rather than conservative treatment. Splenectomy and distal pancreatectomy is a safe choice. Spleen preserving distal pancreatectomy although attractive in principle is technically difficult and is associated with the risk of intraoperative hemorrhage and postoperative fistula. Pancreaticogastrostomy is the author's preferred technique of internal drainage as it obviates the need for multiple anastomoses unlike in Roux-en-Y pancreaticojejunostomy.

Pancreatico-duodenectomy has a very high mortality rate, and drainage and diversion in emergency seems to be a better option.

SUMMARY

The diagnosis and management of pancreatico-duodenal injuries are challenging. In an unstable patient with abdominal trauma emergent life-saving laparotomy must be expeditiously performed. Retroperitoneal structures must be examined in all trauma patients undergoing a laparotomy—particularly with periduodenal or central hematoma, retroperitoneal bile staining or crepitus. Control of hemorrhage and spillage are the only goals and time consuming reconstructions should be deferred in an unstable patient. In stable patients, it is possible to achieve preoperative diagnosis with contrast enhanced CT scan. Principles of repair of duodenal injury involve closure of wound whenever possible, diversion of chyme and bile from the site of injury, provision for postoperative jejunal feeding and drainage of the injured area.

Pancreatic injury needs intervention only if the duct is disrupted, which can be diagnosed on MR cholangiopancreatography and in a suitable case, endoscopic pancreatic stenting should be attempted. Nonoperative management of ductal disruption in the absence of stenting is associated with prolonged hospital stay as compared to the surgical intervention. Principles of surgical management of pancreatic injury with ductal disruption involve resection or internal drainage of the distal stump with closure of the proximal stump and drainage of the area. Patients must be closely watched for complications like infected collection, pseudocyst and fistula.

REFERENCES

1. Asensio JA, Petrone P, Roldán G, Pak-art R, Salim A. Pancreatic and duodenal injuries. Complex and lethal. Scand J Surg. 2002;91(1):81-6.
2. Jurkovich GJ. Injuries to the pancreas and duodenum in ACS Surgery: Principles and Practice BC Decker Inc. (Publishers) 2008.
3. Boffard KD (Ed). Manual of Definitive Surgical Trauma Care, 3rd edition, London: Hodder Arnold; 2011.
4. Bokhari F, Phelan H, Holev AR, Brautigam AR, Collier B, Como JJ, et al. EAST guidelines for the diagnosis and management of pancreatic trauma, 2009.
5. Subramanian A, Dente CJ, Feliciano DV. The management of pancreatic trauma in the modern era. Surgical Clinica of North Amerca. 2007;87:1515-32.
6. Arkovitz MS, Johnson N, Garcia VF. Pancreatic trauma in children: mechanisms of injury. J Trauma. 1997;42(1):49-53.
7. Abdominal and Pelvic Trauma in Advanced Trauma Life Support® Student Course Manual, 9th edition. © 2012 American College of Surgeons.
8. Ergene U, Coşkun F, Eray O, Gokçe O, Fowler J, Haciyanli M, et al. Current value of peritoneal tap in blunt abdominal trauma. Eur J Emerg Med. 2002;9(3):253-7.
9. Holmes JF, Offerman SR, Chang CH, Randel BE, Hahn DD, Frankovsky MJ, et al. Performance of helical computed tomography without oral contrast for the detection of gastrointestinal injuries. Ann Emerg Med. 2004;43(1):120-8.
10. Ragozzino A, Manfredi R, Scaglione M, De Ritis R, Romano S, Rotondo A. The use of MRCP in the detection of pancreatic injuries after blunt trauma. Emerg Radiol. 2003;10(1):14-8.
11. Gilliams AR, Kurzawinski T, Lees WR. Diagnosis of duct disruption and assessment of pancreatic leak with dynamic secretin stimulated MR cholangiopancreatography. American Journal of Roentgenology. 2006;186:499-506.
12. Rogers SJ, Cello JP, Schecter WP. Endoscopic retrograde cholangiopancreatography in patients with pancreatic trauma. Trauma. 2010;68(3):538-44.
13. Moore EE, Cogbill TH, Malangoni MA, Jurkovich GJ, Champion HR, Gennarelli TA, et al. Organ injury scaling II: pancreas, duodenum, small bowel, colon and rectum. J Trauma. 1990;30:1427-9.
14. Degiannis E, Boffard K. Duodenal injuries. British Journal of Surgery. 2000;87:1473-9.
15. Okamoto H, Fujii H. Traumatic pancreatitis-Endoscopic and Surgical Management in Pancreatitis-Treatment and Complications, Prof. Louis Rodrigo (Ed), ISBN 978-953-51-0109-3, In Tech Available from: http://www.intechopen.com/books/panreatitis-treatment-and-complications/-traumatic-pancreatitis-endoscopic-and-surgical-managements.
16. Hamidian Jahromi A, D'Agostino HR, Zibari GB, Chu QD, Clark C, Shokouh-Amiri H. Surgical versus nonsurgical management of traumatic major pancreatic duct transection: institutional experience and review of the literature. Pancreas. 2013;42(1):76-87.

CHAPTER 48

Pancreas and Islet Transplantation

Rakesh Rai

Pancreas Transplant

INTRODUCTION

Type I diabetes mellitus is an autoimmune condition which results in selective destruction of beta cells in the islets of Langerhans.[1] According to International Diabetes Federation (IDF) in 2011, more than 366 million people had diabetes worldwide, which led to 4.6 million deaths each year. The highest incidence of diabetes is now reported from Indian subcontinent. The reported prevalence of diabetes in adults between the ages of 20 and 79 is as follows: India 8.31%, Bangladesh 9.85%, Nepal 3.03%, Sri Lanka 7.77% and Pakistan 6.72%.[2] In India, age-related prevalence of diabetes is significantly higher than several other countries.[3]

Due to recent advances in the management of type 1 diabetes mellitus (T1DM) the incidence of kidney failure has decreased over time. Earlier 15% of patients who survive with diabetes for 30 years developed renal dysfunction[4] now it is less than 8%.[5] The advantages of accurate glycemic control on the progression of renal disease have been well accepted in the Diabetes Control and Complications Trial (DCCT)[6] and Epidemiology of Diabetes Interventions and Complications (EDIC)[7] Trial.

The aim of pancreas transplantation is to restore a physiological control by providing Beta cells especially for type 1 diabetes where they have been destroyed by an autoimmune process. Such a control of glucose metabolism may result in stopping or even reversing the secondary complications of diabetes, i.e. neuropathy, nephropathy, retinopathy, microangiopathy and macroangiopathy.[8]

HISTORY

Experimental pancreatic transplantation in animals started in 1890 and demonstrated success in the treatment of insulin dependent diabetes mellitus.[9] The first successful simultaneous kidney and pancreas transplantation was performed by W.D. Kelly and Richard Lillehei from the University of Minnesota in 1966.[10] Between 1967 and 1973, 12 transplants were done at University of Minnesota but nearly all of them got rejected before completing the first year.

Other than rejection management of exocrine secretions of pancreas was another major problem. During 1970s three different procedures were being used for drainage of pancreatic exocrine secretions: (1) enteric drainage (ED), (2) urinary drainage (UD) into the ureter or (3) directly into the bladder (BD). In 1978, Dubernard et al.[11] reported a technique of injecting neoprene, a synthetic polymer in the pancreatic duct of the segmental pancreas graft. In 1983, Hans Sollinger[12] at the University of Wisconsin reported draining segmental graft pancreatic duct to the bladder. The advantage of this technique was that urinary amylase could be easily monitored and decrease in urinary amylase served as a sensitive, though nonspecific, marker of rejection. Another significant event in the early 80s was introduction of cyclosporine for immunosuppression[13] which led to significant improvement in outcome of transplants. The main disadvantage of bladder drainage was chronic problem of urinary tract infections, hematuria, acidosis, dehydration that required conversion to enteric drainage in 10–15% of bladder drained recipients.

Thus in 1984, Starzl et al.[14] reintroduced the technique of enteric drainage.

Till 1991 venous drainage of pancreas was in systemic vein mainly iliac vein. In 1992 Rosenlof et al.[15] from the University of Virginia and Shokouh-Amiri group[16] from University of Tennessee described the technique where portal vein of the graft was anastomosed with the portal vein of the recipient.

Living donors pancreas transplant using Segmental graft was first introduced in 1979 in University of Minnesota[17] and laparoscopic distal pancreatectomy of the donor was introduced in

2001 at the same center.[18] In India, a case of simultaneous kidney-pancreas transplant was reported in 2005.[19]

INDICATION OF PANCREAS TRANSPLANT

Pancreas transplantation is carried out in patients with type 1 diabetes and in selected group of type 2 diabetes who are on insulin and have renal failure.

While selecting patients for pancreas transplant the risk and benefit has to be carefully weighed as it is not an immediate life-saving procedure. The need for lifetime immunosuppression immediate complications of the procedure and frequent interventional surveillance (such as protocol biopsies) has to be considered.

The most common indications for pancreas transplant are as follows:

Patients with diabetes who have end organ damage, like diabetic nephropathy, retinopathy, neuropathy, or those with incapacitating emotional or clinical problems associated with insulin therapy.[8] Patients with hypoglycemic unawareness are also candidates for pancreas transplant even in absence of other complications of diabetes.[20]

Only 10% of cases are performed as pancreas transplantation alone (PTA) in patients with very labile and problematic diabetes or in patients with hypoglycemic unawareness or other diabetic complications without proteinuria. Majority (about 75%) of pancreatic transplantations are done simultaneously with kidney transplantation in patients with diabetic nephropathy with renal failure. Both organs are from the same donor and this is referred to as simultaneous pancreas-kidney (SPK) transplantation. About 15% of pancreas transplantations follow kidney transplant (PAK).

The total number of pancreas transplantations in the US reported to IPTR/UNOS from December 16, 1966, through December 31, 2010 was 25,030. In 2010, 7% of pancreas transplant was for type 2 diabetes.[21]

Patient with diabetes and chronic renal dysfunction has multiple treatment options. Selection of procedure will depend on multiple factors including waiting time for renal or pancreatic graft. Before deciding on treatment choice following assessment should be undertaken (Flow chart 1).

- Has the patient got any living donor for kidney transplant?
- How severe and debilitating are the diabetes related symptoms and how is the glycemic control with best diabetic care available?
- Patient needs to understand the increased risk of mortality (2%) and pancreatic graft loss (10–15%) in the first year if SPK is done rather kidney transplant alone.
- Waiting time for a cadaver SPK graft?

Flow chart 1 Therapeutic approach to the patient with type 1 diabetes mellitus (T1DM) with glomerular filtration rate (GFR) <30 mL/min[22]

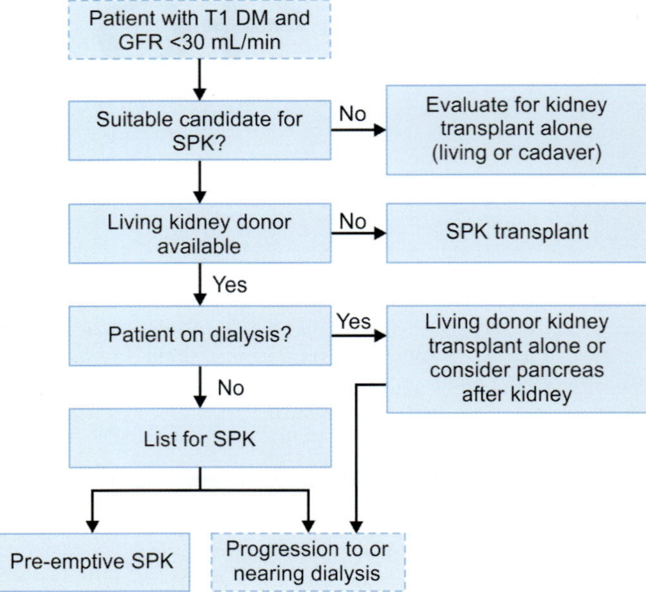

CADAVERIC PANCREAS TRANSPLANTATION

Selection of Cadaver Donor

Majority of pancreas graft comes from brain dead cadaver donor worldwide. Although pancreas grafts from donation after cardiac death (DCD) donors can be successfully transplanted. In 2010, only 4% of pancreatic graft came from DCD donors as per International Pancreas Transplant Registry (IPTR) data. Cadaver pancreatic donation is based on ABO compatibility and on a documented negative cross match. In SPK transplants HLA matching is not critical but for solitary pancreas transplants the degree of match affects graft survival.[23]

Contraindications for pancreas donation include presence of acute or chronic pancreatitis, active infection or malignancy, hepatitis C virus (HCV), human immunodeficiency virus (HIV), hepatitis B surface antigen (HBsAg) positive donor, proven diabetes mellitus, severe pancreatic steatosis edema, previous pancreatic surgery and intra-abdominal sepsis.

An ideal pancreas donor is in age from 10 to 40 years, weigh from 30 to 80 kg and have sustained brain death due to a traumatic etiology. With increasing experience in pancreas transplantation, some of the earlier contraindications for pancreas donation have become mere risk factors for a successful outcome. According to International Pancreas Transplant Registry data, the following variables: (1) donor age above 40 years; (2) cardiovascular or cerebrovascular cause of brain death and (3) cold ischemia time greater than 24 hours, are associated with an increased incidence of pancreas allograft thrombosis.

Donor age as a risk factor for pancreatic graft thrombosis is debatable. Some studies have suggested that it is an independent risk factor for graft loss[24] and thrombosis,[25] whereas others have shown it may only be a factor indirectly, that is, a surrogate for other factors including a "cause of death other than trauma.[26] Either way, it would be prudent to consider limiting donors of advanced age, especially when the same patients have other risk factors, which in conjunction with their age, would almost certainly increase the incidence of thrombosis and reduce overall graft survival.

In pancreatic transplant, donor obesity has been shown to increase the risk of surgical infections, thrombosis, overall technical failure and short-term graft survival.[27] Other donor risk factors include hemodynamic instability with massive volume resuscitation involving catecholamine therapy and a cerebrovascular cause of death.[25] Due to these criteria, in 2004, only 21%

of the available deceased donor in Unites States were used as pancreas donor as per the IPTR report.

Donor Surgery

Procurement of pancreas must be done by a team well experienced in pancreatic retrieval. It is very important that suitability of pancreas graft is assessed by examination of pancreas in donor by an experienced pancreas transplant surgeon. Organs demonstrating gross fibrosis, with a firm or "woody" texture of the parenchyma, typically are not accepted. Surgeon needs to have a solid knowledge of anatomical variants of intra-abdominal vessels, which is of great importance in case of multi-organ procurement. It must be remembered that even in presence of vascular anomalies, combined liver, kidney and whole-organ pancreaticoduodenal retrieval can be safely done. Harvesting techniques used are adjusted to the anatomical vascular variants and hemodynamic status of the donor and require proper identification, dissection and cannulation of the vascular pedicles.[28]

Long midline incision is used. Next step is exploration which involves verification of the vascular anatomy of the upper abdomen (mainly variant of hepatic arterial anatomy like origin of right hepatic artery arising from the superior mesenteric artery (SMA) or the left hepatic artery from the left gastric artery). Pancreatic head is supplied by the superior pancreaticoduodenal artery from the celiac trunk and the inferior pancreaticoduodenal artery from the SMA. Splenic artery, SMA and dorsal pancreatic artery have to be preserved for the vascular restoration.

The next step consists in the mobilization of the right colon, by retroperitoneum exposure and Kocher maneuver, with subsequent mobilization of the pancreatic head. Incision of the gastrohepatic ligament is performed with proper care to save accessory hepatic arterial branch from left gastric artery. The operation is continued with the dissection of the common hepatic artery, gastroduodenal artery, splenic artery, left gastric artery and portal vein. An accessory hepatic branch from the SMA, which runs along the right side of the portal vein, should be looked for. The stomach is mobilized by incising the gastrocolic ligament. The short gastric vessels, the right gastroepiploic artery, and right gastric artery are ligated and divided.

The mobilization of the pancreas begins with spleen mobilization. Spleen is used as a handle to move the pancreas (Fig. 1) without touching pancreas (no touch technique). No touch procurement of the pancreas is meant to avoid the capsule damage of the organ, which could result in fluid leakage during pancreatic perfusion.

The pancreas is medially retracted by sharp dissection, detaching it from left kidney and adrenal gland and abdominal aorta. The SMA, the splenic and gastroduodenal arteries are preserved for adequate perfusion of the pancreas with preservation solution. The left gastric artery is ligated but avoiding the ligation of the accessory arterial branch to the liver. The infrarenal aorta and inferior vena cava are dissected up to their bifurcations. The aorta at bifurcation or one of the common iliac arteries is taped and is used for cannulation. Portal vein is cannulated via the inferior mesenteric vein (IMV). The inferior mesenteric artery is ligated. For cross clamping control, the aorta is taped sub-diaphragmatically, after sharp dissection and incision of diaphragmatic crura and periaortic serosa, and retroaortic blunt dissection. The lavage of duodenum is given using betadine solution through nasogastric tube. Then first and the fourth segment of the duodenum is divided using linear stapler.

The fast technique is preferred in a hemodynamic unstable or non-heart-beating donor and also in liver pancreas en bloc harvesting. The fast technique begins with infrarenal abdominal aorta cannulation and then supraceliac aorta is prepared for cannulation. Organs are retrieved en bloc to minimize retrieval time.

Once ready for perfusion Heparin 300 IU per kg is given IV. The iliac arteries are tied, the isolated supraceliac aorta is clamped or tied and perfusion of chilled preservative solution is started through aortic cannula and through IMV. Infrarenal IVC is divided for flush out. The amount of perfusate varies according to the preservative solution used. The two most commonly used preservative solutions are Histidine-Tryptophan-Ketoglutarate (HTK) solution and University of Wisconsin (UW) solution. In a retrospective analysis performed by Becker et al.[29] there was no significant difference between HTK and University of Wisconsin (UW) solution. The pancreas is packed with sterile ice for quick topical cooling.

Immediately after initiation of the infusion, the mesentery root together with the superior mesenteric vessels is stapled. At the end of perfusion, the gastroduodenal and splenic arteries are ligated and divided. The portal vein is divided at the upper border of the pancreas so that a stump of PV is with the pancreatic graft and rest goes with liver. The graft is removed. Donor vessels (common iliac artery and vein with bifurcation) are retrieved.

Backbench Surgery

Before implanting the pancreatic graft it is important to prepare the pancreatic graft in the backbench ready for implantation. Excessive fat surrounding the pancreas should be removed. The SMA stump is dissected and vascular branches at the inferior border of pancreas are ligated to prevent bleeding postreperfusion. Excess of duodenum at both ends is resected and both distal and proximal stump is reinforced by sutures. Reconstruction of arterial supply is done by anastomosis of the donor iliac Y-graft as in Figures 1 and 2. External iliac branch is anastomosed to the pancreatic graft superior mesenteric and internal iliac branch to splenic artery (Figs 1 and 2).

Recipient Evaluation

The recipient undergoes detailed evaluation to diagnose coexisting medical problems which might need treatment to optimize patient condition before transplant. The tests should include detailed assessment of cardiac profile as these patients have severe diabetes. Specific blood tests include C-peptide level to establish insulin deficiency. Certain unique problem with pancreas recipient need detailed evaluation as they may have impact on post-transplant outcome.

Diabetic Retinopathy

Diabetic retinopathy is nearly an invariable accompaniment of patients with end-stage renal disease (ESRD) with diabetes. It is important to ensure that these patients with visual impairment have adequate help to take care of their graft.

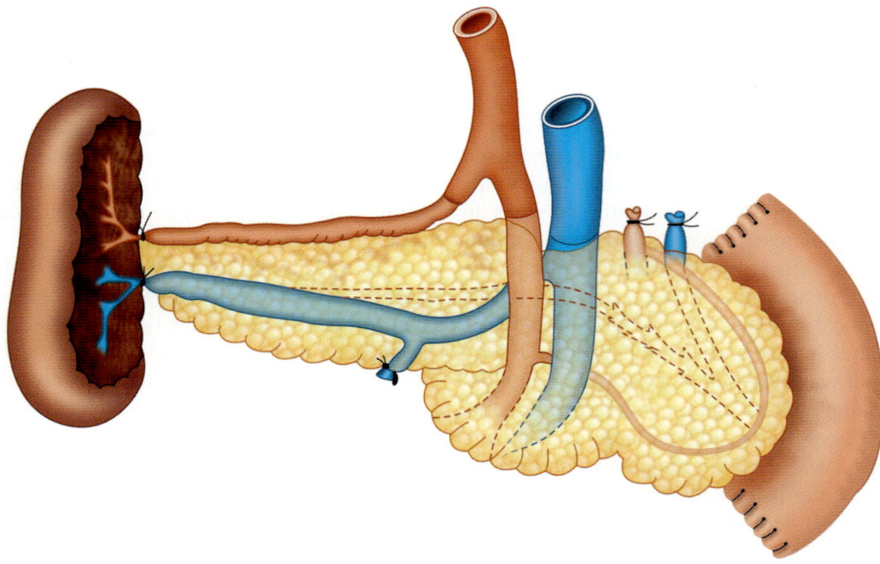

Figure 1 Extension graft on graft artery and vein on backbench

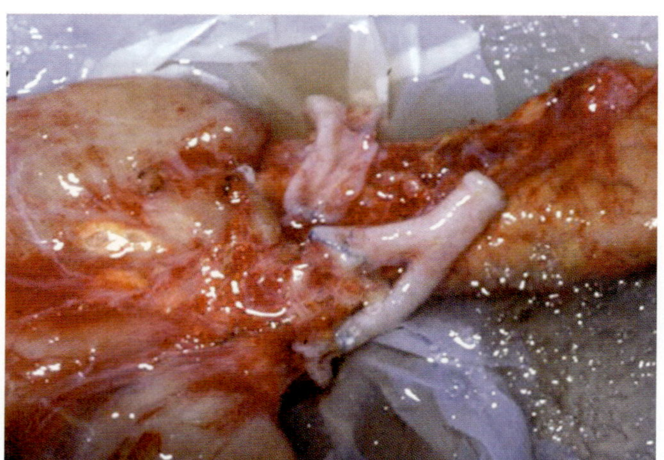

Figure 2 Backbench procedure

Gastroparesis

Many patients with long standing diabetes have significant gastroparesis. These patients may need treatment with prokinetic agents such as metoclopramide and erythromycin or other prokinetic agents.

Coronary Artery Disease

Coronary artery disease (CAD) is the most significant comorbidity in patients with type I diabetes with diabetic nephropathy. Associated neuropathy in many of these may cause silent myocardial ischemia. These patients have a nearly 50-times increased risk of cardiovascular events compared to the general population. All these patients should undergo cardiac evaluation with stress test, echocardiography or angiography as significant coronary stenosis (>50%) is seen in 45–55% patients.

Stroke

Rate of strokes and transient ischemic attacks are higher in diabetics with ESRD. Deaths related to cerebral vascular disease are approximately twice as common in patients with diabetes compared to patients without diabetes once ESRD has occurred.

Peripheral Vascular Disease

Somatosensory neuropathy and peripheral vascular disease is commonly seen in diabetic patients. These patients frequently have foot ulcers and if not properly cared for, may land up with amputation of a lower limb.

Autonomic Neuropathy

Autonomic neuropathy is manifests as cystopathy, gastropathy and orthostatic hypotension. Pancreatic drainage into bladder in SPK or pancreas alone may be a problem. Vesicoureteral reflux and high post-void residual volumes increases the incidences of infection and graft pancreatitis.

Dysregulation of vascular tone leads to orthostatic hypotension and recumbent hypertension. In patients with bladder drained pancreas there is also a predisposition toward volume depletion. This renders control of blood pressure a difficult task in post-transplant phase.

Motor and Sensory Neuropathies

These neuropathies are commonly encountered in long-standing diabetics. This makes rehabilitation difficult after transplantation.

Mental or Emotional Illnesses

Depression and neuroses are commonly present in severe diabetic. These illnesses need to be diagnosed and appropriately treated to make sure a high degree of medical compliance post-transplant.

Recipient Surgery

In a case of SPK transplant the pancreas transplant can be done before or after kidney transplant. The kidney transplant is done in the left iliac fossa with a separate incision usually with extraperitoneal approach and renal vessels are anastomosed to iliac vessels.

For pancreatic graft a midline incision is used and pancreas is usually placed intraperitoneally. Right side is preferred as right iliac artery is in more superficial position. Venous anastomosis is constructed before the arterial anastomosis because short portal vein of the graft may limit movements needed for venous reconstruction.

The option of venous drainage is either into systemic venous (SV) or portal venous (PV) system. Graft portal vein may be anastomosed to recipient SMV (PV) or recipient iliac vein/ IVC (SV). PV drainage which simulates the normal drainage was thought to be more physiological. Over the years systemic venous drainage has become more popular and a recent study has demonstrated that SV and PV drainage methods provide similar long-term outcome regarding graft survival, graft function, rejection rate and metabolic profile.[30] In a study of International Pancreas Registry in 2010, PV drainage accounted for only 18% in SPK and PAK and for 10% in PTA.[21] The arterial reconstruction is by anastomosing right common iliac to donor iliac Y graft. After finishing the arterial and venous reconstructions, the graft is reperfused. Bleeding around the margins of the graft is quite brisk and hemostasis should be meticulously done. It may otherwise lead to hypotension and renal damage. This hypotension can be avoided by adequate infusion of crystalloid and blood. Following perfusion of the graft the duodenal patch is anastomosed to a loop of Jejunum or to a Roux-en-Y loop or to native duodenum (duodenoduodenostomy) (Fig. 3).

The exocrine secretion can also be drained to the recipient bladder (BD) by anastomosing duodenum to bladder. The preferred approach these days for the duct drainage is enteric drainage. In a study of ITR in 2010, ED was used in 91% of SPK, 89% of PAK and 85% of PTA patients.[21]

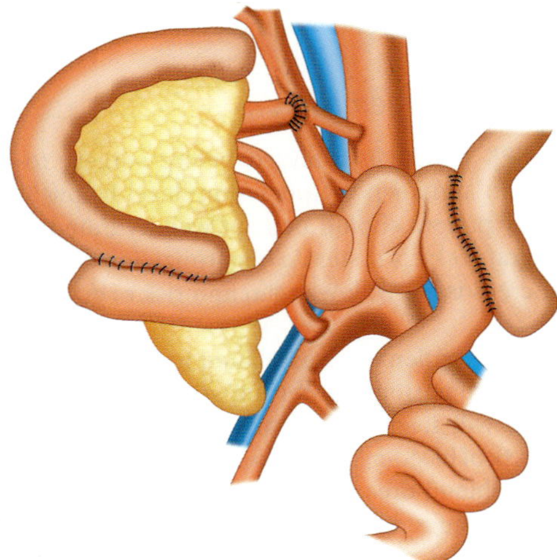

Figure 3 Portal—enteric drainage of pancreas graft

Bladder drainage is associated with chronic complications such as recurrent urinary tract infections, chemical cystitis and urethritis, urethral stricture and perineal excoriations, dehydration, hyperchloremic metabolic acidosis, recurrent hematuria, bladder stones and recurrent graft pancreatitis.[31] In early days of pancreas transplant BD was used as the graft function could be monitored with urinary amylase. Hyperglycemia is preceded by a decrease in amylase as an indication of pancreatic graft rejection. For bladder drainage SPK transplants, when rejection affected both pancreas and kidneys, rejection can be diagnosed by rise in creatinine as decline in urine amylase occurs later. Thus in isolated pancreas transplant bladder drainage is frequently used.

Due to technical reasons portal venous drainage means that bladder drainage cannot be chosen and vice versa. This is because the pancreas is directed cephalad for portal venous drainage which makes bladder drainage nearly impossible. Drains are usually placed near pancreas to monitor leaks or bleeding.

The other technical variations in pancreas transplant is use of extra-peritoneal approaches for pancreas graft that allows for easier arterial anastomosis and percutaneous biopsies.[32,33]

COMPLICATIONS OF PANCREAS TRANSPLANT

Surgical Complications

In major transplant centers in the world the rate of surgical complications have gone down up to 8%.[34] Some of the surgical complications, like reflux pancreatitis, recurrent cystitis, hematuria, duodenocystostomy leakage, are unique to bladder drained pancreas graft and about one-fourth of these cases necessitate conversion to enteric drainage.

Vascular Thrombosis

It occurs in 3–10% and in majority of cases will lead to graft loss.[35] Mostly vascular thrombosis is due to technical problem in view of multiple vascular anastomoses in pancreas transplant. The known causes of vascular injury that leads to thrombosis include rotation during back table arterial reconstruction, intimal damage due to accidental handling and over distention during flushing. The other important factors contributing to vascular thrombosis are—death due to cardiocerebrovascular reason, higher donor age, high volume fluid resuscitation leading to graft edema, donor instability, sirolimus use, hypercoagulable state of the recipient and use of HTK as the preservative solution, especially when cold ischemia exceeds 12 hours.[34]

Graft pancreatitis or rejection can cause venous thrombosis or it may be secondary to arterial thrombosis. Venous thrombosis may occur due to technical reasons, extension grafts or hypercoagulable state. Heparin is usually given for 5–7 days and thereafter aspirin can be continued. In known hypercoagulable states or second transplants warfarin should be continued in the postoperative phase. Usually graft thrombosis is suspected when blood sugars suddenly start rising and a Doppler study will pick up the vascular problem. Rarely radiological intervention may open up the thrombosed segment but mostly these cases need laparotomy for graft removal.

Leak

Leak from enteric anastomosis usually presents with abdominal pain, signs of peritonitis and rising white cell count. Many factors may contribute to anastomotic leak including technical errors, ischemia of the pancreatic head (because of vascular events, severe acute rejections, pre-existing atherosclerosis in the donor), re-exploration for another cause, duodenal edema at the time of reconstruction, intra-abdominal bleeding, and cytomegalovirus (CMV) infections. Revascularization of the gastroduodenal artery or even the gastroepiploic artery may avert ischemia of the pancreatic head and C loop of duodenum.[36] Most of the time suspected leak will be confirmed by a CT scan and will need a laparotomy. Unless it is a localized leak and patient is stable it will need graft removal. In case of duodenocystostomy, drainage of bladder and abdominal drain may help or bladder drainage can be converted to enteric drainage.

Pancreatitis

Poor graft handling leads to early pancreatitis. Cold ischemia for more than 12 hours, HTK as the preservative and poor graft from the donor is also the culprit.[31] Ischemic and reperfusion injury are seen as graft edema and diffuse or focal fat necrosis near the graft. Uncommon cause of acute pancreatitis can be CMV or other viral infections which should be treated by ganciclovir or other antiviral agents. Pancreatitis may result from urine reflux in bladder drained pancreas. Usually it is diagnosed due to abdominal pain with rising amylase and lipase while the endocrine function of the graft is preserved. Graft pancreatitis may cause similar complications as in the native pancreatitis and needs to be treated similarly. Peripancreatic sterile fluid, pseudocyst, pancreatic ascites, pancreatic fistula, bleeding and arteriovenous thrombosis can all be seen, which are treated accordingly. Severe pancreatitis with necrosis may require necrosectomy or even graft pancreatectomy.

Bleeding

Bleeding is not uncommon following this operation. Inadequate hemostasis of the graft, technical errors in vascular anastomosis and heparin overdose may cause bleeding. Activated PTT should be done to diagnose heparin overdose and if required, treated with protamine sulfate. Delayed bleeding (2 weeks to several months) is usually due to pseudoaneurysm of the infected vascular anastomoses or due to severe pancreatitis. Postoperative uncontrolled hypertension may also cause bleeding from vascular anastomoses which is usually transient and is controlled spontaneously with control of hypertension.

Patients with enteric drainage may have gastrointestinal bleeding. Bleeding can occur from any of the anastomotic sites or mucosal ulcers. Mucosal ulcers may occur due to rejection, ischemia or CMV infection.[37] The control of bleeding may require angiography and intervention or may require laparotomy.

Lymphocoele

Due to dissection around SMV and iliac vessels lymph collection around the graft is common. Sometimes it may be large volume chylous drain. Most of the time lymphatic drain settle down with conservative treatment but occasionally may lead to graft dysfunction. The best way to prevent them is to do a meticulous dissection and all lymphatics should be ligated.

Immunological Complication

Acute Rejection

Incidence of acute rejection has decreased progressively over the years and is now around 10–20%.[38] Clinical symptoms are seen in approximately 5–20% of patients with pancreas graft rejection. Rejection is highest in PTA recipients and the lowest incidence is in SPK patients. Immunoprotective effect of the renal graft or earlier diagnosis of the rejections with better therapeutic response may be responsible.

Urine amylase has been used in bladder drained patients most widely as a rejection marker which precedes hyperglycemia. In SPK transplant rising creatinine is a marker of both renal and pancreas rejection as isolated pancreas rejection is rare. Many centers now do protocol biopsy of the pancreatic graft to detect rejection at an early stage.[39]

Simultaneous pancreas-kidney transplant does not require HLA matching. In PTA and PAK categories however, HLA matching has remained important. Treatment of acute rejection involves increasing the dose of base line immunosuppression as well as pulse methylprednisolone therapy. If rejection does not improve it will require thymoglobulin or use of T-cell depleting antibodies.

Chronic Rejection

Incidence of chronic rejection is around 11% for PAK and PTA and lowest for SPK (3.7%).[40] In chronic rejection the pancreas architecture is distorted and acini is replaced with fibrous tissue. Patients develop progressive hyperglycemia and finally will require insulin therapy. There is no treatment for chronic rejection but recently sirolimus has been used in this condition.[41]

Other Complications

Other infective complications are common to all types of solid organ transplantation. Some of the complications are related to underlying diabetes like gastroparesis, poor visual acuity (accelerated retinopathy) and peripheral neuropathy.

Postoperative Management

Usually the SPK patient is dialyzed before surgery to optimize platelet function and keep the potassium level below 5.5 meq/L. During surgery patient should be kept well hydrated and before clamping of graft vessels systemic heparinization should be done because pancreas is a low flow organ and risk of graft thrombosis is high.

Majority of the patients are extubated in the operation theatre and do not require postoperative ventilation. Hypotension should be avoided as will lead to graft thrombosis and hypertension increases the risk of bleeding. For monitoring of graft function lipase, amylase, serum blood urea nitrogen, creatinine, along with blood sugar levels are required. Some centers also do daily US Doppler to document arterial and venous flow in the graft. Creatinine clearance and urine protein, C-peptide levels, and HbA1c can be periodically obtained to assess long-term graft function.

Immunosuppression

Many centers use routine induction therapy using either—thymoglobulin or IL2 blockers. Maintenance immunotherapy consists of calcineurin inhibitor, mycophenolic acid and steroid.

Outcome of Pancreas Transplant

The total number of pancreas transplantations in the US reported to IPTR/UNOS from December 16, 1966, through December 31, 2010 was 25,030. In the meantime more than 10,000 pancreas transplants were done outside US mainly in Europe.

As per IPTR data the survival rate of DD pancreas transplants has reached more than 95% at 1 year in all 3 categories (SPK, PTA, PAK) for transplantations performed in 2009. Five years unadjusted patient survival rate is 87% in SPK, 83% in PAK, and 89% in PTA. Overall 10 year survival was 70% and in PTA recipients 82%. The functioning kidney is important for survival in patients with SPK and PAK patients. With kidney graft failure the RR of death increased to almost 17-fold, in SPK and PAK recipients. The duct management technique did not impact patient survival. A large study, published recently, described 5, 10 and 20 year patient survival for SPK recipients was 89, 80, and 58%, respectively.[42]

Pancreas transplantation improves hypoglycemic unawareness and diabetes-related quality of life.[43]

PANCREAS TRANSPLANTATION AND EFFECT ON SECONDARY COMPLICATIONS OF DIABETES

After pancreas transplantation HBA1C level declines indicating improved glycemic control. Lipid profile and hepatic glucose production is also normalized and counter-regulatory effects of glucagon to hypoglycemia is inhibited.[8]

Nephropathy

Bohman et al.[44] in 1985 demonstrated that in recipients of pancreas transplant the development of diabetic glomerulopathy was prevented. Although glomerulopathy is not reversed, normoglycemia also stabilizes the diabetic glomerulopathy and decreases proteinuria. In PAK transplantation the renal graft may survive longer as improved glucose metabolism prevents accelerated diabetic glomerulopathy. Some studies show that an early PTA may preserve renal function and can reverse the lesions of diabetic nephropathy over many years.[45]

Retinopathy

Effect on diabetic retinopathy is usually not as significant as on nephropathy. In over 30% of patients retinopathy will deteriorate if it is in an advanced proliferative phase. Progression of retinopathy may be stabilized after three years of pancreatic transplantation.[46] An early pancreas transplant will prevent progression of diabetic retinopathy.

Neuropathy

Studies have proven improvement in nerve function post-pancreas transplant in patients who achieved normoglycemic state.[47] This improvement was more obvious for somatic than for autonomic nerve functions and was maintained even after 10 years.

Living Donor Pancreas Transplant

First living donor pancreas transplant was carried out at the University of Minnesota in 1979.[48] First successful SKP was also performed at the same institution in 1994.[49]

The rationale for living donor pancreas transplant has changed over time. Earlier in the era of cyclosporine and azathioprine living donor pancreas had better result due to its immunologic advantage. Since introduction of tacrolimus and mycophenolate in mid 1990s the survival rate of cadaveric pancreas transplant improved significantly because of reduced rate of graft loss from rejection. Thus most of the centers in west have access to enough cadaveric pancreatic graft for indications of isolated pancreas transplant as in PA or PAK. Thus indication of living donor isolated pancreas transplant is—in severely sensitized (panel reactive antibody >80%) recipient who is unlikely to receive a cadaveric donation; patient has a non-diabetic identical twin or a 6-antigen-matched sibling and must avoid high dose immunosuppression.[50] Majority of the living donor pancreas transplant is SPK waiting list for which is longer. About 40% of these listed patients in US die within 4 years of enlisting for cadaver SPK transplant.

Donor Selection

Living pancreas donor under goes general medical check-up and assessment of pancreatic endocrine function. In living related donors no other sibling or family members can be diabetic. Donor must be at least 10 years older than the age at which the intended recipient was diagnosed if they are related. Potential donors with a history of gestational diabetes are also excluded.[51]

To evaluate the status of pancreas in donor specific tests include serum amylase and lipase, fasting blood sugar and fasting HbA1c determination. Potential donors should also have oral glucose tolerance tests and studies to determine their insulin secretion and functional insulin secretory reserve.

Living Donor Surgery

Distal pancreas is harvested without spleen and splenic artery, and splenic vein is preserved for vascularization of the graft. It is most important to handle the pancreas gently and to do a meticulous dissection to diminish the incidence of pancreatitis postperfusion in the graft as well as in the donor post surgery.

Recipient Surgery

The splenic artery and vein are anastomosed to the recipient external iliac vessels. Duct drainage can be either in bladder or a Roux-en-Y loop of jejunum sutured to the pancreatic stump.

Results

Living donor distal pancreatectomy has little morbidity and most of the centers do it laparoscopically. The long-term risk of diabetes is there and that's why it is important to select donor after a detailed metabolic evaluation. Among 103 living pancreas transplant donor only three donors did not remain normoglycemic in center with the largest experience of living donor pancreas.[52] Living related pancreatic grafts have slightly increased risk of thrombosis in view of smaller vessels compared to cadaveric graft. Rejection is less common after living donor transplant. The recipient survival rate is better than cadaver pancreas transplant with 1 year and 5 year survival of 100% reported by experienced center.[53]

Although results of living donor pancreas transplant have improved significantly we need to remember that these results are from centers where they have accumulated huge experience of cadaver pancreas transplant. The pancreas transplant is not immediate life-saving like liver transplant, thus use of living donor for such transplant needs to be carefully assessed.

Islet Transplantation

The obvious drawbacks of whole organ pancreas transplant is—major surgery with a high complication rate and the need for lifelong immunosuppression.

The advantage of islet transplantation is avoidance of the major surgery needed for whole pancreas transplantation. However, like pancreas transplants, isolated islets are susceptible to immunologic rejection despite maintenance immunosuppression.

Serious work on islet replacement began in the early 1970s on rodents demonstrating reversal of diabetes after islet transplant.[54] But the first clinical transplant was achieved only in 1989.[55]

The foremost advantage of Islet transplant is safety. According to the Collaborative Islet Transplant Registry (CITR) report, islet transplantation has 20-fold lower morbidity risk than pancreatic transplants.[56] Another advantage of islet transplantation is use of pancreas which are not suitable for whole pancreas transplant.[57]

The problem of islet transplantation is short lived insulin production from islets. This is due to the fact that during the isolation process and after transplantation, an important number of the islets is lost, which determines the use of multiple donors in order to achieve an insulin free status.[58] The standard donor-to-recipient ratio for islet transplantation is presently 2–4:1, in contrast to a ratio of 1:1 for whole-pancreas transplantation. A human pancreas contains 0.3–1.5 x 10^6 islets per pancreas but at present only 30–50% can be isolated with a viability of 65% following isolation.[59]

The rejection of islet cells cannot be diagnosed early thus cannot be treated on time. All this lead to poor outcome and islet transplants was not accepted as replacement of whole pancreas transplant. In a trial of 65 patients conducted by the Edmonton group in 2004, only 10% of the patients remained insulin-independent at 5 years, although partial graft function persisted in 80% of the patients.[60] A recent study from the group of Minnesota has shown high rates of islet engraftment, with 50% insulin independence at 5 years similar to vascularized pancreas transplantation.[61]

Donor above 50 years who are not considered suitable for whole pancreas graft should be considered for islet transplantation. Due to the declining pool of donors, even donors 65–70 years old are accepted for islet transplantation, as marginal donors, under the condition of obtaining a greater number of islets from multiple donors. Pediatric donors and young donors less than 18 years may be a good candidate for whole pancreatic graft but due to the existence of a denser extracellular matrix structure isolating islet may be cumbersome procedure.

It is known that the obese patients (BMI over 30), with no history of diabetes, represent a better group of islet donors than lean patients, because beta cell mass is increased in accordance with increased need of obesity-associated insulin. Thus isolated beta cell mass is proportional to the donor weight. In many islet transplant centers, BMI of the donor must be over 22 for islet donation.

The success of islet transplantation depends on a careful selection of the recipient as well as high quality isolation procedure of the harvested pancreas. Recipients with low insulin requirement will be better candidate for islet transplant as they will need less number of beta cells. The graft procurement for islet isolation from cadaver donor should be done with same meticulous dissection as in whole pancreas transplant so that graft does not get damaged during procurement. After retrieval pancreas is transported in preservative solution to the laboratory where islet isolation will be carried out. The accepted cold ischemia time for the whole pancreas transplantation is a maximum 18–24 hours, and for islet transplantation maximum 8–12 hours, with an optimum time less than 8 hours.

Once islet isolation procedure is completed in the laboratory islets are injected in the portal vein either by interventional radiologist by US guided portal vein puncture or by a surgeon through small abdominal incision and direct injection in portal vein. Patient may require multiple injections of islets for glycemic control. Patients require immunesuppressants as in whole pancreas graft.

The islet transplantation is evolving and at present the indications for islet transplantation are not well defined. Patients who benefit the most from transplantation are still uncertain. The major limiting factor is more than one sitting of islet transplantation to achieve insulin independence. Islet yield and islet engraftment need to be improved, and new islet specific immunosuppression regimen needs to be designed to improve islet survival and function. Limitation in islet cell donors also remains a hindrance to islet transplantation. Stem cells as a source of islets in future would be keenly watched. Research is underway and treatment of diabetes and its secondary complications may become revolutionized in future.

REFERENCES

1. Eisenbarth GS. Type I diabetes mellitus. A chronic autoimmune disease. New Engl J Med. 1986;314(21):1360-8.
2. Unwin N, Whiting D, Guariguata L, Ghyoot G, Gan D. Diabetes Atlas, 5th edition. Brussels, Belgium: International Diabetes Federation; 2011.
3. Ali MK, Narayan KM, Tandon N. Coronary heart disease: current perspectives. Indian J Med Res. 2010;132(11):584-97.
4. Krolewski M, Eggers PW, Warram JH. Magnitude of end-stage renal disease in IDDM: a 35 year follow-up study. Kidney Int. 1996;50:2041-6.
5. Finne P, Reunanen A, Stenman S, Groop PH, Grönhagen-Riska C. Incidence of end-stage renal disease in patients with type 1 diabetes. JAMA. 2005;294(14):1782-7.
6. The effect of intensive treatment of diabetes on the development and progression of long-term complications in insulin-dependent diabetes mellitus. The Diabetes Control and Complications Trial Research Group [no authors listed]. N Engl J Med. 1993;329:977-86.
7. Writing Team for the Diabetes Control and Complications Trial/ Epidemiology of Diabetes Interventions and Complications

Research Group. Sustained effect of intensive treatment of type 1 diabetes mellitus on development and progression of diabetic nephropathy: the Epidemiology of Diabetes Interventions and Complications (EDIC) study. JAMA. 2003;290:2159-67.
8. White AS, Shaw AJ, Sutherland D. Pancreas transplantation. Lancet. 2009;373(9677):1808-17.
9. Burke GW, Ciancio G, Sollinger HW. Advances in pancreas transplantation. Transplantation. 2004;77:(9 Suppl):S62-7.
10. Kelly WD, Lillehei RC, Merkel FK, Idezuki Y, Goetz FC. Allotransplantation of the pancreas and duodenum along with the kidney in diabetic nephropathy. Surgery. 1967;61(6):827-37.
11. Dubernard JM, Traeger J, Neyra P, Touraine JL, Tranchant D, Blanc-Brunat N. A new method of preparation of segmental pancreatic grafts for transplantation: trials in dogs and in man. Surgery. 1978;84(5):633-9.
12. Sollinger HW, Kamps D, Cook K. Segmental pancreatic allotransplantation with high-dose cyclosporine and low-dose prednisone. Transplant Proc. 1983;15:2997-3000.
13. Squifflet JP, Gruessner RW, Sutherland DE. The history of pancreas transplantation: past, present and future. Acta Chir Belg. 2008;108(3):367-78.
14. Starzl TE, Iwatsuki S, Shaw BW Jr, Greene DA, Van Thiel DH, Nalesnik MA, et al. Pancreaticoduodenal transplantation in humans. Surg Gynecol Obstet. 1984;159(3):265-72.
15. Rosenlof LK, Earnhardt RC, Pruett TL, Stevenson WC, Douglas MT, Cornett GC, et al. Pancreas transplantation. An initial experience with systemic and portal drainage of pancreatic allografts. Ann Surg. 1992;215(6):586-95.
16. Shokouh-Amiri MH, Gaber AO, Gaber LW, Jensen SL, Hughes TA, Elmer D, et al. Pancreas transplantation with portal venous drainage and enteric exocrine diversion: a new technique. Transplant Proc. 1992;24(3):776-7.
17. Sutherland DE, Goetz FC, Najarian JS. Living-related donor segmental pancreatectomy for transplantation. Transplant Proc. 1980;12(4 Suppl 2):19-25.
18. Gruessner RW, Kandaswamy R, Denny R. Laparoscopic simultaneous nephrectomy and distal pancreatectomy from a live donor. J Am Coll Surg. 2001;193(3):333-7.
19. Guleria S, Aggarwal S, Bansal VK, Varma MC, Kashyap L, Tandon N, et al. The first successful simultaneous pancreas-kidney transplant in India. Natl Med J India. 2005;18(1):18-9.
20. Cryer PE. Hypoglycemia-associated autonomic failure in diabetes. Am J Physiol Endocrinol Metab. 2001;281:E1115-21.
21. Angelika C. Gruessner. Update Pancreas Transplantation: Comprehensive Trend Analysis of 25,000 Cases Followed Up Over the Course of Twenty-Four Years at the International Pancreas Transplant Registry (IPTR). Rev Diabet Stud. 2011;8(1):6-16.
22. Wiseman AC. The role of kidney-pancreas transplantation in diabetic kidney disease. Curr Diab Rep. 2010;10(5):385-91.
23. Sutherland DE, Gruessner R, Gillingham K, Moudry-Munns K, Dunn D, Brayman K, et al. A single institution's experience with solitary pancreas transplantation: a multivariate analysis of factors leading to improved outcome. Clin Transpl. 1991:141-52.
24. Sousa MG, Linhares MM, Gonzalez AM, Rangel EB, Melaragno C, Sá JR, et al. Multivariate analysis of risk factors for early loss of pancreas grafts among simultaneous pancreas-kidney transplants. Transplant Proc. 2010;42(2):547-51.
25. Troppmann C, Gruessner AC, Benedetti E, Papalois BE, Dunn DL, Najarian JS. Vascular graft thrombosis after pancreatic transplantation: univariate and multivariate operative and non-operative risk factor analysis. J Am Coll Surg. 1996;182(4):285-316.
26. Humar A, Ramcharan T, Kandaswamy R, Gruessner RW, Gruessner AC, Sutherland DE. Technical failures after pancreas transplants: why grafts fail and the risk factors—a multivariate analysis. Transplantation. 2004;78(8):1188-92.
27. Humar A, Ramcharan T, Kandaswamy R, Gruessner RW, Gruessner AG, Sutherland DE. The impact of donor obesity on outcomes after cadaver pancreas transplants. Am J Transplant. 2004;4(4):605-10.
28. Wunderlich H, Brockmann JG, Voigt R, Rauchfuss F, Pascher A, Brose S, et al. DTG procurement guidelines in heart beating donors. Transpl Int. 2011;24(7):733-57.
29. Becker T, Ringe B, Nyibata M, Meyer zu Vilsendorf A, Schrem H, Lück R, et al. Pancreas transplantation with histidine-tryptophan-ketoglutarate (HTK) solution and University of Wisconsin (UW) solution: is there a difference? JOP. 2007;8(3):304-11.
30. Bazerbachia F, Selznera M, Marquez MA, Norgatea A, Aslania N, McGilvraya ID. Portal venous versus systemic venous drainage of pancreas grafts: impact on long-term results. Am J Transplant. 2012;12(1):226-32.
31. Han DJ, Sutherland DE. Pancreas transplantation. Gut Liver. 2010;4(4):450-65.
32. Boggi U, Vistoli F, Signori S, Del Chiaro M, Campatelli A, Amorese G, et al. A technique for retroperitoneal pancreas transplantation with portal-enteric drainage. Transplantation. 2005;79(9):1137-42.
33. Kahn J, Iberer F, Kniepeiss D, Duller D, Jakoby E, Tscheliessnigg K. Retroperitoneal pancreas transplantation with systemic-enteric drainage—case report. Clin Transplant. 2008;22(5):674-6.
34. Troppmann C. Complications after pancreas transplantation. Curr Opin Organ Transplant. 2010;15(1):112-8.
35. Goodman J, Becker YT. Pancreas surgical complications. Curr Opin Organ Transplant. 2009;14(1):85-9.
36. Nghiem DD. Revascularization of the gastroepiploic artery in pancreas transplant. Transplant Int. 2008;21(8):774-7.
37. Nikeghbalian S, Bahador A, Salahi H, Kakaei F, Kazemi K, Dehghani M. Non-marginal donor C-loop ulcers as a cause of gastrointestinal bleeding after pancreas transplantation: three case reports. Transplant Proc. 2009;41(7):2930-2.
38. Singh RP, Stratta RJ. Advances in immunosuppression for pancreas transplantation. Curr Opin Organ Transplant. 2008;13(1):79-84.
39. Gaber LW. Pancreas allograft biopsies in the management of pancreas transplant recipients: histopathology review and clinical correlations. Arch Pathol Lab Med. 2007;131(8):1192-9.
40. Humar A, Khwaja K, Ramcharan T, Asolati M, Kandaswamy R, Gruessner RW. Chronic rejection: the next major challenge for pancreas transplant recipients. Transplantation. 2003;76(6): 918-23.
41. Matias P, Araujo MR, Romão JE Jr, Abensur H, Noronha IL. Conversion to sirolimus in kidney-pancreas and pancreas transplantation. Transplant Proc. 2008;40(10):3601-5.
42. Wai PY, Sollinger HW. Long-term outcomes after simultaneous pancreas-kidney transplant. Curr Opin Organ Transplant. 2011;16(1):128-34.
43. Suresh KK, Patel BM, Markatos A, Nghiem DD, Marcus RJ. Quality of life after organ transplantation in type 1 diabetics with end-stage renal disease. Clin Transplant. 2006;20(1):19-25.
44. Bohman SO, Tyden G, Wilczek H, Lundgren G, Jaremko G, Gunnarsson R. Prevention of kidney graft diabetic nephropathy by pancreas transplantation in man. Diabetes. 1985;34(3):306-8.
45. Sutherland DE, Gruessner RW, Dunn DL, Matas AJ, Humar A, Kandaswamy R. Lessons learned from more than 1,000 pancreas transplants at a single institution. Ann Surg. 2001;233(4):463-501.
46. Chow VC, Pai RP, Chapman JR, O'Connell PJ, Allen RD, Mitchell P. Diabetic retinopathy after combined kidney pancreas transplantation. Clin Transplant. 1999;13(4):356-62.
47. Navarro X, Sutherland DE, Kennedy WR. Long-term effects of pancreatic transplantation on diabetic neuropathy. Ann Neurol. 1997;42(5):727-36.
48. Sutherland DE, Goetz FC, Najarian JS. Living-related donor segmental pancreatectomy for transplantation. Transplant Proc. 1980;12(4 Suppl 2):19-25.

49. Gruessner RW, Sutherland DE. Simultaneous kidney and segmental pancreas transplants from living related donors—the first two successful cases. Transplantation. 1996;61(8):1265-8.
50. Sibley S, Seaquist ER. Diabetes mellitus: classification and epidemiology. Transplantation of the pancreas. New York: Springer-Verlag; 2004.
51. Gruessner RW, Kendall DM, Drangstveit MB, GruessnerAC, Sutherland DE. Simultaneous pancreas-kidney transplantation from live donors. Ann Surg. 1997;226(4):471-80.
52. Humar A, Gruessner G, Sutherland D. Living related donor pancreas and pancreas-kidney transplantation. Br Med Bull. 1997;53(4):879-91.
53. Gruessner RW, Kendall DM, Drangstveit MB, Gruessner AC, Sutherland DE. Ann Surg. 1997;226(4):471-80.
54. Ballinger WF, Lacy PE. Transplantation of intact pancreatic islets in rats. Surgery. 1972;72(2):175-86.
55. Scharp DW, Lacy PE, Santiago JV, McCullough CS, Weide LG, Boyle PJ, et al. Results of our first nine intraportal islet allografts in type 1, insulin dependent diabetic patients. Transplantation. 1991;51(1):76-85.
56. Sá JR, Gonzalez AM, Melaragno CS, Saitovic D, Franco DR, Rangel EB. Transplante de pâncreas e ilhotasemportadores de diabetes melito. Arquivos Brasileiros de Endocrinologia & Metabologia. 2008;52(2):355-66.
57. Rother KI, Harlan DM. Challenges facing islet transplantation for the treatment of type 1 diabetes mellitus. J Clin Invest. 2004;114(7):877-83.
58. Kandaswamy R, Sutherland DER. Pancreas versus islet transplantation in diabetes mellitus: how to allocate deceased donor pancreata? Transplantation Proceedings. 2006;38(2):365-7.
59. Plesner A, Verchere CB. Advances and challenges in islet transplantation: islet procurement rates and lessons learned from suboptimal islet transplantation. Journal of Transplantation. 2011;2011:979527.
60. Ryan EA, Paty BW, Senior PA, Bigam D, Alfadhli E, Kneteman NM. Five-year follow-up after clinical Islet transplantation. Diabetes. 2005;54(7):2060-9.
61. Barton FB, Rickels MR, Alejandro R, Hering BJ, Wease S, Naziruddin B, et al. Improvement in outcomes of clinical islet transplantation: 1999-2010. Diabetes Care. 2012;35(7):1436-45.

SECTION 5

Gallbladder and Bile Ducts

CHAPTER 49

Gallbladder and Bile Ducts: Anatomy and Physiology

Satyajit Godhi, PK Mishra

INTRODUCTION

Gallbladder is one organ which has long been in the public domain and imagination. Cholecystectomy is one of the most common operations in the whole world. Those who have experienced the gallbladder pain would certainly testify to the utility of this operation. Gallbladder cancer is taking almost epidemic proportions in the northern parts of India. Bile duct stones and malignancies are also common clinical problems. This chapter is a brief reminder of the origin of gallbladder and bile ducts, their anatomy and physiology. It would help us to understand the formation of gallstones and the subtle nuances involved in the operations on gallbladder and bile duct.

EMBRYOLOGY OF GALLBLADDER AND BILIARY SYSTEM

Liver and biliary passages are derived from the hepatic bud. This bud arises from the gut at the junction of foregut and midgut. It is derived from endoderm.

Liver primodium appears at the distal end of foregut as an outgrowth at 25 days approximately. This outgrowth is called hepatic diverticulum or liver bud. This diverticulum penetrates the septum transversum. The hepatic cell strands penetrate the septum. The bile duct is formed by the narrowing of the communication between duodenum and hepatic diverticulum. The bile duct gives rise to pars cystica which forms the future gallbladder and cystic duct (Figs 1A to E).

The hepatic bud proximal to the pars cystica forms the bile duct. Bile duct at first opens on the ventral aspect of the developing duodenum. The duodenum has a differential growth which eventually causes the bile duct to open dorsomedially.[1]

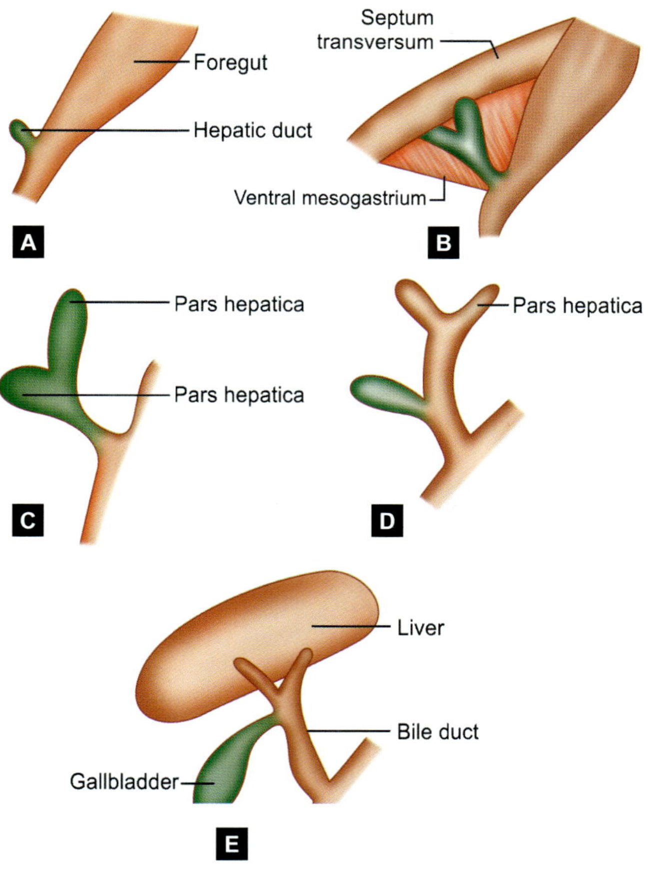

Figures 1A to E Development of gallbladder

ANATOMY OF GALLBLADDER

The gallbladder is located on the undersurface of segment V in the right lobe of the liver. The gallbladder is separated from the liver by the cystic plate. Cystic plate arises from Glisson's capsule and is in continuity with hilar plate of liver (Fig. 2).[2]

The gallbladder varies from 7 cms to 10 cms in length and from 2.5 cms to 3.5 cms in width.[3] Capacity of gallbladder is 50–60 mL.

Gallbladder has 4 parts: fundus, body, infundibulum and neck.

Histology of Gallbladder

Gallbladder has 3 layers (Fig. 3)

1. The mucous membrane
2. The muscularis
3. The adventitia (serosa)

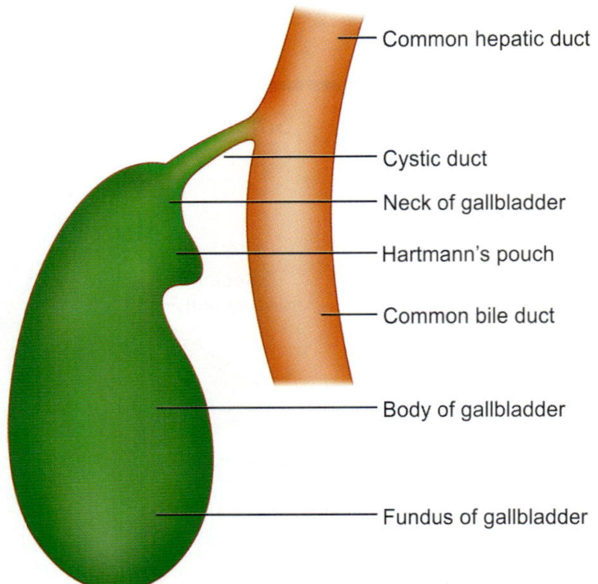

Figure 2 Normal anatomy of gallbladder

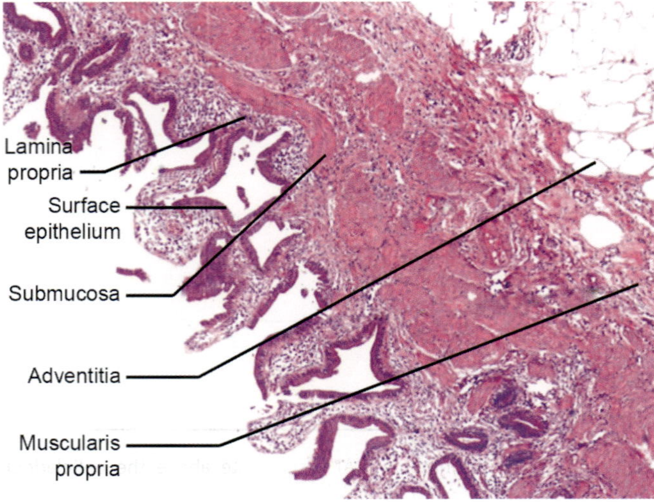

Figure 3 Picture depicting normal histology of gallbladder

Mucous Membrane

Mucosa has rugae at resting phase. All epithelial cells are columnar cells with basal nucleus. They have absorptive and secretory function. Lamina propria also contains lymphatics, elastic fibers, loose connective tissue and occasionally mast cells and macrophages.

Muscularis

Gallbladder does not have a submucosa. External to the mucosa is a layer of smooth muscle. The muscularis is made up of collagenous tissue, elastic fibers, ganglia and some smooth muscle fibers. Rokitansky-Aschoff sinuses are invaginations of epithelium into the lamina propria, muscle and subserosal connective tissue. 40% of normal gallbladder and all inflamed gallbladders have them.[3] Ducts of Luschka are tiny bile ducts found in muscle layer in 10% of normal gallbladder.

Adventitia or Serosa

The gallbladder is located on the inferior surface of the liver. Outer aspect of gallbladder has well-formed serosa which is continuous with the peritoneal layer. Serosa contains blood vessels and lymphatics. The normal thickness of gallbladder wall is 3 mm.

Cystic Duct

The infundibulum of the gallbladder continues as the cystic duct and runs medial and inferior to join the common hepatic duct. The cystic duct is typically 1–3 mm in diameter and can range from 1cm to 6 cm in length. Spiral mucosal folds, referred to as valves of Heister, are present in the mucosa of the cystic duct.[2]

Extrahepatic Biliary Anatomy

The right and left duct unite anteriorly to the right branch of portal vein to form the common hepatic duct (CHD). The CHD unites with the cystic duct to form the common bile duct (CBD), which runs through the head of pancreas to enter the second part of duodenum.

The right duct branches into an anterior and posterior sectoral duct soon after its entrance into liver. Thus the right duct has a short extrahepatic course (<1 cm).

The left hepatic duct enters the liver at the umbilical fissure. In contrast to the right duct, the left duct after its formation has a 2–3 cm of extrahepatic length. It runs along the base of quadrate lobe before it enters the liver.

Lowering the hilar plate (i.e., connective tissue enclosing the left hepatic elements and Glisson's capsule) at the base of the quadrate lobe provides great exposure to both the biliary hilum and the extrahepatic portion of the left hepatic duct.[2]

Common Bile Duct

The cystic duct unites with the CHD to form the CBD. In the hepatoduodenal ligament hepatic artery lies lateral to CBD and portal vein lies posterior to it. CBD then courses posterior to pancreas and enters the second part of duodenum (medial aspect).

The CBD is approximately 8 cm in length. The normal diameter of the CBD ranges from 4 mm to 9 mm with a mean of 6 mm. CBD is considered enlarged if the duct diameter exceeds 6 mm on ultrasound.

The retroduodenal portion of the CBD passes behind the first portion of the duodenum, lateral to the portal vein and anterior to the inferior vena cava (IVC). The intrapancreatic portion of the CBD traverses the posterior aspect of the pancreas in a tunnel or groove to enter the second portion of the duodenum, where it is usually joined by the pancreatic duct. The intraduodenal portion of the CBD passes obliquely through the duodenal wall to enter the duodenum at the papilla of Vater.

The course henceforth is divided into

- Retroduodenal
- Intrapancreatic
- Intraduodenal

The retroduodenal CBD runs anterior to IVC. The intrapancreatic CBD unites with the pancreatic duct. The intraduodenal CBD enters the duodenum at the ampulla of Vater.

Pancreatobiliary Junction

The union of CBD and pancreatic duct is variable

- Union can be outside the duodenal wall to form a long common channel
- Union can be within the duodenal wall to form short common channel
- The two structures may rarely enter the duodenum independently through separate orifices

Abnormal pancreatobiliary junction contributes in the pathogenesis of choledochal cysts. A long common channel causes reflux of pancreatic juice leading to inflammatory ectasia and dilation.[4] Two distinct anomalous pancreaticobiliary junctions have been identified: *type 1*: in which major pancreatic duct joins the side of the CBD and *type 2*: in which the main pancreatic duct is joined from the side by CBD. Type 2 anomalous junction is more likely to result in pancreatitis anatomically (Chiijiwa and Koga 1993).

Histology of Extrahepatic Biliary Ducts

The extrahepatic bile ducts contain a columnar mucosa surrounded by a connective tissue layer (Fig. 4). Muscle fibers in the bile duct are sparse and discontinuous. The muscle fibers are longitudinal, although occasional circular fibers are observed. The distal CBD begins to develop a muscle layer in the intrapancreatic portion of the duct, which becomes prominent at the sphincter of Oddi.

Intrahepatic Ducts

An understanding of intrahepatic ductal anatomy is obviously important and vital to the performance of a high biliary anastomoses for cholangiocarcinoma (Klatskin tumors), an intrahepatic bilioenteric bypass, and complex hepatic resections such as caudate lobectomy, and left and right trisegmentectomy. The lobar and segmental anatomy of the liver is determined by the sequential branching of the portal vein, hepatic artery and biliary tree. More specifically, bile ducts are usually situated superior to its complementary portal vein branch, while the hepatic artery lies inferiorly.

The right and left hepatic ducts drain the right and left lobe of liver. The left hepatic duct drains segment II, III and IV. Right hepatic duct divides into anterior and posterior segmental ducts. Anterior segmental duct drains segment V and VIII, posterior division drains segment VI and VII.

Biliary drainage of the caudate lobe is less predictable. Conceptually, the caudate lobe has three distinct areas—a right part, a left part and the caudate process. In some instances three separate bile ducts may be present. The caudate process represents a narrow bridge of tissue that connects the caudate to the right lobe (segment V).[2] Majority of the times caudate lobe is drained by both the right and left ducts by 1–4 small ducts. Exclusive drainage to left duct is seen only in 15% cases and to the right duct in 5% cases.

Hilar Plate

The hilar plate is made up of connective tissue and separates the biliary confluence from liver. It is avascular and can be dissected to gain an access to the confluence (Fig. 5).

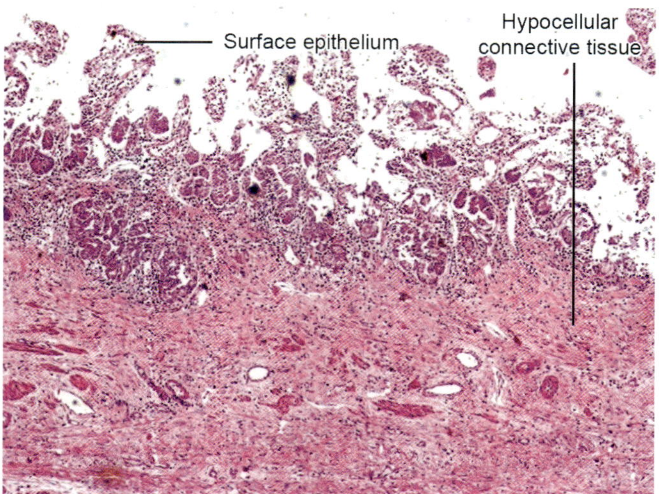

Figure 4 Histological picture of extrahepatic bile ducts

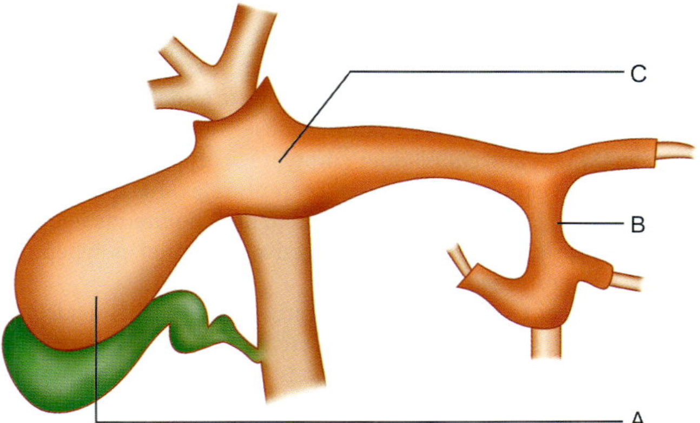

Figure 5 Hilar plate anatomy—(A) cystic plate above the gallbladder (B) hilar plate above the umbilical part of portal vein (C) Hilar plate above the biliary confluence

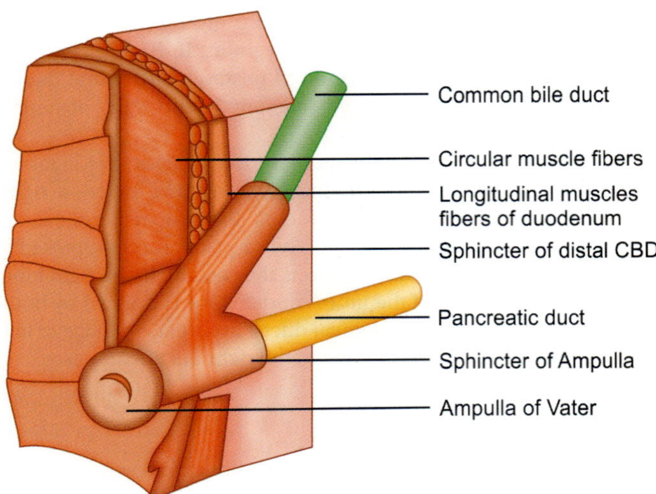

Figure 6 Sphincter of Oddi

Sphincter of Oddi

Sphincter of Oddi encloses the distal bile duct and the pancreatic duct (Fig. 6). The sphincter is made up of both circular and longitudinal muscle fibers. It has separate sphincters for the distal bile duct, the pancreatic duct and the ampulla. The common channel is usually less than 1 cm. If the common channel is longer than 1.0 cm or the biliary and pancreatic ducts open separately into the duodenum, pathologic biliary or pancreatic problems are likely to develop. The entire sphincter mechanism is actually composed of four sphincters containing both circular and longitudinal smooth muscle fibers. The four sphincters are the superior and inferior sphincter choledochus, the sphincter pancreaticus, and the sphincter of the ampulla.

Sphincter of Oddi Physiology and Functional Issues

Sphincter of Oddi is a high pressure zone. The basal pressures are higher than the duodenal and CBD/pancreatic pressure. The amplitude of contractions is 130 mm of hg with a frequency of 4/min. These are antegrade contractions, but few of them can be retrograde.

The neural and hormonal factors control sphincter of Oddi. During fasting, gallbladder filling occurs due to tonically contracted sphincter of Oddi. It relaxes during phase 3 of migrating motor complex (MMC) and gallbladder emptying takes place.

The cholecystokinin (CCK) and secretin relax the sphincter of Oddi following meals. Nonadrenergic and noncholinergic neurons also relax the sphincter using vasoactive intestinal polypeptide (VIP) as a neurotransmitter.

Sphincter of Oddi dysfunction represents a benign acalculus obstruction to the flow of biliary or pancreatic secretions through the pancreatobiliary junction. It is known by many names: ampullary stenosis, papillary stenosis, papillitis and postcholecystectomy syndrome. They present with classic pancreatobiliary pain. This pain is defined by Rome 2 criteria as upper abdominal pain typically post prandial in nature and associated with nausea.[5]

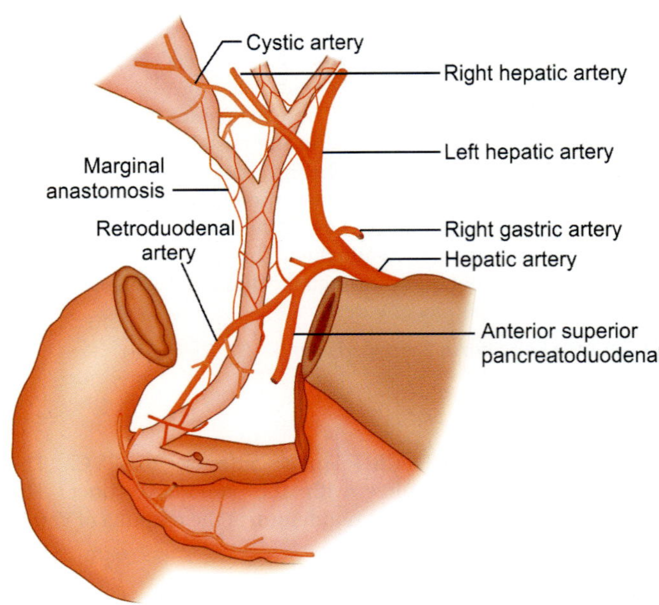

Figure 7 Blood supply of the CBD

Vascular Anatomy

The right and left hepatic duct and upper part of CHD have a common blood supply i.e. from right and left hepatic arteries and cystic artery. The supra-duodenal CBD receives blood supply originating both superiorly and inferiorly (Fig. 7). Superiorly the supply is from cystic and right and left hepatic arteries and inferiorly from posterior superior pancreaticoduodenal and retroduodenal arteries. The majority of blood supply (60%) comes from inferiorly. CBD has these arteries running around it at 3 o'clock and 9 o'clock position. The blood supply to the retroduodenal and intrapancreatic bile duct is from the retroduodenal and pancreaticoduodenal arteries.

The cystic artery arises from the right hepatic artery and runs in the Calot's triangle. It can also arise from other arteries like common hepatic, left hepatic, superior mesenteric and gastroduodenal.

The cystic artery supplies the cystic duct and gallbladder. It supplies the gallbladder with a superficial branch and a deep branch. Common relation of right hepatic artery to the CBD is that it lies posterior to it (85%). Occasionally, right hepatic artery may arise from superior mesenteric artery and course through the medial aspect of Calot's triangle where it might be injured. Thus, recognition of variations in biliary and vascular anatomy is important. These should be looked for, to avoid inadvertent injuries to important structures.

Venous Drainage

- The hepatic veins drain the superior surface of gallbladder.
- One or two cystic veins drain the rest of gallbladder. These veins join the veins draining the hepatic duct and enter the liver.
- Portal vein drains the lower part of bile duct.

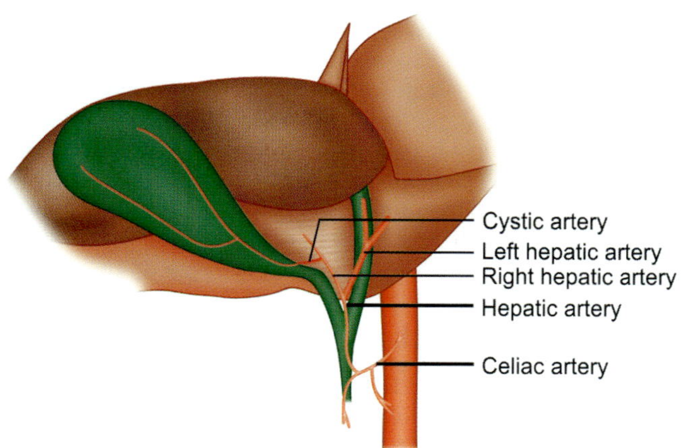

Figure 8 Calot's triangle

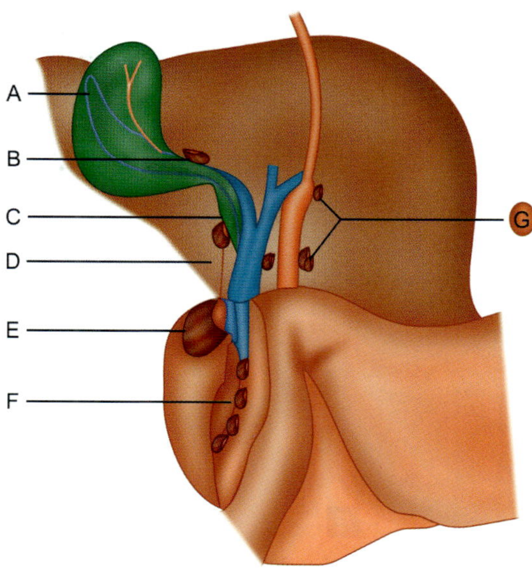

Figure 9 Lymphatic drainage of gallbladder (A) Collecting lymphatic trunks on wall of gallbladder, (B) Cystic node, (C) Uninterrupted lymph vessel sending in lower nodes, (D) Node of hiatus (E) Superior pancreaticoduodenal node, (F) Posterior pancreaticoduodenal nodes, (G) Nodes along hepatic artery

Calot's Triangle

Jean-Francois described the Calot's triangle in his thesis in 1891 (Fig. 8). It was an isosceles triangle. The modern definition though has changed. The triangle contains the cystic artery and often right branch of hepatic artery. The boundaries are:

- CHD forms the left border
- Cystic duct forms the inferior border
- Under surface of liver forms the right upper border.

Lymphatic Drainage of Gallbladder

The collecting trunks course through the medial and lateral wall of gallbladder. Most of the collecting trunks on the medial wall terminate in the cystic node. The collecting trunks on the lateral wall of the gallbladder, usually pass along the right border of the neck of the organ and extend uninterrupted to end in the pericholedochal nodes.

Three pathways define the lymphatic drainage of gallbladder.

- The cholecysto-retropancreatic pathway: The lymphatics run along the CBD to reach the retroportal node which is the main terminal node of this pathway.
- The cholecysto-celiac pathway: Lymphatics reach the celiac nodes across the hepatoduodenal ligament.
- The cholecysto-mesenteric pathway: Lymphatics reach the superior mesenteric root travelling along the portal vein.

Final lymph node where these pathways meet is the interaortocaval node near the left renal vein. Extensive connections between the various sets of lymph vessels can lead to direct spread to interaortocaval nodes from pericholedochal nodes (Fig. 9).

ANOMALIES OF GALLBLADDER AND BILIARY APPARATUS

Anomalies of Hepatic Ducts

An effort should always be made to define the intrahepatic anatomy based on preoperative imaging since failure to do so may result in unwanted complication. The more common type of each of the anomalies will be described in more detail below.

Common hepatic duct is formed by the union of right anterior and posterior sectoral ducts (57–68%) of cases. Variations do exist though. Triple confluence is seen in 15% cases. And in about 20% cases right sectoral duct (either anterior or posterior) unite with the CHD distally. If this situation is not recognized it can be very dangerous and represents a common cause of injury during laparoscopic cholecystectomy. In 5% cases right posterior sectoral duct unites with the intraparenchymal portion of left hepatic duct. Failure to appreciate this anomaly prior to right or left hepatectomy, can lead to significant postoperative problems. Some authorities believe that this anomaly represents the most common intrahepatic biliary variations (Figs 10A to F). In 1.5–3% of patients, the cystic duct joins at the union of all the ducts or with one of the right hepatic ducts.

Accessory ducts do exist to confuse the anatomy. These ducts drain a small segment of liver and unite with the cystic duct, CHD, CBD or gallbladder. These ducts can course through the Calot's triangle and can be injured easily during cholecystectomy. Cholecystohepatic ducts are small biliary ducts that emerge from the liver to enter the hepatic surface of the gallbladder directly. If a cholecystohepatic duct is discovered during surgery, it should be ligated to avoid a postoperative bile leak.

Cystic Duct Anomalies

In 1976, Benson and Page described five ductal anomalies to be careful about during performance of a cholecystectomy (Figs 11A to E). Of these five anomalies, three involve abnormalities in the length, course or insertion of the cystic duct into the CHD. The cystic duct may run parallel to the CHD for a variable distance, or it may wrap around the CHD to form a left-sided union. Parallel cystic ducts occur in 15% of individuals, whereas spiral cystic

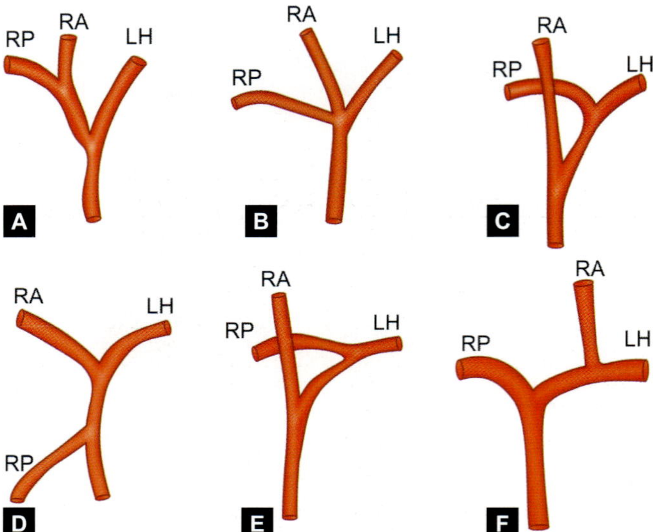

Figures 10A to F Variations of anatomy of intrahepatic ducts (A) Normal anatomy. (B) Triple confluence, (C) Ectopic drainage of right anterior duct into common bile duct, (D) Ectopic drainage of right posterior duct into common bile duct, (E) Ectopic right posterior duct drainage into left hepatic duct, (F) Ectopic right anterior duct drainage into left hepatic duct

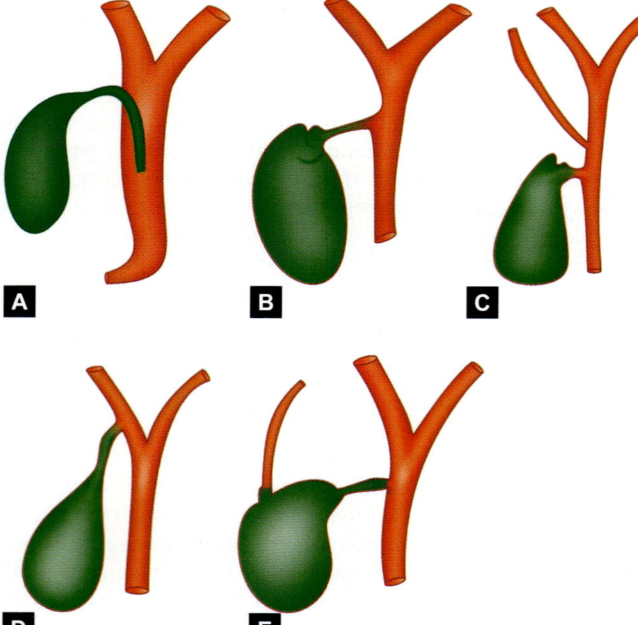

Figures 11A to E Cystic duct anomalies (A) Low insertion of cystic duct, (B) Normal anatomy, (C) Accessory right hepatic duct inserting into CHD, (D) Cystic duct insertion into right hepatic duct, (E) An accessory cystic duct draining the body of gallbladder

ducts are found in approximately 8%. The parallel or spiral cystic duct may be normal in length or may course downward in the hepatoduodenal ligament for a considerable distance before forming a low union with the common hepatic duct. In both situations, the cystic duct is usually closely adhered to the CHD by a sheath of connective tissue.

The cystic duct can have anomalous drainage into right duct or any segmental duct. A trifurcation may also form when the cystic duct unites with the right and left hepatic duct. This anomaly is dangerous as the right hepatic duct may undergo ligation mistaking it for a cystic duct. Occasionally, the gallbladder may join the CHD with a short or virtually nonexistent cystic duct. During ligation of a short cystic duct, care must be taken not to compromise the lumen of the CBD.

Gallbladder Anomalies

The anomalies of gallbladder are given in Table 1.

Anomalies of the gallbladder are usually of minimal clinical significance by themselves. They are as follows.

Abnormal Formation

Phrygian cap or folded fundus: Phrygian cap incidence is 2–6%. This anomaly of formation is the most common of the gallbladder. Phrygian cap occurs more commonly in women. The phrygian cap deformity is created by an infolding of a septum between the body and the fundus. The gallbladder functions normally, and this anomaly is not an indication for cholecystectomy.

Bilobulated gallbladder: This is an exaggerated form of the above.

Hourglass gallbladder: This anomaly can be seen in children as well as adults. In children it is congenital and it does not require any treatment. In adults it is seen with chronic cholecystitis and should be removed if causing biliary symptoms.

Diverticulum of the gallbladder: Congenital diverticula of the gallbladder are rare. They may occur in any part of gallbladder. These diverticula are clinically insignificant unless they become the site of disease like stones, become acutely inflamed or even perforate. Hartmann pouch is an acquired diverticulum of the infundibulum or neck of the gallbladder. This pouch projects from the convexity of the gallbladder neck and may be closely adherent to the CBD. Hartmann pouch is associated with pathologic conditions of the gallbladder, especially those involving prolonged obstruction to gallbladder emptying.

Table 1: Anomalies of the gallbladder

1. *Formation*
    - Phrygian cap
    - Bilobed gallbladder
    - Hourglass gallbladder
    - Diverticulum of the gallbladder
    - Rudimentary gallbladder
2. *Number*
    - Absence of gallbladder
    - Duplication of the gallbladder
3. *Position*
    - Floating gallbladder
    - Intrahepatic gallbladder
    - Left sided gallbladder
    - Transverse gallbladder
    - Retrodisplaced gallbladder

Rudimentary gallbladder: It can be seen in children as well as adults. If seen in children, it is due to hypoplasia and does not require any treatment. If seen in adults then it is due to cholecystitis and might merit removal if symptomatic.

Abnormal Number

Hypoplasia or agenesis of gallbladder: Complete absence of gallbladder occurs when the cystic duct end fails to expand. The incidence of agenesis of gallbladder is 10–65 per 100,000.[6] CBD stones and duct dilatations are common in these patients.

Double gallbladder: Duplicated gallbladder is seen in 1 in 4000 persons. A true duplicated gallbladder has two separate cavities drained by its own cystic duct and supplied by its own cystic artery. There are two varieties: (1) the ductular type, in which each gallbladder has its own cystic duct and (2) a nonductular type in which the two ducts gradually merge into a common cystic duct before emptying into the CBD. The gallbladder itself may be seen as two distinct organs at variable distances apart or may outwardly have the appearance of a single organ. Each cavity may function normally or become diseased independently of the other. Duplication of the gallbladder is clinically unimportant and generally requires no treatment (Figs 12A to E).

Rarely, a gallbladder may be found in an abnormal location. This type of gallbladder requires no treatment unless it causes symptoms. Five different conditions are recognized: floating, intrahepatic, left-sided, transverse and retrodisplaced.

Abnormal Position of Gallbladder

Intrahepatic gallbladder: These gallbladders pose a lot of difficulty during cholecystectomy.

Transposition or left-sided gallbladder: Gallbladder bed may be placed in the left lobe of liver or between the two lobes.

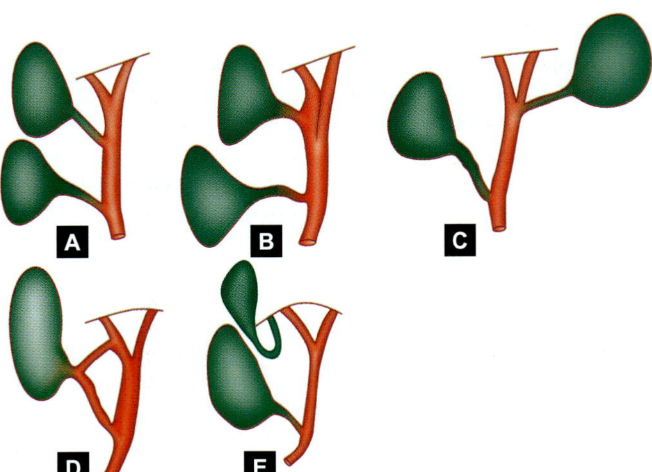

Figures 12A to E Types of duplicated gallbladder: (A) Duplicated gallbladder with duplicated cystic duct; (B) Duplicated gallbladder with one cystic duct draining into the CHD and the other draining into CBD; (C) Duplicated gallbladder with one cystic duct on either side of CBD; (D) Single gallbladder with duplicated cystic duct—one draining into the CHD and the other draining into CBD; (E) Duplicated gallbladder with one cystic duct draining into intrahepatic ducts and the other into CBD

Transverse gallbladder: Gallbladder is positioned horizontally in the transverse fissure of the liver.

Retrodisplaced gallbladder: Retrodisplacement of the gallbladder is a condition in which the organ is not situated in the gallbladder fossa but is bound to another portion of the liver or freely suspended from the liver with the fundus extending posteriorly.

Floating gallbladder: A floating gallbladder has been reported to occur in approximately 5% of persons. In this condition, the gallbladder is completely surrounded by peritoneum and is attached to the undersurface of the cystic fossa by the peritoneal reflection from the liver. Such a gallbladder may undergo torsion around its pedicle. Torsion of the gallbladder requires operative detorsion and removal of the gallbladder, which may be infarcted as a result of occlusion of its blood vessels.

Anomalies of Common Bile Duct

Several variations of CBD malposition and duplication have been described:

- CBD opening into antrum
- CBD into gastric fundus
- CBD independently into duodenum
- Two CBDs opening into duodenum
- A bifurcating CBD, one into duodenum, another into stomach
- A bifurcating CBD with both branches entering the duodenum; and
- A septate CBD, with two openings of the single duct into the duodenum.

The mere presence of these anomalies does not produce symptoms, and their clinical importance rests solely on their recognition and on the avoidance of injury during an operation.

Vascular Anomalies

Arterial variations are more common than ductal variations (Figs 13A to H). Hepatic artery and cystic artery variations are very common (50%). An accessory cystic artery may cause inadvertent bleeding during cholecystectomy and should be identified and clipped whenever it exists.

The caterpillar hump occurs in 15% of cases. The right hepatic artery humps in a semicircular shape and gives the cystic artery. Here it lies very close to the cystic duct. If not identified during cholecystectomy, the right hepatic artery may be clipped.

GALLBLADDER PHYSIOLOGY

"What's the gallbladder's favorite rock band???
The Rolling Stones"

To understand the pathophysiology of gallstone disease it is essential to know the physiology of bile formation.

Bile Formation

Bile has 2 main functions:

- Bilirubin and cholesterol are excreted in bile
- Lipids and fat soluble vitamins are absorbed in presence of bile.

Major component of bile is water. It makes up around 95% of bile. Bilirubin, bile salts, phospholipids and cholesterol make the other components of bile.

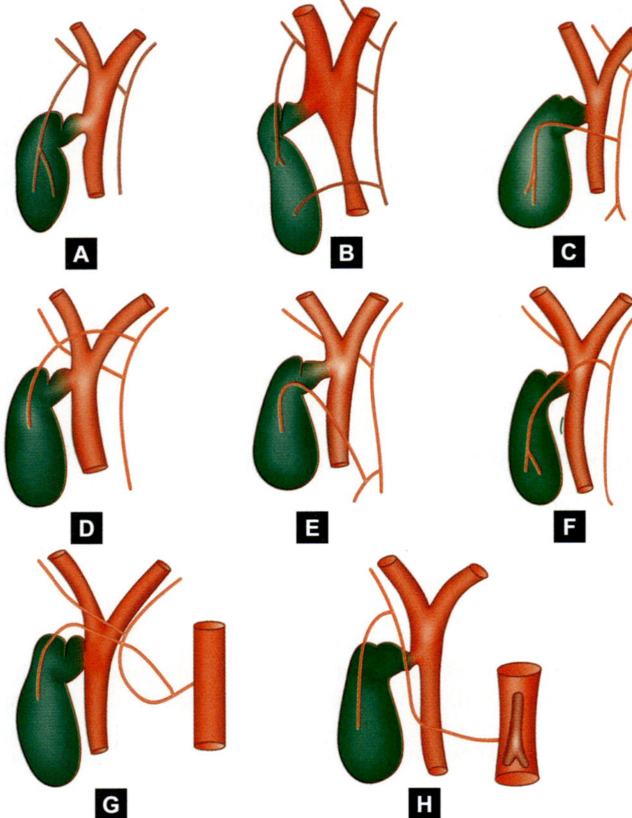

Figures 13A to H Variations in the vascular anatomy of the biliary system (A) Normal anatomy, (B) Double cystic artery, (C) Cystic artery going across main bile duct anteriorly, (D) Cystic artery originating from left hepatic artery, (E) Cystic artery originating from gastroduodenal artery, (F) Cystic artery arising from right hepatic artery and going anteriorly across the CHD, (G) Cystic artery arising from celiac axis, (H) Cystic artery arising from replaced right hepatic artery

Cholic and chenodeoxycholic acid (primary bile acids) gets conjugated with taurine and glycine which then undergo bacterial alteration to form secondary bile salts. Deoxycholate and lithocolate form the secondary bile salts. The lipids are absorbed due to the presence of bile salts.

Bile Composition[3]

Lecithin forms 95% of phospholipids. Cholesterol synthesized by liver forms the major solute of bile (Table 2). About 1,000 mL of bile is secreted daily by the liver. The flow of bile depends on:

- Neurogenic
- Hormonal
- Chemical control
- Neurogenic: Bile secretion increases with vagal stimulation and decreases with splanchnic stimulation.
- Hormonal: The water and electrolyte secretion in bile is increased by certain hormones like secretin, gastrin, CCK and glucagon. This in turn increases the bile flow.
- Chemical: Bile salts play an important part in controlling the volume of bile. Bile salts are returned to the liver by the enterohepatic circulation.

Table 2: Composition of hepatic and gallbladder bile

Characteristics	*Hepatic bile*	*Gallbladder bile*
Na	160	270
K	5	10
Cl	90	15
HCO_3	45	10
Ca	4	25
Mg	2	4
Bilirubin	1.5	15
Proteins	150	200
Bile acids	50	150
Phospholipids	8	40
Cholesterol	4	18
Total solids	-	125
pH	7.8	7.2

Bile Salt Secretion

Bile is secreted by the liver cells or the hepatocyte. The canalculi drain this bile into biliary channels leading to the main bile ducts. Bile salts play an important role in bile flow by generating the osmotic force. Daily bile salt production is 500–600 mg.

Cholesterol is the source of bile acids. It has 2 major pathways:

1. A classic pathway produces cholic acid
2. Alternate pathway that results in the synthesis of chenodeoxycholic.

Bile acids always circulate in a bound state. This binding is with lipoproteins and albumin. Bile salt uptake into the hepatocytes is through the space of Disse. There are 2 processes to mediate the same:

1. *Sodium-dependent*
2. *Sodium-independent*

Intracellular bile acid transport occurs by two mechanisms:

1. By bile acid binding proteins
2. Vesicular transport.

Rate limiting step of bile salt secretion is the transportation of bile salts across the canalicular membrane. It is an adenosine 5'-triphosphate (ATP) dependent active transport.

Enterohepatic Circulation

Always 95% of bile salts get absorbed in the ileum and via portal vein reaches back to the liver. Enterohepatic cycle occurs 6–10 times daily. The daily loss of bile salt in feces is around 600 mg. Cholate and chenodeoxycholate are acted upon by the bacterial flora in colon and are converted into deoxycholate and lithocholate.

Diseases involving the terminal ileum will lead to excessive losses of bile salts. This is compensated by an increase in production of bile salts.

Cholesterol Saturation

Cholesterol does not dissolve in bile. Micelles maintain the cholesterol in solution. Micelles are a phospholipid-cholesterol complex. Bile salts have two portions: hydrophobic and hydrophilic. In solution, the hydrophilic end is outward. Cholesterol gets added to the hydrophobic end with the help of phospholipids. Cholesterol is retained in solution in an aqueous medium. Majority of cholesterol exists in vesicles. Vesicles are bilayered made of cholesterol and phospholipids. The vesicles are unilamellar in their simplest and smallest forms, but multi-lamellar forms do exist. Crystal precipitation occurs when the capacity of these vesicles gets saturated to transport cholesterol. The solubility is dependent on the concentration of cholesterol, bile salts and phospholipids.

Bilirubin Metabolism

Heme is a degraded product of RBC's by the reticuloendothelial system. Majority of the bilirubin is from heme (80–85%). Rest is from the breakdown of hepatic hemoproteins.

Heme is converted to biliverdin by hemeoxygenase. Biliverdin gets reduced to bilirubin by biliverdin reductase. Bilirubin then binds to albumin. The toxic bilirubin undergoes esterification and gets converted into monoconjugated and diconjugated derivatives. Conjugated bilirubin is then excreted into the duodenum.

Bile Flow

Total bile produced daily is about 1 litre. Water and electrolytes get absorbed. Gallbladder stores bile during starvation and releases the same during a meal. Along with storage gallbladder also absorbs water and electrolytes to concentrate bile. Gallbladder capacity is about 40–50 mL. The gallbladder mucosa has the greatest absorptive capacity per unit of any structure in the body.

GALLBLADDER FUNCTION

During fasting state gallbladder concentrates and store hepatic bile. The gallbladder has absorptive, secretory, and motor capabilities. Absorption of water is an active process. The gallbladder's mucosa actively secretes glycoproteins and hydrogen ions. The mucin gel protects the gallbladder cell membrane from the luminal bile. Hepatic bile has a higher pH than gallbladder bile. This is due to the acidification by the gallbladder.

Absorption

The concentration process of bile occurs by active Na-Cl transport by the gallbladder epithelium. Water is passively absorbed. The concentration of calcium in gallbladder bile is influenced by serum calcium, hepatic bile calcium, gallbladder water absorption, and the concentration of organic substances such as bile salts in gallbladder bile.

However, the absorption of bilirubin, cholesterol, phospholipids, and bile salts is minimal compared with that of water. The organic compounds are significantly concentrated by the normal absorptive process that occurs in the gallbladder. Unconjugated bile salts are absorbed more readily than conjugated bile salts and may actually damage the gallbladder's mucosa, causing a nonselective increase in absorption of other solutes. Thus, increased absorption of unconjugated bile salts, caused by bacterial deconjugation or mucosal inflammation, may impair cholesterol solubility and therefore promote cholesterol gallstone formation.

Secretion

The epithelial cells secrete glycoprotein and hydrogen ions. Prostaglandins stimulate gallbladder mucin secretion. The hydrogen ions released from gallbladder epithelium, acidify the bile. Calcium remains soluble in the acidic environment. This acidification process lowers gallbladder pH from 7.1–7.3. Compared with gallbladder bile, the bile secreted by the liver is slightly alkaline, pH 7.5–7.8.

Motility

The ampulla contracts facilitating gallbladder filling. The pressure in the CBD is 10–15 mm. This is due the contracted ampullary sphincter. Release of stored bile from the gallbladder occurs with gallbladder contraction and sphincter of Oddi relaxation following a meal. CCK empties the gallbladder in response to a meal. About 60% of it is emptied within 30–40 minutes of meal when stimulated by eating. Gallbladder refilling takes next 60–90 minutes.

REFERENCES

1. Inderbirsingh. Human embryology, 7th edition. New Delhi: Macmillan India limited; 2006. pp. 186-8.
2. Hesham AAbdeldayem(2013). Hepatic Surgery. Available from www.intechopen.com/books/hepatic-surgery/essential-functional-hepatic-and-biliary-anatomy-for-the-surgeon. [Accessed April 2015].
3. Henry A Pitt, Thomas R Gadacz. Anatomy, embryology, anomalies and physiology. In: Henry A, Charles J Yeo (Eds). Shackleford's Surgery of the alimentary tract. 7th edition. Philadelphia: Elsevier Sanders; 2013. pp. 1286-303.
4. Leslie HB, Lucy EH. Surgical and radiologic anatomy of the liver, biliary tract and pancreas. In William RJ (Ed). Blumgart's Surgery of the Liver, Biliary Tract and Pancreas. 5th edition. Philadelphia: Elsevier Saunders; 2012. pp. 31-57.
5. Seetharam P, Rodrigues G. Sphincter of Oddi and its Dysfunction. Saudi J Gastroenterol. 2008;14(1):1-6.
6. Kasi PM, Ramirez R, Rogal SS, Littleton K, Fasanella KE. Gallbladder agenesis. Case Rep Gastroenterol. 2011;5(3):654-62.

CHAPTER 50

Imaging of Liver and Biliary Tract

Ankur Arora, Sunil Kumar Puri

INTRODUCTION

While clinical evaluation is the mainstay of patient management, definitive treatment of hepatobiliary disorders requires a specific diagnosis. Thus radiological imaging has a critical role in the diagnostic work up of the patients, and this becomes especially important when the clinical findings are nonspecific or equivocal. Any radiological examination should be contemplated following a thorough clinical and laboratory workup of the patient. This includes eliciting a detailed clinical history and a meticulous medical examination. It is essential that the radiological investigations are ordered judiciously; when there is a reasonable chance that it might influence the clinical management. The patient should not be subjected to a series of investigations in the hope that at least some test would yield positive results. This not only increases the financial burden but also causes distress to the patient. For judicious use of imaging, a fundamental knowledge regarding the advantages, drawbacks and appropriate indications of the diverse modalities is imperative. It goes without saying that examinations without ionizing radiation should be given precedence wherever feasible, especially in the pregnant and pediatric population.[1]

A variety of imaging modalities can be used to investigate the liver and biliary tract. The most widely used modality is ultrasound (US), which apart from being readily available, is affordable and free of radiation. A positive US examination often mandates further imaging work-up, which is mostly via computed tomography (CT) or magnetic resonance imaging (MRI) or both.[2] Fluoroscopic imaging procedures are mostly reserved for performing minimally invasive therapeutic (interventional) procedures. These procedures include endoscopic cholangiopancreatography, percutaneous transhepatic cholangiography, percutaneous transarterial chemoembolization of tumors, angioplasty of hepatic artery stenosis, etc. All these interventional techniques have proven to be very helpful in the treatment of varied clinical conditions ranging from obstructive jaundice to some of the life threatening diseases such as hepatic malignancies.[1-3]

GALLBLADDER IMAGING

Congenital Pathology

Gallbladder Duplication

Congenital duplication of the gallbladder is rare with a reported incidence of 1 in 4,000–5,000 persons. According to Boyden's classification (Panel-B) gallbladder duplication can be classified into: a bifid gallbladder with a common neck or complete duplication with common (Y-shaped) or separate (H-shaped) cystic ducts. Gallbladder duplication can be well-recognized at MRI as well as magnetic resonance cholangiography (MRCP) as presence of two pear-shaped cystic structures in the gallbladder fossa (Figs 1A and B).[4] Preoperative identification of gallbladder duplication is crucial to avoid intraoperative perplexity and long-term complication of a missed second gallbladder. Furthermore, precise depiction of the biliary anatomy is vital for appropriate surgical planning and avoidance of inadvertent injury to the biliary tract.[5] Attendant complications such as cholelithiasis, cholecystitis, and obstructive jaundice that may be associated with gallbladder duplication can also be picked with high sensitivity and specificity with MRCP imaging.[4-8]

Inflammatory Lesions

Acute Cholecystitis

Patients with acute cholecystitis generally present with pain in right upper abdomen, nausea or vomiting and occasionally, jaundice.

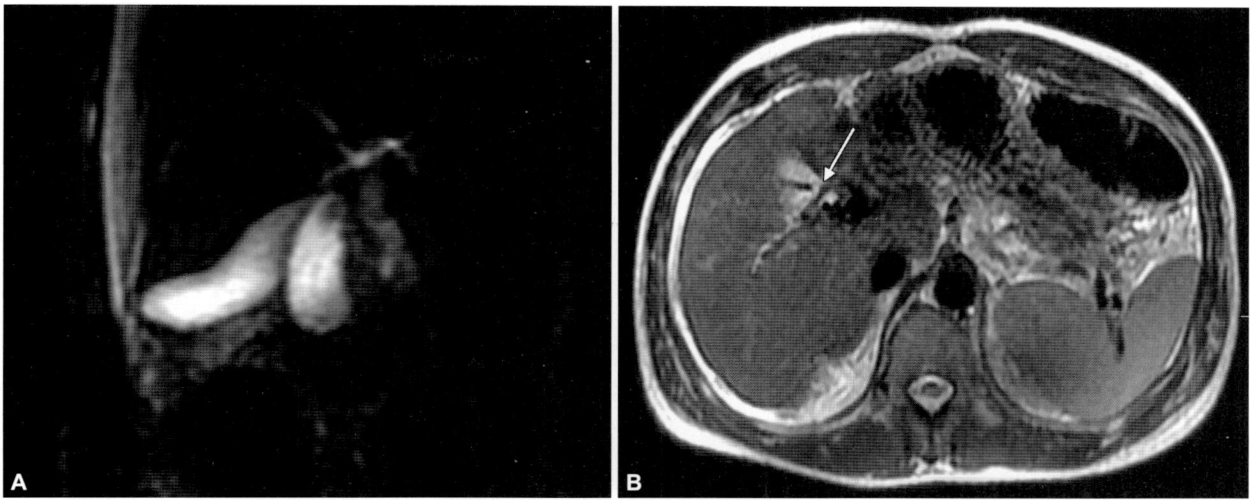

Figures 1A and B (A) Thick slab 2D-MRCP sequence displaying gallbladder duplication; (B) Axial T2-weighted MRI showing a common neck of the two gallbladder moieties (arrow)

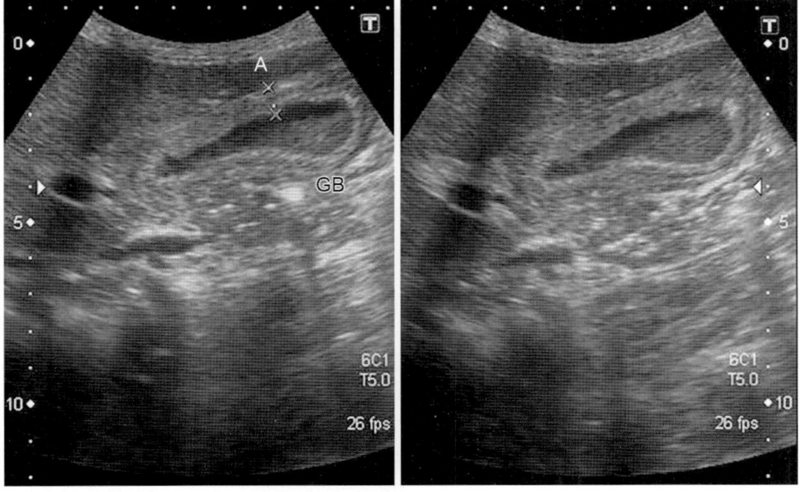

Figure 2 Gray scale ultrasound image showing edematous circumferential gallbladder wall thickening and pericholecystic fluid in a patient with acute cholecystitis. Also note thick intraluminal echoes in keeping with gallbladder sludge. The sonographic Murphy's sign was positive

Of the patients with right upper quadrant pain up to 20–35% are found to have acute cholecystitis. US is considered the initial imaging modality of choice for the work-up of patients presenting with right upper quadrant pain and suspected biliary tract disease.[3,9-14] As per the American College of Radiology (ACR) appropriateness criteria, US is recommended as the most appropriate imaging modality for acute cholecystitis. The presence of gallstones (seen as echogenic foci within the gallbladder lumen causing dense posterior shadowing) along with a positive sonographic Murphy's sign has a 92% positive predictive value for acute cholecystitis. A positive sonographic Murphy's sign refers to elicitation of point tenderness over the inflamed gallbladder upon application of pressure by the US probe. Other signs such as gallbladder wall thickening (>3–5 mm), wall edema and pericholecystic fluid on US have a sensitivity and specificity of greater than 80% (Fig. 2).[10-14] CT and MRI is usually reserved for cases where the US imaging manifestations are equivocal. Also, CT and MRI are crucial for the delineation of complications such as gangrenous cholecystitis, gallbladder perforation, pericholecystic abscess formation, etc. (Fig. 3).[9,11,15,16] Also, MRI is considered better for the delineation of stones in the gallbladder neck and/or the cystic duct. Imaging also helps to exclude other differentials of right upper quadrant pain such as liver abscess, subphrenic collection, nephrolithiasis, right sided pleural effusion etc. Cholescintigraphy, in the current era, is usually reserved as a contemporary imaging test primarily when the sonography findings are equivocal. Moreover, it is also used

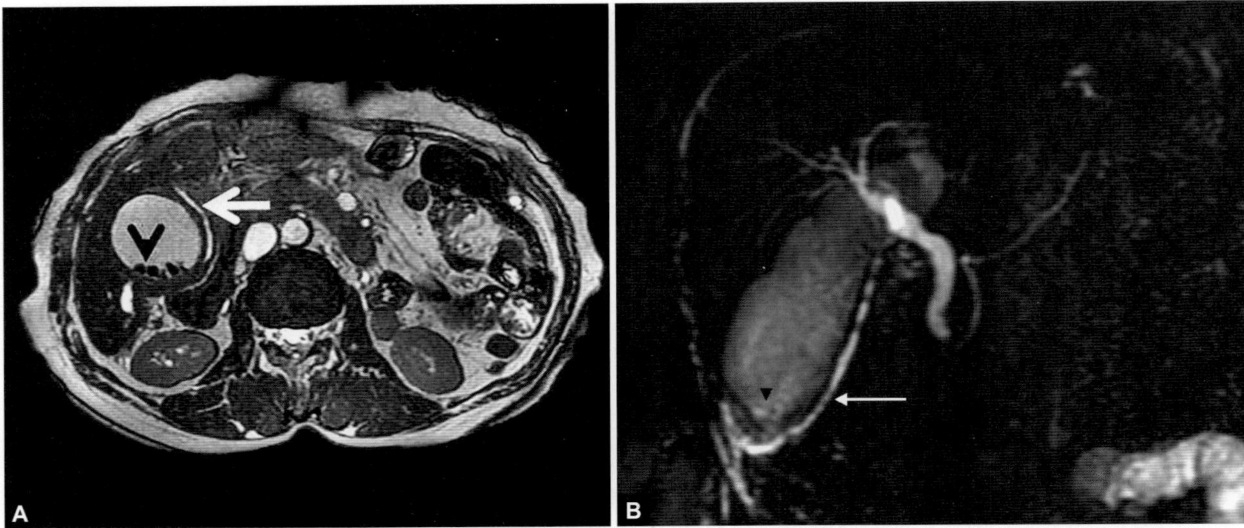

Figures 3A and B (A) Axial FIESTA and (B) thick slab 2D-MRCP sequences showing gallbladder stones (arrowhead) with pericholecystic fluid (arrow) in a 50-year-old lady with acute cholecystitis

in critically sick patients with suspected cholecystitis (on other imaging studies), but whose medical condition and high surgical risk demand the highest level of certainty of the diagnosis.[12]

Chronic Cholecystitis

Recurrent episodes of gallbladder inflammation result in progressive scarring of its walls resulting in a thickened and fibrosed gallbladder with loss of contractility and near-total obliteration of the lumen. On US imaging, this manifests as what is popularly known as the wall-echo-shadow (WES) complex or the "double arc sign" (Fig. 4).[3,17] The two echogenic (bright) arcs of the WES complex represent the adjacent gallbladder wall and the echogenic gallstone, respectively, which are separated by a thin anechoic (dark) layer of residual intraluminal bile.[17] Cholescintigraphy is useful for confirming chronic cholecystitis by delineating the following manifestations such as delayed accumulation of isotope by the gallbladder, irregular luminal filling, and/or the presence of photopenic areas.[12]

Gangrenous Cholecystitis

Akin to uncomplicated cholecystitis, those with gangrenous cholecystitis also show gallbladder wall thickening and attendant gallstones and biliary sludge. However, typically the severity of inflammation is severe and degree of wall thickening and distension relatively more. US feature suggestive of the diagnosis includes presence of intraluminal membranes which represents ischemic necrosis and sloughing of the mucosal layer.[15] Also, fibrinous exudates from the gallbladder walls can manifest as intraluminal membranes. As compared to CT, the intraluminal membranes are better delineated on US examination. However, CT is considered more specific and is able to show patchy areas of lack of mural enhancement reflecting areas of mural necrosis. These changes may be accompanied with pericholecystic abscess formation, intraluminal hemorrhage and/or intramural air (Figs 5A and B).[18-20]

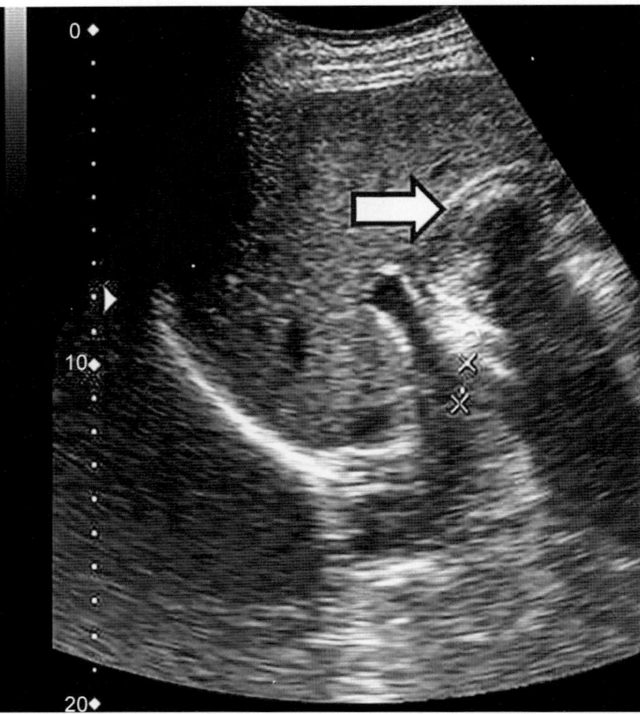

Figure 4 Transabdominal US showing wall-echo-shadow complex (double arc sign) in a patient with chronic calculus cholecystitis (arrow)

Gallbladder Perforation

The inflammatory changes in up to 5–10% of patients with acute cholecystitis can progress and lead to gallbladder perforation. Owing to the least vascular supply, the gallbladder fundus is usually the most common site to give way. Gallbladder perforation is usually subacute ensuing formation of a complex (peri) cholecystic fluid abscess—which may remain confined to the gallbladder wall,

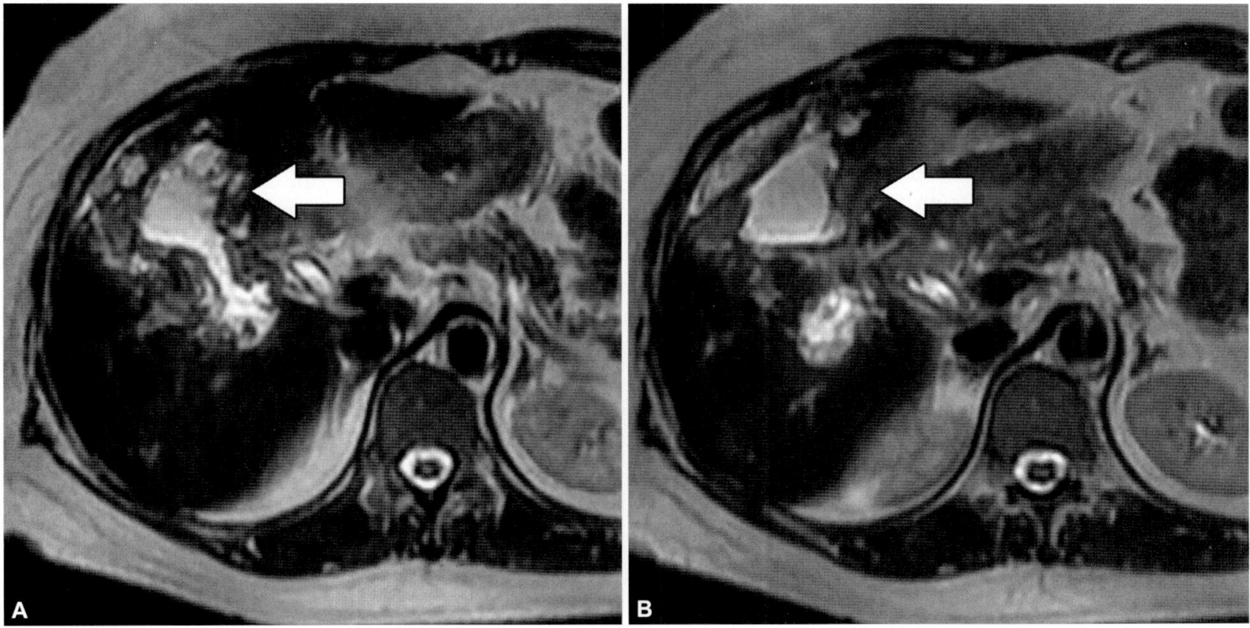

Figures 5A and B Axial T2-weighted MRI in a pyrexic patient with right hypochondial pain showing sloughed-off gallbladder walls in keeping with gangrenous cholecystitis

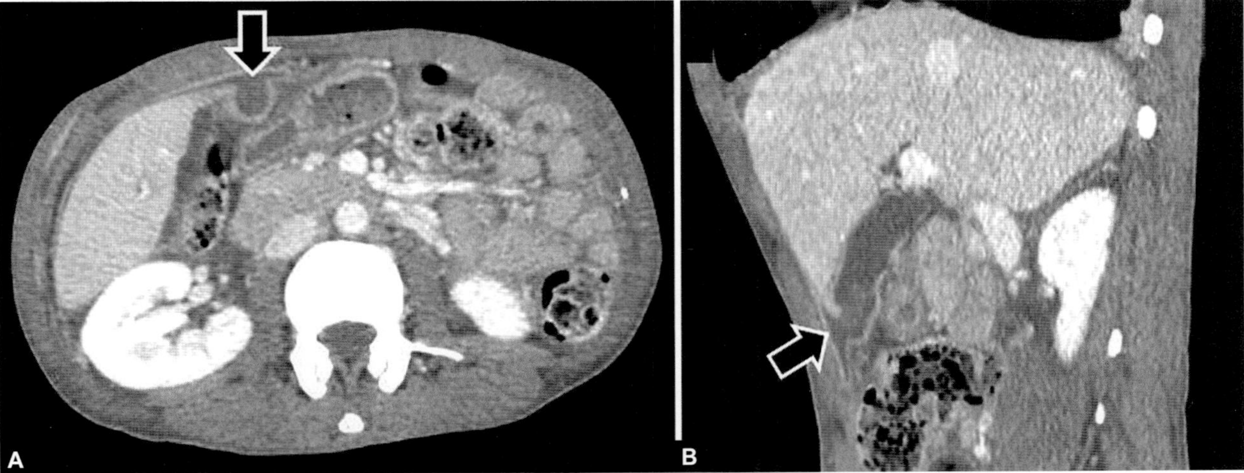

Figures 6A and B (A) Axial and (B) Sagittal contrast enhanced CT showing focal discontinuity in the gallbladder walls suggesting gallbladder perforation (arrow) with attendant pericholecystic/perihepatic fluid collection

or may extend into the pericholecystic space, adjacent hepatic parenchyma or the peritoneal cavity. On imaging three subtypes of gallbladder perforation have been described including localized perforation, cholecystoenteric fistula, and free intraperitoneal rupture resulting in biloma formation and acute gallbladder perforation can cause biliary leak and biliary peritonitis (Figs 6A and B).[11,20] Although US can suggest the possibility of gallbladder peroration by depicting a complex fluid collection in the vicinity of an inflamed but collapsed gallbladder, CT is generally required for confirmation and to ascertain the exact extent of the disease. However, a mural defect is appreciable in only 70% of patients on contrast enhanced CT or MRI.[11,20]

Gallbladder Empyema

Gallbladder empyema refers to distension of gallbladder with purulent material (pus) and is also known by the name of suppurative cholecystitis. It is a complication of calculus cholecystitis and is often clinically indistinguishable from uncomplicated cholecystitis. On US imaging, intraluminal echogenic pus can be indistinguishable from gallbladder sludge. Similarly, on CT the purulent material may display high attenuation similar to that of sludge. AT times, MRI using heavily T2-weighted sequences may aid in distinguishing pus from sludge by depicting fluid-fluid level and layering of purulent bile along the dependent wall of the gallbladder (Figs 7A and B).[4,11]

Emphysematous Cholecystitis

Emphysematous cholecystitis is a rare but severe form of acute cholecystitis which is characterized by the presence of air within the gallbladder. It constitutes less than 1% of cases of acute cholecystitis and is usually secondary to infection with anaerobic organisms (for e.g., *Clostridium* sp, *E. coli, Staphylococcus, Streptococcus,* etc.) and can be rapidly fatal. The disease typically affects elderly men (contrasting other form of cholecystitis) often with a background of longstanding diabetes mellitus. The reported incidence of gallbladder gangrene and perforation in emphysematous cholecystitis are 75% and 25% respectively.[11,21-23] Diagnosis of emphysematous cholecystitis is largely dependent upon imaging and the disease usually does not manifest with alarming clinical signs of sepsis, often remaining indistinguishable from uncomplicated acute cholecystitis. CT is considered as the image modality of choice and based upon the imaging manifestations the disease can be staged as stage I, II and III. Stage I is characterized by the presence of intramural air, stage II by the presence of intraluminal air and stage III is associated with extension of air into the pericholecystic space (Figs 8A and B).[21-23]

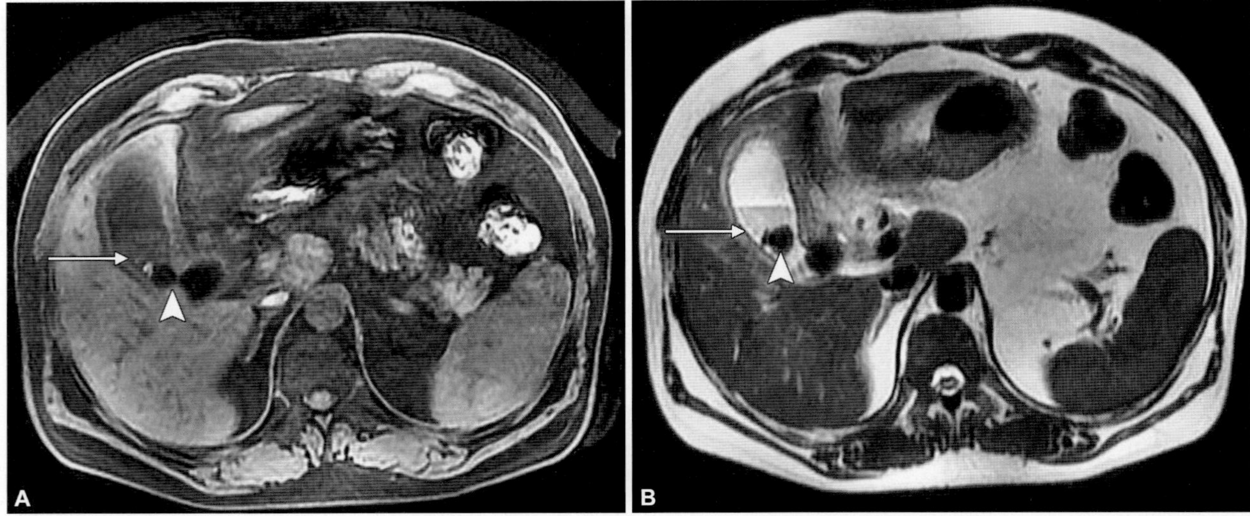

Figures 7A and B (A) Axial T1-weighted and (B) T2-weighetd MRI showing cholelithiasis (arrowhead) with edematous gallbladder wall thickening and intraluminal fluid-fluid level (arrow) in a patient with acute gallbladder empyema

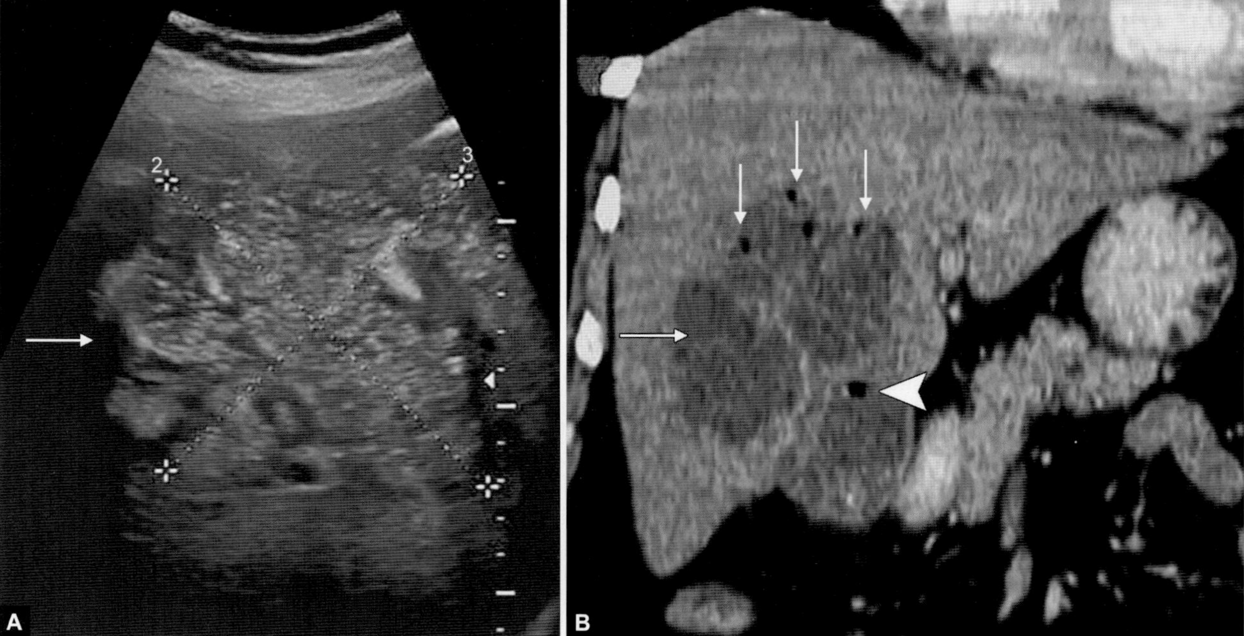

Figures 8A and B (A) Transabdominal US showing a complex heteroechoic lesion in the gallbladder fossa (B) Coronal contrast-enhanced CT showing inflamed gallbladder with intraluminal sir speck (arrowhead). There is large contiguous hepatic abscess (thick arrow) with multiple air specks (thin arrows)

Xanthogranulomatous Cholecystitis

It is well-known that the imaging features of gallbladder carcinoma and xanthogranulomatous cholecystitis can overlap substantially and can be indistinguishable. But, more recently reports have underscored that certain cross sectional imaging manifestations, if present, can provide high prospective diagnostic accuracy of xanthogranulomatous cholecystitis.[24-29] Uchiyama et al. found in their study population of 32 cases, that the CT features of the continuous mucosal enhancement together with gallstones in a patient with chronic gallbladder disease were highly suggestive of xanthogranulomatous cholecystitis.[25] Goshima et al. reported that when at least three of the five CT findings (diffuse wall thickening; a continuous mucosal enhancement; intramural hypoattenuating nodules; absence of macroscopic liver invasion; and absence of intrahepatic bile duct dilatation) were observed in combination, the sensitivity, specificity, and accuracy of differentiating xanthogranulomatous cholecystitis from carcinoma were 83%, 100% and 91%, respectively.[28] More recently, the diagnostic accuracy of multidetector computed tomography (MDCT) for differentiating xanthogranulomatous cholecystitis from early-stage gallbladder cancer was studied by Chang et al.[24] They reported that early mural enhancement was more common in GB cancer probably suggesting a differential enhancement pattern between inflammatory pathology and gallbladder carcinoma. Although inflammation also increases local blood, angiogenesis is deficient in inflammation, which could explain why early perfusion is less in xanthogranulomatous cholecystitis than in patient with gallbladder cancer. However, this differential enhancement pattern warrants further studies for validation.

Acalculous Cholecystitis

Acalculous cholecystitis is typically seen in an ICU setting in those who are critically ill, or in postoperative or post trauma patients. Additionally, those with diabetes mellitus, underlying malignancy, vasculitis, cardiac failure or cardiac arrest are at high risk. Bile stasis and gall blader ischemia are central in its pathogenesis. US is usually the first test used in the evaluation of acalculous cholecystitis. It not only has a good sensitivity and specificity for diagnosing acalculous cholecystitis but can also help exclude alternative diagnoses—most importantly calculus cholecystitis. US findings suggestive of acalculous cholecystitis include unusually distended gallbladder (>5 cm), exhibiting smooth wall thickening (>3–5 mm), with presence of pericholecystic fluid, positive Murphy's sign, and/or intraluminal sludge (in the absence of gallstones).[2,3] Untreated cases may go in for complications such as gangrene, perforation, and pericholecystic abscess formation. Although CT can be used to confirm the diagnosis, MR is generally avoided in lieu of patient's clinical condition. However, cholescintigraphy can be performed in equivocal cases as it has a high specificity of 100% although the sensitivity is only 67%.[11,30,31]

Noninflammatory Lesions

Adenomyomatosis

Adenomyomatosis is a common nonneoplastic and noninflammatory condition of the gallbladder which is seen in up to 5% of all cholecystectomy specimens. As the name suggests, it

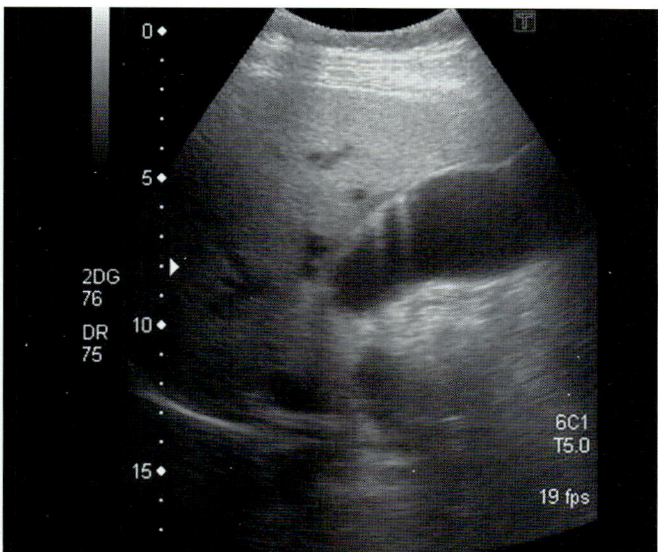

Figure 9 Transabdominal US showing comet-tail artifacts emanating from the gallbladder walls suggesting adenomyomatosis

refers to a hyperplastic pathology of the gallbladder wherein there is excessive epithelial proliferation with resultant invaginations (Rokitansky-Aschoff sinuses) into a hypertrophied muscularis propria.[32-36] Majority of patients remain asymptomatic and the disease is usually incidentally picked up during imaging evaluation for other reasons, and therefore requires no specific treatment. However, cases where differentiation from gallbladder carcinoma is challenging are subjected to cholecystectomy. Morphologically, the disease can be classified into three morphologic types: diffuse, segmental and fundal adenomyomatosis. Accordingly, the disease manifests as gallbladder wall thickening which may be generalized, annular, segmental, or localized fundal (adenomyoma) in localization. On US, gallbladder wall thickening in adenomyomatosis can be confused for malignancy if the characteristic anechoic intramural diverticulae are not visualized. These anechoic structures represent the dilated Rokitansky-Aschoff sinuses and may display comet-tail reverberation echoes—which are an imaging hallmark of the disease on sonography (Fig. 9). However, the changes of adenomyomatosis are best discernible on MRCP sequences or heavily T2-weighted MR sequence which displays these bile-filled intramural Rokitansky-Aschoff sinuses assuming a pearl-necklace appearance (Fig. 10). On CT, following intravenous contrast administration the epithelial lining of the Rokitansky-Aschoff sinuses enhances and is seen as rim-enhancement of small cystic intramural collections referred to as the CT rosary sign.[32-36]

Malignant Lesions

Gallbladder Carcinoma

Globally, carcinoma gallbladder is one of the most common biliary malignancies. It is the fifth most common gastrointestinal (GI) malignancy. Some of the risk factors for gallbladder carcinoma are long standing cholelithiasis, chronic cholecystitis, chronic biliary

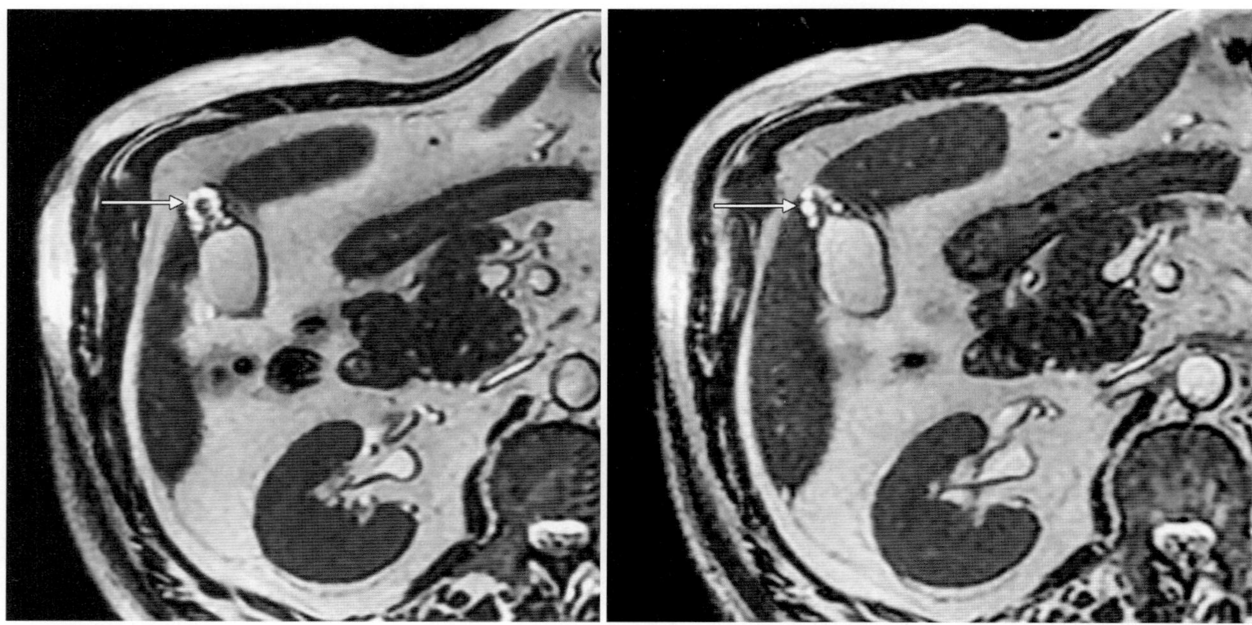

Figure 10 Axial FIESTA sequence showing classical pearl-necklace appearance secondary to dilated intramural diverticulae seen at the gallbladder fundus (arrow)

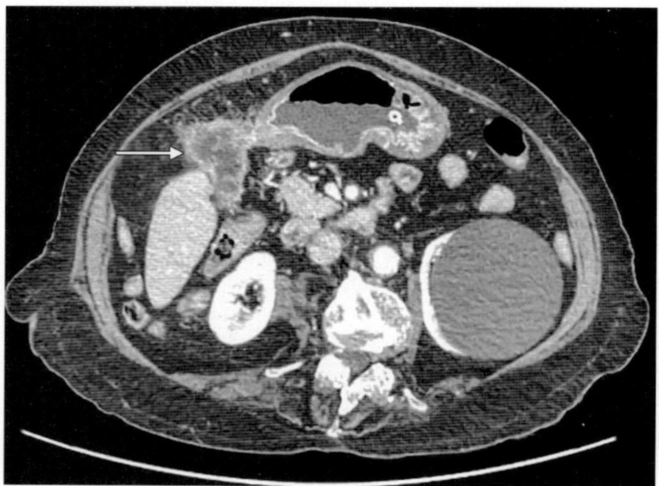

Figure 11 Axial contrast enhanced CT in an elderly female with gallbladder cancer showing irregular heterogeneously enhancing gallbladder wall thickening with infiltration of the pericholecystic fat (arrow)

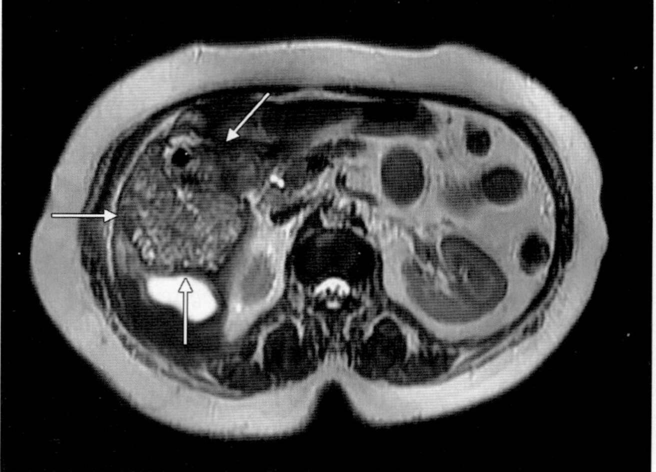

Figure 12 Axial T2-weighted MRI showing a large heterogeneous mass lesion replacing the gallbladder (arrows). Note is made of a dark stone within the gallbladder lumen

infections (*Opisthorchis viverrini, Salmonella typhi*), primary sclerosing cholangitis (PSC), anomalous pancreaticobiliary junction, and porcelain gallbladder. Although carcinoma gallbladder can have diverse imaging appearances, it can be broadly classified into three types: focal or diffuse gallbladder wall thickening, intraluminal polypoid mass lesion (usually >10 mm), or an ill-defined infiltrative mass replacing the gallbladder (Figs 11 to 13).[37-42]

On US, smooth symmetrical gallbladder wall thickening suggests a benign etiology, whereas carcinoma causes irregular, asymmetric or marked hypoechoic wall thickening which may be seen infiltrating the adjacent hepatic parenchyma. On CT or MRI, carcinomatous wall thickening typically demonstrates avid arterial phase enhancement which persists or becomes isodense or isointense to the hepatic parenchyma on the portal venous phase. Other imaging manifestation favoring gallbladder carcinoma includes contiguous hepatic infiltration, hepatic metastases, locoregional or retroperitoneal lymphadenopathy, and biliary obstruction at the level of the porta hepatis. Contrast enhanced CT or MRI is especially useful for staging of the disease and to ascertain lesion respectability.[37-39,42] Presence of invasion of the main portal vein, the hepatic artery, or multiple extrahepatic organs marks

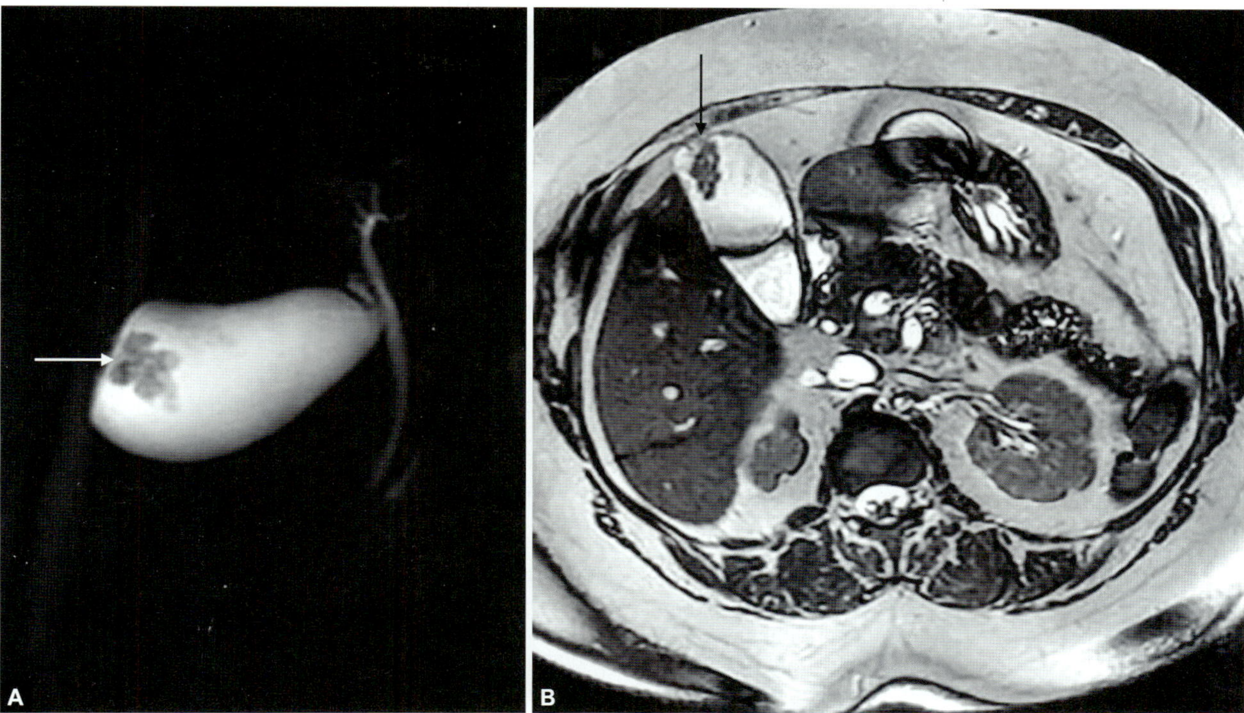

Figures 13A and B (A) Thick slab 2D-MRCP and (B) axial FIESTA sequence showing a polypoid mass projecting within the gallbladder lumen (arrow)

the disease as T4 as per the American Joint Committee on Cancer staging manual for gallbladder carcinoma. The presence of enlarged cystic, hilar, pericholedochal, periduodenal, peripancreatic and superior mesenteric nodes suggest lymphatic spread. This may be seen in up to 50% patients. Presence of interaortocaval and more distant nodes is considered metastatic or M1 disease. FDG PET-CT can detect occult sites of metastatic disease which may not yet be identifiable on routine CT or imaging, however, it may still fail to pick up small volume peritoneal disease or subcentimetric peritoneal lesions.[40]

BILIARY TRACT IMAGING

Congenital Bile Duct (Choledochal) Cysts

Imaging not only plays a crucial role in the diagnosis but also an important role in preoperative planning of patients with choledochal cysts. On imaging, choledochal cysts appear as unusual dilatation of the common bile duct (CBD) with or without involving the intrahepatic biliary radicles. The cyst may assume a cystic or a fusiform morphology and occasionally can assume gigantic sizes containing as much as 5–10 liters of bile. Often, US is used as the initial imaging modality followed by CT or MRI. MR cholangiography is considered the noninvasive imaging modality of choice for the evaluation of congenital choledochal cysts and associated biliopancreatic abnormalities (e.g., anomalous biliopancreatic junction) (Fig. 14).[43-50] Attendant complications such as intrabiliary stones, cholangitis-related liver abscesses, or concomitant carcinoma can be depicted with high degree of sensitivity. MDCT examination of the abdomen with reformatted images is another vital technique to exquisitely delineate the anatomic details of the biliary tract and the pancreaticobiliary duct union. Although endoscopic retrograde cholangiopancreatography (ERCP) can delineate better the pancreaticobiliary junction it is limited by its invasive nature and potential risk of procedure related complications such as pancreatitis, perforation, etc. Currently, the role of ERCP has been limited to those cases where MRCP visualization of the terminal CBD or the pancreaticobiliary

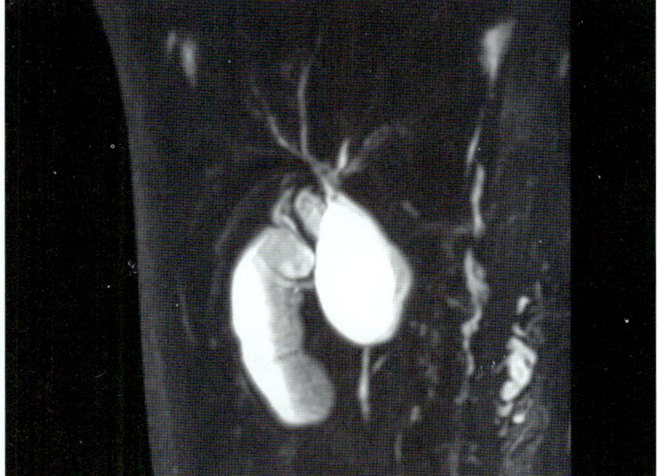

Figure 14 Thick slab MRCP sequence showing fusiform dilatation of the extrahepatic bile ducts in a 10-year old girl in keeping with Todani type-I choledochal cyst

junction is suboptimal, or when a therapeutic procedure is contemplated.[43-50]

Stone Disease

It is estimated that up to 15% of patients who undergo cholecystectomy have bile duct stones and despite of the advancement in imaging detection of small bile duct stones continues to remain challenging. US which is the usually the first imaging modality used to image the hepatobiliary system has an overall sensitivity of only 21–63% for detecting bile duct stones. This is primarily secondary to limited sonographic window often due to overlying gas shadows, variant biliary anatomy, and/or absence of bile duct dilatation which may be associated with almost 50% of patients harboring bile duct stones. If visible, bile duct stones typically appear as intrabiliary echogenic foci often with dense posterior shadowing. Contrasting US, MRCP is considered the noninvasive imaging modality of choice which has a reported sensitivity and specificity of 89–100% and 83–100%, respectively, when thinner sections (<3 mm) are used (Figs 15A and B). However, for stones smaller than 3 mm the sensitivity of MRI can be as low as 50%.[50] Also, MRCP is especially helpful in patients where ERCP and PTC have failed, or in patients with anastomotic site stricture at biliary-enteric anastomosis in whom ERCP is not feasible. On MRCP, intrabiliary stones are seen as low-signal-intensity filling defects within high-signal-intensity bile, with or without attendant biliary dilatation. Apart from stones, hemobilia and pneumobilia can also appear as low-signal-intensity filling defects within high-signal-intensity bile, and in such instances CT is considered superior for reliably differentiating them from each other.[48]

Bile Leak

For confirming bile leaks or differentiating bilomas from other perihepatic fluid collections, dynamic MRI of the biliary system can be performed using hepatocyte-specific contrast agents which are preferentially excreted into bile. These contrast agents, such gadoxetate disodium or mangafodipir trisodium, in addition to providing anatomic information also provides us with functional details that can be used to identify bile leaks and bile collections. T1-weighted MRCP images obtained 20 minutes after intravenous administration of hepatocyte-specific contrast agents usually provide excellent delineation of the biliary tract and/or identification of biliary leak, if any.[51]

Inflammatory Disorders

Infectious Cholangitis

The most characteristic imaging manifestations of infectious cholangitis include circumferential bile duct wall thickening that shows increased enhancement following intravenous contrast administration. This can be appreciated on CT as well as MRI, though better discernible on post gadolinium fat-suppressed T1-weighted MR images (Figs 16A and B). In addition, streaky periportal hyperintensity may be evident on T2-weighted images. Advanced disease may also show wedge-shaped hyperintense areas in the liver hepatic parenchyma. Predisposing factors for infectious cholangitis include partial or complete obstruction of the biliary tract which can be best evaluated with MR cholangiography.[52,53]

Recurrent Pyogenic Cholangitis

Recurrent pyogenic cholangitis (or oriental cholangiohepatitis) is characterized by intrahepatic bile duct stones, strictures and recurrent episodes of infection. Recurrent infections and hepatic lithiasis in turn predisposes the patient to multiple liver abscesses, further duct injury and strictures, and in advanced cases, progressive liver parenchymal damage, hepatic fibrosis and cirrhosis, and portal hypertension. MRCP is the preferred noninvasive imaging tool which can help to localize the involved bile ducts and

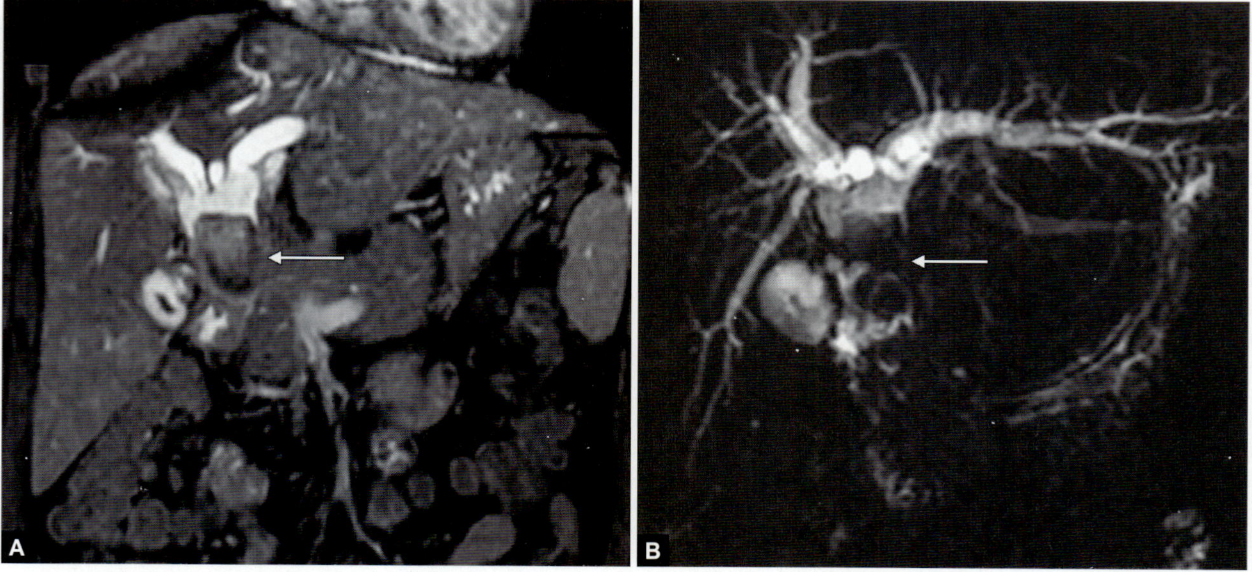

Figures 15A and B (A) Coronal FIESTA and (B) thick slab 2D-MRCP sequence showing a large intraductal calculus within the mid extrahepatic bile duct causing biliary obstruction and upstream intrahepatic bilobar biliary dilatation

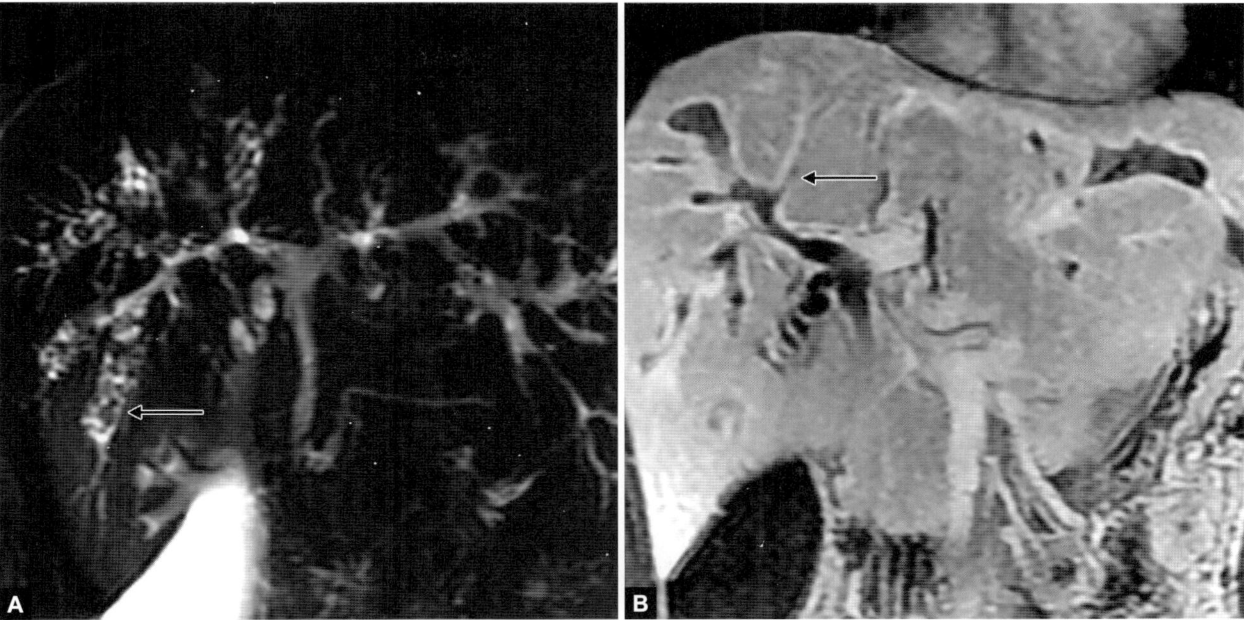

Figures 16A and B (A) Thick slab 2D-MRCP sequence showing bilobar intrahepatic biliary dilatation with multiple intraductal filling defects suggesting hepatic lithiasis; (B) Contrast-enhanced coronal T1-weighted MRI showing enhancing bile duct walls in keeping with acute cholangitis

determine the disease severity. Imaging manifestations include extrahepatic and central intrahepatic bile duct dilatation with multiple intrahepatic bile duct stones and concomitant stricture of the intrahepatic bile ducts.[54-56] Often there is accompanying thickening of the bile duct walls, and hepatic abscesses during an acute episode. Long standing disease is associated with atrophy of the liver segments that contain intrabiliary stones.

Primary Sclerosing Cholangitis

Typical imaging manifestations of primary sclerosing cholangiopathy include randomly distributed multifocal biliary strictures alternating with segmental ectasias giving rise to a "beaded" appearance to the intrahepatic biliary radicles. While both small as well as large ducts are involved in 75% of the patients, isolated small duct involvement is seen in 15% and of large ducts alone in 10% of the patients.[57-59] The intra-as well as extrahepatic bile ducts frequently show annular wall thickening and progressive fibrosis of bile duct walls causes peripheral "pruning" of the biliary radicles. Conventionally, invasive ERCP has been considered the gold standard imaging modality for diagnosing PSC; although, now MRCP has proven itself to be a useful noninvasive alternative (Fig. 17). Also, MRI in patients with PSC has the advantage of allowing concomitant assessment of the hepatic parenchyma and extrahepatic association.[57,58] It is crucial to not to miss cholangiocarcinoma in patients with PSC as this can be seen in as many as in 10–15% of the patients. Imaging manifestations suggesting malignant transformation include: hilar mass, irregular high-grade biliary narrowing or bile duct stricture with shouldered margins, disproportionate upstream biliary dilatation, rapid progression of strictures, atrophy of affected liver segments, and the presence of intraluminal polypoid lesions. Recently, certain studies have suggested that FDG PET can be useful in confirming the suspicion of cholangiocarcinoma in patients with PSC, although larger studies have been recommended for validation of these results.[57-59]

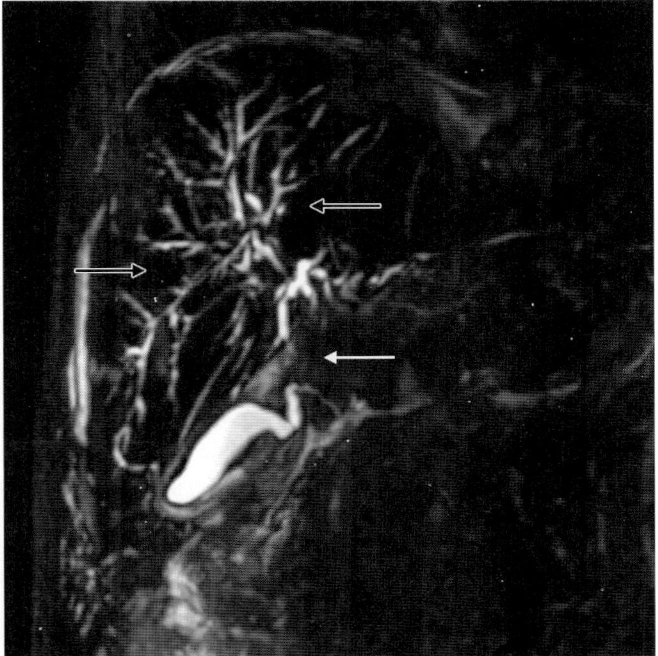

Figure 17 3D-MRCP sequence displaying characteristic imaging manifestations of sclerosing cholangitis in the form of multifocal biliary strictures alternating with segmental ectasias involving the bilobar intrahepatic biliary radicals (black arrows). In addition, there is narrowing of the extrahepatic bile duct (white arrow)

Bile Duct Tumors

Benign Bile Duct Adenoma

Bile duct adenomas are highly uncommon and the neoplasm can involve the intra- as well as extrahepatic bile duct. Extrahepatic adenomas are seen as an intrabiliary polypoid mass with or without upstream biliary dilatation. On imaging, the neoplasm can be mistaken for bile duct stones or a polypoid cholangiocarcinoma.[60]

Precancerous Tumor

Biliary Intraepithelial Neoplasia

These are flat or micropapillary tumors which are undetectable by means of routine imaging techniques such as US, CT and MRI. They are usually encountered during pathological evaluation of surgical specimens following excision for hepatolithiasis.[60]

Intraductal Papillary Mucinous Neoplasm of Bile Duct (IPMN-B)

Intraductal papillary mucinous neoplasm of bile ducts (IPMN-Bs) are increasingly diagnosed tumors of the biliary tree which encompasses the previously reported biliary papilloma and papillomatosis. They are considered premalignant which can be associated with invasive carcinomas or can progress to frank intraductal-growing variety of cholangiocarcinomas. As the name suggests IPMN-B is characterized by intraductal papillary or villous growth of biliary epithelium. Depending upon the lesion size, the tumor may or may not be visible on conventional imaging. However, the most constant feature seen on imaging is focal or generalized dilatation of the intrahepatic or extrahepatic bile duct with the involved bile duct showing disproportionate dilatation. The biliary dilatation has been ascribed to the copious amount of mucin which the tumor produces. MRI including MRCP is undoubtedly superior to CT for delineating the intraductal popypoidal mass owing to its higher soft tissue resolution. Apart from conventional MR sequences diffusion weighted imaging has shown promising results for differentiating a benign IPMN-B from those associated with invasive carcinoma as the latter tend to show restricted diffusion. Vascular invasion and locoregional lymphnodal enlargement should prompt the consideration of progression to intraductal cholangiocarcinoma.[60]

Malignant

Cholangiocarcinoma

Cholangiocarcinoma is a slow-growing adenocarcinoma arising from the biliary epithelium seen predominantly in males in their sixth and seventh decades of life. It usually occurs as a complication of choledochal cyst, primary sclerosing cholangitis, intrahepatic stone disease or liver fluke infections. Three primary growth patterns are recognized including mass forming, periductal infiltrating and intraluminal. Based on anatomical location, they can be classified into intrahepatic (10%), hilar or Klatskin's tumors (25–30%) and extrahepatic (60–65%).[61,62] On imaging, intrahepatic mass-forming cholangiocarcinoma appears as a well-defined hypodense lobulated mass which shows enhancement of the periphery, which contains viable cells, on the arterial phase while the fibrous center of the tumor remains unenhanced. In the equilibrium phase, the center of the tumor may show varying degree of enhancement. Focal intrahepatic biliary dilatation with atrophy of segments drained by these ducts and retraction of overlying liver capsule may be seen. On MRI, the center of the tumor is more hypointense than the periphery on T2-weighted images reflecting the fibrous stroma (Figs 18A and B). Periductal infiltrating type of

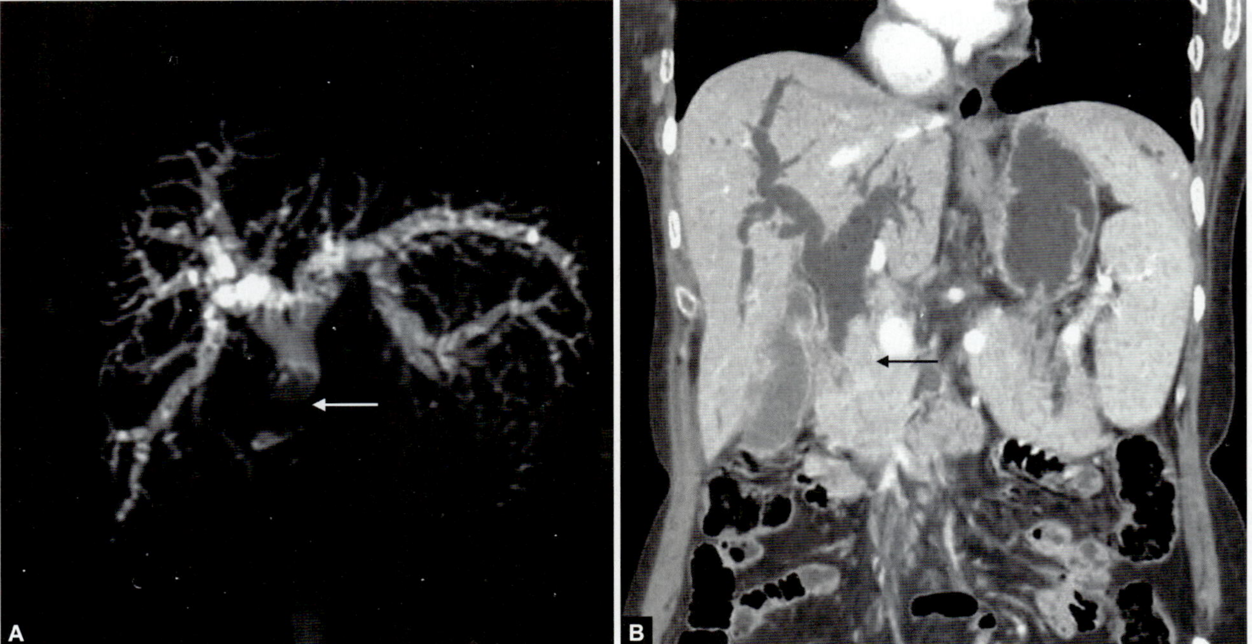

Figures 18A and B (A) Thick slab 2D-MRCP sequence showing a lobulated intraductal filling defect. (B) Contrast-enhanced coronal CT of the same patient showing an enhancing mass occluding the lower bile duct

cholangiocarcinoma develops along the bile ducts in an elongated, branching pattern causing irregular narrowing of the involved ducts with peripheral ductal dilatation. Whereas intraductal tumors are polypoidal or sessile lesions that show papillary growth within the bile duct lumen seen as an intraductal filling defect on MRCP or ERCP study.[61-63] Some of these tumors can produce large amounts of mucin causing disproportionate dilatation of biliary system.

HEPATIC IMAGING

Hepatic Trauma

Liver is affected in approximately 20–30% of cases of blunt abdominal trauma making it the second most commonly injured abdominal organ overall. The posterior segments of right lobe are most frequent involved. The pattern of injuries ranges from parenchymal contusions to central and subcapsular hematoma and intraparenchymal lacerations with or without capsular involvement. Contrast-enhanced CT is the imaging modality of choice for accurate detection and characterization of hepatic injuries (Figs 19A and B, and 20A and B).[64-66] Lacerations appear as low-density linear or stellate defects usually paralleling the course of hepatic vasculature. Hematomas are commonly associated with lacerations seen as relatively ill-defined areas of low attenuation. Delayed complications include bilomas, abscess formation, hemobilia and vascular complications such as pseudoaneurysm and arterioportal fistulas. US is mainly reserved for serial assessment of lesions and detection of delayed complications. Owing to advancements in imaging techniques and intensive

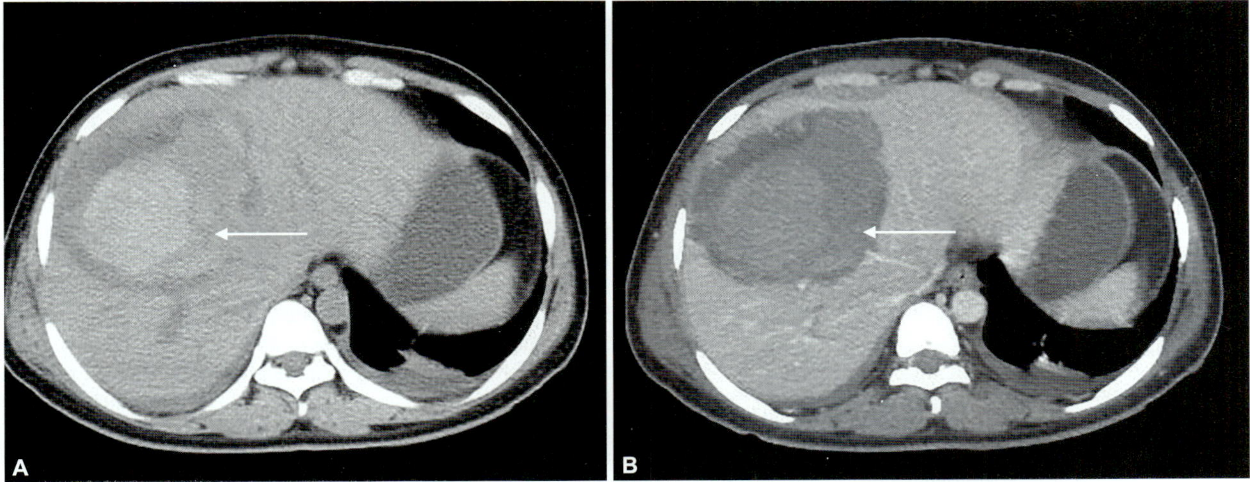

Figures 19A and B (A) Axial unenhanced and (B) contrast-enhanced CT showing a large intraparenchymal hematoma in the right liver lobe in a young male following high speed road traffic accident

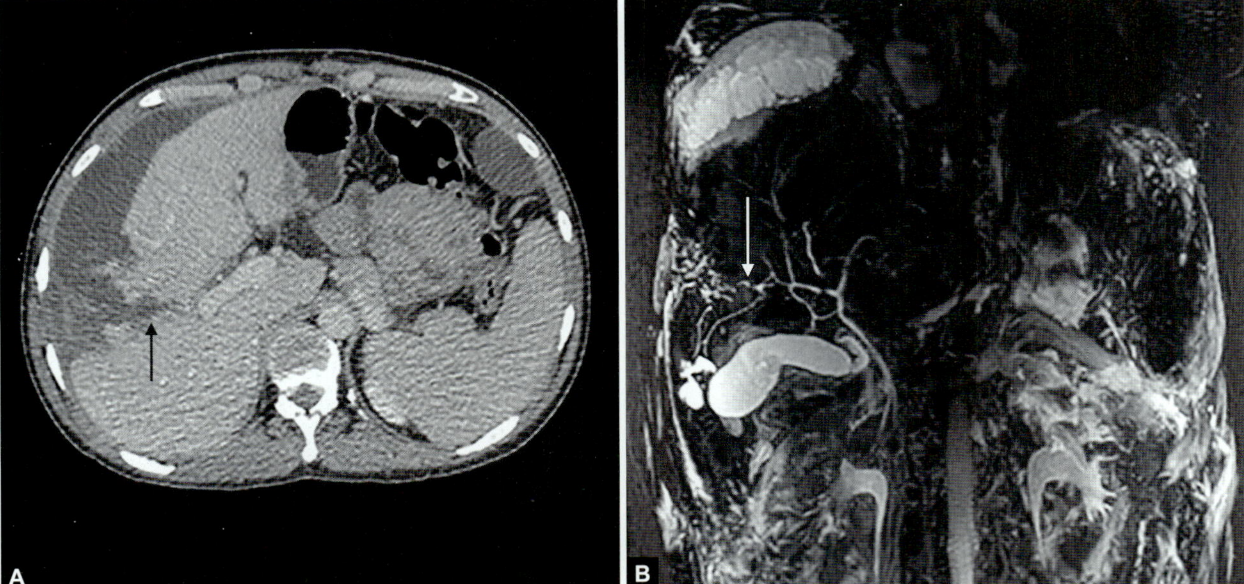

Figures 20A and B (A) Axial contrast-enhanced CT showing a hypoattenuating linear laceration extending from the liver capsule up to the liver hilum (arrow). (B) Follow-up MRCP of the same patient shows extension of the laceration up to the biliary tree. Note a large biloma in the right subphrenic space

care management, there has been a paradigm shift towards conservative management in hepatic trauma in recent years. If active contrast extravasation or traumatic vascular malformations are seen on imaging, angiographic assessment and intervention should be done. Complex perihilar injuries in hemodynamically unstable patients are managed more aggressively.[65,66]

Hepatic Infections

Pyogenic Abscess

Bacterial abscesses usually develop secondary to hematogenous dissemination (of either GI infection via the portal vein or septicemia via the hepatic artery) or ascending cholangitis from benign or malignant biliary obstruction. *Escherichia coli* is the most common bacterium involved although over one-half of liver abscesses are polymicrobic. Depending on the amount of liquefaction, the appearance at US may range from a predominantly cystic lesion with thick, irregular walls to a more solid appearing mass with varying degrees of internal echoes and debris. At contrast enhanced CT, abscesses appear relatively well-defined and hypoattenuating. Rim enhancement is relatively uncommon. They may have smooth margins with a single unilocular lesion or irregular contour and internal septa with a complex lesion (Figs. 21A and B). On MRI, they have variable signal intensity on T1 and T2 weighted images depending on their protein and fluid content.

Amebic Abscess

Amebic liver abscess is the most common extraintestinal complication of amebiasis. It is common in tropical zones with maximum prevalence seen in Indian subcontinent, the Far-East, Africa and Central and South America. Colonic trophozoites travel via the portal vein and invade the liver parenchyma. Frequently solitary, the abscess is located most commonly in the right lobe. On imaging, it may be often difficult to distinguish pyogenic and amoebic abscesses. However clinical course in combination with serology is usually diagnostic. An amebic abscess on US may appear as a round or oval hypoechoic lesion typically located near the liver capsule with fine low-level internal echoes and absence of a prominent abscess wall.[67,68] At contrast-enhanced CT, it usually appears as a well-defined lesion with thick enhancing walls and a characteristic perilesional zone of edema. Extension to chest wall, pleural cavity and adjacent viscera is relatively more commonly associated with amoebic abscesses as compared to pyogenic abscesses. At MRI, amebic abscesses cavities are generally seen as hypointense on T1 and hyperintense on T2-weighted images. Perilesional edema is seen on T2-weighted MR images in 50% of cases.[67,68]

Hydatid Disease

Hydatid disease caused by *Echinococcus granulosus* or *Echinococcus multilocularis* is dog-borne zoonoses with a worldwide distribution. Humans are accidental hosts who get infected by ingesting food or water infested with dog feces. The larval stage of the tapeworm pierces the enteric walls and reaches the liver through the portal venous system which is the most common organ to get involved (75% cases). Imaging manifestations of hepatic hydatid disease depends on the stage of cyst growth.[69-71] Gharbi has classified hepatic hydatid cysts into five subtypes. Type 1 are indistinguishable from simple cysts on imaging (25–40%) whereas type 2 is characterized by what is popularly referred to as "water lily" sign secondary to a floating intracystic detached endocyst. Type 3 shows a multivesicular morphology and a honeycomb appearance with multiple daughter cysts filling up the mother cyst (Figs 22A and B). Type 4 is a complex lesion that shows an irregular

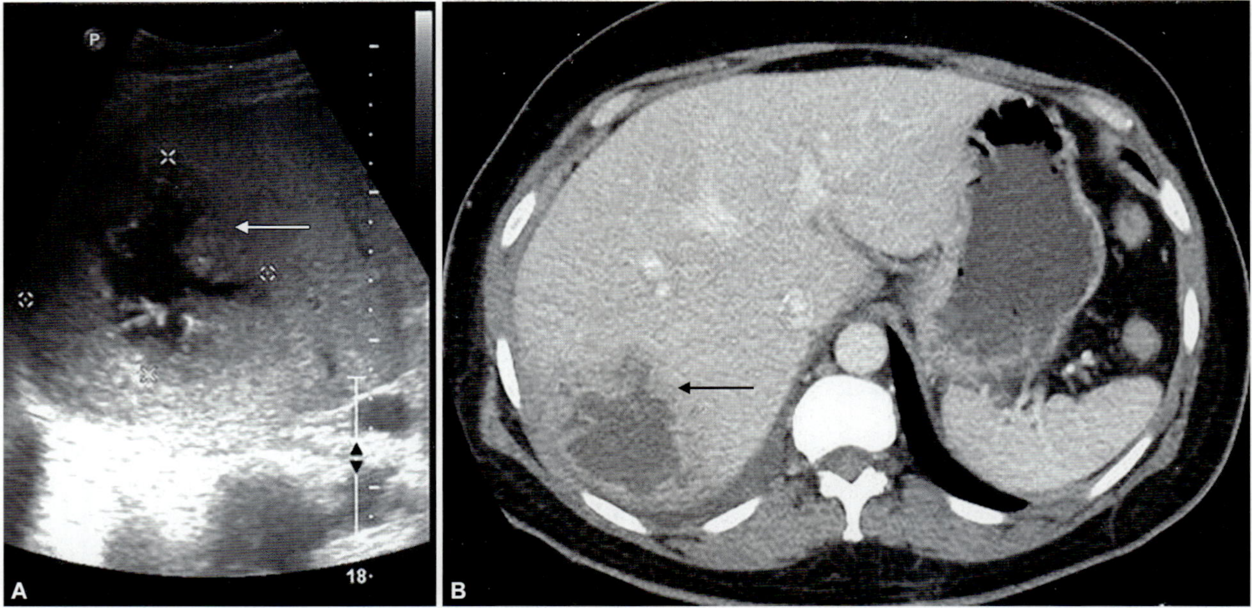

Figures 21A and B (A) Transabdominal US showing a necrotic abscess with central liquefaction in the right liver lobe (B) Contrast enhanced CT of the same patient showing a fluid-attenuation abscess with thick edematous enhancing walls

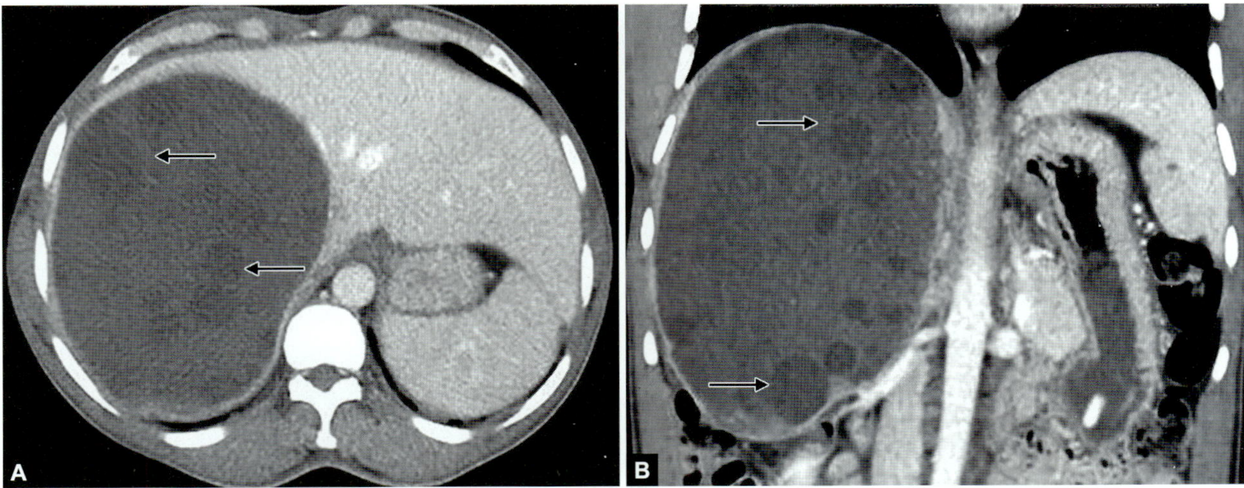

Figures 22A and B Axial and coronal CT sections showing a large cystic liver lesion in the right lobe displaying 'honeycomb' morphology secondary to multiple variable-sized hypodense daughter cysts (arrows)

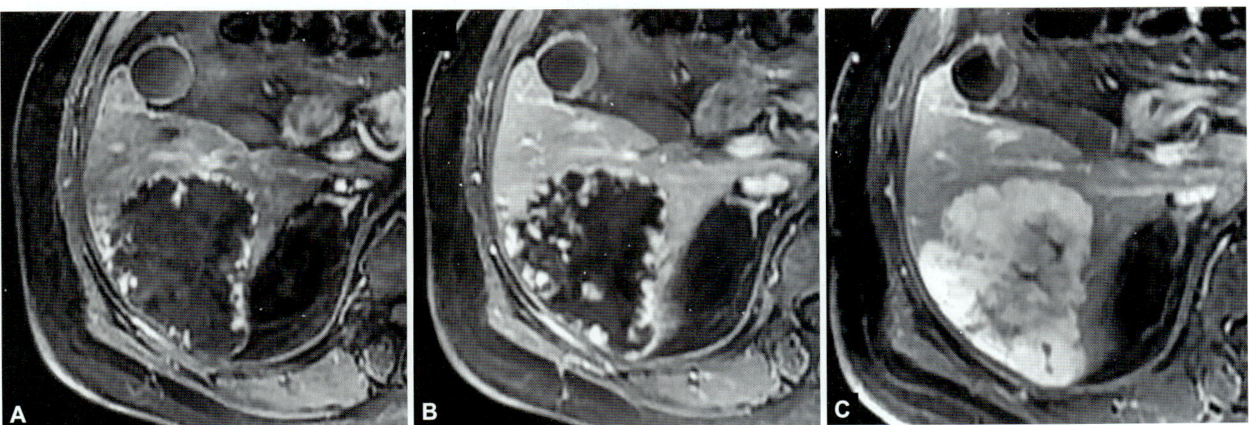

Figures 23A to C Axial dynamic contrast enhanced MRI showing a well-marginated subcapsular liver lesion displaying (A) discontinuous peripheral nodular contrast enhancement on arterial phase (B) progressive centripetal fill-in on portal venous and (C) equilibrium phase

appearance and pseudotumoral appearance often difficult to distinguish from other neoplasms. Type 5 lesion shows partial or complete calcification. One of the most common complications of hepatic hydatid cysts is cystobiliary fistulous communication or rupture into the biliary tree which is present in as many as 5–25% of cases. Those cysts located near to the liver hilum are at a higher risk for developing a cystobiliary communication.

Benign Hepatic Tumors

Hemangioma

Hemangiomas are the most common benign neoplasm of the liver and the second most common hepatic tumors exceeded in incidence only by metastases. Pathologically, the tumor is composed of large, thin-walled, blood-filled vascular spaces lined by epithelium and separated by fibrous septa. Small hemangiomas (<2 cm) are asymptomatic and seen in all age groups with a female predominance. Giant cavernous hemangiomas are by definition lesions greater than 10 cm in size and may cause symptoms by pressure effect, hemorrhage or arteriovenous shunting. Posterior segment of right lobe are most commonly affected with a predilection for subcapsular location adjacent to vessels. On sonography, hemangiomas appear as an echogenic lesion with sharp geographic margins. On CT and MRI it is seen as a well-defined lesion showing peripheral discontinuous enhancement on the arterial phase images and centripetal fill-in of contrast on the subsequent phases (Figs 23A, B and C). On MRI the lesions are hypointense on T1 and hyperintense on T2 WI. The typical contrast enhancement characteristics, sharp geographic margins, lack of deformity of liver surface, superficial location and lack of displacement of vessels help in differentiating it from other liver lesions.[72-74]

Focal Nodular Hyperplasia

Focal nodular hyperplasia (FNH) is the second most common benign tumor of liver after hemangioma. Congenital vascular malformation leads to hepatocyte hyperplasia is the proposed to be the underlying cause for its formation. Hormonal influence may also be a factor as it is more common in middle aged females. The lesion contains hepatocytes, bile duct elements and Kupffer cells. It is usually found incidentally on imaging but up to one-third can be symptomatic. On sonography, owing to its isoechoic nature, it may be visible only due to its mass effect on vessels. CT demonstrates a hypodense lesion often located in subcapsular location deforming the adjacent liver contours. Stellate-shaped central scar may be appreciated in some cases as a low-density area. Post contrast administration, the lesion shows early enhancement with steady decrease in attenuation appearing isodense to liver in the portal venous phase. Central scar, if present, remains hypodense till the portal venous phase but then accumulates contrast, appearing hyperdense on equilibrium phase images. On MRI, both the lesion and the scar are hypointense on T1 and hyperintense on T2 weighted imaging (Figs 24A to E).[75-78]

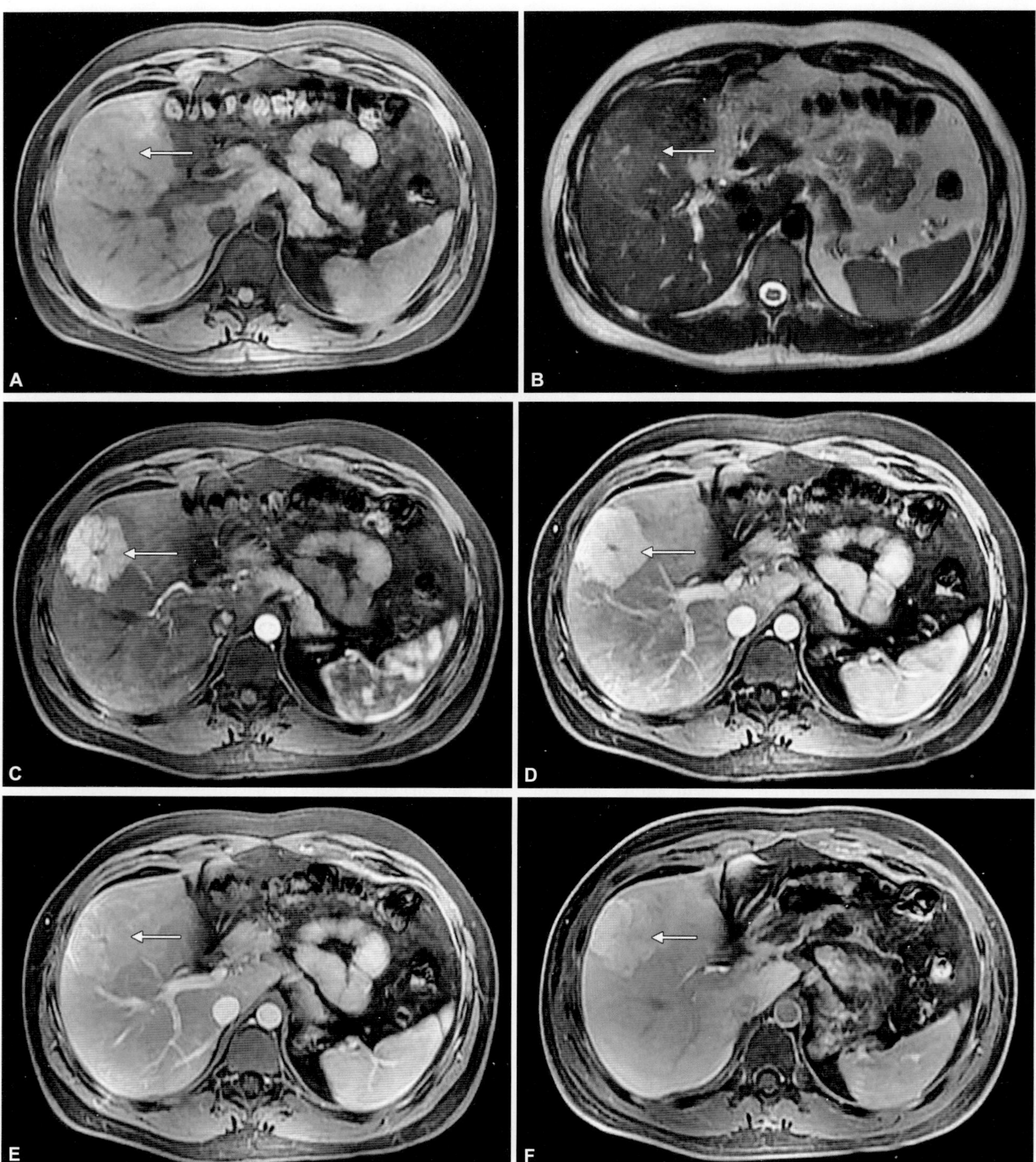

Figures 24A to E Axial T1-weighted (A) and T2-weighted (B) MRI showing a nearly isointense nodular mass lesion in the right lobe. The lesion shows avid enhancement following intravenous (hepatocyte-specific) contrast administration on hepatic arterial (C) and portal venous (D) phase (E). The lesion becomes isointense on equilibrium phase and shows contrast retention on 1-hour delayed scan (F). Findings typical for FNH

Hepatocellular Adenoma

Adenomas are rare benign tumors containing well-differentiated hepatocytes that lack bile ducts and portal triads. Kupffer cells are occasionally present but are nonfunctional. Majority are solitary (70–80%) and occur typically in young (<40 years) female patients. Predisposing factors include use of oral contraceptive in female and anabolic steroid in male patients and presence of glycogen storage disease. Spontaneous intralesional and peritoneal hemorrhage can rarely require emergency intervention. On sonography, adenomas appear as a well-circumscribed tumor with predominantly echogenic appearance due to intra tumoral fat and glycogen. Intralesional anechoic areas may be seen due to hemorrhage and scar tissue. CT demonstrates as hypo to isodense lesion showing moderate enhancement on arterial phase images with washout and enhancement similar to that of surrounding liver parenchyma on portal venous and delayed phase images. On MRI the lesions are iso to hyperintense on T1 and hyperintense on T2 weighted imaging.[79-83]

Lipomatous Tumors

Lipomatous hepatic tumors include lipomas, angiomyolipomas and myelolipomas depending upon the cellular composition. None of them have malignant potential. They occur in 10% of patients with tuberous sclerosis and renal angiomyolipomas. Most are asymptomatic and discovered incidentally. On sonography they appear as well-defined echogenic tumors indistinguishable from hemangiomas or focal fatty infiltration. The lipomatous nature of these tumors can be demonstrated on CT. Enhancement ranges from none in pure lipomas to significant in angiomyolipomas. On MRI, fat containing tumors appear hyperintense on both T1 and T2 weighted imaging comparable to the signal intensity of subcutaneous and retroperitoneal fat. Chemical shift imaging may be used to differentiate pure lipomas from tumors with mixed cellularity such as angiomyolipomas and myelolipomas.[84,85]

Infantile Hemangioendothelioma

Infantile hemangioendotheliomas account for more than 12% of childhood liver tumors. Majority are seen within the first 6 months of life with a female preponderance. It is a benign vascular tumor comprised of vascular channels formed by proliferating endothelial cells. Presenting signs include abdominal mass, hepatomegaly or high output congestive heart failure due to arteriovenous shunting within the lesion. Lesions on US can have a variable appearance ranging from highly echogenic, hypoechoic to anechoic with echogenic septa. Doppler demonstrates characteristic changes in the hepatic arteries and veins. The celiac axis and common hepatic artery are dilated and the caliber of the abdominal aorta reduces below the origin of the celiac axis. Hepatic veins draining the lesion may be prominent. On CT hypodense, well-defined homogenous masses are seen with evidence of calcifications in up to 40% of lesions. Lesions demonstrate early peripheral enhancement with centripetal progression of enhancement on equilibrium phase. The appearance on MRI is that of a heterogeneous, predominantly hyperintense mass on T2 weighted imaging due to the presence of hemorrhage, necrosis and fibrosis.[86-88]

Mesenchymal Hamartoma

Mesenchymal hamartomas account for 7% of all primary hepatic tumors in pediatric population. These are usually seen in children below 2 years of age with a male preponderance. On sonography, these usually present as a well-marginated multilocular cystic mass with echogenic septa, typically in the right lobe of liver. The internal septae may enhance on contrast administration. On MRI, cystic components are hyperintense on T2 weighted imaging and stromal components appear hypointense on T1.[89-91]

Malignant Hepatic Tumors

Hepatocellular Carcinoma

Hepatocellular carcinoma (HCC) is the most common primary malignant hepatic neoplasm worldwide. Risk factors include Hepatitis B and C infection, alcoholic cirrhosis, primary hemochromatosis and exposure to carcinogens including aflatoxin. More than 80% of HCC's occur in cirrhotic livers. Three patterns of tumor growth are seen: solitary (50%), diffuse infiltrative (30%) and multinodular tumor (20%). In Asia, HCC usually presents as a well-defined mass, either solitary or multifocal, associated with cirrhosis. In the west, it usually presents as a diffusely infiltrating mass associated with alcoholic cirrhosis. Majority of small HCCs (<2 cm) are hypoechoic on US while the larger ones are either heterogeneous or echogenic. A less common pattern is diffuse parenchymal involvement with disorganization of normal echopattern. They have a high propensity to invade the portal and hepatic veins. Color Doppler demonstrates intralesional vascularity. On CT solitary or multiple low attenuating lesions are seen which may show areas of fat density within. On administration of intravenous contrast, lesions demonstrate intense heterogeneous enhancement on arterial phase images. During portal venous phase there is rapid washout of contrast and the lesion becomes hypodense to normal liver. On equilibrium phase images, enhancing pseudocapsule may be demonstrated in some cases (Figs 25A and B). Severely dysplastic nodules do not show rapid washout while metastatic lesions only show peripheral enhancement and hence can be readily differentiated. On MRI HCCs are usually hypointense on T1 and hyperintense on T2 weighted imaging.[92,93] Diffusion-weighted MRI (DWI) is an innovative technique that acquires image contrasts based on differences in the water molecule diffusion between different tissues. DWI is especially useful for improving lesion detection (Figs 26A and B), predicting the histological grade and for ascertaining treatment response and recurrence in patients with HCC.[94] Contrast-enhanced US is similar to CT and MRI for delineating HCC hypervascularity. Because a substantial proportion of patients with advanced chronic liver disease can have attendant renal dysfunction, contrast-enhanced US can be a safer alternative to contrast-enhanced CT and MRI not only for detection but also for guiding ablative procedures such as RF ablation (Fig. 27).[95] Perfusion CT can deliver quantitative data regarding tumor vascularity (perfusion) and is usually reserved for assessing hemodynamic changes to antiangiogenic therapy (with sorafenib) in the treatment of HCC. However, exposure to high doses of ionizing radiation limits its use in routine clinical practice.[94]

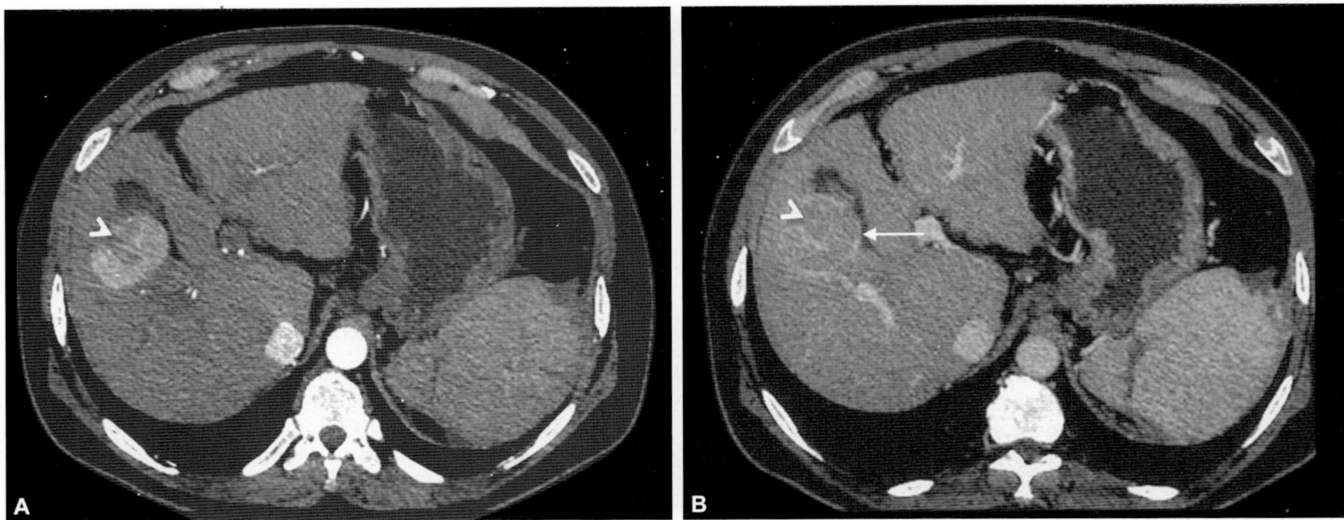

Figures 25A and B Axial arterial-phase (A) and portal venous-phase CT (B) of a chronic hepatitis-B carrier with HCC. Note the typical manifestation of HCC i.e. arterial hypervascularity with subsequent washout (arrowheads) and an enhancing capsule (arrow)

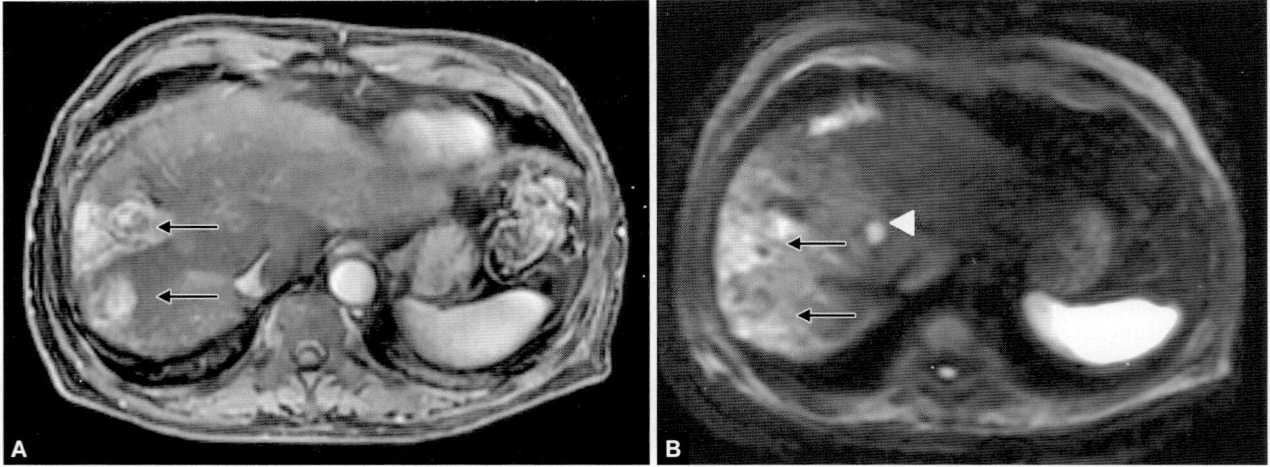

Figures 26A and B (A) Arterial phase contrast-enhanced MRI showing multifocal hyperenhancing HCC in right lobe (black arrows). (B) Diffusion weighted imaging demonstrates an additional lesion in caudate lobe which was not well discernible on contrast study

Fibrolamellar Carcinoma

Fibrolamellar carcinoma is a slow-growing tumor seen in young adults that usually arises in healthy liver. It usually presents as a large, solitary, encapsulated, circumscribed liver mass. Central scar may be seen in up to 60% of cases. The scar may calcify (33–55%) and is a major radiological clue to the diagnosis. A lobulated predominantly hyperechoic mass is seen on US. Central hyperechoic areas with foci of shadowing may be visualized consistent with central scar and calcification within the scar. On CT, it is seen as a well-defined, lobulated hypodense lesion which shows heterogeneous enhancement on arterial and venous phases (Figs 28A to D). Scar enhances on delayed images. MRI demonstrates a T1-hypointense and T2 hyperintense lesion. Scar, being fibrous in nature remains hypointense on both T1 and T2 weighted imaging (as opposed to the scar of FNH which appears hypointense on T1 and hyperintense on T2 weighted images). Portal vein invasion, necrosis and hemorrhage are much less common than classical HCC making these tumors frequently resectable with a better prognosis.[96,97]

Hepatoblastoma

Hepatoblastoma is the most common primary malignant hepatic neoplasm of childhood. It usually presents within the first 3 years of life as a painless abdominal mass with history of weight loss, jaundice and raised alpha-fetoprotein (AFP) levels. On imaging, the tumor is frequently seen as a large, inhomogeneous, predominantly echogenic mass on US. The tumor may sometimes show varying degrees of internal calcification. Internal anechoic

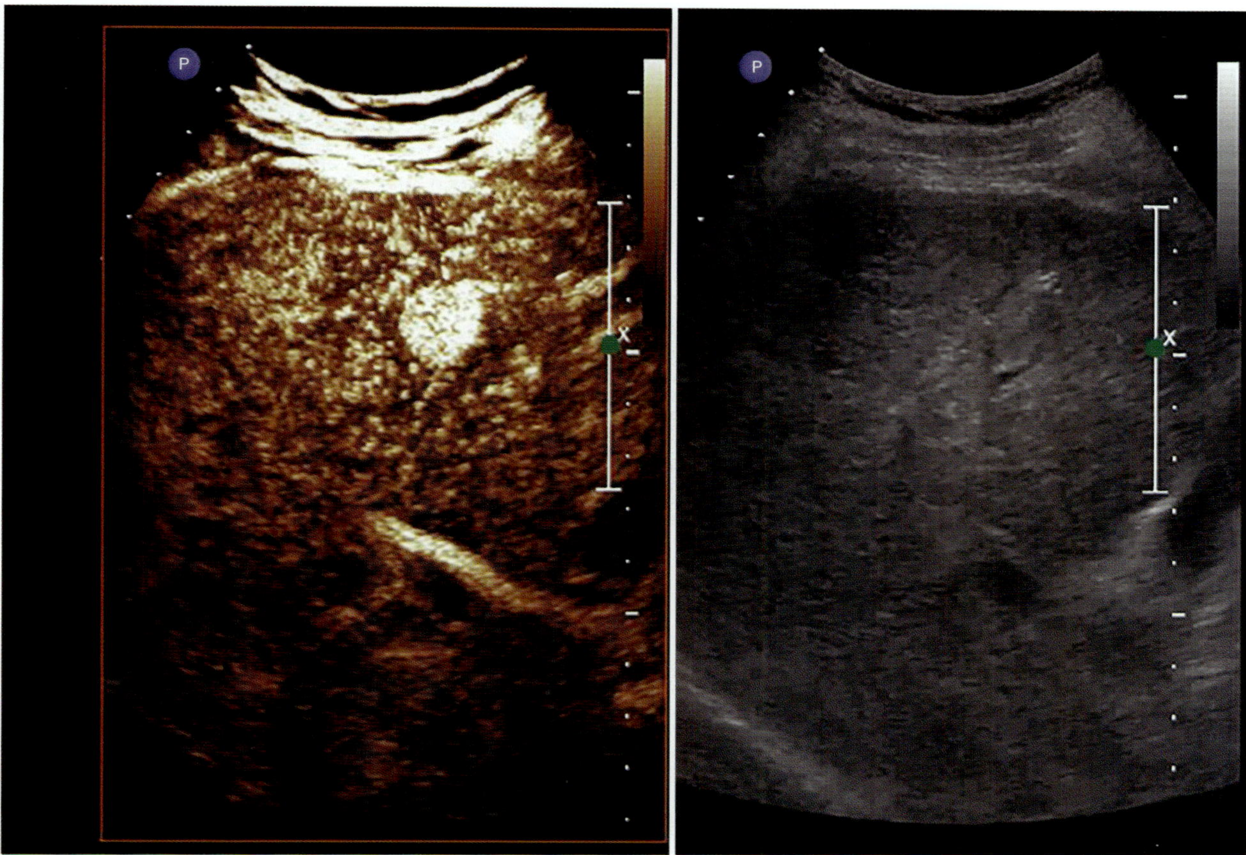

Figure 27 Side-by-side arterial-phase contrast-enhanced and grayscale US images obtained prior to radiofrequency ablation of HCC in a patient with alcohol-related liver disease. Note the lesion is not discernible on grayscale US, however, shows avid enhancement following contrast administration

areas due to necrosis and a lobular pattern due to septations may also be seen. On CT, the neoplasm tends to be relatively well-defined and hypoattenuating. It shows varying degrees of enhancement following intravenous contrast administration. Invasion of portal vein and vena cava may be demonstrated (Fig. 29).[98,99]

Epithelioid Hemangioendothelioma

Epithelioid hemangioendothelioma is a rare low-grade malignant tumor of vascular origin seen commonly in adult females. The tumor tends to be multiple with the nodular lesions coalescing in the subcapsular area over the course of disease. On sonography, it is seen as nonspecific well-defined peripheral hypoechoic masses. Nonenhanced CT depicts multiple hypodense subcapsular nodules sometimes with calcification and overlying capsular retraction. On the arterial phase contrast enhanced CT, subtle peripheral enhancement may be seen surrounding a low attenuation fibrous core. Retraction of the overlying capsule is a characteristic common finding and should raise the possibility of this tumor. The lesions tend to be hypointense on T1 weighted imaging and often show a thin peripheral dark rim. On T2 weighted images lesions appear heterogeneously hyperintense. Moderate peripheral and delayed central enhancement is encountered following intravenous gadolinium administration.[100,101]

Angiosarcoma

Hepatic angiosarcoma is a rare tumor seen in elderly (fifth to seventh decade of life) and is relatively more common in men. Risk factors include exposure to thorotrast, vinyl chloride and arsenic and its clinical presentation is nonspecific and may include weight loss and vague abdominal pain. It usually presents as multiple lesions scattered in the liver. These lesions are unencapsulated and contain blood filled cystic spaces. On US, these appear hyperechoic and may show anechoic areas due to necrosis and/or hyperechoic areas secondary to fresh hemorrhage. Unenhanced CT demonstrates a nonspecific low attenuation pattern while following contrast administration marked peripheral enhancement similar to hemangioma can be encountered.[102] On MRI, the lesions tend to be hypointense on T1 and heterogeneously hyperintense on T2 weighted imaging. Fluid levels may be present indicating internal hemorrhage. Dynamic contrast enhanced MRI shows enhancement pattern similar to hemangioma however it's unusual for hemangiomas to be heterogeneous on T2WI.[102]

Metastases

Metastatic lesions of liver are far more common than primary hepatic malignancies—the most common primary sites being the colon, stomach, pancreas and breast. Patients usually present with

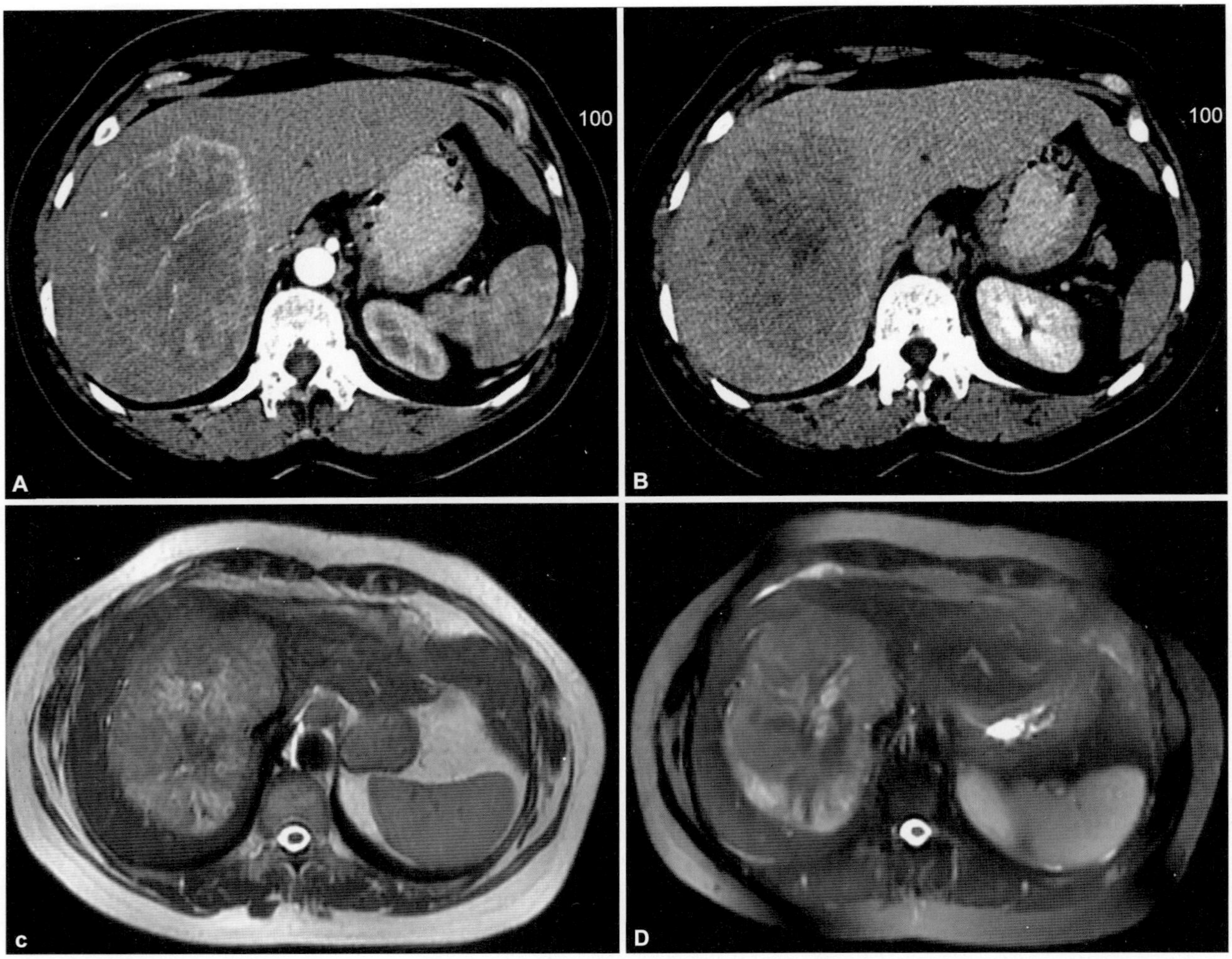

Figures 28A to D (A and B) Arterial and equilibrium phase CT in a young female showing a hypervascular liver mass showing contrast washout (C and D) On T2-weighted the mass appears hyperintense and shows a central scar

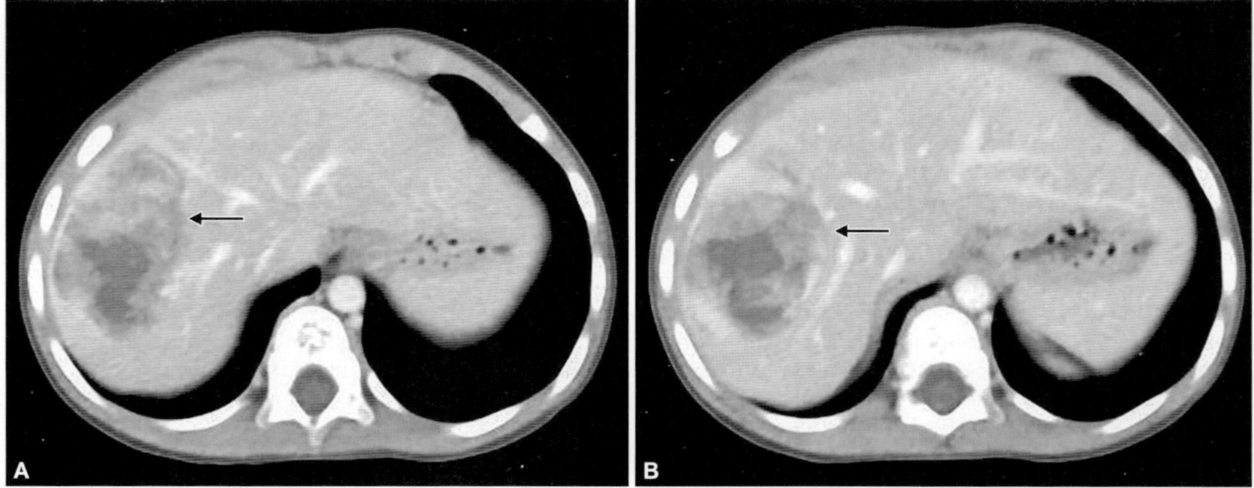

Figures 29A and B Axial contrast-enhanced CT in a 4-year-old boy with hepatoblastoma showing a large mixed attenuation heterogeneous mass in the right lobe

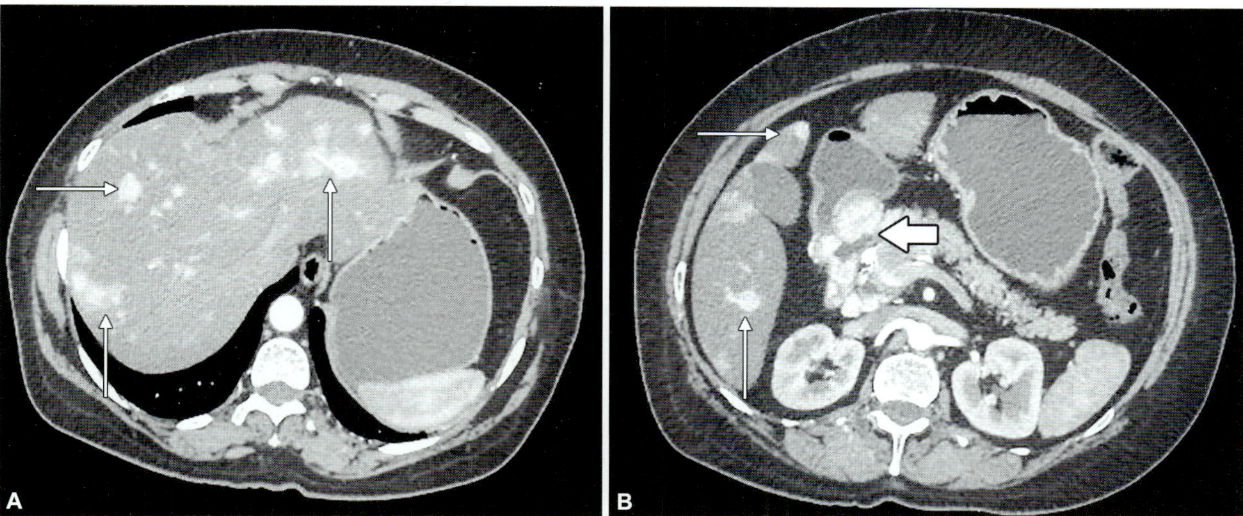

Figures 30A and B (A and B) Axial arterial-phase contrast-enhanced CT showing multiple hypervascular liver metastases (thin arrows) in a patient with duodenal neuroendocrine carcinoma (thick arrow)

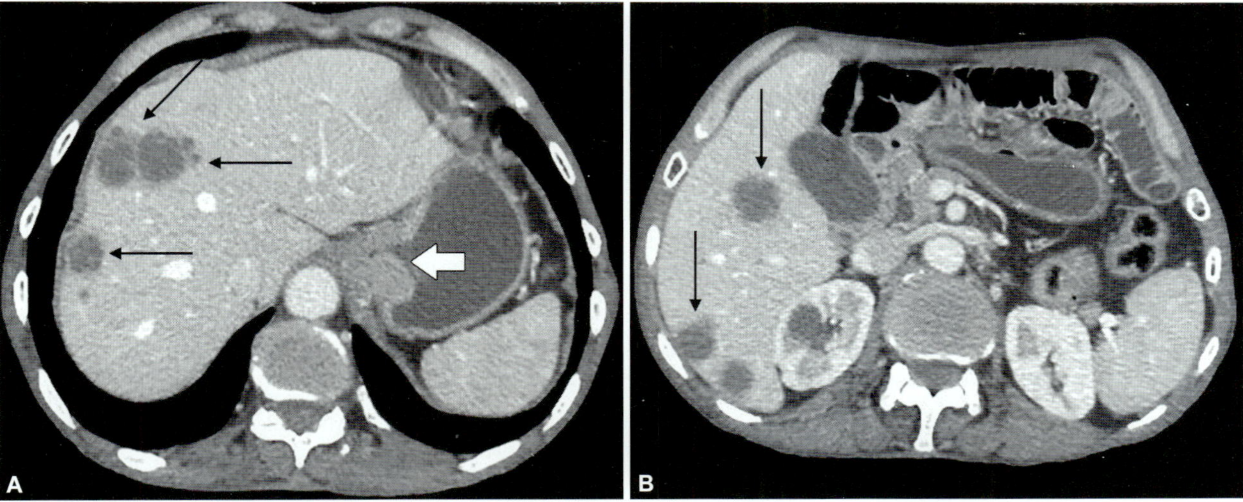

Figures 31A and B (A and B) Axial contrast-enhanced CT showing multiple hypovascular metastatic liver lesions (thin arrows) in a patient with gastric carcinoma (thick arrow)

hepatomegaly, ascites, jaundice and deranged liver function tests. The lesions are most commonly seen as hypoechoic nodules with no distal shadowing or enhancement on US. Hyperechoic metastases are often seen with colonic and GI malignancies and with vascular metastases from islet cell tumors, carcinoid, choriocarcinomas and renal cell carcinomas. Echogenic lesion with hypoechoic halo (bull's eye or target sign) indicates an aggressive tumor commonly seen with bronchogenic carcinomas. Calcification can be seen with mucinous metastases from colon and ovary whereas cystic metastases are seen with adenocarcinomas of pancreas, ovary and colon. On CT most metastatic lesions are hypodense to the liver parenchyma, whereas some are indistinguishable from normal liver. Small lesions tend to be nodular and homogeneous while large ones are more irregular, heterogeneous and ill-defined. Following contrast administration, hypovascular lesions may have an enhancing rim on arterial phase images with or without incomplete centripetal fill-in on delayed phase (Figs 30A and B). In contrast, hypervascular tumors show moderate to intense peripheral ring enhancement immediately during the arterial phase that persists during the portal venous phase (Figs 31A and B). MRI usually depicts the lesions as hypointense on T1 and hyperintense on T2WI.[103,104]

REFERENCES

1. Crownover BK, Bepko JL. Appropriate and safe use of diagnostic imaging. Am Fam Physician. 2013;87(7):494-501.
2. Rubens DJ. Hepatobiliary imaging and its pitfalls. Radiol Clin North Am. 2004;42(2):257-78.
3. Rubens DJ. Ultrasound Imaging of the Biliary Tract. Ultrasound Clin. 2007;2(3):391-413. DOI:10.1016/j.cult. 2007.08.007.
4. Catalano OA, Sahani DV, Kalva SP, Cushing MS, Hahn PF, Brown JJ, et al. MR imaging of the gallbladder: a pictorial essay. Radiographics. 2008;28(1):135-55.

5. Mulholland D, McEntee G, McCormack O, Geoghegan TW. Double trouble - duplication of the gallbladder requiring repeat laparoscopic cholecystectomy. Ir Med J. 2012;105(10):346-7.
6. Causey MW, Miller S, Fernelius CA, Burgess JR, Brown TA, Newton C. Gallbladder duplication: evaluation, treatment, and classification. J Pediatr Surg. 2010;45(2):443-6. doi: 10.1016/j.jpedsurg.2009.12.015.
7. Desolneux G, Mucci S, Lebigot J, Arnaud JP, Hamy A. Duplication of the gallbladder. A case report. Gastroenterol Res Pract. 2009;2009:483473. doi: 10.1155/2009/483473.
8. Pitiakoudis M, Papanas N, Polychronidis A, Maltezos E, Prassopoulos P, Simopoulos C. Double gall-bladder--two pathologies: a case report. Acta Chir Belg. 2008;108(2):261-3.
9. O'Connor OJ, Maher MM. Imaging of cholecystitis. AJR Am J Roentgenol. 2011 Apr;196(4):W367-74. doi: 10.2214/AJR.10.4340.
10. Smith EA, Dillman JR, Elsayes KM, Menias CO, Bude RO. Cross-sectional imaging of acute and chronic gallbladder inflammatory disease. AJR Am J Roentgenol. 2009;192(1):188-96. doi: 10.2214/AJR.07.3803.
11. Shakespear JS, Shaaban AM, Rezvani M. CT findings of acute cholecystitis and its complications. AJR Am J Roentgenol. 2010;194(6):1523-9. doi: 10.2214/AJR.09.3640.
12. Tulchinsky M, Colletti PM, Allen TW. Hepatobiliary scintigraphy in acute cholecystitis. Semin Nucl Med. 2012;42(2):84-100. doi: 10.1053/j.semnuclmed.2011.10.005.
13. Pinto A, Reginelli A, Cagini L, Coppolino F, Stabile Ianora AA, Bracale R, et al. Accuracy of ultrasonography in the diagnosis of acute calculous cholecystitis: review of the literature. Crit Ultrasound J. 2013;5 Suppl 1:S11. doi: 10.1186/2036-7902-5-S1-S11.
14. Kiewiet JJ, Leeuwenburgh MM, Bipat S, Bossuyt PM, Stoker J, Boermeester MA. A systematic review and meta-analysis of diagnostic performance of imaging in acute cholecystitis. Radiology. 2012;264(3):708-20. doi: 10.1148/radiol.12111561. Epub 2012 Jul 12.
15. Corr P. Sonography of gangrenous cholecystitis. J Emerg Trauma Shock. 2012;5(1):82-3. doi: 10.4103/0974-2700.93112.
16. An C, Park S, Ko S, Park MS, Kim MJ, Kim KW. Usefulness of the tensile gallbladder fundus sign in the diagnosis of early acute cholecystitis. AJR Am J Roentgenol. 2013;201(2):340-6. doi: 10.2214/AJR.12.9919.
17. Rybicki FJ. The WES sign. Radiology. 2000; 214(3):881-2.
18. Wu CH, Chen CC, Wang CJ, Wong YC, Wang LJ, Huang CC, et al. Discrimination of gangrenous from uncomplicated acute cholecystitis: accuracy of CT findings. Abdom Imaging. 2011;36(2):174-8. doi: 10.1007/s00261-010-9612-x.
19. Charalel RA, Jeffrey RB, Shin LK. Complicated cholecystitis: the complementary roles of sonography and computed tomography. Ultrasound Q. 2011;27(3):161-70. doi: 10.1097/RUQ.0b013e31822a33e8.
20. Fuks D, Mouly C, Robert B, Hajji H, Yzet T, Regimbeau JM. Acute cholecystitis: preoperative CT can help the surgeon consider conversion from laparoscopic to open cholecystectomy. Radiology. 2012 Apr;263(1):128-38. doi: 10.1148/radiol.12110460.
21. Sunnapwar A, Raut AA, Nagar AM, Katre R. Emphysematous cholecystitis: Imaging findings in nine patients. Indian J Radiol Imaging. 2011;21(2):142-6. doi: 10.4103/0971-3026.82300.
22. Miyahara H, Shida D, Matsunaga H, Takahama Y, Miyamoto S. Emphysematous cholecystitis with massive gas in the abdominal cavity. World J Gastroenterol. 2013;19(4):604-6. doi: 10.3748/wjg.v19.i4.604.
23. Huang HS, Chuang CH, Yang PJ. Abnormal gas in the gallbladder: emphysematous cholecystitis. J Emerg Med. 2013;45(2):254-5. doi: 10.1016/j.jemermed.2011.05.087. Epub 2013 Jun 12.
24. Chang BJ, Kim SH, Park HY, Lim SW, Kim J, Lee KH, et al. Distinguishing xanthogranulomatous cholecystitis from the wall-thickening type of early-stage gallbladder cancer. Gut Liver. 2010;4(4):518-23. doi: 10.5009/gnl.2010.4.4.518.
25. Uchiyama K, Ozawa S, Ueno M, Hayami S, Hirono S, Ina S, et al. Xanthogranulomatous cholecystitis: the use of preoperative CT findings to differentiate it from gallbladder carcinoma. J Hepatobiliary Pancreat Surg. 2009;16(3):333-8. doi: 10.1007/s00534-009-0067-9.
26. Shuto R, Kiyosue H, Komatsu E, Matsumoto S, Kawano K, Kondo Y, et al. CT and MR imaging findings of xanthogranulomatous cholecystitis: correlation with pathologic findings. Eur Radiol. 2004;14(3):440-6.
27. Parra JA, Acinas O, Bueno J, Güezmes A, Fernández MA, Fariñas MC. Xanthogranulomatous cholecystitis: clinical, sonographic, and CT findings in 26 patients. AJR Am J Roentgenol. 2000;174(4):979-83.
28. Goshima S, Chang S, Wang JH, Kanematsu M, Bae KT, Federle MP. Xanthogranulomatous cholecystitis: diagnostic performance of CT to differentiate from gallbladder cancer. Eur J Radiol. 2010;74(3):e79-83. doi: 10.1016/j.ejrad.2009.04.017.
29. Enomoto T, Todoroki T, Koike N, Kawamoto T, Matsumoto H. Xanthogranulomatous cholecystitis mimicking stage IV gallbladder cancer. Hepatogastroenterology. 2003;50(53):1255-8.
30. Bortoff GA, Chen MY, Ott DJ, Wolfman NT, Routh WD. Gallbladder stones: imaging and intervention. Radiographics. 2000;20(3):751-66.
31. Ahvenjarvi L, Koivukangas V, Jartti A, Ohtonen P, Saarnio J, Syrjala H, et al. Diagnostic accuracy of computed tomography imaging of surgically treated acute acalculous cholecystitis in critically ill patients. J Trauma. 2011;70(1):183-8. doi: 10.1097/TA.0b013e3181cf7e6a.
32. Ching BH, Yeh BM, Westphalen AC, Joe BN, Qayyum A, Coakley FV. CT differentiation of adenomyomatosis and gallbladder cancer. AJR Am J Roentgenol. 2007;189(1):62-6.
33. Joo I, Lee JY, Kim JH, Kim SJ, Kim MA, Han JK, et al. Differentiation of adenomyomatosis of the gallbladder from early-stage, wall-thickening-type gallbladder cancer using high-resolution ultrasound. Eur Radiol. 2013;23(3):730-8. doi: 10.1007/s00330-012-2641-9.
34. Haradome H, Ichikawa T, Sou H, Yoshikawa T, Nakamura A, Araki T, et al. The pearl necklace sign: an imaging sign of adenomyomatosis of the gallbladder at MR cholangiopancreatography. Radiology. 2003;227(1):80-8.
35. Owen CC, Bilhartz LE. Gallbladder polyps, cholesterolosis, adenomyomatosis, and acute acalculous cholecystitis. Semin Gastrointest Dis. 2003;14(4):178-88.
36. Chao C, Hsiao HC, Wu CS, Wang KC. Computed tomographic finding in adenomyomatosis of the gallbladder. J Formos Med Assoc. 1992;91:467-9.
37. Lim KS, Peters CC, Kow A, Tan CH. The varying faces of gallbladder carcinoma: pictorial essay. Acta Radiol. 2012;53(5):494-500. doi: 10.1258/ar.2012.110684.
38. Kim SJ, Lee JM, Kim H, Yoon JH, Han JK, Choi BI. Role of diffusion-weighted magnetic resonance imaging in the diagnosis of gallbladder cancer. J Magn Reson Imaging. 2013;38(1):127-37. doi: 10.1002/jmri.23956.
39. Li B, Xu XX, Du Y, Yang HF, Li Y, Zhang Q, et al. Computed tomography for assessing resectability of gallbladder carcinoma: a systematic review and meta-analysis. Clin Imaging. 2013;37(2):327-33. doi: 10.1016/j.clinimag.2012.05.009.
40. Albazaz R, Patel CN, Chowdhury FU, Scarsbrook AF. Clinical impact of FDG PET-CT on management decisions for patients with primary biliary tumours. Insights Imaging. 2013;4(5):691-700. doi: 10.1007/s13244-013-0268-2.
41. Furlan A, Ferris JV, Hosseinzadeh K, Borhani AA. Gallbladder carcinoma update: multimodality imaging evaluation, staging,

and treatment options. AJR Am J Roentgenol. 2008;191(5):1440-7. doi: 10.2214/AJR.07.3599.
42. Levy AD, Murakata LA, Rohrmann CA. Gallbladder carcinoma: radiologic-pathologic correlation. Radiographics. 2001;21(2): 295-314.
43. Lee HK, Park SJ, Yi BH, Lee AL, Moon JH, Chang YW. Imaging features of adult choledochal cysts: a pictorial review. Korean J Radiol. 2009;10(1):71-80. doi: 10.3348/kjr.2009.10.1.71.
44. Sacher VY, Davis JS, Sleeman D, Casillas J. Role of magnetic resonance cholangiopancreatography in diagnosing choledochal cysts: Case series and review. World J Radiol. 2013;5(8):304-12. doi: 10.4329/wjr.v5.i8.304.
45. Mortelé KJ, Rocha TC, Streeter JL, Taylor AJ. Multimodality imaging of pancreatic and biliary congenital anomalies. Radiographics. 2006;26(3):715-31.
46. Brancatelli G, Federle MP, Vilgrain V, Vullierme MP, Marin D, Lagalla R. Fibropolycystic liver disease: CT and MR imaging findings. Radiographics. 2005;25(3):659-70.
47. Krausé D, Cercueil JP, Dranssart M, Cognet F, Piard F, Hillon P. MRI for evaluating congenital bile duct abnormalities. J Comput Assist Tomogr. 2002;26(4):541-52.
48. O'Connor OJ, O'Neill S, Maher MM. Imaging of biliary tract disease. AJR Am J Roentgenol. 2011;197(4):W551-8. doi: 10.2214/AJR.10.4341.
49. Watanabe Y, Nagayama M, Okumura A, Amoh Y, Katsube T, Suga T, et al. MR imaging of acute biliary disorders. Radiographics. 2007;27(2):477-95.
50. Yeh BM, Liu PS, Soto JA, Corvera CA, Hussain HK. MR imaging and CT of the biliary tract. Radiographics. 2009 Oct;29(6):1669-88.
51. Gupta RT, Brady CM, Lotz J, Boll DT, Merkle EM. Dynamic MR imaging of the biliary system using hepatocyte-specific contrast agents. AJR Am J Roentgenol. 2010 Aug;195(2):405-13.
52. Bilgin M, Shaikh F, Semelka RC, Bilgin SS, Balci NC, Erdogan A. Magnetic resonance imaging of gallbladder and biliary system. Top Magn Reson Imaging. 2009;20(1):31-42. doi: 10.1097/RMR.0b013e3181b48aa2.
53. Greenfield NP, Azziz AS, Jung AJ, Yeh BM, Aslam R, Coakley FV. Imaging late complications of cholecystectomy. Clin Imaging. 2012;36(6):763-7. doi: 10.1016/j.clinimag.2012.01.024.
54. Heffernan EJ, Geoghegan T, Munk PL, Ho SG, Harris AC. Recurrent pyogenic cholangitis: from imaging to intervention. AJR Am J Roentgenol. 2009;192(1):W28-35. doi: 10.2214/AJR.08.1104.
55. Wani NA, Robbani I, Kosar T. MRI of oriental cholangiohepatitis. Clin Radiol. 2011;66(2):158-63. doi: 10.1016/j.crad.2010.06.017.
56. Tsui WM, Chan YK, Wong CT, Lo YF, Yeung YW, Lee YW. Hepatolithiasis and the syndrome of recurrent pyogenic cholangitis: clinical, radiologic, and pathologic features. Semin Liver Dis. 2011;31(1):33-48. doi: 10.1055/s-0031-1272833.
57. Menias CO, Surabhi VR, Prasad SR, Wang HL, Narra VR, Chintapalli KN. Mimics of cholangiocarcinoma: spectrum of disease. Radiographics. 2008;28(4):1115-29.
58. Elsayes KM, Oliveira EP, Narra VR, Abou El Abbass HA, Ahmed MI, Tongdee R, et al. MR and MRCP in the evaluation of primary sclerosing cholangitis: current applications and imaging findings. J Comput Assist Tomogr. 2006;30(3):398-404.
59. Vitellas KM, Keogan MT, Freed KS, Enns RA, Spritzer CE, Baillie JM, et al. Radiologic manifestations of sclerosing cholangitis with emphasis on MR cholangiopancreatography. Radiographics. 2000;20(4):959-75
60. Joo I, Lee JM. Imaging bile duct tumors: pathologic concepts, classification, and early tumor detection. Abdom Imaging. 2013; 38(6):1334-50.
61. Lim JH. Cholangiocarcinoma: morphologic classification according to growth pattern and imaging findings. AJR Am J Roentgenol. 2003;181(3):819-27.
62. Chung YE, Kim MJ, Park YN, Choi JY, Pyo JY, Kim YC, et al. Varying appearances of cholangiocarcinoma: radiologic-pathologic correlation. Radiographics. 2009;29(3):683-700.
63. Sainani NI, Catalano OA, Holalkere NS, Zhu AX, Hahn PF, Sahani DV. Cholangiocarcinoma: current and novel imaging techniques. Radiographics. 2008;28(5):1263-87
64. Richards JR, McGahan JP, Pali MJ, Bohnen PA. Sonographic detection of blunt hepatic trauma: hemoperitoneum and parenchymal patterns of injury. J Trauma. 1999;47(6):1092-7.
65. Poletti PA, Mirvis SE, Shanmuganathan K, Killeen KL, Coldwell D. CT criteria for management of blunt liver trauma: correlation with angiographic and surgical findings. Radiology. Aug 2000; 216(2):418-27.
66. Yamamoto F, Pu Y, Igimi H, Kojima T, Witt JL, Yamamoto S. MR imaging of traumatic hepatic laceration: evaluation and course of healing after surgery. Abdom Imaging. 1993;18(3):253-7.
67. Mortelé KJ, Segatto E, Ros PR. The infected liver: radiologic-pathologic correlation. Radiographics. 2004;24(4):937-55.
68. Mathieu D, Vasile N, Fagniez PL, Segui S, Grably D, Lardé D. Dynamic CT features of hepatic abscesses. Radiology. 1985; 154(3):749-52.
69. Pedrosa I, Saíz A, Arrazola J, Ferreirós J, Pedrosa CS. Hydatid disease: radiologic and pathologic features and complications. Radiographics. 2000;20(3):795-817.
70. Lim JH. Parasitic diseases in the abdomen: imaging findings. Abdom Imaging.2008;33(2):130-2.
71. Mortele KJ, Ros PR. Cystic focal liver lesions in the adult: differential CT and MR imaging features. Radiographics. 2001;21(4):895-910.
72. Dickie B, Dasgupta R, Nair R, Alonso MH, Ryckman FC, Tiao GM, et al. Spectrum of hepatic hemangiomas: management and outcome. J Pediatr Surg. 2009;44(1):125-33.
73. Yamashita Y, Ogata I, Urata J, Takahashi M. Cavernous hemangioma of the liver: pathologic correlation with dynamic CT findings. Radiology. 1997;203(1):121-5.
74. Klotz T, Montoriol PF, Da Ines D, Petitcolin V, Joubert-Zakeyh J, Garcier JM. Hepatic haemangioma: Common and uncommon imaging features. Diagn Interv Imaging. 2013;94(9): 849-59.
75. Hussain SM, Terkivatan T, Zondervan PE, Lanjouw E, de Rave S, Ijzermans JN, et al. Focal nodular hyperplasia: findings at state-of-the-art MR imaging, US, CT, and pathologic analysis. Radiographics. 24(1):3-17.
76. Ferlicot S, Kobeiter H, Tran van nhieu J, Cherqui D, Dhumeaux D, Mathieu D, et al. MRI of atypical focal nodular hyperplasia of the liver: radiology-pathology correlation. AJR Am J Roentgenol. 2004;182(5): 1227-31.
77. Seale MK, Catalano OA, Saini S, Hahn PF, Sahani DV. Hepatobiliary-specific MR contrast agents: role in imaging the liver and biliary tree. Radiographics. 2009;29(6): 1725-48.
78. Mortele KJ, Praet M, Van vlierberghe H, de Hemptinne B, Zou K, Ros PR. Focal nodular hyperplasia of the liver: detection and characterization with plain and dynamic-enhanced MRI. Abdom Imaging. 2002;27(6):700-7.
79. Ichikawa T, Federle MP, Grazioli L, Nalesnik M. Hepatocellular adenoma: multiphasic CT and histopathologic findings in 25 patients. Radiology. 2000;214(3):861-8.
80. Paulson EK, McClellan JS, Washington K, Spritzer CE, Meyers WC, Baker ME. Hepatic adenoma: MR characteristics and correlation with pathologic findings. AJR Am J Roentgenol. 1994;163(1): 113-6.
81. Faria SC, Iyer RB, Rashid A, Whitman GJ. Hepatic adenoma. AJR Am J Roentgenol. 2004;182(6):1520.
82. Hussain SM, Van den bos IC, Dwarkasing RS, Kuiper JW, den Hollander J. Hepatocellular adenoma: findings at state-of-the-art magnetic resonance imaging, ultrasound, computed tomography and pathologic analysis. Eur Radiol. 2006;16(9): 1873-86.

83. Grazioli L, Federle MP, Brancatelli G, Ichikawa T, Olivetti L, Blachar A. Hepatic adenomas: imaging and pathologic findings. Radiographics. 2001;21(4):877-92.
84. Basaran C, Karcaaltincaba M, Akata D, Karabulut N, Akinci D, Ozmen M, et al. Fat-Containing Lesions of the Liver: Cross-Sectional Imaging Findings with Emphasis on MRI. AJR Am J Roentgenol. 2005;184(4):1103-10.
85. Roberts JL, Fishman EK, Hartman DS, Sanders R, Goodman Z, Siegelman SS.Lipomatous tumors of the liver: evaluation with CT and US. Radiology. 1986;158(3):613-7.
86. Woodward PJ, Sohaey R, Kennedy A, Koeller KK. From the archives of the AFIP: a comprehensive review of fetal tumors with pathologic correlation. Radiographics. 25(1): 215-42.
87. Roos JE, Pfiffner R, Stallmach T, Stuckmann G, Marincek B, Willi U. Infantile hemangioendothelioma. Radiographics. 2003;23(6): 1649-55.
88. Kassarjian A1, Zurakowski D, Dubois J, Paltiel HJ, Fishman SJ, Burrows PE. Infantile hepatic hemangiomas: clinical and imaging findings and their correlation with therapy. AJR Am J Roentgenol. 2004;182(3):785-95.
89. Stanley P, Hall TR, Woolley MM, Diament MJ, Gilsanz V, Miller JH et al. Mesenchymal hamartomas of the liver in childhood: sonographic and CT findings. AJR Am J Roentgenol. 1986;147(5):1035-9.
90. Ye BB, Hu B, Wang LJ, Liu HS, Zou Y, Zhou YB, et al. Mesenchymal hamartoma of liver: magnetic resonance imaging and histopathologic correlation. World J. Gastroenterol. 2005;11(37):5807-10.
91. Anil G, Fortier M, Low Y. Cystic hepatic mesenchymal hamartoma: the role of radiology in diagnosis and perioperative management. Br J Radiol. 2011;84(1001):e91-4.
92. Willatt JM, Hussain HK, Adusumilli S, Marrero JA. MR Imaging of hepatocellular carcinoma in the cirrhotic liver: challenges and controversies. Radiology. 2008;247(2):311-30.
93. Parente DB, Perez RM, Eiras-Araujo A, Oliveira Neto JA, Marchiori E, Constantino CP, et al. MR imaging of hypervascular lesions in the cirrhotic liver: a diagnostic dilemma. Radiographics. 2012;32(3):767-87.
94. Joo I, Choi BI. New paradigm for management of hepatocellular carcinoma by imaging. Liver Cancer. 2012;1(2):94-109.
95. Rajesh S, Mukund A, Arora A, Jain D, Sarin SK. Contrast-enhanced US-guided radiofrequency ablation of hepatocellular carcinoma. J Vasc Interv Radiol. 2013;24(8):1235-40.
96. Smith MT, Blatt ER, Jedlicka P Strain JD, Fenton LZ. Best cases from the AFIP: fibrolamellar hepatocellular carcinoma. Radiographics. 2008;28(2):609-13.
97. Mclarney JK, Rucker PT, Bender GN, Goodman ZD, Kashitani N, Ros PR. Fibrolamellar carcinoma of the liver: radiologic-pathologic correlation. Radiographics. 1999;19(2):453-71.
98. Dachman AH, Pakter RL, Ros PR, Fishman EK, Goodman ZD, Lichtenstein JE. Hepatoblastoma: radiologic-pathologic correlation in 50 cases. Radiology. 1987;164(1):15-9.
99. King SJ, Babyn PS, Greenberg ML, Phillips MJ, Filler RM. Value of CT in determining the resectability of hepatoblastoma before and after chemotherapy. AJR Am J Roentgenol. 1993;160(4):793-8.
100. Earnest F, Johnson CD. Case 96: Hepatic epithelioid hemangio-endothelioma. Radiology. 2006;240(1):295-8.
101. Lyburn ID, Torreggiani WC, Harris AC, Zwirewich CV, Buckley AR, Davis JE, et al. Hepatic epithelioid hemangioendothelioma: sonographic, CT, and MR imaging appearances. AJR Am J Roentgenol. 2003;180(5):1359-64.
102. Peterson MS, Baron RL, Rankin SC. Hepatic angiosarcoma: findings on multiphasic contrast-enhanced helical CT do not mimic hepatic hemangioma. AJR Am J Roentgenol. 2000;175(1):165-70.
103. Namasivayam S, Martin DR, Saini S. Imaging of liver metastases: MRI. Cancer Imaging. 2007;7:2-9.
104. Danet IM, Semelka RC, Leonardou P, Braga L, Vaidean G, Woosley JT, et al. Spectrum of MRI appearances of untreated metastases of the liver. AJR Am J Roentgenol. 2003;181(3):809-17.

CHAPTER 51

Endoscopic Retrograde Cholangiopancreatography in Biliary and Pancreatic Diseases

Zaheer, D Nageshwar Reddy

BACKGROUND

Endoscopic retrograde cholangiopancreatography (ERCP) was first introduced in the late 60's,[1] followed by introduction of endoscopic sphincterotomy in 1974.[2] Since then, ERCP has grown from a diagnostic procedure to a primarily therapeutic one for both pancreatic and biliary diseases. The main reason for this evolution is that diagnostic modalities have been developed that are less invasive than ERCP but possess similar sensitivity and specificity for diseases of the pancreaticobiliary system.[3] Imaging techniques like endoscopic ultrasonography (EUS) and magnetic resonance cholangiopancreatography (MRCP) have largely replaced diagnostic ERCP. These modalities, in combination with essential clinical information helps in selecting patients appropriate for ERCP.

ENDOSCOPIC RETROGRADE CHOLANGIOPANCREATOGRAPHY: ROLE IN DIAGNOSIS OF PANCREATICOBILIARY DISORDERS

Endoscopic retrograde cholangiopancreatography has been used widely in past to diagnose various pancreaticobiliary disorders like choledocholithiasis, sphincter of Oddi dysfunction (SOD), primary sclerosing cholangitis (PSC), chronic pancreatitis, etc. These disorders also included congenital malformations of biliary (choledochal cysts, biliary atresia, abnormal pancreaticobiliary union) as well as pancreatic ducts (pancreas divisum, annular pancreas). However as mentioned before, the role of diagnostic ERCP in these diseases has reduced dramatically since the availability of safer techniques (EUS/MRCP). As a general rule, ERCP is performed in most of these cases only if a therapeutic intervention is expected.

In the following section, we will discuss the present scope of diagnostic ERCP and some of the recent advances which supplement diagnostic ERCP.

INDICATIONS OF DIAGNOSTIC ENDOSCOPIC RETROGRADE CHOLANGIOPANCREATOGRAPHY

- Ampullary mass—duodenal or distal biliary/pancreatic sampling during ERCP can help in making a definitive diagnosis of ampullary mass (adenoma/adenocarcinoma/carcinoid tumor)
- Common bile duct (CBD) strictures—Sampling during ERCP can help distinguishing between inflammatory/benign strictures [chronic pancreatitis, choledocholithiasis, PSC, or autoimmune pancreatitis (AIP) related] from malignant ones (pancreatic adenocarcinoma or distal cholangiocarcinoma)
- Pancreatic strictures—chronic pancreatitis or pancreatic malignancy
- Sphincter of Oddi dysfunction (SOD)—Biliary or pancreatic

PANCREATICOBILIARY STRICTURES

Endoscopic retrograde cholangiopancreatography plays an important role in acquiring tissue sample in patients with obstructive jaundice especially when pancreaticobiliary malignancy is suspected. Main tissue sampling methods include—fine needle aspiration cytology, brush cytology and intraductal forceps biopsy.[4] Although ERCP is still the initial approach for cytopathological sampling of biliary strictures, due to paucicellular nature of cholangiocarcinoma and submucosal pattern of tumor growth, the sensitivity of brush cytology remains low (37–56%).[5-7] Novel adjunctive techniques to improve the sensitivity of brush cytology include—digital image analysis (DIA) and fluorescent in situ hybridization (FISH). In recent studies, routine cytology in combination with FISH had significantly higher sensitivity for pancreaticobiliary strictures than cytology alone.[8]

Other recent developments in evaluating indeterminate biliary strictures include the use of chloangioscopy,[9] endoscopic ultrasound—FNA,[10] intraductal ultrasound[11] and confocal laser endomicroscope.[12]

ENDOSCOPIC DIAGNOSIS OF BILIARY TRACT DISEASE: RECENT ADVANCES

Digital Image Analysis and Fluorescent in situ Hybridization

A number of strategies have emerged to improve the sensitivity of brush cytology, including—FISH, DIA, mutation analysis and immunohistochemistry testing. DIA technique uses special stains to evaluate for the presence of aneuploidy and quantifies nuclear DNA while chromosomal polysomy is detected by FISH using fluorescent probes. In a recent study the presence of polysomy of chromosome 3, 7, or 17 by FISH increased the sensitivity of brush cytology from 21% to 58%, and when the deletion of 9p21 was included, sensitivity became 89%.[13]

Cholangioscopy

Cholangioscopy (Figs 1A and B) is a noninvasive endoscopic method that allows direct visual diagnostic evaluation of the bile duct and directed biopsies as required. Since its initial description about 35 years ago, per oral cholangioscopy has undergone significant advancements. The original "mother-baby" endoscopes had a number of drawbacks including limited scope tip maneuvrability, requirement of two endoscopists and fragility. They are now being replaced by single operator cholangioscopy systems which overcome most of these limitations. It allows visually directed intrabiliary biopsies and has an emerging role in the assessment of indeterminate biliary strictures. In a recent multicenter study, and in our own experience cholangioscopy was safe and highly successful in diagnosing indeterminate biliary strictures.[14,9] Identification of the surface structure and vessels of the lesions by narrow band imaging (NBI) cholangioscopy may further improve results of cholangioscopy in biliary strictures.[15-17] Potential therapeutic applications of cholangioscopy include treatment of problematic bile duct stones through the use of laser or electrohydraulic lithotripsy,[14,18] ablation of cholangiocarcinoma with radiofrequency ablation (RFA) and in guiding the passage of a guide wire across difficult biliary strictures.[19,20]

Confocal Laser Endomicroscopy

Confocal laser endomicroscopy (CLE) is a technique which provides real time microscopic images of tissues. A CLE probe can be used during ERCP or through the working channel of a duodenoscope under fluoroscopic guidance. It enables real-time microscopic visualization of strictures during an on-going ERCP. A recent multicenter study, found probe based CLE to be highly accurate for indeterminate pancreaticobiliary strictures.[21]

THERAPEUTIC ENDOSCOPIC RETROGRADE CHOLANGIOPANCREATOGRAPHY IN PANCREATICOBILIARY DISORDERS

Endoscopic sphincterotomy forms the mainstay of most therapeutic ERCPs. It is a complex procedure that involves deep cannulation of the bile duct followed by severance of the SOD by electrocautery using endoscopic as well as fluoroscopic guidance. The primary indications for endoscopic sphincterotomy include extraction of CBD or pancreatic duct stones, enablement of endotherapy (tissue

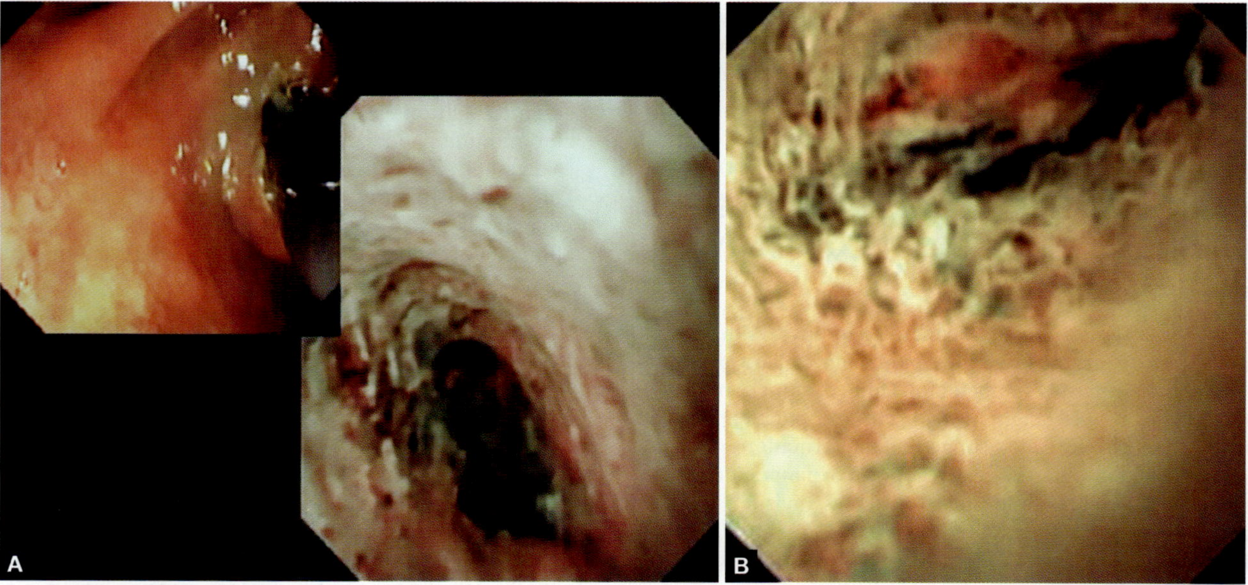

Figures 1A and B (A) Cholangioscopic views of cholangiocarcinoma showing a nodular lesion with thick circuitous vessels; (B) NBI cholangioscopy showing abnormal mucosal vessels

sampling, stent placement and stricture dilation) and treatment of papillary stenosis. Main complications include bleeding (4%), cholangitis (2%), pancreatitis (1%) and perforation in (1%).[22]

Indications of Therapeutic Endoscopic Retrograde Cholangiopancreatography in Biliary Disorders

- Bile duct stones
- Postoperative bile leaks
- Bile duct strictures—benign and malignant
- SOD dysfunction
- Biliary ascariasis (acute cholangitis, failure of pharmacological therapy, persistent infestation in biliary tree)

Choledocholithiasis

The sensitivity and specificity of ERCP for diagnosis of choledocholithiasis is approximately 95%, however it is seldom used for this purpose in the era of less invasive techniques like EUS and MRCP, which are equal in accuracy to ERCP.[3,23] In our center we use an EUS based approach to confirm CBD stones, before proceeding to ERCP as it can avoid unnecessary ERCP in about 40–50% of cases.[24]

Endoscopic treatment for CBD stones includes endoscopic sphincterotomy and stone extraction with soft Fogarty-type balloons or wire baskets. It has a successful outcome in more than 90% of cases.[25] Needle knife papillotomy may be used when standard cannulating techniques fail. It is especially useful for stones impacted in papilla and in patients with altered anatomy (e.g. bilroth II).

Endoscopic balloon dilatation is another treatment option for CBD stones. Since there is no need to cut the sphincter (in contrast to sphincterotomy), it may be a safer alternative in the presence of coagulopathy. However the relative risk of post ERCP pancreatitis is higher than sphincterotomy.

In patients with concomitant gallstones and CBD stones single stage procedure (laparoscopic cholecystectomy with CBD exploration) has been found equivalent in safety to two-stage procedure (ERCP and laparoscopic cholecystectomy).[26]

Endoscopic Therapy in Difficult Common Bile Duct Stones

In 10–15% cases, bile duct stones can be difficult to remove by ERCP.[27] Factors commonly linked with failure include multiple stones, diameter of more than 1 cm and altered biliary anatomy. Patients who fail conventional endoscopic measures can undergo extracorporeal shock wave lithotripsy (ESWL), endoscopic papillary large balloon dilatation with or without endoscopic sphincterotomy, electrohydraulic, mechanical or laser lithotripsy or surgical treatment.

Endoscopic papillary large-balloon dilation (EPLBD) dilates CBD after sphincterotomy using a 12–20 mm controlled radial expansion (CRE) balloon. Balloon size should not be larger than the CBD and of same diameter as the stone. Complications (10–15%), include pancreatitis, mild-to-moderate cholangitis and bleeding.[28] A recent multicenter study concluded that EPLBD is a reasonable alternative option when standard endoscopic techniques fail to remove stones.[29]

Table 1: Etiologies of benign biliary strictures

1. Post-surgery—Laparoscopic or open cholecystectomy*
   Biliary anastomosis (liver transplantation, biliary-enteric anastomosis)*
2. Nonsurgical—Chronic pancreatitis*
   - Autoimmune cholangiopathy
   - Primary sclerosing cholangitis*
   - Infections (tuberculosis, viral, parasitic)
   - Choledocholithiasis
3. Others—Ischemia (intrahepatic infusion of chemotherapy agents, vascular injuries, hepatic artery thrombosis)
   - Post-endoscopic biliary sphincterotomy
   - Trauma

*Relatively common causes.

Among other options, ESWL can be used for large impacted stones that cannot be safely extracted by endoscopy, stones proximal to biliary strictures, intrahepatic stones, stones with Mirizzi's syndrome compressing the common hepatic duct (Figs 2A and B) and cystic duct remnant stones. In a recent large Indian study, ESWL achieved a total CBD clearance in about 85% patients with difficult bile duct stones (stones not amenable to extraction by the standard technique of sphincterotomy followed by use of a Dormia basket or balloon)[30].

There is no role of routine biliary stenting in successful endotherapies for bile duct stones. However endoscopic biliary stenting may be required in very old patients, those with serious co-morbidities where other endoscopic or surgical procedures may confer unacceptably high risks, and if ductal clearance cannot be achieved during ERCP or in between procedures in patients who require more than one session for ductal clearance.[31]

Acute Cholangitis

Acute cholangitis occurs due to a combination of bacterial proliferation and bile duct obstruction. It manifests as jaundice, fever with chills and right upper quadrant pain (Charcot's triad). Urgent biliary decompression is mandatory in severe cholangitis.[32] Biliary stent or nasobiliary drain placement, with or without biliary sphincterotomy are the available options.

Bile Leaks

Bile leaks can occur following surgery (cholecystectomy, liver transplantation, and major liver surgery) or after hepatobiliary trauma. Endoscopic treatment includes biliary stenting, biliary sphincterotomy, or nasobiliary drainage and is usually effective. It reduces the pressure gradient between the biliary tree and the duodenum to promote preferential bile flow into the duodenum and to allow for leak sealing. Biliary sphincterotomy alone is effective for mild leaks, while biliary stenting may be required for 4–6 weeks for severe leaks or in case of stricture, contraindication to sphincterotomy, or inadequate contrast drainage after sphincterotomy.[33] In a prospective study from India, endoscopic therapy was found to be safe and effective in the management of bile leaks and fistulae after surgery with equal efficacy for sphincterotomy with endoprosthesis or endoprosthesis alone.[34]

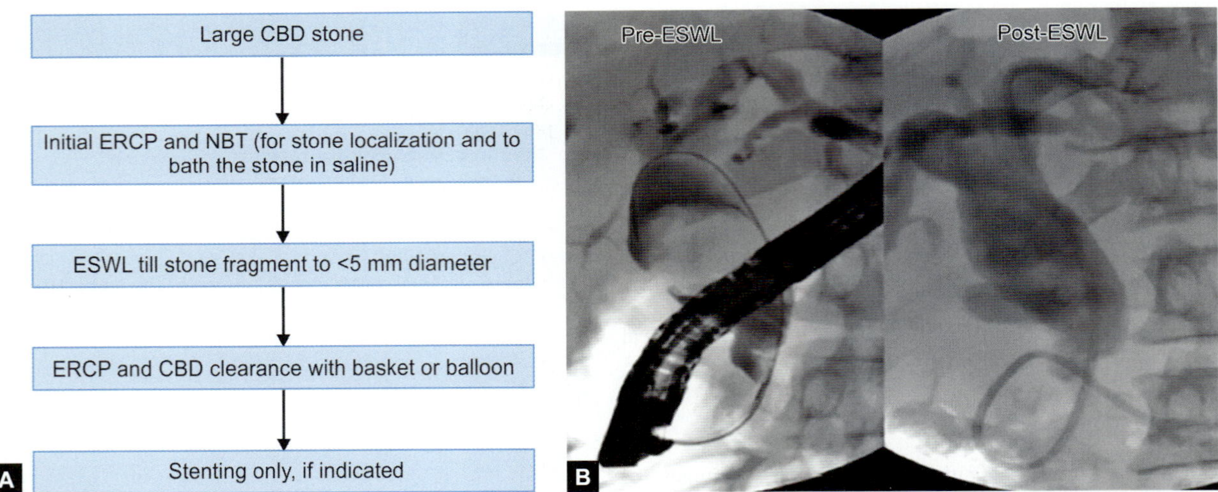

Figures 2A and B (A) Protocol for ESWL of large common bile duct calculi (B) Large common bile duct calculi with narrow distal common bile duct. Good fragmentation achieved with extracorporeal shockwave lithotripsy

Abbreviations: CBD, common bile duct; ERCP, endoscopic retrograde cholangiopancreatography; NBT, nasobiliary tube; ESWL, extracorporeal shockwave lithotripsy; ESWL, extracorporeal shockwave lithotripsy.

Endoscopic Retrograde Cholangiopancreatography in Benign Biliary Strictures

Benign biliary strictures (BBS) have different etiologies (Table 1), each with different natural course and responses to therapeutic ERCP.

The management of BBS (especially post cholecystectomy and chronic pancreatitis-related) has evolved from placement of a single plastic stent (PS) to serial placement of multiple plastic stents across the stricture. Better results are achieved with multiple, large bore stents placed side-by-side for long periods (at least 1 year). The number of stents are increased gradually and exchanged every 3–4 months.[35] More recently, the role of fully covered self-expanding metal stents (FCSEMS) is evolving with encouraging results.[36-39] In a prospective multicenter study, BBS resolved in about 90% of cases when FCSEMS was used as a primary or second line approach with a recurrence rate of about 7% on mean follow-up for 15 months.[38] Further randomized, prospective studies are needed to assess the efficacy, long-term safety and cost-effectiveness of FCSEMS before routine use can be recommended for BBS.

Prognosis and duration of treatment of BBS is determined by etiology of stricture, location and characteristics. Strictures which are distally located, at anastomotic site and with etiology other than chronic calcifying pancreatitis, respond better to endotherapy.

Although there is no randomized trial comparing the efficacy of surgical vs. endoscopic management for BBS, few nonrandomized studies show equal efficacy in both groups.[40-42] Endoscopic stenting of BBS is now first-line therapy at many centers (including ours) because of its less invasive approach, low morbidity and convenience. The choice and option of surgery depends upon patient preference, expertise at the treating center as well as the presence of co morbidities.

Chronic Pancreatitis-related Biliary Strictures

Due to fibrotic pancreatic tissue, biliary strictures secondary to chronic pancreatitis are more resilient to endoscopic treatment. However, sequential placement of multiple plastic stents (10 Fr) improves outcome in these patients with response rate of up to 90%.[42,43] The results with FCSEMS are encouraging as well, though the response may be less than in other BBS.[37,38]

Primary Sclerosing Cholangitis

Primary sclerosing cholangitis (PSC) is characterized by multifocal stricturing and ectasia of the biliary tree. Endoscopic therapy has the potential to relieve symptoms (jaundice, pruritus and abdominal pain) and prolong transplant free survival especially in those with one or more dominant stricture.[44,45] Endotherapy involves dilation of the dominant stricture with a balloon, with or without temporary placement of a biliary stent (1–2 weeks).[46] There are two important considerations to be made prior to endoscopic therapy in patients with PSC—aggressively ruling out malignancy (cholangiocarcinoma) in the presence of a dominant stricture and avoiding unnecessary endoscopic intervention in absence of symptoms or a dominant biliary stricture.

Autoimmune Cholangiopathy

Autoimmune cholangiopathy can occur as an isolated disease or more commonly as a part of AIP with intrahepatic, proximal extrahepatic or intrapancreatic biliary strictures. Oral steroids are the mainstay of treatment and endoscopic stent can be placed to temporarily relieve biliary obstruction while awaiting response to corticosteroids.[47]

Endoscopic Management of Malignant Biliary Obstruction

Endoscopic retrograde cholangiopancreatography is of both diagnostic and therapeutic value in malignant biliary strictures. Maligant biliary obstruction commonly occurs due to cholangiocarcinoma, carcinoma of gallbladder, or pancreatic head malignancies.

Endoscopic biliary drainage is an effective palliation therapy for most patients with malignant biliary obstruction. Biliary drainage in these patients improves quality of life, as well as ability to tolerate chemotherapy (palliative or neoadjuvant). The choice of stents (plastic versus. self-expandable metal stent), depends on the management plan and life expectancy of the patients. Plastic stents or nasobiliary drains (in hospitalized patients) can be used until diagnostic analyses and management decisions have been finalized. Metal stents provide longer patency rates and are more cost effective[48] and indicated if patients are not candidates for surgery or liver transplantation. Recent guidelines advocate metal stents if the life expectancy is more than 4 months.[49]

Though endoscopic biliary drainage is preferred in most patients, percutaneous approach may yield higher success rate and low level of procedure-related cholangitis in those with type 3 or 4 hilar cholangiocarcinomas.[50]

Biliary stenting is also indicated in potentially resectable malignant obstruction where neoadjuvant treatment is to be given. It is also required for patients with acute cholangitis, or in patients with severe pruritus.

Novel Endoscopic Techniques for Palliation of Cholangiocarcinoma

New endoscopic methods to improve quality of life and survival in patients with cholangiocarcinoma are evolving.

Photodynamic therapy (PDT) is a new technique which uses a photosensitizing agent, which gets preferentially deposited in malignant tumors which are actively proliferating. Subsequently red laser light is used for photoactivation. This leads to generation of reactive oxygen species and selective tumor-cell death. There was dramatic increase of median survival time in two randomized controlled trials when PDT was compared to patients receiving only endoprosthetic stenting (16.4 months versus 3.3 months).[51,52]

Radiofrequency ablation (RFA) within the bile duct causes local coagulative necrosis. In a recent pilot study of 21 patients with malignant obstructive jaundice RFA was found to be safe and effective.[53] However, further randomized controlled trials are required to establish cost effectiveness, improved survival and self-expandable metallic stent patency, cost-effectiveness, and survival advantages if any.

Sphincter of Oddi Dysfunction

Sphincter of Oddi (SOD) dysfunction is classified into two types: the biliary type and the pancreatic type which are sub-classified as type I, II, III on the basis of symptoms, laboratory tests and radiological imaging.[54] Endoscopic sphincterotomy is the main stay of treatment and provides greatest benefit for type I SOD followed by type II and least in type III.

ENDOSCOPIC RETROGRADE PANCREATOGRAPHY (ERP) IN PANCREATIC DISORDERS

Indications of Endoscopic Retrograde Pancreatography

- Acute pancreatitis: ERCP has no role in acute pancreatitis, with the exception of gallstone pancreatitis (selected patients).
- Chronic pancreatitis: Treatment of pancreatic ductal stones and strictures, duct disruption and communicating pseudocysts. Diagnostic ERP prior to endotherapy can be done in these settings.
- Idiopathic recurrent pancreatitis: Identification and management of various causes of idiopathic recurrent pancreatitis like pancreatic SOD, pancreas divisum, anomalous pancreatico-biliary union and intraductal papillary mucinous neoplasm (IPMN).[55]
- Prophylaxis: Prophylactic placement of pancreatic stents to reduce the incidence of post-ERCP pancreatitis in high risk settings.[56]
- As a useful adjunct in diagnosis of AIP. The four key features of AIP identified in a recent multicenter study are (i) long (>1/3 the length of the pancreatic duct) stricture; (ii) lack of upstream dilatation from the stricture (<5 mm); (iii) multiple strictures; and (iv) side branches arising from a strictured segment.[57]
- Pancreatic cancer: Management of malignant biliary stricture in pancreatic malignancies.

Endoscopic Retrograde Cholangio-pancreatography in Acute Pancreatitis

Endoscopic Retrograde Cholangiopancreatography in Acute Gallstone Pancreatitis

Several randomized studies have compared urgent ERCP with sphincterotomy versus conventional treatment in the management of gallstone pancreatitis.[58-60] Differences in the designs of these studies do not allow direct comparisons. A recent systemic review, concluded that ERCP/ES (endoscopic sphincterotomy) is indicated in patients with acute biliary pancreatitis (ABP) and coexisting cholangitis and/or persistent cholestasis. However consensus is lacking on the role of routine early ERCP/ES in patients with predicted severe ABP.[61]

Recurrent Acute Pancreatitis

There are multiple factors associated with recurrent episodes of acute pancreatitis of which some are amenable to endoscopic therapy including pancreas divisum, SOD dysfunction, choledochocele and ampullary neoplasms.

The prevalence of SOD in unexplained recurrent acute pancreatitis is about 40%, making it the most common cause of pancreatitis identified in this group.[62] Endoscopic sphincterotomy (biliary or dual) forms the mainstay of treatment. Long-term results of endoscopic sphincterotomy in SOD, show a recurrence rate of about 50%.[63] However controversy continues, whether SOD causes acute recurrent pancreatitis especially in the present era when genetic mutations are increasingly being recognized in recurrent pancreatitis. Moreover, only a few studies have evaluated the efficacy of endoscopic sphincterotomy in SOD.[63]

Intraductal papillary mucinous neoplasms can present as recurrent acute pancreatitis. It has a classic "fish eye" appearance on ERCP with dilated ampulla extruding mucin. Pancreaticoscopy in addition to ERCP can be utilized to directly visualize and sample suspicious lesions in IPMN.[55]

Pancreas Divisum

Failure of the dorsal and ventral pancreatic ducts to fuse during embryogenesis results in pancreas divisum. There is relative outflow obstruction due to major part of pancreatic exocrine secretions draining through the relatively small dorsal duct of Santorini and minor papilla. Endotherapy for pancreas divisum consists of minor papillotomy with or without subsequent placement of 3 or 5 French stents into the minor pancreatic duct. The outcome of endotherapy is good in selected patients with pancreas divisum. Acute recurrent pancreatitis type respond significantly better (81.2%) as compared to chronic pancreatitis-type (68.8%).[64]

Pancreatic Duct Leak

Pancreatic duct leak (PL) is a well-known complication of acute pancreatitis, chronic pancreatitis, trauma or pancreatic surgery. Patients who suffer from PL may manifest with pancreatic pseudocyst (PPC), pancreatic ascites, pleural effusion or internal and external fistulas. ERP not only confirms the site and size of PL but also bridge the site of disruption by placing a stent into upstream duct. However, in patients with complete duct disruption, endoscopic therapy can be challenging. In such cases only those patients will respond, who have a very short gap between these two disconnected ducts and the endoscopist is able to traverse the guidewire and put the plastic stent to bridge the ducts.[65,66]

Endoscopic Retrograde Cholangio-pancreatography in Chronic Pancreatitis

Role in Diagnosis

Endoscopic retrograde pancreaticography (ERP), has often been used in past to diagnose and treat chronic pancreatitis. The Cambridge system classifies chronic pancreatitis into equivocal, mild, moderate and marked categories according to the ERP changes in main pancreatic duct and number of side branches involved.[67] However the drawbacks of diagnostic ERP are threefold—it provides no information about parenchymal changes, it is insensitive for early stage chronic pancreatitis and there is substantial risk of post ERP pancreatitis (10–15%). For the same reason, and with the availability of less invasive techniques like MRCP and EUS, ERP is now seldom used for diagnostic purposes unless therapeutic intervention is being considered. The main utility of ERP in the setting of chronic pancreatitis is endotherapy for strictures or stones of the main pancreatic duct.

In the following section we will discuss the role of ERCP in managing chronic pancreatitis and associated complications. Chronic pancreatitis related biliary strictures have been discussed earlier in this chapter.

Endotherapy in Chronic Pancreatitis

Chronic pancreatitis (CP) is a disease characterized by progressive and irreversible damage to the pancreas and majority of the patients present with pain as the dominant symptom. Endotherapy is primarily directed towards the control of pain and management of complications associated with CP. Pain in CP is multifactorial, of which endotherapy is well-established for patients with ductal strictures, calculi, ductal disruption and biliary strictures. Although several randomized trials have shown the superiority of surgical treatment over endotherapy with regards to durability of pain relief in painful chronic pancreatitis,[68-70] these trials had methodological flaws with suboptimal endotherapy. Therefore, further studies are required before these results can be applied to clinical practice. Endotherapy offers many distinct advantages over surgery:

- High success rate in properly selected patients[71-73]
- Low morbidity[71,73]
- Procedure can be repeated without undue morbidity as associated with repeat surgery
- Age is not considered a barrier
- Failed endotherapy does not hinder subsequent surgery
- Endoscopic approach can also predict the response to surgical therapy.[30]

Endoscopic Management of Pancreatic Ductal Strictures and Stones

Strictures of main pancreatic duct (MPD) are frequently seen as consequence of CP and could be due to inflammation, fibrosis or rarely malignancy. Before proceeding to endotherapy for MPD strictures, malignancy should always be kept in mind and should be ruled out with appropriate imaging whenever clinically suspected[74] (e.g., elderly patients with significant weight loss, isolated PD stricture with no other stigmata of chronic pancreatitis). Endotherapy for MPD strictures usually consists of stricture dilation with a graduated dilating catheter or balloon dilators followed by placement of large bore stents (7–10 Fr). Stents may be exchanged routinely (3–6 months) or on-demand based on recurrence of symptoms.[75] Definitive removal of stents is done when there is adequate outflow of contrast across the stricture or a 5–6 Fr stent can be easily passed through the stricture. Strictures refractory to the standard endoscopic treatment can be addressed by placing multiple plastic stents or fully covered self-expanding metal stents.[76,77] However the long-term safety and efficacy of these modalities (especially self-expanding metal stents) remains to be seen in future studies.

Endotherapy for ductal calculi includes extraction with dormia basket or balloon trawl following endoscopic pancreatic sphincterotomy (for small stones <5 mm in size) and fragmentation with ESWL (>5 mm size) prior to extraction or spontaneous expulsion from the MPD. ESWL is now accepted as the standard of care in the management of large PD calculi not amenable to routine endotherapy. A recent systemic review of 11 series (1,149 patients) and a meta-analysis of 17 studies (491 patients) showed that ESWL is useful for clearing MPD stones and for decreasing pain.[78,79] Our own single center study of over 1,000 patients shows complete clearance in 76% patients and partial clearance in another 17% patients following ESWL and endotherapy for large calculi.[73]

Overall long-term benefits of endotherapy (ERCP and ESWL) can be expected in about two-thirds of patients. However surgery may be ultimately required in up to a quarter of these.[73,75] Factors predicting good response to endotherapy include—calcifications/strictures located in head of pancreas, short duration of symptoms, complete MPD clearance and cessation of tobacco and alcohol following endotherapy.[75]

- Ideal candidates for endotherapy
  - Single strictures in the head
  - Calculi in the head or body

- Poor candidates for endotherapy
  - Isolated strictures in tail or multiple strictures
  - Isolated calculi in tail
  - Extensive calculi in head, body and tail
  - Poor compliance for repeat procedures (when required)
- Drawbacks of endotherapy
  - Multiple sessions may be required (especially in case of strictures)
  - Up to one quarter of cases may finally require surgery
  - Small duct disease does not respond well to endotherapy
  - Pain in chronic pancreatitis is multifactorial including-neurogenic inflammation, visceral nerve sensitization, central nerve sensitization, oxidative stress of which intraductal hypertension is only a part managed with endotherapy

Pseudocyst

Pancreatic pseudocyst (PPC) in CP is the result of disruption of the MPD or its side branches. Disruption generally follows obstruction by stone or stricture. Drainage of symptomatic pseudocysts is indicated and can be done by transmural (transgastric or transduodenal) or transpapillary route. Transpapillary drainage is reserved for small cysts (<6 cm size) and those in communication with the MPD.[80] The advantages of this technique are that non bulging pseudocysts can be treated and there is minimum risk of enteric perforations and vascular injury. However, the risk of infection and stent induced pancreatic ductal damage are the major limitations.

SUMMARY

The horizon of ERCP has expanded in last few decades, despite its replacement by other modalities (MRCP/EUS) for diagnostic purposes in pancreaticobiliary disorders. Diagnostic ERCP is now limited to tissue acquisition from pancreaticobiliary ductal system. DIA and FISH are promising tools that improve the accuracy of brush cytology, and may soon find a place in the diagnostic algorithms of indeterminate biliary strictures. Cholangioscopy and pancreaticoscopy further add to the diagnostic and therapeutic capabilities of ERCP.

Major advancements in therapeutic ERCP include the evolving role of FCEMS in benign pancreaticobiliary strictures and the expanded use of EUS-guided biliary and pancreatic ductal cannulation in patients with difficult anatomy. Initial results with locoregional therapy of cholangiocarcinoma (RFA/PDT) are encouraging, though the time is not yet ripe to recommend these routinely.

Attempts to reduce the incidence of post ERCP pancreatitis (prophylactic PD stenting/rectal NSAIDs/wire guided cannulation) have met with great success and should reduce the morbidity associated with this procedure.

REFERENCES

1. McCune WS, Shorb PE, Moscovitz H. Endoscopic cannulation of the ampulla of Vater: a preliminary report. Ann Surg 1968;167(5):752-6.
2. Kawai K, Akasaka Y, Murakami K, Tada M, Koli Y. Endoscopic sphincterotomy of the ampulla of Vater. Gastrointest Endosc 1974;20(4):148-51.
3. Cohen S, Bacon BR, Berlin JA, Fleischer D, Hecht GA, Loehrer PJ, et al. National Institutes of Health State-of-the-Science Conference Statement: ERCP for diagnosis and therapy, January 14-16, 2002. Gastrointest Endosc. 2002;56(6):803-9.
4. Papachristou GI, Smyrk TC, Baron TH. Endoscopic Retrograde Cholangiopancreatography Tissue Sampling:When and How? Clin Gastroenterol Hepatol. 2007;5(7):783-90
5. Lee JG, Leung JW, Baillie J, Layfield LJ, Cotton PB. Benign, dysplastic, or malignant-making sense of endoscopic bile duct brush cytology:results in 149 consecutive patients. Am J Gastroenterol 1995;90(5):722-6.
6. Glasbrenner B, Ardan M, Boeck W, Preclik G, Möller P, Adler G. Prospective evaluation of brush cytology of biliary strictures during endoscopic retrograde cholangiopancreatography. Endoscopy 1999;31(9):712-7.
7. Fogel EL, deBellis M, McHenry L, Watkins JL, Chappo J, Cramer H, et al. Effectiveness of a new long cytology brush in the evaluation of malignant biliary obstruction:a prospective study. Gastrointest Endosc 2006;63(1):71-7
8. Smoczynski M, Jablonska A, Matyskiel A, Lakomy J, Dubowik M, Marek I, et al. Routine brush cytology and fluorescence in situ hybridization for assessment of pancreatobiliary strictures. Gastrointest Endosc. 2012 Jan;75(1):65-73
9. Ramchandani M, Reddy DN, Gupta R, Lakhtakia S, Tandan M, Darisetty S, et al. Role of single-operator peroral cholangioscopy in the diagnosis of indeterminate biliary lesions: a single-center, prospective study. Gastrointest Endosc. 2011;74(3):511-9.
10. Levy MJ, Heimbach JK, Gores GJ. Endoscopic ultrasound staging of cholangiocarcinoma. Curr Opin Gastroenterol. 2012;28(3):244-52.
11. Meister T1, Heinzow HS, Woestmeyer C, Lenz P, Menzel J, Kucharzik T, et al. Intraductal ultrasound substantiates diagnostics of bile duct strictures of uncertain etiology. World J Gastroenterol. 2013;19(6):874-81.
12. Meining A, Chen YK, Pleskow D, Stevens P, Shah RJ, Chuttani R, et al. Direct visualization of indeterminate pancreaticobiliary strictures with probe-based confocal laser endomicroscopy: a multicenter experience. Gastrointest Endosc. 2011;74(5):961-8.
13. Gonda TA, Glick MP, Sethi A, Poneros JM, Palmas W, Iqbal S, et al. Polysomy and p16 deletion by fluorescence in situ hybridization in the diagnosis of indeterminate biliary strictures. Gastrointest Endosc. 2012;75(1):74-9.
14. Chen YK, Parsi MA, Binmoeller KF, Hawes RH, Pleskow DK, Slivka A, et al. Single-operator cholangioscopy in patients requiring evaluation of bile duct disease or therapy of biliary stones. Gastrointest Endosc. 2011;74(4):805-14.
15. Itoi T, Neuhaus H, Chen YK. Diagnostic value of image-enhanced video cholangiopancreatoscopy. Gastrointest Endosc Clin N Am. 2009;19(4):557-66.
16. Gupta R1, Lakhtakia S, Santosh D, Anuradha S, Tandan M, Ramchandani M,et al. Narrow band imaging cholangioscopy in hilar cholangiocarcinoma. Indian J Gastroenterol. 2010;29(2): 78-80.
17. Itoi T, Sofuni A, Itokawa F, Tsuchiya T, Kurihara T, Ishii K, et al. Peroral cholangioscopic diagnosis of biliary-tract diseases by using narrow-band imaging (with videos). Gastrointest Endosc. 2007;66(4):730-6.
18. Seelhoff A, Schumacher B, Neuhaus H. Single operator peroral cholangioscopic guided therapy of bile duct stones. J Hepatobiliary Pancreat Sci. 2011;18(3):346-9.
19. Parsi MA, Guardino J, Vargo JJ. Peroral cholangioscopy-guided stricture therapy in living donor liver transplantation. Liver Transpl. 2009;15(2):263-5.
20. Parsi MA. Peroral cholangioscopy-assisted guidewire placement for removal of impacted stones in the cystic duct remnant. World J Gastrointest Surg. 2009;1(1):59-61.

21. Meining A, Chen YK, Pleskow D, Stevens P, Shah RJ, Chuttani R, et al. A Direct visualization of indeterminate pancreaticobiliary strictures with probe-based confocal laser endomicroscopy: a multicenter experience. Gastrointest Endosc. 2011;74(5):961-8.
22. Vaira D, D'Anna L, Ainley C, et al. Endoscopic sphincterotomy in 1000 consecutive patients. Lancet. 1989;2(8660):431-4.
23. Tse F, Liu L, Barkun AN, Armstrong D, Moayyedi P. EUS: a meta-analysis of test performance in suspected choledocholithiasis. Gastrointest Endosc. 2008;67(2):235-44.
24. Buscarini E, Tansini P, Vallisa D, Zambelli A, Buscarini L. EUS for suspected choledocholithiasis: do benefits outweigh costs? A prospective, controlled study. Gastrointest Endosc. 2003;57(4): 510–8.
25. Strömberg C, Nilsson M. Nationwide study of the treatment of common bile duct stones in Sweden between 1965 and 2009. Br J Surg. 2011;98(12):1766-74
26. Lu J, Cheng Y, Xiong XZ, Lin YX, Wu SJ, Cheng NS. Two-stage vs single-stage management for concomitant gallstones and common bile duct stones. World J Gastroenterol. 2012;18(24):3156–66.
27. ASGE Standards of Practice Committee, Maple JT, Ikenberry SO, Anderson MA, Appalaneni V, Decker GA, et al. The role of endoscopy in the management of choledocholithiasis. Gastrointest Endosc. 2011;74(4):731-44.
28. Ersoz G, Tekesin O, Ozutemiz AO, Gunsar F. et al. Biliary sphincterotomy plus dilation with a large balloon for bile duct stones that are difficult to extract. Gastrointest Endosc. 2003;57(2):156-9.
29. Attasaranya S, Cheon YK, Vittal H, Howell DA, Wakelin DE, Cunningham JT, et al. Large-diameter biliary orifice balloon dilation to aid in endoscopic bile duct stone removal: a multicenter series. Gastrointest Endosc. 2008;67(7):1046-52.
30. T andan M1, Reddy DN, Santosh D, Reddy V, Koppuju V, Lakhtakia S, et al. Extracorporeal shock wave lithotripsy of large difficult common bile duct stones: efficacy and analysis of factors that favor stone fragmentation. J Gastroenterol Hepatol. 2009; 24(8):1370-4.
31. Lee DK, Jahng JH. Alternative methods in the endoscopic management of difficult common bile duct stones. Dig Endosc 2010; 22 Suppl 1: S79-S84
32. Takada T, Strasberg SM, Solomkin JS, Pitt HA, Gomi H, Yoshida M, et al.TG13: Updated Tokyo Guidelines for the management of acute cholangitis and cholecystitis. J Hepatobiliary Pancreat Sci. 2013;20(1):1-7.
33. Sandha GS, Bourke MJ, Haber GB, Kortan PP. Endoscopic therapy for bile leak based on a new classification: results in 207 patients. Gastrointest Endosc. 2004;60(4):567-74
34. Agarwal N, Sharma BC, Garg S, Kumar R, Sarin SK. Endoscopic management of postoperative bile leaks. Hepatobiliary Pancreat Dis Int. 2006;5(2):273-7.
35. Costamagna G, Pandolfi M, Mutignani M, Spada C, Perri V. Long-term results of endoscopic management of post-operative bile duct strictures with increasing number of stents. Gastrointest Endosc. 2001;54(2):162-8.
36. Park do H, Lee SS, Lee TH, Ryu CH, Kim HJ, Seo DW, et al. Anchoring flap versus flare end, fully covered self-expandable metal stents to prevent migration in patients with benign biliary strictures: a multicenter, prospective, comparative pilot study. Gastrointest Endosc. 2011;73(1):64-70
37. Tarantino I, Mangiavillano B, Di Mitri R, Barresi L, Mocciaro F, Granata A, et al. Fully covered self-expandable metallic stents in benign biliary strictures: a multicenter study on efficacy and safety. Endoscopy. 2012;44(10):923-7.
38. Poley JW, Cahen DL, Metselaar HJ, van Buuren HR, Kazemier G, van Eijck CH, et al. A prospective group sequential study evaluating a new type of fully covered self-expandable metal stent for the treatment of benign biliary strictures. Gastrointest Endosc. 2012; 75(4):783-9.
39. Kao D1, Zepeda-Gomez S, Tandon P, Bain VG. Managing the post-liver transplantation anastomotic biliary stricture: multiple plastic versus metal stents: a systematic review. Gastrointest Endosc. 2013;77(5):679-91.
40. Davids PH, Tanka AK, Rauws EA, van Gulik TM, van Leeuwen DJ, de Wit LT, et al. Benign biliary strictures. Surgery or endoscopy? Ann Surg. 1993;217(3):237-43.
41. De Palma GD, Persico G, Sottile R, Puzziello A, Iuliano G, Salvati V, et al. Surgery or endoscopy for treatment of postcholecystectomy bile duct strictures? Am J Surg. 2003;185(6):532-5.
42. Catalano MF, Linder JD, George S, Alcocer E, Geenen JE. Treatment of symptomatic distal common bile duct stenosis secondary to chronic pancreatitis: comparison of single vs. multiple simultaneous stents. Gastrointest Endosc. 2004;60(6):945-52.
43. Craig PI. Role of endoscopic stenting for biliary strictures in chronic pancreatitis. Dig Endosc. 2012;24 Suppl 1:38-42.
44. Gluck M, Cantone NR, Brandabur JJ, Patterson DJ, Bredfeldt JE, Kozarek RA. A twenty-year experience with endoscopic therapy for symptomatic primary sclerosing cholangitis. J Clin Gastroenterol. 2008;42(9):1032-9.
45. Gotthardt DN1, Rudolph G, Klöters-Plachky P, Kulaksiz H, Stiehl A. Endoscopic dilation of dominant stenoses in primary sclerosing cholangitis: outcome after long-term treatment. Gastrointest Endosc. 2010;71(3):527-34.
46. Aljiffry M, Renfrew PD, Walsh MJ, Laryea M, Molinari M. Analytical review of diagnosis and treatment strategies for dominant bile duct strictures in patients with primary sclerosing cholangitis. HPB (Oxford). 2011;13(2):79-90.
47. Ghazale A, Chari ST, Zhang L, Smyrk TC, Takahashi N, Levy MJ, et al. Immunoglobulin G4-associated cholangitis: clinical profile and response to therapy. Gastroenterology. 2008;134(3): 706-15.
48. Moss AC, Morris E, Leyden J, MacMathuna P. Do the benefits of metal stents justify the costs? A systematic review and meta-analysis of trials comparing endoscopic stents for malignant biliary obstruction. Eur J Gastroenterol Hepatol. 2007;19(12):1119-24
49. Khan SA, Davidson BR, Goldin RD, Heaton N, Karani J, Pereira SP, et al. Guidelines for the diagnosis and treatment of cholangiocarcinoma: an update. Gut. 2012;61(12):1657-69.
50. Paik WH, Park YS, Hwang JH, Lee SH, Yoon CJ, Kang SG, et al. Palliative treatment with self-expandable metallic stents in patients with advanced type III or IV hilar cholangiocarcinoma: a percutaneous versus endoscopic approach. Gastrointest Endosc. 2009;69(1):55-62.
51. Ortner ME, Caca K, Berr F, Liebetruth J, Mansmann U, Huster D, et al. Successful photodynamic therapy for nonresectable cholangiocarcinoma: a randomized prospective study. Gastroenterology. 2003;125(5):1355–63.
52. Zoepf T, Jakobs R, Arnold JC, Apel D, Riemann JF. Palliation of non resectable bile duct cancer: improved survival after photodynamic therapy. Am J Gastroenterol. 2005;100(11):2426-30.
53. Steel AW, Postgate AJ, Khorsandi S, Nicholls J, Jiao L, Vlavianos P, et al. Endoscopically applied radiofrequency ablation appears to be safe in the treatment of malignant biliary obstruction. Gastrointest Endosc. 2011;73(1):149-53.
54. Hogan WJ, Geenen JE. Biliary dyskinesia. Endoscopy 1988;20 Suppl 1:179-83
55. Yasuda K, Sakata M, Ueda M, Uno K, Nakajima M. The use of pancreatoscopy in the diagnosis of intraductal papillary mucinous tumor lesions of the pancreas. Clin Gastroenterol Hepatol. 2005;3 (7 Suppl 1):S53-7.
56. Choudhary A, Bechtold ML, Arif M, Szary NM, Puli SR, Othman MO, et al. Pancreatic stents for prophylaxis against

post-ERCP pancreatitis: a meta-analysis and systematic review. Gastrointest Endosc. 2011;73:275-82.

57. Sugumar A, Levy MJ, Kamisawa T, Webster GJ, Kim MH, Enders F, et al. Endoscopic retrograde pancreatography criteria to diagnose autoimmune pancreatitis: an international multicentre study. Gut. 2011;60(5):666-70.
58. Neoptolemos JP, Carr-Locke DL, London NJ, Bailey IA, James D, Fossard DP. Controlled trial of urgent endoscopic retrograde cholangiopancreatography and endoscopic sphincterotomy versus conservative treatment for acute pancreatitis due to gallstones. Lancet 1988;2(8618):979-83
59. Fan ST, Lai ECS, Mok FP, Lo CM, Zheng SS, Wong J. Early treatment of acute biliary pancreatitis by endoscopic papillotomy. N Engl J Med. 1993;328(4):228.
60. Fölsch UR, Nitsche R, Ludtke R, Hilgers RA, Creutzfeldt W. Early ERCP and papillotomy compared with conservative treatment for acute biliary pancreatitis. N Engl J Med. 1997;336(4):237-42.
61. van Geenen EJ, van Santvoort HC, Besselink MG, van der Peet DL, van Erpecum KJ, Fockens P, et al. Lack of Consensus on the Role of Endoscopic Retrograde Cholangiography in Acute Biliary Pancreatitis in Published Meta-Analyses and Guidelines: A Systematic Review. Pancreas. 2013;42(5):774-80.
62. Fischer M, Hassan A, Sipe BW, Fogel EL, McHenry L, Sherman S, et al. ERCP and manometry findings in 1,241 idiopathic pancreatitis patients. Pancreatology. 2010;10(4):444-52.
63. Wehrmann T. Long-term results (>10 years) of endoscopic therapy for sphincter of Oddi dysfunction in patients with acute recurrent pancreatitis. Endoscopy. 2011;43(3):202-7.
64. Liao Z, Gao R, Wang W, Ye Z, Lai XW, Wang XT, et al. A systematic review on endoscopic detection rate, endotherapy, and surgery for pancreas divisum. Endoscopy. 2009 May;41(5):439-44.
65. Varadarajulu S, Noone TC, Tutuian R, Hawes RH, Cotton PB. Predictors of outcome in pancreatic duct disruption managed by endoscopic transpapillary stent placement. Gastrointest Endosc. 2005;61(4):568-75
66. Telford JJ, Farrell JJ, Saltzman JR, Shields SJ, Banks PA, Lichtenstein DR, et al. Pancreatic stent placement for duct disruption. Gastrointest Endosc. 2002;56(1):18-24.
67. Axon AT, Classen M, Cotton PB, Cremer M, Freeny PC, Lees WR. Pancreatography in chronic pancreatitis: international definitions. Gut. 1984;25(10):1107-12.
68. Díte P, Ruzicka M, Zboril V, Novotný I. A prospective, randomized trial comparing endoscopic and surgical therapy for chronic pancreatitis. Endoscopy. 2003;35(7):553-8.
69. Cahen DL, Gouma DJ, Nio Y, Rauws EA, Boermeester MA, Busch OR, et al. Endoscopic versus surgical drainage of the pancreatic duct in chronic pancreatitis. N Engl J Med. 2007;356(7):676-84.
70. Cahen DL, Gouma DJ, Laramée P, Nio Y, Rauws EA, Boermeester MA, et al. Long-term outcomes of endoscopic vs surgical drainage of the pancreatic duct in patients with chronic pancreatitis. Gastroenterology. 2011;141(5):1690-5.
71. Rösch T, Daniel S, Scholz M, Huibregtse K, Smits M, Schneider T, et al. Endoscopic treatment of chronic pancreatitis: a multicenter study of 1000 patients with long-term follow-up. Endoscopy. 2002;34(10):765-71.
72. Gabbrielli A, Pandolfi M, Mutignani M, Spada C, Perri V, Petruzziello L, et al. Efficacy of main pancreatic-duct endoscopic drainage in patients with chronic pancreatitis, continuous pain, and dilated duct. Gastrointest Endosc. 2005;61(4):576-81.
73. Tandan M, Reddy DN, Santosh D, Vinod K, Ramchandani M, Rajesh G, et al. Extracorporeal shock wave lithotripsy and endotherapy for pancreatic calculi-a large single center experience. Indian J Gastroenterol. 2010;29(4):143-8.
74. Kalady MF, Peterson B, Baillie J, Onaitis MW, Abdul-Wahab OI, Howden JK, et al. Pancreatic duct strictures: identifying risk of malignancy. Ann Surg Oncol. 2004;11(6):581-8.
75. Delhaye M, Matos C, Deviere J. Endoscopic technique for the management of pancreatitis and its complications. Best Pract Res Clin Gastroenterol. 2004;18(1):155-81.
76. Costamagna G, Bulajic M, Tringali A, Pandolfi M, Gabbrielli A, Spada C, et al. Multiple stenting of refractory pancreatic duct strictures in severe chronic pancreatitis: long-term results. Endoscopy. 2006;38(3):254-9.
77. Moon SH, Kim MH, Park do H, Song TJ, Eum J, Lee SS, et al. Modified fully covered self-expandable metal stents with antimigration features for benign pancreatic-duct strictures in advanced chronic pancreatitis, with a focus on the safety profile and reducing migration. Gastrointest Endosc. 2010;72(1):86-91.
78. Nguyen-Tang T, Dumonceau J-M. Endoscopic treatment in chronic pancreatitis, timing, duration and type of intervention. Best Pract Res Clin Gastroenterol. 2010;24(3):281-98.
79. Guda NM, Partington S, Freeman ML. Extracorporeal shock wave lithotripsy in the management of chronic calcific pancreatitis: a meta-analysis. JOP. 2005;6(1):6-12.
80. Catalano MF, Geenen JE, Schmalz MJ, Johnson GK, Dean RS, Hogan WJ, et al. Treatment of pancreatic pseudocysts with ductal communication by transpapillary pancreatic duct endoprosthesis. Gastrointest Endosc. 1995;42(3):214-8.

CHAPTER 52

Gallstone Disease

Avinash Supe, Ramkrishna Prabhu

INTRODUCTION

"It is unfortunate that so few appreciate from what small causes diseases come", Charles Mayo 1902. Though this was the dictum 100 years ago, now there is enough evidence that most incidentally discovered, clinically silent gallstones rarely have clinical significance. Gallstones are diagnosed today more commonly, mainly as a result of the widespread use of ultrasonography (USG) for the evaluation of patients for unrelated or vague abdominal complaints. In India, out of 800 million adult populations, approximately 15% (120 millions) have gallstones. Gallbladder calculus disease is a common surgical problem with a high prevalence in our North Indian population (4.3%). This prevalence of gallstones is less than that in developed world. Gallstone disease prevalence varies in our country, the highest being in Punjabis (North Indians) and the lowest in South Indians. Besides regional influence, dietary differences are also likely to be responsible for this regional variation. Gallstones in North India were predominantly cholesterol and those from South India were predominantly pigment gallstones.[1] Incidence among Indian population was, Punjabi (7.4%), Gujaratis (7.4%), Bengalis (4.4%) and South Indians (1.8%). The reason for this striking difference in the type of gallstones in the two regions is not clear, but again may be due to dietary differences or genetic predisposition. There was no significant difference between the ages of gallstone patients from South India and North India.[2]

PATHOGENESIS OF GALLSTONES

Normal Bile

It contains in addition to bile salts and bile pigments many other components like cholesterol and phospholipids in a dissolved state. Any disequilibrium in the soluble components cause precipitation of these and are responsible for stone formation. In India, most commonly found stones are black pigment stones, cholesterol stones and brown pigment stones:

Black Pigment Stones

These stones are commonly found in patients with hemolytic states like red blood cell (RBC) wall abnormality, e.g. hereditary spherocytosis, hemoglobinopathies and thalassemia. These stones mainly comprise of calcium salts of bilirubinate, phosphate and carbonate. These are also found in subclinical hemolytic states like liver cirrhosis and inflammatory bowel disease, e.g. Crohn's disease.

Brown Pigment Stones

These stones are mainly composed of calcium bilirubinate, cholesterol and proteins. They are softer and are associated with chronic infection and contain bacterial products. Bacteria in bile duct produce various chemical and organic products which form nidus for stone formation. Parasites such as round worm or its parts (eggs) may initiate such stone formation.

Cholesterol Stones

Mechanisms of cholesterol lithogenesis include biliary cholesterol hypersecretion, supersaturation of bile with cholesterol, nucleation of crystals and formation of gallstones. Disequilibrium in the soluble cholesterol leads to supersaturation of bile with cholesterol causing nucleation of cholesterol crystals.

CLINICAL PRESENTATIONS AND DECISION-MAKING IN GALLSTONE DISEASE

A longitudinal follow-up study of asymptomatic gallstones showed that over 20-year period only 18% of patients developed biliary pain and mean yearly probability of development of 2% during first, 5 years, 1% during second, 5 years, 0.5% during third, 5 years.[3] Most patients live and die with their gallstones having never caused pain or other medical problems.

Asymptomatic Gallstones

Selective Cholecystectomy

There is lot of literature on performing laparoscopic cholecystectomy (LC) in select subgroup of patients with asymptomatic cholelithiasis, who are at greater risk for the development of symptoms or complications.[1,4]

The definite indications[5] include:

- Suspicion or risk of malignancy
- Gallstones associated with gallbladder polyps greater than 1 cm in diameter
- Calcified or porcelain gallbladder
- Some ethnic groups or subjects living in areas with high prevalence of gallbladder cancer associated with gallstones (Uttar Pradesh and Bihar in North India, American Indians, Mexican Americans, Colombia, Chile, Bolivia)
- Presence of large (>3 cm) gallstones
- Asymptomatic cholelithiasis associated with choledocholithiasis
- Transplant patients (before or during transplantation)
- Chronic hemolytic conditions (sickle-cell anemia)
- As a part of bariatric surgery.

The relative indications include:

- Increased risk of conversion from asymptomatic to symptomatic disease
- Life expectancy more than 20 years
- Calculi more than 2 cm in diameter
- Calculi less than 3 mm and patent cystic duct
- Nonfunctioning gallbladder
- Diabetes mellitus
- Vague dyspeptic symptoms in the presence of gallstones
- Aortic aneurysm.

The questionable indications are:

- Patients living in an area remote from medical facilities and
- Incidental (concomitant) cholecystectomy during another abdominal operation.

Three indications are discussed in detail as relevant to India:

1. *Gallbladder carcinoma:* Though gallbladder cancer is uncommon in many parts of developed world it is commonly seen local population of North and South America (especially Chile), and in the Maori region of New Zealand. In India, it is higher in East Uttar Pradesh and Bihar. The incidence of gallstones is high in these regions and could be due to presence of cholesterol lithogenic genes. The risk of gallbladder cancer increases by four times in patients with gallstones. Approximately, four out of five patients developing gallbladder carcinoma have larger gallstones or gallbladder polyps larger than 10 mm in diameter. Though prophylactic cholecystectomy is not advised for all asymptomatic patients, it is strongly recommended for select subgroup of patients where gallbladder cancer is prevalent Kapoor et al. have argued against "routine" prophylactic cholecystectomy while conceding that considering higher incidence of gallbladder carcinoma in endemic areas of North India, prophylactic cholecystectomy may be considered for a young woman who has a large gallstone or gallbladder packed with stones.[6] Prophylactic cholecystectomy is indicated in patients with gallbladder polyps larger than 10 mm in diameter and in patients with large gallstones (>3 cm).
2. *Chronic hemolytic syndromes:* Sickle cell disease (SCD) is common in parts of India. Patients suffering from chronic hemolytic syndromes like SCD are at 58% increased risk for gallstone development at a young age due to repeated hemolytic crises. Two-thirds of these patients are likely to develop symptoms.[7] The onset of gallstones at a young age in SCD raises the lifetime risk of biliary complications. Therefore, cholecystectomy for asymptomatic cholelithiasis is advisable in SCD patients.
3. *Diabetes:* Diabetic patients with asymptomatic gallstones were recommended for cholecystectomy.[8] This was based on concern that they will be at risk of developing complications (such as infected bile, gangrenous changes and perforation of the gallbladder), more than normal populations. Pain is masked in diabetics due to autonomic neuropathy and hence, there can be delay in diagnosis. Therefore, diabetics were considered a high-risk group and prophylactic cholecystectomy was recommended. However, other researchers have shown benign course of gallstones in diabetics with low risk of major complications.[9] The cumulative percentage symptoms and complications of gallstones were found to be similar among diabetic patients. Therefore, there is no clear benefit of prophylactic cholecystectomy in diabetic patients with asymptomatic gallstones. Surgery neither appears to increase the duration nor improve the quality of life. It may, in fact, reduce it.[10] Early elective cholecystectomy is advocated once symptoms develop.

Concomitant Cholecystectomy

Concomitant cholecystectomy for asymptomatic cholelithiasis (diagnosed either preoperatively or intraoperatively) during a planned abdominal operation is a common clinical scenario. Several studies showed a high (up to 70%) incidence of symptoms and/or complications from the biliary system (such as biliary colic, acute cholecystitis, jaundice) in patients with asymptomatic cholelithiasis following laparotomy for unrelated conditions (bariatric surgery, transplant and other interventions). Cholecystectomy was required in a large percentage (up to 40%) of these patients within 1 year of the initial operation.[11] The aim of incidental cholecystectomy in such cases is to prevent postoperative cholecystitis or the later development of symptoms.

Addition of cholecystectomy does not portend added risk to the patient. Cholecystectomy related complications can be avoided by using proper surgical technique, including adequate exposure, by performing an uncomplicated primary operation, and by appropriate patient selection taking into account comorbidities and general health. Obviously, this strategy is not recommended for high-risk patients, with significant comorbidity, where a minimal operating and anesthesia time is advisable for an uneventful recovery. The performance of concomitant cholecystectomy may be more difficult in case of a pelvic (gynecologic) procedure, because it may require an additional or extended incision. However, this poses no problem if the pelvic procedure is conducted laparoscopically.

Acute Cholecystitis

Acute cholecystitis is associated with right upper quadrant pain, fever and leukocytosis associated with gallbladder inflammation, usually related to gallstone disease. The initial Tokyo Guidelines of 2007 were revised in 2013 (TG13) and is used to diagnose acute cholecystitis.

Criteria for Acute Cholecystitis

A. local signs of inflammation, etc.:
   (1) Murphy's sign, (2) RUQ mass or pain or tenderness
B. Systemic signs of inflammation, etc.:
   (1) Fever, TG13 diagnostic (2) Elevated C-reactive protein (CRP), (3) Elevated white blood cell (WBC) count
C. Imaging findings:
   (1) Imaging findings characteristic of acute cholecystitis
   (2) Suspected diagnosis: One item in A + one item in B
   (3) Definite diagnosis: One item in A + one item in B + C
   (Acute hepatitis, other acute abdominal diseases, and chronic cholecystitis should be excluded: RUQ - Right upper abdominal quadrant, CRP - C-reactive protein, WBC - white blood cell).[12]

Severity Assessment Criteria for Acute Cholecystitis

They were classified as:

- "Severe" (Grade III) acute cholecystitis, if accompanied by dysfunctions in any one of the following organs/systems:
  - Cardiovascular dysfunction: Hypotension requiring treatment with dopamine more than or equal to 5 µg/kg/min or any dose of dobutamine
  - Neurological dysfunction: Decreased level of consciousness
  - Respiratory dysfunction: Arterial oxygen partial pressure/fractional inspired oxygen (PaO_2/FiO_2) ratio less than 300
  - Renal dysfunction: Oliguria, creatinine more than 2.0 mg/dL
  - Hepatic dysfunction: Prothrombin time-International normalized ratio (PT-INR) more than 1.5
  - Hematological dysfunction: Platelet count less than 100,000/mm^3
- "Moderate" (Grade II) acute cholecystitis is accompanied by any one of the following conditions:
  - Elevated WBC count (>18,000/mm^3)
  - Palpable tender mass in the right upper abdominal quadrant
  - Duration of complaints more than 72 hours
  - Marked local inflammation (gangrenous cholecystitis, pericholecystic abscess, hepatic abscess, biliary peritonitis, emphysematous cholecystitis)
- "Mild" (Grade I) acute cholecystitis does not meet the criteria of "Severe (Grade III)" or "Moderate (Grade II)" acute cholecystitis. Grade I can also be defined as acute cholecystitis in a healthy patient with no organ dysfunction and only mild inflammatory changes in the gallbladder, making cholecystectomy a safe and low-risk operative procedure.

The distribution of severity grading varies as follows: 39.3–68.5% of the cases were classified as Grade I, 25.5-59.5% as Grade II and 1.2-6% as Grade III.[13,14]

Sensitivity and Specificity of Criteria Considered in TG13

Acute cholecystitis is characterized by Murphy's sign which has a sensitivity of 50-60% and specificity of 79%[13] or 96%.[14] Sonography in acute cholecystitis is cost-effective, accurate and fast and should be carried out for diagnosis.[15] The sensitivity of USG in acute inflammation is high and is up to 90-95%[16] and hence is preferred in emergency.[19-21] Other radiological features that support diagnosis of acute cholecystitis are wall thickening (5 mm or greater), pericholecystic fluid or direct probe tenderness (ultrasonographic Murphy's sign). Computed tomography scan in patients with of acute cholecystitis has revealed features such as gallbladder distention (41%), gallbladder wall thickening (59%), pericholecystic fat density (52%) and pericholecystic fluid collection (31%).[17]

Laparoscopic cholecystectomy is now the gold standard of treatment of acute cholecystitis. There is still some on-going debate with respect to timing of intervention. There are strong proponents of early intervention. Guller et al. concluded that delayed surgery after admission resulted in higher conversion rates, doubled the risk for postoperative complications and a significantly longer period of postoperative hospitalization. The rate of reoperation was more than 4-fold greater in patients who were operated on or after day 6, compared with patients who were operated on the day of admission.[23,24] The Cochrane review of 2006 stated that, there was no statistically significant difference between the two groups for any of the outcomes including bile duct injury and conversion to open cholecystectomy. In the delayed group 17.5% underwent emergency laparoscopic cholecystectomy due to non-resolving or recurrent cholecystitis and 45% of these had to undergo conversion to open procedure. The total hospital stay was about three days shorter in the early group compared with the delayed group.[18] The authors also recommend laparoscopic surgery in acute cholecystitis should be performed within 96 hours after the onset of symptoms with a higher threshold for conversion for performing a safe surgery.

Gangrenous Cholecystitis

Severe acute inflammation of the gallbladder can progress to necrosis if left untreated. This represents a serious condition that eventually leads to gallbladder perforation, peritonitis or abscess formation. The gangrenous gallbladder is also at increased risk for rupture during cholecystostomy. Some of these imaging findings can be present in cases of acute uncomplicated cholecystitis as well. Notably, the Murphy sign may be absent in patients with severe complicated cholecystitis.

Imaging findings that suggest gangrenous cholecystitis;

- Sonolucencies or striations in gallbladder wall with ultrasound
- Intramural fluid collections on computed tomography or magnetic resonance imaging (MRI)
- Sloughed membranes in the gallbladder lumen

- Pericholecystic abscess
- Disruption of the gallbladder wall
- Lack of gallbladder wall enhancement on computed tomography or MRI
- Hepatic hyper-enhancement adjacent to gallbladder on computed tomography or MRI
- Rim sign on Tc-99m iminodiacetic acid derivative scan.

Emphysematous Cholecystitis

Emphysematous cholecystitis represents a severe form of cholecystitis that occurs with or without coexistent cholelithiasis. The perforation rate is relatively high with this condition, and patients should be managed with urgent cholecystectomy. Diabetics are particularly prone to this disease. The diagnosis is made when gas is identified within the wall of the gallbladder in a patient with suspected cholecystitis. Gas can be present within the gallbladder lumen in such cases, although intraluminal gas can also be introduced via other means such as gas can be present within the gallbladder lumen such as endoscopic retrograde cholangiopancreatography (ERCP). When severe, the abnormal gas collections can be visible in the right upper quadrant on abdominal radiographs. Intramural gas is readily identified on computed tomography images as areas of very low attenuation within the gallbladder wall. MRI is relatively insensitive to the detection of small amounts of gas, although a sufficient amount of gas manifests on MR images as areas of susceptibility artifact. With ultrasound, intramural gas appears as echogenic foci with posterior acoustic shadowing or reverberation artifact. Emphysematous cholecystitis must be kept in mind when the gallbladder cannot be visualized in the setting of suspected acute cholecystitis.

Empyema Gallbladder

In case of acute cholecystitis (associated with gallstone disease, gallbladder cancer or acalculous cholecystitis) gallbladder cavity fills with infected material or frank pus. This can progress to patchy gangrene or micro perforation, macro perforation, or, rarely, cholecysto-duodenal fistula. Patients at increased risk for cholecystitis include those with diabetes, immunosuppression, obesity or hemoglobinopathies.

The clinical history of a patient with empyema of the gallbladder is similar to that of a patient with acute cholecystitis (from which the empyema derives). Patients with empyema gallbladder present with pain, high-grade fever and rigors may have masking effect and do not overtly have symptoms. On examination, these patients have high fever (temperature, >101°F), and mild tachycardia. Superficial palpation reveals mild to moderate tenderness in right upper abdomen. A positive Murphy sign is present with a palpable, inflamed and distended gallbladder. Patient will perforation presents with high fever (temperature ≥103°F), rigors, hypotension and severe tachycardia.

Intravenous antibiotic therapy based on local culture trends and immediate decompression (cholecystostomy-percutaneous or operative) and/or cholecystectomy is procedure of choice. Though surgical decompression and cholecystectomy is the standard, in patients who are hemodynamically unstable or unfit due to comorbidity, cholecystostomy may arrest septic process and save patients life.

Laparoscopic cholecystectomy in gangrenous and edematous inflamed gallbladder is difficult but is achievable with experience. Intraoperative decompression of tense gallbladder may make the procedure simpler. The conversion-to-open and complication rates are variable as per experience of individual. Laparoscopic subtotal cholecystectomy should be carried out if there is severe inflammation precludes safe dissection.[19]

Chronic Cholecystitis

Chronic cholecystitis results from chronic irritation or repeated episodes of acute inflammation leading to mural fibrosis. Chronic cholecystitis can be asymptomatic, is usually associated with gallstones, and is commonly found in cholecystectomy specimens after surgery for symptomatic cholelithiasis. When sufficiently severe, it can manifest on imaging studies as gallbladder wall thickening in the presence of gallstones. Features present with acute cholecystitis, such as pericholecystic fluid, gallbladder distention, Murphy sign and hyperemia are absent in chronic cholecystitis, although acute and chronic cholecystitis may coexist.

Cholescintigraphy is often normal in the setting of chronic cholecystitis, although delayed (>1 h) filling of the gallbladder is seen in some patients. Patients with symptomatic chronic cholecystitis may demonstrate a low gallbladder ejection fraction.

Xanthogranulomatous Cholecystitis (XGC)

Xanthogranulomatous cholecystitis is a rare inflammatory disease of the gallbladder characterized by a focal or diffuse destructive inflammatory process, with accumulation of lipid laden macrophages, fibrous tissue, and acute and chronic inflammatory cells.[20] Incidence of XGC among cholecystitis patients ranges from 0.7% in the USA to up to 10% in India and Japan. In an Indian study mean age was 44–63 and was nine times more common in women.[21,22] Xantho Granulomatous Cholecystitis occurs due to extravasation of bile into the gallbladder wall from rupture of Rokitansky-Aschoff sinuses or by ulcers in mucosa.[22] This results into inflammatory reaction in the interstitial tissue, leading to the formation of xanthoma cells. XGC is associated with cholelithiasis and can coexist with gallbladder carcinoma in a small minority of cases. The imaging features of XGC include wall thickening and the presence of xanthogranulomatous foci within the wall. These manifest as areas of decreased echogenicity on sonography and low attenuation on computed tomography imaging.

Radiographic Features of Xanthogranulomatous Cholecystitis

Ultrasound

- Diffuse or focal gallbladder wall thickening l
- Intramural nodules hypo-echoic
- Loss of fat plane between gallbladder and liver
- Associated gallstones.

Computed Tomography

- Intramural nodules (hypo-attenuated) small
- Poor or heterogeneous contrast enhancement
- Local infiltration or other complications, such as perforation, abscess formation or formation of fistulous tracts.

Magnetic Resonance Imaging

- Mucosal lining integrity and a high signal intensity with T2-weighted imaging.

As with acute cholecystitis, early enhancement of the adjacent liver parenchyma may occur with XGC. Because XGC can extend into the liver and have associated enlarged hepatoduodenal lymph nodes, it can closely mimic gallbladder carcinoma. Although the distinction between XGC and gallbladder carcinoma on imaging examinations can be difficult, some imaging findings can suggest XGC. In particular, a well-defined internal gallbladder border with continuous luminal surface enhancement and the presence of intramural hypo-echoic (US), low-attenuation (computed tomography) or high-signal-intensity (T2-weighted MRI) areas should prompt consideration of this entity.

Xanthogranulomatous cholecystitis is difficult to diagnose either preoperatively or intraoperatively and definite diagnosis depends exclusively on pathological examination. Firm adhesions of the gallbladder to neighboring organs and tissues are common and lead to difficulty in surgical treatments. A resectable carcinoma of gallbladder cannot be left unresected. Simultaneously, many patients of XGC undergo unnecessary radical cholecystectomy with multi-visceral resections. Although many criteria have been proposed for differentiation of these two entities, none has a high sensitivity and specificity. Whenever, XGC is suspected frozen biopsy should be carried out to differentiate XGC from carcinoma of the gallbladder (coexistence of gallbladder cancer 2.3–13.3%).

Xanthogranulomatous cholecystitis creates difficulty at laparoscopy and therefore, any preoperative suspicion of XGC should cause the clinician to consider open cholecystectomy, though there are papers to the contrary.[23]

Gallstones and Pancreatitis

Acute Pancreatitis

Bile duct stones are smaller in case of pancreatitis than in obstructive jaundice (multivariate analysis identified old age and small stones as independent risk factors for pancreatitis).[24] Patients at risk of stone migration and thereby pancreatitis and jaundice have large cystic ducts (>4 mm) that can be detected by ultrasound assessment. Gallbladder motility was stronger in pancreatitis patients than in patients with uncomplicated symptomatic gallstones. The potential benefit of prophylactic cholecystectomy in this patient category has yet to be explored.[25]

Chronic Pancreatitis

There is a possible connection between gallstones and chronic pancreatitis. The mechanism of pancreatic damage in gallstone patients is inflammation. Gallstones or sludge in gallbladder or bile duct system can induce relapsing inflammation, bacterial cholecystitis, cholangitis and papillitis. Gallstone pancreatitis with its complications can lead to chronic changes in pancreas. Stones impact at the ampulla during passage to duodenum.[26,27] Higher pancreatic duct pressure, leads to pancreatic juice regurgitation results into pancreatic auto digestion. Pareja et al.[28] studied anatomical changes in pancreatic duct with MRI, 5 years after the episode of pancreatitis, and found scarring lesions. Gallstones and abnormal bile or pancreatic duct can influence pancreatic secretion function.[29] Other factors that can cause chronic pancreatitis are alcohol misuse, microlithiasis and obstruction of pancreatic duct.[30,31] Ampullary stenosis,[32] sphincter of Oddi (SO) dysfunction and increased pancreatic ductal pressure[33] are also associated with chronic pancreatitis. Therefore, there are many causes for idiopathic pancreatitis other than genetic mutation.

Gallstones and Gallbladder Cancer

Chronic inflammation can rarely lead to calcium deposit in gallbladder wall which is commonly called as "porcelain gallbladder". Porcelain gallbladder was associated with cancer in about quarter of cases. However, recent reports refute such an association. Asymptomatic patients with porcelain gallbladder is advised cholecystectomy for prevention of cancer.

Chronic bacterial infections such as *Salmonella typhi* also carriers 8- to 12-fold increased risk chronic inflammation with 6% developing gallbladder cancer. However others feel that chronic typhoid careers do not have such risk of developing cancer.[34]

Laparoscopic Cholecystectomy

Since the first laparoscopic cholecystectomy was performed by Mouret in 1987 (Lyon, France), it has revolutionized management of gallstones as well as general surgery all over the world. Laparoscopic cholecystectomy has become now gold standard for treating gallstones.

Most cholecystectomies are now performed laparoscopically, contraindicated only by severe conditions (sepsis, acute pancreatitis, biliary enteric fistula, end-stage portal hypertension, medical contraindications). Even laparoscopic cholecystectomy for acute cholecystitis is now performed routinely. In the first 24–48 hours soft edema may even make dissection easier. Beyond that time, the subacute gallbladder with woody edema and a thick hepatoduodenal ligament can be both tough and dangerous. Minimally invasive procedures should reduce patient discomfort yet maintain the efficacy and safety of surgical gold standards such as open cholecystectomy. Laparoscopic cholecystectomy allows a quick return to normal activities, if it can be done without complications.

Difficult Cholecystectomy: Factors Predicting Overall Operative Difficulty

Clinical Factors

- Acute cholecystitis with or without empyema of the gallbladder
- Stones in common bile duct (CBD)
- Previous abdominal surgery or abdominal pathology
- Cirrhosis
- Age more than 65 years
- Male patients
- Patients with a body mass index more than 27.2 kg/m^2.

Ultrasonographic Factors

- Thickness of the gallbladder wall more than 4 mm and mass, if any
- Contracted gallbladder

- Pericholecystic collection
- Size of stones: A stone at least 20 mm in diameter, a gallbladder empty of bile and packed with stones
- Stone impaction in Hartman's pouch
- Dilatation of CBD wider than 6 mm
- Status of liver and pancreas
- Presence of adhesions.

Ultrasound impression may be incorrect and a case labeled "difficult" on USG may be straightforward at laparoscopy. Provided a surgeon has an honest awareness of his own capability and keeps patient safety uppermost, he should be prepared to convert to open surgery. Conversion to open surgery is not a complication; rather it is an expression of the degree of maturity and humility necessary for surgery.

Preoperative prediction of a difficult laparoscopic cholecystectomy can help the patient as well as the surgeon prepare better for the intraoperative risk and the risk of conversion to open cholecystectomy. Significant predictors of conversion to open cholecystectomy are body mass index more than 30 kg/m^2, male gender, past history of acute cholecystitis or acute pancreatitis, past history of upper abdominal surgery and gallbladder wall thickness exceeding 3 mm.[35]

Laparoscopic cholecystectomy comprises four clear steps:

1. Creation of pneumoperitoneum and insertion of all trocars.
2. Separation of all adhesions to the gallbladder and the surrounding liver, with exposure of the peritoneal fold in which the cystic duct and artery are situated.
3. Dissection and skeletonization of the cystic duct and cystic artery and occlusion and division of these structures.
4. Excision and extraction of the gallbladder and closure of incisions.

Preoperative

- Preoperative evaluation of cardiac and pulmonary function.
- Intraoperative monitoring with cardiogram, oxygen saturation and end-tidal carbon dioxide.

Position

- Leg abduction position (European method): Legs are abducted and surgeon stands in center facing patient's abdomen. The table is tilted 30^0 head up and right side up. Television monitor is placed on the right side of the patient. The fundus lies free. The neck is retracted towards the midclavicular port. The porta hepatis is gently lifted to provide counter traction.
- Classical supine position (British or American method): Supine position with head high and right tilts. The fundus is retracted both above liver and laterally. The neck is retracted towards the midclavicular port. Surgeon stands on left of patient.

Access to Peritoneal Cavity

- Parts are prepared and draped.
- The peritoneum is accessed via closed pneumoperitoneum followed by insertion of optical port. (10 mm subumbilical port). Veress needle is passed through a small subumbilical incision. The access to peritoneum is confirmed with either syringe aspiration or drop test or negative pressure test. In case of adhesions open method of visual guided insertion of the trocars is done. There are now many modern devices such as a sliding olive or fixation sutures or blunt obturator which minimize injuries and air leaks.
- Some surgeons prefer open access to peritoneum. Umbilicus is lifted with a Lanz forceps or towel clip. A 1 cm vertical or transverse incision is made in subumbilical region. Subcutaneous tissue is dissected. Umbilical tube is felt as tout vertical structure. An incision is made into umbilical tube to access into peritoneum. Blunt trocar is used to enter the peritoneum.

Laparoscopic Inspection

- Previously heated telescope 0° or 30° is attached to endocamera (sterile or inside transparent sterile plastic sleeve), light cable is attached to the telescope, and the system is "white balanced". The telescope is then inserted down the optic port.
- The surgeon, standing on the patient's left or between the legs, operates through the 10 mm epigastric and the 5 mm right paraumbilical port. The assistant retracts through the 5 mm right anterior axillary line port. A 5 mm left subcostal port may be added, if retraction of a large left lateral lobe is necessary. The 30° scope is between the surgeon's hands giving an optimal eye, camera and hand orientation.
- Laparoscopic inspection has three objectives:
  1. Detection of inadvertent injuries caused during insertion of scope
  2. Exclusion of additional unsuspected intra-abdominal pathology.
  3. Assessment of the feasibility of laparoscopic cholecystectomy.

Decision-Making

- The decision on technical feasibility is influenced by experience of the surgeon in laparoscopic surgery. The cases are divided into:
  - Easy: Minimal intraperitoneal fat and gallbladder floppy and nonadherent. All structures readily identified.
  - Difficult: Obese patients with fat laden cystic duct, large stone load with difficulty in grasping, inflammation, adhesions or abnormal anatomy. Experienced surgeon needed.
  - Uncertain feasibility: Dense adhesions, cystic pedicle not visualized or adherence to CBD, trial dissection is indicated. If dissection does not clearly identify structures, onversion to open surgery must be done.
  - Unsuitable cases: Severe acute cholecystitis or gangrene or phlegmon in porta hepatis or Mirrizzi's syndrome or varices around gallbladder abandon lap procedure.

Dissection and Clipping of Cystic Duct

- The fundus of the gallbladder is elevated progressively as adhesions gently peeled down toward the infundibulum and Hartmann's pouch. A tensely distended gallbladder should be aspirated through the fundus initially to allow grasping, reduce the risk of spillage and ease removal through a trocar site. The fundus grasper is placed over the puncture site. The infundibulum is exposed, grasped, and retracted to the left (never upward or vertically).

- Dissection is begun on the left side of the infundibulum where there are usually no vital structures (when an accessory or replaced right hepatic artery is present (in 15% of individuals) it may lie to the right of the bile duct). Dissection is carried around the neck of the infundibulum as Hartmann's pouch is retracted to the right. The cystic duct is isolated at the junction. The key to avoid injury to ducts is "hug the gallbladder" i.e. remain close to the gallbladder wall while dissection.
- The peritoneum on the left side of the gallbladder is dissected further to expose the cystic artery, the combined visualization of the artery and duct being called the critical view.
- The normal relationships of the common hepatic and right hepatic ducts and the right hepatic artery are shown. The first clip is placed at the cystic duct or infundibulum junction to prevent passage of stones during subsequent manipulation. Hartmann's pouch is retracted laterally to separate the cystic duct from other ductal structures and both tips of the clip applier must be visible before closing. If there is inadequate length of cystic duct for safe clipping, the cystic artery may be clipped and divided first to allow the cystic duct to unkink and lengthen.
- A cystic duct cholangiogram may be performed, if indicated.
- If cholangiogram is normal or not done, Hartmann's pouch is relaxed downward to ensure that there is no tension on the common duct before placing the proximal clips.
- Usually three large medium (gray) sized clips are placed on cystic duct. Two clips are put on proximal side while one clip in put on distal side. In case duct is very broad, first confirm that it is cystic duct and not CBD and then put a knot with 2-0 or 3-0 vicryl.

Isolation of Cystic Artery and Clipping of Artery

- The cystic artery is dissected far enough onto the gallbladder to ensure that it is not a caterpillar hump or aberrant right hepatic that turns back into the liver. Both deep and superficial branches should be looked for. The vessel is clipped proximally and distally and divided. If the vessel is damaged before clipping or escapes, the magnified stream of blood looks far more alarming than it is life threatening. The camera should be immediately pulled back to avoid being obscured by blood and an atraumatic broad grasper should be used to gain temporary control. Clear identification of all structures is essential before placing any clip to avoid damaging nearby bile ducts.
- The cystic duct is also transected using the hook scissors, visualizing the tip of the bottom blade before cutting.

Dissection of Gallbladder from Fossa

- The infundibulum is elevated to tense the areolar connections of gallbladder to the liver bed and cautery is carefully used to divide the tissue without burning liver. Steady state tension must be maintained as the tissue yields.
- When the gallbladder is held by its last attachment, the elevated and exposed gallbladder bed is checked for hemostasis.

Removal of Gallbladder and Closure

- The gallbladder is detached and may be removed directly through a port site. A cleaner and safer option to avoid rupture, spillage and possible infection is to place the gallbladder in a retrieval bag to pull it through a 10 mm puncture site. Large stones may need to be crushed through the neck of the gallbladder or the fascia may need to be incised to extract the bag.
- Pneumoperitoneum is slowly deflated. Port sites are closed with subcuticlar stitches including fascial layers with 1-0 vicryl.
- Pitfalls leading to devastating major duct injury include tenting of the common duct (upper left), inadequate dissection and misidentification of ducts (upper right) and blind hemostasis (lower).

Operative management of common duct stones should only be undertaken if the operator has advanced skills. Small stones (<4 mm) are likely to pass on their own and ERCP in skilled hands is capable of removing 95% of larger stones, with or without lithotripsy. These factors should be weighed against the risks of laparoscopic common duct exploration. An attractive and increasingly used alternative to laparoscopic choledochotomy is transcystic common duct exploration. The majority of cystic ducts can be adequately widened with controlled balloon dilatation to admit the choledochoscope and basket.

Extraction of Gallbladder

The gallbladder is extracted through the 10.0 mm or 11.0 mm port. Extraction within a bag is recommended as it prevents stone loss and prevents wound contamination (both for bacteria as well as tumor cells in unsuspected cancers).

Closure of Port Wounds

Before closure of port wounds, one must inspect operative area, especially cystic artery and duct stumps, gallbladder bed and other adjoining area for bleeding and injuries. If there is bile spillage, irrigation of operative area with saline is done until returning fluid is clean. Port wounds are closed with absorbable (polyamide or PDS) sutures. All port wounds may be infiltrated with long-acting local anesthetic for postoperative pain relief.

Common Ending for All Methods

- Hemostasis in the gallbladder fossa is confirmed. If bile spillage, then lavage with saline
- Look for Saint's triad
- Drainage after cholecystectomy is as per surgeon's choice. Most surgeons today do not drain. In suspected or problematic cases Ryle's tube (size 12/14) is usually introduced as drain from lateral port and removed after 24 hours unless there is continuing blood or bile leak.

Specimen of gallbladder is sent for histopathology.

Complications

On Table

Damage

- Blood vessels: Cystic artery
  - Right hepatic artery
- Rupture gallbladder: Biliary peritonitis
- Subcostal nerve

- Liver, stomach, duodenum, transverse colon while retracting
- Common bile duct/right hepatic duct leads to stricture. (blind use of hemostat to catch cystic artery or use of excessive cautery)
- Inclusion of common hepatic duct/ common bile duct in cystic duct ligature
- Damage to blood vessels or duct because of anomalous position.

Bleeding from Gallbladder Fossa

- Treatment: Pressure with sponge, gel foam pack, under running or cauterize.

Early

- Reactionary hemorrhage due to slipping of ligature
- Biliary leak leading to peritonitis
- Subhepatic or subphrenic or intraperitoneal abscess
- Ascending cholangitis leading to intrahepatic abscess
- Pancreatitis because of blockage of ampulla of Vater by sludge
- Obstructive jaundice because of retained stone
- Biliary fistula or biloma: Drain malfunctioning may form accumulation of bile that goes behind the liver. Hence, the liver is pushed to the left therefore; inferior vena cava is kinked leading to decreased venous return and hypotension. This is characterized by upper abdominal or chest pain, tachycardia and persistent low blood pressure (Waltman-Walters syndrome). Acute Coronary Thrombosis. Immediate USG and drain the collection or reposit the drain.
- Wound infection or dehiscence.

Late

- Postcholecystectomy syndrome
  Signs and symptoms remain as:
  - Stone is retained
  - Large stump of cystic duct
  - Cystic duct neuroma
  - Bile duct strictures leading to obstructive jaundice
  - Incisional hernia.

Bleeding can occur from avulsion of the cystic artery, from injury to the hepatic artery or the liver bed. Usually the cystic artery can be clipped, if it is partially avulsed. Major vascular injuries to the portal vein, vena cava, or aorta are rare (prevalence, 0.11%) and require prompt exploratory laparotomy.

CONCLUSION

Laparoscopic cholecystectomy has been accepted all over the world over last two decades. This has definitely benefited patients for early recovery, minimal pain and less hospital time. There is evidence of increased bile duct injury in the laparoscopic era, which should be assiduously avoided.

FURTHER READING

1. Cuscheri A, Berci G. Laparoscopic Biliary Surgery. Oxford: Blackwell Scientific Publications; 1990.
2. Cuschieri A, Croce E, Faggioni J, Croce E, Lacy A, Toouli J, et al. EAES multicenter prospective randomized trial comparing two-stage vs single-stage management of patients with gallstone disease and ductal calculi. Surg Endosc. 1999:13:952-7.
3. Nathanson LK, Shimi S, Cuschieri A. Laparoscopic cholecystectomy: the Dundee technique. Br J Surg. 1991;78:155-9.
4. Udwadia TE. Laparoscopic surgery in Developing Countries. New Delhi: Jaypee Brothers; 1997. p. 92.

REFERENCES

1. Tandon RK, Thakur VS, Basak AK, Lal K, Jayanthi V, Nijhawan S. Pigment gallstones predominate in South India. Indian J Gastroenterol. 1994;13(Suppl 1):81(A-E6).
2. Tandon RK. Prevalence and type of biliary stones in India. World J Gastroenterol. 2000;6(Suppl 3):4-5.
3. Lowenfels AB, Domellöf L, Lindström CG, Bergman F, Monk MA, Sternby NH. Cholelithiasis, cholecystectomy and cancer: a case control study in Sweden. Gastroenterology. 1982;83:672-6.
4. Mulvihill SJ. Surgical management of gallstone disease and postoperative complications. Semin Gastrointest Dis. 2003;14:237-44.
5. Sakorafas GS, Milingos D, Peros G. Asymptomatic cholelithiasis: is cholecystectomy really needed? A critical reappraisal 15 Years after the introduction of laparoscopic cholecystectomy. Dig Dis Sci. 2007;52:1313-25.
6. Kapoor VK. Cholecystectomy in patients with asymptomatic gallstones to prevent gallbladder cancer—the case against. Indian J Gastroenterol. 2006;25:152-4.
7. Serafini AN, Spoliansky G, Sfakianakis GN, Montalvo B, Jensen WN. Diagnostic studies in patients with sickle cell anemia and acute abdominal pain. Arch Intern Med. 1987;147:1061-2.
8. Patino JF, Quintero GA. Asymptomatic cholelithiasis revisited. World J Surg. 1998;22:1119-24.
9. Del Favero G, Caroli A, Meggiato T, Volpi A, Scalon P, Puglisi A, et al. Natural history of gallstones in non-insulin-dependent diabetes mellitus. A prospective 5-year follow-up. Dig Dis Sci. 1994;39: 1704-7.
10. Ahmed A, Cheung RC, Keeffe EB. Management of gallstones and their complications. Am Fam Physician. 2000;61:1673-80,1687-8.
11. Bragg LE, Thompson JS. Concomitant cholecystectomy for asymptomatic cholelithiasis. Arch Surg. 1989;124:460-2.
12. Yokoe M, Takada T, Strasberg SM, Solomkin JS, Mayumi T, Gomi H, etal. New diagnostic criteria and severity assessment of acute cholecystitis in revised Tokyo guidelines. J Hepatobiliary Pancreat Sci. 2012;19(5):578-85.
13. Trowbridge RL, Rutkowski NK, Shojania KG. Does this patient have acute cholecystitis? JAMA. 2003;289:80-6.
14. Halasz NA. Counterfeit cholecystitis, a common diagnostic dilemma. Am J Surg. 1975;130:189-93.
15. Ralls PW, Colletti PM, Lapin SA, Chandrasoma P, Boswell WD, Ngo C, et al. Real-time sonography in suspected acute cholecystitis. Prospective evaluation of primary and secondary signs. Radiology. 1985;155(3):767-71.
16. Hunt DR, Chu FC. Gangrenous cholecystitis in the laparoscopic era. Aust NZ J Surg. 2000;70:428-30.
17. Fidler J, Paulson EK, Layfield L. CT evaluation of acute cholecystitis: findings and usefulness in diagnosis. AJR. 1996;166:1085-8.
18. Gurusamy KS, Samraj K. Early versus delayed laparoscopic cholecystectomy for acute cholecystitis. Cochrane Database Syst Rev. 2006;(4):CD005440.
19. Philips JA, Lawes DA, Cook AJ, Arulampalam TH, Zaborsky A, Menzies D, et al. The use of laparoscopic subtotal cholecystectomy for complicated cholelithiasis. Surg Endosc. 2008;22(7):1697-700.
20. Jessurun J, Albores-Saavedra J. Gallbladder and extrahepatic biliary ducts. In: Anderson's pathology, Damjanov I, Linder J (Eds). St. Louis: CV Mosby; 1996. p. 1859.
21. Roberts KM, Parsons MA. Xanthogranulomatous cholecystitis: clinicopathological study of 13 cases. J Clin Pathol. 1987;40(4): 412-7.

22. Goodman ZD, Ishak KG. Xanthogranulomatous cholecystitis. Am J Surg Pathol. 1981;5(7):653-9.
23. Kwon AH, Matsui Y, Uemura Y. Surgical procedures and histopathologic findings for patients with xanthogranulomatous cholecystitis. J Am Coll Surg. 2004;199(2):204-10.
24. Venneman NG, Buskens E, Besselink MG, Stads S, Go PM, Bosscha K, et al. Small gallstones are associated with increased risk of acute pancreatitis: potential benefits of prophylactic cholecystectomy? Am J Gastroenterol. 2005;100(11):2540-50.
25. Venneman NG, Renooij W, Rehfeld JF, VanBerge-Henegouwen GP, Go PM, Broeders IA, et al. Small gallstones, preserved gallbladder motility, and fast crystallization are associated with pancreatitis. Hepatology. 2005;41(4):738-46.
26. Joergensen A, Thuesen B. Chronic obstructive pancreatitis associated with gallstone in a child. Acta Chir Scand. 1983;149:805-6.
27. Kelly TR, Swaney PE. Gallstone pancreatitis: the second time around. Surgery. 1982;92:571-5.
28. Pareja E, Mir J, Artigues E, Martínez V, Fabra R, Trullenque R. Acute biliary pancreatitis: does the pancreas change morphologically in the long term? Pancreatology. 2005;5:59-64.
29. Wakabayashi A, Saito S, Nishii T, Takeda Y, Mori R. Comparison of pancreatic dysfunction in chronic alcoholic pancreatitis and chronic gallstone pancreatitis. Gastroenterol Jpn. 1976;11:133-40.
30. Suda K, Takase M, Fukumura Y, Suzuki F, Jim A, Kakinuma C, et al. Histopathologic difference between chronic pancreatitis animal models and human chronic pancreatitis. Pancreas. 2004; 28:e86-9.
31. Tanaka T, Miura Y, Matsugu Y, Ichiba Y, Ito H, Dohi K. Pancreatic duct obstruction is an aggravating factor in the canine model of chronic alcoholic pancreatitis. Gastroenterology. 1998;115: 1248-53.
32. Gu ZY, Zhang KH. Chronic pancreatitis in China: etiology and management. World J Surg. 1990;14:28-31.
33. Okazaki K, Yamamoto Y, Nishimori I, Nishioka T, Kagiyama S, Tamura S, et al. Motility of the sphincter of Oddi and pancreatic main ductal pressure in patients with alcoholic, gallstone-associated, and idiopathic chronic pancreatitis. Am J Gastroentero. 1988;83:820-6.
34. Matsukura N, Yokomuro S, Yamada S, Tajiri T, Sundo T, Hadama T, et al. Association between Helicobacter bilis in bile and biliary tract malignancies: H. bilis in bile from Japanese and Thai patients with benign and malignant diseases in the biliary tract. Jpn J Cancer Res. 2002;93:842-7.
35. Nachnani J, Supe AN. Prediction of difficult laparoscopic cholecystectomy. Indian J Gastroenterol. 2005;24:16-8.

CHAPTER 53

Current Management of Common Bile Duct Stones

Jagdish Chander, Anubhav Vindal

INTRODUCTION

During the age of open cholecystectomy, treatment options for common bile duct stones (CBDS) were relatively straightforward. The scenario however changed with the introduction and adoption of laparoscopic cholecystectomy in 1980s, and till date, there is no consensus on the management of CBDS diagnosed either preoperatively, intraoperatively or in the postoperative period. The various accepted management strategies that have been described in the preoperative period include preoperative endoscopic extraction using endoscopic retrograde cholangiopancreatography (ERCP); in the intraoperative setting include removal during open CBD exploration, endoscopic extraction using ERCP with or without endoscopic sphincterotomy or laparoscopic removal of CBDSs; and in the postoperative period include endoscopic extraction with ERCP with endoscopic sphincterotomy.

HISTORY

In early 19th century, biliary tract surgery mainly consisted of percutaneous extraction of stones and creation of bilio-cutaneous fistulae, a replica of the natural course of untreated bile duct stones. The introduction of anesthesia in surgery paved the way for formal biliary surgery and Carl Langenbuch performed the first cholecystectomy in 1882. Soon thereafter, Ludwig Courvoisier removed a gallstone through a choledochotomy in 1890, in what can be termed as the first surgery on CBD.[1] Thorton and Abbe also reported removal of CBDS through choledochotomy.[2]

The start of biliary tract imaging in 1932 with intraoperative cholangiography by Mirizzi was a pivotal step in the history of biliary surgery.[1] The imaging helped in reducing unnecessary and unindicated CBD explorations, and at the same time was instrumental in decreasing the incidence of retained CBDS after CBD exploration.

The introduction of endoscopic modalities in the seventies for diagnosis and treatment of CBDS with ERCP and endoscopic sphincterotomy proved to be a boon in the management of CBDS. The endoscopic methods gained popularity very quickly and became the modality of choice for managing CBDS.[2]

George Berci was instrumental in direct visualization of the biliary ducts by inventing and popularizing the rigid and flexible choledochoscopy in the late 1970s.[1] Soon, intraoperative choledochoscopy was adopted widely and this helped to further reduce the incidence of retained stones by an additional 10–15%.[3,4]

In the age of open surgery, the treatment of CBD calculi was pretty streamlined with standard protocols defined for specific clinical situations. If there was a suspicion of CBDS intraoperatively, the biliary tree was imaged using intraoperative cholangiography. If CBDSs were found, they were removed through a choledochotomy. With the arrival of laparoscopic cholecystectomy as a treatment modality for gallstones, the biliary world turned upside down.

Patients undergoing laparoscopic cholecystectomy and suspected of having CBDS preoperatively were investigated using ERCP, which was both diagnostic, as well as therapeutic (in the form of endoscopic sphincterotomy). Soon this became the standard of care for patients undergoing laparoscopic cholecystectomy to avoid intraoperative conversion to open procedure. Similarly, intraoperatively diagnosed CBDS during laparoscopic cholecystectomy were managed with postoperative ERCP and endoscopic sphincterotomy as were CBDS discovered in the postoperative period.[5,6]

As the complications of ERCP and endoscopic sphincterotomy were recognized, efforts were made to find a safer alternative. It was also thought desirable to be able to treat the gallstones and the CBDS in a single sitting as in the open era, which was not possible with the endoscopic means. This led the laparoscopic surgeons to devise laparoscopic CBD exploration through the cystic duct in early 1990s. The CBDS were removed using modalities like hydrostatic lavage, trawling with wire baskets or biliary balloon catheters, extraction with cystic duct dilation, balloon dilation of the ampulla, stone retrieval with wire baskets under direct vision using biliary endoscopy and in situ lithotripsy. Almost concurrently, the technique of laparoscopic CBD exploration using a choledochotomy was also described.[6] This technique was the laparoscopic replica of the open procedure that many surgeons were well versed with. The trans-choledochotomy approach was found to be especially useful in cases where the stone size was too large, or the stones were too many or the cystic duct morphology was unfavorable for the transcystic route.

INCIDENCE

Common bile duct stones are found in about 3–18% of patients undergoing laparoscopic cholecystectomy for gallstones.[7,8] Unless actively sought for, these may be very easily missed, as a large percentage of these are totally asymptomatic.[9]

CLINICAL PRESENTATION

The signs and symptoms of CBDS are pleomorphic and may vary from completely asymptomatic patients to life threatening serious complications such as cholangitis or pancreatitis.[9]

It is estimated that the CBDS may be asymptomatic in 5.2–12% of patients.[10] Biliary colic is a very common presentation of CBDS with pain in right hypochondrium or epigastrium lasting in duration from several minutes to several hours. There may be associated nausea and vomiting. Other common presentation of CBDS includes obstructive jaundice with pale stools and dark-coloured urine.[9]

Common bile duct stones can also present in the form of life threatening complications. Acute obstructive cholangitis occurs when there is superadded infection of the bile ducts in the presence of biliary obstruction.[9] The patient may present with the classic symptoms of Charcot's triad or the less common but serious Reynold's pentad.[9] Acute obstructive cholangitis has a mortality rate of 10–20% despite the advancements in treatment.[11] Gallstone pancreatitis is another serious and often fatal complication of CBDS that is seen due to the obstruction of the distal CBD that serves as a common channel for the bile as well as the pancreatic secretions.

DIAGNOSTIC INVESTIGATIONS

The preoperative workup for suspected CBDS should include a meticulous history, biochemical tests including liver function tests (LFTs) and transabdominal ultrasonography (TAS). This screening may avoid unnecessary further detailed preoperative or intraoperative evaluation on patients classified to be at low risk of harboring CBDS (no jaundice, normal LFTs and a normal biliary tree on USG with CBD diameter <9 mm).[12]

The patients determined to be at a high risk for CBDS need to be investigated further. Magnetic resonance cholangiopancreatography (MRCP) or ERCP can confirm or refute the presence of CBDS preoperatively. However, ERCP should not be used solely as a diagnostic modality, but only when an intervention is required on the biliary tree.[12]

LABORATORY TESTS

Patients exhibiting the symptoms suspicious for CBDS need further investigations to evaluate the presence of CBDS.[13] LFTs can be used as a screening tool for CBDS. Raised serum bilirubin, alkaline phosphatase and gamma-glutamyl transpeptidase (GGT) are often seen in biliary obstruction but have low sensitivity and specificity.[14] Most frequent anomalies are elevated serum GGT and ALP in symptomatic CBDS patients.[9] To predict the likelihood of CBDS laboratory studies must be used in addition to imaging modalities.[14]

IMAGING MODALITIES

Transabdominal Ultrasonography

It is often the first as well as an important screening investigation in suspected CBDS patients.[9] TAS has a sensitivity between 25% and 63% and a specificity of nearly 95% for detection of CBDS. Its accuracy is operator dependent and also depends on the dilation of the CBD.[9,13]

Endoscopic Retrograde Cholangiopancreatography

Endoscopic retrograde cholangiopancreatography (ERCP) was considered as the gold standard investigation for the detection of CBDS. It is now rarely used for diagnosis, and is now almost exclusively used as a therapeutic tool.[13] ERCP has a sensitivity of 90–95% and a specificity of 92–98% for CBDS.[13,15] However, ERCP has a significant associated morbidity (12–18%) and mortality rate (1%).[16]

Percutaneous Transhepatic Cholangiography

It is an invasive procedure where the intrahepatic biliary system is cannulated under radiological guidance followed by instillation of dye through a percutaneously placed needle. It is not the initial modality of choice but is a useful alternative. Indications for percutaneous transhepatic cholangiography (PTC) include patients with previous gastric surgery, distal impacted CBDS that not amenable to ERCP or in patients with cholangiohepatitis and multiple intrahepatic stones.[17]

Endoscopic Ultrasound

Introduction of an ultrasound probe through an endoscope into the second half of the duodenum captures ultrasound images of the CBD directly by placing the transducer against the medial duodenal wall. With absence of subcutaneous fat and bowel gas, the image quality is excellent.[18] The proximity of the transducer to the area of interest also allows the use of high frequency, which further contributes to the enhanced image resolution. Sensitivity of endoscopic ultrasound (EUS) is between 95–97%, while specificity varies from 95–98%.[18,19] This is much better than TAS for CBDS detection. Despite being less invasive with minimal morbidity its sensitivity is comparable to the diagnostic ERCP.[18]

Magnetic Resonance Cholangiopancreatography

Magnetic resonance cholangiopancreatography is an accurate, noninvasive diagnostic tool for interrogating the biliary system.[20] The biggest advantage of this imaging modality is that there is no need for any contrast agent. However, the disadvantages include lower resolution compared to ERCP, inability to perform the study in patients with implants and claustrophobia causing problems to some patients.[20,21] MRCP, unlike ERCP, is only a diagnostic and not a therapeutic modality. MRCP had an overall sensitivity of 95% and a specificity of 97% in a meta-analysis of 67 trials.[21]

Intraoperative Cholangiography

First described by Mirizzi, this imaging modality involves instillation of contrast into the biliary tree through the cystic duct, which is then screened under fluoroscopy for any filling defects suggestive of CBDS. Use of intraoperative cholangiography (IOC) routinely is still contentious. While some authors support routine IOC, others favor selective IOC in high risk patients, and still others report no advantages of IOC.[12] It has a sensitivity of 98% and specificity of 94% for detection of CBDS[22] and can be done during open or laparoscopic cholecystectomy. However, it may give erroneous results due to the presence of air bubbles mimicking stones in the CBD, failure to fill the biliary tree properly and spasm of the sphincter of Oddi. Reports have shown that this procedure reduces retained stones and CBD injuries.[9,12,22] Operative time is lengthened by approximately 15 minutes and it may lead to cholangitis.[12,22]

Intraductal Ultrasonography

With technological advancements in the ultrasound probes, the developments of small caliber intraductal ultrasound mini probes (about 2 mm) have been made possible. These can be channeled through endoscopes directly into the bile or pancreatic ducts. Intraductal ultrasonography (IDUS) provides better image resolution than standard EUS as these probes operate at higher frequencies (12–30 MHz) than standard EUS. Acoustic coupling is optimized due to the fact that the CBD is fluid filled and only slightly larger in caliber than the probe.

Although the utility of IDUS for CBDS has been reported, its place in the management and decision-making in patients of CBDS has not been clearly elucidated.[23] IDUS is useful for small residual stones remaining in the CBD after endoscopic lithotripsy.[23,24] IDUS is specifically reported to be of use in patients with a dilated CBD and suspected small CBDS especially when ERCP is not diagnostic.[24]

MANAGEMENT OPTIONS

No consensus exists regarding the ideal management of gallstones and CBDS. CBDSs can be detected preoperatively, intraoperatively or postoperatively. Consequently the management options are quite varied especially in the present era of advanced laparoendoscopic techniques.

The following management strategies are available:

- Endoscopic sphincterotomy with stone extraction followed by laparoscopic cholecystectomy.
- Simultaneous endoscopic stone extraction with laparoscopic cholecystectomy.
- Combined laparoscopic cholecystectomy and CBD exploration (LCBDE).
- Open cholecystectomy with CBD exploration.
- Endoscopic sphincterotomy postcholecystectomy.

Other methods that may be less frequently used are extracorporeal shockwave lithotripsy (ESWL), laser lithotripsy, electrohydraulic lithotripsy (EHL) and dissolution solutions.

Every procedure has its advantages and disadvantages and there is a broad overlap between the indications for an ideal management option in a particular clinical scenario.

The decision of how to manage and treat CBDS is based on the availability of local modalities and expertise. The most frequently used modalities of treating CBDS are:

- Preoperative or postoperative ERCP with endoscopic sphincterotomy (gallstones and CBDS treated in a two-stage procedure).
- Open or laparoscopic CBD exploration and stone clearance with cholecystectomy (single stage procedure).

Several randomized controlled trials have shown similar success rates for both these treatment modalities.[25,26] However, it has been reported that single stage management of gallstones and CBDS has lesser morbidity and mortality (7% and 0.19%) compared with staged endoscopic management (13.5% and 0.5%).[26]

Open Common Bile Duct Exploration

Open surgery for CBDS had been the traditional treatment for management of this disorder. However, with the advent of laparoscopic surgery in general, and laparoscopic CBD exploration in particular, fewer than ever procedures are being done through the open approach worldwide.[27] The advantages offered by the laparoscopic approach over the open approach include, among many others, lesser postoperative pain and discomfort for the patient, faster postoperative recovery and significantly shorter hospital stay. The patients are able to return to the activities of daily living much faster compared to the open technique. However, there still remain few situations in which the open route is preferable over the laparoscopic approach, and these include non-availability of the expertise/equipment for laparoscopic surgery, unfavorable biliary anatomy, large impacted stones in the CBD and other general contraindications to laparoscopic surgery.[12,27]

Preoperative Endoscopic Retrograde Cholangiopancreatography

The success rate of preoperative ERCP for CBDS clearance is 87–97% but this modality has the drawback that it treats only CBDS and a separate procedure is needed for treating gallstones. Moreover, ERCP is not possible in 3–10% of patients and up to 25% of patients need more than one session of ERCP for complete stone clearance.[26,28] The procedure is also associated with serious complications like duodenal perforation, bleeding, cholangitis, pancreatitis and bile duct injury and has considerable morbidity (5–11%) and mortality rates (0.7–1.2%).[26,28] Long-term follow-up of up to 70 months has confirmed that the 75–84% patients are symptom free after ERCP and endoscopic sphincterotomy.[29]

Intraoperative Endoscopic Retrograde Cholangiopancreatography

The use of ERCP for removal of CBDS during an open or laparoscopic cholecystectomy is another option, most commonly described for stones in the common hepatic or intrahepatic ducts. The modality is effective but has the drawbacks of logistic and technical difficulties. A trained endoscopist along with the specialized endoscopy equipment has to be available in the OT during the procedure. The supine position used for the primary surgical procedure may not be optimal for the endoscopic procedure, thereby resulting in difficulties in identification and cannulation of the papilla.[26,28]

Postoperative Endoscopic Retrograde Cholangiopancreatography

Postoperative ERCP is done for unsuspected CBDS found during laparoscopic cholecystectomy when the expertise to perform laparoscopic CBD exploration is not available. The patients are usually taken up for ERCP in the same admission and the success rates of removal of stones vary from 55% to 80%.[28] However, the dangers include all the complications of ERCP and the problem of managing CBDS in case ERCP fails to extract CBDS, necessitating a third procedure.[26,28]

Laparoscopic Common Bile Duct Exploration

Laparoscopic CBD exploration was first reported in 1991.[1,2] Berci and Morgenstern, in 1994, described laparoscopic extraction of CBDS in a multi-institutional SAGES study.[30] In 1999, Cuschieri et al. reported that the laparoscopic one stage management of gallstones CBDS is the preferable option in fit patients.[31] However, the popularity and acceptance of this procedure worldwide has been limited.

For the transcystic exploration, a balloon angioplasty catheter (8 Fr) is used to dilate the cystic duct and CBDSs are visualized using either IOC and fluoroscopy or directly through a choledochoscope. CBDSs are removed using trawling with wire baskets or balloon catheters or are flushed into duodenum by saline lavage under hydrostatic pressure.[30]

For the transcholedochal route, a choledochotomy is made in the supraduodenal part of the CBD. Intraoperative choledochoscopy is usually performed to remove the CBDS under vision (Fig. 1) and to ensure complete removal. An additional 5-mm epigastric port is placed for choledochoscopy of the distal CBD (Figs 2 and 3).[32] The CBDS are extracted using a Dormia basket (Fig. 4). Impacted stones are fragmented using intracorporeal lithotripsy with Holmium laser, and the fragments can be pushed into the duodenum by flushing.[32]

Closure of the CBD can be done in several ways depending on the merits of each case. In cases of concern, drainage of CBD is advised. This may be due to suspicion of residual debris, excessive manipulation of the ampulla or severe inflammation. The drainage can either be in the form of an external drainage (T-tube), or internal drainage (endobiliary stent).[32] In cases with no residual debris or any inflammation of the CBD, primary closure of the duct without any drainage is preferred. Choledochotomy is closed using continuous sutures of 4-0 polygalactin, although some surgeons may prefer an interrupted closure.[32] Where the CBD is more than 20 mm in diameter and/or impacted stones not amenable to removal, laparoscopic choledochoduodenostomy is performed creating a stoma of at least 20 mm, using single layer of interrupted sutures of 3-0 polygalactin.[32,33]

The success of laparoscopic CBD exploration is determined by factors like the surgical expertise, proper equipment, biliary anatomy and the number and size of CBDS. The success rates for LCBDE are reported to be between 85% and 95% with a morbidity rate of 4–16% and mortality of 0–2%.[32,34] A meta-analysis of 1,762 CBDE patients from 19 studies showed a success rate of 80%, morbidity of 4–16% and a mortality of 0–2.7%.[35] Also, the transcystic route is reported to have a recovery similar to laparoscopic cholecystectomy as it does not involve opening of CBD (Table 1).[34,35]

The authors have reported their own experience of laparoscopic CBD exploration, which is the largest series published from southeast Asia.[32] Most of patients in this series had stones between 5–15 mm in size and multiple in number. As a result of the large average stone size and number, transcholedochal route was used

Table 1: Laparoscopic transcystic common bile duct exploration (LTCBDE) versus laparoscopic choledochotomy[32]

	LTCBDE	*Lap choledochotomy*
Skill	Endoscopy	Lap suturing
Stones (number)	<8	Any number
Stone size (mm)	<9	Any size
Stone location	Distal to cystic duct	Entire duct
CBD diameter (mm)	Any	>9
Drain	Optional	Suggested
Contraindication	Friable cystic duct	Small-diameter CBD
	Intrahepatic stones	
	Multiple, large stones	
Advantages	No T-tube	T-tube for postoperative access
	Shorter hospital stay	
	Quick	
Disadvantages	Equipment	Lap suturing
	Intensive new skills required	T-tube

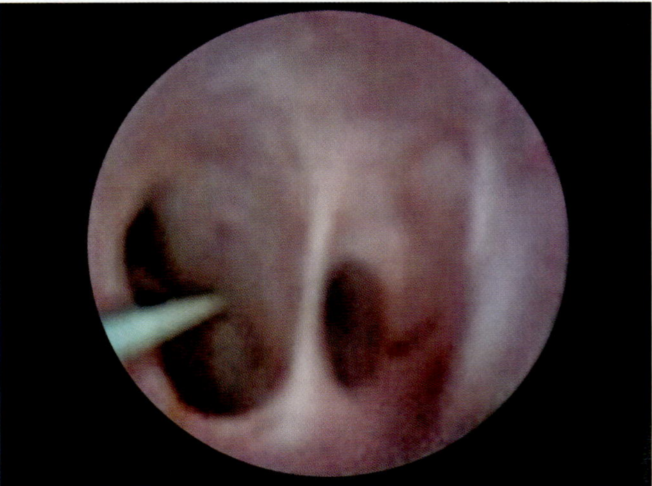

Figure 1 Intraoperative check choledochoscopy—proximal common hepatic duct with the confluence of left and right hepatic ducts during a transcholedochal laparoscopic common bile duct exploration

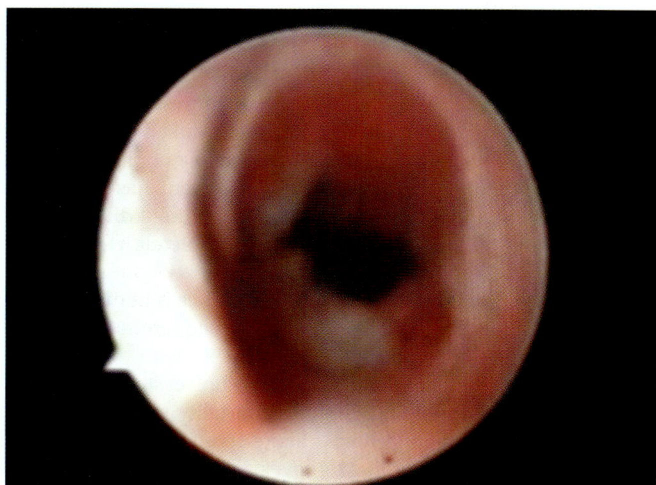

Figure 2 Intraoperative check choledochoscopy—distal common bile duct showing the ampulla opening passively under hydrostatic pressure during a trans-choledochal laparoscopic common bile duct exploration

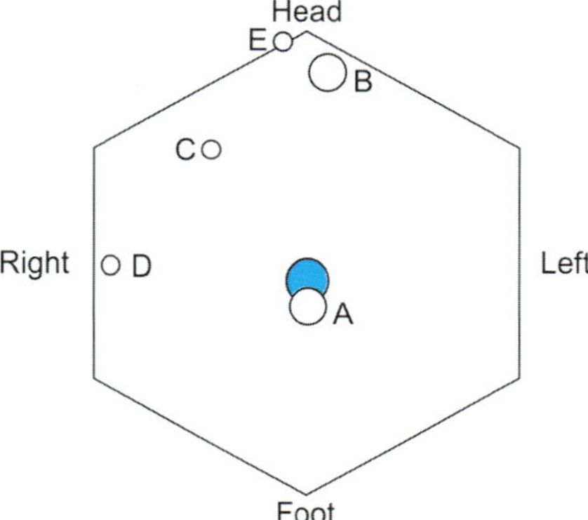

Figure 3 Schematic diagram showing typical port placement for laparoscopic common bile duct exploration – A: 10 mm camera port, B: 12 mm surgeon's right hand port, C: 5 mm surgeon's left hand port, D: 5 mm assistant port, E: 5 mm port for choledochoscopy of distal common bile duct

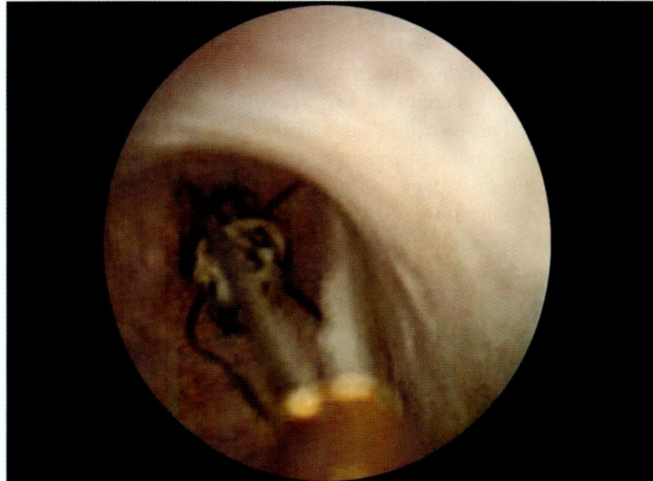

Figure 4 Intraoperative choledochoscopic view during transcholedochal laparoscopic common bile duct exploration. The common bile duct stone has been trapped by the dormia basket and is ready for extraction

in the majority of patients. The average duration of surgery was 139.9 ± 26.3 (range- 90-205 minutes) and the conversion rate was 4% which is one of the lowest reported in the published literature.[32] Fifteen percent of the patients had nonfatal postoperative complications. There were three cases of retained stones (2%), all of which were managed effectively with postoperative ERCP. The average postoperative stay was 4.6 ± 4.1 days.[32]

The authors believe that LCBDE is an ideal method of CBDS removal as it preserves the sanctity of sphincter of Oddi.[32,36] Unlike ERCP there is no reflux cholangitis or recurrent stones due to sphincter damage. One-stage management of CBDS with laparoscopy treats both gallstones and CBDS in single sitting compared with endoscopic staged procedures.[27,35] Compared to two staged procedure it has low morbidity and mortality and can be even performed as day care procedure.

The mean number of interventions required for complete clearance of CBD is also lesser in LCBDE compared to ERCP for clearance of CBD (1.23 vs 1.45).[26,31]

Extracorporeal Shock Wave Lithotripsy

Extracorporeal shock wave lithotripsy was first used for treating gallstones in 1980s after its success in the treatment of renal calculi.[9] This modality is most commonly used in conjunction with ERCP to fragment the larger stones into small pieces that are more amenable to extraction by endoscopic means. The use of this modality has not gained popularity outside Europe, where the duct clearance rates of 83–90% have been reported.[9,12]

Dissolution Techniques

These solutions are instilled either directly into the biliary tree or administered orally, absorbed by GIT and then secreted in the bile. They do not cause irritation of the biliary tree and are not toxic. The disadvantage of this treatment modality is the long duration lasting several weeks.[37] The most commonly used solvents are urso-deoxy-cholic acid and cheno-deoxy-cholic acid which only dissolve cholesterol-containing stones. Methyl-tert-butyl-ether is another cholesterol solvent that has faster dissolution rates, but has higher hepatic toxicity. These agents have been successfully reported to prevent recurrence of gall bladder microlithiasis in the western population where about 85–95% of patients have cholesterol stones, unlike India, where mixed stones, which are not amenable to dissolution by these agents, are the most common variety.[9] Combining dissolution therapy with endoscopic modalities or lithotripsy have been reported to have better outcomes.[9,12,37]

Percutaneous Extraction

This technique is used for nonoperative extraction of CBDS when ERCP has failed or has not been possible due to an altered anatomy and an inaccessible papilla. As a preliminary procedure, a percutaneous transhepatic cholangiography is performed and the stones are visualized. Percutaneous transhepatic balloon dilatation of the papilla is then performed and the stones are pushed into the duodenum using a balloon catheter.[38] If the stone diameter is larger than 1.5 cm, then the stones can be broken down using lithotripsy before they are pushed into the duodenum. The procedure has a success rate of 80–96% in CBDS and in 55–61.5% in intrahepatic stones.[38] Complications described for this procedure include cholangitis, subcapsular biloma, subcapsular hematoma, subcapsular abscess, bile peritonitis, duodenal perforation and CBD perforation.[38]

ENDOSCOPIC VERSUS LAPAROSCOPIC REMOVAL

Endoscopic retrograde cholangiopancreatography with or without endoscopic sphincterotomy for success requires an experienced and skilled endoscopist.[26] A practical problem is that even after ERCP, endoscopic sphincterotomy is not always possible, and when endoscopic sphincterotomy is successful the CBD may not always be cleared of stones.[25,26]

The endoscopic procedures have a considerable cost, morbidity and mortality associated with them. It has been reported that ERCP increases the total treatment cost to twice that of LCBDE.[26] The reported stone clearance rates with ERCP and endoscopic sphincterotomy are 65–75% after one session and 85–92.5% after three sessions.[39] The patients with retropancreatic biliary stenosis, Mirizzi's syndrome or an altered anatomy, such as Billroth II bypass or intradiverticular papilla or abnormal location of papilla have decreased success rates with endoscopic means.[26,39]

As discussed earlier, endoscopic modalities have a morbidity of 7.6–13.5% and carry the risk of serious and life threatening sequelae like bleeding, perforation, pancreatitis, cholangitis, delayed stricture of sphincter, residual/recurrent stones, papillary stenosis, along with a reported mortality of 0.4–0.55%.[25,26]

Preoperative ERCP also causes bacterial contamination of the distal CBD.[12,26] Post-endoscopic sphincterotomy recurrent stones are bilirubinate type regardless of the type of initial stones, indicating a role of reflux with infection due to sphincter ablation.[12,25,26] Post-endoscopic sphincterotomy stricture with CBD dilatation also causes stasis of bile and recurrent stone formation.[26,39] Late papillary stenosis is seen in 10–33% of patients, with recurrent stone formation and consequent cholangitis.[9,26]

With advancements in technology, laparoscopic CBD exploration has become safe, efficient, and cost-effective.[40] Randomized trials comparing two-stage procedures (preoperative or postoperative ERCP/endoscopic sphincterotomy and laparoscopic cholecystectomy) with one stage procedures (laparoscopic cholecystectomy with LCBDE) have shown similar success rates.[30,31,39] Laparoscopic CBD exploration has clearance rates between 75% and 95%, morbidity of around 10%, and mortality of approximately 1.5%.[30,32,40] Patients undergoing LCBDE had a significantly shorter hospital stay and lower hospital cost compared with those treated with a two-stage procedure.[30,31,39] Cuschieri et al. have advocated that LCBDE is preferable for fit patients, whereas endoscopic means may be more suited for high-risk patients.[31] The reported average morbidity and mortality rates for preoperative endoscopic sphincterotomy followed by laparoscopic cholecystectomy is 13% and 2% respectively whereas that after LCBDE is 8% and 1% respectively.[12,30,39]

CURRENT SCENARIO

Stones Diagnosed Preoperatively

The general trend of management of preoperatively diagnosed CBDSs has been by ERCP with stone extraction with stenting if indicated, followed by laparoscopic cholecystectomy. However, single stage LCBDE is emerging as a primary and cost-effective treatment modality with less morbidity.[30,31,39]

In elderly and unfit patients, ERCP and stone extraction from the CBD is the initial and probably the definitive treatment. It is also the initial treatment in patients presenting with jaundice, cholangitis or severe pancreatitis. Laparoscopic cholecystectomy is undertaken once the condition of the patient has improved. Biliary stenting is advocated for patients with large dilated CBD, multiple impacted stones or stones not completely removed by ERCP.[12]

For patients who are fit for surgery, the choice is between single stage operative exploration of CBD or a sequential approach, i.e. preoperative or postoperative ERCP with endoscopic sphincterotomy along with laparoscopic cholecystectomy. ERCP has a morbidity rate of 5–9.8% and a mortality rate of 0.3–2.3%, mostly due to post-procedural acute pancreatitis, duodenal perforation and bleeding.[31] Moreover it causes injury to the sphincter of Oddi which should be avoided in patients younger than 60 years of age.[26,32,36]

Recent studies show that single-stage management of CBDS with LCBDE has lower morbidity and mortality and has lower costs with a shorter hospital stay.[26,39] It treats both gallstones and CBDS in single sitting compared with sequential procedures, and can also be performed as a day care procedure.[40] LCBDE also preserves the function of sphincter of Oddi thereby preventing potential complications such as cholangitis and recurrent stones associated with sphincter damage and resultant bile reflux.[26,32,36]

Performing ERCP along with laparoscopic cholecystectomy has inherent logistic problems concerning the availability of an endoscopist and endoscopy equipment in the operating theatre whenever needed. Post-laparoscopic cholecystectomy ERCP has the disadvantage of needing an additional procedure in patients where the endoscopic modality fails to retrieve the CBDS.[36]

Specialist centers for laparoscopic surgery advocate the treatment of both gallstones and CBDS in a single sitting by the laparoscopic approach.[30-32,36] However, no consensus has been achieved regarding the best approach (laparoscopic or endoscopic) because LCBDE has not been adopted widely till now due to the advanced laparoscopic skills needed for the same. In situations where there are difficulties in performing a combined laparoendoscopic procedure or the laparoscopic experience is limited, it is safer to perform an ERCP followed by cholecystectomy.[36]

A number of studies have reported the mid-long-term results of LCBDE, with excellent results reported up to 15 years post surgery.[27,41-44] These studies have also pointed out the advantage of the laparoscopic approach over the endoscopic approach in maintaining an intact sphincter of Oddi, thus obviating the drawbacks of bile reflux in the lower end of the CBD in the long term. This is especially more important in case of young patients, where the incidence of post-procedural bacteriobilia and recurrent stones have been linked to loss of the function of sphincter and the accompanying reflux into the lower end of the CBD.[27,44]

Stones Discovered Intraoperatively

The available options are: (a) total laparoscopic clearance, (b) combined laparoendoscopic treatment, (c) conversion to open CBD exploration and (d) post-cholecystectomy ERCP.

If the surgeon is experienced the most appropriate treatment would be a total laparoscopic approach. Several cohort studies published from the western countries have shown that two-thirds of the stones detected by IOC can be removed via the transcystic approach.[45] However, this may not be true in Asian population where the CBDS are often large, multiple and densely impacted in the CBD. For patients in whom transcystic extraction of CBDS fails, laparoscopic choledochotomy has been advocated. However, this approach is possible only when the CBD diameter is more than 9 mm, and requires the skills for laparoscopic suturing for closure of choledochotomy.

Martin et al. concluded in their systematic review that transcystic LCBDE is the recommended procedure for CBDS discovered intraoperatively.[26] In situations where this is not possible either due to the unavailability of expertise or due to stone characteristics, postoperative endoscopic sphincterotomy should be the most suitable option.

The other alternative that has been described for intraoperatively diagnosed CBDS is delayed treatment. An endobiliary stent can be introduced into the CBD through the cystic duct and passed through the sphincter of Oddi.[26] This would then facilitate endoscopic access to the bile duct for postoperative clearance by endoscopic sphincterotomy.

Stones Discovered Postoperatively

These patients are best managed by endoscopic clearance, which is considered as the least morbid procedure. Failure rates of up to 10% have been reported.[26,31] In these situations the treatment options are either laparoscopic or open exploration of the CBD depending on the surgical expertise and resources at disposal.

LAPAROENDOSCOPIC SINGLE-SITE SURGERY

Laparoendoscopic single-site (LESS) surgery has emerged as an alternative to conventional laparoscopic surgery with some proven benefits.[46] Many clinical applications of LESS surgeries have been reported in the fields of gynecology, urology and general surgery. Although laparoscopic CBD exploration has a high rate of stone clearance rate and low morbidity and mortality, this technique requires the acquisition of suturing and knot tying skills.[46] Suturing and ligation are more difficult in LESS surgery, compared to conventional laparoscopic surgery due to the angle limitations.

ROBOTIC

Recent developments in LCBDE have focused mainly on introducing robotically assisted surgery and new imaging modalities.[47] After the da Vinci robotic system (Intuitive Surgical, Sunnyvale, CA, USA) was approved for general surgical procedures by the FDA, many studies have reported its use in biliary surgery. However, the robotically assisted LCBDE may still be considered investigational as its actual advantage and cost-effectiveness for this indication is yet to be proven.

CONCLUSION

The best treatment for CBDS is the one that is simple, reliable, readily available and cost-effective for most patients. As the technology for laparoscopic surgery advances along with ever increasing experience, skills and techniques of laparoscopic surgeons, LCBDE is being recognized as a feasible and safe option for management of CBDS in fit patients. This modality has the benefits of avoiding all the potential complications associated with ERCP and endoscopic sphincterotomy and keeps the sphincter anatomically intact, particularly in young patients. Moreover, the benefits of minimally invasive surgery can be extended to the subset of patients with large and/or multiple CBDS which are otherwise unfit for ERCP and endoscopic sphincterotomy and have to undergo open procedures for stone removal.

REFERENCES

1. Beal JM. Historical perspective of gallstone disease. Surg Gynecol Obstet. 1984;158:181-9.
2. Meade RH. The development of surgery of the gall bladder and the bile ducts. In: Meade RH (Ed). Introduction to the History of General Surgery. Philadelphia: WB Saunders; 1968. pp. 223-37.
3. Berci G, Shore M, Morgenstern L, Hamlin A. Choledochoscopy and operative fluorocholangiography in the prevention of retained bile duct stones. World J Surg. 1978;2:411-27.
4. Rattner DW, Warshaw AL. Impact of choledochoscopy on the management of choledocholithiasis: experience with 499 common duct explorations at the Massachusetts General Hospital. Ann Surg. 1981;194:76-9.
5. Fletcher DR. Changes in the practice of biliary surgery and ERCP during the introduction of laparoscopic cholecystectomy to Australia: their possible significance. Aust N Z J Surg. 1994;64: 75-80.
6. DePaula AL, Hashiba K, Bafutto M. Laparoscopic management of choledocholithiasis. Surg Endosc. 1994;8:1399-403.
7. Lacitignola S, Minardi M. Management of common bile duct stones: a ten-year experience at a tertiary care center. JSLS. 2008;12: 62-5.
8. Riciardi R, Islam S, Canete JJ, Arcand PL, Stoker ME. Effectiveness and long-term results of laparoscopic common bile duct exploration. Surg Endosc. 2003;17(1):19-22.
9. Caddy GR, Tham TCK. Symptoms, diagnosis and endoscopic management of common bile duct stones. Best Prac Res Clin Gastroenterol. 2006;20(6):1085-101.
10. Rosseland AR, Glomsaker TB. Asymptomatic common bile duct stones. Eur J Gastroenterol Hepatol. 2000;12(11):1171-3.
11. Kuo CH, Changchien CS, Chen JJ, Tai DI, Chiou SS, Lee CM. Septic acute cholecystitis. Scand J Gastroenterol. 1995;30(3):272-5.
12. Cho CS, D'Angelica MI. Bile duct exploration and biliary-enteric anastomosis. In: Blumgart LH (Ed). Surgery of the Liver, Biliary Tract, and Pancreas, 5 edition. Pennsylvania, USA: Elsevier-Saunders; 2012. pp. 470-80.
13. Lahmann BE, Adrales G, Schwartz RW. Choledocholithiasis—principles of diagnosis and management. Current Surg. 2004;61(3): 290-3.
14. Sgourakis G, Dedemadi G, Stamatelopoulos A, Leandros E, Voros D, Karaliotas K. Predictors of common bile duct lithiasis in laparoscopic era. W J Gastroenterol. 2005;11(21):3267-72.
15. NIH state-of-the-science statement on endoscopic retrograde cholangio-pancreatography (ERCP) for diagnosis and therapy. NIH Consensus and State-of-the-Science Statements. 2002;19(1):1-26.
16. Christensen M, Matzen P, Schulze S, Rosenberg J. Complications of ERCP: a prospective study. Gastrointest Endosc. 2004;60(5): 721-31.
17. Tse F, Barkun JS, Barkun AN. The elective evaluation of patients with suspected choledocholithiasis undergoing laparoscopic cholecystectomy. Gastrointest Endosc. 2004;60(3):437-48.
18. Sivac MV Jr. EUS for bile duct stones: how does it compare with ERCP? Gastrointest Endosc. 2002;56:S175-7.

19. Tse F, Liu L, Barkun AN, Armstrong D, Moayyedi P. EUS: a meta-analysis of test performance in suspected choledocholithiasis. Gastrointest Endosc. 2008;67(2):235-44.
20. Hallal AH, Amortegui JD, Jeroukhimov IM. Magnetic resonance cholangiopancreatography accurately detects common bile duct stones in resolving gallstone pancreatitis. J Am Col Surg. 2005;200(6):869-75.
21. Romagnuolo J, Bardou M, Rahme E, Joseph L, Reinhold C, Barkun AN. Magnetic resonance cholangiopancreatography: a meta-analysis of test performance in suspected biliary disease. Ann Int Med. 2003;139(7):547-57.
22. Griniatsos J, Karvounis E, Isla AM. Limitations of fluoroscopic intraoperative cholangiography in cases suggestive of choledo-cholithiasis. J Laparoendosc Adv Surg Tech. 2005;15(3):312-7.
23. Endo T, Ito K, Fujita N. The clinical significance of intraductal ultrasonography for patients with suspected common bile duct stones. Gastrointest Endosc. 2007;65:AB217.
24. Kubota Y, Takaoka M, Yamamoto S. Diagnosis of common bile duct calculi with intraductal ultrasonography during endoscopic biliary cannulation. J Gastroenterol Hepatol. 2002;17(6):708-12.
25. Clayton ESJ, Connor S, Alexakis N, Leandros E. Meta-analysis of endoscopy and surgery versus surgery alone for common bile duct stones with the gall bladder in situ. Br J Surg. 2006;93(10):1185-91.
26. Martin DJ, Vernon DR, Toouli J. Surgical versus endoscopic treatment of bile duct stones. Cochrane Database Syst Rev. 2006;19(2):CD003327.
27. Grubnik VV, Tkachenko AI, Ilyashenko VV, Vorotyntseva KO. Laparoscopic common bile duct exploration versus open surgery: comparative prospective randomized trial. Surg Endosc. 2012;26:2165-71.
28. Shojaiefard A, Esmaeilzadeh M, Ghafouri A, Mehrabi A. Various techniques for the surgical treatment of common bile duct stones: a meta review. Gasteroenterol Res Pract. 2009:840208.
29. Schreurs WH, Vles WJ, Stuifbergen WHNM, Oostvogel HJM. Endoscopic management of common bile duct stones leaving the gall bladder in situ: a cohort study with long-term follow-up. Dig Surg. 2004;21(1):60-4.
30. Berci G, Morgenstern L. Laparoscopic management of common bile duct stones. A multi-institutional SAGES study. Society of American Gastrointestinal Endoscopic Surgeons. Surg Endosc. 2004;8:1168-74.
31. Cuschieri A, Lezoche E, Morino M, Croce E, Lacy A, Toouli J, et al. EAES multicenter prospective randomized trial comparing two-stage vs single-stage management of patients with gallstone disease and ductal calculi. Surg Endosc. 1999;13:952-7.
32. Chander J, Vindal A, Lal P, Gupta N, Ramteke VK. Laparoscopic management of CBD stones: an Indian experience. Surg Endosc. 2011;25:172-81.
33. Chander J, Mangla V, Vindal A, Lal P, Ramteke VK. Laparoscopic choledochoduodenostomy for biliary stone disease: a single-center 10-year experience. J Laparoendosc Adv Surg Tech A. 2012;22(1):81-4.
34. Thompson MH, Tranter SE. All-comers policy for laparoscopic exploration of the common bile duct. Br J Surg. 2002;89(12):1608-12.
35. Guruswamy KS, Samraj K. Primary closure versus T-tube drainage after laparoscopic common bile duct exploration. Cochrane Database Syst Rev. 2007;1:CD005641.
36. Tang CN, Tsui KK, Ha JP, Siu WT, Li MK. Laparoscopic exploration of the common bile duct: 10-year experience of 174 patients from a single centre. Hong Kong Med J. 2006;12:191-6.
37. Kelly E, Williams JD, Organ Jr KH. A history of the dissolution of retained choledocholithiasis. Am J Surg. 2000;180(2):86-98.
38. Ozcan N, Kahriman G, Mavili E. Percutaneous transhepatic removal of bile duct stones: results of 261 patients. Cardiovasc Intervent Radiol. 2012;35(3):621-7.
39. Urbach DR, Khajanchee YS, Jobe BA, Standage BA, Hansen PD, Swanstrom LL. Cost-effective management of common bile duct stones: a decision analysis of the use of endoscopic retrograde cholangiopancreatography (ERCP), intraoperative cholangiography, and laparoscopic bile duct exploration. Surg Endosc. 2001;15:4-13.
40. Topal B, Aerts R, Penninckx F. Laparoscopic common bile duct stone clearance with flexible choledochoscopy. Surg Endosc. 2007;21:2317-21.
41. Costi R, Mazzeo A, Tartamella F, Manceau C, Vacher B, Valverde A. Cholecystocholedocholithiasis: a case-control study comparing the short- and long-term outcomes for a "laparoscopy first" attitude with the outcome for sequential treatment (systematic endoscopic sphincterotomy followed by laparoscopic cholecystectomy). Surg Endosc. 2010;24:51-62.
42. Li MKW, Tang CN, Lai ECH. Managing concomitant gall bladder stones and common bile duct stones in the laparoscopic era: a systematic review. Asian J Endosc Surg. 2011;4:53-8.
43. Petelin JB. Laparoscopic common bile duct exploration. Lessons learnt from >12 years experience. Surg Endosc. 2003;17:1705-15.
44. Riciardi R, Islam S, Canete JJ, Arcand L, Stoker ME. Effectiveness long-term results of laparoscopic common bile duct exploration. Surg Endosc. 2003;17:19-22.
45. Nathanson LK, O'Rourke NA, Martin IJ, Fielding GA, Cowen AE, Roberts RK, et al. Postoperative ERCP versus laparoscopic choledochotomy for clearance of selected bile duct calculi: a randomized trial. Ann Surg. 2005;242:188-92.
46. Shibao K, Higure A, Yamaguchi K. Laparoendoscopic single-site common bile duct exploration using the manual manipulator. Surg Endosc. 2013;27:3009-15.
47. Alkhamesi NA, Davies WT, Pinto RF, Schlachta CM. Robot-assisted common bile duct exploration as an option for complex choledocholithiasis. Surg Endosc. 2013;27:263-6.

CHAPTER 54

Cholangitis

Gourdas Choudhuri, Pawan Rawal

DEFINITION

Cholangitis is a clinical diagnosis based on symptoms and signs of systemic sepsis originating from the biliary tract. This is a bacterial infection superimposed on an obstruction of the biliary tree. It was first described as a serious, life-threatening entity in 1850s by Jean-Martin Charcot. Other terms used are ascending cholangitis and suppurative cholangitis.

ETIOPATHOGENESIS OF CHOLANGITIS

Bile is usually sterile. Normal pressure in common bile duct (CBD) is 8–12 cm H_2O. Biliary tree is normally protected because there is normal flow of bile to flush, the sphincter of Oddi prevents backflow from the small intestine (mechanical), and bile salts have bacteriostatic properties. Factors required for cholangitis are biliary obstruction, increased biliary pressure and presence of microorganisms.

Causes of biliary obstruction can be:

- Choledocholithiasis
- Obstructive tumors:
  - Periampullary and Pancreatic cancer
  - Cholangiocarcinoma
  - Carcinoma Gallbladder
  - Adjoining organs, lymph nodal
- Benign strictures:
  - Post Cholecystectomy
  - Inflammatory
  - Extramural compression-tubercular
  - Sclerosing cholangitis
- Others:
  - Endoscopic retrograde cholangiopancreatography (ERCP) and other interventions
  - Acquired immune deficiency syndrome (AIDS) and infections that complicate HIV disease (i.e. cryptosporidium or microsporidium)
  - Parasites that infect the biliary tract like Ascaris, Clonorchis sinensis, Opisthorchis and *Fasciola hepatica.*[1]

Common bile duct (CBD) stones, benign biliary strictures and neoplasms are the common etiological factors.[2,3] Less commonly it results from biliary tree manipulation, or biliary sludge. An Indian study reported that 70% of the patients with acute cholangitis had CBD stones and 21% had malignancy.[4] Frequent endoscopic and radiological interventions have also led to an increase in incidence of cholangitis in malignant biliary obstruction.[5] Parasites, hemobilia and hereditary abnormalities may also rarely cause obstruction and cholangitis.

Biliary obstruction reduces defense to bacteria, increases intestinal permeability and causes disruption of intestinal integrity. It also increases small bowel bacterial colonization. Bacteria reach the biliary tract from duodenum by retrograde ascent from duodenum or from portal vein or rarely via hepatic artery or lymphatic. Pressure in the biliary channels disrupts the hepatocellular junctions, and spreads the infection. Pressure in the biliary tree is directly correlated with endotoxemia.

Severity of biliary obstruction is not proportionate to incidence of cholangitis. In fact, partial obstruction has a higher rate of infection and cholangitis than complete obstruction. For this reason obstruction from calculus disease is associated with a much higher rate of cholangitis than neoplastic and fixed obstruction.

Most common organisms responsible for cholangitis are aerobes including *E. Coli, K. pneumonia, Enterobacter species, Proteus species, Pseudomonas species* and *S. faecalis.* Anaerobes include *Cl. perfringens, B. fragilis, Anaerobic cocci, Fusobacterium* and *Actinomyces species.* Infection with anaerobes causes a more severe infection than aerobes.[6] Combination of aerobic and anaerobic bacteria cause a more serious cholangitis with rapid deterioration.

DIAGNOSIS OF CHOLANGITIS

Clinical presentation of cholangitis varies from mild, intermittent and self-limiting disease to acute suppurative cholangitis (severe) form which behaves as fulminant potentially life threatening septicemia.

Charcot's triad classically comprises of right upper quadrant pain, fever and jaundice seen in 50–70% of patients. Additional clinical features of hypotension and alteration of consciousness constitute the Reynold's pentad. Individually, fever, abdominal pain and jaundice are seen in 90%, 70%, and 60% patients respectively.[7,8] In the older age groups, cholangitis may not present with the typical clinical features, which sometimes leads to a delay in diagnosis. In this subset of patients, abnormal liver enzymes are a clue to the diagnosis.[9] Other symptoms may be pruritus acholic or hypocholic stools and malaise. Chills resulting from intermittent bacteremia are prominent in some of patients. Tenderness in right upper quadrant is seen on examination in two-thirds of cases.

Presentation with acute renal failure, hypotension, associated chronic liver disease, inflammatory bowel disease, higher age, cholangitic abscesses and failure to respond to medical management is associated with higher morbidity and mortality rates.

Diagnosis

Early diagnosis and therapy is as important as the close watch on treatment response. Diagnosis of acute cholangitis is suspected clinically. Imaging and laboratory investigations are helpful to differentiate it from other conditions with similar presentation like acute cholecystitis, hepatic abscesses, and pancreatitis and diverticulitis.

Laboratory Values

In complete blood counts, 80% of patients have leukocytosis (WBC >10,000). Patients with severe sepsis and having neutropenia have poor prognosis. Hyperbilirubinemia (88–100%) and increased serum alkaline phosphatase (>80%) is seen in these patients. Bilirubin levels depend on duration and severity of obstruction and are more in malignant etiology. Calcium levels may be low if pancreatitis is also present. Aminotransferase enzymes are elevated to around 1,000 U/L. GGT is a sensitive marker of choledocholithiasis. Amylase may be elevated in one third cases of lower CBD obstruction. Blood cultures are positive in 20–30%.

Imaging

Ultrasonography

Ultrasound is a sensitive for detecting cholelithiasis but only about 50% sensitive for CBD stone. Distal CBD stone are especially obscured by duodenum and bowel gas. However the indirect evidence of common bile duct stones can be inferred from common bile duct (CBD) dilatation (diameter >6 mm). CBD dilatation on ultrasound is associated with high prevalence of CBD stone. Dilated CBD is found on ultrasound in 64% patients of cholangitis. It is a rapid diagnostic procedure and can be done at bedside. Screening of whole abdomen especially liver, pancreas can be done reliably. False negative rates are 10–20% and thus a normal US does not rule out cholangitis. It can also detect complications like empyema, liver abscess and perforation.

Computed Tomography

Contrast-enhanced computed tomography (CECT) is better than ultrasonography for detecting the level of biliary obstruction and delineating its cause. CT cholangiography increases detection of biliary pathology and CBD stones (sensitivity 95%). It can detect other lesions like liver abscess, periampullary and pancreatic tumors and rule out other focus of infection like diverticulitis, pyelonephritis, mesenteric ischemia and ruptured appendix. Problems with CT include contrast sensitivity, radiation exposure and poor delineation of gallstones.

Magnetic Resonance Cholangiopancreatography

Magnetic resonance imaging (MRI) and magnetic resonance cholangiopancreatography (MRCP) detect choledocholithiasis, neoplasms, strictures, biliary dilations. It has a sensitivity of 81–100% and specificity of 92–100% of choledocholithiasis. It is minimally invasive with high accuracy and also avoids invasive procedure like ERCP in approximately 50% of patients. Problem with MRCP include that it cannot sample bile, test cytology and remove stone or obstruction like ERCP. MRI may take long time in a closed gantry and gives claustrophobia to some patients. It is unsuitable for unstable patients and should not be done in patients with pacemaker, implants and prosthetic valves.

Endoscopic Retrograde Cholangiopancreatography

Endoscopic retrograde cholangiopancreatography (ERCP) is gold standard for diagnosis of CBD stones, chronic pancreatitis, periampullary and duodenal tumors, and sphincter of Oddi dysfunction. It is the therapeutic option when CBD stone are identified. It is associated with potential complications like pancreatitis, cholangitis, and perforation of duodenum or bile duct and bleeding. Since ERCP has potential for serious complications ERCP should not be used solely as a diagnostic modality. In the present day, CECT, US, MRI-MRCP and endoscopic ultrasound have largely replaced ERCP for diagnostic purposes. ERCP should be used discreetly only when there is high likelihood of therapeutic intervention.

Endoscopic Ultrasound

Endoscopic ultrasound (EUS) is fast catching up as an accurate means to assess pancreatobiliary pathology. A normal EUS has high negative predictive value for bile duct stones and virtually rules out the necessity of ERCP.

Other Tests

Blood Culture

Aerobic blood cultures are reported to be positive in about 20–30% of patients.[10] These reveal single organisms predominantly.

Bile Culture

The results of aerobic bile cultures are more impressive with positive yield of around 70%.[11] Bile cultures as contrasted to the blood cultures are more often polymicrobial.

TREATMENT

General Supportive Care

Initial treatment starts with resuscitation, monitoring and stabilization if patient is unstable, correction of electrolytes and coagulopathy, and broad spectrum appropriate antibiotics after obtaining blood cultures.

One should have high index of suspicion for the diagnosis of cholangitis and has to consider cholangitis in all patients with sepsis, especially in the presence of abnormal liver function tests and cholestasis.

About 80–90% of patients with mild cholangitis start improving with medical therapy. Those who do not show an early response should quickly undergo endoscopic or surgical decompression of biliary system. In severely ill patients, decompression should be immediate.

Antibiotics

Empiric broad-spectrum antibiotics (Table 1) should be started after blood cultures are drawn. The choice of antibiotic is based on the clinical picture, severity of infection, age of patient, history of intervention, or surgery, and is usually based on local resistance patterns. Ampicillin (2 g/4h IV) plus gentamicin (4–6 mg/kg IV daily) can be the initial choice but the disadvantages are limited anaerobic coverage, frequent microbial resistance, and nephrotoxicity. The piperacillin/tazobactam combination is a good alternative to the ampicillin/gentamicin combination. In severely ill patients, carbapenems, imipenem/cilastatin, ertapenem, or meropenem can be used and will cover gram negative, enterococcus and anaerobes. Levofloxacin (500 mg IV qD) can be used for impaired renal functions. 80% of patients can be managed conservatively 12–24 hours of antibiotics. Generally, antibiotic therapy is given for 7–10 days.[12]

Factors modifying the efficacy are type of biliary obstruction, hepatocellular disease, bacteremia, spectrum of activity against common pathogens and bactericidal activity of antibiotic in bile.

Table 1: In vitro activity: antibiotics

Drug	*Pseudo-monas*	*Entero-bacter*	*S. fecalis*	*B. fragilis*	*Other anaerobes*
Ampi/Amoxy	----	+	+++	±	+++
Piperacillin	+++	++	++	++	+++
Cefotaxime	---	+++	---	+	++
Imepenem	+++	+++	---	+	+++
Amino-glycoside	+	+++	----	---	---
Metronidazole	---	----	---	+++	+++

Biliary Drainage

If patients respond well to initial management, drainage can be performed semi electively in next 24–48 hours. If medical therapy fails, mortality rate is almost 100% without decompression. Presence of persistent pain, hypotension, fever, mental confusion should lead to prompt biliary drainage. In any case biliary drainage remains the cornerstone of treatment of cholangitis because cholangitis will not resolve fully in the presence of mechanical obstruction. There are three dominant methods of biliary drainage—endoscopic, percutaneous and surgical.

Endoscopic Biliary Drainage

Endoscopic biliary drainage by ERCP is the optimal procedure for biliary drainage. Other than allowing drainage, ERCP helps in defining ductal anatomy, identifying simultaneous pathology, collecting bile sample for cytology and microbiology and taking biopsy (such as in ampullary tumors). Studies have shown it to be superior to percutaneous drainage in terms of length of hospitalization, and overall success rate. In acute cholangitis ERCP involves endoscopic sphincterotomy with stone extraction, nasobiliary drain (NBD) placement and stent insertion.[13,14] One of above three procedures can be performed depending upon the clinical condition of patient. In hemodynamically unstable patients, it is not necessary to clear the CBD of stones and just the placement of nasobiliary drain or stent to establish drainage is sufficient. In very sick or unstable patients, a nasobiliary catheter/drain is preferred as it allows for a short procedure time, continuous negative pressure suctions and allows for repeated lavage of the biliary system.[15-17] Stone clearance or other definitive procedure can be performed after the condition of the patient has improved. ERCP has therapeutic mortality of 4.7% and morbidity of 10% which is lower than surgical decompression. Intraductal pressure can be increased by forceful injection of contrast during biliary cannulation which should be avoided or minimized. EUS guided drainage can be performed in cases where papillary access to common bile duct is not possible.

Percutaneous Transhepatic Cholangiography

Percutaneous drainage is a reasonable option for decompressing the biliary tract in unstable patients who are less likely to withstand ERCP. It can be performed under local anesthesia. With some expertise biliary ducts can be cannulated even when not dilated. Overall success rate of this procedure approaches 95–98% in patients who have biliary ductal dilation 70–80% in patients who do not have biliary ductal dilation.[18] It is an alternative when ERCP expertise is lacking or the selective access to common bile duct not possible because of previous bowel surgery, tumor or other reasons.

A combined or 'rendezvous' technique can be performed wherein radiologist provides a guide wire through the percutaneous drain that can be pulled up by the duodenoscope using a snare or forceps thus establishing access for CBD stent placement.

Surgery

Emergency surgery has high morbidity and mortality. It has therefore been replaced by nonoperative biliary drainage.[19,20]

Once patient is out of the septicemia phase, early elective surgery should be done. Surgical exploration of CBD can be done conventionally or laparoscopically depending on the expertise. Difficult or impacted stones are removed along with cholecystectomy. Elective surgery has low morbidity and mortality compared with emergency surgery.

In emergency surgery, doing choledochotomy alone carries lower morbidity and mortality compared with performing both CBD exploration and cholecystectomy. Surgery should be tailored according to the operative findings and condition of the patient.

REFERENCES

1. Liu LX, Harinasuta KT. Liver and intestinal flukes. Gastroenterol Clin North Am. 1996;25:627-36.
2. Agarwal N, Sharma BC, Sarin SK. Endoscopic management of acute cholangitis in elderly patients. World J Gastroenterol. 2006;12:6551-5.
3. Lipsett PA, Pitt HA. Acute cholangitis. Surg Clin North Am. 1990;70:1297-312.
4. Agarwal N, Sharma BC, Sarin SK. Endoscopic management of acute cholangitis in elderly patients. World J Gastroenterol. 2006;12:6551-5.
5. Lorenz R, Herrmann M, Kassem AM, et al. Microbiological examinations and in-vitro testing of different antibiotics in therapeutic endoscopy of the biliary system. Endoscopy. 1998;30:708-12.
6. Reiss R, Eliashiv A, Deutsch AA. Septic complications and bile cultures in 800 consecutive cholecystectomies.World J Surg. 1982;6:195-9.
7. Horton J, Bilhartz L. Gallstone disease and its complications. In: Feldman M, Friedman L, Sleisenger M (Eds). Sleisenger and Fordtran's gastrointestinal and liver disease: pathophysiology, diagnosis, management. Philadelphia: WB Saunders; 2002. pp. 1065-90.
8. Hanau LH, Steigbigel NH. Acute (ascending) cholangitis. Infect Dis Clin North Am. 2000;14:521-46.
9. Rahman SH, Larvin M, McMahon MJ, et al. Clinical presentation and delayed treatment of cholangitis in older people. Dig Dis Sci. 2005;50(12):2207-10.
10. Lee WJ, Chang KJ, Lee CS, Chen KM. Surgery in cholangitis: bacteriology and choice of antibiotic. Hepatogastroenterology. 1992;39:347-9. 11. Bae WK, Moon YS, Kim JH, et al. Microbiologic study of the bile culture and antimicrobial susceptibility in patients with biliary tract infection. Korean J Gastroenterol. 2008;51:248-54.
12. Dooley JS, Hamilton-Miller JM, BrumfittW, et al. Antibiotics in the treatment of biliary infection. Gut. 1984;25:988-98.
13. Sugiyama M, Atomi Y. Treatment of acute cholangitis due to choledocholithiasis in elderly and younger patients. Arch Surg. 1997;132:1129-33.
14. Sugiyama M, Atomi Y. The benefits of endoscopic nasobiliary drainage without sphincterotomy for acute cholangitis. Am J Gastroenterol. 1998;93:2065-8.
15. Chopra KB, Peters RA,O'Toole PA, et al. Randomised study of endoscopic biliary endoprosthesis versus duct clearance for bile duct stones in high-risk patients. Lancet. 1996;348:791-3.
16. Lee DW, Chan AC, Lam YH, et al. Biliary decompression by nasobiliary catheter or biliary stent in acute suppurative cholangitis: a prospective randomized trial. Gastrointest Endosc. 2002;56:361-5.
17. Sharma BC, Kumar R, Agarwal N, et al. Endoscopic biliary drainage by nasobiliary drain or by stent placement in patients with acute cholangitis. Endoscopy. 2005;37:439-43.
18. Burke DR, Lewis CA, Cardella JF, et al. Quality improvement guidelines for percutaneous transhepatic cholangiography and biliary drainage. J Vasc Interv Radiol. 2003;14:S243-6.
19. Lai EC, Tam PC, Paterson IA, et al. Emergency surgery for severe acute cholangitis: the high risk patients. Ann Surg. 1990;211:55-9.
20. Raraty MG, Finch M, Neoptolemos JP. Acute cholangitis and pancreatitis secondary to common duct stones: management update. World J Surg. 1998;22:1155-61.

CHAPTER 55

Biliary Atresia

Yogesh Kumar Sarin, Sushmita Nitin Bhatnagar

INTRODUCTION

Biliary atresia is a progressive fibro-obliterative pan-ductular cholangiopathy affecting varying degrees of both extrahepatic and intrahepatic biliary tree resulting in obstructive bile flow, cholestasis and jaundice in neonates.[1-3] Without treatment, progressive hepatic fibrosis leads to cirrhosis, portal hypertension, liver failure, failure to thrive, malnutrition and death by the age of 2 years.[1,2] More than four decades ago, in the year 1959, Morio Kasai described the first successful portoenterostomy, which gave forth a ray of hope for the biliary atresia patients. However, even today, biliary atresia continues to be a formidable challenge for the pediatric surgeons all over the world. The surgical management comprises of a Kasai portoenterostomy (KPE) at an appropriate age followed by a liver transplant in as many as 85% of long-term survivors. The two procedures are thus sequential with KPE being the bridge to liver transplant for most.

EPIDEMIOLOGY

There is extensive geographic variation across the world from about 1 in 5,000 births in Taiwan to about 1 in 20,000 in Northern Europe, with no apparent seasonal variation and equal gender preponderance.[4-6] Regional variation can also be noticed within a country and this may be attributed to inherent racial differences within a national population.[6]

ANATOMICAL CLASSIFICATION OF BILIARY ATRESIA

The anatomical classification given by the Japanese Society of Pediatric Surgeons has bearing on the management and the outcome. Biliary atresia is classified into three types based on the most proximal level of occlusion of the extrahepatic biliary tree:[1]

1. Type 1 (about 5%)—Obstruction is at the level of the common bile duct (CBD); the proximal biliary tree is patent (Fig. 1) and may be dilated like a cyst (Fig. 2). The gall bladder may contain bile. These cysts have been further classified into cloudy type, mixed type and treelike type.[7]

   A proportion of Type 1 biliary atresia infants, especially those presenting late may have intrahepatic bile lakes (Fig. 3) and these patients are more susceptible to postoperative cholangitis because of stasis within these bile lakes.
2. Type 2 (about 2%)—Biliary duct is obstructed at the level of the common hepatic duct (CHD). The atresia extends till the

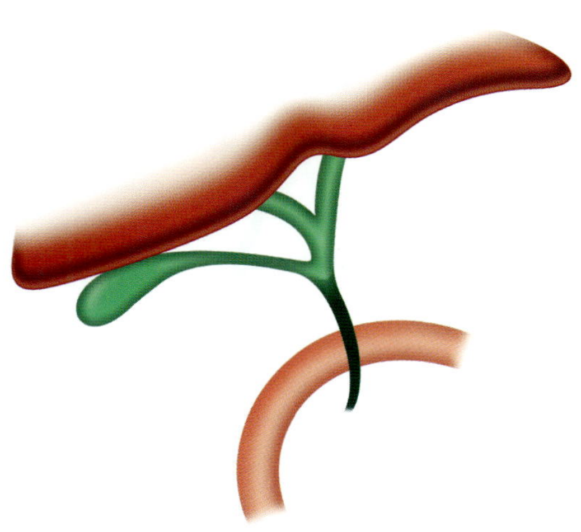

Figure 1 Type 1 biliary atresia

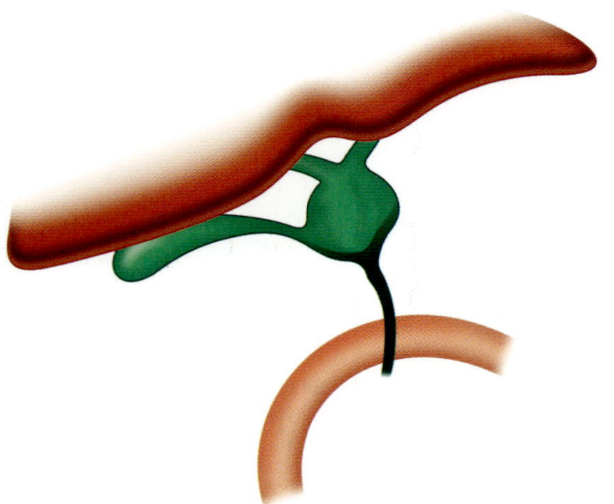

Figure 2 Type 1 biliary atresia with cyst

confluence; the proximal right and left hepatic ducts have a lumen (Fig. 4).

In Types 1 and 2 biliary atresia, although intrahepatic bile ducts are preserved to some extent, they are irregular and non-dilated.

3. In Type 3 (>90%)—The atresia extends into the porta hepatis—no macroscopic or visible extrahepatic bile ducts at the porta. Additional cystic dilatation of the extrahepatic bile duct remnants may be present. The intrahepatic bile ducts are grossly abnormal with numerous small ductules coalescing at the porta hepatis (Fig. 5).

Out of all Type 3 biliary atresias, ~20% have a normal gall bladder and a patent CBD (subtype a) as shown in cholangiogram (Fig. 6). These babies often have a good-sized gall bladder containing a few milliliter of crystal-clear mucus, which on the preoperative US scan may misguide about the preoperative diagnosis of biliary atresia.

About 5–15% of Type 3 biliary atresia infants may have a mucous containing cysts at the porta, which on direct contrast

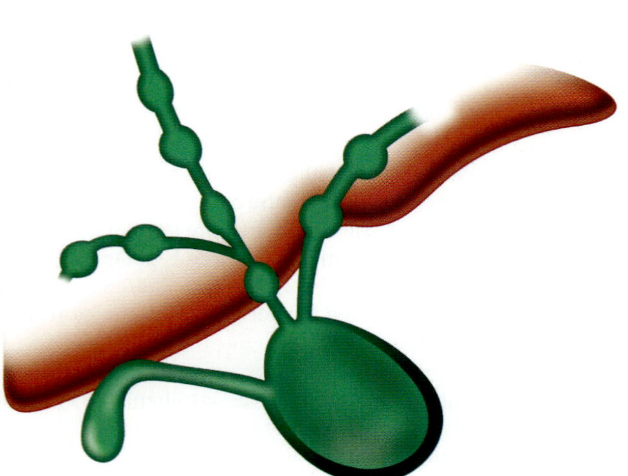

Figure 3 Type 1 biliary atresia with intrahepatic bile lakes

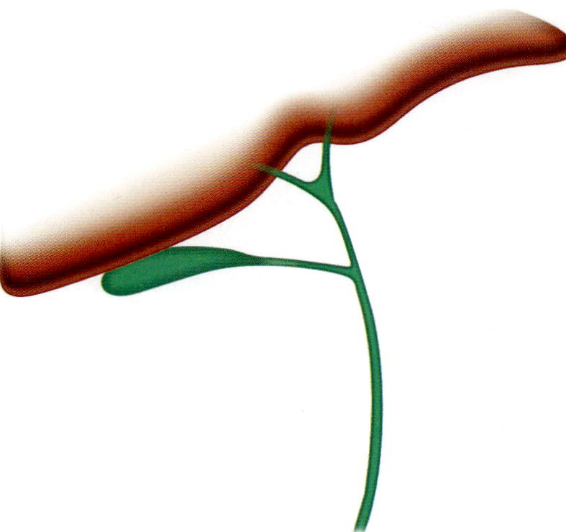

Figure 5 Type 3 biliary atresia

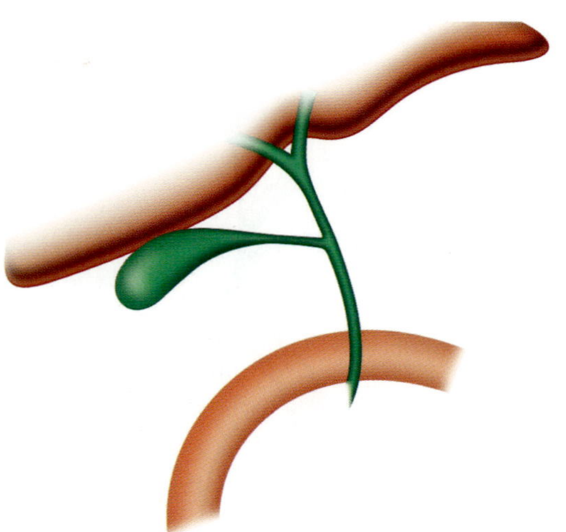

Figure 4 Type 2 biliary atresia

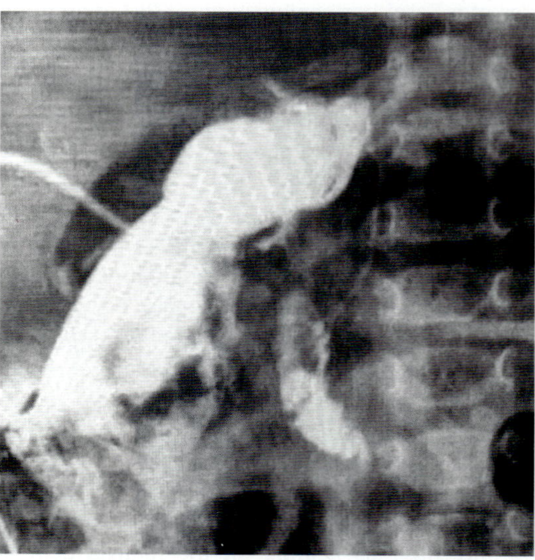

Figure 6 Type 3 biliary atresia with patent CBD

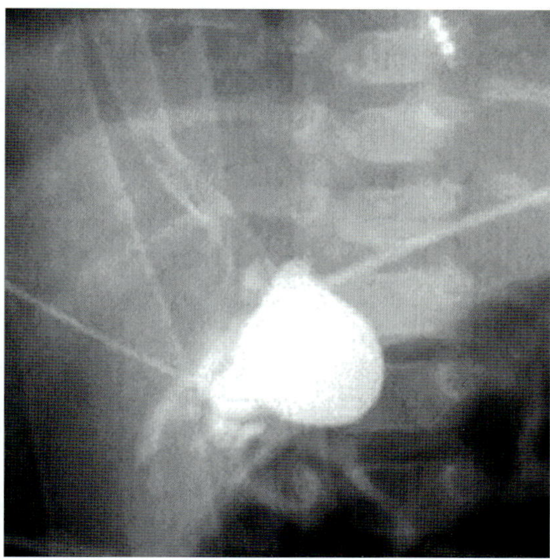

Figure 7 Type 3 biliary atresia with mucous cyst at porta

injection show no communication with intrahepatic biliary duct system (Fig. 7).

Approximately 4% of Type 3 biliary atresia patients have hypoplastic portal plate; these have poor outcome following KPE.

ETIOLOGICAL CLASSIFICATION OF BILIARY ATRESIA

Based on underlying etiology, biliary atresia is classified in two groups.

Embryonic/Congenital/Developmental Form

The onset of disease is prenatal; however, manifest at the time of birth. There is female preponderance.[6] This group includes two subgroups of patients.

Patients with Syndromic Biliary Atresia

This subgroup represents 10–20% of all biliary atresia patients in the western world[4] and includes biliary atresia splenic malformation (BASM) syndrome,[8] cat-eye syndrome[9] and also those where associated malformations appear more random (e.g. esophageal atresia, malrotation, jejunal atresia).[10,11]

Biliary atresia splenic malformation occurs due to an early embryologic insult (30–35 days).[10] BASM syndrome patients have a group of anomalies including preduodenal portal vein, intestinal malrotation, asplenia/polysplenia, absent inferior vena cava, situs inversus, cardiac malformations and pancreatic malformations; situs inversus is seen in about half of the patients.[10] The extrahepatic biliary remnant is sparse, non-inflamed with a missing CBD, and a central and symmetric liver. Etiology is not clearly known, although mutations of the CFC-1 gene and maternal diabetes have been suggested possible etiologies of BASM.[12,13]

In a recent study, in both syndromic and non-syndromic biliary atresia, cholangiocyte cilia showed distinct abnormalities of activity and shape, suggesting it to be a form of ciliopathy.[14]

Cystic Biliary Atresia[9,15]

These biliary atresia patients have cystic structure at porta hepatis in the presence of otherwise obliterated biliary tract. Lal et al.[16] have subclassified cystic biliary atresia (CBA) into three groups according to the cholangiographic anatomy: Group A—Type 3 biliary atresia with extrahepatic cyst; Group B—Type 1 or 2 biliary atresia with extrahepatic biliary cyst and Group C—Type 1 or 2 biliary atresia with both extrahepatic and intrahepatic biliary cysts.

Acquired or Perinatal Form

The onset of occlusion of biliary ductal system in this group is much more controversial, and some authorities believe that, at the time of birth, bile duct can be normal and patent however become occluded secondarily by virally mediated damage for instance [e.g. cytomegalovirus (CMV) associated biliary atresia].[10] The term "evolving biliary atresia" has been also used in this context.[17]

However, the largest subgroup of biliary atresia (probably representing about three-fourths of all biliary atresia patients) is the one with isolated (or idiopathic) biliary atresia where no developmental or infective etiology could be demonstrated.[10] It is a heterogeneous subgroup demonstrating variation in extent of inflammation, time of presentation and obliteration of biliary tree.

CLINICAL FEATURES

Biliary atresia is usually suspected when an otherwise healthy term neonate, conjugated jaundice persisting beyond 14 days of age with dark urine and acholic stools. As time passes, the infant would show signs of failure to thrive due to fat malabsorption,[6] which will also manifest with deficiency of the fat-soluble vitamins A, D, E and, most importantly, K. Due to this, infants may predisposed to bleeding tendency, even intracranial hemorrhage. Infants presenting within 3 months from birth may not show clinical findings of cirrhosis and portal hypertension such as esophageal varices, splenomegaly or ascites; however, these features are invariably present in infants beyond 100 days.[10] As compared to other neonatal cholestatic diseases, such as Alagille syndrome or α-1-antitrypsin deficiency, the cirrhosis occurs comparatively early in biliary atresia.[10]

DIAGNOSIS

Differential diagnosis of neonatal cholestasis is extensive and includes various metabolic, infectious, structural, genetic and toxic conditions (Table 1). Typical laboratory findings of biliary atresia include moderate to high conjugated hyperbilirubinemia, mildly to moderately elevated serum aminotransferases, raised glutamyltransferase, and variably preserved serum markers of hepatic synthetic function. Biliary atresia should be suspected in all infants with extended neonatal jaundice beyond 14 days of age and conjugated hyperbilirubinemia. In those with conjugated bilirubin over 20 μmol/L (1.2 g/dL) or over 20% of the total

Table 1: Differential diagnoses of biliary atresia

1. Bile flow obstruction a. Intrahepatic cholestasis—persistent i. Idiopathic neonatal hepatitis ii. Alagille syndrome (arteriohepatic dysplasia) iii. Intrahepatic biliary hypoplasia or paucity of intrahepatic bile ducts (non-syndromic) iv. Byler's disease (progressive familial intrahepatic cholestasis) b. Intrahepatic cholestasis—recurrent i. Familial benign recurrent cholestasis associated with lymph-edema (Aagenaes syndrome) ii. Congenital hepatic fibrosis iii. Caroli's disease c. Extrahepatic disorders i. Choledochal cyst ii. Spontaneous perforation of the common bile duct iii. Non-syndromic hypoplasia of biliary tract iv. Neonatal sclerosing cholangitis v. Tumors vi. Bile duct stenosis vii. Bile plug syndrome viii. Choledocholithiasis ix. Portal lymphadenopathy
2. Hepatic cell injury a. Infections i. Bacterial ii. Viral 1. Rubella 2. Coxsackie 3. Cytomegalovirus (CMV) 4. Herpes 5. Hepatitis A, B. 6. Reovirus—Type 3 iii. Parasitic 1. Toxoplasmosis iv. Idiopathic neonatal hepatitis b. Metabolic disorders c. Cardiovascular disorders d. Toxic i. Parenteral nutrition ii. Drugs e. Chromosomal disorders f. Miscellaneous including genetic disorders i. Rotor syndrome ii. Dubin-Johnson syndrome

Source: Adapted from Refs. 3 and 20.

bilirubin, further assessment is recommended without a delay.[18] Additional diagnostic modalities include abdominal ultrasound, radioisotope excretion scan, liver histology and operative findings with intraoperative cholangiography.

It is well known that the most important factor determining the surgical outcome is the age at the time of surgery.[4,19] Therefore, any delay in the diagnostic work-up is unwarranted.

Ultrasonography

An absent, or hypoplastic gall bladder, with no evidence of distension between feeds are the typical findings of biliary atresia on ultrasound, although a few patients may have a normal gall bladder as mentioned above. Gall bladder could also be seen in early obliterative phase in evolving biliary atresia. Presence of proximal and intrahepatic biliary tract dilatation rules out biliary atresia. Presence of a CBA could be confused for choledochal cyst (CDC). The cystic component in CBA is usually smaller and may or may not contain bile as compared to CDC. Rarely, CDC may be present in association proximal atresia of the biliary tract.[20-22] A more specific but still controversial feature is presence of hyperechogenic liver hilum, the so-called "triangular cord sign.[23] It is believed to represent the solid proximal biliary vestige in front of portal vein bifurcation. Some authors believe it to be extremely specific and accurate for biliary atresia,[24] others are not convinced.[25]

Coarse liver echo texture, presence of cirrhotic changes, ascites, and splenomegaly on USG are all indicative of advanced disease, which helps in prognosticating the disease.

Cystic biliary atresia may be picked up at antenatal US scan, typically at around 20 weeks gestation;[26] this should mandate a postnatal US and timely referral. Much importance should not be given to non-visualization of gall bladder on 2nd trimester ultrasound.[27]

Duodenal Intubation

Simple placement of a nasoduodenal tube and failure to aspirate bile over 24 hours is an easy bedside test to make the diagnosis of biliary atresia that has very high sensitivity and specificity.[28]

Radioisotope Scan

A radioisotope labeled hepatobiliary excretion scan such as HIDA or DISIDA scan is often done in an infant suspected of biliary atresia. DISIDA scores over HIDA in its ability to provide a greater concentration in bile, faster to perform and being more reliable than HIDA in patients with bilirubin levels more than 20 mg/dL. The scan typically shows fair to good hepatic uptake (depending on the status of the liver) combined with absent excretion of the isotope in the gut even after 24 hours. These are non-specific findings for biliary atresia, and conditions resulting in intrahepatic cholestasis such as alagille syndrome associated with hypoplastic biliary tree may also show reduced hepatic excretion. Normal hepatic excretion of the isotope rules out biliary atresia with a great certainty, but non-excretion of isotope does not categorically conclude about the presence of biliary atresia. Various cholagogues such as ursodeoxycholic acid (UDCA) (20–30 mg/kg/day in 2–3 divided doses for 48–72 hours), betamethasone (2.5 mg/kg/day for 5 days) and phenobarbitone (5 mg/kg/day for 5 days) have been used singly or in combination to prime the infant's liver before radioisotope scan;[29-31] they improve the diagnostic accuracy of the scan.

Liver Biopsy

Liver histology is obtained by percutaneous biopsy (FNAC/trucut). Typical histological findings in biliary atresia include proliferation of bile duct, varying degrees of portal fibrosis, absence of sinusoidal fibrosis, cholestasis and inflammation. The extent of liver fibrosis varies from mild portal tract fibrosis to bridging fibrosis and cirrhosis. Sporadically, giant cell transformation is observed, impeding differentiation between biliary atresia and neonatal hepatitis, particularly in early course of the disease. Positive predictive value of biopsy for biliary atresia is high (near 90%).[32,33] In CMV associated biliary atresia patients, CMV inclusion bodies may be seen on biopsy. This investigation becomes essential in the setting where clinical picture and imaging studies are not very confirmatory of biliary atresia. International normalized ratio (INR) must be in acceptable range before liver biopsy is performed.

Other Tests

For liver fibrosis, AST/platelet ratio index has been used as an alternative of biopsy in several liver diseases, including biliary atresia.[10] Macroscopic cirrhosis evident at laparotomy could also predict with reasonable sensitivity and specificity using a cutoff value of 1.2. This ratio is known to increase with increasing age at surgery. It is much higher in the CMV associated biliary atresia patients.

Presently, instead of full laparotomy, there are two methods of achieving cholangiography: endoscopic retrograde cholangio-pancreatography (ERCP) or laparoscopy. ERCP has been used selectively when results in radioisotope excretion scan and liver biopsy are doubtful;[34,35] admittedly this investigation has not been reported from any Indian center. Direct puncture of the gall bladder on laparoscopy is also relatively simpler way of performing cholangiogram.[36,37] Occasionally, if there is any doubt of the diagnosis at the time of operation, intraoperative cholangiography is performed before KPE.

SCREENING FOR BILIARY ATRESIA

In India and many other developing countries, there is a considerable delay before a baby with suspected biliary atresia attends health care system for definitive surgery. The average age of patients that are fortunate to reach an experienced pediatric surgeon is 3.5 months[20] in contrast to countries like the UK and Japan where the average age is 2 months. The delay occurs at two levels. First level delay occurs before seeking medical attention, which is usually of 4–5 weeks. Easily observable ominous signs in a jaundiced infant, like high colored urine and acholic stools, are rarely taken seriously by parents. Numerous factors are responsible including misapprehensions of parents, remote health center, and ignorance of health care workers. Countries like Japan and Taiwan have developed a large-scale screening programs including stool color card that helped to decrease the average age for diagnosis and referral of biliary atresia. This has abridged their time to surgery, with the median age at KPE being less than 50 days in Taiwan.[5] In the USA, in a well-baby examination clinic, primary care providers are educated to track all infants with jaundice at the 2-week and to get a total and direct bilirubin if the jaundice persists for more than 2–3 weeks or if the infant has pale stools, dark urine or hepatomegaly.[38]

Second-level delay occurs in getting time-consuming investigations. It is a general practice to investigate a patient of conjugated hyperbilirubinemia to exclude medical causes thus losing out optimal time in the management of biliary atresia. If patients present early, ideally all investigations to exclude disorders that mimic biliary atresia should be done within 2-weeks, prior to subjecting the baby to diagnostic laparoscopy/mini-laparotomy and proceed to KPE if indicated.

Surgery

The front line surgical treatment in biliary atresia remains KPE however when KPE fails or deterioration of liver function occurs after initially successful establishment of bile flow, liver transplant serves as a salvage treatment. Portoenterostomy provides adequate bile flow and relief of jaundice both clinically and biochemically ensuing prolonged survival with their native liver in many children. Majority of children ultimately require liver transplant, delaying it into later childhood, adolescence or even in adulthood may be beneficial in several ways. As the child grows, availability of potential liver graft donors increases and technical demands of liver transplant decreases thereby reducing the surgical complications. In addition, the side effects of life-long immunosuppressive therapy is reduced.

PORTOENTEROSTOMY

Preoperative optimization of the coagulation profile of the patient is very important; often fresh frozen plasma is administered for few days prior to surgery, along with gut preparation to reduce the incidence of postoperative cholangitis. Broad-spectrum antibiotics should be administered at the time of induction of anesthesia, and appropriate measures are undertaken to avoid intraoperative hypothermia.

Most centers perform KPE through laparotomy. Surgery begins with a small right subcostal incision and inspection of the liver and gall bladder. In the most common type of biliary atresia, the gall bladder is atretic/hypoplastic and there is no scope for intraoperative cholangiogram. The incision is then extended to generous transverse upper abdominal or Chevron incision. The liver may be exteriorized after division of triangular and coronary ligaments so that the porta literally faces the surgeon; this facilitates a thorough portal dissection. Liver exteriorization may be associated with a fall in CVP and blood pressure, which responds to a fluid bolus to fill up the intravascular volume.

To get the necessary porta exposure, some divide and extract only the left lobe, whereas others leave the liver in situ but sling the portal pedicles. The abdominal cavity is carefully inspected for associated anomalies, e.g. BASM. The gall bladder is taken down, and the peritoneum on the anterior and lateral surface of hepatoduodenal ligament is incised. The fibrotic cord anterior to the portal vein is carefully dissected circumferentially and lifted up. As it is dissected proximally, it often fans out into a cone of fibrous tissue cranial to the portal bifurcation.

The fibrous mass of tissue, which represents the atretic extrahepatic biliary tree, is dissected off the right hepatic artery. The right hepatic artery is followed cranially till it bifurcates into anterior and posterior branches and these branches enter the liver parenchyma. For optimal portal dissection on the left side, a bridge of liver tissue between segment III and IV is divided with cautery. This exposes the umbilical point, i.e. the junction of the umbilical ligament with the left portal vein in the recess of Rex (Fig. 8).

After having dissected the fibrous cone from the hepatic arteries, the plane of dissection is deepened to dissect the fibrous cone of portal remnant from the portal vein. Numerous portal vein tributaries are seen to enter the fibrous portal remnant and into the caudate lobe of liver. They are transfixed with 6-0 prolene

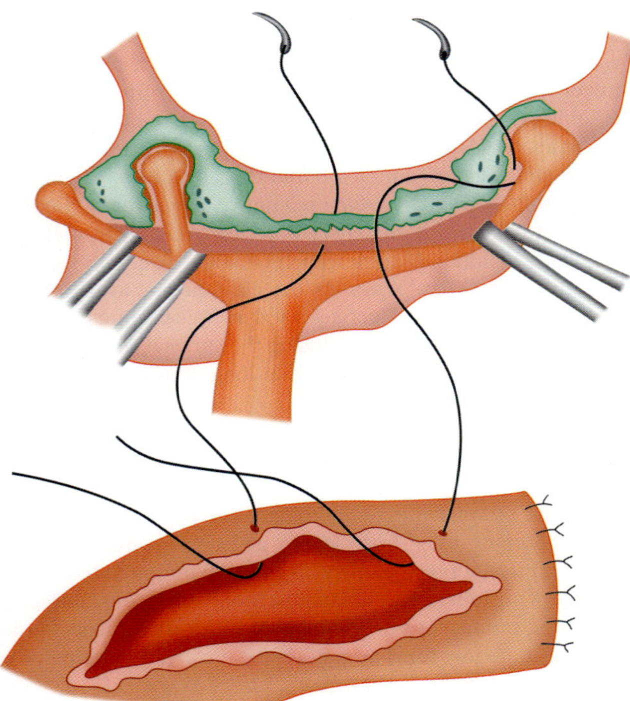

Figure 8 Portal dissection during KPE

and divided. This frees the portal vein completely, which could be now lifted off completely so as to expose the superior border of the caudate lobe of liver, which is the posteroinferior limit of transection of the fibrous portal remnant (Figs 9A to C).

The fibrotic portal plate is incised sharply parallel to and at level of the liver capsule. Coring of liver parenchyma is not recommended as it leads to unnecessary bleeding and fibrosis. The use of cautery is avoided at this step; instead the cleared porta hepatis is gently packed with adrenaline soaked pledgets. The liver is replaced into the abdomen at this stage. A retrocolic 40 cm jejunal Roux-en-Y limb is anastomosed to the cleared porta hepatis. Care should be taken to keep the blind end of the roux loop short. The abdominal drain is retained for ~5 days for occasional excretion of ascites.

Laparoscopic approach of Kasai operations continue to be reported by minimally invasive enthusiasts, but this has not been taken up on a regular basis by the high volume centers performing the standard KPE in the world. Laparoscopic Kasai surgery does not offer much to the child apart from an adhesion-free abdominal cavity for the transplant surgeon and a better scar. In view of rarely comparable results, major centers from China and Germany have reverted to the standard open approach.[39,40] This may be due to difficulties with portal plate dissection using presently available laparoscopic instruments.

One might consider hepatic portocholecystostomy (HPC) if they found a patent native gall bladder and CBD and also HPC does have the advantage of abolishing postoperative cholangitis.[41] However, revisions for repeated biliary obstruction have been reported with a poorer long-term outcome with HPC compared with a standard Roux-en-Y loop (Fig. 10).[42]

Types 1 and 2 biliary atresias, typically manifesting as CBA known to have better long-term outcomes, would allow a hepaticojejunostomy to be performed.[9,43,44] However, it is better to dissect it higher and clear the portal plate to perform a standard KPE even in these patients.

One of the authors (Sushmita Nitin Bhatnagar) has attempted using duodenum instead of Roux-en-Y jejunal loop to createbilio-enteric anastomosis similar to that used for CDC, but long-term results of this procedure are not known.

COMPLICATIONS

The most common problem leading to end-stage liver disease is failure of KPE and continuation of the natural history of biliary atresia. Portal hypertension may develop rapidly in such a situation resulting in ascitis formation, splenomegaly and esophageal varices. Such infants obviously need urgent consideration for liver transplant. There are some specific complications, which may occur after KPE in biliary atresia patients who have done relatively better.

Complications such as ascending cholangitis and portal hypertension may occur even after successful KPE suggested by clearance of jaundice and serum bilirubin within normal range.

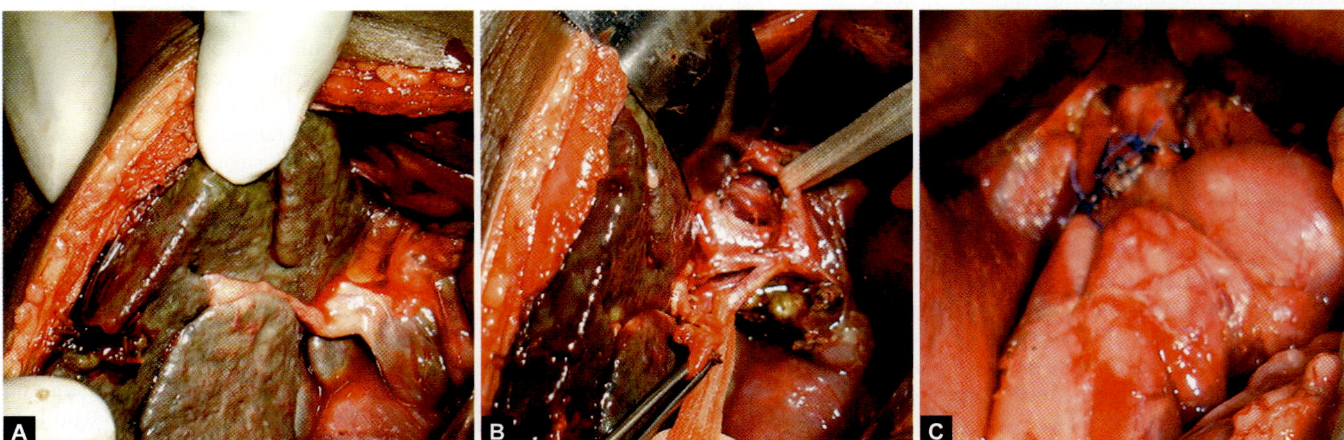

Figures 9A to C Intraoperative photographs of portal dissection and portoenterostomy during KPE

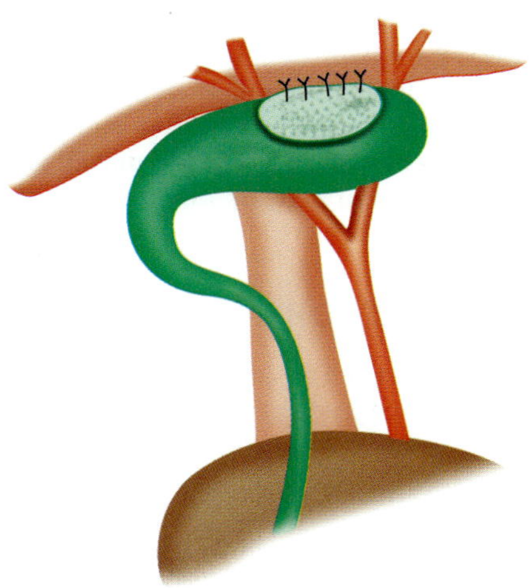

Figure 10 Portocholecystostomy

Cholangitis

Kasai portoenterostomy predisposes to ascending cholangitis, and it is seen in up to 50% of large series.[45,46] It occurs most often early after KPE and may present with abdominal pain, fever, worsening jaundice, acholic stools and elevated inflammatory parameters associated with variable increase in serum bilirubin and aminotransferases. It should be treated aggressively with broad-spectrum intravenous antibiotics effective against Gram-negative organisms [e.g. gentamicin, meropenem, Tazocin (piperacillin/tazobactam)].

Intrahepatic Biliary Lakes

Recurrent cholangitis may be associated with intrahepatic cystic dilatations known as biliary lakes; presence of multiple biliary lakes associated with cholangitis is a bad prognostic sign.[47] Intrahepatic biliary lakes (some call them cysts) could be simple or complicated and could be single or multiple. Simple lakes are not associated with cholangitis and can be left alone. The complicated multiple lakes are problematic as recurrent or persistent cholangitis indicate poor prognosis and need for transplant.

Portal Hypertension and Esophageal Varices

At the time of KPE, portal venous pressure is abnormally high in about 70% of biliary atresia infants and it is caused by increasing liver fibrosis.[48] It correlates with age at KPE, level of bilirubin, and US-measured spleen size; however, it is a poor predictor of outcome of KPE or variceal development.[48] It is clearance of jaundice and perhaps more importantly slowing down of the hepatic fibrotic process post-KPE, rather than the early state of the liver that determines variceal formation.[49]

Bleeding is unusual before 9 months of age as varices takes time to develop. It occurs usually from 2 to 3 years. Variceal bleeding after failed KPE with compromised liver function leads to rapid deterioration of general condition. Using endoscopic surveillance, children surviving beyond 2 years about 60% will have definite varices and of these about 20–30% will bleed.[50,51] It is recommended that each child with biliary atresia should have yearly surveillance upper endoscopies for esophageal varices and if varices are encountered prophylactic sclerotherapy should be done. The presence of significant red wale sign in grade II/III esophageal varices and obvious (usually lesser curve) gastric varices usually prompt prophylactic endoscopic treatment.[51]

The treatment of bleeding varices in emergency particularly includes the use of vasopressin (e.g. terlipressin) or somatostatin analogs (e.g. octreotide), but sometimes a Sengstaken-pattern tube needs to be used.[52] Most varices in biliary atresia can be treated endoscopically with banding or in the very young injection sclerotherapy.[50] This is all necessary in those with reasonable restoration of liver function; however, those who are still significantly jaundiced will require liver transplant. Oral propranolol (1–2 mg/kg/day) has been used as prophylaxis of bleeding in some children with cirrhosis caused by biliary atresia.[53] Shunt surgery have been also advocated for patients older than 6 or 7 years of age.[54]

Ascites

This is mainly due to portal hypertension but other contributory factors are hypoalbuminemia and hyponatremia. It also predisposes to spontaneous bacterial peritonitis. Conventional management includes a salt restricted diet, fluid restriction and the use of diuretics particularly spironolactone. It is often seen in settings of malnutrition and end-stage liver disease. A high calorie, high protein diet is advisable.[10]

Malignancy

Because of ongoing cirrhosis, all patients should be kept in regular follow-up in view of small risk of hepatic malignancy.

ADJUVANT THERAPY FOR BILIARY ATRESIA

Adjuvant medical therapy is commonly used for 6–12 months post-KPE. The presumed rationale of adjuvant medications includes prevention of postoperative cholangitis, stimulation of bile flow and reducing hepatic inflammation and progressive fibrosis associated with biliary atresia, though it needs to be emphasized that the effectiveness of either of these in preventing postoperative cholangitis has not been proved by any randomized controlled trial.

Antibiotics

Most centers use low dose oral antibiotic prophylaxis for 3 months or longer in order to decrease frequency of cholangitis. Variable antimicrobial preparations (amoxicillin, cephalexin, trimethoprim) and their combinations are used while there are little published data to support one antibiotic over another.

Corticosteroids

Many centers employ prednisolone in the dose of 2–5 mg/kg/day for variable period of time (usually day 7 to day 28) after KPE. Besides having anti-inflammatory and immunomodulatory properties, steroids enhance bile salt dependent bile flow.[55,56] However, a meta-analysis has concluded that there is no significant effect of steroids on jaundice clearance or need for liver transplant.[57]

Ursodeoxycholic Acid

Oral UDCA has been known to stimulate bile flow and to have liver immunomodulatory protective effects. An early trial from the USA in early 1990s suggested some clinical and biochemical benefit.[58] One prospective French study[59] had successfully used using UDCA (25 mg/kg/day in three divided doses) in discontinuation/ reintroduction method. In an Indian study,[60] UDCA administration was found beneficial in increasing bile flow and reducing cholangitis in only those patients who had biliary ductules more than 50 microns in size at porta hepatis.

Antiviral Drugs

Some authors have suggested using antivirals such as valganciclovir in patients CMV associated biliary atresia.[61] CMV hepatitis with a high urinary viral load if left untreated causes irreversible hepatic cirrhosis and failure of appropriate bile flow in spite of an optimal surgery.

LIVER TRANSPLANTATION

The most common indication for liver transplant in children is biliary atresia. Most patients require liver transplant during infancy or the first years of life. Failed KPE and refractory growth failure are the most common indications for liver transplant among children with biliary atresia. Other indications related to advanced or end stage liver disease includes variceal bleeding, refractory ascites, progressive cholestasis, recurrent cholangitis, intractable pruritus, deterioration of hepatic function and hepatopulmonary syndrome, etc.[2,62] Usually most of the children with failed KPE are transplanted after development of these complications. Another important issue is small recipient size that mandate employment of technical variant grafts, mainly segments II and III from adult donors. Associated severe cardiac malformations may preclude liver transplant from treatment of biliary atresia.

The technical challenges during liver transplant among children with biliary atresia and previous KPE are small recipient size, hepatic arterial and biliary reconstruction, limited intra-abdominal space and adhesions.[62] Significant vascular and/or intestinal malformations due to BASM may be encountered in ~10% of recipients with biliary atresia. Intraoperatively, careful placement of a technical variant graft is necessary to prevent twisting of vascular structures.

Intra-abdominal adhesions especially after failed KPE and portal hypertension may predispose to intestinal perforations during dissection.[63] The overall incidence of biliary complications is relatively high (25%).[64,65] Hepatic arterial complications occur in 15% and portal venous complications in 8% of children undergoing liver transplant for biliary atresia respectively.[64-66] Reoperations are common (50%) after liver transplant for biliary atresia and mainly performed after transplantation of a technical variant graft for postoperative hemorrhage.[3]

Patient with cirrhosis at presentation, KPE can be occasionally beneficial; however, prediction of benefit is difficult. These infants have a highest risk of postoperative morbidity. Primary liver transplant is an option in such patients.[10]

There are very few centers in India that have considerable experience in liver transplant for biliary atresia. Due to high cost of treatment, infections, inability to support long-term care, and non-availability of expertise, acceptance of liver transplant for biliary atresia in India has been slow.[65] It is hoped that all physicians and surgeons dealing with such patients would start considering this treatment modality.

PROGNOSTIC FACTORS

There are various factors that are identified as important, although the outcome in largely unpredictable in each case.

Age at Kasai Portoenterostomy

If a bile-obstructed liver is left alone, then delayed surgery will be associated with worse outcomes of KPE in terms of native liver survival as the liver ultimately becomes cirrhotic and unsalvageable.[66] It is important to note that even in the congenital forms of biliary atresia, the injurious inflammation and liver fibrosis begin at the time of birth—not before.[67] The effect of age on outcome is neither simple nor linear and depends crucially on the type and variant of biliary atresia.[10] In a UK study, the age-effect was noted to be more pronounced in the patients with congenital biliary atresia (BASM and CBA patients). There was barely any major harm done until about 90 days of age in those with isolated biliary atresia;[68] an Indian center also had similar experience.[69]

Type of Biliary Atresia

There is improved outcome in Types 1 and 2 as compared with Type 3 biliary atresia and CBA compared with non-cystic biliary atresia.[9,66,68] This may be due to presence of few connections between the intrahepatic and extrahepatic bile ducts and ductules. Infants with BASM have a worse prognosis, and typically their remnants are fairly scanty.[10] Prognosis of infants with CMV associated biliary atresia is worst of all due to the ongoing immunologic destruction of intrahepatic biliary ductules.

Liver Histology and Biliary Remnant: Anatomical Effect

Microscopic size of resected biliary remnants has been good predictor of outcome; however, prospective evaluation of the macroscopic features of the hepatobiliary elements like hardness of the liver, presence of ascites, etc. being relatively poor predictors.[70] Older series suggested that better outcome has been correlated with those showing large ductules (>300 μm);[71] the converse is also true so that minimal or no ductules in the remnant is predictive of poor prognosis.[72,73] Of the Indian studies, the Mumbai group reported that children with ductular size more than 200 μm have a good prognosis.[69]

As regards the liver histology, the extent of liver fibrosis at the time of KPE is a strong negative predictor of outcome.[26] A study from AIIMS, New Delhi,[74] concluded that parameters such as bile ductule proliferation, bile duct inflammation, higher degree of cholestasis, hepatocellular alteration are significantly correlated with poor surgical outcome. Other factors such as portal edema and high-grade hepatic fibrosis showed an inclination toward poor outcome but did not reach statistical significance. Giant cell transformation and ductal plate malformation did not show any association with surgical outcomes in this center, whereas a study from Kolkata reported that a higher degree of fibrosis at the time of KPE and presence of ductal plate malformation were related to a significantly poorer clinical outcome.[75]

Postoperative Biochemical Results

After KPE, serum bilirubin is the strongest predictor of outcome. Normal serum bilirubin level within few months after KPE predicts favorable long-term outcome.[1,2] However, preoperative liver function tests have been known not to have any effect on the outcome.[69]

Post-KPE Intrapulmonary AV Shunts

The development of intrapulmonary arteriovenous shunts after KPE is a poor prognostic factor and can be useful in deciding priority that which patient will need liver transplant.[76]

Manganese Toxicity

A study from AIIMS, New Delhi, a risk of latent manganese toxicity in patients with biliary atresia who have undergone KPE was identified.[77] Brain MRI and serial monitoring of whole blood manganese assay can be used for early detection of these complications. This tool can be used to prognosticate after KPE and in selecting patients who will need a liver transplant on a priority basis.

Centralization: Who Should Do the Kasai Portoenterostomy?

Centralization has improved results in biliary atresia as experience of a particular center counts. Presently in England and Wales, there are only three authorized centers where all biliary atresia patients are managed.[10] Smaller European countries, such as Finland[78] and Denmark,[79] have also adopted this approach. In Finland, centralization has clearly improved nationwide and institutional outcomes of biliary atresia in terms of clearance of jaundice and native liver survival, although the age at KPE has remained unchanged.[78] There has been an increased awareness of the need to improve collaboration and communication between centers in other countries too (e.g. France, United States and Canada).[80-82] However, such an arrangement is a far-fetched dream for our country.

OVERALL SURVIVAL

Ten-year survival rate in the original Kasai series from Sendai for the first 63 patients treated from 1953 to 1967 was 10%; for 44 cases from 1968 to 1972 was 27%; and for 61 cases from 1973 to 1977 was 48%.[83] Of these, about two-thirds were jaundice free (<20 μmol/L). If we discuss global outcomes, only 10–20% of all patients undergoing KPE during infancy survive into adulthood with their native liver;[2,66] these patients would be jaundice free, free from recurrent cholangitis and clinically symptomatic PHT, near normal growth, would be gainfully employed and would be able to parent children, though the liver enzymes and the liver histology may continue to show derangement. For the remaining 85% patients, liver transplant seems to be the ultimate reality by the time they reach adulthood. With the advent of a complementary system of surgical treatment (KPE followed by liver transplant), the overall 5-year and 10-year survival rates close to 90% have been reported from Europe.[84] Actuarial native liver 5-year survival rates of about 60% have been reported from Finland.[85] At present, the liver transplants for biliary atresia survivors are undertaken in very few centers in our country and those centers are inaccessible for common man due to the prohibitive costs involved. Improvements in the donor organ pool and early detection of the need for liver transplant are also desirable. Unless we improve in all the above-cited areas, the results in biliary atresia would continue to be dismal.

FUTURE CONSIDERATIONS

Hepatocyte growth factor activator inhibitor (HAI-1 and HAI-2) are over expressed in the liver in cholangiopathies with ductular reactions and are probably implicated in hepatic differentiation and liver fibrosis; they could be investigated as disease markers and effective pharmacologic methods could be developed against them;[86] this may alter the natural history of the disease. Infusion of hepatic progenitor cell transplantation through hepatic artery[87] and infusion of bone marrow derived autologous stem cells[88] have also been described. These modalities may hold the future of management of biliary atresia. Very recently, an interesting hypothesis of treating biliary atresia non-surgically has been put forward.[89]

REFERENCES

1. Hartley JL, Davenport M, Kelly DA. Biliary atresia. Lancet. 2009;374:1704-13.
2. Basset MD, Murray KF. Biliary atresia. Recent progress. J Clin Gastroenterol. 2008;42:720-9.
3. Pakarinen MP, Rintala RJ. Surgery of biliary atresia. Scand J Surg. 2011:100:49-53.
4. Chardot C, Carton M, Spire-Bendelac N, Le Pommelet C, Golmard JL, Auvert B. Epidemiology of biliary atresia in France: a national study 1986-96. J Hepatol. 1999;31:1006-13.
5. Hsiao CH, Chang MH, Chen HL, Lee HC, Wu TC, Lin CC, et al. Universal screening for biliary atresia using an infant stool color card in Taiwan. Hepatology. 2008;47:1233-40.
6. Livesey E, Cortina Borja M, Sharif K, Alizai N, McClean P, Kelly D, et al. Epidemiology of biliary atresia in England and Wales (1999-2006). Arch Dis Child Fetal Neonatal Ed. 2009;94:F451-5.
7. Nio M, Sano N, Ishii T, Sasaki H, Hayashi Y, Ohi R. Long-term outcome in type I biliary atresia. J Pediatr Surg. 2006;41:1973-5.
8. Davenport M, Tizzard SA, Underhill J, Mieli-Vergani G, Portmann B, Hadzić N. The biliary atresia splenic malformation syndrome: a 28-year single-center retrospective study. J Pediatr. 2006;149: 393-400.
9. Caponcelli E, Knisely AS, Davenport M. Cystic biliary atresia: an etiologic and prognostic subgroup. J Pediatr Surg. 2008;43:1619-24.
10. Davenport M. Biliary atresia: clinical aspects. Semin Pediatr Surg. 2012;21:175-84.
11. Kataria R, Kataria A, Gupta DK. Spectrum of congenital anomalies associated with biliary atresia. Indian J Pediatr. 1996;63:651-4.
12. Davit-Spraul A, Baussan C, Hermeziu B, Bernard O, Jacquemin E. CFC1 gene involvement in biliary atresia with polysplenia syndrome. J Pediatr Gastroenterol Nutr. 2008;46:111-2.

13. Davenport M, Savage M, Mowat AP, Howard ER. The biliary atresia splenic malformation syndrome. Surgery. 1993;113:662-8.
14. Chu AS, Russo PA, Wells RG. Cholangiocyte cilia are abnormal in syndromic and non-syndromic biliary atresia. Mod Pathol. 2012;25:751-7.
15. Arora A, Patidar Y, Khanna R, Alam S, Rastogi A, Negi SS. Cystic biliary atresia: confounding and intriguing. J Pediatr. 2012; 161:562.
16. Lal R, Prasad DK, Krishna P, Sikora SS, Poddar U, Yachha SK, et al. Bilairy atresia with "cyst at porta": management and outcome as per the cholangiograhic anatomy. Pediatr Surg Int. 2007;23:773-8.
17. Mohanty S, Shah I, Bahtnagar S. Evolving biliary atresia with cytomegalovirus. Indian Pediatr. 2011;48:644-6.
18. Sokol RJ, Shepherd RW, Superina R, Bezerra JA, Robuck P, Hoofnagle JH. Screening and outcomes in biliary atresia: summary of a national institute of health workshop. Hepatology. 2007;46: 566-81.
19. Ohi R. Biliary atresia. A surgical perspective. Clin Liver Dis. 2000;4:779-804.
20. Gupta R, Nagdeve NG, Sarin YK. Neonatal surgical jaundice revisited. Indian J Pediatr. 2005;72:415-23.
21. Obaidah A, Dhende NP, Mane SB, Acharya H. Biliary atresia associated with choledochal cyst. Afr J Paediatr Surg. 2009;6:61-2.
22. Sinha S, Sarin YK. Extra hepatic biliary atresia associated with choledochal cyst—A diagnostic dilemma in neonatal obstructive jaundice. J Neonat Surg. 2013;2:11.
23. Park WH, Choi SO, Lee HJ, Kim SP, Zeon SK, Lee SL. A new diagnostic approach to biliary atresia with emphasis on the ultrasonographic triangular cord sign: comparison of ultrasonography, hepatobiliary scintigraphy, and liver needle biopsy in the evaluation of infantile cholestasis. J Pediatr Surg. 1997;32:1555-9.
24. Humphrey TM, Stringer MD. Biliary atresia: US diagnosis. Radiology. 2007;244:845-51.
25. Mittal V, Saxena AK, Sodhi KS, Thapa BR, Rao KL, Das A, et al. Role of abdominal sonography in the preoperative diagnosis of extrahepatic biliary atresia in infants younger than 90 days. Am J Roentgenol. 2011;196:W438-45.
26. Hinds R, Davenport M, Mieli-Vergani G, Hadzić N. Antenatal presentation of biliary atresia. J Pediatr. 2004;144:43-6.
27. Shen O, Rabinowitz R, Yagel S, Gal M. Absent gall bladder on fetal ultrasound: prenatal findings and postnatal outcome. Ultrasound Obstet Gynecol. 2011;37:673-7.
28. Miesheri IV, Kasat LS, Kumar A, Bahety G, Kothary P. Duodenal intubation and test for bile—a reliable method to rule out biliary atresia. Pediatr Surg Int. 2002;18:392-5.
29. Gupta DK, Charles AR, Srinivas M, Dave S, Bal CS. Betamethasone plus phenobarbitone prior to hepatobiliary scintigraphy increases diagnostic accuracy in infants with jaundice. Indian J Pediatr. 2001;68:1039-41.
30. Poddar U, Bhattacharya A, Thapa BR, Mittal BR, Singh K. Ursodeoxycholic acid-augmented hepatobiliary scintigraphy in the evaluation of neonatal jaundice. J Nucl Med. 2004;45:1488-92.
31. Shah I, Bhatnagar S, Rangarajan V, Patankar N. Utility of Tc99m-Mebrofenin hepato-biliary scintigraphy (HIDA scan) for the diagnosis of biliary atresia. Trop Gastroenterol. 2012;33:62-4.
32. Rastogi A, Krishnani N, Yachha SK, Khanna V, Poddar U, Lal R. Histopathological features and accuracy for diagnosing biliary atresia by prelaparotomy liver biopsy in developing countries. J Gastroenterol Hepatol. 2009;24:97-102.
33. Russo P, Magee JC, Boitnott J, Bove KE, Raghunathan T, Finegold M, et al. Design and validation of the biliary atresia research consortium histologic assessment system for cholestasis in infancy. Clin Gastroenterol Hepatol. 2011;9:357-62.
34. Petersen C, Meier PN, Schneider A, Turowski C, Pfister ED, Manns MP, et al. Endoscopic retrograde cholangiopancreaticography prior to explorative laparotomy avoids unnecessary surgery in patients suspected for biliary atresia. J Hepatol. 2009;51:1055-60.
35. Shanmugam NP, Harrison PM, Devlin J, Peddu P, Knisely AS, Davenport M, et al. Selective use of endoscopic retrograde cholangiopancreatography in the diagnosis of biliary atresia in infants younger than 100 days. J Pediatr Gastroenterol Nutr. 2009;49:435-41.
36. Shah AA, Sitapara M, Sjah AV. Laparoscopy in diagnosis of prolonged neonatal jaundice. Indian Pediatr. 2002;39:1138-42.
37. Nose S, Hasegawa T, Soh H, Sasaki T, Kimura T, Fukuzawa M. Laparoscopic cholecystocholangiography as an effective alternative exploratory laparotomy for the differentiation of biliary atresia. Surg Today. 2005;35:925-8.
38. Sokol RJ, Mack C, Narkewicz MR. Pathogenesis and outcome of biliary atresia: recent concepts. J Pediatr Gastoenterol Nutr. 2003;37:4-22.
39. Wong KK, Chung PH, Chan KL, et al. Should open Kasai portoenterostomy be performed for biliary atresia in the era of laparoscopy? Pediatr Surg Int. 2008;24:931-3.
40. Ure BM, Kuebler JF, Schukfeh N, Engelmann C, Dingemann J, Petersen C. Survival with the native liver after laparoscopic versus conventional Kasai portoenterostomy in infants with biliary atresia: a prospective trial. Ann Surg. 2011;253:826-30.
41. Chandrasekheram VV. Surgical treatment of biliary atresia with patent distal extrahepatic bile ducts: is portocholecystostomy the right choice. J Indian Assoc Pediatr Surg. 2009;14:24-6.
42. Zhao R, Li H, Shen C, Xiao X. Hepatic portocholecystostomy (HPC) is ineffective in the treatment of biliary atresia with patent distal extrahepatic bile ducts. J Invest Surg. 2011;24:53-8.
43. Davenport M, Kerkar N, Mieli-Vergani G, Mowat AP, Howard ER. Biliary atresia: the King's College Hospital experience (1974-1995). J Pediatr Surg. 1997;32:479-85.
44. Superina R, Magee JC, Brandt ML, Healey PJ, Tiao G, Ryckman F, et al. The anatomic pattern of biliary atresia identified at time of Kasai hepatoportoenterostomy and early postoperative clearance of jaundice are significant predictors of transplant-free survival. Ann Surg. 2011;254:577-85.
45. Ernst van Heurn LW, Saing H, Tam PK. Cholangitis after hepatic portoenterostomy for biliary atresia: a multivariate analysis of risk factors. J Pediatr. 2003;142:566-71.
46. Ecoffey C, Rothman E, Bernard O, Hadchouel M, Valayer J, Alagille D. Bacterial cholangitis after surgery for biliary atresia. J Pediatr. 1987;111:824-9.
47. Watanabe M, Kaneko TH, Komuro H, Komuro H, Hirai M, Inoue S, et al. Intrahepatic biliary cysts in children with biliary atresia who have had a Kasai operation. J Pediatr Surg. 2007;42:1185-9.
48. Shalaby A, Makin E, Davenport M. Portal venous pressure in biliary atresia. J Pediatr Surg. 2012;47:363-6.
49. Kang N, Davenport M, Driver M, Howard ER. Hepatic histology and the development of esophageal varices in biliary atresia. J Pediatr Surg. 1993;28:63-6.
50. Stringer MD, Howard ER, Mowat AP. Endoscopic sclerotherapy in the management of esophageal varices in 61 children with biliary atresia. J Pediatr Surg. 1989;24:438-42.
51. Duché M, Ducot B, Tournay E, Fabre M, Cohen J, Jacquemin E, et al. Prognostic value of endoscopy in children with biliary atresia at risk for early development of varices and bleeding. Gastroenterology. 2010;139:1952-60.
52. Eroglu Y, Emerick KM, Whitingon PF, Alonso EM. Octreotide therapy for control of acute gastrointestinal bleeding in children. J Pediatr Gastroenterol Nutr. 2004;38:41-7.
53. Sökücü S, Süoglu OD, Elkabes B, Saner G. Long-term outcome after sclerotherapy with or without a beta-blocker for variceal bleeding in children. Pediatr Int. 2003;45:388-94.

54. Ohi R, Mochizuki I, Komatsu K, Kasai M. Portal hypertension after successful hepatic portoenterostomy in biliary atresia. J Pediatr Surg. 1986;21:271-4.
55. Meyers RL, Book LS, O'Gorman M, Jackson WD, Black RE, Johnson DG, et al. High dose steroids, ursodeoxycholic acid and chronic intravenous antibiotics improve bile flow after Kasai procedure in infants with biliary atresia. J Pediatr Surg. 2004;38:406-11.
56. Petersen C, Harder D, Melter M, Becker T, Wasielewski RV, Leonhardt J, et al. Postoperative high-dose steroids do not improve mid-term survival with native liver in biliary atresia. Am J Gastroenterol. 2008;103:712-9.
57. Sarkhy A, Schreiber RA, Milner RA, Barker CC. Does adjuvant steroid therapy post-Kasai portoenterostomy improve outcome of biliary atresia? Systematic review and meta-analysis. Can J Gastroenterol. 2011;25:440-4.
58. A-Kader HH, Santangelo JD, Setchell KDR, et al. The effects of ursodeoxycholic acid therapy in biliary atresia: a double blind, randomized, placebo controlled trial. Pediatr Res. 1993;33:97A.
59. Willot S, Uhlen S, Michaud L, Briand G, Bonnevalle M, Sfeir R, et al. Effect of ursodeoxycholic acid on liver function in children after successful surgery for biliary atresia. Pediatrics. 2008;122:e1236-41.
60. Mohanty MK, Gupta SD, Bhatnagar V. Surgical outcome in relation to duct size at porta hepatis and the use of cholagouges in patients with biliary atresia. Trop Gastroenterol. 2010;31:184-9.
61. Shah I, Bhatnagar S. Biliary atresia any cytomegalovirus and response to valganciclovir. Indian Pediatr. 2012;49:484-6.
62. Schneider BL, Mazariegos GV. Biliary atresia: a transplant perspective. Liver Transpl. 2007;13:1482-95.
63. Diamond IR, Fecteau A, Millis JM, Losanoff JE, Ng V, Anand R, et al. Impact of graft type on outcome in pediatric liver transplantation. Ann Surg. 2007;246:301-10.
64. Anderson CD, Turmelle YP, Lowell JA, Nadler M, Millis M, Anand R, et al. The effect of recipient-specific surgical issues on outcome of liver transplantation in biliary atresia. Am J Transpl. 2008;8:1-8.
65. Rao S, D'cruz AL, Aggarwal R, Chandrashekhar S, Chetan G, Gopalkrishnan G, et al. Pediatric liver transplantation: a report from a pediatric surgical unit. J Indian Assoc Pediatr Surg. 2011;16:2-7.
66. Serinet M-O, Wildhaber BE, Broué P, Lachaux A, Sarles J, Jacquemin E, et al. Impact of age at Kasai operation on its results in late childhood and adolescence: a rational basis for biliary atresia screening. Pediatrics. 2009;123:1280-6.
67. Makin E, Quaglia A, Kvist N, Petersen BL, Portmann B, Davenport M. Congenital biliary atresia: liver injury begins at birth. J Pediatr Surg. 2009;44:630-3.
68. Davenport M, Caponcelli E, Livesey E, Hadzic N, Howard E. Surgical outcome in biliary atresia: etiology affects the influence of age at surgery. Ann Surg. 2008;247:694-8.
69. Sanghai SR, Shah I, Bhatnagar S, Murthy A. Incidence and prognostic factors associated with biliary atresia in western India. Ann Hepatol. 2009;8:120-2.
70. Davenport M, Howard ER. Macroscopic appearance at portoenterostomy—a prognostic variable in biliary atresia. J Pediatr Surg. 1996;31:1387-90.
71. Howard ER, Driver M, McClement J, Mowat AP. Results of surgery in 88 consecutive cases of extrahepatic biliary atresia. J R Soc Med. 1982;75:408-13.
72. Tan CE, Davenport M, Driver M, Howard ER. Does the morphology of the extrahepatic biliary remnants in biliary atresia influence survival? A review of 205 cases. J Pediatr Surg. 1994;29:1459-64.
73. Pape L, Olsson K, Petersen C, von Wasilewski R, Melter M. Prognostic value of computerized quantification of liver fibrosis in children with biliary atresia. Liver Transpl. 2009;15:876-82.
74. Gupta L, Gupta SD, Bhatnagar V. Extrahepatic biliary atresia: correlation of histopathology and liver function tests with surgical outcomes. J Indian Assoc Pediatr Surg. 2012;17:147-52.
75. Roy P, Chatterjee U, Ganguli M, Banerjee S, Chatterjee SK, Basu AK. A histopathological study of liver and biliary remnants with clinical outcome in cases of extrahepatic biliary atresia. Indian J Pathol Microbiol. 2010;53:101-5.
76. Agarwal GS, Saxena A, Bhatnagar V. The development of intrapulmonary arteriovenous shunts as a poor prognostic factor following surgery for biliary atresia. Trop Gastroenterol. 2009;30:110-2.
77. Agarwal GS, Sharma R, Bhatnagar V. Assessment of latent manganese toxicity as a prognostic factor following surgery for biliary atresia. Eur J Pediatr Surg. 2008;18:22-5.
78. Lampela H, Ritvanen A, Kosola S, Koivusalo A, Rintala R, Jalanko H, et al. National centralization of biliary atresia care to an assigned multidisciplinary team provides high-quality outcomes. Scand J Gastroenterol. 2012;47:99-107.
79. Kvist N, Davenport M. Thirty-four years' experience with biliary atresia in Denmark: a single center study. Eur J Pediatr Surg. 2011;21:224-8.
80. Superina R, Magee JC, Brandt ML, Healey PJ, Tiao G, Ryckman F, et al. The anatomic pattern of biliary atresia identified at time of Kasai hepatoportoenterostomy and early postoperative clearance of jaundice are significant predictors of transplant-free survival. Ann Surg. 2011;254:577-85.
81. Serinet MO, Broué P, Jacquemin E, Lachaux A, Sarles J, Gottrand F, et al. Management of patients with biliary atresia in France: results of a decentralized policy 1986-2002. Hepatology. 2006;44:75-84.
82. Schreiber RA, Barker CC, Roberts EA, Martin SR, Alvarez F, Smith L, et al. Biliary atresia: the Canadian experience. J Pediatr. 2007;151:659-65.
83. Ohi R. Biliary atresia: long-term results of hepatic portoenterostomy. In: Howard ER (Ed). Surgery of Liver Disease in Childhood. London: Butterworth-Heinemann; 1991. pp. 60-71.
84. Davenport M, Ong E, Sharif K, McClean P, Hadzic N, Kelly DA. Biliary atresia in England and Wales: results of centralization and new benchmark. J Pediatr Surg. 2011;46:1689-94.
85. Pakarinen MP, Lampela H, Gylling H, Miettinen TA, Koivusalo AI, Nissinen MJ. Surrogate markers of cholesterol metabolism in children with native liver after successful portoenterostomy for biliary atresia. J Pediatr Surg. 2010;45:1659-64.
86. Huang HP, Chang MH, Chen YT, Hsu HY, Chiang CL, Cheng TS, et al. Persistent elevation of hepatocyte growth factor activator inhibitors in cholangiopathies affects liver fibrosis and differentiation. Hepatology. 2012;55:161-72.
87. Khan AA, Parveen N, Mahaboob VS, Rajendra Prasad A, Ravindra Prakash HR, Venkateswarlu J, et al. Management of hyperbilirubinemia in biliary atresia by hepatic progenitor cell transplantation through hepatic artery: a case report. Transplant Proc. 2008;40:1153-5.
88. Sharma S, Kumar L, Mohanty S, Kumar R, Datta Gupta S, Gupta DK. Bone marrow mononuclear stem cell infusion improves biochemical parameters and scintigraphy in infants with biliary atresia. Pediatr Surg Int. 2011;27:81-9.
89. Raveenthiran V. Long-term survival of biliary atresia without any surgery: lessons learnt from lamprey. J Neonat Surg. 2014;3:19.

CHAPTER 56

Choledochal Cysts

Sundeep Singh Saluja, Mohammed Nayeem, Vaibhav Varshney

INTRODUCTION

Choledochal cysts (CDCs), more appropriately called bile duct cysts, encompass a group of diseases manifested by cystic dilatation of the biliary ductal system, which may be extrahepatic, intrahepatic or both.

DEMOGRAPHICS

Bile duct cysts account for approximately 1% of all benign biliary disease.[1] The reported clinical incidence ranges from 1 in 13,000 to 1 in 2 million patients.[2] CDCs may be symptomatic at any age. About 25% of cases are diagnosed during infancy and 60% before the age of 10 years.[3] Ten percent of CDCs are found in patients over the age of 40 years.

Choledochal cysts of the same type in family members have been reported but no hereditary pattern or genetic predisposition has been found. CDC is more common in orient particularly Japan. CDCs with exception of choledochoceles are four times more common in females.[4] The significance of the predilection for females is unclear, although sex hormones have never been implicated.

Choledochal cysts may be associated with other anomalies of the biliary tree, including biliary atresia, gall bladder duplication, accessory hepatic ducts or congenital hepatic fibrosis. Hypoplastic or polycystic kidneys may also be rarely found.

CLINICAL FEATURES

Choledochal cysts are typically recognized serendipitously in adults during imaging for some unrelated disease process. In symptomatic patients, the types of symptoms are related to the age at presentation and the morphology of the bile duct cyst. Patients with cystic morphology of the CDC present early with symptoms of jaundice or an abdominal lump, whereas those with fusiform dilatation are likely to present with abdominal pain.[5]

Recurrent upper abdominal pain, fever and jaundice are the most common initial symptoms. Nearly in 50% of the patients the symptoms are initially attributed to gallstones, cholecystitis or acid peptic disease and as many as 10–50% may have undergone cholecystectomy or other surgical procedure before a correct diagnosis is made.[6] The mean duration from development of symptoms to diagnosis and treatment in adults (age >16 years) is a considerably long 6 years.[7]

A palpable abdominal lump is rare in adults and if present, malignancy within the cyst must be ruled out. Significant weight loss is also unusual, and if present a majority of patients (70%), will have an associated malignancy.

Infants characteristically present with obstructive jaundice (70%) either with or without abdominal pain. Vomiting, abdominal mass and failure to thrive may also be present. Older children present more often with abdominal pain. The classic oft quoted triad of jaundice, pain and an abdominal mass is found in approximately one-third of children and only in 5–10% of adults.

CLASSIFICATION

Alonso-Lej[8] and colleagues (1959) first proposed the classification of extrahepatic bile duct cysts into three types:

Type I: A fusiform or saccular dilation of the common hepatic or common bile duct (CBD),

Type II: A supraduodenal diverticulum of the common hepatic or bile duct, and

Type III: An intraduodenal diverticulum of the distal common bile duct also known as choledochocele.

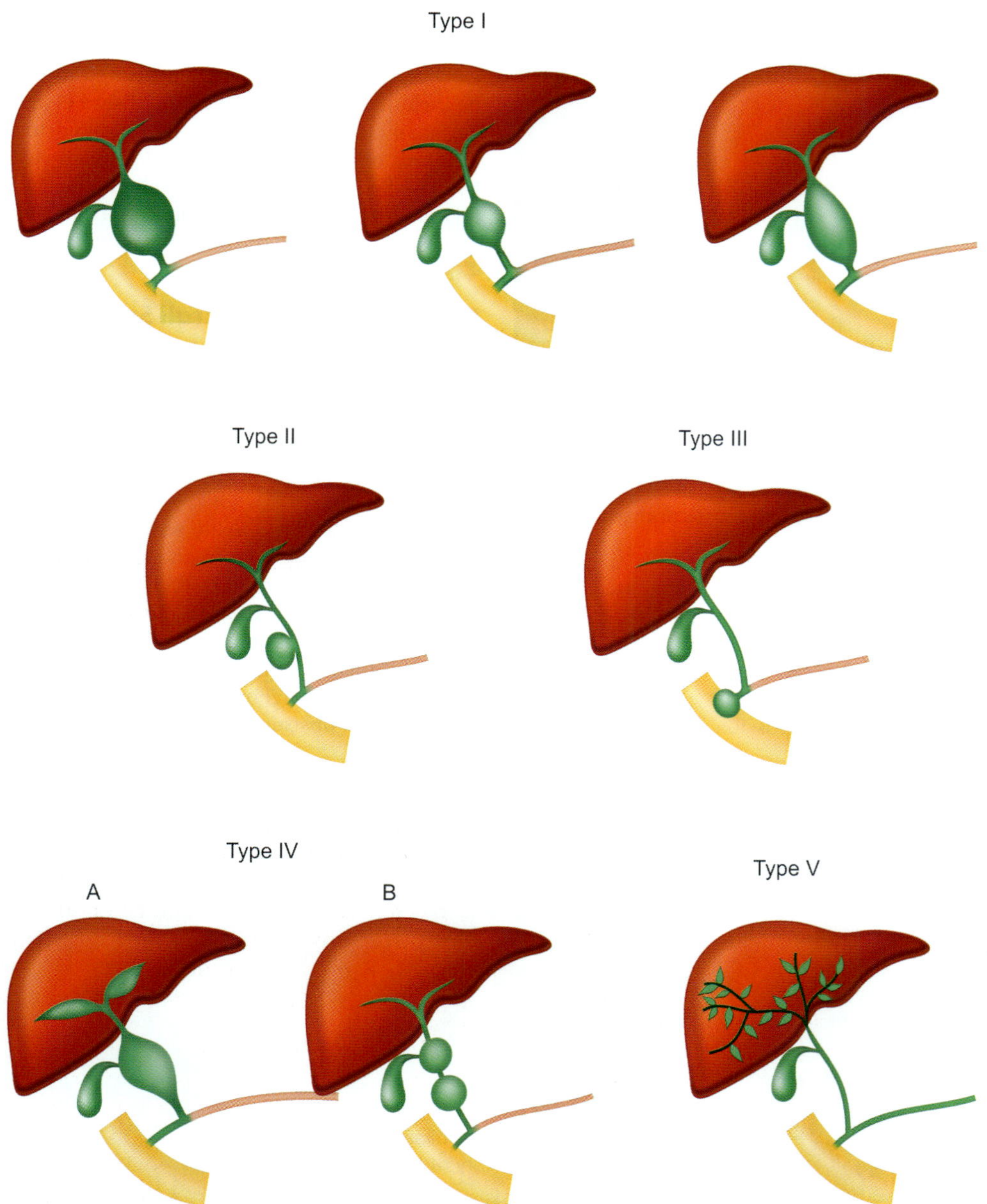

Figure 1 Schematic diagram showing Todani's classification of choledochal cyst

Caroli[9] (1958) and colleagues described a syndrome of multiple intrahepatic bile duct cysts both in the absence and presence of extrahepatic cysts. Todani[10] et al. (1977) modified the original Alonso-Lej classification system by recognizing and including the intrahepatic cyst variants (Type IV-A, B and Type V cysts) (Fig. 1).

Type IVA cysts are multiple intrahepatic and extrahepatic dilatations.

Type IVB cysts refer to multiple dilatations of the extrahepatic biliary tree only, described radiologically as a string of beads or bunch of grapes appearance.

Intrahepatic dilatation which resolves after excision of an extrahepatic bile duct cyst (Type I) must be distinguished from true cystic dilatation of the intrahepatic ducts (Type IV) which tends to persist.[11] The treatment of bile duct cysts is dictated by the location of the cyst and not its configuration; therefore, the more detailed classification schemes proposed have found little favor and are not in use.

The frequency of bile duct cysts is Type I CDC (79%), followed by Type IV (13%), then Type III, or choledochocele (4%), Type II (2.6%) and Type V or Caroli disease (<1%). The distribution of cyst types is similar in adults and children, except that more Type IV cysts are seen in adults leading to speculation that the cysts may not be congenital always but may also develop later in life.

Visser[11] and colleagues have suggested that the classification by Todani is inaccurate. They classified cysts based on histologic

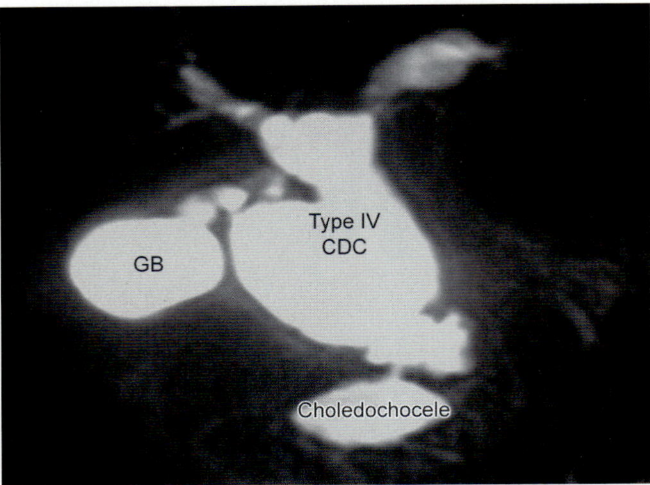

Figure 2 MRCP image of mixed variety of choledochal cyst

findings that Type I cysts contain no biliary mucosa, Type II lesions closely resemble duplication cysts, Type III cysts are lined by duodenal mucosa, and Type V lesions or Caroli's disease are associated with hepatic fibrosis.

They state that Todani's classification grouped together separate disease entities, marked by possible differing etiologies, surgical options and complication profiles. They postulate that the rare Caroli disease (Type V), choledochoceles (Type III) and CBD diverticula (Type II) are unrelated to CDCs and should not be included in the classification. Mishra et al. also suggested that Todani's classification could be modified to include increasing numbers of variations in the CDC. Mixed variants (Fig. 2) could be classified as Type VI CDC while cystic duct dilatation can be included in Type II. This would help in comparing the results across the board and provide new solutions.[12]

Caroli Disease and Caroli Syndrome

The term *Caroli disease* has been broadly applied to describe any patient with multiple intrahepatic bile duct cysts, regardless of the presence of extrahepatic bile duct cysts. Caroli disease (Figs. 3A and B) is characterized by saccular dilation of the intrahepatic bile ducts and may be associated with renal tubular disorder and/or pancreatic cysts.

Caroli syndrome, usually seen in children, is inherited in an autosomal recessive pattern and is more common than the Caroli disease. It is characterized by dilation of the intrahepatic bile ducts, periportal fibrosis leading to cirrhosis, and portal hypertension (PHT). The "central dot sign" seen on ultrasound and CT/MR is a dilated duct surrounding a portal bundle and is characteristic although not pathognomonic of Caroli disease as it may also be seen in biliary obstruction.

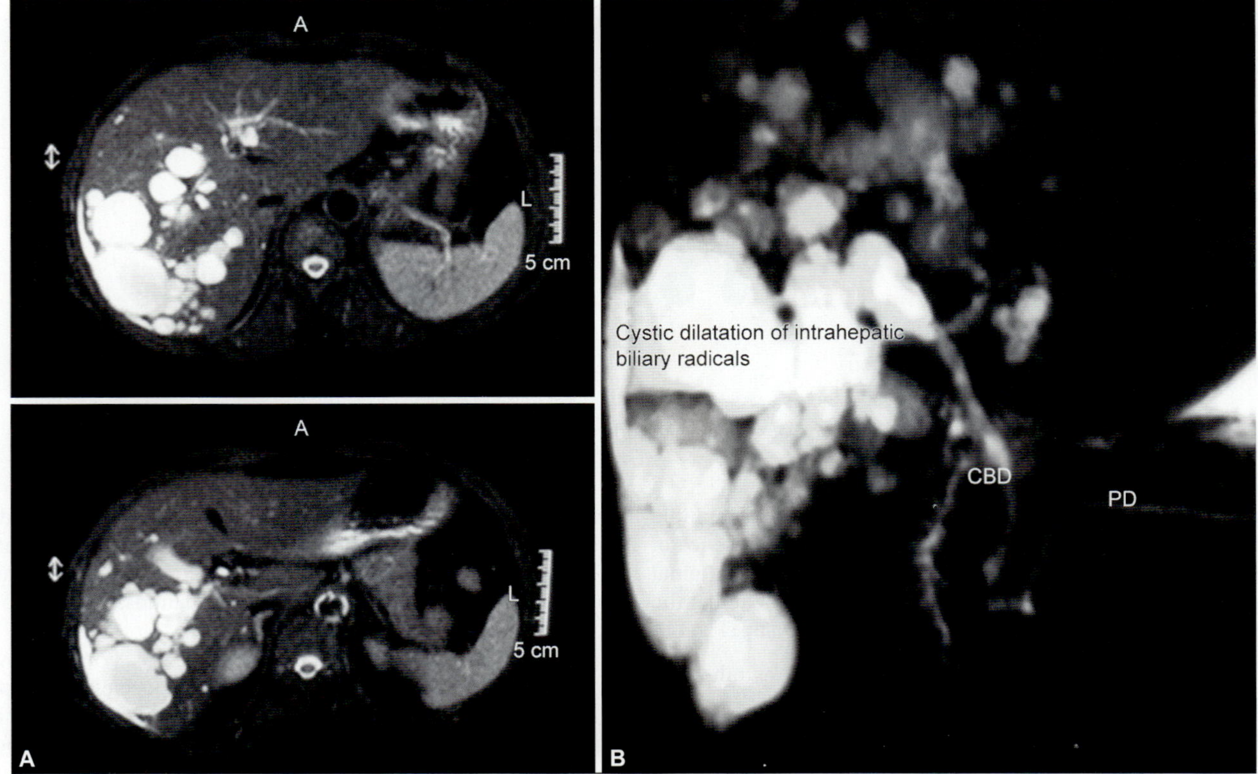

Figures 3A and B (A) Axial section of contrast enhanced CT scan showing cystic dilatation of intrahepatic biliary radicals suggestive of Caroli disease; (B) MRCP image showing cystic dilatation of bilateral intrahepatic radicals with normal common bile duct suggestive of Caroli's disease

PATHOPHYSIOLOGY

The most favored and widely accepted hypothesis of the origin of bile duct cysts is the long common channel theory (Babbitt).[13] An anomalous pancreaticobiliary ductal junction (APBDJ) wherein the terminal common bile duct and the pancreatic duct unite well outside the duodenal wall, creating a long common channel (defined as >10 mm in children and >15 mm in adults) is frequently associated with the CDCs. APBDJ being not surrounded by the normal sphincter mechanism, encourages reflux of pancreatic juice (which is at a higher pressure 30–50 cm H_2O) into the biliary tree (resting pressure 25–30 cm H_2O) leading to inflammation, ectasia and, ultimately, to dilation.

This theory although confirmed in various experimental studies, cannot be responsible for the cystic dilatation alone as an APBDJ is detected in only 57–96% of patients.[14] The role of other factors postulated in the pathogenesis include, obstructed CBD, dysmotility of the sphincter of Oddi, oligoganglionosis of the distal CBD producing a functional obstruction and proximal dilatation analogous to achalasia or to Hirschsprung's disease.

Kimura has divided APBDJ into two types which are clinically relevant for the surgeon. In the first type, the main pancreatic duct joins the common bile-duct just below the site of cystic dilatation. In the second type, the distal narrow end of the CDC joins the main pancreatic duct (Fig. 4).[15] It is important to recognize this anatomic variation of the pancreaticobiliary ductal junction to avoid damage to the pancreatic duct during cyst excision.

Komi et al.[16] gave another classification for APBDJ based on angle of union of CBD and pancreatic duct (Fig. 5).

Type I: The ducts join each other at a right angle:
- IA without dilatation of common channel
- IB with dilatation of common channel

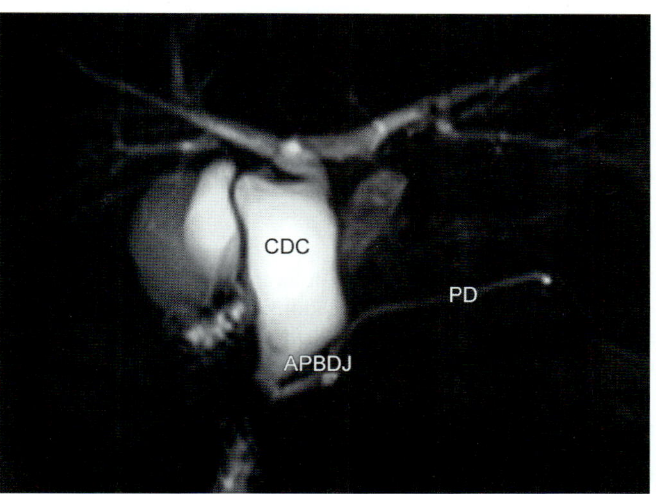

Figure 4 MIP image of MRCP showing Type IV choledochal cyst with BP type of APBDJ according to Kimura classification

Type II: The ducts join each other at an acute angle:
- IIA without dilatation of common channel
- IIB with dilatation of common channel

Type III: Comprises of a complex pattern of accessory pancreatic ducts with or without intricate duct networks:
- IIIA classic pancreas divisum with biliary dilation
- IIIB is characterized by the absence of the Wirsung's duct
- IIIC1 tiny communication exists between the main duct and the accessory duct

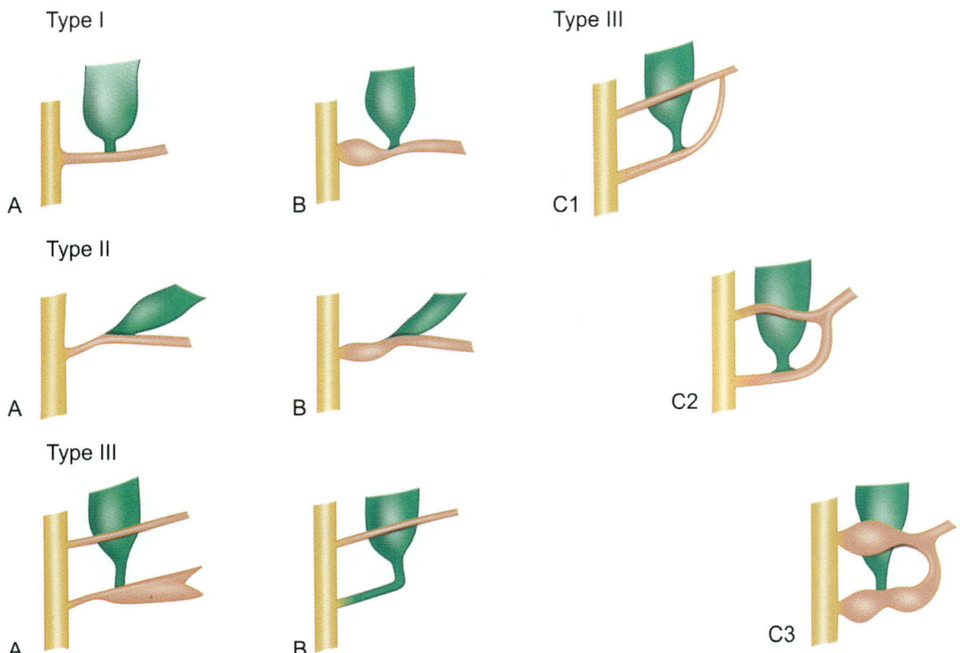

Figure 5 Schematic diagram showing types of abnormal pancreatic biliary duct junction (APBDJ) according to Komi's classification

- IIIC2 comprises of common channel made up of common and accessory duct of equal caliber
- IIIC3 total or partial dilatation of the ductal system.

They suggested that patients with dilated common channel (IB, IIB, IIIC3) can have relapsing pancreatitis leading to chronic pancreatitis due to formation of protein plug after CDC excision.

COMPLICATIONS

In contrast to children, CDCs in adults are associated with a higher incidence of cyst related complications. These include cystolithiasis, hepaticolithiasis, cholangitis, pancreatitis, malignancy and cirrhosis with PHT.

Cystolithiasis

Cystolithiasis is the most frequent complication of bile duct cysts, found in up to 70% of adults. This is in contrast to the low prevalence of cystolithiasis in children. Most intracystic stones are soft, earthy, and brown in appearance secondary to long standing bile stasis. Hepatolithiasis usually occurs with Type IV bile duct cysts or due to stricture of the previous cyst-enteric anastomosis. Membranous or septal stenosis of the major lobar bile ducts is usually present at the confluence of Type IV cysts and must be excluded in all patients with hepatolithiasis (Fig. 6).

Pancreatitis

Clinical acute pancreatitis is present in nearly 30% of patients with CDCs.[17] It is usually acute, mild and often relapsing. The risk of pancreatitis has been directly related to cyst size and presence of an APBDJ (90% in patients with cysts of 5 cm or larger versus 9% in those with smaller cysts).[18] The other risk factors associated with increased incidence of pancreatitis include long (>21 mm) and wide (>5 mm) common channel, a wide (>2.5 mm) proximal pancreatic duct, presence of filling defects in the common channel and presence of pancreatic duct anomaly (ansa pancreatica type, loop type and divisum type). Some patients with bile duct cysts develop pancreatitis although they have normal pancreaticobiliary anatomy.

Very high amylase levels are usually found in the bile within the cysts. In infants, hyperamylasemia is not seen within the bile owing to pancreatic immaturity. However, biliary concentrations of other pancreatic enzymes lipase, elastase, and trypsin are significantly elevated in infants with CDC.

Most patients with associated pancreatitis improve on conservative management. Subsequently the cyst excision is performed in an elective setting.

Pseudopancreatitis[19]

Pseudopancreatitis also known as biochemical pancreatitis is manifested by only raised serum amylase. It may be found in up to 70% of patients, particularly children and results from either diffusion of pancreatic amylase through the denuded epithelium of the cyst, or from cholangiovenous reflux of amylase-rich fluid by high choledochal pressure.

Chronic Pancreatitis

Chronic pancreatitis associated with bile duct cysts is rare with only a few cases reported in literature.[20] Pancreatic insufficiency seldom occurs. The amalgam of protein plug and pancreatic calculus in the dilated common channel or the pancreatic duct is likely responsible for recurrent bouts of acute pancreatitis, leading to chronic pancreatitis in some patients (Fig. 7). Simultaneous excision of the cyst along with Frey's procedure or longitudinal pancreaticojejunostomy is usually curative in symptomatic patients.[21]

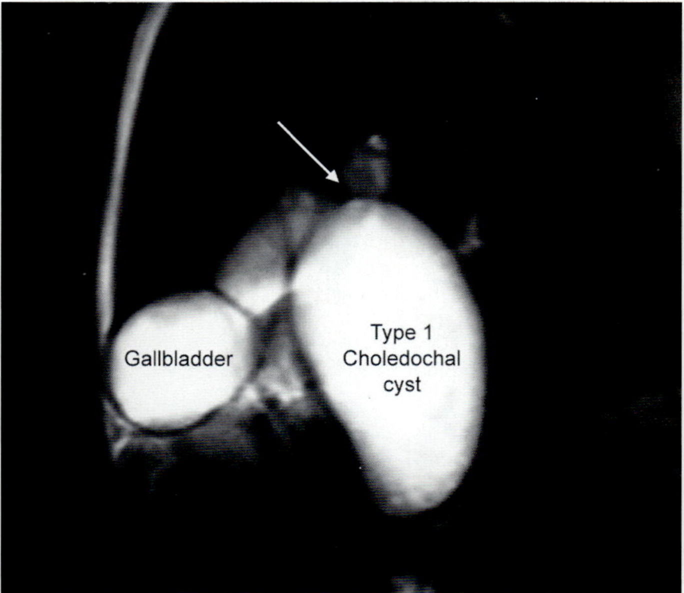

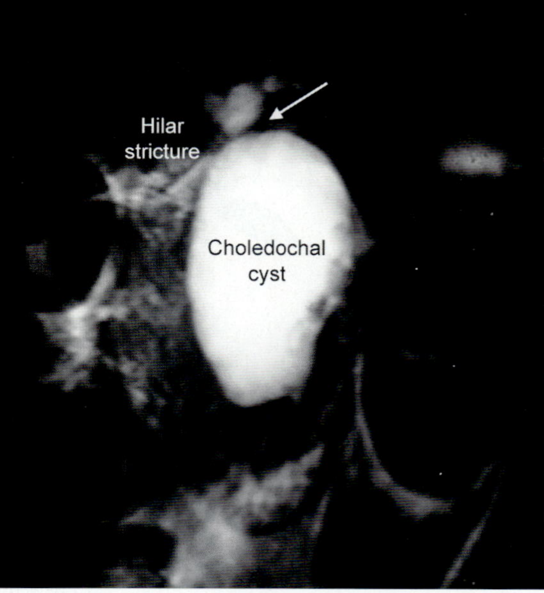

Figure 6 MIP images of MRCP showing choledochal cyst with hilar stricture (arrows)

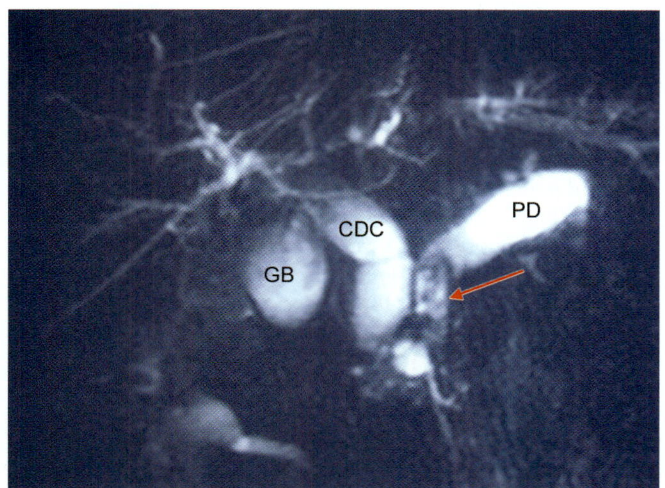

Figure 7 MRCP image showing dilated CBD with minimal intrahepatic dilated radicals and dilated main pancreatic duct along with stones at proximal end suggestive of choledochal cyst with chronic pancreatitis

Cholangitis and Intrahepatic Abscesses

Solitary large intrahepatic abscess may result from recurrent cholangitis. They occur predominantly in the left lobe of liver and may be related partly to the acute angle made by the left main duct.

Cirrhosis

Nearly 15% of adults with CDCs present with cirrhosis or hepatic fibrosis secondary to chronic biliary obstruction.[22] PHT may result from secondary biliary cirrhosis (SBC) or fibrosis, portal vein thrombosis from local compression of the portal vein by the cyst, or Caroli disease associated congenital hepatic fibrosis.[23] PHT in adults generally is preceded by numerous operations for cyst drainage.[24] Although the pericholedochal tissues are very vascular, hypervascularity is most often limited to the ductal wall and rarely precludes excision.[25] Presence of hepatosplenomeagly, jaundice, hematemesis, malena or ascites should raise the suspicion of PHT in patients with CDC (Fig. 8). The cause responsible for development of PHT determines whether the surgical intervention will be beneficial.

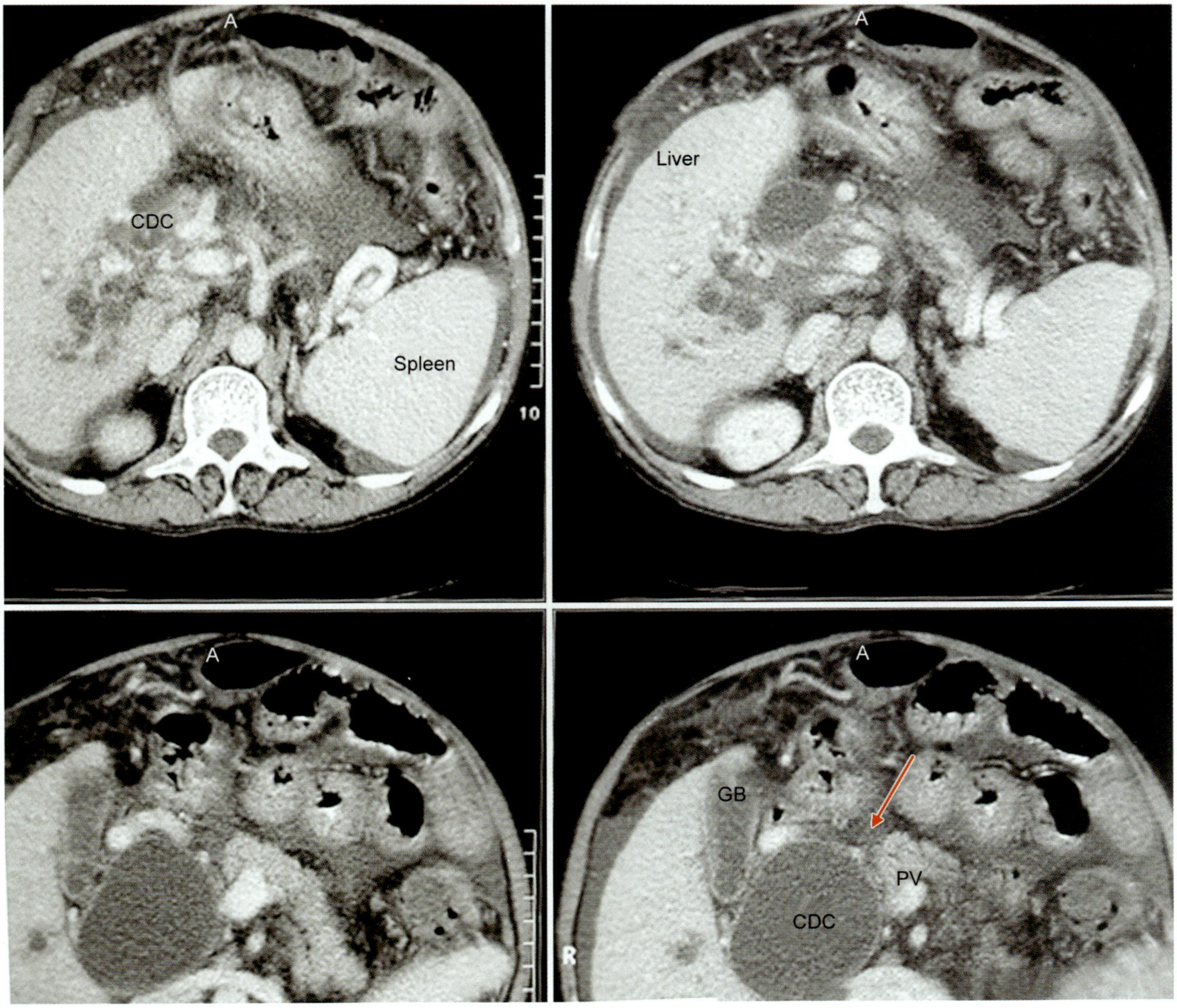

Figure 8 Axial sections of contrast enhanced CT scan showing dilated CBD with dilated portal vein, enlarged spleen and periportal collaterals (red arrow) suggestive of choledochal cyst with portal hypertension

Cyst Perforation

Cyst perforation is a rare complication limited to children up to 4 years of age and pregnant women.[26] Spontaneous perforation may occur in any part of the cyst and may be difficult to differentiate from spontaneous perforation of the bile duct. Perforations may be single or multiple and there is no relationship between the cyst size and rupture. Definitive surgery is usually possible at the time of diagnosis, although temporary external drainage of the cyst is a safer option with delayed surgery once the inflammation has subsided.[27]

Malignancy

Kasai[28] was the first to report the increased incidence of bile duct carcinoma arising in bile duct cysts and proposed surgical excision. The diagnosis of malignancy arising in a CDC is often delayed. All symptoms are usually attributed to CDC until the patient develops significant weight loss. The age related cancer risk has been reported to be 0.7% in the first decade, 7% in the second decade and 14% after 20 years of age.[29]

The mean age[30] of patients with cancer associated with bile duct cysts is 32 years, which is about two decades earlier than the general population. Malignancy arising in a bile duct cyst has also been reported in children and therefore early diagnosis and treatment is essential. Malignancies may be associated with any type of CDC, although the incidence is higher in Types I, IV and V cysts. In Type I cystic dilatations the malignancy often develops in the cyst wall, whereas in Type I fusiform dilatations the gall bladder is the most common site.

Malignancies commonly associated with CDCs include cholangiocarcinoma, adenocarcinoma, squamous cell carcinoma, gall bladder carcinoma, hepatocellular carcinoma and pancreatic carcinoma. Indeed, only 57% of tumors are intracystic.[31] Tumors are most frequently found in the posterior wall of CDCs. Cholangiocarcinoma is the most common malignancy associated with bile duct cysts, and its incidence is approximately 20 times greater than the incidence of bile duct carcinoma in the general population.[32]

The prognosis of malignant CDCs when detected at the time of operation is poor. Delay in diagnosis, advanced stage at presentation, tumor multicentricity and intra-abdominal seeding from previous operations preclude curative resection.

The risk of malignancy increases to as high as 50% in patients with a prior internal drainage procedure without cyst excision and occurs at a mean of 10 years postoperatively.[33] It is therefore recommended that any patient who had an internal drainage procedure to treat a CDC or has a residual cyst should have the cyst excised, irrespective of the presence or absence of symptoms.

The incidence of malignancy even after cyst excision has been estimated at 0·7%.[34] Incompletely excised extrahepatic ducts, dilated intrahepatic bile ducts, biliary-enteric anastomosis and the terminal common bile duct have all been affected underscoring the importance of long-term surveillance. Type IVA cysts in particular, owing to the presence of dilated intrahepatic ducts need intense lifelong surveillance

DIFFERENTIAL DIAGNOSIS

Other causes of common bile duct obstruction must be excluded. In infants, cystic form of biliary atresia and CDCs may have similar presentations. Tc[99] hepatobiliary iminodiacetic acid (HIDA) scan is helpful in differentiating biliary atresia from CDC in jaundiced neonates, both of which can present as cyst at the porta. HIDA scan will show emptying of contrast into bowel with CDC, whereas retention of contrast in biliary atresia.

Other abdominal cystic lesions that may mimic CDC in adults include ovarian, mesenteric, hepatic or renal cyst. A hydronephrotic kidney or pancreatic pseudocyst causing obstructive jaundice can also occasionally be confused with a CDC on ultrasound.

Prenatal diagnosis: CDCs can be detected as early as 15 weeks of gestation by an observant sonologist. Most of the CDCs diagnosed intrauterine are found to be Type I variants. Infants with CDC particularly if symptomatic with mass or jaundice should be treated with early surgery (preferably within 3 months).

IMAGING

Ultrasound scan is the preferred initial diagnostic study and will identify a dilated segment of the common bile duct with an abrupt change between the dilated portion and the normal duct. Ultrasound fails to identify choledochoceles because of the small size of these cysts and the bowel gas hampering the view of the terminal common bile duct.

Direct cholangiography in the form of endoscopic retrograde cholangiopancreatography (ERCP) or percutaneous transhepatic cholangiography (PTC) though accurate in defining the type of CDC and the associated APBDJ, is invasive and rarely required. Its therapeutic capability is limited only to choledochoceles. Sometimes the diagnosis of CDC is made in retrospect during ERC extraction of bile duct stones. All such patients who have an ERCP should have a stent placed in the bile duct to prevent post-procedure cholangitis. ERCP may overestimate the size of the duct due to filling of contrast under pressure.

Magnetic resonance cholangiopancreatography (MRCP) is now the accepted "gold standard" for visualizing a bile duct cyst across all age groups and particularly in pregnant women. It is though limited in its ability to clearly define the pancreaticobiliary junction (diagnostic accuracy 69%).

Liver function tests may be deranged, normal or show an isolated rise in alkaline phosphatase. Esophagogastroscopy should be done particularly in adults to look for varices and signs of PHT.

HISTOPATHOLOGY

The wall of the CDC is usually thickened because of recurrent attacks of clinical/subclinical cholangitis. The wall is typically composed of fibrous tissue with few disrupted elastic fibers and attenuated smooth muscle layer. The mucosa of the cyst shows ulcerated cuboidal epithelium. Typical biliary mucosal lining is not seen. The degree of inflammation to the cyst wall is directly correlated with age, as infants and small children rarely have inflammation in the cyst. Liver histology may be normal or show mild periportal fibrosis or sometimes even biliary cirrhosis. The epithelial lining may be ulcerated, or show epithelial metaplasia or dysplasia, especially in long standing cases.

FORME FRUSTE

Mere presence of pancreaticobiliary malunion with minimal or no cystic biliary dilatation has been termed "forme fruste" of CDC (Lilly et al.[35]). The optimal treatment for such cases in adults is controversial ranging from simple cholecystectomy alone to bile duct excision. However, in children the extrahepatic bile duct should probably be excised, because of the risk of malignancy over an extended period of time.

It is important to differentiate patients with dilated CBD from CDC especially when they have normal alkaline phosphatase and CBD diameter is 10–12 mm. More such cases are being reported with advent of MRCP. One needs to consider age of patient, presence of symptoms, past history, presence or absence of ABPDJ and imaging before making a final diagnosis. Past history of pancreatitis or deranged LFT suggestive of passed CBD stone, post cholecystectomy, and presence of perivaterian, viral infection and small periampullary tumour diverticulum in absence of ABPDJ are among important causes for dilated CBD with normal SAP. In patients with raised SAP with dilated CBD definitive cause of obstruction should be considered and investigated accordingly. A subgroup of patients with no such history, normal alkaline phosphatase and mild dilation of CBD without ABPDJ may be labeled as obscure CBD dilatation.

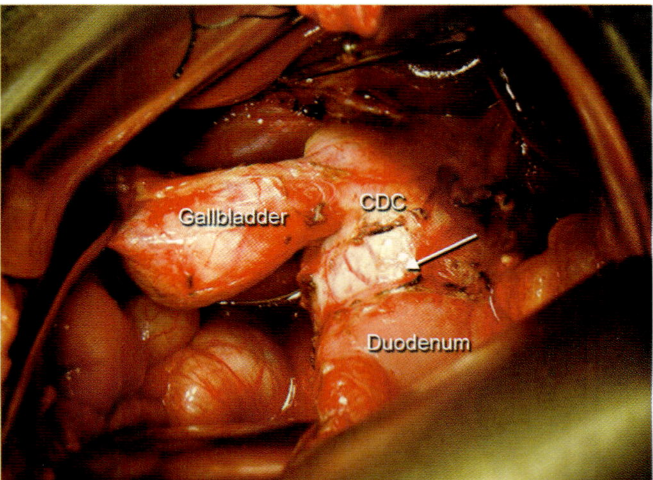

Figure 9 Operative picture showing initial step in cyst excision where lower part of the cyst is being separated from first part of duodenum (arrow)

SURGICAL MANAGEMENT

Golden McWhorter[36] in 1924 performed the first successful complete excision of a CDC and restored biliary continuity using hepaticoduodenostomy.

Factors to consider before surgical treatment of patients with CDC include age, presenting symptoms, cyst type, previous biliary surgery, intrahepatic strictures, hepatic atrophy/hypertrophy complex, biliary cirrhosis, PHT and presence of synchronous biliary malignancy.

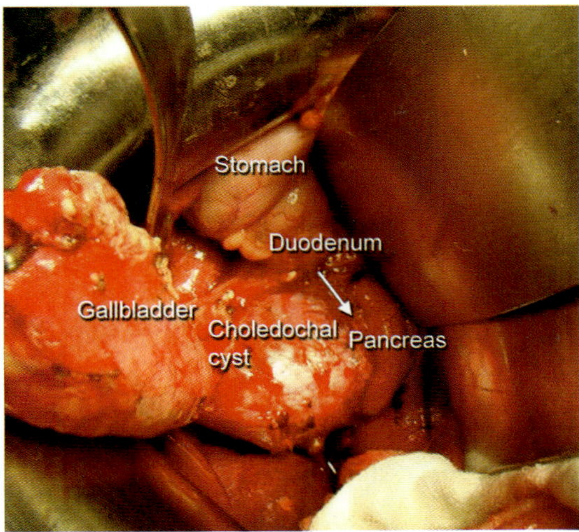

Figure 10 Operative picture showing cyst wall is being separated from pancreatic tissue (arrow) to reach the lower limit

TECHNIQUE

The gall bladder is mobilized from its bed and the cyst dissected away from the hilar structures. A sample of bile is aspirated from the cyst for culture and measurement of pancreatic amylase concentrations and a liver biopsy is taken. Hepatic artery and the portal vein are isolated before dissection of the posterior cyst wall to prevent their injury. While dissecting the lower end of the cyst, first step is to divide peritoneal layer between duodenum and supraduodenal part of cyst (Fig. 9). Next make a plane between intrapancreatic portion of cyst and surrounding pancreatic tissue (Fig. 10). Avoid dissection between duodenal pancreatic grooves which may result in excessive bleeding. The intrapancreatic portion of the cyst is separated from the pancreas dissecting along the loose areolar tissue between these structures. Meanwhile as the dissection is completed the cyst can be looped which helps in further dissection (Figs 11A and B). The cyst is transected distally within the head of the pancreas over sewing the distal common bile duct just above its junction with the pancreatic duct with fine monofilament suture. Once the lower end is divided, cyst is dissected off the surrounding structures in the porta hepatis. The cyst is divided at the level of the common hepatic duct bifurcation and the extrahepatic cyst completely excised. The upper limit is ascertained after dividing the anterior wall of CBD (Fig. 12). This method allows inspection of the hilar confluence from inside to avoid any damage to duct above the confluence. Any dilated proximal intrahepatic ducts or strictures are inspected and cleared of debris. The left hepatic duct is opened, and a wide hilar bilioenteric mucosa-to-mucosa anastomosis is constructed with a Roux loop of jejunum (Figs 13A and B). Ducts, if not repeatedly inflamed, are thin walled. A fine suture like polygalactin 4-0 is used for hepaticojejunostomy. The hepaticojejunostomy stoma is widened by an incision along the lateral wall of the left duct. Ohi et al.[37] recommend the removal of the area of relative stenosis between the common hepatic duct and the intrahepatic bile duct cyst to achieve free drainage of bile from the liver. It is recommended to position the hepatic arteries posterior to the bilioenteric anastomosis to reduce the risk of injury in case of re-exploration.

LILLY TECHNIQUE

Occasionally dense inflammation from previous surgery or cholangitis makes complete excision of the cyst difficult and dangerous. Lilly[38] advocated excising the anterolateral wall of the

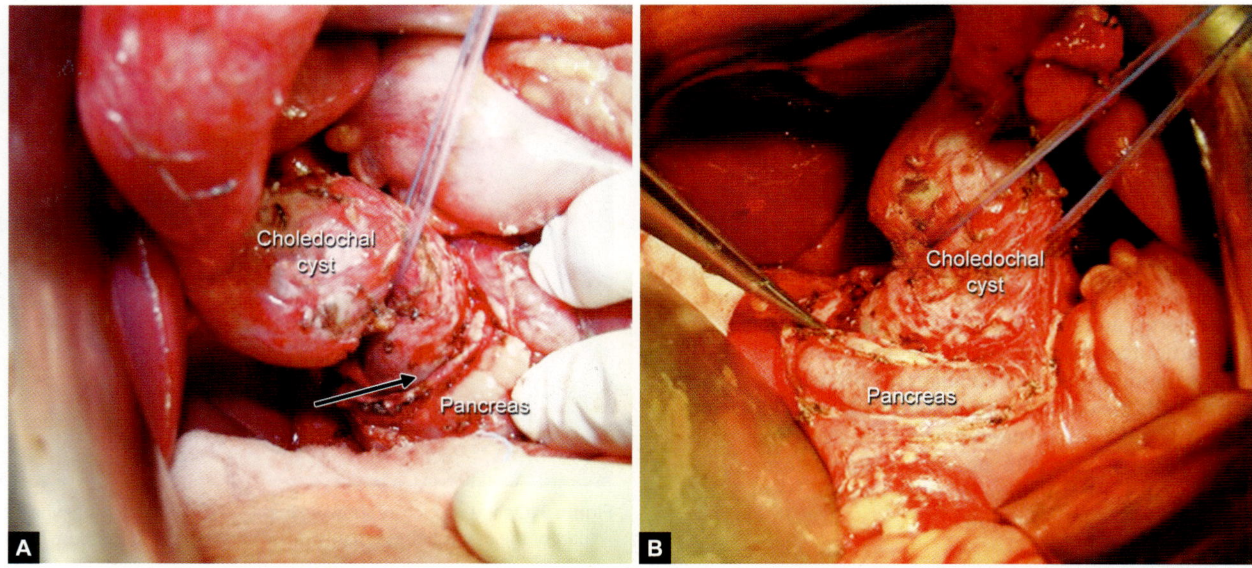

Figures 11A and B (A) Operative picture showing cyst has been looped to facilitate intrapancreatic dissection (black arrow); (B) Operative picture showing near completion of intrapancreatic cyst dissection

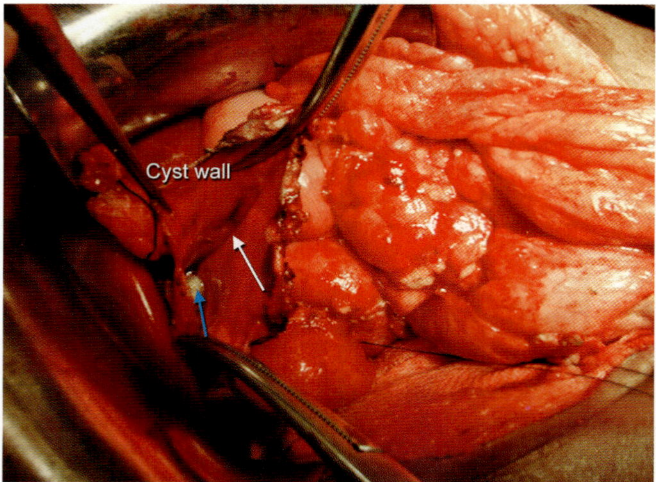

Figure 12 Operative picture showing anterior wall of cyst wall being divided to expose opening of ducts at hepatic hilum (white arrow). Intracystic stone (blue arrow) removed

cyst with excision of only the mucosa of the posteroinferior wall (intramural dissection). It helps to avoid inadvertent damage to the posteriorly placed portal vein and the hepatic arteries which may be adherent due to pericystic inflammation.

BILIARY RECONSTRUCTION (HEPATICOJEJUNOSTOMY VS HEPATICODUODENOSTOMY)

Type I Cysts

Biliary reconstruction following cyst excision with hepaticojejunostomy has been found to be superior to hepaticoduodenostomy, as the incidence of long-term complications is significantly increased with a duodenal anastomosis. Roux-en-Y hepaticojejunostomy is associated with a complication rate of 7% as compared to 42% with hepaticoduodenostomy. Hepaticoduodenostomy carries a higher risk of bile reflux, gastritis, esophagitis and ulceration. Cholangitis is a concern especially in patients with intrahepatic dilated ducts, and hence this procedure is not routine, being performed only in select patients with Type IVA cysts.

Mobility of the duodenum is another limiting factor and restricts its use in some patients particularly in those with complicated cyst. However, reconstruction by hepaticoduodenostomy is more physiologic, avoids complications associated with the Roux-en-Y and allows postoperative endoscopic access to the anastomosis if strictures or stones occur. The residual cyst biliary mucosa is accessible to direct visualization by endoscopy and is helpful in long-term surveillance. The other technical factors influencing the choice of hepaticoenterostomy (Roux-en-Y hepaticojejunostomy vs hepaticoduodenostomy) include aberrant hilar duct and arterial anatomy, duct size and presence of strictures.

Type II Cysts

The preferred surgical approach for Type II cysts is excision of the cyst with preservation of the CBD. The technique involves excision of the cyst and closure of the defect primarily if small or over a T tube if the defect in the neck of the cyst at its junction with the common duct is large. The defect in the CBD is closed transversely and not longitudinally to avoid narrowing of the bile duct lumen. Complete excision has been reported along with hepaticojejunostomy though no potential advantage has been observed over excision alone.

Type III Choledochal Cysts

Type III choledochal cysts are also called choledochoceles owing to similar morphology and postulated etiology to ureteroceles. They are difficult to distinguish from duplication cysts of the duodenum

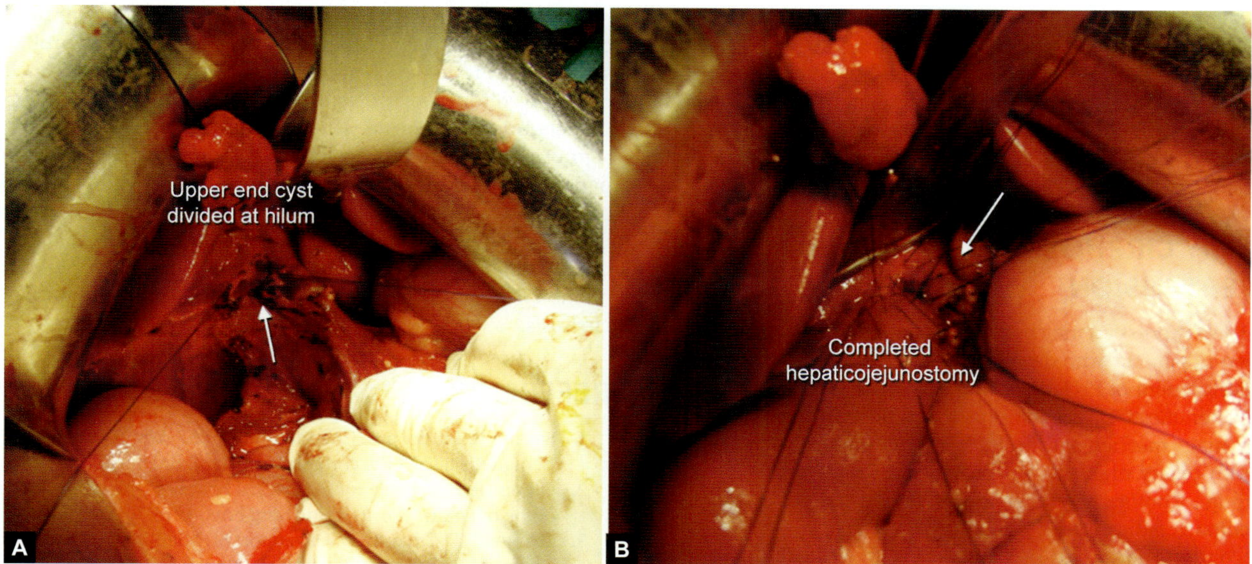

Figures 13A and B (A) Operative picture showing hepatic hilum with opening of right and left hepatic duct (white arrow) after choledochal cyst has been excised; (B) Peroperative picture showing hepatic hilum after hepaticojejunostomy has been performed

unless mucosal lining is histologically examined. Although the outer lining of the cyst is always lined by duodenal mucosa, the inner lining can be either duodenal or biliary epithelium. Duplication cysts may have similar imaging characteristics as choledochoceles and are sometimes very difficult to differentiate. A muscular wall is present in duplication cysts and absent in choledochoceles and is better characterized on endo-ultrasound. Choledochoceles cause obstructive jaundice in one-fourth and pancreatitis in approximately one-third of cases.[39]

These lesions are usually symptomatic, but if asymptomatic it may be justifiable not to operate as it is not certain that the lesion is a choledochocele or a duodenal duplication cyst or some other lesion. Secondly, the mucosal lining of these cysts is usually duodenal and not biliary and as a consequence, carcinoma is exceedingly rare with only three cases reported in literature.[40] The procedure of choice for smaller choledochoceles (<3 cm) is ERCP because endoscopic papillotomy is potentially therapeutic.[41] Transduodenal excision with reimplantation of the CBD and pancreatic duct into the duodenum has been recommended for larger (>3 cm) choledochoceles.[42] Damage to the major pancreatic duct is the major source of operative morbidity and mortality. Identification of the duct of Wirsung is important before transduodenal cyst excision or sphincteroplasty because of numerous pancreatic biliary ductal variations.

Type IV Cysts

For Todani Type IVA CDC, excision with Roux-en-Y hepatico-jejunostomy has been recommended, as for Type I cyst. If intrahepatic cysts are localized to one lobe and the cysts are complicated by stones, strictures or intrahepatic abscesses, the affected lobe should be resected. For Type IVB cysts, excision and reconstruction with a Roux-en-Y hepaticojejunostomy has been practiced. The extrahepatic component of Type IVA and IVB cysts is approached as for a Type I bile duct cyst. Transduodenal sphincteroplasty may be required along with Roux-en-Y hepaticojejunostomy for the treatment of Type IVB cysts, which have a choledochocele component. Any stenosis, membranous or bridge like should be excised circumferentially to their base for Type IVA cysts. Long-term results of the treatment of Type IVB cysts in adults are similar to those of Type I CDCs.

For diffuse complicated intrahepatic cysts involving both lobes of the liver or complicated by cirrhosis, access loop can be added to the Roux-en-Y hepaticojejunostomy for approach to the biliary tree for diagnosis and treatment. Liver transplantation should be considered in such cases and is curative.

Type V Cysts

In Type V, Caroli's disease excision of the cyst is not possible and surgical treatment is not indicated. Ursodiol on a prophylactic basis to reduce biliary sludge, stasis, and cholangitis might be helpful. Any stenosis in the distal bile duct should be dealt with by endoscopic means. Caroli's disease is characterized by recurrent episodes of cholangitis and hospital stays, with a consequent loss of quality of life and productive capacity, often ending in death due to uncontrolled infection. Endoscopic drainage of the bile duct, percutaneously or surgically, is palliative and not a good long-term solution for these patients. Hepatic resection for some unilateral intrahepatic ductal cysts has been therapeutic in some cases when recurrent cholangitis cannot be managed by any other means. Orthotopic liver transplantation is an effective curative option for the treatment of patients with Caroli's disease particularly when complicated with hepatic failure.

LAPAROSCOPIC CHOLEDOCHAL CYST EXCISION

Laparoscopic bile duct cyst excision was first described by Farello et al.[43] in 1995 in a pediatric patient with a Type I CDC. Several case reports and small series have since followed demonstrating feasibility with reasonable outcomes. Palanivelu[44] reported the largest series (35 patients) of laparoscopic treatment of bile duct cysts of which 16 were adults. Conversion rate to open procedure was low and postoperative complications occurred in 14%, with no operative mortality. Laparoscopic excision of CDCs though feasible is technically challenging and should be limited to centers with experience in advanced laparoscopy and hepatobiliary surgery.

BILIARY CIRRHOSIS AND PORTAL HYPERTENSION

Portal decompression may be required not uncommonly before cyst excision in patients who develop PHT. The mechanism responsible for development of PHT determines whether surgical intervention may be beneficial. Direct compression of the portal vein is reported as the main mechanism in children and surgical excision of the cyst with biliary drainage has been shown to reverse PHT in this subgroup. Another cause reported in children is presence of congenital hepatic fibrosis.

Secondary biliary cirrhosis and unrelated cirrhosis are the main reasons responsible for development of PHT in adults. Since there is higher morbidity and mortality after cyst excision in presence of PHT, patients without any evidence of biliary obstruction with definitive evidence of cirrhosis due to other cause can be managed conservatively.

Management of patients with SBC will depend upon the child status, presence of portal vein thrombosis and amount of collaterals around the cyst. Decompression of cyst may prevent further deterioration of liver function and may even improve if not completely reverse the cirrhotic changes.

Surgical decompression appears to be more effective than endoscopic stenting. Endoscopic drainage may have a place as temporizing measure in patients not fit for surgery. Prolonged endoscopic drainage may be associated with complications like stent blockage and require stent change. Therefore patient should be considered for definitive surgical treatment once endoscopic stenting improves the liver function and reduces the surgical risk in these patients. Preoperative preparation includes correction of coagulation status, improvement of albumin level, control of ascites and varices. Although decompression by Roux-en-Y drainage can result in adequate long-term functional result in 60–70% cases, the excision and hepaticojejunostomy remains the treatment of choice.

Portal decompression may be required before biliary reconstruction especially in presence of portal vein thrombosis and collaterals along the hepatoduodenal ligament. On the other hand, shunt may further deteriorate the liver function by diverting the portal flow especially in child C status. Liver transplantation should be offered to patients with Child C cirrhosis.[24] TIPS may be used for portal decompression and the cyst excision can be undertaken 4–6 weeks after portosystemic shunting. For patients with Caroli disease and PHT liver transplantation is indicated though cyst drainage or partial liver resection with or without TIPS may provide temporary relief.

FOLLOW-UP

Although all patients with biliary cysts require lifelong follow-up, those with Type IV cysts in which cyst parts that have not been removed fully and those with an APBDJ should be subjected to more intense long-term surveillance.

Postoperatively, patients have problems mainly with recurrent cholangitis. There is a small but definite potential problem of stenosis of the hepaticojejunostomy, and these patients should be followed for life with serial liver function tests and abdominal ultrasound. Elevation of alkaline phosphatase may be the only sign of partial biliary obstruction in an otherwise asymptomatic patient. Mild increase in alkaline phosphatase with no significant biliary ductal dilatation on imaging may be closely followed. Significant rise in liver enzymes particularly in presence of any ductal dilatation would require percutaneous or endoscopic dilation of the anastomosis or reoperation to prevent future biliary cirrhosis.

REFERENCES

1. Saxena R, Pradeep R, Chander J, Kumar P, Wig JD, Yadav RV, et al. Benign disease of the common bile duct. Br J Surg. 1988;75:803-6.
2. Olbourne NA. Choledochal cysts: a review of the cystic anomalies of the biliary tree. Ann R Coll Surg Engl. 1975;56:26-32.
3. Stringer MD, Dhawan A, Davenport M, Mieli-Vergani G, Mowat AP, Howard ER. Choledochal cysts: lessons from a 20 year experience. Arch Dis Child. 1995;73:528-31
4. Stain SC, Guthrie CR, Yellin AE, Donovan AJ. Choledochal cyst in the adult. Ann Surg. 1995;222:128-33.
5. Miyano T, Yamataka A. Choledochal cysts. Curr Opin Pediatr. 1997;9:283-8.
6. Gigot J, Nagorney D, Farnell M, Moir C, Ilstrup D. Bile duct cysts: a changing spectrum of disease. J Hepatobiliary Pancreat Surg. 1996;3:405-11.
7. Lipsett PA, Pitt HA, Colombani PM, Boitnott JK, Cameron JL. Choledochal cyst disease. A changing pattern of presentation. Ann Surg. 1994;220:644-52.
8. Alonso-Lej F, Rever WB, Pessagno DJ. Congenital choledochal cysts, with a report of 2, and an analysis of 94 cases. Int Abstr Surg. 1959;108:1-30.
9. Caroli J, Soupault R, Kossakowski J, Plocker L, Paradowska. La dilatation polykisliquecongenitale des voiesbiliariesintrahepatiques. Essai de classification. Semnares des Hopitaux de Paris. 1958;34: 488-95.
10. Todani T, Watanabe Y, Narusue M, Tabuchi K, Okajima K. Congenital bile duct cysts: classifications, operative procedures, and review of thirty-seven cases including cancer arising from choledochal cyst. Am J Surg. 1977;134:263-9.
11. Visser BC, Suh I, Way LW, Kang SM. Congenital choledochal cysts in adults. Arch Surg. 2004;139:855-60.
12. Mishra PK, Ramaswamy D, Saluja SS, Patil N, Chandrashekhar S. Unusual variants of choledochal cyst: how to classify. Am Surg. 2013;79(4):E162-4.
13. Babbitt DP. Congenital choledochal cysts: new etiological concept based on anomalous relationships of common bile duct and pancreatic bulb. Annal Radiol (Paris). 1969;12:231-40.
14. Iwai N, Tokiwa K, Tsuto T, Yanagihara J, Takahashi T. Biliary manometry in choledochal cyst with abnormal choledocho-pancreatico ductal junction. J Pediatr Surg. 1986;21:873-6.
15. Kimura K. Studies in 28 cases of congenital cystic dilatation of the common bile duct in adults: roentgenological features and a union between the choledochus and the main pancreatic duct. Jpn J Gastroenterol. 1976;71:401-14.
16. Komi N, Takehara H, Kunitomo K, Miyoshi Y, Yagi T. Does the type of anomalous arrangement of pancreaticobiliary ducts influence the surgery and prognosis of choledochal cyst? J Pediatr Surg. 1992;27(6):728-31.
17. Nagorney DM, McIlrath DC, Adson MA. Choledochal cysts in adults: clinical management. Surgery. 1984;96:656-63.

18. Swisher SG, Cates JA, Hunt KK, Robert ME, Bennion RS, Thompson JE, et al. Pancreatitis associated with adult choledochal cysts. Pancreas. 1994;9:633-7.
19. Todani T, Urushihara N, Watanabe Y, Toki A, Uemura S, Sato Y, et al. Pseudopancreatitis in choledochal cyst in children: intraoperative study of amylase levels in the serum. J Pediatr Surg. 1990;25:303-6.
20. Saluja SS, Nayeem M, Sharma BC, Mishra PK. Management of choledochal cysts and their complications. Am Surg. 2012;78(3):284-90.
21. Saluja SS, Mishra PK, Nayeem M, Nag HH. Choledochal cyst with chronic pancreatitis: presentation and management. JOP. 2010;11(6):601-3.
22. Nicholl M, Pitt HA, Wolf P, Cooney J, Kalayoglu M, Shilyansky J, et al. Choledochal cysts in western adults: complexities compared to children. J Gastrointest Surg. 2004;8:245-52.
23. Martin LW, Rowe GA. Portal hypertension secondary to choledochal cyst. Ann Surg. 1979;190:638-9.
24. Chaudhary A, Dhar P, Sachdev A. Reoperative surgery for choledochal cysts. Br J Surg. 1997;84:781-4.
25. Saluja SS, Mishra PK, Sharma BC, Narang P. Management of choledochal cyst with portal hypertension. Singapore Med J. 2011;52(12)e239-43.
26. Bostanoglu S, Besim H, Erverdi N, Korkmaz A. Ruptured choledochal cyst. HPB Surg. 2000;2:57-9.
27. Hewitt PM, Kriege JE, Bornman PC, Terblanche J. Choledochal cyst in pregnancy: a therapeutic dilemma. J Am CollSurg. 1995;181: 237-40.
28. Kasai M, Asakura Y, Taira Y. Surgical treatment of choledochal cyst. Ann Surg. 1970;172(5):844-51.
29. Voyles CR, Smadja C, Shands WC, Blumgart LH. Carcinoma in choledochal cysts. Age-related incidence. Arch Surg. 1983;118: 986-8.
30. Ono J, Sakoda K, Akita H. Surgical aspect of cystic dilatation of the bile duct: an anomalous junction of the pancreaticobiliary tract in adults. Ann Surg. 1982;195:203-8.
31. Flanigan DP. Biliary carcinoma associated with biliary cysts. Cancer. 1977;40:880-3.
32. Flanigan DP. Biliary cysts. Ann Surg. 1975;182:635-43.
33. Goto N, Yasuda I, Uematsu T, Kanemura N, Takao S, Ando K, et al. Intrahepatic cholangiocarcinoma arising 10 years after the excision of congenital extrahepatic biliary dilation. J Gastroenterol. 2001;36:856-62.
34. Watanabe Y, Toki A, Todani T. Bile duct cancer developed after cyst excision for choledochal cyst. J Hepatobiliary Pancreat Surg. 1999;6:207-12.
35. Lilly JR, Stellin GP, Karrer FM. Formefruste choledochal cyst. J Pediatr Surg. 1985;20:449-51.
36. McWhorter GL. Congenital cystic dilatation of the common bile duct. Report of a case, with cure. Archives of Surgery. 1924;8: 604-26.
37. Ohi R, Yaoita S, Kamiyama T, Ibrahim M, Hayashi Y, Chiba T. Surgical treatment of congenital dilatation of the bile duct with special reference to late complications after total excisional operation. J Pediatr Surg. 1990;25(6):613-7.
38. Lilly JR. The surgical treatment of choledochal cyst. Surg Gynecol Obstet. 1979;149:36-42.
39. Kamisawa T, Yoshiike M, Egawa N, Surata K, Okamoto A, Matsukawa M. Classification of choledochocele. Hepatogastroenterology. 2005;52(61):29-32.
40. Horaguchi J, Fujita N, Kobayashi G, Noda Y, Ito K, Takasawa O. Clinical study of choledochocele: is it a risk factor for biliary malignancies? J Gastroenterol. 2005;40(4):396-401.
41. Martin RF, Biber BP, Bosco JJ, Howell DA. Symptomatic choledochoceles in adults: endoscopic retrograde cholangio-pancreatography recognition and management. Arch Surg. 1992;127:536-9.
42. Masetti R, Antinori A, Coppola R, Coco C, Mattana C, Crucitti A, et al. Choledochocele: changing trends in diagnosis and management. Surg Today. 1996;26:281-5.
43. Farello GA, Cerofolini A, Rebonato M, Bergamaschi G, Ferrari C, Chiappetta A. Congenital choledochal cyst: video-guided laparoscopic treatment. Surg Laparosc Endosc. 1995;5(5):354-8.
44. Palanivelu C, Rangarajan M, Parthasarathi R, Amar V, Senthilnathan P. Laparoscopic management of choledochal cysts: technique and outcomes—a retrospective study of 35 patients from a tertiary center. J Am Coll Surg. 2008;207(6):839-46.

CHAPTER 57

Bile Duct Injury, Biliary Fistula and Benign Biliary Stricture

Sundeep Singh Saluja, Nilesh Patil, Neeraj Goel

Bile Duct Injury

INTRODUCTION

Bile duct injury (BDI) is an important health problem since it often affects people in their most productive years. As most of these injuries are iatrogenic, they carry a medicolegal implication. These injuries can occur during various surgeries varying from cholecystectomies to gastric or hepatic surgeries. The most common cause of BDI is cholecytectomy which can be open or laparoscopic. Rarely, BDI can also occur following abdominal trauma.

These injuries, if not treated properly, can lead to life threatening complications like secondary biliary cirrhosis and portal hypertension (PHTN). In the era of liver transplantation there appears to be a conceptual change in management of bile duct injuries (BDIs). Early surgery can be offered now in selected group of patients especially when referred immediately after injury.

POST-CHOLECYSTECTOMY BILE DUCT INJURY

Cholecystectomy is the most common cause of BDI. With the advent of the laparoscopic cholecystectomy the incidence (0.85%) of the BDI has increased two to three times when compared with open cholecystectomy (0.3%).[1] In a review of over 125,000 cholecystectomies, an incidence of 0.52% has been reported for the major BDIs.[1] Even a higher rate of injury has been reported with single incision laparoscopic cholecystectomy.[2] It has been shown that biliary injuries sustained during laparoscopic cholecystectomy are more likely to present earlier, more often associated with persistent bile leaks, and usually closer to the porta hepatis as compared to open surgery.[3,4]

Mechanism of Injury

The most common mechanism of injury during laparoscopic cholecystectomy is the *misidentification of the CBD* for cystic duct leading to complete transection of CBD, often with some part of the biliary tree.

Other less common causes of injury include excessive use of cautery resulting in *thermal injury*, application of multiple clips for *bleeding in the Calot's triangle*, deep *dissection into GB bed* or *ischemia* of CBD secondary to extensive circumferential dissection, when mistaken for cystic duct.

Small *bile leaks* may occur after inadvertent injury to a subvesical duct in GB bed, which may be present in 20–50% of cases. Another important site for biliary leak is from the *cystic duct stump*. Bile leak from the cystic duct stump more commonly results from the distal CBD obstruction caused by a *retained CBD stone* with resultant blow out of cystic duct stump. In addition, it may occur due to thermal injury, pressure necrosis from a metal clip, inadequate ligation or sloughing of the ligature.

Factors Predisposing to Bile Duct Injury

Learning curve: This question has been frequently discussed. An inverse relationship has been noted between the incidence of BDI versus number of cases performed by the operating surgeon.[5,6] But not all surgeons agree; there are reports showing that there is no change in the incidence of the BDI over time.[7] BDI does continue to occur in the hands of experienced surgeons.

Certain factors, pertaining to *technical difficulties* and *certain anomalies*, have also been observed as a factor predisposing to BDI.

Anomalies such as following may mislead the surgeon resulting in injury to the bile duct:

- A very short or long tortuous cystic duct
- Sessile gallbladder
- Aberrant anatomy of the bile ducts (Fig. 1A)
- Cystic artery anomalies like caterpillar hump.

Certain *pathologies* that may cause technical difficulties to the surgeon while performing cholecystectomy and may result in injury of the biliary system. These are

- Acute cholecystitis, empyema GB, small contracted GB, thick walled gallbladder, intrahepatic gallbladder, Mirizzi's syndrome (Fig. 1B) (including cholecystoenteric fistula)
- Obliteration of Calot's triangle.

Prevention of the Injury

It is foremost to decrease the burden of this problem.

Certain points should be kept in mind while performing cholecystectomy. Doing this may reduce the chances of injury.

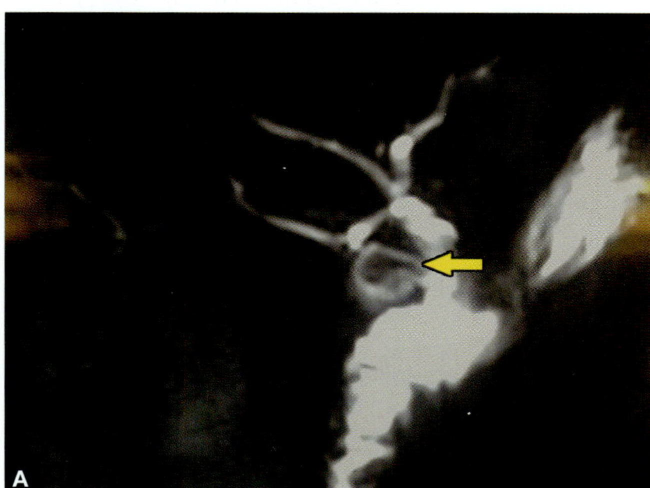

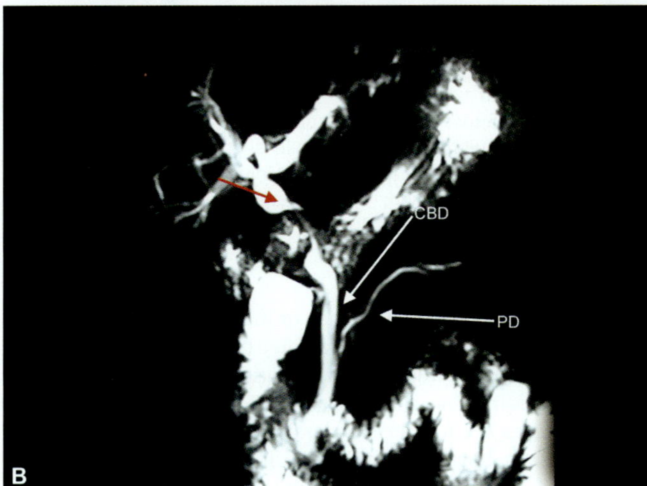

Figures 1A and B (A) Aberrant anatomy: low insertion of right posterior sectoral duct (RPSD); (B) MRCP image shows a calculus in gallbladder neck compressing the common hepatic duct and causing proximal biliary dilatation suggestive of Mirizzi syndrome

- No clipping should be done before critical view of safety is achieved. Critical view of safety is defined as when only two tubular structures, i.e. cystic artery and duct are seen along with liver seen clearly in the background.
- Excessive use of electrocautery at Calot's triangle or near CBD should be avoided. Also care needs to be exercised to prevent inadvertent collateral injury due to long length of the bare portion of the dissector. Instruments need to be regularly checked for chipping off of insulations.
- Always stay close to the gallbladder and no attempt should be made to identify the cystic duct-common bile duct junction.
- In case of difficult dissection at Calot's triangle (frozen triangle) the technique of subtotal cholecystectomy should be used.
- Gallbladder should be carefully dissected off of the bed as reckless dissection lead to an uncontrolled bleeding and injury to subvesical duct and even to segment V duct.
- Once clips are applied, their security should be ensured. No electrocautery should be used to for cutting the structures once clips have been deployed as heat is conducted further beyond from the area of interest.
- If bleeding occurs one should not put clamps blindly as it might lead to BDI.
- Intraoperative cholangiography (IOC): Role of IOC in prevention of BDI is controversial. If one can define the bile duct before clipping it is expected that the incidence of BDI should decrease. Large population based studies have shown lower incidence of BDI in cases where IOC was performed. They also report a lower incidence of BDI by surgeons who routinely perform IOC.[8,9] There is evidence that IOC can lead to identification of BDI when it occurs more often,[8] but its role in prevention of BDI is still controversial. Moreover, IOC is technically demanding and its interpretation is totally subjective. Injury can occur while performing IOC itself. The incidence of BDI has been very low in large series of laparoscopic cholecystectomy not routinely using IOC.[10]

Nugent et al.[11] reported an incidence of 0.43% of missed CBD stones when IOC was performed with strict criteria. It implies that unnecessary IOCs will be performed in many patients. The IOC should be applied selectively in following cases: (a) those with raised bilirubin and/or alkaline phosphatase levels; (b) those having history of jaundice; (c) if one finds dilated CBD or palpate stones in CBD; (d) or when there is unclear or aberrant anatomy. In first two conditions preoperative magnetic resonance cholangiopancreatography (MRCP) may obviate the need of IOC.

Classification

The outcome of BDI is dependent on the type and location of injury. Therefore there is a need of a classification that covers both therapeutic and prognostic implications of BDI. Till now various classifications have been proposed to define the type of BDI. In fact, most classifications are based on the mechanism and varying types of injuries involving the extrahepatic bile ducts ranging from minor cystic duct leaks to complete transection, including excision of the CBD, with or without a concomitant vascular injury.[1,12-14] But the main drawback of all these classifications is that they do not take into consideration the role of various factors that influence the outcome of BDI. These include condition of patient, associated vascular injuries, the timing of recognition of injury, presence of biliary fistula, PHTN, atrophy/hypertrophy complex, and any

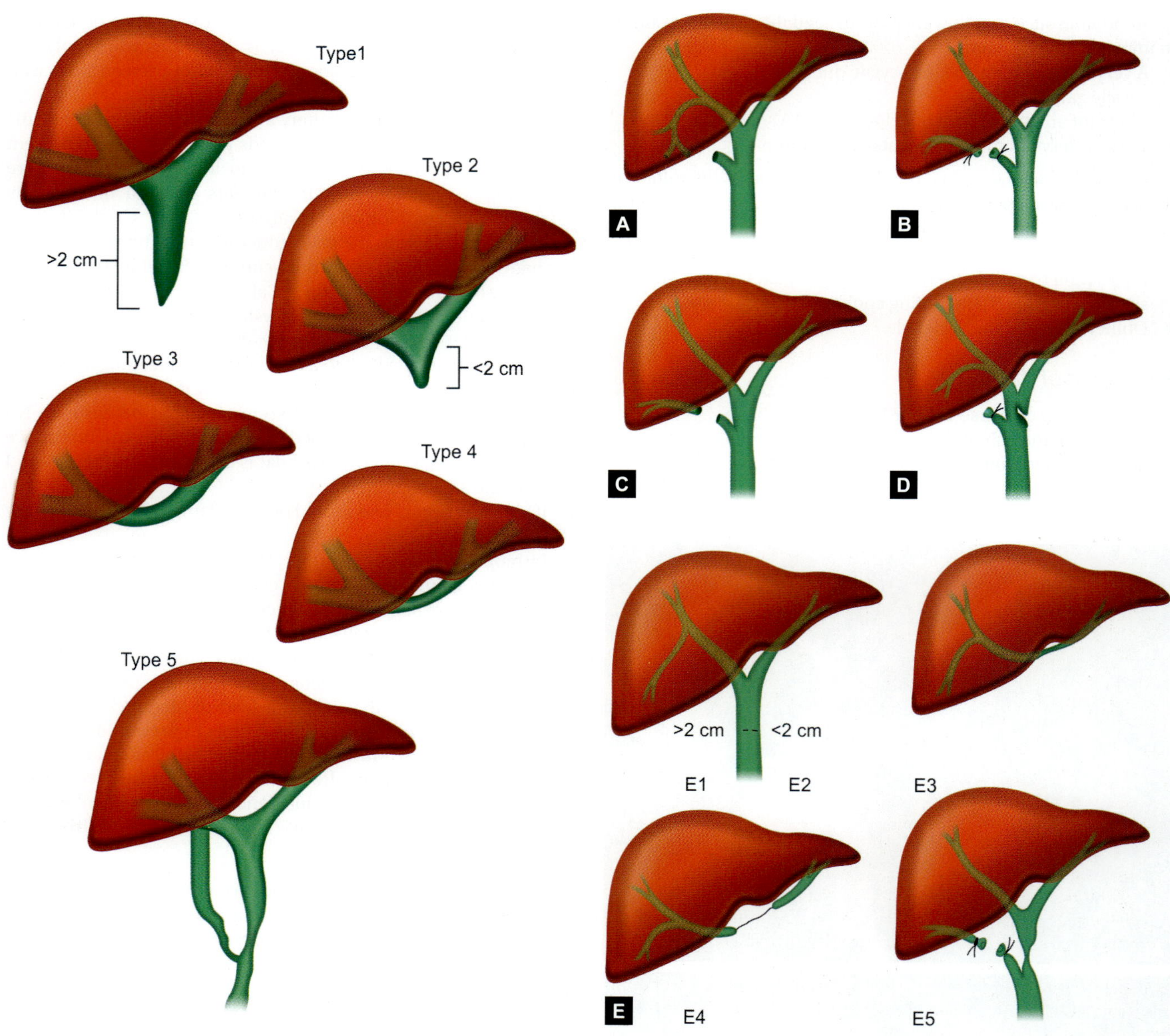

Figure 2 Bismuth's classification. Type 1: Low common hepatic duct stricture: common hepatic duct stump >2 cm; Type 2: High common hepatic duct stricture: common hepatic duct stump <2 cm; Type 3: Hilar stricture with no common hepatic duct but confluence formed; Type 4: No confluence with separation of right and left hepatic duct; and Type 5: Stricture of aberrant hepatic duct with or without stricture of common hepatic duct

Figures 3A to E Strasberg's classification: (Type A) Bile leak from minor duct still in continuity with common bile duct; (Type B) Aberrant duct injury with ligation; (Type C) Aberrant duct injury with leak and continuity with bile duct not maintained; (Type D) Lateral injury to extrahepatic bile duct and (Type E1–E5): Same as Bismuth Types I–V

previous repairs. Therefore, there is no universally accepted classification that is comprehensive in terms of combining all relevant factors affecting long-term outcome.

Bismuth and Strasberg classifications are most widely used all over the world. The Bismuth classification[15] was proposed before the laparoscopic era (Fig. 2). It stratifies the patients with an established biliary stricture based on the level of BDI. It is an excellent classification in terms of outcome of BDI and for planning the operative repair. The main drawback of this classification is that it does not take into consideration the entire spectrum of injuries especially the bile leaks which may or may not be associated with stricture formation. This lacuna was filled by Strasberg classification that came in 1995.[1] Strasberg classification stratifies laparoscopic biliary injuries into five categories from Type A to E (Figs 3A to E). Type E injuries are further subclassified into E1 to E5 according to the Bismuth classification system. It is based on mechanisms and technical errors. Other commonly used classifications in the clinical practice are Csendes Classification[16] (Table 1), Academic Medical Center (AMC) Amsterdam Classification of Bile Duct Injuries[17] (Table 2) and Stewart Way Classification (Fig. 4).[12]

Table 1: Csendes classification	
I	Small duct, RHD, CHD
II	Cystic-CBD junction
III	Partial or complete section of CBD
IV	Resection

Abbreviations: RHD, right hepatic duct; CHD, common hepatic duct; CBD, common bile duct.

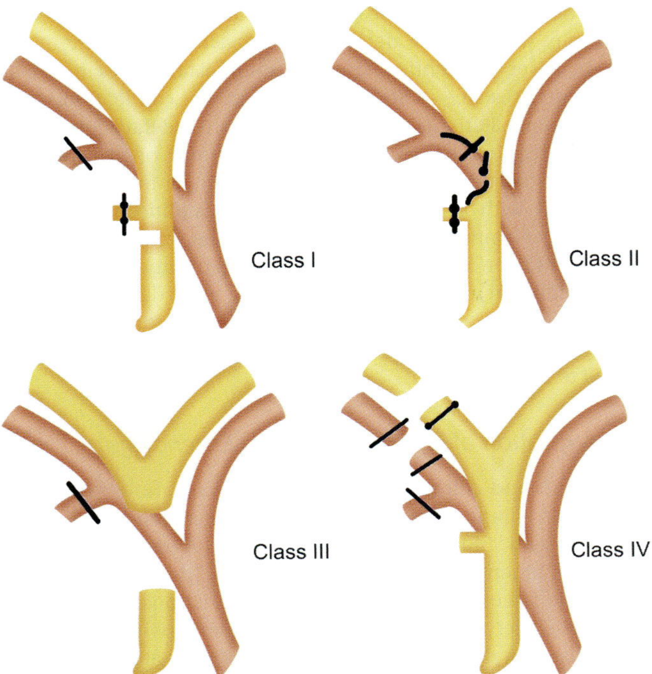

Figure 4 Stewart Way classification: (Class I) CBD mistaken for cystic duct but recognized; cholangiogram incision of cystic duct extended into CBD; (Class II) Lateral damage to common hepatic duct from cautery or clips placed on duct; associated bleeding, poor visibility; (Class III) CBD mistaken for cystic duct, not recognized; CBD, CHD, RHD, LHD transected or resected and (Class IV) RHD mistaken for cystic duct, RHA mistaken for cystic artery, RHD and RHA transected; lateral damage to the RHD from cautery or clips placed on ducts

Table 2: Academic Medical Center (AMC) Amsterdam classification of bile duct injuries	
A	Leakage from cystic or peripheral hepatic radicles
B	Major hepatic duct injury with leakage from common hepatic duct or aberrant segmental extrahepatic branch of right hepatic duct
C	Common hepatic duct stricture without leakage
D	Complete transaction of common hepatic duct

Recently, the European Association for Endoscopic Surgery (EAES) composite, all-inclusive, nominal classification anatomic, time of detection, mechanism (ATOM)[18] has combined 15 different classifications available in the literature for better guidance to therapeutic indications for iatrogenic BDI following cholecystectomy. But it is very exhaustive and complex. In addition it does not give any idea regarding the progression in severity of the injury as provided by Bismuth's classification system.

Clinical Presentation

Bilioma

When the bile leak occurs in the absence of drain, the resultant collection of bile into the peritoneal cavity may be either localized or generalized. The localized collection of bile is known as a bilioma. How symptomatic is the bilioma, will depend upon the presence or absence of infection in the bilioma. In the absence of infection, patients usually present with non-specific symptoms such as abdominal pain or localized abdominal distension, persistent vomiting, or uneasiness. The important examination findings are tachycardia and mild icterus. Patients with infected biliomas, in addition to above findings, have fever and signs and symptoms related to localized inflammation in the peritoneal cavity.

The free leakage of bile into the peritoneal cavity in the absence of drain results in either *biliary ascites* or *biliary peritonitis*. When the bile is sterile, the peritoneal cavity fails to evoke an inflammatory reaction. It leads to a collection of large amount of bile in the peritoneal cavity without features of peritonitis. Free leak of the infected bile within the peritoneal cavity leads to development of signs and symptoms of biliary peritonitis such as fever, tachycardia, tachypnea and generalized abdominal distension with guarding and rigidity. Patients with biliary peritonitis or biliary ascites can have mild jaundice secondary to absorption of bile from the peritoneal cavity.

Patients with bilioma constitute an important subgroup since patients in this group can develop biliary peritonitis and sepsis. This situation can be life threatening. Patients in this subgroup who may develop sepsis constitute one of the most important causes for early mortality.[19]

External Biliary Fistula

An abnormal communication between bile duct and abdominal wall (outside) is defined as external biliary fistula (EBF). The EBF may be either controlled or uncontrolled. In controlled fistula, there is adequate external drainage of the bile through the drain or from the drain site/wound without any significant intra-abdominal collection. While, uncontrolled EBF is associated with intra-abdominal bile leak and collection along with inadequate external drainage, resulting in either localized or generalized peritonitis with sepsis. In addition, cholangitis with or without cholangiolar abscesses can occur secondary to ascending infection to further complicate the course of the EBF. The presence of skin excoriation at the fistula site suggests concomitant enteric leak. Since bile alone does not contain any digestive enzymes, it does not cause any skin excoriation. The features of cholestasis are usually absent in the initial phase of the EBF. They start appearing during the healing phase of fistula when fistula closes and stricture is formed secondary to fibrosis.

The clinical implications of EBF depends upon the daily output of bile leak, duration of the fistula, whether complete or partial transection of bile duct has occurred and presence or absence of concomitant biliary infection. Total loss of bile from the fistula site may be tolerated up to 3 weeks as body can compensate for this loss till this time. However, prolonged high output fistula in absence of replacement therapy may result in fluid and electrolyte imbalance. It results in metabolic acidosis as sodium loss is usually greater than that of chloride loss. In initial stages the serum potassium level is low, but with severe fluid losses hyperkalemia can occur secondary to low output renal failure. Electrolyte changes may result in drowsiness and vasomotor collapse. Fat soluble vitamin deficiency may occur due to lack of bile from the GI tract required for their absorption. In addition, total biliary loss can cause disruption of the intestinal barrier function with resultant bacterial translocation. Also, in neglected cases it may result in protein and calorie malnutrition with weight loss.

Bile Duct Ligation/Clipping (Figs 5A and B)

Patients with bile duct ligation often present early with painless progressive cholestatic jaundice without any symptoms related to bile leak. Retained CBD stones and missed carcinoma should be kept in mind as differential diagnosis for patients presenting with jaundice in the early postoperative period after cholecystectomy. Cholangitis can develop in these patients if there are retained CBD stones or subsequent to endoscopic intervention. In addition, prolonged complete CBD obstruction can lead to liver failure.

Early versus Delayed Presentation

Recognition of BDI at the time of occurrence is of paramount importance. Only about 20–30% of injuries are diagnosed at the time of initial surgery.[20] Intraoperatively, the possible *tell-tale signs*, which can help in recognition of the injury early are detection of clear bright-yellow thin watery bile in the dissection field, vertically downward retraction of divided duct (which was presumed as cystic duct) behind the duodenum and inability to free the gallbladder after division of clipped cystic duct.

Bile duct injuries following laparoscopic cholecystectomy are more likely to be detected earlier as compared to open cholecystectomy, possibly due to differences in the pattern of injuries between the two approaches and increased awareness of the potential for injury at the time of laparoscopic cholecystectomy.[1,3] The major BDIs (Type E) are more likely to be recognized intraoperatively. But, they can sometimes remain undiagnosed until few days postoperatively, when they present with major bile leak (if not clipped) or jaundice (clipping). The minor injuries (Types A, C and D) are usually missed intraoperatively and most of the time, they present with bile leak within first week of surgery.

Patients with complete ligation or clipping of the CBD usually present early with progressive cholestatic jaundice. In addition, when the drain is placed peroperatively, BDI missed during surgery may present with bile in drain fluid within 24–48 hours. High index of suspicion is required in the absence of drain because such patients may present with subtle symptoms. These patients should be evaluated with LFTs and USG abdomen. The neglected cases may present in a delayed fashion with either bilioma or EBF. In cases, presenting late, the manifestations of bile leak varies with presence or absence of factors that can lead to septic complications. Patients with uncontrolled EBF, delayed detection of BDI, preoperative endoscopic intervention or concomitant biliary obstruction (partial/complete) with infection present more often with septic complications. In addition, sepsis can also occur secondary to concomitant vascular injury, resulting in ischemia of liver. Sepsis is the most important cause of morbidity and mortality in early phase of BDI. Thus, early detection of BDI and prompt institution of management is essential to decrease the septic complications and hence, the morbidity and mortality related to BDI.

Differentiation of Biliary Injury from Enteric Injury

Duodenum and colon may get injured during cholecystectomy. These enteric injuries especially duodenal can lead to diagnostic difficulty with EBF. The output from a duodenal fistula will have dark green bile, raised amylase levels (due to presence of pancreatic juice) and will cause skin excoriations at fistula site due to presence of activated digestive enzymes, while the output from biliary fistula is a golden yellow bile with low amylase content and does not cause skin excoriations. Colonic injury causes more purulent fistula output and it will have feculent odor. In doubtful cases, oral dye study is a simple investigation to localize the site of injury. Methylene blue mixed in fluid or charcoal given orally or by Ryle's tube can help in differentiating an enteric fistula from the biliary fistula at bedside.

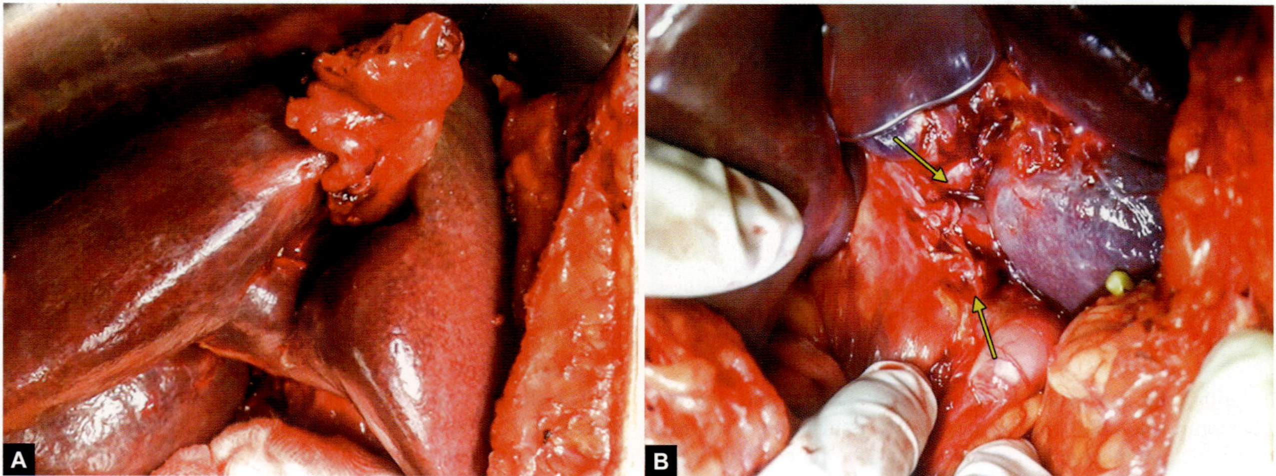

Figures 5A and B (A) Operative picture showing enlarged cholestatic liver in a patient with complete ligation; (B) Operative picture of the same patient showing clip at lower and upper end of CBD (yellow arrows). A spilled gallstone is also seen

Evaluation

All patients should be evaluated with a detailed history and comprehensive examination. It is important to review the operative details and discuss with the primary surgeon whenever possible, if the patient has been referred from another hospital. Previous US, CECT and operative recording, if available, should be reviewed. It is important to review the histology of the gallbladder from the previous operation. Patient with carcinoma of gallbladder are sometimes not recognized by an inexperienced surgeon. Liver function tests, renal function tests, hemogram, and a coagulation profile should be obtained, besides screening for HIV, HCV and HBs Ag. Evaluation and management sometimes go hand in hand depending on the condition of the patient.

USG abdomen: It is easily available, cost effective and noninvasive investigation for initial evaluation of patients with BDI. It provides the information about: (a) presence of intra-abdominal collection or free fluid with or without internal echoes; (b) dilatation of biliary radicles and CBD to assess the level of block/injury, presence of pneumobilia or stones in the biliary system; (c) concomitant assessment of vascular injuries using Doppler. It also helps in performing a percutaneous drainage of biliomas.

The main disadvantages of USG are: (a) it is an operator dependent assessment; (b) it fails to provide all the anatomical details, especially in the early postoperative period with tender operated areas; (c) it may not be reliable in presence of distended and dilated bowel loops and in obese patients.

CT Scan: Contrast enhanced CT scan of abdomen with oral contrast gives the following information (Fig. 6): (i) anatomical details of biliomas; (ii) vascular injury and integrity of the hilar arcade; (iii) any signs of liver ischemia and intrahepatic cholangiolar abscesses; (iv) dilatation of biliary radicles; (v) any associated enteric injury. It also helps in guided drainage of biliomas.

The CT scan abdomen is indicated if patient is having uncontrolled fistula or if early surgery is contemplated and one has to assess the associated vascular injury if present. It is also indicated in cases where patient has a sentinel bleed and one suspects a pseudoaneurysm.

Figure 6 Sagittal section of CT scan showing a large collection in subhepatic, lesser omentum and left suprahepatic region in a patient undergone cholecystectomy suggestive of biloma

Both USG and CT do not provide precise anatomical information on the type and extent of biliary injury.

Cholangiography

IOC (Fig. 7)

If the BDI is detected on table, precise surgical exploration and demonstration of biliary tree by intraoperative cholangiogram help in evaluating extent and type of BDI. It provides road map of biliary tree and helps in planning treatment accordingly. If the gallbladder is in situ, IOC is done through the cystic duct or else biliary anatomy can be assessed by a needle cholangiogram, performed through the CBD. Care should be taken while performing IOC to avoid additional injury to the biliary tree.

ERCP (Fig. 8)

It is a good investigation for delineation of the biliary tree. However, it has no value in BDIs where the biliary enteric continuity is lost

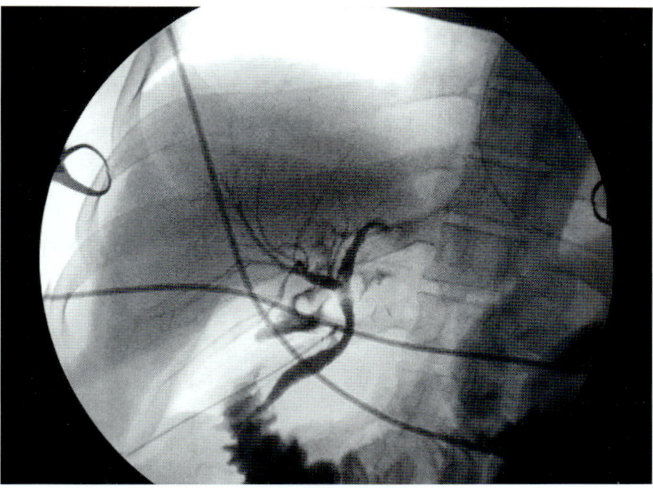

Figure 7 An intraoperative cholangiogram performed through cystic duct stump showing the complete biliary tree

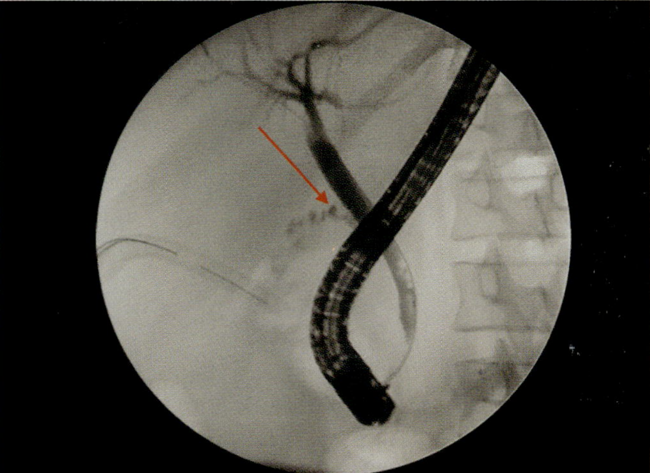

Figure 8 ERCP image showing common bile duct, hepatic duct and intrahepatic biliary radicles with leak of dye from the cystic duct stump in to peritoneal cavity along with drain in situ suggestive of Type A injury

and also in patients with isolated duct injuries (Types B and C). In the present era of MRCP, it is more commonly used with therapeutic intention, as it is an invasive procedure associated with a definite morbidity and mortality. Unnecessary ERCP can introduce infection into biliary system. ERCP is indicated in patients with biliary fistula when clinical investigations suggest that bilioenteric continuity is not lost.

MRCP (Figs 9A to D)

Magnetic resonance cholangiopancreatography has been accepted as the gold standard for assessment of the biliary tree. It is a valuable modality in the evaluation of BDI.[21-23] It gives a better cholangiogram than CECT and does not require any contrast (useful in patients with renal failure). When compared to ERCP and PTC, MRCP is a noninvasive investigation and can be safely performed on patients who are already sick or having deranged coagulation profile. In addition, the peripheral biliary radicles are visualized better than by the direct cholangiography.[24] Also, in a single study it provides additional information in the form of images of liver, any intra-abdominal collection, vascular injury or PHTN. It is best suited for patients with more proximal BDIs with separation of right and left hepatic ducts, undilated biliary system, "isolated" ducts and biliary obstruction at multiple levels. Limitations of MRCP are that it does not have any therapeutic potential, is more expensive and is less widely available. Also, it can miss minor bile leakage and in case of bilioma or metal clips the MRI picture may not be clear. In addition, the length of stricture may appear longer as the biliary system immediately below a tight stricture may be collapsed.

PTC (Fig. 10)

Presently, it has a limited role in evaluation of BDIs. It can be performed when MRCP is not available and ERCP or a fistulogram fail to demonstrate the complete biliary system. It may also be performed during drainage of isolated biliary radicles in the presence of cholangitis, during dilatation of strictured

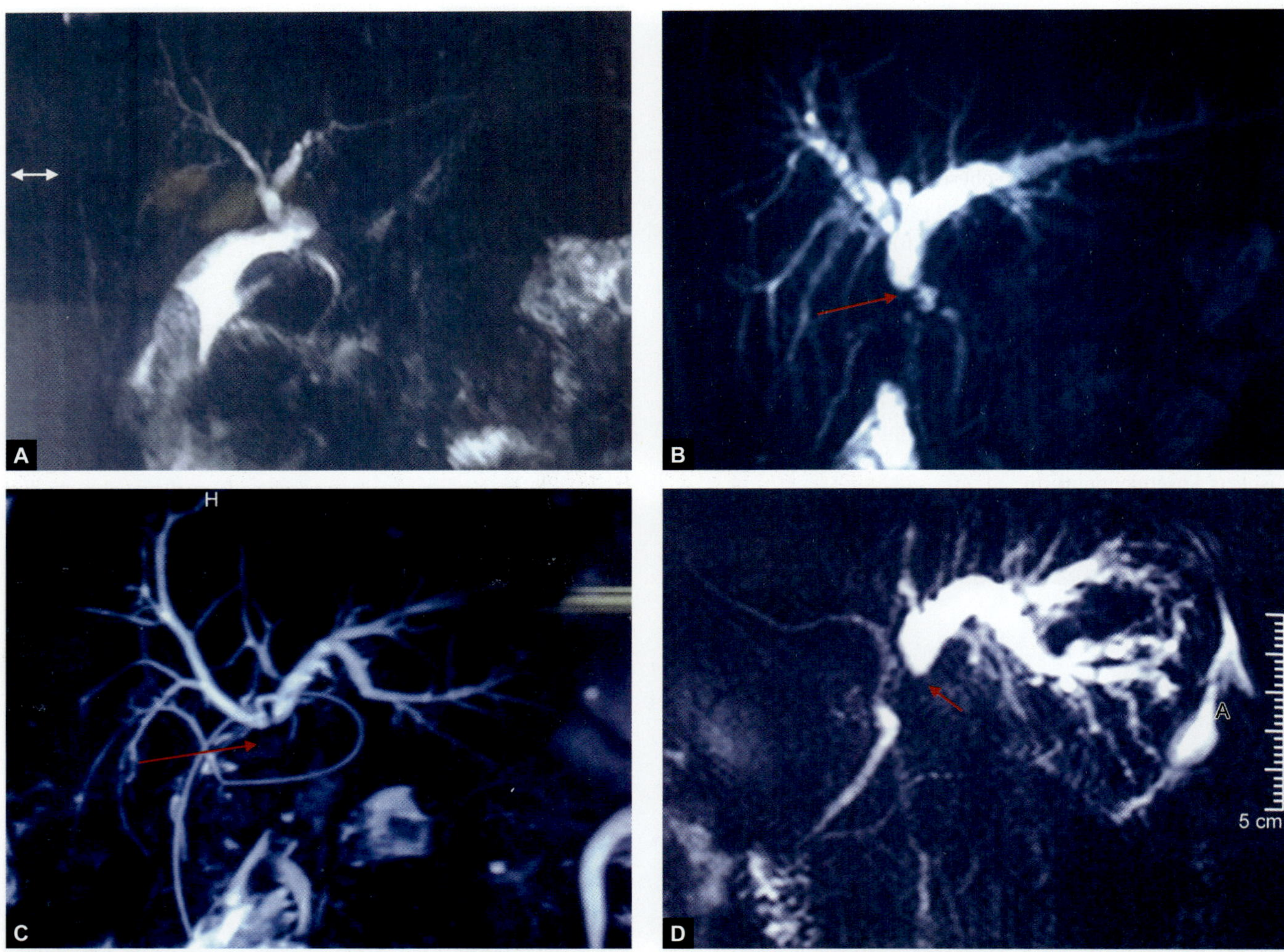

Figures 9A to D (A) MRCP image showing leak at the level of cystic duct stump with both proximal and distal biliary ducts delineated suggestive of Type A or D injury; (B) MRCP image showing dilated bilateral IHBRD along with stricture below hilum (arrow). The confluence is formed. There is loss of segment with normal distal CBD. Suggestive of Bismuth Type 2/1 stricture; (C) MRCP image showing dilated bilateral IHBRD along with stricture at hilum. The confluence is not formed with left and right duct separated suggestive of Bismuth Type 4 stricture; (D) MRCP image showing dilated left-sided IHBRD along with stricture in left hepatic duct while the right system and common bile duct are normal suggestive of Bismuth Type 5 stricture

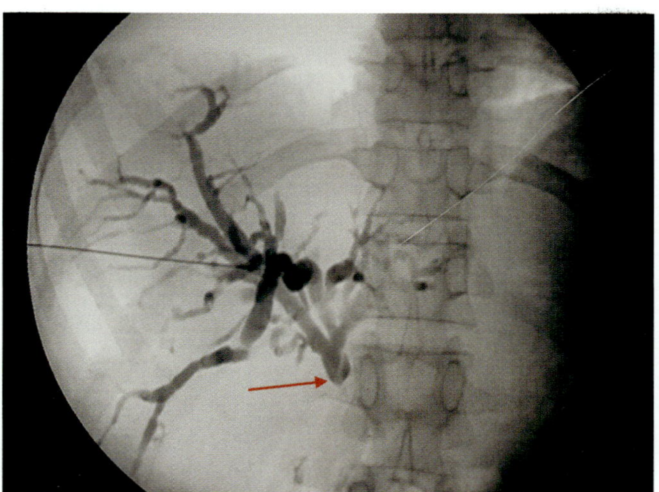

Figure 10 Percutaneous transhepatic cholangiogram showing bilateral IHBRD with stricture just below confluence (arrow)

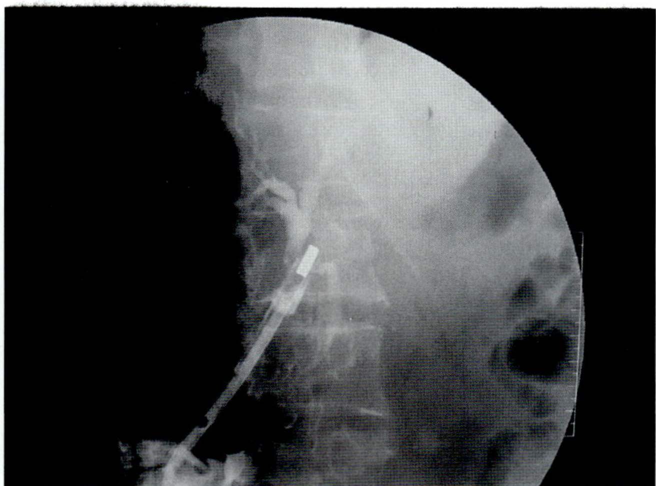

Figure 11 Fistulogram showing a tract communicating to biliary system below confluence. Both left and right duct are visualized without any abscess cavity suggestive of controlled fistula

hepaticojejunostomy or when preoperative catheter placement is planned while repairing a high biliary injury with persistent EBF along with undilated biliary system. Another important indication for PTC would be when PTBD is contemplated to stabilize the patient with long standing biliary stricture with deranged live function or renal function along with secondary biliary cirrhosis. Preoperative drainage may help in recovery of liver function before contemplating definitive repair. It is comparable to MRC with regards to image quality, detection of intrahepatic bile duct dilatation, assessment of the level of injury, and detection of abnormalities such as intraductal calculi, cholangitic liver abscesses, and atrophy of liver lobes.[21] The main disadvantages of PTC are that it is an invasive procedure with a finite risk of complications, needs patient preparation before the procedure and should be done a day before surgery to avoid any infective complication. It is not patient friendly as introduction of catheter causes pain and discomfort to the patient. Also, in the presence of EBF/bilioma, the underlying stricture and distal CBD may be masked/not visualized due to leakage of contrast through fistula site. Isolated bile ducts can also be missed on PTC.

Tubogram and Fistulogram (Fig. 11)

Tube cholangiography should be performed through a T-tube (if placed earlier) in the CBD before its removal. It may reveal retained CBD stones, biliary injury or stricture, or sometimes tumor. Findings of T-tube cholangiogram helps in planning the treatment of these conditions.

Fistulogram, performed through surgically or percutaneously placed drain, is a simple and cost effective investigation for delineation of biliary tree, where facilities for MRCP or ERCP are not available. But the limitations of fistulogram are that it may fail to visualize the biliary tree in the presence of bilioma. Sometimes it may not show all the ducts or entirely fail to delineate the biliary tree. Introduction of infection is also a problem. Prophylactic antibiotics should be given before performing a tubogram or fistulogram to minimize the risk of bacteremia and associated infective complications.

Scintigraphy

Hepatobiliary iminodiacetic acid (HIDA) scanning is helpful in the diagnosis of bile leakage in the absence of drain.[25] One important use of HIDA scan is in a symptomatic patient shortly after cholecystectomy in whom imaging does not show significant collection so as to suggest BDI. Also, it gives the information about adequacy of external drainage (whether uncontrolled or controlled EBF) and the bilioenteric continuity. In addition, hold up in particular liver segments may suggest an "isolated" bile duct (Type B injury). However, it lacks specificity in relation to biliary anatomy, the level of the leak or the cause of bile leak and sometimes it may fail to demonstrate biliary enteric continuity in the presence of high output EBF.

Management

Bile duct injuries and bile leaks require a multidisciplinary approach for their optimum management. The role of endoscopist, intervention radiologist and surgeon should be complementary to each other in treating these patients.

Initial management of patients with bile leak should be directed at controlling the sepsis, drainage of biliomas or abscesses and control of any bleed if present. The on-going bleed from pseudoaneurysm should be controlled by angioembolization with help of interventional radiologist. Biliary peritonitis with sepsis and bleeding from pseudoaneurysm are the important causes of mortality in the early phase which emphasizes the early diagnosis and referral for these patients.[19]

Management of Bilioma

Bile collections should be evaluated with adequate imaging, preferably with *CT abdomen* as it has a better sensitivity compared to ultrasonography (96% vs 70%) in detecting the fluid collections.[26] Biliomas and biliary ascites can be drained by *image-guided PCD insertion*. Sometimes multiple catheters may be required for an adequate drainage. Drainage should be done via close suction drainage bag system under a low pressure. This helps in reducing the cavity of bilioma and formation of controlled fistula. Patient should be reassessed with USG to check the position of the catheter and any residual collection. In due course, the controlled EBF will develop preferentially through one catheter and other catheters can be removed once their drainage output becomes minimal.

Laparotomy may be needed in some patients with: (a) diffuse biliary peritonitis, (b) biliomas which are not amenable to PCD such as multiple/multiseptate intra-abdominal collections and large biliomas with internal necrotic material/debris and those, (c) who failed per cutaneous drainage. The incision (right subcostal or midline) should be planned depending upon the locations of biliomas on preoperative imaging.

The following principles should be followed during laparotomy:

- Minimal and careful adhesiolysis
- Avoid enteric injury
- Drainage of all biliomas seen on imaging
- No attempt should be made at definitive repair
- Thorough peritoneal lavage with copious amounts of warm saline
- Insertion of multiple large subhepatic drains

In addition to drainage of intra-abdominal collections, *control of sepsis* requires administration of parenteral broad spectrum antibiotics, covering enteric organisms. Later antibiotics can be modified depending upon the culture sensitivity report. Also, large cholangiolar abscesses in the liver may need aspiration or percutaneous drainage.

The bilioma may end up either as *EBF and biliary stricture once fistula* closes. They are then managed accordingly.

Management of EBF

Every effort should be made to convert an *uncontrolled bile leak into a controlled EBF* with tube drainage of intra-abdominal collections either by percutaneous approach or laparotomy. Based on bile culture sensitivity reports, *parenteral antibiotics* should be administered to control infection. *Fluid and electrolyte balance maintenance* is one the cornerstone of management in these patients. It is often ignored and leads to fatal complications. The ringer lactate solution is the most appropriate replacement fluid for the bile losses. Total loss of bile from the fistula site may be tolerated up to 3 weeks as body can compensate for this loss till this time. However, prolonged high output fistula results in fluid and electrolyte imbalance in absence of replacement therapy. *Nutritional support* is another essential component of management of such patients. Patient should be well nourished so as to have a good outcome while contemplating definitive surgery. Enteral feeding is preferred mode of feeding. Parenteral nutrition may be needed in the presence of associated enteric leak or if oral intake is less (calorie intake <1,500 kcal/day). In addition, bile refeeding could decrease the endotoxemia and nutritional manifestations secondary to prolonged bile loss. **Coagulation defects** should be monitored in such patients. Depleted body stores of vitamin K due to prolonged bile loss should be corrected with administration of vitamin K 10 mg intramuscularly daily for 3–5 days. Patients with significantly deranged coagulation profile despite vitamin K supplementation, who require any intervention, may need transfusion of fresh frozen plasma before the procedure. *Skin protection*: Appropriate measures should be taken to protect the skin at the fistula site. Biliary fistula sites are easier to maintain unlike enteric fistula sites as there are no activated enzymes present that cause severe skin excoriations if not protected. Simple stoma bag application around the tube draining bile is sufficient for skin protection.

Once the controlled EBF is established, appropriate imaging should be performed to assess the fistula origin, type and extent of the injury and presence/absence of biliary enteric continuity. MRI or MRCP is the investigation of choice to delineate the above-mentioned information. Fistulogram is a cheap alternative to MRCP in such patients but it should be carefully interpreted as described above.

Fistula Closure

Usually type of the injury decides the fistula closure. Bile leaks in the presence of biliary enteric continuity such as those from the cystic ducts, subvesical duct and most lateral injuries heal over a short period of time, while fistula from major injuries such as larger lateral defect in the CBD or Type E injuries and Type C injury may take longer time to heal or they may not heal at all. Also, fistula closure may be facilitated by endoscopic or percutaneous transhepatic biliary interventions.

Few studies have reported inferior results following biliary repair in the presence of persistent EBF.[27] So some authors prefer to wait till fistula heals. There is no consensus in the literature on the optimal duration of waiting before a definitive repair in patients of biliary stricture with concomitant EBF. About two-thirds of EBFs (even in complete BDI) are closed by 6–12 weeks. In a study by Mishra et al., the average time for fistula closure was 60 days (range: 5–240 days). They also reported good outcome in 11 patients with persistent fistula, who underwent definitive repair with hepaticojejunostomy after a median interval of 3 months (range: 3–6 months) after BDI. Thus, it is sensible to wait for a minimum of 3 months and a maximum of 6 months following index surgery. This allows the optimization of patient, fistula to heal/get controlled, inflammation and edema to subside, the level of the injury to demarcate, and the ducts to dilate and mature to improve the success of definitive repair. Waiting beyond 6 months may place the patient at risk of SBC due to repeated cholangitis and calorie and protein malnutrition due to prolonged bile loss.[19]

Definitive Management

Endoscopic Treatment

Endoscopic treatment in the form of a sphincterotomy, stenting or both is a good option for treating EBF in patients with preserved biliary-enteric continuity (Strasberg Type A or D injury). It is more suitable for patients with infrahilar leaks and small defect in the CBD. Also, the underlying cause of fistula such as retained CBD stones, papillary stenosis, small growth in the ampullary region can be tackled with endoscopic therapy. Thus, it facilitates the closure of the fistula and in addition, biliary stenting relieves the cholangitis, if present. de Reuver PR et al.[28] reported 97% and 89% success rate of stenting for cystic duct leak and bile duct leak respectively. However, endoscopic treatment is associated with limitations of morbidity due to its complications, repeated interventions and frequent follow-up which has significant impact on the cost and QOL of patients. So, it is prudent to delay the endoscopic intervention for 3–6 weeks to allow the spontaneous healing of the fistula. In addition, the timing of the endoscopic treatment can be decided depending upon the daily output and the trend of biliary fistula. Once the fistula has healed, the stent should be removed and patients are followed up with liver function tests at regular intervals to detect the changes suggestive of stricture formation.

Percutaneous Transhepatic Biliary Catheterization

It is rarely indicated in management of postcholecystectomy EBF. The main indication is when preoperative catheter placement is planned while repairing a high biliary injury with persistent EBF and an undilated biliary system. Misra S et al.[29] reported success rate of 60% with percutaneous treatment while treating post-laparoscopic cholecystectomy biliary injuries. The main complications of percutaneous approach are catheter related complications in addition to those mentioned for endoscopic treatment. Rarely patients may require combined percutaneous and endoscopic approach, also known as "rendezvous technique" for the management of biliary leaks/fistulas.

Surgical Treatment

As previously mentioned, laparotomy may be required in case of biliary peritonitis or in some patients for drainage of intra-abdominal collections to establish a controlled EBF.

Definitive surgical treatment is usually required for patients with *complete transection of CBD (Type E)* or *sectoral duct (Type B injury)*. The patients with *Type D injury* managed initially with endoscopic treatment can develop stricture later during life. These patients usually have stent placement during initial endoscopy. They may either go for endoscopic stent therapy or surgical definitive repair as discussed in biliary stricture management.

Hepaticojejunostomy is the procedure of choice for patients with complete transection of bile duct. Single-layer, mucosa to mucosa, tension free anastomosis to healthy bile duct tissue and use of absorbable sutures during hepaticojejunostomy are associated with good outcome.[30] It can be extended over left hepatic duct at the base of segment 4 to obtain the adequate length of anastomosis with wide drainage of bile duct in case of Type 3 or 4 injuries.

Timing of Repair

Early versus Delayed Repair

General condition of the patient, presence or absence of local inflammation and availability of the expertise are key determinants for the timing of repair. However, the optimal timing of definitive repair remains controversial.

Many authors[17,31-35] advise delayed repair for BDI because during early repair it is difficult to assess the extent of ischemic damage and performing a high biliary anastomosis in the presence of inflammation and non-dilated ducts may result in an high restricture rate. Also, the mucosa of the injured bile ducts starts recovering at around 3 weeks and 6 months is the time when it heals completely. In addition, delayed repair has shown excellent long-term outcomes with a very low risk of mortality.[36]

With the experience and results of liver transplantation and improvement in expertise, gadgets and perioperative care it is believed that early repair can be performed in patients with complete transection of the bile duct. The definition of optimum early repair varies among different studies. In the study of de Reuver et al.,[33] 2 patients who underwent surgery within 2 days of laparoscopic cholecystectomy did not experience complications and they believed that surgical repair can be performed within 2–3 days of BDI when the sepsis and peritoneal contamination are absent and there is fair chance of successful outcome. Thomson et al.[31] reported cost savings, decreased morbidity, mortality and hospital stay with immediate repair. Sicklick JK[37] from John's Hopkins group reported no difference in outcome between patients who underwent repair at an early (<1 month after referral), intermediate (1–12 months) or delayed (>12 months) time. However, Sahajpal AK et al.[38] revealed significantly high stricture rate with repairs in the intermediate period (72 hours to 6 weeks). They concluded that repairs should be undertaken either in the immediate (0–72 hours) or delayed (>6 weeks) periods after laparoscopic cholecystectomy as acute inflammation related to recent surgical intervention is maximal during this period of 72 hours to 6 weeks following laparoscopic cholecystectomy. In addition, Birmingham group[39] argued that outcomes after immediate (on table repair) and early repairs (<21 days) were comparable to late repairs (>21 days) when performed by a specialist. Recently, our group reported favorable outcome in 5 patients of acute BDI who were repaired within 48 hours.[19]

There is consensus that the initial repair is associated with highest success rate, if it is performed by an experienced hepatobiliary surgeon. Therefore, early repair demands immediate recognition of injury and early referral to a tertiary care center. It appears to be a favorable option in patients with a low level injury, who are hemodynamically stable and there is no evidence of uncontrolled biliary fistula and sepsis. However, it is wiser to delay the repair in the presence of higher injuries with loss of confluence, concomitant vascular injury, significant diathermy injury or on-going sepsis. Patients with complete bile duct ligation or clipping should be repaired immediately irrespective of the timing of detection, as delaying repair can increase the morbidity and mortality in these patients.

It is important to note that timing of surgical repair does not influence success rate if the repair is performed in an experienced center in a patient with an optimal general condition.[40,41]

Operative Management of Injuries Which are Recognized Immediately (Figs 12A and B)

Review of literature, as well as our experience, suggests that if BDI is detected on table or within 24–48 hours and the patient is in a reasonable condition (hemodynamically stable, no inflammation/sepsis and no evidence uncontrolled bile leak) immediate repair can be contemplated by specialist surgeon. It is associated with excellent outcome and decreases the morbidity associated with the injury.[32] The first attempt at repair is the best attempt as there is loss of some length of healthy duct at each subsequent repair therefore such cases should be performed by specialist surgeon. Heise et at.[42] evaluated 175 patients with BDI and reported that the number of attempted repairs before referral was a significant predictor of poor outcome.

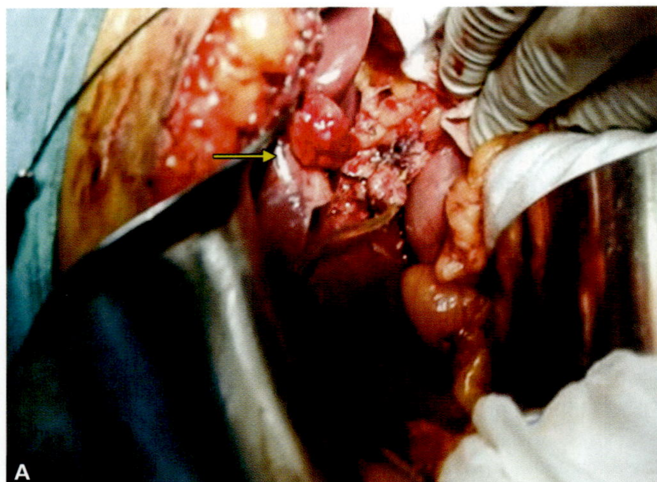
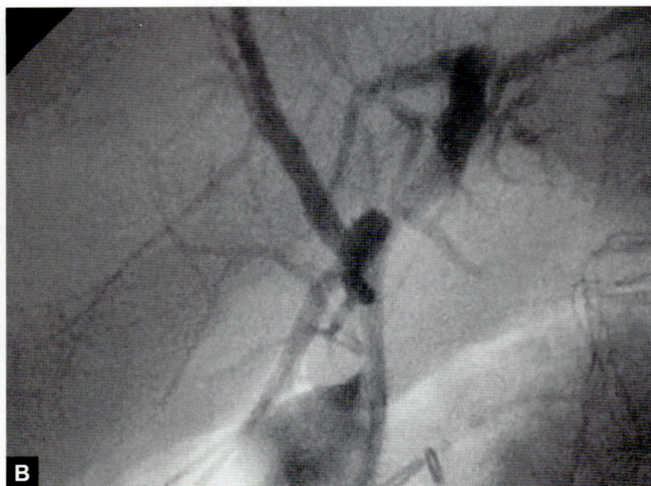

Figures 12A and B (A) Acute bile duct injury: drainage tube within transected CBD; (B) Intraoperative cholangiogram of the patient with acute bile duct injury

If the expertise is not available, thorough lavage with copious amounts of warm saline should be given and subhepatic space is drained by large bore drains to convert BDI into a controlled EBF. Also, ongoing bleeding if present should be controlled. No attempt should be made to clip or ligate the duct as it leads to the necrosis of the duct and bile leak. Patient should then be transferred to tertiary care center. In the review of 88 patients with BDI, by Stewart and Law,[30] only 17% of repairs performed by a primary surgeon were successful compared with 94% of those performed by a specialist biliary surgeon, and the hospital stay was three times longer when managed by a non-specialist surgeon (78 vs 222 days). The morbidity and mortality of those treated by a primary surgeon as compared to a specialist surgeon were 58% and 1.6% versus 4% and 0%, respectively.

The procedure needs to be *converted to open* while repairing a biliary injury. Leaks from cystic duct stump or small ducts in liver bed are managed with ligation of offending duct during surgery. *Primary repair* with fine absorbable sutures and *drainage of subhepatic* space is a good surgical option for patients with partial injury to CBD/CHD without tissue loss. Closure over T-tube is controversial. There is no comparative studies in the literature on primary closure with or without a T-tube following BDI. Thety et al.[43] reported higher stricture rate with use of T-tube during a choledochocholedochostomy as compared to repair without a T-tube in liver transplantation (25% vs 11%). *Partial injuries with a large defect* in the bile duct should be treated with hepaticojejunostomy.

Hepaticojejunostomy is the preferred procedure for patients with *complete transection* of bile duct. Single-layer, mucosa to mucosa, tension free anastomosis to healthy bile duct tissue and use of absorbable sutures during hepaticojejunostomy are associated with good outcome.[30] It can be extended over left hepatic duct at the base of segment 4 to obtain the adequate length of anastomosis with wide drainage of bile duct. *End-to-end repair* may be considered in patients with BDI which is detected on table, duct diameter more than 4 mm, with no extensive tissue loss and no local inflammation.[44,45] In these group of patients, Jabłońska et al.[44] reported comparable long-term results and quality of life to that after hepaticojejunostomy. In addition, according to Reuver et al.[45] complications (stricture or leakage) following end-to-end repair can be adequately managed by endoscopic or percutaneous drainage in the majority of patients (66%) and reconstructive surgery after complicated end-to-end anastomosis is a procedure with relative low morbidity and no mortality.

Role of Laparoscopy

It has *limited role* in the management of BDIs. Minor bile leaks such as *leaks from the cystic duct or sub-vesical duct, when detected intraoperatively* can be tackled laparoscopically.[46] In addition, in experienced hands, patients with minor tear in CBD/CHD might benefit from laparoscopic repair. In case of bilioma, when the facilities/expertise of PCD is not available, laparoscopy may be considered for drainage. But it requires general anesthesia and is technically difficult in the presence of inflammatory reactions and unclear anatomy, leading to failure to achieve adequate drainage. Also, repeated laparoscopy can further increase the morbidity in an already sick patient. In addition, it has potential for malpractice litigation.

Vasculobiliary Injuries (Fig. 13)

Strasberg and Helton[47] defined vasculobiliary injury (VBI) as "an injury to both a bile duct and a hepatic artery and/or portal vein; the BDI may be caused by operative trauma, be ischemic in origin or both, and may or may not be accompanied by various degrees of hepatic ischemia".

Concomitant injury of hepatic artery has been seen in 12–40% of patients of BDI[47-49] and it may present as occlusion, pseudoaneurysm, or complete disruption.[37] Right hepatic artery is the most commonly involved vessel in VBI. It can go unnoticed in most patients as it may not cause any significant ischemia because intact portal blood flow and rapid development of collateral circulation between the left and right hepatic arteries through the hilar plate may compensate for blood flow to affected hepatic tissue.[50-52]

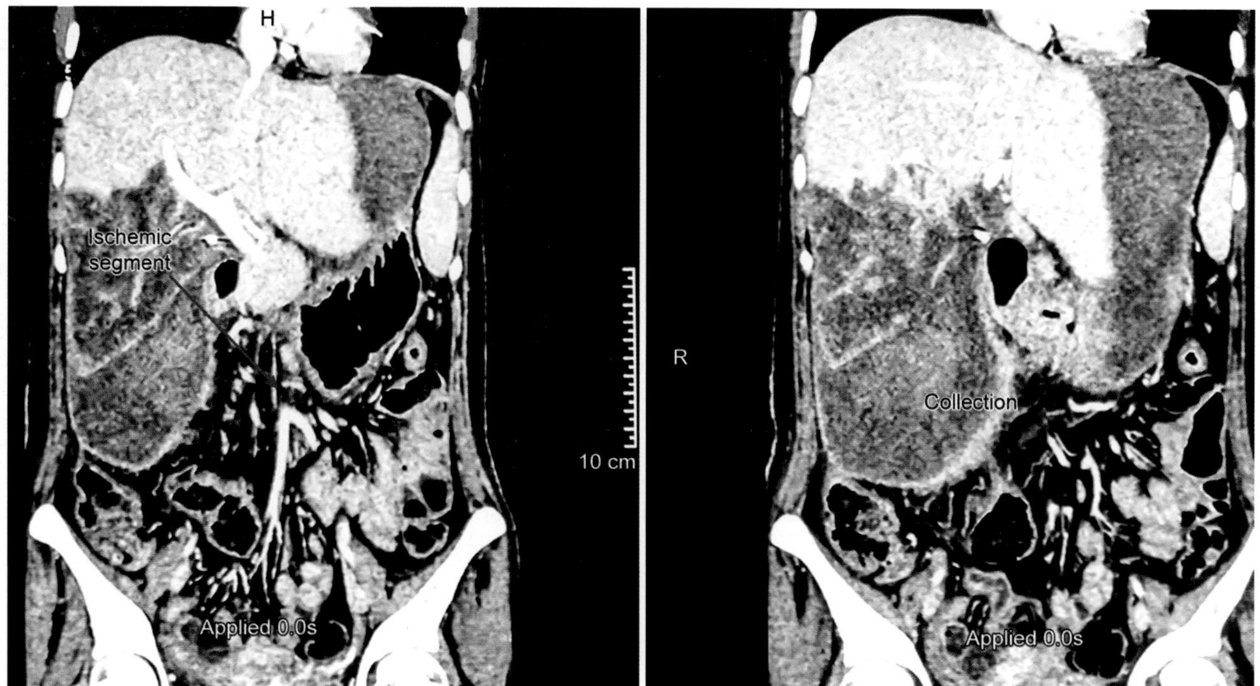

Figure 13 CECT scan section showing loss of normal enhancement pattern in segments 5 and 6 with a collection after cholecystectomy suggestive of vasculobiliary injury

When an early repair of BDI is planned, evaluation of vascular injury is very important. Patients with history of significant bleed during initial surgery, high BDI (Strasberg E3 to E5) and those with previous attempt to repair have a higher chance of concomitant vascular injury. Nowadays, CT or MR angiography are preferred over invasive angiography for evaluation.

Management of vascular injury depends on the *timing of recognition of injury, associated liver ischemia and availability of expertise.* If the RHA injury is detected *early (on table or within 4 days)* and expertise is available, repair of arterial injury should be considered (if distal arterial stump can be dissected) and concurrent biliary injury is also repaired.[48,53,54] If *restoration* of arterial flow is *not technically possible* but the biliary confluence and the hilar arcade is intact, *hepaticojejunostomy* should be performed with a Hepp-Couinaud technique to avoid postoperative anastomotic stricture.[55]

When the patient presents *late (>4 days)*, there is no need to attempt arterial repair and associated biliary injury should be tackled in a delayed fashion. Some authors advocated to ignore the arterial injury irrespective of the timing of detection, as RHA ligation in a normal liver does not produce any severe consequences.[56-58] Angio-embolization is safe and effective to control the delayed hemorrhage secondary to pseudoaneurysm. In the prospective study by Alves et al.[49] and the largest study by Stewart et al.[58] there was no difference in the mortality between the patients with isolated BDI and combined VBI. In both the studies, overall morbidity remained same if the repair was performed by a specialist surgeon. In addition, Alves et al.[49] reported 93% success rate when biliary repair was performed by a Hepp-Couinaud technique. Neither of these studies revealed any difference in anastomotic stricture rate between the two groups. However, Sarno G et al.[59] reported poor outcome following BDI repair in patients with concomitant VBI and/or sepsis.

Right hepatic artery VBI may cause hepatic infarction in about 10% of patients especially in patients with associated proximal BDI (E4 or E5)[47] which may require either resection of ischemic segments or liver transplantation[60] for acute liver failure. In a literature review, Truant et al.[61] reported higher hepatectomy rate in patients of combined arterial and Strasberg E4 or E5 injury, with satisfactory long-term outcomes despite high postoperative morbidity. Also, hepatic arterial and Strasberg E4 and E5 injuries were independent factors associated with hepatectomy.

Portal vein is less prone to injury as compared to right hepatic artery and therefore only few case series are reported in the literature. In 4% of patients it may be associated with concomitant arterial injury.[59] Portal vein injury leads to either rapid hepatic ischemia or slow atrophy. If it is recognized intraoperatively and expertise is available, portal vein can be repaired provided patient is hemodynamically stable. Ligation of portal vein may be required in hemodynamically unstable patients or in complex injuries. Thrombolytic and anticoagulation therapy is safe and effective in patients who present early with thrombosis of portal vein.[62] Liver transplantation may be considered in patients with either rapid deterioration secondary to liver infarction during acute phase or chronic liver failure in late period.[62]

Sectoral Duct Injuries (Figs 14A and B)

The right posterior sectoral duct (RPSD) is particularly prone to injury during cholecystectomy, when there is low insertion of RPSD into either the cystic duct or the common hepatic duct.[63] Incidence of RPSD injury during laparoscopic cholecystectomy

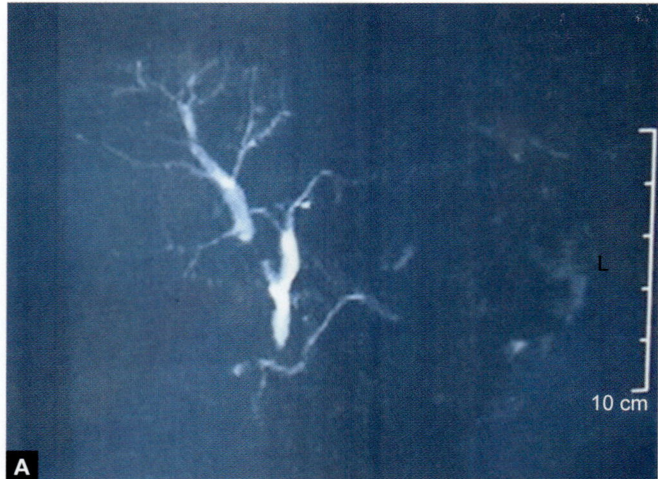

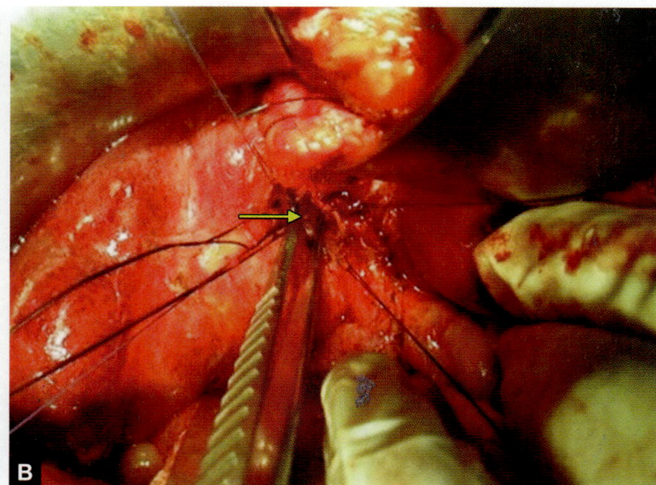

Figures 14A and B RPSD injury (Strasberg type B): (A) MRCP picture; (B) Intraoperative picture showing repair

varies from 6% to 9%.[64] Limited information is available in the literature regarding diagnosis and management of injuries of RPSD. If recognized intraoperatively, immediate repair should be performed by specialist hepatobiliary surgeon when the size of RPSD is adequate (>3 mm), suggesting drainage from a significant portion of liver parenchyma. When these patients present late, there are controversies in the literature regarding its management. Strasberg Type B injuries may remain asymptomatic or present with sectoral cholangitis. The latter may require either drainage or resection depending upon the presence or absence of atrophy of liver segments drained by RPSD. The trend of fistula output may guide the management of these Type C injuries.[65] Surgical intervention may be considered in patients with large fistula output or persistence of fistula beyond 6–12 weeks. Patients with low output fistula or decreasing trend of fistula may be treated conservatively.

Biliary Fistula

INTRODUCTION

Biliary fistula is defined as any abnormal communication between biliary tree and its part with another epithelial lining. These communications can be either internal or external. They can be spontaneous or iatrogenic. Internal biliary fistulae are rare and spontaneous. External biliary fistulae are more common and iatrogenic in majority of cases.

EXTERNAL BILIARY FISTULA

They occur following a variety of surgeries varying from cholecystectomies to gastric or hepatic surgeries. The extent of biliary injury, the patient's general condition, the timing of recognition and the availability of experienced hepatobiliary surgeon are the key determinants of good long-term outcome. Inadequate treatment can lead to sepsis in the early phase and PHTN or secondary biliary cirrhosis in the late phase. These complications can lead to high mortality. In addition, EBF may be controlled or uncontrolled depending upon the adequacy of external drainage.

Causes of External Biliary Fistula

Post-cholecystetomy EBF

(see above)

Traumatic

Biliary tact injury is a *rare consequence* of blunt and penetrating trauma to abdomen. The majority have *associated injury* to other organs especially liver, pancreas and duodenum. In addition, 10% of patients may an associated hepatic vascular injury in HDL. Blunt trauma causes sudden de-acceleration leading to either disruption in bile duct, usually at the supra-pancreatic portion or intra-mural/extra-biliary hematoma compressing the bile duct, while penetrating trauma can involve any part of the biliary tract. Also, the concomitant vascular interruption can cause ischemic injury to biliary tract in both the blunt and penetrating trauma.

Clinical presentation varies with the type of injury: *bilioma* or *biliary peritonitis* are the common mode of presentation in patients with tear in the bile duct, while biliary stricture secondary to hematoma or ischemia causes delayed onset jaundice. *Imaging findings* are usually nonspecific. In acute setting, CT scan reveals intra-peritoneal collections/free fluid, associated injury in liver/pancreaticoduodenal complex, or hematoma in HDL. In patients with biliary stricture, dilatation of biliary radicles proximal to level of stricture with or without atrophy-hypertrophy of the liver segments will be seen on either CT or MRI.

Management: Gallbladder injury is usually treated with cholecystectomy either at the time of initial surgery or after damage control laparotomy. During damage control surgery, injury to biliary tree can be best controlled with abdominal drains or insertion of T-tubes as definitive repair in the setting of sepsis or shock has poor outcome. In addition, percutaneous drainage is required for patients presenting with localized biliomas. Simple drainage alone will close the majority of biliary leaks from the intrahepatic biliary radicles although persistent bile leak after liver injury sometimes may require either endoscopic intervention or fistulojejunostomy. At a later date, when the patient has returned to optimal physiological state, injuries to the extrahepatic biliary tract is managed best with Roux-en-Y hepaticojejunostomy (RYHJ).[66] It gives excellent long-term outcome as the majority of the trauma related injuries are of low level as compared to those after laparoscopic cholecystectomy. Endoscopic management is possible in intrahepatic and partial extrahepatic biliary injuries, especially to tackle the prolonged high output biliary fistula. Also, it may be considered as an initial treatment option for patients with infrahilar stricture.[66] Hepatic resection is mainly required in the circumstances of unreconstructable biliary injury. But, in acute setting, the resections should be performed as a staged procedure following damage control surgery.

Post-gastrectomy

Biliary injury may occur during partial gastrectomy, especially when the pyloric region or duodenal bulb is deformed due to scarring caused by peptic ulcer or by malignancy. The duodenal contracture decreases distance between the ampulla and the pylorus, which places the biliary tree in a vulnerable position. When the surgeon tries to mobilizes the first part of duodenum for secure closure of duodenal stump in Billroth II gastrectomy or for anastomosis to the gastric remnant in a Billroth I reconstruction, the plane of dissection is carried out caudally between the medial wall of duodenum and pancreatic head. This maneuver causes injury to the bile duct or the confluence of bile duct and pancreatic duct. Another mechanism for biliary or ampullary injury is mobilization of duodenum by Kocher's maneuver in a wrong plane, i.e. between the pancreas and duodenum instead of mobilizing pancreaticoduodenal complex from the IVC.

Clinical presentation: These biliary injuries presents as a biliary fistula in the immediate postoperative period or in a delayed manner with the symptoms of a stricture. If the injury is recognized intraoperatively, it should be repaired immediately. The isolated BDI can be managed with either choledochoduodenostomy (CDD) or Roux-en-Y choledochojejunostomy (CDJ).[67] The ampullary injury can be tackled with anastomosing either ductal confluence or the bile duct and pancreatic duct individually over the stents to the advanced duodenal stump, the afferent limb of a Billroth II gastrojejunostomy or the Roux-en-Y loop.[68] Rarely, pancreaticoduodenectomy may be required for complex ampullary injury or extensive duodenal devascularization.

Following Common Bile Duct Exploration

A biliary fistula may occur after open or laparoscopic exploration of the CBD. It can manifest as persistent bile drainage either through the T-tube or following its removal. Patients with primary closure of CBD after exploration may present with either controlled or uncontrolled bile leak depending upon the presence or absence of drain, placed intraoperatively. The most common cause is retained CBD stones. The distal CBD block due to papillary stenosis or rarely, malignancy can also cause persistent biliary fistula following CBD exploration. The management depends upon the underlying cause of obstruction.

Following Biliary Enteric Anastomosis

External biliary fistula can occur after any biliary enteric anastomosis, but it is important to differentiate the biliary leak from the enteric leak. De Castro et al.[69] reported bile leak rate of 2.3% following hepaticojejunostomy. Many studies[69-71] have reported various *risk factors* for bile leakage such as a body mass index greater than 35 kg/m^2, endoscopic biliary drainage, anastomosis of the segmental bile ducts, low serum albumin level, higher ASA grade, preoperative radiochemotherapy, preoperative low cholinesterase levels, biliary complications after liver transplantation necessitating a hepaticojejunostomy and simultaneous liver resection.

The patient usually present with bile leak through the drain, which is placed intraoperatively. In the absence of drain, it can result in formation of bilioma or frank biliary peritonitis. The technical factors such as suture line disruption or failure to include a significant biliary radicle into the anastomosis cause bile leak early in the postoperative period. However, bile leaks secondary to abscess or ischemia, causing disruption of the sutures usually become evident in a delayed manner. Most of the controlled leaks respond to *conservative management*, but in the presence of leak, healing occurs by excessive fibrosis, leading to increased risk of anastomotic stricture. Patients presenting with biliomas or biliary peritonitis may require either percutaneous or operative intervention respectively to establish a controlled EBF.

Following Liver Resection

Recently, the ISGLS has standardized the definition of bile leak as a bilirubin level in a drain 3 times the serum concentration on or after POD 3 or the need for radiologic or operative intervention from a biliary collection or bile peritonitis.[72]

The various large series[73,74] have reported bile leak of 2.5–33% following hepatic resection. The incidence varies with the type, extent and reason for liver resection. Capussotti et al.[73] reported no significant difference in bile leak rates for benign versus malignant tumors. But, higher biliary leak rates were found after hepatic resections for intrahepatic cholangiocarcinoma. In addition, no significant difference was found in leak rates for nonanatomical versus anatomical resections. The tumors, which are deeply located requiring major hepatectomy and dissection close to the major bile duct/hilar plate, are associated with increased risk of postoperative bile leak.[73,75] Anatomical anomalies of the biliary tree, especially intrahepatically, poorly vascularized liver segments or bile duct and prolonged operative times are the potential favoring factors. Also, the incidence of bile leak is higher following central hepatectomy, left sided hepatectomies and caudate lobe resections.[73-75] The concomitant bile duct resection and bilioenteric anastomosis increase the bile leak rate.[75] The leak rate is not affected by the method of liver transection. Cochrane database systematic review reported no significant difference in the bile leak rates following different parenchymal transection techniques.[76]

Intraoperatively, any leaking ducts during or after transection should be identified and carefully ligated. IOC and transcystic injection of air, saline, fat emulsion, methylene blue, indigocarmine, or ICG helps to identify biliary leaks. There is no sufficient evidence regarding the role of topical sealants (such as fibrin glue) and omental wrapping in prevention of bile leak from the resection margin. Only one randomized trial has reported lower drain bilirubin levels following use of fibrin glue.[77] Nagano et al.[78] classified postoperative bile leaks after hepatic resection into four types, which has significant implications on management.

Type A: Minor leaks from small biliary radicles on the liver transection surface
Type B: Leaks from the major bile duct branches on the liver transection surface
Type C: Injury to the main duct commonly near the hilum
Type D: Leakage due to a transected duct disconnected from the main duct.

Type A leaks usually close spontaneously with external drainage alone, while Types B and C leaks may require ERCP and stenting along with drainage of biliomas.

Type D leaks usually require bilio enteric anastomosis. If the draining segment is not significant, fibrin glue occlusion or acetic acid ablation can be helpful. Sometimes surgical excision of the excluded segment may be required.

Spontaneous External Fistulization

Neglected gallstones disease can lead to spontaneous cholecystocutaneous fistula. But over last five decades only few cases have been reported due to early diagnosis and treatment. The commonest location of fistula is the right upper quadrant of the abdomen. However, other sites such as umbilicus, right inguinal region, gluteal region or chest wall also have been described.

After Interventions

Percutaneous interventions such as PTC, PTBD or liver biopsy can lead to an EBF. In addition, obstruction of the cystic duct or distal CBD can result in persistent EBF after percutaneous or surgical cholecystostomy for empyema GB. The underlying cause of obstruction decides the management.

INTERNAL BILIARY FISTULA

They are rare and usually occur spontaneously. The incidence is reported to be less than 2%.[79] Patients with internal biliary fistula are increased risk of BDI, as these are usually recognized intraoperatively. The operating surgeon should be aware of these conditions and a proper preoperative diagnosis should be made to avoid intraoperative difficulty.

Biliobiliary Fistula

Mirizzi syndrome is caused by a large impacted stone in the gallbladder neck or infundibulum, causing extrinsic compression of the CHD with or without associated fistula. Beltran MA[80] classified Mirizzi syndrome into four types depending up on the presence or absence of fistula and the extent of destruction of CHD. Patients of Mirizzi syndrome are usually females in fifth to seventh decade and present with obstructive jaundice. Sometimes they can present with acute cholecystitis or cholangitis. Findings of USG and CT are non-specific but may be suggestive of Mirizzi syndrome in presence of dilated proximal biliary radicles only. The diagnostic accuracy of cholangiography (ERCP/MRCP) ranges from 50% to 90%. But, most patients are diagnosed intraoperatively.

Management: ERCP and stenting helps in controlling cholangitis. Surgical management is required and its extent is decided by the type of Mirizzi syndrome. Type I can be managed by cholecystectomy or subtotal cholecystectomy alone, while biliary reconstruction is often required in Types II, III and IV.[81] Although laparoscopic treatment of Mirizzi syndrome has been described,[82] low threshold for conversion should be exercised due to high risk of BDI. Intraoperatively, frozen section of the gallbladder should be performed, as malignancy may be found in up to 25% of patients.[83]

Biliary Enteric Fistula

Chronic neglected gallstone disease can lead to biliary enteric fistula. The most frequent variety is cholecystoduodenal (55–75%), followed by cholecystocolic fistula (15–30%).[84] Other less common fistula sites are cholecystogastric, choledochoduodenal and cholecystojejunal. Choledochoduodenal fistula develops most commonly due to posterior erosion of the ulcer in the first part of the duodenum. Nowadays, due to effective medical management of peptic ulcer disease, these are rarely reported. Cholecystoduodenal fistula usually remains clinically silent or can produce vague abdominal symptoms. However, passage of the large stone can cause gallstone ileus. The site of the obstruction in gallstone ileus may be distal ileum, colon (usually in the presence of stricture) or pyloroduodenal region (Bouveret syndrome). In contrast to cholecystoduodenal fistula, cholecystocolic fistula presents with unexpected change from the mild biliary colic to acute attacks. At the time of acute attack, most of the patients will have cholangitis. In addition, nausea, weight loss and steatorrhea may be present due to bile acid loss. Sometimes the irritant effect of bile acids on the colonic mucosa may cause severe choleretic diarrhea. Surgical management requires cholecystectomy with resection of the fistula tract. Laparoscopic management is not widely used, although it has been described.[85]

intravascular Fistulization

Hemobilia

It may originate from biliary tree, gallbladder and liver. Bleeding usually occurs periodically and can range from occult to clinically significant bleed. The source of significant bleed is usually arterial, although venous bleed can be massive in case of PHTN. The most frequent cause is trauma either accidental or iatrogenic. It is important to mention that postcholecystectomy pseudoaneurysms secondary to operative trauma can cause bile leaks and massive hemobilia in the early phase and bile duct strictures as a late complication.[86-88] Other causes are inflammatory conditions including gallstone disease, vascular disorders and hepatobiliary malignancies. Minor hemobilia remains asymptomatic except for chronic anemia due to fibrinolytic activity of the flowing bile causing dissolution of blood clots. Rapid bleed presents with GI hemorrhage, in the form of either melena (90%) or hemetemesis (60%), biliary colic in 70% of patients and jaundice in 60% of patients.[89,90] In suspected cases, initial evaluation should be with upper GI endoscopy to confirm the diagnosis and to rule out other causes. The cross sectional imaging either CT or MRI will reveal blood in the biliary system and also the underlying cause. When the arterial source is identified, selective angioembolization is the mainstay of treatment. Bile duct obstruction due to hemobilia can be successfully managed with endoscopic approach in most of the patients.

Bilhemia

Bile can enter into blood stream through the abnormal fistulization between the obstructed biliary system and the low pressure venous system (portal vein, hepatic veins or IVC). Though the incidence of clinically significant bilhemia is very low, but if it occurs can lead to catastrophic complications in the form of pulmonary embolization of bile or sepsis.[91] The causes are abdominal trauma, iatrogenic injury secondary to percutaneous transhepatic interventions and insertions of biliary stents/ TIPS and rarely venous erosion of gallstones. The characteristic diagnostic feature of bilhemia is rapidly progressing jaundice and marked direct hyperbilirubinemia without elevation of liver enzymes. The site of fistula is most accurately diagnosed by cholangiography by endoscopic or transhepatic approach. In addition, the diagnosis can be made on hepatobiliary scintigraphy.[92] The management should aim at relieving biliary obstruction by endoscopic or percutaneous approach, which can lead to spontaneous closure of fistula. Also, successful closure of the fistula by insertion of covered stents or angiographic coil embolization has been described.[93,94]

Intrathoracic Fistulization

The site of fistulization within the thoracic cavity may be either the pleural space or the bronchial tree. It can be iatrogenic due to external drainage procedures or secondary to parasitic diseases (amebic or echinococcal), biliary obstruction with suppuration and thoracoabdominal trauma. Patients present with pain in the right upper abdomen, pleuritic type chest pain and sometimes only difficulty in breathing.[95] In addition, patients with bronchobiliary fistula (BBF) have yellow productive sputum with bitter taste.[96] Also, signs and symptoms of systemic inflammation may be present. Imaging will reveal sub-phrenic collection, right sided pleural effusion, or consolidation in the affected bronchopulmonary segment in case of BBF. ERC, PTC or fistulogram will show the exact site of the fistula. Management is that of underlying etiology. Endoscopic or percutaneous occlusion of the fistula can be attempted and surgery should be reserved for refractory cases.[97]

Benign Biliary Stricture

INTRODUCTION

Bile duct strictures have diverse causes, each with different natural histories and management strategies. But, most frequently they are the eventual result of the BDIs; which in majority of cases are iatrogenic. Early detection, appropriate evaluation and management at the experienced centers are the key determinants for good long-term outcome. Neglected cases may develop recurrent cholangitis, biliary cirrhosis and PHTN, which can increase the morbidity and mortality.

CLASSIFICATION OF BENIGN BILIARY STRICTURES

Iatrogenic

- Open or laparoscopic cholecystectomy
- Post-transplant
- Biliary-enteric anastomosis
- ERCP related: Biliary sphincterotomy, dilation and stenting
- Percutaneous therapy for malignancies
- Radiation therapy.

Traumatic

- Blunt and penetrating abdominal trauma.

Ischemic

- Hypotension
- Hepatic artery thrombosis or stenosis
- Prolonged organ ischemia during transplant: warm and cold ischemic times
- Portal biliopathy.

Inflammatory

- Stone related: Choledocholithiasis, Mirizzi syndrome
- Chronic pancreatitis
- Primary sclerosing cholangitis
- Autoimmune cholangiopathy
- Vasculitis: systemic lupus erythematosus, Behcet disease.

Infectious

- Recurrent pyogenic cholangitis
- Parasites: Ascaris lumbricoides, Clonorchis sinensis and Opisthorchis viverrini
- Granulomatous: Tuberculosis, histoplasmosis
- Viral: Cytomegalovirus, human immunodeficiency virus

Post-cholecystectomy Benign Biliary Stricture

After BDI, as with other injuries, an inflammatory process sets in and the ultimate healing occurs by fibrosis as at other places. Healing is affected by the associated vascular injury, type of injury and amount of sepsis and local inflammation. But whatever the case may be, the net result is fibrosis, scar formation and scar contracture. This contracture results in stricture and formation of what is known as benign biliary stricture (BBS). But not all injuries will lead to BBS. Approximately 30–60% of the BDIs will develop BBS requiring intervention.[15]

PRESENTATION

These patients usually present *late with obstructive jaundice* with or without EBF. Patients with *internal fistulization* or *strictures following sectoral duct injury* may present with unexplained fever, anorexia and general debility due to repeated cholangitis.

Flow chart 1 DDs of various sequelae following post-cholecystectomy BDI

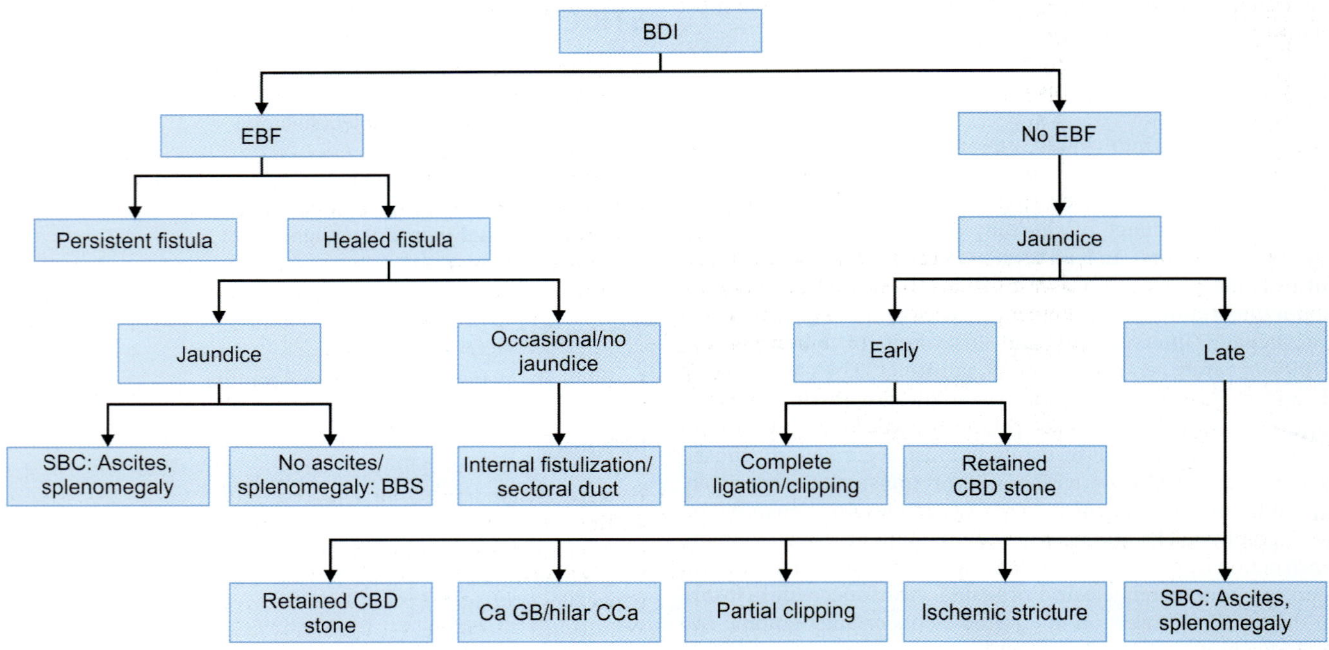

Neglected cases present with secondary biliary cirrhosis: change of complexion due to excessive pigmentation, significant weight loss and signs and symptoms of liver cell failure. In an analysis by Mishra et al.[19] out of 41 patients with BBS, 12 patients presented with progressive jaundice immediately after index surgery, while 22 were diagnosed within 2 years, 6 after 2 years and 1 case as late as 14 years after surgery. In addition, 6 patients presented with PHTN within 24–48 months after BDI. In a study published from SGPGI comprising 300 patients of BBS—the median time to presentation was 7 months, 70% patients had jaundice, 70% had recent or past history of cholangitis. About 22% had EBF and 3.7% had PHTN (Flow chart 1).[40]

Differentiation between Benign and Malignant Strictures

It is important to differentiate BBS from malignant stricture as they may present in similar way. As compared to benign stricture, patients with malignant stricture are older and more commonly have anorexia and weight loss.[98] Previous biliary surgery plays an important role in deciding the nature of the lesion as BBS are most commonly secondary to iatrogenic BDI. In a prospective study by Saluja et al.[98] out of 34 patients who had a past history of cholecystectomy, 27 had a benign stricture and 7 had a malignant stricture. In addition patients with malignant stricture usually have uneventful postoperative course with no bile leak or fistula and present with jaundice late, i.e. few weeks to months usually within a year following cholecystectomy.[99] In case of a delayed presentation, i.e. 1–2 years after uneventful cholecystectomy does not completely rule out BBS from a denovo malignancy, as in the study by Mishra et al.[19] Six patients presented after 2 years, while 1 case as late as 14 years after surgery. In such cases level of jaundice, tumor marker and imaging findings help in deciding the nature of block.

Also, malignant strictures tend to have complete obstruction with higher levels of bilirubin and alkaline phosphatase as compared to benign conditions.[98] Serum CA19-9 levels also help in differentiating benign stricture from malignant one. Saluja et al.[98] reported sensitivity of 45.5% and specificity of 88% with CA 19-9 level of more than 100 U/L in predicting the malignant strictures. But it has low predictive value in case of biliary obstruction and cholangitis, which also results in high CA 19-9 levels. However, following biliary decompression, its serum level falls in a benign condition but not in malignant structure. Thus, it is important to repeat a CA19-9 assay, 2–3 weeks following relief of jaundice.[100]

Magnetic resonance cholangiopancreatography has a better sensitivity and specificity than CT in predicting nature of the stricture.[98] On imaging, irregular duct wall thickening suggestive of a mass lesion, rim-like contrast enhancement in either the arterial or portal phase, high stricture with or without separation of right and left hepatic ducts, long stricture with an irregular margin, higher and asymmetric proximal dilatation, associated lymph node enlargement more than 1 cm and vascular invasion more favorably suggest a malignant stricture[98,99,101] (Figs. 15A to C). In addition, EUS guided FNA or brush cytology by endoscopic or percutaneous approach can sometimes help in difficult situation, but a negative result does not negate the presence of a malignancy.

Sequelae of Biliary Stricture

The BBS can lead to development of certain complications such as:

Cholangitis: Obstructed biliary system is prone to get infected and can result in recurrent cholangitis. Cholangiolitic abscesses are not uncommon in these patients. Recurrent cholangitis delays the surgical management, can result in stone formation and also increases the risk of PHTN. Cholangitis should be managed with appropriate antibiotic therapy. Sometimes in case of non-resolving

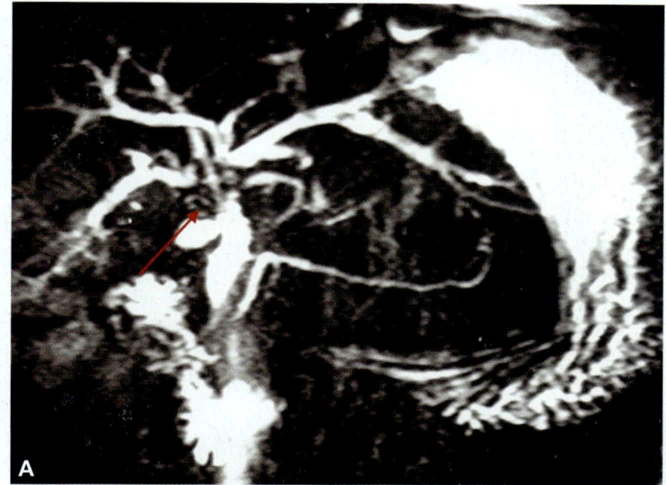

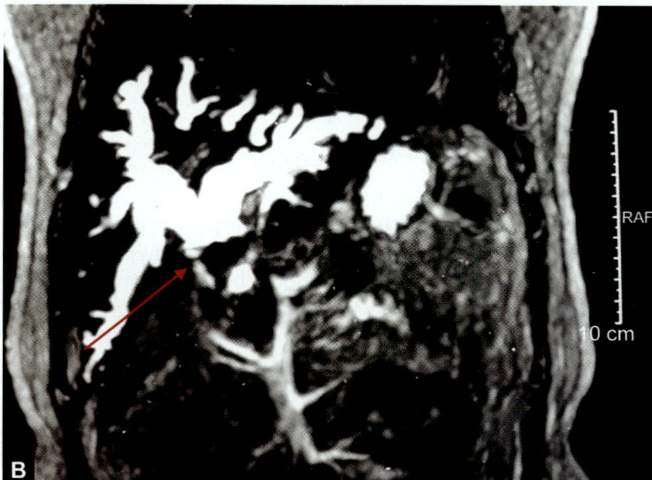

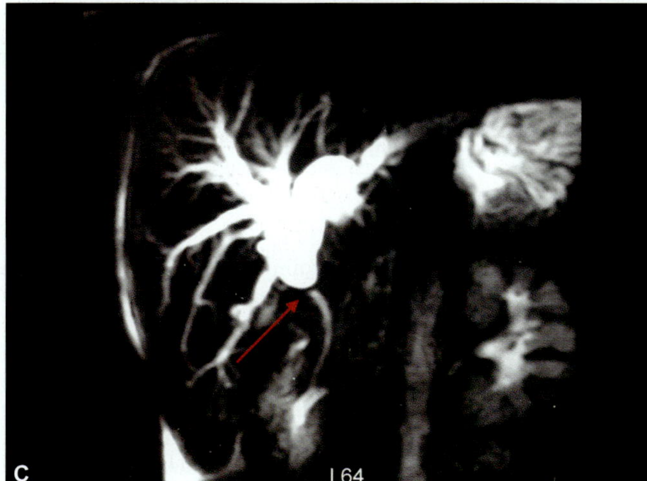

Figures 15A to C (A) MRCP image showing a stricture with separation of duct with non-formation of confluence (arrow); (B) MRCP image with abrupt cut off with irregular margin (arrow). Both these features are suggestive of a malignant stricture; (C) MRCP image showing a stricture with abrupt cut off just below confluence with smooth margins suggestive of a benign stricture

cholangitis, a biliary drainage in form of PTBD is required. In addition, abscesses not responding to biliary drainage may require percutaneous aspiration or PCD.

Portal hypertension: Approximately 15–20% patients of BBS develop PHTN.[102] It may develop as a result of secondary hepatic fibrosis, direct injury to the portal vein, or due to pre-existing liver disease. Patients of BBS usually have latent PHTN without clinical, radiological or endoscopic evidence of PHTN.[103] Overt PHTN is present in patient with long standing strictures with history of recurrent cholangitis, redo hepaticojejunostomy and rarely in patients with portal vein injury. It is important to rule out portal biliopathy secondary to PHTN in patients with blocked portal vein with collaterals in hepatoduodenal ligament. These patients may require shunt surgery before contemplating hepaticojejunotomy for biliary stricture. Presence of collaterals with patent portal vein increases the difficulty of surgery and the postoperative morbidity but does not contraindicate the surgery. Biliary repair can be done with acceptable morbidity.[102] Reversal of PHTN secondary to resolution of fibrosis has been reported after hepaticojejunostomy for BBS.[103]

Atrophy of the liver (Figs 16A and B): Atrophy of the liver is generally associated with vascular injury especially portal vein injury, although prolonged biliary obstruction can itself lead to atrophy-hypertrophy of the liver. Atrophy of single or multiple segment(s) may be associated with sectoral duct injury. In addition, atrophy-hypertrophy complex may develop due to secondary biliary cirrhosis. Presence of atrophy-hypertrophy increases the difficulty of surgery due to hilar rotation and also the chances of recurrent strictures.[104]

Secondary biliary cirrhosis (SBC): Untreated biliary strictures can lead to secondary biliary cirrhosis eventually. Sikora et al.[104,105] reported that almost all patients will have some degree of fibrosis and approximately 18% will have cirrhosis. It has more rapid course from the time of injury compared to other forms of cirrhosis and also nodular regeneration is less common. Progression is halted and liver function may recover if obstruction is relieved. However, hepatic insult can be irreversible at later stages and progress into cirrhosis in spite of biliary decompression. It is associated with adverse outcomes after surgical drainage for relief of biliary obstruction due to high risk surgical candidates, increased incidence of postoperative complications such as liver failure or hemorrhage and increased mortality.

INVESTIGATIONS

Laboratory investigations: These include routine hematological, biochemical (LFT, KFT) and coagulation profile of the patients. LFT usually reveals hyperbilirubinemia of varying intensity with raised alkaline phosphatase levels in almost all the patients. Leukocytosis may be present in the event of cholangitis. In case of EBF bile should always be sent for culture and sensitivity.

Ultrasonography: It is the initial investigation of choice in patients presenting with obstructive jaundice. It shows intrahepatic biliary radical dilatation (IHBRD), along with level of block with high sensitivity and specificity. It can also show cholangitic liver abscesses, atrophy-hypertrophy of liver lobes and intrahepatic stones which can complicate the disease process. Doppler signals

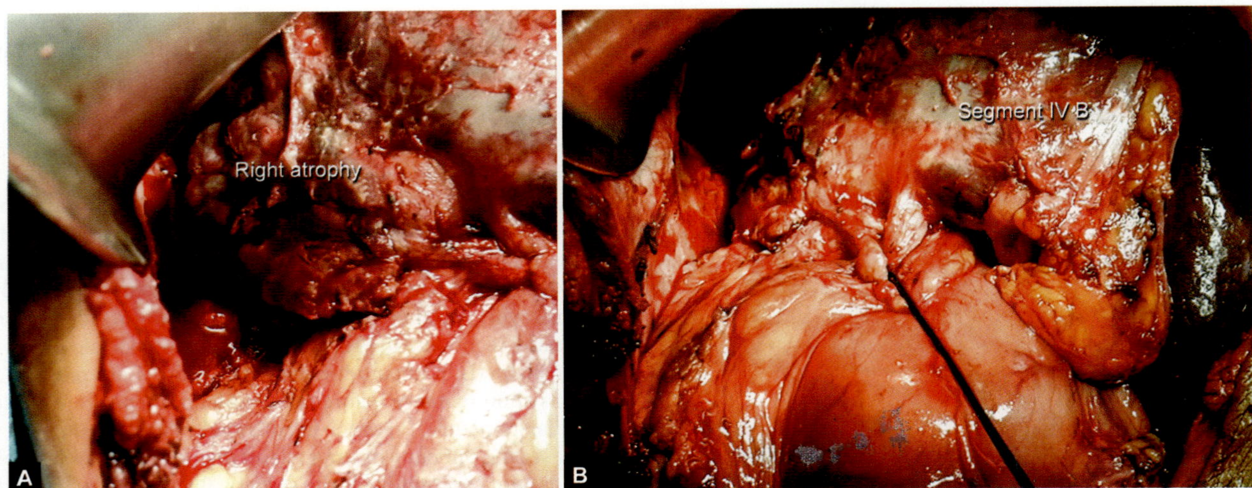

Figures 16A and B (A) Sagittal section of CECT showing right lobe atrophy with left lobe hypertrophy in a patient of bile duct stricture secondary to bile duct injury; (B) Intraoperative pictures of the same patient with right atrophy and left hypertrophy as a sequel of bile duct injury

can help in identifying the PHTN, presence of collaterals and the arterial system.

Cholangiography: Cholangiography is essential to ascertain the type of stricture and for planning of the surgery. MRCP is the investigation of choice for delineating the BBS as it can show the complete biliary tree and the level of stricture. In addition, it can reveal the atrophy, hypertrophy, IHBRD, intra-ductal calculi and cholangitic liver abscesses. Invasive procedures like percutaneous transhepatic cholangiography (PTC) are not anymore indicated except in instances when preoperative catheter placement is being planned. In case of associated EBF a fistulogram or drainogram may be done. But it is seldom done as there is an increased risk of biliary sepsis and secondly it may not show all the ducts. Endoscopic retrograde cholangiography (ERC) is indicated only with therapeutic intent. It is considered in selected cases (infrahilar and partial strictures) with therapeutic intention.

Upper GI endoscopy should be performed only in patients with long standing biliary obstruction to rule out varices secondary to PHTN.

MANAGEMENT

Before going on for surgery the surgeon should be able to answer the following questions:

- What is the level of stricture?
- Are there any associated vascular injuries?
- Is there any atrophy-hypertrophy complex associated?
- Is there any sepsis in any form like cholangitis or abscesses?
- Is there any EBF?
- Is there any PHTN?
- Can malignancy be ruled out?

The post-cholecystectomy biliary strictures are usually dealt with surgically which remains the gold standard treatment option. Recent advances in the endoscopic management have made endoscopic stenting as an alternative treatment option in selected cases with varying degree of success.

Operative Management

Once the surgeon has all the answers to the above questions he may proceed with surgery. Before taking the patient for surgery, the biochemical, hematological and coagulation parameters should be corrected if deranged. Antibiotics should be started preoperatively and should continue postoperatively. If a high stricture is seen, preoperatively percutaneously placed transhepatic stents may be used for identifying the ducts for anastomosis during surgery although we have never resorted to the same.

The aim of the surgery is to do bilioenteric anastomosis for flow of bile into the GIT. The success rate of surgical management is reported around more than 90%.[40]

The aim of the surgical repair is tension free bilioenteric mucosa to mucosa anastomosis.

The basic surgical principles are:

- Exposure of the healthy ducts draining the whole liver
- Freshening the mucosal edges for future anastomosis
- Creation of mucosa to mucosa RYHJ.

Operative Procedure

Right subcostal incision is most commonly used incision which may be converted to bilateral subcostal as required. Subhepatic adhesions are taken down and an effort is made to identify the hilum. Care should be taken to avoid injury to the colon and duodenum which are most of the time adherent to the undersurface of the liver. If the patient has an EBF with drain in situ, it helps in guiding the surgeon to the fistulous communication and the strictured area. Similar to the drain, the surgical clips also help identify the stricture site. In case of PHTN the difficult dissection is further complicated by the presence of the collaterals in hepatoduodenal area.

Intraoperative cholangiography (Fig. 17) should be performed whenever there is difficulty in identifying the biliary radicals. Hilar plate should be lowered to expose the confluence of the hepatic ducts and extrahepatic part of the left duct especially in Types 3 and 4 strictures. At all the times the biliary anatomy should be

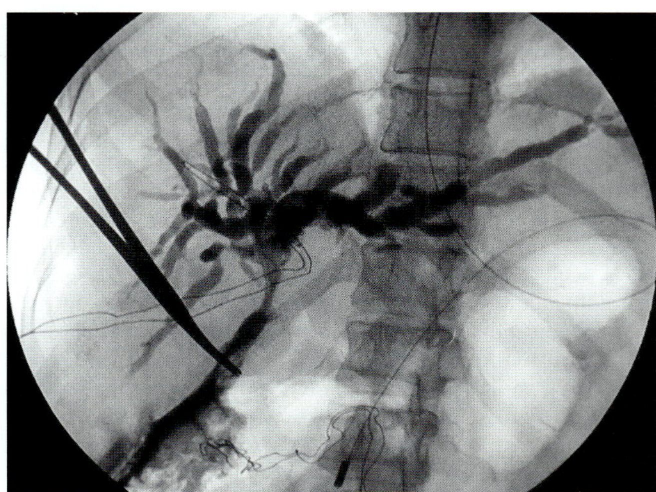

Figure 17 Intraoperative cholangiogram performed in a difficult stricture showing both left and right ductal system

correlated with the cholangiographic picture. The aim is to reach a healthy non-fibrotic area of the bile ducts. The anastomosis is straightforward in cases of Types I and II strictures, but in cases of higher strictures dissection is difficult and requires some special maneuvers. Sometimes in complex strictures the hepatotomy may be required in the gallbladder fossa to expose the right duct or a resection of a segment may be required to expose the ducts. Scar tissue is not required to be excised unless cholangiocarcinoma is suspected. Once the anastomotic site is defined, a RYHJ is done. A wide anastomosis is preferred (usually 1.5–2 cm). This is required in consideration of future contracture at the anastomosis. In case on dissection a sectoral duct is seen separately, a septoplasty is performed to make one stoma. Sometimes it may not be possible to do a septoplasty, in such a case one should perform two separate anastomosis. Utmost care should be taken to preserve the arterial supply which might be already compromised. The anastomosis is done with Blumgart-Kelly technique.[106] The anastomosis should be high irrespective of the level of the BBS. In cases of high strictures some alternative procedures may be required such as:

- Longmire procedure[107]: Hepaticojejunostomy to the cut surface of the liver
- Smith mucosal graft[108]
- Portoenterostomy.

These procedures are not frequently done and are not recommended because of high restricturing rates and morbidity. Hepatectomy may be useful in these circumstances. In case of atrophy-hypertrophy complex especially involving the right sectoral duct and right lobe, a formal right hepatectomy with left RYHJ is more acceptable than attempting usual RYHJ.

A liver biopsy (both wedge and needle) from both the lobes should be taken in Type 4 stricture to assess the grade of liver fibrosis.

Finally, liver transplantation is an alternative treatment option for end stage liver disease.

Transanastomotic stents: Routine use of transanastomotic stents is not followed by most surgeons. Surgeons use stents in selected cases such as when anastomosis is performed in nondilated ducts (<5 mm) or friable ducts. If percutaneous catheters are already in place they can be advanced across the anastomosis. Alternatively drain can be placed in retrograde fashion through the bile duct into the hepatic parenchyma with the help of a wire or probe. These stents are placed in such a way that they help in obtaining a postoperative cholangiogram. They may be kept in situ for longer duration even up to a year.

Access loop: Some surgeons have described the access loop[109] where end of the jejunal loop used for RYHJ is sutured to the parieties and marked with radiopaque markers. This loop can be accessed by the endoscopist in future if the need arises. But with radiological expertise of percutaneous transhepatic access, the access loop is rarely used.

Vascular consideration: Most experienced centers will not be attempting vascular reconstruction during the definitive repair for BBS. PHTN makes the dissection difficult at the hilum due to the presence of collaterals.[102] Sometimes the dissection may be so difficult that procedure may be abandoned altogether. In such cases a preoperative shunt is done followed by RYHJ.

Results of Surgical Repair

The results of operative repairs of BBS are difficult to analyze because of the non-uniformity in the reported surgical series. BBS after laparoscopic cholecystectomies are said to have an inferior outcomes as compared to open because of more complex nature of injuries and inflammation and subsequent fibrosis.[110] The results are assessed by MacDonald Classification in most series. The serum bilirubin and alkaline phosphatase levels fall significantly within 1–2 weeks after surgery. Negi SS[111] reported that basal values of liver function tests and degree of hepatic fibrosis are the most important predictors of abnormal recovery pattern of liver function following adequate biliary decompression in patients with post-cholecystectomy bile duct stricture. Thus, advanced hepatic fibrosis may be the actual cause of abnormal liver function tests, despite a patent hepaticojejunostomy. In absence of underlying liver parenchymal damage, a persistently elevated serum bilirubin levels and alkaline phosphatase levels on follow-up are the earliest indicators of stricture hepaticojejunostomy, while normal bilirubin but elevated ALP levels indicate undrained segment of liver. Also, sometimes the abnormal stasis in Roux loop can cause symptoms and deranged liver function tests. HIDA scan is a good investigation in the follow-up of these patients, as it evaluates both liver function and patency of the hepaticojejunostomy (Table 3).

Operative mortality has been reported from 0.6% to 1.7%.[37,40] The hospital stay in most cases varies from 5 to 10 days.[37] Postoperative complications are reported in range of 30–40%.[37,40]

Table 3: MacDonald classification

Grade A	Normal liver function test (LFT), asymptomatic
Grade B	Mild elevation of LFT, asymptomatic
Grade C	Abnormal LFT, cholangitis, pain
Grade D	Surgical revision or dilatation required

The most commonly reported complications are cholangitis, intra-abdominal abscesses and bile leaks. Failure rates of 10–19% have been reported even from high volume centres.[32,37]

Factors Deciding Successful Repair

A study from the SGPGI reported preoperative bilirubin, attempted bilioenteric anastomosis before referral, cirrhosis, PHTN, repair in the presence of EBF and spontaneous bilioenteric fistula as risk factors for failure of surgical repair for BBS.[27] Chaudhary et al.[31] found early surgery (<3 weeks) to be associated with poor outcome But, Injury-repair interval, preoperative stenting, and duration of postoperative stenting were not found to influence the outcome of repair in the series of McDonald et al.[112] and Pellegrini et al.[113]Bansal et al.[114] from AIIMS, New Delhi, demonstrated that level of injury at or above the confluence, prior attempted repair, associated vascular injury and delay in referral were associated with poorer outcomes in long-term follow-up. In addition, Sarno et al.[72] described poor outcome following BDI repair in patients with concomitant VBI and/or sepsis. However, our group[19] could not find any such factor affecting outcome following repair for BBS as poor outcome was seen in only 4% of our patients. A longer follow-up, especially in Types 3 and 4 strictures, is however necessary before these results are accepted. Delayed repair, complete delineation of biliary anatomy and mucosa-to-mucosa anastomosis in all cases attributed to these excellent results. Thus, early referral, complete characterization of the injury, definitive repair in the absence of inflammation and performance of a wide mucosa-mucosa biliary enteric anastomosis are the key determinants of good long-term outcome. Also, favorable outcome could be achieved in most of the patients with restricture by combination of percutaneous dilatation and revision surgery.

Liver Transplantation

Rarely prolonged biliary obstruction can result in progression of secondary biliary fibrosis into true cirrhosis. In these patients, liver transplantation should be taken into consideration as a substitute to biliary reconstruction. Majority of these patients will have complex BDIs with failed multiple previous attempts at biliary repair.[115] It is difficult surgical procedure compared to other indications due to previous attempts at biliary reconstruction. Although it is associated with increased duration of surgery and blood loss, morbidity and long-term results are usually similar to liver transplant performed for other indications.[116]

Nonoperative Management

With advances in endoscopy, nonoperative management using stents has been attempted and shown to be effective by the gastroenterologist. As described earlier the healing occurs by fibrosis after following a cascade of angiogenesis and re-epithelialization. By performing endoscopic dilatation of the scarred tissue there is a hematoma formation and this may further increase the fibrosis and scarring. In addition, Dunkin et al.[117] reported that stent insertion itself results in chronic inflammation of the biliary system within 4 weeks. Thus the long-term patency may be compromised.

Endoscopic balloon dilatation with stenting is utilized in the treatment protocol for endoscopic management. Stents are exchanged at an interval of 3–12 months. With this protocol Davids et al.[118] reported the endoscopic therapy results to be at par with the surgical hepaticojejunostomy. Early complications were more common with surgical treatment but total numbers of complications during the therapy were more common in the endoscopic group. Costamagna et al.[119] used a more intensive protocol of putting as many stents as could be fitted in the dilated ducts, which at 3 months were removed and replaced with an increasing number of stents. They reported a success rate of ~90% with complication (cholangitis) in only one patient at a follow-up period of 49 months. Other studies[120,121] also reported good results over a long period. Bregmann et al.[120] followed their patients up for 9 years (n=44). Only 59% could complete the treatment and 47% were stricture free with a short stent removal to restricture period. Vitale et al.[121] avoided endoscopic therapy in cases with biliary strictures longer than 2 cm or a lateral wall defect larger than one half the bile duct diameter with a concomitant bile leak. Importantly the endoscopic dilatation was used mostly in cases of Types I and II where there is some biliary continuity.

The surgical series discussed above have reported success rates of more than 90%. Tocchi et al.[122] while comparing surgical and endoscopic therapy reported excellent results in 17 of 22 patients managed surgically and 16 of 20 patients managed endoscopically. They concluded by saying that hepaticojejunostomy is the best procedure for BBS with evidence that endoscopic stenting can be an alternative strategy. Recently, Fatima[123] from Mayo Clinic concluded that endoscopic treatment policy may be used in selected patients who deny surgery, are not optimal surgical candidates, or in whom stricture develops following a surgical repair. But in simplification it can be said that endoscopy therapy requires prolonged duration of treatments with multiple endoscopic procedures with a fair success rates at relatively shorter follow-up periods. Likewise evidently surgery is a proper answer for complex strictures with excellent success rates and acceptable morbidity. It is one time answer to the problem. In short, the nonoperative treatment needs to be individualized and offered to patients who are motivated enough to adhere to the treatment protocol.

Benign Biliary Stricture Due to Other Causes

Secondary to Peptic Ulcer Disease

Penetrating posterior duodenal ulcer can cause lower end CBD stricture due to extrinsic compression, resulting from edema and fibrosis associated with ulcer. Now, such complication is rarely seen due to advent of acid reducing agents and anti *H. pylori* therapy. Sometimes deeply placed sutures to control the bleeding from duodenal ulcer can lead to a delayed distal CBD stricture. Most patients are males possibly due to the higher incidence of peptic ulcer disease in men.[124]

These patients usually present with jaundice with or without cholangitis, addition to ulcer related symptoms. Jaundice may be transient or persistent. Also, they may have associated sign and symptoms related to gastric outlet obstruction. MRCP will reveal a long smooth stricture in the distal common duct without any signal void. Upper GI endoscopy and barium meal will show ulcer itself, deformed pyloroduodenal region, edematous duodenal mucosal folds with luminal narrowing and helps in ruling out malignancy.

Management is aimed at underlying ulcer disease. Transient biliary obstruction that occurs due to inflammatory edema during acute attack of ulcer disease usually subsides with conservative medical management. However, fixed biliary obstruction secondary to ulcer related fibrosis and symptoms of cholangitis require a surgical intervention. For the ulcer, vagotomy and drainage in the form of gastrojejunostomy is preferred as antrectomy will be more morbid procedure with an increased risk of both BDI and postoperative duodenal stump leak due to difficulty in its closure.[125] At the same time, biliary bypass is performed either with CDD or Roux-en-Y CDJ depending upon the length of the stricture and status of the duodenum.

Secondary to Chronic Pancreatitis

The incidence of biliary obstruction secondary to stricture in patients with chronic pancreatitis range from 3% to 29%.[126] Biliary obstruction more commonly develops in patients with advanced stages of chronic pancreatitis, since these patients have a higher incidence of endocrine and exocrine insufficiency as reported by Kalvaria et al.[127] It results from recurrent acute inflammatory episodes leading to periductal fibrosis and subsequent stricture. The acute attack of pancreatitis resulting in edema at sphincter of Oddi and a pseudocyst compressing CBD may also cause biliary obstruction. Symptoms usually subside with resolution of the acute attack and pseudocyst, although low grade residual obstruction may remain.

Biliary obstruction in chronic pancreatitis has a varied clinical presentation from an incidental finding (17%) to overt jaundice (30–50%) and cholangitis (10%).[126] Jaundice may be transient, recurrent or persistent. Although pain is the cardinal clinical feature in these patients, biliary obstruction has minimal influence of the painful symptoms of chronic pancreatitis.[128] Laboratory tests most frequently reveal elevation of alkaline phosphatase level. Transient hyperbilirubinemia is classically seen during acute exacerbation in chronic pancreatitis. However, hyperbilirubinemia may become persistent when there is fixed obstruction of distal CBD due to cicatrization. On imaging, CT abdomen provides an accurate delineation of morphological changes in pancreas, including pseudocyst, while MRCP shows pancreatic ductal abnormalities more precisely and also reveals long and smooth stricture in the distal CBD. Sometimes, the "bent knee" and "hourglass" configurations of the CBD are seen on MRCP in chronic pancreatitis with biliary obstruction. Every effort should be made preoperatively to differentiate between benign and malignant stricture on the basis of clinical, laboratory (including serum CA 19-9 level) and imaging findings. In doubtful cases, EUS guided FANC or endoscopic brush cytology may help, although they cannot disprove the malignancy completely. Surgical exploration and intraoperative trucut biopsy and frozen section analysis are the additional tools to differentiate these two clinical entities.

Indications of biliary drainage in chronic pancreatitis with biliary obstruction (Frey et al.[129]) are:

- Symptomatic cholangitis or infected bile.
- Biliary cirrhosis (biopsy proven)
- CBD stones in association with common bile duct stricture
- Inability to rule out cancer of the pancreas
- Progression of the common bile duct stricture based on radiological assessment of increased dilatation of the common and intrahepatic bile ducts
- Persistent jaundice for over a month
- Persistently elevated alkaline phosphatase (>3 × normal levels >1 month).

Management of isolated elevation of alkaline phosphatase in chronic pancreatitis with biliary obstruction is controversial. Some authors[126,129] recommend biliary drainage in these patients due to long-term risk of secondary biliary cirrhosis (7.3%). But in the study reported by Stahl et al.,[130] out of 20 patients with isolated elevation of alkaline phosphatase, only one patient required biliary drainage during the median follow-up of 3.8 years. Also in our series (Saluja et al.[131]) none of the 15 patients with asymptomatic elevation of SAP developed complications of biliary obstruction during a median follow-up of 3 years. In addition, out of these 15 patients, 10 patients underwent only pancreatic drainage, and none of them developed complications of biliary obstruction during the follow-up period. So, biliary drainage for isolated raised alkaline phosphatase in patients who require pancreatic drainage is not required. From these three studies, it is wiser to consider serial follow-up in patients with asymptomatic elevation of alkaline phosphatase in patients of chronic pancreatitis with biliary obstruction.

Endoscopic Management

Endoscopic therapy has a limited role in managing these patients as many studies have reported poor long term outcome with increased risk of stent related complications such as blockage and migration.[132,133] Recently, Regimbeau et al.[134] reported better long-term success rate with surgery as compared to endoscopic management (65% vs 12% at 24 months). Also, Chaudhary et al.[135] reported more complications (infections) with a longer hospital stay for patients undergoing first-line endoscopy before surgery.

Surgical Management

Pancreatic head resection and bilioenteric bypass are the options for surgical management of biliary obstruction in chronic pancreatitis.

Pancreatic head resection: Pancreaticoduodenectomy is preferred in patients with high suspicion of malignancy, while in inflammatory head mass, both pancreaticoduodenectomy and Frey's procedure have been used with similar long-term results.[136] In addition, during Frey's procedure, if IOC reveals residual biliary obstruction, a bilioenteric bypass needs be performed. However, CBD reinsertion into resection cavity of Frey's procedure is not widely practiced as it is associated with a higher stricture recurrence rate as reported by Cataldegirmen et al.[137]

Bilioenteric Bypass

The options for bilioenteric bypass are cholecystojejunostomy, CDD, Roux-en-Y CDJ. Cholecystojejunostomy is not advocated as it is associated with long-term failure rate of up to 23%.[138] Both CDD and CDJ are effective biliary drainage procedures. However, the choice between these depends up on the various factors such as size of CBD, length of CBD stricture, presence of duodenal obstruction and coexistence of other pancreatic complications requiring operative treatment.[131] Addition of these biliary enteric anastomoses to pancreatic drainage procedure, does not increase the risk of major complications and also the low risk of postoperative pancreatic fistula.[139]

REFERENCES

1. Strasberg SM, Hertl M, Soper NJ. An analysis of the problem of biliary injury during laparoscopic cholecystectomy. J Am Coll Surg. 1995;180:101-25.
2. Joseph M, Phillips MR, Farrell TM, Rupp CC. Single incision laparoscopic cholecystectomy is associated with a higher bile duct injury rate: a review and a word of caution. Ann Surg. 2012;256:1-6.
3. Chaudhary A, Manisegran M, Chandra A, Agarwal AK, Sachdev AK. How do bile duct injuries sustained during laparoscopic cholecystectomy differ from those during open cholecystectomy? J Laparoendosc Adv Surg Tech A. 2001;11:187-91.
4. Sikora SS, Kumar A, Das NR, Sarkari A, Saxena R, Kapoor VK. Laparoscopic bile duct injuries: spectrum at a tertiary-care center. J of Laproendosc Adv Surg Tech. 2001;A11:63-8.
5. Gigot J, Etienne J, Aerts R, Wibin E, Dallemagne B, Deweer F, et al. The dramatic reality of biliary tract injury during laparoscopic cholecystectomy: an anonymous multicenter Belgian survey of 65 patients. Surg Endosc. 1997;11:1171-8.
6. Woods MS, Traverso LW, Kozarek RA, Tsao J, Rossi RL, Gough D, et al. Characteristics of biliary tract complications during laparoscopic cholecystectomy: a multi-institutional study. Am J Surg. 1994;167:27-33.
7. Adamsen S, Hansen OH, Funch-Jensen P, Schulze S, Stage JG, Wara P. Bile duct injury during laparoscopic cholecystectomy: a prospective nationwide series. J Am Coll Surg. 1997;184:571-8.
8. Fletcher ER, Hobbs MS, Tan P, Valinsky LJ, Hockey RL, Pikora TJ, et al. Complications of cholecystectomy: risks of the laparoscopic approach and protective effects of operative cholangiography. A population based study. Ann Surg. 1999;229:449-57.
9. Flum DR, Dellinger EP, Cheadle A, Chan L, Koepsell T. Intraoperative cholangiography and risk of common bile duct injury during cholecystectomy. JAMA. 2003;289(13):1639-44.
10. Hamad MA, Nada AA, Abdel Atty MY, et al. Major biliary complications in 2714 cases of laparoscopic cholecystectomy without intraoperative cholangiography: a multicentre retrospective study. Surg Endosc. 2011;25:3747-51.
11. Nugent N, Doyle M, Mealy K. Low incidence of retained common bile duct stones using a selective policy of biliary imaging. Surgeon. 2005;3(5):352-6.
12. Stewart L, Robinson TN, Lee CM, Liu K, Whang K, Way LW. Right hepatic artery injury associated with laparoscopic bile duct injury: incidence, mechanism, and consequences. J Gastrointest Surg. 2004;8:523-31.
13. Lau WY, Lai ECH. Classification of iatrogenic bile duct injury. Hepatobiliary Pancreat Dis Int. 2007;6:459-63.
14. Bektas H, Schrem H, Winny M, Klempnauer J. Surgical treatment and outcome of iatrogenic bile duct lesions after cholecystectomy and the impact of different clinical classification systems. Br J Surg. 2007;94(9):1119-27.
15. Bismuth H, Lazorthes F. 83rd Congress of the French Surgical Society (Paris, 21-24 September 1981): second report—operative injuries of the common biliary duct. J Chir (Paris). 1981;118:601-9.
16. Csendes A, Navarrete C, Burdiles P, Yarmuch J. Treatment of common bile duct injuries during laparoscopic cholecystectomy: endoscopic and surgical management. World J Surg. 2001;25: 1346-51.
17. Bergman JJ, van den Brink GR, Rauws EA, de Wit L, Obertop H, Huibregtse K, et al. Treatment of bile duct lesions after laparoscopic cholecystectomy. Gut. 1996;38:141-7.
18. Fingerhut A, Dziri C, Garden OJ, Gouma D, Millat B, Neugebauer E, et al. ATOM, the all-inclusive, nominal EAES classification of bile duct injuries during cholecystectomy. Surg Endosc. 2013;27(12):4608-1.
19. Mishra PK, Saluja SS, Nayeem Md, et al. Bile duct injury—from injury to repair: an analysis of management and outcome. Indian J Surg. DOI 10.1007/s12262-013-0915-3.
20. Way LW, Stewart L, Gantert W, Liu K, Lee CM, Whang K, et al. Causes and prevention of laparoscopic bile duct injuries: analysis of 252 cases from a human factors and cognitive psychology perspective. Ann Surg. 2003;237:460-9.
21. Coakley FV, Schwartz LH, Blumgart LH, Fong Y, Jarnagin WR, Panicek DM. Complex postcholecystectomy biliary disorders: preliminary experience with evaluation by means of breath-hold MR cholangiography. Radiology. 1998;209:141-6.
22. Chaudhary A, Negi SS, Puri SK, Narang P. Comparison of magnetic resonance cholangiography and percutaneous transhepatic cholangiography in the evaluation of bile duct strictures after cholecystectomy. Br J Surg. 2002;89(4):433-6.
23. Ragozzino A, De Ritis R, Mosca A, Iaccarino V, Imbriaco M. Value of MR cholangiography in patients with iatrogenic bile duct injury after cholecystectomy. Am J Roentgenol. 2004;183:1567-72.
24. Hall-Craggs MA, Allen CM, Owens CM, Theis BA, Donald JJ, Paley M, et al. MR cholangiography: clinical evaluation in 40 cases. Radiology. 1993;189(2):423-7.
25. Shinhar S, Nobel M, Shimonov M, Antebi E. Tc99m-HIDA scintigraphy versus endoscopic retrograde cholangiopancreatography in demonstrating bile leaks after laparoscopic cholecystectomy. J Nucl Med. 1998;39:1802-4.
26. Lee CM, Stewart L, Way LW. Postcholecystectomy abdominal bilecollections. Arch Surg. 2000;135:538-44.
27. Pottakkat B, Vijayahari R, Prakash A, Singh RK, Behari A, Kumar A, et al. Factors predicting failure following high bilio-enteric anastomosis for post-cholecystectomy benign biliary strictures. J Gastrointest Surg. 2010;14:1389-94.
28. de Reuver PR, Rauws EA, Vermeulen M, Dijkgraaf MG, Gouma DJ, Bruno MJ. Endoscopic treatment of post-surgical bile duct injuries: long term outcome and predictors of success. Gut. 2007;56(11):1599-605.
29. Misra S, Melton GB, Geschwind JF Venbrux AC, Cameron JL, Lillemoe KD. Percutaneous management of bile duct strictures and injuries associated with laparoscopic cholecystectomy: a decade of experience. J Am Coll Surg. 2004;198(2):218-26.
30. Stewart L, Way LW. Bile duct injuries during laparoscopic cholecystectomy. Factors that influence the results of treatment. Arch Surg. 1995;130:1123-8.
31. Chaudhary A, Chandra A, Negi SS, Sachdev A. Reoperative surgery for postcholecystectomy bile duct injuries. Dig Surg. 2002;19:22-7.
32. Schmidt SC, Langrehr JM, Hintze RE, Neuhaus P. Long-term results and risk factors influencing outcome of major bile duct injuries following cholecystectomy. Br J Surg. 2005;92(1):76-82.
33. de Reuver PR, Grossmann I, Busch OR, Obertop H, van Gulik TM, Gouma DJ. Referral pattern and timing of repair are risk factors for complications after reconstructive surgery for bile duct injury. Ann Surg. 2007;245(5):763-70.
34. Walsh RM, Henderson JM, Vogt DP, Brown N. Long-term outcome of biliary reconstruction for bile duct injuries from laparoscopic cholecystectomies. Surgery. 2007;142(4):450-7.
35. Murr MM, Gigot JF, Nagorney DM, Harmsen WS, Ilstrup DM, Farnell MB. Long term results of biliary reconstruction after laparoscopic bile duct injuries. Arch Surg. 1999;134(6):604-10.

36. Kapoor VK. Management of bile duct injuries: a practical approach. Am Surg. 2009;75:1157-60.
37. Sicklick JK, Camp MS, Lillemoe KD, Melton GB, Yeo CJ, Campbell KA, et al. Surgical management of bile duct injuries sustained during laparoscopic cholecystectomy: perioperative results in 200 patients. Ann Surg. 2005;241(5):786-95.
38. Sahajpal AK, Chow SC, Dixon E, Greig PD, Gallinger S, Wei AC. Bile duct injuries associated with laparoscopic cholecystectomy: timing of repair and long-term outcomes. Arch Surg. 2010;145(8): 757-63.
39. Perera MT, Silva MA, Hegab B, Muralidharan V, Bramhall SR, Mayer AD, et al. Specialist early and immediate repair of post-laparoscopic cholecystectomy bile duct injuries is associated with an improved long-term outcome. Ann Surg. 2011;253(3):553-60.
40. Sikora SS, Pottakkat B, Srikanth G, Kumar A, Saxena R, Kapoor VK. Post cholecystectomy benign biliary strictures—long-term results. Dig Surg. 2006;23:304-12.
41. Stewart L, Way LW. Laparoscopic bile duct injuries: timing of surgical repair does not influence success rate. A multivariate analysis of factors influencing surgical outcomes. HPB (Oxford). 2009;11(6):516-22.
42. Heise M, Schmidt SC, Adler A, Hintze RE, Langrehr JM, Neuhaus P. Management of bile duct injuries following laparoscopic cholecystectomy. Zentralbl Chir. 2003;128:944-51.
43. Thethy S, Thomson BNJ, Pleass H, Wigmore SJ, Madhavan K, Akyol M, et al. Management of biliary tract complications after orthotopic liver transplantation. Clin Transplant. 2004;18:647-53.
44. Jabłońska B, Lampe P, Olakowski M, Górka Z, Lekstan A, Gruszka T. Hepaticojejunostomy vs. end-to-end biliary reconstructions in the treatment of iatrogenic bile duct injuries. J Gastrointest Surg. 2009;13:1084-93.
45. de Reuver PR, Busch OR, Rauws EA, Lameris JS, van Gulik TM, Gouma DJ. Long-term results of a primary end-to-end anastomosis in peroperative detected bile duct injury. J Gastrointest Surg. 2007;11:296-302.
46. Wills VL, Jorgensen JO, Hunt DR. Role of relaparoscopy in the management of minor bile leakage after laparoscopic cholecystectomy. Br J Surg. 2000;87(2):176-80.
47. Strasberg SM, Helton WS. An analytical review of vasculobiliary injury in laparoscopic and open cholecystectomy. HPB (Oxford). 2011;13:1-14.
48. Li J, Frilling A, Nadalin S, Paul A, Malagò M, Broelsch CE. Management of concomitant hepatic artery injury in patients with iatrogenic major bile duct injury after laparoscopic cholecystectomy. Br J Surg. 2008;95:460-5.
49. Alves A, Farges O, Nicolet J, Watrin T, Sauvanet A, Belghiti J. Incidence and consequence of an hepatic artery injury in patients with postcholecystectomy bile duct strictures. Ann Surg. 2003;238:93-6.
50. Mays ET, Wheeler CS. Demonstration of collateral arterial flow after interruption of hepatic arteries in man. N Engl J Med. 1974;290:993-6.
51. Bengmark S, Rosengren K. Angiographic study of the collateral circulation to the liver after ligation of the hepatic artery in man. Am J Surg. 1970;119:620-4.
52. Vellar ID. The blood supply of the biliary ductal system and its relevance to vasculobiliary injuries following cholecystectomy. Aust N Z J Surg. 1999;69:816-20.
53. Bachellier P, Nakano H, Weber JC Lemarque P, Oussoultzoglou E, Candau C, et al. Surgical repair after bile duct and vascular injuries during laparoscopic cholecystectomy: when and how? World J. Surg. 2001;25:1335-45.
54. Gupta N, Solomon H, Fairchild R, Kaminski DL. Management and outcome of patients with combined bile duct and hepatic artery injuries. Arch Surg. 1998;133:176-81.
55. Pulitanò C, Parks RW, Ireland H, Wigmore SJ, Garden OJ. Impact of concomitant arterial injury on the outcome of laparoscopic bile duct injury. Am J Surg. 2011;201(2):238-44.
56. Tzovaras G, Dervenis C. Vascular injuries in laparoscopic cholecystectomy: an underestimated problem. Dig Surg. 2006;23: 370-4.
57. Halasz NA. Cholecystectomy and hepatic artery injury. Arch Surg. 1991;126:137-8.
58. Stewart L, Robinson TN, Lee CM, Liu K, Whang K, Way LW. Right hepatic injury associated with laparoscopic bile duct injury: incidence, mechanism and consequences. J Gastrointest Surg. 2004;8:523-31.
59. Sarno G, Al-Sarira AA, Ghaneh P, Fenwick SW, Malik HZ, Poston GJ. Cholecystectomy-related bile duct and vasculobiliary injuries. British Journal of Surgery. 2012;99:1129-36.
60. DeSantibañes E, Ardiles V, Gadano A, Palavecino M, Pekolj J, Ciardullo M, et al. Liver transplantation: the last measure in the treatment of bile duct injuries. World J Surg. 2008;32:1714-21.
61. Truant S, Boleslawski E, Lebuffe G, Sergent G, Pruvot FR. Hepatic resection for post-cholecystectomy bile duct injuries: a literature review. HPB. 2010;12:334-41.
62. Wang Z, Yu L, Wang W, Xia J, Li D, Lu Y, et al. Therapeutic strategies of iatrogenic portal vein injury after cholecystectomy. J Surg Res. 2013;185(2):934-9.
63. Meyers WC, Peterseim DS, Pappas TN, Schauer PR, Eubanks S, Murray E, et al. Low insertion of hepatic segmental duct VII-VIII is an important cause of major biliary injury or misdiagnosis. Am J Surg. 1996;171(1):187-91.
64. Babel N, Sakpal SV, Paragi P, Wellen J, Feldman S, Chamberlain RS. Iatrogenic bile duct injury associated with anomalies of the right hepatic sectoral ducts: a misunderstood and underappreciated problem. HPB Surg. 2009;2009:153269.
65. Perera MT, Monaco A, Silva MA, Bramhall SR, Mayer AD, Buckels JA, et al. Laparoscopic posterior sectoral bile duct injury: the emerging role of nonoperative management with improved long-term results after delayed diagnosis. Surg Endosc. 2011;25(8): 2684-91.
66. Mishra PK, Saluja SS, Nag HH, Goel N, Jain A, Kujur D. Isolated extrahepatic bile duct injury after blunt trauma abdomen. Am Surg. 2012;78(9):1014-6.
67. Dixon JA, Morgan KA, Adams DB. Management of common bile duct injury during partial gastrectomy. Am Surg. 2009;75(8): 719-21.
68. White TT, Sanderson ER, Morgan A. Injury to the sphincter of Oddi in the course of gastric and duodenal surgery. Am J Surg. 1967;114(2):247-53.
69. de Castro SM, Kuhlmann KF, Busch OR, van Delden OM, Laméris JS, van Gulik TM, et al. Incidence and management of biliary leakage after hepaticojejunostomy. J Gastrointest Surg. 2005;9(8):1163-71.
70. Zafar SN, Khan MR, Raza R, Khan MN, Kasi M, Rafiq A, et al. Early complications after biliary enteric anastomosis for benign diseases: a retrospective analysis. BMC Surg. 2011;11:19.
71. Antolovic D, Koch M, Galindo L, et al. Hepaticojejunostomy—analysis of risk factors for postoperative bile leaks and surgical complications. J Gastrointest Surg. 2007;11(5):555-61.
72. Koch M, Garden OJ, Padbury R, Rahbari NN, Adam R, Capussotti L, et al. Bile leakage after hepatobiliary and pancreatic surgery: a definition and grading of severity by the International Study Group of Liver Surgery. Surgery. 2011;149(5):680-8.
73. Capussotti L, Ferrero A, Viganò L, Sgotto E, Muratore A, Polastri R. Bile leakage and liver resection: where is the risk? Arch Surg. 2006;141(7):690-4.
74. Yamashita Y, Hamatsu T, Rikimaru T, Tanaka S, Shirabe K, Shimada M, et al. Bile leakage after hepatic resection. Ann Surg. 2001;233(1):45-50.

75. Lo CM, Fan ST, Liu CL, Lai EC, Wong J. Biliary complications after hepatic resection: risk factors, management, and outcome. Arch Surg. 1998;133(2):156-61.
76. Gurusamy KS, Pamecha V, Sharma D, Davidson BR. Techniques for liver parenchymal transection in liver resection. Cochrane Database Syst Rev. 2009;(1):CD006880.
77. Boonstra EA, Molenaar IQ, Porte RJ, de Boer MT. Topical haemostatic agents in liver surgery: do we need them? HPB (Oxford). 2009;11(4):306-10.
78. Nagano Y, Togo S, Tanaka K, Masui H, Endo I, Sekido H, et al. Risk factors and management of bile leakage after hepatic resection. World J Surg. 2003;27(6):695-8.
79. Reisner RM, Cohen JR. Gallstones: a review of 1001 reported cases. Am Surg. 1994;60:441-6.
80. Beltran MA, Csendes A, Cruces KS. The relationship of Mirizzi syndrome and cholecystoenteric fistula: validation of a modified classification. World J Surg. 2008;32:2237-43.
81. Beltran MA. Mirizzi syndrome: history, current knowledge and proposal of a simplified classification. World J Gastroenterol. 2012;18(34):4639-50.
82. Yeh C, Jan Y, Chen M. Laparoscopic treatment for Mirizzi syndrome. Surg Endosc. 2003;17:1573-8.
83. Redaelli CA, Buchler MW, Schilling MK, Krähenbühl L, Ruchti C, Blumgart LH, et al. High coincidence of Mirizzi syndrome and gallbladder carcinoma. Surgery. 1997;121:58-63.
84. Petrowsky H, Clavien P. Biliary fistula, gallstone ileus, and Mirizzi's syndrome. In: Clavien PA, Baillie J (Eds). Diseases of the Gallbladder and Bile Ducts: Diagnosis and Treatment, 2nd edition. Malden (MA): Blackwell Publishing; 2008. pp. 239-51.
85. Gentileschi P, Forlini A, Rossi P, Bacaro D, Zoffoli M, Gentileschi E. Laparoscopic approach to cholecystocolic fistula: report of a case. J Laparoendosc Surg. 1995;5:413-7.
86. Dogru O, Cetinkaya Z, Bulbuller N, Camci C, Aygen E. Hemobilia: a rare complication of laparoscopic cholecystectomy. Surg Endosc. 2003;17:1495-6.
87. Srinivasaiah N, Bhojak M, Jackson R, Woodcock S. Vascular emergencies in cholelithiasis and cholecystectomy: our experience with two cases and literature review. Hepatobiliary Pancreat Dis Int. 2008;7:217-20.
88. Madanur MA, Battula N, Sethi H, Deshpande R, Heaton N, Rela M. Pseudoaneurysm following laparoscopic cholecystectomy. Hepatobiliary Pancreat Dis Int. 2007;6:294-8.
89. Sandblom P. Hemobilia (Biliary Tract Hemorrhage). Springfield (MA): Charles C Thomas; 1972.
90. Kim KH, Kim TN. Etiology, clinical features, and endoscopic management of hemobilia: a retrospective analysis of 37 cases. Korean J Gastroenterol. 2012;59:296-302.
91. Sandblom P, Jakobsson B, Lindgren H, Lunderquist A. Fatal bilhemia. Surgery. 2000;127:354-7.
92. Francois D, Walrand S, Van Nieuwenhuyse JP, de Ville de Goyet J, Pauwels S. Hepatobiliary scintigraphyin a patient with bilhemia. Eur J Nucl Med. 1994;21:1020-3.
93. Struyven J, Cremer M, Pirson P, Jeanty P, Jeanmart J. Posttraumatic bilhemia: diagnosis and catheter therapy. AJR Am J Roentgenol. 1982;138:746-7.
94. Rankin RN, Vellet DA. Portobiliary fistula: occurrence and treatment. Can Assoc Radiol J. 1991;42:55-9.
95. Gugenheim J, Ciardullo M, Traynor O, Bismuth H. Bronchobiliary fistulas in adults. Ann Surg. 1988;207:90-4.
96. Poullis M, Poullis A. Biliptysis caused by a bronchobiliary fistula. J Thorac Cardiovasc Surg. 1999;118:971-2.
97. Singh B, Moodley J, Sheik-Gafoor MH, Dhooma N, Reddi A. Conservative management of thoracobiliaryfistula. Ann Thorac Surg. 2002;73:1088-91.
98. Saluja SS, Sharma R, Pal S, Sahni P, Chattopadhyay TK. Differentiation between benign and malignant hilar obstructions using laboratory and radiological investigations: a prospective study. HPB (Oxford). 2007;9(5):373-82.
99. Sharma A, Behari A, Sikora SS, Kumar A, Saxena R, Kapoor VK. Post-cholecystectomy biliary strictures: not always benign. J Gastroenterol Hepatol. 2008;23(7 Pt 2):e63-6.
100. Mann DV, Edwards R, Ho S, Lau WY, Glazer G. Elevatedtumour marker CA19-9: clinical interpretation and influence of obstructive jaundice. Eur J Surg Oncol. 2000;26:474-9.
101. Choi SH, Han JK, Lee JM, Lee KH, Kim SH, Lee JY, et al. Differentiating malignant from benign common bile duct stricture with multiphasic helical CT. Radiology. 2005;236(1):178-83.
102. Agarwal AK, Gupta V, Singh S, Agarwal S, Sakhuja P. Management of patients of postcholecystectomy benign biliary stricture complicated by portal hypertension. Am J Surg. 2008;195(4):421-6.
103. Ibrarullah M, Sikora SS, Agarwal DK. "Latent" portal hypertension in benign biliary obstruction. HPB Surg. 1996;9(3):149-52.
104. Pottakkat B, Vijayahari R, Prasad KV, Sikora SS, Behari A, Singh RK, et al. Surgical management of patients with post-cholecystectomy benign biliary stricture complicated by atrophy-hypertrophy complex of the liver. HPB (Oxford). 2009;11(2):125-9.
105. Sikora SS, Srikanth G, Agrawal V, Gupta RK, Kumar A, Saxena R, et al. Liver histology in benign biliary stricture: fibrosis to cirrhosis and reversal? J Gastroenterol Hepatol. 2008;23:1879-84.
106. Blumgart LH, Kelly CJ. Hepaticojejunostomy in benign and malignant high bile duct stricture—approaches to the left hepatic ducts. Br J Surg. 1984;71:257-61.
107. Longmire WP, Sandford MC. Intrahepatic cholangiojejunostomy with partial hepatectomy for biliary obstruction. Surgery. 1948;128:264-76.
108. Wexler MJ, Smith R. Jejunal mucosal graft: a sutureless technic for repair of high bile duct strictures. Am J Surg. 1975;129(2):204-11.
109. Al-Ghnaneim R, Benjamin IS. Long term outcomes of hepaticojejunostomy with routine access loop formation following iatrogenic bile duct injury. Br J Surg. 2002;89:1118-24.
110. Lillemoe KD, Martin SA, Cameron JL, Yeo CJ, Talamini MA, Kaushal S, et al. Major bile duct injuries during laparoscopic cholecystectomy. Follow-up after combined surgical and radiologic management. Ann Surg. 1997;225(5):459-68.
111. Negi SS, Chaudhary A. Analysis of abnormal recovery pattern of liver function tests after surgical repair of bile duct strictures. J Gastroenterol Hepatol. 2005;20(10):1533-7.
112. McDonald MI, Farnell MB, Nagorney D, Ilstrup DM, Kutch JM. Benign biliary strictures: repair and outcome with a contemporary approach. Surgery. 1995;118:582-91.
113. Pellegrini CA, Thomas MJ, Way LW. Recurrent biliary stricture—pattern of recurrence and outcome of surgical therapy. Am J Surg.1984;147:175-80.
114. Bansal VK, KrishnaA, Misra MC, et al. Factors affecting short-term and long-term outcomes after bilioenteric reconstruction for post-cholecystectomy bile duct injury: experience at a tertiary care centre. Indian J Surg. DOI 10.1007/s12262-013-0880-x.
115. de Santibañes E, Ardiles V, Gadano A, Palavecino M, Pekolj J, Ciardullo M. Liver transplantation: the last measure in the treatment of bile duct injuries. World J Surg. 2008;32(8):1714-2.
116. Lubikowski J, Chmurowicz T, Post M, Jarosz K, Białek A, Milkiewicz P, et al. Liver transplantation as an ultimate step in the management of iatrogenic bile duct injury complicated by secondary biliary cirrhosis. Ann Transplant. 2012;17(2):38-44.
117. Dunkin BJ, Marks JM, Singh J, Lash RH, Ponsky JL. Short-term endobiliary stenting results in chronic inflammation of the porcine extrahepatic biliary system. Surg Laparosc Endosc Percutan Tech. 2000;10:275-7.

118. Davids PH, Tanka AK, Rauws EA, et al. Benign biliary strictures. Surgery or endoscopy? Ann Surg. 1993;217:237-43.
119. Costamagna G, Pandolfi M, Mutignanin M, Spada C, Perri V. Long term results of endoscopic management of bile duct strictures with increasing number of stents. Gastrointest Endosc. 2001;54:162-8.
120. Bregman JJ, Burgemeister L, Bruno MJ, Rauws EA, Gouma DJ, Tytgat GN, et al. Long term follow up after biliary stent placement for post operative bile duct stenosis. Gastroinetst Endosc. 2001;54: 154-61.
121. Vitale GC, Tran TC, Davis BR, Vitale M, Vitale D, Larson G. Endoscopic management of postcholecystectomy bile duct strictures. J Am Coll Surg. 2008;206:918-25.
122. Tocchi A, Mazzoni G, Liotta G, Costa G, Lepre L, Miccini M, et al. Management of benign biliary strictures: biliary enteric anastomosis vs. endoscopic stenting. Arch Surg. 2000;135(2):153-7.
123. Fatima J, Barton JG, Grotz TE, Geng Z, Harmsen WS, Huebner M, et al. Is there a role for endoscopic therapy as a definitive treatment for post-laparoscopic bile duct injuries? J Am Coll Surg. 2010;211: 495-502.
124. Hutchings VC, Wheeler JR, Puestow CB. Choledochoduodenal fistula complicating duodenal ulcer. AMA Arch Surg. 1956;73:598.
125. Glick S. Benign non-traumatic stricture of the common bile-duct owing to penetrating duodenal ulcer. Br J Surg. 1971;58(12):918-20.
126. Abdallah AA, Krige JE, Bornman PC. Biliary tract obstruction in chronic pancreatitis. HPB (Oxf). 2007;9:421-8.
127. Kalvaria I, Bornman PC, Marks IN, Girdwood AH, Bank L, Kottler RE. The spectrum and natural history of common bile duct stenosis in chronic alcohol induced pancreatitis. Ann Surg. 1989;210:608-13.
128. Kahl S, Zimmermann S, Genz I, Schmidt U, Pross M, Schulz HU, et al. Biliary strictures are not the cause of pain in patients with chronic pancreatitis. Pancreas. 2004;28:387-90.
129. Frey C, Suzuki M, Isaji S. Treatment of chronic pancreatitis by obstruction of the bile duct or duodenum. World J Surg. 1990;14: 59-69.
130. Stahl TJ, Allen MO, Ansel HJ, Vennes JA. Partial biliary obstruction caused by chronic pancreatitis. An appraisal of indications for surgical biliary drainage. Ann Surg. 1988;207:26-32.
131. Saluja SS, Kalayarasan R, Mishra PK, Srivastava S, Chandrasekar S, Godhi S. Chronic pancreatitis with benign biliary obstruction: management issues. World J Surg. 2014;38(9):2455-9.
132. Farnbacher MJ, Rabenstein T, Ell C, Hahn EG, Schneider HT. Is endoscopic drainage of common bile duct stenoses in chronic pancreatitis up-to-date? Am J Gastroenterol. 2000;95:1466-71.
133. Kahl S, Zimmermann S, Genz I, Glasbrenner B, Pross M, Schulz HU, et al. Risk factors for failure of endoscopic stenting of biliary strictures in chronic pancreatitis: a prospective follow-up study. Am J Gastroenterol. 2003;98:2448-53.
134. Regimbeau JM, Fuks D, Bartoli E, Fumery M, Hanes A, Yzet T, et al. A comparative study of surgery and endoscopy for the treatment of bile duct stricture in patients with chronic pancreatitis. Surg Endosc. 2012;26(10):2902-8.
135. Chaudhary A, Negi SS, Masood S, Thombare M. Complications after Frey's procedure for chronic pancreatitis. Am J Surg. 2004;188: 277-81.
136. Strate T, Bachmann K, Busch P, Mann O, Schneider C, Bruhn JP, et al. Resection vs. drainage in treatment of chronic pancreatitis: long-term results of a randomized trial. Gastroenterology. 2008;134:1406-11.
137. Cataldegirmen G, Bogoevski D, Mann O, Kaifi JT, Izbicki JR, Yekebas EF. Late morbidity after duodenum-preservingpancreatic head resection with bile duct reinsertion into theresection cavity. Br J Surg. 2008;95:447-52.
138. Vijungco J, Prinz R. Management of biliary and duodenal complications of chronic pancreatitis. World J Surg. 2003;27: 1258-70.
139. Cauchy F, Regimbeau JM, Fuks D, Balladur P, Tiret E, Paye F. Influence of bile duct obstruction on the results of Frey's procedure for chronic pancreatitis. Pancreatology. 2014;14(1):21-6.

CHAPTER 58

Primary Sclerosing Cholangitis

Siddharth Srivastava

INTRODUCTION

Primary sclerosing cholangitis (PSC) is a chronic, progressive cholestatic liver disease of unidentified etiology and poorly understood pathogenesis. It is characterized by ongoing inflammation, fibrosis and strictures of intrahepatic and extrahepatic bile ducts culminating to biliary cirrhosis. Liver transplant for survival essentially emphasizes lack of drugs or such treatment which could reverse the pathogenic mechanism. These patients are prone to develop cholangiocarcinoma (CCA), colorectal cancer (CRC) and pancreatic carcinoma.[1] In other words PSC is a potentially fatal precancerous disorder. Ten-year survival is about 65% and prognosis is poorer with onset of jaundice.[2] Asymptomatic PSC and small duct PSC (PSC variant solely involving bile ducts at the microscopic level) have a better long-term prognosis. PSC is often difficult to diagnose and challenging to treat.

EPIDEMIOLOGY

Primary sclerosing cholangitis is uncommon in India and Southeast Asia. There are only case series from India on PSC. Highest prevalence is reported from northern Europe. Age of onset of PSC varies from childhood (<10 years) to 70–80 years of age.[3] PSC is mainly a disease of young adults in the 3rd and 4th decade of life. There are no systematic studies on epidemiology of PSC. Reported incidence from systematic review of eight studies was 0.77 per 100,000 person-years with median age of 41 years.[4] Peak prevalence (16.2/100,000) is reported from western Sweden along with increasing inflammatory bowel disease (IBD)-associated PSC, large duct PSC, and PSC without IBD, also small-duct PSC among males.[5] PSC prevalence is increased among first-degree relatives of patients with PSC.

CURRENT PATHOGENETIC CONCEPTS IN PRIMARY SCLEROSING CHOLANGITIS

Concepts in pathogenesis of PSC are largely marred by lack of animal model. Histopathologically PSC is characterized by concentric periductal fibrosis involving medium to large bile ducts culminating in strictures and end stage liver disease.[6] Multiple theories are postulated for pathogenesis of PSC, following have been proposed as putative mechanisms involved in pathogenesis of PSC.

- As PSC and ulcerative colitis are closely related immune mediated destruction of liver may be linked to leaky gut. Primary injury seems to be directed against cholangiocytes leading to obliterative changes.[7] Multiple other putative mechanisms possibly play a role as majority of PSC is associated with ulcerative colitis (>90%) but only around 10% of ulcerative colitis is associated with PSC.
- Portal pyemia leading to "toxic bile" may be contributory in pathogenesis of PSC.
- Ischemic injury to bile ducts might activate the vicious cycle of obliterative changes in bile ducts and hence to perpetuation of PSC.
- Genetic factors as outlined by genome wide association studies (GWAS) (Fig. 1).

Gut liver axis: Increased intestinal permeability due to altered gut barrier function leads to lymphocyte activation and increased number of lymphocytes in portal circulation. Several extra-intestinal manifestations of IBD are correlated with disease activity.[8] These manifestations are result of activated effector cells recruitment from the gut. Some manifestations are not related to disease activity of IBD and may develop even after proctocolectomy which is possibly because of circulating long-living gut-derived

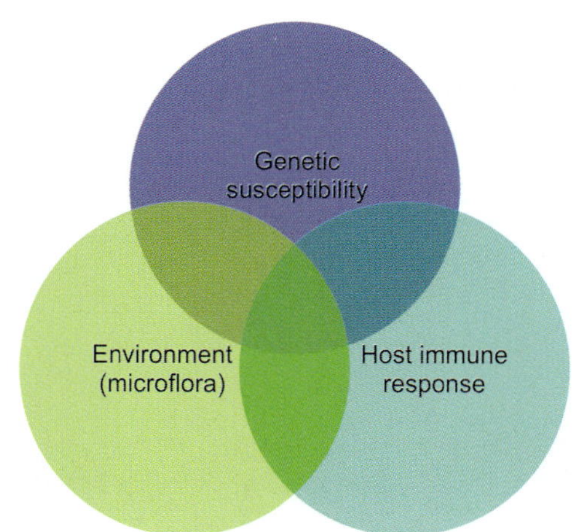

Figure 1 Interplay between host and environmental factors in primary sclerosing cholangitis

memory lymphocytes.[8] To support the gut liver axis hypothesis it is postulated that circulating perinuclear anti-neutrophil cytoplasmic antibodies (p-ANCA) is result of cross reactions between tubulin beta 5 and intestinal bacterial antigens.[9]

The "toxic bile" concept: There are contradictory reports regarding this hypothesis. Although mice studies showed evidence of bacterial infection and hence toxic bile in knock out models.[10,11] Some studies found increased risk of portal venous bacteremia in PSC; subsequent reviews, however, did not confirm the same.[12,13]

Genetics: Genetic predisposition is implicated in IBD and PSC. First degree relatives of PSC have higher risk for developing PSC and also IBD without PSC compared with the general population.[14] Recent Norwegian study found strong associations near the extended HLA complex on chromosome 6p21 and weaker associations at the GPC5/GPC6 (GPC, glypican) region on 13q31 as well as genetic loci on 3p21 and 2q35, which have been implicated in genetic susceptibility to IBD.[15] Other genes implicated in PSC include:

- ABCB4 or PXR (nuclear xenobiotic receptor) variants.
- Bile salt export pump (BSEP) and MDR3 variant segregation and haplotypes.[16]
- TGR5, the G-protein coupled bile acid receptor.[7,15,17]
- Ulcerative colitis susceptibility loci REL, IL2 and CARD9.[18-22]

MANIFESTATIONS

Clinical Features

No specific features are attributed to PSC. Majority of patients are asymptomatic and PSC is usually diagnosed as part of evaluation of abnormal liver function tests in setting of ulcerative colitis.[12,23,24] Commonest symptom reported is fatigue, pathogenesis of which is poorly understood. Other clinical features include pruritus, right upper quadrant pain, weight loss, fever and chills.[12] Severe pruritus warrants liver transplantation.

Laboratory evaluation reveals predominantly cholestatic pattern of liver injury, i.e. elevated serum alkaline phospatase and γ-glutamyl transferase with or without hyperbilirubinemia. Serum albumin levels are usually normal except when end stage liver disease has set in or acute exacerbation of IBD. Transaminases are typically elevated but usually less than 300 IU/mL.

Natural History

Primary sclerosing cholangitis is progressive destructive disease; survival without liver transplant is about 10–12 years from the time of diagnosis of disease.

Autoantibodies in Primary Sclerosing Cholangitis

Primary sclerosing cholangitis is more like immune mediated destruction of bile ducts. Multiple antibodies are seen in PSC, these include: Hypergammaglobulinemia in about third of patients, increased IgM levels in about 50% of patients, p-ANCA in 30–80% of cases and human leukocyte antigen DRw52a.[25,26] Anti-mitochondrial antibodies (AMA) are characteristically absent in PSC. Angulo et al. found that 97% patients with PSC were positive for at least one autoantibody, while 81% were positive for more than or equal to 3 antibodies.[27] Antibodies do not correlate with prognosis.

Radiology

Diagnosis of PSC is established by radiographic techniques only. Cholangiography is gold standard for diagnosing PSC.[28,29] Ultrasonographic evaluation of biliary tract is usually normal or reveals non-specific changes in bile ducts which include wall thickening and focal bile duct dilations.[30] Gall bladder also may show changes of cholecystitis, stones, sludge or mass in gall bladder. Mass is most often malignant. Ultrasound is also important to look for changes of chronic liver disease and portal hypertension.

Computed tomography usually shows findings similar to ultrasonographic findings; none of changes in USG or CT are diagnostic for PSC.

Depending upon changes in cholangiography, PSC is classified into classic PSC or small duct PSC. Cholangiography can be done either noninvasively by magnetic resonance cholangiopancreatography (MRCP) (Fig. 2) or invasively by endoscopic retrograde cholangiopancreatography (ERCP) (Fig. 3)

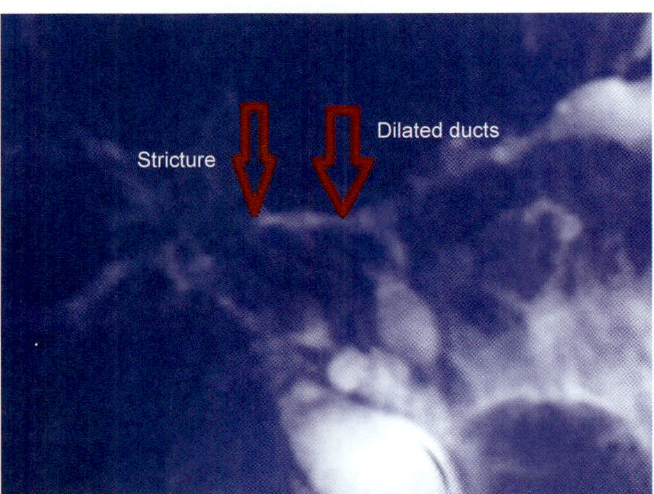

Figure 2 MRCP images showing strictures in primary sclerosing cholangitis

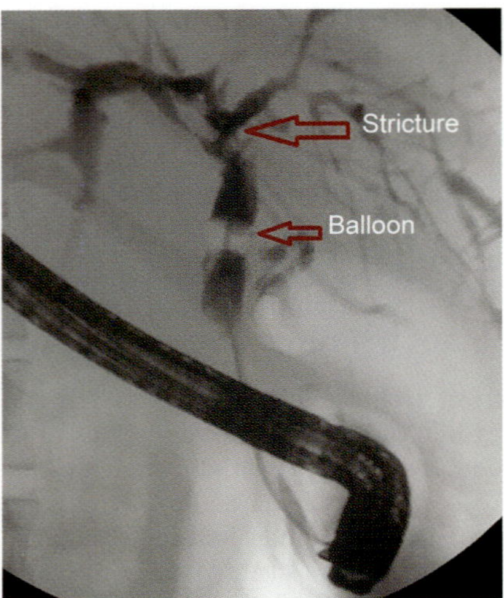

Figure 3 ERCP images showing multiple strictures and dilatations

or by percutaneous transhepatic cholangiogram (PTC). ERCP is still the diagnostic test of choice and due to invasiveness MRCP is usually first test in diagnosis of PSC. Recent meta-analysis of six studies found, the sensitivity and specificity of MRCP in diagnosing PSC as 86% and 94%, respectively. MRCP reveals focal stricturing and resultant dilatations giving characteristic beaded pattern.

Classic Primary Sclerosing Cholangitis

Classic PSC shows strictures, dilatations and sometimes pruning of bile ducts. PSC can involve all parts of biliary tree. Lee et al. demonstrated that 87% of patients have both intrahepatic and extrahepatic bile ducts involvement,11% have only intrahepatic bile ducts involved while extrahepatic ducts are involved in only 2% cases.[31] Up to 40% patients have gall bladder and cystic duct abnormalities.[32] Gall bladder involvement is more common in extrahepatic bile duct involvement. Gall bladder mass if present is predominantly malignant.[32]

Small Duct Primary Sclerosing Cholangitis

Specifically includes condition with clinical, biochemical and histopathologic features of PSC in absence of cholangiographic alterations.[3] Small proportion about 15% of PSC cases fall in this category and 22% of these may progress to large duct variety over follow-up of 72 months, signifying importance of repeat cholangiography in patients of small duct PSC.[33] Small duct PSC has favorable long-term prognosis and lower risk of CCA as compared to classic PSC.[33]

Liver Biopsy

Controversies exist over role of liver biopsy in diagnosing PSC. American Association for Study on Liver Diseases (AASLD) does not favor liver biopsy in diagnosing PSC.[30] Liver biopsy is advocated in small duct PSC where index of suspicion is high but cholangiography does not show characteristic changes of PSC. Biospy however is important for staging, and to exclude other or coexisting liver diseases.

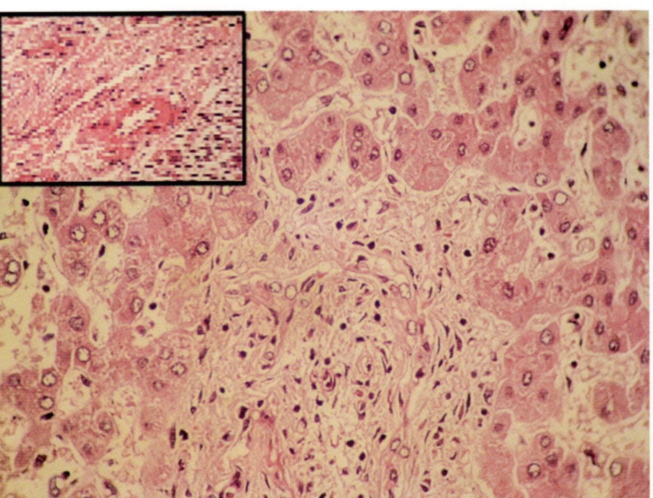

Figure 4 Liver biopsy of case of PSC. H & E stained slide showing fibrosis of portal tract with sparse lymphocytic inflammation with sclerosed bile duct (x10). Inset showed characteristic concentric fibrosis. (x40)
Source: Dr. RK Saran, Department of Pathology.

Histologically (Fig. 4) disease starts from portal triads gradually progressing to involve hepatic parenchyma. Disease is classified into four stages similar to primary biliary cirrhosis (PBC):[34]

- Stage I: Limited to portal triads with enlargement, edema, and scarring, and mononuclear cell infiltration with some piecemeal necrosis and damage to isolated bile ducts. Although proliferation of bile ducts may be seen but inflammation is less dense as compared to PBC.
- Stage II: Disease extends into the liver parenchyma.
- Stage III: Bridging fibrosis.
- Stage IV: Cirrhosis.

Pathognomonic feature in liver biopsy is onion skin-type periductal fibrosis encountered rarely.[31] Fibro-obliterative cholangitis, the other feature is not only specific for PSC but also seen in PBC, ductopenic rejection after liver transplant, biliary obstruction and intra-arterial chemotherapy.[34]

CAUSES OF SECONDARY SCLEROSING CHOLANGITIS

Primary sclerosing cholangitis should be contemplated only after all secondary causes have to be ruled out. List below is not exhaustive but contains diseases to be ruled out. These diseases cause destruction of the biliary tree leading to biliary cirrhosis. Biochemical and cholangiographic features are similar to PSC. These causes include:[30]

- Chronic bacterial cholangitis
- Infectious or ischemic cholangiopathy
- Cholangiocarcinoma
- Choledocholithiasis
- Diffuse intrahepatic metastases
- Eosinophilic cholangitis
- Intra-arterial chemotherapy
- Mast cell cholangiopathy
- Portal hypertensive biliopathy

Flow chart 1 Complications of PSC

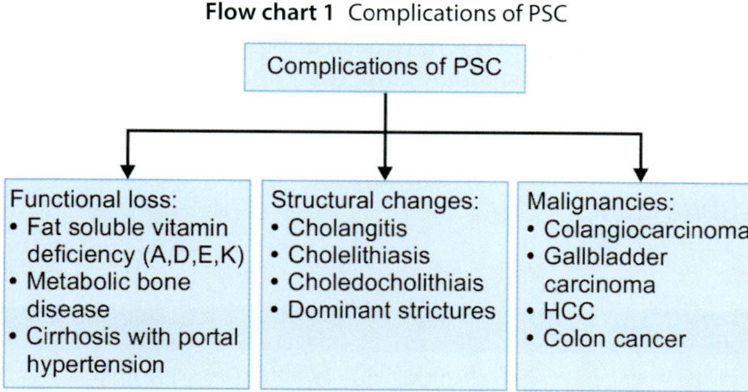

- Recurrent pancreatitis
- Recurrent pyogenic cholangitis
- Surgical biliary trauma

COMPLICATIONS OF SECONDARY SCLEROSING CHOLANGITIS

Complications of PSC can be grouped into (Flow chart 1):
- Due to functional loss
- Due to structural changes in biliary tree
- Malignancies

MALIGNANCIES IN PRIMARY SCLEROSING CHOLANGITIS

Malignancies with increased risk as compared to general population are tabulated in Table 1.

PROGNOSIS

Many prognostic models have been used for predicting mortality in PSC. Mayo model is best used for predicting survival in patients with PSC. For transplant allocation MELD is used. Components of Mayo score include age, serum bilirubin, AST, serum albumin levels and presence of variceal bleed.

Mayo score is available online on URL mentioned, it is complex and difficult to use in routine clinical practice. Rough guide to assess prognosis is if patient is non-icteric then survival without transplant is about 15–20 years and in patients with icterus is 10–12 years.

Mayo model for predicted survival in primary sclerosing cholangitis:[35]

$$R = 0.03\ [\text{age (yrs)}] + 0.54_e\ [\text{bilirubin (mg/dL)}] + 0.54_e\log\ [\text{AST (IU/L)}] + 1.24\ [\text{variceal bleeding } (0 = \text{no}/1 = \text{yes})] - 0.84\ [\text{albumin (g/dL)}].$$

Survival function coefficient [$S_o(t)$]:

1 year = 0.963
2 years = 0.919
3 years = 0.873
4 years = 0.833

Calculated Patient Survival[35]

Probability of survival at time t years is calculated as $S(t) = S_o(t)^{\exp(R-1.00)}$

MANAGEMENT

Management of PSC is difficult as disease is relentlessly progressive. Management largely is aimed at:
- Retardation of progression of disease.
- Management of complications arising due to disease progression.

Thus treatment is required to control steatorrhea, pruritus and fatigue. *Pruritus* can be controlled with cholestyramine 4 g TID. This drug binds other drugs hence should be given cautiously. Other drugs used for pruritus are rifampin (150 mg BID), anticholinergics, phenobarbital, naloxone and methylprednisolone. Metabolic diseases due to lack of fat soluble vitamins should also be monitored and treated. Vitamin levels should be monitored and supplemented. Osteoporosis is difficult to manage in late stages of PSC as there is no proven medical therapy.

Fact that many drugs have been tried in patients with PSC proves that none is effective in retarding or halting the disease progression. Following is the list of drugs tried in management of patients with PSC:
1. Ursodeoxycholic acid (UDCA)
2. Glucocorticoids
3. Cyclosporine
4. Methotrexate
5. Vancomycin
6. Azathioprine and 6-mercaptopurine
7. Tacrolimus
8. D-penicillamine
9. Etanercept

Of all the drugs listed only UDCA was approved by FDA in management of PSC but 2010 recommendations did not favor use of UDCA for the same. None of the drugs have proven to retard or halt progression of PSC or prolong transplant free survival.

Ursodeoxycholic Acid

In normal human being UDCA constitutes about 3% of bile acid pool. No drug so far alters the natural history of disease. Of these UDCA is the most extensively studied. Although 15 mg/kg/day of UDCA, showed efficacy in improving biochemical abnormalities and hepatic inflammation, but no improvement in overall survival

Table 1: Malignancies in primary sclerosing cholangitis

Cholangiocarcinoma	*GB cancer*	*HCC*	*Colorectal cancer*	*Ca pancreas*
Lifetime incidence 10–15% 50% diagnosed with diagnosis of PSC or within 1 year CA19-9 best tumor marker	Lifetime incidence 2% Annual USG recommended Cholecystectomy if mass lesion seen	Lifetime incidence 2%	More common in PSC with ulcerative colitis than ulcerative colitis alone Surveillance colonoscopy recommended every 1–2 years	Up to 14 times higher risk

or transplant free survival.[5-9,36-39] Results of controlled trials on UDCA are summarized in Table 2.

High-dose UDCA

As there was no definite improvement with standard dose UDCA several pilot studies with high dose were done defined as 20–30 mg/kg/day with premise of improvement in all parameters.[18-21] Studies on high dose UDCA have been discussed in Table 3.

Overall data from standard dose trials and high dose trials are encouraging in the form of improvement in biochemistry and symptoms but this did not translate into need for liver transplant or survival benefit. Hence, no consensus could be made about use of UDCA in PSC.

Table 2: Results of controlled trials on UDCA

Author	*Year*	*N*	*Dose*	*Duration*	*Biochemical response*	*Symptom response*	*Histologic response*
Beuers et al.[40]	1992	14	13–15 kg/kg/day	1 year	Yes	No	Yes
Stiehl et al.[41]	1994	20	750 mg/day	3 month	Yes	No	Yes
De Maria et al.[42]	1996	59	600 mg/day	2 years	No	NA	No
Lindor et al.[43]	1997	105	13–15 mg/kg/day	2.2 years	Yes	No	No
Van Hoogstraten et al.[44]	1998	48	10 mg/kg/day	2 years	Yes	No	No
Okolicsanyi[45]	2003	86	8–13 mg/kg/day	Retrospective	Yes	Yes	NA

Table 3: Studies on high dose UDCA

Author	*Year*	*N*	*Dose*	*Duration*	*Biochemical response*	*Symptom response*	*Histologic response*
Harnois et al.[46]	2001	30	25–30 kg/kg/day	1 year	Yes	NA (improved survival)	NA
Mitchell et al.[47]	2001	26	20 mg/kg/day	2 years	Yes	No	Yes
Olsson et al.[48]	2005	219	17–23 mg/day	5 years	Yes	No	NA

Table 4: Studies of UDCA plus therapies

Author	*Year*	*N*	*Therapy*	*Duration*	*Biochemical response*	*Symptom response*	*Histologic response*
Lindor et al.[49]	1996	19	13–15 kg/kg/day UDCA + Methotrexate 0.25 mg/kg/week	2 year	No diff with UDCA alone	No	No
Stiehl et al.[50]	1997	65	750 mg/day UDCA + ERCP	45 months	Yes	NA, improved survival	NA
Schramm et al.[51]	1999	15	500–750 mg/day UDCA + Azathioprine 1–1.5 mg/kg/day initially	41 months	Yes	Yes	Yes
Van Hoogstraten et al.[52]	2000	18	12 mg/kg/day UDCA + budesonide 3 or 9 mg/day or prednisolone 10 mg/day	8 weeks	Yes in pred group	Yes in pred group	NA
Sterling et al.[53]	2004	25	13–15 mg/kg/day UDCA ± MMF 2000 mg/day	2 years	Yes (No diff from UDCA alone)	NA	No
Farkkila et al.[54]	2004	80	15 mg/kg/day UDCA ± Metronidazole 600–800 mg/day	3 years	Yes	NA	No

UDCA Plus Therapies

As no substantial benefit could be demonstrated there was interest in combination therapies especially with antifibrotic therapies like colchicines, mycophenolate, methotrexate, steroids and even ERCP. Table 4 summarizes studies of UDCA plus therapies.

ENDOSCOPIC THERAPY

Endoscopic therapy can be tried in a subset of patients with dominant extrahepatic biliary stricture. Well defined patient characteristics favoring endoscopic therapy is lacking.[55-57] One of the largest series included 125 patients revealed a dominant stricture in the common bile duct and/or right or left hepatic duct only in 56 patients (45%).[58] Furthermore, patients who do not have a stricture at baseline may develop a stricture over time.

In another study of 104 patients, clinical improvement reported in 35% and 70% respectively after diagnostic and therapeutic ERCPs. Although LFTs improved after diagnostic and therapeutic ERCPs, bilirubin levels decreased only in the therapeutic group. Authors concluded that endoscopic therapy in dominant strictures with high serum bilirubin were predictors of clinical and laboratory improvement. Total complication rates were equivalent between diagnostic and therapeutic ERCPs but severe complications were more common in the therapeutic group.[59]

Endoscopic treatment of dominant strictures improves outcomes is still debatable and has not been evaluated in controlled trials. In a study involving 125 patients, 56 with a dominant stricture, none of which were treated,[60] after mean follow-up of 1 year there was no change in measures of cholestasis, suggesting that the dominant strictures did not contribute significantly to cholestasis. It was speculated that endoscopic therapy should not be undertaken routinely even if stricture is dominant. A lot of reports recently have contradicted this study and have documented clinical and radiographic improvement following endoscopic dilation.[60-65] Recent report of 32 patients treated endoscopically, the majority were treated with short-term placement of a 10 French plastic stent, and removed after a mean of 11 days,[65] total follow-up was 3 years. Cholestatic complaints improved in 83% after a mean of 2 months while serum bilirubin returned to normal in 12 of 14 patients. Only 40% of patients required additional endoscopic intervention while 60% did not require any additional intervention during follow-up.

Before considering endoscopic therapy following factors should be considered:

- Therapeutic ERCP should only be performed at centers with experience in PSC management.
- Always exclude CCA.
- Antibiotic prophylaxis should be given although these patients remain at some risk of cholangitis even if prophylaxis is given. In a series of 168 patients with PSC and 981 without PSC who had at least one ERCP in preceding year, cholangitis was significantly higher in the PSC group despite routine prophylactic use of antibiotics (4.0% vs 0.2%).[66]

LIVER TRANSPLANTATION

Primary sclerosing cholangitis is the fourth most common indication of liver transplant. For patients with advanced PSC this is the only effective treatment. Liver transplant indications in PSC include intractable ascites with muscle wasting and encephalopathy, bleeding from varices or portal gastropathy and recurrent cholangitis. One of the problems is obliterative inflammation similar to PSC in the transplanted liver. This is seen in up to 20% of patients in several series. In patients of PSC with ulcerative colitis, clonic inflammation may show improvement but the risk of malignancy remains same or worse. Surveillance with colonoscopy is thus mandatory.

REFERENCES

1. Bergquist A, Ekbom A, Olsson R, Kornfeldt D, Lööf L, Danielsson A, et al. Hepatic and extrahepatic malignancies in primary sclerosing cholangitis. J Hepatol. 2002;36(3):321-7.
2. Bambha K, Kim WR, Talwalkar J, Torgerson H, Benson JT, Therneau TM, et al. Incidence, clinical spectrum, and outcomes of primary sclerosing cholangitis in a United States community. Gastroenterology. 2003;125(5):1364-9.
3. Karlsen TH, Schrumpf E, Boberg KM. Update on primary sclerosing cholangitis. Dig Liver Dis Off J Ital Soc Gastroenterol Ital Assoc Study Liver. 2010;42(6):390-400.
4. Molodecky NA, Kareemi H, Parab R, Barkema HW, Quan H, Myers RP, et al. Incidence of primary sclerosing cholangitis: a systematic review and meta-analysis. Hepatology. 2011;53(5):1590-9.
5. Lindkvist B, Benito de Valle M, Gullberg B, Björnsson E. Incidence and prevalence of primary sclerosing cholangitis in a defined adult population in Sweden. Hepatol Baltim Md. 2010;52(2):571-7.
6. Portmann BC, Nakanuma Y, Burt AD (Eds). MacSween's Pathology of the Liver. Philadelphia: Churchill Livingstone Elsevier; 2007. pp. 517-81.
7. Hirschfield GM, Heathcote EJ, Gershwin ME. Pathogenesis of cholestatic liver disease and therapeutic approaches. Gastroenterology. 2010;139(5):1481-96.
8. Eksteen B, Miles AE, Grant AJ, Adams DH. Lymphocyte homing in the pathogenesis of extra-intestinal manifestations of inflammatory bowel disease. Clin Med Lond Engl. 2004;4(2):173-80.
9. Terjung B, Söhne J, Lechtenberg B, Gottwein J, Muennich M, Herzog V, et al. p-ANCAs in autoimmune liver disorders recognise human beta-tubulin isotype 5 and cross-react with microbial protein FtsZ. Gut. 2010;59(6):808-16.
10. Fickert P, Fuchsbichler A, Wagner M, Zollner G, Kaser A, Tilg H, et al. Regurgitation of bile acids from leaky bile ducts causes sclerosing cholangitis in Mdr2 (Abcb4) knockout mice. Gastroenterology. 2004;127(1):261-74.
11. Fickert P, Wagner M, Marschall H-U, Fuchsbichler A, Zollner G, Tsybrovskyy O, et al. 24-norUrsodeoxycholic acid is superior to ursodeoxycholic acid in the treatment of sclerosing cholangitis in Mdr2 (Abcb4) knockout mice. Gastroenterology. 2006;130(2): 465-81.
12. Broomé U, Olsson R, Lööf L, Bodemar G, Hultcrantz R, Danielsson A, et al. Natural history and prognostic factors in 305 Swedish patients with primary sclerosing cholangitis. Gut. 1996;38(4):610-5.
13. Chapman RW, Arborgh BA, Rhodes JM, Summerfield JA, Dick R, Scheuer PJ, et al. Primary sclerosing cholangitis: a review of its clinical features, cholangiography, and hepatic histology. Gut. 1980;21(10):870-7.
14. Bergquist A, Montgomery SM, Bahmanyar S, Olsson R, Danielsson A, Lindgren S, et al. Increased risk of primary sclerosing cholangitis and ulcerative colitis in first-degree relatives of patients with primary sclerosing cholangitis. Clin Gastroenterol Hepatol Off Clin Pract J Am Gastroenterol Assoc. 2008;6(8):939-43.
15. Karlsen TH, Franke A, Melum E, Kaser A, Hov JR, Balschun T, et al. Genome-wide association analysis in primary sclerosing cholangitis. Gastroenterology. 2010;138(3):1102-11.

16. Pauli-Magnus C, Kerb R, Fattinger K, Lang T, Anwald B, Kullak-Ublick GA, et al. BSEP and MDR3 haplotype structure in healthy Caucasians, primary biliary cirrhosis and primary sclerosing cholangitis. Hepatol Baltim Md. 2004;39(3):779-91.
17. Hov JR, Keitel V, Laerdahl JK, Spomer L, Ellinghaus E, ElSharawy A, et al. Mutational characterization of the bile acid receptor TGR5 in primary sclerosing cholangitis. PloS One. 2010;5(8):e12403.
18. Janse M, Lamberts LE, Franke L, Raychaudhuri S, Ellinghaus E, Muri Boberg K, et al. Three ulcerative colitis susceptibility loci are associated with primary sclerosing cholangitis and indicate a role for IL2, REL, and CARD9. Hepatol Baltim Md. 2011;53(6): 1977-85.
19. Juran BD, Atkinson EJ, Schlicht EM, Larson JJ, Ellinghaus D, Franke A, et al. Genetic polymorphisms of matrix metalloproteinase 3 in primary sclerosing cholangitis. Liver Int Off J Int Assoc Study Liver. 2011;31(6):785-91.
20. Satsangi J, Chapman RW, Haldar N, Donaldson P, Mitchell S, Simmons J, et al. A functional polymorphism of the stromelysin gene (MMP-3) influences susceptibility to primary sclerosing cholangitis. Gastroenterology. 2001;121(1):124-30.
21. Wiencke K, Louka AS, Spurkland A, Vatn M, Schrumpf E, Boberg KM, et al. Association of matrix metalloproteinase-1 and -3 promoter polymorphisms with clinical subsets of Norwegian primary sclerosing cholangitis patients. J Hepatol. 2004;41(2): 209-14.
22. Folseraas T, Karlsen TH. To MMP or not to MMP: a role for matrix metalloproteinase 3 in primary sclerosing cholangitis? Liver Int Off J Int Assoc Study Liver. 2011;31(6):751-4.
23. Tischendorf JJW, Hecker H, Krüger M, Manns MP, Meier PN. Characterization, outcome, and prognosis in 273 patients with primary sclerosing cholangitis: a single center study. Am J Gastroenterol. 2007;102(1):107-14.
24. Mendes FD, Levy C, Enders FB, Loftus EV, Angulo P, Lindor KD. Abnormal hepatic biochemistries in patients with inflammatory bowel disease. Am J Gastroenterol. 2007;102(2):344-50.
25. Zetterquist H, Broomé U, Einarsson K, Olerup O. HLA class II genes in primary sclerosing cholangitis and chronic inflammatory bowel disease: no HLA-DRw52a association in Swedish patients with sclerosing cholangitis. Gut. 1992;33(7):942-6.
26. Prochazka EJ, Terasaki PI, Park MS, Goldstein LI, Busuttil RW. Association of primary sclerosing cholangitis with HLA-DRw52a. N Engl J Med. 1990;322(26):1842-4.
27. Angulo P, Peter JB, Gershwin ME, DeSotel CK, Shoenfeld Y, Ahmed AE, et al. Serum autoantibodies in patients with primary sclerosing cholangitis. J Hepatol. 2000;32(2):182-7.
28. Dave M, Elmunzer BJ, Dwamena BA, Higgins PDR. Primary sclerosing cholangitis: meta-analysis of diagnostic performance of MR cholangiopancreatography. Radiology. 2010;256(2):387-96.
29. Angulo P, Lindor KD. Primary sclerosing cholangitis. Hepatol Baltim Md. 1999;30(1):325-32.
30. Chapman R, Fevery J, Kalloo A, Nagorney DM, Boberg KM, Shneider B, et al. Diagnosis and management of primary sclerosing cholangitis. Hepatol Baltim Md. 2010;51(2):660-78.
31. Lee YM, Kaplan MM. Primary sclerosing cholangitis. N Engl J Med. 1995;332(14):924-33.
32. Buckles DC, Lindor KD, Larusso NF, Petrovic LM, Gores GJ. In primary sclerosing cholangitis, gall bladder polyps are frequently malignant. Am J Gastroenterol. 2002;97(5):1138-42.
33. Björnsson E, Olsson R, Bergquist A, Lindgren S, Braden B, Chapman RW, et al. The natural history of small-duct primary sclerosing cholangitis. Gastroenterology. 2008;134(4):975-80.
34. Scheuer PJ. Ludwig Symposium on biliary disorders--part II. Pathologic features and evolution of primary biliary cirrhosis and primary sclerosing cholangitis. Mayo Clin Proc. 1998;73(2):179-83.
35. Kim WR, Therneau TM, Wiesner RH, Poterucha JJ, Benson JT, Malinchoc M, et al. A revised natural history model for primary sclerosing cholangitis. Mayo Clin Proc. 2000;75(7):688-94.
36. Molodecky NA, Myers RP, Barkema HW, Quan H, Kaplan GG. Validity of administrative data for the diagnosis of primary sclerosing cholangitis: a population-based study. Liver Int Off J Int Assoc Study Liver. 2011;31(5):712-20.
37. Vierling JM. Animal models for primary sclerosing cholangitis. Best Pract Res Clin Gastroenterol. 2001;15(4):591-610.
38. Loftus EV, Harewood GC, Loftus CG, Tremaine WJ, Harmsen WS, Zinsmeister AR, et al. PSC-IBD: a unique form of inflammatory bowel disease associated with primary sclerosing cholangitis. Gut. 2005;54(1):91-6.
39. Trauner M, Fickert P, Wagner M. MDR3 (ABCB4) defects: a paradigm for the genetics of adult cholestatic syndromes. Semin Liver Dis. 2007;27(1):77-98.
40. Beuers U, Spengler U, Kruis W, Aydemir U, Wiebecke B, Heldwein W, et al. Ursodeoxycholic acid for treatment of primary sclerosing cholangitis: a placebo-controlled trial. Hepatol Baltim Md. 1992;16(3):707-14.
41. Stiehl A, Walker S, Stiehl L, Rudolph G, Hofmann WJ, Theilmann L. Effect of ursodeoxycholic acid on liver and bile duct disease in primary sclerosing cholangitis. A 3-year pilot study with a placebo-controlled study period. J Hepatol. 1994;20(1):57-64.
42. De Maria N, Colantoni A, Rosenbloom E, Van Thiel DH. Ursodeoxycholic acid does not improve the clinical course of primary sclerosing cholangitis over a 2-year period. Hepatogastroenterology. 1996;43(12):1472-9.
43. Lindor KD, Kowdley KV, Luketic VAC, Harrison ME, McCashland T, Befeler AS, et al. High-dose ursodeoxycholic acid for the treatment of primary sclerosing cholangitis. Hepatol Baltim Md. 2009;50(3):808-14.
44. Van Hoogstraten HJ, Wolfhagen FH, van de Meeberg PC, Kuiper H, Nix GA, Becx MC, et al. Ursodeoxycholic acid therapy for primary sclerosing cholangitis: results of a 2-year randomized controlled trial to evaluate single versus multiple daily doses. J Hepatol. 1998;29(3):417-23.
45. Okolicsanyi L, Fabris L, Viaggi S, Carulli N, Podda M, Ricci G. Primary sclerosing cholangitis: clinical presentation, natural history and prognostic variables: an Italian multicentre study. The Italian PSC Study Group. Eur J Gastroenterol Hepatol. 1996;8(7):685-91.
46. Harnois DM, Angulo P, Jorgensen RA, Larusso NF, Lindor KD. High-dose ursodeoxycholic acid as a therapy for patients with primary sclerosing cholangitis. Am J Gastroenterol. 2001;96(5):1558-62.
47. Mitchell SA, Bansi DS, Hunt N, Von Bergmann K, Fleming KA, Chapman RW. A preliminary trial of high-dose ursodeoxycholic acid in primary sclerosing cholangitis. Gastroenterology. 2001; 121(4):900-7.
48. Olsson R, Boberg KM, de Muckadell OS, Lindgren S, Hultcrantz R, Folvik G, et al. High-dose ursodeoxycholic acid in primary sclerosing cholangitis: a 5-year multicenter, randomized, controlled study. Gastroenterology. 2005;129(5):1464-72.
49. Lindor KD, Jorgensen RA, Anderson ML, Gores GJ, Hofmann AF, LaRusso NF. Ursodeoxycholic acid and methotrexate for primary sclerosing cholangitis: a pilot study. Am J Gastroenterol. 1996;91(3):511-5.
50. Stiehl A. Primary sclerosing cholangitis: the role of endoscopic therapy. Semin Liver Dis. 2006;26(1):62-8.
51. Schramm C, Schirmacher P, Helmreich-Becker I, Gerken G, zum Büschenfelde KH, Lohse AW. Combined therapy with azathioprine, prednisolone, and ursodiol in patients with primary sclerosing cholangitis. A case series. Ann Intern Med. 1999;131(12):943-6.
52. Van Hoogstraten HJ, Vleggaar FP, Boland GJ, van Steenbergen W, Griffioen P, Hop WC, et al. Budesonide or prednisone in

combination with ursodeoxycholic acid in primary sclerosing cholangitis: a randomized double-blind pilot study. Belgian-Dutch PSC Study Group. Am J Gastroenterol. 2000;95(8):2015-22.
53. Sterling RK, Salvatori JJ, Luketic VA, Sanyal AJ, Fulcher AS, Stravitz RT, et al. A prospective, randomized-controlled pilot study of ursodeoxycholic acid combined with mycophenolate mofetil in the treatment of primary sclerosing cholangitis. Aliment Pharmacol Ther. 2004;20(9):943-9.
54. Färkkilä M, Karvonen A-L, Nurmi H, Nuutinen H, Taavitsainen M, Pikkarainen P, et al. Metronidazole and ursodeoxycholic acid for primary sclerosing cholangitis: a randomized placebo-controlled trial. Hepatol Baltim Md. 2004;40(6):1379-86.
55. Naitoh I, Zen Y, Nakazawa T, Ando T, Hayashi K, Okumura F, et al. Small bile duct involvement in IgG4-related sclerosing cholangitis: liver biopsy and cholangiography correlation. J Gastroenterol. 2011;46(2):269-76.
56. Falk RJ, Jennette JC. Anti-neutrophil cytoplasmic autoantibodies with specificity for myeloperoxidase in patients with systemic vasculitis and idiopathic necrotizing and crescentic glomerulonephritis. N Engl J Med. 1988;318(25):1651-7.
57. Terjung B, Herzog V, Worman HJ, Gestmann I, Bauer C, Sauerbruch T, et al. Atypical antineutrophil cytoplasmic antibodies with perinuclear fluorescence in chronic inflammatory bowel diseases and hepatobiliary disorders colocalize with nuclear lamina proteins. Hepatol Baltim Md. 1998;28(2):332-40.
58. Terjung B, Spengler U, Sauerbruch T, Worman HJ. "Atypical p-ANCA" in IBD and hepatobiliary disorders react with a 50-kilodalton nuclear envelope protein of neutrophils and myeloid cell lines. Gastroenterology. 2000;119(2):310-22.
59. Enns R, Eloubeidi MA, Mergener K, Jowell PS, Branch MS, Baillie J. Predictors of successful clinical and laboratory outcomes in patients with primary sclerosing cholangitis undergoing endoscopic retrograde cholangiopancreatography. Can J Gastroenterol J Can Gastroenterol. 2003;17(4):243-8.
60. MacCarty RL, LaRusso NF, Wiesner RH, Ludwig J. Primary sclerosing cholangitis: findings on cholangiography and pancreatography. Radiology. 1983;149(1):39-44.
61. May G, Bender C, LaRusso N, Wiesner R. Nonoperative dilatation of dominant strictures in primary sclerosing cholangitis. Am J Roentgenol. 1985;145(5):1061-4.
62. Lee JG, Schutz SM, England RE, Leung JW, Cotton PB. Endoscopic therapy of sclerosing cholangitis. Hepatol Baltim Md. 1995;21(3):661-7.
63. Gaing AA, Geders JM, Cohen SA, Siegel JH. Endoscopic management of primary sclerosing cholangitis: review, and report of an open series. Am J Gastroenterol. 1993;88(12):2000-8.
64. Van Milligen de Wit AW, van Bracht J, Rauws EA, Jones EA, Tytgat GN, Huibregtse K. Endoscopic stent therapy for dominant extrahepatic bile duct strictures in primary sclerosing cholangitis. Gastrointest Endosc. 1996;44(3):293-9.
65. Ponsioen CY, Lam K, van Milligen de Wit AW, Huibregtse K, Tytgat GNJ. Four years experience with short term stenting in primary sclerosing cholangitis. Am J Gastroenterol. 1999;94(9):2403-7.
66. Bangarulingam SY, Gossard AA, Petersen BT, Ott BJ, Lindor KD. Complications of endoscopic retrograde cholangiopancreatography in primary sclerosing cholangitis. Am J Gastroenterol. 2009;104(4):855-60.

CHAPTER 59

Recurrent Pyogenic Cholangitis

Sukanta Ray

INTRODUCTION

Recurrent pyogenic cholangitis (RPC) was first described as a separate clinical entity by Digby in 1930s.[1] He noticed that the incidence of intrahepatic biliary calculus is frequent in Hong Kong than European countries. In 1950s, Cook coined the term "recurrent pyogenic cholangitis" to describe the condition as a repeated infection of the biliary system with formation of stones and strictures.[2] The synonyms associated with this condition include oriental cholangitis, Asiatic cholangiohepatitis, oriental cholangiohepatitis, Hong Kong disease,[3] Chinese biliary obstruction syndrome,[4] etc. RPC is more common in Southeast Asian countries, but as a result of growing Asian immigration, it is being increasingly encountered in the West. During the 1960s, RPC was the most frequent hepatobiliary disease in Queen Mary Hospital in Hong Kong. Since then, the incidence of RPC has been decreasing in the East Asia, possibly due to improvement of socioeconomic conditions and Westernization of diet.

PATHOGENESIS

The pathogenesis of this condition is poorly understood. Infection probably starts in the small biliary radicles by bowel microorganisms. Even under normal circumstances, organisms may reach the biliary radicles but clinical infection does not occur. When the infection is severe or caused by virulent organisms, the host defense mechanism is overwhelmed and pathogenic mechanisms are initiated. In severe enteric infection, a condition common in malnourished population of Asia, virulent organism may enter the portal vein. Infection by flukes and worms with associated malnutrition may reduce the capacity of the liver to eliminate enteric organisms effectively.

Once the organisms gain a foot hold in the liver, infection starts in the cholangioles and spreads to rest of the portal triads. The hepatocytes may undergo vacuolation and later necrosis in severe infection and hence the name cholangiohepatitis. Early on normal morphology can be restored but frequent severe infection lead to fibrosis of the intrahepatic ducts with stone and stricture formation. The calculi formed in RPC are pigmented bilirubinate stones. In human beings, the major portion of bilirubin is excreted in the bile as bilirubin di-glucuronide or mono-glucuronides. In the presence of beta-glucuronidase, bilirubin glucuronide is hydrolyzed into free bilirubin and glucuronic acid. Normally calcium is secreted in the bile and when it combines with carboxyl radical of free bilirubin, insoluble calcium bilirubinate is formed. Normal bile is free of organism and glucuronidase activity. In RPC, bile culture is frequently positive and usually yields *Escherichia coli, Enterococcus fecalis* or other enteric bacteria. *E. coli* infection has intense beta-glucuronidase activity. Calcium secretion in the bile increases in presence of biliary tract infection. This coupled with intense hydrolysis of bilirubin glucuronides by beta-glucuronidase of *E. coli* leads to formation of multiple biliary calculi classically seen in RPC.[5]

Infection by *Clonorchis sinensis* and *Ascaris lumbricoides* are still regarded as causally significant.[6] Evidence against causal role of clonorchis is that RPC remains prevalent in countries like Philippines where clonorchis is absent and in Japan RPC is declining despite endemic infection of clonorchis. Also, clonorchis ova are isolated from the stool in only 25% patients with RPC and ascariasis is present in only 5% cases.[7]

PATHOLOGY

In acute stage, liver is soft, congested, bile stained and prone to bleeding during mobilization. In long-standing cases, due to repeated biliary sepsis, the surface of the liver is scarred and there is dense adhesion formation between the liver surface and the adjoining parietal peritoneum, stomach and the diaphragm (Figs. 1A and B). Isolated left lobe (40%) is more commonly affected than the right (20%) while involvement of both ducts is found in 40%. In long-standing cases, the affected lobe may be destroyed. There is atrophy of the affected lobe with compensatory hypertrophy of the opposite lobe. On palpation, the stones within the dilated bile duct in the atrophic segment are easily palpable. Occasionally, the underlying lobe is so destroyed by the recurrent episodes of cholangiohepatitis that what remains is the cavernous biliary sac with minimal surrounding liver parenchyma. The cavernous sac often contains biliary muds and stones (Fig. 2).

The pathologic hallmark of RPC is progressive, periportal fibrosis with recurrent cholangiohepatitis. In the early stage, the histological feature of acute episode is similar to that of acute bacterial cholangitis. In the early lesions the lumen of the small bile ducts is filled with pus. There is marked dissociation of the liver cells by polymorphonuclear infiltration of the sinusoids together with Kupffer cell hyperplasia. In the lobules around the affected duct there is varying degree of cellular necrosis. Resolution of the underlying inflammation leads to dense round cell infiltration, which is then replaced by fibrous tissue. In the larger intrahepatic ducts, the duct wall becomes inflamed, ulcerated, and destroyed together with formation of cholangitic abscesses. Resolution results in dense fibrosis and relative stricture formation. Repeated attacks of severe infection and resolution lead to permanent damage of the duct wall and the ducts remain dilated. The relative stricture then becomes a true localized stricture. These strictures are most commonly found at the site of ductal confluence. The stones in RPC are bilirubinate stones (brown pigmented stone). They are soft, earthy, and friable and crumble when pressed between the fingers.

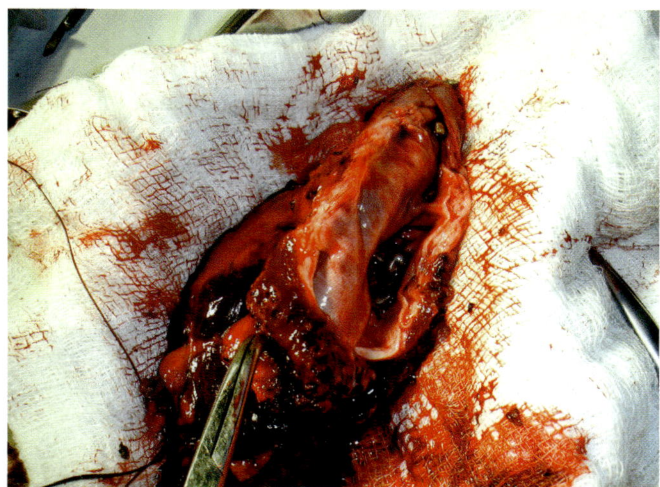

Figure 2 Left hepatectomy specimen showing cavernous sac formation with few stones

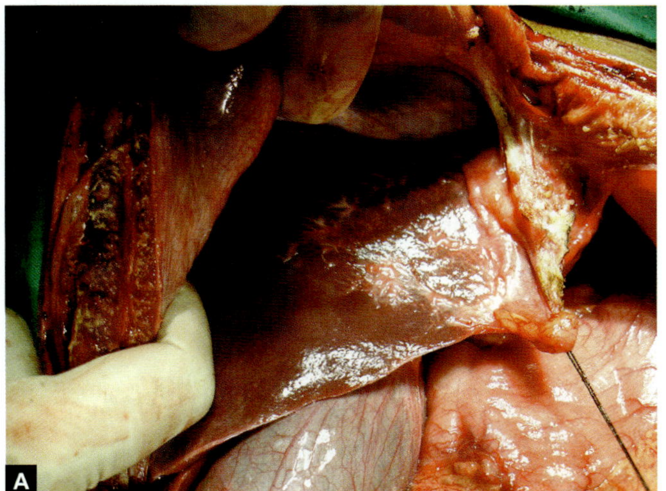

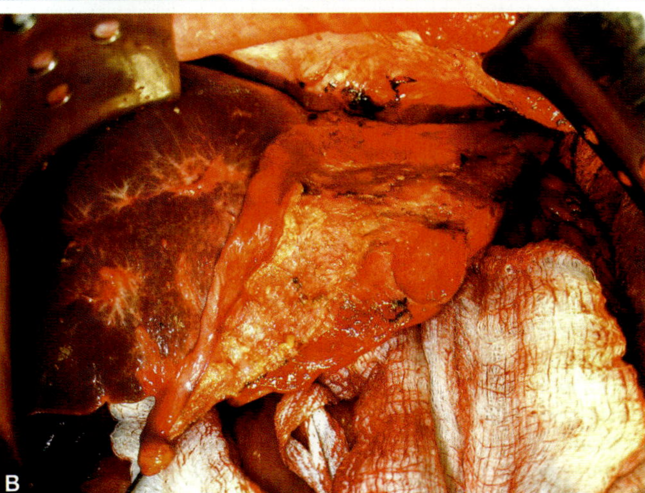

Figures 1A and B Extensive adhesion with parietal wall and scar on the surface of the left lobe of liver

The gallbladder in these patients is usually thin-walled and distended. The incidence of gallstone ranges between 15% and 40%.[8] Macroscopically the gallbladder looks normal but histological examination shows low grade chronic cholecystitis. Enlarged lymph nodes can be found in the gastrohepatic ligament.

CLINICAL PRESENTATION

The usual age of presentation is in the 3rd to 4th decade of life. There is no sex predilection. It usually affects the lower socioeconomic classes. The symptoms of RPC are similar to that of acute cholangitis like right hypochondrial and epigastric pain, fever and jaundice. The pain is constant and seldom colicky, and lasts for hours. It often radiates to back. Nausea is seen frequently but vomiting is uncommon. Jaundice is absent or mild due to partial obstruction of the bile ducts. Patients often notice passage of tea color urine. Fever is spiky in nature. Constant fever indicates development of liver abscess. Weight loss is unusual. But significant weight loss in patients with RPC may need evaluation for intrahepatic cholangiocarcinoma.

In acute stage, the patient looks restless and unwell with tinge of jaundice. Abdominal examination may reveal scar of previous surgery. A history of previous biliary tract surgery is found in more than 50% of cases.[9] Tenderness with varying degree of guarding is found in the epigastrium or right upper abdomen. Marked tenderness may imply underlying abscess. Deterioration of abdominal signs and worsening hemodynamic parameters during conservative management may pinpoint the need for urgent biliary decompression. The liver is enlarged in about 60% of patients and spleen is palpable in 25% of cases of RPC.

INVESTIGATIONS

Both hematological and biochemical tests do not distinguish RPC from other causes of biliary obstruction and infection. Liver function tests (LFTs) show mild to moderate elevation of bilirubin with marked elevation of serum alkaline phosphatase and gamma-glutamyltransferase (GGT). Patients may have normal LFT particularly during quiescent phase.

Imaging studies are required for establishing diagnosis, assessment of the extent of disease, associated complications and formulation of treatment plans. Ultrasonography (USG) is the first line of investigation. It can demonstrate the presence of intrahepatic and extrahepatic stones, size of ducts, liver abscess, biloma and solid liver mass. Color Doppler may be useful for assessment of portal venous hemodynamics. The disadvantage of USG is that it is observer dependent. It fails to differentiate intrahepatic stones from pneumobilia. In some cases, the amorphous and small stones may form biliary cast, and in this case highly reflective echoes and posterior acoustic shadows are absent making USG interpretation difficult. Computed tomography removes this bias. It confirms the information given by USG besides precisely distinguish pneumobilia from intrahepatic stones. Non-contrast scan is important to avoid a false negative interpretation. Atrophy-hypertrophy complex, parenchymal changes in long-standing cases, and volumetric assessment of liver are best done by computed tomography scan (Fig. 3) and is essential before liver resection. USG and computed tomography scan do not provide sufficient details of the ductal anatomy. Cholangiography, in the form of endoscopic retrograde cholangiopancreatography (ERCP) and/or percutaneous transhepatic cholangiography (PTC), is essential for the detail delineation of entire biliary tract. We generally prefer ERCP first because it is both diagnostic and therapeutic. Moreover, external biliary tree is affected in more than 50% cases of RPC. The classical cholangiogram will show dilated extrahepatic duct with "truncated tree" appearance of the intrahepatic ducts. PTC is preferred when a stone or stricture prevents the filling of the intrahepatic ducts or when ERCP is technically not feasible as in cases of previous biliary enteric by-pass surgery or in presence of Bilroth II reconstruction. Similar to USG, computed tomography scan and direct cholangiography, magnetic resonance cholangiopancreatograpgy (MRCP) is a sensitive modality for delineation of ductal and hepatic parenchymal changes in RPC. Strictures and stones are best seen in T2-weighted images (Fig. 4). Moreover volume and contour changes of liver are also seen in MRI. MRCP is better than ERCP for delineation of intrahepatic ductal dilatation and stones, because intrahepatic stricture may prevent the filling of intrahepatic branches. In addition to ductal lesions, associated complications like intrahepatic cholangiocarcinoma, liver abscess are also detected by MRI. Nowadays MRCP has replaced ERCP or PTC in situations where therapeutic procedure is not mandatory.

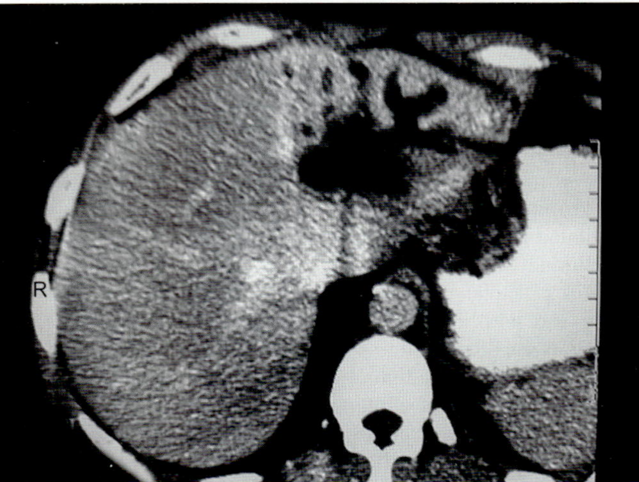

Figure 3 CT scan of abdomen showing dilated intrahepatic biliary radical of left lobe with atrophy of the left lobe

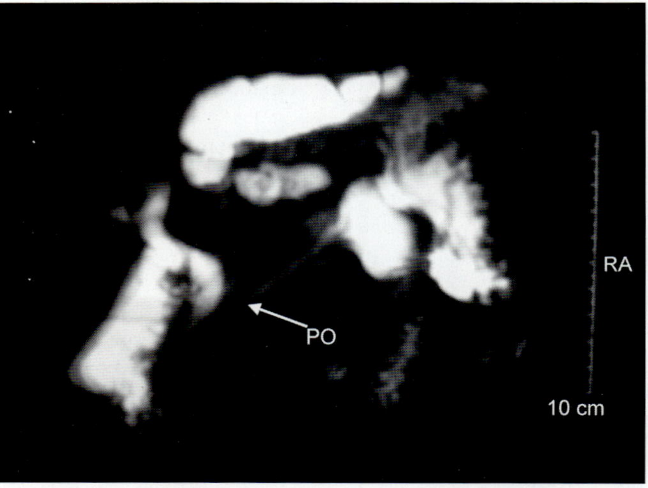

Figure 4 MRCP showing hugely dilated left ductal system with stricture at its junction with the right duct

MANAGEMENT

Management of Acute Episode

Recurrent pyogenic cholangitis patients have repeated episodes of acute cholangitis which would settle on conservative management in the majority of the cases. About 35% of patients require urgent intervention for peritonitis due to ruptured liver abscess, perforated gangrenous gallbladder or those with septicemic shock despite adequate conservative measures.[10] The initial approach to any acute episode is to control infection with commencement of intravenous fluid, antibiotics and analgesics. The patient should be monitored closely for signs of deterioration. Those responding to conservative treatments will show a reduction of abdominal pain, fall in body temperature and disappearance of tachycardia within 48 hours. If there is no obvious improvement, the possibility of undrained biliary system or liver abscess should be considered and biliary decompression should be done urgently before the patient deteriorates and dies due to irreversible septicemia and multiorgan failure. An urgent USG abdomen should be performed to detect the extent of lithiasis and the presence of liver abscess. The best way to drain biliary system is to perform ERCP. No attempt is made to obtain a complete cholangiogram or to take out all stones. The biliary system is decompressed with a nasobiliary drainage. Once the condition of the patient is improved and stabilized, check cholangiogram with endoscopic stone removal should be performed. If part of the biliary system cannot be decompressed due to impacted stones or stricture, ERCP alone may not be adequate and the patient will need percutaneous transhepatic biliary drainage (PTBD). Occasionally open surgery is required to deal with peritonitis as a result of perforated gallbladder, ruptured liver abscess or where facilities for urgent ERCP and PTBD is not available. The most expedient way to decompress CBD is to place a large bore (16 Fr) T tube. Intrahepatic strictures can be dilated to get a free flow of bile. Sometimes concomitant PTBD may be necessary in acute setting. During exploration of CBD, high pressure syringing should be avoided as this may escalate bacteremia and only gentle irrigation should be done. Following gentle saline wash of CBD, a Fogarty catheter is passed down the CBD into the duodenum to check the patency of the lower end of CBD. Stone impacted in the lower end of CBD may not require removal in emergency situation unless there is associated acute pancreatitis. In acute pancreatitis, it is extracted by transduodenal sphincteroplasty. Postoperatively the patients improve dramatically. In patients with septic shock, an extended recovery and intensive care unit support may be required.

Definitive Management

The definitive management of RPC requires a multidisciplinary team approach to establish satisfactory biliary drainage, remove all stones and to resect a non-functioning segment of liver which may serve as a focus of infection.

Role of Minimally Access Approach

Once the acute episode has settled, more definitive treatment via endoscopic or under radiological guidance can be performed. Stones confined to CBD and CHD can be removed via ERCP with dormia basket. Large stones can be crushed or fragmented with mechanical lithotripter or by laser prior to their removal. ERCP can be used as a sole modality for intrahepatic stones in high risk surgical patients. Using mother-baby scope, the complete stone removal rate is about 64%.[11] Intrahepatic calculi within dilated biliary ducts usually lie proximal to a stricture. The stricture can be dilated sufficiently to allow complete removal of stones. The immediate overall success rate of complete stone clearance with balloon dilatation in a series of 57 patients was 94.5%.[12] The main complications of dilation therapy include septicemia, hemobilia and restenosis. In patients with PTBD catheter in situ, the tract can be dilated to allow dormia basket stone retreival under fluoroscopic guidance or by flexible twin channel choledochoscope. Under direct vision, the stones can be fragmented with electrohydraulic lithotripter and the fragments can be removed with a basket. Intrahepatic strictures can be dilated or stented. Percutaneous choledochoscopy in a large study (n=245) was shown to have stone clearance rate of 85.3%. However, the overall rate for stone recurrence and/or cholangitis over a mean follow-up of 10.3 years was 63.2%.[13,14] In a further study that compared percutaneous choledochoscopy with hepatectomy for hepatolithiasis, both treatments were found to satisfactory for stone clearance, but recurrence in the percutaneous choledochoscopy group was much higher (31.5%) than in the hepatectomy group (5.6%).[15] Thus percutaneous choledochoscopy has high recurrence rate and cannot be suggested as a definitive treatment in low-risk patients.

Role of Surgery

Before embarking on definitive surgery, it is mandatory to have a vivid knowledge of the extent of lithiasis, unilobar or bilobar distribution, associated strictures with or without concomitant liver atrophy.

In the presence of predominantly extrahepatic disease, simple exploration of CBD with intraoperative choledochoscopy will suffice. We routinely remove gallbladder for two reasons: (1) histologically it shows low grade inflammation and (2) if sphincter of Oddi is destroyed or bypassed, gallbladder will permanently remain in a collapsed state. The placement of large bore T tube will allow postoperative imaging of the biliary tree and residual stone may be removed through the matured T tube tract. If the bile duct is markedly dilated and the patient had history of two or more number of operations in the bile duct, biliary-enteric bypass procedure should be considered.

In the presence of both intrahepatic and extrahepatic disease, complete stone extraction may be difficult particularly when stones are impacted behind a stricture or within an angulated duct like right posterior or left medial segmental ducts. After CBD exploration and removal of all stones from extrahepatic biliary tree, choledochoscopy should be performed to rule out stricture at the junction of left and right hepatic ducts. Stricture, if present should be dilated. The ducts are then flushed with normal saline to remove stones and muds. The right and left lobes of the liver are gently massaged in between the flushing. This maneuver normally helps to discharge and dislodge more mud and stones from the intrahepatic ducts. Once the effluent is clear, choledochoscopy is repeated and any residual stone can be retrieved with a dormia basket. Sometimes electrohydraulic lithotripsy may be required to fragment large impacted stones. Direct hepatotomy to remove intrahepatic stone may sometimes be necessary but this can be bloody particularly when the stone is deeply situated.

When hepaticojejunostomy is done, access loop should be performed. It helps to access the biliary tract percutaneously. The end of the access loop can be placed intraperitoneally, can be placed under the skin, can be opened as stoma, or can be anastomosed with the stomach. When access loop is made it should have a short and straight course from the anterolateral abdominal wall to the biliary-enteric anastomosis. Via this access loop, recurrent stones can be removed and strictures can be dilated without surgery.

Hepatic resection should be reserved for patients where resection carries no obvious additional morbidity or mortality compared to CBD exploration and stone clearance alone. It is required in patients with multiple liver abscesses, significant hepatic atrophy and fibrosis or concurrent intrahepatic cholangiocarcinoma, which may occur in 3–5% of patients treated conservatively.[16,17] Most commonly performed hepatectomy in RPC is left lateral segmentectomy. In more extensive disease, the medial segment of the left lobe may be affected due to tight stricture in the left hepatic duct which can be best treated by left hepatectomy. Liver resection for right sided disease is unusual in RPC. In a published series of 172 patients of hepatolithiasis, liver resection was performed in 37% cases, of which left lateral segmentectomy and left hepatectomy accounted for 90.5% of cases. Right hepatectomy was performed in only one patient.[18] The overall mortality of hepatic resection in RPC is low (<2%) but the morbidity, such as wound infection, subphrenic collection, biliary fistula and sepsis is significantly high (approximately 30%). High rate of infective complications can be explained by the presence of positive bile culture in more than 90% of cases.

Liver transplantation is indicated in patients with bilateral extensive disease associated with secondary biliary cirrhosis, portal hypertension, liver failure and bleeding esophageal varices. Vascular adhesion from previous surgery and significant portal hypertension makes recipient hepatectomy difficult and potentially hazardous.[19]

Outcome of Different Modalities of Treatments

With the use of multidisciplinary approaches, stone clearance rate has improved markedly. Overall stone clearance rate is more than 90%. Results of treatment depend on the extent of lithiasis, presence of portal hypertension, treatment modalities, and the duration of follow-up. Cheon et al. have shown in their long-term follow-up study (median follow-up—8 years) that nonoperative therapy, residual stones, biliary cirrhosis, biliary stricture and bilobar disease were associated with recurrent stones and/or cholangitis after treatment.[20] Similarly, Lee et al. have shown that overall rates for residual stones, stone recurrence and biliary sepsis recurrence were 21.2%, 16.5% and 21.2%, respectively, during a median follow-up of 45.4 months.[21] Overall hepatectomy achieves superior outcomes with minimal residual stones, postoperative cholangitis and recurrences compared to percutaneous, endoscopic treatments.[22,23]

Overall, 10–20% of patients may die of the disease and its complications. This is due to failure to eliminate the disease with resultant cholangitis, liver damage, secondary biliary cirrhosis and cholangiocarcinoma.

REFERENCES

1. Digby KH. Common duct stones of liver origin. Br J Surg. 1930;17: 578-91.
2. Cook J, Hou PC, Ho HC, McFadzean AJ. Recurrent pyogenic cholangeitis. Br JSurg. 1954;42(172):188-203.
3. Mage S, Morel AS. Surgical experience with cholangiohepatitis (Hong Kong disease) in canton Chinese. Ann Surg. 1965;162: 187-90.
4. Harrison-Levy A. The biliary obstruction syndrome of the Chinese. Br J Surg.1962;49:674-85.
5. Maki T. Pathogenesis of calcium bilirubinate gallstone: role of E. coli, beta-glucuronidase and coagulation by inorganic ions, polyelectrolytes and agitation. Ann Surg. 1966;164(1):90-100.
6. Rana SS, Bhasin DK, Nanda M, Singh K. Parasitic infestations of the biliary tract. Curr Gastroenterol Rep. 2007;9(2):156-64.
7. Ong GB. A study of recurrent pyogenic cholangitis. Arch Surg. 1962;84:199-225.
8. Federle MP, Cello JP, Laing FC, Jeffrey RB Jr. Recurrent pyogenic cholangitis in Asian immigrants. Use of ultrasonography, computed tomography, and cholangiography. Radiology. 1982;143(1):151-6.
9. Liu CL, Fan ST, Wong J. Primary biliary stones: diagnosis and management. World J Surg. 1998;22(11):1162-6.
10. Fan ST, Lai EC, Mok FP, Choi TK, Wong J. Acute cholangitis secondary to hepatolithiasis. Arch Surg. 1991;126(8):1027-31.
11. Okugawa T, Tsuyuguchi T, K C S, Ando T, Ishihara T, Yamaguchi T, et al. Peroral cholangioscopic treatment of hepatolithiasis: long-term results. Gastrointest Endosc. 2002;56(3):366-71.
12. Jeng KS, Yang FS, Ohta I, Chiang HJ. Dilatation of intrahepatic biliary strictures in patients with hepatolithiasis. World J Surg. 1990;14(5):587-92.
13. Huang MH, Chen CH, Yang JC, Yang CC, Yeh YH, Chou DA, et al. Longterm outcome of percutaneous transhepatic cholangioscopic lithotomy for hepatolithiasis. Am J Gastroenterol. 2003;98:2655-62.
14. Chen C, Huang M, Yang J, Yang C, Yeh Y, Wu H, et al. Reappraisal of percutaneous transhepatic cholangioscopic lithotomy for primary hepatolithiasis. Surg Endosc. 2005;19:505-9.
15. Otani K, Shimizu S, Chijiiwa K, Ogawa T, Morisaki T, Sugitani A, et al. Comparison of treatments for hepatolithiasis: hepatic resection vs. cholangioscopic lithotomy. J Am Coll Surg. 1999;189:177-82.
16. Bergman S, Di Carlo A, Chaudhury P, Blum C, Nahal A, Metrakos P. Recurrent pyogenic cholangitis in a white woman. Can J Surg. 2007;50(5):E9-10.
17. Al-Sukhni W, Gallinger S, Pratzer A, Wei A, Ho CS, Kortan P, et al. Recurrent pyogenic cholangitis with hepatolithiasis—the role of surgical therapy in North America. J Gastrointest Surg. 2008;12(3):496-503.
18. Fan ST, Lai EC, Wong J. Hepatic resection for hepatolithiasis. Arch Surg. 1993;128(9):1070-4.
19. Strong RW, Chew SP, Wall DR, Fawcett J, Lynch SV. Liver transplantation for hepatolithiasis. Asian J Surg. 2002;25(2): 180-3.
20. Cheon YK, Cho YD, Moon JH, Lee JS, Shim CS. Evaluation of long-term results and recurrent factors after operative and nonoperative treatment for hepatolithiasis. Surgery. 2009;146(5): 843-53.
21. Lee KF, Chong CN, Ng D, Cheung YS, Ng W, Wong J, et al. Outcome of surgical treatment for recurrent pyogenic cholangitis: a single-centre study. HPB (Oxford). 2009;11(1):75-80.
22. Li SQ, Liang LJ, Peng BG, Lai JM, Lu MD, Li DM. Hepaticojejunostomy for hepatolithiais: a critical appraisal. World J Gastroenterol. 2006;12:4170-4.
23. Uchiyama K, Kawai M, Ueno M, Ozawa S, Tani M, Yamaue H. Reducing residual and recurrent stones by hepatectomy for hepatolithiasis. J Gastrointest Surg. 2007;11:626-30.

CHAPTER 60

Gallbladder Polyps

Biju Pottakkat

INTRODUCTION

Gallbladder polyps are lesions that project into the gallbladder lumen. Gallbladder polyps can be benign or malignant and some benign lesions can be premalignant. Majority are diagnosed on ultrasonography and/or in cholecystectomy specimens. Most of them are benign. The true incidence is unknown. The prevalence of gallbladder polyps by ultrasonography in random populations is 4.5–6.1% and are equally distributed in both sexes.[1,2] The diagnosis is usually made in the middle age. Attempt to identify malignant lesions among the wide range of polypoid lesions in the gallbladder dominates all management guidelines of polypoid lesions in gallbladder.

RISK FACTORS FOR GALLBLADDER POLYPS

Various population based studies have been done to identify the risk factors for the development of gallbladder polyps. In healthy people, male gender, hepatitis B surface antigen positivity, past history of acute cholecystitis and low serum levels of high density lipoprotein-C are found to be associated with higher risk of development of gallbladder polyps.[3,4] Metabolic syndrome has been found to be associated with gallbladder polyp in Korean population.[5] But none of these factors was found to be independently predicting to categorize as risk factor for development of polyp. Gardners syndrome and Peutz-Jeghers syndrome are found to be associated with adenomatous polyp of the gallbladder.[6-8]

PATHOLOGICAL TYPES

Gallbladder polyps are classified according to pathology. Gallbladder may harbor benign and malignant lesions but the incidence of benign gallbladder polyps is more than malignant polyps. Among benign lesions, non-neoplastic predominates. Cholesterol polyps are the most common gallbladder polyps followed by adenomas (Table 1).

In a series of 540 gallbladder specimens, adenomyomatosis (3%), cholesterol polyp (6%), adenoma (1.3%), invasive adenocarcinoma (2.2%) and cystadenocarcinoma (0.2%) constituted the spectrum of polypoid lesions.[9] In areas where the incidence of gallbladder carcinoma (GBC) is more than 1%, the proportion of malignancy among the polypoid lesions may be up to 26%.[10] Non-neoplastic polyps are generally smaller compared to neoplastic polyps. Cholesterol polyps are generally small, single and have no malignant potential. Adenomas are mostly solitary and have malignant potential. They are pedunculated and single and are associated with stones. Tubular and papillary are the most common types of adenomas. Adenomyomatosis although benign has to be considered as premalignant.[11]

Table 1: Types of gallbladder polyps

Benign	*Malignant*
• Cholesterolosis • Cholesterol polyps • Inflammatory polyps • Hyperplastic polyps • Adenoma • Myoma • Papilloma • Fibroma • Lipoma • Hemangioma • Granular cell tumor • Xanthogranuloma • Heterotopic gastric tissue • Heterotopic intestinal tissue	• Carcinoma • Carcinoid tumors • Sarcoma • Mucinous cystadenoma • Adenoacanthoma

MORPHOLOGY

Polypoid lesions of the gallbladder can be of three morphological types: (1) pedunculated, (2) sessile or (3) mass forming. Majority of polyps are pedunculated and solitary. Cholesterol polyps and hyperplastic polyps are pedunculated whereas carcinomas are sessile or mass forming.[12] Adenomas can be of either type. In a series of 97 polypoid lesions of the gallbladder, carcinoma was noted in 9 (13%) of the 67 pedunculated lesions and in 10 (33%) of the 30 sessile lesions.[13] In a report of 124 patients in European population, solitary polyps were found in 52.4%, two polyps in 16.1%, three polyps in 6.5%, several polyps in 22.6% and multiple polyps in 2.4%.[2] Some lesions can be seen as floating on imaging.

PRESENTING FEATURES

Patients with gallbladder polyps are generally asymptomatic. The diagnosis is usually made on ultrasonography and on cholecystectomy specimens. Rare presentations with acute cholecystitis and biliary colic can occur due to obstruction of the cystic duct and consequent cholecystomegaly. Gallstones can coexist with gallbladder polyp. The reported incidence of gallstones is 47.1% in cases of non-neoplastic epithelial polyp and 48% in adenoma.[14] Biliary pain in a patient with gallbladder polyp in the absence of stones should be presumed to be caused by the polyp itself whereas it is prudent to consider gallstones as the cause of symptoms in patients with gallstones and gallbladder polyp. As symptoms unequivocally necessitate cholecystectomy, it is not important to attribute the pain either to stones or to polyp. In patients with gallbladder polyps and symptoms other than biliary colic, risk of malignancy is high.

DIAGNOSIS

Diagnosis of gallbladder polyp is usually made on an abdominal ultrasonography. In a sonographically diagnosed gallbladder polyp, other modalities are mainly used for categorization of the polyp before deciding management. Increasing usage of abdominal contrast enhanced computed tomography has also contributed to the increased incidental detection of gallbladder polyps. The categorization of gallbladder polyp can be done by a variety of modalities including ultrasonography, computed tomography and magnetic resonance imaging. Endoscopic ultrasonography (EUS) and positron emission tomography (PET) are also being used for categorization.

Ultrasonography

Transabdominal Ultrasonography

Most of the gallbladder polyps are detected on ultrasonography. Polyps are visualized as immobile lesions in the lumen of the gallbladder attached to the wall with variable echo features which further depends on the type of polyp (Fig. 1). Echogenicity is more in small cholesterol polyps whereas neoplastic polyps are hypoechoic. Absence of echogenicity has no direct relation with malignancy. Small stones impacted in the gallbladder wall may have the same sonographic features of a gallbladder polyp. Transabdominal ultrasonography has intermediate sensitivity and high specificity for detection of gallbladder polyps. The size of the polyp as assessed by the ultrasonography can be a bench mark for follow-up but sometimes the size may not be matching with that in computed tomography or at operation. Ultrasonography will help to select the patients with gallbladder polyps who require further investigations or follow-up. The sensitivity and specificity of ultrasonography for polyps less than 1 cm was 20% and 95%, and for polyps more than 1 cm was 80% and 99%, respectively.[15] In a series of 13,278 gallbladder specimens, French et al. reported a 1.2% incidence of gallbladder polyps out of which only 50% were diagnosed on transabdominal ultrasonography although the specificity was 98%.[16] The accuracy of ultrasonography in diagnosing polyps less than 1 cm was poor.[15] A significant proportion of ultrasonography detected polyps may not be confirmed on surgical specimens.[17] Layers of the gallbladder wall and its relation with polyp can be assessed by ultrasonography. As the cytological diagnosis of gallbladder polyp is not required for management decisions except in suspected unresectable gallbladder cancer, fine needle aspiration cytology (FNAC) is not advised in polypoid lesions of the gallbladder. Malignant foci in the gallbladder polyp are usually missed on FNAC. FNAC can give a specific diagnosis only in cholesterol polys by detecting foamy histiocytes.[18]

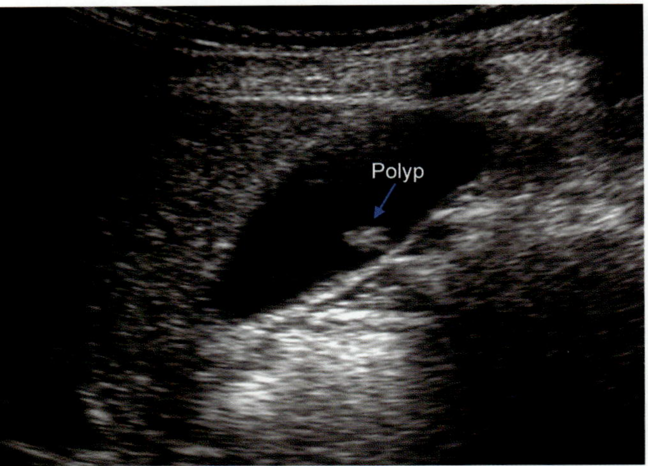

Figure 1 Gallbladder polyp seen as a non-echogenic shadow on ultrasonography

Harmonic and Contrast Ultrasonography

Harmonic ultrasonography differentiates true lesions from biliary sludge because of its increased vascularity, and the difference in vascularity in true lesions is more a function of size than the pathology.[19,20] Harmonic imaging will give precise information about the wall of the gallbladder and also about the size of the polyp. Contrast ultrasonography uses the vascular pattern to differentiate between benign and malignant polyps. Diffuse and branched vascularity is more consistent with cancer and can be used as an adjunct in diagnosing GBC.[21,22]

Endoscopic Ultrasonography

Endoscopic ultrasonography is considered more accurate than transabdominal ultrasonography in differentiating neoplastic from non-neoplastic polyps but the accuracy is less in lesions less than 10 mm.[23] Hypoechoic foci were seen in 91% of neoplastic polyps whereas only 11% of the non-neoplastic polyps showed hypoechoic foci.[24] Hyperechoic spots and multiple microcysts are features of cholesterol polyps and adenomyomatosis, respectively.[25] The role of EUS in gallbladder polyps is limited to situations in which a transabdominal ultrasonography cannot rule out a neoplasia[26] in patients in whom it is suspected. Contrast enhancement technique can also be added with EUS.

Computed Tomography

Computed tomography is indicated in ultrasonography detected polyps which are large and when the suspicion of gallbladder cancer is high. In high incidence areas of gallbladder cancer, the threshold for computed tomography should be kept low. In non-contrast computed tomography, malignant lesions appear hyperdense whereas benign lesions appear isodense.[27] Contrast enhanced computed tomography is superior to non-enhanced computed tomography in detecting gallbladder polyps. In polyps less than 20 mm detected on ultrasonography, the detection rate of unenhanced computed tomography was 40% whereas enhanced computed tomography detected all lesions.[28] The morphology of the lesion can be delineated in more detail by computed tomography which gives insights into categorization of a polyp. About 91% of the sessile lesions detected on computed tomography are neoplastic compared to 30% of pedunculated lesions.[29] Floating lesions can also be seen on computed tomography. All polypoid lesions with infiltration of layers of the gallbladder wall or infiltration to the liver on ultrasonography should undergo a computed tomography because of the likelihood of carcinoma. In a comparative study, the diagnostic sensitivities for malignancy were 90% for harmonic ultrasonography, 86% for EUS and 72% for computed tomography.[30]

Magnetic Resonance Imaging

Magnetic resonance imaging is not usually recommended for evaluation of a gallbladder polyp unless a contrast computed tomography is contraindicated as in conditions like renal failure. With increasing usage of magnetic cholangiopancreatography (MRCP) for biliary pathologies, the incidental reporting of gallbladder polyps are increasing. Biliary dilatation in a gallbladder polyp on ultrasonography can be an indication for magnetic resonance imaging and MRCP. Most of the malignant gallbladder polyps are highly hyperintense whereas benign lesions are less intense or hypointense.[31] Positive signal rate with diffusion-weighted magnetic resonance imaging (DWI-MRI) has been found to be more with malignant gallbladder lesions than with benign gallbladder lesions.[32]

Positron Emission Tomography

Fluoro-deoxy glucose PET (FDG-PET) scan to differentiate neoplastic polyps from non-neoplastic polys can be used but a hot spot can be considered as a risk factor for malignancy only in polyps more than 1 cm size.[33] The reported sensitivity to detect malignancy was 75% and specificity was 88% for PET scan in gallbladder tumors.[34] The information provided by PET scan is not much useful in clinical management as diagnostic and management dilemmas are mostly encountered in polyps less than 1 cm.

PREDICTORS OF MALIGNANCY

Gallbladder cancer can morphologically present as polyp and gallbladder polyp can harbor focus of malignancy. Although the incidence of GBC is rare, its detection at an advanced stage and poor survival make it one of the aggressive cancers. A significant proportion of symptomatic cancers of the gallbladder are incurable and reasonable survival can be expected in asymptomatic patients with malignant gallbladder polyps. Malignant polyps are generally early GBCs and hence their detection increases the resectability rate of GBC. Polyps less than 1 cm rarely become malignant. Metaplasia-dysplasia-carcinoma sequence exists in the development of GBC[35] and possibly in the conversion of benign polyps to GBC. Age more than 60 years and size of the polyp more than 10 mm were the only factors found to be independently predicting risk for GBC in large series,[36,37] a finding consistent with the published literature. The risk of malignancy in polys more than 1 cm is 34–88%.[38] Polyps greater than or equal to 10 mm had a 24.2 times greater risk of malignancy than polyps less than 10 mm.[39] In areas where the incidence of GBC is high, increased gallbladder wall thickness is a risk factor for malignancy. Sessile polyps are more likely to be malignant than pedunculated polyps,[40] and single lesions are more likely to be malignant than multiple lesions. There was significant difference in prevalence of malignancy in gallbladder polyp among patients with Indian ethnic background (5.5%) compared to Caucasian patients (0.08%).[41] High geographical incidence of GBC, association of genetic syndromes, primary sclerosing cholangitis, growth rate of polyp, hypoechoic foci on ultrasonography, association with gallstones more than 10 mm in size, hot spot on PET scan and high vascularity of polyp on imaging are factors found to be associated with malignant polyps. A combination of a polyp and a stone can be considered more as a risk factor for GBC than as an association.

MANAGEMENT OF GALLBLADDER POLYP

Considerable heterogeneity exists among practitioners regarding treatment and surveillance protocols.[42] National guidelines does not exist for management of gallbladder polyps. Society of American Gastrointestinal and Endoscopic Surgeons (SAGES) recommends laparoscopic cholecystectomy for larger, especially single, polyps or those with associated symptoms with watchful waiting for small (<5 mm) asymptomatic polyps (Level II grade B evidence).[43]

Management decisions can be made in most of the gallbladder polyps based upon the findings of transabdominal ultrasonography examination. The three main indications for operation in a gallbladder polyp are symptoms, associated stones and risk of malignancy. Size of the polyp on ultrasound is the most important predictor of management decisions because it correlates well with the symptoms and also with the risk of malignancy. All patients with gallbladder polyps more than 10 mm need cholecystectomy. Polyps less than 10 mm are rarely symptomatic, risk of malignancy is low and hence only follow-up is required. All patients with symptomatic gallbladder polyps should undergo cholecystectomy irrespective of the size. Symptoms may persist in some patients even after cholecystectomy. The justification for cholecystectomy is directed toward prevention of a possible malignant conversion and also to detect a malignant focus in a polyp at pathology.

In areas where incidence of GBC is high, an alternate approach has to be followed. A thick gallbladder wall seen with polyp is an indication for surgical management. The presence of risk factors for GBC like female sex, solitary gallbladder stone, stone size more than 10 mm, etc. are to be given due importance before selecting the option of surveillance. Patients with gallbladder polyps coming from areas where the incidence of GBC is high have to be explained about the increased risk of malignancy.

The routine use of laparoscopic approach for cholecystectomy for gallbladder diseases has changed the approach to gallbladder polyps as well. Minimally symptomatic patients and multiple associated factors for GBC can be considered as an indication for cholecystectomy. In all doubtful polyps, the benefits of a laparoscopic cholecystectomy outweigh its possible demerits and the threshold for operation should be kept low. In situations where the need for a specialized imaging to detect malignancy in a polyp arise, the option of a laparoscopic cholecystectomy and pathological examination has to be considered as an alternative and it has nearly 100% specificity for diagnosis. A preoperatively detected malignant gallbladder polyp necessitates and open approach rather than laparoscopic. A gallbladder polyp should be examined grossly immediately after removing the specimen and any suspicion of malignancy mandates a frozen section pathology examination.

SURVEILLANCE OF GALLBLADDER POLYPS

For polyps less than 6 mm, regular follow-up ultrasonography can be avoided.[44,45] In a series of 467 patients of gallbladder polyps analyzed by Cairns V et al., only 6.6% had shown increase in size; only 3.7% had malignancy and increase in size of the polyp was a risk factor for malignancy.[46] This study showed that a surveillance policy could prevent 5.4 GBC per 1,000 individuals per year. A follow-up study of gallbladder polyps detected on a prospective ultrasound examination in 34 patients could not identify any significant increase in size or malignant change over seven years.[47] If the patient is not a suitable candidate for surveillance, laparoscopic cholecystectomy can be offered for lesions more than 5 mm.

REFERENCES

1. Jorgensen T, Jensen KH. Polyps in the gallbladder. A prevalence study. Scand J Gastroenterol. 1990;25:281-6.
2. Kratzer W, Schmid A, Akinli AS, Thiel R, Mason RA, Schuler A, et al. Gallbladder polyps: prevalence and risk factors. Ultraschall Med. 2011;32(Suppl 1):S68-73.
3. Yang HL, Kong L, Hou LL, Shen HF, Wang Y, Gu XG, et al. Analysis of risk factors for polypoid lesions of gallbladder among health examinees. World J Gastroenterol. 2012;18(23):3015-9.
4. Xu Q, Tao LY, Wu Q, Gao F, Zhang FL, Yuan L, et al. Prevalences of and risk factors for biliary stones and gallbladder polyps in a large Chinese population. HPB (Oxford). 2012;14(6):373-81.
5. Park EJ, Lee HS, Lee SH, Chun HJ, Kim SY, Choi YK, et al. Association between metabolic syndrome and gallbladder polyps in healthy Korean adults. J Korean Med Sci. 2013;28(6):876-80.
6. Brevet M, Brehant O, Dumont F, Regimbeau JM, Dupas JL, Chatelain D. Adenomatous polyposis of the gallbladder and Gardner's syndrome. A rare association. Gastroenterol Clin Biol. 2007;31(4):425-7.
7. Wada K, Tanaka M, Yamaguchi K, Wada K. Carcinoma and polyps of the gallbladder associated with Peutz-Jeghers syndrome. Dig Dis Sci. 1987;32(8):943-6.
8. Yamamoto M, Nakajo S, Tahara E. Gallstones in gallbladder diseases. Acta Pathol Jpn. 1989;39(9):582-5.
9. Terada T. Histopathologic features and frequency of gallbladder lesions in consecutive 540 cholecystectomies. Int J Clin Exp Pathol. 2013;6(1):91-6.
10. Terzi C, Sökmen S, Seçkin S, Albayrak L, Uğurlu M. Polypoid lesions of the gallbladder: report of 100 cases with special reference to operative indications. Surgery. 2000;127(6):622-7.
11. Pellino G, Sciaudone G, Candilio G, Perna G, Santoriello A, Canonico S, et al. Stepwise approach and surgery for gallbladder adenomyomatosis: a mini-review. Hepatobiliary Pancreat Dis Int. 2013;12(2):136-42.
12. Furukawa H, Takayasu K, Mukai K, Inoue K, Kyokane T, Shimada K, et al. CT evaluation of small polypoid lesions of the gallbladder. Hepatogastroenterology. 1995;42(6):800-10.
13. Ishikawa O, Ohhigashi H, Imaoka S, Nakaizumi A, Kitamura T, Sasaki Y, et al. The difference in malignancy between pedunculated and sessile polypoid lesions of the gallbladder. Am J Gastroenterol. 1989;84(11):1386-90.
14. Yamamoto M, Nakajo S, Tahara E. Gallstones in gallbladder diseases. Acta Pathol Jpn. 1989;39(9):582-5.
15. Akyürek N, Salman B, Irkörücü O, Sare M, Tatlicioğlu E. Ultrasonography in the diagnosis of true gallbladder polyps: the contradiction in the literature. HPB(Oxford). 2005;7(2):155-8.
16. French DG, Allen PD, Ellsmere JC. The diagnostic accuracy of transabdominal ultrasonography needs to be considered when managing gallbladder polyps. Surg Endosc. 2013;27(11):4021-5.
17. Konstantinidis IT, Bajpai S, Kambadakone AR, Tanabe KK, Berger DL, Zheng H,et al. Gallbladder lesions identified on ultrasound. Lessons from the last 10 years. J Gastrointest Surg. 2012;16(3):549-53.
18. Wu SS, Lin KC, Soon MS, Yeh KT. Ultrasound-guided percutaneous transhepatic fine needle aspiration cytology study of gallbladder polypoid lesions. Am J Gastroenterol. 1996;91(8):1591-4.
19. Inoue T, Kitano M, Kudo M, Sakamoto H, Kawasaki T, Yasuda C, et al. Diagnosis of gallbladder diseases by contrast-enhanced phase-inversion harmonic ultrasonography. Ultrasound Med Biol. 2007;33(3):353-61.
20. Pasławski M, Krupski W, Złomaniec J. The value of ultrasound harmonic imaging in the diagnostics of gallbladder cholesterol polyps. Ann Univ Mariae Curie Sklodowska Med. 2004;59(2):293-7.
21. Hattori M, Inui K, Yoshino J, Miyoshi H, Okushima K, Nakamura Y, et al. Usefulness of contrast-enhanced ultrasonography in the differential diagnosis of polypoid gallbladder lesions. Nihon Shokakibyo Gakkai Zasshi. 2007;104(6):790-8.
22. Tsuji S, Sofuni A, Moriyasu F, Itokawa F, Ishii K, Kurihara T, et al. Contrast-enhanced ultrasonography in the diagnosis of gallbladder disease. Hepatogastroenterology. 2012;59(114):336-40.
23. Cheon YK, Cho WY, Lee TH, Cho YD, Moon JH, Lee JS, et al. Endoscopic ultrasonography does not differentiate neoplastic from non-neoplastic small gallbladder polyps. World J Gastroenterol. 2009;15(19):2361-6.
24. Cho JH, Park JY, Kim YJ, Kim HM, Kim HJ, Hong SP, et al. Hypoechoic foci on EUS are simple and strong predictive factors for neoplastic gallbladder polyps. Gastrointest Endosc. 2009; 69(7):1244-50.
25. Akatsu T, Aiura K, Shimazu M, Ueda M, Wakabayashi G, Tanabe M, et al. Can endoscopic ultrasonography differentiate nonneoplastic from neoplastic gallbladder polyps? Dig Dis Sci. 2006;51(2): 416-21.
26. Sugiyama M, Atomi Y, Yamato T. Endoscopic ultrasonography for differential diagnosis of polypoid gallbladder lesions: analysis in surgical and follow up series. Gut. 2000;46(2):250-4.
27. Shindoh N. CT findings of the small polypoid lesions of the gallbladder (2 cm or less PLG): differentiation between benign

and malignant disease on unenhanced CT. Nihon Igaku Hoshasen Gakkai Zasshi. 1996;56(3):102-8.
28. Furukawa H, Takayasu K, Mukai K, Inoue K, Kyokane T, Shimada K, et al. CT evaluation of small polypoid lesions of the gallbladder. Hepatogastroenterology. 1995;42(6):800-10.
29. Furukawa H, Kosuge T, Shimada K, Yamamoto J, Kanai Y, Mukai K, et al. Small polypoid lesions of the gallbladder: differential diagnosis and surgical indications by helical computed tomography. Arch Surg. 1998;133(7):735-9.
30. Jang JY, Kim SW, Lee SE, Hwang DW, Kim EJ, Lee JY, et al. Differential diagnostic and staging accuracies of high resolution ultrasonography, endoscopic ultrasonography, and multidetector computed tomography for gallbladder polypoid lesions and gallbladder cancer. Ann Surg. 2009;250(6):943-9.
31. Irie H, Kamochi N, Nojiri J, Egashira Y, Sasaguri K, Kudo S. High b-value diffusion-weighted MRI in differentiation between benign and malignant polypoid gallbladder lesions. Acta Radiol. 2011;1;52(3):236-40.
32. Ogawa T, Horaguchi J, Fujita N, Noda Y, Kobayashi G, Ito K, et al. High b-value diffusion-weighted magnetic resonance imaging for gallbladder lesions: differentiation between benignity and malignancy. J Gastroenterol. 2012;47(12):1352-60.
33. Lee J, Yun M, Kim KS, Lee JD, Kim CK. Risk stratification of gallbladder polyps (1–2 cm) for surgical intervention with 18F-FDG PET/CT. J Nucl Med. 2012;53(3):353-8.
34. Koh T, Taniguchi H, Yamaguchi A, Kunishima S, Yamagishi H. Differential diagnosis of gallbladder cancer using positron emission tomography with fluorine-18-labeled fluoro-deoxyglucose (FDG-PET). J Surg Oncol. 2003;84(2):74-81.
35. Meirelles-Costa AL, Bresciani CJ, Perez RO, Bresciani BH, Siqueira SA, Cecconello I. Are histological alterations observed in the gallbladder precancerous lesions? Clinics (Sao Paulo). 2010;65(2):143-50.
36. Park JK, Yoon YB, Kim YT, Ryu JK, Yoon WJ, Lee SH, et al. Management strategies for gallbladder polyps: is it possible to predict malignant gallbladder polyps? Gut Liver. 2008;2(2):88-94.
37. Kwon W, Jang JY, Lee SE, Hwang DW, Kim SW. Clinicopathologic features of polypoid lesions of the gallbladder and risk factors of gallbladder cancer. J Korean Med Sci. 2009;24(3):481-7.
38. Bang S. Natural course and treatment strategy of gallbladder polyp. Korean J Gastroenterol. 2009;53(6):336-40.
39. Park JY, Hong SP, Kim YJ, Kim HJ, Kim HM, Cho JH, et al. Long-term follow up of gallbladder polyps. J Gastroenterol Hepatol. 2009;24(2):219-22.
40. Kwon W, Jang JY, Lee SE, Hwang DW, Kim SW. Clinicopathologic features of polypoid lesions of the gallbladder and risk factors of gallbladder cancer. J Korean Med Sci. 2009;24(3):481-7.
41. Aldouri AQ, Malik HZ, Waytt J, Khan S, Ranganathan K, Kummaraganti S, et al. The risk of gallbladder cancer from polyps in a large multiethnic series. Eur J Surg Oncol. 2009;35(1):48-51.
42. Marangoni G, Hakeem A, Toogood GJ, Lodge JP, Prasad KR. Treatment and surveillance of polypoid lesions of the gallbladder in the United Kingdom. HPB (Oxford). 2012;14(7):435-40.
43. SAGES Guideline Committee. SAGES guidelines for the clinical application of laparoscopic tract surgery, section H-gallbladder polyps. January 2010. Available at http://www.sages.org/publications/id/06/.
44. Pedersen MR, Dam C, Rafaelsen SR. Ultrasound follow-up for gallbladder polyps less than 6 mm may not be necessary. Dan Med J. 2012;59(10):A4503.
45. Corwin MT, Siewert B, Sheiman RG, Kane RA. Incidentally detected gallbladder polyps: is follow-up necessary?—Long-term clinical and US analysis of 346 patients. Radiology. 2011;258(1):277-82.
46. Cairns V, Neal CP, Dennison AR, Garcea G. Risk and cost-effectiveness of surveillance followed by cholecystectomy for gallbladder polyps. Arch Surg. 2012;147(12):1078-83.
47. Kratzer W, Haenle MM, Voegtle A, Mason RA, Akinli AS, Hirschbuehl K, et al. Ultrasonographically detected gallbladder polyps: a reason for concern? A seven-year follow-up study. BMC Gastroenterol. 2008;8:41.

CHAPTER 61

Carcinoma Gallbladder

Asit Arora, PK Mishra

INTRODUCTION

First ever description of carcinoma gallbladder was provided by Maximilian Stoll, an Austrian physician from Vienna in 1777. Even after two centuries the nihilistic and pessimistic attitude toward gallbladder cancer persists and not so without reason. Due to non-specific symptomatology, patients usually present late leading to very low resectability and 5-year survival rates.[1] It is the most common malignancy of biliary tract[2] but with peculiar geographic and ethnic distribution and a complex interplay of multiple host, environmental, dietary and genetic risk factors.[3] Significant advances in the fields of epidemiology, tumor biology, imaging, surgical techniques and chemoradiotherapy have brought a degree of optimism in the management of this otherwise unforgiving and fatal disease.

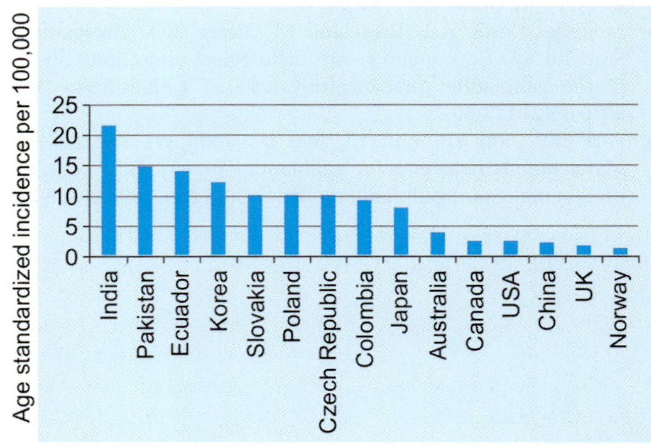

Figure 1 Incidence of gallbladder cancer in select geographic areas

EPIDEMIOLOGY

There is a wide variation in the incidence of gallbladder cancer across the world. Highest reported incidence is from North India (21.5/100,000 in females) followed by Pakistan. Other geographic areas with reported high incidence of gallbladder cancer are Japan, Korea, East European countries like Slovakia, Poland and Czech Republic. Latin American countries, like Columbia, Peru and Chile, have also reported high incidences. To the contrary low incidences are seen in the continents of North America and Australia and most of the Europe (Fig. 1).[3]

A strong female preponderance is observed in almost all populations. This difference is more striking in high incidence regions like Columbia and Pakistan where male: female ratio of 1:5 have been reported but in most of areas including India 1: 2–3 is the usual ratio.[3,4]

Gallbladder cancer incidence increases with age in both males and females with peak incidence in sixth and seventh decade. In high incidence areas like India, many patients are seen in fourth and fifth decades. Higher parity, older age at menarche and younger age at first birth have been implicated as risk factors for increased incidence of gallbladder cancer in females. Though rare, cases have been reported in young and even in children.[5,6]

With the advent of sophisticated imaging techniques and laparoscopy, widespread use of ultrasound and increased availability of cholecystectomy the incidence and mortality of gallbladder cancer have decreased in certain parts of the world. Analysis have shown that age standardized mortality of gallbladder carcinoma (GBC) in women have decreased by 30% in the USA and Europe.[3] But incidence and fatality remain high in high incidence areas like India, Chile and Japan.

Table 1: Risk factors for gallbladder cancer

Host factors	Age[3,9] Socioeconomic status[9] Gender[3,10] Family history of gallbladder cancer[3] Ethnicity
Factors promoting inflammation and stasis	Gallstones[3,9,11-13] Anomalous pancreaticobiliary duct junction (APBDJ)[3,14,15] *Salmonella* and *Helicobacter* infection[3,16,17] Obesity[3] Multiple pregnancy[3,11,18] Porcelain gallbladder[13,19]
Factors promoting mutation	Smoking[3] Chemical exposure—oil, textile and paper industry[3,13] pesticides heavy metals
Dietary factors	Vit B6, C and E deficiency[3,12] High calorie, carbohydrate, red meat, red chilli and pepper intake[3,12] Low vegetable, fiber and fruit intake[3,12]
Gallbladder polyp	Adenomatous polyp[18]

Incidence has increased in North as well as traditionally low incidence areas of South India. Mean annual percentage change in age standardized rates in India ranged from 1.0% to 8.1% over a period of 1998–2006.[7]

ETIOLOGY

Carcinoma gallbladder is a multifactorial disease with a complex interplay of various risk factors which interacts in an additive manner to give rise to high incidence as well as early age of onset.[8] Various risk factors that have been implicated can be classified as in Table 1.

Prevalence of multiple etiological factors leads to increased incidence of GBC. In North India and various other high incidence areas like Latin America along with high prevalence of gallstone various other factors coexist. Poor socioeconomic status, poor sanitation, high incidence of salmonella and helicobacter infections, nutritional deficiencies, high parity, presence of pollutants like pesticides in drinking water and thus in bile in presence of gallstone provide a fertile ground for growth of this fatal disease.[20-23] This also explains low incidence of gallbladder cancer in western population despite high prevalence of gallstones.[24]

Two main pathways for genesis of gallbladder cancer exist. Metaplasia → dysplasia → carcinoma pathway and adenoma → carcinoma pathway. Unlike other hollow viscus the dysplasia carcinoma pathway is the predominant one. Gallstone leads to a chronic inflammatory state and superadded recurrent infections lead to metaplasia, dysplasia and over 10–15 years carcinoma.[25] Gallstones by far is the strongest risk factor for gallbladder cancer.[3,13] Any factor that leads to stasis and thus gallstone formation is also a risk factor for GBC (Flow chart 1).

Gallbladder packed with stones, stones more than 3 cm in size, cholesterol stones and symptomatic stone are associated with higher risk of developing malignancy.[26,27]

Flow chart 1 Cancer pathway in gallbladder cancer

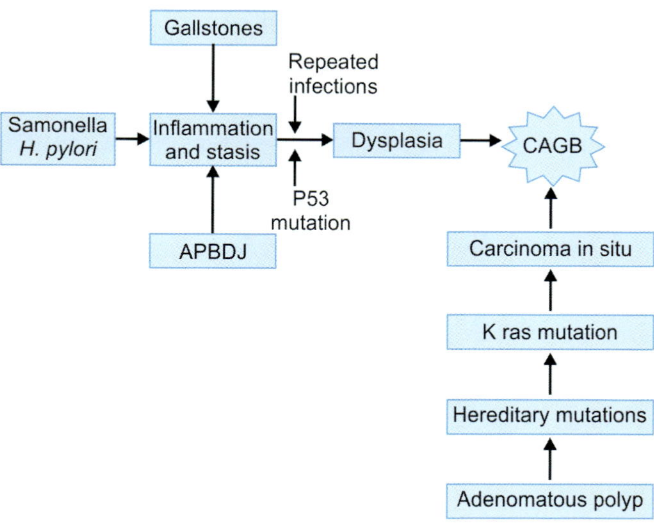

Anomalous pancreaticobiliary ductal junction is an important etiological factor for gallbladder cancer especially in Japan and Korea where its prevalence is high. Due to the malunion, which allows continuous reflux of pancreatic juice into biliary tree, there is persistent inflammation and bile stasis leading to formation of carcinoma via dysplasia pathway.[28] Papillary tumor is specially associated with APBDJ.[29] Meta-analysis on relationship of APBDJ and gallbladder cancer showed statistically significant higher incidence of APBDJ in GBC patients than in control population (10.60% vs 1.76%, OR: 7.41, 95% CI: 5.03 to 10.87, $p<0.00001$). Also the age of GBC patients with APBDJ was 10 years younger as compared to those without. Cholecystectomy is recommended for patients with APBDJ, without congenital dilatation of common bile duct even in the absence of gallstones.[15]

Gallbladder polyp is a common entity seen in up to 0.3–12% cases.[30,31] Majority of these polyps are benign with no malignant potential. Adenoma carcinoma sequence is rare but has been reported. Polyps more than 1 cm have been shown to have substantial risk of malignancy. Age more than 50, solitary polyps, biliary type symptoms, documented increase in size during follow-up and polyps in setting of PSC are also considered as risk factors and are indications for cholecystectomy in patients with gallbladder polyp (Flow chart 2).[32-34]

GENETICS IN GALLBLADDER CANCER

Multiple *genetic mutations* and molecular abnormalities have been identified in patients of gallbladder cancer. Most dominant one is mutation of p53 gene which is seen in more than 50% of cases. p53 gene is seen frequently in human cancers. It is known to play a role in maintaining the genomic integrity of cells. K-Ras mutation has been observed in up to 40–50% cases but is more commonly seen in patients with APBDJ. Two major pathways K-Ras related to hyperplasia-dysplasia-carcinoma and TP53 gene related to cholecystitis-dysplasia-carcinoma in situ invasive carcinoma have been identified. Other less common mutations are p21 and p16 gene mutations which are associated with poorer outcome. Various other aberrations like over expression of COX-2, VEGF

Flow chart 2 Management algorithm for gallbladder polyp

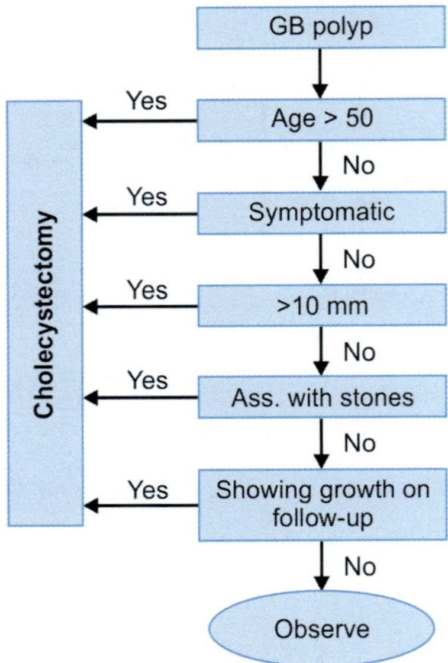

Flow chart 3 Lymphatic pathway for gallbladder

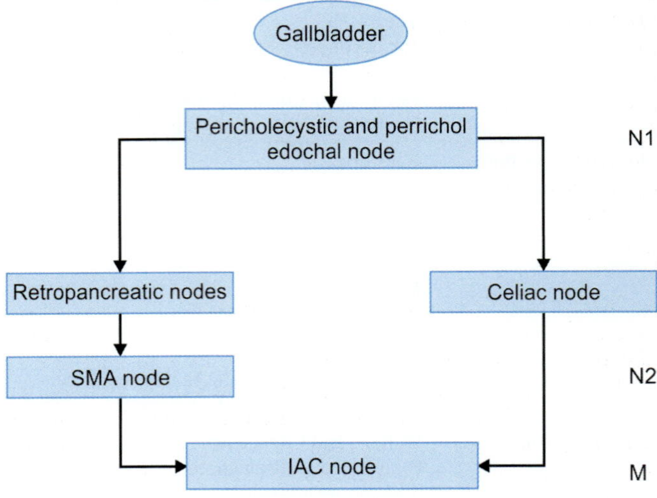

and heparanase have also been reported in literature. Fragile Histidine Triad (FHIT) a tumor suppresser gene has also been reported to be inactivated in this cancer. Allelic loss at FHIT locus has been reported from Chile which has high incidence of gallbladder cancer.

RELEVANT ANATOMY OF GALLBLADDER

It is important to mention the peculiarities of gallbladder wall which is pertinent to the management of gallbladder cancer. Conspicuous absence of muscularis mucosae and submucosa and thin layered muscularis propria and lamina propria allows early and easy access of malignant cells to adjacent structures and lymph nodes. Gallbladder is covered by serosa all around except at the liver bed where cystic plate separates these two structures. This plane is utilized to dissect gallbladder during cholecystectomy, and thus results in tumor violation in all but T1a tumors making it an inappropriate surgery for these tumors. Gallbladder is located in an area, close to hepatic hilum and having close juxtaposition to duodenum and hepatic flexure of colon. Tumor arising from fundus and body of gallbladder have propensity to invade liver, colon and duodenum requiring multivisceral resections at many instances. Similarly due to proximity to porta hepatis in general and right portal pedicle in particular the tumors arising from neck and infundibulum have early infiltration to these structures mandating a major hepatic resection and CBD excision to achieve complete tumor clearance.

Lymphatic drainage of gallbladder is into pericholedochal nodes. From here lymph takes two pathways (Flow chart 3). First via retropancreatic node into superior mesenteric arteries (SMA) node and finally into interaortocaval (IAC) nodes and second from retroportal to celiac into IAC node. There can be involvement of IAC node directly without either celiac or retro-pancreatic SMA lymph nodal basin involvement. This is important as involvement of IAC node is considered as metastatic thus requiring proper assessment of IAC region preoperatively with CT scan and intraoperatively with a wide kocherization maneuver to rule out any lymph node metastasis in this region before proceeding to resection of tumor.

PATHOLOGY

Fundus is the most dependent part of gallbladder in erect position and most prone for stagnation and not surprisingly is the most common site of malignancy.[35] Grossly the tumors have been classified as in Table 2. Infiltrative variety is the most common and aggressive one. It has a propensity to spread along the wall of the gallbladder and involve CBD early. Papillary tumor has intraluminal growth pattern with minimal infiltration to adjacent structure and thus has best prognosis. Histologically, adenocarcinoma is the most common type accounting for 90% of cases.[36,37] Other rare varieties like lymphoma, sarcoma and melanoma have also been reported.[35] Majority of the gallbladder cancers are poorly differentiated type highlighting the aggressiveness of this tumor.

Table 2: Classification of the tumors

Location[35]	Fundus—60% Body—30% Neck—10%
Gross[36]	Infiltrative Nodular Combined infiltrative nodular Papillary Combined papillary infiltrative
Histology[35]	Adenocarcinoma—90% Adenosquamous/squamous Neuroendocrine Sarcoma Lymphoma Melanoma
Grade[37]	Well-differentiated Moderately differentiated Poorly differentiated Undifferentiated

CLINICAL FEATURES

Gallbladder cancer can remain silent for a long duration of time. Even when it is symptomatic, early presentation mimics cholecystitis and is ignored by many. Most common presenting feature of gallbladder cancer is pain which is present in 54-97% cases. Ominous signs like anorexia and weight loss in an elderly with right hypochondriac pain should alert an astute clinician to this etiology.

A subset of patients present with palpable lump which is a predictor of advanced disease. At examination patient's general condition should be assessed closely. Presence of jaundice, supraclavicular lymph node should be carefully ascertained. Presence of supraclavicular lymph node is often missed in these patients. Presence of this finding with FNAC confirmation may obviate further expensive evaluation. Abdominal examination can reveal gallbladder mass and liver enlargement. In advanced cases features of gastric outlet obstruction, emaciation and ascites may be seen. Splenic enlargement should also be ascertained. Per rectal examination is mandatory to look for Blumer's shelf.

Presentation of gallbladder cancer as jaundice is not unusual. It is seen in 30-50% cases.[38,39] Jaundice could be because of direct infiltration of bile duct, lymph nodal compression or associated CBD stones. Presence of jaundice due to infiltration or lymph nodal disease is an ominous feature and decreases the chances of resection.[40] Surgical resection (R0) improves survival in patients with gallbladder cancer.

As gallbladder has close anatomical association with duodenum and hepatic flexure of colon, their involvement in advanced gallbladder cancer is not uncommon. This subset of patient may presents as gastric oulet obstruction and colonic obstruction respectively. Ascites, fixed pain to back, emaciation are ominous features indicating terminal disease. Presentation of GBC has not changed over the last century and most patients still present with advanced disease only.[41]

Investigation

Appropriate assessment both for diagnosis and staging of gallbladder cancer is mandatory before commencement of any treatment. In early stages gallbladder cancer may mimic cholecystitis not only clinically but also radiologically and if subjected to cholecystectomy leads to suboptimal treatment and a lost opportunity to deliver a meaningful survival to this most favorable patient group. Every attempt should be made to establish accurate diagnosis and staging of this disease and radiology is corner stone of this. Various modalities available to us are USG, CT, MRI, PET and EUS.

Radiologically, gallbladder cancer presents in three forms: (1) mass replacing the gallbladder, (2) thickening of the gallbladder wall and (3) polypoidal intraluminal growth with a frequency of 40-65%, 20-30% and 15-25% respectively.

Ultrasound is a freely available, cost effective and usually first line investigation for gallbladder disease. It is a very sensitive investigation for advanced disease. Heterogeneous predominantly hypoechoic mass in gallbladder is the usual finding. In early cases asymmetrical thickening of gallbladder wall, discontinuous mucosa and submucosal echolucency are subtle features that should raise a suspicion of malignant change. Ultrasound has a sensitivity of only 53% in these early cancers.[42] Ultrasound is also very poor in identifying lymph node metastasis in HDL region and distant metastasis. Newer high frequency 7 MHz probes with compound imaging, speckle reduction imaging and harmonious techniques have resulted in better resolution and have achieved a diagnostic accuracy of 85% in differentiating between benign and malignant etiologies.[43]

CT Scan

Dual phase contrast enhanced CT scan is the mainstay of the diagnostic evaluation of gallbladder cancer (Figs 2A and B). The tumor is usually hypodense on plain CT, with no or minimal enhancement on contrast administration. About 40% of lesions may show hypervascular foci of enhancement equal to or greater than that of liver after intravenous contrast administration.[44,45] Peripheral intense irregular enhancement may occur in large gallbladder cancers during the early arterial phase. This enhancement may be retained in fibrous stromal components during the portal venous and delayed phases aiding in differentiation from large central

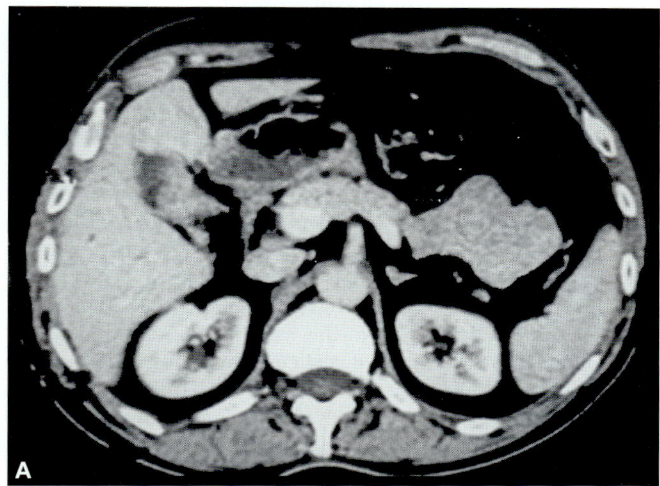

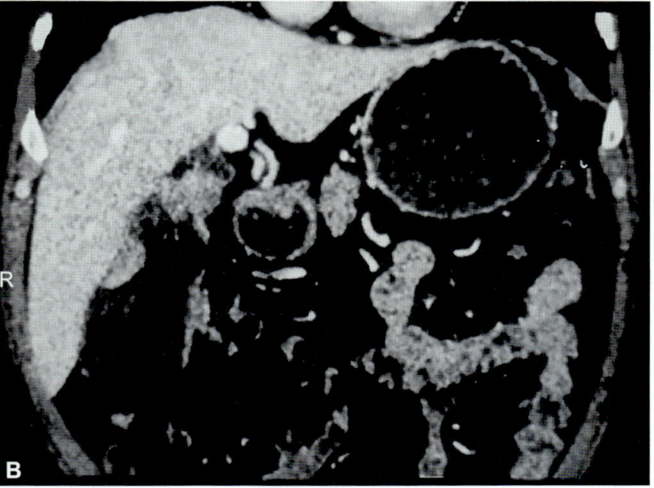

Figures 2A and B CECT showing gallbladder cancer with hypodense mass with minimal enhancement: (A) Carcinoma gallbladder involving fundus and body; (B) Carcinoma gallbladder involving body and neck

hepatocellular carcinomas, which have a greater tendency to washout contrast material.[46]

Most difficult scenario is to differentiate early GBC which presents as gallbladder wall thickening only, from benign etiology like chronic cholecystitis. Investigators have looked upon the enhancement pattern of gallbladder wall on Multi Detector CT scan. The important findings that are suggestive of malignant etiology are enhancing thick inner layer of the gallbladder wall, stronger enhancement of the inner layer than of liver parenchyma, thin outer layer less than or equal to 3.4 mm, irregular contour of the affected wall and focal involvement in the decreasing order of importance.[47] Accuracy of MDCT in differentiating T1 lesion from T2 and above is around 94% whereas it decreases to 89.9% when it comes to differentiating T2 lesions from T3 and above. The overall accuracy for T staging when compared with final pathological staging is 83.9%. It has also been shown that combining multiplanar reconstruction (MPR) images with axial images improve the accuracy of T staging of MDCT from 71.7% to 84.9%, as MPR images reduce the partial volume effect seen in axial cuts hence improving the accuracy.[48] MPR images can also be used to see CBD and portal vein involvement (Fig. 3). To detect overall resectability of gallbladder cancer CT scan has a sensitivity, specificity and accuracy of 67%, 100% and 85% respectively. It is a highly reliable test for detecting vascular invasion both arterial and portal venous. But it over stages duodenal infiltration, T staging in papillary tumors and malignant change in presence of inflammatory pathologies like cholecystitis.[48,49] Limitation of the CT scan in detecting peritoneal metastasis is well known. MDCT have increased the sensitivity to pick peritoneal metastasis to 85–93% from 63–79% in conventional CT scan. Accurate assessment of lymph nodal metastasis is an important component of staging the disease. A rounded shape, heterogenous architecture and a size more than 1 cm of the lymph nodes is indicative of involvement. However, histological confirmation should be done whenever possible. CT scan has a sensitivity of only 36% and 47% respectively for N1 and N2 nodes.[50] But for IAC and para-aortic nodes (Fig. 4) sensitivity of CT scan reaches nearly 100%.[49] This is an important distinction as N1 and N2 nodes are considered as regional nodes and even when detected intraoperatively will not preclude a surgical resection, whereas aortocaval nodes are considered metastatic and if detected preoperatively can avoid an unnecessary laparotomy.

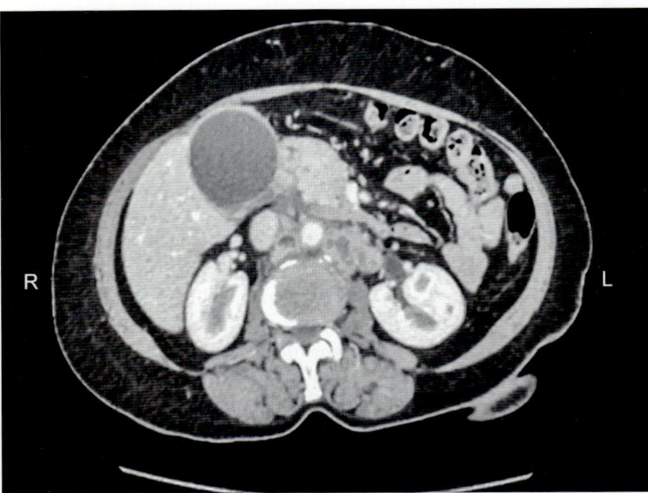

Figure 4 Enlarged inter aortocaval and para-aortic nodes in a patient of gallbladder cancer suggestive of metastatic disease

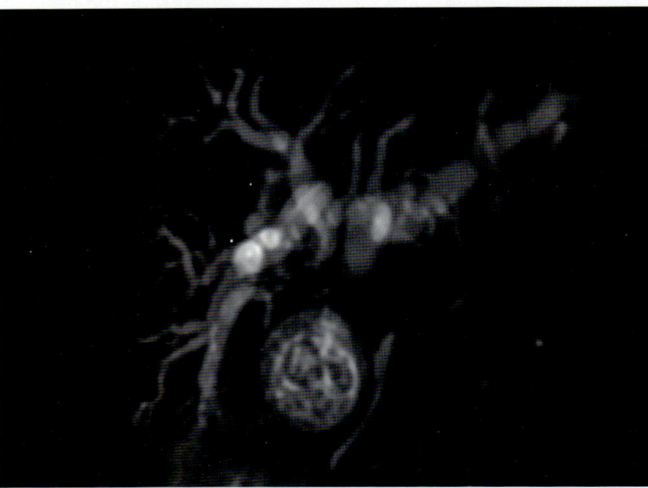

Figure 5 MRCP picture showing a gallbladder neck mass infiltrating CHD involving the primary confluence resulting in hilar separation, distal CBD is seen. Gallbladder is distended

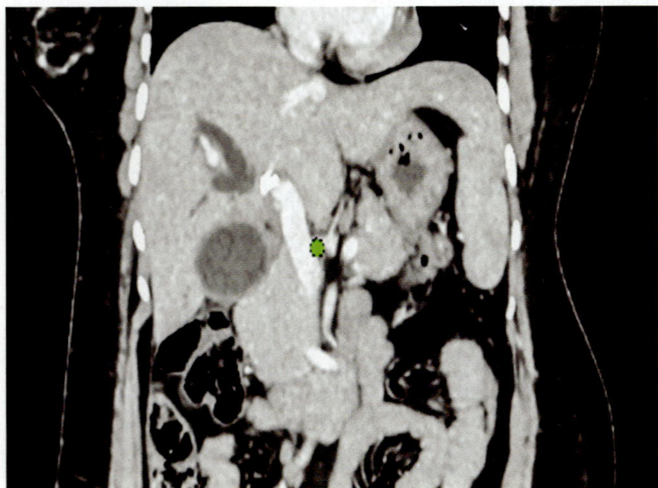

Figure 3 MPR reconstruction of CT images showing a GB neck mass causing hilar block and resultant IHBRD in right lobe. PTBD catheter is seen draining the left lobe

MRI and MRCP

Even though the CT scan is the first line modality for evaluation of gallbladder cancer, use of MRI has increased in recent times. At present it is indicated in jaundiced patients and in cases of diagnostic problems (Fig. 5). A typical gallbladder cancer appears as hypointense to isointense on T1 weighted image and hyperintense on T2 weighted image.[51] MRI has shown a sensitivity of 70–100% for liver invasion and 60–75% for lymph node metastasis, but it does not add to the findings of CT scan in staging gallbladder

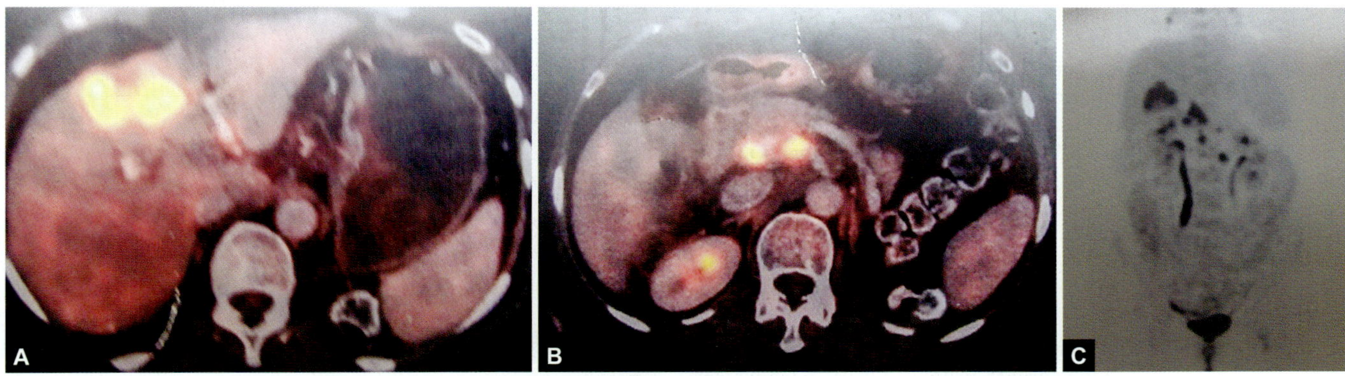

Figures 6A to C Showing PET CT for carcinoma gallbladder. (A) Uptake seen in gallbladder. (B) Uptake in aortocaval nodes. (C) Uptake seen in GB, aortocaval and retroperitoneal lymph nodes

cancer.[52,53] Improvement in the technology have expanded the application of MRI in gallbladder cancer as well. One of the noteworthy changes is the use of diffusion weighted MR imaging (DWI). Its use has been evaluated in thick walled gallbladders to differentiate benign from malignant etiologies. Positive signal rate with DWI was significantly higher in gallbladder cancer (78% as compared to benign gallbladder disease 22%; $p<0.001$). This new technique has offered some help in solving this difficult problem.[54] MR cholangiography is indispensable for evaluation of biliary tree and it helps in surgical planning in patients with biliary tract invasion.

PET

Role of PET scan is not very well defined in gallbladder cancer and at best is controversial. Although gallbladder cancer is an FDG avid lesion and lights up on PET scan (Figs 6A to C), not much data exists to support its routine use. PET has been used in four different scenarios in the context of gallbladder cancer. First for staging and assessing resectability of primary gallbladder cancer, second in incidental gallbladder cancer before re-resection, thirdly in thick walled gallbladder with suspected malignancy in differentiating benign from malignant etiology. Postoperatively, it is used in follow-up for detection of recurrent disease. With the increasing use of adjuvant and neoadjuvant therapies it may also be used for response assessment, like in other malignancies.

Initial studies evaluating role of PET on biliary malignancies including small number of carcinoma gallbladder (14 and 31 cases) reported that i.e. 14 and 31cases reported that surgical plan was changed in 17% and 23% cases respectively in these two studies by detection of distant metastasis by the virtue of PET scan.[55,56] PET does not offer any advantage over MDCT in detecting primary disease but for distant metastasis PET-CT has a higher sensitivity (94.7% vs 63.2%, $p=0.02$).[57] Roles of PET-CT have also been investigated in incidental gallbladder cancer before re-resection. In a study of 92 patients of incidental gallbladder cancer, MDCT had a sensitivity, PPV and accuracy of 100%, 85.5% and 87.5% respectively as compared to 100%, 91.3% and 91.6% for PET-CT in defining resectability. PET-CT could detect occult metastasis in some patients where MDCT was normal.[58] Usefulness of PET in differentiating benign and malignant lesions in setting of thick walled gallbladder has also been described in some studies.[59,60] In a study by Oe et al. three out of four patients with thick walled gallbladder having PET uptake turned out to be GBC whereas none without uptake had malignancy.[59] There are limited data for its routine use for surveillance or for detection of recurrence in follow-up.

Even though there is some evidence that PET may improve preoperative staging, due to small number of studies with very limited cases any definitive conclusion on the value of PET cannot be made. Cost of the study remains a major issue for its routine use. Larger studies are required to better define the role of PET in gallbladder cancer.

Endoscopic Ultrasound

Endoscopic ultrasound (EUS) has been inducted in routine workup protocols of various pancreatic and ampullary lesions but its role in gallbladder malignancy is still investigatory. As the experience is growing with this modality, it is being more frequently used for evaluation of gallbladder cancer and its likely resectability. Malignancy in polypoidal lesions of gallbladder, EUS guided FNA from gallbladder mass, evaluation of CBD obstruction and the lymph nodes, assessment of portal vein involvement and evaluation of IAC node (Fig. 7) and its FNA have been some areas where EUS has made an impact.[61,62]

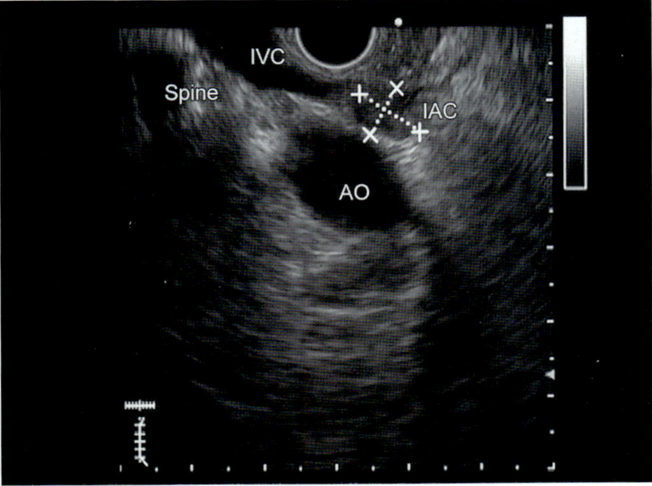

Figure 7 Inter aortocaval lymph node on endoscopic ultrasound

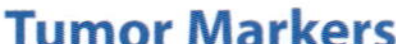

Tumor Markers

CA19-9 and CEA are commonly used tumor markers in pancreaticobiliary malignancies, but have been poorly studied in the context of GBC. Their utility is very limited as far as screening and diagnosis is concerned. Also their role in prognostication and follow-up is poorly defined. More studies with large numbers of patients are needed to better define the role of tumor markers in GBC.

Staging

Various staging systems have been used in past years. Nevin's classification was one of the earliest, proposed in 1976 which was later modified in 1990 by Donohue et al.[63,64] A simple and easy to use classification fell out of favor as it was too simple for increasing complexities of management of GBC.

Modified Nevin Classification

Stage 1	Carcinoma in situ
Stage 2	Mucosal or muscular invasion
Stage 3	Direct liver infiltration
Stage 4	Lymph nodal metastasis
Stage 5	Distant metastasis

TNM classification is the most widely used classification system in the present times. Seventh edition of AJCC classification was proposed in 2010.[65]

Tumor

TX	Primary tumor cannot be assessed
T0	No evidence of primary tumor
Tis	Carcinoma *in situ*
T1	Tumor invades lamina propria or muscular layer
T1a	Tumor invades lamina propria
T1b	Tumor invades muscular layer
T2	Tumor invades perimuscular connective tissue; no extension beyond serosa or into liver
T3	Tumor perforates the serosa (visceral peritoneum) and/or directly invades the liver and/or one other adjacent organ or structure, such as the stomach, duodenum, colon, pancreas, omentum or extrahepatic bile ducts
T4	Tumor invades main portal vein or hepatic artery or invades at least two extrahepatic organs or structures

Node

NX	Regional lymph nodes cannot be assessed
N0	No regional lymph node metastasis
N1	Metastases to nodes along the cystic duct, common bile duct, hepatic artery, and/or portal vein
N2	Metastases to periaortic, pericaval, SMA and/or celiac artery lymph nodes

Metastasis

M0	No distant metastasis
M1	Distant metastasis

Clinical Staging

Stage	*T*	*N*	*M*
0	Tis	N0	M0
I	T1	N0	M0
II	T2	N0	M0
IIIA	T3	N0	M0
IIIB	T1–3	N1	M0
IVA	T4	N0–1	M0
IVB	Any T	N2	M0
	Any T	Any N	M1

Most important changes made in AJCC 7 from AJCC 6 was segregation of regional lymph node into two station N1 and N2, N1 comprised of nodes in hepatoduodenal ligament, i.e. pericholecystic, pericholedochal, periportal and hepatic artery nodes, whereas celiac, periduodenal, peripancreatic and SMA nodes are now classified as N2 nodes. Changes have been made in stage grouping so as to better correlate with patient out come and resectability rates. Locally unresectable T4 lesions are classified as stage IVa now, which was classified as stage III in 6th edition. N2 disease is clubbed along with M1 disease in stage IVb. There has been some criticism of this new staging system. Even though segregation of N1 and N2 has helped in better correlation of staging to survival and prognostication, the fact that N2 disease has been clubbed along with M1 disease is contested by some authors. Up to 19% 3-year survival has been shown in N2 disease as compared to none in M1.[66] Similarly difference in survival has been observed in T1-T2N1 versus T3-N1 which in present staging system has been clubbed together. Also clubbing retropancreatic nodes with celiac and SMA nodes in N2 category is objectionable to many investigators especially Japanese, as retropancreatic nodes are considered as regional nodes and good survival is expected after their resection.

SURGICAL MANAGEMENT

Gallbladder cancer is an aggressive disease, usually presenting late. Surgery is the only potentially curative treatment option. Surgical resections can range from liver wedge resections to the more formidable extended right hepatectomies or hepato-pancreaticoduodenectomy. Thus, a proper patient selection and preoperative preparation is paramount prior to surgery. It should be ensured that the patient has a good performance status before he/she is subjected to a major surgery. A stair climbing test or a breath holding test is a good tool to assess general fitness. Patient's nutritional status should also be checked in preoperative assessment, serum albumin being one of the astute markers for the same. Any patient with suboptimal condition should be optimized prior to surgery. Dietary counseling should be done to provide high protein and adequate calorie diet. Adequate emphasis should be laid on teaching them incentive spirometry prior to surgery.

Patients should be screened for comorbid conditions which, if present, need to be optimized prior to surgery. Patients presenting with jaundice may require rehydration, correction of coagulopathy and treatment of infection which should be looked into diligently. A good surgical outcome depends primarily upon a meticulous preoperative assessment and patient selection otherwise a wonderfully performed surgery may end up in a catastrophe.

PREOPERATIVE PREPARATION

- ECOG status
- Incentive spirometer and steam inhalation
- Nutritional status and dietary counseling
- Jaundiced patient—(a) Inj. vitmain K × 3 doses, (b) adequate hydration and (c) need for preoperative drainage (d) assessment of future liver remnant and need for portal vein embolization
- Taking care of comorbid condition like diabetes/hypertension/asthma.

INCIDENTAL GALLBLADDER CANCER

Incidental gallbladder cancer is seen in 0.27–2.1% of cholecystectomy specimens.[67,68] These incidentally detected cancers could be *true incidental tumors* in which neither preoperative imaging studies nor intraoperative findings and inspection of cut surface of gallbladder mucosa raised any suspicion of malignancy. These tumors are identified only during histopathological evaluation of resected gallbladder. These are usually very early tumors. A *missed carcinoma gallbladder* is an incidentally detected tumor in which potential pointer toward malignancy has been overlooked on imaging studies and/or on intraoperative findings. These tumors are more advanced than true incidental tumors and even T2 and T3 tumors have been missed. An *unsuspected gallbladder cancer* is one when preoperatively there is no suspicion of malignancy but intraoperative findings are suggestive of malignancy or cutting open the cholecystectomy specimen reveals malignancy. Management of unsuspected gallbladder cancer is just like a primary gallbladder cancer, i.e. a radical resection with lymphadenectomy. If the capabilities of such a resection are not available a surgeon should be called or the patient should be referred to a specialized center.

In a scenario where malignancy of gallbladder comes to light after cholecystectomy by histopathological assessment of the gallbladder further treatment is directed by the pathological stage and resection margin status. In a T1a tumor a simple cholecystectomy is curative if the cystic duct margin is negative.[69,70] In T2 and T3 disease undergoing completion of radical surgery, residual disease is seen in liver bed in 10.4% and 36.4% patients and lymph nodal disease is seen in 31.3% and 45.5% cases respectively.[71] Aggressive re-resection with lymphadenectomy is required in any tumor T2 and beyond. Cystic duct margin status dictates the need for CBD excision. If the cystic duct margin is positive at the time of re-resection CBD should be excised, routine CBD excision is of no added advantage.

There has been some controversy in past regarding management of T1b tumors. Five-year survival up to 95% after simple cholecystectomy was reported in some earlier studies,[72] but more recent reports with large number of patients have shown a rather poor survival in this subset of patients undergoing a simple cholecystectomy. Most of the patients experience a survival benefit by re-resection in this subgroup also. In a study of 72 patients with incidental T1b gallbladder cancer of which 23 underwent completion radical cholecystectomy showed a 5-year survival benefit of 42% versus 79% in favor of the resection group.[73,74] T1b tumors have also been shown to have lymphatic and venous invasion and thus also requires radical re-resection.[75] A decision analysis study done for radical re-resection in T1b showed significant survival benefit across the age groups and is thus strongly recommended.[76]

Another bone of contention is port site excision during completion radical surgery for incidental GBC after laparoscopic cholecystectomy. Port site recurrences have been known to occur in incidental gallbladder cancer and incidence has been reported to be as high as 14–30%.[77] It is both because of direct contamination of wound during gallbladder extraction and indirect spread via pneumoperitoneum. Gallbladder perforation occurring during cholecystectomy leading to bile spillage also increases the risk of port site recurrences.

Port site recurrence could be associated with peritoneal dissemination and metastasis at other sites or it could be an isolated occurrence also, former being the more common outcome.[78-81] Port site excision during completion radical surgery is practiced but not universally accepted as there is no definitive evidence to either accept or refute this practice. Some authors do not believe in routine port site excision, in a study from MSKCC comprising 113 patients of incidental GBC, 69 underwent port site excision and 44 did not. There was no improvement in survival or disease recurrence.[82] A study by Fuks et al. showed similar results. In that study no survival benefit was found in 54 of 148 patients with incidental GBC undergoing port site excision.[83] Both these authors concluded that port site excision should not be mandatory at the time of completion radical cholecystectomy. But in instances where port site recurrence is an isolated phenomenon port site excision will improve overall survival and it also helps in prognostication and better staging.[80,81]

Role of staging laparoscopy (Fig. 8) is well established in primary GBC but is not well defined in incidental GBC. Butte et al. reported a yield of 4.3% in detecting disseminated disease.[84] Since the risk of dissemination increases with increasing T stage, positive margins and poorly differentiated tumor targeting these lesions are likely to increase the yield.[82]

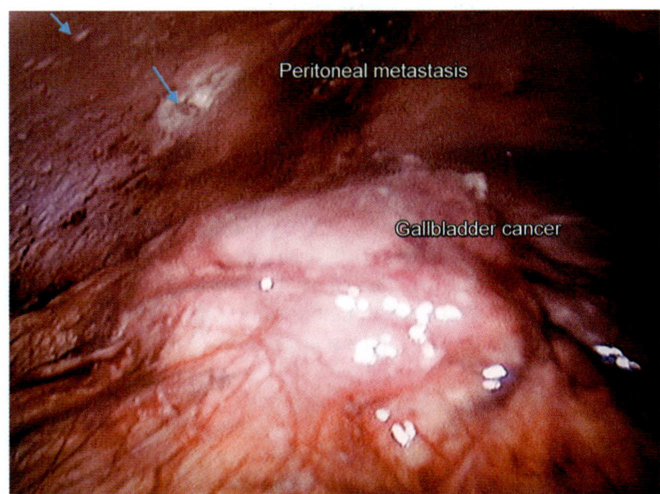

Figure 8 Multiple peritoneal mets on staging laparoscopy

In summary, treatment of incidental gallbladder cancer is determined by the histopathological assessment of gallbladder. Cholecystectomy itself is curative for T1a tumor. For all other tumors completion radical cholecystectomy with regional lymphadenectomy should be performed. Cystic duct margin status decides the need for CBD excision which is required in positive duct margins. Before embarking on a radical resection a thorough preoperative assessment of disease status should be performed. Contrast enhanced CT scan to look for any site of distant metastasis is required. PET-CT has shown to be useful by detecting metastatic disease missed by CT scan.[58] Staging laparoscopy has low yield but in high risk patients like T2, T3 tumors, positive margins and poor differentiation it should be done. Role of port site excision is controversial but favored by many.

Primary Gallbladder Cancer

From the point of view of management, primary gallbladder cancer may be divided into early, locally advanced and metastatic gallbladder cancer. Early gallbladder cancer is one where tumor is confined to gallbladder wall, i.e. T1 and T2 lesions. These tumors have a low lymph node metastasis and good 5-year survival rates. Many of T1 tumors are detected incidentally after cholecystectomy especially T1a tumors which are mostly identified on histopathological examination of resected gallbladder. It is the definitive procedure for these very early tumors. But for T1b and T2 tumors, radical resection with negative margins along with regional lymphadenectomy is the standard of care.

Locally advanced tumors are the ones in which tumor has gone beyond the confines of the gallbladder to invade liver, adjacent organs like duodenum, colon, bile ducts or the vascular structures like hepatic artery or portal veins. These tumors have high incidence of lymph node metastasis, relatively poor resectability and 5-year survival rates. Traditionally aggressive surgical approach was not pursued in majority of these patients. Last decade has witnessed a change in the philosophy in surgical fraternity. Favorable results with extensive resections like multivisceral resection, hepato-pancreatoduodenectomy, extensive liver resections for hilar block have brought a sea change in the management of these advanced lesions. Metastatic tumors on the other hand are managed with best supportive care.

Role of Staging Laparoscopy in Primary GBC

Staging laparoscopy should be an integral part of management of GBC (Fig. 8). It has a potential to detect disseminated disease missed on CT or MRI and thus obviating a non-therapeutic laparotomy, as most of these patients do not require a surgical palliative procedure. In a large prospective study of 409 patients of primary gallbladder cancer from GB Pant Hospital, New Delhi,[85] staging laparoscopy detected disseminated disease in 95 cases with an overall yield of 23.20%. It prevented non-therapeutic laparotomy in 55.9% of unresectable tumors further highlighting the importance of staging laparoscopy in GBC.

Extent of Lymphadenectomy

An adequate oncologic resection requires an en bloc removal of tumor along with its regional lymph nodes, but in case of gallbladder cancer extent of regional lymphadenectomy remains controversial.

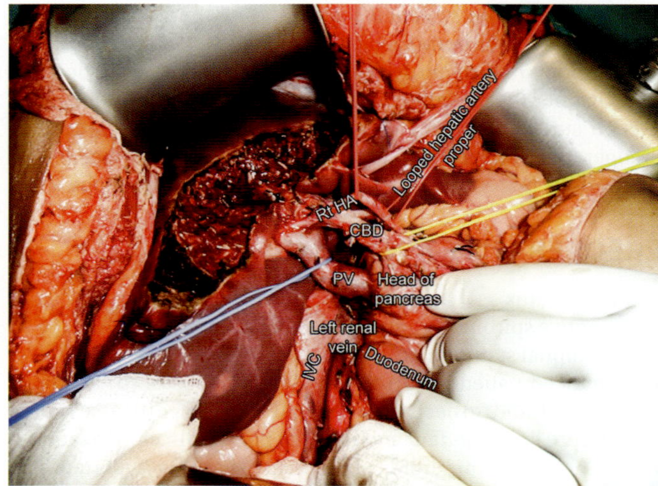

Figure 9 Extended portal lymphadenectomy--en block removal of nodes from hepatic hilum to below including pericholedochal nodes, periportal and retroportal nodes, common hepatic artery and hepatic artery proper nodes till the right of the celiac artery and posterosuperior pancreaticoduodenal node

Reason for non-standardization of extent of lymphadenectomy are firstly the perception of poor survival in node positive patients therefore aggressive lymphadenectomy is not pursued by all and secondly because of differences in practice in east and west.

From the description in previous section we know the lymph flows from gallbladder via first echelon nodes (cystic and pericholedochal nodes) into second echelon nodes (hepatic artery, retroportal and posterosuperior pancreaticoduodenal nodes) and finally into para-aortic nodes (Fig. 10).[86]

In east, specially Japanese surgeons define extent of lymphadenectomy as en bloc removal of nodes from hepatic hilum to below including pericholedochal nodes, periportal and retroportal nodes, common hepatic artery and hepatic artery proper nodes till the right of the celiac artery (also known as posterior hepatic node) and posterosuperior pancreaticoduodenal node which they term as extended portal lymphadenectomy (Fig. 9).[87,88] On the other hand the prevalent practice in west is to do HDL lymphadenectomy and general feeling is that patients with lymph nodes beyond N1 should not undergo resection.[89]

Further confusion is added by difference in staging system. AJCC 7 classification puts retroportal, hepatic artery and retropancreatic nodes as N2 node along with celiac and SMA nodes. Whereas in Japanese classification HA, PV and retropancreatic nodes are 2nd echelon node and nodes beyond these are 3rd echelon nodes, i.e. celiac and SMA nodes are classified separately. En bloc lymphadenectomy of 1st and 2nd echelon lymph nodes as per Shirai et al.[87] seems to be the more rational approach. In an analysis of 152 patients undergoing radical surgery for gallbladder cancer, 130 underwent R0 resection. Out of these 130 patients receiving R0 resection 68 were node negative while 62 were node positive and disease specific survival differed according to nodal status ($p<0.001$). Twenty-two patients with R0 and node positive status had more than 5-year survival, whereas 5-year survival in node positive patients in western series is a rarity. Adequate lymph node yield in GBC should be more than 6 nodes.[90,91] Lymph node

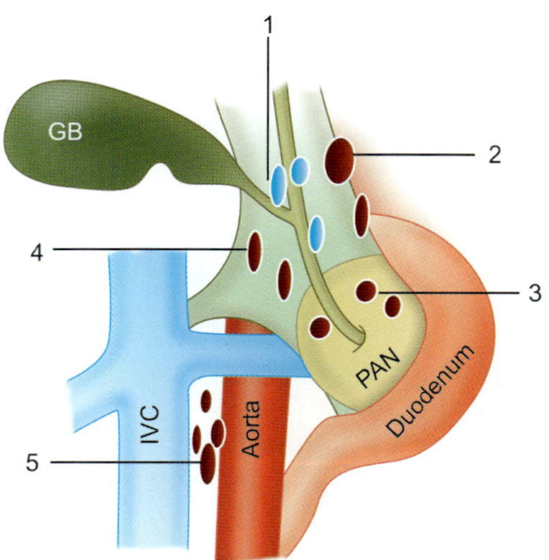

Figure 10 (1) Pericholedochal nodes; (2) hepatic artery nodes; (3) posterosuperiorpancreatico duodenal nodes; (4) retroportal nodes; (5) inter-aortocaval nodes

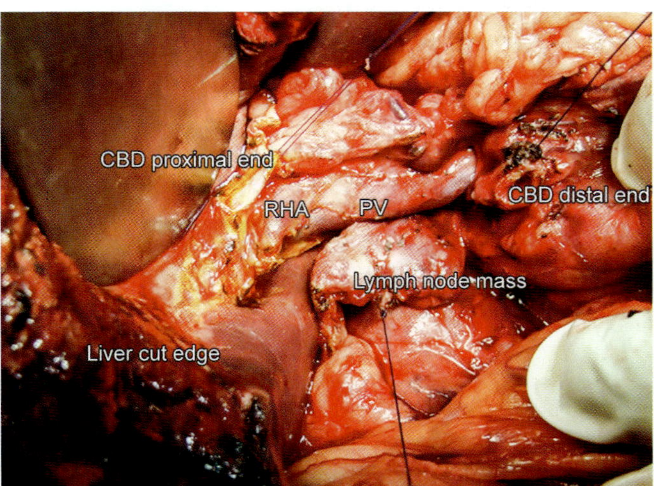

Figure 11 Gallbladder cancer involving CBD; radical cholecystectomy with CBD excision; cut upper and lower end CBD is seen marked with suture. Other suture at hepatoduodenal lymph nodal mass. Hepatoduodenal tissue and lymph nodes being cleared

yield is suboptimal in most western series[90,92] as compared to east where extended portal lymphadenectomy is performed[87] and it is cited as one of the reasons for better survival in node positive patients in Japanese series.

There also exists a difference in opinion *whether to excise CBD* for the sole purpose of facilitating lymphadenectomy. Role of CBD excision to achieve negative margins (Fig. 11) is well accepted, but routine CBD excision with lymphadenectomy is debatable. Shimizu et al. proposed routine CBD excision with radical cholecystectomy. In their analysis of 50 patients 30 had involvement of HDL and 24 of these patients did not have preoperative jaundice. As per their results CBD excision is required to attain R0 resection even in patients without jaundice or apparent CBD involvement.[93] Another reason cited for routine CBD excision is risk of ischemic damage and stricture formation. During aggressive lymphadenectomy 3'o clock and 9'o clock arteries, posterosuperior pancreaticoduodenal artery and small branches of right hepatic artery may be sacrificed leading to ischemic strictures.[94] CBD excision also facilitates lymphadenectomy allowing more complete and thorough lymphadenectomy.[87] To the contrary, some authors do not advocate routine CBD excision as it adds up to morbidity without improving survival or increasing lymph node yield.[95,96] This controversy is still far from over. Prevalent practice in India is to perform CBD excision only in cases of cystic margin positivity or frank infiltration in jaundiced patients. Role of pancreatic resection for lymphadenectomy and tumor clearance is discussed later in the chapter.

Extent of Hepatic Resection

Some form of liver resection is must for tumors T1b and beyond. Unlike lymphadenectomy where aggressiveness is the call of the day, moderation is the order in extent of liver resection. The goal of liver resection is to achieve R0 status and more extended resections are not warranted otherwise.[96] Tumors which are limited to gallbladder wall or with minimal liver infiltration a wedge resection of liver (Fig. 12) with a tumor free margin of 1-2 cm are adequate. A formal bisegmentectomy (seg IVb & V) (Figs 13A to D) may be required for tumors with greater liver infiltration where a wedge resection may compromise the margin status. Formal bisegmentectomy also offers a benefit of decreased blood loss and bile leak. More extended resections like an extended right hepatectomy (Figs 14A to D) may be required in instances where limited resection is not likely to provide an R0 resection. Situations like extensive liver infiltration, involvement of portal pedicle and CAGB with jaundice due to bile duct infiltration may require extensive liver resection to attain an R0 status and must be pursued in fit patients with localized disease.

Management of Locally Advanced Tumors

Locally advanced tumors are those which have gone beyond the confines of gallbladder wall, infiltrating into liver and/or

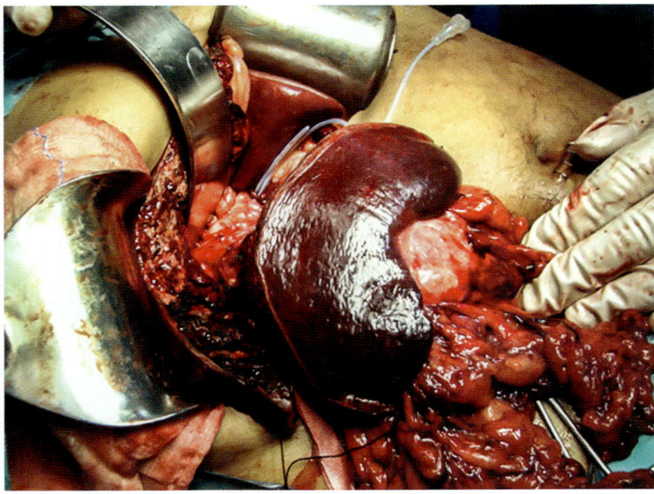

Figure 12 Liver wedge with GB and adherent omentum

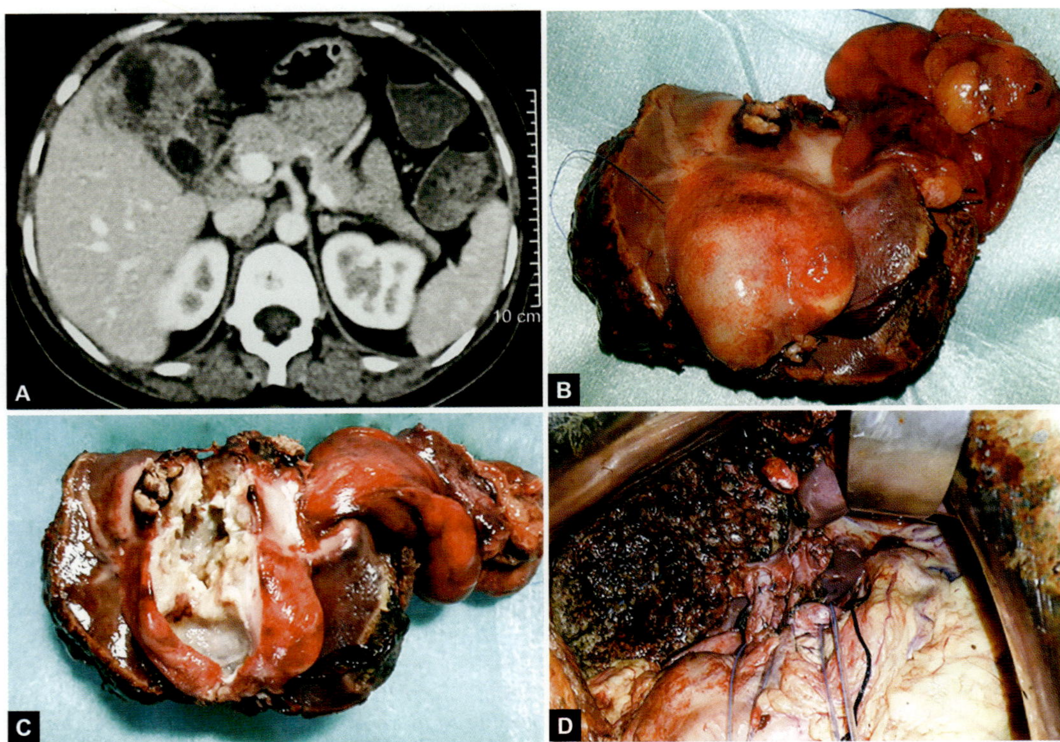

Figures 13A to D Gallbladder cancer with bisegmentectomy: (A) CT scan showing mass involving fundus of gallbladder; (B) Segment 4b, 5 resection; (C) Opened up gallbladder showing tumor in body and fundus. Cystic duct is clear (tied); (D) Lymphadenectomy in progress

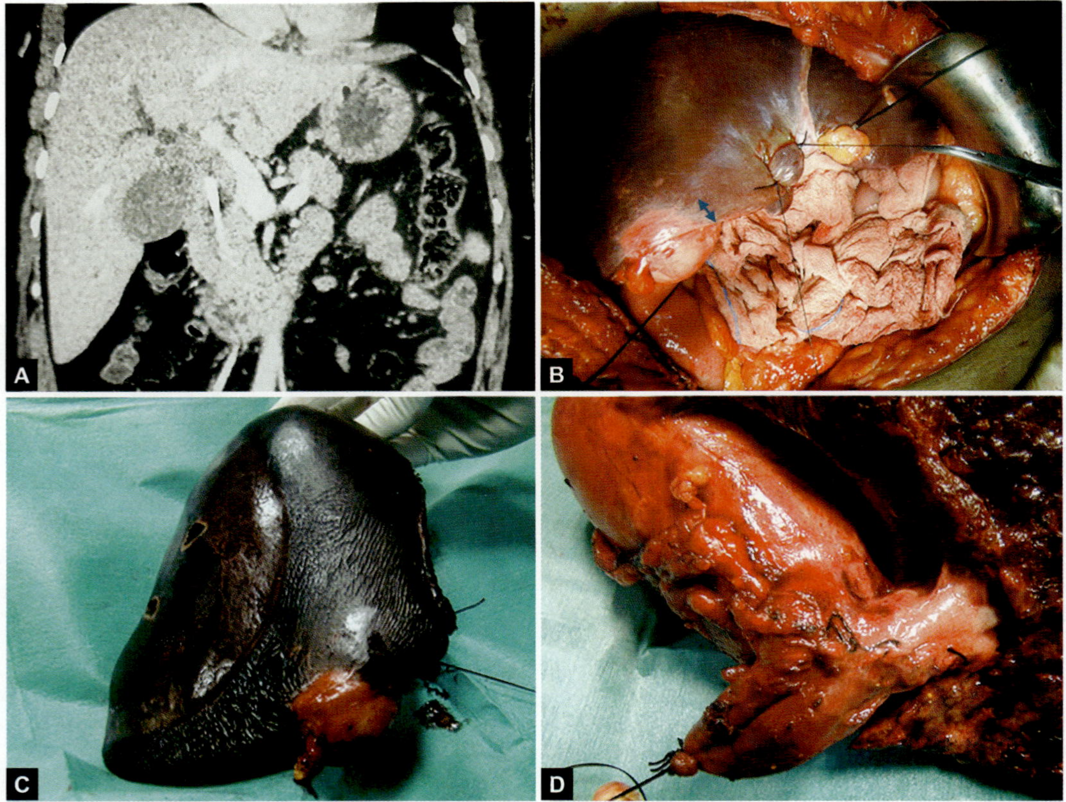

Figures 14A to D Right trisegmentectomy: (A) CT showing tumor involvement of CBD with stent *in situ*; (B) Right PV and hepatic artery tied in preparation for resection. Arrow shows demarcation line; (C) Resected liver with gallbladder. Two sites of frozen biopsy are seen; (D) Resected CBD and gallbladder

extrahepatic structures like colon, duodenum, extrahepatic bile duct, portal vein and hepatic artery. On the basis of liver infiltration these tumors have been divided as liver bed type—which has predominant involvement of liver away from porta hepatis, and hepatic hilum type which spread toward the hilum involving hilar structures early.[97,98] R0 resection can be achieved with segment IVb, V resection for liver bed type tumors whereas hepatic hilum type tumors invariably requires major hepatic resections like extended right hepatectomy to obtain clear margins.[99] Miyazaki further classified advanced GBC on the basis of involvement of liver and adjoining structures into four subtypes:[100]

Type I	Hepatic invasion ± gastrointestinal invasion
Type II	Bile duct invasion ± gastrointestinal invasion
Type III	Hepatic and bile duct invasion ± gastrointestinal invasion
Type IV	Gastrointestinal invasion without hepatic or bile duct invasion

In this series Type I tumors had highest resectability rates with better 5-year survival which reached statistical significance. Authors proposed that Type I tumors should be pursued aggressively for radical surgery as it yields most favorable outcome.[100] At most centers surgery in not very aggressively pursued for T4 tumors as patients rarely achieve long-term survival even after radical surgery. More recently, this popular belief has been challenged especially by Japanese centers claiming good 5-year survival rates in even stage IV tumors. Kondo et al. reported their experience of 72 patients with stage IV disease who underwent surgery with curative intent. Eleven of these patients had survived for more than 3 years. But this aggressive approach was associated with 19% postoperative mortality and significant morbidity.[101,102] Similarly Nishio et al. reported 12% 5-year survival among 166 stage IV patients undergoing surgery with a hospital mortality of 14%.[103] Even though some meaningful survival can be achieved in stage IV cancers, it comes with a cost of high mortality and morbidity. This means that a very good patient selection is required so that the surgery could be offered to those who are likely to be benefitted most by it. There have been attempts to identify predictors of survival in stage IV patients. Presence of vascular invasion and need for portal vein resection, presence of liver metastasis, extended right hepatectomy in cholestatic liver and involvement of non-regional lymph nodes have all been associated with increased postoperative mortality and morbidity and poor survival even after surgery. Specific issues like surgery in GBC with jaundice, role of vascular resection and HPD will be discussed in detail.

Role of Hepatopancreatoduodenectomy

Combining hepatectomy with pancreaticoduodenectomy is termed as HPD (Fig. 15). One of the most formidable procedures done for carcinoma gallbladder, it was initially described by Takasaki. Since then many centers have reported their experience of this high risk and potentially morbid procedure with yet unclear benefits.

Indications of HPD in context of gallbladder cancer are: (1) direct infiltration of duodenum and pancreas with tumor; (2) extensive peripancreatic lymphnodes which cannot be cleared without PD; (3) diffuse biliary involvement; (4) last and

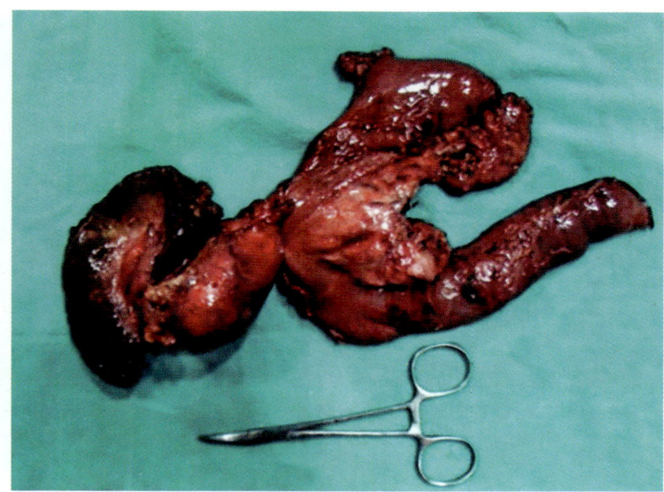

Figure 15 Hepatopancreatoduodenectomy specimen

the most controversial one is to allow complete retropancreatic lymphadenectomy. HPD for the last indication is practiced in some centers across Japan and has not shown any clear survival benefits. Direct infiltration of duodenum and pancreas does not always merits HPD as R0 resection is achieved in cases with limited involvement of duodenum and pancreas by performing duodenal sleeve (Figs. 16A to C) and pancreatic wedge resections. An HPD can be avoided in these instances as a limited resection achieving an R0 resection not only decreases the complication rates but also does it without any increase in the recurrence rates.

HPD is associated with high morbidity and mortality. Various centers have reported morbidity rates from 60% to 71% and mortality rates from 6.3% to 30%, most of which are attributable to liver failure and pancreatic fistula.[104-108] Pancreatic fistula rates are higher in HPD as pancreas is almost always soft with non-dilated pancreatic duct. Associated hepatectomy leads to a large dead space allowing pancreatic secretion to stagnate. This allows more contact of pancreatic secretions with surrounding tissue leading to higher incidence of complications. Liver failure rates also increase as a "vicious cycle" of liver failure-infection-liver failure sets in which is propagated by underlying pancreatic anastomotic leaks. Various modifications have been tried to decrease the complication rates. Preoperative PVE, preoperative biliary drainage and control of infection, limiting the extent of hepatectomy, external drainage of pancreatic duct and two stage pancreaticojejunostomy have shown to decrease the complication rates.[109,110]

Survival benefits of HPD are still not very clear. Though some researchers have shown survival advantage with many 5-year survivors, others did not find any benefit at all. Reasons for such varied results are: (1) difference in the indication of HPD; (2) R0 resection rates. R0 resection rates vary from as low as 20% to 58% resulting in difference in survival. Similarly HPD done for direct tumor infiltration of duodenum or pancreas yield better results when compared to HPD done for extensive retropancreatic lymph nodal involvement. Despite advances in surgical techniques and perioperative care, HPD still carries a high morbidity and mortality and thus should be used with great caution only in select group of patient.

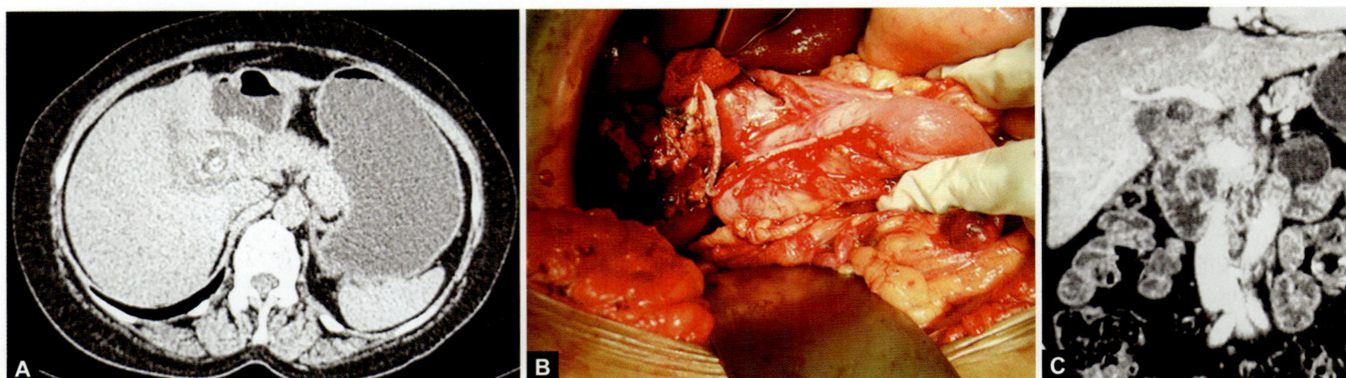

Figures 16A to C GBC with duodenal involvement. (A) CECT arterial phase axial section showing obliteration of plane between GBC and duodenum. (B) At operation, stomach and duodenum separated with sleeve resection. (C) Same thing seen in coronal section in portal phase.

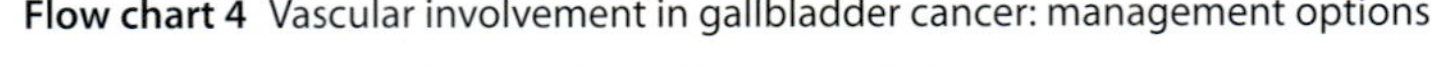

Flow chart 4 Vascular involvement in gallbladder cancer: management options

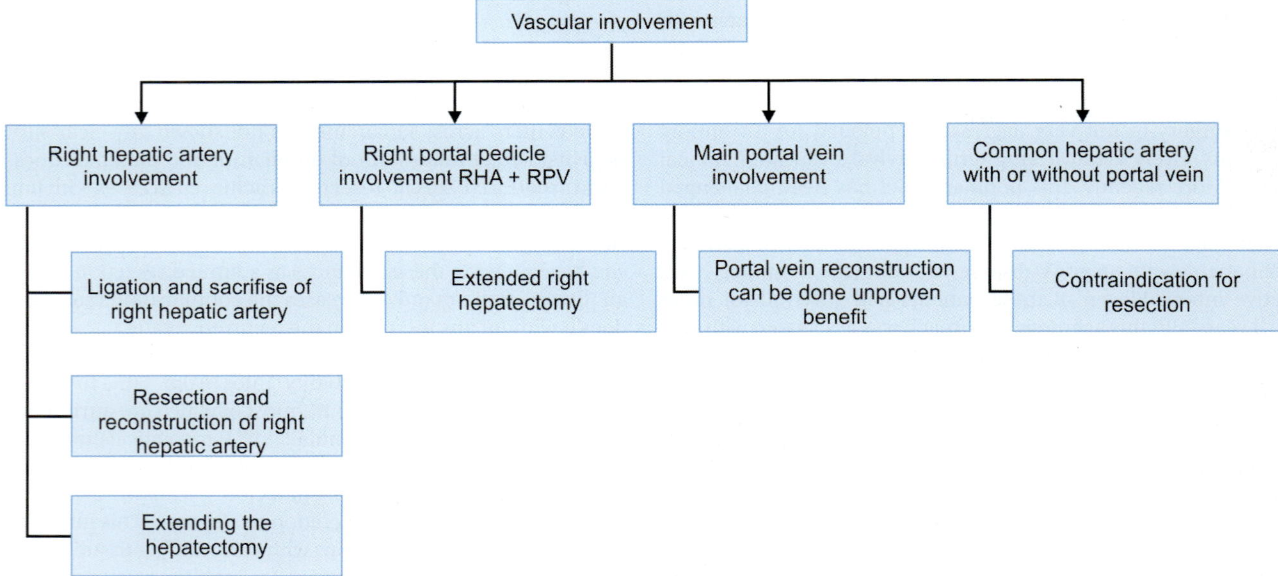

Role of Vascular Resection in Locally Advanced GBC

Due to the location of gallbladder, vascular involvement, especially right portal pedicle involvement is not infrequent. Some advanced tumors also involve the main portal vein and common hepatic artery. But unlike hilar cholangiocarcinomas where vascular reconstruction is well established, its role in gallbladder cancer is still controversial. Vascular involvement in GBC can be classified as above (Flow chart 4) and management can be tailored accordingly.

Involvement of the right hepatic artery can be managed with excision and reconstruction of the vessel or simply ligation and sacrificing the right hepatic artery provided the right portal vein is patent with normal flow.[111] One should be careful in cholestatic liver with high jaundice while exercising the ligation alone as an option. Whereas the involvement of right portal pedicle means an extended resection in the form of either right trisegmentectomy or segment IVA sparing trisegmentectomy is required. Treatment of tumors with involvement of *main portal vein* is controversial. Proponents of aggressive surgery advocate resection and reconstruction of portal vein provided an R0 status can be achieved.[112,113] But presence of portal vein involvement is a poor prognostic factor and portal vein reconstruction is an independent risk factor for in hospital mortality.[110] Chijiiwa et al. reported that survival of patients with portal vein and hepatic artery invasion that underwent resection was similar to the patients who did not undergo surgery.[114] Simultaneous involvement of portal vein and hepatic artery is considered as contraindication for surgery by most groups.[115] Vascular resection for main portal vein and common hepatic artery cannot be advocated routinely for advanced gallbladder cancer and should be used with caution.

GALLBLADDER CANCER WITH JAUNDICE

Patients with jaundice and gallbladder cancer present a unique and difficult problem. Jaundice in patients due to bile duct infiltration indicates a pT3/4 disease (AJCC VIIth edition). It has been one of the banes of patients of gallbladder cancer. It is seen in 25–50% patients of GBC. MRI-MRCP is required besides CECT, for assessment of the site of block and for planning of resection. These patients also require assessment of future liver remnant and additional measures to enhance the same. PTBD is required to decrease the jaundice in these patients. Usually left lobe is drained. In case of jaundice not coming down or cholangitis due to obstructed right lobe additional drains may be required. In case the future liver remnant is small, portal vein embolization may also be required. Liver functions are required to be optimized before any resection is contemplated.

Most of these patients are unresectable with advanced disease at presentation. In others, by the time they come up for resection, either their disease has advanced or the condition has deteriorated. At surgery, they require extended resections but the prognosis remains dismal in most series.

First large series specifically addressing the problem of jaundice in patients of GBC was from Memorial Sloan Kettering.[116] Out of 240 patients of GBC 82 (34%) had jaundice. While there was no difference in explorations of patients with or without jaundice (67% vs 66%) resectability in jaundiced patients was 7% compared to 41% without jaundice. Among 6 resected patients, none survived 2 years compared to 21% in the non-jaundiced group. Median survival of jaundiced patients with GBC was only 6 months. They concluded that routine exploration of jaundiced patients in GBC is not warranted.

Regimbeau et al.[117] reporting for the French study group investigated prognostic value of jaundice in their 110/429 cases of GBC. They reported that 1 and 3 year survival for resected and non-resected jaundiced patients with GBC was 48% and 19% and 31% and 0% respectively. They concluded that R0 resection did not increase the overall survival in all resected patients, but R0 resection increased median survival in the subgroup of N0 patients (20 months vs 6 months, p=0.01). Overall resectability was 45% in their jaundiced patients with GBC. Kaneoka et al.[118] found curative resection to be possible in 30% and 75% of patients with or without jaundice. Patients who had nodal metastasis with bile duct infiltration had only 5.9% 3-year survival. In node negative patients survival was 14.3% and 65.6% in patients with and without bile duct infiltration.

Recently, articles mainly from Japan, have suggested that aggressive resection can lead to long-term survival.[110,118-120] However, when jaundiced patients with GBC are specifically analyzed survival is limited. Nishio et al.[121] from Nagoya University, Japan, reported on 100 cases of pT3/4 N0/1 M0 disease. Five-year and median survival for pathologically involved and uninvolved CBD was 23% and 54% and 1.5 years and 15.4 years respectively. Their mortality was 11% and 28 patients underwent portal vein resection. When combined with resection of adjacent organ (pancreas, colon and stomach) 5-year survival was 16% but median survival was only 0.8 years. Importantly, 12 patients survived more than 5 years, 6 of whom had lymph node involvement as well. They concluded that although challenging, R0 resection should be done in these patients especially when it did not entail adjacent organ resection. In this series cases were analyzed for involvement of CBD and not for jaundice. Shimizu et al.[93] have analyzed that all patients with hepatoduodenal infiltration do not have preoperative jaundice. In their series of GBC patients with hepatoduodenal infiltration, only 12% (6/50) cases had preoperative jaundice. All the jaundiced patients had direct extramural spread to CBD associated with worse prognosis. Thus jaundice may represent a higher level of hepatoduodenal ligament involvement than microscopic positivity of CBD in resected specimens.

D'Angelica et al.[96] reported 21% 5-year survival in their gallbladder cancers with clinically involved CBD. Chan et al.[122] from Taiwan reported no difference in survival between jaundiced and non-jaundiced patients of carcinoma gallbladder though results in both groups were equally dismal. They also concluded that beneficial effect of non-curative resection for definitively improving survival was limited. Endo et al.[123] investigated 22 patients of GBC with hepatoduodenal invasion and compared them to 36 patients with no hepatoduodenal invasion. Portal vein reconstruction, hepatic lobectomy and pancreaticoduodenectomy were frequently used to achieve R0 resection. Five-year survival for the hepatoduodenal invasion positive and negative patients was 10.6% and 46.6% respectively. However, their study was also based on pathological hepatoduodenal invasion and not on clinical jaundice.

We analyzed our 270 cases of admitted gallbladder (2003–2011) cancer recently. Out of these, 117 (43%) had jaundice. Spurred by the Japanese articles aggressive strategy for resection, whenever possible, has been followed by us in view of the poor results with chemotherapy in patients of GBC. Out of 117, six patients who had bile duct stone as cause of jaundice were excluded. The mean age was 49.4 years (range 25–76 years). There were 76 (68%) females. Of these 111 patients evaluated, 51 patients (46%) had metastatic disease. Preoperative workup after admission revealed distant metastasis in 7 patients while in rest 44 metastatic disease was diagnosed at operation. Among 60 patients with locally advanced disease, 25 patients were considered unresectable/inoperable when reassessed after preoperative biliary drainage. Either their disease had progressed (unresectable n=6) or their general condition had deteriorated (inoperable n=19) to preclude surgical intervention in these patients. Of the remaining 35 patients, 17 underwent curative resection while rest had palliative treatment.

Five patients had right trisegmentectomy while others had radical cholecystectomy with or without CBD resection. R0 resection was achieved in all our patients. There were two postoperative deaths. The cause of death was respiratory complication and liver failure in one each. The overall morbidity was 41% and mean hospital stay was 12.2 days (range 6–30 days). Among 5 patients with trisegmentectomy, 2 patients died (ARDS n=1, postoperative liver failure n=1) while another 2 had prolonged hospital stay due to grade B liver failure. The long-term survival of these 3 survivors was of 8, 12 and 14 months. Duration of jaundice (>2 months), bilirubin level more than 15 mg% and duodenal infiltration had negative impact on resectability.

The mean survival of patients that underwent curative resection was 14 months while median survival was 12 months. Only 2 patients are surviving for more than 3 years.

In unresectable locally advanced group, the median survival was 6 months. In the metastatic group follow-up was available for 28 patients. The median survival was only 4 months. Only 1 patient survived for 20 months.

Our results show that GBC patients with jaundice have advanced and usually, unresectable disease. Some of these patients may possibly benefit from an oncological en mass liver, portal vein and

CBD resections with pancreaticoduodenectomy. However, most patients are adjudged unfit for such massive undertaking. This may be especially so, when a multi-visceral resection is required due to involvement of duodenum or colon. When survival of only 2 patients for more than 3 years is seen in light of postoperative mortality of 2 patients, perspective becomes even starker. This is in line with conclusion drawn by other authors.[116,117,124] Median survivals of our resected patients was only 12 months. Survival was not different in our patients with or without lymph node involvement. Since the number of patients finally resected is small, meaningful subgroup analysis was not possible.

In view of this, a pragmatic approach needs to be evolved. Technical feasibility of extended resections including portal vein resection has been shown by some Japanese studies. It seems apparent that better survival and cure are seen in only resected group of patients. On the basis of our experience and analysis of literature we conclude that jaundice is a poor prognostic factor in patients of GBC. While R0 resection should be tried in GBC patients with jaundice, resectability is low for patients of GBC with jaundice. Although, few long-term survivals have been achieved with aggressive resections their overall survival remains dismal. Patients of GBC with high jaundice, requiring multiorgan visceral resection or having node positive disease should be carefully weighed before any extensive surgery.

ROLE OF CHEMOTHERAPY AND RADIOTHERAPY IN GALLBLADDER CANCER

Though surgery is the sole modality which offers long-term survival in gallbladder cancer, even after optimal surgery recurrence rates are high. A significant proportion of patients are beyond realms of surgery and many more present as metastatic disease (Figs 17 and 18), making role of chemotherapy and radiotherapy very significant. Chemotherapy and radiotherapy can be used in three settings: (1) palliative, (2) adjuvant and (3) neoadjuvant

Palliative Therapy

5-FU was the initial chemotherapeutic agent of choice but it failed to show any benefit. 5-FU was as good as best supportive care for unresectable gallbladder cancer.[125] Focus was then shifted to gemcitabine, but as a single agent it also failed to show any significant results. Combination of gemcitabine with platinum based drugs (cisplatin and oxaliplatin) brought about some meaningful results. ABC-2 trial published in 2010 enrolled 410 patients of which 149 were cancer gallbladder patients. Patients treated with combination of gemcitabine and cisplatin showed overall survival of 3.6 months more than those treated with gemcitabine alone. No difference was noted between the responses for GBC versus cholangiocarcinoma.[126] Another RCT of 81 patients was reported from AIIMS, New Delhi, comparing gemcitabine and oxaliplatin combination to 5-FU alone or best supportive care. There was a median OS of 9.5, 4.6 and 4.5 months and a response rate of 30.7%, 14.3% and 0% respectively.[125] Gemcitabine + oxaliplatin have a similar response rate to Gemcitabine + cisplatin with less toxicity.[127] Radiotherapy does not have much role in this setting.

Adjuvant Therapy

5-FU failed to show any impact on survival as a single agent in adjuvant therapy. Since gemcitabine and oxaliplatin has shown positive response in unresectable patients its role as adjuvant therapy was investigated but there is no conclusive evidence to support its use as an adjunct to surgery.[128,129] There is conflicting data for the use of radiation as an adjuvant therapy as one study showed a survival benefit for node positive and T2 or greater disease whereas the other showed no response what so ever.[130,131] Role of adjuvant chemoradiation is more keenly studied. Wang et al. in a retrospective analysis compared 126 patients receiving adjuvant chemotherapy to a matched group of 126 patients receiving adjuvant chemoradiation. They observed a benefit in chemoradiation arm, but this study has been criticized for its retrospective nature, poor quality of surgery (low R0 resection rates, incomplete lymphadenectomy) and very low overall survival of 11 months which is well below historic control.[132] Mayo experience of adjuvant therapy was published in 2009, of 73 patients of gallbladder cancer undergoing resection 25 received chemoradiotherapy (50.4 CGy radiation + 5-FU based chemotherapy), and showed a survival advantage in patients

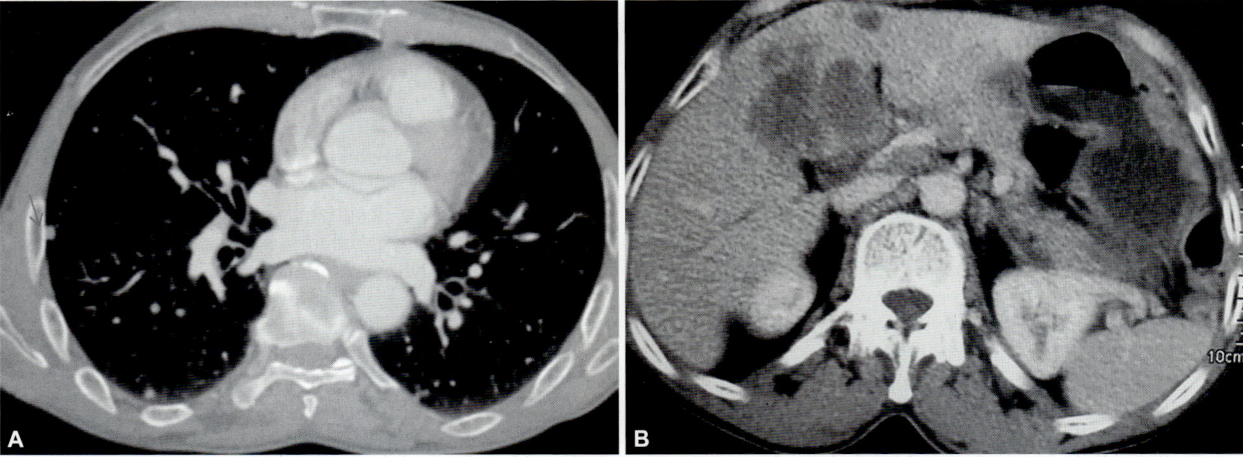

Figures 17A and B CECT showing multiple pulmonary and liver metastasis

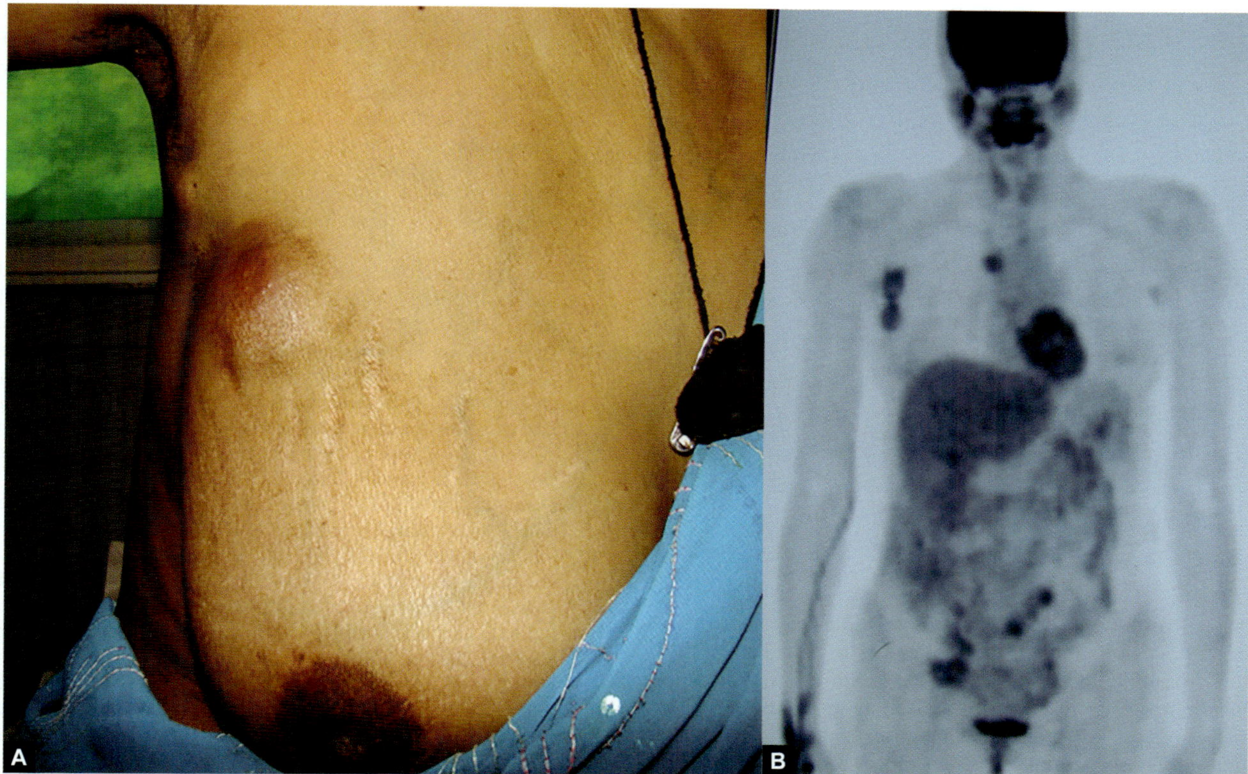

Figures 18A and B Patient of laparoscopic cholecystectomy with gallbladder cancer with port site metastasis. Patient developed intraperitoneal, axillary and mediastinal lymph node metastasis: (A) Axillary metastasis; (B) PET scan of same lady showing metastatic sites

receiving adjuvant treatment. Adequacy and radicality of surgery was questioned for this series as well.[133] To the contrary a study from Korea by Kim et al. which included 166 patients of GBC did not find any benefit of adding adjuvant therapy to an adequately performed surgery irrespective of T & N staging of tumor.[134]

It is apparent that in case of less than optimal surgery (incomplete lymphadenectomy or positive or close margins) adjuvant chemoradiation may provide survival advantage but its role after an oncologically appropriate resection is still not clear.

Neoadjuvant Treatment

Most of the patients by the time they seek medical advice have tumors grown beyond the scope of surgery. Apparent response seen in gallbladder cancer in palliative setting has prompted researchers to investigate role of neoadjuvant treatment. The first evidence of benefit was provided by a report from Tata Memorial Hospital, Mumbai, where they reported an excellent response of neoadjuvant chemoradiation (gemcitabine + 57 Gy radiation) in 3 patients with adenocarcinoma of gallbladder. Two patients showed complete metabolic and radiologic response and 1 patient showed complete pathological response on evaluation of resected specimen.[135] Similarly Kato et al. reported a retrospective series of 22 cases of locally advanced biliary tract cancers including both gallbladder cancer and cholangiocarcinomas. These patients received weekly gemcitabine therapy for 3 weeks followed by 1 week gap and surgery. Of 22 patients, 8 achieved significant response and were resected (36.4%) of which 4 had R0 resections.[136] These initial results are promising, suggesting some role of neoadjuvant chemotherapy or chemoradiation for locally advanced tumors in good risk patients but more studies with large number of patients are required before we can draw any conclusion.

Palliative Therapy for Gallbladder Cancer

Palliative treatment assumes as important a role as curative treatment for GBC. Most of the patients' present late thus curative treatment cannot be offered, and are symptomatic with pain, jaundice or bowel obstruction (colonic or duodenal) requiring some form of palliation.

Most important symptom requiring palliation is pain which should be treated adequately with opioid or non-opioid analgesics to provide acceptable quality of life.

Jaundice is seen in 30–50% of cases as presenting symptom and many more may present with jaundice as the disease progresses. Jaundice requires palliation when leading to intractable pruritis or cholangitis and also prior to administering chemotherapy. Surgical palliation of jaundice is almost never recommended, endoscopic (Fig. 19) and percutaneous approaches can both be utilized as per the availability of technical expertise and anatomy of biliary block. Saluja et al. in an RCT reported that percutaneous approach is more successful in providing drainage (89% vs 41%; $p<0.001$) and also offers better palliation in hilar blocks as compared to endoscopic approach.[137] However, self-expanding metal stent (SEMS) was not used in the endoscopic approach in this study.

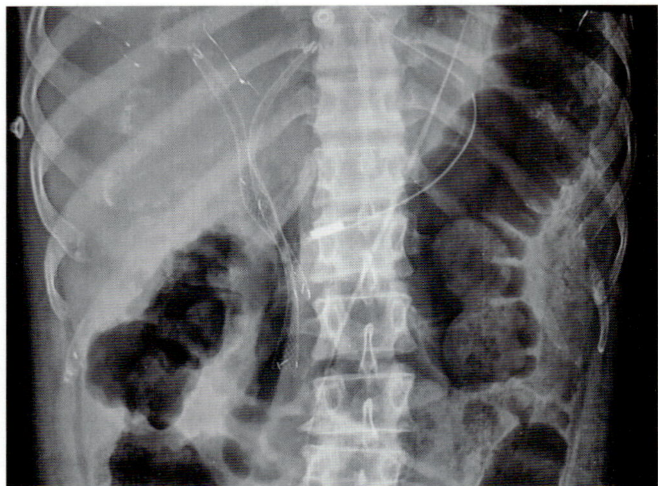

Figure 19 Bilateral self expanding metal stent for palliation of gallbladder cancer

Bowel obstruction (duodenum and colon) can be seen in advanced stages of gallbladder cancer due to proximity of these structures to gallbladder resulting in direct infiltration. Endoscopic stenting may relieve duodenal obstruction in selected patients but many may require surgical palliation especially in colonic obstruction. These patients have very poor outcome with high mortality and morbidity post-surgery.

Coeliac Plexus Block for Pain

Pain is the most important symptom requiring palliation in gallbladder cancer. Systemic analgesic therapy is the first line of treatment but many patients do not get optimal relief with it. Just like gallbladder cancer, unresectable pancreatic cancer also present with pain and celiac plexus neurolysis has been studied in the setting of pancreatic cancers in various retrospective studies and few RCTs demonstrating better pain relief with similar or decreased opiod requirement.[138] Unfortunately no such data exist for gallbladder cancer. There is no report in literature regarding the use of percutaneous or EUS guided celiac plexus neurolysis in gallbladder cancer. As the visceral pain originating from gallbladder and liver also travels cephalad via celiac plexus, CPN holds promise in this setting as well but studies need to be conducted to demonstrate its efficacy. Chemotherapy in palliative setting can be administered to good risk patients. Gemcitabine with cisplatin or oxaliplatin may offer some survival advantage.

REFERENCES

1. Batra Y, Pal S, Dutta U, Desai P, Garg PK, Makharia G, et al. Gallbladder cancer in India: a dismal picture. J Gastroenterol Hepatol. 2005;20:309-14.
2. Wistuba II, Gazdar AF. Gallbladder cancer: lessons from a rare tumour. Nat Rev Cancer. 2004;4:695-706.
3. Randi G, Franceschi S, La Vecchia C. Gallbladder cancer worldwide: geographical distribution and risk factors. Int J Cancer. 2006;118:1591-602.
4. Randi G, Malvezzi M, Levi F, Ferlay J, Negri E, Franceschi S, et al. Epidemiology of biliary tract cancers: an update. Ann Oncol. 2009;20:146-59.
5. De Aretxabala X, Roa I, Araya JC, Burgos L, Flores P, Wistuba I, et al. Gallbladder cancer in patients less than 40 years old. Br J Surg. 1994;81(1):111.
6. Muduly DK, SatyanarayanaDeo SV, Shukla NK, Kallianpur AA, Prakash R, Jayakrishnan T. Gallbladder cancer in a child: a rare occurrence. J Can Res Ther. 2012;8:653-4.
7. Murthy NS, Rajaram D, GauthamMS, Shivraj NS, Pruthvish S, George PS, et al. Trends in incidence of gallbladder cancer—Indian scenario. Gastrointestinal Cancer: Targets and Therapy. 2011;1:1-9.
8. Dutta U, Nagi B, Garg PK, Sinha SK, Singh K, Tandon RK. Patients with gallstones develop gallbladder cancer at an earlier age. Eur J Cancer Prev. 2005;14:381-5.
9. Dutta U, Garg PK, Kumar R, Tandon RK. Typhoid carriers among patients with gallstones are at increased risk for carcinoma of the gallbladder. Am J Gastroenterol. 2000;95:784-7.
10. Lazcano-Ponce EC, Miquel JF, Munoz N, Herrero R, Ferrecio C, Wistuba II, et al. Epidemiology and molecular pathology of gallbladder cancer. CA Cancer J Clin. 2001;51:349-64.
11. Diehl AK. Epidemiology of gallbladder cancer: a synthesis of recent data. J Natl Cancer Inst. 1980;65:1209-14.
12. Rustagi T, Dasanu CA. Risk factors for gallbladder cancer and cholangiocarcinoma: similarities, differences and updates. J Gastrointest Cancer. 2012;43(2):137-47.
13. Lai CH, Lau WY. Gallbladder cancer—a comprehensive review. Surgeon. 2008;6:101-10.
14. Hu B, Gong B, Zhou DY. Association of anomalous pancreaticobiliary ductal junction with gallbladder carcinoma in Chinese patients: an ERCP study. Gastrointest Endosc. 2003;57:541-5.
15. Deng YL, Cheng NS, Lin YX, Zhou RX, Yang C, Jin YW, et al. Relationship between pancreaticobiliary maljunction and gallbladder carcinoma: meta-analysis. Hepatobiliary Pancreat Dis Int. 2011;10(6):570-80.
16. Roa I, Ibacache G, Carvallo J, Melo A, Araya J, De Aretxabala X, et al. Microbiological study of gallbladder bile in a high risk zone for gallbladder cancer. Rev Med Chil.1999;127:1049-55.
17. Misra V, Misra SP, Dwivedi M, Shouche Y, Dharne M, Singh PA. Helicobacter pylori in areas of gastric metaplasia in the gallbladder and isolation of H. pylori DNA from gallstones. Pathology. 2007;39:419-24.
18. Liu B, Beral V, Balkwill A, Million Women SC. Childbearing, breastfeeding, other reproductive factors and the subsequent risk of hospitalization for gallbladder disease. Int J Epidemiol. 2009;38:312-8.
19. Khan ZS, Livingston EH, Huerta S. Reassessing the need for prophylactic surgery in patients with porcelain gallbladder: case series and systematic review of the literature. Arch Surg. 2011;146(10):1143-7.
20. Dutta U, Poornachandra KS. Gallbladder polyps: how to pick up the sinister ones. J Gastroenterol Hepatol. 2009;24:175-8.
21. Misra V, Misra SP, Dwivedi M, Shouche Y, Dharne M, Singh PA. Helicobacter pylori in areas of gastric metaplasia in the gallbladder and isolation of H. pylori DNA from gallstones. Pathology. 2007;39: 419-24.
22. Bertran E, Heise K, Andia ME, Ferreccio C. Gallbladder cancer: incidence and survival in a high-risk area of Chile. Int J Cancer. 2010;127:2446-54.
23. Unisa S, Jagannath P, Dhir V, Khandelwal C, Sarangi L, Roy TK. Population-based study to estimate prevalence and determine risk factors of gallbladder diseases in the rural gangetic basin of North India. HPB (Oxford). 2011;13:117-25.
24. Attili AF, De Santis A, Capri R, Repice AM, Maselli S. The natural history of gallstones: the GREPCO experience. The GREPCO Group. Hepatology.1995;21:655-60.
25. Roa I, de Aretxabala X, Araya JC, Roa J. Preneoplastic lesions in gallbladder cancer. J SurgOncol. 2006;93(8):615-23.

26. Diehl AK. Gallstone size and the risk of gallbladder cancer. JAMA.1983;250:2323-6.
27. Lowenfels AB, Walker AM, Althaus DP, Townsend G, DomellofL. Gallstone growth, size, and risk of gallbladder cancer: an interracial study. Int J Epidemiol 1989;18:50-4.
28. Wistuba II, Gazdar AF. Gallbladder cancer: lessons from a rare tumour. Nat Rev Cancer. 2004;4:695-706.
29. Nuzzo G, Clemente G, Cadeddu F, Ardito F, Ricci R, Vecchio FM. Papillary carcinoma of the gallbladder and anomalous pancreaticobiliary junction. Report of three cases and review of the literature. Hepatogastroenterology. 2005;52:1034-8.
30. Jørgensen T, Jensen KH. Polyps in the gallbladder. A prevalence study. Scand J Gastroenterol. 1990;25:281-6.
31. Lin WR, Lin DY, Tai DI, Hsieh SY, Lin CY, Sheen IS, et al. Prevalence of and risk factors for gallbladder polyps detected by ultrasonography among healthy Chinese: analysis of 34 669 cases. J Gastroenterol Hepatol. 2008;23:965-9.
32. Morera-Ocón FJ, Ballestín-Vicente J, Calatayud-Blas AM, de Tursi-RispoliLC, Bernal-Sprekelsen JC. Surgical indications in gallbladder polyps. Cir Esp. 2013;91(5):324-30.
33. Bang S. Natural course and treatment strategy of gallbladder polyp. Korean J Gastroenterol. 2009;53(6):336-40.
34. Sarkut P, Kilicturgay S, Ozer A, Ozturk E, Yilmazlar T. Gallbladder polyps: factors affecting surgical decision. World J Gastroenterol. 2013;19(28):4526-30.
35. Albores-Saavedra J, Henson D. Tumors of the gallbladder and extrahepatic bile ducts. Atlas of Tumor Pathology, Series II, Fascicle, 22 edition. Bethesda, MD: Armed Forces Institute of Pathology; 1986. pp. 28-123.
36. Sumiyoshi K, Nagai E, Chijiiwa K, Nakayama F. Pathology of carcinoma of the gallbladder. World J Surg. 1991;15:315-21.
37. Henson DE, Albores-Saavedra J, Corle D. Carcinoma of the gallbladder: histologic types, stage of disease, grade, and survival rates. Cancer. 1992;70:1493-7.
38. Hawkins WG, DeMatteo RP, Jarnagin WR, Ben-PoratL, Blumgart LH, Fong Y. Jaundice predicts advanced disease and early mortality in patients with gallbladder cancer. Ann Surg Oncol. 2004;11(3): 310-5.
39. Dwivedi M, Misra SP, Misra V. Clinical and ultrasonographic findings of carcinoma of gallbladder in Indian patients. J Assoc Physicians India. 2000;48(2):192-5.
40. Agarwal AK, Mandal S, Singh S, Bhojwani R, Sakhuja P, Uppal R. Biliary obstruction in gallbladder cancer is not sine qua non of inoperability. Ann Surg Oncol. 2007;14(10):2831-7.
41. Grobmyer SR, Lieberman MD, Daly JM. Gallbladder cancer in the twentieth century: single institution's experience. World J Surg. 2004;28(1):47-9.
42. Tsuchiya Y. Early carcinoma of the gallbladder: macroscopic features and US findings. Radiology. 1991;179:171-5.
43. Jang JY, Kim SW, Lee SE, Hwang DW, Kim EJ, Lee JY, et al. Differential diagnostic and staging accuracies of high resolution ultrasonography, endoscopic ultrasonography, and multidetector computed tomography for gallbladder polypoid lesions and gallbladder cancer. Ann Surg. 2009;250(6):943-9.
44. Franquet T, Montes M, Ruiz de Azua Y, Jimenez FJ, Cozcolluela R. Primary gallbladder carcinoma: imaging findings in 50 patients with pathologic correlation. Gastrointest Radiol. 1991;16:143-8.
45. Yun EJ, Cho SG, Park S, Park SW, Kim WH, Kim HJ, et al. Gallbladder cancer and chronic cholecystitis: differentiation with two phase spiral CT. Abdom Imaging. 2004;29:102-8.
46. Furlan A, Ferris JV, Hosseinzadeh K, Borhani AA. Gallbladder carcinoma update: multimodality imaging evaluation, staging, and treatment options. AJR Am J Roentgenol. 2008;191(5):1440-7.
47. Kim SJ, Lee JM, Lee JY, Kim SH, Han JK, Choi BI, et al. Analysis of enhancement pattern of flat gallbladder wall thickening on MDCT to differentiate gallbladder cancer from cholecystitis. AJR Am J Roentgenol. 2008;191(3):765-71.
48. Kim SJ, Lee JM, Lee JY, Choi JY, Kim SH, Han JK, et al. Accuracy of preoperative T-staging of gallbladder carcinoma using MDCT. AJR Am J Roentgenol. 2008;190(1):74-80.
49. Kalra N, Suri S, Gupta R, Natarajan SK, Khandelwal N, Wig JD, et al. MDCT in the staging of gallbladder carcinoma. AJR Am J Roentgenol. 2006;186(3):758-62.
50. Ohtani T, Shirai Y, Tsukada K, Muto T, Hatakeyama K. Spread of gallbladder carcinoma: CT evaluation with pathologic correlation. Abdom Imaging. 1996;21:195-201.
51. Levy AD, Murakata LA, Rohrmann CA. Gallbladder carcinoma: radiologic-pathologic correlation. Radio Graphics. 2001;21: 295-314.
52. Schwartz LH, Black J, Fong Y, Jarnagin W, Blumgart L, Gruen D, et al. Gallbladder carcinoma: findings at MR imaging with MR cholangiopancreatography. J Comput Assist Tomogr. 2002;26(3): 405-10.
53. Rao ND, Gulati MS, Paul SB, Pande GK, Sahni P, Chattopadhyay TK. Three-dimensional helical computed tomography cholangiography with minimum intensity projection in gallbladder carcinoma patients with obstructive jaundice: comparison with magnetic resonance cholangiography and percutaneous transhepatic cholangiography. J Gastroenterol Hepatol. 2005;20(2):304-8.
54. Ogawa T, Horaguchi J, Fujita N, Noda Y, Kobayashi G, Ito K, et al. High b-value diffusion-weighted magnetic resonance imaging for gallbladder lesions: differentiation between benignity and malignancy. J Gastroenterol. 2012;47(12):1352-60.
55. Petrowsky H, Wildbrett P, Husarik DB, Hany TF, Tam S, Jochum W, et al. Impact of integrated positron emission tomography and computed tomography on staging and management of gallbladder cancer and cholangiocarcinoma. J Hepatol. 2006;45(1):43-50.
56. Corvera CU, Blumgart LH, Akhurst T, DeMatteo RP, D'Angelica M, Fong Y, et al. 18F-fluorodeoxyglucose positron emission tomography influences management decisions in patients with biliary cancer. J Am Coll Surg. 2008;206(1):57-65.
57. Lee SW, Kim HJ, Park JH, Park DI, Cho YK, Sohn CI, et al. Clinical usefulness of 18F-FDG PET-CT for patients with gallbladder cancer and cholangiocarcinoma. J Gastroenterol. 2010;45(5):560-6.
58. Shukla PJ, Barreto SG, Arya S, Shrikhande SV, Hawaldar R, Purandare N, et al. Does PET-CT scan have a role prior to radical re-resection for incidental gallbladder cancer? HPB (Oxford). 2008;10(6):439-45.
59. Oe A, Kawabe J, Torii K, Kawamura E, Higashiyama S, Kotani J, et al. Distinguishing benign from malignant gallbladder wall thickening using FDG-PET. Ann Nucl Med. 2006;20(10):699-703.
60. Nishiyama Y, Yamamoto Y, Fukunaga K, Kimura N, Miki A, Sasakawa Y, et al. Dual-time-point 18F-FDG PET for the evaluation of gallbladder carcinoma. J Nucl Med. 2006;47(4):633-8.
61. Kim HJ, Lee SK, Jang JW, Kim TG, Ryu CH, Park do H, et al. Diagnostic role of endoscopic ultrasonography-guided fine needle aspiration of gallbladder lesions. Hepatogastroenterology. 2012;59(118):1691-5.
62. Kim HJ, Park JH, Park DI, Cho YK, Sohn CI, Jeon WK, et al. Clinical usefulness of endoscopic ultrasonography in the differential diagnosis of gallbladder wall thickening. Dig Dis Sci. 2012;57(2):508-15.
63. Nevin JE, Moran TJ, Kay S, King R. Carcinoma of the gallbladder: staging, treatment, and prognosis. Cancer. 1976;37(1):141-8.
64. Donohue JH, Nagorney DM, Grant CS, Tsushima K, Ilstrup DM, Adson MA. Carcinoma of the gallbladder. Does radical resection improve outcome? Arch Surg. 1990;125(2):237-41.
65. Edge SB, American Joint Committee on Cancer, American Cancer Society. AJCC Cancer Staging Handbook: From the AJCC Cancer Staging Manual, 7th edition. New York: Springer; 2010.

66. Oh TG, Chung MJ, Bang S, Park SW, Chung JB, Song SY, et al. Comparison of the sixth and seventh editions of the AJCC TNM classification for gallbladder cancer. J Gastrointest Surg. 2013;17(5): 925-30.
67. Kwon AH, Imamura A, Kitade H, Kamiyama Y. Unsuspected gallbladder cancer diagnosed during or after laparoscopic cholecystectomy. J Surg Oncol. 2008;97(3):241-5.
68. Darmas B, Mahmud S, Abbas A, Baker AL. Is there any justification for the routine histological examination of straightforward cholecystectomy specimens? Ann R Coll Surg Engl. 2007;89(3):238-41.
69. Yamaguchi K, Tsuneyoshi M. Subclinical gallbladder carcinoma. Am J Surg. 1992;163(4):382-6.
70. Shirai Y, Yoshida K, Tsukada K, Muto T, Watanabe H. Early carcinoma of the gallbladder. Eur J Surg. 1992;158(10):545-8.
71. Pawlik TM, Gleisner AL, Vigano L, Kooby DA, Bauer TW, Frilling A, et al. Incidence of finding residual disease for incidental gallbladder carcinoma: implications for re-resection. J Gastrointest Surg. 2007;11(11):1478-86.
72. Ouchi K, Mikuni J, Kakugawa Y, Organizing Committee, The 30th Annual Congress of the Japanese Society of Biliary Surgery. Laparoscopic cholecystectomy for gallbladder carcinoma: results of a Japanese survey of 498 patients. J Hepatobiliary Pancreat Surg. 2002;9(2):256-60.
73. Dong Do You, Hyung Geun Lee, Kwang Yeol Paik, Jin Seok Heo, Seong Ho Choi, Dong Wook Choi. What is an adequate extent of resection for T1 gallbladder cancers? Ann Surg. 2008;247:835-8.
74. Goetze TO, Paolucci V. Immediate re-resection of T1 incidental gallbladder carcinomas: a survival analysis of the German Registry. Surg Endosc. 2008;22:2462-5.
75. Ouchi K, Owada Y, Matsuno S, Sato T. Prognostic factors in the surgical treatment of gallbladder carcinoma. Surgery. 1987; 101(6):731-7.
76. Abramson MA, Pandharipande P, Ruan D, Gold JS, Whang EE. Radical resection for T1b gallbladder cancer: a decision analysis. HPB (Oxford). 2009;11(8):656-63.
77. Paolucci V. Port site recurrences after laparoscopic cholecystectomy. J Hepatobiliary Pancreat Surg. 2001;8(6):535-43.
78. Z'graggen K, Birrer S, Maurer CA, Wehrli H, Klaiber C, Baer HU. Incidence of port site recurrence after laparoscopic cholecystectomy for preoperatively unsuspected gallbladder carcinoma. Surgery. 1998;124(5):831-8.
79. Paolucci V, Schaeff B, Schneider M, Gutt C. Tumor seeding following laparoscopy: international survey. World J Surg. 1999;23(10):989-95; discussion 996-7.
80. Nakagawa S, Tada T, Furukawa H, Abe M, Hatakeyama K. Late-type recurrence at the port site of unexpected gallbladder carcinoma after a laparoscopic cholecystectomy: report of a case. Surg Today. 2000;30(9):853-5.
81. Suzuki K, Kimura T, Hashimoto H, Nishihira T, Ogawa H. Port site recurrence of gallbladder cancer after laparoscopic surgery: two case reports of long-term survival. Surg Laparosc Endosc Percutan Tech. 2000;10(2):86-8.
82. Maker AV, Butte JM, Oxenberg J, Kuk D, Gonen M, Fong Y, et al. Is port site resection necessary in the surgical management of gallbladder cancer? Ann Surg Oncol. 2012;19(2):409-17.
83. Fuks D, Regimbeau JM, Pessaux P, Bachellier P, Raventos A, Mantion G, et al. Is port-site resection necessary in the surgical management of gallbladder cancer? J Visc Surg. 2013;150(4):277-84.
84. Butte JM, Gönen M, Allen PJ, D'Angelica MI, Kingham TP, Fong Y, et al. The role of laparoscopic staging in patients with incidental gallbladder cancer. HPB (Oxford). 2011;13(7):463-72.
85. Agarwal AK, Kalayarasan R, Javed A, Gupta N, Nag HH. The role of staging laparoscopy in primary gallbladder cancer—an analysis of 409 patients: a prospective study to evaluate the role of staging laparoscopy in the management of gallbladder cancer. Ann Surg. 2013;258(2):318-23.
86. Shirai Y, Yoshida K, Tsukada K, Ohtani T, Muto T. Identification of the regional lymphatic system of the gallbladder by vital staining. Br J Surg. 1992;79:659-62.
87. Shirai Y, Wakai T, Sakata J, Hatakeyama K. Regional lymphadenectomy for gallbladder cancer: rational extent, technical details, and patient outcomes. World J Gastroenterol. 2012;18(22):2775-83.
88. Shimada H, Endo I, Fujii Y, Kamiya N, Masunari H, Kunihiro O, et al. Appraisal of surgical resection of gallbladder cancer with special reference to lymph node dissection. Langenbecks Arch Surg. 2000;385(8):509-14.
89. Benson AB, Abrams TA, Ben-Josef E, Bloomston PM, Botha JF, Clary BM, et al. NCCN clinical practice guidelines in oncology: hepatobiliary cancers. J Natl Compr Canc Netw. 2009;7:350-91.
90. Ito H, Ito K, D'Angelica M, Gonen M, Klimstra D, Allen P, et al. Accurate staging for gallbladder cancer: implications for surgical therapy and pathological assessment. Ann Surg. 2011;254(2): 320-5.
91. Negi SS, Singh A, Chaudhary A. Lymph nodal involvement as prognostic factor in gallbladder cancer: location, count or ratio? J Gastrointest Surg. 2011;15(6):1017-25.
92. Coburn NG, Cleary SP, Tan JC, Law CH. Surgery for gallbladder cancer: a population-based analysis. J Am Coll Surg. 2008;207: 371-82.
93. Shimizu Y, Ohtsuka M, Ito H, Kimura F, Shimizu H, Togawa A, et al. Should the extrahepaticbile duct be resected for locally advanced gallbladder cancer? Surgery. 2004;136:1012-7; discussion 1018.
94. Ishizuka D, Shirai Y, Hatakeyama K. Ischemic biliary stricture due to lymph node dissection in the hepatoduodenal ligament. Hepatogastroenterology. 1998;45:2048-50.
95. Pawlik TM, Gleisner AL, Vigano L, Kooby DA, Bauer TW, Frilling A, et al. Incidence of finding residual disease for incidental gallbladder carcinoma: implications for re-resection. J Gastrointest Surg. 2007;11(11):1478-86; discussion 1486-7.
96. D'Angelica M, Dalal KM, DeMatteo RP, Fong Y, Blumgart LH, Jarnagin WR. Analysis of the extent of resection for adenocarcinoma of the gallbladder. Ann Surg Oncol. 2009;16(4):806-16.
97. Ogura Y, Tabata M, Kawarada Y, et al. Effect of hepatic invasion on the choice of hepatic resection for advanced carcinoma of the gallbladder: histologic analysis of 32 surgical cases. World J Surg. 1998;22:262-7.
98. Nagai H, Kuroda A, Morioka Y, et al. Modes of spread of gallbladder carcinoma: A study of autopsied cases (in Japanese). Tan to Sui (J BilPancr). 1983;4:1227.
99. Yamaguchi K, Chijiiwa K, Shimizu S, Yokohata K, Tsuneyoshi M, Tanaka M. Anatomical limit of extended cholecystectomy for gallbladder carcinoma involving the neck of the gallbladder. Int Surg. 1998;83:21-3.
100. Miyazaki M, Ito H, Ambiru S, Shimizu H, Togawa A, Gohchi E, et al. Radical surgery for advanced gallbladder carcinoma. Br J Surg. 1996;83:478-81.
101. Kondo S, Nimura Y, Kamiya J, Nagino M, Kanai M, Uesaka K, et al. Factors influencing postoperative hospital mortality and long-term survival after radical resection for stage IV gallbladder carcinoma. World J Surg. 2003;27(3):272-7.
102. Kondo S, Nimura Y, Kamiya J, Nagino M, Kanai M, Uesaka K, et al. Five-year survivors after aggressive surgery for stage IV gallbladder cancer. J Hepatobiliary Pancreat Surg. 2001;8(6):511-7.
103. Nishio H, Nagino M, Ebata T, Yokoyama Y, Igami T, Nimura Y. Aggressive surgery for stage IV gallbladder carcinoma; what are the contraindications? J Hepatobiliary Pancreat Surg. 2007;14(4): 351-7.
104. Sakamoto Y, Nara S, Kishi Y, Esaki M, Shimada K, Kokudo N, et al. Is extended hemihepatectomy plus pancreaticoduodenectomy justified for advanced bile duct cancer and gallbladder cancer? Surgery. 2013;153(6):794-800.

105. Lim CS, Jang JY, Lee SE, Kang MJ, Kim SW. Reappraisal of hepatopancreatoduodenectomy as a treatment modality for bile duct and gallbladder cancer. J Gastrointest Surg. 2012;16(5):1012-8.
106. Wakai T, Shirai Y, Tsuchiya Y, Nomura T, Akazawa K, Hatakeyama K. Combined major hepatectomy and pancreaticoduodenectomy for locally advanced biliary carcinoma: long-term results. World J Surg. 2008;32(6):1067-74.
107. Kaneoka Y, Yamaguchi A, Isogai M. Hepatopancreatoduodenectomy: its suitability for bile duct cancer versus gallbladder cancer. J Hepatobiliary Pancreat Surg. 2007;14(2):142-8.
108. Sasaki R, Itabashi H, Fujita T, Takeda Y, Hoshikawa K, Takahashi M, et al. Significance of extensive surgery including resection of the pancreas head for the treatment of gallbladder cancer—from the perspective of mode of lymph node involvement and surgical outcome. World J Surg. 2006;30(1):36-42.
109. Hasegawa K, Kokudo N, Sano K, Seyama Y, Aoki T, Ikeda M, et al. Two-stage pancreatojejunostomy in pancreaticoduodenectomy: a retrospective analysis of short-term results. Am J Surg. 2008;196(1):3-10.
110. Kondo S, Nimura Y, Kamiya J, Nagino M, Kanai M, Uesaka K, et al. Factors influencing postoperative hospital mortality and long-term survival after radical resection for stage IV gallbladder carcinoma. World J Surg. 2003;27(3):272-7.
111. Sakamoto Y, Sano T, Shimada K, Kosuge T, Kimata Y, Sakuraba M, et al. Clinical significance of reconstruction of the right hepatic artery for biliary malignancy. Langenbecks Arch Surg. 2006;391:203-8.
112. Nimura Y, Hayakawa N, Kamiya J, Maeda S, Kondo S, Yasui A, et al. Combined portal vein and liver resection for carcinoma of the biliary tract. Br J Surg. 1991;78:727-31.
113. Kondo S, Nimura Y, Hayakawa N, Kamiya J, Nagino M, Uesaka K. Extensive surgery for gallbladder cancer. Br J Surg. 2002;89:179-84.
114. Chijiiwa K, Kai M, Nagano M, Hiyoshi M, Ohuchida J, Kondo K. Outcome of radical surgery for stage IV gallbladder carcinoma. J Hepatobiliary Pancreat Surg. 2007;14(4):345-50.
115. Kobayashi A, Oda T, Fukunaga K, Sasaki R, Ohkohchi N. Invasion of the hepatic artery is a crucial predictor of poor outcomes in gallbladder carcinoma. World J Surg. 2012;36(3):645-50.
116. Hawkins WG, DeMatteo RP, Jarnagin WR, Ben-Porat L, Blumgart LH, Fong Y. Jaundice predicts advanced disease and early mortality in patients with gallbladder cancer. Ann Surg Oncol. 2004;11(3):310-5.
117. Regimbeau JM, Fuks D, Bachellier P, Le Treut YP, Pruvot FR, Navarro F, et al. Prognostic value of jaundice in patients with gallbladder cancer by the AFC-GBC-2009 study group. Eur J Surg Oncol. 2011;37(6):505-12.
118. Kaneoka Y, Yamaguchi A, Isogai M, Harada T, Suzuki M. Hepatoduodenal ligament invasion by gallbladder carcinoma: histologic patterns and surgical recommendation. World J Surg. 2003;27(3):260-5.
119. Todoroki T, Takahashi H, Koike N, Kawamoto T, Kondo T, Yoshida S, et al. Outcomes of aggressive treatment of stage IV gallbladder cancer and predictors of survival. Hepatogastroenterology. 1999;46(28):2114-21.
120. Nakamura S, Suzuki S, Konno H, Baba S, Baba S. Outcome of extensive surgery for TNM stage IV carcinoma of the gallbladder. Hepatogastroenterology. 1999;46(28):2138-43.
121. Nishio H, Ebata T, Yokoyama Y, Igami T, Sugawara G, Nagino M. Gallbladder cancer involving the extrahepatic bile duct is worthy of resection. Ann Surg. 2011;253(5):953-60.
122. Chan KM, Yeh TS, Yu MC, Jan YY, Hwang TL, Chen MF. Gallbladder carcinoma with biliary invasion: clinical analysis of the differences from nonbiliary invasion. World J Surg. 2005;29(1):72-5.
123. Endo I, Shimada H, Fujii Y, Sugita M, Masunari H, Miura Y, et al. Indications for curative resection of advanced gallbladder cancer with hepatoduodenal ligament invasion. J Hepatobiliary Pancreat Surg. 2001;8(6):505-10.
124. Sikora SS, Singh RK. Surgical strategies in patients with gallbladder cancer: nihilism to optimism. J Surg Oncol. 2006;93(8):670-81.
125. Sharma A, Dwary AD, Mohanti BK, Deo SV, Pal S, Sreenivas V, et al. Best supportive care compared with chemotherapy for unresectable gallbladder cancer: a randomized controlled study. J Clin Oncol. 2010;28:4581-6.
126. Valle J, Wasan H, Palmer DH, Cunningham D, Anthoney A, Maraveyas A, et al. Cisplatin plus gemcitabine versus gemcitabine for biliary tract cancer. N Engl J Med. 2010;362:1273-81.
127. Sharma A, Mohanti B, Raina V, Shukla N, Pal S, Dwary A, et al. A phase II study of gemcitabine and oxaliplatin (Oxigem) in unresectable gallbladder cancer. Cancer Chemother Pharmacol. 2010;65:497-502.
128. Park HS, Lim JY, Yoon DS, Park JS, Lee DK, Lee SJ, et al. Outcome of adjuvant therapy for gallbladder cancer. Oncology. 2010;79:168-73.
129. Glazer ES, Liu P, Abdalla EK, Vauthey JN, Curley SA. Neither neoadjuvant nor adjuvant therapy increases survival after biliary tract cancer resection with wide negative margins. J Gastrointest Surg. 2012;16:1666-71.
130. Wang SJ, Fuller CD, Kim JS, Sittig DF, Thomas Jr CR, Ravdin PM. Prediction model for estimating the survival benefit of adjuvant radiotherapy for gallbladder cancer. J Clin Oncol. 2008;26:2112-7.
131. Mayo SC, Shore AD, Nathan H, Edil B, Wolfgang CL, Hirose K, et al. National trends in the management and survival of surgically managed gallbladder adenocarcinoma over 15 years: a population-based analysis. J Gastrointest Surg. 2010;14:1578-91.
132. Wang SJ, Lemieux A, Kalpathy-Cramer J, Ord CB, Walker GV, Fuller CD, et al. Nomogram for predicting the benefit of adjuvant chemoradiotherapy for resected gallbladder cancer. J Clin Oncol. 2011;29:4627-32.
133. Gold DG, Miller RC, Haddock MG, Gunderson LL, Quevedo F, Donohue JH, et al. Adjuvant therapy for gallbladder carcinoma: the Mayo clinic experience. Int J Radiat Oncol Biol Phys. 2009;75:150-5.
134. Kim WS, Choi DW, You DD, Ho CY, Heo JS, Choi SH. Risk factors influencing recurrence, patterns of recurrence, and the efficacy of adjuvant therapy after radical resection for gallbladder carcinoma. J Gastrointest Surg. 2010;14:679-87.
135. Engineer R, Wadasadawala T, Mehta S, Mahantshetty U, Purandare N, Rangarajan V, et al. Chemoradiation for unresectable gallbladder cancer: time to review historic nihilism? J Gastrointest Cancer. 2011;42:222-7.
136. Kato A, Shimizu H, Ohtsuka M, Yoshidome H, Yoshitomi H, Furukawa K, et al. Surgical resection after downsizing chemotherapy for initially unresectable locally advanced biliary tract cancer: a retrospective single-center study. Ann Surg Oncol. 2013;20(1):318-24.
137. Saluja SS, Gulati M, Garg PK, Pal H, Pal S, Sahni P, et al. Endoscopic or percutaneous biliary drainage for gallbladder cancer: a randomized trial and quality of life assessment. Clin Gastroenterol Hepatol. 2008;6(8):944-50.
138. Wyse JM, Chen YI, Sahai AV. Celiac plexus neurolysis in the management of unresectable pancreatic cancer: when and how? World J Gastroenterol. 2014;20(9):2186-92.

CHAPTER 62

Cholangiocarcinoma

Rajan Saxena, Himanshu Yadav

INTRODUCTION

Cholangiocarcinoma (CCA) is an uncommon cancer, accounting for only 2% of all reported malignancies.[1] This tumor, a more serious undertaking in hepatobiliary surgery, at times, presents serious diagnostic challenges contrasting with benign strictures, and the debate finally gets settled only after surgical excision and histological examination.

LOCATION

It may arise anywhere along the biliary system: hilar CCA accounts for 40–60% of these tumors, distal CCA 20–30%, and intrahepatic CCA 10%. Less than 10% CCA are multifocal.[2,3] Newer classification schemes have put forth the definition of perihilar cholangiocarcinoma (PHC) as "tumors located in the extrahepatic biliary tree proximal to the origin of the cystic duct".[4] As no clear cut boundary has been defined between extrahepatic and intrahepatic bile ducts, PHC can be divided into two types of tumors: (1) "extrahepatic" type, arising from the large hilar bile duct and (2) "intrahepatic" type, which has an intrahepatic component with invasion of the hepatic hilus.

ETIOLOGY

The known risk factors include primary sclerosing cholangitis (PSC), hepatolithiasis, choledochal cyst, prior operative transduodenal sphincteroplasty, and chronic biliary parasitic infestation. Numerous teratogens have been implicated in its pathogenesis including agents like thorotrast, asbestos, dioxin and nitrosamines. Most common age at presentation is in the 7th and 8th decades of life. CCA afflicts males slightly more frequently than females.

PATHOLOGY

Three major subtypes of extrahepatic CCAs are recognized: (1) sclerosing, (2) nodular and (3) papillary. Most common is the sclerosing type, usually hilar in location, and characterized by circumferential ductal thickening with periductal fibrosis and inflammation. The nodular type is a firm tumor extending irregularly into the duct lumen. The papillary type, a soft and friable tumor typically projecting into the duct lumen in a pedunculated fashion, is usually distal in location and associated with higher resectability and more favorable outcomes.

Their pattern of growth is insidiously longitudinal, and tumor spread beyond grossly negative margins is well known, demanding careful attention to margins at surgery to ensure complete tumor resection. The desmoplastic response accompanying these tumors can render the analysis of needle biopsy specimens challenging and highly susceptible to sampling error.

Regarded earlier as a locally aggressive neoplasm, CCA is known to have perineural and lymphovascular spread; at presentation up to one-third of patients have nodal metastases, and distant metastases are not uncommon. The World Health Organization has classified carcinomas of extrahepatic bile ducts based on their histologic characteristics (Box 1).[5]

HILAR CHOLANGIOCARCINOMA

Clinical Presentation

Most common presentation of extraheptic CCA is jaundice which may be intermittent in papillary variant. Other symptoms are quite non-specific like-anorexia, weight loss, abdominal pain and pruritus. These symptoms are seen in about 33% of patients. In contrast to distal CCA, overt jaundice may not be a part of the initial

BOX 1 The World Health Organization classification of carcinomas of extrahepatic bile ducts

- Adenocarcinoma
- Papillary adenocarcinoma
- Adenocarcinoma, intestinal type
- Adenocarcinoma, gastric foveolar type
- Mucinous adenocarcinoma
- Clear cell adenocarcinoma
- Signet-ring cell carcinoma
- Adenosquamous carcinoma
- Squamous cell carcinoma
- Small cell (oat cell) carcinoma
- Large cell neuroendocrine carcinoma
- Undifferentiated carcinoma
- Biliary cystadenoma

presentation of hilar CCA, especially if unilateral or segmental duct is involved. In such patients pruritus antedates clinical jaundice, sometimes by weeks and months. An isolated elevation of serum alkaline phosphatase may serve as a useful pointer to the diagnosis. However, most patients ultimately become jaundiced. Without manipulations of biliary tract cholangitis is rare, although bactibilia is seen in up to one-third patients.[2,6-8]

Examination findings may provide useful clues regarding the level of biliary tract obstruction. Most patients with extrahepatic biliary cancers have hepatomegaly but patients with hilar CCA tend to have a non-palpable gallbladder in contrast to those with distal cancers. Portal hypertension is rare and is seen in cases of long standing bile duct obstruction or involvement of portal vein or both.[9]

Differential Diagnosis

Alternative diagnoses are possible in 10–15% of patients.[10] A search should always be made for such conditions because it has a bearing on treatment and ultimate outcome.

Carcinoma Gallbladder

Gallbladder carcinoma causing hilar obstruction via intraductal spread may be difficult to distinguish from hilar CCA. Radiological findings of an irregular gallbladder wall thickening, segment IV and V infiltration, selective involvement of the right portal pedicle and obstruction below the hilum may indicate a gallbladder carcinoma.

Mirizzi Syndrome

The pericholecystic and periductal inflammation from a large impacted stone at gallbladder neck can obstruct the proximal bile duct. It may be sometimes become difficult to differentiate from a CCA (Figs 1A and B).[11-13] This may be associated with xanthogranulomatous cholecystitis in a number of patients.

Choledocholithiasis

Uncommonly, choledocholithiasis can obstruct the biliary confluence in the absence predisposing conditions. However, one must also be mindful of the fact that both these conditions can coexist and the presence of choledocholithiasis should not detract one from further investigations.

Other Benign Focal Strictures (Malignant Masquerade)

There is an important subgroup of patients who present with hilar strictures without a history of PSC, who present with focal strictures at the hilum.[10,14-16] Because of the considerable diagnostic overlap, hilar CCA must be the leading differential diagnosis till disproved on exploration. The results of biliary crush cytology percutaneous needle biopsy may be misleading, and a surgical exploration is the best modality to resolve diagnostic dilemmas in this setting.[17]

Diagnosis

In an appropriate clinical setting with a focal stenotic lesion on radiology a presumptive diagnosis of hilar CCA can be made.[10]

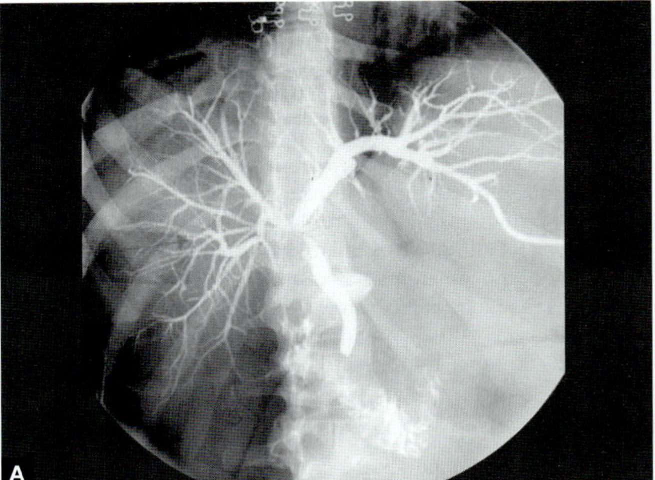

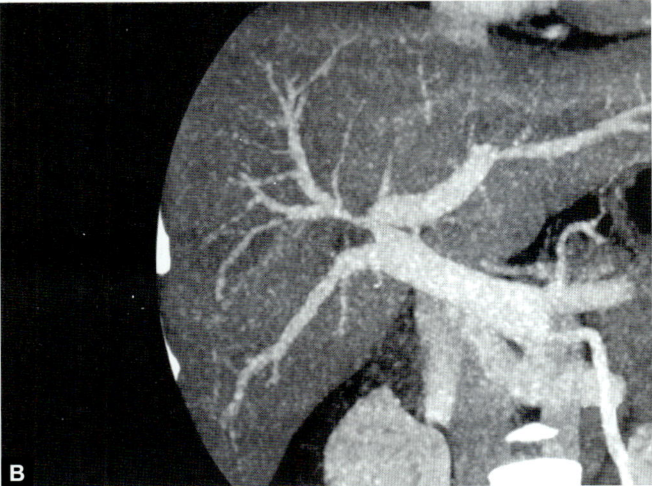

Figures 1A and B (A) Direct cholangiogram (PTBDgram) in a patient with a preoperative working diagnosis of Mirizzi syndrome with carcinoma gallbladder. The patient had presented with features of cholangitis and a serum bilirubin level 28 mg/dL; (B) CT reconstruction images of the same patient showing constriction of the right anterior sectoral portal vein. Operative and histopathological findings however confirmed that the patient had Mirizzi syndrome with Xanthogranulomatous cholecystitis

It is not mandatory to preoperatively confirm the malignancy histologically and attempts to do so are not justified. Tumor markers like serum carbohydrate antigen 19-9 (CA 19-9) and carcinoembryonic antigen (CEA) have had little diagnostic value, besides being fallacious in jaundiced patients.[7]

Imaging

Duplex ultrasound: A dedicated ultrasound study can show the level of biliary obstruction fairly accurately. Other information deciphered is extension into bile ducts, periductal tissues and vessels (with the use of Doppler signal).[18-20] Thus it is quite useful in assessing resectability. A study involving 63 patients using duplex US predicted portal vein involvement in 93% of cases (specificity and positive predictive value being 99% and 97% respectively)[21] which was comparable to angiography with computed tomographic angioportography (90% sensitivity, 99% specificity, and 95% positive predictive value).

Triple phase computed tomographic scan abdomen: Computed tomographic scan images are recorded in three distinct phases—(1) the arterial, (2) pancreatic and (3) portal venous phase after injection of intravenous contrast. Such imaging can tell the level of obstruction, vascular involvement, and liver atrophy.

The typical finding on computed tomography is dilatation of the biliary radicles in both the right and left lobes with non-union of the dilated ducts at the hilum. CCA should be suspected if there is an abrupt end to the biliary dilatation without a visible mass, especially if it occurs between the hilum and the pancreatic head. Radiological descriptions have described hilar CCA as *infiltrating, exophytic,* and *polypoid* types. Infiltrating hilar CCA is the most common type of CCA. On computed tomography usually there is a focal thickening of the duct wall which may obliterate the lumen. Such thickening will only be evident when thin cuts are taken from the area of interest. Biliary dilatation proximal to the tumor will be present and the appearance may mimic a benign stricture or obstruction secondary to a stone. Thin-section computed tomography targeted to this area, however, may reveal wall thickening or a small intraluminal mass consistent with tumor.

Exophytic CCA on computed tomography appears similar to peripheral CCA as a mass with peripheral rim enhancement. The polypoid type on computed tomography is seen as an intraductal soft-tissue mass which can result in expansion of the duct lumen. It may be multifocal involving both intrahepatic as well as extrahepatic bile ducts. However, one must acknowledge that owing to significant subepithelial spread, radiological descriptions may underestimate the actual extent of CCA.

Computed tomography is a useful modality for assessing vascular involvement. Compression, narrowing, encasement or occlusion usually indicates involvement of adjacent vascular structures (Figs 2A and B). Enhancement of liver parenchyma peripheral to a CCA may be altered as a result of portal vein invasion. Increased enhancement of the liver parenchyma distal to the tumor on bolus-enhanced computed tomography and decreased enhancement of the same area on computed tomography arterioportography is suspicious of portal vein invasion. Lobar atrophy is also well recognized on computed tomographic scans. Long standing bile duct obstruction may cause moderate atrophy of the ipsilateral lobe. But associated portal venous obstruction may cause rapid and severe atrophy of the affected lobe. In addition to nodal involvement, distant metastases also are amenable to detection by computed tomography.

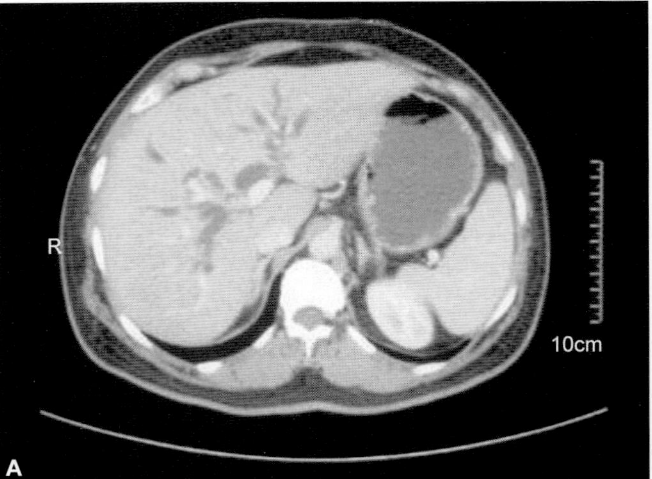

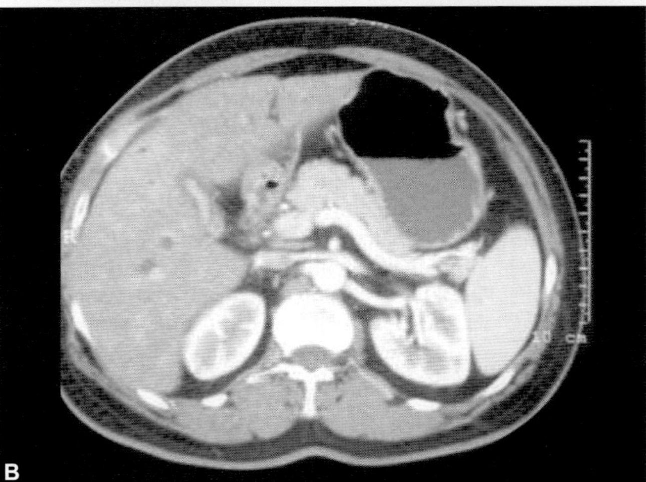

Figures 2A and B (A) Portal venous phase images in a patient with hilar cholangiocarcinoma showing involvement of the right anterior sectoral portal vein as it courses through the mass; (B) Note the collapsed gallbladder consistent with the diagnosis of hilar cholangiocarcinoma

Magnetic resonance imaging (MRI): Several studies have shown the utility of magnetic resonance cholangiopancreaticogram (MRCP) in evaluating patients with biliary obstruction.[22-24] MRCP identifies the tumor and the level of biliary obstruction. It also identifies the isolated and obstructed ducts. MRCP in combination with magnetic resonance angiography (MRA) and magnetic resonance portovenogram (MRPV) provide same information as the contrast enhanced computed tomography.

Endoscopic Approaches

Percutaneous transhepatic cholangioscopy: Percutaneous transhepatic cholangioscopy (PTCS) allows macroscopic examination of the bile duct and histopathologic examination by obtaining biopsy specimens. Some investigators have suggested that PTCS should be used for early diagnosis of hilar CCA and preoperative assessment of the extent of tumor.[25,26] It is particularly useful in the preoperative definitive diagnosis of more difficult CCA located not only in the extrahepatic bile duct but also in the intrahepatic bile ducts.[27-32]

However, specificity of histological examination alone is low. Nevertheless, even in such cases (false negatives) macroscopic findings of "tumor vessels" can be a useful aid in diagnosis. According to Kim et al., this finding could be detected in 61% malignant bile duct strictures, and most cases showing tumor vessels were malignant.[33] In addition, it has been reported that by combining the results of histological examination and tumor vessels, the specificity increases.[33]

Mapping biopsy defines the proximal and distal extension of the tumor for superficially spreading CCA and is helpful in designing a curative resection.[27,32,34-36] In cases of mucin-producing intrahepatic CCA, percutaneous transhepatic biliary drainage (PTBD) followed by PTCS is important in evaluating the progress of cancer along the bile ducts and in treatment planning.[37-39]

Endoscopic ultrasound: Endoscopic ultrasound (EUS) often offers valuable access for tumor and lymph node biopsy.[40,41] It is increasingly being used to assess the extent of tumor. It may be helpful by providing tissue sample through fine-needle aspiration (FNA). It complements the endoscopic and percutaneous transhepatic approaches. This is particularly relevant among patients considered for liver transplantation because the Mayo Clinic protocol and other modified Mayo protocols exclude all patients with lymph node metastases.[42-45] Eloubeidi et al.[46] reported a diagnostic sensitivity of 86% with EUS-FNA. However, another group reported the diagnostic sensitivity to be ~45%.[47] EUS-FNA is especially useful in patients with negative brush cytology and forceps biopsy findings.

Intraductal ultrasonography: Intraductal ultrasonography (IDUS) is an emerging imaging modality for the evaluation of a variety of biliary disorders.[48,49] Although it does not provide definite diagnoses, the characterization of biliary structures provided by IDUS can be used in combination with other diagnostic approaches to develop appropriate therapeutic strategies.[50-53] A recent study reported an increased accuracy of endoscopic retrograde cholangiopancreatography (ERCP) with the use of IDUS. The accuracy to differentiate the benign from malignant stricture increased from 58% to 90%.[54] The same has been confirmed by others also.[55,56]

Brush cytology and forceps biopsy: Brush cytology is the most common tissue sampling technique in patients with suspected bile duct strictures with a sensitivity of 30–60% (for malignant strictures). It is generally safe, requires little time, and is technically easier compared to forceps biopsy. For diagnosing malignant strictures the forceps biopsy carries a sensitivity of 43–81%. Forceps biopsy is more time consuming and less widely used, but it provides a sample of subepithelial stroma.[57-59] It was reported recently that with combined approach (brush cytology and forceps biopsy) the diagnostic sensitivity increased to only 60.3% from respective sensitivities of 41.4% and 53.4% respectively.[60]

Fluorescence in situ hybridization: The incidence of aneuploidy in bile duct cancers is 80%.[61] Fluorescence in situ hybridization (FISH) identifies these malignant cells by detecting aneuploidy and deletion of the locus 9p21. This technique has found only limited clinical utility in the evaluation of hilar CCA.

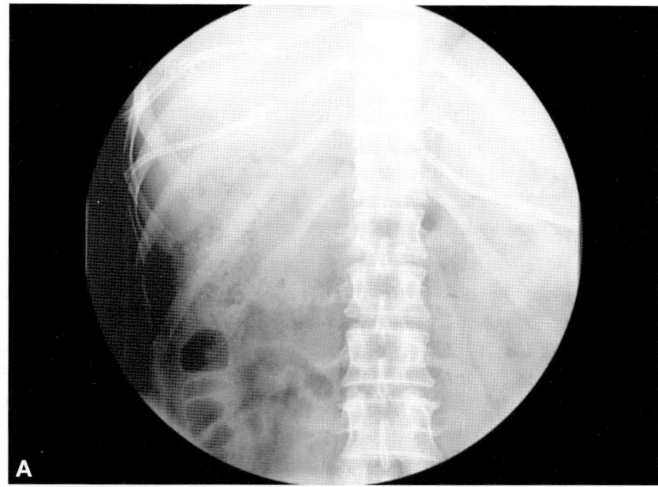

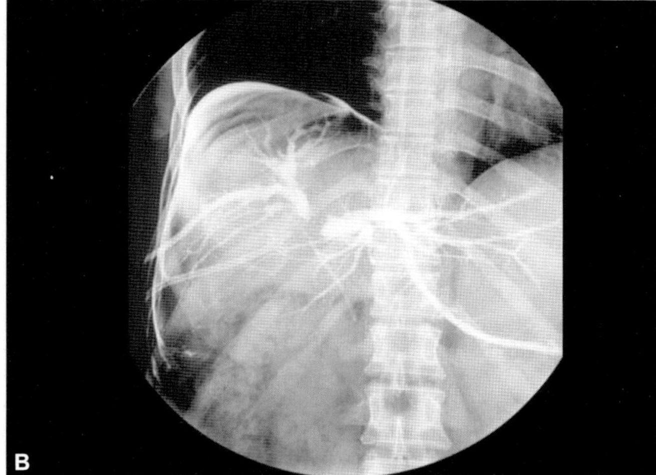

Figures 3A and B (A) Plain image of a patient showing three PTBDs in situ who had undergone preoperative biliary drainage; (B) PTBDgram shows a mass sitting at the hilum causing separation of the secondary confluence

Direct cholangiography: Direct cholangiogram maps the location of the tumor and the biliary extent. In the appropriate clinical setting, ERCP can effectively provide biliary drainage, although it comes with a higher risk of cholangitis. PTBD is an effective method of relieving jaundice and also an important diagnostic modality. It can accurately assess the extent of intrahepatic bile duct involvement (Figs 3A and B).[7,62-64]

Staging laparoscopy: Despite advances in imaging, occult metastases are detected in almost one-third of patients with hilar CCA at laparotomy. Staging laparoscopy, therefore, avoids the high morbidity of a non-therapeutic laparotomy.

FDG-PET: FDG PET may identify occult metastatic disease or advanced regional lymphadenopathy (N2 disease) in a significant proportion of patients. However, the exact role of this modality has not been defined in the setting of hilar CCA.[65-67]

Preoperative Evaluation

Assessment of Resectability

There are four crucial determinants of resectability:

1. Extent of tumor within the biliary tree
2. Vascular involvement
3. Hepatic lobar atrophy
4. Metastatic disease.

Cholangiography is extremely useful in assessing the extent of tumor within the biliary tree. The radial spread of these tumors can be better assessed using cross-sectional imaging modalities. In addition to vascular involvement, these modalities also are useful in assessing lobar atrophy and intra-abdominal metastases. With improvement in imaging softwares, these modalities can be extremely useful in liver volumetry. Patients with lobar atrophy and an adequate liver remnant may be directly offered liver resection, without the need for preoperative biliary drainage.[68] The various criteria for non-resectability among patients with hilar CCA have been listed in Box 2.

Preoperative Biliary Drainage

Most of the available evidence suggests that routine preoperative biliary drainage for optimizing patients prior to surgery is not indicated as it does not reduce operative morbidity or mortality. This fact has been borne out in several prospective randomized studies.[69-73] A meta-analysis also concluded that preoperative biliary drainage increased the surgical morbidity.[74] However, it may be useful in patients with biliary sepsis, advanced malnutrition and when a major liver resection is contemplated. In addition, preoperatively placed catheters may help difficult biliary dissections at proximal bile duct region, and they may aid in the placement of long-term transhepatic stents.

Percutaneous transhepatic biliary drainage procedure has traditionally been used for the purpose of biliary drainage among these patients. However, endoscopic modalities have increasingly come up and several centers have reported good results with this modality.

Endoscopic retrograde biliary drainage preserves intestinal bile flow which is more advantageous.[75] It carries shorter hospital stay, has more patient comfort and lower procedure related morbidity and mortality. If multiple ducts are manipulated (instrumentation) and not drained thereafter; there is a fair chance of cholangitis. Follow-up assessment with regards to segmental duct involvement is also made difficult by the endobiliary stent placement.[76-79] Segmental ducts cannot be cannulated accurately.

BOX 2 Criteria for nonresectability among patients with hilar cholangiocarcinoma

Patient factors:

- Medically unfit for operation
- Cirrhosis/portal hypertension

Local factors:

- Hepatic duct involvement up to secondary radicles bilaterally
- Encasement or occlusion of the main portal vein proximal to its bifurcation
- Atrophy of one lobe with encasement of contralateral portal vein branch
- Atrophy of one lobe with contralateral involvement of secondary biliary radicles

Distant disease:

- Histologically proven metastases to lymph node groups beyond the hepatoduodenal ligament (celiac, para-aortic, retropancreatic)
- Histologically proven metastases to liver, lung or peritoneum

Certain guiding principles should be followed. The drainage is usually done in the predicted future liver remnant (FLR).[80,81] Left hepatic duct should be intubated in cases where FLR cannot be predicted preoperatively with certainty. Multiple drainage catheters may be required in case of segmental isolation of the intrahepatic ducts.[82,83]

It is not uncommon for segmental cholangitis to develop in patients with endoscopic or transhepatic biliary drainage catheters and in such cases affected ducts should be drained urgently.[84,85]

Resuscitation and control of infection is required before surgical intervention in patients with biliary tract sepsis.

Preoperative portal vein embolization: When functioning residual liver volume becomes a concern following a planned major liver resection, augmentation of the residual liver volume is frequently required. The concern is more pronounced in jaundiced patients being submitted to an extended liver resection. To obviate the risk of postoperative liver failure, preoperative portal vein embolization (PVE) is used selectively to enhance liver volume, but after decompressing the biliary tree. There are two recognized methods of PVE—the transhepatic route and the transileocolic route. The percutaneous transhepatic route is preferred over the transileocolic approach, as it avoids a laparotomy.[86-88] PVE does translate into a significant hypertrophy of the contralateral lobe, especially if done properly in cases of hilar CCA.

Associating liver partition and portal vein ligation for staged hepatectomy (ALPPS) is the other approach for inducing significant liver hypertrophy to extend the boundaries for liver resection in patients where the tumor would be considered unresectable. This approach, however, has no place in the management of hilar CCA.

Vascular Involvement and Resectability

Arterial anatomy: Unilateral involvement of the hepatic artery is compatible with resection.[89] Although a debatable issue, selected cases with more extensive arterial involvement are also being taken up for surgery. This surge has been fuelled by advances made in the field of liver transplantation and the reported low mortality rates with arterial reconstruction in recent literature.

Portal Venous Anatomy

Main portal vein invasion may not allow complete resection and long-term outcomes may not be very good but still it is not an absolute contraindication for resection of hilar CCA.[89,90-92] Reasonable long-term results have been reported with portal vein resection for advanced biliary cancer.[93-96]

Preoperative Staging

Although the tumor-node-metastasis (TNM) classification is the gold standard for many cancers, it has limited utility when applied to hilar CCA, where local factors are crucial in predicting the natural history and choosing therapy. The systems most commonly used to evaluate PHC in most parts of the world are the modified Bismuth-Corlette system, the American Joint Committee on Cancer (AJCC)/Union for International Cancer Control (UICC) TNM classification, the Memorial Sloan-Kettering Cancer Center (MSKCC) classification and the recent DeOliviera's classification.[5,97-99]

The fact that numerous classification schemes have been utilized for hilar CCA indicates that none of them have been able to cover all the aspects of this disease.

Bismuth-Corlette System

This classification is based on the extent of ductal involvement by tumor alone (Fig. 4).[97] It does not predict resectability or survival. It does not provide information on lymph node involvement, distant metastases, vascular encasement and atrophy of a part of the liver. Its applicability may be changed by the anatomic variation in biliary tree which is common.

TNM Classification for Extrahepatic Bile Duct Tumors

This system is based on the pathological findings (Table 1). In the seventh edition of AJCC Cancer Staging, extrahepatic biliary tract adenocarcinoma has been included and carcinoid and sarcomas have been excluded.[100,101] This system also takes into account the histological grading.

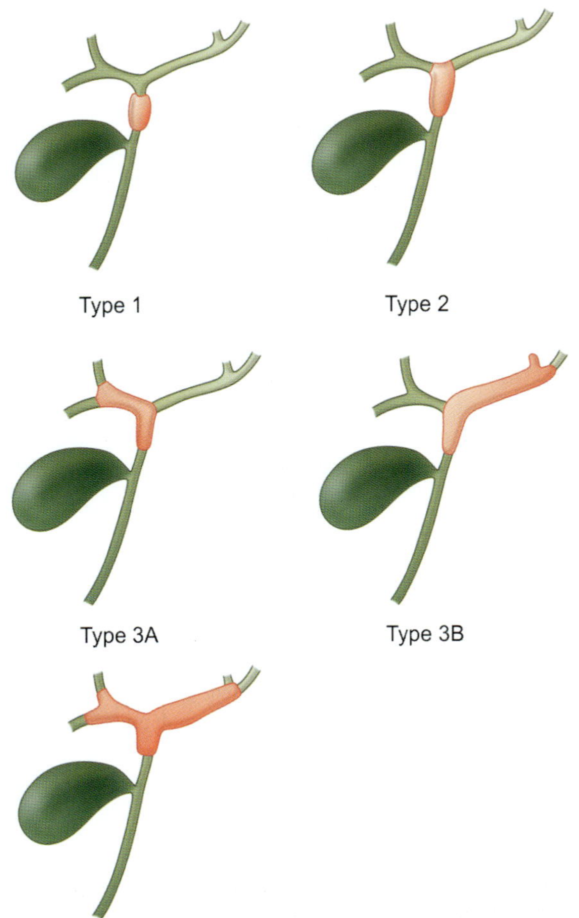

Figure 4 Bismuth-Corlette classification for hilar cholangiocarcinoma

Table 1: TNM classification of extrahepatic bile duct tumors according to the AJCC/UICC 7th edition

Primary tumor (T)	
TX	The primary tumor cannot be assessed
T0	No evidence of a primary tumor
Tis	Carcinoma in situ
T1	The tumor is confined to the bile duct histologically
T2a	The tumor invades the surrounding adipose tissue beyond the wall of the bile duct
T2b	The tumor invades the adjacent hepatic parenchyma
T3	The tumor invades unilateral branches of the portal vein or hepatic artery
T4	The tumor invades the main portal vein or its branches bilaterally, the common hepatic artery, the second-order biliary radicles bilaterally, or the unilateral second-order biliary radicles with contralateral portal vein or hepatic vein involvement
Regional lymph nodes (N)	
NX	Regional lymph nodes cannot be assessed
N0	No regional lymph node metastasis
N1	Regional lymph node metastasis (cystic duct, common bile duct, hepatic artery and portal vein)
N2	Metastasis to periaortic, pericaval, superior mesentery artery and/or celiac artery nodes
Distant metastasis (M)	
M0	No distant metastasis
M1	Distant metastasis
Stage grouping	
Stage 0	Tis N0 M0
Stage I	T1 N0 M0
Stage II	T2a-T2b N0 M0
Stage IIIA	T3 N0 M0
Stage IIIB	T1-T3 N1 M0
Stage IVA	T4 Any N M0
Stage IVB	Any T N2 M0 Any T Any N M1

Histological grading: Gx (no assessment), G1 (well differentiated), G2 (moderately differentiated), G3 (poorly differentiated), or G4 (undifferentiated).

Being a pathological system it can be used postoperatively only; thereby limiting its utility in the preoperative settings.

MSKCC Classification

In an attempt to predict respectability, Jarnagin and colleagues (2001) proposed a system based on: (1) extent of tumor within the biliary tree, (2) vascular involvement and (3) lobar atrophy. It is preoperative clinical staging system which does not take into consideration N or M status (Table 2).[99] In a series of 87 patients this system correlated closely with respectability and median survival.[99,102]

Table 2: Tumor staging according to the MSKCC classification

Tumor stage (T) description	
T1	The tumor involves the biliary confluence with unilateral involvement up to secondary biliary radicles. There is no portal vein involvement or liver atrophy.
T2	The tumor involves the biliary confluence with unilateral involvement up to secondary biliary radicles. There is ipsilateral portal vein involvement or ipsilateral hepatic lobar atrophy.
T3	The tumor involves the biliary confluence with bilateral involvement up to secondary biliary radicles, unilateral extension to secondary biliary radicles with contralateral portal vein involvement, unilateral involvement up to secondary biliary radicles with contralateral hepatic lobar atrophy, or main/bilateral portal vein involvement.

More detailed information on vessel invasion is currently crucial for adequate preoperative and surgical staging.[103]

Classification by International Cholangiocarcinoma Group (DeOliviera's Classification)

DeOliviera et al. (2011) proposed a classification scheme to overcome the limitations of the above mentioned classifications (Table 3).[104] This system takes into account some parameters from previous staging systems. Connotation "B" has been used for Bismuth-Corlette system. Based on recent data showing better prognosis for smaller tumors (including outcomes of liver transplantation for liver limited disease), cut off value of 3 cm has been taken for T3.[42,99,105] A separate subgroup of mixed type of tumor has been added among the macroscopic subtypes.[35,106-108]

Vascular involvement and liver remnant volume are the other key areas that have been addressed in this classification. Tumor involving more than 180 degree of vessel circumference is generally indicative of vascular involvement. Most of this evidence comes from patients with pancreatic cancer where tumor involvement exceeding 180 degree of vessel circumference translated into 80–100% probability of vascular involvement. Similar data were reported for the portal vein and hepatic artery in a small series of PHC patients.[109]

Liver atrophy and remnant liver hypertrophy are crucial factors in predicting resectability. As the definition of liver atrophy and minimum residual liver volume acceptable varies among centres,[110-112] this system uses volume (V) as the percentage of the total volume or body weight ratio. Underlying diseases (fibrosis, non-alcoholic steatohepatitis or PSC) is denoted by the letter "D".

Information about the lymph node status is based on Japanese Society of Biliary Surgery classification.[113] Nodal status N1 has been modified to denote positive periportal or hepatic artery lymph nodes and N2 for positive para-aortic lymph nodes.[114] Metastases, including liver and peritoneal metastases, are graded according to the TNM classification.[5]

Surgical Treatment

Objectives

- Complete tumor excision with negative histological margins (R0 resection)
- Relief of symptoms related to biliary obstruction
- Restoration of biliary continuity.

Table 3: Proposed classification system by DeOliviera[104]

Label	*Side/Location**	*Description*
Bile duct (B)†		
B1	Common bile duct	
B2	Hepatic duct confluence	
B3 R	Right hepatic duct	
B3 L	Left hepatic duct	
B4	Right and left hepatic duct	
Tumor size (T)		
T1	<1 cm	
T2	1–3 cm	
T3	≥3 cm	
Tumor form (F)		
Sclerosing	Sclerosing (or periductal)	
Mass	Mass-forming (or nodular)	
Mixed	Sclerosing and mass-forming	
Polypoid	Polypoid (or intraductal)	
Involvement (>180°) of the portal vein (PV)		
PV0	No portal involvement	
PV1	Main portal vein	
PV2	Portal vein bifurcation	
PV3 R	Right portal vein	
PV3 L	Left portal vein	
PV4	Right and left portal veins	
Involvement (>180°) of the hepatic artery (HA)		
HA0	No arterial involvement	
HA1	Proper hepatic artery	
HA2	Hepatic artery bifurcation	
HA3 R	Right hepatic artery	
HA3 L	Left hepatic artery	
HA4	Right and left hepatic artery	
Liver remnant volume (V)		
V0		No information on the volume needed (liver resection not foreseen)
V%	Indicate Segments	Percentage of the total volume of a putative remnant liver after resection
Underlying liver disease (D)		
Fibrosis		
Nonalcoholic steatohepatitis		
Primary sclerosing cholangitis		
Lymph nodes (N)‡		
N0	No lymph node involvement	
N1	Hilar and/or hepatic artery lymph node involvement	
N2	Periaortic lymph node involvement	
Metastases (M)§		
M0	No distant metastases	
M1	Distant metastases (including liver and peritoneal metastases)	

*"R" indicates right, and "L" indicates left.
†Based on the Bismuth classification.
‡Based on the Japanese Society of Biliary Surgery classification.
§Based on the TNM classification.

Types of Operations

Bile duct resections: Bile duct resections involve removal of the hilar ducts with the extrahepatic biliary system up to the upper border of duodenum and all fat, fascia and lymphatics in the hepatoduodenal ligament. Local bile duct resection is possible when the disease has not extended into the liver and when vascular involvement is absent. A bile duct margin of 5 mm constitutes R0 resection in such cases. However, this is only applicable to Bismuth-Corlette types 1 and 2 without concomitant vascular involvement. Local complete resections are inferior to en bloc partial hepatectomy with respect to long-term survival (Fig. 5).[115]

One particular clinical situation wherein well defined guidelines are lacking is a mid-common bile duct (CBD) CCA without vascular involvement, especially when an adequate margin can be achieved both proximally and distally. In such cases the likelihood of leaving behind residual disease with a local resection has to be balanced with the morbidity of performing a hepatopancreaticoduodenectomy. This issue has not been addressed in the literature, but local extrahepatic bile duct resection may be useful for such patients.

Bile duct resections combined with hepatic or vascular resections: Hepatic resections may be required either (i) when the disease has extended into the right or left hepatic ducts (Bismuth-Corlette type 3a or 3b) or (ii) when the right or left portal vein is involved by tumor.

Liver Resection Alone

Most patients with a separated confluence require an en bloc caudate lobectomy. Anatomical reasons are the primary basis of this approach and available evidence indicates that caudate lobectomy does translate into superior oncologic outcomes.[116-119]

In patients without vascular involvement, parenchyma conserving liver resection (PCLR) or Central hepatectomy or Taj Mahal resection may be a useful option.[120] It is prudent to maintain the blood supply and venous drainage to the remnant part in this demanding approach. Bilateral biliary reconstruction is required and it produces two resection surfaces. Caudate lobectomy is mandated in all these patients to achieve oncologic clearance. The major advantage is the preservation of functioning liver tissue. Therefore, despite its technical challenges, PCLR may be an attractive alternative in selected cases of advanced hilar CCA in which an extended liver resection is contraindicated due to the small amount of remaining liver tissue.

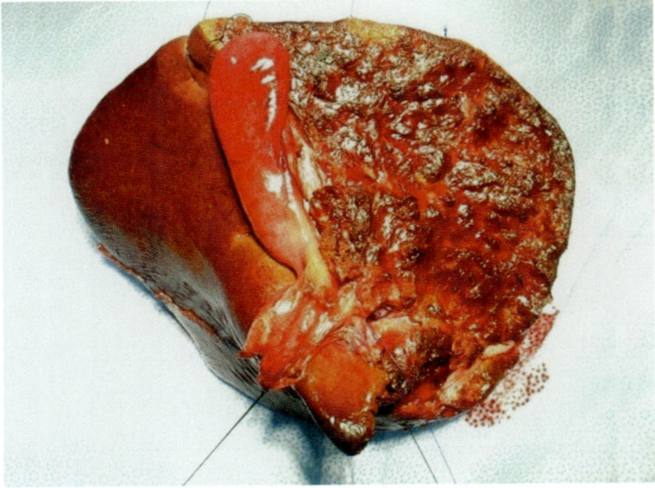

Figure 5 Extended right hepatectomy specimen in a patient with hilar cholangiocarcinoma

Formal major hepatectomies are required in following instances

Liver resection	*For tumors*
Right hepatectomy	1. Involving right anterior and posterior sectoral ducts (with segment IV duct spared) 2. Involving the right hepatic artery
Right trisectionectomy	Involving right hepatic duct and segment IV duct
Left extended resection	Involving the left intrahepatic ducts and right anterior sectoral duct

Liver Resection with Vascular Resection and Reconstruction

Portal vein resection and reconstruction: It should be done only in cases where portal vein bifurcation is inseparably adherent to tumor. It is carried out during the hilar dissection prior to hepatic parenchymal transaction. Direct end-to-end anastomosis of the main trunk of the portal vein and the left branch is carried out and such anastomosis is usually possible during right-sided resections.[95,121] An autologous graft (usually the external iliac vein) is required during portal vein reconstruction, between the right portal vein and the main trunk during left-sided resections.

Hepatic arterial resection: With the increasing experience with the liver transplantation, performance of hepatic artery resection and reconstruction has been facilitated. The utility of this approach could not be established in the study conducted by Miyazaki, where there were no long-term survivors.[122] Recent studies by Nagino et al. have shown encouraging results with major hepatectomy involving simultaneous resections and reconstructions of the portal vein and hepatic artery performed with an acceptable mortality rate of 2% and with a 5-year survival rate of 30%. The relevance of hepatic artery resection is still debatable, and issue will only be laid to rest once the results of ongoing trials are available.

Hepatopancreatoduodenectomy

The survival benefit of a hepatopancreatoduodenectomy (HPD) has been hindered by the number of patients and a high rate of mortality ranging from 13% to 60%. Even today, HPD for biliary cancer remains controversial and is the most challenging operation employed by hepatobiliary surgeons.

Ebata et al. a mortality rate of only 2.4%, and the overall 5-year survival rate of 37.4%.[123] HPD offers an improved chance of survival in selected patients The role of super-extended resection, i.e. hepatoligamentopancreatoduodenectomy (HLPD + en bloc resection of hepatoduodenal ligament) is still under evaluation.

Liver transplant—current status: Orthotopic liver transplantation (OLT) is a promising modality for the treatment of intrahepatic and hilar CCA, because of its radicality and the ability to treat underlying liver disease. The early experience with OLT was fraught with high recurrence rates and poor survival. The survival of patients with incidentally diagnosed small tumor (<1 cm) with no lymph nodal involvement, is similar to patients undergoing liver transplantation for chronic liver disease with no tumor diagnosed in the explant.[124] These results did indicate that excellent results can be achieved in highly selected patients with early stage disease.

Neoadjuvant therapy with subsequent liver transplantation has increasingly been used among patients with unresectable hilar CCA or hilar CCA arising in the setting of PSC. A protocol of initial neoadjuvant chemoradiotherapy followed by liver transplant was initially adopted at the University of Nebraska for tumors deemed unresectable.[125] The Mayo group were able to achieve encouraging results following adoption of a similar protocol. No difference in survival was reported among patients undergoing living donor versus deceased donor liver transplant. These results do compare favorably to survival after OLT for chronic liver disease and for hepatocellular carcinoma. Inherent within this approach are the considerable morbidity of neoadjuvant therapy and a unique set of complications not usually encountered with transplantation alone.

Heimbach et al. (2006) reviewed the experience at Mayo Clinic and found that only 17% had documented recurrences after transplantation, with a mean follow-up of 32 months.[42] Pridictors of recurrence:

Clinical factors: Prior cholecystectomy, older patient age, CA19-9 greater than 100 at the time of transplantation, an extended waiting time between conclusion of neoadjuvant therapy and OLT and a visible mass on cross-sectional imaging.

Pathologic findings: Residual CCA larger than 2 cm, perineural invasion and high-grade histology.

Adjuvant Therapy

Most of the data regarding adjuvant therapy come from small non-randomized trials consisting of only a limited number of patients. So far there is no convincing evidence to support the routine role of adjuvant or neoadjuvant radiation therapy.[126]

A Phase III randomized study also did not find any benefit of adjuvant systemic 5-fluorouracil (5-FU) and mitomycin C.[127]

Palliation

Palliative care has a significant role in the management of patients with hilar CCA as most patients are not suitable candidates for surgery. Patients whose tumors are deemed unresectable on table can be offered a Segment 3 bypass, provided that the drained liver segment is not atrophic. In selected circumstances bypass to a right sided duct can also be considered. We have described a triple bypass procedure for patients with gallbladder carcinoma with gastric outlet obstruction (Fig. 6).[128] These patients survived for variable periods ranging from 3 months to 17 months. A similar procedure can be used for patients with unresectable hilar CCA.

As a part of palliative care, biliary decompression should be considered for relief of a specific symptom (intractable pruritus, cholangitis) or among potential candidates for chemotherapy/radiotherapy. Endoscopic biliary drainage offers several advantages over PTBD. However, the former approach is not feasible in all patients and PTBD with subsequent placement of a self-expandable metallic endoprosthesis offers good palliation.

In the absence of disseminated disease, patients with locally advanced tumors have been treated with external beam radiation therapy with or without intraluminal brachytherapy. Although postulated to improve stent patency rates among patients undergoing biliary decompression, survival benefit of external radiation or intraluminal brachytherapy has not yet been convincingly demonstrated.[129]

Ortner et al. have reported their experience with photodynamic therapy among patients who had not responded to endoscopic stenting.[130] However, the reported zero mortality for the procedure comes with several caveats. First, the mortality related to endoscopic stenting was not considered and the reason for biliary drainage was not specified. Second, the reasons for non-resectability were not discussed. Finally, the reported median survival (439 days) in the setting of advanced disease is hard to interpret.

Whether or not palliative chemotherapy should be administered is still debatable.

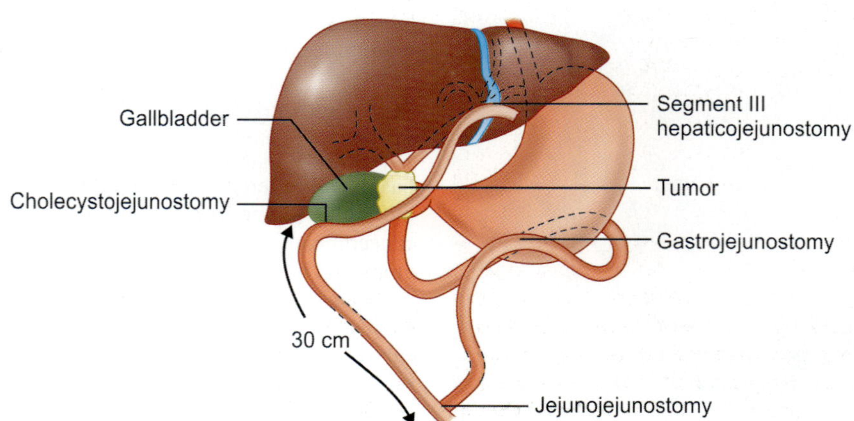

Figure 6 Diagrammatic representation of the triple bypass procedure for obstructing carcinoma of the neck of gallbladder

DISTAL CHOLANGIOCARCINOMA

Clinical Presentation

History

Patients with distal CCA mimic patients with other periampullary malignancies. Painless progressive jaundice is the most common presentation. However, patients with the papillary variant may present with intermittent jaundice. Less than one-third patients present with abdominal pain, weight loss, fever or pruritus.

Examination

Among patients with painless progressive jaundice as a consequence of extrahepatic biliary malignancy, the finding of a palpable gallbladder may provide a useful pointer to the site of the lesion.

Investigations

Cross-sectional Imaging modalities are extremely useful in diagnosing these neoplasms. A triphasic MDCT scan can be used to assess vascular involvement and uncover any metastatic disease. Most of these tumors are small at presentation and a mass may not be apparent on imaging. Dilated extrahepatic duct terminating abruptly in distal part without concomitant dilatation of main pancreatic duct is the typical finding in such a case (Fig. 7). MRCP can provide useful images of the distal bile duct similar to computed tomography and without the need for an invasive procedure like ERCP.

Endoscopic retrograde cholangiopancreatography may be useful in ruling out the presence of choledocholithiasis in cases where a doubt exists. It also provides information regarding the level of obstruction and may delineate the lesion, thereby establishing its site of origin (biliary vs pancreatic). But with the advent of MRCP this is required less frequently. PTC is less often used in the management of distal bile duct tumors.

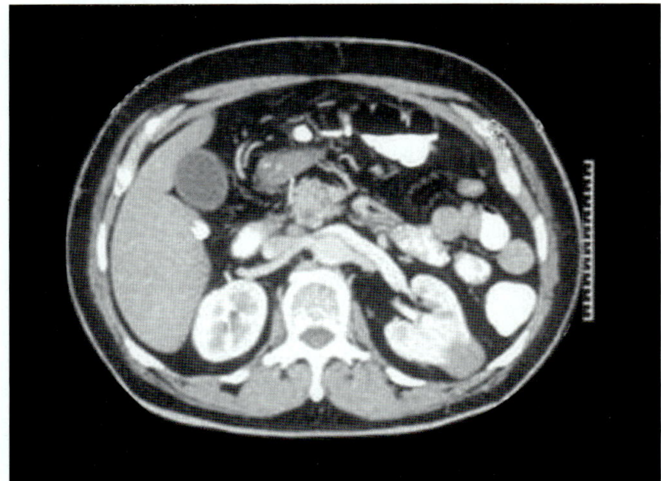

Figure 7 CT image suggestive of distal cholangiocarcinoma in a patient with obstructive jaundice. EUS done in the same patient suggested a distal CBD stone and ERC clearance was achieved

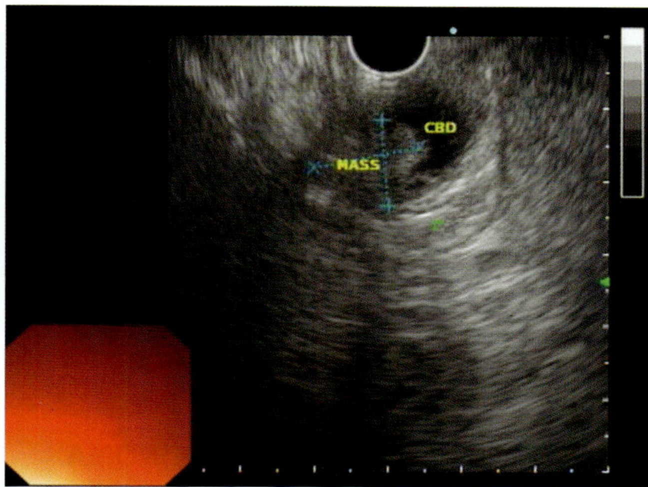

Figure 8 EUS image of a patient with distal cholangiocarcinoma

Endoscopic ultrasound typically images extrahepatic bile duct strictures well, and can be a useful aid in diagnosis particularly in those cases where ERC findings are indeterminate (Fig. 8). EUS findings of an irregular outer edge of the bile duct wall, or a bile duct wall thickness of more than 3 mm, are associated with malignancy in indeterminate biliary strictures, but not diagnostic. EUS-FNA may establish the diagnosis of indeterminate biliary strictures with a sensitivity ranging between 77% and 89% in prior ERC negative cases.[46,131]

In patients with a clinical presentation consistent with CCA and a distal CBD stricture, histologic confirmation of malignancy is generally unwarranted and often unrewarding—in fact, any attempts at proving a malignant etiology in an adult with an unprovoked obstruction at the lower end of CBD with convincing exclusion of stone disease only needlessly delays the appropriate treatment which is surgical extirpation of the affected area. In 9 out of 10 instances, the obstruction is proved malignant at histopathology. The caveat is that stone disease has to be absolutely ruled out with a EUS examination.

Treatment

Pancreaticoduodenectomy is the mainstay of surgical treatment of these tumors. Compared with patients with pancreatic cancer, those with distal CCA are more often amenable to resection, less often have positive resection margins, and less frequently have lymph node involvement.[2,132,133] Most of the published series have reported 5-year survival rates of up to 40% among patients with distal CCA who underwent a curative resection, which is better than the survival of most patients with pancreatic cancers.

Negative resection margin is the most important determinant of long-term survival. Lymph node status is an additional predictor of long-term survival. Fong et al. found that positive nodes confer a 6.7 times greater likelihood of recurrence and death.[132] Wade et al. had survivors beyond 3 years with involved regional lymph nodes. Similarly Nakeeb et al. reported that tumor differentiation and lymph node status are independent predictors of survival.[2,134]

Palliation: Endoprosthesis versus Surgical Bypass

Endoprosthesis: In patients, who are not candidates for surgery, biliary endoprosthesis placement is a viable option and the results are better than for endoprosthesis placed to relieve hilar blocks.[135]

Surgical bypass: Is more appropriate for patients with an expected life span of more than 6 months. In those patients who are deemed unresectable on table, a biliary bypass may be considered. Our own policy is to affect a surgical bypass in stented patients who have a locally advanced disease precluding a resection because those surviving a year with stents frequently need hospitalization for repeated stent blockade and recurrent cholangitis. Such operations for a palliative biliary bypass have acceptable levels of morbidity and mortality when performed in high volume centers.

INTRAHEPATIC CHOLANGIOCARCINOMA (PERIPHERAL CHOLANGIOCARCINOMA)

Intrahepatic CCA (IHC) is the second most common primary liver tumor. Most of these tumors occur in patients without a background of chronic liver disease. It also remains an important differential diagnosis for evaluation of isolated metastases (of unknown origin) to liver.

Clinical Presentation

Most patients are asymptomatic, and these tumors are mostly uncovered incidentally or during the course of evaluation of deranged liver function tests. In those with symptoms, abdominal pain is common. Jaundice is also not infrequently seen and is usually a consequence of compression or invasion of biliary confluence by a centrally located tumor. Examination findings are mostly unremarkable, except for the presence of a palpable mass in larger lesions.

Evaluation

Serum α-fetoprotein levels are generally normal in these patients. Serum CA 19-9 levels may be elevated, but are not diagnostic.

Percutaneous biopsy is not as specific as in patients with hepatocellular carcinoma and search should be made to look for an occult primary with metastatic disease. This workup should include endoscopy (upper and lower), along with computed tomography of chest, abdomen and pelvis.

Cross-sectional imaging (computed tomography, MRI) provides useful information regarding the extent of tumor (intrahepatic and extrahepatic), as well as vascular and biliary involvement. Search should also be made to look for small satellite lesions while dealing with these neoplasms. If CCA arises peripherally in the liver parenchyma, it usually presents as well-defined mass with typical peripheral biliary dilatation distal to the tumor. Rarely, a diffusely infiltrating or sclerosing type can occur. The mass is usually heterogeneous but hypodense relative to the liver on unenhanced scans. There may be areas of altered attenuation in the mass because of the presence of mucinous material or necrosis. With intravenous contrast, heterogeneous enhancement is seen, often peripherally. The differential diagnostic considerations of such a mass would include hepatocellular carcinoma, biliary cystadenoma or cystadenocarcinoma, and metastases. Hepatocellular carcinoma is much more common than CCA and typically arises in cirrhotic livers. The serum α-fetoprotein is usually not elevated in CCA, but the bilirubin may be higher than typically seen with hepatocellular carcinoma. In addition, if intrahepatic biliary dilatation is associated with the mass, then IHC should be suspected over hepatocellular carcinoma. Portal vein invasion occurs less frequently with IHC than with hepatocellular carcinoma grossly. However, microscopically, portal vein invasion is common (89–90%). Biliary cystadenoma and cystadenocarcinoma may mimic this form of CCA, but they are usually more cystic than is CCA. Finally, metastases may have a similar appearance to this form of CCA and are far more common. Percutaneous needle biopsy is usually the only definite way to differentiate these lesions. If required, preoperative percutaneous biliary drainage may be required to decompress the FLR.

Treatment

Complete resection is the treatment of choice in patients who are fit to undergo surgery. Patients with distant metastatic disease or multiple intrahepatic metastases are not candidates for surgery. Patients with satellite lesions and lymph node involvement are not candidates for curative resection, but palliative resection can still be undertaken in patients with complications including bleeding and biliary obstruction. Even palliative resection in this setting can be undertaken with acceptable results in high volume centers. However, metastatic disease to celiac or retroperitoneal nodes is considered a contraindication to resection.

Role of liver transplant: In patients with peripheral or central CCA in the setting of chronic liver disease, if the tumor is picked up on routine screening in patients with cirrhosis, and provided there is no lymph node involvement or distant disease, liver transplant is a viable therapeutic option, with good survival results.

REFERENCES

1. Kuwayti K, Baggenstoss AH, Stauffer MH, Priestley JT. Carcinoma of the major intrahepatic and the extrahepatic bile ducts exclusive of the papilla of vater. Surg Gynecol Obstet. 1957;104:357-66.
2. Nakeeb A, Pitt HA, Sohn TA, Coleman J, Abrams RA, Piantadosi S, et al. Cholangiocarcinoma: a spectrum of intrahepatic, perihilar, and distal tumors. Ann Surg. 1996;224:463-75.
3. Jarnagin W. Cholangiocarcinoma of the extrahepatic bile ducts. Semin Surg Oncol. 2000;19:156-76.
4. Nagino M. Perihilar cholangiocarcinoma: a surgeon's viewpoint on current topics. J Gastroenterol. 2012;47(11):1165-76.
5. Edge SB, Byrd DR, Compton CC, Fritz AG, Greene FL, Trotti III A. Perihilar bile ducts. In: AJCC Cancer Staging Handbook, 7th edition. Chicago, IL: Springer; 2012. p. 718.
6. Farley DR, Weaver AL, Nagorney DM. "Natural history" of unresected cholangiocarcinoma: patient outcome after noncurative intervention. Mayo Clin Proc. 1995;70:425-9.
7. Pitt HA, Dooley WC, Yeo CJ, Cameron JL. Malignancies of the biliary tree. Current Prob Surg. 1995;32:1-90.
8. Hochwald SN, Burke EC, Jarnagin WR, Fong Y, Blumgart LH. Preoperative biliary stenting is associated with increased post-operative infectious complications in proximal cholangio-carcinoma. Arch Surg. 1999;134:261-6.
9. McPherson GA, Benjamin IS, Hodgson HJ, Bowley NB, Allison DJ, Blumgart LH. Preoperative percutaneous transhepatic biliary drainage: the results of a controlled trial. Br J Surg. 1984;71:371-5.

10. Wetter LA, Ring EJ, Pellegrini CA, Way LW. Differential diagnosis of sclerosing cholangiocarcinomas of the common hepatic duct (Klatskin tumors). Am J Surg. 1991;161:57-63.
11. Baer HU, Matthews JB, Schweizer WP, Gertsch P, Blumgart LH. Management of the Mirizzi syndrome and the surgical implications of cholecystcholedochal fistula. Br J Surg. 1990;77:743-5.
12. Callery MP, Strasberg SM, Doherty GM, Soper NJ, Norton JA. Staging laparoscopy with laparoscopic ultrasonography: optimizing respectability in hepatobiliary and pancreatic malignancy. J Am Coll Surg. 1997;185:33-9.
13. Cabooter M, Sas S, Laukens P. Mirizzi syndrome. Ned Tijdschr Geneeskd. 1990;134:708-11.
14. Hadjis NS, Collier NA, Blumgart LH. Malignant masquerade at the hilum of the liver. Br J Surg. 1985;72:659-61.
15. Saldinger PF, Blumgart LH. Resection of hilar cholangiocarcinoma—A European and United States experience. J Hepatobiliary Pancreat Surg. 2000;7:111-4.
16. Verbeek PC, van Leeuwen DJ, de Wit LT, Reeders JW, Smits NJ, Bosma A, et al. Benign fibrosing disease at the hepatic confluence mimicking Klatskin tumors. Surgery. 1992;112:866-71.
17. Rabinovitz M, Zajko AB, Hassanein T, Shetty B, Bron KM, Schade RR, et al. Diagnostic value of brush cytology in the diagnosis of bile duct carcinoma: a study in 65 patients with bile duct strictures. Hepatology. 1990;12:747-52.
18. Gibson RN, Yeung E, Thompson JN, Carr DH, Hemingway AP, Bradpiece HA, et al. Bile duct obstruction: radiologic evaluation of level, cause and respectability. Radiology. 1986;160:43-7.
19. Hann LE, Greatrex KV, Bach AM, Fong Y, Blumgart LH. Carcinoma of the hepatic hilus: sonographic findings. Am J Roentgenol. 1997;167:1017-21.
20. Okuda K, Ohto M, Tsuchiya Y. The role of ultrasound, percutaneous transhepatic cholangiography, computed tomographic imaging, and magnetic resonance imaging in the preoperative assessment of bile duct cancer. World J Surg. 1988;12:18-26.
21. Bach AM, Hann LE, Brown KT, Getrajdman GI, Herman SK, Fong Y, et al. Portal vein evaluation with US: comparison to angiography combined with CT arterial portography. Radiology. 1996;201:149-54.
22. Guthrie JA, Ward J, Robinson PJ. Hilar cholangiocarcinomas: T2 weighted spin echo and gadolinium enhanced FLASH MR imaging. Radiology. 1996;201:347-51.
23. Lee MG, Lee HJ, Kim MH, Kang EM, Kim YH, Lee SG, et al. Extrahepatic biliary diseases: 3D MR cholangiopancreaticography compared with endoscopic retrograde cholangiopancreaticography. Radiology. 1997;202:663-9.
24. Schwartz LH, Coakley FV, Sun Y, Blumgart LH, Fong Y, Panicek DM. Neoplastic pancreaticobiliary duct obstruction: evaluation with breath-hold MR cholangiopancreaticography. AJR Am J Roentgenol. 1998;170:1491-5.
25. Seo DW, Lee SK, Yoo KS, Kang GH, Kim MH, Suh DJ, et al. Cholangioscopic findings in bile duct tumors. Gastrointest Endosc. 2000;52:630-4.
26. Nimura Y, Kamiya J, Kondo S, Nagino M, Uesaka K, Oda K, et al. Aggressive preoperative management and extended surgery for hilar cholangiocarcinoma: Nagoya experience. J Hepatobiliary Pancreat Surg. 2000;7:155-62.
27. Nimura Y, Shionoya S, Hayakawa N, Kamiya J, Kondo S, Yasui A. Value of percutaneous transhepatic cholangioscopy (PTCS). Surg Endosc. 1988;2:213-9.
28. Nimura Y, Kamiya J, Hayakawa N, Shionoya S. Cholangioscopic differentiation of biliary strictures and polyps. Endoscopy. 1989;21(Suppl. 1):351-6.
29. Seo DW, Lee SK, Yoo KS, Kang GH, Kim MH, Suh DJ, et al. Cholangioscopic findings in bile duct tumors. Gastrointest Endosc. 2000;52:630-4.
30. Tischendorf JW, Krüger M, Trautwein C, Duckstein N, Schneider A, Manns MP, et al. Cholangioscopic characterization of dominant bile duct stenoses in patients with primary sclerosing cholangitis. Endoscopy. 2006;38:665-9.
31. Nimura Y, Hayakawa N, Kamiya J, Kondo S, Shionoya S. Hepatic segmentectomy with caudate lobe resection for bile duct carcinoma of the hepatic hilus. World J Surg. 1990;14:535-44.
32. Nimura Y. Staging of biliary carcinoma: cholangiography and cholangioscopy. Endoscopy. 1993;25:76-80.
33. Kim HJ, Kim MH, Lee SK, Yoo KS, Seo DW, Min YI. Tumor vessel: a valuable cholangioscopic clue of malignant biliary stricture. Gastrointest Endosc. 2000;52:635-8.
34. Nimura Y, Hayakawa N, Toyoda S, Iyomasa Y, Nakazawa S. Percutaneous transhepatic cholangioscopy. Stomach Intestine. 1981;16:681-9.
35. Kato M, Nimura Y, Kamiya J, Kondo S, Nagino M, Miyachi M, et al. Carcinoma of the common bile duct with superficial spread to the intrahepatic segmental bile ducts: a case report. Am Surg. 1997;63:943-7.
36. Iwahashi N, Hayakawa N, Yamamoto H, Maki A, Kawabata Y, Murayama A, et al. Mucosal bile duct carcinoma with superficial spread. J Hepatobil Pancreat Surg. 1998;5:221-5.
37. Sakamoto E, Nimura Y, Hayakawa N, Kamiya J, Kondo S, Nagino M, et al. Clinicopathological studies of mucin-producing cholangiocarcinoma. J Hepatobil Pancreat Surg. 1997;4:157-62.
38. Sakamoto E, Hayakawa N, Kamiya J, Kondo S, Nagino M, Kanai M, et al. Treatment strategy for mucin-producing intrahepatic cholangiocarcinoma: value of percutaneous transhepatic biliary drainage and cholangioscopy. World J Surg. 1999;23:1038-44.
39. Sano T, Kamiya J, Nagino M, Uesaka K, Kondo S, Kanai M, et al. Macroscopic classification and preoperative diagnosis of intrahepatic cholangiocarcinoma in Japan. J Hepatobil Pancreat Surg. 1999;6:101-7.
40. DeWitt J, Misra VL, Leblanc JK, McHenry L, Sherman S. EUS-guided FNA of proximal biliary strictures after negative ERCP brush cytology results. Gastrointest Endosc. 2006;64:325-33.
41. Harewood GC. Endoscopic tissue diagnosis of cholangiocarcinoma. Curr Opin Gastroenterol. 2008;24:627-30.
42. Heimbach JK, Gores GJ, Haddock MG, Alberts SR, Pedersen R, Kremers W, et al. Predictors of disease recurrence following neoadjuvant chemoradiotherapy and liver transplantation for unresectable perihilar cholangiocarcinoma. Transplantation. 2006;82:1703-7.
43. Rea DJ, Heimbach JK, Rosen CB, Haddock MG, Alberts SR, Kremers WK, et al. Liver transplantation with neoadjuvant chemoradiation is more effective than resection for hilar cholangiocarcinoma. Ann Surg. 2005;242:451-8.
44. Robles R, Figueras J, Turrion VS, Margarit C, Moya A, Varo E, et al. Spanish experience in liver transplantation for hilar and peripheral cholangiocarcinoma. Ann Surg. 2004;239:265-71.
45. Kadry Z, Mullhaupt B, Renner EL, Bauerfeind P, Schanz U, Pestalozzi BC, et al. Living donor liver transplantation and tolerance: a potential strategy in cholangiocarcinoma. Transplantation. 2003;76:1003-6.
46. Eloubeidi MA, Chen VK, Jhala NC, Eltoum IE, Jhala D, Chhieng DC, et al. Endoscopic ultrasound-guided fine needle aspiration biopsy of suspected cholangiocarcinoma. Clin Gastroenterol Hepatol. 2004;2:209-13.
47. Byrne MF, Gerke H, Mitchell RM, Stiffler HL, McGrath K, Branch MS, et al. Yield of endoscopic ultrasound-guided fine needle aspiration of bile duct lesions. Endoscopy. 2004;36:715-9.
48. Tamada K, Inui K, Menzel J. Intraductal ultrasonography of the bile duct system. Endoscopy. 2001;33:878-85.
49. Levy MJ, Vazquez-Sequeiros E, Wiersema MJ. Evaluation of the pancreaticobiliary ductal systems by intraductal US. Gastrointest Endosc. 2002;55:397-408.

50. Tamada K, Ido K, Ueno N, Kimura K, Ichiyama M, Tomiyama T. Preoperative staging of extrahepatic bile duct cancer with intraductal ultrasonography. Am J Gastroenterol. 1995;90:239-46.
51. Tamada K, Ido K, Ueno N, Ichiyama M, Tomiyama T, Nishizono T, et al. Assessment of portal vein invasion by bile duct cancer using intraductal ultrasonography. Endoscopy. 1995;27:573-8.
52. Tamada K, Ido K, Ueno N, Ichiyama M, Tomiyama T, Nishizono T, et al. Assessment of hepatic artery invasion by bile duct cancer using intraductal ultrasonography. Endoscopy. 1995;27:579-83.
53. Tamada K, Nagai H, Yasuda Y, Tomiyama T, Ohashi A, Wada S, et al. Transpapillary intraductal US prior to biliary drainage in the assessment of longitudinal spread of extrahepatic bile duct carcinoma. Gastrointest Endosc. 2001;53:300-7.
54. Stavropoulos S, Larghi A, Verna E, Battezzati P, Stevens P. Intraductal ultrasound for the evaluation of patients with biliary strictures and no abdominal mass on computed tomography. Endoscopy. 2005;37:715-21.
55. Tamada K, Tomiyama T, Wada S, Ohashi A, Satoh Y, Ido K, et al. Endoscopic transpapillary bile duct biopsy with the combination of intraductal ultrasonography in the diagnosis of biliary strictures. Gut. 2002;50:326-31.
56. Vazquez-Sequeiros E, Baron TH, Clain JE, Gostout CJ, Norton ID, Petersen BT, et al. Evaluation of indeterminate bile duct strictures by intraductal US. Gastrointest Endosc. 2002;56:372-9.
57. Ponchon T, Gagnon P, Berger F, Labadie M, Liaras A, Chavaillon A, et al. Value of endobiliary brush cytology and biopsies for the diagnosis of malignant bile duct stenosis: results of a prospective study. Gastrointest Endosc. 1995;42:565-72.
58. Pugliese V, Conio M, Nicolo G, Saccomanno S, Gatteschi B. Endoscopic retrograde forceps biopsy and brush cytology of biliary strictures: a prospective study. Gastrointest Endosc. 1995;42:520-6.
59. Kubota Y, Yamaguchi T, Tani K, Takaoka M, Fujimura K, Ogura M, et al. Anatomical variation of pancreatobiliary ducts in biliary stone diseases. Abdom Imaging. 1993;18:145-9.
60. Weber A, von Weyhern C, Fend F, Schneider J, Neu B, Meining A, et al. Endoscopic transpapillary brush cytology and forceps biopsy in patients with hilar cholangiocarcinoma. World J Gastroenterol. 2008;14:1097-101.
61. Bergquist A, Tribukait B, Glaumann H, Broome U. Can DNA cytometry be used for evaluation of malignancy and premalignancy in bile duct strictures in primary sclerosing cholangitis? J Hepatol. 2000;33:873-7.
62. Pitt HA, Nakeeb A, Abrams RA, Coleman J, Piantadosi S, Yeo CJ, et al. Perihilar cholangiocarcinoma: postoperative radiotherapy does not improve survival. Ann Surg. 1995;221:788-98.
63. Kondo S, Hirano S, Ambo Y, Tanaka E, Okushiba S, Morikawa T, et al. Forty consecutive resections of hilar cholangiocarcinoma with no postoperative mortality and no positive ductal margins: results of a prospective study. Ann Surg. 2004;240:95-101.
64. Nimura Y. Surgical anatomy of the biliary ducts. In: Rossi P (Ed). Biliary Tract Radiology. Berlin: Springer-Verlag; 1997. pp. 21-30.
65. Anderson CD, Rice MH, Pinson CW, Chapman WC, Chari RS, Delbeke D. Fluorodeoxyglucose PET imaging in the evaluation of gallbladder carcinoma and cholangiocarcinoma. J Gastronintest Surg. 2004;8:90-7.
66. Fritscher-Ravens A, Bohuslavizki KH, Broering DC, Jenicke L, Schäfer H, Buchert R, et al. FDG PET in the diagnosis of hilar cholangiocarcinoma. Nucl Med Commun. 2001;22:1277-85.
67. Kluge R, Schmidt F, Caca K, Barthel H, Hesse S, Georgi P, et al. Positron emission tomography with [(18)F] fluoro-2-deoxy-D glucose for diagnosis and staging of bile duct cancer. Hepatology. 2001;33:1029-35.
68. Kennedy TJ, Yopp A, Qin Y, Zhao B, Guo P, Liu F, et al. Role of preoperative biliary drainage of liver remnant prior to extended liver resection for hilar cholangiocarcinoma. HPB (Oxford). 2009;11:445-51.
69. Hatfield AR, Tobias R, Terblanche J, Girdwood AH, Fataar S, Harries-Jones R, et al. Preoperative external biliary drainage in obstructive jaundice: a prospective controlled trial. Lancet. 1982;2:896-9.
70. Lai EC, Tompkins RK, Mann LL, Roslyn JJ. Proximal bile duct cancer: quality of survival. Ann Surg. 1994;205:111-8.
71. McPherson GA, Benjamin IS, Hodgson HJ, Bowley NB, Allison DJ, Blumgart LH. Preoperative percutaneous transhepatic biliary drainage: results of a controlled trial. Br J Surg. 1984;71:371-5.
72. Pitt HA, Gomes AS, Lois JF, Mann LL, Deutsch LS, Longmire WP Jr. Does preoperative percutaneous biliary drainage reduce operative risk or increase hospital cost? Ann Surg. 1985;201:545-52.
73. Kloek JJ, van der Gaag NA, Aziz Y, Rauws EA, van Delden OM, Lameris JS, et al. Endoscopic and percutaneous preoperative biliary drainage in patients with suspected hilar cholangiocarcinoma. J Gastrointest Surg. 2010;14:119-25.
74. Pisters PW, Lee JE, Vauthey JN, Evans DB. Comment and perspective on Sewnath and colleagues' recent meta-analysis of the efficacy of preoperative biliary drainage for tumors causing obstructive jaundice. Ann Surg. 2003;237:594-5.
75. Clements WD, Diamond T, McCrory DC, Rowlands BJ. Biliar drainage in obstructive jaundice: experimental and clinical aspects. Br J Surg. 1993;80:834-42.
76. Andersen JR, Sørensen SM, Kruse A, Rokkjaer M, Matzen P. Randomized trial of endoscopic endoprosthesis versus operative bypass in malignant obstructive jaundice. Gut. 1989;30:1132-5.
77. Chang WH, Kortan P, Haber GB. Outcome of patients with bifurcation tumors who undergo unilateral versus bilateral hepatic duct drainage. Gastrointest Endosc. 1998;47:354-62.
78. Liu CL, Lai EC, Fan ST. Endoscopic retrograde cholangiopancreatography and endoscopic endoprosthesis insertion in patients with Klatskin tumors. Arch Surg. 1998;133:293-6.
79. Rerknimitr R, Kladcharoen N, Mahachai V, Kullavanijaya P. Results of endoscopic biliary drainage in hilar cholangiocarcinoma. J Clinical Gastroenterol. 2004;38:518-23.
80. Kawasaki S, Imamura H, Kobayashi A, Noike T, Miwa S, Miyagawa S. Results of surgical resection for patients with hilar bile duct cancer: application of extended hepatectomy after biliary drainage and hemihepatic portal vein embolization. Ann Surg. 2003;238:84-92.
81. Seyama Y, Kubota K, Sano K, Noie T, Takayama T, Kosuge T, et al. Long term outcome of extended hemihepatectomy for hilar bile duct cancer with no mortality and high survival rate. Ann Surg. 2003;238:73-83.
82. Nagino M, Hayakawa N, Nimura Y, Dohke M, Kitagawa S. Percutaneous transhepatic biliary drainage in patients with malignant biliary obstruction of the hepatic confluence. Hepatogastroenterology. 1992;39:296-300.
83. Nimura Y, Kamiya J, Kondo S, Nagino M, Kanai M. Technique for inserting multiple biliary drainage and management. Hepatogastroenterology. 1995;42:323-31.
84. Iyomasa S et al. Successful management of preoperative cholangitis by percutaneous transhepatic biliary drainage: case report of advanced gallbladder carcinoma with severe cholangitis. J Hepatobiliary Pancreat Surg. 1994;1:424-8.
85. Sakamoto E, Nimura Y, Hayakawa N, Kamiya J, Kondo S, Nagino M, et al. Case of bile duct carcinoma of the hepatic hilus with segmental obstructive cholangitis. Hepatogastroenterology. 1995;42:501-5.
86. De Baere T, Roche A, Vavasseur D, Therasse E, Indushekar S, Elias D, et al. Portal vein embolization: utility for inducing left hepatic lobe hypertrophy before surgery. Radiology. 1993;188:73-7.
87. Kinoshita H, Sakai K, Hirohashi K, Igawa S, Yamasaki O, Kubo S. Preoperative portal vein embolization for hepatocellular carcinoma. World J Surg. 1986;10:803-8.
88. Makuuchi M, Thai BL, Takayasu K, Takayama T, Kosuge T, Gunvén P, et al. Preoperative portal embolization to increase the safety of major hepatectomy for hilar bile duct carcinoma: a preliminary report. Surgery. 1990;107:521-7.

89. Williamson BW, Blumgart LH, McKellar NJ. Management of tumors of the liver: combined use of arteriography and venography in the assessment of resectability especially in hilar tumors. Am J Surg. 1980;139:210-5.
90. Blumgart LH, Hadjis NS, Benjamin IS, Beazley R. Surgical approaches to cholangiocarcinoma at confluence of hepatic ducts. Lancet. 1984;1:66-70.
91. Hoevels J, Ihse J. Percutaneous transhepatic portography in bile duct carcinoma: correlation with percutaneous transhepatic cholanhiography and angiography. Fortesch Roentgenstr. 1979;131: 140-50.
92. Launois B, Campion JP, Brissot P, Gosselin M. Carcinoma of the hepatic hilus: surgical management and the case for resection. Ann Surg. 1979;190:151-7.
93. Ebata T, Nagino M, Kamiya J, Uesaka K, Nagasaka T, Nimura Y. Hepatectomy with portal vein resection for hilar cholangio-carcinoma: audit of 52 consecutive cases. Ann Surg. 2003;238: 720-7.
94. Miyazaki M, Ito H, Nakagawa K, Ambiru S, Shimizu H, Shimizu Y, et al. Aggressive surgical approaches to hilar cholangiocarcinoma: hepatic or local resection? Surgery. 1998;123:131-6.
95. Nimura Y, Hayakawa N, Kamiya J, Maeda S, Kondo S, Yasui A, et al. Combined portal vein and liver resection for carcinoma of the biliary tract. Br J Surg. 1991;78:727-31.
96. Sakaguchi S, Nakamura S. Surgery of the portal vein in resection of cancer of the hepatic hilus. Surgery. 1986;99:344-9.
97. Bismuth H, Nakache R, Diamond T. Management strategies in resection for hilar cholangiocarcinoma. Ann Surg. 1992;215:31-8.
98. Bismuth H, Corlette MB. Intrahepatic cholangioenteric anastomosis in carcinoma of the hilus of the liver. Surg Gynecol Obstet. 1975;140:170-8.
99. Jarnagin WR, Fong Y, DeMatteo RP, Gonen M, Burke EC, Bodniewicz BJ, et al. Staging, resectability, and outcome in 225 patients with hilar cholangiocarcinoma. Ann Surg. 2001;234:507-17.
100. Sobin LH, Gospodarowicz MK, Wittekind, C. TNM Classification of Malignant Tumors, 7th edition. New York, NY: John Wiley & Sons; 2009.
101. Sobin LH. TNM: principles, history, and relation to other prognostic factors. Cancer. 2001;91:1589-92.
102. Burke EC. Hilar cholangiocarcinoma: patterns of spread, the importance of hepatic resections for curative operation, and a presurgical clinical staging system. Ann Surg. 1998;228:385-94.
103. Kondo S, Takada T, Miyazaki M, Miyakawa S, Tsukada K, Nagino M, et al. Guidelines for the management of biliary tract and ampullary carcinomas: surgical treatment. J Hepatobiliary Pancreat Surg. 2008;15:41-54.
104. DeOliveira ML, Cunningham SC, Cameron JL, Kamangar F, Winter JM, Lillemoe KD, et al. Cholangiocarcinoma: thirty-one-year experience with 564 patients at a single institution. Ann Surg. 2007;245:755-62.
105. Ito F, Agni R, Rettammel RJ, Been MJ, Cho CS, Mahvi DM, et al. Resection of hilar cholangiocarcinoma: concomitant liver resection decreases hepatic recurrence. Ann Surg. 2008;248:273-9.
106. Sakamoto E, Nimura Y, Hayakawa N, Kamiya J, Kondo S, Nagino M, et al. The pattern of infiltration at the proximal border of hilar bile duct carcinoma: a histologic analysis of 62 resected cases. Ann Surg. 1998;227:405-11.
107. Igami T, Nagino M, Oda K, Nishio H, Ebata T, Yokoyama Y, et al. Clinicopathologic study of cholangiocarcinoma with superficial spread. Ann Surg. 2009;249:296-302.
108. Nimura Y. Staging cholangiocarcinoma by cholangioscopy. HPB (Oxford). 2008;10:113-5.
109. Okumoto T, Sato A, Yamada T, Takase K, Matsuhashi T, Tsuda M, et al. Correct diagnosis of vascular encasement and longitudinal extension of hilar cholangiocarcinoma by four-channel multidetector-row computed tomography. Tohoku J Exp Med. 2009;217:1-8.
110. Clavien PA, Petrowsky H, DeOliveira ML, Graf R. Strategies for safer liver surgery and partial liver transplantation. N Engl J Med. 2007;356:1545-59.
111. Nagino M, Ando M, Kamiya J, Uesaka K, Sano T, Nimura Y. Liver regeneration after major hepatectomy for biliary cancer. Br J Surg. 2001;88:1084-91.
112. Makuuchi M, Thai BL, Takayasu K, Takayama T, Kosuge T, Gunven P, et al. Preoperative portal embolization to increase safety of major hepatectomy for hilar bile duct carcinoma: a preliminary report. Surgery. 1990;107:521-7.
113. Japanese Society of Biliary Surgery. General Rules for Surgical and Pathological Studies on Cancer of Biliary Tract, 5th edition. Tokyo, Japan: Kanehara; 2003.
114. Sakamoto Y, Sano T, Shimada K, Kosuge T, Kimata Y, Sakuraba M, et al. Clinical significance of reconstruction of the right hepatic artery for biliary malignancy. Langenbecks Arch Surg. 2006;391:203-8.
115. Jarnagin WR, Bowne W, Klimstra DS, Ben-Porat L, Roggin K, Cymes K, et al. Papillary phenotype confers improved survival after resection for hilar cholangiocarcinoma. Ann Surg. 2005;241: 703-12.
116. Cheng QB, Yi B, Wang JH, Jiang XQ, Luo XJ, Liu C, et al. Resection with total caudate lobectomy confers survival benefit in hilar cholangiocarcinoma of Bismuth type III and IV. Eur J Surg Oncol. 2012;38(12):1197-203.
117. Song SC, Choi DW, Kow AW, Choi SH, Heo JS, Kim WS, et al. Surgical outcomes of 230 resected hilar cholangiocarcinoma in a single centre. ANZ J Surg. 2013;83:268-74.
118. Cho MS, Kim SH, Park SW, Lim JH, Choi GH, Park JS, et al. Surgical outcomes and predicting factors of curative resection in patients with hilar cholangiocarcinoma: 10-year single-institution experience. Gastrointest Surg. 2012;16:1672-9.
119. Kow AW, Wook CD, Song SC, Kim WS, Kim MJ, Park HJ, et al. Role of caudate lobectomy in type III A and III B hilar cholangiocarcinoma: a 15-year experience in a tertiary institution. World J Surg. 2012;36:1112-21.
120. Ramesh H, Kuruvilla K, Venugopal A, Lekha V, Jacob G. Surgery for hilar cholangiocarcinoma: feasibility and results of parenchyma-conserving liver resection. Dig Surg. 2004;21:114-22.
121. Ebata T, Nagino M, Kamiya J, Uesaka K, Nagasaka T, Nimura Y. Hepatectomy with portal vein resection for hilar cholangio-carcinoma: audit of 52 consecutive cases. Ann Surg. 2003;238: 720-7.
122. Miyazaki M, Kato A, Ito H, Kimura F, Shimizu H, Ohtsuka M, et al. Combined vascular resection in operative resection for hilar cholangiocarcinoma: does it work or not? Surgery. 2007;141:581-8.
123. Ebata T, Yokoyama Y, Igami T, Sugawara G, Takahashi Y, Nimura Y, et al. Hepatopancreatoduodenectomy for cholangiocarcinoma: a single center review of 85 consecutive patients. Ann Surg. 2012;256:297-305.
124. Goss JA, Shackleton CR, Farmer DG, Arnaout WS, Seu P, Markowitz JS, et al. Orthotopic liver transplantation for primary sclerosing cholangitis. A 12-year single center experience. Ann Surg. 1997;225:472-81.
125. Sudan D, DeRoover A, Chinnakotla S, Fox I, Shaw B Jr, McCashland T, et al. Radiochemotherapy and transplantation allow long-term survival for nonresectable hilar cholangiocarcinoma. Am J Transplant. 2002;2:774-9.
126. Cameron JL, Pitt HA, Zinner MJ, Kaufman SL, Coleman J. Management of proximal cholangiocarcinoma by surgical resection and radiotherapy. Am J Surg. 1990;38:610-5.
127. Takada T, Amano H, Yasuda H, Nimura Y, Matsushiro T, Kato H, et al. Is postoperative adjuvant chemotherapy useful for gallbladder carcinoma? A phase III multicenter prospective randomized controlled trial in patients with resected pancreaticobiliary carcinoma. Cancer. 2002;95:1685-95.

128. Saxena R, Sikora SS, Kaushik SP. A triple bypass procedure for advanced carcinoma of the neck of gallbladder. British Journal of Surgery. 1995;82:394-5.
129. Bowling TE Galbraith SM, Hatfield AR, Solano J, Spittle MF. A retrospective comparison of endoscopic stenting alone with stenting and radiotherapy in non-resectable cholangiocarcinoma. Gut. 1996;39:852-5.
130. Ortner MA, Liebetruth J, Schreiber S, Hanft M, Wruck U, Fusco V, et al. Photodynamic therapy of nonresectable cholangiocarcinoma. Photodynamic Therapy: Gastroenterology. 1998;114:536-42.
131. Fritscher-Ravens A, Broering DC, Knoefel WT, Rogiers X, Swain P, Thonke F, et al. EUS-guided fine-needle aspiration of suspected hilar cholangiocarcinoma in potentially operable patients with negative brush cytology. Am J Gastroenterol. 2004;99:45-51.
132. Fong Y, Blumgart LH, Lin E, Fortner JG, Brennan MF. Outcome of treatment for distal bile duct cancer. Br J Surg. 1996;83:1712-5.
133. Yeo CJ, Cameron JL, Sohn TA, Lillemoe KD, Pitt HA, Talamini MA, et al. Six hundred fifty consecutive pancreaticoduodenectomies in the 1990s: pathology, complications and outcomes. Ann Surg. 1997;226:248-57.
134. Wade TP, Prasad CN, Virgo KS, Johnson FE. Experience with distal bile duct cancer in US Veterans Affairs Hospitals: 1987-1991. J Surg Oncol. 1997;64:242-5.
135. Becker CD, Glättli A, Maibach R, Baer HU. Percutaneous palliation of malignant obstructive jaundice with the Wallstent endoprosthesis: follow up and reintervention in patients with hilar and non-hilar obstruction. J Vasc Interv Radiol. 1993;4:597-604.

Index

Page numbers followed by *f* refer to figure, *fc* to flow chart and *t* refer to table

B

D

E

F

G

H

J

K

L

M

N

O

P

W

X

Z

TEXTBOOK OF
SURGICAL GASTROENTEROLOGY

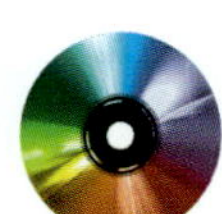

System requirements:

- Operating System—Windows Vista or above
- Web Browser—Internet Explorer 8 or above, Google Chrome and Mozilla Firefox
- Essential plugins—Java and PDF Reader
  - Facing problems in viewing content—it may be, your system does not have java enabled
  - You can test Java and download PDF reader by using the links from the help section of the **CD/DVD**

Accompanying **DVD-ROMs** is playable only in Computer and not in DVD player. CD/DVD has autorun function—it may take few seconds to load on your computer. If it does not work for you, then follow the steps below to access the contents manually:

- Click on my computer
- Select the CD/DVD drive and click open/explore—this will show list of files in the CD/DVD
- Find and double click file—"launch.html"

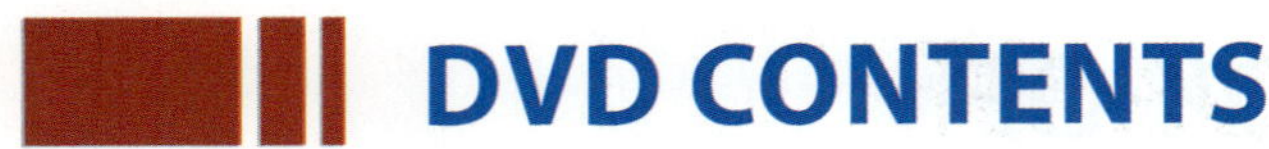

DVD CONTENTS

(Videos have no voice over)

TEXTBOOK OF
SURGICAL GASTROENTEROLOGY

VOLUME 2

Editor

PK Mishra

MS PhD

Professor

Govind Ballabh Pant Institute of
Postgraduate Medical Education and
Research

New Delhi, India

Foreword

Samiran Nundy

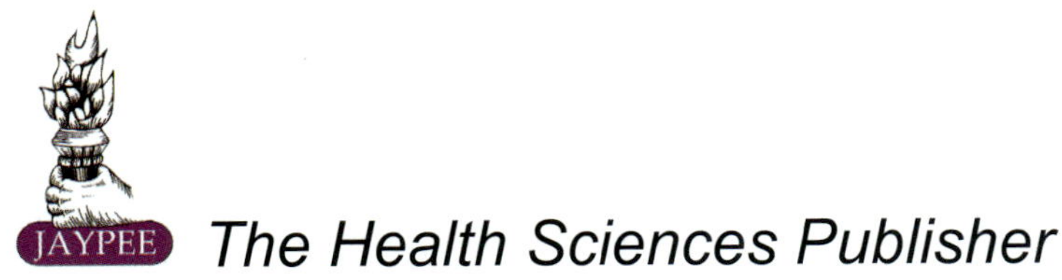

New Delhi | London | Philadelphia | Panama

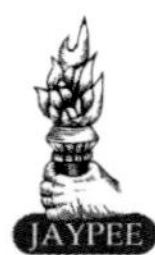

Jaypee Brothers Medical Publishers (P) Ltd.

Headquarters
Jaypee Brothers Medical Publishers (P) Ltd.
4838/24, Ansari Road, Daryaganj
New Delhi 110 002, India
Phone: +91-11-43574357
Fax: +91-11-43574314
E-mail: jaypee@jaypeebrothers.com

Overseas Offices
J.P. Medical Ltd.
83, Victoria Street, London
SW1H 0HW (UK)
Phone: +44-20 3170 8910
Fax: +44(0) 20 3008 6180
E-mail: info@jpmedpub.com

Jaypee-Highlights Medical Publishers Inc.
City of Knowledge, Bld. 237, Clayton
Panama City, Panama
Phone: +1 507-301-0496
Fax: +1 507-301-0499
E-mail: cservice@jphmedical.com

JP Medical Inc.
325, Chestnut Street
Suite 412
Philadelphia, PA 19106, USA
Phone: +1 267-519-9789
E-mail: support@jpmedus.com

Jaypee Brothers Medical Publishers (P) Ltd.
17/1-B, Babar Road, Block-B, Shaymali
Mohammadpur, Dhaka-1207
Bangladesh
Mobile: +08801912003485
E-mail: jaypeedhaka@gmail.com

Jaypee Brothers Medical Publishers (P) Ltd.
Bhotahity, Kathmandu, Nepal
Phone: +977-9741283608
E-mail: kathmandu@jaypeebrothers.com

Website: www.jaypeebrothers.com
Website: www.jaypeedigital.com

Inquiries for bulk sales may be solicited at: jaypee@jaypeebrothers.com

Textbook of Surgical Gastroenterology (2 Volumes)

First Edition: **2016**

ISBN: 978-93-5152-998-9

Printed at Replika Press Pvt. Ltd.

Contents

VOLUME 1

SECTION 1 General

SECTION 2 Esophagus

SECTION 3 Stomach, Duodenum, Small Intestine and Retroperitoneum

SECTION 4 Pancreas

SECTION 5 Gallbladder and Bile Ducts

VOLUME 2

SECTION 6 Liver

SECTION 7 Spleen

SECTION 8 Colon, Rectum and Anal Canal

SECTION 9 Liver Transplantation

SECTION 10 Miscellaneous

SECTION 6

Liver

CHAPTER 63

Surgical Anatomy of the Liver

Supriyo Ghatak, Anshuman Ray

INTRODUCTION

Precise knowledge of hepatic anatomy is a must for successful performance of operation on liver. It is the largest gland and the second largest organ of the body preceded only by the skin. The volume of the liver is variable in accordance with body size, age and sex. It weighs around 1,500 g, contributing 2.5% of the adult weight. The size of liver increases steadily (from childhood) and stabilizes at the age of 18 years. After middle age it starts decreasing slowly once again.[1]

Structurally, the liver is a wedge shaped highly vascular organ, reddish brown in color, soft in consistency and moves with respiration. Its major bulk is located in the right hypochondrium (right lobe) but it reaches to upper part of the epigastrium and adjoining part of the left hypochondrium (left lobe). It lies protected under the ribcage, under the diaphragm. The upper border of the liver is at 4th/5th intercostal space.

The peritoneum envelops the whole of the liver except on the posterior aspect. At this area, called the Bare area, peritoneal layers separate to form left triangular ligament and the coronary ligament. The right leaf of the lesser omentum joins the left layer of the falciform ligament to form the upper and lower layers of the left triangular ligament respectively. The right triangular ligament is formed by the right layer of the falciform ligament and posterior peritoneum to form the right triangular ligament.

EMBRYOLOGY

An out-pouching (hepatic bud or diverticulum) from the terminal part of the primitive foregut develops into the liver and bile ducts. This hepatic diverticulum or liver bud rapidly proliferates and penetrates the septum transversum. The connection between foregut and primordial liver further narrows down and forms bile ducts. Cystic duct and gallbladder originate from a small ventral bud from the bile duct. The presence of the hepatic mesenchyme derived from the septum transversum is essential for the differentiation of the endodermal cells of the hepatic bud into hepatocytes.

Notch signaling seems to have a role in mediating the decision as to whether a hepatoblast becomes a hepatocyte or a cholangiocyte. Mutations in *NOTCH* ligand *JAGGED1* or in the receptor *NOTCH2* are associated with autosomal dominant *Alagille Syndrome* with a dearth of bile ducts. Throughout prenatal development, hepatocytes proliferate mainly by autocrine mechanisms. However, postnatally, migration and proliferation of hepatocytes require extraneous growth factors, viz. *Hgf* and *Egf*.[2]

The epithelial liver cords differentiate into plates of liver cells that branch and anastomose with one another and form the liver parenchyma. Cardiogenic mesoderm, endothelium, and the septum transversum mesenchymal cells emit growth factor signals, viz. *Vegfs*, *Bmps* and *Fgfs* that are required for liver parenchymal development.[2]

In addition to the development of the fibroareolar stroma of the liver mesenchyme of the septum transversum also gives rise to the hematopoietic cells, Kupffers cells and connective tissue cells. The growth of the liver plates within the septum transversum disturbs the longitudinal course of the vitelline and umbilical veins. Eventually these vessels break up into the capillary network and join secondarily with the hepatic sinusoids which develop in situ between the plates of the liver cells.

The portion of the ventral mesogastrium which is between the diaphragm, ventral abdominal wall and the liver is thinned out as the coronary, triangular and falciform ligaments of the liver. The umbilical vein gets obliterated and persists as the ligamentum teres hepatis in the falciform ligament.

The part of the ventral mesogastrium extending from the liver to the stomach and the foregut part of the duodenum persists as the lesser omentum. The mesoderm on the surface of the liver differentiates into visceral peritoneum except on its cranial surface. Bare area of the liver is not covered by the peritoneum and is in contact with the diaphragm. It is clothed by the Glisson's hepatic capsule developed from the ventral mesogastrium.

The extensive enlargement of the liver in the intrauterine life is attributed partly to an abundance of oxygenated blood, which stimulates its profuse growth as well as the hematopoietic function of the fetal liver. Hematopoiesis attains its maximal activity in the liver toward 6–7th months. This activity regresses rapidly in the last 2 months of pregnancy, and only a few disseminated hematopoietic islands remain at birth. One group of transcription factors important in facilitation of the hepatic functions near birth from a hematopoietic organ to a metabolic and detoxifying organ is the *hepatic nuclear factor (Hnf)* family. Other transcription factors that are involved in the maturation and functional change of the liver include *C/EBPα, OncostatinM, Hgf* and *Tgfβ*.[2]

ARCHITECTURE OF THE LIVER

The structure of the liver in terms of a functional unit may be visualized as:

i. Classic lobule
ii. Portal lobule
iii. Liver acinus.

The alterations in the initial arrangement of the liver cells as portal lobules to the classical liver lobules suggest that primarily the liver is exocrine in function, but in the later part of development it shows greater importance as an endocrine organ. The structural components of the liver include:

- *Parenchyma:* Consists of structured arrangement of hepatocytes. In children up to 6 years, the liver cells are arranged in two plates while in adult they are normally one cell thick and separated by sinusoidal capillaries.
- *Connective tissue stroma:* Continuous with the Glisson's capsule and establish a passageway for lymphatics, nerves, vessels and bile ducts.
- *Sinusoidal capillaries (sinusoids):* Form the vascular channels amid the hepatocytes.
- *Perisinusoidal spaces of Disse:* In between the sinusoidal endothelium and hepatocytes.

Classic Lobule

The classic lobule is the accustomed way to outline the hepatic architecture based on the circulation of the hepatic artery and portal vein within the organ. It consists of anastomosing single plate of hepatocytes, separated by a sinusoidal arrangement. Mixed arterial and portal blood flows in these sinusoids to perfuse the cells and drain into a large terminal *central vein* at the center of the lobule.

The basic structure of the hepatic lobules is hexagonal with portal triads at the angles and central vein at the center. The cells are arranged in the form of plates which radiate to the peripheries from the central vein. These *portal triads* consist of branches of the hepatic artery and portal vein and branches of the bile duct system. However, it is a misnomer because one or more vessels of the lymphatic drainage system of the liver always travel with the vein, artery and the bile duct. At the edges of the portal canal, between the connective tissue and the hepatocytes, is a small periportal connective tissue space which is known as the *Space of Mall*.[3]

Portal Lobule

The model of a portal lobule allows a structural comparison of the exocrine function of the liver to that of other exocrine glands. The morphologic axis of the portal lobule is the interlobular bile duct of the portal triad of the "Classic lobule". It is formed by drawing imaginary lines in between the closest central veins to the portal triad that approximately define a triangular block of tissue that includes those portions of three classic lobules that separates the bile that drains into its axial duct.

Liver Acinus

This concept allows a description of the exocrine secretory function of the liver comparable to that of the portal lobule. The liver acinus represents the smallest functional unit of the hepatic parenchyma that delivers the best correlation of perfusion, metabolic activity and hepatic pathology. In a two dimensional view the liver acinus occupies parts of adjacent classic lobules whose short axis is between the portal triads lying along the border of two classical lobules. Line joining the two central veins closest to short axis constitutes the long axis.

The hepatocytes in each liver acinus are described as being arranged in three concentric elliptical zones surrounding the short axis.[3]

Zone 1 is closest to the short axis and corresponds to the periphery of the classic lobules.

Zone 2 lies intermediate to zone 1 and zone 3.

Zone 3 is farthest from the short axis and closest to the central vein. This zone corresponds to the most central part of the classic lobule that surrounds the terminal hepatic vein.

The zonation is vital due to vascular perfusion pattern of the hepatocytes. It helps interpret the degeneration, regeneration, ischemic and toxic exposure of the liver parenchyma. Cells in zone 1 are the first to receive oxygen, nutrients and toxins from the sinusoidal blood and are the first to show morphologic changes after bile duct occlusion (bile stasis). These cells are also the last to die if circulation is impaired and the first to regenerate. Cells in zone 3 are the first to show fat accumulation and centrilobular ischemic necrosis in situations of reduced perfusion and the last to respond to toxic substances and bile stasis. Cells in zone 2 have functional and morphologic characteristics intermediate to the two zones.[3]

Perisinusoidal Space of Disse

The *perisinusoidal space of Disse* is the pathway for liver secretion other than bile. It lies between the basal surfaces of endothelial and Kupffer cells lining the sinusoids and the hepatocytes. It receives lipoproteins and proteins synthesized in the hepatocytes. Plasma from this space drains to the *Space of Mall*, to enter the lymphatic capillaries and travel with portal triads to the hilum of the liver.

Ito cells (stellate cells) which are primarily the storehouses for vitamin A (in the form of retinyl esters within cytoplasmic lipid droplets) are found in perisinusoidal space.[3] In chronic inflammation or cirrhosis, stellate cells lose their lipid and vitamin A storage capability and exhibit characteristics of myofibroblasts that synthesize and deposit types I and III collagen within the perisinusoidal space resulting in liver fibrosis. During cell contraction, the cytoplasmic desmin and α-actin filaments of the

Ito cells increase the vascular resistance within the sinusoids by constricting the vascular channels, leading to portal hypertension. Moreover, the stellate cells play a role in reconstructing the extracellular matrix subsequent to hepatic impairment.[3]

SURGICAL ANATOMY

Anatomical Lobes of the Liver

Topographically liver is divided into four lobes: (1) right, (2) left, (3) quadrate and (4) caudate. The attachment of the falciform ligament on the anterosuperior surface separates the liver into a larger right lobe and a smaller left lobe (Fig. 1). On the visceral surface quadrate lobe is demarcated by gallbladder fossa, porta hepatis and ligamentum teres hepatis. The caudate lobe is marked by the groove of the inferior vena cava (IVC), porta hepatis and ligamentum venosum.

Functional anatomy of the liver: What described above does not help in understanding the functional independence of the liver segments. The functional anatomy was well elucidated by Couinaud in 1959. The following discussion is based on the same.

The three major hepatic veins divide the liver into four sectors (Fig. 2). The planes in which hepatic veins travel are called portal scissurae. Cantlie's line divides the liver in two functional parts, right and left and they are independent in terms of arterial, portal supply and biliary drainage. Externally this plane is marked from the gallbladder fossa to the left of the IVC. It is this plane in which middle hepatic vein travels. The plane containing the right and left hepatic vein is called the right and left portal scissurae respectively.

The liver is placed in the right upper quadrant in such a plane that right lobe is oriented more anteroposteriorly and the left lobe more mediolaterally. Therefore the right and the left scissurae divide the right lobe into anterior and posterior sectors and left lobe into anteromedial and posterolateral sectors respectively. The right portal scissura from the right margin of the IVC and follows the upper layer of the coronary ligament to a point on the inferior margin about midway between gallbladder fossa and the right margin of the liver.

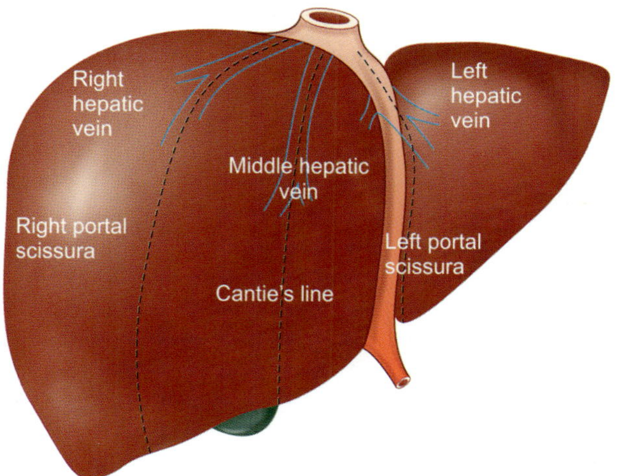

Figure 2 Three scissurae of the liver

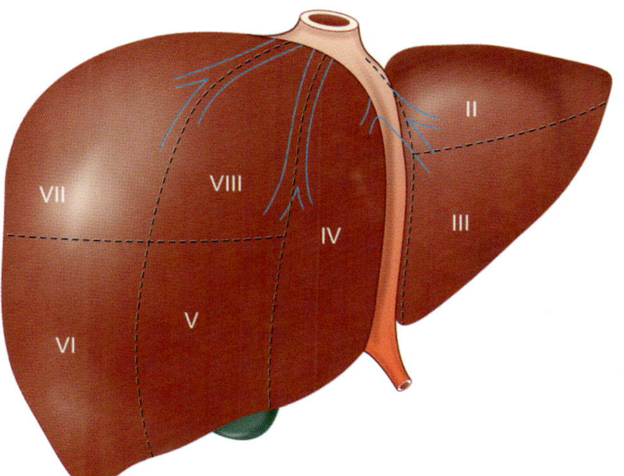

Figure 3 Segment-based anatomy of the liver

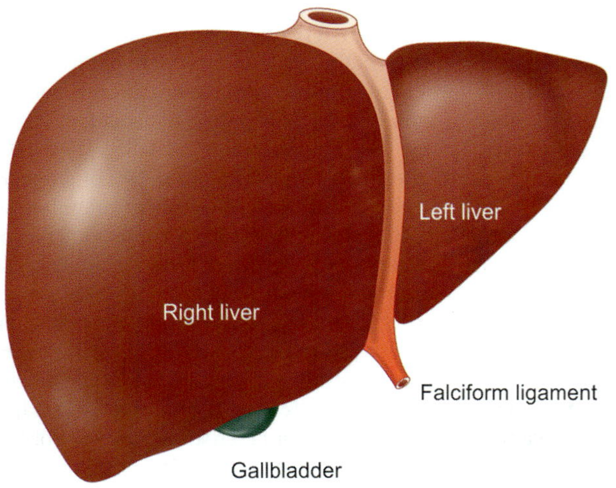

Figure 1 The classical description of liver anatomy

Each sector is subdivided into segments based on their independent portal triad (containing a branch of portal vein and hepatic artery and drained by a tributary of a bile duct). There are eight segments. Falciform ligament divides the left anterior sector into a median segment (segment IV or the quadrate lobe), and a lateral segment or segment III. Left posterolateral sector contains only one segment, i.e. segment II. Segment IV is subdivided into superior segment IVa and inferior segment IVb by the portal branches (Figs 3 and 4).

The caudate lobe or segment I lies posteriorly straddling the vena cava with a constant left portion and variable right portion as caudate process. Caudate lobe receives blood supply from both the left and right portal triads and drained by tributaries into both bile ducts. It drains directly into the vena cava via short hepatic veins. It is possible to individually remove each of these segments without jeopardizing the vascular flow or biliary drainage of the remaining segments.

The Brisbane terminology of hepatic anatomy and resection is given in Table 1.

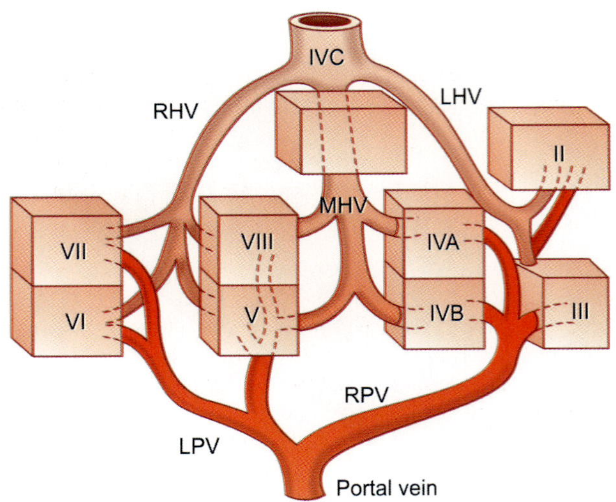

Figure 4 The schematic representation of various segments of the liver in relation to portal vein tributaries and hepatic venous tributaries

Table 1: The Brisbane 2000 terminology of hepatic anatomy and resection from the Terminology Committee of the International Hepato-Pancreato-Biliary Association. Available at: *www.ihpba.org* (liver resection guidelines)

Terminology	*Segments*
Right anterior section	V, VIII
Right posterior section	VI, VII
Left lateral section	II, III
Left medial section	IV
Left hepatic lobe	II, III, IV
Right hepatic lobe	V, VI, VII, VIII

HEPATIC VASCULATURE

The liver has a dual blood supply, approximately 70% from portal vein and 30% from the hepatic artery and in a similar ration oxygen is supplied by these systems.

The portal vein along with the artery and bile duct enters the liver with the tough Glissonian sheath around it. This point is important to differentiate a portal vein tributary from a hepatic vein tributary as the latter lacks this sheath. Sinusoids are the place where exchange of substances between blood and hepatocytes occurs. The sinusoids lead to a central vein that in turn empties into sublobular veins. Blood ultimately drains into the vena cava through the hepatic veins.

Portal Vein

The portal vein is about 7–10 cm long and between 0.8 and 1.4 cm in diameter. Superior mesenteric vein and splenic vein join behind the neck of the pancreas to form portal vein. It is without any valves therefore the pressure anywhere in the portal venous system will remain the same. It lies posterior to bile duct and the hepatic artery in the hepatoduodenal ligament and in general this arrangement continues within the liver too. The portal vein bifurcates into right and left branches just outside the liver at porta. The right branch is short and lies anteriorly to the caudate process of the caudate lobe. Before entering into the parenchyma of the liver the right branch gives off a branch to caudate lobe, this branch has to be actively searched for before encircling the right branch during porta dissection to prevent troublesome bleeding. On entering the liver parenchyma right branch soon divides into the anterior and posterior segmental branches. Each segmental branch further divides into superior and inferior subsegmental branches to serve the respective parenchymal subsegments.

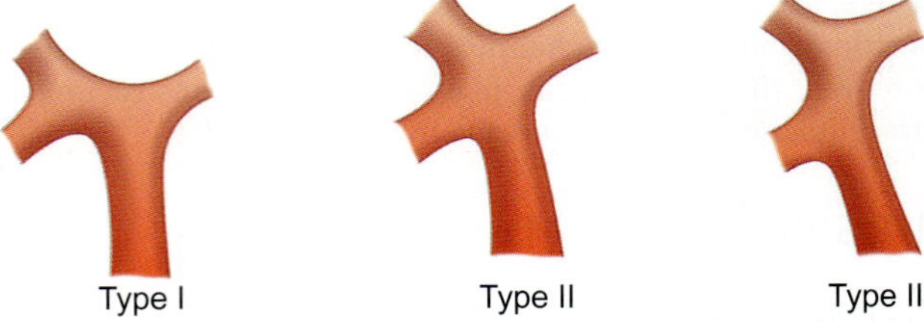

Figure 5 Variations in portal vein confluence

In 88.8% of cases there is a short right branch (type I), other less common variations are trifurcation of right anterior (type II), right posterior and left branch and right anterior branch arising from left branch (type III) (Fig. 5).[4]

The left portal vein is longer and its course can be divided into transverse and umbilical parts. A branch to caudate lobe is given by the transverse part after which it turns anteriorly at the umbilical fissure. It terminates in a cul-de-sac joining with the ligamentum teres. From there the left branch divides into medial and lateral segmental branches, each dividing into superior and inferior subsegmental branches.

Hepatic Artery

The *hepatic artery* carries oxygenated blood to the lower hilum of the liver. It arises most of the times from celiac trunk (86%), but may arise from the superior mesenteric artery (2.9%), the aorta (1.1%) or the left gastric artery.[5] It courses at along the superior border of pancreas. After giving off the gastroduodenal artery it continues as proper hepatic artery and turns upward toward the liver hilum in the hepatoduodenal ligament. Here it lies to the left of bile duct and anterior to the portal vein. It divides into right and left hepatic artery. The right branch usually turns behind the hepatic duct and in front of the portal vein to enter the liver. In the triangle between cystic duct and common bile duct (hepatocystic triangle) it gives off cystic artery.

Aberrant hepatic arteries are found in about 45% of subjects.[6] Sometimes they are in addition to the conventional branches and called "accessory" whereas sole supplying aberrant branches are called "replaced" arteries. In surgeries of liver or surrounding organs preoperative arterial reconstructions on CT scans provide clear path of these arteries. Left hepatic artery may originate from the left gastric artery in approximately 25-30% of cases.[5,7] During surgery lesser omentum needs to inspected and palpated to detect this variation. Right hepatic artery may arise from superior mesenteric artery in 17% of cases in which case it travels posteriolaterally to the common bile duct in the hepatoduodenal ligament.[7] While encircling the bile duct this variant needs to be protected to prevent ischemia to the right side of the liver.

Hepatic Vein

Three major hepatic veins drain obliquely to the inferior vena from the posterosuperior surface of the liver. The right hepatic vein is of larger caliber than the middle and left hepatic veins and has a shorter (1 cm) extrahepatic portion. The middle and left hepatic veins usually join together to form a common channel that runs extrahepatically for about 2 cm before emptying into the left side of the anterior surface of the IVC. There are 5-50 short hepatic veins draining from the posterior surface of the liver directly to the IVC, some of them may be large and surgically significant in graft implantation during liver transplantation. The middle vein anatomy is also very important in liver transplantation. Most commonly (70%) observed pattern is equal drainage from segments IV, V and VIII via large branches that join to form the middle hepatic vein. During living donor operation large branches (>5 mm) from segments V or VIII should be preserved and reimplanted for venous outflow preservation during right liver graft harvesting.

The umbilical vein runs beneath the falciform ligament between the left and middle hepatic veins and usually empties into the left hepatic vein.

Intrahepatic Bile Duct

The left hepatic duct drains the segments II, III and IV, whereas the segments V-VIII are drained by right hepatic duct. The orientation of the bile ducts and portal vein is the same as at the hepatoduodenal ligament, i.e. duct is above the portal vein. The caudate lobe is unique as it drains into both right and left hepatic ducts via several ducts. The left hepatic duct has a longer extrahepatic course and at the base of the quadrate lobe (segment IV) joins with the short right duct. The confluence usually lies anterior to the portal vein bifurcation. As describe earlier the confluence is in the Glisson's sheath with the portal vein. It fuses with the connective tissue at the base of the quadrate lobe known as hilar plate. This plate can be raised to expose the extrahepatic bile duct during surgery.

Lymphatics

There are two lymphatic networks in the liver. Superficial one is located within the Glisson's capsule and lymph flows to the internal thoracic artery and mediastinal lymph nodes, across the bare area of liver or foramen of Morgagni. Some lymphatics flow toward paracardial lymph nodes and celiac lymph nodes. Majority of the lymphatics reach the hilar lymph nodes, from there toward aortic nodes. The deep network either follows the hepatic veins and reaches the lateral phrenic nerve nodes or follows the portal vein branches and reaches the hilum.

PHYSIOLOGICAL CONSIDERATIONS

The hepatobiliary system exhibits several structural and physiological features that conduct a vast range of biochemical & metabolic activities, synthesizing and sharing substrates and energy between different metabolic systems.

The liver is especially important in preserving a normal blood glucose concentration mainly by contributing to storage of glycogen, gluconeogenesis as well as conversion of galactose and fructose to glucose.

Almost every cell of the body can metabolize fat but fatty acid β-oxidation, synthesis of phospholipids, cholesterol and most lipoproteins, viz. VLDL/LDL/HDL, occur mainly in the liver. In protein metabolism liver synthesizes and deaminates amino acids, forms urea for removal of ammonia and forms essentially 90% of all plasma proteins with the exception of part of the gamma globulin.[8,9]

The liver is an important site for uptake, storage and distribution of vitamins and nutrients. Liver has vitamin A stores which can run for approximately 10 months, vitamin B12 for at least 1 year and vitamin D for 3-4 months.[8] When vitamin A levels in the blood decrease, the liver mobilizes its storage sites in the hepatic stellate cells. Vitamin A is then released into the circulation in the form of retinol bound to retinol binding protein (RBP). The liver plays an important role in vitamin D metabolism by converting vitamin D3 to D25 hydroxycholecalciferol, the predominant form of circulating vitamin D.[3]

Except for the iron in hemoglobin of the blood, by far the greatest proportion of iron is stored in the liver. It synthesizes almost all glycoproteins involved in iron transport and metabolism such as haptoglobin, transferrin and hemopexin.[3] The Apoferritin-ferritin system of the liver acts as iron storage medium within the hepatocyte cytoplasm in the form of ferritin and acts as buffer.

Liver forms the coagulation components including fibrinogen, prothrombin, Factor VII as well vitamin K required in hepatic synthesis of prothrombin and several clotting factors.

Since the liver serves as the first station for most nutrients absorbed across the gastrointestinal tract, it serves as a filtration port for degradation of non-hydrophilic drugs, hormones and toxins into more soluble forms by oxidation and conjugation so that the final conjugated product can be easily eliminated by the kidney. Finally, liver forms a major route of calcium excretion into the bile and through feces.[9]

As an endocrine gland, the liver modifies the structure and function of many hormones, viz. thyroxine, growth hormone, insulin and glucagon while the exclusive exocrine function of liver is production of bile.

Bilirubin Metabolism

Bilirubin pigment is primarily a degraded product, formed by breakdown of hemoglobin in macrophages of the spleen and bone marrow, and to a lesser extent by Kupffer cells of hepatic sinusoids. The hemoglobin released from destruction of senescent erythrocytes is phagocytosed and converted by the reticuloendothelial system of the body. The first substrate formed is biliverdin which is rapidly reduced to unconjugated bilirubin and gradually released from the macrophages into plasma. This bilirubin immediately combines strongly with plasma albumin and is transported to the liver where it is absorbed from the plasma in the Space of Disse. Bilirubin is rendered water soluble by conjugation of 80% of the bilirubin with glucuronic acid by the enzyme glucuronyl transferase to form bilirubin glucuronide, and 20% with sulfate and other substances. In these forms the bilirubin is excreted from the hepatocytes by an active transporter known as multidrug resistance protein 2 (MRP 2)[9] into the bile canaliculi and then into the intestine.

In the intestine, almost half of the conjugated bilirubin is converted by bacterial action into urobilinogen. The intestinal mucosa is relatively permeable to unconjugated bilirubin and urobilinogen. There is an enterohepatic circulation of bile pigment as part of the urobilinogen is reabsorbed into the capillaries of the intestine and drain into the portal system. As the blood containing reabsorbed urobilinogen passes along the sinusoids of the liver, the urobilinogen is taken up by the hepatocytes. Most of it is re-excreted into the intestine and approximately 5% is excreted into the urine. Oxidized form of it in urine is known as urobilin and correspondingly oxidized form in feces is stercobilin.

Disorders of bilirubin metabolism will result in either conjugated hyperbilirubinemia (Dubin-Johnson and Rotor's syndrome), or unconjugated hyperbilirubinemia (Crigler-Najjar Type II and Gilbert's syndromes).

There is said to be an enterohepatic circulation of steroid hormones as well. The hormones produced by the adrenal cortex and the sex glands are constantly absorbed from the blood by hepatocytes and metabolized to different extents which are partly secreted into the bile. Some hormone may be subsequently reabsorbed into the bloodstream from the bile in the intestine.[8]

REFERENCES

1. Standring S, Borley NR (Eds). Liver. Gray's Anatomy: The Anatomical Basis of Clinical Practice, 40th edition. Spain: Churchill Livingstone Elsevier; 2011. p. 1163.
2. Schoenwolf GC, Bleyl SB, Brauer PR, Francis West PH. Larsen's Human Embryology, 4th edition. Churchill Livingstone Elsevier; 2009. p. 449.
3. Ross MH, Pawlina W. Histology: A Text & Atlas,5th edition. Philadelphia: Lippincott Williams & Wilkins; 2006. pp. 579-86.
4. Couinaud C. Surgical Anatomy of the Liver Revisited. 1989.
5. Van Damme JP, Bonte J. The Branches of the Celiac Trunk. Acta Anat. 1985;122:110-4.
6. Smith R, Suzuki T, Nakayasu A, Kauabe K, et al. (Eds). Surgical significance of anatomic variations of the hepatic artery. Am J Surg. 1971;122:505-12.
7. Michels NA. Newer anatomy of the liver and variant blood supply and collateral circulation. Am J Surg. 1966;112:337-47.
8. Hall JE. The Liver as an organ. Guyton & Hall's Text Book of Medical Physiology, 12th edition. Philadelphia: Elsevier Saunders; 2011. pp. 839-41.
9. Barett KE, Barman S, Boitano S, Brooks HL. Transport & metabolic functions of liver. Overview of gastrointestinal function & regulation. Ganong's Review of Medical Physiology, 23rd edition. Tata McGraw Hill; 2010. pp. 438,479-83.

CHAPTER 64

Liver Function Tests

Kaushal Madan, Pankaj Tyagi

INTRODUCTION

Liver is large organ and carries out multitude of functions including synthesis, metabolism, detoxification and excretion of several intrinsic and extrinsic compounds. Thus, diseases of the liver can result in changes in amounts of a large variety of substances in the body fluids. Hence, a careful measurement and interpretation of these chemicals can provide useful information about the presence, severity, nature and etiology of liver injury or dysfunction. Also, serial measurements may allow assessment of the course of liver disease and monitoring of therapy. However, because of the large functional capacity of the liver, some tests may remain normal till very late in the course of liver disease.

Liver function tests (LFTs) may be broadly classified as tests depicting hepatocyte injury, tests demonstrating cholestasis, tests depicting liver synthetic capacity and tests assessing metabolic capacity of the liver (Box 1).

BOX 1 Points to remember regarding LFT

- Single part of LFT is not the representative of whole LFT
- Always order full LFT at baseline
- Many time serial LFTs are required to make meaningful conclusion
- High bilirubin alone without any other abnormality will not represent hepatobiliary abnormality

TESTS DEPICTING HEPATOCYTE INJURY

Hepatocytes injury induces a release of hepatocellular enzymes into the blood, either due to disruption of these cells or through leakage across the cell membrane, leading to elevation of blood level of these enzymes. Estimation of their blood levels provides an excellent initial screening tool for assessing the presence of liver injury. The enzymes most commonly measured are the aminotransferases [aspartate aminotransferase (AST) or serum glutamic oxaloacetate transaminase (SGOT), alanine aminotransferase (ALT) or serum glutamic pyruvate transaminase (SGPT) and alkaline phosphatase (ALP)]. These enzymes are normally present in the blood in small quantities. Elevation of their serum levels is a function of increase in the rate of their release into the serum from the damaged liver cells. Differential pattern and degree of liver enzyme elevation may provide a clue to the etiology of liver injury, and may at times provide information that guides therapy and prognosis.

Aminotransferases

The elevation of these enzymes usually signifies hepatic necroinflammation. But these enzymes are also present in other body tissues, such as skeletal and cardiac muscle, kidneys, brain, lungs, leucocytes and erythrocytes. So, a rise in these enzymes may not necessarily point toward the presence of liver disease. Rise of ALT has greater specificity for hepatobiliary disease than that of AST. Thus, elevation of AST levels alone (without ALT elevation) with no other evidence of hepatobiliary disease should prompt a search for non-hepatic causes, such as ischemic cardiac damage, myositis, myopathies and hemolysis.

Although, conventionally the upper limit for these enzymes have been described as 30–40 IU/L, several recent studies have suggested lower cut-offs. Recent studies have suggested that in chronic hepatitis C and non-alcoholic fatty liver disease, current ALT cut-offs miss people with minimal to mild necroinflammation, who may be at future risk of progressive liver disease. It has therefore been proposed that lower ALT cut-offs [30 international units per liter (IU/L) for men and 19 IU/L for women] should be used because of their superior sensitivity in identifying patients with liver disease.[1,2] But, there is a need to find out the best cut-offs of ALT for different populations since they may vary with different geographical area and population structure.[3]

Table 1: Common causes of severe, moderate and mild elevations of AST and ALT		
Very high aminotransferases	*Moderate elevation of aminotransferases*	*Mild elevations of aminotransferases*
Acute viral hepatitis	Acute viral hepatitis	Chronic viral hepatitis
Drug-induced liver injury	Drug-induced liver injury	Non-alcoholic fatty liver disease
Ischemic hepatitis	Ischemic hepatitis	Drug-induced liver injury
	Alcoholic hepatitis	Metabolic liver diseases
	Autoimmune hepatitis	Autoimmune hepatitis
	Metabolic liver diseases	Granulomatous hepatitis
	Biliary obstruction	Congestive heart failure

Peak of Aminotransferase Elevation

The peak levels of and pattern of aminotransferase elevation provides some useful diagnostic and prognostic clues (Table 1).

Very high levels of AST and ALT (10–20 times the upper limit of normal) are usually seen in patients with severe hepatocellular necroinflammation induced by hepatitis viruses, hepatotoxic drugs [drug induced liver injury (DILI)] and liver ischemia. But, lower degrees of liver enzyme elevation do not exclude these conditions. Also, the extent of elevation of aminotransferases does not correlate with the extent of liver injury or prognosis. In fact, rapidly declining levels of aminotransferases may be a poor prognostic sign in patients with fulminant hepatitis, possibly reflecting a low viable liver cell mass.

Moderate elevation of AST and ALT (5–10 times the upper limit of normal) may be seen in patients with acute viral hepatitis, drug-induced liver injury, alcoholic hepatitis and autoimmune hepatitis. In acute alcoholic hepatitis, the aminotransferase levels are usually up to 300 IU/L; the reason for this is unclear, since patients with alcoholic liver disease (ALD) and superimposed acute viral or drug-induced hepatitis have higher ALT levels. Some patients with acute bile duct obstruction due to a common bile duct stone may have aminotransferase levels up to 10 times the upper limit of normal or even higher; however, this elevation is associated with rising ALP, and quickly reverts to normal.

Mild elevations of AST and ALT (1.5–5 times upper limit of normal) can be seen in a large number of conditions such as chronic viral hepatitis, DILI, alcoholic hepatitis, autoimmune hepatitis, non-alcoholic fatty liver disease, metabolic and storage disorders of the liver (Wilson's disease, hemochromatosis, alpha-1-antitrypsin deficiency), obstructive jaundice, cirrhosis, congestive heart failure, granulomatous hepatitis and in some patients with acute viral hepatitis. All conditions which cause very high aminotransferases can also cause mild elevation in these enzymes.

Pattern of Aminotransferase Elevation

In most diseases with primarily liver involvement, ALT levels are elevated to a greater degree than the AST levels, that is, the AST/ALT ratio is less than 1.0. Since AST is present in tissue other than liver, AST may be higher than ALT in conditions which primarily involve other AST producing tissues. So, higher AST levels (higher than ALT), may be of cardiac origin (myocardial infarction), RBC origin (hemolysis) or skeletal muscle origin (myositis or after vigorous muscular activity). Ratio of AST/ALT also exceeds 1.0 in patients with ALD, Wilson's disease and cirrhosis of any cause. The high AST/ALT ratio is particularly useful in suggesting that alcohol is the cause of liver disease. ALT levels of up to 300 IU/L with AST/ALT ratio of more than 1.0 is suggestive of ALD; the specificity increases further if the ratio is 3.0 or higher.[4] The high AST/ALT ratio in ALD is related to the deficiency of pyridoxal-5-phosphate, which is more important for ALT activity than for AST activity, in patients with ALD. Further, AST preferentially binds to immunoglobulin A (IgA) than to immunoglobulin G (IgG) or immunoglobulin M (IgM); since ALD is associated with increased IgA levels, the consequent excess of AST-IgA complexes may result in a higher AST/ALT ratio.[5] Among patients with chronic hepatitis C and non-alcoholic fatty liver disease, a high AST/ALT ratio suggests the presence of advanced fibrosis or cirrhosis. Patients with Wilson's disease may have an AST/ALT ratio more than or equal to 4.0, possibly due to associated hemolysis (which causes extrahepatic AST to rise) caused by excess copper in the blood.

ALT Elevation in Preoperative Setting

Hepatologists are frequently called upon for clearing patients who have been detected to have elevated AST and ALT levels during preoperative work-up. The abnormal measurement may represent an evolving condition, a stable finding or the recovery phase of an illness. For instance, elevation of aminotransferases may be the first biochemical abnormality in patients with acute viral hepatitis, with rise in serum bilirubin lagging behind by about a week. In some patients, serum bilirubin levels may remain normal or below the level associated with jaundice (anicteric hepatitis). Thus, mild elevation of aminotransferases in the absence of jaundice may represent an early phase of evolving acute hepatitis. In other patients, the ALT elevation may represent a transient and insignificant finding, which normalizes within a few days to week. Thus, to resolve the significance of an elevated ALT level, it is essential to retest ALT levels at least twice.

Surgery in patients with acute viral hepatitis is associated with a very high mortality.[6,7] Similar high mortality has been reported in patients operated during acute alcoholic hepatitis.[8] So, serial testing, if suggestive of an evolving acute hepatitis, elective surgeries should be deferred till the hepatitis recovers. All such patients should be tested for acute hepatitis viral markers (IgM anti-HAV, IgM anti-HEV, HBsAg, IgM anti-HBc and anti-HCV).

Flow chart 1 Algorithm for work-up of transaminase elevation deteted preoperatively

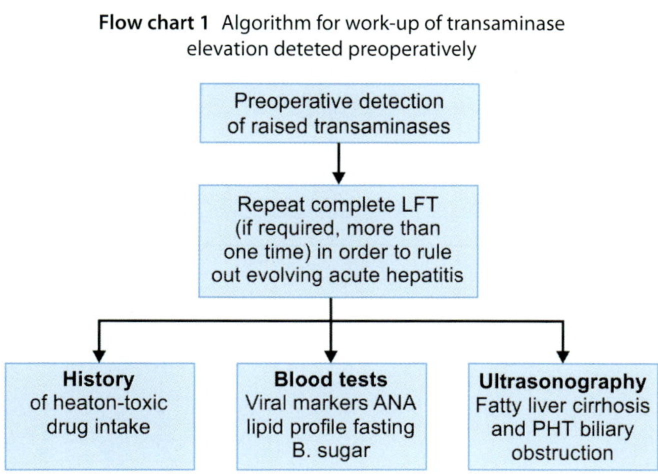

Careful history should be taken to rule out use of hepatotoxic drugs. If aminotransferase levels show persistent mild elevation, the most likely causes include chronic viral hepatitis B or C, DILI or non-alcoholic fatty liver disease (NAFLD).[9] Anti-nuclear antibodies (ANA) and a lipid profile should be done to screen for autoimmune hepatitis and fatty liver. An ultrasound of the upper abdomen should also be done, in order to rule out the presence of biliary obstruction and to look for evidence of fatty liver, cirrhosis and portal hypertension (PHT). Flow chart 1 outlines the plan for patients detected to have raised aminotransferases in the preoperative period.

Postoperative morbidity and mortality rates in these patients depend on the nature and severity of the underlying liver disease. Patients with chronic hepatitis (viral or autoimmune or NAFLD) who do not have cirrhosis are low risk for perioperative complications and therefore can be cleared for surgery. Those who have cirrhosis are at an increased risk of postoperative decompensation. In patients with liver cirrhosis, the postoperative mortality increases as liver function deteriorates. Thus, in addition to viral markers and history of drug intake, an ultrasonography should be done to look for evidence of cirrhosis or PHT. Child-Turcotte-Pugh (CTP) score and model for end-stage liver disease (MELD) score provide useful methods of risk assessment and stratification. The mortality rates among patients with liver cirrhosis undergoing non-liver surgery have been described to be 10% in CTP class A patients to 80% among patients with CTP class C.[10] However, subsequent studies from centers with experience liver transplantation have demonstrated lower mortality rates. A retrospective review of 100 cirrhotics, mortality was 2%, 12% and 12% in patients with CTP class A, B and C respectively. MELD more than or equal to 15 was associated with a mortality of 29% and in addition if the serum albumin was below 2.5 g% the mortality was 60%.[11] In a recent study of 772 patients with liver cirrhosis undergoing major gastrointestinal or non-gastrointestinal surgery, MELD was a good predictor of 30-day postoperative mortality (5.7% for score <8 and 50% for score >20).[12] Thus there may be different cut-offs described by different investigators, but the essence is that patients with advanced liver dysfunction (measured variously by CTP score, MELD score, low albumin, ascites, presence of PHT) are associated with poor outcomes following non-transplant surgery.

Table 2: Common causes of raised aminotransferases in the postoperative period
Hepatotoxic drugs
Sepsis
Hepatobiliary damage
Ischemic hepatitis
Viral hepatitis

Elevated Aminotransferases Detected in the Postoperative Period

The work-up of the raised aminotransferases in the postoperative period is similar to the work-up outlined above; however, the etiologies differ (Table 2).

TESTS INDICATING CHOLESTASIS

Alkaline Phosphatase[13]

Alkaline phosphatase is a serum enzyme whose level in the serum comes from the liver as well as other organs, including bone, placenta and intestines. The normal range for levels of this enzyme varies according to the measurement technique used (e.g. 3–13 King-Armstrong units or 21–85 IU/L); the range may also vary between laboratories.

Alkaline phosphatase is invariably raised in most or all cases of extrahepatic biliary obstruction or intrahepatic cholestasis. The retained bile acids due to cholestasis stimulate the *de novo* synthesis of ALP from the liver, which then leaks into the serum. The bile acids also cause disruption of hepatic organelles, leading to leakage of ALP into the circulation.[14,15] In general, ALP levels are higher in biliary obstruction due to malignant causes; however, significant overlap of ALP levels with benign causes of obstruction makes this an unreliable etiologic indicator. In patients with benign causes of biliary obstruction (such as common bile duct stones, benign biliary strictures, etc.), intrahepatic cholestasis due to viral or drug-induced liver injury, primary biliary cirrhosis, primary sclerosing cholangitis and some infiltrative liver disorders, ALP levels are raised up to four times the upper limit of normal. Lesser degrees of ALP rise are non-specific and may occur in many hepatocellular disorders such as viral hepatitis without cholestasis, liver congestion (congestive heart failure, hepatic venous outflow tract obstruction), ALD and infiltrative liver disorders. So, lower degrees of ALP rise may not be able to differentiate between cholestatic liver injury and hepatitic liver injury.

Alkaline phosphatase may rise in certain physiological conditions. Placental release of ALP may cause a rise in this enzyme up to 2–3 times upper limit of normal during the third trimester of pregnancy. In adolescents, ALP levels are often up to three times the upper limit of normal in adults, due to release of the enzyme from growing bone tissue.

An isolated ALP rise needs further evaluation to determine whether it is related to a hepatobiliary disorder or arises from another organ. Nearly 70% of detectable serum activity of ALP arises in liver and bone, which produce different isoenzymes of ALP. Polyacrylamide gel electrophoresis can separate the different isoenzymes as can be heat lability of hepatic ALP. However, these tests are not practical and not usually available in clinical laboratories. The third (most commonly used and most practical) method for ascertaining whether the rise in serum ALP is due to some hepatobiliary disorder is to measure the activity of another enzyme which is also raised in cholestasis and is more specific for hepatobiliary disorders. Examples of such enzymes include gamma-glutamyl transpeptidase (GGT), 5'-nucleotidase and leucine aminopeptidase; their levels rise in parallel with those of ALP in patients with hepatobiliary disease. ALP levels are markedly decreased in patients with fulminant Wilson's disease.[16]

Gamma-glutamyl Transpeptidase

Elevated levels of GGT are found in diseases of the liver, biliary tract and pancreas. The normal range is 0–30 IU/L. The most important clinical utility of measuring GGT is to determine whether elevated ALP is of hepatobiliary origin or of bone origin, because GGT is not elevated in bone diseases. High GGT may also be used as a marker of surreptitious alcohol intake since alcohol induces hepatic microsomal GGT. For this reason, GGT levels may also be elevated in patients who have been taking microsomal enzyme inducing drugs such as phenobarbitone or phenytoin.[17]

Once cholestasis is suspected because of a raised ALP or GGT, the level of obstruction should be determined by imaging modalities. Ultrasound is the best for initial screening. Subsequently, a magnetic resonance cholangiopancreatography (MRCP) can be ordered to confirm the level of block and its etiology. Liver biopsy may be required in some patients to confirm certain intrahepatic causes of cholestasis, such as primary biliary cirrhosis, primary sclerosing cholangitis, drug induced cholestasis or vanishing bile duct syndrome (Box 2). Flow chart 2 outlines the approach to a patient with raised ALP.

BOX 2 Points to remember regarding ALP/GGT

- Hepatobiliary source of ALP should be confirmed by documenting raised GGT
- Cholestasis where GGT may be normal are:
  - Benign recurrent intrahepatic cholestasis
  - Intrahepatic cholestasis of pregnancy
- GGT has the highest negative predictive value than other component of LFT for detecting bile duct stones in patients undergoing laparoscopic cholecystectomy
- Investigation of choice in cases of increase ALP/GGT is abdominal USG

Flow chart 2 Algorithm for work-up for raised alkaline phosphatase

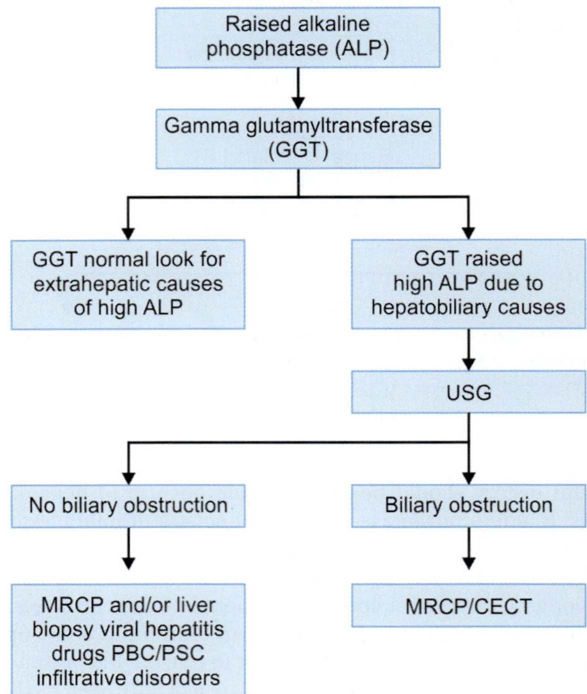

TESTS DEPICTING LIVER SYNTHETIC CAPACITY

Liver is the manufacturing unit for many proteins in the body, some of which can be measured in the serum. Of these, serum albumin and prothrombin are synthesized exclusively in the hepatocytes. Hence, the measurement of serum albumin levels and prothrombin time (PT) are extensively used for assessing the synthetic capacity of the liver.

Albumin

Albumin, synthesized by the hepatocytes, a serum protein, whose half-life is about 3 weeks. The normal serum levels are between 3.5 and 4.5 g/dL. The serum levels are a function of the rates of its synthesis and degradation, and the volume of its distribution. In the context of hepatobiliary disease, low serum albumin usually signifies presence of chronic liver disease with significant loss of hepatocyte function. The levels are usually normal in patients with acute liver disorders, such as acute viral hepatitis, drug-induced liver injury and obstructive jaundice. In these disorders, the detection of low serum albumin level usually suggests the presence of an underlying chronic liver disease which might have recently decompensated because of a superimposed acute insult. Patients with acute liver failure may also rapidly develop low albumin levels due to loss of hepatocytes and enhanced catabolism.[18] Among patients with chronic hepatitis, low albumin levels are seen only when they develop advanced cirrhosis.

Hypoalbuminemia, in the absence of other signs of liver dysfunction, may occur due to protein loss from the intestines (e.g. in intestinal tuberculosis, inflammatory bowel disease, intestinal lymphomas, intestinal lymphangiectasia, etc.), kidneys (nephrotic syndrome, diabetic nephropathy) or other sites (extensive burns), or reduced protein intake (malnutrition) or absorption (malabsorptive states) or even due to severe catabolic states (sepsis). Low albumin has been shown to be associated with high morbidity and poor wound healing after the surgery.[19]

Prothrombin Time and International Normalized Ratio

All the clotting factors, except factor VIII, are synthesized in the liver. PT measurement, depends on the activity of clotting factors I (fibrinogen), II (prothrombin), V, VII and X with the rate of conversion of prothrombin to thrombin serving as the rate-limiting step. The result is expressed in seconds, and is compared to that with a control plasma specimen. Prolongation of PT by more than 4 seconds beyond the control indicates that the patient is at risk of bleeding. The PT may also be expressed as international normalized ratio (INR), which is now the internationally accepted way of expressing the results. This takes into account and corrects for variations in the composition of the tissue extract (thromboplastin) used and allows for comparison of results across different laboratories. Since prothrombin has a short half-life of about 6–7 hours, abnormal PT is an early indicator of liver cell failure.

Prothrombin time or international normalized ratio is a very useful prognostic indicator in several liver diseases. Thus, INR is an integral part of calculation of the CTP score and MELD score, which are used to prognosticate patients with cirrhosis; higher scores signifying shorter survival without liver transplantation. The MELD score is derived from a mathematical calculation based on INR, serum bilirubin and serum creatinine levels. It is a good indicator of short-term (3 months) mortality, and is currently used for the purpose of donor liver allocation for liver transplantation in several countries.[20] MELD is now used for predicting mortality/survival in a variety of causes of end stage liver diseases. Prolonged PT and/or INR is also a poor prognostic indicator in patients with acute liver failure (acetaminophen related as well as that due to non-acetaminophen causes)[21] and ALD. In the latter condition, it is included as a component of Maddrey's index, which has been shown to predict 30-day mortality in acute alcoholic hepatitis.[22] In patients with acute viral hepatitis, a prolonged PT may indicate an impending acute liver failure.

Prolonged PT can also occur due to non-liver related causes. Prothrombin, as also other clotting factors (VII, IX and X), requires vitamin K for its activation. Hence, conditions associated with deficiency of vitamin K (a fat-soluble vitamin), such as fat malabsorption, obstructive jaundice and intake of antibiotics that alter intestinal flora (intestinal flora is a source of vitamin K) can lead to a prolonged PT. However, prolonged PT due to vitamin K deficiency improves on administration of vitamin K. This simple test can be used to distinguish between prolongation of PT caused by parenchymal liver dysfunction and by deficiency of vitamin K.

Patients undergoing percutaneous procedures such as liver biopsy, percutaneous transhepatic biliary drainage, transhepatic hepatic vein angioplasty, and splenic puncture should have a normal PT/INR and these procedures should be deferred, if the PT is prolonged by more than 3 seconds or INR is more than 1.5. If the procedures are required urgently, then INR should first be corrected either by vitamin K administration or by transfusion of fresh frozen plasma.

TESTS ASSESSING METABOLIC CAPACITY OF THE LIVER

These tests provide information on various metabolic compartments—the capacity of the liver to clear, transport or metabolize and then excrete endogenous or exogenous substances. The hepatic turnover of a test substance is determined by liver blood flow, diffusion of the substance between the sinusoidal blood and the hepatocyte, hepatocyte uptake at the basolateral membrane, the metabolic capacity of liver parenchyma and the efficacy of canalicular transport systems. The "functional liver cell mass" is responsible for the processing and excretion of the substance. This assessment appears more physiological than the biochemical parameters or organ failure assessment especially in patients who are left with a precariously reduced mass of functionally active hepatocytes. Tests that assess the metabolic capacity can be divided into blood based (measurement of substrate or metabolite in the blood) or breath based (measurement of the metabolite in exhaled breath). They can also be referred to as quantitative liver function tests (Q-LFTs). Nowadays, Q-LFTs are very rarely applied in clinical practice and their use is restricted to a few specialized centers.

Bilirubin

The simplest test in this category is the serum bilirubin (endogenous molecule) which is taken up, conjugated and excreted in the bile. Bilirubin is formed by catabolism of heme-containing substrates in the reticuloendothelial system (mainly liver and spleen). From here, it is transported to the hepatocytes, where it is taken up and conjugated with glucuronic acid and excreted in the bile. Endogenous nature of bilirubin, its uptake, metabolism and excretion of bilirubin by liver cells, and ease of measurement make it eminently suitable for use as a liver function test without administration of any external agent. However, it has a limited sensitivity for detecting mild liver dysfunction and its levels may be elevated in some conditions with intact liver function.

Bilirubin circulates in the blood in two forms, namely: (1) direct reacting (conjugated form, which is water soluble and therefore capable of renal excretion) and (2) indirect reacting (unconjugated form, which is poorly water soluble and therefore not excreted in urine) fractions. With the measurement techniques in common use, indirect-reacting bilirubin appears to account for almost all the circulating bilirubin. The bilirubin levels in healthy persons are usually below 1 mg/dL; clinically detectable jaundice usually requires levels exceeding 2–3 mg/dL.

Raised bilirubin levels may represent excessive production, diminished hepatic uptake, impaired conjugation or reduced excretion of bilirubin from the hepatocytes, or may be related to regurgitation of conjugated bilirubin from the damaged hepatocytes or bile ducts. From the diagnostic viewpoint, the causes of hyperbilirubinemia may be classified as those that cause predominantly unconjugated hyperbilirubinemia (with more than 80% of serum bilirubin in unconjugated form) and those that cause predominantly conjugated hyperbilirubinemia (with more than 50% of bilirubin in conjugated form) (Table 3).

The level of total bilirubin may be of some help in etiological differential diagnosis. In patients with pure hemolytic diseases, the bilirubin level is usually less than 5 mg/dL. This is related to an extremely large capacity of the hepatocytes to take up bilirubin so that the liver uptake is not a rate-limiting step in bilirubin metabolism. Similarly, in Gilbert's syndrome, the peak bilirubin level almost invariably remains below 4–5 mg/dL.

In general, patients with benign or incomplete biliary obstruction have lower serum bilirubin levels than those with malignant biliary obstruction. In obstructive jaundice, most of the accumulated bilirubin is in the conjugated form which can be easily excreted through the kidneys; thus, the bilirubin levels tend to plateau at about 35–40 mg/dL. Levels higher than this in patients with conjugated hyperbilirubinemia usually suggest coexisting renal failure or hemolysis.

Table 3: Common causes of hyperbilirubinemia

Unconjugated hyperbilirubinemia	*Conjugated hyperbilirubinemia*
Excessive bilirubin production: • Hemolytic disorders • Ineffective erythropoiesis • Resorption of large hematoma *Impaired bilirubin uptake by hepatocytes:* • Drugs: rifampicin and probenecid *Impaired bilirubin conjugation:* • Congenital unconjugated hyperbilirubinemia: – Gilbert's syndrome – Crigler-Najjar syndrome type I – Crigler-Najjar syndrome type II *Neonatal jaundice*	*Hepatocellular:* • Viral hepatitis • Drug-induced hepatitis • Alcoholic hepatitis • Autoimmune hepatitis • Sepsis • Intrahepatic cholestatic disorders *Obstructive jaundice:* • Benign: – Common bile duct stones – Intrahepatic stones – Bile duct strictures – Primary sclerosing cholangitis – Choledochal cyst • Malignant: – Carcinoma gallbladder – Cholangiocarcinoma – Carcinoma head of pancreas – Periampullary carcinoma *Congenital conjugated hyperbilirubinemia:* • Dubin-Johnson syndrome • Rotor's syndrome

In patients who have prolonged biliary obstruction, serum levels of bilirubin may decline slowly even after successful relief of obstruction. This is related to covalent bonding of conjugated bilirubin to albumin (delta bilirubin), which has a circulation half-life similar to that of albumin (2–3 weeks).

The level of bilirubin elevation may also have prognostic value in some conditions, such as acute liver failure, acute alcoholic hepatitis and liver cirrhosis (serum bilirubin is part of the prognostic scores). In patients with liver cirrhosis, serum bilirubin levels form an important component of the widely used prognostic indices like the CTP score and the MELD score. Even in cholestatic liver disorders such as primary biliary cirrhosis and primary sclerosing cholangitis, serum bilirubin level is an important determinant of the need for liver transplantation. In contrast, in patients with acute viral hepatitis, the prognostic significance of bilirubin levels appears to be limited, if any.

Dye Tests

These tests involve the administration of known amount of a particular exogenous dye followed by measurement of its blood levels after fixed time interval(s). The dye is taken up by the hepatocytes, and is either conjugated [sulfobromophthalein sodium (BSP)] or excreted unchanged [indocyanine green (ICG)]. Concentration of the dye remaining in the circulation thus provides a quantitative estimate of the degree of hepatic dysfunction.

These tests are however fairly non-specific, and are therefore deranged in a variety of liver disorders. These thus have little value in differential diagnosis of liver disorders. One clinical situation where BSP excretion test is of some diagnostic value is in differentiating Dubin-Johnson syndrome from Rotor's syndrome. In the former, plasma BSP concentration shows an initial rapid decline followed by a secondary rise 45–90 minutes later, whereas in the latter the initial decline is much slower and there is no secondary increase.[23]

Indocyanine Green Test

The ICG is an organic anionic dye that after intravenous injection is cleared exclusively by the liver and 97% of the administered dose is excreted unchanged in to the bile. It remains in the intravascular space and exclusively taken up by the liver and its transport capacity localized in the sinusoidal liver cell membrane. After excretion, it is not reabsorbed in the intestine. The ICG clearance and retention at 15 minutes in patients with CLD are thought to reflect the degree of sinusoidal capillarization (one of the earliest changes in liver fibrogenesis, intrahepatic portovenous shunt and alteration in liver blood flow (Ohwada). It gives an important estimate of the functional liver reserve, since only the functional liver mass will be able to clear the administered dose of ICG.

Conventionally ICG was used to assess hepatic blood flow using the Fick's principle. It has more commonly been used for assessing the risk of liver failure following hepatic resection. For this purpose, retention of the administered dose is measured at 15 minutes after a bolus intravenous injection. If the retention at 15 minutes is less than 15%, it suggests good hepatic function, since the liver was able to clear most of the injected concentration. However, it involves taking a blood sample and measuring the concentration in a lab. In patients undergoing liver resection, ICG retention test is a good indicator of functional liver reserve and can guide the volume of liver that can be resected. ICG retention of less than 15% at 15 minutes suggests a low risk of postoperative liver failure after hepatic resection and has been shown to be reproducible; it should be carried out wherever facilities are available.[24] The group from Hong Kong describes a cut-off of less than 14% and less than 22% for ICG 15 (ICG retention at 15 minutes) to guide major and minor liver resection respectively.[25] The Japanese surgeons follow a decision tree based on presence and absence of ascites, serum bilirubin levels and the ICG 15 values to decide the volume of liver that can be resected. This is called Makuuchi's criteria. In patients who have no ascites and the serum bilirubin level is less than 1, ICG15 values of less than 10%, 10–19%, 20–29%, 30–39% and more than or equal to 40% are used to guide major hepatectomy or trisegementectomy, left lobectomy, subsegmentectomy, limited resection and enucleation resepectively.[26]

As a recent innovation ICG clearance can also be monitored non-invasively using pulse spectrophotometry, and can be used as a handy bedside tool for predicting liver reserve in perioperative setting.[27] De Liquori et al. used the LiMON (Pulsion Medical Systems, Munich, Germany) device for pulse spectrophotometric measurement of ICG plasma disappearance rate (ICG-PDR) in 37 patients undergoing liver resection. It was demonstrated that the postoperative day 1 ICG-PDR correlated well with bilirubin levels on day 1, 5 and 10 as well as with serum albumin levels on day 5 and 10.[28] ICG-clearance correlates with the Child-Pugh classification, galactose elimination capacity, BSP elimination and with the results of the aminopyrine breath test in cirrhotic patients. However, it has not been used routinely in clinical practice because of its high cost and limited availability.

MEGX Test

Cytochrome P-450 system metabolizes the drug lignocaine to its metabolite monoethylglycinexylidide (MEGX). Serial measurement of serum levels of MEGX after intravenous administration of lignocaine is thus a good measure of the functional capacity of the liver. Abnormalities in the MEGX test have been shown to correlate well with liver insufficiency. Among cirrhotic patients undergoing hepatic resection for liver cancer, MEGX test has been shown to predict the occurrence of postoperative complications.[29] This test may also be used to select optimal donors for liver transplantation.

Breath Tests to Assess Hepatic Functions

Breath testing with ^{13}C-labeled substrates could provide a safe, noninvasive means for evaluating hepatic metabolism in correlation with liver function. ^{13}C is a stable, non-radioactive isotope, which can be incorporated into a specific location within a test substrate and later released as $^{13}CO_2$ when the compound is metabolized by the liver. Ideally, the ^{13}C-compound should be exclusively metabolized by liver microsomes, orally administered and rapidly absorbed. The ratio of $^{13}C/^{12}C$ is measured in exhaled breath within 20–60 minutes. Some examples are ^{14}C aminopyrine breath test, ^{13}C phenylalanine breath test (PheBT) and ^{13}C galactose breath test (GBT).[30,31] But most of the available tests are cumbersome, labor intensive and expensive and therefore cannot be used routinely for day to day assessment of critically ill patients.

^{13}C-methacetin is another such substrate which is metabolized by the microsomal mixed function oxygenase, cytochrome P450 1A2. It is a derivative of phenacetin and it undergoes O-demethylation into acetaminophen and formaldehyde. The formaldehyde after two more successive oxidative steps releases $^{13}CO_2$. The resultant $^{13}CO_2$ can be measured in the exhaled breath. The amount of metabolized methacetin indicates the residual liver function. Methacetin is a safe molecule for human consumption.[32-35]

The problem with most currently available ^{13}C based breath tests is the method for detection of exhaled $^{13}CO_2$. The gold standard, isotopic ratio mass spectrometry (IRMS), is very cumbersome, time consuming and inconvenient for the patients and therefore cannot be used routinely on a day to day basis. To circumvent this problem, a new method has been developed by Exhalenz Bioscience (Modi'in, Israel) which utilizes the molecular correlation spectrometry (MCS) to analyze the ratio of exhaled $^{13}CO_2/^{12}CO_2$. This method has been validated against the gold standard of IRMS.[36]

Exhalenz has developed a molecular correlation spectrometer, based on specific optical-radiation emission and absorption by $^{13}CO_2$ and $^{12}CO_2$ gases. Based on MCS, the Breath ID® device continuously measures $^{13}CO_2$ and $^{12}CO_2$ concentrations from the patient's breath and establishes the $^{13}CO_2/^{12}CO_2$ ratio. Results are displayed in real time on the screen and are printed after the completion of the test.

^{13}C-methacetin breath test (MBT) has been used earlier also for assessing liver functional capacity in a variety of clinical situations,[37,38] but as has been mentioned earlier, due to the short comings of the conventional method of detection of inhaled ^{13}C, it did not become very popular. MBT with breath ID has recently been used in clinical studies and has shown that it can effectively assess liver function in both acute and chronic liver diseases. Around 184 treatment naïve HCV patients, 74 NAFLD patients and 74 healthy controls were assessed with ^{13}C-MBT. In both HCV and NAFLD patients, all MBT parameters correlated with fibrosis stage ($p<0.0001$).[39] The noninvasive ^{13}C-MBT was evaluated for its use in the follow-up of 15 patients with acute severe liver disease during different phases of their illness. During the acute phase of the illness, clinical improvement and normalization of biochemical parameters were accompanied by progressive improvement of ^{13}C-MBT scores in all patients.[40]

This test thus holds promise for routine, bedside use in assessing residual liver function among patients with a variety of liver diseases and liver failure and can also be used as a predictive tool in such patients as well as a tool to assess suitability for hepatic resection among cirrhotics.

All these tests of functional liver capacity may be more sensitive than bilirubin but are more invasive, more cumbersome to perform and lack specificity. Thus, their use has been limited to specialized centers and to research studies. However, in future, these may be used as noninvasive tools for measuring residual liver reserve in patients with chronic liver disease with the aim of obviating liver biopsy.

CONCLUSION

In conclusion, biochemical evaluation of liver function requires a battery of several easily performed tests. This usually includes a combination of serum enzymes (indicating hepatocellular necroinflammation and/or cholestasis), serum bilirubin and tests of synthetic capacity (serum albumin and PT), forming a cheap and sensitive panel to screen for liver function abnormalities. Proper interpretation of these tests can provide a lot of useful information regarding diagnosis, severity and prognosis of various liver disorders and may help avoid more expensive and cumbersome tests (Box 3).

BOX 3 Specific surgical conditions and LFT derangement

- Acute cholecystitis:
  - Mild elevation of bilirubin and AST/ALT can occur
  - If elevated then get USG abdomen to rule out CBD stone
- Biliary pancreatitis:
  - High ALT suggests CBD stone in biliary pancreatitis
  - Biliary sepsis, CBD stone (evidenced by cholestatic LFT picture) is an indication of ERCP
- Surgical procedures can be done safely in liver disease, if MELD score is <14 or in child A status

REFERENCES

1. Prati D, Emanuela T, Zanella A, Toree ED, Butelli S, Vecchio ED, et al. Updated definitions of healthy ranges for serum alanine aminotransferase levels. Ann Intern Med. 2002;137:1-9.
2. Kim HC, Nam CM, Jee SH, Han KH, Oh DK, Suh II. Normal serum aminotransferase concentration and risk of mortality from liver diseases: prospective cohort study. Br Med J. 2004;328:983-8.
3. Ruhl CE, Everhart JE. Upper limits of normal for alanine aminotransferase activity in the United States population. Hepatology. 2012;55:447-54.
4. Cohen JA, Kaplan MM. The SGOT/SGPT ratio: an indicator of alcoholic liver disease. Dig Dis Sci. 1979;24:835-8.

5. Tameda M, Shirak K, Ooi K, Takase K, Kosaka Y, Nobori T, et al. Aspartate aminotransferase-immunoglobulin complexes in patients with chronic liver disease. World J Gastroenterol. 2005;11:1529-31.
6. Harville DD, Summerskill WH. Surgery in acute hepatitis: causes and effects. JAMA. 1963;184:257-61.
7. Powell-Jackson P, Greenway B, Williams R. Adverse effects of exploratory laparotomy in patients with unsuspected liver disease. Br J Surg. 1982;69:449-51.
8. Greenwood SM, Leffler CT, Minkowitz S. The increased mortality rate of open liver biopsy in alcoholic hepatitis. Surg Gynecol Obstet. 1972;134:600-4.
9. Madan K, Batra Y, Panda SK, DattaGupta S, Haxari S, Jha JK, et al. Role of polymerase chain reaction and liver biopsy in the evaluation of patients with asymptomatic trasnaminitis: implications in diagnostic approach. Journal of Gastroenterol Hepatol. 2004;19:1291-9.
10. Nicoll A. Surgical risk in patients with cirrhosis. Journal of Gastroetnerol and Hepatol. 2012;27:1569-75.
11. Telem DA, Schiano T, Goldstone R, Han DK, Buch KE, Chin EH, et al. Factors that predict outcome of abdominal operations in patients with advanced cirrhosis. Clin Gastroenterol Hepatol. 2010;8:451-7.
12. Teh SH, Nagorney DM, Stevens SR, Offord KP, Therneau TM, Plevak DJ, et al. Risk factors for mortality after surgery in patients with cirrhosis. Gastroenterology. 2007;132:1261-9.
13. Siddiqui A, Kowdley KV. Approach to a patient with elevated serum alkaline phosphatase. Clin Liver Dis. 2012;16:199-229.
14. Kaplan MM, Righetti A. Induction of rat liver alkaline pahsphatase: the mechanism of the serum elevation in bile duct obstruction. J Clin Invest. 1970;49:508-16.
15. Kaplan MM. Serum alkaline phosphatase: another piece is added to the puzzle. Hepatology. 1986;6:526-8.
16. Shaver WA, Bhatt H, Combes B. Low serum alkaline phosphatase activity in Wilson's disease. Hepatology. 1986;6:859-63.
17. Goldberg DM. Structural, functional and clinical aspects of gamma-glutamyl transferase. CRC Crit Rev Lab Sci. 1980;12:1-58.
18. Dhiman RK, Makharia GK, Jain S, Chawla Y. Ascites and spontaneous bacterial peritonitis. Am J Gastroenterol. 2000;95: 233-8.
19. Uppal S, Al-Niaimi A, Rice LW, Rose SL, Kushner DM, Spencer RJ, et al. Preoperative hypoalbuminemia is an independent predictor of poor perioperative outcomes in women undergoing open surgery for gynecologic malignancies. Gynecol Oncol. 2013:131(2):416-22.
20. Kamath PS, Kim WR. Advanced Liver Disease Study Group. The model for end-stage liver disease (MELD). Hepatology. 2007;45:797-805.
21. Cholongitas E, Theocharidou E, Vasionopoulou P, Betrosian A, Shaw S, Patch D, et al. Comparison of the sequential organ failure assessment score with the King's College Hospital criteria and the model for end-stage liver disease score for the prognosis of acetaminophen-induced acute liver failure. Liver Transpl. 2012;18:405-12.
22. Maddrey WC, Boitnott JK, Bedine MS. Corticosteroid therapy of alcoholic hepatitis. Gastroenterology. 1978;75:193-99.
23. Shani M, Gilon E, Ben-Ezzer J, Shiba C. Sulfobromophthalein tolerance test in patients with Dubin-Johnson syndrome and their relatives. Gastroenterology. 1970;59:842-7.
24. Frazakas J, Mandli T, Ther G, Arkossy M, Pap S, Fule B, et al. Evaluation of liver function for hepatic resection. Transplant Proc. 2006;38:798-800.
25. Fan ST. Liver functional reserve estimation: state of the art and relevance for local treatments: the eastern perspective. J Hepatobiliary Pancreat Sci. 2010;17:380-4.
26. Makuuchi M, Kosuge T, Takayama T, Yamazaki S, Kakazu T, Miyagawa S, et al. Surgery for small liver cancers. Semin Surg Oncol. 1993;9:298-304.
27. Ohwada S, Kawate S, Hamada K, Yamada T, Sunose Y, Tsutsumi H, et al. Perioperative real-time monitoring of indocyanine green clearance by pulse spectrophotometry predicts remnant liver functional reserve in resection of hepatocellular carcinoma. Br J Surg. 2006;93:339-46.
28. de Liguori Carino N, O'Reilly DA, Dajani K, Ghaneh P, Poston GJ, Wu AV. Perioperative use of the LiMON method of indocyanine green elimination measurement for the prediction and early detection of post-hepatectomy liver failure. Eur J Surg Oncol. 2009;35:957-62.
29. Ravaioli M, Grazi GL, Principe A, Ercolani G, Cescon M, Gardini A, et al. Operative risk by the lidocaine test (MEGX) in resected patients for HCC on cirrhosis. Hepatogastroenterology. 2003;50:1552-5.
30. Opekun AR, Klein PD, Graham DY. [13C] amionpyrine breath test detects altered liver metabolism caused by low dose oral contraceptives. Dig Dis Sci. 1995;40:2417-22.
31. Hsieh CB, Yu CY, Tzao C, Chu HC, Chen TW, Hsieh HF, et al. Prediction of the risk of hepatic failure in patients with portal vein invasion hepatoma after hepatic rsection. Eur J Surg Oncol. 2006;32:72-6.
32. Ciccocioppo R, Candelli M, Di Francesco D, Ciocca F, Taqlieri G, Armuzzi A, et al. Study of liver function in healthy elderly subjects using the 13C-methacetin breath test. Aliment Pharmacol Ther. 2003;17:271-7.
33. Krumbiegel P, Gunther K, Faust H, Mobius G, Hirschberg K, Schneider G. Nuclear medicine liver function tests for pregnant women and children.1. Breath tests with 14C-methacetin and 13C-methacetin. Eur J Nucl Med. 1985;10:129-33.
34. Krumbiegel P, Stolz L, Herbarth O, Braun W, Boehm G, Kausch S, et al. Is the [15N] methacetin liver function test suited to estimate environmental effects on the maturity of neonates? Cent Eur J Public Health. 1994;2:49-51.
35. Matsumoto K, Suehiro M, Iio M, Kawabe T, Shiratori Y, Okano Y, et al. [13C] methacetin breath test for evaluation of liver damage. Dig Dis Sci. 1987;32:344-8.
36. Goetze O, Selzner N, Fruehauf H, Fried M, Gerlach T, Mullhaupt B. 13C-methacetin breath test as a quantitative liver function test in patients with chronic hepatitis C infection: continuous automatic molecular correlation spectroscopy compared to isotopic ratio mass spectrometry. Alimnet Pharmacol Ther. 2007;26:305-11.
37. Schneider A, Caspary WF, Saich R, Dietrich CF, Sarrazin C, Kuker W, et al. 13C-Methacetin breath test shortened: 2 point measurements after 15 minutes reliably indicate the presence of liver cirrhosis. J Clin Gastroenterol. 2007;41:33-7.
38. Pterolati A, Festi D, De Berardinis G, Colaiocco-Ferrante L, Di Paolo D, Tisone G, et al. 13C-Methacetin breath tests for monitoring hepatic function in cirrhotic patients before and after liver transplantation. Alimentary Pharmacology and Therapeutics. 2003;18:785-90.
39. Lalazar G, Braun M, Ben Ari Z, et al. The non-invasive 13C-methacetin breath test accurately detects liver fibrosis in patients with chronic HCV infection or non-alcoholic fatty liver disease. J Hepatol. 2007;46:S209.
40. Lalazar GSM, Hajaj TR, Margalit M. Use of a 13C-methacetin breath test (MBT) for follow-up of patients with acute liver disease. J Hepatol. 2006;44:S63.

CHAPTER 65

Approach to a Patient with Jaundice

R Surendran, Paari Vijayraghavan

INTRODUCTION

Jaundice (icterus) (derived from French word *jaune* meaning yellow) refers to excess of bile pigments in the serum and tissues leading to yellowish discoloration of skin, mucus membrane and sclera. Jaundice is clinically apparent when the serum bilirubin exceeds 2–3 mg/dL. It is a symptom of myriad of diseases ranging from benign causes, e.g. Gilbert syndrome requiring no specific treatment to very aggressive disease, e.g. pancreatic cancer where early diagnosis and treatment is the only way to cure, if any.

Based on the underlying etiology, causes of jaundice can be prehepatic, hepatic and posthepatic. The "*medical jaundice*" is usually associated with either excess production of the bilirubin pigment or defect in the hepatic metabolism of the same while the "*surgical jaundice*" (also referred to commonly as obstructive jaundice) is usually referred to the conditions causing the obstruction to the flow of the bile in the major biliary passages. While prehepatic and hepatic causes are usually medical (thus the collective term of medical jaundice for these causes), posthepatic causes are due to causes amenable to surgical (or endoscopic) intervention (thus surgical jaundice, Box 1). Cholestasis refers to impaired formation or flow of bile, and may result from problem at any level from the basolateral membrane of the hepatocytes to the ampulla of Vater. Surgical jaundice or obstructive jaundice would be the main focus of this chapter.

BOX 1 Causes of jaundice (obstructive)

Progressive:
- Carcinoma gallbladder
- Hilar cholangiocarcinoma
- Periampullary carcinoma
- Pancreatic carcinoma
- Cystic tumor pancreas (head)
- Chronic pancreatitis
- Benign biliary stricture (post-cholecystectomy)

Intermittent:
- Choledocholithiasis
- Primary sclerosing cholangitis
- Choledochal cyst
- Biliary parasites (ascariasis)
- Papillary tumor gallbladder/bile duct
- Hydatid cyst with biliary communication
- Ampullary carcinoma
- Mirizzi syndrome

PATHOPHYSIOLOGY OF OBSTRUCTIVE JAUNDICE

Bile secretion from the liver serves multiple functions like digestion and absorption of lipids, elimination of toxins and detoxifications products, drug excretion, etc. Bile is the principal route of excretion for cholesterol, bilirubin and many hormones. In obstructive jaundice, the excretion is blocked and two kinds of pathophysiologic effects are seen. First type of effect is due to absence of bile constituents in the intestines (bile salts, bilirubin derivatives and lipids). Second type is due to their overflow into the systemic circulation. Stools are pale as less bilirubin derived pigments (urobilinogen) reaches the intestine. Prolonged and severe biliary obstruction leads to malabsorption and steatorrhea and leads to deficiencies of fat-soluble vitamins (particularly A, K and D). Vitamin K deficiency causes prolonged prothrombin time. Vitamin D and Calcium malabsorption can cause osteoporosis or osteomalacia in patients with prolonged cholestasis. As conjugated bilirubin is water soluble, it is excreted in the urine and urine becomes dark in obstructive jaundice. Pruritus is usually associated with high levels of circulating bile salts. Cholesterol and phospholipid retention produces hyperlipidemia despite fat malabsorption (although increased liver synthesis and decreased plasma esterification of cholesterol also contribute); Triglyceride levels are usually seen to be normal. Abnormal, low-density lipoprotein called lipoprotein X may be seen in the circulation.

APPROACH TO A PATIENT WITH JAUNDICE

For the surgeon the most important question while evaluating a patient with jaundice is whether the patient has medical or surgical jaundice. Importance of a careful history, clinical examination and basic laboratory test and its careful interpretation cannot be underestimated as an accurate diagnosis can be established in 75% of cases based on above.[1] Yellowish discoloration may be seen in hyper beta carotenemia due to excess ingestion of food containing beta carotene like carrots; this condition is associated with yellow discoloration of skin but not sclera and normal serum bilirubin levels but is seldom seen in darker skinned races.

CLINICAL FEATURES

A careful history, physical examination, routine biochemical and hematological tests are required during evaluation. Presence of abdominal pain, fever, rigors usually indicates surgical jaundice while anorexia, myalgia, malaise, nausea, aversion to smoking may indicate viral or drug induced hepatitis. History of prior hepatobiliary surgery (to rule out biliary stricture) or any other abdominal surgery (to rule out liver metastases), history of any other surgery or hospitalization, blood transfusion, injection, tattooing, etc. (to rule out hepatitis), prior history of jaundice, family history of jaundice, history of alcoholism are important during evaluation.

Patient with prior history of calculus biliary tract disease may develop recurrent/retained stones, known case of chronic pancreatitis may develop biliary stricture or pancreatic carcinoma, and prior cholecystectomy may develop benign/malignant biliary stricture presenting as jaundice.

Painful intermittent jaundice specially in association with fever (suggestive of cholangitis) is seen more commonly with benign conditions like stone while relatively painless progressive jaundice usually indicates malignant biliary tract obstruction. Cholangitis in such cases is usually after some endobiliary intervention.

Examination should focus specifically for the presence of anemia, lymph nodes, pedal edema, ascites, signs of chronic liver disease (palmar erythema, spider nevi, splenomegaly, dilated vein on the anterior abdominal wall, flapping tremors, etc.), scratch marks, abdominal lump, palpable gallbladder, etc.

Clinical Pearls from the History and Presentation

- Long standing jaundice usually indicates a medical cause like primary biliary cirrhosis, autoimmune hepatitis, hemolytic anemia or Gilbert's syndrome while most of the surgically treatable conditions like choledocholitiasis or malignancies typically come to medical attention within shorter span of time after the onset of jaundice.
- Fluctuating jaundice may sometimes be seen in choledocholitiasis (stone may block and then get passed away or due to "ball valve effect") or small periampullary tumor when spontaneous resolution of jaundice can occur due to sloughing of the tumor causing transient malena.
- Sometimes the jaundice may be associated with pain in the upper abdomen, high grade fever with chills and rigors—the clinical syndrome of "Charcot's triad" which indicates suppurative cholangitis. In more severe cases, the patient may have hypotension and mental status changes to complete the "Reynolds's pentad". Suppurative cholangitis is usually associated with benign conditions like choledocholitiasis or iatrogenic biliary injury/stricture than malignant causes of biliary obstruction like cholangiocarcinoma or carcinoma of head of pancreas.
- "Painless progressive jaundice" is typically associated with malignant biliary obstructions like carcinoma of head of pancreas, periampullary carcinoma, carcinoma of neck of gallbladder or hilar cholangiocarcinoma ("Klatskin tumor"). The malignant causes of jaundice are usually associated with significant recent loss of weight and anorexia, though the above symptoms may be present in medical conditions also.
- Presence of pruritus points toward the cholestatic cause of jaundice, not necessarily "surgical jaundice". The "medical conditions like primary biliary cirrhosis, autoimmune hepatitis can be associated with pruritus as is the case with malignant obstruction to the biliary passages or choledocholitiasis.
- History of an upper abdomen surgery (typically cholecystectomy) should give rise to the suspicion of iatrogenic biliary injury leading to stricture of the biliary tract. Typically these patients may have a history of bile leak in the surgical drains in the postoperative period which would have resolved.
- Presence of the episodic triad of symptoms of jaundice, pain abdomen and malena in a patient who has history of trauma to the liver or any iatrogenic interventions like liver biopsy should alert one to the possibility of hemobilia—where the bleeding from the hepatic arterial source into the biliary passages causes clot to cause obstructive jaundice.
- Choledochal cyst can manifest as combination of any of the following symptoms: jaundice, pain, cholangitis, lump or symptoms of portal hypertension. This condition is predominantly seen in children and young adults but can also uncommonly be seen in older patients.
- Other rarer causes of jaundice in developing countries include biliary parasitosis (Ascariasis, clonorchis).
- In general, very severe jaundice (s. bilirubin > 20 mg/dL) is more often seen with malignant causes of obstructive jaundice than the benign ones, though it is not a rule.
- Obstructive jaundice is associated with high colored ("cola colored") urine due to presence of conjugated bilirubin filtered by kidney into the urine from the blood. Jaundice associated with hemolytic anemia is not associated with such high colored urine (acholuric jaundice) due to presence predominantly of unconjugated bilirubin in serum which is not filtered by the kidneys.
- One of the very striking features of obstructive jaundice is the presence of severe pruritus in these patients; scratch marks all over the body and the associated "shining nails" may be seen in many patients.
- Jaundice with severe pallor may indicate hemolytic anemia with choledocholitiasis (usually associated with pain) or may indicate periampullary malignancy with GI blood loss from ulceration of the lesion (painless).
- Jaundice in a severely malnourished patient may be due to underlying malignancy like carcinoma of gallbladder, head

of pancreas, extensive liver metastasis or may indicate an advanced decompensated chronic liver disease. Interestingly, it is often seen that patients with hilar cholangiocarcinoma and periampullary malignancy do not present with very severe malnutrition.

- Presence of left supra-clavicular lymph nodal mass along with jaundice indicates advanced biliary-pancreatic tract malignancy or associated advanced liver metastasis.
- Abdomen examination may be unremarkable in many of cases of obstructive jaundice. Hepatomegaly may be appreciated due to enlarged cholestatic liver; uncommonly large palpable hepatocellular carcinoma may be associated with jaundice—due to liver volume replacement, biliary tumor embolus or compression on the major bile ducts in the hilum.
- Distended gallbladder may be palpable in malignant biliary obstructions at or below the level of cystic duct insertion into bile duct but not in benign causes like choledocholithiasis (Courvoisier's rule). In some instances the palpable gallbladder may be due to a large gallbladder carcinoma involving the fundus region or a neck mass causing obstruction.
- Ill-defined upper midline lump associated with jaundice may be associated with a large carcinoma in head of pancreas or rarely inflammatory pseudotumors associated with acute exacerbation of chronic pancreatitis. Typically, most of the carcinoma of head of pancreas presenting with palpable lump turns out to be far advanced for surgical resection.
- Presence of splenomegaly in a jaundiced patient may be due to hemolytic anemia, portal hypertension, infiltrative diseases or splenic vein thrombosis.
- Ascites in these patients may be pointer toward advanced malignancy or chronic liver disease with portal hypertension.

INVESTIGATIONS (FLOW CHART 1)

Laboratory Investigations

Complete liver function test should be obtained. Raised serum bilirubin confirms the presence of jaundice while predominant rise in conjugated bilirubin with increased serum alkaline phosphatase (>3 times the upper limit of normal) indicates cholestatic jaundice especially if gamma-glutamyl transferase (GGT) is also raised. Serum glutamic-pyruvic transaminase (SGPT) and serum glutamic oxaloacetic transaminase (SGOT) are predominantly raised in hepatitis. However, in acute biliary obstruction, these enzymes may be raised up to 20 times normal even before significant increase in serum alkaline phosphates. These enzymes are also raised in cholangitis. A high serum bilirubin at presentation may be indicative of malignant biliary obstruction. Serum bilirubin level more than 100 mmol/L (5.9 mg/dL) has 72% sensitivity and 87% specificity in differentiating benign from malignant obstructive jaundice, and specificity further increases to 97% when level is more than 250 mmol/L (14.7 mg/dL).[2] Jaundice is not always detected

Flow chart 1 Approach to obstructive jaundice

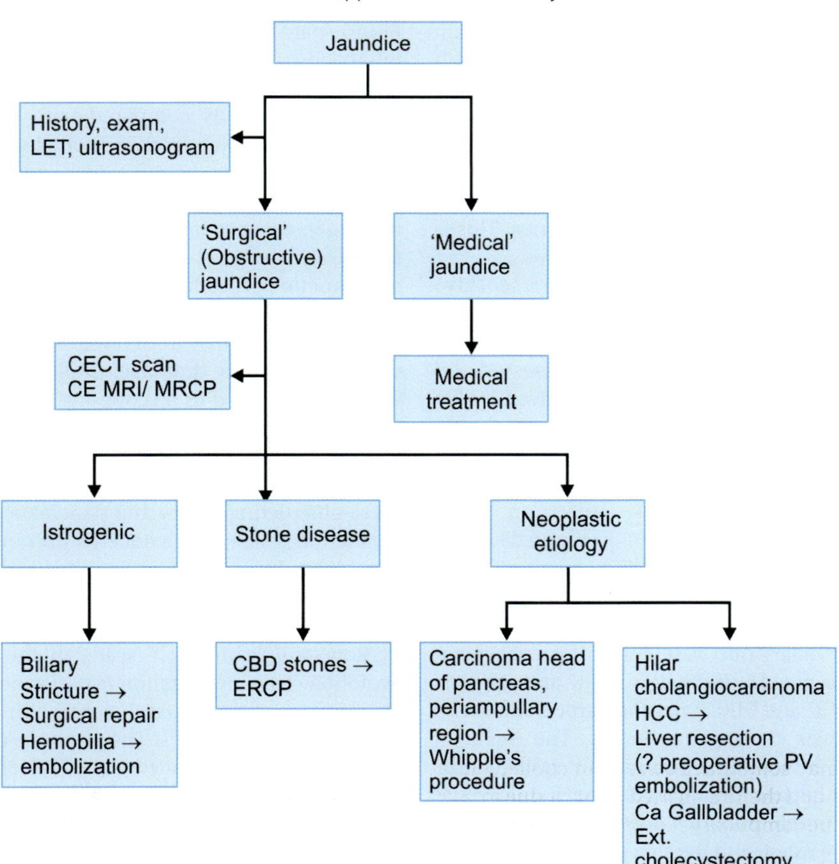

by the patients. Comparatively, pain or fever may nece ssitate the patient to consult earlier. Hence, patients with stone disease present earlier and jaundice is also less severe. Jaundice in common bile duct (CBD) stones may sometimes fluctuate with disimpaction or complete obstruction. Cholangitis can lead to sudden increase in bilirubin with raised enzymes in biliary strictures or stone disease. This differs from steadily progressive nature of jaundice in malignant obstruction. Leucocytosis is seen with cholangitis, acute alcoholic hepatitis and also in malignant diseases. Serum albumin and prothrombin time may be altered in chronic hepatocellular or obstructive jaundice.

Tumor marker CA19-9 may also give some clue regarding the nature of biliary obstruction. Serum level of CA19-9 more than 70 u/mL is usually indicates malignant cause of obstructive jaundice with a sensitivity of 82% and specificity of 85%.[3] Higher values and acute cholangitis seen in benign obstruction are related to raised bilirubin level, and CA19-9 in such cases falls after biliary drainage. On the other hand serum CA19-9 level remains elevated in malignant biliary obstruction even after drainage.

Imaging

Ultrasound (US) is usually the initial imaging modality of choice due to wider availability and low cost. It is 55–91% sensitive and 82–95% specific in diagnosing biliary obstruction. However, it is observer dependent; assessment may be suboptimal in the presence of bowel gases, in obese patients, and in the presence of fibrotic liver where firm liver does not allow biliary dilatation. Once biliary dilatation is confirmed in the patient having obstructive jaundice, further evaluation will focus on the identification of its cause. Certain underlying causes (e.g. CBD stone, pancreatobiliary malignancy with liver metastases) can be very well assessed on USG only and may obviate further imaging. Majority of other causes will require further imaging. US will also show presence of ascites, portal hypertension, lymph nodal enlargement and liver infiltration. Coupled with Doppler it may give valuable information regarding status of portal vein, superior mesenteric vein (SMV) and hepatic arteries. This is especially important in malignancies and bile duct injuries.

Contrast enhanced CT scan of the abdomen is 63–96% sensitive and 93–100% specific in diagnosing biliary obstruction. In addition to detecting the biliary obstruction, its cause (carcinoma gallbladder, periampullary malignancy, etc.) can be assessed and staged at the same time. It gives all the information given by the US besides being more accurate. Spatial and anatomic resolution is better and the visual information is of great help for the surgeon in planning the surgery. Triple phase CT scan remains the most informative modality.

MRI/MRCP is 82–100% sensitive and 92–95% specific in detecting biliary obstruction. It is 70–98% sensitive in differentiating benign from malignant biliary stricture.[4,5] Features suggestive of malignant biliary stricture include presence of mass, long irregular stricture and asymmetric dilatation. For biliary tract assessment it is considered to be superior to other imaging. However, it is costly and may not be universally available. MRI and MRCP may be particularly useful in planning surgery for hilar cholangiocarcinoma. The extent of intrahepatic biliary ductal involvement, presence of ipsilateral or contralateral portal vein or hepatic arterial involvement and the site of hepatic lobar atrophy ("intrahepatic bile ductular crowding") are essential in determining the extent and the side of the liver resection required. MRCP also is useful in confirming the presence and the number of CBD stones when the information may not be forthcoming on an ultrasonogram due to various factors like bowel gas. MRCP is also useful in mapping the anatomical details in cases of iatrogenic biliary strictures before surgical repair. But the accuracy of MRCP in gauging the exact grade of iatrogenic stricture is far from satisfactory; it is found to be especially inaccurate in assessing higher grade strictures like Bismuth grades III and above and percutaneous transhepatic cholangiography (PTC) may be more accurate in delineating such higher grade biliary strictures. The obvious drawback of the PTC over MRCP is its invasive nature and expertise required to perform the procedure and should be considered only when very essential information for surgical planning is not forthcoming with MRCP or a preoperative biliary drainage is required. Biliary-enteric anastomosis such as choledochojejunostomy, hepaticojejunostomy and Billroth 2 anastomosis make endoscopic retrograde cholangiopancreatography (ERCP) difficult or impossible. In these patients MRCP is the imaging modality of choice for the work-up of biliary obstruction.

Endoscopic retrograde cholangiopancreatography may be useful when other imaging modalities are uninformative. However, its diagnostic use has decreased considerably with the availability of MRCP and other noninvasive imagings. Brush cytology, bile sample and tissue biopsy can also be taken during ERCP. Cholangio-carcinoma diagnosis on brush cytology samples may be enhanced by addition of florescence in-situ hybridization (FISH) for polysomies to the routine cytological examination. Also an option of biliary drainage is an advantage of this modality, though it is invasive and has complication.

Of late *endoscopic ultrasonography (EUS)* and EUS guided biopsies are being increasingly used to assess the periampullary biliary obstructions and gallbladder malignancies. Endosonogram also has shown almost equal or better sensitivity in picking up CBD stones as compared with conventional MRCP. With increasing experience this modality appears very promising to give diagnostic benefits over and above the conventional ERCP in assessing periampullary lesions. With the above array of diagnostic armamentarium, the ERCP is now being more selectively used in obstructive jaundice; essentially it is only when a therapeutic procedure like internal biliary drainage is indicated for acute cholangitis or intense hyperbilirubinemia that an ERCP is considered. Biopsy of the lesion may also be done at the same time as the biliary drainage. Cholangioscopes are now available which can be used as a scope-inside scope/mother-baby scopes. Using the cholangioscopes it is possible to directly visualize the obstructing lesions inside the biliary ducts and pancreatic ducts and targeted biopsy can be taken.[1] Despite the ability to target these obstructing biliary and pancreatic lesions using these latest generation scopes, the concerns do remain about the yield from such procedures. Surgical decision-making is seldom altered by the availability of the histopathology of these obstructing lesions, which in vast majority of cases require surgical intervention.

Role of *FDG-PET CT* scans in the HPB area is still under evolution. This investigation is performed to detect any abnormal uptake of the ^{18}Flurodeoxyglucose for the cellular metabolism of the tumor or its secondaries. The presence of Glucose-6-phosphatase enzyme in the hepatocytes and the cells of well differentiated hepatocellular carcinomas serve to metabolize the ^{18}F-FDG used in these scans and hence do not concentrate this tracer and are not well detected by the scan; gallbladder and biliary tumors are also not very FDG avid but adenocarcinoma of head of pancreas and pancreatic neuroendocrine tumors are more FDG avid and the investigation may be more useful in these lesions.[6]

To summarize, patients with jaundice should be evaluated thoroughly. History taking and physical examination remain integral part of their evaluation; imaging and laboratory tests can supplement clinical evaluation to reach a correct diagnosis. Proper selection of correct imaging modality out of widely available array of modalities is important.

REFERENCES

1. Lidofsky SD. Jaundice. In: Feldman M, Friedman LS, Brandt LJ (Eds). Sleisanger & Fordtran's Gastrointestinal and Liver Disease, 9th edition. 2010. pp. 323-35.
2. Garcea G, Ngu W, Neal CP, Dennison AR, Berry DP. Bilirubin levels predict malignancy in patients with obstructive jaundice. HPB (Oxford). 2011;13(6):426-30.
3. Morris-Stiff G, Teli M, Jardine N, Puntis MC. CA19-9 antigen levels can distinguish between benign and malignant pancreaticobiliary disease. Hepatobiliary Pancreat Dis Int. 2009;8(6):620-6.
4. Saluja SS, Sharma R, Pal S, Sahni P, Chattopadhyay TK. Differentiation between benign and malignant hilar obstructions using laboratory and radiological investigations: a prospective study. HPB (Oxford). 2007;9(5):373-82.
5. Tsukada K, Takada T, Miyazaki M, Miyakawa S, Nagino M, Kondo S, et al. Diagnosis of biliary tract and ampullary carcinomas. J Hepatobiliary Pancreat Surg. 2008;15(1):31-40.
6. Garcea G, Ong SL, Maddern GJ. The current role of PET-CT in the characterization of hepatobiliary malignancies. HPB (Oxford). 2009;11(1):4-17.

CHAPTER 66

Liver Abscess

Mihir K Mohapatra, Satya Prasad Samantaray, Vedavyas Mohapatra

INTRODUCTION

Abscesses in the liver fall into two broad types: (1) pyogenic liver abscess (PLA) and (2) amebic liver abscess (ALA); the later caused by the parasite *Entameba histolytica*. Early diagnosis with ultrasonography (US) and computed tomography (CT) and treatment with percutaneous aspiration and drainage procedures have added to improvement in morbidity and mortality.

PYOGENIC LIVER ABSCESS

Mortality related to PLA brought awareness for this condition. Surgical drainage with antibiotics[1] and subsequently percutaneous drainage[2] has improved outcomes of treatment. Diabetes is the major predisposing disease and it can develop as a primary liver abscess without predisposing hepatobiliary disease. CT and US have contributed to early and proper detection. Whereas at turn of the nineteenth century the patient with PLA used to be a male in 20s or 30s with pylephlebitis from an intra-abdominal source of infection such as appendicitis or diverticulitis, nowadays such patients are elderly males (in 60s) with a hepatobiliary pathology which could be either malignant or benign.[3-5]

Etiology and Pathogenesis

Ascending infection of the biliary tree associated with obstruction is the most common cause identified for PLA.[6] Intrahepatic stone is responsible in Asian countries[7,8] whereas cholangiocarcinoma (among malignancies) is more common in the West.[9] Biliary intervention and stenting have also contributed to PLA. Acute appendicitis and diverticulitis can lead to portal pyemia and be causes for PLA, though their incidence is decreasing. Blood borne spread from bacterial endocarditis and bacteremia can also lead to PLA. Liver abscess due to trauma or interventions like radiofrequency ablation and percutaneous ethanol injection may predispose to infection and development of PLA. Direct extension of infection from adjacent viscera may be another source for them. Cryptogenic PLA is one without any identifiable cause and constitute 25% of all liver abscesses. Abscess less than 2 cm in diameter is called a microabscess. Most often they coalesce to form a larger one. Right lobe is the commoner site for liver abscess.

Clinical Presentation

To start with liver abscess presents with vague symptoms like fever, fatigue, malaise, myalgia, loss of appetite. But typically pain right upper quadrant, fever and generalized malaise points to a liver abscess. When it is a secondary abscess, the features of the primary disease like biliary obstruction or hepatobiliary malignancy get added to the other symptoms.

Diagnosis

Raised white cell count and anemia along with raised transaminases and alkaline phosphatase are frequent findings, while elevated bilirubin is less common and may indicate underlying biliary obstruction. Low albumin level is present in long standing disease. Laboratory tests alone cannot contribute to the diagnosis. Plain X-ray chest and abdomen, ultrasound and CT are radiological tests contributing to the diagnosis. Chest X-ray may show a raised right dome of diaphragm, pleural effusion, lung collapse or subdiaphragmatic air-fluid levels.[6]

Ultrasound is the preferred imaging test with a reported sensitivity of 83–95%.[9,10] The PLA in its early stage is hyperechoic without distinct margin. With formation of pus it looks like a walled of hypoechoic space occupying lesion. Underlying biliary disease like intrahepatic or extrahepatic stones, dilation of the bile ducts can be detected by ultrasound. Added Doppler scan should be done to evaluate portal vein patency and exclude solid tumor.

CT scanning is useful for detecting microabscess and has a sensitivity of 93–100%.[6,11] The abscess looks like a central hypodense lesion and peripheral enhancement[12] during the portal phase. It also helps in detecting any associated abdominal disease like appendicitis or diverticulitis. Plural effusion or spontaneous rupture of the abscess can also be detected by CT scan.

On magnetic resonance imaging (MRI) scan the PLA looks like any other fluid containing lesion. Magnetic resonance cholangiopancreatography may help in identifying the level of any associated biliary obstruction. Isotope scan has limited role in the diagnosis of PLA.

Microbiology

Percutaneous aspiration and culture for bacteria show the monomicrobial and polymicrobial nature of the infections.[13-15] *Escherichia coli, Klebsiella, Enterococcus* and *Bacteroides* species are the most commonly isolated organisms in PLA. Klebsiella pneumoniae is responsible in Asian countries.[16] Those associated with blood borne organisms have isolate of *Staphylococcus aureus* or *Streptococcus* and tend to be solitary. Gram stain in addition to blood culture is useful in planning initial treatment.

Treatment

The principle of treatment is drainage like abscess of any site. Drainage is done either percutaneously or by open surgery. Appropriate antibiotic guided by the culture report and treatment of the underlying disease are steps of management for PLA.

About 33–55% of liver abscess are polymicrobial in nature.[13-15] Treatment with antibiotics should be started while waiting for the culture report and it should have broad-based coverage. Results of causes of PLA reported should be helpful in deciding the choice of initial antibiotics. Gram-negative and anaerobic bacteria like bacteroides[17] are isolated when the source is intra-abdominal whereas Gram-negative bacteria are isolated in biliary tract disorders. Therefore an extended spectrum beta-lactams like penicillins (piperacillin-tazobactam, ticarcillin-clavulanate, ampicillin-sulbactam), carbapenems (imipenem, meropenem, ertapenem), or second-generation cephalosporins with or without metronidazole are good initial antibiotics of choice. This can be modified later after the culture and sensitivity reports are obtained from the aspirate and blood cultures. Prolonged treatment with a 4–6 weeks course of antibiotic is necessary, out of which 2–3 weeks, it should be given by parenteral route.[18]

Percutaneous aspiration and/or catheter drainage along with antibiotic therapy is established as the mainstay of treatment for PLA.[19,20] Preference of aspiration over catheter drainage, as reported, would depend on factors like location, number, size and viscosity of the content of the abscess. Inadequate drainage sometimes requires repositioning or placement of extra catheters to evacuate the abscess cavity. As far as possible transpleural intercostal catheter placement should be avoided because it contaminates the pleural cavity and adds to morbidity. If there is persistent drainage of bile through the catheter, indicating communication with a bile duct endoscopic sphincterotomy and stenting may be necessary. Treatment for the underlying cause of biliary obstruction will require modification of the approach.

Surgical Drainage

Indications for surgical drainage: (1) failure of medical management or (2) failure of percutaneous drainage or its complications like bleeding, peritonitis; (3) surgery may be the initial approach where the source control is needed along with drainage; (4) rupture of the abscess with peritonitis; (5) associated biliary obstruction; (6) drainage with partial liver resection if there is destruction of the liver parenchyma or an associated malignant tumor.

Extended subcostal or upper midline incision is given. Appendicitis or diverticulitis are dealt with, if present. Following exploration of the peritoneal cavity, the abscess in the liver is localized, aspirated and drained at its most dependent part. The aspirate is sent for Gram staining and culture, sensitivity test. Breaking the loculations should be gentle, because sometimes intrahepatic portal structure wrapped in Glisson's capsule traverse across the cavity and injuring them will cause bleeding and bile leakage. Multiple catheters are placed inside the cavity before closer of the abdomen for drainage. They can be used for irrigation or contrast studies if necessary.

Summary

There is a definite risk of recurrence and mortality. Recurrence rates vary from 2% to 23.8% and mortality rate vary from 3% to 30%. Mortality is high in patients with associated medical diseases like renal failure, malignancy, cirrhosis and in the elderly.

Though diabetes is a known risk factor, mortality is not high in them. Patients with leucocytosis, hypoalbuminemia, jaundice, prolonged prothrombin time and raised serum creatinine are at a high risk of death, so also are those with anaerobic and multidrug resistant isolates.

AMEBIC LIVER ABSCESS (ALA)

Entameba hystolytica is a parasite which causes amebiasis. Liver is the common site of extraintestinal amebiasis and liver abscess develops in 3–9% of the infected population. Tropical Asia and Africa have a high prevalence, among which India and Mexico have very high prevalence. Poor hygiene and sanitation make population in these countries vulnerable to this infection. Males in 30s to 40s, often alcoholics, are more often seen to be affected.

Entameba hystolytica has a cyst and a trophozoite form. Cysts are the infective from transmitted by fecal-oral route via water and food. They are destroyed by heat and drying.

Etiology and Pathogenesis

The quadrinucleated cysts survive the acidic secretion of the stomach and trophozoites are released in the small intestine where excystation occurs in alkaline secretion. In the large intestine the trophozoite multiplies and cysts are produced. Cecum is the site of amebic colitis. ALA is caused by trophozoite entering the portal blood flow after penetrating the colonic mucosa and localizing in the liver, mostly the right lobe. Neutrophil destruction caused by the invasion and lysis, destroys hepatocytes by its cytotoxic mediators and if the destruction continues affecting a large area, the abscess develops. The content is chocolate color, viscous exudate described as "anchovy sauce pus" (Fig. 1). This pus is sterile and does not contain ameba which are present at the margins of the lesion.

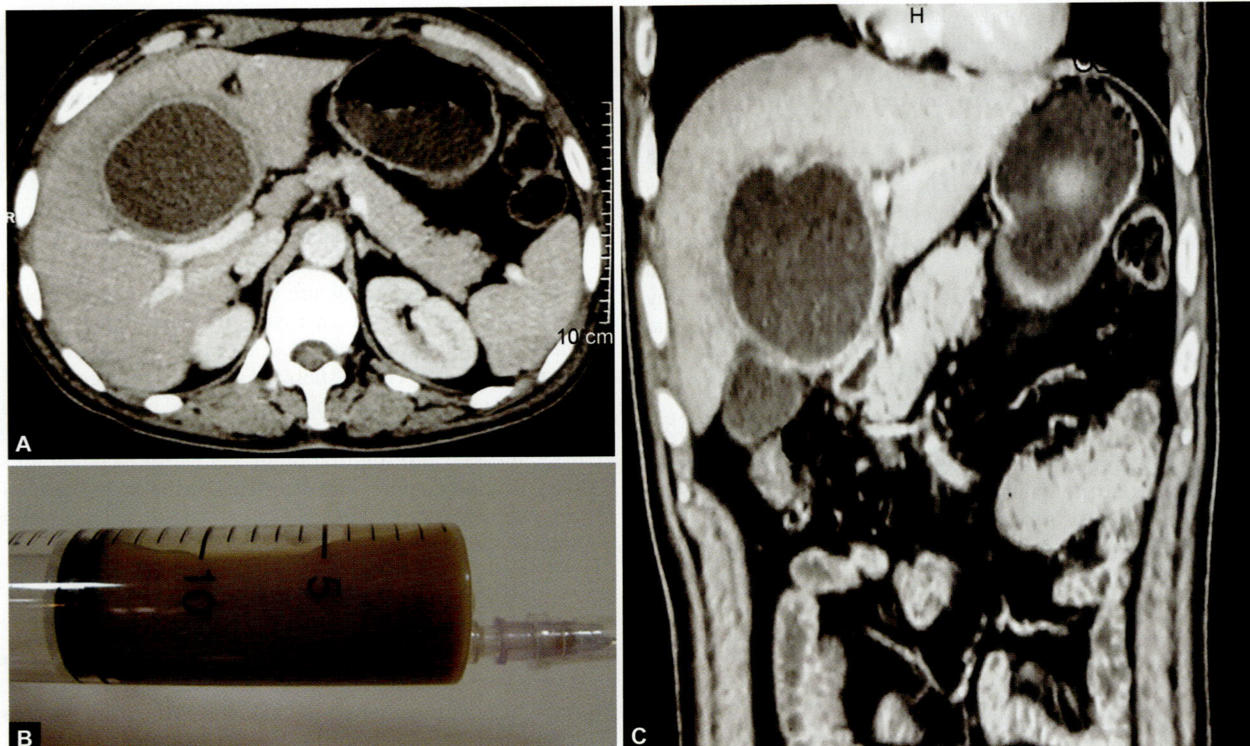

Figures 1A to C Amebic liver abscess. (A and B) CT scan axial and coronal sections with a single well-defined abscess with enhancing wall. (C) Anchovy sauce aspirate

Polymorphonuclear leucocyte gathers around the trophozoite in the early stage and later macrophages, lymphocytes and epitheloid cells surround them, which contribute to the formation of granuloma.

Clinical Features

Amebiasis has an insidious course and may cause diarrhea and dysentery and pain abdomen. An attack of gastroenteritis leading to fever and pain right upper quadrant of abdomen is common with the ALA. When irritating the diaphragm right lower chest pain in present. Pain is in the epigastrium if the abscess is in the left lobe and a large abscess might cause jaundice due to compression or erosion of the biliary tree.

Soft tender hepatomegaly with intercostal tenderness is present on examination. Right basal lung signs as of pleural effusion or lung abscess may be present.[21] When compared with PLA, patients with ALA are young males with solitary right lobe lesion.[22] History of intestinal amebiasis precedes the attack, accompanied by a high amebic serology.

Laboratory Findings

It is recommended that three stool samples collected over 10 days should be examined under light microscopy[23] for detection of trophozoite when there is dysentery.

Raised leucocyte count with raised alanine aminotransferase is seen frequently in acute form of the abscess. In about 70% cases the alkaline phosphatase levels are high.

The overall accuracy of serologic test for ALA is 95%. Indirect hemagglutination assay and ELISA (enzyme-linked immunosorbent assay) are the two most commonly used tests to detect amebic antibody. Antibodies are detected 7–10 days after unset of the illness. If serologic titer is below 1:256, a PLA is likely.

Imaging

A plain X-ray abdomen shows an enlarged liver shadow. Chest X-ray is abnormal with elevated right dome of diaphragm. Pleural effusion on right side and basal consolidation is seen in about half of the patients. Ultrasound shows a solitary hypoechoic lesion in the right lobe of liver and is accurate in 90% cases.[24] CT shows a well-defined, round, fluid containing lesion in the liver (Fig. 1) and is the preferred imaging study.[25] The wall enhances with contrast with a peripheral zone of edema. MRI has no specific advantage over CT. With each of the three, guided biopsy and aspiration can be done.

Resolution of the lesion on imaging takes about a year and in 90% cases complete resolution occurs.[26]

Treatment

Drug treatment constitutes the main modality of therapy for ALA. Nitroimidazole compounds like metronidazole, ornidazole, tinidazole compounds are used as the first line of drugs. Metronidazole is used in a dose of 500–750 mg three times a day, either orally or intravenously for 5–10 days. The side effects are nausea, vomiting and metallic test. It is contraindicated in the first trimester of pregnancy.

Dihydroemetine, a parenteral drug given intramuscularly or subcutaneously is used in rupture ALA and can be combined with metronidazole. It is contraindicated in patients with cardiac and muscular diseases.

Chloroquin is another drug in ALA and is given orally. The dosage is 1 g. (600 mg base) for 2 days and then 500 mg (300 mg base) per day for the rest of the duration of 3 weeks.

Percutaneous aspiration is done in addition to metronidazole therapy if the patient is sick, there is impending rupture or bacterial superinfection. When communication with the biliary systems is present, endoscopic papillotomy and stenting is undertaken. These lesions are usually larger in size and may present with jaundice.

Surgery is indicated for established or impending rupture, or failure of catheter drainage. If it has ruptured into the pleural cavity, inter costal tube drainage is done. During open drainage emetine hydrochloride in saline may be instilled into the cavity. Post drainage, these patients require intravenous metronidazole and a broad spectrum antibiotic.

Complications

Rupture in to the chest and pericardium and abdominal viscera can occur. Large size and left lobe abscesses are more prone for rupture. In the chest it can rupture into the bronchus, lungs,[27] pericardium and pleural cavity and in the abdomen into the peritoneal cavity, stomach or colon.

Outcome

Overall mortality for ALA is 5%. The risk increases with raised bilirubin, hypoalbuminemia, larger and multiple abscesses, rupture and diabetes.[28] The patients are usually young males, living in poor sanitary surroundings. Compared with PLA, ALA is solitary, in the right lobe and less often accompanied by jaundice. On Amebic serology, titers are higher than 1:256. Medical treatment is adequate in majority and percutaneous drainage is less often indicated in contrast to PLA. Improvement in sanitation and healthy habits helps in preventing amebic infection in the community.

REFERENCES

1. Ochsner A, DeBakey M, Murray S. Pyogenic abscess of the liver. Am J Surg. 1988;40:292.
2. McFadzean AJ, Chang KP, Wong CC. Solitary pyogenic abscess of the liver treated by closed aspiration and antibiotics; a report of 14 consecutive cases with recovery. Br J Surg. 1953;41:141.
3. O'Farrell N, Collins CG, McEntee GP: Pyogenic liver abscesses: diminished role for operative treatment. Surgeon. 2010;8:192.
4. Mezhir JJ, Fong Y, Jacks LM, Getrajdman GI, Brody LA, Covey AM, et al: Current management of pyogenic liver abscess: surgery is now second-line treatment. J Am Coll Surg. 2010;210:975-83.
5. Meddings L, Myers RP, Hubbard J, Shaheen AA, Laupland KB, Dixon E, et al. A population-based study of pyogenic liver abscesses in the United States: incidence, mortality, and temporal trends. Am J Gastroenterol. 2010;105:117-24.
6. Seeto RK, Rockey DC. Pyogenic liver abscess. Changes in etiology, management, and outcome. Medicine (Baltimore) 1996;75:99-113.
7. Chou FF, Sheen-Chen SM, Chen YS, Chen MC. Single and multiple pyogenic liver abscesses: clinical course, etiology, and results of treatment. World J Surg 1997;21:384; discussion 388-9.
8. Chu KM, Fan ST, Lai EC, Lo CM, Wong J. Pyogenic liver abscess. An audit of experience over the past decade. Arch Surg. 1996;131: 148-52.
9. Huang CJ, Pitt HA, Lipsett PA, Osterman FA Jr, Lillemoe KD, Cameron JL, et al. Pyogenic hepatic abscess. Changing trends over 42 years. Ann Surg. 1996;223:600-7; discussion 607-9.
10. Alvarez JA, Gonzalez JJ, Baldonedo RF, Sanz L, Carreño G, Jorge JI. Single and multiple pyogenic liver abscesses: etiology, clinical course, and outcome. Dig Surg. 2001;18:283-8.
11. Saini S. Imaging of the hepatobiliary tract. N Engl J Med 1997;336:1889-94.
12. Benedetti NJ, Desser TS, Jeffrey RB. Imaging of hepatic infections. Ultrasound Q. 2008;24:267-78.
13. Mohsen AH, Green ST, Read RC, McKendrick MW. Liver abscess in adults: ten years experience in a UK centre. QJM. 2002;95:797-802.
14. Alvarez Perez JA, Gonzalez JJ, Baldonedo RF, Sanz L, Carreño G, Junco A, et al. Clinical course, treatment, and multivariate analysis of risk factors for pyogenic liver abscess. Am J Surg. 2001;181: 177-86.
15. Rahimian J, Wilson T, Oram V, Holzman RS. Pyogenic liver abscess: recent trends in etiology and mortality. Clin Infect Dis. 2004;39:1654-9.
16. Wang JH, Liu YC, Lee SS, Yen MY, Chen YS, Wang JH, et al. Primary liver abscess due to Klebsiella pneumoniae in Taiwan. Clin Infect Dis. 1998;26:1434-8.
17. Johannsen EC, Sifri CD, Madoff LC. Pyogenic liver abscesses. Infect Dis Clin North Am. 2000;14:547-63.
18. Ng FH, Wong WM, Wong BC, Kng C, Wong SY, Lai KC, et al. Sequential intravenous/oral antibiotic vs. continuous intravenous antibiotic in the treatment of pyogenic liver abscess. Aliment Pharmacol Ther. 2002;16:1083-90.
19. Branum GD, Tyson GS, Branum MA, Meyers WC. Hepatic abscess. Changes in etiology, diagnosis, and management. Ann Surg. 1990;212:655-62.
20. Yu SC, Ho SS, Lau WY, Yeung DT, Yuen EH, Lee PS, et al. Treatment of pyogenic liver abscess: prospective randomized comparison of catheter drainage and needle aspiration. Hepatology. 2004;39: 932-8.
21. Loulergue P, Mir O. Pleural empyema secondary to amebic liver abscess. Int J Infect Dis. 2009;13:e135-6.
22. Lodhi S, Sarwari AR, Muzammil M, Salam A, Smego RA. Features distinguishing amoebic from pyogenic liver abscess: a review of 577 adult cases. Trop Med Int Health. 2004;9:718-23.
23. Fotedar R, Stark D, Beebe N, Marriott D, Ellis J, Harkness J. Laboratory diagnostic techniques for Entamoeba species. Clin Microbiol Rev. 2007;20:511-32.
24. Reid-Lombardo KM, Khan S, Sclabas G. Hepatic cysts and liver abscess. Surg Clin North Am. 2010;90:679-97.
25. Radin DR, Ralls PW, Colletti PM, Halls JM. CT of amebic liver abscess. AJR Am J Roentgenol. 1988;150:1297-301.
26. Blessmann J, Khoa ND, Van An L, Tannich E. Ultrasound patterns and frequency of focal liver lesions after successful treatment of amoebic liver abscess. Trop Med Int Health. 2006;11:504-8.
27. Stanley Jr SL. Amebiasis. Lancet. 2003;361:1025-34.
28. Hughes MA, Petri Jr WA. Amebic liver abscess. Infect Dis Clin North Am. 2000;14:565-82.

CHAPTER 67

Hydatid Disease of Liver

Eppa Vimalakar Reddy, Mohan N, Ramesh Ardhnari

INTRODUCTION

Hydatid disease is an important zoonotic infection of humans caused by genus Echinococcus and the family Taeniidae. It is transmitted to human being by ingestion of food and water contaminated by (cestodes) eggs of tapeworm excreted in the feces of infected dogs and sheep. The problem is endemic in certain parts of the world where people are in close contact with such animals.[1-3]

In human, four species have been identified to cause different types of echinococcal infection:

1. *Echinococcus oligarthrus*—polycystic echinococcosis
2. *Echinococcus vogeli*—polycystic echinococcosis
3. *Echinococcus granulosus*—cystic echinococcosis
4. *Echinococcus multilocularis*—alveolar echinococcosis

Echinococcus granulosus is the most common variety while multilocularis is the most aggressive variety. *E. granulosus* is located in viscera mainly liver and lung. *E. multilocularis* and *E. vogeli* are located mainly in liver while *E. oligarthrus* is primarily located in muscles.

EPIDEMIOLOGY

Around the globe 65 million people are affected by this disease causing a major economic burden. The prevalence is very high in southern South America, Australia, parts of Africa, central Asia and zones of Soviet Union that lie in temperate zones. In India, 100–200/100,000 persons are affected annually, majority being from Kashmir, Andhra Pradesh, Tamil Nadu and Central India.[4]

Life Cycle of *Echinococcus granulosus* (Fig. 1)

The primary hosts are predators like canine and intermediate hosts are preys like sheep. Human beings are accidental, intermediate hosts. Infection is acquired by ingestion of food or water contaminated with eggs of the parasite. In the duodenum, larvae are released and they migrate to the liver by penetrating mucosa through the mesenteric vessels. In 70% of cases, liver is the primary site of filter and in 15–30% of cases lung acts as the second filter. After lodging in an organ, larvae develop into cysts, which grow at a rate of 1–3 cm/year. The cysts become clinically evident when they reach large sizes.[3] Sometimes the eggs penetrate the circulation and spread via blood stream to other organs like lung, spleen, kidney, brain or bone.

HYDATID CYST STRUCTURE (FIG. 2)

The cyst wall contains three layers:

1. Outer fibrous capsule called pericyst formed due to host reaction. It is present in liver and spleen while absent in lung and brain. Vascular structures and biliary radicals remain intact in this adventitial layer for a quite a period while cyst is growing.
2. Chitinous middle layer (laminated membrane) called ectocyst easily separable from the pericyst. It is 1–2 mm thick. It supports the endocyst and protects the cyst from bile, enzymes and bacteria. It is permeable to water, K^+, urea and Ca^+
3. Germinal inner layer called endocyst. The endocyst is the only living portion, which secretes hydatid fluid and forms brood capsules which eventually becomes daughter cysts.
4. Hydatid fluid is colorless, odorless clear fluid in an uncomplicated cyst. The color changes to bile stained in cyst with biliary communication, purulent in infected cyst and turbid in

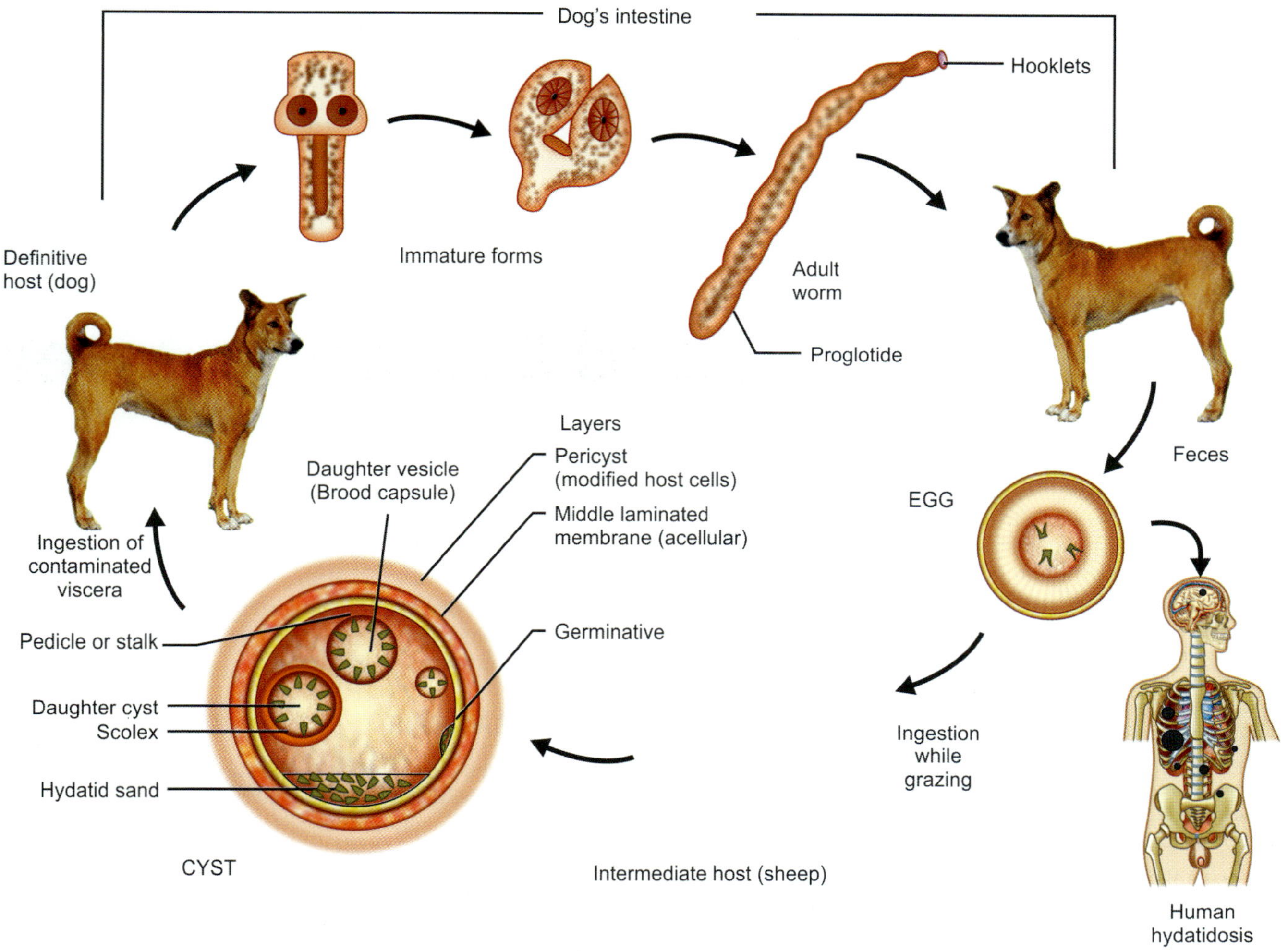

Figure 1 Life cycle of *Echinococcus granulosus*

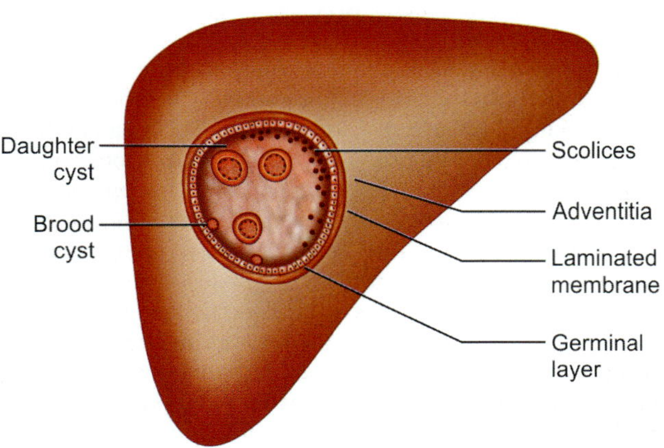

Figure 2 Diagram showing different parts of hydatid cyst of liver

degenerated cyst. The cyst pressure are as high as 70 cm of water in viable cyst which decreases to as low as 0 cm in dead cyst.

NATURAL HISTORY AND CLINICAL FEATURES

Cyst with size less than 5 cm and uncomplicated cyst are usually asymptomatic. When growth of cyst occurs, it produces a mass effect causing vague upper abdomen pain and discomfort. Acute abdominal pain usually occurs either when cyst is infected or it ruptures into the peritoneal cavity. In some cases the cyst may compress the biliary radicals and cause obstructive jaundice. More commonly jaundice occur when there cyst biliary communication with major ducts. The cyst may then rupture leading to various complications. The growth phase is followed by a phase of ageing and involution, in which scolices and daughter cysts replace the hydatid fluid ultimately leading to calcification of the advential wall. Fully calcified wall is impermeable to all nutrients, and oxygen may eventually lead to death of cyst.

COMPLICATIONS OF HYDATID CYST OF THE LIVER

- Allergic manifestations
- Intrabiliary rupture of hydatid cyst:
  - Into right hepatic duct: 55–60%
  - Into left hepatic duct: 25–30%
  - Into rest of biliary system: 8–11%

It is most common complication of hydatid liver cyst. This may be either occult when it ruptures into the minor ducts (10–37%) in which cystic fluid alone drains into biliary tree or frank when ruptures into major ducts (3–17%) in which daughter cysts also drain. Rupture into the major ducts manifests as obstructive jaundice or cholangitis (Fig. 3).[5-7] The risk for cyst biliary communication is reported to be higher in patients with mutilocular cyst, patients having raised alkaline phosphatase preoperatively, cyst located near biliary bifurcation, male patients and size of cyst more than 10 cm.

1. Rupture into the thorax: In 0.6–16% of cases, liver hydatid may rupture into the pulmonary system due to pulmonary erosion. If the patient develops bronchobiliary fistula, they develop cyst and bile expectoration, otherwise they present with cough and dyspnea.[6-10] Cyst located in posterior superior part of liver are prone to rupture into thorax (Fig. 4).
2. Rupture into the peritoneum (Figs 5A and B): Rarely (1–8%) free rupture of cyst can happen in large cysts, which may lead on to anaphylactic reactions presenting as fever, pain, nausea, vomiting, urticaria and secondary echinococcosis.[11-13] It can present as acute abdomen with abdominal signs. Diagnostic peritoneal lavage is highly specific in diagnosing hydatid rupture into peritoneal cavity.

Other complications:

3. Portal hypertension due to budd chiari syndrome[14]
4. Vascular erosions

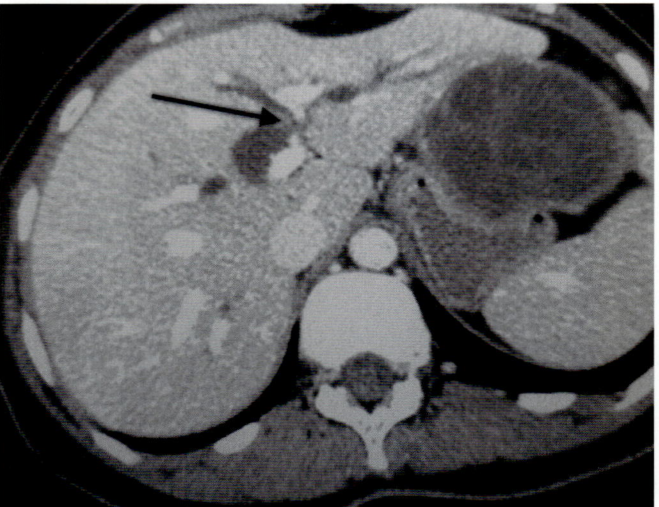

Figure 3 Axial section CT scan abdomen showing dilated intrahepatic radicles on left lobe along with a cyst partially decompressed into left biliary system (arrow). Another cyst located in the left lobe hanging from segment 3 also seen

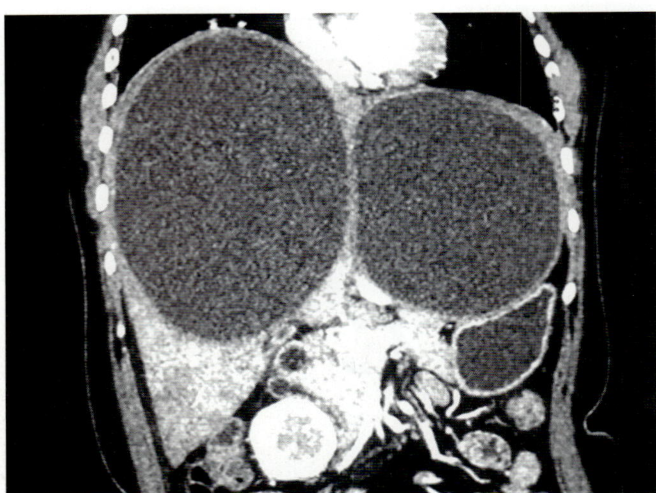

Figure 4 Sagittal section CT scan of abdomen showing two large hydatid cysts. The right lobe cyst located in the segment 7 & 8 growing toward diaphragm. Such cysts are prone to rupture into pleural cavity

5. Erosions into digestive system leading to hydatid emesis and hydatid enterica
6. Fistulization to skin.

INVESTIGATIONS

The combination of imaging techniques and serology are required to form a definitive diagnosis of hydatid cyst. Laboratory tests other than serology are usually normal. Liver function tests are deranged in patients having cyst biliary communication. They may have raised serum bilirubin, and alkaline phosphates. Raised serum transaminases and high total leukocyte counts (TLC) suggest cholangitis in these patients. Occasionally they may have high eosinophil count (>3%). These are nonspecific in endemic areas.

SEROLOGY AND IMMUNOLOGICAL TESTS

They are used for diagnosis, post-treatment follow-up and epidemiological surveillance. Recent and past infections can be diagnosed by detecting specific IgM and IgG antibodies to the parasite respectively. ELISA, indirect immune fluorescence assay (IFA) and counter immunoelectrophoresis (CIEP) are the tests used widely in clinical practice. Among them ELISA and IFA being highly sensitive (90–95%) and CIEP being highly specific (100%) and sensitive (80–90%).[1,3,15] In postoperative follow-up circulating hydatid antigen is used for detection of residual or recurrent disease. CIEP is useful for post-treatment follow-up unlike ElLISA as circulating IgG antibodies may present up to 4 years after surgery therefore can give false positive result. Casoni test is no more used due to hypersensitivity reactions and low sensitivity.

In order to detect antibody response to parasite, several hydatid antigens have been extracted and used for serological diagnosis. The most specific native antigens for the immune-diagnosis of cystic Echinococcosis include hydatid fluid antigen B (AgB) and antigen 5 (Ag5) from *E. Granulosus*.[16] Western blot using these antigens is useful for diagnosis and post-treatment follow-up with sensitivity of 95% and specificity of 100%.

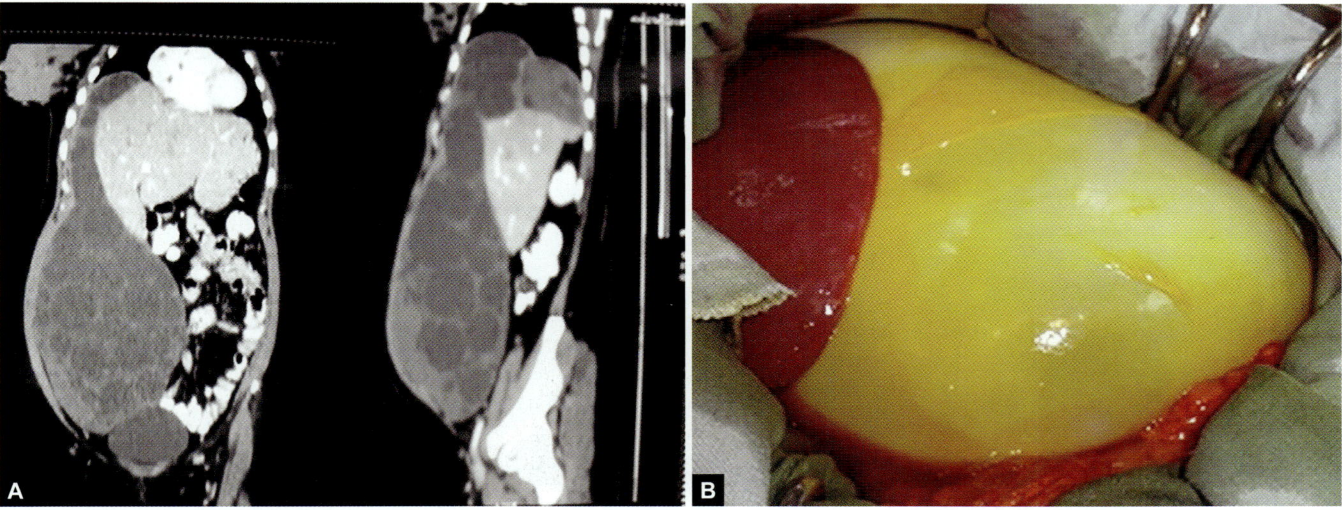

Figures 5A and B (A) Sagittal section CT of abdomen showing a hydatid cyst with multiple daughter cysts arising from segment 6 and growing inferiorly down to pelvis. Such cysts are prone to rupture into peritoneal cavity; (B) Intraoperative picture showing hydatid ruptured into peritoneal cavity occupying most of the peritoneal cavity

IMAGING TECHNIQUES

Plain Radiographs

X-ray abdomen and chest are nondiagnostic, with only nonspecific signs like curvilinear or ring like calcifications and elevation of hemidiaphragm. A dead parasite is seen as a complete calcification.

Ultrasonography

Ultrasonography (USG) (Fig. 6) of abdomen is useful in screening and establishing the diagnosis. It has a diagnostic accuracy of 90%. Ultrasound shows hydatid sand which moves freely with position, daughter cysts as localized thickening, undulating membrane seen as a water lily sign and calcification as the diagnostic features. It is also useful for performing percutaneous treatment and post-treatment follow-up. Gharbi et al. classified hydatid cyst based on ultrasound features (Table 1).

Table 1: Gharbi classification on ultrasonography features of hydatid cyst[17]

Type	*Ultrasound appearance*
I	Pure fluid collection
II	Fluid collection with a split wall (*detached membrane*)
III	Fluid collection with septa and/or *daughter cysts*
IV	Heterogeneous echo pattern (*Hyperechoic with high internal echoes*)
V	Reflecting walls (Cyst with reflecting calcified thick wall)

Figure 6 Ultrasound of abdomen showing Gharbi type II hydatid cyst liver

Sometimes biliary obstruction due to cyst or cystobiliary communication can also be detected by USG. Recently WHO has standardized the classification based on ultrasound features.[18]

CL type usually corresponds to early stage of development. They are *active* single cysts with well-defined wall and liquid content. It is difficult to differentiate them from simple biliary cyst. Cysts are fertile.

CE1 types are simple cysts that contain hyperechogenic material known as hydatid sand. They are *active* and fertile. Presence of hydatid sand is known as snow flake sign. It has a visible cyst wall.

CE2 types are multivesicular cysts that contain daughter cyst which give them a spoke wheel or a honeycomb like appearance. They are active type and fertile in nature.

CE3 types are degenerating cysts that have partial or total detachment of laminated membrane known as water lily or water snake sign. They still contain some viable protoscolices and known as *transition* type.

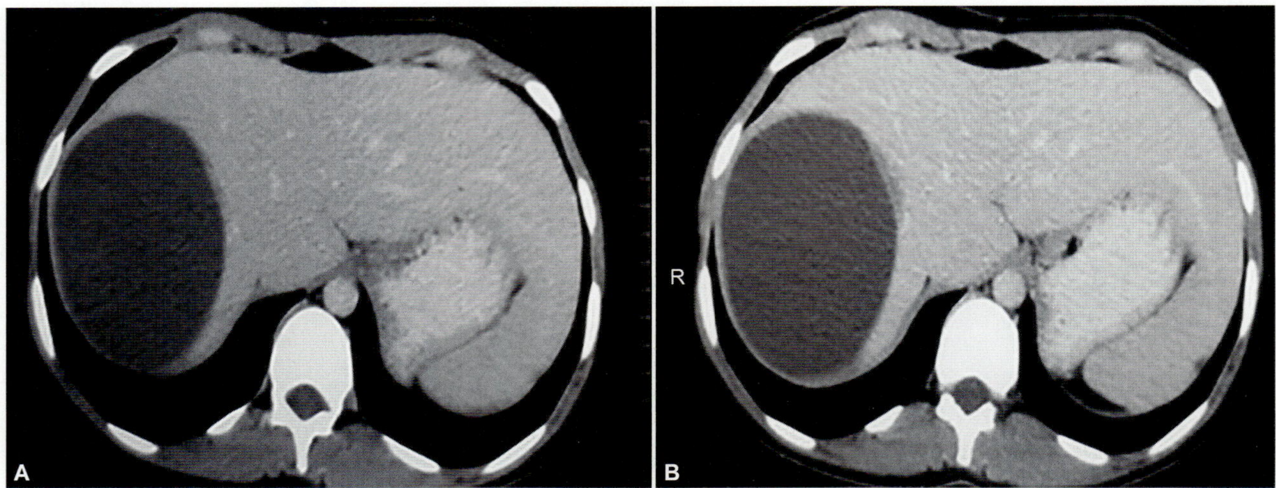

Figures 7A and B (A and B) Axial sections of CT scan showing cystic lesion without any debris or membrane or daughter cysts located segment 6 suggestive of CL type of hydatid cyst

CE4 types occur when degeneration is advanced and are classified as *inactive* type. They may be calcified. They have both cystic and solid component therefore a heterogeneous appearance without any visible daughter cysts.

CE5 type cysts contain amorphous mass like matrix giving it a solid appearance. They have a calcified wall and are *inactive* and *infertile* variety.

The classification allows uniform nomenclature to different stages of cyst for comparison of various management strategies.

Computed Tomographic Scan (Figs 7 to 10)

Computed tomographic scan helps to know the size, location and number of cysts. The sensitivity of CT scan is as high as 100%. It also helps in diagnosing complications like cystobiliary communication, intraperitoneal and intrathoracic rupture. For Gharbi type I and type IV cysts diagnosis, CT scan is better than ultrasound. In the planning of surgery, CT scan is a definitely indicated to know the relation with the vascular structures and future liver remnant.[19,20]

Magnetic Resonance Imaging (MRI) Scan

Hydatid cyst appears a low intensity lesion on T2-weighted MRI scan. This characteristic sign on MRI is due to collagen rich laminated membrane. MRI does not score over CT scan in routine diagnosis of hydatid cyst.[21] It is useful in patients with cyst biliary communication. Magnetic resonance cholangiopancreatography

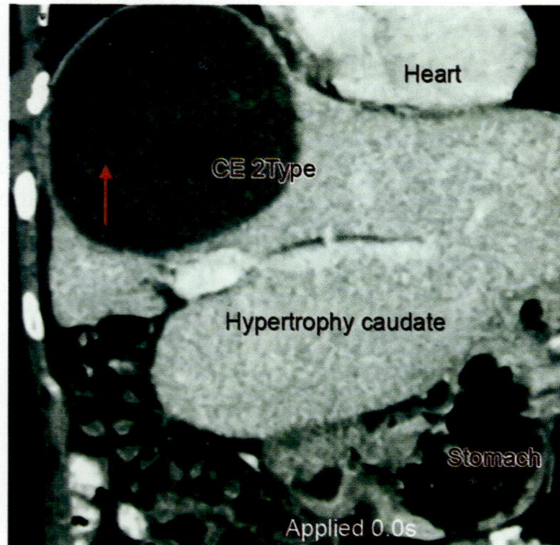

Figure 8 Axial section of CT scan showing cystic lesion located in segment 7 of liver containing debris (arrow) depicting hydatid sand suggestive of CE type I hydatid cyst

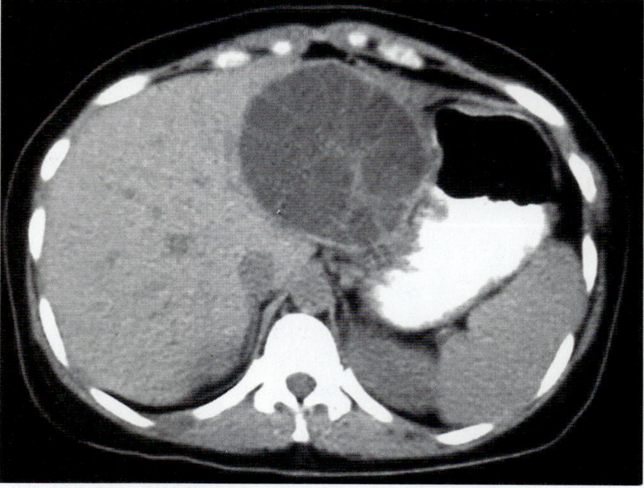

Figure 9 Axial section of CT scan showing cystic lesion located in segments 2 and 3 of liver containing multiple daughter cysts giving honeycomb or spoke-wheel appearance suggestive of CE type II hydatid cyst

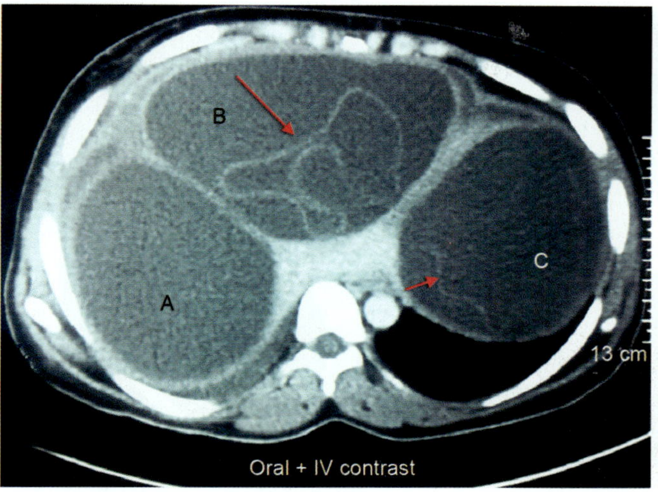

Figure 10 Axial section of CT scan showing multiple cystic lesions in both lobe of liver. Cyst labeled B and C has typical membrane (arrow) known as water lily sign suggestive of CE type III hydatid cyst

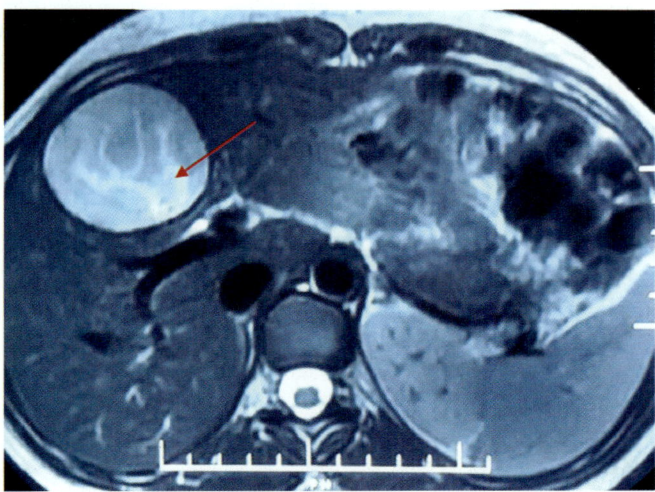

Figure 11 Axial section of T2-weighted MRI scan showing cystic lesion in liver with membranes suggestive of hydatid cyst liver

(MRCP) detects cystobiliary communication better than CT (Fig. 11).

Endoscopic Retrograde Cholangiopancreatography

Primary benefit of an endoscopic retrograde cholangiopancreatography (ERCP) would be the clearance of CBD prior to surgery, but it also detects cystobiliary communication akin to MRCP.[22] It is indicated in patients presenting with cholangitis.

Direct Cholangiography

Suspicion of an intrabiliary communication during surgery needs an intraoperative cholangiography.

TREATMENT

The Consensus Statement of WHO-IWGE in 2009 suggested image-based and stage specific treatment options for management of hydatid cyst.[22] The various treatment options available are:

- Surgery
- Percutaneous treatment (PT)
- Chemotherapy
- Watchful waiting.

Surgery

The surgery remains the mainstay of treatment for hydatid liver disease.

Indications

- Large size cysts with multiple daughter cysts
- Single cysts located superficially that may rupture
- Infected cysts
- Those having with cystobiliary communication
- Cysts exerting pressure on adjacent organs.

Contraindications

- Calcified asymptomatic cysts are also known as dead cyst
- Small cysts less than 5 cm especially when located deep within parenchyma of liver.

Surgical procedures may be classified as either conservative methods or radical procedure. The principle for treatment are—total removal of the cyst, avoidance of spillage, management of cystobiliary communication and management of residual cavity.[23-25]

Proposed advantages for radical procedures:

A. Total removal of cyst and exocysts is associated with the lowest recurrence rate.
B. Chemotherapy after radical removal of intact cyst may not be required.
C. The use of intraoperative scolicidal agents is not required if the cyst is not entered.
D. The chance of biliary fistula and cavity related complications is low.
E. Calcified cysts can be removed.
F. In expert hands mortality and morbidity are low.

Proposed disadvantages for radical procedures:

A. Not all cysts are suitable for radical surgery. A large cyst adherent to major vascular structures can be difficult to resect and can result in mortality in a benign condition.
B. It requires technical expertise and a set up with specific equipment aiding in radical surgery that may not be available everywhere.

Radical procedures have lower complication rate related to cyst cavity and lower recurrences but many authors consider them inappropriate, claiming that intraoperative risks are too high for a benign disease.[26] Therefore decision regarding radical procedure should be based on availability of expertise, performance status of the patients, location of the cyst and presence of cyst related

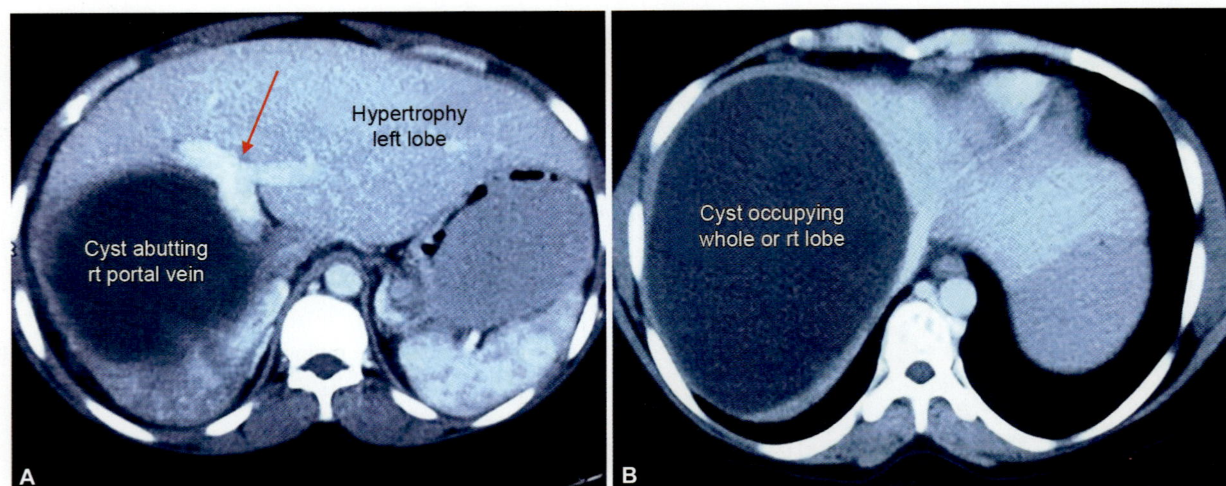

Figures 12A and B Axial section CT scan showing: (A) cyst in close relation with portal pedicle or (B) a cyst occupying almost whole of the right lobe. Such cysts are risk of intraoperative complication such as bleeding if radical procedures are contemplated for them

complications. If the expertise are available and cyst is located away from major vascular structures or occupying whole lobe with minimal resection of normal lobe and adequate residual liver volume radical procedure can contemplated. Centrally located cysts are usually not suitable for cystopericystectomy especially when in close relation to portal pedicle (Figs 12A and B).

Incision and Protection

The choice of incision depends upon location of cyst, presence of extrahepatic cyst and cyst related complication. The subcostal incision with midline or bilateral subcostal extension allows adequate exposure in most cases. Midline incision is preferred in patients with left lobe cyst, abdominal hydatidosis and cyst perforated into peritoneal cavity. For adequate protection, the surrounding area is packed with saline soaked sponges followed by protoscolicidal soaked sponges except small most prominent area from where cyst is evacuated (Fig. 13).

Conservative Technique

These are technically simple, safe and are used for uncomplicated hydatid cysts, but are associated with higher rate of postoperative complications compared to radical procedures.[27]

The principles of conservative management include controlled evacuation of cyst contents and management of the residual cavity including biliary communication if any.

Controlled Evacuation of Cyst (Figs 14A and B)

It includes avoiding spillage of contents, inactivate cyst contents and carefully evacuate the cyst contents. Minimal mobilization of cyst and liver before evacuation avoids iatrogenic injury to cyst and inadvertent spillage of contents. Cone described by Saidi et al. is useful in providing safe drainage. They are not useful in posterior-superior cyst. Laparoscopic trocars are useful for insertion and evacuation of cyst. High pressure suction is introduced through trocar to evacuate, and gas port is used to introduce the scolicidal agent.

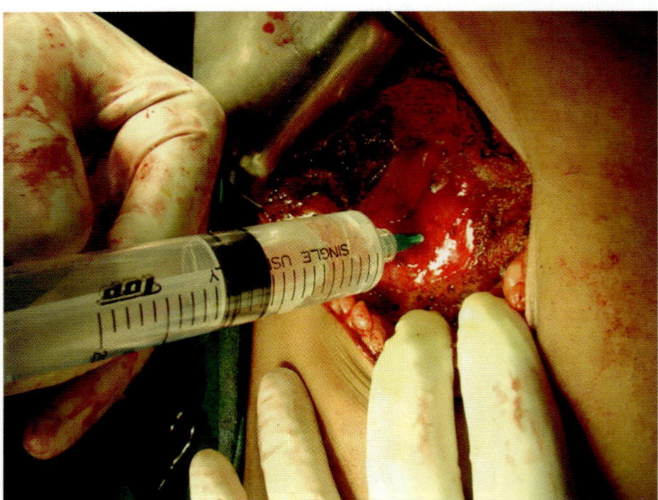

Figure 13 Intraoperative picture showing how cyst is aspirated with adequate protection before starting deroofing and evacuation of cyst. The colorless nature of fluid is typical of hydatid without any biliary communication

Protoscoicidal agent: It should not be injected in bile stained cyst. Various agents available are:

- *Hypertonic saline*: It is the most commonly use scolicidal. Various conc 3–30% are available. Solution (20%) is used and is kept for at least 6 minutes for optimal result.
- *Cetrimide (0.5%) and chlorhexidine (0.05%)* combined solution for 5 minutes is also an effective scolicidal. The important side effects include metabolic acidosis and methemoglobinemia.
- *Absolute alcohol* is useful scolicidal used by interventional radiologist for percutaneous treatment. It is not effective on scolices inside daughter cyst and ineffective if dilution occurs. Major side effects include caustic cholangitis and potential for fire accident due to inflammable nature especially in presence of cautery.

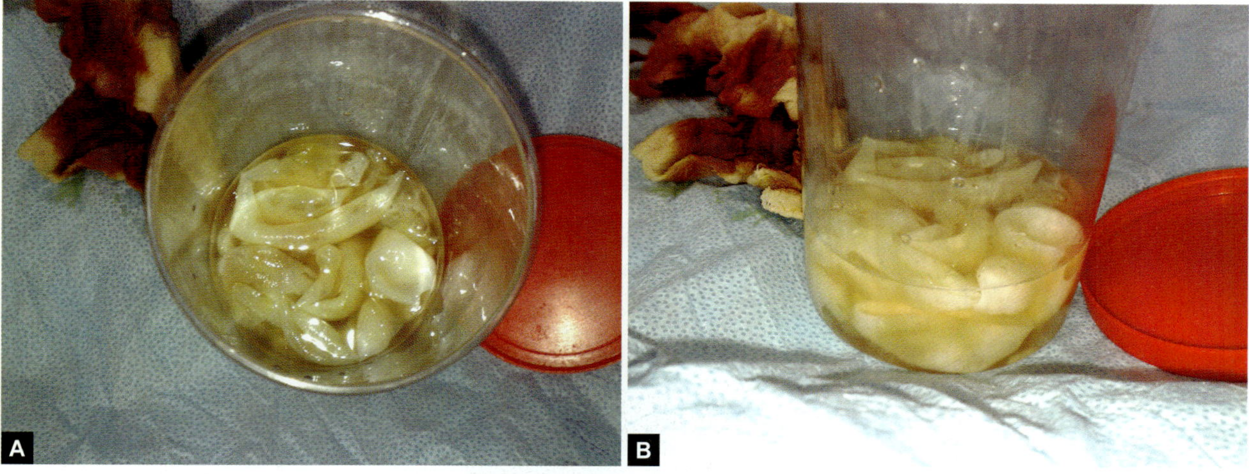

Figures 14A and B (A and B) Intraoperative picture showing evacuation of daughter cysts

- *Povidine iodine:* About 10% is easily available and effective scolicidal. The side effects include caustic cholangitis. It colors the cyst wall therefore may make difficult to identify cyst biliary communication.

Management of the residual cavity:

- *External tube drainage:* After deroofing, evacuation and sterilization of the cyst cavity one or more drains are left in place. Commonly used in infected cyst and cyst biliary communication. Most commonly used method. It is usually combined with partial pericystectomy (Fig. 15).
- *Leaving the cyst open:* Large, shallow cavities that cannot be obliterated may be left open or covered with an omental flap sutured to the rim.
- *Capsulorrhaphy:* Sterilized cyst cavity is filled with saline solution and closed by approximating the edges with running absorbable sutures. This is done in small, non-infected and non-calcified cysts only. The drawbacks are lack of access for peritoneal absorption and risk for secondary endogenous infection.
- *Omentoplasty:* A viable omental flap is developed and placed into the remaining cyst cavity. If the cavity is deep and has a large volume, a closed-system drain is placed alongside the omentum. It is the only technique that has preventive effect on postoperative bile leakage. Combined options like partial capitonnage plus omentoplasty are also used in very large cysts (Figs 16A and B).
- *Capitonnage:* It is approximation of cyst wall by suturing to obliterate the cavity. One technique is infolding the redundant pericyst wall from the depths of the pericyst with layers of sutures. An alternate technique is circular suturing from the depth of the pericyst toward the surface. It is not possible when the volume of pericyst is large (Fig. 17).
- *Marsupialization:* It is external drainage of the cyst by suturing the opening on the pericyst to the abdominal wall. It has been abandoned because bleeding from the cyst and infection were frequent and morbidity was high.
- *Introflexion:* Folding in and approximating opposite edges of the pericyst and suturing them in place.
- *Myoplasty:* Rectus muscle and diaphragm muscle flaps have been used to obliterate cyst cavity in complex situations.

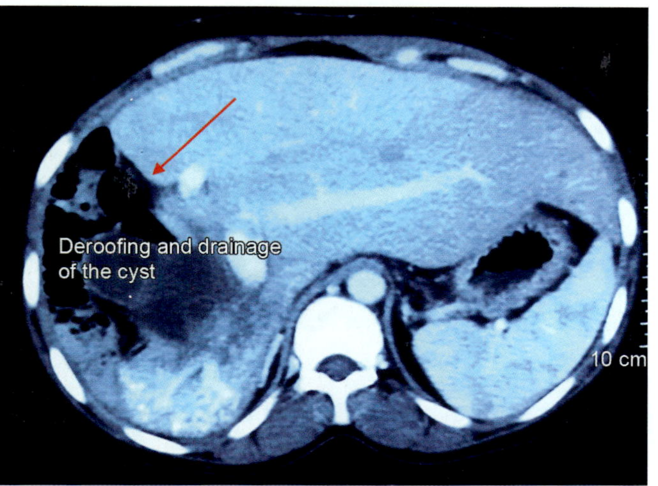

Figure 15 Axial section of postoperative CT scan (6 months later) of a patient who underwent partial cyst excision with cyst evacuation showing residual cavity after drainage with no evidence of recurrence

Radical Surgical Procedures

Radical surgical procedures include complete removal of cyst along with pericyst with or without adjacent parenchyma. The radical operations include anatomic and non-anatomic liver resection, pericystectomy or cystectomy.

A. *Cystectomy:* The simplest radical procedure is cystectomy which includes removal of hydatid cyst with laminar layer. After cystectomy the residual cavity needs to be managed by any one of the methods, as mentioned previously.
B. *Pericystectomy:* It also known as radical cystectomy, total pericystetcomy or cystopericystectomy. Removal of complete cyst with compressed surrounding liver parenchyma is called pericystectomy (Figs 18A and B). Closed cystopericystectomy is complete removal of cyst without opening the cyst. Cavitron ultrasonic aspirator is useful in identifying the plane between pericyst and liver parenchyma. This helps in avoiding injury

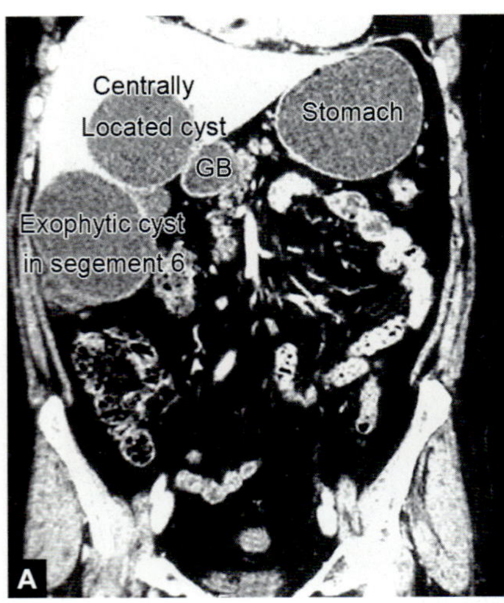

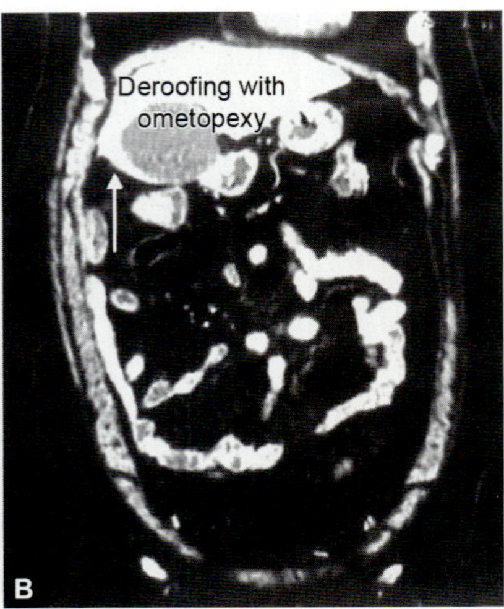

Figures 16A and B (A) Sagittal section of preoperative CT scan of a patient with two large cysts one located peripherally with exophytic component suitable for cystoprostatectomy and second located centrally close to portal pedicle. (B) Postoperative scan of same patient showing cystopericystectomy done for peripheral lesion and drainage and omentopexy (arrow) for central lesion

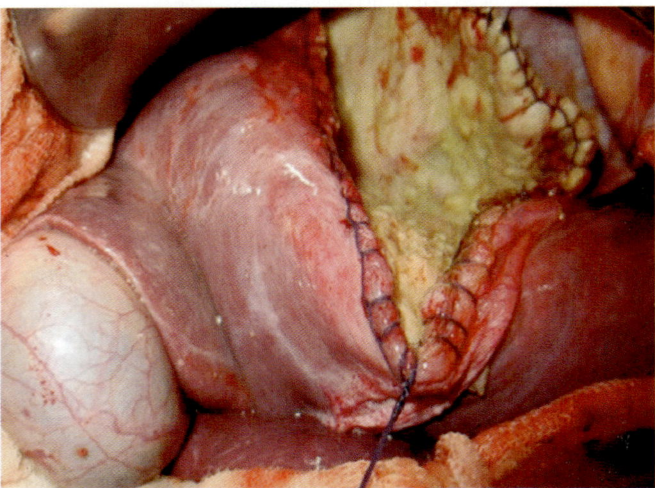

Figure 17 Intraoperative picture showing Capitonnage after drainage procedure

to vessels and bile duct adjacent to the cyst. It should be used away from pericyst to avoid any fracture on to the cyst. In open technique, cyst is opened or needle aspirated to decrease the size of the cyst and allow safe handling during its complete removal.

C. *Hepatic resections:* Anatomical or non-anatomical hepatectomies are the best modality to eradicate the complete disease especially when ectocyst are present. But for a benign disease, in a smaller set up the morbidity will overweigh the benefits. Non-anatomical liver resection is preferred for peripherally located cyst especially when cut surface is smaller with wedge resection. It also decreases the chances of ischemia in surrounding area. Formal hepatectomy is performed when large multilocular cyst occupies most part of left or sometimes right lobe and there is hypetrophy of the remnant liver and can safely achieved (Figs 19A and B).

Laparoscopic Management of Hydatid Cysts[28-30]

The minimally invasive management of hydatid disease is emerging with the advancement of technology and expertise in minimal invasive surgery. Apart from the routine advantages of laparoscopy, such as low morbidity, shorter hospital stay and faster recovery, due to high magnification, better control of cyst cavity and detection of biliary fistula were observed. In the setting of cystobiliary communication, centrally located cyst, very large cyst (>15 cm) and calcified cyst laparoscopy is not of much use. Compared to open surgery, risk of spillage of cyst contents while evacuating is more in laparoscopy.

Supraumbilical port is mostly used as camera port. Surrounding area is packed with scolicidal agent soaked gauze packs. Cyst is punctured using trocar and evacuate cyst using high pressure suction device. Gas port is used instill the scolicidal agent while another laparoscope can inserted into the cyst to have magnified view of cavity. This may help in removal of daughter cyst and identify the cyst biliary communications.

Complications of Surgery

A. *Morbidity:* The most common complication following surgery is biliary leakage (6–28%), but most of them close spontaneously. Any bile leak regardless of amount is defined as bile leakage. When patient is having persistent bile leakage for more than 10 days, it is defined as biliary fistula. Endoscopic treatment is the mainstay of management in such cases. Around 4–27% of cases, the bile leak might persist and require an endoscopic sphincterotomy.[31,32] Stent placement or nasobiliary stent may be added to the endoscopic sphincterotomy. Ideal method is not known. The success rate is reported between 83–100%. Other complication like infection of the residual cavity, especially for large hydatid cysts, can also occur.
B. *Mortality:* A mortality rate of 0.9–3.6% is noted after surgical management.
C. Recurrence failure to achieve permanent control of treated cyst is defined as local recurrence. Appearance of new cyst in the peritoneal cavity is defined as disseminated disease. The recurrence rate is higher with conservative type of surgical therapy or intraoperative spillage, accounting for 11.3% within 5 years. Use of ineffective scolicidal agent, overlooked or ectocyst and remnant cyst materials are other causes for recurrence. CIEP and western blotting test are useful in identification of recurrence.

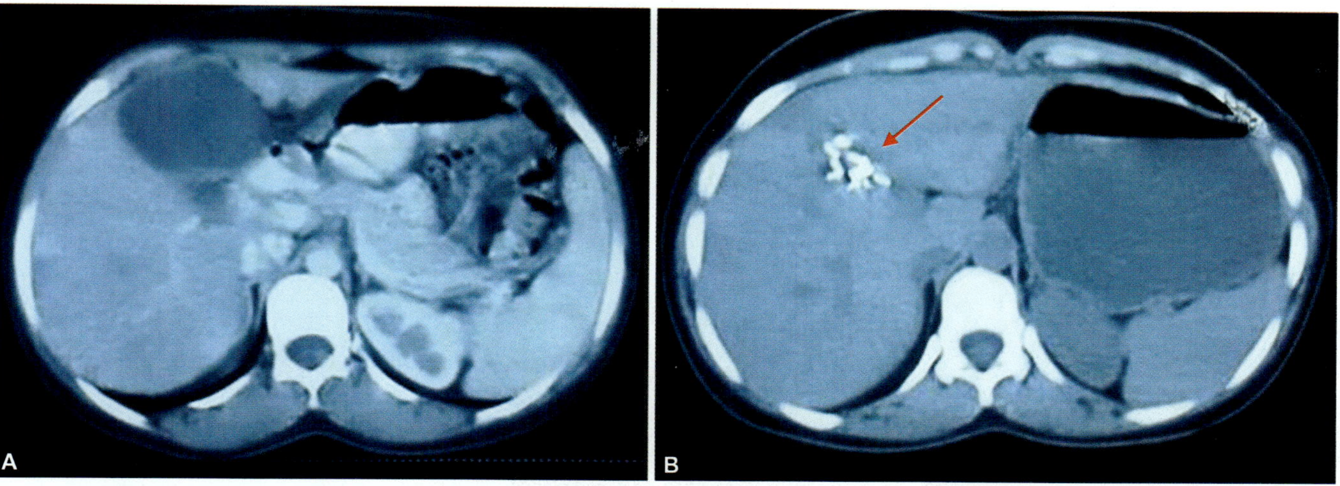

Figures 18A and B (A) Axial section of preoperative CT scan of a patient showing a hydatid cyst located in segment 3. (B) Axial section of postoperative scan of same patient who underwent cystoprostatectomy shows clip without any recurrent cyst

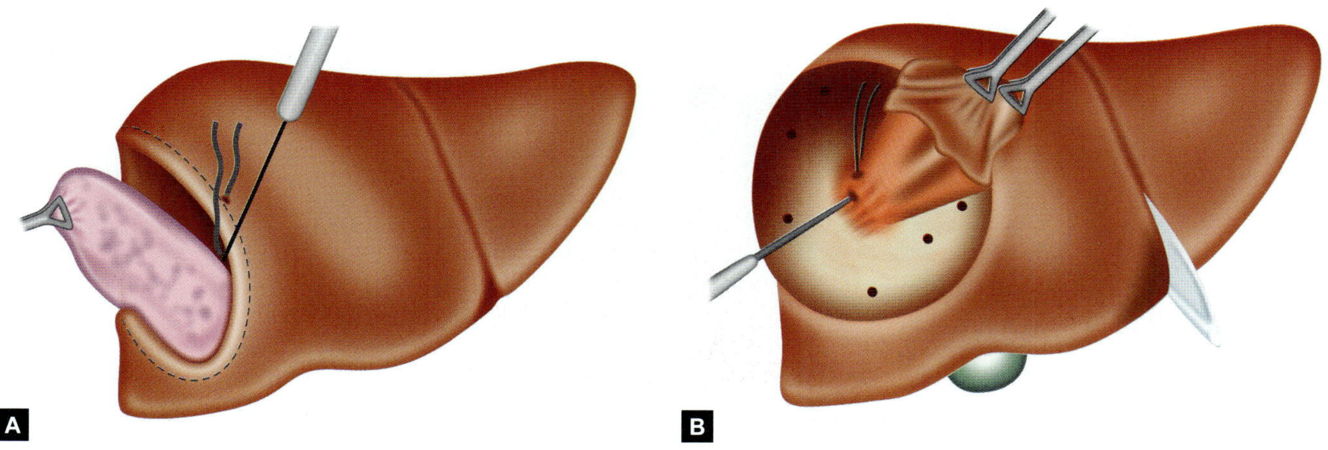

Figures 19A and B (A) Radical surgery: Partial cystectomy. (B) Technique of the pericystectomy

Percutaneous Treatment of Hydatid Cyst (Figs 20A to F)

Percuatneous approach known as puncture-aspiration-injection-reaspiration (PAIR), i.e. puncture, aspiration of cyst content, injection of protoscoicidal agent and reaspiration of the fluid, was proposed by Tunisian team in 1986. In this treatment albendazole prophylaxis is begun 1 week before the procedure and medication is continued for 3–4 weeks thereafter. The cyst is carefully punctured with a fine needle transhepatically under ultrasound guidance. Cyst fluid is aspirated as much as possible; scolicidal agent is injected and after 10 minutes reaspirated. Commonly used scolicidal agents are hypertonic saline (20%) and 95% alcohol. The agents used previously were 10% povidone-iodine, 10% formaline, 5% chlorhexidine gluconate, cetavlon, silver nitrate, 3% hydrogen peroxide. In view of caustic sclerosing cholangitis these agents are seldom used now.[33] WHO recommends PAIR as an effective alternative to surgery in CE1 and CE3 type and selected type CE2 cyst. Complicated cysts, cysts with many daughter cysts or large volume cysts are indications for PAIR modifications:

A. PAIR catheter technique described by Akhan et al. The procedure is similar except that catheter is left in situ for drainage for 24 hours. If there is no biliary drainage then absolute alcohol is injected and kept for 20 minutes. The cysts larger than 6 cm are considered to treat by catheterization technique rather than PAIR.
B. Double puncture, aspiration and injection (D-PAI) technique.
C. Percutaneous evacuation of cyst content (PEVAC) technique is used for multivesicular cyst wherein after aspiration and catheter placement then catheter is upgraded to allow insertion of suction device to evacuate the cyst content. Subsequently catheter is kept on drainage and removed once there is no drainage.
D. Modified catheter aspiration (MoCAT) technique.

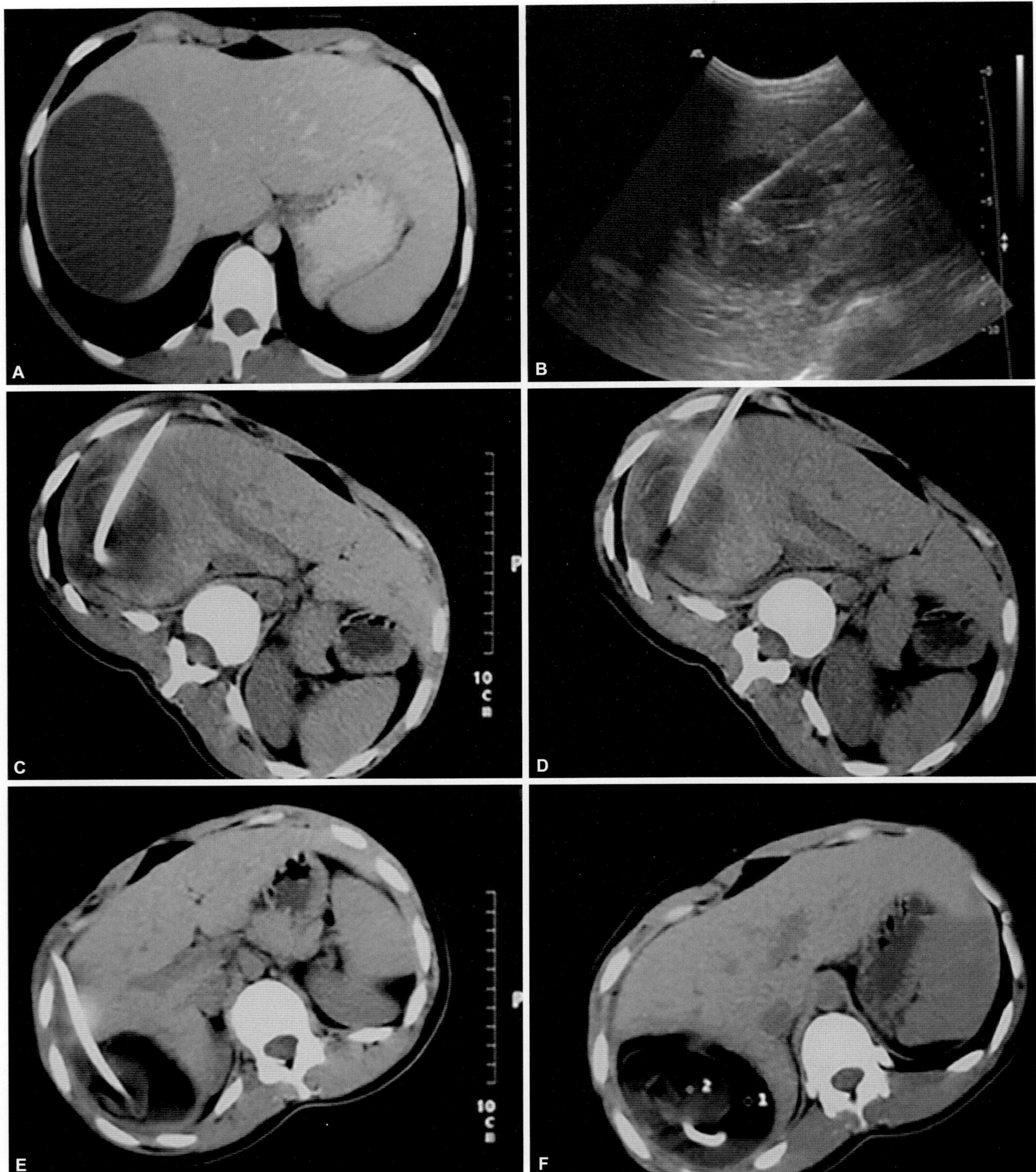

Figures 20A to F (A) Axial section CT scan showing type CL cyst suitable for PAIR. (B) Ultrasound image showing USG guided placement of needle. (C and D) CT image showing placement of pigtail catheter and evacuation of cyst. (E and F) CT image showing cyst completely evacuated

WHO Guidelines for PAIR:[34]

- Indications:
  - CE1 type anechoic cyst >5 cm size
  - CE 3 type
  - Selected CE2 type, i.e. if daughter cysts are accessible to puncture
  - Infected cysts
  - Patients who either refuse surgery or if surgery is contraindicated
  - Recurrent who relapse after surgery
  - Children >3 years and pregnant women
  - Patients who fail to respond to chemotherapy alone
- Contraindications for PAIR:
  - Cyst that are inaccessible to puncture or puncture is risky
  - Cyst having cystobiliary communication
  - Dead or calcified cyst
  - Uncooperative patients.

Khuroo et al.[35] in their study showed disappearance of cysts in 88% cases using percutaneous approach along albendazole coverage (10 mg/kg body weight) for 8 weeks. They found that efficacy of percutaneous treatment was similar to that surgical treatment at 2 years follow-up. The advantages of percutaneous drainage include a shorter hospital stay and a lower complication rate.

Chemotherapy for Hydatid Disease of Liver

The drugs widely used for medical management of hydatid disease belong to benzimidazole carbamates group. The commonly used ones are mebendazole and albendazole. They act by penetrating the cyst wall and their active metabolites persist within the cyst. Among these albendazole seems to be more effective.[36,37]

Indications

- Perioperative period especially along with conservative surgical procedure
- Disseminated disease (Figs 21A and B)
- Along with percutaneous treatment
- Inoperable patients.

Contraindications

- Chronic liver disease
- Early pregnancy.

Side Effects

Albendazole therapy: Pain in abdomen, nausea and vomiting, headache, pruritis, rashes, dizziness and alopecia (reversible). Occasionally, patients can have raised transaminases, leucopenia and eosinophilia.

Dosing Schedules WHO Recommendation

- Preoperative treatment should be started at least 4 days before surgery
- Postoperative treatment to prevent recurrence:
  - Intraoperative spillage 3–4 cycles of 4 weeks course and 2 weeks interval is recommended. For maximum benefit minimum recommended period is 3 months and maximum for 6 months
  - Uncomplicated cyst 3–8 weeks treatment
- Inoperable cases—as primary treatment—continuous 6 months treatment without interruption preferred
- Preoperative treatment to make the cyst non-viable requires at least 3 months of treatment.

In a study by Wen et al. it was observed that cyst was viable in 8% patients undergoing treatment compared to 100% in those without treatment. In another review, Dziri et al.[38] tried to provide evidence-based answers to some important aspects on management of hydatid cyst. They suggested that chemotherapy is not the ideal treatment for uncomplicated hydatid liver cyst when used alone, and the level of evidence was too low to help in choosing between

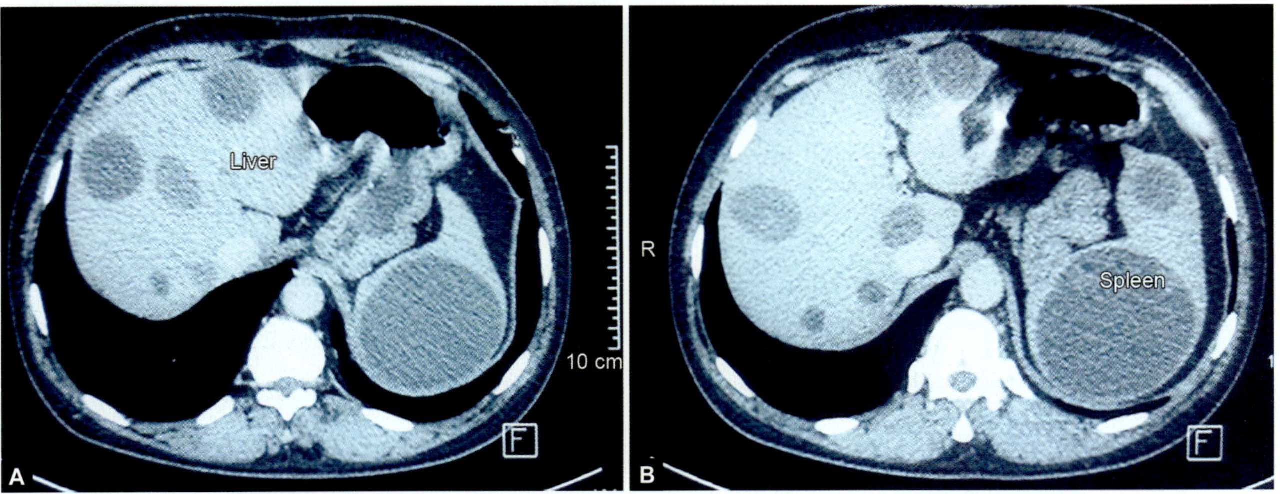

Figures 21A and B (A and B) Axial section of CT scan showing multiple cysts in liver and spleen suggestive of disseminated disease. This patient also had cyst in lung

radical or conservative treatment. Percutaneous drainage plus albendazole proved to be safe and effective in selected patients.

Watchful Waiting

Wait and watch policy is followed in inactive CE4-CE5 cysts that are asymptomatic and uncomplicated less than 5 cm CL type.

Treatment of Hydatid Cysts Rupture into the Biliary Tracts

Principle: The contents of cyst usually do not spontaneously drain into the biliary system if the communication is less than 5 mm. These can be managed by suturing under the vision. The contents of cyst including membranes and debris enter into biliary tree in more than 65% of cases in patients having communication larger than 5 mm. These patients require early surgical intervention else cholangitis and abscess formation may occur and septicemia may set in.

Identification of Communication

Careful inspection allows identification of the orifice of bile leakage around 10–15% of the patients. Placement of clean dry sponge on the cavity for few minutes helps in identifying small communications especially in difficult locations such as posterior located cysts. Intraoperative cholangiography through cystic duct is useful identifying the leaks. Radio-opaque dye or methylene blue is injected.

Treatment of Cystobiliary Communication (Figs 22 and 23)

A. *Direct suture:* Small less than 5 mm communication can close directly using absorbable 4,0 or 5,0 polyglactin sutures. Placement of omentum helps in further reducing the risk of postoperative bile leak.
B. *T-tube drainage of defect:* Whenever radical surgery is not performed and partial cystopericystectomy is contemplated, the defect is treated by a method called transparieto-hepatic fistulization which is described by Perdromo et al. They place a T-tube in one of the branches of intrahepatic radicals and other intracystic.[39] The tube is kept for 4–6 weeks and removed after cholangiography (Fig. 24).
C. *Internal drainage technique:* It was described by Goinard.[40] It is useful in patients with centrally located cyst with a large fistula. In such patients partial pericystectomy is done to reduce the size of residual cavity, followed by suturing of the margin of pericyst and placement of T-tube in the CBD. A drain is placed in the cyst cavity for 5–8 weeks and removed after cholangiography.
D. *CBD exploration and T-tube placement:* Supraduodenal CBD exploration is performed in all patients with major duct communication. Cholecystectomy should be added in these patients. All debris and membranes should be removed and CBD is closed over T-tube.[41] It allows external drainage of bile in the immediate postoperative period and help in performing cholangiography to cessation of bile leak. The tube is removed 4–6 weeks after surgery.

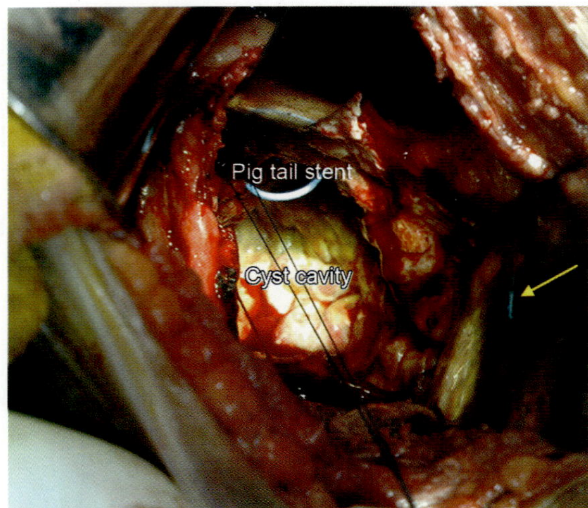

Figure 22 Intraoperative picture of patient with hydatid cyst with biliary communication. Patient underwent preoperative ERCP and stent placement seen as catheter with the cyst cavity. Patient underwent partial cystectomy with cavity showing bile staining

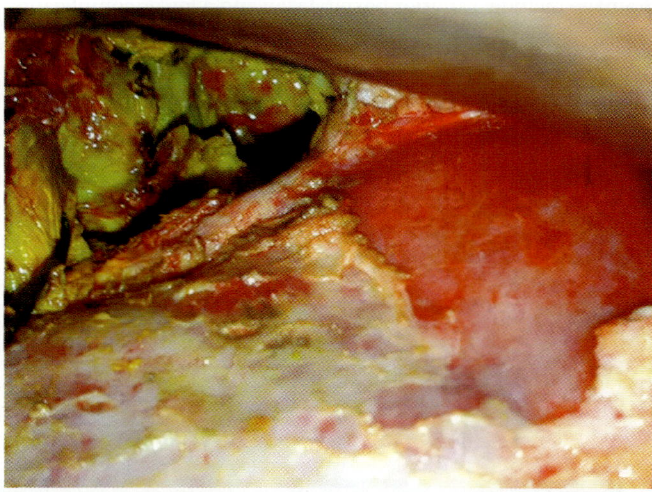

Figure 23 Intraoperative photograph of cyst located in superior segment of right lobe underwent deroofing. Cyst cavity shows bile staining and underwent external drainage

E. *Performing radical surgery* reduces the risk for biliary fistula in patients suspected to have biliary communication.

HYDATID AT OTHER SITES

Hydatid Cyst of Lung (Figs 25A to C)

Epidemiology and Mode of Spread

Lung is the second most common site after liver with occurrence of 20–30% of all hydatid cysts.[42,43] In 4–25% of patients there may be concomitant lung and liver involvement. It can be primary site when hematogenous spread occurs bypassing the liver during larval stage of Echinoccocus or secondary following rupture of

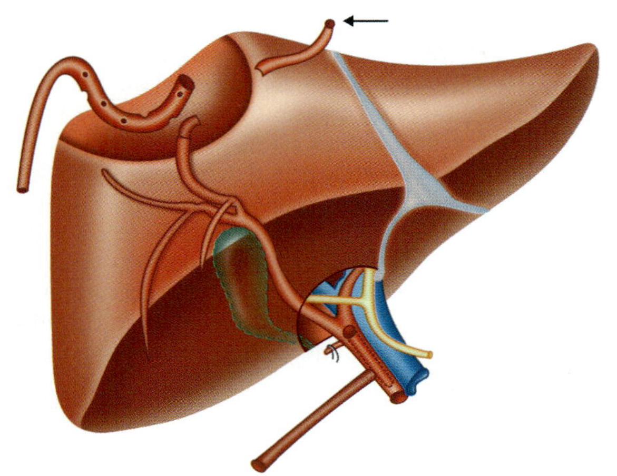

Figure 24 Diagram depicting transparietohepatic fistulization (perdromo)

hepatic hydatid or rarely cardiac hydatid disease. Right lung is more commonly affected with predilection for lower lobe.[44] Multiple unilateral or bilateral involvement is less common as compared to single unilateral involvement.[45,46] Extrapulmonary intrathoracic hydatid cysts are rare with reported incidence of 5.4%[47] and pleural cysts are most frequently found among them.[48] Pulmonary hydatid cysts grow rapidly due to presence of negative intrathoracic pressure, the greater elasticity of lung tissue and absence of pericyst.

Clinical Presentation

The clinical presentation depends upon the size and the location of the cyst. They may remain clinically silent in 10–37% of cases.[45,46] Cough, chest pain and dyspnea are frequently seen among the symptomatic patients.[44] The risk of rupture reported in the literature varies from 8% to 55% while anaphylaxis is very rare (0–0.3%).[44] Intrabronchial rupture can lead to hemoptysis, expectoration of purulent sputum mixed with cyst contents and segmental or lobar pneumonia along with other constitutional symptoms. Hydropneumothorax, pleural effusion or empyema may develop following rupture into the pleural cavity.

Diagnosis

Eosinophilia is seen in 20–34% of cases[44] with a limited diagnostic role, while the yield of serological test is low (65%) in pulmonary hydatid cysts.[49] Chest X-ray is the preferred initial radiological investigation in diagnosis. CT chest precisely delineates the morphological characteristics of the cyst, its location and extent and associated complications. USG abdomen and echocardiography are useful in patients with suspected secondary lung hydatid disease. The differential diagnoses include primary malignant tumor, secondaries (for multiple cysts) and lung abscess. Also, mediastinal tumors and aortic aneurysm may be confused with juxtamediastinal cysts.

Treatment

Antihelminthic drugs are considered in patients with anatomically inaccessible cysts, poor surgical risk and recurrent disease. In addition they are used as adjunct therapy to percutaneous and surgical interventions. The management of pulmonary hydatid cyst is mainly surgical and the approach is decided by the location of the cyst. The preferred approach for unilateral cyst is lateral thoracotomy. Staged thoracotomy with interval of 2 months or a median sternotomy are preferred approaches for bilateral disease. When two-staged surgery is planned for combined pulmonary and abdominal hydatidosis, the priority is given to lung disease to avoid potential chest complications in uncomplicated cases. Recently, thoracophrenotomy or sternophrenotomy is becoming popular to approach these combined hydatid cysts in a single session. Usually parenchyma preserving procedures, such as cystotomy with or without capitonnage, enucleation and pericystectomy, are preferred.[46,50] All bronchial openings should be located carefully during hyperinflation and closed with sutures. Segmentectomy, lobectomy and pneumonectomy can be considered in patients with cyst occupying more than 50% of the lobe, associated severe lung suppuration not responding to conservative treatment or multiple unilocular cysts.[44] In addition, total cyst excision is preferred choice for cases with extrapulmonary intrathoracic hydatid cyst.

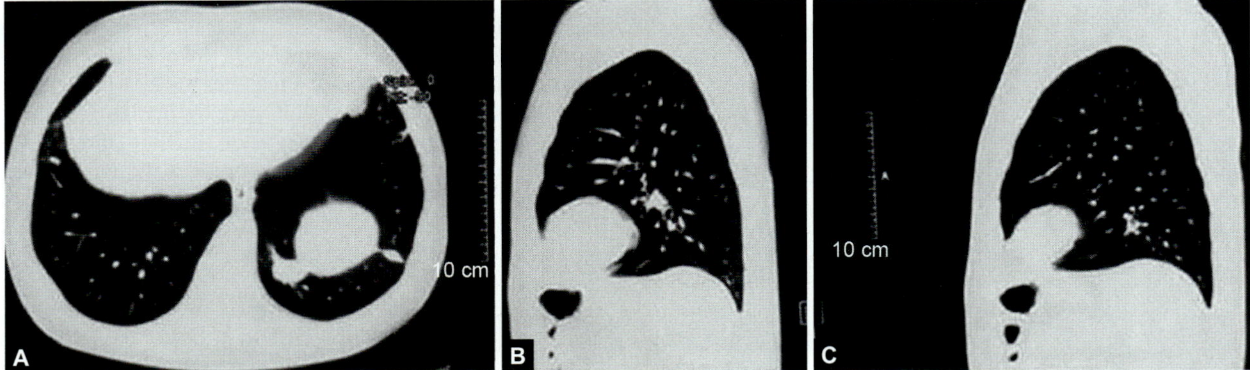

Figures 25A to C (A to C) Axial image CT chest showing hydatid cyst in lower lobe left lung. Sagittal section also cyst in lower lobe lung

Hydatid Cyst of Spleen (Fig. 26)

Epidemiology and Mode of Spread

In 1790, Berlot reported first splenic hydatidosis in his autopsy findings.[51] Spleen is the third most common site involved by Echinoccocus following liver and lung.[52-54] Involvement of spleen is rare in patients with hydatid disease with reported incidence varies from 0.5% to 4%.[55] In endemic areas, hydatid cyst constitutes 50–80% of all splenic cysts.[56] In 20–30% of cases, there may be concomitant liver and/or lung involvement.[57,58] Splenic hydatid cysts are usually solitary. Multiple cysts are found in 25–33% of patients. Infestation of the spleen occurs primarily by an arterial route after passing through liver and lungs. Sometimes spleen may get infected through retrograde flow from portal vein in case of portal hypertension. Secondary disease can occur due to systemic dissemination or intraperitoneal spread following rupture of any extrasplenic hydatid cyst.

Clinical Features

Due to its slow growth, it remains asymptomatic for many years and in up to 30% of cases, it is diagnosed incidentally.[59] Symptoms depend upon the location of the cyst. They are secondary to compression over adjacent organs, rupture (either spontaneous or post-traumatic), superadded infection, hemorrhage within the cyst or fistulization into neighboring viscera. Patients frequently present with dull aching pain in the left upper abdomen. Other symptoms include fullness in upper abdomen, referred pain to left shoulder and back, left sided pleuritic chest pain, difficulty in breathing, early satiety, constipation or pressure symptoms over left kidney. Rarely, it may present as acute abdomen secondary to rupture with hemoperitoneum,[60] anaphylactic shock, gastrointestinal bleed,[61] hypersplenism[62] or portal hypertension.[63] Physical examination usually reveals either a lump in the left upper quadrant or splenomegaly.

Diagnosis

The important differential diagnoses of splenic hydatid cyst are pancreatic pseudocyst, splenic abscess, splenic hematoma, and other cystic neoplasms of the spleen. Laboratory evaluation shows eosinophilia in only 25% of cases.[64] CT abdomen alone or in combination with USG usually establishes the diagnosis in majority of the patients. Imaging findings depend upon the age of cyst and associated complications. They vary from simple unilocular cyst to complicated cyst with or without calcifications. MRI may be helpful in patient with negative serology and indeterminate USG and CT findings. Serological tests for echinococcosis such as immune-electrophoresis, indirect hemagglutination (IHA), complement fixation test and enzyme-linked immunosorbent assay (ELISA) can be useful for diagnosis and follow-up for recurrence.[65] The personal history, presence of daughter cysts, calcification and associated lesion in the liver and other organs are important clues for successful diagnosis.

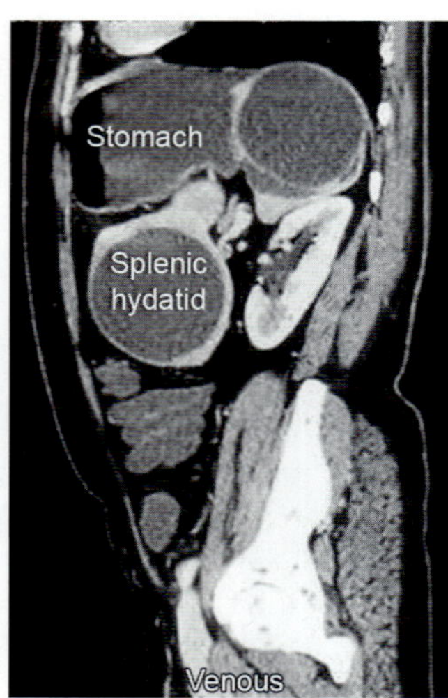

Figure 26 Sagittal section CT scan showing multiple cysts in the spleen suggestive of hydatid spleen

Treatment

At present treatment options available are medical, minimally invasive such as PAIR and surgery. As most of the antihelminthic medication are absorbed poorly from GI tract, there role as a primary treatment modality remains controversial. The benefits of medical therapy are seen in patients with secondary splenic hydatid cyst, undergoing spleen-conserving surgery, recurrent disease, or complications and as a pre and post PAIR or surgical treatment prophylaxis. Small asymptomatic cysts also can be treated conservatively with antihelminthic drugs. PAIR has been found effective in patients who deny surgery or are poor surgical candidates, type I or II cysts and cysts less than 5 cm in size.[66,67] Surgical treatment has been accepted as a gold standard for splenic hydatid cyst. Total splenectomy is optimal treatment for multiple cysts, large cysts (involving >75% of the spleen), cysts located near hilum or intraparenchymally as it is associated with very low rate of recurrence. Spleen preserving procedures such as partial splenectomy, enucleation, deroofing of the cyst, or external drainage may preferred in patients with infected cysts, superficial cysts or cysts located at the upper or lower poles. In addition, these techniques are primarily used in children and in cases with severe pericystic adhesions to prevent septic complications.

Hydatid Cyst of Pancreas (Figs 27 and 28)

Epidemiology and Mode of Spread

It is important to consider a hydatid cyst in the differential diagnosis of cystic lesions of the pancreas, especially in patients from the endemic areas. Pancreatic involvement by hydatid disease is rare with reported incidence of less than 1%.[68] The pancreas is most commonly infested by hematogenous route. Other reported modes of infestation include direct invasion through pancreatobiliary ducts, peripancreatic lymphatics and retroperitoneum.[69] Pancreatic hydatid cysts are usually solitary. They are more commonly found in the head region (57%) as compared to body (24%) and tail (19%).[70]

Clinical Features

It remains asymptomatic in some cases for long duration. Such patients are usually diagnosed incidentally while investigating for other clinical conditions. The location within the pancreas

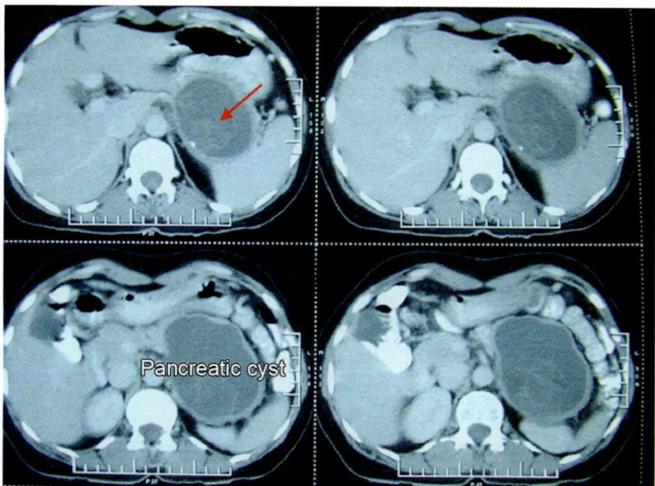

Figure 27 Axial sections of CT scan showing cyst lesion in body tail pancreas with membrane suggestive pancreatic hydatid

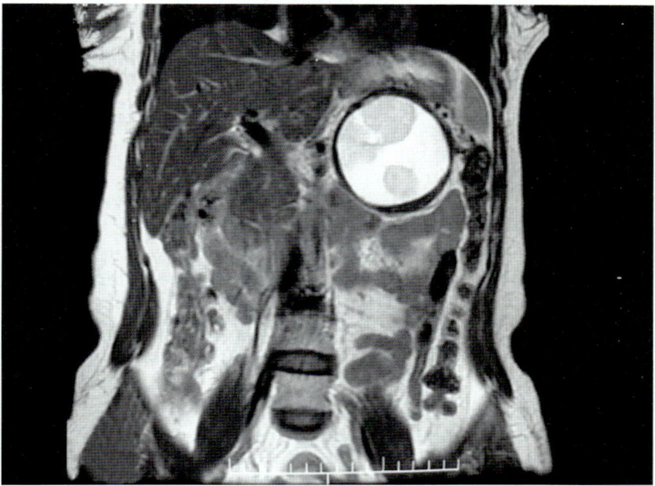

Figure 28 Sagittal view of MRI scan of same patient showing daughter cyst in cyst located in region pancreatic body tail suggestive of pancreatic hydatid

and size of the cyst mainly decides the clinical presentation in symptomatic patients. Cysts located in head region can lead to pancreatitis and obstructive jaundice due to impingement on or fistulization into pancreatic duct and CBD respectively. Less commonly it may present with epigastric mass or gastric outlet obstruction.[71] Body and tail hydatid cysts frequently remain clinically silent until they grow large enough to cause early satiety due to gastric compression[71] or left sided portal hypertension secondary to splenic vein compression.[72] Sometimes pancreatic hydatid cysts may get infected and present with either nonspecific symptoms such as anorexia and weight loss or acute abdomen following its spontaneous rupture into peritoneal cavity.[71,72] In addition, erosion of pancreatic hydatid cyst into adjacent hollow viscera has been reported in the literature.[71,72]

Diagnosis

The differential diagnoses include pseudocyst, choledochal cyst (especially in children with hydatid cyst in head of pancreas), congenital pancreatic cysts and cystic tumors of pancreas. The role of USG is limited in evaluating pancreatic cysts due to its retroperitoneal location and bowel gas. CT abdomen is excellent in delineating size of the cyst, its location and extent and any cyst wall calcification. As compared to CT, MRI abdomen with MRCP provides the relationship between the cyst and pancreaticobiliary ducts more precisely. Endoscopic ultrasonography (EUS) is less commonly used. But it helps to differentiate hydatid cyst from other cystic lesions of pancreas as it is capable of characterizing the cyst more accurately and also allows aspiration of the cyst fluid for analysis. In addition, EUS can show the relation between the cyst and pancreatic duct accurately. The positivity rate of the serological tests in extrahepatic hydatid cysts is low as compared to that of intrahepatic hydatid cysts (54% in pancreatic hydatid cysts).[73] However, serological tests can used complementary to imaging findings especially in cases with recurrent disease.

Treatment

Cholangitis and pancreatitis can be treated with ERCP and stent insertion. The role of PAIR in management of pancreatic hydatid cyst is limited due to high risk of cyst perforation and associated complications as compared to solid organs such as liver and spleen. Surgical treatment is most preferred and the decision of appropriate surgical procedure mainly depends up on the location of cyst within pancreas and its relation to pancreaticobiliary ductal system. Prophylactic antihelminthic medications must be given for 2–4 weaks prior to any surgical intervention in order to reduce the risk of anaphylaxis and postoperative recurrence. Pancreatic head cyst without pancreatic or biliary ductal communication can be treated with deroofing or partial cystectomy with external drainage or enucleation. Some patients with complicated cysts, when cystic neoplasm cannot be ruled out preoperatively may require pancreaticoduodenectomy. Cysts with ductal communication are drained internally into stomach, duodenum or jejunum. Intraoperatively cholangiography or cystogram may delineate the ductal communication. Distal pancreatectomy with or without splenectomy (depending up on the involvement of spleen) is the most appropriate surgical modality for the cysts located in the body and tail. Central pancreatectomy may also be considered for hydatid cyst in the neck or body of pancreas.[74]

REFERENCES

1. Moro P, Schantz PM. Echinococcosis: a review. International Journal of Infectious Diseases. 2009;13:125-33.
2. Nunnari G, Pinzone MR, Gruttadauria S, Celesia BM, Madeddu G, Malaguarnera G, et al. Hepatic echinococcosis: clinical and therapeutic aspects. World J Gastroenterol. 2012;18(13):1448-58.
3. Khanfar N. Hydatid disease: a review and update. Current Anaesthesia & Critical Care. 2004;15:173-83.
4. Falguni Parikh. Echinococcosis—cut to cure but what about control? JAPI. 2012;60:9-10.
5. Eckert J, Deplazes P. Biological, epidemiological, and clinical aspects of echinococcosis, a zoonosis of increasing concern. Clin Microbiol Rev. 2004;17(1):107-35.

6. Zaouche A, Haouet K, Jouini M, El Hachaichi A, Dziri C. Management of liver hydatid cysts with a large biliocystic fistula: multicenter retrospective study. Tunisian Surgical Association. World J Surg. 2001;25(1):28-39.
7. Gharbi HA, Mnif J, Ben Abdallah M, Abdelmoula M, Hammou-Jeddi A. Epidemiology of hydatic cyst in Tunisia. Results of investigation by abdominal echography on 3116 inhabitants of Menzel Bourguiba area. Médecineet Maladies Infectieuses. 1986;16(3):151-6.
8. Sakhri J, Ben Ali A, Letaief R, DerbelF, Dahmen Y, Ben HadjHmida R. Les kysteshydatiques du foierompusdansle thorax: aspects diagnostiques et thérapeutiques. J Chir (Paris). 1996;133:437-41.
9. Kilani T, Daoues A, Horchani H, Sellami M. Place de la thoracotomiedans les complications thoraciques des Kysteshydatiques du foie. Ann Chir Thorac Cardiovasc. 1991;45:705-10.
10. Caporale A, Frittelli P, Della Casa U, Rengo M, Agrò GA, Mosillo L, et al. Surgical treatment of hydatid cysts of the hepatic dome ruptured into the thoracic cavity. G Chir. 1990;11:23-8.
11. Karakaya K. Spontaneous rupture of a hepatic hydatıd cyst into the peritoneum causing only mild abdominal pain: a case report. World J Gastroenterol. 2007;13(5):806-8.
12. Acharya AN, Gupta S. Peritoneal hydatidosis: a review of seven cases. Tropical Gastroenterology. 2009;30(1):32-4.
13. İlhanÇiftçi, HüseyinYılmaz. Hepatic hydatid cyst and intraperitoneal free hydatid cyst. Eur J Gen Med. 2012;9(Suppl 1):50-2.
14. Emre A, Arioğul O, Alper A, Okten A, Uras A, Yalçin S. Hydatid Cysts of Liver and Portal Hypertension. HPB Surgery. 1990;2:129-33.
15. Zhang W, Li J, McManus DP. Concepts in immunology and diagnosis of hydatid disease. Clin Microbiol Rev. 2003,16(1):18-36.
16. Zhang W, McManus DP. Recent advances in the immunology and diagnosis of echinococcosis. FEMS Immunol Med Microbiol. 2006;47:24-41.
17. Gharbi HA, Hassine W, Brauner MW, Dupuch K. Ultrasound examination of the hydatic liver. Radiology. 1981;139:459-63.
18. WHO Informal working group on Echinococcosis. International classification of ultrasound images in cystic echinococcosis for application in clinical and field epidemiological settings. Acta Trop. 2003;85(2):253-61.
19. Torricelli P, Martinelli C, Biagini R, Ruggieri P, De Cristofaro R. Radiographic and computed tomographic findings in hydatid disease of bone. Skelet Radiol. 1990;19(6):435-9.
20. Kalinova K. Imaging (ultrasonography, computed tomography) of patients with hydatid liver disease. Bulgarian Journal of Veterinary Medicine. 2007;10(1):45-51.
21. Lim JH. Parasitic diseases in the abdomen: imaging findings. Abdom Imaging. 2008;33:130-2.
22. Brunetti E, Kern P, Vuitton DA. Expert consensus for the diagnosis and treatment of cystic and alveolar echinococcosis in humans. Acta Trop. 2010;114(1):1-16.
23. Magistrelli P, Masetti R, Coppola R, Messia A. Surgical treatment of hydatid disease of liver: a 20 year experience. Arch Surg. 1991;126:518-23.
24. Balik AA, Başoğlu M, Celebi F, Oren D, Polat KY, Atamanalp SS, et al. Surgical treatment of hydatid disease of the liver review of 304 cases. Arch Surg. 1999;134:166-9.
25. Silva MA, Mirza DF, Bramhall SR, Mayer AD, McMaster P, Buckels JA. Treatment of hydatid disease of the liver. Evaluation of a UK experience. Dig Surg. 2004;21:227-34.
26. Rinaldi F, Brunetti E, Neumayr A, Maestri M, Goblirsch S, Tamarozzi F. Cystic echinococcosis of the liver: a primer for hepatologists. World J Hepatol. 2014;6(5):293-305.
27. Skroubis G, Vagianos C, Polydorou A, Tzoracoleftherakis E, Androulakis J. Significance of bile leaks complicating conservative surgery for liver hydatidosis. World J Surg. 2002;26:704-8.
28. Saglam A. Laparoscopic treatment of liver hydatid cysts. Surg Lap Endosc. 1996;6:16-21.
29. Ertem M, Karahasanoglu T, Yavuz N, Erguney S. Laparoscopically treated liver hydatid cysts. Arch Surg. 2002;137:1170-3.
30. Hasan HM, El-Sayed OM. Laproscopic treatment of liver hydatid cyst. Journal of Medicine and Biomedical Sciences. 2010; ISSN: 2078-0273.
31. Ersan O, Yusuf B. Endoscopic therapy in the management of hepatobiliary hydatid disease. J Clin Gastrienterol. 2002;35:160-74.
32. Saritas U, Parlak E, Akoglu E, Sahin B. Effectiveness of endoscopic treatment modalities in complicated hepatic hydatid disease after surgical intervention. Endoscopy. 2001;33:858-63.
33. Ben Amor N, Gargouri M, Gharbi HA, Golvan YJ, Ayachi K, Kchouck H. Trial therapy of inoperable abdominal hydatid cysts by puncture. Ann Parasitol Hum Comp. 1986;61:689-92.
34. PAIR: Puncture, Aspiration, Injection, Re-Aspiration—An option for the treatment of Cystic Echinococcosis World Health Organization. WHO/CDS/CSR/APH/2001.6.
35. Khuroo MS, Wani NA, Javid G, Khan BA, Yattoo GN, Shah AH, et al. Percutaneous drainage compared with surgery for hepatic hydatid cysts. N Engl J Med. 1997;337:881-7.
36. Aktan AO, Yalin R. Preoperative albendazole treatment for liver hydatid disease decreases the viability of the cyst. Eur J Gastroenterol Hepatol. 1996;8:877-9.
37. Blanton RE, Wachira TM, Zeyhle EE, Njoroge EM, Magambo JK, Schantz PM. Oxfendazole treatment for cystic hydatid disease in naturally infected animals. Antimicrob Agents Chemother. 1998;42:601-5.
38. Dziri C, Haouet K, Fingerhut A. Treatment of hydatid cyst of the liver: where is the evidence? World J Surg. 2004;28:731-6.
39. Perdromo R, Morelli R, Carrquiry L, Chifflet J, Berragalli L. Cholédocostomietranshépaticokystique en cas de kystehydatiqueouvertdans les voiesbiliaires. Presse Med. 1977;6:747-9.
40. Giordano G, Angrisano A, Palazzo P, et al. Surgical treatment of hydatid cyst of the liver: pericystectomy or resection. Personal experience. Int J Surg Sci. 1999;6:113-7.
41. Elbir O, Gundogdu H, Caglikulekci M, Kayaalp C, Atalay F, Savkilioglu M, et al. Surgical treatment of intrabiliary rupture of hydatid cysts of liver: comparison of choledochoduodenostomy with T-tube drainage. Dig Surg. 2001;18:289-93.
42. Eroğlu A, Kürkçüoğlu C, Karaoğlanoğlu N, Tekinbaş C, Kaynar H, Onbaş O. Primary hydatid cysts of the mediastinum. Eur J Cardiothorac Surg. 2002;22:599-601.
43. Pieters G, Van den Spiefel A, Demeester P. Le kyste hydatiquepulmonaire. Acta Chir Belg. 1976;75:55s-66.
44. Harlaftis NN, Aletras HA, Symbas PN. Hydatid disease of thelung. In: Shields TW, LoCicero J III, Ponn RB, Rusch VW (Eds). General Thoracic Surgery. Philadelphia: Lippincott Williamsand Wilkins; 2005. pp. 1298-308.
45. Burgos R, Varela A, Castedo E, Roda J, Montero CG, SerranoS, et al. Pulmonary hydatidosis: surgical treatment and follow-up of 240 cases. Eur J Cardiothorac Surg. 1999;16:628-34.
46. Shehatha J, Alizzi A, Alward M, Konstantinov I. Thoracic hydatid disease: a review of 763 cases. Heart Lung Circ. 2008;17:502-4.
47. Thameur H, Chenik S, Abdelmoulah S, Bey M, Hachicha S, Chemingui M, et al. Thoracic hydatidosis: a review of 1619 cases. Rev Pneumol Clin. 2000;56:7-15.
48. Oğuzkaya F, Akçali Y, Kahraman C, Emiroğullari N, Bilgin M, Sahin A. Unusually located hydatid cysts: intrathoracic but extrapulmonary. Ann Thorac Surg. 1997;64:334-7.
49. Biava MF, Kurès L. Biological diagnosis of echinococcosis. Rev Prat. 1990;40:201-4.
50. Dogan R, Yüksel M, Çetin G, Süzer K, Alp K, Kaya S, et al. Surgical treatment of hydatid cysts of the lung: report on 1055 patients. Thorax. 1989;44:192-9.

51. Muro J, Ortiz-Vázquez J, Miño G, Sanmartín P. Angiographic localization of hydatid cyst of the spleen. Rev Clin Esp. 1969;115:433-8.
52. Safioleas M, Misiakos E, Manti C. Surgical treatment for splenic hydatidosis. World J Surg. 1997;21:374-7.
53. Safioleas M, Misiakos EP, Kakisis J, Manti C, Papachristodoulou A, Lambrou P, et al. Surgical treatment of human echinococcosis. Int Surg. 2000;85:358-65.
54. Mazumdar A, Singh G, Gupta NM. Primary splenic hydatid in adults. Trop Gastroenterol. 2000;21:78-9.
55. Humphreys WG, Johnston GW. Splenic cysts: a review of 6 cases. Br J Surg. 1979;66:407-8.
56. Gharaibeh KI. Laparoscopic excision of splenic hydatid cyst. Postgrad Med J. 2001;77:195-6.
57. Prousalidis J, Tzardinoglou K, Sgouradis L, Katsohis C, Aletras H. Uncommon sites of hydatid disease. World J Surg. 1998;22:17-22.
58. Ratych RE. Tumours, cysts and abscesses of spleen. In: Cameroon JL (Ed). Current Surgical Therapy, 4th edition. St Louis: Mosby; 1992. pp. 518-21.
59. Schwartz SI. Principles of Surgery, 7th edition. New York: McGraw-Hill Companies; 1999. pp. 1395-435.
60. Erel S, Kilicoglu B, Kismet K, Gollu A, Akkus MA. Peritoneal hydatid cyst perforation: a rare cause of emergency abdominal surgeries. Adv Ther. 2008;25(9):943-50.
61. Teke Z, Yagci AB, Atalay AO, Kabay B. Splenic hydatid cyst perforating into the colon manifesting as acute massive lower gastrointestinal bleeding: an unusual presentation of disseminated abdominal echinococcosis. Singapore Med J. 2008;49(5):e113-6.
62. Raman PG, Mulye R, Ganguly D. A case of hydatid cyst in spleen with hypersplenism. J Assoc Physicians India. 1995;43:797-8.
63. Sahu SK, Srivastava R, Bahl DV, Sachan PK. Primary hydatid cyst of the spleen: a rare site of presentation. Internet J Surg. 2008;14:1.
64. Abu-Eshy SA. Some rare presentations of hydatid cyst (*Echinococcus granulosus*). J R Coll Surg Edinb. 1998;43:347-52.
65. Carmena D, Benito A, Eraso E. The immunodiagnosis of *Echinococcus multilocularis* infection. Clin Microbiol Infect. 2007;13:460-75.
66. Zerem E, Nuhanović A, Caluk J. Modified pair technique for treatmentof hydatid cysts in the spleen. Bosn J Basic Med Sci. 2005;5(3):74-8.
67. Ormeci N, Soykan I, Palabiyikoğlu M, Idilman R, Erdem H, BektaşA, et al. A new therapeutic approach for treatment of hydatidcysts of the spleen. Dig Dis Sci. 2002;47(9):2037-44.
68. Ibis C, Albayrak D, Altan A. Primary hydatid disease of pancreas mimicking cystic neoplasm. South Med J. 2009;102:529-30.
69. Wani RA, Wani I, Malik AA, Parray FQ, Wani AA, DarAM. Hydatid disease at unusual sites. Int J Case Reposts Images. 2012;3:1-6.
70. Ozmen MM, Moran M, Karakahya M, Coskun F. Recurrent acute pancreatitis due to a hydatid cyst of the pancreatic head: a case report and review of the literature. JOP 2005;6:354-8.
71. Trigui A, Rejab H, Guirat A, Mizouni A, Amar MB, Mzali R, et al. Hydatid cyst of the pancreas About 12 cases. Ann Ital Chir. 2013;84:165-70.
72. Szanto P, Goian I, Al Hajjar N, Badea R, Seicean A, Manciula D, et al. Hydatid cyst of the pancreas causing portal hypertension. Maedica (Buchar). 2010;5:139-41.
73. Akbulut S, Yavuz R, Sogutcu N, Kaya B, Hatipoglu S, Senol A, et al. Hydatid cyst of the pancreas: report of an undiagnosed case of pancreatic hydatid cyst and brief literature review. World J Gastrointest Surg. 2014;6(10):190-200.
74. Shah OJ, Robbani I, Zargar SA, Yattoo GN, Shah P, Ali S, et al. Hydatid cyst of the pancreas. An experience with six cases. JOP. 2010;11:575-81.

CHAPTER 68

Imaging and Intervention in Hemobilia

Shivanand Gamanagatti, Prasad Thotton Veedu

INTRODUCTION

Phenomenon of bleeding within or into the biliary tree has been recognized as a cause for massive upper gastrointestinal hemorrhage (UGIH) from early seventeenth century.[1] The term hemobilia was coined for this entity by Sandblom in 1948.[2] Since then several reports of hemobilia can be found in literature. It is an unusual cause of UGIH which occurs due to an abnormal vascular communication with biliary tree. The site of bleeding can be intrahepatic or extrahepatic biliary tract, gallbladder, pancreas or the ampulla of vater. The severity of hemobilia depends on the type of pathological process, the vessel involved and nature of vascular lesion.

ETIOLOGY (TABLE 1)

Hemobilia can be a complication of many hepatobiliary disorders. Most cases of hemobila are seen in setting of trauma.[3,4] Among traumatic causes, iatrogenic injuries to hepatobiliary tract top the list. It includes complications arising from hepatobiliary surgery, percutaneous hepatic procedures, endoscopic procedures and endovascular procedures. Road traffic accidents and assaults are the common modes of accidental trauma and it may cause blunt or penetrating injury in abdomen. Other causes include tumors, infection, cholelithiasis, vascular lesions and coagulopathy.[5,6]

Table 1: Common causes of hemobilia

Trauma: • Blunt • Penetrating
Iatrogenic: • Liver biopsy • PTC/PTBD • Cholecystectomy • Hepatectomy • Other surgeries
Inflammation: • Gallstone disease • Cholecystitis • Ascariasis • Liver abscess • Pancreatitis
Tumors: • Cholangiocarcinoma • HCC • Carcinoma gallbladder
Vascular: • Coagulopathy • Vascular malformations

PRESENTATION

The classical clinical triad of hemobilia includes biliary colic, obstructive jaundice and gastrointestinal bleeding which is seen in only less than 20% of patients. Most of them present with UGIH and abdominal pain. The symptoms depend also on the rate of intrabiliary bleeding. Slow bleeding into biliary tree enhances clot formation which further causes stasis of bile with jaundice and biliary colic.[7] Patients can also develop cholangitis, cholecystitis and pancreatitis as a complication of biliary obstruction at various levels.

MECHANISM[7,8]

Anatomical fistulous communication between a vessel and biliary tract is essential for hemobilia to occur. Simultaneous injury of vessel and bile ducts are more likely because of their close and parallel course in liver. Portal venous injury is an unusual cause of hemobilia because of low pressure gradient with biliary tree imparting faster hemostasis. However, arterial lesions with high pressure flow have high likelihood of significant bleeding.

Vascular injury during percutaneous hepatic procedures such as liver biopsy, percutaneous transhepatic biliary drainage (PTBD) and percutaneous transhepatic cholangiography (PTC) can cause inadvertent injury to branches of hepatic artery. This can result in vascular injury, pseudoaneurysms or arteriobiliary fistulas and patients present with periodic gastrointestinal bleeding and abdominal colic with or without jaundice. Risk factors, like ascites, coagulopathy, cirrhosis and transplanted liver, increase the chance of significant hemobilia. Liver biopsy with small caliber needle has the least chance (<1%) although many procedures are done without image guidance. PTC is reported to have an incidence of hemobilia up to 4%. PTBD procedures have the highest risk (2–10%) because of the high caliber of tubes deployed and pre-existing bile stasis. Selection of ducts away from hilum and avoiding major vessels with real time ultrasonographic guidance can decrease the risk. Minor hemobila which is common after PTBD is usually controlled by conservative measures.

Hepatobiliary surgeries can inadvertently injure hepatic arteries and cystic artery. Laparoscopic procedures have higher reported incidence of vascular injuries. Inefficient ligation of cystic artery during cholecystectomy is also found to be a frequent cause for hemobilia. Exploration of bile ducts for biliary stones is also very prone for vascular injury, as the vessels are running close to ducts. Postoperative check cholangiogram may show clots in bile ducts as filling defects confusing them with retained stones.

Penetrating injury in abdomen can cause direct vascular and hepatic injuries and can result in hemobilia. Although such cases are managed with surgical intervention routinely, the injured intraprenchymal vessels can continue to bleed and result in complications. Blunt abdominal trauma can cause shearing injury to liver parenchyma, blood vessels and bile ducts. Nowadays, cases of blunt abdominal trauma are primarily managed by conservative method unless there are specific surgical indications. Lower grade liver lacerations and hematomas are generally managed non-operatively. In such cases the intrahepatic hematomas and collections can expand and get communicated to biliary tree to result in hemobilia. As more and more cases of blunt abdominal trauma are managed conservatively the incidence of hemobilia also increases. Gallbladder injury which is seen in up to 2% trauma cases is also reported to cause hemobilia. Selective angioembolization of hepatic arterial branches is the best prophylactic method in such settings.

Inflammatory disorders can cause vascular injury by enzymatic erosion of vessel walls. Cholecystitis can be complicated by injury of hepatic and cystic arteries to form pseudoaneurysms. Splenic artery lesions are also observed as a complication of necrotizing pancreatitis. Hemobilia is also observed in few cases of liver abscesses. Occasionally, gallstone diseases also get complicated with vascular erosions and hemobilia. Parasitic infestation of bile duct as in ascariasis and hydatid cysts of liver can also present with hemobilia.

Primary and secondary tumors of liver or gallbladder can cause bleeding into bile ducts and gallbladder. It happens when these tumors invade bile ducts. Cholangiocarcinoma and gallbladder carcinoma are the common malignancies in that group. Most of the time hemobilia caused by tumors is mild and occult and results in chronic secondary anemia.

Among the primary vascular disorders hepatic artery aneurysm is the most common cause of hemobilia. Others include arteriovenous malformations, angiodysplasia and hemangiomas.

DIAGNOSIS (FIGS 1 TO 3)

Hemobilia has to be considered in the differential diagnosis when UGIH is associated with biliary symptoms. It should also be suspected in any patient with history of recent or remote liver trauma or instrumentation presenting with UGIH. The diagnostic and management approach in these patients depends on the mode and severity of presentation.

Endoscopy

First investigation of choice for any UGIH is esophagoduodenoscopy. It can rule out other common causes of gastrointestinal hemorrhage such as varices, erosions and malignancies. Demonstration of bleeding from duodenal ampulla (of vater) is diagnostic for hemobilia. As the bleeding is intermittent and slow, endoscopy might be negative in up to 10% of cases. Also, the etiology of hemobilia cannot be well evaluated with endoscopy and additional investigations are required.

Ultrasonography

Ultrasonography (USG) has very poor sensitivity in assessing hemobilia. It may visualize the primary etiology such as pseudoaneurysms (with Doppler), intrahepatic collections, cholecystitis and gallstones. More commonly USG shows the secondary signs of hemobilia such as clot in biliary tract or gallbladder and biliary dilatation.

Computed Tomography

Computed tomography (CT) scan is highly accurate in assessing the etiology and complications of hemobilia. CT angiography is highly sensitive in picking vascular lesions like pseudoaneurysms, arteriovenous malformations and arteriobiliary fistulas. It is also accurate in evaluating parenchymal injury, collections and inflammatory changes.

Angiography

Digital subtraction angiography (DSA) is presently the gold standard in evaluating patients with hemobilia. It is the procedure of choice after endoscopy in hemodynamically unstable patients. The findings observed in angiography are active bleeding into biliary tree and vascular lesions like aneurysms.

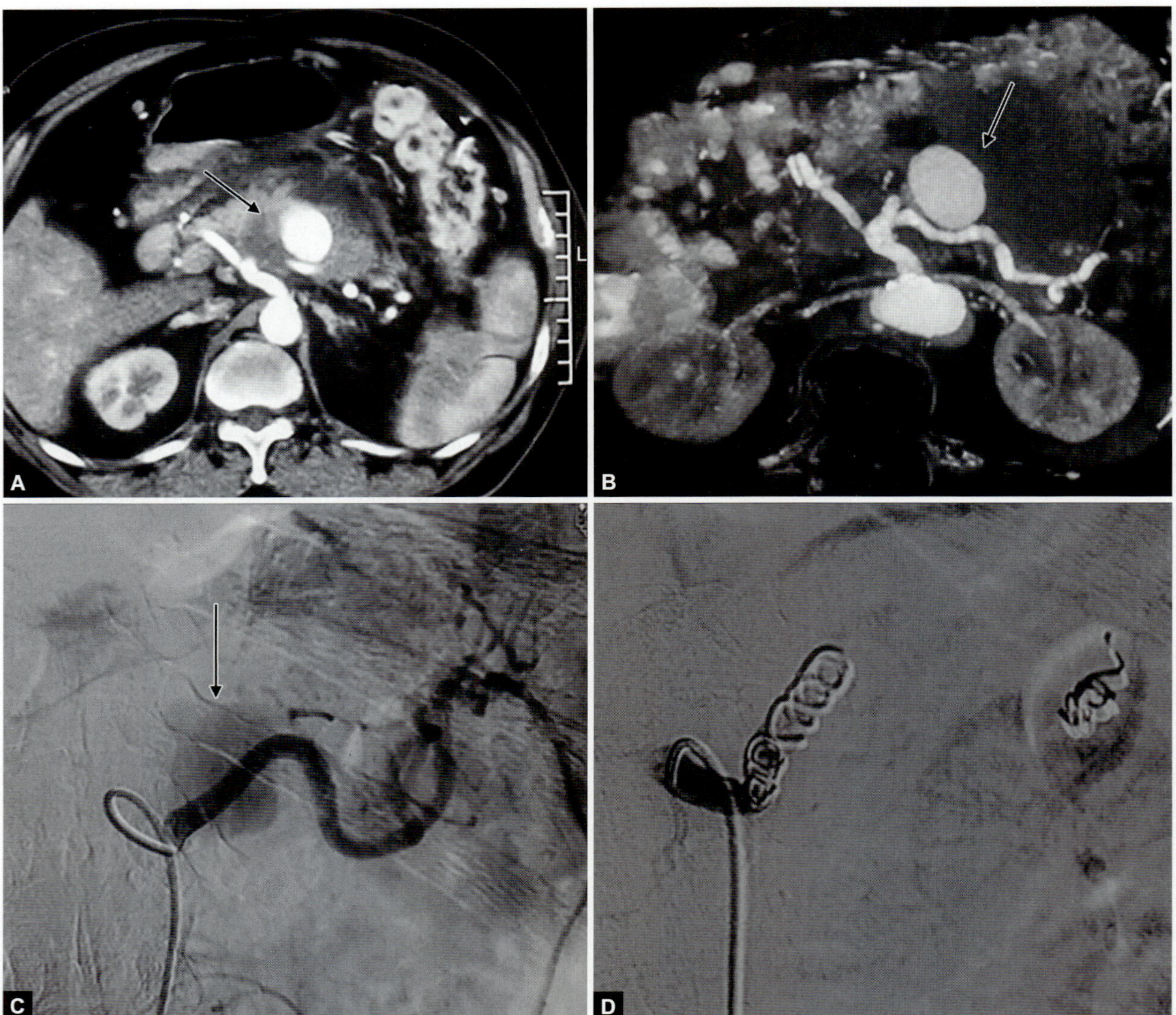

Figures 1A to D Elderly male presented with hemetemesis/hemobilia on endoscopy: (A) CT angiographic arterial phase, (B) MIP images and (C) splenic arteriography showing pseudoaneurysm (arrow) arising from proximal splenic artery. Coil embolization is performed across the neck of pseudoaneurysm, (D) post-embolization angiography is showing coils in splenic artery with nonopacification of pseudoaneurysm

TREATMENT

Management of patients with hemobilia involves resuscitation, arrest of bleeding and relieving biliary obstruction. The treatment options are angiographic embolization, surgery and conservative approach.

Role of Interventional Radiology

Advantage of angiography is in combining therapeutic measures with diagnostic technique.[8,9] Superselective catheterization of bleeding vessel or feeding vessel to aneurysm is done whenever possible. The culprit vessel is embolized with gelatin sponge, steel coils or glue (Figs 1 to 3). Selective approach decreases the risk of significant hepatic necrosis as long as portal vein is patent. When a major vessel is involved, stenting can also be deployed to control the bleeding while maintaining the vessel patency.

Role of Surgery

The surgical procedures include ligation of involved vessels (especially in extrahepatic source of bleeding) and resection of liver segments (for intrahepatic lesions). With the advent of improved angiographic techniques and hardwares, surgery is indicated only if the patient is not fit for angiography or angiographic embolization has failed to control the bleeding. Bipolar ligation is usually employed. Rarely, resection of the vascular segment with anastomosis may be done. When the surgical option is

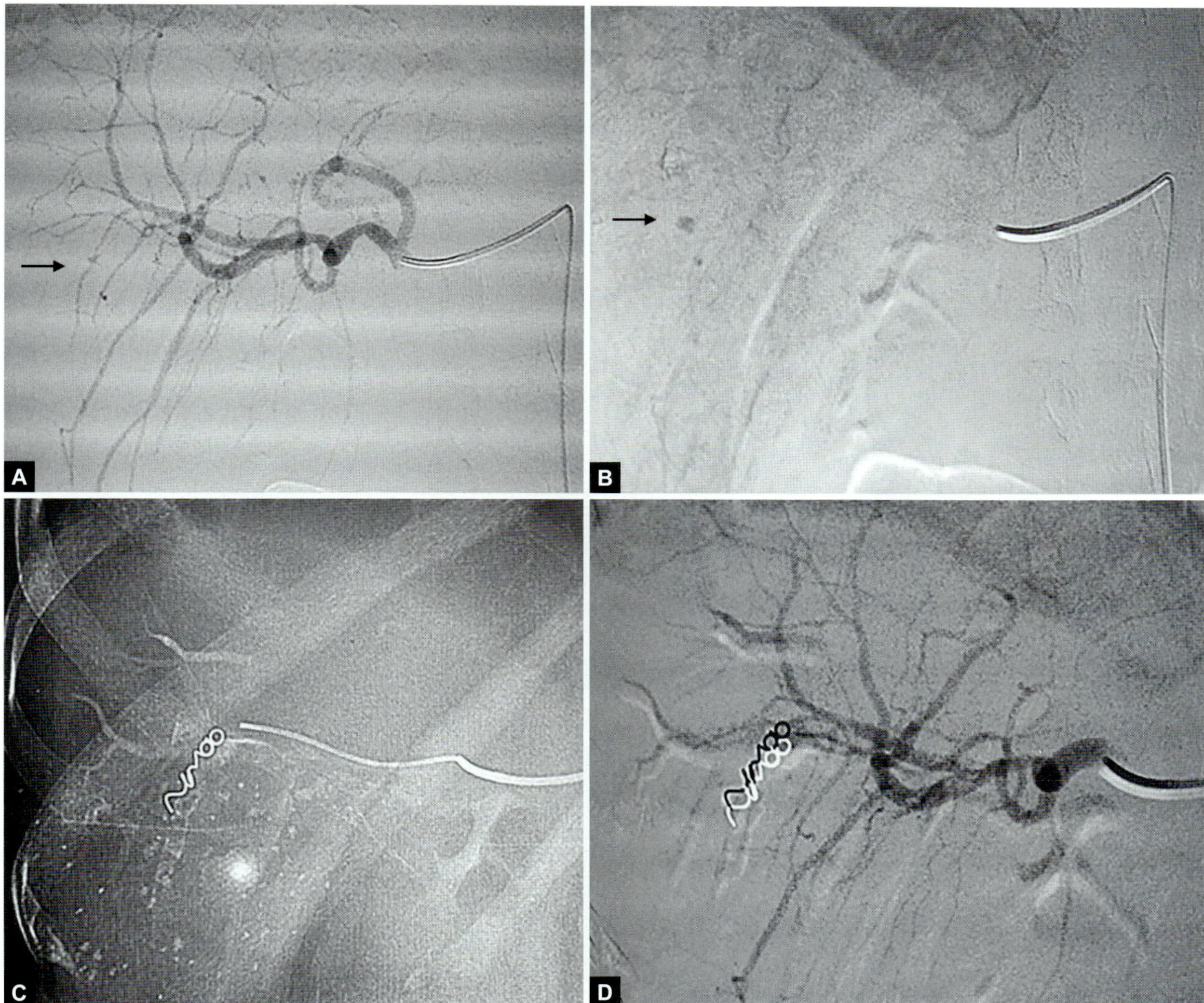

Figures 2A to D Patient presented with hemobilia after liver biopsy. (A and B) Right hepatic artery angiogram is showing small pseudoaneurysm (arrows) arising from distal branch. (C) After selective cannulation, coil is deployed in the feeding branch and (D) post-embolization run showing non-opacification of aneurysm

exercised, mostly the patient has had multiple bleeds, is depleted and hemodynamically unstable. There may be limited access due to previous disease or surgery (e.g. Whipple's procedure) and consequent adhesions. Rapid control of bleeding vessel is the main aim and is achieved by under running the vessel with few prolene sutures.

Biliary Tract Management

In patients with PTBD presenting with bleeding into the catheters, cholangiography is to be done after resuscitating the patient. Cholangiography can delineate the communication (biliary-venous or biliary-arterial). In case of venous bleeding catheter repositioning or upgradation will stop the bleeding by tamponade. In case of arterial bleeding angiographic embolization may be required. To relieve biliary obstruction by clots, ERCP and clot aspiration can be performed. When percutaneous catheters are in place, irrigation of catheters will be enough to lyse and flush off the clots.

Hemosuccus pancreaticus: Bleeding into pancreatic duct and through ampulla of vater into GI tract is known as hemosuccus pancreaticus. It is usually seen as a complication of pancreatitis or pancreatic tumors. Pseudoaneurysm of celiac trunk or splenic artery (Fig. 1) is the usual culprit lesion. Patients usually present with abdominal pain, UGIH and hyperamylasemia with history of acute or chronic pancreatitis. The diagnostic work up and management is similar to hemobilia. Angiographic embolization is the treatment of choice.

Bilhemia denotes the reverse of hemobilia with bile entering the blood pool through a communication to hepatic veins or portal vein. Most of the patients have distal biliary obstruction

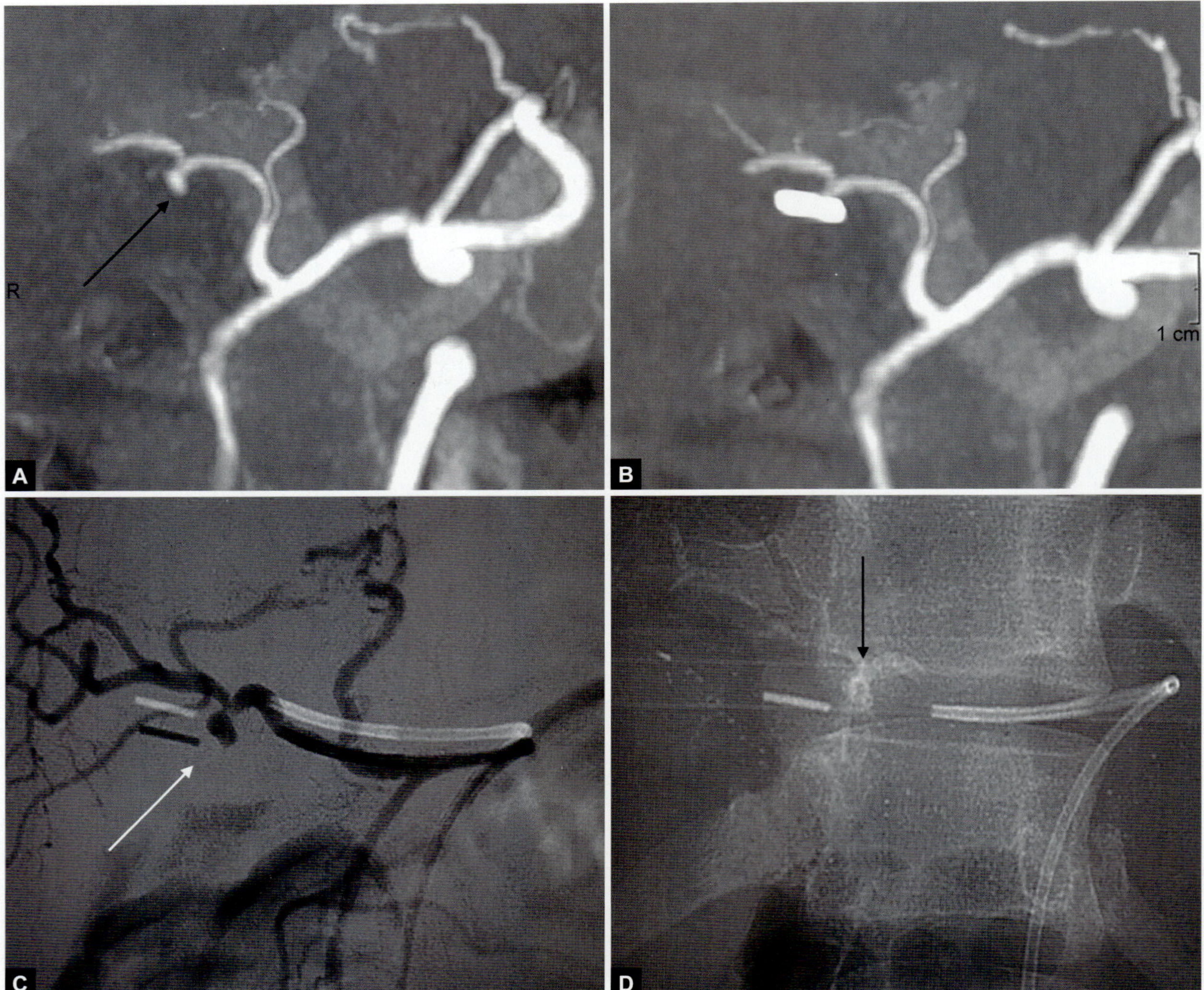

Figures 3A to D Post-laparoscopic cholecystecomy patient presented with hemetemesis; endoscopy showed bleeding from ampulla: (A and B) Coronal MIP images of CT angiography in arterial phase and (C) DSA-Hepatic angiography are showing pseudoaneurysm (arrows) at the level of surgical clips. The aneurysm is embolized with glue mixed with lipiodol. (D) Post-embolization radiograph showing glue cast in the aneurysm (arrow)

increasing the intrabiliary pressure gradient compared to venous system. Treatment aims at relieving biliary obstruction either by endoscopic sphincterotomy or percutaneous approach.

REFERENCES

1. Glisson F. Anatomia Hepatis, 1st edition. Amsterdam: Janssonium and Weyerstraten; 1654.
2. Sandblom P. Hemorrhage into the biliary tract following trauma; traumatic hemobilia. Surgery. 1948;24(3):571-86.
3. Green MH, Duell RM, Johnson CD, Jamieson NV. Haemobilia. Br J Surg. 2001;88(6):773-86.
4. Merrell SW, Schneider PD. Hemobilia—evolution of current diagnosis and treatment. West J Med. 1991;155(6):621-5.
5. Kim KH, Kim TN. Etiology, clinical features, and endoscopic management of hemobilia: a retrospective analysis of 37 cases. Korean J Gastroenterol Taehan Sohwagi Hakhoe Chi. 2012;59(4): 296-302.
6. Goodnight JE, Blaisdell FW. Hemobilia. Surg Clin North Am. 1981;61(4):973-9.
7. Sandblom P, Mirkovitch V, Saegesser F. Formation and fate of fibrin clots in the biliary tract: a clinical and experimental study. Ann Surg. 1977;185(3):356-66.
8. Yopp A. Hemobilia and bihemia. Blumgart's Surgery of the Liver, Biliary Tract, and Pancreas, 5th edition. Philadelphia: Saunders Elsevier; 2012. pp. 1832-44.
9. Srivastava DN, Sharma S, Pal S, Thulkar S, Seith A, Bandhu S, et al. Transcatheter arterial embolization in the management of hemobilia. Abdom Imaging. 2006;31(4):439-48.

CHAPTER 69

Hepatic Trauma

Rajan Chaudhry, Anuj Sharma

INTRODUCTION

The liver is an organ of enigma and since time immemorial severe liver injuries have posed the most difficult problems for managing the injured. Advances in the development of trauma surgery have led to improved outcomes following liver injury. The initial enthusiasm of surgeons who attempted formal major hepatic resections for liver injuries was later replaced by disappointment as the results with this aggressive approach were far from satisfactory. Subsequent understanding of the injured patient's physiology led to a shift toward damage control in most severe trauma victims. Appreciation of good outcomes following less invasive surgery in patients with liver and splenic injuries subsequently favored nonoperative management of patients with such injuries especially with easy availability of cross sectional imaging and minimally invasive technologies.[1-3] With a paradigm shift toward nonoperative management, most hepatic injuries are successfully observed and managed conservatively (Table 1). In addition, the mortality from hepatic injury has declined over the past several decades.[4-8] The reasons for the decrease in mortality for hepatic trauma over the past 25 years are the following:

- Improved results with packing and reoperation
- Use of arteriography and embolization
- Advances in operative techniques for major hepatic trauma
- Decrease in the number of hepatic venous injuries undergoing surgery.

Patients with blunt hepatic injury may present either as hemodynamically stable (who can be observed) or hemodynamically unstable, requiring urgent laparotomy to control hemorrhage from a major hepatic injury. But because most injuries to the liver are minor (grade I or II), most blunt hepatic injuries can be safely observed.[3,5-14] On the other hand, as many as two-thirds of higher-grade hepatic injuries (grades III, IV, V) may require laparotomy for control of hemorrhage.[2,4,9,15-18] Even at busy trauma centers, high-grade hepatic injuries, particularly juxtahepatic venous injuries, are uncommon. Thus, operations required for liver injury can be challenging both in decision-making and operative techniques.

Table 1: Liver organ injury scale

Grade		*Description*
I	Hematoma Laceration	Subcapsular, <10% surface area Capsular tear, <1 cm parenchymal depth
II	Hematoma Laceration	Subcapsular, 10%–15% surface area; intraparenchymal, <10 cm in diameter 1–3 cm parenchymal depth, <10 cm in length
III	Hematoma Laceration	Subcapsular, >50% surface area or expanding; ruptured subcapsular or parenchymal hematoma >3 cm parenchymal depth
IV	Hematoma	Parenchymal disruption involving 25%–75% of hepatic lobe or 1–3 Couinaud segments within a single lobe
V	Laceration Vascular	Parenchymal disruption involving >75% of hepatic lobe or >3 Couinaud segments within a single lobe Juxtahepatic venous injuries; i.e., retrohepatic vena cava/central major hepatic vein
VI		Hepatic avulsion

Source: Moore EE, Pachter HL. Organ injury scaling: spleen, liver and kidney. J Trauma. 1995;38:323-4.

MECHANISM OF INJURY

The liver is suspended by superior attachments to the diaphragm, and anterior attachments of the coronary ligaments, triangular ligaments and the falciform ligament. It is also attached to the lesser curve of the stomach.[19] Deceleration injuries result in tears at these sites of fixation. A deceleration injury often causes a fracture between the posterior and the anterior segments of the right lobe. A crushing mechanism or a focused blunt injury to the right upper quadrant compresses the ribs onto the liver causing a stellate-type laceration across the dome extending onto the anterior surface of the right lobe, often termed a "bear-claw injury". Anterior-posterior forces can produce a split-liver, often through the line of Cantlie. In general, blunt trauma more commonly affects the right hepatic lobe. It is also pertinent to mention that high velocity missile injuries to the liver usually have a dramatic presentation and abdominal exploration is a rule rather than an exception.

CLINICAL PRESENTATION AND DIAGNOSIS

Patients with abdominal trauma who are unstable at presentation or become unstable in the trauma center despite resuscitative efforts should be taken immediately to the operation theater for laparotomy. In contrast, the stable patient should undergo a rapid physical examination and portable chest radiography. Although outward signs of injury are nonspecific and the absence of such findings do not exclude injury, seatbelt signs or other marks, regions of tenderness, and obvious penetrating wounds must be noted. Patients with a seatbelt sign have a 3.1-fold higher incidence of liver injury than those patients presenting without a seatbelt sign.[20] Right-sided rib fractures or pulmonary contusion should also raise suspicion for hepatic injury.

The focused assessment by ultrasound for trauma (FAST) has become a routine diagnostic tool for trauma surgeons. Unstable patient with a positive FAST is transported immediately to the operation theater for laparotomy.

Computerized tomography (CT) is the standard diagnostic modality for stable trauma patients with a suspected abdominal injury. The inherent advantage of an in-house CT scanner cannot be over emphasized and can be extremely invaluable in certain circumstances. CT has sensitivity in excess of 92% with a specificity of 98.7% for detection of liver injury.[4,10,21] CT can identify type and grade of liver injury, the severity of hemoperitoneum and whether there is active bleeding or only clotted blood. CT scan also detects other associated intraperitoneal and retroperitoneal injuries, including splenic, renal, bowel, chest trauma and pelvic fractures.

The American Association for the Surgery of Trauma (AAST) published a liver injury scale (Table 1) with the aim to categorize severity of hepatic trauma uniformly.[22] This scale is useful both as a descriptive tool and as a prognostic indicator across various groups of patients.

Basically the AAST Liver Injury Scale translates into three types of injuries as far as the operating surgeon is concerned:

1. Superficial parenchymal injuries requiring nothing more than a simple suture or use of a local hemostatic technique.
2. Deep parenchymal injury or extensive parenchymal disruption, which can be packed.
3. Deep injury involving major vascular structures, which requires special maneuvers for control of bleeding. These often carry a poor prognosis.

The approach to each type of injury depends on the patient's hemodynamic stability and the cumulative physiologic insult.

NONOPERATIVE MANAGEMENT

The current approach to hepatic trauma has evolved to nonoperative management in more than 80% of cases.[2,4-6,9,13,20,23] Several contributing factors have been recognized:

- Experience that more than 50% of liver injuries stop bleeding spontaneously.[9,24]
- The precedence of successful nonoperative management in pediatric patients.[1,25]
- Knowledge that the liver has tremendous capacity to heal after injury.[26,27]
- Improvements in liver imaging with CT.[28-31]

Criteria for nonoperative management include hemodynamic stability, absence of other abdominal injuries that mandate laparotomy, immediate availability of resources including a fully staffed operating room, if required and a watchful and alert surgeon. In general, any patient who is stable enough to have a CT scan performed is likely to be successfully managed nonoperatively. Grades I and II hepatic injuries should be observed in ICU setting with serial hematocrit evaluations and bed rest. Higher-grade injuries in stable patients should be observed in an intensive care unit setting with optimization of all coagulation factors.

The current reported success rate of nonoperative management of hepatic trauma ranges from 82% to 100%.[12,13,21-23,30,32-34] About a quarter of patients with blunt hepatic injury of grade IV or higher-grade managed nonoperatively will require some intervention because of complications.[25,26,31,34,35] Interventional radiology may be needed to perform an angiogram and embolization for bleeding or to percutaneously drain an abscess or biloma. An endoscopic retrograde cholangiopancreatogram (ERCP) and stent placement may be required for biliary leak. Even when such complications of the liver injury develop, only 15% require operative intervention. Hepatic artery angiography with embolization is an important tool for the stable patient with contrast extravasation who is being managed nonoperatively. It can also be invaluable for the postoperative patient who has been stabilized by perihepatic packing or who has rebled after an initial period of stability. Angioembolization has a greater than 90% success rate in the control of bleeding with a low risk of rebleed and a reduction in the required volume of transfusion.[18,32,36]

Bile leaks are common (6–20% of cases) following nonoperative management of liver injuries. Biliary complications are variable in their time of presentation and may require multiple treatment strategies. Ultrasound, CT and MRI scans are used to diagnose a biloma, whereas a hepatobiliary iminodiacetic acid scan is used to show an active bile leak. Most collections can be managed by simple ultrasound or CT guided percutaneous drainage. Approximately one-third of patients with a biloma require ERCP and stent placement in addition to radiologic drainage to manage on going bile leak.

A less common complication is hemobilia, caused by an abnormal communication between an intrahepatic blood vessel, usually an artery, and the biliary tree. The incidence after trauma is less than 3% and is more often associated with blunt trauma than with penetrating injuries. Hemobilia presents as gastrointestinal bleeding with or without abdominal pain and jaundice caused by occlusion of bile ducts by blood clots. Angiography permits precise identification and selective embolization of the appropriate branch vessel as opposed to the surgical alternative of ligation of a main hepatic artery or hepatic resection, thereby preserving more functional hepatic parenchyma.[33] Table 2 lists complications of nonoperative management.

Reported predictors of failure of nonoperative management include hypotension on admission, high CT grades of injury, and the need for blood transfusion. It is now regarded that hemodynamically stable patients with intraperitoneal contrast extravasation and hemoperitoneum in six compartments on CT are at high risk for the need of operation after blunt hepatic trauma.[34]

The risk for failure of nonoperative management approaches 96% in the presence of: (1) a splenic (Fig. 1) or renal injury with a positive FAST result; (2) an estimated amount of free fluid on CT of greater than 300 mL and (3) the requirement for blood transfusion.[23] If all of these factors are absent, the risk for nonoperative management failure is only 2%. Needless to say, it is imperative that in the absence of diagnostic facilities like CT scan and angiography, and patients whose access to tertiary care is compromised, the threshold for conversion to operative management should be low.

Table 2: Complications of nonoperative management
1. Ongoing bleeding
2. Biloma
3. Biliary fistula
4. Intra-abdominal abscess
5. Hepatic abscess
6. Hemobilia
7. Liver necrosis
8. Missed hollow viscus injury
9. Abdominal compartment syndrome

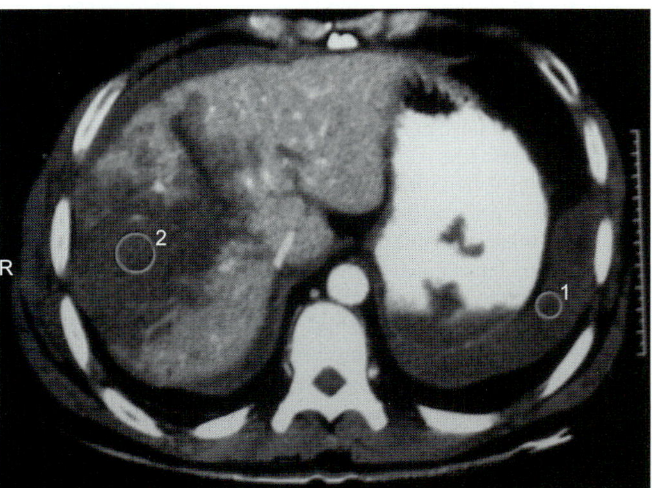

Figure 1 Large area of parenchymal contusion in right lobe liver which is unperfused after contrast injection. Subcapsular collections (hemorrhages) are seen around liver and spleen (*Source:* Sundeep Jain, Fortis, Jaipur)

NON-OPERATIVE MANAGEMENT OF PENETRATING LIVER TRAUMA

The success of non-operative management for blunt hepatic trauma in the 1990s, led to attempts to extend the concept to penetrating injuries. Although conservative management of stab wounds to the abdomen, including the liver, has been practiced for years, application of this approach to gunshot wounds is controversial. Clearly, nonoperative management of hepatic gunshot wounds must be applied carefully and selectively and is not currently the standard of care.[24] Success hinges on complete CT delineation of the entire bullet trajectory within the liver and the ability to reliably exclude injury to adjacent hollow organs, especially the right colon.

OPERATIVE MANAGEMENT

Operations for liver injury are necessary in the setting of complex hepatic injury and generally indicated for hypotension and significant bleeding; these operations are often challenging. In part, because of this difficulty, paradigm shifts have occurred in the operative approach to hepatic trauma. Before World War II, "house surgeons advocated expectant or conservative treatment, or no treatment at all for the majority of wounds of the liver." During World War II, drainage of liver injuries and abandonment of the use of gauze packs decreased mortality from 30% to 17%. Temporary packing and damage control with the goals to control bleeding and limit gastrointestinal contamination with an abbreviated laparotomy have made resurgence and are invaluable when appropriately used. It is critical that surgical bleeding is controlled before truncating any operation on the liver.[25-28]

Anesthesiologists must ensure that blood products are already in the room. The massive transfusion protocol should be followed and the blood bank should be ahead of the patient's needs for packed red blood cells and other blood products. Adequate vascular access and arterial blood pressure monitoring are essential. It is necessary to have venous access above the diaphragm. Resuscitation fluids infused under pressure through femoral access will exacerbate hepatic venous bleeding, at times dramatically so. Massive transfusion protocols should be activated early to prevent any delay in resuscitation with blood products.

As with every trauma laparotomy, the patient should be widely prepped, chin to knees and table to table laterally. A generous midline incision is made. For injuries to the right lobe or right hepatic vein, a transverse incision branched to the right of the midline incision is essential.[29] Self-retaining retractors are helpful. The most easily and quickly applicable retractor in the patient exsanguinating from a liver injury is the Rochard or Thompson retractor.

The four quadrants are quickly packed with swabs. This allows the anesthesiologist to achieve effective intraoperative resuscitation. The lower quadrants are unpacked first, the bowel is quickly examined and contamination is quickly temporized. The left upper quadrant is evaluated next. If an injury to the spleen is noted, it is removed. The right upper quadrant packs can then be removed to allow evaluation of the liver injury.

If significant liver bleeding is seen, initial methods to temporize the hemorrhage can also be diagnostic. The liver should first be manually compressed. How this is conceptualized and performed is important. Packs placed in an anterior-posterior axis will often

Table 3: Surgical goals in the management of liver injuries
1. Control hemorrhage
2. Control bile leak
3. Debride/Resect devitalized liver
4. Drainage

distract the injured liver further and worsen the bleeding. The lobes of the liver must be compressed back to normal position, essentially back towards midline. Simultaneously, the liver is pushed toward the diaphragm. Maintenance of this anatomic compression by the first or second assistant is critical to reduce bleeding as the surgeon assesses the liver injury or mobilizes the liver. Perihepatic packing can help to maintain this tamponade. Most minor venous bleeding and small lacerations to the parenchyma can be temporized by this technique. Hemostatic agents such as surgical, thrombin-soaked gel foam, or fibrin glue are useful adjuncts. The argon beam coagulator is also an effective means of hemostasis in this case. Omentum can be placed over the liver defect as a more permanent packing method. If these simple maneuvers are effective, the operation should be truncated in the lines of damage control laparotomy and the patient should be shifted to the intensive care unit for further resuscitation (Table 3).

In an unstable patient, delay to control hemorrhage will negatively affect outcome. As an independent predictor of outcome, the mortality doubles (25–50%) as the patient's transfusion requirement increases from 10 to 20 units of packed red blood cells. Ideally, the bleeding should be staunched as early as possible within this time frame. Avoidance of hypothermia, acidosis and coagulopathy is best accomplished by early control of hemorrhage. Once the decision has been made to operate on an unstable patient with a known or suspected liver injury, the procedure of choice is often damage-control laparotomy. The goals of a damage-control laparotomy are twofold: (1) to control hemorrhage and (2) to control contamination. Perihepatic packing will control bleeding in up to 80% of patients undergoing laparotomy and allow for transfer to the intensive care unit for resuscitation and warming. Folded laparotomy packs are inserted over the diaphragmatic surfaces of the liver, never within a laceration, to promote a tamponade effect. Underpacking or inappropriate packing leads to worsened patient outcomes.[28] Excessive packing can also be detrimental, leading to renal vein and vena caval compression and subsequent abdominal compartment syndrome.

If hemorrhage continues in the operation theater, the Pringle maneuver should be applied with placement of an atraumatic vascular clamp across the porta hepatis. If this controls the bleeding, an injury to a branch of the portal vein or hepatic artery is the likely source. A major injury to the hepatic veins or vena cava is less likely. However, when the Pringle maneuver fails to control bleeding from within a liver injury or dark venous bleeding persists from behind a hepatic lobe, a juxtahepatic venous injury is likely. If simple sutures and compression are performed and bleeding is still profuse, experienced judgment is crucial to decide whether to proceed with further exploration and attempted repair or perihepatic packing (Table 4).

Once the decision is made to perform a major operation, adequate exposure of the liver is essential. Injury high in the dome of the liver will likely require mobilization of the right lobe.

Table 4: Golden rules for the surgeon dealing with liver trauma
1. Do not take the patient to the operation theater, unless clearly indicated
2. In hemodynamically unstable patients, do only what is essential to stop bleeding at the first operation. If simple measures work, pack and truncate the operation (damage control)
3. If major resection is required, the decision must be made early in the operation
4. Once you are committed to a major resection, technical/clinical expertise and speed are critical
5. Plan delayed resection in selected patients

The falciform and triangular ligaments are taken down with simultaneous compression of the liver. If the midline incision has not been extended to a subcostal incision, it can be extended at this time.

Hepatotomy and selective vascular ligation is one technique for management of major hepatic venous, portal venous, and arterial injuries. With Pringle control, the injured portion of the liver is further fractured with the surgeon's finger or with a Kelly clamp or the stapling devices to allow direct ligation of the bleeding vessels. This must be done early and expediently in the operation.

Nonanatomical resection refers to removal of injured parenchyma along the line of the injury rather than along a standard anatomic plane. In many cases, this involves the completion of an already extensive avulsion injury. Vascular stapling devices are the most rapid means of dividing tissue and controlling major veins. As with elective hepatic surgery, the stapling devices have been a major advance in the treatment of hepatic trauma.

Anatomic resection involves removal of injured liver segments along standard anatomic places.[19,31,35] Hepatic resection of an injured segment of the liver definitively controls bleeding, potential bile leak, and removes devitalized tissue. However, its role in the management of liver injury remains controversial.

The mortality for liver resection was 80% in 1900s. Advances in operative technique, better understanding of liver anatomy and technologic advances (diagnostic and operative) have now made hepatic resection routine and safe in many centers. Strong and colleagues reported a liver related mortality of 8% and hepatic complication rate of 19% following liver resection for trauma.[37]

It is not essential to perform liver resection at the first laparotomy, if bleeding has been effectively controlled. The mortality for grades IV and V hepatic injuries, which generally comprise only 15% of liver injuries, is greater than 50% in most series.[4,8,15,18,38,39] As a rule, these patients are hypotensive on presentation and require urgent laparotomy. The corollary is that most blunt hepatic injuries requiring urgent surgery are hemodynamically unstable patients, with grade IV (Figs 2 and 3) or V injury, a third of whom have an associated hepatic vascular injury. Exsanguination is the cause of death, usually on the operating table. Grade V hepatic injury has two subtypes, which are very different in anatomy and outcome. A grade V laceration is parenchymal disruption involving more than 75% of the hepatic lobe or more than three couinaud segments within a single lobe. The patients may be hemodynamically stable and some will do well with nonoperative management. A grade V vascular injury is a juxtahepatic venous injury (retrohepatic inferior vena cava). These patients are

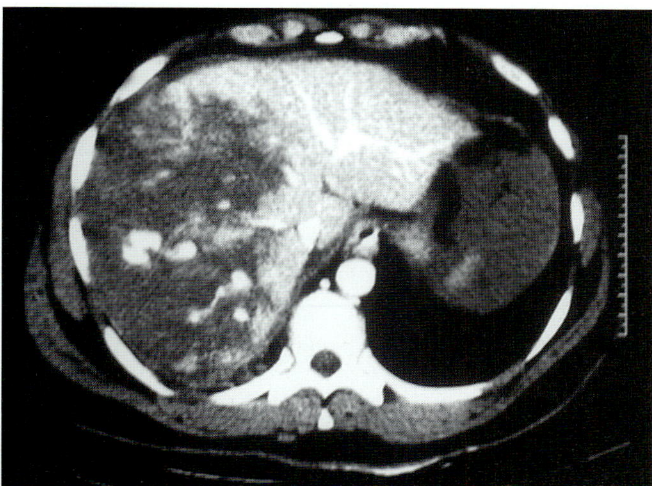

Figure 2 Large grade IV hepatic contusion with focal pooling of contrast suggestive of active bleeding (*Source:* Sundeep Jain, Fortis, Jaipur)

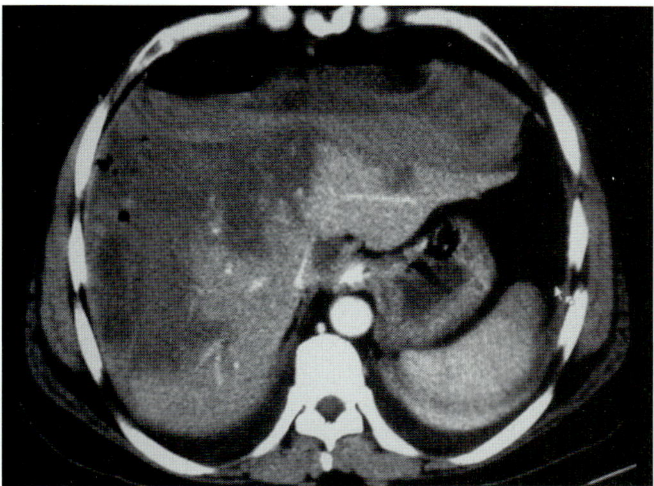

Figure 3 Extensive bilobar grade IV hepatic contusions with parenchymal and subcapsular air. Spleen also shows subcapsular hemorrhage (*Source:* Sundeep Jain, Fortis, Jaipur)

exsanguinating and require urgent operation in almost all cases. These hepatic venous and retrohepatic injuries are technically difficult to manage in the operating room and carry 50–80% mortality in most series, particularly following blunt injury. Presumably, high-grade liver injury from a blunt mechanism produces more severe parenchymal disruption than penetrating injury from low velocity civilian weapons.[4,14,39-42]

Approach to juxtahepatic injuries may require total vascular isolation of the liver by clamping the suprahepatic IVC, the suprarenal IVC and the porta hepatis.[35] The liver can then be fully mobilized allowing exposure of the venous injuries followed by primary repair or ligation. Rapid control of the suprahepatic IVC can be obtained by incising the peritoneum between the esophagus and IVC at the diaphragm, following the plane between the crura and the esophagus to the patient's left and caudate lobe/IVC on the patient's right. The plane can be followed with the index finger around and then encircling the suprahepatic IVC. Another technique for rapid control of the suprahepatic IVC is incision in the central diaphragm/pericardium and a vascular clamp placed on the intrapericardial IVC. Venovenous bypass or the atriocaval shunt in the management of these injuries is generally not advocated. Adequate exposure through sufficient incisions (broad subcostal, Mercedes Benz or midline with right subcostal extension), self-retaining retractors, and help from surgeons experienced in hepatic surgery are necessary and sufficient. Assistance from an experienced liver or liver transplant surgeon is invaluable in these cases.

If the decision is made to truncate the operation after initial damage control, the abdomen is temporarily closed with a rapid skin closure silo technique or a laparotomy created with use of a Bogota bag, zippers or even a negative-pressure vacuum-assisted closure dressing, and the patient is transferred to the intensive care unit. Aggressive resuscitation and warming are required to correct coagulopathy. On the other hand, maintenance of a low central venous pressure may minimize hepatic bleeding and swelling. Once the patient has been stabilized, re-exploration and possible definitive repair in the operation theater must be planned.

Suggested end points of resuscitation include a systemic lactate concentration less than 2.5 mmol/L, base deficit less than 4 mmol/L, core temperature greater than 35°C and an internationalized normalized ratio of less than 1.25. Optimal timing for pack removal is controversial. Caruso and colleagues showed that rebleeding from the liver was significantly increased when packs were removed within 36 hours rather than waiting until after 36 hours. In addition to rebleeding, packing for liver trauma has also been associated with increased rates of abdominal sepsis and bile leaks. Nicol and colleagues demonstrated that the duration of packing is not associated with these complications and that a second-look laparotomy should only be performed after 48 hours.[27] There is reasonable evidence that we generally return these patients to the operating room for pack removal 48 hours after damage-control laparotomy.[27,28] Management algorithm is given as Flow chart 1.

SUMMARY

A multidisciplinary approach to the management of hepatic injuries has evolved over the last few decades, but the basic principles of trauma continue to be observed. Diagnostic and therapeutic endeavors are chosen based mainly on the stability of the patient. Stable patients with reliable examinations and available resources can be managed nonoperatively. Unstable patients belong to the operation theater and should never be taken to the CT scanner. Once in the operating room, simple maneuvers are attempted first followed by an early decision to proceed with resection if necessary. More experienced liver surgeons are invaluable resources when they are available. Interventional radiological techniques can prevent and treat complications of nonoperative and operative management of liver injuries. Successful management of patients with complex liver trauma depends on aggressive correction of hypothermia, coagulopathy, and acidosis, rapid critical decision-making and experienced judgment. Nonoperative management of hemodynamically stable patients with blunt hepatic injury has become the standard method of care; however, this conservative approach often requires the use of adjunctive measures to manage sequelae and complications. Hemodynamically unstable patients with a bleeding liver require emergency laparotomy, although most

Flow chart 1 Management algorithm

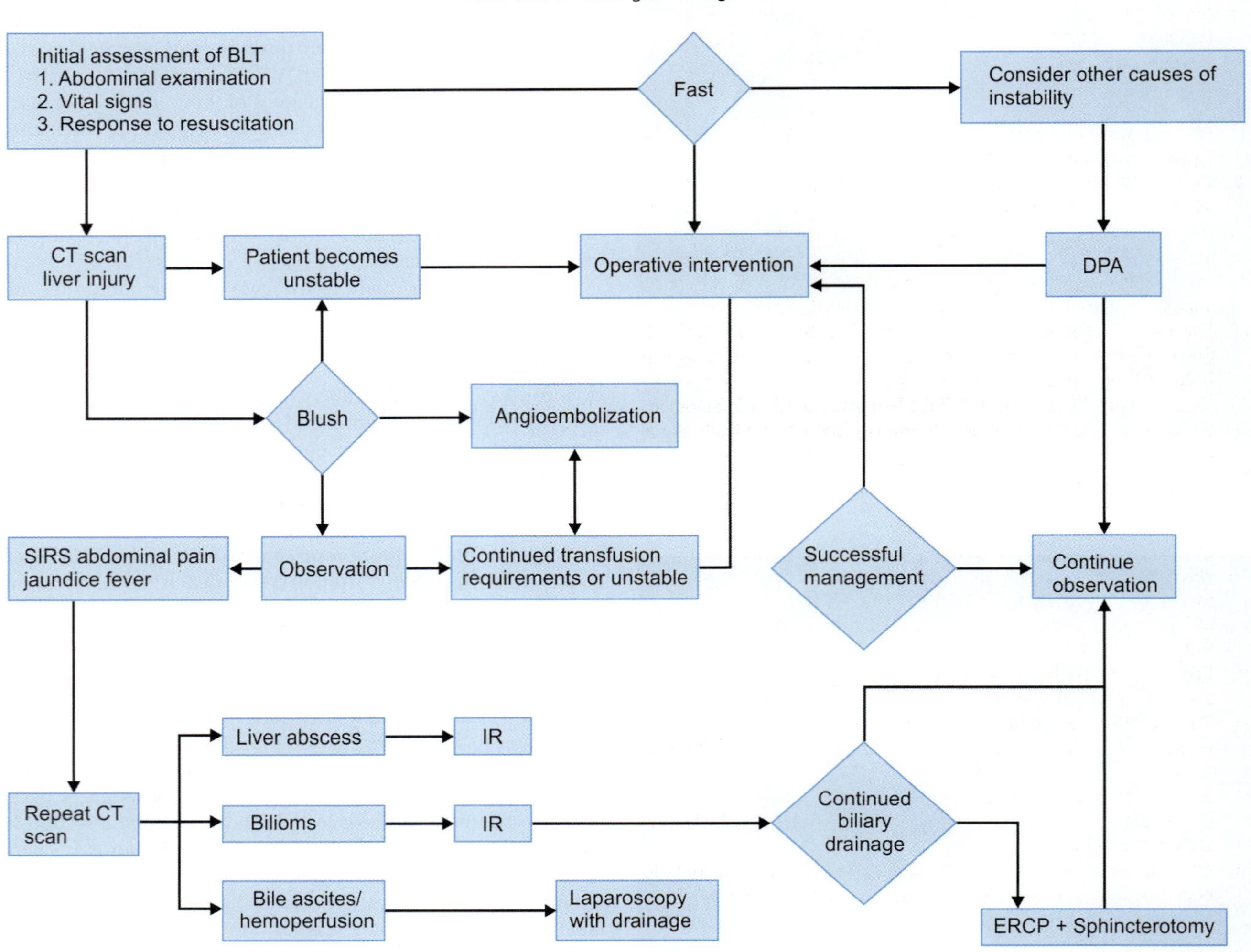

patients with significant hemorrhage can and should be managed by packing. Liver resection, either anatomic or nonanatomic, should be used in appropriate patients with complex liver injury and can be accomplished with low morbidity and mortality. The stapling devices and clear understanding of hepatic anatomy facilitate operative management.

REFERENCES

1. Ong CC. Primary hepatic artery embolization in pediatric blunt hepatic trauma. J Pediatr Surg. 2012;47(12):2316-20.
2. Hoff WS, Holevar M, Nagy KK, Patterson L, Young JS, Arrillaga A, et al. Practice management guidelines for the evaluation of blunt abdominal trauma: the EAST practice management guidelines work group. J Trauma. 2002;53:602-15.
3. Menegaux F, Langlois P, Chigot JP. Severe blunt trauma of the liver: study of mortality factors. J Trauma. 1993;35:865-9.
4. Pop PA. Hepatic trauma management in polytraumatised patients. Chirurgia (Bucur). 2012;107(5):591-7.
5. Allard MA, Dondero F, Sommacale D, Dokmak S, Belghiti J, Farges O. Liver packing during elective surgery: an option that can be considered. World J Surg. 2011;35:2493-8.
6. Blecher GA. Hepatoportal fistula in an 83-year-old male, presenting with hematemesis 52 years after blunt trauma. Surg Laparosc Endosc Percutan Tech. 2013;23(2): e84-6.
7. Polanco P, Leon S, Pineda J, Puyana JC, Ochoa JB, Alarcon L, et al. Hepatic resection in the management of complex injury to the liver. J Trauma. 2008;65(6):1264-9.
8. Pachter HL, Spencer FC, Hofstetter SR, Liang HG, Coppa GF. Significant trends in the treatment of hepatic injuries. Experience with 411 injuries. Ann Surg. 1992;215:492-500.
9. Swift C. Non-operative management of liver trauma. J R Army Med Corps. 2012;158(2): 85-95.
10. Trunkey DD. Hepatic trauma: contemporary management. Surg Clin North Am. 2004;84:437-50.
11. Richardson JD, Franklin GA, Lukan JK, Carrillo EH, Spain DA, Miller FB, et al. Evolution in the management of hepatic trauma: a 25-year perspective. Ann Surg. 2000;232:324-30.
12. Moore EE, Shackford SR, Pachter HL. Organ injury scaling: spleen, liver and kidney. J Trauma. 1995;38:323-4.
13. Beal SL. Fatal hepatic hemorrhage: an unresolved problem in the management of complex liver injuries. J Trauma. 1990;30(2):163-9.
14. Asensio JA, Demetriades D, Chahwan S, Gomez H, Hanpeter D, Velmahos G, et al. Approach to the management of complex hepatic injuries. J Trauma. 2000;48:66-9.

15. Leppäniemi AK, Mentula PJ, Streng MH, Koivikko MP, Handolin LE. Severe hepatic trauma: nonoperative management, definitive repair, or damage control surgery? World J Surg. 2011;35:2643-9.
16. Badger SA, Barclay R, Campbell P, Mole DJ, Diamond T. Management of liver trauma. World J Surg. 2009;33:2522-37.
17. Velmahos GC, Toutouzas KG, Radin R, Chan L, Demetriades D. Nonoperative treatment of blunt injury to solid abdominal organs: a prospective study. Arch Surg. 2003;138(8):844-51.
18. Carillo EH, Spain DA, Wohltmann CD, Schmieg RE, Boaz PW, Miller FB, et al. Interventional techniques are useful adjuncts in nonoperative management of hepatic injuries. J Trauma. 1999;46:619-22.
19. Skandalakis JE, Skandalakis LJ, Skandalakis PN, Mirilas P. Hepatic surgical anatomy. Surg Clin North Am. 2004;84:413-35.
20. Sharma OP, Oswanski MF, Kaminski BP, Issa NM, Duffy B, Stringfellow K, et al. Clinical implications of the seat belt sign in blunt trauma. Am Surg. 2009;75(9):822-7.
21. Fang JF, Wong YC, Lin BC, Hsu YP, Chen MF. The CT risk factors for the need of operative treatment in initially hemodynamically stable patients after blunt hepatic trauma. J Trauma. 2006;61(3):547-53.
22. Sclafani SJ, Shaftan GW, McAuley J, Nayaranaswamy T, Mitchell WG, Gordon DH, et al. Interventional radiology in the management of hepatic trauma. J Trauma. 1984;24:256-62.
23. Mohr AM, Lavery RF, Barone A, Bahramipour P, Magnotti LJ, Osband AJ, et al. Angiographic embolisation for liver injuries: low mortality, high morbidity. J Trauma. 2003;55:1077-81.
24. Madding GF, Kennedy PA. Trauma to the Liver. Philadelphia: WB Saunders; 1971.
25. Krige JEJ, Bornman PC, Terblanche J. Liver trauma in 446 patients. S Afr J Surg. 1997;1:10-5.
26. Caruso DM, Battistella FD, Owings JT, Lee SL, Samaco RC. Perihepatic packing of major liver injuries. Arch Surg. 1999;134: 958-63.
27. Nicol AJ, Hommes M, Primrose R, Navsaria PH, Krige JE. Packing for control of hemorrhage in major liver trauma. World J Surg. 2007;31(3):569-74.
28. Aydin U, Yazici P, Zeytunlu M, Coker A. Is it more dangerous to perform inadequate packing? World J Emerg Surg. 2008;14(3):1.
29. Berney T, Morel P, Huber O, Zurbuchen P, Mentha G. Combined midline-transverse surgical approach for severe blunt injuries to the liver. J Trauma. 2000;48:349-53.
30. Loverland JA, Boffard KD. Damage control in the abdomen and beyond. Br J Surg. 2004;91:1095-101.
31. Liau KH, Blumgart LH, DeMatteo RP. Segment-oriented approach to liver resection. Surg Clin North Am. 2004;84:543-61.
32. Misselbeck TS, Teicher EJ, Cipolle MD, Pasquale MD, Shah KT, Dangleben DA, et al. Hepatic angioembolization in trauma patients: indications and complications. J Trauma. 2009;67(4):769-73.
33. Forlee MV, Krige JE, Welman CJ, Beningfield SJ. Haemobilia after penetrating and blunt liver injury: treatment with selective hepatic artery embolisation. Injury. 2004;35(1):23-8.
34. Croce MA, Fabian TC, Spiers AP, Kudsk KA. Traumatic hepatic artery pseudoaneurysm with hemobilia. Am J Surg. 1994;138: 235-8.
35. Abdalla EK, Noun R, Belghiti J. Hepatic vascular occlusion: which technique? Surg Clin North Am. 2004;84:563-85.
36. Wahl WL, Ahrns KS, Brandt MM, et al. The need for early angiographic embolisation in blunt liver injuries. J Trauma. 2002;52: 1097-101.
37. Strong RW, Lynch SV, Wall DR, Liu CL. Anatomic resection for severe liver trauma. Surgery. 1998;123:251-7.
38. Duane TM, Como JJ, Bochicchio GV, Scalea TM. Reevaluating the management and outcomes of severe blunt liver injury. J Trauma. 2004;57:494-500.
39. Buckman RF Jr, Miraliakbari R, Badellino MM. Juxtahepatic venous injuries: a critical review of reported management strategies. J Trauma. 2000;48:978-84.
40. Chen RJ, Fang JF, Lin BC, Hsu YP, Kao JL, Chen MF. Factors determining operative mortality of Grade V blunt hepatic trauma. J Trauma. 2000;49:886-91.
41. Chen RJ, Fang JF, Lin BC, Jeng LB, Chen MF. Surgical management of juxtahepatic venous injuries in blunt hepatic trauma. J Trauma. 1995;38:886-90.
42. Cogbill TH, Moore EE, Jurkovich GJ, Feliciano DV, Morris JA, Mucha P. Severe hepatic trauma: a multicenter experience with 1335 liver injuries. J Trauma. 1988;28:1433-8.

CHAPTER 70

Approach to Space-occupying Lesion of Liver

Nilesh Patil, PK Mishra

INTRODUCTION

Space-occupying lesion (SOL) in a liver is a clinical dilemma for the physician. The incidence is increasing because of increasing use of various diagnostic modalities as well as an increasing incidence of primary and secondary hepatic malignancies. Liver SOLs may be detected during investigation of a clinical complaint or incidentally in the course of investigation of some unrelated problem or during a routine check-up. Incidentally detected liver SOLs have been termed as *incidentalomas*. Liver SOLs are truly a diagnostic challenge and their accurate diagnosis requires systematic and multidisciplinary approach by treating surgeon, radiologist and pathologist. With the appropriate interpretation of clinical history and examination, laboratory and imaging findings, it is possible to determine the exact nature of the lesion in majority of the patients. Correct diagnosis avoids delay in the management of malignant lesions and allows the optimal treatment of benign lesions in the form of reassurance, regular follow-up or surgical removal. Imaging of liver and biliary tree has been covered separately. This chapter gives a brief outline of the imaging modalities for the liver SOLs and their characteristic features. Attempt is to outline an algorithmic approach toward the liver SOLs.

HISTORY AND PHYSICAL EXAMINATION

It is critical to review the clinical history and examination findings, as the appropriate correlation between these findings and imaging features helps in narrowing the differential diagnoses for liver SOLs. The factors of clinical concern in the patient's history are *age, gender, history of malignancy, drug and alcohol usage and associated medical conditions*. Consideration of *age and gender* of patient gives some clues in evaluating the cause of liver SOL. Hepatoblastoma is known to occur exclusively in pediatric population. Although hepatocellular carcinoma (HCC) tends to occur in 5th or 6th decade, fibrolamellar HCC is found typically in younger individuals. HCC occurs more commonly in men, while certain liver tumors, such as hemangioma, hepatic adenoma, focal nodular hyperplasia (FNH), are more frequently found in females. The possible factors though to be associated with male predominance of HCC are *alcohol abuse, smoking* and also the hormonal factors. Hepatic neoplasia has been linked to steroid usage. The use of *oral contraceptive pills* has been associated with hepatic adenoma, FNH, epitheloid hemangioendothelioma and possibly hepatoma.[1] In addition the association between administration of *anabolic steroids* and neoplastic hepatic lesions has been described. Few studies have demonstrated strong linkage between cumulative exposure of *vinyl chloride* and development of malignant hepatic lesions such as angiosarcoma.[2,3] *Radiation exposure* either accidental or as a part of cancer treatment can cause liver injury and subsequently increased risk of neoplasia such as lymphoma.[4] In addition, administration of *systemic chemotherapy* can result in focal accumulation of fat in liver which may appear as a new SOL on imaging. The liver is a frequent site of metastases due to favorable intrahepatic milieu and drainage of GI tract through portal vein into liver. It has been seen that 35–50% of patients with colorectal cancer develop liver secondary at some point in their disease.[5] In addition, some primary malignancies such as breast cancer, malignant melanoma have propensity to metastasize to the liver. But, in patients with hematological malignancies, the liver SOLs may develop due to primary or extramedullary hematopoiesis or they may be due to multiple fungal abscesses as a result of immunosuppression. Thus despite a high degree of suspicion all aspects need to be considered when a liver SOL is detected in patients with previous history of malignancy. In addition to history of malignancy, other medical diseases may also have significance pertaining to evaluation of liver SOL. Among them the most important is the *presence of cirrhosis*, which is commonly due to either *viral or alcoholic* hepatitis. The etiology of cirrhosis may have important bearing on the biological features of malignant liver SOL, e.g. HCC secondary to HCV related cirrhosis are more frequently multifocal and are more likely associated with intrahepatic recurrences, while those associated with HBV are usually large and solitary.[6,7] HCC may develop many years after the beginning of fibrotic changes in about 40% of patients with *primary biliary cirrhosis*.[8] In addition to cirrhosis, patients suffering from hemochromatosis, autoimmune hepatitis or Wilson's disease are also at increased risk for HCC. Thus, high index of suspicion is required while evaluating liver SOL in these patients. However, fibrolamellar HCC is usually not associated with history of either hepatitis or cirrhosis. Similarly, patients with history of *PSC* or the associated disease such as *ulcerative colitis, Caroli's syndrome*, liver fluke infestation and *hepaticolithiasis* are at increased risk of cholangiocarcinoma, which can present as a liver SOL. Also, there may be few patients with underlying predisposing conditions for certain liver SOLs, e.g. hepatic adenoma in *glycogen storage disorder*, hemangiomas in various *genetic syndromes* with angiomatous malformations. In addition, patients with family history of *young onset diabetes mellitus* may be predisposed to hepatic adenomatosis.

Among the clinical symptoms, abdominal pain is usually non-specific. Symptoms such as fever may be of value in diagnosis of inflammatory lesions such as liver abscesses or sometimes granuloma or inflammatory pseudotumor; however, it can also be related to malignant liver SOL. Other symptoms, e.g. painless cholestatic jaundice, are more suggestive of underlying malignancy such as cholangiocarcinoma. In addition, constitutional symptoms such as fatigue, anorexia and weight loss points more toward the malignant cause. Also, symptoms indicative of certain paraneoplastic syndromes are also helpful in narrowing the differential diagnoses for underlying malignant etiology. Symptoms such as cough and hemoptysis, breast lump, GI bleeding, any mass in abdomen, abnormal menstrual history and any history of previous malignancy should also be explored with suitable questions.

Physical examination may reveal features of portal hypertension (PHT) due to underlying chronic liver disease (CLD) such as splenomegaly, ascites, caput medusa or spider angiomas. In addition, some benign SOLs and advanced malignancy can lead to palpable hepatomegaly, which may be nodular in multifocal lesions. Also, the associated generalized lymphadenopathy may give an important clue toward lymphoma causing secondary hepatic infiltration. Complete physical examination including supraclavicular node, abdomen and chest, and per rectal examination should be carried out in each case. Per-vaginal examination is done as necessary.

LABORATORY TESTS

The findings of laboratory tests will be complementary to the history and physical examination. It may reveal raised bilirubin levels, active hepatitis and thrombocytopenia secondary to CLD with PHT or positive serology (in case of liver abscess/hydatid cyst). The role of tumor markers is limited in the differential diagnosis of liver SOLs because of reported low sensitivity in case of small volume disease and also low specificity. But, their raised levels correlate with the tumor burden, including extrahepatic disease and help in prognostication of the outcome. The trend in AFP level is more helpful than one time measurement in early diagnosis of HCC in patient with underlying HBV or HCV related chronic hepatitis. The raised CA 19-9 levels in the absence of cholangitis and/or biliary obstruction can be useful in diagnosis of cholangiocarcinoma. The CEA level is useful for evaluating patients with colorectal cancers. Serum chromogranin A or 24-hour urinary 5-hydroxyindoleacetic acid levels are useful in evaluating patients with neuroendocrine tumors. In addition, raised serum lactate dehydrogenase levels along with generalized lymphadenopathy may suggest liver infiltration by lymphoma.

IMAGING TECHNIQUES

The selection of an appropriate imaging modality for evaluation of liver SOL should be based on the diagnostic accuracy of the test, safety of the patient and the cost effectiveness of the imaging technique. In the various modalities attention is paid to detection, size and multiplicity of the lesion. It is evaluated whether it is cystic or solid. Vascularity pattern is assessed. Whether the lesion is displacing or invading the surrounding liver parenchyma, ductular and vascular structures is also seen. Nature of the baseline liver is also assessed.

Main modalities for assessment of liver SOLs are ultrasound, MRI and CT scan. These are discussed below. Their advantages and disadvantages are summarized in Table 1. In addition, the different imaging features of various benign and malignant liver SOLs are outlined in Table 2.

Ultrasound

Ultrasound abdomen is frequently preferred as the initial imaging modality for the evaluation of the lesions in the liver because of its low cost, wide availability, lack of radiation and the high spatial resolution with inherent tissue contrast. Focal liver masses are better detected than the diffuse hepatic disease. Also, the lesions of 1 cm or more in size can be visualized easily. Important step in predicting the risk of malignancy for a liver SOL is to establish whether or not the lesion is cystic or solid. As it evaluates the masses based on the differential acoustic impedance relative to the surrounding tissues, USG is an excellent modality for defining the lesion as either cystic or solid. Doppler imaging can provide additional information by the flow characteristics of the lesion. The diagnostic appearance of simple cyst on USG consists of smooth wall with echo free contents and absence of impedance to transmission of sound waves (Fig. 1). For small cysts, USG is more accurate than CT. In addition, the hydatid cysts produce a characteristic appearance with the internal daughter cysts (Fig. 2). The most common SOL in liver, a cavernous hemangioma, is usually hyperechoic often with lack of impedance to transmission of sound waves. Such a lesion is frequently less than 3 cm in size. If the lesion is more than 3 cm, the appearance is atypical or the hypervascular metastasis is suspected, further evaluation is needed with contrast imaging for confirmation. The other differential diagnoses for hyperechoic lesion on USG are focal area of fatty degeneration and rarely hepatic adenoma, particularly in case of storage disorder. Both the primary and secondary carcinoma within the liver can produce various appearances on USG, including an isoechoic or hypoechoic pattern depending up on the degree of vascularity and the presence/absence of degenerative

Table 1: Advantages and disadvantages of imaging modalities

Imaging modality	*Advantages*	*Disadvantages*
Ultrasound	• Low cost • Wide availability • Portability • Lack of ionizing radiation • Excellent technique for evaluating the lesion as either cystic or solid • Provide additional information by Doppler imaging • Can detect associated biliary dilatation or gallbladder disease	• Operator dependent • Limited view of field • Poor image quality in case of obesity and deeply seated lesions • Can miss small lesions • May not characterize solid lesions adequately
CT	• Can detect focal lesions ≥1 cm in size, diffuse liver disease and calcification • Provide anatomical details of focal liver lesion • Adequate visualization of adjacent organs and retroperitoneum • Good reproducibility • Suitable for obese patients • Short scanning time with a large area of coverage • Good image quality and multiphasic image acquisition with IV contrast agents • Post-processing formats allow 3D visualization • Reduced motion artifacts	• Lack of portability • Hazards of ionizing radiation • IV contrast agents—nephrotoxicity and sensitivity reactions • Specialized protocol and expert radiologist in case of MDCT • Cannot adequately characterize small lesions <1 cm in size
MRI	• Lack of ionizing radiation • Excellent soft tissue contrast resolution • Accurate detection of fluid containing lesions and biliary radicles • Better characterization of small liver lesions ≤1 cm • Better differentiation of benign versus malignant liver lesions due to various pulse sequences and different hepatobiliary specific contrast agents	• High cost • Lack of wide availability and portability • Long scanning time • Motion artefacts • Not suitable for patients with cardiac pacemakers, ventilated patients and less cooperative patients • Difficult for surgeons to interpret

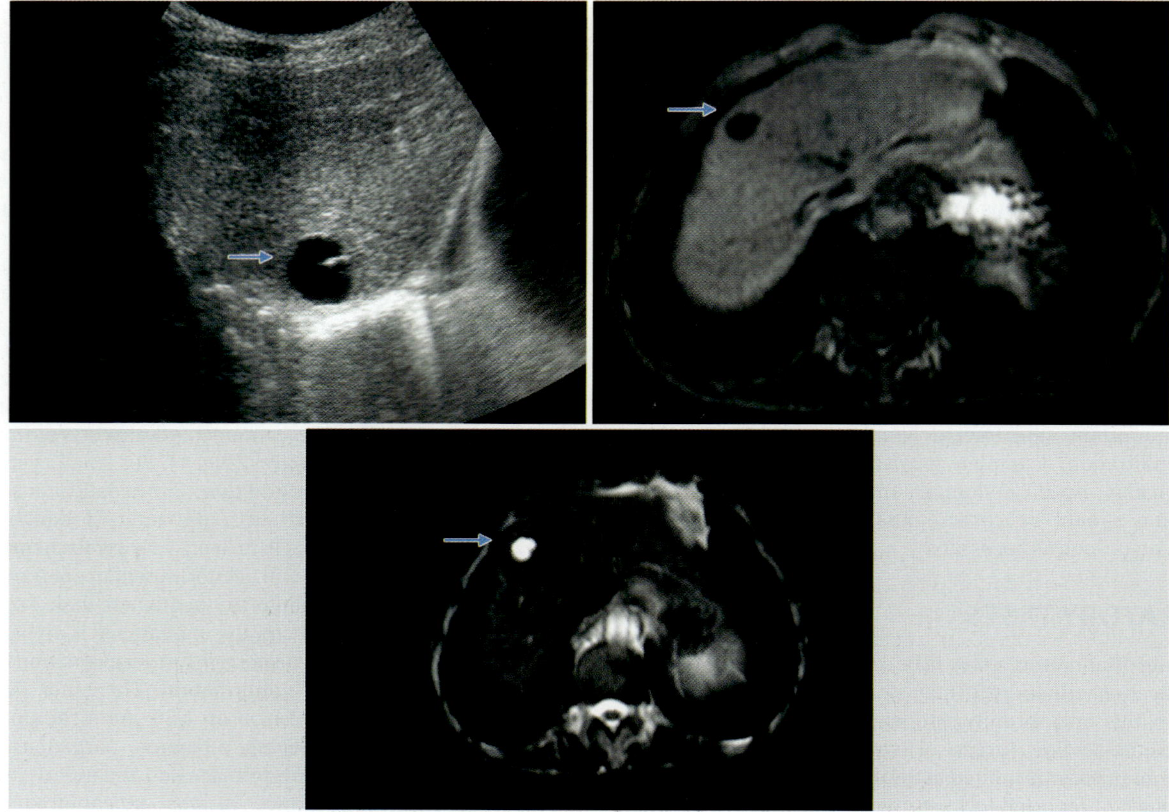

Figure 1 USG, T1W and T2W axial image in a 60-year-old male. USG shows well defined anechoic lesion, seen as hypointense on T1WI and hyperintense on T2WI

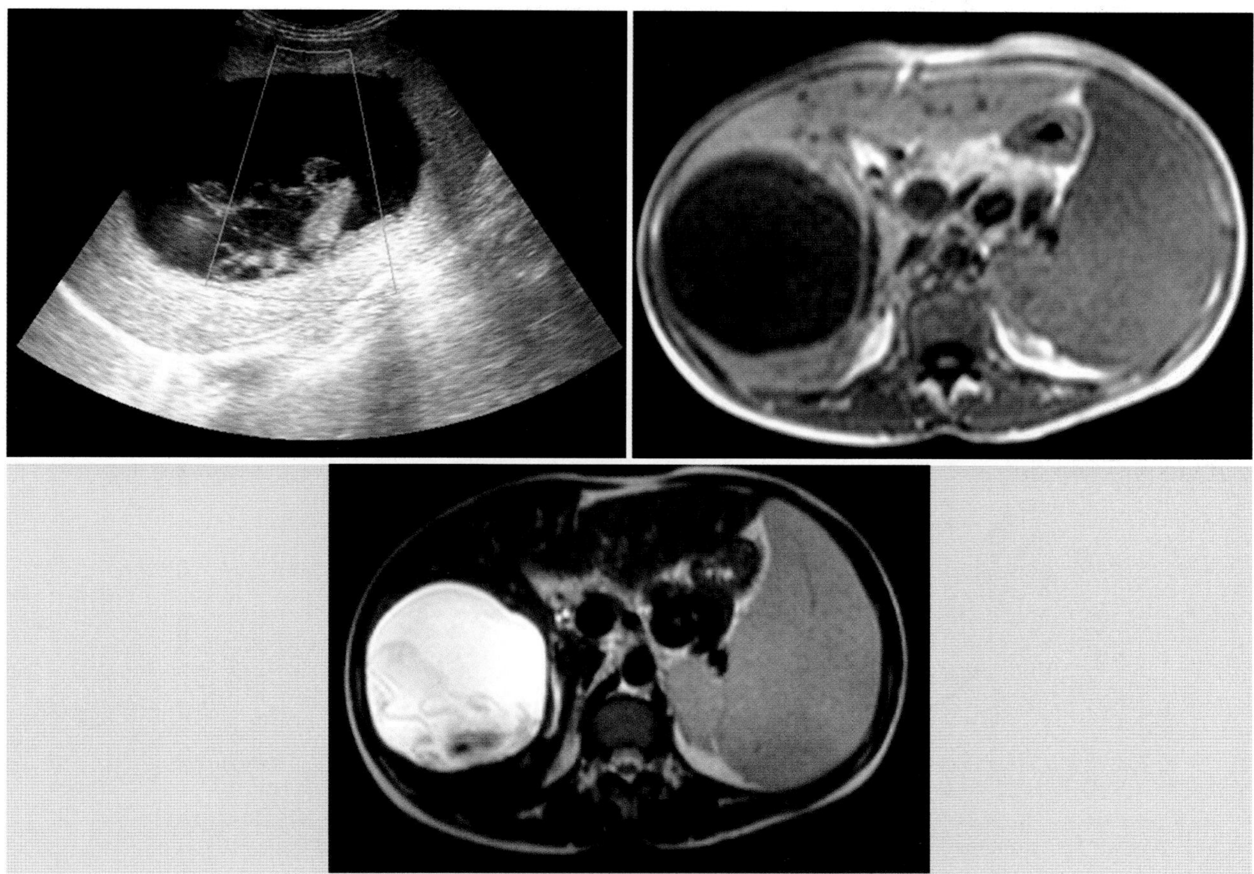

Figure 2 USG, TIWI, T2WI in a 20-year-old female with positive hydatid serology. USG shows anechoic lesion with posterior acoustic enhancement and internal membranes. The lesion is seen as hypointense on T1WI and hyperintense on T2WI with collapsed internal membranes

changes. Necrotic tumors can mimic cysts or abscesses. But, the classical bull's eye appearance is highly suggestive of a metastatic lesion. Similarly, some benign lesions of the liver such as FNH and hepatocellular adenoma may be either isoechoic or hypoechoic on USG. Thus, because of the varied and confusing origin of isoechoic and hypoechoic lesions, further confirmation with contrast imaging technique is needed in majority of hypoechoic and isoechoic lesions. In addition to focal liver lesions, USG can easily detect the associated biliary dilatation, gall bladder disease and some diffuse liver abnormalities such as cirrhosis and fatty liver. As compared to other cross sectional imaging, USG has few important limitations such as restricted view of field, significant image degradation in case of obesity and operator dependency.

Recently, after the invention of microbubble contrast agents, CEUS allows to perform real time dynamic assessment of SOLs of liver in the different phases of hepatic blood flow. The typical enhancement pattern for a given liver lesion on CEUS increases the ability to characterize the different liver masses, allowing definitive diagnosis in most of the patients. Some series has shown the diagnostic reliability of over 80% with CEUS for classifying the focal liver lesions less than 20 mm and even the lesions less than 10 mm. Large studies[9,10] have reported a diagnostic accuracy of over 90% for CEUS in differentiating benign from malignant focal liver lesions. In addition, the prospective multicenter DEGUM Study[9] and also the two recent meta analyses[11,12] have shown that CEUS is equivalent to CT and MRI for the diagnosis of focal lesions in the liver. Also, the EFSUMB recommendations[13] has included the CEUS in the evaluation algorithm for focal liver lesions in cirrhotic patients as well as in non-cirrhotic patients with lesions more than 2 cm in size that develop during a follow-up regimen. The Asian Pacific Association for the Study of the Liver recommendations[14] on HCC validates that the sensitivity of CEUS is similar to that of dynamic CT or MRI in the diagnosis of HCC. But, limitation of the CEUS are lack of display of a complete field, more operator dependency on patient specific factors and need to focus on a single lesion in cases with multiple focal lesions. Also, premature destruction of the microbubbles because of the high mechanical index of the lesion can lead to faulty late phase contrasting. Cysts and calcifications, which lacks contrast enhancement may be wrongly interpreted as malignant infiltration. The degenerative process in large tumors (>5 cm) can lead to perfusion changes and thus the imaging characteristics. In addition, steatosis or CLD decreases the sensitivity of CEUS, while poor signals from the deeply seated lesion can affect the detection of its vascularity.

Table 2: Different imaging features of various benign and malignant liver SOLs

Liver SOL	*Clinical features and laboratory findings*	*USG*	*CT*	*MRI*	*Other features*
Simple cyst	• Usually asymptomatic, but RUQ pain or fullness, if large • May be associated with polycystic kidney disease	• Sharply marginated • Anechoic with posterior acoustic shadowing	• Water attenuated and lacks calcification on non-contrast CT • Do not enhance on contrast CT	• Homogeneous lesions • Hypointense on T1-weighted images • Markedly hyperintense on T2-weighted images • Lack enhancement on contrast MRI	
Biliary cystadenoma	• Middle-aged women • Majority are asymptomatic	• Irregular wall with papillary growths • Internal septations forming loculi	• Heterogeneous on non-contrast CT • Thickened irregular wall with intra-mural nodules and rarely calcifications • Enhancing internal septae and mural nodules on contrast enhanced CT	• May appear heterogeneous • T1: Hypointense • T2: Hyperintense • Absence of biliary communication on MRCP	
Hydatid cyst	• Positive serological result and clinical history	• May appear similar to SHC • Progress to develop daughter cysts in periphery, thick and calcified walls, hyperechoic/hypoechoic contents	• Hypodense lesion • Calcified walls, septae, daughter cysts in the periphery • Enhancing hypervascular pericyst	• T1: Hypointense • T2: Hyperintense • Surrounding hypointense rim on T2-weighted images • Daughter cysts in the periphery • Membranes seen as floating linear structures	
Bile duct hamartoma (von Meyenburg complexes)	• Usually asymptomatic	• Hypoechoic or anechoic small nodules <1.5 cm in size with distal acoustic enhancement • Sometimes small hyperechoic cystic lesions with comet-tail echoes may also be seen	• Multiple hypoattenuating lesions, typically <1.5 cm in size and irregular outlined • Lack contrast enhancement	• Multiple hypointense lesions on T1-weighted images • Strongly hyperintense lesions on T2-weighted images • Lack biliary communication on MRCP	
Abscess	• Older age group • Associated with underlying hepatobiliary or GI pathology, diabetes mellitus • Fever, sepsis	• In early stage hyperechoic without distinct margins • Hypoechoic space occupying lesion with formation of pus	• In acute stage: clustering of small hypodense lesions • Chronic stage: thick wall lesion with homogeneous hypodensity • On contrast CT: double target sign: perilesional edema with enhancing peripheral rim	• Homogeneous low signal intensity on T1-weighted MR images • Homogeneous hyperintensity on T2-weighted images • Contrast MRI: similar CT	

Contd...

Contd...

Liver SOL	*Clinical features and laboratory findings*	*USG*	*CT*	*MRI*	*Other features*
Hemangioma	• Females (20–50 years) • Usually asymptomatic • Rarely thrombocytopenia in few cases	• Homogeneous, hyperechoic, smooth outline, absence of halo sign • On Doppler: low flow	• Noncontrast CT: hypoattenuating • Contrast CT: <2 cm—homogeneously enhancing on arterial and portal venous phase imaging and >2 cm—peripheral nodular enhancement on arterial phase images with centripetal filling in the delayed phase	• Sharply marginated and homogeneous • Typically hypointense on T1-weighted images • Markedly hyperintense on T2-weighted images • Contrast MRI: enhancement similar to that seen in CT	• Technetium-99m-labeled red blood scintigraphy: highly specific for hemangioma >1.5 cm
FNH	• Females (30–40 years) • Usually asymptomatic • Remain stable in size	• Homogeneous isoechoic or hypoechoic • Central hyperchoic area with arterial signals on Doppler study	• Non-contrast CT: hypodense or isodense and central hypodense scar (rarely calcified) • Contrast CT: homogeneous enhancement on the arterial phase, isodense on portal venous phase and hyperdense scar on delayed phase	• Typically isointense on T1-weighted images • Isointense to slightly hyperintense on T2-weighted images • Central scar: hypointense on T1 and markedly hyperintense on T2-weighted scans • Contrast MRI: enhancement similar to that seen in CT	• Hyperintense or isointense on hepatobiliary phase MRI with liver-specific contrast • Hot spot on Technetium-99m sulfur colloid nuclear scan
Hepatic adenoma	• Young adult women • Strongly associated with prolonged oral contraceptive use	• Heteroechoic • Hyperechoic if steatotic but anechoic center if hemorrhage or necrosis	• Lacks central scar • Non-contrast CT: hypoattenuating due to the presence of intracellular lipid, old hemorrhage or necrosis, or may be hyperattenuating due to recent hemorrhage or large amounts of glycogen; and large adenomas may be heterogeneous • Contrast CT: homogeneous enhancement on arterial phase (less than FNH) and isodense on venous phase	• Hyperintense on T1 and isointense or hyperintense on T2-weighted images • Loss of signal on out of phase T1-weighted images	• Hypointense on hepatobiliary phase MRI with liver-specific contrast
Nodular regenerative hyperplasia	• Rarely symptomatic • Associated with immunological and hematological disorders, cardiac and pulmonary disorders, several drugs and toxins, neoplasias, and organ transplantation	• Normal liver with multiple isoechoic or hyperechoic nodules	• Nonenhancing sub-centimetre nodules, sometimes hypodense	• Hyperintese on T1-weighted images • Variable intensity on T2-weighted images	• Definitive diagnosis is made by biopsy only

Contd...

Contd…

Liver SOL	*Clinical features and laboratory findings*	*USG*	*CT*	*MRI*	*Other features*
HCC	• Suspected if cirrhosis or chronic viral hepatitis are present • Other risk factors such as hemochromatosis, autoimmune hepatitis or Wilson's disease • Positive viral serology • Raised AFP levels	• Small HCC <3 cm often hypoechoic, but may be hyperechoic if there is fatty change • Tumor >3 cm: mosaic or mixed pattern	• On non-contrast CT: hypodense due to necrosis and/or fat • On contrast CT: robust enhancement in arterial phase, wash out in portal venous phase and relatively hypodense in delayed phase	• Variable intensity on T1-weighted images • Hyperintense on T2-weighted images • Contrast MRI: enhancement pattern similar to CT	
Fibrolamellar HCC	• Adults younger than 40 years • No predisposing risk factors • Normal AFP levels	• Well-defined mass with lobulated margins and mixed echogenicity • Central scar: central area of hyperechogenicity	• On non-contrast CT: hypodense mass and coarse calcifications within central scar • On contrast CT: heterogeneous arterial phase enhancement, variable enhancement pattern in portal venous phase and delayed phase, and central scar lacks enhancement	• Hypointense to isointense on T1-weighted images • Slightly hyperintense on T2-weighted sequences • Central scar: hypointense on T1- and T2-weighted images • Contrast MRI: enhancement pattern similar to CT	
Intrahepatic cholangiocarcinoma	• Elderly male patient • History of PSC or the associated disease such as ulcerative colitis, Caroli's syndrome, liver fluke infestation and hepaticolithiasis • Exposure to chemical agents such as vinyl chloride • Raised CA 19-9 levels	• Hypoechoic mass lesion • May be associated with segmental or lobar biliary ductal	• Non-contrast CT: heterogenous mass lesion with sub-capsular retraction and segmental or lobar biliary ductal dilation • Contrast CT: peripheral rim enhancement in arterial phase, progressive non-globular central enhancement in portal venous phase and central pooling of the contrast in delayed phase; presence of satellite nodules and vascular encasement	• Isointense to hypointense on T1-weighted images • Hyperintense on T2-weighted images and associated segmental or lobar biliary ductal dilation • Contrast MRI: enhancement pattern similar to CT	

Contd…

Contd…

Liver SOL	*Clinical features and laboratory findings*	*USG*	*CT*	*MRI*	*Other features*
Metastasis	• History of extrahepatic malignancy • Elevated CEA levels if colorectal • Elevated chromogranin or urinary 5-HIAA levels if neuroendocrine	• Hypoechoic lesions on USG	• Hypodense on non-contrast CT • Contrast CT: weak peripheral heterogeneous rim like enhancement in arterial phase (homogeneous enhancement in case of hypervascular metastasis), hypodense in portal venous phase (peripheral wash out, i.e. hypointense rim in case of hypervascular metastasis) and hypodense on delayed phase	• Hypointense on T1-weighted images • Hyperintense on T2-weighted images • Signal loss on heavily T2-weighted images • Contrast MRI: enhancement pattern similar to CT	
Hepatic epithelioid hemangioendothelioma	• Occurs in young females • Possible association with oral contraceptives • Non-specific symptoms and laboratory profiles • >85% of patients have multifocal bilobar lesions	• Variable pattern of echogenicity	• On plane CT: multiple irregular hypodense nodules, predominant subcapsular location, coalescence of nodules forming confluent masses tumor calcification in 20% of cases • Contrast CT: minimal enhancement in arterial phase, rim-like enhancement in portal venous phase and gradual centripetal fill in enhancement in delayed phase	• Low signal intensity on T1-weighted MR images • Homogeneous or target shaped high signal intensity on T2-weighted MR images	• Homogeneous or target shaped low signal intensity on hepatobiliary phase MRI with liver-specific contrast
Hepatic angiosarcoma	• Elderly male patients • History of exposure to Thorotrast, vinyl chloride, arsenic, androgenic steroids such as methyltestosterone as well as long-term use of oral contraceptives • Can present as multiple lesions or a solitary large mass	• Inhomogeneous echogenicity • Small lesions appear isoechoic and well-defined • Large lesions appear hypoechoic ill-defined	• On plane CT: hypodense lesion • Contrast CT: peripheral irregular enhancement in arterial phase, centripetal filling of contrast agent in the portal phase and complete wash out in delayed phase (black hole sign) • Some cases may have a diffuse "flash-fill", a "reverse hemangioma" enhancement pattern or mixture of centripetal and centrifugal enhancement patterns	• Hypointense on T1-weighted images • Hyperintense on T2-weighted images • Contrast MRI: enhancement pattern similar to CT	

Computed Tomography

CT can easily detect a liver SOL of 1 cm or more in size and also the diffuse liver disease. Nowadays, CT is commonly used for the preoperative diagnosis, staging, treatment planning and follow-up of patients with suspected hepatic neoplasms. Many studies on CT has reported high sensitivity (65–93%) and specificity (75–90%) for detecting primary and metastatic hepatic neoplasms.[15,16] The advantage of CT over USG is to provide anatomical details of the focal liver lesion including its segmental position and relationship to vessels and, with IV cholangiography contrast medias, the biliary radicles. Also, it gives good visualization of the adjacent organs and the retroperitoneum. As compared to USG, it is more reproducible and better suited for obese patients. After the introduction of MDCT it is possible to acquire large anatomical volumes in a short scanning time with thin sections without any increased radiation dose. It has high special as well as temporal resolution. In addition, it has led to multiphasic image acquisition after intravenous contrast administration, decreased motion artefacts, and the ability to generate high resolution 2D and 3D image reformations in any desired plane. Also, in a single examination it provides detailed information on the number, size, distribution and vascularity of the liver lesions, which plays vital role in clinical decision-making and planning the treatment. Most of the liver tumors are best visualized in the hepatic venous phase, because of their predominant arterial supply, causing maximum attenuation difference between the enhancing liver parenchyma (fed by portal vein) and hypoattenuating liver masses. The non-contrast phase can allow the characterization of hepatic lesion which are having attenuation higher (iron, glycogen, calcification or hemorrhage) or lower (edema, fat or necrosis) than hepatic parenchyma. Also, due to higher water content, the neoplastic masses are usually hypoattenuating during unenhanced phase compared to normal bright liver parenchyma. The hepatic arterial phase acquisition is crucial for certain liver tumors such as FNH, hepatocellular adenoma, HCC, and hypervascular liver metastases; which receive substantial arterial supply. In the hepatic arterial phase, these tumors are detected as hyperattenuating lesions relative to the poorly enhanced adjacent liver parenchyma. But they may be obscured during hepatic venous phase due to progressive hepatic enhancement from the portal vein. The lesion needs to be differentiated from vascular lesions such as aneurysms/pseudoaneurysms and arterioportal shunts. In addition, the delayed phase is acquired about 3–10 minutes following the initiation of contrast injection. The key role of delayed phase is in the diagnosis of liver masses with either predominant component of fibrosis such as cholangiocarcioma or hepatic masses containing central scar or effect of blood pooling such as cavernous hemangioma (Fig. 3). During the delayed phase, these lesions show prolonged contrast enhancement relative to the surrounding liver parenchyma.

When fatty infiltration occurs focally, differentiating it from metastases and other lesions may be challenging. As it does not cause fat density lesion, the absolute attenuation values on CT are not reliable indicators. However, there are several diagnostic features that help in differentiation such as their location adjacent to gall bladder fossa and falciform ligament near segments II, III and IV, absence of local mass effect or contour abnormalities and normal course of vessels through the fatty area. These lesions may show improvement on follow-up imaging. Similarly, alterations of the dual vascular supply of the liver can cause parenchymal perfusion disorders such as "transient hepatic attenuation differences" (THAD), THAD corresponds to focal increase in arterial flow when the portal venous flow decreases. Thus, focal areas of liver parenchymal enhancement occur during the arterial phase of contrast enhanced CT. These perfusion disorders may be mistaken for other "flash filling" lesions such as hemangiomas, adenomas, HCC, hypervascular metastases or arterioportal shunts (Fig. 3). Both malignant and benign liver lesions produce THADs through surrounding parenchymal perfusion due to increase in primary arterial flow (siphoning effect) (causing multisegmental THAD), by compression/infiltration/thrombosis of a portal venous branch resulting in decreased portal blood flow (causing wedge shaped THAD) or by arterioportal shunting resulting in flow diversion. However, THAD can also be seen in the absence of a mass lesion due to thrombosis of portal venous branch, anomalous arterial blood supply, arterioportal shunts (congenital

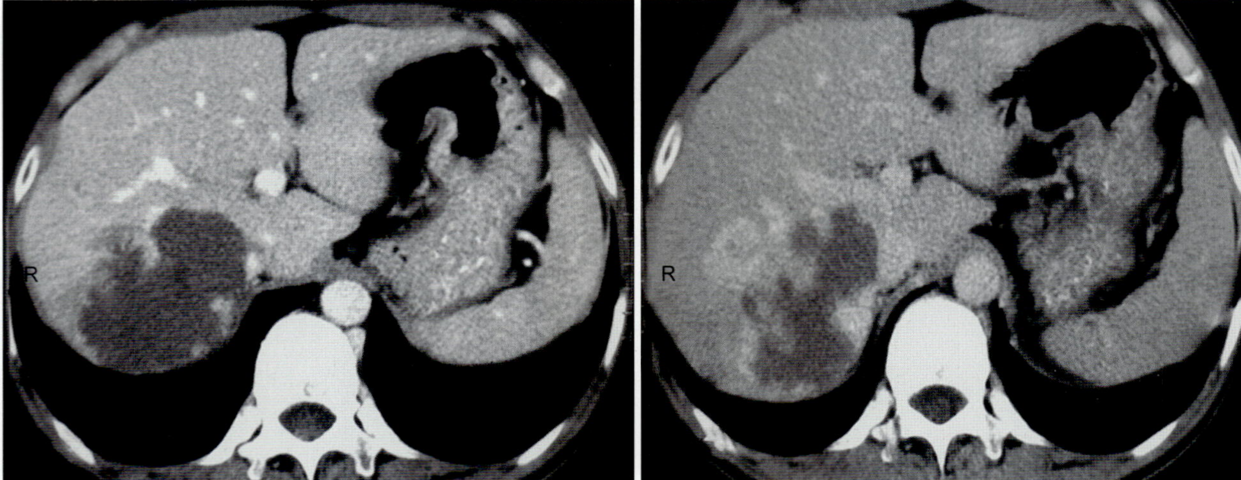

Figure 3 Peripheral nodular enhancement with gradually increasing centripetal filling suggestive of hemangioma

or traumatic), collateral vessels in superior vena cava obstruction, cholecystitis or pancreatitis. Sometimes right sided heart failure, Budd-Chiari syndrome and long standing biliary obstruction can result in diffuse THADs due to abnormal attenuation near the portal triads.

The drawbacks of CT are lack of portability, radiation exposure and contrast induced nephropathy. The important limitation of the CT is that it may not adequately characterize liver lesions less than 1 cm in size because of a partial volume effect. In addition CT protocol requires optimization of several factors including iodine concentration and volume, timing and injection rate of contrast administration and also the scanning delay following the start of contrast injection. The rapid initial contrast enhancement may be missed as a result of predetermined scan delay. Also, sometimes erroneous diagnoses may be made on the basis of hepatic venous phase enhancement patterns due to diffusion of the contrast medium into interstitium and later slow wash out.

Magnetic Resonance Imaging

Recently some authors have advocated MRI as the modality of choice for noninvasive evaluation of liver SOL because of the wide spread use of rapid imaging sequences, allowing breath-hold imaging of liver in less than 20 seconds and also marked reduction in the cost per test.[17,18] The advantages of MRI over CT include better soft tissue contrast resolution, higher sensitivity to contrast agents based on the gadolinium and perfect visualization of fluid containing structures such as cystic lesions and biliary tree. It is superior to CT in characterizing small liver lesions and also differentiating benign versus malignant liver lesions with diagnostic reliability of over 90%. Because of the lack of ionizing radiation, it preferred in children and young adults and in patients requiring follow-up imaging The MRI depicts the nature of tissue based upon the density of hydrogen protons and hence the water content. Similar to CT, it also delineates the architecture of lesion, its degree of heterogeneity and its relationship to vascular and biliary structures. The MRI protocol for liver examination consists of pulse sequences which evaluate T1 and T2 contrast appearances of the different tissues and the additional multiphasic dynamic imaging similar to MDCT after IV administration of contrast agents.[19] There are three categories of contrast agents:

1. *Extracellular fluid agents:* These are most commonly used and are gadolinium based. They depend upon differential blood flow for characterization of the lesion. In addition, they shorten the T1 relaxation time, leading to increased signal intensity on T1-weighted images. These agents are usually nephrotoxic at high doses.
2. *Hepatobiliary specific agents:* These are also gadolinium based and their uptake by hepatocytes allows delayed imaging which does not need to be accurately timed. Also, bile ducts are visualized on delayed imaging as result of varying degree of biliary excretion of these agents. The benefit of these agents is the ability to differentiate hepatic adenoma from FNH and also they are useful in diagnosis of HCC and metastasis. But it is important to note that even with these agents it may not be possible to differentiate benign lesions from well differentiated HCC.
3. *Reticuloendothelial agents:* Superparamagnetic iron oxide particles are currently used reticuloendothelial agents. Kupffer cells within the normal liver parenchyma phagocytose these particles, resulting in T2 signal loss. So normal liver tissue appears as low signal on T2-weighted images as compared to hepatic tumors, which usually lack Kupffer cells. But, currently these agents are not widely used because of their high cost and intolerance by the patients.

The fat sensitive chemical shift gradient-echo imaging sequence with in-phase and opposed phase acquisitions helps in differentiating focal fat deposition or focal fat sparing. It also helps in detection of fat containing benign and malignant focal liver lesions and the lesions on the background of diffuse fatty infiltration.[20] Recently, the emerging tool for the investigation of liver SOL is diffusion weighted MRI. On diffusion weighted MRI, malignant lesions appear brighter as they show restricted diffusion. But, restricted diffusion alone is not specific for malignancy. When combined with contrast enhanced MRI, it increases accuracy for detection of malignant liver lesions. Although MRI is safe, its use is limited in patients with cardiac pacemakers, ventilated patients and less cooperative patients; and unlike CT, MRI is not good for detection of calcification.

On T1-weighted images the benign liver lesions, e.g. cysts (Fig. 1), hemangiomas and majority of the metastases, are hypointense compared to liver, while on T2-weighted images both the lesions are hyperintense to spleen. On heavily T2-weighted sequences cysts and hemangiomas remain hyperintense, but metastatic lesion show signal loss. But it is important to note that mucinous adenocarcinoma can retain hyperintensity on heavily T2-weighted images due to presence of low viscosity mucin with high water content. The common focal hepatocellular lesion such as FNH, hepatic adenoma, focal steatosis and HCC are usually isointense to hyperintense relative to liver on T1-weighted sequences. FNH contains central scar which is hyperintense relative to liver on T2-weighted images and also shows delayed enhancement after administration of gadolinium, while scar in the fibrolamellar HCC remains hypointense on T2-weighted image and lacks delayed enhancement (Fig. 4). Unlike FNH, hepatic adenoma does not have central scar and surrounding liver loses signal intensity on opposed phase imaging due to steatosis. Focal steatosis lose signal intensity on opposed phase imaging, while cyst, hemangiomas and secondaries do not, as they do not contain fat. Unlike focal steatosis, siderotic nodules lose signal intensity on an in-phase imaging compared to corresponding opposed phase image. Majority of the focal liver lesions detected in clinical practice are hyperintense relative to liver on T2-weighted images. Focal liver lesions which show T2 hypointensity include siderotic nodules, necrosis, hemorrhage and intralesional fibrosis. On T2-weighted images, in patients with known cirrhosis or primary malignancy, a focal liver lesion that is isointense to spleen should be considered malignant until proven otherwise.

Suspicious Features of Malignancy on CT or MRI

The infiltrative margins with surrounding liver parenchyma often suggests malignant liver lesion, while benign masses usually have a well-defined parenchymal interface. A malignant focal liver lesion may show either diffuse heterogenous enhancement or an enhancing rim. A hypoattenuating or hypointense halo surrounding the lesion is also highly indicative of malignancy. However, it can be seen with hepatic adenoma. The hypervascular tumors such as HCC and hypervascular secondary frequently show peripheral wash out on delayed images, but it can be found

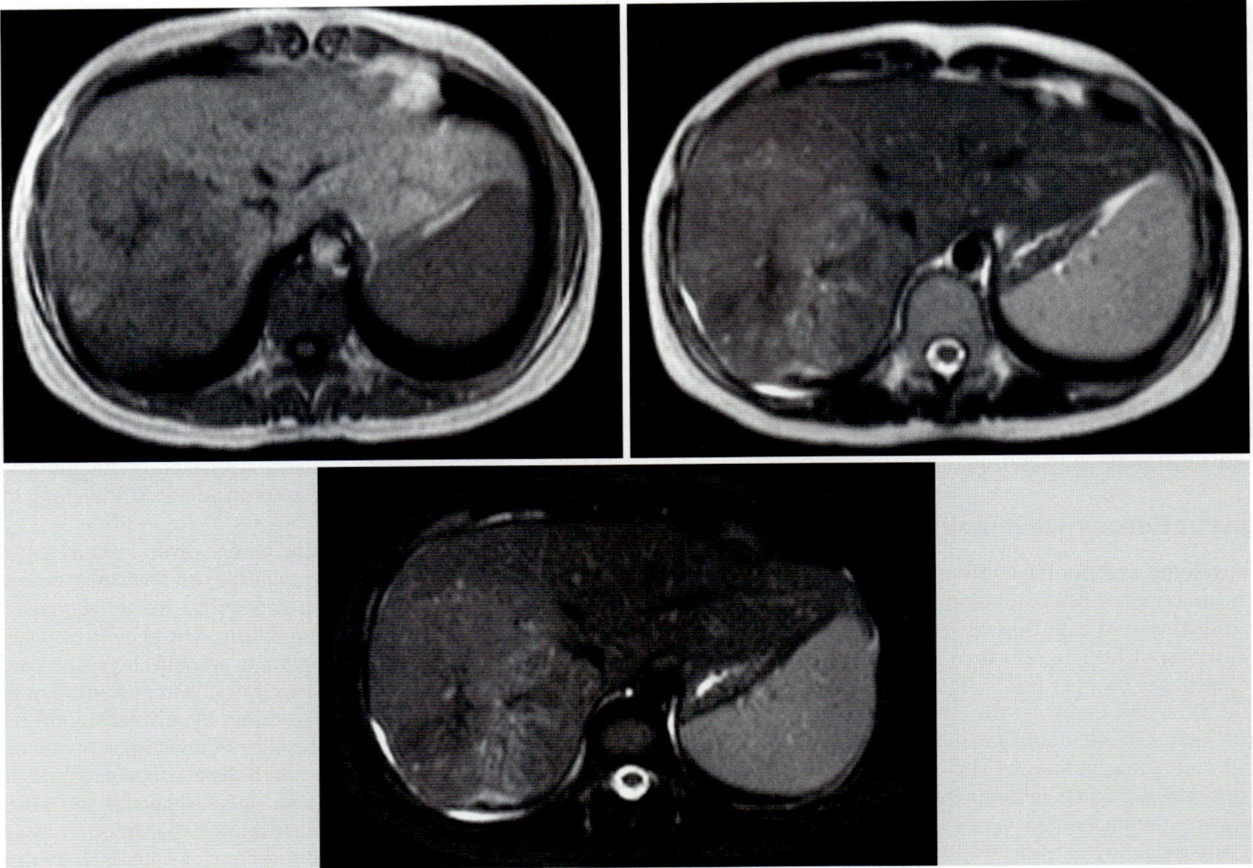

Figure 4 T1W, T2W, T2W fat-sat in a 20-year-old female patient with abdominal pain. Lesion appears hypointense on T1W and hyperintense on T2W and T2W fat-sat with a hypointense scar. Fibrolamellar HCC

in cholangiocarcinoma and other metastases. The presence of vascular invasion is also consistent with a malignant neoplasm and is more commonly found with primary hepatic malignancy than secondary. As compared to malignant liver masses, benign lesions are usually sharply marginated, homogenous, lack enhancement and have low attenuation up to about 20 HU. Also, in a retrospective series of patients of hepatic resection for the suspected malignancy, lesion size less than 4 cm and stability over time correlated well with a benign pathology.[21]

Other Imaging

Although USG, CT or MRI have largely replaced radioisotope scanning, scintigraphy carried out with radiolabeled tracers sometimes helps in delineating the biological nature of the focal liver lesion. Technetium-99m sulfur colloid may aid in the diagnosis of FNH because it detects the Kupffer cells within these lesions. But, the concentration of sulfur colloid may also occur in regenerative nodules, focal hepatic steatosis, and some hepatocellular adenomas. Hepatobiliary scanning with technetium-99m diethyl-iminodiacetic acid can also detect FNH. It appears as a hot spot within the liver on the delayed images due to abnormal biliary drainage, resulting in delayed excretion of the agent. Technetium-99m-labeled red blood scintigraphy can establish the diagnosis of hemangioma as small as 1.5 cm, but CT and MRI are adequate in majority of cases. Similarly, although USG or CT can secure the diagnosis of liver abscess in majority of the patients, gallium scanning plays a role in patients with chronic sepsis of unknown origin, where focal increase in radioactivity may indicate inflammatory collection. In addition scintigraphy performed with radiotracers having affinity for somatostatin receptors may detect unexpected lesions in lymph nodes and in extrahepatic location in patient with suspected focal liver lesions of neuroendocrine origin on cross sectional imaging.

Positron emission tomography (PET) scanning with F-18 FDG identifies carcinomas because of increased glucose utilization in malignant tissue. Also, the biological aggressiveness of tumors can be defined as the poorly differentiated lesions have greater activity than the well-differentiated variety. Thus, it can further characterize the focal liver lesion detected by USG, CT or MRI. However, it is of limited value in specifying the lesions less than 1 cm. In addition, it does not provide anatomical details of the lesion, for which it needs to be supplemented by CT or MRI. In case of malignant liver SOL with unknown primary, body FDG/PET scanning can reveal an index primary malignancy or additional extrahepatic or intrahepatic secondary. A recent meta-analysis has reported a diagnostic performance rate of 37% with FDG-PET in detecting primary tumor.[22,23] FDG/PET has shown a sensitivity and specificity of more than 90% in detecting liver metastases, particularly from colorectal cancers and it can alter the management in up to 40% of the patients.[24,25] But false negative result may occur with small lesions less than 1 cm, necrotic masses originating from cancers with mucinous or neuroendocrine component and some inflammatory lesion particularly the granulomatous ones. Recently, gallium-68 Dotatate PET has been found to be more sensitive in detecting low grade neuroendocrine tumors than F-18 FDG PET.[26] Clinical utility of FDG-PET is still disputed in diagnostic work up of primary liver tumors. FDG/PET has low sensitivity (only 55%) in detecting HCC as compared to that of CT (90%).[27] If the HCC lesion shows FDG uptake, it may be useful for staging, as FDG avid HCCs are often poorly differentiated and more likely to metastasize. In case of cholangiocarcinoma, FDG-PET is good for recognizing intrahepatic cholangiocarcinoma, especially nodular type more than 1 cm in size, but it has low sensitivity in detecting infiltrating variety.[28,29]

IMAGE-GUIDED BIOPSY

Due to improved quality of the imaging methods, the clinical utility of image guided biopsy has decreased over last few years. With combination of clinical history, appropriate biochemical investigations and modern imaging technique, it is possible to characterize a focal liver lesions in over 90% of cases under the right clinical circumstances. The clinical context and imaging characteristics decide whether or not to perform a tissue diagnosis. A tissue diagnosis may be needed before deciding a therapeutic option, if the clinical factors and imaging characteristics are not definitive. It should not be used indiscriminately as it has definite disadvantages.

The diagnostic accuracy of the image guided biopsy depends upon many factors and even under optimal conditions, it is only up to 90%.[30,31] In case of small liver lesions, there is about 10% false negative rate due to difficulty in targeting the lesion. In addition, with benign lesions, there is a significant risk of false positive malignant diagnoses.[32] Few authors have reported discordance rate of 34–40% between the histologies of biopsy and surgical preparation.[33] As image guided biopsy is associated with non-negligible risk (<2%) of needle track tumor seeding, it should be avoided in potentially resectable or transplantable primary or metastatic hepatic malignancy if the imaging features are clinically reliable. Also, it has morbidity of 0.5% and a mortality of 0.05%.[33] Although image guided biopsy appears to be safe, even such a small risk of morbidity and mortality is not acceptable if it does not alter the diagnosis or management. Biopsy is still relevant however for the differential diagnosis of malignant liver lesions, especially before a palliative chemotherapy for inoperable or technically unresectable cancer.

DIAGNOSTIC APPROACH

Ultrasonography of abdomen is the preferred initial imaging modality for the study of liver SOL because of the wide availability, low cost and high safety profile. USG alone might be sufficient to diagnose common benign liver lesions such as cysts and hemangiomas with confidence. If the lesion is solid, indeterminate or a complex cyst on USG, it needs further characterization with CT or MRI. CT is preferred over MRI due to its wide availability, lower cost and robustness in uncooperative patients. In addition, CT is easy to perform and interpret with expertise. MRI is usually used as an alternate reference modality when CT fails to reveal a correct diagnosis. However, in children or young adults or patients with renal impairment in whom serial follow-up examination is required, MRI may replace CT because of the lack of hazards of ionizing radiation and intravenous contrast media. If these imaging modalities fail to establish the diagnosis, further evaluation is done with either interval follow-up imaging or confirmatory imaging test such as MRI with liver specific contrast agents. Radionuclide scanning may be used in place of MRI with contrast in patients with renal dysfunction or in centers where facilities of MRI are not available. If the imaging features are diagnostic or highly indicative of malignancy, further plan of action includes initiation of appropriate therapeutic option for cancer or biopsy if histological diagnosis is required. However, if imaging findings are still equivocal, further management options are serial follow-up imaging, biopsy or surgical resection. The choice of the optimal option in a given clinical context is decided by number of factors including age of the patient, general fitness, severity of complaints, presence or absence of risk factors, patient's wishes, cost and availability of equipment, experience of the radiologist and preference of the treating surgeon.

INCIDENTAL LIVER SOL

Incidental liver masses are increasingly recognized because of the wide availabilities and use of advanced imaging modalities. They are detected during evaluation for unrelated clinical problem or cross sectional imaging done for screening purposes. The autopsy studies from the Western population has found benign liver lesions in up to 52% of patients.[34] They are detected in 7.2–33% of patients when investigated by CT.[35,36] The reports from the Asian countries have described 2.3–6.2% prevalence of incidental focal liver lesions on USG screening at a population level.[37,38] After recognition of the incidental liver mass, it is difficult for the treating physician to achieve a balance between the potential risk associated with the lesion and the value of further evaluation and management. The clinician can suggest a safe and effective plan of action based on the careful consideration of patient factors and imaging features. The first step after recognition of incidental liver mass must always be to get a detailed history and physical examination. Factors such as size, number, morphology and existence of liver parenchymal pathology should be considered while evaluating imaging features.

It is important to consider following three clinical scenarios in diagnostic work up patients with incidentally detected focal liver lesions.

1. *Incidental focal liver lesions in healthy patients:* As majority of these lesions tend to be benign, the principal aim of imaging should be to establish a firm diagnosis to circumvent the unnecessary evaluation and management and also to decrease the patient's anxiety. In a study of 64 patients of incidental liver lesions, Little et al. found hemangioma in 50% of patients, FNH in 7/64 patients, adenoma in 5/64 patients and a malignant tumor in 11/64 patients. Malignancy was not detected in any of the lesions less than 3 cm.[39] In majority of the patients, the modern imaging techniques provide a definite diagnosis of benign lesions including cysts, hemangiomas, focal steatosis and FNH. However, in some cases with indeterminate or equivocal imaging findings, a liver biopsy may be needed to elucidate the nature of a liver lesion.

2. *Incidental focal liver lesions in patients with cirrhosis:* The single most important predisposing factor for HCC is the cirrhosis from various etiologies. In a cirrhotic liver, more than 80% of the detected focal liver lesions more than or equal to 2 cm are HCC. Even for lesions less than 20 mm, the proportion rests effectively above 50%.[40] In the DEGUM multicenter studies, HCC constituted 76.6% of focal liver lesions in hepatic cirrhosis patients as opposed to only 6.1% in patients without cirrhosis. The other lesions such as regeneration nodes, metastases, hemangioma and cholangiocellular carcinoma were significantly more infrequent than HCC.[41] Imaging modalities such as CEUS, CT or MRI play a crucial role in the diagnosis of HCC. Arterial enhancement and "wash out" on later phases are the characteristic imaging features that differentiate HCC (Fig. 5) from other benign, cirrhosis-associated nodules such as regenerative nodules and dysplastic nodules (Figs 6 to 8).

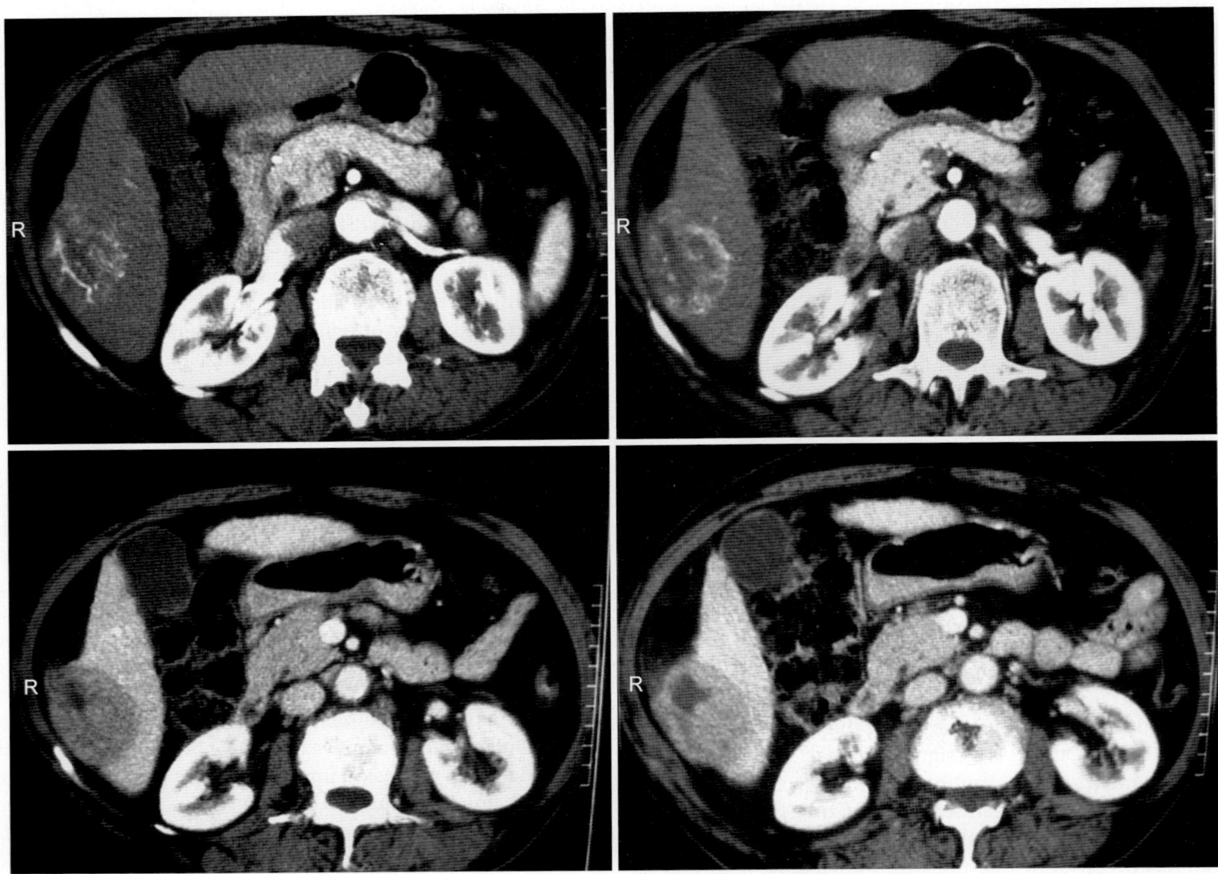

Figure 5 Arterial enhancement and portal phase washout in an HCC

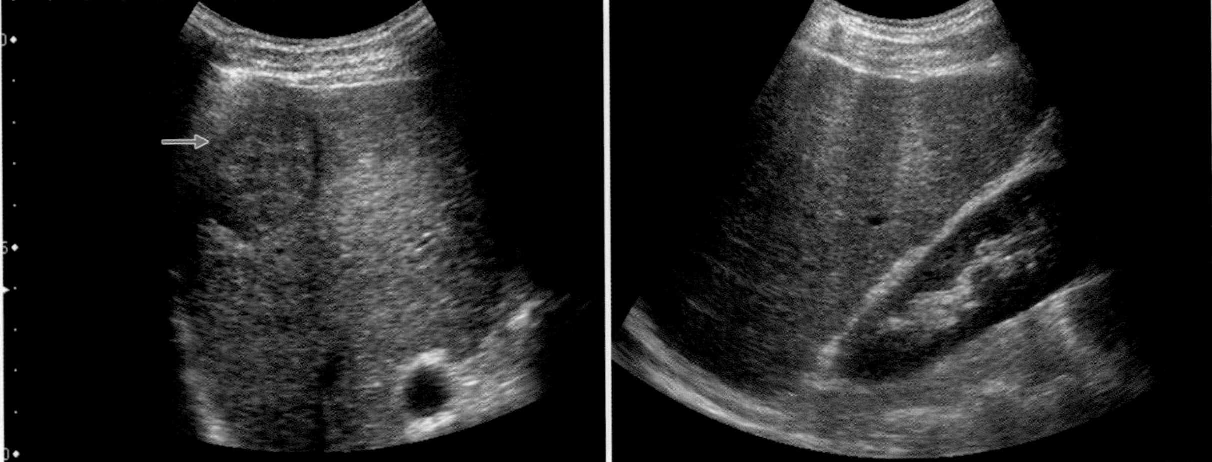

Figure 6 USG in a 67-year-old male shows a hypoechoic mass with a more hypoechoic rim. Note nodularity of hepatic contour

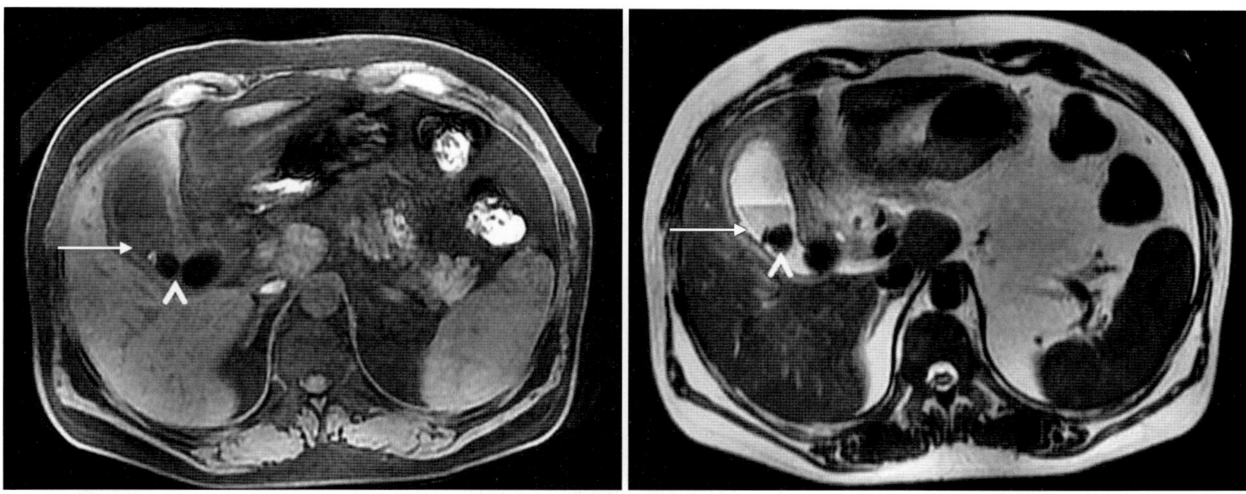

Figure 7 CECT (triple phase) of the same patient (Fig. 6) shows moderate arterial phase enhancement showing washout on delayed phase with liver cirrhosis

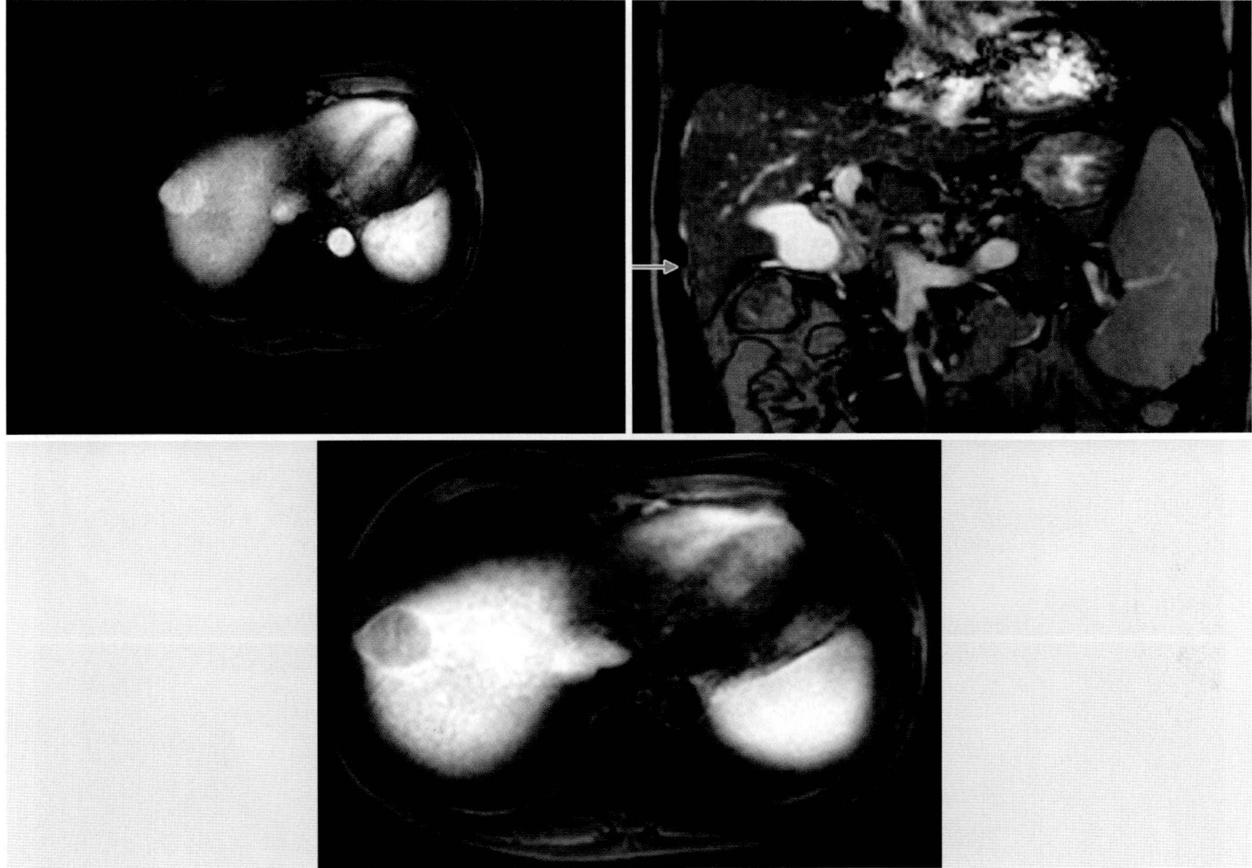

Figure 8 Same case as Figures 6 and 7. Balanced coronal and dynamic MRI in the same patient suggestive of dysplastic nodule in a cirrhotic liver

These imaging features have a high positive predictive value, but a relatively low negative predictive value. Small well differentiated HCCs may be missed during arterial phase as they receive minimal arterial supply. But these lesions tend to remain hypovascular comparative to liver in later phases. The arterioportal shunts and hemangiomas, particularly if less than 2 cm in size, also show similar arterial enhancement like HCC. However, unlike HCC, they show persistent enhancement in the portal venous and/or delayed phase. For HCC, the specificity of CT is superior to MRI (93% vs 82%), but reverse is true as regards to sensitivity (85% to 68%).[42] Overall MRI is considered superior to CT for HCC less than 2 cm the choice depends up on the available expertise, breath hold time and patient's preference. In addition MRI can characterize regenerative nodules and dysplastic nodules. The regenerative nodules are usually less than 1 cm and isointense in both T1-weighted and T2-weighted images, while dysplastic nodules show homogenous hyperintensity on T1-weighted images and hypointensity on T2-weighted images. But, unlike HCC, both lesions are never hyperintense on T2-weighted images and lack arterial enhancement. Biopsy of a lesion or, in case of a small lesion less than 1 cm, imaging follow-up may be considered if imaging findings are equivocal to rule out HCC in a cirrhotic patient.

3. *Incidental focal liver lesions in patient with known primary malignancy:* Metastasis is the most common hepatic malignant neoplasm as liver is a common site of secondary (Figs 9 and 10). In the patients with history of primary malignancy, the

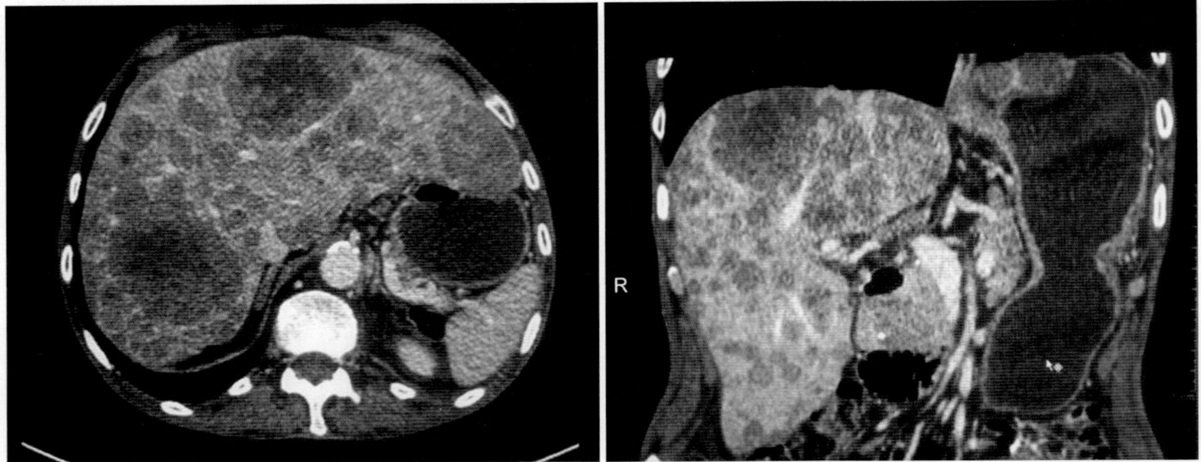

Figure 9 Multifocal hypodense liver metastases

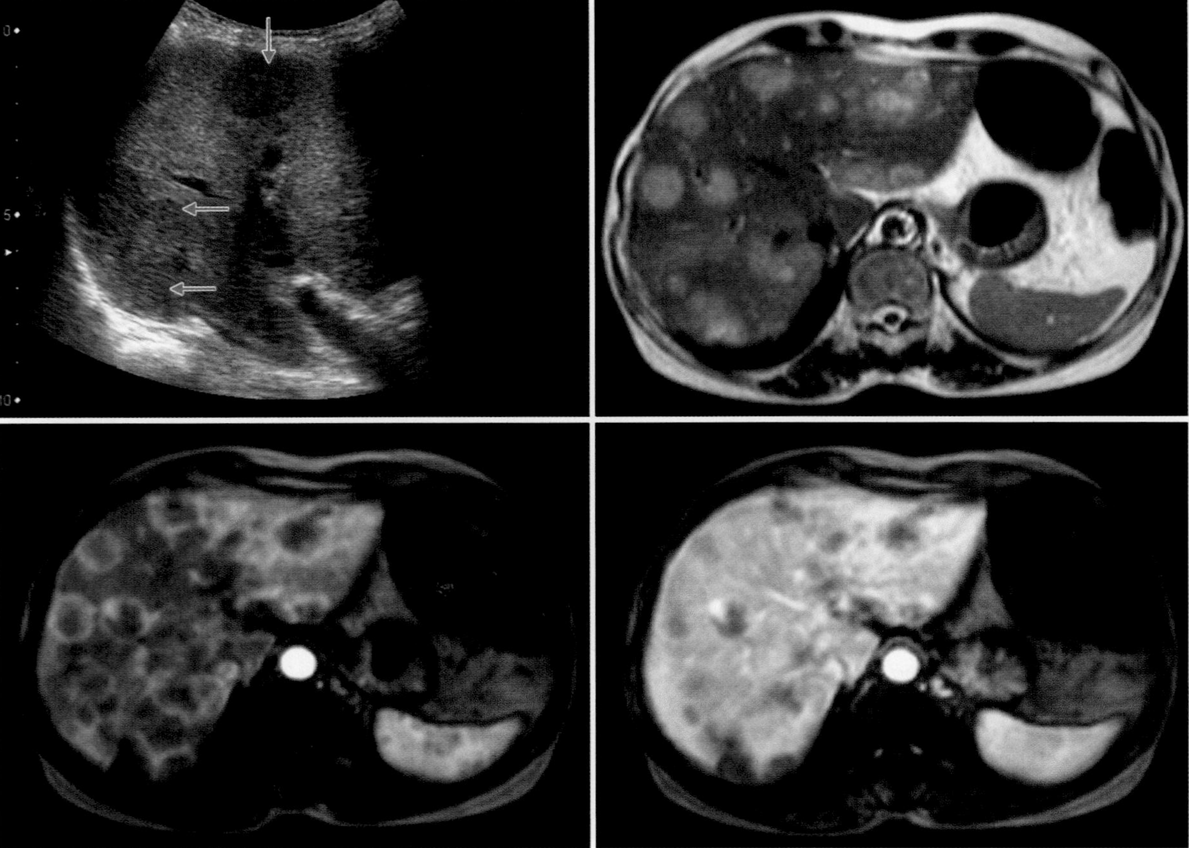

Figure 10 Multiple hypoechoic lesions in a 48-year-old female follow-up case of periampullary carcinoma. T2W axial and arterial and venous phase of Dynamic MRI reveals multiple lesions showing progressive peripheral enhancement

probability of being a metastasis is significantly higher for the focal liver lesion. However, it should be kept in mind that only 50–90% of lesions found on imaging with a maximal diameter of 15 mm are actual secondaries.[43,44] Due to increasing use of thin section acquisition during contrast enhanced CT, the smaller hepatic lesion (<15 mm) are increasingly detected. However, these lesions often create a diagnostic dilemma during work up of these patients as they are difficult to characterize on CT.[43,44] The suspicion of cancer in these "too small to characterize" (TSTC) lesions depends upon the several factors including the number of such lesions and the origin of primary. About 65% of single lesions of size less than 15 mm are benign[43,44] and the likelihood of malignancy increases with increasing number of TSTC lesions.[45] In addition, a large study from MSKCC, TSTC lesions were seen in 12.7% of patients and the most common primary site was breast (22%) followed by colorectal cancers (14%) and lymphoma (4%).[46] Based upon the possible impact on management, these lesions may be evaluated further with either follow-up with close interval imaging or additional imaging such as MRI. As compared to CT, MRI gives auxiliary useful data for characterization of these lesions, e.g. signal intensity based on T2-weighted images, better detection of lesion specific enhancement patterns and also the functional information with the use of liver specific contrast agents.

Recently the American College of Radiologists Incidental Findings Committee (ACRFC) has proposed guidelines for the evaluation and management of incidentally detected hepatic masses on abdominal CT.[47] It depends upon the level of risk for every individual to develop a significant liver lesion and the imaging features of a mass lesion. First, the patients are classified into risk groups depending upon the clinical factors such as age, known primary malignancy, cirrhosis and/or other risk factors. Secondly, the lesions are stratified based on the size—large (>1.5 cm diameter), small (between 0.5 cm and 1.5 cm in diameter) or very small (<0.5 cm in diameter). Finally, lesions are characterized radiologically. The lesions may have a benign appearance, be strongly enhancing on arterial phase or may show features that are suspicious for malignancy.

It is very difficult to characterize the lesions less than 5 mm. The risk stratification decides the further management in these patients. ACRFC considers that these very small lesions are more likely to be benign in low and average risk patients and do not need further follow-up or investigation.

The larger lesions more than 15 mm are easy to characterize radiologically. In this group, robustly enhancing lesions with benign imaging characteristics are usually hemangioma, FNH or THAD. However, due to concern of malignancy, the committee recommends follow-up, further evaluation or biopsy in patients with

Flow chart 1 Liver SOL on USG abdomen

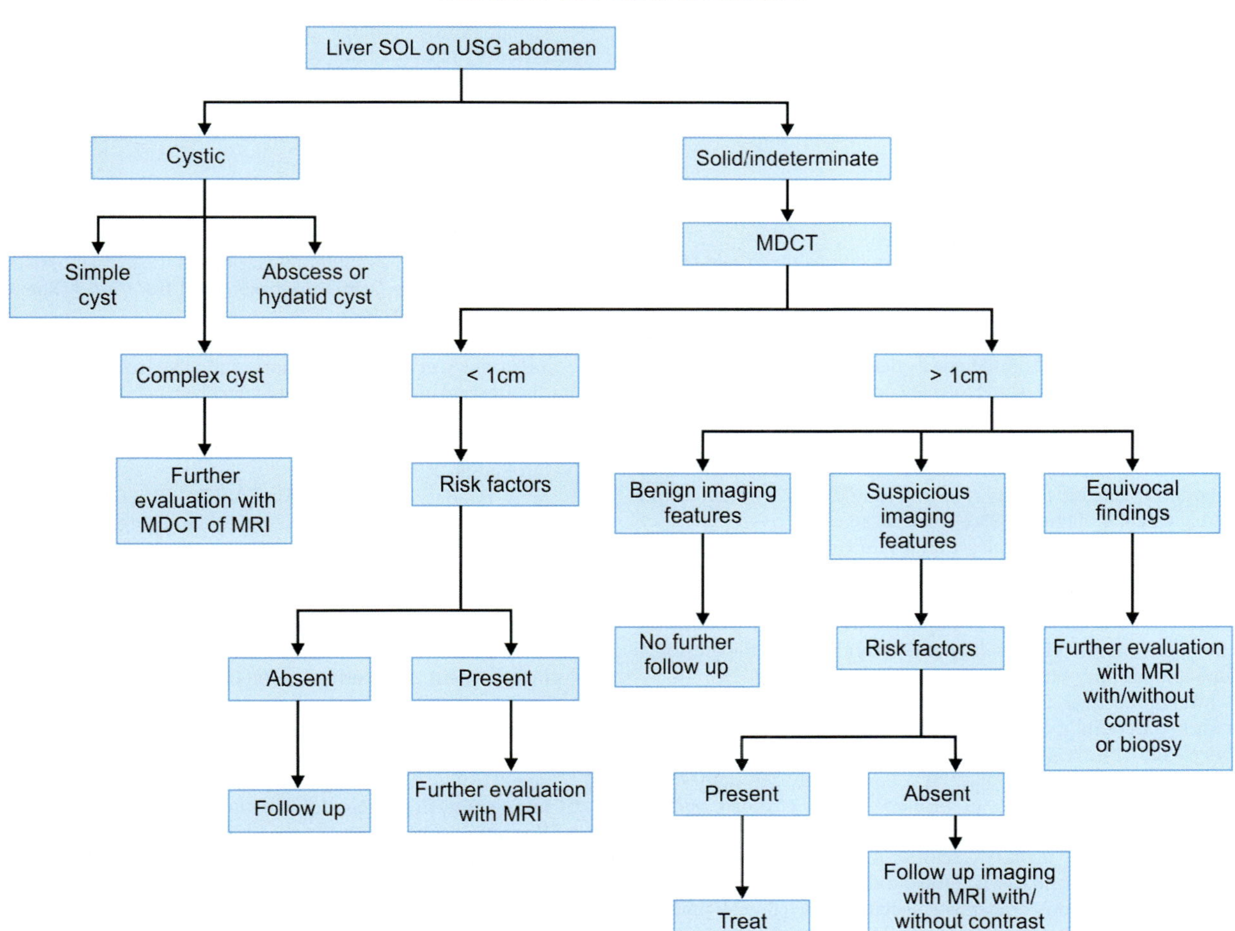

robustly enhancing lesions without benign imaging characteristics. Low attenuation lesions with benign imaging features do not need further follow-up. Management of patients with suspicious imaging features is decided by the risk stratification.

Strongly enhancing lesions between 5 and 15 mm suggest a hepatic hemangioma in a low or average risk patient, but creates the anxiety of a hypervascular malignancy in a high risk patient. If these small lesions lack contrast enhancement, one should look for either benign or suspicious imaging features.

The committee recommends follow-up imaging in high risk patients with either very small lesion or strongly enhancing small lesions and also in all suspicious small lesions. The interval of follow-up imaging is decided by the risk group of patient. It also suggest further evaluation with additional imaging, preferably MRI with contrast or biopsy in strongly enhancing small lesions in high risk patients, large suspicious lesions and strongly enhancing large lesions that lack benign features.

SUGGESTED ALGORITHM FOR EVALUATION OF LIVER SOL

Suggested algorithm for evaluation of liver SOL has been shown in Flow chart 1.

Risk factors: Known primary malignancy, risk factors for HCC/cholangiocarcinoma, raised tumor markers, use of oral contraceptives/anabolic steroids.

ACKNOWLEDGMENTS

Image courtesy: Dr Poonam Narang, Director Professor, GB Pant, New Delhi.

REFERENCES

1. Klatskin G. Hepatic tumors: possible relationship to use of oral contraceptives. Gastroenterology. 1977;73(2):386-94.
2. Creagh TM, Rubin A, Evans DJ. Hepatic tumours induced by anabolic steroids in an athlete. J Clin Pathol. 1988;41(4):441-3.
3. Simonato L, L'Abbe KA, Andersen A, Belli S, Comba P, Engholm G, et al. A collaborative study of cancer incidence and mortality among vinyl chloride workers. Scand J Work Environ Health. 1991;17(3):159-69.
4. Lawrence TS, Robertson JM, Anscher MS, Jirtle RL, Ensminger WD, Fajardo LF. Hepatic toxicity resulting from cancer treatment. Int J Radiat Oncol Biol Phys. 1995;31(5):1237-48.
5. Pawlik TM, Choti MA. Surgical therapy for colorectal metastases to the liver. J Gastrointest Surg. 2007;11(8):1057-77.
6. Yamanaka N, Tanaka T, Tanaka W, Yamanaka J, Yasui C, Kuroda N, et al. Correlation of hepatitis virus serologic status with clinicopathologic features in patients undergoing hepatectomy for hepatocellular carcinoma. Cancer. 1997;79(8):1509-15.
7. Schwartz M. Liver transplantation: the preferred treatment for early hepatocellular carcinoma in the setting of cirrhosis? Ann Surg Oncol. 2007;14(2): 548-52.
8. Jones DE, Metcalf JV, Collier JD, Bassendine MF, James OF. Hepatocellular carcinoma in primary biliary cirrhosis and its impact on outcomes. Hepatology. 1997;26(5):1138-42.
9. Strobel D, Seitz K, Blank W, Schuler A, Dietrich C, von Herbay A, et al. Contrast-enhanced ultrasound for the characterization of focal liver lesions—diagnostic accuracy in clinical practice (DEGUM multicenter trial). Ultraschall Med. 2008;29:499-505.
10. Trillaud H, Bruel JM, Valette PJ, Vilgrain V, Schmutz G, Oyen R, et al. Characterization of focal liver lesions with SonoVue-enhanced sonography: international multicenter-study in comparison to CT and MRI. World J Gastroenterol. 2009;15:3748-56.
11. Guang Y, Xie L, Ding H, Cai A, Huang Y. Diagnosis value of focal liver lesions with SonoVue®-enhanced ultrasound compared with contrast-enhanced computed tomography and contrast-enhanced MRI: a meta-analysis. J Cancer Res Clin Oncol. 2011; 137:1595-605.
12. Xie L, Guang Y, Ding H, Cai A, Huang Y. Diagnostic value of contrast-enhanced ultrasound, computed tomography and magnetic resonance imaging for focal liver lesions: a meta-analysis. Ultrasound Med Biol. 2011;37:854-61.
13. Claudon M, Cosgrove D, Albrecht T, Bolondi L, Bosio M, Calliada F, et al. Guidelines and good clinical practice recommendations for contrast enhanced ultrasound (CEUS)—update 2008. Ultraschall Med. 2008;29:28-44.
14. Omata M, Lesmana LA, Tateishi R, Chen PJ, Lin SM, Yoshida H, et al. Asian Pacific Association for the Study of the Liver consensus recommendations on hepatocellular carcinoma. Hepatol Int. 2010;4:439-74.
15. Matsuo M, Kanematsu M, Inaba Y, Matsueda K, Yamagami T, Kondo H, et al. Pre-operative detection of malignant hepatic tumours: value of combined helical CT during arterial portography and biphasic CT during hepatic arteriography. Clin Radiol. 2001;56(2):138-45.
16. Kehagias D, Metafa A, Hatziioannou A, Mourikis D, Vourtsi A, Prahalias A, et al. Comparison of CT, MRI and CT during arterial portography in the detection of malignant hepatic lesion. Hepatogastroenterology. 2000;47(35):1399-403.
17. Kwee TC, Basu S, Cheng G, Alavi A. FDG PET/CT in carcinoma of unknown primary. Eur J Nucl Med Mol Imaging. 2010;37:635Y644.
18. Neto JA, Elazzazzi M, Altun E, Semelka RC. When should abdominal magnetic resonance imaging be used? Clin Gastroenterol Hepatol. 2008;6:610-5.
19. Semelka RC, Martin DR, Balci NC. Magnetic resonance imaging of the liver: how I do it. J Gastroenterol Hepatol. 2006;21:632-7.
20. Basaran C, Karcaaltincaba M, Akata D, Karabulut N, Akinci D, Ozmen M, et al. Fat-containing lesions of the liver: cross-sectional imaging findings with emphasis on MRI. Am J Roentgenol. 2005;184:1103-10.
21. Shimizu S, Takayama T, Kosuge T, Yamamoto J, Shimada K, Yamazaki S, et al. Benign tumors of the liver resected because of a diagnosis of malignancy. Surg Gynecol Obstet. 1992;174(5):403-7.
22. Kwee TC, Kwee RM. Combined FDG-PET/CT for the detection of unknown primary tumors: systematic review and meta-analysis. Eur Radiol. 2009;19:731Y744.
23. Kwee TC, Basu S, Cheng G, Alavi A. FDG PET/CT in carcinoma of unknown primary. Eur J Nucl Med Mol Imaging. 2010;37:635Y644.
24. Orlacchio A, Schillaci O, Fusco N, Broccoli P, Maurici M, Yamgoue M, et al. Role of PET/CT in the detection of liver metastases from colorectal cancer. Radiol Med. 2009;114(4):571-85.
25. Desai DC, Zervos EE, Arnold MW, Burak WE Jr, Mantil J, Martin EW Jr, et al. Positron emission tomography affects surgical management in recurrent colorectal cancer patients. Ann Surg Oncol. 2003;10(1):59-64.
26. Putzer D, Gabriel M, Kendler D, Henninger B, Knoflach M, Kroiss A, et al. Comparison of (68)Ga-DOTA-Tyr(3)-octreotide and (18)F-fluoro-L-dihydroxyphenylalanine positron emission tomography in neuroendocrine tumor patients. Q J Nucl Med Mol Imaging. 2010;54(1):68-75.
27. Khan MA, Combs CS, Brunt EM, Lowe VJ, Wolverson MK, Solomon H, et al. Positron emission tomography scanning in the evaluation of hepatocellular carcinoma. J Hepatol. 2000;32(5): 792-7.

28. Sacks A, Peller PJ, Surasi DS, Chatburn L, Mercier G, Subramaniam RM. Value of PET/CT in the management of primary hepatobiliary tumors, part 2. AJR Am J Roentgenol. 2011;197:W260YW265.
29. Jadvar H, Henderson RW, Conti PS. [F-18]fluorodeoxyglucose positron emission tomography and positron emission tomography: computed tomography in recurrent and metastatic cholangiocarcinoma. J Comput Assist Tomogr. 2007;31:223Y228.
30. Caturelli E, Solmi L, Anti M, Fusilli S, Roselli P, Andriulli A, et al. Ultrasound guided fine needle biopsy of early hepatocellular carcinoma complicating liver cirrhosis: a multicentre study. Gut. 2004;53:1356-62.
31. Wee A. Fine needle aspiration biopsy of hepatocellular carcinoma and hepatocellular nodular lesions: role, controversies and approach to diagnosis. Cytopathology. 2011;22:287-305.
32. Young NA, Mody DR, Davey DD. Misinterpretation of normal cellular elements in fine-needle aspiration biopsy specimens: observations from the College of American Pathologists Interlaboratory Comparison Program in Non-Gynecologic Cytopathology. Arch Pathol Lab Med. 2002;126:670-5.
33. Loss M, Zülke C, Obed A, Stöltzing O, Schlitt HJ. Surgical therapy of benign liver tumors. Chirurg. 2008;79(8):722-8.
34. Karhunen PJ, Penttilä A, Liesto K, Männikkö A, Möttönen M. Benign bile duct tumours, non-parasitic liver cysts and liver damage in males. Journal of Hepatology. 1986;2(1):89-99.
35. Devine AS, Jackson CS, Lyons L, Mason JD. Frequency of incidental findings on computed tomography of trauma patients. West J Emerg Med. 2010;11:24-7.
36. Völk M, Strotzer M, Lenhart M, Techert J, Seitz J, Feuerbach S. Frequency of benign hepatic lesions incidentally detected with contrast-enhanced thin-section portal venous phase spiral CT. Acta Radiol. 2001;42:172-5.
37. Rungsinaporn K, Phaisakamas T. Frequency of abnormalities detected by upper abdominal ultrasound. J Med Assoc Thai. 2008;91:1072-5.
38. Lu SN, Wang LY, Chang WY, Chen CJ, Su WP, Chen SC, et al. Abdominal sonographic screening in a single community. Gaoxiong Yixue Kexue Zazhi. 1990;6:643-6.
39. Little JM, Richardson A, Tait N. Hepatic dystychoma: a five year experience. HPB Surg. 1991;4:291-7.
40. Bruix J, Sherman M. Management of hepatocellular carcinoma: an update. Hepatology. 2011;53:1020-2.
41. Seitz K, Greis C, Schuler A, Bernatik T, Blank W, Dietrich CF, et al. Frequency of tumor entities among liver tumors of unclear etiology initially detected by sonography in the noncirrhotic or cirrhotic livers of 1349 patients. Results of the DEGUM multicenter study. Ultraschall Med. 2011;32:598-603.
42. Colli A, Fraquelli M, Casazza G, Massironi S, Colucci A, Conte D, et al. Accuracy of ultrasonography, spiral CT, magnetic resonance, and alpha-fetoprotein in diagnosing hepatocellular carcinoma: a systematic review. Am J Gastroenterol. 2006;101:513-23.
43. Jones EC, Chezmar JL, Nelson RC, Bernardino ME. The frequency and significance of small (less than or equal to 15 mm) hepatic lesions detected by CT. AJR Am J Roentgenol. 1992;158:535-9.
44. Laghi F, Catalano O, Maresca M, Sandomenico F, Siani A. Indeterminate, subcentimetric focal liver lesions in cancer patients: additional role of contrast-enhanced ultrasound. Ultraschall Med. 2010;31:283-8.
45. Jones EC, Chezmar JL, Nelson RC, Bernardino ME. The frequency and significance of small (less than or equal to 15 mm) hepatic lesions detected by CT. AJR Am J Roentgenol. 1992;158(3):535-9.
46. Schwartz LH, Gandras EJ, Colangelo SM, Ercolani MC, Panicek DM. Prevalence and importance of small hepatic lesions found at CT in patients with cancer. Radiology. 1999;210(1):71-4.
47. Berland LL, Silverman SG, Gore RM, Mayo-Smith WW, Megibow AJ, Yee J, et al. Managing incidental findings on abdominal CT: white paper of the ACR incidental findings committee. J Am Coll Radiol. 2010;7:754-73.

CHAPTER 71

Benign Liver Tumors

Sudeep R Shah

INTRODUCTION

Abdominal imaging modalities have rapidly increased in type resolution and quality. Scans are increasingly ordered for minor symptoms including for routine "health checks". This has led to detection of many solid organ lesions, the vast majority of which are benign. This provides diagnostic and treatment challenges to radiologists and surgeons alike.

Benign liver lesions may be solid or cystic. This chapter focuses on solid lesions as cysts are covered elsewhere.

Key issues that need to be addressed are: is this truly a pathological lesion, is it really benign, establishing an accurate diagnosis, prognostication, weighing the benefits of surgery versus observation for these lesions and accordingly planning treatment or follow-up.

The recent rise in laparoscopic surgery has led to a large number of resections for these lesions, however the need for resection should not be influenced by ease of surgery or rapidity of recovery.

The common benign solid lesions are hemangioma, focal nodular hyperplasia and hepatic adenoma. The major discussion focuses on these lesions.

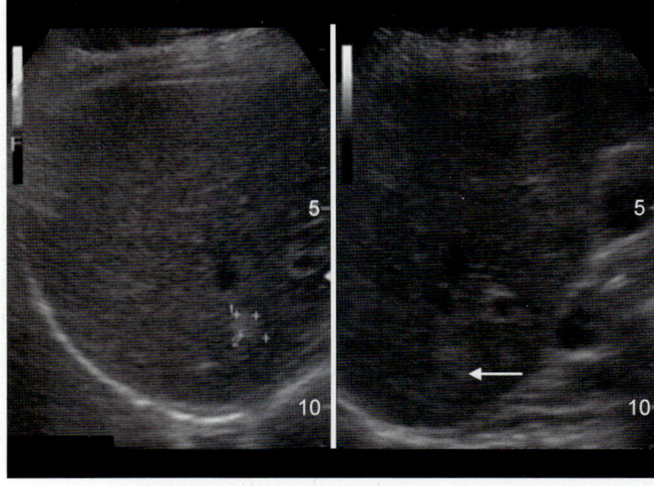

Figure 1 Ultrasonography showing a hyperechoic small liver lesion typical of hemangioma

HEMANGIOMA

Cavernous liver hemangioma is the most common solid lesion seen in all age groups.[1] The prevalence may be as high as 20%. The majority are easy to diagnose. They are characteristically uniform and bright (hyperechoic) on ultrasonography and usually less than 2 cm in size (Fig. 1). Growth is usually imperceptibly slow and these rarely cause symptoms.

Hemangiomas greater than 5 cm are often referred to as giant hemangiomas. In spite of this size, symptoms are rare. Very occasionally, hemangiomas may grow in size to weigh many kilograms and lead to abdominal symptoms owing to their sheer bulk. These need resection for quality of life. Rarely large lesions may present with a chronic disseminated intravascular coagulation like picture with bleeding tendencies and low platelets, this is known as the Kasabach Merritt syndrome. The Blumgart Bornmann Terblanche syndrome presents with fever and abdominal pain. Traumatic rupture is extremely rare and restricted to case reports.[2] Fear of rupture is not an indication for surgery. Iatrogenic injury may be caused by enthusiastic Trucut® biopsy for diagnosis.

Rarely, pain may result from infarction or bleeding within. Occasionally, liver hemangiomas may be multiple, often with similar lesions in other organs. They may be associated with hereditary hemorrhagic telangiectasis, the Osler Weber Rendau Syndrome.

Though estrogen receptors have been demonstrated and some lesions show increasing size with pregnancy and involution with menopause, there is no role for hormonal manipulation, nor are oral contraceptives contraindicated.

When incidentally detected, these lesions may be observed. The screening sonologist can predict hemangiomas with great confidence. Doubts are raised in case the lesion does not have the typical appearance on sonography,[3] i.e. a variegated appearance. Further, if there is a background underlying liver disease, these should be viewed with suspicion. If the lesion is new, i.e. not seen on previous imaging or has shown an increase in size on serial sonography, further imaging is indicated. If a large lesion is seen, it is better to obtain confirmatory imaging with computed tomography scan or magnetic resonance imaging (MRI).

The multphasic contrast computed tomography appearance is typical showing a cotton wool appearance at the periphery which fills up in the venous and delayed phase till the complete lesion is uniformly contrast rich (Fig. 2). MRI has a higher accuracy.[4] These lesions are hypointense on T1 (Fig. 3A) and hyperintense on T2 weighted imaging - the lightbulb sign (Fig. 3B). Contrast shows enhancement patterns as seen on computed tomography scan (Fig. 4). Diffusion weighted imaging (DWI) has been used to differentiate between benign and malignant lesions. Hemangiomas appear bright, not through restricted diffusion but through T2 shine through.

On imaging, several atypical features may be seen. Flash fill hemangiomas show intense early enhancement, but no washout in contrast to hepatocellular carcinoma (HCC). Alternately, there may be a very slow fill. Degeneration may cause hyalinization or calcification. Involution and fibrosis may be present. HCC, hypervasular metastasis and hemangioendotheliomatosis may be mistaken of atypical hemangiomas.

Formerly Tc99 labeled red blood cells (RBC) single photon emission computed tomography (SPECT) scan[5] was used in diagnosis (Fig. 5), however it adds little to modern computed tomography or MRI scans.

As long as there is certainty in diagnosis, the vast majority may be conserved. In case of atypical features on imaging, it is prudent to do serial ultrasonography to demonstrate constancy of size. In case of symptomatic hemangiomas, parenchyma preserving surgery is indicated. Enucleation[6] may be sufficient even in giant hemangiomas (Fig. 6) and is facilitated by a cavitron ultrasonic

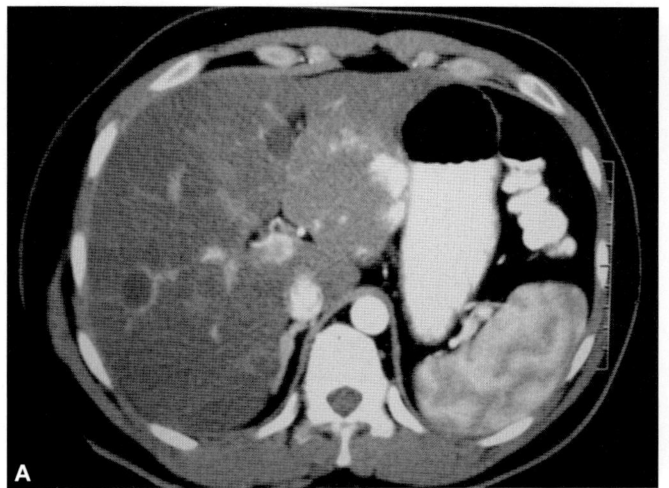

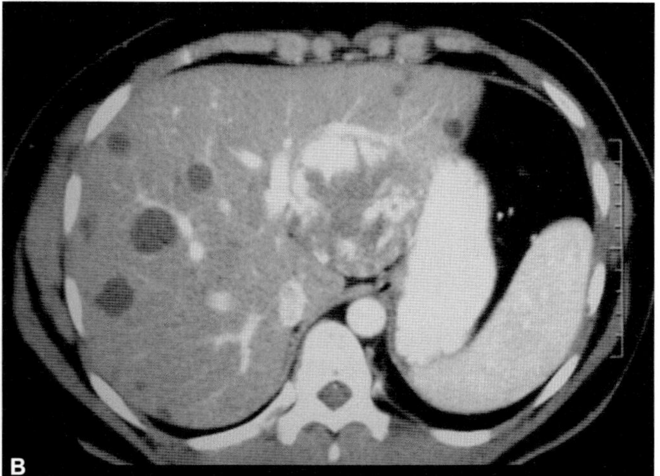

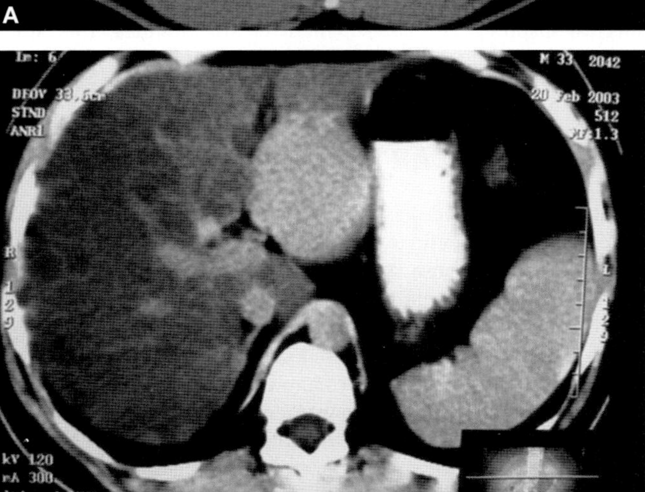

Figures 2A to C Contrast-enhanced computed tomography scan of a patient; (A) Arterial phase; (B) Venous phase; (C) Delayed phase showing peripheral to central complete filling of hemangioma. Incidental liver cysts are seen in right lobe

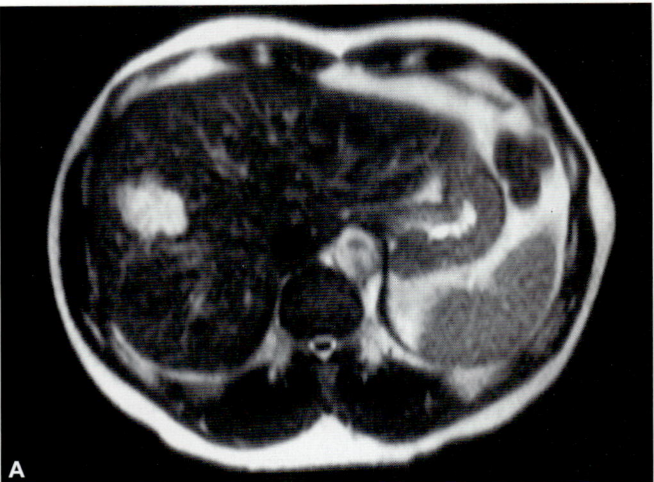

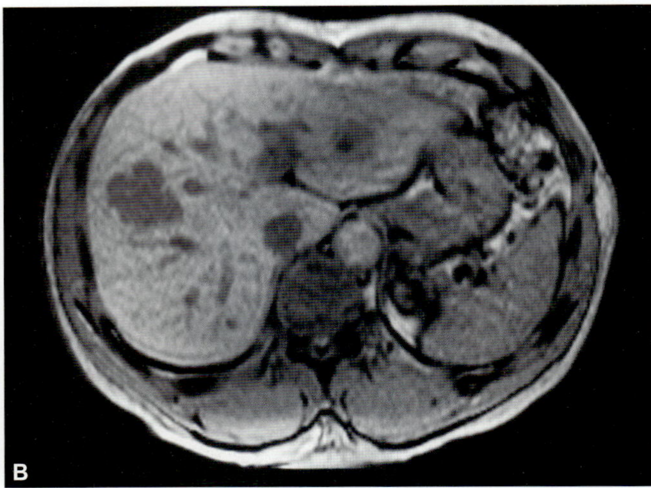

Figures 3A and B Magnetic resonance imaging scan of right lobe hemangioma showing the lesion to be; (A) Hypointense in T1 phase; (B) Hyperintense in the T2 phase

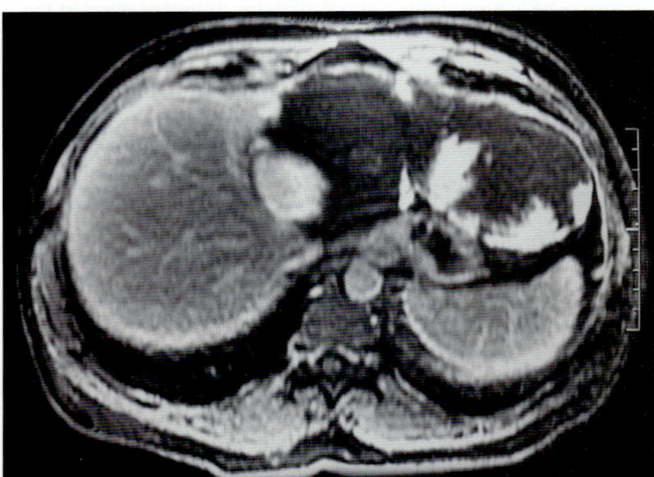

Figure 4 Magnetic resonance imaging with contrast showing the cloud like enhancement at the periphery

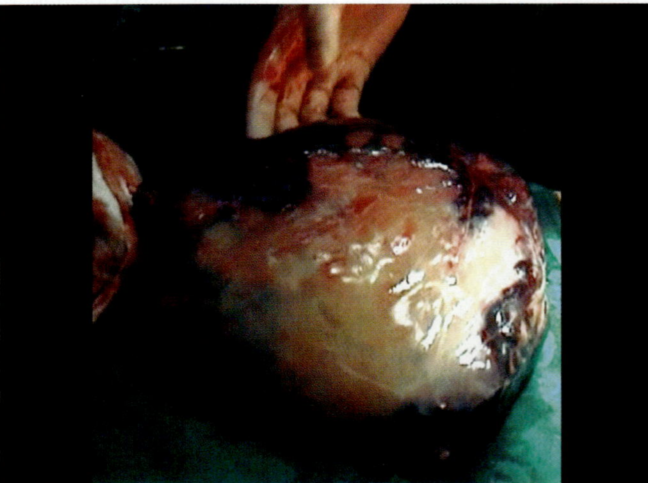

Figure 6 Specimen of symptomatic giant hemangioma weighing 4 kg enucleated

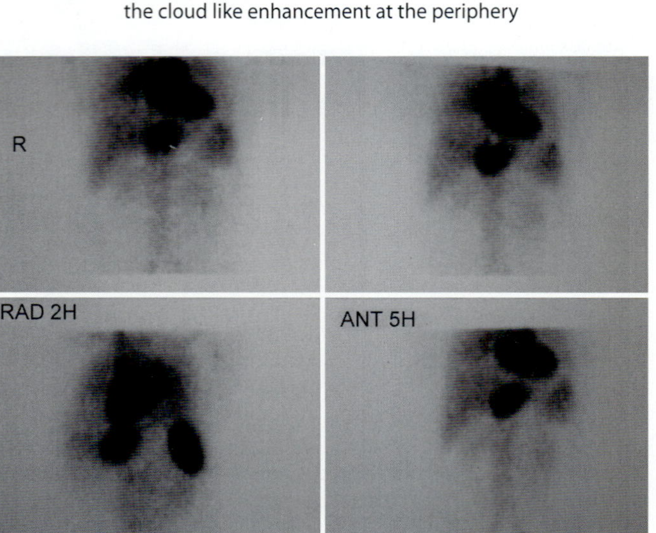

Figure 5 Tc99 RBC tagged scan showing filling up of left lobe hemangioma seen in Figure 1

surgical aspirator (CUSA) which clearly defines the small peripheral feeding vessels. As this is a slow filling cavernous lesion, angioembolization has absolutely no role.

FOCAL NODULAR HYPERPLASIA

Focal nodular hyperplasia (FNH) is a variation of normal development,[7] a nodular lesion around a central artery which supplies the lesion in a stellate manner (Fig. 7). The hepatocytes are arranged in a normal pattern with drainage into hepatic veins. There is no portal venous supply but show normal biliary excretion unlike any other liver lesion. These lesions are always benign and do not undergo malignant transformation. These lesions are hormone dependent and usually occur in women of childbearing age, though rarely they may present in young children and in men. Children subjected to chemotherapy are more prone to these lesions.[8]

Computed tomography scan shows typical arterial enhancement with a feeding vessel, except for the central scar (Fig. 8). The scar shows delayed enhancement. MRI[4] shows hypointensity to

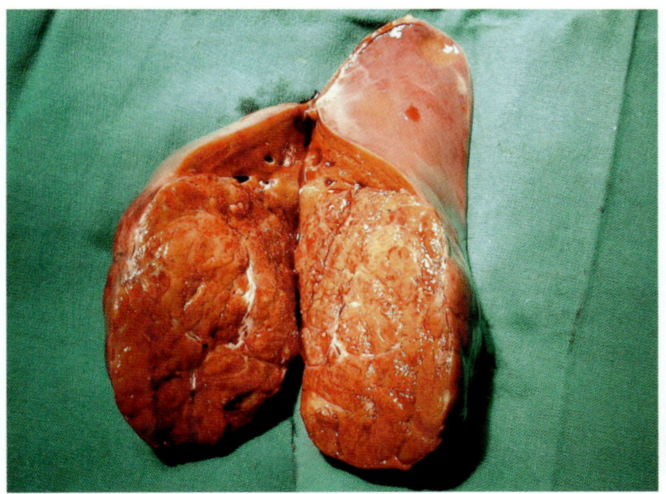

Figure 7 Resected specimen of focal nodular hyperplasia showing central scar

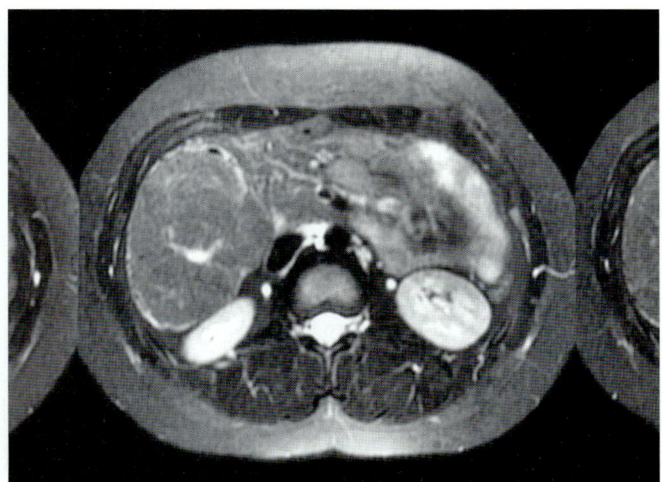

Figure 9 Magnetic resonance imaging liver T2 phase showing scar enhancement in focal nodular hyperplasia

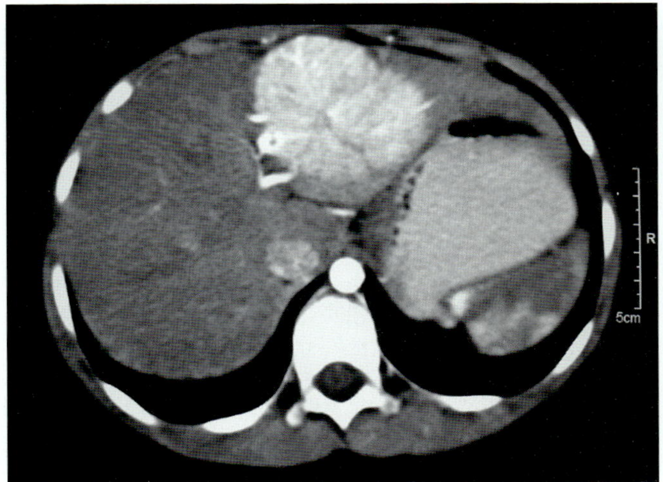

Figure 8 Contrast-enhanced computed tomography scan showing intensely arterially enhancing focal nodular hyperplasia with central scar

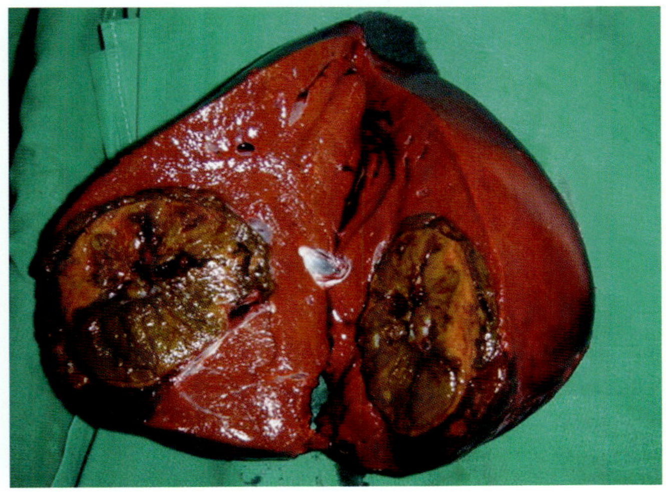

Figure 10 Specimen of hepatic adenoma showing well encapsulated fat rich lesion with necrosis and bile staining due to hepatocyte function and absence of biliary canaliculi

isointensity in T1 and hyperintensity to isointensity in T2 phase with the scar showing hypointensity and hyperintensity (Fig. 9). Owing to the presence of Kupffer cells, they appear hypointense with agents like super paramagnetic iron oxide (SPIO). Similarly, they take up Tc99 sulfur colloid unlike Kupffer cell deficient lesions like HCC and metastasis. Atypical FNH do not have a central scar and should be monitored carefully.

Once diagnosed, FNH can be invariably conserved. Current recommendations even permit oral contraceptive use[9] under monitoring in patients with FNH. Surgery is reserved for the rare symptomatic case or those with diagnostic dilemma.

HEPATIC ADENOMA

These are a group of lesions which lead to considerable diagnostic and therapeutic dilemmas. These well encapsulated lesions consist of a monoclonal proliferation of hepatocytes without normal lobular architecture and reduced Kupffer cells.[7] Often there is considerable fat deposition in these lesions (Fig. 10). Hemorrhage is common and there is a risk of rupture. Malignant transformation within hepatic adenomas has been described.

These are hormone dependent tumors and, if seen in women on hormone supplementation, may regress on stoppage of treatment. Similarly, they are associated with use of anabolic steroids in men.

Recently, molecular genetic studies have led to a subclassification of hepatic adenomas into four types.[10] Type 1 has inactivation of hepatocyte nuclear factor alfa. Type 2 has mutations activating beta catenin. Type 3 lacks both these mutations, however shows inflammation and Type 4 has no distinguishing molecular or morphologic features. Type 2 has high risk of malignant transformation. Type 1 with steatosis may be associated with maturity onset diabetes of youth, Type 3.

Multiple (>10) adenomatosis is a rare syndrome. Rarely liver transplantation[11] has been performed for this as well as for risk of malignant change in livers studded with these lesions.

Hepatic adenomas present as usually solitary solid lesions which may be hyperechoic on sonography if fat rich (Fig. 11). Hemorrhage may lead to a variegated appearance. On computed tomography scan they are well encapsulated and may be arterially enhancing however they are isointense on the venous phase and do not show a washout unlike HCCs. MRI may show hyper isointensity or hypointensity in T1 and T2 phase, however, fat rich lesions lose signal in the out phase of the MRI (Fig. 12). On gadolinium contrast MR, they are hypointense.[4] Nuclear imaging shows uptake with biliary tracer like HIDA or mebrofenin and no excretion.

Surgery is usually advised as rupture is a common complication and there is a rare risk of malignant transformation.

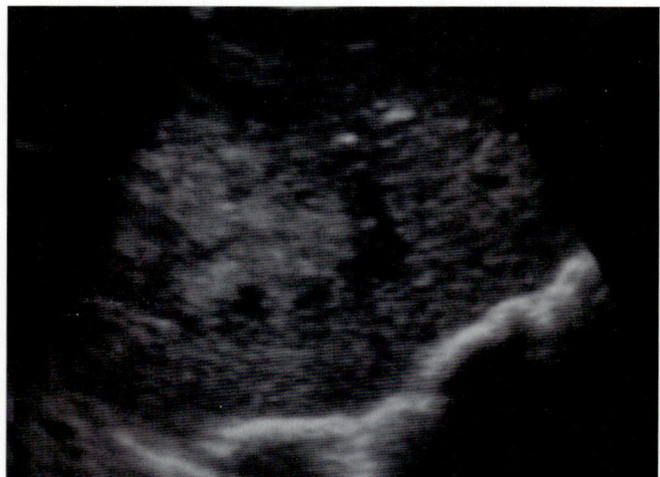

Figure 11 Intraoperative ultrasonography of hepatic adenoma showing hyperechoic fat rich lesion

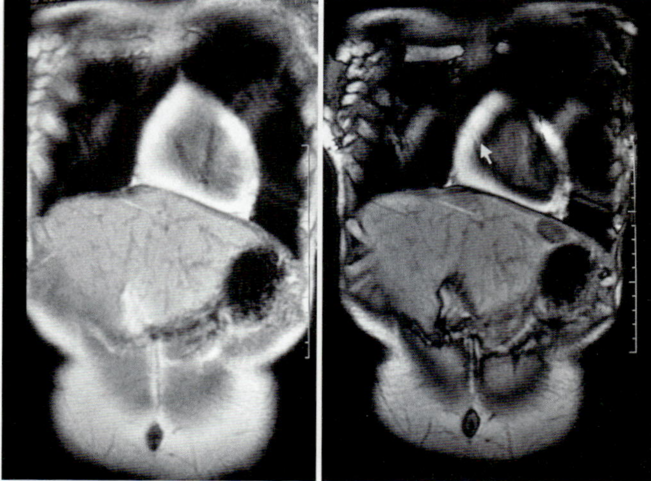

Figure 12 Photograph of magnetic resonance imaging monitor showing in phase (left) and out phase (right). The fat laden lesion loses signal in the out phase and is well seen

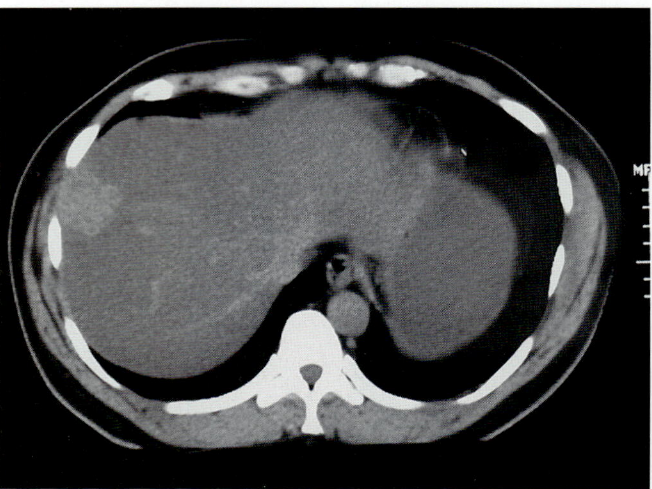

Figure 13 Fat sparing: plain computed tomography scan showing a severely fatty liver where the fat spared area stands out mimicking a lesion. Note how the veins can be seen even in the absence of contrast

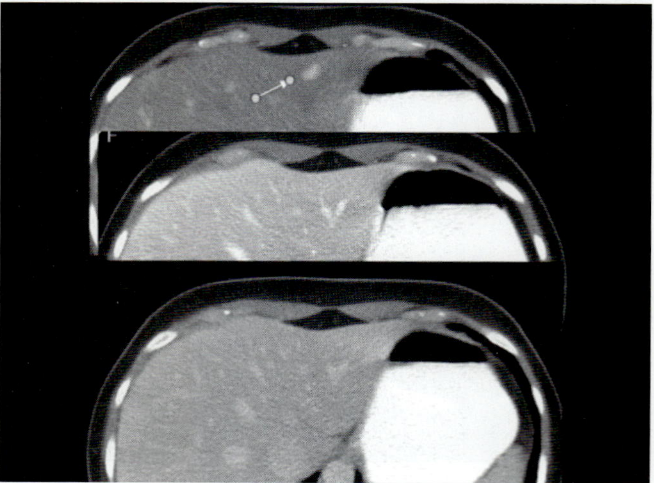

Figure 14 Contrast-enhanced computed tomography showing a transient hepatic attenuation difference in the arterial phase (top). The lesion is not seen in the venous and late phases (middle and bottom)

RARE LESIONS

Focal fat deposits or fat sparing may mimic lesions on imaging (Fig. 13). These are seen at the periphery or near the root of the falciform ligament and are easily sorted by looking at all phases of the scan. Transient hepatic attenuation difference (THAD) lesions are diagnosed by the characteristic wedge shape small areas of arterial enhancement not evident in other phases (Fig. 14).

Mesenchymal hamartomas are rare solid-cystic lesions seen mainly in children. They may grow to a very large size and merit resection due to pressure symptoms.

Hepatic angiomyolipomas are liver lesions far rarer than those seen in the kidney. They contain fat, smooth muscle and blood vessels. They drain into hepatic veins and the vessel of drainage may be demonstrated. Fat content can be demonstrated on computed tomography and MRI. If the diagnosis is made with

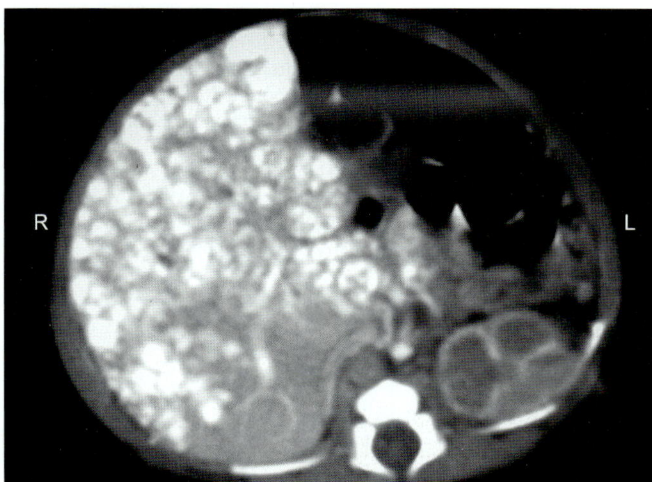

Figure 15 Hemangioendotheliomatosis in a 3-month-old child presenting with cardiac failure

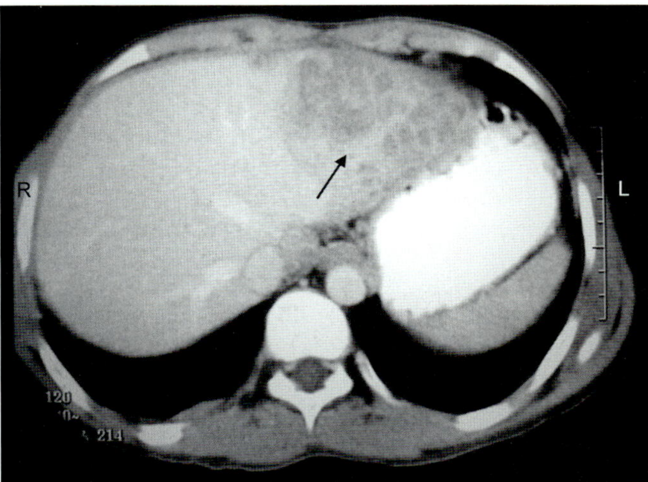

Figure 16 Left lobe liver lesion of tuberculosis showing variegated appearance. The left hepatic vein is running through it (arrow) rather than being displaced or obliterated

certainty, these can be conserved, however, there is a small chance of rupture.

Hepatic hemangioendotheliomas (Fig. 15) are rare multiple vascular lesions in children which may result in cardiac failure due to shunting of blood.

A large number of these resolve with time. Temporarily high dose steroids and alpha interferon are useful to control symptoms. Hepatic artery embolization may help, though is challenging to perform in infants. Rarely, liver transplant is required.[12]

Hepatic lipomas are rare. They show low Hounsfield units on computed tomography and have absolutely no enhancement with contrast.

Liver tuberculosis (Fig. 16) may present as focal lesions in the liver.[13] The confluent granulomas mimic a solid lesion. The characteristic feature is that the vessels are not displaced by the lesion but pass within it. This is a rare situation where biopsy is useful and saves surgery. Lesions resolve well with anti tubercular therapy.

Primary perivascular epitheloid tumor of liver (PEComa) [14] is a rare tumor with malignant potential. These are arterially enhancing without venous washout and hypo intense on MRI T1 phase and hyperintense on T2 phase. These are generally resected due to malignant potential. Histologically they are characterized by clear epitheloid and spindle cells arranged around vessels.

Bile duct adenomas and biliary rests (von Myenburgh complex) are small lesions which are often picked up on diagnostic laparoscopy in the subcapsular lesion. The frozen section diagnosis on this is important as they may be mistaken for metastasis.

SUMMARY OF MANAGEMENT

If there is a suspicion of any diagnosis other than a benign lesion, contrast-enhanced computed tomography or MRI is used as a discriminating tool. Positron emission tomography (PET) scan has little role as absence of uptake may be seen even in HCCs. Monitoring with serial imaging is recommended, if atypical features are seen. Liver biopsy has a small role due to sampling error as well as the difficulty in differentiation between well differentiated HCC and adenomas. Biopsy may be dangerous in hemangiomas.

The majority of patients can be reassured and left alone as the diagnosis can be made with confidence.

Serial imaging with ultrasonography is extremely useful in conservative management of these lesions to reassure the patient and the surgeon.

Indications for surgery are risk of malignant potential, symptoms or unsure diagnosis versus primary tumor.

Resection can often be performed laparoscopically.[15] Energy sources such as the harmonic scalpel or Ligasure™ vessel sealing device facilitate easy resection. Parenchyma preserving resections are encouraged as long as malignancy is not suspected. Ease of surgery should not be used as an excuse for resection.

REFERENCES

1. Choi BY, Nguyen MH. The diagnosis and management of benign hepatic tumors. J Clin Gastroenterol. 2005;39:401-12.
2. Donati M, Stavrou GA, Donati A, Oldhafer KJ. The risk of spontaneous rupture of liver hemangiomas: a critical review of the literature. J Hepatobiliary Pancreat Sci. 2011.
3. Jang HJ, Kim TK, Lim HK, Park SJ, Sim JS, Kim HY, et al. Hepatic hemangioma: atypical appearances on CT, MR imaging, and sonography. AJR Am J Roentgenol. 2003;180:135-41.
4. Cogley JR, Miller FH. MR imaging of benign focal liver lesions. Radiol Clin North Am. 2014;52:657-82.
5. el-Desouki M, Mohamadiyeh M, al-Rashed R, Othman S, al-Mofleh I: Features of hepatic cavernous hemangioma on planar and SPECT Tc-99m-labeled red blood cell scintigraphy. Clin Nucl Med. 1999;24:583-9.
6. Gedaly R, Pomposelli JJ, Pomfret EA, Lewis WD, Jenkins RL. Cavernous hemangioma of the liver: anatomic resection vs. enucleation. Arch Surg 1999;134:407-11.
7. Rebouissou S, Bioulac-Sage P, Zucman-Rossi J. Molecular pathogenesis of focal nodular hyperplasia and hepatocellular adenoma. J Hepatol 2008;48:163-70.
8. Masetti R, Colecchia A, Rondelli R, Martoni A, Vendemini F, Biagi C, Prete A, Festi D, Lima M, Pession A: Benign hepatic nodular lesions after treatment for childhood cancer. J Pediatr Gastroenterol Nutr. 2013;56:151-5.

9. Mathieu D, Kobeiter H, Maison P, Rahmouni A, Cherqui D, Zafrani ES, et al. Oral contraceptive use and focal nodular hyperplasia of the liver. Gastroenterology. 2000;118:560-4.
10. Dhingra S, Fiel MI. Update on the new classification of hepatic adenomas: clinical, molecular, and pathologic characteristics. Arch Pathol Lab Med. 2014;138:1090-7.
11. Ercolani G, Grazi GL, Pinna AD. Liver transplantation for benign hepatic tumors: a systematic review. Dig Surg. 2010;27:68-75.
12. Mistry AM, Gorden DL, Busler JF, Coogan AC, Kelly BS. Diagnostic and therapeutic challenges in hepatic epithelioid hemangioendothelioma. J Gastrointest Cancer. 2012;43:521-5.
13. Desai CS, Josh AG, Abraham P, Desai DC, Deshpande RB, Bhaduri A, Shah SR: Hepatic tuberculosis in absence of disseminated abdominal tuberculosis. Ann Hepatol. 2006;5:41-3.
14. Cheung TT, Trendell-Smith N, Poon RT. Primary perivascular epithelioid cell tumour (PEComa) of the liver. BMJ Case Rep. 2013;2013.
15. Fallahzadeh MK, Zibari GB, Hamidian Jahromi A, Chu Q, Shi R, Shokouh-Amiri H. Laparoscopic versus open liver resection for benign and malignant solid liver tumors: a case-matched study. J Laparoendosc Adv Surg Tech A. 2013;23:908-11.

CHAPTER 72

Malignant Neoplasms of Liver

S Sudhindran

HEPATOCELLULAR CARCINOMA

Hepatocellular carcinoma (HCC) is the most common malignant tumor of the liver. It is an aggressive tumor, the median survival being 6–20 months. It is usually diagnosed late in the course. Worldwide, HCC stands third amongst the causes of cancer-related death.[1] Because of the high incidence of Hepatitis B and C in Asian countries, the prevalence of HCC is high in the region. However, most global epidemiological data ranks India as a low incidence area for HCC.[2] This is almost certainly due to the lack of good quality publications on HCC from India.

In Western countries, incidence of HCC has almost trebled over the three decades from 1985.[3,4] Furthermore, its prevalence is likely to rise globally in the coming years, in parallel with the increase in its epidemiological factors, such as aging population, alcoholic cirrhosis, virus infection and nonalcoholic fatty liver disease.

Risk Factors

Approximately, 80% of HCC develop on the background of cirrhosis, therefore the risk factors of HCC are the same as for chronic liver disease. They broadly include Hepatitis B and C cirrhosis, alcoholic cirrhosis, nonalcoholic steatosis (mostly due to obesity or type 2 diabetes, i.e. the metabolic syndrome), genetic hemochromatosis, α-1 antitrypsin deficiency, primary biliary cirrhosis and autoimmune hepatitis. Virtually, all cases of HCC in childhood and approximately, 50% of all cases of HCC are caused by chronic Hepatitis B virus (HBV) infection. In chronic HBV infection, HCC can develop even without cirrhosis, the virus being able to integrate into the host genome and cause mutagenesis.[5]

Aflatoxin produced by *Aspergillus* fungus, which commonly contaminates peanuts, soybeans and corn,[6] is the most common environmental factor.

Prevention of Hepatocellular Carcinoma

The hepatitis B vaccine is safe and effective and should ideally be given to all newborns and persons at risk of infection. There is evidence that antiviral therapy such as lamivudine in Hepatitis B surface antigen-positive (HBsAg-positive) patients can substantially reduce the risk of development of HCC.[7] A risk reduction of up to 75% has been reported after use of interferon based therapy which could result in sustained viral response.[8] Vitamin K2 causes cell cycle arrest thereby arresting the hepatoma cell growth. It has been used as a preventive agent in a recent study suggesting its possible beneficial role.[9] In patients with nonalcoholic liver disease, control of risk factors such as obesity, type II diabetes and dyslipidemia and increasing aerobic exercise can help prevent development of cirrhosis and HCC. Few studies have indicated there may be risk reduction by coffee drinking.[10]

Clinical Features

Symptoms of HCC are nonspecific and merely reflect those of the underlying chronic liver disease. A known cirrhotic patient developing decompensation in the form of ascites, encephalopathy or jaundice, should raise the suspicion of HCC. This may indicate that the tumor might have extended into the portal vein or biliary tract.

Other symptoms may be abdominal pain, early satiety, weight loss or palpable lump (Fig. 1). Other uncommon presentations include obstructive jaundice caused by invasion of the biliary tree, tumor rupture causing intraperitoneal bleed, fever secondary to tumor necrosis and liver abscess. Very rarely, secretion of abnormal proteins by the HCC, like insulin-like growth factor-II, erythropoietin, parathyroid hormone (PTH)-related protein or vasoactive intestinal peptide (VIP) could result in paraneoplastic manifestations, such as

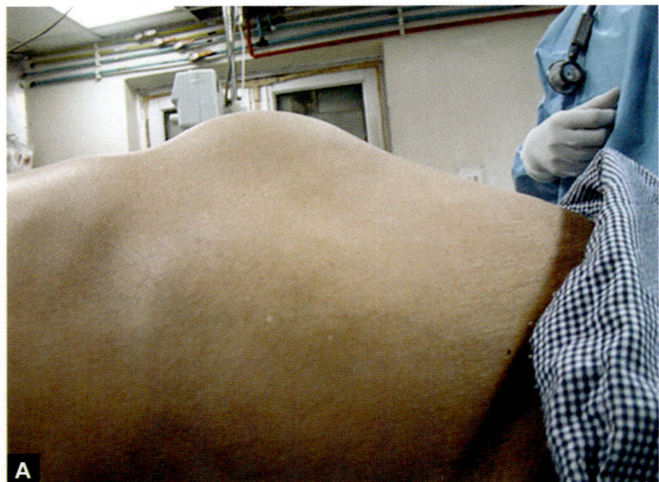

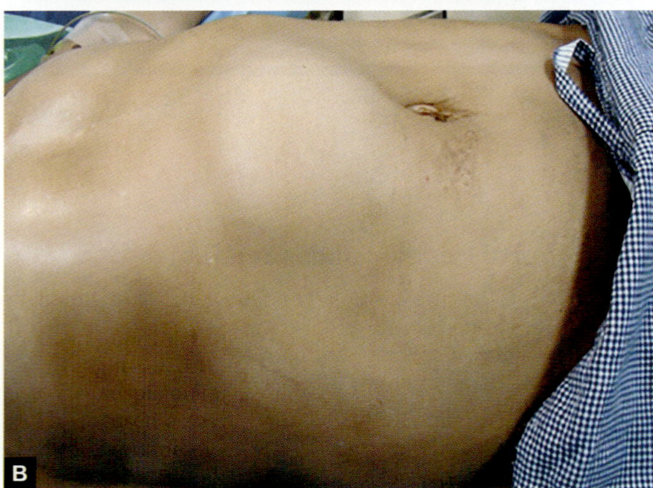

Figures 1A and B Two views showing a projecting mass from left lobe of liver

hypoglycemia, erythrocytosis, hypercalcemia or watery diarrhea, respectively.

There is no physical finding specific to HCC. Physical examination often exposes the chronic liver disease and associated portal hypertension. Hepatomegaly may be present or a bruit may be heard over the liver. Laboratory examination is again usually nonspecific and may show thrombocytopenia, hypoalbuminemia, hyperbilirubinemia, hypoprothrombinemia, anemia or electrolyte disturbances.

Extrahepatic spread is present at the time of diagnosis in about 10% of cases. Metastases are more common in patients with tumors more than 5 cm, multiple tumors and those with vascular invasion. The most common site of metastases is to the lung followed by intra-abdominal lymph nodes, bone and adrenal gland. Brain metastases are rare overall.

Diagnosis

Diagnosis of HCC depends predominantly on biochemical markers and radiology. Histological confirmation is required only in doubtful cases.

The most commonly used marker for HCC is serum alpha-fetoprotein (AFP). AFP is a glycoprotein which is normally produced by the fetal liver and yolk sac. Elevated serum AFP occurs in pregnancy and also in gonadal tumors and in gastric cancer. A rise in serum AFP in a patient with cirrhosis points to the development of HCC. A level of greater than 200 mcg/L (normal is between 10 mcg/L and 20 mcg/L) in a high-risk patient is diagnostic of HCC. The serum AFP level additionally appeared to be an independent prognostic factor and predictor of survival in HCC. Approximately, 40% of patients of HCC will have normal levels of AFP. Furthermore, AFP levels may be elevated in acute or chronic viral hepatitis.

Other tumor markers of HCC include Des gamma carboxy prothrombin (otherwise known as PIVKA-II or prothrombin induced by Vitamin K absence or antagonism), AFP L3 (or lens culinaris agglutinin-reactive fraction of AFP), glypican 3 and plasma micro RNA expression.

On ultrasound HCC may have poorly-defined margins, irregular and coarse internal echoes. Small tumors appear hypoechoic. Sometimes, HCC may have similar echotexture as rest of the liver, thereby making the distinction difficult. Visualization of the lesions below the diaphragm, in obese patients and with bowel gases may be difficult. The sensitivity of ultrasound for diagnosing HCC is around 65% and specificity 90%.[11,12] Recently, contrast has been used in ultrasonography (USG) which may improve the accuracy of USG. Because of the low positive predictive value, an additional investigation is required to confirm the presence of HCC in a suspicious lesion observed on ultrasound.

Vast majority of HCC can be diagnosed from contrast-enhanced cross-sectional imaging, either multidetector computed tomography (MDCT) or magnetic resonance imaging (MRI). HCC receives its blood supply from hepatic artery but liver as such is perfused mainly by the portal vein. This characteristic is used by the four-phase MDCT (unenhanced, arterial, portal venous, delayed venous shown in Figure 2) or dynamic contrast-enhanced MRI which have established a classic imaging profile of HCC. On the arterial phase acquired approximately 20 seconds after intravenous contrast injection, when the contrast opacifies the hepatic artery, the tumor will enhance due to their hepatic arterial supply and appear white against the darker liver ("white on black"). On the portal phase acquired 40 seconds later, as the contrast reaches the portal vein, the normal liver will enhance and appear white whilst the tumor will now appear relatively black due to absence of portal venous supply. The "black on white" appearance of the tumor is accentuated in the delayed venous phase too, acquired 60–90 seconds after contrast injection. This arterial phase enhancement with venous washout is typical of HCC.

Hepatocellular carcinoma are hyperintense on T1 and hypointense on T2 weighted images of MRI. It has same sensitivity as that of computed tomography (CT). MRI angiography may yield same information as contrast-enhanced computed tomography (CECT). Superparamagnetic iron oxide (SPIO) particles when used with gadolinium-based contrast agents, so called double contrast MRI, increase the sensitivity of MRI for detection of HCC.[13]

[18F] fluorodeoxyglucose (FDG) positron emission tomography (PET) scanning has a role in detection of primary HCCs, tumor staging, assessing response to therapy, and for

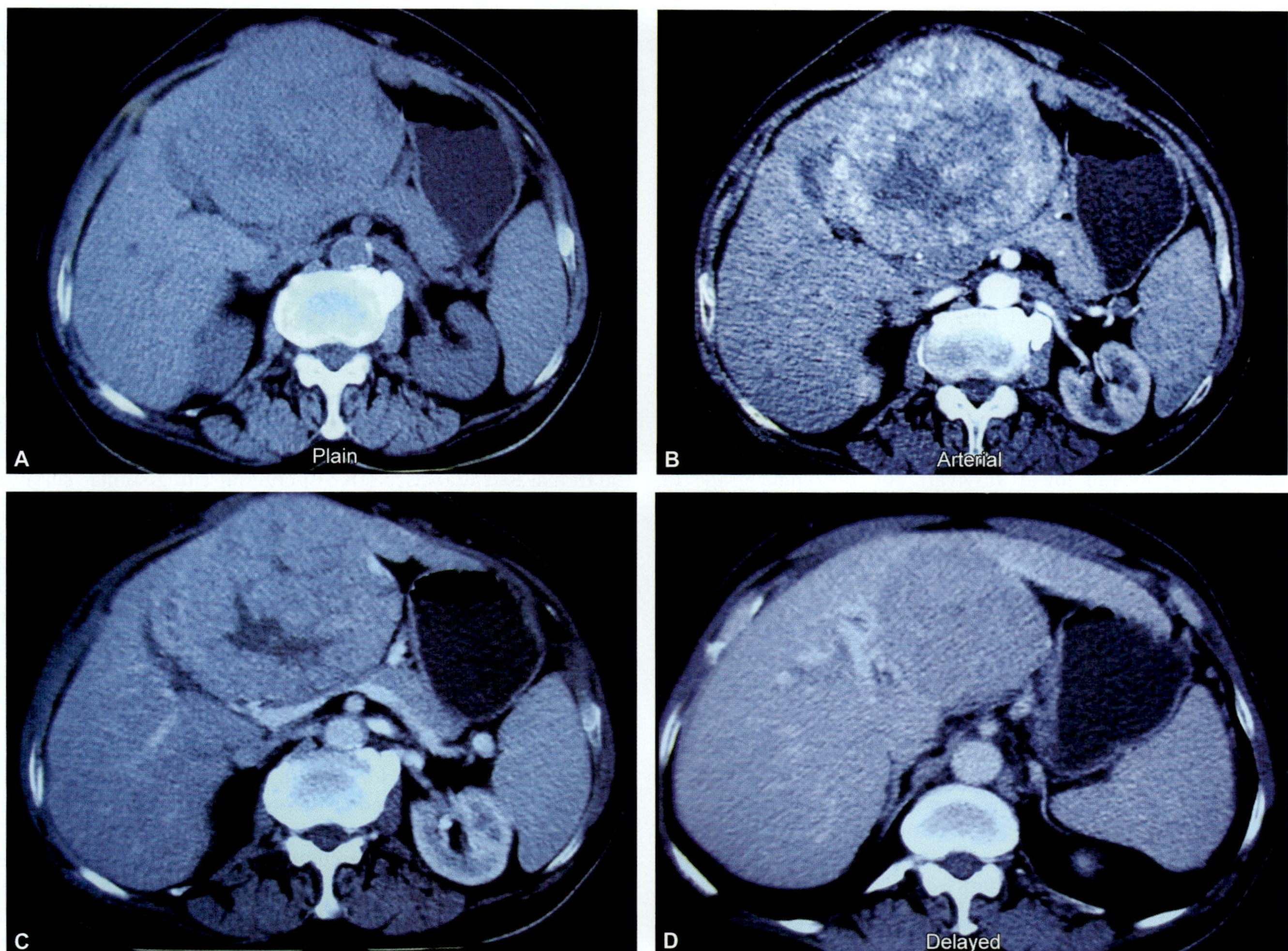

Figures 2A to D Plain film, early arterial phase, venous phase and delayed phase showing characteristic changes in a hepatocelluar carcinoma

predicting prognosis. However, only 55–65% of tumors are positive by PET scanning, with high-grade tumors generally having greater FDG avidity as assessed by higher standardized uptake values (SUV) than lower grade lesions. This variability limits the utility of PET scanning for diagnostic purposes. PET has a greater sensitivity for detection of distant metastases than other imaging modalities. Nonetheless, sensitivity is limited for lesions less than or equal to 1 cm and false-positive and false-negative results are also problematic. FDG avidity may correlate with therapeutic efficacy for treatments with non-avid tumors showing better prognosis.[14,15]

The only way to effectively diagnose HCC in a timely fashion is to enroll patients who are at high risk for development of this tumor in a regular surveillance program. Most practice guidelines recommend surveillance by 6 monthly ultrasound and AFP although evidence supporting its effectiveness in improving the survival of participants is modest.[11,16,17] Using the commonly employed 200 ng/mL cutoff point, the sensitivity of AFP is only around 20% but has specificity in excess of 90%.[18] Ultrasound has a sensitivity of approximately 65% and a specificity of 90% for early detection of HCC.[11]

The approach to diagnosis and surveillance of HCC outlined in a consensus statement issued by the American Association for the Study of Liver Diseases:[11,12]

- Nodules less than 1 cm found on surveillance ultrasound should be followed with serial ultrasounds at 3–6 months interval for assessment of growth. If no growth is seen over next 2 years routine surveillance should be performed thereafter.
- Lesions larger than 1 cm in diameter should be evaluated with dynamic MRI or MDCT. If the appearance is typical for HCC, no further investigation is required. If the picture is not typical of HCC, a second study (CT or MRI) or biopsy should be performed.
- Percutaneous biopsy should be done in cases of diagnostic dilemma and it is thought the results might alter the plan of management. Complications are bleeding and needle track seeding which has been reported to be in the tune of 3%.[19]
- Staining for tumor markers including cluster of differentiation 34 (CD34), cytokeratin 7 (CK7), glypican 3, heat shock protein [(HSP)-70] and glutamine synthetase can help characterize lesions that are not clearly HCC on microscopy. If the biopsy is negative for HCC, repeat imaging be done at 3–6 monthly

intervals until the nodule either disappears, enlarges, or displays diagnostic characteristics of HCC. If the lesion enlarges but remains atypical for HCC a repeat biopsy is recommended.

Staging

A number of systems have been proposed to predict the prognosis for HCC, none of which has been universally adopted. The four most commonly used schemes are the tumor-node-metastasis (TNM), Okuda, Barcelona systems and the Cancer of the Liver Italian Program (CLIP) score.[20-25] These variably incorporate four features that have been recognized as being important determinants of survival: the size of tumor, the severity of underlying liver disease, extension of the tumor into adjacent structures and the presence of metastases. Other factors influencing survival include whether patients are living in high-incidence versus low-incidence areas (high incidence areas having overall lower survival), the histologic grade of differentiation, and levels of serum AFP level at diagnosis.

There is no hard evidence that one staging system is superior to the other in predicting the survival of patients with HCC. The American Joint Committee on Cancer (AJCC) TNM staging which is a purely pathologic system predicts prognosis better than do clinical systems when assessing the outcomes of resection. The Barcelona Clinic Liver Cancer (BCLC) staging classification is perhaps the most widely accepted.[22,23] It comprises five stages that are based upon the size and number of the primary lesion, performance status, Child-Pugh class to assess liver function, vascular invasion and extrahepatic spread. Very early-stage (stage 0 or tumors <2 cm with normal liver function) and early-stage (stage A or single lesion <5 cm or 3 nodules each <3 cm) comprise patients with good performance status that are suitable for radical therapies such as resection or transplantation. Intermediate stage (stage B) patients have multinodular HCC; advanced stage (stage C) patients have vascular invasion and/or extrahepatic spread. These patients are candidates for ablative therapies and not resection. Patients with stage D disease have advanced liver disease or poor performance status, have an extremely poor prognosis and treatment should be for symptom control.

Treatment

There are two potentially curative treatment options for HCC-resection (Fig. 3) and liver transplantation. Liver transplantation is probably the best if possible as it will remove all the at risk parenchyma, but due to lack of organs it is not possible for every patient. Live donor liver transplantation (LDLT) can provide solution to this problem. Unfortunately, up to 80% of patients will also not be fit for resection or transplantation because of tumor extent and poor performance status. Due to this combination of surgery and local directed therapies or tumor ablation [Radio Frequency Ablation (RFA), percutaneous ethanol injection (PEI)], transarterial chemoembolization (TACE), radiation therapy, and systemic therapy, has been used.

Liver transplantation achieves resection of the malignant tumor with the widest possible margins and restores the liver function to normalcy. However, early experience with transplantation for patients with unresectable HCC was disappointing with tumor recurring in up to 80% of patients, and long-term survival rates well below that of patients transplanted for nonmalignant disease. Survival of patients undergoing liver transplantation for conditions other than HCC, and have small HCC in explanted liver, is not different from patients who had transplants for benign diseases.[26] This finding changed the philosophy of liver transplantation for HCC. The landmark study of Mazzaferro in 1996 established orthotopic deceased-donor liver transplantation as a viable option for the treatment of HCC.[27] They showed that when transplantation was restricted to patients with "early HCC" (so called Milan criteria that include single lesion ≤5 cm or three separate lesions none >3 cm, no evidence of gross vascular invasion, and no regional nodal or distant metastases), a 4-year survival rate of 75% could be achieved. The tumor recurrence was much less compared to partial liver resection. Milan criteria are currently widely accepted world over but are too restrictive. University College San Francisco expanded this criterion to include solitary tumor up to 6.5 cm or three or fewer nodules with the largest lesion of 4.5 cm and total tumor diameter of 8 cm for liver transplantation [University of California, San Francisco (UCSF) criteria] citing similar survival achieved using their criteria when compared to Milan's.[28] Subsequently, many other criteria have been proposed from different units from North America, Europe and Asia, all claiming good survival following liver transplantation. It must be noted that there are no adequate data in literature backing any other criteria to validate long-term survival results comparable to those satisfying Milan criteria. Histopathologic grading and presence of microvascular invasion are two important adverse prognostic factors.

Long waiting times for liver grafts has offset the survival benefit of liver transplantation for HCC patients. During this waiting period there is a risk of tumor progression which may decrease the survival. To prevent tumor growth during waiting period "bridging" treatments like resection, percutaneous ablation, and TACE are adopted. LDLT can avoid the waiting period and therefore is emerging as a viable solution to the graft shortage. However, the potential risk of donor hepatectomy and relatively higher biliary complication in the recipients need to be considered in offering such treatment. Furthermore, live donor liver grafts are often small for size and the subsequent acute-phase injury, regeneration and angiogenesis might increase the chance of tumor recurrence. Some have postulated that higher recurrence rates after LDLT may reflect the fact that longer wait times for a deceased donor organ permits the dropout of those patients with poor biology who are destined to have an early recurrence.

Another major disadvantage following liver transplantation is the need for lifelong immunosuppression with its attendant risks. Newer immunosuppressive drugs from the category mammalian target of rapamycin (m-TOR) inhibitors like sirolimus and everolimus have antitumor activity as well. These drugs may have the advantage of "hitting two birds with one stone" after liver transplantation for HCC.

Liver resection (Fig. 3) is a first-line curative treatment in a patient with adequate functional reserve who has anatomically resectable solitary or multifocal HCC. The ideal patient for resection has a solitary HCC confined to the liver no evidence of invasion of the hepatic vasculature or portal hypertension, and well-preserved hepatic function.

Long-term relapse-free survival rates average 40% or better and 5-year survival rates as high as 80% are reported in carefully selected patients. No size criterion has been in vogue for selection of patients for resection. Invasion of portal or hepatic vein radicals,

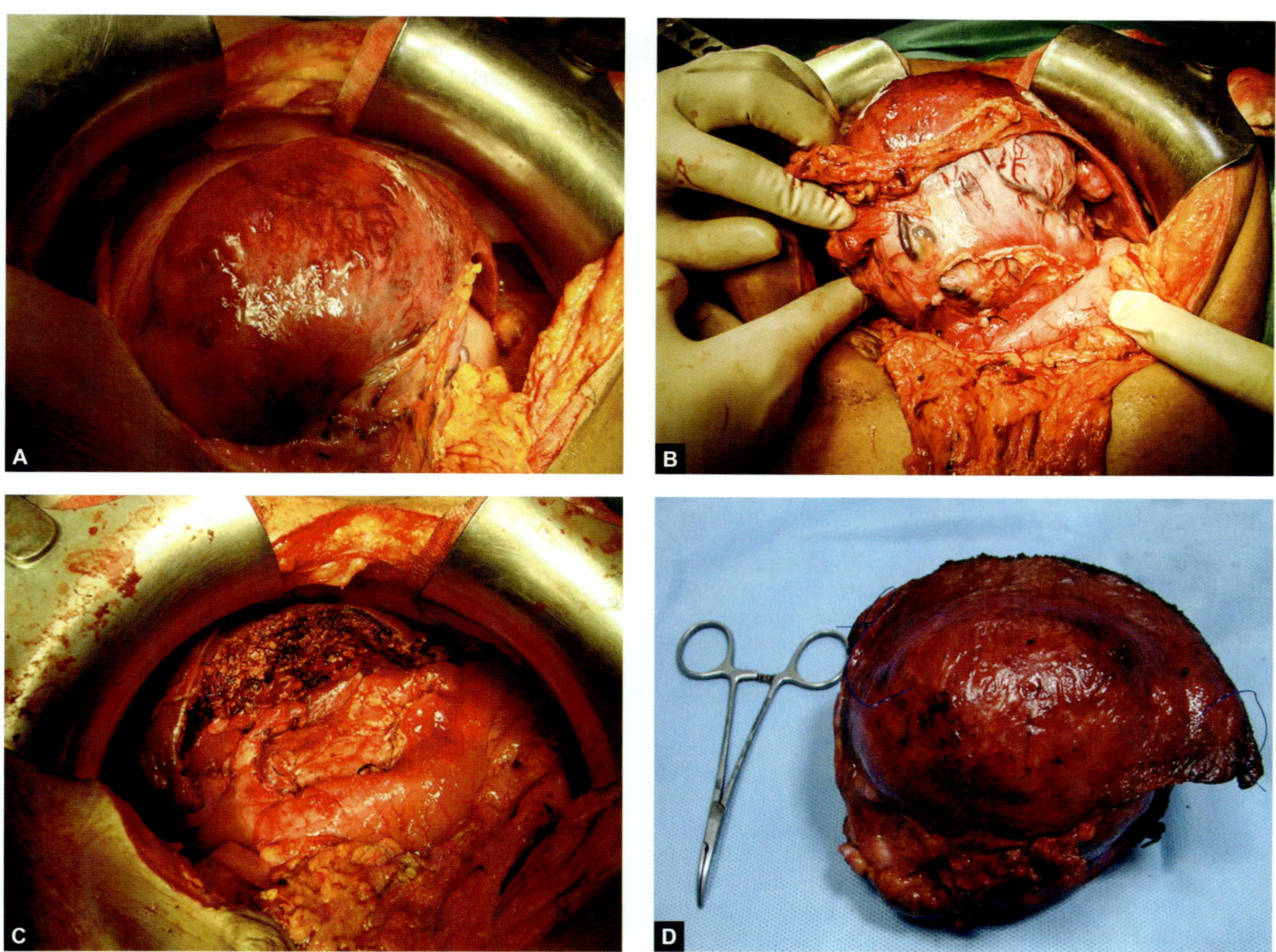

Figures 3A to D Same patient as in Figures 1 and 2. Operative appearance and the resected tumor

nodal and distant metastasis and invasion of adjacent structures are poor prognostic factors.

The mortality rate after hepatic resection is approximately 5% at major centers but morbidity remains high at 30–40%. Major complications such as liver failure, bile leak and bleeding occurs in less than 5% nowadays but minor complications such as postoperative ascites, wound infection and pneumonia remain common. Open surgery is the conventional approach for liver resection but recently laparoscopic hepatectomy is gathering pace in major centers.

Although the rare situation of tumor rupture of an HCC suggests a high likelihood of peritoneal seeding and a poor outcome from resection, this is not inevitable. The most common approach in such cases is initial control of bleeding (which may require transarterial embolization or emergency surgery) followed by a formal staging evaluation, and a subsequent attempt at resection.

Salvage Transplants

Initial hepatic resection for selected patients with small tumors and adequate liver function and subsequent liver transplant in case of tumor recurrence or deteriorating liver function is termed salvage liver transplant. The rationale for such an approach is that liver resection, although associated with a higher recurrence rate does offer cure for some patients who will then not compete for the already scarce deceased donor liver graft.

Nonsurgical Modes

Unfortunately, due to advanced disease or poor performance status at the time of diagnosis or both, the majority of patients with HCC can only be offered one of the following nonsurgical methods of treatment:

Radiofrequency ablation (RFA): It involves the use of conversion of ultrasonic energy to heat energy to desiccate the tissue. A high frequency alternating current moves from the tip of an electrode into the tissue surrounding that electrode. As the ions within the tissue attempt to follow the change in the direction of the alternating current, their movement results in frictional heating of the tissue. Cells die at a temperature more than 60°C. The necrosis starts appearing around the electrode. This can be done percutaneously or more recently laparoscopic probes have also been available recently for the procedure. This procedure is useful for candidates who do not meet resectability criteria but still have their disease confined to the liver. An ideal lesion will be less than 4 cm, not superficially located and away from the major vessels and bile ducts. The best outcomes are in patients with a single tumor less than 4 cm in diameter.[29] Morbidity (primarily pleural effusion and peritoneal bleed) is approximately 10% and procedure related mortality is 0%–0.3%. Survival rates of up to 70% have been reported for tumors less than 2 cm which is comparable to surgical resection.

Percutaneous ethanol or acetic acid ablation (PEI): It was the favored minimally invasive method for HCC before the advent of RFA.[30] Repeated injections are required. It is a low cost procedure which requires minimal equipment. Good results have been shown at many institutions sometimes supplanting RFA. Necrosis rates of 90%–100% for tumors less than 2 cm but reduces for tumors more than 2 cm. Acetic acid may produce similar results with fewer side effects. Five-year survival of up to 50% as been reported in Child-Pugh A patients.

Transarterial chemoembolization: HCCs derive its blood supply majorly from hepatic arteries. TACE eliminates the tumor's blood supply and administers cytotoxic chemotherapy directly to the tumor. In TACE chemotherapeutic agent is injected into the hepatic artery with or without lipiodol or a procoagulant material. Lipiodol is an oily contrast agent that promotes intratumoral retention of chemotherapy drugs. A more recent method of chemoembolization involves the use of drug-eluting polyvinyl alcohol microspheres called as "beads", which seems to cause less toxicity with similar efficacy. Simultaneous or sequential occlusion of the hepatic artery until stagnation of blood flow to the tumor occurs may result in greater antitumor efficacy than chemotherapy alone. TACE is used for unresectable HCCs that are not amenable to RFA or other local treatments. It is commonly used as a "bridging therapy" prior to transplant. Bland particle embolization alone (i.e. without chemotherapy) has also been used for both unresectable and locally recurrent HCC. Absolute contraindications to this technique include the absence of hepatopetal portal blood flow (including portal vein thrombosis), encephalopathy, and biliary obstruction. Relative contraindications include serum bilirubin more than 2 mg/dL, aspartate aminotransferase more than 100 unit/L, tumor burden involving more than 50% of the liver, cardiac or renal insufficiency, ascites, recent variceal bleed, or significant thrombocytopenia. Postembolization syndrome (which consists of fever, abdominal pain and ileus) is common and seen in up to 50% of patients. Extensive tumor necrosis is seen in up to 50% of patients. Complete response is achieved in only 2% of patients. The improvement in survival in treated patients ranges from 20%–60% at 2 years.

Radiation therapy: Liver is an extremely radiosensitive organ. As a whole, the liver can only tolerate about 20 Gy. HCC is a radiosensitive tumor. Stereotactic body radiation therapy (SBRT) is a technique in which a limited number of high dose radiation fractions are delivered to a small, precisely-defined target using multiple, nonparallel radiation beams. This targeting allows treatment of tumors less than 5 cm in either a single or limited number of dose fractions.

Radioembolization: As in TACE where chemotherapeutic agents are injected with lipiodol, in radioembolization, radiolabelled lipiodol or radiotagged glass microspheres are injected into hepatic arteries supplying the tumor. The radioisotopes used are, iodine-131 (131I), labeled lipiodol or yttrium-90 (90Y)-tagged glass microspheres. Early reports suggest that radioembolization is safe and induces objective responses in patients with unresectable HCC.[31] However, longer-term follow-up of these studies and additional experience is needed.

Systemic therapy: Study of heart and renal protection (SHARP) trial in 2007 demonstrated significant survival benefit for for sorafenib (a multitargeted tyrosine kinase inhibitor) over supportive care alone in patients with advanced HCC.[32,33] Sorafenib monotherapy has now become the new reference standard systemic treatment for advanced HCC (especially HBV-associated HCCs). The data available is for Child-Pugh A patients majorly. Data is scarce for Child-Pugh B. Therefore, at present sorafenib has not been recommended in these patients and improvement in survival should be carefully evaluated.

Hepatocellular carcinoma is relatively chemotherapy resistant tumor. Therefore, cytotoxic chemotherapy has not been used routinely. This may be in part due to the high rate of expression of drug resistance genes, including p-glycoprotein, glutathione-S-transferase, heat shock proteins and mutations in p53.

INTRAHEPATIC CHOLANGIOCARCINOMA

Intrahepatic cholangiocarcinomas (IHCC) is the second most common primary tumor of the liver. Current nomenclature defines IHCC as tumor arising from biliary epithelium of the ducts proximal to main right and left hepatic ducts.

Risk Factors

Intrahepatic cholangiocarcinomas usually occurs in the six or seventh decade. It occurs more frequently in men.[34] Primary sclerosing cholangitis (PSC) is strongly associated with cholangiocarcinoma, the cumulative incidence being 1.5% per year. The risk is higher in patients of inflammatory bowel disease. In these patients, the 10- and 20-year rates for cholangiocarcinoma are 15% and 30% respectively. Congenital fibrocystic diseases of the biliary tree like Caroli's syndrome, congenital hepatic fibrosis and choledochal cysts has about 15% risk of malignant change in the early adult years where average age at diagnosis is around 35 years.[35,36] Biliary papillomatosis can turn malignant in nearly 80%.[37] Parasitic infections like clonorchis and opisthorchis genera predisposes to cholangiocarcinoma of the intrahepatic bile ducts. Additionally, there is evidence of strong association between chronic intrahepatic stone disease or recurrent pyogenic cholangitis and cholangiocarcinoma.[38-40] Several occupations, including auto, rubber, chemical and wood-finishing industries as well as exposure to the radiologic contrast agent thorotrast are associated with increased risk for cholagiocarcinoma. Chronic liver disease particularly those secondary to Hepatitis B virus and Hepatitis C virus have also been found as risk factor for IHCC.[40,41]

Pathology

More than 90% of cholangiocarcinomas are adenocarcinomas (well-differentiated and mucin-producing type), with squamous cell carcinoma being responsible for most of the remaining cases.

Rarely small cell carcinoma and sarcoma can occur. IHCC can be mass-forming tumors (with tendency for localized vascular invasion), periductal tumors (infiltrative along peribile duct tissues) or intraductal variant (characterized by papillary or granular growth within the lumen).

Clinical Features and Diagnosis

Intrahepatic cholangiocarcinomas usually present with dull right upper quadrant pain and weight loss, an elevated serum alkaline phosphatase and normal or slightly elevated serum bilirubin levels. This is distinctly different from extrahepatic cholangiocarcinoma, which usually present with obstructive jaundice. IHCC is usually detected on imaging as a space occupying liver lesion atypical for HCC. The primary differential diagnosis is metastases, which need to be excluded.

Certain tumor markers like carcinoembryonic antigen (CEA) and cancer antigen (CA) 19-9 have been best studied in this context. CA 19-9 has limited specificity in diagnosis as it is frequently elevated in various benign pancreaticobiliary conditions causing cholangitis or cholestasis as well as in other malignancies, including pancreatic cancer. CA 19-9 cutoff value of more than or equal to 40 U/mL has almost 80% sensitivity and specificity for malignant disease in patients with neither cholangitis nor cholestasis.[42] In cholestasis or cholangitis, a cutoff value more than or equal to 300 U/mL increases the specificity to nearly 90% but at the expense of decreased sensitivity (approximately 40%).[42] Biliary CEA concentration maybe elevated approximately 5-fold in patients with cholangiocarcinoma compared to those with benign strictures.[43]

Radiological Evaluation

On ultrasound scan, IHCC appear as hypoechoic mass lesion. On Doppler, it appears hypovascular with minimal internal blood flow. Ultrasound also may be useful in diagnosis of advanced disease, like presence of ascites, vascular invasion, liver metastases and lymphadenopathy.

The typical appearance of IHCC in contrast-enhanced triple phase computed tomography is a hypodense lesion with peripheral or rim enhancement in arterial phase with no discernible portal venous phase washout. The central area of the tumor typically remains hypovascular. Computed tomography image typically shows peripheral biliary dilatation around the tumor. The arterial enhancement may rarely be intense and global, mimicking HCC.[44,45] Computed tomography is highly sensitive in distinguishing benign from malignant intrahepatic bile duct strictures, ruling out metastatic disease affecting regional lymph nodes, peritoneum, or lung fields and visualizing the pertinent nodal basins.

On MRI scan IHCC appear as hypointense lesions on T1-weighted images that are hyperintense on T2-weighted images. T2-weighted images may also show central hypointensity corresponding to areas of fibrosis, characteristic of IHCC. Pooling of contrast on delayed images is suggestive of a peripheral cholangiocarcinoma.[46]

Positron emission tomography scan detects cholangiocarcinoma because of the high glucose uptake by the malignant cholangiocytes. Although PET detects mass forming nodular IHCC, it is less helpful for infiltrating types. The importance of PET scan is in identifying occult metastases and regional lymph node involvement where it has a sensitivity of 50% and specificity of 80%.[47,48] PET may also have a possible role in screening patients with PSC for the presence of cholangiocarcinoma and as a diagnostic tool after resection to detect recurrence. Limitations are high false positivity in patients with biliary tract infections or inflammatory processes (as in PSC) and high false negative values with mucinous tumors.[49]

Treatment

Mainstay of treatment for IHCC is resection with negative margin, but IHCC usually present at an advanced stage. If untreated, median survival for IHCC is less than 12 months whilst 5-year survival rates for patients who undergo complete (R0) resection range between 30% and 65%.[50,51]

Criteria for resectability of IHCC include:

- Absence of nodal metastases beyond the hepatoduodenal ligament (i.e. celiac or periaortic nodes) or liver or distant metastases
- Absence of invasion of the portal vein or main hepatic artery (although some centers support en bloc resection with vascular reconstruction)
- Absence of extrahepatic adjacent organ invasion
- Adequate remnant liver with good inflow, outflow and biliary drainage
- Absence medical comorbidities that precludes resection.

Regional lymph node metastasis, although an indicator of poor outcome, is not necessarily an absolute contraindication to surgery. Nevertheless, data is minimal regarding the benefits of lymphadenectomy for IHCC except that it may provide better staging and a resultant spuriously improved survival due to "stage migration". We do not perform a routine portal lymph node dissection for peripheral localized tumor but do perform lymphadenectomy with centrally located tumors in which an extrahepatic bile duct resection is required to maximize the margin. Some patients may require preoperative portal vein embolization to permit contralateral lobe hypertrophy and a margin-negative resection.

Following R0 resection, there is as yet no evidence for benefit for adjuvant therapy. For patients with positive margins, options may include re-resection, radiofrequency or microwave ablation and fluoropyrimidine or gemcitabine-based chemotherapy. Many centers suggest chemoradiotherapy rather than chemotherapy alone following either a margin-positive or node-positive resection.

In locally advanced unresectable or metastatic disease, the treatment options are fluoropyrimidine or gemcitabine-based chemotherapy, chemoradiotherapy or supportive care. A partial response of 10% and 20% is seen with systemic chemotherapy. Large unresectable tumors can turn potentially resectable and should be considered in such cases. Concerning the efficacy of hepatic artery infusion chemotherapy or of biological agents like sorafenib, the response rate reported so far is not impressive.

The most important prognostic factors following resection are margin status and lymph node involvement. Five-year survival is significantly better in patients with clear negative margin compared to positive margin. Other bad prognostic factors include vascular invasion and multiple tumors. IHCC in patients with PSC have dismal prognosis.[52]

For palliation, biliary stenting is usually not required, unlike in extrahepatic cholangiocarcinoma, since jaundice is rarely a presenting symptom, except in tumor compressing hilum. Other symptoms to be palliated in these patients are capsular stretch pain and massive ascites. Tumor ablation by radiofrequency or microwave ablation, transarterial chemoembolization or radioembolization can be used in palliative settings.

Role of liver transplantation in IHCC is a controversial topic. Although good 5-year survival of up to 80% for early-stage hilar cholangiocarcinoma has been reported from various centers in selected cases following neoadjuvant chemoradiation, it should only be performed as part of a randomized trial.[53,54]

OTHER RARE PRIMARY MALIGNANT TUMORS OF LIVER

These make up less than 10% of all primary malignant tumors of the liver and include the following:

Fibrolamellar HCC is a distinct variety of HCC that predominates in young adults. It carries a more favorable prognosis when compared to classical HCC. The tumor may be associated with focal nodular hyperplasia (FNH) and sometimes has a morphologic appearance at imaging that is difficult to distinguish from FNH. A central scar like lesion may be seen in both tumors, but calcifications indicate fibrolamellar HCC. Fibrolamellar HCC does not express AFP but high serum vitamin B12 binding capacity and elevated neurotensin values in serum can be found. Fibrolamellar HCC can also express aromatase which may result in clinically manifest steroid action, such as gynecomastia. Although resection maybe feasible in the majority and recommended as the first line therapy, the risk of recurrence is close to 50%. Close follow-up with contrast computed tomography scan following resection is necessary.

Mixed or combined HCC-cholangiocarcinoma (HCC-CC) represents an uncommon group of primary liver carcinomas presenting features of hepatocelullar and cholangiocellular epithelial differentiation. It is probably a variant of HCC with cholangiocellular features. Detailed investigations of histology, immunohistochemistry and ribonucleic acid (RNA) expression have added considerably to better understanding of these tumors and their features of biphenotypic differentiation. The survival pattern reflects that of the traditional HCC.

Other very rare malignant tumors include angiosarcoma, undifferentiated embryonal sarcoma, primary hepatic malignant tumor with rhabdoid features, leiomyosarcoma, primary neuroendocrine tumor of liver, non-Hodgkin's lymphoma of liver and adult hepatoblastoma.

REFERENCES

1. Parkin DM, Bray F, Ferlay J, Pisani P. Estimating the world cancer burden: Globocan 2000. Int J Cancer. 2001;94:153-6.
2. World Health Organization. 2008. International Agency for Research on Cancer. GLOBOCAN. [Online] Available from http://globocan.iarc.fr [Accessed May, 2015].
3. El-Serag HB, Mason AC. Rising incidence of hepatocellular carcinoma in the United States. N Engl J Med. 1999;340:745-50.
4. Bosetti C, Levi F, Boffetta P, Lucchini F, Negri E, La Vecchia C. Trends in mortality from hepatocellular carcinoma in Europe, 1980-2004. Hepatology. 2008;48:137-45.
5. McGlynn KA, London WT. The global epidemiology of hepatocellular carcinoma: present and future. Clin Liver Dis. 2011;15(2):223-43, vii–x.
6. Chen CJ, Wang LY, Lu SN, Wu MH, You SL, Zhang YJ, et al. Elevated aflatoxin exposure and increased risk of hepatocellular carcinoma. Hepatology. 1996;24(1):38-42.
7. Liaw YF, Sung JJ, Chow WC, Farrell G, Lee CZ, Yuen H, et al. Lamivudine for patients with chronic hepatitis B and advanced liver disease. N Engl J Med. 2004;351:1521-31.
8. Di Bisceglie AM, Shiffman ML, Ever- son GT, Lindsay KL, Everhart JE, Wright EC, et al. Prolonged therapy of advanced chronic hepatitis C with low-dose peginterferon. N Engl J Med. 2008;359:2429-41.
9. Habu D, Shiomi S, Tamori A, Takeda T, Tanaka T, Kubo S, et al. Role of vitamin K2 in the development of hepatocellular carcinoma in women with viral cirrhosis of the liver. JAMA. 2004;292:358-61.
10. Larsson SC, Wolk A. Coffee consumption and risk of liver cancer: a meta-analysis. Gastroenterology. 2007;132:1740-5.
11. Bruix J, Sherman M. Management of hepatocellular carcinoma. Hepatology. 2005;42:1208-36.
12. Bruix J, Sherman M. Management of hepatocellular carcinoma an update. Hepatology. 2011;53:1021-23.
13. Yoo HJ, Lee JM, Lee MW, Kim SJ, Lee JY, Han JK, et al. Hepatocellular carcinoma in cirrhotic liver: double-contrast- enhanced, high-resolution 3.0T-MR imaging with pathologic correlation. Invest Radiol. 2008;43:538-46.
14. Kornberg A, Küpper B, Tannapfel A, Büchler P, Krause B, Witt U, et al. Patients with non-[18 F]fludeoxyglucose-avid advanced hepatocellular carcinoma on clinical staging may achieve long-term recurrence-free survival after liver transplantation. Liver Transpl. 2012;18:53-61.
15. JH, Park JY, Kim do Y, Ahn SH, Han KH, Seo HJ, et al. Prognostic value of 18F-FDG PET for hepatocellular carcinoma patients treated with sorafenib. Liver Int. 2011;31:1144-9.
16. Zhang BH, Yang BH, Tang ZY. Randomized controlled trial of screening for hepatocellular carcinoma. J Cancer Res Clin Oncol. 2004;130:417-22.
17. Chen JG, Parkin DM, Chen QG, Lu JH, Shen QJ, Zhang BC, et al. Screening for liver cancer: results of a randomized controlled trial in Qidong, China. J Med Screen. 2003;10:204-9.
18. Trevisani F, D'Intino PE, Morselli-Labate AM, Mazzella G, Accogli E, Caraceni P, et al. Serum alpha-fetoprotein for diagnosis of hepatocellular carcinoma in patients with chronic liver disease: influence of HBsAg and anti-HCV status. J Hepatol. 2001;34:570-5.
19. Silva MA, Hegab B, Hyde C, Guo B, Buckels JA, Mirza DF. Needle track seeding following biopsy of liver lesions in the diagnosis of hepatocellular cancer: a systematic review and meta-analysis. Gut. 2008; 57:1592-6.
20. American Joint Committee on Cancer. American Joint Committee on Cancer Staging Manual, 7th edition. In: Edge SB, Byrd DR, Compton CC, et al (Eds). New York: Springer; 2010. p. 175.
21. Okuda K, Ohtsuki T, Obata H, Tomimatsu M, Okazaki N, Hasegawa H, et al. Natural history of hepatocellular carcinoma and prognosis in relation to treatment. Study of 850 patients. Cancer. 1985;56:918-28.
22. Llovet JM, Brú C, Bruix J. Prognosis of hepatocellular carcinoma: the BCLC staging classification. Semin Liver Dis. 1999;19:329-38.
23. Forner A, Reig ME, de Lope CR, Bruix J. Current strategy for staging and treatment: the BCLC update and future prospects. Semin Liver Dis. 2010;30:61-74.
24. A new prognostic system for hepatocellular carcinoma: a retrospective study of 435 patients: the Cancer of the Liver Italian Program (CLIP) investigators. Hepatology. 1998;28:751-5.
25. Chevret S, Trinchet JC, Mathieu D, Rached AA, Beaugrand M, Chastang C, et al. A new prognostic classification for predicting

survival in patients with hepatocellular carcinoma. Groupe d'Etude et de Traitement du Carcinome Hépatocellulaire. J Hepatol. 1999;31:133-41.

26. Iwatsuki S, Starzl TE, Sheahan DG, Yokoyama I, Demetris AJ, Todo S, et al. Hepatic resection versus transplantation for hepatocellular carcinoma. Ann Surg. 1991;214:221-8.
27. Mazzaferro V, Regalia E, Doci R, Andreola S, Pulvirenti A, Bozzetti F, et al. Liver transplantation for the treatment of small hepatocellular carcinomas in patients with cirrhosis. N Engl J Med. 1996;334:693-9.
28. Yao FY, Ferrell L, Bass NM, Watson JJ, Bacchetti P, Venook A, et al. Liver transplantation for hepatocellular carcinoma: expansion of the tumor size limits does not adversely impact survival. Hepatology. 2001;33:1394-1403.
29. Livraghi T, Meloni F, Di Stasi M, Rolle E, Solbiati L, Tinelli C, et al. Sustained complete response and complications rates after radiofrequency ablation of very early hepatocellular carcinoma in cirrhosis: Is resection still the treatment of choice? Hepatology. 2008;47:82-9.
30. Cho YK, Kim JK, Kim MY, Rhim H, Han JK. Systematic review of randomized trials for hepatocellular carcinoma treated with percutaneous ablation therapies. Hepatology. 2009;49:453-9.
31. Sangro B, Bilbao JI, Boan J, Martinez-Cuesta A, Benito A, Rodriguez J, Panizo A, et al. Radioembolization using 90Y-resin microspheres for patients with advanced hepatocellular carcinoma. Int J Radiat Oncol Biol Phys. 2006;66:792-800.
32. Llovet JM, Ricci S, Mazzaferro V, Hilgard P, Gane E, Blanc JF, et al. Sorafenib in advanced hepatocellular carcinoma. N Engl J Med. 2008;359:378-90.
33. Cheng AL, Kang YK, Chen Z, Tsao CJ, Qin S, Kim JS, et al. Efficacy and safety of sorafenib in patients in the Asia-Pacific region with advanced hepatocellular carcinoma: a phase III randomized, double-blind, placebo-controlled trial. Lancet Oncol. 2009;10:25-34.
34. Henson DE, Albores-Saavedra J, Corle D. Carcinoma of the extrahepatic bile ducts. Histologic types, stage of disease, grade, and survival rates. Cancer. 1992;70:1498-501.
35. Khan SA, Thomas HC, Davidson BR, Taylor-Robinson SD. Cholangiocarcinoma. Lancet. 2005;366:1303-14.
36. Scott J, Shousha S, Thomas HC, Sherlock S. Bile duct carcinoma: a late complication of congenital hepatic fibrosis. Case report and review of literature. Am J Gastroenterol. 1980; 73:113.
37. Lee SS, Kim MH, Lee SK, Jang SJ, Song MH, Kim KP, et al. Clinicopathologic review of 58 patients with biliary papillomatosis. Cancer. 2004;100:783-93.
38. Chen MF. Peripheral cholangiocarcinoma (cholangiocellular carcinoma): clinical features, diagnosis and treatment. J Gastroenterol Hepatol. 1999;14:1144-9.
39. Su CH, Shyr YM, Lui WY, P'Eng FK. Hepatolithiasis associated with cholangiocarcinoma. Br J Surg. 1997;84:969-73.
40. Sorensen HT, Friis S, Olsen JH, Thulstrup AM, Mellemkjaer L, Linet M, et al. Risk of liver and other types of cancer in patients with cirrhosis: nationwide cohort study in Denmark. Hepatology. 1998;28:921-5.
41. Welzel TM, Graubard BI, El-Serag HB, Shaib YH, Hsing AW, Davila JA, et al. Risk factors for intrahepatic and extrahepatic cholangiocarcinoma in the United States: a population-based case-control study. Clin Gastroenterol Hepatol. 2007;5:1221-8.
42. Kim HJ, Kim MH, Myung SJ, Lim BC, Park ET, Yoo KS, et al. A new strategy for the application of CA19-9 in the differentiation of pancreaticobiliary cancer: analysis using a receiver operating characteristic curve. Am J Gastroenterol. 1999;94:1941-6.
43. Nakeeb A, Lipsett PA, Lillemoe KD, Fox-Talbot MK, Coleman J, Cameron JL, et al. Biliary carcinoembryonic antigen levels are a marker for cholangiocarcinoma. Am J Surg. 1996;171:147-52.
44. Valls C, Gumà A, Puig I, Sanchez A, Andía E, Serrano T, et al. Intrahepatic peripheral cholangiocarcinoma: CT evaluation. Abdom Imaging. 2000;25:490-6.
45. Choi SH, Han JK, Lee JM, Lee KH, Kim SH, Lee JY, et al. Differentiating malignant from benign common bile duct stricture with multiphasic helical CT. Radiology. 2005;236:178-83.
46. Manfredi R, Barbaro B, Masselli G, Vecchioli A, Marano P. Magnetic resonance imaging of cholangiocarcinoma. Semin Liver Dis. 2004;24:155-64.
47. Kim YJ, Yun M, Lee WJ, Kim KS, Lee JD. Usefulness of 18F-FDG PET in intrahepatic cholangiocarcinoma. Eur J Nucl Med Mol Imaging. 2003;30:1467-72.
48. Kluge R, Schmidt F, Caca K, Barthel H, Hesse S, Georgi P, et al. Positron emission tomography with [(18)F]fluoro-2-deoxy-D-glucose for diagnosis and staging of bile duct cancer. Hepatology. 2001;33:1029-35.
49. Prytz H, Keiding S, Björnsson E, Broomé U, Almer S, Castedal M, et al. Dynamic FDG-PET is useful for detection of cholangiocarcinoma in patients with PSC listed for liver transplantation. Hepatology. 2006;44:1572-80.
50. Choi SB, Kim KS, Choi JY, Park SW, Choi JS, Lee WJ, et al. The prognosis and survival outcome of intrahepatic cholangiocarcinoma following surgical resection: association of lymph node metastasis and lymph node dissection with survival. Ann Surg Oncol. 2009;16:3048-56.
51. Endo I, Gonen M, Yopp AC, Dala l KM, Zhou Q, Klimstra D, et al. Intrahepatic cholangiocarcinoma: rising frequency, improved survival, and determinants of outcome after resection. Ann Surg. 2008;248:84-96.
52. Kaya M, de Groen PC, Angulo P, Nagorney DM, Gunderson LL, Gores GJ, et al. Treatment of cholangiocarcinoma complicating primary sclerosing cholangitis: the Mayo Clinic experience. Am J Gastroenterol. 2001;96:1164-9.
53. Schwartz JJ, Hutson WR, Gayowski TJ, So-rensen JB. Liver transplantation for cholangiocarcinoma. Transplantation. 2009;88:295-8.
54. Rea DJ, Heimbach JK, Rosen CB, Haddock MG, Alberts SR, Kremers WK, et al. Liver transplantation with neoadjuvant chemoradiation is more effective than resection for hilar cholangiocarcinoma. Ann Surg. 2005;242:451-8.

CHAPTER 73

Liver Metastases

Sanjay Govil, Ashwin Rammohan

Treatment of liver metastases with surgery appears at first to be counter intuitive. Perhaps in no other disease is assessment of tumor biology more important than in the surgical treatment of liver metastases. Patients with oligometastases, that appear months to years after treatment of the primary, that remain relatively static in size and number over a period of observation, and for which complementary non-surgical treatments are effective, are most likely to benefit from resection. Because of the potential complexity of decision-making for these patients, attempts have been made to develop clinical scoring systems, and these patients are best treated under the care of multidisciplinary committees. The overwhelming prevalence of colorectal cancer (CRC) means that clinical experience is greatest for colorectal liver metastases (CRLM), followed closely by neuroendocrine liver metastases and then by a host of noncolorectal nonendocrine liver metastases (NCNELM).

Colorectal Liver Metastases

INTRODUCTION

Colorectal cancer is the third most common cancer in men and second most common in women worldwide. The liver is often the first and only site of metastasis in 30–40% of patients. Approximately 20–25% of new cases have liver metastases at diagnosis and an additional 40–50% will develop them during their lifetime, usually within 3 years of initial diagnosis of the primary.[1] Median survival without treatment is less than 8 months although patients with solitary metastases may survive longer.[2] Even so, 5-year survival without treatment is exceptional (below 5%), whereas a number of studies demonstrate a median survival at 5 years of 30% (range 15–67%) with surgical treatment.[3] Early diagnosis and treatment of CRLM is therefore essential.

DIAGNOSIS

Radiology

Patients who undergo surgery for CRC should ideally undergo CT scan of the chest, abdomen and pelvis prior to operation in order to detect synchronous metastases.[1] However, the additional yield of CT chest in patients with normal chest X-ray is only 5%.[4] Patients who undergo emergency surgery should be adequately imaged as soon as possible therafter.[1] Ultrasonography is inadequate to detect liver metastases.[5] A CT scan should ideally be performed annually for at least the first 3 years of follow-up, and certainly once within the first 2 years.[1]

Contrast CT scan of the abdomen detects 68–91% liver metastases (70% in lesions below 1 cm diameter),[5] but accuracy varies depending on the equipment and technique. High resolution scans with maximum intensity technique and volumetric three-dimensional rendering are most accurate. Narrowing CT scan slice thickness below 2–4 mm causes degradation of image quality without improving accuracy.[6] Small CRLM appear hyperdense in the arterial phase. Larger tumors may show a hyperdense rim but are mostly hypodense in the arterial phase and are completely hypodense in the venous phase.[6] CT scans are best examined in the venous phase and images viewed on a high contrast liver window to detect CRLM (Fig. 1).

Although multidetector computed tomography (MDCT) is the most commonly used diagnostic modality, MRI using liver-specific contrast agents [particularly super-paramagnetic iron oxide (SPIO)] is considered most accurate to detect lesions smaller than 1 cm diameter,[6,7] but is not widely available. MRI is more sensitive

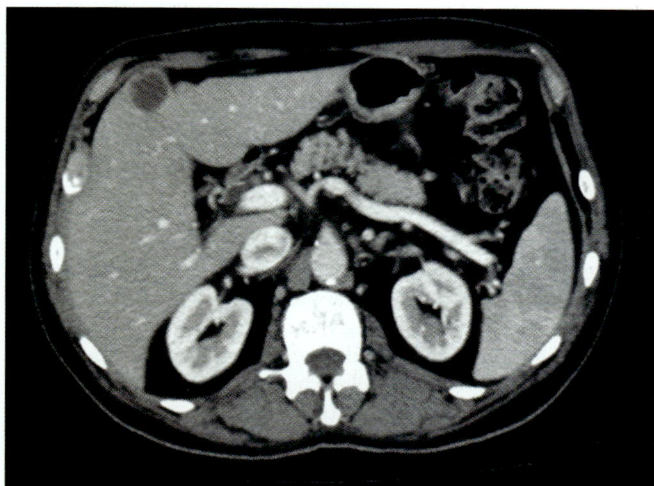

Figure 1 Typical hypodense appearance of a solitary colorectal liver metastasis in segment IV viewed in the portal venous phase of a CT scan

even than CT arterioportograhy and has less false positives, apart from being noninvasive.[6,7]

Addition of metabolic imaging using fluorodeoxyglucose (FDG) PET/CT is more sensitive than US, CT or MRI in detecting CRLM on a per-patient basis, but is equivalent to MRI on a per-lesion basis.[6,7] PET/CT is recommended to stage disease once liver metastases have been detected. The addition of PET/CT to the evaluation of CRLM alters the clinical management of approximately 25–30% patients. The combination of PET with functional MRI would probably provide the greatest accuracy in diagnosing CRLM.

Finally, the use of contrast enhanced intraoperative ultrasound may further increase accuracy but is highly operator dependent.[6]

Role of CEA

CEA is elevated in up to 90% of patients with CRLM, although this may not happen till late in the course of the disease.[8] The role of limiting follow-up after CRC resection to serial CEA measurements is unproven, although a fall in CEA levels after resection of the CRC followed by a rising level is indicative of metastasis.[1]

Biopsy

Biopsy is unnecessary when the diagnosis of CRLM is not in doubt; however, it may be necessary sometimes.[1] It should be used with caution because, although reports of tumor seeding after FNAC are rare, one study has reported seeding after 5 of 51 biopsies.[9] The need for biopsy is best decided after discussion in a multidisciplinary team meeting.

SURGERY

Approximately 20–30% of patients with CRLM are suitable for resection. Surgery provides the best chance of long-term survival for these patients, with several studies reporting 5-year survivals of 25–44% (compared with approximately 10–11% 5-year survival with chemotherapy alone) and operative mortality between 0–6%.[1] The median cancer-specific survival after resection of CRLM is 42.5 months.[10,11]

Surgery may be considered in patients in whom the residual liver volume after resection with adequate margin (R0) is at least two contiguous liver segments with adequate vascular inflow and outflow as well as biliary drainage. Tumor should not involve the common hepatic artery, main portal vein or celiac and para-aortic lymph nodes, and any extrahepatic disease detected on preoperative imaging should be amenable to either synchronous or subsequent resection. Earlier recommendations as to the number and location of metastases are no longer relevant although a greater number of metastases will influence long-term survival adversely.[12]

Margins

Earlier studies reported inferior results with surgical margins below 1 cm[13] (45% vs 23% 5-year survival). Presently a positive margin is defined as being less than 1 mm from the tumor margin. Patients with margins varying from 1 mm to 10 mm from the tumor edge showed no difference in recurrence rates.[12,14] However, a margin positive status resulted in significantly poorer survival, particularly in patients who also had a poor morphological response to neoadjuvant chemotherapy.[14] The aim of resection is therefore to achieve an R0 resection while preserving parenchyma by performing segmental or non-anatomical resections when possible rather than extended resections.[15]

Hilar Lymph Nodes

The presence of hilar lymph node metastases is clearly an adverse prognostic sign with 5-year disease free survival of about 11% and overall 5-year survival of 18%.[16] The positive predictive value (PPV) of CT scan to detect enlarged hilar lymph nodes is only 56%, and even intraoperative evaluation has a PPV of only 43%.[17] The only accurate technique of diagnosing hilar nodal metastases is therefore by performing hilar lymphadenectomy as part of the resection. When diagnosed preoperatively, there is evidence to show that patients who respond to neoadjuvant chemotherapy may still benefit from resection.[16] Patients diagnosed on H&E stain of the lymphadenectomy specimen have a poorer outcome compared to those on whom the diagnosis was made on immunohistochemistry.[18] Those with involvement of the nodes along the common hepatic artery (station 8) had poorer outcomes than those with hilar nodes (station 12).[16,18]

Increasing Resectability

Neoadjuvant Chemotherapy

Neoadjuvant chemotherapy for initially unresectable CRLM that are expected to become resectable by downsizing is given the term "Conversion Therapy". Conversion therapy is successful in approximately 20–30% of patients and is able to provide 5-year survivals in the range of 30–35%.[19] This comes at the expense of chemotherapy associated parenchymal dysfunction that may result in postoperative liver failure if inadequately addressed, and the problem of the "disappearing metastasis".

Hepatic arterial infusion chemotherapy using either floxuridine or oxaliplatin into the hepatic artery combined with systemic chemotherapy has been used by some centers to treat initially unresectable CRLM with bilobar disease.[20,21] The results from uncontrolled cohort studies are very exciting with 92% of chemotherapy naive patients undergoing a complete or partial response and 43% undergoing successful surgery with a median survival of 40 months from port placement. Sixteen percent of patients who had initially failed chemotherapy also became amenable for resection and achieved a 5-year survival of 56% versus 0 for those who did not undergo surgery. These results need to be confirmed using randomized controlled trials.

Approximately 9–24% of CRLM undergo a complete radiological response (CRR) after neoadjuvant chemotherapy.[22] However, the correlation between CRR and complete pathological response is poor. Between 17% and 69% of "disappearing liver metastases" show residual tumor at pathology, and therefore should be resected whenever possible. One-third to half of these lesions are detected at laparotomy, with a combination of clinical examination and intraoperative ultrasound. The reason for the disappearance of DLM can be hepatic steatosis (which masks the hypodense liver metastasis), location of the metastasis at a subcapsular location or near the falciform ligament (where lesions may be missed by preoperative imaging), reduction in the size of the lesion below the resolution of the scanner, and true pathological response. MRI is more likely to detect metastases that have disappeared on CT scan.

Chemotherapy with oxaliplatin, irinotecan and bevacizumab induces parenchymal injury that has a negative impact on the functional reserve of the liver.[23] Oxaliplatin causes hepatic sinusoidal obstruction syndrome (blue liver, Fig. 2) similar to that seen in veno-occlusive disease. It induces sinusoidal dilatation and hepatocyte atrophy, which in more severe cases may be associated with perisinusoidal fibrosis and nodular regenerative hyperplasia. These changes are at least partially reversible over a period of 4–6 weeks, and occur less commonly with concomitant use of bevacizumab. Irinotecan causes hepatic steatosis and steatohepatitis [yellow liver, chemotherapy associated steatohepatitis (CASH)], the implications of which are a greater degree of postoperative liver dysfunction and a higher incidence of disappearing liver metastases. These changes are also partially reversible over 4–6 weeks. There is some evidence to suggest that the use of greater than 6–8 cycles of chemotherapy is more likely to be associated with hepatic parenchymal injury. Bevacizumab interferes with wound healing and surgery is to be avoided for 8 weeks after completion of therapy. Whenever surgery for CRLM is planned after neoadjuvant chemotherapy, it should be delayed 4–8 weeks to allow the parenchyma to recover and the future functional liver remnant should not be below 30% of total liver volume.

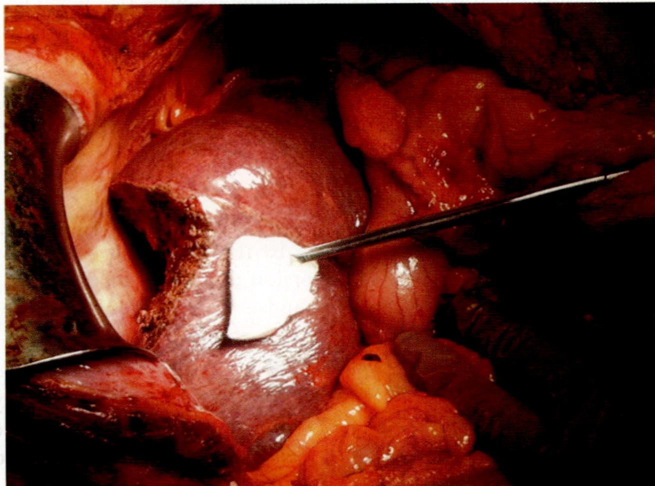

Figure 2 "Blue liver" caused by sinusoidal obstruction due to oxaliplatin therapy. The patient has undergone a bisegmentectomy VII/VIII

Portal Vein Embolization/Ligation[24,25]

Embolization of portal vein branches into the segments of the liver that are planned for resection result in compensatory hypertrophy of the future liver remnant by approximately 30% (20–46%) over a period of 2–8 weeks. The degree of improvement in function is believed to be greater than the degree of parenchymal hypertrophy. This procedure is therefore useful when the FLR is below 25–30% of the total liver volume or the ratio of the FLR to body weight is below 0.5. It is usually performed percutaneously and transhepatically but can also be performed by cannulation of one of the ileocolic veins using an incision in the right iliac fossa, or by laparoscopic access. When performed percutaneously it is usually done under local anesthesia using an ipsilateral approach (through the lobe of the liver that is to be resected) so as to avoid potential injury to the FLR. A variety of embolic agents such as gelatin sponge, polyvinyl alcohol, lipiodol, cyanoacrylate glue and embolization coils may be used. The portal vein may also be ligated surgically, especially as a component of the two-stage hepatectomy.

Portal vein embolization (PVE) is well tolerated by patients. Post-embolization nausea and vomiting are rare. More than 50% patients do not show any changes in liver function. If transaminases do become elevated, they peak at levels below three times normal at 3 days after the procedure and normalize within 7 days. Coagulation parameters do not alter. Complications of the procedure are infrequent (liver hematoma, progressive portomesenteric thrombosis and tumor progression while waiting for hypertrophy) and mortality was not reported from a review of 1,088 patients who underwent this procedure.

Staged Hepatectomy[26,27] *(Figs 3A and B)*

Two-stage hepatectomy is a technique that may be used to treat patients with bilobar CRLM in whom a single operation may not permit an adequate sized liver remnant. It may be performed in two ways—the latter being more common. In the first, as many metastases as safely possible are removed in the first stage. Sufficient time is then allowed for the remaining liver to hypertrophy. Interval chemotherapy is used to downstage tumor further, and then all residual tumors are resected or ablated in the second stage procedure. The second, more favored technique, involves a first stage in which all tumors are removed from the planned future liver remnant. Portal vein ligation may be performed to the more involved lobe that is to be resected in the second stage, thereby allowing the FLR to hypertrophy further. Chemotherapy may be used in the interval between the two stages to minimize growth of residual tumor. The second stage is then performed when it is felt that the FLR is of adequate size and function.

A recent review of 12 studies comprising 488 patients who were planned for two-stage resection from among 4,940 patients who underwent surgery for CRLM found that 77% of patients completed both stages of the procedure. Interval tumor progression was the most common cause for abandoning the procedure but other causes included poor performance status, and inadequate hypertrophy

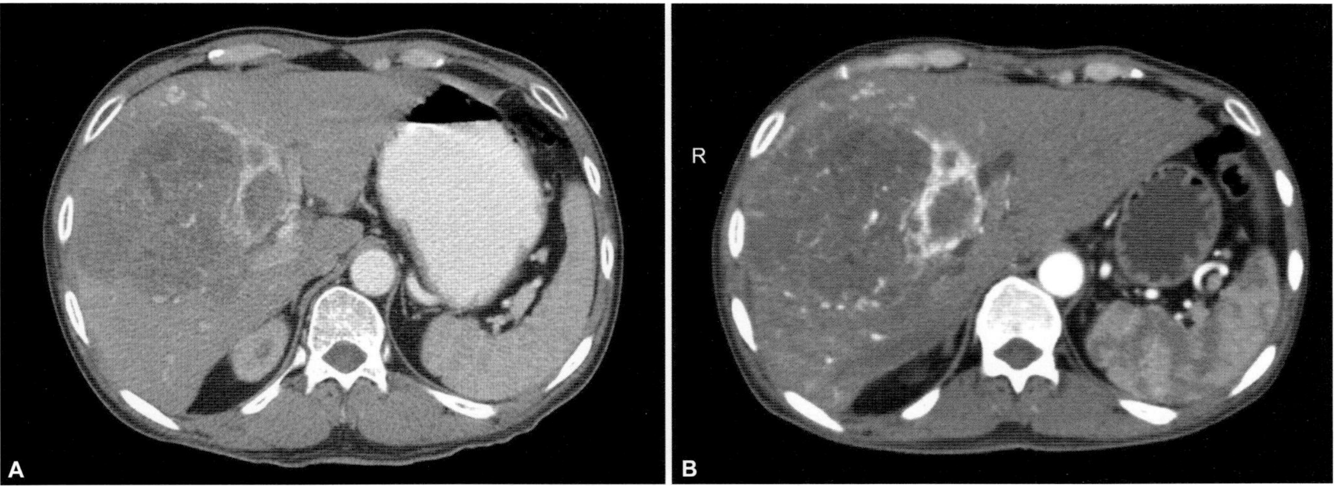

Figures 3A and B GI stromal tumor metastasis treated by 2-stage hepatectomy. (A) Stage 1 involved laparoscopic metastatectomy and right portal vein ligation. (B) Stage 2 consisted of right trisectionectomy

of the remnant. The first stage was usually a minor resection (>3 segments in only 4%) that was performed synchronously with resection of the primary in 30% patients. Most patients (78%) underwent portal vein ligation in the first procedure and more than two-thirds received interval chemotherapy. The second-stage procedure was performed a median of 99 days after the first (range 32–210 days). It was most often a major hepatectomy and was associated with twice the morbidity of the first stage resection (33% vs 14%). The median 3- and 5-year overall survival after this procedure was 60% and 48%. The median disease free survival was 37 months versus 16 months in those who were unable to complete the second stage.

Predictors of failure to complete the second stage procedure included older age, postoperative complications after the first stage, CEA above 200 ng/mL before PVE, a higher mean number of tumors and greater exposure to chemotherapy prior to the first stage. Factors associated with better survival after two-stage resection include: (1) fewer than 6 metastases, (2) absence of extrahepatic disease, (3) adjuvant chemotherapy after second hepatectomy and (4) R0 resection margin.

Portal Vein Ligation with in-situ Split[28,29]

In a recent German multicenter study, Schnitzbauer and colleagues used a modification of the two-stage hepatectomy, designated the "associated liver partition with portal vein ligation staged hepatectomy" (ALPPS). This procedure requires parenchymal transection just to the right of the umbilical fissure with simultaneous right portal vein ligation during the first stage of the operation, followed about a week later by completion right trisectionectomy. The ALPPS procedure resulted in a median increase in volume of the left lateral segment of 74% within 9 days with necrosis of segment IV, but was associated with postoperative bile leak in five and death in three of 25 patients.

The precise role and value of ALPPS are yet to be determined. Its greatest advantage is the degree of hypertrophy and the rapidity of its onset are unparalleled, although right PVE with additional segment 4 vein embolization may produce hypertrophy that is closely comparable. Obviously this procedure is really only appropriate in the context of a right or left trisectionectomy.

Ex-vivo Resections[30]

Centrally located tumors that involve the inferior vena cava or the hepatic veins adjacent to the vena cava are a technical challenge to resect. These patients usually need to be operated upon under total vascular exclusion (TVE) to prevent massive blood loss. The duration of vascular exclusion often exceeds the maximum permissible warm ischemia time tolerated by the liver, particularly when vascular reconstructions are necessary as part of the resection. Liver hypothermia (28°C) greatly prolongs the ability of this organ to withstand TVE. Additional techniques that may extend the benefits of hypothermic TVE are *ante-situm* and *ex-vivo* resections with autotransplantation. *Ex-vivo* resections entail complete removal of the diseased liver including transection of the hepatic vascular inflow and bile duct, and then reimplantation with reconstruction of these structures. However, the morbidity of this procedure is high and the mortality as much as 30%. The *ante-situm* technique allows preservation of the vascular inflow, which is only occluded, thereby minimizing the procedural risk. These techniques are very rarely necessary.

Liver Transplantation[31,32]

A recent publication by Hagness et al. from Norway has rekindled the debate about liver transplantation for unresectable, multiple bilobar CRLM. Transplantation was performed for CRLM in the 1990s and achieved 1- and 5-year survivals of 62% and 18%. However, it was abandoned because of the high rate of recurrence and shortage of organs. The Hagness study reports on outcomes from 21 selected patients and has no control arm. Although the estimated 1- and 5-year survivals were 95% and 60%, essentially all patients had developed extrahepatic tumor recurrence within 2 years of transplantation. None of the patients received postoperative chemotherapy but did receive mTOR inhibitor Sirolimus for immunosuppression. Recurrences were treated with

Table 1: Standard chemotherapy regimens for colorectal liver metastases			
Folfox Regimen (Repeat 2 weekly over 12 cycles)			
Day 1 5 FU bolus 400 mg/m^2 over 2–4 minutes		Day 2 5 FU bolus 400 mg/m^2 over 2–4 minutes	
Leucovorin 200 mg/m^2 over 2 hours	5 FU infusion 600 mg/m^2 over 22 hours	Leucovorin 200 mg/m^2 over 2 hours	5 FU infusion 600 mg/m^2 over 22 hours
Oxaliplatin 85 mg/m^2 over 2 hours			
Folfiri Regimen (Repeat twice weekly over 12 cycles)			
Day 1		Day 2	
Irinotecan 180 mg/m^2 over 1.5 hours		5 FU 400 mg/m^2 bolus followed by 2400 mg/m^2 infusion over 46 hours	
Folinic acid 400 mg/m^2 over 2 hours			
Capeox Regimen (Repeat 3 weekly for 8 cycles)			
Capecitabine 1000 mg/m^2 twice daily for 2 weeks			
Oxaliplatin 135 mg/m^2 over 2 hours			

surgery or ablation so that at a median of 27 months, 33% of patients were tumor free. High tumor load, interval between primary surgery and transplant, and progressive disease on chemotherapy were identified as prognostic factors. This procedure remains highly controversial essentially for the same reasons as before.

SYSTEMIC CHEMOTHERAPY

Randomized trials confirm that systemic chemotherapy improves survival in patients with unresectable CRLM, and as discussed earlier a proportion of these patients may become operable after chemotherapy.[33,34]

Perioperative chemotherapy consists of enough neoadjuvant chemotherapy to assess tumor response, generally 8–12 weeks, followed by a full course of adjuvant chemotherapy after resection. Some trials include hepatic intra-arterial chemotherapy as well.

There is Level 1 evidence to suggest that perioperative chemotherapy prolongs disease free survival, progression free survival and to a lesser extent overall survival in patients with CRLM at the expense of slightly higher non-lethal postoperative complications.[35,36] It also reduces the risk of non-therapeutic laparotomy.[36] An additional benefit is that the response to chemotherapy is assessable and patients who progress on chemotherapy may avoid an unnecessary operation. There is evidence that response rates to chemotherapy in initially resectable liver only disease may be a surrogate marker for subsequent liver resection rates with curative intent.[37]

The decision on whether or not to use neoadjuvant chemotherapy for resectable CRLM is therefore contentious and may need to be individualized. Neoadjuvant chemotherapy may be beneficial in patients with more than 4–6 tumors, extrahepatic disease or in those in whom even a minor reduction in size may make the surgery less challenging (obviate the need to resect a vascular structure), and is perhaps best avoided in the elderly, obese patients, diabetics and those with a borderline liver remnant. In others, the need for preoperative chemotherapy may be decided on the basis of a departmental protocol.

Many units around the world are now going for upfront surgery when the CRLM is resectable and using chemotherapy as an adjuvant with excellent results.[38]

The most commonly used chemotherapy regimens that are recommended currently are FOLFOX, CAPEOX or FOLFIRI[39,40] (Table 1), often in combination with bevacizumab or cetuximab. Response to chemotherapy is to be assessed once every 2–3 months, ideally by PET/CT. Tumors that respond poorly to oxaliplatin based regimes may respond well to irinotecan based regimens, and vice versa. FOLFOXIRI combines both drugs, is very toxic, may be poorly tolerated but is under evaluation—particularly in patients who have received FOLFOX within the past 12 months.

Anti VEGF and Anti EGFR targeted antibodies increase the efficacy of chemotherapy. Bevacizumab (anti VEGF) is an appropriate biological agent to add onto any of the chemotherapeutic regimens. It has the added benefit of protecting the liver from the sinusoidal obstruction syndrome caused by oxaliplatin. Newer anti VEGF antibodies such as aflibercept and regorafenib are under evaluation. Anti EGFR antibodies such as panitumumab and cetuximab are similarly effective—but only in patients with wild type k-ras in tumor tissue.[40]

ABLATIVE THERAPY[41]

Ablative therapies such as radiofrequency, cryoablation or microwave ablation have the potential to provide equivalent survival to surgical resection in carefully selected patients. Patients with up to five tumors, each of which is smaller than 3 cm in diameter may be selected for ablation in patients unsuitable for resection. The aim should be to provide an ablation margin of 5 mm, and these patients need to be followed aggressively with contrast CT or MR to identify residual or recurrent tumor that may occur in between 10% and 40% of patients. There are no prospective controlled studies comparing survival after ablation and resection; retrospective studies show varied, but generally inferior results.

Ablation is perhaps best used as an adjunct to destroy small deeply placed tumors so as to conserve liver parenchyma. Laparoscopic or open surgical ablations are generally more effective than percutaneous techniques that are limited by access.

SYNCHRONOUS LESIONS[42,43]

Approximately 20–25% of patients with CRC will have liver metastases diagnosed at the time of initial presentation and can potentially have both bowel and liver tumors treated simultaneously. Despite the possible benefits in terms of cost, traditionally such patients have been treated with staged resections, and have received chemotherapy between their two operations.

The reason for this is that a number of studies found a higher morbidity and mortality associated with synchronous resections, particularly when the nature of the liver resection was complex. The risk of anastomotic leak and its related mortality was particularly significant. Also, overall survival after synchronous resection was considerably worse than after staged resection. This was believed to be due to the interval between the two resections allowing tumor biology to manifest, occult lesions to become apparent and tumor response to chemotherapy to become evident.

More recently, studies from Mayo Clinic and Memorial Sloan-Kettering demonstrated that synchronous resections could be performed with no greater morbidity and mortality than staged resections. However, the size and number of tumors were less, and there were fewer major resections in the synchronous resection group. Also there were a greater number of right hemicolectomies in this group. The hospital stay and cost of treatment were lower in the synchronous resection group with survival figures comparable to those with staged resections.

Synchronous resections should not be attempted during emergency operations for CRC. Nor should they be performed when the liver is compromised with cirrhosis or when a major hepatectomy is warranted. They should be performed only when surgery for both the primary and the secondary are easy and likely to be uncomplicated.

Liver metastases should not be biopsied routinely at the first operation because there is a high risk of tumor seeding following this procedure.

FOLLOW-UP AFTER LIVER RESECTION[1,39]

Approximately 60% of patients will develop recurrence following resection of CRLM. Of these 20% will recur only within the liver and be suitable for re-resection. Ninety percent of these will become apparent within the first 2 years after initial resection. Re-resection, although technically more demanding, can be performed with a morbidity, mortality and potential for survival similar to the first resection. Therefore it is prudent to follow these patients carefully. The NCCN recommendations for follow-up are: (1) CEA every 3 months for 2 years and every 6 months for the next 3–5 years. (2) CT of the chest, abdomen and pelvis every 3–6 months for 2 years and every 6–12 months up to a total of 5 years and (3) Colonoscopy in 1 year; if no adenoma then after 3 years, and every 5 years thereafter.

Neuroendocrine Liver Metastases

INTRODUCTION[44-47]

Neuroendocrine tumors (NETs) include both carcinoid tumors which arise from the enterochromaffin cells of the GI tract, as well as pancreatic neuroendocrine cells. Most patients with NET have liver metastases. Although estimates vary widely (10–85%), approximately 40% of patients with ileal carcinoids, 80% of those with cecal carcinoids and 30–85% of pancreatic NETs will have liver metastases at presentation. Approximately 10% of patients will present with liver metastases without an apparent primary. Of those who do not have neuroendocrine liver metastases (NELM) at presentation, an additional 25% will develop them during their lifetime.

Table 2: Grading of neuroendocrine tumors

	Mitoses	*Ki 67 Index*
G1	Less than 2/10 HPF	Less than 3%
G2	2–20/10 HPF	3–20%
G3	More than 20/10 HPF	More than 20%

Patients most often present with symptoms as a consequence of the mass effect of the tumor at the site of origin or metastasis (bowel obstruction, GI bleed, abdominal pain), but 25–50% may have functional tumors that present with specific symptoms caused by the proteins they release (such as facial flushing and diarrhea in carcinoids).

Neuroendocrine tumor is generally believed to be an indolent tumor when compared to other tumors from the same site (i.e. adenocarcinoma) and GI NET has a relatively more indolent course than pancreatic NET. However, once liver metastases occur, 5-year survival drops from 75–100% to 13–54%. Median survival once liver metastases develop is 2–4 years without treatment. Tumor grade (G1-3) using the number of mitoses per high power field and the Ki67 index (Table 2) plays an extremely important part in determining survival and treatment options. G1 tumors are extremely indolent and benefit from therapeutic interventions for metastases, while G3 tumors are aggressive and may respond only to chemotherapy.

Staging

In contrast to CRLM, NELM are hyperdense on MDCT scan, particularly in the arterial phase (Figs 4 and 5). Serum Chromogranin A will help in confirming the diagnosis. Hormone studies may help to diagnose specific functioning tumors. Core Needle Biopsy is helpful to determine tumor grade prior to decision-making.

Apart from CT and MR, which have a similar accuracy as for CRLM, patients with NELM should undergo somatostatin receptor scintigraphy (SRS), which is very effective at detecting tumors that express somatostatin receptor 2 on their surface. Only poorly differentiated NET is avid for FDG during PET scan. Gallium labeled somatostatin analogs when combined with PET-CT (68 Ga-DOTATOC PET/CT) increase the diagnostic sensitivity by about 30% over conventional scanning and results in a change in the clinical management of 33–77% NET patients. Apart from helping to stage the disease, SRS also helps to identify patients who may benefit from somatostatin-receptor based radiotherapy.

Surgery[44-47]

Surgery, when possible, is consistently shown to provide a survival benefit to patients with NELM. A recent systematic review considering 29 studies (between 1980 and 2009) found a 5-year OS of 70.5% (range 31–100%) and a 5-year progression free survival of 29% (range 6–66%).[48]

Frilling et al.[49] described three patterns of NELM distribution on imaging that help to determine the nature of optimum surgical treatment. Type I (20–25%): an isolated lesion of any size;

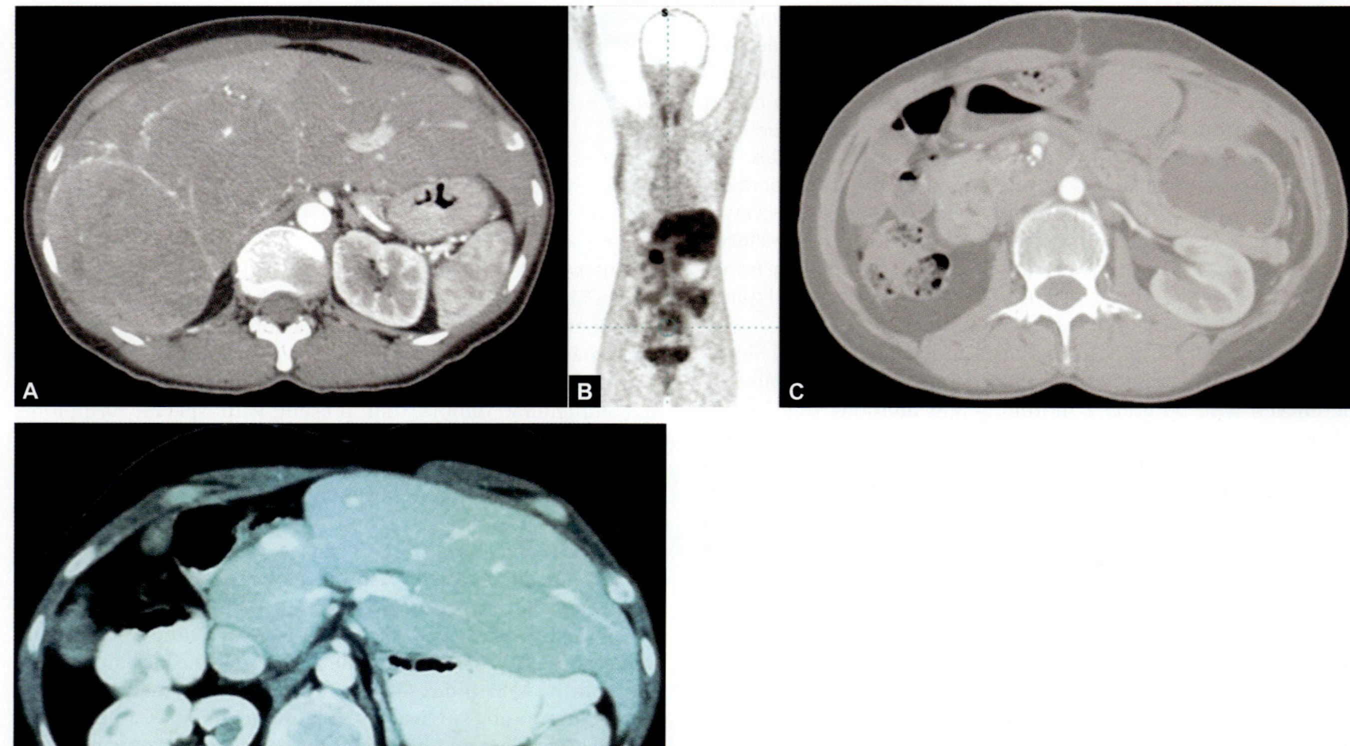

Figures 4A to C (A) Large neuroendocrine metastasis to liver. The patient underwent right trisectionectomy. The primary site was not detected at laparotomy. (B) Primary site in duodenum infiltrating head of pancreas detected at follow-up 8 months later on PET CT. The patient underwent pancreaticoduodenectomy. (C) Two years after completion of pancreaticoduodenectomy and adjuvant chemotherapy

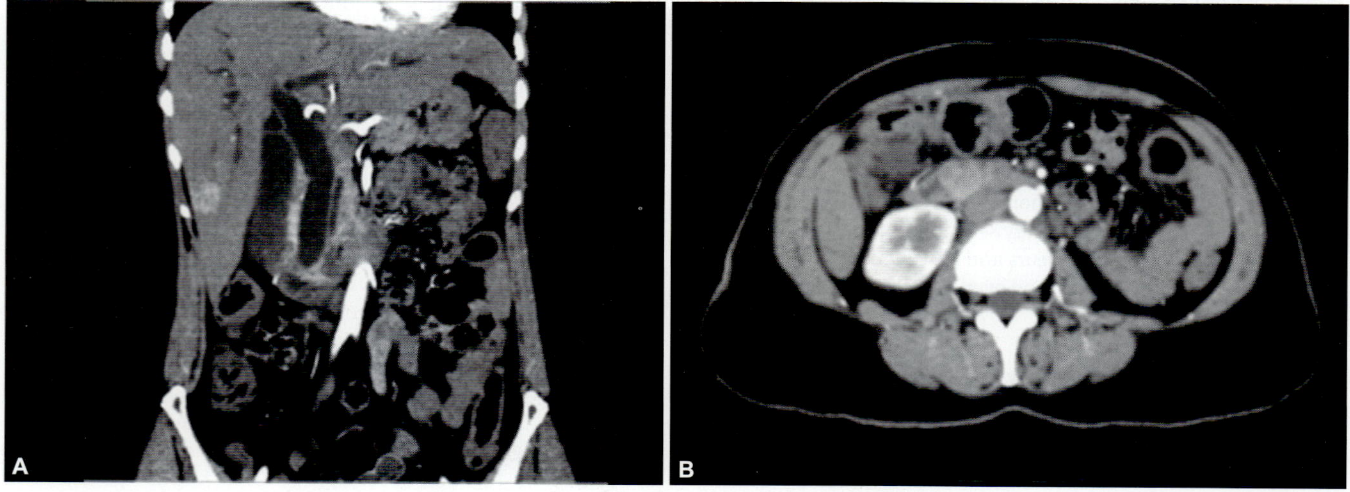

Figures 5A and B (A) Typical hyperdense neuroendocrine liver metastasis in segment 6 with a pancreatic primary obstructing the bile duct. (B) Axial view of the pancreatic primary neuroendocrine tumor. The patient was treated with pancreaticoduodenectomy and metastatectomy

Type II (10–15%): a large focus of metastatic bulk with smaller surrounding lesions, always with involvement of both lobes of the liver and Type III (60–70%): widely disseminated metastatic spread with involvement of both hemilivers and essentially no normal liver parenchyma appreciable on preoperative imaging. Patients in Type I or Type II may be candidates for hepatic resection—particularly those with Grade 1 or Grade 2 tumors, in whom extrahepatic disease has already been resected or can be resected simultaneously, and when there is no significant carcinoid induced cardiac disease (right atrial pressure below 15 mm Hg). Overall 15–50% patients will be candidates for surgical resection.

Mayo et al.[50] reported a multicenter trial including 339 patients with median survival of 125 months, and 5- and 10-year survivals of 74% and 51% respectively. These results have been duplicated at other centers as well. In this study patients with symptomatic, hormonally functional tumors who underwent R0 or R1 resection had the maximum benefit from resection. Contrary to conventional wisdom, patients who underwent R1 resection benefit significantly from resection; 53.7% patients in the Mayo study had R1 resections. However, R0 resection does provide additional benefit over R1 resection (5-year disease recurrence of 10% vs 75%) and concerted attempts should be made to achieve this.[51]

Most patients will have need for resection of tumor from both sides of the liver. The treatment options are therefore multiple metastasectomies, or staged resections combined with radiofrequency ablation or intra-arterial therapies, in an attempt to spare parenchyma. Although some earlier studies suggested that debulking disease improves survival in these patients, this procedure should be used selectively. Symptomatic patients, particularly those with hormonally active tumors are the most likely to benefit from debulking procedures, when greater than 80–90% of the disease can be removed.[52] Surgical treatment of asymptomatic patients with bilateral NELM is highly controversial. Treatment in this setting needs to be highly individualized, using combinations of all the different treatment modalities available, and is best decided upon after discussion at a multidisciplinary meeting.

Radiofrequency or Microwave ablation as a primary modality of treatment provides relief in symptomatic patients, usually with individual tumors below 5 cm in diameter. Studies have reported laparoscopic ablation of 12–15 tumors at one sitting. However, follow-up revealed 50–80% recurrence at 3 years. The role of ablation is suited for use in combination with surgical resection and also for treatment of small recurrences after resection.[44]

Published reports on repeat resections provide survival figures similar to primary resections but selection of these patients is highly individualized and no clear indications for repeat resection have been outlined in any of the studies.[44] Once again, it stands to reason that symptomatic patients with dominant tumor masses that have failed other treatment options might gain maximum benefit from second resections.

Liver transplantation may be considered for more extensive, but relatively stable disease in whom either resection or debulking of more than 90% of liver disease is not feasible, there is no extrahepatic disease, and in whom the primary has been resected at least 1 year prior to consideration of transplant—particularly in those who have failed nonoperative treatment. Gedaly et al.[53] reported the results of 150 patients who underwent transplantation over a 10-year period using information from the UNOS database. They found the 1-, 3- and 5-year survivals to be 81%, 65% and 49% respectively—no different from patients with hepatocellular carcinoma. Le Treut et al.[54] reported an operative mortality of 14% and 5-year survival of 47% in 85 patients with NELM after LT. Other studies have a much smaller number of patients (<20) and report 5-year survival after LT as 67–90%; disease free survival is however low, at 20–48%. Operative mortality in some of these studies were very high but was almost restricted to patients who underwent resection of their primary tumor at the same time as transplantation. Most centers select patients with low grade disease (Ki67 index below 2, or at most 5%). Poorer outcomes were associated with patients older than 55 years of age, hepatomegaly, those who underwent synchronous major extrahepatic resections, and those with pancreatic or duodenal primaries. Mazzaferro et al.[55] could achieve a 90% overall survival and 77% recurrence free survival at 5 years by defining specific criteria for indication of liver transplant in the setting of NELM: (a) well-differentiated NETs (low-grade functioning or nonfunctioning), (b) a prior curatively resected primary tumor drained by the portal system (thereby excluding pulmonary and rectal primaries), (c) less than or equal to 50% metastatic involvement of the liver, (d) good response or stable disease for a minimum of 6 months prior to transplantation and (e) age below 50 years.

Intra-arterial Therapies and Peptide Receptor Radionuclide Therapy[44-47]

Nonendocrine liver metastases should respond well to intra-arterial therapies because they arterially enhance on CT scan and derive most of their blood supply from the hepatic artery. They have been shown to retard tumor growth as well as provide symptom control, particularly in hormonally active tumors. The intra-arterial treatments available include transarterial chemoembolization (TACE), bland embolization (TAE), embolization with drug eluting beads and transarterial radioembolization (TARE) using either resin beads (sirspheres) or glass beads (theraspheres). Peptide receptor radionuclide therapeutic (PRRT) agents such as Y^{90} or Lu^{177} DOTATOC target somatostatin receptors on the tumor cell, and may be administered either intravenously or into the hepatic artery. All these agents provide similar outcomes, and are most suitable for Frilling Type III NELM, or patients with recurrent disease.

TAE and TACE can improve patient symptoms and shrink tumor, showing a complete or partial response for symptoms, circulating biomarkers and imaging in 73–100%, 57–91% and 33–35% patients respectively. The median survival is 24–32 months. Moreover, there is no evidence that TACE is superior to TAE. Doxorubicin or streptozotocin is the cytotoxic agent usually used for TACE; streptozotocin was found to be more efficacious in a recent retrospective study. TAE or TACE are contraindicated in cases of complete portal vein thrombosis and hepatic insufficiency. TACE using drug eluting beads has been shown to be associated with a high incidence of bilomas in patients with NELM and has fallen into disfavor.

TARE using beads with Yttrium (Y^{90}) is a more commonly used alternative when there is portal vein thrombosis or liver insufficiency, although it is more expensive than TACE. TARE is less commonly associated with post-embolization syndrome, and more likely to permit repeated treatments when compared to TACE or TAE. Patients undergoing radioembolization should also have preprocedural evaluation for hepatopulmonary shunts (by macroaggregated albumin scans) to ensure minimal extrahepatic delivery of Yttrium or Lutetium.

Peptide receptor radionuclide therapeutic is most appropriate for patients with extrahepatic disease along with NELM as their effect, when administered intravenously is systemic and not limited to hepatic artery territory.

Mayo et al.[56] reported a large heterogenous series of 753 patients treated with PPRT or surgery. The PPRT patients tended to have greater tumor load, extrahepatic disease or an unknown primary site. However, they identified a subgroup of 118 patients with matching tumor load and clinical characteristics, 52 patients received intra-arterial therapies while 66 patients underwent surgery. Analysis of this subgroup found that resection provided greater survival benefit than IAT (median survival of 38.8 vs 84 months), that symptomatic high volume liver disease (>25% liver volume replaced by disease) was best treated by surgery (median survival 87 vs 51 months), but both treatments were equivalent in the treatment of asymptomatic high-volume liver disease (median survival 16.7 vs 18.5 months). They concluded that in view of the survival advantage, low volume disease and high volume symptomatic disease should preferably be treated by resection/ablation, while high volume asymptomatic disease should be treated by IAT.

External Radiotherapy[44]

Newer forms of external radiotherapy such as stereotactic radiotherapy may be useful to treat small, asymptomatic oligometastases, although perhaps their greatest indication may be in the palliation of symptomatic metastases. Data on outcomes with this form of treatment are very limited, and with the availability of numerous other less expensive therapies, external radiation is rarely used.

Other Medical Therapies[44-46]

Systemic therapies, such as long acting somatostain analogs, chemotherapy and targeted biological therapies may be used as adjuncts to surgery and the intra-arterial therapies for NELM. They will be discussed in detail in the chapter on Neuroendocrine Tumors.

Long acting somatostatin analogs such as octreotide LAR/lanreotide are useful to control hormone related symptoms from these tumors, but have also been shown to stabilize disease in about two-thirds of patients with Grade 1 tumors—particularly in those with a small tumor burden (<10% liver replacement) or after resection. New agents like pasireotide have a 30–40 times greater affinity to somatostatin receptors than lanreotide, and may be effective even after lanreotide is no longer so.

mTOR inhibitors such as everolimus, and tyrosine kinase inhibitors of vascular and epidermal growth factors like sunitinib and bevacizumab are similarly effective. These drugs may be used in patients with extensive disease but with minimal symptoms.

Systemic chemotherapy is useful against symptomatic high grade tumors. Streptozotocin and temozolomide are effective single agents against NELM. Cisplatinum and etoposide are used in combination therapy. Flow chart 1 provides an overview of the treatment of NELM.

Noncolorectal Nonendocrine Liver Metastases[57,58]

The surgical treatment of NCNELM needs to be highly individualized. Treatment of tumors from breast, GI stromal, urological, adrenal and gynecological malignancies is estimated to provide greater than 30% 5-year survival. On the other hand many GI cancers, metastatic squamous cancers from the lung and head and neck have poor outcomes with less than 15% 5-year survival and melanomas have an intermediate survival.

Adam et al.[44] developed a scoring system that may help to determine the anticipated benefit from resection of NCNELM.

Flow chart 1 Algorithm for management of neuroendocrine liver metastases

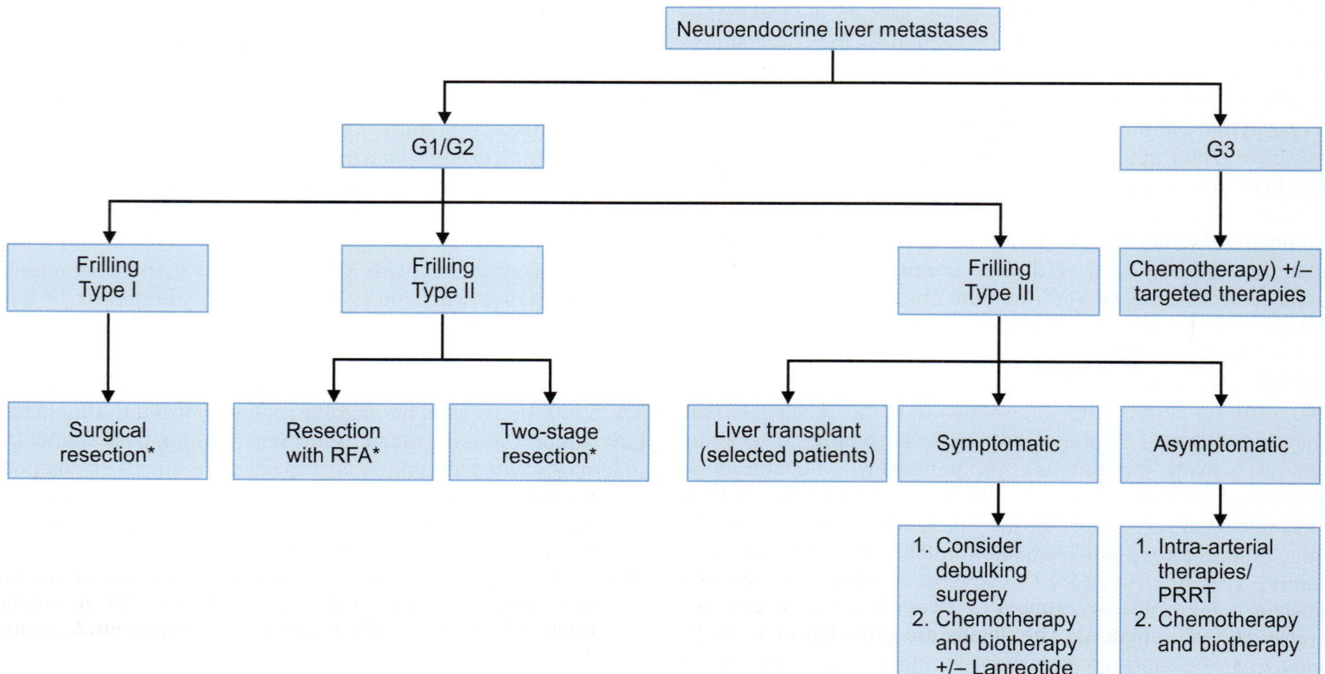

* Add Lanreotide in case of R1/R2 resection or if patient has hormone related symptoms

Table 3: Author's personal experience with surgery for liver metastases

	Colorectal		*Neurendocrine*		*Others*	*Total*
	Sync	*Meta*	*Sync*	*Meta*		
Right lobectomy	1	5	0	2	2	10
Left lobectomy	2	4	0	1	2	9
Bisegmentectomy						
Segments 2 & 3	2	2	1	1	1	7
Segments 5 & 6		1	1		2	4
Segments 7 & 8		1				1
Segments 6 & 7	1				1	2
Segmentectomy	1					1
Central hepatectomy		1		1		2
Right trisectionectomy		1				1
ALPPS left trisectionectomy		1				1
2-stage hepatectomy		1		1		2
Metastatectomy	3	7*	1		1	12

* Four of these procedures were performed in conjunction with either a left hepatectomy or bisegmentectomy, or as part of a 2-stage resection.

Numeric scores were given for six sets of variables. One point was assigned for the presence of each of the following factors: extrahepatic metastases present prior to or at the time of hepatectomy, major hepatectomy and R2 resection. Absence of these factors resulted in an assignment of 0 points for these categories. Two factors (patient age and length of disease free interval between treatment of the primary tumor and diagnosis of metastases) were stratified on a 3-point scale. Patient's less than 30 years of age were assigned 0 points while those 30–60 years of age were assigned 1 point and patients older than 60 years were assigned 2 points. Patients with a disease free interval greater than 24 months were assigned 0 points while those with a disease free interval between 12 and 24 months were assigned 1 point and patients with a disease free interval less than 12 months were assigned 2 points. Finally, the primary tumor characteristics (site and histology) were stratified on a 4-point scale. Patients with breast primary tumors were assigned 0 points, patients with squamous histology were assigned 2 points, and patients with melanoma were assigned 3 points. All other patients were assigned 1 point.

Based on this system, a scale of 0–10 points was obtained with an estimated 5-year survival decreasing from 69% for patients with 0 points to 0% for patients with 10 points. Estimated 5-year survival was over 30% for patients having 0–3 points, 10–30% for those having 4–6 points, and less than 10% for those having more than 6 points.

PERSONAL EXPERIENCE

Between 2006 and 2013, the author has performed 48 liver resections for liver metastases (Table 3). Of these 30 were for CRLM (10 synchronous, 20 metachronous), 9 for neuroendocrine metastases and 9 for noncolorectal nonendocrine metastases (3 breast, 3 GI stromal tumors, 1 head & neck, 1 adrenal, 1 cystadenoma pancreas). The details are provided in Table 2. There was one mortality (synchronous right hepatectomy with right hemicolectomy from anastomotic leak) and 2 patients had transient bile leaks.

REFERENCES

1. Garden OJ, Rees M, Poston GJ, Mirza D, Saunders M, Ledermann J, et al. Guideline for resection of colorectal cancer liver metastases. Gut. 2006;55(Suppl III):iii1-8.
2. Lahr CJ, Soong SJ, Cloud G, Smith JW, Urist MM, Balch CM. A multifactorial analysis of prognostic factors in patients with liver metastases from colorectal carcinoma. J Clin Oncol. 1983;1:720-6.
3. Simmonds PC, Primrose JN, Colquitt JL, Garden OJ, Poston GJ, Rees M. Surgical resection of hepatic metastases from colorectal cancer: a systematic review of published studies. Br J Cancer. 2006;94:982-99.
4. Kronawitter U, Kemeny NE, Heelan R, Fata F, Fong Y. Evaluation of chest computed tomography in the staging of patients with potentially resectable liver metastases from colorectal carcinoma. Cancer. 1999;86:229-35.
5. Ward BA, Miller DL, Frank JA, Dwyer AJ, Simmons JT, Chang R, et al. Prospective evaluation of hepatic imaging studies in the detection of colorectal metastases: correlation with surgical findings. Surgery. 1989;105:180-7.
6. Xu LH, Cai SJ, Cai GX, Peng WJ. Imaging diagnosis of colorectal liver metastases. World J Gastroenterol. 2011;17:4654-9.
7. Floriani I, Torri V, Rulli E, Garavaglia D, Compagnoni A, Salvolini L, et al. Performance of Imaging modalitiesin diagnosis of liver metastases from colorectal cancer: a systematic review and meta-analysis. J Magn Reson Imaging. 2010;31:19-31.
8. McCall JL, Black RB, Rich CA, Harvey JR, Baker RA, Watts JM, et al. The value of serum carcinoembryonic antigen in predicting recurrent disease following curative resection of colorectal cancer. Dis Colon Rectum. 1994;37:875-81.
9. Jamison RL, Donohue JH, Nagorney DM, Rosen CB, Harmsen WS, Ilstrup DM. Hepatic resection for metastatic colorectal cancer results in cure for some patients. Arch Surg. 1997;132:505-10.
10. Rees M, Tekkis PP, Welsh FK, O'Rourke T, John TG. Evaluation of long-term survival after hepatic resection for metastatic colorectal cancer: a multifactorial model of 929 patients. Ann Surg. 2008;247:125-35.
11. Fong Y, Fortner J, Sun RL, Brennan MF, Blumgart LH. Clinical score for predicting recurrence after hepatic resection for metastatic

colorectal cancer: analysis of 1001 consecutive cases. Ann Surg. 1999;230:309-18; discussion 18-21.
12. Pawlik TM, Scoggins CR, Zorzi D, Abdalla EK, Andres A, Eng C, et al. Effect of surgical margin status on survival and site of recurrence after hepatic resection for colorectal metastases. Ann Surg. 2005;241(5):715-22; discussion 722-4.
13. Hughes KS, Simon R, Songhorabodi S, Adson MA, Ilstrup DM, Fortner JG, et al. Resection of the liver for colorectal carcinoma metastases: a multi-institutional study of patterns of recurrence. Surgery. 1986;100:278-84.
14. Andreou A, Aloia TA, Brouquet A, Dickson PV, Zimmitti G, Maru DM, et al. margin status remains an important determinant of survival after surgical resection of colorectal liver metastases in the era of modern chemotherapy. Ann Surg. 2013;257:1079-88.
15. von Heesen M, Schuld J, Sperling J, Grünhage F, Lammert F, Richter S, et al. Parenchyma-preserving hepatic resection for colorectal liver metastases. Langenbecks Arch Surg. 2012;397:383-95.
16. Adam R, de Haas RJ, Wicherts DA, Aloia TA, Delvart V, Azoulay D, et al. Is hepatic resection justified after chemotherapy in patients with colorectal liver metastases and lymph node involvement? J Clin Oncol. 2008;26:3672-80.
17. Rau C, Blanc B, Ronot M, Dokmak S, Aussilhou B, Faivre S, et al. Neither preoperative computed tomography nor intra-operative examination can predict metastatic lymph node in the hepatic pedicle in patients with colorectal liver metastasis. Ann Surg Oncol. 2012;19:163-8.
18. Bennett JJ, Schmidt CR, Klimstra DS, Grobmyer SR, Ishill NM, D'Angelica M, et al. Perihepatic lymph node micrometastases impact outcome after partial hepatectomy for colorectal metastases. Ann Surg Oncol. 2008;15:1130-6.
19. Adam R, Wicherts DA, de Haas RJ, Ciacio O, Lévi F, Paule B, et al. Patients with initially unresectable colorectal liver metastases: is there a possibility of cure? J Clin Oncol. 2009;27:1829-35.
20. Kemeny NE, Melendez FD, Capanu M, Paty PB, Fong Y, Schwartz LH, et al. Conversion to resectability using hepatic artery infusion plus systemic chemotherapy for the treatment of unresectable liver metastases from colorectal carcinoma. J Clin Oncol. 2009;27(21):3465-71.
21. GoéréD, Deshaies I, de Baere T, Boige V, Malka D, Dumont F, et al. Prolonged survival of initially unresectable hepatic colorectal cancer patients treated with hepatic arterial infusion of oxaliplatin followed by radical surgery of metastases. Ann Surg. 2010;251(4):686-91.
22. Ferrero A, Langella S, Russolillo N, Vigano' L, Lo Tesoriere R, Capussotti L. Intraoperative detection of disappearing colorectal liver metastases as a predictor of residual disease. J Gastrointest Surg. 2012;16:806-14.
23. Robinson SM, Wilson CH, Burt AD, Manas DM, White SA. Chemotherapy associated liver injury in patients with colorectal liver metastases: a systematic review and meta-analysis. Ann Surg Oncol. 2012;19:4287-99.
24. Liu H, Zhu S. Present status and future perspectives of preoperative portal vein embolization. Am J Surg. 2009;197:686-90.
25. Lim C, Farges O. Portal vein occlusion before major hepatectomy in patients with colorectal liver metastases: rationale, indications, technical aspects, complications and outcome. J Visc Surg. 2012;149:e86-96.
26. Chua TC, Liauw W, Chu F, Morris DL. Summary outcomes of two-stage resection for advanced colorectal liver metastases. J Surg Oncol. 2013;107:211-6.
27. Jaeck D, Oussoultzoglou E, Rosso E, Greget M, Weber JC, Bachellier P. A two-stage hepatectomy procedure combined with portal vein embolization to achieve curative resection for initially unresectable multipleand bilobar colorectal liver metastases. Ann Surg. 2004;240:1037-51.
28. Schnitzbauer AA, Lang SA, Goessmann H, Nadalin S, Baumgart J, Farkas SA, et al. Right portal vein ligation combined with *in situ* splitting induces rapid left lateral liver lobe hypertrophy enabling two-staged extended right hepatic resection in small-for-size settings. Ann Surg. 2012;255:405-14.
29. Govil S. Rapid improvement in liver volume induced by portal vein ligation and staged hepatectomy: the ALPPS procedure. HPB (Oxford). 2012;14:874.
30. Govil S. Liver resection under hypothermic total vascular exclusion. Indian J Gastroenterol. 2013;32:222-6.
31. Foss A, Adam R, Dueland S. Liver transplantation for colorectal liver metastases: revisiting the concept. Transpl Int. 2010;23:679-85.
32. Hagness M, Foss A, Line PD, Scholz T, Jørgensen PF, Fosby B, et al. Liver transplantation for nonresectable liver metastases from colorectal cancer. Ann Surg. 2013;257:800-6.
33. Simmonds PC. Palliative chemotherapy for advanced colorectal cancer: systematic review and meta-analysis. Colorectal Cancer Collaborative Group. BMJ. 2000;321:531-5.
34. Jonker DJ, Maroun JA, Kocha W. Survival benefit of chemotherapy in metastatic colorectal cancer: a meta-analysis of randomized controlled trials. Br J Cancer. 2000;82:1789-94.
35. Weiser M, Sauerland S, Arnold D, Schmiegel W, Reinacher-Schick A. RPeri-operative chemotherapy for the treatment of resectable liver metastases from colorectal cancer: a systematic review and meta-analysis of randomized trials. BMC Cancer. 2010;10:309-22.
36. Nordlinger B, Sorbye H, Glimelius B, Poston GJ, Schlag PM, Rougier P, et al. Perioperative chemotherapy with FOLFOX4 and surgery versus surgery alone for resectable liver metastases from colorectal cancer (EORTC Intergroup trial 40983): a randomised controlled trial. Lancet. 2008;371(9617):1007-16.
37. Folprecht G, Grothey A, Alberts S, Raab HR, Köhne CH. Neoadjuvant treatment of unresectable colorectal liver metastases: correlation between tumour response and resection rates. Ann Oncol. 2005;16:1311-9.
38. Nanji S, Cleary S, Ryan P, Guindi M, Selvarajah S, Grieg P, et al. Up-front hepatic resection for metastatic colorectal cancer results in favorable long-term survival. Ann Surg Oncol. 2013;20:295-304.
39. National Comprehensive Cancer Network (NCCN) guidelines. Available at: www.nccn.org.
40. Schwarz RE, Berlin JD, Lenz HJ, Nordlinger B, Rubbia-Brandt L, Choti MA. Systemic cytotoxic and biological therapies of colorectal liver metastases: expert consensus statement. HPB (Oxford). 2013;15:106-15.
41. Minami Y, Kudo M. Radiofrequency ablation of liver metastases from colorectal cancer: a literature review. Gut Liver. 2013;7:1-6.
42. Moug S, Horgan P. The role of synchronous proceduresin the treatment of colorectal liver metastases. Surg Oncol. 2007;16:53-8.
43. Pathak S, Sarno G, Nunes QM, Poston GJ. Synchronous resection for colorectal liver metastases: the future. Eur J Surg Oncol. 2010;36:1044-6.
44. Mayo SC, Herman JM, Cosgrove D, Bhagat N, Kamel I, Geschind JH, et al. Emerging approaches in the management of patients with neuroendocrine liver metastasis: role of liver-directed and systemic therapies. J Am Coll Surg. 2013;216:123-34.
45. Rossi RE, Massironi S, Spampatti MP, Conte D, Ciafardini C, Cavalcoli F, et al. Treatment of liver metastases in patients with digestive neuroendocrine tumors. J Gastrointest Surg. 2012;16:1981-92.
46. Baccetti S, Bertozzi S, Londero AL, Uzzau A, Pasqual EM. Surgical treatment and survival in patients with liver metastases from neuroendocrine tumors: a meta-analysis of observational studies. Int J Hepatol. 2013;2013:235040.
47. Jagannath P, Chhabra D, Shrikhande S, Shah R. Surgical treatment of liver metastases in neurendocrine neoplasms. Int J Hepatol. 2012:782672.

48. Saxena A, Chua TC, Perera M, Chu F, Morris DL. Surgical resection of hepatic metastases from neuroendocrine neoplasms: a systematic review. Surgical Oncology. 2012;21:e131-41.
49. Frilling A, Li J, Malamutmann E, Schmid KW, Bockisch A, Broelsch CE. Treatment of liver metastases from neuroendocrine tumours in relation to the extent of hepatic disease. Br J Surg. 2009;96: 175-84.
50. Mayo SC, de Jong MC, Bloomston M, Pulitano C, Clary BM, Reddy SK, et al. Surgical management of hepatic neuroendocrine tumor metastasis: results from an international multi-institutional analysis. Ann Surg Oncol. 2010;17:3129-36.
51. Gomez D, Malik HZ, Al-Mukthar A, "Hepatic resection for metastatic gastrointestinal and pancreatic neuroendocrine tumours: outcome and prognostic predictors," International Hepato-Pancreato-Biliary Association. 2007;9(5):345-51.
52. Sarmiento JM, Heywood G, Rubin J, Ilstrup DM, Nagorney DM, Que FG. Surgical treatment of neuroendocrine metastases to the liver: a plea for resection to increase survival. J Am Coll Surg. 2003;197:29-37.
53. Gedaly R, Daily MF, Davenport D, McHugh PP, Koch A, Angulo P, et al. Liver transplantation for the treatment of liver metastases from neuroendocrine tumors: an analysis of the UNOS database. Arch Surg. 2011;146:953-8.
54. Le Treut YP, Grégoire E, Belghiti J, Boillot O, Soubrane O, Mantion G, et al. Location of the primary tumor and liver size are predictors for survival after liver transplantation for endocrine metastases. An 85-case French multicentric series. Am J Transplant. 2008;8:1205-13.
55. Mazzaferro V, Pulvirenti A, Coppa J. Neuroendocrine tumors metastatic to the liver: how to select patients for liver transplantation? J Hepatol. 2007;47:460-6.
56. Mayo SC, de Jong MC, Bloomston M, Pulitano C, Clary BM, Reddy SK, et al. Surgery versus intra-arterial therapy for neuroendocrine liver metastasis: a multicenter international analysis. Ann Surg Oncol. 2011;18:3657-65.
57. Adam R, Chiche L, Aloia T, Elias D, Salmon R, Rivoire M, et al. Hepatic resection for noncolorectal nonendocrine. liver metastases: analysis of 1452 patients and development of a prognostic model. Ann Surg. 2006;244:524-35.
58. Groeschl RT, Nachmany I, Steel JL, Reddy SK, Glazer ES, de Jong MC, et al. Hepatectomy for noncolorectal non-neuroendocrine metastatic cancer: a multi-institutional analysis. J Am Coll Surg. 2012;214:769-77.

CHAPTER 74

Perioperative Management in Patients with Biliary Tract and Liver Disease

Ankur Garg, Sanjay Singh Negi

INTRODUCTION

The field of hepatobiliary surgery has undergone tremendous transformations over the years. The overall outcomes of hepatobiliary surgery both in terms of morbidity and mortality have improved despite more aggressive and extensive surgery being performed nowadays. These changes are a result of improvement in the perioperative management and technical developments both in the field of surgery and anesthesia.

Due to improved survival of patients with liver diseases surgical intervention is performed more frequently in these patients now than previously. Perioperative risk in these patients needs to be accurately assessed. Optimal outcome depends both on the underlying liver disease as well as the type of procedure performed. Surgery can be of formidable risk in certain conditions (Box 1). The Child-Pugh classification (Child-Turcotte-Pugh score) and the model for end-stage liver disease (MELD) score give a reasonable assessment of perioperative mortality but cannot replace careful preoperative preparation and postoperative monitoring. Formidable procedures in these patients have essential morbidity. Important thing is to recognize them quickly and manage expeditiously. Encephalopathy, ascites, renal dysfunction and coagulopathy should be optimized preoperatively. Perioperative management of these patients covers all the three aspects of preoperative, intraoperative and postoperative care and optimization. Major issues in these areas are tabulated in Box 2.

GENERAL ASSESSMENT AND PREOPERATIVE PREPARATION

The successful outcome of any surgical intervention depends on the patient's ability to tolerate and recover from the stress of the procedure. Such tolerance and performance needs to be assessed and if required optimized before surgery. Although there are many objective criteria on which to base such an assessment, the subjective impression of an experienced and circumspect clinician could be remarkably accurate. The need of thorough history cannot be overemphasized and should be inclusive of any personal or family accounts of liver disease. Even a distant or vague history of hepatitis or jaundice should indicate the need for specific laboratory testing. Also of particular relevance is a history of recent weight loss, exercise intolerance, shortness of breath, smoking, gastrointestinal bleeding, prior surgery or delayed wound healing. In addition to a meticulous general physical evaluation, a focused examination should seek evidence of chronic liver disease such as temporal wasting, scleral icterus, jugular venous distension, supraclavicular adenopathy, diminished breath sounds at the lung bases, gynecomastia, spider angiomata, palmar erythema, splenomegaly, a firm liver edge, peripheral edema or asterixis.

Basic laboratory tests should include a complete blood count, as well as a comprehensive metabolic panel and coagulation profile. Frequently, in elective circumstances, abnormalities may be corrected before surgery. The potential need for intraoperative transfusion should be anticipated during any liver or biliary operation. The use of blood and blood products during liver resection for cancer has been associated with increased rate of recurrence, more postoperative complications and overall worse survival, but transfusion may be unavoidable in major resections.[1] If anemia is absent and a delay is acceptable, then autologous blood donation may be an option. Autologous donation has been associated with an improved prognosis in patients with cirrhosis undergoing resection of hepatocellular carcinoma who are likely to need transfusion.[2] Although there is less evidence with autologous transfusion, the use of banked blood has long been controversial from the standpoint of immune function versus recurrence of malignancy.[3,4] Thrombocytopenia correlates well with portal

Box 1: Contraindications to elective surgery in patients with liver disease

- Acute liver failure
- Acute renal failure
- Acute viral hepatitis
- Alcoholic hepatitis
- Cardiomyopathy
- Hypoxemia
- Severe coagulopathy (despite treatment)

hypertension and diminished hepatocellular function.[5] Although hypersplenism may be associated with a reduction in any of the formed blood elements, a low platelet count is most common.

Abnormalities in electrolytes and intravascular volume are common in patients with liver or biliary tract disease. Patients may display dilutional hyponatremia with peripheral edema and third-space fluid accumulation compounded by hypoalbuminemia. Hypokalemia may result from increased urinary excretion, even with the use of a potassium-sparing diuretic such as spironolactone. Severe hyponatremia should be corrected slowly with free water restriction, albumin infusion, treating sepsis and by discontinuing diuretics. Vaptans are new drugs that are sometimes required for treatment of resistant hyponatremia. Supplemental oral or intravenous potassium may be required to correct hypokalemia. Diminished renal function is often associated with liver disease. Serum blood urea nitrogen and creatinine should be measured, and consideration also should be given to assessment of urine electrolytes and 24-hour creatinine clearance. Ominous signs of hepatorenal syndrome should be sought and treated as it represents a major risk to any contemplated surgical procedure.[6]

Coagulation testing should include a partial thromboplastin time, a prothrombin time (PT), and an international normalized ratio (INR). An additional assessment of fibrinolytic activity requires measuring fibrin degradation products and fibrinogen. Identified abnormalities may better inform preoperative discussion of risks and may prove useful to the anesthesia team. Finally, thorough assessment of cardiopulmonary function should be performed. An electrocardiogram is indicated in patients with previous heart disease and generally appropriate in those older than age 35–40 years, depending on the magnitude of the contemplated procedure. Further, cardiac evaluation may be indicated depending on the history, physical examination, or electrocardiogram abnormalities. For older patients undergoing major hepatic surgery, a cardiac stress test is almost always indicated. In high-risk patients, cardiac catheterization may be advisable. Formal pulmonary function testing should be based on history or clinical findings. Room air-blood gas analysis should be performed in those with significant pulmonary risk factors such as smoking, chronic cough, or shortness of breath.

NUTRITIONAL STATUS AND INTERVENTION

Poor nutritional status is associated with a diminished immune response, an increased susceptibility to infection, poor wound healing, increased risk of organ dysfunction and generally suboptimal outcomes. Despite the significance of nutritional status, none of the many different available methods for its assessment are ideal. The history and physical examination are probably still the most important. Comparison of the patient's current

Box 2: Perioperative issues in patients with biliary tract and liver disease

Preoperative

- General assessment
- Nutrition
- Coagulopathy
- Jaundice
- Issues pertaining to degree of liver damage or hepatic functional reserve and adequate future remnant liver volume
- Renal

Intraoperative

- Anesthesia considerations
- Operative considerations

Postoperative

- Postoperative care
- Post-hepatectomy liver failure

and premorbid state is essential, as an individual who otherwise appears to be of normal weight or build may have started from a baseline of obesity or greater muscular physique. Overt cachexia is common in patients with cirrhosis or malignancy, but more subtle signs of temporal and thenar wasting may be overlooked if not specifically sought.

Objective evaluation of nutritional status includes measurement of serum albumin or other visceral proteins (prealbumin or transferrin), triceps skin fold thickness, total lymphocyte count, and indirect calorimetry. Some of these tests are cumbersome, costly, and not widely available, and none has proven superior to the judgment of an experienced clinician.[7] Characteristics of patients at higher risk include serum albumin less than 3.0 g/dL, weight loss of 10%–15% over a period of 3–4 months, serum transferrin level less than 200 mg/dL, energy to injected skin antigens, functional impairment for ordinary tasks and lack of ability to carry out functional tests to normal capacity such as hand dynamometry.[8] Protein-calorie malnutrition (PCM) due to deficiency of proteins as well as calories is seen in 65–90% of patients with advanced chronic liver disease and in nearly 100% of liver transplant candidates.[9,10] In a prospective cross-sectional study, Padillo et al. evaluated patients with benign and malignant biliary obstructive diseases and identified PCM in 82% of these jaundiced patients. Micronutrient deficiencies may not present with overt cachexia but can have serious consequences in these patients. The duration of jaundice correlated with worsening malnutrition, and patients with malignant obstruction were more likely to have moderate or severe malnutrition than those with benign obstruction.[11,12] A number of studies suggest that serum albumin alone may be the best predictor of morbidity for a range of types of major abdominal surgery.[13,14]

Enteral and parenteral nutritional supplementation with both enteral and parenteral formulas has been used for decades in an effort to improve surgical outcomes.[15] Total parenteral nutrition (TPN) is chosen when the otherwise-preferred enteral route cannot be used. Based on the veterans affairs cooperative study, a minimum of 2 weeks of TPN is required to obtain nutritional enhancement and improve outcomes in severely malnourished patients.[13] Although mildly malnourished patients also showed improvement, it was at the cost of significant increases in noncatheter-related nosocomial infections that negated the benefit. Preoperative TPN has often been found to increase rather than decrease surgical risks.[16] Despite best intentions, patients with cirrhosis or protein and calorie malnutrition resulting from obstructive jaundice are only rarely able to make significant improvement in preoperative nutritional status with a course of enteral supplementation even with detailed instructions. Although decompression of the biliary tree in jaundiced patients can stimulate appetite and calorie intake, the effect is usually insufficient to improve surgical outcome.

Early enteral nutrition in both trauma and burn patients attenuates the inevitable hypercatabolic response.[17] Both animal and human studies have shown that enteral nutrition prevents small bowel disuse atrophy and subsequent bacterial translocation, septic complications, and multisystem organ failure.[18-21] Patients with cirrhosis and biliary obstruction demonstrate reduced capacity to clear translocating bacteria, although the basis for this dysfunction remains to be fully established.[22,23] However, nutritional optimization can offset some of these problems if not wholly.

COAGULOPATHY

Among the potential complications of liver disease, acute hemorrhage is particularly dangerous (Boxes 3 and 4). Diminished synthetic capacity for factors II, VII, IX and X can be recognized by prolongation of the INR or prothrombin time. Whether because of intrinsic parenchymal dysfunction or extrahepatic biliary obstruction, cholestasis further contributes to coagulopathy by inhibiting absorption of vitamin K, on which many clotting factors functionally depend. Thrombocytopenia is also associated with chronic liver disease and is a result of portal hypertension and hypersplenism. The degree of thrombocytopenia appears to roughly correlate with the severity of portal hypertension and cirrhosis. The manifestations of hypersplenism may be improved by transjugular intrahepatic portosystemic shunt (TIPS).[24,25]

Coagulopathy in patients with liver and biliary tract disease is to be treated on the basis of the underlying pathology. Coagulopathy due to malnutrition, biliary obstruction or bacterial overgrowth can be corrected by parenteral vitamin K administration. Active bleeding due to coagulopathy caused by parenchymal injury requires fresh frozen plasma (FFP) for correction. In such patients, FFP should also be transfused before invasive procedures. It is important to realize that more FFP may be required in patients with chronic liver disease than in those with coagulopathy from unrelated causes.[2] Cryoprecipitate is useful in severe coagulopathy with hypofibrinogenemia. It also avoids volume overload. When platelet count is below 50,000/mL single donor or pooled platelets may be required for either active bleeding or any invasive procedure. The use of recombinant factor VIIa, thrombopoietin, antithrombin III, prothrombin complexes and 1-deamino-8-D-arginine vasopressin for correction of coagulopathy and thrombocytopenia, is currently under evaluation.[26]

Box 3: Role of liver in coagulation system

- Synthesis of coagulation factors
- Absorption of vitamin K (II, VII, IX, X)
- Clearance of activated coagulation factors
  - Fibrinogen degradation products
  - Plasminogen activators
- Control of coagulation and thrombosis
  - Antithrombins
  - Protein C and S via vitamin K

Box 4: Consequence of liver disease on coagulation

- Predisposition to disseminated intravascular coagulation
- Accelerated or decreased fibrinolysis
- Thrombocytopenia
- Qualitative defects
  - Platelet function
  - Dysfibrinogenemia
- Fluid overload, dilutional thrombocytopenia
- Increased susceptibility to infection (in turn aggravating the above effects directly or indirectly)

BILIARY OBSTRUCTION AND ROLE OF PREOPERATIVE BILIARY DRAINAGE

Patients with obstructive jaundice are at risk for hepatocellular injury and impaired liver function. Obstructive jaundice leads to hyperbilirubinemia which leads to many alterations, including decreased fat absorption, impaired digestion and hepatic dysfunction. There may be biliary infection and endotoxemia. Nephropathy, hepatorenal syndrome may occur with end stage liver disease. Decreased fat absorption leads to impaired absorption of fat soluble vitamins, immunodeficiency and coagulopathy. There is a plethora of literature on preoperative biliary drainage (PBD) in patients undergoing pancreatoduodenectomy (PD) or hepatic resection and the following paragraphs will highlight the literature available till date.

Preoperative Biliary Drainage in Patients Undergoing Pancreatoduodenectomy

Pancreatic and periampullary cancers commonly present with obstructive jaundice. Surgical resection is the most important intervention for cure.[27-29] PBD reverses the impact of obstruction and was introduced to improve postoperative outcome. In several retrospective and experimental studies PBD reduced morbidity and mortality.[30-33] However, a systematic review and two meta-analyses of randomized trials showed that direct surgery without PBD had lesser complications.[34,35] Procedure for PBD itself was a major source of morbidity. Despite this, PBD became part of the protocol for treatment of these cancers at several centers.[36-38] In 2010, New England Journal of Medicine published data for the randomized control trial (RCT), preoperative drainage versus direct surgery.[39] Patients with bilirubin between 2.3 mg/dL and 14.6 mg/dL were randomized to either direct surgery within a week or PBD for 4–6 weeks followed by surgery (Figs 1 and 2). Drainage was successful in 94% with complications in 46% of the patients. The surgical complication rate was 47% in the drained group versus 37% in the direct group. Severe complications were also more in the preoperative drainage group although length of stay and mortality were similar in the two groups. Authors therefore cautioned against preoperative drainage. In this study, patients with bilirubin more than 15 were excluded where the maximum benefits of a preoperative drainage could be seen. Also, complication rate for endoscopic retrograde

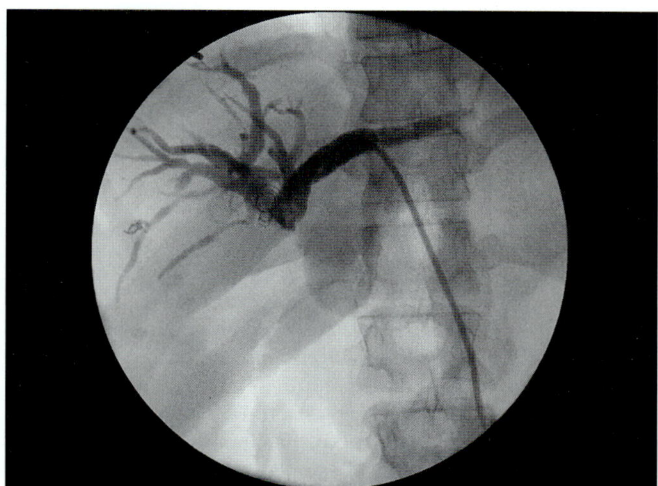

Figure 1 Unilateral (left-sided) percutaneous transhepatic biliary drainage with right-sided portal vein embolization performed in a patient with gall bladder cancer and hilar block

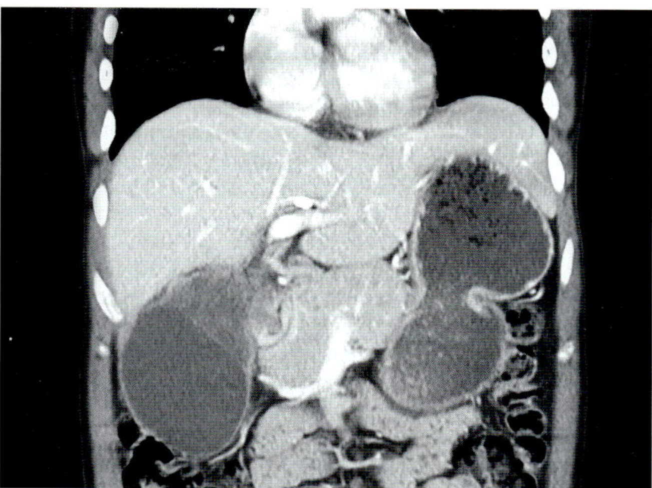

Figure 2 Compensatory hypertrophy of left hemi-liver, 4 weeks after percutaneous transhepatic biliary drainage and portal vein embolization, in the same patient

cholangiopancreatography (ERCP) (46%) was substantially more than other studies (5%–10%).[40-42] Taking all this into consideration one can conclude that there is no benefit from routine PBD in patients undergoing pancreatoduodenectomy. At what level of bilirubin stenting should be done remains controversial. However, there are certain circumstances when it has a definite role, like in patients requiring optimization or nutritional improvement, patients who are selected for neo-adjuvant therapy and patients having preoperative renal dysfunction. It is needless to say that patients who have preoperative cholangitis must undergo stenting. The choice of drainage route is endoscopic in such patients.

Preoperative Biliary Drainage in Patients Undergoing Hepatic Resection

Biliary drainage in patient planned for hepatic resection is mainly indicated in patients with hilar or mid bile duct block. However, these patients have distinctive peculiarities compared with patients of pancreatoduodenectomy. In patients of malignant biliary obstruction undergoing hepatic resection postoperative mortality is almost 10% which is mainly due to hepatic failure.[43] Patients with perihilar cholangiocarcinoma often require extended liver resection. In perioperative assessment accurate preoperative assessment of future liver remnant (FLR) volume and of liver function is mandatory. There is no clear consensus regarding PBD prior to hepatic resection, though it is uniformly agreed to perform PBD in presence of acute cholangitis and in patients' who are expected to have small FLR and are thus candidates for portal vein embolization (PVE).

Hepatic resection in jaundiced patients is associated with higher morbidity and mortality rates due to hemorrhages, sepsis, subphrenic abscesses from biliary fistulae and liver failure in several studies.[44-48] Several studies from Eastern centers advocated PBD to reduce these complications and to increase the resectability.[49-53] Seyama and Makuuchi[54] used preoperative drainage in all their jaundiced patients who were candidates for major bilio-hepatic resection. Authors used drainage in the FLR and the liver resection was performed after the hepatic function was fully restored. Various other studies mainly from the eastern centers and few European centers recommend PBD for perihilar block planned for hepatic resection.[55-60] Studies performed on pathophysiology of jaundice have supported role of PBD. These studies have shown that cholestatic livers were more susceptible to ischemia/reperfusion hepatic damage. Reperfusion and ischemia triggered inflammation and decreased antioxidant activity causing increased activation of coagulation and fibrinolysis.[61,62] A clinical study showed that obstructive cholestasis is associated with a procoagulant state, despite impaired vitamin K-dependent coagulation factor synthesis, which can be reversed by biliary drainage.[63]

In contrast, there is a contrary view which states that PBD is not required and is associated with increased risk of postoperative morbidity with risk of making potentially resectable lesion unresectable in view of increased waiting period postbiliary drainage. Figueras et al.[64] did not find any significant differences in mortality rate (1/11 vs 2/9) or postoperative morbidity (100% vs 66%) in patients of major hepatectomies with or without preoperative drainage. They recommended early surgical resection to avoid deterioration of patient by jaundice. Systematic review in 2011 by Liu et al. also did not find PBD to be beneficial in patients of hilar cholangiocarcinoma.[65] Postoperative complication and infection rates were significantly increased in percutaneous transhepatic biliary drainage (PTBD) group compared with direct surgery. Ferrero et al.[66] in their study also found the septic complications to be increased in the drained patients (40% vs 17%, $P = 0.044$).

To conclude there is divergence of opinion on PBD in jaundiced patients undergoing a major hepatectomy. The need to perform PBD prior to liver resection can be mandated based on surgeon or center policy. Large multicenter RCT is required to reach consensus and recommendations.

It is now safe to say that there is no convincing evidence to support routine PBD. The benefits accrued by PBD are probably nullified by its inherent complications.[67] Alterations of glycogen metabolism, impaired hepatic and renal functions, decreased cell-mediated immunity, increased circulating endotoxins and depressed synthesis of homeostasis factors are the direct result of biliary obstruction, which can potentially jeopardize an operative procedure success, by increasing postoperative mortality and morbidity.[68] The PBD to reduce bilirubin level is a natural recourse to avoid such complications. The percutaneous PTBD in itself can induce inflammatory changes in the bile duct thereby increasing the risk of postoperative biliary anastomotic leak with infectious complications. The clogging of drainage tube and undrained segments can lead to cholangitis. PTBD is one of the most common causes of hemobilia as a result of iatrogenic injury to the peribiliary vascular structure. The anatomical proximity of biliary ducts to the branches of portal and hepatic arterial vasculature, vascular injury not uncommonly accompanies PTBD. In the majority of cases the injury is related to portal venous branches which get controlled after insertion of tubes. On the other hand arterial injuries, though uncommon can call for further intervention in the form of angiographic embolization.[66] Implantation metastases along the catheter tract have been rare but lethal complications. It can preclude surgery in otherwise resectable tumors. The exact rate remains unknown, however, in a study by Sakata et al.[69] it was reported in up to 6% of cases after PTBD. Survival after the detection of implantation metastasis is generally poor. For this reason most Japanese surgeons have stopped doing PTBD for preoperative biliary decompression and have switched over to placing nasobiliary drainage catheters.

HEPATIC FUNCTIONAL RESERVE AND PORTAL VEIN EMBOLIZATION

The question of assessing functional reserve of the liver is central to the idea of successful major liver surgery. However, no reliable single test exists to assess functional hepatic reserve, and in particular, the adequacy of the postoperative remnant liver.[70] Although often not a major concern when the liver is otherwise healthy or the extent of the planned resection is smaller, assessment of functional reserve becomes critical when a major resection such as trisegmentectomy is required or when underlying liver disease is present in order to avoid a lingering postoperative hepatic failure and death.[71] In the field of liver transplantation, the term small-for-size syndrome describes the analogs situation in which an allograft is of inadequate functional capacity.[72] A number of modalities assessing liver function are available[73] including measurement of the clearance of indocyanine green (ICG), a high first-pass, metabolized drug that is excreted into bile. The rate of ICG clearance correlates with hepatocyte function and hepatic blood flow. Biliary ICG excretion corresponds with hepatic adenosine triphosphate (ATP) level and a decrease may reflect a diminution in post resection regenerative capacity. The true clinical usefulness of ICG clearance remains questionable. Over the years a number of other tests have also been employed, including nuclear imaging of the asialoglycoprotein receptor, hippurate ratio determination, the aminopyrine breath test, caffeine-clearance test, galactose-elimination capacity, arterial ketone body ratio, monoethylglycinexylidide, trimethadione and single-photon emission computed tomography.[74] The current best and most commonly used method is volumetric analysis based on axial imaging. It has been suggested that resection of less than 60% of non-tumor-bearing liver is generally acceptable for non-cirrhotic livers. When greater than 60% resection is required, preoperative PVE may be used to increase the size of the anticipated remnant liver.[74] It has been reported that 90% of patients develop hepatic dysfunction, if less than 26% of normal liver remains after trisegmentectomy for colorectal hepatic metastases.[75] Volume assessment is most appropriate when there is no underlying parenchymal disease. Any degree of fibrosis, inflammation or fatty infiltration effectively diminishes the remnant function. In patients with frank cirrhosis, even a small segmental resection may result in hepatic failure.[76] Combining major extrahepatic surgery [e.g. pancreatoduodenetomy/gastrectomy/abdominoperineal resection (APR) or anterior resection] with a major hepatectomy also can precipitate postoperative liver failure.

Portal vein embolization was described by Kinoshita et al. in 1986 and is recommended, if an insufficient functional liver mass is anticipated postoperatively. Postoperative cholestasis, impaired synthetic function and fluid retention may occur in the presence of small FLR. Preoperative PVE induces hypertrophy of the non-embolized liver segments of the FLR by redirecting the portal flow to the segments to be preserved. Recent studies have confirmed the efficacy of PVE, enabling many previously unresectable patients to undergo potentially curative hepatic resection.[77,78] PVE is now considered the standard of care prior to major hepatectomy in many hepatobiliary centers worldwide.[79]

Portal vein embolization can be performed by: (A) transhepatic contralateral approach, (B) Transhepatic ipsilateral approaches, (C) percutaneous transjugular approach and (D) transileocolic venous approach. Transhepatic approaches are used most commonly because of their technical ease. The transhepatic contralateral approach embolizes the portal vein by approaching it via portal radicle in the FLR. This approach may cause injury to the liver lobe to be preserved. For this reason the transhepatic ipsilateral approach has become popular. Hepatic lobe to be resected is traversed in this which is a potentially safer alternative.[80] Percutaneous transjugular approach is technically possible but the experience remains limited.[81] The intraoperative transileocolic venous approach requires laparotomy and anesthesia. It was the initial approach used but now rarely employed. It is used only when combined with some other synchronous procedure requiring laparotomy.[82]

To select patients for PVE one must consider several factors. Patients weight and body surface area, extrahepatic disease, portal hypertension, functional liver remnant and the state of the underlying liver. Complexity of the liver resection and any associated surgery (like pancreatic resection or APR) must be borne in mind.[83,84] Although true FLR limit remains controversial most guidelines suggest a minimum FLR of more than 40, more than 30 and more than 25% for cirrhotic, diseased and normal liver respectively.[85,86]

Portal vein thrombosis, hemorrhage, hemobilia, hepatic failure, nontargeted embolization and subcapsular hematoma have been reported after PVE. In two studies by Di Stefano et al. and Kodama et al.[80,87] reported complication rate after PVE was 12.8% and 14.9% respectively. Increase in FLR has been reported by various authors. Ribero et al.[77] described FLR volume increased from an average of 290 cm^3 before PVE to 440 cm^3 after PVE. The difference between the FLR before and after PVE was 8.8%. In the study by Nagino et al.[78] the calculated volume of the non-embolized hepatic lobe increased from an average of 361 cm^3 before PVE to 460 cm^3 after PVE. The volumetric ratio calculated by the authors, increased from 33% to 43% on an average. Maximal increase occurred in the first 3 weeks and is similar to several recent studies (Figs 1 and 2).[78-89]

Impact of PVE was studied in a recent meta-analysis by Abdulkhir et al. [88] On analyzing 1088 patients of PVE (both percutaneous and transileocolic approaches) success rate was more than 95% and 85% underwent laparotomy for resection. The increase in FLR volume was significantly greater in patients who underwent PVE using a percutaneous compared to transileocolic approach (11.9% vs 9.7%). Major complications were observed in only 2.2% of the patients.

Farges et al.[89] compared the outcomes of 55 patients who underwent right hepatectomy with (n = 28) or without (n = 27) preoperative PVE in a prospective nonrandomized study. Patients with underlying hepatic disease gained from PVE, with a shorter hospital stay and decreased number of postoperative complications. In contrast patients with normal liver did not benefit from PVE. Study was criticized for lack of randomization and the relatively large FLR in several of the patients without underlying hepatic disease who underwent PVE. This again highlighted the need for judicious use of this technique with proper patient selection. Fears of increase in tumor growth have also been expressed. Judiciously used, PVE allows more patients with previously unresectable disease to become surgical candidates and decrease postoperative morbidity.[79]

RENAL FUNCTION STATUS

Renal dysfunction in patients with obstructive jaundice is a well-established phenomenon. Acute renal failure (ARF) occurs in approximately 8–10% of patients undergoing surgery for treatment of obstructive jaundice and contributes to mortality in 70–80% of those who develop ARF. Jaundice without underlying liver disease (i.e. accumulated bile acids/salts), depresses cardiac function, decreases systemic vascular resistance, causes natriuresis and diuresis resulting in volume depletion. All these factors contribute to prerenal type of renal dysfunction. Increased levels of endotoxin and altered nitric oxide levels have deleterious effects on systemic vasculature as well as renal microcirculation leading to acute tubular damage. Infection (cholangitis), surgical intervention triggers events (increased endotoxemia, hypotension) resulting in further damage to renal function.[90,91] Preventive measures include adequate hydration, measures to decrease endotoxemia (viz. supplementation of bile salts, administration of lactulose, prophylactic antibiotics),[92] or internal biliary drainage. Theoretically, internal biliary drainage seems very apt and has been recommended in patients with obstructive jaundice and impaired renal function.[93]

INTRAOPERATIVE MANAGEMENT

Anesthesia Considerations

In addition to the altered hemodynamics, coagulopathy and other systemic effects of liver disease, the hepatic metabolism of many routinely used drugs poses a challenge for intraoperative management. The half-life of drugs cleared by the liver can be significantly prolonged and can thus alter dosage, duration of action and lipid solubility. Ascites or edema present in cirrhotics can increase the volume of distribution. Conversely, in patients with a history of chronic alcohol use, an increased capacity for enzymatic metabolism may result in larger drug requirements during surgery. Because hepatic impairment also leads to decreased serum albumin concentrations, drugs that are usually protein bound may be present at increased plasma concentrations and give rise to an exaggerated response.

Surgical manipulation of the liver significantly increases the hepatic oxygen extraction ratio in connection with splanchnic vasoconstriction.[94] However, portal blood flow can be preserved despite a 20%–60% reduction in blood pressure, provided that the cardiac index is maintained during sodium nitroprusside hypotension.[95] Therefore, a well-planned anesthesia that includes the aforementioned considerations and makes use of the now accepted low central venous pressure technique will allow the greatest success. Low central venous pressure maintained during anesthesia avoids vena cava distention and facilitate hepatic mobilization and dissection of the retrohepatic cava and hepatic veins.[96,97] This is a different outlook from crystalloid fluid loading in the pre-resection phase. The goal in the loading method is to account for expected blood loss by dilutional bleeding. On the contrary, this technique can lead to more blood loss by distending the cava and making venous repair more difficult. Blood loss of more than 5 L has been associated with excess mortality.[98] Consequently, if central venous pressure is lowered from 15 mm Hg to 3 mm Hg, caval blood loss from an injury can be theoretically reduced by a factor of 5. This pressure decrease requires fluid restriction until the resection is completed. Therefore, minimal preoperative fluid is given, and small boluses are used to maintain blood pressure. This strategy requires the close availability of a rapid infusion system to provide emergency fluid and blood infusion. Although a low intraoperative urine volume may result, this is not necessarily associated with an increased incidence of postoperative renal failure.[97] The need for effective communication between the surgeon and anesthesiologist cannot be overemphasized.

Inhalational agents such as isoflurane and desflurane have been studied extensively and found to be safe in patients with liver disease. They both undergo negligible hepatic metabolism and result in no free radical formation.[99] Isoflurane maintains better hepatic blood flow and the hepatic artery buffer response than any other volatile anesthetic.[100] In contrast, halothane and other halogenated hydrocarbons must be avoided. Although halothane is a good general anesthetic for most patients, halothane hepatitis may occur from a single exposure,[101] and multiple exposures can result in fulminant hepatic failure. Although the exact cause remains unclear, hypoxic, metabolic or immunologic mechanisms are likely.[102]

The use of local anesthesia should be encouraged, especially for small procedures. Amide-linked local anesthetics undergo hepatic metabolism and should be used with caution. Regional anesthesia is an excellent adjunct, and continuous epidural catheter placement can enhance pain control in the intraoperative and postoperative period. The problem with the widespread use of regional anesthesia in this population is hemostatic impairment, which contraindicates spinal or epidural puncture.

Operative Considerations

Although preparation for surgery is the key to success, some special intraoperative factors must be considered, as well as the basic tenets of abdominal surgery. Adequate exposure is critical, and proper consideration must be given to the type and extent of the incision. Extension of the incision should be performed whenever safety requires. A dependable self-retaining retractor system is essential.

A variety of methods to limit intraoperative blood loss can be employed. The most common method used to limit blood loss during liver resection is either intermittent or continuous clamping of the portal triad (Pringle maneuver). Use of this technique is limited by the degree of underlying parenchymal disease. A normal liver may tolerate up to a total cumulative clamping time of 1 hour, but a diseased liver will tolerate much less. The use of total vascular occlusion during major liver resection may be feasible but should be discussed well in advance with the anesthesiologist. Venovenous bypass may be a useful adjunct in selected circumstances, such as in patients with large tumors involving the vena cava. Consideration of the placement of feeding tubes for postoperative alimentation should be given. Wound closure can be performed by any standard method but special consideration should be given to those patients with ascites or those at risk for its development.

Postoperative Considerations

Postoperatively, cirrhotic patients may develop hepatic decompensation, including ascites, encephalopathy, coagulopathy, worsening jaundice and renal dysfunction. In presence of any of these features supportive therapy should be immediately started. Rising bilirubin indicates liver failure. Bilirubin can sometimes be elevated due to blood transfusions, infections or resorption of extravasated blood. The prothrombin time is the single best indicator of hepatic synthetic function. Hypoglycemia may occur in patients with decompensated cirrhosis or acute liver failure as a result of depleted hepatic glycogen stores and impaired gluconeogenesis. Serum glucose levels may be erratic and require close monitoring especially when postoperative liver failure is suspected. Careful attention should be paid to the assessment of intravascular volume, which is often difficult in the setting of extravascular volume overload. Intravascular volume maintenance minimizes the risk of hepatic and renal under-perfusion. On the other hand, infusion of too much crystalloid may lead to acute hepatic congestion, increased venous oozing and pulmonary edema, and also cause postoperative ascites, peripheral edema and wound dehiscence. Renal function must be monitored closely. When renal dysfunction is found, the cause should be established and treatment initiated.

Liver failure following hepatectomy is a dreaded complication and a major cause of post-hepatectomy mortality.[103] Post-hepatectomy liver failure (PHLF) is mainly dependent on quality and volume of remnant liver (FLR). Incidence varies from 0% to 2% after resection in normal livers but can reach 7% after major hepatectomy. PHLF in the case of resections on cirrhotic liver ranges from 0% to 10% after limited resection and reaches over 30% after major hepatectomies.[104] International Study Group of Liver Surgery (ISGLS) definition of PHLF is postoperatively acquired deterioration in the ability of the liver to maintain its synthetic, excretory and detoxifying functions, which are characterized by an increased INR and concomitant hyperbilirubinemia on or after postoperative day (POD) 5. Increased INR and hyperbilirubinemia are defined according to the normal range of cut-off levels of the local laboratory. In patients with preoperatively increased INR or increased serum bilirubin concentration, PHLF is defined by an increasing serum bilirubin concentration and increasing INR on or after POD 5 compared with the values of the previous day. Furthermore, the need for clotting factors such as fresh frozen plasma (FFP) to maintain normal INR on or after

Table 1: Grading of post-hepatectomy liver failure[106]

Grade A	PHLF resulting in abnormal laboratory parameters but requiring no change in the clinical management of the patient.
Grade B	PHLF resulting in a deviation from the regular clinical management but manageable without invasive treatment.
Grade C	PHLF resulting in a deviation from the regular clinical management and requiring invasive treatment.

Abbreviation: PHLF, post-hepatectomy liver failure.

Table 2: Risk factors associated with post-hepatectomy liver failure[104,105,108]

Patient-related	• Age of >65 years old • High American Society of Anesthesiology score (ASA), • Malnutrition • Male gender • Diabetes
Liver parenchyma-related	• Cirrhosis and portal hypertension • Long-standing cholestasis • Non-alcoholic steatohepatitis (NASH) • Neo-adjuvant chemotherapy
Liver volume-related	• FLR <20% • Standardized liver volume ratio – <20%, in normal livers – <40%, in cirrhosis (Child A and early B).

Abbreviation: FLR, future liver remnant.

POD 5 in combination with hyperbilirubinemia is considered PHLF.[106] According to Balzan et al., PHLF is characterized by the combination of prothrombin time index less than 50% and serum bilirubin more than 50 µmol/L (i.e. 2.9 mg/dL) on POD 5.[107] Grading of PHLF is given in Table 1. Commonly associated risk factors are tabulated in Table 2.

Prevention of PHLF can be achieved with many measures such as PVE, two-stage hepatectomy, portal vein ligation and in situ splitting, preservation of the hepatic venous outflow, in situ hypothermic perfusion of the liver, splenic artery embolization and hemi-portocaval shunt.[107] Treatment options mainly aim at early identification and supportive management. This includes identification of source of infection, appropriate antimicrobial therapy, recognition of any vascular complication (arterial or venous thrombosis), drainage of intra-abdominal collection, adequate hydration to maintain optimal intravascular volume, nutrition as per requirement, avoidance of hepatotoxic and nephrotoxic drugs, anti-encephalopathy measures, organ support as and when indicated, orthotopic liver transplant especially in nononcologic setting.[108,109]

REFERENCES

1. Cescon M, Vetrone G, Grazi GL, Ramacciato G, Ercolani G, Ravaioli M, et al. Trends in perioperative outcome after hepatic resection. Ann Surg. 2009;249:995-1002.
2. Kato K, Nomoto S, Sugimoto H, Kanazumi N, Takeda S, Nakao A. Autologous blood storage before hepatectomy for hepatocellular carcinoma. Hepatogastroenterology. 2009;56:802-7.

3. Busch OR, Hop WC, Hoynck van Papendrecht MA, Marquet RL, Jeekel J. Blood transfusions and prognosis in colorectal cancer. N Engl J Med. 1993;328:1372-6.
4. Marik PE. The hazards of blood transfusion. Br J Hosp Med. 2009;70:12-5.
5. Pluta A, Gutkowski K, Hartleb M. Coagulopathy in liver diseases. Adv Med Sci. 2010;55:16-21.
6. Venkat D, Venkat KK. Hepatorenal syndrome. South Med J. 2010;103:654-61.
7. Jeejeebhoy KN, Baker JP, Wolman SL, Wesson DE, Langer B, Harrison JE, et al. Critical evaluation of the role of clinical assessment and body composition studies in patients with malnutrition and after total parenteral nutrition. Am J Clin Nutr. 1982;35:1117-27.
8. Sax HC, Souba WW. Enteral and parenteral feedings. Guidelines and recommendations. Med Clin North Am. 1993;77:863-80.
9. Lautz HU, Selberg O, Körber J, Bürger M, Müller MJ. Protein–calorie malnutrition in liver cirrhosis. Clin Investig. 1992;70:478-86.
10. DiCecco SR, Wieners EJ, Wiesner RH, Southorn PA, Plevak DJ, Krom RA. Assessment of nutritional status of patients with end-stage liver disease undergoing liver transplantation. Mayo Clin Proc. 1989;64:95-102.
11. Padillo F, Rodríguez Mf, Hervas A, Miño G, Sitges-Serra A, Pera-Madrazo C. Nutritional assessment of patients with benign and malignant obstructions of the biliary tract. Rev Esp Enferm Dig. 1999;91:622-9.
12. Padillo FJ, Andicoberry B, Muntane J, Lozano JM, Miño G, Sitges-Serra A, et al. Factors predicting nutritional derangements in patients with obstructive jaundice: Multivariate analysis. World J Surg. 2001;25:413-8.
13. Veterans Affairs Total Parenteral Nutrition Cooperative Study Group: Perioperative total parenteral nutrition in surgical patients. N Engl J Med. 1991;325:525-32.
14. Kudsk KA, Tolley EA, DeWitt RC, Janu PG, Blackwell AP, Yeary S, et al. Preoperative albumin and surgical site identify surgical risk for major postoperative complications. JPEN J Parenter Enteral Nutr. 2003;27:1-9.
15. Moore EE, Jones TN. Benefits of immediate jejunostomy feeding after major abdominal trauma—a prospective, randomized study. J Trauma. 1986;26:874-81.
16. Archer SB, Burnett RJ, Fischer JE. Current uses and abuses of total parenteral nutrition. Adv Surg. 1996;29:165-89.
17. Mochizuki H, Trocki O, Dominioni L, Brackett KA, Joffe SN, Alexander JW. Mechanism of prevention of post burn hypermetabolism and catabolism by early enteral feeding. Ann Surg. 1984;200:297-310.
18. Cerra FB, Cheung NK, Fischer JE, Kaplowitz N, Schiff ER, Dienstag JL, et al. Disease-specific amino acid infusion (F080) in hepatic encephalopathy: A prospective, randomized, double-blind, controlled trial. JPEN J Parenter Enteral Nutr. 1985;9:288-95.
19. Alverdy JC, Saunders J, Chamberlin WH, Moss GS. Diagnostic peritoneal lavage in intra-abdominal sepsis. Am Surg. 1988;54:456-9.
20. Qiu JG, Delany HM, Teh EL, Freundlich L, Gliedman ML, Steinberg JJ, et al. Contrasting effects of identical nutrients given parenterally or enterally after 70% hepatectomy: Bacterial translocation. Nutrition. 1997;13:431-7.
21. Alverdy J, Holbrook C, Rocha F, Seiden L, Wu RL, Musch M, et al. Gut-derived sepsis occurs when the right pathogen with the right virulence genes meets the right host: Evidence for in vivo virulence expression in Pseudomonas aeruginosa. Ann Surg. 2000;232:480-9.
22. Zulfikaroglu B, Zulfikaroglu E, Ozmen MM, Ozalp N, Berkem R, Erdogan S, et al. The effect of immunonutrition on bacterial translocation, and intestinal villus atrophy in experimental obstructive jaundice. Clin Nutr. 2003;22:277-81.
23. Chuang JH, Shieh CS, Chang NK, Chen WJ, Lin JN. Role of parenteral nutrition in preventing malnutrition and decreasing bacterial translocation to liver in obstructive jaundice. World J Surg. 1993;17:580-5.
24. Karasu Z, Gurakar A, Kerwin B, Hulagu S, Jazzar A, McFadden R, et al. Effect of transjugular intrahepatic portosystemic shunt on thrombocytopenia associated with cirrhosis. Dig Dis Sci. 2000;45:1971-6.
25. Youssef WI, Salazar F, Dasarathy S, Beddow T, Mullen KD. Role of fresh frozen plasma infusion in correction of coagulopathy of chronic liver disease: A dual phase study. Am J Gastroenterol. 2003;98:1391-4.
26. Kaul VV, Munoz SJ. Coagulopathy of liver disease. Curr Treat Option Gastroenterol. 2000;3:433-8.
27. Guidelines for the management of patients with pancreatic cancer periampullary and ampullary carcinomas. Gut. 2005;54:Suppl 5:v1-16.
28. de Groen PC, Gores GJ, LaRusso NF, Gunderson LL, Nagorney DM. Biliary tract cancers. N Engl J Med. 1999;341:1368-78.
29. Phoa SS, Reeders JW, Rauws EA, De Wit L, Gouma DJ, Laméris JS. Spiral computed tomography for preoperative staging of potentially resectable carcinoma of the pancreatic head. Br J Surg. 1999;86:789-94.
30. Van der Gaag NA, Kloek JJ, de Castro SM, Busch OR, van Gulik TM, Gouma DJ. Preoperative biliary drainage in patients with obstructive jaundice: history and current status. J Gastrointest Surg. 2009;13:814-20.
31. Klinkenbijl JH, Jeekel J, Schmitz PI, Rombout PA, Nix GA, Bruining HA, et al. Carcinoma of the pancreas and periampullary region: palliation versus cure. Br J Surg. 1993;80:1575-8.
32. Trede M, Schwall G. The complications of pancreatectomy. Ann Surg. 1988;207:39-47.
33. Kimmings AN, van Deventer SJ, Obertop H, Rauws EA, Huibregtse K, Gouma DJ. Endotoxin, cytokines, and endotoxin binding proteins in obstructive jaundice and after preoperative biliary drainage. Gut. 2000;46:725-31.
34. Wang Q, Gurusamy KS, Lin H, Xie X, Wang C. Preoperative biliary drainage for obstructive jaundice. Cochrane Database Syst Rev. 2008;3:CD005444.
35. Sewnath ME, Karsten TM, Prins MH, Rauws EJ, Obertop H, Gouma DJ. A meta-analysis on the efficacy of preoperative biliary drainage for tumors causing obstructive jaundice. Ann Surg. 2002;236:17-27.
36. Lillemoe KD. Preoperative biliary drainage and surgical outcome. Ann Surg. 1999;230:143-4.
37. Sewnath ME, Birjmohun RS, Rauws EA, Huibregtse K, Obertop H, Gouma DJ. The effect of preoperative biliary drainage on postoperative complications after pancreaticoduodenectomy. J Am Coll Surg. 2001;192:726-34.
38. Pisters PW, Hudec WA, Hess KR, Lee JE, Vauthey JN, Lahoti S, et al. Effect of preoperative biliary decompression on pancreaticoduodenectomy-associated morbidity in 300 consecutive patients. Ann Surg. 2001;234:47-55.
39. van der Gaag NA, Rauws EA, van Eijck CH, Bruno MJ, van der Harst E, Kubben FJ, et al. Preoperative biliary drainage for cancer of the head of the pancreas. N Engl J Med. 2010;362:129-37.
40. Tsujino T, Isayama H, Koike K. Preoperative drainage in pancreatic cancer. N Engl J Med. 2010;362:1343-4.
41. Baron TH, Kozarek RA. Preoperative biliary stents in pancreatic cancer—proceed with caution. N Engl J Med. 2010;362:170-2.
42. Chen VK, Arguedas MR, Baron TH. Expandable metal biliary stents before pancreaticoduodenectomy for pancreatic cancer: a Monte-Carlo decision analysis. Clin Gastroenterol Hepatol. 2005;3:1229-37.
43. Nagino M, Kamiya J, Uesaka K, Sano T, Yamamoto H, Hayakawa N, et al. Complications of hepatectomy for hilar cholangiocarcinoma. World J Surg. 2001;25:1277-83.

44. Lai EC, Chu KM, Lo CY, Mok FP, Fan ST, Lo CM, et al. Surgery for malignant obstructive jaundice: analysis of mortality. Surgery. 1992;112:891-6.
45. Su CH, P'Eng FK, Lui WY. Factors affecting morbidity and mortality in biliary tract surgery. World J Surg. 1992;16:536-40.
46. Clements WD, Diamond T, Mc Crory DC, Rowlands BJ. Biliary drainage in obstructive jaundice: experimental and clinical aspects. Br J Surg. 1993;80:834-42.
47. Su CH, Tsay SH, Wu CC, Shyr YM, King KL, Lee CH, et al. Factors influencing postoperative morbidity, mortality, and survival after resection for hilar cholangiocarcinoma. Ann Surg. 1996;223:384-94.
48. Cherqui D, Benoist S, Malassagne B, Humeres R, Rodriguez V, Fagniez PL. Major liver resection for carcinoma in jaundiced patients without preoperative biliary drainage. Arch Surg. 2000;135:302-8.
49. Nagino M, Nimura YM. Perihilar cholangiocarcinoma with emphasis on presurgical management. In: Blumgart LH (Ed). Surgery of the liver, biliary tract and pancreas, 4th edition. Philadelphia, PA: Saunders Elsevier; 2006. pp. 804-14.
50. Miyagawa S, Makuuchi M, Kawasaki S. Outcome of extended right hepatectomy after biliary drainage in hilar bile duct cancer. Arch Surg. 1995;130:759-63.
51. Ebata T, Nagino M, Kamiya J, Uesaka K, Nagasaka T, Nimura Y. Hepatectomy with portal vein resection for hilar cholangiocarcinoma: audit of 52 consecutive cases. Ann Surg. 2003;238:720-7.
52. Seyama Y, Kubota K, Sano K, Noie T, Takayama T, Kosuge T, et al. Long-term outcome of extended hemihepatectomy for hilar bile duct cancer with no mortality and high survival rate. Ann Surg. 2003;238:73-83.
53. Nagino M, Takada T, Miyazaki M, Miyakawa S, Tsukada K, Kondo S, et al. Preoperative biliary drainage for biliary tract and ampullary carcinomas. J Hepatobiliary Pancreat Surg. 2008;15:25-30.
54. Seyama Y, Makuuchi M. Current surgical treatment for bile duct cancer. World J Gastroenterol. 2007;13:1505-15.
55. Nimura Y. Preoperative biliary drainage before resection for cholangiocarcinoma (Pro). HPB (Oxford). 2008;10:130-3.
56. Lee SG, Song GW, Hwang S, Ha TY, Moon DB, Jung DH, et al. Surgical treatment of hilar cholangiocarcinoma in the new era: the Asan experience. J Hepatobiliary Pancreat Sci. 2010;17:476-89.
57. Arakura N, Takayama M, Ozaki Y, Maruyama M, Chou Y, Kodama R, et al. Efficacy of preoperative endoscopic nasobiliary drainage for hilar cholangiocarcinoma. J Hepatobiliary Pancreat Surg. 2009;16:473-7.
58. Kawakami H, Kuwatani M, Onodera M, Haba S, Eto K, Ehira N, et al. Endoscopic nasobiliary drainage is the most suitable preoperative biliary drainage method in the management of patients with hilar cholangiocarcinoma. J Gastroenterol. 2011;46:242-8.
59. Hirano S, Kondo S, Tanaka E, Shichinohe T, Tsuchikawa T, Kato K, et al. Outcome of surgical treatment of hilar cholangiocarcinoma: a special reference to postoperative morbidity and mortality. J HepatobiliaryPancreat Sci. 2010;17:455-62.
60. Kloek JJ, van der Gaag NA, Aziz Y, Rauws EA, van Delden OM, Lameris JS, et al. Endoscopic and percutaneous preoperative biliary drainage in patients with suspected hilar cholangiocarcinoma. J Gastrointest Surg. 2010;14:119-25.
61. Kloek JJ, Marsman HA, van Vliet AK, Gouma DJ, 4rv extra van Gulik TM. Biliary drainage attenuates postischemic reperfusion injury in the cholestatic rat liver. Surgery. 2008;144:22-31.
62. Kloek JJ, Levi M, Heger M, van der Loos CM, Gouma DJ, van Gulik TM. Cholestasis enhances liver ischemia/reperfusion-induced coagulation activation in rats. Hepatol Res. 2010;40:204-15.
63. Kloek JJ, Heger M, van der Gaag NA, Beuers U, van Gulik TM, Gouma DJ, et al. Effect of preoperative biliary drainage on coagulation and fibrinolysis in severe obstructive cholestasis. J Clin Gastroenterol. 2010;44:646-52.
64. Figueras J, Llado L, Valls C, Serrano T, Ramos E, Fabregat J, et al. Changing strategies in diagnosis and management of hilar cholangiocarcinoma. Liver Transpl. 2000;6:786-94.
65. Liu F, Li Y, Wei Y. Preoperative biliary drainage before resection for Hilar cholangiocarcinoma: whether or not? A systematic review. Dig Dis Sci. 2011;56:663-72.
66. Ferrero A, Lo Tesoriere R, Viganò L, Caggiano L, Sgotto E, Capussotti L, et al. Preoperative biliary drainage increases infectious complications after hepatectomy for proximal bile duct tumor obstruction. World J Surg. 2009;33:318-25.
67. Qiu YD, Bai JL, Xu FG, Ding YT. Effect of preoperative biliary drainage on malignant obstructive jaundice: a meta-analysis. World J Gastroenterol. 2011;17:391-6.
68. Li Z, Zhang Z, Hu W, Zeng Y, Liu X, Mai G, et al. Pancreaticoduodenectomy with preoperative obstructive jaundice: drainage or not. Pancreas. 2009;38:379-86.
69. Sakata J, Shirai Y, Wakai T, Nomura T, Sakata E, Hatakeyama K. Catheter tract implantation metastases associated with percutaneous biliary drainage for extra hepatic cholangiocarcinoma. World J Gastroenterol. 2005;11:7024-7.
70. Garcea G, Ong SL, Maddern GJ. Predicting liver failure following major hepatectomy. Dig Liver Dis. 2009;41:798-806.
71. Garcea G, Maddern GJ. Liver failure after major hepatic resection. J Hepatobiliary Pancreat Surg. 2009;16:145-55.
72. Emond JC, Renz JF, Ferrell LD, Rosenthal P, Lim RC, Roberts JP, et al. Functional analysis of grafts from living donors. Implications for the treatment of older recipients. Ann Surg. 1996;224:544-52.
73. Manizate F, Hiotis SP, Labow D, Roayaie S, Schwartz M. Liver functional reserve estimation: State of the art and relevance to local treatments. Oncology. 2010;78:131-4.
74. Mullin EJ, Metcalfe MS, Maddern GJ. How much liver resection is too much? Am J Surg. 2005;190:87-97.
75. Shoup M, Gonen M, D'Angelica M, Jarnagin WR, DeMatteo RP, Schwartz LH, et al. Volumetric analysis predicts hepatic dysfunction in patients undergoing major liver resection. J Gastrointest Surg. 2003;7:325-30.
76. van den Broek MA, OldeDamink SW, Dejong CH, Lang H, Malagó M, Jalan R, et al. Liver failure after partial hepatic resection: Definition, pathophysiology, risk factors and treatment. Liver Int. 2008;28:767-80.
77. Ribero D, Abdalla EK, Madoff DC, Donadon M, Loyer E M, Vauthey JN. Portal vein embolization before major hepatectomy and its effects on regeneration, resectability and outcome. Br J Surg. 2007;94:1386-94.
78. Nagino M, Kamiya J, Nishio H, Ebata T, Arai T, Nimura Y. Two hundred forty consecutive portal vein embolizations before extended hepatectomy for biliary cancer: surgical outcome and long-term follow-up. Ann Surg. 2006;243:364-72.
79. Avritscher R, de Baere T, Murthy R, Deschamps F, Madoff DC. Percutaneous transhepatic portal vein embolization: rationale, technique, and outcomes. Semin Intervent Radiol. 2008;25:132-45.
80. Kodama Y, Shimizu T, Endo H, Miyamoto N, Miyasaka K. Complications of percutaneous transhepatic portal vein embolization. J Vasc Interv Radiol. 2002;13:1233-7.
81. Perarnau JM, Daradkeh S, Johann M, Deneuville M, Weinling P, Coniel C. Transjugular preoperative portal embolization (TJPE): a pilot study. Hepatogastroenterology. 2003;50:610-3.
82. Makuuchi M, Thai BL, Takayasu K, Takayama T, Kosuge T, Gunvén P, et al. Preoperative portal embolization to increase safety of major hepatectomy for hilar bile duct carcinoma: a preliminary report. Surgery. 1990;107:521-7.
83. Abdalla EK, Hicks ME, Vauthey JN. Portal vein embolization: rationale, technique and future prospects. Br J Surg. 2001;88:165-75.

84. Abdalla EK, Barnett CC, Doherty D, Curley SA, Vauthey JN. Extended hepatectomy in patients with hepatobiliary malignancies with and without preoperative portal vein embolization. Arch Surg. 2002;137:675-80.
85. Vauthey JN, Abdalla EK, Doherty DA, Gertsch P, Fenstermacher MJ, Loyer EM, et al. Body surface area and body weight predict total liver volume in Western adults. Liver Transpl. 2002;8:233-40.
86. Denys AL, De Baere T, Doenz F. Portal vein embolization: a plea for strict patient selection. AJR Am J Roentgenol. 2006;187:W125.
87. Di Stefano DR, de Baere T, Denys A, Hakime A, Gorin G, Gillet M, et al. Preoperative percutaneous portal vein embolization: evaluation of adverse events in 188 patients. Radiology. 2005;234:625-30.
88. Abulkhir A, Limongelli P, Healey AJ, Damrah O, Tait P, Jackson J, et al. Preoperative portal vein embolization for major liver resection: a meta-analysis. Ann Surg. 2008;247:49-57.
89. Farges O, Belghiti J, Kianmanesh R, Regimbeau JM, Santoro R, Vilgrain V, et al. Portal vein embolization before right hepatectomy: prospective clinical trial. Ann Surg. 2003;237:208-17.
90. Green J, Better OS. Systemic hypotension and renal failure in obstructive jaundice-mechanistic and therapeutic aspects. J Am Soc Nephrol. 1995;5:1853-71.
91. Clarke DL, Pillay Y, Anderson F, Thomson SR. The current standard of care in the periprocedural management of the patient with obstructive jaundice. Ann R Coll Surg Engl. 2006;88:610-6.
92. Pain JA, Cahill CJ, Gilbert JM, Johnson CD, Trapnell JE, Bailey ME. Prevention of postoperative renal dysfunction in patients with obstructive jaundice: a multicentre study of bile salts and lactulose. Br J Surg. 1991;78:467-9.
93. Dumonceau JM, Tringali A, Blero D. European society of gastrointestinal endoscopy endoscopy. biliary stenting: indications, choice of stents and results: European Society of Gastrointestinal Endoscopy (ESGE) clinical guideline. 2012;44:277-98.
94. Whittle BJ, Moncada S. Nitric oxide: The elusive mediator of the hyperdynamic circulation of cirrhosis? Hepatology. 1992;16:1089.
95. Chauvin M, Bonnet F, Montembault C, Lafay M, Curet P, Viars P, et al. Hepatic plasma flow during sodium nitroprusside-induced hypotension in humans. Anesthesiology. 1985;63:287-93.
96. Cunningham JD, Fong Y, Shriver C, Melendez J, Marx WL, Blumgart LH. One hundred consecutive hepatic resections. Blood loss, transfusion and operative technique. Arch Surg. 1994;129:1050-6.
97. Melendez JA, Arslan V, Fischer ME, Wuest D, Jarnagin WR, Fong Y, et al. Perioperative outcomes of major hepatic resections under low central venous pressure anesthesia: Blood loss, blood transfusion, and the risk of postoperative renal dysfunction. J Am Coll Surg. 1998;187:620-5.
98. Yanaga K, Kanematsu T, Takenaka K, Matsumata T, Yoshida Y, Sugimachi K. Hepatic resection for hepatocellular carcinoma in elderly patients. Am J Surg. 1988;155:238-41.
99. Elliott RH, Strunin L. Hepatotoxicity of volatile anaesthetics. Br J Anaesth. 1993;70:339-48.
100. Trey C, Lipworth L, Chalmers TC, Davidson CS, Gottlieb LS, Popper H, et al. Fulminant hepatic failure. Presumable contribution to halothane. N Engl J Med. 1968;279:798-801.
101. Neuberger JM. Halothane and hepatitis. Incidence, predisposing factors and exposure guidelines. Drug Saf. 1990;5:28-38.
102. Hubbard AK, Roth TP, Gandolfi AJ, Brown BR, Webster NR, Nunn JF. Halothane hepatitis patients generate an antibody response toward a covalently bound metabolite of halothane. Anesthesiology. 1988;68:791-6.
103. Poon RT, Fan ST, Lo CM, Liu CL, Lam CM, Yuen WK, et al. Improving perioperative outcome expands the role of hepatectomy in management of benign and malignant hepatobiliary diseases: analysis of 1222 consecutive patients from a prospective database. Ann Surg. 2004;240:698-708.
104. Golse N, Bucur PO, Adam R, Castaing D, Sa Cunha A, Vibert E. New paradigms in post-hepatectomy liver failure. J Gastrointest Surg. 2013;17:593-605.
105. Truant S, Oberlin O, Sergent G, Lebuffe G, Gambiez L, Ernst O, et al. Remnant liver volume to body weight ratio ≥0.5%: a new cut-off to estimate postoperative risks after extended resection in noncirrhotic liver. J Am Coll Surg. 2007;204:22-33.
106. Rahbari NN, Garden OJ, Padbury R, Brooke-Smith M, Crawford M, Adam R, et al. Posthepatectomy liver failure: a definition and grading by the International Study Group of Liver Surgery (ISGLS). Surgery. 2011;149:713-24.
107. Hammond JS, Guha IN, Beckingham IJ, Lobo DN. Prediction, prevention and management of post-resection liver failure. Br J Surg. 2011;98:1188-200.
108. Kishi Y, Abdalla EK, Chun YS, Zorzi D, Madoff DC, Wallace MJ, et al. Three hundred and one consecutive extended right hepatectomies. Transactions of the Meeting of the American Surgical Association. 2009;127:171-9.
109. van den Broek MA, Olde Damink SW, Dejong CH, Lang H, Malagó M, Jalan R, et al. Liver failure after partial hepatic resection: definition, pathophysiology, risk factors and treatment. Liver Int. 2008;26:767-80.

CHAPTER 75

Liver Resection

Girish K Pande, Sujoy Pal

INTRODUCTION AND HISTORY

For many years, the liver was considered a mysterious organ with complex anatomy, a bewildering array of physiological functions and an extraordinary capacity to regenerate. The enormous capacity of the liver to regenerate was first recognized by the Greeks. They have a legend which says that Prometheus stole fire from the Gods and gave it to man. For this, he was punished by Zeus and was chained to a rock. An eagle came and ate his liver by day and it regenerated by night. So, the eagle would return every day to feed on his liver. Despite the fact that the regenerative capacity of liver was recognized thousands of years ago, modern day liver surgery evolved only over the last six decades.

The liver, which was once considered an "untouchable" organ by surgeons, is now amenable to all kinds of surgical procedures. These can range from a minor wedge resection to complex segmental and lobar resections with an acceptable morbidity and mortality. Perhaps no other field of modern surgery has seen such an extraordinary amalgamation of anatomical knowledge, physiological principles, use of modern technology and the art of surgical technique.

The earliest hepatic surgery was performed for trauma. Langenbuch was credited with the first liver resection for a tumor in 1888. In 1891, Wendell performed the first successful major hepatic resection using selective hilar ligation of inflow vessels.[1] Hepatic inflow occlusion was first used by James Hogarth Pringle an Australian born British surgeon in 1908. The further developments made various liver diseases amenable to surgical treatment, either by resection of the liver or transplantation. The refinements in surgical technique coupled with microvascular reconstruction expanded the horizon of liver transplantation making the implantation of a lobe or even a segment of liver possible. In fact, this has opened up the field of living donor transplantation of the liver where a part of the liver is taken from a living donor and transplanted into another person. The first such successful procedure was performed by Professor Russell Strong in Brisbane in 1989.[2]

INDICATIONS FOR LIVER RESECTION

- Cysts
- Primary liver tumors such as hepatocellular carcinoma (HCC) and fibro lamellar HCC
- Primary biliary tumors especially Klatskin tumors
- Secondary liver tumors, e.g. colorectal, neuroendocrine
- Complex liver abscesses both amoebic and pyogenic
- Hydatid disease of the liver
- Large hemangiomas
- Caroli's disease
- Inflammatory pseudotumors
- Refractory hepatolithiasis
- Major liver trauma
- For liver transplantation

SURGICAL ANATOMY AND NOMENCLATURE

The external surface of the liver has markings which helped anatomists to divide it into four lobes: right, left, quadrate and caudate. This division did not take into account the distribution of the hepatic artery, portal venous and the biliary radicles which drain the liver. The surgical and functional anatomy of the liver was studied by pioneers such as James Cantlie,[3] McIndoe and Counsellor[4] and the French surgeon-anatomist Couinaud.[5] They used embryological concepts[6] as the basis to define the anatomy of the liver as follows:

- Primary division of the liver into the right and left side is based on invasion by a single liver mass of the right- and left-sided vitelline veins (the portal vein predecessors).

- Hepatic artery and bile ducts develop much later than the venous circulation. The secondary divisions of these structures correspond to the portal branching on the right side. However, on the left side they branch into two equally sized branches that run into the developing masses of liver tissue on either side of the intrahepatic portion of umbilical vein and provide an arterial and biliary watershed that lies in a plane passing through the umbilical fissure.
- Moulding of the liver is caused by extrahepatic structures which contribute to the lobularity and external shape of the liver.

The American authors classified the liver on the basis of the biliary and arterial anatomy while the French anatomist, Couinaud, based his description on the distribution of the portal pedicles and the location of the hepatic veins. Couinaud's description of the functional anatomy of the liver was based on resin casts of the bile ducts, portal, arterial and hepatic vein branches of more than 100 livers which helped him to decipher a pattern of distribution of these structures within the liver. His description is very detailed and is followed by most surgeons.

As per Couinaud's description[5] there are three hepatic veins (right, middle and left) which drain the liver and join the suprahepatic inferior vena cava (IVC). These hepatic veins lie in three different planes which are termed as portal scissurae (viz. right, middle and left scissurae containing the right, middle and left hepatic veins (LHVs) respectively (Fig. 1). The main scissura, also known as Cantlie's line, is occupied by the middle hepatic vein (MHV) and divides the liver into the functional right and left hemilivers. It also demarcates the vascular watershed between the right and left portal pedicles. The right hemiliver is the larger of the two functional halves comprising between 55% and 60% of the total liver mass. There is no surface marking for the main portal scissura. However, we can deduce this by imagining a plane that passes through a line joining the middle of the gall bladder bed anteroinferiorly to the left of the suprahepatic IVC posterosuperiorly.

The three portal scissurae, occupied by the three hepatic veins, divide the liver into four sectors (Fig. 2). Each of these sectors receives an independent portal pedicle and, hence, has been termed as portal sector. The various planes in which portal pedicles run are called hepatic scissurae, none of which have any natural surface marking, except for the umbilical fissure on the left side and

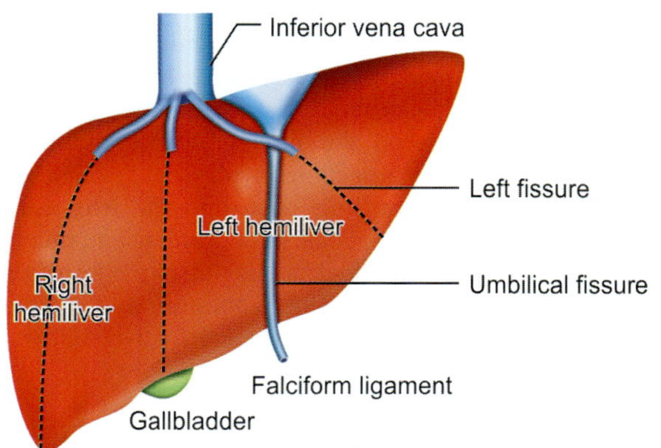

Figure 1 Surface marking of the liver showing the surface markings of the three portal fissures (scissurae) in which the three hepatic veins lie thereby dividing the liver into four portal sectors

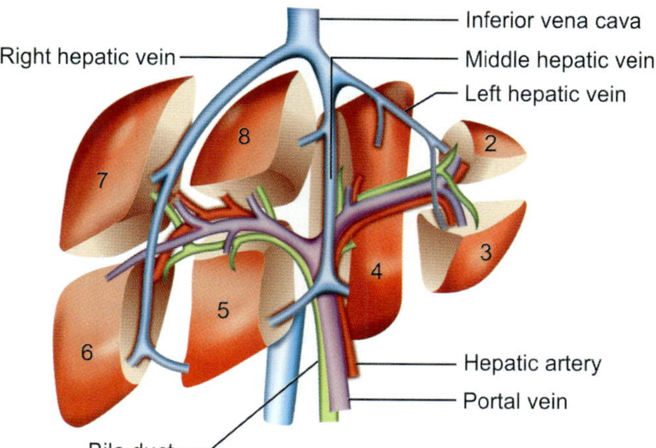

Figure 2 An exploded view of the liver showing the various segments and branching pattern of the main portal vein and the location of the main hepatic veins

occasionally the Rouviere's sulcus on the right side. The Rouviere's sulcus is a deep groove on the inferior surface of the liver to the right of the gall bladder bed. It contains the right posterior sector pedicle. It is also known as incisura dextra of Gans and is present in about 70% of the cases.[7] During laparoscopic cholecystectomy, this sulcus marks a very convenient landmark. It is important to make sure that all the dissection during laparoscopic cholecystectomy is done above this sulcus. Failure to do so can result in damage to the bile duct. The right hemiliver is divided by the right portal scissura [which contains the right hepatic vein (RHV) into an anteromedial (right anterior] and a posterolateral (right posterior) sector. Each of these two sectors is further divided into two segments. The right anterior sector is divided into segment V and VIII, and the right posterior sector into segments VI and VII. Each of these segments receives an independent portal pedicle (Fig. 2).

The left hemiliver is divided into two sectors by the LHV (lying in the left portal scissura) the anterior and posterolateral sector. But, because of the unique umbilical portion of the left portal vein (which lies at the base of the umbilical fissure) the left anterior sector is divided into two segments: medially segment IV (quadrate lobe) and laterally segment III, representing the anterior part of the morphologic left lobe. The posterior sector (posterolateral part) consists of only one segment, and is labeled as segment II (an exception to the nomenclature wherein each sector comprises of two segments). Thus, in total, there are seven segments making the two hemilivers. The segment IV has been further divided into segment IVa and segment IVb, on the basis of a transverse plane passing through the liver at the level of portal bifurcation.[8]

The segment I of liver (so called caudate lobe) rests in a plane posterior to the portal structures and anterior to the IVC. It extends on both sides of the IVC. This segment comprises of the caudate lobe proper which lies mainly on the left side of IVC, the right paracaval portion (also sometimes called segment IX)[9] and a tongue-like projection going to the right which is called as caudate process. From an anatomical point of view, the segment 1 is unique and autonomous because its vascular inflow and outflow are independent of the portal branching pattern and the three major hepatic veins. It receives blood supply from the left as well as the right portal pedicle. The main supply is from the left portal vein and left hepatic artery by one or two branches at the base of the umbilical fissure. It drains directly into the retrohepatic IVC through several small veins (usually 4; range 1-9). Similar to the blood supply, two to three biliary ducts from the caudate lobe proper drain separately at the confluence or into the main left and right hepatic ducts. The bile ducts from the caudate process drain into the right posterior sectoral bile duct.

It is important to realize the anatomic and surgical importance of the fibrous Glisson's capsule which covers the liver and extends into it as sheaths around the hepatic ducts and the branches of hepatic arteries and portal vein. Thus, within the hepatic substance, the individual components of the segmental portal pedicles need not be dissected individually and can be isolated along with the sheath and ligated en masse.[10] These sectoral or segmental pedicles can be approached, either anteriorly (i.e. after the division of liver parenchyma along the various portal scissurae) or posteriorly from behind the porta hepatis (Fig. 2).[11]

Despite a detailed anatomical description by several workers, the terminology used for describing various types of resections has not been consistent and uniform. For example, a right lobectomy may mean a right hemihepatectomy or may denote an extended right hepatectomy. To overcome this confusion in nomenclature of hepatic anatomy and liver resections, the scientific committee of the IHPBA (International Hepato-Pancreato-Biliary Association) created a terminology committee in 1998. The recommendations of the committee were adopted at the World Congress of the IHPBA in Brisbane in 2000 and were termed "The Brisbane 2000 terminology of liver anatomy and resections".[12] These guidelines recommend naming the resection based on the first, second and third order divisions of the bile duct and hepatic artery and are described in detail in Table 1.

CURRENT CONCEPTS OF LIVER REGENERATION

A normal human liver tolerates resections of up to 70% of its functioning mass. This capacity of the mammalian liver to regenerate has been known to mankind for over a millennium. Much of what we know about the kinetics and the basis of liver regeneration is based on the partial hepatectomy models in rats and dogs.[13] Newer experimental models incorporating a portocaval shunt have shed further light on this enigmatic aspect of the liver.[14,15] The acquired knowledge indicates that liver growth is dependent on a multifactorial and multistep process involving interplay of growth-stimulating and growth-inhibiting factors.

At any given time only a few hepatocytes retain the ability to replicate (1 in 20,000). This changes rapidly whenever the functional mass of the liver is reduced by either surgical resection or chemical toxins. After partial hepatectomy between 60% and 90% of the resting hepatocytes abandon "G0" phase to reach the mitotic phase within 24 hours and the process is complete in 7–10 days.[16,17]

Interestingly, all the liver cells do not divide at the same time and rather follow a sequence. The hepatocytes divide first followed by the bile duct cells. This if followed by the Kupffer cells and stellate cells and lastly the endothelial cells. The division of hepatocytes occurs from the periportal to the pericentral area of the liver in the form of a wave. The cells surrounding the central vein are the last to divide. The timing varies in different species.[18] While the process is complete in 7–10 days in the rat, in humans the process is much slower. There is rapid regeneration in the first 2 weeks after hepatectomy. The process then slows down and stops about 6–12 months later. Initially, the liver lobules are larger and the cell plates thicker. Later remodeling takes place and finally, the regenerated liver is similar to the original liver.[19]

Following a 70% liver resection the entire portal blood flow is diverted through the remaining one-third of the liver thus tripling the blood flow. This and other events are the trigger for signaling pathways.[20] One of the first events is an increase of uPA (urokinase-like plasminogen activator).[21] This contributes to remodeling of the extracellular matrix in the liver and the release of growth factors. The proliferation step is guided by a combination of cytokines and growth factors. The most prominent among the growth factors is the hepatocyte growth factor (HGF).[22] Another growth factor involved in the process is the epidermal growth factor (EGF). This is secreted by the Brunner's glands of the duodenum and is present in portal blood. Multiple signaling pathways are involved in the process, the most important being HGF and its receptor cMET. Other agents that play a role include transforming growth factor (TGF) alpha, tumor necrosis factor (TNF), interleukin 6, norepinephrine, bile acids, serotonin, components of complement, leptin and insulin.

One of the most intriguing aspects of liver regeneration is the termination of the process. The number of hepatocytes produced as a result of regeneration often exceeds the original. A wave of apoptosis then occurs at the end of regeneration and the number of cells closely approximates the original number. Livers from larger animals transplanted into smaller ones decrease in size while the opposite is also true. This has raised the concept of a "hepatostat" control system which ensures that the weight of the liver remains optimal for that creature. The process is not well understood but it is speculated that the reassembly of extracellular matrix and sinusoidal capillary network results in matrix driven signaling which results in termination of regeneration.[23]

PREOPERATIVE EVALUATION

The decision to resect either primary or secondary hepatic malignancy is based on a determination that the lesions are resectable from an anatomic viewpoint and the residual liver would be enough to cope with the physiological needs of life. One should also ensure that the primary malignancy is controlled, there is no metastatic disease outside the liver and there is no evidence of decompensated cirrhosis. In cases where oncological principles are not of any concern, (e.g. benign lesions such as hemangiomas, adenomas, etc.) the above statement remains equally applicable as they would also require anatomic resections. Considering these aspects, the preoperative evaluation of a patient undergoing liver resection involves a detailed clinical and laboratory assessment with regard to the liver function, nutritional and performance status, renal, cardiac and pulmonary function, and a detailed radiological imaging of the liver from the surgical point of view. The clinical, laboratory and radiological evaluation also aims at predicting postoperative liver failure.

Clinical Examination

This is directed to look for malnutrition, performance status, any stigmata of chronic hepatocellular dysfunction, presence and depth of jaundice, presence of ascites and evaluation of liver size or

Table 1: International Hepato-Pancreato-Biliary Association Brisbane liver terminology

1 *First-order division*

Anatomical Term	Couinaud segments referred to	Term for surgical resection	Diagram (pertinent area is shaded)
Right Hemiliver **OR** *Right Liver*	*Sg 5-8(+/-Sg1)*	*Right Hepatectomy* **OR** *Right Hemihepatectomy* (stipulate +/-segment 1)	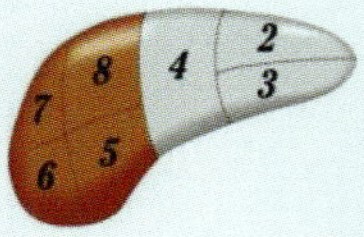
Left Hemiliver **OR** *Left Liver*	*Sg 2-4 (+/-Sg1)*	*Left Hepatectomy* **OR** *Left Hemihepatectomy* (stipulate +/-segment 1)	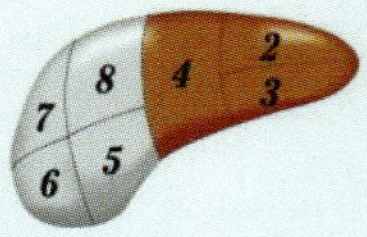

Border or watershed: The border or watershed of the first order division which separates the two hemilivers is a plane which intersects the gallbladder fossa and the fossa for the IVC and is called the midplane of the liver.

2 *Second-order division*

(second-order division based on bile ducts and hepatic artery)

Anatomical Term	Couinaud segments referred to	Term for surgical resection	Diagram (pertinent area is shaded)
Right Anterior Section	*Sg 5,8*	Add (-ectomy)to any of the anatomical terms as in *Right anterior sectionectomy*	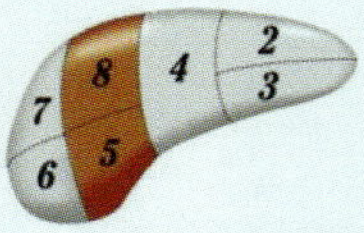
Right Posterior Section	*Sg 6,7*	*Right posterior sectionectomy*	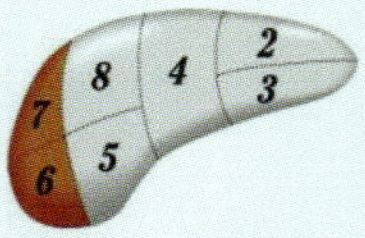
Left Medial Section	*Sg 4*	*Left medial sectionectomy* **OR** *Resection segment 4* (also see Third order) **OR** *Segmentectomy 4* (also see Third order)	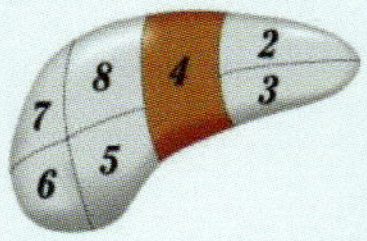
Left Lateral Section	*Sg 2,3*	*Left lateral sectionectomy* **OR** *Bisegmentectomy 2,3* (also see Third order)	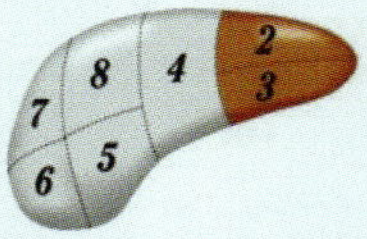

Other "sectional" liver resections

Anatomical Term	Couinaud segments referred to	Term for surgical resection	Diagram (pertinent area is shaded)
	Sg 4-8 (+/-Sg1)	*Right Trisectionectomy* *(preferred term)* **or** *Extended Right Hepatectomy* **or** *Extended Right Hemihepatectomy* (stipulate +/-segment 1)	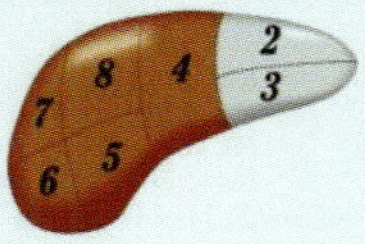
	Sg 2,3,4,5,8 (+/-Sg1)	*Left Trisectionectomy* *(preferred term)* **or** *Extended Left Hepatectomy* **or** *Extended Left Hemihepatectomy* (stipulate +/-segment 1)	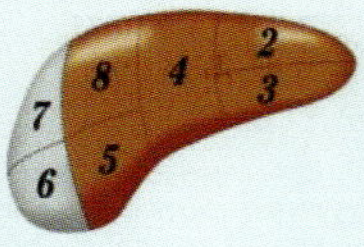

Border or watershed: The borders or watersheds of the sections are planes referred to as the *right and left intersectional planes.* The left intersectional plane passes through the umbilical fissure and the attachment of the falciform ligament. There is no surface marking of the right intersectional plane.

Contd...

Contd...

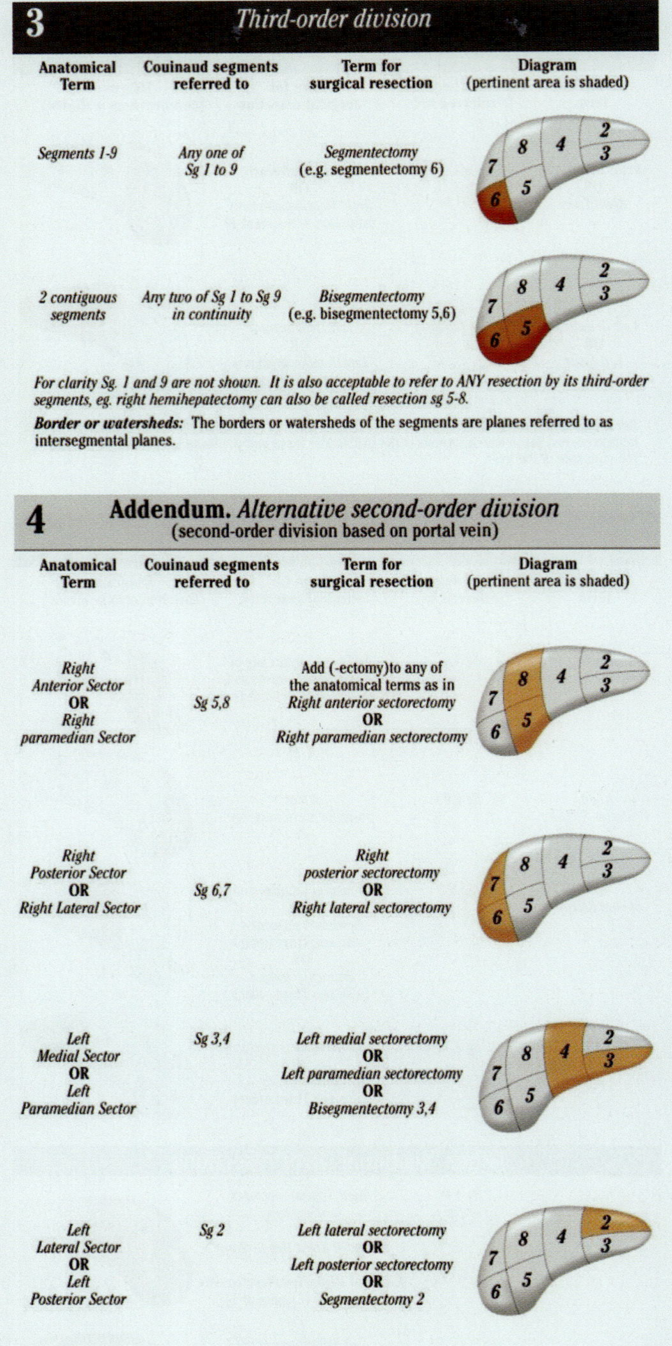

3 *Third-order division*

Anatomical Term	Couinaud segments referred to	Term for surgical resection	Diagram (pertinent area is shaded)
Segments 1-9	*Any one of Sg 1 to 9*	*Segmentectomy* (e.g. segmentectomy 6)	
2 contiguous segments	*Any two of Sg 1 to Sg 9 in continuity*	*Bisegmentectomy* (e.g. bisegmentectomy 5,6)	

For clarity Sg. 1 and 9 are not shown. It is also acceptable to refer to ANY resection by its third-order segments, eg. right hemihepatectomy can also be called resection sg 5-8.

Border or watersheds: The borders or watersheds of the segments are planes referred to as intersegmental planes.

4 **Addendum.** *Alternative second-order division* (second-order division based on portal vein)

Anatomical Term	Couinaud segments referred to	Term for surgical resection	Diagram (pertinent area is shaded)
Right Anterior Sector **OR** *Right paramedian Sector*	*Sg 5,8*	Add (-ectomy)to any of the anatomical terms as in *Right anterior sectorectomy* **OR** *Right paramedian sectorectomy*	
Right Posterior Sector **OR** *Right Lateral Sector*	*Sg 6,7*	*Right posterior sectorectomy* **OR** *Right lateral sectorectomy*	
Left Medial Sector **OR** *Left Paramedian Sector*	*Sg 3,4*	*Left medial sectorectomy* **OR** *Left paramedian sectorectomy* **OR** *Bisegmentectomy 3,4*	
Left Lateral Sector **OR** *Left Posterior Sector*	*Sg 2*	*Left lateral sectorectomy* **OR** *Left posterior sectorectomy* **OR** *Segmentectomy 2*	

Right anterior sector and Right anterior section are synonyms. Right posterior sector and Right posterior section are synonyms. Left medial sector and Left medial section are NOT synonyms and are NOT exchangeable terms. They do not describe the same anatomic areas. Left lateral sector and Left lateral section are also NOT synonyms and are NOT exchangeable terms.

Border or watersheds: The border or watersheds of second-order division based on PV are called right and left intesectoral planes. These have no surface markings.

span, surface and consistency. If presence of portal hypertension is suspected an upper gastrointestinal endoscopy is required to look for varices. The signs of IVC obstruction (lower limb edema, engorged veins on the trunk) indicate the likelihood of IVC involvement either by the tumor thrombus or by direct invasion.

Laboratory Investigations

The liver function test (LFT) looks at enzymes released from the hepatocytes [alanine aminotransferase (ALT) and aspartate aminotransferase (AST)] and those from the bile canaliculi (alkaline phosphatase and gamma-glutamyl transpeptidase). It also looks at the synthetic function of the liver by assessing the total proteins and albumin. An important component is the prothrombin time which is one of the first tests to be deranged in chronic liver disease. This test is helpful in determining the degree of liver dysfunction and differentiating obstructive from hepatocellular jaundice. Patients with hepatocellular jaundice are not good candidates for liver resection. The etiology of hepatocellular disorder can be determined by immunological markers of viral hepatitis B and C, markers for primary biliary cirrhosis and autoimmune chronic active hepatitis and tumor markers such as alpha fetoprotein and des-gamma-carboxyprothrombin[24] in HCC. Serological markers of fibrolamellar HCC are neurotensin and vitamin B12 binding protein. However, their levels are rarely assessed in the management of these tumors. Chromogranin A levels can help to monitor recurrence of carcinoid and other neuroendocrine tumors.

Assessment of Preoperative Functional Status of the Liver

The prediction of postoperative liver function following a major liver resection is crucial especially in patients with underlying cirrhosis and hepatocellular dysfunction. Patients with cirrhosis and chronic active hepatitis have limited hepatic reserve and an impaired ability to regenerate following resection. Therefore, they have a higher chance of developing postoperative liver failure. The preoperative recognition of cirrhosis may alter the intended surgical plan in favor of lesser resections or, in some instances, liver transplantation. A needle biopsy of the remaining liver may be required to confirm cirrhosis or grade the severity of necroinflammatory process in an underlying chronic active hepatitis. A Child-Pugh score, which is based on the clinical and biochemical profile of the patient helps to predict the likelihood of postoperative liver failure and the operative mortality. The reported mortality in patients with Child's A status is 1–2%. However, this can dramatically rise to 10%–50% in those with Child's B and C cirrhosis.[25] Further assessment of liver function in patients with cirrhosis of the liver has been advocated using indocyanine green (ICG) clearance. ICG retention of 10–14% at 15 minutes is considered safe for a major hepatectomy.[26] However, a study from Hong Kong suggests that liver resection can be performed in selected cirrhotic patients with ICG clearance between 15% and 35% with an acceptable morbidity and mortality.[27] Though ICG clearance is routinely used by Japanese workers, its utility remains unproven in non-cirrhotic patients.[26,28] The various other tests described for evaluating liver function such as the aminopyrine breath test, bromsulphalein (BSP) retention test, galactose elimination and xylidide test[29] have not been adopted into routine clinical practice. In general, non-cirrhotic patients who have a large space occupying lesion (SOL), in the absence of any abnormalities of routine biochemical LFTs, are amenable to major resection without any undue risk for post-resection liver failure. As a rule extended resections are precluded in a cirrhotic patient or in a patient with atrophic left lobe (segments II and III). With good patient selection and an adaptation of surgical technique to preserve as much functional liver tissue as possible, selected patients with Child's A cirrhosis can safely undergo segmental hepatic resections.[30,31]

The MELD score (model for end-stage liver disease) was devised as a prognostic measure of short-term mortality in patients with cirrhosis undergoing radiological procedures.[32] The MELD score is derived from a complex formula that uses three biochemical parameters—the serum total bilirubin concentration, serum creatinine concentration and international normalized ratio (INR). The formula for the MELD score is MELD = $9.57 \times \log_e(\text{Cr mg/dL}) + 3.78 \times \log_e(\text{total Bil mg/dL}) + 11.20 \times \log_e(\text{INR}) + 6.43$.[33] A score between 6 and 40 is assigned. It has been found that a score above 9 is associated with increasing morbidity and mortality following liver resection.

Assessment of Patient-related Factors

Apart from the preoperative status of the liver, certain patient-related factors adversely affect the perioperative course and outcome. These include poor performance status, low albumin levels (<3 g/dL) and old age (>65 years).[8,34] Presence of diabetes mellitus and hepatic steatosis decrease the regenerating capacity of the liver and this can lead to a higher incidence of postoperative hepatic dysfunction. The presence of diabetes mellitus is also an independent risk factor for postoperative morbidity and decreased long-term recurrence free survival in patients undergoing major hepatic resection for HCC.[35] Renal function should also be assessed and is a prognostic factor in the postoperative recovery. A score has been developed using multivariate logistic regression analysis to predict postoperative acute renal failure. This uses the preoperative parameters of age, gender, preexisting chronic renal dysfunction, cardiovascular disease, diabetes and bilirubin and ALT levels. It was found that elevated ALT, preexisting cardiovascular disease, chronic renal failure and diabetes were the strongest predictors of postoperative acute renal failure.[36]

Radiological Imaging

In addition to its diagnostic role, radiologic imaging is used to study the liver parenchyma, biliary tree and the relation of the tumor with the inflow (hepatic artery, portal vein) and outflow vessels (hepatic veins and IVC). The detailed imaging has a direct bearing on the decision to operate and the surgical approach. It has been well documented that patients with large primary tumors (>10 cm), multicentricity and infiltration of major vessels have a low resectability rate and poor long-term survival.[8,37] In addition, preoperative estimation of the liver volume with estimates of the likely extent of liver resection and the remaining liver parenchyma, using volumetric analysis based on computed tomography scan, helps in predicting postoperative liver function.[26]

The common modes of liver imaging used are computerized tomography, ultrasonography, magnetic resonance imaging (MRI) and positron emission tomography (PET).

Computerized Tomography

Multi-detector row helical computed tomography scanners have improved the speed of acquisition of images, resolution and the ability to scan the liver during different phases of contrast injection. Normally, the computed tomography scan is performed in the portal phase when a survey is undertaken. However, a staging examination is required when liver resection is being contemplated. In these situations, quadruple-phase examinations are performed. This includes a non-contrast phase, followed by an arterial phase, portal venous phase and lastly the delayed phase. The computed tomography scan has a 93% sensitivity and 100% specificity for detecting liver metastases.[38] It is preferred over the ultrasound scan because it is much less operator-dependent, reproducible and more readily interpretable.[39,40] Also, to study the rest of the abdomen in a single breath hold it gives better information as compared to ultrasonography and MRI.[41] In cirrhotic patients with suspicion of HCC ultrasound is a good screening tool. However, it is not very accurate in detecting small HCC in cirrhotic livers.[42] In this situation contrast-enhanced computed tomography or MRI is preferred. The sensitivity of these techniques ranges from 40% to 70%.[43,44] The arterial phase shows early uptake and quick washout of the contrast occurs during the portal phase. Regenerative nodules on the other hand usually do not take up contrast.[45]

The disadvantage of the computed tomography scanner is the high dose of radiation and poor characterization of lesions smaller than 1 cm. Computed tomography fluoroscopy is a new technique that can help in taking liver biopsies under computed tomography guidance.[46]

Ultrasonography

Conventional ultrasound scanner is considered as the hepatologist's stethoscope due to its widespread availability, mobility, low-cost, real-time imaging and absence of radiation. It is excellent to characterize liver cysts. However, it is not as sensitive as computed tomography in picking up solid focal lesions of the liver, especially the smaller (<1 cm) and superficial ones. However, it is useful in evaluating the biliary tree in patients with obstructive jaundice, for a guided liver biopsy to rule out cirrhosis, for instilling alcohol in tumors and for percutaneous portal vein cannulation and embolization. Doppler ultrasonography is helpful to evaluate the splenoportal vascular axis, hepatic veins and IVC with fair degree of accuracy.[47,48] By the identification of efferent tumor vessels and characterization of intratumoral blood flow, Doppler ultrasonography is helpful in differentiating between a HCC and a hyperplastic nodule.

The development of laparoscopic ultrasonography has allowed better and more accurate tumor staging in patients with primary and secondary liver tumors and helped to avoid unnecessary laparotomy, in a select group of patients. In a study on staging laparoscopy and laparoscopic ultrasonography in 50 patients with potentially resectable liver tumors, laparoscopy precluded curative surgery in 46% of the patients,[49] while laparoscopic ultrasonography identified tumors not visible at laparoscopy in 33% of patients, and provided additional information for more accurate staging in 42% of patients. With the use of above investigations, the resectability rate was 93% compared to 58% in patients in whom operative assessment was undertaken without laparoscopy. The use of laparoscopy is likely to expand with the advent of laparoscopic liver resections.[50] Endoscopic ultrasound (EUS) helps in studying the left lobe of liver and taking biopsies and fine needle aspirates.[51] Ultrasonography-contrast agents are now being deployed and may improve the diagnosis of various liver lesions.[52]

Although not strictly a preoperative investigation, intraoperative ultrasound (IOUS) has been proven to be a useful tool for the evaluation of liver. As IOUS has better resolution due to higher frequency probes (7.5–10 MHz), it helps in better detection of occult hepatic metastases when combined with bimanual digital palpation.[53] Further, the IOUS aids in mapping the relationship of hepatic tumors to major vessels such as the hepatic veins, and helps in avoiding inadvertent injury to them during liver resection. Altogether, the evaluation of the extent of tumor, the confinements imposed by its vascular relations, and the detection of occult metastasis helps in surgical decision making. Bismuth demonstrated that IOUS made a difference in the operative decision making in 24 out of 31 (77%) patients with metastatic gastrointestinal cancer and in 21 out of 79 (27%) patients with primary liver tumors.[54] In addition, for patients in whom segmental resections are planned, IOUS allows selective cannulation of the second and third order branches of the portal vein and delineation of anatomical segments by using vital staining.[55]

MRI and MRCP

Magnetic resonance imaging is probably the best imaging modality for detection and characterization of liver tumors. Many studies have shown that a contrast-enhanced MRI is superior to contrast-enhanced computed tomography and non-contrast MRI in staging liver examinations.[56] Breath hold three-dimensional (3D) imaging and rapid half-Fourier acquisition can image the liver in a single breath hold. Gadolinium diethylene-triamine-penta-acetic-acid (DTPA) is a contrast agent similar to the iodinated contrast agents used in computed tomography scans. It is used to differentiate liver tumors and for magnetic resonance angiography. Mangafodipir, gadobenate and gadodexate (Primovist) are taken up by hepatocytes and ferrum oxides are taken up by Kupffer cells. Iron oxides decrease the intensity of the normal liver on T2 weighted images. The metastases or tumors which do not contain Kupffer cells stand out because their signal is unchanged. However, better images are obtained when hepatocyte-specific T1 contrast agents are used.[57]

Patients with cholangiocarcinoma or gall bladder cancer planned for liver resection require imaging of the biliary system, especially of the proximal biliary tree. Japanese workers preferred percutaneous transhepatic cholangiography (PTC) to accurately map the intrahepatic extent of cholangiocarcinoma prior to surgical resection.[58] In addition, the delineation of biliary anatomy to identify anomalies of intrahepatic biliary radicals, especially on the right side where the right posterior sectoral duct may join the left hepatic duct,[59] is important in patients undergoing extended left hepatectomies (ELH) so as to avoid intraoperative biliary injuries. The advent of magnetic resonance cholangiopancreatography (MRCP) has allowed safe biliary imaging without the inherent risk of infection and other complications related to PTC and endoscopic retrograde cholangiopancreatography (ERCP) due to their invasiveness.

Although the role of angiography, to define the hepatic arterial anatomy and its anomalies before undertaking liver resection, has diminished with the advent of computed tomography angiography, the angiographic techniques are often used for therapeutic purposes such as selective tumor embolization, chemoembolization for advanced or unresectable tumors and for palliation in patients unfit for surgery.[60]

PET Scans

Positron emission tomography is now increasingly being used to detect liver secondaries. The principle of this test is that tumor cells have a higher metabolic rate compared to their surrounding structures. Therefore, they take up more glucose. This uptake is identified with ^{18}F-fluoro-2-deoxy-Dglucose (FDG) PET.[61] Its advantage is a high sensitivity and the chance to image the whole body in a single scan. While this procedure is sensitive any increased metabolic area can give similar uptakes. PET–CT combines the PET scan with computed tomography images taken at the same time to localize the location of increased uptake. PET is not very useful in detecting HCC and its detection of liver metastases is similar to MRI.[62]

Liver Volumetry

Pre-resection and postresection liver volumes can be calculated to a high degree of accuracy using computed tomography scans and MRI scans. Liver volumetry is useful in selecting patients for liver resection and helps to reduce complications.[63]

The minimal volume of normal, non-cirrhotic liver that has to be left behind is suggested to be between 25% and 30%.[64,65] It is now recognized that the required remnant liver volume is determined by the functional status of the remaining liver parenchyma. Major liver resection is less well tolerated in patients with cirrhosis[66] or steatosis of the liver.[67] Also, post-chemotherapy nodular regenerative hyperplasia is considered not to have the same functional capacity as normal liver tissue. Hence, volumetry alone will not help to determine which patients are safe for surgery in these groups. A dynamic functional liver test using a combination of volumetry and ICG clearance may be required in these patients. In patients with HCC and underlying chronic liver disease, a remnant liver volume of more than 250 mL/m^2 has been considered safe. Interestingly, liver volumetry can now be performed using software on a personal computer.[68]

Portal Vein Embolization Prior to Major Hepatic Resections

This technique, developed by Kinoshita et al. in 1986 aims at causing compensatory hypertrophy of the left lobe by embolizing the right portal vein.[69] This decreases the risk of postoperative liver failure in patients undergoing resection of the right lobe of liver, especially if the left lobe is small. Under sonographic and fluoroscopic guidance a tributary of the right portal vein is entered transhepatically.[70] Using the Seldinger technique, the right portal vein is cannulated and then embolized using a 1:4 mixture of cyanoacrylate glue and lipiodol emulsion. The lipiodol contrast permits accurate and selective embolization and also allows visualization of the "portal cast" on subsequent plain radiographs. After embolization the patient remains in hospital for a few days and the LFT and clinical condition is monitored daily. Repeat computed tomography scanning is preformed 4 weeks after the procedure and compared with a pre-embolization computed tomography to determine the extent of compensatory hypertrophy of the left lobe volumetrically. The hepatic resection is performed once optimal hypertrophy has occurred. Volumetric measurements have shown that the portal vein embolization induces compensatory hypertrophy of the remnant liver ranging from 24% to 54% over a period of 4–6 weeks, thus allowing hepatectomy to be performed safely.[71] So far, this technique has had no significant morbidity and is feasible in 90% of the cases being considered for major resections.[70] In those patients, where portal vein embolization is not possible under radiological guidance, it can be performed surgically, through a right iliac fossa incision, using the ileocolic vein and guiding the catheter into the right portal vein under fluoroscopic assistance.[72]

PREOPERATIVE PREPARATION

The preoperative preparation aims at vigorous chest physiotherapy, deep breathing exercises, incentive spirometry and parenteral or enteral hyperalimentation with high protein content to attain the best possible general condition for a major operation. A randomized trial has shown that perioperative parenteral hyperalimentation, using branched chain amino acid (BCAA) and medium chain triglyceride infusions, in cirrhotic patients with HCC undergoing liver resection, significantly reduced the incidence of postoperative septic complications.[73,74] To decrease the gut-derived endotoxin load in patients with cirrhosis and those with obstructive jaundice, bowel preparation using mechanical cleansing (bowel washes, enemas) and topical antibiotics, is initiated well in time before the scheduled day of operation. Jaundiced patients are hydrated well with intravenous crystalloids over a period of 2–3 days.[75] Prothrombin time is corrected using vitamin K injections. A broad-spectrum parenteral antibiotic regimen is started on the day of operation, before the patient is shifted to the operating room and is continued for 3–5 days depending on the postoperative course.

TECHNIQUES OF LIVER TRANSECTION

Operative blood loss during liver resection had been the main fear in the surgeon's mind and was an important reason for the liver to be considered an untouchable organ. Presently, the amount of blood loss and its influence on the postoperative course is well recognized in patients undergoing major liver resections.[76,77] Excessive hemorrhage can increase the risk of operative morbidity and mortality. It also leads to perioperative blood transfusion which causes immunosuppression. This in turn jeopardizes long-term survival after resection of liver malignancies because the associated immunosuppression leads to a higher risk of tumor recurrence.[78,79] The operative blood loss is likely to occur during the dissection phase while isolating inflow and outflow vessels, during the parenchymal transection, or during the revascularization phase (i.e. after the clamp on the inflow vessels is released) of the procedure. During the dissection phase, meticulous technique helps in avoiding excessive hemorrhage. IOUS can be used to determine the location and branching pattern of major vessels to avoid damaging them. During the parenchymal division the bleeding occurs from the arterial and portal branches, and from the hepatic veins and their tributaries.

Low Central Venous Pressure

It has been noticed that most of the bleeding occurs from branches of the hepatic veins. In fact, reducing the central venous pressure (CVP) to around 5 cm water helps to reduce the bleeding.[80] The low CVP is achieved by a combination of change of posture, restriction of fluids and use of diuretics, vasodilators and agents such as isoflurane that cause vasodilation. The patient is placed in a 15° Trendelenburg position to help protect the brain. There is a risk of air embolism when a low CVP is maintained. However, clinically significant air embolism is seldom seen. Wang et al. showed in a randomized controlled trial (RCT) that low CVP (2–4 mm Hg) during liver transection resulted in significant reduction in blood loss and hospital stay as compared to normal CVP.[81]

Delineation of the Proper Transection Plane

It is important to define the correct plane for liver transection. This helps to provide a proper tumor free margin and prevents inadvertent damage to important biliary and vascular structures. The first step is to study the computed tomography scan and plan the resection well. IOUS helps to define the limits of the tumor and position of intrahepatic portal and hepatic vein pedicles. It can be used to mark the transection plane on the surface. During surgery it is important to ensure the correct plane of transection is maintained. To achieve it the liver should be mobilized completely. This is done by dividing the falciform ligament, the right triangular ligament and the left triangular ligament. This helps to rotate the liver and orient the surgeon to the correct plane of transection.

Methods of Liver Transection

Hepatic resection was associated with a mortality of 10–20% in the 1980s.[82] It has been reduced to less than 5% in most major centers now.[83] Various methods can be utilized to transect the liver as detailed below:

Finger Fracture or Clamp Crushing

The liver capsule is divided with diathermy and the parenchyma is crushed between the surgeon's fingers. Vascular and bile duct structures feel like a "band" and are divided between ligatures. The technique was described by Lin in 1960[84] and modified by Ton That Tung in 1963 who occluded the portal pedicle and then transected the liver by finger fracture.[85] Lin later modified his technique and used the Kelly clamp to crush the liver and delineate the vascular and biliary channels.[86] It is now a widely used technique for liver resection.[87]

Water Jet Transection

This technique was first used in 1980s and uses a pressurized jet of water to fragment the liver tissue and expose the vascular and ductal structures.[88] Water jets using a pressure of 20,000–55,000 pounds/square inch (PSI) are used in industry to cut steel. This jet has been modified for the medical industry. Typically, the jet uses a pressure of 30–40 bar with a nozzle of 0.1 mm. This is combined with a suction device which clears the surgical field of blood and hepatocytes. The capsule is incised with a diathermy and the water jet is applied on the liver parenchyma, rapidly moving it along the dissection line. In a randomized trial, comparing cavitron ultrasonic surgical aspirator (CUSA) and water jet with about 30 patients in each arm, water jet was found to reduce blood loss, blood transfusion and transection time compared to CUSA.[89] The water jet has not become very popular because of the fear of splash back of the water from the tissues. There is also a risk of contamination of the operation theater and dissemination of cancer cells. Hand pieces for laparoscopic work have also been designed.

Ultrasonic Dissection

These devices use low frequency ultrasonic waves between 23 kHz and 36 kHz. These waves are generated by a piezoelectric transducer incorporated in the hand piece of the instrument. These waves cause an implosion of cells that have high water content by vaporizing the intracellular water. This occurs by the formation of vacuoles in the cell which resonate with the vibrating tip of the instrument. This process is called cavitation. Connective tissue contains less water than the hepatocytes and fat. Hence, the cavitation effect keeps the vessels and bile ducts intact while fragmenting the fat and hepatocytes. The ultrasonic dissectors (Fig. 3) (e.g. CUSA, CUSA-Tyco healthcare, Mansfield, MA, USA) have an integrated irrigation and aspiration system which allows removal of cell debris during transection. Cirrhotic livers need higher vibration settings. Some authors have shown lower blood loss and better results when comparing CUSA with clamp crush technique[90] while others have shown no difference.[91]

Harmonic Scalpel

The ultrasonic shear (harmonic scalpel, ethicon endo-surgery, Cincinnati, OH, USA) uses ultrasonically activated shears which vibrate at a frequency of 55.5 KHz over a 50–100 μm arc. This movement dissects the liver parenchyma. Also, the small blood vessels between the blades are sealed by coagulation which occurs due to protein denaturation as a result of destruction of hydrogen bonds. This is similar to whisking an egg to denature the protein. Blood vessels 3–5 mm in diameter are sealed by this mechanism (up to 7 mm in the newer instruments). This instrument has the advantage that it can be used for laparoscopic liver resection and

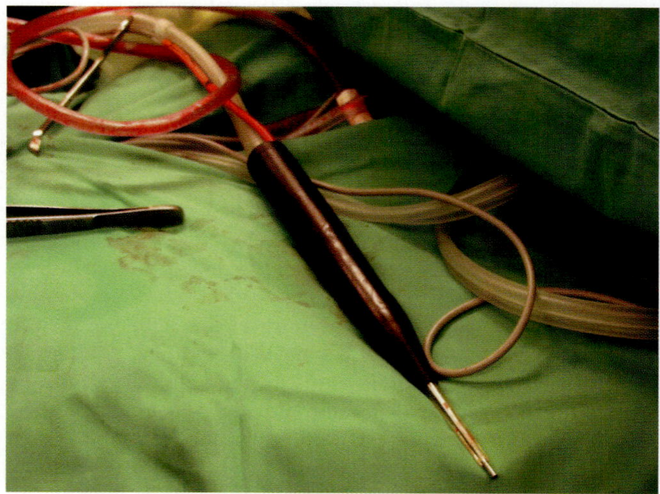

Figure 3 The CUSA probe with the suction, irrigation and ultrasonic dissector tip

also for tough tissue such as the cirrhotic liver. The instrument may have a limitation in dissection of large vessels such as portal or hepatic veins because it will not be able to seal large vessels. In this situation, it can be combined with the CUSA to dissect large vessels and reduce blood loss.[92] A study reported no bile leakage in 46 cases[93] while another suggested a significantly increased bile leak suggesting that the harmonic scalpel may not seal bile ducts well.[94]

Ligasure

This is an ingenious system for sealing blood vessels. The Ligasure system (Covidien) uses a combination of pressure and energy to seal the blood vessels. The heat generated from the bipolar energy causes the fusion of collagen and elastin in the walls of the vessel with the creation of a permanent sealed zone. The system is computer controlled and detects the thickness of tissue to be coagulated and automatically defines the amount of energy required and the delivering time. An acoustic signal informs the surgeon when the vessel is sealed and it can be divided. The seal zone shows a translucent appearance that is easy to recognize. There is no dissipation of heat beyond the jaws of the instrument. This instrument can seal blood vessels up to 7 mm. For liver transection it can be used as a clamp crush technique or better in combination with CUSA to dissect the liver parenchyma and seal the blood vessels and bile ductules with Ligasure. A RCT showed that Ligasure combined with the clamp crush technique resulted in lower blood loss and faster transection compared to conventional technique of electric diathermy or Ligasure for controlling vessels in the transection plane.[95]

Tissue Link Dissecting Sealer

The thermal effect generated by ionic agitation caused by radiofrequency generator system can also be used to coagulate tissue. The tissue link dissecting sealer is a new technology developed for liver transection using saline linked radiofrequency energy (tissue link medical Inc., Dover, NH, USA). In this instrument, radiofrequency energy (480 KHz) is focused near the tip of the instrument and conveyed to the tissue using saline. The instrument can be used to transect the liver and seal it simultaneously. It can also be used laparoscopically.

Radiofrequency-Assisted Liver Transection

A Cool-tip™ radiofrequency electrode (radionics Inc., Burlington, MA, USA) is inserted along the transection plane 1–2 cm apart. Radiofrequency energy is then applied for 1–2 minutes. This results in cylinders of coagulated tissue which are then cut with a scalpel. The technique is simple but has the disadvantage of leaving a 1 cm wide necrotic tissue at the edge of the remnant liver. Preliminary results with the use of this device show low blood loss.[96,97]

Use of Vascular Staplers in Liver Transection

The conventional technique to divide the stump of the portal vein or the hepatic veins was to use a vascular clamp, divide the vessel and suture the cut end. The danger, especially with the hepatic vein, was that the clamp could slip resulting in massive hemorrhage and air embolism. Vascular staplers make this task safer and faster.[98] They can also be used to divide the liver parenchyma.[99] Care should be taken while applying the vascular stapler at the inflow especially in large tumors close to the confluence. If not applied with care there is a risk of narrowing or occluding the hepatic duct confluence. With staplers there is an increased risk of bile leak because the staples are not very effective in sealing small bile ducts.

Different surgeons have different preferences when it comes to the choice of transection technique. While CUSA is the technique most commonly used, some studies have shown that clamp crushing or water jet is better and faster.[91] Recently, a randomized trial compared clamp crushing, CUSA, hydrojet and dissecting sealer for liver transection with 25 patients in each group.[100] The study found that clamp crushing was associated with the fastest transection speed, lowest blood loss and lowest blood transfusion requirement. Furthermore, clamp crushing was the most cost-effective technique. However, the Pringle maneuver (inflow control) was used in the clamp crush technique and not used with the other techniques. This may have affected the results especially blood loss.

TECHNIQUES OF VASCULAR CONTROL

Earlier attempts at reducing hemorrhage during the parenchymal transection included Lin's clamp to mechanically compress the liver and the inflow occlusion at porta hepatis pioneered by James Hogarth Pringle. Later, as the liver anatomy was better understood and the experience in liver surgery expanded better techniques to reduce operative blood loss evolved. With the currently available techniques majority of the classical liver resections can be performed without the need for a blood transfusion. Broadly, these techniques can be grouped into three types:

1. Ligation of inflow and outflow vessels for hemihepatectomies
2. The liver hanging maneuver
3. Methods of temporary vascular control.

Ligation of Inflow and Outflow Vessels for Hemihepatectomies

This technique, first described by Lortat-Jacob for a right hemihepatectomy in 1952, involves the ligation of right portal pedicle and the RHV before-hand to reduce the blood loss[75] during parenchymal transection.[101] With the preliminary inflow vascular control a line of demarcation appears allowing accurate parenchymal division (Fig. 4). The extrahepatic ligation of RHV is relatively a difficult step, especially in patients with large tumors encroaching on to RHV and suprahepatic IVC. Careful division of the short veins draining the caudate lobe to the IVC helps to lift up the liver from the IVC and expose the junction of the RHV and IVC. The extrahepatic isolation of RHV needs to be carried out judiciously avoiding any injury to RHV and IVC which can lead to a fatal massive hemorrhage or an air embolism.[102]

Bismuth combined both the abovementioned techniques to eliminate their relative disadvantages and advocated a preliminary hilar dissection to isolate and apply a clamp or tourniquet on the concerned portal pedicle, followed by mobilization of the liver off the IVC.[103] The next step involved parenchymal transection along the line of demarcation followed by the ligation of portal structures distal to the tourniquet and corresponding hepatic vein, toward the end of parenchymal division.

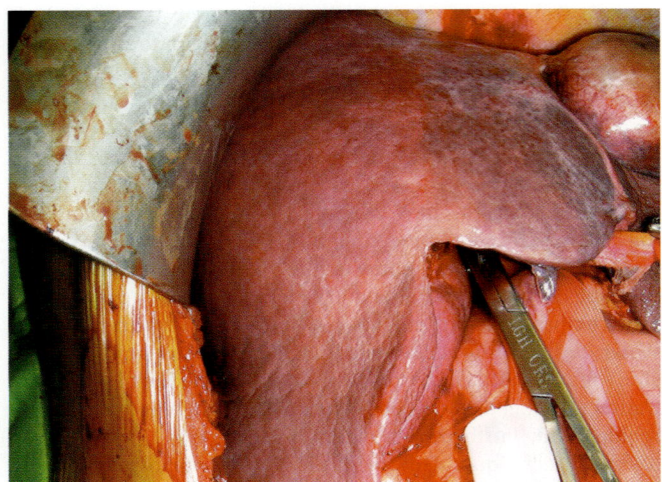

Figure 4 Picture showing the demarcation line between the left and right livers after the left Inflow system has been clamped

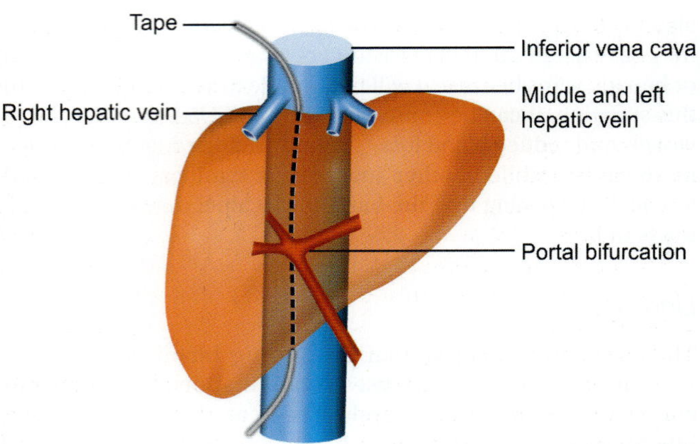

Figure 5 Diagram showing the position of the tape across the anterior surface of the retrohepatic inferior vena cava that can be used to perform liver resection using the "hanging maneuvre". The diagram shows the position of the tape for a right or a left hepatectomy. It can be altered to perform other types of resections such as right and left trisectionectomies

Liver Hanging Maneuver (LHM)

When there is a large tumor in the right lobe of liver extrahepatic control of the hepatic veins becomes difficult. The veins can be damaged in an attempt to mobilize the liver; there is risk of tumor dissemination due to excessive handling and hypotension due to pressure on the vena cava during manipulation of the tumor. To circumvent these problems, the "anterior approach" (AA) was proposed by Ozawa in 1992[104] and later developed by practitioners in Hong Kong.[105] This unconventional approach consists of parenchymal transection without prior mobilization of the liver. The blood loss is less because mobilization of the right lobe of liver becomes easier after it has been transected. Because this is a "no touch" technique tumor dissemination is also reduced. The cumulative survival of these patients is better than conventional surgery.[105]

The drawback of the anterior approach is that the liver cannot be lifted up for manual control of bleeding. To overcome this, the Hanging maneuver was developed. In this procedure, the liver is lifted by a tape passed between the anterior surface of the vena cava and the liver, thereby providing effective vascular control, in order to make the anterior approach safer and easier (Fig. 5).[106]

The most important step of the LHM is the dissection along the anterior aspect of the retrohepatic IVC. The existence of a longitudinal avascular plane between the IVC and the liver makes this maneuver feasible. The presence of a constant avascular channel located at the 10–11 o'clock position along the anterior wall of the retrohepatic IVC has been confirmed by many authors.[107,108] The technique has been further modified for safety by the use of "guided" dissection using IOUS. Another technique is the "upside down" technique where the dissection in the avascular plane is carried out from the upper end downward. The dissection near the major hepatic veins is therefore under vision. A Double tape technique allows the passage of two tapes in the retrohepatic area. They are pulled in opposite directions during transection of the liver resulting in excellent hemostasis during transection.[109]

Methods of Temporary Vascular Control

These techniques involve occlusion of inflow vessels alone or occlusion of both the inflow and outflow vessels ranging from total inflow occlusion to hemihepatic, sectoral and segmental inflow occlusions. The experience from liver transplantation allowed total hepatic vascular exclusion (THVE) for the resection of large tumors reducing the operative blood loss to a minimum. With the advent of IOUS, selective occlusion of portal vein branches with balloon catheters became possible. Further, the addition of in vivo hypothermic liver perfusion after THVE helped prolong the safe ischemia time for complex liver resections.

The following description briefly refers to the details of these techniques and their merits and demerits:

Total Inflow Occlusion: The Pringle's Maneuver (PM)

The most commonly used method to occlude the inflow vessels, involves clamping of the entire portal pedicle at the hepatoduodenal ligament and is effective in minimizing the blood loss during the parenchymal transection in all types of liver resections.[110] A broad atraumatic vascular clamp or a tourniquet around the hepatoduodenal ligament is used to effect the occlusion. A temporary occlusion may also be achieved manually by applying firm pressure using the thumb and finger. A left hepatic artery originating from the left gastric artery should always be looked for which, if present, needs separate occlusion to achieve complete inflow control.

Hepatic Tolerance and Preconditioning

Hemodynamically Pringle's maneuver initiates an increase in systemic vascular resistance, mean arterial pressure (about 20%) and heart rate with a fall in pulmonary arterial pressure and cardiac output (<10%). These changes revert within a few minutes of declamping and are well tolerated for up to 60 minutes of clamping time, by patients with normal liver[111,112] and up to 30 minutes by patients with Child's A cirrhosis.[113,114] Some studies have indicated that an extended clamping time ranging between 75 and 90 minutes is safely tolerated by the healthy liver without any significant increase in the postoperative morbidity.[115,116] Further, if Pringle's maneuver is used intermittently (15–20 minutes clamping time with 5 minutes declamping) the occlusion time can be extended to 90–120 minutes in patients with normal livers.[117] In patients with cirrhotic liver, intermittent Pringle's maneuver (PM) for 45 minutes has been used.[118] In a RCT, it has been shown that intermittent inflow control can be prolonged and is safer in patients with steatosis and chronic liver disease. No major difference in blood loss has been shown during continuous and intermittent clamping methods.

Clavien et al. have shown that an initial period of ischemia for 10 minutes followed by reperfusion for 10 minutes protects the liver against subsequent prolonged ischemia.[119] It is called preconditioning of the liver. The benefit of preconditioning, however, was shown only for 30 minutes of continuous clamping. Use of intermittent clamping may combine the advantages of preconditioning with the potential for unhurried surgery, providing time for complex resection with low blood loss (particularly in patients with abnormal underlying liver).

In fact the technique of preconditioning has been shown to be advantageous in living donors undergoing graft harvest.[120] The authors showed that intermittent clamping during donor hepatectomy was well tolerated by the donor and the graft. There was no difference in graft function as compared to procedures performed without hepatic pedicle clamping.

Hemihepatic Vascular Occlusion (HHVO)

This was first described by Makuuchi et al. to limit the ischemic damage only to the side of the liver to be resected.[121] The technique is especially useful in patients with cirrhosis or those with obstructive jaundice, where the liver is more susceptible to ischemic damage. The approach to the hepatic pedicle can be extrahepatic or intrahepatic.

Extrahepatic approach: A cholecystectomy is performed prior to hilar dissection. The hilar dissection involves the isolation of the ipsilateral hepatic artery and portal vein in the hilum of the liver. These are then divided using a stapler or suture ligated. The bile duct is usually controlled during transection in the substance of the liver. The technique is time consuming and can result in damage to contralateral bile duct or vessels.

Intrahepatic approach: This technique is called the Glissonian sheath approach as suggested by Launois and Jamieson.[10] It is known that the hepatic artery, bile duct and portal vein travel within the liver in a well formed single sheath (Fig. 6). This is an extension of the Glisson's capsule which surrounds these structures as they enter the liver at the hilum. Thus within the liver these three structures can be isolated and ligated en masse within the sheath. Outside the liver there is no such sheath hence the structures have to be ligated individually. This technique can be performed by two approaches: In the posterior approach[11] hepatotomies are created anterior and posterior to the hilus on the side of transection. A finger or blunt clamp is passed around the pedicle which is encircled using a sling. In the anterior approach, the liver parenchyma is divided from anterior to posterior till the pedicle is seen and encircled.[10] Both approaches can be helped by the use of IOUS to show the position of the pedicles.

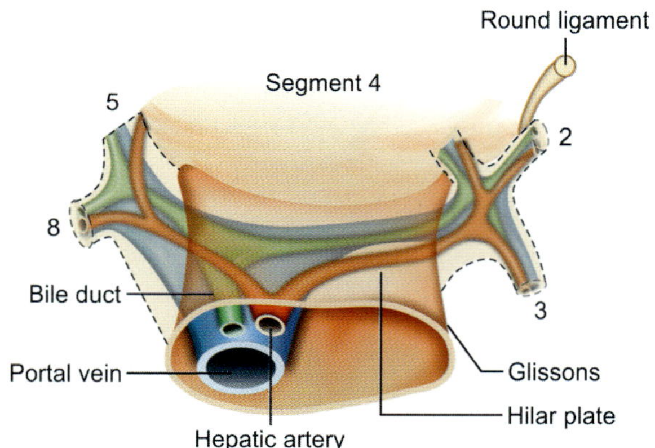

Figure 6 The Glisson's capsule seen enveloping the portal triad bifurcation near the porta hepatis developing into a right sided and a left sided portal pedicle containing the portal vein, hepatic artery and bile duct

The advantage of HHVO over Pringle's maneuver is that it prevents splanchnic congestion and prolonged aggravation of portal hypertension. Following Pringle's maneuver, asymptomatic hyperamylasemia has been observed in patients with chronic liver disease, presumably due to prolonged pancreatic venous congestion. It does not occur when HHVO is employed.[122] In patients where Pringle's maneuver is to be avoided, HHVO can be applied in an alternating fashion on the left and right portal pedicles, especially when there are two planes of parenchymal transection (e.g. mesohepatectomy).

Selective Occlusion of Segmental Sectoral Portal Branches

This is accomplished by dissecting the desired sectoral and segmental portal pedicles using a perihilar posterior intrahepatic approach (Fig. 6).[11] After lowering the hilar plate, the liver tissue is bluntly pushed away to reach the superior surface of the hilar confluence. A vascular tape is placed around the desired branch (right or left) of the main portal pedicle. Traction on this tape brings the looped structures to a more superficial and extrahepatic position. The right sheath is then dissected further to reach the sectoral and segmental pedicles using a CUSA and cutting into the liver parenchyma along the lines 1 and 2 as shown in Fig. 7. The first branch encountered just behind the gall bladder bed is the sheath of segment VI. The right anterior sectoral sheath (to segments V and VIII) is encountered coursing upward. The further differentiation between the individual sheaths of segment V and VIII is accomplished by opening the main fissure deeper into the liver parenchyma, close to the hilum. The right posterior sectoral sheath is seen in Rouviere's sulcus, when present, or dissected by transecting the liver parenchyma along the line 2 (Fig. 7). The segment VII sheath sometimes remains buried as it passes posteriorly into the liver substance.

For selective isolation on the left side, a similar approach is used at the base of umbilical fissure. The left main sheath is dissected from the base of quadrate lobe extrahepatically. The pedicles to segment IVa and b are encountered on the right of the umbilical fissure. The sheath to segment III is superficial as compared to that of segment II and can be dissected out in the vicinity of left-sided attachments of the ligamentum teres to the left portal vein.

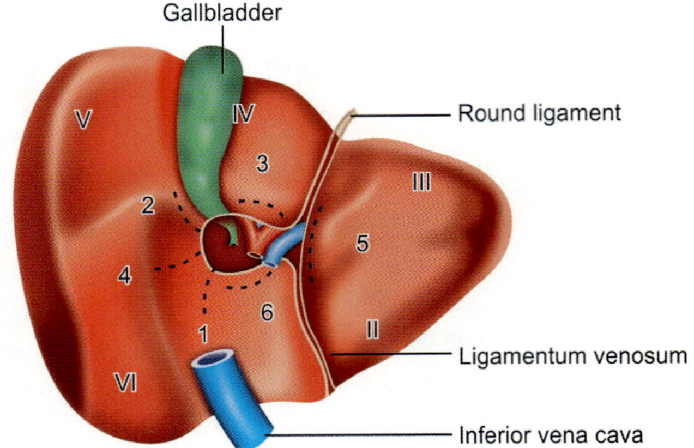

Figure 7 Sites for perihilar hepatotomy in portal pedicle isolation. The diagram shows the undersurface of the liver. The dashed lines indicate sites for hepatotomy. Incision at 3 allows lowering of the Hilar plate; incisions at 1 and 2 allow control of the right main portal pedicle; incisions at 1 and 4 allow control of the Right posterior sectoral pedicle; incisions at 2 and 4 allow control of the right anterior sectoral pedicle; incisions at 3 and 5 allow control of the left portal pedicle and incision at 6 allows dissection of the short branches from the left portal pedicle supplying the caudate lobe

In some patients, especially with cirrhosis and portal hypertension and those who have undergone a prior operation or transarterial chemoembolization (TACE), the hilar dissection to isolate vessels selectively becomes tedious and a time consuming procedure. In such cases, balloon catheters have been used to selectively occlude the desired branch of the portal vein at its bifurcation or sectoral and segmental level. The balloon catheter is placed into the portal vein under the IOUS guidance, either by needle puncture of the liver or by introducing through a tributary of the ileocolic vein. After confirmation of the tip of the balloon catheter, the desired branch of portal vein is occluded. The injection of a dye (methylene blue, indigo carmine) through this catheter is helpful in marking the surface area of a particular segment thus facilitating accurate parenchymal transection.[55,123] As the arterial supply is not occluded arterial bleeding does occur and may require temporary clamping of the hepatic artery.

Total Hepatic Vascular Exclusion

This technique was described by Heaney[124] and later extensively applied by Huguet.[125] It refers to the combined occlusion of the inflow and outflow vessels of liver. The surgical preparation for THVE includes the following steps:

- Division of all the ligaments of liver and its complete mobilization from the diaphragm and the retroperitoneum
- Dissection and looping of suprahepatic IVC
- Dissection and looping of infrahepatic IVC above the right adrenal vein or after ligating the adrenal vein in the suprarenal portion of the IVC
- Preparation of the hepatoduodenal ligament for the Pringle's maneuver
- Occlusion of any other accessory or indirect vascular connections of the liver especially an accessory left hepatic artery, inferior phrenic artery and vein.

Total hepatic vascular exclusion, unlike Pringle's maneuver, induces hemodynamic intolerance in 10-15% of patients and may have to be abandoned.[121,126] Hence, a preliminary trial clamping is performed to assess the patient's ability to tolerate the THVE. Usually, there is a 25% reduction in the pulmonary arterial pressure, 40% decrease in cardiac index and a marked increase in peripheral vascular resistance. This requires an invasive monitoring of arterial blood pressure, CVP, pulmonary arterial pressure, cardiac index and arterial blood gases by the anesthetist. On trial clamping, after adequate preloading, if there is a more than 30% decrease of arterial blood pressure and a more than 50% decrease of cardiac index, THVE is better abandoned.[127] The clamping and declamping sequence in THVE is as follows:

- Test Pringle's maneuver for 5 minutes with adequate fluid infusion for volume loading.
- Trial clamping of the infrahepatic IVC and, if this is tolerated, the clamping of suprahepatic IVC followed by the resection.
- At the end of the resection, any air if present is evacuated from the IVC and the clamps are removed in a sequence reverse to that of their placement (i.e. first the suprahepatic IVC clamp followed by the infrahepatic IVC clamp and finally the clamp used for Pringle's maneuver).

In an attempt to make THVE more useful, several modifications of the original THVE technique have been proposed. Heaney et al.[124] recommended concomitant clamping of the supraceliac aorta with the aim of further limiting blood loss, preserving hemodynamic stability and reducing the splanchnic congestion. This entails significant risk of inducing renal and intestinal ischemia along with injury to the aorta itself, especially, when the latter is atherosclerotic. Alternatively, instead of aortic clamping, venovenous bypass can be used to divert blood flow from the lower limbs and the portal vein into an axillary or subclavian vein, to maintain adequate venous return to the heart while the THVE is in place.[128] Another technical variation in THVE technique incorporates individual isolation and clamping of the hepatic veins, without clamping of the IVC so as to preserve the caval blood flow.[129,130] The latter is not only better tolerated hemodynamically, but also allows intermittent vascular occlusion which is not possible in the original THVE technique.

Total hepatic vascular exclusion is well tolerated by patients with normal livers for up to 60 minutes[131] and in cirrhotics up to 30 minutes.[132] Though THVE involves a complex and time-consuming exercise, it allows safe removal of tumors involving the hepatic veins, retrohepatic IVC or the hepatic vein-caval junction with an acceptable morbidity and mortality (range: 17%–50% and 0%–10% respectively).[132,133]

In Situ Hypothermic Liver Perfusion with Total Hepatic Vascular Exclusion

This technique has been used safely to further extend the ischemia time up to 2.5 hours[134,135] especially when University of Wisconsin (UW) solution is used as the cold perfusate. This has been adopted from the technique followed for an orthotopic liver transplant donor retrieval procedure. Heparinized Ringer's lactate at 4°C can also be used as a cold perfusate. Fortner et al. reported their preliminary experience with this technique in 1974.[136] This technique is useful in patients undergoing complex operative procedures on liver requiring resection and reconstruction of portal vein or hepatic vein and/or IVC for which a period of 60–90 minutes of normothermic ischemia is not adequate.[131] It is important to realize that the specific therapeutic value of this technique has not yet been fully established and the worldwide experience with such a technique remains limited.

Though minor and also some major liver resections can be safely performed, without a prior hepatic vascular occlusion, controlled clinical studies employing vascular exclusion or occlusion techniques have shown that the operative blood loss is significantly reduced.[113,137,138] In one randomized study comparing the operative course of non-cirrhotic patients undergoing liver resections with Pringle's maneuver and those with THVE, the latter was associated with unpredictable hemodynamic intolerance in 14% of patients, a higher incidence of postoperative complications and a longer hospital stay.[139] Therefore, the use of THVE should be restricted to rare circumstances where it is absolutely essential.

BASIC OPERATIVE STEPS

The commonly performed major resections include right and left hemihepatectomies and the corresponding extended hepatectomies. The basic surgical steps required for all the major liver resections are as follows:

- With the patient placed in supine position, a bilateral subcostal incision provides adequate exposure. Use of a Rochard retractor or a chain retractor (Goligher) fixed to a steel frame at the head end of the operating table further enhances the exposure by elevating the costal margins (Figs 8A and B).
- The peritoneal cavity is explored to rule out any extrahepatic disease and liver cirrhosis which may alter the surgical plan.
- Complete mobilization of the liver from its diaphragmatic attachments which involves division of the right and left coronary ligaments and the falciform ligament. This allows the liver to be manipulated for easy access to the portal scissurae.
- Performance of bimanual palpation of the tumor and the rest of liver combined with IOUS examination to rule out satellite deposits or multicentric disease, determine the anatomic extent of the tumor in relation to the three major hepatic veins and localize the structures of concerned portal triad.
- Dissection and preparation of the hepatoduodenal ligament to allow Pringle's maneuver or selective vascular occlusion.
- The right lobe of liver is mobilized off the retrohepatic IVC, in patients requiring right-sided or caudate lobe resections or where the parenchymal transection plane passes through the main scissura. This entails division of small veins which drain the right hemiliver (mainly segment VI and VII) and the caudate lobe directly into the IVC. These veins have been grouped into the upper, middle and inferior retrohepatic veins. Sometimes (in up to 20% individuals), one of the inferior retrohepatic veins, becomes a dominant channel (called as the right inferior hepatic vein) draining the segment VI.[140] This vein needs to be identified and preserved in patients undergoing resection of segment VII alone or in combination with segment VIII, where RHV needs to be sacrificed.
- The next step involves dissection to isolate the concerned hepatic vein or veins extrahepatically, unless it is not possible because of the location of a large tumor. The extrahepatic isolation of MHV and LHV separately is usually not possible as both these veins form a common channel intrahepatically before draining into the IVC in up to 80–90% of cases.[8,102] It has been documented that these veins can be isolated in a majority of cases after complete mobilization of the liver off the IVC.[141]
- Before the parenchymal transection is started, the patient is placed in a 15° Trendelenburg position and the CVP kept below 5 mm Hg. The line of demarcation is marked with electrocautery.
- Preconditioning of the liver is done at this stage by clamping the liver inflow for 10 minutes and then reperfusing the liver for 10 minutes. This maneuver preconditions the liver to further ischemia reperfusion damage. Intermittent inflow occlusion during parenchymal transection can also be practiced.
- Any of the methods described to divide the liver parenchyma may be used. As the parenchymal division progresses deeper, toward IVC, one encounters small branches of portal vein, hepatic artery, the biliary ducts and the tributaries of hepatic vein which are ligated using 3-0 or 4-0 silk (Fig. 9). These vessels can be clipped using metal clips or divided using Ligasure or harmonic scalpel.

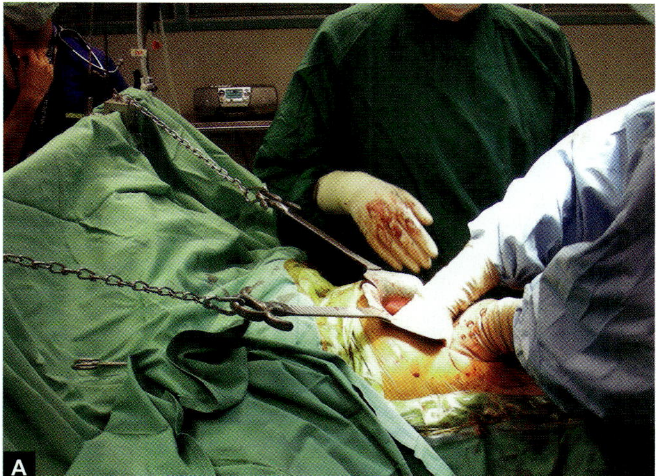

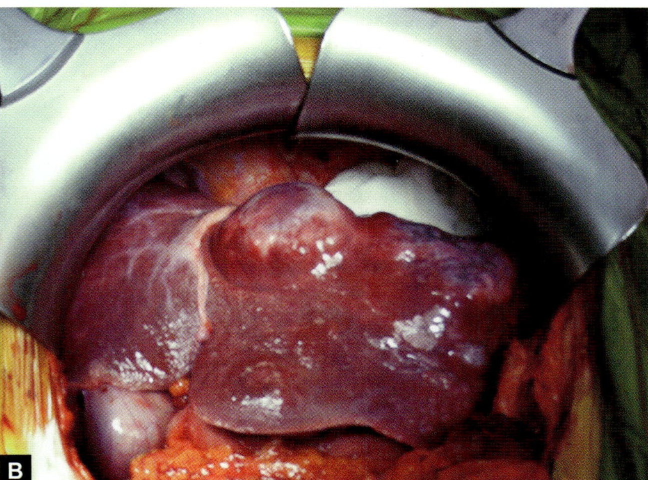

Figures 8A and B (A) The Goligher retraction system with the blades fixed to the table with a chain. The blades help to lift up the rib cage; (B) The retractor gives good views of the liver. The tumor is located in the left lobe of the liver

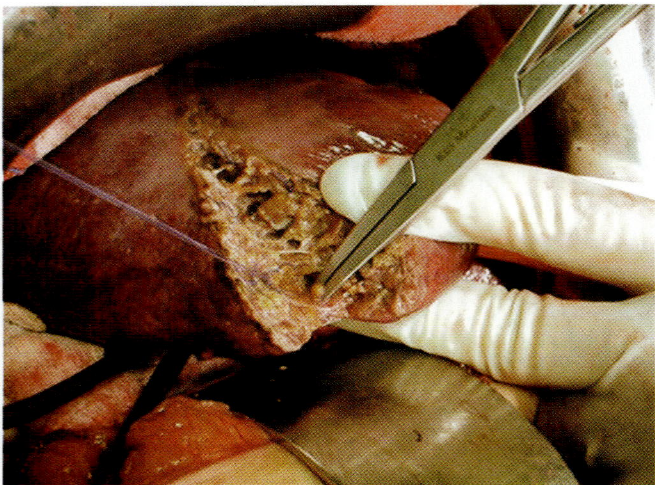

Figure 9 The cavitron ultrasonic surgical aspirator (CUSA) dissects the liver parenchyma leaving the vessels to be ligated

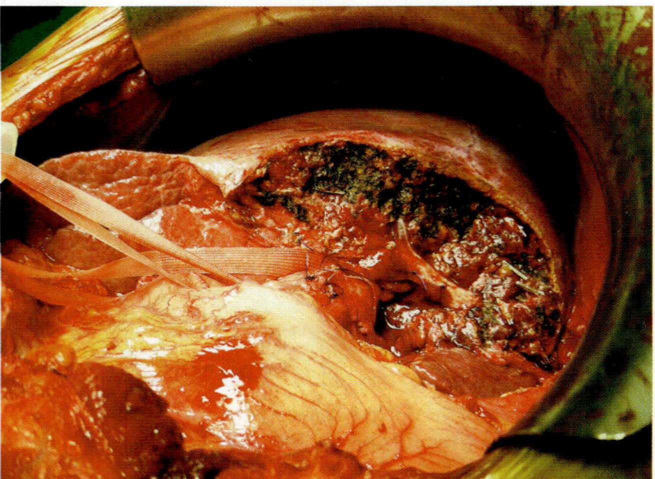

Figure 10 Cut edge of right lobe liver after a left hepatectomy. Middle hepatic vein can be seen in the lower part of the picture on the surface

- After the parenchymal division is completed, the inflow control is released and meticulous hemostasis of the cut surface of the remnant liver is carried out. Bleeding vessels are underrun using 6-0 polydioxanone (PDS) or prolene while the diffuse ooze is controlled using spray diathermy, an argon beam coagulator,[142] fibrin or synthetic surgical glue.[143]
- Once the hemostasis has been achieved, the cut surface of liver is carefully examined (Fig. 10) for bile leak by cannulating the cystic duct with a feeding tube and injecting saline after transiently occluding the distal common bile duct (CBD) with atraumatic clamps or finger pressure. Biliary leak, if present, is repaired or transfixed with fine absorbable sutures. In the event of a large leak, a T-tube may be left in the CBD.
- A closed-drainage system can be safely used to drain out any bile leaks or serous or lymphatic collections which may occur following a major liver resection.[8,144] Following minor liver resections routine drainage may not be necessary.[145]
- When the right lobe of liver is resected it is imperative that the left lobe is anchored to the diaphragm by reconstituting the falciform ligament. If this is not done the liver flops to one side twisting the hepatic veins. This results in acute hepatic venous outflow obstruction and liver failure.

EXTENDED HEPATIC RESECTIONS

Extended hepatic resections namely right and left trisectionectomy (extended right or left hepatectomy) remove a large part of the liver. It is important to ensure that the remaining liver is adequate for the survival of the patient. Most often this is accomplished by embolization of the ipsilateral portal vein. This results in hypertrophy of the contralateral liver. The process takes between 4–6 weeks at which time the liver is imaged again and surgery undertaken if feasible.

Right Trisectionectomy

This is also termed extended right hepatectomy or extended right hemihepatectomy (segments IV to VIII with or without segment I). Extended right hepatectomy, first performed by Starzl in 1980,[146] is indicated for large tumors of right lobe crossing the principal plane and involving the medial segment (IV) of the left hemiliver. The initial steps, including vascular inflow and outflow control, are completed and the dissection in the region of the liver hilum is continued to the base of the umbilical fissure. Branches from the hepatic artery and those of the portal vein supplying the caudate lobe are ligated and divided. This dissection is stopped short of the umbilical fissure. The incision on the liver surface, for parenchymal transection, is made just to the right of falciform ligament and kept well away to the right of the LHV, as it reaches closer to suprahepatic IVC. As the parenchymal transection proceeds the portal pedicles supplying the medial segment (IV) are encountered and ligated. The termination of MHV is tackled within the parenchyma toward the end of parenchymal dissection before it joins LHV to form the common channel or it joins the IVC. After achieving hemo- and biliostasis, the remnant liver is fixed to the under surface of the diaphragm to prevent postoperative torsion of the remnant liver which can lead to hepatic vein out flow obstruction. A right trisectionectomy may or may not include segment 1 resection depending on oncological requirements.

Left Trisectionectomy

This is also termed extended left hepatectomy or extended left hemihepatectomy (segments II, III, IV, V and VIII with or without segment 1). The technique of Left trisectionectomy was first published by Starzl in 1982.[147] Technically, left trisectionectomy is a demanding procedure and is associated with the risk of damaging the biliary ducts due to frequently occurring intrahepatic and extrahepatic biliary anomalies. There is also a risk of injury to the RHV.[148] To map the biliary tree and know the anatomy of right posterior sectoral duct and avoid biliary injuries, biliary imaging is carried out, preferably employing a noninvasive modality such as MRCP. After the initial mobilization of liver, IOUS is used to assess the relations of the tumor with neighboring vessels. The hilar dissection is carried out to isolate the contents of left portal pedicle. The point of division of left portal pedicle is determined by whether segment 1 is involved by tumor or not. If segment I is to be preserved then the contents of left portal pedicle are ligated at the base of umbilical fissure, otherwise close to the hilum. Further, a deeper dissection at the hilum, using CUSA, allows one to isolate and loop the right anterior sectoral pedicle, a trial clamping of which demarcates the anterior and posterior sectors of the right hemiliver. Once the identity of right anterior pedicle is ascertained, the pedicle is ligated and divided. The next step involves the dissection on the suprahepatic IVC to isolate and ligate the MHV and LHV. The liver surface is marked for parenchymal transection along the line of demarcation. The plane of parenchymal transection extends from the anterior border of the RHV and passes horizontally, parallel and just anterior to the right portal scissura well to the right of the gall bladder fossa. During the parenchymal division a Pringle's maneuver is usually required to keep the field dry. This enables the dissection to stay in the proper plane avoiding an inadvertent damage to the RHV. The remnant liver presents an en face raw surface area.

Left trisectionectomy is associated with two major problems, significant blood loss which occurs during parenchymal transection and the risk of injury to biliary radicals resulting in postoperative biliary fistula and/or stricture. Avoidance of biliary complications centers on the approach to control the right anterior sector pedicle with preservation of the posterior sectoral vessels and duct. However, sometimes the isolation of right anterior sectoral pedicle is difficult when the tumor is large and distorts the hilar anatomy or impinges on the hilar bifurcation. With adequate preoperative evaluation and meticulous technique, the procedure can be performed with acceptable morbidity and mortality in expert hands.[148]

Mesohepatectomy

This involves the resection of segments IV, V and VIII. It can also be termed central hepatectomy (right anterior sectionectomy + left medial sectionectomy). The concept of mesohepatectomy originated from the need to conserve more of normal liverparenchyma after a major resection, especially in patients with cirrhosis.[149] It was first described by McBride and Wallance.[150] This procedure is indicated in patients with a tumor involving segments IV, V and VIII with intact main left and right posterior portal pedicle as well as RHV and LHV. The procedure is, usually, performed using an intermittent hepatic inflow occlusion or alternating the HHVO to minimize blood loss during the parenchymal transection. Cholecystectomy is done first and the right anterior and posterior portal pedicles are dissected. On the right side, transection of the liver parenchyma is performed along the line of demarcation between the right anterior and posterior sectors. On the left side, the parenchyma is divided in a similar fashion as in a right trisectionectomy. The right anterior portal pedicle is then dealt with at the end of the transection. The postoperative recovery is usually fast. The operative mortality after mesohepatectomy varies between 5-10% with long-term survival rates comparable to that of an extended resection.[148,149,151]

Transverse Hepatectomy

Transverse hepatectomy involves the en bloc removal of hepatic segments IVb, V and VI (Fig. 11) in continuity along with the gall bladder through the transverse scissura.[152] Hilar dissection is carried out and extended to the umbilical fissure. The vessels and ducts to the segment IVb are ligated and divided. The cystic duct and artery are ligated and divided while the gall bladder is left in situ. On the right of the falciform ligament the parenchymal transection is started to the midpoint of anterior surface of segment IV, which

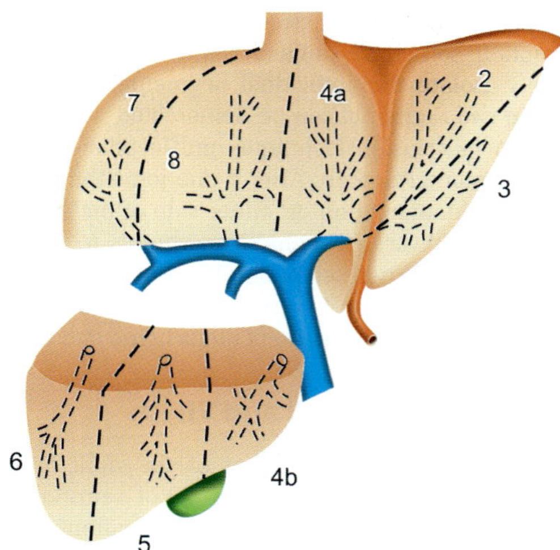

Figure 11 Transverse hepatectomy involving removal of the segments IVb, V and VI en bloc with the gallbladder

corresponds to the portal bifurcation. Subsequent parenchymal transection continues along the transverse scissura, which runs almost at right angles to the longitudinal body axis on to the point of portal ramifications, towards the right border of liver splitting the hepatic segments IVb from IVa, V from VIII and VI from VII. Numerous large branches of the right and MHV are encountered in this plane which are ligated and divided. The crucial step includes the identification and preservation of both the right anterior and posterior portal pedicles and preservation of segmental pedicles to segments VII and VIII while ligating the pedicles of the segments to be removed. Such a resection is usually performed on patients with gall bladder carcinoma and occasionally in those with multiple metastatic tumor deposits in these segments, to ensure an adequate margin of resection without sacrificing liver parenchyma.

SEGMENT-ORIENTED RESECTIONS OF THE LIVER

A segment-oriented approach to liver resection is particularly useful in cirrhotic patients with HCC and those undergoing repeat liver resections or bilobar resections for metastatic disease.[55,153,154] In addition to the preservation of normal liver parenchyma, segmental resections allow safe and oncologically complete removal of the targeted lesion. The inflow control is achieved with an intermittent Pringle maneuver along with the isolation of segmental or sectoral pedicles, if technically possible.

Resections of Segments V and VIII

The anatomic location of segment VIII makes its isolated removal one of the most technically demanding procedures of various mono-segmentectomies. Inflow control is obtained by isolating the right anterior sectoral portal pedicle. The RHV is clamped temporarily, if easily approachable from the suprahepatic aspect, and carefully preserved as it drains the remaining right posterior sector. For the resection of right anterior section (segments V and VIII) the parenchyma is transected through the principal scissura medially and right scissura toward right, anterior to the RHV.[155] For an isolated resection of segment V or VIII, accurate demarcation between the two segments is sometimes difficult, as it is not always possible to separately isolate the individual segmental portal pedicles. However, the two segments can be demarcated using transportal balloon catheter-occlusion technique and instillation of dye into the desired segmental branch. Also, if one joins the midpoints of both the lines of demarcation on either side of the sector, on the anterior surface of liver, it roughly corresponds to the anatomic boundary between the two segments. The raw surface left behind after segment VIII resection is nearly as large as that following a hemihepatectomy and requires meticulous hemo and biliostasis.

Resection of Segments VI and VII

This requires complete mobilization of the right lobe off the retrohepatic IVC along with the division of retrohepatic veins that drain directly into the IVC. For mono-segmental resections of either segment, the plane of parenchymal transection is just posterior to the right portal scissura. The RHV is identified and can be sacrificed in isolated segment VII resections if an inferior RHV is present to drain segment VI. Otherwise it is preserved, as far as possible, unless invaded by the tumor. Inflow occlusion is achieved by clamping the right posterior sectoral portal pedicle.

Left Lateral Sectionectomy (Segments II and III)

Isolated resections of segments II or III are rarely required, as the lesions in this region are better managed by a left lateral sectionectomy. Inflow control is achieved by isolation of the pedicles to segments II and III within the umbilical fissure to the left of the umbilical portion of the left portal vein. The LHV is controlled and divided either extrahepatically or at the end of the parenchymal transection. The line of parenchymal division is maintained strictly to the left of the falciform ligament to avoid injuring the portal supply to segment IV.

Left Medial Sectionectomy (Segment IV Resection)

Although isolated segment IV resections are uncommon, resection of segment IVb is often a part of either a mesohepatectomy or a transverse hepatectomy. Sometimes, in patients with cholangiocarcinoma, segment IV is resected along with segment I.[58] The initial step in all segment IV resections involves mobilization of the ligamentum teres and falciform ligament along with the division of a bridge of liver tissue that frequently connects the undersurface of segment IVb to segment III. The hilar plate is lowered to expose the left portal pedicle up to the base of umbilical fissure. For the removal of entire segment, all the portal branches to the right of the umbilical fissure are ligated and divided, while only the distal ones need ligation for the resection of segment IVb. The parenchymal transection is carried out to the right of the falciform ligament on the left side and in the principal plane on the right side. In the principal plane, tributaries draining into MHV are dealt with, carefully preserving the MHV by keeping the dissection slightly to the left of the principal plane. Once, both the sides of parenchymal divisions are complete, a transverse incision is made close to the suprahepatic IVC to join the posterior ends of the previous lines of parenchymal transection. The rest of the parenchymal division is completed, taking care of the remaining tributaries to MHV and the specimen removed. For segment IVb resections, the transverse incision is made corresponding to the level of portal bifurcation on the anterior surface of liver.

Caudate Lobe (Segment I) Resection

Three approaches to segment I resection have been described;[156] (1) isolated caudate lobectomy: when lesion is mainly located in the caudate lobe proper, (2) combined resection of the caudate lobe along with left or right hemiliver by using either a right-sided or a left-sided approach: for large infiltrating lesions of segment I for hilar cholangiocarcinomas and (3) transhepatic anterior approach with splitting of liver parenchyma along the main portal scissura: when the lesion is large or occupies the paracaval portion of caudate lobe. After full mobilization of liver and lowering the hilar plate, the inflow control is achieved by ligating the arterial and portal branches arising at the hepatic hilum and the umbilical fissure. Suprahepatic dissection is done to get control of the MHV and LHV to avoid injury to these veins. Also if injury to these veins does occur it can be managed easily. Such an injury can occur during resection of large caudate lobe tumors.[156,157] The right lobe of the liver is lifted off its fossa and rotated toward the left. The dissection is carried out between the liver and the IVC beginning from below and the retrohepatic veins are carefully dissected, ligated and divided individually (Figs 12A and B). A similar

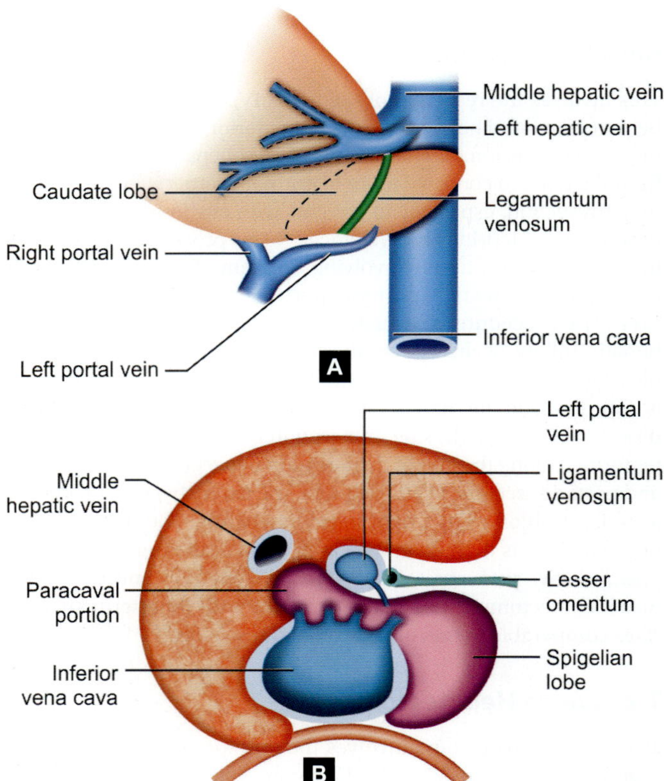

Figures 12A and B (A) Schematic diagram showing relationship of the caudate lobe with major vascular structures; (B) Cross-section of the liver showing the close relationship of the paracaval portion of the caudate lobe to the middle hepatic vein, the major blood supply from the left portal vein and venous drainage into anterior aspect of the retrohepatic inferior vena cava

dissection is required from the left after mobilizing the left lobe and rotating it to the right. The bridge of liver parenchyma between the base of segment IV and left side of segment VII is divided and the specimen removed. For a very large tumor arising in caudate lobe, performing a left hepatectomy may facilitate its removal.

Two major series involving 66 caudate lobe resections,[157,158] in isolation or with associated segments, have reported a morbidity of approximately 40% and a mortality ranging between 7% and 10%. In another large study on various types of segment-oriented resection in 79 patients, Billingsley et al.[153] reported the operative morbidity and mortality of 26% and 2.5%, respectively.

Resections for Live-related Liver Transplantation (LRLT)

The anatomical and surgical principles involved in segmental resections of liver have been applied to the field of LRLT as well. The amount of liver to be removed from the donor depends upon the age and the size of the recipient. Usually, the graft is harvested from a healthy adult and implanted into a child. For this purpose, most centers use the left lateral segment. However, right hemiliver grafts have also been transplanted.[159-163]

The donor is selected after performing ABO compatibility and a detailed preoperative evaluation of the status of liver and its vascular anatomy. The surgical techniques for harvesting right hemiliver or left hemiliver grafts do not differ from that of the classical right or left hepatectomy operation.

The harvesting of left lateral segment requires the initial portal dissection to identify the left hepatic artery and left portal vein. The branches to segment I and IV are carefully ligated and divided. The left hepatic duct is isolated but not divided until the parenchymal dissection is completed. The LHV is isolated and looped with a sling. The parenchymal transection is performed on the right of the falciform ligament. After the completion of parenchymal dissection, the left hepatic artery, the left branch of the portal vein, and the LHV are clamped in that order and the left lateral segment excised. The hemo- and biliostasis is achieved on the cut surface of the donor liver. At the end of operation, segment IV may appear dusky and is left without worry and the abdomen is closed. Another technique which is rarely done involves removal of the entire left hemiliver (segments II, III and IV) and subsequent resection of segment IV on the bench.[164] Careful surgery coupled with the use of autologous blood transfusion minimizes the blood loss to less than 500 mL and avoids the need of heterologous blood transfusion. The major donor morbidity include biliary leaks and sub-phrenic collections.[162,163]

Postoperative Management

The postoperative care of patients with liver resection requires an understanding of liver physiology and common problems that can occur in these patients. To achieve good results, it is imperative that the patients are selected carefully and meticulous techniques are used intraoperatively to minimize blood loss, as both the amount of blood loss and blood transfused influence the occurrence of postoperative liver failure. The hematocrit is maintained around 30% during surgery and between 25% and 30% in the postoperative period, taking care to maintain hemodynamic stability at all times. These important issues following liver resection are discussed.

Fluid and Electrolyte Management

After liver resection maintenance of adequate fluid balance and renal function is important. Cirrhotic patients develop ascites, vasodilatation and hypotension. The intravascular volume should be restored with colloids rather than crystalloids. Preoperative ascites is a contraindication to major liver resection. Postoperative ascites is controlled with salt restriction (<2 g/day), potassium sparing and loop diuretics, fluid and electrolyte replacement and albumin infusions. Uncontrolled ascites may lead to wound dehiscence, pulmonary complications as well as sepsis, and may require repeated large volume paracentesis.

Hyperlactemia and hypophosphatemia are common derangements following liver resection. The stressed liver is not able to metabolize lactate and high lactate levels in the postoperative period suggest a poor prognosis. Hence, lactate free fluids may be used in the postoperative period.[165]

Hypophosphatemia is common after liver resection. The mechanism is not clear. It is believed that regenerating hepatocytes use up phosphate. Another theory is that increased loss of phosphate in the urine mediated by chemicals called phosphatonins is responsible for this phenomenon. Low phosphate levels result in impaired energy metabolism and cause dysfunction in many organ systems. The treatment is to replace phosphate by oral and parenteral route in the postoperative period.[166,167]

Nutrition

In the early postoperative period emphasis is laid on early ambulation, chest physiotherapy and early institution of oral feeding. The preoperative hyperalimentation and resumption of early feeding in the postoperative period helps in faster recovery and is likely to reduce the morbidity due to sepsis and ascites. Patients are in a catabolic state after liver resection and require glucose and other nutrients. Non-cirrhotic patients with adequate reserves should be started on early oral or enteral feeds. However, malnourished patients and those with cirrhosis or steatosis need nutritional supplements. This should preferably be given by the enteral route. It has been shown that early enteral feeding results in significantly lower wound and catheter related infection as compared to parenteral infection.[168] Infectious complications in these patients were also lower. Total parenteral nutrition (TPN) supplements on the other hand showed no benefit.[169]

Liver disease alters the amino acid metabolism resulting in low levels of BCAAs (leucine, isoleucine and valine) and elevated circulating levels of aromatic amino acids and methionine. Randomized trials have shown that supplementation with BCAA in patients with advanced cirrhosis resulted in better nutritional status and lower rate of complications.[170,171] In a randomized study on cirrhotic patients undergoing liver resections for HCC, prolonged feeding with an oral formulation of BCAA solution for a period of one year after the surgery helped the patients to gain weight with an improvement in biochemical liver function parameters and reduced the incidence of neuropsychiatric complications.

Glycemic Control

Hyperglycemia occurs in the postoperative period due to surgical stress. Strict control of blood sugar levels in this period results in better outcomes.[172] Many techniques of control of blood sugar have been used. Fisette et al. have shown that the hyperinsulinemic-normoglycemic clamp technique reduces postoperative liver dysfunction, infections and complications when compared to insulin sliding scale.[173]

Coagulopathy

After liver resection there is an increase in INR and decrease in platelet counts and fibrinogen.[174,175] This peaks between days 2 and 5 because of decreased production of coagulation factors by the liver and increased consumption.

Pain Management

Good pain relief after liver resection allows early mobilization and better respiratory function. Opioids (morphine and fentanyl) are used commonly but one should be aware of their side-effects. In cirrhotic patients and those with major liver resections metabolism of opioids and benzodiazepines is slow. The size of liver resection has been correlated to the impairment of opioid metabolism.[176]

Epidural analgesia reduces chest infection, duration of ileus and provides better pain control.[177] However, there is risk of epidural hematoma, spinal cord injury and epidural abscess with these catheters. This risk is increased in patients with coagulopathy. Its use may be associated with increased transfusion requirements.[178] Intravenous acetaminophen can be used in a maximal dose of 2 g/day in patients with hepatic impairment.

Local anesthetic can be instilled into the wound by placing catheters in the musculofascial layer of the subcostal wound (On-Q® PainBuster® system). This can be combined with the use of patient controlled analgesia and results in lower use of morphine and better pain control in the postoperative period.[179,180]

Postoperative Infection

Infection in the postoperative period results in increased morbidity mortality after liver resection.[181] Factors that predispose to infection are obesity, preoperative biliary drainage, extent of hepatic resection, operative blood loss, comorbid conditions and postoperative bile leak.[182,183]

The antibiotic regimen is aimed at broad-spectrum coverage, consisting of newer cephalosporins, aminoglycosides and metronidazole. Any indication of postoperative sepsis is managed aggressively with bacterial or fungal culture and sensitivity tests on blood, ascitic fluid, intra-abdominal collection, pulmonary secretions and urine. Stress induced by sepsis may lead the patient, especially the one with postoperative liver dysfunction, into liver failure and irreversible multiorgan failure. The common septic complications include infected bile collections, subphrenic abscesses and bacterial peritonitis. Most of the biliary collections are manageable by percutaneous drainage. Those which do not resolve due to a persistent leak from major bile ducts, require an endoscopic papillotomy and a temporary biliary stenting.

It has been shown that early institution of enteral nutrition preserves the gut barrier function and reduces infectious complications after liver resections.[184] Use of probiotics has also been shown to reduce infections.

Thromboprophylaxis

Between 15% and 40% of surgical patients suffer venous thromboembolism in the postoperative period.[185] There is a fear that prophylactic anticoagulation in liver resection patients may lead to increased bleeding. This is not the case.[186] In fact, it has been shown that liver resection patients are hypercoagulable. The reduced volume of liver produces less coagulant factors. However, it also produces less anticoagulant factors such as protein S, protein C and antithrombin III. Levels of Von Willebrand factor and factor VIII increase probably due to trauma. This combined with lower anticoagulant levels produces a hypercoagulable state. Use of thromboprophylaxis on the night of surgery is associated with lower VTE incidence and no increase in blood transfusions.[186,187] Unless, there is a high risk of bleeding, pharmacologic thromboprophylaxis should be started on the day of surgery.

Portal Hypertension

Although portal vein pressure rises after any major liver resection,[188] the occurrence of postoperative variceal bleeding does not correlate with the extent of resection or the preoperative grade of the varices and is unpredictable. The risk of variceal bleeding remains high within the first postoperative month. In case of postoperative variceal bleed, the management requires an immediate endoscopic sclerotherapy (EST) or variceal-band ligation (EVL). Most authors recommend preoperative control of large varices (grade III and IV) with either EVL or EST, prophylactically, especially in those patients who have had a prior bleed.[189,190] Others have performed portocaval shunt at the time of liver resection to prevent variceal bleeding.[191-193] However, a portocaval shunt should be avoided as the postoperative liver regeneration depends on the amount of portal blood flow.

Liver Failure

The management protocol varies between patients with cirrhosis and those without. In the postoperative period, 10%–15% patients with cirrhosis develop liver failure, 40%–80% develop ascites and 6%–10% develop variceal bleeding. Sepsis and intra-abdominal bleeding can occur in 3%–5% of cases.[194] Postoperative liver failure is the most important and common cause of in-hospital mortality, followed by variceal hemorrhage and sepsis. The signs of postoperative liver failure include progressive hyperbilirubinemia with normal transaminases, glucose intolerance or refractory hypoglycemia, progressive ascites and mental obtundation. A thorough search is made to look for and treat predisposing factors such as the presence of sepsis, dyselectrolytemia and diuretic toxicity. There is little that can be done, once liver failure occurs, except for supportive measures such as administration of lactulose and high dose topical antibiotics to diminish the gut-derived endotoxin load.[195] Nutrition is maintained with low protein diet (<50 g/day). The prognosis is dismal once liver failure sets in, resulting in most of postoperative in-hospital or delayed deaths (within up to 6 months) after discharge.[194,196]

Operative Mortality

In the current scenario, operative mortality associated with liver resection in patients without cirrhosis is less than 5%.[197] In patients with cirrhosis the mortality can range from 10% to 15%.[198] Most patients leave hospital between days 5 and 10 after the operation. LFTs show a rise of AST and ALT in the first few days after a liver resection. These levels soon normalize. The early rise of alkaline phosphatase and gamma glutamyl transferase (GGT) levels signals regeneration in the postoperative period and should not be mistaken for biliary obstruction.

NEW DEVELOPMENTS

Laparoscopic Liver Resections

The first laparoscopic liver resections were performed in 1992.[199] The technique of laparoscopy is now being increasingly used for liver resections. The common indications are benign tumors of the liver, malignant liver resections and living donor hepatectomy.

There are three approaches used for minimally invasive liver resection. These include pure laparoscopic surgery, hand-assisted laparoscopic surgery and a hybrid approach. In the latter, liver mobilization and some of the transection is done laparoscopically and the procedure is completed by open surgery.[200]

Indications

Laparoscopic liver resections were initially used for benign tumors. However, Nguyen et al. reviewed the experience of laparoscopic liver resections in 2009.[201] They found that 50% resections were for malignant lesions, and 1.7% for donor hepatectomies. Of the resections 75% were performed totally laparoscopically, 17% hand-assisted and 2% were hybrid. The most common liver resection was a wedge resection or segmentectomy (45%) followed by anatomical left lateral sectionectomy (20%), right hepatectomy (9%) and left hepatectomy (7%).

Resection of lesions by laparoscopic approach, which are 5 cm or less, located in segment 2-6 has been suggested in the Louisville statement on the International position on laparoscopic surgery.[202] There is a learning curve and it has been suggested that this can be overcome with 60 cases for minor hepatectomy.[203]

Laparoscopic Major Hepatectomy

Several centers are now performing major liver resections laparoscopically. O'Rourke from Brisbane reported a series of 12 laparoscopic right hepatectomies in 2004.[204] Recently, 210 major hepatic resections from 6 major centers were reviewed (136 right and 74 left).[205] The selection criteria for major hepatectomy included lesions smaller than 5 cm well beyond lines of transection, non-cirrhotics or well compensated cirrhotics, grade I or no esophageal varices, platelet count more than 80,000/mL and an American Society of Anesthesiologists (ASA) score of three or less. Mean operative blood loss was 300 mL with a 12% conversion rate. Some authors have reported use of the liver hanging technique where the liver is mobilized laparoscopically and a small subcostal incision is used to complete the transection of the liver.[206]

Intraoperative and Postoperative Benefits of Laparoscopic Liver Resection

One of the benefits of laparoscopic liver resection is reduced blood loss during surgery. This is due to two reasons. The first is the better visualization and control of small blood vessels during transection of the liver. The second is the effect of pneumoperitoneum which creates a tamponade effect due to increased pressure on the hepatic and portal venules. There are no prospective RCTs of laparoscopic vs open hepatectomy. However, a review of nonrandomized series by Reddy et al. has shown that laparoscopic liver resection is associated with less operative blood loss, less postoperative pain and narcotic requirement and a shorter length of hospital stay with comparable postoperative morbidity and mortality to open liver resection.[200] The width of resection margin between laparoscopic and open liver resections is similar[207] with one study showing wider margins in the laparoscopic group.[208]

Safety of Laparoscopic Liver Resections

A multi-institutional European study reported their experience of laparoscopic liver resections for HCC.[209] A total of 163 liver resections were performed (74% in cirrhotics). The median blood loss was 250 mL, conversion to open surgery was 9.2%. The mortality rate was 1.2% and morbidity 11.6%. For colorectal liver metastases open conversion rates range from 4% to 20%. Mortality rates range from 0% to 2% and morbidity from 5% to 20%.[200]

Robotic Liver Resections

Laparoscopic liver surgery has been a major advance in surgical technique. However, it has inherent limitations. The degree of movement is limited, there is a fulcrum effect against the port, amplification of tremor, awkward ergonomics and the surgeon has to adapt to a two-dimensional image. Robotic surgery eliminates all these limitations and is surgeon friendly.

Advantages of Robotic Surgery

The first robotic cholecystectomy was performed by Himpens et al. in 1997.[210] They used a da Vinci robotic prototype. The advantages of the robotic system are that the surgeon can be seated for long periods of time. The da Vinci robot has three arms with EndoWrist® instruments which provide considerable freedom of movement. The tremor is reduced. It provides three-dimensional imaging, real time radiographic correlation and easy suture manipulation in tight places.[211-214] The ability to lock instruments in place such as vascular clamps gives time for the anesthetic and surgical teams to prepare the next step if bleeding occurs.[214]

Robotic liver surgery requires two surgeons namely the patient side surgeon and the console surgeon. The patient side surgeon should be highly skilled in laparoscopic surgery and should be able to manage harmonic scalpel, CUSA, ligasure and clipping and stapling devices. They should be able to install and change robotic arms and instruments. It has been suggested that mastering the robot requires at least 10 procedures in robot-assisted laparoscopic surgery.[215] The learning curve may be shorter than laparoscopic liver surgery because of better imaging, more freedom of movement and better ergonomics.

Results of Robotic Liver Resections

Ho et al. reviewed 25 publications with 217 patients overall who had undergone robotic liver resections.[216] Two studies compared robotic surgery to conventional or laparoscopic surgery.[217,218] The number of patients in each study ranged from 1 to 70. All studies used the da Vinci robot system (Intuitive, Sunnyvale, CA).

The most common indications for robotic surgery were wedge resection or segmentectomy (37.7%) followed by right hepatectomy (21.6%) and left lateral segmentectomy (20.8%). Five or six ports were used (three for the robotic working arm, one for the robotic camera, and one or two for the assistant working port). The camera port was usually placed in the umbilical or right paraumbilical area. Liver transection was performed using harmonic device, bipolar cautery or CUSA. The facility to use running suture for hemostasis provided a considerable advantage over conventional laparoscopic surgery. Conversion was reported in 4.6% cases. There was no surgical mortality. The morbidity was 20.3%. The two comparative studies reported a similar rate of complications during robotic liver resection compared to conventional laparoscopic procedures.[217,218]

While it has been shown that robotic surgery is feasible and safe for selected procedures long-term results need to be reported. More importantly cost-effectiveness of the procedure needs to be established because of the prohibitive cost of the instrument and the equipment used.

REFERENCES

1. Meyers WC, Jones RS (Eds). Textbook of liver and biliary surgery. Philadelphia: JB Lippincott; 1990.
2. Strong R, Lynch S, Ong T, Matsunami H, Koido Y, Balderson G. Successful liver transplantation from a living donor to her son. N Engl J Med. 1990;322:1505-7.
3. Cantlie I. On a new arrangement on the right and left lobes of the liver. Proc Anat Soc Great Britain, lreland. 1897;32:4-9.
4. Mcindoe AH, Counseller VS. The bilaterality of the liver. Arch Surg. 1927;15:589-94.
5. Couinaud C. Surgical anatomy of the liver revisited. Paris: Maugein & Cie. 1989:123-34.
6. Strasberg SM. Terminology of liver anatomy and liver resections: coming to terms with hepatic babel. J Am Coll Surg. 1997;184:413-34.
7. Reynaud BH, Coucora vas GO, Giuly JA. Basis to improve several hepatectomy 'techniques involving the surgical anatomy of the lncisura dextra of Gans. Surg Gynaecol Obstet. 1991;172:490-2.
8. Blumgart LH. Liver resection-liver and biliary tumors. Chapter in: Surgery of the liver and biliary tract. Blumgart LH (Ed), 2nd edition. Edinburgh, Churchill Livingstone; 1994. pp. 1495-538.
9. Kumon M. Anatomy of the caudate lobe with special reference of portal vein and bile duct (in Japanese with English abstract). Acta Hepatol Jpn. 1985;12:1193-9.
10. Launois B, Jamieson GG. The importance of Glisson's capsule and its sheaths in the intrahepatic approach to resection of the liver. Surg Gynecol Obstet. 1992;174:7-10.
11. Launois B, Jamieson GG. The posterior intrahepatic approach for hepatectomy or removal of segments of the liver. Surg Gynecol Obstet. 1992;174:155-8.
12. Pang YY. The Brisbane 2000 terminology of liver anatomy and resections. HPB 2000; 2:333-9. HPB (Oxford). 2002;4(2):99.
13. Francavilla A, Polimeno L, Barone M, Azzarone A, Starzl TE. Hepatic regeneration and growth factors. J Surg Oncol. 1993;3:1-7.
14. Starzl TE, Porter KA, Putnam CW. Intraportal insulin protects from the liver injury of portocaval shunt in dogs. Lancet. 1975;2(7947):1241-2.
15. Kam I, Lynch S, Svanas G, Todo S, Polimeno L, Francavilla A, et al. Evidence that host size determines liver size: studies in dogs receiving orthotopic liver transplants. Hepatology. 1987;7:362-6.
16. Grisham JW. A morphological study of deoxyribonucleic acid synthesis and cell proliferation in regenerating liver; autoradiography with thymidine-H3. Cancer Res. 1962;22:842-9.
17. Rabes HM, Wirshing R, Tuczek HV, Iseler G. Analysis of cell cycle compartments of hepatocytes after partial hepatectomy. Cell Tissue Kinet. 1976;6:517-32.
18. Michalopoulos GK. Liver regeneration: molecular mechanisms of growth control. Faseb J. 1990;4:176-87.
19. Sakomoto T, Liu Z, Murase N, Ezure T, Yokomuro S, Poli V, et al. Mitosis and apoptosis in the liver of interleukin-6-deficient mice after partial hepatectomy. Hepatology. 1999;29:403-11.
20. Marubashi S, Sakon M, Nagano H, Gotoh K, Hashimoto K, Kubota M, et al. Effect of portal haemodynamics on liver regeneration studied in a novel portohepatic shunt rat model. Surgery. 2004;136:1028-37.
21. Mars WM, Liu ML, Kitson RP, Goldfarb RH, Gabauer MK, Michalopoulos GK. Immediate early detection of urokinase receptor after partial hepatectomy and its implications for initiation of liver regeneration. Hepatology. 1995;21:1695-1701.
22. Masumoto A, Yamamoto N. Stimulation of DNA synthesis in hepatocytes by hepatocyte growth factor bound to extracellular matrix. Biochem Biophys Res Commun. 1993;191:1218-23.
23. Michalopoulos GK. Liver regeneration. J Cell Physiol. 2007;213:286-300.
24. Imamura H, Matsuyama Y, Miyagawa Y, Ishida K, Shimada R, Miyagawa S, et al. Prognostic significance of anatomical resection and des-gamma-carboxyprothrombin in patients with HCC. Br J Surg. 1999;86:1032-8.
25. van Thiel DH, Hagler NG, Schade RR, Skolnick ML, Heyl AP, Rosenblum E, et al. In vivo hepatic volume determination using sonography and computed tomography. Gastroenterology. 1985;88:1812-7.
26. Okamoto E, Kyo A, Yamanaka N, Tanaka N, Kuwata K. Prediction of safe limits of hepatectomy by combined volumetric and functional measurements in patients with impaired hepatic function. Surgery. 1984;95:586-91.
27. Lam CM, Fan ST, Lo CM, Wong J. Major hepatectomy for hepatocellular carcinoma in patients with unsatisfactory Indocyanine green clearance. Br J Surg. 1999;86:1012-7.
28. Matsumata T, Kanematsu T, Yoshida Y, Furuta T, Yanaga K, Sugimachi K. The indocyanine green test enables prediction of the postoperative complications after hepatic resection. World J Surg. 1987;11:678-81.
29. Friedman LS, Martin P, Santiago JN. Liver function test and objective evaluation of patients with liver disease. In: Zakim D, Boyer TD (Eds). Hepatology, Philadelphia: WB Saunders; 1996;791-833.
30. Bismuth H, Houssin D, Omowski J, Meriggi F. Liver resections in cirrhotic patients: a western experience. World J Surg. 1986;10:311-7.
31. Fan ST, Lai EC, Lo CM, Ng IO, Wong J. Hospital mortality of major hepatectomy for hepatocellular carcinomas associated with cirrhosis. Arch Surg. 1995;130:198-203
32. Malinchoc M, Kamath PS, Gordon FD, Peine CJ, Rank J, ter Borg PC. A model to predict poor survival in patients undergoing transjugular intrahepatic porto-systemic shunts. Hepatology. 2000;31:864-71.
33. Delis SG, Bakoyiannis A, Biliatis I, Athanassiou K, Tassopoulos N, Dervenis C. Model for end-stage liver disease (MELD) score, as a prognostic factor for post-operative morbidity and mortality in cirrhotic patients, undergoing hepatectomy for hepatocellular carcinoma. HPB. 2009;11:351-7.
34. Takenaka K, Shimada M, Higashi H, Adachi E, Nishizaki T, Yanaga K, et al. Liver resection for hepatocellular carcinoma in the elderly. Arch Surg. 1994;129:846-50.
35. Ikeda Y, Shimada M, Hasegawa H, Gion T, Kajiyama K, Shirabe K, et al. Prognosis of hepatocellular carcinoma with diabetes mellitus after hepatic resection. Hepatology. 1998;27:1567-71.

36. Slankamenac K1, Breitenstein S, Held U, Beck-Schimmer B, Puhan MA, Clavien PA. Development and validation of a prediction score for postoperative acute renal failure following liver resection. Ann Surg. 2009;250:720-8.
37. Alderson PO, Adams OF, Mc Neil BJ. Computed tomography, ultrasound and scintigraphy of the liver in patients with colon or breast carcinoma: a prospective comparison. Radiology. 1983;149:225-30.
38. Chezmar JL, Rumancik WM, Megibow AJ, Hulnick DH, Belson RC, Bernardino ME. Liver and abdominal screening in patients with cancer: CT versus MR Imaging. Radiology. 1988;168:43-7.
39. Knopf DR, Torres WE, Fajman WJ, Sones PJ. Liver lesions: comparative accuracy of scintigraphy and computed tomography. AJR. 1982;138:623-7.
40. Yamaguchi A, Ishide T, Nishimura G, Kanno M, Kosaka T, Yonemura Y, et al. Detection by CT during arterial portography of colorectal cancer metastases to the liver. Dis Col Rect. 1991;34:37-40.
41. Hopper KD, Singapuri K, Finkel A. Body CT and oncologic imaging. Radiology. 2000;215:27-40.
42. Vogl TJ, Eichler K, Zangos S, Mack M, Hammerstingl R. Hepatocellular carcinoma: role of imaging diagnostics in detection, intervention and follow-up. Rofo Fortschr Geb Rontgenstr Neuen Bildgeb Verfahr. 2002;174:1358-68.
43. Libbrecht L, Bielen D, Verslype C, Vanbeckevoort D, Pirenne J, Nevens F, et al. Focal lesions in cirrhotic explant livers: pathological evaluation and accuracy of pretransplantation imaging examinations. Liver Transplantation. 2002;8:749-61.
44. Baron RL, Peterson MS. From the RSNA refresher courses: screening the cirrhotic liver for hepatocellular carcinoma with CT and MR imaging: opportunities and pitfalls. Radiographics. 2001;21 Spec No:S117-32.
45. Krinsky GA, Lee VS, Theise ND, Weinreb JC, Rofsky NM, Diflo T, et al. Hepatocellular carcinoma and dysplastic nodules in patients with cirrhosis: prospective diagnosis with MR imaging and explanation correlation. Radiology. 2001;219:445-54.
46. Bissoli E, Bison L, Gioulis E, Chisena C, Fabbris R. [Multislice CT fluoroscopy: technical principles, clinical applications and dosimetry] Radiol Med. (Torino) 2003;106:201-12.
47. Tanaka S, Kitamra T, Fujita M, Kasugai H, Inoue A, Ishiguro S. Small hepatocellular carcinoma: Differentiation from adenomatous hyperplastic nodule with color Doppler flow imaging. Radiology. 1992;182:161-5.
48. Shimamoto K, Sakuma S, Ishigaki T, Ishiguchi T, Itoh S, Fukatsu H. Hepatocellular carcinoma: evaluation with color Doppler US and MRI Imaging. Radiology. 1992;190:741-4.
49. John TG, Greig JD, Crosbie JL. Superior staging of liver tumors with laparoscopy and laparoscopic ultrasound. Ann Surg. 1994;220:711-9.
50. Kathkouda N, Mouiel J. Laparoscopic surgery or the liver. In: Arregui ME, Fitzgibbons RJ, Kathkouda N, McRenean JB, Reich H (Eds). Principles of laparoscopic surgery. New York: Springer-Verlag; 1995:345-55.
51. DeWitt J, LeBlanc J, McHenry L, Ciaccia D, Imperiale T, Chappo J, et al. Endoscopic ultrasound-guided fine needle aspiration cytology of solid liver lesions: a large single-center experience. Am J Gastroenterol. 2003;98:1976-81.
52. Furuse J, Nagase M, Ishii H, Yoshino M. Contrast enhancement patterns of hepatic tumours during the vascular phase using coded harmonic imaging and Levovist to differentiate hepatocellular carcinoma from other focal lesions. Br J Radiol. 2003;76:385-92.
53. Machi J, Isomoto H, Kurohiji T, Yamashita Y, Shirouzu K, Kakegawa T, et al. Accuracy of intraoperative ultrasonography in diagnosing liver metastases from colorectal cancer: evaluation with postoperative follow up results. World J Surg. 1991;15:551-7.
54. Bismuth H, Castaing D, Garden OJ. The use of operative ultrasound in surgery of primary liver tumors. World J Surg. 1987;11:610-4.
55. Makuuchi M, Hasegawa H, Yamazaki S. Ultrasonically guided subsegmentectomy. Surg Gynecol Obstet. 1985;162:346-50.
56. Weinmann HJ, Ebert W, Misselwitz B, Schmitt-Willich H. Tissue specific MR contrast agents. Eur J Radiol. 2003;46:33-44.
57. Oliva MR, Saini S. Liver cancer imaging: role of CT, MRI, US and PET. Cancer Imaging. 2004;4:S42-S6.
58. Nimura Y, Hayakawa N, Kamiya J, Kondo S, Shionoya S. Hepatic segmentectomy with caudate lobe resection for bile duct cancer of the hepatic hilus. World J Surg. 1990;14:535-43.
59. Ger R. Surgical anatomy of the liver. Surg Clin North Am. 1990;69:179-92.
60. Choi BI, Kim HC, Han JK, Park JH, Kim YI, Kim ST, et al. Therapeutic effect of transcatheter oily chemoembolization therapy for encapsulated nodular hepatocellular carcinoma: CT and pathologic findings. Radiology. 1992;182:709-13.
61. Zealley IA, Skehan SJ, Rawlinson J, Coates G, Nahmias C, Somers S. Selection of patients for resection of hepatic metastases: improved detection of extrahepatic disease with FDG PET. Radiographics. 2001;21:S55-69.
62. Yang M, Martin DR, Karabulut N, Frick MP. Comparison of MR and PET imaging for the evaluation of liver metastases. J Magn Reson Imaging. 2003;17:343-9.
63. Schindl MJ, Redhead DN, Fearon KC, Garden OJ, Wigmore SJ. Edinburgh Liver Surgery and Transplantation Experimental Research Group (eLISTER). The value of residual liver volume as a predictor of hepatic dysfunction and infection after major liver resection. Gut. 2005;54:289-6.
64. Shoup M, Gonen M, D'Angelica M, Jarnagin WR, DeMatteo RP, Schwartz LH, et al. Volumetric analysis predicts hepatic dysfunction in patients undergoing major liver resection. J Gastrointest Surg. 2003;7:325-30.
65. Yigitler C, Farges O, Kianmanesh R, Regimbeau JM, Abdalla EK, Belghiti J. The small remnant liver after major liver resection: how common and how relevant? Liver Transpl. 2003;9:S18-25.
66. Fan ST. Methods and related drawbacks in the estimation of surgical risks in cirrhotic patients undergoing hepatectomy. Hepatogastroenterology. 2002;49:17-20.
67. Behrns KE, Tsiotos GG, DeSouza NF, Krishna MK, Ludwig J, Nagorney DM. Hepatic steatosis as a potential risk factor for major hepatic resection. J Gastrointest Surg. 1998;2:292-8.
68. Dello SAWG, van Dam RM, Slangen JJG, van de Poll MCG, Bemelmans MHA, Greve JW, et al. Liver Volumetry Plug and Play: Do It Yourself with Image J. World J Surg. 2007;31:2215-21.
69. Kinoshita H, Sakai K, Hirohashi K, Igawa S, Yamasaki O, Kubo S. Preoperative portal vein embolization for hepatocellular carcinoma. World J Surg. 1986;10:803-8.
70. Azoulay D, Raccuia JS, Castaing D, Bismuth H. Right portal vein embolization in preparation for major hepatic resection. J Am Coll Surg. 1995:181:267-9.
71. Harada H, Imamura H, Miyagawa S, Kawasaki S. Fate of human liver after hemihepatic portal vein embolization: Cell kinetic and morphometric study. Hepatology. 1997;26:1162-70.
72. Makuuchi M, Thai BL, Takayasu K, Takayama T, Kosuge T, Gunvén P, et al. Preoperative portal embolization for increased safety of major hepatectomy in hilar bile duct carcinoma: a preliminary report. Surgery. 1990;107:521-7.
73. Fan ST, Lo CM, Lai EC, Chu KM, Liu CL, Wong J. Perioperative nutritional support in patients undergoing hepatectomy for HCC. N Engl J Med. 1994;331:1547-52.
74. Zeigler TR. Perioperative nutritional support in patients undergoing hepatectomy for HCC. J Parenter Enteral Nutr (JPEN). 1996;20:91-2.

75. Nishizaki T, Takenaka K, Yanaga K, Shimada M, Shirabe K, Matsumata T, et al. Nutritional support after hepatic resection: a randomized prospective study. Hepatogastroenterology. 1996;43:608-13.
76. Matsumata T, Kanematsu K, Shirabe T, Sonoda T, Furuta T, Sugimachi K. Decreased morbidity and mortality rates in surgical patients with hepatocellular carcinoma. Br J Surg. 1990;77:677-80.
77. Thompson HH, Tompkins RK, Longmire WP. Major hepatic resections: a 25 year experience. Ann Surg. 1983;197:375-88.
78. Kooby DA, Stockman J, Ben-Porat L, Gonen M, Jarnagin WR, Dematteo RP, et al. Influence of transfusions on perioperative and long-term outcome in patients following hepatic resection for colorectal metastases. Ann Surg. 2003;237:860-9.
79. Fan ST, Ng IO, Poon RT, Lo CM, Liu CL, Wong J. Hepatectomy for hepatocellular carcinoma: the surgeon's role in long-term survival. Arch Surg. 1999;134:1124-30.
80. Melendez JA, Arslan V, Fischer ME, Wuest D, Jarnagin WR, Fong Y, et al. Perioperative outcomes of major hepatic resections under low central venous pressure anesthesia: blood loss, blood transfusion, and the risk of postoperative renal dysfunction. J Am Coll Surg. 1998;187:620-5.
81. Wang WD, Liang LJ, Huang XQ, Yin XY. Low central venous pressure reduces blood loss in hepatectomy. World J Gastroenterol. 2006;12:935-9.
82. Fortner JG, Blumgart LH. A historic perspective of liver surgery for tumours at the end of the millennium. J Am Coll Surg. 2001;193:210-22.
83. Poon RT, Fan ST, Lo CM, Liu CL, Lam CM, Yuen WK, et al. Improving perioperative outcome expands the role of hepatectomy in management of benign and malignant hepatobiliary diseases: analysis of 1222 consecutive patients from a prospective database. Ann Surg. 2004;240:698-708.
84. Lin TY, Chem KM, Liu TK. Total right hepatic lobectomy for primary hepatoma. Surgery. 1960;48:1048-60.
85. Tung TT. A new technique for operation on the liver. Lancet. 1963:1:192-3.
86. Lin TY. A simplified technique for hepatic resection: the crush method. Ann Surg. 1974;180:285-90.
87. Sun HC, Qin LX, Lu L, Wang L, Ye QH, Ren N, et al. Randomized clinical trial of the effects of abdominal drainage after elective hepatectomy using the crushing clamp method. Br J Surg. 2006;93:422-6.
88. Papachristou DN, Berters R. Resection of the liver with a water jet. Br J Surg. 1982;69:93-4.
89. Rau HG, Wichmann MW, Schinkel S, Butler E, Pickelmann S, Schauer R, et al. Surgical techniques in hepatic resections: Ultrasonic aspirator versus Jet-Cutter. A prospective randomized clinical trial. Zentralbl Chir. 2001;126:586-90.
90. Fan ST, Lai EC, Lo CM, Chu KM, Liu CL, Wong J. Hepatectomy with an ultrasonic dissector for hepatocellular carcinoma. Br J Surg. 1996;83:117-20.
91. Takayama T, Makuuchi M, Kubota K, Harihara Y, Hiu AM, Sano K, et al. Randomized comparison of ultrasonic vs clamp transection of the liver. Arch Surg. 2001;136:922-8.
92. Aldrighetti L, Pulitano C, Arru M, Catena M, Finazzi R, Ferla G. "Technological" approach versus clamp crushing technique for hepatic parenchymal transection: a comparative study. J Gastrointest Surg. 2006;10:974-9.
93. Schmidbauer S, Hallfeldt KK, Sitzmann G, Kantelhardt T, Trupka A. Experience with ultrasound scissors and blades (UltraCision) in open and laparoscopic liver resection. Ann Surg. 2002;235:27-30.
94. Kim J, Ahmad SA, Lowy AM, Buell JF, Pennington LJ, Soldano DA, et al. Increased biliary fistulas after liver resection with the harmonic scalpel. Am Surg. 2003;69:815-9.
95. Saiura A, Yamamoto J, Koga R, Sakamoto Y, Kokudo N, Seki M, et al. Usefulness of LigaSure for liver resection: analysis by randomized clinical trial. Am J Surg. 2006;192:41-5.
96. Weber JC, Navarra G, Jiao LR, Nicholls JP, Jensen SL, Habib NA. New technique for liver resection using heat coagulative necrosis. Ann Surg. 2002;236:560-3.
97. Stella M, Percivale A, Pasqualini M, Profeti A, Gandolfo N, Serafini G, et al. Radiofrequency-assisted liver resection. J Gastrointest Surg. 2003;7:797-801.
98. Fong Y, Blumgart LH. Useful stapling techniques in liver surgery. J Am Coll Surg. 1997;185:93-100.
99. Kaneko H, Otsuka Y, Takagi S, Tsuchiya M, Tamura A, Shiba T. Hepatic resection using stapling devices. Am J Surg. 2004;187:280-4.
100. Lersutel M, Selzner M, Petrowsky S, McCormack L, Clavien PA. How should transection of the liver be performed?: a prospective randomized study in 100 consecutive patients: comparing four different transection strategies. Ann Surg. 2005;242:814-22.
101. Lortat-Jacob JL, Robert HG, Henry L. Un cas d' hepatectomie droite reglee. Momoires de la Academie de-Chirurgie. 1952;78:244-51.
102. Ger R. Surgical anatomy of the hepatic venous system. Clin Anal. 1988;1:15-22.
103. Bismuth H. Surgical anatomy and anatomical surgery of liver. World J Surg. 1982;6:3-9.
104. Ozawa K. Liver Surgery Approached through the Mitochondria. Tokyo: Medical Tribune; 1992. pp. 117-65.
105. Liu CL, Fan ST, Cheung ST, Lo CM, Ng IO, Wong J. Anterior approach versus conventional approach right hepatic resection for large hepatocellular carcinoma: a prospective randomized controlled study. Ann Surg. 2006;244:194-203.
106. Belghiti J, Guevara OA, Noun R, Saldinger PF, Kianmanesh R. Liver hanging manoeuvre: a safe approach to right hepatectomy without liver mobilization. J Am Coll Surg. 2001;193:109-11.
107. Trotovsek B, Belghiti J, Gadzijev EM, Ravnik D, Hribernik M. Anatomical basis of the liver hanging manoeuvre. Hepatogatroenterology. 2005;52:728-30.
108. Meng WC, Shao CX, Mak KL, Lau PY, Yeung YP, Yip AW. Anatomical justification of Belghiti's 'liver hanging manoeuvre' in right hepatectomy with anterior approach. Aust N Z J Surg. 2003;73:407-9.
109. Liddo G, Buc E, Nagarajan G, Hidaka M, Dokmak S, Belghiti J. The liver hanging manoeuvre. HPB (Oxford). 2009;11:296-305.
110. Pringle JH. Notes on the arrest of hepatic haemorrhage due to trauma. Ann Surg. 1908;48:541-9.
111. Delva E, Camus Y, Paugam C, Parc R, Huguet C, Lienhart A. Haemodynamic effects of portal triad clamping in humans. Anaesth Analg. 1987;66:864-8.
112. Huguet C, Gavelli A, Bona S. Hepatic resection with ischaemia of the liver exceeding one hour. J Am Coll Surg. 1994;178:454-8.
113. Nagasue N, Yukaya H, Ogawa Y, Hirose S, Okita M. Segemental and subsegmental resections of the cirrhotic liver under hepatic inflow and outflow occlusion. Br J Surg. 1985;72:565-8.
114. Nagasue N, Yukaya H, Suehiro S, Ogawa Y. Tolerance of the cirrhotic liver to normothermic ischaemia. A clinical study in 15 patients. Am J Surg. 1984;147:772-5.
115. Hannoun L, Jones D, Vaillant JC, Nordlinger B, Parc R. Liver resection with normothermic ischaemia exceeding one hour. Br J Surg. 1993;80:1161-5.
116. Kim YI, Kobayashi M, Aramaki M, Nakashima K, Mitarai Y, Yoshida T. "Early-stage" cirrhotic liver can withstand 75 minutes of inflow occlusion during liver resection. Hepatogastroenterology. 1994;41:355-8.
117. Elias D, Desruennes E, Lasser P. Prolonged intermittent clamping of the portal triad during hepatectomy. Br J Surg. 1991;78:42-4.
118. Dionigi R, Dominioni L, Benevento A, et al. Risultati dell 'i mpiego delle nuove tecnologie nelle resezioni epatiche. Chir Triveneta. 1996;36:4-9.
119. Clavien PA, Yadav S, Sindram D, Bentley RC. Protective effects of ischemic preconditioning for liver resection performed under inflow occlusion in humans. Ann Surg. 2000;232:155-62.

120. Imamura H, Takayama T, Sugawara Y, Kokudo N, Aoki T, Kaneko J, et al. Pringle's manoeuvre in living donors. Lancet. 2002;360:2049-50.
121. Makuuchi M, Mori T, Gunvén P, Yamazaki S, Hasegawa H. Safety of hemihepatic vascular exclusion during resection of the liver. Surg Gynecol Obstet. 1987;164:155-8.
122. Miyagawa S, Makuchhi M, Kawasaki S, Kakazu T. Changes in serum amylase level following hepatic resection in chronic liver disease. Arch Surg. 1994;129:634-8.
123. Shimamura Y, Gunvén P, Takenaka Y, Shimizu H, Akimoto H, Shima Y, et al. Selective portal branch occlusion by balloon catheter during liver resection. Surgery. 1986;100:938-41.
124. Heaney JP, Stanton WK, Halbert OS, Seidel J, Vice T. An improved technic for vascular isolation of the liver: experimental study and case reports. Ann Surg. 1966;163:237-41.
125. Huguet C, Nordlinger B, Galopin JJ, Bloch P, Gallot D. Normothermic vascular exclusion for extensive hepatectomy. Surg Gynecol Obstet. 1978;147:689-93.
126. Delva E, Barberousse JP, Nordlinger B, Ollivier JM, Vacher B, Guilmet C, et al. Hemodynamic and biochemical monitoring during major liver resection with the use of hepatic vascular exclusion. Surgery. 1984;95:309-18.
127. Belghiti J, Noun R. Vascular exclusion techniques in liver resections. In: Forni E, Merrigi F (Eds). Selected topics of HPB Surgery and Medicine, Proceedings of Alpe-Adria Hepatopancreatobiliary Congress, Pavia; 1995. pp. 93-8.
128. Yamaoka Y, Ozawa K, Kumada K, Shimahara Y, Tanaka K, Mori K, et al. Total vascular exclusion for hepatic resection in cirrhotic patients-application of venovenous bypass. Arch Surg. 1992;127:276-80.
129. Emre S, Schwartz M E, Katz E, Miller CM. Liver resection under total vascular isolation-variations on a theme. Ann Surg. 1993;217:15-9.
130. Cherqui D, Malassagne N, Colau PI, Brunetti F, Rotman N, Fagniez PL. Hepatic vascular exclusion with preservation of the caval flow for liver resections. Ann Surg. 1999;230:24-30.
131. Huguet C, Gavelli A, Chieco PA, Bona S, Harb J, Joseph JM, et al. Liver ischaemia for hepatic resection: where is the limit? Surgery. 1992;111:251-9.
132. Emond J, Wachs ME, Renz JF, Kelley S, Harris H, Roberts JP, et al. Total vascular exclusion for major hepatectomy in patients with abnormal liver parenchyma. Arch Surg. 1995;130:824-31.
133. Habib N, Zografos G, Dalla Serra G, Greco L, Bean A. Liver resection with total vascular exclusion for malignant tumors. Br J Surg. 1994;81:1181-4.
134. Pichlmayr R, Grosse H, Hauss J, Gubernatis G, Lamesch P, Bretschneider HJ. Technique and preliminary results of extracorporeal liver surgery (bench procedure) and of surgery on the in situ perfused liver. Br J Surg. 1990;77:21-6.
135. Delreviere L, Hannoun L. In situ and ex situ in vivo procedures for complex major hepatic resections requiring prolonged hepatic vascular exclusion in normal and diseased liver. J Am Coll Surg. 1995;181:272-6.
136. Fortner JG, Shiu MH, Kinne DW, Kim DK, Castro EB, Watson RC, et al. Major hepatic resections using vascular isolation and hypothermic perfusion. Ann Surg. 1974;180:644-52.
137. Kim YI, Nakashima K, Tada I, Kawano K, Kobayashi M. Prolonged normothermic ischaemia of human cirrhotic liver during hepatectomy: a preliminary report. Br J Surg. 1993;80:1566-70.
138. Nuzzo G, Giuliante F, Murazio M, et al. IIclampaggio del ped unculo poriale nelle resezioni epatiche. Chirurgia. 1994;7:576-82.
139. Belghiti J, Noun R, Zante E, Ballet T, Sauvanet A. Portal triad clamping or hepatic vascular exclusion for major liver resection- a controlled study. Ann Surg. 1996;224:155-61.
140. Makuchhi M, Hasegawa H, Yamazaki S, Takayasu K. Four new hepatectomy procedures for resection of the right hepatic vein and preservation of the inferior right hepatic vein. Surg Gynaecol Obstet. 1987;164:69-72.
141. Czerniak A, Ayalon A. A direct approach to the left and middle hepatic veins during left-sided hepatectomy. Surg Gynecol Obstet. 1993;177:303-7.
142. Postema RR, Plaiser PW, Kate FG. Haemostasis after partial hepatectomy using argon beam coagulation. Br J Surg. 1993;80:1563-5.
143. Scheele J. lndikation, tecchnik und ergebnis der Fibrin klebung nach Leberresektionen. In: Scheele J (Ed). Fibrin klebung, Berlin: Springer-Verlag; 1982.
144. Bona S, Gavelli A, Huguet C. The role of abdominal drainage after major hepatic resection. Am J Surg. 1994;167:593-5.
145. Belghiti J, Kabbej M, Sauvanet A, Vilgrain V, Panis Y, Fekete F. Drainage after elective hepatic resection- a randomized trial. Br J Surg. 1993;218:748-53.
146. Starzl TE, Koep LJ, Weil R, Lilly JR, Putnam CW, Aldrete JA. Right trisegmentectomy for hepatic neoplasms. Surg Gynecol Obstet. 1980;150:208-14.
147. Starzl TE, Iwatsuki S, Shaw BW, Waterman PM, Van Thiel D, Diliz HS, et al. Left hepatic trisegmentectomy.Surg Gynecol Obstet. 1982;155:21-7.
148. Blumgart LH, Baer HU, Czerniak A, Zimmermann A, Dennison AR. Extended left hepatectomy: technical aspects of an evolving procedure. Br J Surg. 1993;80:903-6.
149. Wu CC, Ho WL, Chen JT, Tang CS, Yeh DC, Liu TJ, P'eng FK. Mesohepatectomy for centrally located hepatocellular carcinoma: An appraisal of a rare procedure. J Am Coll Surg. 1999;188:508-15.
150. McBride LM, Wallance S. Cancer of the right lobe of liver. Arch Surg. 1972;105:289-96.
151. Hasegawa H, Makuuchi M, Yamazaki S, Gunvén P. Central bisegmentectomy of the liver: experience in 16 patients. World J Surg. 1989;13:786-90.
152. Sugarbaker PS. En bloc resection of segments IVb, V and VI by transverse hepatectomy. Surg Gynecol Obstet. 1990;170:250-2.
153. Billingsley KG, Jarnagin WR, Fong Y, Blumgart LH. Segment-oriented hepatic resection in the management of malignant neoplasms of the liver. J Am Coll Surg. 1998;187:471-81.
154. Takayama T, Makuuchi M. lntraoperative ultrasonography and other techniques for segmental resections. Surg Oncol Clin North Am. 1996;5:261-9.
155. Makuuchi M, Hashikura Y, Kawasaki S, Tan D, Kosuge T, Takayama T. Personal experience of right anterior segmentectomy (segments V & Vlll) for hepatic malignancies. Surgery. 1993;114:52-8.
156. Sasada A, Ataka K, Tsuchiya K, Yamagishi H, Maeda H, Okada M. Complete caudate lobectomy: its definition, indications, and surgical approaches. HPB Surg. 1998;11:87-95.
157. Bartlett D, Fong Y, Blumgart LH. Complete resection of the caudate lobe of the liver: technique and results. Br J Surg. 1996;83:1076-81.
158. Nimura Y, Hayakawa N, Kamiya J, Kondo S, Nagino M, Kanai M. Hilar cholangiocarcinoma-surgical anatomy and curative resection. J Hep Bil Pancr Surg. 1995;2:239-48.
159. Broelsch CE, Whitington PF, Emond JC, Heffron TG, Thistlethwaite JR, Stevens L, et al. Liver transplantation in children from living related donors. Ann Surg. 1991;214:428-38.
160. Makuuchi M, Kawasaki S, Noguchi T, Hashikura Y, Matsunami H, Hayashi K, et al. Donor hepatectomy for living related partial liver transplantation. Surgery. 1993;113:395-402.
161. Chan SC, Fan ST, Lo CM, Liu CL, Wong J. Toward current standards of donor right hepatectomy for adult-to-adult live donor liver transplantation through the experience of 200 Cases. Ann Surg. 2007;245:110-7.

162. Rao PP, Routh D, Naidu CS, Sharma S, Sharma AK, Priyaranjan, et al. Donor outcome in live-related liver transplantation. Medical Journal Armed Forces India. 2014;70:100-4.
163. Soin AS, Kumaran V, Rastogi AN, Mohanka R, Mehta N, Saigal S, et al. Evolution of a reliable biliary reconstructive technique in 400 consecutive living donor liver transplants. J Am Coll Surg. 2010;211:24-32.
164. Heaton ND, Tan KC. Living-related liver transplantation. Chapter in: The practice of liver transplantation. Williams R, Portmann B and Tan KC (Eds). Edinburgh: Churchill-Livingstone; 1995. pp. 153-9.
165. Watanabe I, Mayumi T, Arishima T, Takahashi H, Shikano T, Nakao A, et al. Hyperlactemia can predict the prognosis of liver resection. Shock. 2007;28:35-8.
166. Geerse DA, Bindels AJ, Kuiper MA, Roos AN, Spronk PE, Schultz MJ. Treatment of hypophosphatemia in the intensive care unit: a review. Crit Care. 2010;14:R147.
167. Shor R, Halabe A, Rishver S, Tilis Y, Matas Z, Fux A, et al. Severe hypophosphatemia in sepsis as a mortality predictor. Ann Clin Lab Sci. 2006;36:67-72.
168. Richter B, Schmandra TC, Golling M, Bechstein WO. Nutritional support after open liver resection: a systematic rev iew. Dig Surg. 2006;23:139-45.
169. Hotta T, Kobayashi Y, Taniguchi K, Johata K, Sahara M, Naka T, et al. Evaluation of postoperative nutritional state after hepatectomy for hepatocellular carcinoma. Hepatogastroenterology. 2003;50:1511-6.
170. Marchesini G, Bianchi G, Merli M, Amodio P, Panella C, Loguercio C, et al. Nutritional supplementation with branched-chain amino acids in advanced cirrhosis: a double-blind, randomized trial. Gastroenterology. 2003;124:1792-801.
171. Muto Y, Sato S, Watanabe A, Moriwaki H, Suzuki K, Kato A, et al. Effects of oral branched-chain amino acid granules on event-free survival in patients with liver cirrhosis. Clin Gastroenterol Hepatol. 2005;3:705-13.
172. van den Berghe G, Wouters P, Weekers F, Verwaest C, Bruyninckx F, Schetz M, et al. Intensive insulin therapy in the critically ill patients. N Engl J Med. 2001;345:1359-67.
173. Fisette A, Hassanain M, Metrakos P, Doi SA, Salman A, Schricker T, et al. High-Dose Insulin Therapy Reduces Postoperative Liver Dysfunction and Complications in Liver Resection Patients through Reduced Apoptosis and Altered Inflammation. J Clin Endocrinol Metab. 2012;97:217-26.
174. De Pietri L, Montalti R, Begliomini B, Scaglioni G, Marconi G, Reggiani A, et al. Thromboelastographic changes in liver and pancreatic cancer surgery: hypercoagulability, hypocoagulability or normocoagulability? Eur J Anaesthesiol. 2010;27:608-16.
175. Shontz R, Karuparthy V, Temple R, Brennan TJ. Prevalence and risk factors predisposing to coagulopathy in patients receiving epidural analgesia for hepatic surgery. Reg Anesth Pain Med. 2009;34:308-11.
176. Rudin A, Lundberg JF, Hammarlund-Udenaes M, Flisberg P, Werner MU. Morphine metabolism after major liver surgery. Anesth Analg. 2007;104:1409-14.
177. Werawatganon T, Charuluxanun S. Patient controlled intravenous opioid analgesia versus continuous epidural analgesia for pain after intra-abdominal surgery. Cochrane Data Base Syst Rev. 2005;1:CD004088.
178. Page AJ, Kooby DA. Perioperative management of hepatic resection. J Gastrointest Oncol. 2012;3:19-27.
179. Blackford D, Hewitt P, Pande G, Nguyen H, Chilvers C, Robertson I. Future of analgesia for abdominal laparotomy. ANZ J Surg. 2008;78:527-9.
180. Chan SK, Lai PB, Li PT, Wong J, Karmakar MK, Lee KF, et al. The analgesic efficacy of continuous wound instillation with ropivacaine after open hepatic surgery. Anaesthesia. 2010;65:1180-6.
181. Neal CP, Mann CD, Garcea G, Briggs CD, Dennison AR, Berry DP. Preoperative systemic inflammation and infectious complications after resection of colorectal liver metastases. Arch Surg. 2011;146:471-8.
182. Kaibori M, Ishizaki M, Matsui K, Kwon AH. Postoperative infectious and non- infectious complications after hepatectomy for hepatocellular carcinoma. Hepatogastroenterology. 2011;58:1747-56.
183. Okabayashi T, Nishimori I, Yamashita K, Sugimoto T, Yatabe T, Maeda H, et al. Risk factors and predictors for surgical site infection after hepatic resection. J Hosp Infect. 2009;73:47-53.
184. Yeh DC, Wu CC, Ho WM, Cheng SB, Lu IY, Liu TJ, et al. Bacterial translocation after cirrhotic liver resection: a clinical investigation of 181 patients. J Surg Res. 2003;111:209-14.
185. Geerts WH, Bergqvist D, Pineo GF, Heit JA, Samama CM, Lassen MR, et al. Prevention of venous thromboembolism: American College of Chest Physicians Evidence-Based Clinical Practice Guidelines (8th Edition). Chest. 2008;133:381S-453S.
186. Reddy SK, Turley RS, Barbas AS, Steel JL, Tsung A, Marsh J W, et al. Post-operative pharmacologic thromboprophylaxis after major hepatectomy: does peripheral venous thromboembolism prevention outweigh bleeding risks? J Gastrointest Surg. 2011;15:1602-10.
187. De Pietri L, Montalti R, Begliomini B, Scaglioni G, Marconi G, Reggiani A, et al. Thromboelastographic changes in liver and pancreatic cancer surgery: hypercoagulability, hypocoagulability or normocoagulability? Eur J Anaesthesiol. 2010;27:608-16.
188. Nagasue N, Yukaya H, Ogawa Y, Higashi T. Portal pressure following partial to extensive hepatic resection in patients with and without cirrhosis. Ann Chir Gynaecol. 1983;72:18-22.
189. Kanematsu T, Sugimachi K, Kohno H, Matsumata T, Kobayashi M, Inokuchi K. Minute liver cancer and concomitant esophageal varices: detection and successful surgical treatment. World J Surg. 1981;5:707-11.
190. Ohnishi K, Tanabe Y, Ryu M, Isono K, Yamamoto Y, Usui S, et al. Prognosis of hepatocellular carcinoma smaller than 5 cms in relation treatment: study of 100 patients. Hepatology. 1987;7:1285-90.
191. Nagasue N, Yukaya H, Ogawa Y, Sasaki Y, Chang YC, Niimi K. Clinical experience with 118 hepatic resections for hepatocellular carcinoma. Surgery. 1986;99:694-701.
192. Hasegawa H, Yamazaki S, Makuuchi M, Elias D. [Hepatectomy for hepatocarcinoma on a cirrhotic liver: decision plans and principles of perioperative resuscitation. Experience with 204 cases]. (Article in French). J Chir (Paris). 1987;124:425-31.
193. Harada A, Nonami T, Nakao A, Kurokawa T, Takagi H. Surgical treatment for hepatocellular carcinoma and concomitant esophagogastric varices. Seminars Surg Oncol. 1996;12:193-6.
194. Franco D, Borgonova G. Liver resection in cirrhosis of the liver. Chapter in: Surgery of the liver and biliary tract. Blumgart LH (Ed); 2nd Edition. Edinburgh: Churchill-Livingstone;. 1994:1539-55.
195. van Leeuwen PA, Hong RW, Rounds JD, Rodrick ML, Wilmore D. Hepatic failure and coma after liver resection is reversed by manipulation of gut contents: the role of endotoxin. Surgery. 1991;110:169-74.
196. Takenaka K, Kanematsu T, Fukuzawa K, Sugimachi K. Can hepatic failure after surgery for HCC in cirrhotic patients be prevented? World J Surg. 1990;14:123-7.
197. Tsao JI, Loftus JP, Nagorney DM, Adson MA, Ilstrup DM. Trends in morbidity and mortality of hepatic resection for malignancy. A matched comparative analysis. Ann Surg. 1994;220:199-205.
198. Nagasue N, Kohno H, Chang YC, Taniura H, Yamanoi A, Uchida M, et al. Liver resection for hepatocellular carcinoma. Results of 229 consecutive patients during 11 years. Ann Surg. 1993;217:375-84.
199. Gagner M, Rheault M, Dubuc J. Laparoscopic partial hepatectomy for liver tumor. Surg Endosc. 1992;6:97-8.

200. Reddy SK, Tsung A, Geller DA. Laparoscopic liver resection. World J Surg. 2011;35:1478-86.
201. Nguyen KT, Gamblin TC, Geller DA. World review of laparoscopic liver resection-2804 patients. Ann Surg. 2009;250:831-41.
202. Bluell JF, Cherqui D, Geller DA, O'Rourke N, Lannitti D, Dagher I, et al. The International position on laparoscopic liver surgery: The Louisville Statement, 2008. Ann Surg. 2009:250:825-30.
203. Viagno L, Laurent A, Tayar C, Tomatis M, Ponti A, Cherqui D. The learning curve in laparoscopic liver resection: improved feasibility and reproducibility. Ann Surg. 2009;250:772-82.
204. O'Rourke N, Fielding G. Laparoscopic right hepatectomy: surgical technique. J Gastrointest Surg. 2004;8:213-6.
205. Dagher I, O'Rourke N, Geller DA. Laparoscopic major hepatectomy: an evolution in standard of care. Ann Surg. 2009;250:856-60.
206. Nitta H, Sasaki A, Fujita T, Itabashi H, Hoshikawa K, Takahara T, et al. Laparoscopy-assisted major liver resections employing a hanging technique: the original procedure. Ann Surg. 2010;251:450-3.
207. Dagher I, Di Giuro G, Dubrez J, Lainas P, Smadja C, Franco D. Laparoscopic versus open right hepatectomy: a comparative study. Am J Surg. 2009;198:173-7.
208. Ito K, Ito H, Are C, Allen PJ, Fong Y, DeMatteo RP, et al. Laparoscopic versus open liver resection: a matched-pair case control study. J Gastrointest Surg. 2009;3:2276-83.
209. Dagher I, Belli G, Fantini C, Laurent A, Tayar C, Lainas P, et al. Laparoscopic hepatectomy for hepatocellular carcinoma: a European experience. J Am Coll Surg. 2010;211:16-23.
210. Himpens J, Leman G, Cadiere GB. Telesurgical laparoscopic cholecystectomy. Surg Endosc. 1998;12:1091.
211. Hyung WJ. Robotic surgery in gastrointestinal surgery. Korean J Gastroenterol. 2007;50:256-9.
212. Antoniou SA, Antoniou GA, Koch OO, Pointner R, Granderath FA. Robot-assisted laparoscopic surgery of the colon and rectum. Surg Endosc. 2012;26:1-11.
213. Kitisin K, Packiam V, Bartlett DL, Tsung A. A current update on the evolution of robotic liver surgery. Minerva Chir. 2011;66:281-93.
214. Idrees K, Bartlett DL. Robotic liver surgery. Surg Clin North Am. 2010;90:761-74.
215. Corcione F, Esposito C, Cuccurullo D, Settembre A, Miranda N, Amato F, et al.) Advantages and limits of robot-assisted laparoscopic surgery: preliminary experience. Surg Endosc. 2005;19:117-9.
216. Ho CM, Wakabayashi G, Nitta H, Ito N, Hasegawa Y, Takahara T. Systematic review of robotic liver resection. Surg Endosc. 2013;27:732-9.
217. Ji WB, Wang HG, Zhao ZM, Duan WD, Lu F, Dong JH. Robotic-assisted laparoscopic anatomic hepatectomy in China: initial experience. Ann Surg. 2011;253:342-8.
218. Berber E, Akyildiz HY, Aucejo F, Gunasekaran G, Chalikonda S, Fung J. Robotic versus laparoscopic resection of liver tumours. HPB. 2010;12:583-6.

CHAPTER 76

Non-Cirrhotic Portal Hypertension

Shivraj Bahadur Singh, Vivek Mangla, Sujoy Pal

Extrahepatic Portal Venous Obstruction

INTRODUCTION

Portal hypertension is elevation of portal venous pressures due to any cause. This disease process is usually secondary to an underlying problem resulting in prehepatic, intrahepatic or posthepatic obstruction to portal venous blood flow. In Western countries, cirrhosis represents the most common underlying etiology. In the Indian setting, however, non-cirrhotic causes comprise a significant proportion (40–50%) of patients with portal hypertension, especially so in younger age groups. This subgroup is represented by extrahepatic portal venous obstruction (EHPVO), non-cirrhotic portal fibrosis (NCPF) and hepatic venous outflow tract obstruction (HVOTO). This chapter focuses on EHPVO and NCPF. HVOTO is dealt with elsewhere in this book.

Extrahepatic portal venous obstruction is defined as occlusion of the extrahepatic portal vein regardless of involvement of the intrahepatic portal vein, splenic or mesenteric veins.[1] Thrombosis secondary to cirrhosis or hepatocellular carcinoma is not included. Additionally, isolated occlusion of the splenic or superior mesenteric veins is not considered EHPVO.

Extrahepatic portal venous obstruction is rare in the west but represents a significant disease burden in India.[2] It accounts for 70% of portal hypertension in the pediatric age group.[1,3]

ETIOLOGY

In EHPVO, the thrombosis occurs at the confluence of the superior mesenteric and splenic veins in nearly 95% of patients. Subsequently, collaterals develop around the portal vein resulting in portal cavernoma formation in the gastrohepatic ligament surrounding portal structures entering the liver hilum.

The underlying etiology is yet to be determined but various hypotheses have been suggested.

Infection

Intra-abdominal and umbilical vein sepsis can both result in thrombotic occlusion of the portal vein.[4] In the case of umbilical vein sepsis, a single or multiple episodes of infection can theoretically result in extension of the infected thrombus into the left and subsequently main portal vein resulting in EHPVO. This theory, however, supports this diagnosis in less than 5% of patients indicating that infection is unlikely to be the sole etiology. Similarly, intra-abdominal sepsis or recurrent episodes of gastroenteritis in childhood also predispose to portal vein thrombosis. However, their role in EHPVO remains conjectural.

Along similar lines umbilical vein catheterization can result in thrombosis[5,6] extending into the main portal vein. But evidence of umbilical sepsis, umbilical catheterization and intra-abdominal sepsis is available in only a small percentage of patients with EHPVO[4,7] leaving the majority of patients with an undetermined etiology.

Congenital Defects

In Western series, there has been a correlation between EHPVO and congenital abnormalities resulting in the theory of a congenital etiology. However, this suggestion is not, supported by the available Indian literature where large series have failed to identify such a correlation and most patients with EHPVO do not have other co-existing congenital anomalies.

Hypercoagulable States

Hypercoagulable states are more commonly found in adults. Protein C deficiency is found most commonly followed by protein S.[8] Western series cite a significant proportion of their patients having underlying hypercoagulability[9] but this etiology is unsupported in Indian literature where only 15% of patients have been shown to have some hypercoagulable state.[8]

In keeping with the inadequate evidence in support of any one aetiologic[4,8,10,11] hypothesis, the Asian Pacific Association for the Study of the Liver (APASL) 2006 consensus statement concluded that EHPVO is a heterogeneous disease with only a small proportion of patients having an identifiable etiology, the majority of patients being idiopathic.[1]

PATHOPHYSIOLOGY

Occlusion of the portal vein results in development of a hepatopetal pattern of venous collateralization in an attempt to maintain portal venous blood flow to the liver. Since the portal vein is replaced by surrounding collaterals, the terms portal vein cavernoma and cavernomatous transformation are used. Maintenance of the hepatic portal blood supply results in adequate preservation of the liver structure and function. These collaterals, however, are not sufficient to decompress the portal system resulting in portosystemic collaterals such as esophagogastric, periportal, pericholecystic, retropancreatic, perisplenic, lienorenal and lower rectal varices. Of these, collaterals at the esophagogastric junction are common and clinically important, as variceal bleeding resulting in hematemesis is the most common presentation in these patients.

Collaterals in the hepatoduodenal ligament are often associated with abnormalities of the intrahepatic and/or extrahepatic biliary tree, referred to as portal biliopathy. The abnormalities include localized strictures, dilatation, angulations, wall irregularities, displacement and biliary stones.[10] Compression of the biliary tree by dilated collaterals in Saint's epicholedochal and Petren's paracholedochal venous plexuses were initially believed to effect these changes. However, portal biliopathy is not always completely reversible on portosystemic shunting and it is plausible that ischemia of the bile ducts resulting from long standing extrinsic pressure or venous hypertension could be responsible for these persistent abnormalities.[12]

Clinical Presentation

Patients with EHO are generally children or young adults, most of whom have onset of symptoms in childhood. The most common presentation is recurrent, massive hematemesis and splenomegaly in the absence of liver dysfunction. Morbidity and mortality in these patients is predominantly related to variceal hemorrhage, symptomatic portal biliopathy, hypersplenism and rarely recurrent thrombosis.[13]

Bleeding

In children upper gastrointestinal hemorrhage is the most common presentation. Nearly 70% of patients experience at least one episode of bleeding by the age of 15.[12] In children with untreated EHPVO, rebleeding is the rule rather than the exception with 70% of patients experiencing rebleeding within 3 years of their first bleed.[12] Despite this the individual risk of rebleeding is markedly variable.[13] Bleeding episodes in this patient population are not associated with hepatic decompensation as seen in cirrhosis and the bleeding episodes are well tolerated.[14] This said, the mortality from a single bleeding episode still remains between 7% and 13% in developing countries.[15] In one series from India, of 25 patients with EHPVO, being followed-up without surgery, there was a 100% mortality due to variceal bleeding within 5 years.[16] Added to this, there are risks associated with repeated blood transfusions including risk of transmission of infections. In our surgical series of nearly 1,000 patients, 4% and 2% of patients had hepatitis B and C infection, respectively.[17] The problem is further compounded by the limited facilities for safe blood transfusion in developing countries.

The incidence of gastric varices increases with the duration of portal hypertension and is higher in patients who have previously received endotherapy for esophageal varices.[18-20] Gastric varices are generally more difficult to treat than esophageal varices and tend to have higher rebleeding rates and mortality.

Changes due to portal hypertension are also seen in the colon and rectum with variable extent and severity. Bleeding from these lesions has been reported in 8% of patients and is much more common in patients with EHO than cirrhosis.[21]

Portal hypertensive Gastropathy (PHG) or Portal Hypertensive Colopathy (PHC)

Patients with EHPVO often show changes in the gastric mucosa. A similar mucosal appearance in the colon analogous to PHG in the colon is termed *portal hypertensive colopathy*. Endoscopy reveals a mosaic-like mucosal pattern. It is considered mild when only a mosaic like pattern is seen, and, severe when there are additional discrete red spots. It occurs more often in patients with EHPVO than cirrhosis and more often following endoscopic variceal ligation or sclerotherapy. Both these entities are reversible with successful surgical portosystemic shunts (PSSs).

Splenomegaly

Almost all patients with EHPVO have splenomegaly. Of these, 12–22% have hypersplenism.[22,23] Hypersplenism is defined as cytopenia involving any one or more of the three blood cell lines [hemoglobin (Hb), platelet or leukocyte count] with a normal or hypercellular bone marrow; the cytopenia being reversible following splenectomy. Patients often present with left upper abdominal discomfort or a dragging sensation due to the enlarged spleen. Spleen is variable in size but generally smaller than seen in patients with NCPF. Clinically, significant hypersplenism (7–10%) is associated with recurrent gum bleeds, epistaxis, menorrhagia, easy fatigability and recurrent infections besides recurrent attacks of abdominal pain due to splenic infarcts.[24]

Ascites

During infancy and early childhood, some patients have high portal pressure and poorly developed collateral circulation resulting in ascites, growth failure, and chronic anemia secondary to blood loss. After a variable period of time, recanalization of the thrombosed portal vein and gradual development of collateral venous channels leads to resolution of the ascites and for a period of time, these children may grow and develop in a near normal manner. Ascites may also occur at the time of gastrointestinal bleeding but is transient and usually does not require diuretics.[1]

The diagnosis of EHPVO should be eyed with suspicion in a patient having significant ascites.

Growth Retardation

Growth retardation is commonly seen in children with EHPVO. In India, nearly 50% of children with EHPVO have growth retardation. The severity of this symptom set correlates with the duration of symptoms.[25] Resistance to growth hormone, reduced insulin-like growth factor, mucosal changes secondary to raised portal pressure and hypersplenism are the postulated mechanisms for growth retardation.[26] However, the exact cause remains unknown. Shunt surgery is associated with a spurt in growth in most patients with EHPVO and growth retardation.[25,26]

Portal Biliopathy

This group of symptoms presents more commonly in the adult population with EHPVO and occurs in 5–14% of patients with the rest of the population remaining asymptomatic.[27] The common presentations include recurrent biliary pain, obstructive jaundice and recurrent cholangitis.

INVESTIGATIONS

Hematology

Patients with bleeding or hypersplenism may present with anemia. Reticulocyte count is essential to confirm an adequately functioning bone marrow.

In adults presenting with this disease a prothrombotic state must be ruled out, and patients should be tested for hypercoaguable states including protein C and S deficiency.

Liver Function Tests

Liver function tests are usually normal in these patients. An elevation in alkaline phosphatase and gamma glutamyl transpeptidase (GGT) may suggest the presence of portal biliopathy.

Endoscopy

An upper gastrointestinal endoscopy should be done in all patients to confirm the presence of esophageal varices which occur in 90% of patients. Ectopic varices are uncommon but their incidence increases with time and following endoscopic eradication of esophageal varices. Among ectopic varices, anorectal ones are most common and are generally larger than those found in portal hypertension due to other causes.[21,28] Endoscopy is also useful to assess for variceal regression (which is a surrogate marker for shunt patency) after shunt surgery (Fig. 1). Endoscopic retrograde cholangiopancreatography followed by biliary stenting or nasobiliary drainage is used in the preoperative or nonoperative management of patients with symptomatic portal biliopathy but should not be used solely for diagnostic purposes in this setting.

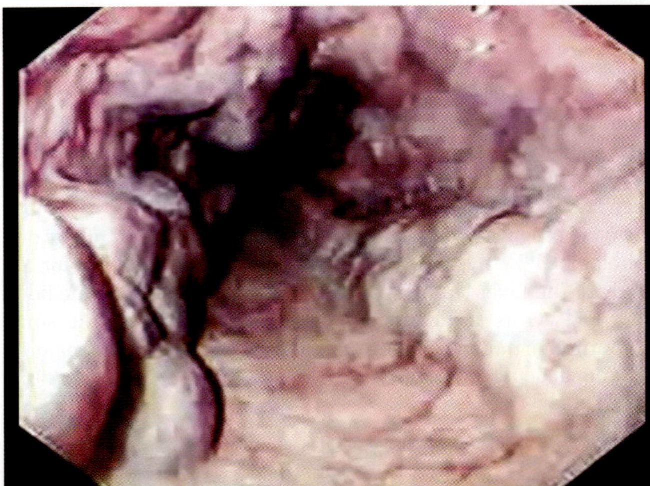

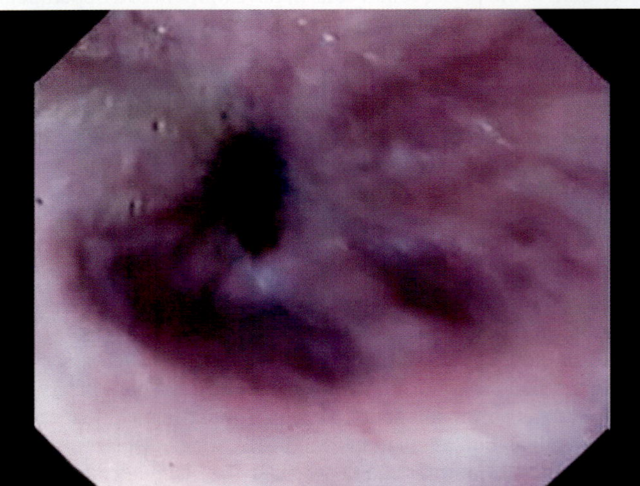

Figure 1 Upper gastrointestinal endoscopy (preshunt and postshunt) showing complete regression of varices on endoscopy following shunt surgery

Radiology

Abdominal Ultrasound with Doppler

Ultrasound is a useful tool in preoperative and postoperative management of EHPVO. It is a reliable noninvasive means of diagnosing a portal cavernoma (Fig. 2), confirming the splenomegaly (Fig. 3) and detecting portal biliopathy by identifying intrahepatic bile duct dilatation. It is also useful in evaluating patency and calibre of the splenic and superior mesenteric veins.

In operative planning, ultrasound confirms the normal anatomical location of the left kidney and the left renal vein before a proximal lienorenal shunt is performed. A Doppler study is also useful in the follow-up of patients after a proximal lienorenal shunt to evaluate shunt patency, wherein, either visualization of the patent shunt or the presence of a dilated left renal vein (indirect evidence) suggests a patent shunt.

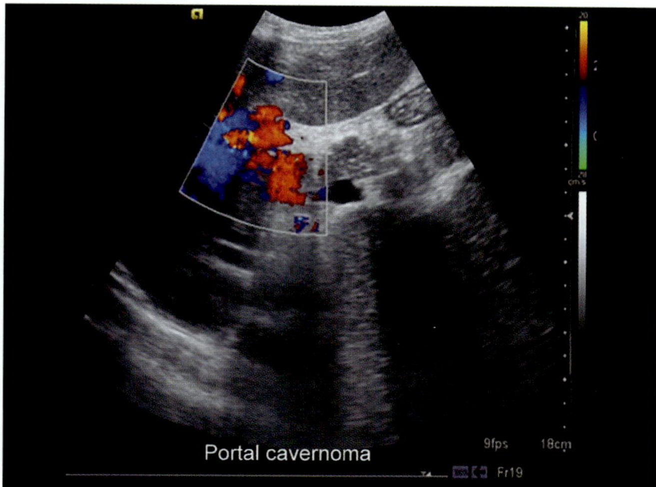

Figure 2 Ultrasound Doppler showing replacement of portal vein by a cavernoma

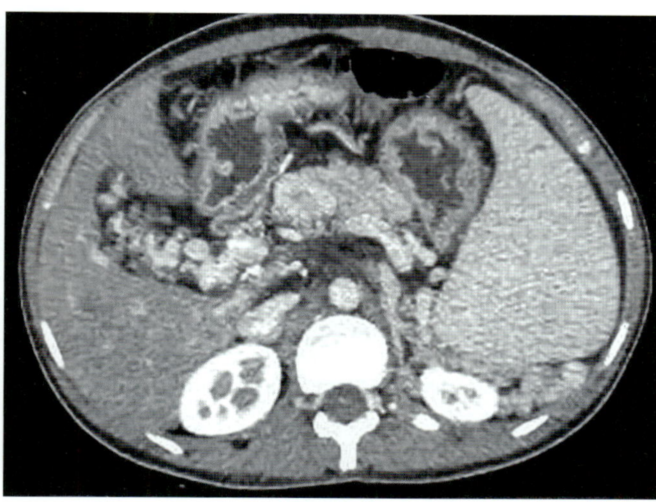

Figure 4 Computed tomography portography showing splenomegaly, portal cavernoma, patent splenic vein and extensive splenorenal collaterals

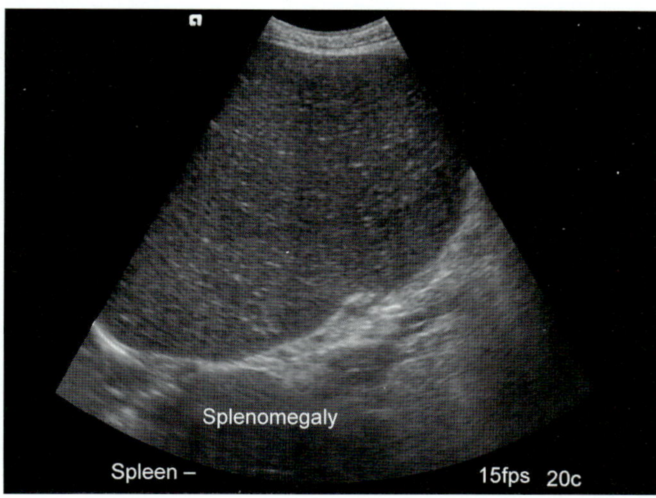

Figure 3 Ultrasound showing splenomegaly

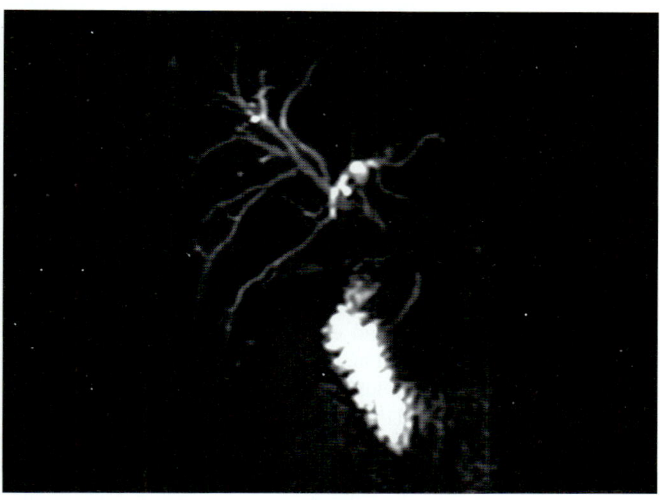

Figure 5 Magnetic resonance cholangiopancreatography showing features of portal biliopathy (*Source:* Dr Ankur Arora, ILBS., New Delhi)

Computed Tomography Portography (Fig. 4)

Computed tomography is highly specific and less operator dependent than ultrasound. However, due to the associated risk from contrast injection and radiation exposure, it is required only when ultrasonography is of suboptimal quality or the portal venous system cannot be evaluated satisfactorily with ultrasonography.

Magnetic Resonance Cholangiopancreatography

Magnetic resonance cholangiopancreatography (MRCP) (Fig. 5) is useful to evaluate patients with suspected portal biliopathy. Biliary abnormailities described include smooth strictures of various lengths and degrees, caliber irregularity, segmental upstream dilatation, ectasia, indentations, displacement and angulations of ducts, clustering of intrahepatic ducts and pruning of intrahepatic ducts.[29,30]

Hemodynamic Studies

Patients with EHPVO have a high intrasplenic pressure. The wedged hepatic venous pressure, which reflects the sinusoidal pressure is normal thus confirming the presinusoidal nature of the portal hypertension in these patients. Measurement of the portal pressure has a very limited role in the clinical management of these patients and therefore should not be done routinely.[1]

Liver Biopsy

Liver biopsy is unnecessary in the routine evaluation and management of patients with EHPVO. In patients with atypical clinical or laboratory features, a liver biopsy may be done to rule out the presence of chronic liver disease. Liver biopsy is essentially normal in patients with EHPVO. It may, however, occasionally show minimal sclerosis of the intrahepatic portal radicles. Other minor changes include minimal fibrosis in the portal tracts and mild focal parenchymal changes. These changes are of little clinical importance.

Patients with portal biliopathy usually have features of cholestasis. There is usually no ductopenia, ductular proliferation or portal triaditis which helps differentiate changes due to portal biliopathy from those due to other primary cholestatic diseases of the liver.

In all patients undergoing surgery, it is advisable to do an intraoperative wedge or needle biopsy of the liver. This allows for baseline histology in the event of future presentations due to liver disease.

Immune Function

Extrahepatic hepatic portal venous obstruction patients have changes in cell mediated immunity including anergy to delayed hypersensitivity skin testing, reduced T-lymphocyte concentrations and mitogen responsiveness. The humoral immunity is normal. Tests for immune function, however, are not routinely indicated in these patients.

Management

The main problem in patients with EHPVO is gastrointestinal bleeding which may result in hemodynamic instability and even death. Some have suggested that children outgrow their disease by adolescence due to the formation of more effective collaterals and therefore require only supportive treatment for bleeding episodes.[31] The weight of current evidence, does not, however support this. Several studies have provided evidence to the contrary.[12,16,32-34] One Indian study by Mitra et al. revealed that among patients with EHPVO who had not bled, 80% bled on follow-up, further, 19% of nonoperated patients died due to gastrointestinal bleeding and 5% of patients in their study died from variceal bleeding while awaiting elective surgery.[24] The aim of treatment is to minimize the risk of life-threatening bleeding from gastrointestinal varices, the alternatives being surgery or endoscopic management. At present, there are no large prospective studies comparing endoscopic and surgical management.

Primary Prophylaxis of Variceal Bleeding

The concept of surgical prophylaxis in the context of portal hypertension is not new. In the setting of cirrhosis with portal hypertension shunt surgery had failed as it had enhanced the occurrence of liver failure in the cohort undergoing prophylactic shunts. Since patients with EHPVO have preserved liver function, between 1976 and 2010, we operated on selected patients with EHPVO, who had no history of variceal bleeding but had "high risk" esophagogastric varices or severe PHG, and/or hypersplenism and came from remote areas with poor access to tertiary healthcare. Following surgery, these patients were prospectively followed-up with regards to mortality, variceal bleeding, encephalopathy and liver function. A total of 114 patients underwent prophylactic operations (proximal splenorenal shunts: 98(86%); esophagogastric devascularization: 16). Postoperative mortality was 0.9%. Among 89 (79%) patients who were followed-up (mean: 60 months), hypersplenism was cured and 6 (6.7%) developed variceal bleeding. The latter were managed successfully by endoscopic treatment. No patient developed overwhelming postsplenectomy sepsis or encephalopathy and 90% were free of symptoms.[23] Therefore, we believe that in selected patients with EHPVO, prophylactic surgery is fairly safe and prevents variceal bleeding in approximately 94% of patients with no occurrence of portosystemic encephalopathy or liver failure. These results have prompted us to recommend prophylactic operations to patients with EHPVO who have not bled but have high-risk varices and/or hypersplenism and poor access to medical facilities.[23]

Acute Bleeding

Therapeutic endoscopy is the treatment of choice in acute bleeding as success rates are as high as 95%.[2-4] Somatostatin (250 μg stat and 250 μg hourly intravenous infusion for 3–5 days) or terlipressin (1–2 mg intravenous stat and repeated every 4–6 h till bleeding stops or up to 3–5 days) are also used as adjuncts in the medical management. Both these drugs can very rarely cause mesenteric ischemia and Terlipressin may precipate myocardial ischemia in susceptible patients hence cautious use is advised.

Surgery is considered a second-line treatment in patients with bleeding refractory to endoscopic therapy.[31] Another indication for emergency surgery is rebleeding after initial control. In patients undergoing emergency surgery, after initial control of bleeding, consideration must be given for a PSS.[35]

Prevention of Rebleeding

Endoscopic variceal sclerotherapy and band ligation: The widespread availability of flexible endoscopes and trained endoscopists has increased the popularity of endoscopic sclerotherapy and variceal ligation for the treatment of varices. With newer advances and more frequent use of band ligation, complications with endoscopic procedures are fewer. Despite endotherapy, the portal pressure remains high resulting in variceal recurrence. Additionally, PHG and portal biliopathy do not resolve and may get aggravated.

The true incidence of variceal recurrence and rebleeding after endotherapy in patients with EHPVO is difficult to ascertain, as most series of patients treated with endotherapy have included both cirrhotic and non-cirrhotic patients. A few studies evaluating the results of endotherapy in a selected group of patients with EHPVO (excluding other causes of portal hypertension) exist (Table 1). This data for endotherapy is largely from small and retrospective studies with a limited follow-up.

Most endoscopic series have failed to recognize portal biliopathy as a long-term complication of EHPVO. There seems to be an association between portal biliopathy and endoscopic therapy and there may be a cause and effect relationship.[7,17] In addition, multiple sessions of endotherapy may be required throughout the life of the patient with consequent morbidity and high costs.

Surgery

Surgical intervention offers a one-time cure for these patients. The surgical options for management of EHPVO can be divided

Table I: Selected series of endotherapy for patients with extrahepatic portal venous obstruction from India

Author (year)	*No. of patients*	*Variceal obliteration rate (%)*	*Sessions required*	*Duration of follow-up (months)*	*Rebleeding (%)*	*Variceal recurrence (%)*	*Remarks*
Chawla (1990)[36]	122	91	Median 5 (2–18)	24 (4–60)	–	16	Nearly 15% lost to follow-up Interval bleeding: 16% Mortality: 5%
Bhargava (1991)[37]	87	92	7.95 ± 2.2	28	111.5		2.3% late mortality due to bleeding 10% complication rate
Yachha (1997)[38]	50	88	Mean 8	19 (12–36)	0	10	Interval bleeding 26%
Poddar (2003)[39]	257	95	Mean 4.5	36 (3–113)	–	17	20% lost to follow up prior to eradication 5 bleed related deaths Nearly 10% required surgery Interval bleeding 10.6% Significant procedure related morbidity
Zargar (2004)[18]	59	91.3	6.3 ± 1.8	10.4–20.1 (mean, 15.1 ± 3.1) years	11.9 at median of 3 years	14	Failure to achieve eradication in 8.7% Surgery in ten patients Procedure-related morbidity 28.9%
Itha (2006)[19]	183	-	8	3.07 ± 1.84 years	7	40	Nearly 8 endotherapy sessions for eradication Only patients achieving variceal eradication included Significant increase in incidence of congestive gastropathy No mortality in patients requiring surgery following failed endotherapy
Thomas (2009)[7]	198/223		-	Median 20 (14–23) years	17.2	20	Only patients with variceal eradication with endotherapy included Failure to recognize the subgroup with failure to eradicate varices and rebleeding Number of patients who bled while on endotherapy not mentioned Surgery in 6% for failed endotherapy 15% esophageal stricture rate requiring dilatation Portal biliopathy in 6%, management unclear No deaths related to varices/endotherapy complications

into PSSs and non-shunt procedures. In non-shunt procedures, the varices or their venous communications are ligated. Devascularization procedures are the only surgical option in patients with a thrombosed splenoportal and mesentericoportal axis and therefore no "shuntable" vein.

Portosystemic Shunts

The preferred surgical option is a PSS.[40-42] Conventional portocaval shunts are unsuitable in this patient population because the portal vein is replaced by a cavernoma therefore an alternative shunt is required.

The PSSs for EHPVO can be selective such as distal splenorenal shunt or non-selective. These include central or proximal lienorenal, side-to-side splenorenal or mesocaval shunts.

The distal splenorenal shunt selectively decompresses gastrooesophageal varices while preserving the hepatopetal blood flow in addition to preserving the spleen. However, there are certain reservations regarding the use of distal or side-to-side splenorenal shunts:

- The hepatic blood flow is preserved even in non-selective shunts in patients with EHPVO.
- Since post-shunt encephalopathy does not occur in EHPVO, performing a selective shunt does not provide any additional benefit.[41,43]
- The distal splenorenal shunt loses selectivity with time due to development of collateral channels between the low pressure gastrosplenic and the high pressure mesenteric portal venous system.
- This procedure is not suited for patients with hypersplenism as up to 40% of patients have persistent hypersplenism following distal splenorenal shunting.[43]

The end-to-side mesocaval shunt (Clatworthy) is an alternative procedure particularly in children because ligation of the inferior vena cava does not result in limb edema in children unlike the case in adults. The so-called "makeshift" shunts, usually done when no shuntable vein is available due to extensive splanchnic thrombosis, may not remain patent for long and are often unsuccessful.[24]

Thus almost all of our patients with EHPVO requiring surgery undergo a proximal lienorenal shunt. After splenectomy, the proximal splenic vein is joined end-to-side to the left renal vein using continuous suturing technique with "growth factor". If the splenic vein is small in caliber an interrupted suturing technique is preferred. Details of the procedure will be discussed in the chapter on operations for portal hypertension.

Results of Shunt Surgery

Shunt surgery has a nearly 1% risk of mortality in the elective setting. Rebleeding occurs in 0–10% patients after surgery.[42-44] Higher rebleeding rates have generally been reported from low volume centers and high volume centers have consistently reporting lower rebleeding rates.[40,45] In India, the elective and emergency mortality rates have been reported to be 0.7% and 10% respectively. The rebleeding rate is about 11% and the actuarial 15-year survival by life-table analysis is 95%. Reversal of hypersplenism is seen in all patients.[40,41]

Long-term studies from experienced centers in the West have shown similar results with the use of shunt surgery in children with EHPVO. Bismuth et al. have reported long-term shunt patency rates of 96%. In this study, no prophylactic shunts were done but all conservatively managed patients developed variceal bleeding.[42] Based on these results, proximal lienorenal shunt (Fig. 6) is advocated for patients with EHPVO in the developing countries.

Table 2 shows summarized results from various series reporting shunt surgery in patients with extrahepatic hepatic portal venous obstruction.

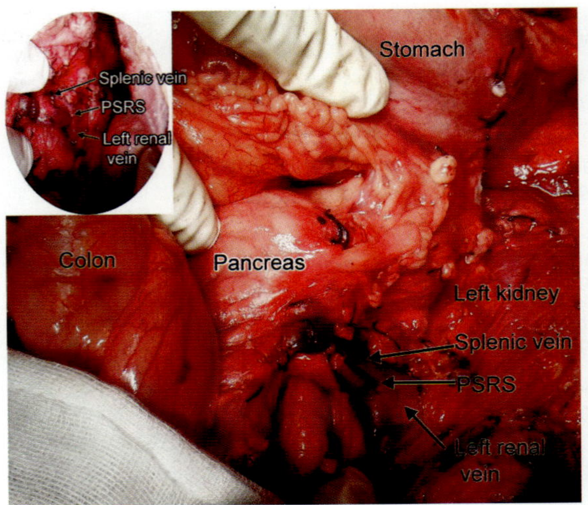

Figure 6 Operative photograph showing proximal splenorenal shunt after completion of shunt surgery
Abbreviation: PSRS, proximal splenorenal shunt.

Mesenterico-Left Portal Vein Bypass (Rex Shunt)

The Rex shunt was initially reported in pediatric liver transplant recipients who developed extrahepatic portal venous thrombosis after liver transplantation.[46,47] Today it is used as an alternative procedure in EHPVO. Superina et al. found 91% shunt patency rates at 7 years with no rebleeding in their study of 34 patients with EHPVO. Significant improvements in left portal vein diameter, left lobe liver size and reversal of hypersplenism have also been reported.[48,49]

Two new series of patients with 65 and 69 patients comparing Rex and PSSs have been recently reported. One of these studies has shown significantly better success rates with PSS compared to Rex Shunt whereas the other study has shown equivocal results.[50,51]

Theoretically, Rex Shunt seems better than PSS. The procedure, however, has certain limitations. It is not applicable to a subgroup of patients in whom either the left portal vein or the superior mesenteric vein is not patent. Use of autologous veins would be preferable but mainly feasible in the pediatric age group and in the others this procedure often entails use of a synthetic graft resulting in a life-long requirement of anticoagulation with its attendant risks. In addition, the expertise for this procedure is available at very few centers.

Table 2: Series reporting portosystemic shunt surgery in patients with extrahepatic portal venous obstruction

Author (year)	*No. of patients*	*Type of shunt*	*Mortality (%)*	*Rebleed (%)*	*Encephalopathy (%)*	*Follow-up (months)*	*Remarks*
Mitra (1978)[24]	10	PSRS, S-S SRS	24	24	0	-	Majority of mortality in emergency cases
Bismuth (1980)[42]	52	PSRS, DSRS, MCS	0	1.9%	0	50	-
Prasad (1994)[40]	160; Elective: 140 Emergency: 20	PSRS, MCS	Overall: 1.9 Elective: 0.7 Emergency: 10	11	0	12–180	95% 15-year survival No OPSI 4 deaths: 2 rebleeding, 1 renal failure, 1 unknown cause 91% follow-up
Orloff (2002)[44]	200	PSRS, MCS, S-S SRS	0	2.5 (all PSRS)	0	-	Surgery for secondary prophylaxis 93% follow up >5 years 83% follow up >10 years Normal liver biopsy in all
Mangla V (2012)[17]	832	PSRS	Overall: 1.2 Elective: 0.9 Emergency: 7	9.4	0	69 (1–408)	75% follow up No OPSI/Encephalopathy 5% emergency procedures 15-year survival ≥96%

Abbreviations: PSRS, proximal splenorenal shunt; S-S SRS, side-to-side splenorenal shunt; MCS, mesocaval shunt; OPSI, opportunistic post-splenectomy infection; DSRS, distal splenorenal shunt.

Esophagogastric Devascularization

About 10% patients with EHPVO have extensive splanchnic venous thrombosis on preoperative or intraoperative evaluation and are, thus, not candidates for a shunt procedure. Esophagogastric devascularization is the only surgical option in a patient with recurrent variceal bleeding and no major shuntable vein.

Various types of transabdominal and transthoracic devascularization procedures have been described for controlling variceal bleeding or for prevention of rebleeding in patients with portal hypertension.[52] Gastric or esophageal transection done as a part of Sugiura's procedure or its various modifications has been shown to reduce rebleeding rates.[53-54]

Hassab's procedure is a transabdominal devascularization procedure entailing devascularisation of the gastroesophageal junction and stomach with splenectomy without gastric or esophageal transection.[55,56] In view of the morbidity in terms of leak and/or strictures at the site of gastric or esophageal transection with Sugiura's procedure or its modifications, many centers prefer a Hassab's procedure with minor modifications for patients with EHPVO deemed unsuitable for shunt surgery. In patients with uncontrolled acute variceal bleeding despite endotherapy, direct ligation of the bleeding varices may be required early during the operation to achieve control of bleeding before proceeding to the remaining part of the procedure. This helps avoid esophageal or gastric transection with the attendant morbidity in terms of leaks and/or strictures. Devascularization procedures can be done through a transabdominal or a transthoracic approach. Patients with EHPVO have extensive collateral vessels and dense vascular adhesions between the spleen and diaphragm especially after endoscopic sclerotherapy. In such patients, a left thoracoabdominal incision offers good exposure for this part of the procedure without any significant increase in morbidity. In most patients, however, a left subcostal incision with or without an upper midline extension provides an adequate exposure. Reversal of hypersplenism occurs after devascularization along expected lines.[43] Since there is no decompression of the portal venous system, the portal pressure following this surgery remains high and consequently changes of portal biliopathy do not reverse.[57] In addition, these patients are at risk of developing ectopic varices and PHG from which bleeding may recur. Even though devascularization obviates the need for further blood transfusions and endotherapy in most patients, a regular follow-up is required for the evaluation and management of problems related to persistent portal hypertension such as rebleeding and portal biliopathy. Our experience with devascularization is described in Table 3.

Table 3: Results of devascularization procedures in extrahepatic portal venous obstruction

Author (year)	Number of patients	Age*	No. of bleeds^	Previous endotherapy	Evaluation for possibility of shunt	Procedure	Operative mortality#	Operating time@	Intra-operative blood loss£	Intra-operative blood transfusion£	Hospital stay&	Follow up$	Post splenectomy sepsis#	Encephalopathy#	Rebleed#	Survival	Late mortality	Remark
Shah (1999)[58]	14	17.2 ± 12.8 (3-48)	2.5 ± 1.3 (1-5)	7 (50)	Yes	Modified Sugiura	0 (0)	Median 240 (150-480)	Median 500 (100-2200)	-	16 ± 5.5 (10-28)	38.4± 22.6 (17-90)	-	-	1 (7.3)	-	0(0)	Symptomatic hypersplenism in none, thrombocytopenia in 3, dragging pain in one, esophageal stricture 2 (14.7%)
Mathur (1999)[59]	46	-	-	-	No	Modified Sugiura	2 (4.4)	-	-	-	-	55.6 ± 31.3 (12-137)	-	0 (0)	3 (7)	5 yr 91%	-	Mixed series of etiology of portal hypertension, data in table for EHPVO patients only
Rao (2004)[43]	7	9 ± 5.36 (2.5-14)	2.3 ± 1.50 (0-4)	7 (100)	Yes	Devascularization without transection	0 (0%)	-	-	-	-	(3–5)	0 (0%)	0 (0%)	0 (0)	-	-	Regression of varices in all 5 patients in whom postop UGIE was done
Roy Choudhury (2007)[60]	14	9.7 ± 1.98 (7-12)	1.8 ± 1.25 (0-3)	14 (100)	No	Hassab's procedure	0 (0%)	210 (-)	-	350 ± 80(-)	-	2.58 ± 1.6 (1-5)	0 (0%)	0 (0%)	0 (0%)	-	-	-
Mangla (2012)[61]	103	20.8 ± 11.0 (3-55)	2.8 ± 2.63 (0-20)	42 (40.8)	Yes	Modified Hassab's procedure	8 (7.8%)	334.4 ± 42.55 (280-410)	781.3 ± 556.74 350-2100)		8.72 ± 6.79 (3-57)	59.67 ± 76.81 (3-355)	0 (0)	0 (0)	14 (20.3)	100%	0 (0)	

*in years, Mean ± S.D. (range); # n, (Percent); $ in months, Mean ± S.D. (range); @ in minutes, Mean ± S.D. (range); & in days, Mean ± S.D. (range); £ in mL, Mean ± S.D. (range); ^Mean ± S.D. (range)

Abbreviations: EHPVO, extrahepatic portal venous obstruction; UGIE, upper gastrointestinal endoscopy.

Comparison of Results of Endotherapy with Surgery

Endoscopic therapy and surgery have similar rebleeding rates in the short-term but achieving this requires multiple endoscopic sessions compared to a single surgical procedure. Management of patients by endoscopic ablation of esophageal varices has the added disadvantage of ectopic variceal formation, namely, gastric, anorectal and more uncommonly duodenal. These ectopic varices may not be amenable to endoscopic management and represent a bleeding risk. A significant increase in the incidence of portal gastropathy and its severity has been reported following sclerotherapy.[36,62] About 4%–12% of these patients may require surgery, some for emergency control of bleeding with its attendant risks.[63]

Further pitfalls of endoscopic therapy are that portal biliopathy remains untreated and may, in fact, worsen after sclerotherapy. Band ligation can result in esophageal ulceration, stricture formation and even perforation. Endotherapy does not address the persistent splenomegaly resulting in persistent hypersplenism and its associated symptoms. Shunt surgery is shown to improve decreased intestinal absorptive capacity,[64] growth retardation,[25] PHG,[65] portal biliopathy[9] and PHC[66] all of which remain untreated following sclerotherapy.[10,67]

Furthermore, with a patent shunt, varices disappear or decrease in size and episodes of variceal bleeding cease.[10,24,40] This reduction in variceal grade can be used as an indirect marker of shunt patency.[68] Real time ultrasound with Doppler has been reported to be an accurate noninvasive method for assessment of shunt patency.[69] Computed tomography portography has also been shown to be a useful tool in the postoperative assessment of shunt patency with a better sensitivity than color Doppler flow imaging. However the direction of blood flow cannot be ascertained by computed tomography imaging.[70]

Postsplenectomy sepsis is rare in patients with EHPVO.[24,40,43] For this reason, we do not recommend routine pneumococcal vaccination prior to the operation. No portosystemic encephalopathy has been reported after shunt surgery in multiple series of patients with EHPVO.[24,40,43] Even detailed evaluation of patients with EHPVO after shunt surgery has failed to detect overt or subclinical encephalopathy.

Improvement in the quality of life and growth parameters has been reported following successful shunt surgery in patients with EHPVO.[26] Prophylactic shunts have been advocated by some authors who believe that almost all patients with EHPVO will bleed some time in their natural course of disease, exposing patients to the associated risks.[23,40,48]

Although prophylactic shunts are not a standard recommendation, they have been performed and found to be

Flow chart 1 Algorithmic approach to management of patients with extrahepatic portal venous obstruction

EHO
Bleeder
Nonbleeder
Doppler/CT
High grade varices
Poor access
Portal biliopathy
Symptomatic hypersplenism
Growth retardation
Low grade varices
Easy access to health care
No biliopathy
No growth retardation
Patent splenic or superior mesenteric vein
Yes
No
Shunt surgery
Symptomatic hypersplenism and/or growth retardaton
Successful
No
Yes
Especially if high grade varices
Yes
No
Endotherapy
Fails
Devascularization
Follow-up

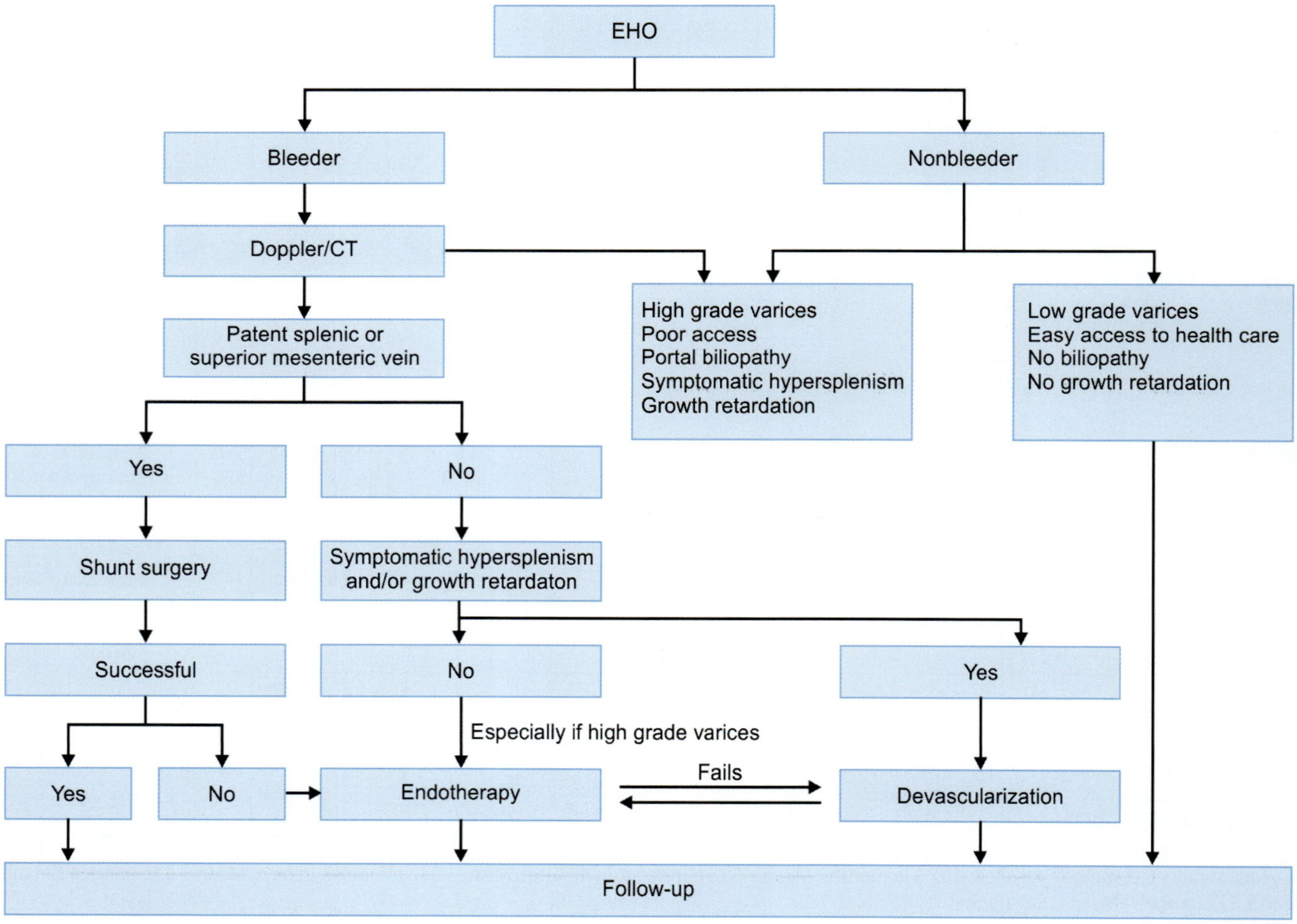

Abbreviations: EHPVO, extrahepatic portal venous obstruction; CT, computed tomography.

useful in selected patients such as those with limited access to health care, those with massive splenomegaly and symptomatic hypersplenism and patients with high-grade varices or symptomatic portal biliopathy.[9,23,42] The superiority of one type of shunt over others has not been conclusively established.

Flow chart 1 outlines our approach to the management of patients with EHPVO.

Portal Biliopathy

Surgical management of portal biliopathy is challenging due to the presence of difficult strictures surrounded by friable collaterals under high pressure. Retrospective studies from two Indian centers have found a high morbidity and mortality in patients who underwent a direct hepaticojejunostomy.[27,66] In patients with shuntable veins, PSSs have been shown to decrease the morbidity of a second stage bilioenteric anastomosis. A significant number of patients may also improve with shunt surgery alone, negating the need for further surgical intervention.[27,67,71,72]

Endoscopic therapy has been recommended as definitive management of patients with EHPVO. The long-term results with endoscopic treatment, however, are not promising with significant procedure related morbidity in terms of bleeding, cholangitis and pancreatitis.

Dhiman et al. showed reversal of portal biliopathy after shunt surgery suggesting that the biliary obstruction was at least partly due to compression by collateral channels.[10] It has been recommended that a PSS should be done before any attempt at bilioenteric anastomosis is planned in EHPVO.[10,27,67,72] We propose the following algorithm for management of patients with EHPVO and portal biliopathy (Flow chart 2).

Flow chart 2 Algorithmic approach to management of patients with portal biliopathy

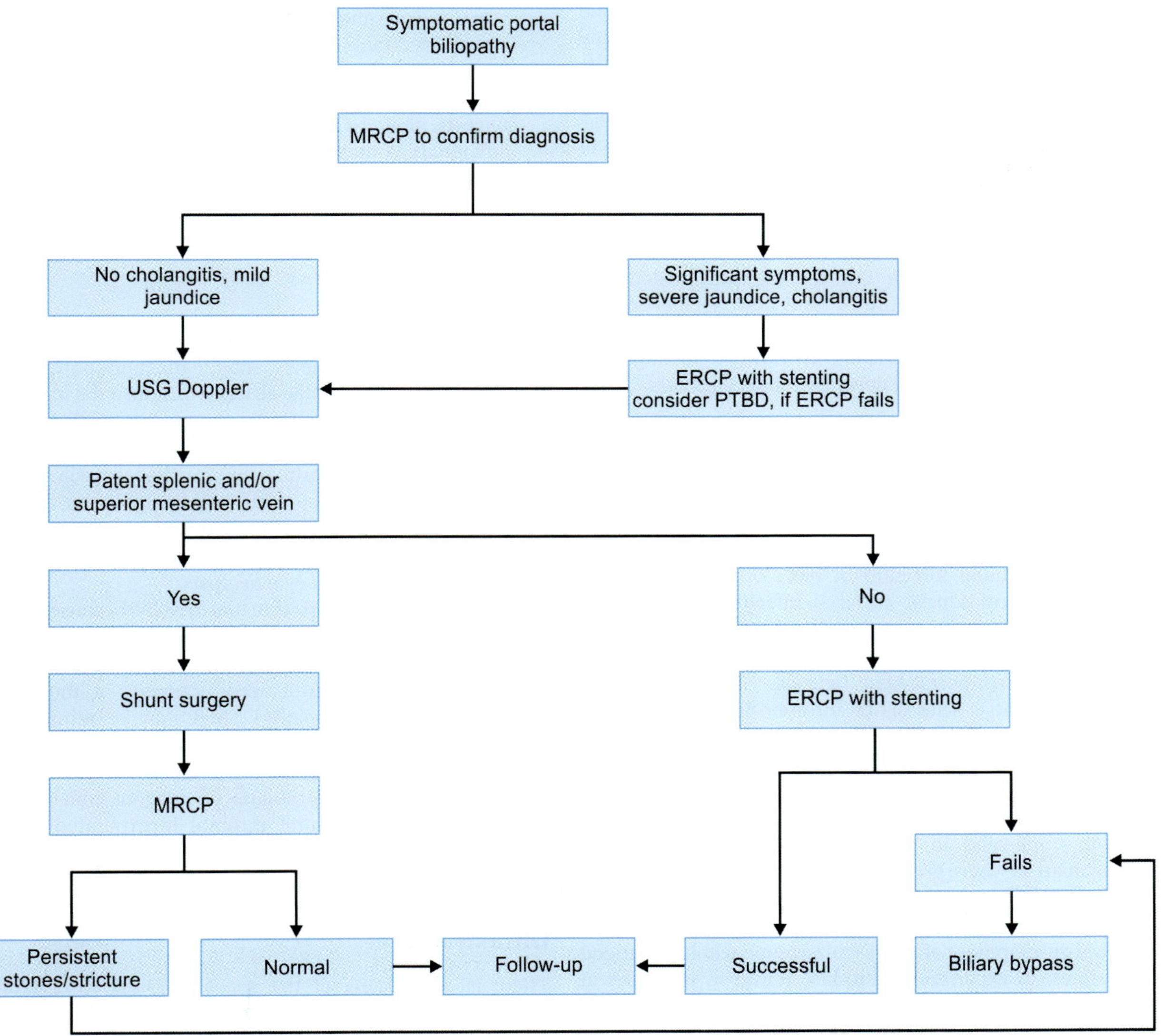

Abbreviations: MRCP, magnetic resonance cholangiopancreatography; ERCP, endoscopic retrograde cholangiopancreatogram; PTBP, percutaneous transhepatic biliary drainage.

Non-Cirrhotic Portal Fibrosis

INTRODUCTION

This disease entity was first described by Banti in 1889 in a group of patients with anemia and splenomegaly without obvious hematological disease.[73] In the late 1950s, the terms "Tropical splenomegaly syndrome" and "Bengal splenomegaly" were used to describe such patients. In the early 1960s, non-cirrhotic adult patients who presented with recurrent episodes of upper gastrointestinal bleeding without ascites or encephalopathy were observed. The term NCPF was first used by Basu et al. (1967) and endorsed by the Indian Council of Medical Research (ICMR) in 1969.[74] A similar condition with subtle differences, reported in Japan, was called idiopathic portal hypertension (IPH).[75]

DEFINITION

The APASL working party on portal hypertension has defined NCPF as a disease of uncertain etiology characterized by periportal fibrosis and involvement of small and medium branches of the portal vein, resulting in the development of presinusoidal portal hypertension with primarily normal liver structure and function.[76] The main portal vein and its primary branches are usually patent and significantly dilated.

EPIDEMIOLOGY

This disease occurs worldwide but the highest incidence is reported from developing countries and low socioeconomic groups. In India, the incidence ranges from 0.9% to 46.7% in series of patients with portal hypertension. Worldwide, including in India, the incidence of NCPF has decreased in recent years.[76]

ETIOPATHOGENESIS

As with EHPVO, there is no identifiable single agent implicated in the etiopathogenesis of NCPF. Several hypotheses have, however, been proposed:

- *Infections:* Abdominal infection at birth or early childhood including umbilical sepsis, bacterial infections or diarrheal episodes leading to portal pyemia and pylephlebitis may result in thrombosis, sclerosis and therefore obstruction of the small and medium sized portal vein radicals. However, whether the primary event is sclerosis or thrombosis is not clear. In experimental studies, similar changes have been reported after injection of dead nonpathogenic bacteria (*E. coli)* into the portal veins of rabbits and dogs.[77]
- *Exposure to chemicals, trace metals and certain drugs:* Arsenic has been implicated in NCPF. Liver biopsies of patients dwelling in areas where ground water levels of arsenic are high show changes similar to NCPF. Liver histology in these patients reveals periportal fibrosis and incomplete septal cirrhosis, with or without development of neovascularization within expanded portal zones. In experimental studies, however, increases in hepatic collagen and hydroxyproline without features of NCPF or portal hypertension have been seen suggesting that arsenic ingestion is not an important factor in the etiopathogenesis of this disease.
  - Various other factors including pica, chronic exposure to vinyl chloride monomers, copper sulphate (vineyard sprayers), and protracted treatment with methotrexate, vitamin A, immunosupression with 6-mercaptopurine, azathioprine and corticosteroids following renal transplantation have been implicated with none being conclusively shown to be involved.[78-80]
  - Altered immunity: Patients with NCPF have a reduced cell-mediated immunity. There is a decrease in T8 cells, alteration in the T4/T8 ratio and increased vascular cell adhesion molecule-1 (VCAM-1) and soluble tumor necrosis factor (TNF) receptor I and II. The role of these changes in the pathogenesis or whether it is the result of the disease process is still unclear. IPH, as reported from Japan, is associated with autoimmune disorders such as systemic lupus erythematosus, progressive systemic sclerosis, thyroiditis and mixed connective tissue disease with elevated anti-ds DNA and antinuclear antibodies. Familial aggregation and a high frequency of HLA-DR3 have also been reported.
  - In one experimental study, injection of splenic extract in pre-sensitized rabbits has been shown to result in development of a NCPF-like picture.
- *Unifying hypothesis:* This hypothesis, proposed from India, suggests that NCPF develops in genetically predisposed individuals. A major thrombotic event at birth or early in life blocks the main portal vein. Subsequently, with repeated microthrombotic events in young adults, the small or medium branches of the portal vein are affected resulting in NCPF.[75]

PATHOLOGY

In NCPF, the liver surface is nodular in 10-15% of patients.[81] Histological analysis shows subhepatic and portal fibrosis in some patients and a notable absence of sinusoidal fibrosis in most patients. Another characteristic feature of NCPF is portal vein dilatation with wall sclerosis and thickening. Thrombi are seen in medium and small portal vein branches, so called obliterative portal venopathy.[82] A deep-core wedge along with a needle biopsy has been recommended.[76] There is usually a variable involvement of portal tracts with mild portal tract edema and lymphocytic infiltration and no hepatocyte necrosis.

Pathology of IPH differs from that of NCPF because of associated autoimmune conditions. There is fibrosis of the portal tracts along with marked but patchy and segmental, subendothelial thickening of the large and medium-sized branches of the portal vein (obliterative portal venopathy). There may be intimal thickening of intrahepatic portal venous channels with obliteration of small portal venules and characteristic emergence of new aberrant portal channels. There may be stigma of previous phlebothrombosis as evident from old mural thrombi incorporated in the wall. Regenerative nodules are characteristically absent differentiating NCPF from cirrhosis.

Ultrastructure

There is a widening of the space of Disse with haphazardly arranged collagen bands in the perisinusoidal space are also seen.[83] Hepatocytes show only a mild change manifested by increase in lysosomes and fat droplets without changes in mitochondria or endoplasmic reticulum.[83]

HEMODYNAMICS

There is a marked elevation in the portal venous pressure, with one pressure gradient noted between the spleen and liver and another between the intrahepatic and wedged hepatic venous pressure[84] suggesting two possible sites of obstruction. However, most researchers believe the site of obstruction to be presinusoidal.[76] In these patients, the hepatic venous pressure gradient is normal or near normal and there is a marked increase in splenic and portal vein blood flow.

NATURAL HISTORY

Little is known about the early stages of this disease. What is known is that these patients have high variceal bleeding rates of 32%–95% with variceal bleeding being the most common cause of death.[77] Mortality from variceal bleeding is, however, lower than in patients with cirrhosis. Ascites is rare and usually associated with upper gastrointestinal bleeding following which it resolves spontaneously. Liver function is well preserved in these patients.

CLINICAL FEATURES

These patients present with episodes of upper gastrointestinal bleeding without hepatic decompensation. Jaundice and hepatic encephalopathy are rare. A massive enlargement of the spleen is present in most patients and causes left upper abdominal pain. Features of hypersplenism are common.

Rarely patients may present with glomerulonephritis or hypoxemia due to pulmonary arteriovenous fistulae.[85] The disease is generally considered to be more common in men compared to women though there is no unanimity on this data.

LABORATORY FEATURES

Hematology

Anemia is common and is usually microcytic and hypochromic due to blood loss. Leucopoenia and thrombocytopenia are common and suggest hypersplenism. These patients may have coagulation and platelet function anomalies, probably mild compensated disseminated intravascular coagulation (DIC) secondary to endotoxemia.[86]

Viral Serology

The frequency of hepatitis B and C in non-transfused patients is the same as in the general population.

Liver Function Tests

These patients have normal liver function tests both qualitative and quantitative.

IMAGING

Ultrasonography is the investigation of choice. The splenoportal axis is dilated and patent with significant thickening of the portal vein and its main branches. Spontaneous lienorenal shunts may be present in 10%–15% of patients.

Computed tomography portography and computed tomography hepatic angiography may help differentiate between NCPF and cirrhosis. It shows a patent and dilated portal vein, huge splenomegaly with usually no ascites and a normal size liver.

Splenoportography was the investigation of choice before Doppler and computed tomography became available. It reveals a markedly dilated portal and splenic veins with "prune tree" appearance of the intrahepatic portal vein branches. There are frequent and extensive collaterals and natural shunts have been reported in about 16% patients with NCPF.[87] in the present era, splenoportography is essentially of historical interest.

ENDOSCOPY

Esophagogastric varices are present in 85%–95% of patients. Varices are more often large (90%) compared to cirrhotic patients (70%). Gastric and anorectal varices are seen more commonly in NCPF than cirrhosis. Portal hypertensive gastropathy (PHG) is uncommon and usually develops after variceal obliteration.

DIFFERENTIAL DIAGNOSIS

Child's A Cirrhosis

Patients with Child's A cirrhosis have normal liver function tests. A disproportionately large spleen with a dilated and thickened portal vein favors NCPF. However, viral serology and finally histology definitively differentiate NCPF from Child's A cirrhosis.

EHPVO

Patients with EHPVO tend to present a decade earlier than those with NCPF. The spleen also tends to be smaller in patients with EHPVO. An ultrasound Doppler clinches the diagnosis with a patent thick walled portal vein being suggestive of NCPF.

Tropical Splenomegaly Syndrome

Portal hypertension is uncommon. Additionally, these patients have elevated serum immunoglobulin M (IgM) levels and high malarial antibody titres.

Idiopathic Portal Hypertension

Patients with idiopathic portal hypertension (IPH) tend to be older in age and women. There is a lower reported incidence of upper gastrointestinal bleeding in this condition with most patients presenting with splenomegaly with or without ascites.[88]

MANAGEMENT

Primary Prophylaxis

Exsanguinating hemorrhage is the most common cause of death in these patients therefore, in large varices, endoscopic ligation may be considered. There is no consensus on the use of β-blockers. One small study from India did, however, find β-blockers and endoscopic variceal ligation to be equally effective in this setting.[76] Balloon occluded retrograde transvenous obliteration (BORTO) is another prophylactic option which may be considered in patients with large gastric varices.[89]

As compared to patients with EHPVO, surgery has a limited role in primary prophylaxis in patients with NCPF. A study from India revealed that although prophylactic shunt surgery has no mortality and can effectively prevent variceal bleeding, it is associated with high long term morbidity (>50%) and consequently prophylactic surgery should not be routinely recommended.[90] These findings are reflected in the recommendations of the APASL working party guidelines on NCPF.[76]

Acute Variceal Bleeding

These patients are managed with endoscopic treatment after initiation of resuscitation and starting pharmacotherapy with somatostatin or terlipressin infusion. Variceal band ligation and endoscopic sclerotherapy have been found to be equally efficacious (95% success). Combination of pharmacotherapy and endotherapy can have an additive effect. Surgery to control variceal bleeding is required in less than 5% of patients and is reserved for patients who fail medical and endoscopic therapy. Failure is defined by continued or recurrent variceal bleeding after two endoscopic treatments during a single admission for acute variceal bleeding.

Prevention of Rebleeding

Nonsurgical treatment: β-blockers and endotherapy have been used extensively for prevention of rebleeding. Endoscopic variceal ligation is considered superior to drugs alone. Cyanoacrylate glue injection for gastric varices is generally recommended. The results from various endotherapy series in patients with NCPF have been summarized in Table 4.

Surgery: Surgery is a good option for patients with frequent rebleeding refractory to endotherapy. Surgery also carries the added advantage of simultaneously treating symptomatic hypersplenism. It is also a good one off option for patients from remote areas for whom medical access is limited. The rebleeding rates are lower with surgery with lesser risk of ectopic varices or PHC.

Surgical options include PSSs and devascularization.[59,81,87] We prefer a proximal lienorenal shunt for prevention of variceal rebleeding. Following shunt surgery, the rebleeding rates are 8% in a series reported from India.[93] But unlike the situation in EHPVO, there is an association of shunt surgery with encephalopathy (up to 13%; clinical and subclinical), nephropathy and myelopathy in NCPF patients. In view of the risk of encephalopathy, devascularization procedures have also been described, the results of which are summarized in Table 5. Postsurgery the long-term cumulative 15-year survival is around 88%, slightly inferior to what is obtained in the cohort of EHPVO patients.[81]

Generally, encephalopathy can be managed medically and only rarely does this cause severe debility. In our experience, three patients with severely debilitating encephalopathy required shunt embolization or ligation. Some patients with NCPF develop severe impairment in liver functions over time.[95,96] In a recent series from India of 402 transplant patients, 5% had NCPF on final histology.[97] Fifty percent of these patients had encephalopathy and 50% had history of spontaneous bacterial peritonitis. Model for end-stage liver disease (MELD) score of patients in this series varied from 9 to 22. This data suggests that a small subset of patients with NCPF can have such significant impairment of liver functions so as to require a liver transplantation.[96]

Endoscopic therapy and PSS surgery are both safe and effective in patients with NCPF for secondary prophylaxis.[76] We prefer a proximal splenorenal shunt in patients with NCPF for prevention of variceal rebleeding. There is insufficient data on the role of

Table 4: Indian series reporting endotherapy in patients with non-cirrhotic portal fibrosis

Author (year)	*n*	*Variceal obliteration rate (%)*	*Sessions required*	*Follow-up (months)*	*Complications (%)*	*Variceal recurrence (%)*	*Rebleeding (%)*	*Bleed related deaths*	*Survival (%)*	*Remark*
Sarin (1986)[91]	31	-	1.6 ± 0.9	17.5±5.7	22.5	22.5	3.3	0	100	Only patients achieving variceal eradication included No late deaths
Bhargava (1989)[92]	60	88	8.43 ± 4.82	28.1 (3 months –5 years)	12	15	28	4	86 *at 5 years*	85% follow up Interval bleeding: 21 episodes Poorer survival in patients with poor liver functions
Bhargava (1991)[37]	83	87	7.33 ± 2.1	37	10	16	23 (prior to eradication)	6	73.6 *at 7 years*	-
Chawla (1997)[93]	72	90.3	5.7 ± 3.0	21.4 +/- 20.4 (1-96)	25	13.9	9.2	2	-	Interval bleeding 17.3%
Dhiman (2002)[87]	45	-	6 ± 3.2		25	14		1	-	21 patients lost to follow up

Table 5: Indian series reporting surgery in patients with non-cirrhotic portal fibrosis

Author (year)	*n*	*Procedure*	*Operative mortality (%)*	*Follow-up (months)*	*Variceal rebleed (%)*	*Remark*
Sama (1971)[94]	16	Splenorenal shunt	6.25	6–48	18.8	
	9	Portocaval shunt	22.2	12–120	-	
	3	Splenectomy with transgastric resection of gastric varices	0	-	33.3	One bleed related death in follow up
Mathur (1999)[59]	22	Modified Sugiura's	4.5	53±34	0	Three late deaths (none bleed-related) 5-year survival: 82%
Pal (2002)[81]	285	PSRS	0.8	-	8	Elective surgery Encephalopathy: 13% 15-year cumulative survival: 88%
Dhiman (2002)[87]	53	Shunt 46, devascularization 7	8	-	-	Encephalopathy: 2%
Pal (2005)[90]	45	PSRS 41 Splenectomy alone: 2 Splenectomy with devasc: 2	0	49 (12–236)	2.6	Surgery as primary prophylaxis 7 patients lost to follow up No bleed-related death 2 deaths on long-term follow-up; 1 unrelated, 1 due to chronic renal failure 47% long-term morbidity (encephalopathy, glomerulonephritis, hypoxemia, ascites requiring diuretics)

Abbreviation: PSRS, proximal splenorenal shunt.

Flow chart 3 Algorithmic approach to evaluation and management of patients with non-cirrhotic portal fibrosis

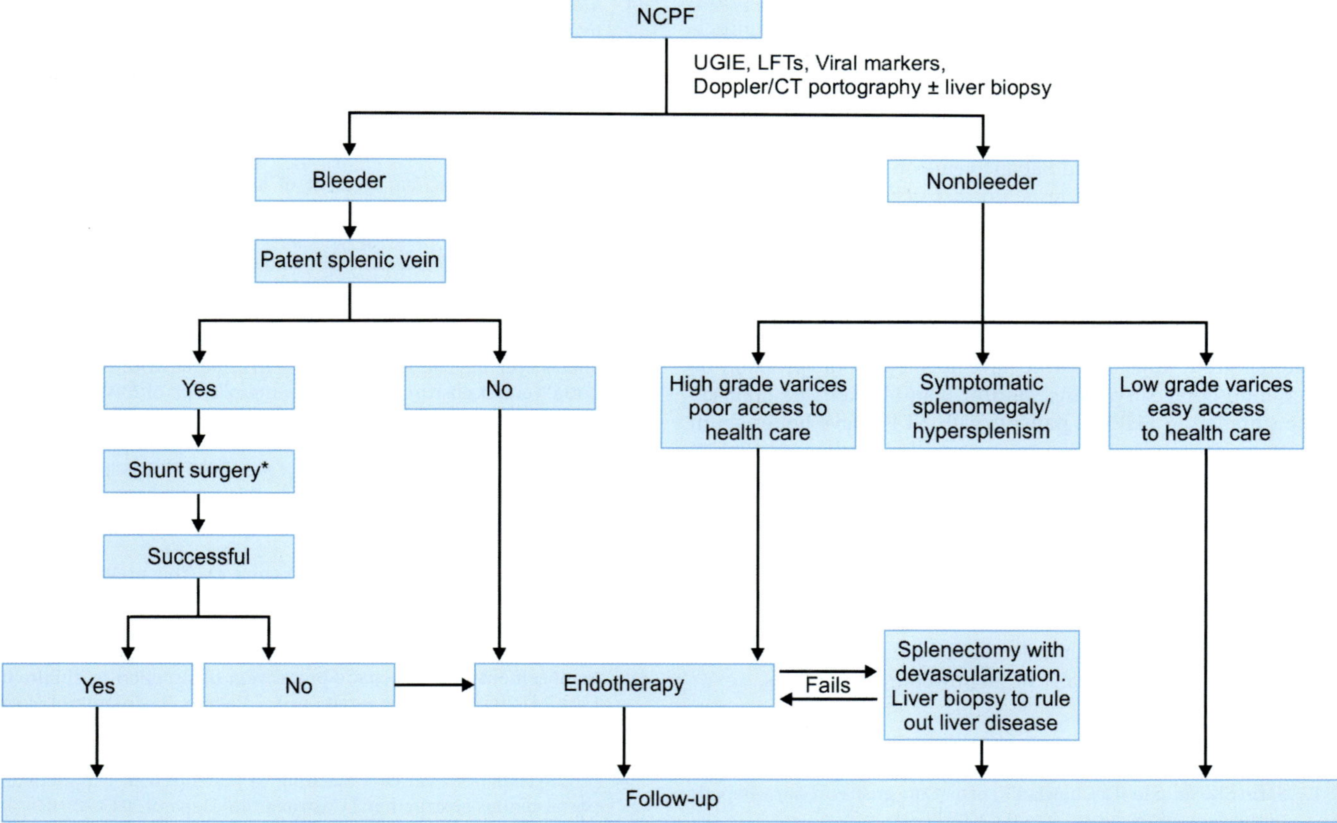

* Consider splenectomy with devascularization, if unsuspected cirrhosis present at surgery

Abbreviations: NCPF, non-cirrhotic portal fibrosis; UGIE, upper gastrointestinal endoscopy; LFTs, liver function tests; CT, computed tomography.

transjugular intrahepatic portosystemic shunt (TIPS) in these patients. We propose the following algorithm for management of patients with NCPF (Flow chart 3).

LIMITATIONS OF AVAILABLE DATA

Limited information is available about the natural course of NCPF. There are no randomized trials available comparing endotherapy with surgery for prevention of rebleeding. There is also no information available regarding whether the complications seen in patients being managed with endotherapy occur in the natural course of disease without intervention.

SUMMARY

Extrahepatic hepatic portal venous obstruction remains a disease of uncertain etiology but affects younger patients who have good liver reserve. In the emergency scenario, endoscopic sclerotherapy or variceal ligation is the treatment of choice for control of variceal bleeding. Shunt surgery (proximal lienorenal shunt), is feasible and safe in most patients and is associated with good long-term outcomes and, in our view, the treatment of choice in the elective setting. Also this can be offered to selected patients with EHPVO for primary prophylaxis from variceal bleeding. Devascularization (Hassab's) remains an option for patients with unshuntable splanchnic vascular anatomy. The problem of portal biliopathy has sinister implications on the long term outcomes of these patients, if left untreated. Many patients with symptomatic portal biliopathy improve with shunt surgery, but a few will require a bilioenteric bypass which is usually rendered safer with a previous portosystemic shunt.

Non-cirrhotic portal fibrosis is a disease characterized by moderate to massive splenomegaly, evidence of portal hypertension, patent splenoportal axis and hepatic veins on Doppler. Normal or near normal liver function tests, normal or near normal hepatic venous pressure gradient and no evidence of parenchymal injury or cirrhosis on liver biopsy are characteristic. The exact etiology still remains obscure. Its incidence over the years has shown a significant decrease in our country. Patients who have had a major upper gastrointestinal bleeding are best managed with proximal lienorenal shunt while those who have not bled should probably be under endoscopic surveillance and/or beta-blockers. As opposed to the situation in EHPVO, patients with NCPF have better shunt patency and may develop 'shunt encephalopathy' in 10–15% of cases which may need medical management. It is unclear whether primary prophylaxis with endotherapy provides any benefit to these patients.

ACKNOWLEDGEMENTS

The authors acknowledge the help of Miss Sarasvati Bahadursingh for help with formatting of algorithm flowcharts and tables.

REFERENCES

1. Sarin SK, Sollano JD, Chawla YK, et al. Consensus on extra-hepatic portal vein obstruction. Liver Int 2006;26:512-9.
2. Sahni P, Parde GK, Nundy S. Extrahepatic portal vein obstruction. Br J Surg 1990;77:1201-2.
3. Fonkalsrud EW, Myers NA, Robinson MJ. Management of extrahepatic portal hypertension in children. Ann Surg 1974;180: 487-93.
4. Yadav S, Dutta AK, Sarin SK. Do umbilical vein catheterization and sepsis lead to portal vein thrombosis? A prospective, clinical, and sonographic evaluation. J Pediatr Gastroenterol Nutr 1993;17:392-6.
5. Clatworthy HW, Jr., Boles ET, Jr. Extrahepatic portal bed block in children: pathogenesis and treatment. Ann Surg 1959;150:371-83.
6. Myers NA, Robinson MJ. Extrahepatic portal hypertension in children. J Pediatr Surg 1973;8:467-73.
7. Thomas V, Jose T, Kumar S. Natural history of bleeding after esophageal variceal eradication in patients with extrahepatic portal venous obstruction; a 20-year follow-up. Indian J Gastroenterol 2009;28:206-11.
8. Bhattacharyya M, Makharia G, Kannan M, Ahmed RP, Gupta PK, Saxena R. Inherited prothrombotic defects in Budd-Chiari syndrome and portal vein thrombosis: a study from North India. Am J Clin Pathol 2004;121:844-7.
9. Sarin SK, Agarwal SR. Extrahepatic portal vein obstruction. Semin Liver Dis 2002;22:43-58.
10. Dhiman RK, Behera A, Chawla YK, Dilawari JB, Suri S. Portal hypertensive biliopathy. Gut 2007;56:1001-8.
11. de Franchis R. Evolving consensus in portal hypertension. Report of the Baveno IV consensus workshop on methodology of diagnosis and therapy in portal hypertension. J Hepatol 2005;43:167-76.
12. Koshy A, Bhasin DK, Kapur KK. Bleeding in extrahepatic portal vein obstruction. Indian J Gastroenterol 1984;3:13-4.
13. Shah SR, Mathur SK. Presentation and natural history of variceal bleeding in patients with portal hypertension due to extrahepatic portal venous obstruction. Indian J Gastroenterol 2003;22:217-20.
14. Maddrey WC, Sen Gupta KP, Mallik KC, Iber FL, Basu AK. Extrahepatic obstruction of the portal venous system. Surg Gynecol Obstet 1968;127:989-98.
15. Bismuth H, Farges O. Cirrhosis and portal hypertension : portal hypertension in children. In : Surgery of the Liver and Biliary Tract. Blumgart LH, ed, Edinburgh : Churchill Livingstone, 1988;1313-1321.
16. Basu AK. Surgical management of juvenile portal hypertension. In: 37th international Pediatric Congress. New Delhi; December 1977.
17. Mangla V, Pal S, George J, Dash NR, Sahni P, Acharya SK, Chattopadhyay TK, Nundy S. Long-term results of proximal splenorenal shunt in patients with extrahepatic portal venous obstruction. (Abstract). HPB 2102;14(s2):267.
18. Zargar SA, Yattoo GN, Javid G, et al. Fifteen-year follow up of endoscopic injection sclerotherapy in children with extrahepatic portal venous obstruction. J Gastroenterol Hepatol 2004;19:139-45.
19. Itha S, Yachha SK. Endoscopic outcome beyond esophageal variceal eradication in children with extrahepatic portal venous obstruction. J Pediatr Gastroenterol Nutr 2006;42:196-200.
20. Sarin SK, Jain AK, Lamba GS, Gupta R, Chowdhary A. Isolated gastric varices: prevalence, clinical relevance and natural history. Dig Surg 2003;20:42-7.
21. Ganguly S, Sarin SK, Bhatia V, Lahoti D. The prevalence and spectrum of colonic lesions in patients with cirrhotic and noncirrhotic portal hypertension. Hepatology 1995;21:1226-31.
22. Abd El-Hamid N, Taylor RM, Marinello D, et al. Aetiology and management of extrahepatic portal vein obstruction in children: King's College Hospital experience. J Pediatr Gastroenterol Nutr 2008;47:630-4.
23. Pal S, Mangla V, Radhakrishna P, et al. Surgery as primary prophylaxis from variceal bleeding in patients with extrahepatic portal venous obstruction. J Gastroenterol Hepatol 2013;28:1010-4.
24. Mitra SK, Kumar V, Datta DV, et al. Extrahepatic portal hypertension: a review of 70 cases. J Pediatr Surg 1978;13:51-7.

25. Sarin SK, Bansal A, Sasan S, Nigam A. Portal-vein obstruction in children leads to growth retardation. Hepatology 1992;15:229-33.
26. Kato T, Romero R, Koutouby R, et al. Portosystemic shunting in children during the era of endoscopic therapy: improved postoperative growth parameters. J Pediatr Gastroenterol Nutr 2000;30:419-25.
27. Khare R, Sikora SS, Srikanth G, et al. Extrahepatic portal venous obstruction and obstructive jaundice: approach to management. J Gastroenterol Hepatol 2005;20:56-61.
28. Chawla Y, Dilawari JB. Anorectal varices—their frequency in cirrhotic and non-cirrhotic portal hypertension. Gut 1991;32:309-11.
29. Khan MR, Tariq J, Raza R, Effendi MS. Portal hypertensive biliopathy: review of pathophysiology and management. Trop Gastroenterol 2012;33:173-8.
30. Chattopadhyay S, Nundy S. Portal biliopathy. World J Gastroenterol 2012;18:6177-82.
31. Dilawari JB, Chawla, Y.K. Treatment of extrahepatic portal venous obstruction. Natl Med J Ind 1998;6:51-4.
32. Bhandarkar PV, Sreenivasa D, Mistry FP, Abraham P, Bhatia SJ. Profile of extrahepatic portal venous obstruction in Mumbai. J Assoc Physicians India 1999;47:791-4.
33. Voorhees AB, Jr., Harris RC, Britton RC, Price JB, Santulli TV. Portal Hypertension in Children: 98 Cases. Surgery 1965;58:540-9.
34. Sood S, Minocha VR. Portal hypertension in children. Indian Pediatr 1989;26:61-71.
35. Nundy S, Tandon, B. N. Emergency operations for bleeding esophageal varices- A case for doing splenectomy and lienorenal shunts. Tropical Gastroenetrology 1980;1:27.
36. Chawla YK, Dilawari JB, Ramesh GN, Kaur U, Mitra SK, Walia BN. Sclerotherapy in extrahepatic portal venous obstruction. Gut 1990;31:213-6.
37. Bhargava DK, Dasarathy S, Sundaram KR, Ahuja RK. Results of endoscopic variceal sclerotherapy: influence of etiology of portal hypertension and hepatic functional status. Gastroenterol Jpn 1991;26 Suppl 3:32-5.
38. Yachha SK, Sharma BC, Kumar M, Khanduri A. Endoscopic sclerotherapy for esophageal varices in children with extrahepatic portal venous obstruction: a follow-up study. J Pediatr Gastroenterol Nutr 1997;24:49-52.
39. Poddar U, Thapa BR, Singh K. Endoscopic sclerotherapy in children: experience with 257 cases of extrahepatic portal venous obstruction. Gastrointest Endosc 2003;57:683-6.
40. Prasad AS, Gupta S, Kohli V, Pande GK, Sahni P, Nundy S. Proximal splenorenal shunts for extrahepatic portal venous obstruction in children. Ann Surg 1994;219:193-6.
41. Pande GK, Reddy VM, Kar P, et al. Operations for portal hypertension due to extrahepatic obstruction: results and 10 year follow up. Br Med J (Clin Res Ed) 1987;295:1115-7.
42. Bismuth H, Franco D, Alagille D. Portal diversion for portal hypertension in children. The first ninety patients. Ann Surg 1980;192:18-24.
43. Rao KL, Goyal A, Menon P, et al. Extrahepatic portal hypertension in children: observations on three surgical procedures. Pediatr Surg Int 2004;20:679-84.
44. Orloff MJ, Orloff MS, Girard B, Orloff SL. Bleeding esophagogastric varices from extrahepatic portal hypertension: 40 years' experience with portal-systemic shunt. J Am Coll Surg 2002;194:717-28; discussion 28-30.
45. Szczepanik AB, Rudowski WJ. Extrahepatic portal hypertension: long-term results of surgical treatment. Ann R Coll Surg Engl 1989;71:222-5.
46. de Ville de Goyet J, Clapuyt P, Otte JB. Extrahilar mesenterico-left portal shunt to relieve extrahepatic portal hypertension after partial liver transplant. Transplantation 1992;53:231-2.
47. de Ville de Goyet J, Gibbs P, Clapuyt P, Reding R, Sokal EM, Otte JB. Original extrahilar approach for hepatic portal revascularization and relief of extrahepatic portal hypertension related to later portal vein thrombosis after pediatric liver transplantation. Long term results. Transplantation 1996;62:71-5.
48. Superina R, Bambini DA, Lokar J, Rigsby C, Whitington PF. Correction of extrahepatic portal vein thrombosis by the mesenteric to left portal vein bypass. Ann Surg 2006;243:515-21.
49. Superina R, Shneider B, Emre S, Sarin S, de Ville de Goyet J. Surgical guidelines for the management of extra-hepatic portal vein obstruction. Pediatr Transplant 2006;10:908-13.
50. Lautz TB, Sundaram SS, Whitington PF, Keys L, Superina RA. Growth impairment in children with extrahepatic portal vein obstruction is improved by mesenterico-left portal vein bypass. J Pediatr Surg 2009;44:2067-70.
51. Guerin F, Bidault V, Gonzales E, Franchi-Abella S, De Lambert G, Branchereau S. Meso-Rex bypass for extrahepatic portal vein obstruction in children. Br J Surg 2013;100:1606-13.
52. Tanner NC. The late results of porto-azygos disconnexion in the treatment of bleeding from oesophageal varices. Ann R Coll Surg Engl 1961;28:153-74.
53. Sugiura M, Futagawa S. Esophageal transection with paraesophagogastric devascularizations (the Sugiura procedure) in the treatment of esophageal varices. World J Surg 1984;8:673-9.
54. Sugiura M, Futagawa S. A new technique for treating esophageal varices. J Thorac Cardiovasc Surg 1973;66:677-85.
55. Hassab MA. Nonshunt operations in portal hypertension without cirrhosis. Surg Gynecol Obstet 1970;131:648-54.
56. Hassab MA. Gastro-esophageal decongestion and splenectomy GEDS (Hassab), in the management of bleeding varices. Review of literature. Int Surg 1998;83:38-41.
57. Kawasaki S, Kidokoro A, Sugiura M, Sanjo K, Idezuki Y. Effects of nonshunting operations on portal venous pressure and hepatic blood flow. Am J Surg 1987;153:295-9.
58. Shah SR, Nagral SS, Mathur SK. Results of a modified sugiura's devascularisation in the management of "unshuntable" portal hypertension. HPB Surg 1999;11:235-9.
59. Mathur SK, Shah SR, Nagral SS, Soonawala ZF. Transabdominal extensive esophagogastric devascularization with gastroesophageal stapling for management of noncirrhotic portal hypertension: long-term results. World J Surg 1999;23:1168-74; discussion 74-5.
60. Subhasis RC, Rajiv C, Kumar SA, Kumar AV, Kumar PA. Surgical treatment of massive splenomegaly and severe hypersplenism secondary to extrahepatic portal venous obstruction in children. Surg Today 2007;37:19-23.
61. Mangla V, Pal S, George J, Dash NR, Sahni P, Chattopadhyay TK, Acharya SK, Nundy S. Long-term results of splenectomy with esophagogastric devascularization in patients with extrahepatic portal venous obstruction. (Abstract). HPB 2012;14(S2):266.
62. Poddar U, Thapa BR, Singh K. Frequency of gastropathy and gastric varices in children with extrahepatic portal venous obstruction treated with sclerotherapy. J Gastroenterol Hepatol 2004;19:1253-6.
63. Stringer MD, Howard ER. Longterm outcome after injection sclerotherapy for oesophageal varices in children with extrahepatic portal hypertension. Gut 1994;35:257-9.
64. Taylor RM, Bjarnason I, Cheeseman P, et al. Intestinal permeability and absorptive capacity in children with portal hypertension. Scand J Gastroenterol 2002;37:807-11.
65. Ryckman FC, Alonso, M.H. Cause and management of portal hypertension in the pediatric population. Clin Liver Dis 2001;15:789-818.
66. Yachha SK, Ghoshal UC, Gupta R, Sharma BC, Ayyagari A. Portal hypertensive gastropathy in children with extrahepatic portal venous obstruction: role of variceal obliteration by endoscopic sclerotherapy and Helicobacter pylori infection. J Pediatr Gastroenterol Nutr 1996;23:20-3.

67. Chaudhary A, Dhar P, Sarin SK, et al. Bile duct obstruction due to portal biliopathy in extrahepatic portal hypertension: surgical management. Br J Surg 1998;85:326-9.
68. Kashyap N, Sharma DP, Mukhopadhyay S, Nundy S, Bhargava S. Evaluation of techniques for assessing portosystemic shunt patency. Indian J Med Res 1983;78:841-6.
69. Rodgers BM, Kaude JV. Real-time ultrasound in determination of portasystemic shunt patency in children. J Pediatr Surg 1981;16:968-71.
70. Gulati MS, Paul SB, Arora NK, Berry M. Evaluation of extrahepatic portal hypertension and surgical portal systemic shunts by intravenous CT portography. Clin Imaging 1999;23:377-85.
71. Mohapatra MK, Mohapatra AK, Acharya SK, Sahni P, Nundy S. Encephalopathy in patients with extrahepatic obstruction after lienorenal shunts. Br J Surg 1992;79:1103-5.
72. Agarwal AK, Sharma D, Singh S, Agarwal S, Girish SP. Portal biliopathy: a study of 39 surgically treated patients. HPB (Oxford) 2011;13:33-9.
73. Banti G. Splenomegallie mit leberizirrhose. Beitrage Zus pathologischen. Anat Algemeinea Pathol 1889;24:21-33.
74. Basu AK, Boyer J, Bhattacharya R, Mallik KC, Sen Gupta KP. Non-cirrhotic portal fibrosis with portal hypertension: a new syndrome. I. Clinical and function studies and results of operations. Indian J Med Res 1967;55:336-50.
75. Sarin SK, Kapoor D. Non-cirrhotic portal fibrosis: current concepts and management. J Gastroenterol Hepatol 2002;17:526-34.
76. Sarin SK, Kumar A, Chawla YK, et al. Noncirrhotic portal fibrosis/ idiopathic portal hypertension: APASL recommendations for diagnosis and treatment. Hepatol Int 2007;1:398-413.
77. Kono K, Ohnishi K, Omata M, et al. Experimental portal fibrosis produced by intraportal injection of killed nonpathogenic Escherichia coli in rabbits. Gastroenterology 1988;94:787-96.
78. Datta DV, Mitra SK, Chhuttani PN, Chakravarti RN. Chronic oral arsenic intoxication as a possible aetiological factor in idiopathic portal hypertension (non-cirrhotic portal fibrosis) in India. Gut 1979;20:378-84.
79. Guha Mazumdar DN, Das Gupta J. Arsenic and non-cirrhotic portal hypertension. J Hepatol 1991;13:376.
80. Nevens F, Fevery J, Van Steenbergen W, Sciot R, Desmet V, De Groote J. Arsenic and non-cirrhotic portal hypertension. A report of eight cases. J Hepatol 1990;11:80-5.
81. Pal S, Desai PR, Rao G, Sahni P, Pande GK. Non-cirrhotic portal fibrosis: results of surgery in 317 consecutive patients over 1 25-year period from an Indian center. (Abstract). Gastroenterology 2002;123 (Suppl 1): T1454:88.
82. Nayak NC, Ramalingaswami V. Obliterative portal venopathy of the liver. Associated with so-called idiopathic portal hypertension or tropical splenomegaly. Arch Pathol 1969;87:359-69.
83. Tandon BN, Lakshminarayanan R, Bhargava S, Nayak NC, Sama SK. Ultrastructure of the liver in non-cirrhotic portal fibrosis with portal hypertension. Gut 1970;11:905-10.
84. Sarin SK, Sethi KK, Nanda R. Measurement and correlation of wedged hepatic, intrahepatic, intrasplenic and intravariceal pressures in patients with cirrhosis of liver and non-cirrhotic portal fibrosis. Gut 1987;28:260-6.
85. Babbs C, Warnes TW, Haboubi NY. Non-cirrhotic portal hypertension with hypoxaemia. Gut 1988;29:129-31.
86. Bajaj JS, Bhattacharjee J, Sarin SK. Coagulation profile and platelet function in patients with extrahepatic portal vein obstruction and non-cirrhotic portal fibrosis. J Gastroenterol Hepatol 2001;16: 641-6.
87. Dhiman RK, Chawla Y, Vasishta RK, et al. Non-cirrhotic portal fibrosis (idiopathic portal hypertension): experience with 151 patients and a review of the literature. J Gastroenterol Hepatol 2002;17:6-16.
88. Sarin SK. Non-cirrhotic portal fibrosis. J Gastroenterol Hepatol 2002;17 Suppl 3:S214-23.
89. Saad WE, Simon PO, Jr., Rose SC. Balloon-occluded retrograde transvenous obliteration of gastric varices. Cardiovasc Intervent Radiol 2014;37:299-315.
90. Pal S, Radhakrishna P, Sahni P, Pande GK, Nundy S, Chattopadhyay TK. Prophylactic surgery in non-cirrhotic portal fibrosis: is it worthwhile? Indian J Gastroenterol 2005;24:239-42.
91. Sarin SK, Sachdev G, Nanda R. Follow-up of patients after variceal eradication. A comparison of patients with cirrhosis, noncirrhotic portal fibrosis, and extrahepatic obstruction. Ann Surg 1986;204: 78-82.
92. Bhargava DK, Dwivedi M, Dasarathy S, Arora A. Endoscopic sclerotherapy for portal hypertension due to extrahepatic obstruction: long-term follow-up. Gastrointest Endosc 1989;35: 309-11.
93. Chawla YK, Dilawari JB, Dhiman RK, et al. Sclerotherapy in noncirrhotic portal fibrosis. Dig Dis Sci 1997;42:1449-53.
94. Sama SK, Bhargava S, Nath NG, et al. Noncirrhotic portal fibrosis. Am J Med 1971;51:160-9.
95. Geramizadeh B, Malek-Hosseini SA, Salahi H, Bahador A, Nikeghbalian S. Liver failure and the need for transplantation in three patients with hepatoportal sclerosis. Transplant Proc 2008;40:3526-8.
96. Isabel Fiel M, Thung SN, Hytiroglou P, Emre S, Schiano TD. Liver failure and need for liver transplantation in patients with advanced hepatoportal sclerosis. Am J Surg Pathol 2007;31: 607-14.
97. Saigal S, Nayak NC, Jain D, et al. Non-cirrhotic portal fibrosis related end stage liver disease in adults: evaluation from a study on living donor liver transplant recipients. Hepatol Int 2011;5:882-9.

CHAPTER 77

Budd-Chiari and Other Vascular Diseases of Liver

Prakash Jain, Shyamkumar N Keshava, Vinu Moses, Venkatramani Sitaram

INTRODUCTION

The Budd-Chiari syndrome (BCS) is a condition where the blood flow out of the liver is either interrupted or reduced.[1] However, when commonly referred to, it is taken to mean a syndrome in which thrombosis of the hepatic veins or inferior vena cava (IVC) inside or above the liver causes the blood flow out of the liver to be affected. This confusion has led to alternate names being considered.[2]

ETIOLOGY

More than 80% of patients with BCS have an underlying disorder, such as malignancy, myeloproliferative disorders or anatomic obstructions causing hepatic venous outflow to be reduced. The underlying common feature in all these conditions is the presence of a hypercoagulable state. Some patients have more than one risk factor.[3]

The American Association for the Study of Liver Diseases suggests that the following points be considered in the evaluation of the etiology for BCS:[4]

- Consider space occupying lesions or malignant tumors compressing or invading the hepatic venous outflow tract and evaluate with abdominal ultrasonography, CT scan or MRI.
- Investigate for ulcerative colitis, celiac disease and systemic diseases.
- Perform hematological work-up for risk factors for thrombosis or a hypercoagulable state.

Myeloproliferative Disorders

More than 50% of all cases of the BCS may have a chronic myeloproliferative condition such as essential thrombocythemia or polycythemia vera, super-imposed on a hypercoagulable state. The blood picture in BCS may be affected by changes seen in portal hypertension such as thrombocytopenia.

The combination of a myeloproliferative disorder (occult or overt) associated with a hypercoagulable state(s) is common.[3] The bone marrow examination of patients with BCS and suspected myeloproliferative conditions will reveal spontaneous erythroid colony formation in the presence of low serum erythropoietin levels, increased megakaryocyte colony growth, and clonal karyotypic abnormalities. It is worthwhile doing this examination even in cases of idiopathic BCS as this can reveal an occult myeloproliferative condition.[5-7]

Janus kinase 2 (JAK2) tyrosine kinase (V617F) mutation is present in nearly all patients with polycythemia vera and chronic idiopathic myelofibrosis.[6] It has also been detected in up to 50–60% of patients with BCS. It is therefore, worthwhile checking for this mutation in patients with BCS to rule out a myeloproliferative condition before labeling them as having an idiopathic etiology.

Infections of the Liver

Some infections, such as liver abscesses, parasitic cysts, mucormycosis and aspergillosis of the liver, can lead to a hypercoagulable state, precipitating BCS.

Benign Liver Lesions

Liver adenomas, cystadenomas or even hemangiomas can also predispose to a hypercoagulable state.

Malignancies

Malignancies can account for up to 10% of BCS cases. Hepatocellular carcinoma (HCC), metastases from adrenal, stomach, lung and pancreatic tumors can result in BCS. These tumors, especially HCC, sarcomas of the IVC or right atrium and renal cell carcinoma extending into the IVC can produce BCS by vascular compression or direct invasion of the hepatic venous outflow tract. In addition, the hypercoagulable state associated with malignancies can also predispose to BCS.[3,7]

Other Hypercoagulable States

A number of other hypercoagulable states have been associated with the BCS. These include:[8]

- G1691A factor V (Leiden) gene mutation, which produces activated protein C resistance. Factor V Leiden mutation is the most common cause of hereditary thrombophilia. Patients with this mutation using oral contraceptive pills (OCPs) are at greater risk of BCS due to the interplay between factors.
- Other hypercoagulable states include:
  - G20210A factor II gene mutation[9]
  - Anti-phospholipid syndrome[10,11]
  - Antithrombin III deficiency[12]
  - Hyperhomocysteinemia[3]
  - Protein C deficiency[13]
  - Protein S deficiency
  - Paroxysmal nocturnal hemoglobinuria[3,14]
  - Hereditary thrombophilia[15]

The possibility of primary BCS being caused by the presence of one or more of these factors is nearly 75%. Combination of risk factors was seen in 25%.[16] Therefore presence of one factor should not deter one from looking at other thrombophilic states.

Vasculitis

Autoimmune vasculitis in Behcet's syndrome may cause BCS. A study of 493 patients with Behcet's revealed that 53 had one or more large vessel thrombosis.[17] Of these 53 patients, there were fourteen who had hepatic vein thrombosis, eight with IVC thrombosis, and two who had both IVC and portal vein thrombosis.

Obstructing Membranous Webs

This condition is called membranous occlusion of the vena cava (MOVC) or short length hepatic vein stenosis (SHVS). These webs are usually considered congenital but can be caused by a myeloproliferative disorder. This condition is more common in Asia and India and is unusual in the West.[7,18,19] Since the problem is anatomic, with resultant partial or complete IVC obstruction, surgical options are available for treatment. The usual causes of BCS are not amenable for operative treatment.[18,20] The obstructing membranous webs are present cephalad to the entrance of the right hepatic vein into the IVC.[20] Surgical approaches to these webs are discussed below.

Oral Contraceptives and Pregnancy

The hypercoagulable state attributed to pregnancy[21] and OCP use,[22] especially those with higher estrogen component is thought to predispose to BCS. The duration of OCP use does not correlate with the risk of developing BCS, nor does the history of prior uneventful pregnancies.[22-24]

Miscellaneous and Idiopathic

These are mainly autoimmune disorders with hypercoagulable states or associated vasculitis. These include systemic lupus erythematosus, mixed-connective tissue disease, Sjögren's syndrome, inflammatory bowel disease, hypereosinophilic syndrome and idiopathic granulomatous venulitis. Other rare causes are protein-losing enteropathy, minimal change nephrotic syndrome, neurofibromatosis, alpha-1 antitrypsin deficiency and some rare familial cases.[25,26] Currently, nearly 15–20% of BCS cases are labeled as idiopathic.[3] It is probable that as more sophisticated and sensitive tests are developed, the etiology of these cases will come under the classification of autoimmune and hypercoagulable states.

Physiological Changes Due to Budd-Chiari Syndrome

While the etiology of BCS may be varied, the symptom complex and physiological changes remain the same. There is post-sinusoidal hypertension presents in the portal system and leads to a clinical picture similar to that caused by liver cirrhosis. However, the cardiopulmonary and indices of systemic vascular resistance such as plasma renin, aldosterone and norepinephrine levels are normal in BCS as opposed to cirrhosis where these are markedly affected. The neurohumoral and plasma volume expansion systems are activated in BCS despite normal systemic vascular resistance.

EPIDEMIOLOGY

Budd-Chiari syndrome is more common in women than in men (2:1). The median age is 35 years (range 13–76 years). The commonest presenting features are ascites and liver enlargement.[27] The commonest site of outflow obstruction is the hepatic veins followed by the IVC and associated portal vein thrombosis in one-third of these patients.[28]

Classification Based on Clinical Presentation

The presentation of BCS can be considered as acute (fulminant, 20%), subacute (40%) or chronic (40%).[7]

Acute Disease

Acute BCS is defined as the presence of abdominal pain, an alanine aminotransferase (ALT) level more than 5 times the upper limit of normal, and liver cell loss at biopsy.[7]

In this situation, patients present with short duration of severe right upper quadrant pain and hepatomegaly. Jaundice and ascites may not be apparent to begin with, but can appear very soon as liver function is rapidly affected. Symptoms are those of fulminant hepatic failure. Upper gastrointestinal bleeding may occur due to varices. Encephalopathy can also occur.

Biochemical tests of liver function are widely abnormal. Elevated serum aminotransferases between 100 and more than 600 IU/mL reflect vascular congestion and resulting ischemic hepatocellular damage. A study has suggested that high levels of ALT (≥5 times the upper limit of normal) reflect acute, severe but potentially reversible ischemic injury.[29] Conversely a slow decline in ALT levels (<50% of starting concentration within 3 days) predicted a poor outcome.

Since the symptoms of BCS are similar to other conditions presenting as fulminant hepatic failure, it is important to rule them out. These conditions include ischemic, viral, toxic and malignant fulminant hepatic failure.

Subacute and Chronic Disease

Subacute BCS is considered when symptoms have been present for several weeks up to 6 months. These symptoms are much less dramatic than the acute form and patients may be asymptomatic till the disease progresses significantly. The clinical presentation depends on the extent, site and exact vessel occlusion and the effectiveness of the collateral circulation. BCS is considered chronic when symptoms have been presented for more than 6 months.[30] Chronic is defined as previous symptoms or hospitalizations, splenomegaly, atrophy or hypertrophy complex of liver lobes and centrilobular fibrosis or cirrhosis on biopsy.

Chronic occlusion of the hepatic veins can cause hypertrophy of the caudate lobe of the liver as it has a venous drainage independent from the rest of the liver. This caudate lobe can hypertrophy and cause compression of the intrahepatic IVC. This extrinsic compression can result in further worsening of the existing outflow obstruction, causing severe ascites and lower limb edema. In addition, the liver remains congested and cirrhosis can develop resulting in portal hypertension and variceal bleeding. Massive ascites, massive hepatomegaly and severe pain can result. However, hepatic encephalopathy is not common, unlike in acute BCS.[31] Hepatopulmonary syndrome can occur as a response by improving collateral supply.

In the subacute and chronic forms of BCS, liver function tests may be slightly deranged with aminotransferases being 2–3 times normal and moderately elevated serum alkaline phosphatase. Clinical jaundice is unusual. It is important to rule out right heart failure and other causes of cirrhosis and portal hypertension.

CLINICAL FEATURES

Acute BCS should be considered in patients with acute hepatic failure and in those with veno-occlusive disease. These patients will usually have hepatomegaly, right upper abdominal pain and ascites, often massive.

Splenomegaly is uncommon seen only in up to 30% of patients, and venous collaterals may be seen on the anterior abdominal wall. It is important to examine for edema of the lower limbs as this, along with distended veins on the back draining upwards, may suggest IVC obstruction. Jugular venous distention, exaggerated venous wave on compression of the liver and other signs of right-sided congestive heart failure are not characteristic of BCS, and may suggest an underlying cardiac cause.

Subacute or chronic BCS should be suspected in patients with known risk factors for BCS and where ascites is the prominent symptom along with liver dysfunction.

Radiological Evaluation

Noninvasive modes of evaluation include ultrasonography with Doppler studies, CT scan or magnetic resonance angiography. The accuracy of noninvasive imaging depends upon the clinical characteristics, duration of disease and the location of the obstruction. Occlusion of the portal vein in patients with BCS limits therapeutic options and has a poor prognosis.[32] The splenic circulation should also be evaluated to exclude associated thrombosis, which is important in prognostication and in planning shunt operations.

Invasive methods include venography which can be considered to be the gold standard as well as arteriography. Additionally, liver biopsy, usually performed during transjugular venography, helps in prognostication. It occasionally helps to decide which subacute BCS patient may benefit from either liver transplantation or shunt operation.

Ultrasound Abdomen with Doppler

This is used to screen for the presence of BCS.[33] Nonspecific findings on ultrasound include hepatomegaly, splenomegaly, ascites, intra-abdominal collaterals, caudate lobe hypertrophy, atrophy of other hepatic lobes and compression or narrowing of the IVC or hepatic veins. These findings are not specific for BCS. Specific findings of focal and segmental stenosis or occlusion of the hepatic veins or IVC are diagnostic of BCS. Ultrasound and Doppler abdomen are the mainstay investigations in the initial diagnosis of BCS, with contrast-enhanced computerized tomography (CECT) and MRI providing little additional direct evidence of BCS.

Contrast-enhanced Computerized Tomography

Contrast-enhanced computerized tomography scanning can reveal the same nonspecific abnormalities seen during ultrasound Doppler examination. Findings specific to BCS on CECT[4] include a delay of filling in the hepatic veins (usually within 60 seconds) or complete absence of filling of the right, middle and left hepatic veins. In addition, contrast is quickly cleared from the caudate lobe; the suprahepatic IVC may be only partially opacified or sometimes not seen at all. A typical appearance of the liver, referred to as flea-bitten appearance can be described, as a result of irregular parenchymal enhancement that occurs in BCS.[4]

Magnetic Resonance Imaging

The presence of hepatomegaly, splenomegaly, ascites, intra-abdominal collaterals, caudate lobe hypertrophy, atrophy of other hepatic lobes, and compression or narrowing of the IVC is also seen on MRI.[34] Comma-shaped intrahepatic collaterals have been described along with reduction in caliber of the main hepatic veins.[34] Contrast-enhanced magnetic resonance venography is sometimes useful in depicting the morphological abnormalities of BCS.[35]

Other investigations such as sulfur-colloid scintigraphy are now mainly of historical interest since they do not contribute anything more than ultrasound Doppler.

Venography

This is considered the gold standard for diagnosis[4] and is indicated if there is doubt of the diagnosis after noninvasive testing. It is performed by accessing the hepatic venous circulation percutaneously, using the internal jugular vein, cephalic vein, or femoral vein routes.

Pressures should be recorded above and below the suspected stenosis or occlusion in the IVC or hepatic veins to determine whether the stenosis or occlusion causes a significant pressure gradient. Once the IVC has been determined to be patent, opacification of each of the individual hepatic veins should be attempted even though it may not be feasible in all patients. Therefore, injection of contrast following balloon occlusion of a specific hepatic vein may facilitate its visualization and also demonstrate the so-called "spider web" pattern characteristic of BCS (this is not standard practice in our institution). This pattern depicts the futile attempts of the liver to form venous collaterals in an attempt to bypass the obstructed hepatic veins.

The advantage of the invasive tests over the noninvasive is that compression or occlusion of the intrahepatic IVC leads to sluggish flow in hepatic veins. As a result, the hepatic veins can be undetectable during ultrasound Doppler studies, although they may be patent and amenable to therapy. Hepatic veins with diffuse compression are usually not treated even if the vein is patent. Invasive tests can detect the presence of these compressed vessels and can produce a more accurate picture of the nature of obstruction. Further, exact pressure gradient readings can help to assess the effectiveness of the therapy and to help prognosticate.

Arteriography

Visceral arteriography is considered important when planning a surgical approach to decompress the congested liver. Patency of the portal, splenic, and mesenteric veins can be determined, and this influences the planned approach. Additionally, tumors involving the liver, IVC, or the hepatic and portal veins can be identified which can sometimes be missed, altering the diagnosis and the planned treatment.

Liver Biopsy

Liver biopsy[36] can be diagnostic of BCS and can be helpful in prognostication[37] and in helping to decide on surgical and other options. This is mainly in the acute or subacute form of the disease where histological features include centrozonal congestion, necrosis and hemorrhage. Large regenerative nodules and obstructive portal venopathy may also be seen.[38] Nonspecific cirrhotic changes may be seen in the chronic form of the disease.

It is often practical to obtain a liver biopsy via the transjugular route during performance of hepatic venography and to avoid the percutaneous approach due the presence of ascites in the majority of patients. If a percutaneous biopsy is what is being considered, it is important to ensure that it is done in patients in whom there is no ascites or after ascites has been medically managed. It is also worthwhile remembering that percutaneous liver biopsy should not be done without ensuring that the coagulation profile is normal. Transjugular liver biopsy should be considered in patients with ascites, abnormal coagulation profile and chronic renal failure.

In determining treatment options, liver biopsy can be helpful. In a situation where cirrhosis has already occurred, patients are less likely to benefit from revascularization procedures in contrast to patients who have predominant features of hepatic congestion but no parenchymal scarring. This can be considered controversial since one study suggested that histologic findings at the time of diagnosis did not predict 5-year survival, although there was a trend to decreased survival among those with central vein thrombosis.[37]

Sometimes liver biopsy from both lobes may be required, as the thrombotic process in BCS may not involve all the hepatic veins resulting in focal or patchy changes. In suitably fit patients, a laparoscopic approach may be considered instead of two percutaneous biopsies.

The American Association for the Study of Liver Diseases (AASLD) recommends performing a liver biopsy only when an obstructed hepatic venous outflow tract has not been demonstrated with noninvasive imaging.[4]

TREATMENT

Treatment of BCS can be medical or surgical. Medical treatment options include transjugular intrahepatic portosystemic shunt (TIPSS) placement, angioplasty and stenting as well supportive care, anticoagulation and thrombolysis. Operative interventions include shunt procedures and liver transplantation. An overview of the treatment options is given in Table 1 at the end.

The choice of a particular approach or combination of approaches depends upon the clinical and anatomic features of the individual patient. The experience of the treating center is also important, as surgical options may be favored in centers without strong interventional radiology experience. Centers which prefer interventional radiological procedures may advocate the sequential invasive procedures which are determined by the clinical response.[39,40] A combined approach may be considered, tailored for individual patients through a multidisciplinary team approach.

Runyon in 2004 and Klein in 2006 stated that irrespective of the treatment option finally decided upon, the aim is to:[41,42]

- Relieve the offending obstruction (bypass or by preventing clot propagation).
- Provide symptom relief and prevent complications related to malnutrition, fluid retention and portal hypertension.
- Restore patency of thrombosed veins.
- Decompress the congested liver.

Medical Therapy

Medical therapy[41] includes symptom relief and nonoperative options for therapy.

Symptom Relief

Fluid retention can be addressed with judicious use of diuretics, fluid restriction and low sodium diet. It is important to monitor electrolytes in these patients. Ascites due to cirrhosis can be more difficult to treat and refractory ascites may be considered an indication for shunt operation or liver transplantation.

Every effort must be made to improve the nutritional status, and specific nutritional supplementation can be offered after a careful diet history and appropriate investigations. A simple way to improve caloric intake is to advise the consumption of multiple, small frequent meals throughout the day, balancing protein and sodium intake with potentially worsening ascites and encephalopathy. Pedal edema can be addressed by use of pressure stockings and foot elevation and in difficult situations, by use of active graded proprietary compression pump devices.

As medical or drug therapy alone does not cure the patient, it is important to evaluate the cause of BCS and treat accordingly. Clot propagation can be slowed or treated by anticoagulation and patients with polycythemia and hypercoagulable states can be administered hydroxyurea and aspirin as appropriate.

Anticoagulation

Sufficient recanalization of occluded vessels with or without development of adequate collateral circulation to avoid the progression of liver disease cannot be guaranteed by anticoagulation alone. However, there are reports of good long-term survival with this alone.

The risk of anticoagulation should also be considered, especially in patients who present with bleeding complications. Patients receiving only medical therapy should be monitored closely for disease progression by monitoring the liver synthetic function parameters. Serial upper gastrointestinal endoscopies to look for varices and sequential liver biopsies becoming less frequent after 3 years or more of stable disease can be considered.

Bleeding complications appear to be common in patients maintained on anticoagulation, emphasizing the need for close follow-up and monitoring of coagulation status, especially during invasive procedures.[43]

One of the largest series of patients with BCS treated medically included 237 patients treated at four centers between 1984 and 2001 of whom 72% received anticoagulation.[28] The authors generated a statistical model predicting categories of disease severity (Classes I to III), which correlated with survival. Independent variables predicting a worse prognosis included the presence of encephalopathy, ascites, an International Normalized Ratio (INR) of more than 2.3, and higher bilirubin concentrations (variables that are notably similar to the Child-Turcotte-Pugh classification except for the absence of albumin). A trend for a benefit of anticoagulation on survival (RR 0.14, 95% CI 0.02–1.21) could only be demonstrated in patients with Class I disease (i.e. less severe disease).

Another retrospective study examined factors associated with prognosis in a series of 120 patients with BCS, 82 of whom had been treated with surgical portosystemic shunts, and 38 of whom had received only medical therapy (with diuretics and anticoagulants).[44] Independent predictors identified on multivariate analysis associated with a worse prognosis included: older age at diagnosis, more severe liver failure and the presence of refractory ascites. Patients with a favorable profile had up to an 80% 5-year survival with medical therapy alone. However, only 13 patients fell into this category.

A subsequent report from the same authors found that (in addition to the predictors described above) prognosis was worse in patients who presented with clinical features suggesting chronic disease.[45] Surgical portosystemic shunting had no apparent benefit on survival.

Medical management alone is considered only for patients with subacute or chronic BCS who have compensated liver disease but are not transplant candidates. However, these patients should be worked up with an aim to offer decompressive therapy before disease progression occurs. Medical therapy is the only option in patients who are unsuitable for radiological intervention and those with poor performance status.

Thrombolytic Therapy

Systemic and locally administered thrombolytic agents have been used in the treatment of BCS although there are no comparative studies to suggest benefit of one method over another.[46] It seems reasonable to consider that since there exist the technical capability[47] to selectively and super-selectively cannulate various vessels, it should be possible to increase the efficacy of the thrombolytic agent by injecting a similar volume to what is injected systemically, close to the clot. Since the volume of medication administered during local infusion causes a comparable coagulopathy to systemic administration, the risk of bleeding is similar.

Thrombolytic treatment can be considered in patients with the acute or subacute form of BCS,[48] in which blood clots are younger than 3–4 weeks. Published experience of successful thrombolysis is limited to small case series and individual reports. Thrombolysis has limited efficacy, and exposes the patient to the risks of thrombolytic therapy (bleeding, stroke and pulmonary embolism). Thrombolytic agents are contraindicated in treating the chronic form of BCS.[49] These clots have matured and thrombolysis will be ineffective. Additionally, such patients may have already developed portal hypertension and thrombolysis in this situation will be catastrophic due to the resulting torrential bleeding.

Role of Interventional Radiology

With increasing expertise and improved technology, the treatment of BCS has seen a shift from operative approaches, to those being driven by interventional radiology techniques. These techniques are also considered minimally invasive and include all procedures that are performed by interventional radiology, including diagnostics.

Angioplasty alone or with placement of a stent and TIPSS is also included and sometimes these can be combined. The results and outcomes have been revolutionary, with declining requirements for operation and transplantation.[50,51] Five-years transplant-free survival rates of 77–100% using an approach involving transvenous and a combination of percutaneous-transvenous approaches or TIPSS have been reported.[51,52]

Angioplasty

In some forms of BCS, the hepatic venous circulation may reveal a focal abnormality that can be treated by balloon angioplasty,[53] such as a membranous web in the IVC which can be dilated (Figs 1 to 4).[54] This is physiological restoration of hepatic venous outflow. Balloon dilation of hepatic veins may also be effective in some patients with short strictured segments.[55] Angioplasty can be combined with thrombolytic therapy in patients in whom there is acute or subacute thrombosis of a single hepatic vein.[55] With angioplasty alone, the major complication is that of reocclusion of the affected vein. To prevent this and to improve the vessel patency rates, deployment of self-expanding metal stent (SEMS) can be performed.[56,57] Once the SEMS has been deployed, it cannot be removed as it embeds into the tissue around. To prevent complications during liver transplantation if

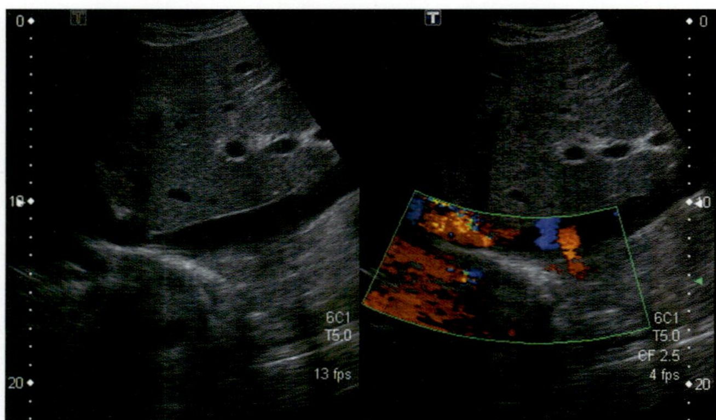

Figure 1 Ultrasound and Doppler imaging of the abdomen reveal a focal tight stenosis of the supra-hepatic stump of the IVC; IVC below the stenosis is dilated. The diagnosis is IVC membranous occlusion

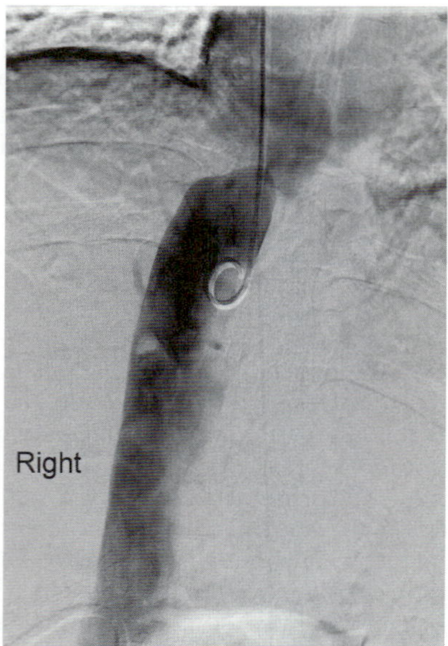

Figure 2 Venography shows an abrupt cut off of the IVC at the suprahepatic stump with a thin jet of contrast into the right atrium

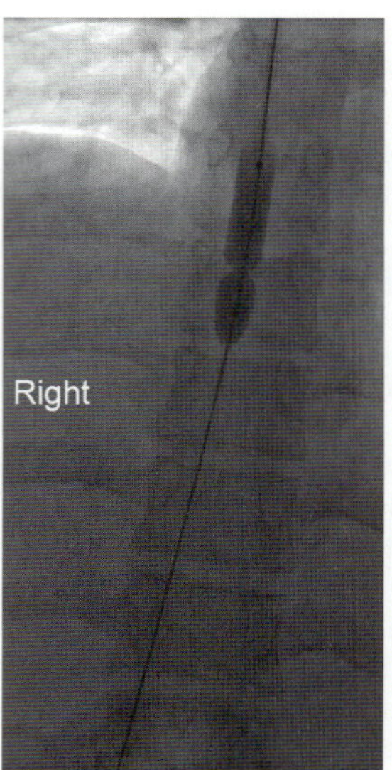

Figure 3 Balloon angioplasty of the web illustrates focal "waisting" of balloon at the level of the IVC web

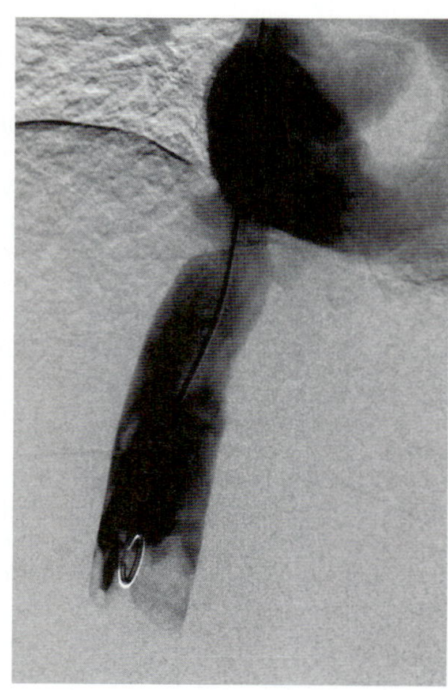

Figure 4 Post-angioplasty venogram shows restoration of lumen in the narrowed segment of IVC with good outflow of contrast across the IVC into the right atrium

required subsequently, the decision to place this should be in consultation with a liver transplant team.

Published experience is limited to small numbers; however, long-term survival with improvement in liver function and reduction of portal hypertension has been reported.[58] This technique, however, has been seen to function more as a stop-gap procedure with most patients ultimately requiring liver transplantation.

TIPSS and Direct Intrahepatic Portosystemic Shunt in Budd-Chiari Syndrome

The rationale for the concept, development and subsequent successful clinical application of TIPSS and direct intrahepatic portosystemic shunt (DIPSS) in BCS is decompression of the congested liver segments through the creation of an alternative venous outflow tract. This is physiological modification of hepatic venous outflow.

The concept of TIPSS is the artificial formation of a low-resistance channel between the hepatic vein (usually the right) and the intrahepatic portion of the portal vein (usually the right branch). The tract created is kept patent by deployment of a covered stent graft, thereby allowing blood to return to the systemic circulation. TIPSS therefore functions like a surgical side-to-side portacaval shunt without requiring a major operation. DIPSS is the creation of a similar portacaval shunt through a puncture in the anterior wall of the retrohepatic IVC (Figs 5 and 6).

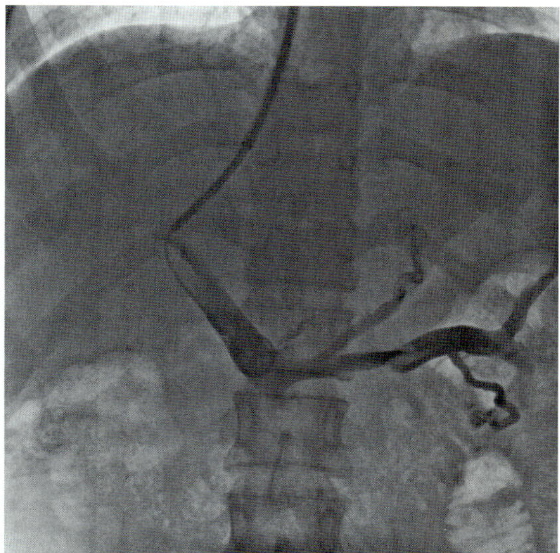

Figure 5 Direct intrahepatic portosystemic shunt in a young woman with history of variceal bleeding. Ultrasound abdomen showed features of chronic liver disease with cirrhosis and BCS with occlusion of all hepatic veins. Through a transjugular venous access, a cannula in the IVC is used to create a parenchymal track between IVC and right branch of portal vein under ultrasound and fluoroscopic guidance. Image shows a portogram after the track is created with hepatofugal flow of contrast into collaterals

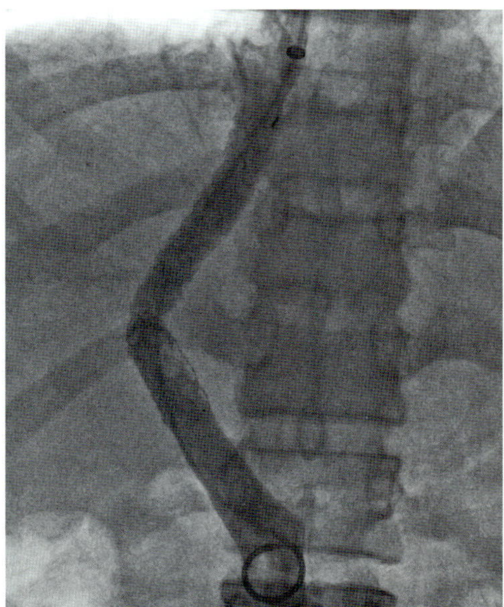

Figure 6 A covered stent is placed across the parenchymal track, with portogram now showing hepatopetal flow and non-visualization of varices

Several reports have shown that TIPSS can be successfully performed in patients with BCS.[59,60] Transplant-free survival at 1 and 5 years after TIPSS has been shown to be 88% and 78%, respectively.[60] A prognostic score based upon age, bilirubin and INR levels predicted a small group of patients expected to have high mortality after TIPSS, who would be better managed by liver transplantation.[60]

There are more than a few problems with this technique. It is not technically possible in all patients. It can sometimes drain only a small portion of the liver. In current practice a covered stent is used in TIPSS/DIPSS. TIPSS/DIPSS are only considered when there are no restorable hepatic veins. Covered PTFE stents as opposed to SEMS are also being used, and are seen by some to be a reason for the popularity of TIPSS.[61]

Pre-TIPSS Evaluation

A cardiac evaluation should be performed prior to TIPSS placement in patients with signs, symptoms, or a history of heart failure, tricuspid regurgitation, cardiomyopathy, or pulmonary hypertension. Evaluation should include an echocardiogram, cardiology consultation, and in some cases, an atrial fluid challenge. In patients who do not have a cardiac history, the appropriate evaluation is less clear. A 2005 guideline from the American Association for the Study of Liver Diseases does not recommend routine echocardiograms prior to TIPSS placement.[62] However, there are those who recommend routine echocardiography because pulmonary hypertension is seen in up to 16% of patients being referred for liver transplantation.[63]

Absolute contraindications:

- Tricuspid regurgitation
- Severe pulmonary hypertension (mean pulmonary artery pressure >45 mm Hg)
- Multiple hepatic cysts
- Uncontrolled systemic infection or sepsis
- Unrelieved biliary obstruction.

Relative contraindications:

- Obstruction of all hepatic veins
- Portal vein thrombosis
- Severe coagulopathy
- Thrombocytopenia (<20,000/mm^3)
- Moderate pulmonary hypertension.

COMPLICATIONS

- Technical complications such as cardiac arrhythmias, inadvertent carotid artery or tracheal puncture, tearing of the liver capsule during attempts to enter the portal vein, creation of a tract between the shunt or the portal vein and the hepatic artery or bile ducts, and extrahepatic puncture of the portal vein.
- The primary complication related to portosystemic shunting is the development of portosystemic encephalopathy (PSE). It usually becomes clinically apparent 2–3 weeks after TIPSS insertion. The occurrence of PSE 6 weeks or more after TIPSS insertion is usually associated with gastrointestinal bleeding.
- Unique TIPSS-related complications such as severe hyperbilirubinemia, hemolytic anemia, TIPSS stenosis and vegetative infections.

It is therefore probably best to use TIPSS when angioplasty and stent placement is not feasible or have failed. TIPSS can also be used as a bridge to transplant in a patient with acute fulminating BCS while waiting for an organ to become available.[64] This must be done correctly to prevent compromising the transplant operation.

PRINCIPLES OF OPERATIONS FOR BUDD-CHIARI SYNDROME

Only principles for offering operation will be discussed here; the reader is referred to a standard text-book of HPB Surgery for the operative surgical steps.

The fundamental goal of operative treatment of BCS is restoration of normal or as near-normal liver function as possible. The choice of operation if all else is equal depends on the state of liver function. If liver dysfunction has not progressed to cirrhosis, decompression of the liver by restoring hepatic venous outflow can often result in significant clinical improvement. This can be accomplished by shunt procedures; many procedures have been described.

Most surgical shunts will drain the portal or mesenteric venous system into the IVC or the right atrium. This allows blood entering the liver through the hepatic arteries to have a low pressure route by which to drain out of the liver. The arterial blood will flow preferentially into the low pressure system and decompress the liver. Even acute hepatocellular necrosis caused by pressure-induced atrophy of hepatocytes will often regress following the successful functioning of decompressive shunt operation.

In cirrhosis or advanced liver dysfunction (elevated prothrombin time and serum bilirubin level, decreased serum albumin), the best option is liver transplantation.

Some advocates of surgical thrombectomy have reported good results when performed with appropriate liver resection. These are not operations for the inexperienced surgeon.[65]

Five-year survival rates after decompressive procedures depend on the state of the preoperation liver function and continued graft function.[66] Five-year survival as high as 90% have been reported in patients who underwent shunt surgery prior to the development of cirrhosis, and whose shunts remained patent.[67,68] These have not been replicated in other centers.[69]

OPERATIVE APPROACHES

Prior to any operation being planned or performed, it is important to identify the thrombotic cause of BCS and to treat it. This will prevent unnecessary operations and complications.

It is safe to say that the evolution and progression of the TIPSS (and DIPSS) procedure has made many operations for BCS obsolete.[60] The number of operations for BCS will further reduce as TIPSS becomes more readily available in a larger number of centers and also because BCS is a rare disease itself. The further subdivision of surgical specialties has meant that many vascular surgeons have no experience with these procedures and hepatobiliary or transplant units may be the only referral centers for these patients. While this is acceptable for subacute and chronic BCS, the lack of a formal functioning referral system in India means that many acute BCS patients will never receive the care they need.

Another reason to involve a transplant team is that the shunt operation may only delay the future need for transplantation. As in the case of the decision to use TIPSS with SEMS, it is important to have a multidisciplinary team approach, preferably with a transplant unit involved. The underlying cause of the thrombotic diathesis should be identified and treated prior to considering a shunt operation.

SHUNT OPERATIONS

Portosystemic shunts (interposition mesocaval, conventional splenorenal, side to side portocaval) will work only if the IVC is patent and there is no significant pressure gradient present between the supra-hepatic and infra-hepatic parts. Additionally, the infra-hepatic IVC pressure should be at least 10 mm Hg lower than the portal pressure.[67] Usually the hypertrophied caudate lobe compresses the retrohepatic IVC. This would then mean that a meso-cavo-right atrial or meso-right atrial shunt is necessary as advocated by Orloff and colleagues.[68,69] The synthetic nature of the graft means that shunt thrombosis is a real problem. Solomon Victor described a retrohepatic cavoatrial shunt through a right posterolateral thoracotomy for pure IVC obstruction. He used a ringed Gore-Tex graft.

PERIOPERATIVE MANAGEMENT AND FOLLOW-UP

Perioperative management of patients undergoing surgical decompression is critical for determining the outcome of the operation.[70] Anticoagulation may be needed for continued shunt patency; this poses risk of bleeding. Evaluation of graft function may be done by regular ultrasound Doppler examinations. CT angiographic evaluation should be considered if there is clinical or biochemical deterioration in patients following shunt operation. If thrombosis of the shunt is present, angiographic treatment through angioplasty or selective thrombolysis may salvage shunt function.

LIVER TRANSPLANTATION

Orthotopic liver transplantation (OLTX) may be the only option for patients with BCS who are not candidates for radiologic or surgical decompression or who have decompensated cirrhosis, either acute or chronic. Patients who develop the BCS as a result of protein S, C, or antithrombin III deficiency may also be cured of their clotting tendency by liver transplantation in an elegant solution, since the transplanted liver will produce normal amounts of these factors.

Survival following OLTX depends upon the underlying cause of the BCS and the patient's condition at the time of the transplant.[71] Survival appears to have improved in recent years with advances in liver transplantation technology and routine use of the model for end-stage liver disease (MELD) score.[72]

One of the largest series of 510 patients compared survival in patients who underwent transplantation after introduction of the MELD score to the pre-MELD era.[72] Three-year graft survival (81% vs 65%) and patient survival (85% vs 73%) was significantly better following introduction of the MELD score. In another large series (248 patients), overall survival was 76%, 71% and 68% at 1, 5 and 10 years respectively.[73] Most deaths (77%) occurred in the first 3 months. The only predictor of mortality was impaired renal function and a history of a shunt. Ten-year survival ranged from 69% to 84% in another series.

Table 1: Overview of treatment options in hepatic venous outflow obstruction

Portosystemic shunting	*Thrombolysis, angioplasty and stenting*	*TIPSS*	*Liver transplantation*
The role of surgical shunts in BCS is controversial. Perioperative mortality has been reported from 0% to 50%. Long-term survival rates after various shunting procedures have been reported to be as high as 90% even at follow-up of 14 years. Comparing surgical shunts to medical or minimally invasive techniques is difficult because data is reprospective, may have significant time bias with sicker patients being managed non-operatively. Shunt procedures are done less frequently so technical inexperience may translate to more morbidity/mortality. Shunts are indicated in patients with reversible liver injury and where TIPSS is not technically feasible (long IVC thrombus). Orloff et al. reported great success with portocaval shunts with 31 of 32 patients alive at 3.5–27 years. In situations where IVC obstruction and/or an infrahepatic to right atrium pressure gradient is present, mesocaval and portocaval shunts may not effectively decompress the liver. Mesocaval with cavoatrial or mesoatrial shunts may be better. Some reports show better long-term outcomes with a pressure gradient of greater than 10 mm Hg between the portal vein and IVC. Murad's multivariate analysis stratified 205 patients with BCS treated by a variety of modalities into three classes and found that surgical shunt and TIPSS was associated with increased mortality as the interval between diagnosis and shunting lengthened. Thus, the high early mortality of the procedure may be balanced by the late beneficial effects of relieving hepatic congestion. *Summary:* The most important pressure gradient is not between the infra- and supra-hepatic vena cava, but between the two vascular structures that are to be connected. Shunts need to be constructed meticulously in carefully selected patients in order to ensure full advantage of these challenging operations.	Systemic thrombolytic therapy is of little value. Catheter-directed thrombolysis with tissue plasminogen activator delivered just proximal to the thrombus is efficacious for acute thrombus which is not completely occlusive. Angioplasty and stenting are additional adjuncts those may be used. Angioplasty often suffers from high reocclusion rates: better place stents in the IVC or hepatic veins. Reports indicate overall shunt patency of 90% with a mean follow-up of more than 45 months. Angioplasty and stenting may have advantages for patients who suffer from BCS due to technical reasons after liver transplantation. *Summary*: Angioplasty and stenting good in membranous BCS (Asian) and in setting of acute thrombus.	For patients who present weeks to months after formation of hepatic vein thrombus, TIPSS is useful in elective and emergent situations. TIPSS effectively decompresses the portal system and may serve as a bridge to transplant. The first report of TIPSS for the treatment of BCS was in 1993. Extended TIPSS with or without thrombolysis can be used in cases of BCS with portal vein thrombosis. Two series with a total of 34 patients showed improved patency and less dysfunction with PTFE covered stents over bare stents. Other series using TIPSS in BCS report eventual transplantation in 10–40% of patients. One series of 61 patients who underwent TIPSS with or without hepatic vein recanalization with angioplasty and stenting showed excellent survival with 40 patients requiring repeated radiological interventions. Additionally it appears that short-length stenosis of hepatic veins is under-recognized and percutaneous recanalization is under-utilized in treating these BCS patients. TIPSS seems to be utilized for the sickest patients, especially those unlikely to survive operation. *Summary*: TIPSS is best for those BCS patients with chronic disease, both electively and emergently. PTFE stents are better and repeat procedures may be required. It is best to discuss with a transplant team prior to performing the procedure.	In BCS and acute fulminant liver failure or cirrhosis and in decompensated disease with poor synthetic function, liver transplantation is the treatment of choice. Compared with patients who receive shunting procedures, transplanted patients maintain higher serum albumin levels and improved synthetic function. Where synthetic deficiencies such as anti-thrombin III or protein C occur, transplantation is an elegant solution to curing these genetic problems. Transplantation is a safe therapeutic option for patients with BCS but should be used judiciously as there are other options open to these patients which may not be there for others on the transplant waiting list. Segev published the largest series of transplantation for BCS which included 510 patients who were divided into three time periods: historical (1987–1997), pre-MELD (1998–2002) and MELD (2002–2006). The study found that TIPSS did not adversely affect graft loss or death over all time periods. The final analysis found that only life support prior to transplantation and prolonged cold ischemia time (4.5 hours) were independent predictors of both graft loss and death. The European Liver Transplant Registry (ELTR) recorded 391 patients from 1968 to 2001 who received transplantation for BCS with a 1-, 5- and 10-year patient survival of 73%, 68% and 63% respectively. The important point that is seen here is that short-term survival in patients with BCS is lower while long-term survival is equivalent to other indications. In Mentha's series of 256 patients undergoing transplantation for BCS multivariate analysis found that only retransplant predictors of mortality to be impaired renal function and a history of a surgical shunt/TIPSS; this group only included patients whose shunts had failed. Comparing Mentha's results with Murad's, those from Mentha's cohort had improved 5-year survival (71%) with transplantation compared with Murad's cohort treated without transplant (42%). Budd-Chiari syndrome following liver transplantation with the piggyback technique is a well-described complication due to impaired venous outflow with a reported incidence of 1–7%. Two retrospective studies were unable to detect a difference in the rate of BCS between the piggyback techniques. The standard technique and analysis of large series did not reveal statistical significance in rates of BCS either with the standard (1.7%) or piggyback (1.5%) technique. Technical factors that have been associated with this complication are inadequate graft size and use of two hepatic veins for the venous anastomosis. The side-to-side variation of the piggyback technique has been associated with a decreased incidence of BCS. For those who develop BCS after transplantation, up to 25–27%, lifelong anticoagulation is recommended. *Summary*: Liver transplantation is the treatment of choice for BCS patients with fulminant hepatic failure or those with cirrhosis and poor synthetic liver function. Attention to technical details may help to avoid BCS after transplantation.

SUMMARY BASED ON AASLD GUIDELINES FOR TREATMENT OF BUDD-CHIARI SYNDROME[4]

The 2009 guidelines from the American Association for the Study of Liver Diseases include the following recommendations for treatment of BCS:

- Correct without delay the underlying risk factor(s) for venous thrombosis.
- Start anticoagulation therapy immediately. Use low molecular weight heparin.
- Change to an oral anticoagulant when clinically appropriate, targeting the INR between 2 and 3.
- Maintain permanent anticoagulation therapy unless a major contraindication is present or complication occurs.
- Treat complications of portal hypertension as recommended for other types of liver disease.
- Check for a venous obstruction amenable to percutaneous angioplasty/stenting in all symptomatic patients and treat accordingly.
- In patients without ongoing improvement on anticoagulation therapy (with or without angioplasty), consider TIPSS.
- Consider liver transplantation if TIPSS insertion fails or does not improve the patient's condition and in those with fulminant hepatic failure.
- Coordinate care with a transplant center.
- Monitor patients with longstanding, well controlled BCS for the late development of hepatocellular cancer[74] and transformation of underlying myeloproliferative disease.

REFERENCES

1. Menon KVN, Shah V, Kamath PS. The Budd-Chiari syndrome. N Engl J Med. 2004;350(6):578-85.
2. Okuda K, Kage M, Shrestha SM. Proposal of a new nomenclature for Budd-Chiari syndrome: hepatic vein thrombosis versus thrombosis of the inferior vena cava at its hepatic portion. Hepatol Baltim Md. 1998;28(5):1191-8.
3. Murad SD, Plessier A, Hernandez-Guerra M, Fabris F, Eapen CE, Bahr MJ, et al. Etiology, management, and outcome of the Budd-Chiari syndrome. Ann Intern Med. 2009;151(3):167-75.
4. DeLeve LD, Valla D-C, Garcia-Tsao G, American Association for the Study Liver Diseases. Vascular disorders of the liver. Hepatol Baltim Md. 2009;49(5):1729-64.
5. Amitrano L, Guardascione MA, Ames PR, Margaglione M, Antinolfi I, Iannaccone L, et al. Thrombophilic genotypes, natural anticoagulants, and plasma homocysteine in myeloproliferative disorders: relationship with splanchnic vein thrombosis and arterial disease. Am J Hematol. 2003;72(2):75-81.
6. Primignani M, Barosi G, Bergamaschi G, Gianelli U, Fabris F, Reati R, et al. Role of the JAK2 mutation in the diagnosis of chronic myeloproliferative disorders in splanchnic vein thrombosis. Hepatology. 2006;44(6):1528-34.
7. Eapen CE, Mammen T, Moses V, Shyamkumar NK. Changing profile of Budd-Chiari syndrome in India. Indian J Gastroenterol. 2007;26:77-81.
8. Shetty S, Ghosh K. Thrombophilic dimension of Budd-Chiari syndrome and portal venous thrombosis—a concise review. Thromb Res. 2011;127(6):505-12.
9. Laposata M. The prothrombin G20210A mutation: a new high-prevalence congenital risk factor for thrombosis. Gastroenterology. 1999;116(1):213-5.
10. Espinosa G, Font J, García-Pagan JC, Tàssies D, Reverter JC, Gaig C, et al. Budd-Chiari syndrome secondary to antiphospholipid syndrome: clinical and immunologic characteristics of 43 patients. Medicine (Baltimore). 2001;80(6):345-54.
11. Saca LF, Szer IS, Henar E, Nanjundiah P, Haddad ZH, Quismorio FP Jr. Budd-Chiari syndrome associated with antiphospholipid antibodies in a child: report of a case and review of the literature. J Rheumatol. 1994;21(3):545-8.
12. Das M, Carroll SF. Antithrombin III deficiency: an etiology of Budd-Chiari syndrome. Surgery. 1985;97(2):242-6.
13. Sugano S, Suzuki T, Makino H, Yanagimoto S, Nishio M, Onmura H, et al. Budd-Chiari syndrome attributed to protein C deficiency. Am J Gastroenterol. 1996;91(4):777-9.
14. Valla D, Dhumeaux D, Babany G, Hillon P, Rueff B, Rochant H, et al. Hepatic vein thrombosis in paroxysmal nocturnal hemoglobinuria. A spectrum from asymptomatic occlusion of hepatic venules to fatal Budd-Chiari syndrome. Gastroenterology. 1987;93(3):569-75.
15. Mohanty D, Shetty S, Ghosh K, Pawar A, Abraham P. Hereditary thrombophilia as a cause of Budd-Chiari syndrome: a study from Western India. Hepatol Baltim Md. 2001;34(4 Pt 1):666-70.
16. Janssen HLA, Meinardi JR, Vleggaar FP, Uum SHM van, Haagsma EB, Meer FJM van der, et al. Factor V Leiden mutation, prothrombin gene mutation, and deficiencies in coagulation inhibitors associated with Budd-Chiari syndrome and portal vein thrombosis: results of a case-control study. Blood. 2000;96(7):2364-8.
17. Bayraktar Y, Balkanci F, Bayraktar M, Calguneri M. Budd-Chiari syndrome: a common complication of Behçet's disease. Am J Gastroenterol. 1997;92(5):858-62.
18. Rector WG Jr, Xu YH, Goldstein L, Peters RL, Reynolds TB. Membranous obstruction of the inferior vena cava in the United States. Medicine (Baltimore). 1985;64(2):134-43.
19. Simson IW. Membranous obstruction of the inferior vena cava and hepatocellular carcinoma in South Africa. Gastroenterology. 1982;82(2):171-8.
20. Mori H, Hayashi K, Amamoto Y. Membranous obstruction of the inferior vena cava associated with intrahepatic portosystemic shunt. Cardiovasc Intervent Radiol. 1986;9(4):209-13.
21. Perarnau J-M, Bacq Y. Hepatic vascular involvement related to pregnancy, oral contraceptives, and estrogen replacement therapy. Semin Liver Dis. 2008;28(3):315-27.
22. Lewis JH, Tice HL, Zimmerman HJ. Budd-Chiari syndrome associated with oral contraceptive steroids. Review of treatment of 47 cases. Dig Dis Sci. 1983;28(8):673-83.
23. Valla D, Le MG, Poynard T, Zucman N, Rueff B, Benhamou JP. Risk of hepatic vein thrombosis in relation to recent use of oral contraceptives. A case-control study. Gastroenterology. 1986;90(4):807-11.
24. Khuroo MS, Datta DV. Budd-Chiari syndrome following pregnancy: report of 16 cases, with roentgenologic, hemodynamic and histologic studies of the hepatic outflow tract. Am J Med. 1980;68(1):113-21.
25. Young ID, Clark RN, Manley PN, Groll A, Simon JB. Response to steroids in Budd-Chiari syndrome caused by idiopathic granulomatous venulitis. Gastroenterology. 1988;94(2):503-7.
26. Valla D, Hadengue A, el Younsi M, Azar N, Zeitoun G, Boudet MJ, et al. Hepatic venous outflow block caused by short-length hepatic vein stenoses. Hepatol Baltim Md. 1997;25(4):814-9.
27. Plessier A, Valla D-C. Budd-Chiari syndrome. Semin Liver Dis 200828259-269 [Internet]. Available from: https://www.orpha.net/data/patho/Pro/en/BuddChiari-FRenPro854v01.pdf.

28. Murad SD, Valla D-C, de Groen PC, Zeitoun G, Hopmans JAM, Haagsma EB, et al. Determinants of survival and the effect of portosystemic shunting in patients with Budd-Chiari syndrome. Hepatology. 2004;39(2):500-8.
29. Rautou P, Moucari R, Cazals-Hatem D, Escolano S, Denié C, Douarin L, et al. Levels and initial course of serum alanine aminotransferase can predict outcome of patients with Budd-Chiari syndrome. Clin Gastroenterol Hepatol. 2009;7(11): 1230-5.
30. Hadengue A, Poliquin M, Vilgrain V, Belghiti J, Degott C, Erlinger S, et al. The changing scene of hepatic vein thrombosis: recognition of asymptomatic cases. Gastroenterology. 1994;106(4):1042-7.
31. De Binay K, Sen S, Biswas PK, Mandal SK, Das D, Das U, et al. Occurrence of hepatopulmonary syndrome in Budd-Chiari syndrome and the role of venous decompression. Gastroenterology. 2002;122(4):897-903.
32. Mahmoud AE, Helmy AS, Billingham L, Elias E. Poor prognosis and limited therapeutic options in patients with Budd-Chiari syndrome and portal venous system thrombosis. Eur J Gastroenterol Hepatol. 1997;9(5):485-9.
33. Gupta S, Barter S, Phillips GW, Gibson RN, Hodgson HJ. Comparison of ultrasonography, computed tomography and 99mTc liver scan in diagnosis of Budd-Chiari syndrome. Gut. 1987;28(3):242-7.
34. Soyer P, Rabenandrasana A, Barge J, Laissy JP, Zeitoun G, Hay JM, et al. MRI of Budd-Chiari syndrome. Abdom Imaging. 1994;19(4):325-9.
35. Lin J, Zhou K-R, Chen Z-W, Wang J-H, Yan Z-P, Wang Y-XJ. Vena cava 3D contrast-enhanced MR venography: a pictorial review. Cardiovasc Intervent Radiol. 2005;28(6):795-805.
36. Cazals-Hatem D, Vilgrain V, Genin P, Denninger M-H, Durand F, Belghiti J, et al. Arterial and portal circulation and parenchymal changes in Budd-Chiari syndrome: a study in 17 explanted livers. Hepatology. 2003;37(3):510-9.
37. Tang TJ, Batts KP, de Groen PC, van Hoek B, Haagsma EB, Hop WC, et al. The prognostic value of histology in the assessment of patients with Budd-Chiari syndrome. J Hepatol. 2001;35(3):338-43.
38. Cazals-Hatem D, Vilgrain V, Genin P, Denninger M-H, Durand F, Belghiti J, et al. Arterial and portal circulation and parenchymal changes in Budd-Chiari syndrome: a study in 17 explanted livers. Hepatol Baltim Md. 2003;37(3):510-9.
39. Plessier A, Sibert A, Consigny Y, Hakime A, Zappa M, Denninger M-H, et al. Aiming at minimal invasiveness as a therapeutic strategy for Budd-Chiari syndrome. Hepatology. 2006;44(5):1308-16.
40. Slakey DP, Klein AS, Venbrux AC, Cameron JL. Budd-Chiari syndrome: current management options. Ann Surg. 2001;233(4): 522-7.
41. Runyon BA. Management of adult patients with ascites due to cirrhosis. Hepatology. 2004;39(3):841-56.
42. Klein AS. Management of Budd-Chiari syndrome. Liver Transpl. 2006;12(S2):S23-8.
43. Rautou P-E, Douarin L, Denninger M-H, Escolano S, Lebrec D, Moreau R, et al. Bleeding in patients with Budd-Chiari syndrome. J Hepatol. 2011;54(1):56-63.
44. Zeitoun G, Escolano S, Hadengue A, Azar N, El Younsi M, Mallet A, et al. Outcome of Budd-Chiari syndrome: a multivariate analysis of factors related to survival including surgical portosystemic shunting. Hepatol Baltim Md. 1999;30(1):84-9.
45. Langlet P, Escolano S, Valla D, Coste-Zeitoun D, Denie C, Mallet A, et al. Clinicopathological forms and prognostic index in Budd-Chiari syndrome. J Hepatol. 2003;39(4):496-501.
46. Min AD, Atillasoy EO, Schwartz ME, Thiim M, Miller CM, Bodenheimer HC Jr. Reassessing the role of medical therapy in the management of hepatic vein thrombosis. Liver Transplant Surg Off Publ Am Assoc Study Liver Dis Int Liver Transplant Soc. 1997;3(4):423-9.
47. Greenwood LH, Yrizarry JM, JW Hallett J, GS Scoville J. Urokinase treatment of Budd-Chiari syndrome [Internet]. http://dx.doi.org/10.2214/ajr.141.5.1057. 2012 [cited 2013 Aug 4]. Available from: http://www.ajronline.org/doi/abs/10.2214/ajr.141.5.1057.
48. Sharma S, Texeira A, Texeira P, Elias E, Wilde J, Olliff SP. Pharmacological thrombolysis in Budd-Chiari syndrome: a single center experience and review of the literature. J Hepatol. 2004;40(1):172-80.
49. Raju GS, Felver M, Olin JW, Satti SD. Thrombolysis for acute Budd-Chiari syndrome: case report and literature review. Am J Gastroenterol. 1996;91(6):1262-3.
50. Wang ZG, Zhang FJ, Yi MQ, Qiang LX. Evolution of management for Budd-Chiari syndrome: a team's view from 2564 patients. Anz J Surg. 2005;75(1-2):55-63.
51. Eapen CE, Velissaris D, Heydtmann M, Gunson B, Olliff S, Elias E. Favourable medium term outcome following hepatic vein recanalisation and/or transjugular intrahepatic portosystemic shunt for Budd-Chiari syndrome. Gut. 2006;55(6):878-84.
52. Han G, Qi X, Zhang W, He C, Yin Z, Wang J, et al. Percutaneous recanalization for Budd-Chiari syndrome: an 11-year retrospective study on patency and survival in 177 Chinese patients from a single center. Radiology. 2013;266(2):657-67.
53. Sparano J, Chang J, Trasi S, Bonanno C. Treatment of the Budd-Chiari syndrome with percutaneous transluminal angioplasty: case report and review of the literature. Am J Med. 1987;82(4):821-8.
54. Yang X-L, Cheng TO, Chen C-R. Successful treatment by percutaneous balloon angioplasty of Budd-Chiari syndrome caused by membranous obstruction of inferior vena cava: 8-year follow-up study. J Am Coll Cardiol. 1996;28(7):1720-4.
55. Fisher NC, McCafferty I, Dolapci M, Wali M, Buckels JA, Olliff SP, et al. Managing Budd-Chiari syndrome: a retrospective review of percutaneous hepatic vein angioplasty and surgical shunting. Gut. 1999;44(4):568-74.
56. Lopez RR Jr, Benner KG, Hall L, Rösch J, Pinson CW. Expandable venous stents for treatment of the Budd-Chiari syndrome. Gastroenterology. 1991;100(5 Pt 1):1435-41.
57. Xue H, Li Y-C, Shakya P, Palikhe M, Jha RK. The role of intravascular intervention in the management of Budd-Chiari syndrome. Dig Dis Sci. 2009;55(9):2659-63.
58. Witte AM, Kool LJ, Veenendaal R, Lamers CB, van Hoek B. Hepatic vein stenting for Budd-Chiari syndrome. Am J Gastroenterol. 1997;92(3):498-501.
59. Ganger DR, Klapman JB, McDonald V, Matalon TA, Kaur S, Rosenblate H, et al. Transjugular intrahepatic portosystemic shunt (TIPS) for Budd-Chiari syndrome or portal vein thrombosis. Am J Gastroenterol. 1999;94(3):603-8.
60. Garcia-Pagán JC, Heydtmann M, Raffa S, Plessier A, Murad S, Fabris F, et al. TIPS for Budd-Chiari syndrome: long-term results and prognostics factors in 124 patients. Gastroenterology. 2008;135(3):808-15.
61. Hernández-Guerra M, Turnes J, Rubinstein P, Olliff S, Elias E, Bosch J, et al. PTFE-covered stents improve TIPS patency in Budd-Chiari syndrome. Hepatol Baltim Md. 2004;40(5):1197-202.
62. Boyer TD, Haskal ZJ. The role of transjugular intrahepatic portosystemic shunt in the management of portal hypertension. Hepatology. 2005;41(2):386-400.
63. Hoeper MM, Krowka MJ, Strassburg CP. Portopulmonary hypertension and hepatopulmonary syndrome. The Lancet. 2004;363(9419):1461-8.
64. Shrestha R, Durham JD, Wachs M, Bilir BM, Kam I, Trouillot T, et al. Use of transjugular intrahepatic portosystemic shunt as a bridge

to transplantation in fulminant hepatic failure due to Budd-Chiari syndrome. Am J Gastroenterol. 1997;92(12):2304-6.

65. Bansky G, Ernest C, Jenni R, Zollikofer C, Burger HR, Senning A. Treatment of Budd-Chiari syndrome by dorsocranial liver resection and direct hepatoatrial anastomosis. J Hepatol. 1986; 2(1):101-12.
66. McDermott WV, Stone MD, Bothe A Jr, Trey C. Budd-Chiari syndrome. Historical and clinical review with an analysis of surgical corrective procedures. Am J Surg. 1984;147(4):463-7.
67. Orloff MJ, Girard B. Long term results of treatment of Budd-Chiari syndrome by side to side portacaval shunt. Surg Gynecol Obstet. 1989;168(1):33-41.
68. Orloff MJ, Daily PO, Orloff SL, Girard B, Orloff MS. A 27-year experience with surgical treatment of Budd-Chiari syndrome. Ann Surg. 2000;232(3):340-52.
69. Pq X, Xx M, Xx Y, Ls F, Xw D, Yf Z, et al. Surgical treatment of 1360 cases of Budd-Chiari syndrome: 20-year experience. Hepatobiliary Pancreat Dis Int. 2004;3(3):391-4.
70. Ringe B, Lang H, Oldhafer KJ, Gebel M, Flemming P, Georgii A, et al. Which is the best surgery for Budd-Chiari syndrome: venous decompression or liver transplantation? A single-center experience with 50 patients. Hepatol Baltim Md. 1995;21(5):1337-44.
71. Campbell DA Jr, Rolles K, Jamieson N, O'Grady J, Wight D, Williams R, et al. Hepatic transplantation with perioperative and long term anticoagulation as treatment for Budd-Chiari syndrome. Surg Gynecol Obstet. 1988;166(6):511-8.
72. Segev DL, Nguyen GC, Locke JE, Simpkins CE, Montgomery RA, Maley WR, et al. Twenty years of liver transplantation for Budd-Chiari syndrome: a national registry analysis. Liver Transpl. 2007;13(9):1285-94.
73. Mentha G, Giostra E, Majno PE, Bechstein WO, Neuhaus P, O'Grady J, et al. Liver transplantation for Budd-Chiari syndrome: a European study on 248 patients from 51 centers. J Hepatol. 2006;44(3):520-8.
74. Moucari R, Rautou P-E, Cazals-Hatem D, Geara A, Bureau C, Consigny Y, et al. Hepatocellular carcinoma in Budd-Chiari syndrome: characteristics and risk factors. Gut. 2008;57(6):828-35.

CHAPTER 78

Cirrhosis and its Complications

Cyriac Abby Philips, SK Sarin

INTRODUCTION

Cirrhosis is derived from the Greek word "κίρρος" meaning tawny. The transformation of normal lobular architecture to one that of nodularity due to angiogenesis, vascular remodeling, sinusoidal capillarization, perisinusoidal fibrosis and loss of metabolic zonation is pertinent to cirrhosis.[1] The development of fibrous bands as well as regenerative nodules in response to chronic inflammation results in portal hypertension (PHT) and end stage liver disease is defined as cirrhosis. The earliest complication of cirrhosis is PHT and this is a result of intrahepatic resistance increment in lieu with a raised hepatic and portal arterial blood flow. Advances in hepatology have changed cirrhosis into an entity that is dynamic and reversible, rather than static and irreversible. This concept has given rise to the fact that cirrhosis is a result of series of critical steps which progress through four stages of clinical, functional and histopathological changes (Table 1). Depending on the type of disease, targeted treatment has shown to control inflammatory process in the liver and helped in prevention of further fibrosis and reversal of cirrhosis; as in antiviral therapy for hepatitis C and hepatitis B, suppression of autoimmunity (in autoimmune hepatitis) or removal of offending agent such as alcohol or iron (in hemochromatosis). Regression of fibrosis can take place in both pre-cirrhotic and cirrhotic livers. This novel ideal led to the evolution of an entity termed "incomplete septal cirrhosis" where in there is thinning and loss of fibrous septa surrounding the nodules with persistence of at least some degree of vascular changes characteristic of cirrhosis.[2]

ETIOLOGY OF CIRRHOSIS

Etiology of cirrhosis varies demographically. The main causes of cirrhosis include chronic viral hepatitis (B and C), alcoholic liver disease, fatty liver diseases, autoimmune hepatitis, chronic biliary diseases and several inherited metabolic disorders. Liver disease due to alcohol consumption and chronic viral hepatitis C infection are the most common causes of cirrhosis in the West, in contrast to Asian and African countries where chronic viral hepatitis B infection is more often seen. Cryptogenic cirrhosis is an entity that is slowly being diagnosed less these days with better detection of hepatitis C and also with the upcoming of non-alcoholic fatty liver disease and steatohepatitis in the recent decade. Multiple risk factors acting in tandem can lead to the development of cirrhosis as seen with age more than fifty, chronic alcohol use, male gender, chronic viral hepatitis C, diabetes mellitus Type 2, insulin resistance, hypertension, dyslipidemia and obesity (syndrome X or metabolic syndrome) in non-alcoholic steatohepatitis. Patients in whom both human immunodeficiency virus and chronic viral hepatitis C infection coexist, progress to fibrosis and cirrhosis much faster than that seen with hepatitis C alone.[3] Other causes include, chronic cholestatic diseases of the liver, primary and

Table 1: Classification of cirrhosis

Histology	*Fl to F3*	*F4*		
Clinical	Non-cirrhotic		Compensated	Decompensated
Symptoms			Varices	Ascites, Encephalopathy Variceal bleeding
Sub Stage		I	II	III/IV
HVPG mm of Hg		> 6	> 10	> 12
Biological	Fibrogenesis Angiogenesis	Scar Cross linking	Thick scar Nodules	Insoluble scar

secondary vascular occlusive diseases, granulomatous diseases, metabolic diseases (Wilsons disease, Hemochromatosis, alpha-1-antityrpsin disease, storage disorders), autoimmune liver diseases, drugs and toxins, and cryptogenic causes.

PATHOPHYSIOLOGY OF CIRRHOSIS

Hepatic fibrogenesis is the central component of progression to cirrhosis (Fig. 1). Fibrosis is the replacement and encapsulation seen in injured tissue by collagen rich scar. Perpetually abnormal wound healing secondary to etiological insult in the hepatic parenchyma result in continued fibrogenesis in liver. The progression and severity of fibrosis depends on the cause of liver disease, environmental and host factors.[4] Progression of fibrosis leading to distortion of hepatic vasculature further leads to arterioportal shunting that result in compromise of exchange between adjacent liver parenchyma and hepatic sinusoids. Loss of endothelial fenestrations on the sinusoids leads to filling of space of Disse with scar tissue (sinusoidal capillarization). The ultimate effect is formation of vascularized fibrotic septa that connect portal tracts and central veins with one another that result in hepatocyte islands formation that are surrounded by fibrotic septa in absence of central veins. This further aggravates hepatocyte dysfunction and increase in intrahepatic resistance progressing to liver failure and PHT. The ultimate effect of altered hepatic vasculature and PHT include splanchnic vasodilatation, vasoconstriction of renal vessels leading to hypoperfusion of kidneys, salt and water retention and increased cardiac output, leading to decompensation features. In liver fibrosis, myofibroblasts are the source of extracellular matrix protein deposition.[5] Myofibroblasts are found only in the injured liver. The activation and proliferation is the key mechanism in development of liver cirrhosis. Hepatic myofibroblasts originate from the hepatic stellate cells and from fibroblasts in the portal areas by way of transdifferentiation. Recently light has also been shed on origin of myofibroblasts from marrow derived stem cells (mesenchymal and circulating fibrocytes) through epithelial to mesenchymal transformation involving hepatocytes and, to some extent, cholangiocytes. Hepatic stellate cells are perisinusoidal cells seen in the subendothelial space between the hepatocytes and sinusoidal endothelial cells. Quiescent stellate cells are expressive

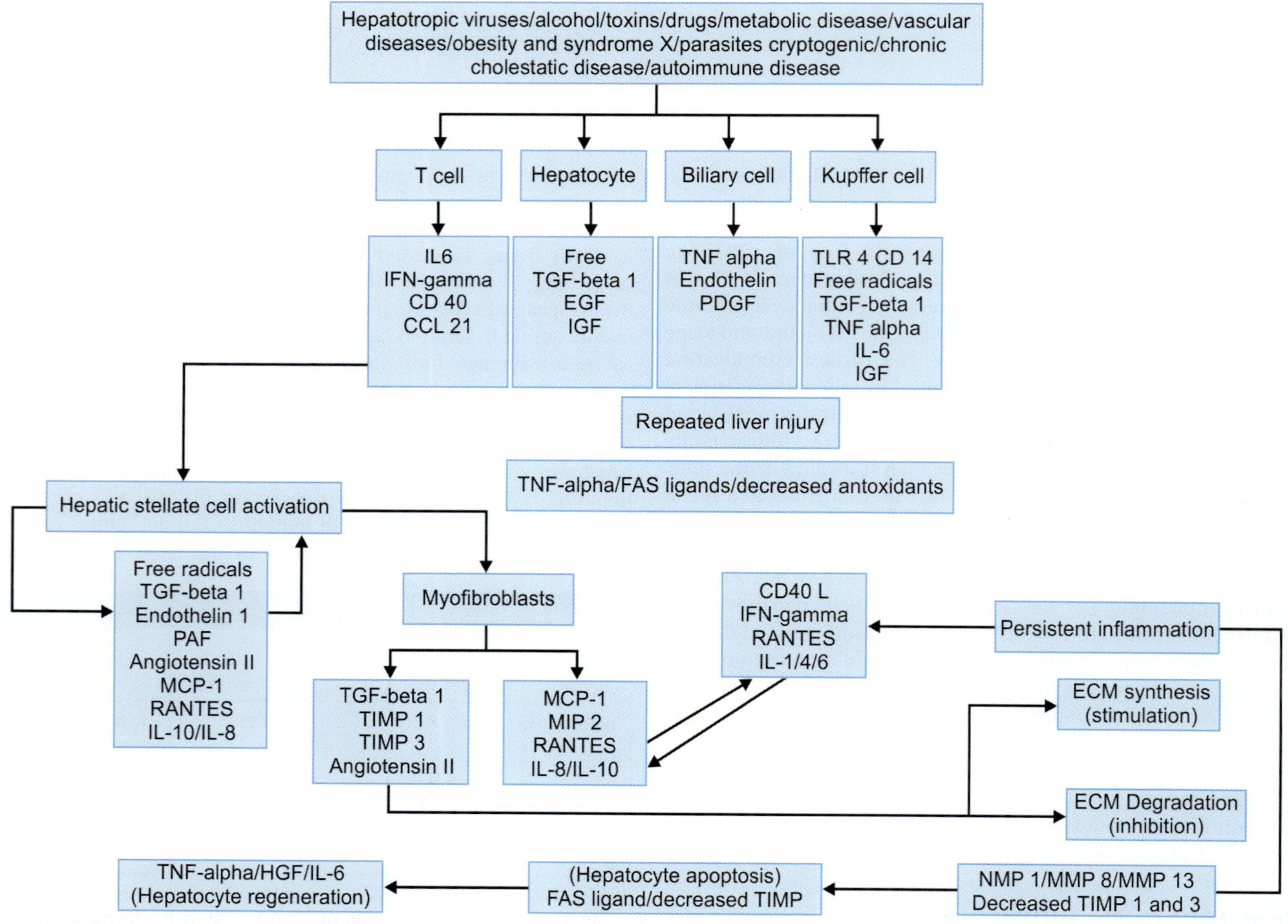

Figure 1 The pathogenesis of liver cirrhosis

Abbreviations: IL 6, interleukine 6; IFN, interferon; TGF, transforming growth factor beta 1; TNF, tumor necrosis alpha; EGF, epidermal growth factor; IGF, insulin growth factor; PDGF, platelet derived growth factor; MCP, monocyte chemoattractant protein; MMP, matrix metalloproteinases; ECM, extracellular matrix; TIMP, tissue inhibitor of metalloproteinase; RANTES, regulated on activation, normal T cell expressed and secreted (CCL5).

of markers that are characteristic of adipocytes like sterol regulatory element binding protein (SREBP) and peroxisome proliferator-activated receptor (PPAR)-gamma and leptin, in contrast to activated stellate cells that express myogenic markers such as myocyte enhancer factor-2, c-myb, and alpha smooth muscle actin. The activated and transformed stellate cells result in aberrant immune response through secretion of cytokines and chemokines that contribute to angiogenesis and upregulation of oxidant stress. Migration of activated stellate cell toward sites of tissue repair along with secretion of large amounts of extracellular matrix take place.[6] Kupffer cells most predominantly secrete platelet-derived growth factor (PDGF), which acts as the predominant mitigating factor for activating stellate cells. The stellate cell related collagen synthesis regulation occur at transcriptional and post-transcriptional level managed by sequences in collagen mRNA at 3' untranslated region. Genetic predisposition to development and progression to fibrosis (slow versus fast fibrosers) have also been delineated in recent studies; a brief summary of which is shown in Table 2. The key cytokines regulating inflammatory responses to liver injury are many. Monocyte chemotactic protein Type 1 (MCP-1) and RANTES modulate and initiate fibrogenesis while IL-10 and interferon alpha act as anti-inflammatory agents.[7] Transforming growth factor-beta 1 (TGF-β) helps in stimulation of matrix protein synthesis and in myofibroblast transformation. PDGF a potent activator upregulated in the fibrotic liver is an important mitogen for stellate cells. Vasodilator cytokines like nitric oxide exert antifibrotic effect while vasoconstrictor cytokines like angiotensin II have opposite effects. Angiotensin II ges de novo generated by activated stellate cells and is also expressed locally in chronically damaged liver parenchyma, resulting in cell migration/proliferation/collagen synthesis and proinflammatory cytokine secretion, mediated by reactive oxygen species generated by non-phagocytic form of NADPH oxidase. The potent vasoconstrictor, Endothelin-1 stimulates fibrogenesis through Type A receptor. Adipokines like leptin is required for stellate cell activation while adiponectin markedly inhibits liver fibrogenesis. This could explain the influence of obesity on fibrosis development in chronic hepatitis C infection. The important intracellular pathways that mediate liver fibrogenesis include c-Jun-terminal kinase pathway, focal adhesion kinase PI3K-Akt signaling pathway, TGF beta-1 pathway which activates SMAD signaling, PPAR-gamma and NF-kB pathway along with the recently identified TLR and cathepsin related signaling pathways.[8] Fibrosis pathophysiology is also dependent on the etiology. In alcohol induced liver fibrosis, alteration of the population of gut bacteria leads to Gram-negative bacterial overgrowth resulting in lipopolysaccharide elevation in portal blood that further activates Kupffer cells through CD14/TLR-4 leading to TNF alpha production and reactive oxidant stress which further promotes neutrophil infiltration and hepatocyte fall out. Whereas in hepatitis C related chronic liver disease, HLA-II directed immune surveillance fails to clear the virus which leads to hepatocyte injury, directly by the viral particle and by dysregulated immune mechanisms leading to recruitment of inflammatory cells that lead to stellate cell activation and collagen deposition. In cholestatic diseases, persistent bile duct damage occurs by way of T lymphocytes and cytokine activity. Biliary epithelial cells (dysfunctional) secrete fibrogenic mediators activating portal myofibroblasts which secrete extracellular matrix leading to excessive collagen deposition.[9] In NAFLD, the two hit model comes into play wherein insulin resistance and hyperglycemia promote elevated serum levels of free fatty acids, leading to hepatic steatosis, and untoward oxidative stress and in the presence of unregulated proinflammatory cytokines come into action promoting hepatocyte apoptosis and inflammatory cell recruitment leading to progressive fibrosis.[10]

Table 2: Genetic mutations predisposing to fibrogenesis in liver cirrhosis

Liver disease	*Candidate genes*
Chronic HCY infection	HFE Angiotensinogen TGF-β1 TNF-α ApoE MEH MCP-I miff MCP-2 Factor V
Alcohol	IL- 10 IL-1β ADH ALDH CYP2E1 TNF-α CTLA-4 TAP2 MnSOD
NASH	HFE Angiotensinogen TGF-β1
PBC	IL-1β TNF-α ApoE
Autoimmune Hepatitis	HLA II

NATURAL HISTORY OF CIRRHOSIS

Natural history of cirrhosis starts off with an asymptomatic phase termed compensated cirrhosis, which then progresses relentlessly to culminate into the symptomatic, decompensated phase. This is marked by the development of complications of PHT and/or liver dysfunction. Portal pressure maybe normal or low in compensated cirrhosis, below the threshold for clinically significant PHT (defined as an HVPG of more than or equal to 10 mm Hg).[11] Development of ascites, encephalopathy, jaundice and/or portal hypertensive gastrointestinal bleeding are features of decompensation. Progression in the decompensated state is accelerated by development of rebleeding episodes, renal impairment such as refractory ascites associated with hepatorenal syndrome (HRS) (Types 1/2/3), hepatopulmonary syndrome (HPS) and sepsis related to spontaneous bacterial peritonitis (SBP).[12] The dreaded complication of hepatocellular carcinoma can complicate cirrhosis at any stage. Median survival of patients of compensated cirrhosis is reported to be as long as 10–12 years with death occurring when transition to decompensation occurs. The median survival of patient at 1 and 2 years after diagnosis of compensated cirrhosis is 95% and 90% respectively. Based on Laennec's cirrhosis classification, three histological stages of cirrhosis have been described and a modification of METAVIR stage 4 of fibrosis was proposed. This staging system (see further) is based on the thickness of fibrous

Table 3: The Child-Turcotte Pugh classification for prognosis in cirrhosis

Criteria	*Points*		
	1	2	3
Encephalopathy	None	Mild to Moderate (I/II)	Severe (III/IV)
Ascites	None	Mild to Moderate (medically controlled)	Severe (refractory)
Bilirubin (mg/dL)	< 2	2-3	> 3
Albumin (g/dL)	> 3.5	2.8-3.5	< 2.8
TNR	< 1.7	1.7-2.3	> 2.3
CLASS	One Year Survival		Two Year Survival
A (5 to 6)	100%		85%
B (7 to 9)	81%		57%
C (10 to 15)	45%		35%
In primary sclerosing cholangitis (PSC) and primary biliary cirrhosis (PBC) the bilirubin reference are changed to reflect the fact that these diseases feature high conjugated bilirubin levels. The upper limit for 1 point is 4 mg/dL and the upper limit for 2 point is 10 mg/dL.			
Dr CG Child and Dr JG Turcotte of the University of Michigan first proposed the scoring system in 1964. It was modified by Pugh et al. in 1972 wherein replacement of Child' criterion of nutritional status with the prothrombin time or TNR was done			

bands and nodule sizes.[13] Overall decompensation occurs at an almost constant rate of 5% per year. The risk of decompensation has been approximately double in patients with esophagogastric varices compared to those without variceal disease. Ascites is the most frequent decompensating event, followed by bleeding, jaundice and encephalopathy. Decompensation is associated with an expected 1 and 3 year survival rate of approximately 60% and 45% respectively. The best prognostic indicator for survival and decompensation are the Child-Turcotte-Pugh (CTP) classification (Table 3), the Model for End Stage Liver Disease (MELD) (Table 4), albumin, HVPG more than or equal to 10 mm Hg and increased body mass index (BMI). Mortality in patients with compensated cirrhosis is around 1-3% per year and significantly increases with evolution to variceal disease. Compensated and decompensated cirrhosis are considered two distinct entities that have characteristic unique clinical course, survival rates, prognostic indicators and causes of death. A four stage system was proposed with subsequent modification into a five stage one–two compensated stages and three decompensated stages (Fig. 2).[14] In *Stage 1* there is absence of esophageal varices in compensated patients. While patients remain in this stage, the 1-year mortality rate is 1.5%. Patients exit this stage at a cumulative rate of 11.9% per year (6.2% because of the development of varices and 4.2% because of decompensation, mostly marked by development of ascites). *Stage 2* is characterized by the presence of esophageal varices with compensated cirrhosis. While patients remain in this stage, the 1-year mortality rate is 2%. Patients leave this stage also by developing decompensation (12.2% per year) mostly characterized by bleeding or ascites. *Stage 3* is characterized by upper digestive bleeding without other decompensating events. While patients remain in this stage, the 1-year mortality rate is 10% per year, significantly higher than in the two former stages. Twenty-one percent of patients also exit this stage by developing other decompensating events (mostly ascites). *Stage 4* is characterized by ascites, jaundice or encephalopathy. In this stage the 1-year mortality rate is 21%, while 10% of patients develop further decompensating events thus transitioning in Stage 5. *Stage 5* is characterized by more than one decompensating event thus indicating a more advanced liver dysfunction. One-year mortality in this stage is 27%. To note, a total of 87% of these patients die within 5 years, mostly after developing further decompensating events. The development of HCC occurs at an almost constant rate of 3% per year and is associated with a worse outcome at whatever stage it develops. For prognostication of cirrhosis, MELD is found to be more reproducible than the Child-Pugh score as there is absence of subjective variables such as ascites and encephalopathy in the former, but its utilization at the bedside is not feasible. The predictive accuracy of MELD score has not been proven to be superior to the Child-Pugh score.[15]

Table 4: The model for end stage liver disease

MELD = 3.78 x ln[serum bilirubin (mg/dL)] + 11.2 x ln[INR] + 9.57 x ln[serum creatinine (mg/dL)] + 6.43
UNOS modification
If the patient has been dialyzed twice within the last 7 days, then the value for serum creatinine used should be 4.0. Any value less than one is given a value of l (i.e. if bilirubin i 0.8 a value of 1.0 is used)
3 month mortality
40 or more—71.3% mortality
30- 39—52.6% mortality
20- 29—19.6% mortality
10-19—6.0% mortality
<9—1.9% mortality

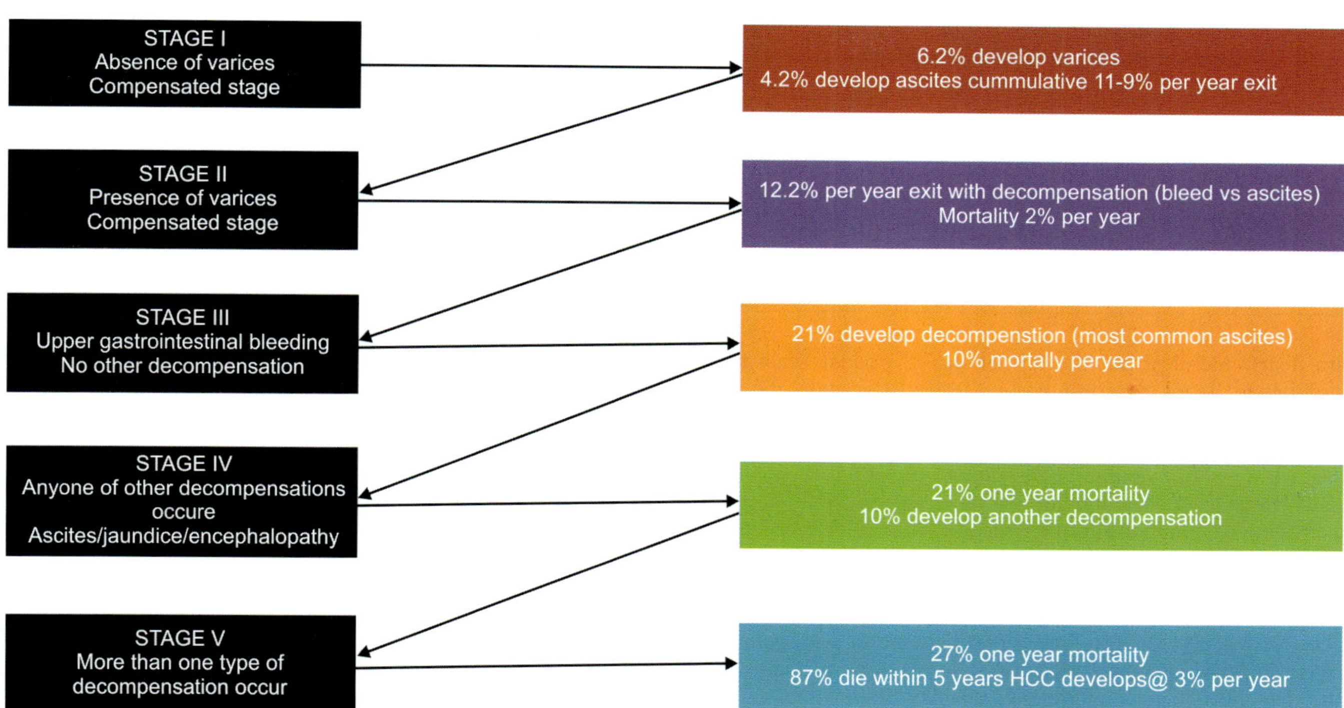

Figure 2 The stages of progression in cirrhosis and their relation to outcomes

ASSESSMENT OF FIBROSIS-CIRRHOSIS

Biopsy is the gold standard for assessment of fibrosis and cirrhosis (advanced fibrosis). Other valuable parameters include serological assessment, hepatic venous pressure gradient (HVPG) evaluation and liver stiffness measurement. The aspartate transaminase (AST) to platelet ration index (APRI) is expressed as a function of the upper limit of normal (ULN) (AST/ULN of AST × 100).[16] As fibrosis increases, AST increases and the platelet count declines. In patients with advanced fibrosis and cirrhosis, this value rises exponentially. Values greater than 1.5 are highly indicative of the same. This test is difficult to apply in patients of no or mild fibrosis. Another serological test for assessment of fibrosis, the fibrotest, uses five hematological markers (alpha 2-macroglobulin, haptoglobulin, gamma glutamyl transpeptidase, total bilirubin and apolipoprotein-alpha-1). These values are however affected by the degree of inflammation in the liver and were mostly tried and tested in patients of hepatitis C virus infection where in the degree of inflammation increased with severity of fibrosis. Sequential Algorithm for Fibrosis Evaluation (SAFE) utilizes APRI and Fibrotest-Fibrosure tests in a sequential manner to test for fibrosis and cirrhosis. Fibroscan utilizes transiet elastography principle whereby sound waves that are pulsed into the liver parenchyma and the speed at which these waves return to the transducer is related to the liver stiffness which increases with increasing fibrosis. This accuracy declines with obesity and is falsely elevated in states of high bilirubin. Magnetic resonance elastography is a more promising tool in comparison to ultrasound elastography.[17] This technique utilizes a vibrating device by which a shear wave is induced in the liver and detection of the shear wave is captured via modified magnetic resonance imager after which a color-coded image is generated corresponding to the wave velocity and hence stiffness, in the organ. In magnetic resonance elastography, a value more than 4.46 kPa indicates cirrhosis (and a value <4.13 indicates no cirrhosis) and a value less than 2.84 appears to exclude presence of significant fibrosis. None of these noninvasive tests can differentiate between advanced bridging fibrosis and cirrhosis or those with no fibrosis from mild fibrosis. An adequate liver biopsy is considered to be 20 mm × 1 mm with 11 portal tracts, which is enough to grade chronic activity.[6] A basic knowledge of various scoring systems is important for understanding liver fibrosis and its progressive implications (Table 5). The METAVIR Scoring System was designed in patients with chronic hepatitis C virus infection. It consists of a grading system and a staging system. The grade (0–4) provides information regarding the activity of inflammation and the Stage (0–4) represents the amount of fibrosis or scarring. The fibrosis score is assigned as: 0 = no scarring; 1 = minimal scarring; 2 = scarring has occurred and extends outside the areas in the liver that contains blood vessels; 3 = bridging fibrosis is spreading and connecting to other areas that contain fibrosis; 4 = cirrhosis or advanced scarring of the liver. The KNODELL Scoring System also known as the histologic activity index (HAI) is a commonly used staging system in liver disease. Currently, the revised KNODELL or ISHAK Scoring System is the most widely used in staging of liver fibrosis. This system corrects the numerical discontinuity seen with other system grading by re-introducing the number 2. In the ISHAK Scoring System which consists of four parameters, the combined score was taken out and parameters of confluent necrosis, including bridging necrosis, were made a separate category for necroinflammatory assessment and further introduction related to minor alterations in semi-quantitative grading of activity was done. To summarize, regarding fibrosis, ISHAK and METAVIR

Table 5: Salient features of fibrosis scores in fibrosis-cirrhosis assessment

Description	*Knodell*	*Metavir*	*Ishak*	*Scheuer*
No fibrosis	0	0	0	0
Portal fibrosis	1	1	1,2	1
Portal fibrosis with septae extending outside portal area		2	2,3	2
Bridging fibrosis	3	3	3,4	3
Cirrhosis	4	4	5,6	4

are nearly identical but the former has a broader scale range and hence better description. In METAVIR system, the term septa is equal to bridging fibrosis in ISHAK. Fibrosis Stage 3 in METAVIR score includes incomplete (developing) cirrhosis. The description of necroinflammatory injury, in METAVIR was more sensitive to severe activity and was more reproducible. Recently, quantitative evaluations through image analysis have been utilized for assessment of liver fibrosis. Digital image analysis can be done variably. The most sensitive among them is the FibroQuant method. Quantification of perisinusoidal fibrosis (SF), portal-periportal and septal fibrosis (PF), portal periportal and septal area (PA) and portal vessel and biliary duct lumen areas (LA) are done automatically. The percentage area of perisinusoidal fibrosis (PSF) is calculated as PSF = 100 × SF/(LA–PA) likewise, percentage area of portal-periportal and septal fibrosis (PPF), PPF = 100 × PF/(PA–LA) and percentage area of portal vessel and biliary duct lumina as PLA = 100 + LA/PA. FibroQuant image processing is a very sensitive and reproducible method of fibrosis quantification and matches with level of HPVG and liver stiffness measurement. The serum proteomics-quantitative analysis of human microfibril-associated protein 4 (MFAP-4) in a study showed MFAP-4 as a novel candidate biomarker which had a high diagnostic accuracy for prediction of non-diseased liver versus cirrhosis/ stage 0 versus Stage 4 fibrosis and Stages 0–3 versus Stage 4 fibrosis. This paves way for a new era in noninvasive diagnosis of fibrosis-cirrhosis.[18,19]

REGRESSION OF CIRRHOSIS

Contrary to older belief, regression of cirrhosis is currently a topic of intense study and hope. Regression is associated with a net decrease in fibrous tissue content. The histologic features that suggest regression of cirrhosis is termed the hepatic repair complex and consists of the following—Absence of shunting vessels expanding from portal tract; Complete or partial restoration of lobular architecture; Lack of ductular proliferation; Central vein or portal tract morphological resurgence and Restoration of enzymatic lobular zonation. Decrease in fibrosis is associated with residual collagen bundles. Shunting new vessels regress as there is decreased angiogenesis. Thinning of septa decreases non-functioning capillaries. The septa become incomplete (incomplete septal cirrhosis) and may disappear. The reappearance of portal tracts and central vein later on takes place, in the absence of portal vein thrombosis. The Laennecs Classification of Cirrhosis (Fig. 3) is the best staging system that takes into consideration, cirrhosis and its regression. In the METAVIR system, Stage 4 classifies cirrhosis. Laennecs system subclassifies this stage into three categories: 4a—Mild cirrhosis; 4b—Moderate cirrhosis; 4c—Severe cirrhosis, based on septal thickness and which correlates well with the portal pressure.[20]

Cirrhosis largely remains asymptomatic as long the patient remains in the compensated state. Patients present with clinical symptoms and signs once cirrhosis is advanced. The most common sign of cirrhosis is ascites (secondary to PHT). Jaundice, constitutional symptoms, including anorexia, fatigue, weakness, and weight loss is seen commonly. Clubbing and hypertrophic osteoarthropathy, Dupuytren's contracture, fetor hepaticus (a sweet, fruity but pungent breath), gynecomastia, firm nodular hepatomegaly, palmar erythema, vascular spiders (spider telangiectasias, spider angiomata), testicular atrophy and splenomegaly (sign of PHT) are also detectable (Fig. 4). Spiders angiomas are not specific for cirrhosis. They also occur during pregnancy, in patients with severe malnutrition, and in healthy persons. As shown by Foutch et al. in 1988, the number and size of vascular spiders have been shown to correlate with the severity of chronic liver disease. Frequency of variceal bleeding was higher when greater than 20 spiders were present and when multiple atypically located lesions were detected. Large spiders (>15 mm) are best associated with large varices and have the strongest association with bleeding. Asterixis or negative myoclonus is associated with irregular myoclonic pauses/lapses affecting various parts of the body and is a disorder of motor control. Lapses are caused by involuntary 50- to 200-msec silent periods appearing in muscles (even antagonistic groups of muscles) which are tonically active. That is, the silent periods and postural lapses occur in muscles that have been contracting for a time whether or not there has been slow shortening or lengthening but probably do not occur during or immediately after a sudden movement at a joint. Young and Shahani classified the involuntary movements as a form of mini-asterixis and the pauses as negative myoclonus. Negative myoclonus is characterized by a brief loss of muscle tone in agonist muscles followed by a compensatory jerk of the antagonistic muscles. Asterixis, posthypoxic myoclonus and stiff man syndrome are examples of negative myoclonus. Even though the exact mechanism underlying asterixis remains elusive, few pathogenic mechanisms have been suggested such as, result of diffuse, widespread derangement of CNS function, a "receptive inattentiveness to incoming information", which could thus result from a dysfunction of the sensorimotor integration occurring in the contralateral parietal lobe and midbrain, an episodic dysfunction within neural circuits concerned with maintenance of sustained or tonic muscle. Nail changes in cirrhosis include Muehrcke's nails (paired horizontal white bands separated by normal color) and Terry's nails (proximal two-thirds of nail plate appears white in comparison to the distal one-third which is red). Cruveilhier-Baumgarten murmur is a venous hum heard on auscultation around the umbilical region, in patients with PHT with extensive caput medusa (per umbilical venous collaterals).[21] Chest X-rays in a patient with cirrhosis can reveal elevation of the diaphragms from gross ascites, the presence of gynecomastia and enlargement of azygos vein because of collateral flow and pleural effusions (hydrothorax) may be evident. Sometimes, large esophageal varices can be seen as soft-tissue mass at the gastroesophageal junction. Ultrasound is a powerful screening tool for cirrhosis. Presence of coarse heterogenous echotexture with segmental atrophy or hypertrophy, a nodular surface, the ratio of caudate lobe width

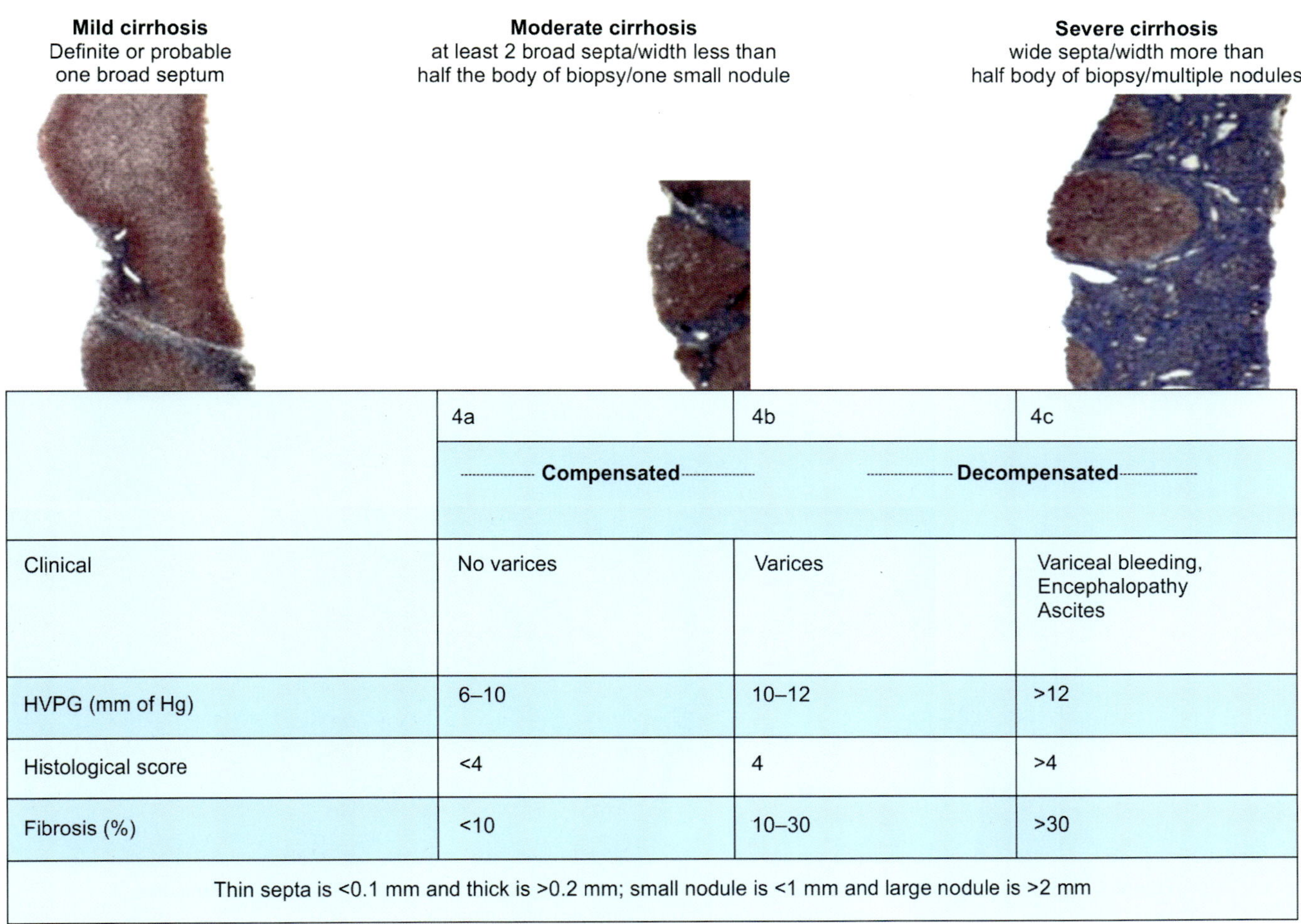

	4a	4b	4c
	Compensated	**Decompensated**	
Clinical	No varices	Varices	Variceal bleeding, Encephalopathy Ascites
HVPG (mm of Hg)	6–10	10–12	>12
Histological score	<4	4	>4
Fibrosis (%)	<10	10–30	>30
Thin septa is <0.1 mm and thick is >0.2 mm; small nodule is <1 mm and large nodule is >2 mm			

Figure 3 Classification of cirrhosis according to Laennec's system and the division of cirrhosis into three stages based on the METAVIR stage 4 modification

to that of right lobe more than 0.65, signs of PHT enlarged portal vein diameter more than 13 mm, expanded superior mesenteric vein and splenic vein diameter more than 10 mm, respiratory variation loss within the superior mesenteric vein, portal vein thrombosis with or without cavernoma formation, reversal to and fro portal venous flow, recanalization of paraumbilical veins with hepatofugal flow within the presence of portosystemic collaterals, most commonly seen splenorenal region, splenomegaly and ascites are major findings for diagnosis of cirrhosis. The Doppler measure of hepatic arterial vascular resistance which is elevated in patients with cirrhosis correlates well with the HVPG or portal pressures. Early cirrhosis does not show morphological changes on CT imaging. Apart from the mentioned features, the presence of a modified caudate lobe width to right lobe width, incorporating the right portal vein instead of main portal vein also yields good diagnostic accuracy. The segmental hypertrophy mentioned above most commonly involves the lateral segments, II and III and segmental atrophy is mostly seen with posterior segments VI and VII and IV (medial segment) of the left lobe. The posterior notch sign (enlarged hilar periportal space), widening of interlobular fissures (generalized) and expansion of the gall-bladder fossa are also important signs in diagnosis of cirrhosis. Cirrhosis secondary to chronic cholestatic jaundice states such as primary biliary cirrhosis or primary sclerosing cholangitis (PSC) reveals pseudotumoral enlargement of caudate lobe associated with atrophy of peripheral hepatic segments that lead to a lobulated or bosselated contour of the liver. The presence of multiple irregular strictures of the intrahepatic and extrahepatic bile ducts is also seen. The presence of striking lace like fibrosis along with regenerative nodules and lymphadenopathy can be seen in early cirrhosis with PHT in primary biliary cirrhosis. Alcoholic cirrhosis presents with shrunken liver in late stages. A tongue like appearance is seen with shrinkage of medial segment IV of left lobe and associated hypertrophy of lateral segments, II and III.[11] Nodular regeneration in the liver can be classified as micronodular (<3 mm in diameter) or macronodular (>3 mm in diameter). In the presence of a siderotic nodule (iron containing regenerative nodule) there is evidence of hyperdensity in the nodule in comparison to the surrounding parenchyma on non-contrast computed tomography. There is no enhancement in regenerative nodules in the arterial phase of contrast imaging and they remain isodense to parenchyma on venous phasing. The most common morphologic presentation seen in cirrhotic patients is a combination of micronodular and macronodular regeneration.[22] The most important complication of cirrhosis is PHT and its related effects.

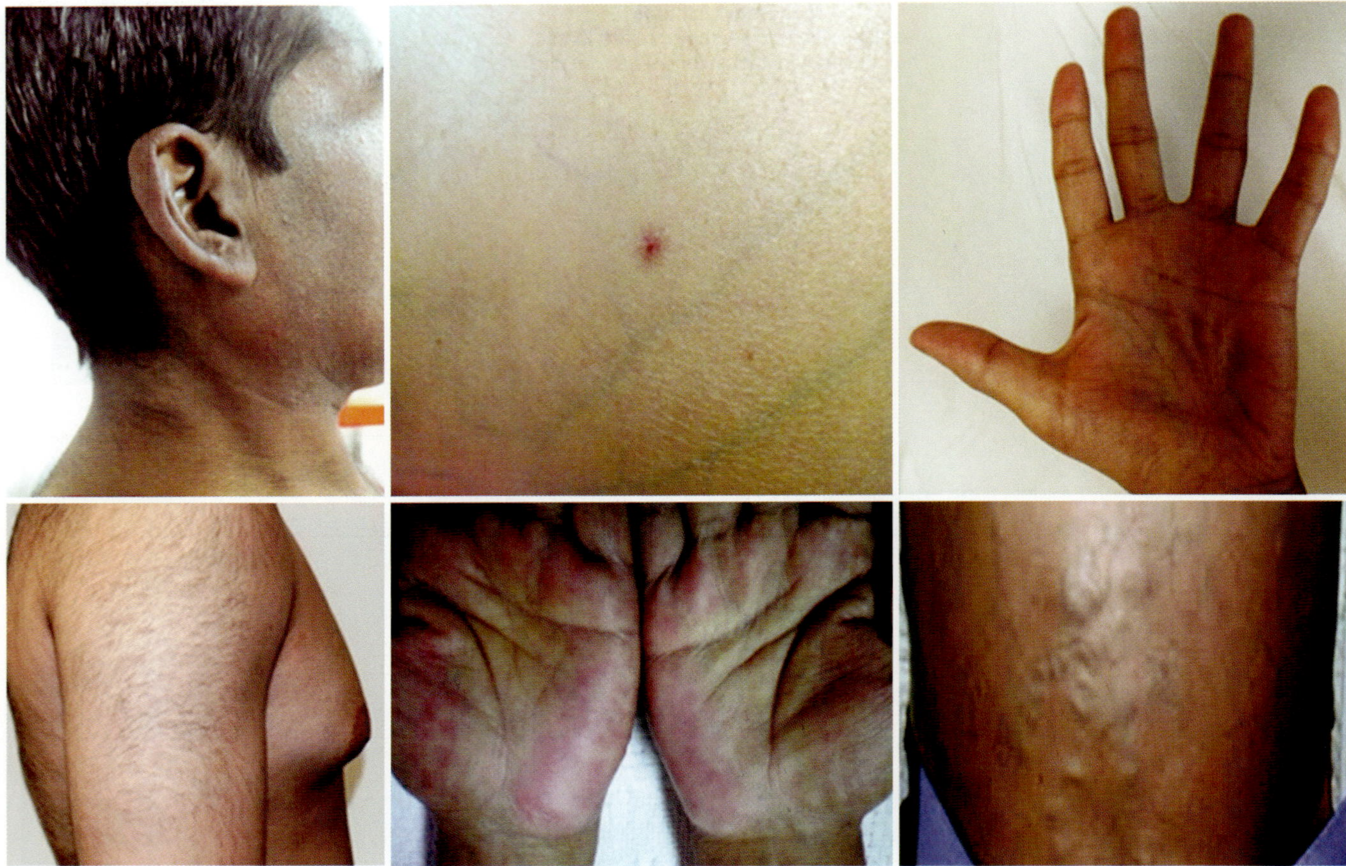

Figure 4 Peripheral IGNS of liver failure. Clockwise from left: parotidomegaly, spider angioma, Dupyutren's contracture, caput medusa, palmary erythema and gynecomastia

PORTAL HYPERTENSION

In PHT, there is increased portosystemic pressure gradient in any portion of the portal venous system. It can be secondary to prehepatic abnormalities, intrahepatic (presinusoidal/sinusoidal/postsinusoidal) and posthepatic. Cirrhosis is the most common cause of PHT. The measurement of wedged hepatic pressure (measure of sinusoidal pressure) minus that of free hepatic venous pressure (measure of systemic pressure) provides the portosystemic gradient known as HVPG. The normal HVPG is 3–5 mm Hg. An HVPG more than 6 mm Hg defines PHT; but an HVPG of 10 mm Hg or greater is known as clinically significant PHT (CSPH). CSPH is important because it predicts the natural course of events in cirrhosis such as occurrence of varices, variceal bleeding, encephalopathy, ascites and decompensation, death after liver resection and HCC development.

The measurement of portal pressure by means of HVPG is performed with fluoroscopy and can be completed in around 10–30 minutes with experience. Clinically, a patient of cirrhosis and PHT presents with ascites, varices or both. Findings of PHT include splenomegaly, portal vein dilatation, portal vein occlusion, collateral vessel formation, thrombocytopenia and ascites with a high serum ascites to albumin gradient (SAGG more than 1.1 g.dL).[23] HVPG is very useful to assess the type of PHT—normal in cases of PHT secondary to prehepatic and presinusoidal causes. Repetitive HVPG measurements can help in monitoring of patients for progression of liver disease and assess for pharmacotherapy (beta blockers) response. The etiology of PHT is shown in Flow chart 1. Goel et al. conducted a study in South Indian adult population in which cryptogenic cirrhosis was the most common cause of PHT in adults, closely followed by alcohol and then chronic viral hepatitis B infection. In patients of cryptogenic cirrhosis who underwent liver biopsy, non-cirrhotic idiopathic PHT was seen predominantly. Ten percent of the adults had vascular disorders of the liver in this particular study. The rates of chronic viral hepatitis related cirrhosis is expected to decline in India in the future and that of non-alcoholic fatty liver disease and alcoholic related cirrhosis are expected to rise secondary to a major change in life style. In cirrhosis, PHT results from three distinct mechanisms. Firstly, mechanical obstruction secondary to fibrosis and compression due to regenerative nodules result in an adynamic component initially. Secondly a functional component occurs due to active contraction of vascular smooth muscle cells and activated stellate cells that account for 30% of increase in intrahepatic pressure. Lastly, an increase in mesenteric vasodilatation results in increased portal blood flow leading to worsening of PHT. The portal pressure gradient is determined by the product of portal blood flow and the vascular resistance that opposes that flow. Ohm's law defines this fact in the equation $\Delta P = Q \times R$, in which delta P is the portal pressure gradient; Q is the flow within the portal system and R is

Flow chart 1 Etiology of portal hypertension

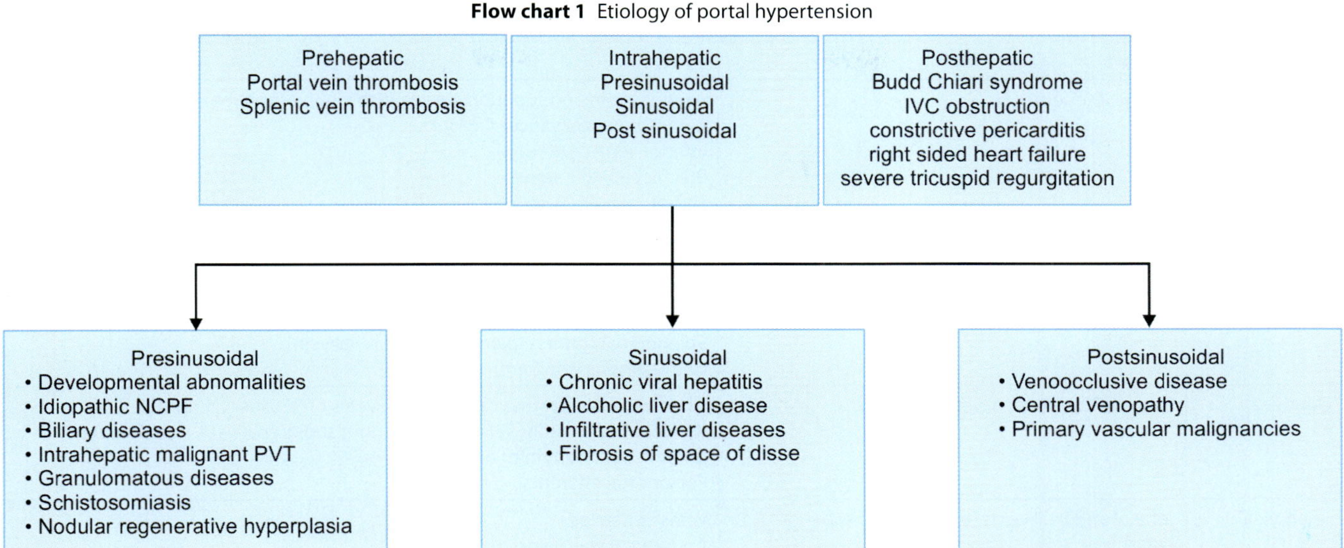

the vascular resistance (the sum of resistance of the portal vein, the hepatic vascular bed and portosystemic collaterals).[24] The portal pressure maybe increased by an increase in portal blood flow, vascular resistance or a combination of both. Increased resistance to portal blood flow can occur at any site within the portal venous system. Contractile addition to resistance occurs at the level of sinusoidal as well as extra-sinusoidal areas, including vascular smooth muscle cells in the small portal venules, activated hepatic stellate cells located in the perisinusoidal space of Disse and hepatic myofibroblasts that compress regenerating nodules or venous shunts inside the fibrous septa. Another factor is the exaggerated responses of vasoconstrictors on hepatic vasculature bed and their increased production. Norepinephrine is usually elevated in decompensated cirrhosis and increases intrahepatic vascular resistance. This gets blunted when prazosin (alpha adrenergic antagonist) is administered. Adrenergic receptors are involved in regulation of intrahepatic resistance in cirrhosis. The hepatic vascular bed in cirrhotic livers forms an exaggerated response to alpha-adrenergic agents through promotion of release of arachidonic acid from plasma membrane through various vasoactive metabolites like prostaglandins, thromboxanes and leukotrienes. Cyclooxygenase is an inducible enzyme that is usually over expressed in proinflammatory states. The hyper response of hepatic vasculature in cirrhosis is associated with over production of thromboxane A2 by cyclooxygenase 1. Increase in thromboxane leads to vasoconstriction in hepatic vasculature. The 5-lipooxygenase derived eicosanoids also add to increase in hepatic vascular resistance. Endothelin receptor A (ET-A) shows high affinity for ET-1 and not ET-3 and ET-B has affinity for both equally. Under the influence of nitric oxide, ET-B receptors on vascular smooth muscles produce vasoconstriction and those on endothelial cells produce vasodilatation. The higher circulating levels of plasma ET-1 and ET-3 increased portal perfusion pressure by way of increment in intrahepatic resistance. Renin angiotensin system activation resulting in angiotensin II increment results in worsening of intrahepatic resistance in cirrhotic patients. The increase in vascular tone in the intrahepatic vasculature is mainly due to endothelial dysfunction. This is due to decreased availability of nitric oxide and an increase in production of vasoconstrictors secreted from the dysfunctional endothelium, such as prostaglandins, reactive oxygen species and thromboxane A2. Reactive oxygen species, that form from unchecked proinflammatory proceses (like superoxide) reacts with NO leading toperoxynitrite formation thereby further decreasing NO bioavailability. Reactive oxygen species also deactivate eNOS by incapacitating its cofactor, tetrahydrobiopterin leading to eNOS uncoupling, leading to oxygen formation instead of NO. In PHT there is increase in blood flow in the splanchnic organs draining into the portal vein. This is a vicious cycle that eventually leads to portal venous system collateral formation that aggravates further PHT. Overproduction of endogenous vasodilators is associated with splanchnic hyperemia and decreased vascular reactivity to vacoconstrictors. Vascular endothelial growth factor (VEGF) dependent neovascularization/angiogenesis in hyperemic splanchnic organs lead to collateral formation that eventually try to decompress portal systemic pressures, but fail ultimately.[25] The development of portal collateral circulation is one of the main complications of PHT. Collateral formation involves opening, dilatation and hypertrophy of pre-existing vascular channels. The collateral circulation is able to carry about 90% of the blood entering the portal system. Splanchnic vasodilatation produces systemic hyperkinetic syndrome, where there is reduction in arterial pressure and peripheral resistance which leads to increased plasma volume and cardiac output. Peripheral vasodilatation leads to activation of endogenous neurohumoral systems that result in sodium and water retention followed by an increase in cardiac index, leading to aggravation and/or complications of PHT.[26]

COLLATERAL SYSTEM IN PORTAL HYPERTENSION (TABLE 6)

Portal hypertension, as described above results in a vicious cycle that involves formation of extensive portosystemic collaterals

Table 6: The main collateral systems in portal hypertension secondary to cirrhosis of the liver

Varices	*Afferent*	*Efferent*
Esophageal	Left gastric vein	Azygous vein and superior vena cava through esophageal and paraesophageal varices (78%) Inferior vena cava (12%) Brachiocephalic veins Left pulmonary veins
Gastric	Left gastric vein Short gastric vein Posterior gastric vein	Superior vena cava through esophageal varices (80%) Gastrorenal shunt (inferior phrenic vein to renal vein 80–85%) Gastrocaval shunt (inferior phrenic vein to inferior vena cava 10–15%) Left gonadal vein Splenorenal shunts (splenic vein and renal vein) Hemiazygous vein (rare)
Duodenal	Pancreaticoduodenal venous arcade	Drain into inferior vena cava through veins of Retzius (via right renal vein, gonadal vein, lumbar vein, iliac vein, right suprarenal vein, right inferior phrenic vein, right inferior adrenal vein) Portoportal efferents
Jejunoileal	Jejunal and Ileal veins (tributaries of superior mesenteric vein)	Veins of Retzius Abdominal wall veins
Colonic	Ileocolic vein Right colic vein Middle colic vein Sigmoid colonic vein	Right gonadal vein Right renal vein Systemic lumbar veins Right renal capsular vein
Rectal	Superior rectal vein (continuation of inferior mesenteric vein)	Inferior rectal vein Middle rectal vein Internal pudental vein Extrinsic and intrinsic rectal venous plexus
Omental	Superior or inferior mesenteric vein	Retroperitoneal or pelvic veins Gastroesophageal varices
Ectopic	Paraumbilical veins (inferior veins of Sappey) Superior veins of Sappey Left umbilical vein Ligamentum teres Left inferior phrenic vein Intercostal vein Right inferior phrenic vein Cystic veins and branches of left gastric veins Diaphragmatic veins (bare area of liver) Ligamentum venosum	Superior epigastric veins Inferior epigastric veins Abdominal wall (Caput Medusae)
Gallbladder	Cystic vein, branch of the right portal vein	Hepatic vein or intrahepatic portal vein Anterior abdominal wall veins
Diaphragmatic	Cardiophrenic varices (collaterals from the paraumbilical vein)	Internal mammary vein

that function to adapt to the increasing portal pressures and capacitate hypertension in the venous system. This adaptiveness largely depends upon the extent and size of the intrahepatic and extrahepatic collateral vascular juncture between the portal and systemic circulation. Left gastric vein, posterior gastric vein/short gastric veins of the portal system which anastomose with esophageal, diaphragmatic, intercostals and azygous minor veins of the systemic circulation form collaterals at the cardia of the stomach whereby they form varices in the lower end of esophagus at its lower end and fundus of the stomach. The middle and inferior hemorrhoidal veins of the caval system form rectal varices with collateral connections with the superior hemorrhoidal vein at the anal region. Collaterals also form in the falciform ligament through the paraumbilical veins and also where the abdominal organs are in contact with retroperitoneal tissues or adherent to the abdominal wall. These collaterals are present from the liver to diaphragm and in the splenorenal ligament and omentum. Other areas of collateral formation include left renal vein via splenic vein or left adrenal vein, left gastric vein, pancreatic vein or diaphragmatic veins. They also develop from veins developing in previous surgical scars or lumbar veins. The collateral blood flow from gastroesophageal varices ultimately reaches the superior vena cava through the azygos-hemiazygos systems.[27]

COMPLICATIONS OF PORTAL HYPERTENSION

Ascites

Ascites is derived from the Greek word, "askos" meaning a wine bag or sac. An important landmark in the progression of cirrhosis and survival of the cirrhotic patient is formation of ascites. Ascites is also a good marker of mortality at 1 year. Ascites secondary to cirrhosis and PHT is seen in 85% of all cases of ascites. Ascites can be of prehepatic and post-hepatic causes. The former includes lymphomatous malignancies, portal vein thrombosis, abdominal injuries, bowel perforation, pancreatitis, granulomatous infections, renal failure and peritoneal carcinomatosis and the latter comprise of severe right sided valvular heart diseases, constrictive pericarditis, hepatic venous outflow obstruction, congestive cardiac failure or severe pulmonary hypertension. Malignant ascites is found in 10% of total cases of ascites. Up to 20% of these have no primary malignancy identified. Pathogenesis of ascites in cirrhosis is multifactorial, even though a hybrid theory cumulating the overflow and underfill theories has been popular.[28] The normal portal vein is approximately 8 cm in length and less than 13 mm in diameter, formed by the union of the splenic and superiors mesenteric veins. In the presence of PHT, the indirect portal pressure, assessed by HVPG rises more than or equal to 6 mm Hg. Ascites formation (Flow chart 2) occurs at 8 mm Hg, clinically significant PHT develops at and above 10 mm Hg, Variceal bleeding risk increases above 12 mm Hg and risk of recurrent varcieal bleed occurs above 20 mm Hg. The vasodilatory substances like nitric oxide and leukotrienes accumulate in the splanchnic circulation and also within the intrahepatic vasculature leading to vasodilatation with resultant hypoperfusion of the renal system. The renin-angiotensin-aldosterone system (RAAS) comes into play after sensing such a dysregulation, leading to aggressive fluid and salt retention. To briefly summaries the RAAS system, renin is secreted from the renal juxtaglomerular apparatus around the proximal nephrons in response to changes in vascular pressures and changes in serum levels of sodium. This converts angiotensinogen (in liver) to angiotensin I, converted to angiotensin II (by angiotensin converting enzyme in lung). Angiotensin II drives fluid retention and mobilization, stimulates thirst drive, releases aldosterone from zona glomerulosa of adrenal cortex and stimulates secretion of vasopressin from posterior pituitary. All these actions lead to excessive accumulation of plasma volume in cirrhosis and PHT. This excess retained blood volume is thought to leak out directly from both liver surface and the mesenteric vessels. The basic pathology behind this leakage is in concordance with Starling's law here in there is overwhelming of reabsorptive capacity of peritoneal surface and lymphatic system as seen by increased hydrostatic pressure, vascular permeability and concurrent decrease in oncotic pressures, in the form of absolute or relative hypoalbuminemia seen in decompensated cirrhosis.[29] The peritoneal cavity normally is decompressed and has a pressure of 5–10 mm Hg, containing around 25–50 mL of serous fluid. The maximum absorption of fluid out of the peritoneum is around 850 mL/day. Continued dysregulatory factors as mentioned above relates to progression and worsening of ascites in cirrhosis. Clinically ascites can present variably. It can occur slowly or suddenly. It can occur with abdominal pain or without pain. Sudden formation can be seen in hepatic or portal vein obstruction or compression of IVC due to trauma or hematoma or in acute liver failure. If associated with pain, it can be simply because of mechanical stretching of peritoneum, presence of bacterial peritonitis or hepatocellular carcinoma or portal vein thrombosis in the setting of cirrhosis. Careful examination should be undertaken to rule out an expanding panniculitis, gaseous distension, solid or cystic lesions of abdomen and loculated ascites. Ascites can be of three grades, clinically. Grade I—when the ascites is diagnosed by way of ultrasound examination, requiring approximately 100 mL of fluid; Grade II—when there is 1,000 mL of fluid in the abdomen, elicited by the shifting dullness on clinical examination and Grade III—when there is gross, tense ascites giving rise to a fluid thrill. Investigational analysis of ascites fluid is of utmost importance.

Flow chart 2 The pathogenesis of ascites in portal hypertension

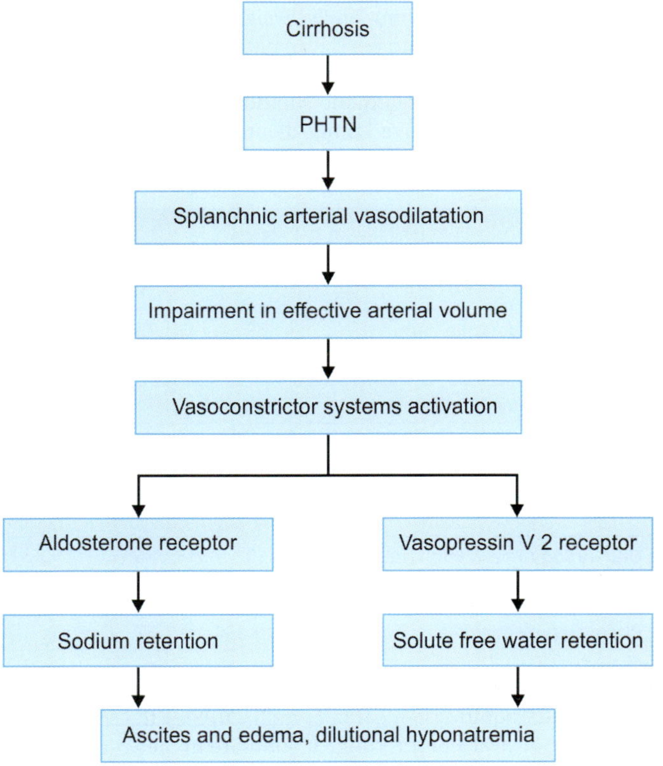

Paracentesis has been well tolerated in patients with platelet counts below 20,000 cells/cumm and an INR as high as 8.7. The only absolute contraindication to paracentesis is severe diffuse intravascular coagulation (DIC). Paracentesis should not be done where there is evidence of hyperfibrinolysis; which can be gauged using three dimensional ecchymosis or hematoma or a euglobin clot lysis time of <120 minutes. Ascites removal can be safely performed once lysis time has normalized on treatment. Bleeding conditions occur in less than 1/1,000 patients who require paracentesis.[30] Even though there is no cut off for parameters of coagulation at which paracentesis is held, many centers utilize the cut off of platelet counts more than 50,000/cu mm and INR of less than 1.5 to perform paracentesis (which practically leads to unwanted massive transfusions in cirrhosis). Ascites tapping is preferred at the left lower quadrant. The abdominal wall in the left lower quadrant, about 3 cm, i.e. 2 finger breadths cephalad and 2 finger breadths medial to the anterior-superior iliac spine, is typically used as the preferred area for paracentesis because it is thinner and with a larger amount of fluid than the midline area. The danger with using the right lower quadrant is that, in the presence of a dilated cecum (due to lactulose therapy) or an appendectomy scar, there is chance of bowel perforation. Inferior epigastric arteries should be avoided as these vessels are located midway between the pubis and anterior superior iliac spines and then run upward in the rectus sheath. A diagnostic paracentesis requires around 30–50 mL of fluid for investigations. Ascitic fluid analysis in all cases should include cell counts and differential, albumin and total protein and ascitic fluid culture, inoculated into blood culture bottles at the bedside itself before antibiotic treatment starts. Other specialized tests that can be done on ascitic fluid can include lactate dehydrogenase (LDH), cytology, amylase, glucose, total protein and triglycerides. Uninfected ascitic fluid is clear to yellow and transparent. An ascitic fluid carcinoembryonic antigen more than 5 ng/mL or ascitic fluid alkaline phosphatase more than 240 U/L is helpful in detecting gut perforation. In normal ascitic fluid the neutrophil count is usually less than 250 cells/mm^3. Molecules such as lactoferrin are not suitable enough for diagnosis of ascitic fluid infections. Patients on peritoneal dialysis require lower thresholds for SBP diagnosis (like neutrophils >50 neutrophils/mm^3). In hemorrhagic ascites, for every 250 RBCs, a correction factor subtracting 1 neutrophil should be followed. A milky ascitic fluid with a high triglyceride level of more than 100–200 mg/dL is chylous. An elevated ascitic fluid amylase level is suggestive for pancreatic ascites. Difference in ascitic fluid albumin in comparison to serum albumin as the SAAG (where ≥1.1 g/dL defines a high albumin gradient) suggests portal-hypertension as a cause with 97% sensitivity. Accuracy is decreased if the serum and ascitic fluid albumin are not drawn at the same time, or if the serum albumin is less than 1.1 g/dL. The ascitic fluid cytology is positive only in peritoneal carcinomatosis with a sensitivity that approaches 96.7%, if three samples are sent (at least 50 mL) and processed without haste. The first sample is positive in 82.8% and at least one of two samples is positive in 93.3%. DNA cytometry or magnetic enrichment improves the sensitivity of cytology but is not widely utilized. Peritoneal carcinomatosis is usually seen in patients who have or who are known to have breast, colon, gastric, or pancreatic primary carcinoma. The sensitivity of fluid smear for mycobacteria is approximately 0% and the sensitivity of fluid culture for mycobacteria is around 50%. Laparoscopy followed by biopsy and mycobacterial culture of tubercles is the most accurate/gold standard method for diagnosing tuberculous peritonitis. Fifty percent of ascitic fluid cultures show bacterial growth when the samples are send using traditional methods like sending a syringe or tube of fluid to the lab in contrast to inoculation of the ascitic fluid into blood culture bottles at bedside in which the culture growth rates go up to 80%. Testing serum for CA125 is not recommended in patients with ascites of any type, especially in those patients of cirrhosis as it is not helpful. The prognostic factors in patients of cirrhosis and ascites is given in Table 7.[31] Treatment modalities are many for ascites in cirrhosis (Fig. 5). A diet consisting of 2 g per day or less of salt (equivalent to 88 mmol per day of sodium) is advocated. Fluid restriction (of about 1–1.5 liters per day) is not necessary unless patients have dilutional hyponatremia (defined as serum sodium less than 130 mEq/L) together with ascites and/or edema. Patients with serum sodium concentration between 130 and 135 mEq/L should be cautious about fluid intake to prevent fluid retention and development of dilutional hyponatremia. In hypervolumic hyponatremia, even levels between 110–120 mmol/L are common and well tolerated. Adherence to a restricted sodium diet can be assessed by measuring 24 hour urinary sodium, which should at least show 78 mmol per day excretion of sodium with resultant weight loss. Spot urine sodium to potassium ratio more than 1 in the setting of weight gain also suggests dietary non-adherence. Patients who do not lose weight and excrete more than 78 mmol sodium/day should be given a higher dose of diuretics. Non-steroidal anti-inflammatory drugs (NSAIDs, that inhibit prostaglandin synthesis leading to constriction of afferent renal arterioles), ACE inhibitors (which inhibit angiotensin converting enzyme, that activate angiotensin II leading to dilatation of efferent arterioles) should be avoided in patients with cirrhotic ascites. This leads to decrease in renal perfusion and promotes renal injury. Classical diuretic use involves spironolactone (aldosterone antagonist) and furosemide (loop diuretic). The former downregulates sodium channels on the apical surface of renal cortical collecting ducts and the latter acts on the sodium-potassium-2-chloride symport inhibitor in ascending limb of loop of Henle. Furosemide has a half-life of around 2 hours and spironolactone, 24 hours. These diuretics are used in the ratio of 100 mg of spironolactone to 40 mg of furosemide. This maintains adequate natriuresis and maintains normokalemia. The increments of spironolactone, starting from 100 mg per day, are done every 5–7 days with 100 mg each time to a maximum of 400 mg per day. Loop diuretic is started at a dose of 40 mg per day with increments of 40 mg per day until a maximum of 160 mg/day. The recommended weight loss during therapy is acceptable at half kilogram per day in patients without edema and one kilogram daily in patients with edema.[32] Tapering and/or cessation of diuretic treatment should be done when serum creatinine increased above 1.5 mg/dL and/or hyponatremia with serum sodium levels less than 120 mmol/L. Side effects of

Table 7: Prognostic factors in patient with cirrhosis and ascites

Parameter		*Median survival (months)*
Mean arterial pressure (mm Hg)	>80	46
	<80	11
Serum creatinine (mg/dL)	1.2 to 1.5	11
	>1.5 4	
Hyponatremia (<130 mEq/L)	No	27
	Yes	7
Urinary sodium excretion (mEq/d)	>10	46
	<10	17
Plasma renin activity	Normal	57
	Increased	6
Plasma norepinephrine	Normal	23
	Increased	13

Treatment strategy for patients with cirrhosis and moderate volume (grade 2) ascites

Start with a low-sodium diet (90 mmol/day) and spironolactone (50–100 mg/day) to reach goal of weight loss: 300–500 g/day. If needed, doses to be increased every 7 days up to 400 mg/day of spironolactone. Furosemide can be added at a starting dose of 20–40 mg/day and subsquently increased to 160 mg day if needed

Treatment strategy for patients with cirrhosis and large-volume (grade 3) ascites

Total paracentesis plus intravenous albumin (8 g per liter of ascites removed) followed by a low-sodium diet (90 mmol/day) and diuretics if patient tolerated them beforehand

Treatment strategy for refractory ascites

Total paracentesis plus intravenous albumin can be performed as needed. Consider use of TIPS in patients with very requent recurrent ascites without severely impaired hepatic function, aged <70 years and no hepatic encephalopathy

Diuretic: Resistant ascites

Ascites that cannot be mobilized or the early recurrence of which cannot be prevented because of a lack of response to sodium restriction and diuretic treatment.

Diuretic: Intractable ascites

Ascites that cannot be mobilized or the early recurrence of which cannot be prevented because of the development of diuretic-induced complications that preclude that use of an effective diuretic dosage.

Requisites for refractoriness

- Treatment duration: Patients must be on intensive diuretic therapy (spironolactone 400 mg/day and furosemide 160 mg/day) for at least 1 week and on a salt-restricted diet of less than 90 mmol/day
- Lack of response: Mean weight loss of <0.8 kg over 4 days and urinary sodium output less than the sodium intake.
- Early ascites recurrence: Reappearance of grade 2 or 3 ascites withing 4 weeks of initial mobilization

Diuretic-induced complication: Diuretic-induced hepatic encephalopathy in the development of encephalopathy in the absence of any other precipitation factor. Diuretic-induced renal impairment is an increase of serum creatinine by >100% to a value >2 mg/dL in patients with ascites responding to treatment. Diuretic-induced hyponatremia is defined as a decrease of serum sodium by >10 mEq/L to a serum sodium of <125 mEq/L. Diuretic induced hypo- or hyperkalemia is defined as a change in serum potassium to <3 mEq/L or >6 mEq/L despite appropriate measures

Figure 5 Management of ascites in cirrhosis

spironolactone such as gynecomastia, sexual dysfunction and allergies to sulfa moiety warrants switch over to alternatives such as amiloride, which is a direct inhibitor of apical sodium channel on principal cells of renal cortical collecting duct. In the event of non-response in higher doses to furosemide, torsemide/bumetanide can be used, which is forty times more potent with a similar side effects profile. Painful gynecomastia can be treated using tamoxifen 20 mg orally twice daily and muscle cramps that can complicate diuretic therapy may need dose reduction. Quinidine at the dose of 400 mg per day has been shown to improve cramps in few case reports and intravenous albumin use, 25 g per week has been shown to reduce the frequency and severity of muscle cramps in patient on diuretic therapy. Vasopressin is secreted from the hypothalamus and stored in the posterior pituitary and released in the event of changes in blood volume and high serum osmolarity. Vasopressin binds to V2 receptors on the basolateral cells of the renal cortical collecting ducts, causes activation of aquaporin 2 channels in the apical surface and promotes free water entry. Tolvaptan is the drug that has been approved for use in volume dysregulated states such as congestive heart failure and syndrome of inappropriate antidiuretic hormone secretion. When serum sodium is less than 135 mmol/L, tolvaptan is started at 15 mg per day and can be titrated up by 15 mg per day to a maximum of 60 mg per day. Improvements in hyponatremia can be observed in 8 hours' time. Even though this has been regarded for use in cirrhosis earlier, current evidence does not recommend its use in advanced liver disease. Effective and rapid treatment of ascites can be achieved through large volume paracentesis (removal of more than 5 L of fluid) where in the fluid can be all removed at once with slow catheter placed drainage. Repeated paracentesis is not associated with increased frequency of infections. Paracentesis induced circulatory dysfunction (PICD) may be seen in 15% of large volume paracentesis sessions and occurs due to unregulated activation of RAAS and down gradation of high pressure baroreceptors with stimulation of non-osmotic hypersecretion of vasopressin, dilutional hyponatremia and free water retention, with associated renal dysfunction. Intravenous albumin replacement of 8 g per liter of fluid removed needs to be done when fluid removal goes beyond 5 liters. Infusions using 5% albumin increases sodium load fivefold. Non-albumin solutions such as hydroxyethyl starch can worsen underlying PHT by causing Kupffer cell swelling. Terlipressin (3 mg intravenous infusion post paracentesis) is a good option in reducing plasma renin activity in large volume paracentesis and is as effective as albumin infusions. It has a half-life of 6 hours and is a vasopressin analog with V1 receptor selectivity and produces vasoconstriction.[33]

Refractory Ascites

Ascites that cannot be controlled adequately by means of dietary sodium restriction, pharmacologic therapy and/or paracentesis modalities is termed refractory. It can occur in 10% of patient with cirrhosis and PHT. Maximal diuretic therapy is defined as spironolactone 400 mg per day plus furosemide 160 mg per day. Non-response to such dosing is termed RESISTANT ascites and intolerance to diuretic therapy, thereby causing refractoriness is termed INTRACTABLE ascites. Type 2 HRS and a low MELD in the presence of advanced cirrhosis is very common to refractory ascites. The use of midodrine, which is an alpha 1 agonist which acts on arterial and venous system, leading to increase in vascular tone, has been described. It has been shown to be as effective as albumin infusion in preventing PICD in patients of refractory ascites on large volume paracentesis sessions. The use of non-selective beta blockers is associated with increased mortality (four times more) in patients of refractory ascites and advanced cirrhosis. Their use results in inhibition of compensatory cardiac output, leading to worsening renal parameters in cirrhosis and predisposing to PICD. Refractory ascites is a strong indication for liver transplantation referral and action. Transjugular intrahepatic portosystemic shunt (TIPSS) is a procedure in which there is establishment of direct continuity (by way of stent, low resistance profile) from a large portal branch to a hepatic vein. This results in by passing of the high resistance cirrhotic parenchymal tissue and decreases resultant complication of severe PHT. TIPSS is used as a bridge to liver transplantation. Recurrent variceal bleeding and refractory ascites with HRS Type 2 are strong indications for TIPSS use in a cirrhotic patient.[34] A MELD of 14 points or less suggests good candidacy for TIPSS and more than 24 points could become deleterious and merits liver transplantation. Contraindication to TIPSS placement include significant right heart failure, pulmonary hypertension, recurrent spontaneous encephalopathy, polycystic liver disease, central hepatocellular carcinoma, active infection such as SBP and severe renal disease. An ideal cirrhotic for TIPSS is one with preserved liver function, such as total bilirubin less than 3 mg/dL, serum sodium level more than 130 mEq/L and a Child score of less than 12, age less than 70 years and MELD score less than 18 without history of spontaneous hepatic encephalopathy, hepatocellular carcinoma or cardiopulmonary diseases. The very rare patient who cannot undergo TIPSS procedure for the indication of refractory ascites, placement of peritoneovenous shunts is an option, even though not utilized widely nowadays. There are two types of peritoneovenous shunts (LaVeen and Denver, both are one-way valve stents, emptying into the superior vena cava). Shunt surgery is contraindicated in loculated ascites, severe coagulopathy, advanced cardiac or renal disease, hemorrhagic and chylous ascites (chances of shunt occlusion is more). Shunt patency is poor with less than 20% at 2 years.

The ALFA pump system (Sequana Medical AG, Zurich, Switzerland) is an experimental device developed for the management of refractory ascites. It is a subcutaneously-implanted, battery-powered peritoneo-vesical shunt that pumps excess peritoneal fluid into the bladder where in the excess ascitic fluid is eliminated through urine. It is currently in phase 3 trials and has been shown to improve 90% of ascites in 40 patients who underwent the procedure. As described above, patients with refractory ascites, have low MELD scores and can remain on the transplant wait list for an extended period of time; a reason for refractory ascites not being given MELD exception status.[35] But it has been shown that mortality of refractory ascites cirrhotics on wait list is more than 20% at 6 months, despite a lower MELD score (less than 21), in the presence of moderate ascites and hyponatremia. Severity of hyponatremia and grade of ascites are independent predictors of mortality for cirrhosis patients with refractory ascites on the wait list. In such a case, the Child status of the patient is a far better index for prognosis of such patients in whom the MELD score is more than 14.

SPONTAENOUS BACTERIAL PERITONITIS

Spontaneous bacterial peritonitis is an infection of the sterile ascitic fluid in the absence of a surgical abdomen or a treatable source of abdominal infection and is of the following types, as shown in (Table 8). In SBP, there is positive bacterial culture positivity in ascites and increase in neutrophils counts to more than or equal to 250 cells/mm^3. The presence of microbiological evidence (monomicrobial) is seen in 60–70% of cases. Culture negative neutrocytic ascites (CNNA) is when there is no evidence of culture positivity in ascites, but there is an increase in neutrophil counts to more than or equal to 250 cell/mm^3. In one-third of such cases, if left untreated, later on shows positive bacterial evidence. Thirty-three to fifty-seven percent of patients with CNNC have positive microbiological evidence in blood cultures. Patients of CNNA and SBP show similar natural courses in the history of cirrhosis, with regards to symptoms and mortality. Thirdly, monomicrobial bacterascites (MNNB), a rare phenomenon among ascites infection is seen when there is positive bacterial culture in ascites without increase in neutrophils counts above the definite limit of 250 cells/mm^3 as is mostly seen with Child A and B cirrhosis patients. Spontaneous recovery occurs in 60–80% of patients and in the rest, it can transform into frank SBP. In MNNB, the use of antibiotics is recommended if the patient is symptomatic or if the culture is persistently positive.[36]

Table 8: Types of bacterial peritonitis seen in cirrhosis

Condition	*Diagnosis*	*Treatment*
Classical SBP	PMNs >250 cells/mm^3 with positive ascitic culture for single organism	Treat with appropriate antibiotics
Culture-negative SBP	PMNs >250 cells/mm^3 with negative ascitic culture	Treat with antibiotics as per classical SBP
Monomicrobial non-neutrocytic bacteriascites	PMNs <250 cells/mm^3 with positive ascitic culture for single organism	If symptomatic, repeat diagnostic tap. Treat if culture remains positive or PMNs >250 cells/mm^3
Ploymicrobial bacteriascites	PMNs <250 cells/mm^3 and culture with multiple organisms	Antibiotics may be required. Treat cause (usually GI perforation during paracentesis)
Secondary bacterial peritonitis	PMNs >250 cells/mm^3 and culture with multiple organisms	Treat with antibiotics and correct underlying cause

The International Ascites Club identifies SBP and CNNA to be similar from a clinical and therapeutic point of view. Infections complicating malignant ascites can also occur spontaneously. Ten to thirty percent of patients admitted to the hospital with ascites have SBP at admission and in 5% of outpatients. Forty to seventy percent of patients develop a second episode of SBP within 1 year and the 1-year survival after an episode of SBP patients is only 30–40% while the 2-year survival is 20%, which in the presence of Child C cirrhosis becomes even lower. The median survival rate after the first episode of SBP in a decompensated cirrhosis patient is 6 months. The most common organism seen is Gram-negative bacteria in 65% of positive culture results of which *Escherichia coli* (*E. coli*) and *Klebsiellae* are the most common and second most common microbes, respectively. Remaining 35% infection is by Gram-positive cocci. Bacteria causing SBP in hospital and non-hospital scenarios are different. While Gram-negative bacteria are responsible for most of hospital acquired SBP, Gram-positive bacteria are responsible for non-hospital related SBP. In contrast to this, among animal models of SBP, Enterococcus faecalis was mostly isolated and SBP was mostly of polymicrobial origin in around half of the cases.[37] Leaky gut in cirrhosis predisposes to bacteremia after which ascites gets infected. Development and progression of SBP depends mostly on the antibacterial opsonin activity of the ascitic fluid which on the other hand positively correlates with the content of total protein in ascites and also the immune status (immunocompetence) of the patient. In the presence of ascites infection, activation of neutrophilic granulocytes occur which migrate into the peritoneal cavity and initiate a complex cytokine cascade, in the wake of increased interleukin-6 and tumor necrosis factor-alpha in the fluid. To briefly put, main reasons for pathogenesis of SBP involves small intestinal bacterial overgrowth (SIBO), increased intestinal permeability, bacterial translocation and immunosuppressed state in cirrhosis. SIBO is a classical association in cirrhosis (more in alcoholic cirrhosis). The SIBO in cirrhotics is mainly due to prolonged intestinal transit, bile secretory abnormality and dysregulation, hypochlorhydria, IgA secretory abnormalities and malnutrition. SIBO is seen in 20–60% of all cirrhosis patients. SIBO is also associated with use of drugs that reduce secretion of hydrochloric acid in the gastric region [proton pump inhibitors (PPI)] and there is a risk of SIBO and hence SBP in cirrhosis patients who take PPIs for long. PHT is one of the main reasons for increased intestinal permeability. Bacterial translocation (organism or bacterial products) in SIBO can be active or passive. They first pass through the mucosal epithelial layer, to the lamina propria, then to mesenteric lymph nodes and extraintestinal sites. It has been shown that translocation occurs when bacterial numbers are high, up to 108 bacteria per 1 g of feces. There are four grades of bacterial translocation. In the grade zero, there is penetration of the mucosa by mechanisms such as active intracellular penetration, diffusion, endocytosis, phagocytosis and absorption by macrophages. In grade one, bacteria and its components enter the mesenteric lymphatic system by centripetal penetration. In grade two, the bacteria and components are present in systemic circulation and organ systems. In grade three, the microorganism and its products overwhelms the host leading to sepsis. Anaerobic organisms lack the ability to translocate across intestinal epithelium, but enterobacteria and staphylococci can pass live, across the mucosal surface.[38] Neutrophilic granulocytosis in ascites show decreased action for chemotaxis in the back ground of decreased opsonin activity in ascites. Patients with reduced total protein content in ascites (less than 1.5 g/dL) are prone to the development of SBP. SBP can present variably in a patient of advanced cirrhosis such as failure of diuretic therapy, worsening or new onset encephalopathy and/or renal dysfunction. Diagnostic paracentesis is warranted in a patient of cirrhosis who present with signs of abdominal or systemic infection (abdominal pain or tenderness, loose stools, fever, acidosis, peripheral leukocytosis or with encephalopathy or worsened renal functions). In SBP, there is worsening of splanchnic vasodilatation in the presence of endotoxemia and decreased effective circulating blood volume. These further result in worsening of renal function and can cause HRS. Positive culture of ascites is seen in 30% of cases of SBP. The level of interleukin 6 was shown to be of help in diagnosing SBP with 100% sensitivity when a limit of 5 ng/mL in fluid was considered. The utilization of ascites pH less than 7.35 or an arterial to ascites pH gradient of more than 0.1 was considered to be diagnostic of SBP. Antibiotic therapy with a third generation cephalosporin, mostly cefotaxime in doses of 2 g with administration every 8 hourly would suffice in treating SBP. Other antibiotics that can be used include a combination of amoxicillin, clavulanic acid or ofloxacin 400 mg may be administered every 12 hours for a period of 7–10 days. Albumin infusion at a dose of 1.5 g/kg in the first day and 1 g/kg on the third day improves survival benefit and prevents chances of kidney injury in these cohort of patients.[39] Albumin is also indicated in the presence of clinical doubt of SBP with blood urea nitrogen more than 30 mg/dL, totoal bilirubin of more than 4 mg/dL and serum creatinine more than 1 mg/dL. Response is gauged by decrement of neutrophils in the ascites by at least 25% from the baseline and in the absence of that, change of antibiotics is warranted. The group of patients who are at risk for SBP include, patients with gastrointestinal bleeding, survivors of SBP and patients with low protein in ascites. Patients who survive the SBP episode should be put on long-term prophylaxis with daily norfloxacin 400 mg dosing and in the presence of contraindication to fluroquinolones or fluroquinolone resistance, trimethoprim/sulfamethoxazole combination can also be offered. Liver transplantation is the definitive management, in the event SBP has occurred in the natural course of the disease. Primary prophylaxis of SBP can be offered to a patient of decompensated cirrhosis when ascites fluid protein is less than 1.1 g/dL along with serum sodium less than 130 mEq/L, blood urea nitrogen more than 25 mg/dL, serum creatinine more than 1.2 mg/dL or Child score more than 9 points with hyperbilirubinemia more than 3 mg/dL[40] (Table 9).

DIFFICULT TO TREAT SPONTANEOUS BACTERIAL PERITONITIS

The in-hospital mortality of SBP is 30% and 1-year mortality is approximately 60%. Severity of SBP can be gauged by, in the presence of upper gastrointestinal bleeds, severe sepsis with multiorgan failure, disseminated intravascular coagulation, a serum bilirubin more than 4 mg/dL, blood urea more than 30 mg/dL, creatinine values more than 1.2 mg/dL, nosocomial etiology of SBP and hemodynamic instability. Nosocomial SBP is considered when the diagnosis of SBP is in a patient who has had

Table 9: Treatment and prophylaxis of spontaneous bacterial peritonitis

Indications for spontaneous bacterial peritonitis (SBP) prophylaxis				
Indicator	*Comments*	*Special considerations*	*Preferred antibiotic therapy*	*Reasonable alternative*
Prior episode (s) of SBP	Indefinite duration unless ascites resolves	Standard therapy	Cefotaxime 2 g IV q8h × 5 days	Ceftriaxone 1 g IV q12h or 2 g IV q24h × 5 days
Advanced liver disease (without prior history of SBP)	Ascitic fluid protein less than 1.5 g/dL and at least one of the following: Serum creatinine ≥1.2 mg/dL Blood urea nitrogen ≥ 25 mg/dL Serum sodium ≤ 130 mEq/L, or Child-Pugh score ≥ 9 +bilirubin ≥ 3 mg/dL	Uncomplicated SBP	Ofloxacin 400 mg PO bid × 8 days is an option	Ciprofloxacin 500 mg PO bid Or Levofloxacin 500 mg PO q24 h
Acute gastrointestinal bleeding	Duration limited to 7 days	Nosocomial SBP	Extended spectrum antibiotics (carbapenems piperacillin-tazobactam)	Depends on local resistance patterns
		Patient receiving fluoroquinolone or trimethoprim-sulfamethoxazole SBP prophylaxis	Cefotaxime 2 g IV q8h × 5 days	Ceftriaxone 1 g IV q12h or 2 g IV q24h × 5 days
		Beta lactam hypersensitivity	Ciprofloxacin 400 mg IV q12h	Levofloxacin 500 mg PO q24 h
		Advanced liver or renal failure: serum creatinine greater than 1 mg/dL, blood urea nitrogen greater than 30 mg/dL or total bilirubin greater than 4 mg/dL	IV Cefotaxime 2 g IV q8h × 5 days plus IV albumin 1.5 g/kg given on day 1 ad 1.0 g/kg given on day 3	

a history of ICU stay during the previous 3 months or had been on prophylactic antibiotics for infection or had antibiotic treatment during previous 3 months or had undergone a recent intervention in the hospital setting. SBP is considered difficult to treat when it is community acquired with a risk of developing kidney injury; nosocomial acquired with high risk of ESBL or MRSA or multidrug resistant bacteria related or recurrent severe SBP as was described above. In the event that SBP is community acquired, the treatment is by standard protocol as for any episode of SBP, but with graded and step wise antibiotic upgradation as per clinical and investigational findings. On the other hand, the nosocomial etiology of SBP needs to be tackled initially with carbapenems with or without glycopeptides use; even though this strategy has not been validated yet. With regards to studies from Europe, the sensitivity of Gram-negative and Gram-positive bacteria is preserved toward carbapenem and glycopeptides and hence these are first empirical choice of antibiotic with necessary modification according to cultures and clinical assessment.[41]

HEPATIC HYDROTHORAX AND SPONTANEOUS BACTERIAL PLEURITIS (EMPYEMA)

Hepatic hydrothorax is defined as pleural effusion greater than 500 mL, in a cirrhotic patient, without an underlying pulmonary or cardiac disease. It has a prevalence in cirrhosis patients of 5–12%. In 85% of cases, the hepatic hydrothorax develops on the right side, 13% occur on the left side and 2% are seen to be bilateral. In majority of cases, ascites is also present. Modest volumes of pleural fluid can cause significant respiratory symptoms, including dyspnea and chest pain in cirrhosis patients as against the good tolerance seen to large ascites collections. Increased total extracellular fluid volume in cirrhosis patients lead to accumulation of fluid in the peritoneal and/or pleural cavities and interstitial tissues. This is mainly dependent on renal sodium reabsorption, fall in effective arterial blood volume and arterial splanchnic vasodilatation. Hypoalbuminemia, decreased colloid osmotic pressure, azygous vein hypertension, leakage of ascites through diaphragmatic defects and trans-diaphragmatic flow of fluid through lymphatic channels are proposed to be pathobiologies operating in patients who develop hepatic hydrothorax. Emerson in 1955, described for the first time, fenestrations in the diaphragm associated with cirrhosis and right sided pleural effusion. Discontinuities in the collagen bundles of the tendinous portion of the diaphragm are seen on microscopic examination of these fenestrations. Intra-abdominal pressure increase, as a result of ascites, coughing, or straining, leads to small herniations (also called pleuroperitoneal blebs) of the peritoneum through these gaps into the pleural cavity. The blebs rupture, forming defects, which are typically less than 1 cm in diameter which allows for free communication between the pleural and peritoneal space, causing hydrothorax. Because of the presence of negative intrapleural pressure, there is one way migration of ascites fluid into the pleural cavity and its entrapment there.[42] In hepatic hydrothorax, accumulation of fluid overwhelms the absorptive capacity of the pleural lymphatics. In the presence of studies that have utilized air, colored dyes or radiolabelled substances, these abnormalities in the diaphragm were clearly delineated. Huang et al. classified hydrothorax anatomically based on the diaphragmatic defects, into four types as below.

Type I: No obvious defect

Type II: Blebs lying on the diaphragm

Type III: Fenestrations in the diaphragm

Type IV: Multiple gaps in the diaphragm

It has been shown in postmortem studies that pleuroperitoneal blebs occur less frequently in the left hemidiaphragm, as it is thicker and more muscular. Real time demonstration of diaphragmatic defects or fenestrations can be easily shown by way of contrast enhanced ultrasonography.[43] Hepatic hydrothorax should be suspected in any cirrhosis patient with PHT presenting with a unilateral pleural effusion, most commonly on the right side. Symptomatic hydrothorax presents with dyspnea, non-productive cough, pleural chest pain, and fatigue due to hypoxemia. The severity of these symptoms depends on the volume of pleural fluid. Unilateral pleural effusions in cirrhotic patients can also occur without clinical or even ultrasonic evidence of ascites (Table 10). An uncomplicated hepatic hydrothorax has a cell count less than 500 cells/mm^3, and the total protein concentration is less than 2.5 g/dL. PHT can also give rise to hepatic chylothorax due to increase in splanchnic lymph flow and subsequent rupture of lymphatic channels in the pleural space. In the presence of a pleuroperitoneal communication, the lymph fluid is diluted by ascites and the triglyceride and lymphocyte counts are usually lower than in other forms of chylothorax, retaining the characteristic of transudate.[44] Recently it has been proposed that the finding of an elevated serum soluble Fas ligand may help distinguish a hepatic hydrothorax from one resulting from heart failure in patients with viral cirrhosis. In cases when hepatic hydrothorax is doubtful as in left sided effusions or in the absence of ascites, intraperitoneal administration of ^{99m}Technitium human serum albumin or ^{99m}Technitium-sulfur colloid can reveal the migration of radioisotope into the pleural cavity within hours thereby confirming the presence of a communication between the pleural and peritoneal spaces (sensitivity and specificity rates of 71% and 100%, respectively). This technique has also been used in the absence of ascites by way of ultrasound guided application of radiolabeled substance in a 500-mL volume of normal saline. Most patients with hepatic hydrothorax have end-stage liver disease and should be considered as potential candidates for orthotopic liver transplantation. Medical management of hydrothorax in decompensated cirrhosis patients is same as that of ascites management with low sodium diet with 70–90 mmol/day, improvement of the nutritional status, diuretic use, (spironolactone, 50–400 mg/day, given in combination with furosemide, 20–160 mg/day) and drugs such as Terlipressin in whom hepatic hydrothorax is refractory to thoracic tube drainage and octreotide treatment along with albumin. Terlipressin administration resulted in both improvement in renal function and successful decrement/resolution of hepatic hydrothorax. Other combination therapies include the use of pleurodesis and TIPSS and treatment with octreotide (Flow chart 3).[45]

Table 10: Characteristics of hepatic hydrothorax

Location	Right sided (85%) Left sided (13%) Bilateral (2%)
Fluid characteristics	• Cell count [<250 polymorphonuclear cells/cumm, uncomplicated] • Protein (<2.5 g/dL) • Pleural fluid/serum total protein ratio (<0.5) • Pleural fluid/serum lactate dehydrogenase (LDH) ratio (>0.6) • Pleural fluid/serum albumin gradient (>1.1) • Pleural fluid/serum bilirubin ratio (<0.6) • pH (>7.4) • Glucose level similar to that of serum

REFRACTORY HYDROTHORAX

As per criteria for refractoriness of ascites, the same is applicable for hydrothorax. The hydrothorax maybe diuretic resistant (poor response to sodium restriction with maximal diuretic dosing) or intractable (diuretic related complications that preclude maximal and responsive dosing). Repeated thoracocentesis is the most effective way of managing refractory hydrothorax.[46] It helps in immediate relief of dyspnea in cirrhotics with large pleural effusions. Natriuresis—that is urine sodium more than 30 mEq/day is important in hepatic hydrothorax management as is with ascites. This natriuretic sign can be evaluated every 2 weeks in patient who develop severe sodium retention (urine sodium less than 10 mEq/day) and step wise up-gradation of diuretics can be tried before billing thee patients are cases of refractory hydrothorax. Pneumothorax is the major complication of thoracocentesis. It occurs at a rate of 7.7% with first session of pleurocentesis to 34.7% during the fourth session. In most cases of pleurocentesis, no more than 2 liters should be removed or until the patient coughs, in view of early re-expansion pulmonary edema and/or hypotension. Other complications associated with pleurocentesis include, pain at puncture, air embolism, soft tissue infection, vasovagal episodes, bleeding diathesis, laceration of the liver or spleen, secondary bacterial empyema and/or subcutaneous emphysema. TIPSS is the treatment of choice in patients of refractory hydrothorax (Figs 5A and B). It leads to symptomatic improvement in 70–80% of patients of refractory hydrothorax and common complications include shunt occlusion and hepatic encephalopathy. TIPSS has also been attributed to have a mortality rate of 20–25% in the first 2 months after placement, mostly attributed to underlying end stage liver disease. TIPSS does not work well with patients who have a MELD score more than 14, bilirubin more than 3 mg/dL, ALT more than 100 IU/L, presence of hepatic encephalopathy pre-TIPSS and in emergency indications for TIPSS (independent predictors of survival post TIPSS). Patients of refractory hydrothorax can also be intervened with surgical procedures like tube thoracostomy with sclerosant injection like talc, leading to obliteration of space between parietal and visceral pleura. In this procedure, the rates of fluid re-accumulation is very high and multiple other complications like fever, empyema, pneumonia, chest pain, wound infection and incomplete re-expansion also occur and hence is not a current recommended modality. Repair of defects in diaphragm using vide assisted thoracoscopy (VATS) has been utilized at many centers around the world. Further advances such as use of pleura and mesh onlay technique to reinforce the

Flow chart 3 Management algorithm of hepatic hydrothorax in cirrhosis

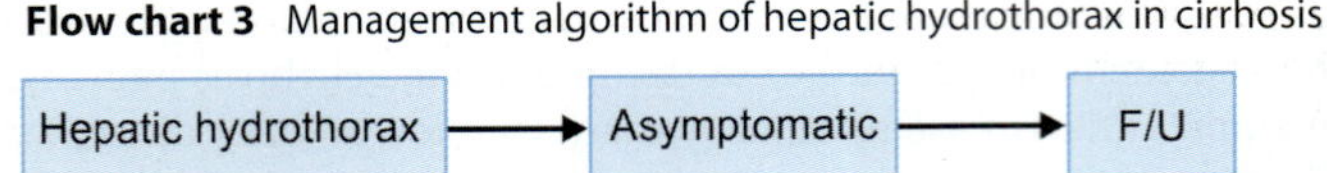

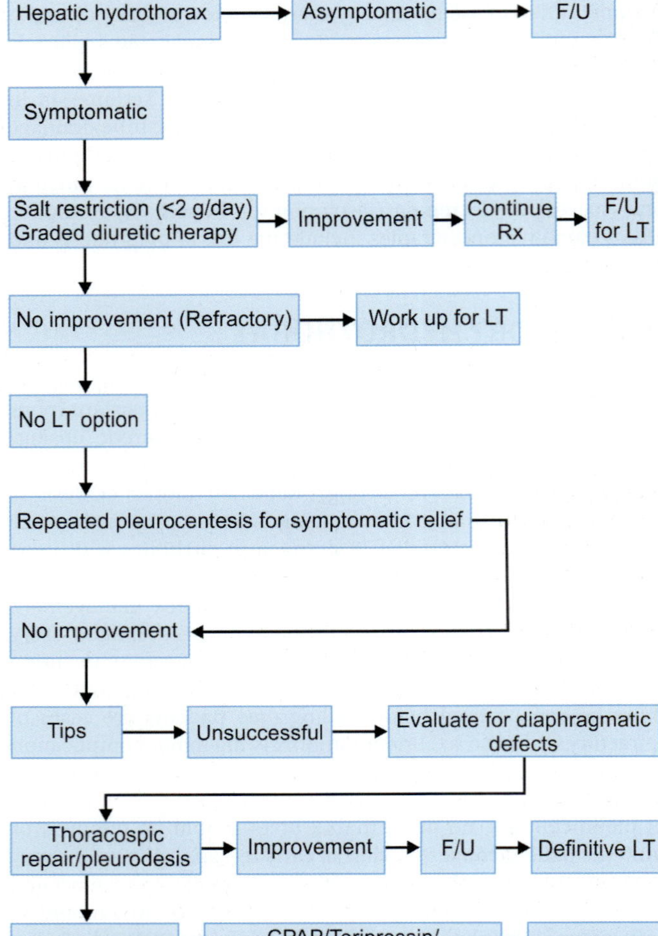

diaphragm have shown benefit in some studies. Peritoneovenous shunting for the treatment of hepatic hydrothorax is currently abandoned. Liver transplantation is an excellent therapeutic option for patients with hepatic hydrothorax, because it offers the choice of curative treatment. Use of nasal continuous airway pressure where in conversion of intrathoracic pressure from negative to positive is a new modality in management of hepatic hydrothorax and is primarily useful in patients of hydrothorax with Pickwikian features (snoring increases intrathoracic negative pressures, worsening hydrothorax).[47]

Spontaneous bacterial empyema currently re-termed as pleuritis (SBPe) is the spontaneous infection of the pleural fluid. Its prevalence is seen in 13% of in-hospital cirrhosis patients with hydrothorax and has an estimated mortality of over 20% in the same admission. It is postulated to occur as a direct spread of bacteria from the peritoneal cavity.[48] In 40% patients of SBPe, there is no associated SBP. SBPe can also occur in the absence of ascites. Another theory regarding its pathogenesis is that transient bacteremia that infects the pleural space. Defective local pleural factors such as low fluid complement levels and low opsonic activity (similar to that seen in ascites that develop SBP) is also seen

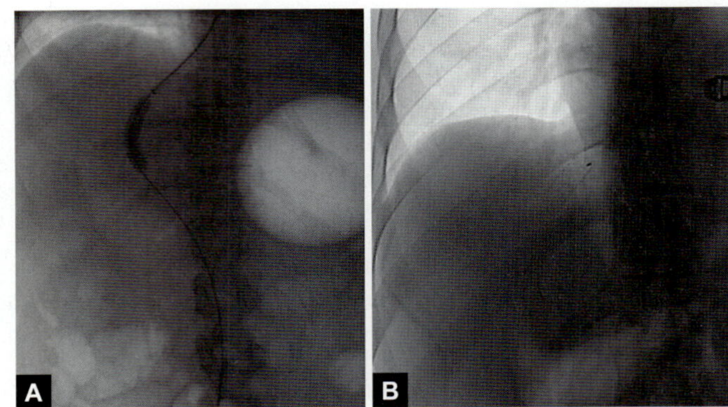

Figures 5A and B Realtime images of transjugular intrahepatic portosystemic shunt procedure. In (B) the TIPS stent is seen *in situ*

in SBPe pathogenesis, which enhances bacterial translocation.

The causative micro-organisms in most cases of SBEM are *E. coli, Streptococcus* species, *Enterococcus* and *Klebsiella,* which are different from that causing SBP.[49] A high Child-Pugh score, decreased pleural fluid total protein and low levels of C3 component in pleural fluid were proved risk factors for the development of SBEM. SBP is also a predictive factor of SBEM. It is recommended to use the pleural fluid total protein concentration in clinical practice to detect those patients at a risk for developing SBEM. The infection of the pleural fluid is frequently associated with few localizing signs. A decompensated cirrhosis patient with hydrothorax who develops fever, pleuritic pain, encephalopathy or unexplained deterioration in renal function should undergo diagnostic thoracocentesis. SBEM is defined when the pleural fluid polymorphonuclear cell count is more than 500 cells/mm^3 or if there is a positive culture with polymorphonuclear cell count more than 250 cells/mm^3 with the exclusion of a parapneumonic effusion. Pleural fluid culture should be performed by inoculating 10 mL pleural fluid into a TSB blood culture bottle at bedside since it contains an opsonin inhibitor that protects bacteria from further complement- or phagocyte-mediated killing. Routine pleural fluid analysis showed limited diagnostic efficacy in the diagnosis of SBEM since LDH, total protein and glucose were not reported to differ significantly between the patients with SBEM and those with non-infected effusion and it did not correlate with neutrophil cell count. Hence, the diagnosis of SBE should not be overlooked when these parameters are found within the expected levels found in the transudate. Treatment of SBPe include intravenous third generation cephalosporin; for example, ceftriaxone 1 g every 12 hours for 7–10 days along with albumin infusions, 1.5 g/kg on day one followed by 1 g/kg on day three. In the presence of poor clinical response, a repeat pleurocentesis is recommended to check for fluid cell response based on which antibiotic modification can be made. Placement of a chest tube should be done in a cirrhotic patient with SBPe. The definitive treatment is by liver transplantation, even when complicated by empyema (Table 11).[50]

VARICEAL DISEASE (FIG. 6)

Variceal bleeding is a major complication of PHT and is a leading cause of death in patients with cirrhosis. Early mortality after an episode of acute variceal bleeding (AVB) remains high (15–24%).[51]

Table 11: Risk factors and diagnostic criteria for spontaneous bacterial empyema (pleuritis) in cirrhosis patients

Risk Factors for Development of SBEM in Cirrhosis
• High Child-Pugh score
• Low serum albumin
• Low pleural fluid protein
• Low pleural fluid C3
• Spontaneous bacterial peritonitis
Diagnostic Criteria of SBEM in Cirrhosis
• Serium/pleural fluid albumin gradient >1.1 g/dL
• Polymorphonuclear leukocyte count >500/mm^3 or positive fluid culture with PMN cell count >250 cells/mm^3
• Absence of pneumonia or a contiguous infection process on chest radiography

Esophageal Varices

Acute esophageal variceal bleed cause approximately 70% of all upper gastrointestinal bleed in cirrhosis. Around 40–50% of variceal bleeds stop spontaneously. Even in the wake of most effective treatments, 25% of patients will still show either a failure to control the bleeding or an early recurrence of the bleeding in the first 6 weeks after the initial bleeding. This risk peaks during the first 5 days, the period in which 40% of all rebleeding occur. Afterwards, it decreases slowly, equaling at 6 week, the risk prior to the bleeding episode. Any death occurring within 6 weeks of admission from the index bleeding should be considered as a bleeding related death. Prognostic indicators of rebleeding known as the "5 day failure" (initial failure to control the acute bleeding and 5 day mortality) include the Child-Pugh and MELD scores or its individual components. Active bleeding at initial endoscopy has also been identified as an important risk factor for 5-day failure. Regarding early mortality, the Child-Pugh class is the main and most constant prognostic indicator.[52] Another independent factor for 6 week mortality is the presence of hepatoellular carcinoma or early rebleeding, as shown in multivariate analysis. Upper GI endoscopy is the gold standard for diagnosing esophageal varices. The platelet count per cubic millimeter to spleen size (maximum bipolar diameter in millimeters by ultrasonography) ratio of more than 909 has a high negative predictive value for the presence of esophageal varices.

Hepatic venous pressure gradient helps in stratifying patients at risk from complications of PHT. PHT is said to be present if the HVPG is greater than 5 mm Hg and is clinically significant when the HVPG is greater than 10 mm Hg (strong predictor of development of varices, events of decompensation, and hepatocellular carcinoma). In patients of AVB, an HVPG of more than 20 mm Hg (measured within 24 hours after admission) is the best predictor of a poor outcome. A reduction in the HVPG to less than 12 mm Hg (post TIPSS) or a reduction of more than 20% from the baseline (on beta blocker, check after 1 month of initiation of treatment) value has a decreased risk of variceal hemorrhage and improved survival. Recently, new statistical approaches on techniques such as classification and regression tree analysis (CART) helps in recognition of prognostic subgroups in cirrhosis patients as targets for interventions.[53] Variceal bleeding is seen in 70% of all upper digestive tract bleeding in portal hypertensive patients. The Asia Pacific Association for the Study of Liver recommended the following terminologies in AVB, in a seminal workshop conducted in the year 2011. The definition of AVB was given as the presence of hemetemesis within the last 24 hours of presentation, and/or ongoing melena, with last melenic stool within last 24 hours. Active bleeding, defined endoscopically, as spurting or oozing from the varix. Failure to control AVB is defined as the failure of combination therapy given with any of the following events that occurred within 48 hours from start of combination therapy (vasoactive agents plus band ligation)—development of fresh hematemesis after 2 hours of therapy or a 2 g drop in Hb (6% drop in hematocrit, if no transfusion is administered); continuous increase in heart rate and decrease of systolic blood pressure with adequate infusion or death. Rebleeding was defined as any new hematemesis (or new melena) after 48 hours of index presentation and after a period of 24 hours of hemodynamic stability. Very early rebleeding was that which occurred between 48 hours and 120 hours from the index presentation. Early rebleeding was one which occurred between 6 days and 42 days from the index bleed and late rebleeding as that occurred after 42 days from the index hemorrhagic episode. Clinically significant rebleeding was defined as rebleeding associated with a decrease of 2 g of hemoglobin if no blood transfusion is given or an ABRI (adjusted blood requirement index) of more than or equal to 0.5 at any time point. Recent bleed referred to a clinically significant bleed which occurred within 6 weeks of presentation and past bleed was a clinically significant bleed which occurred more than 6 weeks after index presentation. They also proposed the use of American College Criteria for severity of blood loss and the APASL severity score for stratifying severity of variceal bleed. Coronary venous collateral vessels are vascular channels in the triangular fatty tissue between the medial wall of the upper gastric body and the posterior margin of the left hepatic lobe, the lesser omentum. A coronary (left gastric) vein larger than 5–6 mm in diameter on Doppler sonograms or CT scans is considered abnormal and is an indicator of PHT and multiple dilated veins 4–6 mm in diameter in the lesser omentum were also considered to be varices. Varices are easily recognized on the basis of their tubular or serpentine configuration, their enhancement with contrast material, and the presence of adjacent collateral vessels. Esophageal varices are enlarged, tortuous veins situated in the wall of the lower esophagus which are formed by communications between the dilated subepithelial and submucosal veins and the dilated venae comitantes of the vagus nerves that lie in the adventitia outside the tunica muscularis. These varices are mostly supplied by the anterior branch of the left gastric vein, whereas the posterior branch of this vein supplies paraesophageal collateral vessels.[54] The paraesophageal varices situated outside the wall of the esophagus in the mediastinum may be confused with esophageal varices. On Doppler sonograms, hepatofugal flow within a patent paraumbilical vein is a reliable indicator of PHT even in the absence of esophageal varices. Among patients with large spontaneous shunts, there is a high frequency of hepatic encephalopathy and a lower frequency of esophageal varices.[55]

Primary Prophylaxis: Prevention of Varices and First Variceal Bleed

Primary prophylaxis of bleeding from esophageal varices is defined as a therapeutic intervention that aims at the prevention of the

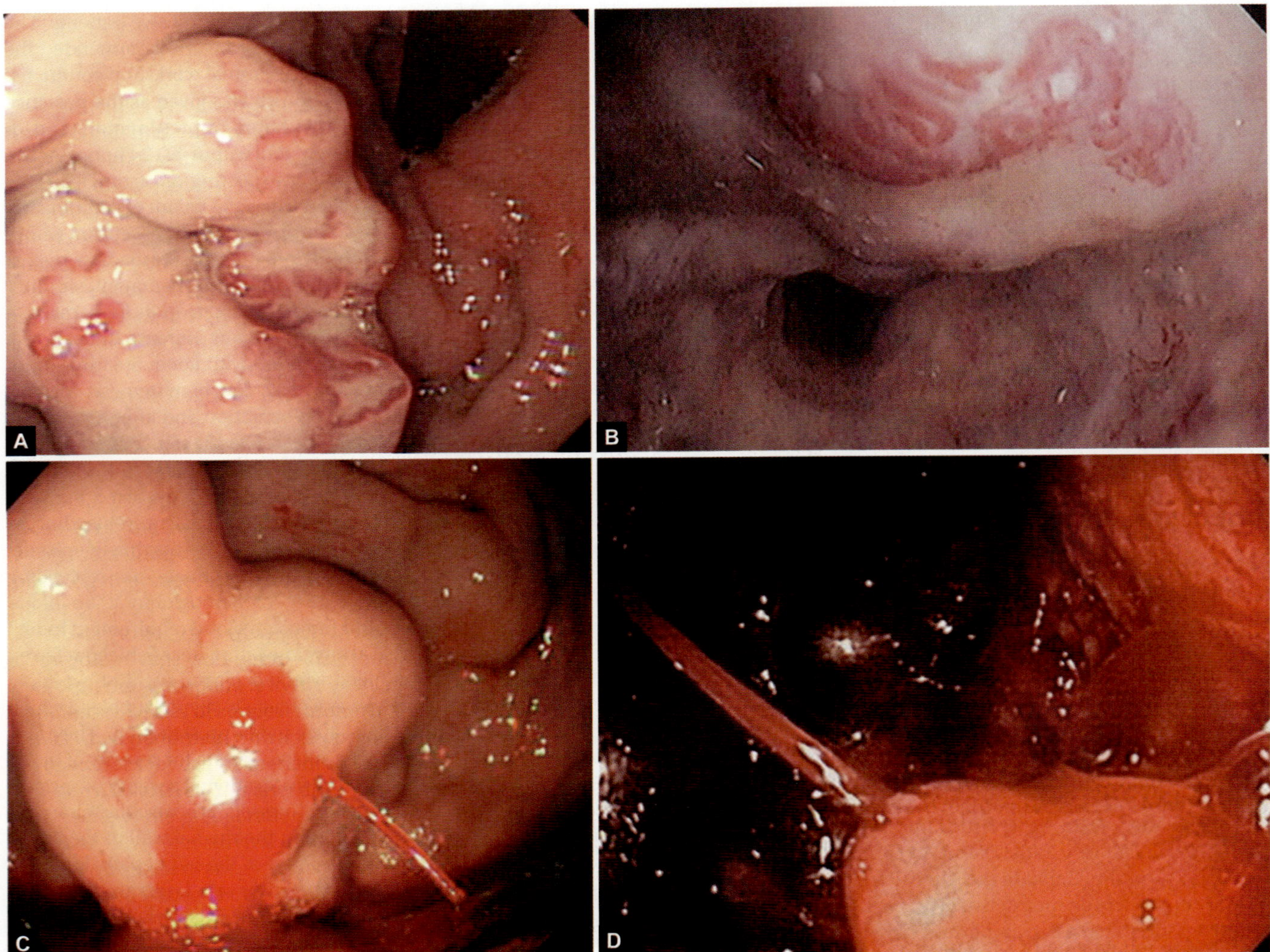

Figures 6A to D Esophagogastric variceal disease in cirrhosis. Clockwise from left—large GOV1 with red color signs; large esophageal varcies with red color signs; bleeding esophageal varices; bleeding gastric varices (active spurter)

first variceal hemorrhage. At the time of the first diagnosis, about half of the patients with liver cirrhosis have esophageal varices. During the course of the disease about 90% of the patients develop esophageal varices. The identification and prophylactic treatment of patients at risk for esophageal bleeding is therefore mandatory. Risk factors for variceal bleeding are the diameter of the varix, presence of red wale signs, HVPG more than 12 mm Hg and an impaired liver function. In patients where there are esophageal varices with a diameter of more than 5 mm, prophylactic treatment should be initiated. Prophylactic treatment is not necessary when only small varices (diameter below 5 mm) are present. The overall incidence of esophageal varices is 5% per year. Esophageal varices tend to increase in size in a linear fashion with an increase in variceal size in 21%, 45% and 66% of the patients after 1.5, 3 and 4.5 years, respectively (the course of the underlying liver disease is a major determinant of variceal progression). The recommendation for surveillance in patients with compensated liver disease and small varices at the screening endoscopy is a follow-up examination after 1-2 years. If the screening endoscopy showed no varices, a follow-up examination after 2-3 years is sufficient in patients with compensated liver disease (Figs 7A and B).[56] Non-selective beta-blockers cause vasoconstriction of the splanchnic circulation by β2-receptor inhibition and decrease cardiac output by β1-receptor blockade. This leads to a decrease in portal venous inflow and thereby lowers portal pressure. Beta-blocker therapy is not effective in preventing gastro-esophageal varices in patients with cirrhosis. Patients with varices at risk of bleeding should receive prophylactic treatment since the risk of bleeding is 30–35% in 2 years. Effective prophylactic treatment reduces the risk of bleeding by about 50%. Not all patients respond to beta-blockers with a reduction of the HVPG. Clinical studies have shown that at most 50% of beta-blocker treated patients achieved a reduction of the HVPG below 12 mm Hg or more than 20% from baseline levels (responders). However, other effects of beta-blocker therapy besides the reduction of HVPG like a decrease in azygous blood flow or a decrease in bacterial translocation from the gut[18] may play a role in the prevention of variceal hemorrhage. Endoscopic sclerotherapy and shunt procedures are obsolete in primary prophylaxis. Standard modalities include drug therapy with non-selective beta-blockers and EBL. The non-cardioselective vasodilating beta-blocker with mild intrinsic anti-$\alpha(1)$-adrenergic activity carvedilol is at least as effective in lowering HVPG as propranolol or nadolol plus nitrate and also as effective as EBL for primary prophylaxis of variceal bleeding. A monotherapy with nitrates or a combination of beta-blockers and nitrates compared to beta-blockers alone has no benefit in primary prophylaxis. Around 20% of patients suffer from intolerable side effects that require discontinuation of the drug. The most important predictor for variceal bleeding in patients on a therapy with beta-blockers is the dose of the drug. All patients tolerating the drug regimen should therefore receive the highest tolerated dose. An effective alternative treatment for primary prophylaxis is EBL. But because of the low costs, ease of administration as well as the absence of procedure-related mortality, nonselective beta-blockers are recommended as first-line treatment for the primary prophylaxis of esophageal variceal bleeding. EBL is recommended in patients with serious side effects or intolerability of beta-blocker therapy as well as in patients with contraindications for drug therapy.[57]

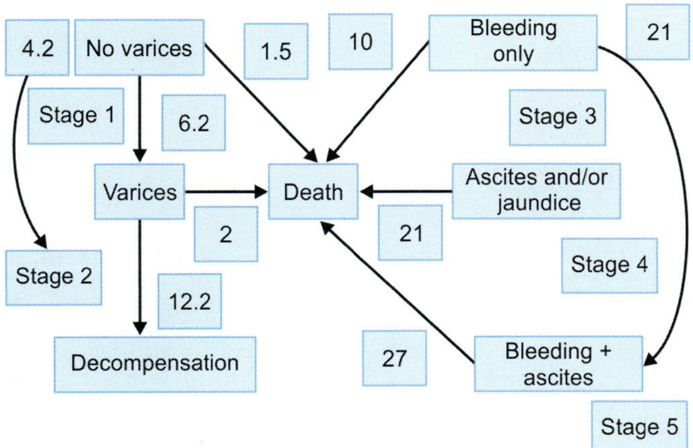

Figure 7A Natural history of variceal disease in cirrhosis in lieu with other decompensation factors, in each stage of cirrhosis

	Class 1	Class 2	Class 3	Class 4
Blood loss	<750	750–1,500	1,500–2,000	>2,000
Blood loss (%)	0–15	15–30	30–40	>40
Systolic BP	No change	Normal	Reduced	Very reduced
Diastolic BP	No change	Raised	Reduced	Very reduced
PR (min)	Slight tachycardia	100–120	120 (thready)	120 (very thready)
RR (min)	Normal	Normal	<20	<20
Mental state	Alert, thirsty	Anxious, aggressive	Anxious, aggressive, or drowsy	Drowsy, aggressive confused, or unconscious

Parameter	Value	Point
Systolic blood pressure	>90 mm Hg and no postural drop	0
	> 90 mm Hg with postural drop	1
	< 90 mm Hg	2
Child Turcotte-Pugh class	A	0
	B	1
	C	2
Platelet count	> 100,000 mm^{-3}	0
		1
Infection	Absent	0
	Present	1
Active bleeding at endoscopy	Absent	0
	Present	1
	Total	Minimum 0, Maximum 7

Figure 7B Scoring for blood loss in acute variceal bleeding (American College Criteria for Blood Loss) and variceal bleeding severity (Asian Pacific Association for Study of Liver Severity Score)

Management of Acute Varcieal Bleed (Figs 8A and B)

During the initial resuscitation in AVB, airway and breathing security should be maintained to prevent bronchial aspiration of stomach contents and blood. Patients in encephalopathy are at highest risk for this, during emergency endoscopy procedures. Endotracheal intubation is mandatory in patients with hepatic encephalopathy grade III and above. Adequate large bore venous access (ideally two) should be made for fluid and blood administration and to maintain adequate mean arterial pressure. The systolic pressure should be maintained at or above 100 mm Hg; the ideal/optimal systolic blood pressure at which endoscopy can be safely performed in 70 mm Hg. Long standing hypotension and inadequate volume resuscitation can result in kidney injury and increase chances of infection, both of which are associated with risk of rebleeding and mortality. Rebound high portal pressures and risk of rebleeding occur when there is over transfusion. The aim of blood transfusion is to maintain hemoglobin levels between 7–8 g/dL except in patients of ischemic heart disease, ongoing bleeds and/or cerebral disease, in which the threshold should be higher. It has been suggested that volume replacement should be done with human albumin fraction or gelatin based colloid which have been associated with less effect on clotting compared to dextran. Similarly, vigorous resuscitation with saline solution should be avoided because it can worsen or precipitate a recurrent variceal hemorrhage and accumulation of ascites and fluid at other extravascular sites.[58] The thrombocytopenia that is usually encountered in these patients is now considered to impair not only primary hemostasis but also thrombin generation but the transfusion of fresh frozen plasma and platelets are not validated yet in larger studies and survival benefit in doing so has not been confirmed yet. The use of recombinant activated factor VII which corrects prothrombin time in cirrhotics has not been beneficial over standard therapy in preventing treatment failure and is not currently recommended. The gold standard for the diagnosis of variceal hemorrhage is endoscopy. Delayed endoscopy (defined as that performed 15 hours after admission) is a risk factor for in-hospital mortality. Current recommendation is to perform an emergent endoscopy within 6 hours of onset of AVB, which has shown to improve survival outcomes. Approximately 20% of cirrhosis patients with AVB have bacterial infections and another 50% will develop infections in hospital. SBP and spontaneous bacteremia are the most common, followed by urinary tract infections and pneumonia, a pattern that is changing with the rise of MDR strains in hospital, leading to pneumonia becoming a common cause these days.

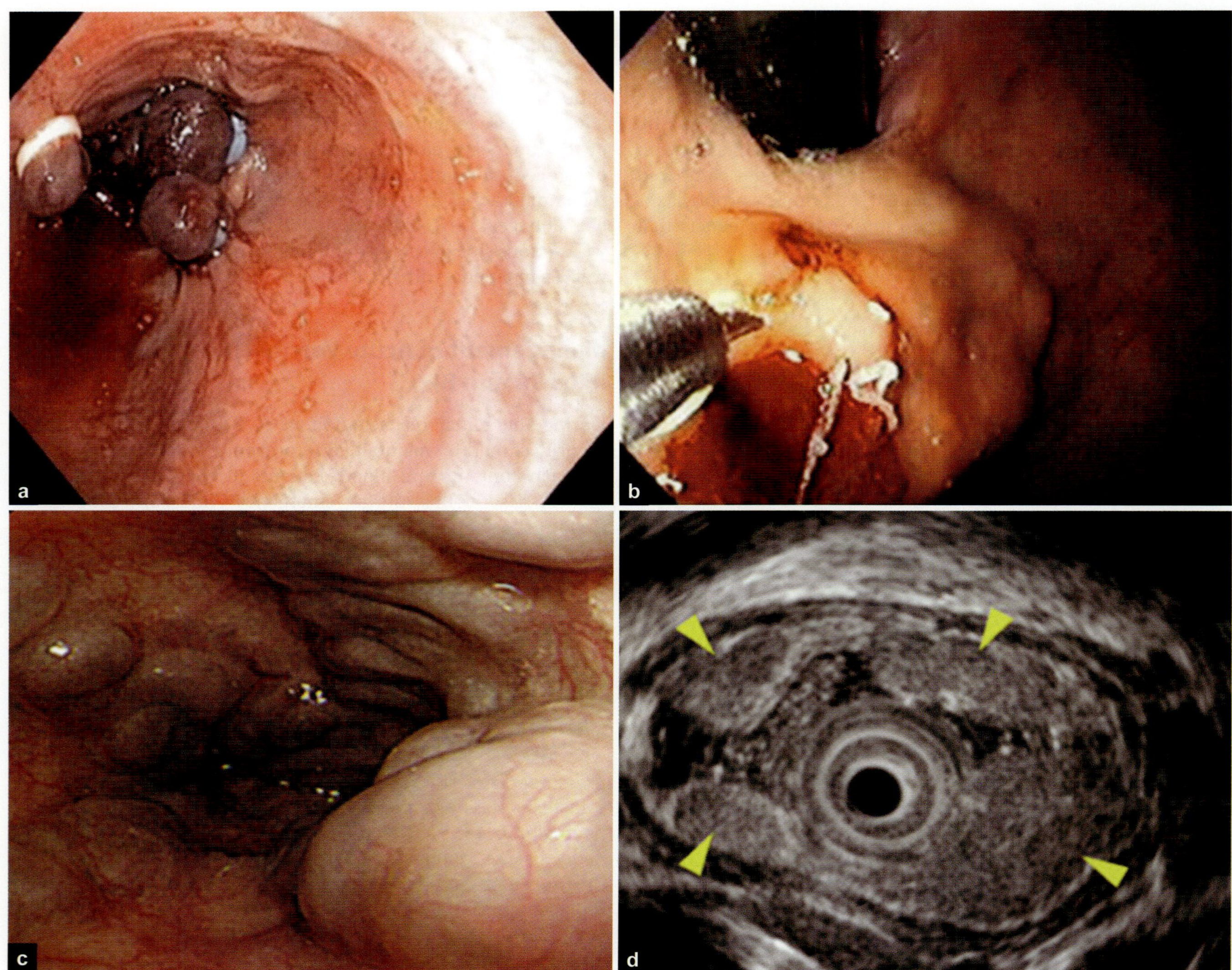

Figure 8A Management of acute variceal bleeding: (a) Endoscopic band ligation; (b) Endoscopic sclerotherapy; (c and d) Endoscopic ultrasonography guided variceal detection for coiling method
Modified from: Jae-Jun Shim. Clin Endosc. 2012 Sep;45(3):324–327.

Infection in the presence of AVB is a poor prognostic marker. Hence early antibiotic therapy improves survival in this cohort of patients. Recommendations currently state that oral norfloxacin, 400 mg twice daily, oral or intravenous for 7 days help decreasing infection rates in the event of AVB. Intravenous ceftriaxone is also a good option. Decrement of portal and variceal pressure can also be done with paracentesis of tense ascites under albumin cover. Kidney injury can occur in 11% of patients with AVB and has a dismal prognosis. The urine output should be maintained at a minimum of 40 mL per hour and those with urine output less than 20 mL per hour has a poor prognosis. After a period of 24 hours has passed, the feeding can be resumed. Treatment with vasoactive drugs alone controls bleeding in up to 83% of patients. Vasoactive drugs should be started as soon as possible, even before diagnostic confirmation. Current guidelines recommend continuing vasoactive drug treatment for 2–5 days, the time frame during which chances of rebleeding is more. Terlipressin is a synthetic analog of vasopressin with longer activity and fewer side effects. It reduces portal pressure and its effects last for about 4 hours after administration. Terlipressin helps in controlling AVB in 75–80% at 48 hours and 67% at day 5. It is the only drug that has been shown to improve survival. On the downside, terlipressin can provoke ischemic complications and severe dysrhythmias. Therefore, it should be used with extreme caution or even avoided in those patients with a history of ischemic heart or cerebral disease, limb or gut vascular disease or heart rhythm disorders. Terlipressin is given as a 2 g bolus dose every 4 hours during the first 2 days. The dose is halved after bleeding is controlled and can be maintained for up to 5 days. Somatostatin also causes splanchnic vasoconstriction at therapeutical doses and has proven to reduce portal pressure and HVPG during active bleeding. Additionally, somatostatin blocks the postprandial increase in portal blood flow and portal pressure. Major side effects with somatostatin are extremely rare. Somatostatin is usually given at a continuous

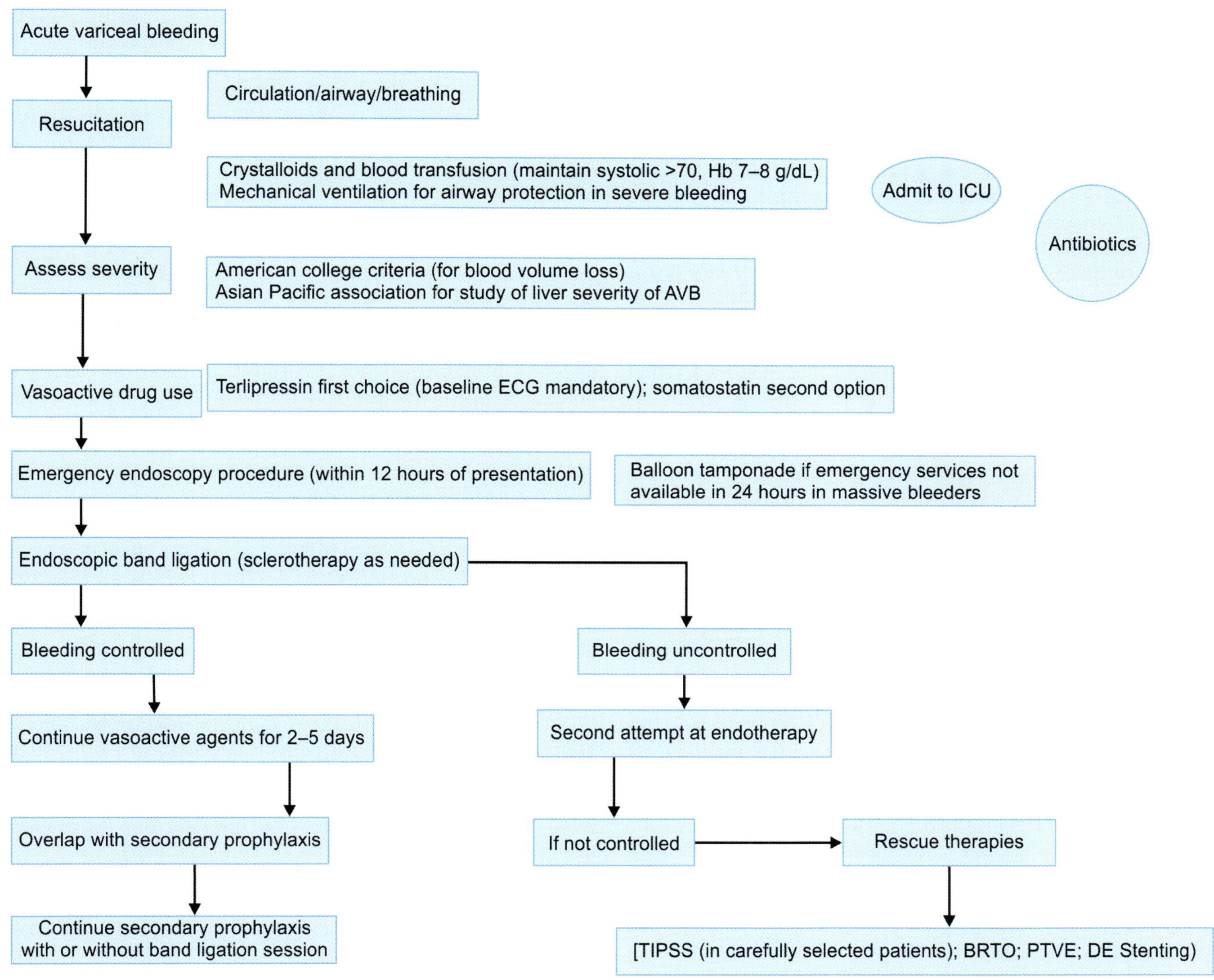

Figure 8B Algorithm for management of acute variceal bleeding
Abbreviations: ICU, intensive care unit; TIPSS, transjugular intrahepatic portosystemic shunt; BRTO, balloon retrograde transvenous obliteration; PTVE, percutaneous transvenous variceal obliteration; DE, Danis Ella stenting

perfusion dose of 250 µg/hour after an initial 250 µg bolus (which can be repeated up to 3 times during the first hour). The infusion should be maintained for 5 days or until a 24 hour period free of rebleeding has been achieved. The use of 500 µg/hour doses has been associated with greater decreases in HVPG, utilized in severe bleeding scenarios. Octreotide is a synthetic analog of natural somatostatin with similar mechanism of action and longer half-life. However, this does not result in longer hemodynamic effects, due to the development of tachyphylaxis. The drug is usually given in continuous infusion of 25–50 µg/hour with an optional initial intravenous or subcutaneous bolus of 50 µg. Vapreotide and lanreotide, two other synthetic somatostatin analogs have equal affinity for somatostatin receptors. The most potent splanchnic vasoconstrictor is vasopressin, which reduces vascular flow to all splanchnic organs and helps in reducing portal venous inflow and thereby, portal pressures. It is also associated adverse effects of cardiac and peripheral ischemia, hypertension, arrhythmias and has a non-tolerance withdrawal rate of 25%. Vasopressin is given at continuous intravenous infusion of 0.2–0.4 U/minute that can be increased to a maximal dose of 0.8 U/minute. It should always be used with intravenous nitroglycerine at a 40–400 µg/minute dose, adjusted to maintain blood pressure above 90 mm Hg. Endoscopic sclerotherapy (EST) alone controls active bleeding in at least 62% of patients.[59] Combined endoscopic and pharmacological therapy improves initial control of bleeding and decreases treatment failure when compared with either one of them alone. The combination endoscopic band ligation (EBL) along with vasoactive drugs is superior to EST-vasoactive drugs in terms of bleeding control. It has also been shown that EBL is better than EST in terms of controlling the initial bleeding and survival and is associated with less adverse events. Studies have shown that EST, but not EBL may induce sustained increases in HVPG which may affect control of bleeding and favor an early recurrence. Emergency EBL may be more difficult to perform in the presence of massive bleeding due to a more reduced field of view compared to EST. Even after current state of the art endoscopic therapy, 10–20% of patients will still experience treatment failure or early rebleeding. Rescue therapies then come into play and becomes a major factor in management of this subset of patients. Current guidelines recommend that failure of the initial combined treatment can be managed with a second attempt at endoscopic therapy. Balloon tamponade is a very effective measure in controlling the acute bleeding. The use of Sengstaken-Blakemore tube when a massive variceal bleeding is suspected allows initial control of bleeding in up to 80% of patients. It is associated with complications such as aspiration, asphyxia due to balloon ligation and esophagus perforation which are associated with a high mortality. Besides, bleeding recurs after deflation in over 50% of cases. Therefore, its use should be restricted to patients with uncontrollable bleeding for a short period of time (<24 hours) as a bridge to a more definitive therapy. Recently, esophageal stents have been proposed as an alternative to balloon tamponade in the initial control of massive variceal hemorrhages. These removable self-expanding devices were able to control initially refractory bleedings in 70–100% patients in three small non-controlled pilot studies. They have the advantage over tamponade of less severe complications and additional protection against early rebleeding since they can be left in place for up to 14 days. Both TIPSS and surgical shunt procedures are extremely effective in controlling variceal bleeding in patients who fail to respond to initial pharmacological and endoscopic therapies. However, the incidence of encephalopathy (50%) and mortality (30% in the first month) are untoward consequences, especially for patients with poor liver function (Child B or C). Final hemostasis with TIPSS is achieved in 90–95% of patients with uncontrolled bleeding. In patients with Child-Pugh score more than 13, early mortality after TIPSS is almost inevitable. For rapid stratification and aggressive sensible management, the patients at higher risk of complication should be rapidly identified. The hemodynamic criteria of HVPG ≥20 mm Hg for patient selection showed that TIPSS significantly reduced rebleeding and mortality without increasing the incidence of encephalopathy.[60] In summary, it is currently recommended to combine pharmacological and endoscopic therapies for the initial treatment of AVB. Vasoactive drugs (preferable somatostatin or terlipressin) should be started as soon as a variceal bleeding is suspected and maintained afterward for 2–5 days. Post stabilization, an emergency endoscopy must be done and endoscopic variceal treatment (ligation as first choice, sclerotherapy if EBL not feasible) should be performed. Antibiotic prophylaxis must be regarded as integral part of the treatment of AVB and should be started at admission and maintained for at least 7 days. In case of failure to control the acute bleeding, rescue therapies should be immediately started. Shunt therapies like TIPSS, are very effective at controlling treatment failures after AVB. In patients who survive the first episode of esophageal hemorrhage, the risk of recurrent bleeding is as high as 60% with a mortality rate of up to 33%. Secondary prophylaxis of variceal bleeding is defined as the prevention of rebleeding from varices. The nonselective beta-blockers propranolol or nadolol are helpful in reduction of the rebleeding risk as well as a reduction in mortality. Addition of nitrates further improves effect. Essential to management is a reduction of the HVPG of at least 20%, even if a reduction below 12 mm Hg. For prophylaxis of recurrent bleeding, sclerotherapy is now replaced widely by EBL. EBL along with medical management brings out the best effect in secondary prophylaxis. In patients who cannot tolerate beta blockers or have contraindications to beta blockers, EBL alone would suffice. TIPSS in comparison to EBL or sclerotherapy proved to have lesser rebleeding rates, albeit at the cost of development of hepatic encephalopathy. Shunt surgery has been shown to be effective in the prophylaxis of rebleeding from esophageal varices. The most important side effects were the incidence of hepatic encephalopathy.

Gastric Varices

Gastric varices (GV) are the second most common cause of upper GI bleed in patients of cirrhosis and PHT. Bleeding GV portend higher morbidity and mortality and is usually more severe than EV bleeding. GV are subtyped into those related to isolated splenic vein thrombosis (SVT) and those secondary to PHT (cirrhotic/non-cirrhotic). The isolated SVT related GV arise from short gastric veins and those due to PHT usually arise from splenorenal or gastrorenal shunts, in association with fundal varices. GV when associated with SVT are difficult to manage and are multiple, because they bleed recurrently through short gastric connections. Pancreatitis related SVT leading to bleeding GV is best managed with splenectomy. Classification of GV is according to Sarin et al. and other classification systems as shown in Figure 9. Sarin classification is based on the location and appearance of varices and another classification, known as the Japanese Vascular Classification, is based on the underlying vascular anatomy.[61] Thirty percent of all cirrhosis patients develop variceal bleeding and 10–20% of these are from GV. Fundal varices (which include Sarin class GOV2 or IGV1) are less common than varices over lesser curvature, i.e. GOV1. The risk of bleeding from incidentally detected fundal varices in cirrhosis is 16%, 36% and 44% at 1 year, 3 years and 5 years, respectively.[62] The drainage of GV into the systemic vasculature is by way of esophageal and paraesophageal varices, inferior phrenic vein or both. These correspond to Sarin classification well. GOV1 usually drains through the former and IGV1 through the latter and GOV2 through both. In the presence of an aberrant gastric vein, an accessory route of drainage forms through which embolic materials can migrate in to portal venous system during procedures such as balloon retrograde transvenous occlusion (BRTO), leading to liver failure.[63] Initial management of GV bleeding includes intravenous access and airway control and overaggressive volume resuscitation should be avoided as it can exacerbate PHT. During endoscopy, clearing the overlying fundal clot using a large-bore lavage tube (Edlich or Ewald Lavage tubes) is advisable. Conventional endoscopic approaches include usage of sclerosants or banding. It is recommended to combine banding with sclerosing therapy to minimize chances of rebleeding. Sengstaken-Blakemore or Minnesota tubes can be used to tamponade these bleeding varices. A target hematocrit level of 21% is acceptable and in the presence of an optimized platelet function a target of 25% for hematocrit is usually appropriate. The portal venous gradient is not very predictive of gastric variceal bleeding. If TIPSS is used as salvage in severe bleeding then it should be accompanied by bland embolization of the GV via a trans-TIPSS technique. BRTO is a good option for patients who are not good candidates for TIPSS (Fig. 10). Cyanoacrylate is the agent used for glue therapy in

Conn classification	Criteria
I	Flat varices–Disappearing when insufflating air within esophagus
II	Varices permanently visible in lumen but appearing in well bands
III	Varices that are extremely prominent in lumen so that they appear to almost occlude the lumen of esophagus when not inflated

NIEC classification	
Size	FI-small, straight FII-medium-occupying <1/3rd of esophageal lumen FIII-large-tortuous, occuping >1/3rd of esophageal lumen
Red color sign (rwm, crs, hcs)	–nt–No RCS Mild–>10 lesions Moderate–>10 lesions Severe–extensive, +nt on all varices

Japanese society classification	Code	Subcategory
Location	L	Longitudinal extent • Ls-Locus superior (above level of tracheal bifurcation) • Lm-Locus medialis (at/near level of tracheal bifurcation) • Li-Locus inferior (within abdominal and lower thoracic esophagus) • Lg-Locus gastric • Lg-c-Gastric varices adjacent to cardia
Form	F	Shape and size F0-Lesions assuming varicose appearance F1-Small, straight F2-Moderately enlarged, beady varices F3-Markedly enlarged, nodular or tumor shaped
Colour	C	Fundamental color Cw-White varices Cb-Blue varices
Red color sign	RC	RC-, +, ++, +++ Red wale markings (RWM) Cherry red spot (CRS) Hematocystic spot (HCS) Telangiectasia (TE +)
Bleeding sign	B	During bleedingspurting, oozing after hemostasis–red plug, white plug
Mucosal finding	E Ul S	Erosion Ulcer Scar

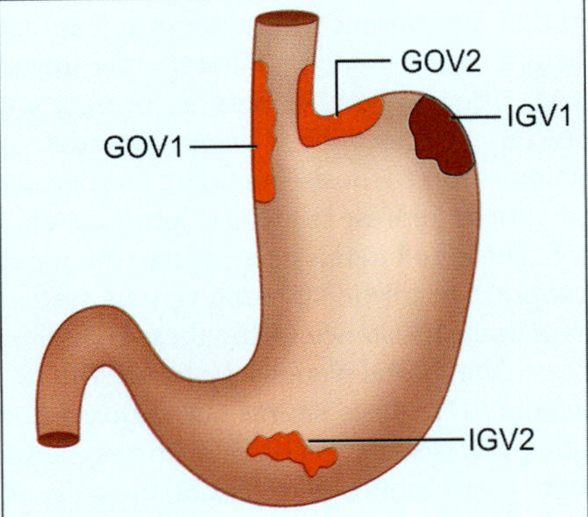

A. Gastroesophageal varices–gastric varices in continuity with esophageal varices
GEV1–along lesser curvature (usually 2 to 5 cm in length)
GEV2–along the greater curvature extending towards the gastric fundus

B. Isolated gastric varices
IGV1–isolated cluster of gastric varices in the gastric fundus
IGV2–isolated gastric varices in other parts of the stomach

Sarin classification of gastric varices

Hashizume classification of gastric varices

Form-three type tortuous (F1), nodular (F2), and tumorous (F3)

Location-five types Anterior (La), posterior (Lp), lesser (Ll) and greater curvature (Lg) of the cardia, and fundic area (Lf)

Color can be white (Cw) or red (Cr)

The glossy, thin-walled focal redness on the varix was defined as red color spot (RC spot)

Figure 9 Various classifications of esophageal and gastric varices

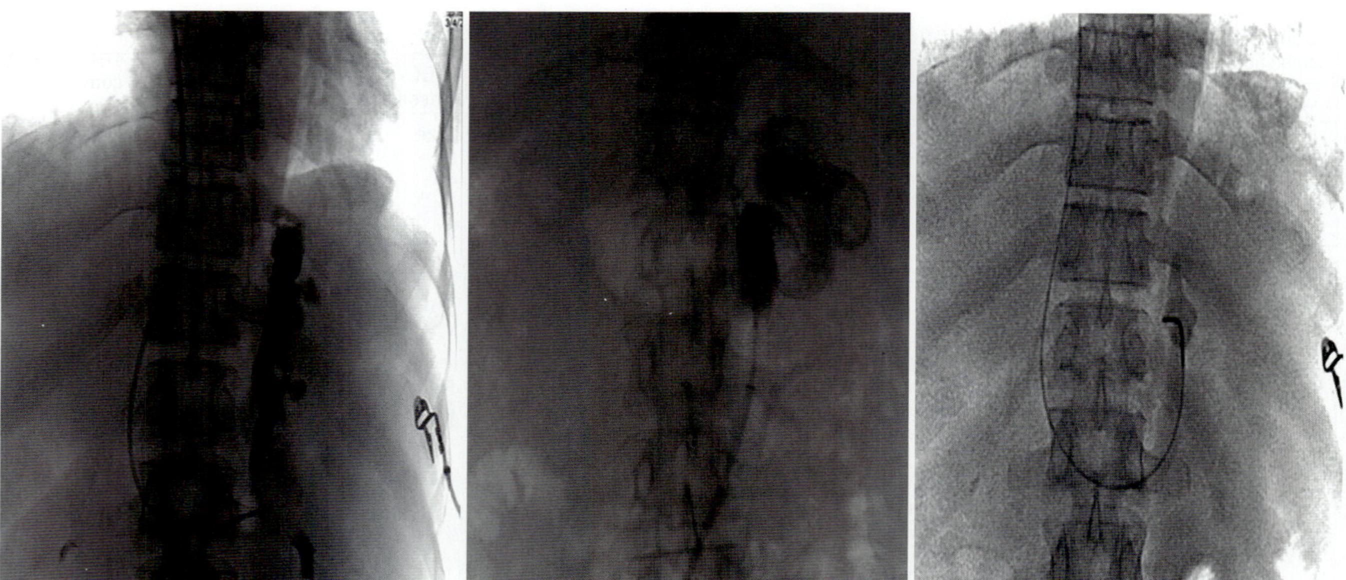

Figure 10 Balloon retrograde transvenous occlusion procedure for management of gastric varices by way of shunt occlusion. The last image shows complete obliteration of gastric varcies

bleeding GV. These agents have a basic monomeric structure that has a reactive cyano (nitrile) group and an alkoxycarbonyl group of different carbon chain length. This therapy is the recommended first-line therapy in bleeding GV. The initial control of bleeding is in the range of 90–100% and rebleeding rates are less than 15.[64] The presence of large systemic shunts must always be looked for before BRTO procedure because shunts are associated with the risk for systemic glue embolism. The characteristics of glue therapy are shown in the Table 3. The initial session of GV endotherapy is always aimed at complete variceal obturation, including tributaries and a reassessment is done 4 weeks later to confirm GV obliteration and/or to treat residual varices. In the event of complete variceal obliteration, repeat endoscopies are performed at 3–6 month intervals. Glue cast is visible for weeks to months after endotherapy and the adverse effects include early glue cast extrusion and associated bleeding, distant glue embolism and post-endotherapy bacteremia and sepsis. The use of endoscopic ultrasonography guided coiling and/or glue injection or combined endoscopic cyanoacrylate injection with angiographic balloon occlusion of shunt can minimize systemic embolization. Thrombin injection and use of fibrin sealants are other modalities for GV bleeding, but thrombin embolization could promote disseminated intravascular coagulation or pulmonary embolism. For GOVs, when most options have failed, then percutaneous transhepatic obliteration could be considered as another treatment option.[65] BRTO (in which sclerosant instillation into gastric varix through a balloon occluding catheter placed through shunt is done) can be used to completely obliterate GOV with lower recurrent bleeding rates. This often results in increased portal pressures after large portosystemic venous shunt occlusion and can aggravate esophageal variceal grading, bleeding and/or worsening of ascites (other adverse effects include fever, pleural effusions and development of EV in 66% of patients). The utility of BRTO is applicable in the presence of gastrorenal shunts, seen in up to 85% of patients with GV. When partial splenic artery embolization before BRTO is done, there is significant reduction in EV formation or worsening of existing EV. Flow chart 4 summarizes the algorithm for management of gastric variceal bleeding.[66-68]

Ectopic Varices (Fig. 11)

Ectopic varices are abnormally dilated veins associated with gastrointestinal mucosa with propensity for gastrointestinal hemorrhage. Sometimes it is also loosely used for portosystemic collaterals in the abdominal wall and retroperitoneum. Ectopic varices are best described as large pressurized portosystemic venous collaterals occurring anywhere in the abdomen except in the gastroesophageal region. They account for up to 5% of all variceal bleeding. They may be present in duodenum, jejunum, ileum, colon, anorectum, peristomal, biliary, peritoneal, retroperitoneal, umbilical, urinary bladder, uterine, ovaries and other locations. Anorectal varices have been reported in approximately 44% of patients with cirrhosis, but only a few become symptomatic.[67] Ectopic varices represent natural portosystemic shunts secondary to PHT. These collaterals occur where the portal venous system is in juxtaposition to the systemic venous system. Under normal circumstances the resistance within these collaterals is high, while it is low in the portal venous system. With the development of intrahepatic PHT, these shunts act to divert flow from the increased intrahepatic vascular resistance. Portosystemic communications through gastroesophageal plexus to azygous-coronary system, hemorrhoidal plexus, recanalized umbilical vein, and pancreatoduodenal venous arcade to inferior vena cava through retroperitoneal veins of Retzius occur to form ectopic varices. Most reported cases of hemorrhage from ectopic varices in the West are associated with intrahepatic PHT in contrast to extrahepatic PHT. Prior abdominal surgery predisposes patients with PHT to develop varices in unusual locations, like urinary bladder, ovaries and bare area of the liver due to adhesions. Ectopic varices can also develop in the absence of PHT due to congenital

Table 12: Glue therapy characteristics in management of gastric variceal bleeding. The endoscopic real time images from left to right shows a large actively bleeding GOV2 into which cyanoacrylate injection is performed, which later on forms a glue cast with stoppage of bleeding

Characteristic	*N-butyl 2-cyanoacrylate*	*Octyl-2-cyanoacrylate*
Mixed with lipidol	Yes	No
Injected volume per puncture site	1:1	N/A
Maximum volume per treatment session	</= 5 mL	</= 10 mL
A dedicated 21-grauge injection catheter is recommeded; Distilled water or normal saline can be used both for catheter priming and flushing of glue		

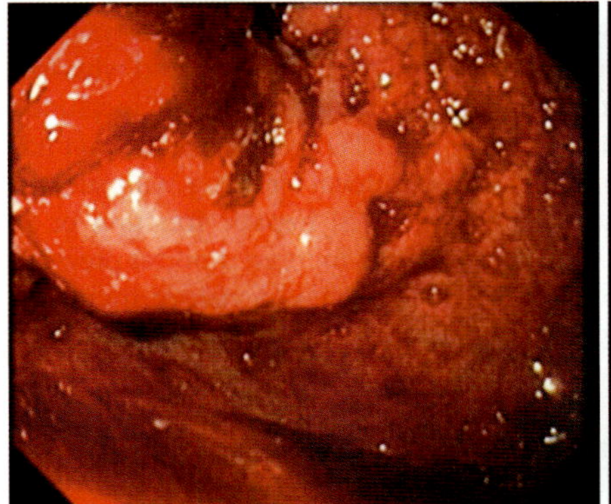
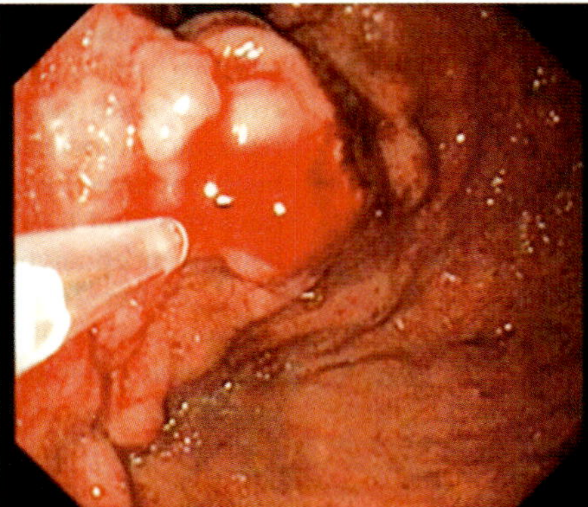
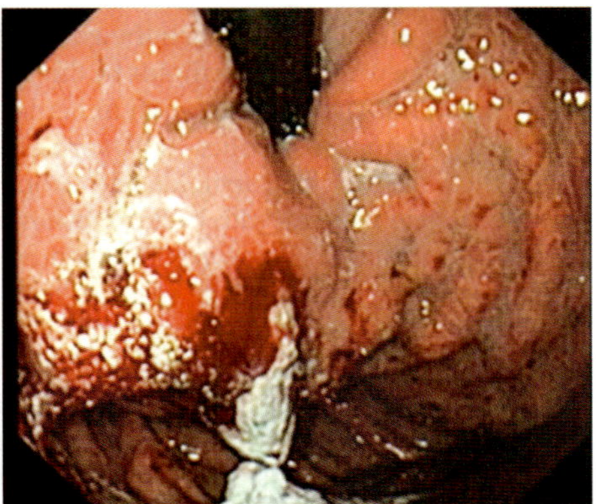

Flow chart 4 Algorithm for management of gastric variceal bleeding

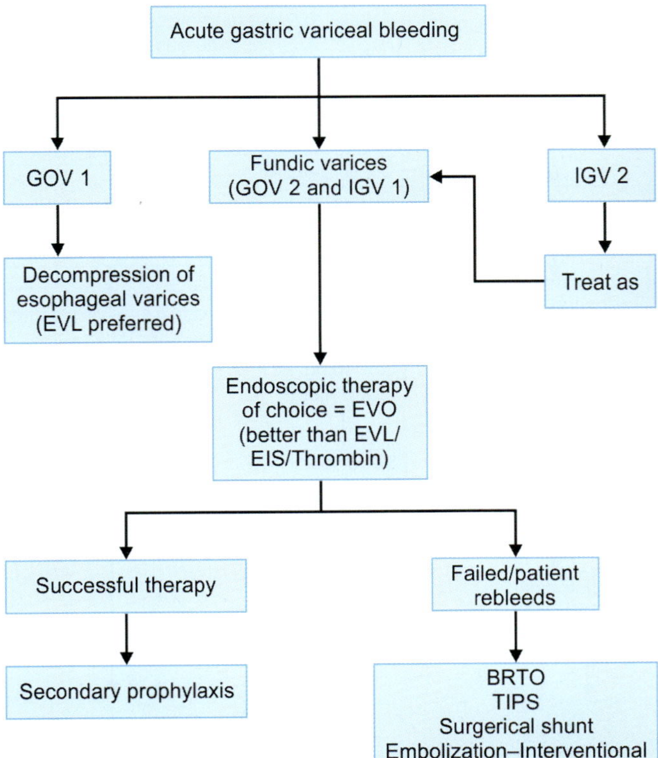

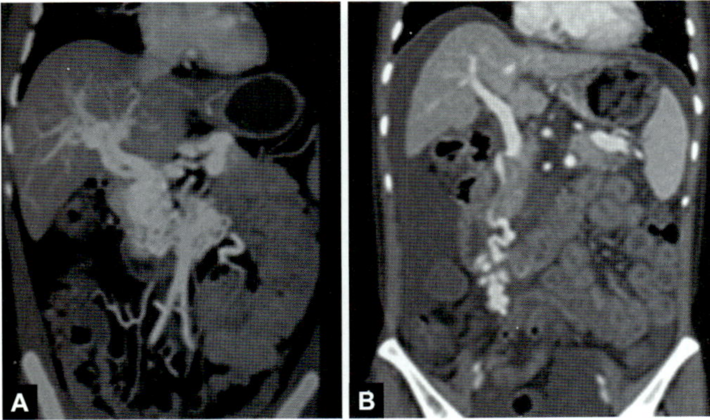

Figures 11A and B Computed tomography of the abdomen showing large ectopic varices near the porta (A) and presence of jejunal ectopic varices (B)

anomalous portosystemic anastomoses, abnormal vessel structures arteriovenous fistulae and as part of rare familial condition or related to thrombosis.[69] Ectopic varices, like GV may bleed at a portosystemic gradient of less than 12 mm Hg. Ectopic varices present in a multitude of ways. They may manifest with mild or massive hematemesis or lower gastrointestinal bleeding; with hematochezia, melena, or intraperitoneal bleeding; urinary bladder varices may present with hematuria and biliary varices with biliary obstruction or hemobilia. Ruptured varices at the right diaphragm can cause hemothoraces and dyspnea. Abdominal wall varices can rupture externally or internally, whereas those located around the falciform ligament, diaphragm, splenic ligament or in the rectovesical region may rupture into the peritoneal cavity, leading to occult, potentially fatal intraperitoneal hemorrhage. Presence of ectopic varices should be strongly considered in patients with known liver disease or stigmata of PHT particularly when both upper and lower endoscopies fail to identify a source of bleeding. Detection of small bowel varices can be accomplished through elective capsule endoscopy, double balloon enteroscopy or push enteroscopy modalities. Hemodynamic assessment of rectal and Biliary varices can be achieved using endoscopic ultrasonography whereas gall bladder, duodenal, umbilical and choledochal varices can also be assessed using color Doppler ultrasonography. Most common cause of duodenal varices is cirrhosis (30%). Such varices develop from collateral veins that begin from portal vein or superior mesenteric vein which drain into inferior vena cava through retroperitoneal veins (veins of Retzius). Variceal bleeding from duodenal sites can lead to severe bleeding and mortality as high as 40% in the first episode. A triad of PHT, hematochezia without hematemesis and prior abdominal surgery characterize bleeding from small intestinal varices.[69] These varices most commonly flow into systemic circulation through the gonadal veins. Rectal varices are distinguished from hemorrhoids by their typical presence above the dentate line. The differentiation of hemorrhoids and anorectal varices is an important one. Anal varices collapse with digital pressure, whereas hemorrhoids do not. The prevalence of hemorrhoids in patients with liver disease is not higher than in the general population. These varices represent a portosystemic collateral pathway between the superior rectal veins of the inferior mesenteric system to the middle and inferior rectal veins of the iliac system. They can be present with mild or uncontrolled hematochezia. Ganguly and coworkers described rectal varices as dilated veins originating more than four centimeters above the anal verge and not contiguous with the anal column or pectinate line. Classification of rectal varices was done endoscopically as Grade1, <3 mm; Grade 2, 3–6 mm and Grade 3, >6 mm. Lower gastrointestinal bleeding secondary to rectal varices was based on three parameters—evidence of rectal varices and fresh blood in rectum, the sigmoid colon should not contain fresh blood and there should be absence of hemorrhoids and/or colopathy. Commonest sites of rectal varices are cecum and rectum and isolated colonic varices are a rarity. Abnormally dilated veins that develop in stomal mucosa with a purplish hue around the stomal region were called ectopic stomal varices, which are commonly found in patients with intrahepatic PHT secondary to PSC and also in patients who undergo ileostomies after proctocolectomy for inflammatory bowel disease associated with PSC. In extrahepatic portal vein thrombosis, gall bladder and common bile duct varices can occur in as many as 30% of patients.[69] The appearance of biliary tree, by direct endoscopic retrograde cholangiopancreatography may mimic that of PSC, and is termed as pseudosclerosing cholangitis. Biliary varices can lead to hemobilia or even catastrophic bleeding diathesis. The urinary bladder wall is an unusual collateral route for venous splanchnic blood flow and these varices may develop after abdominal surgery secondary to adhesions. Bleeding from vesical varices is a rare event in patients with PHT and an unusual cause of hematuria. Other more unusual sites include right diaphragm, splenorenal ligament, splenoparametrial, adnexal, vaginal, umbilical and cutaneous varices leading to unusual clinical signs. The management of ectopic varices and hemoperitoneum secondary to ectopic variceal bleeding is shown in Flow chart 5. The management depends upon location of bleeding, presentation, local physician expertise, and the underlying causes of PHT. Many ectopic varices can be managed by standard endoscopic methods and with the advent of double balloon or push enteroscopy, therapeutic aggressiveness has evolved further. The options include EBL and endoscopic injection sclerotherapy (EST) with different agents including N-butyl-2-cyanoacrylate (NBCA), thrombin or other sclerosants. EBL was found to be superior to EST. Sclerotherapy may lead to deep ulceration, which can lead to rebleeding, stricture formation, or perforation. Combination of two in the form of endoscopic scleroligation (ESL) has shown to be superior with decreased recurrence rates. Multiple options include image-guided direct percutaneous access to varices, antegrade and retrograde sclerotherapy and/or embolotherapy and portosystemic shunts.[70] Transjugular and transhepatic as well as retrograde transjugular or transfemoral venous approaches have been useful. TIPSS have proven more effective in preventing recurrent esophageal variceal rebleeding than endoscopic therapy. It has been shown that a more than 50% reduction in pressure gradient protected patients from rebleeding and even a reduction between 25% and 50% was also effective, with a probability of rebleeding of only 7% and with less risk of encephalopathy and liver failure. Balloon occluded retrograde transvenous obliteration (BRTO) is a technique that has been employed for control of gastric variceal bleeding, with success rates reaching 89% without detriment in hepatic function or in hepatic encephalopathy. However, since increased portal pressure is not addressed by this procedure, there is a risk of increased pressure and bleeding from varices that have not been sclerosed and are at other sites, or development of ascites. Aggravation of esophageal varices is recognized after BRTO of GV. Percutaneous embolization using a transhepatic approach has shown successful

Flow chart 5 Algorithm for management of ectopic variceal bleed and hemoperitoneum secondary to ectopic variceal bleed

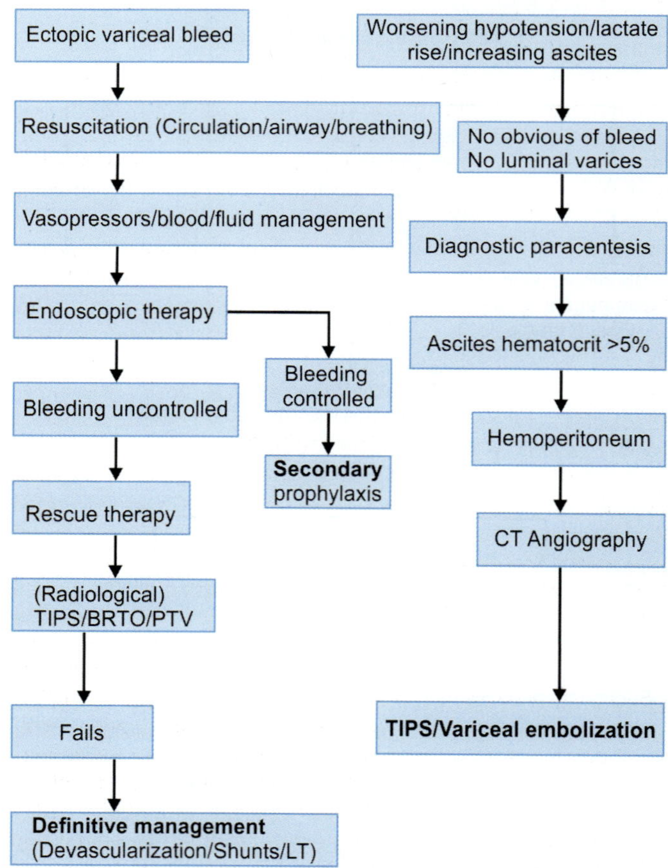

Source: Modified from Sarin and Kumar, Clinics in Liver Diseases (November 2011).

embolization rates that reach 80%, with up to 65% rebleeding rate within 5 month. Its added risks include transhepatic tract bleeding, recurrent hemorrhage due to lack of secondary portal decompression, and added contraindications in ascites patients. Surgery may be considered a salvage option in select patients when endoscopic and interventional radiological procedures have failed. These include distal splenorenal shunts, portocaval shunts, mesocaval shunts and devascularization procedures.[71]

HEPATOPULMONARY SYNDROME

Hepatopulmonary syndrome is defined by the triad that includes liver disease, pulmonary gas exchange abnormalities leading to arterial deoxygenation in the presence of intrapulmonary vasodilatations. It occurs in 4–47% of cirrhosis patients in multiple studies. Fluckiger in 1884 noted the relationship between lung and liver in cirrhosis patient, based on observations in female who had clinical features of cirrhosis, finger clubbing and cyanosis.[72] Kennedy and Knudson, a century later described HPS clinicopathologically as hypoxemia in a cirrhosis patient with intrapulmonary vascular channel dilatations. Presence of underlying liver disease is not mandatory for HPS, as it can be seen in milder form of liver disease, acute forms of liver disease and also in non-cirrhotic patients. HPS is considered an independent risk factor of mortality in cirrhosis patients. Berthelot in 1966 described the pathologic changes associated with HPS as widespread dilatation of pulmonary microvasculature which involved the pulmonary precapillary and alveolar capillary beds. This resulted in ventilation perfusion mismatch, shunting and diffusion limitation, which were the cardinal pathological mechanisms that perpetuated HPS. Over perfusion in the alveolar capillary bed, most importantly in the dependent lower zones, leads to ventilation perfusion mismatch which further worsened with blunted vasoconstrictor response to hypoxemic stimulus. The distance between the oxygen diffusion from the alveolus to the red blood cells in the center of the alveolar capillary bed increases because of pulmonary microvessel dilatation, thereby forming a functional diffusion barrier to gas exchange. This is further worsened by a hyperdynamic circulation secondary to PHT. Nitric oxide (NO) plays a central role in mediating pulmonary vasodilatation, as it plays in systemic and splanchnic vasodilatation in cirrhosis. L-arginine is the substrate from which NO is synthesized, by action of NO synthetase (NOS) which is of three isoforms: (1) inducible (iNOS), (2) endothelial (eNOS) and (3) neuronal (nNOS). The former two are increased in pulmonary capillary bed in cirrhosis patients who develop HPS. iNOS present in the pulmonary intravascular monocytes get activated to produce proinflammatory cytokines such as TNF-α which further leads to upregulation of iNOS. Gut bacterial translocation and bacterial overgrowth leads to endotoxemic effects in the lung by which further proinflammatory cytokines upregulation develops, leading to increment in iNOS. It has been shown that selective gut decontamination with fluroquinolones (norfloxacin) improves iNOS (normalization) upregulation, thereby diminishing HPS expression in animal models. Activation of endothelin-B receptors by endothelin-1 (ET-1, ET-B) leads to NO related vasodilatation in pulmonary vasculature, an effect that selectively occurs in lung bed rather than the systemic vasculature, as a result of increase in eNOS. Carbon monoxide (CO) mediates vasodilation through stimulation of cGMP production in vascular smooth muscle cells. In patients of HPS, there is increase in arterial carboxyhemoglobin leading to augmentation of vasodilatation in pulmonary vessels. Apart from these mechanisms, pulmonary angiogenesis is also implicated in pathogenesis of HPS; this is as a result of accumulation of pulmonary intravascular monocytes (secondary to increased TNF-alpha signaling). In the alveolar-capillary oxygen disequilibrium theory of HPS pathogenesis, the capillary dilatation leads to oxygen molecules from adjacent alveoli being unable to permeate sufficiently to the center of the dilated vessel.[73] Decrease in hemoglobin oxygenation leads to hypoxemia, which can be partially overcome with the use of supplemental oxygen therapy. Only 50% of HPS patients have underlying cirrhosis. Typical symptoms include platypnea (difficulty in breathing in the erect posture) and orthodeoxia (hypoxia worsening in erect posture). Clubbing of digits is commonly seen and severe HPS patients can have cyanosis at rest. Pulse oximetry is the best screening tool for HPS with a value cut off at 97% showing high sensitivity and moderate specificity for PaO_2 of 70 mm Hg. Confirmation can be done by arterial blood gas analysis in sitting and standing position, with patient breathing room air. An increased alveolar to arterial oxygen gradient is a very sensitive indicator of HPS with recommended cut off values for HPS diagnosis being PaO_2 80 mm Hg or $PAaO_2$ of 15 mm Hg, except in patients older than 64 years where in the cut off of PaO_2 of 70 mm Hg or $PAaO_2$ of 20 mm Hg. Alveolar septal capillaries have a normal diameter of 7–15 microns, but in HPS, intrapulmonary capillary dilatation as much as 500 microns have been seen. The intrapulmonary dilatations are of two types in HPS. Type I lesions are most common and are diffuse dilatations at the precapillary level that are close to normal gas exchange units of lung and Type II lesions, which are more discrete and focal, localized dilatations which are rare large arteriovenous communications are seen to be away from the gas exchange units. Clinically types of dilatations are significant because supplementary oxygen improves hypoxemia in Type I but not Type II HPS (where in there is true anatomical shunting present).[73] Assessment of intrapulmonary dilatation are of two types—in the first one, contrast echocardiography is used, most often using microbubbles as the contrast, and in the second, the radioactive lung perfusion scan using macroaggregated albumin (MAA) is used. More sensitivity was seen with bubble contrast echo which is less invasive, easily available and can also exclude intracardiac shunting in comparison to MAA scan. In the former, the saline is shaken vigorously (usually three times) which result in development of microbubbles. This is then injected into an arm vein and the cardiac chambers are observed through trasnthoracic ultrasonography. In the normal situation, the bubbles, which are more than 25 mm in diameter, are trapped in the alveolar capillary bed (vessel diameter of 5–8 mm) and their appearance in left atrium usually after 5–6 cardiac cycles signifies presence of intrapulmonary shunting. If the appearance is within three cardiac cycles in the left chamber (after initial appearance in right chamber), an intracardiac shunt is suspected. In MAA scan, radiolabelled Technitium-99 MAA particles are injected into a peripheral vein and whole body scanning is done to estimate the extrapulmonary shunt fraction. These particles are of 10–90 mm in diameter and are normally removed in the pulmonary circulation and the presence of more than 6% of fraction of MAA particles in the brain is suggestive of pulmonary shunting and presence of

HPS. MAA scan is highly specific, but sensitivity is poor in comparison to contrast echo because it does not detect intracardiac shunting and fails to detect intrapulmonary shunting in the absence of hypoxia. However, it is a useful modality to assess for HPS in the presence of underlying lung disease and is advantageous as it is also quantitative, thereby giving an idea of severity of shunting. Pulmonary angiography is helpful in patients with large arteriovenous shunts and is beneficial because it can also act as a therapeutic option by way of radiological coil embolization of the shunt. The severity of HPS is classified as mild when the PaO_2 is more than or equal to 80 mm Hg, moderate when PaO_2 is less than 80 mm Hg or more than or equal to 60 mm Hg, severe when PaO_2 is less than 60 mm Hg or more than or equal to 50 mm Hg and very severe when PaO_2 is less than 50 mm Hg. Cirrhosis patients with HPS have a 5-year survival rate of 23% without liver transplantation in comparison to 63% 5-year survival in matched cirrhotic controls without HPS. The prognosis is worst when there is severe hypoxia, and most patients with PaO_2 <60 mm Hg die within 6 months. For this reason, cirrhosis patients with HPS associated with PaO_2 <60 mm Hg get MELD exception points and transplant priority.[74] Medical management includes the following: pentoxifylline (PTX) is a nonspecific phosphodiesterase inhibitor that non-specifically inhibits tumor necrosis factor-alpha (TNF-α). It has also other anti-inflammatory properties including inhibition of monocyte chemoattractant protein-1 (MCP-1), macrophage inhibitory protein-1 (MIP-1), interleukin-6 and interleukin-8, decreased expression of adhesion molecules and decreased activation and proliferation of neutrophils. PTX has been widely used in peripheral vascular diseases like intermittent claudication, in vascular dementia and with corticosteroid in alcoholic hepatitis. PTX has mainly two characteristics which justify its use in HPS—one, its inhibitory effect on iNOS leading to subsequent decrease in NO production and two, the newly found PTX effect on downregulation of angiogenesis. Studies have shown the beneficial effect of this medication in improvement of dyspnea, palmar erythema, and cyanosis. PTX therapy was also associated with marked improvement in arterial O_2 pressure, exercise-induced change in oxygen, and decreased median levels of TNF-α without significant adverse reaction. Methylene blue (MB) has been used in medicine as a contrast agent for diagnostic purposes like chromoendoscopy, for the treatment of methemoglobinemia and recently for septic shock due to its inhibitory effect on NO-induced vasodilatation. The vasoconstrictor effect of MB results from its inhibitory influence on activation of soluble guanylate cyclase by NO. There are reported effects of MB in decreasing cardiac output, pulmonary artery pressure and increasing systemic vascular resistance, and pulmonary vascular resistance. Improvement of HPS after intravenous infusion of MB at 3 mg per kilogram has been reported. MB can also be used to improve hypoxemia and reduce post liver transplant complications. The useful effect of MB in improvement of HPS can be attributed to its inhibitory effect on NOS activity and subsequent reduction of NO which is a potent vasodilator of pulmonary vasculature. MB administration has been shown to ameliorate angiogenesis, another main mechanism in HPS, possibly by acting through inhibition of VEGF and PDGF dependent pathways. The treatment of bacterial overgrowth in the gut for the prevention of bacterial translocation may be helpful to control HPS via suppression of NO synthesis. Norfloxacin, an active quinolone antibiotic against Gram-negative bacteria, has been a candidate because of its potential to prevent bacterial translocation. Irrespective of the underlying mechanism, garlic (Allivum sativum) has been used in patients with HPS. Improvement of HPS with *garlic capsule* (once daily for 6 months) was also observed in a pilot trial among 15 patients with HPS. Abrams and Fallon explained that garlic therapy leads to redistribution of pulmonary blood flow to mid and apical portions of lungs as a result of uniform vasodilation. This resulted in an improvement in ventilation/perfusion ratio and HPS. Another probable mechanism is the antiangiogenesis properties of garlic which has been shown in some studies. Targeting NO pathway is supposed to be a therapeutic option in treatment of HPS. In an experimental study, oral administration of an inhibitor of NOS activity, NG-nitro-L-arginine methyl ester (L-NAME), was shown to decrease NO synthesis and prevent HPS in a rat model of cirrhosis. However, inhaled L-NAME was not able to ameliorate HPS in cirrhotic patients despite the decreased NO. *Quercetin* is a major flavonoid in human diet with several beneficial effects on human health. Quercetin has been reported to be effective in decreasing oxidative stress, nuclear translocation of NF-κB, expression of NOS, HO-1, and endothelin B (ET-B) receptor and improvement of HPS. *Mycophenolate mofetil (MMF)* which inhibits NO production shows significant improvement of clinical signs including clubbing, cyanosis, and spider nevi. *Sorafenib,* a multikinase inhibitor targeting several signaling pathways has been successfully used in rat model of cirrhosis for prevention of HPS and shown to reduce alveolar-arterial oxygen gradient and intrapulmonary shunting. *Iloprost* is a synthetic analog of prostacyclin (PGI2) which is frequently used intravenously for the treatment of pulmonary hypertension. Inhaled iloprost is an alternative form of PGI2 which is approved for the treatment of pulmonary hypertension. Inhaled iloprost has been applied for the treatment of HPS in post-transplant period and was outlined to be effective in the improvement of clinical symptoms and hypoxemia. *N-acetyl cysteine,* an inhibitor of reactive oxygen species, has been shown to attenuate HPS in rat models of cirrhosis. *Caffeic Acid Phenethyl Ester (CAPE)* is an antioxidant, anti-inflammatory agent which has shown to reduce NO synthesis and inhibit pulmonary fibrosis. Beneficial effects of CAPE has been shown in rat models where in decreased levels of NO was seen associated with decreased pulmonary vasodilatation. The only curative treatment for HPS is *liver transplantation.* Increased mortality is evident post-transplant when the PaO_2 is less than 50 mm Hg and/or the shunt fraction in more than 20% pretransplant (mortality rate—67%). The ideal transplant window for HPS patients is when the PaO_2 is less than 60% and they receive prioritization for transplant. TIPSS is of no value in improving survival rates in cirrhosis patients with HPS. In some patients with Type II HPS, *intra-arterial coil embolization* helps in improving right to left shunting.[75]

PORTOPULMONARY HYPERTENSION

Pulmonary arterial hypertension (PAH) in the setting of PHT is called portopulmonary hypertension (POPH). The world Symposium on Pulmonary Hypertension, convened at Dana Point in 2008 defined PAH as an increase in mean pulmonary artery pressure (MPAP) to 25 mm Hg, confirmed using right heart catheterization techniques. Mild POPH is when the MPAP is less than 35 mm Hg and is common in patients of cirrhosis. MPAP of 35–45 mm Hg (moderate) and those above 45 mm Hg (severe) is associated with high mortality and procures MELD exception points. Severe

POPH is a contraindication to liver transplantation in the event of no improvement with medical therapy. In the presence of MPAP more than 35 mm Hg the mortality rate post-transplant is 50% and it is 100% if the MPAP is more than 50 mm Hg.[75] A pulmonary vascular resistance (PVR) more than or equal to 240 dyn s cm^{-5} and pulmonary wedge pressure less than or equal to 15 mm Hg is seen in association with POPH. The use of transpulmonary gradient, i.e. TPG which is equal to MPAP—wedge pulmonary pressure is useful for assessment of POPH in the presence of fluid overloaded states. The presence of increased PVR, high pulmonary venous pressure and high cardiac output promotes POPH. Routine screening of cirrhosis patients can reveal an increased right ventricular systolic pressure (RVSP) based on tricuspid regurgitant velocity (measures on echocardiography). RVSP is measured using Bernoulli equation where in, RVSP = 4 × TR^2 (tricuspid regurgitant peak velocity) + RAP (right atrial pressure). The pathophysiology of POPH[76] is shown in Figure 12. POPH is seen in 6–8% of patients with cirrhosis and some studies show that female sex and autoimmune disease were important risk factors for development of POPH. Single-nucleotide polymorphisms of estrogen receptor 1, aromatase, phosphodiesterase 5 (PDE5), angiopoietin 1, and calcium binding protein A4 have been found to predispose cirrhosis patients to POPH. Factors like endothelial remodeling, uncontrolled and dysregulated vasoconstriction, arterial smooth muscle proliferation in association with microvascular thrombosis are involved in pathogenesis of POPH. The histopathology changes of POPH include medial hypertrophy, intimal proliferation and adventitial fibrosis in small muscular pulmonary arteries. The plexiform lesion is a characteristic finding in all forms of PAH. It results from proliferation of endothelial cells, usually in the more distal branches of the pulmonary artery. In situ thrombosis

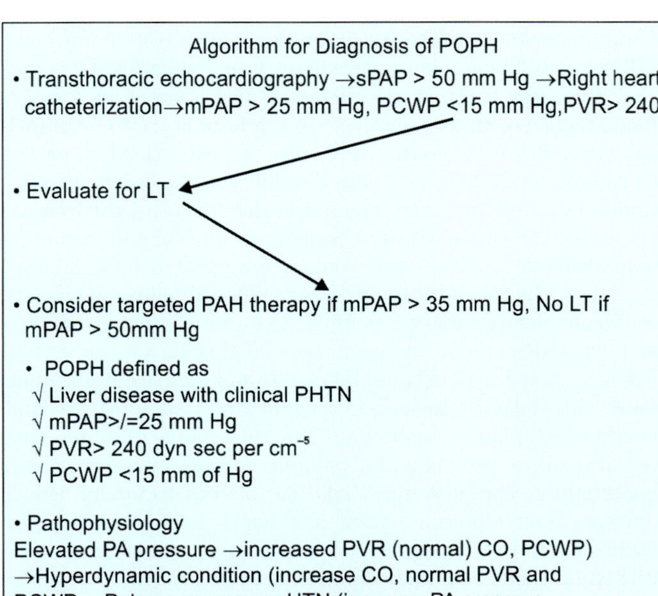

Figure 12 Brief review of portopulmonary hypertension (POPH)
Abbreviations: mPAP, mean pulmonary artery pressure, PCWP, pulmonary capillary wedge pressure; PVR, pulmonary vascular resistance; CO, cardiac output.

in the pulmonary vasculature has been attributed to the loss of endothelial processes that usually prevent clot formation which leads to aggravation of POPH.

Endothelin-1 and IL-6 are elevated in patients of POPH. Exertional dyspnea can be a presenting feature. A loud second heart sound (pulmonic component) is seen in 82% of patients and 61% of patients can have a systolic murmur in the pulmonary region (functional flow murmur).[77] The presence of low cardiac index and increasing severity of cirrhosis (Child C vs A or B) are directly associated with mortality in POPH. The treatment of POPH involves vasodilator therapy to control hemodynamics after which patients are deemed fit to undergo liver transplantation. Prostaglandin use in POPH is justified in the presence of low levels of circulating endogenous prostacyclin. The synthetic prostaglandin I2 (PGI2) or epoprostenol, derived from the metabolism of arachidonic acid, a powerful pulmonary and systemic vasodilator which has potent inhibitor activity of platelet aggregation was approved for management of PAH. The action is mediated through modulation of pulmonary vascular remodeling. The half-life of epoprostenol is 3–5 minutes and it is delivered continuously by a special pump. Adverse effects consist of flushing, vomiting, jaw pain, nausea, diarrhea, vascular access sepsis and flu like illness. In the event of increase in MPAP with a normal to low PVR/TPG, leading to increase in cardiac output, epoprostenol toxicity should be considered. Epoprostenol should then be stopped within 48 hours of liver transplantation and then reintroduced with tapering doses over a period of 2–3 weeks. Teprostinil is another prostanoid which is administered subcutaneously or intravenously or nebulized. The former mode can produce side effects of pain which is dose limiting. Iloprost is an inhaled prostanoid with a short half-life with dosing requirement of six to nine times daily. Non-specific anti-endothelin agents like bosentan or endothelin A antagonist ambrisentan and sitaxsentan are also useful in PAH. The former has limited use in POPH because of idiosyncratic hepatotoxicity and the latter is less toxic. Sildenafil, a phosphodiesterase 5 inhibitor was found have safe utility in a small group of POPH patients. An inotropic and vasodilator milrinone is a useful drug in POPH. It is useful in patients who have associated left ventricular failure with normal systemic blood pressure. Use of beta blockers should be withheld in patients of moderate to severe POPH. MELD exception points of 22 with an increase every 3 months in POPH need to made as long as MPAP remains less than 35 mm Hg and PVR remains less than 400 dyn s cm^{-5}. Schistosoma mansoni infection could be the most common form of POPH in the world. An immune complex deposition mediated hypersensitivity in the lungs promote granulomatous inflammatory changes that lead to pulmonary vascular remodeling leading to pulmonary hypertension as well as PHT (non-cirrhotic POPH).[78,79]

HEPATORENAL SYNDROME

It was Frerichs and Flint who initially noted a relation between end-stage liver disease, ascites and oliguric renal failure that occurred in the absence of histological changes in the kidney. Hecker and Sherlock coined the term HRS. This entity is a reversible functional renal failure which is seen to occur in patients of advanced liver cirrhosis (Types 1, 2 or 3) or in those with fulminant liver failure (Type 4). There occurs a reduction in glomerular filtration rate and renal perfusion without other causes of renal failure. Intense renal vasoconstriction is the hallmark of HRS associated with peripheral vasodilatation. There is preservation of tubular function in the absence of proteinuria or renal histology changes. Type 1 HRS is rapidly progressive and is defined as a doubling of baseline creatinine to more than or equal to 2.5mg/dL or a 50% reduction in creatinine clearance to an ultimate of less than 20 mL/minute within 2 weeks. In Type 2 HRS, there is insidious renal impairment which is moderate, where in the serum creatinine rises to above 1.5 mg/dL. Recently, the definition of acute kidney injury (AKI) has been modified to a serum creatinine rise to above 0.3 mg/dL from baseline in 48 hours or the presence of acute kidney injury network (AKIN) Stage 1 with serum creatinine more than 1.5 mg/dL. HRS is when there is pre-renal AKI which is volume unresponsive. An increase in vasoconstrictor response and a decrement in vasodilator response on renal circulation promote HRS development. Peripheral arterial vasodilatation along with hyperdynamic circulation results in renal vasoconstriction. This is augmented by stimulation of renal sympathetic nervous system and underlying cardiac dysfunction leading to microcirculatory dysfunction, renal hypoperfusion and unregulated cytokine storm in association with vasoactive elements acting on the renal vasculature. An increase in splanchnic circulatory volume in cirrhosis leads to decrease in effective intravascular/circulatory volume secondary to increase in intrahepatic vascular resistance. Hence, a low circulating volume affects downgrading of high pressure baroreceptors in carotid and aortic arch bodies leading to sympathetic nervous system activation and RAAS activation with non-osmotic secretion of vasopressin. A hyperdynamic circulation thus develops with an increase in cardiac output, further leading to decreased systemic vascular resistance and severe vasoconstriction of renal vessels. Progression of this dysregulated circulatory homeostasis, in the event of worsening liver disease, results in further worsening, leading to a viscious cycle that leads to HRS.[80,81] Hepatic sinusoidal pressure increase leads to decrease in sinusoidal blood flow which activates hepatorenal reflex, which further results in renal vasoconstriction. Cardiac dysfunction that is inherent to cirrhosis, as a result of depressed myocardial contractility (at rest/exercise), elevated natriuretic peptide level which leads to diastolic dysfunction and neurohumoral exaggeration leading to myocardial hypertrophy and fibrosis associated with decrease in myocardial adrenergic drive all cause further renal impairment. NO, TNF-α, endotoxemia, endothelin, vasodilatory prostaglandins and glucagon lead to splanchnic vasodilatation with high systemic vascular resistance in end-stage liver cirrhosis leading to low urine sodium excretion and water retention (Flow chart 6).[82]

Precipitating events such as bacterial infections, unregulated large volume paracentesis or variceal bleeding are the cause identified to promote HRS Type 1 in 70–100% of cirrhosis patients. In SBP, the cytokine storm that is dysregulated lead to circulatory disturbances and progressive RAAS activation and dysfunction sympathetic nervous system activation leading to renal vasoconstriction. Eighteen percent of patients with cirrhosis over 1 year and 39% over 5 years have probability of developing HRS Type 1. Hyponatremia, low urine sodium, low plasma osmolality, low mean arterial pressures with high plasma renin activity all contribute to and are risk factors for development of HRS. The diagnosis of HRS is briefly shown in Table 13. Eighty percent of HRS Type 1 patient dies in two weeks and only 10% survive for more than 3 months.[83] This is in contrast to HRS Type 2 in which the median survival is around 6 months. Independent predictor of mortality in HRS is the MELD score, where in a score of more than or equal to 20, predicts death at 1 month and in those with lower score, death within 8 months. Apart from aggressive treatment of precipitating factors, the use of vasopressor with albumin improves survival in HRS 1 patients. The vasopressor therapy can be utilized with terlipressin or alpha adrenergic agonists such as noradrenaline and midodrine with octreotide. Response to therapy is defined as a decrease in serum creatinine level of more than 25% from pretreatment values within 72 hours of start of therapy (or less than 1.5 mg/dL). The goal of such treatment is to achieve the lowest creatinine value as possible. The various types of responses to vasopressor therapy are shown in Table 14. In the event of non-response (non-decrement in serum creatinine or increase in levels of creatinine), with the maximal dose of terlipressin, the treatment has to be stopped within 3–4 days. If the decrement of creatinine is slow, then the therapy needs to be continued until the lowest possible serum creatinine level can be achieved, without untoward side effects of therapy in the long term. Adverse effects of vasopressor, especially ischemic, are seen in around 10% of treated patients.[84] Rebound HRS after stopping of adequate terlipressin therapy is seen in 15% of patients, which eventually, in most cases gets resolved with retreatment with terlipressin. Noradrenaline is given as a continuous infusion, with doses escalated from 0.5 mg per hour to 1.5 mg per hour within 24–48 hours, until an MAP of 80–85 is achieved and urine output is maintained at a minimum of 40 mL per hour. This has been shown to be as effective as terlipressin therapy. Midodrine (2.5 mg 8 hourly, with increments) along with octreotide, 100 microgram subcutaneous 8 hourly is also considered a good option for treatment of HRS Type 1. Low dose dopamine is another good option which is infused over 24 hours and has shown to improve cortical blood flow, glomerular filtration rate (GFR) and urine production (Table 15).[85] Performing TIPSS in HRS Type 2 improves kidney function and survival and also decreases chances of developing HRS Type 1 or Type 2. Renal replacement therapy (RRT) in the form of continuous RRT has been shown to improve outcomes in post-transplant period in patients of HRS Type 1 who develop acute tubular necrosis. Continuous RRT provides gradual correction of hyponatremia, controlled correction of raised intracranial tension and maintains hemodynamic stability and removes unregulated inflammatory cytokines. The use of continuous RRT on decompensated patients on mechanical ventilation is futile. The use of other modalities of renal replacement has been associated with adverse effects such as arterial hypotension, infections and increase in bleeding rates. The molecular adsorbent recirculating system (MARS) and fractionated plasma separation and adsorption (Prometheus) are also useful modalities in patients of liver dysfunction and renal failure. The former is a cell free dialysis technique which removes both albumin bound and water soluble wastes and utilizes albumin enriched dialysate with concomitant continuous RRT use.[86] Patients of HRS Type 1 should be prioritized to attain early liver transplantation. Patients of HRS who undergo liver transplantation have reversibility of renal dysfunction and hence do not need to undergo combined liver and kidney transplantation (SLK). SLK is utilized for patients who are on RRT for more than 6–8 weeks.[87] The criteria for SLK are shown in Table 16.

Flow chart 6 Pathogenesis of hepatorenal syndrome. General mechanisms of HRS development are shown above

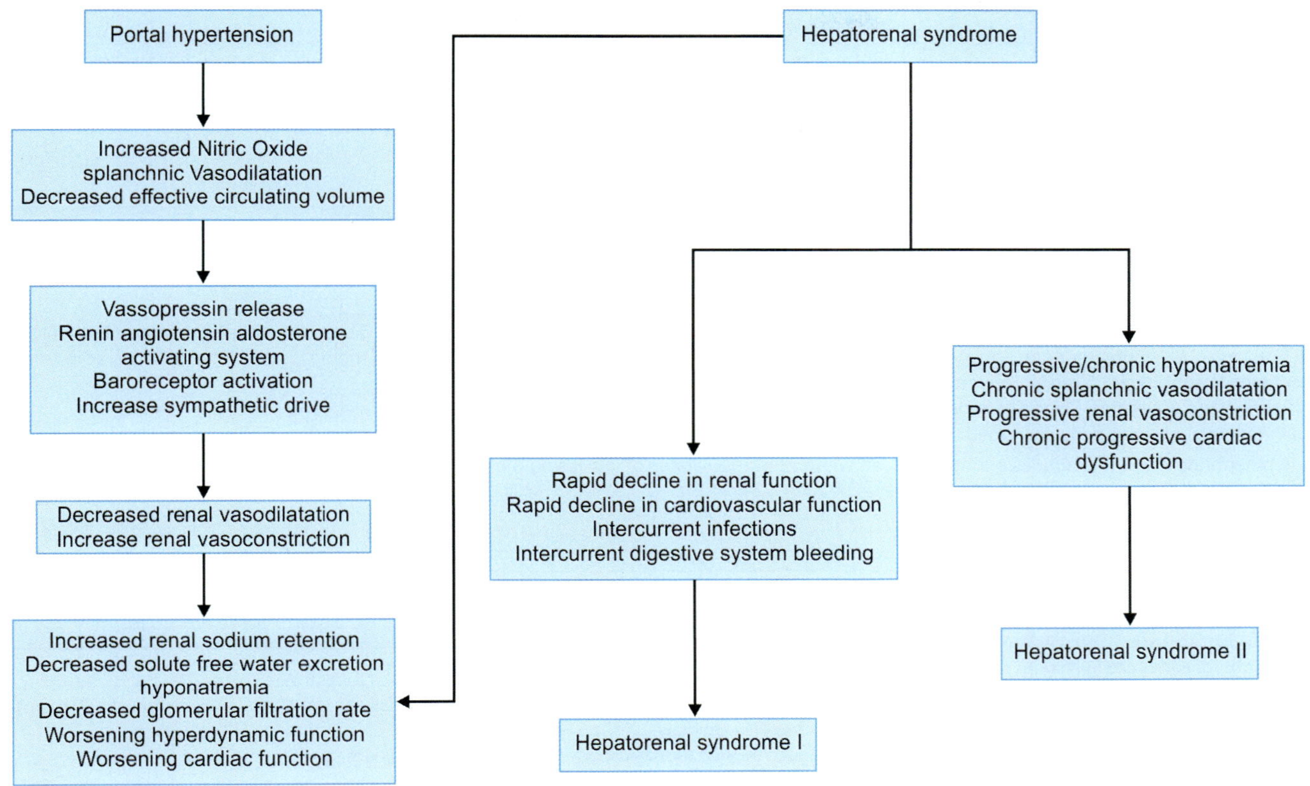

Table 13: Types and diagnosis of hepatorenal syndrome

Parameter	*Definitions [International Club of Ascites – Acute Kidney Injury Criteria (ICA-AKI)]*
Baseline serum creatinine (Cr)	A value obtained in the previous 3 months, when available, can be used as baseline. In patients with more than one value within the previous 3 months, the value closest to the admission time to the hospital should be used. In patients without a previous available value, value on admission should be used as baseline.
Definition of acute kidney injury	Increase in Cr ≥0.3 mg/dL within 48 hours OR A percentage increase Cr ≥50% from baseline which is known, or presumed to have occurred within the prior 7 days
Staging of acute kidney injury	Stage 1: increase in sCr ≥0.3 mg/dL or an increase in sCr ≥1.5-fold to 2-fold from baseline Stage 2: increase in sCr >2-fold to 3-fold from baseline Stage 3: increase of sCr >3-fold from baseline or sCr ≥4.0 mg/dL with an acute increase ≥0.3 mg/dL or initiation of renal replacement therapy
Criteria for hepatorenal syndrome (I)	Diagnosis of cirrhosis and ascites with diagnosis of acute kidney injury according to ICA-AKI criteria – No response after 2 consecutive days of diuretic withdrawal and plasma volume expansion with albumin 1 g per kg of body weight • Absence of shock • No current or recent use of nephrotoxic drugs • No macroscopic signs of structural kidney injury [defined as: – absence of proteinuria (>500 mg/day) – absence of microhematuria (>50 RBCs per high power field), – normal findings on renal ultrasonography]

Modified from: Paolo Angeli, et al. Diagnosis and management of acute kidney injury in patients with cirrhosis: Revised consensus recommendations of the International Club of Ascites. Journal of Hepatology 2015 vol. 62; 968–74.

HEPATIC ENCEPHALOPATHY

Neuropsychiatric manifestation seen in acute and chronic liver disease is termed hepatic encephalopathy. Alterations in intellectual, emotional, behavioral, cognitive, fine motor and psychomotor domains represent hepatic encephalopathy, which is classified as overt hepatic encephalopathy (OHE) or covert [minimal hepatic encephalopathy (MHE)].[88] OHE is detected by bedside clinical tests. MHE requires the use of specific psychometric tests. Modified Parson-Smith scale (West Haven criteria or Conn's Modified scale) classifies hepatic encephalopathy into five grades:

Grade 0: Subclinical encephalopathy; abnormalities only on psychometric testing.

Grade 1: Trivial lack of awareness; shortened attention span.

Table 14: Types of responses in hepatorenal syndrome to medical therapy		
No response	*Partial response*	*Full response*
No regression of AKI	Regression of AKI stage with a reduction of Cr to ≥0.3 mg/dL above the baseline value	Return of Cr to a value within 0.3 mg/dL of the baseline value

Modified from: Paolo Angeli et al. Diagnosis and management of acute kidney injury in patients with cirrhosis: Revised consensus recommendations of the International Club of Ascites. Journal of Hepatology 2015 vol. 62; 968–74.

Table 15: Treatment options in hepatorenal syndrome
Pharmacological options for hepatorenal syndrome
Vasoconstrictors: Terlipressin: 1 mg/4–6 hours intravenously. The dose is increased up to a maximum of 2 mg/4–6 hours after 3 days if there is no response to therapy (defined as a 25% or greater reduction in serum creatinine compared to pretreatment levels). A response to therapy is defined as a decrease in serum creatinine levels below 1.5 mg/dL (133 mol/L). The treatment is usually applied for 5–15 days. Midodrine and octreotide: 7.5 mg of midodrine orally 3 times daily (increased to 12.5 mg 3 times daily if needed) and 100 lg of octreotide subcutaneously 3 times daily (increased to 200 lg 3 times daily if needed). The duration of treatment depends on the effects on serum creatinine. Norepinephrine: 0.5–3 mg/hour as a continuous intravenous infusion aimed at increasing the mean arterial pressure by 10 mm Hg. The treatment is continued until the serum creatinine level decreases below 1.5 mg/dL. Albumin administration: Concomitant administration of albumin and vasoconstrictor drugs (1 g/kg of body weight on day 1 followed by 20–40 g/day).

Table 16: Summary of indications for combined liver-kidney transplantation	
Indications for combined liver-kidney transplant	
Davis et al. (2006)	a. Patients with CKD with a measured creatinine clearance (or preferentially an iothalamate clearance) of ≤30 mL/min b. Patients with AKI and/or HRS on dialysis for ≥6 weeks c. Patients with prolonged AKI with kidney biopsy showing fixed renal damage d. SLK is not recommended in patients with AKI not requiring dialysis
Eason et al. (2007)	a. Patients with ESRD with cirrhosis and symptomatic portal hypertension or hepatic vein wedge pressure gradient ≥10 mm Hg b. Patients with CKD with GFR ≤30 mL/min c. Patients with AKI/HRS with Scr ≥2 mg/dL and dialysis ≥8 weeks d. Patients with evidence of CKD and kidney biopsy demonstrating >30% glomerulosclerosis or 30% fibrosis e. Other criteria recommended are the presence of comorbidities such as diabetes, hypertension, age >65, other preexisting renal disease along with proteinuria, renal size and duration of elevated Scr
OPTN Kidney Transplantation Committee and the Liver and Intestinal Organ Transplantation Committee	a. CKD requiring dialysis with documentation of the CMS form 2728 b. CKD (GFR ≤30 mL/min by MDRD-6 or iothalamate measurement and proteinuria >3 g/day c. Sustained AKI requiring dialysis for 6 weeks or more (defined as dialysis at least twice per week for 6 consecutive weeks) d. Sustained AKI (GFR ≤25 mL/min for 6 weeks or more by MDRD6 or direct measurement) not requiring dialysis e. Sustained AKI: Patients may also qualify for SLK listing with a combination of time in categories (c) and (d) above for a total of 6 weeks (e.g. patients with a GFR <25 mL/min for 3 weeks followed by dialysis for 3 weeks) f. Metabolic disease

Grade 2: Lethargy, disorientation, personality change.

Grade 3: Somnolence to semi stupor; responsive to stimuli, confused.

Grade 4: Coma.

As per the Working Party of Vienna Congress, universal definition and classification of hepatic encephalopathy have been modified to that shown in Figure 13. Pathogenetic processes culminating to hepatic encephalopathy are complicated and multifactorial. Hyperammonemia and low grade persistent inflammation lead to astrocyte swelling. Ammonia, under normal conditions, is eliminated in the form of urea, which is formed in the liver and excreted through the kidneys. Earlier studies by Pavlov, Nencki and Zaleski on dogs, where they utilized portocaval shunt surgery followed by heavy meat predominant diet, showed that experimental animals developed neuropsychiatric manifestations. They termed this "meat intoxication syndrome". Ammonia, as the central role in promoting hepatic encephalopathy was shown by Lockwood and coworkers, as shown in Flow chart 7. Glutamine synthetase present in the endoplasmic reticulum of astrocytes helps in converting glutamate to ammonia and to glutamine. Levels of glutamine increase with liver failure[89,90] which further activates excitatory neuronal function resulting in hepatic encephalopathy and its clinical sequelae, in the acute form, Type A and in the chronic form, Type C in the presence of low grade cerebral edema and mostly neuroinhibitory state where the astrocytes, after prolonged hyperammonemia exposure undergo dysregulated

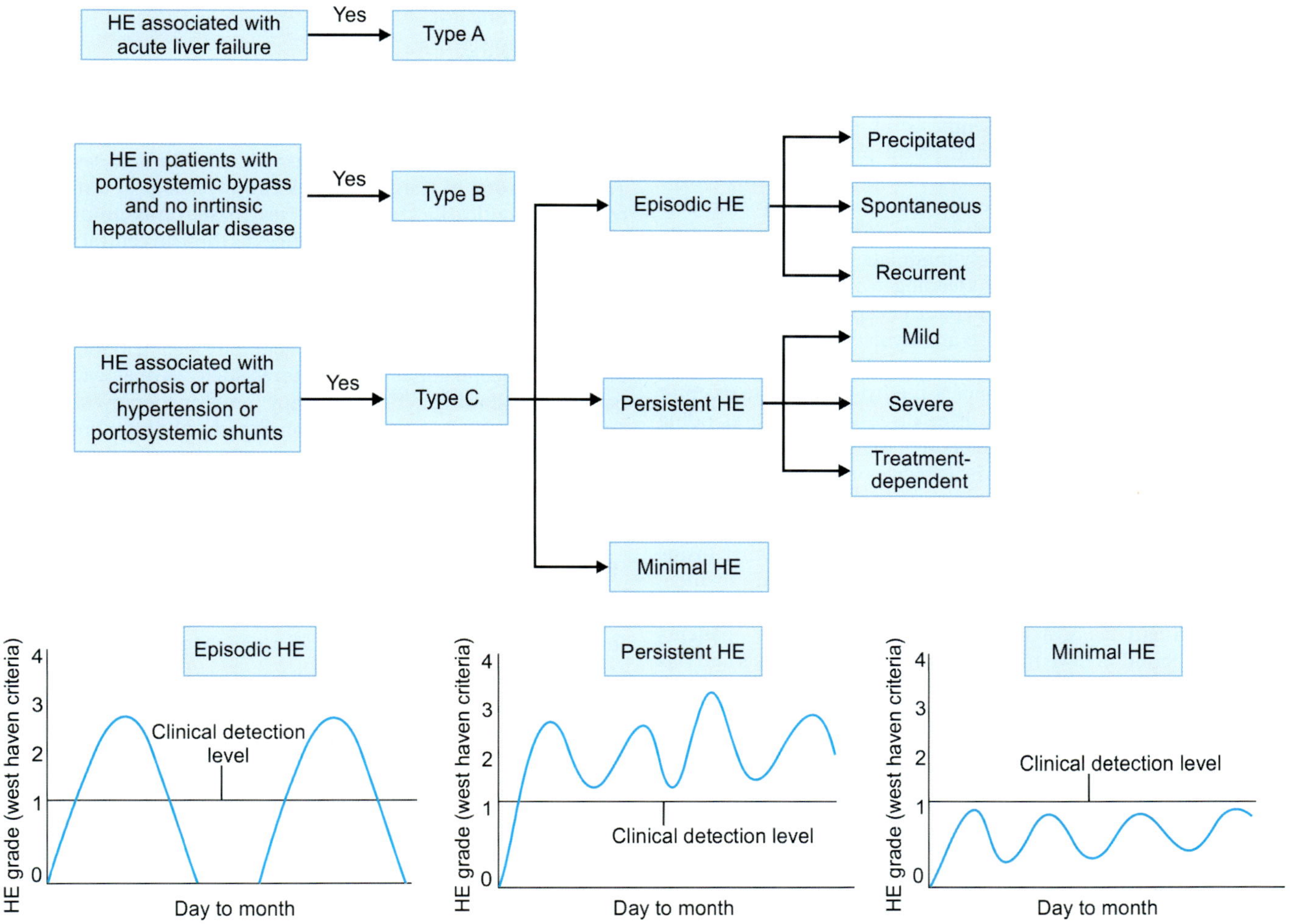

Figure 13 Classification of hepatic encephalopathy and their natural history
Source: Modified from Prakash R, Mullen K. Nature. 2010.

Flow chart 7 Pathogenesis of hepatic encephalopathy

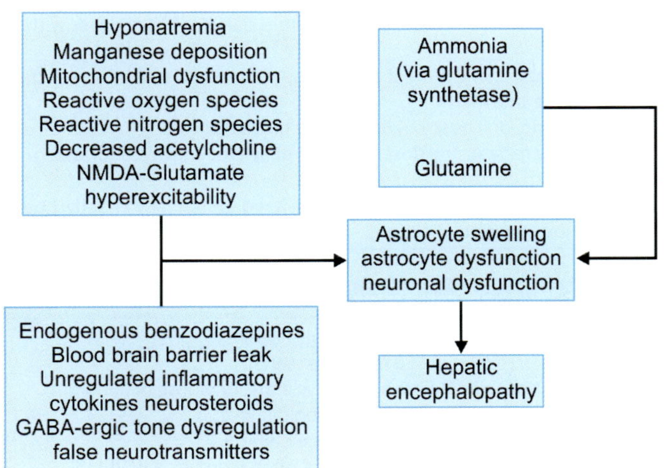

adaptive changes. Myoinositol and taurine are osmolytes that are released from astrocytes which help in compensation of worsening swelling. Further, glutamate receptor activity in post-synaptic region is decreased and the glutamate transporters on the cell membrane get deactivated. Morphometric changes occur and the affected astrocytes become Alzheimer Type II, which are dysfunctional. The complete pathogenesis of hepatic encephalopathy cannot be explained by only hyperammonemia, nor can the improvement or worsening of hepatic encephalopathy be fully described on the basis of ammonia levels. Background inflammatory dysregulation, occurring persistently, in the low grade state plays an important role in development and worsening of hepatic encephalopathy. Proinflammatory cytokines released by dysfunctional astrocytes and microglial cells, such as TNF-α and IL-6, damage the blood brain barrier function and increase fluid phase permeability of endothelial cells in the central nervous system leading to further diffusion of ammonia into astrocytes and microglial cells, leading to a vicious cycle of inflammation and hepatic encephalopathy. The role of neurosteroids in hepatic encephalopathy manifestation has been studied well. Upregulation of peripheral type of benzodiazepine receptors in microglial cells activated under inflammatory conditions lead to increased mitochondrial synthesis of neuroactive steroids synthesized from cholesterol and sterol precursors in gonads, adrenals and brain tissue. Neurosteroid production in brain is mainly by myelinating glial cells. Accumulation of ammonia and manganese in liver dysfunction enhances neurosteroid production. These then positively modulate GABA receptors and increase the entry of chloride ions leading to increase in GABAergic tone (classically seen in Type C hepatic encephalopathy). Reactive nitrogen and oxygen species also are involved in pathogenesis of hepatic encephalopathy. This is independent of calcium levels and happens through activation of N-methyl D-aspartate receptor pathways (NMDA). In chronic liver disease and long standing portosystemic shunting, accumulation of manganese occurs in the basal ganglia leading to changes in astrocytes and Alzheimer Type II cell morphing of normal cells. Such patients develop Parkinsonism features in the background of chronic persistent hepatic encephalopathy and have "Hepatic Parkinsonism". Other toxins implicated in development of hepatic encephalopathy include, mercaptans, false neurotransmitters such as octopamine and short chain fatty acids. Acetylcholinesterase in cirrhosis patients have been found to have higher activity in neuronal cells and has been found to be independent of ammonia levels in promoting hepatic encephalopathy. A common dyselectrolytemia in cirrhosis is hyponatremia which leads to decrease in intracellular organic osmolytes. This also leads to astrocyte swelling, low grade cerebral edema and reactive nitrogen and oxygen species related stress leading to astrocyte dysfunction. For this reason, a low sodium level in cirrhosis patients is an independent predictor of overt hepatic encephalopathy development. The management approach to a cirrhosis patient with hepatic encephalopathy includes excluding other causes of cerebral dysfunction, identifying and treating the precipitating cause and empiric treatment for hepatic encephalopathy.[91] Response to hepatic encephalopathy should occur within 72 hours, in the absence of which, other causes of encephalopathy should be ruled out. Ammonia levels in venous and arterial samples correlate positively with severity of hepatic encephalopathy but serial or routine measurements do not correlate with improvement of worsening of hepatic encephalopathy. Blood for ammonia measurement is collected from a vein without tourniquet application and is transported on ice to the laboratory to be analyzed within 20 minutes. Amodio and coworkers proposed the modified version of West Haven criteria in 2004, by introducing objective scales for the assessment of the individual components. The Hepatic Encephalopathy Scoring Algorithm (HESA) originally described by Hassanein and colleagues is useful in assessment of low grade of hepatic encephalopathy. Neuropsychiatric tests include paper and pencil and computerized tests and are useful in diagnosing subtle cognitive changes in patients of cirrhosis. In psychometric hepatic encephalopathy score or PHES, a battery neuropsychometric tests help in characterizing MHE. The Working Party at the 1998 World Congress of Gastroenterology officially declared this test as the "gold standard" for diagnosis of MHE. This test consists of the following:

- Number connection test A
- Number connection test B
- Serial dotting test
- Line tracing test
- Digit symbol test

Among the computerized psychometric tests, the Inhibitory Control Test is based on target and lure principle. A lure greater than five out of forty attempts detects MHE with high sensitivity. The other group of tests include electrophysiological testing that comprise of critical flicker frequency test (based on assumption that retinal glial cells undergo same changes as those in central nervous system; hepatic retinopathy), in which light pulses, to start with, at a frequency of 60 Hz, gradually reduced by 0.1 Hz per second is shown on the patients eyes. A critical flicker frequency less than 39 Hz is diagnostic of MHE. Electroencephalography testing in the context of hepatic encephalopathy shows three spike wave activities with background slowing.[92,93] Post therapy (empiric therapy, shown in Tables 17 and 18) for hepatic encephalopathy, the ammonia levels usually lag behind clinical improvement. Therapy aims at reducing the production and absorption of ammonia in the gut. This can be achieved by means of using non-absorbable dissacharides that include lactulose and lactitol. These agents promote laxative effect, reduce colonic pH and mucosal uptake of glutamine in gut thereby curbing ammonia production and improving ammonia clearance. Lactulose is either given orally in a conscious patient or through the nasogastric tube or rectally in a patient in coma. The dose ranges from 15 to 30 mL given twice daily to induce two to three soft stools per day. The most common adverse effect is bloating. Excessive lactulose use can result in dehydration, hyponatremia and worsening of hepatic encephalopathy. Empirically antibiotic rifaximin which is minimally absorbed in the gut with few side effects and minimal drug-drug interaction is used. A dose of 500 mg twice daily is used. Neomycin is another antibiotic used that acts by inhibiting mucosal glutaminase in intestine and promotes decreased production of ammonia in gut, by inhibiting ammonia producing coliforms that produce urease. But this has the potential to cause side effects such as ototoxicity, renal dysfunction and intestinal malabsorption. Metabolism of excessively produced

Table 17: Empiric treatment of hepatic encephalopathy

- Lactulose, oral dose of 15–30 mL twice daily
- Rifaximin, oral dose of 550 mg twice daily
- Neomycin, oral dose of 500 mg four times daily (use high doses with caution)
- Metronidazole, oral dose of 250 mg four times daily (recommended only in the short term)
- Vancomycin, oral dose of 250 mg four times daily
- Sodium benzoate, oral dose 5 g twice daily (not approved for use in the USA)
- Flumazenil, intravenous injection of 1–3 mg (potentially effective, but very short duration of action)

Table 18: Long-term management of hepatic encephalopathy

- Lactulose (oral dose of 15–30 mL twice daily)
- Rifaximin (oral dose of 550 mg twice daily)
- Zinc repletion (zinc sulfate and zinc acetate, oral dose of 600 mg)
- Bromocriptine (oral dose of 15–60 mg daily)
- Sodium benzoate (oral dose 5 g twice daily)
- L-ornithine l-aspartate (oral dose of 6 g three times daily)
- Vegetable-based protein diet

ammonia in cirrhosis is taken over by skeletal muscles. In the presence of sarcopenia seen in advanced cirrhosis, ammonia clearance also reduces and this contributes to hyperammonemic episodes. The recommended protein intake in cirrhosis patients is 1.2 g/kg daily and supplemented with branched chain amino acids (BCAAs) and vegetable protein. A BCAA rich snack at midnight is an important aspect of nutritional therapy in cirrhosis patients. BCAAs also improve albumin levels, reduces hospital stay and number of hospitalizations and increase progression free survival in cirrhosis patients. Fiber rich, vegetable based proteins increase the decreases intestinal transit time and increase colonic motility, thereby promoting intestinal nitrogen clearance. A decreased colonic pH occurs whereby ammonia absorption from the gut is prevented. Addition of dairy products to a predominant vegetarian diet decreases adverse effects such as flatulence or bloating. Persistent hepatic encephalopathy requires liver transplantation as the curative option. Portosystemic shunting related hepatic encephalopathy can be treated through interventional methods that utilize shunt closure techniques and are mostly undertaken when the patient is not an ideal candidate for liver transplantation. Artificial devices such as extra-corporeal albumin dialysis using molecular adsorbent recirculating system (MARS) has been recently shown to improve outcomes.[94]

PORTAL HYPERTENSIVE GASTROPATHY

Portal hypertensive gastropathy (PHG) can be seen with cirrhosis and otherwise. Presentations range from acute and massive upper gastrointestinal bleed to insidious blood loss and is classically described endoscopically (Figs 14A to I) as mosaic like pattern resembling snake skin with or without red spots.[95] It is also seen to occur in the small and large intestines of patients with PHT and is called portal hypertensive enteropathy or colopathy respectively. PHG is seen in 20–70% of patients with underlying cirrhosis. There

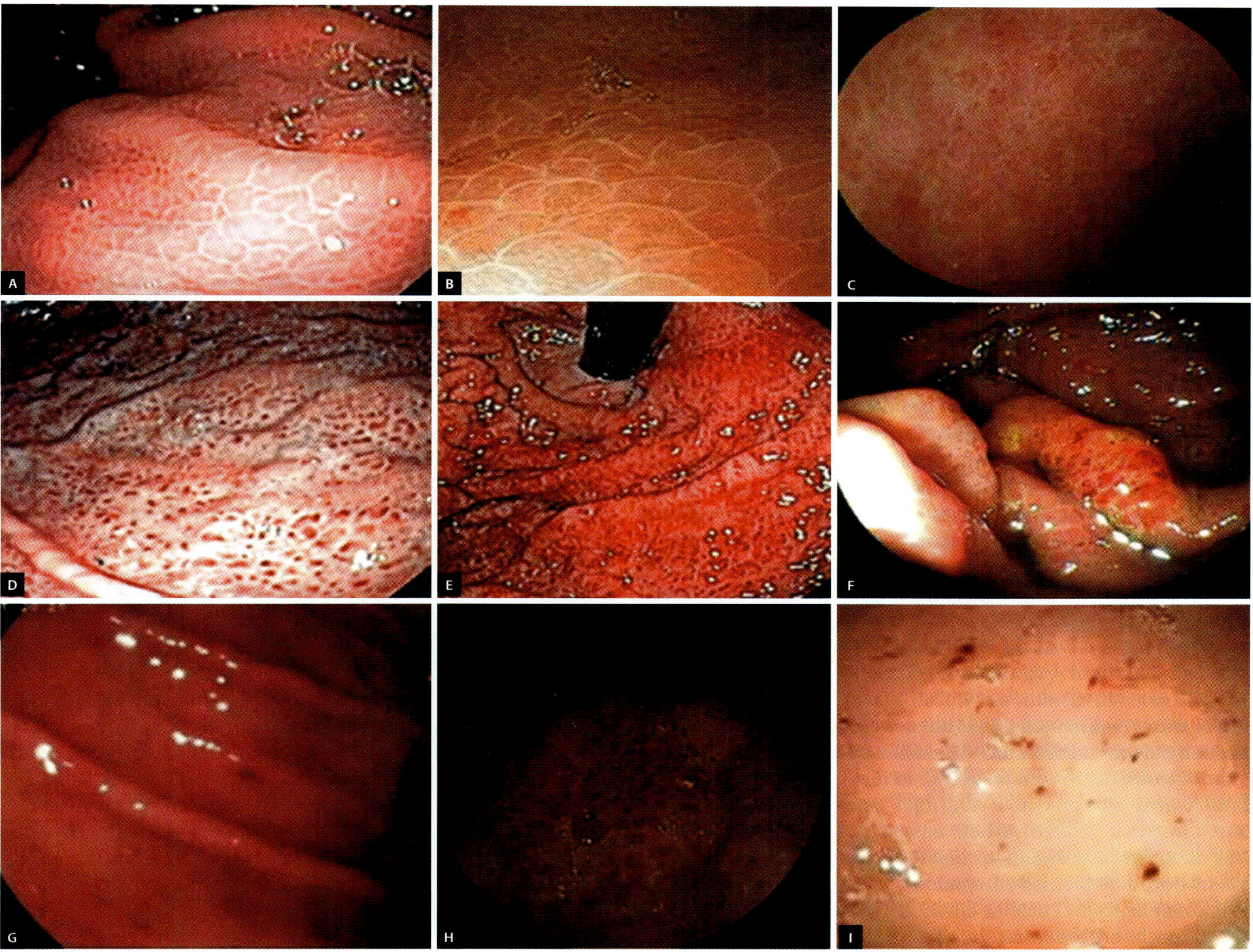

Figures 14A to I Endoscopic appearance of portal hypertensive gastropathy. (A) Corresponds to severe mosaic like pattern as per Baveno system; (B) Severe mosaic like pattern as per New Italian Endoscopic Classification (NIEC); (C) Mild mosaic pattern as per McCormack system; (D) Discrete red spots (McCormack), cherry red spots (NIEC) or red point lesions (Baveno system); (E) Diffuse hemorrhagic lesions (McCormack) or diffuse red spots (NIEC); (F) Superficial reddening (McCormack); (G) Single cherry red spot (NIEC) or isolated red point lesion (Baveno); (H) Confluent red marks as per Baveno system; (I) Inactive black brown spots (NIEC)

is a higher prevalence in Child C cirrhosis patients and in those who undergo sclerotherapy or variceal ligation. Factors that are independently associated with PHG include hypoalbuminemia, high bilirubin and thrombocytopenia. PHG increases with variceal ligation and is seen in the presence of medium and large varices. PHG does not correlate linearly with increased portal pressures, but the latter is the main pathogenetic culprit in development of PHG. Risk factors for PHG that also pertain to pathogenesis include severity of liver disease and *H. pylori* infection.[96] When the total blood flow in the mucosa and submucosa of stomach is increased, increased congestion results in PHG which is dependent on severity of liver disease and PHT. Gastric microcirculatory dysfunction leads to mucosal hypoxia associated with congestive changes that result in epithelial cell disintegrity. This action is mediated by nitric oxide, endothelin-1, proinflammatory cytokines (TNF-α, IL-6), superoxide species and prostaglandins. Diagnosis of PHG is mainly by endoscopy and is based on three classification systems (Table 19). Apart from these, the Baveno System divides mosaic pattern into mild, corresponding to pink mosaic like pattern and severe, corresponding to red mosaic like pattern.[97] Severe PHG is diagnosed when red marks with or without mosaic pattern is seen. Histopathologically, vascular ectasia of mucosal and submucosal veins and capillaries are seen. Biopsy is not needed for diagnosis. An accuracy of above 95% can be attributed to PHG for presence of underlying PHT. Important differential diagnoses include gastric antral vascular ectasia (GAVE), polycythemia, acute gastritis, purpura of the stomach and hereditary hemorrhagic telangiectasias. Progression of PHG is seen in 30% of cases and regression in 20%. Variceal band ligation is associated with faster progression, even though 44% patients show regression with the same.[98] Acute bleeding (significant mortality only in 0.1%) manifestations from PHG occur in 2–12% patients, while chronic bleeding (decrement of more than 2 g/dL of hemoglobin between two time periods, 6 months apart, in a patient who has not acutely bled in the meantime and not on NSAID drugs) occurs in up to 3–26%.[99] Propanolol, the non-selective beta blocker, is the most commonly used pharmacotherapy for PHG management and octreotide (vasopressin/terlipressin also useful) (100 µg bolus followed by 25 µg per hour infusion for 2 days) is useful in acute events. Vitamin E and other antioxidants have been shown to reverse oxidative injury to gastric mucosa in PHG. Thalidomide and prednisolone are also successfully used in case reports for control of bleeding PHG. TIPSS has no role in management of acute or chronic blood loss in PHG. Since mortality and morbidity events are less in patients, secondary to PHG, primary prophylaxis is not needed. Patients with severe PHG without prophylactic indication for treatment of varices can be started on non-selective beta blocker therapy.[100,101]

GASTRIC ANTRAL VASCULAR ECTASIA (FIGS 15A TO D)

Rider and colleagues described GAVE in a patient of chronic iron deficiency anemia which was transfusion dependent. Initially they described it as an erosive gastritis with veno-capillary ectasia.[102] Jabbari and coworkers in 1984 better defined this condition as longitudinal antral folds, converging on the pylorus consisting of visible columns of tortuous red ectatic vasculature. Hyperplasia of mucosa, capillary ectasia, fibromuscular dysplasia of lamina

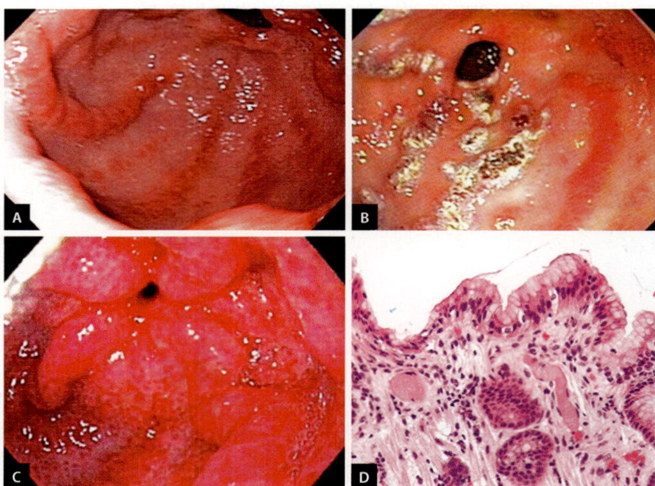

Figures 15A to D Endoscopic appearance and histopathology of gastric antral vascular ectasia. (A) Classical endoscopic appearance as suggested by Jabbari et al. in 1984, the "watermelon stomach"; (B) Endoscopic therapy using argon plasma coagulation over bleeding points in gastric antral vascular ectasia; (C) Diffuse GAVE related bleeding on endoscopic view; (D) Histopathology of GAVE showing diagnostic features of mucosal vascular capillary ectasia, fibrin thrombi in capillaries and fibromuscular hyperplasia of lamina propria. Immunohistochemical staining (not shown here) for vascular markers CD31 and CD34 as well as platelet marker CD61 can be useful in histological differentiation between GAVE and PHG if the morphology is inconclusive on endoscopy

Table 19: Summary of different classification systems of portal hypertensive gastropathy

Classification category	*NIEC system*	*McCormack et al.*	*Tanoue et al.*
Mild	"Mosaic-like pattern" Mild: diffusely pink areola Moderate: flat red spot in center of pink areola Severe: diffusely red areola	Fine speckling or "scarlatina" type of rash Superficial reddening Snake skin pattern	Grade 1: Mild reddening Congestive mucosa
Moderate	Not considered	Not considered	Grade 2: Severe redness and a fine reticular pattern separating areas of raised mucosa
Severe	Red marks—Red lesions of variable diameter, flat or slightly protruding. Discrete or confluent	Cherry red spots, confluent or not Diffuse hemorrhage	Grade 3—Grade 2 plus point bleeding

Table 20: Differences between portal hypertensive gastropathy and gastric antral vascular ectasia

	PHG	*GAVE*
Predominant location	Body and fundus	Antrum
Classic endoscopic appearance	Mosaic like pattern or red marks	Linear red stripes separated by normal mucosa
Histology	Mild to moderate dilation of veins and capillaries of gastric mucosa and submucosa. No changes in vessel Walls	Marked dilation of capillaries and venules in gastric mucosa and submucosa with areas of intimal thickening and thrombi
PHT	Always present	Can be seen without portal hypertension
Associations	Only seen in conditions that cause portal hypertension	Autoimmune and connective tissue diseases (scleroderma, pernicious anemia, hypothyroidsm), liver cirrhosis
Endoscopic therapy	No	Yes, argon plasma coagulation preferred
Response to beta blockers and TIPS	Yes	No

propria, thrombosis, fibrohyalinosis and abnormal spindle cell proliferation and presence of abnormal vessels in the submucosal histopathologically define GAVE. Classical endoscopic appearance is termed "watermelon stomach". Even though traditionally speaking, GAVE is limited to antrum, extra-antral lesions, more so, at the cardia can also be found. The main differential diagnosis of GAVE is antral gastritis.[103] Non-variceal bleeding occur in cirrhosis patients and bleeding GAVE accounts 4% of such cases apart from other presentations such as occult bleeding and transfusion dependent chronic iron deficiency. One of every forty patients of cirrhosis have GAVE and cirrhosis is found in 30% of GAVE patients. Apart from cirrhosis, 62% of autoimmune connective tissue disease patients, 31% patients with Raynaud's phenomenon and 20% of patients with scleroderma have GAVE. It is also seen in chronic renal failure and acute leukemia patients. Non-cirrhotic patients have the classical watermelon GAVE and those with cirrhosis have diffuse GAVE. Females predominate in the non-cirrhotic GAVE group and those with cirrhosis tend to be younger and are males. Main consideration is to differentiate GAVE from PHG, which is shown in Table 20. Patients who harbor GAVE have more severe underlying liver disease, lower serum gastrin levels, higher chances of having prior sclerotherapy and greater blood loss. The gold standard of GAVE diagnosis is through biopsy. The presence of spindle cell proliferation and fibro-hyalinosis are associated with an 85% accuracy in predicting GAVE over PHG. PHT is not found to play a predominant role in development of GAVE[104] and it does not improve with decrease in portal pressures. Rather, achlorhydria and GAVE have been found to correlate positively, independent of presence of cirrhosis. There are various theories in development of GAVE:

- Gastric vessel vasodilatation secondary to gastrin increase
- Gastric vasodilatation secondary to prostaglandin E2 increase
- Serotonin increase that modulate local mileu leading to ectatic changes
- Increase in gastric motility and mechanical stress factors (partial prolapse of loose distal gastric mucosa due to increased peristaltic waves through the pyloric channel leading to accentuation of longitudinal folds promoting fibro-muscular hyperplasia of antrum and ectatic vessel formation.

The treatment is conservative with resuscitative efforts in bleeding GAVE with blood and blood products, iron supplementation in chronic GAVE, some degree of portal pressure reduction (not successful in trials), hormonal manipulation, tranexamic acid in decreasing acute bleeding events, thalidomide (highly effective in case studies) and experimental therapies such as alpha interferon, calcitonin, cyproheptadine were also found to be of use in sporadic case reports. Other useful modalities include sclerotherapy and use of laser and thermal coagulation endoscopically. Neodymium-Ytrium-Aluminium Garnet (Nd-YAG) laser and Argon plasma coagulation has been found to be very effective. This therapy has an added advantage of improvement in hepatic encephalopathy in patients of cirrhosis. In uncontrolled bleeding from GAVE, the only solution is antrectomy which still remains a curative treatment. It is nevertheless a highly morbid procedure in cirrhosis patients with high mortality rates. Other modalities of treatment include surgical portosystemic shunts and TIPSS. Finally it is well known that liver transplantation improves GAVE.[105]

CIRRHOTIC CARDIOMYOPATHY

Appropriate cardiac responses to stimuli is blunted in patients of cirrhosis, a manifestation termed cirrhotic cardiomyopathy (CCM). Arterial hypotension, decreased peripheral vascular resistance and increased cardiac output define this condition. The ventricular contractile response is decreased in patients of cirrhosis in the presence of drugs or exercise that promote it.[106] The specific diagnostic criteria for CCM are show in Tables 21 and 22. An international consensus committee defined CCM as "the chronic cardiac dysfunction in a patient of cirrhosis which is defined by blunted contractile responsiveness to stress and/or altered diastolic relaxation with electrophysiological abnormalities in the absence of known cardiac disease". Prolonged diastole in the presence of normal systolic function, i.e. normal ejection fraction characterizes CCM. The E/A ratio (an index of diastolic filling, which is more common than systolic dysfunction) is abnormal in cirrhotic patients at rest or otherwise. Early rapid filling velocity (E) is usually more than the late filling velocity, which is dependent on the atrial contraction (A). The E/A ratio of less than one reveal a dysfunctional ventricular relaxation. This ratio can also be negative in elderly. On Tissue Doppler imaging, the E', which represents slow velocity high amplitude annular tissue motion (less affected by preload, in conditions where patient is overloaded) and the E ratio is more sensitive in assessing lusitropic dysfunction.

Table 21: Diagnosis of cirrhotic cardiomyopathy
Definition of cirrhotic cardiomyopathy
General definition: • Cirrhotic cardiomyopathy is defined as chronic cardiac dysfunction in patients with cirrhosis, characterized by blunted contractile responsiveness to stress, and/or altered diastolic relaxation with electrophysiological abnormalities, in the absence of known cardiac disease. Diagnostic criteria: • Abnormal systolic contractile responses to stress • Diastolic dysfunction at rest • Absence of clinically significant cardiopulmonary disease Systolic dysfunction (at least one of the following): • Blunted increase in cardiac output with exercise, volume challenge or pharmacological stimuli. – Resting LVEF <55% Diastolic dysfunction (at least one of the following): • E/A ratio (age corrected) <1.0 • Prolonged deceleration time (>200 ms) • Prolonged isovolumic relaxation time (>80 ms) Supportive criteria: • Electrophysiological abnormalities including the following: – Abnormal chronotropic response to stress – Electromechanical uncoupling/dyssynchrony – Prolonged QTc interval • Heart chamber alterations: Enlarged LA, increased LVWT • Increased pro-BNP and BNP • Increased troponin I

Table 22: Salient features of cirrhotic cardiomyopathy
Main features of cirrhotic cardiomyopathy
Systolic dysfunction: • Generally subclinical; can be unveiled by increasing the cardiac afterload, physical exercise, stressful event Diastolic dysfunction: • Revealed by the echocardiographic study of the diastolic transmitral flow pattern; can be unveiled by sudden increases in cardiac preload (e.g. TIPS) • Electrophysiological abnormalities • Chronotropic incompetence • Incapacity of increasing heart rate under physiological or pharmacological adrenergic stimulation • Electromechanical uncoupling • Disruption of the process leading to cardiomyocyte contraction following electrical excitation • Electrocardiographic QT interval prolongation • Due to altered repolarization, needs to be corrected by heart rate; Fredericia's formula (QTc ¼ QT/3HRR) should be used in cirrhosis • Pathological features • Hypertrophy of left ventricle (mainly interventricular septum and posterior wall) • Left atrium dilatation

CCM and associated lusitropic dysfunction improves with ascites fluid mobilization and/or liver transplantation. QT prolongation (due to dysregulated potassium channels that prolong duration of action potential) is the main and most common electrocardiographic change in cirrhosis. Chronotropic incompetence and electromechanical dissociation are also associated conditions. Prolongation of corrected QT is seen to increase with worsening liver disease and with increasing PHT, which correlated with higher plasma norepinephrine levels. QT changes are also associated with sudden death in cirrhosis (independent risk factor). Also, corrected QTc more than 463 milliseconds is an independent predictor of mortality from upper digestive tract bleeding in cirrhosis. In chronotropic incompetence, there is a decreased heart rate response to physiological and pharmacological stimuli in the presence of higher plasma norepinephrine levels in the background of cirrhosis. This inability of the heart to increase rate in response to higher demands result in reduced cardiac output under stress, but high cardiac output under resting conditions. Macrolides and some quinolone drugs (sparfloxacin, moxifloxacin) and domperidone prolong QT and promote chances of ventricular arrhythmias. Cardiac events consist of 15% of deaths in post-liver transplant patients.[107] E/A ratio 28 days after TIPSS procedure has been considered an important predictor of mortality at 1 year. Sepsis related cardiodepression is likened to CCM. QT prolongation in association with electromechanical dys-synchrony (wide dispersion of time interval between QRS onset and mechanical systole) has been shown to be more predominant in patients of cirrhosis. The peripheral vasodilatation and compensatory reduction of negative inotropic mechanisms prevent cirrhosis patients from developing overt heart failure. The molecular basis of CCM include decreased Gs and Gi protein levels, reduction in cAMP generation, uncoupling of beta adrenergic receptor (BAR) complex from G protein, reduced BAR density and decrease in membrane fluidity with impairment in cardiomyocyte function. Increase in circulating endogenous cannabinoids such as anandamide and increased expression of cannabinoid receptors (especially CB1) in endothelial cells due to local cardiac production of the same lead to blunted responses to cardiovascular and stress stimuli also promoting CCM development. Other factors in pathogenesis include increase in TNF-α via NFk-B signaling, iNOS activation and p38 MAPK pathway activity that lead to cardiodepression.[108,109] Serum brain natriuretic peptide level of more than 250 pg/mL has been shown to predict cardiac failure in early post-transplantation period. More than 60% of patients with decompensated cirrhosis have autonomic and cardiovascular dysfunction prior to transplantation. Reversal of QT has been shown in patient's post-liver transplantation. Dobutamine stress echocardiography is a good tool to screen patients of cirrhosis who develop cardiac related complications. A better modality for assessment of CCM is cardiac magnetic resonance imaging (CMRI). The presence of increase in left ventricular mass with increase in left atrial and ventricular end diastolic volumes is the classical finding. Tissue Doppler assessment of cardiac status shows weakness in longitudinal subendocardial fibers which is assessed by measurement of peak left ventricular systolic velocity and strain. The diastolic dysfunction in CCM is also termed "lusitropic dysfucntion", a term that better defines the ventricular relaxation property of cardiac musculature. An increment in myocardial wall stiffness due to myocardial hypertrophy, subendothelial edema and fibrosis lead to increased filling pressures of left ventricle and atrium. Beta blocker therapy improves QT prolongation. Normalization of QT occurs in some patients with the use of beta blockers, but not all. Early period of post-liver transplantation is associated with reversal of QTc. Cirrhosis patients with cardiomyopathy benefit from liver transplantation as no specific treatment other than transplantation exists for this condition.[110-112]

REFERENCES

1. Hytiroglou P, Snover DC, Alves V, Balabaud C, Bhathal PS, Bioulac-Sage P, et al. Beyond "cirrhosis": a proposal from the International Liver Pathology Study Group. Am J Clin Pathol. 2012;137:5-9.
2. Standish RA, Cholongitas E, Dhillon A, Burroughs AK, Dhillon AP. An appraisal of the histopathological assessment of Liver fibrosis. Gut. 2006;55;569-78.
3. Fabris C, Smirne C, Toniutto P, Colletta C, Rapetti R, Minisini R, et al. Usefulness of six non-proprietary indirect markers of liver fibrosis in patients with chronic hepatitis C. Clin Chem Lab Med. 2008;46:253-9.
4. Pinzani M, Rosselli M, Zuckermann M. Liver cirrhosis. Best Pract Res Cli Gastroenterol. 2011;25:281-90.
5. Falize L, Guillygomarc'h A, Perrin M, Lainé F, Guyader D, Brissot P, et al. Reversibility of hepatic fibrosis in treated genetic hemochromatosis: a study of 36 cases. Hepatology. 2006;44:472-7.
6. Martinez SM, Crespo G, Navasa M, Forns X. Noninvasive assessment of liver fibrosis. Hepatology. 2011;53:325-35.
7. Garcia-Tsao G, Friedman S, Iredale J, Pinzani M. Now there are many (stages) where before there was one: in search of a pathophysiological classification of cirrhosis. Hepatology. 2010;51:1445-9.
8. Friedman SL. Mechanisms of hepatic fibrogenesis. Gastroenterology. 2008;134:1655-69.
9. Choi SS, Diehl AM. Epithelial-tomesenchymal transitions in the liver. Hepatology. 2009;50:2007-13.
10. Merat S, Sotoudehmanesh R, Nouraie M, Peikan-Heirati M, Sepanlou SG, Malekzadeh R, et al. Sampling error in histopathology findings of nonalcoholic fatty liver disease: a post mortem liver histology study. Arch Iran Med. 2012;15:418-21.
11. Pinzani M, Rombouts K, Colagrande S. Fibrosis in chronic liver diseases: diagnosis and management. J Hepatol. 2005;42(Suppl):S22-36.
12. Wong VW, Wong GL, Choi PC, Chan AW, Li MK, Chan HY, et al. Disease progression of non-alcoholic fatty liver disease: a prospective study with paired liver biopsies at 3 years. Gut. 2010;59:969-74.
13. Zhao W, Li JJ, Cao DY, Li X, Zhang LY, He Y, et al. Intravenous injection of mesenchymal stem cells is effective in treating liver fibrosis. World J Gastroenterol. 2012;18:1048-58.
14. Kisseleva T, Cong M, Paik Y, Scholten D, Jiang C, Benner C, et al. Myofibroblasts revert to an inactive phenotype during regression of liver fibrosis. Proc Natl Acad Sci USA. 2012;109:9448-53.
15. Friedman SL. Evolving challenges in hepatic fibrosis. Nat Rev Gastroenterol Hepatol. 2010;7:425-36.
16. Seki E, De Minicis S, Osterreicher CH, Kluwe J, Osawa Y, Brenner DA, et al. TLR4 enhances TGF-beta signaling and hepatic fibrosis. Nat Med. 2007;13:1324-32.
17. Dranoff JA, Wells RG. Portal fibroblasts: underappreciated mediators of biliary fibrosis. Hepatology. 2010;51:1438-44.
18. Mani H, Kleiner DE. Liver biopsy findings in chronic hepatitis B. Hepatology. 2009;49:S61-71.
19. Pirovino M, Linder R, Boss C, Kochli HP, Mahler F. Cutaneous spider nevi in liver cirrhosis: capillary microscopical and hormonal investigations. Klin Wochenschr. 1988;66:298-302.
20. Foutch PG, Sullivan JA, Gaines JA, Sanowski RA. Cutaneous vascular spiders in cirrhotic patients: correlation with hemorrhage from esophageal varices. Am J Gastroenterol. 1988;83:723-6.
21. Simonovsky V. The diagnosis of cirrhosis by high resolution ultrasound of the liver surface. Br J Radiol. 1999;72:29-34.
22. Groszmann RJ, Abraldes JG. Portal hypertension. From bedside to bench. J Clin Gastroenterol. 2005;39(Suppl 2):S125-30.
23. Ripoll C, Groszmann R, Garcia-Tsao G, Grace N, Burroughs A, Planas R, et al. Hepatic venous pressure gradient predicts clinical decompensation in patients with compensated cirrhosis. Gastroenterology. 2007;133:481-8.
24. D'Amico G, Garcia-Tsao G, Pagliaro L. Natural history and prognostic indicators of survival in cirrhosis: a systematic review of 118 studies. J Hepatol. 2006;44:217-31.
25. de Franchis R. Revising consensus in portal hypertension: report of the Baveno V consensus workshop on methodology of diagnosis and therapy in portal hypertension. J Hepatol. 2010;53:762-8.
26. Sanyal AJ, Bosch J, Blei A, Arroyo V. Portal hypertension and its complications. Gastroenterology. 2008;134:1715-28.
27. Castera L, Pinzani M, Bosch J. Noninvasive evaluation of portal hypertension using transient elastography. J Hepatol. 2012;56:696-703.
28. Thabut D, Moreau R, Lebrec D. Noninvasive assessment of portal hypertension in patients with cirrhosis. Hepatology. 2011;53:683-94.
29. Monescillo A, Martinez-Lagares F, Ruiz-del-Arbol L, Sierra A, Guevara C, Jimenez E, et al. Influence of portal hypertension and its early decompression by TIPS placement on the outcome of variceal bleeding. Hepatology. 2004;40:793-801.
30. Runyon BA. Management of adult patients with ascites due to cirrhosis. Hepatology. 2004;39:841-56.
31. Gines P, Cardenas A, Arroyo V, Rodes J. Management of cirrhosis and ascites. N Engl J Med. 2004;350:1646-54.
32. Moore KP, Aithal GP. Guidelines on the management of ascites in cirrhosis. Gut. 2006;55(Suppl 6):vi1-12.
33. Gerbes AL, Gulberg V. Progress in treatment of massive ascites and hepatorenal syndrome. World J Gastroenterol. 2006;12:516-9.
34. Leung W, Wong F. Medical management of ascites. Expert Opin Pharmacother. 2011;12:1269-83.
35. Salerno F, Guevara M, Bernardi M, Moreau R, Wong F, Angeli P, et al. Refractory ascites, pathogenesis, definition, and therapy of a severe complication in cirrhotic patients. Liver Int. 2010;30:937-47.
36. European Association for the Study of the Liver, Ginès P, Angeli P, Lenz K, Møller S, Moore K, et al. EASL clinical practice guidelines on the management of ascites, spontaneous bacterial peritonitis, and hepatorenal syndrome in cirrhosis. J Hepatol. 2010;53:397-417.
37. Sigal SH, Stanca CM, Fernandez J, Arroyo V, Navasa M. Restricted use of albumin for spontaneous bacterial peritonitis. Gut. 2007;56:597-9.
38. Thanopoulou AC, Koskinas JS, Hadziyannis SJ. Spontaneous bacterial peritonitis (SBP): clinical, laboratory, and prognostic features. A single-center experience. Eur J Intern Med. 2002;13:194-8.
39. Runyon BA. Management of adult patients with ascites due to cirrhosis: an update. Hepatology. 2009;49:2087-107.
40. Shalimar, Acharya SK. Difficult to treat spontaneous bacterial peritonitis. Trop Gastro. 2013;34(1):7-13.
41. Wiest R, Krag A, Gerbes A. Spontaneous bacterial peritonitis: recent guidelines and beyond. Gut. 2012;61:297-310.
42. Cardenas A, Kelleher T, Chopra S. Review article: hepatic hydrothorax. Aliment Pharmacol Ther. 2004;20:271-9.
43. Lazaridis KN, Frank JW, Krowka MJ, Kamath PS. Hepatic hydrothorax: pathogenesis, diagnosis, and management. Am J Med. 1999;107:262-7.
44. Kinasewitz GT, Keddissi JI. Hepatic hydrothorax. Curr Opin Pulm Med. 2003;9:261-5.
45. Foschi F, Piscaglia F, Pompili M, Corbelli C, Marano G. Real-time contras enhanced ultrasound—a new simple tool for detection of peritoneal-pleural communications in hepatic hydrothorax. Ultraschall Med. 2008;29:538-42.
46. Xiol X, Guardiola J. Hepatic hydrothorax. Curr Opin Pulm Med. 1998;4:239-42.
47. Garcia N Jr, Mihas AA. Hepatic hydrothorax: pathophysiology, diagnosis, and management. Clin Gastroenterol. 2004;38:52-8.
48. Xiol X, Tremosa G, Castellote J, Gornals J, Lama C, Lopez C, et al. Liver transplantation in patients with hepatic hydrothorax. Transp Int. 2005;18:672-5.

49. Takahashi K, Chin K, Sumi K, Nakamura T, Matsumoto H, Niimi A, et al. Resistant hepatic hydrothorax: a successful case with treatment by nCPAP. Respiratory Medicine. 2005,99:262-4.
50. Takayama T, Kurokawa Y, Kaiwa Y, Ansai M, Chiba T, Inoue T, et al. A new technique of thoracoscopic pleurodesis for refractory hepatic hydrothorax. Surg Endosc. 2004;18:140-3.
51. Gluud LL, Krag A. Banding ligation versus beta-blockers for primary prevention in oesophageal varices in adults. Cochrane Database Syst Rev. 2012;8:CD004544.
52. Solà E, Lens S, Guevara M, Martín-Llahí M, Fagundes C, Pereira G, et al. Hyponatremia in patients treated with terlipressin for severe gastrointestinal bleeding due to portal hypertension. Hepatology. 2010;52:1783-90.
53. García-Pagán JC, Caca K, Bureau C, Laleman W, Appenrodt B, Luca A, et al. Early use of TIPS in patients with cirrhosis and variceal bleeding. N Engl J Med. 2010;362:2370-9.
54. Abraldes JG, Villanueva C, Bañares R, Aracil C, Catalina MV, Garci A-Pagán JC, et al. Hepatic venous pressure gradient and prognosis in patients with acute variceal bleeding treated with pharmacologic and endoscopic therapy. J Hepatol. 2008;48: 229-36.
55. Augustin S, Altamirano J, González A, Dot J, Abu-Suboh M, Armengol JR, et al. Effectiveness of combined pharmacologic and ligation therapy in high-risk patients with acute esophageal variceal bleeding. Am J Gastroenterol. 2011;106:1787-95.
56. Bambha K, Kim WR, Pedersen R, Bida JP, Kremers WK, Kamath PS. Predictors of early re-bleeding and mortality after acute variceal haemorrhage in patients with cirrhosis. Gut. 2008;57:814-20.
57. Garcia-Tsao G, Sanyal AJ, Grace ND, Carey W. Prevention and management of gastroesophageal varices and variceal hemorrhage in cirrhosis. Hepatology. 2007;46:922-38.
58. Austin MJ, Shawcross DL. Outcome of patients with cirrhosis admitted to intensive care. Curr Opin Crit Care. 2008;14:202-7.
59. Sarin N, Monga N, Adams PC. Time to endoscopy and outcomes in upper gastrointestinal bleeding. Can J Gastroenterol. 2009;23: 489-93.
60. Dell'Era A, de Franchis R, Iannuzzi F. Acute variceal bleeding: pharmacological treatment and primary/secondary prophylaxis. Best Pract Res Clin Gastroenterol. 2008;22:279-94.
61. Sarin SK, Kumar A. Gastric varices: profile, classification, and management. Am J Gastroenterol. 1989;84(10):1244-9.
62. Trudeau W, Prindiville T. Endoscopic injection sclerosis in bleeding gastric varices. Gastrointest Endosc. 1986;32(4):264-8.
63. Tanihata H, Minamiguchi H, Sato M, Kawai N, Sonomura T, Takasaka I, et al. Changes in portal systemic pressure gradient after balloon-occluded retrograde transvenous obliteration of gastric varices and aggravation of esophageal varices. Cardiovasc Intervent Radiol. 2009;32(6):1209-16.
64. Sarin SK, Mishra SR. Endoscopic therapy for gastric varices. Clin Liver Dis. 2010;14(2):263-79.
65. Irani S, Kowdley K, Kozarek R. Gastric varices: an updated review of management. J Clin Gastroenterol. 2011;45(2):133-48.
66. Procaccini NJ, Al-Osaimi AM, Northup P, Argo C, Caldwell SH. Endoscopic cyanoacrylate versus transjugular intrahepatic portosystemic shunt for gastric variceal bleeding: a single-center U.S. analysis. Gastrointest Endosc. 2009;70(5):881-7.
67. Zhao LQ, He W, Ji M, Liu P, Li P. 64-row multidetector computed tomography portal venography of gastric variceal collateral circulation. World J Gastroenterol. 2010;16(8):1003-7.
68. Mishra SR, Sharma BC, Kumar A, Sarin SK. Primary prophylaxis of gastric variceal bleeding comparing cyanoacrylate injection and beta-blockers: a randomized controlled trial. J Hepatol. 2011;54(6):1161-7.
69. Takaji R, Kiyosue H, Matsumoto S, Okahara M, Tanoue S, Kondo Y, et al. Partial thrombosis of gastric varices after balloonoccluded retrograde transvenous obliteration: CT findings and endoscopic correlation. AJR Am J Roentgenol. 2011;196(3): 686-91.
70. Saleem A, Buttar N, Rajan E, Gostout CJ, Baron TH, Wong Kee Song LM. Efficacy and safety of 2-octyl-cyanoacrylate injection for the treatment of gastric variceal hemorrhage. Gastrointest Endosc. 2011;73(4 Suppl. 1):AB210.
71. Sarin SK, Kumar CKN. Ectopic varices. Clinical Liver Disease. 2012;1:168-72.
72. Rodríguez-Roisin R, Krowka MJ. Hepatopulmonary syndrome—a liver-induced lung vascular disorder. The New England Journal of Medicine. 2008;358(22):2378-87.
73. Pham DM, Subramanian R, Parekh S. Coexisting hepatopulmonary syndrome and portopulmonary hypertension: implications for liver transplantation. J Clin Gastroenterol. 2010;44:e136-40.
74. Gupta S, Castel H, Rao RV, Picard M, Lilly L, Faughnan ME, et al. Improved survival after liver transplantation in patients with hepatopulmonary syndrome. Am J Transplant. 2010;10:354-63.
75. Hadengue A, Benhayoun MK, Lebrec D, Benhamou JP. Pulmonary hypertension complicating portal hypertension: prevalence and relation to splanchnic hemodynamics. Gastroenterology. 1991;100:520-8.
76. Bosch J, Garcia-Pagan JC, Berzigotti A, Abraldes JG. Measurement of portal pressure and its role in the management of chronic liver disease. Semin Liver Dis. 2006;26:348-62.
77. Swanson KL, Krowka MJ. Screen for portopulmonary hypertension, especially in liver transplant candidates. Cleve Clin J Med. 2008;75:121-2, 125-30, 133.
78. Sussman NL, Kochar R, Fallon MB. Pulmonary complications in cirrhosis. Curr Opin Organ Transplant. 2011;16:281-8.
79. Ramsay M. Portopulmonary hypertension and right heart failure in patients with cirrhosis. Curr Opin Anaesthesiol. 2010;23:145-50.
80. Fagundes C, Ginés P. Hepatorenal syndrome: a severe, but treatable, cause of kidney failure in cirrhosis. Am J Kidney Dis. 2012;59:874-85.
81. Arroyo V, Fernandez J, Ginés P. Pathogenesis and treatment of hepatorenal syndrome. Semin Liver Dis. 2008;28:81-95.
82. Verna EC, Brown RS, Farrand E, Pichardo EM, Forster CS, Sola-Del Valle DA, et al. Urinary neutrophil gelatinase-associated lipocalin predicts mortality and identifies acute kidney injury in cirrhosis. Dig Dis Sci. 2012;57:2362-70.
83. Gluud LL, Christensen K, Christensen E, Krag A. Systematic review of randomized trials on vasoconstrictor drugs for hepatorenal syndrome. Hepatology. 2010;51:576-84.
84. Charlton MR, Wall WJ, Ojo AO, Ginés P, Textor S, Shihab FS, et al. Report of the first international Liver Transplantation Society expert panel consensus conference on renal insufficiency in liver transplantation. Liver Transpl. 2009;15:S1-34.
85. Angeli P, Ginés P. Hepatorenal syndrome, MELD score and liver transplantation: an evolving issue with relevant implications for clinical practice. J Hepatol. 2012;57:1135-40.
86. Skagen C, Einstein M, Lucey MR, Said A. Combination treatment with octreotide, midodrine, and albumin improves survival in patients with type 1 and type 2 hepatorenal syndrome. J Clin Gastroenterol. 2009;43:680-5.
87. Rice JP, Skagen C, Said A. Liver transplant outcomes for patients with hepatorenal syndrome treated with pretransplant vasoconstrictors and albumin. Transplantation. 2011;91:1141-7.
88. Ferenci P. Lockwood A, Mullen K, Tarter R, Weissenborn K, Blei AT. Hepatic encephalopathy—definition, nomenclature, diagnosis, and quantification: final report of the working party at the 11th World Congresses of Gastroenterology, Vienna, 1998. Hepatology. 2002;35:716-21.
89. Shawcross DL, Wright G, Olde Damink SW, Jalan R. Role of ammonia and inflammation in minimal hepatic encephalopathy. Metab Brain Dis. 2007;22:125-38.

90. Shawcross DL, Davies NA, Williams R, Jalan R. Systemic inflammatory response exacerbates the neuropsychological effects of induced hyperammonemia in cirrhosis. J Hepatol. 2004;40:247-54.
91. Bajaj JS. Current and future diagnosis of hepatic encephalopathy. Metab Brain Dis. 2010;25:107-10.
92. Bajaj JS, Schubert CM, Heuman DM, Wade JB, Gibson DP, Topaz A, et al. Persistence of cognitive impairment after resolution of overt hepatic encephalopathy. Gastroenterology. 2010;138:2332-40.
93. Román E, Córdoba J, Torrens M, Torras X, Villanueva C, Vargas V, et al. Minimal hepatic encephalopathy is associated with falls. Am J Gastroenterol. 2011;106:476-82.
94. Bajaj JS, Heuman DM, Wade JB, Gibson DP, Saeian K, Wegelin JA, et al. Rifaximin improves driving simulator performance in a randomized trial of patients with minimal hepatic encephalopathy. Gastroenterology. 2011;140:478-87.
95. Sarin SK, Sreenivas DV, Lahoti D, Saraya A. Factors influencing development of portal hypertensive gastropathy in patients with portal hypertension. Gastroenterology. 1992;102:994-9.
96. Primignani M, Carpinelli L, Preatoni P, Battaglia G, Carta A, Prada A, et al. Natural history of portal hypertensive gastropathy in patients with liver cirrhosis. The New Italian Endoscopic Club for the study and treatment of esophageal varices (NIEC). Gastroenterology. 2000;119:181-7.
97. Perini R, Camara P, Ferraz J. Pathogenesis of portal hypertensive gastropathy: translating basic research into clinical practice. Nat Clin Pract Gastroenterol Hepatol. 2009;6:150-8.
98. Karajeh M, Hurlstone D, Stephenson T, Ray-Chaudhuri D, Gleeson D. Refractory bleeding from portal hypertensive gastropathy: a further novel role for thalidomide therapy? Eur J Gastroenterol Hepatol. 2006;18:545-8.
99. Pan WD, Xun RY, Chen YM. Correlations of portal hypertensive gastropathy of hepatitis B cirrhosis with other factors. Hepatobiliary Pancreatic Dis Int. 2002;1:527-31.
100. Yuksel O, Koklu S, Arhan M, Yolcu OF, Ertuğrul I, Odemiş B, et al. Effects of esophageal varices eradication on portal hypertensive gastropathy and fundal varices: a retrospective and comparative study. Dig Dis Sci. 2006;51:27-30.
101. Abraldes JG, Angermayr B, Bosch J. The management of portal hypertension. Clin Liver Dis. 2005;9:685-713.
102. Dulai GS, Jensen DM, Kovacs TO, Grainek IM, Jutabha R. Endoscopic treatment outcomes in watermelon stomach patients with and without portal hypertension. Endoscopy. 2004;36:68-72.
103. Burak KW, Lee SS, Beck PL. Portal hypertensive gastropathy and gastric antral vascular ectasia (GAVE) syndrome. Gut. 2001;49:866-72.
104. Rosenfeld G, Enns R. Argon photocoagulation in the treatment of gastric antral vascular ectasia and radiation proctitis. Curr Endoscop Prac. 2009;23:801-4.
105. Wells CD, Harrison ME, Gurudu SR, Crowell MD, Byrne TJ, Depetris G, et al. Treatment of gastric antral vascular ectasia (watermelon stomach) with endoscopic band ligation. Gastrointest Endosc. 2008;68:231-6.
106. Alqahtani SA, Fouad TR, Lee SS. Cirrhotic cardiomyopathy. Semin Liver Dis. 2008;28:59-69.
107. Wong F. Cirrhotic cardiomyopathy. Hepatol Int. 2009;3:294-304.
108. Møller S, Henriksen JH. Cirrhotic cardiomyopathy. J Hepatol. 2010;53:179-90.
109. Trevisani F, Di Micoli A, Zambruni A, Biselli M, Santi V, Erroi V, et al. QT interval prolongation by acute gastrointestinal bleeding in patients with cirrhosis. Liver Int. 2012;32:1510-5.
110. Mandell MS, Tsou MY. Cardiovascular dysfunction in patients with endstage liver disease. J Chin Med Assoc. 2008;71:331-5.
111. Carey EJ, Gautam M, Ingall T, Douglas DD. The effect of liver transplantation on autonomic dysfunction in patients with end-stage liver disease. Liver Transpl. 2008;14:235-9.
112. Ripoll C, Catalina MV, Yotti R, Olmedilla L, Pérez-Peña J, Lo Iacono O, et al. Cardiac dysfunction during liver transplantation: incidence and preoperative predictors. Transplantation. 2008;85:1766-72.

CHAPTER 79

Artificial Liver Support in Liver Failure

Rakhi Maiwall, Manoj Kumar Sharma

INTRODUCTION

The liver is considered as a complex internal organ which has multitude of functions including storage, synthesis, detoxification and immune modulation. Lack of these functions because of liver failure culminates in life threatening multiorgan dysfunction. Despite improved outcomes in patients with acute liver failure (ALF) following the introduction of liver transplantation in the early 1980s, mortality among these patients has remained high. Organ shortage, which makes it difficult or impossible to perform transplantation in a timely manner, may explain the relative high mortality of 40–50% among these patients.[1] Only 30% of the patients get liver transplantation either because of scarcity of organs or because of factors causing exclusion from the transplant waiting list. Complications and side effects associated with immunosuppression play an important role in the result of liver transplantation for liver failure. A liver support system, on the other hand, may either provide temporary support until an organ becomes available, or ideally replace the failing liver until it can regenerate. Another situation where artificial liver support has been tried is acute on chronic liver failure (ACLF) which has been defined as acute hepatic insult presenting as jaundice (Sr. Bil. ≥5 mg/dL) and coagulopathy [international normalized ratio (INR) ≥1.5], complicated within 4 weeks by ascites and/or encephalopathy in a patient with previously diagnosed or undiagnosed chronic liver disease.[2] The mortality of these patients is very high, almost 50–60%, as majority of these patients succumb to multiorgan failure and die waiting on transplant list.[3] It has always been a challenge to support the failing liver during the crisis caused by the precipitating event as in most of these patients the liver failure is usually reversible. Liver transplantation remains the only treatment modality that can improve survival in patients with both ALF and ACLF. There are two broad types of extracorporeal liver support, i.e. non-cell based and cell-based. Non-cell based systems are nonbiological systems which provide only detoxification function and include hemofiltration, hemodialysis, plasma exchange, charcoal perfusion which were used in the past and more recently include the molecular adsorbent recirculating system (MARS) and Prometheus. Cell-based systems incorporate hepatocytes and hence perform detoxification, biotransformation and synthetic functions and include bioartificial liver, hepatocyte transplantation and xenogenic support.

NON-CELL BASED EXTRACORPOREAL LIVER SUPPORT SYSTEM

Several extracorporeal liver support systems like hemodialysis, plasma exchange, hemofiltration, charcoal perfusion have been utilized earlier with an aim to get rid of the putative toxins and inflammatory cytokines that allow liver to recover or as a bridge to liver transplantation. However, extent of removal of protein-bound toxins is only minor. The accumulation of toxic metabolites plays a crucial role in liver failure and these toxins differ in their physicochemical characteristics (viz. their water solubility, molecular size and protein binding). Each of the conventional extracorporeal procedures which evolved was designed so as to incorporate highest toxin removal efficacy in liver failure by enabling removal of large protein-bound toxins apart from the small water-soluble toxins like ammonia and urea which are removed by the conventional hemodialysis and hemofiltration. As a consequence of this, artificial liver support capable of removing lipophilic substances such as bilirubin (both conjugated as well as unconjugated), bile acids, aromatic amino acids, medium-chain fatty acids, indoles, tryptophan, mercaptans and endogenous benzodiazepines were developed. Later on came the concept of removal of protein-bound toxins via albumin as a substrate for adsorption as in detoxification procedure and hence the concept of albumin dialysis and fractionated plasma separation and adsorption (FPSA) were introduced.[4] A brief description of the currently available artificial liver support therapies is as under:

Peritoneal Dialysis

This is mainly used in patients with ascites who have both renal as well as liver failure, however the efficacy to remove hepatic toxins is limited.[5,6]

Hemodialysis

This also removes predominantly water-soluble toxins by diffusion and as albumin-bound toxins not removed with the conventional hemodialysis, it has limited role in liver failure.

Hemofiltration

This process provides some benefit in liver failure as it allow removal of albumin-bound toxins like ammonia by use of highly permeable membranes. Studies have demonstrated benefit in patients with fulminant hepatitis with hepatic encephalopathy.[7,8]

Continuous Renal Replacement Therapy (CRRT)

In this, permeable membranes are incorporated with a blood pump that allows replacement therapy for extended periods and is associated with good intracranial stability and few cardiovascular complications when compared to hemodialysis and hemofiltration.[9] The blood pump is not required if an arterial line is obtained, wherein it is called continuous arteriovenous hemodialysis (CAVHD). However, with the use of venous lines, a blood pump is required and is called continuous venovenous hemodialysis (CVVHD). CRRT by decreasing intracranial pressure (ICP) help in improving hepatic encephalopathy and in recovery from sepsis by removing the inflammatory cytokines.[10,11] CRRT has not however shown an effect on overall outcome of patients. Primary applications hence include control of elevated ICP in fulminant hepatic failure and management of cerebral edema through removal of middle molecules.[12]

Charcoal Hemoperfusion

In charcoal hemoperfusion, blood containing lipid soluble toxins is made to pass through a charcoal particles cartridge which adsorbs these toxins and is considered better than hemodialysis (HD) or hemofiltration (HF) because of its capability to removed lipid soluble toxins in patients with liver failure. Randomized controlled trials (RCTs) have shown that it may not help in prolonging survival, so not gained any popularity.[13]

Plasma Exchange

This incorporates use of highly permeable plasma filters and use of charcoal columns for adsorption of toxins and hence in patients with liver failure this helps in removal of both water-soluble and lipid-soluble toxins in patients with liver failure. Only few case series exist on plasma exchange which have showed no improvement in neurological function or mortality, in spite of improvement in coagulation parameters and decreased levels of cytokines and endotoxin.[14] Plasma exchange involves removal of liver toxins which is replaced by equivalent amount of fresh frozen plasma. It has been shown to have some clinical benefit but no improvement in survival has been seen. Moreover, it is very costly because of the huge volumes of plasma that is required.

Single Pass Albumin Dialysis

The single pass albumin dialysis (SPAD) procedure is based on the same principle as molecular adsorbent recirculating system (MARS) i.e. of albumin dialysis. In SPAD on one side of a semipermeable membrane toxin-rich blood passes by and on the other side, in counter-current manner an albumin-enriched electrolyte solution flows in the opposite direction. High-flux membranes having relatively small pore size allow passage of smaller compounds freely, however passage of large albumin molecules is hindered. SPAD is a simple procedure which can be performed using continuous venovenous hemofiltration (CVVHDF) machine used for CRRT. In this blood flows through a standard albumin-impermeable high-flux dialyzer and later dialyzed against an albumin-containing dialysate. In SPAD, protein-bound molecules that can pass through the membrane pores are removed. Dialysate is discarded after each passage through the dialyzer or hemofilter that makes it different from MARS. Heparin or citrate is used for anticoagulation. The albumin concentration used in the dialysate is 2% and flow of dialysate is set to 1 L/h in counter-current manner and the albumin consumption is approximately 480 g per 24 hours which increases the cost of the procedure tremendously.

Molecular Adsorbent and Recirculation System

Molecular adsorbent re-circulatory system (MARS) is the most commonly applied artificial liver support that is based on the similar principle as albumin dialysis in SPAD where albumin acts as molecular adsorber. MARS was introduced in 1993 and requires a hemodialysis or hemofiltration and MARS monitoring device. It comprise of a hemofilter (Marsflux filter) with a size selection threshold of less than 60 kDa through which patient's blood is passed. As these are impermeable for albumin and albumin-bound toxins such as unconjugated bilirubin which are retained on the blood side of the membrane. In the secondary circuit, 20% albumin solution act as the dialysate and flow in a counter-direction. Due to concentration gradient across the MARS membrane, toxins in the patient's blood dissociate and bind to the albumin which is there in the secondary circuit. Later in the secondary circuit, water-soluble toxins are removed using high flux filter and the toxin bound albumin solution is next regenerated by passing two adsorbers: an uncoated charcoal adsorber and an anion exchanger resin and finally the cleansed albumin re-enters the hemofilter of the primary circuit. The duration of single MARS session is approximately 6–8 hours, and after that time binding competence of the adsorbers fall significantly and adsorbers need to be replaced in case the session needs to be prolonged. The systemic hemodynamics improves with MARS treatment and hypotension is rarely reported with MARS as compared to Prometheus. This is because the albumin which fills in the secondary circuit is exogenous albumin as compared to Prometheus where the patients' albumin fills in the secondary circuit causing more frequent hemodynamic alterations.[15-17] The frequency of bleeding episodes are reported less frequently with MARS as compared to Prometheus because the membrane pore size is smaller in MARS and hence coagulation factors and large proteins are unable to cross the MARS membrane.[18] For the same reason toxin removal efficacy of Prometheus is proven to be better as compared to MARS as larger molecules which are tightly bound to albumin, i.e. unconjugated bilirubin can cross the Prometheus membrane. A reversible fall in platelet counts and activation of coagulation cascade has been reported with MARS.[19-22] There is only a single study which describes severe bleeding episodes in association with MARS treatment.[21]

Prometheus (FPSA–Fractional Plasma Separation and Adsorption)

Falkenhagen et al. in 1999, introduced FPSA which removes both water-soluble and protein-bound toxins.[23-25] In this system, an albumin-permeable filter with a size selection threshold of approximately 250,000 Dalton (250 kD) is used. This enables removal of both albumin and protein-bound toxins from the blood by a special adsorber within the secondary circuit. Prometheus system includes the FPSA method with high-flux hemodialysis (of the blood) in an extracorporeal detoxification system. Using a usual dialysis catheter, blood with all the toxins passes through the primary extracorporeal circuit where the albumin fraction of the blood is selectively filtered through a specific membrane i.e. Albuflow® which is a polysulfone, albumin-permeable filter and then it enters a secondary circuit where the toxins are adsorbed by two adsorber columns, i.e. a neutral resin adsorber (Prometh® 01), and an anion exchanger (Prometh® 02). After passing through the two adsorber columns, the purified blood enters the primary circuit wherein high-flux dialyzer enables effective removal of water-soluble compounds from patient's blood like a conventional dialysis system. Hypotension is more likely with Prometheus as compared to MARS and SPAD[26] as early in the procedure, there occur an acute decrease in intravascular blood volume as it moves and fills in the extracorporeal circuit. For the same reason a reduction of the colloid osmotic pressure has been reported with Prometheus.[15,18] A reversible decrease in white blood cells (WBC) counts, activation of coagulation similar to MARS has been reported.[27] Prometheus is associated with more loss of anticoagulant and procoagulant proteins because of a larger pore size of the membrane however, these effects have not translated into serious adverse effects and overall its considered a safe therapy. Also toxin removal efficacy has been shown to be superior to MARS.[28,29]

Indications of Extracorporeal Liver Support

- Acute on chronic liver failure complicated by progressive jaundice, renal dysfunction and hepatic encephalopathy
- Acute liver failure
- Severe alcoholic steatohepatitis
- Primary graft dysfunction postliver transplantation
- Post-hepatectomy liver failure
- Intrahepatic cholestasis with intractable pruritus
- Overdoses or intoxication with protein-bound substances.

Therapeutic Effects of Extracorporeal Therapy

Effect on Toxin Removal

Substances which are removed include albumin-bound substances like unconjugated bilirubin, aromatic amino acids, cholic acid, hydrophobic (unbound) substances, like ammonia, phenols, mercaptans, hydrophilic substances including conjugated bilirubin, cytokines [tumor necrosis factor alpha (TNFα), interleukin 6 (IL-6)] and additionally uremic substances and possibly endotoxin. Studies have shown higher competence of Prometheus as compared to MARS in removal of toxins.[16-18]

There have been limited reported data which have looked into artificial liver support systems in ALF patients, as most studies looked into patients with ACLF.

Effect on Hepatic Encephalopathy and Survival

In a meta-analysis of four RCTs, where 67 patients were analyzed and in two nonrandomized trials where 61 patients were used for explorative analysis. In the primary meta-analysis, mortality rate seems comparable between MARS treatment and standard medical treatment [relative risk (RR), 0.56; 95% confidence interval (CI), 0.28–1.14; p 0.11]. Out of four, only one randomized trial showed significant decline in mortality. Also, similar results reported in subgroup analysis of two trials one for ALF and another for ACLF that there is no survival benefit with MARS treatment. However, significant survival benefit noted with MARS treatment after explorative analysis of two nonrandomized trials (RR, 0.36; 95% CI, 0.17–0.76; p 0.007) which could be ascribed to bias in nonrandomized trials and authors of the meta-analysis concluded that MARS treatment in comparison with standard medical therapy (SMT) had no significant survival benefit in liver failure patients.[30] In another systematic review and meta-analysis comparing SMT with extracorporeal artificial and bioartificial liver support a significant survival benefit was seen in patients with ALF (risk ratio 0·70; Z = 1·95; P = 0·05) with number needed to treat (NNT) = 8.[31] In controlled trials by Kantola et al. and Schmidt et al., a significant survival benefit and improvement in systemic hemodynamics was seen with MARS therapy respectively.[32,33] In large multicentric ALF study (presented at American Association for the Study of Liver Disease (AASLD), San Francisco 2008) patients treated with at least three sessions of MARS had significantly improved survival. MARS was used as a bridge to transplantation in this study. In a study by Bergis et al.,[34] use of liver support therapy by FPSA (Prometheus®) was shown to offer a safe way to remove amanita toxin and can avoid the need for liver transplantation. In another trial of 27 patients[35] 85.2% (ALF) and 14.8% (ACLF) treated with Prometheus for 85 applications (median 3 treatments/patient, mean: 6 h) significant decreases in biochemical parameters total bilirubin, ammonia, blood urea nitrogen, creatinine and pH was demonstrated. Four patients (14.8%) received liver transplantation after the treatments; however in nine patients, transplantation was not necessary. Overall survival was 48.1% (4 transplanted and 9 treated patients). FPSA is associated with no hematological complications.

Effect on Systemic Hemodynamics

Laleman et al. randomized 12 patients with ACLF to SMT (n = 6), or MARS with SMT (n = 6). In comparison to SMT, favorable effects of MARS on mean arterial pressure (MAP), systemic vascular resistance index (SVRI), plasma rennin activity (PRA) and nitric oxide (NO) were seen. They showed that MARS treatment improves systemic hemodynamics in these patients.[17]

Effect on Hepatic Encephalopathy, Renal Dysfunction and Survival

Heemann et al. conducted a prospective controlled trial in two centers looked at 24 patients of cirrhosis with acute decompensation with marked hyperbilirubinemia (serum bilirubin >20 mg/dL) who were randomized to receive SMT alone (controls, n = 12) or extracorporeal albumin dialysis (ECAD) (using MARS) in addition (n = 12). In comparison to control, patient treated with ECAD showed significant decrease in plasma bile acids and bilirubin with improvement in encephalopathy and renal function. The procedure was found to be safe, with comparable adverse event profiles in both groups and most importantly, albumin dialysis was associated with a significant improvement in 30-day survival (11 of 12 vs 6 of 12 in controls).[36]

In another study conducted by Sen et al., 18 patients with alcohol-related ACLF due to inflammation-related precipitants randomized to SMT alone, or with MARS therapy over 7 days. In comparison to SMT, encephalopathy improved significantly with MARS (P <01). Renal function and MAP remained unchanged with no significant alteration observed in plasma ammonia and cytokines in either group.[37]

In a prospective, randomized, controlled, multicenter trial to assess the tolerability, efficacy and safety of ECAD using molecular adsorbent recirculating system (MARS, n = 39) and SMT (n = 31) alone. ECAD showed better improvement in hepatic encephalopathy (mean, 34%; median, 30%) when compared with the SMT group (mean, 18.9%; median, 0%) (P = 0.044) and was reached faster and more commonly than in the SMT group (P = 0.045). However, the study was not designed to assess survival.[38]

Rifai et al., in an uncontrolled study showed no improvement in hepatic encephalopathy by Prometheus in patients with ACLF. Animal studies have shown decrease of ICP under extracorporeal liver support. There are no human studies available till date. In an animal study, MARS helped in reduction of ICP in ALF in pigs, another study showed similar results with Prometheus.[39-41]

Hepatorenal syndrome (HRS) is a late complication in cirrhosis and is associated with increased mortality.[42-44] In the large prospective randomized multicentric trial across 10 European countries (HELIOS trial) 145 patients were randomized to SMT + FPSA therapy (n = 77) or SMT; n = 68). During the first 3 weeks of study, FPSA therapy was intended for 8–11 treatments (each having minimum duration of 4 h). Overall survival difference did not reach statistical significance (p = 0.38, log rank test). Twenty-eight patients underwent liver transplantation comprising 15 patients in SMT+FPSA (19.5%) and 13 in SMT (19.1%). In subgroup analysis, FPSA therapy showed a significant survival benefit in patients with HRS type I (p = 0.0 4) or MELD score more than 30 (p = 0.02).[45] In a prospective clinical study by Rifai et al., 10 patients with HRS underwent two consecutive Prometheus treatments. After treatment, statistically significant improvement was noted in serum creatinine and urea levels as well as blood pH. However, the survival was not assessed in this study.[43]

Mitzner et al. looked at multiorgan dysfunction in patients with HRS. Eight HRS patients were treated intermittently 4–14 times (total 47, mean 5.9 ± 3.4) between 4 h and 8 h or single treatment. Apart from improvement in biochemical parameters there was improvement in MAP increased from 71.9 ± 12.8 to 95.6 ± 7.8 Torr (p <0.001), oliguria or anuria, which reverted with treatment and ascites which was present in all patients became undetectable in all. A decrease in encephalopathy was also observed, from 2.8 ± 0.8 to 0.8 ± 0.7 (p < 0.0001), Child's index decreased from 13.25 ± 1.3 to 9.4 ± 1.8 (p < 0.001). Survival rate in the hospital was 62%.[42]

One eighty nine ACLF patients (bilirubin >5 mg/dL and at least one of the following: HRS, hepatic encephalopathy grade II–IV or bilirubin more than 20 mg/dL) were randomized either to MARS (n = 95) or to standard therapy (ST) (n = 94) in the multicentric RELIEF trial.[46] MARS was planned at low doses (around ten 6–8 h sessions during 21 days). No significant differences were noted at inclusion, although precipitating factors like high MELD (>20; 81.7% vs 69.4%; p = 0.07) or spontaneous bacterial peritonitis (SBP) (16.9% vs 7.1%; p = 0.05) were more in the MARS group. A higher fall in the level of serum creatinine and bilirubin with improvement in hepatic encephalopathy (56% vs 39% p = 0.06) was observed in MARS group. The percentage of patients dying within 28 days after treated with MARS or standard therapy was almost similar in the two groups (40.8% vs 40.0%). Age, MELD and SBP were associated with higher mortality (15.9% vs 8.6%; p = 0.1). Survival benefit of MARS was not observed (OR: 0.77, 95% CI: 0.37–1.59).[37]

In 16 French centers, a randomized controlled multicenter trial (The FULMAR study) was conducted in 102 patients to assess the efficacy and safety of MARS in subfulminant and fulminant hepatic failure, 38% of which had paracetamol poisoning. However, a trend toward better 6-month survival was noted in the MARS group: 84.9 vs 75.5%; although not reached to the statistical significance. Due to short pretransplantation study phase, as 68 of the 102 patients were transplanted with a median delay of 16.2 hours between listing and incision, interpretation of results became difficult.[47]

Safety of Currently Available Nonbiological Liver Support Systems

Most of the studies published till date have found it to be safe with few reports of worsening of coagulopathy and sepsis associated with albumin dialysis due to removal of clotting factors causing increase in the risk of bleeding.[27,28]

Other Indications

- For severe alcoholic hepatitis
  In the study by Jalan et al.,[48] eight patients of severe alcoholic hepatitis treated with MARS were studied. Patients with histologically proven cirrhosis, encephalopathy stage 2 and serum bilirubin over 150 mmol/L were included. The biochemical parameters of patients that were resistant or had contraindications to other treatments such as corticosteroids were a serum bilirubin between 225 mmol/L and 708 mmol/L, prothrombin time between 17 s and 38 s, the Child-Pugh score was between 11 and 14, serum creatinine of more than 150 mmol/L in six cases, the Maddrey score was at 39 for one case and between 70 and 190 for the other seven patients,

three had SBP, three had previous gastrointestinal bleeding, and one had pneumonia. Out of these patients who received 3–12 courses of 6 hours MARS treatment, four were alive at 3 months, one was alive after successful liver transplantation performed at 21 days post-MARS, however, four died from multiple organ dysfunction or sepsis within the first 38 days post-MARS. For such severely ill patients, a 50% survival rate at 3 months is encouraging. Extracorporeal liver support has to find its position in the treatment of acute severe alcoholic hepatitis with Maddrey's score of more than 32 in comparison or in combination with other treatments such as steroids[49-51] or pentoxyfilline,[52] or treatments which are already under investigation like anti-TNF agents.[53] There is a need for adequately powered RCTs to define its role further in this group of patients.

- For refractory cholestatic pruritus
  Uncontrolled data exists showing effectiveness of MARS or Prometheus therapy in relieving severe cholestatic pruritus[54-56] however, removal of protein-bound drugs by MARS could be demonstrated in animal studies.[57]

From the available studies, it is apparent that the artificial liver support systems have a definite improvement in removing water-soluble and protein-bound toxins with a consequent improvement in biochemical parameters in patients with acute and ACLF without any major adverse events and other safety issues. Various studies have reported improvement in MAP, hepatic encephalopathy and HRS.

However, there are still many unanswered questions regarding which group of patients would best benefit from therapy, what is the correct time and mode of treatment, efficacy with respect to clinical end points like survival which need to be assessed with effectively powered and well designed RCTs with strict inclusion and exclusion criteria. It also is important to explore the benefit as a bridge to liver transplantation in patients with acute on chronic liver disease who are not candidates for transplantation to allow for potential recovery of critical liver cell mass that is needed and time to recover from the insult caused by the precipitating event.

CELL-BASED THERAPIES

They can be extracorporeal or ex vivo, i.e. the bioartificial liver or in vivo such as hepatocyte transplantation.

Extracorporeal or ex vivo Therapies

Bioartificial Liver

The term bioartificial liver was first introduced by Matsumura in 1987. He perfused a suspension of porcine hepatocytes in an extracorporeal suspension bioreactor composed of 10×10^9 cryopreserved rabbit hepatocytes separated by a membrane which allowed passage of low and middle molecular weight molecules.[58] It is a challenge to develop an ideal bioreactor for the bioartificial liver which should provide a suitable environment enabling growth and metabolism of hepatocytes. An ideal bioreactor should provide adequate bidirectional mass transport between patient's blood (or plasma) and hepatocytes and protect hepatocytes from the immune system of the host. The common structural designs of bioreactors include, (1) flat plate and monolayer;[59-61] (2) hollow fiber;[62-64] (3) perfused beds or scaffolds;[65-69] (4) beds with encapsulated or suspended cells;[70-73] (5) other designs as in compound bioreactors.[74] There are many bioreactors which have undergone clinical trials however, despite all this there is no bioreactor which is commercially available for clinical use. Another important challenge to develop a bioartificial liver is to get an ideal source of hepatocytes. The common source of isolated hepatocytes are firstly primary hepatocytes but the problems are short viability of hepatocytes even under ideal conditions required for their sustenance and the need for these to attach to an extracellular support matrix to evade programmed cell death and the limited availability of human hepatocytes. Most of these are derived from cadaveric livers which are deemed unsuitable for transplantation thus yielding a poor quality of hepatocytes with a consequential lack of maintaining their viability for extended periods of time.[75] To combat these problems, investigators came up with immortalized human hepatocytes which were developed via spontaneous transformation or telomerase constructs introduction or retroviral transfection. The C3A line, a subclone of the HepG2 hepatoblastoma cell line, has been tested clinically in extracorporeal liver assist device (ELAD)™[76-78] The clinical trials have suggested safety without any evidence of tumorigenicity, however when compared to adult porcine hepatocytes, the problems stayed is of decreased levels of ammonia detoxification and urea cycle activity, P450 activity, and amino acid metabolism.[79] The plausible reason for reduced ammonia removal has been recognized as primarily due to reduced expression of its urea cycle genes.[80] To overcome this problem and to enhance the ammonia detoxification activity of C3A hepatocytes, the investigators showed higher ammonia clearance after transfection of glutamine synthetase gene into C3A cells.[81] Another important source of hepatocytes for bioartificial liver is immortalized hepatocytes from normal human hepatocytes as these HepCL cells were functionally alike to primary human fetal hepatocytes and additionally showed no tumorigenicity; and hence a superiority of HepCL to HepG2 cells.[82] Xenogenic cells have also been explored as possible cell source in view of the shortage of human hepatocytes and consequently primary porcine hepatocytes have been tried. These have the advantage of maintaining hepatocyte-specific metabolic functions including ammonia detoxification which was a limitation in using immortalized human hepatocytes.[83] The use of porcine hepatocytes in the bioartificial livers raises serious concerns for a potential for stimulating a humor land cellular immunologic response because of functional mismatch[84] between proteins released by porcine hepatocytes as compared to humans and also transmission of porcine endogenous retrovirus. Till date, however this has not been recognized in the clinically tested bioartificial livers incorporating porcine hepatocytes. Another challenge while making an ideal bioreactor device is to address the important concept of liver zonation. In the normal human liver there exists zonation i.e. as blood travels through the sinusoids, there is decrease in concentration of certain substrates such as oxygen or hormones. There is variation in cells in the periportal zone (close to the branches of the portal vein and hepatic artery) from cells in the perivenous zone (region close to the central vein) in the presence of enzymes, receptors and metabolic capacity, for example, bile formation and urea synthesis which is seen in the periportal zone whereas glutamine synthesis and xenobiotic metabolism is more prevalent in the perivenous zone.

The different bioartificial liver systems which have been tested in clinical trials include:

Academic Medical Center-bioartificial liver (AMC-BAL) bioreactor: The AMC-BAL bioreactor was developed by Chamuleau. In this 100 g of primary porcine hepatocytes bound to a spiral-shaped polyester fabric with integrated hollow fibers were used. In phase I study, 12 patients with ALF underwent multiple treatments with AMC-BAL, total period varying from 4–35 hours, 1 patient recovered liver function without transplantation and 11 were effectively bridged to transplantation. No adverse events were associated with treatment. Only 8 patients finally survived and were alive at a follow up of 6–30 months. The advantage of the AMC-BAL bioreactor is because of its hollow fiber design which ensures a uniform oxygen supply and a direct connection with patient's plasma and hepatocytes in the bioreactor thus maintaining homogeneity in oxygen supply and metabolite accumulation.[85]

Hepat Assist device: This was formed by Demetriou et al. and it used 5X109 to 7X109 cryopreserved porcine hepatocytes. It is a hybrid device wherein an extracorporeal circuit, the porcine hepatocytes are bound to charcoal columns and collagen-coated microcarriers. The basis for using the charcoal columns was to reduce contact of patient's plasma with its toxins from being exposed to the hepatocytes. In a phase I clinical trial, 39 patients with ALF were treated with 90% survival rate at 1 month.[86] There was improvement noted in biochemical parameters as demonstrated by a significant decrease in blood ammonia, bilirubin and creatinine as well as reduction in ICPs. In another multicenter phase II or III prospective RCT in patients with ALF or primary nonfunction, survival rate at 30 days was not significantly different, 73% and 59% respectively.[87]

Modular Extracorporeal Liver Support-bioartificial liver (MELS-BAL) bioreactor: The MELS-BAL system was developed by Igor M. Sauer and coworkers in Charite Virchow Clinic, Berlin, Germany. This device contains fresh primary porcine hepatocytes incorporated in four autonomously functioning hollow fiber capillary compartments (500 g of primary human hepatocytes in each), albumin dialysis (Detox module) and continuous venovenous hemodiafiltration (Dialysis module).[88,89] The advantages of this system are maintenance of a direct contact between plasma and hepatocytes. The MELS bioreactor mimics a hepatic lobules and in addition combines the detoxification devices, however it has been difficult to manufacture because of its complexity. In vitro studies have confirmed hepatocyte-specific function within the MELS device for approximately 2 months thus maintaining functionality for an extended period of time. Eight patients with ALF were studied in a phase I study in 2003 demonstrated safety and all patients being successfully bridged to transplantation and all alive at 3 years. However, the clinical experience with MELS has been limited by unpredictable supply of human hepatocytes, concerns of xenozoonosis and its relative complexity and high cost.[90,91]

Extracorporeal liver assist device (ELAD): This was developed by Sussman et al. This includes conventional hemodialysis with filtration and four ELAD cartridges containing C3A human hepatoblastoma cells (each has 200 g of hepatocytes). These have ability to grow in glucose-deficient medium and for high albumin production, however have inferior metabolic profiles (ureagenesis). The main problem with the use of this device remained issues of safety and oncogenicity because of use of human hepatoblastoma cells. In a RCT, 24 patients of acute alcoholic hepatitis were treated with ELAD and in comparison to control improvement in hepatic encephalopathy and reduction of ammonia and bilirubin was demonstrated, but did not reached to the statistical significance.[92]

Bioartificial liver support system (BLSS): This device is developed by Excorp Medical (Minneapolis, MN). This device uses a single hollow fiber cartridge containing 100 g of primary porcine hepatocytes and to circulate the patient's anticoagulated blood a venovenous bypass system is used.[93] Safety was demonstrated in a phase I trial in which four patients were treated with BLSS[94] and this is an ongoing phase I or II trial safety evaluation at the University of Pittsburgh or UPMC System.

Hepatic spheroid: This is developed by Mayo Clinic called as the Mayo Spheroid Reservoir Bioartificial Liver (SRBAL). In comparison to monolayer hepatocyte culture, the metabolic performance of the hepatocyte spheroids in terms of albumin production and ureagenesis is superior and the metabolically active state is maintained for up to 28 days. The design is simple and it enables support of unlimited number of primary hepatocytes (up to 250 g to 500 g) in high cell density suspension culture which is 2–5 times more than most first-generation devices allowing and sustaining large quantities of hepatocytes in the same reservoir of the extracorporeal circuit. It hence overcomes the pitfalls of the first generation devices wherein the hepatocytes could only be sustained for a few hours due to the death of anchorage dependent hepatocytes in suspension culture. Spheroids hence allow for a greater dose of cells and also enable higher functionality. A newly developed Multi-Shelf Rocker has been built which can create up to 6 L of hepatocyte suspension.[95]

Hence, the common problems with the bioartificial liver is to get a constant yield of functional hepatocytes. Primary human hepatocytes demonstrate a serious loss of viability after repeated freeze-thaw process and are difficult to proliferate efficiently in vitro, use of human liver tumor-derived cell lines, such as GS-HepG2 [glutamine synthetase (GS)], HepG2-GS-3A4 and functional liver cell-4 (FLC-4), in large animal models[81,96-100] however, have not shown consistent results. It has also been argued that it is difficult to replace all liver functions with a single cell line.[101] Secondly and most importantly, the liver is not only formed by hepatocytes but also by other non-parenchymal cells such as stellate cells, kupffer cells and sinusoidal endothelial cells which are in a state of dynamic interaction with each other. To enable this co-culture techniques have therefore been tried.[102] Hence, it is important to design a bioreactor which is akin to in vivo-like hepatic environment. The most important factors which influence this are maintenance of an adequate oxygenation and bile secretion. In the AMC-BAL and the MELS system there was the advantage of an integral oxygenator[102,103] enabling hepatocytes to acquire oxygen from their immediate surroundings. Again, the disadvantage of such an integral oxygenator is lack of self-regulation and an inability to protect from hypoxia and oxygen toxicity. Another strategy is supplementation of perfusion fluids with red blood cell substitutes (e.g. artificial oxygen carriers), such as perfluorocarbons (PFCs) or hemoglobin-based oxygen carriers (HBOCs)[104-106] which have the capability of carrying large amounts of oxygen. The problems are an increased risk of stroke that has been reported with PFCs.[107] To solve the problem of bile secretion it is possible to incorporate an artificial liver device, for instance an albumin dialysis, or plasma exchange.[108,109] However, the problems with this strategy is the lack of clarity on what proportion of bile acids needs to be discarded.

Cell-based in vivo Therapy

With the recent advances in regenerative medicine there is lot of interest in exploring the potential of hepatic stem cells in therapy for liver diseases. The different types of stem cells which are considered eligible for replacement of liver functions include:

Adult and Fetal Liver Stem Cells

Fetal liver stem cells or hepatoblasts are bipotential cells competent of transforming into both hepatocytes and bile ducts. Isolation and culture of these cells has been shown.[110-112] The adult hepatocytes are endowed with an enormous regenerative potential which is mainly seen in response to hepatectomy or chronic injury and is mainly accomplished by hepatic progenitor cells or oval cells which retain the bipotentiality as seen in fetal hepatobalsts.[111] The main drawback of utilizing these cells on a large scale is the difficult isolation and expansion.[113,114]

Bone Marrow-derived Hepatocyte-like Cells

The bone marrow houses three different types of stem cells i.e. mesenchymal stem cells, hematopoietic stem cells or progenitor cells and endothelial progenitor cells. These cells have demonstrated capability of differentiating into functional hepatocytes. Amongst these mesenchymal stem cells which have favorable immunological properties, ease of access, and with their capability for trans-differentiation might become important in stem cell based therapies for treatment of liver diseases.[115]

Human Annex Stem Cells

Human placental tissue can also be an important source of hepatocyte-like cells. These cells contain higher proliferation and differentiation capacity than adult stem cells. Various studies have demonstrated this as an easily available source of pluripotent stem cells, which can be transplanted or used for cell-therapies.[116,117]

Embryonic Stem Cells

Experiments in animal models have shown the therapeutic potential of these cells where the derivatives have showed the ability to colonize the injured liver and works like a mature hepatocytes.[110]

Hepatocyte-like Cells from IPSCs

These have the advantage of becoming source of an unlimited number of hepatocytes and hence would definitely prove useful in all-autologous settings in future. Hepatocyte-like cells which have been derived from these cells have demonstrated ureagenesis, secretion of albumin and even expression of human cytochrome P450 enzymes and hence fit for therapeutic transplantation.[118]

These cell-based therapies have been mainly tried for ALF, ACLF and acute decompensation of chronic liver disease or after liver resection. Hepatocyte transplantation has also shown benefit with a decrease in mortality among patients with decompensated chronic liver disease awaiting liver transplantation and in patients with ALF.[119,120] Almost 30 cases of hepatocyte transplantation have been reported till date. Mesenchymal stem cells have shown good therapeutic potential in ALF.[121] Encapsulation of hepatocytes and mesenchymal stem cells together has shown improvement in liver functions both in vivo and in vitro for acute liver diseases.[122]

Xenotransplantation

The only liver xenotransplantation (xenoTx) was done in a patient with fulminant hepatic failure as a bridge to allotransplant in 1995 by Makowka et al.[123] To facilitate adsorption of anti-pig antibodies, plasmapheresis and ex vivo perfusion of the donor pig kidneys was done and the pig liver was transplanted heterotopically. The pig liver remained functional however, the patient deteriorated and succumbed to brain stem herniation and died after 34 hours after xenoTx. This simply reflects that use of cross-species transplantation could definitely resolve the current challenge of shortage of suitable donor organs.[124,125] If it is at all possible we can have an unlimited supply of organs both on an emergency and an elective basis. However, major impediments in routine application of this in clinical practice have been the unacceptable graft injury caused by immunosuppression which is administered for extended duration. For patients with ACLF, extracorporeal liver perfusion with pig livers, has been tried[126-129] before the advent of liver transplantation with good results and especially improvement in neurological status was demonstrated. Till date, approximately 141 extracorporeal liver perfusions have been done to treat 87 patients with liver failure.[128] In comparison to BAL devices, xenoTx could be a source of more viable and functional hepatocytes, saves time and cost, incorporates the benefits of providing the whole liver functions with all its associated cell types, which are important functional components of the liver.[130] Apart from this, it also enables removal of the patient's necrotic liver and hence the cytokines released which are responsible for aggravation of liver injury and maintain greater hemodynamic instability. Many of these problems also accrue with hepatocyte transplantation. However, challenges of immunogenicity, risk of porcine endogenous retrovirus transmission (PERV) and above all ethical issues remain major hurdles in its routine clinical use.

Auxiliary Liver Transplantation

In this, the donor graft is implanted orthotopically besides the native liver (reduced surgically) or heterotopically inferior to the native liver, however this has been limited by technical issues and complexity of the surgery and hence limiting its utility in centers with specialized expertise for this procedure.[131,132] The advantage of this procedure is that it allows regeneration of the diseased liver and gradually enabling withdrawal of immunosuppression whereby the transplanted liver may involute or be surgically removed.

Hence, despite all the achievements in hepatocyte transplantation and bioartificial liver therapy over the past few decades, there remain major hurdles to its successful application in treating various liver diseases. Stem cells remain important therapeutic targets enabling a future where cell-based therapy would be feasible on a larger scale. Other strategies which could prove helpful include living donor and split liver transplantation, a tissue engineered transplantable liver or a clinical trial of pig liver xenoTx as a bridge to allotransplantation.

REFERENCES

1. Williams R. Classification, etiology, and considerations of outcome in acute liver failure. Semin Liver Dis. 1996;16:343-8.
2. Sarin SK, Kumar A, Almeida JA, Chawla YK, Fan ST, Garg H, et al. Acute-on-chronic liver failure: consensus recommendations of the Asian Pacific Association for the study of the liver (APASL). Hepatol Int. 2009;269-82.
3. Kjaergard LL, Liu J, Als-Nielsen B, Gluud C. Artificial and bioartificial support systems for acute and acute-on-chronic liver failure: a systematic review. JAMA. 2003:289;217-22.
4. Stange J, Ramlow W, Mitzner S, Schmidt R, Klinkmann H. Dialysis against a recycled albumin solution enables the removal of albumin-bound toxins. Artif Organs. 1993;17(9):809-13.
5. Poulos AM, Howard L, Eisele G, Rodgers JB. Peritoneal dialysis therapy for patients with liver and renal failure with ascites. Am J Gastroenterol. 1993;88:109-12.
6. Davenport A. Extracorporeal support for patients with hepatic failure. Hemodial Int. 2003;7:256-63.
7. Davenport A. Hemofiltration in patients with fulminant hepatic failure. Lancet. 1991;338:1604.
8. Opolon P. High permeability membrane hemodialysis and hemofiltration in acute hepatic coma: experimental and clinical aspects. Int J Artif Organs. 1979;3:354-60.
9. Desmet VJ, De Groote J, Van Damme B. Acute hepatocellular failure. A study of 17 patients treated with exchange transfusion. Hum Pathol. 1972;3:167-82.
10. Davenport A, Will EJ, Losowsky MS, Swindells S. Continuous arteriovenous hemofiltration in patients with hepatic encephalopathy and renal failure. Br Med J. 1987;295:1028.
11. Davenport A, Will EJ, Davison AM. Effective renal replacement therapy in patients with combined acute renal and fulminant hepatic failure. Kidney Int. 1993;43:S245-51.
12. Bellomo R, Baldwin I, Cole L, Ronco C. Preliminary experience with high volume hemofiltration in human septic shock. Kidney Int. 1988;53:S182-5.
13. O Grady JG, Gimson AES, O'Brien CJ, Pucknell A, Hughes RD, Williams R. Controlled trialsof charcoal hemoperfusion and prognostic factors in fulminant hepatic failure. Gastroenterology. 1988;94:1186-92.
14. Freeman JG, Matthewson K, Record CO. Plasmapheresis in acute liver failure. Int J Artif Organs. 1986;9:433-8.
15. Krisper P, Stauber R. Technology insight: artificial extracorporeal liver support-how does Prometheus compare with MARS? Nat Clin Pract Nephrol. 2007;3(5):267-76.
16. Krisper P, Haditsch B, Stauber R, Jung A, Stadlbauer V, Trauner M, et al. In vivo quantification of liver dialysis: comparison of albumin dialysis and fractionated plasma separation. J Hepatol. 2005;43(3):451-7.
17. Laleman W, Wilmer A, Evenepoel P, Elst IV, Zeegers M, Zaman Z, et al. Effect of the molecular adsorbent recirculating system and Prometheus devices on systemic haemodynamics and vasoactive agents in patients with acute-on-chronic alcoholic liver failure. Crit Care. 2006;10(4);R108.
18. Evenepoel P, Laleman W, Wilmer A, Elst IV, Zeegers M, Zaman Z, et al. Prometheus versus molecular adsorbents recirculating system: comparison of efficiency in two different liver detoxification devices. Artif Organs. 2006;30(4):276-84.
19. Rifai K. Extracorporeal albumin dialysis. Hepatol Res. 2008;38(S1):S41-5.
20. Doria C, Mandalà L, Smith JD, Caruana G, Scott VL, Gruttadauria S, et al. Thromboelastography used to assess coagulation during treatment with molecular adsorbent recirculating system. Clin Transplant. 2004;18(4):365-71.
21. Bachli EB, Schuepbach RA, Maggiorini M, Stocker R, Müllhaupt B, Renner EL. Artificial liver support with the molecular adsorbent recirculating system: activation of coagulation and bleeding complications. Liver Int. 2007;27(4):475-84.
22. Stadlbauer V, Krisper P, Aigner R, Haditsch B, Jung A, Lackner C, et al. Effect of extracorporeal liver support by MARS and Prometheus on serum cytokines in acute-on-chronic liver failure. Crit Care. 2006;10(6):R169.
23. Rifai K, Ernst T, Kretschmer U, Haller H, Manns MP, Fliser D. Removal selectivity of Prometheus: a new extracorporeal liver support device. World J Gastroenterol. 2006;12(6):940-4.
24. Falkenhagen D, Strobl W, Vogt G, Schrefl A, Linsberger I, Gerner FJ, et al. Fractionated plasma separation and adsorption system: a novel system for blood purification to remove albumin bound substances. Artif Organs. 1999;23:81-6.
25. Vogt G, Schrefl A, Strobl W, Falkenhagen D. Fractionated plasma separation and adsorption system: technical design and safety systems. Proc EMBEC. 1999;37(Suppl. 2):64.
26. Rifai K, Ernst T, Kretschmer U, Bahr MJ, Schneider A, Hafer C, et al. Prometheus–a new extracorporeal system for the treatment of liver failure. J Hepatol. 2003;39(6):984-90.
27. Herget-Rosenthal S, Lison C, Treichel U, Saner S, Pietruck F, Broelsch C, et al. Citrate anticoagulated modified fractionated plasma separation and adsorption: first clinical efficacy and safety data in liver failure. J Am Soc Nephrol. 2003;14:729A.
28. Meijers BK, Verhamme P, Nevens F, Hoylaerts MF, Bammens B, Wilmer A, et al. Major coagulation disturbances during fractionated plasma separation and adsorption. Am J Transplant. 2007;7(9):2195-9.
29. Stange J, Hassanein TI, Mehta R, Mitzner SR, Bartlett RH. The molecular adsorbents recycling system as a liver support system based on albumin dialysis: a summary of preclinical investigations prospective, randomized, controlled clinical trial and clinical experience from 19 centers. Artif Organs. 2002;26:103-10.
30. Khuroo MS, Khuroo MS, Farahat KL. Molecular adsorbent recirculation system for acute and acute-on-chronic liver failure: a meta-analysis. Liver Transpl. 2004;10(9):1099-106.
31. Stutchfield BM, Simpson K, Wigmore SJ. Systematic review and meta-analysis of survival following extracorporeal liver support. Br J Surg. 2011;98(5):623-31.
32. Kantola T, Koivusalo AM, Hockerstedt K, Isoniemi H. The effect of molecular adsorbent recirculating system treatment on survival, native liver recovery, and need for liver transplantation in acute liver failure patients. Transpl Int. 2008;21:857-6.
33. Schmidt LE, Svendsen LB, Sorensen VR, Hansen BA, Larsen FS. Cerebral blood flow velocity increases during a single treatment with the molecular adsorbents recirculating system in patients with acute on chronic liver failure. Liver Transpl. 2001;7:709-12.
34. Bergis D, Friedrich-Rust M, Zeuzem S, Betz C, Sarrazin C, Bojunga J, et al Treatment of Amanita phalloides intoxication by fractionated plasma separation and adsorption (Prometheus®). J Gastrointestin Liver Dis. 2012;21(2):171-6.
35. Sentürk E, Esen F, Ozcan PE, Rifai K, Pinarbaşi B, Cakar N, et al. The treatment of acute liver failure with fractionated plasma separation and adsorption system: Experience in 85 applications. J Clin Apher. 2010;25(4):195-201.
36. Heemann U, Treichel U, Loock J, Philipp T, Gerken G, Malago M, et al. Albumin dialysis in cirrhosis withsuperimposed acute liver injury: a prospective, controlled study. Hepatology. 2002;36(4 pt 1):949-58.
37. Sen S, Davies NA, Mookerjee RP, Cheshire LM, Hodges SJ, Williams R, et al. Pathophysiological effects of albumin dialysis in acute-on-chronic liver failure: a randomized controlled study. Liver Transpl. 2004;10(9):1109-19.
38. Hassanein TI, Tofteng F, Brown RS, McGuire B, Lynch P, Mehta R, et al. Randomized controlled study of extracorporeal albumin

dialysis for hepatic encephalopathy in advanced cirrhosis. Hepatology. 2007;46(6):1853-62.
39. Ryska M, Laszikova E, Pantoflicek T, Ryska O, Prazak J, Koblihova E. Fractionated plasma separation and adsorption significantly decreases intracranial pressure in acute liver failure: experimental study. Eur Surg Res. 2009;42(4):230-5.
40. Rifai K, Ernst T, Kretschmer U, Bahr MJ, Schneider A, Hafer C, et al. Prometheus–a new extracorporeal system for the treatment of liver failure. J Hepatol. 2003;39(6):984-90.
41. Sen S, Rose C, Ytrebø LM, Davies NA, Nedredal GI, Drevland SS, et al. Effect of albumin dialysis on intracranial pressure increase in pigs with acute liver failure: a randomized study. Crit Care Med. 2006;34(1):158-64.
42. Mitzner SR, Stange J, Klammt S, Risler T, Erley CM, Bader BD, et al. Improvement of hepatorenal syndrome with extracorporeal albumin dialysis MARS: results of a prospective, randomized, controlled clinical trial. Liver Transpl. 2000:6(3);277-86.
43. Guevara M, Ginès P. Hepatorenal syndrome. Dig Dis. 2005;23(1):47-55.
44. Rifai K, Ernst T, Kretschmer U, Hafer C, Haller H, Manns MP, et al. The Prometheus device for extracorporeal support of combined liver and renal failure. Blood Purif. 2005;23(4):298-302.
45. Kribben A, Gerken G, Haag S, Herget-Rosenthal S, Treichel U, Betz C, et al. Effects of fractionated plasma separation and adsorption on survival in patients with acute-on-chronic liver failure. Gastroenterology. 2012;142(4):782-9.e3.
46. Bañares R, Nevens F, Larsen FS, Jalan R, Albillos A, Dollinger M, et al. Extracorporeal albumin dialysis with the molecular adsorbent recirculating system in acute-on-chronic liver failure: the RELIEF trial. Hepatology. 2013;57(3):1153-62.
47. Saliba F, Camus C, Durand F, Mathurin P, Delafosse B, Baranque K, et al. Randomized controlled multicenter trial evaluating the efficacy and safety of albumin dialysis with MARS® in patientswith fulminant and subfulminant hepatic failure. Hepatology. 2008;48 (Suppl):377A.
48. Jalan R, Sen S, Steiner C, Kapoor D, Alisa A, Williams R. Extracorporeal liver support with molecular adsorbents recirculating system in patients with severe acute alcoholic hepatitis. J Hepatol. 2003;38:24-31.
49. Ramond MJ, Poynard T, Rueff B, Mathurin P, Theodore C, ChaputJC, et al. A randomized trial of prednisolone in patients with severealcoholic hepatitis. N Engl J Med. 1992;326:507-12.
50. Mathurin P, Mendenhall CL, Carithers RL, Ramond MJ, MaddreyWC, Garstide P, et al. Corticosteroids improve short-term survivalin patients with severe alcoholic hepatitis (AH): individual data analysis of the last three randomized placebo controlled double blind trialsof corticosteroids in severe AH. J Hepatol. 2002;36:480-7.
51. Christensen E. Alcoholic hepatitis: glucocorticosteroids or not? J Hepatol. 2002;36:547-8.
52. Akriviadis E, Botla R, Briggs W, Han S, Reynolds T, Shakil O. Pentoxifylline improves short-term survival in severe acute alcoholichepatitis: a double-blind, placebo controlled trial. Gastroenterology. 2000;119:1637-48.
53. Spahr L, Rubbia-Brandt L, Frossard JL, Giostra E, Rougemont AL, Pugin G, et al. Combination of steroids with infliximab or placebo insevere alcoholic hepatitis: a randomized controlled pilot study. J Hepatol. 2002;37:448-55.
54. Mas A. Treatment of resistant pruritus from cholestasis with albumin dialysis: combined analysis of patients from three centers. J Hepatol. 2010;53(2):307-12.
55. Bellmann R, Freistritzer C, Zoller H, Graziadei IW, Schwaighofer H, Propst A, et al. Treatment of intractable pruritus in druginduced cholestasis with albumin dialysis: a report of two cases. ASAIO J. 2004;50(4):387-91.
56. Rifai K, Hafer C, Rosenau J, Athmann C, Haller H, Peter Manns M, et al. Treatment of severe refractory pruritus with fractionated plasma separation and adsorption (Prometheus). Scand J Gastroenterol. 2006;41(10):1212-7.
57. Sen S, Ytrebø LM, Rose C, Fuskevaag OM, Davies NA, Nedredal GI, et al. Albumin dialysis: a new therapeutic strategy forintoxication from protein-bound drugs. Intensive Care Med. 2004;30(3):496-501 ().48 Parés A, Herrera M, Avilés J, Sanz M, 2006;212-1217.
58. Matsumura K, Guevara G, Huston H, Hamilton W, Rikimaru M, Yamasaki G, et al. Hybrid bioartificial liver in hepatic failure: preliminary clinical report. Surgery. 1987;101:99-103.
59. Shito M, Kim NH, Baskaran H, Tilles AW, Tompkins RG, Yarmush ML, et al. In vitro and in vivo evaluation of albumin synthesis rate of porcine hepatocytes in a flat-plate bioreactor. Artif Organs. 2001;25:571-8.
60. Shito M, Tilles AW, W,lesles71-8332]er in ML, Toner M. Efficacy of an extracorporeal flatplate bioartificial liver in treating fulminant hepatic failure. J Surg Res. 2003;111:53-62.
61. De Bartolo L, Jarosch-Von Schweder G, Haverich A, Bader A. A novel full-scale flat membrane bioreactor utilizing porcine hepatocytes: cell viability and tissue-specific functions. Biotechnol Prog. 2000;16:102-8.
62. Lu HF, Lim WS, Zhang PC, Chia SM, Yu H, Mao HQ, et al. Galactosylated poly (vinylidene difluoride) hollow fiber bioreactor for hepatocyte culture. Tissue Eng. 2005;11:1667-77.
63. Ho Ye S, Watanabe J, Takai M, Iwasaki Y, Ishihara K. High functional hollow fiber membrane modified with phospholipid polymers for a liver assist bioreactor. Biomaterials. 2006;27:1955-62.
64. Sullivan JP, Gordo JE, Palmer AF. Simulation of oxygen carrier mediated oxygen transport to C3A hepatoma cells housed within a hollow fiber bioreactor. Biotechnol Bioeng. 2006;93:306-17.
65. Wen F, Chang S, Toh YC, Arooz T, Zhuo L, Teoh SH, et al. Development of dual-compartment perfusion bioreactor for serial coculture of hepatocytes and stellate cells in poly (lactic-co-glycolic acid)-collagen scaffolds. J Biomed Mater Res B Appl Biomater. 2008;87:154-62.
66. Chen JP, Lin CT. Dynamic seeding and perfusion culture of hepatocytes with galactosylated vegetable sponge in packed-bed bioreactor. J Biosci Bioeng. 2006;102:41-5.
67. Torok E, Vogel C, Lutgehetmann M, MA PX, Dandri M, Petersen J, et al. Morphological and functional analysis of rat hepatocyte spheroids generated on poly(L-lactic acid) polymer in a pulsatile flow bioreactor. Tissue Eng. 2006;12(7):1881-90.
68. Morsiani E, Pazzi P Puviani AC, Brogli M, Valieri L, Gorini P, et al. Early experiences with a porcine hepatocytebased bioartificial liver in acute hepatic failure patients. Int J Artif Organs. 2002;25:192-202.
69. Nakazawa K, Ijima H, Fukuda J, Sakiyama R, Yamashita Y, Shimada M, et al. Development of a hybrid artificial liver using polyurethane foam/hepatocyte spheroid culture in a preclinical pig experiment. Int J Artif Organs. 2002;25:51-60.
70. Dixit V, Gitnick G. The . bioartificial liver: state-of-the-art. Eur J Surg Suppl. 1998;(582):71-6.
71. Kinasiewicz A, Gautier A, Lewiska D, Smietanka A, Legallais C, Weryński A. Three-dimensional growth of human hepatoma C3A cells within alginate beads for fluidized bioartificial liver. Int J Artif Organs. 2008;31:340-7.
72. Murtas S, Capuani G, Dentini M, Manetti C, Masci G, Massimi M, et al. Alginate beads as immobilization matrix for hepatocytes perfused in a bioreactor: a physico-chemical characterization. J Biomater Sci Polym Ed. 2005;16:829-46.
73. David B, Doré E, Jaffrin MY, Legallais C. Mass fluidized bed bioreactor using alginate beads for a future bioartificial liver. Int J Artif Organs. 2004;27:284-93.

74. Gerlach JC, Encke J, Hole O, Müller C, Ryan CJ, Neuhaus P. Bioreactor for a larger scale hepatocyte in vitro perfusion. Transplantation. 1994;58:984-8.
75. Bhogal RH, Hodson J, Bartlett DC, Weston CJ, Curbishley SM, Haughton E, et al. Isolation of primary human hepatocytes from normal and diseased liver tissue: a one hundred liver experience. PLoS ONE. 2011;6(3):e18222.
76. Duan Z, Zhang J, Xin S, Chen J, He D, Brotherton J, et al. Interim results of randomized controlled trial of ELAD™ in Acute on Chronic Liver Disease. Hepatology. 2007;46(4 Suppl 1):1.
77. Ellis AJ, Hughes RD, Wendon JA, Dunne J, Langley PG, Kelly JH, et al. Pilot-controlled trial ofthe extracorporeal liver assist device in acute liver failure. Hepatology. 1996;24(6):1446-51.
78. Millis JM, Cronin DC, Johnson R, Conjeevaram H, Conlin C, Trevino S, et al. Initial experience with the modified extracorporeal liver-assist device for patients with fulminant hepatic failure: system modifications and clinical impact. Transplantation. 2002;74(12):1735-46.
79. Wang L, Sun J, Li L, Mears D, Horvat M, Sheil AG. Comparison of porcine hepatocytes withhuman hepatoma (C3A) cells for use in a bioartificial liver support system. Cell Transplant. 1998;7(5):459-68.
80. Mavri-Damelin D, Damelin LH, Eaton S, Rees M, Selden C, Hodgson HJ. Cells for bioartificialliver devices: the human hepatoma-derived cell line C3A produces urea but does not detoxifyammonia. Biotechnol Bioeng. 2008;99(3):644-51.
81. Enosawa S, Miyashita T, Fujita Y, Suzuki S, Amemiya H, Omasa T, et al. In vivo estimation of bioartificial liver with recombinant HepG2 cells using pigs with ischemic liver failure. Cell transplantation. 2001;10(4-5):429-33.
82. Chen Y, Li J, Liu X, Zhao W, Wang Y, Wang X. Transplantation of immortalized human fetal hepatocytes prevents acute liver failure in 90% hepatectomized mice. Transplantation proceedings. 2010;42(5):1907-14.
83. Bonavita AG, Quaresma K, Cotta-de-Almeida V, Pinto MA, Saraiva RM, Alves LA. Hepatocytexeno transplantation for treating liver disease. Xenotransplantation. 2010;17(3):181-7.
84. Baquerizo A, Mhoya A, Kearns-Jonker M, Arnaout W, Shackleton C, Busuttil R, et al. Characterization of human xenoreactive antibodies in liver failure patients exposed to pig hepatocytes after bioartificial liver treatment. Transplantation. 1999;67:5-18.
85. van de Kerkhove MP, Hoekstra R, Chamuleau RA, van Gulik TM. Clinical application of bioartificial liver support systems. Ann Surg. 2004;240:216-30.
86. Arkadopoulos N, Detry O, Rozga J, Demetriou AA. Liver assist systems: state of the art. Int J Artif Organs. 1998;21:781-7.
87. Demetriou AA, Brown RS, Busuttil RW, Fair J, McGuire BM, Rosenthal P, et al. Prospective, randomized, multicenter controlled trial of a bioartificial liver in treating acute liver failure. Ann Surg. 2004;239:660-7.
88. Sauer IM, Gerlach JC. Modular extracorporeal liver support. Artif Organs. 2002;26:703-6.
89. Pless G, Sauer IM. Bioartificial liver: current status. Transplant Proc. 2005;37:3893-5.
90. Sauer IM, Kardassis D, Zeillinger K, Pascher A, Gruenwald , Pless G, et al. Clinical extracorporeal hybrid liver support--phase I study with primary porcine liver cells. Xenotransplantation. 2003;10:460-9.
91. Sauer IM1, Zeilinger K, Pless G, Kardassis D, Theruvath T, Pascher A, et al. Extracorporeal liver support based on primary human liver cells and albumin dialysis--treatment of a patient with primary graft non-function. 2003;39:649-53.
92. Ellis AJ, Hughes RD, Wendon JA, Dunne J, Langley PG, Kelly JH, et al. Hepatology. 1996;24:1446-51.
93. Mazariegos GV, Patzer JF 2nd, Lopez RC, Giraldo M, Devera ME, Grogan TA, et al. First clinical use of a novel bioartificial liver support system (BLSS). Am J Transplant. 2002;2(3):260-6.
94. Mazariegos GV, Kramer DJ, Lopez RC, Shakil AO, Rosenbloom AJ, Devera M, et al. Safety observations in phase I clinical evaluation of the Excorp Medical Bioartificial Liver Support System after the first four patients. ASAIO J. 2001;47(5):471-5.
95. McIntosh MB, Corner SM, Amiot BP, Nyberg SL. Engineering analysis and development of the spheroid reservoir bioartificial liver. Conf Proc IEEE Eng Med BiolSoc. 2009;2009:5985-8.
96. Davidson AJ, Ellis MJ, Chaudhuri JB. A theoretical approach to zonation in a bioartificial liver. Biotechnol Bioeng. 2012;109(1):234-43.
97. Kanai H, Marushima H, Kimura N, Iwaki T, Saito M, Maehashi H, et al. Extracorporeal bioartificial liver using the radial flow bioreactor in treatment of fatal experimental hepatic encephalopathy. Artif Organs. 2007;31(2):148-51.
98. Enosawa S, Miyashita T, Tanaka H, Li X, Suzuki S, Amemiya H, et al. Prolongation of survival of pigs with ischemic liver failure by treatment with a bioartificial liver using glutamine synthetase transfected recombinant HepG2. Transplant Proc. 2001;33 (1-2):1945-7.
99. Wang N, Tsuruoka S, Yamamoto H, Enosawa S, Omasa T, Sata N, et al. The bioreactor with CYP3A4- and glutamine synthetase-introduced HepG2 cells: treatment of hepatic failure dog with diazepam overdosage. Artif Organs. 2005;29:681-4.
100. Enosawa S, Miyashita T, Saito T, Omasa T, Matsumura T. The significant improvement of survival times and pathological parameters by bioartificial liver with recombinant HepG2 in porcine liver failure model. Cell Transplant. 2006;15:873-80.
101. Chamuleau RA, Deurholt T, Hoekstra R. Which are the right cells to be used in a bioartificial liver? Metab Brain Dis. 2005;20:327-35.
102. Ding YT, Shi XL. Bioartificial liver devices: Perspective on the state of the art. Front Med. 2011;5:15-9.
103. Flendrig LM, la Soe JW, Jörning GG, Steenbeek A, Karlsen OT, Bovée WM, et al. In vitro evaluation of a novel bioreactor based on an integral oxygenator and a spirally wound nonwoven polyester matrix for hepatocyte culture as small aggregates. J Hepatol. 1997;26(6):1379-92.
104. Chen G, Palmer AF. Perfluorocarbon facilitated O(2) transport in a hepatic hollow fiber bioreactor. Biotechnol Prog. 2009;25:1317-21.
105. Chen G, Palmer AF. Mixtures of hemoglobin-based oxygen carriers and perfluorocarbons exhibit a synergistic effect in oxygenating hepatic hollow fiber bioreactors. Biotechnol Bioeng. 2010;105:534-42.
106. Chen G, Palmer AF. Hemoglobin-based oxygen carrier and convection enhanced oxygen transport in a hollow fiber bioreactor. Biotechnol Bioeng. 2009;102:1603-12.
107. Seghatchian J, d Sousa G. An overview of unresolved inherent problems iated ated with red cell transfusion and potential use of artificial oxygen carriers and ECO-RBC: current status/future trends. Transfus Apher Sci. 2007;37:251-9.
108. Xue YL, Zhao SF, Luo Y, Li XJ, Duan ZP, Chen XP, et al. TECA hybrid artificial liver support system in treatment of acute liver failure. World J Gastroenterol. 2001;7:826-9.
109. Ding YT, Qiu YD, Chen Z, Xu QX, Zhang HY, Tang Q, et al. The development develop bioartificial liver and its application in 12 acute liver failure patients. World J Gastroenterol. 2003;9:829-32.
110. Zaret KS, Grompe M. Generation and regeneration of cells of the liver and pancreas. Science. 2008;322(5907):1490-4.
111. Lazaro C, Rhim J, Yamada Y, Fausto N. Generation of hepatocytes from oval cell precursors inculture. Cancer Research. 1998;58:5514-22.
112. Weber A, Touboul T, Mainot S, Branger J, Mahieu-Caputo D. Human fetal hepatocytes: isolation, characterization, and transplantation. Methods Mol Biol. 2010;640:41-55.
113. Schmelzer E, Wauthier E, Reid LM. The phenotypes of pluripotent human hepatic progenitors. Stem Cells. 2006;24(8):1852-8.
114. Haridass D, Yuan Q, Becker PD, Cantz T, Iken M, Rothe M, et al. Repopulation efficiencies of adult hepatocytes, fetal liver

progenitor cells, and embryonic stem cell-derived hepatic cells in albumin-promoter-enhancer urokinase-type plasminogen activator mice. Am J Pathol. 2009;175(4):1483-92.
115. Li H, Zhang B, Lu Y, Jorgensen M, Petersen B, Song S. Adipose tissue-derived mesenchymal stemcell-based liver gene delivery. J Hepatol. 2011;54(5):930-8.
116. Piscaglia AC, Campanale M, Gasbarrini A, Gasbarrini G. Stem cell-based therapies for liver diseases: state of the art and new perspectives. Stem Cells Int. 2010;2010:259461.
117. Di Campli C, Piscaglia AC, Pierelli L, Rutella S, Bonanno G, Alison MR, et al. A human umbilical cord stem cell rescue therapy in a murine model of toxic liver injury. Digestive and liver disease: official journal of the Italian Society of Gastroenterology and the Italian Association for the Study of the Liver. 2004;36(9):603-13.
118. Si-Tayeb K, Noto FK, Nagaoka M, Li J, Battle MA, Duris C, et al. Highly efficient generation ofhuman hepatocyte-like cells from induced pluripotent stem cells. Hepatology. 2010;51(1):297-305.
119. Pareja E, Cortes M, Bonora A, Fuset P, Orbis F, Lopez R, et al. New alternatives to the treatmentof acute liver failure. Transplantation proceedings. 2010;42(8):2959-61.
120. Jin SZ, Meng XW, Sun X, Han MZ, Liu BR, Wang XH, et al. Hepatocyte growth factor promotesliver regeneration induced by transfusion of bone marrow mononuclear cells in a murine acute liver failure model. J Hepatobiliary Pancreat Sci. 2011;18(3):397-405.
121. Parekkadan B, van Poll D, Suganuma K, Carter EA, Berthiaume F, Tilles AW, et al. Mesenchymal stem cell-derived molecules reverse fulminant hepatic failure. PLoS One. 2007;2(9):e941.
122. Shi XL, Zhang Y, Gu JY, Ding YT. Coencapsulation of hepatocytes with bone marrow mesenchymal stem cells improves hepatocyte-specific functions. Transplantation. 2009;88(10):1178-85.
123. Makowka L, Cramer DV, Hoffman A, Breda M, Sher L, Eiras-Hreha G, et al. The use of pig liver xenograft for temporary support of a patient with fulminant hepatic failure. Transplantation. 1995;59:1654-9.
124. Cooper DK, Gollackner B, Sachs DH. Will the pig solve the transplantation backlog? Annu Rev Med. 2002;53:133-47.
125. Cooper DKC, Dorling A, Pierson RN 3rd, Rees M, Seebach J, Yazer M, et al. Alpha 1, 3-galactosyltransferase gene-knockout pigs for xenotransplantation: where do we go from here? Transplantation. 2007;84:1-7.
126. Abouna GM, Garry R, Hull C, Kirkley J, Walder DN. Pig-liver perfusion in hepatic coma. Lancet. 1968;2:590-610.
127. Eiseman B, Liem DS, Raffucci F. Heterologous liver perfusion in treatment of hepatic failure. Ann Surg. 1965;162:329-45.
128. Abouna, GM. Extracorporeal xenogeneic liver perfusion for the treatment of liver failure. In: Cooper, DKC, Kemp E, Platt JL, White DJG (Eds). Xenotransplantation, 2nd edition. Germany: Springer; 1997. pp. 785-92.
129. Chari RS, Collins BH, Magee JC, DiMaio JM, Kirk AD, Harland RC, et al. Brief report: treatment of hepatic failure with ex vivo pig-liver perfusion followed by liver transplantation. N Eng J Med. 1994;331:234-7.
130. Ekser B, Gridelli B, Tector AJ, Cooper DK. Pig liver xenotransplantation as a bridge to allotransplantation: which patients might benefit? Transplantation. 2009:15;88(9):1041-9.
131. Sudan DL, Shaw BW, Fox IJ, Langnas AN. Long-term follow-up of auxiliary orthotopic liver transplantation for the treatment of fulminant hepatic failure. Surgery. 1997;122:771-7.
132. Van Hoek B, de Boer J, Boudjema K, Williams R, Corsmit O, Terpstra OT. Auxiliary versus orthotopic liver transplantation for acute liver failure. EURALT Study Group. European Auxiliary Liver Transplant Registry. J Hepatol. 1999;30:699-705.

CHAPTER 80

Surgery in Acute and Chronic Liver Disease

Shalimar, SK Acharya

INTRODUCTION

Surgical procedures are more often performed on patients with liver diseases nowadays, as compared with the past, because of increased survival of these patients. These surgical procedures may be emergency or elective. Increased mortality and morbidity has been noted after surgery in both acute and chronic liver disease. The risk varies with the severity of liver disease, type of anesthesia and the indication for surgery-whether elective or emergency. In addition, the altered hemostasis (coagulopathy and thrombocytopenia) increases the risk. Child-Turcotte-Pugh (CTP) score and model for end-stage liver disease (MELD) score can help in prognostication of these patients. Evaluation of underlying cause of liver dysfunction should be done in patients in the elective setting. Treatment of the cause and optimization of associated complications including ascites, hepatic encephalopathy, electrolyte imbalance and azotemia prior to surgery improves the prognosis.

APPROACH

It is not uncommon for a patient who is posted for surgery to be found to have an incidentally detected abnormality in liver function tests (LFTs). The abnormality may occur in the form of elevation of bilirubin levels which may be predominantly conjugated or unconjugated, and may occur in isolation or in association with elevation of transaminases.

In any patient with abnormal liver tests, the cause and duration of the abnormality should be assessed. This is essential as the cause of the liver disease can be treated and this also helps is assessing the risk. Table 1 shows the various commonly encountered abnormalities in liver function and their interpretation.

ACUTE AND CHRONIC HEPATITIS

The most common cause of acute hepatitis in India is viral hepatitis. In adults, the most common etiology is hepatitis E, whereas in children it is hepatitis A. Patients who consume alcohol may present as acute alcoholic hepatitis, the presentation of which may be similar to acute viral hepatitis. Other causes of acute hepatitis include drugs such as antitubercular therapy, antiepileptics and paracetamol (which is the most commonly cause in the west but is uncommon in India). Autoimmune liver disease and Wilson's disease may also present acutely. The common causes of chronic liver disease include hepatitis B and C, alcohol, fatty liver, nonalcoholic steatohepatitis (NASH), autoimmune liver disease, primary sclerosing cholangitis, primary biliary cirrhosis and secondary biliary cirrhosis. Table 2 lists the common causes of acute and chronic liver disease.

CLINICAL EVALUATION

The clinical evaluation should include a detailed history regarding the onset of illness. A short history with a prodrome points to a viral etiology, likely hepatitis A or E virus infection. In addition, multiple cases of acute viral hepatitis in the community point to a common source of the infection. Hepatitis A usually affects children and hepatitis E affects adults, as by the time children grow up, they become immune to hepatitis A virus infection. A long history, prior history of jaundice, surgery and blood transfusion in the past, intravenous drug abuse, family history of hepatitis B or liver disease and sexual promiscuity point to a hepatitis B or C etiology. Eliciting history of alcohol intake is important. Family history of chronic liver disease and hepatocellular carcinoma should also be taken.

The examination should include assessment of icterus, presence of ascites and pedal edema, peripheral stigmata of chronic liver

Table 1: Abnormalities of liver function tests and their causes

Liver functions	*Possible causes*
Elevated bilirubin, predominantly conjugated, normal aminotransferases	Sepsis
Elevated bilirubin, predominantly conjugated, elevated aminotransferases	Obstructive jaundice, viral hepatitis
Elevated bilirubin, predominantly unconjugated, normal aminotransferases	Hemolytic anemia, Gilbert's syndrome
Elevated bilirubin, predominantly unconjugated, elevated aminotransferases	Viral hepatitis, Wilson's disease
In addition to deranged bilirubin, aminotransferases presence of hypoalbuminemia	Cirrhosis

disease (palmar erythema, parotid enlargement, especially in alcoholics, loss of axillary and pubic hair, gynecomastia, testicular atrophy, spider nevi, clubbing and caput medusae). The assessment of nutrition and signs of vitamin deficiency should be looked for. The liver span is markedly reduced in acute liver failure whereas the liver is shrunken in chronic liver disease. The presence of an enlarged liver in a suspected chronic liver disease should raise the possibility of underlying alcoholic liver disease, hepatocellular carcinoma, hepatic venous outflow tract obstruction or hemochromatosis.

APPROACH TO A PATIENT WITH TRANSAMINITIS

Acute Viral Hepatitis and Acute Liver Failure

Patients having acute hepatitis, acute liver failure and alcoholic hepatitis are generally considered contraindications to elective surgery. In addition, patients with acute viral hepatitis and transaminitis (etiology not known) should be evaluated prior to the surgery. Once the etiology is treated and the LFTs have normalized, then these patients should be considered for surgery. Box 1 lists the conditions in which surgery is contraindicated.

Persistent Transaminitis and Chronic Hepatitis

A patient with transaminitis should be evaluated for the etiology prior to surgery. Patients with acute liver failure should not be taken up for any surgery apart from liver transplantation. A recent onset elevation of enzyme levels in the presence of a prodrome is suggestive of acute viral hepatitis. There is a risk of decompensation of liver disease after surgery. Patients with persistent transaminitis where the etiology may be chronic viral hepatitis, autoimmune hepatitis, NASH and fatty liver tolerate surgery well, although the risk is more as compared with the general population.

Box 1: List of conditions in which surgery is contraindicated or associated with high risk

1. Acute liver failure
2. Acute renal failure
3. Persistent severe coagulopathy
4. Cardiomyopathy
5. Alcoholic hepatitis
6. Hypoxemia
7. Acute viral hepatitis

Chronic Liver Disease

Scores for Assessing the Risk

The Child class and MELD score are used for assessing the risk. The MELD and the Child scores are complementary. The risk of surgery in cirrhotic patients can be accurately assessed by these scores. The Child score is a sum calculation of 5 variables, namely, bilirubin, albumin, prothrombin time (INR), ascites and encephalopathy. Table 3 gives the various values and the scores. The final score is the sum total of all scores. Child A: 5–6, Child B: 7–9, Child C: 10 or more than.

Risk in Relevance to Child Status

The estimated risk of mortality in cirrhotic patients with cirrhotic patients A (CTP-A) is 10%, CTP-B is 30% and CTP-C is 70%. The risk increases in cases of emergency surgery (Child A: 22%, Child B: 40% and Child C: 100%). The presence of ascites, hydrothorax, hepatopulmonary and/or portopulmonary syndromes exacerbates hypoxia. There is also an increased risk of bacterial infections. A prolonged prothrombin time increases the risk of bleeding. These patients are also at increased risk of hypotension due to the anesthetic drugs, due to changes in the circulation caused by cirrhosis per se. The presence of chronic obstructive airway disease and other comorbidities increase the risk during surgery.

Table 2: Various causes of acute and chronic liver diseases

Acute liver disease	*Chronic liver disease*
Viral hepatitis: Hepatitis A, B, C and E	Fatty liver, NASH
Alcoholic hepatitis	Alcoholic liver disease
Drugs: Antitubercular, antiepileptics, paracetamol	Viral: Hepatitis B, C
	Autoimmune, primary sclerosing cholangitis
	Hepatic venous outflow tract obstruction

Abbreviation: NASH, nonalcoholic steatohepatitis.

Table 3: Child score calculator

Parameter	*1*	*2*	*3*
Total bilirubin (mg/dL)	<2	2–3	>3
Serum albumin	>3.5	2.8–3.5	<2.8
INR	<1.7	1.7–2.3	>2.3
Ascites	None	Mild	Moderate-severe
HE	None	Grade I–II	III–IV

Abbreviations: HE, hepatic encephalopathy; INR, international normalized ratio.

MELD Score in Predicting the Risk

The MELD score can be calculated online at http://www.mayoclinic.org/meld/mayomodel9.html or on various applications available on smart phones. It takes into account 3 parameters; international normalized ratio (INR), serum creatinine levels and bilirubin. It is more effective in assessing the preoperative mortality in hepatic dysfunction. It is objective, has no set cut-off values and each variable is counted for. Therefore, it is said to be more accurate than CTP score. It has been reported that mortality is increased by 1% for each one point increase in MELD score from 5 to 20 and by 2% for each point increase beyond 20. Increasing mortality has been shown with increasing MELD score (5.7% with score <7, 10.3% with 8–11 and 25.4% with score of 12–15). Patient's age and the American society of Anesthesiologists (ASA) classification (on a scale of 1–5) contribute to the risk. An ASA class IV is associated with an increased risk equivalent to addition of 5 MELD points, whereas ASA class V has been associated with a 100% mortality risk.

Other Factors Influencing Outcome of Surgery

The reduced hepatic blood flow, hypoxemia due to ascites, hydrothorax and portopulmonary hypertension and altered drug metabolism are responsible for increased complications. The drugs commonly used in the preoperative and postoperative period may cause worsening of the liver disease. The anesthetic agents and antibiotics can cause hepatotoxicity, benzodiazepines and narcotics increase the risk of hepatic encephalopathy and nonsteroidal anti-inflammatory drugs (NSAIDs) increase the risk of renal failure. In addition, other factors which lead to a poor outcome include older age, low albumin, serum sodium less than 130 mmol/L and intraoperative blood transfusion. Lower gastrointestinal tract surgery carries a higher risk than upper gastrointestinal tract. This may be due to the fact that most such surgeries are carried out in emergency settings and in elderly patients, which are risk factors for poor outcome. Surgeries performed in liver transplant centers with intensive care unit (ICU) facilities are associated with better outcome.

Other Methods to Assess Risk

A number of other tests have been proposed to assess the liver reserve. These include quantitative assessment of liver functions such as galactose elimination capacity, indocyanine green clearance, rate of metabolism of lidocaine to monoethylglycinexylidide (MEGX) and aminopyrine breath test. These tests are performed in specialized centers and require special instruments. However, none of these is superior to Child-Pugh classification, and hence are not widely used.

TYPE OF SURGERY

Higher incidence of gallstones is seen in cirrhotics. Patients with Child A and selected Child B cases without portal hypertension can undergo laparoscopic cholecystectomy. The morbidity and mortality increases with increasing child score. Open cholecystectomy has more postoperative complications as compared to laparoscopic cholecystectomy with similar disease severity. Patients with Child C may be considered for cholecystostomy. In patients undergoing hepatic resection mortality varies from 0% with MELD score less than 8 to 29% among those with MELD score more than 9.

MANAGEMENT

The evaluation of the patients begins in the preoperative period. A careful assessment of the underlying Child status and MELD score helps in assessing the risk of mortality and morbidity. In addition, optimization of the liver function should be done. Flow chart 1 shows the approach to the management of patients with cirrhosis. Mobilization of ascitic fluid should be done prior to the surgery. It reduces the risk of abdominal wall herniation and wound dehiscence. The treatment options include salt restricted diet, diuretics, and large volume paracentesis to completely drain the abdomen and albumin infusion. Electrolyte imbalances and azotemia should be corrected to reduce the risk of encephalopathy after surgery.

Flow chart 1 Approach for management of cirrhotic patient undergoing surgery

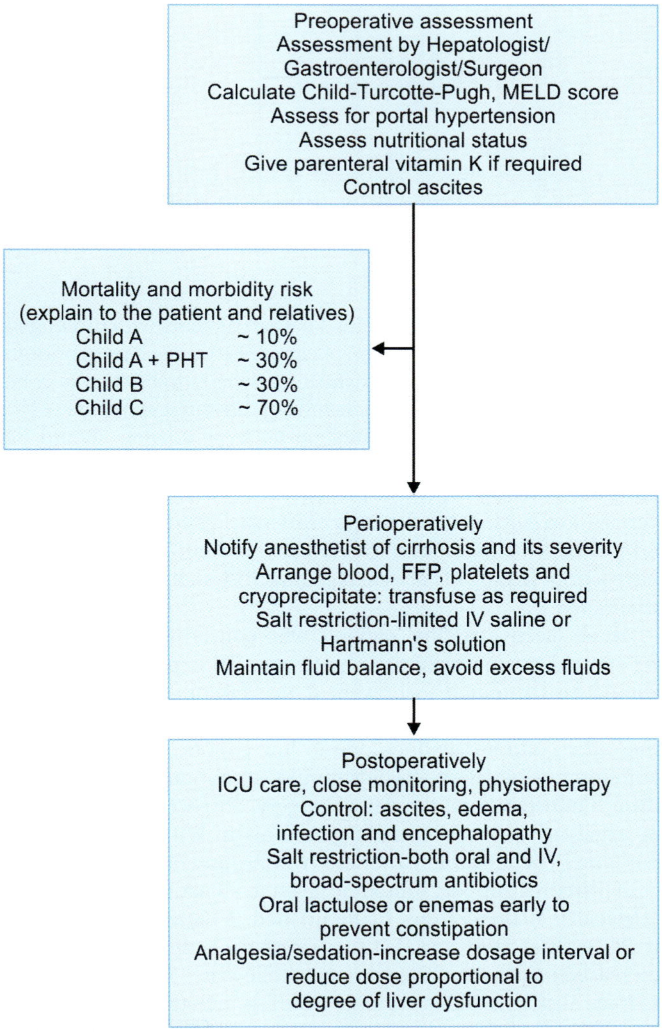

Preoperative assessment
Assessment by Hepatologist/Gastroenterologist/Surgeon
Calculate Child-Turcotte-Pugh, MELD score
Assess for portal hypertension
Assess nutritional status
Give parenteral vitamin K if required
Control ascites

→ Mortality and morbidity risk (explain to the patient and relatives)

Child A	~ 10%
Child A + PHT	~ 30%
Child B	~ 30%
Child C	~ 70%

↓

Perioperatively
Notify anesthetist of cirrhosis and its severity
Arrange blood, FFP, platelets and cryoprecipitate: transfuse as required
Salt restriction-limited IV saline or Hartmann's solution
Maintain fluid balance, avoid excess fluids

↓

Postoperatively
ICU care, close monitoring, physiotherapy
Control: ascites, edema, infection and encephalopathy
Salt restriction-both oral and IV, broad-spectrum antibiotics
Oral lactulose or enemas early to prevent constipation
Analgesia/sedation-increase dosage interval or reduce dose proportional to degree of liver dysfunction

Abbreviations: PHT, pulmonary hypertension; FFP, fresh frozen plasma; IV, intravenous; ICU, intensive care unit; MELD, model for end-stage liver disease

Flow chart 2 Approach to patients with acute and chronic liver disease undergoing surgery

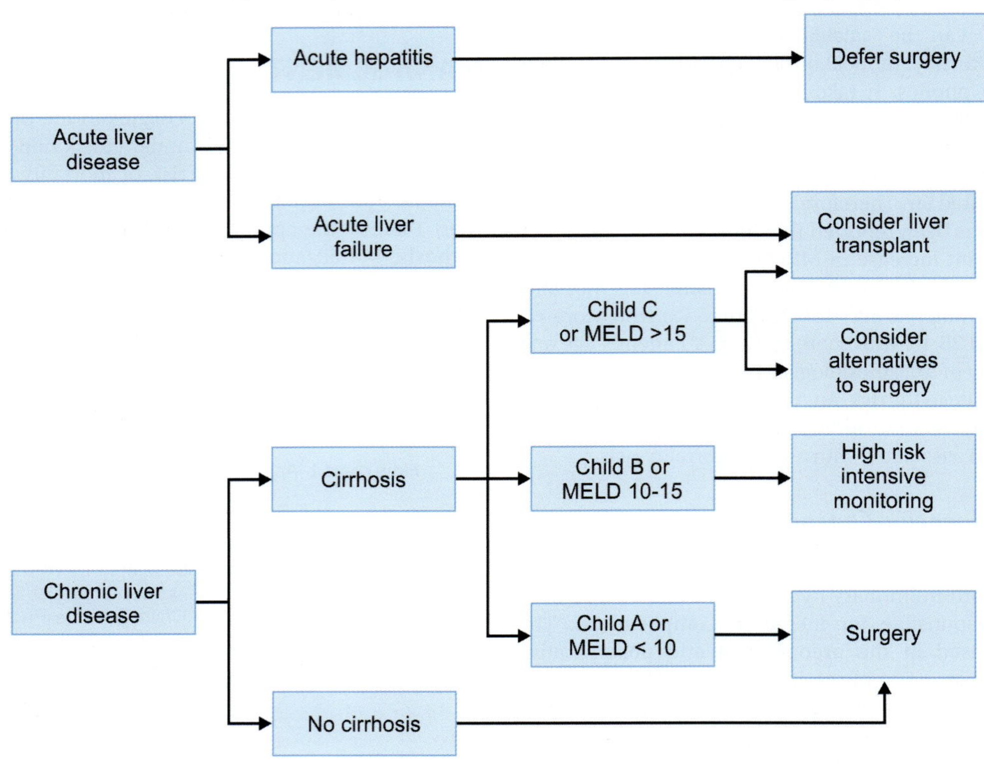

Vitamin K should be given for 3 days to patients with prolonged prothrombin time. Fresh frozen plasma (FFP) may be used prior to or during surgery. Platelet transfusion and cryoprecipitate may be beneficial or required in patients having thrombocytopenia.

An assessment of associated portal hypertension should be done prior to the surgery. The risk of complications in Child A patients increases with the presence of portal hypertension. If varices are present, endoscopic variceal ligation (EVL) and/or nonselective beta-blockers should be considered. In patients who have a prior history of variceal bleeding, EVL should be done prior to surgery.

In an elective setting, patients who consume alcohol should be advised to stop alcohol. In patients with hepatitis B, therapy should be continued to prevent flares. Interferon and ribavirin should be continued in chronic hepatitis C afflicted patients unless there are contraindications due to low counts. In patients with autoimmune hepatitis, steroids should be continued and switched over to injectables on the day of surgery. Surgery may precipitate or aggravate neuropsychiatric symptoms in Wilson's disease; in addition D-pencillamine interferes with wound healing.

Nutritional support should be given to all patients as cirrhotics (especially alcoholics) are malnourished. A reasonable approach is 30–35 kcal/kg/d and 1–1.5 g/kg of proteins per day, to be increased as per the underlying catabolic state. Supplementation of trace elements and fat-soluble vitamins including A, D, E and K should be done. Serum glucose levels should be monitored closely as hypoglycemia may occur (due to depleted glycogen stores).

RECOMMENDATIONS

All the risks should be explained thoroughly to patient before surgery. The Child score and MELD score and overall general state of the patient should be assessed preoperatively to estimate the risk of decompensation during and after surgical procedure. Individualization of care of each patient is required which includes a preoperative assessment, optimization of medical therapy for control of ascites, electrolyte imbalance, management for hepatic encephalopathy and close monitoring in an ICU in the postoperative period. Flow chart 2 highlights the approach to patients with acute and chronic liver disease who are considered for surgery.

BIBLIOGRAPHY

1. Farnsworth N, Fagan SP, Berger DH, Awad SS. Child-Turcotte-Pugh versus MELD score as a predictor of outcome after elective and emergent surgery in cirrhotic patients. Am J Surg. 2004;188(5):580-3.
2. Friedman LS. The risk of surgery in patients with liver disease. Hepatology. 1999;29(6):1617-23.
3. Teh SH, Nagorney DM, Stevens SR, Offord KP, Therneau TM, Plevak DJ, et al. Risk factors for mortality after surgery in patients with cirrhosis. Gastroenterology. 2007;132(4):1261-9.
4. Telem DA, Schiano T, Goldstone R, Han DK, Buch KE, Chin EH, et al. Factors that predict outcome of abdominal operations in patients with advanced cirrhosis. Clin Gastroenterol Hepatol. 2010;8(5):451-7.

SECTION 7

Spleen

CHAPTER 81

Anatomy and Physiology of Spleen

AK Singh, Priya Ranjan

INTRODUCTION

The spleen is the largest reticuloendothelial organ. Spleen was described as a "seat of laughter" by Jewish Talmud in 2nd-6th centuries. Van Leewenhoeck studied the spleen arguing that it played a role in the purification of the blood.[1]

It consists of vascular and lymphoid tissue derived from the primitive mesoderm and is surrounded by a thin capsule. Although present in other mammals, smooth muscle cells are not a feature of the human splenic capsule. The spleen lies in the left hypochondrium underneath the 9th, 10th, and 11th ribs. It measures 7–11 cm in length, and weighs an average of 150 g (normal range 80–300 g). With advancing age, the size of spleen decreases. Normally, it is not palpable under left hypochondrium. Splenomegaly can be seen in various pathological conditions. However, it becomes palpable when its size is at least double the normal. The long axis of spleen runs parallel to the 10th rib (Fig. 1).[1,2]

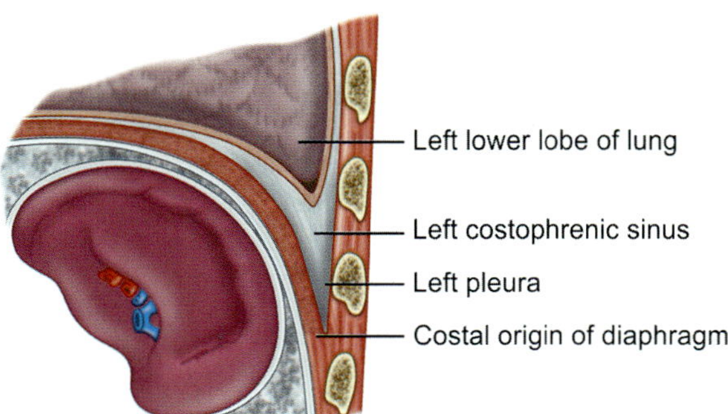

Figure 1 Anatomical location of spleen

The spleen receives at least 5–6% of the cardiac output, i.e. about 300 mL blood per minute.

Approximately 20% of the population has one or more accessory spleens, usually located within the hilar region. The incidence of accessory spleens may be as high as 30% in individuals with hematologic pathologies.[1,2]

EMBRYOLOGY

At 5th week of gestation, stomach appears in the foregut tube as fusiform swelling. It is attached to the dorsal body wall by a fold of mesentery called dorsal mesogastrium and to ventral body wall by ventral mesogastrium. The disproportionate growth and rotation of stomach causes the dorsal mesogastrium to lie in the left of the median plane. At the same process of development, the spleen primordium appears as a mesodermal proliferation between the two leaves of the dorsal mesogastrium. This fetal splenic tissue divides the dorsal mesogastrium into two parts: (1) gastrosplenic ligament (between stomach and spleen) and (2) lienorenal ligament (between left kidney and spleen). The mesenchymal tissue condensed to become spleen and later during development infiltrated by lymphoid tissue (Fig. 2).[2,3]

EMBRYOLOGICAL ANOMALY

Accesory Spleen

This is the most common anomaly of spleen which can be present in 20% of the population. Mostly (>80%) accessary spleen is located at splenic hilum but it can be seen at gastrocolic ligament, pancreatic tail, greater omentum, splenocolic ligament, mesentery, left spermatic cord or left broad ligament in women. In splenectomy for hematological disease, accesory spleen may cause recurrence of symptoms.[1]

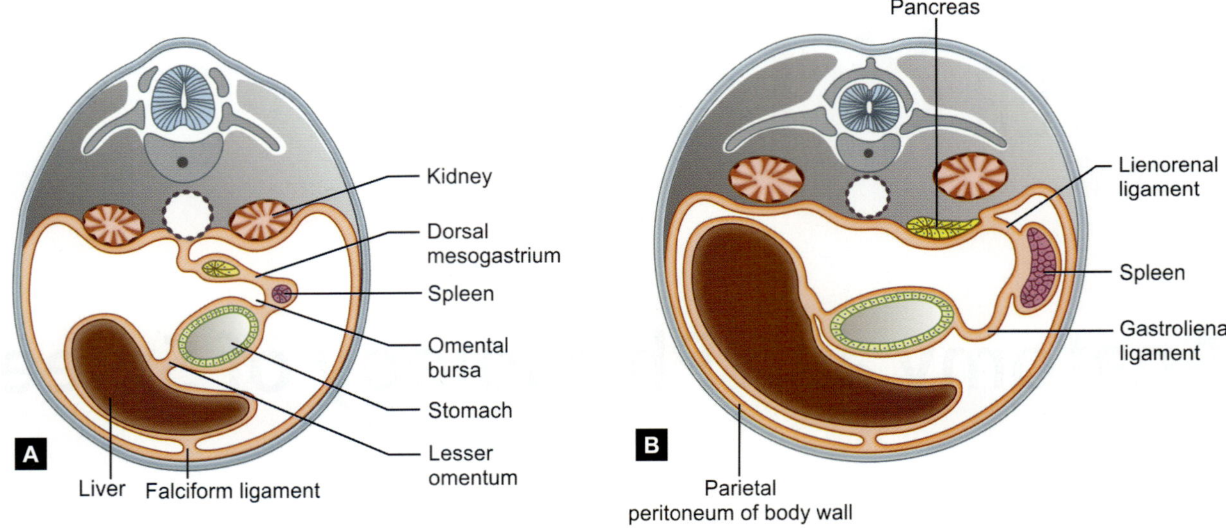

Figure 2 Development of spleen

Asplenia

Congenital absence of spleen can be associated with multiple syndromes.

Wondering Spleen

Spleen is attached with adjacent organ by ligaments like gastrosplenic ligament, lienorenal ligament, phrenosplenic ligaments, splenocolic ligament. Laxity of these supportive ligaments and abnormal length of the splenic vessels can result in excessive splenic mobility. This is known as wandering (ptotic) spleen.[1]

ANATOMY

The spleen is covered by a fibrous capsule. Trabeculae arising from the inner aspect of the capsule divide the spleen into communicating compartments. The splenic parenchyma is composed of the *white pulp* and the *red pulp* based on complex vascular arrangements. The *red pulp* comprises *splenic sinuses* and *sinusoids*, and cellular tissue arranged in thin plates composing the splenic cords. Splenic sinuses are thin walled and large branching vessels. The *white pulp* consists of periarteriolar lymphatic sheaths and lymphoid follicles. Marginal zone is the area between the *white pulp* and the *red pulp* containing lymphatic and macrophages. Seventy-five per cent of spleen volume comprises of the *red pulp* (Fig. 3).[2,4]

The macrophages inside the red pulp remove microorganisms, cellular debris, antigen/antibody complexes and senescent erythrocytes from circulation thus serving as a dynamic filtration system. Blood flow from the splenic artery enters the trabecular arteries from which central arteries supply the *white pulp*. At the terminal part of central arteries, the adventitia is replaced by a periarteriolar lymphoid sheath (PALS) which is T-cell predominant, and at various points these enlarge to form the B-cells splenic follicles. The *white pulp*, with the B-cell lymphoid follicles and the T-cell PALS, along with the lymphoid, non-filtering *red pulp* (both B and T lymphocytes), are responsible for the spleen's immunological function (Fig. 4).[5-7]

Splenic Circulation

Blood enters into the red pulp from the trabecular artery and penicillary arterioles and reaches trabecular veins via two routes, thus defining two types of circulation of spleen. Open circulation and closed circulation. In the "open circulation" blood filters out to sinusoids via the splenic cords while in "closed circulation" the penicillary arterioles directly drain into trabecular veins and do not pass through the splenic sinusoids. The majority of the circulation is the closed circulation which is more rapid circulatory pathway. The trabecular veins collect blood both from "open" and "closed" circulation and eventually drain into splenic vein. The closed circulation has predominance of plasma flow while open flow has more of erythrocytes thus helping in filtration process in the *red pulp*.[8]

TOPOGRAPHY AND RELATIONS

The spleen is located in the left upper quadrant of the abdomen and separated from left pleural cavity by diaphragm; it is related to stomach medially, the left kidney and left adrenal gland posteriorly and the chest wall (the 9th to 11th left ribs) laterally. Pancreatic tail lies in contact with spleen in 30% and within 1 cm of the hilum in 70% of cases.

Spleen is suspended by multiple peritoneal folds to the adjacent organs. These are gastrosplenic ligament, lieno(spleno) renal ligament, splenophrenic ligament, splenocolic ligament and pancreatosplenic ligaments. Short gastric arteries run in the gastrosplenic ligaments (Fig. 5).[1,2]

VASCULAR ANATOMY OF SPLEEN

Arterial Supply

The splenic artery is the main source of arterial blood to spleen. Celiac trunk gives three branches of which splenic artery is the largest of the three branches. Other two branches are the common hepatic and left gastric arteries. Accessory supply

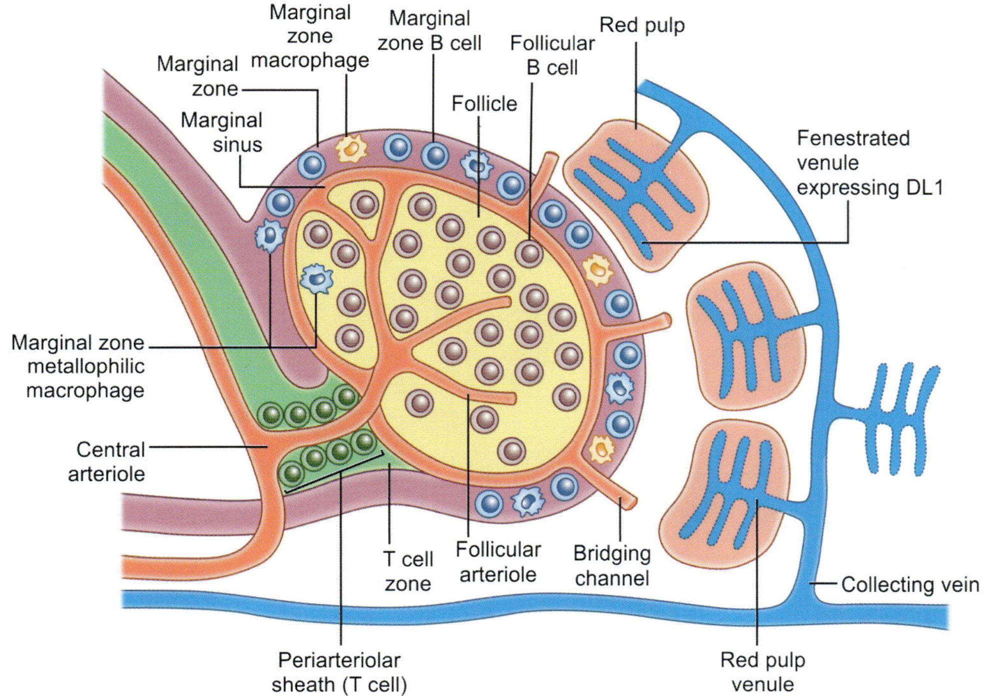

Figure 3 Microscopic anatomy of spleen

is from the left gastroepiploic artery. The splenic artery after originating from the celiac trunk it courses leftward in close relation to the upper border of the pancreas. The splenic artery terminates at splenic hilum by diving into two or three main branches. These branches that penetrate through the hilum of the spleen and further divide into segmental arteries that enters along the splenic trabeculae. These are end arteries and occlusion of one of these arteries usually is associated with infarction of the corresponding region of the spleen. Segmental arteries give rise to trabecular arteries which branches into central arteries.

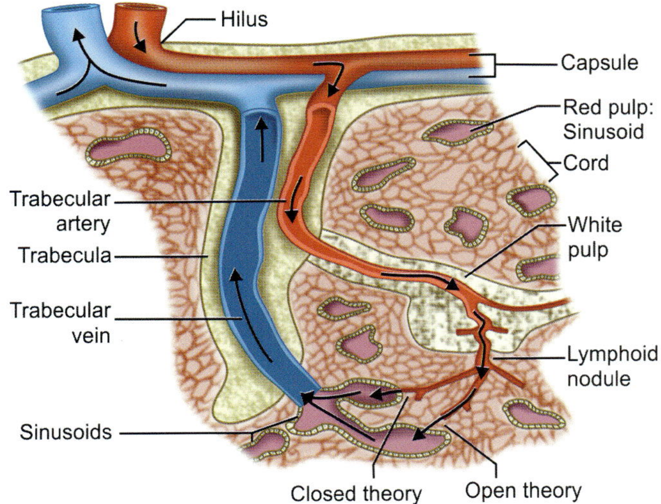

Figure 4 Splenic microcirculation

Short gastric arteries and left gastroepiploic artery originate from splenic artery.

Venous Drainage

Several veins at hilum of spleen join to form the splenic vein. The splenic vein traverses behind the pancreas collecting its tributaries and joins the superior mesenteric vein to form the portal vein. Portal vein is formed behind the neck of pancreas. The inferior mesenteric vein drains mostly in splenic vein but may occasionally join the portal or superior mesenteric vein (Fig. 6).[1,2]

FUNCTIONS OF THE SPLEEN

During early fetal life spleen has a hematopoietic function. It produces both red and white cells during this phase. The hematopoietic function is assumed by bone marrow by the fifth months of gestation, and spleen has no hematopoietic function. In adult, hematopoiesis in spleen is seen in pathological state like myeloproliferative disorders. Mechanical filtration of red cells and immunological function are the most important and dominant functions of spleen in the adult human. These functions of spleen are due to splenic structure and splenic microcirculations.

Mechanical Filtration

It is the most important function of the spleen which removes senescent erythrocytes and deformed erythrocytes from the

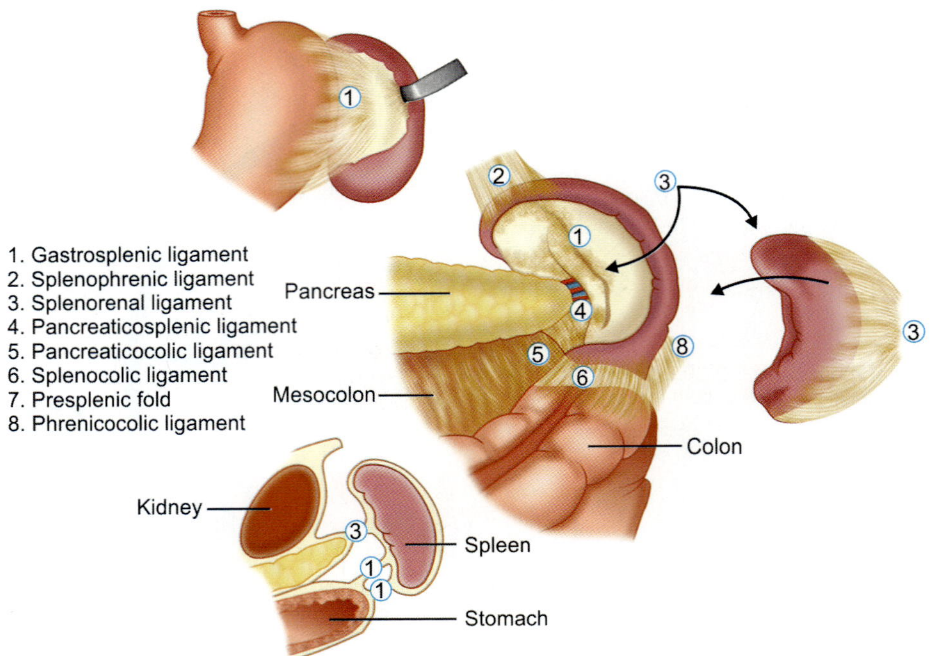

Figure 5 Attachments and anatomical relation of spleen

circulation. It also filters from blood certain pathogens for which we do not have a definite antibody like malaria parasite and capsulated bacteria.

Normal red blood cells being biconcave in morphology deform easily while passing through the splenic microvasculature. In hereditary spherocytosis, red blood cells are biconvex in shape which cannot pass through the splenic microvasculature and gets destroyed. The immature red blood cells also get morphological changes and repair in the spleen including removal of nuclei and excessive cell membrane. Surface aberrations in the erythrocytes such as pits and spurs are also removed by the spleen. In the asplenic condition, Howell-Jolly bodies (nuclear remnant), Pappenheimer bodies (iron granules), Heinz bodies (denatured hemoglobin), target cells (immature cells), spur cells and stippling may appear in peripheral circulation.

The destruction of erythrocytes is called *culling* while the removal of erythrocytic inclusions is termed as pitting. Platelets and leukocytes are not usually removed in the spleen.

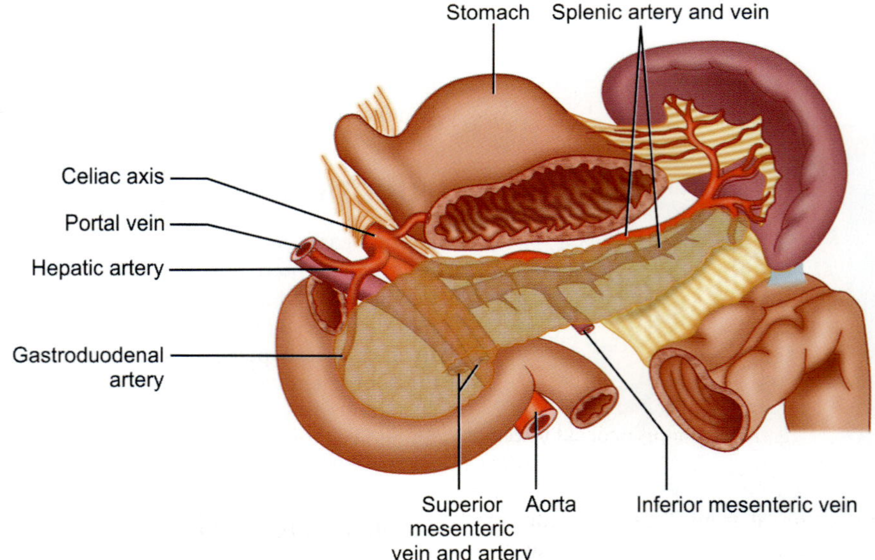

Figure 6 Blood supply and anatomical relation of spleen

Immunological Function

Spleen has an important role in immunological defense and contributes both to humoral and cell mediated immunity. The spleen has a major role in the recognition of antigens, in the production of antibodies, and in the removal from the bloodstream of particles coated with antibodies. The antigens are trapped in periarteriolar lymphatic sheath of the white pulp and present to immunocompetent centers within the lymphoid follicles. This leads to production of antibody by plasma cells (predominantly IgM) and an increase in size of the germinal centers in the lymphoid follicles.

It also produces *opsonin*, *tuftsin* and *properdin*. *Tuftsin* is circulating monocytes which in the red pulp gets converted into macrophages and helps in phagocytic activity of the spleen. *Properdin* helps in initiation of alternate pathways of complement activation. These factors help to clear the bacteria from the circulation especially the encapsulated bacteria like *Haemophilus influenza* and pneumococcus. In asplenic patient, levels of these factors in serum are decreased; activation of alternate pathways of complement system is impaired. These patients have risk of overwhelming post-splenectomy infections (OPSIs).[5-8]

Hypersplenism and Splenomegaly

Splenomegaly refers to enlargement of spleen while hypersplenism refers to decreased in blood component (cytopenia) due to splenic enlargement. In health, spleen causes destruction of damaged blood components. Splenomegaly can lead to rapid destruction of blood components (red blood cells, platelets and white blood cells) leading to anemia, leucopenia, thrombocytopenia or pancytopenia. Hypersplenism is defined as splenic enlargement, a decrease in circulating levels of one or more of the blood lines (anemia, leucopenia, thrombocytopenia or pancytopenia), and a compensatory increase in bone marrow activity in response to the deficiency in the circulating blood elements. Splenectomy in hypersplenism corrects and causes reversal of the low cell counts.[5-7,9]

LATE MORBIDITY AFTER SPLENECTOMY

Overwhelming Postsplenectomy Infection

Spleen contributed both to humoral immunity and cell mediated immunity. Splenectomy causes loss of immunological function of spleen leading to decreased phagocytosis of encapsulated bacteria and parasites. Splenectomy also results in decreased antibody production. These asplenic patients are at risk of OPSI which is a life-threatening fulminant condition. OPSI was initially observed by King and Shumacker in 1952 in infants and children following splenectomy. OPSI is the most common fatal late complication of splenectomy.[10]

Overwhelming post-splenectomy infection can occur at any time after splenectomy. The risk of aggressive pneumococcal infection in splenectomy patients is increased 12–25 times the normal population. Major risk factors for OPSI are age at splenectomy, indication of splenectomy, interval from time of splenectomy and the overall immune status of patient. Children of age less than 2 years are at major developing infection. Splenectomy for a hematological disorder, like hereditary spherocytosis, thalassemia, ITP, autoimmune hemolysis or lymphoma, has more risk of developing OPSI than splenectomy after trauma in adult.[10,11]

Sepsis can be caused by any bacterial or fungal organism but encapsulated organisms like *Streptococcus pneumonia* more frequently cause sepsis in asplenic patients. Even small amount of specific antibody can readily control encapsulated organisms like *S. pneumoniae* which are particularly resistant to phagocytosis. As antibody production is also impaired in these asplenic patients resulting in rapid proliferation of bacteria and overwhelming sepsis. Most frequent organism causing OPSI are *S. pneumoniae* (50–90%), and *S. pyogenes* (25%). *H. influenza and Neisseria meningitidis* are also seen frequently.[10-12]

Early stage of OPSI has nonspecific and mild physical symptoms like fever, fatigue, myalgia, malaise, headache, abdominal pain, diarrhea and vomiting. The clinical symptoms rapidly and fulminantly progress to shock, respiratory distress, hypoglycemia and severe acidosis. Electrolyte abnormalities and disseminated intravascular coagulation may further complicate the clinical situation. These patients have mortality of more than 50% in first 48 hours.[12]

Immunization

Preventive strategy includes vaccination against common organism. Vaccines include the 23-valent pneumococcal polysaccharide vaccine (PPV23), a 7-valent protein conjugated pneumococcal vaccine, meningococcal vaccine and the *H. influenzae* type B vaccine, and the meningococcal vaccine. These cover for most common organisms. All asplenic patients should have vaccination with polysaccharide-based pneumococcal vaccine.[10,13] The Centers for Disease Control and Prevention (CDC) recommends vaccination 2 weeks before surgery with both the meningococcal and pneumococcal vaccines. CDC does not recommend the routine administration of the *H. influenza B* vaccine prior to splenectomy.

In most of the patient with PPV23 vaccination, the antibody titer falls after 5–10 years and revaccination is recommended in high-risk patients every 6 years by CDC, US.

CDC recommendation for revaccination:

1. Routine revaccination of immunocompetent persons who were previously vaccinated with PPV23 is not recommended.
2. Revaccination with PPV23 recommended in high-risk individuals:
   (a) Person vaccinated with 14-valent vaccine and at risk of pneumococcal infection.
   (b) Person vaccinated with PPV23 6-years prior.
   (c) Adults at highest risk with a rapid decline in pneumococcal antibody levels (nephrotic syndrome, renal failure, transplant recipients).
   (d) Children at highest risk (asplenia, nephritic syndrome, sickle cell anemia) who would be 10 years old at revaccination.

In cases of emergency splenectomy, vaccines should be given within 2 weeks of postoperative period.

Antibiotic Prophylaxis

In asplenic patient, especially children, prophylactic antibiotics with penicillin are practiced for initial few years. Efficacy of oral prophylaxis in adults is debatable. However, at onset of febrile illness or onset of rigor, an asplenic patient must take empirically an antibiotic prophylaxis. Empirical treatment with third generation cephalosporin and aminoglycosides is essential in patient with prodromal symptoms and at risk of OPSI.[14] A rational approach may be to provide oral antibiotics to post-splenectomy adults, with instructions to start medication at the onset of a febrile illness and report for immediate medical evaluation. Whether the patient elects to take antibiotic prophylaxis and, because of the risk of OPSI and the extreme level of associated mortality, any asplenic patient who presents with rigors or fever must be started immediately on aggressive empiric antibiotic coverage, even without culture data.

Postsplenectomy Thrombocytosis

The spleen is the primary site for platelets destruction. In normal healthy individual platelet regulation is done in spleen. In hypersplenism the destruction of platelets occurs at rapid rate leading to thrombocytopenia. Similarly after splenectomy the platelet count is increased leading to reactive thrombocytosis. Postsplenectomy platelet count varies between $600 - 1000 \times 10^9$ per liter. It reaches its peak between 7–12 days. Post-splenectomy thrombocytosis is more profound in myeloproliferative disorders. This can result into thrombosis of mesenteric vein, renal vein and portal vein. These patients are also at risk of developing deep venous thrombosis and pulmonary embolism. Prophylactic tab aspirin 150 mg per day has been suggested to prevent thromboembolic phenomenon if count is more the 750×10^9 per liter. Hydroxyurea and anagrelide in combination with aspirin also have been used.[15-18]

REFERENCES

1. Skandalakis JE, Colborn GL, Weidman TA, Foster RS Jr, Kingsnorth AN, Skandalakis LE, et al. Skandalakis' Surgical Anatomy.
2. Standring S (Ed). Gray's Anatomy: The Anatomical Basis of Clinical Practice. Philadelphia: Elsevier Churchill Livingstone; 2008. p. 1225.
3. Sadler TW. Langman's Medical Embryology; 12th edition. Philadelphia: Lippincott Williams & Wilkins; 2012. p. 214.
4. Mebius RE, Kraal G. Structure and function of the spleen. Nat Immunol. 2005;5:606-16.
5. Han J, et al. Spleen. In: Mills SE (Ed). Histology for Pathologists, 3rd edition. Philadelphia: Lippincott Williams and Wilkins; 2007. p. 783.
6. Tablin F, et al. The microanatomy of the mammalian spleen. In: Bowdler AJ (Ed). The Complete Spleen; 2nd edition. Totowa, NJ: Humana; 2002. p. 11.
7. Dailey MO. The immune functions of the spleen. In: Bowdler AJ (Ed). The Complete Spleen; 2nd edition. Totowa, NJ: Humana; 2002. p. 51.
8. Paraskevas F. Lymphocytes and lymphatic organs. In: Greer JP et al. (Eds). Wintrobe's Clinical Hematology, 12th edition. Philadelphia: Lippincott Williams & Wilkins; 2009. p. 300.
9. Molmenti EP, Christensen DO, Nicastro JM, Coppa GF, Villar HV. Anatomy and physiology of the spleen. In: Yeo CJ (Eds). Shackelford's Surgery of the Alimentary Tract, 7th edition. Philadelphia: WB Saunders; 2013. pp. 1610-7.
10. Antonio Di Sabatino, Carsetti R, Corazza GR. Post-splenectomy and hyposplenic states. Lancet. 2011;378:86-97.
11. Okabayashi T, Hanazaki K. Overwhelming postsplenectomy infection syndrome in adults—a clinically preventable disease. World J Gastroenterol. 2008;14(2):176-9.
12. Holdsworth RJ, Irving AD, Cuschieri A. Postsplenectomy sepsis and its mortality rate: actual versus perceived risks. Br J Surg. 1991;78:1031-8.
13. Shatz DV, Romero-Steiner S, Elie CM, Holder PF, Carlone GM. Antibody responses in postsplenectomy trauma patients receiving the 23-valent pneumococcal polysaccharide vaccine at 14 versus 28 days postoperatively. J Trauma. 2002;53:1037-42.
14. Kaplinsky C, Spirer Z. Post-splenectomy antibiotic prophylaxis-unfinished story: to treat or not to treat? Pediatr Blood Cancer. 2006;47:740-1.
15. Buss DH, Cashell AW, O'Connor ML, Richards F 2nd, Case LD. Occurrence, etiology, and clinical significance of extreme thrombocytosis: a study of 280 cases. Am J Med. 1994;96(3):247-53.
16. McIntyre KJ, Hoagland HC, Silverstein MN, Petitt RM. Essential thrombocythemia in young adults. Mayo Clin Proc. 1991;66(2):149-54.
17. Koh KK, Cho SK, Kim SS, Oh BH, Lee YW. Coronary vasospasm, multiple coronary thrombosis, unstable angina and essential thrombocytosis. Int J Cardiol. 1993;41(2):168-70.
18. Murphy S, Peterson P, Iland H, Laszlo J. Experience of the Polycythemia Vera Study Group with essential thrombocythemia: a final report on diagnostic criteria, survival, and leukemic transition by treatment. Semin Hematol. 1997;34(1):29-39.

CHAPTER 82

Splenic Trauma

JK Banerjee

INTRODUCTION

Spleen is the most commonly injured intra-abdominal organ following a blunt trauma. Though spleen is also commonly injured following a penetrating injury to left upper quadrant of abdomen and lower chest, its diagnosis and management is clear cut and is operative in most of the cases. The management of blunt trauma to spleen, however, has undergone important changes in last two to three decades primarily with the goal of preservation of functional splenic tissue. Initially, it shifted from splenectomy to spleen salvage surgery like partial splenectomy and splenorrhaphy, primarily to prevent lifelong risk of severe infections like overwhelming postsplenectomy infection (OPSI). However, over last two decades or so the trend is more for a nonoperative management (NOM) which not only preserves the spleen, but also avoids a major surgery.[1-4] The chances of successful outcome from NOM can be increased further by adjuncts like a transcatheter splenic artery embolization. However, it is very important for the treating surgeon to correctly identify the cases which are appropriate for NOM and to recognize the failures early amongst the cases kept under observation.

SPLENIC ANATOMY AND PHYSIOLOGY, RELEVANT TO TRAUMA

Normally, spleen is a well protected organ by virtue of its location in the left upper quadrant of abdomen beneath the left hemidiaphragm, protected by lower ribs. However, in conditions where spleen is enlarged and extending beyond the protection of costal margin, it is vulnerable to trauma. Normal spleen is a major lymphopoietic organ and carries out the important functions of opsonization of encapsulated organisms. It also takes part in production of opsonins and cellular antigenic response.[5] These have bearing on risk of OPSI in postsplenectomy patients.[6,7]

MECHANISM OF TRAUMA TO SPLEEN

A blunt trauma to spleen commonly occurs following a road traffic accident, due to assault, sports related activities or fall from height. Penetrating injuries are much less common and are commonly due to gun shot or occasionally due to knife assaults. Another common mode of injury is iatrogenic, where a tear in the splenic capsule happens during the surgery on adjacent organs following careless retraction or due to tension on splenic capsule during manipulation.[8]

EVALUATION OF A PATIENT WITH SUSPECTED SPLENIC TRAUMA

History and Clinical Examination

In a blunt trauma of abdomen, an accurate history taking especially about the mode of injury, is extremely important. History of trauma to left upper quadrant or left flank should raise a suspicion of splenic injury. However, it must be remembered that absence of such a history does not exclude splenic injury.

For a penetrating injury to spleen, entry wound may be far away from spleen and depends upon the trajectory of the missile or the impaling agent.

Patient may present with a history of pain in the chest wall on left side, left upper abdomen or may even complain of a pain in left shoulder region (Kehr's sign) due to blood collection near left hemidiaphragm irritating the phrenic nerve. A bruise, abdominal wall contusion or an evidence of fracture of left lower ribs may be a very important clue indicating splenic injury.[9] An attempt must be made to look for any evidence of injury to other intra-abdominal viscera especially rupture of a hollow viscus. Many of the clinical signs of such injury may be masked due to associated neurological injury or inebriated state of the patient.[10]

Diagnostic Work-Up

A plain X-ray film may show rib fracture or medial displacement of gastric bubble in a suspected case of splenic injury. However the following two investigations are used by most of the centers for evaluating a case of blunt injury of abdomen.

FAST

Focused abdominal sonogram for trauma (FAST) is used at the bedside by the treating surgeon and usually is the only evaluation done in a hemodynamically unstable patient. A hypoechoic rim of sub capsular fluid or intraperitoneal fluid around the spleen or in splenorenal recess indicates splenic injury. However, it must be remembered that a negative FAST examination is not sufficient to rule out a splenic trauma (Fig. 1).

CT Scan

Computed tomography scan is commonly done in such patients provided the patient is hemodynamically stable. The computed tomography scan is done with intravenous contrast to look for any active bleeding but may be done without an oral contrast if so required. It is performed using a helical scanner at 10 mm intervals and if an injury is detected, 5 mm cuts are taken through the injured area to delineate the anatomy better (Fig. 2). The computed tomography scan may show subcapsular or intraparenchymal hematoma, or areas of parenchymal disruption of spleen. Active extravasation of contrast implies ongoing bleeding. It may show contrast blush within splenic parenchyma indicating areas of parenchymal disruption or pseudoaneurysm of splenic vessels. It may show hemoperitoneum. Based on the computed tomography findings, the severity of the splenic injury has been graded by the American Association for the Surgery of Trauma (AAST). This is of immense value in the decision making regarding further management especially the NOM.

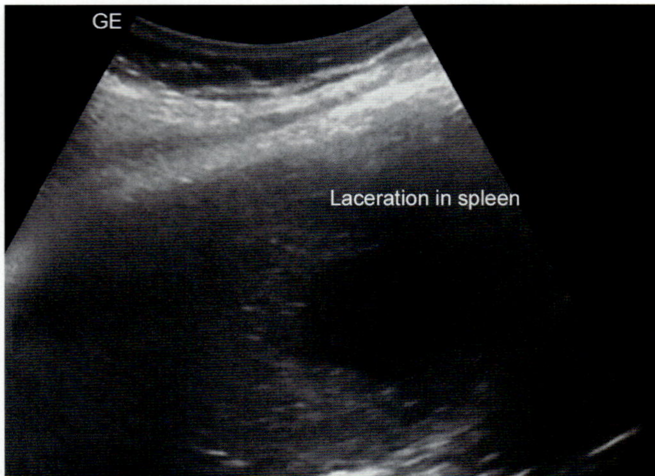

Figure 1 Ultrasonography is the most important investigation for evaluating a blunt injury of abdomen. In such situation, the test should be done at bedside by the treating surgeon (FAST). The investigation can be quick and very informative

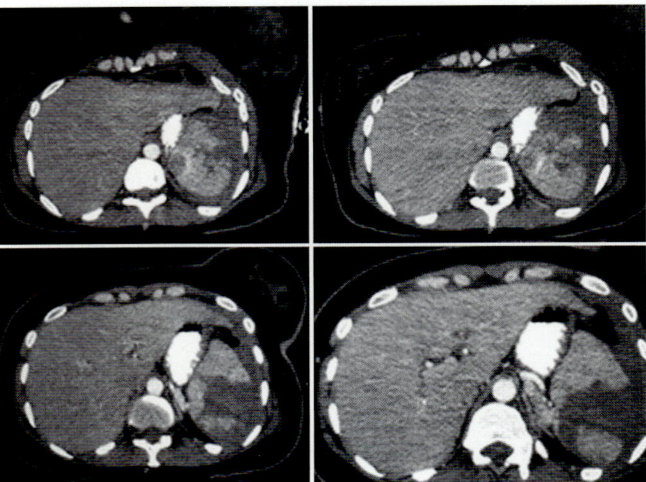

Figure 2 A contrast-enhanced computed tomography scan is the most useful investigation, in hemodynamically stable patients. It can show the anatomical details of the injury required for grading the injury and can also give information about any ongoing active bleeding. This picture also shows additional findings of contusion, hematoma and surgical emphysema on left mammary area and adjacent chest wall

GRADING OF SPLENIC INJURY (AAST SPLEEN INJURY SCALE 1994 REVISION)

The AAST has graded the splenic trauma based on the computed tomography scan findings of the anatomical extent of the injury as under (Fig. 3):

Grade I	Hematoma:	Subcapsular less than 10% of surface area
	Laceration:	Capsular tear less than 1 cm in depth into parenchyma
Grade II	Hematoma:	Subcapsular 10–50% of surface area
	Laceration:	Capsular tear 1–3 cm in depth but not involving a trabecular vessel
Grade III	Hematoma:	Subcapsular more than 50% of surface area or expanding, ruptured subcapsular hematoma or intraparenchymal hematoma 5 cm or expanding
	Laceration:	More than 3 cm in depth or involving trabecular vessels
Grade IV	Laceration:	Involving segmental or hilar vessels with major devasculation, i.e. more than 25% of the spleen
Grade V	Hematoma:	Shattered spleen
	Laceration:	Hilar vascular injury devascularising the spleen

THE APPROACH TO MANAGEMENT

The approach to management varies from institution to institution depending upon multiple factors such as:

- Hemodynamic stability status of the patient
- Grade of injury

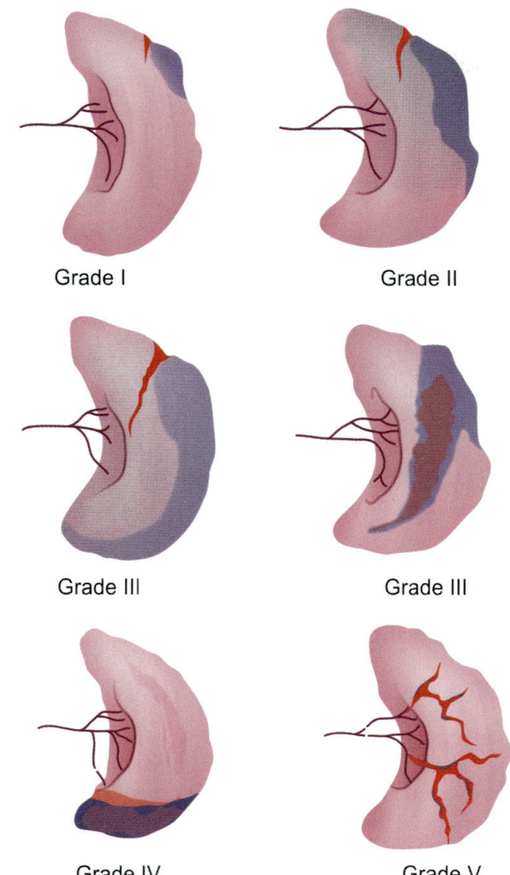

Figure 3 Grading of blunt splenic trauma (AAST grading)

- Presence of associated injuries
- Availability of facilities for evaluation.

Penetrating injuries to the spleen are subjected to surgical exploration due to high incidence of associated visceral injuries. However, in hemodynamically stable isolated penetrating splenic injury a NOM may be followed.

The management of blunt injury cases may be broadly divided into two, depending on their hemodynamic stability status:

Hemodynamically Unstable Patients

Hemodynamic status of the patient is the most important deciding factor about the approach to management. A hemodynamically unstable patient with a positive FAST will require immediate laparotomy to determine the source of intraperitoneal hemorrhage and control it.

Hemodynamically Stable Patients

Management approach of these patients will depend on the grade of injury, evidence of any associated intraperitoneal injury and any associated extra-abdominal injury requiring surgical intervention.

Nonoperative Management

Over a period of time, importance of salvaging the functional splenic tissue in avoiding complications following splenectomy was understood more and more. This initially lead to attempts of spleen salvaging surgery such as partial splenectomy or splenorrhaphy and subsequently to adoption of NOM. This management, however, is not attempted in certain conditions like hemodynamic instability, suspicion of associated intraperitoneal injury, presence of portal hypertension, in higher grade splenic injuries (grade IV or V) and with evidence of active bleeding on computed tomography scan. Certain conditions, like large volume hemoperitoneum (blood seen in both paracolic gutters on computed tomography scan or >250 cc), altered neurological status or injury to spleen with existing pathological condition-which were invariably considered as contraindications of NOM earlier are being increasingly considered for NOM.[11] Grade IV and V are generally not considered for NOM due to their unsuitability for angiographic embolization. Grade IV injuries are occasionally given initial attempt at NOM by arterial embolization provided they do not have any other contraindication for NOM.[12-14]

The NOM requires careful patient selection and availability of adequate facilities in the institute for close monitoring of the patient and emergency intervention like angiographic embolization and surgery. Most of the institutions follow a protocol of initial intensive care and close monitoring in an intensive care unit (ICU) set up which includes bed rest, serial hemoglobin level estimation done at least 6 or 12 hourly, and are kept nil orally in initial 24 hours. If the parameters remain stable further observation is done in a step-down facility for next 4–5 days. There is difference in institutional protocols regarding repeat computed tomography scans during period of observation. Generally, a repeat computed tomography scan is required only in case of deterioration of vital parameters, aggravation of symptoms or in situations where the clinical condition of the patient cannot be assessed fully due to associated neurological obtundation. Though not supported by clinical evidence, yet most of the institution protocols observe the patients with higher grade injury for a longer duration, in comparison to a lower grade injury.[15] Majority of the patients will require an in hospital observation for about 5 days to decide about need for any intervention. Nearly, 90% of the cases failing a NOM will do so within 96 hours of hospital admission.[16]

Those who fail a NOM require some emergency intervention–usually an angiographic embolization or an emergency surgery. An embolization for control of bleeding, if patient can wait till then, is a preferred pursuit in most of the cases. However, it depends upon the infrastructure and the expertise available in the institution. Success rate of angiographic embolization for control of active bleeding due to splenic trauma varies from 57–93%,[14,17-22] depending on various factors including the grade of injury, patient's anatomy, operator's skill and the type of embolization material used. Quick and easy availability of embolization makes significant impact on successful outcome of NOM.[17,23-26]

A NOM cuts out all the risks resulting directly from a major surgical intervention and its complications. In addition, it has the advantage of preservation of spleen. However, in order to achieve a successful NOM, patient may have to have multiple blood transfusions, may require to undergo a potentially dangerous procedure like angiographic embolization, and be at risk of delayed hemorrhage, and missed intra-abdominal injuries or complications arising out of these. The NOM fails in about 6–20% of patients under observation and require emergency surgical intervention.[16,27,28]

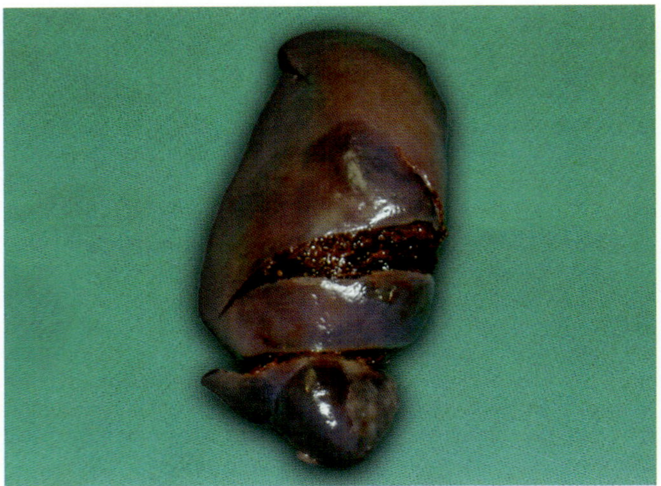

Figure 4 Case of blunt injury to spleen with Grade IV injury. Patient was hemodynamically unstable and required an emergency splenectomy

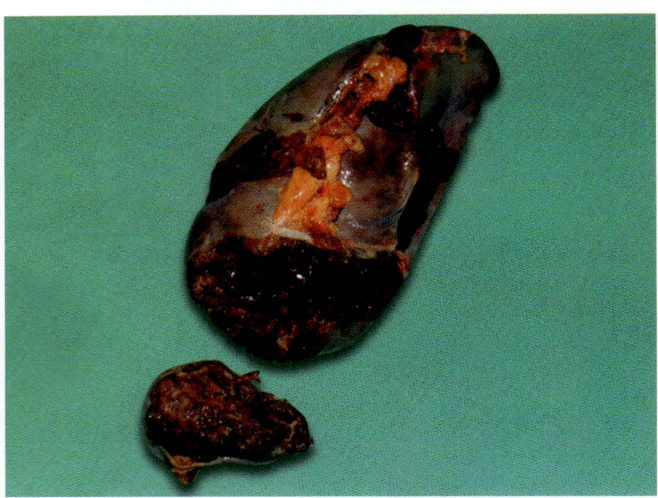

Figure 5 Same case as in Fig. 4. Case of blunt injury to spleen with Grade IV injury

Follow-Up Care of Cases Managed by NOM

On discharge from hospital, patients are advised to avoid contact sports, adventure sports and military combat duties etc. for about 3 months. A repeat follow up computed tomography scan is generally not considered necessary and is advised, 3 months after the injury, only for the specific group of patients who wish to resume the restricted activities and those proceeding to remote areas where health care facilities are limited.[29-31]

Operative management is done for either those who were not considered for NOM, being hemodynamically unstable or those who have failed a NOM. These patients require surgical exploration and depending on the extent of injury, clinical status of the patient and associated injuries, may either undergo a splenic salvage surgery or splenectomy (Figs. 4 and 5). The salvage surgery could be either a partial splenectomy preserving more than half of spleen or a splenorrhaphy.

ASPLENIA AND IMMUNOCOMPETENCE

Since splenectomy causes impaired opsonization of capsulated organisms, these patients require immunization. Vaccination is ideally administered 14 days before a planned splenectomy (due to any reason) or 14 days after an emergency splenectomy.[32,33]

ALGORITHMIC APPROACH TO MANAGEMENT OF SPLENIC TRAUMA

An algorithmic approach to management of splenic trauma, both penetrating and blunt trauma is given in Flowcharts 1 and 2.

Flowchart 1 Algorithmic approach to the management of penetrating injury to spleen

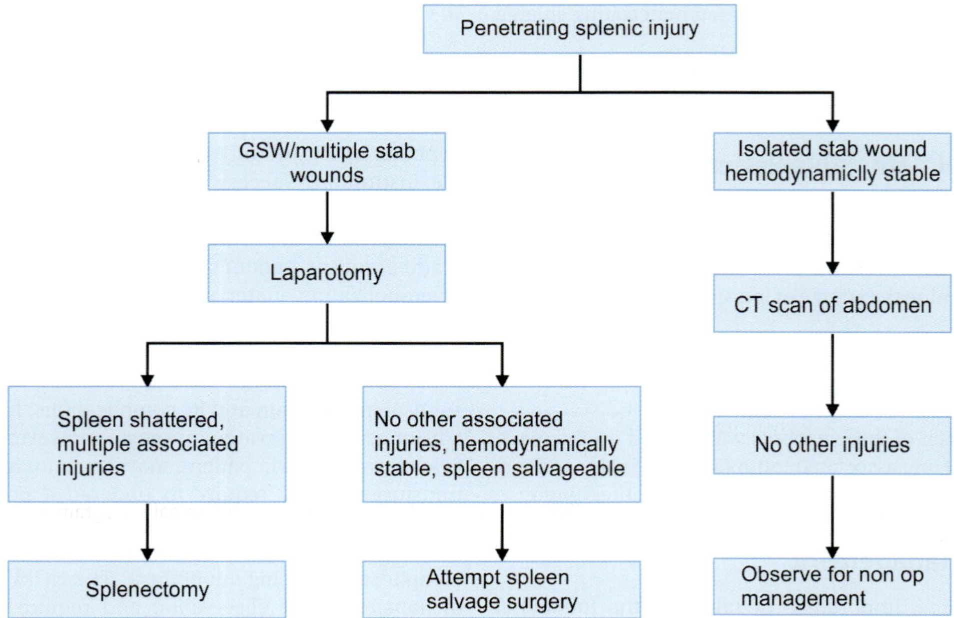

Abbreviations: GSW, gunshot wound; CT, computed tomography.

Flow chart 2 Algorithmic approach to the management of blunt trauma to spleen

Blunt splenic injury

Hemodynamically stable

CT scan of abdomen and pelvis

No injury

Splenic injury present

Gd I and II

Gd III and Gd IV (+/–)

Gd V

Small hemoperitoneum

Large hemoperitoneum

Splenic angiography

No active bleeding

Active bleeding seen

Angiographic embolization

No further bleeding seen

Bleeding continues

Hemodynamically unstable

Abd signs present

No abd signs

USG/FAST

+ve

–ve

Look for other causes of bleeding

Observe for non operative management, do serial hematocrit, if NOM fails

Laparotomy

Abbreviations: Gd, grade; CT, computed tomography; USG, ultrasonography; FAST, focused abdominal sonogram for trauma; NOM, nonoperative management.

REFERENCES

1. Pachter HL, Spencer FC, Hofstetter SR, Liang HG, Hoballah J, Coppa GF. Experience with selective operative and nonoperative treatment of splenic injuries in 193 patients. Ann Surg. 1990;211:583-9.
2. Feliciano DV, Spjut-Patrinely v, Burch JM, Mattox KL, Bitondo CG, Cruse-Martocci P. The alternative. Ann Surg. 1990;211:569-82.
3. Malangoni MA, Cue JI, Fallat ME, Willing SJ, Richardson JD. Evaluation of Splenic injury by computed tomography and its impact on treatment. Ann Surg. 1990;211:592-7.
4. Pachter HL, Hofstetter SR, Spencer FC. Evolving concepts in splenic surgery-splenorrhaphy versus splenectomy and postsplenectomy drainage: experience in 105 patients. Ann Surg. 1981;194:262-9.
5. Lucas CE. Splenic trauma. Choice of management. Ann Surg. 1991;213:98-112.
6. Holdsworth RJ, Irving AD, Cuschieri A. Postsplenectomy sepsis and its mortality rate: actual versus perceived risk. Br J Surg. 1991;78:1031-8.
7. Singer DB. Postsplenectomy sepsis. Perspect Pediatr Pathol. 1973;1:285-311.
8. Merchea A, Dozois EJ, Wang JK, Larson DW. Anatomic mechanism for splenic injury during colorectal surgery. Clin Anat. 2012;25:212-7.
9. Jacoby R, Wisner D. Injury to spleen. In: Feliciano D, Mattox K, Moore E (Eds). Trauma, 6th edition. New York: McGraw-Hill Professional; 2008. pp. 661-73.
10. Salim A, Sangthong B, Martin M, Carlos B, David P, Demetrios D. Whole body imaging in blunt multisystem trauma patients without obvious signs of injury: results of a prospective study. Arch Surg. 2006;141:468-75.
11. Guth AA, Pachter HL, Jacobwitz GR. Rupture of the pathologic spleen: is there a role for nonoperative therapy? J Trauma. 1996;41:214-8.
12. Sclafani SJA, Shaftan GW, Scalea TM, Paterson LA, Kohl L, Kantor A, et al. Nonoperative salvage of computed tomography-diagnosed splenic injuries: utilization of angiography for triage and embolization for hemostasis. J Trauma. 1995;39:818-27.
13. Schurr MJ, Fabian TC, Gavant M, Croce MA, Kudsk KA, Minard G, et al. Management of blunt splenic trauma: computed tomography blush predicts failure of nonoperative management. J Trauma. 1995;39:507-13.
14. Davis KA, Fabian TC, Croce MA, Gavant M, Flick P, Minard G, et al. Improved success in nonoperative management of blunt Splenic trauma: embolization of splenic artery pseudoaneurysm. J Trauma1998;44:1008-13.
15. Fata P, Robinson L, Fakhry SM, Samir M. A survey of EAST member practices in blunt splenic injury: a description of current trends and opportunities for improvement. J Trauma. 2005;59:836-42.
16. Peitzman AB, Heil B, Rivera L, Federle MB, Harbrecht BG, Clancy KD. Blunt Splenic injury in adults: Multi-institutional Study of the Eastern Association for the Surgery of Trauma. J Trauma. 2000;49:177-89.
17. Haan JM, Biffl W, Knudson MM, Davis KA, Oka T, Majercik S, et al. Splenic embolization revisited: a multicenter review. J Trauma. 2004;56:542-7.
18. Bhullar IS, Frykberg ER, Siragusa D, Chesire D, Paul J, Joseph J, et al. Selective angiographic embolization of blunt Splenic traumatic injuries in adults decreases failure rate of non operative management. J Trauma Acute Care Surg. 2012;72:1127-34.
19. Raikhlin A, Baerlocher MO, Asch MR, Myer A. Imaging and transcatheter arterial embolization for traumatic splenic injuries: review of literature. Can J Surg. 2008;51:464-72.
20. Gaarder C, Dormagen FB, Eken T, Skaga NO, Klow NE, Pilgram-Larsen J, et al. Nonoperative management of splenic injuries: improved results with angioembolization. J Trauma. 2006;61: 192-8.
21. Harbrecht BG, Ko SH, Watson GA, Gregory A, Forsythe RM, Rosengart MR, et al. Angiography for blunt splenic trauma does not improve the success rate of nonoperative management. J Trauma. 2007;63:44-9.
22. Smith HE, Biffl WL, Majercik SD, Jednacz J, Lambiase R, Cioffi W. Splenic artery embolization: Have we gone too far? J Trauma. 2006;61:541-49.
23. Haan J, Ilahi ON, Kramer M, Myers J, Scalea T. Protocol-driven nonoperative management in patients with blunt splenic trauma and minimal associated injury decreases length of stay. J Trauma. 2003;55:317-21.
24. Liu PP, Lee WC, Cheng YF, Fan Y, Hsieh PM, Hsieh YM, et al. Use of splenic artery embolization as an adjunct to nonsurgical management of blunt splenic injury. J Trauma. 2004;56:768-73.
25. Rajani RR, Claridge JA, Yowler CJ, Patrick P, Wiant A, Summers JI, et al. Improved outcome of adult blunt Splenic injury: a cohort analysis. Surgery. 2006;140:625-31.
26. Sabe AA, Claridge JA, Rosenblum DI, Lie K, Malangoni MA. The effects of splenic artery embolization on nonoperative management of blunt splenic injury: a 16-year experience. J Trauma. 2009;67:565-72.
27. McIntyre LK, Schiff M, Jurkovich GJ. Failure of nonoperative management of splenic injuries: causes and consequences. Arch Surg. 2005;140:563-69.
28. Bhangu A, Nepogodiev D, Lal N, Bowley DM. Meta-analysis of predictive factors and outcomes for failure of nonoperative management of blunt splenic trauma. Injury. 2012;43:1337-43.
29. Pachter HL, Guth AA, Hofstetter SR, Spencer FC. Changing patterns in the management of splenic trauma: impact of nonoperative management. Ann Surg. 1998;227:708-19.
30. Allins A, Ho T, Nguyen TH, Cohen M, Waxman K, Hiatt JR. Limited value of routine followup CT scans in nonoperative management of blunt liver and splenic injuries. Am Surg. 1996;62:883-6.
31. Lawson DE, Jacobson JA, Spizarny DL, Pranikoff T. Splenic trauma: value of follow up CT. Radiology. 1995;194;97-100.
32. Howdieshell TR, Heffernan D, Dipiro JT. Therapeutic Agents Committee of the Surgical Infection Society. Surgical infection society guidelines for vaccination after traumatic injury. Surg Infect (Larchmt). 2006;7:275.
33. Centers for Disease Control and Prevention (CDC). Updated recommendation from the Advisary Committee on Immunization Practices (ACIP) for revaccination of persons at prolonged increased risk for meningococcal disease. MMWR Morb Mortal Wkly Rep. 2009;58:1042-3.

CHAPTER 83

Splenic Cysts, Tumors and Abscess

Hirdaya H Nag, R Kalayarasan

Splenic cysts, tumors and abscess are uncommon lesions of the spleen. However, they present a significant challenge to diagnosis and management. The understanding that spleen is a vital organ shifted the management of these lesions from splenectomy to spleen preservation whenever possible. In this chapter a brief overview of these uncommon lesions is given.

SPLENIC CYSTS

Splenic cysts are rare, however, with the advancements in imaging technology they are diagnosed with increased frequency. On the basis of presence or absence of true epithelial lining, splenic cysts are classified into *primary (true)* cysts and *secondary (false)* cysts.

Primary (True) Cysts

Primary (true) cysts are further divided into parasitic cyst and non-parasitic cyst.[1]

Parasitic Cysts

These cysts are most common types of the cystic lesions of spleen, accounting for about 75–80% of all cases.[2] Splenic hydatid is the most common parasitic cyst with *Echinococcus granulosus* being the most common causative organism (Fig. 1). Parasite reaches spleen through blood stream, lymphatics or by reflux from portal vein during increase in intra-abdominal pressure. Splenic hydatid may occur in isolation (primary hydatidosis) or as part of disseminated disease (secondary hydatidosis), former usually occur when parasite bypasses liver and lung to infest spleen. Similar to hydatid cyst of the liver they contain inner germinal layer (endocyst), outer laminated layer (ectocyst) and a fibrous capsule (pericyst). Splenic hydatid grows at a rate of 1–2 cm per year.

Non-parasitic Cysts

Non-parasitic cysts of spleen are further classified into congenital and neoplastic cysts. *Congenital* splenic cysts account for 10% of all splenic cysts and arise from invagination of the mesothelium of splenic capsule during development.[3] *Neoplastic* cysts are further classified into epidermoid, dermoid and lymphangiomas. Epidermoid cyst represents 10% of non-parasitic cyst and 90% of all neoplastic cysts of spleen. They are usually benign, and malignant transformation is very rare.[2]

Secondary Cyst or Pseudocyst

Secondary cyst or pseudocyst of spleen usually develops secondary to trauma, although they may develop following splenic infarcts or splenic infection. Post-traumatic pseudocyst results from organization, liquefaction, resorption and encapsulation of intraparenchymal or subcapsular hematoma (Fig. 2). Lack of an epithelial lining and presence of hemosiderin on microscopic examination supports the diagnosis. Post-traumatic pseudocyst is the second most common type of splenic cyst. These cysts are solitary in 75–80% of cases. Clinical differentiation of true cyst and pseudocyst is usually not possible, and diagnosis is usually made at histological examination. Is incidence of such pseudocyst increasing with increasing use of conservative management for splenic trauma?

Splenic cysts can occur at any age but seen most commonly during second and third decades. Splenic cysts commonly present as painless mass in left upper abdomen or detected incidentally, some patients may present as dull, dragging type pain in abdomen. Large cysts (>5 cm) are prone to rupture and may present with acute abdomen. Symptoms due to pressure over surrounding structures are common with large cysts which

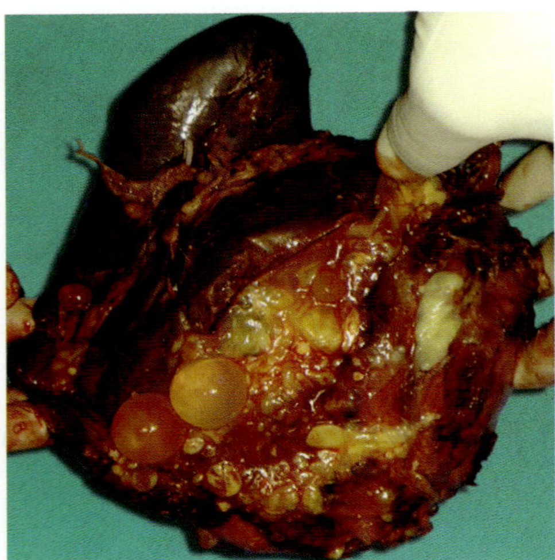

Figure 1 Splenectomy performed for splenic hydatid multiple daughter cysts

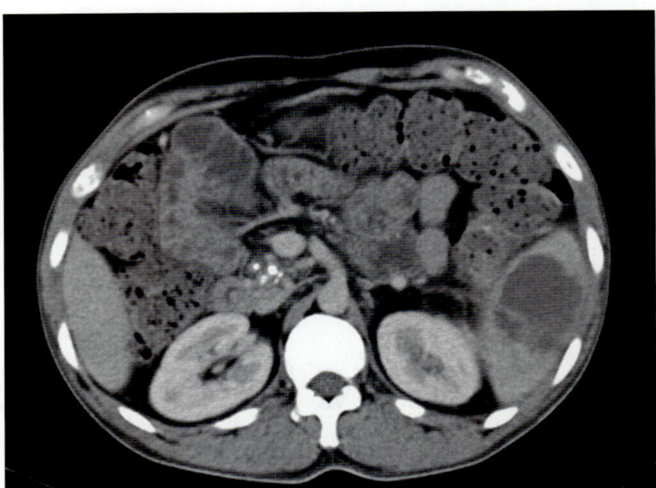

Figure 2 Contrast enhanced CT abdomen of a patient with post-traumatic pseudocyst

include hypertension (left renal artery), urinary symptoms (left kidney or ureteropelvic junction), early satiety (stomach), and respiratory complaints (diaphragm).

Ultrasound abdomen is the initial investigation to determine nature of the splenic mass and to know its solid or cystic nature. True non-parasitic cysts are usually seen as homogenous anechoic lesion, hydatid cyst may appear as unilocular lesion with internal septations, presence of internal debris indicates abscess or pseudocyst. Contrast enhanced computed tomography (CECT) or magnetic resonance imaging (MRI) of the abdomen can further characterize the lesion. Presence of wall calcification, internal septations indicate toward diagnosis of hydatid cyst which can be further confirmed by serological tests. Serum CA 19-9 is often elevated in patients with epidermoid cyst and it can also be used in detecting recurrence after definitive treatment.

Treatment options for splenic cyst include observation, percutaneous drainage, fenestration, marsupialization, partial splenectomy and total splenectomy (Flow chart 1). Observation with serial follow-up using ultrasound abdomen is a reasonable option in patients with small asymptomatic cyst (<5 cm) since risk

Flow chart 1 Algorithm for the management of splenic cysts

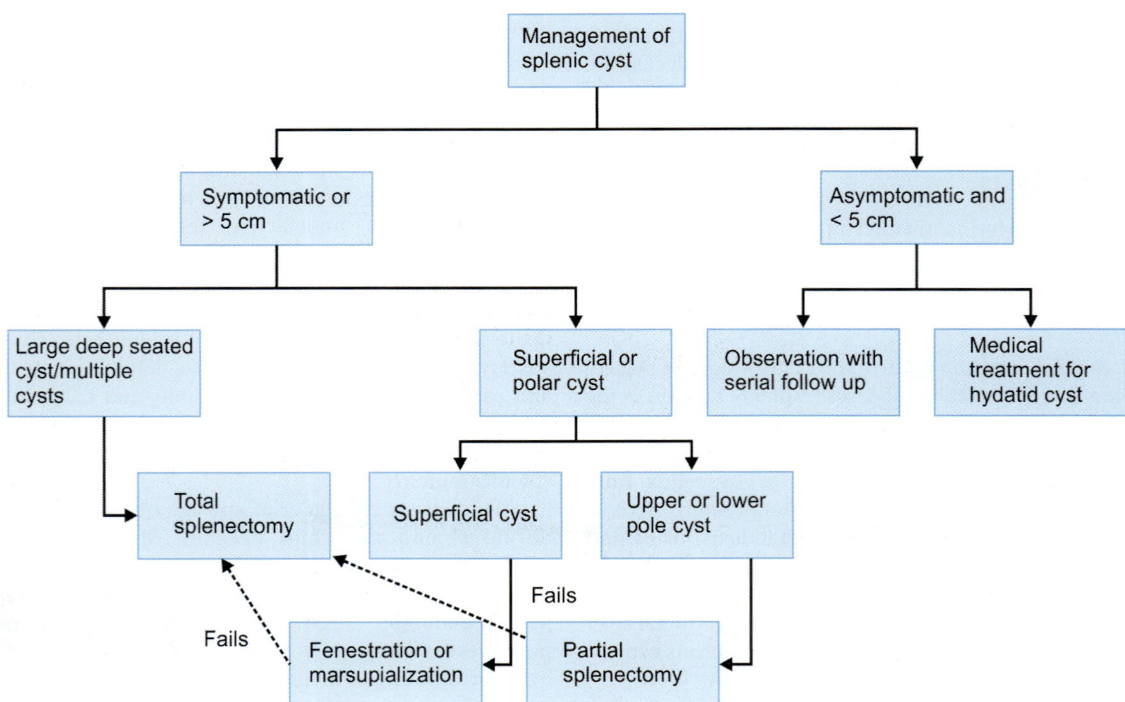

of complications is low and spontaneous resolution may occur with small non-parasitic cyst. Medical treatment with albendazole at 10–15 mg/kg/day in two divided doses for a period of 3–6 months can be effective in small hydatid cyst and intervention is required for cysts larger than 5 cm to prevent complications.[4-6] Percutaneous drainage of cyst with injection of sclerosants is not a preferable option due to high recurrence rate and risk of complications associated with rupture in case of hydatid cyst. Moreover, dense inflammatory reaction induced by the sclerosant injection can make future surgery difficult. Fenestration may be an option for superficial cysts but hydatid cyst should be ruled out beforehand. Fenestration can be done by open, laparoscopic or needlescopic approach and a sufficient portion of cyst wall should be excised to avoid recurrence. Marsupialization is also an option in superficial non-parasitic cysts and it involves partial excision of cyst wall with overrunning of cut edge by a suture. Both fenestration and marsupialization operations are associated with recurrence. Partial splenectomy is ideally suited for polar cysts and preservation of at least 25% of the splenic parenchyma is necessary to avoid immunological dysfunction. In a recent review there was no significant difference in the recurrence rate between total and partial splenectomy for cysts located in one of the poles of spleen. However, a full anatomic knowledge of the splenic vascularization is required in order to avoid intraoperative bleeding and postoperative necrosis of splenic remnant. In majority of the patients splenic artery divides into two to three groups of branches that provide vascularization to the upper pole, intermediate portion and lower pole of the spleen. For performing partial splenectomy, an adequate mobilization of the spleen is achieved by ligating and dissecting the gastrosplenic ligament and short gastric vessels. Splenic vessels are identified and branches directed to the pole to be removed are clamped to produce ischemic line of demarcation. Splenic parenchymal transection can be performed using staplers or energy devices to reduce bleeding. Total splenectomy is indicated for large cysts, deep seated splenic cysts, multiple splenic cysts and as a salvage procedure for patients with uncontrolled bleeding after partial splenectomy. Laparoscopic approach is associated with shorter hospital stay, faster recovery, less postoperative pain and better cosmetic outcomes compared to open splenectomy. To minimize the risk of overwhelming post splenectomy sepsis vaccination against *Streptococcus pneumonia, Neisseria meningitis, Hemophilus influenza* should be administered in the perioperative period.

SPLENIC TUMORS

Splenic tumors are rare and could be lymphoid or non-lymphoid type (Fig. 3). Lymphoid tumors include Hodgkin's and non-Hodgkin's lymphoma. Primary lymphoid tumors are far more common than secondary lymphoid tumors. Most of the non-lymphoid tumors are primary as spleen is uncommon site for metastasis.

Hodgkin's disease is common in young adults and usually present with cervical lymphadenopathy. Ann Arbor classification divides them into four stages and a subscript S is added to every stage for splenic involvement. Historically splenectomy was performed as part of staging laparotomy for stages I and II lymphoma to rule out infradiaphragmatic involvement. However, with advancements in imaging technology staging laparotomy is rarely performed for Hodgkin's disease. Splenic involvement

Flow chart 2 Classification of splenic tumors

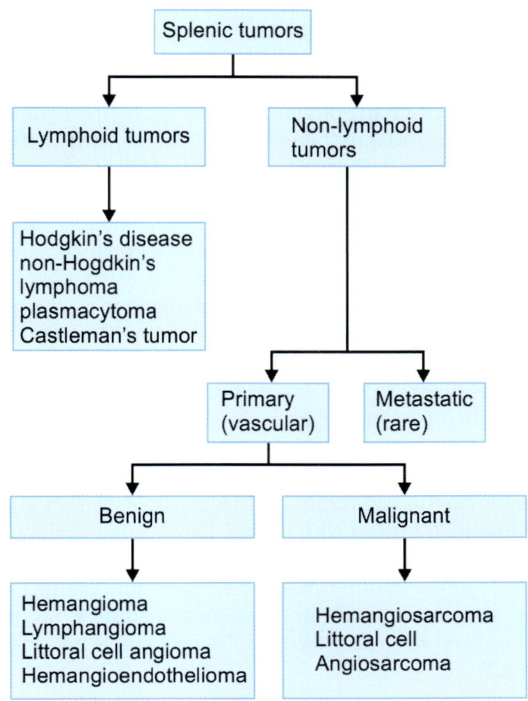

is more common in non-Hodgkin's type of lymphoma, and splenectomy is indicated for symptomatic splenomegaly or hypersplenism. Survival benefit with splenectomy is seen in patients with predominant splenic disease.[7]

Non-lymphoid tumors of spleen usually arise from vascular tissue. *Hemangioma* is the most common vascular neoplasm of spleen. Hemangiomas are usually benign and mostly detected incidentally. They are reported to occur in all age groups, although more common between third and fifth decades and both sexes are affected equally. Hemangiomas are usually solitary and they may be associated with Klippel-Trenaunay-Weber, Beckwith-Weidemann or Turner syndromes.[7] Small hemangiomas are usually asymptomatic, large tumors may present with pain in left upper quadrant, early satiety, abdominal lump and symptoms due to pressure over surrounding viscera. Consumptive coagulopathy may occur due to platelet trapping in cavernous spaces. Rupture is the most common complication although malignant degeneration can also occur rarely (REF). Large size and pressure necrosis of splenic capsule predisposes to splenic rupture, true incidence of splenic rupture is not known but it has been reported in up to 25% in some series.[8] On ultrasound abdomen hemangiomas are seen as hyperechoic solid or complex cystic mass with echogenic calcifications in some patients. Similar to hemangiomas of the liver, splenic hemangiomas show marked contrast enhancement with delayed washout on CECT abdomen. Traditionally patients with symptomatic hemangiomas are managed with open splenectomy although laparoscopic removal has been reported. Partial splenectomy may be performed for polar lesions although other conservative approaches like radiofrequency ablation, angio embolization are also reported with some success.[7,8]

Lymphangiomas of spleen are less common than hemangioma and are detected frequently in children. Clinical presentation can range from an incidental finding to a large symptomatic mass. Large lymphangiomas are usually associated with congenital lymphatic malformations at other sites or organs and occur as part of diffuse lymphangiomatosis.[7,9] Splenic lymphangiomas are frequently subcapsular or trabecular in location, where lymphatics are normally situated. On ultrasound they are seen as hypoechoic mass with occasional internal septations, echogenic debris and tiny wall calcifications. On CECT lymphangiomas appear as hypodense mass with no significant contrast enhancement which differentiates them from hemangioma. Reported complication includes bleeding, infection and rare malignant transformation. Similar to hemangiomas, large symptomatic lymphangioma should be treated by complete excision in the form of total or partial splenectomy. Conservative therapy like percutaneous injection with injection of sclerosant agents is associated with high recurrence rate.[7,9]

Littoral cell angioma is a rare benign neoplasm of "littoral cells" lining the splenic sinusoids. Macroscopically they appear as multiple nodular lesions with no specific imaging characteristics. One-third patients with this rare tumor may be associated with malignant tumors in other parts of the body and about 15% may occur in association with immunological disorders. So, patients with littoral cell angioma need careful evaluation and long-term follow-up.[10]

Hemangiosarcoma (angiosarcoma) is the most common primary malignant tumor of spleen. It occurs in elderly people without gender predilection. Unlike angiosarcomas of the liver, splenic angiosarcoma is not related to exposure to carcinogens like thorium, vinyl chloride or arsenic. Abdominal pain is the most common symptom which may be accompanied by hypersplenism and constitutional symptoms.[11] Splenomegaly with palpable splenic mass is the most common presentation, rupture is also reported in up to 30% of patients.[12] Metastasis is hematogenous and mainly occurs in liver, lung and bone. Differentiation of hemangioma from hemangiosarcoma is essential especially in patients without metastasis. Hemangiosarcoma appear as complex mass with heterogeneous echotexture on ultrasonography. CECT picture of this tumor is of an ill-defined splenic mass with heterogeneous contrast enhancement and areas of necrotic degeneration. Scattered punctate or radial calcification can be found in some cases and metastatic lesions are hypervascular. Splenectomy is the treatment of choice for localized disease as chemotherapy has limited role. Prognosis is poor especially in patients with metastatic disease with overall survival of less than 1 year.[11]

It rarely affects spleen due to inherent features like acute angulation of splenic artery, absence of afferent lymphatics and rhythmic contractions which make spleen an unfavorable destination for metastasis.[13] Common sites of primary tumor are breast, lungs, colon and rectum. Isolated splenic metastasis is rare and usually it is associated with metastasis in other organs. Survival benefit with splenectomy or radiofrequency ablation of isolated splenic metastases has been reported.

SPLENIC ABSCESS

Splenic abscess are uncommon in occurrence but incidence is increasing due to increase in number of immunocompromised patients and increased detection with recent imaging modalities. The most common micro-organisms implicated are *Staphylococcus aureus, Streptococci* and *Escherichia coli*. However, there is marked geographical variation in the microbial profile. *Mycobacterium tuberculosis, Klebsiella pneumoniae* and *Salmonella typhi* were reported as common etiological agents in few series.[14] Fungal abscess are common in immunocompromised patients, common agents are *Candida, Aspergillus, Cryptococcus* and *Blastomyces.*[15] The most common route is hematogenous spread from remote foci or contiguous spread from adjacent organs.[16] Concurrent systemic infection, immunosuppression, splenic trauma, splenic infarction and systemic disorders like diabetes mellitus are common predisposing factors for splenic abscess. IV drug abusers, SABE pts are also predisposed to it.

Fever and abdominal pain are the most common symptoms. The classic triad of fever, left upper quadrant pain and left upper abdomen mass described by Sarr and Zuidema (1982) is seen only in 30–50% of patients.[17] Laboratory parameters suggestive of splenic abscess are leukocytosis and thrombocytosis. Blood cultures is positive in more than 50% and in some cases organism isolated from splenic abscess is different from organism in blood culture.[18]

Ultrasound and CT scan play an important role in the diagnosis and management of splenic abscess. Most common ultrasound finding is anechoic or hypoechoic mass lesion with irregular wall and internal echogenicity.[19] CECT abdomen shows them as a hypodense lesion with peripheral enhancement although contrast enhancement is less prominent than other pyogenic abscesses. Sensitivity and specificity of CECT (90–95%) is better than ultrasound.[15,20,21]

Treatment options include antimicrobials alone, antimicrobials with percutaneous aspiration or drainage and splenectomy. There are no prospective or randomized trials comparing various treatment options. Medical treatment with antimicrobials alone is associated with high mortality and hence recommended only for small abscess (<3 cm) if the clinical response is good.[22] Antimicrobials alone can be effective for abscesses caused by *M. tuberculosis* or fungal organisms.[23-25] However, diagnosis of these abscesses is difficult and usually diagnosis of fungal or tubercular abscess is made after splenectomy. While diagnostic percutaneous aspiration and microbiological culture of the splenic abscess can be useful for the diagnosis of common bacterial organisms it is not very useful for diagnosis of fungal or tubercular abscess. Recent studies have shown that molecular techniques like linear probe assay and serological tests for fungal antigens permit rapid diagnosis and can be performed selectively in patients with high index of suspicion like immunocompromised patients.[23-25] Almost all other cases will require combined therapy including antimicrobials and imaging guided percutaneous aspiration or drainage. Percutaneous aspiration can be therapeutic in small abscess, however, for large abscess (>5 cm) placement of drainage catheter (12 or 14F) is recommended. Complications like bleeding and injury to adjacent organs associated with percutaneous splenic interventions have decreased with advances in imaging technology. The advantages of PCD are less invasive, tolerated well even in critically ill patients, splenic preservation which is critical in children and immunocompromised patients. Main disadvantage with *percutaneous intervention* is treatment failure which is reported in up to 30% of patients. Success rate is higher in solitary, unilocular abscess with well-defined wall and liquefied contents. In some studies percutaneous intervention is used even in patients with multiple abscesses as a bridge to splenectomy. Salvage splenectomy after failed percutaneous interventions has not been associated with significant increase in morbidity and mortality. Current evidence favors combined therapy (antimicrobials + radiological intervention) as a first line of treatment option in splenic abscess. Splenectomy is indicated for failure of conservative treatment, multiple splenic abscesses and splenic abscess in association with other intra-abdominal pathology requiring surgical treatment. Presence of extensive adhesions make splenectomy technically difficult in this condition and early control of splenic artery is recommended to minimize intraoperative bleeding. Intraoperative rupture of splenic abscess should be avoided and in cases with extensive adhesions external drainage of the abscess may be a better option and splenectomy can be performed at a later date, if required. Laparoscopic approach has been successfully employed for splenectomy and drainage of splenic abscess.[26] Prognosis of patients with splenic abscess depends upon number of abscess, underlying pathology and predisposing factors. However, mortality associated with splenic abscess had reduced with the advancements in the diagnosis and use of radiological and minimally invasive approaches.

REFERENCES

1. Martin JW. Congenital splenic cysts. Am J Surg. 1958,96:302-8.
2. Robbin FG, Albert E, Yellin AE, Lingua RW, Craig JR, Turrill FL, et al. Splenic epidermoid cyst. Ann Surg. 1978,87:231-5.
3. Ough YD, Nash HR, Wood DA. Mesothelial cysts of the spleen with squamous metaplasia. Am J Clin Pathol. 1981;76:666-9.
4. Brunetti E, Kern P, Vuitton DA, Writing Panel for the WHO-IWGE. Expert consensus for the diagnosis and treatment of cystic and alveolar echinococcosis in humans. Acta Trop. 2010;114:1-16.
5. Hansen MB, Moller AC. Splenic cysts. Surg Laparosc Endosc Percutan Tech. 2004;14:316-22.
6. Akbulut S, Sogutcu N, Eris C. Hydatid disease of the spleen: single-center experience and a brief literature review. J Gastrointest Surg. 2013;17:1784-95.
7. Morgenstern L, Rosenburg J, Geller SA. Tumors of spleen. Wolrd J Surg. 1985;9:468-76.
8. Morgenstern L, Mc-cafferty L, Rosenburg J, Michel SL. Hamartomas of the spleen. Arch Surg. 1984;119(11):1291-3.
9. Feigenburg Z, Wysenbeek A, Avidor E, Dintsman M. Malignant lymphagiomas of spleen. Isr J Med Sci. 1983;19:202-4.
10. Schneider G, Uder M, Altmeyer K, Bonkhoff H, Gruber M, Kramann B. Littoral cell angioma of the spleen: CT and MR imaging apperarnce. Eur Radiol. 2000;10:1395-400.
11. Aranha GV, Gold J, Grace TB. Hemangiosarcoma of the spleen: report of a case and review of previously reports cases. J Surg Oncol. 1976;8:481-7.
12. Autry JR, Weitzner S. Hemagiosarcoma of the spleen with splontaneous rupture. Cancer. 1975;35:534-9.
13. Lam KY. Metastatic tumors of spleen: a twenty five year clinic pathologic study. Arch Pathol Lab Med. 2000;124:526-30.
14. Phillip GS, Radosevich MD, Lipsett PA. Splenic abscess: another look at an old disease. Arch Surg. 1997;132:1331-5.
15. Farres H, Felsher J, Banbury M, Brody F. Management of splenic abscess in critically ill patients. Surg Laposc Endosc Percutan Tech. 2004;14:49-52.
16. Saadeh AM, Abu-Farsakh NA, Omari HZ. Infective endocarditis and occult splenic abscess caused by Brucella melintesis infection: a case report and review of literature. Acta Cardiol. 1996;51: 279-85.
17. Sarr MG, Zuidema D. Splenic abscess: presentation, diagnosis and treatment. Surgery. 1982;92:480-5.
18. Ng KK, Lee TY, Wan YL, Tan CF, Lui KW, Cheung YC, et al. Splenic abscess: diagnosis and management. Hepatogastroenterology. 2002;49:567-71.
19. Goerg C, Schwerk WB, Georg K. Sonography of focal lesion of the spleen. AJR Am J Roentgenol. 1991;34:661-7.
20. Tikkakoski T, Siniluoto T, Päivänsalo M, Taavitsainen M, Leppänen M, Dean K, et al. Splenic abscess: imaging and intervention. Acta Radiol. 1992;33:561-5.
21. Anuradha S, Singh N, Agarwal S. Splenic abscess: a diversity within. J Indian Acad Clin Med. 2000;1:279-81.
22. Chang KC, Chuah SK, Changchien CS, Tsai TL, Lu SN, Chiu YC, et al. Clinical characteristics and prognostic factors of splenic abscess: a review of 67 cases in a single medical center of Taiwan. World J Gastroenterol. 2006;12(3):460-4.
23. Helton WS, Carrico GJ, Zaveruba PA, Schaller R. Diagnosis and treatment of splenic fungal abscess in the immunocompromised patient. Arch Surg. 1986;121:580-6.
24. Migita M, Kaizu K, Asai M, Yamaguchi K, Ikegami E, Maeda M, et al. Multiple fungal splenic abscesses in a patient with T-acute lymphoblastic leukemia undergoing chemotherapy. Pediatr Int. 2004;46(6):733-5.
25. Jadhav SV, Vyawahare CR, Chaudhari N, Gupta NS, Gandham NR, Misra RN. Primary splenic tubercular abscess in an immunocompromised patient-rapid diagnosis by line probe assay. J Clin Diagn Res. 2013;7(9):1996-8.
26. Rosen M, Brody F, Walsh RM, Tarnoff M, Malm J, Ponsky J. Outcome of laparoscopic splenectomy based on hematologic indication. Surg Endosc. 2002;16:272-9.

CHAPTER 84

Non-Traumatic Splenectomy

Kamal Yadav, Deborshi Sharma

INTRODUCTION

The first recorded splenectomy is credited to Adrian Zacarelli who operated on a 24-year-old Neapolitan woman in 1549. Since then mode and role of splenectomy has changed over the years with many non-traumatic indications being included in the list. In recent years splenectomy has moved toward minimal invasive techniques and splenic preservation.

In 1910, Sutherland and Burghad performed the first splenectomy for treating hereditary spherocytosis.[1] Subsequently, 6 years later Kaznelson advocated splenectomy as treatment for idiopathic thrombocytopenic purpura (ITP).[2] Till Harrinton and his associates[3] opened the door for medical treatment by showing the role of plasma immunoglobulin induced thrombocytopenia in ITP, surgery was regarded as the treatment of choice. Role of steroids and medical management were highlighted by Dameshek and colleagues,[4] in treating hypersplenism with ITP in 1958. Surgical treatment can have remission rates in two-thirds cases while medical treatment with glucocorticoids is effective only in 25% of chronic ITP patients.[5] Surgery is regarded today as a superior form of treatment as it removes both the antiplatelet antibody synthesis and along with the main place of antibody-sensitized platelet destruction.

The first successful laparoscopic splenectomy was reported by Delaitrein 1991.[6,7]

COMMON INDICATIONS

Elective splenectomy is most commonly performed for ITP.[8-10] Pediatric ITP is generally of acute onset and remits spontaneously in about 80% patients within 6 months. In adults ITP is insidious in onset and chronic. Spontaneous remissions in adults are rare. Clinical manifestations of ITP can have a varied range from being symptomless to cutaneous ecchymoses or severe forms of mucosal bleeding or can even present with intracranial bleeding. Thrombocytopenia severity is directly proportional to the severity at the time of presentation with counts of more than 50,000/µl rarely leading to any significant symptoms. Platelet counts below 30,000/µl, any evidence of substantial mucus membrane bleeding, active peptic ulcer and patients with potential for trauma warrants active treatment.[5] Observation without active therapy can be continued in asymptomatic patients with platelet counts above 30,000/µl.

In all cases requiring treatment medical management is always the first approach; Indications of surgery in general are severe thrombocytopenia which is not responding to medical management for 4–6 weeks and patients requiring very high doses of steroids to achieve remission or patients who relapse in spite of high doses and an initial response to steroid therapy.[7] Other types of thrombotic or HIV related purpura may also be treated with splenectomy. It is also indicated for other forms of hemolytic diseases like hereditary spherocytosis, major and intermediate thalassemia with hyperslenism or refractory autoimmune hemolytic anemia.

Selection of surgical candidates and the response rates of treatment along with prognostic factors for success after splenectomy depend on age,[11-13] prior steroid or immunoglobulin therapy and their response,[12,14,15] sequestration of platelets in spleen,[16] and hemorrhagic tendency if any with its severity.[7,13]

Myeloprolifrative disorders may also require a surgical approach. Although pathological staging splenectomy is no longer indicated, splenectomy has shown 75% improvement in the blood parameters in Hodgkin and non-Hodgkin lymphoma or chronic lymphocytic leukemia (Table 1).[17]

Table 1: Common indications of non-traumatic splenectomy

- Primary splenic tumor
- Hereditary spherocytosis
- Primary hypersplenism
- Idiopathic thrombocytopenic purpura
- Splenic vein thrombosis with secondary gastric varices
- Splenic abscess
- Cystic diseases of spleen (Hydatid diseases, etc.) (Figs. 1 and 2)
- Autoimmune hemolytic disease
- Elliptocytosis with hemolysis
- Nonspherocytic congenital hemolytic anemia
- Hodgkin's disease (for staging) and splenic lymphoma
- Thrombotic thrombocytopenic purpura
- Idiopathic myelofibrosis
- Splenic artery aneurysm
- Wiscott-Aldrich syndrome
- Gaucher's disease (Fig. 3)
- Mastocytosis-aggressive disease
- Chronic leukemia
- Macroglobulinemia
- Thalassemia major
- Sickle cell anemia
- Portal hypertension with congestive splenomegaly and hypersplenism
- Felty's syndrome
- Hairy cell leukemia
- Chediak-Higashi syndrome
- Sarcoidosis

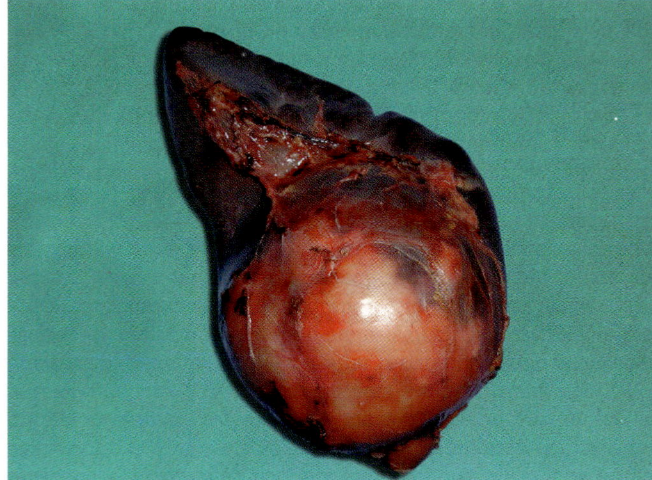

Figure 1 Hydatid spleen at its lower pole

ANATOMY AND PHYSIOLOGY OF SPLEEN

The spleen is an organ shaped like a shoe that lies in the long axis of the tenth rib, extending from the 9th and 11th ribs and is located in the left hypochondrium between the fundus of the stomach and the diaphragm (Fig. 4). It is a highly vascular organ, reddish purple in color with variable size and weight. A healthy spleen is not palpable. During the sixth week of intrauterine life the spleen develops from the cephalic part of dorsal mesogastrium into a number of nodules which later fuse and form the lobulated spleen. Multiple origin is evident by the notch on its superior border.

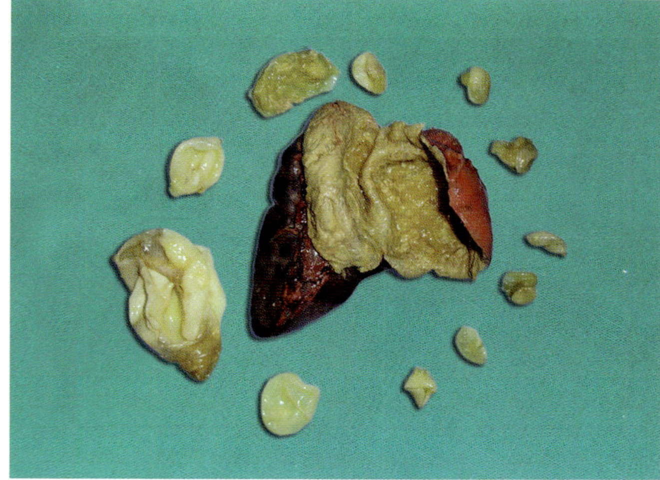

Figure 2 Opened up hydatid cyst with the daughter cysts

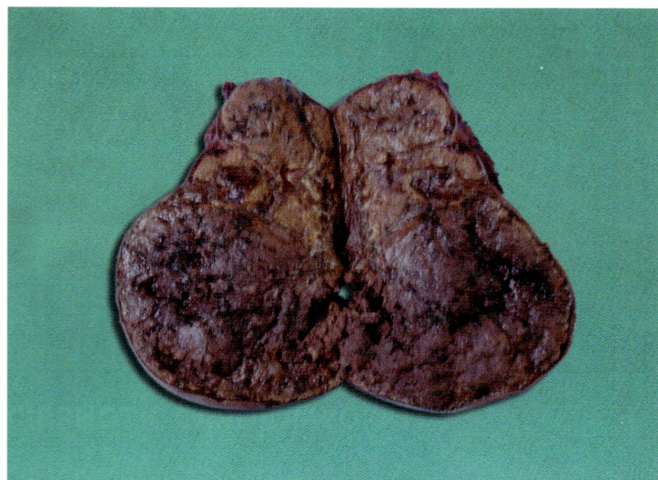

Figure 3 Cut open specimen of Gaucher's disease of spleen

The spleen is anatomically described to have two ends (anterior expanded and posterior rounded), three borders (superior, inferior and intermediate) and two surfaces (diaphragmatic and visceral). The anterior end notches the superior border while the inferior border is a rounded one. The intermediate border points toward the right.

The healthy spleen measures 11 × 7 × 4 cm and weighs 100–250 g.[18] Many differ in the criteria to name "splenomegaly" or "massive splenomegaly" in literature. Mostly accepted splenomegaly is with a splenic length in long axis of more than 15 cm and massive splenomegaly when the long axis exceeds 20 cm on preoperative imaging. Preoperative splenic weight though mentioned as exceeding 500 g to be labeled as splenomegaly can actually only be measured postoperatively hence the criteria of splenic weight has no preoperative role in the choice of surgical procedure.

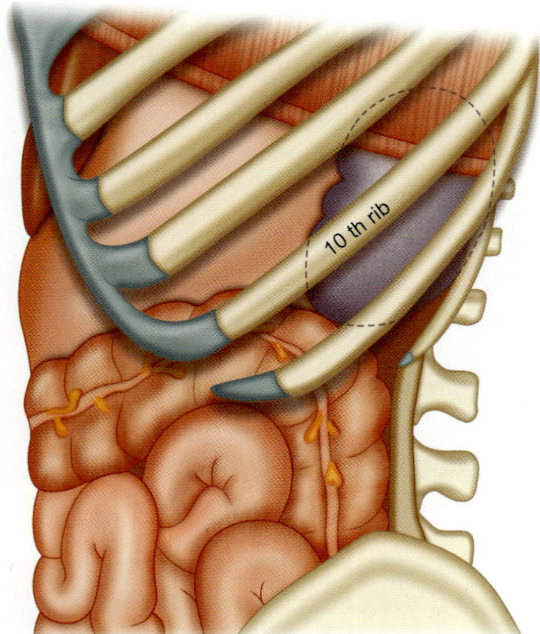

Figure 4 Anatomic position and relations of spleen

ACCESORY SPLEEN

Accessory spleens are made of blood, sinuses and malpighian bodies. It has been classified into two types: (1) a constricted part of the main organ to which it is bound by fibrous tissue is uncommon, and (2) the more common is a distinct, separate mass in 14–30%. The latter is more commonly seen in patients with hematologic disorders. Splenic artery is the main source of blood supply to accessory spleens. They are found in descending order from the hilum of the spleen, gastrosplenic ligament, splenorenal ligament, to the great omentum.[19]

During elective splenectomy hematological diseases, a search for accessory spleens should be conducted every time. They are present in approximately one-third of patients and it might be the source for inadequate response to splenectomy in the treatment of hematologic disease, such as ITP.[19]

PREOPERATIVE EVALUATION

Imaging

The main purpose of any preoperative abdominal imaging is to assess the splenic size, detect accessory spleens if any, and also find concomitant gallstone disease particularly in patients with chronic hemolytic disorders. Ultrasound is useful in assessing the size of the spleen but is regarded as a poor modality for preoperative detection of accessory spleens.[20] Advanced CT machines doing multidetector spiral CT can detect accessory spleens irrespective of their sizes to the tune of 43–100%.[20,21] CT scan can further detect lymph nodes at hilum with surrounding inflammation if any or infarction within the spleen which if present may lead to intraoperative problems.[22]

Preoperative and postoperative splenic scintigraphy can be helpful in some cases however their exact role is not yet clearly defined. Hand held gamma probe should only be used as an adjunct tool for detection of accessory spleens.[18]

Splenic Artery Embolization

Splenic artery can be embolized preoperatively particularly in massive splenomegaly to reduce intraoperative blood loss as well as decrease substantial intraoperative time.[23] However, these procedures come with its own complications like severe pain, shifting or migration of coils to the systemic circulation, ischemic complications and may present with an abscess.[7,23]

PREOPERATIVE PREPARATION

Autoimmune thrombocytopenia with platelet count less than 20,000/µl needs treatment by preoperative steroids or immunoglobulins along with intraoperative platelet infusions after ligation of the splenic pedicle. Platelet count less than 20,000/µl does not preclude laparoscopic splenectomy; however, the complication rates are high. Many surgeons reserve platelet transfusion for counts less than 10,000/µl though a few patients with hereditary spherocytosis and hemolytic anemia might present with hemolytic crisis and which may need transfusions. Immunoglobulins might be an effective but costly affair. Immunoglobulin G (400 mg/kg/day) is administered for 3–5 days, 1 week before surgery.[18]

Overwhelming post-splenectomy infection from encapsulated organisms is a well-established life threatening complication for splenectomised patients. The risk is highest within 2 years; however, one-third of all infection occurs after 5 years of surgery with lifelong risk factor.[18] Mortality rates of such infection are very high. Risk is very high for patients with thalassemia major or sickle cell anemia.[24]

Vaccine for pneumococcus, hemophilus influenza (Type B) and neisseria meningitidis must be administered to all ideally; 15 days prior to elective surgery or immediately after any emergency surgery.[7] Patients with myeloproliferative disorders who have a tendency to develop thrombosis, it is advisable to medicate the patient with low-dose heparin, 5,000 units twice daily, and aspirin on the day before surgery and to continue this regimen for 5 days postoperatively.[19]

TECHNIQUE

Patient Preparation

Nasogastric tube, Foley's catheter and pneumatic compression stockings application are routinely done.

Open Splenectomy

Open splenectomy is the long stay of treatment for many hematological disorders. Spleen is approached by variety of incisions which includes midline approach, subcostal approach and thoracoabdominal approach. Patient is generally in supine position with a small bean bag behind the left lower costal margin. Many prefer a slight lateral position (10°-15°) with table bridge at the level of the subcostal margin. The bridge is further bent down at that level to increase the space between the subcostal margin and umbilicus. This maneuver is helpful in moderately obese individuals when the subcostal approach is taken.

The spleen is attached by avascular ligaments laterally to the diaphragm, kidney and colon which are divided with electrocautery or scissors to deliver the spleen to the middle of the incision. Today most surgeons prefer to use the ultrasonic dissector for such dissections also. One has to be more careful with the gastrosplenic ligaments particularly the superior part, which is divided between ligatures or clips taking proper care of the stomach wall. Splenic vessels at the hilum should be dissected and ligated taking care not injuring the pancreatic tail which tends to fall back once the overlying peritoneal fold is separated. Numerous techniques are described for ligation of the splenic vessels which include two proximal and one distal clamp technique of Federoff, mass double ligature of vessels and using vascular linear stapler which is nowadays in vogue. Author prefers to ligate the splenic artery approaching it through the gastrocolic omentum at the superior border of pancreas, before starting the splenic dissection. This is followed by meticulous dissection at the splenic hilum of the artery and vein which is doubly ligated with silk sutures or clipped with hemoclip and cut separately.

Laparoscopic Splenectomy

Multiport Laparoscopic Splenectomy

Position: Laparoscopic splenectomy is done with the patient in a lateral, hemilateral or supine position which depends on many factors like splenic size, patient body contour, surgical expertise and need of any associated procedures. Initial reports of laparoscopic splenectomy were of "supine" position. It allowed good access to the splenic vessels with superb visualization of the hilar structures. Difficulty arose in dissecting the dorsal structures and the hilar tissue when the pancreatic tail remains close. Any concurrent procedure like cholecystectomy, lymph node biopsy, etc. could be done with ease in this position.[25]

In hemilateral (or semilateral) "hanging or leaning spleen" technique[26] patient is positioned supine with elevated left side by use of bean bags or foam wedges up to a 40°-45° angle from the table surface (Fig. 5). The patient's position is further adjusted according to requirements by maneuvering the table to hemilateral or lateral position. Hemilateral position is preferred for an initial entry to lesser sac and subsequent division of short gastric vessels only to move toward a full lateral position later so that stomach, pancreas and other organs fall medially creating space between the hilum and these organs.[27] Complete lateral approach, (90° left lateral) is considered ideal for allowing safe vascular control,[28] as in this position the spleen remains in its original position due to its diaphragmatic attachments while with the help of gravity stomach, transverse colon, greater omentum and most importantly the pancreatic tail falls down to keep it at a safe distance[29] giving good exposure of the hilar structures.

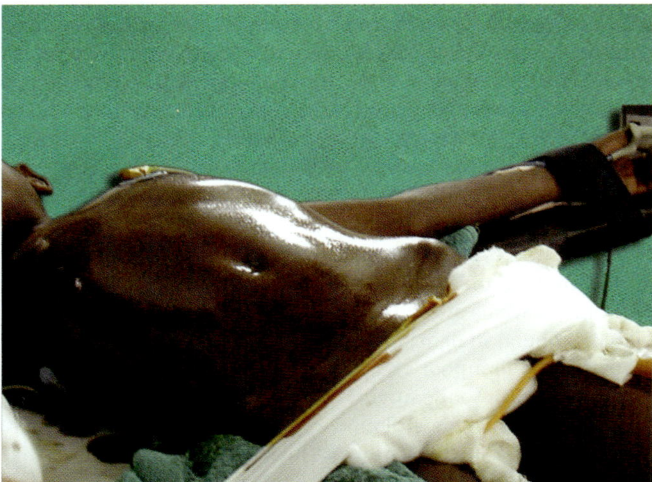

Figure 5 Hanging spleen position during laparoscopic splenectomy

Author prefers the hanging spleen position which is done either by tilting the operation table to the specific site or by using a bean bag. Monitor is placed above the left shoulder facing the surgeon who is standing to the right of the patient.

Port insertion: In the multiport technique initial port is near the umbilicus preferably supraumbilical. However, it depends upon the size of the spleen which is known to grow toward the right lower abdomen. Smaller the spleen, the ports should go toward the subcostal margin while in large spleen it tends to move away. After initial entry, diagnostic laparoscopy is done followed by insertion of other working ports. Working ports should be maintaining triangulation with the camera port which is at the periumbilical area. Hence in a simplified way is to draw an imaginary line from the xiphisternum to umbilicus and laterally extending that line perpendicularly at the umbilicus to the left lumbar region. After the initial periumbilical port, two more 10–12 mm working ports are put about 7–8 cm away from the first port, one on each limbs of the imaginary line. The port on the horizontal imaginary line from the umbilicus to the lumbar region should be preferably 12 mm, which will be able to accommodate the vascular endostapler to be applied later at the splenic hilum. The fourth and fifth ports (5 mm) are inserted further beyond in those two imaginary lines in the epigastrium and lumbar area (left anterior axillary line) to retract a prominent left lobe of liver and hold the greater curve of stomach respectively.

Author prefers to insert the first port at a supine position of the patient which makes it comparatively safe procedure. Tilting the patient is done to the specific position as required by the surgeon and dictated by the size of the spleen, followed by insertion of the other working ports as described above under direct vision. In case the lateral position is made initially, i.e. before first port insertion, large spleen might to fall toward the umbilicus along with the small intestines predisposing them to injury during initial blind entry at the level of umbilicus.

Search for accessory spleen with careful abdominal exploration is done before initiation of any dissection. The stomach has to be retracted toward the right, so that the gastrosplenic, phrenosplenic and the splenocolic ligaments are visible. The greater omentum, and rest of the abdomen are also inspected. The splenic pedicle behind the pancreatic tail is inspected after opening the gastrosplenic ligament. The splenic notch correlates with distribution of the hilar vasculature which can give a fair idea of the level of dissection difficulty and the type of instruments needed to be used later for hilar vasculature.[23]

Literature describes two basic approaches: Anterolateral or hanging spleen technique (introduced by Delaitre and Maignien[6]) and the posterolateral detached spleen technique (described by Gagner et al.[30]).

Dissection proceeds generally in five commonly advocated stages: Careful division of the short gastric vessels, separating the spleen from the colon by dividing the splenocolic ligament, splenic inferior polar vessels ligation followed by vascular control of the hilum and lastly separation of the dorsal (phrenic) attachments of the spleen. The splenocolic ligament should be divided with some amount of connective tissue left on the spleen, so that it can be grasped by surgical assistant, thereby avoiding direct holding of the spleen and preventing any capsular tear.

Splenic hilar vasculature may show many variations; in 1942, Michel's described the following two common variations:[31]

- *Distributed pattern:* The main splenic artery trunk branches into multiple branches about 2–3 cm proximal to the hilum and each of these branches need to be divided or ligated separately. Multiple accessory spleens are commonly found in this distributed type of splenic hilum and is likely to be related to the embryology of accessory spleens (Fig. 6).
- *Magistral pattern:* The splenic artery and veins pedicle enter the hilum as a single structure and can be transacted together using a single application of a 45 mm vascular laparoscopic stapler (Fig. 7).

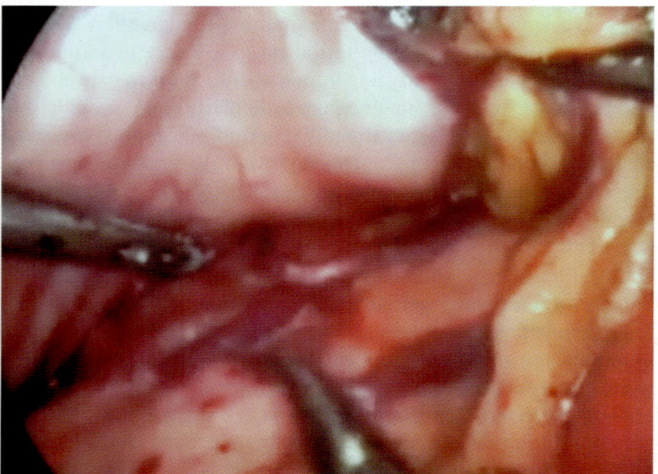

Figure 6 Distributed pattern of blood supply after entering the lesser sac

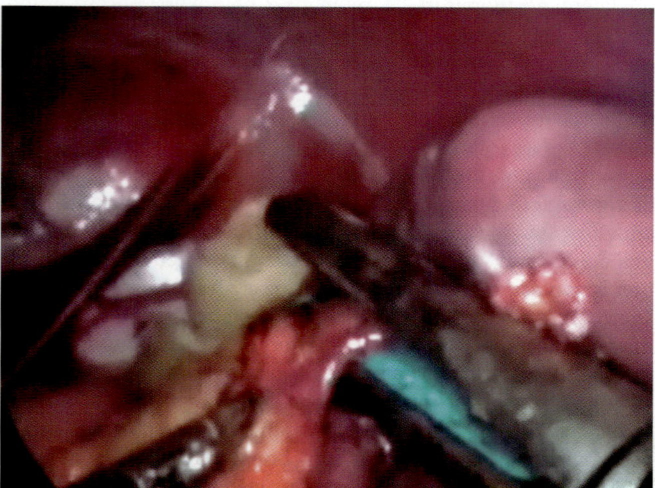

Figure 7 Terminal hilar branches being taken care of by endostapler during laparoscopic splenectomy

After taking control over splenic hilum, the remaining vessels toward the splenic superior pole are divided using ultrasonic shears. After full mobilization of the spleen from diaphragm, it is placed in an endobag by grasping the spleen by its surrounding connective tissue. The spleen is broken into small pieces using either the ovum forceps or sponge holding forceps inside the bag and fragments removed. Outmost care should be taken during this maneuver to avoid spillage of splenic fragments from the sac to prevent splenosis.[7]

Author prefers to make a Pfannensteil incision to take out the spleen in total after inserting it in an endobag. However, in very large spleens this may not be possible and may merit some extent of morcellation.

Risk of hemorrhage in patients with compromised cardiopulmonary function and severe portal hypertension are absolute contraindication for the laparoscopic approach. Other contraindications which can be relative in most cases are a previous history of major abdominal surgery. Morbid obesity is not considered to be a contraindication to laparoscopic splenectomy however it might be difficult as an initial case. On the other hand postsurgical complications like pulmonary embolism, atelectasis or wound infection is less with minimal access surgery.[7] Overall complication rates for laparoscopic splenectomy have been fairly limited at less than 20%.[32-36]

Hand-assisted Laparoscopic Splenectomy

Hand-assisted laparoscopic splenectomy (HALS) is a slight variant of laparoscopic splenectomy where a hand port is used and is preferably done in semi lateral or 45° right lateral decubitus position. HALS has benefits of both minimally access surgery (early recovery, less postoperative pain) and open surgery (tactile feedback, finger dissection, finger retraction, ease of placement of a large spleen into the endobag). Further some difficult situations such as hemorrhage or severe adhesions can be managed promptly using a hand port.

The incision for the hand-assisted procedures is about 7.0–8.0 cm placed in the midline between the xiphisternum and the umbilicus. In case of larger spleens this can cross the mid-line to the right, at Mcburney point or Pfannenstiel site. Pneumoperitoneum is maintained while the non-dominant hand of the operating surgeon is inserted. This hand as expected will take some space inside the abdomen and can also lead to fatigue.

Hand-assisted laparoscopic splenectomy is reported to shorten the operating time, conversion rates are lower with decreased perioperative complications than with pure laparoscopic approach in cases of splenomegaly.[37,38] As a technique it is recommended only for spleens with longitudinal diameter of more than 22 cm, but not for normal sized spleen.[38,39]

Robotic Technology

Massive use of laparoscopic surgery in 1990s stimulated tremendous development in the field of surgery. Laparoscopic surgery also has its problems which are still to be overcome like an unstable camera, inability to bend straight laparoscopic instruments, and 2D imaging, all these lead to a poor ergonomic situation.[40,41] To overcome all these problems, robotic surgery is thought to be capable in bridging the gap.[42] Advantages of Robotic technology are a stable camera platform, depth analysis with 3D imaging, 360° movements like a surgeon's wrist. Robotic surgery can overcome the immobility of using straight laparoscopic instruments, and the surgeon is ergonomically more comfortable operating.[40,43]

Robotic splenectomy and conventional laparoscopic splenectomy nowadays do not have much significant difference in terms of routine intraoperative and postoperative parameters.[44,45] However, duration and cost of surgery were significantly different with more time and cost spent with robotic technology.

Single Port Access Splenectomy

An incision is made at the level of the umbilicus on the left mid-clavicular line. One option is to use multiple trocars, while the other option is to introduce a multiport device after achieving pneumoperitoneum.[46] The principles of the technique are very similar to conventional multiport laparoscopic splenectomy.

It is a greater challenge to work with single access port. Difficulty in maintaining triangulation, Chop-Sticks effect of instruments and lack of space for surgeons and assistants to stand are all reported. Order of the day is to standardize the technique of single port splenectomy as well as to better define the criteria for patient selection is necessary.[47]

Limitation of Laparoscopic Splenectomy

Portal hypertension and liver cirrhosis are always considered to be a contraindication to laparoscopic splenectomy.[48] Portal hypertension along with gastric varices increases the chance of hemorrhage in a patient who is already thrombocytopenic. Morbid obesity and advanced age are no longer regarded as a contraindication for laparoscopic splenectomy.[18] Obesity can have intraoperative difficulties due to less space and bad visualization. However, these patients benefit the most from a minimal access procedure due to lower incidence of wound infection.

Postsplenectomy

The blood smear after splenectomy is characterized by the presence of circulating erythrocytes with Howell-Jolly and Pappenheimer bodies (siderotic granules). Asplenic or hyposplenic patients are particularly susceptible to encapsulated bacteria, such as pneumococcus and malaria. The liver may try to compensate for the loss of the immunologic function of the spleen but it requires an intact complement system and higher antibody production.[19] Preservation of at least 25% of splenic tissue maintains its reticuloendothelial function.[49-51]

Partial Splenectomy

Partial splenectomy for splenic cysts though feasible is not routinely performed due to presumed lack of vascular control of resected splenic tissue. In similar reason trucut biopsy of spleen is also not advocated to assist the diagnosis of malignancy. Radiofrequency generated heat energy can be used to coagulate the resected splenic tissue and biopsy tract, making it technically feasible to do a partial splenectomy and biopsy.[51]

COMPLICATIONS

- Early postoperative bleeding—most common site of bleeding is a short gastric vessel.
- Pneumonia and atelectasis.
- Injury to pancreatic tail while dissecting the hilar vasculature is a potential risk of splenectomy, occurring in 15% or less.[52]
- Overwhelming post-splenectomy sepsis (OPSS). It is less common among adult patients after splenectomy for trauma and non-hematologic disease.
- In unusual cases, the platelet count may rise to very high levels, at times greater than 2 million/mm^3. It requires no specific therapy other than hydration. If medical therapy is thought to be appropriate, a drug that inhibits platelet aggregation, such as acetylsalicylic acid can be used.
- Splenic vein thrombosis, with extension into the portal vein and superior mesenteric vein, is a rare complication, occurring mostly in patients with myeloproliferative disorders or in those with sepsis as a consequence of intra-abdominal abscess.
- One complication that may occur during laparoscopic splenectomy that is rarely seen with open splenectomy is diaphragmatic perforation, which is related to thermal injury during mobilization of the superior pole.[19]

Pancreatic leaks are known to cause hyperamylasemia which can indirectly point toward a pancreatic injury which is one of the commoner complications of splenectomy. Lateral positioning greatly improves visualization and allows atraumatic splenic retraction, but this position can occasionally create an unusual orientation to both the enlarged spleen and to its relation, the pancreatic tail. Using a 45 mm vascular stapler in laparoscopic splenectomy at the hilum may not need dissection of the hilar vasculature thereby reducing chances of vascular injury. However, this may predispose injury to pancreatic tail resulting in its transection. Other pancreatic complications include peripancreatic fluid collection, a pancreatic abscess, or drain fluid rich in amylase, or atypical postoperative pain extending the length of hospitalization.[52]

REFERENCES

1. Sutherland GA, Burghard FF. Treatment of splenic anaemia by splenectomy. Lancet. 1910;2:1819.
2. Kaznelson P. Verschwinden der hamorrhagischendiathesebeieinem-falle von essentiellerthrombopenic (frank) nachMilzexstirpation: Splenogenethrombolytischepupura. WeinKlinWochenschr. 1916; 29;1451.
3. Harrington WJ, Minnich V, Hollingsworth JW, Moore CV. Demonstration of a thrombocytopenic factor in the blood of patients with thrombocytopenic purpura. J Lab Clin Med. 1951;38:1-10.
4. Dameshek W, Rubio F, Mahoney JP, Reeves WH, Burgin LA. Treatment of idiopathic thrombocytopenic purpura (ITP) with prednisolone. JAMA. 1958;166:1805-15.
5. George JN, Woolf SH, Raskob GE, Wasser JS, Aledort LM, Ballem PJ, et al. Idiopathic thromcytopenicpurpura: a practice guideline developed by explicit methods for the American Society of Hematologyu. Blood. 1996;88:3-40.
6. Delaitre B, Maignein B. Splenectomie par voiecoelioscopique 1: Observation. Presse Med. 1991;20:2263.
7. Katkhouda N, Manhas S, Umbach TW, Kaiser AM. Laparoscopic splenectomy. J Laparoendosc Adv Surg Tech A. 2001;11(6):383-90.
8. Brodsky JA, Brody FJ, Walsh RM, Malm JA, Ponsky JL. Laparoscopic splenectomy. Surg Endosc. 2002;16(5):851-4.
9. Heniford BT, Park A, Walsh RM, Kercher KW, Matthews BD, Frenette G, et al. Laparoscopic splenectomy in patients with normal-sized spleens versus splenomegaly: does size matter? Am Surg. 2001;67(9):854-7; discussion 857-8.
10. Targarona EM, Espert JJ, Balagué C, Piulachs J, Artigas V, Trias M. Splenomegaly should not be considered a contraindication for laparoscopic splenectomy. Ann Surg. 1998;228(1):35-9.

11. Akwari OE, Itani KM, Coleman RE, Rosse WF. Splenectomy for primary and recurrent immune thrombocytopenic purpura (ITP). Current criteria for patient selection and results. Ann Surg. 1987;206(4):529-41.
12. DiFino SM, Lachant NA, Kirshner JJ, Gottlieb AJ. Adult idiopathic thrombocytopenic purpura. Clinical findings and response to therapy. Am J Med. 1980;69(3):430-42.
13. Juliá A, Araguás C, Rosselló J, Bueno J, Domenech P, Olona M, et al. Lack of useful clinical predictors of response to splenectomy in patients with chronic idiopathic thrombocytopenic purpura. Br J Haematol. 1990;76(2):250-5.
14. Brennan MF, Rappeport JM, Moloney WC, Wilson RE. Correlation between response to corticosteroids and splenectomy for adult idiopathic thrombocytopenic purpura. Am J Surg. 1975;129(4): 490-2.
15. Law C, Marcaccio M, Tam P, Heddle N, Kelton JG. High-dose intravenous immune globulin and the response to splenectomy in patients with idiopathic thrombocytopenic purpura. N Engl J Med. 1997;336(21):1494-8.
16. Fabris F, Zanatta N, Casonata A, Randy ML, Luzzato G, Girolami A. Response to splenectomy in idiopathic thrombocytopenic purpura: prognostic value of the clinical and laboratory evaluation. Acta Haematol. 1989;81(1):28-33.
17. Cogliandolo A, Berland-Dai B, Pidoto RR, Marc OS. Results of laparoscopic and open splenectomy for nontraumatic diseases. Surg Laparosc Endosc Percutan Tech. 2001;11(4):256-61.
18. Habermalz B, Sauerland S, Decker G, Delaitre B, Gigot JF, Leandros E, et al. Laparoscopic splenectomy: the clinical practice guidelines of the European Association for Endoscopic Surgery (EAES). Surg Endosc. 2008;22(4):821-48.
19. Adrales G, Gadacz TR. The spleen. Maingot's Abdominal Operations, 11th edition. McGraw Hill; 2007. pp. 1075-98.
20. Stanek A, Stefaniak T, Makarewicz W, Kaska L, Podgórczyk H, Hellman A, et al. Accessory spleens: preoperative diagnostics limitations and operational strategy in laparoscopic approach to splenectomy in idiopathic thrombocytopenic purpurapatients. Langenbecks Arch Surg. 2005;390(1):47-51.
21. Napoli A, Catalano C, Silecchia G, Fabiano P, Fraioli F, Pediconi F, et al. Laparoscopic splenectomy: multi-detector row CT for preoperative evaluation Radiology. 2004;232(2):361-7.
22. Heniford BT, Matthews BD, Answini GA, Walsh RM. Laparoscopic splenectomy for malignant diseases. Semin Laparosc Surg. 2000;7(2):93-100.
23. Poulin EC, Thibault C, Mamazza J. Laparoscopic splenectomy. Surg Endosc. 1995;9(2):172-6.
24. Bisharat N, Omari H, Lavi I, Raz R. Risk of infection and death among post splenectomy patients. J Infect. 2001;43(3):182-6.
25. Casaccia M, Torelli P, Squarcia S, Sormani MP, Savelli A, Troilo B, et al. Laparoscopic splenectomy for hematologic diseases: a preliminary analysis performed on the Italian Registry of Laparoscopic Surgery of the Spleen (IRLSS). Surg Endosc. 2006;20(8):1214-20.
26. Delaitre B, Bonnichon P, Barthes T, Dousset B. Laparoscopic splenectomy. The "hanging spleen technique" in a series of nineteen cases. Ann Chir. 1995;49(6):471-6.
27. Dexter SP, Martin IG, Alao D, Norfolk DR, McMahon MJ. Laparoscopic splenectomy. The suspended pedicle technique. Surg Endosc. 1996;10(4):393-6.
28. Park A, Gagner M, Pomp A. The lateral approach to laparoscopic splenectomy. Am J Surg. 1997;173(2):126-30.
29. Nägeli J, Lange J. Indications, technique and outcome of laparoscopic splenectomy. Ther Umsch. 1997;54(9):510-4.
30. Gagner M, Lacroix A, Prinz RA, Bolté E, Albala D, Potvin C, et al. Early experience with laparoscopic approach for adrenalectomy. Surgery. 1993;114(6):1120-4.
31. Michels NA. Variations in the blood-supply of the liver, gallbladder, stomach, duodenum, pancreas and spleen; 200 dissections. Am J Med Sci. 1948;216(1):115.
32. Targarona EM, Espert JJ, Bombuy E, Vidal O, Cerdán G, Artigas V, et al. Complications of laparoscopic splenectomy. Arch Surg. 2000;135(10):1137-40.
33. Park AE, Birgisson G, Mastrangelo MJ, Marcaccio MJ, Witzke DB. Laparoscopic splenectomy: outcomes and lessons learned from over 200 cases. Surgery. 2000;128(4):660-7.
34. Knauer EM, Ailawadi G, Yahanda A, Obermeyer RJ, Millie MP, Ojeda H, et al. 101 laparoscopic splenectomies for the treatment of benign and malignant hematologic disorders. Am J Surg. 2003;186(5):500-4.
35. Cogliandolo A, Berland-Dai B, Pidoto RR, Marc OS. Results of laparoscopic and open splenectomy for nontraumatic diseases. Surg Laparosc Endosc Percutan Tech. 2001;11(4):256-61.
36. Walsh RM, Heniford BT, Brody F, Ponsky J. The ascendance of laparoscopic splenectomy. Am Surg. 2001;67(1):48-53.
37. Borrazzo EC, Daly JM, Morrisey KP, Fischer E, Belmont M, Hogle NJ, et al. Hand-assisted laparoscopic splenectomy for giant spleens. Surg Endosc. 2003;17(6):918-20.
38. Maartense S, Bemelman WA, Gerritsen van der Hoop A, Meijer DW, Gouma DJ. Hand-assisted laparoscopic surgery (HALS): a report of 150 procedures. Surg Endosc. 2004;18(3):397-401.
39. Kercher KW, Matthews BD, Walsh RM, Sing RF, Backus CL, Heniford BT. Laparoscopic splenectomy for massive splenomegaly. Am J Surg. 2002;183(2):192-6.
40. Ballantyne GH. Robotic surgery, telerobotic surgery, telepresence, and telementoring. Review of early clinical results. Surg Endosc. 2002;16(10):1389-402.
41. Yohannes P, Rotariu P, Pinto P, Smith AD, Lee BR. Comparison of robotic versus laparoscopic skills: is there a difference in the learning curve? Urology. 2002;60(1):39-45.
42. Ballantyne GH, Moll F. The da Vinci telerobotic surgical system: the virtual operative field and telepresencesurgery. Surg Clin North Am. 2003;83(6):1293-304.
43. Stylopoulos N, Rattner D. Robotics and ergonomics. Surg Clin North Am. 2003;83(6):1321-37.
44. Maeso S, Reza M, Mayol JA, Blasco JA, Guerra M, Andradas E, et al. Efficacy of the Da Vinci surgical system in abdominal surgery compared with that of laparoscopy: a systematic review and meta-analysis. Ann Surg. 2010;252(2):254-62.
45. Gelmini R, Franzoni C, Spaziani A, Patriti A, Casciola L, Saviano M Laparoscopic splenectomy: conventional versus robotic approach—a comparative study. J Laparoendosc Adv Surg Tech A. 2011;21(5):393-8.
46. Targarona EM, Lima MB, Balague C, Trias M. Single-port splenectomy: current update and controversies. J Minim Access Surg. 2011;7(1):61-4.
47. Gamme G, Birch DW, Karmali S. Minimally invasive splenectomy: an update and review. Can J Surg. 2013;56(4):280-5.
48. Hellman P, Arvidsson D, Rastad J. HandPort-assisted laparoscopic splenectomy in massive splenomegaly. Surg Endosc. 2000;14:1177-9.
49. Malangoni MA, Dawes LG, Droege EA, Rao SA, Collier BD, Almagro UA. Splenic phagocytic function after partial splenectomy and splenic autotransplantation. Arch Surg. 1985;120(3):275-8.
50. Traub A, Giebink GS, Smith C, Kuni CC, Brekke ML, Edlund D, et al. Splenic reticuloendothelial function after splenectomy, spleen repair, and spleen autotransplantation. N Engl J Med. 1987;317(25):1559-64.
51. Habib NA, Spalding D, Navarra G, Nicholls J. How we do a bloodless partial splenectomy. Am J Surg. 2003;186(2):164-6.
52. Chand B, Walsh RM, Ponsky J, Brody F. Pancreatic complications following laparoscopic splenectomy. Surg Endosc. 2001;15(11): 1273-6.

SECTION 8

Colon, Rectum and Anal Canal

CHAPTER 85

History and Examination in Colorectal Disease

Nikhil Gupta, Shivendra Singh

Gastrointestinal tract is a complex system. Patients with gastrointestinal pathology often have vague symptoms at presentation. They usually presents with a conglomerate of symptoms that characterize a disease process, although a doctor may be able to classify the symptoms according to the site of origin. A thorough history and examination is required to lead to a meaningful diagnosis. Various symptoms with which a patient can present when suffering from colorectal diseases are enumerated below.

BLEEDING PER ANUS

Bleeding per anus is one of the most common symptoms that a colorectal surgeon encounters. Before going into detailed history and characterization, one should ascertain any history of bleeding disorder. History of previous such bleeding, bleeding from other sites and family history should be obtained. Bleeding beyond ligament of Treitz is described as lower gastrointestinal bleed and is covered in detail in the chapter on lower gastrointestinal bleed. Lower gastrointestinal bleed can be divided into minimal amount of bleed or massive bleed. Massive on going bleed mixed with stools may be seen in inflammatory bowel disease. Diverticular disease, vascular malformations and ulcerations may also have severe bleeding. Passage of blood clots indicates colonic origin. Various causes of bleeding per anus are:

- Hemorrhoids—Presents as painless bleeding. Usually occurs as drops of bright red blood after passage of stools. May or may not be associated with some mass coming out which either itself goes back or needs to be reposited back manually. Patient usually gives history of prolonged defecation or constipation. He or she may also be spending significant time defecating.
- Anal fissure—Painful bright red bleeding is characteristic of an anal fissure. Patient usually gives history of bleeding with excruciating pain that lasts for few minutes after the passage of stools. He may also give history of preceding episode of constipation with passage of hard stools. Patients may also complain of perianal itching or irritation.
- Polyps—Polyps are mostly asymptomatic. They may be detected in a patient undergoing colonoscopy for some other cause or symptom. They mostly cause occult bleeding per rectum. Rarely may be cause of minimal bleeding per rectum.
- Proctitis (12%)—It can be inflammatory or associated with inflammatory bowel disease. These patients most commonly present with pain in the lower abdomen which might be colicky or may be associated with other rectal symptoms like tenesmus. Patient may also complain of passage of mucus and few loose stools per day. Inflammatory proctitis may also be associated with fever and pain in abdomen. In a suspected patient of inflammatory bowel disease detailed history needs to be taken. A patient with previous history of irradiation may suffer from radiation proctitis or colitis and may present with bleeding per rectum.
- Rectal ulcer (6%)—Rectal ulcers can present with bleeding, passage of mucus, straining during defecation, and a sense of incomplete evacuation.
- Malignancy (6%)—These patients usually present with alteration of bowel habits. They may also present with bleeding per rectum. It may be mixed with stools or streaked along the walls of stools.
- Diverticular disease—Painless severe bleeding with clots may suggest bleeding from diverticular disease.
- Ischemic colitis (12%)—Painful hematochezia with mild abdominal discomfort.
- Anorectal varices—May be indistinguishable from hemorrhoids. Signs of portal hypertension or liver disease may hold the key.

Once a patient comes with such complaints following history needs to be elucidated:

- Is it fresh (bright red—hematochezia) or contains altered blood (melena)?
  - Bright red bleeding is usually of rectal or anal in origin. Most common cause is hemorrhoids. Only rarely a patient with massive upper gastrointestinal bleed may present with bright red bleeding per anum such a patient is usually hemodynamically unstable.
  - Melena usually occurs when the source of bleeding is from upper gastrointestinal tract or proximal colon. It occurs when 50–100 mL of blood comes in the gastrointestinal tract.
  - Maroon colored stools usually occur when bleeding occurs from proximal colon.
- Is the bleeding painful?
  - Pain during defecation occurs in the setting of an anal fissure. History of constipation and passing of hard stools should also be elucidated.
- Is there any mass coming out?
  - Hemorrhoids may be associated with a mass coming out. Even a patient with anal cancer may give history of a mass coming out per rectum.
  - Another cause of bleeding with mass coming out may be procidentia. Additional history of constipation, difficult evacuation and pain may point toward this diagnosis.
- Is bleeding associated with loose stools?
  - Patients with dysentery may give history of bleeding mixed with stools. It may be associated with pain abdomen.
- Is there history of mucus discharge?
  - Mucus discharge usually occurs in conditions of inflammatory bowel disease. History of pain abdomen, history of extraintestinal manifestations associated with IBD should be elucidated.
  - Even in low lying malignancy, patient may give history of mucus discharge.
- Is the blood mixed with stools or separate from stools?
  - Blood mixed stools usually occur when source of bleeding is from either proximal colon. Patients with left sided lesions have stools with blood streaking the sides.
- History of medication use? Aspirin or warfarin may be prescribed commonly especially to cardiac patients.
- Fever may be seen in typhoid and tuberculosis. Tubercular and typhoid ulcers may be important cause of bleeding in India.
- Any history of bleeding diathesis? Bleeding from other sides or previous history of delayed stoppage of bleeding? Any history of bleeding in other family members?
- Any history of prior colonoscopy
  - Prior polypectomy may cause bleeding from the polypectomy site.
- Any history of pelvic radiation?
  - Radiation proctitis or colitis can cause bleeding per rectum.
- Prior surgery?
  - History of prior surgery may point toward bleeding from anastomotic site.

Clinical assessment in a patient with bleeding per rectum should be done. The most important component of the physical examination is the vital signs, including blood pressure and pulse rate. This can help with assessment of vascular volume status, the severity of the hemorrhage, and the need for aggressive volume resuscitation. Other aspects of the examination may be helpful for determining the potential cause of the bleeding, such as stigmata of liver disease that may suggest underlying cirrhosis and portal hypertension. Various investigative modalities include anoscopy, flexible sigmoidoscopy, colonoscopy, nuclear scintigraphy, angiography, contrast enhanced CT scan of the abdomen or barium enema discussion of which is out of purview of this chapter. Some of these aspects are covered in the chapter on lower gastrointestinal hemorrhage.

LUMP ABDOMEN

Sometimes the patient may present with lump in the abdomen. In adults it is most commonly seen in cases of carcinoma. This is seen in children more often due to intussusception. In the intussusception lump is usually sausage shaped and paraumbilical. It may appear and disappear. Patient may also point to lump formation due to distended sigmoid loop in volvulous of colon or due to an inflammatory mass due to diverticulitis. Ileocecal Koch's and carcinoma cecum form the differential for the right iliac fossa lump. Similarly, lumps may be noticed in left inguinal area from sigmoid and in epigastrium from transverse colon malignancy. Patients with testicular malignancy may present with lump in epigastrium. thus, for all lumps in epigastric region in males, testicular examination is a must.

PERIANAL PAIN

Anorectal pain that occurs during passage of stools and is sharp and agonizing and lasts for few minutes after passage of stools is usually associated with anal fissure. It can be traced to past history of constipation and passage of hard stools. Even excoriation in that region may cause burning pain. Many times, fissures can occur due to excoriation caused by recurrent diarrhea. Patients undergoing chemotherapy and radiation may have recurrent and chronic fissures.

Hemorrhoidal pain is of sudden onset, usually occurring after an episode of difficult defecation. Acutely thrombosed hemorrhoids can be suspected when there is a history of a reduction in pain accompanied by bleeding that occur independent of bowel motions, usually noticed on the undergarment. It usually occurs with a painful lump. It appears as a small swelling in anal canal with a bluish tinge (visible clot shines through the skin).

Pain due to perianal abscess is described as throbbing in nature. It is constant and gradually worsening pain. Pain which increases with coughing or sneezing may be associated with inter-sphincteric abscess. An abscess is typically visible as a localized swelling in the perianal or ischioanal area. Fluctuation, erythema, tenderness, and sporadic skin discoloration may or may not be present because deeper the sepsis, less obvious are the signs.

Tenesmus, which is a symptom complex of straining and the painful urge to defecate without yield, is frequently associated with inflammatory or neoplastic conditions of the anorectum. It is due to rectal mucosal inflammation.

Pain due to levator ani syndrome is a pressure like pain that worsens on sitting and disappears on standing or lying down.

Pain of large bowel usually is colicky in nature and is due to excessive contraction of the distended bowel proximal to source of obstruction and its relationship can be attributed to meals. Pain originating from contractions of right colon usually presents in right side of abdomen and that originating from left colon presents in left side especially in cases of sigmoid or rectal obstruction. However, acute cecal dilatation due to left sided obstruction can cause severe right sided pain.

CHANGE IN BOWEL HABITS

Two most common symptoms a patient presents with are constipation and diarrhea.

Constipation is caused by myriad of symptoms. Underlying metabolic, pharmacologic, endocrine, psychological, and neurologic causes often contribute to the problem.

It can be either primary or secondary. Rome III criteria are used to define constipation. According to Rome III criteria, definition of constipation must include two or more of the following:

(a) Straining during at least 25% of defecations; (b) Lumpy or hard stools in at least 25% of defecations; (c) Sensation of incomplete evacuation for at least 25% of defecations; (d) Sensation of anorectal obstruction/blockage for at least 25% of defecations; (e) Manual maneuvers to facilitate at least 25% of defecations (e.g. digital evacuation, support of the pelvic floor); (f) Fewer than three defecations per week.

History to be elucidated in a patient with constipation:

- Frequency of stools
- Consistency of stools
- Whether associated with pain or bleeding
- Urge to defecate
- Sense of incomplete evacuation
- Use of digital maneuvers
- Any change in dietary habits
- Associated soiling of clothes (constipation may present as fecal incontinence in elderly)
- Alarming symptoms like weight loss, easy fatigability (suggestive of anemia)
- History of drugs causing constipation.

Examination includes a thorough general physical examination including abdominal examination to look for hard lumps in left lower quadrant. Perianal examination and DRE is essential to confirm the presence of hard stools or any underlying etiology. Resting anal tone (which is 70–80% attributed to internal sphincters) if high may be the cause of evacuation disorder. Perianal fissure may be the result of constipation and should be carefully searched for. Careful examination of perineum is a must to detect pelvic floor dyssynergia. If asked to push and bear down, normally anal sphincter and puborectalis should relax and perineum should descend. But if paradoxically they contract or failure of perineum to descend suggests pelvic floor dyssynergia.

History of weight loss or family history of colonic cancer should be elicited.

DIARRHEA

Usually stool consistency is considered as diarrhea according to the patient. But both frequency and consistency have been used to define diarrhea. Three or more bowel movements per day are abnormal. The duration, amount, character and frequency of the diarrhea should be determined. Usually diarrhea is self-limiting. But if it becomes chronic then it needs evaluation. It may be acute or chronic, large volume versus small volume, osmotic versus secretary diarrhea.

Clear watery diarrhea may be from a large secretory rectal villous adenoma. Bloody mucous diarrhea may indicate inflammatory bowel disease. Bloody diarrhea associated with pain abdomen may suggest colitis.

Another important complaint may be alternating diarrhea with constipation. This is a feature of carcinoma of left sided lesions. Most of the lesions of the left side are obstructing. Thus small amounts of retained stool frequently pass beyond the obstruction after an episode of constipation.

MUCUS DISCHARGE

Mucus is produced by the goblet cells of the epithelial lining of colon and rectum. Various conditions that lead to mucus discharge per rectum are:

- Early sign of villous adenoma
- Early indication of colitis
- Chemical irritation
- Occasionally, it may be seen normally.

If mucus is associated with bleeding per rectum, it can be due to underlying malignancy or inflammatory bowel disease.

Discharge of mucus per rectum in a continent patient is abnormal. Underlying rectal prolapse, incontinence, ectropion due to hemorrhoidectomy should be ruled out or due to overflow from rectal villous adenoma. Thus in a patient complaining with mucus discharge local examination along with proctoscopy should be performed. In case of associated mucus discharge and bleeding, colonoscopy should also be performed.

PROLAPSE

Many patients present with a mass coming out per rectum. Various points in the history need to be elucidated in patients presenting with mass coming out:

- Is it related to stools or spontaneous?
  - Spontaneous prolapse is more suggestive of hypertrophied anal papilla or full thickness rectal procidentia.
- Does it reposit back on its own or requires manual reposition?
  - It points toward the magnitude of the problem.
- Is it associated with pain?
- Does the patient have history of constipation?
- Does he/she strain during defecation?
- Is it associated with bleeding?
  - May be due to underlying malignancy.
  - Due to erosion of mucosa from a chronic prolapse.

Perianal examination should be performed to rule out hemorrhoids. If no mass is visible, patient should be asked to squat and apply pressure to look for prolapse. Full thickness prolapse can be differentiated from partial prolapse. As a dictum any prolapse more than 4 cm is full thickness prolapse.

INCONTINENCE

Incontinence is defined as inability to defer the passage of stool to a socially acceptable time and place. Detailed history is required to know the cause:

- History of trauma
- History of irradiation to anal sphincter
- History of any neurological disease

- History of concomitant chronic bowel disease—irritable bowel disease or inflammatory bowel disease.

Urge incontinence is an inability to control the urge to defecate. It is due to external sphincter dysfunction. But inability to control the stools irrespective of urge is suggestive of internal sphincter dysfunction.

Always look for perianal scarring suggestive of trauma or previous surgery. Sensation of skin and wink reflex of corrugator cutis ani should be checked with a light touch. A per rectal examination is required to know the sphincter strength. Patient is also asked to squeeze the finger to know the function of external sphincter.

ABDOMINAL DISTENSION

It can have numerous causes but five "Fs" can summarize most of the causes—(1) feces, (2) flatus, (3) fluid, (4) fetus and (5) fat. Sometimes enlarged organs like hepatomegaly or massive splenomegaly can present as abdominal distension.

All patients should have detailed family history, any history of medications (chronic laxative abuse, NSAID use), any other associated illnesses which might point to systemic manifestations of IBD or portal hypertension.

EXAMINATION

Examination of a patient with colonic and anorectal disorders is a delicate exercise. Patient should be assured and explained about the procedure to secure his co-operation. Colorectal diseases require careful general, abdominal and local examination. Local examination includes examination of perineum as well as per rectal examination. In females, per vaginal examination should also be done wherever required. In patients of lower rectal tumors and rectovaginal fistula it is necessary for assessment and treatment planning.

Inflammatory bowel disease may give rise to skin changes, uveitis, clubbing and arthritis presence of a supraclavicular lymphnode may alter the management of colorectal malignancy.

Systematic abdominal examination is done from xiphoid to symphysis pubis. All four quadrants should be carefully inspected, palpated, percussed and auscultated. Characteristic lumps are seen in various diseases. Their site, tenderness, temperature, movement with respiration, margins, surface, consistency, mobility, shape and size should always be noted. Specific correlation to their history is also important. Groin and external genitalia examination should not be missed. Inguinal lymphadenopathy should be looked for in patients with carcinoma of the rectum and anal canal.

For patients with anorectal complaints, perineal examination should be done. Digital rectal examination (DRE) should be performed in all the cases. Anoscopy complements a well done DRE.

Perineal examination should be systematic and include both inspection and palpation. Patient is asked to lie down in left lateral position with buttocks projecting on the side of the table and knees flexed up and touching the chest. The cheeks of the buttocks should be spread outward to gain exposure of the perianal area. It should be inspected for external hemorrhoids, fissure and anal papilla. If procidentia is suspected, patient should be asked to squat and perform Valsalva maneuver. If pink mucosa bulges or bowel is seen, diagnosis of procidentia is clinched. However, sometimes perineum itself may bulge suggesting weak perineal muscles. Presence of a dimple with granulation tissue surrounding it might point towards fistula in ano.

Palpation of perineum is performed next. Tenderness and fluctuation should be elicited to rule out abscess. Fistula track can be palpated. Per rectal examination is done using a well lubricated finger. Pad of finger is used to palpate the anal mucosa, dentate line. Patient is asked to tighten the grip around the finger to know the strength of the sphincters. Thumb should be inserted in posterior vaginal fourchette for bidigital examination for anterior sphincter defect. Distal rectum is palpated lastly, palpating prostate or cervix anteriorly, any drop metastasis in pouch of Douglas or for any fullness suggestive of fluid collection. Circumferential examination is done to avoid missing any abnormal finding.

In the end, after taking out the finger, finger should be examined for any blood, mucus, pus or stools on the examining finger.

Anoscopy should be done either in prone jack knife position or left lateral decubitus position (Sim's position). Some prefer prone jack knife position because of the view that this position straightens the rectosigmoid allowing the passage of proctosigmoidoscope higher. Sim's position is better acceptable for patient than prone jack knife. After consent, well lubricated anoscope is inserted after inserting pressure with scope on posterior aspect of external sphincter and gently guiding it. If resistance is encountered, patient should be asked to strain as it would relax the sphincters and would allow the examination. The scope is fully inserted and then circumferential visualization of mucosa is done and gently withdrawn allowing visualization of whole mucosa.

Proctosigmoidoscopy should be performed by the treating surgeon himself as this gives immense information required from surgical perspective. Three sizes of rigid proctosigmoidoscopes are available but the standard one used is 25 cm in length which can help inspect up to 20 cm. Thus whole of the rectum and distal most sigmoid can be inspected by it.

BIBLIOGRAPHY

1. Nivatvongs S. Principals and Practice of Surgery for the Colon, Rectum and Anus, 3rd edition. New York: Informa Healthcare; 2007.
2. Savides TJ, Jensen DM. Sleisenger and Fordtran's Gastrointestinal and Liver Disease. Pathophysiology/Diagnosis/Management, 9th edition. Philadelphia: Elsevier; 2010.
3. Yeo CJ, Mathews JB, McFadden DW, Pemberton JH, Peters JH. Shackelford's Surgery of the Alimentary Tract, 7th edition. Philadelphia: Elseviers; 2013.

CHAPTER 86

Imaging in Colorectal Disease

Poonam Narang

INTRODUCTION

Gastrointestinal radiology today has developed far beyond the conventional barium techniques of visualizing the lumen and mucosal lining of bowel. Cross-sectional imaging techniques like computed tomography (CT) and magnetic resonance imaging (MRI) are able to show the bowel wall and its outer tissues, in addition to its lumen. With potential of post-processing of images to highlight various selected densities, presenting multiplanar projections and three-dimensional (3D) reformatting, the imaging based diagnosis has become more convincing than ever before. Despite these advances, barium studies still hold their place in being the best studies for depiction of bowel diseases, considering the easy availability, convenience and cost, especially for countries like ours.

Imaging in colonic and anorectal diseases has always had complementary role to endoscopy[1,2] for detection and diagnosis of pathology. Wherever access to the region of interest is possible, endoscopy provides better diagnostic yield, owing to its additional capability of providing tissue for histopathology. The surface texture and color of the mucosa are the fine visual parameters that no imaging can show, but is the basis of most endoscopic diagnosis.

The colon is well imaged on plain X-rays, barium studies, ultrasonography (USG), computed tomography as well as on MRI; each modality yielding a particular set of information. With the plethora of imaging modalities available, the surgeon is, at times, spoilt for a choice, when requesting a particular exam for a particular condition. This chapter endeavors to fill this gap of matching capabilities of an examination with the expectations of surgeon, rather than providing an exhaustive detail of imaging features of pathologies affecting colon and ano-rectum.

Plain X-rays at present are reserved for bedside examination, and for initial examination for suspected perforation, obstruction, toxic dilatation, trauma, etc. Findings such as dilated small or large bowel loops, air under diaphragm, or other findings of pneumoperitoneum, pneumoretroperitoneum, gasless abdomen, air in bowel wall, etc. readily help a surgeon in a busy emergency room to reach a probable diagnosis.

Barium studies for colon (Fig. 1), unlike the small bowel studies, are sought for the localization of a lesion, as mobility, and overlap of bowel loops is not a problem in colon. Luminal narrowing is best seen on single-contrast studies which are easier to perform, while mucosal detail is best evaluated on double-contrast studies. For diseases, like malrotation, strictures, large masses, diverticular disease, etc. single-contrast studies usually suffice; while for inflammatory bowel disease (IBD), polyps and small masses, Double contrast Barium Enema (DCBE) is preferred, as fine mucosal details may get masked on Single Contrast Barium Enema (SCBE) studies.

Sometimes, when rectal instillation of contrast is not possible or contraindicated, colon can be opacified after oral contrast. It is common practice to evaluate cecum following barium meal follow through (BMFT) by per rectal air insufflation of colon, once the barium has crossed ileocecal junction (ICJ). Postoperatively, colostomy or anastomoses can be evaluated by contrast instillation while visualizing under fluoroscopy.

Abdominal USG can detect large masses, grossly dilated bowel segments and inter-loop or extramural collections on a routine scan. Special scans after colonic cleaning and fluid instillation can diagnose fine ulcers, nodularity, polyps, masses and inflammatory layering of colonic wall. Vascular changes picked up on ultrasound color Doppler imaging (CDI), have shown sensitivity for IBD (Crohn's disease and ulcerative colitis) affecting colon. Endorectal sonography has special capability of assessing the anal sphincter, anorectal fistulae and masses in this region. Locoregional staging of infiltrating anorectal masses can be confidently done by endorectal ultrasound (ERUS), as all

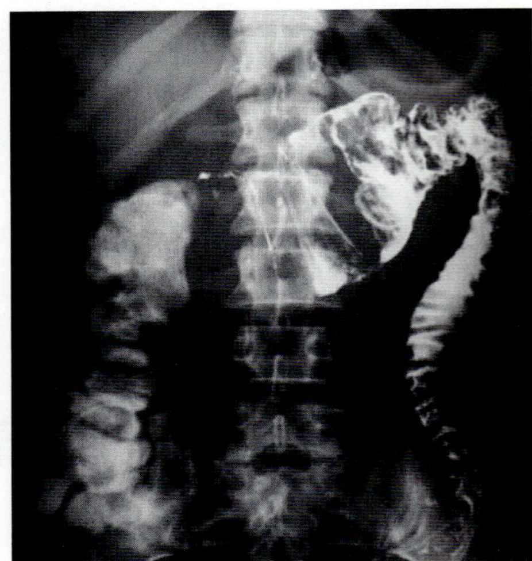

Figure 1 Conventional barium enema showing a nodular stricturing mass involving the splenic flexure

the layers of the rectal walls are clearly visualized as alternating hyperdense and hypodense layers, on high frequency scans performed in such close proximity.

Endorectal ultrasound[3] competes with MRI for local staging of anorectal masses for being the modality of choice for this purpose. Preoperative USG may at times aid the surgeon in completion of clearance of a lesion, especially nodes and liver metastases. However, due to the element of operator dependence and limiting factors like obesity and gas, USG has never been the prime modality of choice, but can be used for answering specific questions within its domain.

Computed tomography becomes the modality of choice wherever information about the extraluminal extent of disease is required for treatment planning (Figs 2 and 3). With advances in computed tomography technology, it is the most sought after study for almost all categories of diseases affecting the large bowl. Obstruction, volvulus, ischemic, inflammatory, neoplastic and post-operative settings, all can justifiably be subjected to computed tomography examination, choosing the correct protocol and preparation.

Low dose plain computed tomography has established its prime place in confirming the diagnosis of appendicitis, diverticulitis, trauma with suspected perforation and even, to some extent in localizing the site of acute lower gastrointestinal bleed. Low dose plain computed tomography is also superior to plain X-rays, in cases of large bowel obstruction due to volvulus, obstructing hernia, strictures or masses. It can better distinguish surgical obstruction from pseudo-obstruction or ileus, information, very important to a busy surgeon in an emergency room.

Colonic computed tomography[2,4] by opacifying the lumen (instilling air, carbon dioxide, positive contrast, methylcellulose) after proper cleansing with purgative, and enema is the best technique for colonic imaging today. Computed tomography colonography or virtual colonoscopy (VC) is the further processing of 3D dataset obtained after computed tomography is performed with the patient in supine and also in prone position. The colonic preparation for virtual colonoscopy has to be meticulous so as to obtain a clean and dry colon. This technique permits an endoluminal 3D viewing of the colonic mucosa akin to an endoscopic visualization (Figs 3 and 4). Screening for polyps, their detection and follow-up can be done by virtual colonoscopy. This technique, has a better patient compliance, as compared to colonoscopy.

Colonic cleansing is of paramount importance for performing a satisfactory computed tomography colonography.[2,5] Colonic preparation can be done with polyetheylene glycol or bisacodyl (wet preparation); or alternatively by sodium phosphate or magnesium citrate (dry preparation). Dry preparation is considered superior for virtual colonoscopy, however care must be taken while using sodium based purgatives in patients with underlying renal or cardiac disease. Air or carbon dioxide at room temperature is used to distend colon. We use dietary fiber restriction and polyethylene glycol enema for cleansing, the night before; and insufflations of room air just prior to imaging for virtual colonoscopy.[6,7] Computed tomography is done in supine

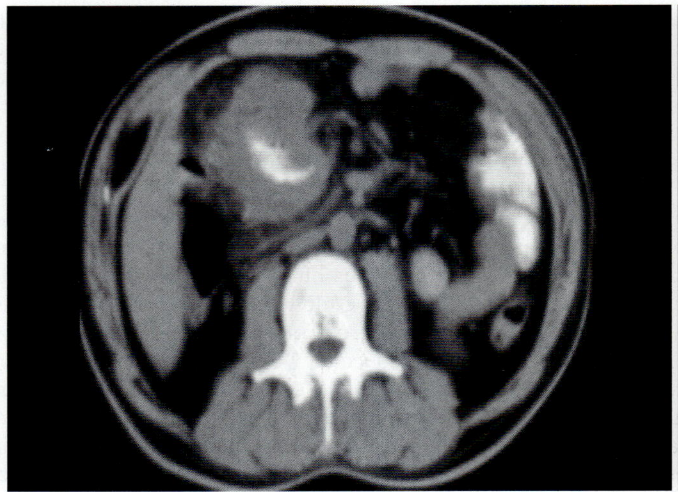

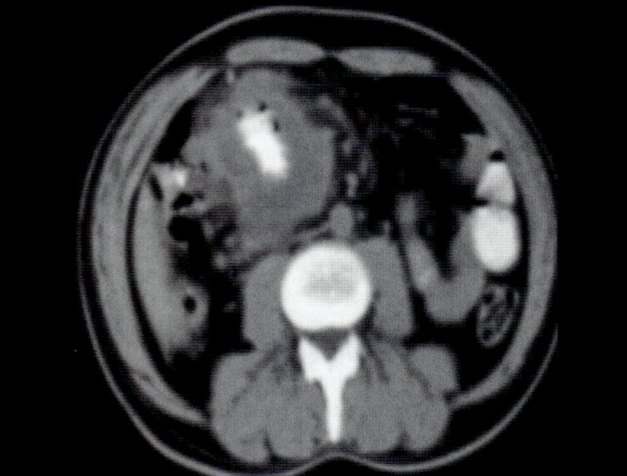

Figure 2 A large mass involving hepatic flexure, with perilesional lymph nodes

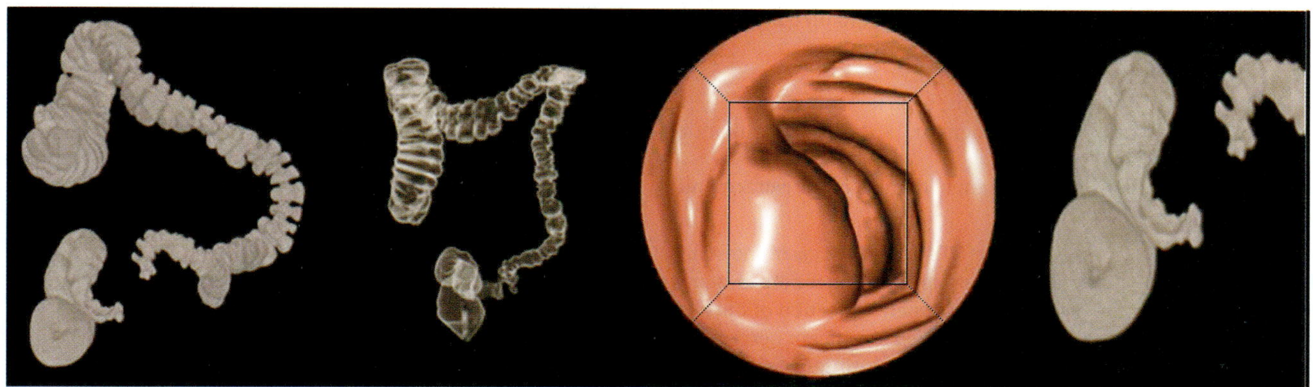

Figure 3 A sigmoid colon mass seen on different image formats of computed tomography colonography

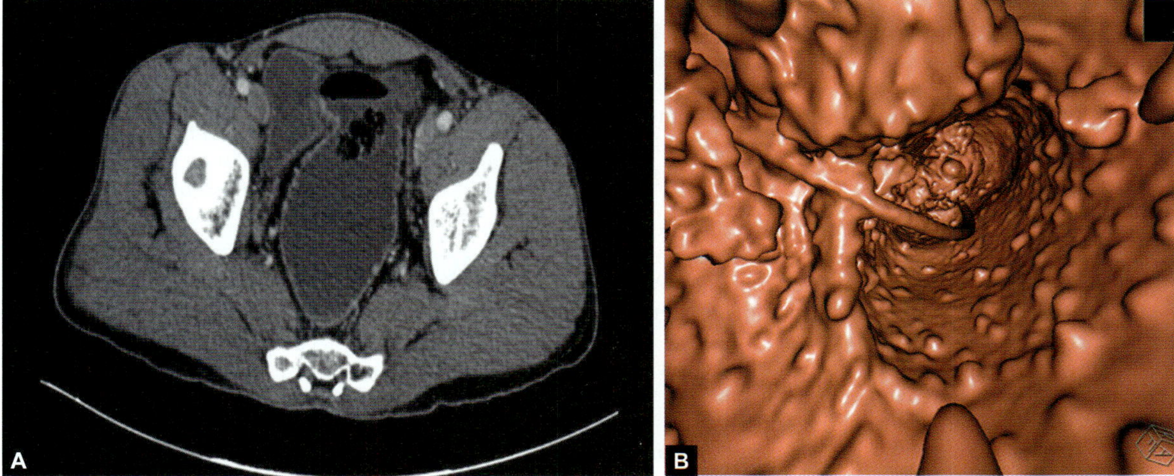

Figures 4A and B Multiple subcentimeter mucosal polyps—barely perceptible on axial computed tomography images, are exquisitely depicted on virtual colonoscopy

and in prone positions using low dose of radiation. Total radiation done can be achieved to be about half that of barium enema. Intravenous contrast improves pick up of smaller polyps. Various two-dimensional or 3D post-processing techniques, then allow multiplanar and endoluminal views. Mimics of polyps that need to be differentiated are adhesion, fecal matter, lipomas, inverted appendiceal stump or deverticulum, prominent ileocecal valve or haustral fold. Pickup for significant polyps (>1 cm) is close to 100% in sensitivity and specificity.

Fecal tagging[6,7] with orally administered barium or water-soluble contrast for a couple of days prior to computed tomography, is another technique that overcomes the tedious process of colonic cleansing. The resultant computed tomography has satisfactory or adequate diagnostic yield even though the pictures are not as "pretty" as those obtained with a clean colon. Any intraluminal colonic projection visualized on fly through images is simultaneously visualized on cross-sectional axial image, to ascertain whether it is a true mucosal lesion or a fecal residue by checking for its "tag" with contrast. Computer software can be used to subtract all contrast tags, so as to obtain a "digitally cleansed colon". This technique is being explored for its use as a readily acceptable screening tool for colonic polyps or masses.

One guideline using computed tomography colonography reporting and data system (C-RADS)[8,9] depicts the clinical decision making based on imaging findings.

- C0: Inadequate study or awaiting prior comparison
  - Inadequate preparation
  - Inadequate insufflations
  - Awaiting prior colon studies for comparison
- C1: Normal colon or benign lesion; continue routine screening
  - No visible abnormality of colon
  - No polyp greater than or equal to 6 mm
  - Lipoma or inverted diverticulum
  - Nonneoplastic finding—e.g. diverticula
- C2: Intermediate polyp or indeterminate finding; surveillance or colonoscopy recommended
  - Intermediate polyp 6–9 mm, less than 3 in number
  - Indeterminate findings, cannot exclude polyp greater than or equal to 6 mm in a technically adequate study

- C3: Polyp, possibly advanced adenoma; follow-up colonoscopy recommended
  - Polyp greater than or equal to 10 mm
  - Greater than or equal to 3 polyps; each 6–9 mm.
- C4: Colonic mass, likely malignant; surgical consultation recommended
  - Lesion compromises bowel lumen, demonstrates extracolonic invasion

Computed tomography angiography (CTA) for lower gastrointestinal bleed has high sensitivity for localization and detection in acute phase and even after the bleeding has stopped. Detection of site and nature of the offending lesion can be done in significant percentage of cases; which is great information for a gastrointestinal surgeon for planning the correct management technique. CTA also detects vascular changes of ischemia, IBD, obstructing hernia and volvulus by showing vascular twisting and altered bowel wall enhancement.

Bowel, because of its contents and mobility, has not been a favorite region for MRI. However, colon and especially anorectal region has proved itself to be worthy of being thus imaged (Fig. 5), after cleansing and luminal distension with appropriate fluid or magnetic resonance contrast.

For imaging of anorectal fistulae magnetic resonance is emerging as the modality of choice, by depicting the tracts with their communications and branching especially on highly T2 weighted thin-slice magnetic resonance in 3D or two-dimensional (2D) with multiplanar capability. Magnetic resonance intravenous contrast also shows inflammatory nature of these tracts and makes them better visible on fat suppressed T1 weighted images. Where available, MRI is the best imaging technique today for preoperative assessment for this condition.

Similarly, locoregional staging of anorectal masses is best done on T2 weighted images for sphincter involvement by the mass lesion, prior to deciding on a sphincter sparing surgery.[10]

Magnetic resonance defecography can be a very rewarding technique for studying sphincter function, even though it use is not encouraged by the radiologist, for obvious reasons.

Where ERUS has a limited access to and around anal and rectal wall, MRI can show involvement of adjacent organs like urinary bladder, seminal vesicles, prostate, mesorectal fascia, vagina and presacral soft tissue, with great confidence. Magnetic resonance colography can also be used in children for studying the colon, when computed tomography has a definite disadvantage of radiation.[10,11]

Postradiotherapy or postoperative changes in colon also provide a setting for MRI to be performed, when distinction of inflammatory changes from recurrence is required.

Nuclear medicine has specific role in imaging malignancies of large bowel. In addition to depiction of the local mass, it provides the best "N" and "M" staging of the lesion by showing physiological hyperactivity in nodes, liver, lungs or bones. It has a better pickup of extrahepatic metastases while it performs poorly for small hepatic lesions. Fusion of CT with PET improves its spatial resolution tremendously, and is currently the most informative imaging for the purpose.

For depiction of acute lower gastrointestinal tract breed, it is standard to advise scintigraphic studies for localization of site, during an active bleed.

In recent year, PET-CT colonography[12,13] has been successfully used to depict the extent of IBD. Infection like tuberculosis, other infective colitides or typhlitis can also be studied by showing uptake of the appropriate radiopharmaceutical. However, this information is more of use when differentiating inflammations from malignancies on the basis of their uptake values, rather than justifying its use for primary diagnosis of colitides.

SPECIFIC DISEASES OF LARGE BOWEL AND THEIR LOGICAL IMAGING FOR SURGICAL DECISION MAKING

Applied Anatomy and Implications for Imaging

Ascending and one-third of transverse colon are derived from midgut while the rest of the distal large bowel represents the embryological hind gut. Congenital variations of rotation can result in left-sided ascending colon and cecum or more commonly a high subhepatic ascending colon; where it needs to

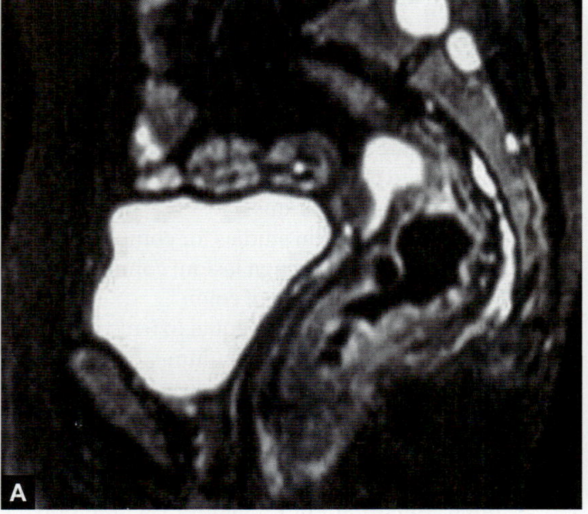

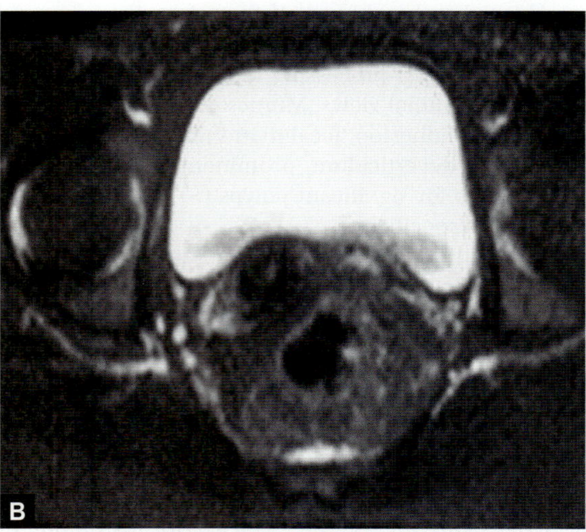

Figures 5A and B Magnetic resonance images showing mesorectal involvement in a case of rectal carcinoma. The tissue planes with vagina are lost

be differentiated from a "pulled up" inflammatory cecal pathology. A left-sided cecum and appendix may result in confusing clinical presentation of appendicitis, when imaging can come to the rescue. Long mesentery responsible for volvulus of sigmoid, may need to be fixed, if it is a recurring problem. Cecal mesentery, if present, is usually the cause for cecal volvulus, owing to its mobility. Plain X-rays (erect and supine) usually suffice to enable the diagnosis to be made. Plain computed tomography, with multiplanar reconstructions in coronal, sagittal or oblique planes, adds confidence to diagnosis. USG and CDI also can show twisted vascular pedicle, if acoustic window permits visualization through gas distended bowel. USG in good operating hands can also be used to look for peritoneal air, in decubitus position, though X-rays are a better way to detect pneumoperitoneum resulting from perforation.

Watershed area of blood supply exists at junction of right two-thirds and left one-third of transverse colon. Even though, branches of superior mesenteric artery (SMA) and inferior mesenteric artery (IMA) anastomose through marginal artery of Drummond and arc of Riolan, this is the site most often involved in hypoperfusion states and ischemia.

Rectum has both mesenteric (IMA) and systemic (branches of internal iliac artery) blood supply. The imaging implication of this fact is, that metastases from rectal masses can show early spread to liver (through mesenteric drainage), as well as to systemic sites (lungs and bones). Colonic malignancies almost always metastasize to liver first.

Colonic wall, unlike the small bowel, has taeniae, as longitudinal muscles resulting in semilunar folds and haustrations. In rectum, the taeniae fuse into a continuous layer and valves appear. The points where muscular walls are penetrated by nutrient vessels are where divecticulosis may occur due to herniation of mucosa and submucosa.

Serosal surface of colon has epiploic, omental fatty appendages, which also have potential for twisting, infarction and inflammation, mimicking diverticulitis and appendicitis both clinically and radiologically.

Mesorectum is the perirectal fat around the rectum, bound externally by thin fascia. On MRI and computed tomography, the invasion of masses beyond the wall can be shown to be extending to and involving the mesorectum, pararectal tissue, obturator muscles, levator ani and other pelvic floor muscles. Their identification is the key to correct locoregional staging for surgical planning.

Colorectal Malignancies

Colonic malignancies are the 3rd most common malignancies, overall and the second most common cause of cancer deaths after lung cancer.

Contribution of dietary and hereditary factors;[6,14,15] presence of preexisting diseases and possible exposures to irritants (e.g. radiation therapy for other pelvic malignancies; chemical irritants like bile salts or acids and neutral sterols) gives this disease, a complex multifactorial genesis. A specific association exists between incidence of colorectal malignancy and exposure to asbestos, printing materials, oils, organic solvents, halogens, metal fumes, paints and dyes. It is rather uncommon in ulcerative colitis, (except in pancolitis); but has higher incidence in setting of Crohn's colitis. The imaging must provide information regarding the presence, type, extent and staging of the lesion. Any synchronous lesions and metastatic deposits also must be looked for.

Immediate postoperative imaging requirements are to look for adequacy of anastomoses, colostomy and inter-loop or retroperitoneal collections. Follow up imaging concerns, that must be addressed, are to look for recurrences, metachronous (5.8%) lesions, metastases; apart from detecting and correctly differentiating radiation induced changes.

Familial adenomatous polyposis (FAP), Turcot Syndrome, juvenile polyposis coli, Cronkhite Canada syndrome, etc. are polyposis conditions of colon where patients develop early colonic malignancy and are usually detected on follow-up and on screening even before symptoms arise, where the conditions are being monitored.

Hereditary non polyposis colorectal carcinoma (Lynch syndrome)[15] accounts for 4–6% of all colorectal malignancies. The prognosis is better than other colonic carcinomas, even though the incidence of metachronous the synchronous lesions is very high in type I. In type II, other organs like endometrium and ovaries also may be involved. Right-sided, young age colonic carcinoma is the most common presentation of Lynch syndrome.

Most colonic malignancies start as an adenomatous polyp.[15,16] It is now recognized that polyps greater than or equal to 1 cm have malignant potential of 5% while those greater than or equal to 2 cm, have 50% chances of being malignant. Other features adding to their malignant potential, are absence of a stalk (i.e. sessile polyps have 50% risk of malignancy); villous architecture of surface and degree of cellular atypia or dysplasia.

Adenoma to adenocarcinoma transition is a slow process, and may take 7–10 years.

Right-sided malignancies are usually large polypoid masses that often outgrow their vascular supply and undergo necrosis. They present late as they do not cause obstructive symptoms. The presentation is usually due to blood loss, anemia or altered bowel habits. Metastatic deposits, at times are the first cause of symptoms.

In contrast, left-sided malignancies are plaque-like or napkin ring or apple-core like, presenting early with obstruction. These tumors are aggressive and infiltrating. Those arising from transverse colon and descending colon are often ulcerative or infiltrative in nature, with early spread to apposing anatomical structures.

Malignancies arising in a setting of IBD are usually mucinous or colloid carcinomas[15] where mucin secreted in the interstitium dissects the walls and helps in extension of the malignancy. On histopathological examination, the mucin component should be more than 50% of the tumors area for diagnosis of mucinous carcinoma to be made. They are often scirrhous plaques and may have fine nodular surface, which may be calcified. The prognosis of these malignancies is worse as compared to adenocarcinoma. At the anorectal junction, squamous cell carcinoma, transitional cell carcinoma and cloacogenic carcinoma may be more frequent as compared to adenocarcinomas.

Other malignancies, like lymphomas, stromal carcinoma, carcinoid, etc. are rare. Metastases from carcinoma breast, ovaries, prostate, lungs, etc. also may present as mass lesions, though rather uncommonly.

The spread of colonic malignancies[17] can occur through direct extension to adjacent fascia or peritoneum or adjacent organs; lymphatic spread to epiploic, paracolic and regional lymph nodes (LNs); and hematogenous spread via portal venous drainage to liver, and to other systemic organs of the body.

Various staging systems[17,18] have evolved from the original staging described by Clithbert and Dukes in 1932 to the current modified Dukes staging suggested by Astler and Coller, which is most commonly used.

- T limited to mucosa
- B1, T extending into but not through muscularis propria
- B2, Tumor penetrating bowel wall without lymph nodes
- C,T with regional lymph nodes
  - C1 Primary Tumour limited to bowel wall
  - C2 Primary Tumour penetrating bowel wall

In 1967, Turnbull introduced stage D, further divided into D1 including fixed and invading adjacent organs and D2 with distant metastases.

Currently, American Joint Committee on Cancer (AJCC) and International Union Against Cancer (UICC) have designated the tumor-node-metastasis (TNM) classification. This is the commonly used alternative method to the modified Dukes.

Both these staging, methods, take into account, the extent of mural invasion which influences prognosis independent of lymph node involvement or distant metastases.

Pri T: Tx To T15 T1 T2 T3 T4 (T4a/T4b)
LN: Nx No N1 N2
Mets: Mx Mo M1
Stage o- Tis; No; Mo
Stage I- T1/T2; No; Mo
Stage II- T3/T4; No; Mo
Stage IIIa- Any T; N1; Mo
Stage IIIb- Any T; N2; Mo
Stage IV- Any T; Any N; M1.

The radiologist has a responsibility to detect, diagnose, stage and prognosticate the disease and guide the surgeon in correct management planning. A complete and accurate assessment of the primary tumor, lymph nodes, local and distant spreads, presence of synchronous lesions is their prime responsibility. Detecting them when they are clinically occult needs meticulous technique and training.

After surgery or other forms of treatment, radiologist has a critical and tougher role of detecting recurrence, residual disease, metachronous and metastatic lesions, besides looking for the other surgical complications like collections, strictures and anastomotic leaks, intussusceptions, etc.

As per recommendations of the American cancer society, beginning at age 50, screening of colorectal cancer should be done according to any one of the following schedules.[8,19,20]

- Yearly fecal occult blood test (FOBT) or fecal immunochemical test (FIT)
- Five yearly flexible sigmoidoscopy
- Yearly FOBT or FIT plus flexible sigmoidoscopy every 5 years
- Double-contrast barium enema (DCBE) every 5 years
- Colonoscopy every 10 years

Fecal occult blood test is the least sensitive for detection of colonic carcinoma (50%) or for colonic polyps (10%) as the bleeding can be intermittent and the polyp is usually over 2 cm in size, for it to bleed regularly.

Flexible sigmoidoscopy has limited access.

Colonoscopy is regarded as the gold standard for measuring the sensitivities of all other techniques, even though it itself lacks due to blind spots behind mucosal folds and around flexures. It has limited patient acceptance and also has a small risk of perforation and hemorrhage, besides being operator dependent for its completion.

Double-contrast barium enema is simple and acceptable,[21] though is only 32% sensitive for polyp detection of less than 0.5 cm, 53% for polyps 0.6–1 cm and 48% for polyps greater than 1 cm (National polyp work group NESH 2000, 342, 1766–72).

Interpretation of DCBE can be done by visualizing the mucosal details in areas filled with barium, where polyps appear as filling defects or projections with pooling of barium at its base or in a small crater or ulcer on the tip. Alternatively barium coated polyps in air filled sections show them as projections on the mucosal relief. Seen enface or in profile their appearance has been given various named signs like Bowlers' Hat (sessile polyps) or Mexican hat (pedunculated polyp) signs. The appearance can also be described as granular or nodular or ulcerated mucosal lesions.

Filling defects like fecal matter, air bubbles and diverticula are mimics that need to be differentiated through meticulous scrutiny of spot films or projections. Direction of dome of filling defect can help differentiate polyps from diverticula where the axis of the dome points away from axis of colon.

This technique has a lot of variables including the state of bowel preparation, fluoroscopy method, area represented in spot films, quality of films, skill of the operator etc. that determine the adequacy of the study.

Criteria[22] for assessing risk of malignancy of a polyp, are based on its lack of pedicle (sessile vs pedunculated); its size (>1 cm); number; presence of basal indentation; and its surface contour.

Pedunculated polyp with stalk greater than 2 cm is likely to be benign with no invasion into adjacent wall.

Presence of basal irregularity and soap bubble or ulcerated surface, signify malignant potential. So called carpet lesions or soap bubble or lacy pattern signifies villous nature of the surface where barium gets entrapped in the fronds, and represents their transition from tubular adenomatous to villous variety.

Detection of a polyp should initiate a search for a synchronous cancer (3.5% chance) or an additional polyp (20%).

Advanced colonic cancers may be short segment annular strictures (Fig. 6), polypoid masses or scirrhous and flat lesions. Irregular, nodular margins resulting in "shouldering" edges to the filling defects in barium columns are the hallmark of malignant stricture where the transition from healthy mucosa to the lesion is rather abrupt.

Ulcerated lesions are also irregular with deep excavating craters and heaped up nodular edges. Saddle lesions involve part of the wall, result in eccentric lumen with nodular margin.

Flat lesions usually occur in the setting of ulcerative colitis and appear as areas of loss of, or change in, mucosal details in that area.

Virtual colonoscopy[4,7] is the new accepted noninvasive method that presents a 3D visualization of the lumen of colon. These surface rendered images are generated from a large amount of data obtained on computed tomography scanning using multislice helical computed tomography.[23] American College of Radiology Imaging Network (ACRIN) study conducted at 15 centers on 2600 asymptomatic patients found that computed tomography colonography has 90% sensitivity and 86% specificity for detection of polyps greater than or equal 1 cm, which is the actual clinically significant size. This has made virtual colonoscopy very popular as a screening tool for early colonic cancer.

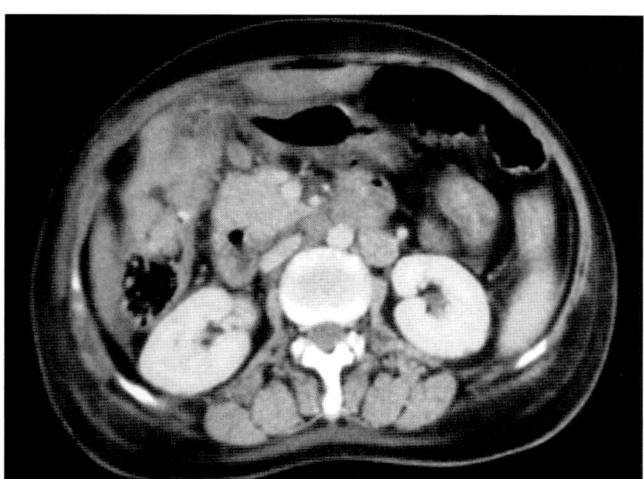

Figure 6 A stricturing mass involving hepatic flexure, showing patchy enhancement, focal calcification suggestive of mucinous or colloid carcinoma. Plane with duodenum is maintained

Computed tomography is also better than barium enema studies, for staging, as it shows the depth of mural invasion, presence of lymph nodal and distant metastases. Treatment planning or prognostication is the preoperative goals of computed tomography or MRI. In cases of obstruction or perforation or fistulous communication or other causes where barium enema is contraindicated, computed tomography is the imaging of choice.

Computed tomography is preferably done after meticulous bowel cleansing and administration of intravenous smooth muscle relaxants and colonic distention with air, water, methylcellulose or contrast. Alternatively, as previously described, fecal tagging may be done if colonic cleansing is not possible, so that any suspected lesion seen on computed tomography can be evaluated to be fecal matter, by the density of its "tag" which is usually barium and has high Hounsfield unit (HU) value.

Normal colonic wall is symmetrical in thickness, measuring 3–6 mm. Focal nodular asymmetric thickening greater than 6 mm, especially when contour or lumen is distorted, signifies the presence of a lesion. Its shape, size surface and invasion, better seen after intravenous contrast, decide its benign versus malignant nature. Computed tomography is poor in visualizing layers of colonic wall separately. Presence of fluid at root of mesentery or engorgement of surrounding mesenteric vasculature, signify an inflammatory etiology like diverticulitis, as against pericolonic lymphatics and lymphnodes which point toward malignancy. Pericolonic lymph nodes are more common in malignancy than in diverticulitis. However, at times this distinction becomes impossible. Care must be taken to evaluate certain areas that are easily overlooked or are difficult to assess on DCBE as well as on computed tomography colonography. Distal rectal lesions may get obscured by catheter hip or by commoner lesions like hemorrhoids or fissures. Small lesions beneath haustral folds may not get noticed. Presence of diverticulosis or previous or present diverticulitis may mimic or obscure filling defects due to small mucosal lesions. Sometimes the barium used may be too dense so that small lesions may get obscured. Insufficient distension, inadequate bowel cleansing, poor mucosal coating by barium are other reasons of false-negative findings.

Lesions involving ileocecal valves too may be missed in early stages. Synchronous lesions are often missed if the observer limits his evaluation to detection or diagnosis of one obvious lesion. As the colorectal cancers are slow growing, it is assumed that if a cancerous lesion is found within 3 years of a previously normal imaging study, the tumor was likely to have been missed.

Local extension to adjacent apposed anatomical structures should be assessed by looking for fat planes between the two, especially in intravenous contrast enhanced images. Structure like seminal vesicles, prostate uterus, vagina, ovaries, bladder and surrounding muscles must be meticulously evaluated for local tumor invasion. Muscles like levator ani, obturator internus, piriformis, coccygeus and glutei are commonly involved by rectosigmoid malignancies. However, loss of fat planes, may overestimate the invasion as vascular or lymphatic engorgement and congestion resulting in edema may also result in apparent loss of fat planes. Extension to or invasion of adjacent pelvic bones or vertebrae or sacrum gives the appearance of what is called a frozen pelvis. Fistulous communications with adjacent organs like bowel loops, urinary bladder and vagina can be identified by contrast filled tracts or by air bubbles or contrast reaching these viscera from colon.

Pericolonic fat enables one to easily look for lymphatic stranding and pericolonic lymph nodes.[24,25] Greater than 1 cm sized nodes are also considered to be metastatic deposits in pericolonic or perirectal regions, a size that is considered insignificant in most other regions in body. Even though, greater than 1 cm inflammatory nodes are common and computed tomography usually cannot distinguish inflammatory from malignant nodes, the lymph nodal staging turns out to be rather accurate when computed tomography N staging is compared with actual post-up staging on Histopathological Examination (HPE). Hence, any nonenhancing perirectal or pericolonic node, irrespective of its size should be considered malignant, for treatment planning.

Liver is the most common site for distant metastases. These lesions are usually hypodense and discreet. Cavitatory, rapidly growing metastases are common in highly malignant lesions. Mucinous carcinoma may give rise to calcified metastases even when the primary is not calcified. Following contrast injection, early peripheral enhancement, uniform enhancement and late hypodense lesions due to washout in portal phase, are commonly seen. Early arterial phase imaging increases the pickup rate by enhancing lesion conspicuity.

Peritoneal spread results in streaking or nodularity, with or without ascites. Computed tomography mostly under estimates (false-negative) early peritoneal metastatic spread. Other sites one must look for, for metastases are the lungs, pleura, adrenals, kidneys and bone marrow. Kruckenberg deposits in ovaries can also occur due to drop metastases in peritoneal cavity.

Computed tomography colonography[7] (Figs 3 and 4) has the following accepted indications for it to be used as the primary imaging modality in setting of colonic malignant lesion.

- Incomplete colonoscopy due to obstructive masses or structure
- Incomplete colonoscopy due to tortuosity, adhesions, diverticular disease or patient intolerance
- Colonoscopy not possible due to anticoagulation therapy or risk of sedation
- Patient refusing colonoscopy.

Contraindications are contrast allergy, possible colonic perforation, acute colitis or diverticulitis; lower gastrointestinal bleeding, complete colonic obstruction, recent colonic surgery or medically unstable patients where colonic preparation is not safe.

Additional extraluminal findings that aid in management also contribute to its superiority over colonoscopy alone.

Working group on virtual colonoscopy has devised C-RADS or computed tomography C-RADS to achieve standardization in reporting.[7,9]

Computed tomography perfusion is a new technique to evaluate malignancies of rectum or colon. Rectal cancers have been shown to have enhanced blood flow (BF) as well as mean transit time (MTT) compared to normal wall. These parameters also help to distinguish potential responders from nonresponders to chemotherapy or radiotherapy. Responders show significant reduction in blood flow and increase in MTT after therapy.[26]

Where computed tomography is the modality of choice for detection and diagnosis of colorectal man lesions, MRI using T2-relaxation-under-spin-tagging (TRUST) are better for T staging as the gutwall can be seen as separate layers of alternating densities; and extent of the invasion of the lesion can be exquisitely depicted. Bowel cleansing still has to be done and intracolonic opacification with air, water or super paramagnetic contrast medium improves visualization. Use of intravenous contrast as well as use of endorectal coils, also improves spatial contrast resolution. Endorectal coils have a very limited depth of view and cannot be used in severely stenosing lesions. They have fallen out of vogue owing to high cost, inconvenience of use and limited additional information they provide.

Optimal MRI[11,12,28] can be done with phased array coils. T1 weight images with fat suppression and intravenous contrast enhancement, preferably in prone position provides adequate information regarding locoregional T and N staging. T2 weight images have become clinically more relevant after the introduction of total mesorectal excision (TME) surgeries for rectal cancer, T2 weight images can depict the merorectal fat, fascia and lymph nodes, better than T1 weight images. Coronal images are preferred for evaluation of sphincter muscles. Liver and bone metastases are also better depicted on MRI than computed tomography especially after Gadolinium contrast. MRI also has a significant role in distinguishing postoperative fibrosis from recurrence of tumor.

Magnetic resonance colonography[27] can also be performed after air insufflation of cleansed colon and administration of spasmolytics. Fast imaging with steady state precession (FISP) 2D/3D, as well as, 3D T1 WI/2D T1 W fast low angle shot (FLASH) are other popular sequences which permit generation of axial, multiplanar and fly through images for evaluation. These have high sensitivity and specificity for significant lesions i.e. greater than or equal to 10 mm, with better soft tissue contrast compared to computed tomography, however, at the expense of lower spatial resolution and more motion artifacts, besides the limitations of imaging times and availability.

Squamous cell carcinomas are rare but may occur in lower rectum, where they are indistinguishable from adenocarcinomas on imaging.

Cloacogenic carcinomas are usually plaque like lesions at anorectal junction, and hence, may be missed on imaging by the catheter tip.

Carcinoid tumors usually present as submucosal masses or polyps inducing intense desmoplastic reaction, resulting in fibrotic kinking of adjacent bowel. Common sites are rectum and cecum. Large hepatic metastases are common at the time of diagnosis.

Mesodermal sarcomas, Kaposi sarcoma, lymphoma and gastrointestinal stromal tumor (GIST) are uncommon tumors in this region. They may have large extramural components, nodulo-polypoidal diffuse lesions or plaques with ulcerations. Other abdominal malignancies with high malignant potential that may metastasize to colon are those from stomach, breast, pancreas and ovaries. Adjacent organs from where contiguous infiltration may occur are stomach, gall bladder, kidney, pancreas and pelvic organs.

Colonic lymphoma is very rare, primary lymphoma being 0.05% of all colonic tumors. Cecum and rectum are commoner sites of involvement. The spectrum of imaging varies from diffuse loss of folds, small nodules to large polyps to large polypoidal masses. Focal strictures, aneurysmal ditatation and ulcero-fistulous lesions are also possible. Extension to terminal items is a feature that helps distinguish cecal lymphoma from adenocarcinoma.

Imaging in Colorectal Bleeding (Lower Gastrointestinal Bleeding)[28,29]

Angiography especially digital subtraction angiography (DSA), used to perform flush aortogram followed by selective and superselective arteriography, is the best technique to image and also treat a large number of appropriate cases of lower gatrointestinal hemorrhage.

For aorta the contrast flow rate is 18–20 mL/sec, for SMA it is 8 mL/sec, while for IMA, a flow rate of 5 mL/sec is adequate.

Rate of active bleeding should be at least 5–6 mL/min for it to be detected on aortogram, and about 0.5–1 mL/min to be detected on selective angiography.

During angiography, extravasation of contrast is seen as puddling or staining that persists beyond capillary or venous phase, and is the direct sign of active bleeding. One must also look for opacified intestinal folds on delayed images. Pseudo-vein appearance occurs, if intraluminal contrast outlines clots already present, due to earlier bleeding. Sometimes, focal spasm of a target vessel provides a clue to the site of hemorrhage.

Slow or intermittent bleeding is better localized on radionuleide studies. 99m Tc sulphur colloid with half-life of 2.5–3 minutes is injected and extravasation in bowel is detected even if rate of hemorrhage is 0.1 mL/min. Low inherent spatial resolution with overlapping structures e.g. flexures with stomach and small intestines sometimes proves a problem for accurate localization

99m Tc labeled red blood cells (RBCs) allows imaging for up to 2 hours after injection. However, this again may be a poor localizer as extravasated isotope can travel in either direction, in the lumen of bowel.

99m Tc pertechnetate scanning is especially used for bleeding Meckel's diverticulum as the traces accumulate in ectopic gastric mucosa.

Multidetector computed tomographic (MDCT) arteriography is today the initial imaging of choice in suspected lower gastrointestinal bleed, unless contraindicated because of contrast related contraindication. It can, in one shot, provide crucial information regarding the site, as well as the offending lesion responsible for the hemorrhage. Its popularity is also attributed to its relative noninvasive nature, and the anatomical detail it provides, in a way that a surgeon can easily interpret. Despite its various limitations, it is the one stop shop for imaging in suspected colonic bleeds, when only the diagnosis is the aim, as no therapeutic procedure can be added to this technique.

Computed tomography, MRI and USG color Doppler studies, all can aid in diagnosing the cause of bleeding, and can be chosen on the basis of suspected outcome, invasiveness of technique and its availability.

Colitis, colonic divecticula, ulcers, angiodysplasias, polyps and masses are the common causes of colorectal bleeding, when hemorroidal and fissural bleedings have been ruled out on proctoscopy.

Most of them are diagnosed and treated on colonoscopy and imaging is rarely required. Angiodysplasias are mucosal telangiectasias, usually involving the right colon. Tuft-like vascular abnormalities seen on arterial phase DSA with early draining vein, are diagnostic of this condition. Malignant lesions may also show similar features on angiography but active bleeding is relatively rare. Incidental nonbleeding telangiectasias, not associated with mass lesions are not treated.

Inflammatory bowel disease and vasculitides show nonspecific generalized findings of dilated tortuous, arteries and mucosal outlining and pooling of extravasated contrast.

Ischemic colitis (occlusive/nonocclusive) may result in submucosal hemorrhages resulting in thumb printing filling defects or thickening of mucosal folds. Arterial phase imaging also shows unenhanced segments corresponding with the occluded arteries. Large collaterals may also be visualized on computed tomography arteriography.

Inflammatory Bowel Disease

Inflammatory bowel disease—ulcerative colitis and Crohn's are two specific diseases of nontubercular intestinal inflammation with extraintestinal manifestations.

Ulcerative colitis is superficial inflammation, starting from rectum and progressing proximally. Terminal items can only be involved as back wash ileitis, if the disease has progressed to cecum as a part of pancolitis.

Crohn's disease is a transmural granulomatous disease involving small bowel more than the large. The disease produces discontinuous lesions rather than continuous ones, fistulae, deep transmural ulcers and lymph nodes' involvement are common features on imaging that help in diagnosing, differentially diagnosing and following-up for assessment of severity, extent of involvement and activity of disease. Imaging also helps in diagnosing extraintestinal complication and response to therapy. DCBE is the imaging of choice for imaging of colonic involvement with IBD. Computed tomography (MDCT) is the cross-sectional imaging of choice for transmural and extraintestinal involvement. Computed tomography perfusion can be done to demonstrate actively inflamed segments (Fig. 7) to plan treatment and to assess response to treatment.

Virtual colonoscopy can suitably replace conventional colonoscopy which may be contraindicated in acute stages where mucosa is friable and there is risk of perforation.[30]

Magnetic resonance imaging and sonography are suitable for follow-up in view of high radiation doses incurred on repeat computed tomography required in these cases. Moreover, MRI can differentiate thick edematous wall due to acute inflammation, from fibrotic thick wall as fibrosis shows low signal on both T1 weight images and T2 weight images.

Bright lumen technique requires colon to be filled with diluted gadolinium (Gd) (with water) while Dark technique requires colon to be filled with plain water. Wall enhancement after intravenous Gd improves visualization of disease extent in dark lumen technique. Wall edema appearing bright on T2 weight images and enhanced bowel after intravenous contrast on TI weight images are the sequences used for assessing activity.

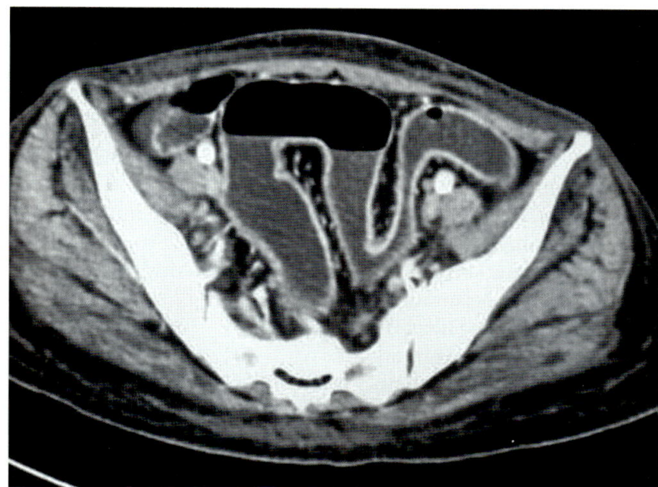

Figure 7 Granulomatous colitis showing pericolonic hyper-vascularity on computed tomography

Colonoscopy or computed tomography for diagnosis and magnetic resonance for follow-up[31,32] is the normal protocol for imaging colonic IBD. USG has emerged with a simple noninvasive technique of hydrocolonic sonography where cleansed colon is filled with water prior to high resolution ultrasound imaging. It can help in visualization of five layers of colonic wall as well as edema or pericolonic inflammation fluid or increased flow on CDI, which are all features of inflammatory hypervascularisation suggestive of activity of the disease. Operator dependence and poor localization of colonic segments on follow-up comparison are the drawbacks.

Positron emission tomography-computed tomography[32,33] can also be utilized for diagnosing as well as for follow-up of IBD of small as well as large bowel. Large bowel PET-CT colonography using 18-FDG shows activity of the disease by accumulating at sites of active inflammation.

In Ulcerative Colitis, earliest imaging feature is the appearance of fine granularity of mucosa, starting at rectum, with evidence of widening of retrorectal-presacral space on DCBE. Shallow ulcers and erosions form with progression to involvement of deeper layers of submucosa. Proximal progression of disease may result in pancolitis, with loss of haustral folds, spasm and narrowing of lumen. Later, inflammatory pseudopolyps may form with associated shortening as well as narrowing of the colon. Fifteen percent cases may show evidence of backwash ileitis, where ileocecal valve is patulous and gaping. Ultrasound, can show layering of colonic wall and flow on CDI in acute stages.

Computed tomography shows intramural changes best. Wall thickening, submucosal fat deposits and patchy enhancement are the additional features specific to the disease process. Target sign is due to this layer of hypodense fat deposit between two enhancing layers of mucosa, lamina propria and muscularis mucosa on the inside and muscularis propria and serosa on the outside. Pericolonic and perirectal fat deposition as well as lymphovascular infiltration is seen in all types of chronic colitides.

Crohn's disease primarily involves small bowel, but can secondarily affect colon as well as other systems.

On the basis of imaging findings, subtypes are recognized to aid clinical management:

- Active inflammatory subtype
  - Mucosal changes: superficial aphthous ulcers, fold thickening.
  - Severe changes: deep ulcers, cobble stone mucosa, wall thickening (comb sign)
- Fibro-stenotic subtype: minimal or severe stenosis.
- Fistulizing or perforating subtype.
  - Deep fissuring ulcers, sinus tracts.
  - Fistulae to adjacent organs.
  - Associated inflammatory mass
- Reparative or Regenerative subtype.
  - Mucosal atrophy, regenerating polyps.

Barium meal follow through or enteroclysis is the initial modality to make the diagnosis, shallow aphthous ulcers which may coalesce are best visualized when double contrast enteroclysis is performed using barium with water, methylcellulose or air. Narrowing or stenosis is eccentric with puckering and retraction of mesentenic border more than the antemesenteric border. A long segment of narrowing gives rise to "string sign" of barium column. Computed tomography is less effective in demonstrating early mucosal findings. Bowel wall thickening is the most common finding on computed tomography. Often involving long segments, it is frequently discontinuous with skip areas. In some cases, mural stratification can be appreciated after intravenous contrast, resulting in double halo or target appearance on cross-section. Rectal sparing in most cases and commoner involvement of small bowel helps differentiate it from ulcerative colitis. Late features of sinuses, fistulae, wall thickening and mesenteric changes are better seen on computed tomography. Mesenteric edema, fatty infiltration, lymphatic and lymphnodal enlargement are the features to be looked for on computed tomography. Large inflammatory masses or abscesses are also better appreciated on computed tomography.

Magnetic resonance enteroclysis with contrast is also a versatile technique for showing the bowel and extra bowel changes. In addition, it helps distinguish between fibrotic and edematous bowel wall thickening so that decision about surgical management can be made. Sino fistulous tracts too can be shown on True-FISP or half-Fourier acquisition single-shot turbo spin-echo (HASTE) sequences. USG using ultrasound contrast or hydrogen peroxide also has been shown to be able to delineate tracts of enterocutaneous fistulae on sonography.[34-36]

Crohn's disease in our country needs differentiation from tubercular disease.[37] Presence of large necrotic lymph nodes, features of peritoneal and mesenteric involvement and ascites, tilt the diagnosis in favor of tuberculosis. Tuberculous colitis is usually associated with ileocecal and small bowel involvement. Segmental colitis, inflammatory strictures and hypertrophic mass like lesions especially in the spacious cecum are the various forms of tubercular involvement. Length of strictures is however shorter in tuberculosis, than that in Crohn's. Anorectal tuberculous usually presents as sinuses, fistulae, fissures and abscesses.

Ischemic colitis can result from arterial or venous causes, both in acute or chronic settings.[38,39] Nonocclusive ischemia due to acute hypovolemic states, affect the watershed zones more and splenic flexure is usually the site of involvement in these cases.

Acute occlusive ischemia usually results from thromboembolic disease, while atherosclerosis or vasculitis is responsible for most cases of chronic ischemia.

Role of imaging is not only to depict the bowel changes, but also to evaluate the offending vascular cause; as well as depiction of collateral circulation. Computed tomography angiography with enteroclysis using negative contrast (water, methylcellulose), is the technique that provides all this information. Computed tomography as well as MRI is able to depict bowel wall changes of thickening, edema and intramural hemorrhages. On ultrasound Doppler examination, main abdominal aorta and its branches can be studied well at their origin. A peak systolic velocity (PSV) of 275 cm/s for SMA or loss of flow signal, are considered significant for intervention.

Nodularity, patchiness or loss of enhancement or submucosal hemorrhages with thumb-printing on the bowel lumen is well appreciated on cross-sectional imaging techniques. Perforation may occur following infarction and necrosis. Air may also be seen dissecting the layers of bowel and even tracking into portal drainage system, a sign with serious irreversible implications. Chronic ischemia may lead to fibrosis and stricture formation.

Appendicitis, Epiploic Appendagitis and Diverticulitis[40-44]

Occlusion of lumen of appendix by an appendicolith, accumulation of fluid, inflammation and ischemia, which may result in periappendiceal fluid or fat stranding; or even perforation and abscess formation; are the stages which imaging should depict to correctly diagnose appendicitis. Equally important is the finding of air or contrast in the lumen of appendix with normal appearing surrounding fat, which confidently rules out appendicitis in a confusing clinical setting.

Ultrasonography of the right iliac fossa, using a graded compression technique to displace overlying bowel gases is a reliable method for initial diagnosis, especially as it can also demonstrate tenderness on probe pressure over the visualized inflamed appendix.[45] Low dose plain spiral computed tomography is a more objective imaging technique acceptable in emergency settings that gives confidence to a clinical diagnosis. Visualization of appendicolith (30–40% cases), arrow head shape of a spastic cecum, with pericecal inflammatory fat stranding, are the features, one relies upon, for a correct diagnosis. Small air pockets or fluid collection with enhancing walls signify perforation and abscess formation respectively.

Epiploic appendages are small fatty appendages on the serosal surface of colon which may get inflamed, due to torsion and ischemia or venous thrombosis. Computed tomography depicts them well as focal pericolic fatty lesions, with inflammatory stranding and a central dense thrombosed vein. Similar focus of pericolonic inflammation can be seen in diverticulitis or even in omental infarction. To make a confident diagnosis of divecticulits, one must look for diverticulae in adjacent colonic segment. Computed tomography not only provides diagnosis of diverticular disease, but also shows its various stages and complications. At times, a differentiation from a colonic malignancy may be difficult especially because perilesional nodes may occur in both conditions.

Inflammatory inter-loop fluid, changes in the root of mesentery or inflammatory stranding of mesentery are changes that point toward an inflammatory pathology.

Tubercular involvement of appendix occurs secondary to cecal tuberculosis. Features of chronic appendicitis may develop secondary to cecal hypertrophy, nodularity or fibrosis.

REFERENCES

1. Goldberg HI, Margulis AR. Gastrointestinal radiology in the United States: An overview of the past 50 years. Radiology. 2000;216(1):1-7.
2. Gluecker TM, Johnson CD, Harmsen WS, Offord KP, Harris AM, Wilson LA, et al. Colorectal cancer screening with CT colonography, colonoscopy and double-contrast barium enema examination: prospective assessment of patient perceptions and preferences. Radiology. 2003;227(2):378-84.
3. Glaser F, Schlag P, Herfarth C. Endorectal ultrasonography for the assessment of invasion of rectal tumours and lymph node involvement. Br J Surg. 1990;77(8):883-7.
4. Dachman AH, Yoshida H. Virtual colonoscopy past, present and future. Radiol Clin North Am. 2003;41:377-93.
5. Rosman AS, Korsten MA. Meta-analysis comparing CT colonography, air contrast barium enema and colonoscopy. Am J Med. 2007;120(3):203-10.e4.
6. Theoni RF, Lanfer I. Polyps and carcinoma of the colon. Textbook of gastrointestinal radiology. In: Gore RM, Levine MS (Eds). Philadelphia: WB Saunders; 2008. pp. 1121-66.
7. Summerton S, Little E, Cappell MS. CT colonography: current status and future promise. Gastroenterol Clin North Am. 2008;37(1):161-89.
8. Mandel JS. Screening for colorectal cancer. Gastrointestinal Clin N Am. 2008;37:97-115.
9. Zalis ME, Barish MA, Choi JR, Dachman AH, Fenlon HM, Ferrucci JT, et al. CT colonography reporting and data system: a consensus proposal. Radiology. 2005;236(1):3-9.
10. Brown G, Radcliffe AG, Newcombe RG, Dallimore NS, Bourne M, Williams GT. Preoperative assessment of prognostic factors in rectal cancer using high-resolution magnetic resonance imaging. Br J Surg. 2003;90(3):355-64.
11. Brown G, Kirkham A, Williams GT, Bourne M, Radcliffe AG, Sayman J, et al. High-resolution MRI of the anatomy important in total mesorectal excision of the rectum. Am J Roentgenol. 2004;182(2):431-9.
12. Kinner S, Antoch G, Bockisch A, Veit-Haibach P. Whole-body PET/CT colonography: a possible new concept for colorectal cancer staging. Abdom Imaging. 2007;32:606-12.
13. Gollub MJ, Akhurst T, Markowitz AJ, Weiser MR, Guillem JG, Smith LM, et al. Combined CT colonography and 18F-FDG PET of colon polyps: potential technique for selective detection of cancer and precancerous lesions. Am J Roentgenol. 2007;188(1):130-8.
14. Mohandas KM, Desai DC. Epidemiology of digestive tract cancers in India. V. Large and small bowel. Indian J Gastroenterol. 1999;18(3):118-21.
15. Gore RM. Colorectal cancer. Clinical and pathological features. Radiol Clin North Am. 1997;35:403-29.
16. Lane N, Fengho CM. The adenocarcinoma sequence in the stomach and colon:I observation on the adenoma as precursor to ordinary large bowel carcinoma. Gastrointestinal Radiology. 1976;1:111-9.
17. Berlin JW, Gore RM, Yaghmai V, Newmark GM, Miller FH. Staging of colorectal cancer. Semin Roentgenol. 2000;35(4):370-84.
18. Johnson RD, Geisinger KR. Colorectal adenocarcinoma: staging and histopathology. Semin Roentgenol. 1996;31(2):94-102.
19. McMahon PM1, Gazelle GS. The case for colorectal cancer screening. Semin Roentgenol. 2000;35(4);325-32.
20. Gelfand DW. Colorectal cancer: screening strategies. Red Clin N Am. 1997;35:431-38.
21. Winawer SJ, Stewart ET, Zauber AG, Bond JH, Ansel H, Waye JD, et al. A comparison of colonoscopy and DCBE for surveillence after polypectomy. National polyp work group. N Engl J Med. 2000;342:1766-72.
22. Bond JH. Diagnosis, treatment, and surveillance for patients with nonfamilial colorectal polyps. Ann Intern Med.1993;119:836-43.
23. Johnson CD, Chen MH, Toledano AY. Accuracy of CT colonography for detection of large adenomas and cancers. N Engl J Med. 2008;359:1207-17.
24. Filippone A, Ambrosini R, Fuschi M, Marinelli T, Genovesi D, Bonomo L. Preoperative T and N staging of colorectal cancer: accuracy of contrast-enhanced multi-detector row CT colonography–initial experience. Radiology. 2004;231(1):83-90.
25. Chung DJ, Huh KC, Choi WJ, Kim JK. CT colonography using 16-MDCT in the evaluation of colorectal cancer. Am J Roentgenol. 2005;184(1):98-103.
26. Beets-Tan RG, Beets GL, Vliegen RF, Kessels AG, Van Boven H, De Bruine A, et al. Accuracy of magnetic resonance imaging in prediction of tumour-free resection margin in rectal cancer surgery. Lancet. 2001;357(9255):497-504.
27. Ajay W, Pelster G, Treichel U, Vogt FM, Debatin JF, Ruehm SG, et al. Dark lumen magnetic resonance colonography; comparison with conventional colonoscopy for the detection of colorectal pathology. Gut. 2003;52:1738-43.
28. Jaeckle T, Stuber G, Hoffmann MHK, Jeltsch M, Schmitz BL, Aschoff AJ. Detection and localization of acute upper and lower gastrointestinal (GI) bleeding with arterial phase multi-detector row helical CT. European Radiology. 2008;18(7):1406-13.
29. Roy-Choudhury SH, Gallacher DJ, Pilmer J, Rankin S, Fowler G, Steers J, et al. Relative threshold of detection of active arterial bleeding: in vitro comparison of MDCT and digital subtraction angiography. AJR Am J Roentgenol. 2007;189(5):W238-46.
30. Horsthuis K, Stokkers CF, Stoker J. Detection of inflammatory bowel disease: diagnostic performance of cross sectional imaging modalities. Abdom Imaging. 2008;33(4):407-16.
31. MacKalski BA, Bernstein CN. New diagnostic imaging tools for inflammatory bowel disease. Gut. 2006;55(5):733-41.
32. Long Sun, Hua Wu, Yong-Song Guan. Colonography by CT, MRI and PET/CT combined with conventional colonoscopy in colorectal cancer screening and staging. World J Gastroenterol. 2008;14(6):853-63.
33. Meisner RS, Spier BJ, Einarsson, Roberson EN, Perlman SB, Bianco JA, et al. Pilot study using PET/CT as a novel, noninvasive assessment of disease activity in inflammatory bowel disease. Inflamm Bowel Dis. 2007;13:993-1000.
34. Schreyer AG, Scheibl K, Heiss P, Feuerbach S, Seitz J. MR colonography in inflammatory bowel disease. Abdominal Imaging. 2006;31(3):302-7.
35. Valette PJ, Rioux M, Pilleul F, Saurin JC, Fouque P, Henry L. Ultrasonography of chronic inflammatory bowel diseases. Eur Radiol. 2001;11(10):1859-66.
36. Sjekavica I, Barbabic-Babic VB, Krznaric Z, Molnar M, Cuković-Cavka S, Stern-Padovan R. Assessment of Crohn's disease activity by Doppler Ultrasound of mesenteric artery and mural arteries in thickened bowel wall: cross-sectional study. Croat Med J. 2007;48;822-30.
37. Lundstedt C, Nyman R, Brismar J, Hugosson C, Kagevi I. Imaging of tuberculosis II. Abdominal manifestations in 112 patients. Acta Radiol. 1996;37(4):489-95.
38. Kim AY, Ha KH. Evaluation of suspected mesenteric ishemia; efficacy of radiology studies Radiol Clin North Am. 2003;41:327-42.
39. Horton KM, Fishman EK. Multidetector CT angiography in the diagnosis of mesenteric ischemia. Radiol Clin North Am. 2007;45(2):275-88.
40. Thoeni RF. CT imaging of colitis. Radiology. 2006;240(3):623-38.

41. Neff CC, vanSonnenberg E. CT of diverticulitis. Diagnosis and treatment. Cello Radiol Clin North Am. 1989;27(4):743-52.
42. Oto A, Ernst RD, Mileski WJ, Nishino TK, Le O, Wolfe GC, et al. Localization of appendix with MDCT and influence of findings on choice of appendectomy incision. AJR Am J Roentgenol. 2006;187(4):987-90.
43. Doria AS, Moineddin R, Kellenberger CJ, Epelman M, Beyene J, Schuh S, et al. US or CT for Diagnosis of Appendicitis in Children and Adults? A Meta-Analysis. Radiology. 2006;241(1):83-94.
44. Garcia Peña BM, Mandl KD, Kraus SJ, Fischer AC, Fleisher GR, Lund DP, et al. Ultrasonography and limited computed tomography in the diagnosis and management of appendicitis in children. JAMA. 1999;282(11):1041-6.
45. Hernandez JA, Swischuk LE, Ange CA, Chung D, Chandler R, Lee S. Imaging of acute appendicitis: US as the primary imaging modality. Pediatric Radiology. 2005;35(4):392-5.

CHAPTER 87

Anal Fistula

BK Jain, PK Garg

INTRODUCTION

Anal fistula is a common anorectal condition which is often managed inadequately. The patient usually reports late due to hesitation on account of involvement of private parts. Intervention by quacks is another important reason for delay in the treatment and deterioration of the condition. Even qualified surgeons are baffled by complex anatomy of anal fistula and its defiance to treatment. The patient often undergoes multiple operations at several hospitals, and yet fails to get relief. Though majority of the anal fistula are simple and can be managed in a straight forward manner; a few other fistulae require attention of surgeons or centers having special interest and expertise in the disease. A small number of fistulae may refuse to heal or continue to recur despite best efforts. A policy of palliative management can provide lasting relief to such patients.

ETIOPATHOGENESIS

The usual anal fistula has its genesis from anal gland infection which develops in intersphincteric space in the anal canal—usually at 6 o clock position at the level of dentate line. The resulting abscess may extend through the intersphincteric space and/or through the internal and/or external sphincter and discharge pus in anal canal as well as through the perianal skin. A remnant of the abscess and the tract which is lined by granulation tissue gives rise to the fistula.[1] These fistulae are known as cryptogenic anal fistulae and this chapter is confined to the management of such fistulae. Other infectious causes include tuberculosis, actinomycosis, amebiasis and sexually transmitted diseases. Neglected pelvic sepsis may present as perianal fistula. The non-infectious causes include inflammatory bowel disease and various anorectal operative procedures. Fistula may occasionally follow sclerotherapy, internal sphincterotomy or closed hemorrhoidectomy.[1] Anal fistula may be the first presenting feature of an underlying anorectal tumor such as squamous cell carcinoma, cloacogenic carcinoma, and adenocarcinoma.

SURGICAL ANATOMY

The length of surgical anal canal is about 4 cm and it extends from anorectal ring to anal verge. The epithelial lining of anal canal is columnar in the upper part and squamous in the lower part. The dentate line, present at about 1.5 cm from the anal verge, marks the level of transition. Anal canal has two sphincters: (1) internal and (2) external. Internal sphincter is the continuation of circular muscle of rectum and has autonomic nerve supply—it is under involuntary control. Voluntary control over defecation is by puborectalis and finally by the external sphincter. The anal glands are situated in the intersphincteric space and their ducts extend through the internal sphincter to open at dentate line. Figure 1 shows the diagrammatical representation of anorectal region. Fistulae are most commonly derived from cryptoglandular disease. Lymph nodal tissue is present near anal crypts which explain their involvement in Crohn's disease and tuberculosis. Paravisceral compartment is present lateral to sphincter muscles. This compartment is divided by levator ani into ischioanal and pelvic space. The lower portion of ischioanal space is called perianal space. The pelvic space between levator ani and pelvis peritoneum is known as supralevator space. Fascial spaces are also present posterior to anal canal: superficial and deep post anal space. Infections can reach these spaces and form abscess. Ischioanal space is commonly involved; infection can ascend through the levator ani to reach supralevator space.

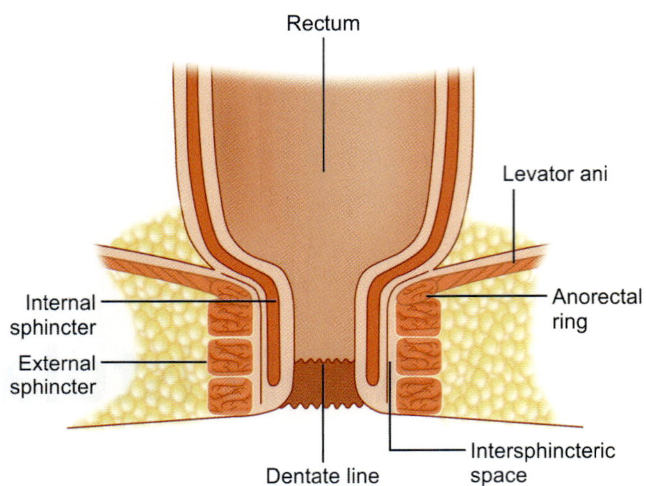

Figure 1 Anatomy of anorectum relevant to anal fistula

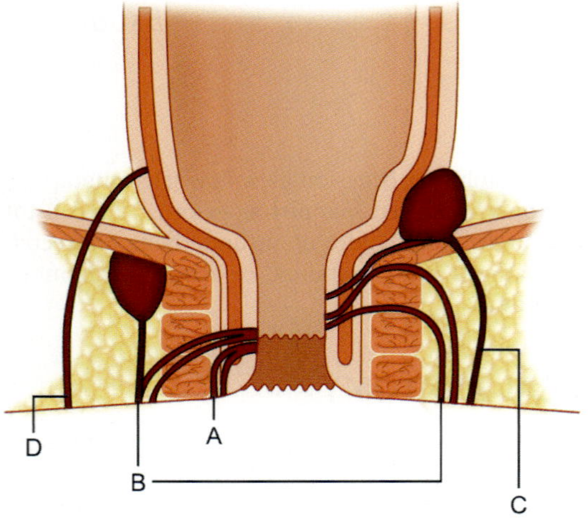

Figure 2 Park's classification of anal fistula: (A) Intersphincteric fistula, (B) Trans-sphincteric fistula, (C) Suprasphincteric fistula, (D) Extrasphincteric fistula

CLASSIFICATION

Parks,[2] in 1976, classified anal fistula according to the fistula tract and its association with the external and internal anal sphincter as shown in Figure 2. The external sphincter is regarded as the keystone for classification.

Intersphincteric fistula: The tract begins at dentate line then tracks through the internal sphincter and intersphincteric space to end at perianal skin or perineum. Secondary tracts in between the sphincters extending superiorly may be seen.

Transsphincteric fistula: The tract passes through both internal and external sphincter and ends at the skin. It can be low or high.

Suprasphincteric fistula: The tract passes through internal sphincter, then loops over the puborectalis to pass through the levator ani muscle and terminates at the skin.

Table 1: Criteria for classification as high and low anal fistula

Study	*Criteria for low fistula*	*Criteria for high fistula*
Mishra et al.,[3] 2013	Internal opening below anorectal ring	Internal opening above anorectal ring
Bleier & Moloo,[4] 2011	Involves small or none of external sphincter	External sphincter is involved
Van koperen et al.,[5] 2007	Involves lower third of external sphincter	Involves upper two-thirds of external sphincter or higher

Extrasphincteric fistula: The tract passes external to external sphincter connecting rectum to perianal skin. It is a rare type of fistula. It may develop after trauma, Crohn's disease, pelvic inflammation, or rupture of supralevator extension into the rectum.

The anal fistula can also be classified as low and high fistula according to the location of internal opening of the fistula in relation to the dentate line in anal canal, and/or the course of fistula tract in relation to the anal sphincters[3-5] (Table 1).

Mishra et al.[3] classified fistula into high and low on the basis of location of internal opening in relation to anorectal ring. This criterion has limitations. Large number of anal fistula, with tracts involving upper sphincter, have internal opening at dentate line. These anal fistulae will be erroneously categorized as low by this criteria.

Anal fistula has been more appropriately classified as simple and complex. Majority of anal fistula consist of a primary tract extending between an external opening and an internal opening and involving lower part of the sphincters. These fistulae can be cured by a simple operation—fistulotomy or fistulectomy. This group includes subcutaneous, intersphincteric or low transsphincteric fistulae and can be categorized as simple anal fistula (SAF). These fistulae are associated with low possibility of recurrence and anal incontinence following surgery.

The other category is complex anal fistula (CAF). These fistulae cannot be cured by a simple fistulotomy or fistulectomy operation. There may be one or more features which are responsible for complexity of the fistulae: (a) internal opening located in upper anal canal or rectum, (b) high primary tract involving larger portion of sphincter (>1/3), (c) high secondary tracts or abscesses in relation to upper anal canal or lower rectum, (d) a horseshoe tract (e) sphincter weakness due to surgery, trauma or disease. The high transsphincteric fistula, suprasphincteric fistula, and any fistula with high secondary tract or abscess fall in this category. All recurrent fistulae are also included under this category. Sometimes, the external opening or the internal opening is not discernable; such cases are also difficult to manage. It is interesting to note that a fistula may persist in absence of a patent internal opening, though internal opening is considered to be reason for persistence of a fistula. Deep seated sepsis in intersphincteric, extrasphincteric, or supralevator space must be the cause of persistence of these fistula despite absence of communication of the tract with anal canal.

According to American Gastroenterological Association, anal fistula is categorized as complex in the following situations:[4]

- A high tract that traverses more than 30-50% of the external sphincter
- An anterior location in a female

- Multiple tracts
- Preexisting incontinence
- Recurrent fistula
- Local irradiation
- Chronic diarrhea
- Fistula involving other organs
- Associated disease, for example, tuberculosis or Crohn's disease.

Surgical management of CAF carries higher risks of delayed healing, failure of treatment, fecal incontinence, and/or recurrence.

CLINICAL PRESENTATION

Commonly, the patient complains of purulent discharge from the perianal region. There may be a history of an abscess which burst spontaneously or was surgically drained. The discharge may cease temporarily due to closure of external opening. This is usually followed by a painful swelling which may again discharge pus and the pain is relieved. In neglected cases, multiple external opening may be found, some of them being situated far away from anus—in scrotum or in gluteal region.

Sometimes, the patient presents with pain in anus and recurrent pus discharge from anus. No external opening is detected. On digital rectal examination (DRE), an internal opening may be found at dentate line. Swelling or induration may be found in relation to anal canal or lower rectum due to associated abscess.

CLINICAL ASSESSMENT

Information regarding associated comorbid conditions like diabetes mellitus or diseases affecting immunity is important. Details of previous surgery—drainage of perianal abscess or surgery for anal fistula should be sought. In woman, history of difficult or complicated labor is noteworthy. Disturbance in anal continence is not usual in patients with anal fistula. However, a discrete enquiry should be made regarding incontinence for flatus, liquid stool, or solid stool and its frequency. This is particularly important in patients who have undergone surgery for anal fistula earlier.

A careful and diligent examination of the perineum yields most of the information required by the surgeon for the management of the patient. Any scar in the perineum should be noted as it may provide a clue about the nature of surgery performed earlier. During inspection, the number and location of the external openings should be noted. Their distance from anus should be recorded. Granulation tissue, skin tag, or a papilla may obscure the external opening. At times, the external opening is obliterated and it may be seen as a scar on the skin (Figs 3A to D). Lax and patulous anus or pouting mucosa suggests possibility of sphincter dysfunction.

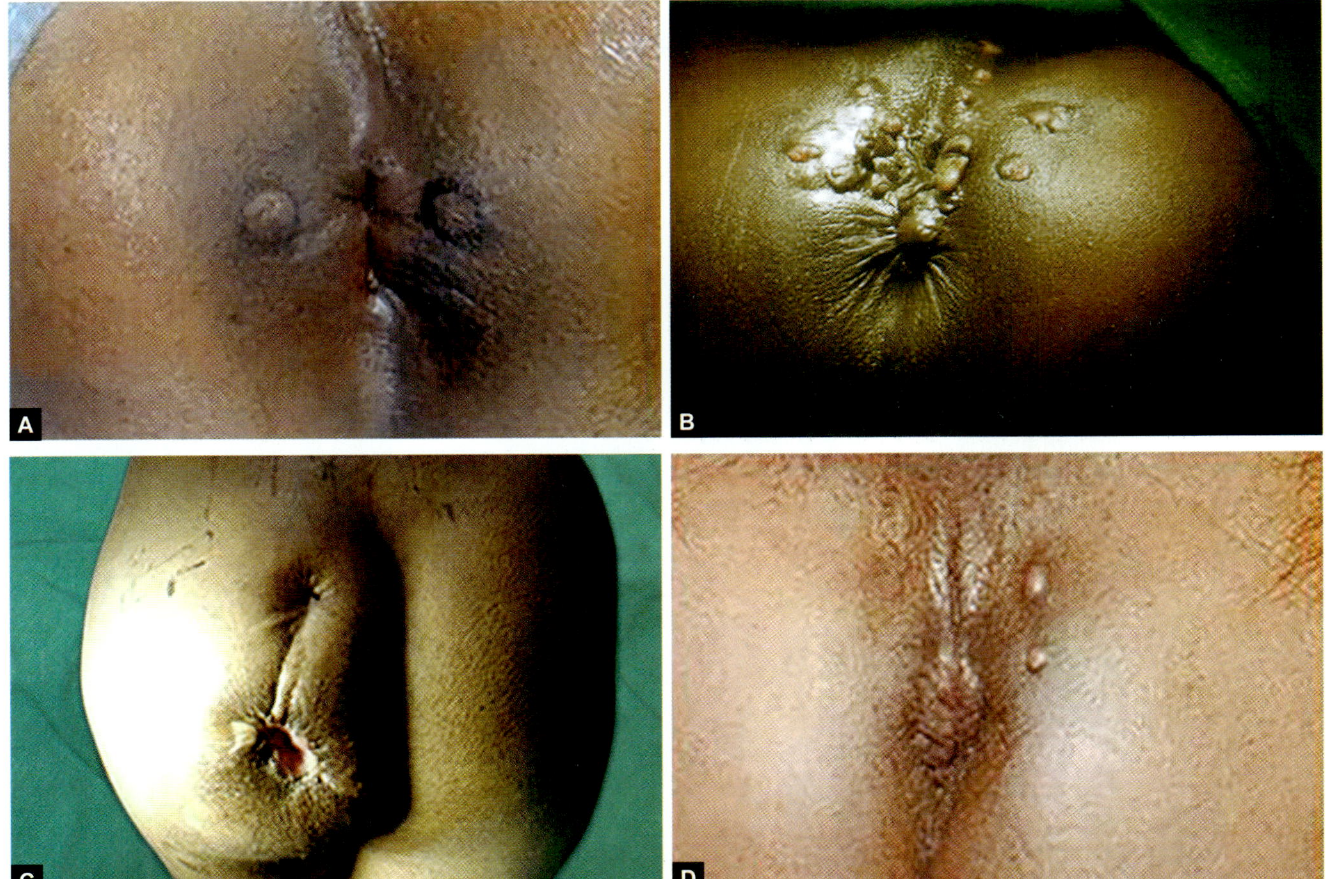

Figures 3A to D (A) Two external openings; (B) Multiple external openings; (C) Previous multiple attempts of surgery; (D) Obliterated external opening

The area around the external opening should be palpated with index finger to ascertain presence of a palpable fistula tract and its direction. In SAF, the tract are usually superficial and can be palpated throughout its length—extending from external opening to the anus. The direction of a palpable tract indicates the location of internal opening in the anal canal (Figs 4A to C).

The resting anal tone and tone on voluntary contraction of anal sphincter should be assessed during DRE. A note should be made about the length of the anal canal. In several patients, the anal canal is unusually short. This may be a result of chronic inflammation and fibrosis. One should be careful in dividing the sphincters during surgery in such patients. The location and the number of the internal openings should be noted. There is only a single internal opening in most of the patients. The most common location is 6 o clock at dentate line in the anal canal. This is true for most of the CAF also. The next common site for internal opening is a point on dentate line radial to the external opening. It may be difficult to locate the internal opening in a few patients. Exploring the suspected area with a rubbing movement of pulp of the index finger helps to identify the pit and the induration around it. A mental note should be made about the distance of internal opening from the anal verge and the anorectal junction. The distance between the internal opening and the anorectal junction may provide an estimate of the amount of sphincter beyond the fistula tract.

A careful DRE can also disclose the deep extent of the disease process in case of CAF. The anorectal junction is usually felt as a soft shelf/edge/rim when the finger tip is moved from anus to rectum. In cases, where the inflammatory process has reached the apex of ischioanal fossa and/or deep postanal space, the anorectal junction is felt as a firm shelf/edge/rim. The supralevator abscess is felt as indurated swelling abutting rectum just superior to anorectal junction. Occasionally a polypoid swelling is felt in rectum just above the anorectal junction. Possibility of a chronic submucous abscess in relation with a high intersphincteric tract should be considered in such situations.

DRE is very useful in assessing the complexity of the anal fistula and in deciding the need for specialized investigations. A single external opening, a single internal opening at dentate line, completely palpable fistula tract, and absence of a palpable abnormality in upper anal canal/lower rectum almost makes sure that one is dealing with a SAF and specialized imaging is not required.

INVESTIGATIONS

As stated earlier, a diligent perineal examination with an educated finger is sufficient to discover most of the information required for the management of the anal fistula. However, several imaging techniques are available for evaluation of anal fistula: fistulogram,

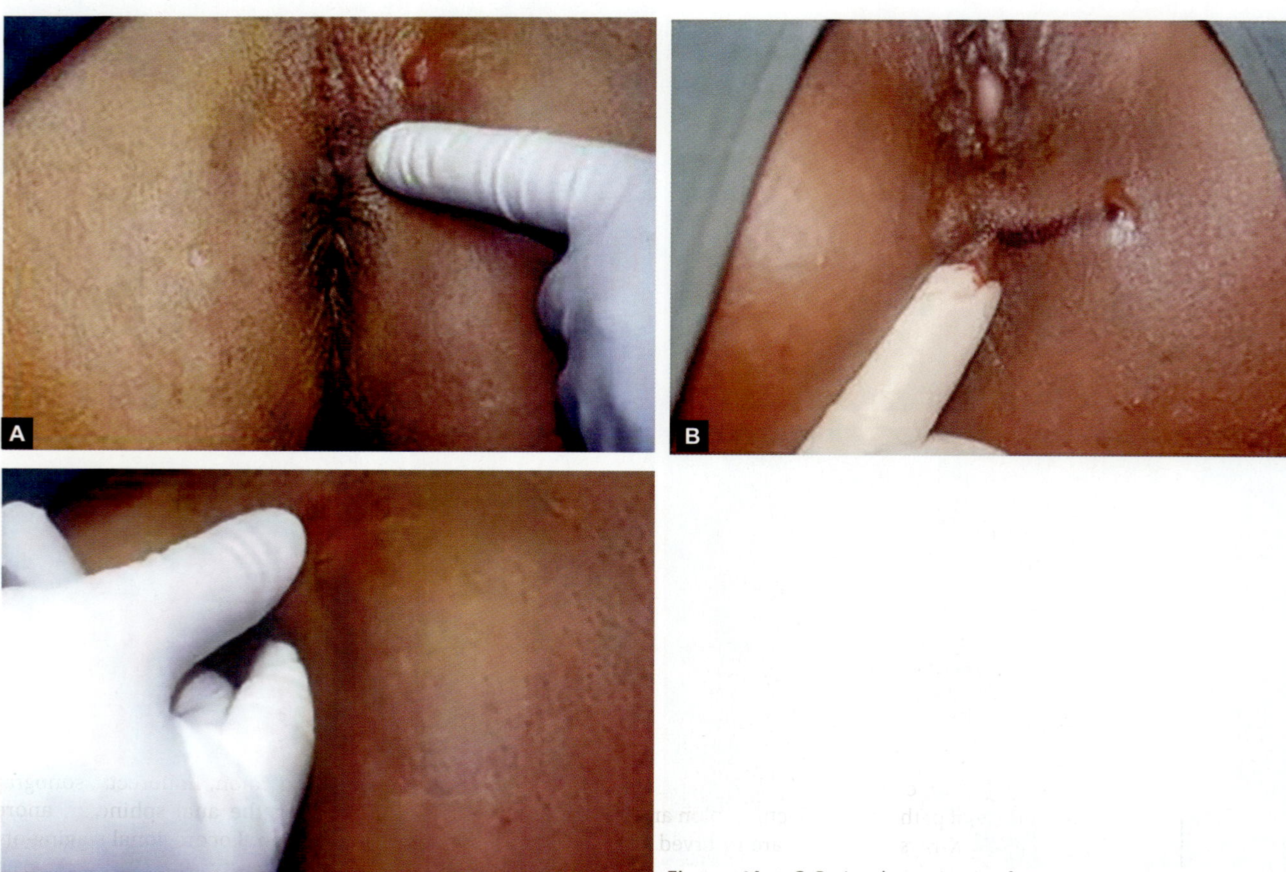

Figures 4A to C Perineal examination for assessing palpability of the fistula tract and locating internal opening

anal endosonography, magnetic resonance imaging (MRI) and computed tomography (CT) fistulography. Microbiology of the underlying infection and histopathology of the fistula tract complete the work-up of a fistula.

IMAGING

As defined earlier, SAF is associated with a single internal and a single external opening, completely palpable tract; and there is no palpable abnormality in upper anal canal or lower rectum. Such fistula can be managed without using imaging modalities. Imaging plays an important role in assessing the topography in patients with CAF, recurrent anal fistula—where the normal perianal anatomy has been distorted by sepsis or previous surgery—and in selected patients with inflammatory bowel disease. Two important questions are required to be answered in such patients before planning treatment. Firstly, can the fistula tract be safely laid open without causing anal incontinence? In other words; how much sphincter would be required to be divided during surgery? Secondly, what is the location and extent of coexisting abscesses and secondary tracts? This knowledge is essential to ensure adequate surgical eradication of infected foci and prevention of recurrence. A number of imaging modalities are available to answer these two questions. It is of utmost importance to understand the merits and demerits of each investigation; this will help in selecting the investigation judiciously. Unnecessary investigations will only add to the cost of the treatment and inconvenience to the patient without providing any value addition.

Fistulography

This is a contrast based study which is used to assess the extent of the fistula tract. After intubation of external opening with small caliber tube, water soluble radiocontrast agent is injected under minimal pressure. Radiographs are obtained in anterior-posterior and if necessary in oblique and lateral projections.

Fistulography is plagued with a number of drawbacks; its description is being included merely for the sake of completion. One of the common problems is failure of primary and secondary tract to fill adequately with contrast agent—this can happen when tracts are closed by debris, pus or granulation tissue. Excessive contrast agent leakage, from either external opening or internal opening, also prohibits filling of primary or secondary tracks with the contrast agent. Fistulography fails to depict these non-opacified tracts which are missed. Similarly higher tracts are not opacified in as high as 44% of patients while horse shoe extensions are missed in 33% patients.[6] A major drawback of fistulography is non-visualization of sphincter muscle complex; hence the relation of fistula tract with sphincter complex cannot be ascertained (Figs 5A and B). It may be extremely difficult to decide whether a fistula tract is intersphincteric or extrasphincteric, or an extension is infralevator or supralevator in position. Similarly, the internal opening is difficult to be located precisely. The injected contrast agent leaks from internal opening into anal canal and travels to rectum. Show of the dye in the rectum is erroneously reported as evidence of high internal opening in the rectum.

Fistulography causes considerable discomfort to the patient, adds to the cost of the treatment, and delays the treatment. It does not provide reliable information regarding topography of the anal fistula. It is not recommended for investigating anal fistula.

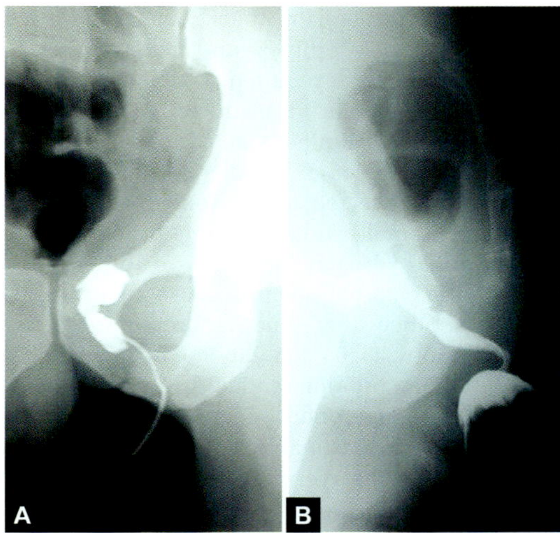

Figures 5A and B Conventional fistulograms

Anal Endosonography

Endoluminal ultrasonography was initially developed for the staging of anorectal cancer; soon its role widened to include benign diseases as well. The examination is well tolerated by the patients and can be done quickly. Imaging of the anal canal and surrounding tissues is done with a rotating endo-probe with 360° real-time scanning of the anus using 10 Mhz transducer. Internal biopsy channel can be used to take biopsy of any suspicious areas.

The patient is placed in the left lateral position. After a careful inspection of the perianal area and DRE, the endo-probe is gently eased into the anal canal to reach distal rectum. As the endo-probe is withdrawn slowly—three levels of anal canal are identified. First is the upper level which is recognized by the U-shaped puborectalis, second is the mid anal canal identified by concentric appearance of internal and external anal sphincter and third part is the lowest part of anal canal marked by the presence of fibers of the superficial external sphincter without the presence of internal sphincter. The internal sphincter is visualized as a black hypoechoic (due to high water content) ring approximately 2-4 mm thick. The subepithelial tissue including the submucosa and hemorrhoidal plexus is seen as a hyperechoic ring between the transducer and the internal sphincter. The external sphincter is displayed as a broad, mixed echogenicity, cylindrical band, approximately 5-8 mm in thickness.[7]

Anal endosonography is considered to be helpful in delineating the internal opening as it is usually positioned right at the probe surface; however, a tract extending till anal mucosal surface is rarely seen. Internal opening is usually appreciated as a hypoechoic spot in the intersphincteric area abutting the internal sphincter which also has a corresponding defect. A breach in the subepithelial layer—suggestive of internal opening—may also be seen rarely. Anal endosonography is particularly useful in identifying intersphincteric fistula as they do not extend beyond intersphincteric space; transsphincteric fistula is also shown by tracts traversing across the external sphincter to reach the ischioanal fossa. Anal endosonography has a high spatial resolution which makes it particularly useful in detecting a small intersphincteric abscess.

However, there are several drawbacks of anal endosonography which limit its use in complex and recurrent anal fistula where other modalities are required to define the topography. Penetration of high frequency transducer is limited beyond the external sphincter which limits its ability to image supralevator space and ischioanal fossa. Anal endosonography cannot reliably differentiate infected tracts from fibrosis which limits its use in recurrent anal fistula. Attempts to identify the fistula tract by injecting hydrogen peroxide or other sonography agents through the external opening cause acoustic shadowing which mimics another tract. Another important drawback of anal endosonography is its inability to image coronal plane which makes it difficult to differentiate supralevator lesion from infralevator lesion. Anal endosonography is highly operator dependent and requires reasonable skill and experience; there are high chances of inter-observer variation. Anal endosonography is a useful investigation, though its wider role in complex and recurrent anal fistula necessitates further research.[8,9]

Magnetic Resonance Imaging

In recent years, MRI has emerged as the leading modality for the preoperative assessment of anal fistula.[10,11] An adequate MRI requires external as well as endoluminal phased array coils. Endoluminal coils are not widely available; however, imaging with external coil also produces good images. The external anal sphincter is appreciated as hypointense on T1W, T2W and fat-suppressed T2W images; it is bounded laterally by the fat of ischioanal fossa. The internal sphincter is hypointense on T1W and T2W TSE images but is seen as hyperintense on fat-suppressed T2W images. Internal sphincter further enhances on post-gadolinium T1W images. Levator ani muscle is well appreciated in coronal image which is helpful to differentiate between supralevator and infralevator lesions (Fig. 6). The puborectalis ring is seen as a condensation of the external sphincter superior fibers. It further merges with the levator plate superiorly. This is important to remember that the anal canal is 45° angulated from the vertical in the sagittal plane. Hence anal canal and fistula track may not be correctly evaluated in straight axial and coronal images. Oblique axial and coronal images oriented orthogonal and parallel to the anal canal, respectively should therefore be obtained.

There are several advantages of MRI: its orthogonal display of the perineum and lower pelvis along with its superior contrast resolution allows faithful reproduction of the topography of fistula tracts. Layers of the anal sphincter are anatomically delineated. The major benefit of MRI is its ability to clearly display the fistula tract as T2W images (TSE and fat-suppressed) provide good contrast between the hyperintense fluid in the tract and the hypointense fibrous wall of the fistula. The site at which the track crosses the sphincter and the presence of horse shoeing is best seen on axial images. Abscesses can also be well seen with post-gadolinium images. Axial images also help to locate the primary tract (ischioanal or intersphincteric). Disruption of the external sphincter distinguishes transsphincteric fistula from an intersphincteric one. The internal opening of the fistula is also best seen in this plane. The axial view also delineates the horseshoe tracts (Fig. 6). In patients with contrast sensitivity diffusion-weighted MRI with T2W imaging can be very useful.

St James's University Hospital MRI classification of perianal fistulae consists of five grades; grade 1, simple linear intersphincteric fistula; grade 2, intersphincteric with abscess or secondary track; grade 3, transsphincteric; grade 4, transsphincteric with abscess or secondary track in ischioanal fossa; grade 5, supralevator and translevator. This relationship has important surgical implications: grades 1 and 2 fistulae do not have involvement of ischioanal or ischiorectal fossa and the disease is confined to the sphincter complex. Grades 3 and 4 have involvement of ischioanal fossa by a fistula tract or abscess related to transsphincteric disease. The fistula tract traverses the levator plate in grade 5. The authors highlighted that this classification deals not only with the demonstration of the primary fistulous track but also with secondary ramifications and associated abscesses. They further concluded that this system is easy to use because it utilizes axial anatomic landmarks familiar to radiologists (Table 2).[10]

Presently, MRI has become the imaging technique of choice for an accurate and noninvasive preoperative assessment of anal fistula.

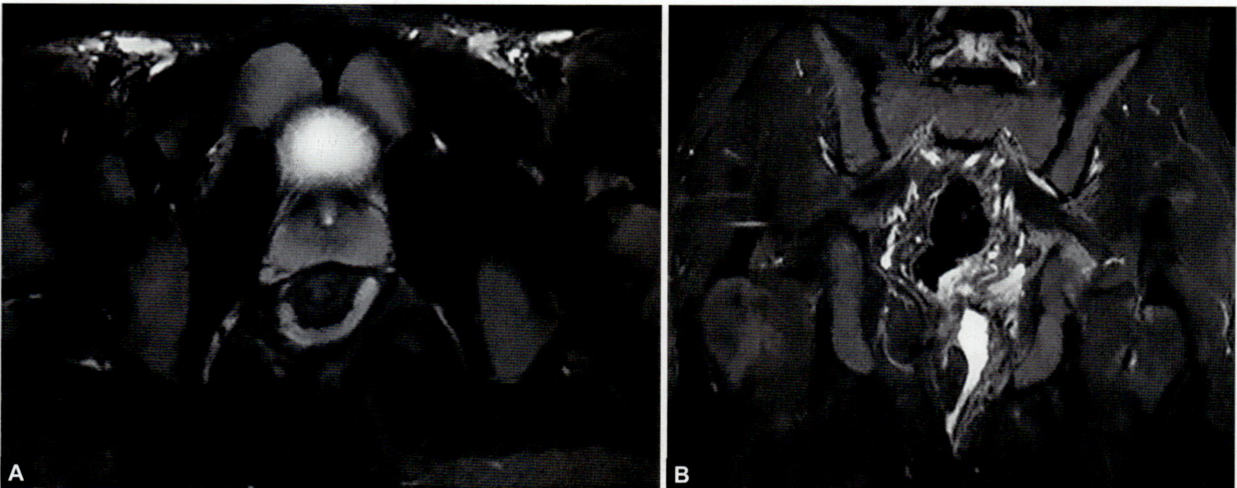

Figures 6A and B (A) MRI T2W axial view showing horseshoe tract; (B) MRI showing fistula tract in right ischiorectal fossa with supralevator extension

Table 2: St James's University Hospital MRI classification of perianal fistulae[10]

Grade	Description
0	Normal appearance
1	Simple linear intersphincteric fistula
2	Intersphincteric fistula with intersphincteric abscess or secondary fistula track
3	Transsphincteric fistula
4	Transsphincteric fistula with abscess or secondary track within the ischiorectal or ischioanal fossa
5	Supralevator and translevator disease

MR fistulography precisely defines the fistula with its secondary tracts or abscesses along with its relation to adjoining structures.

Computed Tomography

Computed tomography fistulography is an upcoming radiological investigation in the preoperative assessment of anal fistula (Figs 7A and B). Since the attenuation values of fibrosis, fistula and sphincter muscles are quite similar, the utility of CT fistulography was limited earlier. Now newer generation of multidetector row CT with its isotropic voxels is expected to improve the results of CT fistulography. The presence of fat in ischioanal fossae helps in evaluating the inflammatory changes. There is scarcity of literature regarding the role of CT fistulography—further research in this modality may clear the air in future.

ANAL MANOMETRY

The use of sphincter pressure testing is not commonly used in patients with anal fistulae. Anal manometry provides information on internal and external sphincter function. Eighty-five percent of the resting anal pressure is the result of internal sphincter activity. Resting pressure provides a useful guide as to how much of the internal anal sphincter can be safely divided. Voluntary contraction provides a measurable assessment of external sphincter and puborectalis activity. Preoperative anal manometry is advisable in patients who have clinical suspicion of decreased anal tone; it will help documenting the anal tone objectively.

SIGMOIDOSCOPY AND COLONOSCOPY

Endoscopy is used to identify underlying inflammatory bowel disease. It is used when the diagnosis is suspected on the basis of physical examination, a history of recurrent or multiple fistulae, or occurrence in young patients.

MICROBIOLOGICAL INVESTIGATIONS

A variety of bacteria *E. coli*, Staphylococcus, Klebseilla, Proteus, Enterococcus, etc. are grown from the pus retrieved from the anal fistula. In addition anaerobic bacteria are also involved. It is desirable that a sample of pus should be obtained on the first hospital visit for smear examination, Gram staining, Ziehl-Neelsen staining, and culture and antibiotic sensitivity. The report would guide the selection of the most appropriate antibiotic as requirement would be different in infections with staphylococcus and enteric bacteria. This may also help to identify tuberculosis.

BIOPSY

Preoperative biopsy is advised if the discharge is particularly glary or mucinous rather than seropurulent. Tissue may be obtained from the edge of the external opening or by curettage of the superficial part of the tract. Rectal biopsy is done if the diagnosis of Crohn's disease is suspected. Anal carcinoma has been reported to masquerade as anal fistula clinically. Histopathological examination of the tract may reveal granulomatous inflammation. For the pathologist it is hazardous to make an etiological diagnosis on the basis of morphology of the granulomas alone—whether

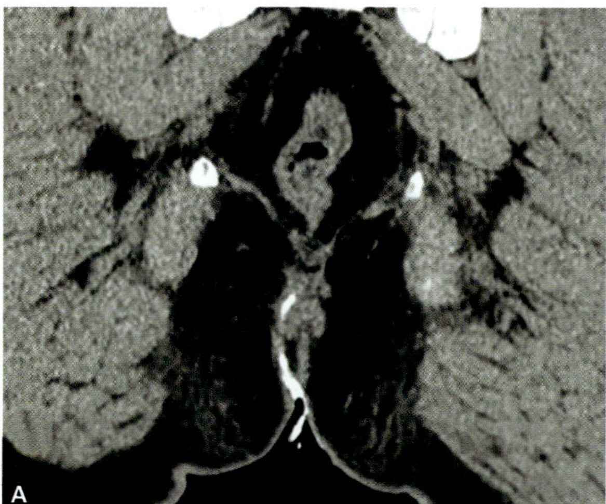

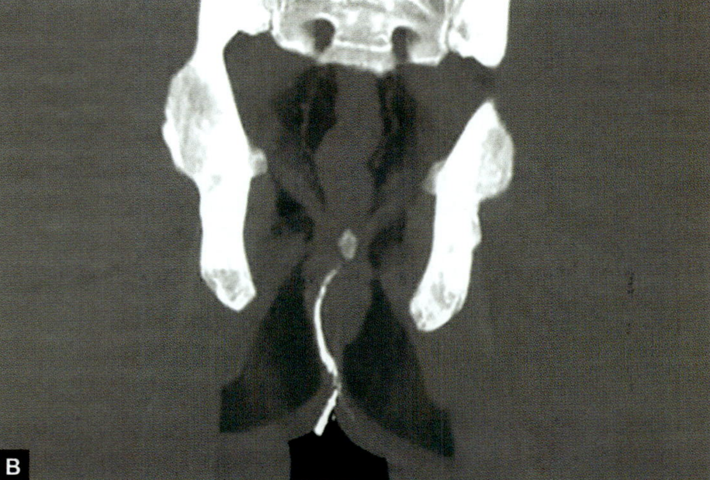

Figures 7A and B (A) Coronal MPR and (B) coronal MIP of MDCT fistulography images show right hyperdense linear infralevator trans-sphincteric tract curving medially and crossing the external sphincter, intersphincteric plane and the internal sphincter

they are composed of epithelioid cells, giant cells or both. Given that the fistula is a conduit for intestinal contents to the perianal skin, the most common granulomas seen on histopathological examination of anal fistula tracts are foreign-body granulomas; and foreign bodies can often be demonstrated in these granulomas. Although uncommon in the Indian subcontinent, other conditions with granulomatous inflammation such as Crohn's disease, and hidradenitis suppurativa may be considered. Granulomatous inflammation may occasionally be seen at the advancing edge of anal carcinoma; however, it is unlikely that the excised tissue will be representative of only the granulomatous component. Other granulomatous disorders such as those of fungal etiology, or syphilis, may be theorized. Staining for acid-fast bacilli is not likely to be rewarding in the absence of caseation necrosis; however, culture and new diagnostic techniques may hold promise.

In summary, because foreign body granulomas are common in the region, evidence of tuberculosis elsewhere in the body should be sought before assigning tuberculosis as the cause of the fistula. If caseous necrosis is seen, diligent search for acid-fast bacilli in multiple sections must be carried out.

MANAGEMENT

The most crucial issue before planning the management of anal fistula in an individual patient is to categorize the fistula as simple or complex fistula. The clinical assessment and imaging—in selected cases—help to assess complexity of the fistula. The treatment methods can be classified into: (i) sphincter sparing methods: fibrin glue, collagen plug, ligation of intersphincteric fistula tract (LIFT), video assisted anal fistula treatment (VAAFT), anocutaneous advancement flap (AAF) and mucosal advancement flap (MAF), (ii) sphincter compromising methods; cutting seton, kshar sutra and fistulotomy. It is difficult to identify the most suitable method by comparing published results (Table 3). The reports differ in respect of number of patients, patient selection, disclosure of type of fistula, period of follow-up, outcome and reporting of complications.[3,5,12-42]

Before commencement of the treatment the surgeon must discuss with the patient the disease process; the complexity of the fistula, options and proposed treatment; possibility of multiple procedure; and likely outcome including development of incontinence, failure of healing, and recurrence, etc. It is wise to offer the patient an option to obtain a second opinion.

Fistulotomy/Fistulectomy

Fistulotomy is the most effective surgical treatment for SAF. A simple fistula, as defined above, involves less than one-third or half of the inferior part of anal sphincters and is not associated with high secondary tract or abscesses. Clinical findings: a single external opening and a single internal opening at dentate line; tract palpable through perianal skin; absence of palpable swelling or induration in relation to anal canal or lower rectum on DRE, indicate SAF. SAF on occasion may be associated with more than one external openings which are situated closely. The tracts from these external openings join each other in the subcutaneous tissue resulting in a common single tract which proceeds further toward the internal opening. A closed/scarred external opening may not allow passage of a probe into the fistula tract. In these cases, a circular incision is made around the external opening and deepened. Sharp dissection is undertaken around the fistula tract which feels like a cord. The tract is divided transversely at a distance of 1–2 cm from the skin. Now, the lumen of the tract is exposed which can be cannulated to perform a dye test. A probe can be negotiated into the tract before proceeding with fistulotomy. The laid open fistula tract should be curetted to remove granulation tissue; any residual spot of granulation tissue needs further exploration to detect a secondary tract. Marsupialization of the fistulotomy wound (approximation of cut edges of fistula tract with the skin) further reduces the size of open wound and facilitates postoperative management and results in early healing[11] (Figs 8A to G). Fistulectomy is another conventional approach to tackle SAF; it involves complete excision of fistula tract thereby eliminating risk of missing secondary tracts and providing complete tissue for histopathological examination. The resulting wound is larger as compared to operative wound following fistulotomy. A regimen of perioperative antibiotics is sufficient for surgery in case of SAF.

Triple Procedure

Complex anal fistula is not amenable to straight forward treatment such as fistulotomy. Presence of a high fistula tract involving large part of anal sphincters, abscesses in high locations—sublevator, supralevator and deep post anal space—and secondary/horseshoe tracts do not allow a single procedure to succeed. Each of these elements needs attention individually. The authors employ a "Triple procedure" comprising of partial fistulectomy/fistulotomy, laying open and drainage of deep seated abscesses/secondary tracts and usage of cutting seton for management of CAF.[43]

Table 3: Outcome of various surgical procedures

Procedure	*Follow-up (Months)*	*Healing (%)*	*Recurrence (%)*	*Incontinence (%)*	*Reference*
Fibrin glue	06–67	10–81	25–30	0	3, 5, 13, 14
Collagen plug	03–93	32–76	5–59	0	15–22
Fistulotomy	03–12	88–100	4–12	5–12	12, 23–26
LIFT	3–9	61–83	17–28	0	27–31
AAF	6–32	46–98	3–11	0–30	32–35
MAF	19–72	63–97	3–69	15–23	36–40
VAAFT	0–9	73.1–82	NA	NA	41–42

Abbreviation: NA, not available/not stated

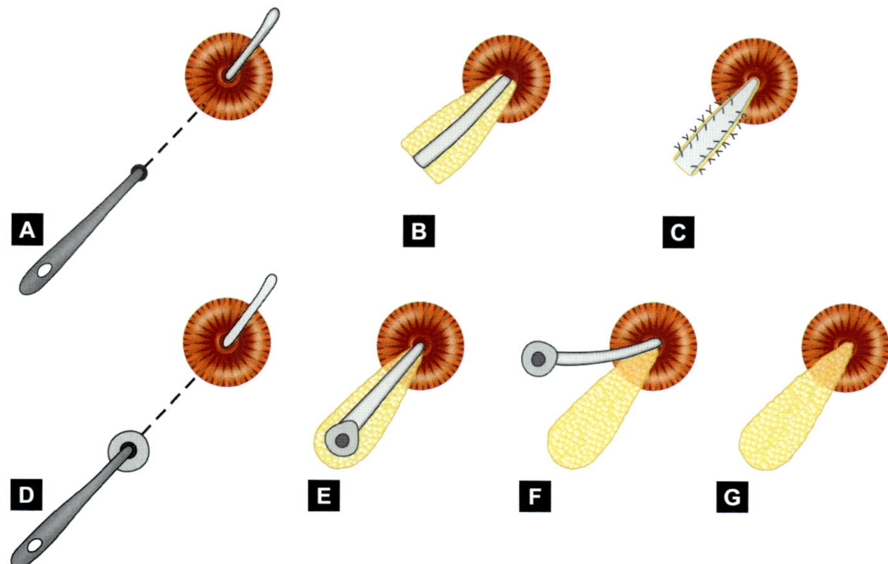

Figures 8A to G Fistulotomy: (A) Malleable probe in the tract, incision over the tract; (B) The fistula tract laid open; (C) Marsupialization by suturing edge of the tract to the skin. Fistulectomy: (D) Incision encircles the external opening also, (E and F) The fistula tract being dissected by sharp dissection; (G) Resulting wound which is larger

Partial Fistulectomy/Fistulotomy

The first step of the procedure is intraoperative assessment of the fistula. The external opening, palpable tract, internal opening, palpable swelling/induration in anal canal or lower rectum are looked for. A dye test is carried out by inserting a moist gauze piece in anorectum, and injecting gently methylene blue through external opening. Staining of the gauze confirms presence and patency of internal opening.

At this stage, the fistula tract is probed with a malleable probe gently and carefully. During probing, a finger should be kept in the anal canal/rectum to monitor the position of the tip of the probe. No force should be applied while passing the probe, slight rotation of the probe may allow the probe to negotiate the tract. The direction and extent of passage of fistula provide valuable information regarding the topography of the tract. In a low fistula, the probe forms an acute angle with the skin and the tip may come out through the internal opening. In contrast, the probe makes almost a right angle with the skin in case of high fistula. The tip of the probe stops where the tract acutely changes direction. The passage of the probe may also be stalled if the tract is communicating with an abscess cavity. The tip of the probe may be felt at the level of rectum by the finger kept in the anorectum; this finding suggests supralevator extension of fistula.

Incision is planned according to the location of the external opening, the extent of the tract, and the plan of surgery. In case the external opening is situated laterally, it is prudent to plan a semicircular incision in perianal skin beyond the extent of external sphincter. If fistulectomy is planned, the incision should go around the external opening. If fistulotomy is planned, the incision should pass through the lumen of the tract (Fig. 9). In case the external opening is situated in posterior midline, it should be explored through a mid line incision extending from the anus to the tip of coccyx. The fistula tract is followed, by sharp dissection, from the external opening to the point where it enters the sphincters or levator ani. In case of fistulectomy, the tract is to be amputated at this level. In case of fistulotomy, all the granulation tissues lining the tracts are scrapped with the help of a curette. The remaining tract extending to internal opening through the sphincters is also explored and curetted if possible. Even if external opening is situated far away from anus, the incision, made at the outer limit of external sphincter, will meet the tract in the depth of the wound, where the tract is laid open. The lateral part of the tract is curetted and the granulation

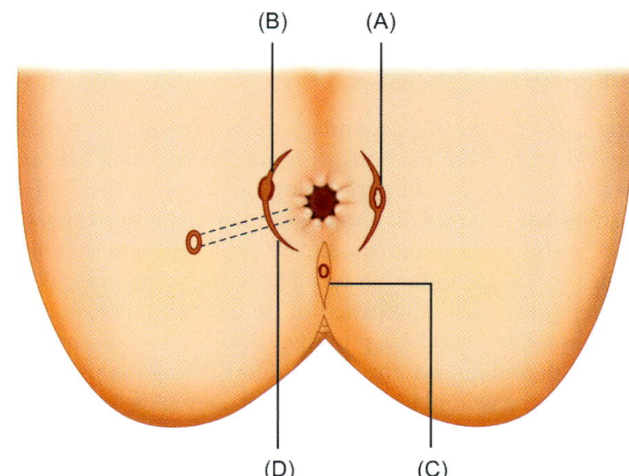

Figure 9 (A) Incision for fistulectomy encircling the external opening, (B) incision for fistulotomy passing through the external opening, (C) incision for posterior fistula, (D) tract from distant external opening being intersected by the incision

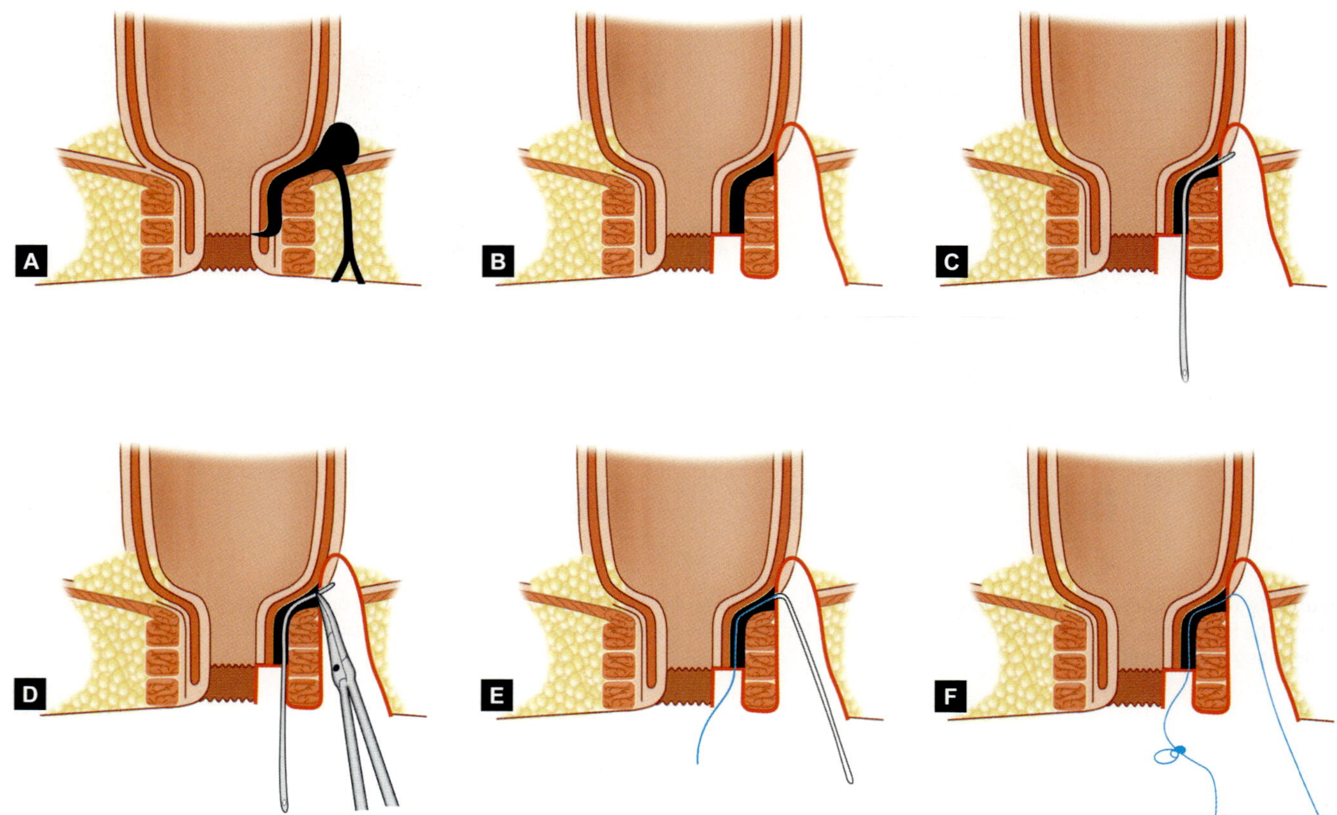

Figures 10A to F (A) Complex anal fistula—suprasphincteric fistula with supralevator collection; (B) Deroofed abscess following partial fistulectomy and drainage of abscess, (C to E) A long, slim, curved artery forceps is passed into the fistulectomy/fistulotomy wound and the tip of the malleable probe is located and caught by the artery forceps and pulled out of the wound. Seton which is threaded in the eye of malleable probe also comes out of the wound; (F) Looped seton is being tied around the sphincter

tissue is removed; the medial part is traced up to the sphincters/levator ani. Division of the lower part of internal sphincter below the internal opening is done to lay open the intersphincteric space affected by anal gland sepsis. The excised fistula tract/granulation tissue is sent for histopathology examination.

Drainage of the Abscess

During fistulectomy, the secondary tracts are identified by show of the dye as their connections with the primary tract are severed during dissection. While performing fistulotomy, the laid open tract should be curetted to remove granulation tissue. Any residual spot of granulation tissue should be explored with a probe for presence of a secondary tract. The sublevator, supralevator, and deep post anal abscesses, or secondary/horseshoe tracts are diligently searched by probing. These abscesses/horseshoe tracts are deroofed and curetted. Wide drainage is provided by landscaping the wound into a skin based cone (Figs 10A to C).

Seton Placement

Seton placement in CAF needs special mention. Silk, nylon, polypropylene, vascular loop, etc. are used as seton. The seton is placed in the fistula tract with the help of a malleable probe. In high transsphincteric fistula and suprasphincteric fistula, the tract takes an acute turn in direction at the level of sphincters. Hence, a probe cannot be negotiated from the external opening to the internal opening in an ordinary way. Indiscrete attempt to negotiate the tract is likely to cause false passage. In such cases, a malleable probe is passed from the internal opening and negotiated up to the highest point of the tract where it is halted due to change in the direction of the tract. Now a long, slim, curved artery forceps is passed into the fistulectomy/fistulotomy wound and the tip of the probe is located and caught by the artery forceps and pull out of the wound. A seton is threaded in the eye of the probe and pull through the tract (Figs 10D and E). The seton

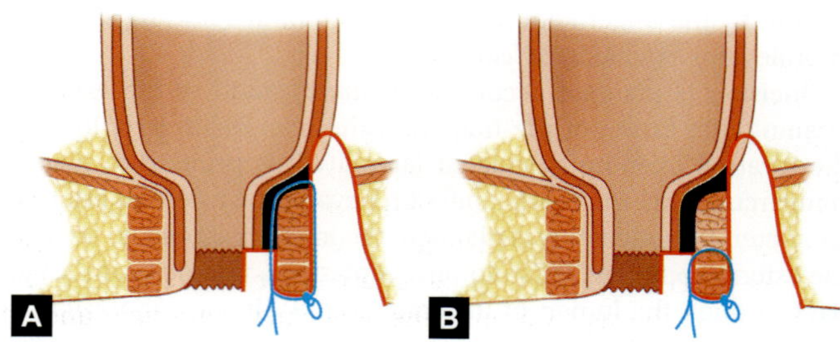

Figures 11A and B Cutting seton—gradual cutting of sphincter with cephalad healing of wound

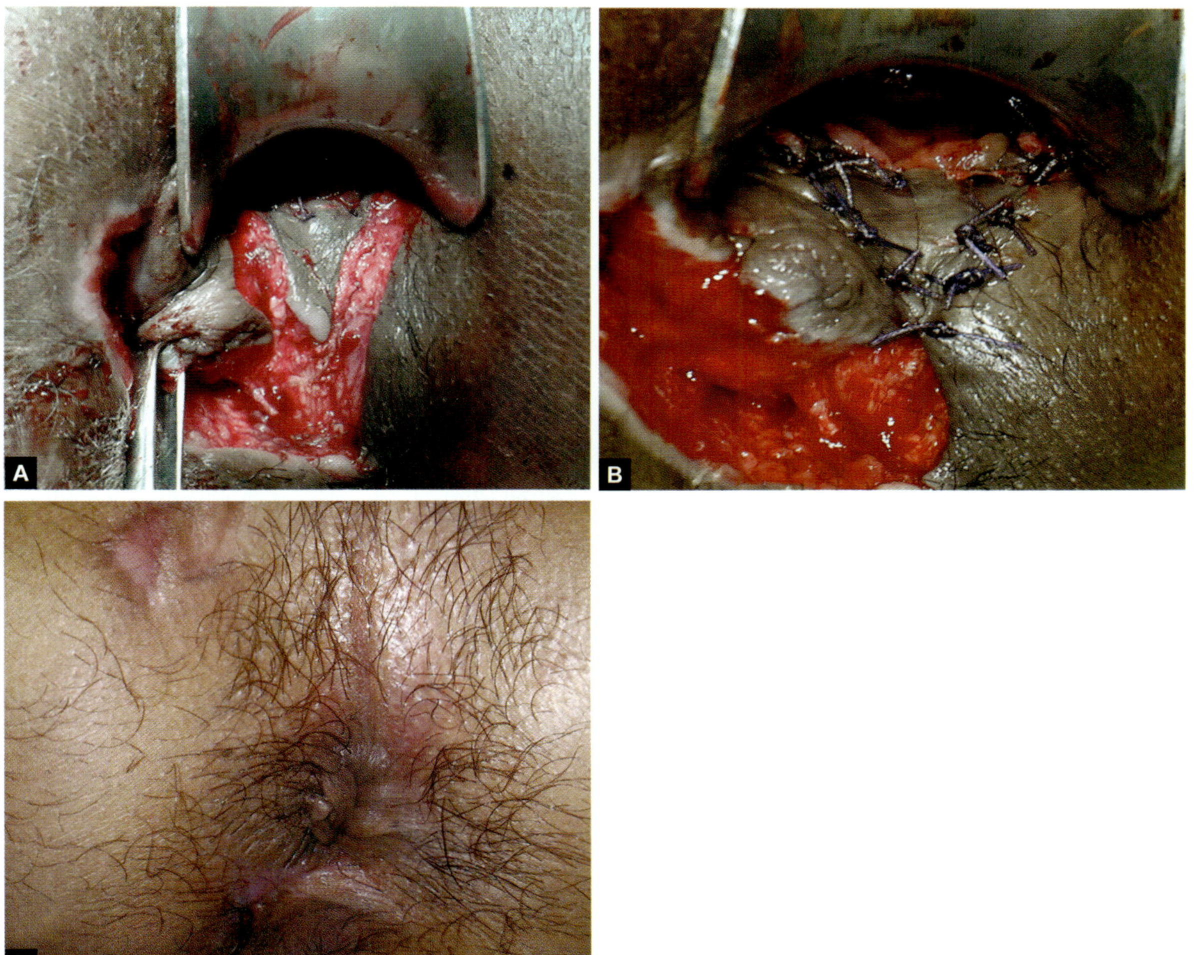

Figures 12A to C Operative images of anocutanoeus advancement flap

is tied around the sphincters tightly to allow gradual cutting of the sphincters (Fig. 11). In patients, in whom the internal opening is not discernable, the third component of the triple procedure—seton placement—cannot be undertaken, and the operative wound is allowed to heal under supervision.

The gradual division of the sphincter by the seton allows fibrosis to occur, and limits retraction of sphincter and anal incontinence. The seton becomes loose as the sphincters are cut and it needs to be tightened or changed at an interval of 1–2 weeks, until the whole sphincter is divided. Looped seton facilitates change of seton as an outpatient procedure.[44] The division of sphincter by cutting seton may take several weeks. The process can be hastened by performing a delayed fistulotomy—division of the sphincter encircled by the seton—about 3 weeks after the index procedure. Cutting seton may not be suitable when the whole sphincter is involved and its cutting may lead to disturbing fecal incontinence. In such cases, the seton is loosely tied as drainage seton and sepsis are allowed to be controlled before a definitive procedure like AAF and MAF is used to close the internal opening of the fistula. It is desirable the sepsis around the anal canal is brought under control by drainage of abscesses, antibiotics, and use of seton in such situations.[45]

Anocutaneous Advancement Flap

The patient is advised liquid diet for 1 day prior to surgery, and the bowel is prepared by an osmotic laxative like polyethylene glycol. An inverted U-shaped or a V-shaped incision is made in the anoderm and the perianal skin. A flap consisting of dermis, subcutaneous fat, and a few fibers of internal sphincter is raised. The proximal part of the tract is curetted or excised and the internal opening is closed by approximating the sphincter by interrupted absorbable sutures. The mobilized flap is now moved over the internal opening and sutures to the mucosa and underlying sphincter. The flap is mobile and can be advanced up to 2 cm without tension (Figs 12A to C).

The success of the procedure depends of the viability of the flap. Patients with two or more previous operations have poor outcome of AAF. This may be due to fibrosis and scarring in the area caused by previous surgery.[34,35] The patient is advised bed rest, liquid diet, antibiotics and bowel movements are avoided for next 3 days.

Mucosal Advancement Flap

A small transverse elliptical incision is made around the internal opening. The fistula tract is cored out up to and through the external sphincter. The internal opening is closed with interrupted absorbable sutures. Two oblique incisions are made upward from the either end of the elliptical wound, and a rectal flap consisting of mucosa, submucosa, and some fibers of circular muscle is developed. The flap extends up to 5 cm cephalad to the internal opening. The flap is mobilized downward to cover the internal opening and it is sutured to the mucosa/anoderm distal to the internal opening. The patent distal tract or the fistulotomy wound drains the operated area. It has been demonstrated that partial thickness flaps have better results than mucosal advancement flaps.[37] Pretreatment with non-cutting seton or diverting stoma increases success rate to 97%. The creation of a stoma is, however, a too radical step for the management of anal fistula.

OTHER NEWER TECHNIQUES

Last two decades have witnessed a number of techniques being mushroomed in and around the corner of the world for the management of anal fistula. These newer techniques have shown very good healing rates at some centers; however, these techniques are plagued with a number of limitations—the results of these techniques could not be reproduced uniformly at even high volume centers; most of these studies involving these techniques did not have separate patient groups for SAF and CAF, thereby limiting the possibility of assessment of their real value in the management of CAF.

Fibrin Glue

Fibrin glue was first reported to be used for anal fistula in early 1980s. In this technique, a mixture of fibrinogen and thrombin is prepared and is injected into the fistula tract after curettage. The probable mode of action is stimulation of pluripotent cells and growth of fibroblasts which seal the tract. These fibroblasts then lay down collagen and extracellular matrix. However, most of the treatment failure cases occur in first three months.[16] Both shorter fistula tracts (<3.5 cm in size) and longer tend to recur more as they do not hold the glue.[13] Complications include abscess formation and formation of new fistula tracts. Reported success rate of anal fistula varies from 10% to 60% in CAF and 81.3% in SAF (Table 3). The recurrence rates noted vary from 25% to 30%. Though most of these studies had a small sample size which cast doubt to its real value, it is worthwhile exploring this option in view of its sphincter saving nature. The high cost of fibrin glue limits its wide spread use.

Collagen Plug

Collagen plug is a biomaterial derived from submucosa of small intestine of swine. It is pliable but strong tissue which acts as a framework for host cells to repair damaged tissues. The defect of the fistula tract is bridged using a biocompatible material and which acts as a scaffold for fibroblasts to help in tissue healing. The tract is first explored and thoroughly irrigated with diluted hydrogen peroxide. A probe is passed through the external opening to emerge at the internal opening. The apex of the plug is then tied to the probe which has been brought out through the internal opening and the plug is pulled out from the external opening. The plug is then cut to fit the tract and secured to the internal opening, thus incorporating it with the mucosa of anorectum, close to internal opening. The healing rates and recurrence rate ranged from 32% to 76% and 5% to 58.8% respectively in the previously reported studies; no incontinence was seen postoperatively (Table 3).

LIFT (Ligation of Intersphincteric Fistula Tract)

This procedure was first described by Rojanashkul[46] from Thailand in 2007. Internal opening is identified through gentle probing of the tract or injection of water through the external opening. The intersphincteric plane is entered through a curvilinear incision at the site of the tract. The tract is hooked with a small right angled clamp after identification. After the intersphincteric tract is identified and dissected out, it is ligated close to the internal sphincter. Secure ligation of the intersphincteric tract abutting the internal opening is the key to success. The tract lateral to the suture site is divided and is excised. Rest of the cavity is thoroughly curetted and all the infected granulation tissues are removed. The open defect at the external anal sphincter is sutured through the intersphincteric wound. Finally, the wound is closed loosely. The excised fistulous tract is sent for histopathological examination. This technique is a sphincter saving procedure. Rojanashkul[46] et al. conducted the study in 18 patients out of which one was suprasphincteric and four were high transsphincteric fistulae. Seventeen patients (94.4%) had successful healing. According to him, recurrence is a major concern. The healing rates reported by the studies vary from 61% to 83% with recurrence in 16.7% to 28%. (Table 3) Since this procedure does not cause anal incontinence and has good healing rate, it can be used for complex anal fistulae.

VAAFT (Video-Assisted Anal Fistula Treatment)

VAAFT was first described by Merinero et al in the year 2012. It is a composite procedure involving fibreoptic fistuloscopy, curettage, irrigation of the fistula tract, closure of the internal opening using a small curved stapler and drainage of the tract through the external opening. They included 74 patients (75.5%) of high transsphincteric fistula, 9 patients (9.2%) of extrasphincteric fistula, 6 patients (6.2%) of suprasphincteric fistula, and 9 patients (9.2%) of horseshoe fistula. They reported that the primary healing was achieved in 72 patients (73.5%) within 2–3 months. They also highlighted that the procedure requires specialized and costly equipment.[41] Another study to evaluate VAAFT was conducted by Schwandner et al; they included patients of anal fistulae with Crohn's disease. The authors reported a success rate of 82% after a mean follow-up of 9 months.[42] Though VAAFT seems a promising surgical technique, there is paucity of evidence to recommend this method of treatment at present.

PALLIATION FOR REFRACTORY FISTULA

Some fistulae fail to heal or recur despite best efforts in best hands. No treatment has cent percent success rate. More aggressive treatment may damage/scar the sphincter to the extent that the cure may become worse than the disease itself. It is possible to barter multiple and distant external openings for a single external opening lying close to anus and to control recurrent sepsis by draining the fistula tract with a permanent seton.[47] A judiciously performed triple procedure—with deployment of a loose seton—can achieve this objective. The seton allows the pus to drain, prevents abscess formation and extension of the disease to deeper planes. All surgeons should realize this end point and not subject the patient to repeated and futile operations.

REFERENCES

1. Agrawal V, Garg PK, Jain BK, Mishra K, Mohanty D. Amoebic anal fistula: new insight in a old disease. Acta Med Indones. 2014;46:131-3.
2. Parks AG, Gordon PH, Hardcastle JC. A classification of fistula in ano. Br J Surg. 1992;79:195-205.
3. Mishra A, Shah S, Nar AS, Bawa A. The Role of fibrin glue in the treatment of high and low fistulae in ano. J Clin Diagn Res. 2013;7:876-9.
4. Bleier JI, Moloo H. Current management of cryptoglandular fistula-in-ano. World J Gastroenterol. 2011;17:3286-91.
5. van Koperen PJ, Wind J, Bemelman WA, Slors JF. Fibrin glue and transanal rectal advancement flap for high transsphincteric perianal fistulae; is there any advantage? Int J Colorectal Dis. 2008;23:697-701.
6. Kujipers HC, Schulpen T. Fistulography for fistula-in-ano. Is it useful? Dis Colon Rectum. 1985;28:103-5.
7. Mortensen N. Rectal and anal endosonography. Gut. 1992;33:148-9.
8. Fernández-Frías AM, Pérez-Vicente F, Arroyo A, Sánchez-Romero AM, Navarro JM, Serrano P, et al. Is anal endosonography useful in the study of recurrent complex fistula-in-ano? Rev Esp Enferm Dig. 2006;98:573-81.
9. Deen KI, Williams JG, Hutchinson R, Keighley MR, Kumar D. Fistulas in ano: endoanal ultrasonographic assessment assists decision making for surgery. Gut. 1994;35:391-4.
10. Morris J, Spencer JA, Ambrose NS. MR imaging classification of perianal fistulas and its implications for patient management. Radiographics. 2000;20:623-35.
11. Vanbeckevoort D, Bielen D, Vanslembrouck R, Van Assche G. Magnetic resonance imaging of perianal fistulas. Magn Reson Imaging Clin N Am. 2014;22:113-23.
12. Jain BK, Vaibhaw K, Garg PK, Gupta S, Mohanty D. Comparison of a fistulectomy and a fistulotomy with marsupialization in the management of a simple anal fistula: a randomized, controlled pilot trial. J Korean Soc Coloproctol. 2012;28:78-82.
13. Venkatesh KS, Ramanujam P. Fibrin glue application in treatment of recurrent anal fistulae. Dis Colon Rectum. 1999;42:1136-9.
14. Damin DC, Rosito MA, Contu PC, Tarta C. Fibrin glue in the management of complex anal fistula. Arq Gastroenterol. 2009;46:300-3.
15. Blom J, Husberg-Sellberg B, Lindelius A, Gustafsson UM, Carlens S, Oppelstrup H, et al. Results of collagen plug occlusion of anal fistula: a multicentre study of 126 patients. Colorectal Dis. 2014;16(8):626-30.
16. Cintron JR, Abcarian H, Chaudhry V, Singer M, Hunt S, Birnbaum E, et al. Treatment of fistula-in-ano using a porcine small intestinal submucosa anal fistula plug. Tech Coloproctol. 2013;17:187-91.
17. Ellis CN, Rostas JW, Greiner FG. Long-term outcomes with the use of bioprosthetic plugs for the management of complex anal fistulae. Dis Colon Rectum. 2010;53:798-802.
18. McGee MF, Champagne BJ, Stulberg JJ, Reynolds H, Marderstein E, Delaney CP. Tract length predicts successful closure with anal fistula plug in cryptoglandular fistulae. Dis Colon Rectum. 2010;53:1116-20.
19. Lenisa L, Espìn-Basany E, Rusconi A, Mascheroni L, Escoll-Rufino J, Lozoya-Trujillo R, et al. Anal fistula plug is a valid alternative option for the treatment of complex anal fistula in the long term. Int J Colorectal Dis. 2010;25:1487-93.
20. Wang JY, Garcia-Aguilar J, Sternberg JA, Abel ME, Varma MG. Treatment of transsphincteric anal fistulae: are fistula plugs an acceptable alternative? Dis Colon Rectum. 2009;52:692-7.
21. Christoforidis D, Pieh MC, Madoff RD, Mellgren AF. Treatment of transsphincteric anal fistulae by endorectal advancement flap or collagen fistula plug: a comparative study. Dis Colon Rectum. 2009;52:18-22.
22. van Koperen PJ, D'Hoore A, Wolthuis AM, Bemelman WA, Slors JF. Anal fistula plug for closure of difficult anorectal fistula: a prospective study. Dis Colon Rectum. 2007;50:2168-72.
23. Linsey I, Smiglin-Humphreys MM, Cunningham C, Mortensen N, George B. A randomized controlled trial of fibrin glue vs. conventional treatment for anal fistula. Dis Colon Rectum. 2002;45:1608-15.
24. Ratto C, Litta F, Parello A, Zaccone G, Donisi L, De Simone V. Fistulotomy with end-to-end primary sphincteroplasty for anal fistula: results from a prospective study. Dis Colon Rectum. 2013;56:226-33.
25. Ho YH, Tan M, Leong AF, Choen F. Marsupialization of fistulotomy wounds improves healing: a randomized controlled trial. Br J Surg. 1998;85:105-7.
26. Kronborg O. To lay open or excise a fistula-in-ano: a randomized trial. Br J Surg. 1985;72:970.
27. Sileri P, Giarratano G, Franceschilli L, Limura E, Perrone F, Stazi A, et al. Ligation of the intersphincteric fistula tract (LIFT): a minimally invasive procedure for complex anal fistula: two-year results of a prospective multicentric study. Surg Innov. 2013;21(5):476-80.
28. Campbell ML, Abboud EC, Dolberg ME, Sanchez JE, Marcet JE, Rasheid SH. Treatment of refractory perianal fistulae with ligation of the intersphincteric fistula tract: preliminary results. Am Surg. 2013;79:723-7.
29. Liu WY, Aboulian A, Kaji AH, Kumar RR. Long-term results of ligation of intersphincteric fistula tract (LIFT) for fistula-in-ano. Dis Colon Rectum. 2013;56:343-7.
30. Ooi K, Skinner I, Croxford M, Faragher I, McLaughlin S. Managing fistula-in-ano with ligation of the intersphincteric fistula tract procedure: the Western Hospital experience. Colorectal Dis. 2012;14:599-603.
31. Shanwani A, Nor AM, Amri N. Ligation of the intersphincteric fistula tract (LIFT): a sphincter-saving technique for fistula-in-ano. Dis Colon Rectum. 2010;53:39-42.
32. Amin SN, Tierney GM, Lund JN, Armitage NC.V-Y advancement flap for treatment of fistula-in-ano. Dis Colon Rectum. 2003;46: 540-3.
33. Jun SH, Choi GS. Anocutaneous advancement flap closure of high anal fistulae. Br J Surg. 1999;86:490-2.
34. Zimmerman DD, Briel JW, Gosselink MP, Schouten WR. Anocutaneous advancement flap repair of transsphincteric fistulae. Dis Colon Rectum. 2001;44:1474-80.
35. Sungurtekin U, Sungurtekin H, Kabay B, Tekin K, Aytekin F, Erdem E, et al. Anocutaneous V-Y advancement flap for the treatment of complex perianal fistula. Dis Colon Rectum. 2004;47: 2178-83.
36. Muhlmann MD, Hayes JL, Merrie AE, Parry BR, Bissett IP. Complex anal fistulae: plug or flap? ANZ J Surg. 2011;81:720-4.
37. Khafagy W, Omar W, El Nakeeb A, Fouda E, Yousef M, Farid M. Treatment of anal fistulae by partial rectal wall advancement flap or mucosal advancement flap: a prospective randomized study. Int J Surg. 2010;8:321-5.
38. Van der Hagen SJ, Baeten CG, Soeters PB, van Gemert WG. Long-term outcome following mucosal advancement flap for high perianal fistulae and fistulotomy for low perianal fistulae: recurrent

perianal fistulae: failure of treatment or recurrent patient disease? Int J Colorectal Dis. 2006;21:784-90.
39. Van der Hagen SJ, Baeten CG, Soeters PB, Beets-Tan RG, Russel MG, van Gemert WG. Staged mucosal advancement flap for the treatment of complex anal fistulae: pretreatment with noncutting Setons and in case of recurrent multiple abscesses a diverting stoma. Colorectal Dis. 2005;7:513-8.
40. Golub RW, Wise WE Jr, Kerner BA, Khanduja KS, Aguilar PS. Endorectal mucosal advancement flap: the preferred method for complex mucosal advancement flap: the preferred method for complex cryptoglandular fistula-in-ano. J Gastrointest Surg. 1997; 1:487-91.
41. Meinero P, Mori L. Video-assisted anal fistula treatment (VAAFT): a novel sphincter-saving procedure for treating complex anal fistulae. Tech Coloproctol. 2011;15:417-22.
42. Schwandner O. Video-assisted anal fistula treatment (VAAFT) combined with advancement flap repair in Crohn's disease. Tech Coloproctol. 2013;17:221-5.
43. Jain BK, Garg PK. Triple procedure for complex anal fistula. Tech Coloproctol. 2014;19:47-50.
44. Jain BK, Gupta A. Simple method of tightening cutting setons (correspondence), Br J Surg. 1995;82:996-1004.
45. Garg PK, Jain BK. Seton drainage in high anal fistula. Int J Colorectal Dis. 2011;26:1495.
46. Rojanashkul A, Pattanaarun J, Sahakitrungruang C, Tantiphlachiva K. Total anal sphincter saving technique for fistula-in-ano; the ligation of intersphincteric fistula tract. J Med Assoc Thai. 2007;90: 581-6.
47. Jain BK, Garg PK. Palliation for refractory anal fistula-an honorable respite. Int J Colorectal Dis. 2014;30:857-8.

CHAPTER 88

Rectal Prolapse

Rajinder Parshad, Kamal Kataria, Saurabh Singhal, Kamlesh Kumar

INTRODUCTION

Rectal prolapse is a debilitating condition known since ancient times[1] and entails circumferential protrusion of all layers of rectum through anal canal. The exact etiology and an ideal surgical treatment continue to elude the clinicians. This is evident from the fact that many etiological theories have been proposed and many surgical procedures are in vogue. The rectal prolapse may be full thickness when there is protrusion of the entire rectal wall through the anal canal or it may be protrusion of only rectal mucosa. Occult rectal prolapse or internal intussusception refers to a condition when rectal wall has prolapsed but doesn't come out through anus.[2,3] Some view it as an end point of the spectrum that begins with internal intussusception and progresses through mucosal prolapse to a full thickness rectal prolapse. In this chapter we shall briefly review the current thinking and evidence with regard to the etio-pathogenesis and management of patients with rectal prolapse. The discussion shall be restricted to the management of adult patients with complete rectal prolapse.

History

The Egyptian and Greek civilizations were familiar with this disease and the earliest written documentation of rectal prolapse was found in Ebers Papyrus of 1500 B.C. Further evidence exists in the form of a preserved mummy (400–500 B.C.) with a rectal prolapse.[1]

The treatment modalities used in historic times were barbaric and included hanging the person by the heels and shaking the person followed by application of 'caustic potass' and binding the thighs for few days, burning the anus in an attempt to cause scarring to rectal mucosa, application of powdered dry dung of dog fed on bones and use of specially carved sticks during defecation to prevent prolapse. More gentle treatment options used were wearing of breeches and truss made of leather and iron wings.[4]

Pathopysiology

In the modern era various anatomical and functional causes have been postulated to be associated with the development of rectal prolapse and the treatment options have also evolved as the understanding of possible mechanisms has improved. Some of the salient hypotheses related to development of rectal prolapse are listed in Table 1.

Two theories have dominated the thinking with regard to cause of rectal prolapse.

Sliding Hernia Theory

This theory was propounded by Moschowitz in 1912 who proposed that rectal prolapse is a sliding hernia which develops due to weakness in the transversalis fascia secondary to increased intra-abdominal pressure.[10] Sigmoid and occasionally small bowel lying within a deep cul-de sac along with acute angulation of recto sigmoid was thought to result in excessive straining at defecation eventually culminating in herniation through a weakened pelvic floor (Fig. 1).[4,15] This concept led to attempts at repair of rectal prolapse by obliterating the deep pouch of Douglas but the results were dismal.[4,16]

Intussusception Theory

Salmon in 1931 hypothesized intussusception to be the cause of rectal prolapse.[1,5] It is believed that rectal prolapse starts as circumferential intussusception 6–8 cm above the anal verge

Table 1: Various theories to explain pathophysiology of rectal prolapse

Year Author	*Proposed causes*	*Remarks*
1831, Salmon[5]	• Intussusception of colon in the upper part of rectum	Devadhar (1965) and Broden and Snellman (1968) by means of cineradiography and defecating proctograms confirmed the Intussusception theory.[6,7]
1847, Bodenhamer[8]	1. Increased intra-abdominal pressure 2. The anal sphincter weakness s 3. Less curved intestine and imperfect development of some of the contiguous supporting structures	
1903, Tuttle[9]	• Described the structures that support the rectum in the lower, middle and upper part and attributed procidentia to the weakening and destruction of the supports along with some force capable of dislodging the rectum from its position.	
1912, Moschcowitz[10]	• Proposed the sliding hernia theory and stated that rectal prolapse is similar to the "hernie par glissement".	Pantanowitz and Levine in 1975 provided radiological evidence of sliding hernia theory by means of strategically placed metallic clips on the prolapsed rectum.[11]
1920, Todd[12]	• Stressed the Importance of the lateral rectal stalks in upholding the rectum.	
1939, Pemberton and Stalker[13]	• Proposed that rectal prolapsed occurs due to "loosely attached rectum".	
1942, Graham[14]	• Supported the Moschcowitz's hypothesis and suggested that rectal proplapse results from a sliding hernia of the anterior wall of rectum at the level of the cul-de-sac or rectovesical pouch.	

and eventually everts through the anus (Fig. 2). This is the most popular theory and has been subsequently confirmed in the modern times by radiological studies employing cine radiography and defecography. However, there are studies that suggest that asymptomatic intussusception exists and not all, found to have intussusception, progress to overt rectal prolapse.[17,18]

Figure 1 Sliding hernia theory; showing herniation of small bowel at weak pelvic floor through cul-de sac

From anatomic point of view, pelvic floor is the major support to the pelvic viscera. it is a combination of several muscles, including pelvic diaphragm and urogenital diaphragm, attached to the lower sacro-pelvic cavity and fashioned like a sling around pelvic viscera thus providing the sphincter functions to urethra, anal canal and vagina. The levator ani along with fibres of puborectalis muscle loop around lower rectum and give stability and continence mechanism to rectum.[10,19] Inferior rectal branches of pudendal nerve innervate above mentioned muscles along with external anal sphincter and thus significantly contribute towards support and continence mechanisms. The weakening of these supports structures either congenitally or secondary to trauma,

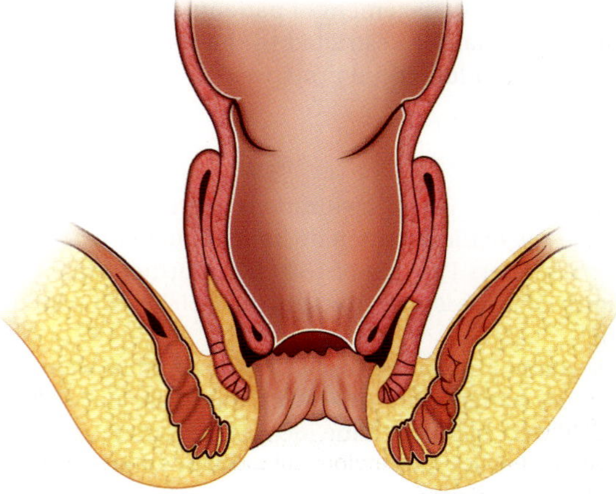

Figure 2 Intussusception theory; hypothesized that rectal prolapse starts as circumferential intussusception above the anal verge

obstetric injury or surgical procedures has been considered to play an important role in the pathophysiology of rectal prolapse. Some of the other factors associated with rectal prolapse include loose fixation of mesorectum to the sacrum, straightening of the rectum and the anorectal angle, lax lateral ligaments, pudendal nerve injury,[20] a non-relaxing puborectal muscle,[21] colonic dysmotility and chronic constipation. Long standing constipation with chronic straining causes stretching of pelvic floor support and forces anterior wall of the upper rectum into rectal lumen. This may accentuate the already present subclinical form of rectal prolapse. Obstetric trauma due to too much exertion during child birth may also tear pelvic supports leading to prolapse of pelvic organs. Some of the factors associated with rectal prolapse are listed in Table 2.

Epidemiology

The incidence of rectal prolapse in Indian population is not known. Elsewhere it is reported to be an uncommon disorder with incidence rates of 2.5 to 4.2 per 100,000 population.[31,32] Peak incidence is at extremes of ages. Pediatric population shows no sex predilection.[22,24,33] Women suffer more than men with a female to male ratio ranges from 6:1 to 10:1.[15,34,35] Although it is believed that multiparity contributes to rectal prolapse, as many as one third female patients are nulliparous.[15] Moreover age distribution is also different in women and men. Men present in their twenties and thirties while women present commonly after sixth decade with peak in seventh decade.[36] Children and young adults are more likely to have associated psychiatric disorders like autism, developmental delays and on multiple psychiatric medications for other disorders.[27]

Clinical Evaluation

History

A detailed history and physical examination helps in reaching the diagnosis of rectal prolapse. Most patients of rectal prolapse present with mass per rectum which may appear spontaneously or while defecation or straining due to other reasons. The mass may spontaneously reduce after defecation or may have to be manually reduced. Patients may also present with various non-specific symptoms that include abdominal pain or discomfort, feeling of incomplete evacuation, fecal incontinence, chronic constipation, mucous discharge and perianal itching. Bleeding and pain may occur in long standing prolapse with ulcers due to repeated friction injury to bowel mucosa. Patient may also give history of chronic constipation and obstructed defecation necessitating digital manipulations to help with defecation. The most common symptoms besides prolapse include rectal bleeding (75–100%), fecal incontinence (50–75%) and constipation (25–50%). Other symptoms include pain, urinary incontinence, mucous diarrhoea and associated vaginal vault prolapse. Worsened quality of life is reported by 100% of the patients with rectal prolapse.[21] Careful documentation of associated incontinence or constipation is important for proper treatment planning.

Table 2: Etiology of Rectal prolapse

Various factors associated with rectal prolapse[22-30]
Chronic constipation (15–65%)
Extremes of age, <3 years and >50 years of age
Female gender
Multiple vaginal deliveries, excessive exertion while labour
Chronic straining due to heavy manual labour, chronic cough, COPD
Severe psychiatric disease requiring neuroleptics and antidepressants, dementia
Neurological deficits due to spinal compression syndromes, cauda equina, multiple sclerosis, stroke
Pelvic floor dysfunction e.g. patulous anus, diastasis of levator ani, abnormal perineal descent
Anatomical defects of pelvic viscera

Examination

Rectal prolapse is seen as the full thickness protrusion of rectum through anal aperture which may be persistently present or may occur at the time of straining. If there is doubt of rectal prolapse but it is not seen on physical examination then the patient may be asked to strain while on a toilet seat or in squatting position and this usually makes the prolapse evident. A full thickness rectal prolapse (Figs 3A and B) should be differentiated from mucosal prolapse, prolapsed hemorrhoids (Figs 4A and B) and other conditions such as polyps or rectal neoplasms. While rectal prolapse is concentric, internal haemorrhoids have radial pattern. Examination should include the evaluation of the status of rectal mucosa for any ulcers, length of prolapsed segment, anal sphincter tone and any other associated pathology. Concomitant rectocele, cystocele or uterine prolapse should be looked for at the time of initial evaluation. Solitary rectal ulcer may be seen in about 10–15% patients on proctoscopic examination.[21] Patient should be evaluated for performance status which is a key factor in determining the choice of surgical approach.

Evaluation

Rectal prolapse is primarily a clinical diagnosis. Investigation help in detecting associated conditions which may be contributing to the prolapse or concomitant pathologies that may need to be addressed. It may be remembered that results of many tests are compromised by prolapse and hence should be interpreted cautiously.[21]

Colonoscopy and proctoscopy rules out associated colorectal pathology such as a neoplasm or hemorrhoids or solitary rectal ulcer. Considering that many patients with rectal prolapse are elderly it is prudent do colonoscopy. Colonoscopy may also give an idea about redundant sigmoid though barium enema is considered superior to colonoscopy in this regard. These are most often the only adjunctive investigations easily available in our country in most hospitals. Other investigations are not readily available in our set up and even where available are recommended to be used selectively.[21]

Defecography, also known as defecation proctography, is indicated in patients, in whom a prolapse cannot be demonstrated physically.[15,21] Radiopaque material is instilled into rectum and x-ray pictures are taken. A continuous fluoroscopic record is known as Cine-radiography and may be done with contrast

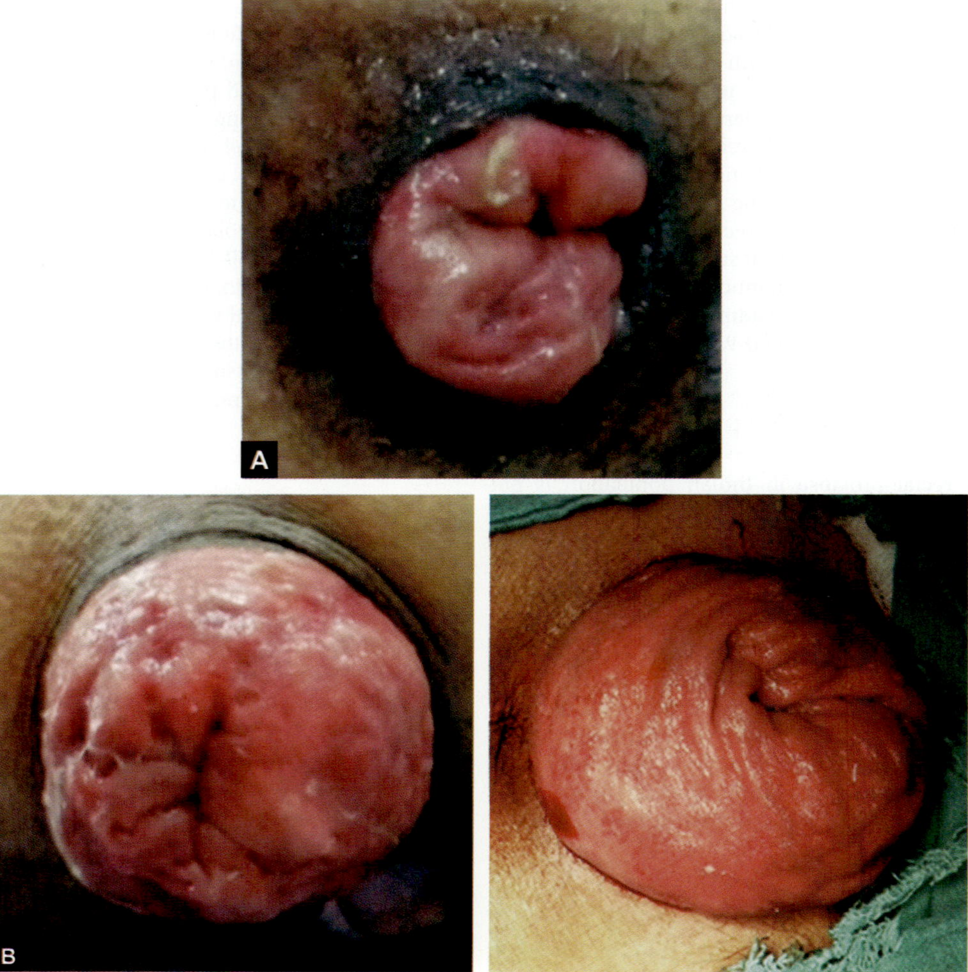

Figures 3A and B Rectal prolapse: (A) Mucosal prolapse; (B) Full thickness prolapse

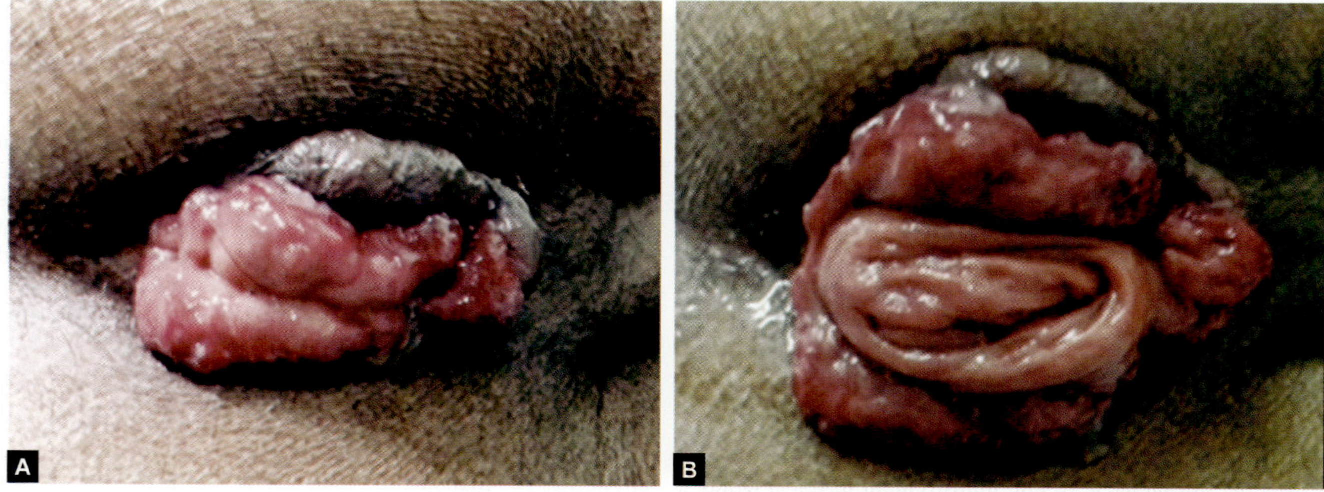

Figures 4A and B (A) Prolapse hemorrhoids; (B) Prolapsed hemorrhoids with rectal prolapse

in rectum, urinary bladder and vagina to rule out concomitant rectocele, cystocele or vaginal vault prolapse.[37]

Dynamic pelvic MRI is a novel approach with no contrast or radiation. MRI allows dynamic visualizations of all three compartments of pelvic floor. This can be done in two ways – a) sitting MR defecography, or b) supine dynamic MRI. Both techniques show equivalent results.[38] MRI helps in visualization of pelvic organs and their supports and helps in pre-operative planning of complex cases.

Anorectal physiologic testing may be done to assess associated functional disorders such as constipation and fecal incontinence and may help in choosing the operative procedure or predicting post-operative outcome. Patients with chronic constipation may benefit from colonic transit studies to look for colonic inertia and if present such patients may benefit from resectional procedures. The presence of pelvic floor dyssynergia on the other hand may be candidates for post-operative biofeedback.[21]

Patients with associated fecal incontinence may benefit from endorectal ultrasound or MRI which may show sphincter abnormalities.[21,38] Anorectal manometry helps to identify patients at high risk of developing post-operative incontinence while abnormal pudendal nerve terminal motor latency test suggests a possibility of higher rate of post-operative incontinence.[15,21] Having said that it has been observed in many studies that neither manometry nor nerve conduction studies reliably predict post-operative function[39] further confirming the ill understood nature of the disease.

Management

Management of rectal prolapse is primarily operative but nonoperative treatment may have some role in selected cases.

Non-operative Treatment

Nonoperative management may be indicated in limited number of patients who are very poor candidates for surgery, have short life expectancy and those patients who are not consenting for surgery. Adequate dietary fluids and fibres are indicated to avoid constipation. A minimum of 2 liters of fluids and 30 g of fibers are recommended. Inciting agents and drugs causing constipation should be avoided. Some authors have used biofeedback therapy and pelvic floor exercises. Biofeedback is useful in intussusception without external prolapse. Non-operative management has variable success rates in patients with incontinence or obstructed defecation.[40] Management of incarcerated rectal prolapse includes sedation, trendelenburg position and manual reduction of rectal prolapse after application of salt or sugar solution topically over prolapsed part to decrease edema.[41]

Surgical Treatment

An ideal surgical treatment should be safe, complete and provide durable resolutions of symptoms. In literature, more than 100 different procedures or modifications have been described. The choice of operation has evolved with evolution of technology, better anaesthesia facilities and improvement in understanding of pathophysiology of rectal prolapse. With every new procedure, the initial results are described as encouraging however the long-term results don't support the initial findings. A meta-analysis published in 2006 aimed at evaluating the accuracy of published recurrence rate following rectal prolapse surgery concluded that published recurrence rates differed nearly by 47% from the actuarial rates.[42]

The surgical approaches have broadly been divided into abdominal or perineal approaches. Though surgeon's preferences and experience play an important role, the type of approach mainly depends on the health status of patient, presence of comorbidities, patient's age, anal tone and associated functional dysfunctions like constipation or fecal incontinence.[43] Generally elderly and debilitated patients are offered a perineal procedures and the abdominal approaches are preferred in younger and healthier patients. Laparoscopic abdominal approach is gaining popularity among current surgeons and robotic approach has also been attempted by some. It is not possible to describe every single operation that has been tried for rectal prolapse and therefore a brief review of some important surgical approaches is given below.

Perineal Approaches

Perineal approaches have been traditionally preferred for patients who are considered unfit for laparotomy. They have the advantage of less incidence of constipation but are associated with a higher recurrence rate.[44-46] Commonly used perineal procedures are Delorme (anorectal mucosectomy with muscular plication), perineal proctosigmoidectomy (Altemeier operation) and Thiersch operation (anal encirclement). The most widely used perineal procedure in UK is Delorme's while in US, it is Altemeier's proctosigmoidectomy.[47-49]

Thiersch Operation (Anal Encirclement) (Fig. 5)

Thiersch in 1891 described anal encirclement with a silver wire through two perianal incisions 180 degree apart to prevent prolapse. This operation was supposed to act by producing a mechanical barrier and caussing scarring and fibrosis around the wire. Though simple and minimally invasive it was marred by

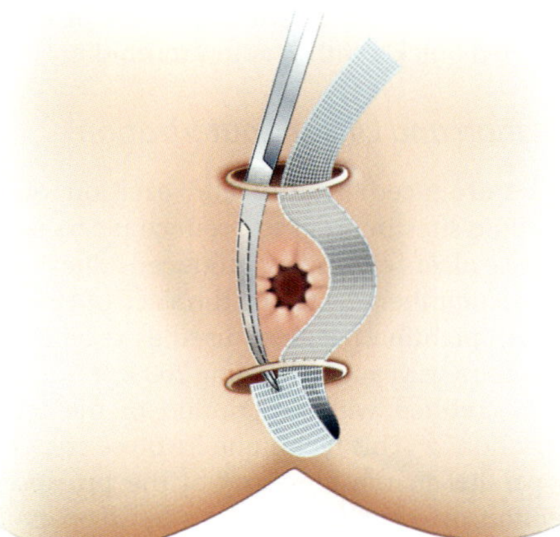

Figure 5 Thiersch operation—Anal encirclement

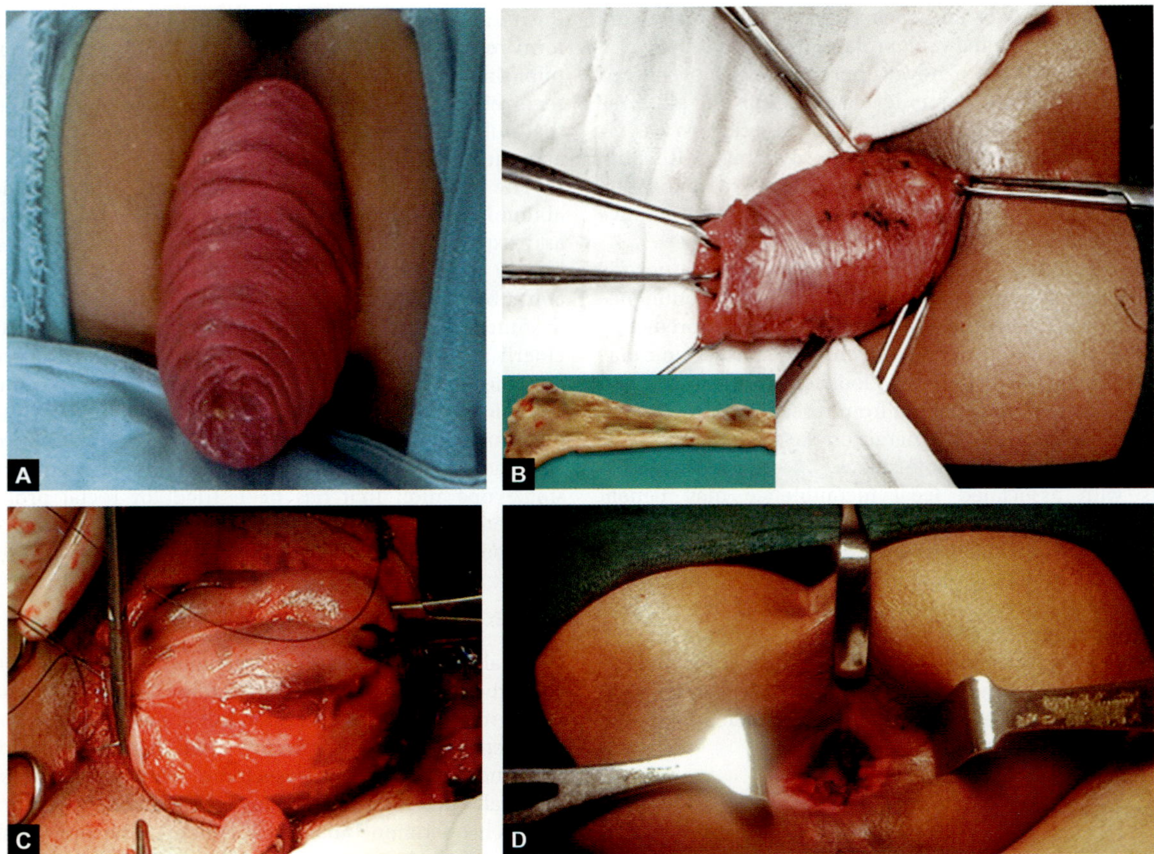

Figures 6A to D Delorme's procedure. (A) The prolapsed rectum. Note the concentric rings. (B) Mucosa is stripped off from about 1 cm above the dentate line till the apex of the prolapse exposing the underlying muscle layer; inset showing resected mucosa

high recurrence rate and complications such as infection, erosion of foreign body into rectum and fecal impaction.[1] In recent times silver wire has been replaced by materials such as monofilament nylon, silicon elastomer, and a 1.5 cm wide strip of polypropylene mesh.[1] Thiersch operation has only few indications nowadays like bedridden patient with short life expectancy, multiple comorbidities and those who may not tolerate even a perineal resection of rectal prolapse. The advantage of this procedure is that it can be performed quickly with very low morbidity.[1]

Mucosal Plication and Linear Cauterization

In 1923, Gant introduced ligature and excision of prolapsed mucosa at multiple sites in order to produce ulcers secondary to sloughing.[50] These ulcers on healing produced adhesions between mucosa and muscular there by taking the slack out of the mucous membrane. This operation has been used as recently as 2003 in Japan in conjunction with anal encircling 2003.[51]

Gant is also credited with description of the technique of "linear cauterization".[50] This technique involves creation of deep linear burns parallel to the long axis of the prolapsed rectum with the intention of creating adhesions between mucosal and muscle layers. This technique has been combined with plication of exposed muscle layer by El-Sibai and Shafik 2002.[52]

Delorme's Procedure (Figs 6A to D)

Delorme described this procedure in 1900.[53] The original operation included excision of a cylinder of the mucosa of the prolapsed rectum followed by suturing of proximal mucosal edge to the distal edge near the anal orifice. Subsequently longitudinal plication of the muscle layer was added to this operation and this modification constitutes the present day Delormes's procedure. Many other modifications[54,55] have been added to this operation including repair of pelvic floor and fixation of prosthetic strips to the apex of the prolapse which are then tunneled subcutaneously and anchored to the external surface of pelvis.

The Delorme's procedure starts with an injection of diluted epinephrine solution in the submucosal plane of prolapsed rectum followed by incision of mucosa with electrocautery 1 cm proximal to dentate line. The mucosa is then stripped off the rectal wall musculature (Figs 6A to D) toward the apex of redundant bowel. The sutures for muscle plication are taken at a distance of 1 cm and tied after a total of 6–8 rows are completed. Finally both ends of mucosa are anastomosed with absorbable suture. The advantage of Delorme operation is that no bowel resection and anastomosis are needed and the complications of laparotomy are avoided. Further it also obviates the risk of impotence in young males. However the recurrence is reported in 4% to 38%.[4] Complications such as urinary retention, infection, bleeding and fecal impaction are reported in 4–12% of the patients.[15]

Although Delorme's has been usually reserved for medically unfit or elderly patients, there is increasing data to suggest that it may be a good procedure in medically fit young patients.[56] Lieberth et al reported recurrence rate of 8% at a median follow-up of 4.8 years in medically fit young patients (Less than 50 years) undergoing Delorme's operation with no surgery site specific complications. In their series of 76 patients, the overall recurrence rate was 14.5% at a mean follow-up of 3.6 years. More than 70% of patients noted an improvement their symptoms. They argued that by avoiding an abdominal approach the risks of abdominopelvic dissections were eliminated including the risk to reproductive function since neither the presacral nor the lateral pelvic plexuses were exposed. Further, the potential risk of injury to the ovaries and fallopian tubes was also eliminated.[57]

Perineal Proctosigmoidectomy

Mickulicz first described this technique in 1889 and Altemeier popularized it in USA.[19,58] Altemeier considered elongated redundant and thickened mesorectum, sliding hernia and pelvic floor defects to be responsible for rectal prolapse and included repair of levators to full thickness resection of prolapsed bowel through anal approach. The first step is to completely prolapse the redundant rectum and inject a diluted epinephrine solution 1 to 2 cm proximal to the dentate line. Then rectal wall is incised full thickness, circumferentially at the level of injection. The rectum and redundant sigmoid colon with its mesentery are excised and the opening into peritoneal cavity is closed. The bowel continuity is restored by anastomosing colon to the distal rectum. In the end, pelvic floor is repaired by posterior levatorplasty. The reported overall mortality rates ranged from 0% to 5% and recurrence rates from 0% to 16%.[59,60]

Perineal procto-sigmoidectomy has been predominantly used in USA for elderly patients or individuals with comorbidities precluding an abdominal procedure.[60-62] It has also been used for patients with incontinence because a concomitant levatorplasty can be performed.[62,63]

In a recently randomized study, 213 patients were randomized between Altemeier's and Delorme's procedure. With median length of follow up of 36 months, the recurrence rate for Delorme's was 31% compared to 24% in Altemeier's procedure. However the difference was not statistically significant. The incontinence and bowel function improved following both procedures with no difference between the two surgical procedures.[47] Four deaths and four anastomotic leakages were reported after Altemeier's operation.

STARR Procedure

Stapled trans-anal resection of the rectum (STARR) is another perineal procedure which involves use of staplers to perform a full thickness transanal rectal resection. However it has been described only for Obstructed Defecation Syndrome (ODS) and occult prolapse and not for complete rectal prolapse.[64]

Abdominal Approaches

Abdominal operations are aimed at suspension and fixation of rectum with or without the resection of redundant sigmoid colon. The operations have included rectal mobilization from sacral hollow alone, rectal mobilization with suture fixation to sacral promontory, rectal mobilization with prosthetic material fixation and resection of redundant sigmoid with restoration of bowel continuity with or without fixation of the mobilized rectum.[1]

Suture Rectopexy

Suture rectopexy was first described by Cutait in 1959 and involves mobilization of rectum to the level of coccyx which is then secured to thickened fascia over the sacral promontory using sutures.[65]

The rationale is to fix the rectum at an elevated level and restore the posterior curve of rectum to minimize the effect of increased intraabdominal pressure. Nelson et al in 2001 suggested that even posterior rectal mobilization without division of lateral stalks is enough to produce fibrotic scar to hold the rectum against the sacral curvature.[66] They tied silk sutures to the areolar tissue overlying the presacral fascia in order to induce a foreign body reaction and produce adhesions. Suture rectopexy has been reported to be associated with a recurrence rates from 3–9%,[67-71] improvement in incontinence and a variable effect on constipation ranging from improvement to worsening.[4]

Posterior Rectopexy Using Prosthetics (Fig. 7)

Wells in 1959 used polyvinyl alcohol, Ivalon, to fix the mobilized rectum to the sacrum. Ivalon excites a vigorous fibrotic response, with resultant fixation of the rectum. Ivalon was subsequently abandoned and is no longer used due to the associated complications and experimental study suggesting a possible carcinogenic effect.[1,4] Synthetic nonabsorbable meshes are and lately absorbable meshes have been used instead of Ivalon for posterior fixation with similar efficacy.[1,72-75] The size and shape of the mesh, extent of posterior and anterior mobilization, division or preservation of lateral ligaments and the degree of circumference of rectum to be wrapped by mesh has varied with authors.[73-75] In general at least anterior one third of the rectum should be free of mesh while fixing it to the lateral rectal wall. It has been seen that the preservation of lateral ligaments produces lesser constipation but is associated with slightly

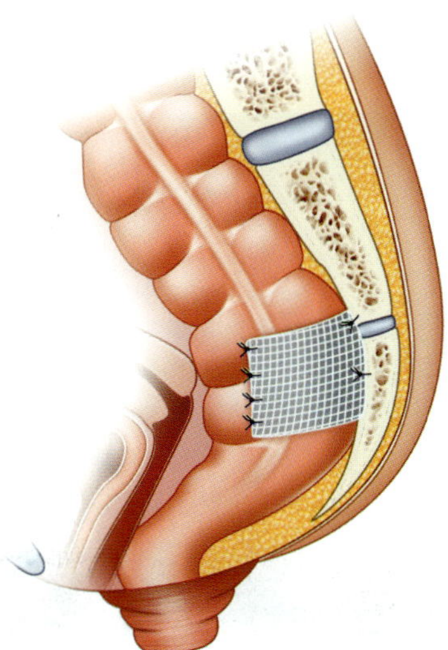

Figure 7 Posterior mesh rectopexy

higher recurrence rates. The practice guidelines for the management of rectal prolapse[15] suggests that the division of lateral stalks during dissection is associated with worsening constipation possibly due to denervation of rectum from neural efferents that reside in lateral ligaments. However there are studies that do not corroborate this concept.[15] Well's repair and other posterior synthetic mesh repairs have been improvement in continence ranging from 3–40%. The procedure gives mixed results with respect to constipation and the general feeling is that it is better avoided in patients with severe constipation. These procedures have been performed with a mortality ranging from 0–1% and recurrences ranging from 0–6%. One of the chief concerns with insertion of foreign material has been sepsis which has been reported in 2–16%[4] of patients. The other complications include formation of hematoma during posterior mobilization, injury to the autonomic nerve plexus leading to erectile and reproductive dysfunction and erosion of the foreign body through rectum (Figs 8A to C).[4] This procedure has been well adapted in laparoscopic era and continues to enjoy popularity.

Anterior Rectopexy

Orr, in 1947, suspended the rectum using strips of fascia lata attached to each side of rectum and fixed to fascia above promontory thus obliterating the deep cu de sac.[76] A modification of this procedure was used by Loyuge (Orr-Loyuge procedure) who added rectal mobilization in the plane of mesorectum down to levator ani without disturbing the lateral ligaments and suspended the rectum by strips of nylon.[77] He reported a mortality of less than 1% and a recurrence rate of 4.3% in 253 patients.

Ripstein devised a form of mesh rectopexy (Fig. 9) based on concepts of loss of normal posterior curve of rectal tube and atrophic pelvic supports to the rectum. He first described, in 1952,[78] the repair of anterior pelvic floor defect using a sling of fascia lata around rectum fixed to the sacral promontory thus restoring the normal posterior curvature of rectum. This followed the posterior mobilization of rectum, excision of pouch of Douglas and repair of levator ani complex. Later, he modified the procedure and introduced use of synthetic mesh anteriorly fixed to rectum and posteriorly sutured to presacral fascia below sacral promontory without pelvic floor repair.[79] This procedure is commonly considered as standard Ripstein procedure. Although this procedure was associated with very low mortality rates (0–2.8%) and recurrence rates (0–13%), complications were seen in almost 50% patients ranging from obstruction, hematoma formation, adhesions and mesh invasion and migration.[1,80] This led him to abandon the anterior wrap and with McMahan he further published a modification of the procedure in 1987[80] in which mesh was placed posteriorly to sacrum and fixed to lateral rectal wall

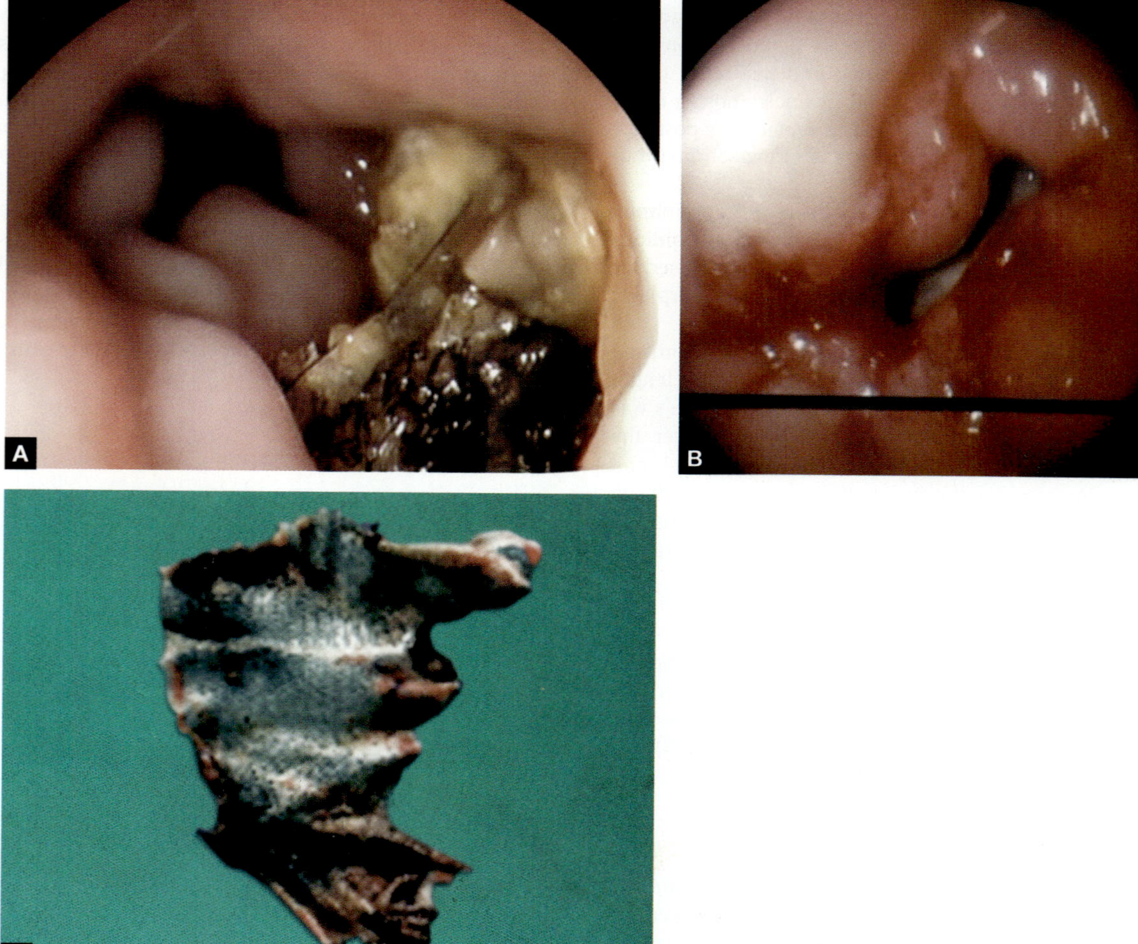

Figures 8A to C Complication of posterior mesh rectopexy

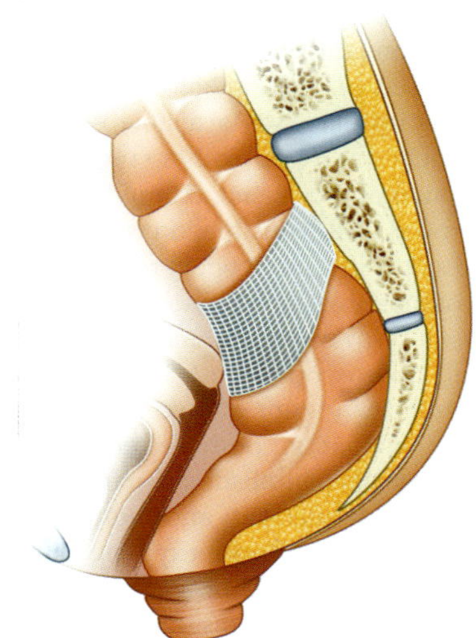

Figure 9 Anterior rectopexy (Ripstein procedure)

keeping a gap between mesh ends anteriorly. Tjandra et al[27] in 1993 published their experience with anterior rectopexy as described by Ripstein using loosely applied encircling Teflon mesh in 142 patients and reported 8% recurrence with improvement in fecal incontinence in about half the patients. The results were not encouraging with respect to constipation with 57% reporting persistent constipation and 15 patients developed new constipation. A review of Ripstein procedure in 1,111 patients[81] revealed a recurrence rate of 2.3% with 183 complications directly related to sling. The commonest complications include fecal impaction (74, 6.7%), pre sacral bleeding (29, 2.6%), stricture (20, 1.8%), pelvic abscess (17, 1.5%), small bowel obstruction (15, 1.4%) and impotence (9, 0.8%).

The modern day ventral mesh rectopexy has been pioneered by D'Hoore[82,83] (Fig. 6) who described a laparoscopic approach aimed at correction of intussusception and obliteration of a deep cul-de-sac. The procedure includes placement of two 12 mm laparoscopic ports at umbilicus (for camera) and at right lower quadrant while two 5 mm ports at left lower quadrant and left lateral abdominal wall. The procedure begins with an inverted 'J' incision (Fig. 10A) from sacral promontory along the right rectal wall and is carried forwards along the rectovesical pouch or pouch of Douglas towards the left. Care is taken to preserve the right hypogastric nerves and the right ureter. Denonvillier's fascia is incised and rectovaginal septum is widely opened down to the pelvic floor. The redundant pouch of Douglas, if any, may be resected. No rectal mobilization, posterior dissection or transaction of lateral rectal ligaments is attempted. A 3 × 17 cm Marlex mesh is sutured to the anterior rectal wall and fixed without traction to the sacral promontory (Fig. 10B). Care should be taken to reduce the prolapse while suturing the mesh. An associated vaginal wall prolapse can be corrected by elevating the posterior vaginal wall and suturing it to the same strip of mesh. Mesh is completely covered by resuturing the incised peritoneum over the mesh (Fig. 10C).

Preservation of nerves, avoidance of rectal mobilization and preservation of lateral ligaments is aimed at improving the postoperative rectal motility, decreasing the incidence of constipation and eliminating the risk of impotence. In addition the procedure is supposed to be associated with less possibility of pelvic sepsis and erosion.[83]

The procedure has been predominantly performed in females and long term results were published. A recurrence rate of 3.6% and a morbidity of 7% has been reported. There was no perioperative mortality nor any mesh infection or erosion.[83]

A systematic review on ventral rectopexy with total 728 patients in 12 non randomized case series reported recurrence rates ranging from 0 to 15.4% with a crude recurrence rates of 3.4%.[84] Morbidity rate ranged from 1.4 to 47%, commonest being port site or incisional hernias and urinary tract infection and postoperative bleed. Four patients had mesh related complications including one case of mesh infection, one case of

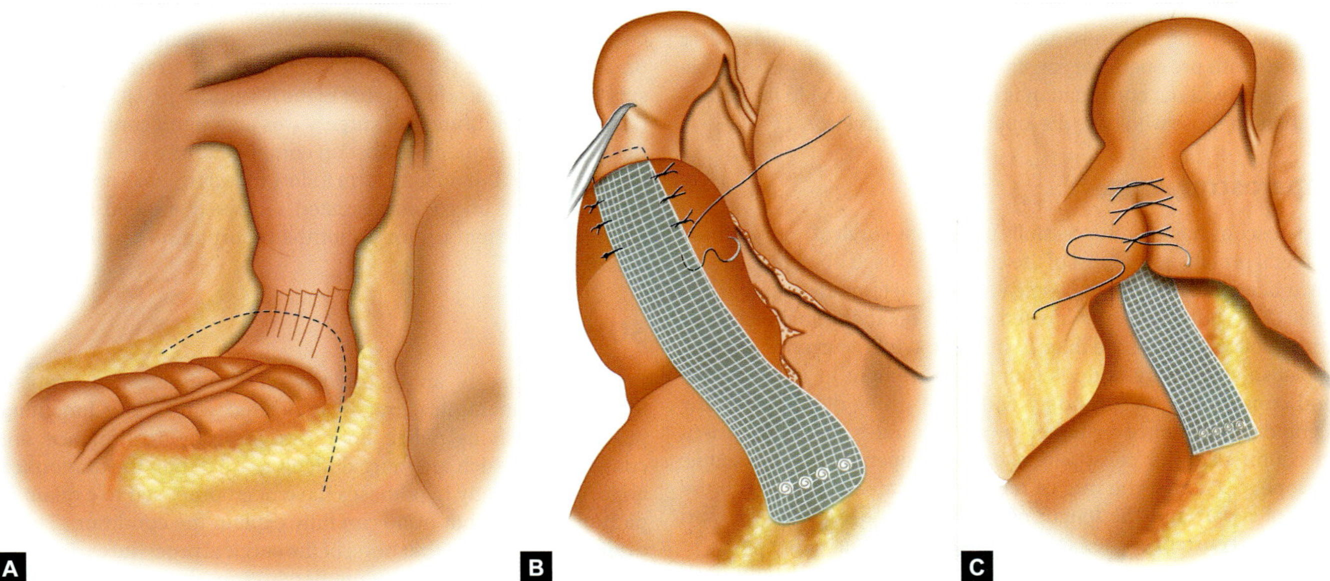

Figures 10A to C Ventral rectopexy as described by D'Hoore. (A) Inverted 'J' shaped incision from sacral promontory along the right rectal wall extending across the pouch of Douglas; (B) Mesh is sutured to anterior rectal wall and fixed to sacral promontory; (C) Peritoneum is closed over the mesh

mesh erosion and two cases of mesh detachment. There were three perioperative mortalities. Overall weighted mean decrease in constipation rate was reported to be 23.9% and in fecal incontinence was 44.9%.

Resection

Sigmoid resection and anterior resection have also been proposed to deal with rectal prolapse with constipation.[85] The idea is to remove redundant sigmoid and create adhesions between mobilized rectum and sacrum. However these operations are not popular as standalone procedures. Studies have reported increasing recurrence with passage of time, serious complications such as anastomotic leak and loss of continence if anastomosis is performed low in pelvis.[25,86]

Resection and Rectopexy

The addition of sigmoid resection to rectopexy (the Frykman-Goldberg procedure) combines the advantage of rectal mobilization which provides suspension and fixation of rectum and removal of redundant sigmoid colon that helps in improving the constipation.[87] It has been postulated that redundant sigmoid leads to kinking of rectosigmoid junction once the rectum is fixed and resection avoids this by straightening the rectosigmoid angle thus relieving the outlet obstruction.[4] Fixation is usually performed using sutures. Only few studies have used mesh rectopexy.[4,28,88-94] Presence of foreign material in the event of an anastomotic leak can prove detrimental and is best avoided in our view. Major complications are reported in 0–20%[15] of patients and are secondary to either anastomotic leak or obstruction. A meta-analysis[97] of open resection rectopexy comprising 7 studies published between 1985 and 1999 and a follow up ranging from 17 to 98 months showed a recurrence rate of 0 to 8.3%.[95] Postoperative improvement in incontinence ranged from 11 to 90%, and the rate of constipation improved in 18 to 56%. No worsening of incontinence or constipation was described after the intervention. The improvement in constipation and continence however was not significant on quantitative analysis using the random effect model. Cochrane review and Practice guidelines suggest that resection does improve constipation and that resection rectopexy may be considered in patients with pre operative constipation and rectal prolapse. Its role in patients without constipation is not established and in fact it may not benefit those who have pre-operative incontinence.[15,98]

Laparoscopy

Laparoscopy has been successfully used in the surgical management of rectal prolapse and most of the commonly used open procedures have been adapted laparoscopically. In a meta-analysis published in 2012,[97] Cadeddu et al evaluated studies on abdominal rectopexy with a follow-up of more than 16 months. With recurrence of rectal prolapse as primary endpoint and improvement in incontinence and constipation as secondary end points, they did not find any significant difference in either recurrence rates or improvement in continence and constipation between open and laparoscopic rectopexy. Though the rate of recurrence varied according to the type of repair and the length of follow-up, most studies showed that the recurrence rates for rectal prolapse after either open or laparoscopic surgery are below 10%.[99] The laparoscopic approach seems to be associated with faster recovery.

A long-term follow up study on laparoscopic suture rectopexy in 179 patients predominantly comprising of females (174 females and 5 males) reported on the outcome of laparoscopic suture rectopexy.[100] Follow up data was available on 172 patients and revealed 10 recurrences at 5-year with a crude recurrence rate of 6% and 10-year actuarial recurrence rate of 20%. Continence and quality of life improved while constipation was unchanged. A meta-analysis on laparoscopic suture rectopexy revealed a recurrence rate of 0 to 7% with postoperative improvement in incontinence ranging from 50 to 82% and improvement in constipation from 0 to 69%.[97]

The results of laparoscopic mesh rectopexy are similar to those of open rectopexy in terms of recurrence rates and relief of incontinence and constipation. Both posterior and ventral mesh procedures have been accomplished laparoscopically with an added advantage of early recovery and reduced hospitalization. The mortality for laparoscopic rectopexy ranged between 0% and 3%,[4] with recurrence rates of 0 to 7.14%.[97]

D'Hoore et al published their results on laparoscopic ventral mesh rectopexy (LVR) in 42 patients in 2004 and subsequently on 109 patients in 2006.[82,83] They reported a recurrence rate of 3.6%. Sixteen of 19 patients with pre-operative constipation improved with worsening in 2 patients. Incontinence improved in 28 of 31 patients.[82]

Resection and rectopexy has also been successfully performed laparoscopically with recurrence rates similar to open surgery.[97] An analysis of 6 studies in which laparoscopic resection and rectopexy using sutures was performed in 244 patients reported no recurrences. Improvement in incontinence was 38–100% of patients and constipation was reported to improve in 8–76% individuals with some reporting worsening of continence and constipation.[97,101] The quantitative analysis showed improvement in incontinence after operation while there was no significant improvement in constipation.

Robotic Surgery for Rectal Prolapse

A few centers have begun utilizing the robot for rectopexy in patients with rectal prolapse but the numbers available in contemporary literature are too low to draw any conclusion. Heemskerk et al conducted a comparative study between conventional (CR, n=14) or robot-assisted (RR, n=19) laparoscopic surgery.[102] Cost of surgery was significantly higher in the RR group ($p<0.05$) than in the CR group. The duration of surgery was also significantly higher in the RR group. Immediate post op complications were comparable in both groups but no long term follow up was done. Another study by Munz et al on robotic assisted rectopexy studied 6 patients and followed them up for 6 months reporting no recurrences or constipation.[103]

SUMMARY

Rectal prolapse is an ill understood condition. The problem is not only anatomical but is associated with many functional problems such as pelvic floor dyssynergia, incontinence and constipation which are more difficult to treat than the anatomical abnormality. Many hypotheses have been proposed to explain its pathophysiology but none can fully explain the condition. This is evident from the fact that none of the surgical procedures designed based on different theories completely cures the condition and no single procedure is suited to all.

A detailed history and examination remains the cornerstone in the diagnosis of rectal prolapse. It is imperative to document history of concomitant symptoms of constipation and fecal incontinence besides other organ prolapse since they may have a bearing on the choice of surgery. Digital rectal examination should be done for evaluation of anal sphincter tone and rule out concomitant anorectal pathology such as polyps, neoplasm or solitary rectal ulcer. Proctoscopy and colonoscopy are important to identify concomitant rectal pathologies. Other tests like defecography or cineradiography should be done in selected patients as and when required.

The surgical treatment, in rectal prolapse, is aimed at restoring the normal anatomy and to improve the associated incontinence or constipation. It is particularly very difficult to correct the associated constipation keeping the recurrence rates to the minimum. The review of literature suggests that some procedures may be better suited to deal with associated functional abnormality and therefore an attempt should be made to tailor the choice of surgery to individual's requirements.

Among the perineal procedures, Delorme's procedure has generally been reserved for elderly patients but it should be considered for medically fit young patients, particularly males, to avoid the risk of impotence. Further, it is also devoid of risk of anastomotic leak associated with Altemeier's procedure. As discussed above, a randomized study did not show any statistically significant difference in recurrence rates or functional improvement between Delorme's and Altemeier's procedures.

Sigmoid resection with suture rectopexy appears to be the preferred option for patients with prolapse and preoperative constipation. Preservation of lateral ligaments during lateral mobilization appears to be beneficial in patients with constipation.

The Ripstein procedure is best avoided since it is associated with high morbidity and Ripstein himself switched over to posterior mesh rectopexy.

The posterior mesh rectopexy continues to enjoy popularity and appears to be a good option in patients who have poor anal tone or low anal resting pressures with or without incontinence and do not have preoperative constipation.

The laparoscopic ventral rectopexy, described by D'Hoore, has shown good results. Since it preserves lateral ligaments and hypogastric nerve plexus and there is no posterior rectal mobilization, it has the potential to avoid complications associated with traditional mesh rectopexy such as impotence and constipation. However, the experience in male patients is very limited and the procedure has been predominantly used in females.

Laparoscopic approach is suitable for all patients ideal for abdominal approach and having no anesthetic contra-indications. As discussed before, laparoscopy has successfully been adapted to most commonly used abdominal procedures with results similar to open techniques. It is advisable that the laparoscopic approach should be attempted after having gained sufficient proficiency in laparoscopic surgery. Use of 3D-laparoscopic cameras and robot may further refine the minimally invasive operations.

REFERENCES

1. Wu JS. Rectal prolapse: a historical perspective. Curr Probl Surg 2009;46:602-716.
2. Jacobs LK, Lin YJ, Orkin BA. The best operation for rectal prolapse. Surg Clin North Am. 1997;77:49-70.
3. Felt-Bersma RJ, Cuesta MA. Rectal prolapse, rectal intussusception, rectocele and solitary ulcer syndrome. Gastroenterol Clin North Am. 2001;30:199-222.
4. Gourgiotis S, Baratsis S. Rectal prolapse. Int J Colorectal Dis. 2007; 22:231-243.
5. Salmon F. Practical Observations on Prolapsus of the Rectum. London: Whittaker, Treacher and Arnot, Ave-Maria Lane; 1831; chapter I, p. 8.
6. Devadhar DSC. A new concept of mechanism and treatment of rectal procidentia. Dis Colon Rectum. 1965;8:75-7.
7. Brodén B, Snellman B. Procidentia of the rectum studied with cineradiography: a contribution to the discussion of causative mechanism. Dis Colon Rectum. 1968;11:330-47.
8. Bodenhamer W. Prolapsus ani. In: Practical Observations on Some of the Diseases of the Rectum, Anus and Contiguous Textures; giving their Nature, Seat, Causes, Symptoms, Consequences, and Prevention; especially addressed to the Nonmedical Reader. Cincinnati: A.G. Sparhawk; 1847; chapter IX, pp. 76-9.
9. Tuttle JP. Prolapse of the rectum, procidentia intestini recti. In: A Treatise on Diseases of the Anus, Rectum and Pelvic Colon. New York: D. Appleton and Company; 1903; chapter XVII, pp. 667-710.
10. Moschcowitz AV. The pathogenesis, anatomy, and cure of prolapse of the rectum. Surg Gynecol Obstet. 1912;15:7-21.
11. Pantanowitz D, Levine E. The mechanism of rectal prolapse. South African J Surg. 1975;13:53-6.
12. Todd TW. Anatomical considerations in the rectal prolapse of infants. Ann Surg. 1920;71:163-7.
13. Pemberton J deJ, Stalker LK. Surgical treatment of complete rectal prolapse. Ann Surg. 1939;109:799-808.
14. Graham RR. The operative repair of massive rectal prolapse. Ann Surg. 1942;115:1007-14.
15. Varma M, Rafferty J, Buie WD. Practice Parameters for the Management of Rectal Prolapse. Dis Colon Rectum. 2011;54:1339-1346.
16. Porter N. A physiological study of the pelvic floor in rectal prolapse. Ann R Coll Surg Engl. 1961;31:379-404.
17. Sun WM, Read NW, Donnelly TC et al. A common pathophysiology for full thickness rectal prolapse, anterior mucosal prolapse and solitary rectal ulcer. Br J Surg. 1989;76:290-295.
18. Mellgren A, Schultz I, Johansson C, Dolk A. Internal rectal intussusception seldom develops into total rectal prolapse. Dis Colon Rectum. 1997;40:817-820.
19. Mikulicz J. Zur operativen behandlung dis prolapsus recti et coli invaginati. Arch Klin Chir. 1988;38:74-97.
20. Parks AG, Swash M, Urich H. Sphincter denervation in anorectal incontinence and rectal prolapse. Gut. 1977;18:656-665.
21. Bordeianou L, Hicks CW, Kaiser AM, Alavi K, Sudan R, Wise PE. Rectal Prolapse: An Overview of Clinical Features, Diagnosis, and Patient-Specific Management Strategies. J Gastrointest Surg. 2014;18(5):1059-1069.
22. Madiba TE, Baig MK, Wexner SD. Surgical management of rectal prolapse. Arch Surg. 2005 Jan;140(1):63-73.
23. Hiltunen KM, Matikainen MJ, Auvinen O, Hietanen P. Clinical and manometric evaluation of anal sphincter function in patients with rectal prolapse. Am J Surg. 1986;151:489-492.
24. Jacobs LK, Lin YJ, Orkin BA. The best operation for rectal prolapse. Surg Clin North Am. 1997;77:49-70.
25. Cirocco WC, Brown AC. Anterior resection for the treatment of rectal prolapse: a 20-year experience. Am Surg. 1993;59:265-269.
26. Keighley MR, Shouler PJ. Abnormalities of colonic function in patients with rectal prolapse and faecal incontinence. Br J Surg. 1984;71:892-895.
27. Mann CV, Hoffman C. Complete rectal prolapse: the anatomical and functional results of treatment by an extended abdominal rectopexy. Br J Surg. 1988;75:34-37.

28. Tjandra JJ, Fazio VW, Church JM, et al. Ripstein procedure is an effective treatment for rectal prolapse without constipation. Dis Colon Rectum. 1993;36:501-507.
29. Marceau C, Parc Y, Debroux E, et al. Complete rectal prolapse in young patients: psychiatric disease a risk factor of poor outcome. Colorectal Dis. 2005;7:360.
30. Mellgren A, Bremmer S, Johansson C, et al. Defecography. Results of investigations in 2,816 patients. Dis Colon Rectum 1994;37:1133.
31. Patel SM, Lembo AJ. Constipation: Rectal prolapse and solitary rectal ulcer syndrome. In: Sleisenger and Fordtan's Gastrointestinal and Liver Disease, 8th, Feldman M. (Ed), Saunders Elsevier, Philadelphia 2006. Vol. 1, p. 230.
32. Kairaluoma MV, Kellokumpu IH. Epidemiologic aspects of complete rectal prolapse. Scand J Surg. 2005;94:207.
33. Wassef R, Rothenberger DA, Goldberg SM. Rectal prolapse. Curr Probl Surg. 1986;23:397-451.
34. Van Geluwe B, Wolthuis A, D'Hoore A. Laparoscopy for pelvic floor disorders. Best Pract Res Clin Gastroenterol. 2014 Feb;28(1):69-80.
35. Van Geluwe B, Wolthuis A, Penninckx F, D'Hoore A. Lessons learned after more than 400 laparoscopic ventral rectopexies. Acta Chir Belg. 2013;113:103-6.
36. Bharucha AE. Pelvic floor: anatomy and function. Neurogastroenterol Motil. 2006;18(7):507-519.
37. Maglinte DD, Hale DS, Sandrasegaran K. Comparison between dynamic cystocolpoproctography and dynamic pelvic floor MRI: pros and cons: which is the "functional" examination for anorectal and pelvic floor dysfunction? Abdom Imaging. 2013 Oct;38(5):952-73.
38. Law YM, Fielding JR. MRI of Pelvic Floor Dysfunction: Review. AJR Am J Roentgenol. 2008 Dec;191(6 Suppl):S45-53.
39. Felt-Bersma RJ, Tiersma ES, Cuesta MA. Rectal prolapse, rectal intussusception, rectocele, solitary rectal ulcer syndrome, and enterocele. Gastroenterol Clin North Am. 2008;37:645-668.
40. Hamalainen KJ, Raivio P, Antila S, Palmu A, Mecklin JP. Biofeedback therapy in rectal prolapse patients. Dis Colon Rectum. 1996 Mar;39(3):262-5.
41. Coburn WM 3rd, Russel MA, Hofstetter WL. Sucrose as an aid to manual reduction of incarcerated prolapse. Ann Emerg Med. 1997;30:347.
42. DiGiuro G, Ignjatovic D, Brogger J, Bergamaschi R, et al. How accurate are published recurrence rates after rectal prolapse surgery? A meta-analysis of individual patient data. Am J Surg. 2006;191:773-8.
43. Brown AJ, Anderson JH, McKee RF, Finlay IG. Strategy for selection of type of operation for rectal prolapse based on clinical criteria. Dis Colon Rectum. 2004;47:103-107.
44. Watts JD, Rothenberger DA, Buls JG, Goldberg SM, Nivatvongs S. The management of procidentia: 30 years experience. Dis Colon Rectum. 1985;28:96-102.
45. Pescatori M, Interisano A, Stolfi VM, Zoffoli M. Delorme's operation and sphincteroplasty for rectal prolapse and fecal incontinence. Int J Colorectal Dis. 1998;13:223-227.
46. Whitlow CB, Beck DE, Opelka FG, Gathright JB Jr, Timmcke AE, Hicks T. Perineal repair of rectal prolapse. J La State Med Soc. 1997; 149:22-26.
47. Senapati A, Gray RG, Middleton LJ, Harding J, Hills RK, Armitage RCM, Buckley L, Northover JMA. PROSPER: a randomised comparison of surgical treatments for rectal prolapse. Colorectal Dis. 2013 Jul;15(7):858-68.
48. Tekkis PP, Senagore AJ, Delaney CP, Fazio VW. Evaluation of the learning curve in laparoscopic colorectal surgery:comparison of right-sided and left-sided resections. Ann Surg. 2005;242:83-91.
49. Lagasse RS. Anesthesia safety: model or myth? A review of the published literature and analysis of current original data. Anesthesiology. 2002;97:1609-17.
50. Gant SG. Procidentia ani, recti, and sigmoidae. In: Diseases of the Rectum, Anus and Colon, Including the Ileocolic Angle, Appendix, Colon, Sigmoid Flexure, Rectum, Anus, Buttocks, and Sacrococcygeal Region, Vol II. Philadelphia: W.B. Saunders, Co.; 1923; chapter XXXVII, pp. 37-8.
51. Yamana T, Iwadare J. Mucosal plication (Gant-Miwa procedure) with anal encircling for rectal prolapse-a review of the Japanese experience. Dis Colon Rectum. 2003;46(Suppl):S94-S99.
52. El-Sibai O, Shafik AA. Cauterization-plication operation in the treatment of complete rectal prolapse. Tech Coloproctol. 2002;6:51-4.
53. Delorme R. Sur le traitment des prolapses du rectum totaux pour l'excision de la muscueuse rectale ou rectocolique. Bull Mem Soc Chir Paris. 1900;26:499-518.
54. Lechaux JP, Lechaux D, Perez M. Results of Delorme's procedure for rectal prolapse: advantages of a modified technique. Dis Colon Rectum. 1995;38:301-307.
55. Williams NS, Giordano P, Dvorkin LS, Huang A, Hetzer FH, Scott SM. External pelvic rectal suspension (The Express Procedure) for full-thickness rectal prolapse: evolution of a new technique. Dis Colon Rectum. 2005;48:307-16.
56. Watts AMI, Thompson MR. Evaluation of Delorme's procedure as a treatment for full-thickness rectal prolapse. Br J Surg. 2000; 87:218-222.
57. Lieberth M, Kondylis LA, Reilly JC, Kondylis PD. The Delorme repair for full-thickness rectal prolapse: a retrospective review. Am J Surg. 2009 Mar;197(3):418-423.
58. Altemeier WA, Culbertson WR, Schwengerdt C et al. Nineteen years' experience with the one-stage perineal repair of rectal prolapse. Ann Surg. 1971;173:993-1006.
59. Agachan F, Reissman P, Pfeifer J et al. Comparison of three perineal procedures for the treatment of rectal prolapse. South Med J. 1997; 90:925-932.
60. Prasad ML, Pearl RK, Abcarian H et al. Perineal proctectomy, posterior rectopexy and post anal levator repair for the treatment of rectal prolapse. Dis Colon Rectum. 1986;29:547-552.
61. Williams JG, Rothenberger DA, Madoff RD, Goldberg SM. Treatment of rectal prolapse in the elderly by perineal rectosigmoidectomy. Dis Colon Rectum. 1992;35:830-834.
62. Johansen OB, Wexner SD, Daniel N et al. Perineal rectosigmoidectomy in the elderly. Dis Colon Rectum. 1993;36:767-772.
63. Takesue Y, Yokoyama T, Murakami Y et al. The effectiveness of perineal rectosigmoidectomy for the treatment of rectal prolapse. Surg Today. 1999;29:290-293.
64. Farouk R, R Bhardwaj R, Phillips RKS, Dehn T. Stapled Transanal Resection of the Rectum (STARR) for the Obstructed Defaecation Syndrome. Ann R Coll Surg Engl. May 2009;91(4):287-291.
65. Cutait D. Sacro-promontory fixation of the rectum for complete rectal prolapse. Proc R Soc Med. 1959;52:105.
66. Nelson R, Spitz J, pearl RK et al. What role does full rectal mobilization alone play in the treatment of rectal prolapse? Tech Coloproctol. 2001;5:33.
67. Briel JW, Schouten WR, Boerma MO. Long-term results of suture rectopexy in patients with fecal incontinence associated with incomplete rectal prolapse. Dis Colon Rectum. 1997;40:1228-1232.
68. Carter AE. Rectosacral suture fixation for complete rectal prolapse in the elderly, the frail and the demented. Br J Surg. 1983;70:522-523.
69. Graf W, Karlbom U, Pahlman L, Nilsson S, Ejerblad S. Functional results after abdominal suture rectopexy for rectal prolapse or intussusception. Eur J Surg. 1996;162:905-911.
70. Khanna AK, Misra MK, Kumar K. Simplified sutured sacral rectopexy for complete rectal prolapse in adults. Eur J Surg. 1996;162:143-146.
71. Novell JR, Osborne MJ, Winslet MC, Lewis AA. Prospective randomized trial of Ivalon sponge versus sutured rectopexy for fullthickness rectal prolapse. Br J Surg. 1994;81:904-906.

72. Calne RY. Ivalon wrap operation for rectal prolapse. Proc R Soc Med. 1966;59:127-8.
73. Morgan CN, Porter NH, Klugman DJ. Ivalon (polyvinyl alcohol) sponge in the repair of complete rectal prolapse. Br J Surg. 1972;59:841-6.
74. Penfold JCB, Hawley PR. Experiences of Ivalon-sponge implant for complete rectal prolapse at St. Marks Hospital, 1960-70. Br J Surg. 1972;59:846-8.
75. Allen-Mersh TG, Turner MJ, Mann CV. Effect of abdominal Ivalon® rectopexy on bowel habit and rectal wall. Dis Colon Rectum. 1990;33:550-3.
76. Orr TG. A suspension operation for prolapse of the rectum. Ann Surg. 1947;126:833-837.
77. Loygue J, Nordlinger B, Cunci O et al. (1984). Rectopexy to the promontory of the treatment of rectal prolapse: report of 257 cases. Dis Colon Rectum. 27:356-359.
78. Ripstein CB. Treatment of massive rectal prolapse. Am J Surg. 1952;83:68-71.
79. Ripstein CB. Surgical care of massive rectal prolapse. Dis Colon Rectum. 1965;8:34-8.
80. McMahan JD, Ripstein CB. Rectal prolapse. An update on the rectal sling procedure. Am Surg. 1987 Jan;53(1):37-40.
81. Gordon PH, Hoexter B. Complications of the Ripstein Procedure. Dis Colon Rectum. 1978 May-Jun;21(4):277-280.
82. D'Hoore A, Cadoni R, Penninckx F. Long-term outcome of laparoscopic ventral rectopexy for total rectal prolapse. BJS 2004;91:1500-1505.
83. D'Hoore A, Penninckx F. Laparoscopic ventral recto(colpo)pexy for rectal prolapse: surgical technique and outcome for 109 patients. Surg Endosc. 2006;20:1919-1923.
84. Samaranayake CB, Luo C, Plank AW, Merrie AE, Plank LD, Bissett IP. Systematic review on ventral rectopexy for rectal prolapse and intussusception. Colorectal Dis. 2010 Jun;12(6):504-12.
85. Azimuddin K, Khubchandani IT, Rosen L et al. Rectal prolapse: a search for the best operation. Am Surg. 2001; 67:622-627.
86. Schlinkert RT, Beart RW Jr, Wolff BG, Pemberton JH. Anterior resection for complete rectal prolapse. Dis Colon Rectum. 1985 Jun;28(6):409-412.
87. Frykman HM. Abdominal proctopexy and primary sigmoid resection for rectal procidentia. Am J Surg. 1955;90:780-789.
88. Yakut M, Kaymakciioglu N, Simsek A et al. Surgical treatment of rectal prolapse: a retrospective analysis of 94 cases. Int Surg. 1998;83:53-55.
89. Luukkonen P, Mikkonen U, Järvinen H. Abdominal rectopexy with sigmoidectomy vs rectopexy alone for rectal prolapse: a prospective, randomised study. Int J Colorectal Dis. 1992;7: 219-222
90. Sayfan J, Pinho M, Alexander-Williams J, Keighley MRB. Sutured posterior abdominal rectopexy with sigmoidectomy compared with Marlex rectopexy rectal prolapse. Br J Surg. 1990;77:143-145.
91. Galili Y, Rabau M. Comparison of polyglycolic acid and polypropylene mesh for rectopexy in the treatment of rectal prolapse. Eur J Surg. 1997;163:445-448.
92. Himpens J, Cadière GB, Bruyns J, Vertruyen M. Laparoscopic rectopexy according to Wells. Surg Endosc. 1999;13:139-141.
93. Watts JD, Rothenberger DA, Buls JG, Goldberg SM, Nivatvongs S. The management of procidentia: 30 years experience. Dis Colon Rectum. 1985;28:96-102.
94. Huber FT, Stein H, Siewert JR. Functional results after treatment of rectal prolapse with rectopexy and sigmoid resection. World J Surg. 1995;19:138-143.
95. Deen KI, Grant E, Billingham C, Keighley MRB. Abdominal resection rectopexy with pelvic floor repair versus perineal rectosigmoidectomy and pelvic floor repair for fullthickness rectal prolapse. Br J Surg. 1994;81:302-304.
96. Kim D-S, Tsang CB, Wong WD et al. Complete rectal prolapse: evolution of management and results. Dis Colon Rectum. 1999;42:460-469.
97. Cadeddu F, Sileri P, Grande M, De Luca E, Franceschilli L, Milito G. Focus on abdominal rectopexy for full-thickness rectal prolapse: meta-analysis of literature. Tech Coloproctol. 2012 Feb;16(1):37-53.
98. Tou S, Brown SR, Malik AI, Nelson RL. Surgery for complete rectal prolapse in adults. Cochrane Database of Systematic Reviews 2008, Issue 4. Art. No.: CD001758.
99. Kariv Y, Delaney CP, Casillas S et al. Long-term outcome after laparoscopic and open surgery for rectal prolapse: a case-control study. Surg Endosc. 2006;20:35-42.
100. Foppa C, Martinek L, Arnaud JP, Bergamaschi R. Ten-year follow-up after laparoscopic suture rectopexy for full-thickness rectal prolapse. Colorectal Dis. 2014 Jun 19. doi: 10.1111/codi.12689. [Epub ahead of print]
101. Lechaux D, Trebuchet G, Siproudhis L, Campion JP. Laparoscopic rectopexy for full-thickness rectal prolapse: a single-institution retrospective study evaluating surgical outcome. Surg Endosc. 2005;19:514-518.
102. Heemskerk J, de Hoog DE, van Gemert WG, Baeten CG, Greve JW, Bouvy ND. Robot-assisted vs. conventional laparoscopic rectopexy for rectal prolapse: a comparative study on costs and time. Dis Colon Rectum. 2007 Nov;50(11):1825-30.
103. Munz Y, Moorthy K, Kudchadkar R, Hernandez JD, Martin S, Darzi A, Rockall T. Robotic assisted rectopexy. Am J Surg. 2004 Jan;187(1):88-92.

CHAPTER 89

Rectovaginal Fistula

Ashok Kumar, Rakesh Kumar Singh

INTRODUCTION

Rectovaginal fistulas are abnormal epithelial lined connections between the rectum and vagina. It accounts for approximately 5% of all anorectal fistulas.

ETIOPATHOGENESIS

Obstetric Cause

The most common cause of a rectovaginal fistula is obstetric trauma. Most common contributing factor is prolonged second stage of labor with ischemic necrosis of the rectovaginal septum. Other risk factors include a high forceps delivery, shoulder dystocia, midline episiotomy and third- or fourth-degree perineal laceration[1,2] Rectovaginal fistula after vaginal delivery occurs more commonly in underdeveloped countries because of lack of prompt access to appropriate health care facilities. Among obstetric fistulas, 74% are vesicovaginal, 21% are combined vesicovaginal and rectovaginal and 5% are rectovaginal alone.

Inflammatory Bowel Disease

More commonly associated with Crohn's disease because of transmural inflammation. Crohn's disease is associated with rectovaginal fistula in more than 10% of women with the disease.[3] The incidence of Crohn's rectovaginal fistula is more common in patients with Crohn's colitis and women who had hysterectomy before. Ulcerative colitis is rarely associated with rectovaginal fistula.

Infection

Abscesses in the rectovaginal septum and anterior horseshoe anorectal abscesses may result in rectovaginal fistulas. Diverticulitis is more commonly associated with a colovaginal than rectovaginal fistula and occurs almost exclusively in women who have undergone a prior hysterectomy. Other infectious etiologies include tuberculosis, lymphogranuloma venereum, human immunodeficiency virus (HIV) and cytomegalovirus (CMV).

Postoperative Complications

Rectovaginal fistula can result as a postoperative complication after a variety of rectal, vaginal and pelvic operations, including hysterectomy, low anterior resection with stapled anastomosis, ileal pouch-anal anastomosis (IPAA), procedure for prolapse and hemorrhoids (PPH), stapled transanal rectal resection (STARR), and pelvic mesh placement for pelvic organ prolapse. Fistula developing after LAR is due to entrapment of vaginal wall in staple line or a manifestation of anastomotic leakage, which occurs in up to 13% of women after low anterior resection for rectal cancer. Risk factors include low anastomosis, stapled anastomosis and preoperative radiotherapy.[4] In IPAA, early pouch-vaginal fistulas are a manifestation of anastomotic leakage, pelvic sepsis, ischemia or tension on the anastomosis, whereas late fistulas are more commonly caused by unsuspected Crohn's disease.[5]

Malignancy

Rectovaginal fistulas may be a part of presenting symptom of malignancy of cervix, rectum, uterus or vagina because of direct involvement. This may be a presentation of recurrent disease but may also occur after radiation therapy. Incidence of rectovaginal fistulas is as high as 18% in patients who received external beam radiotherapy in addition to interstitial brachytherapy for an advanced gynecologic malignancy.[6]

Other Causes

Less common causes of rectovaginal fistulas include congenital fistulas, fecal impaction, long-standing pessary usage, sexual assault, ergotamine suppository usage, autoimmune disease (Behçet's disease).

PRESENTATION

Symptoms are dependent on the location, size and etiology of the rectovaginal fistula. The chief presenting complaint is the passage of stool or air per vagina. Foul-smelling vaginal discharge with recurrent vaginitis or urinary tract infections may be the presenting complaint. In women with rectovaginal fistulas from an obstetric injury, patients may have fecal incontinence. Associated symptoms, such as diarrhea, abdominal pain, or mucous discharge, are suggestive of inflammatory bowel disease (IBD).

EXAMINATION

Examination is required to confirm the presence of a rectovaginal fistula, to determine the size and location of the rectovaginal fistula, to assess the state of the anal sphincter, and to search for signs of an underlying disease state, such as an acute infection, Crohn's disease, irradiation injury, or a neoplastic process. Most often, the fistula is palpable and/or visualized easily via rectovaginal examination and proctosigmoidoscopy (Fig. 1). Stool may be seen in the vagina. Small fistulous opening may appear only as a depression or a pit-like defect. Gentle probing may be necessary to reveal the fistula. Examination with one finger in the rectum and one in the vagina (Bimanual examination) assists in assessing the surrounding tissues and the bulk (usually quite attenuated) of the rectovaginal septum. If a fistula is not seen on initial examination but is suspected on clinical grounds, a variety of bedside maneuvers like Tampons test or Air leak test may be performed to diagnose the fistula. A tampon placed in the vagina and a dilute methylene blue enema instilled in the rectum, with care not to contaminate the string of the tampon. Tampons are removed after 15–20 minutes. The presence of methylene blue on the tampon confirms the fistula is present and open. Another method is Air leak test. The patient placed in the lithotomy position. Water is placed in the vagina, and air is insufflated into the rectum with a sigmoidoscope. The presence of air bubbles in the vagina indicates a fistula.

EVALUATION

Low rectovaginal fistulas are generally straightforward to demonstrate on physical examination. Middle and high fistula are also mostly demonstrated on physical examination or bedside tests. Imaging studies (transrectal ultrasound with use of hydrogen peroxide, vaginography and magnetic resonance imaging) occasionally may be necessary to outline the rectovaginal fistula and to exclude underlying disease states, involvement of other parts of the bowels, or fistulas concomitant with other organs. It is essential to assess the anatomy and function of the sphincter muscles (by endoanal USG, anal manometry and pudendal nerve terminal motor latency), especially in patients who have a rectovaginal fistula resulting from obstetric injury or who have fecal incontinence. Prolonged pudendal nerve terminal motor latency is associated with poorer outcome of repair.[7-10] Endoscopic evaluation may be required if high suspicion of IBD.

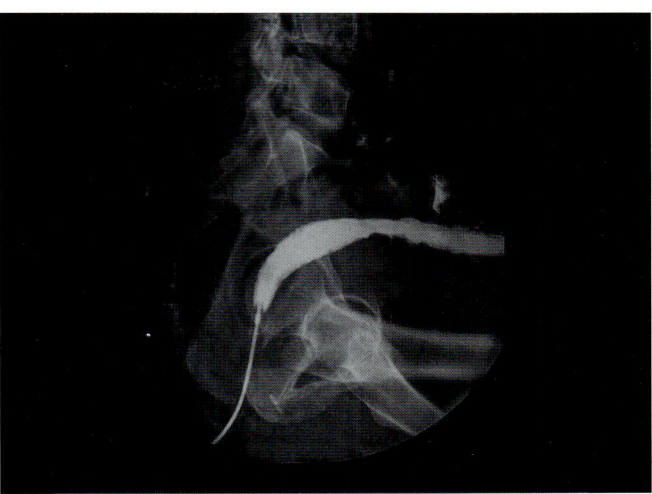

Figure 1 Rectal contrast study to demonstrate the fistula

CLASSIFICATION

Rectovaginal fistulas may be classified on the basis of location, size and etiology (Table 1).

TREATMENT

Conservative Treatment

Few small fistulas may close spontaneously after obstetric trauma in the immediate postpartum period. Hyperbaric oxygen may be associated with successful healing in patients with rectovaginal fistulas from obstetric trauma.[11] Medical therapy, particularly immunomodulation, is associated with healing of rectovaginal fistulas in patients with Crohn's disease.

Table 1: Classification

On the basis of location:	*On the basis of size (diameter):*	*Simple fistula:*
Low: When located at or just slightly above the dentate line with the vaginal opening just inside the vaginal fourchette *High:* When the vaginal opening is behind or near the cervix *Middle:* When located between the high and low sites	*Small:* <0.5 cm *Medium:* 0.5–2.5 cm *Large:* >2.5 cm	Obstetric trauma Infection Relatively small *Complex fistulas:* IBD Irradiation Cancer Failed prior repairs Complications of surgery

SURGICAL OPTIONS FOR RECTOVAGINAL FISTULA

Timing of Surgery

The timing of repair for a rectovaginal fistula caused by obstetric trauma is controversial. If recognized at the time of delivery, it is advisable to repair at the time of the delivery, with the help of expert. In general, surgery for rectovaginal fistulas may be performed as long as the surrounding tissues are soft and pliable. The convention, particularly for fistulas of obstetric origin, has been to wait approximately 3 months, to maximize the condition of the surrounding tissues and also since a small percentage of fistulas close spontaneously in the immediate postpartum period. For patients whose previous repair has failed, a waiting period of 3–6 months has been advocated that permits some healing of the surrounding tissues and often decreases the size of the fistula (Table 2).[12]

Table 2: Different approach for repair of the rectovaginal fistula

A. Local repair

Perineal approach:
- Conversion to complete perineal laceration with layer closure
- Excision of fistula with layer closure ± muscle interposition
- Transperineal repair with layered closure
- Sphincteroplasty
- Fistulotomy

Vaginal approach:
- Layered closure
- Advancement flap
- Use of Martius flap

Transanal approach:
- Advancement flap
- Advancement sleeve flap

Transsphincteric approach (York-Mason):
Sliding flap advancement:
- Anterior rectal wall (noble)
- Mucosa and partial-thickness internal sphincter (Laird)
- Mucosa and full-thickness internal sphincter (Lowry)
- Endorectal type.

B. Transabdominal repair (Sphincter-preserving)
- Without bowel resection, mobilization and division of fistula with closure in layers
- With bowel resection and interposition
- Pull-through procedures
- Low anterior resection—transsacral, EEA stapler
- Abdominoperineal resection
- Fecal diversion (colostomy)
- Sleeve anastomosis (Parks)
- On-lay patch anastomosis (Bricker)

C. Tissue transposition
- Bulbocavernosus (Martius)
- Gluteus maximus
- Gracilis
- Rectus abdominis
- Rectus femoris
- Sartorius
- Adductor longus

D. Miscellaneous
- Colpocleisis
- Collagen fistula plug with button
- Injection of fibrin sealant
- Repair with interposition of bioprosthetics
- Purse-string closure

LOCAL REPAIR

A standard method of local repair is excision of the fistula with a layer closure. This can be accomplished through a vaginal, rectal, perineal or transsphincteric approach, which can be accompanied by the interposition of vascularized pedicles of muscle, if necessary.

Fistulotomy

Simple fistulotomy and drainage, with lying open of the entire tract, work well for an anovaginal fistula, but when used to treat a rectovaginal fistula, partial or total incontinence results. So simple fistulotomy is not advocated for repair of rectovaginal fistulas.

Conversion to Complete Perineal Laceration (Perineoproctotomy) with Layer Closure

The entire rectovaginal fistulous tract, including the perineal body and adjacent sphincter is excised (Figs 2A to F). The vaginal wall is separated from the remains of the perineal body, and a two- or three-layer closure is performed. This procedure can be completed in one stage or two stages. Healing rate is 98–100%.

Transperineal Repair with Layered Closure

This procedure essentially involves an overlapping sphincteroplasty. It corrects any underlying sphincter defect and provides good muscle bulk to interpose in the rectovaginal septum. It may be performed as the sole procedure or combined with sliding flap repair. It is indicated for simple rectovaginal fistulas with an associated sphincter defect. The fistula is identified. After injection of saline with epinephrine to facilitate the dissection, a curvilinear incision is made in the perineum around the anus, and the edges of the external and internal sphincter muscles are identified and mobilized. Scar tissue is usually left in place on the muscle and not debrided. Fistula is identified, and the dissection is carried cephalad, separating the rectum and vagina for several centimeters until soft pliable tissue is reached. It is important to adequately separate the rectum and vagina at the site of the fistula and to extend the dissection cephalad for 1–2 cm. The levator muscles are identified and plicated.[13,14] The perineal skin may be either closed loosely or left open. The vaginal mucosa is left open for drainage. Sphincteroplasty for rectovaginal fistula is associated with success rates of 65–100%.[13,15-17]

Sliding Flap Advancement

The sliding flap repair for the treatment of patients with rectovaginal fistulas was first reported by Noble[18] in 1902. He used Advancement of the anterior rectal wall. In 1948, Laird[19] described the use of a flap of mucosa, submucosa and some fibers of the internal sphincter. Lowry[20] advocated the use of a flap of mucosa, submucosa and the full thickness of the internal sphincter. The procedure is generally used for patients with simple low fistulas who have not had previous repairs. Patients with rectovaginal fistula from obstetric injuries (without an associated sphincter

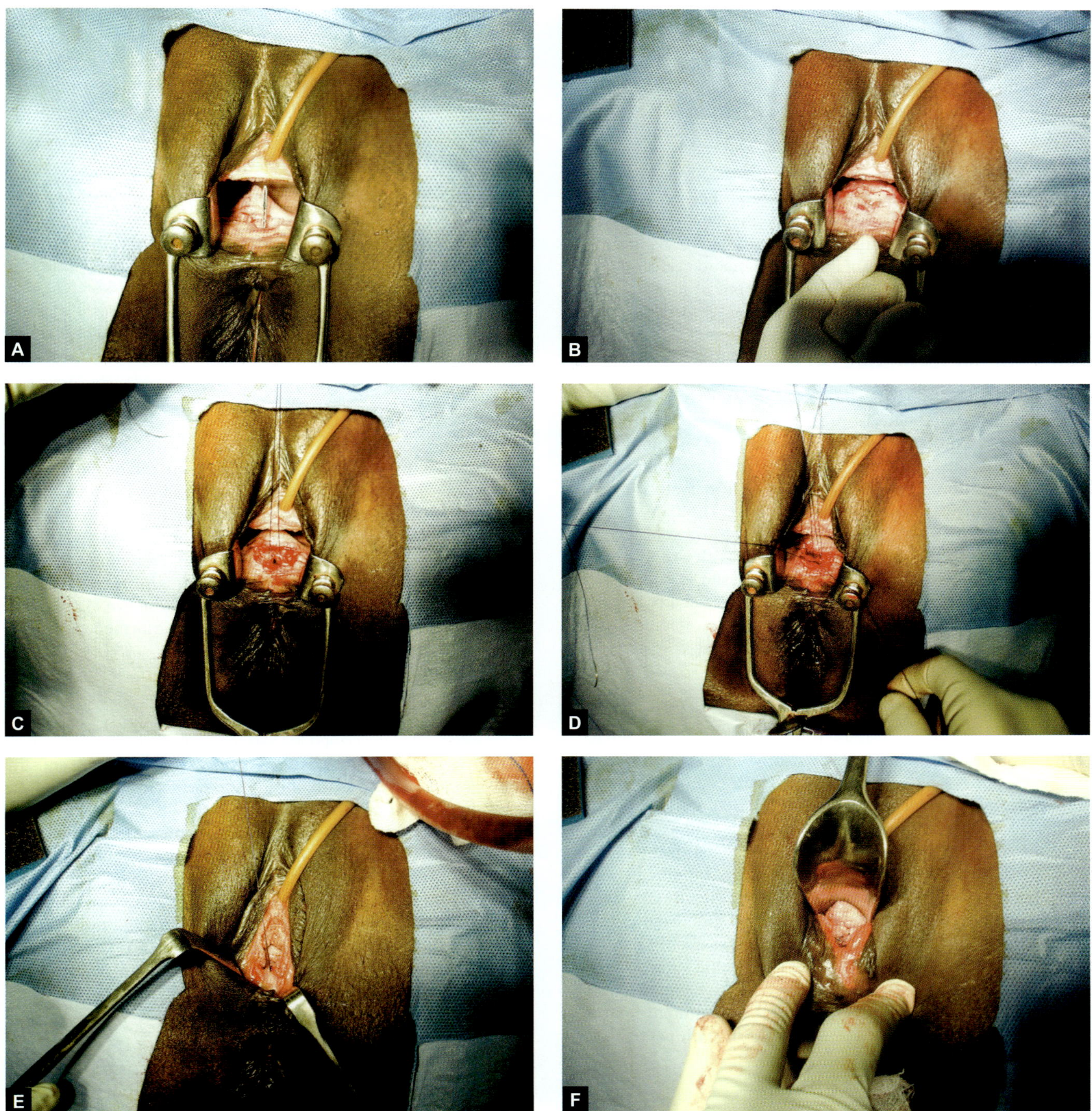

Figures 2A to F Transvaginal layered closure of fistula. (A) Midlevel rectovaginal fistula - probe in to the vagina; (B) Finger in the rectum - exposing the fistulous opening in the vagina; (C to E) Suture closure of the fistulous opening after refreshening the edges; (F) Advancement of the vaginal mucosal flap over the closed fistulous opening

defect) and patients with Crohn's rectovaginal fistulas without associated proctitis are good candidates for sliding flap repair.

Under general anesthesia, the patient is placed in the prone jack-knife position with the buttocks spread by tape. Injections of 0.5% lidocaine (Xylocaine) or 0.25% bupivacaine with 1:200,000 epinephrine solutions are injected along the planned routes of dissection. The rectal flap is mobilized at least 4 cm cephalad to the fistula. The base of the flap should be approximately two times the width of the apex of the flap to ensure adequate blood supply. The flap, consisting of mucosa, submucosa, and part of circular muscle, is raised from the apex to the base. The cut edge of the circular muscle is mobilized laterally to approximate in the midline without tension. Hemostasis is achieved. The mobilized circular muscle then is reconstructed with 2-0 absorbable sutures. Hemostasis is checked before advancement of the flap. Excess flap, including the rectovaginal fistula, is excised. The flap is sutured with 3-0 absorbable sutures at the apex and along each side of the flap. The vagina is left open for drainage. If the patient is incontinent or has a sphincter defect, a concomitant sphincteroplasty is performed. The success rate varies from 43% to 100%. Factors responsible for differing success rates after sliding flap repair include number of previous repairs, whether the initial or ultimate success rate was reported, the presence of a concomitant sphincter, the cause of the rectovaginal fistula, the heterogeneity of the patient groups and variations in surgical technique. Common causes of flap failure include ischemia of the flap and hematoma and/or the development of infection under the flap.

Transvaginal Techniques of Local Repair

A transvaginal approach for sliding flap may also be used to repair rectovaginal fistulas. This approach addresses the fistula from the lower pressure vaginal side. Concomitant sphincteroplasty can be performed if needed. The procedure is performed in the lithotomy position. An incision is made in the posterior vaginal wall by the introitus, and the flap is raised. The flap should be wide enough to ensure good blood supply and mobility. This approach may be advantageous in patients with Crohn's disease (because non diseased, pliable vaginal tissue is used to form the flap, and there is no dissection in the diseased rectum) and in patients with pouch-vaginal fistulas after ileoanal pouch construction.

ADVANCEMENT SLEEVE FLAP

This procedure was described by Simmang[21] to repair a rectovaginal fistula associated with a stricture in Crohn's disease. The operation is performed either in the lithotomy or jack-knife position. Electrocautery is used to circumferentially incise the mucosa. Dissection is started in the submucosal plane by circumferentially incising the mucosa just distal to the palpable stricture. After reaching above the sphincter complex dissection is deepened through the muscle layer to encompass the full thickness of the rectum. Sufficient rectum is mobilized to enable a tension free rectoanal anastomosis. Vaginal opening is closed posteriorly with polyglactin synthetic absorbable sutures. Vaginal mucosa is left open to provide drainage. Rectoanal anastomosis is performed carefully. Loop ileostomy and concomitant treatment of intra-abdominal Crohn's disease is done in conjunction.

TRANSABDOMINAL REPAIR

Local repairs and flap advancements are generally difficult to use for high rectovaginal fistulas. If the fistula is due to irradiation change, neoplasm, or IBD with concomitant intra-abdominal disease, a transabdominal approach should be preferred. Multiple abdominal procedures have been descried. The simplest of these repairs involves mobilization of the rectovaginal septum, division of the fistula, and a layered closure of the rectal and vaginal defects without bowel resection with or without interposition of a live pedicle of tissue when normal tissues are available for the layered repair. In presence of abnormal local tissues (IBD, irradiation, diverticulitis or a neoplasm), bowel resection (like low anterior resection or sleeve advancement anorectoplasty) is most often required. Sphincter-sacrificing bowel resections such as abdominoperineal resection or even pelvic exenteration may sometimes require for patients with neoplasm-induced rectovaginal fistulas.

Radiation-induced Rectovaginal Fistulas

Rectovaginal fistula secondary to radiation injuries are not amenable to local repair because of vascular damage to the remaining tissues. Therefore the repair has to deliver normal vascularized tissue to the region. Two well-known procedures are coloanal sleeve anastomosis as first reported by Parks[22] and Onlay Patch Anastomosis described by Bricker and Johnston.[23] If patients are poor operative risks they may be treated better by a permanent colostomy.

Coloanal Sleeve Anastomosis

This involves complete mobilization of the colon so that nonirradiated bowel can be brought down to the anal canal. The rectum is mobilized down to just beyond the level of the rectovaginal fistula and divided at that point. The irradiated colon is resected. Then, from a perineal approach, the mucosa is stripped off the underlying muscle until the entire remaining rectum is denuded of all mucosa, leaving a rectal muscle tube. Next, the normal colon is threaded through the muscle sleeve. As per anal anastomosis of the colon to the anal canal is performed at the level of the dentate line.

Onlay Patch Anastomosis

This procedure is described for fistulas that involve large portions of the vagina. The procedure involves mobilization of the rectosigmoid and exposure of the fistula. After transaction of the rectosigmoid, an end stoma is formed. The distal rectosigmoid is rotated down then the open end is anastomosed to the debrided edges of the fistula opening in the rectum. After healing has been confirmed with radiographic studies, the proximal sigmoid is sutured in end-to-side fashion to the loop in the rectosigmoid. The advantage of this procedure is that posterior rectal mobilization and entry into the presacral space are not necessary. Disadvantage is that a portion of the diseased rectum is left in place for the anastomosis and it is technically difficult surgery.

Role of Fecal Diversion

For a patient who is a poor medical risk and cannot tolerate major surgery, simple fecal diversion with either a loop ileostomy or colostomy may provide good symptomatic relief and reasonable quality of life. Fecal diversion may be done as part of coloanal anastomosis or Bricker onlay patch anastomosis. Patients whose multiple previous local repairs have failed may also benefit from fecal diversion as an adjunct to primary repair or as a primary procedure. Patients with irradiation induced rectovaginal fistulas or rectovaginal fistulas associated with a *non-resectable* malignancy, especially if they are poor operative risks, may be treated best by a permanent totally diverting colostomy. When dealing with high, complicated rectovaginal fistulas caused by irradiation, neoplasm, active IBD, and active infectious processes, a preliminary colostomy may be a useful. After a diverting colostomy has been established, direct repair of the rectovaginal fistula can be deferred as long as 6–12 months until local tissues are normal.

TISSUE INTERPOSITION PROCEDURES

Tissue interposition for the treatment of patients with rectovaginal fistula is intended to interpose normal well vascularized healthy tissue between suture lines. Different types of tissues have been used, such as the gracilis, sartorius and gluteus maximus muscles. Most commonly used are the bulbocavernosus muscle and gracilis muscle. This technique was first described by Martius[24] in 1928 and was originally used for the repair of vesicovaginal fistulas. It is also useful for radiation-induced rectovaginal fistulas, large obstetric fistulas, those for which previous repairs have failed, and selected pouch-vaginal fistulas after restorative proctocolectomy. The gracilis muscle is also used for interposition. The gracilis is mobilized and brought through a tunnel with care to preserve the neurovascular bundle. An overall healing rate per patient of gracilic transposition is 50–92%.[25] Technique of Martius graft:[26] vertical incision is made over the labia majora and extended ventrally and laterally to include a non-hair-bearing, oval shaped, patch of skin from the medial thigh. The Martius bulbocavernosus fat pad is then mobilized by grasping the edges of the skin with Allis clamps and sharply dissecting the fat pad from the undersurface of the labia majora. Next, the full-thickness skin patch is elevated and sharply dissected from its bed but it is left attached to the bulbocavernosus fat pad. The graft and skin are then passed through the Martius tunnel and attached to the vaginal wall defect with multiple absorbable fine sutures. The vulgar and thigh defects are then closed with interrupted absorbable sutures. Dyspareunia, patient's self-perception of the appearance of the graft site and decreased sensation or numbness of the graft site are major concern.[27]

MISCELLANEOUS

Fibrin Glue

The advantage of fibrin glue for treatment of fistulas is that it can be done without significant complications. This technique has high failure rate because the tract is generally too short to hold the glue for any length of time.[28] Modified technique like closure of the internal opening and use of intra-adhesive antibiotics has not improved the outcome.[29] Fibrin glue as an adjunct with other procedures such as endorectal advancement flap have failure rate similar to endorectal advancement flap alone. Presently, the technique is generally not used for rectovaginal fistulas.

Collagen Fistula Plug with Button

Use of collagen plug for rectovaginal fistulas has been associated with a high failure rate because of early dislodgement of the plug from the short tract. The plug has been modified with a button to potentially obviate this problem.[30] The success rate of button fistula plug is still low with all failure due to dislodgement of plug. The fistula plug is an option in patients with rectovaginal fistulas without an associated sphincter defect or associated incontinence.

Bioprosthetics

Bioprosthetic mesh (made from porcine intestinal submucosa) can be used as an interposition graft to repair rectovaginal fistulas. In a study,[31] patients who underwent advancement flap and placement of an interposition graft of bioprosthetic material had lower recurrence rate (19%) than women who underwent advancement flap repair without mesh (34%). But this was not randomized trial and had small number of patients.

Rectovaginal Fistula in Crohn's Disease

Treatment of rectovaginal fistulas associated with Crohn's disease is demanding. Operative intervention is avoided if symptoms are mild. On the other hand, severely symptomatic patients may require proctectomy.[32] Improvements in medical therapy have led to better prognosis for rectovaginal fistulas in patients with Crohn's disease.[33] Endorectal advancement flap has a success rate of 60–70% and is considered the preferred technique for rectovaginal fistula repair in Crohn's where rectum is comparatively normal.[34,35] However, nearly 50% may need additional surgical treatment and failure is still high. Patients with severe refractory proctitis and rectovaginal fistula may require proctectomy with fistula repair and permanent ostomy. Immunomodulators are associated with successful healing.

RECURRENT RECTOVAGINAL FISTULA

The causes of recurrent rectovaginal fistula include obstetrical injury, fistula following ileal pouch-anal anastomosis for ulcerative colitis, indeterminate colitis, Crohn's disease and cryptoglandular disease. Most recurrent rectovaginal fistulas are complex fistula. Management of recurrent rectovaginal fistula is difficult. Underlying pathology and the previous repair should be considered to decide the optimum treatment. Advancement flap can be used successfully for recurrent rectovaginal fistulas. Haray et al.,[36] described an operative technique that combines the standard endoanal advancement flap procedure with a diamond-shaped cutaneous flap advancement into the vagina for recurrent rectovaginal fistula. Pye et al.[37] described Surgisis mesh repair for recurrent rectovaginal fistula. In this repair Surgisis mesh is interposed between rectal and vaginal walls. Fistula tract is identified and vagina is dissected from the rectum about 2 cm above the fistula. The rectal side of the repair is done in two layers with first layer of PDS 2/0 sutures followed by a second continuous Lembert suture of number 1 polyglactin. This folds the rectal mucosa over the fistula tract. Surgisis mesh is cut to size, approximately 5x5 cm, placed in the rectovaginal space, and held with five 3-0 PDS sutures at each corner of the mesh and in the middle. Vaginal mucosa is finally closed over the mesh with a continuous number 1 polyglactin (Vicryl) suture.

REFERENCES

1. Goldaber KG, Wendel PJ, McIntire DD, Wendel GD Jr. Postpartum perineal morbidity after fourth-degree perineal repair. Am J Obstet Gynecol. 1993;168(2):489-93.
2. Venkatesh KS, Ramanujam PS, Larson DM, Haywood MA. Anorectal complications of vaginal delivery. Dis Colon Rectum. 1989;32(12):1039-41.

3. Radcliffe AG, Ritchie JK, Hawley PR, Lennard-Jones JE, Northover JM. Anovaginal and rectovaginal fistulas in Crohn's disease. Dis Colon Rectum. 1998;31(2):94-9.
4. Matthiessen P, Hansson L, Sjodahl R, Rutegård J. Anastomotic-vaginal fistula (AVF) after anterior resection of the rectum for cancer—occurrence and risk factors. Colorectal Dis. 2010;12(4):351-7.
5. Heriot AG, Tekkis PP, Smith JJ, Bona R, Cohen RG, Nicholls RJ, et al. Management and outcome of pouch-vaginal fistulas following restorative proctocolectomy. Dis Colon Rectum. 2005;48(3):451-8.
6. Kasibhatia M, Clough RW, Montana GS, Oleson JR, Light K, Steffey BA, et al. Predictors of severe gastrointestinal toxicity after external beam radiotherapy and interstitial brachytherapy for advanced or recurrent gynecologic malignancies. Int J Radiat Oncol Biol Phys. 2006;65(2):398-403.
7. Tsang CB, Madoff RD, Wong WD, Rothenberger DA, Finne CO, Singer D, et al. Anal sphincter integrity and function influences outcome in rectovaginal fistula repair. Dis Colon Rectum. 1998;41(9):1141-6.
8. Saclarides TJ. Rectovaginal fistula. Surg Clin North Am. 2002;82(6):1261-72.
9. Sultan AH, Kamm MA, Hudson CN, Thomas JM, Bartram CI. Anal-sphincter disruption during vaginal delivery. N Engl J Med. 1993;329(26):1905-11.
10. Yee LF, Birnbaum EH, Read TE, Kodner IJ, Fleshman JW. Use of endoanal ultrasound in patients with rectovaginal fistulas. Dis Colon Rectum. 1999;42(8):1057-64.
11. Dohgomori H, Arikawa K, Nobori M, Tonari M. Hyperbaric oxygenation for rectovaginal fistula: a report of two cases. J Obstet Gynaecol Res. 1999;25(5):343-4.
12. Halverson AL, Hull TL, Fazio VW, Church J, Hammel J, Floruta C, et al. Repair of recurrent rectovaginal fistulas. Surgery. 2001;130(4):753-7.
13. Tsang CB, Madoff RD, Wong WD, Rothenberger DA, Finne CO, Singer D, et al Anal sphincter integrity and function influences outcome in rectovaginal fistula repair. Dis Colon Rectum. 1998;41(9):1141-6.
14. Baig MK, Zhao RH, Yuen CH, Nogueras JJ, Singh JJ, Weiss EG, et al Simple rectovaginal fistulas. Int J Colorectal Dis. 2000;15(5-6):323-7.
15. Wise WE Jr, Aquilar PS, Padmanabhan A, Meesig DM, Arnold MW, Stewart WR, et al Surgical treatment of low rectovaginal fistulas. Dis Colon Rectum. 1991;34(3):271-4.
16. Athanasiadis S, Oladeinde I, Kuprian A, Keller B. Endorectal advancement flap-plasty vs. transperineal closure in surgical treatment of rectovaginal fistulas: a prospective long-term study of 88 patients. Chirurg. 1995;66(5):493-502.
17. MacRae HM, McLeod RS, Cohen Z, Stern H, Reznick R. Treatment of rectovaginal fistula that has failed previous repair attempts. Dis Colon Rectum. 1995;38(9):921-5.
18. Noble GH. A new operation for complete laceration of the perineum designed for the purpose of eliminating danger of infection from the rectum. Trans Am Gynecol Soc. 1902;27:357.
19. Laird DR. Procedures used in treatment of complicated fistulas. Am J Surg. 1948;76(6):701-8.
20. Lowry AC, Thorson AG, Rothenberger DA, Goldberg SM. Repair of simple rectovaginal fistulas: influence of previous repairs. Dis Colon Rectum. 1988;31(9):676-8.
21. Simmang CL, Lacey SW, Huber PJ Jr. Rectal sleeve advancement: repair of rectovaginal fistula associated with anorectal stricture in Crohn's disease. Dis Colon Rectum. 1998;41(6):787-9.
22. Parks AG, Allen CL, Frank JD, McPartlin JF. A method of treating postirradiation rectovaginal fistulas. Br J Surg. 1978;65(6):417-21.
23. Bricker EM, Johnston WD. Repair of postirradiation rectovaginal fistula and stricture. Surg Gynecol Obstet. 1979;148(4):499-506.
24. Martius H. Die operative Wiederherstellung der vollkommen fehlenden Harnröhre und des Schliessmuskels derselben. Zentralbl Gynäk. 1928;52:480.
25. Lefevre JH, Bretagnol F, Maggiori L Alves A, Ferron M, Panis Y, et al. Operative results and quality of life after gracilis muscle transposition for recurrent rectovaginal fistula. Dis Colon Rectum. 2009;52(7):1290-5.
26. Margolis T, Elkins TE, Seffah J, Opuro-Addo HS, Fort D. Full-thickness Martius grafts to preserve vaginal depth as an adjunct in the repair of large obstetric fistulas. Obstet Gynecol. 1994;84(1): 148-52.
27. Petrou SP, Jones J, Parra RO. Martius flap harvest site: patient self-perception. J Urol. 2001;167(5):2098-9.
28. Abel ME, Chiu YS, Russell TR, Volpe PA. Autologous fibrin glue in the treatment of rectovaginal and complex fistulas. Dis Colon Rectum. 1993;36(5):447-9.
29. Singer M, Cintron J, Nelson R, Orsay C, Bastawrous A, Pearl R, et al. Treatment of fistulas-in-ano with fibrin sealant in combination with intra-adhesive antibiotics and/or surgical closure of the internal fistula opening. Dis Colon Rectum. 2005;48(4):799-808.
30. Schwandner O, Fuerst A, Kunstreich K, Scherer R. Innovative technique for the closure of rectovaginal fistula using Surgisis mesh. Tech Coloproctol. 2009;13(2):135-40.
31. Ellis CN. Outcomes after repair of rectovaginal fistulas using bioprosthetics. Dis Colon Rectum. 2008;52:1084-8.
32. Loffler T, Welsch T, Muhl S, Hinz U, Schmidt J, Kienle P, et al. Long-term success rate after surgical treatment of anorectal and rectovaginal fistulas in Crohn's disease. Int J Colorectal Dis. 2009;24(5):521-6.
33. El-Gazzaz G, Hull T, Mignanelli E, Hammel J, Gurland B, Zutshi M, et al. Analysis of function and predictors of failure in women undergoing repair of Crohn's related rectovaginal fistula. J Gastrointest Surg. 2010;14(5):824-9.
34. Radcliffe AG, Ritchie JK, Hawley PR, Lennard-Jones JE, Northover JMA. Anovaginal and rectovaginal fistulas in Crohn's disease. Dis Colon Rectum. 1988;31(2):94-9.
35. Sher ME, Bauer JJ, Gelernt I. Surgical repair of rectovaginal fistulas in patients with Crohn's disease: transvaginal approach. Dis Colon Rectum. 1991;34(8):641-8.
36. Haray PN, Stiff G, Foster ME. New option for recurrent rectovaginal fistulas. Dis Colon Rectum. 1996;39(4):463-4.
37. Pye PK, Dada T, Duthie G, Phillips K. Surgisis trade mark mesh: a novel approach to repair of a recurrent rectovaginal fistula. Dis Colon Rectum. 2004;47(9):1554-6.

CHAPTER 90

Rectourethral Fistula

Nitesh Patidar, MS Ansari, Ashok Kumar

INTRODUCTION

A rectourethral fistula (RUF) is an abnormal opening between the rectum and urethra that results in pneumaturia, fecaluria and leakage of urine from the rectum.[1]

Rectourethral fistulas are rare; it may be either congenital or acquired and are difficult to treat. Congenital fistulas are often associated with other anorectal anomalies, whereas acquired fistulas may result from trauma, iatrogenic rectal injury during pelvic surgery, anterior rectal wall biopsy, infectious conditions, Crohn's disease and malignancy, especially prostate cancer.[2,3] RUF is a condition encountered in men almost exclusively because in female patients, the vagina sits between the urethra and the rectum and thus protects against RUF.

ETIOLOGY

Culp and Calhoon[4] classified RUFs in five groups on the basis of etiology: (1) congenital, (2) iatrogenic, (3) traumatic, (4) neoplastic and (5) inflammatory. Some of them are discussed hereunder.

Congenital

The incidence of congenital RUF is more than that of acquired fistulas (5,000:1).[5] It is more common in boys and is frequently accompanied by other anorectal anomaly.

Iatrogenic

Acquired RUF may occur in surgery for prostatic disorders, radiotherapy, cryotherapy, anorectal surgery and urethral instrumentation. Radical retropubic prostatectomy is most common procedure which causes RUF. The risk of RUF increases in patients with history of surgery for benign prostatic hyperplasia, radiotherapy and rectal surgery.[6] Incidence of rectal injury in open radical prostatectomy is 0.5–9% whereas in laparoscopic and robotic prostatectomy the incidence is 1–2.7%.[7] Immediate repair of the injury results in excellent outcome without long-term sequelae in the majority of patients.

Incidence of RUF after cryoablation of prostate is between 0.5% and 2%.[8] Higher rate of RUF have been reported when cryotherapy is used as salvage treatment. RUF has also been reported after radiotherapy for prostate cancer. Both external beam radiotherapy and brachytherapy can lead to RUF. Incidence of RUF after brachytherapy is 0.4%. RUF may also occur after high-intensity focused ultrasound treatment (HIFU)[9] for prostate cancer.

Traumatic

Traumatic RUF is often seen in wartime injuries and is accompanied with extensive urethral injury which leads to extensive stricture. Muneer Al-Ali et al. reported 30 men with RUFs of traumatic origin. Surgical repair of traumatic RUF is very challenging. As this condition is very uncommon, no single procedure has become the technique of choice.[10]

CROHN'S DISEASE

In Crohn's disease, the incidence of RUF is approximately 0.3%. Fistulae due to Crohn's disease are complex, and treatment should be individualized. Success of RUF repair in cases of radiation injury and Crohn's disease tends to be lower than in patients with other causes of RUF.[11]

PRESENTATION

Rectourethral fistula may manifest with pneumaturia, fecaluria, rectal bleeding, rectal voiding, leakage or watery diarrhea, and often severe rectal and pelvic pain. Patients may also present with intra-abdominal abscess, sepsis and necrotizing fasciitis, particularly if the diagnosis is delayed.

DIAGNOSIS

Rectourethral fistulas are commonly debilitating and resistant to repeated repair procedures. Therefore, careful preoperative staging evaluation and fecal and urinary diversion are almost universally recommended. Diversion of fecal and urinary streams from the fistula allows inflammation to improve or resolve before repair. Diversion alone is sufficient therapy to allow a small, nonradiated fistula to heal in approximately 20–25% of cases.[6]

Definitive diagnosis of RUF can be made using voiding cystourethrography (VCUG) (Fig. 1) or retrograde urethrography. VCUG helps in delineation of exact location and size of RUF.[6] Lateral films should be taken to visualize small fistula.

CT scan of the abdomen and pelvis in cases of sepsis and suspected abscess should be done. Diagnostic studies should be postponed in the presence of fever or sepsis and undertaken only after proximal urinary diversion, administration of intravenous antibiotics and resolution of the acute process.

Cystoscopy, proctoscopy and examination under anesthesia are necessary to determine tissue necrosis or extent of radiation damage surrounding the fistula, the fistula size and location, the rectal sphincter condition and evidence of associated urethral or bladder neck stricture. It is also important to assess bladder capacity and compliance, which both may be impaired by radiation. Video urodynamic study (VUDS) is excellent for assessment of storage abnormalities; however, in some cases the fistula may be large enough to preclude the accumulation of fluid in the bladder. In these situations, the surgeon must rely on the visual assessment of bladder distensibility at the time of cystoscopy. When the bladder is extremely contracted or fibrotic, preservation of the bladder is not likely to provide a functional outcome. Consideration of the rectal sphincter function should also be made by anal manometry if any doubt about its competence exists.

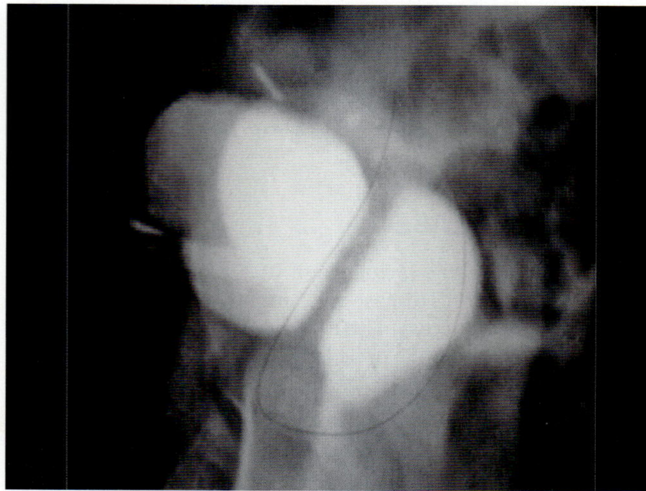

Figure 1 Voiding cystourethrogram (VCUG) showing rectourethral fistula

Table 1: Approaches to RUF repair

I.	Perineal
II.	Posterior sagittal
III.	Transanal
IV.	Anterior transanorectal
V.	Transabdominal
VI.	Combined abdominoperineal

MANAGEMENT

Rectourethral fistula can be managed with conservative and surgical treatment. Majority of the cases need surgical repair while very few close spontaneously with conservative treatment. Spontaneous closure of post-prostatectomy fistula may be seen with catheter drainage and total parenteral nutrition. Fecal diversion is required in some cases. A number of surgical approaches with single and staged repairs have been reported. Initial fecal diversion and later staged repair of all RUF has been proposed by some authors.[12] Some fistula may heal spontaneously with this approach. Single stage repair has the advantage of decreased morbidity and low treatment cost. Small fistula which is not associated with infection or abscess can be managed with single stage repair. Similarly, some small iatrogenic fistula can be treated with this approach. Staged repair is appropriate for large fistula, radiation induced fistula, RUF with infection and in immunocompromised patients.

The various approach described for repair of RUF are depicted in Table 1.

These repairs can be performed either open or by laparoscopic/endoscopic method.

PERINEAL APPROACH

A perineal approach to RUF is suitable for fistulas that are small and low in position. In addition various interpositional flaps, e.g. gracilis muscle, penile skin, pedicled dartos muscle, levator muscle and bladder can be used with this approach with excellent results (Figs 2A to C). Goodwin described principles for successful repair of fistula which include complete excision of fistula, elevation of flaps on rectal and urinary sides of fistula, closure with non-overlapping suture lines and interposition of levator ani muscles if possible.[13] Limited exposure and risk of urinary incontinence are disadvantages of this approach.

An inverted U-shaped incision in the perineum is carried well forward onto the scrotum where the skin and tunica dartos are loose. The plane behind the bulbar urethra is opened by dividing its attachment to the perineal body, which is continued cranially until the track of the fistula can be seen, divided and ligated. The divided ends of the fistula must be covered with some healthy tissue. A catheter is left in the urethra.

POSTERIOR-SAGITTAL APPROACH (FIGS 3A TO D)

This approach was described by Kraske in 1885. A posterior midline incision was made which was extended on left side over the paramedian aspect of coccyx and sacrum. Coccygectomy and

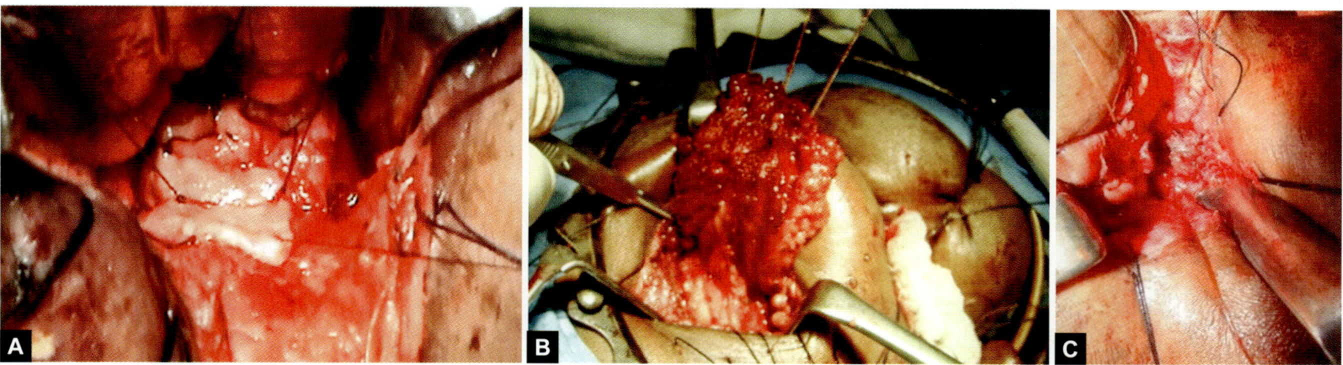

Figures 2A to C (A) Buccal mucosa graft; (B) Harvesting gluteus maximus; (C) Gluteus maximus interposition

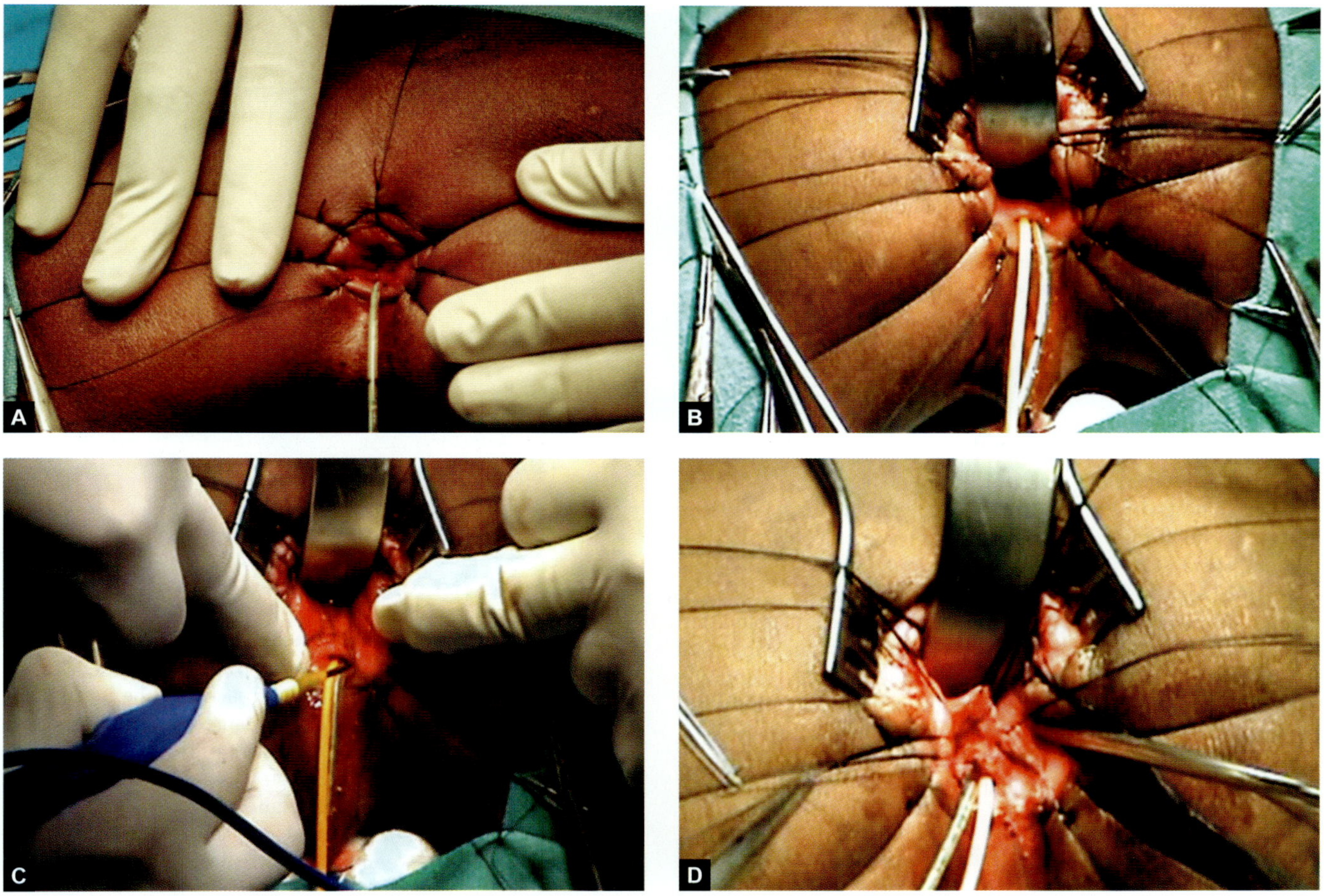

Figures 3A to D Posterior sagittal approach. (A) Rectourethral fistula in prone Jack-knife position; (B) Visualization of fistulous tract; (C) Circumscribing fistula; (D) Mobilized fistulous tract

partial sacrectomy were also done. Fecal continence is preserved in this approach by not dividing the sphincters and lateral sweeping of the rectum bring about resection and reanastomosis of a tumor-bearing rectal segment. Advantages of this approach are excellent exposure and preservation of sphincter mechanism. Excision of sacral segment and surrounding muscles, nerves and ligaments is a disadvantage.[14]

TRANS-SPHINCTERIC APPROACH

York-Mason[15] popularized the posterior midline transrectal transsphincteric approach. In this procedure all sphincters were divided to obtain a direct access to fistula. Advantages of this technique are dissection in virgin planes, rapid access and excellent exposure of fistula, minimal blood loss, preservation of

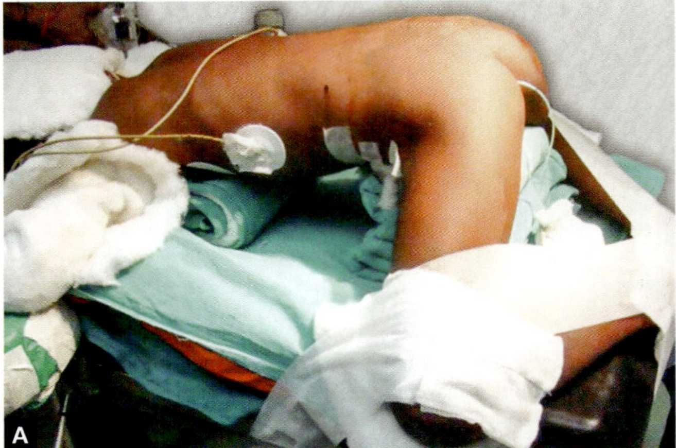

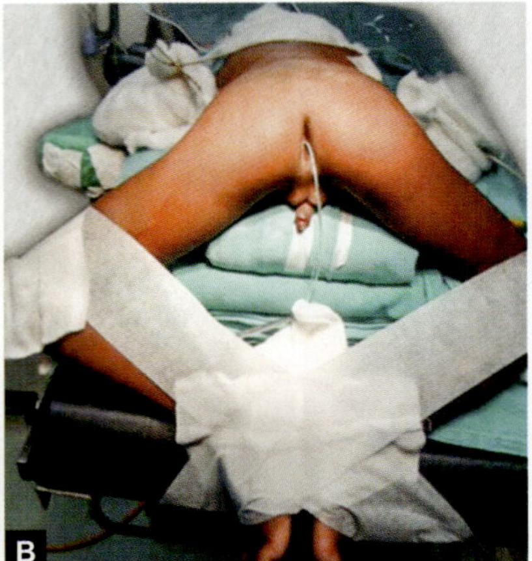

Figures 4A and B Jack-knife position. (A) Lateral view and (B) AP view

erectile function and urinary continence and low morbidity. The patient is placed in prone, jack knife position (Figs 4A and B) and the buttocks taped laterally. An incision is made from the tip of the coccyx to the anal verge. Posterior anal sphincter and rectal mucosa divided and direct access to fistula obtained. Sphincter muscles are carefully tagged for later reconstruction. An incision is made around fistula and planes are developed between the wall of the rectum and the urinary tract. Fistula is excised and urethra is closed. Full thickness rectal wall closure is done in "vest over pants" fashion. Finally posterior rectal wall and sphincter muscle repair are done. Urethral catheter is usually kept for 2 weeks.

TRANSANAL APPROACH

Transanal approach does not involve division of the anal sphincter. The Latzko procedure is a type of transanal approach. In lithotomy position cystoscopy is done to localize the site of fistula and then dilatation and retraction of the anus is done to expose the fistula in rectum. An incision is made in rectal mucosa all around the fistula and rectal mucosa between fistula and circular incision is removed. Fistula is closed with absorbable sutures followed by closure of muscle layer and rectal mucosa. This technique is suitable for low fistula only and poor exposure and restricted movement of instruments are other disadvantages.[16,17] Parks & Motson described a modification of transanal technique using a full thickness flap of anterior rectal wall.[18]

ANTERIOR TRANSANORECTAL APPROACH

Anterior transanorectal approach was described by Gecelter.[19] This technique uses a midline perineal incision and anterior incision of sphincter. Fistulous tract is excised and multilayered repair is done. This approach provides good exposure; allows tissue interposition and continence preservation (Fig. 5).

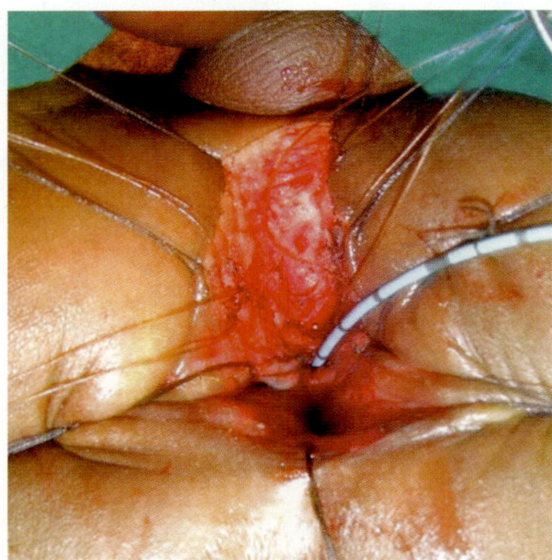

Figure 5 Anterior transanorectal approach

COMBINED ABDOMINOPERINEAL APPROACH

A transabdominal approach has the advantage of availability of omentum for a flap but has disadvantage of poor exposure in deep pelvis, risk of fecal and urinary incontinence and morbidity of laparotomy.[20,21]

A combined abdominoperineal approach may be used, when other simpler techniques have failed. An anterior perineal incision is made behind the prostate to expose the fistula. The presence of a urethral catheter greatly facilitates the dissection, which is continued above the fistula into the plane of the pelvic dissection.

The abdomen is explored, the pelvis is entered and the dissection proceeds between the front of the rectum and the back of the prostate until the perineal dissection is reached. A pedicle omental patch is mobilized based on the right gastroepiploic artery and of sufficient length to reach the perineum. If the omentum cannot be used, a partial rectus abdominis flap and a gracilis interposition are alternative sources of well vascularized tissue. The urethral and rectal defects are closed and omentum, rectus muscle or gracilis is sutured between the two closure sites.

ENDOSCOPIC APPROACH

Wilbert[22] described combined endoscopic closure of RUF. In this technique excision of the fistula and suturing was done endoscopically through transrectal approach and simultaneous transurethral fulguration of urethral side of fistula was done.

MISCELLANEOUS METHODS

Fibrin Glue

Venkatesh & Ramanujam,[23] in their prospective study reported the efficacy of fibrin glue in management of anorectal fistulas. Bardari et al. described use of biological glue (Glubran®) to close one prostato-perineal fistula and one persistent neobladder-ileal fistula.[24] The results of these isolated reports are encouraging. Fibrin glue can be applied in outpatient setting and has no significant procedural complication. It can be used for management of recurrent fistula as an alternative to surgery.

Perineal Pedicled Dartos Flap

Youssef et al.[25] reported use of perineal subcutaneous dartos pedicled flap in RUF. After excision of fistula, flap was interposed between repaired rectum and urethra. No fistula recurrence was reported.

Outcome Following Repair of RUF

The results of various approaches and their outcome have been shown in Table 2.

Table 2: Summary statistics for types of surgical repair, tissue flap usage and primary outcomes[26]

Sl no.	*Study (year)*	*Total RUF patients*	*Transanal repairs*	*Transabdominal repairs*	*Trans-sphincteric repairs*	*Transperineal repairs*	*Tissue flap*	*Gracilis flap*	*Omental flap*	*Dartos and other flaps*	*Successful RUF closure*	*RUF recurrence or persistence*
1	Netsch et al. (2011)	8	2	5	0	1	5	1	4	0	8	0
2	Rouanne et al. (2011)	10	0	0	10	0	0	0	0	0	10	0
3	Samplaski et al. (2011)	13	0	0	0	13	13	13	0	0	12	1
4	Thomas et al. (2010)	13	0	0	0	7	4/7	0	0	4	6/7	1/7
5	Vanni et al. (2010)	74	0	0	0	74	74	68	0	6	68	6
6	Abdalla (2009)	8	0	0	0	8	5	0	0	5	8	0
7	Kasiraeian et al. (2009)	12	0	0	12	0	0	0	0	0	9	3
8	Spahn et al. (2009)	5	0	0	0	5	5	0	0	5	4	1
9	Ulrich et al. (2009)	26	0	0	0	26	26	26	0	0	26	0
10	Ghoniem et al. (2008)	25	0	0	0	25	25	25	0	0	25	0
11	Gupta et al. (2008)	10	0	0	0	10	10	10	0	0	10	0
12	Wexner et al. (2008)	36	0	0	0	36	36	36	0	0	28	8
13	Crippa et al. (2008)	8	0	0	7	0	0	0	0	0	6/7	1/7
14	Varma et al. (2007)	8	0	0	0	8	8	0	0	8	6	2
15	Barisic & Krivokapic (2006)	6	3	0	3	0	0	0	0	0	3	3
16	Lane et al. (2006)	22	0	15	1	1	4/17	2	2	0	15/17	2/17
17	Larson et al. (2005)	10	0	2	0	2	1/4	N/A	N/A	N/A	3/4	1/4
18	Moreira et al. (2004)	11	0	7	3	0	10/10	3	7	0	9/10	1/10
19	Culkin & Ramsey (2003)	5	0	0	5	0	5	0	0	5	4	1
20	Garofalo et al. (2003)	23	14	2	3	0	0	0	0	0	13/19	6/19
21	Zmora et al. (2003)	11	0	0	0	11	11	11	0	0	9	2
22	Nyam et al. (1999)	16	2	3	2	6	3/13	N/A	N/A	N/A	9/13	4/13
23	Youssef et al. (1999)	12	0	0	0	12	12	0	0	12	12	0
24	Al-ali et al. (1997)	30	1	3	11	1	2/16	0	2	0	14/16	2/16
25	Bukowski et al. (1995)	7	0	3	2	1	3/6	1	2	0	4/6	2/6
26	Trippitelli et al. (1985)	7	0	7	0	0	7	0	6	1	7	0

REFERENCES

1. Elliott SP, McAninch JW, Chi T, Doyle SM, Master VA. Management of severe urethral complications of prostate cancer therapy. Journal of Urology. 2006;176(6):2508-13.
2. Renschler TD, Middleton RG. 30 years of experience with York-Mason repair of recto-urinary fistulas. J Urol. 2003;170:1222-5.
3. Vidal Sans J, Palou Redorta J, Pradell Teigell J, Banus Gassol JM. Management and treatment of eighteen rectourethral fistulas. Eur Urol. 1985;11:300-5.
4. Culp OS, Calhoon HW. A variety of rectourethral fistulas: experiences with 20 cases. J Urol. 1964;91:560-71.
5. Endo M, Hayashi A, Ishihara M, Maie M, Nagasaki A, Nishi T, et al. Analysis of 1,992 patients with anorectal malformations over the past two decades in Japan. Steering Committee of Japanese Study Group of Anorectal Anomalies. J Pediatr Surg. 1999;34:435-41.
6. McLaren RH, Barrett DM, Zincke H. Rectal injury occurring at radical retropubic prostatectomy for prostate cancer: etiology and treatment. Urology. 1993;42:401-5.
7. Smith AM, Veenema RJ. Management of rectal injury and rectourethral fistulas following radical retropubic prostatectomy. J Urol. 1972;108:778-9.
8. Zippe CD. Cryosurgery of the prostate: technique and pitfalls. Urol Clin North Am. 1996;23:147-63.
9. Uchida T, Sanghvi NT, Gardner TA, Koch MO, Ishii D, Minei S, et al. Transrectal high-intensity focused ultrasound for treatment of patients with stage T1b-2n0m0 localized prostate cancer: a preliminary report. Urology. 2002;59(3):394-8.
10. Al-Ali M, Kashmoula D, Saoud IJ. Experience with 30 posttraumatic rectourethral fistulas: presentation of posterior transsphincteric anterior rectal wall advancement. J Urol. 1997;158:421-4.
11. Cools P, Vanderputte S, Van der Stighelen Y, Colemont L, Denis B. Rectourethral fistula due to Crohn's disease. Acta Urol Belg. 1996;64:47-8.
12. Shin PR, Foley E, Steers WD. Surgical management of rectourinary fistulae. Journal of American College of Surgeons. 2000;191(5): 547-53.
13. Goodwin WE, Turner RD, Winter CD. Rectourinary fistula: principles of management and a technique of surgical closure. J Urol. 1958;80:246-54.
14. Kilpatrick FR, Mason AY. Postoperative recto-prostatic fistula. Brit J Urol. 1969;41:649-51.
15. Wood TW, Middleton RG. Single-stage transrectal transsphincteric (modified York-Mason) repair of rectourinary fistulas. Urology. 1990;35(1):27-30.
16. Fazio VW, Jones IT, Jagelman DG, Weakley FL. Rectourethral fistulas in Crohn's disease. Surgery Gynecology and Obstetrics. 1987;164(2):148-50.
17. Dreznik Z, Alper D, Vishne TH, Ramadan E. Rectal flap advancement—a simple and effective approach for the treatment of rectourethral fistula. Colorectal Disease. 2003;5(1):53-5.
18. Parks AG, Motson RW. Peranal repair of rectoprostatic fistula. Brit J Surg. 1983;70:725-6.
19. Gecelter L. Anterior transanorectal approach for posterior urethral strictures. S Afr J Surg. 1972;10:189-93.
20. Bukowski TP, Chakrbarty A, Powell IJ, Frontera R, Perlmutter AD, Montie JE. Acquired rectourethral fistula: method of repair. J Urol. 1995;153:730-3.
21. Nyam DC, Pemberton JH. Management of iatrogenic rectourethral fistula. Diseases of the Colon and Rectum. 1999;42(8):994-9.
22. Wilbert DM, Buess G, Bichler KH. Combined endoscopic closure of rectourethral fistula. J Urol. 1996;155:256-8.
23. Venkatesh KS, Ramanujam P. Fibrin glue application in the treatment of recurrent anorectal fistulas. Dis Colon Rectum. 1999;42:1136-9.
24. Bardari F, D´Urso L, Muto G. Conservative treatment of iatrogenic urinary fistulas: the value of synoacrylic glue. Urology. 2001;58(6):1046-8.
25. Youssef AH, Fath Alla M, El-Kassaby AW. Perineal subcutaneous dartos pedicled flap as a new technique for repairing urethrorectal fistula. J Urol. 1999;161:1498-500.
26. Hechenbleikner EM, Buckley JC, Wick EC. Acquired rectourethral fistulas in adults: a systematic review of surgical repair techniques and outcomes. Dis Colon Rectum. 2013;56(3):374-83.

CHAPTER 91

Fecal Incontinence

Abhijit Chandra, Noushif M, Saket Kumar

INTRODUCTION

Fecal incontinence is an often neglected condition, which leads to psychological debilitation and social isolation along with decreased quality of life of patients. Due to social stigma attached patients often hide the history and it also escapes attention of health care professionals and family members. Currently there is no consensus on the definition of fecal incontinence and involuntary loss of liquid or solid stool for the duration of 30 days or more is generally used to define the entity, whereas the loss of control over passage of gas along with fecal soiling is defined as partial incontinence. The reported prevalence of fecal incontinence is between 9.6% and 24%.[1] With time, knowledge about pathophysiology and risk factors for fecal incontinence have evolved but therapeutic options are yet to provide optimum results.

PATHOPHYSIOLOGY

To understand the pathogenesis of fecal incontinence it is required to have a thorough knowledge of normal mechanism of fecal continence. Normal bowel continence mandates the proper functioning of the sphincters, anorectal angle and the rectal sensation and compliance. The anorectal angle created by the sling of puborectalis muscle is the prime factor for maintaining gross continence. The angle between rectum and the anal canal is usually between 90° and 105°. During voluntary contractions this can be narrowed down to as acute as 60° to ensure continence. On the other hand relaxation of puborectalis muscle during the act of defecation can broaden the angle to as wide as 120–180°. The anal sphincter complex is equally important for normal fecal continence. It has two parts: (1) the internal (involuntary) sphincter and (2) the external (voluntary) sphincter. The internal sphincter which is made up of smooth muscle fibers results in 60% of anal resting pressure, whereas the external sphincter which is made up of voluntary striated muscle generates squeeze pressure 50–100% above the resting pressure and aids in delaying the defecation voluntarily.[2]

Appropriate rectal sensation is mandatory for maintaining normal continence and any alteration may lead to fecal impaction and subsequent overflow incontinence. Compliance of the rectum and its storage capacity along with inbuilt neural reflex are also necessary in ensuring continence. Both sympathetic and parasympathetic nerves innervate anorectal sphincter complex. The puborectalis muscle and the external sphincters receive the nerve supply from pudendal nerve. The rectoanal inhibitory reflex (RAIR) prepares the anal canal for defecation as it leads to relaxation of internal sphincter whenever there is rectal distention.[3] This reflex also helps in differentiating gas versus liquid or solid stool by enabling anal mucosa to sense the contents of rectum.

CLASSIFICATION/SCORING

Classification of fecal incontinence is based on primary symptom, nature of leakage and the underlying primary etiology. Multiple factors underscore the pathophysiology of fecal incontinence, and in majority of patients there are more than one contributing factors (Flow chart 1).[3-5] In patients with normal anal sphincter, fecal incontinence might result from a failure to maintain anal pressure during rectal distension or a reduced rectal adaptation to filling.[6,7]

Since the first scoring system for fecal incontinence by Browning and Parks, several other score indices followed but are yet to be validated. Wexner et al.[8] developed an incontinence scoring system (Cleveland Clinic Incontinence Score) which incorporated consistency and frequency of incontinence with the use of pads and life style alteration. The Fecal Incontinence Severity Index (FISI) measures the severity of incontinence that occurs from “2 or more

Flow chart 1 Causes of fecal incontinence

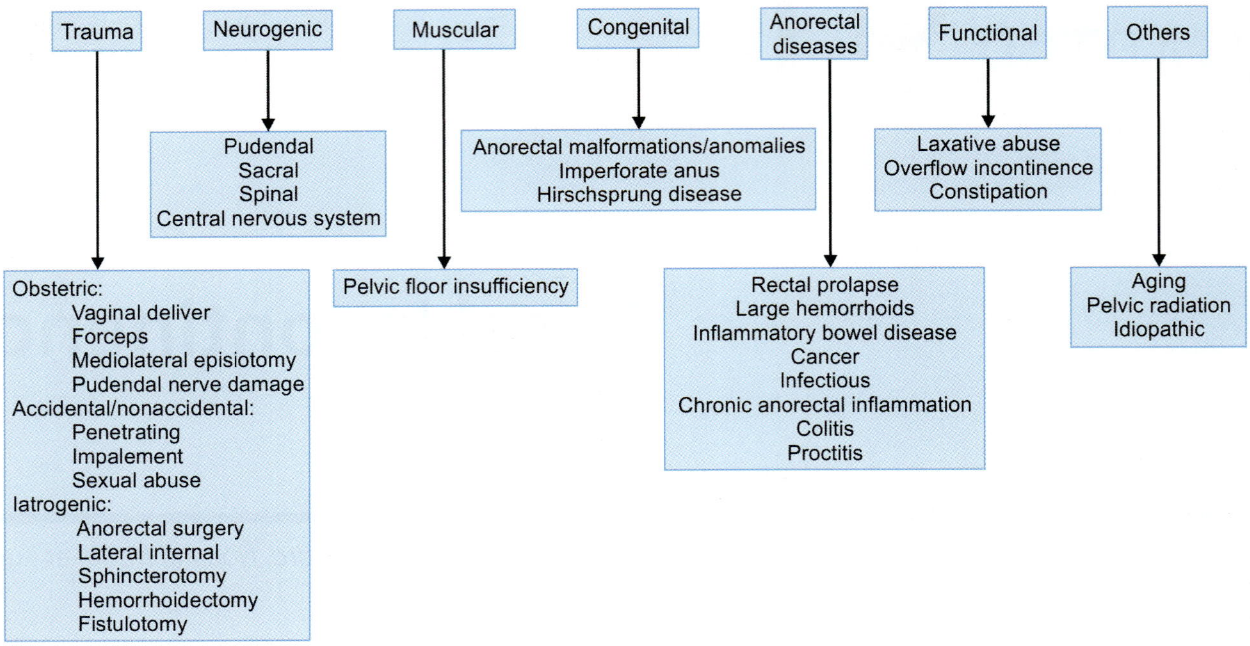

Table 1: St Mark's Hospital Incontinence Score

	Never	*Rarely*	*Sometimes*	*Weekly*	*Daily*
Incontinence for solid stool	0	1	2	3	4
Incontinence for liquid stool	0	1	2	3	4
Incontinence for gas	0	1	2	3	4
Alteration in lifestyle	0	1	2	3	4
		No		*Yes*	
Need to wear a pad or plug		0		2	
Taking constipating medicines		0		2	
Lack of ability to defer defecation for 15 minutes		0		4	

Never—no episodes in the past four weeks
Rarely—1 episode in the past four weeks
Sometimes—>1 episode in the past four weeks but <1 a week
Weekly—1 or more episodes a week but <1 a day
Daily—1 or more episodes a day
Add one score from each row:
Minimum score = 0 = perfect continence
Maximum score = 24 = totally incontinent

Source: Vaizey CJ, Carapeti E, Cahill JA, Kamm MA. Prospective comparison of fecal incontinence grading systems. Gut.1999;44:77-80.

times per day", "once per day", "2 or more times per week", "once a week" to "1-3 times per month". Fecal incontinence may also be classified as either passive or urgent. Passive is when incontinence occurs without awareness, and urgent is when patient is unable to hold defecation. Use of anti-diarrheal drugs may also mask incontinence, taking both these factors into account, Vaizey et al.[9] developed the St. Mark's hospital incontinence score (Table 1) which is widely used nowadays. These tools allow severity to be assessed objectively and thereby also allow treatment progress to be monitored.

EVALUATION

History and Physical Examination

Fecal incontinence is just a sign or a symptom and each patient should be evaluated thoroughly to unearth the underlying cause. A thorough history and physical examination with specific questions directed at exact symptoms are usually required as most patients find it very embarrassing topic to discuss. To improve detection, history should focus on incontinent symptoms, use of protective pads, medical and surgical history, general bowel habits and quality of life.

Perineum should be examined for skin changes, fecal soilage, scars, hemorrhoids, fistula or abscess. Digital rectal examination should be performed to evaluate sphincter defect, resting tone, squeezing pressure, anorectal mass or prolapsed rectum.[10] Pelvic floor weakness should be ruled out by assessing perineum for perineal descent. Vaginal examination may reveal rectoceles, cystoceles, enteroceles or vaginal prolapse which is an important cause for anterior compartment weakness. During digital rectal examination proper assessment of anal sphincters and puborectalis muscle is important as it can tell about sphincter defects, paradoxical contractions or old stigmata of obstetric injury. Perianal sensation and the anocutaneous "wink reflex" serve a simple assessment of neurological function.

Endoscopy

Proctosigmoidoscopy and colonoscopy play a role in patients with new-onset fecal incontinence or recent changes in bowel habits. They specifically aid to rule out organic causes like tumors or inflammation.[5]

Endoanal Ultrasound

An important adjunct for fecal incontinence evaluation in patients with suspected sphincter defects, endoanal ultrasound (EUS) has a crucial role in obstetric trauma. EUS (frequency 6.5–10 MHz) demonstrates the internal (hypoechoic) and external (hyperechoic) sphincters and their anatomical details (length and width). EUS can also demonstrate any scar tissue (mixed echogenicity), lesions or defects in the sphincters (Fig. 1). Additionally, perineal body thickness can be measured with values less than 10 mm considered abnormal. However, the sensitivity and specificity are dependent on the examiner.

Magnetic Resonance Imaging

Pelvic magnetic resonance imaging (MRI) with an endocoil can delineate anorectal sphincter complex nicely, picking up any defect or atrophy of sphincters which may be causing incontinence. Dynamic MRI for the assessment of pelvic floor disorders has also come in use recently. A major drawback of dynamic MRI in fecal incontinence is that the evaluation is performed in supine position rather than sitting.[11]

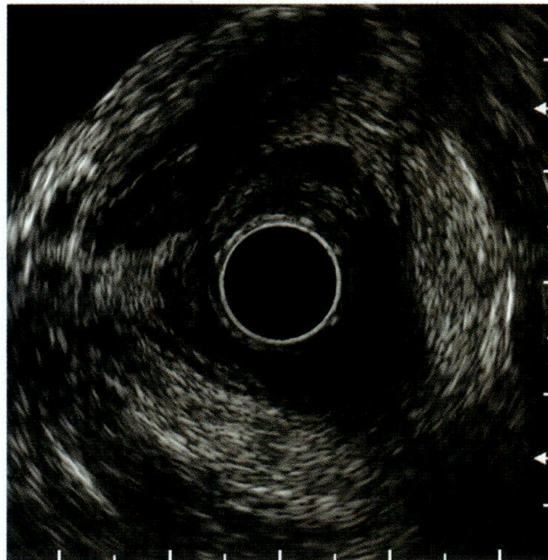

Figure 1 Endoanal ultrasound showing sphincter disruption (internal and external) anteriorly with posterior retraction of muscles following obstetric trauma

Defecography

Defecography provides contrast radiological picture of the dynamic rectal evacuation. It not only provides a real time assessment of anorectal angle, but it can also detect any intussusception or rectocele. Additional information regarding perineal descent and rectal emptying is also readily available. Its use is limited by the interobserver variation, high levels of radiation and the inability to hold the contrast by many patients. The role of defecography in evaluating patients with fecal incontinence is to rule out suspected overflow incontinence and obstructed defecation. MR defecography is emerging as a new tool for this purpose, with ability to visualize all the three perineal compartments simultaneously.

Anorectal Manometry

Functional assessment of anorectum is important especially in the absence of overt "organic disease". Manometry evaluates the anal resting pressure using a "pull-through" technique. Voluntary squeeze pressure and RAIR are measured during simulated defecation and rectal compliance and sensory thresholds are measured using latex balloon distension. Most prevalent method of anorectal manometry is multichannel water-perfused catheters, which measures the resistance to the flow of water to deduce pressure readings. Although there is no direct correlation between clinical symptoms, continence and manometric measurements, it provides reproducible results for individual examiners. Manometry is also helpful to monitor treatment responce.[3,5] The new high-resolution manometry with "3D analysis" provides more precise measurements.[12]

Pudendal Nerve Terminal Motor Latency

This is the time gap between the stimulation of pudendal nerve at the ischial tuberosity and the contraction of pelvic floor muscles which is usually 2.0±0.2 ms. Pudendal neuropathy results in a delayed response and it can be used to predict the outcome of anterior overlapping sphincteroplasty. However, pudendal nerve terminal motor latency (PNTML) testing has not shown to correlate with success after sacral nerve stimulation (SNS) for fecal incontinence.[13]

MANAGEMENT

Nonoperative

Initial management of fecal incontinence includes appraisal of predisposing factors, exclusion of fecal impaction and regulation of bowel habits. Impacted stool may require manual disimpaction and regular enemas. Pharmacotherapy is an important adjunct which includes[14] bulking agents, constipating agents and laxative regimens. Antidiarrheal agents like loperamide or diphenoxylate increases stool firmness by slowing transit and thereby improve symptoms in patients with mild to moderate incontinence. Loperamide is also a sphincter agonist that can increase sphincter pressure. These drugs are often best used prophylactically in patients with limited ability to defer evacuation, and have been shown to improve diarrhea-associated fecal incontinence.

Regulation of bowel pattern and bowel "retraining" is important. Dietary changes like increased fiber and water intake may lead to bulkier, more solid stools that they may evacuate completely. This can be further facilitated by the use of enemas or rectal irrigation to empty the rectum.

Biofeedback

Biofeedback is a retraining program which aims at enhancing sensory and motor functions of anorectum and thus improving continence. It utilizes various stimulus like auditory, visual and many others in order to better patients awareness of rectal distension and improve his/her sphincter contractions. Published studies have shown success rates between 50% and 90%, both in adults and children. A half to 1 hour training session on every 7–14 days is usually performed.[3] Biofeedback has not been proved to be superior to other conservative approaches.[15] Maximum benefits are derived in patients with lesser degree of neuropathic incontinence or with partial sphincter defects, whereas efforts on biofeedback are usually futile for patients with totally denervated pelvis or those with decreased rectal capacity from surgery. Biofeedback should only be considered for highly motivated patients as it is a time consuming and labor-intensive procedure.[3]

Sacral Nerve Stimulation

Sacral nerve stimulation or neuromodulation is performed by placing electrodes in the sacral foramina and stimulating roots of S2, S3, S3 nerves, thus producing contractions of levator ani muscle and external anal sphincter. In the initial stage of this procedure temporary electrodes are placed for 2 weeks to assess its suitability and efficacy. More than 50% decrease in the incontinence episodes is defined as improvement and for such patients permanent electrodes are placed which can be kept for as long as 8 years. A multicenter prospective randomized trial of the use of SNS has shown success rate of over 80% at 3 years follow-up.[16] SNS has been employed in cases with sphincter damage of over more than 50% circumference, but with long-term reports of recurrence.[17] Complications like lead migration, pain and infection leading to explantation of the stimulator have been reported, though rare (5%). SNS has also been shown to be superior to artificial bowel sphincter (ABS) due to the better continence and decreased outlet obstruction rates. SNS is currently indicated for patients with neurogenic incontinence and intact anal sphincters.

OPERATIVE PROCEDURES

Sphincteroplasty

Sphincteroplasty works best for traumatic sphincter defects which may be iatrogenic or secondary to obstetric trauma. It can be performed by apposition, overlapping or plication. Overlapping sphincteroplasty, initially described by Parks et al.[18] is preferred when adequate remnant sphincter is present. Anterior or posterior plication to reduce the anal orifice is also effective at times. No study has demonstrated superiority of one repair to other. Even though the short-term success rates for anterior graciloplasty at 1 year were report to be 80%, but long-term follow-up revealed that less than half of the patients remained fully continent.[3] Zutshi et al.[19] noticed that at 10 year follow-up none of the patients had complete control over stool and flatus, and the overall fecal incontinence severity scores were also higher, but it did not correlate well with quality of life scores.[19] Reports on redo-sphincteroplasty also claims 50% success rates.[20]

Graciloplasty

Gracilis muscle transposition was developed by Pickrell in 1952. This procedure utilizes full length of gracilis muscle which is mobilized in a manner to preserve its innervation and vascularity and tunneled subcutaneously to create a neoanal sphincter (Figs 2A to D).[3] Procedure consists of placing the gracilis muscle around the anal canal and suturing it to the ischial tuberosity. Both right and left gracilis may be used but right is usually preferred. Lithotomy position is used after good bowel preparation. First the gracilis is mobilized with a thigh incision taking care of its neurovascular supply at the proximal end. A wide tunnel is created to pass it into the perineal area. Transverse anterior and posterior incisions are given to create space around the anal canal. Gracilis muscle is then passed anticlockwise beneath the anterior and posterior raphe to encircle the anal canal. It is sutured to the opposite ischial tuberosity after adducting the legs. *Double graciloplasty* has been used by some where both gracilis muscles are mobilized and sutured to each other in a similar fashion. Gracilloplasty is a technically difficult procedure and the results have been quite variable.

Interest in the procedure was renewed with the introduction of electrical stimulation by means of an implantable pulse generator.[21] Electrical stimulation converts the gracilis from predominantly type 2 (fast-twitch, fatigable) to predominantly type 1 (slow twitch, fatigue-resistant) muscle fibers. The stimulator maintains the tonic contraction of the transposed muscle, thereby providing continuous sphincter function. Defecation is effected by turning the stimulator off with a hand-held programmer. The success rate of *dynamic graciloplasty* varies from 40% to 80%; however, the operative morbidity is high. Indications of graciloplasty include a young patient with large sphincter defect not suitable for primary repair, or who have a failed repair. Similar procedure utilizing gluteus maximus with pudendal innervation has been described by Sato et al.;[22] however, long-term results have not been promising.

Artificial Bowel Sphincter

Artificial bowel sphincter (ACTICON; American Medical Systems, MN) consists of silicon cuff which encircles anal canal and a control pump which is attached to a pressure regulating balloon. The cuff is kept in an inflated state to act like a sphincter. In order to facilitate defecation, silicon cuff is deflated with the help of control pump which drives fluid from silicon cuff to balloon.[3] ABS is usually indicated in patients with intractable incontinence in whom standard therapies including surgery have failed. Though ABS has shown up to 85% improvement in fecal incontinence, results are marred with high explant rates.[23]

Bulking Agents

To enhance continence by injecting biomaterial in anal canal in an attractive proposition and the work done on this concept have

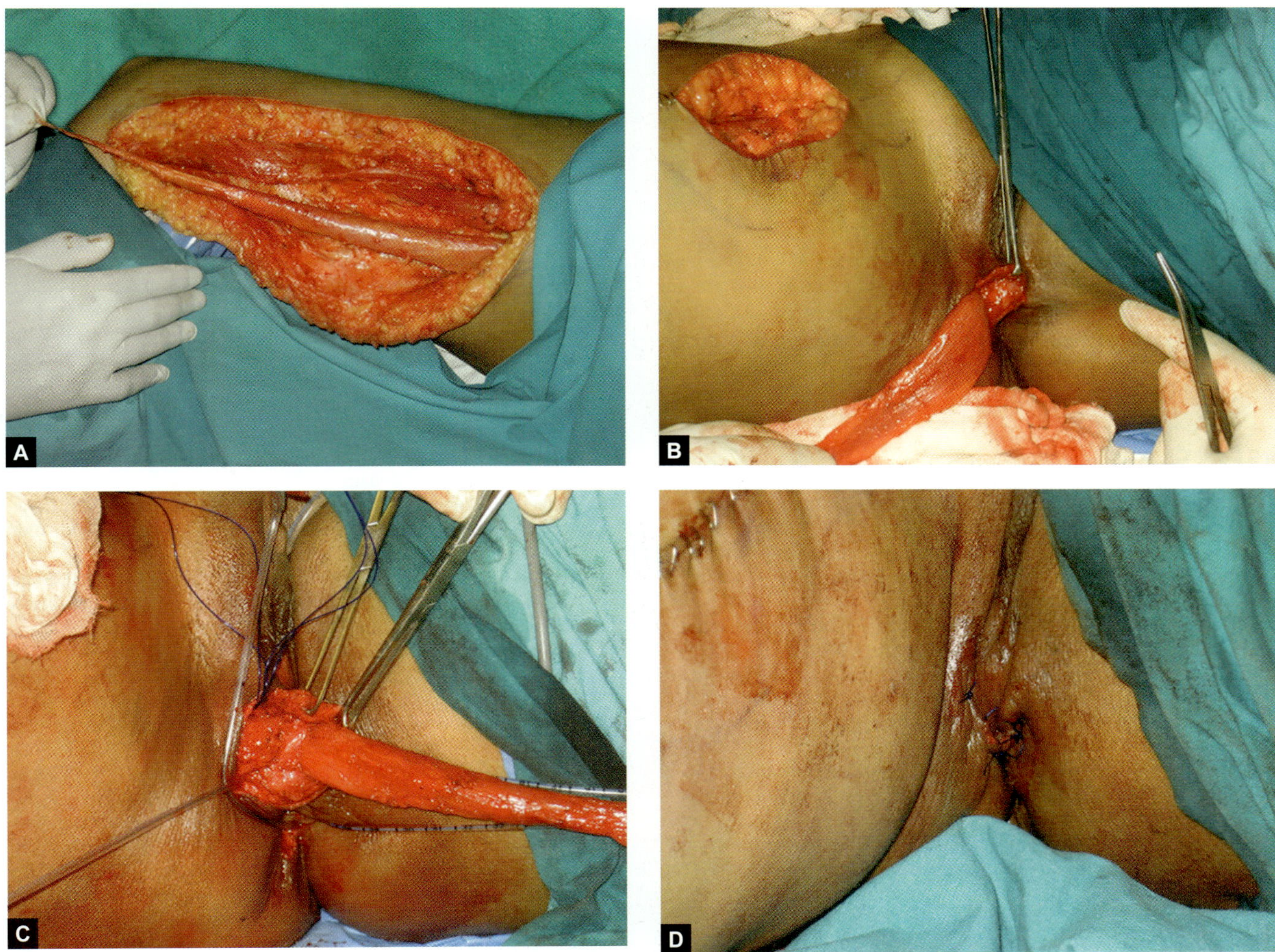

Figures 2A to D (A) Gracilis mobilized with intact neurovascular supply; (B) Gracilis tunneled into perineum; (C) Gracilis being passed beneath the raphe to encircle anal canal; (D) Perineal and thigh wounds sutured (completed repair)

yielded good results in up to 50% of patients. However, this effect is short lived and most patients required multiple injections. Currently, this modality of treatment should be limited to a clinical trial setting and short-term results are encouraging.[24]

Radiofrequency

Radiofrequency has been postulated to work by creating thermal lesions in muscular layer which by healing process leads to tightening of these muscles. However, the data is not convincing enough and the results are at best conflicting.[25]

Fecal Diversion

The term "end stage fecal incontinence" is used when the patient is left with a permanent abdominal stoma as the only option for fecal management. Fecal diversion via a colostomy or ileostomy, though a failure of fecal incontinence treatment, has to be considered for certain patients with intractable incontinence like in severe perianal trauma or pelvic floor denervation.

INDIAN EXPERIENCE

Reports regarding incidence, spectrum and management of fecal incontinence from India are scant in literature. A retrospective analysis of the spectrum of abnormalities on anorectal manometry in patients with fecal incontinence showed a significantly higher incidence of external sphincter defect in females as compared to males, though anal resting pressure, length of the high pressure zone and tolerability to intrarectal balloon distension were comparable.[6]

Fecal incontinence was multifactorial in etiology with obstetric injuries a major contributing factor, as home deliveries are common in the Indian subcontinent.[6,26] Compared to West, a permanent abdominal stoma is less acceptable in Indian population primarily because of attached social stigma, lack of awareness and inadequate stoma care facilities.[27]

Use of pedicled antropyloric valve as an alternative to anorectal sphincter in end stage fecal incontinence was reported recently by us.[27-29] Initial outcomes following the procedure were better for patients with benign conditions or intact sensate anorectum (sphincter trauma) as compared with those having their anorectal sphincter excised. The pyloric smooth muscle behaves as a tonic sphincter when removed from gastrointestinal continuity with a mean resting pressure of 25 mm Hg.[29] Postoperative incontinence scores were satisfactory with better quality of life.[27]

CONCLUSION

Fecal incontinence, though not life threatening, remains a clinical challenge and alternatives for a permanent colostomy are far from perfect. Newer diagnostic and therapeutic techniques along with better understanding of pathophysiology have improved the outcomes in the minority of patients who seek treatment for fecal incontinence.

REFERENCES

1. Halland M, Talley NJ. Faecal incontinence: mechanisms and management. Curr Opin Gastroenterol. 2012;28:57-62.
2. Zhao X, Pasricha PJ. Novel surgical approaches to faecal incontinence: neurostimulation and artificial anal sphincter. Curr Gastroenterol Rep. 2003;5:419-24.
3. Hayden DM, Weiss EG. Faecal incontinence: etiology, evaluation, and treatment. Clin Colon Rectal Surg. 2011;24:64-70.
4. Leung FW. Treatment of faecal incontinence—review of observational studies (OS) and randomized controlled trials (RCT) related to injection of bulking agent into peri-anal tissue. J Interv Gastroenterol. 2011;1:202-6.
5. Probst M, Pages H, Riemann JF, Eickhoff A, Raulf F, Kolbert G. Fecal incontinence: part 4 of a series of articles on incontinence. Dtsch Arztebl Int. 2010;107:596-601.
6. Korah AT, Misra A, Kumar S, Ghoshal UC. Manometric spectrum of faecal incontinence in a tertiary care center in northern India. Trop Gastroenterol. 2010;31:165-8.
7. Siproudhis L, Bellissant E, Pagenault M, Mendler MH, Allain H, Bretagne JF, et al. Faecal incontinence with normal anal canal pressures: where is the pitfall? Am J Gastroenterol. 1999;94:1556-63.
8. Jorge JMN, Wexner SD. Etiology and management of faecal incontinence. Dis Colon Rectum. 1993;36:77-97.
9. Vaizey CJ, Carapeti E, Cahill JA, Kamm MA. Prospective comparison of faecal incontinence grading systems. Gut. 1999;44:77-80.
10. Poirier M, Abcarian H. Faecal incontinence. In: Cameron JL (Ed). Current Surgical Therapy. Philadelphia, PA: Mosby Elsevier; 2008. pp. 285-91.
11. Dann EW. Magnetic resonance defecography: an evaluation of obstructed defecation and pelvic floor weakness. Semin Ultrasound CT MR. 2008;29:414-9.
12. Fruehauf H, Fox MR. Anal manometry in the investigation of faecal incontinence: totum pro parte, not pars pro toto. Digestion. 2012;86:75-7.
13. Brouwer R, Duthie G. Sacral nerve neuromodulation is effective treatment for faecal incontinence in the presence of a sphincter defect, pudendal neuropathy, or previous sphincter repair. Dis Colon Rectum. 2010;53:273-8.
14. Omar MI, Alexander CE. Drug treatment for faecal incontinence in adults. Cochrane Database Syst Rev. 2013;6:CD002116.
15. Norton C, Cody JD. Biofeedback and/or sphincter exercises for the treatment of faecal incontinence in adults. Cochrane Database Syst Rev. 2012;7:CD002111.
16. Wexner SD, Coller JA, Devroede G, Hull T, McCallum R, Chan M, et al. Sacral nerve stimulation for faecal incontinence: results of a 120-patient prospective multicenter study. Ann Surg. 2010;251: 441-9.
17. Matzel KE. Sacral nerve stimulation for faecal incontinence. What has been achieved (current status). Acta Chir Iugosl. 2010;57:67-72.
18. Parks AG, McPartlin JF. Late repair of injuries of the anal sphincter. Proc R Soc Med. 1971;64:1187-9.
19. Zutshi M, Tracey TH, Bast J, Halverson A, Na J. Ten-year outcome after anal sphincter repair for faecal incontinence. Dis Colon Rectum. 2009;52:1089-94.
20. Vaizey CJ, Norton C, Thornton MJ, Nicholls RJ, Kamm MA. Long-term results of repeat anterior anal sphincter repair. Dis Colon Rectum. 2004;47:858-63.
21. Baeten CG, Geerdes BP, Adang EM, Heineman E, Konsten J, Engel GL, et al. Anal dynamic graciloplasty in the treatment of intractable faecal incontinence. N Engl J Med. 1995;332:1600-5.
22. Sato T, Konishi F, Kanazawa K. Anal sphincter reconstruction with a pudendal nerve anastomosis following abdominoperineal resection: report of a case. Dis Colon Rectum. 1997;40:1497-503.
23. Gurusamy KS, Marzouk D, Benziger H. A review of contemporary surgical alternatives to permanent colostomy. Int J Surg. 2005;3:193-205.
24. Maeda Y, Laurberg S, Norton C. Perianal injectable bulking agents as treatment for faecal incontinence in adults. Cochrane Database Syst Rev. 2013;2:CD007959.
25. Ruiz D, Rodrigo A, Hull T, Efron JE, Wexner SD. Does the radiofrequency procedure for faecal incontinence improve quality of life and incontinence at 1-year follow up? Dis Colon Rectum. 2010;53:1041-6.
26. Chase S, Mittal R, Jesudason MR, Nayak S, Perakath B. Anal sphincter repair for faecal incontinence: experience from a tertiary care centre. Indian J Gastroenterol. 2010;29:162-5.
27. Chandra A, Kumar A, Noushif M, Gupta V, Singh D, Kumar M, et al. Perineal antropylorus transposition for end-stage faecal incontinence in humans: initial outcomes. Dis Colon Rectum. 2013;56:360-6.
28. Bansal V, Bhutani R, Doval D, Kumar K, Pande P, Kumar G. Neo adjuvant chemoradiotherapy and rectal cancer: can India follow the West? J Cancer Res Ther. 2012;8:209-14.
29. Chandra A, Ghoshal UC, Gupta V, Jauhari R, Srivastava RN, Misra A, et al. Physiological and functional evaluation of the transposed human pylorus as a distal sphincter. J Neurogastroenterol Motil. 2012;18:269-77.

CHAPTER 92

Ulcerative Colitis

Praneeth Moka, Govind K Makharia

INTRODUCTION

Inflammatory bowel disease (IBD) is a group of idiopathic, chronic, inflammatory diseases of intestine and they occur because of interaction between genetic, environmental and immunological factors.[1] IBD consists of two main categories of the diseases namely: (1) ulcerative colitis and (2) Crohn's disease. In ulcerative colitis, the disease is limited to the colon and it involves predominantly colonic mucosa and submucosa. In Crohn's disease, any part of the gastrointestinal tract from mouth to anus can be involved and the inflammation in the intestine may be transmural. While the involvement of the colon is symmetrical and continuous in patients with ulcerative colitis, skip lesions and discontinuous lesions are characteristic of Crohn's disease[1] (Table 1). About 10% of patients with IBD cannot be categorized either into ulcerative colitis or Crohn's disease, they are called IBD unclassified. In their natural course of evolution, IBD unclassified may ultimately evolve into either ulcerative colitis or Crohn's disease.

EPIDEMIOLOGY

The prevalence and incidence of ulcerative colitis vary according to the ethnicity and geographic location of the population.[1] In countries where the prevalence of IBD is low, ulcerative colitis is more common than Crohn's disease and in countries where the prevalence of IBD is high, Crohn's disease tends to be the dominant sub-type of IBD.[2] While both incidence and prevalence of ulcerative colitis and Crohn's disease have generally stabilized in countries having high prevalence of IBD; however, in countries where IBD is emerging, ulcerative colitis is the predominant disease.[2-4] Studies from Asian countries suggest that the incidence and prevalence rates of IBD in Asia-Pacific region are lower compared to that in Europe and North America, they however are increasing rapidly.[4-14] In India, the prevalence and incidence of ulcerative colitis are 44.3/100,000 and 6.02/100,000, respectively.[11]

Inflammatory bowel disease in the west is characteristically seen with a bimodal age distribution pattern with first peak between 20–39 years and a second smaller peak at the age of 60–79 years. Such bimodal distribution of age however has not been consistently observed in Asian studies.[4,7] The onset of the disease may be delayed and some patients might present at age more than 60 years also. In North America and Europe, the distribution of ulcerative colitis is equal in both men and women at all ages. A male predominance has been reported in patients with ulcerative colitis from a few Asian countries.[4]

PATHOGENESIS OF INFLAMMATORY BOWEL DISEASE

Inflammatory bowel disease is result of complex interplay of genetic, environment and immune factors. IBD represents a state of excessive immune response, which may be targeted against an innocuous or pathogenic microorganism. Studies on animal models of IBD suggest that in genetically susceptible host, commensal bacteria can induce an inappropriate state of inflammation akin to IBD.

Genetic Factors

Variability of prevalence of IBD amongst various ethnic groups, and the increased risk amongst the family members of patients with IBD suggest an important role of genetic factors in the pathogenesis of IBD. The risk of IBD is 2–13 folds higher in offspring of patients with IBD as compared with that in the general population.[15-18] This predisposition in the offsprings can be attributed to either the shared environment or the genetic factors. Recently genome

Table 1: Differences between ulcerative colitis and Crohn's disease

Features	*UC*	*CD*
Clinical:		
Bloody diarrhea	Almost always	50%
Abdominal pain	Less severe	Very common, more severe
Intestinal obstruction	Very uncommon	Common
Perianal disease	None	20–30%
Fever	Occasional	More common
Growth retardation in children	Less marked	More marked
Nutritional deficiency	Less common	More common
Site of the disease:		
Colon	Always	In two-thirds
Terminal Ileum	5–10%	In two-thirds
Small intestine	Never	In two-thirds
UGI tract	Never	Occasional
Rectum involvement	Almost always	In 50% patients
Endoscopic/Radiological features:		
Involvement	Diffuse, continuous	Skip lesions, discontinuous
Type of ulcer	Superficial	Deep
Longitudinal ulcer	Never	Characteristic, present in 30%
Cobblestoning lesions	Never	Characteristic, present in 30%
Stricture	None	Yes
Fistula	Never	Yes
Pathological features:		
Type of involvement	Mucosa and submucosa	Transmural
Granuloma	None/rare	Non caseating granuloma
Fibrosis	None	Yes
Mesenteric thickening	None	Yes
Fibrofatty proliferation	None	Yes

wide association studies have provided information regarding various genetic loci and the overall disease pathogenesis. Analyses of these genes and genetic loci suggest important role for several pathways such as barrier function, epithelial restitution, innate immune regulation, microbial defense, reactive oxygen species (ROS) generation, regulation of adaptive immunity, autophagy, endoplasmic reticulum stress and some metabolic pathways associated with cellular homeostasis.[15-21] Nearly 30% of genetic loci are shared between ulcerative colitis and Crohn's disease.[15-17]

The first susceptibility locus for Crohn's disease was identified in 2001 as NOD2 (nucleotide binding oligomerization domain 2 gene), also called CARD15 (caspase recruitment domain 15). Missense mutation and frame-shift mutation of NOD2/CARD15 gene were found to be associated with Crohn's disease.[16] Both heterozygosity and homozygosity for this mutation are associated with the increased risk for Crohn's disease. In patients with Crohn's disease with associated mutated NOD2, there is a lower activation of NF-κB in the mononuclear cells, and higher expression in inflamed tissues. Surprisingly, NOD2/CARD15 gene has not been found to be associated with Crohn's disease in the Chinese and Indian population.[4]

Microbial Flora

Clinical and experimental observations suggest that intestinal bacterial microbiota is involved in the pathogenesis of IBD. Crohn's disease and ulcerative colitis preferentially involve the bacteria-rich areas of intestine, i.e. terminal ileum and colon. In the animal models for IBD, germ free mice do not develop inflammation, but after bacterial introduction, intestinal inflammation rapidly develops. These evidences highlight the role of bacterial flora in the development of IBD. The interaction between commensal flora and defensive responses of the host at the mucosa may have an important role in the generation and sustenance of inflammation in IBD.[22-24]

The defect in innate immunity or hyper-responsive immune response against non-pathogenic bacteria may be responsible for the chronic low grade inflammation.[24] On the other hand, there may be alteration in the gut flora in IBD, and the loss of protective bacteria may lead to overgrowth of pathogenic bacteria. The exact pathogenesis is still to be defined, but more than one mechanism may be acting in an individual patient.

Microbes induce intestinal inflammation by adhering to intestinal epithelial cells, or by the secretion of proinflammatory cytokines or enterotoxins. Dysbiosis, a breakdown in the balance between protective and harmful intestinal bacteria, can lead to the diseased state. There are a few observations as regards to microbial flora in patients with IBD: (a) a decrease in the bacterial diversity; (b) decrease in abundance of protective bacteria such as Firmicutes (specifically Lachnospiraceae) and Bacteroides; and (c) a relative abundance of pathogenic bacteria such as Proteobacteria and Actinobacteria.[25-28] Firmicutes and Bacteroides are known to produce short chain fatty acids, which provide nutrition to colonocytes, and therefore a reduction in the concentrations of these two bacteria is adverse to colonocytes.

The integrity of the normal epithelial barrier, with its tight junctions and mucin glycoproteins, may be compromised by genetic variations in key molecular determinants leading to a diminished reparative response to injury such as NSAIDs. The products of the luminal commensal bacteria or dietary antigens may stimulate the mucosal immune system to produce chronic or recurrent inflammation of the intestine. Activation of classic antigen-presenting cells (e.g. dendritic cells) by the antigens promotes the differentiation of T-lymphocytes into type-1 helper T cells (Th1) in patients with Crohn's disease and type-2 helper T cells (Th2) in patients with ulcerative colitis.[25-37]

Smoking is other environmental factor, which may be contributing to the etiology of IBD. Ulcerative colitis is more common among non-smokers. After cessation of smoking, within first 2 years, risk of developing ulcerative colitis is higher.[37] On the other hand, Crohn's disease is more common in current smokers.

CLINICAL MANIFESTATIONS

The symptoms of ulcerative colitis vary according to the extent of the disease. The extent of the disease is classified according to Montreal classification (Table 2).[38] The cardinal symptoms of ulcerative colitis are bloody diarrhea, urgency, tenesmus, passage of mucus, and lower abdominal pain. Almost 95% of patients present with episodes of bloody diarrhea, and in the absence of these symptoms, diagnosis of ulcerative colitis should be reconsidered. Most patients at time of presentation recall presence of these symptoms in the past; though few patients can present with acute onset of severe bloody diarrhea. Urgency and tenesmus (feeling of incomplete evacuation) are due to rectal inflammation and loss of rectal capacitance; which leads to desire for defecation, even with the small amount of the stool in the rectum. Diarrhea in the setting of ulcerative colitis is due to several mechanisms including rectal irritability, failure of absorption of salt and water, increase in mucosal permeability, and increased colonic motility. A few patients, especially those with proctitis, may complain of constipation.[1,12]

Table 2: Extent of the disease (ulcerative colitis) according to the Montreal classification

E1	Proctitis
E2	Left-sided extending up to splenic flexure
E3	More extensive disease

Abdominal pain in patients with ulcerative colitis occurs generally during the active phase of the disease. Abdominal pain in them is usually localized to infraumbilical region and left iliac fossa. Persistent pain and worsening in the severity of pain in a patient with active ulcerative colitis should suggest an impending complication such as toxic megacolon or perforation. Anemia and pedal edema are seen in patients with severe and continuous disease, and are due to blood and albumin loss through the inflamed colon. Patient with ulcerative colitis may lose weight because of a catabolic state during active phase of the disease and poor nutritional intake.

Physical signs depend upon the severity of the disease. Patients with severe disease can have tachycardia, fever, anemia, signs of weight loss and malnutrition. Abdomen may be tender in these patients, and the bowel sounds are usually normal or increased. Absence of bowel sound with distension of abdomen is an ominous sign and suggests presence of toxic megacolon. Patients with mild clinical disease may appear normal, and may not have any significant clinical signs.

Anemia, leukocytosis and thrombocytosis reflect an active phase of the disease. Anemia is generally secondary to iron deficiency because of chronic blood loss, anemia of chronic disease, or drug induced (azathioprine, sulfasalazine) bone marrow suppression. During acute exacerbation of the disease, patients may have metabolic alkalosis, hypokalemia and elevated blood urea nitrogen. High ESR and C reactive protein also suggest presence of active disease.[1]

EXTRAINTESTINAL MANIFESTATIONS OF ULCERATIVE COLITIS

Fifteen to fifty percent of patients with ulcerative colitis have extraintestinal manifestations. Some of these symptoms can be quiet distressing. The extraintestinal manifestations of IBD are described in Table 3.[4,12] The most common extraintestinal manifestation of ulcerative colitis is peripheral arthropathy characterized by asymmetrical, pauciarticular (affecting <5 joints) large joints (knees, elbows and ankles) involvement. Such arthritis parallels activity of the disease with self-limiting episodes. Other type of arthropathy involves several small joints independent of disease activity and may have persistent symptoms. Isolated sacroiliitis is detected in 10–15% of patients. Ankylosing arthritis occurs in 1–2% of patients with ulcerative colitis. HLA-B27 is positive in majority of these.

Uveitis and episcleritis occur in 5–8% of patients and are the most common ocular manifestations associated with ulcerative colitis. Glucocorticoid ocular drops should be promptly administered to prevent progression to blindness. Patients receiving corticosteroids may be at higher risk of osteoporosis and osteonecrosis of hips. Fatty liver is found in 60% of patients with severe ulcerative colitis. Primary sclerosing cholangitis is seen in

Table 3: Extraintestinal manifestation of IBD

Joints	Peripheral arthritis
	Ankylosing spondylitis
	Sacroilitis
Skin, mucous membrane	Erythema nodosum
	Pyoderma gangrenosum
	Aphthous ulcers
Hepatobiliary	Fatty liver
	Pericholangitis
	Primary sclerosing cholangitis
	Gallstones
	Autoimmune hepatitis
	Cholangio carcinoma
Ocular	Conjunctivitis
	Episcleritis
	Uveitis
Hematological	Agranulocytosis
	Hemolytic anemia
Renal	Oxalate stone
	Amyloidosis
Nutritional	Macronutrient deficiency Micronutrient deficiency

3% of ulcerative colitis patients. It follows a progressive course after many years of stable disease and is independent of the underlying disease. The dermatological manifestations mainly are erythema nodosum and pyoderma gangrenosum. The lesions of pyoderma gangrenosum occur on trunk or extremities and can manifest or persist despite inactive bowel disease.

DIAGNOSTIC CRITERIA

There is no single gold standard test for the diagnosis of either ulcerative colitis or Crohn's disease. The diagnosis of ulcerative colitis is based on a combination of clinical, endoscopic, histological and radiological features. An infectious cause of the colonic inflammation should be ruled out.[1,39-44]

EVALUATION OF PATIENTS WITH ULCERATIVE COLITIS

A detailed history should be taken from each patient including duration of symptoms, severity of symptoms, remissions and relapses, and medication history (including non-steroidal anti-inflammatory drugs and antibiotics). History of appendectomy, smoking, family history and recent incidences of infectious gastroenteritis should be asked for. A complete physical examination including perineal and perianal examination should be done.[1,39-44]

Full blood count, liver function tests, C reactive protein and erythrocyte sedimentation rate do not have diagnostic value, but can be useful for assessing the activity of the disease. A persistently raised serum alkaline phosphatase should prompt a thought toward a possibility of associated primary sclerosing cholangitis and osteomalacia.

Fecal calprotectin may be used to differentiate IBD from functional diarrhea.[45] Microbiological testing for Clostridium difficile toxin should be done during acute exacerbation. A possibility of CMV superinfection should be considered and excluded specially in those patients with IBD who respond poorly to steroid.

Anti neutrophilic cytoplasmic antibody (ANCA), anti Saccharomyces cerevisiae antibody (ASCA) are useful adjunctive tests to distinguish between ulcerative colitis and Crohn's disease in patients with known IBD. ANCA is associated with ulcerative colitis and ASCA is associated with Crohn's disease. There is insufficient information at present to recommend the use of these serologic tests to screen patients with undiagnosed gastrointestinal symptoms for IBD in general population. Patients with undifferentiated colitis who is ANCA negative and ASCA positive is likely to progress to Crohn's disease, whereas those with ANCA positive and ASCA negative are likely to develop ulcerative colitis.

INVESTIGATIONS FOR THE DIAGNOSIS AND EXTENT OF THE DISEASE

Endoscopic Examination

The best investigation for diagnosis and evaluation of the extent of ulcerative colitis is colonoscopy. Through colonoscope, one can examine the nature of the lesion, activity of the lesion and extent of the disease. Colonoscopy should be avoided or carefully performed by experienced endoscopists during episode of acute severe disease because of high risk of perforation. Changes of ulcerative colitis are typically seen in the rectum, and progress proximally in a symmetrical, circumferential pattern to the variable extent. Endoscopic findings of ulcerative colitis vary from edema, loss of vascularity, granularity, friability of the mucosa, spontaneous bleeding and ulcerations. Depending upon the mucosal appearance, the severity of ulcerative colitis can be classified as mild (loss of vascular pattern, erythema, granularity, mild friability), moderate (erosions and moderate friability) and severe (ulcerations and spontaneous bleeding) (Figs 1A to C). For the diagnosis of ulcerative colitis, even a sigmoidoscopic examination is sufficient; however, every patient with IBD should have a complete evaluation of the whole colon in order to know the extent of the disease and for differentiation from Crohn's disease. Rectal sparing, aphthous ulcers, skip lesions, a cobblestone pattern (areas of longitudinal ulcerations surrounded by areas of submucosal edema) are the feature typically described in Crohn's disease. In patients with long standing inflammation and healing, colonoscopy may reveal pseudopolyps.[1,39-44]

Imaging Studies

Radiology has a limited role in the management of patients with ulcerative colitis. Abdominal plain X-ray should be done in patients with acute severe colitis to rule out toxic megacolon or intestinal perforation. Bowel wall is seen as edematous and irregular in severe

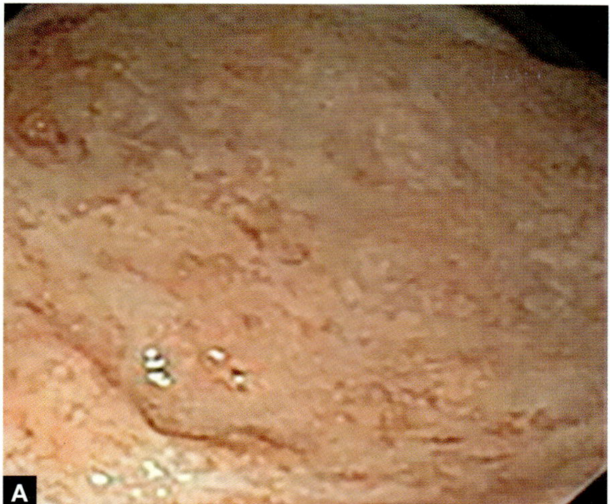

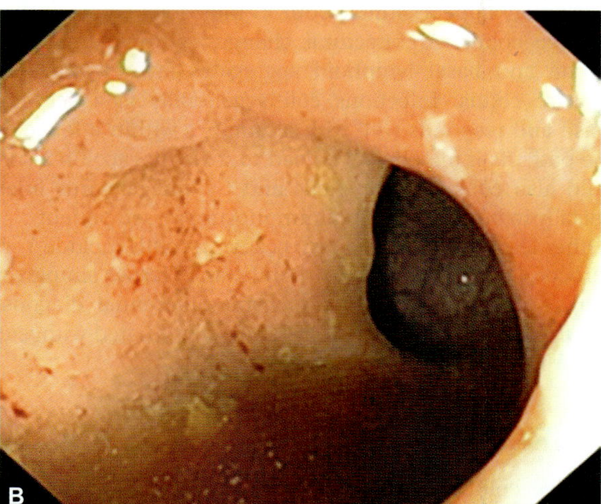

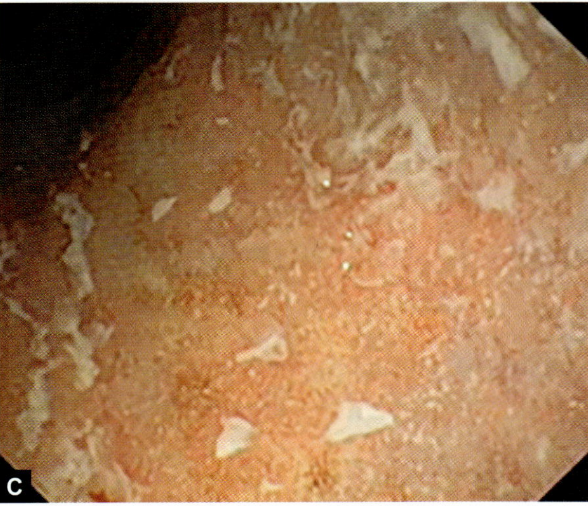

Figures 1A to C Colonoscopic image showing: (A) A normal mucosa of the colon; (B) Loss of vascular pattern and erythema suggesting mild colitis; (C) Loss of vascular pattern, and friability suggesting moderate colitis and loss of vascular pattern, erythema and superficial ulcerations suggesting severe colitis

disease. Inflamed colons seldom contain feces. The presence of colonic dilation of more than 6 cm suggests toxic megacolon.

The use of barium enema in the diagnosis of IBD has generally been abandoned; it however has a role in certain situations. In patients with colonic narrowing due to stricture or malignancy, where proximal examination may be difficult, barium enema may provide essential information regarding the length, location and diameter of the stricture. Moreover, involvement of mucosa proximal to the stricture can also be evaluated. Earliest sign of ulcerative colitis on barium enema is fine mucosal granularity. With increasing severity, mucosal lining become thickened and irregular and superficial and deep ulcers can appear. The colonic haustral folds may be lost in long-standing disease, but may be normal or thickened in patients with shorter duration of the disease.

PATHOLOGY

Grossly, the mucosa in mild ulcerative colitis looks edematous and hyperemic. As disease progresses, colonic mucosa is studded with visible punctate ulcers. Epithelial regeneration gives rise to pseudopolyps. A characteristic appearance of longstanding ulcerative colitis is atrophic and featureless colonic mucosa, accompanied by narrowing and shortening of the colon.[1,39-44]

Biopsies should be taken from different regions of the colon, from rectum to distal ileum for a reliable diagnosis of IBD. In ulcerative colitis, the inflammation is characteristically restricted to the mucosa and submucosa of the colon; while in Crohn's disease, the inflammation may involve all the four layers (transmural) of the intestine. Therefore lesions in the ulcerative colitis are generally superficial and deep in Crohn's disease (Table 1). The histological characteristic, especially the density of inflammatory cells, differ during the active phase of the disease and during the phase of remission. Histologic features of chronic ulcerative colitis include alteration of crypt architecture (e.g. branching crypts with marked deviation of crypt axis from perpendicular, variation in crypt size and/or shape, crypt dropout, foreshortening of crypts, with bases of crypts lifted off muscularis mucosae), increased chronic inflammatory cells (e.g. lymphocytes, plasma cells, especially below the base of crypts—basal plasmacytosis—may be accompanied by more generalized mucosal plasmacytosis) in lamina propria. Neutrophils are not present in colonic mucosa normally. Histologic features of active ulcerative colitis include neutrophilic inflammation, crypt abscesses. Cryptitis and crypt abscesses may be present in infectious colitis and is not pathognomonic of ulcerative colitis. The severity of inflammation on histologic examination may not be directly related to the severity of disease on endoscopy in at least some patients. The biopsies should be evaluated for epithelial dysplasia and colonic mitosis especially if the duration of ulcerative colitis is longer.

Assessment of the Activity of the Disease

The natural history of IBD is that of remission and relapses of the disease. The severity of IBD is generally assessed using clinical parameters, systemic manifestations, mucosal appearance and global impact of the disease on the individual's quality of life. The most commonly used clinical disease activity assessment criteria

Table 4: Truelove and Witt's criteria for of severity of ulcerative colitis

Variables	*Mild*	*Severe*	*Fulminant*
Stools (number/day)	<4	>6	>10
Blood in the stool	Intermittent	Frequent	Continuous
Temperature (°C)	Normal	>37.5°C	>37.5°C
Pulse (per minute)	Normal	90–100	>100
Hemoglobin	Normal	<75% of normal	Transfusion requirement
ESR (mm/hour)	<30	>30	>30
S. albumin (g/dL)	Normal	<3.0	<3.0

Moderate disease includes features of both mild and severe disease.

Table 5: Ulcerative colitis disease activity index

Variables	*Frequency*	*Scores*
Number of stools	Normal	0
	>1–2 than normal	1
	>3–4 than normal	2
	>4 than normal	3
Rectal bleeding	No bleeding	0
	Mild	1
	Moderate	2
	Severe	3
Mucosal friability	No friability	0
	Mild friability	1
	Moderate friability	2
	Exudation and spontaneous bleeding	3
Physician Global Assessment	Normal	0
	Mild	1
	Moderate	2
	Severe	3

UCDAI Score: Normal<2; Mild>2–<4; Moderate>4–<8; Severe>8.

for ulcerative colitis are Truelove and Witt's criteria and Ulcerative Colitis Disease Activity Index (Tables 4 and 5).[1,39-45]

Assessment for the Extent of the Disease

The extent of the ulcerative colitis is limited to only rectum (proctitis) in 20%, rectum and sigmoid (proctosigmoiditis) in 30–40%, splenic flexure (left sided colitis) in 30–40% and 20–30% of patients have pancolitis or extensive colitis.[1,4,12] All patients should undergo evaluation for the extent of the disease using colonoscopy.[1,4,12,39-46]

DIFFERENTIAL DIAGNOSIS

Infectious colitis including amebic colitis is not only an important differential diagnosis of first episode of ulcerative colitis but it may also lead to exacerbation of ulcerative colitis in remission. Salmonella, Shigella and Campylobacter are the most common organisms causing infectious colitis. Abdominal pain and a more acute onset are seen in infectious colitis compared to the flare up of ulcerative colitis. The sigmoidoscopic appearance of the colonic mucosa may appear similar both in infectious colitis and active ulcerative colitis. Architectural changes, chronic inflammatory infiltrate and basal lymphoid aggregates favor a diagnosis of ulcerative colitis. Infectious colitis generally is a self-limiting disease and responds well with antibiotics within a few days. In some patients it may however lead to toxic megacolon also. One should also consider *C. difficile* and Cytomegalovirus infection especially in hospitalized and immunosuppressed patient.

Other less common organisms causing colitis include Yersinia enterocolitica, Aeromonas hydrophila, and Herpes simplex virus. Crohn's disease also is an important differential diagnosis of ulcerative colitis and these two can be differentiated with features listed in Table 1.

NATURAL HISTORY

Ulcerative colitis is a disease characterized by remissions and relapses in almost 80% of the subjects. Mild to moderate disease is seen at first attack in 50%. Severe disease is seen in 6–19% of patients at presentation.[47-51] After the initial flare up, 40–65% subjects have an intermittent and 5–10% of patients have a chronic course.[48-51] About 10% of patients may require colectomy during the initial severe attack.[49] Disease extension follows in 10–30% of ulcerative colitis patients who had earlier presented with proctitis or proctosigmoiditis 10 years after diagnosis.[52,53] The colectomy rate is the highest (10%) in the first year of diagnosis, 3% in the second year and 1% per year thereafter. Overall 24% at 10 years and 30% at 25 years will likely have colectomy.[50]

Before the introduction of glucocorticoids, mortality for a severe attack of colitis used to be 35%. This has now been reduced to less than 2%. Long-term survival for ulcerative colitis patients is similar to age-matched controls.[54-57]

MANAGEMENT

Drugs Used in Inflammatory Bowel Disease

5-Aminosalicylates (5-ASA)

Sulfasalazine and the newer 5-ASA are first line therapy for the treatment of ulcerative colitis. Sulfasalazine has two components: (1) 5-ASA moiety and (2) sulfapyridine joined by an azo-bond.[58]

It reaches colon in intact form where it is cleaved by bacterial enzyme azoreductase releasing sulfapyridine and 5-ASA moieties. The sulfapyridine is responsible for most of the drug's toxicity due to its systematic absorption. The 5-ASA component is the active therapeutic component.[59,60] As 5-ASA is the active compound, but when administered by mouth, it is rapidly absorbed into the jejunum and consequently does not get into the colon. Therefore, various delivery systems have been used to obtain high concentrations of the drug in the colonic lumen. The first method is to coat 5-ASA with a resin or a semipermeable membrane that is pH-sensitive and the second is to link 5-ASA with another molecule by an azo-bond. Mesalamines (Mesacol, Tidocol) are coated with Eudragit S, which dissolve at pH 7.0 or higher, whereas salofalk or claversal are coated with Eudragit L.[61] Pentasa is mesalamines within a semipermeable membrane that releases the drug at luminal pH of more than 6.0 in time release manner.

Sulfasalazine and 5-ASA are anti-inflammatory agents that interfere with the production of arachidonic acid by affecting the thromboxane and lipoxygenase synthesis pathways. Although the precise mechanism of action of the medications in the treatment of IBD is not known, sulfasalazine and the 5-ASA also may have an immune-modulatory effect.[61] Sulfasalazine and the newer 5-ASA preparations are effective treatment for mild-to-moderate ulcerative colitis. Sulfasalazine and mesalamines controls disease activity and induces remission in approximately 70% of patients. Oral mesalazine generally acts in 2–4 weeks-time. Sulfasalazine and the 5-ASA formulations are also effective for maintenance of remission of ulcerative colitis.[62-64]

Corticosteroids

Corticosteroids have been evaluated thoroughly in IBD patients. Besides their non-specific effects on cellular and humoral immune functions, corticosteroids impede the production of cytokines and inflammatory mediators and improve the sense of well-being. Systemic corticosteroids are effective treatment for moderate to severe ulcerative colitis and for controlling acute exacerbations.[65] Topical corticosteroids are delivered rectally and are effective treatment for distal colitis. Several modifications of the glucocorticoid backbone have been developed to maximize the mucosal delivery and enteric anti-inflammatory effects while minimizing systemic side effects. Budesonide is a corticosteroid with extensive first-pass hepatic metabolism. Its targeted delivery via pH and time-dependent formulation to the ileum and right colon reduces side effects compared to other systemic corticosteroids.

Immunosuppressants: Azathioprine and 6-mercaptopurine

Azathioprine (AZA) and 6-mercaptopurine (6-MP) are immunomodulators that are effective for the treatment of steroid dependent ulcerative colitis. After absorption, AZA is non-enzymatically converted to 6-MP, which is then metabolized to the active end product, 6-thioguanine nucleotide. The 6-thioguanine nucleotides inhibit ribonucleotide synthesis and exhibit anti-proliferative effects on activated lymphocytes. These agents have a direct anti-inflammatory effect that is due to suppression of T-cell function and natural killer cell activity. The usual doses are 2.0–2.5 mg/kg/day for azathioprine and 1.0–1.5 mg/kg/day for 6-MP.[65] Idiosyncratic or allergic type reactions to AZA include pancreatitis, fever, rash, arthralgia, diarrhea and nausea. Non-allergic type reactions include bone marrow suppression, infection and hepatitis.[65] AZA or 6-MP induced pancreatitis usually occurs within the first few weeks of treatment and resolves on discontinuation of the drug. Profound leucopenia can develop suddenly and unpredictably. It is recommended that each patient on azathioprine should be monitored. Full blood count and liver function tests should be done every 2–4 weeks initially for 2 months and then every 4–8 weeks.

Cyclosporine

Cyclosporine is a lipophilic peptide that deters the proliferation and activation of T-helper cells by interfering with interleukin (IL)-2 production. It also decreases recruitment of cytotoxic T cells and inhibits production of IL-3, IL-4, tumor necrosis factor (TNF)-α, and interferon-γ.[65] In contrast to 6-MP and AZA, intravenous cyclosporine has an onset of action within days. Compiled results from 20 uncontrolled trials showed a benefit of cyclosporine for patients with severe ulcerative colitis failing steroids. Of the 185 patients treated with cyclosporine, 68% initially avoided colectomy, but only 42% had a sustained response after discontinuing therapy.[66] In a randomized, placebo-controlled trial, 20 patients with severe ulcerative colitis failing intravenous steroids were randomized to either intravenous cyclosporine (4 mg/kg/day) or placebo.[67] Nine of the eleven (82%) patients treated with cyclosporine achieved a response by day 7 compared with none of the patients in the placebo group. At the 6 month follow-up, only 59% maintained a response on oral cyclosporine and approximately 30% required colectomy.[67,68]

The oral microemulsion form of cyclosporine (Neoral) has similar bioavailability compared with intravenous cyclosporine and is more effective than the standard low-dose oral formulations.[69] Monitoring cyclosporine blood levels is required to reduce the chance of toxicity. Potential toxicity limits the use of cyclosporine and common side effects include paresthesias, hypertrichosis, tremor, hypertension, nausea, gingival hyperplasia, vomiting, headaches, nephrotoxicity and seizures.

Biological Agents

With understanding of the initiating and amplifying components of the inflammatory response in patients with IBD, novel therapeutic approaches have evolved.[33,34] We now have the ability to interrupt both proximal (e.g. lymphocyte or cytokine mediated) and distal (e.g. arachidonic acid derivatives—leukotrienes, platelet activating factor) inflammatory cascade. As is anticipated from the experience with steroids and cyclosporine, the more proximal the inhibition, more potential for systemic immune compromise. Thus the present therapy which is evolving is more target specific neutralization of an inflammatory cytokines (anti-TNF-α), and inhibition of specific lymphocytic population. TNF is a key inflammatory cytokine and mediator of intestinal inflammation.[69] There are three ant-TNF agents presently in use. Infliximab is a murine human chimeric monoclonal antibody, adalimumab is a human monoclonal antibody, and certolizumab pegol is a pegylated monoclonal antigen binding fragment (Fab') to TNF-α.[70-72] Golimumab, a humanized anti-TNF agent has been recently approved for induction and maintenance of remission of ulcerative colitis. Anti-TNF therapy is effective in patients with refractory moderate-severe ulcerative colitis. Infliximab has a 66% response rate, twice that of the placebo. At week 30, the response rate was 53% and remission rate 33%, with similar rates at 1 year. Mucosal healing was seen in 51% of patients treated with infliximab.[1,39-45,70,71]

Probiotics in Ulcerative Colitis

Probiotics have been used in induction of remission of active disease and maintenance of remission; however, evidences are not sufficient to recommend probiotics for routine use.[73] Probiotics especially VSL#3 has been found to be effective in both inducing remission in active pouchitis and maintenance of remission in pouchitis.[74,75]

Management of Ulcerative Colitis

The goals of management of ulcerative colitis are to induce remission, maintain remission, prevent complications and improve quality of life. The treatment of ulcerative colitis needs to be individualized. Treatment depends upon the extent of the disease (proctitis, left sided colitis and pancolitis), activity of the disease (active phase, remission phase) and steroid dependency (Flow chart 1). The choice of treatment for many patients in India depends substantially on the cost and affordability of treatment regimens.[1,39-45] A study from Mumbai found that 80% of patients with IBD were non-adherent to treatment (defined as taking <80% of the dose advised). Non-adherent patients were 3 times more likely to develop a relapse as compared to those who adhered to medicines.[76]

Induction of Remission

Mild to moderate proctitis and left sided colitis: Delivery of the anti-inflammatory drugs directly to the inflamed segment is the best option. Topical route delivers a higher amount of the drug directly to the involved mucosa. Systemic absorption of drug is minimized with less systemic adverse effects. Therefore, a disease distal to the splenic flexure is best treated with topical suppositories, foams, enemas and gel depending upon the extent of the disease. Patient preference regarding route of drug delivery should also be considered. Enemas of 5-ASA and suppositories are effective first-line therapies for patients with left sided colitis and ulcerative proctitis. Patients with left sided colitis can also be treated by oral 5-ASA but they are less effective than topical 5-ASA compounds.[1,39-45]

Mild to moderately active extensive colitis: Mild to moderately active extensive colitis is initially managed with oral 5-ASA compounds in the doses up to 3.2–4.8 g/day. Once-daily dose of 5-ASA or newer, controlled-release formulations, such as multi-matrix 5-ASA (1.2 g tablets) are effective and promote adherence to treatment. For those patients who do not respond to only oral 5-ASA, a combined

Flow chart 1 Management algorithm of ulcerative colitis

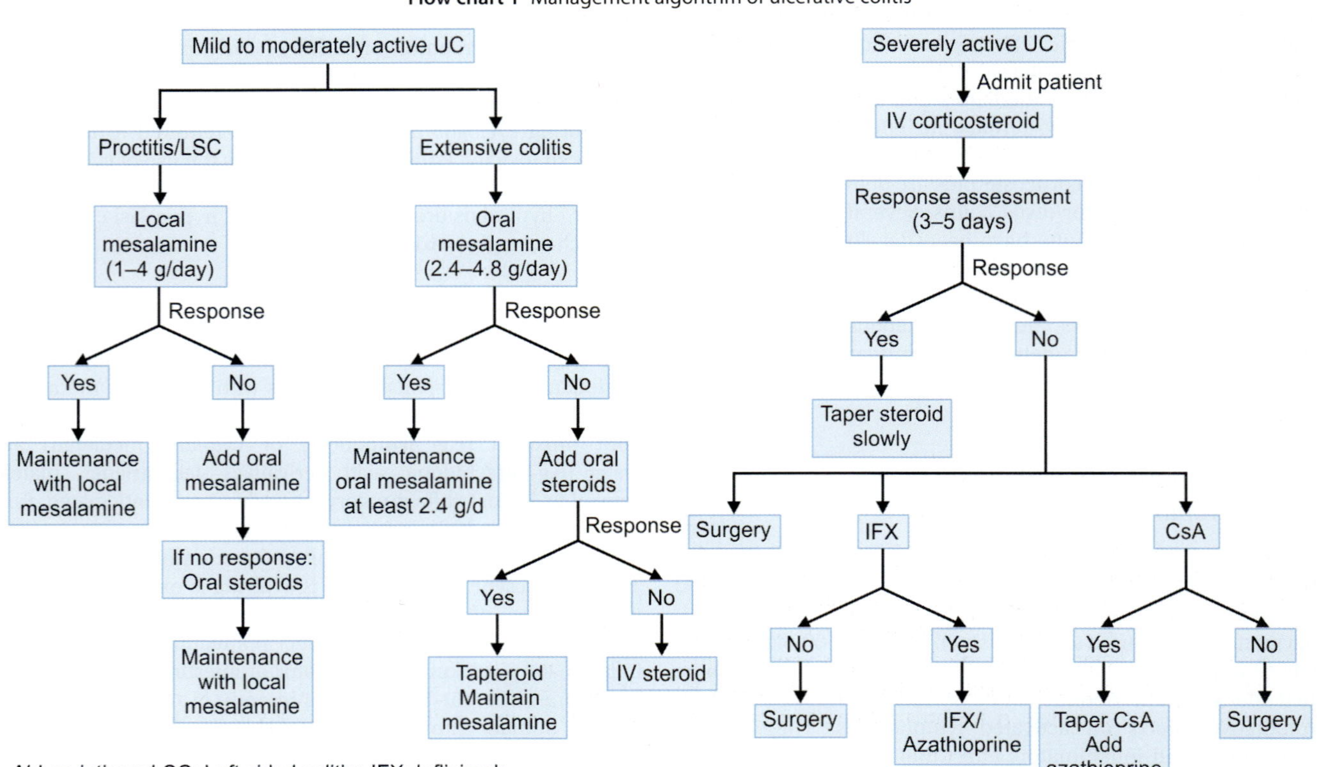

Abbreviations: LSC: Left sided colitis; IFX: Infliximab

oral and topical 5-ASA is superior to oral mesalamine alone. Clinical (and endoscopic) remission can occur in up to 64% within 2 weeks.[1,39-45]

Severely active ulcerative colitis: Patients with mild-to-moderate ulcerative colitis that is refractory to topical therapy or oral therapy and those with moderate to severe disease should be treated with oral glucocorticoids. Patients who have failed to respond to maximal oral treatment with a combination of 5-ASA and/or steroids those who present with severe/fulminant disease should be admitted for intensive intravenous corticosteroids (hydrocortisone 400 mg/day) therapy. The patient should be monitored for number and consistency of stool, amount of blood in the stool, vital signs and abdominal signs (fullness, abdominal tenderness, rebound tenderness and bowel sound). Therefore a constant vigil on the overall condition of the patient is mandatory. Hemogram, ESR, C-reactive protein, serum electrolytes and serum protein should be repeated at every 2–3 days. If on an initial abdominal radiography, the diameter of transverse colon is found to be dilated (>5.5 cm), then abdominal skiagram should be repeated every day. Anticholinergic, anti-diarrheal agents and opioid drugs are best avoided as they can precipitate colonic dilatation. NSAID can worsen disease activity. Most patients are generally on mesalamines, mesalamines may be continued once oral intake resumes.[1,39-44] Infections such as *C. difficile*, Cytomegalovirus infection or other parasitic infections should be excluded. No improvement or deterioration after 3–5 days of intravenous steroids is an indication to start immediate rescue treatment. Continued frequency of stools with fecal blood and elevated levels of CRP after 3 days of corticosteroids indicate no improvement. Surgery, infliximab and cyclosporine are all effective rescue treatments for these patients.[39-45,77,78] Treatment should be customized for each patient, strategically taking into account comorbidities, age, extent of disease and ongoing treatment at the time of relapse. Patients given cyclosporine after failed azathioprine are more likely to need colectomy than are those who have not received azathioprine. Cyclosporine gives good (60–80%) short-term clinical response in steroid-refractory ulcerative colitis. However, use of this drug is limited by serious adverse events and lower efficacy for maintenance of colectomy-free remission in the long term. Cyclosporine is first given intravenously at doses of 2 mg/kg/day and is then converted to an oral microemulsion at doses of 5–10 mg/kg. Cyclosporine dose is titrated to maintain trough serum concentrations of the drug between 200 and 400 ng/mL. Infliximab is also highly effective given intravenously at a dose of 5 mg/kg at weeks 0, 2 and 6. Up to two-thirds of patients with acute severe colitis respond to either infliximab or cyclosporine. Patients who do not respond to either infliximab or cyclosporine should undergo surgical intervention[79,80] (Figs 2A to D).

Immediate surgical referral is necessary if there is evidence of toxic megacolon (transverse colon diameter >5.5 cm, or cecum >9 cm). In toxic megacolon, perforation occurs in 30–45% of cases. Signs of perforation and toxicity may be masked by steroid therapy. Early surgery should be undertaken. In selected patients with mild colonic dilatation, an expectant conservative management can be continued if clinical, laboratory or radiological signs remain stable. In those with toxic megacolon, colonic decompression can be augmented by frequent change in posture to knee elbow position.

Maintenance of Remission

After achieving remission, the goal is to sustain the symptom-free status with various medications. Glucocorticoids have no place in maintenance therapy, because of their side effects over long term. First-line therapy for the maintenance of remission is oral or topical mesalamine. Both oral and rectal 5-ASA are superior to placebo for preventing relapse in patients with distal disease. The appropriate doses of 5-ASA compounds for maintenance of remission of ulcerative colitis are 1,600–2,400 mg of mesalazine, and 2,000 mg sulfasalazine.[39-44]

Patients who relapse while on oral 5-ASA, those who are steroid-dependent, and those with severe ulcerative colitis who need induction therapy with cyclosporin or tacrolimus are candidates for immunosuppressive therapy such as azathioprine, or 6-MP. Azathioprine is given at 2–2.5 mg/kg/day and 6-MP at 1.0–1.5 mg/kg/day. Infliximab is effective for maintenance of remission and is steroid-sparing in patients who are unable to maintain remission while on azathioprine or 6-MP. Most patients will require maintenance treatment for life long.

All patients with IBD who require immunosuppressive medications should be screened for HBV, HCV, HIV and tuberculosis.

Colonic Cancer in Ulcerative Colitis

Carcinomas occur in patients of ulcerative colitis who have had the disease for 10 years. The cancers have a tendency to rapidly metastasize, be multicentric and are atypical in its appearance. The risk of colorectal cancer increases by 0.5–1% per year. Regular surveillance is required. Because of the increased risk of colorectal cancer, guidelines recommend that patients with ulcerative colitis should undergo annual or biannual surveillance colonoscopy after 8–10 years with multiple biopsies taken from all regions.[39-44] Data from a cross-sectional study of ulcerative colitis patients from Vellore showed the CRC risk to be 0% at 10 years, 2.3% at 20 years and 5.8% for disease duration more than 20 years.[81]

Surgery for Ulcerative Colitis

Patients of ulcerative colitis who may require surgery for IBD should be jointly managed by a surgeon and a gastroenterologist. Surgery is an important component in the treatment algorithm of ulcerative colitis and early consultation is recommended especially for acute severe ulcerative colitis that requires hospitalization. Five to twenty percent of patients with ulcerative colitis require colectomy. The decision to operate is best taken in a joint consultation of gastroenterologist, surgeon and the patient. The type of surgery is dependent on the indication and the patient's condition. The indications may be classified as emergency (exsanguinating hemorrhage, intestinal perforation and severe colitis unresponsive to intensive medical treatment) and elective (steroid dependent disease, steroid refractory disease, documented, intolerable side effects of drugs and unaffordability of medical treatment or strongly suspected/confirmed carcinoma). Optimal results depend upon expertise of the surgical team, timely consultation, the clinical setting and patient selection. The

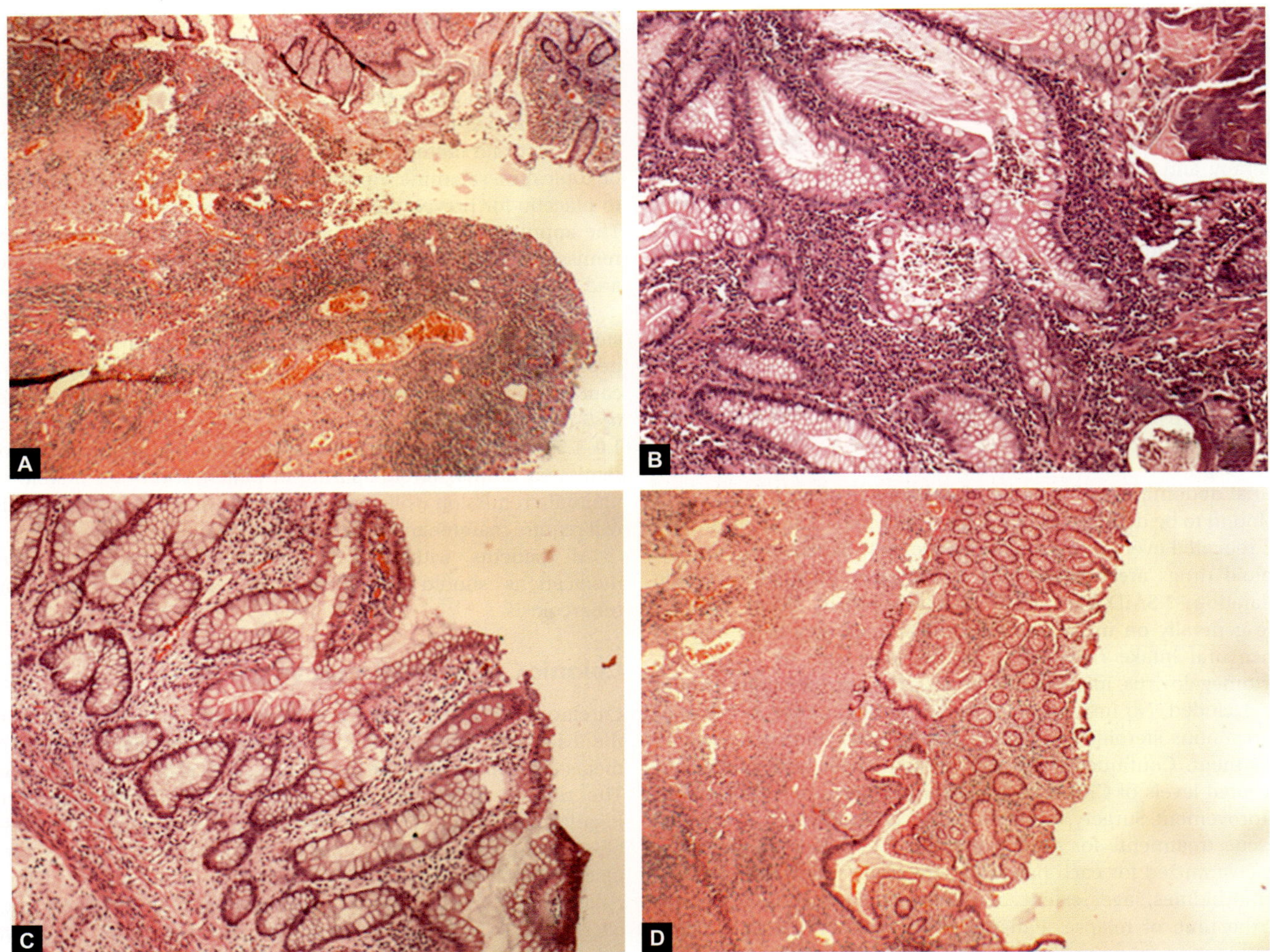

Figures 2A to D Microphotograph of histology of a patient with UC showing: (A) Ulceration of the surface of the mucosa; (B) Crypt abscess; (C and D) chronic changes such as crypt distortion and crypt branching

patient's age, previous intestinal or anal surgery, obesity, patient occupation, liver disease and cancer risk should all be considered. When indicated, the gold standard elective surgery for ulcerative colitis is proctocolectomy with ileal pouch anal anastomosis (IPAA) and this should be performed in a specialized center. In emergency situations (such as toxic megacolon), abdominal colectomy with ileostomy and closure of the rectum (Hartman's operation) or mucous fistula is the procedure of choice. Leaving the rectum in place permits subsequent proctectomy with ileal pouch-anal anastomosis. Emergency proctocolectomy may also be required for uncontrollable hemorrhage. IPAA should not be performed on patients with toxic colitis due to excessively high complication rates. In addition, patients who are on combination immunosuppressive therapy that includes infliximab may benefit from a three-stage IPAA. Patients should be advised that an ileostomy may be required if a continence preserving procedure fails or is not technically possible.[39,44,78,82,83]

Acute complications of IPAA include anastomotic leak, sepsis, injury to local structures including pelvic nerves. The incidence of pouchitis, the most common long-term complication of IPAA, can be as high as 40%. In 10–20% of cases, pouchitis becomes chronic. Symptoms of pouchitis include increased stool frequency, urgency, incontinence and perianal discomfort. Treatment of pouchitis consists primarily of antibiotics (metronidazole, rifaximin, ciprofloxacin) probiotics can be effective for preventing recurrence. Pouch failure, requiring pouch excision or permanent diversion, occurs in 8–10% of patients. Probiotics especially VSL#3 has been found to be very effective in both inducing remission in active pouchitis and maintenance of remission in pouchitis.

Continence preserving surgical procedures are associated with a small risk of urinary and sexual dysfunction; the risk is greatest in patients who require extensive reoperative pelvic surgery. Postoperative impotence and retrograde ejaculation are observed in approximately 1.5% and 4% of men, respectively, while transient dyspareunia occurs in about 7% of women. Decreased fertility is also frequent in women after IPAA.

Fertility and Pregnancy in Ulcerative Colitis

Although fertility in inactive IBD is unaffected, active disease diminishes the fertility. The reasons for decreased fertility in

IBD include inflammatory changes in the female reproductive system during active phase of the disease, local sepsis, pelvic surgery, prior surgery and reversible decrease in sperm motility by sulphasalazine.[84-86] The frequency of abortions, preterm deliveries, cesarean sections, congenital abnormalities and birth weight is no different in patients with IBD compared with non-IBD controls as seen in a prospective study including 332 pregnant women with IBD (145 with Crohn's disease and 187 with ulcerative colitis) from 12 European countries. Women who have IBD are more likely to have a cesarean section, especially those with Crohn's disease.[84] If pregnancy is planned, patient should be counseled to conceive during remission phase of the disease and should continue their maintenance medication. Patients should maintain normal weight, have good nutrition and take calcium, iron and folate supplements. Maternal and fetal health depends on adequate disease control during pregnancy. Patients with ulcerative colitis who are pregnant, should continue to take mesalamine for maintaining remission. If Azathioprine had been instituted well prior to pregnancy, it should be continued. Mesalamine, prednisolone and azathioprine are safe in pregnancy. Pregnant women with IBD should be managed jointly by a gastroenterologist and obstetrician. Patients with acute severe disease or other life-threatening complications of disease should be managed in the similar fashion as the non-pregnant patient. Optimal management of maternal IBD is the key to the best fetal outcome. The mode of delivery should be carefully considered. The mode of delivery is best guided by the obstetric indications rather that of the IBD.[85,86]

Acute exacerbations during pregnancy should be treated with drugs recognized to be safe in pregnancy. Corticosteroids tend to be safe in pregnancy as placental 11-hydroxygenase converts steroids to less active metabolites. Methotrexate and Thalidomide should be avoided during pregnancy.[85,86]

BREASTFEEDING

5-ASA and corticosteroids are safe during breastfeeding. Azathioprine metabolites have not been found in babies exclusively breastfed by mother receiving thiopurines. Therefore most clinicians believe that women should not stop thiopurines during breastfeeding. Methotrexate should be avoided during breastfeeding.

NUTRITION IN INFLAMMATORY BOWEL DISEASE

Nutritional care is an important consideration in the long-term management of IBD. Protein calorie malnutrition is seen in up to 85% of hospitalized patients with exacerbations of IBD. These patients have malnutrition of both macronutrients and micronutrients.[1,39-44] Anemia is a common complication of IBD. Iron deficiency and anemia of chronic disease are the commonest causes of anemia in IBD, though folate and vitamin B12 deficiency may occur. Drug-induced anemia secondary to AZA, 6-MP or sulfasalazine also occurs. Patients with IBD should have at least annual hemoglobin check. The nutritional status of these patients should be assessed and optimum nutritional therapy should be provided to them.[39-44,87]

Osteoporosis is quite common in patients with IBD. Systemic inflammation secondary to active colitis and recurrent or chronic use of high dose corticosteroids are risk factors for osteoporosis. Optimal nutrition, calcium and vitamin D intake, weight-bearing exercise, cessation of smoking and minimization of the use of corticosteroids are recommended.

Because glucocorticoids are mainstay of treatment of patients with IBD, it is important to recognize the effects of glucocorticoids on bone remodeling. Corticosteroids increase the risk of bone loss, especially in the initial months of treatment, by impairing osteoblast function, inducing apoptosis of osteoblasts, reducing intestinal calcium absorption and increasing renal excretion of calcium. Patients at risk for osteoporosis should receive calcium and vitamin D supplementation. Younger men and premenopausal women should have a daily intake of at least 1,000 mg from either supplementation or through diet. Older men and women require at least 1,500 mg of calcium, Vitamin D intake of 400–800 IU/day should be adequate for healthy individuals, but patients with intestinal malabsorption and housebound patients may need an increased amount.

REFERENCES

1. Danese S, Fiocchi C. Ulcerative colitis. N Engl J Med. 2011;365:1713-25.
2. Loftus EV Jr. Clinical epidemiology of inflammatory bowel disease: incidence, prevalence, and environmental influences. Gastroenterology. 2004;126:1504-17.
3. Yang SK, Loftus EV Jr, Sandborn WJ. Epidemiology of inflammatory bowel disease in Asia. Inflamm Bowel Dis. 2001;7:260-70.
4. Ahuja V, Tandon RK. Inflammatory bowel disease in the Asia-Pacific area: a comparison with developed countries and regional differences. J Dig Dis. 2010;11:134-47.
5. Yang S-K, Yun S, Kim J-H, Park JY, Kim HY, Kim Y-H, et al. Epidemiology of inflammatory bowel disease in the Songpa-Kangdong district, Seoul, Korea, 1986–2005: a KASID study. Inflamm Bowel Dis. 2008;14:542-9.
6. Chow DKL, Leong RWL, Tsoi KKF, Ng SSM, Leung W, Wu JCY, et al. Long-term follow-up of ulcerative colitis in the Chinese population. Am J Gastroenterol. 2009;104:647-54.
7. Ling K-L, Ooi C-J, Luman W, Cheong W-K, Choen FS, Ng H-S. Clinical characteristics of ulcerative colitis in Singapore, a multiracial city-state. J Clin Gastroenterol. 2002;35:144-8.
8. Whelan G. Epidemiology of inflammatory bowel disease. Med Clin North Am. 1990;74:1-12.
9. Farrokhyar F, Swarbrick ET, Irvine EJ. A critical review of epidemiological studies in inflammatory bowel disease. Scand J Gastroenterol. 2001;36:2-15.
10. Garland CF, Lilienfeld AM, Mendeloff AI, Markowitz JA, Terrell KB, Garland FC. Incidence rates of ulcerative colitis and Crohn's disease in fifteen areas of the United States. Gastroenterology. 1981;81:1115-24.
11. Sood A, Midha V, Sood N, Bhatia AS, Avasthi G. Incidence and prevalence of ulcerative colitis in Punjab, North India. Gut. 2003;52:1587-90.
12. Makharia GK, Ramakrishna BS, Abraham P, Choudhuri G, Misra SP, Ahuja V, et al. Indian Society of Gastroenterology Task Force on Inflammatory Bowel Disease. Survey of inflammatory bowel diseases in India. Indian J Gastroenterol. 2012;31:299-306.
13. Niv Y, Abuksis G, Fraser GM. Epidemiology of ulcerative colitis in Israel: a survey of Israeli kibbutz settlements. Am J Gastroenterol. 2000;95:693-8.
14. Mangat BK, Evaschesen C, Lee T, Yoshida EM, Salh B. Ethnic variation in the annual rates of adult inflammatory bowel disease in hospitalized patients in Vancouver, British Columbia. Can J Gastroenterol. 2011;25:73-7.

15. Orholm M, Fonager K, Sørensen HT. Risk of ulcerative colitis and Crohn's disease among offspring of patients with chronic inflammatory bowel disease. Am J Gastroenterol. 1999;94:3236-8.
16. Halme L, Paavola-Sakki P, Turunen U, Lappalainen M, Farkkila M, Kontula K. Family and twin studies in inflammatory bowel disease. World J Gastroenterol WJG. 2006;12:3668-72.
17. Khor B, Gardet A, Xavier RJ. Genetics and pathogenesis of inflammatory bowel disease. Nature. 2011;474:307-17.
18. Ng SC, Tsoi KKF, Kamm MA, Xia B, Wu J, Chan FKL, et al. Genetics of inflammatory bowel disease in Asia: systematic review and meta-analysis. Inflamm Bowel Dis. 2012;18:1164-76.
19. Naser SA, Arce M, Khaja A, Fernandez M, Naser N, Elwasila S, et al. Role of ATG16L, NOD2 and IL23R in Crohn's disease pathogenesis. World J Gastroenterol WJG. 2012;18:412-24.
20. Duerr RH, Taylor KD, Brant SR, Rioux JD, Silverberg MS, Daly MJ, et al. A genome-wide association study identifies IL23R as an inflammatory bowel disease gene. Science. 2006;314:1461-3.
21. Kuballa P, Huett A, Rioux JD, Daly MJ, Xavier RJ. Impaired autophagy of an intracellular pathogen induced by a Crohn's disease associated ATG16L1 variant. PloS One. 2008;3:e3391.
22. Rutgeerts P, Goboes K, Peeters M, Hiele M, Penninckx F, Aerts R, et al. Effect of faecal stream diversion on recurrence of Crohn's disease in the neoterminal ileum. Lancet. 1991;338:771-4.
23. D'Haens GR, Geboes K, Peeters M, Baert F, Penninckx F, Rutgeerts P. Early lesions of recurrent Crohn's disease caused by infusion of intestinal contents in excluded ileum. Gastroenterology. 1998;114:262-7.
24. Gersemann M, Wehkamp J, Stange EF. Innate immune dysfunction in inflammatory bowel disease. J Intern Med. 2012;271(5):421-8.
25. Ventham NT, Kennedy NA, Nimmo ER, Satsangi J. Beyond gene discovery in inflammatory bowel disease: the emerging role of epigenetics. Gastroenterology. 2013;145:293-308.
26. D'Haens GR, Geboes K, Peeters M, Baert F, Penninckx F, Rutgeerts P. Early lesions of recurrent Crohn's disease caused by infusion of intestinal contents in excluded ileum. Gastroenterology. 1998;114:262-7.
27. Ley RE, Turnbaugh PJ, Klein S, Gordon JI. Microbial ecology: human gut microbes associated with obesity. Nature. 2006;444:1022-3.
28. Frank DN, St Amand AL, Feldman RA, Boedeker EC, Harpaz N, Pace NR. Molecular-phylogenetic characterization of microbial community imbalances in human inflammatory bowel diseases. Proc Natl Acad Sci USA. 2007;104:13780-5.
29. Kett K, Rognum TO, Brandtzaeg P. Mucosal subclass distribution of immunoglobulin G-producing cells is different in ulcerative colitis and Crohn's disease of the colon. Gastroenterology. 1987;93:919-24.
30. Scott MG, Nahm MH, Macke K, Nash GS, Bertovich MJ, MacDermott RP. Spontaneous secretion of IgG subclasses by intestinal mononuclear cells: differences between ulcerative colitis, Crohn's disease and controls. Clin Exp Immunol. 1986;66:209-15.
31. Snook JA, de Silva HJ, Jewell DP. The association of autoimmune disorders with inflammatory bowel disease. Q J Med. 1989;72:835-40.
32. Das KM, Dasgupta A, Mandal A, Geng X. Autoimmunity to cytoskeletal protein tropomyosin. A clue to the pathogenetic mechanism for ulcerative colitis. J Immunol. 1993;150:2487-93.
33. Baumgart DC, Carding SR. Inflammatory bowel disease: cause and immunobiology. Lancet 2007;369:1627-40.
34. Baumgart DC, Sandborn WJ. Inflammatory bowel disease: clinical aspects and established and evolving therapies. Lancet. 2007;369:1641-57.
35. Strober W, Fuss IJ. Proinflammatory cytokines in the pathogenesis of inflammatory bowel diseases. Gastroenterology. 2011;140:1756-67.
36. Kaser A, Blumberg RS. Autophagy, microbial sensing, endoplasmic reticulum stress, and epithelial function in inflammatory bowel disease. Gastroenterology. 2011;140:1738-47.
37. Rosenfeld G, Bressler B. The truth about cigarette smoking and the risk of inflammatory bowel disease. Am J Gastroenterol. 2012;107:1407-8.
38. Silverberg MS, Satsangi J, Ahmad T, Arnott ID, Bernstein CN, Brant SR, et al. Toward an integrated clinical, molecular and serological classification of inflammatory bowel disease: report of a Working Party of the 2005 Montreal World Congress of Gastroenterology. Can J Gastroenterol. 2005;19(Suppl A):5A-36A.
39. Ramakrishna BS, Makharia GK, Abraham P, Ghoshal UC, Jayanthi V, Agarwal BK, et al. Indian Society of Gastroenterology Task Force on Inflammatory Bowel Diseases. Indian Society of Gastroenterology consensus on ulcerative colitis. Indian J Gastroenterol. 2012;31:307-23.
40. Ooi CJ, Fock KM, Makharia GK, Goh KL, Ling KL, Hilmi I, et al. Asia Pacific Association of Gastroenterology Working Group on Inflammatory Bowel Disease. The Asia-Pacific consensus on ulcerative colitis. J Gastroenterol Hepatol. 2010;25:453-68.
41. Bernstein CN, Fried M, Krabshuis JH, Cohen H, Eliakim R, Fedail S, et al. World Gastroenterology Organization Practice Guidelines for the diagnosis and management of IBD in 2010. Inflamm Bowel Dis. 2010;16:112-24.
42. Dignass A, Eliakim R, Magro F, Maaser C, Chowers Y, Geboes K, et al. Second European evidence-based consensus on the diagnosis and management of ulcerative colitis part 1: definitions and diagnosis. J Crohns Colitis. 2012;6:965-90.
43. Ramakrishna BS, Makharia GK, Abraham P, Ghoshal UC, Jayanthi V, Agarwal BK, et al. Indian Society of Gastroenterology Task Force on Inflammatory Bowel Diseases. Indian Society of Gastroenterology consensus on ulcerative colitis. Indian J Gastroenterol. 2012;31:307-23.
44. Ooi CJ, Fock KM, Makharia GK, Goh KL, Ling KL, Hilmi I, et al. Asia Pacific Association of Gastroenterology Working Group on Inflammatory Bowel Disease. The Asia-Pacific consensus on ulcerative colitis. J Gastroenterol Hepatol. 2010;25:453-68.
45. Dignass A, Lindsay JO, Sturm A, Windsor A, Colombel JF, Allez M, et al. Second European evidence-based consensus on the diagnosis and management of ulcerative colitis part 2: current management. J Crohns Colitis. 2012;6:991-1030.
46. Pera A, Bellando P, Caldera D, Ponti V, Astegiano M, Barletti C, et al. Colonoscopy in inflammatory bowel disease. Diagnostic accuracy and proposal of an endoscopic score. Gastroenterology. 1987;92(1): 181-5.
47. Hendriksen C, Kreiner S, Binder V. Long term prognosis in ulcerative colitis—based on results from a regional patient group from the county of Copenhagen. Gut. 1985;26:158-63.
48. Stonnington CM, Phillips SF, Zinsmeister AR, Melton LJ 3rd. Prognosis of chronic ulcerative colitis in a community. Gut. 1987;28:1261-6.
49. Rao SS, Read NW, Brown C, Bruce C, Holdsworth CD. Studies on the mechanism of bowel disturbance in ulcerative colitis. Gastroenterology. 1987;93:934-40.
50. Langholz E, Munkholm P, Davidsen M, Binder V. Course of ulcerative colitis: analysis of changes in disease activity over years. Gastroenterology. 1994;107:3-11.
51. Bitton A, Sewitch MJ, Peppercorn MA, deB Edwardes MD, Shah S, Ransil B, et al. Psychosocial determinants of relapse in ulcerative colitis: a longitudinal study. Am J Gastroenterol. 2003;98:2203-8.
52. Ayres RC, Gillen CD, Walmsley RS, Allan RN. Progression of ulcerative proctosigmoiditis: incidence and factors influencing progression. Eur J Gastroenterol Hepatol. 1996;8:555-8.
53. Powell-Tuck J, Ritchie JK, Lennard-Jones JE. The prognosis of idiopathic proctitis. Scand J Gastroenterol. 1977;12:727-32.
54. Ritchie JK, Powell-Tuck J, Lennard-Jones JE. Clinical outcome of the first ten years of ulcerative colitis and proctitis. Lancet. 1978;1: 1140-3.

55. Broström O, Monsén U, Nordenwall B, Sörstad J, Hellers G. Prognosis and mortality of ulcerative colitis in Stockholm County, 1955-1979. Scand J Gastroenterol. 1987;22:907-13.
56. Card T, Hubbard R, Logan RFA. Mortality in inflammatory bowel disease: a population-based cohort study. Gastroenterology. 2003;125:1583-90.
57. Winther KV, Jess T, Langholz E, Munkholm P, Binder V. Survival and cause-specific mortality in ulcerative colitis: follow-up of a population-based cohort in Copenhagen County. Gastroenterology. 2003;125:1576-82.
58. Baron JH, Conell AM, Lennard-Jones JE, Jones FA. Sulphasalazine and salicylazosulphadimidine in ulcerative colitis. Lancet. 1962;1(7239):1094-6.
59. Azad Khan AK, Piris J, Truelove SC. An experiment to determine the active therapeutic moiety of sulphasalazine. Lancet. 1977;2(8044):892-5.
60. Van Hees PA, Bakker JH, van Tongeren JH. Effect of sulphapyridine, 5-aminosalicylic acid, and placebo in patients with idiopathic proctitis: a study to determine the active therapeutic moiety of sulphasalazine. Gut. 1980;21:632-5.
61. Sandborn WJ, Hanauer SB. Systematic review: the pharmacokinetic profiles of oral mesalazine formulations and mesalazine pro-drugs used in the management of ulcerative colitis. Aliment Pharmacol Ther. 2003;17:29-42.
62. Hanauer SB. Medical therapy for ulcerative colitis 2004. Gastroenterology. 2004;126:1582-92.
63. Sutherland L, Macdonald JK. Oral 5-aminosalicylic acid for maintenance of remission in ulcerative colitis. Cochrane Database Syst Rev. 2006;(2):CD000544.
64. Sutherland L, Macdonald JK. Oral 5-aminosalicylic acid for induction of remission in ulcerative colitis. Cochrane Database Syst Rev. 2006;(2):CD000543.
65. Lichtenstein GR, Abreu MT, Cohen R, Tremaine W, American Gastroenterological Association. American Gastroenterological Association Institute technical review on corticosteroids, immunomodulators, and infliximab in inflammatory bowel disease. Gastroenterology. 2006;130:940-87.
66. Sandborn WJ. A critical review of cyclosporine therapy in inflammatory bowel disease. Inflamm Bowel Dis. 1995;1:48-63.
67. Lichtiger S, Present DH, Kornbluth A, Gelernt I, Bauer J, Galler G, et al. Cyclosporine in severe ulcerative colitis refractory to steroid therapy. N Engl J Med. 1994;330:1841-5.
68. Actis GC, Aimo G, Priolo G, Moscato D, Rizzetto M, Pagni R. Efficacy and efficiency of oral microemulsion cyclosporin versus intravenous and soft gelatin capsule cyclosporin in the treatment of severe steroid-refractory ulcerative colitis: an open-label retrospective trial. Inflamm Bowel Dis. 1998;4:276-9.
69. Siegel SA, Shealy DJ, Nakada MT, Le J, Woulfe DS, Probert L, et al. The mouse/human chimeric monoclonal antibody cA2 neutralizes TNF in vitro and protects transgenic mice from cachexia and TNF lethality in vivo. Cytokine. 1995;7:15-25.
70. Rutgeerts P, Sandborn WJ, Feagan BG, Reinisch W, Olson A, Johanns J, et al. Infliximab for induction and maintenance therapy for ulcerative colitis. N Engl J Med. 2005;353:2462-76.
71. Sandborn WJ, van Assche G, Reinisch W, Colombel J-F, D'Haens G, Wolf DC, et al. Adalimumab induces and maintains clinical remission in patients with moderate-to-severe ulcerative colitis. Gastroenterology. 2012;142:257-265. e1-3.
72. Sandborn WJ, Feagan BG, Marano C, Zhang H, Strauss R, Johanns J, et al. Subcutaneous golimumab induces clinical response and remission in patients with moderate to severe ulcerative colitis. Gastroenterology. 2014;146(1):85-95.
73. Mimura T, Rizzello F, Helwig U, Poggioli G, Schreiber S, Talbot IC, et al. Once daily high dose probiotic therapy (VSL#3) for maintaining remission in recurrent or refractory pouchitis. Gut. 2004;53:108-14.
74. Gionchetti P, Rizzello F, Helwig U, Venturi A, Lammers KM, Brigidi P, et al. Prophylaxis of pouchitis onset with probiotic therapy: a double-blind, placebo-controlled trial. Gastroenterology. 2003;124:1202-9.
75. Sanders ME, Guarner F, Guerrant R, Holt PR, Quigley EM, Sartor RB, et al. An update on the use and investigation of probiotics in health and disease. Gut. 2013;62:787-96.
76. Bhatt J, Patil S, Joshi A, Abraham P, Desai D. Self-reported treatment adherence in inflammatory bowel disease in Indian patients. Indian J Gastroenterol. 2009;28:143-6.
77. Ford AC, Moayyedi P, Hanauer SB. Ulcerative colitis. BMJ. 2013;346:f432.
78. Van Assche G, Vermeire S, Rutgeerts P. Management of acute severe ulcerative colitis. Gut. 2011;60:130-3.
79. Laharie D, Bourreille A, Branche J, Allez M, Bouhnik Y, Filippi J, et al. Groupe d'Etudes Thérapeutiques des Affections Inflammatoires Digestives. Ciclosporin versus infliximab in patients with severe ulcerative colitis refractory to intravenous steroids: a parallel, open-label randomised controlled trial. Lancet. 2012;380:1909-15.
80. Levesque BG, Sandborn WJ. Infliximab versus ciclosporin in severe ulcerative colitis. Lancet. 2012;380:1887-8.
81. Venkataraman S, Mohan V, Ramakrishna BS, Peter S, Chacko A, Chandy G, et al. Risk of colorectal cancer in ulcerative colitis in India. J Gastroenterol Hepatol. 2005;20:705-9.
82. Burger D, Travis S. Conventional medical management of inflammatory bowel disease. Gastroenterology. 2011;140:1827-37.
83. Ordás I, Eckmann L, Talamini M, Baumgart DC, Sandborn WJ. Ulcerative colitis. Lancet. 2012;380:1606-19.
84. Bortoli A, Pedersen N, Duricova D, D'Inca R, Gionchetti P, Panelli MR, et al. Pregnancy outcome in inflammatory bowel disease: prospective European case-control ECCO-EpiCom study, 2003-2006. Aliment Pharmacol Ther. 2011;34:724-34.
85. Selinger CP, Leong RW, Lal S. Pregnancy related issues in inflammatory bowel disease: evidence base and patients' perspective. World J Gastroenterol. 2012;18:2600-8.
86. Habal FM, Huang VW. Review article: a decision-making algorithm for the management of pregnancy in the inflammatory bowel disease patient. Aliment Pharmacol Ther. 2012;35:501-15.
87. Wagner IJ, Rombeau JL. Nutritional support of surgical patients with inflammatory bowel disease. Surg Clin North Am. 2011;91:787-803.

CHAPTER 93

Surgery for Ulcerative Colitis

Rohin Mittal, Benjamin Perakath

INTRODUCTION

While medical management is central to the treatment of ulcerative colitis, surgical therapy has its own key role to play. When performed at the right time and for the correct indications, surgery can provide cure while preventing significant morbidity and sometimes even mortality. The consequences of delaying surgery, when indicated, can be grave, leading to significant morbidity, prolonged hospitalization, increased costs and even death in some instances.[1] About 20–30% of patients with ulcerative colitis will need surgery at varying points of time during the course of their disease.[2]

INDICATIONS FOR SURGERY

Indications for surgery in ulcerative colitis can be broadly divided into two: emergency and elective.

Surgery on an emergent basis is indicated in the following clinical settings:

- Acute fulminant colitis
- Toxic megacolon
- Colonic perforation
- Colonic hemorrhage.

Indications for surgery in an elective setting include:

- Intractable disease
- Presence of dysplasia or malignancy
- Severe extraintestinal manifestations
- Certain other special individualized circumstances.

SURGICAL OPTIONS

The various surgical options available in ulcerative colitis include:

- Panproctocolectomy with ileal pouch anal anastomosis (IPAA)
- Panproctocolectomy with permanent end ileostomy
- Subtotal colectomy with ileostomy
- Panproctocolectomy with continent Koch's ileostomy
- Abdominal colectomy with an ileorectal anastomosis.

While the first two are performed routinely on an elective basis, the most common emergency operation performed is subtotal colectomy with ileostomy. Proctocolectomy with continent ileostomy and abdominal colectomy with ileorectal anastomosis are not performed routinely for ulcerative colitis anymore, and are mentioned here only for completion and historical interest. These will not be discussed further in this chapter.

EMERGENCY SURGERY FOR ULCERATIVE COLITIS

Indications for Emergency Surgery

Acute Fulminant Colitis

Patients with acute fulminant colitis present with frequent diarrhea (≥10 episodes of loose stools/day) associated with crampy abdominal pain. There are associated systemic symptoms like fever, leucocytosis, anemia and high erythrocyte sedimentation rate (ESR) (>30).[3] They may also have continuous bleeding from the colon, are anorexic and have lost significant amount of weight recently. These patients are at a high risk for developing complications like toxic megacolon, colonic perforation and bleeding, and need immediate hospital admission to a high dependency setting.[4,5] Management of acute fulminant colitis does not change, irrespective of the length of colon involved, and all patients are managed alike.[5]

In these patients, clinical examination should be repeated every 4–6 hours to look for signs of peritonitis and perforation. Close monitoring of vital signs, and monitoring the frequency and nature of stools is essential. Investigations performed should include a full blood count (to look for leucocytosis and anemia), electrolytes, renal function tests, liver function tests, ESR and C-reactive protein (CRP). A plain radiograph of the abdomen should be taken to document colonic distension. Patients should be kept nil by mouth, and a nasogastric tube used for decompression if the colonic diameter is more than 5.5 cm in the transverse colon. Medical therapy includes high dose intravenous steroids (intravenous prednisolone or methylprednisolone) and broad-spectrum antibiotics. Rolling maneuvers every 2 hours or the knee elbow position may help in certain cases, by redistributing the gas in the colon.[6,7] Blood investigations are repeated every 12-24 hours to look for worsening or improvement.

Patients not improving by the third day on medical management can be given a trial of cyclosporine or infliximab,[8] or may be directly taken up for surgery.[9] Cyclosporine, while it may induce remission, is not useful for maintaining remission and the patient needs to be started on alternative medical therapy as well.[10,11] Infliximab, if showing a response, may be used for maintaining long-term remission in these patients.[12] Patients not responding to cyclosporine or infliximab within 4-7 days, or worsening on these medications, are candidates for urgent surgery.[4]

At any point in time during the management of acute fulminant colitis, if the patient shows signs of clinical deterioration (development of peritonitis, toxic megacolon, uncontrolled hemorrhage, or worsening clinical or laboratory parameters), immediate colectomy is warranted and conservative therapy should be abandoned. The operation of choice in this setting is a subtotal colectomy with an end ileostomy, which is discussed in detail later.

The management of acute fulminant colitis is outlined in Flow chart 1.

Flow chart 1 Management of acute fulminant colitis

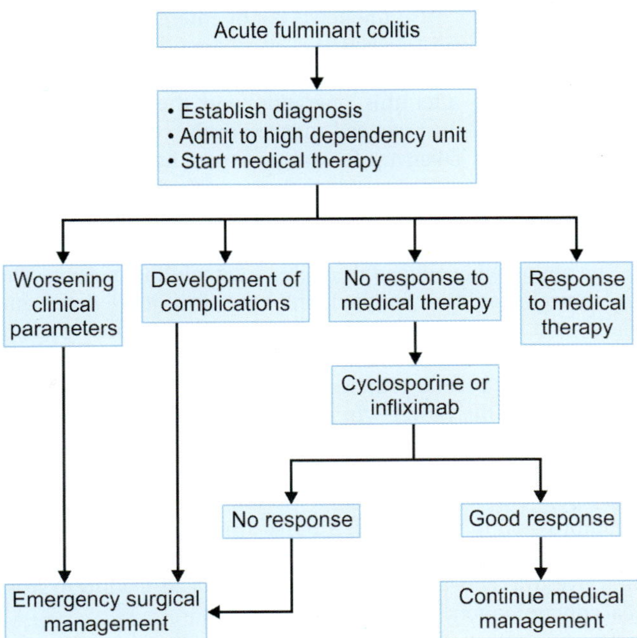

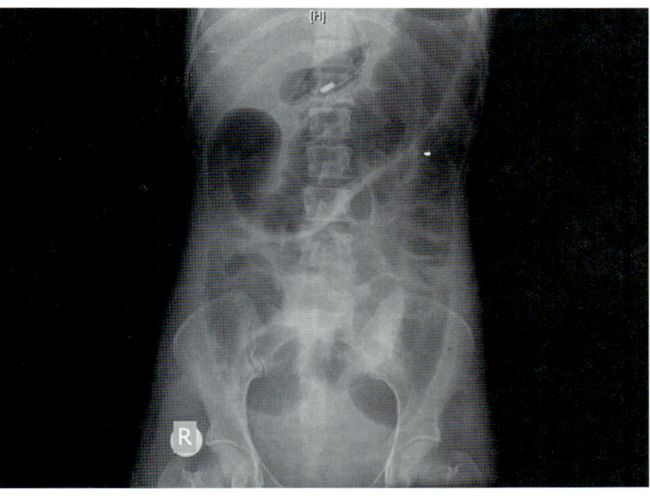

Figure 1 Toxic megacolon: Plain X-ray abdomen, supine film

Toxic Megacolon

Toxic megacolon is defined as total or segmental dilatation of the colon (transverse colon diameter >6 cm or cecal diameter >9 cm) (Fig. 1), without any obstruction, and with systemic toxicity.[13] Often toxic megacolon develops on a background of acute fulminant colitis (5-10%).[14] Precipitating factors include use of antidiarrheal medications, narcotics, anticholinergics or antidepressants.

Although initial therapy in toxic megacolon is medical, surgical treatment may be needed in up to 50% of patients.[13] Initial management is similar to acute fulminant colitis, with the patient being admitted in a high dependency setting and monitored closely. High dose steroids and antibiotic therapy is started. Intermittent rolling manoeuvres[7] or the knee elbow position[6] may be useful, as they redistribute the gas and help in its expulsion. Infliximab may also be tried in the acute setting of toxic megacolon, with some positive results.[15,16] Persistence of symptoms without any improvement after 3 days, or worsening of symptoms, is an indication for colectomy.[16] Medical management may be continued for up to 7 days, if the patient shows signs of improvement.[17] Increasing colonic diameter, presence of colonic wall edema (thumbprinting) (Figs 2A and B) or air in the colonic wall (pneumatosis) imply impending perforation and need urgent colectomy. The operation of choice in this setting is again a subtotal colectomy with an end ileostomy.

Colonic Perforation

With early recognition and treatment of fulminant colitis and toxic megacolon, colonic perforation is becoming increasingly rare in ulcerative colitis. In most cases, it is secondary to untreated toxic megacolon.[18] However, it must be borne in mind that colonic perforation can occur in the absence of colonic dilatation.[19] Clinical presentation is with signs of peritonitis on a background of fulminant colitis.[20] Free intraperitoneal air may be seen on a plain radiographs (Figs 3A and B). Intra-abdominal walled off abscesses are also common. These patients are gravely ill and need urgent colectomy. Mortality varies from 27-57%.[18,19]

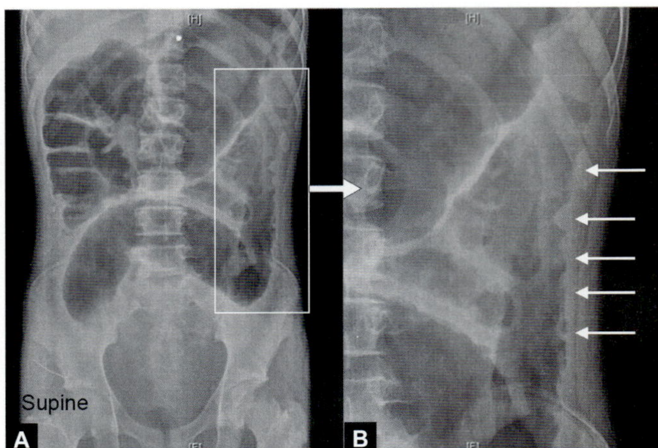

Figures 2A and B Thumbprinting on a background of toxic megacolon. This implies impending perforation

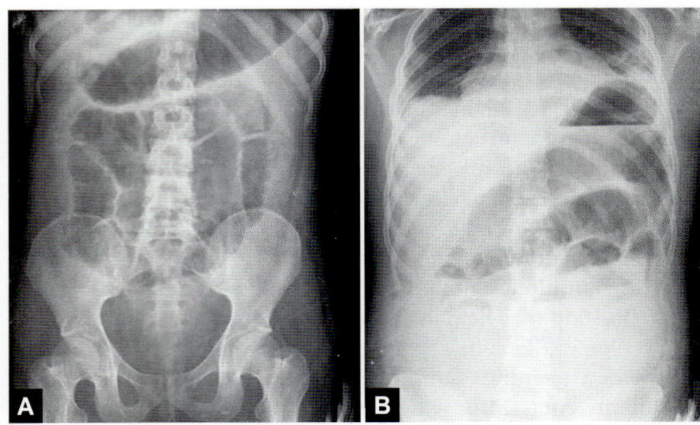

Figures 3A and B Colonic perforation on a background of toxic megacolon. Note the dilated colon on the supine film and the pneumoperitoneum under the left hemidiaphragm on the erect film

Colonic Hemorrhage

Severe colonic hemorrhage requiring colectomy is extremely rare, occurring in 0–4.5% of the patients and is more common in Crohn's disease.[21] Massive hemorrhage is usually secondary to diffuse mucosal ulceration. If the hemorrhage persists despite maximal medical therapy, a colectomy is warranted. Most patients respond to subtotal colectomy, although a slight risk of continuing hemorrhage is present.[22]

Preoperative Preparation for Emergency Surgery

Patients presenting for emergency surgery for ulcerative colitis are seriously ill. They are malnourished and often immunosupressed. Anemia, electrolyte disturbances, coagulopathy, fluid depletion and altered liver and renal functions are common. Careful attention to each of these, and their preoperative optimization, goes a long way in reducing postoperative morbidity and mortality.

Anemia should be corrected along with any accompanying electrolyte disorders and dehydration. A good urine output is often an indicator of adequate fluid resuscitation. Coagulopathy can be corrected by giving parenteral vitamin K along with fresh frozen plasma as needed. All patients should receive venous thromboembolism prophylaxis with injectable heparin or low molecular weight heparin, along with anti-embolism stockings and intermittent pneumatic compression. All patients should also receive therapeutic broad-spectrum antibiotics.

Most of these patients are on many medications including steroids and other immunosuppressants. Most immunosuppressants can be safely stopped before surgery with the exception of steroids. Oral steroids should be converted to parenteral, and can be gradually tapered after surgery. Specific complications of these immunosuppressive drugs like leucopenia, nephrotoxicity and hepatotoxicity should be anticipated, specifically looked for and optimized.

Most patients are extremely malnourished and need support with total parenteral nutrition (TPN).[23] TPN should be started as soon as feasible and continued postoperatively till adequate oral intake has been achieved. A good overlap between oral intake and TPN should be achieved.

An ileostomy should be marked preoperatively. It should be sited so as to be easily accessible, away from bony projections and not hidden in skin creases. Ileostomy bag should be easily applicable at these sites. An enterostomal therapist, if available, can help in choosing an ideal site for an ileostomy.

Patient counseling and a detailed discussion with the patient on the need for emergent surgery are vital to the success of the operation. The patient should be made aware of the disease state, the planned line of management and expected outcomes. Counseling for a postoperative stoma and its need are vital. Support from a good enterostomal therapist in this regard is invaluable.

Subtotal Colectomy with End Ileostomy

This is the procedure of choice for patients presenting for emergency surgery in ulcerative colitis.[24] A subtotal colectomy can be completed in a speedy fashion in an unstable patient, thus reducing morbidity. Also the pelvis is not entered, thus avoiding complications of rectal resection. This operation also leaves the option of restorative proctocolectomy (RPC) at a later date.[25] Patients improve after this operation and the residual rectal disease can usually be managed conservatively.

The patient is taken up for surgery once he has been fully optimized (to the extent possible in the given time). Under general anesthesia, the patient is positioned in a modified Lloyd Davies position (Fig. 4). This allows access to the rectum if required.

The abdomen is opened through a long midline incision. The large bowel should be handled with care since it is dilated and friable, and can perforate easily. If the colon is grossly dilated, attempt should be made to decompress it through the rectum. Introduction of a rectal catheter on low suction is often adequate to decompress the bowel.[22] In case that is unsuccessful and the colon is grossly dilated with air, it can be decompressed with a fine bore intravenous cannula attached to suction, introduced in the right colon. This leads to minimal contamination and satisfactory decompression in most cases. A purse string suture with a sump suction placed through it should be avoided as the purse string often gives way and the suction often gets blocked, leading to gross fecal contamination.[22]

The first step is to look at the extent of colonic involvement and determine the presence of a perforation. While presence of

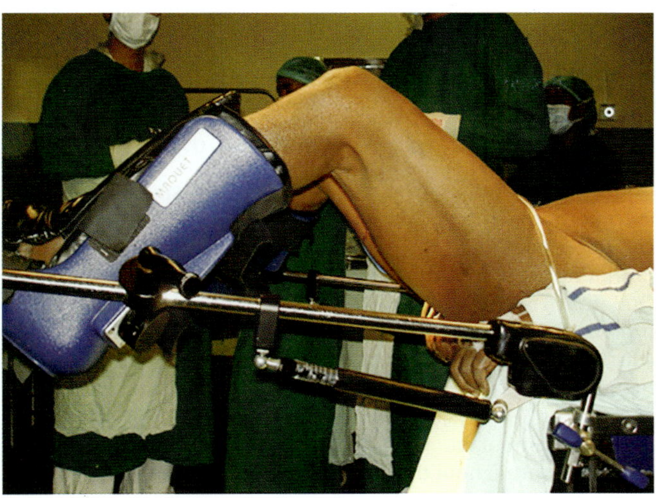

Figure 4 The Lloyd Davies position with Allen stirrups: This facilitates dissection as well as easy changing of position of the legs during the operation

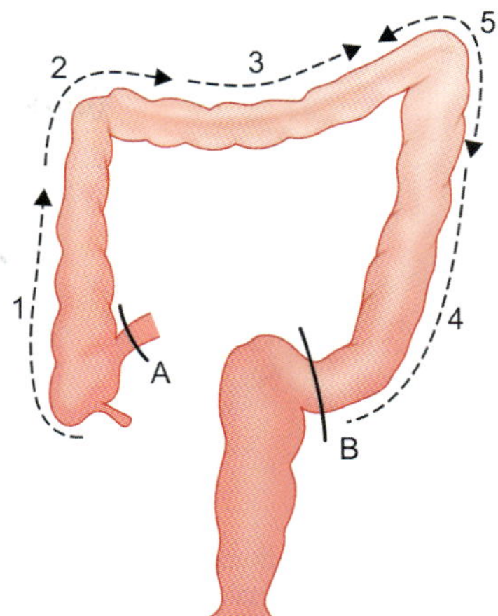

Figure 5 Sequence of mobilization and extent of resection in subtotal colectomy. Note that proximal resection is at the ileocecal junction (A) and distal resection in the distal sigmoid colon (B)

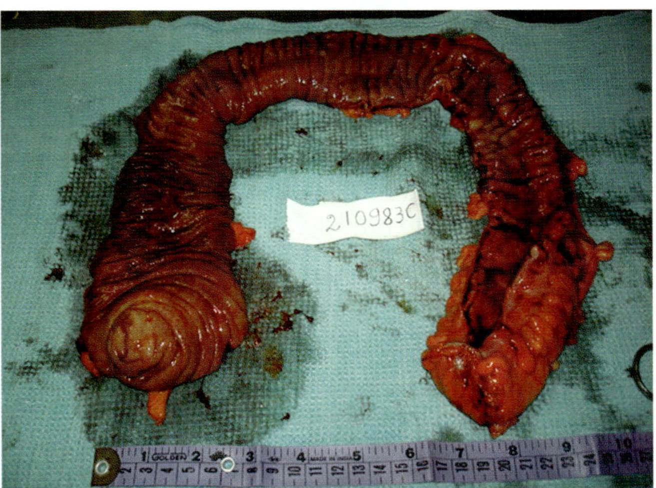

Figure 6 Subtotal colectomy in a case of fulminant acute colitis not responding to medical management. Note that the ileum is transected at the ileocecal junction such that there is virtually no ileum in the specimen

fecal contamination indicates an obvious perforation, presence of omentum adherent to a part of the large bowel with surrounding inflammation is an indication of a sealed off perforation. In such situations, one should not try and mobilize the omentum away, but rather resect it along with the specimen. The small bowel should be inspected to look for small bowel involvement and rule out a missed Crohn's disease.

Colectomy is commenced by mobilizing the right colon from its lateral attachments. Dissection is usually not difficult as the planes are edematous. Care should be taken to avoid a duodenal injury at this point. Next the hepatic flexure is taken down and the transverse colon mobilized. The decision to take the omentum in the specimen or not is based on the suspicion of a perforation. If there is a suspected perforation, being sealed by the omentum, the omentum is taken with the specimen; otherwise it can be left behind.

Next the sigmoid colon is mobilized after dissecting it off its congenital adhesions to the lateral abdominal wall. This dissection is carried upward to the descending colon which is mobilized from lateral to medial along the peritoneal reflection (white line of Toldt). Care must be taken to preserve the left gonadal vessels and left ureter. Lastly, the splenic flexure is mobilized and the whole colon is free. The sequence and extent of division is shown in Figure 5.

Vascular division need not be at the origin of the vessels, unless malignancy is suspected. It is important that the ileocolic artery is not ligated, but preserved. This is extremely important as this would be the blood supply of the pouch, if RPC is planned at a later date. The middle colic, left colic and sigmoid branches are sequentially ligated, preserving the inferior mesenteric artery.

Proximal bowel transection is at the level of the ileocecal junction and distal transaction a few cm proximal to the rectosigmoid junction (Fig. 6). If the distal end is planned to be brought out as a mucous fistula, the distal resection is more proximal in the sigmoid, thus allowing the colon to come to the surface. Both these transections may be done with the help of a stapler or may be hand sewn.

The proximal end is brought out as end ileostomy through the premarked trephine in the right iliac fossa. The choice between suturing the distal sigmoid or rectal stump or bringing it out as a mucous fistula depends on the degree of rectal inflammation.[26] One option is to close the rectal stump and leave it inside, tacking it to the anterior abdominal wall[27] (Fig. 7A). This has been our usual practice too. In cases where the stump is friable and sutures are cutting through, a distal mucous fistula may be created (Fig. 7B). Another method of managing the rectal stump is to close it over a Foley's catheter, which is brought out through the lower edge of the wound to create a controlled fistula. This method is, however, not popular as it leads to mucous discharge from the lower end of the wound, which is a nuisance to the patient.

No drainage is usually necessary, and the abdomen is closed.

Key Points

- Gentle handling of the colon is required, as it is friable and perforates easily.

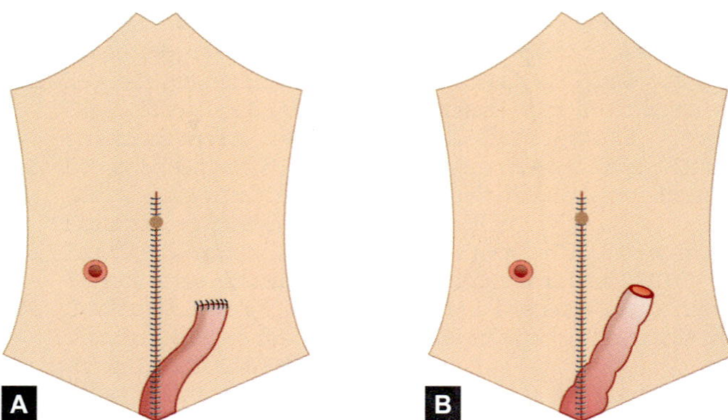

Figures 7A and B (A) Hartman's procedure where the distal stump is sutured and tacked to the abdominal wall; (B) Mucous fistula from the distal end of the sigmoid colon. Note that the mucous fistula is brought out at a site parallel to the ileostomy and not at the midline wound

- The ileocolic artery should be preserved, as it is crucial at the second stage pouch procedure.
- The ileum should be transected as distal as possible, close to the ileocecal junction. This is again crucial to the success of a future ileoanal pouch. Also resection of the terminal ileum can lead to significant nutritional imbalance.
- The pelvis should not be entered, and a long rectal stump left behind. Again this makes a future pouch easier, and reduces the morbidity of the present surgery.
- If a distal mucous fistula is planned, it is preferable to bring it out lateral to the wound, at the site of a marked colostomy, rather than at the lower end of the wound.
- When the rectal stump is closed, it should be marked with a polypropylene suture for easy identification during subsequent surgery. It may also be tacked to the anterior abdominal wall for easy identification. This should be well documented in the operation notes.
- The residual rectal stump usually requires topical treatment. In cases where a mucous fistula has been performed, this can be delivered both antegrade and retrograde.

Laparoscopic Subtotal Colectomy

There has been growing interest in laparoscopic emergency subtotal colectomy for ulcerative colitis. While it offers advantages such as better body image, faster recovery and less postoperative pain, one should bear in mind that subtotal colectomy is an advanced laparoscopic procedure. It requires advanced laparoscopic skills and equipment and involves operating in all quadrants of the abdomen. This can be achieved via complete laparoscopy, laparoscopic assisted techniques and even hand assisted techniques.[28]

Advantages of the laparoscopic approach include less postoperative pain, faster return of bowel function and early discharge.[29] The rates of major complications, and subsequent restorative ileal pouch are similar in both groups.[30] In an analysis of pooled data from 1975 to 2007, conversion rate was found to be 3.4%.[31]

In summary, provided the expertise and equipment is available, laparoscopic subtotal colectomy can be offered to patients with ulcerative colitis, in the urgent setting.

Postoperative Care and Complications

Good postoperative care is essential for speedy recovery, to minimize complications, and for early recognition of complications, when they occur. Adequate analgesia is essential to minimize pain, allow good respiration and early ambulation. Oral intake is started as soon as feasible and gradually increased. If preoperative TPN was started, it is continued till oral intake is adequate. Antibiotics are stopped early, if there was no perforation. In the presence of perforation, antibiotics are continued for a total duration of 5–7 days. Urinary catheter can be removed once the patient is ambulant. Venous thromboembolism prophylaxis is continued throughout the hospital stay. The patient is taught how to manage his stoma.

The most common complication after this operation is small bowel obstruction and postoperative ileus, occurring in about 20% of patients.[31] In most cases, this can be managed conservatively.

Patients are at increased risk of infection, including wound infection/dehiscence (18.6%)[31] and intra-abdominal abscesses (17.8%).[31] This should be anticipated and actively looked for. All infections should be drained and treated with appropriate antibiotics.

A complication specific to subtotal colectomy is distal stump blowout (6.7%).[31] This can present as an intra-abdominal or a pelvic abscess, with high spiking fever and foul smelling rectal discharge. Some patients may just present with low-grade sepsis, failure to thrive and prolonged ileus. Management includes laparotomy, drainage and washout in some patients, while others may be managed conservatively with radiology guided drainage and antibiotics.

Other complications include venous thromboembolism, bleeding and ileostomy related complications.

Follow-up

All patients need close follow up after a subtotal colectomy. The residual rectal stump often needs topical therapy. This is in the form of enemas or foams, and may be delivered antegrade in patients with a distal mucous fistula. Steroids can be tapered in most patients and ultimately stopped.

In about 85% of the patients, an elective proctectomy and an IPAA can be achieved once the patient improves.[29] In a few cases, there may be severe proctitis, not responding to medical therapy, and these need a completion proctectomy alone.

ELECTIVE SURGERY FOR ULCERATIVE COLITIS

Indications for Elective Surgery

Intractable Disease

Elective surgery is indicated when ulcerative colitis is deemed to be intractable to medical therapy. The definition of intractable disease is ever changing, especially with recent advances in medical therapy and introduction of new drugs like infliximab. However, persistence with medical therapy when the disease does not respond, with the sole aim of avoiding a colectomy is futile and can lead to serious harm.[1] The following are some of the scenarios where the disease is considered intractable:

- Persistence of symptoms despite high dose steroid therapy (steroid-refractory disease).
- Dependence on steroids to maintain remission (steroid-dependent disease).
- Worsening of symptoms when on maximal medical treatment.
- Significant treatment related complications (such as long-term complications of corticosteroids, azathioprine induced neutropenia, etc.).

It must be mentioned here that young adults with failure to thrive despite maximal medical therapy, even when in remission, may be a special group of patients who may benefit from colectomy.[32] Treatment in this group should be individualized, and decision for surgery taken after detailed discussion with the patient and his family. A discussion with the treating gastroenterologist preferably at an inflammatory bowel disease multidisciplinary team (IBD MDT) meeting is strongly recommended in these cases.

Presence of Dysplasia or Malignancy

Any patient found to have colonic dysplasia in the setting of ulcerative colitis is a candidate for surgical resection.[33] This is aimed at preventing colonic carcinoma from developing. Risk of colonic malignancy in a patient having an adenoma with low-grade dysplasia varies from 10–30% and with high-grade dysplasia about 30–40%.[34] If the dysplasia is associated with a lesion or a mass (DALM), the risk of malignancy is closer to 80%.[34] Patients not willing for surgery in such circumstances should be warned about the high risk of subsequent colorectal malignancy (13% 5 years incidence)[35] and kept on close surveillance.

In the presence of a proven malignancy, surgical resection and further management is guided by the nature of the malignancy and oncological principles. Surgery, if planned, in these cases, should involve a total colectomy, with or without an ileal pouch formation. Decision for pouch is taken depending on site of lesion, extent and grade of disease.

Long-standing Disease

The risk of colorectal malignancy in patients with ulcerative colitis increases with duration of disease. While the risk is low in the first 8–10 years after diagnosis, it significantly increases thereafter. This risk is estimated to be about 0.5 to 1% per year after the first decade of the disease.[36] Hence patients with long standing disease should be offered prophylactic colectomy, even if no precancerous lesion is detected on surveillance, to prevent further cancer from developing. The extent of colitis (pancolitis) but not the severity of colitis has an increased risk of malignancy.

Severe Extraintestinal Manifestations

Colectomy for intractable extraintestinal manifestations of ulcerative colitis is rarely indicated.[37] However in certain cases of severe extraintestinal manifestations, a colectomy may reduce symptoms. Erythema nodosum, life threatening thromboembolic complications, associated hemolytic anemia and arthralgia of small joints show improvement after a colectomy.[37] Ankylosing spondylitis, pyoderma gangrenosum and large joint arthritis do not show improvement with colectomy. The clinical course of sclerosing cholangitis is also not changed by colectomy.

Special Considerations for Surgery

Some other special factors to take into consideration, especially in resource poor environments are:

- Cost of medical therapy: While medical management of ulcerative colitis may alleviate symptoms in a majority of patients, it entails significant recurring costs. In a resource poor environment, this may lead to significant financial burden on the patient and family. Surgical treatment of ulcerative colitis is associated with long-term economic benefits and reduced costs.
- Access to medical care: In patient living in remote locations, rapid access to good quality health care may not be feasible, and drugs may not be available readily. In these patients, due consideration should be given to surgical management.
- Follow-up and surveillance: In patients who are unable to follow-up on a regular basis, and are unable to follow the surveillance guidelines, due consideration should be given to surgical therapy.
- Surgical treatment obviates the need for continued medical therapy, regular surveillance and reduces complication rates. Therefore, in these special circumstances, surgical therapy may be offered to patients in lieu of medical therapy.

It is important that in these special circumstances, the plans are individualized and clearly discussed with the patient and his relatives, and with the treating gastroenterologist. These cases are also preferably discussed in an IBD MDT.

Inflammatory Bowel Disease Multidisciplinary Team

The IBD MDT is formed with an aim to provide better care to patients with IBD, and thereby improve outcomes. It is a forum consisting of medical gastroenterologists, colorectal surgeons, radiologists, pathologists, enterostomal therapists, dieticians and specialist nurses, who usually meet once a week. All patients with IBD, not responding to standard care should be discussed in this forum, and a collective management plan made. This helps in early identification of patients who may be potential candidates for surgical management, as well as patients who may not need surgery at present. An IBD MDT therefore, is a key component in providing better care for patients with ulcerative colitis.

Surgical Options in the Elective Setting

The following surgical options are routinely used in an elective setting for the management of ulcerative colitis.

- Proctocolectomy with Ileal pouch-anal anastomosis (IPAA) Restorative ProctoColectomy (RPC)
- Subtotal colectomy with Hartman's or mucus fistula
- Proctectomy with IPAA (in patients who have undergone previous subtotal colectomy)
- Panproctocolectomy with permanent ileostomy.

The choice of operation depends on various factors which are outlined subsequently. All of the above mentioned operations may be performed via an open or laparoscopic approach. With modern advancements in technology, single incision laparoscopic surgery and robotic surgery are becoming increasingly popular, and have been reported in literature.[38-40] However, these are yet to be used in routine clinical practice.

PREOPERATIVE ASSESSMENT AND PREPARATION

A detailed preoperative assessment is essential before undertaking any procedure for ulcerative colitis, as these are associated with significant morbidity. Optimization of all associated risk factors goes a long way in minimizing complications.

For patients planned for RPC, a detailed history of continence and previous perianal procedures should be taken. In women, obstetric history and details of previous vaginal births (including episiotomies and perineal tears) should be elicited. Formal assessment of sphincter function using anorectal manometry and incontinence scores like the Vaizey or the Wexner score should be used.

Blood investigations before surgery include a complete blood count, liver function tests, renal function tests and electrolytes. These help to identify anemia, immunosuppression and associated renal dysfunction and dyselectrolytemia. ESR and CRP should be checked to assess disease activity.

Medical therapy for ulcerative colitis should be continued till surgery.

All patients should receive preoperative antimicrobial prophylaxis and venous thromboembolism prophylaxis. Bowel preparation is not indicated. An ileostomy should be planned and an appropriate site marked in conjunction with an enterostomal therapist. Patients should be counseled about the operation, its benefits and complications and the need and implications of an ileostomy. Enhanced recovery pathways, if in place, should be explained to the patient.

Operating Room Adjuncts

The following equipment is of great help in performing an IPAA:

- Allen stirrups (Fig. 4): These can be adjusted intra operatively and are invaluable in performing an IPAA. With the help of these stirrups, a modified Lloyd Davies position can be maintained during the abdominal dissection, and the patient moved to lithotomy for the perineal dissection, without any breach in sterile technique.
- Headlight (Fig. 8): This is also of great help, especially when dissecting deep in the pelvis during abdominal rectal mobilization, and during the perineal part of the operation.
- Antislip mattress and shoulder pads: These have been designed to prevent the patient from slipping back during steep Trendelenberg positioning. This not only helps prevent patient injury, but also makes the perineal dissection easier.
- Retractors: A long pelvic retractor like the St. Marks retractor (Fig. 9) is helpful during pelvic dissection. A Lone Star retractor (Fig. 10) is also very helpful in the perineal dissection during the intersphincteric dissection, if planned.
- Other equipment: Long diathermy tips, patient warming devices, warm intravenous fluids and pneumatic compression devices are useful adjuncts to minimize the trauma of surgery.

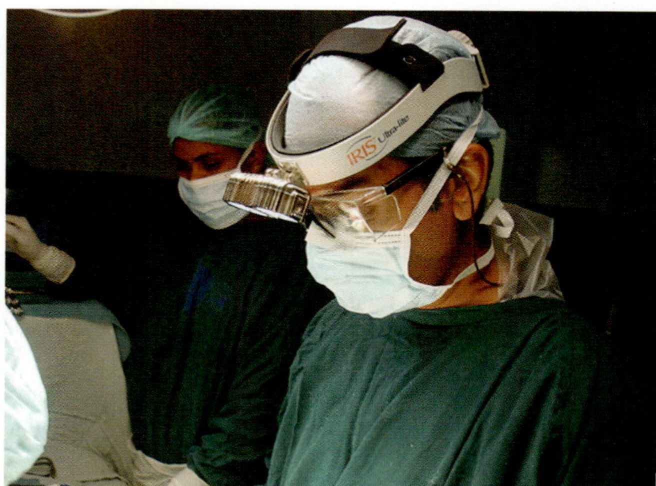

Figure 8 A good headlight is invaluable in emergency and elective surgery for ulcerative colitis

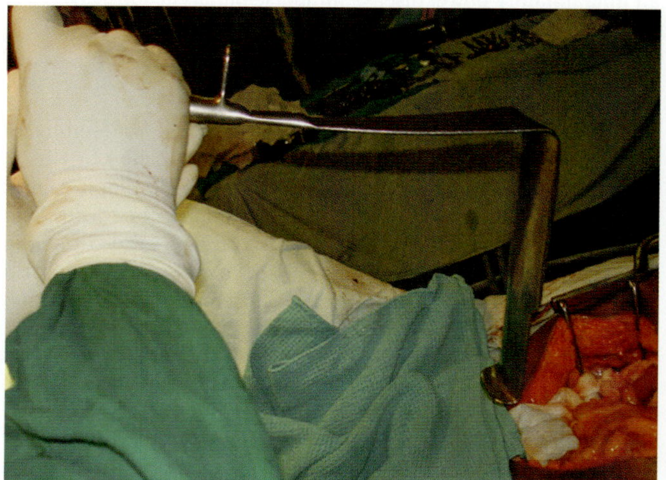

Figure 9 The St. Marks retractor is a better retractor than the Deaver's for rectal mobilization

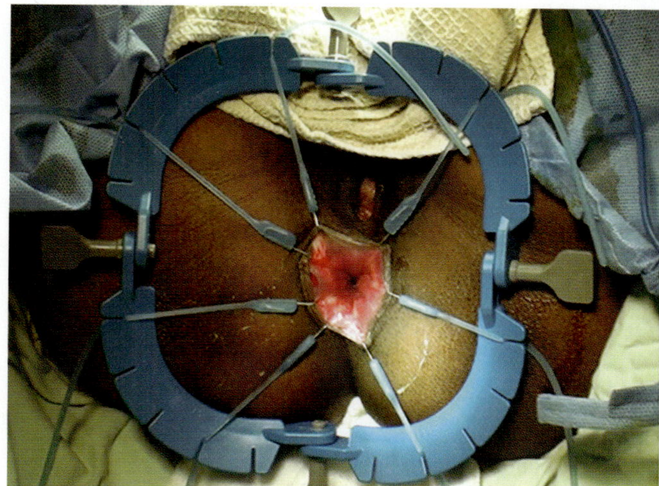

Figure 10 The "Lone Star" retractor helps to evert the anus and helps in the intersphincteric dissection

Choice of Operation

The decision to perform an IPAA or a proctocolectomy with end ileostomy is a major one, as one procedure promises near normal passage of stools compared to a permanent stoma. Factors which need to be taken into consideration while making this decision include:

- Age of the patient: The normal sphincter mechanism becomes weak with age and many elderly patients suffer from varying levels of incontinence.[41] If incontinence is detected at any point, an IPAA should be avoided, as resultant function will not be satisfactory.
- Previous perianal surgery: Patients who have undergone previous perianal surgery may suffer from varying degrees of incontinence. This has to be objectively assessed before an IPAA. Also surgical planes may be obliterated, thus making an IPAA more difficult to perform.
- Previous intestinal surgery: Constructing a pouch may be technically challenging in patients who have undergone previous small bowel resection, especially terminal ileal or ileocecal resection. The pouch may not reach the pelvic floor at times, and various complex techniques may need to be used. This has to be kept in mind before embarking on this procedure in such individuals.
- Obstetric History: This is vital in all female patients. Details of previous vaginal deliveries and perineal tears and episiotomies should be gathered. Many women suffer from sphincter injury, either occult or obvious, and have varying degrees of incontinence[(42)]. One has to be careful in offering an IPAA to such patients. IPAA may have an effect on fertility. Thus this issue needs to be discussed with the female patient of child bearing age.
- Pre-existing anal incontinence: Pre-existing anal incontinence from any cause will lead to poor outcomes after an IPAA. This has to be subjectively and objectively assessed (history, anal manometry and incontinence scoring) before offering the procedure.
- Obesity: Obesity makes an IPAA technically more demanding.[43] In obese, short males with a narrow pelvis, an IPAA is technically difficult to perform and the pouch may not reach the pelvic floor. Failure rates of a pouch are higher in obese individuals.
- Comorbid illness and nutritional status: Presence of other medical comorbidities like liver disease and renal dysfunction increase morbidity and decision to do an IPAA should be carefully weighed against its possible complications. An IPAA should also not be offered to patients with poor nutritional status, as complication rates are higher.
- Active anal disease: Patients with active anal disease such as fistulae, perianal abscesses etc. are not candidates for an IPAA.
- Risk of cancer: If the risk of having a colorectal malignancy is high at the index operation, many surgeons would not offer a pouch at the primary sitting. The patient can be offered a proctocolectomy with an end ileostomy, or a second stage pouch, once the malignancy is treated completely. An IPAA is contraindicated in patients with middle or lower one-third rectal cancer.
- Primary sclerosing cholangitis (PSC): Patients with PSC are a special group of patients who need individualized work up before being considered for an IPAA. Patients with well controlled PSC can undergo IPAA in the primary setting. Patients with poorly controlled or advanced PSC may be candidates of subtotal colectomy with an orthotopic liver transplant. They may be considered for an IPAA once the liver function has recovered.[44]

The surgeon must always keep in mind that although a RPC is desirable and is the ultimate goal in surgical therapy for ulcerative colitis, a well performed proctocolectomy with permanent ileostomy often provides a better quality of life than a poorly functioning pouch with all its complications.

Also, one should keep in mind that a pouch should not be offered to a patient when the diagnosis is in doubt, i.e. the disease may actually represent Crohn's disease or indeterminate colitis. It is wiser to perform a subtotal colectomy in such instances and wait.

Restorative Proctocolectomy with Ileal Pouch Anal Anastomosis

The aim of RPC in ulcerative colitis is complete removal of the disease, while preserving continence. From being a high morbidity and mortality operation in its early days, RPC has come a long way in becoming the standard of care in current surgical management of ulcerative colitis.

The essential steps in a RPC are:

- Complete abdominal colectomy
- Complete rectal mobilization and proctectomy (with or without Mucosectomy)
- Creation of an ileal reservoir (pouch)
- Ileal reservoir (pouch) to anal anastomosis (IPAA).

Each of these steps is described in detail below.

Abdominal Colectomy

The patient is positioned in the modified Lloyd Davies position (Fig. 4), preferably in Allen stirrups. The abdomen is opened via a long midline incision. A thorough abdominal examination is performed with particular attention to the small bowel, to rule out small bowel involvement and possible Crohn's disease. Mobilization of the colon is started from the right colon, which is mobilized in a lateral to medial fashion, followed by the hepatic flexure. Care should be taken to identify the right ureter and the duodenum and prevent trauma to these structures.

Next the omentum is mobilized off the transverse colon and the transverse colon is mobilized. This is followed by mobilization of the sigmoid colon, descending colon and then the splenic flexure. Care should be taken to preserve the left ureter and the left gonadal vessels during left colon and sigmoid mobilization.

Vascular division for ulcerative colitis need not be at the base of the vessels, unless malignancy is suspected. Care should be taken to preserve the ileocolic artery as this will be the artery supplying the ileal pouch. Terminal ileal resection should be as close to the ileocecal junction as possible.

Complete Rectal Mobilization and Proctectomy (With or Without Mucosectomy)

Once the abdominal colonic mobilization is complete, the rectal dissection is started. The patient is positioned in steep Trendlenberg position and all the small bowel is packed away in the upper abdomen with the help of mops. Dissection of the rectum is started by mobilizing the sigmoid colon and extending the peritoneal incision into the pelvis on both sides. The posterior dissection is performed first. Dissection plane is kept just behind the mesorectum, taking care to preserve the presacral nerves. Dissection in this plane also helps in not breaching the presacral fascia, which can lead to troublesome bleeding. This dissection is carried down till the tip of the coccyx. This is followed by lateral dissection where both the lateral attachments of the rectum are divided. This can usually be achieved by diathermy, and there is no need to separately ligate the middle rectal artery which runs in this lateral attachment. The anterior dissection is commenced by dividing the peritoneal reflection anteriorly and developing a plane between the rectum and the seminal vesicle and prostate in males and the cervix and vagina in females. This entire dissection should be carried down to the pelvic floor on all sides. One should adhere to the mesorectal plane, for it avoids bleeding and also helps in autonomic nerve preservation. At this point the rectum has been completely mobilized and is free on all sides.

Mucosectomy versus No Mucosectomy

Ileal pouch anal anastomosis can be performed by two methods:

- Stapled IPAA, where the rectum is stapled off at the pelvic floor and a stapled anastomosis performed between the ileal pouch and the stapled anal stump.[45]
- Hand sewn IPAA, where there is an additional mucosectomy performed transanally, to remove all rectal mucosa, and a hand sewn anastomosis is performed between the pouch and the dentate line.

Proponents of mucosal resection claim that this procedure removes all rectal mucosa, thus reducing future chances of any residual or recurrent disease, as well as future development of malignancy. However, a mucosectomy results in significant sphincter damage and therefore resultant anal function and continence may be inferior to the stapled technique.[46,47]

The stapled technique, on the other hand, is relatively easy to perform and as mentioned, results in less sphincter dysfunction. Also, this technique leads to preservation of the anal transition zone, which also helps in better sphincter function. The theoretical risk of disease recurrence and cancer development in the remnant rectal mucosa is extremely small.[25] Thus most surgeons, including us, routinely perform a stapled rectal transection and IPAA.

Technique of Mucosectomy

If a mucosectomy is to be performed, it is begun once the rectum is completely mobilized and transected, usually with scissors at the anorectal junction. The legs are repositioned to lithotomy and a perineal operator and scrub nurse scrub in. The "Lone Star" or other anal retractor is positioned and the dentate line identified. The mucosa is divided just proximal to the dentate line and dissected off the internal sphincter with diathermy. Some surgeons prefer to infiltrate the submucosal plane with saline or adrenaline and use scissor dissection. The mucosa is removed from distal to proximal till the transected end at the anorectal junction. The open end can then be closed with a purse string suture to enable a stapled pouch-anal anastomosis or stapled across for a double-stapled anastomosis.

Creation of a Pouch

The next stage in the operation is the creation of a pelvic reservoir from the ileum (the ileal pouch). Over the years, various designs of the pouch have been proposed, but few are in common practice. The most common pouch used today, including what we use commonly, is the J pouch, the construction of which will be discussed in detail. Other pouch designs include the W pouch and the S pouch which are rarely used and are mentioned only in brief. The difference in outcomes with various pouch designs is minimal, and the J pouch is easy to construct and technically simple, making it the most popular pouch design.[33]

The J pouch: The J pouch is created with two limbs of the terminal ileum forming a loop joined together by a side to side anastomosis (Fig. 11). The terminal ileum (after closing its distal end) is folded onto itself with two 15 cm loops, and the apex is inspected to make sure it reaches the pelvic floor. An opening is made at the apex of the pouch and a stapling device used to create a side to side anastomosis. Two to three firings of a conventional stapler may be required to make the pouch. Alternatively, the pouch may be hand sewn after opening both the limbs of the ileum and suturing them together. Once the pouch is created, a Foleys catheter is introduced in the pouch and saline instilled (around 250 mL) to check for leaks and pouch capacity.

Using larger lengths of the ileum to make the pouch does not enhance function and has similar outcomes.[33]

In cases where there is difficulty in making the apex of the pouch reach the anal canal, the following maneuvers can be tried:[33]

- Dividing the ileocolic artery
- Making windows in the terminal ileal mesentery
- Scoring out the peritoneum over the terminal ileal mesentery on both sides
- Dividing the apex of the pouch and making a spout, either antiperistaltic or isoperistaltic
- Converting to an S pouch design.

As mentioned, the J pouch is relatively simple to construct, is quick and offers good outcomes. Hence, this is the most popular pouch design today.

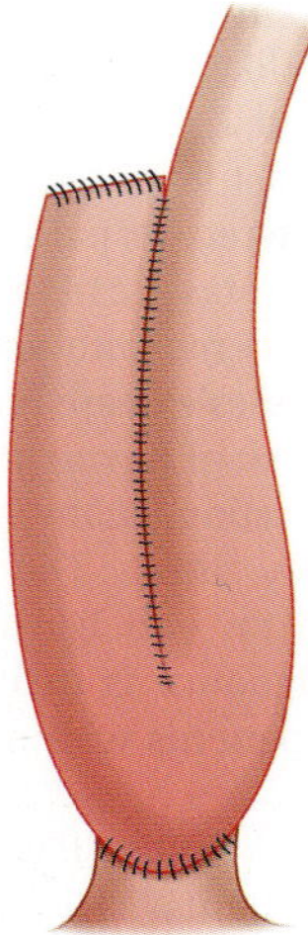

Figure 11 The J pouch, made from two limbs of ileum

The W pouch: The W pouch is constructed from four 12 cm lengths of the terminal ileum folded together in a W fashion and sutured (Fig. 12). The W pouch has a similar diameter to the rectal ampulla and sits well in the pelvis. It also provides the most volume for the length of ileum used. However, it is difficult to construct and is bulky, and in individuals with a narrow pelvis (e.g. obese males) it may be difficult to place this pouch. Some surgeons use it in female patients with a broad gynecoid pelvis, but routine use of the W pouch has fallen out of favor.

The S pouch: The S pouch is constructed from the terminal 30 cm of ileum, by folding it into an S shape and leaving a 5 cm efferent spout (Fig. 13). The main advantage of the S pouch lies in patients where the J pouch does not reach the anal canal. In such cases, the spout of the pouch helps anastomosis of the ileum to the anal canal. However, problems of the pouch include improper emptying and need for self-catheterization. These problems can be reduced by making a shorter spout and by leaving behind a smaller rectal cuff.[33] However, construction of an S pouch is technically challenging, and has again fallen out of favor for routine use as it does not offer any particular advantage over the J pouch.

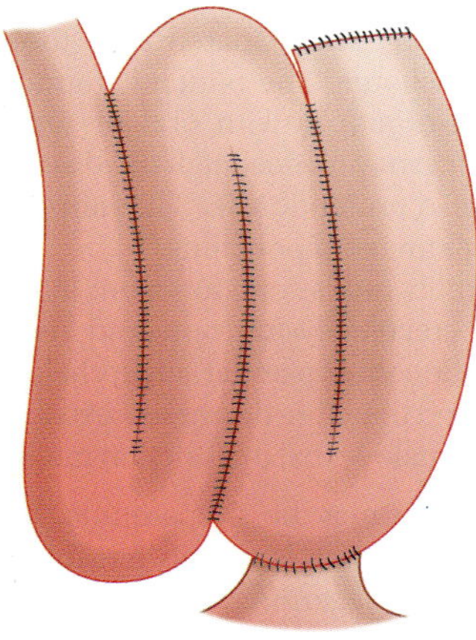

Figure 12 The W pouch, made from four limbs of ileum

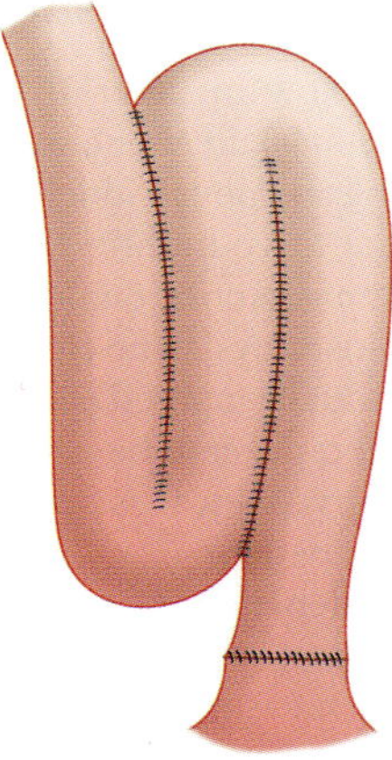

Figure 13 The S pouch, made from three limbs of ileum (note the efferent spout)

Ileal Reservoir (Pouch) to Anal Anastomosis (IPAA)

If a mucosectomy has been performed, the pouch is placed in the pelvis, and a pouch to dentate line anastomosis is performed transanally.

If a stapled anastomosis is to be performed, the opening at the apex of the pouch is used to introduce the anvil of the circular stapler which is kept in place with a purse string suture. The stapler is introduced transanally and a stapled anastomosis performed with an end to end stapler. The anastomosis is checked for leaks with a saline air leak test.

Use of a Covering Ileostomy

A covering ileostomy is usually recommended after an IPAA.[25] This is with a view to reduce morbidity, if the distal IPAA leaks.

While deciding on performing an ileostomy, one has to balance the complications of an ileostomy[48] with the consequences of an anastomotic leak in the absence of a diverting ileostomy. Since, a diverting ileostomy in these cases is more proximal than usual, it can lead to significant dehydration and electrolyte losses. This is in addition to other stomal complications like retraction, prolapse, ischemia and skin excoriation. However, the consequences of a leak in the absence of an ileostomy may be disastrous, eventually sometimes leading to pouch failure or excision. There are many reports of one stage IPAA without the use of a diverting ileostomy,[49,50] but this has not been tested in randomized controlled trials. Most centers in the world, including ours continue to use a protective ileostomy for an IPAA, with a one stage procedure being offered to a select few. Patient who are malnourished, on steroids, or have had a complicated operation are certainly not candidates for a one stage IPAA.

Laparoscopic Restorative Proctocolectomy

With advances in technology, skills and laparoscopic equipment, laparoscopic RPC can now be safely performed for ulcerative colitis. However, laparoscopic RPC requires advanced laparoscopic skills, and involves operating in all quadrants of the abdomen.

While early evidence suggested that laparoscopic surgery did not offer any advantage, while increasing operating times,[51,52] recent studies have demonstrated that laparoscopic RPC offers benefits such as better cosmesis, less pain, earlier return of bowel function, earlier discharge from the hospital, fewer adhesions, a lower incidence of ventral hernia formation and infertility.[53-55] However, functional outcomes are related to the pouch and therefore similar in both the laparoscopic and open group.[54,56] A recent meta-analysis comparing laparoscopic and open surgery for ulcerative colitis observed that the operating times were similar, patients undergoing laparoscopic surgery were able to tolerate oral intake earlier, and had a shorter hospital stay.[57] A recent Cochrane review comparing open and laparoscopic RPC concluded that there were no significant differences in complications, reoperation or readmission rates and mortality.[58]

In short, laparoscopic RPC offers advantages to the patient with no additional morbidity. However, it requires special skills and equipment and should only be done by people trained in advanced laparoscopy.

Single incision laparoscopic proctocolectomy and pouch is now a reality.

POSTOPERATIVE MANAGEMENT AND COMPLICATIONS

Postoperatively, all patients should receive adequate analgesia and venous thromboembolism prophylaxis. Continuing prophylactic antibiotics in the postoperative period is not required. Oral diet is started as soon as the patient tolerates it, and a fast track protocol can be followed. Close monitoring for complications is essential to recognize them early and minimize morbidity.

Some of the complications of RPC with IPAA are discussed below.

- Anastomotic leak: This is one of the most feared complications of an IPAA and often leads to pouch failure and excision. The leak rate can vary from 5–19%.[59] It most often presents as a pelvic abscess with signs of systemic sepsis. Clinical examination may reveal a defect in the anastomotic line and a computed tomography scan reveals a pelvic abscess. Treatment includes drainage of the abscess (percutaneous or via laparotomy).[60] If the dehiscence is large, pouch takedown may be needed. Even if the pouch is left in situ, pouch failure rates are high as the resultant pouch is stiff and noncompliant and functions poorly.
- Anastomotic stricture: An anastomotic stricture can develop in up to 38% of patients with an IPAA, and is severe in 17%.[61] Risk factors for stricture formation include anastomotic dehiscence, use of a small size stapling gun (25 mm)[62] and tension on the anastomosis. Unrecognized Crohn's disease may also lead to strictures, and should be ruled out with the help of biopsies from the stricture site. Strictures may be managed with dilatation, on in some cases need resection with pouch advancement.[63]
- Pouch vaginal fistulas: This complication can occur in two ways. The first is the development of an anastomotic leak with a pelvic abscess, which is then drained or finds its way out through the vagina, leading to fistula formation. The other is a technical error where a part of the vaginal wall has been incorporated into the anastomosis, thus creating a pouch vaginal fistula. Unrecognized Crohn's disease can also lead to fistulization, and should be ruled out with the help of biopsies.

Patients present with fecal discharge per vaginum. Treatment is surgical and involves using a transvaginal approach to cover the defect with a full thickness vaginal flap[64] In extreme cases, it may even require resection of the pouch

- Small bowel obstruction: This is the most common complication after an IPAA, occurring in 15–40% of the patients.[33] It is mostly secondary to adhesions and responds to conservative management. If this fails, operative intervention with adhesiolysis may be needed. Sometimes obstruction may be secondary to the afferent limb folding onto the pouch or herniating behind the pouch. In such cases, the afferent limb should be tacked to the abdominal wall after release.
- Rectal mucosal inflammation and dysplasia: In cases where a stapled IPAA has been performed, the residual rectal mucosa may become inflamed and sometimes even develop dysplasia. This usually responds to topical therapy. In a few cases, resistant to topical therapy, transanal excision of the inflamed mucosa with pouch advancement may be needed.[65]
- Pouchitis: Pouchitis or inflammation of the pouch can develop in 16–48% of the patients.[60] This is usually nonspecific. The exact etiology of pouchitis is not clear but various theories like mucosal ischemia, stasis and bacterial imbalance, mucosal inflammation and reactivation of disease have been proposed. The incidence of pouchitis increases with time.[66]

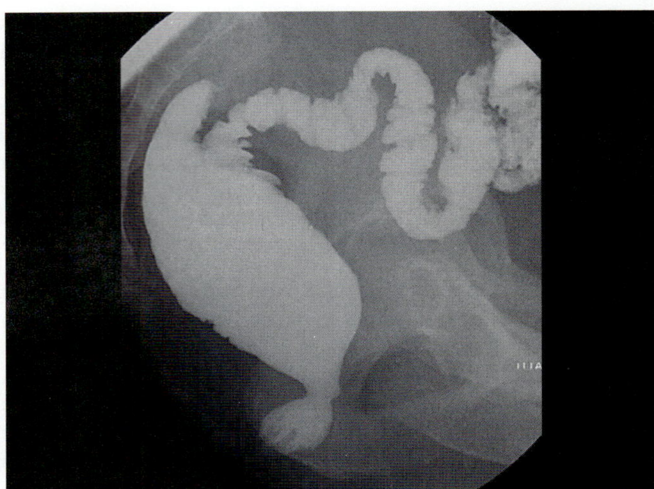

Figure 14 Pouchogram, done before stoma closure reveals a good volume J pouch with good compliance and no anastomotic leak

Patients present with increased stool frequency with mucopurulent discharge. The pouch is found to be inflamed on examination. Treatment is with oral or topical metronidazole. Cyclical antibiotics may be needed if the disease does not respond to metronidazole. A probiotic VSL#3 has also been used with some success in the treatment of pouchitis.[66]

- Effects on fertility and sexual function: In males, pelvic surgery can lead to erectile dysfunction and retrograde ejaculation. Dissecting in the correct plane at surgery helps in autonomic nerve preservation and therefore decreases sexual dysfunction. Current rates of severe male sexual dysfunction range form 2–4%.[33]

In females, there may be dyspareunia, and fertility may be adversely affected.[67,68] This is usually a result of pelvic adhesions. There is controversy regarding the best method for delivery in patients post IPAA. There are groups in favor of both Caesarean section and vaginal delivery, with no clear benefit in each.[60]

Follow-up and Ileostomy Closure

All patients require follow up after IPAA. Once the patient is discharged, they are seen again after 6 weeks to 3 months to check for anastomotic healing and pouch function. Our practice has been to do a pouchogram at three months (Fig. 14) to look for pouch compliance, size and anastomotic dehiscence. If these parameters are satisfactory, the ileostomy can be closed.

Steroids can be gradually tapered and stopped after colectomy. All other medical therapy can be stopped immediately after colectomy. Pouch surveillance is required and has to be individualized for every patient.[25]

Pouch function is dependent on various factors like pouch design, pouch compliance, capacity and anal tone and function.[69] Stool consistency and measures to alter this have no effect on pouch function.[70] Patients on an average pass 3–4 stools per day. Some patients may experience some seepage or incontinence, especially with liquid stools.

Proctocolectomy with End Ileostomy

This operation is offered in the elective setting to patients not fit for a pouch procedure. The essential steps of this operation are similar to the initial steps of a RPC. The complete abdominal colectomy and rectal mobilization is the same as that of a RPC. Perineal dissection starts with a circumanal incision just beyond the anal verge to enter the intersphincteric plane. Once the specimen has been delivered, the external sphincter is brought together and closed, followed by skin. This process of intersphincteric dissection helps prevent a big perineal wound with its attendant complications like infection and wound breakdown.

Stoma Counseling and Life with a Stoma

All patients undergoing a permanent ileostomy should be counseled preoperatively about the stoma and a stoma marked preoperatively. Help from a trained enterostomal therapist is invaluable in this regard. The patients should be provided ample opportunity to clear all doubts about stomas, and if possible even meet a few other patients living with a stoma. A dedicated ostomy clinic to manage postoperative stoma problems, with an enterostomal therapist in charge, can be a useful resource for such patients.

CONCLUSION

Surgery for ulcerative colitis has come a long way over the past few decades. With the advent of RPC, we have moved from the era of just removal of the diseased bowel (panprotocolectomy) to the era where preserving continence has become the primary objective of surgery for ulcerative colitis. With continued advances in technology and the advent of laparoscopic and robotic surgery, the scenario is likely to change again with a greater impetus on reducing morbidity and improving quality of life and body image.

REFERENCES

1. Randall J, Singh B, Warren BF, Travis SP, Mortensen NJ, George BD. Delayed surgery for acute severe colitis is associated with increased risk of postoperative complications. Br J Surg. 2010;97(3):404-9.
2. Leijonmarck CE, Persson PG, Hellers G. Factors affecting colectomy rate in ulcerative colitis: an epidemiologic study. Gut. 1990;31(3):329-33.
3. Satsangi J, Silverberg MS, Vermeire S, Colombel JF. The Montreal classification of inflammatory bowel disease: controversies, consensus, and implications. Gut. 2006;55(6):749-53.
4. Mowat C, Cole A, Windsor A, Ahmad T, Arnott I, Driscoll R, et al. Guidelines for the management of inflammatory bowel disease in adults. Gut. 2011;60(5):571-607.
5. Kornbluth A, Sachar DB, Practice Parameters Committee of the American College of Gastroenterology. Ulcerative colitis practice guidelines in adults: American College Of Gastroenterology, Practice Parameters Committee. Am J Gastroenterol. 2010;105(3): 501-23; quiz 24.
6. Panos MZ, Wood MJ, Asquith P. Toxic megacolon: the knee-elbow position relieves bowel distension. Gut. 1993;34(12):1726-7.
7. Present DH, Wolfson D, Gelernt IM, Rubin PH, Bauer J, Chapman ML. Medical decompression of toxic megacolon by "rolling". A new technique of decompression with favorable long-term follow-up. J Clin Gastroenterol. 1988;10(5):485-90.
8. Halfvarson J, Jarnerot G. Treatment of choice for acute severe steroid-refractory ulcerative colitis is remicade. Inflamm Bowel Dis. 2009;15(1):143-5.
9. Becker JM, Stucchi AF. Treatment of choice for acute severe steroid-refractory ulcerative colitis is colectomy. Inflamm Bowel Dis. 2009;15(1):146-9.
10. Cohen RD. How should we treat severe acute steroid-refractory ulcerative colitis? Inflamm Bowel Dis. 2009;15(1):150-1.
11. Moskovitz DN, Van Assche G, Maenhout B, Arts J, Ferrante M, Vermeire S, et al. Incidence of colectomy during long-term follow-up after cyclosporine-induced remission of severe ulcerative colitis. Clin Gastroenterol Hepatol. 2006;4(6):760-5.
12. Jarnerot G, Hertervig E, Friis-Liby I, Blomquist L, Karlen P, Granno C, et al. Infliximab as rescue therapy in severe to moderately severe ulcerative colitis: a randomized, placebo-controlled study. Gastroenterology. 2005;128(7):1805-11.
13. Fazio VW. Toxic megacolon in ulcerative colitis and Crohn's colitis. Clin Gastroenterol. 1980;9(2):389-407.
14. Greenstein AJ, Sachar DB, Gibas A, Schrag D, Heimann T, Janowitz HD, et al. Outcome of toxic dilatation in ulcerative and Crohn's colitis. J Clin Gastroenterol. 1985;7(2):137-43.
15. Dayan B, Turner D. Role of surgery in severe ulcerative colitis in the era of medical rescue therapy. World J Gastroenterol. 2012;18(29):3833-8.
16. Meier J, Sturm A. Current treatment of ulcerative colitis. World J Gastroenterol. 2011;17(27):3204-12.
17. Caprilli R, Vernia P, Latella G, Torsoli A. Early recognition of toxic megacolon. J Clin Gastroenterol. 1987;9(2):160-4.
18. Heppell J, Farkouh E, Dube S, Peloquin A, Morgan S, Bernard D. Toxic megacolon. An analysis of 70 cases. Dis Colon Rectum. 1986;29(12):789-92.
19. Greenstein AJ, Barth JA, Sachar DB, Aufses AH. Free colonic perforation without dilatation in ulcerative colitis. Am J Surg. 1986;152(3):272-5.
20. Metcalf AM. Elective and emergent operative management of ulcerative colitis. Surg Clin North Am. 2007;87(3):633-41.
21. Robert JR, Sachar DB, Greenstein AJ. Severe gastrointestinal hemorrhage in Crohn's disease. Ann Surg. 1991;213(3):207-11.
22. Keighly MRB, Williams NS (Eds). Surgery of the Anus, Rectum and Colon, 3rd Edition. WB Saunders, London 2007.
23. Salinas H, Dursun A, Konstantinidis I, Nguyen D, Shellito P, Hodin R, et al. Does preoperative total parenteral nutrition in patients with ulcerative colitis produce better outcomes? Int J Colorectal Dis. 2012;27(11):1479-83.
24. Hyman NH, Cataldo P, Osler T. Urgent subtotal colectomy for severe inflammatory bowel disease. Dis Colon Rectum. 2005;48(1):70-3.
25. Dignass A, Lindsay JO, Sturm A, Windsor A, Colombel JF, Allez M, et al. Second European evidence-based consensus on the diagnosis and management of ulcerative colitis part 2: current management. J Crohns Colitis. 2012;6(10):991-1030.
26. Trickett JP, Tilney HS, Gudgeon AM, Mellor SG, Edwards DP. Management of the rectal stump after emergency sub-total colectomy: which surgical option is associated with the lowest morbidity? Colorectal Dis. 2005;7(5):519-22.
27. Carter FM, McLeod RS, Cohen Z. Subtotal colectomy for ulcerative colitis: complications related to the rectal remnant. Dis Colon Rectum. 1991;34(11):1005-9.
28. Watanabe K, Funayama Y, Fukushima K, Shibata C, Takahashi K, Sasaki I. Hand-assisted laparoscopic vs. open subtotal colectomy for severe ulcerative colitis. Dis Colon Rectum. 2009;52(4):640-5.
29. Strong SA. Management of acute colitis and toxic megacolon. Clin Colon Rectal Surg. 2010;23(4):274-84.
30. Chung TP, Fleshman JW, Birnbaum EH, Hunt SR, Dietz DW, Read TE, et al. Laparoscopic vs. open total abdominal colectomy for

severe colitis: impact on recovery and subsequent completion restorative proctectomy. Dis Colon Rectum. 2009;52(1):4-10.
31. Teeuwen PH, Stommel MW, Bremers AJ, van der Wilt GJ, de Jong DJ, Bleichrodt RP. Colectomy in patients with acute colitis: a systematic review. J Gastrointest Surg. 2009;13(4):676-86.
32. Berger M, Gribetz D, Korelitz BI. Growth retardation in children with ulcerative colitis: the effect of medical and surgical therapy. Pediatrics. 1975;55(4):459-67.
33. Yeo CJ, McFadden DW, Pemberton JH, Peters JH. Shackelford's Surgery of the Alimentary Tract. 7th edition. Saunders; 2013.
34. Gorfine SR, Bauer JJ, Harris MT, Kreel I. Dysplasia complicating chronic ulcerative colitis: is immediate colectomy warranted? Dis Colon Rectum. 2000;43(11):1575-81.
35. Kisiel JB, Loftus EV, Harmsen WS, Zinsmeister AR, Sandborn WJ. Outcome of sporadic adenomas and adenoma-like dysplasia in patients with ulcerative colitis undergoing polypectomy. Inflamm Bowel Dis. 2012;18(2):226-35.
36. Ekbom A, Helmick C, Zack M, Adami HO. Ulcerative colitis and colorectal cancer. A population-based study. N Engl J Med. 1990;323(18):1228-33.
37. Goudet P, Dozois RR, Kelly KA, Ilstrup DM, Phillips SF. Characteristics and evolution of extraintestinal manifestations associated with ulcerative colitis after proctocolectomy. Dig Surg. 2001;18(1):51-5.
38. Bulian DR, Knuth J, Krakamp B, Heiss MM. Restorative restproctectomy as single-port surgery through the ostomy site in a three-stage procedure. Surg Endosc. 2012;26(12):3688-90.
39. Pedraza R, Patel CB, Ramos-Valadez DI, Haas EM. Robotic-assisted laparoscopic surgery for restorative proctocolectomy with ileal J pouch-anal anastomosis. Minim Invasive Ther Allied Technol. 2011;20(4):234-9.
40. Abarca F, Cologne KG, Francescatti A, Brand MI, Saclarides TJ. Incisionless laparoscopic total proctocolectomy with ileal J-pouch anal anastomosis. Am Surg. 2011;77(7):929-32.
41. Kang HW, Jung HK, Kwon KJ, Song EM, Choi JY, Kim SE, et al. Prevalence and predictive factors of fecal incontinence. J Neurogastroenterol Motil. 2012;18(1):86-93.
42. Sultan AH, Kamm MA, Hudson CN, Thomas JM, Bartram CI. Anal-sphincter disruption during vaginal delivery. N Engl J Med. 1993;329(26):1905-11.
43. Canedo JA, Pinto RA, McLemore EC, Rosen L, Wexner SD. Restorative proctectomy with ileal pouch-anal anastomosis in obese patients. Dis Colon Rectum. 2010;53(7):1030-4.
44. Poritz LS, Koltun WA. Surgical management of ulcerative colitis in the presence of primary sclerosing cholangitis. Dis Colon Rectum. 2003;46(2):173-8.
45. Kmiot WA, Keighley MR. Totally stapled abdominal restorative proctocolectomy. Br J Surg. 1989;76(9):961-4.
46. Sagar PM, Holdsworth PJ, Johnston D. Correlation between laboratory findings and clinical outcome after restorative proctocolectomy: serial studies in 20 patients with end-to-end pouch-anal anastomosis. Br J Surg. 1991;78(1):67-70.
47. Kirat HT, Remzi FH, Kiran RP, Fazio VW. Comparison of outcomes after hand-sewn versus stapled ileal pouch-anal anastomosis in 3,109 patients. Surgery. 2009;146(4):723-9.
48. Feinberg SM, McLeod RS, Cohen Z. Complications of loop ileostomy. Am J Surg. 1987;153(1):102-7.
49. Sagar PM, Lewis W, Holdsworth PJ, Johnston D. One-stage restorative proctocolectomy without temporary defunctioning ileostomy. Dis Colon Rectum. 1992;35(6):582-8.
50. Gorfine SR, Gelernt IM, Bauer JJ, Harris MT, Kreel I. Restorative proctocolectomy without diverting ileostomy. Dis Colon Rectum. 1995;38(2):188-94.
51. Wexner SD, Johansen OB, Nogueras JJ, Jagelman DG. Laparoscopic total abdominal colectomy. A prospective trial. Dis Colon Rectum. 1992;35(7):651-5.
52. Schmitt SL, Cohen SM, Wexner SD, Nogueras JJ, Jagelman DG. Does laparoscopic-assisted ileal pouch anal anastomosis reduce the length of hospitalization? Int J Colorectal Dis. 1994;9(3):134-7.
53. Marcello PW, Milsom JW, Wong SK, Hammerhofer KA, Goormastic M, Church JM, et al. Laparoscopic restorative proctocolectomy: case-matched comparative study with open restorative proctocolectomy. Dis Colon Rectum. 2000;43(5):604-8.
54. Dunker MS, Bemelman WA, Slors JF, van Duijvendijk P, Gouma DJ. Functional outcome, quality of life, body image, and cosmesis in patients after laparoscopic-assisted and conventional restorative proctocolectomy: a comparative study. Dis Colon Rectum. 2001;44(12):1800-7.
55. Hull TL, Joyce MR, Geisler DP, Coffey JC. Adhesions after laparoscopic and open ileal pouch-anal anastomosis surgery for ulcerative colitis. Br J Surg. 2012;99(2):270-5.
56. Polle SW, Dunker MS, Slors JF, Sprangers MA, Cuesta MA, Gouma DJ, et al. Body image, cosmesis, quality of life, and functional outcome of hand-assisted laparoscopic versus open restorative proctocolectomy: long-term results of a randomized trial. Surg Endosc. 2007;21(8):1301-7.
57. Tan JJ, Tjandra JJ. Laparoscopic surgery for ulcerative colitis-a meta-analysis. Colorectal Dis. 2006;8(8):626-36.
58. Ahmed Ali U, Keus F, Heikens JT, Bemelman WA, Berdah SV, Gooszen HG, et al. Open versus laparoscopic (assisted) ileo pouch anal anastomosis for ulcerative colitis and familial adenomatous polyposis. Cochrane Database Syst Rev. 2009(1):CD006267.
59. Meagher AP, Farouk R, Dozois RR, Kelly KA, Pemberton JH. J ileal pouch-anal anastomosis for chronic ulcerative colitis: complications and long-term outcome in 1310 patients. Br J Surg. 1998;85(6):800-3.
60. Francone TD, Champagne B. Considerations and complications in patients undergoing ileal pouch anal anastomosis. Surg Clin North Am. 2013;93(1):107-43.
61. Lewis WG, Kuzu A, Sagar PM, Holdsworth PJ, Johnston D. Stricture at the pouch-anal anastomosis after restorative proctocolectomy. Dis Colon Rectum. 1994;37(2):120-5.
62. Kirat HT, Kiran RP, Lian L, Remzi FH, Fazio VW. Influence of stapler size used at ileal pouch-anal anastomosis on anastomotic leak, stricture, long-term functional outcomes, and quality of life. Am J Surg. 2010;200(1):68-72.
63. Fazio VW, Tjandra JJ, Lavery IC, Church JM, Milsom JW, Oakley JR. Long-term follow-up of strictureplasty in Crohn's disease. Dis Colon Rectum. 1993;36(4):355-61.
64. Burke D, van Laarhoven CJ, Herbst F, Nicholls RJ. Transvaginal repair of pouch-vaginal fistula. Br J Surg. 2001;88(2):241-5.
65. Fazio VW, Tjandra JJ. Transanal mucosectomy. Ileal pouch advancement for anorectal dysplasia or inflammation after restorative proctocolectomy. Dis Colon Rectum. 1994;37(10):1008-11.
66. Van Assche G, Dignass A, Bokemeyer B, Danese S, Gionchetti P, Moser G, et al. Second European evidence-based consensus on the diagnosis and management of ulcerative colitis part 3: special situations. J Crohns Colitis. 2013;7(1):1-33.
67. Gorgun E, Remzi FH, Goldberg JM, Thornton J, Bast J, Hull TL, et al. Fertility is reduced after restorative proctocolectomy with ileal pouch anal anastomosis: a study of 300 patients. Surgery. 2004;136(4):795-803.
68. Olsen KO, Joelsson M, Laurberg S, Oresland T. Fertility after ileal pouch-anal anastomosis in women with ulcerative colitis. Br J Surg. 1999;86(4):493-5.
69. O'Connell PR, Pemberton JH, Brown ML, Kelly KA. Determinants of stool frequency after ileal pouch-anal anastomosis. Am J Surg. 1987;153(2):157-64.
70. Ambroze WL, Pemberton JH, Bell AM, Brown ML, Zinsmeister AR. The effect of stool consistency on rectal and neorectal emptying. Dis Colon Rectum. 1991;34(1):1-7.

CHAPTER 94

Crohn's Disease

Saurabh Kedia, Vineet Ahuja

Diagnosis of Crohn's Disease

INTRODUCTION

Crohn's disease (CD) is an immunological disorder of gastrointestinal tract which occurs as a result of multifaceted interaction of host immune system, genetic and environmental factors and microbiota.[1] The incidence of CD is on rise in developing countries like India.[2] Diagnosis of CD becomes difficult in countries like India which are endemic for tuberculosis as differentiating CD and intestinal tuberculosis (ITB) still remains an uphill task.[3] First part of this section will cover the approach to diagnosis of CD and the latter part deals on differentiation between CD and ITB.

DIAGNOSIS OF CROHN'S DISEASE

There is no single gold standard for diagnosis of CD. CD is diagnosed on the basis of combination of clinical features, and endoscopic, radiologic and histologic findings.

Clinical Features

The common presenting symptoms of a patient with CD include chronic diarrhea, pain abdomen, bleeding per rectum, recurrent episodes of subacute intestinal obstruction, fever, anorexia, weight loss and perianal fistulae.[4-7] Extraintestinal features which predominantly include musculoskeletal, ocular and dermatologic manifestations may occur simultaneously with active CD or may occur before the onset of CD.[8] CD may also present acutely in some patients, and acute terminal ileitis can mimic acute appendicitis.

Patients should be inquired about above mentioned symptoms including the duration, frequency and severity of these symptoms. In addition, history should also be taken about medications, appendicectomy, family history and smoking. Examination should include thorough general physical examination, abdominal examination for any palpable mass or tenderness, oral inspection and perineal and digital rectal examination.

Laboratory Investigations

Initial laboratory tests should include a complete hemogram, kidney and liver function tests, blood sugar, and markers of inflammation such as erythrocyte sedimentation rate (ESR) or C-reactive protein (CRP). CRP has been shown to correlate with disease activity of CD, and may change with changes in disease activity.[9,10] Other biomarkers of disease activity include fecal calprotectin and fecal lactoferrin.[11] However, based upon current evidence these markers have a better role in predicting relapse than establishing diagnosis.[12] Serologic tests such as anti-Saccharomyces cerevisiae antibodies (ASCA) and antineutrophil cytoplasmic antibody (ANCA) have not been found to be useful in diagnosing CD.[13] In addition to these investigations, skin test (Mantoux) or serologic test (Quantiferon Gold) for tuberculosis should also be obtained, the role of which will be discussed in the later section. Serologies for hepatitis B and C and human immunodeficiency virus (HIV) should also be done as these patients may require immunosuppression.

Endoscopy

Ileocolonoscopy with biopsies is the investigation of choice for the diagnosis of CD.[14,15] Common colonoscopic appearances in CD include discontinuous involvement of colon, longitudinal ulcers, cobblestoning, aphthous ulcers and perianal lesions (Fig. 1). Scoring endoscopic severity by various indices is not routine in clinical practice and is limited to clinical studies. Full colonoscopy should be avoided in presence of severe, active disease as it is associated with high chances of bowel perforation. Therefore,

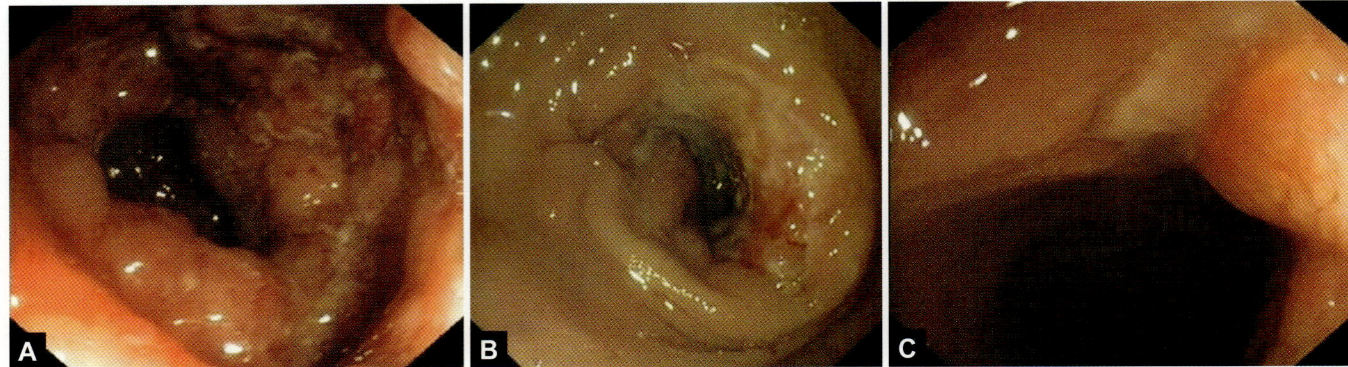

Figures 1A to C Colonoscopic images of patients with Crohn's disease. (A) Cobblestoning; (B) Stricture with ulcer; (C) Longitudinal ileal ulcer

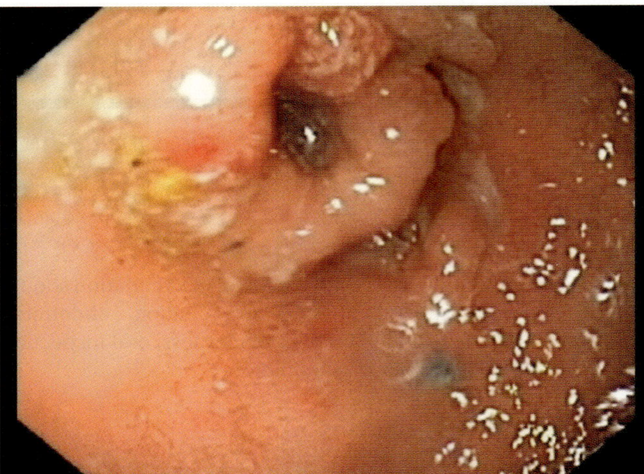
Figure 2 Duodenal stricture in a patient with Crohn's disease

limited flexible sigmoidoscopy with minimal air insufflation is the procedure of choice in these circumstances.

Upper gastrointestinal endoscopy is recommended in patients with suspected upper gastrointestinal symptoms (esophageal, gastric or duodenal CD, Fig. 2). In pediatric patients, upper gastrointestinal endoscopy with gastric biopsies should be done in all patients suspected to have CD.

Capsule endoscopy (CE) (Fig. 3) may detect lesions in small bowel that may be missed by standard endoscopic techniques and imaging.[16] Capsule endoscopy has a better yield than other diagnostic techniques for small bowel [Computed tomography (CT) enteroclysis/enterography and Barium enteroclysis].[17] Capsule endoscopy has a very high sensitivity in detecting small bowel lesions and a normal capsule endoscopy has a high negative predictive value in excluding the diagnosis of CD. However, subtle lesions demonstrated on capsule endoscopy have been seen in 10% of healthy individuals, thus limiting the specificity of capsule endoscopy. Therefore, capsule endoscopy is recommended in patients who have a high probability of having CD and standard endoscopic and radiologic techniques are normal. Capsule endoscopy can also be used to determine the extent of disease cases of proven CD as well as define mucosal healing in patients on therapy. Capsule endoscopy is contraindicated in patients with strictures or fistulas. Therefore, assessment of patency with either patency capsule or with barium or computed tomography enterography is recommended before performing capsule endoscopy.

Double or single balloon enteroscopy (antegrade/retrograde) has the advantage of obtaining biopsies from suspicious lesions, as well as performing therapeutic procedures such as stricture dilatation and retrieval of retained capsules.[18,19]

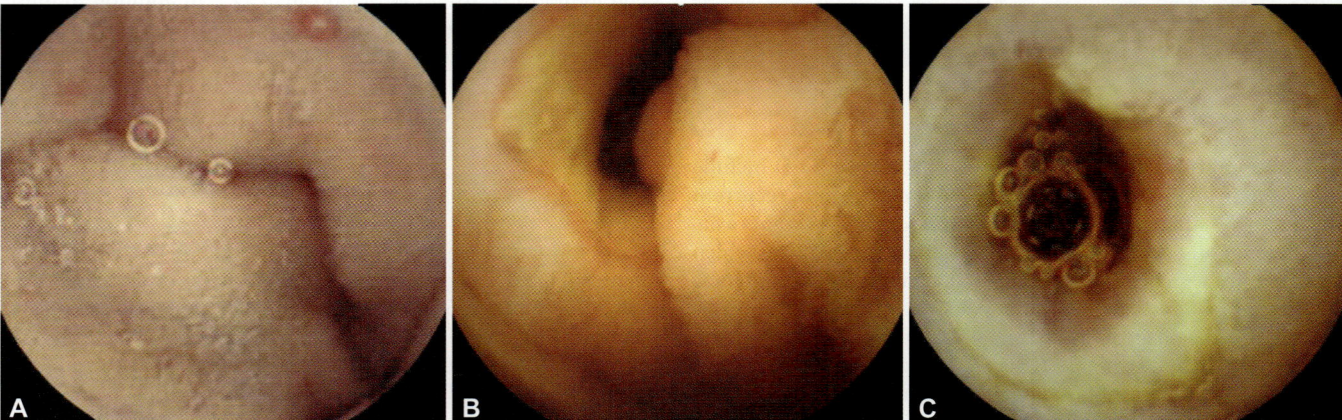

Figures 3A to C Capsule endoscopy images in patients of Crohn's disease. (A) Aphthous ulcer; (B) Deep ulcer; (C) Stricture

Therefore, endoscopic procedures are useful in establish diagnosis of CD, determining the extent of disease, and in assessment of mucosal healing in patients on therapy.

Histology

Histology is an important adjunct to the diagnostic algorithm of CD. Histology is important in both diagnosis as well as assessment of disease activity.[20] Ideally multiple biopsies should be obtained from multiple sites (normal as well as abnormal) for a definite diagnosis.[21] Biopsies should be obtained from the anastomotic site and the neo-terminal ileum to diagnose endoscopic recurrence.

The histologic features which are useful in the diagnosis of CD can be architectural and inflammatory.[22] These can either be observed in mucosal biopsy specimen or surgical samples.

Findings which are seen in mucosal biopsies include:

- Architectural abnormalities: Include crypt distortion (nonparallel crypts, variable diameter or cystically dilated crypts), crypt shortening, crypt branching (>2 branched crypts), decreased crypt density and irregular mucosal surface. Presence of these abnormalities in more than 10% of the crypts is considered significant.[23]
- Inflammatory features include focal or patchy inflammation, basal plasmacytosis, increased intraepithelial lymphocytes, transmucosal inflammation, focal cryptitis, aphthoid ulcers, disproportionate submucosal inflammation, mucin preservation at sites of active inflammation, nerve fiber hyperplasia, proximal location of ulceration and architectural distortion, metaplasia (pseudopyloric in ileum and paneth cell in colon) and granulomas. Of these, most important are focal or patchy inflammation and granulomas.
  - Focal or patchy inflammation: It implies either a focal increase in cellularity with a normal background or an abnormal background with a patchy cellularity.
  - Granulomas:[24] These are a collection of epitheliod histiocytes (macrophages) with vaguely defined outlines. Presence of necrosis and giant cells is rare in these granulomas. In addition, the granulomas in CD are usually small (<200 micron), discrete and small in number (<5 in number). Submucosal granulomas and granulomas distant from active crypt injury are considered characteristic of CD. The granulomas are more frequently seen in large as compared to small bowel, and are more commonly seen in younger patients with shorter disease duration. Granulomas can also be seen in mesenteric lymph nodes along with intestinal wall, but the presence of granulomas in lymph nodes only is against the diagnosis of CD.

Presence of granulomas or focally-enhanced gastritis in gastric biopsies is also a characteristic of CD.

Features which are exclusive to surgical biopsies include:

- Transmural inflammation
- Submucosal expansion by fibromuscular hyperplasia
- Fissures
- Transmural lymphoid aggregates
- Nerve hyperplasia in submucosa.

There is limited data on histologic assessment of disease activity in CD. Presence of neutrophils in association with epithelial injury may be considered as a marker of disease activity in CD.

Radiologic Procedures

Radiologic studies are integral part of diagnostic algorithm of CD (Flow chart 1).[25] Imaging can evaluate segment of gastrointestinal tract inaccessible to endoscopic techniques, mainly small bowel.[26] Secondly, with the advent of cross-sectional imaging techniques and multiplanar reconstructions with computed tomography and magnetic resonance imaging (MRI), imaging can also assess transmural and extraluminal aspects of CD. In addition to playing a role in diagnosis of CD, imaging can also help in differentiation of CD from ulcerative colitis (UC) and ITB. Imaging can also differentiate active from inactive CD as well as assess complications of CD such as abscesses, fistulae, perforations, obstructing strictures and toxic megacolon. Pelvic MRI can provide detailed assessment of perianal complications of CD.[27] There is limited data on the use of MRI or computed tomography for the evaluation of colonic CD.[28]

Barium Studies

On barium studies, a long segment of terminal ileum involvement, with skip lesions and preservation of the cecum and the valve is considered characteristic of CD. Other findings on barium would include long segment small bowel strictures, greater number of involved segments, linear, curvilinear, or spiculated areas of ulceration along the mesenteric border of the small bowel with resultant retraction of the bowel wall, leading to pseudodiverticula and pseudosacculation of the antimesenteric bowel wall.

Cross-sectional Imaging

Computerized tomography (CT) scans with enterography or MRI with enterography have become an critical tool as it can show the location of the disease in the intestine, lymph nodes, peritoneum, mesentery, solid organs and even the retroperitoneum. It is also advantageous in assessing the inflammatory process and extent of the disease. Inflammatory activity can be assessed on the basis of wall thickness and enhancement of the bowel wall.[29] Features of CD include symmetrical bowel wall thickening, fibrofatty proliferation of the mesentry known as "creeping fat", regional mesenteric nodes measuring 3–8 mm and enlarged mesenteric vascular bundles in the involved mesentry known as the comb sign (Fig. 4).

Both computed tomography and MRI have similar diagnostic accuracy. However, MRI is costlier and more time consuming than computed tomography, where as computed tomography has a risk of radiation, which may be appreciable with repeated examinations. Therefore, MRI is considered especially in young individuals where repeated examinations are anticipated. Computed tomography and MRI examinations can either be done with administration of contrast orally (enterography) or through nasojejunal tube placed under fluoroscopy (enteroclysis) to achieve adequate bowel distension. Although bowel distension is superior with enteroclysis, the diagnostic accuracy is similar with both enterography and enteroclysis.[30,31] Enteroclysis may be indicated in cases where proximal small bowel needs to be assessed.

Both computed tomography and MRI can equally assess the extramural complications of CD. Classically, the star sign can be seen on magnetic resonance enterography in cases with fistula formation around the structured bowel segment.[32]

Flow chart 1 Diagnostic algorithm of Crohn's disease

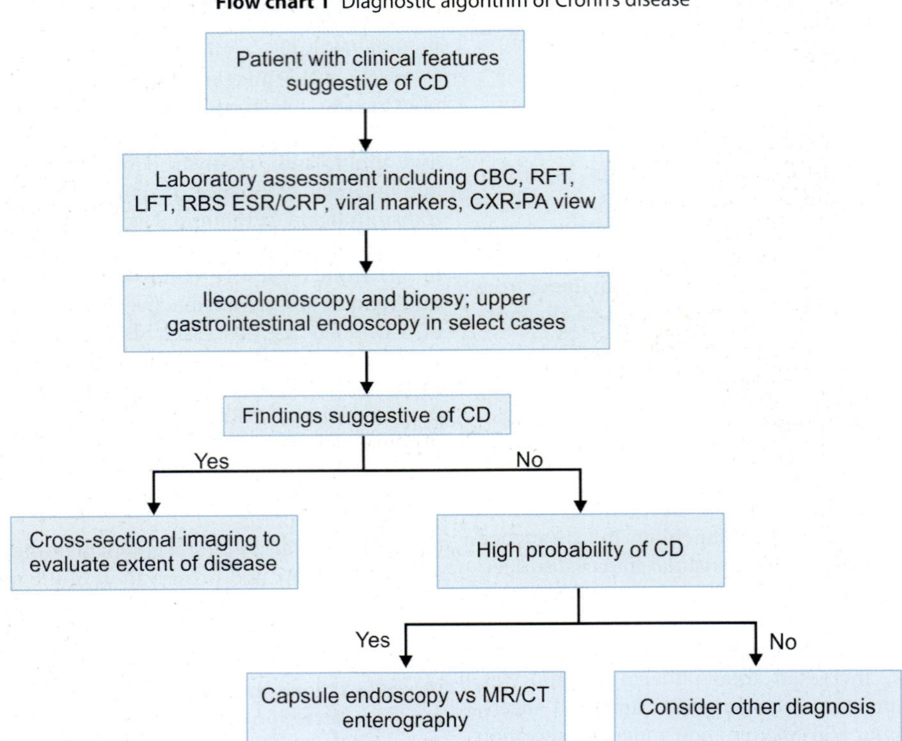

Abbreviations: CD, Crohn's disease; CBC, complete blood count; RFT, renal function test; LFT, liver function test, RBS, random blood sugar; ESR, erythrocyte sedimentation rate; CRP, C-reactive protein; CXR-PA, chest X-ray-posterioranterior; MR, magnetic resonance; CT, computed tomography.

Differentiation of Crohn's Disease from Intestinal Tuberculosis

Intestinal tuberculosis and CD resemble closely in terms of clinical, radiological, endoscopic, surgical and histological features. Differentiation of these two disorders is often an enigma and remains a source of consternation for clinicians, endoscopists, pathologists as well as radiologists. In case of misdiagnosis of CD antituberculosis therapy (ATT) may be delayed and treatment with steroids or monoclonals can further be disastrous. On the other hand, ATT given for CD can give unnecessary toxicity and delay its treatment. This highlights the necessity to establish diagnosis before mounting any empirical therapy. Gradually, increasing incidence of CD in an endemic zone of tuberculosis has further compounded the problem in India.

Clinical Features

Fever and ascites are most common in ITB while prolonged duration of illness, diarrhea, hematochezia and extraintestinal manifestations (EIM) are more commonly seen in CD. In one study, about an 85% accuracy in predicting CD could be reached based on the history of hematochezia, diarrhea and protracted duration of symptoms, and absence of fever.

However, both diseases can have an insidious onset with prolonged duration of undiagnosed illness. Secondly, ITB can also involve several extraintestinal sites with associated immunological phenomena. Thus, extraintestinal signs of CD should be cautiously interpreted in areas of endemic tuberculosis. Although fistulization is one of the important features of CD, enteroenteric, enterocutaneous and perianal fistulas have also been described in ITB. Thus, there is considerable overlap in the features of these two diseases (Table 1).

Extraintestinal Manifestations

In a study from Delhi[8] in 1652 patients (1146 UC, 303 CD, 203 ITB), frequency of any EIM was 33.2%, 38.3%, and 14.3% in ulcerative colitis, CD, and ITB patients, respectively. Relative to ITB, CD patients had higher frequencies of peripheral arthropathy ($p<0.001$), aphthous stomatitis ($p=0.01$), any EIM ($p<0.001$), and multiple EIMs ($p<0.001$).

Site of Involvement

The site of involvement suggests that ITB is seen more in right side of colon and follows a decreasing trend on moving from right to left side of colon. Rectosigmoid is significantly more frequently involved in CD when compared to colonic tuberculosis (Table 2).

Endoscopy

Longitudinal ulcers, aphthous ulcers, cobblestone appearance and anorectal involvement were more common in patients with CD compared to patients with ITB in a recent Korean study.[37] On the other hand, ITB usually has less than four segments involved, transverse ulcers and more scars and a patulous ileocecal valve (Table 3). Evaluation of small bowel with "video capsule

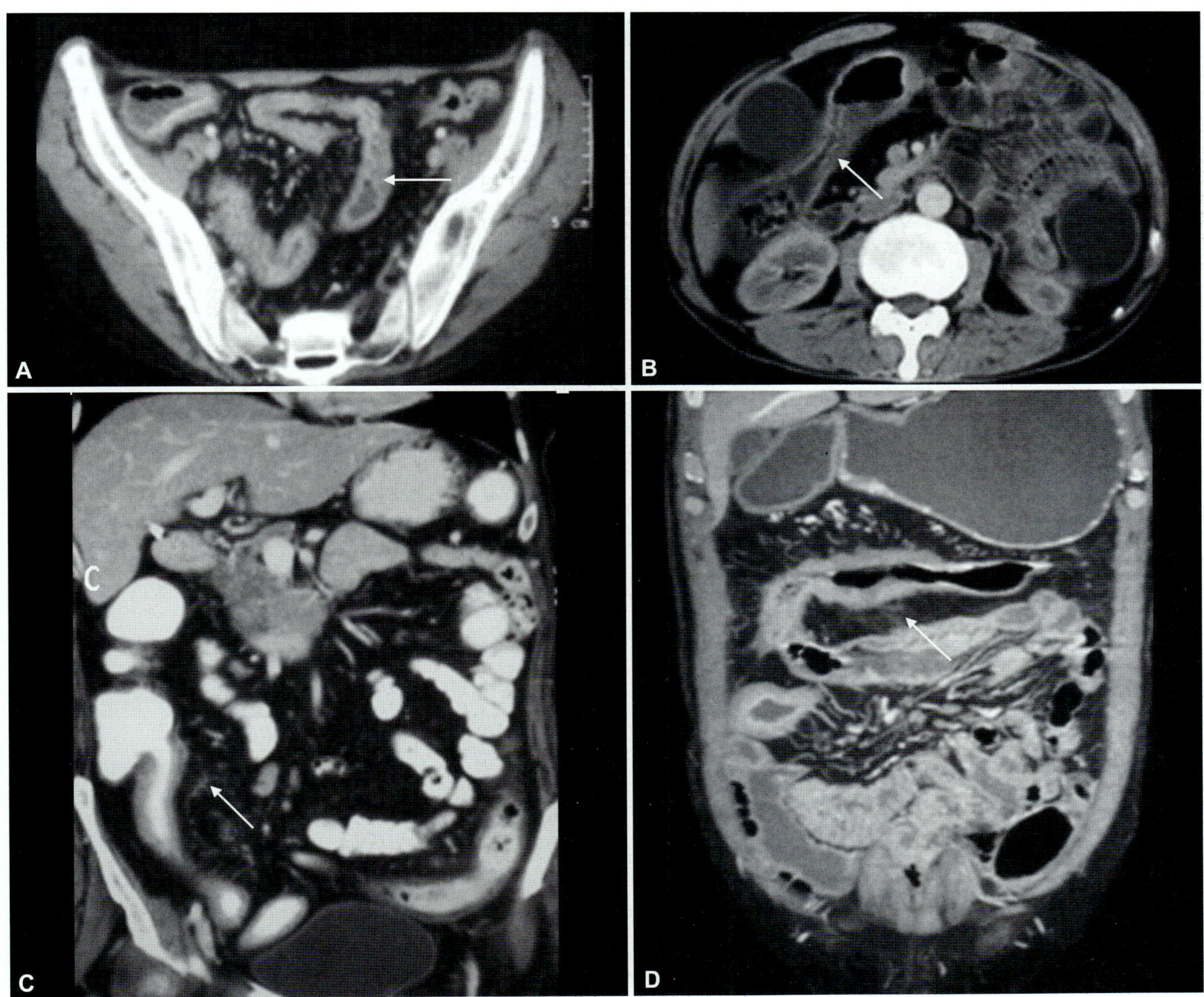

Figures 4A to D Computed tomography features in patients with Crohn's disease. (A) Long-segment terminal ileal involvement with mural stratification and comb sign; (B) Long-segment transverse colon stricture with mural stratification and fat proliferation; (C) Isolated long-segment terminal ileal involvement with mural stratification and fat proliferation; (D) Long-segment transverse colonic stricture with fat proliferation and comb sign

endoscopy" shows that ulcers in ITB are small (1–2 cm), transverse and shallow with irregular "geographic" border. Ulcers in CD are deeper and longitudinal.

Pathology

Features seen more frequently, in ITB include confluent granulomas, multiple granulomas, large granuloma size, ulcers lined by bands of epitheloid histiocytes and disproportionate mucosal inflammation with submucosal granulomas. On the other hand, in CD single granulomas are seen with foci of inflammation. Architectural distortion is seen little farther away from the site of granulomatous inflammation.

Polymerase chain reaction (PCR) for mycobacterial DNA has been used for the differential diagnosis of ITB and CD in several retrospective studies (Table 4). PCR on paraffin embedded formalin fixed colonoscopic biopsy specimen were reported positive in 22% (13/60), 45% (18/40), 64% (25/39), 75% (27/36) of ITB patients while 0% (0/30), 0% (0/26) and 5% (1/20) positivity was seen in CD cases. PCR detection was not influenced by presence of granuloma suggesting that PCR may be worthwhile in histologically inconclusive cases.

Serological Tests

Several recent studies have concluded that the serological markers, such as the perinuclear and the cytoplasmic variants [perinuclear anti-neutrophil cytoplasmic antibodies (p-ANCA) and cytoplasmic antineutrophil cytoplasmic antibodies (c-ANCA)], antineutrophil cytoplasmic antibodies and the immunoglobulin A (IgA) and IgG

Table 1: Differentiating clinical features between intestinal tuberculosis and Crohn's Disease in various case series

Clinical features	*Amarapurkar et al*[33]		*Makharia et al*[34]		*Zhou et al*[35]		*Li et al*[36]	
	CD (26)	*ITB (26)*	*CD (53)*	*ITB (53)*	*CD (30)*	*ITB (30)*	*CD (130)*	*ITB (122)*
Duration of symptoms (months)	58.1	7.2	53.3	23.4			31	16
Chronic diarrhea	69	35	85	38	36	30	66	47
Hematochezia	31	4	68	17	20	10	32	7
Fever	23	69	28	41	23	36	30	43
Weight loss	69	73	55	83	86	93	71	76
Abdominal pain	65	85	70	90	90	100	86	81
Intestinal obstruction	19	12	41	55			28	10
Growth retardation	8	0	–	–				
Ascites	8	35	–	–			7	35
Abdominal lump	8	15	–	–	53	60		
Extraintestinal features	62	23	45	13				
Constipation	–	–	8	49				
Perianal disease	–	–	30	8				
Loss of appetite	–	–	51	70				
Weakness fatigue	–	–	66	70				

Abbreviations: CD, Crohn's disease; ITB, intestinal tuberculosis. All figures are in percentages.

Table 2: Differentiating site of involvement between intestinal tuberculosis and Crohn's Disease in various case series

Site of involvement	*Amarapurkar et al*[33]		*Makharia et al*[34]		*Li et al*[36]	
	CD (26)	*ITB (26)*	*CD (53)*	*ITB (53)*	*CD (130)*	*ITB (122)*
Stomach	0	8	6	2		
Duodenum	4	8	6	4		
Jejunum	4	8	9	0		
Ileum	39	77	24	15	66	60
Ileocecal area	77	81	89	92	55	75
Ascending colon	69	81	64	43	46	62
Descending colon	38	19	60	24	34	25
Sigmoid colon			66	11	45	23
Rectum	31	73	62	19	38	16
Anal canal	8	4	15	4		
Esophagus	0	4				

Abbreviations: CD, Crohn's disease; ITB, intestinal tuberculosis. All figures are in percentages.

subtypes of anti-*Saccharomyces cerevisiae* antibodies, were not accurate in discerning ITB from CD.[42,43] Therefore, these tests do not have role for distinguishing between ITB and CD and should not be depended upon for this purpose.

Tuberculin Skin Test

The value of tuberculin skin test (TST) in ITB is unknown, plus the diagnostic value varies among different regions. Reading TST requires another visit and may also have observer bias. Negative result may be seen in immunocompromised and does not preclude a latent Koch's. Positive value may however, aid in decision for tubercular prophylaxis.

Quantiferon Tuberculosis Gold Test

Interferon (IFN)-gamma based assays have been developed to assess latent tuberculosis (TB) which has been approved by Food and Drug Administration (FDA).[44] These assays measure the amount of IFN-gamma released by T-cells on exposure to these antigens in vitro. IFN-gamma based assay has no cross-reaction with non-tuberculous mycobacteria or (Bacillus Calmette-Guérin)

Table 3: Differentiating endoscopic features between intestinal tuberculosis and Crohn's Disease in various case series

Endoscopy	*Amarapurkar et al*[33]		*Makharia et al*[34]		*Li et al*[36]		*Lee et al*[37]	
	CD (26)	*ITB (26)*	*CD (53)*	*ITB (53)*	*CD (130)*	*ITB (122)*	*CD (44)*	*ITB (44)*
Skip lesions	23	8	66	17	-	-		
Erythema	-	-	26	9	-	-		
Friability	-	-	26	0	-	-		
Aphthous ulcers	35	19	55	13	54	44	82	20
Linear ulcers	58	23	30	8	55	8	41	2
Deep ulcers	-	-	34	51	-	-		
Superficial ulcers	-	-	55	17	-	-		
Nodularity	-	-	25	49	49	33		
Cobblestoning	58	23	17	0	28	2	34	7
Stricture	31	19	-	-	-	-	20	18
Neoplasm-like appearance	0	8	-	-	-	-		
Fistula	12	0	-	-	-	-		
Pseudopolyps	35	19	-	-	-	-	27	52
Fewer than four segments involved	-	-	-	-	-	-	18	82
Anorectal lesions	-	-	-	-	-	-	84	9
Ileocecal lesions	-	-	-	-	-	-	88	91
Patulous ileocecal valve	-	-	-	-	-	-	9	36
Transverse ulcers	-	-	-	-	-	-	25	66

Abbreviations: CD, Crohn's disease; ITB, intestinal tuberculosis. All figures are in percentages.

Table 4: Intestinal tuberculosis (ITB) versus Crohn's disease (CD): Comparison of histological parameters

	Pulimood et al[38]		*Pulimood et al*[39]		*Kirsch et al*[40]		*Jin et al*[41]	
	ITB (20)	*CD (20)*	*ITB (33)*	*CD (31)*	*ITB (18)*	*CD (25)*	*ITB (52)*	*CD (26)*
Caseous necrosis	40	0	36	0	22	0	27	0
Confluent granulomas	60	0	42	3	50	0	46	8
‡5 Granulomas/biopsy site	40	0	45	0	44	24	-	-
‡10 Granulomas/biopsy site	-	-	-	-	33	0	-	-
Large granulomas	90	5	51	0	67	8	75	19
Submucosal granulomas	45	5	39	6	44	12	-	-
Ulcers lined by bands of epitheloid histiocytes	45	5	61	0	61	8	-	-
Disproportionate submucosal inflammation	65	5	-	-	67	10	-	-
Architectural distortion distant to granulomatous inflammation	-	-	0	62	-	-	-	-

Abbreviations: CD, Crohn's disease; ITB, intestinal tuberculosis. All figures are in percentages.

BCG and is thus advantageous over TST. However, these assays need to be further proven in larger studies in areas of high-TB prevalence and in the immunocompromised host. In a recent meta-analysis IFN-γ release assays (IGRA) had a sensitivity of 74% and a specificity of 87% in differentiating ITB and CD.[45]

Radiology

Classically, ileocecal area is the most common segment involved in patients with ITB, noted in up to 90% of cases,[44,46] whereas isolated involvement of the ileocecal region has been rarely associated with CD. In CD, usually there is involvement of the ileum with sparing of the ileocecal valve.[47] CD has been reported to be a multifocal disease whereas ITB is usually a unifocal disease. In a retrospective study of 17 patients with CD, 64.7% patients had multifocal disease.[48] Strictures are one of the common findings reported in ITB, they being short, concentric and smooth in outline with significant prestenotic dilatation.[49] In a study of 265 patients with small bowel tuberculosis, strictures were the most common radiologic finding seen in 62.7% cases. The strictures and

Table 5: Comparison of computed tomography findings in patients with Crohn's disease and intestinal tuberculosis

	CD (n = 54) *Numbers (%)*	*ITB (n = 50)* *Numbers (%)*	*P value*
Site of Involvement:			
Left colon^	12 (22.2)	3 (6)	0.02
Rest of colon#	17 (31.5)	10 (20)	0.18
Ileocecal area+	23 (42.6)	35 (70)	0.01
Rest of small intestine*	29 (53.7)	25 (50)	0.71
Type of involvement:			
Length of segment:			<0.01
Short	17 (21.5)	36 (72)	
Long	37 (68.5)	14 (28)	
Thickness:			0.20
Concentric	52 (96.3)	45 (90)	
Asymmetric	2 (3.7)	5 (10)	
Mural stratification	11 (20.4)	8 (16)	0.56
Skip lesions	34 (63)	21 (42)	0.03
No of segments:			0.09
<3	39 (72.2)	43 (86)	
>3	15 (27.8)	7 (14)	
Stricture:			
Short (<3)	13 (24.1)	16 (32)	0.37
Long (>3)	9 (16.7)	7 (14)	0.71
Wall enhancement	50 (92.6)	48 (96)	0.46
Others:			
Mesenteric changes:			
Comb sign	24 (44.4)	10 (20)	0.01
Fat proliferation	10 (18.5)	6 (12)	0.36
Fat stranding	7 (13)	10 (20)	0.33
Lymph nodes:			
Size:			
<1 cm	18 (33.3)	17 (34)	0.94
>1 cm	1 (1.9)	10 (20)	<0.01

* - rest of small intestine includes jejunum, ileum excluding the terminal ileum
+ - ileocecal area includes terminal ileum just adjacent to the ileocecal valve or contiguous terminal ileal and cecal involvement
# - rest of colon includes cecum (without contiguous terminal ileal involvement), ascending colon, transverse colon
^ - left colon includes descending colon, sigmoid colon, rectum
Abbreviations: CD, Crohn's disease; ITB, intestinal tuberculosis.

involved segments in CD are typically long. Park et al. reported long-segment involvement of bowel to be significantly more common in patients with CD compared to patients with ITB. On cross-sectional imaging, CD is characterized by mural thickening with stratification along with mesenteric vascular engorgement and fibrofatty proliferation.[25] Large hypodense lymph nodes with peripheral enhancement and hypodense centers have characteristically been described with ITB. In a previous study of 27 patients analyzing the differentiation of CD and ITB based on computed tomography, the lymph nodes were noted to be larger in patients with ITB and one-third of them had necrotic centers. Bowel loop displacement was found to be caused by lymphadenopathy in patients with ITB in this study.[50] In a recent study published from our center[51] (54 CD, 50 ITB) left colonic involvement, ileocecal involvement, long-segment involvement, comb sign, presence of skip lesions, involvement of more than 3 segments and more than 1 cm sized lymph nodes were significantly different between CD and ITB. On multivariate analysis, ileocecal involvement, long-segment involvement and presence of lymph node more than 1 cm were statistically significant. Based upon the latter 3 variables a risk score (with values ranging from 0–3) was generated, with scores 0, 1 having specificity of 100%, 87% respectively and positive predictive value (PPV) of 100%, 76% respectively for ITB and scores 2, 3 having specificity of 68%, 90% respectively and PPV of 63%, 80% respectively for CD (Table 5).

Role of Immunological Markers

Forkhead box P3 (FOXP3+) cells are thymus derived regulatory T cells which control the inflammation induced by T effector cells.

In a study from our center frequency of $FOXP3^+$ cells in peripheral blood in ITB as compared to CD patients was significantly increased (37.6% vs 23.6%, p<0.001). Percentage of $FOXP3^+CD4^+$ cells in colonic biopsies were significantly increased in ITB as compared to CD (38.55 vs 12.5%, p<0.001). Receiver operating characteristic (ROC) curve showed that a value more than 32.54% for $FOXP3^+$ cells in peripheral blood could differentiate between CD and ITB with a sensitivity of 75% and a specificity of 90.6%. Therefore, phenotypic enumeration of peripheral $CD4^+CD25^+FOXP3^+$ regulatory T cells (Treg cells) may differentiate ITB from CD with a high diagnostic specificity.[52]

CONCLUSION

Although, there are several differences in clinical, endoscopic, histologic and radiologic features, between CD and ITB, there is also considerable overlap between each of these features. Therefore, there is still no gold standard to differentiate between ITB and CD. Often the clinicians have to resort to trial of antitubercular therapy and subsequently classify the patients as having ITB or CD based on the response to (ATT).

REFERENCES

1. Duchmann R, Kaiser I, Hermann E, Mayet W, Ewe K, Meyer zum Büschenfelde KH. Tolerance exists towards resident intestinal flora but is broken in active inflammatory bowel disease (IBD). Clin Exp Immunol. 1995;102:448-55.
2. Ahuja V, Tandon RK. Inflammatory bowel disease in the Asia-Pacific area: a comparison with developed countries and regional differences. J Dig Dis. 2010;11:134-47.
3. Pulimood AB, Amarapurkar DN, Ghoshal U, Phillip M, Pai CG, Reddy DN, et al. Differentiation of Crohn's disease from intestinal tuberculosis in India in 2010. World J Gastroenterol. 2011;17(4):433-43.
4. Sands BE. From symptom to diagnosis: clinical distinctions among various forms of intestinal inflammation. Gastroenterology. 2004;126(6):1518-32.
5. Burgmann T, Clara I, Graff L, Walker J, Lix L, Rawsthorne P, et al. The Manitoba Inflammatory Bowel Disease Cohort Study: prolonged symptoms before diagnosis–how much is irritable bowel syndrome? Clin Gastroenterol Hepatol. 2006;4(5):614-20.
6. Farmer RG, Hawk WA, Turnbull RB. Clinical patterns in Crohn's disease: a statistical study of 615 cases. Gastroenterology. 1975;68(4 Pt 1):627-35.
7. Schwartz DA, Loftus EV, Tremaine WJ, Panaccione R, Harmsen WS, Zinsmeister AR, et al. The natural history of fistulizing Crohn's disease in Olmsted County, Minnesota. Gastroenterology. 2002;122(4):875-80.
8. Singh B, Kedia S, Konijeti G, Mouli VP, Dhingra R, Kurrey L, et al. Extraintestinal manifestations of inflammatory bowel disease and intestinal tuberculosis: Frequency and relation with disease phenotype. Indian J Gastroenterol. 2015;34(1):43-50.
9. Fagan EA, Dyck RF, Maton PN, Hodgson HJ, Chadwick VS, Petrie A, et al. Serum levels of C-reactive protein in Crohn's disease and ulcerative colitis. Eur J Clin Invest. 1982;12(4):351-9.
10. Vermeire S, Van Assche G, Rutgeerts P. C-reactive protein as a marker for inflammatory bowel disease. Inflamm Bowel Dis. 2004;10(5):661-5.
11. D'Inca R, Dal PE, Di LV, Ferronato A, Fries W, Vettorato MG, et al. Calprotectin and lactoferrin in the assessment of intestinal inflammation and organic disease. Int J Colorectal Dis. 2007;22(4):429-37.
12. Tibble JA, Sigthorsson G, Bridger S, Fagerhol MK, Bjarnason I. Surrogate markers of intestinal inflammation are predictive of relapse in patients with inflammatory bowel disease. Gastroenterology. 2000;119(1):15-22.
13. Reese GE, Constantinides VA, Simillis C, Darzi AW, Orchard TR, Fazio VW, et al. Diagnostic precision of anti-Saccharomyces cerevisiae antibodies and perinuclear antineutrophil cytoplasmic antibodies in inflammatory bowel disease. Am J Gastroenterol. 2006;101(10):2410-22.
14. Coremans G, Rutgeerts P, Geboes K, Van den Oord J, Ponette E, Vantrappen G. The value of ileoscopy with biopsy in the diagnosis of intestinal Crohn's disease. Gastrointest Endosc. 1984;30(3):167-72.
15. Nahon S, Bouhnik Y, Lavergne-Slove A, Bitoun A, Panis Y, Valleur P, et al. Colonoscopy accurately predicts the anatomical severity of colonic Crohn's disease attacks: correlation with findings from colectomy specimens. Am J Gastroenterol. 2002;97(12):3102-7.
16. Voderholzer WA, Beinhoelzl J, Rogalla P, Murrer S, Schachschal G, Lochs H, et al. Small bowel involvement in Crohn's disease: a prospective comparison of wireless capsule endoscopy and computed tomography enteroclysis. Gut. 2005;54(3):369-73.
17. Hara AK, Leighton JA, Heigh RI, Sharma VK, Silva AC, De Petris G, et al. Crohn disease of the small bowel: preliminary comparison among CT enterography, capsule endoscopy, small-bowel follow-through, and ileoscopy. Radiology. 2006;238(1):128-34.
18. Seiderer J, Herrmann K, Diepolder H, Schoenberg SO, Wagner AC, Göke B, et al. Double-balloon enteroscopy versus magnetic resonance enteroclysis in diagnosing suspected small-bowel Crohn's disease: results of a pilot study. Scand J Gastroenterol. 2007;42(11):1376-85.
19. Oshitani N, Yukawa T, Yamagami H, Inagawa M, Kamata N, Watanabe K, et al. Evaluation of deep small bowel involvement by double-balloon enteroscopy in Crohn's disease. Am J Gastroenterol. 2006;101(7):1484-9.
20. Dejaco C, Osterreicher C, Angelberger S, Püspök A, Birner P, Poetzi R, et al. Diagnosing colitis: a prospective study on essential parameters for reaching a diagnosis. Endoscopy. 2003;35:1004-8.
21. Jenkins D, Balsitis M, Gallivan S, Dixon MF, Gilmour HM, Shepherd NA, et al. Guidelines for the initial biopsy diagnosis of suspected chronic idiopathic inflammatory bowel disease. The British Society of Gastroenterology Initiative. J Clin Pathol. 1997;50:93-105.
22. Tanaka M, Saito H, Fukuda S, Sasaki Y, Munakata A, Kudo H, et al. Simple mucosal biopsy criteria differentiating among Crohn's disease, ulcerative colitis, and other forms of colitis Measurement of validity. Scand J Gastroenterol. 2000;35:281-6.
23. Schumacher G, Kollberg B, Sandstedt B. A prospective study of first attacks of inflammatory bowel disease and infectious colitis. Histologic course during the 1st year after presentation. Scand J Gastroenterol. 1994;29:318–32.
24. Bernades P, Hecketsweiler P, Benozio M, Descos L, Geffroy Y, Hemet J, et al. Proposition d'un système de critères pour le diagnostic des entérocolite inflammatoires cryptogénétiques (maladie de Crohn et Rect colite Hémorragique). Gastroentérol Clin Biol. 1978;2:1047-54.
25. Will JS, Lobis IF, Denstman FJ. Crohn's disease: state of the art. Radiology. 1997;202:597-610.
26. Caroline DF, Freidman AC. The radiology of inflammatory bowel disease. Med Clin North Am. 1994;78:1353-85.
27. Chapple KS, Spenser JA, Windsor AC, Wilson D, Ward J, Ambrose NS. Prognostic value of magnetic resonance imaging in the management of fistula-in-ano. Dis Colon Rectum. 2000;43:511-6.
28. Horton KM, Corl FM, Fishman EK. CT evaluation of the colon: Inflammatory disease. Radiographics. 2000;20:388-418.
29. Reittner P, Goritschnig T, Petritsch W, Doerfler O, Preidler KW, Hinterleitner T, et al. Multiplanar spinal CT enterography in patients with Crohn's disease using a negative oral contrast material: initial results of a noninvasive imaging approach. Eur Radiol. 2005;12:2253-7.
30. Wold PB, Fletcher JG, Johnson CD, Sandborn WJ. Assessment of small bowel Crohn disease: noninvasive peroral CT enterography compared with other imaging methods and endoscopy feasibility study. Radiology. 2003;229(1):275-81.

31. Negaard A, Paulsen V, Sandvik L, Berstad AE, Borthne A, Try K, et al. A prospective randomized comparison between two MRI studies of the small bowel in Crohn's disease, the oral contrast method and MR enteroclysis. Eur Radiol. 2007;17(9):2294-301.
32. Herrmann KA, Michaely HJ, Seiderer J, Ochsenkuehn T, Reiser MF, Schoenberg SO. The "star-sign" in magnetic resonance enteroclysis: a characteristic finding of internal fistulae in Crohn's disease. Scand J Gastroenterol. 2006;41(2):239-41.
33. Amarapurkar DN, Patel ND, Rane PS. Diagnosis of Crohn's disease in Indiawhere tuberculosis is widely prevalent. World J Gastroenterol. 2008;14(5):741-6.
34. Makharia GK, Srivastava S, Das P, Goswami P, Singh U, Tripathi M, et al. Clinical, endoscopic, and histological differentiations between Crohn's disease and intestinal tuberculosis. Am J Gastroenterol. 2010;105(3):642-51.
35. Zhou ZY, Luo HS. Differential diagnosis between Crohn's disease and intestinal tuberculosis in China. Int J Clin Pract. 2006;60(2): 212-4.
36. Li X, Liu X, Zou Y, Ouyang C, Wu X, Zhou M, et al. Predictors of clinical and endoscopic findings in differentiating crohn's disease from intestinal tuberculosis. Dig Dis Sci. 2011;56(1):188-96.
37. Lee YJ, Yang SK, Byeon JS, Myung SJ, Chang HS, Hong SS, et al. Analysis of colonoscopic findings in the differential diagnosis between intestinal tuberculosis and Crohn's disease. Endoscopy. 2006;38(6):592-7.
38. Pulimood AB, Peter S, Ramakrishna B, Chacko A, Jeyamani R, Jeyaseelan L, et al. Segmental colonoscopic biopsies in the differentiation of ileocolic tuberculosis from Crohn's disease. J Gastroenterol Hepatol. 2005;20(5):688-96.
39. Pulimood AB, Peter S, Rook GW, Donoghue HD. In situ PCR for Mycobacterium tuberculosis in endoscopic mucosal biopsy specimens of intestinal tuberculosis and Crohn disease. Am J Clin Pathol. 2008;129(6):846-51.
40. Kirsch R, Pentecost M, Hall Pde M, Epstein DP, Watermeyer G, Friederich PW. Role of colonoscopic biopsy in distinguishing between Crohn's disease and intestinal tuberculosis. J Clin Pathol. 2006;59(8):840-4.
41. Jin XJ, Kim JM, Kim HK, Kim L, Choi SJ, Park IS, et al. Histopathology and TB-PCR kit analysis in differentiating the diagnosis of intestinal tuberculosis and Crohn's disease. World J Gastroenterol. 2010;16(20):2496-503.
42. Ghoshal UC, Ghoshal U, Singh H, Tiwari S. Anti-Saccharomyces cerevisiae antibody is not useful to differentiate between Crohn's disease and intestinal tuberculosis in India. J Postgrad Med. 2007;53(3):166-70.
43. Makharia GK, Sachdev V, Gupta R, Lal S, Pandey RM. Anti-Saccharomyces cerevisiae antibody does not differentiate between Crohn's disease and intestinal tuberculosis. Dig Dis Sci. 2007;52(1):33-9.
44. Marshall JB. Tuberculosis of the gastrointestinal tract and peritoneum. Am J Gastroenterol. 1993;88:989-99.
45. Chen W, Fan JH, Luo W, Peng P, Su SB. Effectiveness of interferon-gamma release assays for differentiating intestinal tuberculosis from Crohn's disease: a meta-analysis. World J Gastroenterol. 2013;19(44):8133-40.
46. Lundstedt C, Nyman R, Brismar J, Hugosson C, Kagevi I. Imaging of tuberculosis. II. Abdominal manifestations in 112 patients. Acta Radiol. 1996;37:489-95.
47. Chernish SM, Maglinte DD, O'Connor K. Evaluation of the small intestine by enteroclysis for Crohn's disease. Am J Gastroenterol. 1992;87:696-701.
48. Ching ASC, Mak HKF, Lai CKC, Ip CB, Cheung HS. Imaging features of Crohn's Disease in Chinese People: A Preliminary Study. J HK Coll Radiol. 2002;5:162-9.
49. Nagi B, Sodhi KS, Kochhar R, Bhasin DK, Singh K. Small bowel tuberculosis: enteroclysis findings. Abdom Imaging. 2004;29:335-40.
50. Makanjuola D. Is it Crohn's disease or intestinal tuberculosis? CT analysis. Eur J Radiol. 1998;28:55-61.
51. Kedia S, Sharma S, Nagi B, Mouli VP, Aananthakrishnan A, Dhingra R, et al. CT based predictive model for differentiation of Crohn's disease from Intestinal tuberculosis. Indian J Gastroenterol. 2015;34(2):135-43.
52. Ahuja V, Subodh S, Tuteja A, Mishra V, Garg SK, Gupta N, et al. Genome-wide gene expression analysis for target genes to differentiate patients with intestinal tuberculosis and Crohn's disease and discriminative value of FOXP3 mRNA expression. Gastroenterol Rep (Oxf). 2015 May 11. pii: gov015.

Management of Crohn's Disease

GOALS OF MANAGEMENT

Crohn's disease (CD) is an inflammatory disorder of gastrointestinal tract which occurs as a result of focal, transmural granulomatous inflammation and is characterized with specific, clinical and pathological features.[1] The natural history of CD is characterized by remissions and relapses. Chronic intestinal inflammation in CD cannot be cured medically or surgically and therefore, classically, the treatment goals have been induction and maintenance of clinical remission. However, with advances in therapy and better understanding of the pathophysiology of disease, the therapeutic goals are being redefined. The newer therapeutic goals include induction and maintenance of mucosal healing,[2] reduction in surgeries and hospitalizations and improvement in quality of life. Treatment of CD depends upon the phenotype (disease extent, location and behavior), disease severity and extraintestinal complications.

ASSESSMENT OF DISEASE ACTIVITY

Disease activity is established on the basis of clinical parameters, systemic features and the impact of disease on the individual's quality of life.[3] In the absence of single gold standard, there are multiple indices for measuring disease activity, which have been used in clinical trials. However, because of complexity there use is minimal in clinical practice. Of these, CD activity index (CDAI)[4] is the most commonly used activity index (Table 6). It is based on eight-weighted variables which take into account the symptoms over the last 7 days. The CDAI score ranges from 0–600. Remission is defined as CDAI less than 150, mild disease activity as CDAI between 150 and 219, moderate disease activity as CDAI between 220 and 449, and severe disease activity as CDAI more than 450.

WORKING DEFINITION FOR THE PRACTICING PHYSICIAN

American College of Gastroenterology had formed a more clinical working definition for measuring CD activity. This enables the clinician to guide therapy in an appropriate manner. An individual is in symptomatic remission (corresponding to CDAI <150) when the patient is asymptomatic and has no evidence of active disease. Individuals with mild to moderate disease

Table 6: Crohn's disease activity index

Variable no	*Variable description*	*Multiplier*
1	No. of liquid or soft stools (each day for 7 days)	2
2	Abdominal pain, sum of 7 daily ratings (0 = none, 1 = mild, 2 = moderate, 3 = severe)	5
3	General well-being, sum of 7 daily ratings (0 = generally well, 1 = slightly under par, 2 = poor, 3 = very poor, 4 = terrible)	7
4	Number of listed complications [arthritis or arthralgia, iritis or uveitis, erythema nodosum or pyoderma gangrenosum or aphthous stomatitis, anal fissure or fistula or abscess, other fistula, fever over 37.8°C (l00°F)]	20
5	Use of diphenoxylate or loperamide for diarrhea (0 = no, 1 = yes)	30
6	Abdominal mass (0 = no, 2 = questionable, 5 = definite)	10
7	Hematocrit [males, 47-Hct (%); females, 42-Hct (%)]	6
8	Body weight (1-weight/standard weight) × 100 (add or subtract according to sign)	1

activity (corresponding to CDAI 150–219) are ambulatory and able to tolerate oral nutrition without any sign of dehydration, systemic symptoms like high fever, abdominal tenderness, abdominal lump, intestinal obstruction, or more than 10% weight loss. Individuals considered to have moderate to severe disease (corresponding to CDAI 220–449) are those with more prominent systemic symptoms like fever, significant weight loss, abdominal pain or tenderness, intermittent nausea or vomiting (without obstructive findings), or significant anemia. Finally, those individuals considered to have severe or fulminant disease (corresponding to CDAI >450) are patients with persistent symptoms like high grade fever, vomiting, evidence of intestinal obstruction, peritonitis, cachexia or evidence of an abscess.

PHENOTYPIC CLASSIFICATION OF CROHN'S DISEASE

Crohn's disease was phenotypically classified according to age of onset (A), disease location (L) and disease behavior (B) by Vienna classification. There have been modifications in each of the categories of Vienna classification which is now known as Montreal classification. Montreal classification is listed in Table 7.

Table 7: Montreal classification of Crohn's disease

Age: • A1 • A2 • A3	 • <16 years • 17–40 years • >40 years
Location: • L1 • L2 • L3 • L4	 • Ileal • Colonic • Ileocolonic • Isolated upper gut disease
Behavior: • B1 • B2 • B3 • P	 • Non-stricturing, non-penetrating • Stricturing • Penetrating • Perianal disease modifier

MANAGEMENT

Symptom Assessment

Before deciding to start therapy for CD other conditions which may cause symptoms that resemble those of active CD should be excluded. These include intestinal infections, bacterial overgrowth, lactose intolerance, irritable bowel syndrome and side effects of medicines. In individuals with absence of any obvious mucosal inflammation or ulceration as determined endoscopically or radiologically aforementioned diagnoses should be considered.

General Considerations

Therapy depends upon disease severity, location, behavior and associated complications; and is individualized according to patients' response and tolerance to intervention. Treatment for active disease should be continued till remission is achieved. There should be evidence of clinical improvement within 2–4 weeks of therapy, with maximal improvement evident by 12–16 weeks. As 75% of patients relapse within 1 year of stopping therapy after induction of remission, maintenance therapy should be considered after remission is achieved. In patients not responding to one therapy, alternative therapy should be considered depending upon the clinical status. Surgery is considered in obstructing lesions, suppurative complications, medically intractable disease or neoplastic or preneopalstic lesions.

Disease location is important for medications which have targeted delivery systems such as sulfasalazine, mesalamine, and enteric coated budesonide. For other agents, the therapeutic activity is independent of disease location and occurs throughout the gastrointestinal tract. Figure 5 describes various agents used in induction therapy of CD.

Mild-to-Moderate Crohn's Disease

- 5-aminosalicylic acid (ASA): In two large randomized controlled trials, sulfasalazine was proven to be superior over placebo for up to 16 weeks in patients with active colonic CD.[5,6] Although sulfasalazine was less effective than steroids about 50% patients achieved clinical remission. Further, in a meta-analysis of three large trials, mesalamine

4 g/day showed a statistically significant but non-clinically relevant difference as compared with placebo.[7] Rectal 5-ASA preparations have never been evaluated in controlled trials in patients with colonic CD. There is no role of 5-ASA formulations in the management of patients with small intestinal or ileocolonic CD. Therefore, among the 5-ASA formulations only sulfasalazine has a role in the induction of remission in patients with left colonic CD.

- Antibiotics: Metronidazole in a dose of 10–20 mg/kg/day was found useful in a proportion of patients who did not respond to sulfasalazine.[8] Antitubercular therapy (ATT) was not found to be useful in induction of remission in patients with active CD.[9]
- Budesonide: Controlled release budesonide in a dose of 9 mg daily was found to be more effective than placebo or mesalamine in patients with distal ileal or right colonic CD.[10] Budesonide is, therefore recommended as the first line therapy for patients with mild to moderately active distal ileal or right colonic CD.
- Prednisolone: In patients who do not respond to first line therapy or in patients with moderate CD with systemic symptoms prednisolone should be used.
- Infliximab (IFX) should be reserved for patients with steroid-resistant or steroid-refractory disease.

Moderate-to-Severe Crohn's Disease

- Patients with moderate to severe CD are treated with steroids (Prednisolone) to induce remission. In patients with infection or abscess, appropriate antibiotics and/or drainage of abscess is required. There have been no appropriate studies to evaluate proper doses or dosage schedule of steroids in management of CD. Clinical remission is achieved in approximately 50–70% patients treated with prednisolone at a dose of 0.5–0.75 mg/kg/day (up to 40 mg) over a period of 8–17 weeks.[11] After a clinical response has been achieved, steroids are tapered according to response of patient, usually by 5–10 mg every twice weekly. Owing to increased risk of osteoporosis associated with both glucocorticoids and CD, baseline dual-energy X-ray absorptiometry (DEXA) scan and supplementation with calcium and vitamin D is recommended.[12]
- Remission can also be achieved with azathioprine (AZA) and 6-mercaptopurine (6-MP), however, thiopurines require an average of 16 weeks to derive optimal efficacy.[13]
- Parenteral methotrexate (MTX) at a dose of 25 mg subcutaneous or intramuscular once a week has also been found to be effective at inducing remission in steroid and thiopurine refractory cases.[12] However, lower doses of MTX have not been found to be effective.
- Infliximab, the chimeric monoclonal antibody against tumor necrosis factor-alpha (TNF-α) is effective in attaining remission in patients with moderate to severe CD refractory to steroids or immunomodulators. Approximately, 60% of patients achieve a clinical response and 40% achieve clinical remission after 4 weeks of single 5 mg/kg infusion.[14] However, the currently recommended schedule for induction of remission is a regimen of three infusions at 0, 2 and 6 weeks followed by maintenance therapy. Other biological agents which have been used in the therapy of CD include adalimumab, certolizumab and natalizumab (Table 8). Infliximab monotherapy and infliximab in combination with AZA was found to be more effective than AZA alone in treatment of patients with moderate to severe CD who failed to respond to first line agents and were naïve to biologics [study of biologic and immunomodulator naive patients in Crohn's disease (SONIC) trial].[15]

Fulminant Disease

Patients with persistence of symptoms despite induction with oral steroids or biologics and patients presenting with persistent fever, pain abdomen, evidence of intestinal obstruction, peritonitis, or abscess should be hospitalized. In patients running high grade fever or those with peritoneal signs, a cross-sectional imaging of the abdomen [computed tomography (CT) vs magnetic resonance imaging (MRI)] is warranted to exclude presence of an abscess. Abscess requires immediate drainage. Once an abscess or any other infective focus has been excluded in patients who are nonresponders to oral steroids parenteral steroids [IV (intravenous) hydrocortisone 100 mg ter die sumendum (TDS) to quater in die (QID)] are administered in divided doses.[16] Nutritional support through elemental feeding or parenteral nutrition (depending upon patients' clinical status) is indicated in patients unable to maintain adequate nutritional requirements. In patients with obstructive symptoms, it is important to differentiate between inflammatory narrowing versus fibrotic strictures or adhesions. Computed tomography enterography or magnetic resonance enterography may help differentiate inflammatory from fibrotic strictures (Fig. 4).

Top-down Therapy (Fig. 6)

Recent evidence as generated by the step-up top-down (SUTD) trial indicates that earlier use of biologics and immunosuppressants would improve clinical outcomes.[17] This study compared the effectiveness of early use of combined immunosuppression with

Table 8: Route of administration and doses of various biologics used in the treatment of Crohn's disease

	Infliximab	*Adalimumab*	*Certolizumab*	*Natalizumab*
Type	Chimeric monoclonal antibody	Fully human monoclonal antibody	Humanized pegylated Fab fragment	Anti-α4-integrin
Route	IV	SC	SC	IV
Induction dose	5 mg/kg at 0, 2, 6 weeks	160 mg at week 0, 80 mg at week 2	400 mg at week 0, 2, and 4	300 mg at 0, 4, 8 weeks
Maintenance dose	5 mg/kg every 8 weeks	40 mg every 2 weeks	400 mg every 4 weeks	300 mg every 4 weeks

Abbreviations: IV, intravenous; SC, subcutaneous.

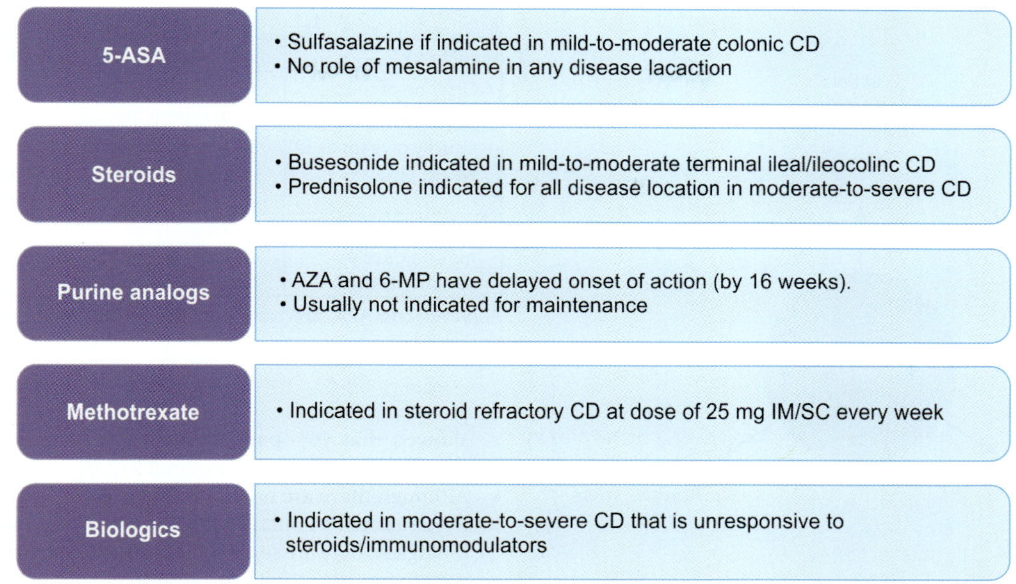

Figure 5 Role of various pharmacological agents in the induction of remission in Crohn's disease
Abbreviations: CD, Crohn's disease; ASA, aminosalicylic acid; AZA, azathioprine; 6-MP, 6-mercaptopurine

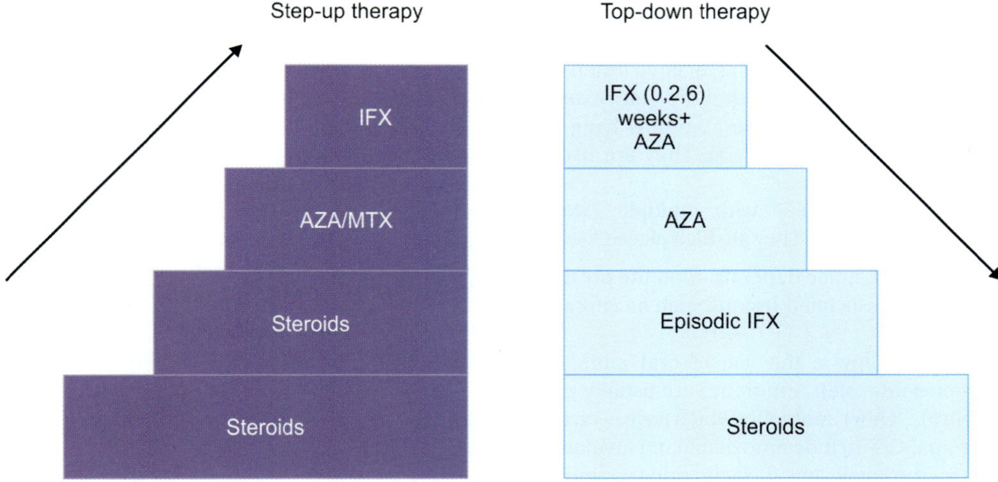

Figure 6 Step-up and top-down therapy in management of Crohn's disease.
Abbreviations: IFX, infliximab; AZA, azathioprine; MTX, methotrexate

infliximab plus AZA ("top-down" therapy) with conventional "step-up" therapy in patients with active CD. The primary outcome measure was remission without corticosteroids or surgery at weeks 26 and 52. At week 26, 60% of patients in the top-down group were in remission without corticosteroids and surgery as compared with 35.9% of patients in the step-up group (P = 0.006). The difference was significant between the two groups up to week 52. Importantly, endoscopic examination revealed that 73.1% of patients receiving top-down therapy had no mucosal ulcers after 2 years compared with only 30.4% of patients receiving step-up therapy.

However, it may be too early to universally treat all patients with CD with a top-down approach. Therefore, it is important to identify a subgroup of patients with an aggressive disease course who may derive the maximum benefit from top-down approach. Beaugerie et al. in a prospective validation cohort of 302 patients identified three independent risk factors at diagnosis which were predictive of a subsequent 5-year disabling CD course (Fig. 7).[18] Patients with two risk factors have a high likelihood of having a disabling course.

Management of Fistulizing Crohn's Disease

Fistulizing disease is seen in one-third of patients with CD. Perianal fistulae are seen in 12% of patients with isolated ileal disease, 15% with ileocolonic disease, 41% with colonic disease, and 92% with colonic disease involving rectum.

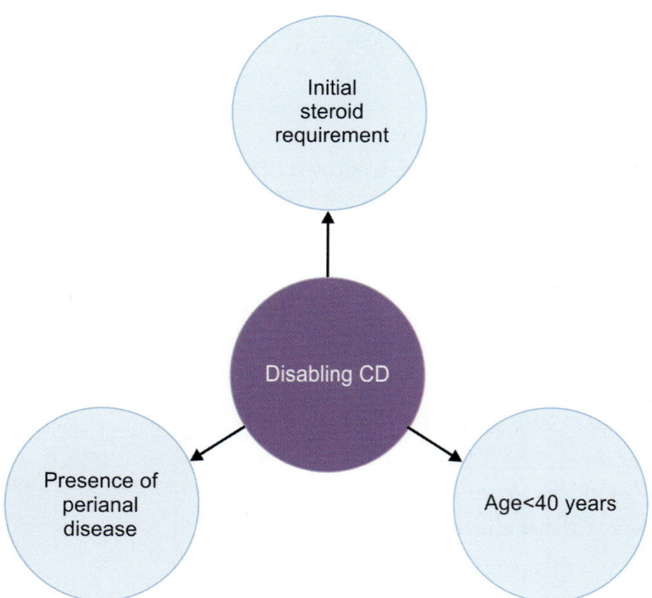

Figure 7 Independent risk factors for disabling Crohn's disease
Abbreviation: CD, Crohn's disease

Perianal fistulae can be classified into simple or complex fistulae depending upon the number of opening and associated lesions.

- Simple fistulae: These are fistulae with only one external opening and no associated abscess. These are low lying and are the most common fistulae seen in CD. They are usually associated with rectal disease.
- Complex fistulae: They are fistulae with multiple external openings and associated abscesses. They are high placed fistulae.

The treatment for perianal fistulae depends upon the presence or absence of infection, and associated lesions such as abscesses (Table 9).

- First line of medical therapy is the use of oral antibiotics (quinolones and metronidazole). Antibiotics are usually given for 8–12 weeks (Table 9).[19] Other antibiotics which have been used in treatment of perianal CD include amoxicillin or clavulanate, trimethoprim sulfamethoxazole, levofloxacin, minocycline and tetracycline.
- There are few uncontrolled series which have reported benefits from short-term treatment with cyclosporine or tacrolimus in patients with perianal CD.[20,21] However, long-term data are lacking, and most patients require subsequent maintenance therapy with AZA or 6-MP. Although several reports from Europe and North America describe long-term improvement with AZA or 6-MP in perianal disease, there are no controlled trials for the same.[22] Similarly, MTX has also shown benefit in some uncontrolled studies, although it has not been prospectively evaluated in a controlled trial.[23]
- The current gold standard for management of fistulizing CD is the use of Infliximab. A placebo controlled trial for induction of remission demonstrated a 62% clinical response, and 46% remission in patients who were nonresponders to prior therapy with antibiotics, corticosteroids, or immunomosupressants.[24] Maintenance therapy trial in responders to induction therapy showed that 46% patients receiving infliximab continued to respond at week 54 as compared to 23% in the placebo group.[25]
- Although there are no controlled trials or uncontrolled studies for treatment of internal fistulae with immunosuppressants or biologics, there are several case series which have demonstrated benefit from MTX with or without infliximab.

Table 9: Medical therapy in fistulizing Crohn's disease

Antibiotics	*Immunomodulators*	*Biologics*
• First line of therapy	• AZA and 6-MP used in long-term therapy	• Current gold standard
• Usually give for 8–12 weeks	• MTX shown benefit in some case series	• Useful for both induction and maintenance
• Quinolones and metronidazole commonly used	• Few reports on cyclosprine and tacrolimus	• Response rate up to 60%

Abbreviations: AZA, azathioprine; MTX, methotrexate; 6-MP, 6-mercaptopurine

Maintenance Therapy in Crohn's Disease

As CD is a lifelong disease and 75% patients have a disease relapse within a year of induction with steroids, maintenance therapy is recommended in majority of patients with CD. However, the length of maintenance therapy in CD is difficult to predict because of the inability to predict individual course of disease, compliance, treatment costs, and long-term drug safety. Agents which have been found to be useful in the maintenance of CD include immunomodulators (AZA, 6-MP and MTX) and biologics. There is no role of 5-ASA agents, steroids, calcineurin inhibitors and antibiotics in the maintenance. As a maintenance agent, budesonide was shown to be effective at 6 mg/day, only for 3 months (supported by a randomized placebo-controlled trial) to 6 months (pooled analysis). Therefore, longer use with budesonide for maintenance cannot be recommended.

Maintenance with Immunomodulators (Purine Analogs and MTX)

Azathiopurine at doses of 2.0–2.5 mg/kg and 6-MP at a dose of 1.5 mg/kg have been shown to be effective at maintaining remission for, at least, 4 years in patients with CD.[26] Blood counts should be monitored frequently early in the course of treatment and at every 3 months in the long-term because of the risk of delayed bone marrow suppression. Pancreatitis may occur in approximately 3–15% of patients, several weeks after initiating therapy and it recurs with reintroduction of either AZA or 6-MP.[27] Neoplasia other than lymphoma, has not been observed with the use of thiopurines in the treatment of IBD.[28] Another rare form of natural killer T cell, hepatosplenic lymphoma has recently been described with AZA therapy either alone or in combination with infliximab.[29] Parenteral MTX at a dose of 15 mg/week has also been shown to maintain remission.[30] Regarding the length of maintenance therapy, it is advisable to continue therapy for 4–5 years. Data beyond 5 years are lacking. Therefore, if patients wish therapy can be stopped after 5 years. However, on relapse immunomodulators should be promptly re-started and therapy should be continued indefinitely.

Maintenance with Biologics

- Scheduled infusions of infliximab at a dose of 5 mg/kg every 8 weeks have been shown to be effective at maintaining remission in both luminal and fistulizing CD.[31] Scheduled therapy has been shown to be more effective than episodic dosing, and it has also been associated with prolonged mucosa healing. Secondly, scheduled therapy is less immunogenic than episodic therapy.
- Can biologics be combined with immunomodulators for maintenance: SONIC trial tried to resolve this issue. This trial included 508 patients with moderate to severe CD who were naïve to biologics and immunomodulators. Patients were randomized to three groups: AZA alone, infliximab alone, and AZA + IFX. At week 26, the proportion of patients in corticosteroid-free clinical remission was significantly greater with IFX-plus-AZA combination therapy and infliximab monotherapy compared with AZA monotherapy (57%, 44% and 31%, respectively). Similarly, proportion of patients with mucosal healing at week 26 was also highest in the combination therapy group. In the SONIC extension phase, a similar trend of efficacy was observed in the three treatment groups at week 50. However, long-term continuation of combination therapy offers no benefit as was shown in an open label randomized control trial. In this trial, patients who had controlled disease more than 6 months after the start of 5 mg/kg infliximab and immunosuppressives were randomized to continue or to stop immunosuppressives, while all patients received scheduled infliximab maintenance therapy for 104 weeks. Patients who continued treatment with immunosuppressives had similar rates of change in infliximab dosing or stopping treatment with infliximab when compared with patients who discontinued immunosuppressives. The endoscopic healing was also similar between both the groups.
- Length of maintenance with infliximab: The benefits of infliximab have been shown to be sustained over a period of more than 4 years. In an observational study of 614 consecutive CD patients, 63% patients were able to sustain clinical benefit over a median follow-up of 55 months.
- However, infliximab can be stopped in some patients as was shown in infliximab diSconTinuation in CD patients in stable Remission on combined therapy with Immunosuppressors (STORI) trial.[32] In this trial, patients who had received scheduled infliximab and immunosuppressants for at least 1 year and were in steroid free clinical remission for more than 6 months were randomized to continue or discontinue infliximab. After 1 year of discontinuation more than 50% patients were in remission. Secondly, patients who relapsed were successfully retreated with infliximab. This trial also suggested predictive factors for relapse after infliximab discontinuation. In a simplified model, it was suggested that out of 6 factors (Box 1) presence of less than 2 factors was associated with a 14–16% relapse rate over 1 year.

Infliximab and Tuberculosis

There is fivefold increased risk of tuberculosis reactivation with infliximab. It usually occurs after a median of 12 weeks of infliximab therapy. Flowchart 2 suggests an algorithm for infliximab therapy in a patient with active tuberculosis (TB) or previous exposure to TB.

BOX 1 Factors predicting relapse after stopping biologics

- No previous surgical resection
- Male gender
- Hemoglobin level ≤14.5 g/L
- Leukocyte count >6 X 10^9/L
- hs-CRP ≥5 mg/L
- Fecal calprotectin ≥300 µg/g

Abbreviations: hsCRP, high sensitive C-reactive protein.

Role of Surgery

Up to 75% of patients with CD will ultimately require surgery. Unlike ulcerative colitis (UC), surgery in CD is not curable as there is a high chance of postoperative recurrence. Therefore, surgery in CD is meant for treating the complications and improvement in quality of life of the patient.

Indications of Surgery (Fig. 8)

Surgery in CD can be emergency or urgent or can be elective. Emergency procedures are indicated in cases of intestinal perforation, rupture of an abscess, massive uncontrolled hemorrhage, fulminant Crohn's colitis with or without toxic megacolon, and severe perianal sepsis. Elective procedures take into account various factors such as nutritional status, patient willingness, nature of the disease and medical and surgical history. Elective surgery is indicated in stricturing disease, fistulizing disease (both internal fistulae and perianal disease) and failure of medical therapy and malignancy.

Surgical Procedures

Emergency or Urgent Procedures

- *Intra-abdominal abscess:* The procedure is usually started with percutaneous drainage, intravenous antibiotics and parenteral nutrition. Definitive surgery is performed several weeks later when it is safe to undertake the procedure. Urgent open surgery and drainage of abscess and abdominal cavity is undertaken in undrained abscesses or failed to drain abscesses. Definitive surgery with bowel removal is done a few weeks later.
- *Fulminant Crohn's colitis:* With fulminant colitis, the conservative management is intensified with steroids + parenteral nutrition + antibiotics. Infliximab should be considered. If there is no improvement in 7 days, conservative approach should be stopped and urgent surgery should be performed. With toxic megacolon, the intensification of treatment should continue for no more than 72 hours. Surgical help should be sought, if there is no positive response within 72 hours.
- *Severe perianal sepsis:* This condition requires aggressive intravenous antibiotics and parenteral nutrition along with drainage of abscess and ostomy.
- *Massive uncontrolled hemorrhage:* Massive uncontrolled hemorrhage is a rare complication of CD and occurs in approximately 1% patients. Unlike UC, massive hemorrhage in CD usually occurs from a single site where an ulcer has eroded into a large vessel. Hence a pre-operative angiography is advised to localize the bleeding point and embolize, if feasible. Surgery is only indicated in case of uncontrolled bleeding.

Flow chart 2 Infliximab treatment in patients with exposure to tuberculosis

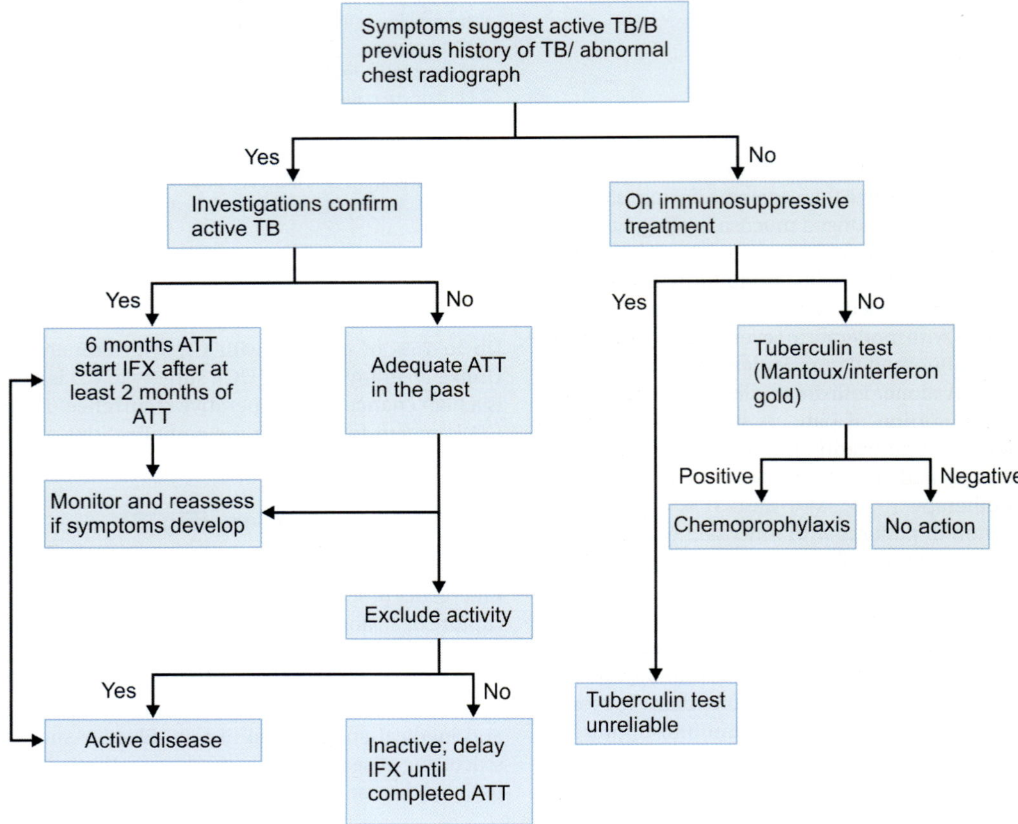

Abbreviations: TB, tuberculosis; IFX, infliximab; ATT, antitubercular therapy.

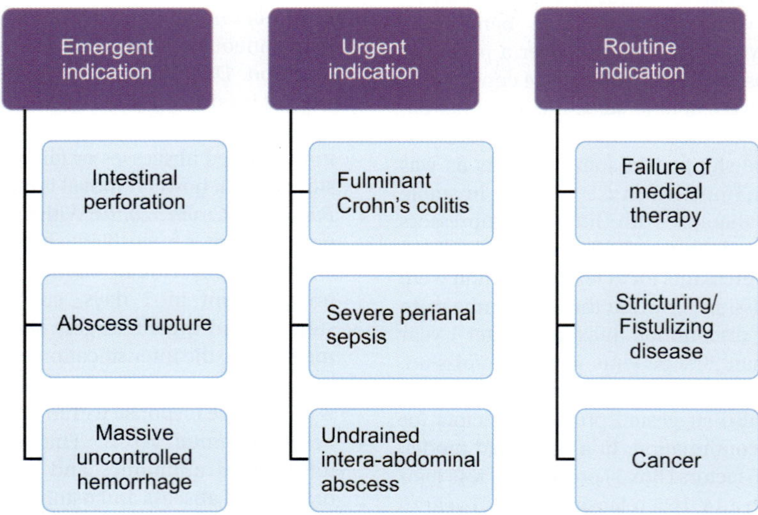

Figure 8 Indications for surgery in Crohn's disease

Elective Procedures

Small bowel Crohn's disease: Common indications for surgery in small bowel CD include structuring disease causing obstruction, internal fistulae and abscesses and small bowel cancer.

Stricturing disease: It is important to find out the type of stricture (inflammatory, fibrotic or anastomotic) as the management depends upon the etiology of stricture. Bowel stricturing usually results in obstructive symptoms. Acute obstruction usually settles with conservative therapy. Further therapy depends upon the type of stricture. Quantitative C-reactive protein and magnetic resonance (MR) enteroclysis help in determining, if the stricture has more of an inflammatory component. Inflammatory stricture would respond to medical therapy, and endoscopic dilatation may be useful in some cases. Endoscopic dilatation is recommended for anastomotic stricture. Fibrotic strictures usually do not respond to medical therapy and surgery is indicated. The general indications for surgery are: two or more episodes of partial recurrent bowel obstruction within a year, failure to discontinue steroid therapy after 12–16 weeks or doses of prednisolone more than 15 mg/day are required for more than 3–6 months following an obstructive episode. Resection or stricturoplasty is performed in most of the cases. Bypass procedures are now out dated and only indication for bypass procedure is gastrojejunostomy for duodenal CD.

- *Stricturoplasty:* The rationale behind this technique is that it corrects obstruction as well as preserves the functional intestinal length. It is, therefore indicated when there are multiple skip lesions or patients have had multiple resections in the past. With small bowel strictures less than 10 cm in length, conventional stricturoplasty (Heineke–Mikulicz stricturoplasty form), which is the most widely accepted form, is considered appropriate. For longer strictures, up to 25 cm in length, side-to-side stricturoplasty (Finney stricturoplasty) is considered appropriate. Stricturoplasty for colonic disease is not generally recommended as often the adjoining mucosa is also involved.
- *Resection and anastomosis*: It is usually indicated either in single strictures or when there are multiple short segment strictures and the remaining bowel length is sufficient to avoid short bowel syndrome. There is no surgical technique that can reduce the risk of postoperative recurrent CD and the technique depends upon the surgeon's choice. Presence of histologic disease at resection margin is not predictive for a greater risk of recurrence.

Surgery for Crohn's colitis: The most common indication for surgery in large bowel CD is failure of medical therapy. The type of surgery depends upon the extent of involvement. There is no role of stricturoplasty in large bowel CD.

- In case of rectal sparing and absence of perianal disease the recommended procedure is colectomy with ileorectal anastomosis.
- In patients with pancolitis and/or perianal disease total proctocolectomy is recommended. The major complication of this surgery is the risk of an unhealed perineal wound, which may occur in up to 20% of the patients.

Perianal CD: There is a combined role of medical as well as surgical therapy in the management of perianal fistulizing CD. The initial step in fistula therapy should be the drainage of abscesses and dilatation of anorectal strictures. In addition, assessment of fistula may be done with examination under anesthesia or MRI of pelvis or endoscopic ultrasound. The surgical procedures which have been found useful include:

- Seton placement: Seton is a silk string or a rubber band which is used to either create a scar tissue around part of the sphincter muscle before cutting it with a knife, or allow it to slowly cut all the way through the muscle over the course of several weeks. The principle behind seton placement is that unless the feeding abscess or infection is drained completely no fistula will close permanently. After the fistula is partially excised the external opening has a tendency to close faster than the internal opening. As the internal opening is inside either an abscess cavity or anus or rectum early closure of external orifice would trap the infection inside and result in recurrent abscess formation. Therefore, by keeping the fistula tract patent and draining for a longer time seton allows for gradual and complete drainage of infection, and thus healing of the fistula. A seton may stay in place for as long as 3–12 months.
- Fistulotomy: Fistulotomy requires probing by the surgeon to find internal opening of the fistula. After this the surgeon cuts the internal opening of the fistula, scrapes and flushes out the infected tissue, stitches its sides to the sides of the incision in order to lay open the fistula. Fistulotomy may be done in two stages, if a significant amount of sphincter muscle must be cut or if the entire channel is not found. Fistulotomy is usually recommended for low fistulae as laying open high fistulae may involve a large amount of external sphincter and this entails the risk of incontinence. Promising alternatives with limited experience for high placed fistulae include: long-term seton, fibrin glue, fibrin plug or flap advancement procedure.
- About 10% patients with perianal fistulizing CD may require proctectomy and permanent ileostomy.

Postoperative Recurrence

Unlike UC, surgery in CD is not curative as disease inexorably recurs. Postoperative clinical recurrence rates are 30% at 3 years and 60% at 1 year. Endoscopic recurrence usually precedes clinical recurrence with a recurrence rate of 65–0% at 1 year and 80–100% at 3 years. Further clinical recurrence is best predicted by endoscopic recurrence. Factors predicting early postoperative recurrence are listed in Box 2.[33]

Therefore, endoscopic examination of the anastomotic site is recommended within 6 months of surgery. This categorizes the risk and severity of postoperative recurrence. Rutgeerts endoscopic score predicts post-operative recurrence (Table 9). An endoscopic grade of 0–2 suggests a lower recurrence risk and a higher score predicts a greater risk of disease recurrence.

Evidence is continuously growing in favor of postoperative therapy to prevent recurrence of disease. Although early trials demonstrated benefits with more than 3 g/day of mesalamine which would reduce the risk of recurrence for up to 3 years, more recent controlled trials have been less supportive.[34] Short-term metronidazole at high doses (20 mg/kg) and ornidazole at 1 g/day for a year have also been shown to reduce the likelihood of recurrence for up to 1 year. Steroids (prednisolone or budesonide) have not been found to effective in reducing the risk of postoperative recurrence. Recent trials have demonstrated benefits with immunosuppressant (AZA/6-MP) as compared with placebo and mesalamine.[35] Recently, infliximab has also shown efficacy in the prevention of both clinical and endoscopic postoperative recurrence.[36]

BOX 2 Factors predicting early postoperative recurrence in Crohn's disease

- Smoking
- Extent >100 cm
- Fistulizing disease
- Shorter preoperative disease duration
- Previous surgery

Table 9: Endoscopic scoring system for postoperative recurrence in Crohn's disease

Grade	*Endoscopic findings*
0	No lesions in distal ileum
1	<5 aphthous lesions
2	>5 aphthous lesions with normal mucosa between the lesions, or skip areas of larger lesions, or lesions confined to ileocolonic anastomosis (i.e. <1 cm in length)
3	Diffuse aphthous ileitis with diffusely inflamed mucosa
4	Diffuse inflammation with already larger ulcers, nodules, and/or narrowing

Algorithm for Management of Crohn's Disease (Fig. 9)

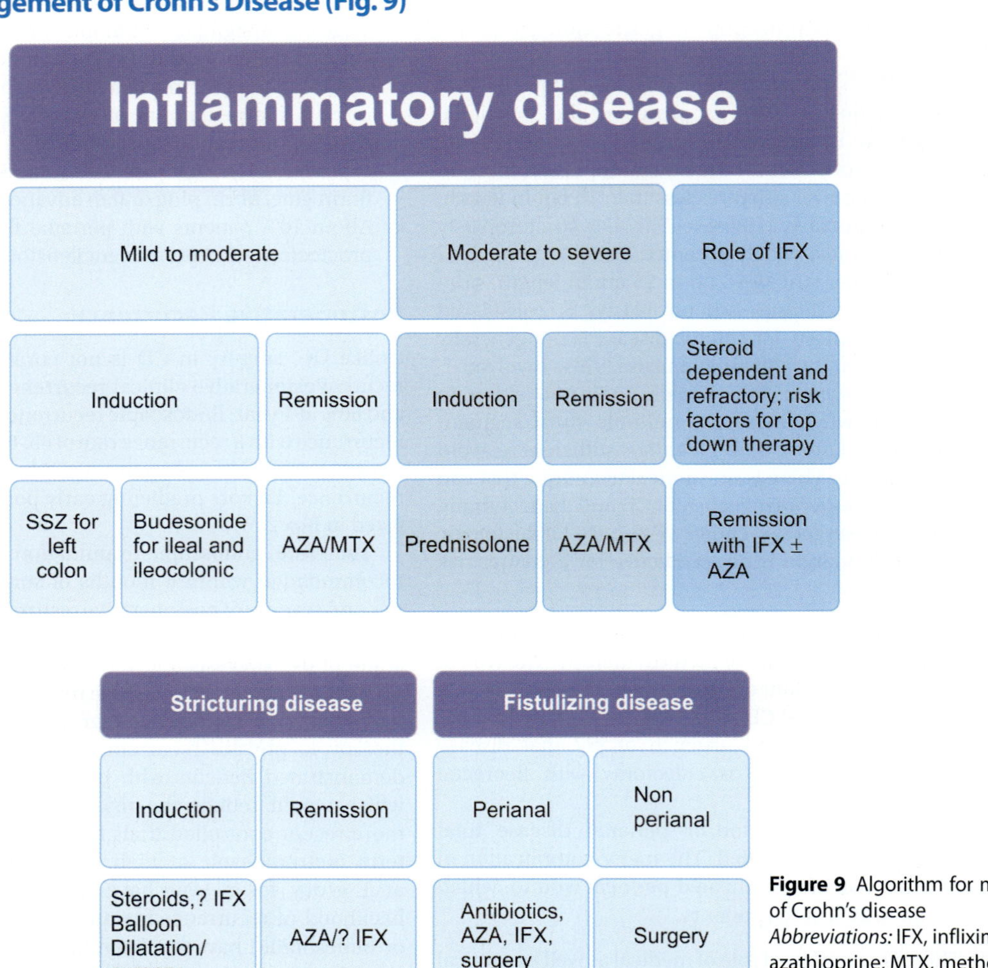

Figure 9 Algorithm for management of Crohn's disease
Abbreviations: IFX, infliximab; AZA, azathioprine; MTX, methotrexate; SSZ, sulfasalazine.

REFERENCES

1. Sands BE. From symptom to diagnosis: clinical distinctions among various forms of intestinal inflammation. Gastroenterology. 2004;126:1518-32.
2. Geboes K, Rutgeerts P, Opdenakker G, Olson A, Patel K, Wagner CL, et al. Endoscopic and histologic evidence of persistent mucosal healing and correlation with clinical improvement following sustained infliximab treatment for Crohn's disease. Curr Med Res Opin. 2005;21:1741-54.
3. Sandborn WJ, Feagan BG, Hanauer SB, Lochs H, Löfberg R, Modigliani R, et al. A review of activity indices and efficacy endpoints for clinical trials of medical therapy in adults with Crohn's disease. Gastroenterology. 2002;122:512-30.
4. Sostegni R, Daperno M, Scaglione N, Lavagna A, Rocca R, Pera A. Review article: Crohn's disease: monitoring disease activity. Aliment Pharmacol Ther. 2003;17(Suppl 2):11-7.
5. Summers RW, Switz DM, Sessions JT, Becktel JM, Best WR, Kern F, et al. National Cooperative Crohn's Disease Study: results of drug treatment. Gastroenterology. 1979;77(4 Pt 2):847-69.

6. Malchow H, Ewe K, Brandes JW, Goebell H, Ehms H, Sommer H, et al. European Cooperative Crohn's Disease Study (ECCDS): results of drug treatment. Gastroenterology. 1984;86(2):249-66.
7. Hanauer SB, Stromberg U. Oral Pentasa in the treatment of active Crohn's disease: a meta-analysis of double-blind, placebo-controlled trials. Clin Gastroenterol Hepatol. 2004;2:379-88.
8. Sutherland L, Singleton J, Sessions J, Hanauer S, Krawitt E, Rankin G, et al. Double blind, placebo controlled trial of metronidazole in Crohn's disease. Gut. 1991;32:1071-5.
9. Selby W, Pavli P, Crotty B, Florin T, Radford-Smith G, Gibson P, et al. Two-year combination antibiotic therapy with clarithromycin, rifabutin, and clofazimine for Crohn's disease. Gastroenterology. 2007;132:2313-9.
10. Thomsen OO, Cortot A, Jewell D, Wright JP, Winter T, Veloso FT, et al. A comparison of budesonide and mesalamine for active Crohn's disease. International Budesonide–Mesalamine Study Group. N Engl J Med. 1998;339:370-4.
11. Rutgeerts P, Loferg R, Malchow H, Lamers C, Olaison G, Jewell D, et al. A comparison of budesonide with prednisolone for active Crohn's disease. N Engl J Med. 1994;331:842-5.
12. Bernstein CN, Leslie WD, Leboff MS. AGA technical review on osteoporosis in gastrointestinal diseases. Gastroenterology. 2003;124(3):795-841.
13. Sandborn W, Sutherland L, Pearson D, May G, Modigliani R, Prantera C. Azathioprine or 6-mercaptopurine for inducing remission of Crohn's disease. Cochrane Database Syst Rev. 2000;(2):CD000545.
14. Targan SR, Hanauer SB, van Deventer SJ, Mayer L, Present DH, Braakman T, et al. A short-term study of chimeric monoclonal antibody cA2 to tumor necrosis factor alpha for Crohn's disease. Crohn's Disease cA2 Study Group. N Engl J Med. 1997;337:1029-35.
15. Colombel JF, Sandborn WJ, Reinisch W, Mantzaris GJ, Kornbluth A, Rachmilewitz D, et al. Infliximab, azathioprine, or combination therapy for Crohn's disease. N Engl J Med. 2010;362:1383-95.
16. Kornbluth A, Marion JF, Salomon P, Janowitz HD. How effective is current medical therapy for severe ulcerative and Crohn's colitis? An analytic review of selected trials. J Clin Gastroenterol. 1995;20(4):280-4.
17. D'Haens GR. Top-down therapy for Crohn's disease: rationale and evidence. Acta Clin Belg. 2009;64(6):540-6.
18. Beaugerie L, Seksik P, Nion-Larmurier I, Gendre JP, Cosnes J. Predictors of Crohn's disease. Gastroenterology. 2006;130(3):650-6.
19. Bernstein LH, Frank MS, Brandt LJ, et al. Healing of perineal Crohn's disease with metronidazole. Gastroenterology. 1980;795:357-65.
20. Egan LJ, Sandborn WJ, Tremaine WJ. Clinical outcome following treatment of refractory inflammatory and fistulizing Crohn's disease with intravenous cyclosporine. Am J Gastroenterol. 1998;93:442-8.
21. Fellermann K, Ludwig D, Stahl M, David-Walek T, Stange EF. Steroid-unresponsive acute attacks of inflammatory bowel disease: immunomodulation by tacrolimus (FK506). Am J Gastroenterol. 1998;93:1860-6.
22. Rutgeerts P. Review article: treatment of perianal fistulizing Crohn's disease. Aliment Pharmacol Ther. 2004;20(Suppl 4):106-10.
23. Mahadevan U, Marion JF, Present DH. Fistula response to methotrexate in Crohn's disease: a case series. Aliment Pharmacol Ther. 2003;18(10):1003-8.
24. Present DH, Rutgeerts P, Targan S, Hanauer SB, Mayer L, van Hogezand RA, et al. Infliximab for the treatment of fistulas in patients with Crohn's disease. N Engl J Med. 1999;340(18):1398-405.
25. Sands BE, Anderson FH, Bernstein CN, Chey WY, Feagan BG, Fedorak RN, et al. Infliximab maintenance therapy for fistulizing Crohn's disease. N Engl J Med. 2004;350:876-85.
26. Pearson DC, May GR, Fick G, Sutherland LR. Azathioprine for maintaining remission of Crohn's disease. Cochrane Database Syst Rev. 2000;(2):CD000067.
27. Lichtenstein GR, Abreu MT, Cohen R, Tremaine W; American Gastroenterological Association. American Gastroenterological Association Institute technical review on corticosteroids, immunomodulators, and infliximab in inflammatory bowel disease. Gastroenterology. 2006;130:940-87.
28. Kandiel A, Fraser AG, Korelitz BI, Brensinger C, Lewis JD. Increased risk of lymphoma among inflammatory bowel disease patients treated with azathioprine and 6-mercaptopurine. Gut. 2005;54:1121-5.
29. Navarro JT, Ribera JM, Mate JL, Granada I, Juncà J, Batlle M, et al. Hepatosplenic T-gammadelta lymphoma in a patient with Crohn's disease treated with azathioprine. Leuk Lymphoma. 2003;44: 531-3.
30. Lemann M, Zenjar T, Bouhnik Y, Cosnes J, Mesnard B, Rambaud JC, et al. Methotrexate in Crohn's disease: long-term efficacy and toxicity. Am J Gastroenterol. 2000;95(7):1730-4.
31. Hanauer SB, Feagan BG, Lichtenstein GR, Mayer LF, Schreiber S, Colombel JF, et al. Maintenance infliximab for Crohn's disease:the ACCENT I randomized trial. Lancet. 2002;359(9317):1541-9.
32. Louis E, Vernier-Massouille G, Grimaud J, et al. Infliximab discontinuation in Crohn's disease patients in stable remission on combined therapy with immunosuppressors: a prospective ongoing cohort study. Gastroenterology. 2009;136:A-146.
33. Yamamoto T. Factors affecting recurrence after surgery for Crohn's disease. World J Gastroenterol. 2005;11(26):3971-9.
34. Camma C, Giunta M, Rosselli M, Cottone M. Mesalamine in the maintenance treatment of Crohn's disease: a meta-analysis adjusted for confounding variables. Gastroenterology. 1997;113:1465-73.
35. Hanauer SB, Korelitz BI, Rutgeerts P, Peppercorn MA, Thisted RA, Cohen RD, et al. Postoperative maintenance of Crohn's disease remission with 6-mercaptopurine, mesalamine, or placebo: a 2-year trial. Gastroenterology. 2004;127(3):723-9.
36. Regueiro MMD, Schraut WMDP, Baidoo LMD, et al. Infliximab for prevention of Crohn's Disease (CD) recurrence after ileal resection. Am J Gastroenterol. 2008;103(Suppl):S412.

CHAPTER 95

Surgery for Crohn's Disease

Benjamin Perakath

INTRODUCTION

Crohn's disease (CD) is a chronic inflammatory bowel disease that can affect any part of the intestine, from the mouth to the anus. The role and effectiveness of surgery for CD have been questioned in the past and have gained a bad reputation. Hence the medical gastroenterologists are reluctant to refer patients for surgery, even when indicated. It must be emphasized that surgery for CD is highly specialized and individualized, and should be performed only in centers with experience in managing such patients. When operated on by experts for the right indications, results are good, with patients achieving relief of symptoms and improvement of nutritional and general status.[1] Because it is a chronic relapsing disease, recurrence is common and most patients will require reoperation in 8–10 years. However, quality of life is much improved in the interval.

PRINCIPLES OF SURGERY IN CROHN'S DISEASE

The type of operation will depend on the site of involvement and the particular patient's previous surgical history. It also depends on the type of disease the patient has, e.g. fistulizing or obstructing.

Extent of Resection

As CD affects different sites of the bowel at different times, the extent of resection has to be balanced against adequate excision of diseased bowel. The required margins of resection have always been controversial, with some authors favoring wide margins proximal and distal to palpable disease. Others have shown closer margins are adequate.[2] Most experts now aim to preserve as much bowel as possible. Microscopic disease at the resection margins does not seem to affect local recurrence rates (Figs 1A and B).

Mode of Anastomosis

There is a general feeling that anastomoses in CD are prone to leak. This is not borne out by the evidence. Leak rates in CD with hand-sewn end to end anastomoses may have a higher leak rate as compared to side to side or end to side anastomoses. Others have shown no difference in the leak rates between stapled and hand-sewn anastomoses.[3] Some authors feel that anastomoses should be wide and, therefore, side to side to decrease anastomotic recurrence, but evidence does not support this belief.[4]

Measurement of Bowel Length

As re-resections in CD are not uncommon, it is vital to measure the length of bowel resected and also the length of bowel remaining. A convenient way of doing this is to use a length of suture 30 cm long. The suture is placed over unstretched bowel from the duodenojejunal (DJ) flexure repeatedly, to the point of interest and the length of bowel measured and recorded in the operation notes, preferably with a diagram to aid the surgeon at the next operation. In our country, where patients move from surgeon to surgeon, this is vital. A copy of the operation notes should ideally be given to the patient.

Assessment of Strictures

However good preoperative imaging may be assessment of strictures has to be done at laparotomy. A dominant proximal stricture on contrast study does not permit assessment of downstream strictures. The most convenient way of distinguishing significant from non-significant strictures is to "trawl" a Foley's bulb inflated to 2 cm diameter through an enterotomy. Strictures that do not allow this balloon to pass need to be dealt with surgically, either by resection or by stricturoplasty.

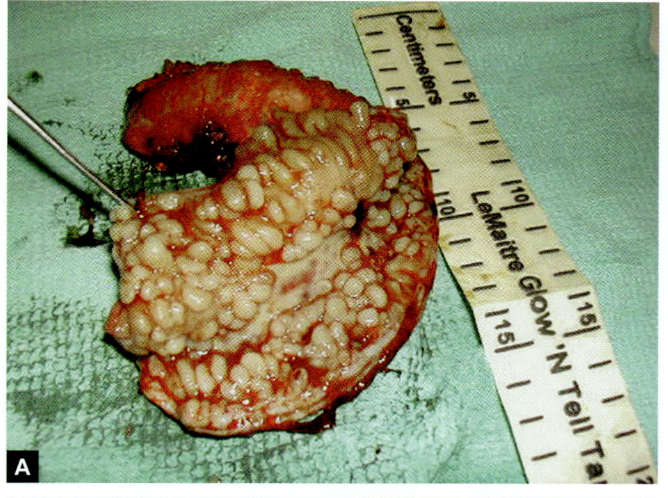

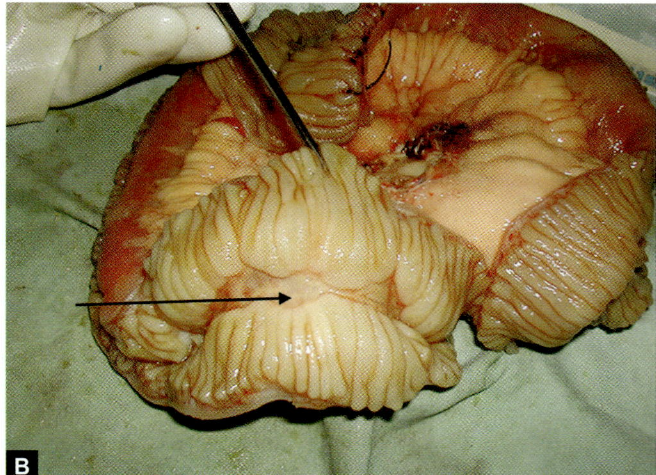

Figures 1A and B (A) Typical cobblestoning in Crohn's disease, (B) Typical Crohn's ulcer in small bowel: Longitudinal, on mesenteric border

ILEOCECAL DISEASE

Ileocecal disease in a young patient is best resected. This will necessitate at least a limited right hemicolectomy.

FISTULATING DISEASE (FIGS 3A AND B)

The diseased segment requires resection. The fistula is usually disconnected in the process of dissecting out the involved loops of bowel. The non-diseased loop does not require resection, and suture of the fistula usually suffices. Fistulae to the skin are dealt with likewise. Granulation tissue in the fistulous tract will require to be curetted.

BYPASS OPERATIONS

Bypass of obstructing lesions should be avoided for fear of missing a malignancy, or of malignancy developing in the diseased segment.

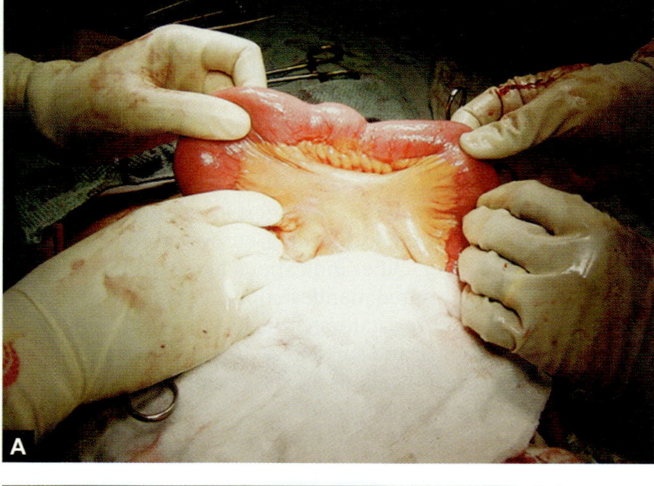

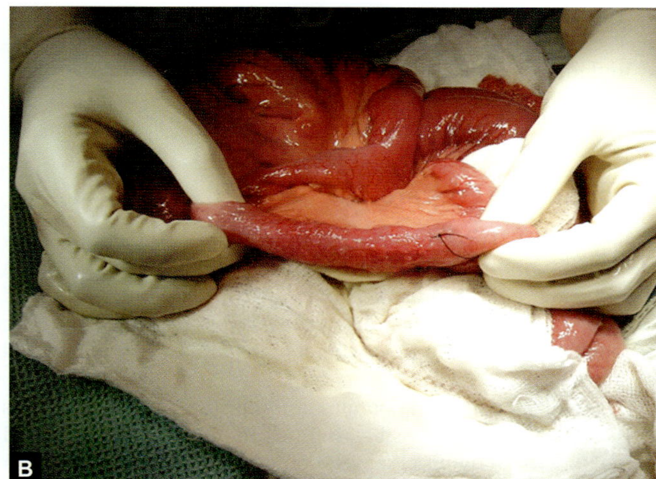

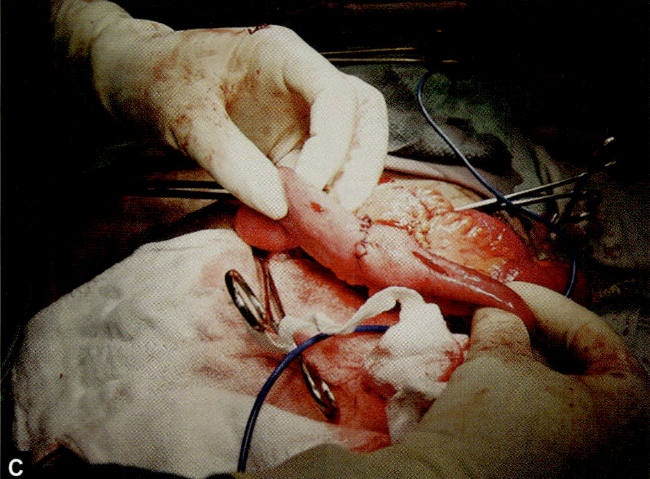

Figures 2A to C (A) Typical Crohn's strictures of small bowel, (B) Diseased segment of small bowel marked for stricturoplasty, (C) Stricturoplasty completed

COLONIC CROHN'S DISEASE

There is controversy regarding management of segmental colonic CD. Segmental resections as well as subtotal colectomy have been advised.[5]

Indications for Surgery

Surgery for CD is synonymous with surgery for complications of CD. Thus obstruction, perforation, bleeding, etc. would constitute some indications for surgery. Other indications like growth retardation in children, extra-intestinal manifestations and failure of medical management (steroid resistant/steroid dependent) require close dialog between medical and surgical gastroenterologist.

The following are indications for surgery in CD:

- Obstruction-fibro-stenotic lesions
- Perforation
- Fistulae
- Hemorrhage
- Carcinoma
- Inflammatory mass and abscess
- Growth retardation
- Failure of medical management.

Preoperative Preparation

Patients with CD who require surgery are often malnourished. This is often a combination of poor nutrition due to abdominal pain and chronic intestinal obstruction and chronic intra-abdominal sepsis. Enteroenteric fistulae can result in malabsorption secondary to exclusion of varying lengths of bowel and bacterial overgrowth.

A varying period of preoperative optimization for surgery results in better outcomes. If possible, steroids should be weaned off and stopped. Intra-abdominal sepsis should be treated with antibiotics and percutaneous drainage. Enteral or parenteral nutrition for a few weeks will bring the serum albumin to 3G/L or more. A balance has to be struck between prolonged preoperative preparation and unrelieved symptoms. These measures undoubtedly result in better outcomes and have considerably improved success rates in this group of poor risk patients.

Site Specific Operations

Gastroduodenal Crohn's Disease

This usually occurs in association with CD at other sites, and fortunately is rare, occurring in 2–4% of cases. The classical teaching for treating such disease surgically has been to bypass the segment by performing a gastrojejunostomy with vagotomy or a Roux-en-Y duodenojejunostomy. Some authors favor stricturoplasty of duodenal lesions,[6] which eliminates complications like stasis, marginal ulceration, recurrent obstruction and fistula formation. Stricturoplasty in this situation would mean a Heinecke-Miculicz or Finney stricturoplasty. Ultimately, the decision to bypass or to do a stricturoplasty would depend on the part and extent of duodenum involved. One must always keep the possibility of a malignancy in a stricture in mind and any suspicious areas should be biopsied and frozen section obtained.

Small Bowel Crohn's Disease (Figs 1A and B)

The small bowel is the most frequently involved part of the GI tract in CD. Conservation of bowel length is the prime principle to be followed whatever the type of lesion or its location.

The most common indication for surgery is obstruction, often at the ileocecal area. Surgery for CD was revolutionized when it was realized that stricturoplasties could be safely performed through diseased bowel without leaks or fistulae, and with amelioration of symptoms.[7] The easiest and most common stricturoplasty performed is the Heinecke-Miculicz stricturoplasty (Figs. 2A to C), where the stricture is incised longitudinally to 1-2 cm beyond the stricture and the defect closed transversely with interrupted sutures (Figs 2A to C). An isolated lesion is usually amenable to excision. A short segment of bowel with multiple strictures close to each other is also ideally resected. In situations where bowel has already been resected previously and further resection is unsafe, a side to side isoperistaltic stricturoplasty is recommended (Michelassi).Strictures far apart from each other with normal intervening bowel are best treated by multiple stricturoplasties. There should be at least 5 cm between stricturoplasties to avoid bunching up of bowel. Stricturoplasty is contraindicated in the following situations:

- Perforation
- Active inflammation
- Multiple strictures in a short segment
- Stricture close to site of resection
- Colonic strictures
- Suspicion of cancer
- Hypoalbuminemia.

The principles outlined above need to be followed in dealing with jejunoileal CD, i.e. conservation of length, complete mobilization, measurement of bowel, etc.

When bowel is resected, management of the mesentery can be challenging. There is often thickened and inflamed mesentery that requires division between clamps with suture ligature of the mesenteric vessels. Modern energy sealing devices have made this tedious part of the operation easier and quicker. Grossly involved bowel is resected close to the palpable edge of the involved bowel. Continuity is restored with an end to end or side to side anastomosis, either hand-sewn or stapled.

Fistulating Disease (Figs 3A and B)

Small bowel CD may fistulate into various organs. This occurs in about 5% of patients with CD. These fistulae may be internal into other intra-abdominal organs or external, to the skin. The principle of surgery for fistulating disease is to resect the diseased bowel from which the fistula arises and to close the defect in the organ to which the fistula is formed. Therefore, an ileovesical fistula would require resection of diseased ileum and closure of the defect in the bladder. Resection of the secondarily involved organ is seldom necessary, but may be required with large defects.

Internal fistulae in themselves are often asymptomatic and many do not require surgical intervention. Surgery is indicated for recurrent symptoms like urinary tract infections, malabsorption due to bypass of long segments of bowel, etc. Chronic moderate/large volume discharge from external fistulae to the skin may also require surgical intervention.

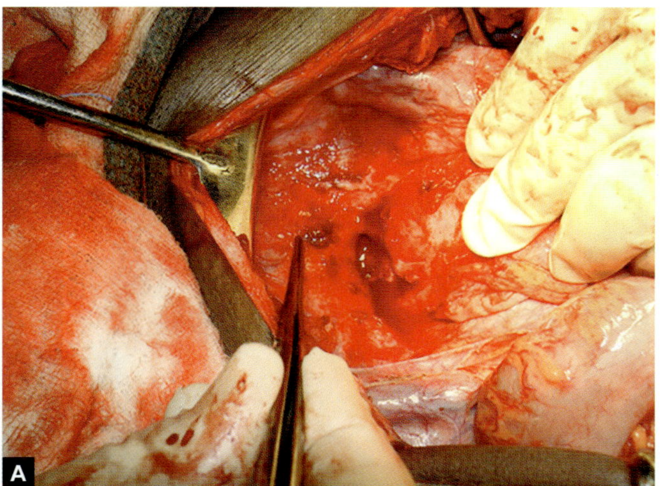

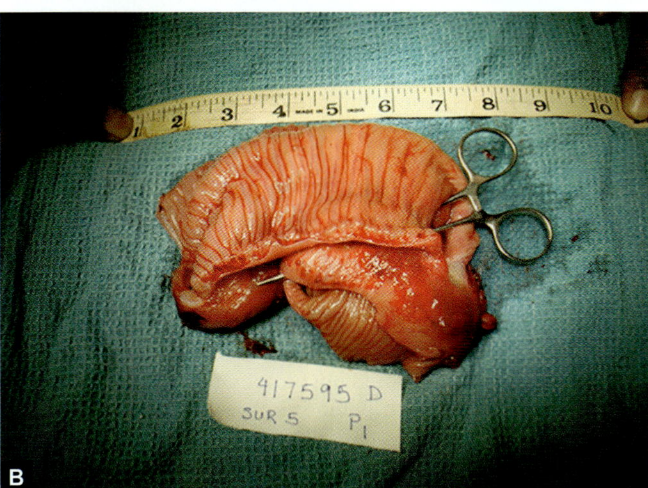

Figures 3A to B (A) Internal fistula in CD between sigmoid colon and bladder, (B) Internal fistula in CD

Intra-abdominal Abscesses

These are often small and indolent, and do not require drainage. Abscesses related to diseased bowel being resected are automatically drained during dissection. Large collections are best drained percutaneously and preoperatively. Occasionally, surgery is required for open drainage of abscesses. Percutaneous drainage prior to elective resection of bowel is said to minimize the extent of bowel resection.

ILEOCOLIC DISEASE

Ileocolic disease is the most common presentation of CD. In a young patient, this is best resected by a limited ileocolic resection (limited right hemicolectomy). This often mimics acute appendicitis and is discovered at surgery. Often an appendicectomy alone is done, and symptoms persist. A discerning surgeon will be able to diagnose Crohn's, if experienced. If technical competence to do an emergency right hemicolectomy is lacking, the case must be referred to

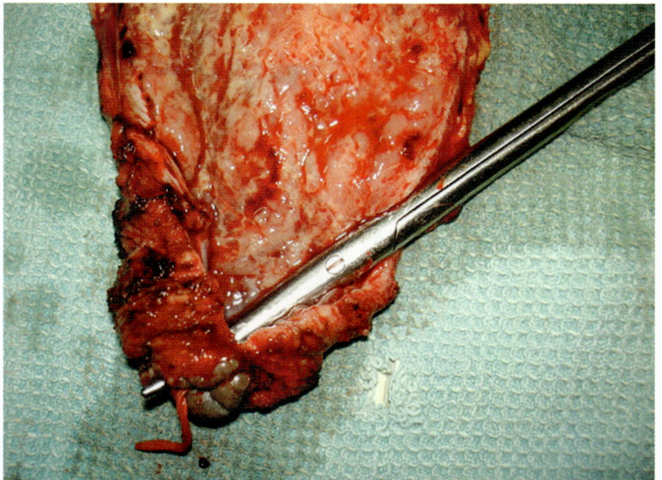

Figure 4 Proctectomy in CD

an expert. Very rarely, in the presence of a fixed phlegmon, a temporary ileocolic bypass maybe necessary.

COLONIC CROHN'S DISEASE

Colonic CD occurs in up to 30% of patients. This may be isolated, or more often, combined with CD at other sites. In the colon, it may be segmental or diffuse, with or without rectal involvement.

Symptoms that require surgical intervention are intractable diarrhea, strictures causing obstruction or preventing complete colonoscopy, dysplasia and risk of cancer, and internal fistulae. The extent of resection depends on the site and extent of disease. As mentioned above, ileocolic disease requires at least a limited right hemicolectomy. If the ascending colon is involved, a formal right hemicolectomy is mandatory. Segmental resections may be performed for isolated disease in the transverse or descending colon. For pancolitis, a subtotal colectomy may be necessary. Unlike in ulcerative colitis, restorative proctocolectomy is not recommended in CD for fear of pouchitis and CD developing in the pouch. The fear of living with a permanent ileostomy is one of the reasons; such patients are not optimally managed in India. In patients with rectal sparing, colectomy and ileorectal anastomosis is an option. Severe rectal disease alone will require proctectomy. The cumulative risk of proctectomy is 8.4% at 10 years and 17.5% after 20 years. A descending colostomy is preferred to a low rectal anastomosis in CD after proctectomy alone, for fear of anastomotic leak or reoperation, low in the pelvis at a later date, for recurrence. Rectal disease may manifest as perianal disease. In general, perianal disease is managed conservatively as far as possible, but when associated with rectal disease, necessitates proctectomy. The perineal approach should be in the intersphincteric plane, to decrease chances of impaired wound healing and non-healing sinuses. The indications for proctectomy (Fig. 4) include:

- Failed medical and conservative surgical therapy
- Multiple previous operations with sphincter damage
- Severe intractable proctitis
- Severe disease with complex fistulae
- Fistula associated carcinoma.

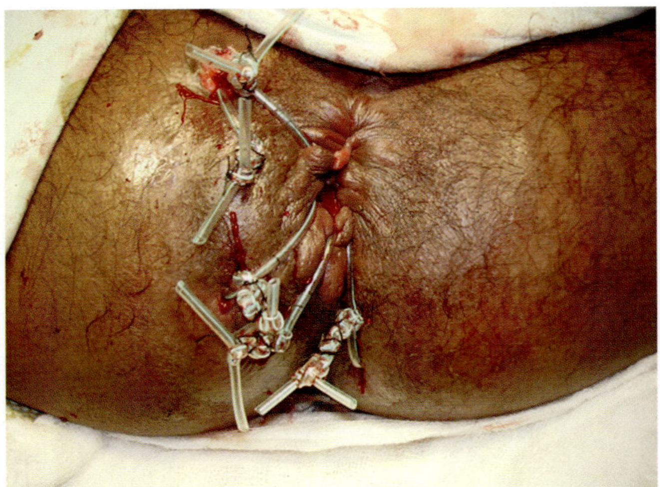

Figure 5 Multiple anal fistulae in CD treated with multiple setons

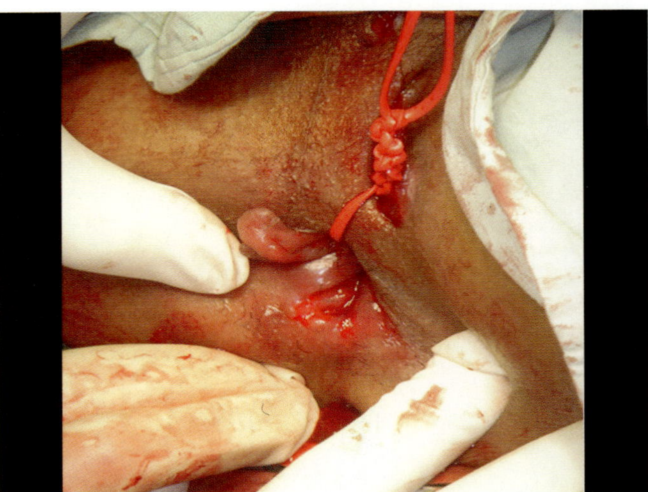

Figure 6 Typical fissures in CD. Note edematous skin tag and associated fistula

HEMORRHAGE

Fortunately, this is a rare complication of CD. Acute severe colonic bleeding will need emergency, subtotal colectomy and ileostomy. Chronic small bowel blood loss will require resection of diseased bowel. Intraoperative enteroscopy is a useful adjunct to detect hitherto unsuspected sources of bleeding.

PERIANAL DISEASE

Perianal CD is seen in 20–30% of patients. It may be the first manifestation of the disease, even before the bowel is involved (45% of patients). Further, it may be indistinguishable from cryptoglandular perianal disease initially. Perianal CD may present as one or more of the following:

- Fistulae (Fig. 5)
- Fissures (Fig. 6)
- Hemorrhoids
- Abscess
- Ulcers
- Strictures
- Skin tags
- Carcinoma.

Perianal CD should be suspected if perianal disease does not subside with routine management or with unusual presentations like atypical fissures, complex fistulae, indurated hemorrhoids, intestinal or extra-intestinal symptoms.

Crohn's fistula should be suspected if there are unusual external openings, if the bladder or vagina is involved, if there are multiple openings and associated fissures or abscesses. The problem with these fistulae which distinguish them from cryptoglandular fistulae is that they recur, and are associated with sphincter damage and incontinence. Surgical management is conservative. As far as possible, fistulotomy should be avoided and the fistulae managed with long-term setons, combined with medical therapy. These loose setons avoid a stoma, are long term, provide drainage and are often found to be well accepted by patients.[8] Other surgical options include fistulotomy, endorectal advancement flaps (contraindicated with proctitis), fibrin glue, plugs and eventually, if all else fail and if there is proctitis, proctectomy.

Fissures in CD are often atypical-multiple, with edematous skin tags, non-healing and, surprisingly, painless. These are managed nonoperatively as far as possible. A tailored lateral anal sphincterotomy may be performed if necessary, provided there is no proctitis. Skin tags should be left alone and not excised for fear of the non-healing wound.

Abscesses are treated by incision and drainage.

Hemorrhoids in CD should not be operated on.

Anal ulcers in CD are painful and are managed medically. Surgical intervention is to be strictly avoided.

Anorectal strictures, if inflammatory may be amenable to dilatation. Fibrotic strictures, if short and annular may also respond to dilatation. Overzealous dilatation is to be avoided to prevent sphincter damage. Ultimately, proctectomy may be required. Diversion as a temporary option can be considered.

Carcinoma supervenes in 0.7% of long standing cases and is treated as any other low rectal or anal cancer.

LAPAROSCOPIC SURGERY

Laparoscopic surgery for CD has been shown to be feasible and safe in expert hands. It improves short term outcomes without compromising long-term results.[9] Since patients with CD are young and may need reoperations, laparoscopic surgery is an attractive proposition. However, there are important differences between laparoscopic surgery for CD and laparoscopic surgery for cancer. The medial to lateral approach may be impossible with thickened and friable mesentery. Loss of tactile feedback can result in segments of involved bowel being missed. Bowel may need to be exteriorized for palpation. Small bowel may not move out of the field due to adhesions or thickened mesentery. Operating times are longer. Benefits include lower wound complication rates, including incisional hernias, faster recovery, and less adhesive intestinal obstruction. Meta analyses have shown similar long-term outcomes in both groups.

CMC EXPERIENCE

There were 850 patients with proven CD requiring admission for medical management in this institution over a 13 year period (1996–2009).

Ninety-five of these patients who fulfilled our criteria were admitted under the surgical team. Eighty-eight patients required resection Seven did not undergo resection. Of these, one patient had a psoas abscess complicating ileocecal disease and underwent laparotomy and drainage. One patient underwent laparotomy and enterotomy for biopsy which was closed as a stricturoplasty. Five patients had a prior ileocecal resection with a covering ileostomy which was closed; review of the earlier resection histology confirmed CD.

Of the 95 cases, 87 came from a different state and 74 had travelled in excess of a thousand kilometers to receive surgical treatment.

The age at operation ranged from 12 to 76 years (mean 41.2 years).

The average age at diagnosis was 39.7 (range 12–76 years).

There were 65 men (68.4%) and only 30 women (31.6%) M:F ratio was 2.2:1.

The average duration of symptoms prior to diagnosis was 4.4 years (range 0–33 years). Only 28 of these patients were known to have CD preoperatively, for the remainder (67), the diagnosis was only established on the basis of the operative findings.

The 28 known cases of CD included 5 cases that had previous operations. One had sepsis in the right iliac fossa and one in the subhepatic space. They had undergone appendicectomy and cholecystectomy respectively. They continued to have intra-abdominal sepsis and were found to have ileocecal and hepatic flexure CD respectively. Of the others, one had a previous ileocolectomy and two others had ileocecal resection. Details of previous surgery were not available in one patient. Five patients had undergone intestinal resection and ileostomy elsewhere and had now presented for closure ileostomy. Seventeen other cases had radiological or endoscopic evidence of CD which was initially non-obstructive and were hence treated medically.

The clinical features were abdominal pain (n=64, 67%), vomiting (n=35, 37%), weight loss (n=31, 33%), chronic anemia (n=17, 18%), perianal fistulae (n=8, 9%).

Ten patients had a fistula: Ileocutaneous fistula in ileocecal disease (n=5), ileosigmoid fistula in ileocecal disease (n=1), anovaginal fistula (n=1) and ileovesical fistula (n=3) with a large pelvic abscess in ileocecal disease presenting with septic shock. Three other patients also had an abscess: ileocecal disease and a psoas abscess, jejunoileal disease and an intra-abdominal abscess and hepatic flexure disease with subhepatic abscess. Eight patients had perianal disease at the time of admission, five were quiescent and three had an abscess needing surgical drainage.

Six patients presented as emergencies: Three with intestinal obstruction, one with gastrointestinal hemorrhage and three in septic shock with extensive intra-abdominal sepsis. The patients in shock died of overwhelming sepsis in 3 days after operation. These patients underwent resection for ileocecal disease. Another patient presenting with intestinal obstruction also died in the immediate postoperative period secondary to Guillain-Barre syndrome. One patient died of chronic myeloid leukemia 3 years after surgery. These were the five deaths in the series.

Twenty-five patients had been assumed elsewhere to have had intra-abdominal tuberculosis. Since none had improved despite compliance to therapy, they were reinvestigated. CD was diagnosed based on radiological and laparotomy criteria. Preoperative intestinal radiology was performed on 75 patients: contrast studies n=33, ultrasound n=39, CT n=31 and MRI n=2. In 73 of these 75 patients (98%), the diagnosis of CD was established by radiological criteria. Only 47 patients underwent colonoscopy which revealed colonic disease (segmental) in 15, ileal ulcers/terminal ileal cobblestone mucosa in 12: colonoscopy was diagnostic in only 20 of 47 examinations (43%). Four patients with albumin levels less than 2 had intra-abdominal sepsis at the time of presentation.

Surgical procedures were multiple in 12 patients (13%). The operations included stricturoplasty in 9 (eight in combination with small bowel resection), small bowel resection in 43, ileocecal resection in 32, segmental colectomy in 5 and subtotal colectomy in 10.

Postoperative complications excluding the three deaths mentioned above included anastomotic bleeding in one patient requiring relaparotomy and refashioning of the anastomosis, a proximal small bowel perforation (presumably from a diathermy burn) requiring relaparotomy and exteriorization as a proximal stoma and laparotomy for adhesive obstruction in a third. Two patients underwent laparotomy and stoma due to a postoperative anastomotic leak. One patient had intra-abdominal sepsis managed conservatively. Two patients underwent relaparotomy and washout for postoperative collection. There were seven wound infections.

Disease confined to the duodenum alone was not seen. Disease involving the jejunum alone was seen in 10(10%). Involvement of the jejunum with other sites was seen in 24(25%) patients.

Likewise ileal disease alone was recorded in 27(29%) and ileal involvement in combination with other sites was seen in 30(32%). Diffuse small bowel disease was seen in 12(13%). The ileocecal region was the dominant disease site in 28(30%). The colon was the dominant site in 13(14%).

Complicated disease resulting in perforation, abscess or fistula was found in 14 patients (15%).

One patient presented with a cecal malignancy for which he underwent right hemicolectomy.

Sixty patients (67%) have been seen on follow-up. For those who have been reassessed the mean duration of follow-up was 2 years (1–11 years). None have required reoperation for recurrence, two have had operations to reverse a temporary stoma, one patient has undergone a subsequent incisional hernia repair and four have symptoms from perianal disease. Maintenance treatment provided by the gastroenterologists was provided for all except one of these patients. The patient with malignancy was treated with adjuvant chemotherapy.

Thus, surgery for Crohn's disease provides useful improvements in quality of life for patients with complications of CD that cannot be managed by medical therapy.

REFERENCES

1. Delaney CP, Kiran RP, Senagore AJ, O'Brien-Ermlich B, Church J, Hull TL, et al. Quality of life improves within 30 days of surgery for Crohn's disease. J Am Coll Surg. 2003;196(5):714-21.
2. Fazio VW, Marchetti F, Church M, Goldblum JR, Lavery C, Hull TL, et al. Effect of resection margins on the recurrence of Crohn's disease in the small bowel. A randomized controlled trial. Ann Surg. 1996;224(4):563-71.

3. Choy PY, Bissett IP, Docherty JG, Parry BR, Merrie A, Fitzgerald A. Stapled versus handsewn methods for ileocolic anastomoses. Cochrane Database Syst Rev. 2011;7(9):CD004320. doi: 10.1002/14651858.CD004320.pub3.
4. Simillis C, Purkayastha S, Yamamoto T, Strong SA, Darzi AW, Tekkis PP. A meta-analysis comparing conventional end-to-end anastomosis vs. other anastomotic configurations after resection in Crohn's disease. Dis Colon Rectum. 2007;50(10):1674-87.
5. Prabhakar LP, Laramee C, Nelson H, Dozois RR. Avoiding a stoma: role for segmental or abdominal colectomy in Crohn's colitis. Dis Colon Rectum.1997;40(1):71-8.
6. Worsey MJ, Hull T, Ryland L, Fazio V. Strictureplasty is an effective option in the operative management of duodenal Crohn's disease. Dis Colon Rectum.1999;42(5):596-600.
7. Dietz DW, Fazio VW, Laureti S, Strong SA, Hull TL, Church J, et al. Strictureplasty in diffuse Crohn's jejunoileitis: safe and durable. Dis Colon Rectum. 2002;45(6):764-70.
8. Scott HJ, Northover JM. Evaluation of surgery for perianal Crohn's fistulas. Dis Colon Rectum. 1996;39(9):1039-43.
9. Tan JJ, Tjandra JJ. Laparoscopic surgery for Crohn's disease: a meta-analysis. Dis Colon Rectum. 2007;50(5):576-85.

CHAPTER 96

Colonic Polyps and Polyposis Syndromes

Brundaban Nahak, Debasis Misra, Shivaram Prasad Singh

INTRODUCTION

Polyp is a descriptive term for any mucosal elevation. Colonic polyps are classified into two major categories: (1) neoplastic and (2) nonneoplastic on the basis of cellular dysplasia (Table 1). Polypoidal submucosal lesions are not considered true polyps. These include lipomas, lymphoid polyps and colitis cystica profunda.

NONNEOPLASTIC POLYPS

Nonneoplastic polyps include a number of disparate entities; juvenile polyps, hyperplastic polyps, mucosal polyps, inflammatory polyps and Peutz-Jeghers polyps are examples of nonneoplastic polyps.

Hyperplastic Polyps

Hyperplastic polyps are usually small in size and sessile. They cannot be differentiated from small adenomatous polyps during colonoscopy. Hyperplastic polyps are made up of elongated colonic crypts; the epithelial cells are arranged to produce a papillary configuration, and they are made up of well-differentiated absorptive and goblet cells. The cell division is restricted to the base of the crypts. These polyps are believed to be a result of sluggish movement of the epithelial cells along the crypt, which occurs in association with the failure of timely shedding of the mature cells.

During colonoscopic examination, hyperplastic polyps can be seen in 9–10% of asymptomatic patients with increasing frequency in older age.[1,2] Smokers have a higher risk for developing hyperplastic polyps.[3] Although hyperplastic polyps do not have significant malignant potential, they have a predilection for persons with a strong family history of colorectal cancer.[4] The hyperplastic polyps are removed during colonoscopy, since it is impossible to differentiate hyperplastic polyps from serrated or neoplastic polyps by mere gross appearance during colonoscopy. However, following polypectomy, they should be followed up by colonoscopy after 10 years.[5]

Serrated Polyps

Serrated polyps have characteristics of both hyperplastic and adenomatous transformation. They consist of:[6]

- Hyperplastic polyps (subtypes: goblet cell and microvesicular)
- Traditional serrated adenoma (TSA)
- Sessile serrated adenoma (SSA).

About 10–20% of colorectal carcinomas are now presumed to evolve through this alternative, serrated pathway. Aberrant DNA methylation plays a central role in this pathway.[7] They are also the precursor lesions for polyps seen in hyperplastic polyposis.[8] TSAs usually located in the distal colon are generally pedunculated. On histology, they have adenomatous dysplasia (crypt serration). The s SSAs differ from the TSA pathogenetically; in addition to DNA methylation, they also have extensive BRAF mutations which are absent in TSAs.[8]

In a large multicenter study, the colon previous study assessed the prevalence of serrated polyps and their association with synchronous advanced neoplasia. Serrated polyps were found in 20.8%; while 6.5% had proximal serrated polyps and 1.8% had large serrated polyps (LSPs). Both the proximal serrated polyps and LSPs were associated with advanced neoplasia.[9] Further, in serrated polyps, an increased risk of malignancy is associated with; polyp size greater than or equal to 10 mm, multiplicity, SSA histology, presence of associated dysplasia and a proximal location.[10]

Mucosal Polyps

Mucosal polyps are excrescences of tissue that are normal histologically. They are small in size and constitute 10–20% of polyps on colonoscopy.

Table 1: Classification of colonic mucosal polyps

Neoplastic		*Non-neoplastic*
Benign polyp	Malignant polyp	
Adenoma: • Tubular • Tubulovillous • Villous	*Noninvasive carcinoma*: • Carcinoma in situ • Intramucosal carcinoma Invasive carcinoma	• Peutz-Jeghers polyp • Inflammatory polyp • Hyperplastic polyp • Mucosal polyp • Juvenile polyp

Juvenile Polyps (Retention Polyps)

Juvenile polyps are primarily hamartomatous polyps possessing dilated cystic glands with excess of lamina propria. On histology, there are distended, mucus-filled glands, with edematous lamina propria and inflammatory cell infiltration. They are usually seen in children in the first decade, and are typically pedunculated and solitary, the diameter varying from 3 mm to 2 cm (Fig. 1A). They are usually asymptomatic, but may prolapse during defecation or sometimes slough, resulting in considerable blood loss. Single Juvenile polyps neither recur nor have malignant potential. However, when they are multiple polyps, there is increased risk of cancer development, either because of presence of adenomatous epithelium in some polyps or due to the existence of coexisting adenoma.[11]

Peutz-Jeghers Polyps

The Peutz-Jeghers polyp is a hamartoma. In these lesions, the glandular epithelium is buttressed by a network of smooth muscle arising from the muscularis mucosae. In Peutz-Jeghers polyps, the lamina propria is normal (not excessive). When there are multiple polyps along with the extraintestinal manifestations, the condition is labeled as Peutz-Jeghers syndrome.

Inflammatory Polyps

Inflammatory polyps are pseudopolyps, which form when there is healing and regeneration associated with chronic inflammation. They may be large and solitary, or may form mucosal bridges that span the lumen (Fig. 1B). Besides inflammatory bowel disease, they can occur following any severe colitis, including amebic colitis, ischemic colitis or bacterial dysentery. Cap polyposis is an uncommon variety of inflammatory polyps; these polyps have an exudative fibrinopurulent cap on their surface.[12] Although these polyps by themselves do not have intrinsic neoplastic potential; however, they are frequently seen in diseased colons with a high predilection for developing colonic cancer (ulcerative colitis), and therefore have to be differentiated from neoplastic polyps. Occasionally, a large pseudopolyp can even produce obstruction of lumen.

NEOPLASTIC POLYPS

Adenomatous polyps can be sessile or pedunculated, and are composed of benign neoplastic epithelium. They are of three types:

1. Tubular adenomas that have an intricate complex of branching adenomatous glands.
2. Villous adenomas in which the adenomatous glands appear as long, finger-like projections.
3. Tubulovillous (villoglandular) adenomas with features of both tubular adenomas and villous adenomas.

Adenomas are categorized as tubular if greater than or equal to 80% of the glands are branching and tubular, and as villous if greater than or equal to 80% of the glands are villiform.[13] Tubular adenomas constitute up to 86%; tubulovillous 8–16% and villous adenomas 3–16% of all adenomas (Figs 2A and B).[14] Tubular adenomas are generally not large and reveal only mild dysplasia on histology unlike the villous adenomas which are usually large and associated with more severe dysplasia. Larger adenomas are generally more common in the distal colon;[3,14] in the elderly,[3,15] and in areas with high prevalence of colon cancer.[1]

Diminutive polyps measuring less than or equal to 5 mm are commonly detected during endoscopy. Of these, the hyperplastic polyps have a predilection for distal colon, especially the sigmoid colon and rectum, while adenomas predominate in the other parts of the colon.[16] Approximately, a third to half of the diminutive polyps are adenomatous, with villous architecture and malignant

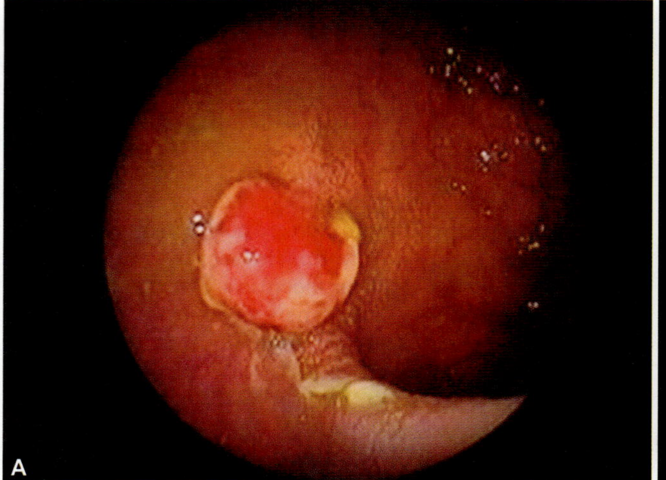

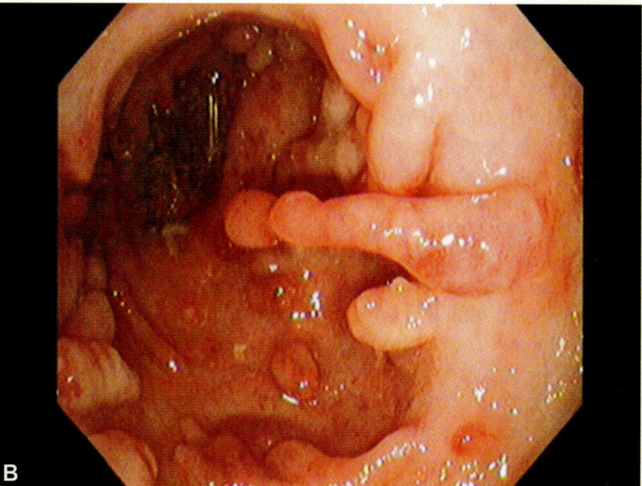

Figures 1A and B Colonoscopic images: (A) Juvenile polyp; (B) Inflammatory colonic pseudopolyps
Source: Dr Md Ibrarullah, MS, M Ch, Bhubaneswar

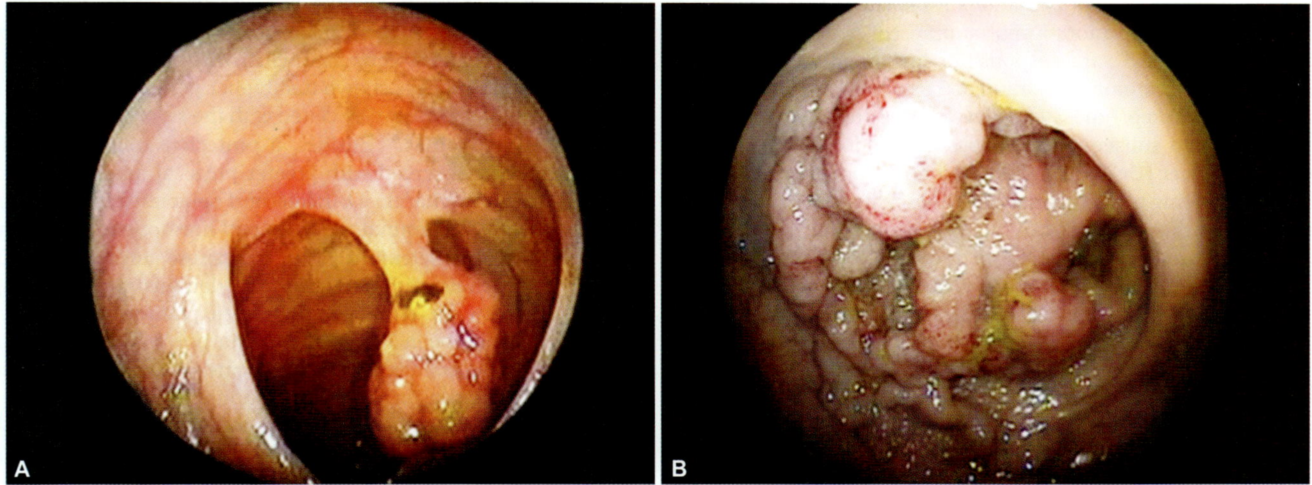

Figures 2A and B Colonoscopic images: (A) Pedunculated villous adenoma; (B) Large rectal tubulovillous adenoma
Source: Dr Md Ibrarullah, MS, M Ch, Bhubaneswar

potential in 1-4.4%.[17-19] Besides, up to a third of the subjects also have a synchronous proximal adenoma .[20]

Adenomas are characterized according to their most dysplastic focus, into low-grade dysplasia and high-grade dysplasia. Low-grade dysplasia includes both mild and moderate dysplasia, while high-grade dysplasia includes both severe dysplasia and carcinoma in situ.[14] In invasive carcinoma (malignant polyps), neoplastic cells invade the muscularis mucosae. Seventy to eighty-six percent of adenomatous polyps have mild dysplasia, 18-20% have moderate dysplasia and 5-10% have severe dysplasia; only about 5-7% have invasive carcinoma.[21] Factors which correlate with malignant potential of adenomas include its size, histology and degree of dysplasia. Villous adenomas with high-grade dysplasia and diameter greater than 1 cm are designated as adenomas with advanced pathology (AAP).

Adenoma Variants

Flat Adenomas

These can be either flat or minimally raised with diameter more than twice its thickness. They constitute up to 12% of all adenomas.[22] Flat adenomas are more likely to possess high-grade dysplasia and early cancer.[23,24]

Serrated Adenomas

In serrated adenomas, the colonic crypts have a saw-tooth, serrated configuration, with features of both adenomatous and hyperplastic polyps.

Aberrant Crypts

They are small, slightly raised dysplastic foci within normal mucosa and are considered, the earliest detectable preneoplastic lesions. These crypts are elliptical and irregular. The dysplastic aberrant crypts prevalent in flat and depressed neoplasms often have mutations in the adenomatous polyposis coli (*APC*) gene.[25,26]

Pathogenesis

There are four molecular pathways for colorectal cancer carcinogenesis:[27]

1. Adenoma-carcinoma sequence
2. Hereditary microsatellite instability
3. Serrated pathway
4. Epidermal growth factor receptor

The adenoma-carcinoma sequence is the most accepted one (Fig. 3). It is assumed that monoclonal expansion of an abnormal cell leads to unicryptal adenoma, and subsequently there is polyclonal transformation of the adenomatous cell population.

Adenoma-Carcinoma Hypothesis: It has been observed that the prevalence of adenomas in any region often parallels the prevalence of colonic carcinoma.[1] Further, the age of development of adenomas generally precedes the age at development of colonic cancers by about a decade.[28] These evidences suggest that most colonic carcinomas develop in previously benign adenomas. However, the most robust evidence in favor of this hypothesis is the fact that all familial adenomatous polyposis (FAP) patients sooner or later develop colorectal carcinoma.

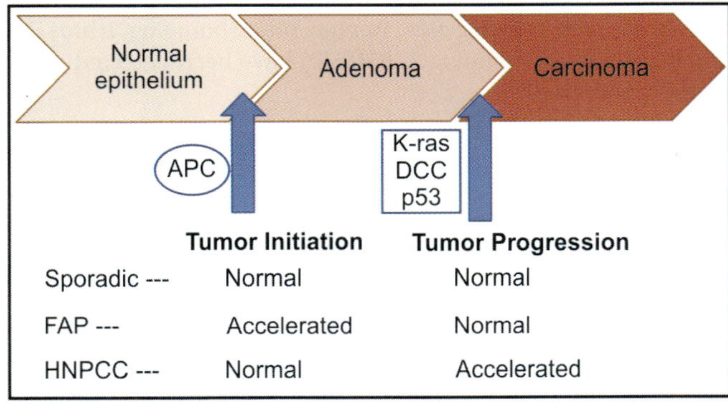

Figure 3 Pathways of colonic carcinogenesis

The molecular genetic alterations especially those associated with oncogene's activation, tumor suppressor genes inactivation and stability genes[29] are responsible for transformation from adenomas to carcinomas. Mutation or loss of the *APC* gene on the long arm of chromosome 5 is believed to be the key initial step. This is followed subsequently by loss of function of "deleted in colorectal cancer (DCC) gene" situated on chromosome 18q and other neighboring tumor suppressor genes. Later on, 17p deletion also occurs in the adenoma-carcinoma progression.[30]

Tumor initiation is the process of development of an adenoma. The process of progression from adenoma to cancer is *tumor progression*. In FAP, an *APC* allele is inherited as germline mutation from an affected parent, while the other is a somatic mutation. Although FAP patients develop polyps at a relatively younger age, but once adenoma formation occurs, they have the usual progression to carcinoma. On the contrary, the adenoma progression phase is considerably hastened in hereditary nonpolyposis colorectal cancer.

Epidemiology

Those with family history of colorectal carcinoma often develop adenomas at a very early age.[31] The prevalence of adenomatous polyps in any population depends on the risk for colonic carcinoma in that region and may be as high as 30–40% in high risk populations.[32] Advanced age is associated with a higher risk of adenoma development, more proximal distribution of colonic polyps, an increased propensity for multiple polyps, larger polyps and greater dysplasia.[2,33-35] Besides, males have an increased risk of adenomas and AAP as compared to women.[36,37] Further, colonic polyps in the left colon harbor high grade dysplasia more often than polyps elsewhere.[38]

Risk Factors

Both genetic predisposition and environmental factors contribute to the propensity to develop adenomas in the colon.

Genetics

Risk factors include genetic predisposition such as inheritance as in FAP and nonpolyposis (HNPCC) colonic cancer syndromes as well as having a first-degree relative affected by colonic adenoma or carcinoma. Up to 10–30% of colonic carcinomas may be familial,[31,39] and germline mutations of *APC* and other genes implicated in the *APC* pathway, including *β-catenin* and *AXIN1* and DNA mismatch repair genes, human mutL homolog 1(hMLH1) and human mutS homolog 2 (hMSH2) have been detected in the majority of them.[40]

Dietary and Lifestyle Risk Factors

Increased adenoma risk is seen in the obese and is also associated with excess consumption of fat and alcohol, and cigarette smoking.[41] A Korean study showed that obese males had an increased predilection for developing colorectal adenomatous polyps; this association was not seen in females.[42] A recent study has also associated stress with the development of colorectal polyps.[43]

Although a previous study[44] had shown a 27% lower risk in persons with high fiber intake, prospective trials of dietary fiber supplementation were inconclusive.[45] An analysis of the Nurses' Health Study has shown that higher poultry intake during adolescence was inversely associated with the risk of development of colorectal adenomas.[46] Besides, a protective role for colonic polyps has been observed with greater physical activity, greater intake of calcium, vitamin D, folate and selenium, ingestion of nonsteroidal anti-inflammatory drugs and hormone replacement therapy (HRT), and selenium.[47-49] A Taiwanese study on plasma homocysteine levels and colonic polyps demonstrated a strong association between the two.[50] Besides, *Helicobacter pylori* infection has also been linked to colonic polyps; prevalence of gastritis due to *Helicobacter pylori* was greater in those with colonic polyps: both hyperplastic as well as adenomatous polyps.[51]

There is an evidence to show that use of Aspirin can reduce risk of development of colonic polyps; an absolute risk reduction of 6.7% was seen with aspirin use in a meta-analysis.[52] Aspirin acts by inhibiting cyclooxygenase enzymes resulting in reduction of cellular proliferation and angiogenesis, and enhancement of apoptosis. Another study comparing DFMO (Difluoromethylornithine) in combination with sulindac in adenoma showed a decrease in recurrence following polypectomy.[53] This is probably mediated through suppression of abnormally expressed polyamine levels in the rectal mucosa. Further, use of statins too has been shown to confer protection.[54]

Conditions Associated with Adenomatous Polyps

There is increased predisposition for adenoma development in persons is as follows:

- Ureterosigmoidostomy:[55] This may be the consequence of *N*-nitrosamines generated from urinary amines; up to 29% may develop colonic neoplasms after a mean latent period of two to three decades.
- Cholecystectomy:[56] Increased delivery of bile acids into colon augments colonocyte proliferative activity; however, results of studies have been inconsistent.
- Acromegaly:[57] The prevalence of adenomatous polyps is as high as 14–35% and is a consequence of increased growth hormone and/or insulin-like growth factor (IGF)-1 levels.[58]
- Bacteremia and endocarditis caused by *S. bovis* have also been associated with colorectal adenomas and cancer, and even with FAP.[59]
- John Cunningham virus (JCV), an oncogenic polyomavirus has also been associated with increased incidence of colonic adenomas and carcinomas.[60]

Clinical Features

Colonic polyps are generally asymptomatic and are often detected during screening. Some of them are often discovered during evaluation of unexplained anemia. Of those having symptoms, the most common symptom is rectal bleeding. Other presentations include constipation, diarrhea, flatulence and intermittent intussusceptions, leading to cramping abdominal pain. Large distal colonic adenomas especially villous adenomas may cause secretory diarrhea with considerable water and electrolyte depletion.[61]

Investigations

Fecal Occult Blood Testing (FOBT)

Overt rectal bleeding occurs in less than a tenth of the patients, and over a third shows positive FOBT.[62]

Fecal Immunochemical Testing (FIT)

This has yielded increased specificity over guaiac-based testing and the great advantage is that it does not require dietary restrictions. The ability to detect large adenomas and adenomas especially with villous component was better with FIT compared to FOBT.[63]

Sigmoidoscopy

This can detect only distal adenomas, but this often gives a wrong assurance as polyps in the proximal colon are more common in those without a family history of colonic carcinoma. In a study, two-thirds of all persons with right colonic adenoma had a normal sigmoidoscopic examination.[64]

Barium Enema

The larger the size of the polyp, the greater is the detection rate. In the National Polyp Study, while the rate for detecting adenomas less than 6 mm was 32%, it was 48% for adenomas greater than 10 mm.[65]

Colonoscopy

A full colonoscopy is considered the gold standard for detection of adenomas; however, the procedure is fraught with some limitations which include:

- The cecum cannot be reached in about 10% colonoscopies
- Colonoscopy can easily miss neoplasms at flexures or under folds
- Detection rate depends on the scope withdrawal time[66]
- Colonoscopy queue position impacts detection rate.

Adenomas that are missed on colonoscopy are generally small.[67] Besides, digital chromoendoscopy with magnification may allow improved evaluation of the mucosal surface.[68] However, endoscopic classification of polyp type using these specialized imaging techniques is not yet standardized. Hence, histopathological assessment is still the gold standard for classification of polyps.[69]

Computed Tomography Colonography

A helical or spiral CT scan can generate two-dimensional as well as three-dimensional images of the colon and rectum. A large study demonstrated 90% sensitivity for polyps greater than 1 cm, but 78% for polyps 6–9 mm in diameter.[70] Besides, it is unable to detect smaller polyps consistently. In another study, 11% more polyps were discovered on CT colonography following a colonoscopic examination.[71]

Altered Human DNA in Stool

This is a novel noninvasive method for detection of adenoma. It detects altered human DNA in stool with a sensitivity of 57% for adenomas greater than or equal to 1 cm and 73% for those with size greater than or equal to 2 cm. A study reported, 83% sensitivity for high-grade dysplasia.[72] Further, studies are necessary to assess the efficacy of this novel screening technique.

Natural History

The progression from adenoma to carcinoma is fortunately quite slow and takes many years. Smaller polyps not only take a longer duration to advance to cancer, but may sometimes not change in size. The risk of progression to cancer is about 2.5% at 5 years, 8% at 10 years and 24% at 20 years following detection of adenoma.[73] Although there are rare reports of polyp regression, the conventional norm is to remove any polyp which is detected.

Treatment

A full colonoscopy is mandatory before treatment because at least one synchronous adenoma or carcinoma have been found in up to 50% of colons especially in the elderly.[27,74] Increasing age, family history of colorectal carcinoma and male sex are associated with enhanced detection of advanced proximal neoplasia.[35,75]

It should be emphasized that mere biopsy of a polyp is not enough to rule out cancer, and hence, polypectomy is essential. Piecemeal excision may be sometimes required to remove a sessile polyp. Poor visualization of the stalk in a giant polyp presents with technical difficulties in snare positioning. Endoscopic submucosal dissection has also been attempted in such cases.[76] Following piecemeal resection, it is prudent to perform a colonoscopy after 3–6 months for assessing completeness of the resection. Polyps that are not suitable for endoscopic resection should undergo a surgical excision.

MANAGEMENT OF THE MALIGNANT POLYP

Malignant polyps may even after adequate endoscopic polypectomy have residual cancer, or there may be involvement of lymph nodes in a tenth of the cases.[77] Haggitt and colleagues proposed a classification for malignant polyps on the basis of the depth of invasion:[78]

- Level 0: Carcinoma without invasion of muscularis mucosae
- Level 1: Carcinoma with invasion across muscularis mucosae into submucosa but restricted to the head of the polyp
- Level 2: Carcinoma with invasion up to level of neck of polyp
- Level 3: Carcinoma with invasion of any segment of stalk
- Level 4: Carcinoma with invasion into the bowel wall submucosa below the polyp pedicle but above the muscularis propria.

Endoscopic polypectomy alone is sufficient therapy for:

- Adenomatous polyps harboring in situ carcinoma
- Pedunculated adenomas with invasive carcinoma which is well or moderately differentiated
- Polypoid carcinomas without submucosal involvement.

A "difficult polyp" is regarded as: (1) size greater than 3 cm, sessile or pedunculated (Is/Ip); (2) polyp morphology (classification of Paris 2003), especially the large sessile-serrated lesions and flat type II lesions IIa-c flat, flat depressed, laterally spreading tumors and (3) assessment of the grade of malignancy is difficult before removal. Chromoendoscopy can assist in distinguishing the milder grade malignancy from advanced flat and depressed type II lesions.[79] Unfavorable features are a poorly differentiated polyp, invasion of the submucosa, vessels or lymphatics, and positive polypectomy margin. In the absence of these features, one can be said to be cured by endoscopic polypectomy alone. However, the presence of one or more unfavorable features can significantly increase the chance of an adverse outcome.[80]

Postpolypectomy bleeding can occur, and is seen more often in the older patients, following piecemeal polypectomy, additional sedation, and in the presence of diverticulosis and intraprocedural bleeding.[81]

Polyp Recurrence

Following polypectomy, the overall risk of recurrence of adenoma development is approximately 20% at 5 years and this may go up to 50% after 15 years; however, these are usually small with lesser dysplasia.[82] Greater age, multiple adenomas (>5), larger polyps (diameter >1 cm), proximal location and villous histology with severe dysplasia usually favor the likelihood of recurrence.[83-85]

Colorectal Cancer Incidence and the Effect of Polypectomy

The national polyp study involved 1,418 patients undergoing polypectomy; the patients were followed postpolypectomy for an average duration of 5.9 years. Only 5 cancers were detected during this period amounting to a significant reduction when compared to the historical reference groups.[86]

Surveillance Colonoscopy

A consensus recommendation for postpolypectomy surveillance by the U.S. Multi-Society Task Force on Colorectal Cancer and the American Cancer Society is outlined in Table 2.[87] Patients who have a negative index colonoscopy should be followed up with colonoscopy at 10 years' interval.

Table 2: Postpolypectomy surveillance recommendations

Colonoscopy findings	*Timing of surveillance colonoscopy*
Small rectal hyperplastic polyps	10 years (treat as normal)
1 or 2 small (<1 cm) tubular adenomas with only LGD	5–10 years (individualized)
3–10 adenomas, any adenoma ≥1 cm, or any adenoma with villous histology or HGD	3 years (to be repeated after 5 years, if normal finding or low risk adenoma)
>10 adenomas detected during one examination	<3 years (individualized)
Suggestive of HNPCC	2–3 years (or more frequent)
Sessile adenoma removed in piecemeal fashion	2–6 months (individualized)

Abbreviations: LGD, low-grade dysplasia; HGD, high-grade dysplasia; HNPCC, hereditary nonpolyposis colorectal cancer.

COLONIC POLYPOSIS SYNDROMES

The term gastrointestinal polyposis is used when there are several polypoid lesions arising from the gastrointestinal tract. Most of these syndromes are inherited, and their importance lies in the increased colon cancer risk. The inherited gastrointestinal poylposis syndromes have been enlisted in Table 3. Hyperplastic polyposis syndrome, Cronkhite-Canada syndrome and Lymphomatous polyposis are noninherited conditions.

Table 3: Classification of inherited gastrointestinal polyposis syndromes

Adenomatous polyposis syndromes	*Hamartomatous polyposis syndromes*
Familial adenomatous polyposis (FAP) *Variants of FAP*: • Gardner's syndrome • Turcot's syndrome • Attenuated adenomatous *polyposis coli* Familial tooth agenesis syndrome Bloom's syndrome *MUTYH* (mutY homolog) polyposis (*MYH* polyposis)	Peutz-Jeghers syndrome Juvenile polyposis *PTEN hamartoma tumor syndromes*: • Cowden's disease • Bannayan-Ruvalcaba-Riley syndrome *Rare hamartomatous polyposis syndromes*: • Hereditary mixed polyposis syndrome • Intestinal ganglioneuromatosis and neurofibromatosis • Devon family syndrome • Basal cell nevus syndrome

Familial Adenomatous Polyposis

Familial adenomatous polyposis is the most extensively analyzed inherited gastrointestinal polyposis syndrome. In this, a mutated *APC* allele is inherited from an affected parent, and the polyposis develops when the second allele, also is mutated or lost. FAP is inherited as an autosomal dominant disorder, and there is 80–100% penetrance. The estimated prevalence of FAP is between 1 in 5,000–7,500.[88] The gene implicated for FAP has been localized to the 5q21–q22 region.[89]

The *APC* protein not only plays a crucial role in cell proliferation, migration, and differentiation, but is also involved in apoptosis and chromosomal segregation.[90] This binds to β-catenin, which is responsible for maintaining cell-cell junctions. Mutations in the β-catenin-binding region of *APC*, allow β-catenin to act synergistically with other transcription factors and up-regulate target genes. *APC* mutations also produce abnormalities in chromosomal segregation with resulting in chromosomal instability. The key characteristics of the different variants of the adenomatous polyposis syndromes are summarized in Table 4.

Clinical Features

Classical FAP is manifested by the progressive appearance of hundreds to thousands of adenomatous polyps in the colon (Fig. 4). In a large series of FAP patients, the mean age for start

Table 4: Adenomatous polyposis syndromes

Syndrome	*Gene mutation*	*Polyps including extracolonic polyps*	*Extraintestinal abnormalities*
Classic FAP	*APC* (usually truncated protein)	Gastric (30–100%; usually fundic gland polyp), duodenal adenomas (60–90%), jejunal adenomas (40%) and ileal adenomas (60–90%)	Mandibular osteomas, exostosis, dental abnormalities
Gardner variant of FAP	*APC*	Same as FAP	Osteomas; fibromas, desmoid tumors, CHRPE, epidermoid cysts, sebaceous cysts, lipomas, thyroid and adrenal tumors
Turcot variant of FAP	*APC* DNA MMR	Colonic adenomas (fewer than in classic FAP)	Medulloblastoma, CHRPE, glioblastoma multiforme
Attenuated FAP	*APC* 5′ and 3′ regions	Colonic adenomas (< 100; proximal colon), duodenal adenomas and gastric fundic gland polyps	Mandibular osteomas (rare)
Familial tooth agenesis	*Axin2* (*APC* pathway)	Colonic adenomas and hyperplastic polyps	Agenesis of teeth
Bloom's syndrome	*BLM*	Colonic adenomas	Small stature, male sterility, facial erythema/telangiectasia, leukemia, lymphoma, adenocarcinomas
MUTYH polyposis	*MUTYH (MYH)*	Colonic adenomas (5–100), duodenal polyposis and gastric cancer	CHRPE, osteomas

Abbreviations: CHRPE, congenital hypertrophy of the retinal pigment epithelium; MMR, mismatch repair; *MUTYH* (mutY homolog).

of polyps was 25 years, and onset of symptoms was 33 years. Besides, while the average age at diagnosis of adenomas was 36 years, this was 39 years for malignancy, and 42 years for death from malignancy. Overall, 90% of the FAP cases were diagnosed before the patients attained the age of 50 years.[91] Histologically, all varieties of adenomas are seen: tubular, tubulovillous and villous adenomas. Colorectal carcinoma is an inexorable sequel in all cases of FAP, and it generally occurs after a gap of 10–15 years after commencement of polyposis.

In FAP, polyps also appear in the stomach and small bowel; the gastric polyps can be present in 30–100%, and these are generally small sessile hyperplastic polyps of fundic glands. Dysplasia may be seen in large polyps and duodenal polyposis.[92] Following proctocolectomy, as there is prolongation of survival in FAP patients, there occurs an increase in incidence of gastric carcinoma.[93] Ninety percent patients with FAP also develop duodenal adenomas, incidence gradually increasing with age.[94] There is an increased predilection of adenomas to affect the periampullary region, which can lead to pancreatic or biliary obstruction. Besides, FAP patients especially with stages III and IV duodenal polyposis (the Spigelman classification),[95] also have an increased incidence of carcinoma of duodenum.[93] The Spigelman classification is based on the size, the numbers and histology of the polyps, and also on the severity of dysplasia. Further, jejunal adenomas and ileal adenomas are also seen in FAP patients.

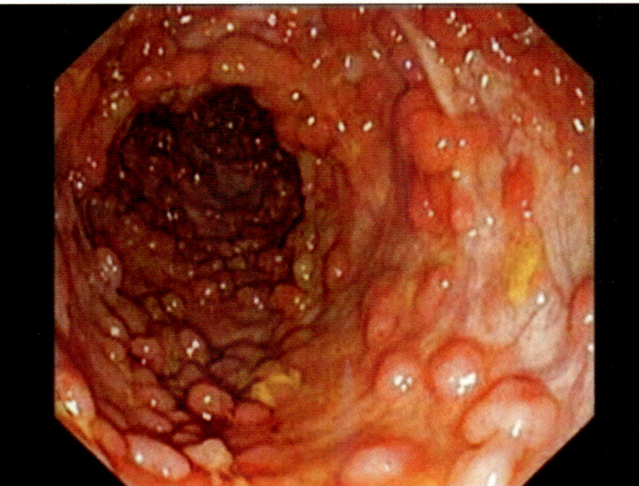

Figure 4 Colonoscopic image of adenomatous polyposis
Source: Dr Asutosh Mohapatra, MD, DM, Bhubaneswar

Another association of the FAP is the occurrence of desmoid tumors, which is a consequence of uninhibited growth of mesenteric fibroblasts. Desmoid tumors can occur spontaneously, as well as after prophylactic proctocolectomy. They can cause intestinal obstruction or constrict vascular structures especially arteries, veins and ureters. These are found in 4–32% of FAP patients.[96] The absolute risk of desmoids in FAP patients is about 2.56/1,000 person-years.[97] Early colectomy and female gender are associated with more desmoids. This is the reason why some experts opine that colectomy should be delayed in young female FAP patients.[98] A few studies have shown that treatment with Sulindac, tamoxifen and progesterone can result in partial shrinkage of desmoids.[99,100]

Treatment

Surgery: The optimal treatment of FAP is total proctocolectomy with ileostomy, or a restorative proctocolectomy with ileal pouch-anal anastomosis. A meta-analysis revealed that, in comparison to restorative proctocolectomy, ileorectal anastomosis had reduced frequency and incontinence but paradoxically, the patients had greater fecal urgency.[101] Both the surgical procedures have similar rates of adverse effects including sexual dysfunction, and other adverse postoperative sequelae.

It is of paramount importance to inform and educate the patients regarding the hazards of subtotal colectomy with ileorectal anastomosis as the patient remains at risk for carcinoma. Besides, the outcome in patients who develop rectal cancer is also very not good. Finally, it has been observed that the risk for rectal cancer is almost three times higher in FAP patients with mutation after codon 1,250 compared to patients with mutations before this codon. Although, this may help identify patients for subtotal colectomy, these patients must be willing to comply with rigorous follow-up.

The gastric polyps are usually hyperplastic. They do not necessitate surgical removal. On the contrary; since, the duodenal and ampullary polyps are usually neoplastic, they need rigorous surveillance and endoscopic polypectomy. Ampullary cancers should be treated with pancreatoduodenectomy (Whipple procedure).

Medical Treatment

For the small rectal adenomatous polyps, various treatments have been tried. Ascorbic acid has been tried in FAP patients following subtotal colectomy with ileorectal anastomosis without any consistent benefits.[102] Similarly, calcium supplementation has also been futile in these patients.[103] In a trial, 58 FAP patients were treated with a cocktail of ascorbic acid (4 g/day), α-tocopherol (vitamin E, 400 mg/day), and supplemental fiber (22.5 g/day). A modest effect was observed 2 years after therapy.[104] Sulindac, an NSAID (nonsteroidal anti-inflammatory drug) has been evaluated in multiple trials and has been shown to decrease the number and size of colorectal adenomas in FAP patients.[35] This favorable benefit might result from the high levels of COX-2 (cyclooxygenase-2) expression which prevents apoptosis. Sulindac induced inhibition can lead to adenoma regression;[105] this effect on reducing adenomas was reversible on discontinuation of the drug.[106] Another study has also demonstrated that Celecoxib, a selective COX-2 inhibitor reduces the number of duodenal adenomas.

Screening

Sooner or later, all FAP patients develop cancer of the colon. Besides, 5–12% would also develop duodenal or periampullary carcinoma. As a consequence, it is recommended that all FAP patients should have an annual screening sigmoidoscopy from the first decades onward, and an upper gastrointestinal endoscopy from the third decade onward. Besides, since family members of FAP patients have greater risk of pancreatic, thyroid and CNS tumors including hepatoblastoma,[107-109] screening should also be advised for them.

Hamartomatous Polyposis Syndromes

These are a cluster of familial syndromes in which the affected patients have multiple hamartomatous polyps arising from the gastrointestinal tract. The progression of these polyps to cancer is poorly understood. It is believed to involve the lamina propria leading to the development of epithelial cancers ("landscaper phenomenon"). The key features of the different familial hamartomatous polyposis syndromes are summarized in Table 5.

There is an increased risk of development of malignancy in patients with various hamartomatous polyposis syndromes. Hence, these patients should be screened at intervals depending on the relative risk of cancer development. The screening recommendations for the common hamartomatous polyposis syndromes (Peutz -Jeghers syndrome) and juvenile polyposis are outlined in Table 6.

Noninherited Polyposis Syndromes

Cronkhite-Canada Syndrome

In this syndrome, there are diffuse hamartomatous gastrointestinal polyposis, alopecia, dystrophic fingernails, hyperpigmentation of the skin, diarrhea, abdominal pain, weight loss and malnutrition.[110] Middle-aged or older patients often present with chronic diarrhea and protein, losing enteropathy. Up to 96% can have polyps located throughout gastrointestinal tract.[110] In these patients, the risk of developing colonic carcinoma and adenomas is about 9% and 40% respectively.[111] Various treatments including antibiotics, anabolic steroids, glucocorticoids and operative resections have been attempted albeit with limited success. Surprisingly, sustained nutritional support seems the determining element in treatment outcome.

Hyperplastic Polyposis Syndrome (HPS)

In hyperplastic polyposis syndrome, there are multiple hyperplastic colonic polyps. In about 5% patients with HPS, family history of HPS is present; the remaining cases appear to be sporadic.

The World Health Organization (WHO) has defined this entity as follows:

- At least five histologically proven hyperplastic polyps of which two are greater than 20 mm, or,
- Any number of hyperplastic polyps present proximal to sigmoid colon, with a first-degree relative with hyperplastic polyposis,
- More than 30 hyperplastic polyps that are distributed throughout the colon and rectum.

In a study from Japan, although the overall prevalence was low, 30% patients had coexistence of HPS with colorectal cancer.[112] These patients should have colonoscopic surveillance at intervals of 1–3 years, but selective cases may need surveillance at shorter intervals, for example in AAPs.

Lymphomatous Polyposis

Both Hodgkin's and non-Hodgkin's lymphoma can present as multiple lymphomatous polyps of the gastrointestinal tract.[113] Further, a host of pathologic variants of these lymphomas, including "immunoproliferative small intestinal disease," can also present as polyposis of gastrointestinal tract.

Hereditary Nonpolyposis Colon Cancer (HNPCC)

Lynch I and II syndromes are inherited in an autosomal dominant disease pattern. Three to five percent of all colorectal cancers are

Table 5: Familial hamartomatous polyposis syndromes

Syndrome	*Polyps*	*Other features*	*Genetic mutation*
Peutz-Jeghers syndrome	Hamartomatous polyps in stomach, small intestine and colon	Pigmentation in mouth, hands, feet Pancreatic and breast cancer Ovarian sex cord tumors Sertoli tumors of the testes Airway polyps Colon and esophageal cancer	*STK11/ LKB1*
Juvenile polyposis	Juvenile polyps in stomach, small intestine and colon Adenomas and hyperplastic polyps also.	Congenital abnormalities Colonic carcinoma in some families	*MADH4, BMPR1A*
Bannayan-Ruvalcaba-Riley syndrome	Juvenile polyps in stomach, small intestine and colon	Macroencephaly and developmental delay Pigmentation over penis	*PTEN*
Neurofibromatosis	Neurofibromas	von Recklinghausen's disease (MEN 2B)	*NF1* *RET*
Cowden's disease	Hamartomas with disorganized muscularis mucosae Hamartomas in stomach and colon	Trichilemmomas and papillomas Benign and malignant breast Uterine and thyroid disease	*PTEN*

Abbreviations: GI, gastrointestinal; MEN, multiple endocrine neoplasia.
Screening Recommendations for Hamartomatous Polyposis Syndromes[108,109]

Table 6: Cancer risk and screening recommendations for the common hamartomatous polyposis syndromes

Cancer risk	*Screening recommendations*
Peutz-Jeghers syndrome	
All gastrointestinal cancers (2–13%)	• Colonoscopy every 3 yearly; start at teen age or start of symptoms; interval depending on number of polyps; upper GI endoscopy, every 2 years to start at age 10 years
Small intestine (RR, 13)	• Annual hemoglobin and small bowel series or enteroscopy every 2 years starting at age 10 years
Pancreatic cancer (RR, 100)	• EUS or abdominal US every 1–2 years; start at age 30 years
Breast cancer (RR, 8.8)	• Annual breast examinations along with mammogram every 2–3 years starting at age 25 years
Uterine cancer; ovarian cancer (RR, 8.0)	• Annual pelvic examinations, pap smear and pelvic US starting at age 20 years
Sertoli cell tumor of testis (Uncommon)	• Annual testicular examination beginning at age 10 years and US of testis, if feminizing features
Juvenile Polyposis	
Colon cancer (< 50%) Gastric, duodenal cancer (Rare)	• Colonoscopic recommendation is same as FAP • Upper GI endoscopy, every 3 years to be commenced in early teens

Abbreviation: RR, relative risk.

HNPCC.[114] In these cases, there is an early onset of colorectal cancers, predominantly in the proximal colon with often synchronous and metachronous cancers. In Lynch I syndrome, there is colonic carcinoma in proximal colon at a pretty young age. In Lynch II syndrome, in addition to colorectal cancer, there is risk of extracolonic cancers, especially cancers of endometrium, ovaries, stomach, small intestine, pancreas and ureters. Genes which have been implicated for the development of this syndrome include *hMSH2*, *hMLH1*, *hMSH6* and *hPMS2* genes.[115]

The diagnosis of HNPCC is based on a detailed and meticulous family history. Various criteria have been laid down. The most important of them is the Amsterdam criteria (1990).[116] There should be at least three relatives with colonic cancer, in addition to all of the following:

- One of the affected patient is a first-degree relative of the other two affected patients
- Two consecutive generations have to be affected
- One of the cases of colonic cancer must be diagnosed before age 50 years
- FAP should be excluded.

The modified Amsterdam criteria (1999) is quite similar to the earlier, with the modification that there should be at least three relatives with HNPCC associated cancer (colorectal cancer, cancer of the endometrium, small bowel and ureter) instead of only colonic carcinoma.

The Bethesda criteria for diagnosis of HNPCC included the Amsterdam criteria or one of the following:[117]

- Two cases of HNPCC-associated cancer in a single patient (synchronous or metachronous)
- Colon cancer and a first-degree relative with HNPCC-associated cancer and/or colonic adenoma (cancer diagnosed before the age of 45 years and adenoma before the age of 40 years)

- Colonic or endometrial cancer diagnosed before the age of 45 years
- Proximal colonic cancer with an undifferentiated histology (solid-cribriform) or signet-cell pattern diagnosed before the age of 45 years
- Adenomas diagnosed before the age of 40 years.

HNPCC patients have 70–80% lifetime risk for developing colorectal cancer and 30–60% risk for endometrial cancer. Hence, all HNPCC patients should be subjected to annual colonoscopy and annual transvaginal ultrasound or endometrial aspirate starting at 20–25 years.

REFERENCES

1. Correa P. Epidemiology of polyps and cancer. In: Morson BC (Ed). The pathogenesis of colorectal cancer. Philadelphia: WB Saunders; 1978. pp. 126-52.
2. Rex DK, Lehman GA, Hawes RH, Ulbright TM, Smith JJ. Screening colonoscopy in asymptomatic average-risk persons with negative fecal occult blood tests. Gastroenterology. 1991;100(1):64-7.
3. Lieberman DA, Prindiville S, Weiss DG, Willett W. Risk factors for advanced colonic neoplasia and hyperplastic polyps in asymptomatic individuals. JAMA. 2003;290(22):2959-67.
4. Liljegren A, Lindblom A, Rotstein S, Nilsson B, Rubio C, Jaramillo E. Prevalence and incidence of hyperplastic polyps and adenomas in familial colorectal cancer: correlation between the two types of colon polyps. Gut. 2003;52(8):1140-7.
5. Winawer SJ, Zauber AG, Fletcher RH, Stillman JS, O'brien MJ, Levin B, et al. Guidelines for colonoscopy surveillance after polypectomy: a consensus update by the US multi-society task force on colorectal cancer and the American cancer society. CA Cancer J Clin. 2006;56(3):143-59.
6. Snover D, Ahnen D, Burt R, Odze RD. Serrated polyps of the colon and rectum and serrated polyposis. WHO Classification of Tumours of the Digestive System, 4th edition. Lyon: IARC; 2010.
7. Patai ÁV, Molnár B, Tulassay Z, Sipos F. Serrated pathway: alternative route to colorectal cancer. World J Gastroenterol. 2013:19(5):607-15.
8. East JE, Saunders BP, Jass JR. Sporadic and syndromic hyperplastic polyps and serrated adenomas of the colon: classification, molecular genetics, natural history, and clinical management. Gastroenterol Clin North Am. 2008;37(1):25-46.
9. Alvarez C, Andreu M, Castells A, Quintero E, Bujanda L, Cubiella J, et al. Relationship of colonoscopy-detected serrated polyps with synchronous advanced neoplasia in average-risk individuals. Gastrointest Endosc. 2013;78(2):333-41.
10. Carballal S, Moreira L, Balaguer F. Serrated polyps and serrated polyposis syndrome. Cir Esp. 2013;91(3):141-8.
11. Nugent KP, Talbot IC, Hodgson SV, Phillips RK. Solitary juvenile polyps: not a marker for subsequent malignancy. Gastroenterology. 1993;105(3):698-700.
12. Gohonot M, Colombel JF, Wolschies E, Quandalle P, Gower P, Lecomte-Houcke M, et al. Cap polyposis occurring in the postoperative course of pelvic surgery. Gut. 1994;35(11):1670-2.
13. Jass JR, Sobin LH. World Health Organization. Histological Typing of Intestinal Tumours, 2nd edition. New York: Springer-Verlag; 1989.
14. O'Brien MJ, Winawer SJ, Zauber AG, Gottlieb LS, Sternberg SS, Diaz B, et al. The national polyp study: patient and polyp characteristics associated with high-grade dysplasia in colorectal adenomas. Gastroenterology. 1990;98(2):371-9.
15. Johannsen LG, Momsen O, Jacobsen NO. Polyps of the large intestine in Aarhus, Denmark: an autopsy study. Scand J Gastroenterol. 1989;24(7):799-806.
16. Tedesco FJ, Hendrix JC, Pickens CA, Brady PG, Mills LR. Diminutive polyps: histopathology, spatial distribution, and clinical significance. Gastrointest Endosc. 1982;28(1):1-5.
17. Ryan ME, Parent K, Wyman JB, et al. Significance of diminutive colorectal polyps in 3282 flexible sigmoidoscopic examinations. Gastrointest Endosc. 1985;31:A149.
18. Weston AP, Campbell DR. Diminutive colonic polyps: histopathology, spatial distribution, concomitant significant lesions, and treatment complications. Am J Gastroenterol. 1995;90(1):24-8.
19. Church JM. Clinical significance of small colorectal polyps. Dis Colon Rectum. 2004;47(4):481-5.
20. Blue MG, Sivak MV, Achkar E, Matzen R, Stahl RR. Hyperplastic polyps seen at sigmoidoscopy are markers for additional adenomas seen at colonoscopy. Gastroenterology. 1991;100(2):564-6.
21. Shinya H, Wolff WI. Morphology, anatomic distribution, and cancer potential of colonic polyps. Ann Surg. 1979;190(6):679-83.
22. Kubota O, Kino I, Kimura T, Harada Y. Nonpolypoid adenomas and adenocarcinomas found in background mucosa of surgically resected colons. Cancer. 1996;77(4):621-6.
23. Saitoh Y, Waxman I, West AB, Popnikolov NK, Gatalica Z, Watari J, et al. Prevalence and distinctive biologic features of flat colorectal adenomas in a North American population. Gastroenterology. 2001;120(7):1657-65.
24. Tsuda S, Veress B, Toth E, Fork FT. Flat and depressed colorectal tumours in a southern Swedish population: a prospective chromoendoscopic and histopathological study. Gut. 2002;51:550-5.
25. Schoen RE, Mutch M, Rall C, Dry SM, Seligson D, Umar A, et al. The natural history of aberrant crypt foci. Gastrointest Endosc. 2008;67(7):1097-102.
26. Hurlstone DP, Karajeh M, Sanders DS, Drew SK, Cross SS,. Rectal aberrant crypt foci identified using high-magnification-chromoscopic colonoscopy: biomarkers for flat and depressed neoplasia. Am J Gastroenterol. 2005;100(6):1283-9.
27. Lynch HT, Knezetic J, Lanspa S. Diagnosing lynch syndrome in absence of colorectal cancer. Expert Opin Med Diagn. 2012;6(6):485-8.
28. Muto T, Bussey HJR, Morson BC. The evolution of cancer of the colon and rectum. Cancer. 1975;36(6):2251-70.
29. Vogelstein B, Kinzler KW. Cancer genes and the pathways they control. Nat Med. 2004;10(8):789-99.
30. Baker SJ, Preisinger AC, Jessup JM, Paraskeva C, Markowitz S, Willson JK, et al. p53 gene mutations occur in combination with 17p allelic deletions as late events in colorectal tumorigenesis. Cancer Res. 1990;50(23):7717-22.
31. Burt RW. Colon cancer screening. Gastroenterology. 2000;119(3):837-53.
32. Rickert RR, Auerbach O, Garfinkel L, Hammond EC, Frasca JM, Adenomatous lesions of the large bowel: an autopsy survey. Cancer. 1979;43(5):1847-57.
33. Pickhardt PJ, Choi JR, Hwang I, Butler JA, Puckett ML, Hildebrandt HA, et al. Computed tomographic virtual colonoscopy to screen for colorectal neoplasia in asymptomatic adults. N Engl J Med. 2003;349(23)2191-200.
34. Imperiale TF, Ransohoff DF, Itzkowitz SH, Turnbull BA, Ross ME. Fecal DNA versus fecal occult blood for colorectal-cancer screening in an average-risk population. N Engl J Med. 2004;351(26):2704-14.
35. Levin TR, Palitz A, Grossman S, Conell C, Finkler L, Ackerson L, et al. Predicting advanced proximal colonic neoplasia with screening sigmoidoscopy. JAMA. 1999;281(17):1611-7.
36. Villavicencio RT, Rex DK. Colonic adenomas: prevalence and incidence rates, growth rates, and miss rates at colonoscopy. Semin Gastrointest Dis. 2000;11(4):185-93.
37. Regula J, Rupinski M, Kraszewska E, Polkowski M, Pachlewski J, Orlowska J, et al. Colonoscopy in colorectal-cancer screening for detection of advanced neoplasia. N Engl J Med. 2006;355(18):1863-72.

38. Zare-Mirzaie A, Abolhasani M, Aryamanesh A. Left sided colorectal adenomatous polyps have more risk for high grade dysplasia. Acta Med Iran. 2013;51(3):172-7.
39. Imperiale TF, Glowinski EA, Lin-Cooper C, Larkin GN, Rogge JD, Ransohoff DF. Five-year risk of colorectal neoplasia after negative screening colonoscopy. N Engl J Med. 2008;359(12):1218-24.
40. Fearnhead NS, Wilding JL, Winney B, Tonks S, Bartlett S, Bicknell DC, et al. Multiple rare variants in different genes account for multifactorial inherited susceptibility to colorectal adenomas. Proc Natl Acad Sci USA. 2004;101(45):15992-7.
41. Kahi CJ, Rex DK, Imperiale TF. Screening, surveillance, and primary prevention for colorectal cancer: a review of the recent literature. Gastroenterology. 2008;135(2):380-99.
42. Lee JY, Kwak SM, Myung SK, Jee SH. Obesity and colorectal adenomatous polyps: a cross-sectional study in Korean adults. Obesity (Silver Spring). 2014;22(2):518-25.
43. Ashktorab H, Hassanzadeh NH, Taylor T, Williams C, Brim H, Mellman T, et al. Role of life events in the presence of colon polyps among African Americans. BMC Gastroenterol. 2013;13(1):101.
44. Peters U, Sinha R, Chatterjee N, Subar AF, Ziegler RG, Kulldorff M, et al. Prostate, lung, colorectal, and ovarian cancer screening trial project team. Dietary fibre and colorectal adenoma in a colorectal cancer early detection programme. Lancet. 2003; 361(9368):1491-5.
45. Ferguson LR, Harris PJ. The dietary fibre debate: more food for thought. Lancet. 2003;361(9368):1487-88.
46. Nimptsch K, Bernstein AM, Giovannucci E, Fuchs CS, Willett WC, Wu K. Dietary intakes of red meat, poultry, and fish during high school and risk of colorectal adenomas in women. Am J Epidemiol. 2013;178(2):172-83.
47. Lieberman DA, Prindiville S, Weiss DG, Willett W. Risk factors for advanced colonic neoplasia and hyperplastic polyps in asymptomatic individuals. JAMA. 2003;290(22):2959-67.
48. Song JH, Kim YS, Yang SY, Chung SJ, Park MJ, Lim SH, et al. Physical activity and other lifestyle factors in relation to the prevalence of colorectal adenoma: a colonoscopy-based study in asymptomatic Koreans. Cancer Causes Control. 2013;24(9):1717-26.
49. Hawk ET, Levin B. Colorectal cancer prevention. J Clin Oncol. 2005;23(2):378-91.
50. Chen FP, Lin CC, Chen TH, Tsai MC, Huang YC. Higher plasma homocysteine is associated with increased risk of developing colorectal polyps. Nutr Cancer. 2013;65(2):195-201.
51. Sonnenberg A, Genta RM. Helicobacter pylori is a risk factor for colonic neoplasms. Am J Gastroenterol. 2013;108(2):208-15.
52. Cole BF, Logan RF, Halabi S, Benamouzig R, Sandler RS, Grainge MJ, et al. Aspirin for the chemoprevention of colorectal adenomas: meta-analysis of the randomized trials. J Natl Cancer Inst. 2009;101(4):256-6.
53. Meyskens FL, McLaren CE, Pelot D, Fujikawa-Brooks S, Carpenter PM, Hawk E, et al. Difluoromethylornithine plus sulindac for the prevention of sporadic colorectal adenomas: a randomized placebo-controlled, double-blind trial. Cancer Prev Res. 2008;1(1):32-8.
54. Broughton T, Sington J, Beales IL. Statin use is associated with a reduced incidence of colorectal adenomatous polyps. Int J Colorectal Dis. 201328(4):469-76.
55. Stewart M, Macrae FA, Williams CB. Neoplasia and ureterosigmoidostomy: a colonoscopic survey. Br J Surg. 1982;69(7):414-6.
56. Neugut AI, Murray TI, Garbowski GC, Forde KA, Treat MR, Waye JD, et al. Cholecystectomy as a risk factor for colorectal adenomatous polyps and carcinoma. Cancer. 1991;68(7):1644-7.
57. Delhougne B, Deneux C, Abs R, Chanson P, Fierens H, Laurent-Puig P, et al. The prevalence of colonic polyps in acromegaly: a colonoscopic and pathological study in 103 patients. J Clin Endocrinol Metab. 1995;80(11):3223-6.
58. Rokkas T, Pistiolas D, Sechopoulos P, Margantinis G, Koukoulis G. Risk of colorectal neoplasm in patients with acromegaly: a meta-analysis. World J Gastroenterol. 2008;14(22):3484-9.
59. Sharara AI, Abou HT, Malli A, El-Halabi MM, Hashash JG, Ghaith OA, et al. Association of Streptococcus bovis endocarditis and advanced colorectal neoplasia. A case-control study. J Dig Dis. 2013;14(7):382-7.
60. Burnett-Hartman AN, Newcomb PA, Potter JD. Infectious agents and colorectal cancer: a review of Helicobacter pylori, Streptococcus bovis, JC virus, and human papillomavirus. Cancer Epidemiol Biomarkers Prev. 2008;17(11):2970-9.
61. Shnitka TK, Friedman MHW, Kidd EG, et al. Villous tumors of the rectum and colon characterized by severe fluid and electrolyte loss. Surg Gynecol Obstet. 1961;112:609.
62. Macrae St F, John DJ. Relationship between patterns of bleeding and hemoccult sensitivity in patients with colorectal cancers or adenomas. Gastroenterology. 1982;82:891-8.
63. Ou CH, Kuo FC, Hsu WH, Lu CY, Yu FJ, Kuo CH, et al. Comparison of the performance of guaiac-based and two immunochemical fecal occult blood tests for identifying advanced colorectal neoplasia in Taiwan. J Dig Dis. 2013;14(9):474-83.
64. Lucendo AJ, Guagnozzi D, Angueira T, González-Castillo S, Fernández-Fuente M, Friginal-Ruiz AB. The relationship between proximal and distal colonic adenomas: is screening sigmoidoscopy enough in the presence of a changing epidemiology? Eur J Gastroenterol Hepatol. 2013;25(8):973-80.
65. Winawer SJ, Stewart ET, Zauber AG, Bond JH, Ansel H, Waye JD, et al. A comparison of colonoscopy and double-contrast barium enema for surveillance after polypectomy. N Engl J Med. 2000;342(24):1766-72.
66. Barclay RL, Vicari JJ, Doughty AS, Johanson JF, Greenlaw RL. Colonoscopic withdrawal times and adenoma detection during screening colonoscopy. N Engl J Med. 2006;355(24):2533-41.
67. Rex DK. Maximizing detection of adenomas and cancers during colonoscopy. Am J Gastroenterol. 2006;101(12):2866-77.
68. Yoshida Y, Matsuda K, Sumiyama K, Kawahara Y, Yoshizawa K, Ishiguro H, et al. A randomized crossover open trial of the adenoma miss rate for narrow band imaging (NBI) versus flexible spectral imaging color enhancement (FICE). Int J Colorectal Dis. 2013;28(11):1511-6.
69. Schachschal G, Mayr M, Treszl A, Balzer K, Wegscheider K, Aschenbeck J, et al. Endoscopic versus histological characterisation of polyps during screening colonoscopy. Gut. 2014;63(3):458-65.
70. Johnson CD, Chen MH, Toledano AY, Heiken JP, Dachman A, Kuo MD, et al. Accuracy of CT colonography for detection of large adenomas and cancers. N Engl J Med. 2008;359(12):1207-17.
71. Pullens HJ, van Leeuwen MS, Laheij RJ, Vleggaar FP, Siersema PD. CT-colonography after incomplete colonoscopy: what is the diagnostic yield? Dis Colon Rectum. 2013; 56(5):593-9.
72. Lidgard GP, Domanico MJ, Bruinsma JJ, Light J, Gagrat ZD, Oldham-Haltom RL, et al. Clinical performance of an automated stool DNA assay for detection of colorectal neoplasia. Clin Gastroenterol Hepatol. 2013;11(10):1313-8.
73. Stryker SJ, Wolff BG, Culp CE, Libbe SD, Ilstrup DM, MacCarty RL. Natural history of untreated colonic polyps. Gastroenterology. 1987;93(5):1009-13.
74. Langevin JM, Nivatvongs S. The true incidence of synchronous cancer of the bowel. A prospective study. Am J Surg. 1984;147(3):330-3.
75. Imperiale TF, Wagner DR, Lin CY, Larkin GN, Rogge JD, Ransohoff DF, et al. Risk of advanced proximal neoplasms in asymptomatic adults according to the distal colorectal findings. N Engl J Med. 2000;343(3):169-74.
76. Choi YS, Lee JB, Lee EJ, Lee SH, Suh JP, Lee DH, et al. Can endoscopic submucosal dissection technique be an alternative

treatment option for a difficult giant (≥30 mm) pedunculated colorectal polyp? Dis Colon Rectum. 2013;56(5):660-6.
77. Wilcox GM, Anderson PB, Colacchio TA. Early invasive carcinoma in colonic polyps: a review of the literature with emphasis on the assessment of the risk of metastasis. Cancer. 1986;57(1):160-71.
78. Haggitt RC, Glotzbach RE, Soffer EE, Wruble LD. Prognostic factors in colorectal carcinoma arising in adenomas: implications for lesions removed by endoscopic polypectomy. Gastroenterology. 1985;89(2):328-36.
79. Jung M. The 'difficult' polyp: pitfalls for endoscopic removal. Dig Dis. 2012;30(Suppl 2):74-80.
80. Coverlizza S, Risio M, Ferrari A, Rossini FP. Colorectal adenomas containing invasive carcinoma: pathologic assessment of lymph node metastatic potential. Cancer. 1989;64(9):1937-47.
81. Wu XR, Church JM, Jarrar A, Liang J, Kalady MF. Risk factors for delayed postpolypectomy bleeding: how to minimize your patients' risk. Int J Colorectal Dis. 2013;28(8):1127-34.
82. Neugut AI, Jacobson JS, Ahsan H, Santos J, Garbowski GC, Forde KA, et al. Incidence and recurrence rates of colorectal adenomas: a prospective study. Gastroenterology. 1995;108(2):402-8.
83. Kronborg O, Hage E, Adamsen S, Deichgraeber E. Follow-up after colorectal polypectomy: II. Repeated examinations of the colon every 6 months after removal of sessile adenomas and adenomas with the highest degree of dysplasia. Scand J Gastroenterol. 1983;18(8):1095-9.
84. Martinez ME, Sampliner R, Marshall JR, Bhattacharyya AK, Reid ME, Alberts DS. Adenoma characteristics as risk factors for recurrence of advanced adenomas. Gastroenterology. 2001;120(5):1077-83.
85. Martinez ME, Baron JA, Lieberman DA, Schatzkin A, Lanza E, Winawer SJ, et al. A pooled analysis of advanced colorectal neoplasia diagnoses after colonoscopic polypectomy. Gastroenterology. 2009;136(3):832-41.
86. Winawer SJ, Zauber AG, Ho MN, O'Brien MJ, Gottlieb LS, Sternberg SS, et al. Prevention of colorectal cancer by colonoscopic polypectomy. N Engl J Med. 1993;329(27):1977-81.
87. Winawer SJ, Zauber AG, Fletcher RH, Stillman JS, O'brien MJ, Levin B, et al. Guidelines for colonoscopy surveillance after polypectomy: a consensus update by the US multi-society task force on colorectal cancer and the American cancer society. CA Cancer J Clin. 2006;56(3):143-59.
88. Bussey HJR, Veale AMO, Morson BC. Genetics of gastrointestinal polyposis. Gastroenterology. 1978;74(6):1325-30.
89. Bodmer WF, Bailey CJ, Bodmer J, Bussey HJ, Ellis A, Gorman P, et al. Localization of the gene for familial adenomatous polyposis on chromosome 5. Nature. 1987;328(6131):614-6.
90. Oving IM, Clevers HC. Molecular causes of colon cancer. Eur J Clin Invest. 2002;32(6):448-57.
91. Bussey HJR. Familial polyposis coli. Baltimore: Johns Hopkins University Press; 1975.
92. Bianchi LK, Burke CA, Bennett AE, Lopez R, Hasson H, Church JM. Fundic gland polyp dysplasia is common in familial adenomatous polyposis. Clin Gastroenterol Hepatol. 2008;6(2):180-5.
93. Park JG, Park KJ, Ahn YO, Song IS, Choi KW, Moon HY, et al. Risk of gastric cancer among Korean familial adenomatous polyposis patients. Report of three cases. Dis Colon Rectum. 1992;35(10):996-8.
94. Debinski HS, Spigelman AD, Hatfield A, Williams CB, Phillips RK,. Upper intestinal surveillance in familial adenomatous polyposis. Eur J Cancer. 1995;31A(7-8):1149-53.
95. Vasen HF, Moslein G, Alonso A, Aretz S, Bernstein I, Bertario L, et al. Guidelines for the clinical management of familial adenomatous polyposis (FAP). Gut. 2008;57(5):704-13.
96. Sturt NJH, Gallagher MC, Bassett P, Philp CR, Neale KF, Tomlinson IP, et al. Evidence for genetic predisposition to desmoid tumors in familial adenomatous polyposis independent of the germline APC mutation. Gut. 2004;53(12):1832-6.
97. Gurbuz AK, Giardiello FM, Petersen GM, Krush AJ, Offerhaus GJ, Booker SV, et al. Desmoid tumors in familial adenomatous polyposis. Gut. 1994;35(3):377-81.
98. Durno C, Monga N, Bapat B, Berk T, Cohen Z, Gallinger S, et al. Does early colectomy increase desmoid risk in familial adenomatous polyposis? Clin Gastroenterol Hepatol. 2007;5(10):1190-4.
99. Lanari A. Effect of progesterone on desmoid tumors (aggressive fibromatosis). N Engl J Med. 1983;309(24):1523.
100. Klein WA, Miller HH, Anderson M, DeCosse JJ. The use of indomethacin, sulindac, and tamoxifen for the treatment of desmoid tumors associated with familial polyposis. Cancer. 1987;60(12):2863-8.
101. Aziz O, Athanasiou T, Fazio VW, Nicholls RJ, Darzi AW, Church J, et al. Meta-analysis of observational studies of ileorectal versus ileal pouch-anal anastomosis for familial adenomatous polyposis. Br J Surg. 2006;93(4):407-17.
102. Bussey HJR, DeCosse JJ, Deschner EE, Eyers AA, Lesser ML, Morson BC, et al. A randomized trial of ascorbic acid in polyposis coli. Cancer. 1982;50(7):1434-9.
103. Stern HS, Gregoire RC, Kashtan H, Stadler J, Bruce RW, Long-term effects of dietary calcium on risk markers for colon cancer in patients with familial polyposis. Surgery. 1990;108(3):528-33.
104. DeCosse JJ, Miller HH, Lesser ML. Effect of wheat fiber and vitamins C and E on rectal polyps in patients with familial adenomatous polyposis. J Natl Cancer Inst. 1989;81(17):1290-7.
105. Prescott SM, White RL. Self-promotion? Intimate connections between APC and prostaglandin H synthase-2. Cell. 1996;87(5):783-6.
106. Giardiello FM, Yang VW, Hylind LM, Krush AJ, Petersen GM, Trimbath JD, et al. Primary chemoprevention of familial adenomatous polyposis with sulindac. N Engl J Med 2002;346(14):1054-9.
107. Brosens LA, Keller JJ, Offerhaus GJ, Goggins M, Giardiello FM. Prevention and management of duodenal polyps in familial adenomatous polyposis. Gut. 2005;54(7):1034-3.
108. Burt RW. Colon cancer screening. Gastroenterology. 2000;119(3):837-53.
109. Vasen HF, Moslein G, Alonso A, Aretz S, Bernstein I, Bertario L, et al. Guidelines for the clinical management of familial adenomatous polyposis (FAP). Gut. 2008;57(5):704-13.
110. Daniel ES, Ludwig SL, Lewin KJ, Ruprecht RM, Rajacich GM, Schwabe AD, et al. The Cronkhite-Canada syndrome: an analysis of the pathologic features and therapy in 55 patients. Medicine (Baltimore). 1982;1(5):293-309.
111. Calva D, Howe JR. Hamartomatous polyposis syndromes. Surg Clin North Am. 2008;88(4):779-81.
112. O'Briani DS, Kennedy MJ, Daly PA, O'Brien AA, Tanner WA, Rogers P, et al. Multiple lymphomatous polyposis of the gastrointestinal tract. A clinicopathologically distinctive form of non-Hodgkin's lymphoma of B-cell centrocytic type. Am J Surg Pathol. 1989;13(8):691-9.
113. Miwata T, Hiyama T, Oka S, Tanaka S, Shimamoto F, Arihiro K, et al. Clinicopathologic features of Japanese hyperplastic/serrated polyposis syndrome. J Gastroenterol Hepatol. 2013;28(11):1693-738.
114. Lynch HT, de la Chapelle A. Hereditary colorectal cancer. N Engl J Med. 2003;348(10):919-32.
115. Lynch HT, de la Chapelle A. Genetic susceptibility to nonpolyposis colorectal cancer. J Med Genet. 1999;36(11):801-18.
116. Vasen HF. Clinical diagnosis and management of hereditary colorectal cancer syndromes. J Clin Oncol. 2000;18(21Suppl): 81S-92S.
117. Umar A, Boland CR, Terdiman JP, , Syngal S, de la Chapelle A, Rüschoff J, et al. Revised Bethesda guidelines for hereditary nonpolyposis colorectal cancer (Lynch syndrome) and microsatellite instability. J Natl Cancer Inst. 2004;96(4):261-8.

CHAPTER 97

Colorectal Cancer: An Overview

Ashok Kumar, Puneet Puri

INTRODUCTION

The colorectal cancer (CRC) is prevalent worldwide with highest burden in western world. The CRC has been the prototype for understanding the genetic mechanisms involved in the cancer. The therapeutic strategies involving chemoradiotherapy have been extensively studied on patients with CRC. This chapter includes an overview regarding etiopathogenesis and management of CRC.

EPIDEMIOLOGY

The worldwide incidence of CRC is highly variable. The maximal incidence being in the Europe and Australia and lowest occurrence in South Central Asia.[1] The CRC is the third most common cancer in the United States. Worldwide it is the third most common cause of cancer related death.[2] The risk of CRC increases with increase in age. There has occurred a constant rise in incidence of colorectal carcinoma over three decades from 1970s till 2000. This can partly be attributed to increase in old population in western world. In the last decade incidence of CRC has got reduced slightly. This fall is contributed by reduction in occurrence of distal cancers.[3] The reduction of incidence can be due to intensive screening program which help to detect the premalignant lesions at the earliest before invasive malignancy develops. The CRC incidence in India matches the lowest rates worldwide. The rates of rectal cancers are higher than that of colon cancer as per data from hospital registries in India.[3-5] There are little variations in incidence of CRC in various parts of Indian subcontinent. The incidence of rectal cancers is higher in rural India.[6,7]

ETIOLOGY

Colorectal cancer can occur in sporadic, hereditary and familial forms. The sporadic form is the most common form of CRC which occurs in elderly individuals without family history. The hereditary forms occur in younger individual with positive family history. The examples include familial adenomatous polyposis (FAP) and hereditary nonpolyposis colon cancer (HNPCC)/Lynch syndrome. The basic differences between the two forms of CRC are highlighted in Table 1.

Despite above mentioned differences the genetics of cancer initiation and progression shares common pathways in both forms of CRC.

Various risk factors have been detected which play role in occurrence of CRC. The interaction between the genetic factors and environmental factors is the basis of occurrence of cancer, determines its biological behavior and consequently cancer related death and post-therapy survival.

Age is the most common non-modifiable risk factor. The CRC is a disease of old population usually occurring in the 6th or 7th decade. Bimodal occurrence of CRC has been appreciated.[8] Juvenile variety occurs more commonly in non-white population whereas adult form occurs more frequently in white population. The juvenile variety is having more aggressive biological behavior, comprising of mucinous carcinoma in three-fourths of cases. There is no associated family history in juvenile variety.

Genetic Mutations

Patients with hereditary polyposis syndromes have increased risk of developing CRCs. Due to "global field defect" malignancy can occur in the polyp or at a different site in the colon. The villous adenoma has highest incidence of harboring malignancy and risk exceeds 50% when size is more than 2 cm. FAP has 100% risk of developing invasive carcinoma if no surgical intervention is offered. The patients with Lynch syndrome have 80% risk of developing malignancy over lifetime.

Table 1: Differences between hereditary and sporadic forms of CRC

Parameters	*Hereditary colorectal cancer*	*Sporadic colorectal cancer*
Age at onset	Younger, usually in 2nd to 3rd decade	5th to 7th decade
Family history	Present	Absent
Genetic mutations	Limited to tumor cells	Present in all cells of individual
Multifocal/multiple tumors	Common	Rare

Patients previously treated for sporadic CRC are always at a higher risk of developing metachronous cancer or polypoidal lesion. Approximately 6% of patients with sporadic colon cancer develop metachronous cancer.[9]

Family History of Colon Cancer

The familial form of CRC is characterized by occurrence of CRC before the age of 50 years and posing the first degree relatives of the affected individual to an increased risk of development of colonic malignancy. The risk increases with rise in number of affected relatives as shown in Table 2.[10]

Inflammatory Bowel Disease

The risk of malignancy is proportionate to duration and extent of disease. The risk is similar in ulcerative colitis and Crohn's disease if disease duration and extent are matched.[11] The risk of malignancy gets doubled with each successive decade of disease duration, i.e. 5% after first decade, 10% after second decade and 20% after third decade. The malignancy is more common in patients with pancolitis. The development of strictures also predispose to malignancy especially in the right colon.

Table 2: Familial CRC: Risk stratification according to degree and number of affected relative

Familial setting	*Risk of colon cancer*
General population (USA)	6%
One first degree relative with colon cancer	Two-fold to threefold increased
Two first degree relatives with colon cancer	Three-fold to fourfold increased
First degree relative with colon cancer diagnosed less than or equal to 50 year	Three-fold to fourfold increased
One second or third degree relative with colon cancer	1.5 fold increased
Two second or third degree relatives with colon cancer	Two-fold to three-fold increased
One first degree relative with adenomatous polyp	Two-fold increased

Note: The first degree relatives: Parents, siblings, children. *The second degree relatives:* Uncles, aunts and grandparents; *The third degree relatives:* Great-grandparents, cousins.

Modifiable Risk Factors

i. *Dietary habits:* Dietary fats and fiber deficient diets are implicated in CRC development. High total fat intake, saturated fats and cholesterol are associated with increased risk of colorectal carcinoma.[12] The consumption of red meat, low fiber diet are associated with high incidence of CRC and CRC risk can be reduced by consumption of fiber rich diet.
ii. *Alcohol intake:* Alcohol intake has been associated with increased risk of distal colonic carcinoma.[13]
iii. *Smoking, sedentary life style, obesity* are associated with higher incidence of colonic cancer.

GENETICS OF COLORECTAL CANCER

The various genes are categorized into three subtypes: (1) proto-oncogenes, (2) tumor suppressor genes, (3) mismatch repair genes (MMR). The mutations of all the three types are involved in colorectal carcinogenesis. The accumulation of mutants of these genes leads to phenotypic expression of polyps and eventually carcinoma.

Proto-oncogenes

These are constitutive genes also named as "Housekeeping" genes which are routinely expressed for maintenance of cellular functions. The mutations of these genes lead to "gain of function" leading to uncontrolled cellular proliferation and consequent neoplasia. The mutation in single allele of gene is sufficient to produce phenotypic expressions. The examples of proto-oncogenes involved in CRC are growth factors (EGF, TGF, IGF), growth factor receptors, signal transducers, transcription factors. The *ras* proto-oncogene located on chromosome no 12 is one of the earliest affected in the carcinogenetic sequence.

Tumor Suppressor Genes

These are known as "gatekeeper" genes. In health, these are regulators of cell cycles by inhibiting the expression of growth promoters. Their biallelic mutations render the cell autonomous and hence unregulated proliferation. The most common studied tumor suppressor gene is *APC* gene which is located on 5q21. The product of *APC* gene binds intracytoplasmic beta-catenin. The germline mutations lead to expression of hereditary condition known as "familial adenomatous polyposis". The detailed studies of *APC* gene have defined a mutation cluster region where majority of truncation mutations occur leading to variety of phenotypic expressions of FAP and extraintestinal manifestations, e.g. Gardner syndrome characterized by FAP in association with mandibular and skull osteoma, periampullary carcinoma and mesenteric desmoids. Even up to 85% sporadic CRCs do exhibit the truncation mutations of *APC* genes. Another tumor suppressor gene involved in colorectal carcinogenesis is the p53 gene known as "guardian of the genome". The colorectal tumors with preserved p53 functions are thought to have survival benefits.

Mismatch Repair Genes (MMR)

These are involved in base excision-repair of mismatched nucleotides in genes, hence also known as "caretaker" genes. The loss of function of such genes leads to accumulation of mismatched base pairs. The examples of this category of genes are *hMLH1, hMSH2, hMSH3, hMSH6*. The defect in mismatch repair genes is associated with hereditary nonpolyposis colon cancer (HNPCC).

The adenoma-carcinoma model of carcinogenesis proposed by Fearon and Vogelstein is the basic step in understanding the colorectal carcinogenesis. The earliest implicated gene is *APC* and earliest phenotypic expression is the aberrant crypt formation. The unregulated growth leading on to accumulation of epithelial cells lead to polyp formation and persistent occurrence of mutations lead to adenoma formation which progresses through early, intermediate and late adenoma and eventually lead to intraepithelial neoplasm and carcinoma. Even carcinoma follows orderly steps of progressive involvement of colonic wall (basement membrane invasion, lamina, submucosa, muscularis propria, serosa) and nodal involvement and eventually distant metastasis. The polypoidal lesions (sessile as well as pedunculated) harboring the carcinoma are classified into five levels (Level 0–4) according to Haggit's classification.[14] The Haggit's classification determines the chances of regional lymph node involvement according to depth of invasion, differentiation of tumor and presence of poor prognostic variables and helps to decide appropriate management of these cancerous polyps.

CLINICAL FEATURES OF COLON CANCER

Colorectal cancer can have sporadic presentation or as hereditary syndromes. The sporadic presentation is the commonest form without positive family history. Despite similar genetic and molecular basis of colon and rectal carcinoma there are variations in their diagnostic and therapeutic algorithms.

The symptoms of colonic carcinoma are varied and depend on multiple factors:

(a) Anatomical location of tumor: The tumors of right colon are proliferative with ulceration of overlying mucosa leading to occult blood loss and unexplained anemia. Less frequently bleeding from right colonic tumor can lead to melena. Unexplained anemia in an adult male and non-menstruating female must raise the suspicion of carcinoma right colon. Due to capacious bowel lumen and soft consistency of fecal matter obstructive symptoms are less common with right sided colonic tumors. Tumors of left colon are of constricting nature leading to constipation. These usually present with recent alteration in bowel habits. The left colonic tumors can present with hematochezia or blood mixed with stools. Sigmoid tumors can lead to sigmoid volvulus.

(b) Extent of involvement of bowel lumen: The left colonic lesions are more prone to obstruction due to narrow diameter of left colon, constricting nature of left colonic growth and solid consistency of fecal matter. Patients initially have episodes of subacute obstruction (colicky abdominal pain, obstipation and abdominal distension relieved after passage of flatus and motion) which are relieved due to forceful peristalsis overcoming the obstruction. Once the diameter is reduced to a critical level acute large bowel obstruction ensues leading to fecal loading and dilatation of colon proximal to site of obstruction. In presence of competent ileocecal valve (which prevents the reflux of colonic contents into terminal ileum) there occurs closed loop colonic obstruction leading to extreme cecal dilatation. The persistent closed loop obstruction can cause critical ischemia and eventual perforation of cecum with fecal contamination of peritoneal cavity leading to peritonitis and septic shock and multiorgan failure. The full thickness bowel involvement with tumor necrosis can lead to tumor perforation. In presence of incompetent ileocecal valve small bowel gets dilated and in addition to other features of obstruction patient has feculent vomiting.

(c) Involvement of adjacent structures: The involvement of retroperitoneal structures like ureters can lead to backpressure changes and hydroureteronephrosis. The unilateral hydroureteronephrosis is usually silent and does not lead to derangement of renal functions. The involvement of duodenum by hepatic flexure of transverse colon growths can lead to duodenal obstruction. The involvement of urinary bladder by cecal and sigmoid carcinoma can lead to colovesical fistula. The involvement of parieties produces somatic pain.

(d) Metastasis: Patients with disseminated CRC present with cachexia, ascites and features of carcinoma peritonei.

CLINICAL FEATURES OF RECTAL CARCINOMA

Rectal cancer can develop de novo or on background of polyposis syndromes or inflammatory bowel disease. The most common symptom of rectal cancer is fresh bleeding per rectum. The symptom is usually attributed wrongly to benign anorectal diseases like hemorrhoids or fissure in ano and leads to delay in the diagnosis.

The features are site specific. The Upper rectal cancers present with constipation and fresh bleeding per rectum. Obstructive lesions have suprapubic pain with abdominal distension. Middle rectal cancers have characteristic sense of incomplete evacuation due to distension of rectal ampulla by growth and mucus. Due to accumulation of mucus with blood in the rectum, patient can have "early morning spurious diarrhea" containing mucus and blood only. Copious mucus production in large villous adenoma of rectum can present with malnutrition due to protein loss along with dyselectrolytemia. Hard growths can lead to pipe like or tape like stools. Patient can have tenesmus that is defined as repeated painful urge to defecate but without yield. The lower rectal growths when encroach upon dentate line present with pain during defecation. The involvement of sphincter complex presents with fecal incontinence. There can be per rectal protrusion of associated rectal polyps. The adjacent structural involvement can cause rectovesical or rectouterine/rectovaginal fistulae. The involvement of lateral pelvic plexus can lead to neurogenic bladder and retrograde ejaculations, impaired penile erection in males. The sacral plexus involvement leads to deep pelvic/perineal pain radiating to posterior surface of thighs. The colloid carcinoma of rectum and that associated with inflammatory bowel disease can have multiple perianal fistulous openings. The lymph nodal involvement in lower rectal cancer can lead to enlarged superficial inguinal nodes.

Apart from general examination, digital rectal examination is most important in assessment of rectal carcinoma. Tumors are assessed to define distance from anal verge, anterior versus posterior rectal wall involvement, luminal compromise by tumor and mobility of tumor.

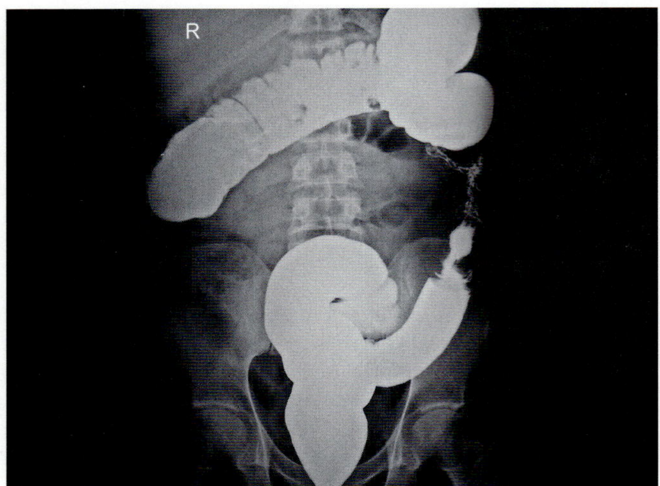

Figure 1 Barium enema-Descending colon Ca

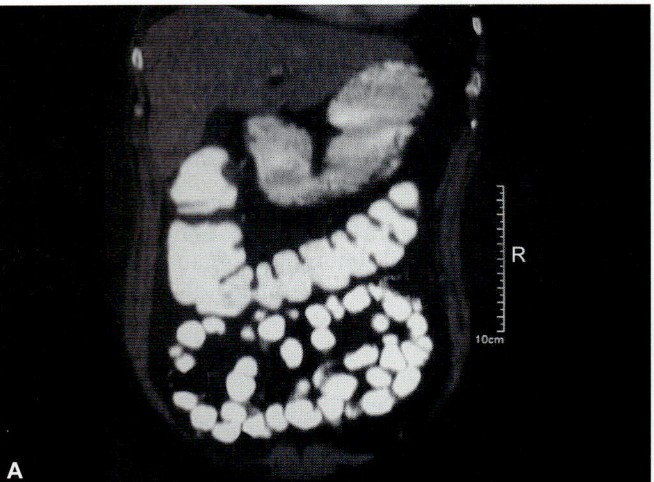

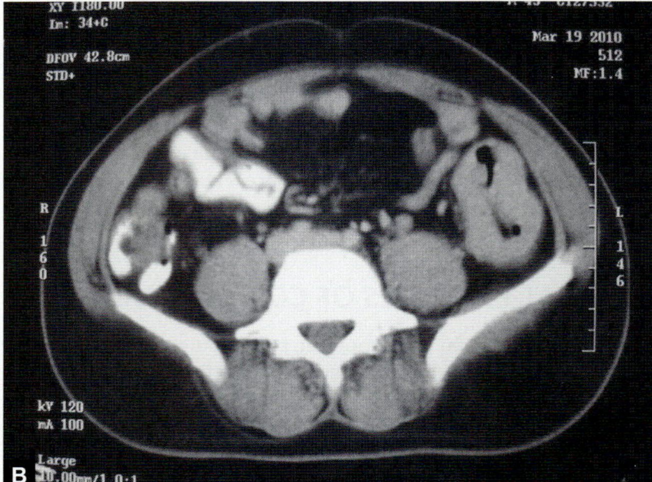

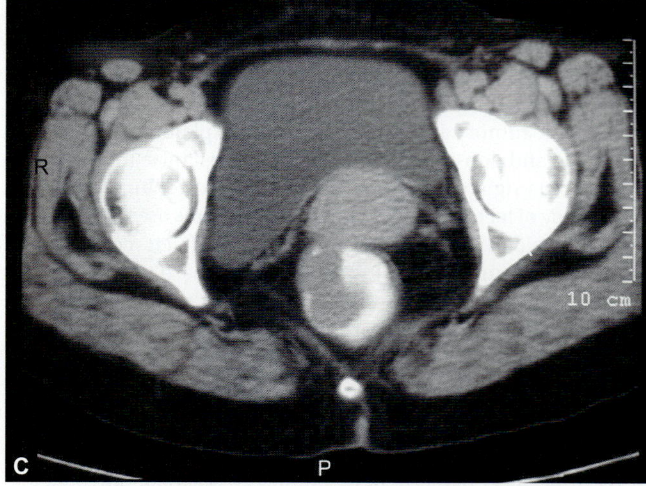

Figures 2A to C (A) CT-Growth at splenic flexure; (B) CT Axial cut-Stricuring lesion in descending colon; (C) CT-growth in lower rectum

DIAGNOSIS OF COLONIC CANCER

Colonoscopy is the gold standard for diagnosis of colon cancer. Colonoscopic biopsy helps to establish histological diagnosis of malignancy. The differentiation of tumor helps to provide biological behavior of tumor. Colonoscopy helps in direct visualization of entire colon to look for synchronous malignancy or polyps. Colonoscopic guided tattooing of colonic lesions can help in their localization during surgery.

Double contrast barium enema can diagnose colonic lesion but subsequent colonoscopy is required to have histological diagnosis and to look for synchronous lesions (Fig. 1).

Virtual colonoscopy or CT colonography is used to diagnose colonic tumors in patients in whom colonoscopy cannot be performed. The virtual colonoscopy requires colonic preparation similar to that for videocolonoscopy. The fecal matter in the colon can interfere with interpretations of virtual colonoscopy.

The contrast enhanced CT scan is used to assess the relation and extent of adjacent organ involvement. Positive oral and rectal contrast is used to opacify the small and large bowel. The CT scan helps to preoperative plan the need of adjacent organ resection (Figs 2A and B).

Role of magnetic resonance imaging (MRI): The MRI by endorectal coils is being frequently used to stage the rectal cancer but its use in colonic lesion has yet not been clinically validated.[15] The inherent advantage of better delineation of layers of bowel wall and multiplanar imaging is overshadowed by movement artifacts due to respiratory movement and bowel peristalsis. At present MRI is being used in metastatic colonic malignancy to assess liver lesions.

Staging of colorectal cancer: The TNM staging of CRC by American Joint committee on cancer (AJCC) 7th edition is universally accepted.[16] The "T" stage increases according to the depth of invasion of bowel wall by tumor. In situ carcinoma can be intraepithelial or intramucosal but is limited by muscularis mucosae. The T4 lesions include tumor invading visceral peritoneum (perforated carcinoma) as well as the other organs. The invasion of other part of large bowel is also considered as other organ involvement. Nodal staging "N" stage is based on number of involved regional lymph nodes. The clinical or pathological stages are marked by prescript "c" and "p" respectively. The prescript "y" denotes that patient has been provided neoadjuvant therapy. The lymphatic, vascular and perineural invasion are represented by L,V and PN (Boxes 1 and 2).

BOX 1 TNM classification by 7th edition of AJCC[16]

PRIMARY TUMOR (T)

- TX Primary tumor cannot be assessed
- T0 No evidence of primary tumor
- Tis Carcinoma *in situ*: intraepithelial or invasion of lamina propria*
- T1 Tumor invades submucosa
- T2 Tumor invades muscularis propria
- T3 Tumor invades through the muscularis propria into pericolorectal tissues
- T4a Tumor penetrates to the surface of the visceral peritoneum[1]
- T4b Tumor directly invades or is adherent to other organs or structures[1]*

REGIONAL LYMPH NODES (N)

- NX Regional lymph nodes cannot be assessed
- N0 No regional lymph node metastasis
- N1 Metastasis in 1-3 regional lymph nodes
- N1a Metastasis in 1 regional lymph node
- N1b Metastasis in 2-3 regional lymph nodes
- N1c Tumor deposit(s) in the subserosa, mesentery, or nonperitonealized pericolic or perirectal tissues without regional nodal metastasis
- N2 Metastasis in 4 or more regional lymph nodes
- N2a Metastasis in 4-6 regional lymph nodes
- N2b Metastasis in 7 or more regional lymph nodes

PRIMARY TUMOR (T)

- M0 No distant metastasis
- M1 Distant metastasis
- M1a Metastasis confined to one organ or site (e.g. liver, lung, ovary, nonregional node)
- M1b Metastases in more than one organ/site or the peritoneum

BOX 2 Stage distribution of colorectal carcinoma according to TNM classification

Anatomic stage	**Prognostic groups**		
Stage	**T**	**N**	**M**
0	Tis	NO	MO
I	T1	NO	MO
	T2	NO	MO
IIA	T3	NO	MO
IIB	T4a	NO	MO
IIC	T4b	NO	MO
IIIA	T1-T2	N1/N1C	MO
	T1	N2a	MO
IIIB	T3-T4a	N1/N1C	MO
	T2-T3	N2a	MO
	T1-T2	N2b	MO
IIIC	T4a	N2a	MO
	T3-T4a	N2b	MO
	T4b	N1-N2	MO
IVA	Any T	Any N	M1a
IVB	Any T	Any N	M1b

The colorectal tumors involving full thickness colonic wall and contiguous adjacent organ involvement without nodal disease are grouped in stages I and II. The regional lymph node involvement denotes stage III of CRC. Presence of distant metastasis denotes stage IV. For accurate staging of CRC at least 12 nodes must be examined.[17]

Treatment Strategy of Colonic Carcinoma

The management of CRC involves multidisciplinary approach involving coloproctologist, radiation and medical oncologist and radiologist. The treatment strategies for colonic and rectal cancers are variable. The rectum is relatively fixed than colon and confined to a closed bony pelvis. Hence providing radiotherapy is feasible in rectal cancer. The colonic wall can also tolerate radiotherapy up to 55 Gy but due to close proximity of small bowel and mobility of colon makes it unsuitable for receiving appropriate fixed dose of radiotherapy without side effects. Surgery is the main stay of treatment for CRC. The extent of colonic resections is guided by vascular supply and lymphatic drainage of involved colonic segment. The right colon along with proximal two-thirds of transverse colon is derivative of mid-gut and is supplied by superior mesenteric territory (ileocolic, right colic and middle colic branches of superior mesenteric artery). The distal one-third of transverse colon and left colon is derived from hindgut and is supplied by inferior mesenteric territory (left colic, sigmoid branches) (Figs 3A and B). The intramural lymphatic spread in colon occurs up to 2 cm and this forms the basis of minimum 5 cm resection margin in colonic carcinoma. But actual length of resected bowel is determined by vascular pedicle division required for adequate lymphatic drainage. The lymphatic drainage of colon follows an orderly pattern. The lymphatics from submucosal layer of colon traverse the muscularis propria and form subserosal plexus and thereafter lymphatics travel sequentially to four nodal stations in centripetal manner. The epicolic nodes are present on the wall of colon. The paracolic lymph node chain is present along the marginal artery. The intermediate group is located along the vascular pedicles in the mesocolon. The principal nodes are present at the route of superior and inferior mesenteric vessels. Thereafter lymphatics enter the cisterna chyli.

The outline of surgical resections for colonic cancers are summarized in Table 3.

Management of obstructed colonic carcinoma: The left colonic lesions are usually at risk of causing bowel obstruction. An emergency surgery is performed entailing resection of appropriate colonic segment with or without primary anastomosis. However, primary anastomisis is usually not preferred. After colonic resection the proximal end is brought out as end colostomy and distal end is either closed (Hartmann procedure) or brought on surface as distal mucus fistula. The primary anastomosis can be considered after on table colonic lavage via appendicular stump or terminal ileum. Recently with availability of self-expanding metal stents these patients are initially subjected to stenting to relieve the acute obstruction followed by definitive resection as elective surgery.

Role of adjuvant therapy: The role of adjuvant chemotherapy is well established in node positive disease, i.e. stage III. Chemotherapy is also advised in stage IIc cancers and cancers with poor prognostic markers like lymphatic and vascular invasion, presence of aneuploidy. Various regimens are available containing 5-Fluorouracil (5-FU), folinic acid along with either oxaliplatin or irinotecan. Various combinations used are Folfox, Folfiri and Capeox. Capecitabine is oral analog of 5-FU and is being frequently used. The adjuvant chemotherapy has shown increased disease free and overall survival as well as recurrence rates are reduced.

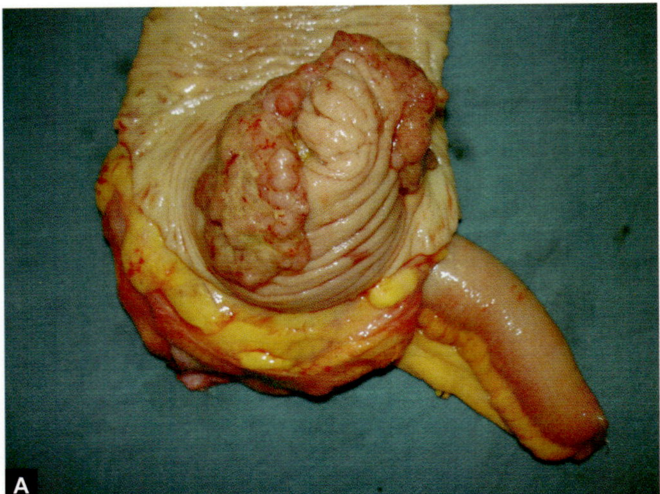

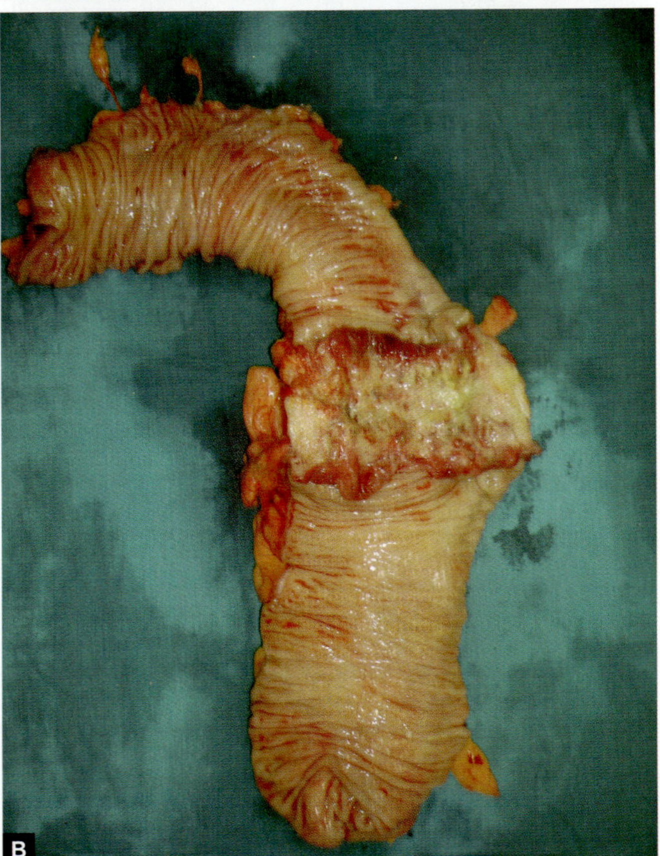

Figures 3A and B (A) Right hemicolectomy specimen-growth in cecum; (B) Extended left hemicolectomy specimen-ulcerated lesion in descending colon

Role of VEGF/EGFR antagonists: These are targeted therapy for CRC. The vascular endothelial growth factor (VEGF) targeted drugs include Bevacizumab (Avastin) and ziv-aflibercept (Zaltrap).These drugs act by inhibiting the neoangiogenesis vital for nutrition of tumor cells.

Epidermal growth factor is a trophic factor for growth of tumor cells. The monoclonal antibodies to its receptor (cetuximab and penitumumab). These drugs are used for metastatic colorectal carcinoma usually in combination of other chemotherapeutic agents. Approximately 40% colorectal malignancies harbor mutations of *K-ras* rendering these drugs to be ineffective in these patients.

Diagnosis and Management of Rectal Cancers

The anatomical proximity of rectum to anal verge makes it feasible for digital examination. The provisional diagnosis of rectal cancer can be made up to 80% cases.[18] The digital rectal examination should be complemented with proctoscopy to assess the location, extent of involvement, mobility, fixity of tumor as well as to assess the sphincter function. Even if low rectal lesion is assessable by proctoscopic biopsy, full colonoscopic examination is done to rule out synchronous lesions.

Imaging of rectal cancer: Endoscopic ultrasound (EUS), MRI with endorectal coil and computerized tomography with rectal contrast (CT) are extensively used for assessing the transmural extent of rectal cancer and to look for regional and distant disease. The endosonoprobes are of high frequency and project sound waves perpendicular to longitudinal axis of rectum. The EUS characterizes bowel wall into five layers of alternating echogenicity. The EUS can better delineate T1 and T2 lesions. The contrast enhanced EUS using microbubble contrast agents can help to delineate lymph nodes. The MRI with endorectal coil is more useful to assess T3 and T4 lesions. The MRI and EUS have comparable sensitivity and specificity and should be used as initial modalities to assess T stage.[19] Post-neoadjuvant treatment high resolution MRI is a good modality for response assessment. The pathological complete response correlates well with that of diffusion weighted MRI.[20] The patients are stratified into low risk, intermediate risk and high risk and treatment is tailored to specific risk strata (Fig. 2C).

Treatment of rectal cancer: The rectal cancer is managed by combined modality treatment. The early rectal lesions T1 can be managed by transanal endoscopic microsurgery (TEMS). TEMS offers better visualization of middle and upper rectal tumors and hence makes their resection more precise and easy.[21] The survival benefits are similar for TEMS and conventional transanal excision.[22]

Neoadjuvant Treatment

The combined modality treatment incorporating surgery, chemotherapy and radiotherapy is the cornerstone of treatment of rectal cancer. The basis of this multimodality treatment has its roots in the fact that 25–50% of T3, T4 and node positive rectal cancers develop locoregional and distant recurrences after surgery alone. Various studies have established that use of combined modality treatment helps in improving the local control rates. The impact on overall survival is variable. There has been debate regarding the sequence of components of multimodality management. The neoadjuvant therapy and subsequent surgery is the approach being used worldwide. The neoadjuvant chemoradiotherapy has inherent advantage of reduced tumor seedling at the time of surgery, improved respectability in previously unresectable locally advanced disease and better chances of sphincter preservation even in lower third rectal cancers. Small bowel gets prevented from excessive exposure to radiation while delivering radiotherapy in preoperative setting

Table 3: Extent of colonic resection according to site of tumor location

Tumor location	*Surgical resection*	*Vascular pedicle division*	*Length of bowel resected*
Cecum and ascending colon	Right hemicolectomy	Ileocolic, right colic, right branch of middle colic	Terminal 6 inches of ileum, right colon and proximal transverse colon
Hepatic flexure	Extended right hemicolectomy	Ileocolic, right colic and middle colic	Terminal 6 inches of ileum, right colon and proximal 2/3rd of transverse colon
Descending colon	Left hemicolectomy	Left colic vessel, sigmoid vessels	Distal 1/3rd of transverse colon and descending colon
Splenic flexure	Extended left hemicolectomy	Left colic and left branch of middle colic	Mid transverse colon and descending colon
Sigmoid colon	Sigmoidectomy	Inferior mesenteric after origin of left colic	Sigmoid colon

Table 4: Preoperative short course radiotherapy versus long course chemoradiation

	Short course	*Long course*
Eligible clinical stage	cT1-3/N0	cT3-4 and/or N+
Treatment schedule	Only RT-5 Gy/fraction x 5 days (25 Gy)	RT 1.8 Gy/fraction over 5–6 weeks (45–50.4 Gy) with concurrent 5-FU based chemotherapy
Interval between RT and surgery	5 days	4–8 weeks
Concurrent chemotherapy	No	Yes
Improved local control	Yes	Yes
Sphincter preservation	No	Yes

whereas due to postoperative adhesions bowel rests in the field and hence gets unnecessary exposure.

There are two approaches being used as neoadjuvant therapy. The European countries use short course radiotherapy whereas others use long course radiotherapy with concurrent chemotherapy. The various trials using preoperative use of radiotherapy as short course preoperative therapy (SCPRT) have established the benefits in terms of reduced local recurrence rates.[23-25] The local control rates and survival benefits are similar in two approaches.[26,27] The definitive surgery is performed 6–8 weeks after the completion of long course chemoradiotherapy. The Table 4 depicts the comparison between the two strategies.[28]

Surgical treatment: Surgery is the only curative modality of treatment for rectal cancer. The various surgical procedures for rectal cancer can be categorized as sphincter preserving surgeries including anterior resection, low and ultralow anterior resection and intersphincteric resection. The abdominoperineal resection entails removal of growth along with sphincter complex with permanent end colostomy.

Patients undergoing surgery for rectal cancer must be counseled for stoma which may be either temporary or permanent. Patients are trained for stoma care by stoma specialist nurses. They should also be advised to interact with ostomates for better understanding and psychological support.

Principles of surgical procedures for rectum: Rectum is having a cuff of loose areolar tissue known as mesorectum. The mesorectum contains fat, lymphatics and blood vessels and is covered by fascia propria of rectum. There is "Holy Plane" existing between fascia propria or the rectum and presacral fascia. The dissection in this plane forms the basis of total mesorectal excision (TME), which is the standard method of rectal cancer surgery. TME, if performed correctly, minimizes bleeding as well as prevents the neural injuries. Various studies have recommended 5 cm distal mesorectal excision for upper rectal tumors and total mesorectal excision for middle and lower rectal cancers (Fig. 4).[29,30]

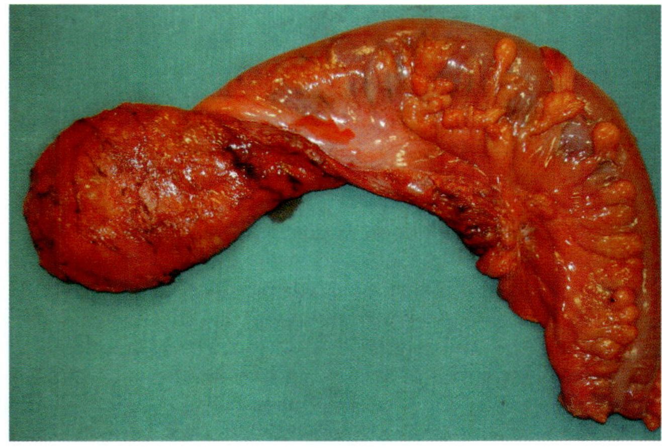

Figure 4 Resected TME specimen for low rectal cancer

Surgical Lay Out Including Neoadjuvant Treatment for Stagewise Disease

Patients with T1 and T2 lesion without nodal disease can be subjected to surgery alone without preoperative therapy. Patients with T3 lesions with or without nodal disease should be subjected to preoperative therapy either short course preoperative radiotherapy (SCPRT) or long course preoperative chemoradiotherapy (CTRT) followed by surgery and adjuvant therapy when indicated. Patients with low lying rectal cancers with involvement of sphincters or involving the levator Ani muscles or nodal disease outside the mesorectum should preferably be subjected to long course preoperative CTRT followed by surgery and then adjuvant therapy.[28]

Need for Proximal Diversion (Either Ileostomy or Transverse Colostomy)

Diversion is not required routinely, but it should be judiciously used in select group of patients, which are as follows:

- Anastomosis less than 7 cm from anal verge
- TME
- Male gender
- Obese patient
- Straight coloanal anastomosis
- Technical mishap during surgery
- Preoperative CTRT
- Significant intraoperative bleeding and hypotension.

Reconstruction after Sphincter Saving Resection

Several techniques of reconstruction have been described with studies reporting superiority of one over the other in terms of functional outcome. However, long-term data does not indicate better quality of life with any one technique over the other.

- Straight colorectal anastomosis
- Straight coloanal anastomosis
- Colonic pouch anal anastomosis
- Coloplasty.

Adjuvant therapy: The role of adjuvant chemotherapy still remains controversial. Nonetheless, the routine practice is to add 4-6 months of postoperative adjuvant chemotherapy using 5-FU, Leucovorin and Oxaliplatin (FOLFOX) in patients who have received preoperative radiation or chemoradiation.

Adjuvant treatment with chemotherapy is associated with significant reduction in local failure but without any survival advantage.[28] Only half to two-thirds of patient could complete the planned postoperative chemotherapy. The clear indications of adjuvant chemotherapy are patient with nodal disease, T3 and T4 lesions with lymphovascular and perineural invasion and patients with positive circumferential resection margin. In routine practice adjuvant therapy is used in patients who have received preoperative radiotherapy or chemoradiation.

SUMMARY

Colorectal cancer is one of the most common cancers leading to cancer related mortality. Various possible and probable factors are implicated in its etiopathogenesis. The role of genetic markers is well established and syndromic forms are characterized. The pathogenetic pathways have been studied in detail and have bearing on management with hereditary CRCs. The diagnostic modalities and treatment strategies are variable for colonic and rectal malignancies. The management protocols involve multimodality approach. The surgery is the only curative treatment. The surgical principals have sound embryological and anatomical basis like TME. The role of chemoradiotherapy is well established. The timings of chemoradiotherapy in relation to surgery have recently been studied in great details and have bearing on local disease control.

REFERENCES

1. Ferlay J, Shin HR, Bray F, Forman D, Mathers C, Parkin DM. Estimates of worldwide burden of cancer in 2008: GLOBOCAN 2008. Int J Cancer. 2010;127:2893-917.
2. Shibuya K, Mathers CD, Boschi-Pinto C, Lopez AD, Murray CJ. Global and regional estimates of cancer mortality and incidence by site: II. Results for global burden of disease 2000. BMC Cancer. 2002;2(1):37.
3. Rabeneck L, Davila JA, El-serag HB. Is there a true "shift" to the right colon in the incidence of colorectal cancer? Am J Gastroenterol. 2003;98(6):1400-9.
4. Curado MP, Edwards B, Shin HR, et al. (Eds). Cancer Incidence in Five Continents, Volume IX. IARC Scientific Publication, No 160 IARC, Lyon; 2007.
5. National Cancer Registry Programme. Accessed at: http://www.icmr.nic.in/ncrp/cancer_reg.htm
6. Yeole BB. Trends in cancer incidence in esophagus, stomach, colon, rectum and liver in males in India. Asian Pac J Cancer Prev. 2008;9:97-100.
7. Swaminathan R, Selvakumaran R, Esmy PO, Sampath P, Ferlay J, Jissa V, et al. Cancer pattern and survival in a rural district in South India. Cancer Epidemiol. 2009;33:325-31.
8. Avni A, Feuchtwanger MM. Juvenile versus adult colonic cancer: distinct different etiologic factors. Dis Colon Rectum. 1984;27:842.
9. Herald RJ. Synchronous and metachronous carcinoma of the colon and rectum. Ann R Coll Surg Engl. 1990;72:172-4.
10. Burt RW. Colon cancer screening. Gastroenterology. 2000;119: 837-53.
11. Sacher DB. Cancer in Chron's disease: dispelling the myths. Gut. 1994;35:1507.
12. Miller AB, Howe GR, Jain M, Craib KJ, Harrison L. Food items and food groups as risk factors in a case-control study of diet and colorectal cancer. Int J Cancer. 1983;32:155-61.
13. Sharpe CR, Siemiatycki J, Rachet B. Effects of alcohol consumption on the risk of colorectal cancer among men by anatomical subsite (Canada). Cancer Causes Control. 2002;13:483-91.
14. Haggit RC, Glotzbach RE, Soffer EE, Wruble LD. Prognostic factors in colorectal carcinoma arising in adenomas: implications for lesions removed by endoscopic polypectomy. Gastroenterology. 1985;89;328-36.
15. Hahn P. Biliary system, pancreas, spleen and alimentary tract. In: Stark DD, Bradley Jr WG (Eds). *Magnetic Resonance Imaging.* St Louis, MO: Mosby; 1999. pp. 471-502.
16. Edge SB, Byrd DR, Compton CC, et al. AJCC Cancer Staging Manual, 7th edition. New York: Springer-Verlag; 2010.
17. Compton CC, Greene FL. The staging of colorectal cancer: 2004 and beyond. CA Cancer J Clin. 2004;54:295-308.
18. McSherry CK, Cornell GN, Glenn F. Carcinoma of the colon and rectum. Ann Surg. 1969;169:502-9.
19. Bipat S, Glas AS, Slors FJ, Zwinderman AH, Bossuyt PM, Stoker J. Rectal cancer: local staging and assessment of lymph node involvement with endoluminal US, CT, and MR imaging—a meta-analysis. Radiology. 2004;232:773-83.
20. Barbaro B, Fiorucci C, Tebala C, Valentini V, Gambacorta MA, Vecchio FM, et al. Locally advanced rectal cancer: MR imaging and prediction of response after preoperative chemotherapy and radiation therapy. Radiology. 2009;250:730-9.

21. Touzios J, Ludwig KA. Local management of rectal neoplasia. Clin Colon Rectal Surg. 2008;21:291-9.
22. Christoforidis D, Cho HM, Dixon MR, Mellgren AF, Madoff RD, Finne CO. Transanal endoscopic microsurgery versus conventional transanal excision for patients with early rectal cancer. Ann Surg. 2009;249:776-82.
23. Folkesson J, Birgisson H, Pahlman L, Cedermark B, Glimelius B, Gunnarsson U. Swedish rectal cancer trial: long lasting benefits from radiotherapy on survival and local recurrence rate. J Clin Oncol. 2005;23:5644-50.
24. Peeters KC, Marijnen CA, Nagtegaal ID, Kranenbarg EK, Putter H, Wiggers T, et al. The TME trail after a median follow-up pf 6 years: increased local control but no survival benefit in irradiated patients with respectable rectal carcinoma. Ann Surg. 2007;246:693-701.
25. Sebag-Montefiore D, Stephens RJ, Steele R, Monson J, Grieve R, Khanna S, et al. Preoperative radiotherapy versus selective postoperative chemoradiotherapy in patients with rectal cancer (MRC CR07 and NCIC-CTG C016): a multicentre, randomized trial. Lancet. 2009;373:811-20.
26. Bujko K, Nowacki MP, Nasierowska-Guttmejer A, Michalski W, Bebenek M, Pudełko M, et al. Sphincter preservation following preoperative radiotherapy for rectal cancer: report of a randomized trial comparing short-term radiotherapy vs. conventionally fractionated radiotherapy. Radiother Oncol. 2004;72:15-24.
27. Ngan S, Fischer R, Goldstein D, et al. A randomized trail comparing local recurrence (LR) rates between short course (SC) and long course (LC) radiotherapy (RT) for clinical T3 rectal cancer: an Intergroup (TROG, AGITG, CSSANZ, RACS). Proc Am Soc Clin Oncol. 2010;28:15s.
28. Kabra V, Goel V, Kumar A. Management of rectal cancer; current status. Roshan Lall Gupta's Recent Advances in Surgery. 2013.
29. Saunders B. The nurse's role in the care of patients with stoma. Br J Clin Pract. 1976;30:81-2.
30. Guidelines for the Management of Colorectal Cancer, 3rd edition. Issued by The Association of Coloproctology of Great Britain and Ireland; 2007.

CHAPTER 98

Colectomy for Colon Cancer

Ashok Kumar, Sunil T

INTRODUCTION

Colorectal cancer is the third most common cancer with a life time risk of 6%. Surgery in the form of colectomy is the main treatment modality for colon cancer with or without chemotherapy. Novel therapies have surfaced in the recent times which include monoclonal antibodies. Present chapter describes the operative details of various types of colectomies performed for colon cancer.

PREOPERATIVE PREPARATION

Assessment of Preoperative Nutritional Status

There are controversies regarding preoperative blood transfusion in colorectal cancer. We prefer to keep the hemoglobin values above 7 g/dL. The ideal time to transfuse would be 2 days prior to the planned surgery. In a patient with poor preoperative nutritional status (low hemoglobin and low albumin), it is wiser to create a stoma rather than restoration of continuity. Distal stump should be brought out as mucus fistula to prevent stump leak and its subsequent complications.

Preoperative Chest X-rays

It is important in identifying pre-existing pulmonary disease and rarely pulmonary metastasis.

Preoperative Tattooing of the Polyps

It helps in identifying smaller lesion during the surgery and is especially useful in laparoscopic surgery.

Marking of Stoma and its Consent

Preoperative counselling and obtaining consent should be a routine practice. Nothing can replace a proper preoperative stomal site marking.

Deep Venous Thrombosis Prophylaxis

The patients receive deep venous thrombosis (DVT) prophylaxis, the evening before surgery. They are advised to ambulate. Anti-DVT garments are used during the procedure. The prophylaxis is continued postoperatively and early ambulation is stressed upon.

Preoperative Bowel Preparation

This has been one of the areas of controversies in colorectal surgery. There is no role for mechanical bowel preparation (MBP) for right colon resections. The debate surrounds around the left colon and rectal resections. Randomized controlled trials and meta-analysis suggests that MBP can be omitted safely. Despite no scientific data favoring its use, many surgeons use MBP during laparoscopic colorectal surgery due to ease in bowel handling.

Antibiotics

The practice of giving peroral antibiotic preparations is to be abandoned according to the existing literature. Three doses of intravenous antibiotic combination which includes cephalosporin and Metrogyl are given an hour prior to incision followed by two postoperative doses.

A second intraoperative dose is given, if the surgery is prolonged for more than 4 hours. Further antibiotic doses are not necessary. In cases of anastomotic leak and intra-abdominal sepsis, therapeutic antibiotic regimens are instituted.

Relevant Anatomy

The surgeon should be familiar with the anatomy of the ureters and pelvic nerves to prevent complications associated with their injury. In colonic resections, the ureter is related to the ileocecal region in the right and the sigmoid colon in the left. It can be appreciated as a whitish tubular structure with streaks of blood vessels on it and do have peristaltic activity. After taking off from the renal pelvis, the ureters are related to the gonadal vessels, which also help to identify the ureters. The gonadal vessels cross the ureter medial to lateral approximately at the level of origin of inferior mesenteric artery. The key of preserving the ureter is to stay close to the colon. If underlying psoas muscle is denuded of its fascia, then we have to think of ureteric injury (Fig. 1).

PRINCIPLES OF SURGERY

- *Margins:* The minimal proximal and distal margin of 5 cm is necessary for a colonic tumor.
- *Clearance of lymph nodes:* The latest National Comprehensive Cancer Network (NCCN) Guidelines recommend a minimum of 12 lymph nodes to be harvested for adequate staging purpose.
- *Colon resection:* Type of colonic resection depends on the site of lesion. Resections are based on vascular supply of the colon.

Position of Patient

Supine or lithotomy position.

Incision

- Midline
- Paramedian
- Pfannenstiel.

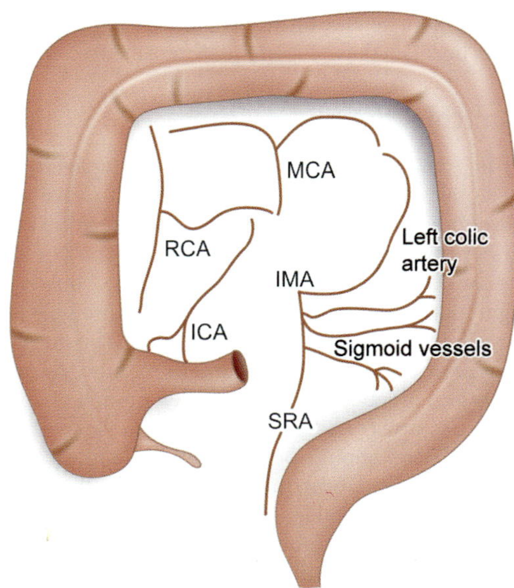

Figure 1 The colonic anatomy
Abbreviations: ICA, ileocolic artery; RCA, right colic artery; MCA, middle colic artery; LCA, left colic artery; SRA, superior rectal artery.

Anesthesia

General anesthesia is the anesthesia of choice. Epidural catheter is placed for postoperative analgesia.

STEPS OF OPERATION

The patient is placed in supine position with anti-DVT garments and adequate paddings to the pressure points. Foley's catheter is inserted. Midline incision is the most preferred one.

To prevent dissemination due to intraoperative handling, various techniques, including wound protection devices tying the proximal and distal margins of the bowel to be resected and minimal handling of the tumor, are advised. There are no randomized controlled trials (RCTs) to support any of the measures. There is no evidence to recommend intraoperative use of tumoricidal solutions.

After entering the abdominal cavity, evidence for dissemination are looked for. In case of gross metastasis, procedure has to be abandoned except for those undergoing surgery for either obstruction or bleeding where a palliative resection may be considered. Findings such as tumor site, extent, adjacent organ infiltration, obstruction and perforation are noted. Rest of the large bowel is felt for synchronous tumors. Lymph node involvement is noted. Greater omentum is palpated not only for peritoneal deposits, but also for enlarged lymph nodes. Skip metastasis are known to occur in colonic cancers (Table 1).

Right Hemicolectomy

The abdomen is opened by vertical midline incision and looked for dissemination. A self retaining retractor is placed and small bowel is packed to the left upper quadrant. The terminal ileum and cecum is retracted medially and upward by the assistant who stands on the left side of the patient. This makes the parietal peritoneum stretched, which could be incised to free the terminal ileum and cecum from the retroperitoneum. This step also helps to prevent ureteric and gonadal vessel injury. Attention is now drawn toward the white line of Toldt, which is incised to free the colon from its lateral attachments. The fibroareolar tissues are divided close to the mesocolon to prevent from entering the Gerota's fascia, which usually happens during the early part of the learning curve. The next structure to be safeguarded is the duodenum. The hepatic flexure is taken down and gastrocolic ligament in the proximal transverse colon is divided.

Once the mobilization is completed, vascular pedicles are isolated with accompanying lymphatics. The right branch of the middle colic artery, ileocolic artery and the right colic artery are ligated at their origin and divided. Care should be taken not to injure the superior mesenteric vein and duodenum during this step. The 15 cm of distal ileum and distal part of the specimen are divided either with stapler or between clamps. End to end or side to side ileocolic anastomosis between the distal ileum and transverse colon is performed. The author's choice is to oversew the staple line with 3–0 silk/prolene, and perform a side to side two layered anastomosis with inner 3-0 vicryl and outer silk/prolene. The mesenteric window is closed. Hemostasis is secured and abdomen is closed in layers.

Extended Right Hemicolectomy

This procedure is performed for tumors of the hepatic flexure. The initial steps are similar to right hemicolectomy. After

Table 1: Resection of colon according to the site of the lesion

Site of tumor	*Vessels ligated*	*Procedure*	*Comment*
Cecum	Ileocolic, right colic and right branch of middle colic artery	Right hemicolectomy	
Ascending colon	Ileocolic artery, right colic artery and right branch of middle colic artery	Right hemicolectomy	
Hepatic flexure	Ileocolic artery, right colic artery and middle colic artery	Extended right hemicolectomy	
Transverse colon	Middle colic artery, peripheral branches of right colic artery and left colic artery close to the tumor	Transverse colectomy	Alternatively, extended right hemicolectomy can be done
Splenic flexure	Middle colic artery, left colic artery and proximal sigmoid branches	Extended left hemicolectomy	Conventional left hemicolectomy can also be performed
Descending colon	Left colic artery and sigmoidal branches	Left hemicolectomy	More radical approach includes ligation of left colic, sigmoidal vessels and IMA
Sigmoid	Sigmoidal branches	Sigmoidectomy	Alternatively IMA after the take off of left colic artery can be divided

mobilizing the hepatic flexure, further dissection is continued till proximal two-thirds of the transverse colon with adequate margin is free from the gastrocolic attachments. The middle colic vessels are taken close to the root and suture is transfixed. Bowel ends are transected by applying stapler. Anastomosis is done by the side to side technique (Fig. 2).

Transverse Colectomy

Transverse colectomy is an alternative procedure to extended right hemicolectomy for the tumors involving the mid transverse colon without lymph nodes in the right or left colic vessels. The hepatic flexure is mobilized and the lesser sac is opened. The greater omentum is divided close to the greater curvature of the stomach.

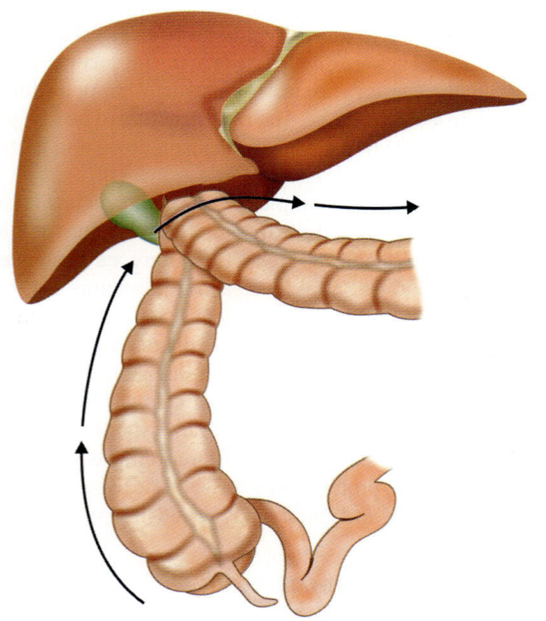

Figure 2 Right hemicolectomy, incision along the line of Toldt

The gastroepiploic vessels and associated lymphatics are included in the specimen. The splenic flexure is taken down carefully after dividing the lienocolic ligament. The middle colic vessels are divided at the base. The specimen is removed and anastomosis is done after dividing at the distal ascending colon and proximal descending colon.

Extended Left Hemicolectomy

This is indicated for the tumors of the distal transverse colon, splenic flexure and proximal descending colon. The distal transverse colon and splenic flexure are mobilized by opening the lesser sac and dividing the lienocolic ligament. The proximal descending colon is mobilized. The middle colic vessels, left colic artery and the proximal sigmoidal vessels are ligated and divided. The anastomosis is done between the right colon and the sigmoid colon or rectum.

The right colon, hepatic flexure and the gastrocolic attachments may have to be taken down for adequate tension free anastomosis.

Left Hemicolectomy

Tumors in the descending colon are managed with left hemicolectomy. The abdomen is entered by a vertical midline incision extending liberally upward. This helps to access the spleen well and hence prevent its accidental injury. The left side of the patient is elevated for better vision, and the small bowel is packed to the right iliac fossa. The left colic artery, sigmoidal vessels and superior rectal artery are ligated and divided. The anastomosis is between the distal transverse colon and the rectum. A conservative approach is also practiced in which the left branch of middle colic artery, left colic artery and proximal sigmoid vessels are ligated. The decision made should be according to the location of the tumor. The gastrocolic omentum is divided in the left side and the splenic flexure is taken down. The dissection continues along the line of Toldt and the sigmoid is mobilized. The inferior mesenteric artery (IMA) is divided, leaving 1–2 cm of stump. The inferior mesenteric vein is divided close to the inferior border of pancreas. After resection, anastomosis is done by hand-sewn method or can be done with staplers.

Total Colectomy

The term subtotal colectomy is also used and includes the resection of colon with preservation of the rectum. The indications in the setting of malignancy are:

- Synchronous colonic tumors (rectum should be uninvolved)
- Familial adenomatous polyposis with or without cancer with rectal sparing
- Hereditary nonpolyposis colorectal cancer
- Obstructed left colonic malignancy with proximal perforation or gross bowel dilatation.

The patient is placed in lithotomy position. The abdomen is opened by a liberal vertical midline incision and looked for signs of dissemination. The mobilization starts from the right colon. After reaching the distal transverse colon, attention is given to mobilize the sigmoid. Sigmoid is mobilized from the lateral attachments initially and then medially after identifying the left ureter. The origin of the IMA is identified and the vessel is ligated leaving at least 1 cm stump. This will help in preserving the autonomic nerves. All the vessels including ileocolic, right colic, middle colic, left colic and superior rectal artery are ligated. Anastomosis can be done, either by hand-sewn technique or by using staplers.

Table 2: Operative complications in colonic resections

General complications	*Intraoperative complications*	*Specific complications*
Chest infection	Ureteric injury (1.1%)	Surgical site infection (3–16%)
Superficial thrombophlebitis	Duodenal, small bowel injury	Abdominal wound dehiscence (3–21%)
Deep vein thrombosis	Splenic injury (<1%)	Anastomotic leak (7–15%)
Urinary tract infection	Intraoperative bleeding	Intra-abdominal collection
	Peroneal nerve injury	Postoperative ileus
	Tumor perforation	Postoperative small bowel obstruction (3%)
		Bladder dysfunction (20–30%)
		Sexual dysfunction
		Anastomotic stricture (0–1.1%)
		Incisional hernia

Minimally Invasive Colectomy

Minimally invasive colectomy has come up in a big way recently. The advantages are small incision and better cosmesis, less pain, early ambulation, early feeding and early discharge. On the other hand, the cost of the procedure, increased operative times and learning curve may offset many of the advantages. The feasibility of laparoscopic colorectal resections has been proved by recent trials. The fear of increased port site recurrences was alleviated by these studies. It is also recommended to have an experience of 20 laparoscopic colonic procedures before performing a laparoscopic colorectal surgery.

The contraindications for minimally invasive colectomies are:

- Obstruction
- Perforation
- Pregnancy
- Large tumors
- Adjacent organ infiltration.

Single Incision Laparoscopic Surgery (SILS) Colectomy

In the last few years, small series of SILS colectomy have also surfaced. The challenges of triangulation are dealt with flexible instruments. Flexible camera and straight dissectors, and energy sources like harmonic scalpel are preferred by majority of the surgeons. Most of the cases were of inflammatory bowel disease (IBD), and early colonic cancers constituting a few. Selecting a non-obese patient is the key for success in SILS during the learning curve. The specimen has less mesenteric fat and hence delivered out through a small incision.

The patient is placed in Trendelenburg position. A 3 cm umbilical incision is made and the port is placed. Right to left approach is preferred by most for total colectomy in case of IBD. Rest of the procedure is like that of minimally invasive colectomy.

The probable advantages of SILS colectomy are early ambulation, less pain, better cosmesis, less wound complications and a short hospital stay. These are yet to be proven by RCTs.

POSTOPERATIVE CARE AND COMPLICATIONS

Early ambulation, good analgesia and early feeding are the key to early discharge. DVT prophylaxis is continued postoperatively. Ryle's tube is removed immediately after the surgery except for patients in bowel obstruction. Urinary catheter and central venous access are removed as early as possible.

Antibiotics are given for two more doses postoperatively unless other indications exist (Table 2).

BIBLIOGRAPHY

1. Corman ML. Colon and Rectal Surgery, 5th edition. Philadelphia: Lippincott Williams & Wilkins; 2005.
2. Fleshman JW, Wolff BG. The ACRS Textbook of Colon and Rectal Surgery. New York: Springer; 2007.
3. Gordon PH, Nivatvongs S. Principles and Practices of Surgery for the Colon, Rectum and Anus, 3rd edition. Informa Healthcare; 2007.
4. Keighley MRB, Williams NS. Surgery of the Anus, Rectum and Colon, 3rd edition. London: WB Saunders; 2008.

CHAPTER 99

Surgery for Carcinoma Rectum

Shivendra Singh, Nikhil Gupta, Suhar Kumar

SURGICAL PERSPECTIVE

Surgery forms the foundation of the multimodality management of the carcinoma rectum. Surgical management of the carcinoma rectum, however, faces the unique problems of the anatomical constraints in the pelvis and proximity to important structures, such as ureters, bladder, prostate, vagina, iliac vessels and sacrum. The general oncological principles of the complete resection of the primary tumor, its lymphatic bed, and other involved organs apply to the surgical resection of rectal carcinoma as well.

HISTORICAL NOTES

Even though colostomy as a diversion procedure is known from the antiquity, Alexis Littre (French anatomist) is credited with the concept of colostomy. Amussat (French surgeon, 1839) popularized colostomy for obstructing rectal lesions. The first documentation of a resection procedure for carcinoma rectum was by Lisfranc, a transanal approach mostly for low-lying lesions. The first person to perform abdominoperineal resection (APR) was Czerny in 1894 whose procedure was later modified by Miles[1] in 1908, whereas the transabdominal resection with the restoration of continuity was first reported by Reybard.

TREATMENT OF RECTAL CANCER

The treatment of rectal cancer is multimodal. It depends on the site of the tumor and stage of the disease. It involves the use of chemotherapy, radiation and surgery. Surgery remains the gold standard treatment option for rectal cancer.

Surgical Approaches

A variety of surgical approaches have been defined for rectal cancer based on the location and extent of the tumor.

These include local procedures, such as endoscopic polypectomy, transanal excision, fulguration and more invasive procedures like anterior or low anterior resection (LAR) with total mesorectal excision (TME) andAPR.

General Guidelines for Surgery based on TNM Staging (Fig. 1)

Local Excision

There are four approaches to local excision:
1. Trans-sphincteric
2. Transcoccygeal
3. Transanal
4. Transanal endoscopic microsurgery (TEM)
   a. Transanal minimally invasive surgery (TAMIS)

Indications

- No evidence of lymphadenopathy on pretreatment imaging
- Mobile, nonfixed
- <30% circumference involved
- <3 cm in size
- Within 8–10 cm of anal verge
- Well to moderately differentiated tumor
- T1 lesion, few T2 lesions
- No lymphovascular or perineural invasion

Trans-sphincteric

First described by Mason, it is performed in prone position. Incision extends from just lateral to sacrococcygeal joint up to the anal verge with all the muscles separated to reach the rectum. It is the less favored technique in view of significant post-op incontinence.

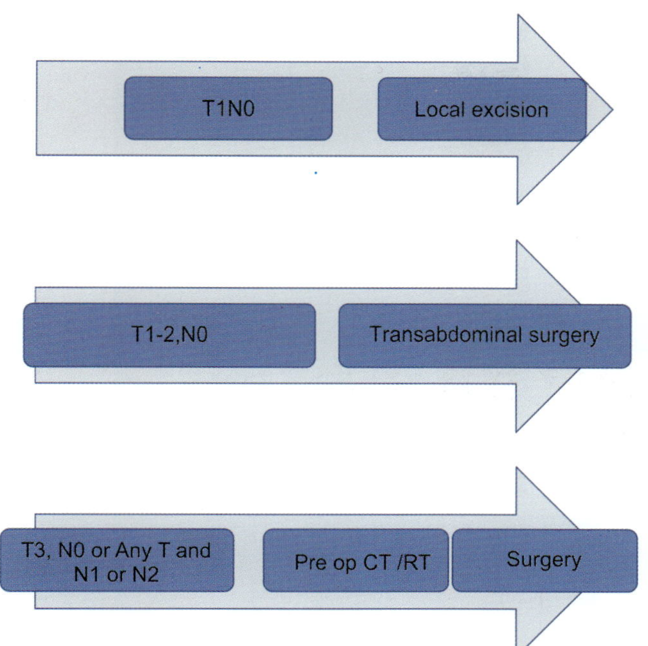

Figure 1 General guidelines for surgery based on TNM staging

Transcoccygeal Excision

The transcoccygeal excision, originally popularized by Kraske, is a procedure used for lesions within the middle or distal third of the rectum on the posterior wall and rarely on the anterior wall. Patient is placed in prone jack knife position. After excising skin and subcutaneous tissue, the coccyx is removed from the sacrococcygeal joint, and the levator ani muscles are separated. Thus, the rectum is reached and can easily be mobilized. Lesions need to be removed with at least 1 cm of margin all around the sides. The posterior approach is advantageous as the mesorectal tissue and perirectal nodes adjacent to the tumor can be removed en bloc with the tumor.

Transanal Excision

Tumors amenable to this approach usually lie within 3 to 5 cm above the dentate line (Fig. 2).

Potential complications of this procedure include fecal impaction, retention of urine, urinary tract infections, infections in the perirectal and ischiorectal spaces, and delayed hemorrhage.

There are a few technical limitations of the conventional transanal technique in patients with distal rectal lesions, patients with deep buttock clefts leading to poor visualization, inadequate margins, and specimen fragmentation.

Transanal Enodoscopic Microsurgery

It was devised by professor GehardBuess[2, 3] from Germany. TEM has two components as follows:

1. **Operating instruments:** Operating rectoscope, stereoscope, and modified laparoscopic instruments for cutting and suturing.

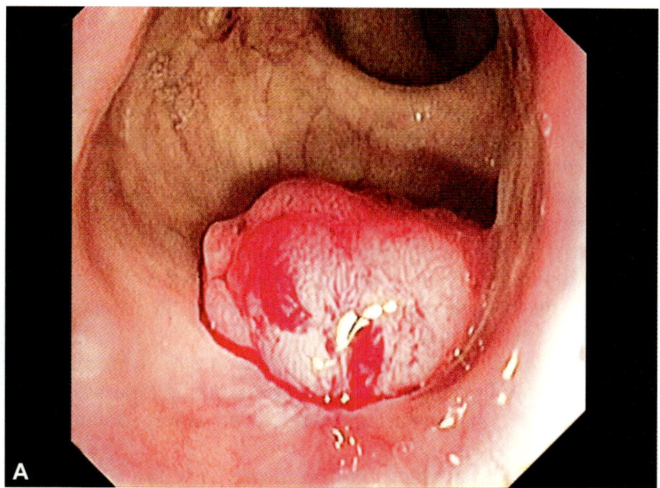

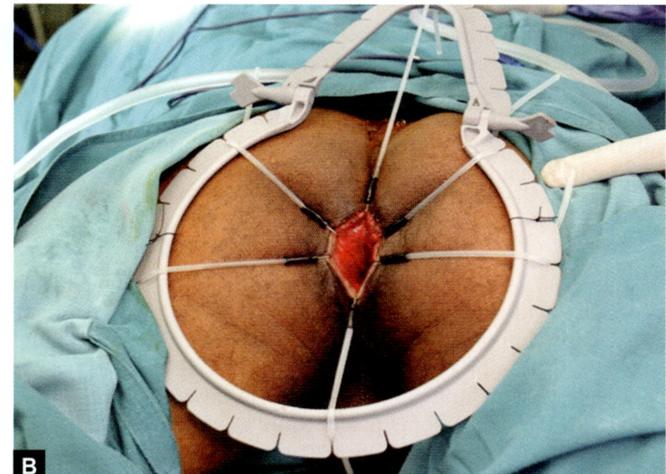

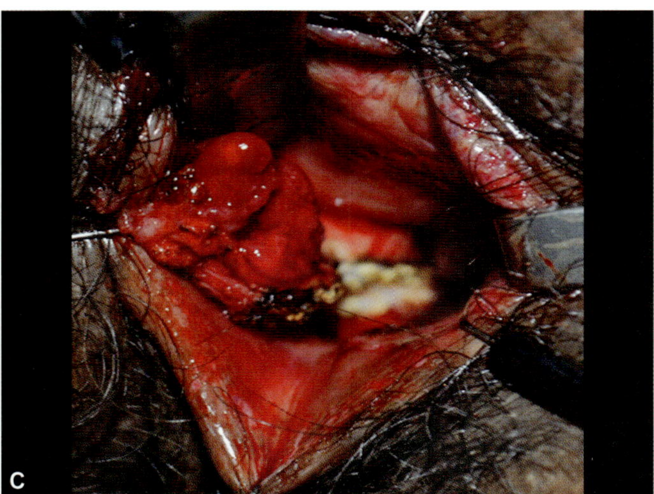

Figures 1A to C Lesion in lower rectum; (B) LINA star retractor to retract the anal verge for adequate exposure; (C) Lesion being removed after local excision

2. **Endosurgical unit**: It provides suction, irrigation, and continuous monitoring of intrarectal pressure.

Gentle anal dilatation is done after lubrication and rectoscope is inserted. Once securely positioned, the rectoscope provides an airtight seal. The rectum is inspected after air insufflation. It is maneuvered for the best visualization of the lesion. It is then attached to the operating table. It has got a port for air insufflation and smoke evacuation and four other ports for camera and three for laparoscopic instrument insertion. The margin of resection should be 10 mm in cases of invasive carcinoma; the resection bed for lesions below the peritoneal reflection may be left open or closed. However, all intraperitoneal defects need to be closed.

The complication rates vary from 10% to 30%, which include hemorrhage and peritoneal breach necessitating laparotomy[5,6,7]. No significant change in the continence level has been documented till date.

The overall recurrence rate following TEM for T1 lesion is 1–11%,[8,9,10] The recurrence rate for a T2 lesion is up to 18% with surgery only and up to 8%[10,11] after adjuvant chemoradiation. In case of unfavorable features like muscle or lymphovascular invasion or involved margins are found after TEM, radical surgery is advocated. Most of the studies now suggest that TEM should be reserved for lesions restricted to mucosa and upper one-third of submucosa only. This invasion can be preoperatively assessed accurately by endorectal ultrasound.

TAMIS

In spite of 30 years since its introduction, TEM has not been able to achieve widespread popularity due to its following features: costly and complex instrumentation, steep learning curve, and specialized training to learn TEM. Thus, TAMIS being cheaper and used with existing gel ports or single incision laparoscopic surgery (SILS) instruments has become a promising alternative to TEM. Moreover, in TAMIS 360° maneuverability is present compared to 220° with TEM (Fig. 3). Indications of TAMIS are similar to those of TEM. It is used for benign adenomas, cT1 lesions with no nodal metastasis, or in patients with radiologically complete response following neoadjuvant treatment to confirm mural sterilization (yT0).

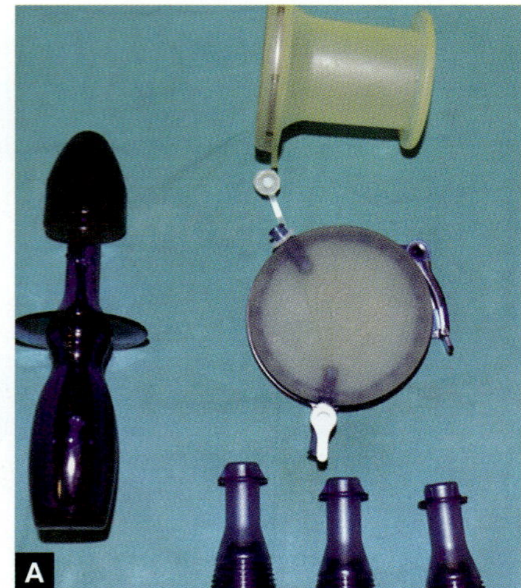

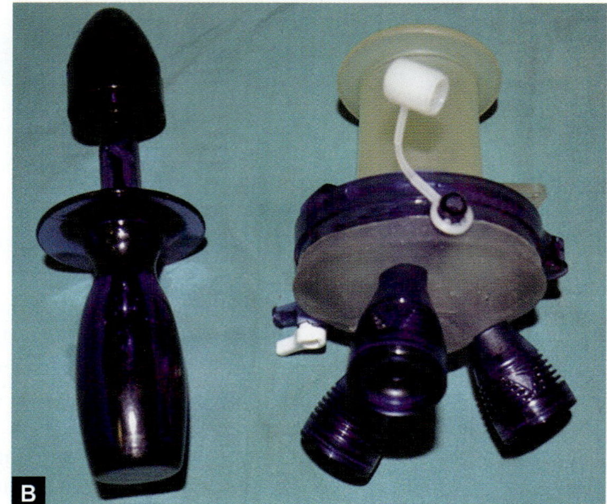

Figures 3A and B Instruments for TAMIS; (B) TAMIS plunger with ports

Fulguration

It uses electrocoagulation that kills the tumor by creating a full thickness scar at the tumor site. This local procedure is used more for historical interest as most of the centers have abandoned it. The main drawback of this procedure is that no specimen is available for histopathological examination. It is reserved for patients with limited life expectancy.

Radical Surgeries for Locally Advanced Rectal Cancers

Radical surgery remains the treatment of choice for locally advanced rectal cancers. It involves the removal of the part of bowel with its lymphovascular pedicle. Factors that determine the exact procedure and prognosis are following: the distance of the tumor from the anal verge, bulk of growth, status of anal sphincters, general condition of the patient, and circumstances whether surgery is being performed in elective or emergency setting. Various abdominal procedures can be classified into two major categories:

1. Sphincter preserving (Fig. 4)
    a. Anterior resection
    b. LAR
    c. Ultra LAR
    d. Hartmann's resection
2. Abdominoperineal resection (APR).

Concept of Total Mesorectal Resection

The basic concept of dissection for a surgeon is pursuing in the planes between embryologically separate organs or tissues. In the rectum, this plane so often described as the "holy plane," is behind the hind gut and a complete fatty and lymphovascular structure surrounding it, which is constituted by the mesorectum. The mesorectum is the fatty envelope surrounding the posterior and lateral aspect of the retroperitoneal rectum. This envelope prevents the tumor spread laterally by confining it. Thus, performing the tumor resection with its complete mesorectal

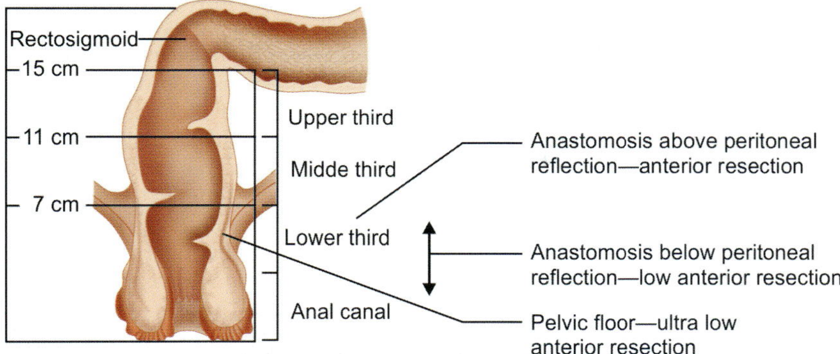

Figure 4 Various rectal resections

envelope reduces the incidence of local recurrence. Moreover, it is a more physiologic``al plane as it is avascular and can be performed even with sharp dissection. TME is performed for middle and lower rectal cancers. For patients with upper rectal cancers, Partial Mesorectal Excision is performed which involves the excision of the mesorectum 5 cm distal to the distal most point of tumor. TME is now considered to be the standard of care for patients with mid- and low rectal cancers.

Basic Steps of Transanal Endoscopic Microsurgery

1. Manual palpation and inspection.
2. High ligation of the inferior mesenteric vessels: The inferior mesenteric artery (IMA) is ligated distal to the origin of the left colic artery (LCA) so as to spare the sympathetic nerve plexus, and the vein is divided above its last tributary close to the pancreas at its inferior border.
3. Posterior dissection of rectum: The sigmoid and upper rectum are lifted anteriorly causing the areolar tissue to spread out and thin peritoneal reflection is visible just anterior to the sacral promontory. This peritoneal reflection is incised and holy plane entered. Sharp dissection either with scissors or diathermy is then started distally, making sure that the plane of dissection is posterior to the superior rectal artery. During this dissection, the hypogastric plexus can be seen dividing posteriorly and coursing above the promontory. Pulsations of the superior rectal artery can be seen anteriorly in the mesorectum. In between this plane, dissection is continued distally till a relatively firm fascia is encountered near the S3 level. This is rectosacral fascia that needs to be incised. Once this is incised, the holy plane opens up and dissection is done till the coccyx. It is continued till the pelvic floor is visible. Failure to recognize this fascia may end up in either entering the mesorectum or bleeding from the sacral venous plexus.
4. Lateral dissection of the rectum: Even though there are some controversies regarding their existence, majority believe that lateral ligaments are constant anatomical structures in terms of components as well as location. Lateral ligaments constitute neuro-lymphovascular pathways from the lower rectum toward the iliac lymph nodes. Middle rectal arteries, lymphatic vessels, the rectal branches from the pelvic plexus, endopelvic fascia, and connective tissue constitute the components of this pathway.
5. Anterior dissection of the rectum: Giving posterior traction to the rectum and anterior traction to the bladder stretches the peritoneum which needs to be incised. Further traction opens up the areolar tissue between seminal vesicles and the rectum in males. In males, there is Denonvilliers fascia between the rectum and the seminal vesicle. It usually comprises two layers. In patients with benign disorders, the plane of dissection can be posterior to this fascia. But in patients with malignancy especially anterior rectal tumors, the plane of dissection should be anterior to Denonvilliers fascia. Care must also be taken in the distal part of this dissection to avoid damage to the neurovascular bundle of the (Walsh) inferior hypogastric plexus which lies just posterior to prostate. Damage to these nerves may cause impotence.

TME Plus

It involves the removal of structures in continuity with the TME which are directly involved due to palpable cancer spread: the levators, ischiorectal fossa, and perianal skin.

Pelvic Autonomic Nervous System

Disturbances of the bladder and sexual function are well-known squeal of rectal cancer surgery. Three common sites of operative injury are: the superior hypogastric plexus, the inferior hypogastric plexus, and the pelvic plexus.

The superior hypogastric nerve forms a plexus around the origin of the IMA and descends into the pelvis crossing the common iliac artery at the level of the first sacral vertebra and then descends into the pelvis along the lateral pelvic wall. Injury can occur while lymph node dissection or while ligating the IMA. If injury occurs high up, it can result in retrograde ejaculation. Thus, ligation of IMA should be done distal to the origin of LCA to prevent the injury.

Another potential site of injury may be observed while dissecting the mesosigmoid from the gonadal vessels and ureter. Here both the superior and inferior hypogastric nerve plexuses descend into the pelvic cavity. Injury to the hypogastric nerves in the retroperitoneal space along the peritoneal reflection of the sigmoid mesentery may result in ejaculatory dysfunction.

The inferior hypogastric nerve forms the pelvic nerve plexus at the lateral pelvic wall with the parasympathetic sacral nerve arising from the 2nd, 3rd and 4th sacral cavities. Numerous tiny neurovascular bundles traversing from the pelvic nerve plexus to the genitalia cross the seminal vesicle in the 10 and 2 o'clock positions. Plane between the inferior hypogastric nerve fibers and the rectal proper fascia is the accurate plane in the pelvic cavity to avoid injury to the neurovascular bundle. These injuries could result in temporary or permanent bladder and/or erectile dysfunction.

Sphincter Preserving Resections

Basic Concepts

1. Complete mobilization of the descending colon and splenic flexure to gain length for anastomosis in the depth of the pelvis
2. No tension in the anastomosis
3. Mesorectum and rectum are divided at the same level
4. Resection of the primary tumor along with the adjacent mesorectal tissue

Anterior Resection for Upper Rectal Cancer

It involves the resection of the bowel 5 cm distal to the tumor just above the peritoneal reflection with partial mesorectal excision. High ligation of IMA is done. The LCA and sigmoid are mobilized. Proximal resection of the bowel usually occurs 5 cm proximal to the tumor taking all the lymphatic tissue along with the specimen.

Low Anterior Resection (LAR) for Mid- and Low-Rectal Cancer

LAR is performed for tumors involving the middle rectum or the lower rectum, and anastomosis is done with the rectum below the peritoneal reflection. The introduction of staplers has helped in achieving a safe anastomosis below the peritoneal reflection even at the level of the pelvic floor. All these patients should have a diverting ileostomy.

The procedure involves TME with a 1 cm tumor-free distal margin following preoperative combined-modality therapy. However, in patients undergoing primary surgery at least the 2 cm margin is recommended.

Colorectal Reconstruction

The rectum may be reconstructed with sutures or staples and with an end-to-end, side-to-end technique.

End to end approach: The anvil is removed from the stapler and placed into the distal end of the colon, which is cleared over the edge of the anvil to avoid stapling through any vascular appendices epiploicae. The stapler is placed transanally and up the rectum. The pin is opened and positioned so that it peeks out just anterior or posterior to the staple line. Avoid coming directly through the staple line because it will tear as the staples catch on the plastic bar. The pointed pin is removed, and a long Kelly clamp is used to hold the anvil pin and is inserted into the stapler cartridge. The stapler is tightened completely (making sure that the bowel loops are aligned properly), fired, and then gently removed. The presence of two intact "doughnuts" is confirmed. The anastomosis is palpated from below and then air injected transanally with saline instilled into the pelvis to look for an air leak.

Post proctectomy, up to one-third of the patients may suffer from what is termed as "anterior resection syndrome." Patients may experience defecation problems with 3 or more bowel movements per/day. Bowels may be irregular with clustering of motions. It may be ill formed with gas and may be accompanied by urgency and incontinence. This is because the normally large capacity compliant rectum is replaced by a less compliant segment of descending or sigmoid colon. Radiation, anastomotic leak, and sphincter damage have also been implicated in the etiology.

In order to counteract this condition of anterior resection syndrome, surgeons have tried various strategies to improve the bowel function. This consists of various methods to better retain stool contents in the neorectum. This includes the following:

1. **Colonic J-pouch anal anastomosis**: The formation of a 6–8 cm colonic J-pouch, constructed from the descending colon by a single longitudinal firing of a linear cutting stapling instrument, is effective in improving stool frequency. Colonic J–pouches of various sizes have been constructed. A 6 cm pouch has less rectal evacuation problems compared to a 9 cm pouch.[12] Patients with a small 6 cm colonic J-pouch have a median of 3 bowel movements a day compared to a median of 6 bowel movements per day for patients with straight anastomosis, at 1 year after surgery. But this benefit was lost after a median follow-up of 2 years as patients with a 6 cm colonic J-pouch and those with straight coloanal anastomosis had similar bowel frequency at about 1 bowel movement a day.[13] Thus, J-pouch gives an immediate benefit in bowel movements with similar long-term results.
2. **Transverse coloplasty pouch**: A transverse coloplasty pouch is designed to "interrupt antegrade colonic peristalsis." One of the problems of the J-pouch is that it is bulky and a narrow pelvis may prevent it from reaching the distal rectum for a secure anastomosis. On the other hand, the transverse coloplasty pouch being less bulky can be an alternative for patients with narrow pelvis. A 7–8 cm longitudinal incision is made between the taenia along the antimesenteric side of the descending colon, starting 4 cm above the distal cut end. The incision is closed transversely with a continuous/ interrupted single layer of seromuscular absorbable suture. The coloplasty "pouch" is then hand sewn or stapled to the anorectal stump.

Side-to-End Anastomosis

The side-to-end colorectal anastomosis was first described by J W Baker in 1950.[14] It can be done with the help of a stapler or can be done entirely by the hand-sewn technique.

Side-to-end anastomosis is functionally similar to the 8 cm colonic J-pouch except a better neorectal evacuation in <15 min in the colonic J-pouch group at 6 months duration.

There is a randomized controlled trial going at our Center comparing the incidence of anterior resection syndrome in patients with side-to-end colorectal anastomosis versus the transverse coloplasty pouch.

Protective Diversion

Routine diversion with either colostomy or loop ileostomy is recommended for patients undergoing LAR. It is not recommended following the anterior resection. However, it should be considered in:

- Patients who have received neoadjuvant radiation
- Incomplete doughnut
- Anastomosis is not satisfactory or a positive leak test
- Poor general condition of the patient

Ultra Low Anterior Resection

It is indicated for patients with tumors of the lower one-third of the rectum. It involves resecting the whole rectum up to the anal canal with anastomosis done with anal canal at or below the pelvic floor. It can also be done by the stapled or hand-sewn technique. Anastomosis lies at 3-4 cm from anal verge. Diverting stoma is done in all the cases.

Intersphincteric Proctectomy with Colonic Pouch to Anal Anastomosis

Intersphincteric resection (ISR) is indicated in patients whose tumors are close to the anorectal ring but have not invaded the external sphincter muscle, intersphincteric groove, or pelvic floor. Various authors have used different criteria to choose a patient for ISR. Some consider a patient with tumor which is 2-3 cm from the dentate line, wheras others use the criteria of 1.5-3 cm from that line. This is based on the fact that, if the muscular rectal tube is followed distally, it ends on the anoderm in the intersphincteric groove at the anal verge. It can be further divided into partial ISR and complete ISR, depending upon whether the partial or whole internal sphincter is removed (Fig. 5). This surgery involves the removal of the upper part of the internal sphincter; hence, there will be some functional changes in the continence. Absolute contraindications for ISR are the involvement of external sphincter and the pelvic floor. The patient needs to be motivated, with a well-functioning sphincter and normal pre-operative continence.

Surgical Steps

Majority of the authors consider the perineal approach for ISR. Very few use the abdominal approach for it. Incision is given at the dentate line and the intersphincteric plane can be directly entered if complete internal sphincteric resection is planned. If partial sphincteric resection is planned, then mucosectomy is done and the plane entered cranially preserving the partial internal sphincter. Anastomosis is done using the hand-sewn technique taking the proximal colon through the rectal cuff in case of partial ISR. Diverting stoma is a must in all patients following ISR.

Immediate major side effects of ISR are the following: anastomotic leak, pelvic sepsis, and intestinal obstruction. Long-term complications include the following: poor continence, nocturnal leakage of stools, and rarely anastomotic stricture.

Resection Margins

Distal Margin

The optimal distal margin of resection is still controversial. In the rectum, the first line of lymphatic spread is upward along the major vessels, but for tumors below the peritoneal reflection, the spread can occur distally via intra or extramural lymphatics. At present, a distal mural margin of 2 cm is considered the standard for rectal cancer resections. A distal margin of 1 cm is accepted for low rectal tumors, if it is necessary to avoid an APR, because distal intramural spread occurs over 1 cm in only 4-10% of the cases.

Radial Margins

Studies have demonstrated that obtaining the negative circumferential radial margin (CRM) is far more critical than the proximal and distal margins. The radial margin has shown to be the independent predictive marker of local recurrence and survival. It has been defined as the presence of a tumor or a metastatic lymph node within 1-2 mm of CRM. Factors responsible for positive CRM are as follows: the advanced tumor stage and the poor surgical technique. Use of neoadjuvant chemoradiation in patients with T2 and above or node positive tumors would decrease the incidence of positive CRM. Use of TME and careful anterior dissections of anteriorly lying tumors should be done to prevent positive CRM.

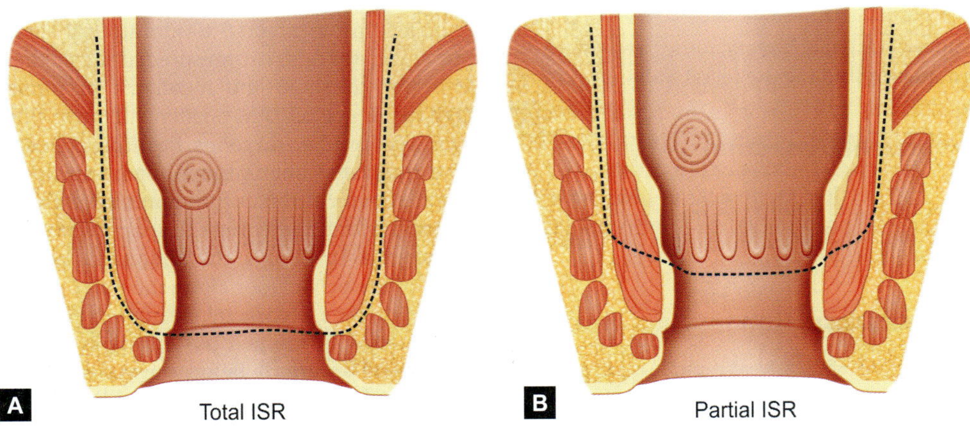

Figures 5A and B Intersphincteric resection (A) Total ISR; (B) Partial ISR

Hartmann' S Procedure

First described by Dr. Henri Albert Hartmann in 1921, it involves the resection of the rectosigmoid colon with the creation of an end colostomy.

The most common indication is when a colonic resection is needed and a primary anastomosis cannot be safely done, for example, in a hemodynamically unstable patient or in a severely immunocompromised or malnourished patient. Other less common indications are patients undergoing emergency surgery for perforation, bleeding, or obstruction, and in a patient who cannot undergo a long operation.

The high morbidity associated with this procedure is largely due to the poor general condition of the patient. This includes stoma complications in the form of stoma retraction, prolapse, or general complication of wound healing.[15]

Abdominoperineal Resection (APR)

Also known as **the Miles procedure**, it involves complete anorectal excision along with the mesorectum by combined dissection through the abdomen and perineum with the formation of a permanent end colostomy. The abdominal approach can be done by laparoscopy as well.

The indications of APR are as follows:

1. **Absolute**
   a. Gross involvement of the anal sphincter
   b. Distal margin of at least 1 cm cannot be achieved from the dentate line
   c. Poor sphincter tone.
2. **Relative**
   a. Old age (doubtful sphincter tone)
   b. Men with a history of prostate cancer treated by either external-beam radiation therapy, brachytherapy seed implantation, or radical prostatectomy
   c. Unable to train the individual after ultra LAR
   d. Patients with extensive diverticulosis or previous left colectomy due to the lack of a sufficient healthy bowel
   e. Low-lying anaplastic or poorly differentiated cancers
   f. Persistent or recurrent epidermoid carcinomas of the anal canal (after initial chemotherapy and radiation)
   g. For some rare lesions of the anorectum (e.g., melanoma)
   h. For sarcomas that arise from the levator ani that involve the anal canal
   i. For locally advanced (i.e., bulky) rectal tumors,
   j. For some chordomas infiltrating the rectal wall

Technique of Abdominal Dissection

The abdominal part of dissection is similar to LAR, with the only difference being that the proximal bowel is resected before commencing the perineal dissection.

Technique of Perineal Dissection

The anal canal is first closed with a heavy purse-string suture placed circumferentially around the anal canal just outside the intersphincteric groove. Incision is made encompassing perineal body anteriorly and extending up to coccyx posteriorly, and ischial tuberosities laterally (roughly 3 cm all around the anal verge). The incision is then carried through the dermis into the ischiorectal fat.

Posterior Dissection

Anococcygeal ligament is exposed and sharply incised. The external sphincter and levator muscles are traversed to enter the pelvis. Once entered posteriorly, dissection is continued laterally.

Lateral Dissection

The levator muscles are divided just lateral to the puborectalis band so that enough cuff is left to close the pelvic floor which is necessary to avoid perineal bowel herniation.

Anterior Dissection

The rectum is pulled through the perineal wound to provide traction. Anterior fibers of the external sphincter muscle are divided to expose superficial and deep transverse perineal muscles. The medial fibers of the puborectalis and pubococcygeus muscles, rectourethralis muscle, visceral fascia, and remaining lateral ligaments on either side are divided to completely remove the rectum.

Closure of the Pelvic Floor and Biological Spacers

After hemostasis and irrigation, the perineal floor is closed in two layers: the first layer is the closure of the pelvic floor by approximating the muscles and the second is the closure of the dermis and skin using absorbable sutures after inserting the romovac drain. Attempt is made to fill the pelvis with an omental pedicle, importing neovasculature or fresh blood supply to promote healing in the irradiated field. A rectus muscle or a myocutaneous flap can be used as a biological spacer, which also serves as a means of excluding the small bowel from the pelvis and as a source of neovasculature as well.

Extralevator APR

Even after a properly performed APR, the local recurrence rate has been very high (up to 30%). Performing TME through the abdominal approach till the pelvic floor and resecting the anal canal from perineum result in waist at the level of the pelvic floor leading to a small tissue around the tumor at this site. Moreover, there is no mesorectal fat in the distal anorectum. This may increase the incidence of tumor perforation and high incidence of CRM positivity. Due to this high incidence of local recurrence, surgeons have proposed another technique of extralevator abdominoperineal excision (ELAPE) (Fig. 6). The main aim of this technique is to perform a wide cylindrical excision without opening the space between the tumor and the levator ani. In ELAPE, the abdominal part of TME is stopped short of the pelvic floor along the outer plane of the levator and dissecting the ischiorectal fat in the perineal phase. Mesorectal mobilization is stopped posteriorly at the upper border of the coccyx and anteriorly below the vesicles in males and cervix in females. Then the patient is turned in prone jack knife position. The incision is marked outside the external sphincter from the coccyx posteriorly to perineum anteriorly. Dissection is started

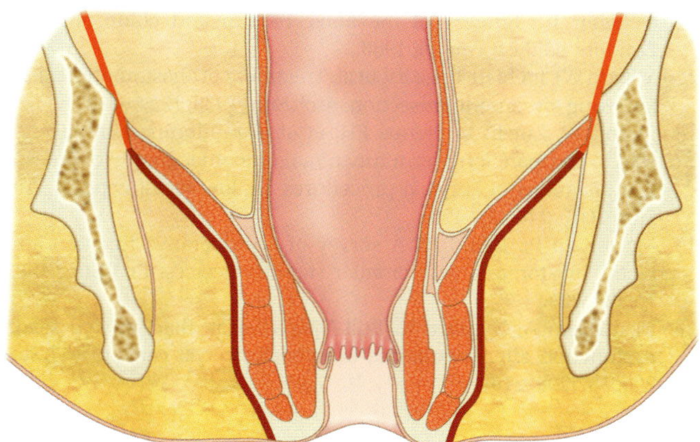

Figure 6 Line diagram showing plane of resection in ELAPE

circumferentially entering just anterior to the coccyx. The coccyx may be incised selectively. The dissection is then continued laterally along the outer plane of the external sphincter, taking the pelvic floor at the level of pelvic side walls. The closure of the perineum can be done either with the help of biological mesh or local flap procedures.

Various reviews and meta-analyses have shown the lower incidence of intraoperative tumor perforations and CRM positivity following the ELAPE procedure. Whether this low incidence is associated with better survival has not been proven till now. On the other hand, ELAPE is associated with a higher incidence of perineal wound healing complications, longer operating times, readmissions, and higher number of wound revisions.

Pelvic Exenteration

In patients with anterior rectal tumors, the tumor may come close to vital structures like prostate making R0 resection impossible. In such patients, pelvic exenteration may be considered. Resection would include APR/LAR along with prostatectomy with or without cystectomy with either wet colostomy or ileal conduit or uretero ureteric or ureterocystostomy. This is known as anterior pelvic exenteration. In females, vagina and uterus help in preventing the urinary involvement. In such patients, combining hysterectomy and vaginectomy with APR may suffice. This is known as posterior pelvic exenteration.

In patients with posteriorly infiltrating tumors, sacrum may be excised along with the rectum. The combination of anterior and posterior pelvic exenteration is termed as total pelvic exenteration.

This treatment option has shown to increase the 5-year survival up to 30–40%.

Complications

Complications of APR

Sexual dysfunction, difficulty in voiding, and urinary incontinence are seen in up to one-third of the patients following TME, prevention of which is dependent on following sound surgical principles as described earlier.

Stomal complications following APR are seen in about 20% of the patients, which include stomal ischemia, hernia, and prolapse.[16] The perineal complications range from 14% to 80%. Minor wound complications include surgical site infections with superficial skin separation and chronic perineal sinus. Major wound complications include deep dehiscence, pelvic abscess, and perineal wound nonhealing and disruptions.

Another common complication following APR is subacute intestinal obstruction. It may occur in 20–40% of the patients.

Complications of Anterior Resection

Anastomotic leak can occur in up to 20% of the patients.[17,18] It usually appears between four and seven days. Symptoms include fever, tachycardia, tachypnea, enterocutaneous fistula, or frank peritonitis. Management includes adequate supportive measures and diversion ileostomy or colostomy in patients who do not respond to conservative measures.

Anterior resection syndrome – frequency, urgency, and soiling[19] – reflects the loss of capacitance and compliance of rectal reservoir. Approximately one-third of the patients have symptoms of urgency and frequency.

In patients who have undergone intersphincteric resection, there is fall in resting anal pressure. These patients may suffer from incontinence although majority of patients have preserved continence (up to 75%).

Effect on sexual function: Infrequent in patients who have undergone standard TME with autonomous nerve preservation. Many series have reported that the preservation of sexual function is significantly better in men less than 60 years (85–90%) than men over 60 years (60–70 %).[20]

REFERENCES

1. Miles WE. A method of performing abdomino-perineal excision for carcinoma of the rectum and of the terminal portion of the pelvic colon (1908).CA Cancer J Clin 1971; 21:361–364.
2. Buess G. Review: Transanal endoscopic microsurgery (TEM). J R Coll Surg Edinb 1993; 38:239–245.
3. Buess G, Kipfmüller K, Hack D, et al. Technique of transanal endoscopic microsurgery. Surg Endosc 1988; 2:71–5.
4. Mason AY. Surgical access to the rectum – a transsphincteric exposure. Proc R Soc Med 1970; 63 Suppl:91–94.
5. Guerrieri M, Baldarelli M, Morino M, et al. Transanal endoscopic microsurgery in rectal adenomas: Experience of six Italian centres. Dig Liver Dis 2006; 38:202–207.
6. Guerrieri M, Baldarelli M, Organetti L, et al. Transanal endoscopoic microsurgery for the treatment of selected patients with distal rectal cancer: 15 years experience. Surg Endosc 2008; 22:2030–2035.
7. Floyd ND, Saclarides TJ. Transanal endoscopic microsurgical resection of pT1 rectal tumors. Dis Colon Rectum 2006; 49: 164–168.
8. Stipa F, Burza A, Lucandri G, et al. Outcomes for early rectal cancer managed with transanal endoscopic microsurgery: A 5-year follow-up study. Surg Endosc 2006; 20:541–545.
9. Maslekar S, Pillinger SH, Monson JR. Transanal endoscopic microsurgery for carcinoma of the rectum. Surg Endosc 2007; 21:97–102.
10. Lezoche E, Guerrieri M, Paganini AM, et al. Transanal endoscopic microsurgical excision of irradiated and nonirradiated rectal cancer. Surg Laparosc Endocsc 1998; 8:249–256.
11. Steele RJ, Hershman MK, Mortensen NJ, et al. Transanal endoscopic microsurgery – initial experience from three centres in the United Kingdom. Br J Surg 1996; 83:207–210.

12. Lazorthes F, Gamagami R, Chiotasso P, et al. Prospective, randomized study comparing clinical resultsbetween small and large colonic J-pouch following coloanalanastomosis. Dis Colon Rectum 1997; 40:1409–1413.
13. Ho YH, Seow-Choen F, Tan M. Colonic J-pouch function at six months versus straight coloanal anastomosis at two years: randomized controlled trial. World J Surg 2001; 25:876–881.
14. Mantyh CR, Hull TL, Fazio VW. Coloplasty in low colorectal anastomosis: Manometric and functional comparison with straight and colonic J-pouch anastomosis. Dis Colon Rectum 2001; 44:37–42.
15. Bass EM, Del Pino A, Tan A, et al. Does preoperative stoma marking and education by the enterostomal therapist affect outcome? *Dis Colon Rectum* 1997; 40:440–442.
16. Goligher JC. Surgery of the anus, rectum and colon, 4th edn. London: BaillièreTindall, 1980.
17. Mileski WJ, Joehl RJ, Rege RV, et al. Treatment of anastomotic leakage following low anterior resection. Arch Surg 1988; 123:968–971.
18. Fazio VW, Zutshi M, Remzi FH, et al. A randomized multicenter trial to compare long-term functional outcome, quality of life, and complications of surgical procedures for low rectal cancers. Ann Surg 2007; 246:481–490.
19. McDonald PJ, Heald RJ. A survey of postoperative function after rectal anastomosis with circular stapling devices. Br J Surg 1983; 70:727–729.
20. Nesbakken A, Nygaard K, Bull-Njaa T, et al. Bladder and sexual dysfunction after mesorectal excision for rectal cancer. Br J Surg 2000; 87:206–210.

CHAPTER 100

Recurrent Rectal Cancer and Pelvic Exenteration

Sundeep Jain, Naresh Jangir

INTRODUCTION

Locoregional disease is the most common type of recurrence after the treatment of rectal cancer. After the curative resection of rectal cancer, the isolated local, combined local and systemic, and systemic recurrence are 4–33%, 7–30%, and 6–19%, respectively.

There are two main factors which affect the type of recurrence: site of rectal cancer and type of resection like abdominoperineal resection (APR) or low anterior resection (LAR). Local recurrence predominates in mid- and low-rectal cancer, while systemic recurrence predominates in upper rectal cancer as in colon cancer. The possible reason of this difference could be the more limited margins of clearance in the pelvis along with the presence of diffuse lymphatic channels in the mesorectum.

Local recurrences after APR and LAR are 12–32% and 7–30%, respectively. The type of initial operation also has a bearing on the extent and resectability of local recurrence. After APR, only 10% of local recurrences are resectable because of the fact that most of these recurrences have a pelvic side wall with or without antero-posterior involvement. On the contrary, after LAR, most of the local recurrences are unfixed, thus being more amenable to surgical re-resection with curative intent.

Recurrent rectal cancer is associated with dismal prognosis without surgical intervention. It has only 6–7 months of median survival without any treatment.[1] Radiotherapy alone gives symptom control in only 30% patients with the survival benefit of up to 12 months only.[2] Thus, radical surgery is the only hope of cure.

Advances in the management of rectal cancer like popularization of total mesorectal excision (TME) and improvement in chemo-radiotherapy regimens have resulted in the decrease in the incidence of loco-regional recurrence from 25–40% to 4–8%.[3] Therefore, surgery is the mainstay of management for most of these patients.[4]

Surgery for such patients is difficult and demanding. It requires a complex procedure, such as pelvic exenteration in the presence of a hostile operative field. TME decreases the chance that recurrence will remain confined to a specific compartment. Previous radiotherapy results into obliterated normal tissue planes, friable tissues, dense adhesions, and extensive fibrosis. This surgical management requires an expertise of specialists, such as urologist, gynecologist, vascular and plastic surgeons, and intensive care specialists. Postoperative morbidity and mortality are as high as 20–60% and 8%, respectively, depending on the complexity of resection.

For these reasons, surgery of recurrent rectal cancers is not commonly performed as is the case with surgery of distant metastases in rectal cancer, such as liver and lung. But the fact remains that surgery remains the only treatment option with a curative potential, and a number of curative resections have increased recently due to improvement in staging, neoadjuvant chemo radiotherapy, surgical expertise, and dedicated centers.

FACTORS RELATED TO INCREASED INCIDENCE OF LOCAL RECURRENCES

These are grouped into three categories as follows.

Anatomical: Positive circumferential or distal resection margins (R1/R2) at primary surgery. In case of neoadjuvant CRT, the negative margin of <1cm is adequate.

Pathological: Degree of lymphovascular invasion, differentiation, and tumor size.

Surgical: High volume centers, LAR, and low serum CEA levels are associated with the lower incidence of local recurrences.

CLASSIFICATION/STAGING

Mayo clinic classified these lesions depending on the presence of pain and the degree of fixation. But currently the most widely used system is anatomical. It depends on the site of recurrence and its anatomical relation to the adjoining structures. It comprises four types: (a) axial, (b) posterior or sacral, (c) anterior, and (d) sidewall or lateral recurrence. This classification is also shown to predict prognosis as lateral recurrences were found to be less likely to be curable than axial or anterior ones.[5]

Axial recurrence includes anastomotic recurrence after LAR, recurrence after local excision procedures like TEMS and perineal recurrence after APR. It affects pelvic organs without invading into bone or sidewalls. Posterior or sacral ones include tumors in presacral space invading sacrum. Anterior recurrences involve genito-urinary organs, and that lateral ones invade ureters, pelvic autonomic nerves, iliac vessels or extend through sciatic foramen.

PRESENTATION

In 70% patients, local recurrence occurs within 2 years and in 85% within 3 years of primary surgery.[6] As up to one-third patients develop asymptomatic recurrence, strict postoperative surveillance is of utmost importance for early detection. It includes the history of bleeding per rectum, change of bowel habits and pelvic pain, and thorough clinical examination including digital rectal/vaginal examination, sigmoidoscopy, and blood investigations like CEA levels.

Mostly the symptoms are disabling in the form of refractory pelvic pain, tenesmus, and malodorous discharge, severely compromising the quality of life.[7] Pain on presentation is directly related to poor prognosis as its severity reflects the degree of fixation in pelvis, which, in turn, is a marker of advanced stage of local recurrence.

MANAGEMENT

It starts with the confirmation of diagnosis and assessment of resectability in terms of attainment of R0 resection with an acceptable level of morbidity and mortality.

It includes thorough history and physical examination to assess patient's fitness and nutritional status (performance status), the presence of comorbidities like diabetes, hypertension, and coronary artery disease. A meticulous physical examination includes lymph node basins, such as supraclavicular and inguinal lymph nodes. If found enlarged, fine needle aspiration cytology (FNAC) of the same should be done. Digital rectal and vaginal examinations, location of recurrent pelvic mass from the anal verge, association of the mass with the surrounding bony structures, and its fixity are important.

Radiological evaluation includes chest x-ray, contrast enhanced computed tomography (CECT) scan, magnetic resonance imaging (MRI), and positron emission tomography-fluorodeoxyglucose (PET-FDG) scan to evaluate the extent of local disease and extra-pelvic metastases. CECT scan has the accuracy of 55–72% in preoperative assessment.[8] It often underestimates the degree of tumor infiltration. MRI, on the other hand, is found to be superior to CECT scan in this setting (accuracy 83%) in determining the feasibility of pelvic exenteration.[9] MRI is also more accurate than CECT in detecting sacral bone and pyriform muscle involvement. But MRI is not reliable in patients with pelvic sidewall involvement and in differentiating radiation changes from tumor involvement. PET-FDG scan is more accurate than CECT and MRI in detecting metastatic disease in extra-pelvic locations.[10]

CONTRAINDICATIONS

A curative intent resection is not advisable under the following circumstances:

1. **Absolute**
   a. Tumor extending through the sciatic foramen
   b. Pelvic sidewall involvement
   c. Common or external iliac vessel involvement
   d. Para-aortic lymph nodes involvement
   e. Involvement of sacrum proximal to S1 (even invasion above S2–S3 is considered as contraindication by some, as it requires internal fixation due to sacro-iliac instability)
   f. Distant metastases
2. **Relative**
   a. Ureteral obstruction
   b. Significant medical comorbidities
   c. Poor surgical candidate with senility or inability to care for stomas

It is important to have tissue diagnosis of pelvic recurrence by colonoscopy or CT-guided biopsy as it is difficult to distinguish fibrosis from local recurrence at pelvic sidewalls. If this is not possible, then watchful waiting is imperative in view of high risk surgery and uncertain diagnosis.

SURGICAL TREATMENT

This includes pelvic exenteration. It is divided into the following types:

1. Total
2. Modified anterior and posterior
3. Composite

Total Pelvic Exenteration

It is defined as the removal of rectum with distal colon, internal reproductive organs, urinary bladder with lower ureters, draining lymph nodes, and pelvic peritoneum (Fig. 1).

Modified Pelvic Exenteration[11,12]

In anterior type (Fig. 2), the rectum is spared. Removal includes the urinary bladder with lower ureters, pelvic peritoneum, reproductive organs, and draining lymph nodes. It maintains the rectum in situ and is, therefore, indicated in pelvic malignancies other than recurrent rectal cancers.

Posterior exenteration (Figs 3 and 4) includes the removal of uterus, cervix, adnexa, posterior vaginal wall, and rectum. The urinary bladder is conserved.

Composite Pelvic Exenteration

It involves bony resections including portions of pubic symphysis, sacrum-coccyx, ischium and ischial pubic rami. Two approaches

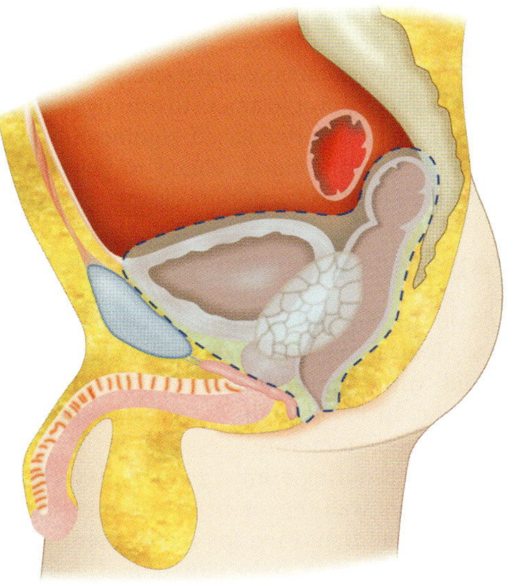

Figure 1 Shaded area showing parts removed for total pelvic exenteration in male patients

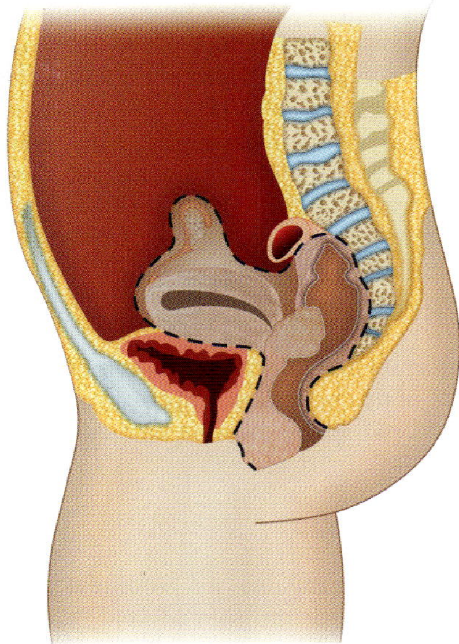

Figure 3 Shaded area showing parts removed in posterior pelvic exenteration

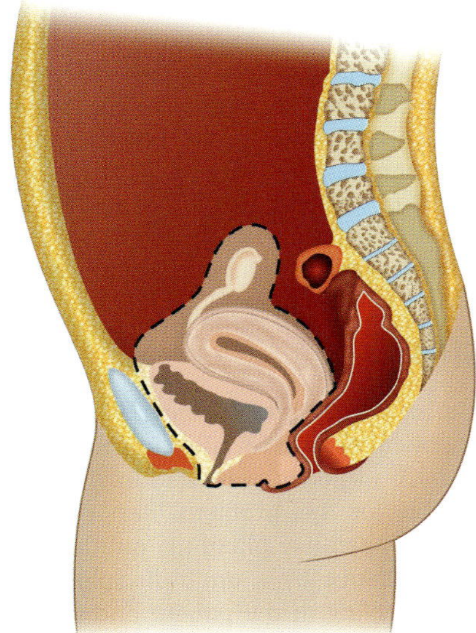

Figure 2 Shaded area showing parts removed in anterior pelvic exenteration

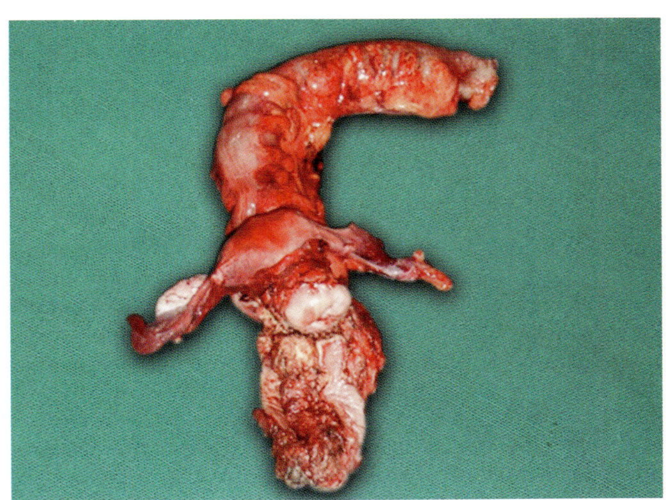

Figure 4 Posterior pelvic exenteration specimen of patient with recurrent rectal cancer involving posterior vaginal wall and cervix

are reported for sacral transaction. In 1981, Wanebo and Marcove[13] described combined an abdominal trans-sacral approach. In this approach, initial dissection is done through the standard anterior approach followed by sacral resection with patient in the prone position. Temple and Ketcham[14] described an approach where an osteotome is used to transect the sacrum from an anterior aspect after the completion of the pelvic dissection and identification of pelvic nerves.

GENERAL PRINCIPLES OF PELVIC EXENTERATION

It starts with the preoperative marking of stomas (colostomy and ileostomy). A surface marking for the level of sacral resection is done. The patient is put in Lloyd-Davis position. An examination under anesthesia is performed followed by cystoscopy and ureteric stenting. Good exposure is paramount and is achieved by long midline incision. The small bowel is completely mobilized to exclude the presence of metastases. If the small bowel loop is found adherent to pelvic mass, it is removed en-bloc. In case ascites is found, the fluid is sent for cytology. Intraoperative differentiation between tumor and radiotherapy-related fibrosis is done using frozen section, and it is often the cause for more radical approaches. Often it takes many hours of exploration before the resectability is ascertained.

In case of urogenital involvement, if only the bladder dome is involved, then partial cystectomy is done. If the bladder trigone and prostate are involved, then total pelvic exenteration with prostatectomy is performed. If there is no urogenital involvement, then the management is decided by the primary procedure. If previous anterior resection has been done, then radical resection outside the plane of primary dissection is done. If previous surgery was APR, then the resection of mass with adherent small bowel loops along with the transperineal approach for perineal recurrence is undertaken. Sometimes distal sacrectomy is also needed.

Currently, there are no guidelines in the literature regarding the extent of lymphadenectomy desirable in this setting.

RECONSTRUCTION PHASE

This is an important and critical phase as it determines the long-term morbidity of this operation. This involves urinary diversion, filling of pelvic dead space, and the reconstruction of vagina in females.

Urinary Diversion

Several options are available as continent and incontinent conduits. The standard is an isolated ileal incontinent conduit. In this, the isolated ileal segment is placed below the intestinal anastomosis. The ureters are anastomosed to one end of the loop and the other end is taken out as ileostomy.

To avoid the need of the permanent ostomy bag, many types of continent conduits were developed. These include Indiana pouch, Koch pouch, Florida pouch, and Miami pouch. The Miami pouch is the most preferred one due to >90% overall long-term continence rates.[15] It is fashioned using the ascending colon, part of the transverse colon and 10 cm of the distal ileum. This gives approximately 650 mL reservoir capacity.

Filling of Pelvic Dead Space

The pelvic dead space predisposes patients to the formation of abscesses, perineal wound problems, fistula, and bowel obstruction. Pelvic floor reconstruction is essential to prevent these complications. It can be accomplished using synthetic absorbable mesh, myocutaneous flaps, or omentum. Use of myocutaneous flaps results in the reduction of dead space. Well vascularized, nonirradiated tissue of the myocutaneous flap replaces the resected skin and leads to good healing. Various types of flaps include rectus abdominis flap, gracilis, and gluteus maximus muscle flap.[16]

Vaginal Reconstruction

It is done either at the time of initial operation or as a delayed procedure. It is done for two reasons. One is that the loss of vagina can be psychological traumatic to the patient and as the other is it being the integral part of healing of perineal wound. This is achieved by various methods including split thickness skin grafts, myocutaneous flaps involving rectus abdominis ,and gracilis muscles.

COMPLICATIONS

Pelvic exenteration has a high incidence of postoperative complications ranging from 32% to 84% with 45% incidence of at least one readmission and 32% additional operative procedure.[17] This high incidence is due to the complexity of surgery and radiotherapy. The complications include bleeding, pelvic abscess, intestinal obstruction, pneumonia, enteroperineal, arterio-ureteral and urinary fistula, perineal hernia, urinary anastomotic stricture, stone formation and urinary sepsis, arterio-ureteral fistula, pelvic abscess, pelvic wound breakdown, myocutaneous flap necrosis, venous thrombosis, depression, and difficulty in adjustment to ostomy care.

The mortality rate has decreased significantly over the last decade.[18] Serious complications related to gastrointestinal and urinary tracts are related to the prior radiotherapy exposure.

PERINEAL SMALL BOWEL FISTULA (PSF)

This is a rare (3.5%) but serious complication after pelvic exenteration. Medical treatment is usually ineffective in this case. It is associated with a mortality rate of 13% and is indicative of disease recurrence in 40% patients.[19] This is mostly seen after total or posterior pelvic exenterations.

Technical aspects during exenteration to prevent PSF includes meticulous intestinal wall repairs before closure, use of ligatures for vessel ligation, and suturing for rectal stump closure rather than clips or staples as they make radiation exposed small bowel loops prone to injuries. Use of omentum and myocutaneous flaps results in decreased rates of PSF.

SURVIVAL

Of all the indications of pelvic exenteration, patients with recurrent rectal cancer have significantly worse five-year survival rates. The survival is affected adversely by the presence of lymph nodal metastases. The reported five-year survival rates are 26–31%.[20] In one of the studies, five-year survival of patients with recurrent rectal cancer was only 20% in comparison to 43% for patients undergoing pelvic exenteration for primary disease.[21]

CONCLUSION

Management of recurrent rectal cancer is a greater challenge than the management of even rectal cancer with liver metastases. Surgery in the form of pelvic exenteration is the only optimum treatment available for this problem. Best results are possible with meticulous preoperative planning, multimodality approach at a center of excellence by a multi-disciplinary team. Proper and adequate counseling of the patient and family members is important to ensure realistic expectations.

OUR EXPERIENCE

In the last 10 years from 2005 till date we have performed resections for rectal cancer in 53 patients. Of these, 40 were LAR (22 laparoscopic LAR), 9 were APR (7 laparoscopic APR), and 5 were pelvic exenterations. We have done exenteration in three patients for advanced rectal cancer. All were posterior exenterations in female patients. In two patients, we did exenteration for recurrent rectal cancer. Both received adjuvant treatment (CRT). One was after 9 months of LAR (open), in which we did posterior exenteration including rectum, uterus, and posterior vaginal wall. The other case was after 18 months of APR (laparoscopic), in which pelvic mass with uterus, posterior vaginal wall along with the ileal loop was resected. All five patients of exenteration had MRI and PET-FDG done along with CEA levels. The average duration of surgery was 5–7 hours with the blood loss of 200–500 mL. Postoperative complications included intestinal obstruction (adhesive) in one and wound infection in other, both managed conservatively. Both were sent for postoperative chemo-radiotherapy. The follow-up of both patients were 6 months and 2 years.

REFERENCES

1. Bakx R, Visser O, Josso J, et al. Management of recurrent rectal cancer: A population based study in greater Amsterdam. World J Gastroenterol 2008; 14:6018–6023.
2. Mirnezami AH, Sagar PM, Kavanagh D, et al. Clinical algorithms for the surgical management of locally recurrent rectal cancer. Dis Colon Rectum 2010; 53:1248–1257.
3. Kapiteijn E, Marijnen CAM, Nagtegaal ID, et al. Preoperative radiotherapy combined with total mesorectal excision for resectable rectal cancer. New England J Med 2001; 345:638–646.
4. Bozzetti F, Bertario L, Rossetti C, et al. Surgical treatment of locally recurrent rectal carcinoma. Dis Colon Rectum 1997; 40:1421–1424.
5. Moore G,. Riedel E, Minsky BD, et al., Adequacy of 1-cm distal margin after restorative rectal cancer resection with sharp mesorectal excision and preoperative combined-modality therapy. Ann Surg Oncol. 2003; 1080–85.
6. Palmer G, Martling A, Cedermark B, Holm T. A population-based study on the management and outcome in patients with locally recurrent rectal cancer. Ann Surg Onc 2007; 14:447–454.
7. Camilleri-Brennan J, Steele RJC. The impact of recurrent rectal cancer on quality of life. Eur J Surg Oncol 2001; 27:349–353.
8. Sasson AR, Sigurdson ER. Management of locally advanced rectal cancer. Surg Oncol 2000; 9:193–204.
9. Popovich MJ, Hricak H, Sugimura K, Stern JL. The role of MR imaging in determining surgical eligibility for pelvic exenteration. AJR Am J Roentgenol 1993; 160:525–531.
10. Smith FW, Heys SD, Evans NT, et al. Pattern of 2-deoxy-2-[18F]-fluro-D-glucose accumulation in liver tumours: Pri-mary, metastatic and after chemotherapy. Nucl Med Commun 1992; 13: 193–195.
11. Magrina JF, Stanhope CR, Weaver AL. Pelvic exenterations: Supralevator, infralevator, and with vulvectomy. Gynecol Oncol 1997; 64:130–135.
12. Magrina JF. Types of pelvic exenterations: A reappraisal. Gynecol Oncol 1990; 37:363–366.
13. Wanebo HJ, Marcove RC. Abdominal sacral resection of locally recurrent rectal cancer. Ann Surg 1981; 194:458–471.
14. Temple WJ, Ketcham AS. Sacral resection for control of pelvic tumors. Am J Surg 1992; 163:370–374.
15. Salom EM, Penalver MA. Pelvic exenteration and recon-struction. Cancer J 2003; 9:415–424.
16. Shibata D, Hyland W, Busse P, et al. Immediate reconstruction of the perineal wound with gracilis muscle flaps following abdominoperineal resection and intraoperative radiation therapy for recurrent carcinoma of the rectum. Ann Surg Oncol 1999; 6: 33–37.
17. Kakuda JT, Lamont JP, Chu DZ, et al. The role of pelvic exenteration in the management of recurrent rectal cancer. Am J Surg 2003; 186:660–664.
18. Goldberg JM, Piver MS, Hempling RE, et al. Improvements in pelvic exenteration: Factors responsible for reducing morbidity and mortality. Ann Surg Oncol 1998; 5:399–406.
19. Turrini O, Guiramand J , Moutardier V, et al. Perineal small bowel fistula after pelvic exenteration for cancer: Technical guidelines for perineal fistula. Ann Surg Oncol 2006; 13:1622–1626.
20. Salo JC, Paty PB, Guillem J, et al. Surgical salvage of recurrent rectal carcinoma after curative resection: A 10-year experience. Ann Surg Oncol 1999; 6:171–177.
21. Hafner GH, Herrera L, Petrelli NJ. Patterns of recurrence after pelvic exenteration for colorectal adenocarcinoma. Arch Surg 1991; 126:1510–1513.

CHAPTER 101

Minimally Invasive Colorectal Cancer Surgery

Subhash Mishra, Mohd. Qaleem, Purak Mishra, Deepak Govil

Minimally invasive surgery (MIS) has been in existence since as early as 1795, when Dr. Bozzini[1] developed the *Lichtleiter,* a crude endoscope, which used a candle as illumination, for exploring intracavitary organs through external orifices. It has taken a giant leap in the past two decades and has been successfully applied across multiple disciplines. An important transition toward minimal access surgery was the acceptance of laparoscopic cholecystectomy over conventional open cholecystectomy by general surgeons. With the establishment of laparoscopic cholecystectomy as the "gold standard," surgeons all over the world started advocating laparoscopic surgical techniques for various surgical conditions.

In last two decades, there has been a rapid evolution toward minimally invasive approaches for colorectal surgery. The first report of laparoscopic colectomy came from Jacobs et al.[2] in 1991. Initially, due to oncological concerns, the use of laparoscopic surgery was doubtful, whereas it was comfortably used by the surgeons for benign cases. Randomized control trials clearly demonstrated that in experienced hands, laparoscopic surgery for colon cancer can produce equivalent results and similar oncologic resections as compared to open surgery. Laparoscopy has established itself as a procedure of choice for colonic malignancy, but similar evidence is lacking in terms of rectal cancer. Laparoscopic pelvic surgery is technically demanding as it requires skills to do an oncologically sound total mesorectal excision (TME) while working in a confined limit of narrow pelvis. Serious doubts were raised regarding the safe oncological margins and outcomes. Studies also confirm that the short-term benefits and long-term results (level I evidences) are still lacking. Numerous studies are underway like Japan Clinical Oncology Group (JCOG) 0404 trial, American College of Surgeons Oncology Group (ACOSOG) Z6051 in the United States, the COLOR II trial of Europe, Canada, and Korea.

Laparoscopic colorectal surgery is technically very demanding involving a long steep learning curve, but it lacks tactile sensation. As compared to open surgery, the laparoscopic approach in colorectal diseases is accompanied by lower abdominal wall insult, lower postoperative pain, better cosmetic results, and faster recovery and improved outcome. New technologies are developed by surgical innovators and industry for even less invasive approaches because of the acceptance of minimally invasive procedures by both patients and surgeons. In the mid 1990s, a novel concept was born. As open colorectal surgery very much depends on the hands' movement, surgeons or their assistants place their one hand inside the abdominal cavity through a small incision, while pneumoperitoneum is maintained and operation is performed through video laparoscopy. It was called "hand-assisted laparoscopic surgery" or HALS. Single-incision laparoscopic surgery (SILS) is associated with few incisions. Robotic techniques are popularized in other specialities, such as urology and gynaecology, due to the ease of working in the confined space of pelvis. Natural orifice transluminal endoscopic surgery (NOTES) in colorectal disease has still not fully transpired, but advances in transitional techniques and instrumentation may allow specimen extraction through natural orifice following laparoscopic colectomy.

Although laparoscopy provides better visualization and access to the pelvis compared to open conventional methods, still working in a narrow pelvis, adequate sigmoid traction, manoeuvring the instruments to get a perpendicular staple line, along with the need for oncologically sound TME, requires considerable training, skills, and optimal instruments. For this reason, advancement in newer techniques is continuously taking place as a result of its demand and here is the place where robotics can play a significant role. Various techniques of MIS which are continuously applied in colorectal fields have been discussed in the following sections.

LAPAROSCOPIC SURGERY

In laparoscopic colorectal surgery, a specialized camera and several laparoscopic instruments are inserted through several small incisions. In general, all ports should be separated by 4 finger breadths (Figs 1 and 2). Pneumoperitoneum is created by insufflating carbon dioxide (CO_2) into the peritoneal cavity that creates a working space to perform the operation. During surgery to get necessary exposure, the operating table is tilted in various directions that allow intra-abdominal organs to fall away from the area of dissection. The performance of a laparoscopic colon resection requires instruments that will allow the gentle handling of small and large bowels, for example, 5 mm atraumatic Babcock graspers. A vessel sealant device permits the efficient division of vascularized structures within the abdomen. Other instruments required are laparoscopic scissors, traumatic/atraumatic dissectors.

Right/left hemicolectomy, total and subtotal colectomy/proctocolectomy, anterior resection, abdominoperineal resection, and rectopexy are being increasingly done with the help of laparoscopic surgery as surgical skills are increasing. The dissection of the mesocolon and the mesentery can be done either from medial to lateral side or in the reverse direction. Medial to lateral side dissection is preferred by most laparoscopic surgeons as in this they can identify, dissect and ligate the vessels properly at the base and also the adjoining lymph nodes. The ureter can be seen and well protected.

Laparoscopic intestinal resection includes the mobilization and removal of a long floppy segment of the colon, ligation of large vessels, and restoration of bowel continuity. After completing the mobilization and division of blood supply, the colonic segment is exteriorized through a small skin incision for extracorporeal resection and anastomosis that is later placed back into the abdomen. A wound protector is used to prevent the cut skin and subcutaneous tissue from contamination and contact with tumour tissues. With experience, intracorporeal resection and hand sewn or stapled anastomosis can be performed with ease.

The following are the advantages and disadvantages of laparoscopic colectomy.

1. Advantages:[3]
   - Better cosmesis
   - Less postoperative pain
   - Early return of bowel function
   - Shorter hospital stay
2. Disadvantages:
   - Longer operating-room times.
   - Lack of tactile feedback.
   - Technically demanding and long learning curve
   - Need of endostaplers and vessel sealing devices

Laparoscopic colon resections are performed with increasing frequency throughout the world. The technique of laparoscopic colectomy has a long learning curve[4] because of the advanced laparoscopic skills it entails, and, hence, is the place of alternative procedures like laparoscopic-assisted procedures and HALS.

The initial bodies of literature comparing laparoscopic and open surgeries for colon cancer treatment have reported high recurrence rates at wound and port sites, raising doubts over the oncologic efficacy of laparoscopy. Large randomized trials that followed were, therefore, attentive to oncologic outcomes, such as positive resection margins, number of lymph nodes harvested, and recurrence rates at port sites. None of the trials showed any difference between the open and laparoscopic procedures regarding these outcomes. Only in the COLOR trial, there were more recurrences in the abdominal wall observed following laparoscopy than those in open surgery for colon cancer (five at the port site and two at the tumour extraction site), but the difference was not significant ($p = 0.09$).

In 2011, Huang and colleagues[5] conducted a meta-analysis including six clinical trials ($n = 1033$) that evaluated the efficacy of laparoscopic surgery in rectal cancer treatment. Three-year overall survival ($p = 0.11$, 4 trials) and disease-free survival ($p = 0.11$, three trials) were not significantly different after laparoscopy or open surgery. After a follow-up ranging from 32.8 to 112.5 months, local recurrence rates after laparoscopic and open surgery were not statistically different ($p = 0.21$, four trials). No difference was either observed between laparoscopy and open surgery for the mean number of lymph nodes harvested ($p = 0.43$, five trials); positive circumferential resection margins were also similar (7.9% v. 5.4%, $p = 0.63$, five trials).

In 2011, Ohtani and colleagues[6] conducted a meta-analysis comparing the oncologic efficacy of laparoscopic and open surgery for rectal cancer. Twelve trials were included ($n = 2095$), and results showed no difference between the two procedures for the oncologic outcomes measured.

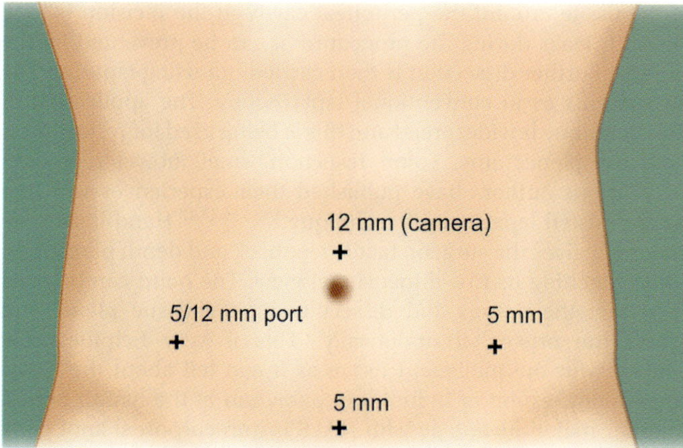

Figure 1 Position of ports for laparoscopic hemicolectomy

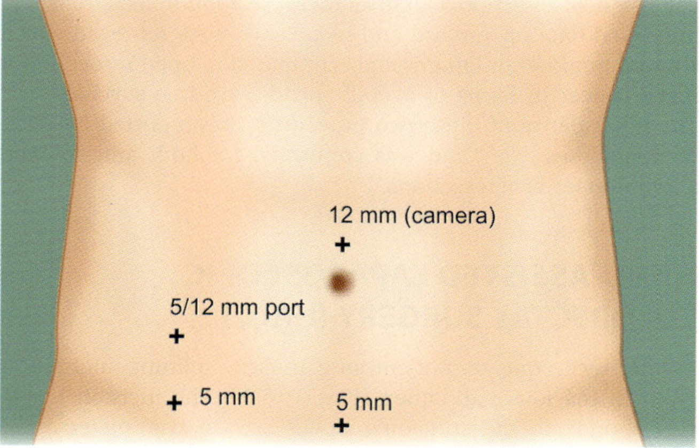

Figure 2 Position of ports for laparoscopic AR

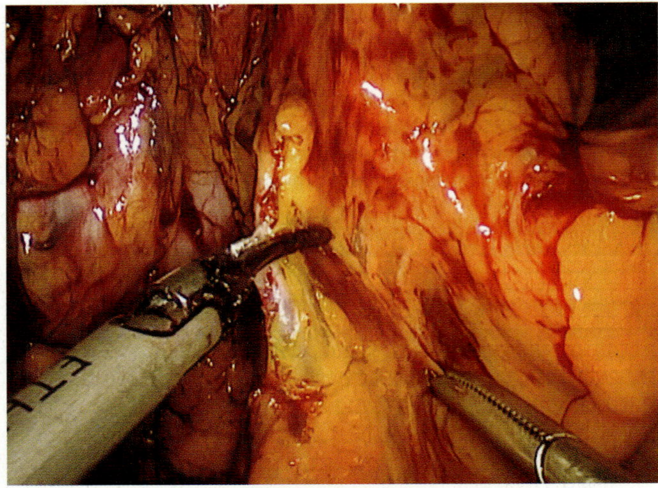

Figure 3 Laparoscopic instruments being used in colorectal surgery

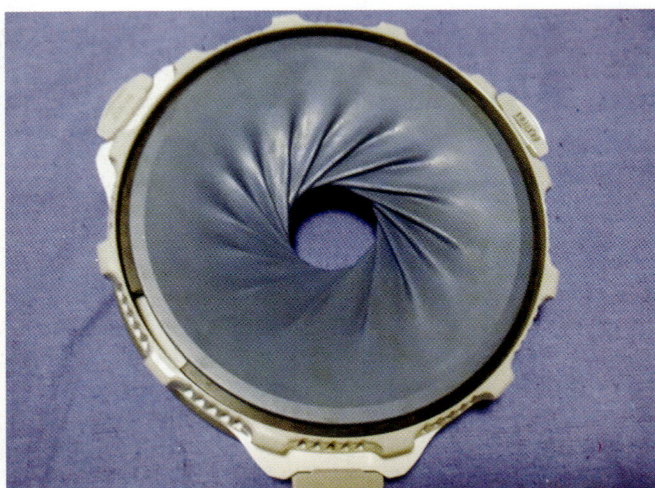

Figure 5 Hand port

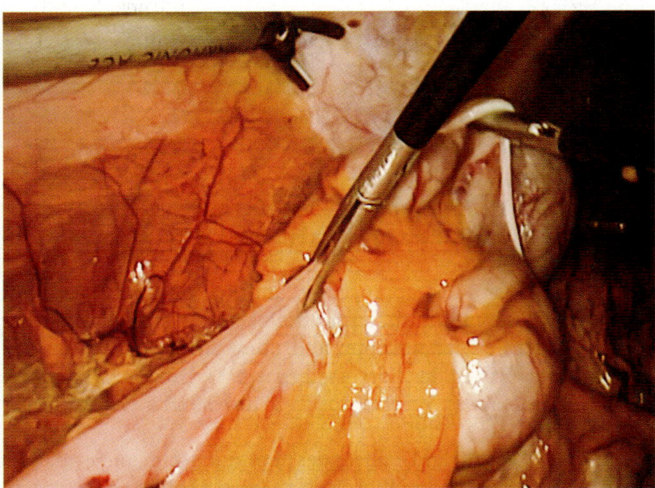

Figure 4 Laparoscopic colorectal surgery

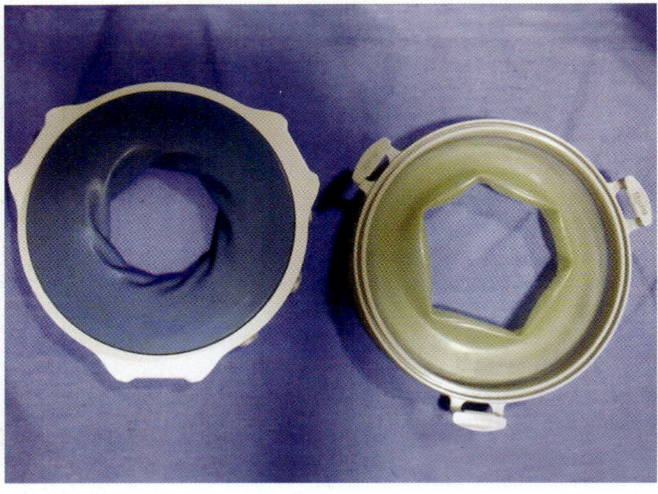

Figure 6 Hand ports

Trials evaluating the laparoscopic procedure for rectal cancer had generally lower power than those evaluating laparoscopic colon cancer resection. Out of all these, six randomized trials that presented data on survival and recurrence were retrieved which showed noninferior laparoscopic compared to open resection for rectal cancer in terms of overall and disease-free survival.[7,8,9,10] The equivalence of these two procedures is supported by three meta-analyses,[11,12,13] and was confirmed for both anterior and abdominoperineal resections.[7]

HAND-ASSISTED LAPAROSCOPIC COLORECTAL SURGERY (HALC)

In this technique, a 7–8-cm-long muscle splitting incision is given in the lower abdomen (Figs 3 to 7). The incision length corresponds to the surgeon's gloves size in centimeters. The exact site of incision depends on the location of pathology. The surgeon places his nondominant gloved hand inside the abdomen. Pneumoperitoneum is maintained by the elasticity of the tissue around the peritoneal cavity. If the incision is long and CO_2 leaks during the procedure, it can be prevented by the sutures. Further dissection is then carried out using laparoscopic instruments as in conventional laparoscopy. The application of this technique is widespread and this is being used for procedures, such as splenectomy, colon resection, small bowel resection, etc. Various authors have published their experiences with the hand-assisted laparoscopic technique.[14,15,16,17,18] Hand inside the abdomen gives the surgeon tactile feedback and depth perception while watching its two-dimensional view. The hand can be used to retract the tissues and dissect along the tissue plane, and reflect the organs atraumatically. This is very helpful while dealing with the malignant tissue as it can tell about the tissue consistency, extent of induration, palpation of the lymph nodes. Another major advantage with HALS is intracorporeal knot tying and suturing. All these things not only contributed to the short

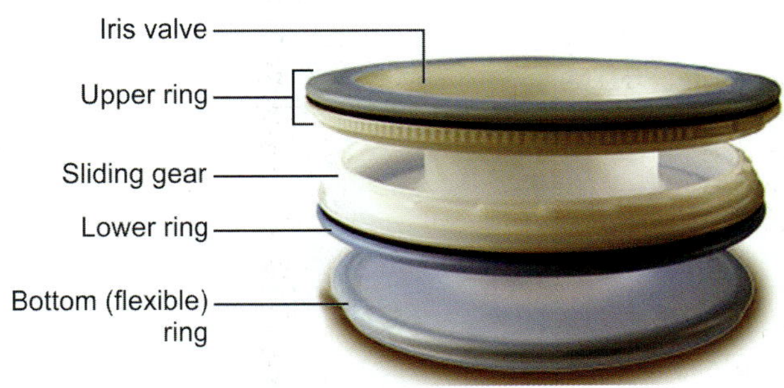

Figure 7 Different parts of hand port

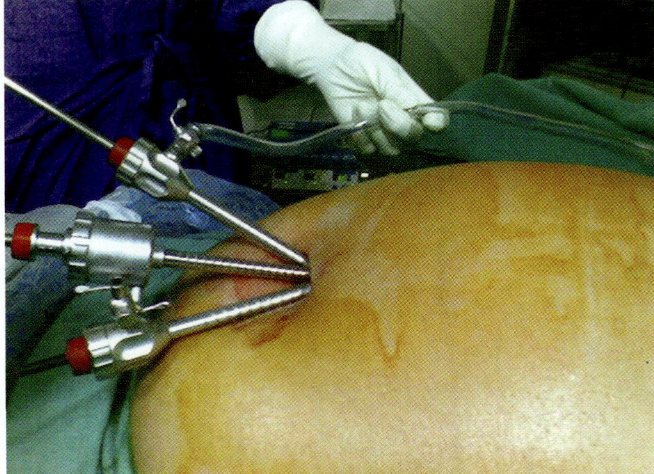

Figure 8 Single incision with direct access surgery

operative time but also a sense of confidence, familiarity, and security to the surgeon, which, in turn, leads to the early learning of the procedure in comparison to the conventional laparoscopy. Another major benefit of the hand inside the abdomen is in a situation where sudden unexpected bleeding occurs. With the HALS technique, it can be stopped immediately and effectively. Hand access port device sites can be used as a portal for the construction of extracorporeal anastomoses, specimen retrieval, and laparoscopic trocar sites. The latter permits the selective use of HAL and laparoscopically assisted (LA) techniques during the same operation at various times.[19]

As with all new ideas, this technique also faced severe criticism from the laparoscopic colorectal surgeons. First, it was said that hand inside the abdomen is against the concept of minimal invasive surgery. It was told to be more traumatizing to a patient as incision was given at the beginning of the procedure. Cosmetically, it was inferior to laparoscopy, so will not be received well by the patients. Second, the major problem with this technique was maintaining the pneumoperitoneum. It was almost impossible to maintain the pneumoperitoneum with the hand inside the abdomen. The hand port devices that were subsequently invented the so-called first generation devices also could not maintain the pneumoperitoneum effectively and that earned a bad name for HALS. Another major factor that prevented the widespread use of HALS was related to ergonomics. It can hinder the view and certain manoeuvres, especially if the patient is thin and surgeon's hand is large. One hand inside the abdomen and other outside the abdomen, holding the long laparoscopic instruments is a very awkward position. It causes hand fatigue, especially if the procedure is long lasting. All these things led to the disregard of this new technique, and it did not gain popularity. In the following few years with the introduction of new devices termed as second generation devices (sleeveless devices) which maintain pneumoperitoneum effectively and the slow progress of advanced laparoscopy, HALS was once again revisited. Several authors published their results, showing the feasibility and short-term benefits of HALS.[20] These authors proved that HALS is better than open surgery and equivalent to laparoscopic assisted surgery. It is a hybrid procedure that not only preserves the principle of the minimal invasive procedure but also gives the advantages of both open and laparoscopic surgeries. It was much easier to learn. HALS gradually established its feasibility, safety, and utility not only in colorectal surgery, but also in other fields like donor nephrectomy and splenectomy.

For the comparison of HALS and open surgery for the treatment of colorectal disease, authors[21] collected studies that were preserved over the past 17 years, and the meta-analysis of 12 studies was done that included 1,362 patients. The conversion rate of the HALS procedure to laparotomy was 2.66%. Incision length, intra-operative blood loss, recovery of intestinal function, and wound infection rate were less in the HALS group as compared to those in the open surgery group. However, no significant differences were noted in operating time, complications, such as urinary tract infection, pneumonia, and anastomotic leaks, total hospitalization cost, and mortality between the groups. The disadvantage of HALS is that a small number of patients may be converted to laparotomy and the oncologic safety and long-term prognosis are not clear. Hence, HALS provides minimal invasion, less blood loss, faster recovery, reduced length of hospitalization without an increase in costs.

In a Cochrane Systematic Review,[22] three randomized controlled studies that met the inclusion criteria (n=189) were included for the comparison of HALS to conventional laparoscopy. No statistically significant difference in operative time or complication rate was noted; however, conversion rates were significantly decreased in patients undergoing hand-assisted surgery. Similar results were noted in meta-analysis reporting. There was a statistically significant decrease in conversion rates among the hand-assisted group with no differences in operating time or peri-operative complication rates.

SINGLE INCISION LAPAROSCOPIC SURGERY

The evolution of the single incision laparoscopic surgery (SILS) was based on better cosmesis and minimizing the trauma and complications of multiport laparoscopy, such as less pain, less infection, less chances of incisional hernia, and less adhesion formation (Fig. 8). Although there is confusion regarding the nomenclature of SILS, it can be divided by the methods of access into three categories:

1. **Single incision single port surgery**: In this method, a single incision is given at umbilicus and a specialized access port is inserted which permits 3–4 trocars.
2. **Single incision multiple port surgery**: In this method, all trocars are inserted transumbilically. Due to this, multiple facial

defects in close proximity are formed and can theoretically raise the concern about incisional hernia.

3. **Single incision direct access surgery**: In this technique, instruments are directly inserted through the abdominal wall along the side of the central telescope. This technique requires specialized articulating instruments.[23]

The technical issues involved in SILS are the site of incision, choice of instruments and telescope, and type of the ports. Most surgeons preferred the umbilical incision, 30° telescope, and conventional laparoscopic instruments. Various commercially available access ports are GelPort Appllied Medical, USA, SILS (Covidien, USA), R Port and Tri Port (Advanced Surgical Concepts Ltd, Ireland), the Uni-X (USA), SSL(Ethicon, USA), Air Seal (Surgiquest, Orange, CT, USA), X-Cone, and Endo-Cone (Karl storz, Germany). Their use depends on individual choice.[24]

Whichever technique is used, the basic principal of colonic surgery remains the same as in open surgery. After operation, specimen is removed through the incision. Facial defect is closed traditionally.

The reported advantages associated with single incision are as follows: less pain, less infection, better cosmesis, less internal adhesions, and early recovery.

Disadvantages associated with the SILS are as follows: technical difficulty with lack of space outside the abdomen causing clashes of instruments, difficulty with retraction of organs, and loss of proprioception due to crossed instruments. Another major issue involved is the learning curve. Although the use of the access port and the articulation of curved flexible instruments have reduced these problems to some extent, then one must require these additional innovative instruments.

SILS is yet to establish itself in the field of colorectal surgery. There are case reports and series which showed that this technique is safe and feasible. In a review article, Makino Tomoki et al., involving 21 studies and 447 patients, from 1983 to 2011 (level 2–4 evidence), showed that single incision laparoscopic colorectal surgery is safe and feasible, and despite some technical difficulties, it is associated with potential benefits over conventional laparoscopy and hand-assisted colorectal surgery.[25]

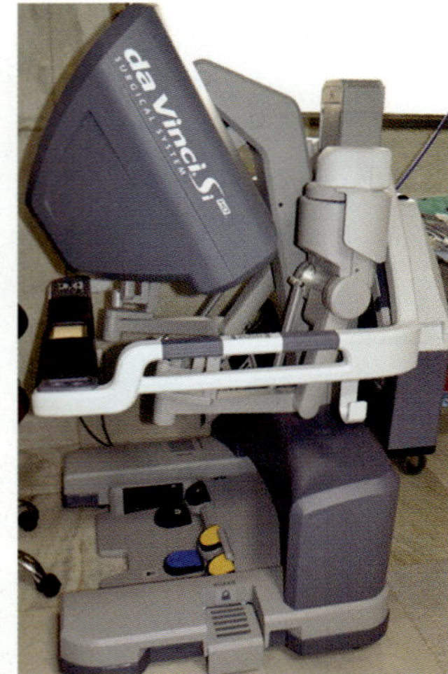

Figure 9 Robotic surgeon's console with hand, foot controls and 3D vision

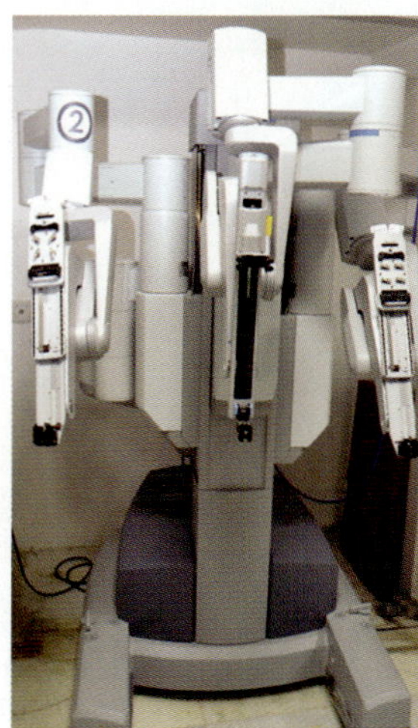

Figure 10 Robot with camera and other arms

ROBOTIC SURGERY

Robot-assisted MIS surgery is gaining acceptance for use in colorectal surgery, especially for cases involving rectal surgery (Figs 9 to 12). The automated endoscopic system for optimal positioning (AESOP) was the first robot used in general surgery (Computer Motion, Santa Barbara, CA, USA). In United States, the FDA-approved first telerobotic manipulation system for intra-abdominal surgery was the da Vinci® robotic system (Intuitive Surgical Inc., Sunnyvale, CA, USA). The da Vinci® robotic system was designed to conquer the limitations of open conventional surgery and laparoscopy. It has three components. First is surgeon's console or master manipulator. Second is a surgical cart or a slave manipulator that has four robotic arms. The third unit is for holding the camera and insufflation instruments. Surgery is performed by manipulating the robotic control on the console by the surgeon. Three-dimensional images are provided to a surgeon by a binocular camera system inserted through the laparoscopic port.

In comparison to laparoscopy, the robotic system provides three-dimensional imaging, filter physiologic tremor, downscale movements (5:1–2:1), and perform intuitive movements between the surgeon's hand and four robotic arms. A camera is held by the central robotic arm and the rest of the arms hold the surgical instruments. The precise dissection and intracorporeal suturing of the da Vinci® system is provided by the endowrist function at the tip of robotic arms, which provide 7 degrees of freedom, 180° articulation, and 540° of rotation. The general concern that we need to know about advance laparoscopy before we can venture into robotic surgery is really a myth as we only have to be well versed with basic laparoscopy like placing ports and pneumo-insufflation before we go for robotic surgery. Surprisingly, the learning curve for the robotic procedure is not as steep as advanced laparoscopy. Suturing with robotics is also much simpler than laparoscopy. There are certain drawbacks associated with the robotic system. Tissue damage may occur due to the lack of tactile and tensile feedback. This can be minimized by highly magnified, 3D visual

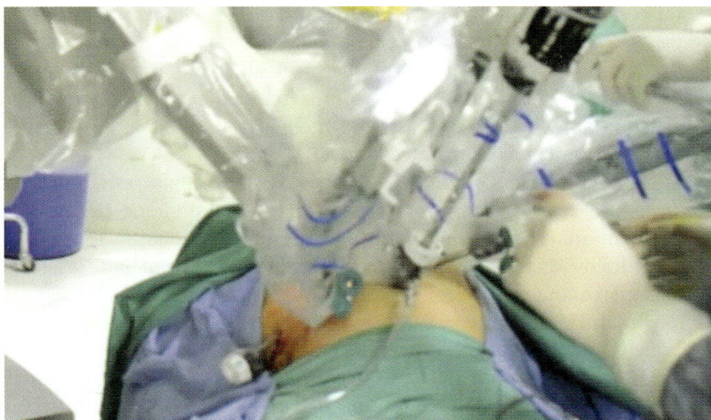

Figure 11 Robotic arms connecting with established ports in abdomen

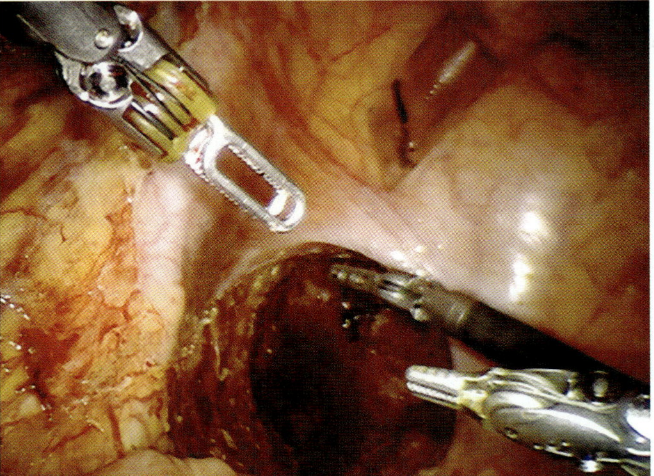

Figure 12 Creation of mesorectal window with robotic arms during rectal surgery

experience. Another important drawback is the time-consuming nature of docking and undocking of the robotic cart from the patient. This can be serious if emergency conversion is required in case of bleeding, although all these things take much less time with the experience of the OT staff. Another major drawback cited is the cost of the robotic system and the cost of the consumables and disposables for the patient.

During robotic surgery, the surgeon is seated at a console, using minimal force controllers while viewing the procedure through an ideally positioned three-dimensional (3D) imaging system. While no direct comparisons for surgeon strain exist between robotics and either laparoscopic or open surgery, few experts would argue that the robotic system is less physically taxing. In fact, robotics may allow surgeons to have longer, more productive careers.

Recent investigations[26,27] comparing open approach with laparoscopy for colorectal cancer have revealed better short-term operative outcomes with similar oncologic outcomes. MIRASAGES consensus[28] stated that the robotic surgery enables more and more surgeons to involve in advanced MIS with less effort as compared to laparoscopic surgery. The surgical robotic system allowed more MIS by overcoming the steep learning curve, especially for rectal cancer surgery.

In 2006, Pigazzi et al. first reported about the robotic TME for rectal cancer.[29] They compared robotic TME with laparoscopic TME for short-term outcomes and concluded that low anterior resection with TME and autonomic nerve preservation was feasible with the robotic approach. Later, they reported a series of 39 patients with primary rectal cancer[30 and] concluded that robotic-assisted surgery for rectal cancer could be performed safely.

In 2007, Baik et al.[31] reported the first Asian experience of robotic TME for rectal cancer patients. After that, they reported combined robotic TME, total abdominal hysterectomy for rectal cancer, and uterine myoma.[32] They concluded that simultaneous robotic surgeries with the da Vinci® system were safe and feasible. In August 2006, the first Asian case of robotic abdominoperineal resection was performed in Hong Kong[33] and other types of robotic general surgeries began to be reported.[34,35]

Spinoglio et al.[36] in 2008 reported their early experience of robotic colorectal surgeries. Fifty robotic resections were compared with 161 cases of laparoscopic resections. They concluded that, although robotic colonic resection took longer operative time, it was feasible and safe.

Baik et al.[37] in 2006 compared 18 robotic low anterior resection with 18 laparoscopic low anterior resection in a prospective randomized controlled trial. The short-term outcome of the pilot study was published in 2008. They showed that robotic low anterior resection is safe, feasible, and have better mesorectal grade, though they could not find statistical differences between the groups.

In a systemic review[38] of 39 case series, right and left/sigmoid colectomies by the robotic approach provided acceptable results in terms of operative morbidity (13.4 and 15.1%, respectively) and open conversion (1.1 and 3.8%, respectively). Robot-assisted anterior resection was associated with adequate lymph node retrieval (14.3, mean), low conversion rate (0.4%), and morbidity (9.7%).

In a meta-analysis[39,40] comparing robotic and laparoscopic surgeries reported that in the robotic group, the conversion rate to open was significantly lower than that with laparoscopic surgery. No significant differences were noted in intra-operative time, length of hospital stay, time to resume regular diet, postoperative morbidity and mortality, and the oncological accuracy of resection. In terms of early postoperative outcomes and complication profile, robotic colorectal surgery has no advantages over the standard laparoscopic approach. It has a shorter learning curve but increased operative time and cost. The resection of rectal cancer is advantageous due to its lower conversion rates even in distal rectal tumors, patients who had neoadjuvant chemoradiotherpy and obese individuals. An improved outcome is also noticed in circumferential resection margin positivity, preservation of autonomic function, and leak rates. The robotic approach has proved its safety profile in both colonic and rectal surgery and addressed most of the shortcomings of the standard laparoscopic surgery. However, the cost involved may restrict its use to patients with challenging rectal cancer and in specialist centers.

NATURAL ORIFICE TRANSLUMINAL ENDOSCOPIC SURGERY (NOTES)

NOTES is an upcoming approach that combine endoscopic and laparoscopic techniques to diagnose and treat abdominal pathology, and avoid abdominal incisions and incision-related complications.[41,42] The peritoneal cavity can be accessed via mouth, anus, or possibly vagina. Current research in the United States has been confined to animal models, but limited human experience is available where transoral, transgastric appendectomies have been performed. In colorectal surgery, this has been utilized in extracting specimen using normal orifices like transvaginal extraction of specimen.

The introduction of the minimal invasive approach in colorectal surgery has changed the entire scene how surgery is performed. Since the first laparoscopic colorectal surgery in 1991, laparoscopic colorectal surgery has come a long way. It would be prudent to say that minimally invasive colorectal surgery (whether laparoscopic or robotic) is here to stay. It has advantages of less pain, patients comfort, and early return to work. With experienced hands, it provides the same oncological results as with conventional surgery. HALS can be used for difficult cases. Conversion can be done from the laparoscopic procedure to HALS than conventional open procedures. Robotic surgery is feasible and definitively has place in colorectal lesions requiring low or ultra-low anterior resection and intersphincteric resections, more so in male patients with narrow pelvis and bulky tumors.

MIS is the future of colorectal cancer surgery and will soon be the gold standard.

REFERENCES

1. Georgeson KE, Owings E. Advances in minimally invasive surgery in children. *Am J Surg* 2000; 180:362–364.
2. Jacobs M, Verdeja JC, Goldstein HS. Minimally invasive colon resection (laparoscopic colectomy). Surg Laparosc Endosc 1991; 1:144–150.
3. Stocchi L[1], Nelson H, Young-Fadok TM, et al. Safety and advantages of laparoscopic vs. open colectomy in the elderly: Matched-control study. Dis Colon Rectum 2000; 43:326–332.
4. *Avital S[1], Hermon H, Greenberg R, et al.* Learning curve in laparoscopic colorectal surgery: our first 100 patients. *Isr Med Assoc J 2006; 8:683–686.*
5. Huang MJ, Liang JL, Wang H, et al. Laparoscopic-assisted versus open surgery for rectal cancer: A meta-analysis of randomized controlled trials on oncologic adequacy of resection and long-term oncologic outcomes. Int J Colorectal Dis 2011; 26:415–421.
6. Ohtani H, Tamamori Y, Azuma T, et al. A meta-analysis of the short-and long-term results of randomized controlled trials that compared laparoscopy-assisted and conventional open surgery for rectal cancer. J Gastrointest Surg 2011; 15:1375–1385.
7. Jayne DG, Thorpe HC, Copeland J, et al. Five-year follow-up of the Medical Research Council CLASICC trial of laparoscopically assisted versus open surgery for colorectal cancer. Br J Surg 2010;97:1638–1645.
8. Liang X, Hou S, Liu H, et al. Effectiveness and safety of laparoscopic resection versus open surgery in patients with rectal cancer: A randomized, controlled trial from China. J Laparoendosc Adv Surg Tech A 2011; 21:381–385.
9. Ng SS, Leung KL, Lee JF, et al. Long-term morbidity and oncologic outcomes of laparoscopic-assisted anterior resection for upper rectal cancer: Ten-year results of a prospective, randomized trial. Dis Colon Rectum 2009; 52:558–566.
10. Ng SS, Leung KL, Lee JF, et al. Laparoscopic-assisted versus open abdominoperineal resection for low rectal cancer: A prospective randomized trial. Ann Surg Oncol 2008; 15:2418–2425.
11. Huang MJ, Liang JL, Wang H, et al. Laparoscopic-assisted versus open surgery for rectal cancer: A meta-analysis of randomized controlled trials on oncologic adequacy of resection and long-term oncologic outcomes. Int J Colorectal Dis 2011; 26:415–421.
12. Ohtani H, Tamamori Y, Azuma T, et al. A meta-analysis of the short-and long-term results of randomized controlled trials that compared laparoscopy-assisted and conventional open surgery for rectal cancer. J Gastrointest Surg 2011; 15:1375–1385.
13. Anderson C, Uman G, Pigazzi A. Oncologic outcomes of laparoscopic surgery for rectal cancer: A systematic review and meta-analysis of the literature. Eur J Surg Oncol 2008; 34:1135–1142.
14. O'Reilly MJ, Saye WB, Mullins SG, et al. Technique of hand-assisted laparoscopic surgery. J Laparoendosc Surg 1996; 6:239–244.
15. Boland JP, Kusminsky RE, Tiley EH. Laparoscopic mini-laparotomy with manipulation: The middle path. *Min Inv Ther* 1993; 2:63–67.
16. Tierney JP, Oliver SR, Kusminsky RE, et al. Laparoscopic radical nephrectomy with intra abdominal manipulation. *Min Inv Ther* 1994; 3:303–305.
17. Dunn DC. Digitally assisted laparoscopic surgery. Br J Surg 1994; 81:474.
18. Ou H. Laparoscopic-assisted mini laparatomy with colectomy. Dis Colon Rectum 1995; 38:324–326.
19. Meshikhes AW. Controversy of hand-assisted laparoscopic colorectal surgery. World J Gastroenterol 2010; 16:5662–5668.
20. Mooney MJ, Elliott PL, Galapon DB, et al. Hand-assisted laparoscopic sigmoidectomy for diverticulitis. *Dis Colon Rectum* 1998; 41:630–635.
21. Ding J, Xia Y, Liao GQ, et al. Hand-assisted laparoscopic surgery versus open surgery for colorectal disease: A systematic review and meta-analysis. Am J Surg 2014; 207:109–119.
22. Moloo H, Haggar F, Coyle D, et al. Hand assisted laparoscopic surgery versus conventional laparoscopy for colorectal surgery. Cochrane Database Syst Rev 2010;10:CD006585.
23. Sharma A, Dahiya P, Khullar R, et al. Single-incision laparoscopic surgery (SILS) in biliary and pancreatic diseases. Indian J Surg 2012;74
24. Venkatapawankumar C. Different type of single incision laparoscopic ports: Review article. World J Laparosc Surg 2011; 4:47–51.
25. Makino T, Milsom JW, Lee SW. Single-incision laparoscopic surgeries forcolorectal diseases: Early experiences of a novel surgical method. Minim Invasive Surg 2012; 2012:783074.
26. Laparoscopically assisted colectomy is as safe and effective as open colectomyin people with colon cancer Abstracted from: Nelson H, Sargent D, Wieand HS, et al; for the Clinical Outcomes of Surgical Therapy Study Group. A comparison of laparoscopically assisted and open colectomy for colon cancer. N Engl J Med 2004; 350:2050–2059. [Cancer Treat Rev 2004; 30:707–709].
27. Guillou PJ, Quirke P, Thorpe H, et al., MRC Clasicc Trial Group. Short-term endpoints of conventional versus laparoscopic-assisted surgery in patients with colorectal cancer (MRC CLASICC trial): Multicentre, randomised controlled trial. Lancet 2005;365: 1718–1726.
28. Herron DM, Marohn M; SAGES-MIRA Robotic Surgery Consensus Group. A consensus document on robotic surgery. Surg Endosc 2008; 22:313–325.
29. Pigazzi A, Ellenhorn JD, Ballantyne GH, et al. Robotic-assisted laparoscopic low anterior resection with total mesorectal excision for rectal cancer. Surg Endosc 2006; 20:1521–1525.
30. Hellan M, Anderson C, Ellenhorn JD, et al. Short-term outcomes after robotic-assisted total mesorectal excision for rectal cancer. Ann Surg Oncol 2007; 14:3168–3173.
31. Baik SH, Kang CM, Lee WJ, et al. Robotic total mesorectal excision for the treatment of rectal cancer. J Robotic Surg 2007; 1:99–102.
32. Baik SH, Kim YT, Ko YT, et al. Simultaneous robotic total mesorectal excision and total abdominal hysterectomy for rectal cancer and uterine myoma. Int J Colorectal Dis 2008; 23:207–208.

33. Ng SS, Lee JF, Yiu RY, et al. Telerobotic-assisted laparoscopic abdominoperineal resection for low rectal cancer: Report of the first case in Hong Kong and China with an updated literature review. World J Gastroenterol 2007; 13:2514–2518.
34. Kang CM, Chi HS, Hyeung WJ, et al. The first Korean experience of telemanipulative robot-assisted laparoscopic cholecystectomy using the da Vinci system. Yonsei Med J 2007;48:540–545.
35. Choi SB, Park JS, Kim JK, et al. Early experiences of robotic-assisted laparoscopic liver resection. Yonsei Med J 2008; 49:632–638.
36. Spinoglio G, Summa M, Priora F, et al. Robotic colorectal surgery: First 50 cases experience. Dis Colon Rectum 2008;51: 1627–1632.
37. Baik SH, Ko YT, Kang CM, et al. Robotic tumor-specific mesorectal excision of rectal cancer: Short-term outcome of a pilot randomized trial. Surg Endosc 2008; 22:1601–1608.
38. Antoniou SA, Antoniou GA, Koch OO, et al. Robot-assisted laparoscopic surgery of the colon and rectum. Surg Endosc 2012;26:1–11.
39. Trastulli S, Farinella E, Cirocchi R, et al. Robotic resection compared with laparoscopic rectal resection for cancer: Systematic review and meta-analysis of short-term outcome. Colorectal Dis 2012; 14:e134–e156.
40. Aly EH. Robotic colorectal surgery: Summary of the current evidence. Int J Colorectal Dis 2014; 29:1–8.
41. Santos BF, Hungness ES. Natural orifice translumenal endoscopic surgery: Progress in humans since white paper. World J Gastroenterol 2011; 17:1655–1665.
42. Kalloo AN, Singh VK, Jagannath SB, et al. Flexible transgastricperitoneoscopy: A novel approach to diagnostic and therapeutic interventions in the peritoneal cavity. Gastrointest Endosc. 2004; 60:114–117.

CHAPTER 102

Chemotherapy for Colorectal Cancer

Sunil Kumar Gupta

Colorectal cancer (CRC) is the world's third most prevalent cancer with almost 10 lac new cases diagnosed every year.[1] It also stands third in the list of cancers leading to deaths in both men and women. CRC accounts for 10 % of the total cancer burden worldwide with the age-standardized incidence rate of more developed regions 10-fold more than that of India. In the last three decades, CRC has shown an exponential growth with incidence increasing by 2–4 folds in Asian countries, such as China, Japan, South Korea, and Singapore with a concomitant rise in the mortality rates.

WHY COLORECTAL CANCER IN INDIA OCCURS A DECADE EARLIER THAN THE WESTERN POPULATION?

Similar to other cancer types, CRC is often seen a decade earlier in India than its Western counterparts. Four types of colorectal carcinogenesis patterns are well recognized, namely, adenoma-carcinoma sequence, de novo, hereditary nonpolyposis colorectal cancer (HNPCC), and colitic cancer.

A recent study from India found evidence for a possible noncanonical pathway-driven early-onset CRC in India.[4] Analysis has revealed the absence of Wnt and microsatellite instability (MSI) in a large number of early-onset CRC as compared to late onset. Also, the KRAS mutations are seen in much lower frequency in early-onset CRC. These findings suggest that early-onset CRCs in India may follow tumorigenesis pathways distinct from the classical CRC progression sequence suggesting the possible existence of non-canonical tumorigenesis pathways in early-onset CRC.

CLINICAL BIOMARKERS FOR COLORECTAL CANCER

A huge amount of research has been done to identify potential biomarkers than can be used to modulate and individualize treatment regimens. Currently, used biomarkers in clinical practice includes MSI and guanylyl cyclase C (GCC) testing in the adjuvant setting, and KRAS mutation testing for metastatic disease. Some of the recent studies have shown that mutations of KRAS and BRAF genes predict poor response to epidermal growth factor receptor (EGFR) inhibitors.[6]

Novel Biomarker for Colorectal Cancer

1. Hypermethylation of the plasma septin-9 gene which is a non-stool-based screening tool shows promise.[7]
2. Hypermethylation of the DYPD gene (encodes the enzyme dihydropyrimidine dehydrogenase) and the variation of the uridinediphosphate-glucuronosyltransferase 1A (UGT1A1) gene have predictive value for side effects and the efficacy of 5-fluoruracil and irinotecan, respectively.[7]
3. Micro-RNA signatures: Aberrant micro-RNA (miRNA) expression might be of potential use as diagnostic and prognostic biomarker for cancers.[8]
4. Genomic signatures: Identification of a biomarker panel for CRC diagnosis and prognostic signatures for survival.[9]

Adjuvant Treatment of Colorectal Cancer[13–17]

The standard care for the treatment of Dukes C and high-risk Dukes B colon carcinoma is surgical resection with en bloc lymph node dissection, followed by 6 months of adjuvant chemotherapy. The adjuvant treatment of CRC varies with the stage of disease. No adjuvant therapy is needed for stage I disease. For low risk stage II disease, capecitabine or 5FU/LV (fluorouracil/leucovorin) can be considered in an individual patient. FOLFOX is not considered based on the MOSAIC trial and the long-term sequel of oxaliplatin-based therapy. For high-risk stage II disease (poorly differentiated tumor, lymph node sampling <12, vascular or lymphatic or perineural invasion, pT4 stage, clinical presentation with intestinal occlusion or perforation), adjuvant chemotherapy with 5FU/LV, capecitabine, FOLFOX, or CapeOx can be considered because of a small absolute benefit. Combination chemotherapy with oxaliplatin and 5FU has yielded 2–3% additional benefit in 5-year overall survival for stage II CRCs in the recently analyzed NSABP protocol. For stage III patients, adjuvant chemotherapy has proven beneficial and should be administered to all. Here also combination chemotherapy in its various permutations (FLOX, FOLFOX, XELOX) fair better than single-agent 5FU in both OS and DFS. Based on the indirect evidence indicating a benefit for colon cancer in MOSAIC study, oxaliplatin has also been approved for the adjuvant treatment of rectal cancers by the National Comprehensive Cancer Network.

Whilst adjuvant therapy in colon cancer has focused on chemotherapy alone, radiotherapy has emerged as an important component in rectal cancer therapy due to distinct local failure patterns. Randomized studies have demonstrated that neoadjuvant radiotherapy confers overall survival benefit and improved local control for patients with T3 and T4 rectal tumors. The Gastrointestinal Tumor Study Group trial published in 1985 demonstrated that post-operative treatment reduced the risk of local recurrence and improved survival for patients with Dukes B2 and C rectal cancer. This was preceded in 1979 by the NCCTG trial, which demonstrated that RT concurrent with 5FU was superior to RT alone.

The necessity of adjuvant RT in patients undergoing total mesorectal excision (TME) is controversial. However, a benefit for adjuvant RT in TME patients was suggested in a Dutch neoadjuvant trial that randomly assigned 1861 patients with resectable rectal cancer to TME alone or a short course of preoperative RT followed by TME. Other data also support the benefit of adjuvant chemotherapy for patients undergoing TME, even if RT is not administered. Both RT and chemoradiotherapy may also be used to downstage tumors for sphincter-sparing surgery. In instances where neoadjuvant therapy is used, preoperative MRI or endorectal ultrasound (ERUS) is necessary to determine the T stage of tumors. Both these modalities may not, however, accurately determine nodal involvement.

Which Agents Should Not be Used in the Adjuvant Therapy?

Three randomized phase III trials have evaluated the combination of irinotecan to 5FU/LV therapy (PETACC 3, FNCLCC Accord02/ FFCD9802, CALGB 89803). However, all three trials have failed to demonstrate any advantage. Trial evaluating the role of the addition of bevacizumab and cetuximab to FOLFOX in adjuvant setting also failed to show any advantage, even though the exact reasons for these results are still unknown, but it strengthens the belief that locally advanced and metastatic diseases are distinct entities and, thus, must be treated differently.[18]

TREATMENT FOR METASTATIC CRC (mCRC)

The use of monoclonal antibodies in combination with other chemotherapeutic agents has become first line treatment for CRC.[19] In previously untreated metastatic disease, the use of bevacizumab along with irinotecan and/or 5FU significantly improves overall survival.[20] And also for patients who have progressed on previous nonbevacizumab chemotherapeutic regimens, the combination of bevacizumab and FOLFOX offers significant survival advantage. Benefits of bevacizumabin metastatic CRCs occur irrespective of the mutational status of KRAS and BRAF genes. The role of cetuximabs in the first-line treatment in combination with both FOLFIRI and FOLFOX4 in patients with KRAS wild-type tumors has been investigated in some recent trials. The addition of the cetuximab to both of these chemotherapeutic regimens has shown to reduce the risk of disease progression as compared to FOLFIRI or FOLFOX alone. Even the combination of panitumumab and FOLFOX4 or FOLFIRI in the treatment of KRAS wild-type mCRC has been shown to significantly increase progression-free survival in stage III trials as the second-line treatment. Second-line treatment depends on the first-line regimen used. For chemoresistant mCRC, cetuximab or panitumumab is recommended as monotherapy in patients with wild-type KRAS tumors.

IMPROVEMENT IN SURVIVAL AFTER COLORECTAL LIVER METASTASIS (CLM) RESECTION

Fifty percent patients of CRC will eventually develop liver metastasis, with nearly 20–25% presenting with hepatic metastasis at the time of initial diagnosis.[21] Patients of CLM may be segregated into three groups:

1. Those with resectable disease
2. Potentially resectable disease, that is, those whose metastases may become resectable
3. Unlikely to become resectable

Only 10–30% of patients with liver-limited colorectal metastasis are in potentially resectable state at the time of presentation. Patients, whose complete resection of liver metastasis is achieved, experience an impressive 5-year survival of over 50% in some recent studies (range 16–74%). Last two decades have witnessed an improving trend of long-term survival for operable and inoperable mCRC alike. Colorectal liver metastases are best managed with a multidisciplinary team approach. Even an upfront resectable disease may benefit from preoperative chemotherapy in the following ways:

1. Those which progress on preoperative chemotherapy have aggressive disease and are selected out
2. Helps in selecting the best chemotherapeutic drugs in individual patients

However, timing of surgery in these patients receiving preoperative chemotherapy is important. These patients have to be re-evaluated after 4 cycles. If the lesions seem to be in the resectable range, these patients should be offered surgery.

NEW DRUGS APPROVED IN 2012 FOR COLORECTAL CANCER[22–23]

Several targeted agents (Vatalanib, Cediranib, Brivanib, Axitinib, Sunitinib, Regorafenib, Aflibercept AMG-706 etc.), with anti-angiogenic properties have been investigated in mCRC. Among these, Aflibercept and Regorafenib, received the FDA approval as the new targeted agents for the treatment of mCRC in 2012. Aflibercept is a recombinant fusion protein of human VEGF receptors 1 and 2 and Fc portion of the human IgG1 immunoglobulin. It is presently approved for those metastatic CRC patients who are either resistant to or have progressed on oxaliplatin-based regimens and is to be used in combination with FOLFIR. Regorafenib is a new, orally active, multikinase inhibitor of VEGF and PDGF receptors along with additional kinases associated with alternative pathways of angiogenesis and resistance to VEGF-targeted drugs. It has been shown to be beneficial for those mCRC which has progressed after all standard therapies, offering a potential new line of therapy in this treatment-refractory population.

REFERENCES

1. GLOBOCAN 2008 [homepage]. Available from: http://globocan.iarc.fr/factsheet.asp. Last Accessed Nov. 11, 2012.
2. PDCR Reports 2006-2008 [homepage]. Available from: http://ncrpindia.org/Reports/PBCR_2006_2008.aspx. Last Accessed Nov. 11, 2012.
3. Pathy S, Lambert R, Sauvaget C, et al. The incidence and survival rates of colorectal cancer in India remain low compared with rising rates in East Asia. Dis Colon Rectum. 2012;55:900-906.
4. Raman R, Kotapalli V, Adduri R, et al. Evidence for possible non-canonical pathway(s) driven early-onset colorectal cancer in India. Mol Carcinog. 2014;53:E181-E186.
5. Quirke P, Risio M, Lambert R, et al. Quality assurance in pathology in colorectal cancer screening and diagnosis - European recommendations. Virchows Arch. 2011;458:1-19.
6. De Roock W, Biesmans B, De Schutter J, et al. Clinical biomarkers in oncology: Focus on colorectal cancer. Mol Diagn Ther. 2009;13:103-114.
7. Newton KF, Newman W, Hill J, et al. Review of biomarkers in colorectal cancer. Colorectal Dis. 2012;14:3-17.
8. Luo X, Burwinkel B, Tao S, et al. MicroRNA signatures: Novel biomarker for colorectal cancer? Cancer Epidemiol Biomarkers Prev. 2011;20:1272-1286.
9. García-Bilbao A, Armañanzas R, Ispizua Z, et al. Identification of a biomarker panel for colorectal cancer diagnosis. BMC Cancer 2012;12:43.
10. Dewhurst C, Rosen MP, Blake MA, et al. ACR Appropriateness Criteria (®) pretreatment staging of colorectal cancer. J Am Coll Radiol. 2012; 9:775-781.
11. Pickhardt PJ, Hassan C, Halligan S, et al. Colorectal cancer: CT colonography and colonoscopy for detection - systematic review and meta-analysis. Radiology. 2011; 259:393-405.
12. Cohen G, Lecht S, Arien-Zakay H, et al. Bio-imaging of colorectal cancer models using near infrared labeled epidermal growth factor. PLoS One 2012; 7:e48803. doi: 10.1371/journal.pone.0048803.
13. Lancet. Efficacy of adjuvant fluorouracil and folinic acid in colon cancer. International Multicentre Pooled Analysis of Colon Cancer Trials (IMPACT) investigators. Lancet. 1995;345:939-944.
14. American Society of Clinical Oncology. Efficacy of adjuvant fluorouracil and folinic acid in B2 colon cancer. International Multicentre Pooled Analysis of B2 Colon Cancer Trials (IMPACT B2) investigators. J Clin Oncol. 1999;17:1356-1363.
15. Krook JE, Moertel CG, Gunderson LL, et al. Effective surgical adjuvant therapy for high-risk rectal carcinoma. N Engl J Med. 1991;324:709-715.
16. Kapiteijn E, Marijnen CA, Nagtegaal ID, et al. Preoperative radiotherapy combined with total mesorectal excision for resectable rectal cancer. N Engl J Med. 2001;345:638-646.
17. Akasu, T, Moriya, Y, Yoshida, S, et al. Adjuvant oral uracil and tegafur (UFT) improves survival after complete mesorectal excision for pathologic TNM stage III rectal cancer: Results of the National Surgical Adjuvant Study (NSAS)-colorectal cancer (CC)-01 trial (abstract). Proc Am Soc Clin Oncol. 2004;23:251a.
18. Oyan B. Why do targeted agents not work in the adjuvant setting in colon cancer? Expert Rev Anticancer Ther 2012; 12:1337-1345.
19. Edwards MS, Chadda SD, Zhao Z, et al. A systematic review of treatment guidelines for metastatic colorectal cancer. Colorectal Dis. 2012;14:e31-e47.
20. Zinser-Sierra JW, Rodríguez-Ramírez S, Villalobos-Valencia R, et al. Use of bevacizumab in metastatic colorectal cancer: Report from the Mexican opinion and analysis forum on colorectal cancer treatment with bevacizumab (September 2009). Drugs RD. 2011;11:101-111.
21. Kanas GP, Taylor A, Primrose JN, et al. Survival after liver resection in metastatic colorectal cancer: Review and meta-analysis of prognostic factors. Clin Epidemiol. 2012;4:283-301.
22. U.S. Food and Drug Administration [homepage]. Available from: http://www.fda.gov/Drugs/InformationOnDrugs/ApprovedDrugs/ucm314438.htm
23. U.S. Food and Drug Administration [homepage]. Available from: http://www.fda.gov/NewsEvents/Newsroom/PressAnnouncements/ucm321271.htm

CHAPTER 103

Radiotherapy for Colorectal and Anal Carcinoma

Swarupa Mitra

HISTORY OF RADIATION THERAPY IN COLORECTAL CARCINOMA

During the last decade, the management of colorectal cancer has undergone a dramatic change. Since ages, surgery was the principal mode of curative treatment for colorectal cancers. Early-stage diseases were well managed with excision, thus avoiding a major surgery and a colostomy. But unfortunately most of the rectal cancers presented at locally advanced stages and required either abdominoperineal resection (APR) or low anterior resection (LAR). Various clinical researches and studies showed numerous pelvic failures (20–50%)[1] in spite of the extensive surgery. Persistent efforts to decrease local failure rates resulted in several randomized trials evaluating various combinations of chemoradiotherapy in adjuvant settings.[2–4] These trials reflected improved survival and local control with the addition of adjuvant therapies, compared to surgery alone.[5,6] Eventually, by the 1990s, concomitant chemoradiotherapy or CRT adjuvant to radical surgery became the new paradigm of management for colorectal cancers.

It was a known fact that the pelvic failures and local recurrences are determined by the T stage and lymph nodal involvement. About the same period, more studies in the UK and other European countries suggested that if the rectum is not removed with its envelope of mesorectal fascia, it would lead to a subtotal resection and persistence of microscopic tumor cells producing high probability for local recurrence.[7] These observations opened the door for total mesorectal excision (TME). In TME, the adjacent mesorectal tissue containing the regional lymphatics and the superior haemorrhoidal artery pedicle are also removed during radical surgery. Presumably, TME, an extra radical surgery, was supposed to eradicate the need for adjuvant radiation therapy because it not only aimed at the removal of all gross disease, but also at the eradication of microscopic disease, with negative proximal, distal, and circumferential margins. But that was not to be. A large randomized trial from Netherlands soon confirmed that despite the more radical surgery, improvement in local control and recurrence-free survival occurred in stage III patients only with the addition of neoadjuvant radiation.[8] Today, the management of colorectal carcinoma is largely a multimodality approach, with radiation therapy as an integral component of the management.

RADIOTHERAPY FOR RECTAL CARCINOMA

Radiotherapy may largely be given in the following settings.

1. Radical radiotherapy:
   a. Adjuvant: Post-operative radiotherapy and post-operative CRT
   b. Neoadjuvant: Neoadjuvant CRT/radiotherapy alone
2. Palliative radiotherapy.

Adjuvant Postoperative Radiotherapy

Concerns about the high local recurrences prompted scientists to look into options of post-operative treatment with combinations of radiation and/or chemotherapy.

Advantage: An important advantage of post-operative radiation is that the patients with high-risk features on histopathology for local failure only can be selected for adjuvant radiation therapy.

Disadvantage: Surgery renders the tumor bed hypoxic making radiation less effective. Moreover, complications may be higher due to the increased radiation exposure of small bowel loops which comes to lie in pelvis post resection. Also, larger tissue volume is treated, especially in patients undergoing APR where the perineal scar is required to be brought into the radiation field.

Postoperative Chemoradiotherapy

In T3, T4, and node positive patients, surgery alone leads to a 25% local failure rate and thus resulting in a low 40–50% overall survival (OS).[9] With the addition of the CRT local failure rate came down to 10–15% and OS rates increased to 50–60%.[10,11] In view of the large local failures after surgery, clinical researchers followed the patients to understand the role of adjuvant radiation and chemotherapy in reducing recurrence rates. Effect of 5-fluorouracil (5FU) as a radio sensitizer in an animal model was first demonstrated by Heidelberg et al. in 1958. However, it was a decade later that Moertel et al. demonstrated a survival advantage in patients with unresectable GI tract cancers with this combine chemotherapy and radiotherapy approach. This landmark study led to the evaluation of combined chemotherapy and radiotherapy for rectal cancers in adjuvant setting. The National Surgical Adjuvant Breast and Bowel Project (NSABP) R-01 study and the NSABP R-02 study showed that even though combined adjuvant chemotherapy and radiotherapy did not show any survival advantage, there was a trend toward better local control. NSABP R-02 study reported a locoregional failure rate of 13% for chemotherapy alone versus 8% in combine chemotherapy radiotherapy group at 5 years.[11] Two more studies, that is, Gastrointestinal Tumor Study Group (GITSG) and North Central Cancer Treatment Group (NCCTG) studies, revealed improvement in survival with post-operative combined chemoradiotherapy. Adjuvant CRT improved OS to 54% versus 27% in surgery alone arm.[12] Adjuvant CRT also reduced overall recurrence by 34%, local recurrence by 46%, and distant metastasis by 37%. Cancer-related deaths were reduced by 36%, whereas overall death was reduced by 29%. Several such reports finally led to the recommendation by the National Institute of Health Consensus Conference that the combined use of CRT in adjuvant setting is more efficacious than the radiotherapy alone, and that the combined treatment has a better chance of improving survival.[13]

Intergroup 0114[14] study compared various chemotherapy regimens to be given concomitantly with radiation treatment and reached a conclusion that bolus 5FU alone was well tolerated with comparable response. With the addition of Levamisole and/or LV did not seem to provide any benefit to the 5FU.

A question still pending to be answered is that: Is there any group of patients who may not be offered adjuvant treatment after LAR or APR with TME? There are no randomized trials to support, but a few studies carried out at Memorial Sloan-Kettering by MGH Willett et al.[15,16] showed that a few favorable T3N0 patients may be selected for no adjuvant treatment. The favorable features seen were, well differentiated to moderately differentiated tumors, invading <2 mm into the perirectal fat, no lymphovascular invasion (LVI). Such patients have excellent survival and local recurrences of as low as <10% without adjuvant radiation or chemotherapy. There has been no randomized trial to support this outcome.

NEOADJUVANT CHEMOTHERAPY/ RADIOTHERAPY

Over the last four decades there have been a surge of various pre- and post-operative radiotherapy and CRT schedules in order to establish the most appropriate sequence and scheduling of the irradiation and 5FU-based chemotherapy.

Neoadjuvant Radiotherapy

The Uppsala trial which was conducted in Sweden from 1980 to 1985 is the only randomized controlled trial (RCT), which directly compared pre-operative radiotherapy to post-operative radiotherapy. The pre-operative RT arm had a short course radiation of five fractions of 5.1 Gy amounting to 25.5 Gy of total radiation, whereas the post-operative radiotherapy arm had 60 Gy in 30 fractions with a gap of 2 weeks after the delivery of 40 Gy. Even though there was a significant decrease in the local failure rates in pre-operative RT group (13% vs. 22%. p=0.02), it did not translate into a significant 5-year survival advantage (42% vs. 35%). The NSABP R-03 and Intergroup 0147 trials were also designed and started to study the difference between pre- and post-operative radiotherapy, but was prematurely terminated due to poor accrual

Two meta-analyses on this subject also noted reductions in the risk of local recurrence with pre-operative radiotherapy, and it reached levels of statistical significance.[17,18] Where one of the meta-analyses also reported survival benefit, whereas the other did not.[17,18] A systematic review by The Swedish Council of Technology Assessment in Health Care,[19] which included 42 RCTs, 3 meta-analyses, along with many prospective and retrospective studies totaling to 25,351 patients concluded that pre-operative radiotherapy decreased the risk of local failure by 50–70% when it was delivered at a dose above 30 Gy. In the comparison, post-operative radiotherapy decreased the local failure rates by only 30–40% that too with doses higher than that used in pre-operative setting. Neoadjuvant RT also helped improving survival by 10%.[19] A Swedish rectal pre-operative radiation randomized trial conducted from 1987 to 1990 enrolling 1,168 patients in two arms: pre-operative radiotherapy of 25 Gy in 5 days followed by a surgery 1 week later and surgery alone. In both arms, patients had resectable rectal cancers. In this study, the local recurrence rates were 12% versus 27% in the neoadjuvant RT group and in the surgery alone group, respectively, in all stages of tumors. There was also a 10% OS advantage in the neoadjuvant RT group at 9 years (58% vs. 48%; p=0.004).[20]

Thus, pre-operative radiotherapy has been proven to be superior to post-operative radiotherapy in various studies. However, another issue was whether the addition of chemotherapy improved the response rate or not.

Neoadjuvant Radiotherapy versus Neoadjuvant Chemoradiotherapy

Two important studies that compared pre-operative radiotherapy with combined CRT were FFCD 9203 study[21] and the European Organization for Research and Treatment of Cancer (EORTC 22921) study.[22] Both these trials showed results in favor of the pre-operative combined CRT group. Complete pathological response was observed in 11.4% versus 3.1%, and 5-year local failure rates were 5% versus 16.5% in the combined CRT arm and the radiation alone arm, respectively. However, no difference was observed in OS.

In recent years pre-operative CRT has been widely recommended as the standard of care for rectal cancer.

Chemoradiotherapy Regimens

There are variations and diversities in the way chemotherapy has been administered in different trials. 5FU has been used concurrently with radiation because of its proven effect as a radio sensitizer. Many studies have used bolus 5FU, whereas others have used leucovorin along with 5FU during the first and last weeks of radiation. The results of the Intergroup study demonstrating a superiority of low-dose continuous infusion of 5FU have been extrapolated to the neoadjuvant approach.[23] Recently, Capecitabine, an oral fluoropyrimidine pro-drug has been used concomitantly with radiation in two divided doses, 825 mg twice a day. It shows similar efficacy as continuous infusion 5FU[24] and is readily absorbed in the gastrointestinal tract. Capecitabine requires the presence of thymidine phosphorylase (TP) for conversion to the active form of 5FU within the cells. TP is present in higher concentration in tumor cells, particularly colorectal cancer than in normal tissues, and this probably produces the therapeutic advantage for capecitabine when compared with intravenous 5FU.[25] Acute toxicity of diarrhea, stomatitis, nausea, and neutropenia are also somewhat less with capecitabine than with 5FU/leucovorin. However, the incidence of hand/foot syndrome is more with capecitabine.

There have been some recent reports of phase I and phase II trials using oxaliplatin and bevacizumab in neoadjuvant CRT regimen, reporting higher pCR rates.[26]

Neoadjvuant Chemoradiation versus Adjuvant Chemoradiation

Various trials were designed to evaluate the best timing of radiation in cases of rectal cancers. Pre-operative radiotherapy offers the advantage of better local control and less morbidity, more so when combined with pre-operative chemotherapy. Two of the earlier phase III trials, that is, the Radiation Therapy Oncology Group (RTOG 94-01) and the NSABP (R-03) trials comparing pre-operative versus post-operative CRT had to be closed prematurely due to the lack of accrual,[27] but a third study, a phase III CAO/ARO/AIO-94 trial could complete the accrual of 823 T3, T4, or node positive patients.[28] In this study, not only the local control rates, downstaging, acute (27% vs. 40%), and chronic toxicities (14% vs. 24%) were better in the neoadjuvant CRT group, but also there were better sphincter preservation rates (39% vs. 19%) in that group. Complete pathological response was observed in 8% of patients receiving pre-operative chemoradiotherapy, whereas node positivity was seen in 25% and 40% of patients in the pre- and postoperative CRT arms, respectively. Despite these favorable results in the neoadjuvant CRT arm, there was no difference in the OS or disease-free survival. These better outcomes led to pre-operative CRT become the therapeutic approach in rectal cancers.

Advantages of Neoadjuvant Chemoradiation

As shown in various trials, neoadjuvant CRT helps in reducing local recurrence rates and is also less toxic for the patient. It has an added advantage of sterilizing the surgical field and thereby decreasing the tumor seeding during the surgery. The nonviolate tumor bed and well oxygenated cells increase the radiosensitivity and tumor response, thus helping in downstaging, leading to higher rates of complete pathological response and decreased venous, lymphatic, and perineural invasion. All these effects eventually lead to better respectability rates and increased sphincter preservation rates. It has even been observed that response to neoadjuvant CRT predicts OS in locally advanced tumors.

Disadvantage of Neoadjuvant Chemoradiation

Overtreatment of early-stage or undetected metastasis is the most important disadvantage of neoadjuvant treatment protocols, but the present generation of cross-sectional imaging along with endorectal ultrasound allows a very precise pretreatment staging, thus negating this potential disadvantage to a large extent.

Recommended Radiation Treatment

Dose: The recommended dose is 4,500–5,000 cGy in 25:28 fractions of 180 cGy each. A boost to the tumor bed or for positive margins is recommended for patients receiving post-operative radiation to dose of 900 cGy.

Target volumes: The presacral space, the primary tumor site, and for post-APR cases, the perineum and the internal iliac and distal common iliac nodes must be included in the radiation fields.

Conventional Technique

The radiation field should cover 5-cm distal to palpable tumor for pre-operative treatment and about 5 cm below the pre-operative tumor bed in a post-operative patient. If APR has been performed, the distal border reaches below the perineum. Laterally, the portals are extended to a 1.5-cm margin on the pelvic brim.

Anteriorly, a 4-cm margin in front of the rectum is the target. If the tumor has extrarectal extension, then all macroscopic disease as seen on CT scan is encompassed with about a 4-cm margin.

3D conformal radiation therapy: The 3D conformal technique should include the gross tumor volume (GTV) as visualized radiologically along with a 2-cm margin, the clinical tumor volume (CTV), and the nodal drainage areas (Fig. 1). Nodes routinely targeted are the presacral, pelvic mesentery, and internaliliac&& nodes. External iliac nodes may be included for T4 disease. A boost field should include the initial GTV plus 2-cm margin around.

Intensity-modulated radiation therapy: During the 1990s, the development of intensity-modulated radiation therapy (IMRT) brought about a paradigm shift in radiation therapy (Fig. 2). With IMRT highly conformal and irregularly shaped beams are used to plan a conformal dose distribution, delivering high dose to the tumor volume, while minimizing radiation to the normal tissues.[29] The accuracy of IMRT treatment strongly depends on accurate target delineation.

At RGCI&RC, we encourage PET/CT fusion to delineate the target volume. In about one-fourth of patients in our experience, PET detects distant metastases, upstaging the patient and changing the overall management of the patient. Moreover, PET/CT also alters the planning treatment volume (PTV) and radiation treatment plan in a similar proportion of patients.

Time of adjuvant radiation: Post-operative radiation is recommended to begin after 3–6 weeks of surgery.

Concurrent chemotherapy schedules*:* Inj 5FU as 1 g/m^2 per day during the first and fifth weeks of radiotherapy as a 120-hour continuous infusion or tab Capecitabine 825 mg/m^2 twice a day for 5 or 7 days a week for 5 weeks.

Altered fractionation radiation schedules*:* Studies have been carried out with altered fractionation schedules. Hyper fractionated

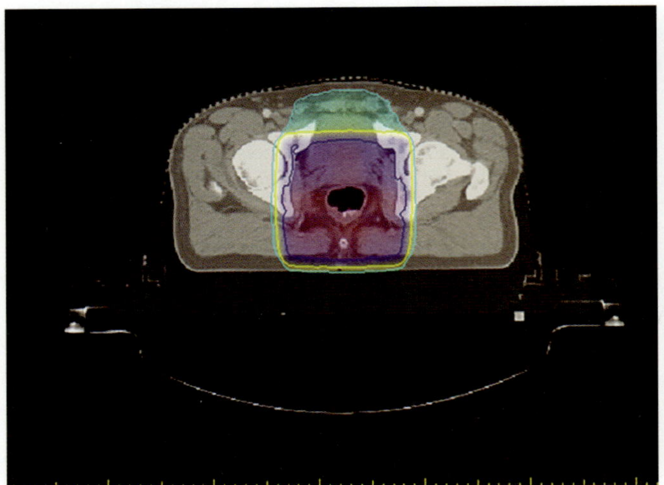

Figure 1 3DCRT planning for rectal carcinoma showing large dose to bladder (RGCI)

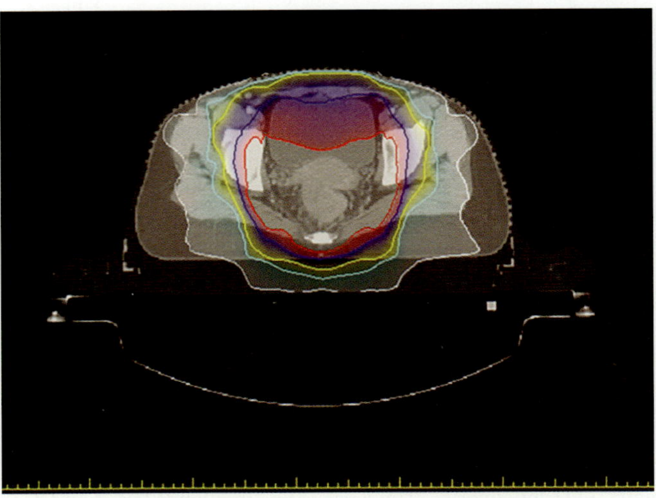

Figure 2 IMRT planning for rectal carcinoma showing sparing of bladder (RGCI)

radiotherapy of 1.2 Gy BID and 50.4 Gy with neoadjuvant chemotherapy was compared with standard fractionation in RTOG 00-12 study. No difference could be elicited in terms of toxicity, tumor response, and downstaging in the two arms. Recently, a phase II randomized study was published, comparing hyper-fractionated radiotherapy with a continuous infusion of 5FU with conventional fractionated radiotherapy with a continuous infusion of 5FU and Irinotecan and local boost of 9–14.4 Gy in both arms. It showed the pCR rates of 30% and 26%, and locoregional recurrences of 16% and 17%, respectively, in favor of the hyper-fractionated arm. The outcome showed that a high pCR is associated with higher dose of radiation, giving a higher rate of R0 resection and hence higher survival.[30]

Short-course Radiotherapy: High-dose per Fraction RT (25 Gy in Five Fractions)

There has been a renewed interest in pre-operative short-course radiotherapy. The Uppsala trial compared short-course pre-operative radiation (25.5 Gy over 5 days) to conventional fractionation post-operative treatment (60 Gy over 8 weeks). Not only the pre-operative treatment was better tolerated, but it also had a lesser local recurrence rate (12% vs. 21%; p=0.02). There were two more such randomized trials: one by Bujko et al.[31] and the other by Ngan et al.[32] with T3 N0 rectal tumors. There were no significant differences in 3-year local recurrence (8% vs. 4%) or 5-year survival (74% vs. 70%). In Table 1, we have shown a comparison of the major trials and their overview.

The long-term results of the Dutch TME trial with short-course radiation has been published recently. It showed significantly improved 10-year survival for stage III patients. Circumferential resection margins were negative in 50% and 40%, respectively, for the neoadjuvant radiotherapy arm versus the surgery only arm, but secondary malignancies were more in the radiation plus surgery arm (14% vs. 9%).[44]

There have been studies comparing the conventional pre-operative radiation (50.4 Gy) to hyper-fractionated short-course pre-operative radiation (5 × 5 Gy) most important being the Polish trial. In view of better pathological response and fewer late complications, most groups now favor conventional chemoradiation protocols worldwide including RGCI.

Contact X-ray Treatment

The chapter would be incomplete without a brief mention of the contact X-rays, which were being used historically in the treatment of rectal cancers. It uses a 50 kV X- ray beam delivered endo-luminally in knee chest position which delivers a very high output of 20 Gy/min needing 2–3 minutes to deliver the entire radiation. It may still prove important in some cases requiring the conservative management of rectal cancers but more robust evidence in support is needed.

Re-irradiation in Carcinoma Rectum

Post-radiotherapy, the local recurrence of rectal cancer poses a formidable challenge, treatment being usually directed toward palliation in the form of diverting colostomy with or without chemotherapy. Re-irradiation of pelvis has traditionally been considered unsafe but lately it has been attempted in a select group of patients providing good symptomatic relief with desired safety. Some of these patients have also been able to undergo a salvage surgery post-irradiation providing a 66% 2-year survival.[45] Reduced-dose radiotherapy, either given daily or with hyper-fractionated dose or with IM-IGRT with or without chemotherapy may be the option in selected patients. These patients should be diligently evaluated for re-resection as it is the preferred option in the irradiated pelvis.

Palliative Treatment of Rectal Cancer

Radiotherapy is frequently used for palliation of both local and metastatic diseases. Local symptoms like bleeding and pain can be very successfully managed with palliative doses of radiation, whereas bony metastases have successfully been palliated by radiopharmaceuticals (samarium-153 and strontium-89).

Table 1: Various short-course radiotherapy randomized trials

	Trial	*Study design*	*No. of patients FU (years)*	*Salient findings*
Stockholm I[33]	5 × 5 Gy with immediate surgery vs surgery alone	849	4.5	No difference in OS. Better disease-specific survival and LRR (11% vs 23%) in radiotherapy arm but higher post-operative mortality (8% vs 2%)
Uppasla[34]	5 × 5.1 Gy with immediate surgery vs postoperative radiotherapy 60 Gy, 2 Gy per fraction	471	5	No difference in OS. Improved LRR (13% vs 22%) and lower rate of late small bowel obstruction (5% vs 11%) with preoperative radiotherapy
StockholmII[35]	5 × 5 Gy with immediate surgery vs surgery alone	557	9	No difference in OS. Fewer LRR (12% vs 25%) and more deaths of intercurrent disease within 6 months of surgery (5% vs 1%) with radiotherapy
Swedish Trial[36,37]	5 × 5 Gy with immediate surgery vs surgery alone	1168	13	Improved OS (38% vs 30%, *p*=0.008) with fewer LRR (9% vs 26%) with EBRT. No increase observed in postoperative morbidity or in late toxicity.
Dutch TME Trial[38,39]	5 × 5 Gy with immediate surgery vs surgery alone (postoperative EBRT 50.4 Gy, 1.8 Gy per fraction for patients with positive CRM or tumor spill). In selective postoperative EBRT arm, 18% were CRM positive although only 11% got RT)	1861	6	No difference in OS in preoperative radiation and in the selective postoperative radiation group. Fewer local recurrences (5.6% vs 10.9%) with preoperative radiotherapy. No downstaging in patients with an interval of <10 days between radiation initiation and TME
MRC CR07[40]	5 × 5 Gy with immediate surgery vs selective postoperative chemoradiation for positive CRM (of patients allocated to the selective postoperative chemoradiotherapy group, 11% were CRM positive although only 70% of them got CRT	1350	3	No difference in overall survival. Significantly improved disease-free survival (80% vs 75%) and LRR (5% vs 11%) with preoperative radiotherapy
Polish Trial[41,42]	5 × 5 Gy with immediate surgery vs chemoradiation (50.4 Gy, 1.8 Gy per fraction + 5-FU/LV) and delayed surgery	312	4	No difference in sphincter preservation. Less acute adverse events with short-course radiotherapy (grade III–IV 3% vs 18%) but more postoperative complications (27% vs 21%). More favorable postoperative pathology with chemoradiotherapy more pathological complete responses (16% vs 1%), fewer positive radial margins (4% vs 13%). No differences in OS, DFS, LRR, and late toxicity
TROG 0104 trial[43]	5 × 5 Gy with immediate surgery vs chemoradiation (50.4 Gy, 1.8 Gy per fraction + 5-FU/LV) and delayed surgery	326	–	Less postradiotherapy acute toxicity with short-course radiotherapy (grade III–IV 1.9% vs 28%). Similar rates of postoperative complications (51% in the short-course group vs. 49% in the chemoradiotherapy group)

Radiotherapy in Metastatic Colorectal Carcinomas

Surgery seems to be the only treatment offering cure in patients with liver metastasis (Tables 1 and 2). But unfortunately only 30% of liver metastasis are amenable to surgical. For inoperable cases, with no extrahepatic disease, a number of regional therapies both ablative and nonablative therapies are offered.

Stereotactic body radiation therapy (SBRT): It is a technique of irradiating extra cranial tumor sites with a high dosage of radiation in 1-6 fractions (Fig. 3). This radiation is delivered in a highly conformal fashion maintaining a steep dose gradient toward surrounding tissue. Multimodal imaging, IGRT, advanced planning, and motion management improve the accuracy of the

Table 2: Ablative and nonablative procedures for metastatic colorectal carcinomas
Thermoablation
Radiofrequency ablation (RFA)
Laser-induced thermotherapy
Microwave ablation
High-intensity focused ultrasound (HIFU)
Cryotherapy
Transarterial chemoembolization (TACE)
Transcatheter arterial embolization (TAE)

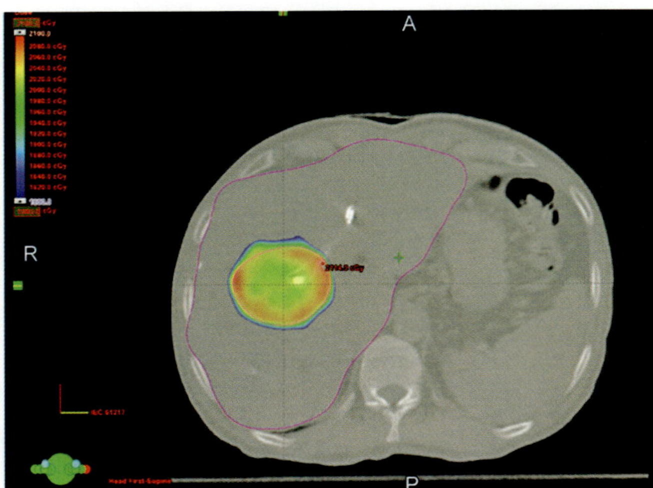

Figure 3 SBRT planning for liver metastasis (RGCI) high dose to lesion and sparing of normal liver

treatment. Local control of liver metastases by the use of SBRT is favorable, with rates ranging from 70% to 100% at 1 year and 60% to 90% at 2 years, which are comparable to the best results achieved in recent phase I and phase II studies on RFA.[46,47]

Inclusion criteria for SBRT are as follows: normal liver functions, ≤5 liver metastasis, <10-cm lesion, and ≥700 cc uninvolved liver. A total prescription dose of 48 Gy or higher in 3 fractions gives good local control. The optimal fractionation is yet to be clearly defined.[48]

Brachytherapy based on CT-guided insertion of iridium-192 high-dose rate sources in the liver with the after-loading technique offers a favorable dose distribution. Severe complications (up to 6–9%) have been reported, which emphasize that brachytherapy should be limited to specialized centers.[49]

Selective internal radiation therapy (SIRT): Yttrium-90 containing micro-beads is utilized to deliver intratumoral radiation by radioembolizing the arterial supply of the liver tumors. It has been used for both focal and diffuse liver metastasis. Some preliminary results have suggested probable benefits in terms of the survival and quality of life.[50] Tumor-free survival of up to 9 months and a median survival of 17.5 months have been reported, but OS remains unchanged.[51] There are no published studies for nonsurgical ablation, but clinical trials combining SBRT with systemic therapy are ongoing.

RADIOTHERAPY IN COLON CARCINOMA

The only curative treatment of colonic adenocarcinoma is resection along with the removal of adjacent lymphatics in the mesentry.[52] However, in certain cases, adjuvant radiation may help in decreasing local recurrences. Unlike rectal carcinoma where the tumor stage is the most important predictor of local failure, both stage and location of tumor are important predictors for colon cancer. Anatomically, the ascending and the descending colons are immobile and close to the retroperitoneal tissues, thereby limiting the extent of surgical dissection. This may give rise to local failures. On the other hand, mid-sigmoid and transverse colon are mobile because of their long mesentries, thereby making resection with wide margins possible, decreasing the chances of local recurrences. High-risk features indicating radiation therapy in colon cancer patients are T4 tumors, tumor location in immobile sites, local perforation, obstruction, and residual disease post-resection.

Table 3: Relative indication for the adjuvant tumor bed
Irradiation with concurrent 5FU-based chemotherapy in colon cancers
(a) Invading adjoining structures or T4 tumors
(b) Those complicated by perforation or fistula
(c) Where incomplete resection is performed

Intraoperative radiation has also been used in addition to EBRT in certain T4 tumors with unknown benefits. For asymptomatic patients with tumor adherent to or invading adjacent structures, the preferred treatment sequence would be pre-operative EBRT plus 5FU-based chemotherapy followed by resection with or without intraoperative electron beam radiation therapy (IOERT) and post-operative systemic therapy.[53] A similar approach would be reasonable for patients with locally recurrent cancers or with regional nodal relapse.

The NCCN 2015 guidelines also recommend adjuvant CRT with 5FU for T4 tumors penetrating to a fixed structure or recurrent disease with IMRT (the fields including the tumor bed as defined by pre-operative imaging and by surgical clips) (Table 3). IOERT boost or external radiotherapy should be considered (10–20 Gy) for such tumors for better local control. To conclude, even though adjuvant radiotherapy has some role to play in colon cancer with residual disease, there is an unproven role of radiation after the curative surgery of colon cancer as per the present data.

CHEMORADIOTHERAPY IN CARCINOMA ANAL CANAL

More than 80% cancers arising from anal and perianal regions are of squamous cell origin. Although rare malignancy, its incidence is increasing especially in immune compromised patients.[54] Other malignancies of the anal canal, such as melanoma, sarcoma, and lymphoma are exceedingly rare.

During the 6th and 7th decades of the last century, the standard treatment for anal canal carcinoma was APR with or without adjuvant radiation.[55] The outcome was poor with a 5-year survival of only 40–70%. Even for early lesions, radical surgical procedures were the only recommended treatment available. In an attempt to preserve the sphincter function and with the growing knowledge of radio responsiveness of these cancers, several hospitals, primarilyin Europe, began to use definitive radiation for the treatment of squamous cell carcinoma of the anal region. Combined CRT gradually emerged as the standard of care since Nigro introduced this approach in 1974 [56] and subsequent phase III trials[57–59] showed higher local control and survival rates by using a combined modality treatment with concomitant radiation and chemotherapy. Today the accepted modality is a radical radiation therapy with concomitantmitomycin C and a continuous infusion of 5FU, given during the first and last weeks of radiation therapy. The optimal radiation dose, schedule, and technique of anal cancer are still being explored.[60] Issues far from resolved are optimal time of treatment, optimal dosing, timing and utility of radiation boost, modalities for response evaluation, allowing planned breaks, and determining the need for salvage surgery. The Radiation Therapy Oncology Group (RTOG) and Eastern Cooperative Oncology Group (ECOG) showed in their randomized trial that the combination of mitomycin C with 5FU and radiation is more effective than 5FU alone with radiation.[61]

Cisplatin as a substitute of mitomycin C has been evaluated in several trials, the largest being the phase III UK Act II trial that presented its reports in 2009.[62] The results concluded that neither the replacement of mitomycin C with cisplatin nor the addition of maintenance chemotherapy after radical chemoradiation affects the complete response rate or decrease the recurrence rates. Any role of neoadjuvant chemotherapy prior to chemoradiation, however, has not been approved by the phase III Intergroup RTOG 98-11 trial or the recently published analysis of the ACCORD 03 trial.[63]

RADIATION THERAPY

Dose and Fractionation

External-beam radiation is delivered as a continuous course at 1.8–2.0 Gy per daily fraction to a total dose of 54–60 Gy in 30–32 fractions.

Treatment break is often necessary for skin intolerance; however, the entire course of radiation should be completed within 5–6.5 weeks, and the break of treatment for skin intolerance should not exceed 10 days in total.

Concomitant chemotherapy is recommended with a continuous infusion of 5FU 1000 mg/m2/day from D1 to D4 and from D29 to D32. Mitomycin C is given at 10 mg/m2 on D1 and D29 in all anal canal carcinomas, except T1N0M0, which can be treated with radiation alone.

The target volume consists of the primary tumor in the anal canal and the posterior pelvic and inguinal nodes. These newer techniques allow a total dose of 60–65 Gy to be planned and delivered over 6–7 weeks, at 1.8–2 Gy per fractions to the primary tumor and the nodal areas. After a dose of 40–45 Gy in 4–5 weeks, the volume is reduced to include the primary tumor with a margin of 2–3 cm to decrease toxicities to the normal tissues around.

In the past,[64,65] this reduced volume was treated after a "gap" of 6–8 weeks with external radiation or an iridium-192 interstitial implant[66,67] and was called as (perineal boost). This gap was contrary to the pivotal principle of radiation oncology, that is, the delivery of a high total fractionated dose without interruptions and without prolongation of the overall treatment time (OTT), particularly in squamous cell carcinomas.[68] Extending OTT has a detrimental impact on local control.[69–71] As a result, enormous concerns were raised on whether the boost given after a gap made any contribution to local control, as tumor repopulation during this period could be hazardous. In a phase II trial, RTOG 92-08, a break of 2 weeks in chemoradiation of anal canal carcinoma resulted in more local recurrences and lower colostomy free survival. Moreover, the Act II trial, showing a higher relapse free survival was inferred to be due to interruption free treatment, 75% at 3 years.

In Europe, however, a split course of radiation is practiced with the use of interstitial implants boost on the tradition of Papillon[72] after the recent studies by European Organization for the Treatment of Cancer (EORTC 22011 and EORTC 22953) limited the gap to 2 weeks.[73,74] Today, IMRT has been accepted as the standard practice for anal canal carcinoma. The only prospective study in this direction was from Kachnic et al. who designed RTOG 0529, a phase II study and showed that the incorporation of dose-painted IMRT (DP-IMRT) reduced grade II combined acute GI and genitourinary adverse events by at least 15% as compared with the conventional radiation/5FU/MMC arm from RTOG 9811.[75]

Management of Lymph Nodes

Nodal metastases should be treated to the same dose as the primary cancer. When lymph nodes are irradiated electively, doses of about 36 Gy in 18 fractions for 3.5 weeks in combination with chemotherapy are recommended. But, on the other hand, doses as low as 24 Gy in 12 fractions in 2.5 weeks have also been used successfully.[76] Although the local control of the involved inguinal nodal areas is excellent, usually about 80%,[77] but the 5-year survival rates are usually 10–20% lower than those without inguinal nodal metastases.[78] Prophylactic or therapeutic radical dissection of the inguino-femoral nodes with or without adjuvant groin radiation is associated with a high risk of morbidity. Hence, the elective irradiation of clinically normal inguinal nodal areas with or without chemotherapy is the preferred treatment. It reduces the risk of late node failure in that area to <5%.[79]

Treatment of Residual or Recurrent Anal Carcinomas

Residual masses at the site of the original anal cancer may take several months to resolve fully after chemoradiation or radiation therapy alone.[80,81] Most studies now recommend biopsy only when persistent cancer is suspected clinically.

Treatment of local residual cancer or recurrence is planned according to the extent of disease, whether locoregional or extra pelvic, and the potential for preserving the anorectal function. Further management with radiation (external beam or brachytherapy) and chemotherapy may still be considered as an option (Figs 4 and 5). But if conservative treatment is not contemplated, surgery, usually APR, should be considered.

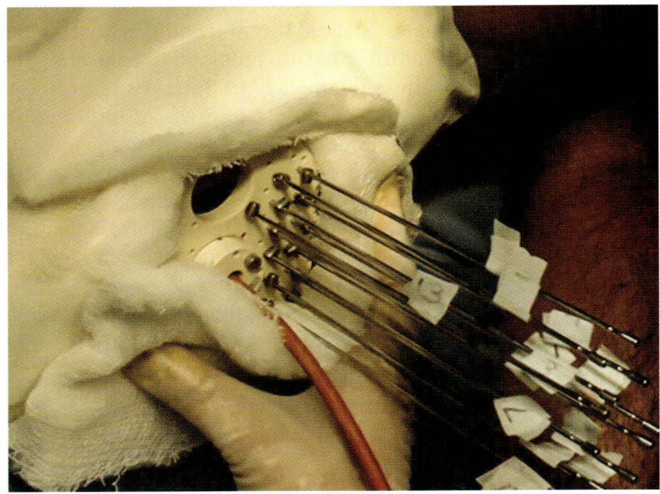

Figure 4 Interstitial brachytherapy for anal canal carcinoma with MUPIT applicator (RGCI)

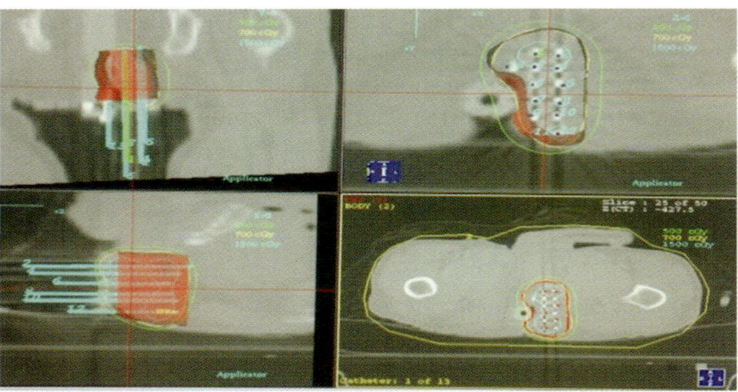

Figure 5 Computerized planning for interstitial brachytherapy for anal canal carcinoma (RGCI)

Perianal Carcinomas

Perianal cancers are a different entity most commonly being squamous cell carcinoma, usually keratinizing and others being basal cell cancers and adenocarcinomas. Wide local excision with a 1-cm margin around is the treatment of choice for all perianal cancers if anal continence can be preserved.[82] Radiation alone or in combination with chemotherapy is also very effective. To treat a small <4 cm perianal cancer with a low risk of regional node metastases by radiation, a dose of 60–66 Gy in 2-Gy fractions over 6 weeks is delivered. A direct enface perineal field is preferred as this reduces the area of skin irradiated. Larger perianal cancers or cancers invading the anal canal should be treated by the same techniques and schedules as used for anal canal cancers along with concomitant chemotherapy.

The regional nodes for the perianal skin are the ipsilateral inguinal nodes. Metastases to the perirectal and pelvic node are uncommon unless the cancer extends to the anal canal. The risk of inguinal node metastases is about 10% for T3 or T4 tumors. Elective bilateral inguinal nodal irradiation may be considered for these tumors, with the inclusion of the pelvic nodes if the anal canal is invaded.

CONCLUSION

Organ conservation with definitive CRT is an effective treatment approach in anal cancer. Stage T1 and early T2 anal canal carcinomas are well controlled with radiation alone, and the addition of chemotherapy is not needed in these patients. Doses in the range of 45–50 Gy with a boost to areas of initial gross disease for a total dose of about 60 Gy are adequate for most of the patients. With larger lesions and involvement of nodes, the addition of chemotherapy improves local control but is associated with more acute toxicity. Elective inguinal irradiation is effective. It can, however, be safely omitted only in patients with stage I disease. Despite the conformal high radiation doses and without any planned treatment interruptions, there still remain some patients who fare relatively poorly. Newer treatment approaches are required to improve the outcomes in these patients.

REFERENCES

1. Rich T, Gunderson LL, Lew R, et al. Patterns of recurrence of rectal cancer after potentially curative surgery. Cancer 1983; 52: 1317–1329.
2. Gastrointestinal Tumor Study Group. Prolongation of the disease free interval in surgically treated rectal carcinoma. N Engl J Med 1985; 312:1465–1472.
3. Krook JE, Moertel CG, Gunderson LL, et al. Effective surgical adjuvant therapy for high-risk rectal carcinoma. N Engl J Med 1991; 324:709–715.
4. Wolmark N, Wieand HS, Hyams DM, et al. Randomized trial of postoperative adjuvant chemotherapy with or without radiotherapy for carcinoma of the rectum: National Surgical Adjuvant Breast and Bowel Project protocol R-02. J Natl Cancer Inst 2000; 92:388–396.
5. Sauer R, Becker H, Hohenberger W, et al. Preoperative versus postoperative chemoradiotherapy for rectal cancer. N Engl J Med 2004; 351:1731–1740.
6. Roh MS, Colangelo LH, O'Connell MJ, et al. Preoperative multimodality multimodality therapy improves disease free survival in patients with carcinoma of the rectum: NSABP R-03. J Clin Oncol 2009; 27:5124–5130.
7. Heald RJ, Moran BJ, Ryall RD, et al. Rectal cancer: The Basingstoke Experience of total mesorectal excision, 1978-97. Arch Surg 1998; 133:894–899.
8. Marijnen CA, van Gijn W, Nagtegaal ID, et al. The TME trial after a median follow-up of 11 years (abstract 1). Presented at the 52nd Annual ASTRO Meeting, November 1, 2010, San Diego, OA.
9. Colorectal Cancer Collaborative Group. Adjuvant radiotherapy for rectal cancer: A systematic overview of 8507 patients from 22 randomised trials. Lancet 2001; 358:1291.
10. Krook JE, Moertel CG, Gunderson LL, et al. Effective surgical adjuvant therapy for high-risk rectal carcinoma. N Engl J Med 1991; 324:709.
11. Wolmark N, Wieand HS, Rockette HE, et al. The prognostic significance of tumor location and bowel obstruction in Dukes B and C colorectal cancer. Findings from the NSABP clinical trials. Ann Surg 1983; 198:743.
12. Prolongation of the disease-free interval in surgically treated rectal carcinoma. Gastrointestinal Tumor Study Group. N Engl J Med 1985;312:1465.
13. NIH Consensus Conference. JAMA 1990; 264:1444–1450.
14. Tepper JE, O'Connell M, Petroni G, et al. Adjuvant postoperative fluorouracil-modulated chemotherapy combined with pelvic radiation therapy for rectal cancer. J Clin Oncol 1997; 15:2030.
15. Merchant NB, Guillem JG, Paty PB, et al. T3N0 rectal cancer: Results following sharp mesorectal excision and no adjuvant therapy. J Gastrointest Surg 1999; 3:642.
16. Willett CG, Badizadegan K, Ancukiewicz M, et al. Prognostic factors in stage T3N0 rectal cancer: Do all patients require postoperative pelvic irradiation and chemotherapy? Dis Colon Rectum 1999; 42:167.
17. Camma C, Giunta M, Fiorica F, et al. Preoperative radiotherapy for resectable rectal cancer: A meta-analysis. JAMA 2000;284:1008.
18. Colorectal Cancer Collaborative Group. Adjuvant radiotherapy for rectal cancer: A systematic overview of 8507 patients from 22 randomised trials. Lancet 2001; 358:1291.
19. Glimelius B, Gronberg H, Jarhult J, et al. A systematic overview of radiation therapy effects in rectal cancer. Acta Oncol 2003; 42: 476–492.
20. Swedish Rectal Cancer Trial. Improved survival with preoperative radiotherapy in resectable rectal cancer. N Engl J Med 1997; 336:980–987.
21. Gerard J, Bonnetain F, Conroy T, et al. Preoperative (preop) radiotherapy (RT) + 5 FU/folinic acid (FA) in T3, 4 rectal cancers: Results of the FFCD 9203 randomized trial. J Clin Oncol 2005; 23:247S (Abstr).
22. Bosset JF, Collette L, Calais G. Chemotherapy with preoperative radiotherapy in rectal cancer. N Engl J Med 2006; 355:1114–1123.

23. O'Connell MJ, Mailliard JA, Kahn MJ, et al. Controlled trial of 5-FU and low-dose leucovorin given for 6 months as postoperative adjuvant therapy for colon cancer. J Clin Oncol 1997;15: 246–250.
24. Di Costanzo F, Sdrobolini A, Gasperoni S. Capecitabine, a new oral fluoropyrimidine for the treatment of colorectal cancer. Crit Rev Oncol Hematol 2000; 35:101.
25. Schild SE, Gunderson LL, Haddock MW, et al. The treatment of locally advanced colon cancer. Int J Radiat Oncol Biol Phys 1997; 37:51–58.
26. Willett CG, Duda DG, di Tomaso E, et al. Efficacy, safety, and biomarkers of neoadjuvant bevacizumab, radiation therapy, and fluorouracil in rectal cancer: A multidisciplinary phase II study. J Clin Oncol 2009; 27:3020–3026.
27. Hyams DM, Mamounas EP, Petrelli N, et al. A clinical trial to evaluate the worth of preoperative multimodality therapy in patients with operable carcinoma of the rectum: A progress report of National Surgical Breast and Bowel Project Protocol R-03. Dis Colon Rectum 1997; 40:131.
28. Sauer R, Becker H, Hohenberger W, et al. Preoperative versus postoperative chemoradiotherapy for rectal cancer. N Engl J Med 2004; 351:1731–1740.
29. Emami B. Medicine of IMRT. In: Mund AJ and Roeske JC, ed. Intensity modulated radiation therapy, a Clinical Perspective. Hamilton Ontario: BC Decker Inc., 2005:75–81.
30. Mohiuddin M, Paulus R, Mitchell E, et al. Neoadjuvant-chemoradiation for distal rectal cancer: 5-year updated results of a randomized phase 2 study of neoadjuvant combine dmodality chemoradiation for distal rectal cancer. Int J RadiatOncolBiol Phys 2013; 86:523–528.
31. Bujko K, Nowacki MP, Nasierowska-Guttmejer A, et al. Sphincter preservation following preoperative radiotherapy for rectal cancer: report of a randomised trial comparing short-term radiotherapy vs conventionally fractionated radiochemotherapy. Radiother Oncol 2004; 72:15–24.
32. Ngan S, Fisher R, Goldstein D, et al. A randomized trial comparing local recurrence (LR) rates between short course (SC) and long course (LC) radiotherapy (RT) for clinical T3 rectal cancer: An Intergroup trial (TROG, AGITG, CSSANZ, RACS). J Clin Oncol 2010; 28: abstract 3509.
33. Stockholm Colorectal Cancer Study Group. Preoperative short-term radiation therapy in operable rectal carcinoma. A prospective randomized trial. Cancer 1990; 66:49–55.
34. Frykholm GJ, Glimelius B, Pahlman L. Preoperative or postoperative irradiation in adenocarcinoma of the rectum: Final treatment results of a randomized trial and evaluation of late secondary effects. Dis Colon Rectum 1993; 36:564–572.
35. Habr-Gama A. Assessment and management of the complete clinical response of rectal cancer to chemoradiotherapy. Colorectal Dis 2006; 8:21–24.
36. Folkesson J, Birgisson H, Pahlman L, et al. Swedish rectal cancer trial: Long lasting benefits from radiotherapy on survival and local recurrence rate. J Clin Oncol 2005; 23:5644–5650.
37. Swedish Rectal Cancer Trial. Initial report from a Swedish multicentre study examining the role of preoperative irradiation in the treatment of patients with resectable rectal carcinoma. Br J Surg 1993; 80:1333–1336.
38. Marijnen CA, Nagtegaal ID, Kapiteijn E, et al. Radiotherapy does not compensate for positive resection margins in rectal cancer patients: Report of a multicenter randomized trial. Int J Radiat Oncol Biol Phys 2003; 55:1311–1320.
39. Peeters KC, Marijnen CA, Nagtegaal ID, et al. The TME trial after a median follow-up of 6 years: Increased local control but no survival benefit in irradiated patients with resectable rectal carcinoma. Ann Surg 2007; 246:693–701.
40. Sebag-Montfiore D, Steele R, Quike P, et al. Short-course preoperative radiotherapy results improves outcome when compared with highly selective postoperative radiochemotherapy. Preliminary results of the MRC CR07 randomised trial. Radiother Oncol 2006; 81:s19 (Abstract).
41. Bujko K, Nowacki MP, Nasierowska-Guttmejer A, et al. Sphincter preservation following preoperative radiotherapy for rectal cancer: Report of a randomised trial comparing short-term radiotherapy vs. conventionally fractionated radiochemotherapy. Radiother Oncol 2004; 72:15–24.
42. Bujko K, Nowacki MP, Nasierowska-Guttmejer A, et al. Long-term results of a randomised trial comparing preoperative short-course radiotherapy vs. preoperative conventionally fractionated chemoradiation for rectal cancer. Br J Surg 2006; 93:1215–1223.
43. Ngan S, Fisher R, Mackay J, et al. Acute adverse events in a randomised trial of short course versus long course preoperative radiotherapy for T3 adenocarcinoma of rectum: A Trans-Tasman Radiation Oncology Group trial (TROG 01.04). Eur J Cancer 2007; 5:237 (Abstract).
44. Marijnen CA, Nagtegaal ID, Van Gijen, et al. Preoperative radiotherapy combined with TME in resectable rectal carcinoma, 12 year follow up of the multicentre randomized controlled TME trial. Lancet Oncol 2011; 12:575–582.
45. Lingareddy V, Ahmad NR, Mohiuddin M. Palliative reirradiation for recurrent rectal cancer. Int J Radiat Oncol Biol Phys 1997; 38:785–790.
46. Lee MT, Kim JJ, Dinniwell R, et al. Phase I study of individualized stereotactic body radiotherapy of liver metastases. J Clin Oncol 2009; 27:1585–1591.
47. Rusthoven KE, Kavanagh BD, Cardenes H, et al. Multi-institutionalphase I/II trial of stereotactic body radiation therapy for liver metastases. J Clin Oncol 2009;27:1572–1578.
48. Høyer M, Swaminath A, Bydder S, et al. Radiotherapy for liver metastases: A review of evidence. Int J Radiat Oncol Biol Phys 2012; 82:1047–1057.
49. Ricke J, Mohnike K, Pech M, et al. Local response and impact on survival after local ablation of liver metastases from colorectal carcinoma by computed tomography-guided highdose-rate brachytherapy. Int J Radiat Oncol Biol Phys 2010; 78:479–485.
50. Nijsen JF, van het Schip AD, Hennink WE, et al. Advances in nuclear oncology: Microspheres for internal radionuclide therapy of liver tumours. Curr Med Chem 2002; 9:73–82.
51. Welsh JS, Kennedy AS, Thomadsen B. Selective internal radiation therapy (SIRT) for liver metastases secondary to colorectal adenocarcinoma. Int J Radiat Oncol Biol Phys 2006; 66:S62–S73.
52. Steele G, Mayer R, Podolsky DK, et al. Cancer of the colon, rectum, and anus. In: Cancer manual, 9th edn. Boston, MA: American Cancer Society, Massachusetts Division, 1996.
53. Gunderson LL, Nelson H, Martenson J, et al. Locally advanced primary colorectal cancer. Intraoperative electron and external beam irradiation +/- 5-FU. Int J Radiat Oncol Biol Phys 1997; 37:601–614.
54. Fenger C, Frisch M, Marti MC, et al. Tumours of the anal canal. In: Hamilton SR, Aaltonen LA, eds. Pathology and genetics of tumours of the digestive system. Lyon: IARC Press, 2000; 145–155.
55. Miles E. A method of performing abdominoperineal excision for carcinoma of the rectum and of the terminal portion of the pelvic colon. *Lancet* 1980; 2:1812–1813.
56. Nigro ND, Vaitkevicius VK, Considine B, Jr. Combined therapy for cancer of the anal canal: A preliminary report. Dis Colon Rectum 1974; 17:354–356.
57. UK Co-ordinating Committee on Cancer Research UKCCCR Anal Cancer Trial Working Party. Epidermoid anal cancer: results from the UKCCCR randomised trial of radiotherapy alone versus radiotherapy, 5-fluorouracil, and mitomycin. Lancet 1996; 348:1049–1054.

58. Bartelink H, Roelofsen F, Eschwege F, et al. Concomitant radiotherapy and chemotherapy is superior to radiotherapy alone in the treatment of locally advanced anal cancer: Results of a phase III randomized trial of the European Organization for Research and Treatment of Cancer Radiotherapy and Gastrointestinal Cooperative Groups. J Clin Oncol 1997; 15:2040–2049.
59. Flam M, John M, Pajak TF, et al. Role of mitomycin in combination with fluorouracil and radiotherapy, and of salvage chemoradiation in the definitive nonsurgical treatment of epidermoid carcinoma of the anal canal: Results of a phase III randomized intergroup study. J Clin Oncol 1996; 14:2527–2539.
60. Lim F, Glynne-Jones R. Chemotherapy/chemoradiation in anal cancer: A systematic review. Cancer Treat Rev 2011; 37:520–532.
61. Flam M, John M, Pajak TF, et al. The role of mitomycin C in combination with 5-fluorouracil and radiotherapy, and of salvage chemoradiation in the definitive nonsurgical treatment of epidermoid carcinoma of the anal canal: Results of a phase III randomized intergroup study. J Clin Oncol 1996; 14:2527–2539.
62. James R, Meadows H, Wan S. ACT II: The second UK phase III anal cancer trail. Clin Oncol (R Coll Radiol) 2005; 17:364–366.
63. Peiffert D, TournierRangeard L, Gerard JP. et al. Induction chemotherapy and intensification of radiation boost in locally advanced anal canal carcinomas: final analysis of randomized UNICANCER ACCORD 03 Trial. J Clin Oncol 2012; 1041–1048.
64. Cummings B, Keane T, Thomas G, et al. Results and toxicity of the treatment of anal canal carcinoma by radiation therapy or radiation therapy and chemotherapy. Cancer 1984; 54:2062–2068.
65. Cummings BJ. Current management of anal canal cancer. Semin Oncol 2005; 32:S123–S128.
66. Eschwege F, Lasser P, Chavy A, et al. Squamous cell carcinoma of the anal canal: Treatment by external beam radiation. Radiother Oncol 1985; 4:145–150.
67. Schlienger M, Krzisch C, Pene F, et al. Epidermoid carcinoma of the anal canal treatment results and prognostic variables. Int J Radiat Oncol Biol Phys 1989; 17:1141–1151.
68. Weber DC, Kurtz JM, Allal AS. The impact of gap duration on local control in anal canal carcinoma treated by split-course radiotherapy and concomitant chemotherapy. Int J Radiat Oncol Biol Phys 2001; 50:675–680.
69. Konski A, Garcia M, John M, et al. Evaluation of planned treatment breaks during radiation therapy for anal cancer: Update of RTOG 92-08. Int J Radiat Oncol Biol Phys 2008; 72:114–118.
70. Cerisoli GL, Ferriri AJ, Cordio S. Role of dose intensity and conservative treatment of anal canal carcinoma: Report of 35 cases. Oncology 1998;55:525–532.
71. Graf R, Wust P, Hilderbrant B, et al. Impact of overall treatment time on local control of anal cancer treated with radiochemotherapy. Oncology 2003; 65:14–22.
72. Papillon J, Montbarbon JF. Epidermoid carcinoma of the anal canal: A series of 276 cases. Dis Colon Rectum 1987; 30:324–333.
73. Bosset JF, Roelofsen F, Morgan DAL, et al. Shortened irradiation schedule, continuous infusion of 5-fluorouracil and fractionation of mitomycin C in locally advanced anal carcinomas. Results of a phase II study of the European Organization for Research and Treatment of Cancer. Radiotherapyand Gastrointestinal Cooperative Groups. Eur J Cancer 2003; 39:45–51.
74. Matzinger O, Roelofsen F, Mineur L, et al. For the EORTC radiation oncology and astrointestinal tract cancer groups. Mitomycin C with continuous fluorouracil or with Cisplatin in combination with radiotherapy for locally advanced anal cancer (European Organisation for Research and Treatmentof Cancer phase II study 22011-40014). Eur J Cancer 2009; 45:2782–2791.
75. Kachnic LA, Winter K, Myerson RJ, et al. RTOG 0529: A phase 2 evaluation of dose-painted intensity modulated radiation therapy in combination with 5-fluorouracil and mitomycin-C for the reduction of acute morbidity in carcinoma of the anal canal. Int J Radiat Oncol Biol Phys 2013; 86:27–33.
76. Cummings BJ, Keane TJ, O'Sullivan B, et al. Epidermoid anal cancer: Treatment by radiation and 5-fluorouracil with and without mitomycin C. Int J Radiat Oncol Biol Phys 1991; 21: 1115–1125.
77. Gerard JP, Chapet O, Samiei F, et al. Management of inguinal lymph node metastases in patients with carcinoma of the anal canal. Experience in a series of 270 patients treated in Lyon and review of the literature. Cancer 2001; 92:77–84.
78. Papillon J. Rectal and anal cancers: Conservative treatment by irradiation. An alternative to radical surgery. Berlin: Springer-Verlag, 1982.
79. Touboul E, Schlienger M, Buffat L, et al. Epidermoid carcinoma of the anal canal. Cancer 1994 ;73:1569–1579.
80. Schlienger M, Touboul E, Mauban S, et al. Resultants du traitment de 286 cas de cancers epidermoides du canal dont 236 par irradiation a visÃ©econservatrice. Lyon Chirurgical 1991; 87:61–64.
81. Tanum G, Tveit K, Karlsen KO, et al. Chemoradiotherapy of anal carcinoma: Tumour response and acute toxicity. Oncology 1993; 50:14–17.
82. Greenall MJ, Quan SHQ, Decosse JJ. Epidermoid cancer of the anus. Br J Surg 1985;72[Suppl]:S97.

SECTION 9

Liver Transplantation

CHAPTER 104

History of Liver Transplantation

Vinay Kumaran

Modern day medicine has increasingly become a field where progress is made incrementally. The magic value p=0.05 holds sway and a new medicine or procedure may show a marginal benefit which requires abstruse statistics to demonstrate. It is rare for a procedure to develop which takes a patient heading for sure death and returns him/her to a normal life. Liver transplant was one such procedure and is still in a state of rapid evolution although the pace at which outcomes are improving seems to be reaching a plateau. The history of liver transplantation makes for interesting reading as it is a story of a few determined individuals who persisted despite initial failures and much criticism to develop the modality into an undisputed standard of care. A perusal of the names in the references indicates the enormous contributions made to the field by Thomas E Starzl and Sir Roy Calne. It is unfortunate that the Nobel Committee looks for single landmark contributions when awarding the prize rather than considering a body of work over a period of time.

The idea of transplanting the liver finds its first mention in 1955, when Welch described transplantation of the liver in dogs.[1] The native liver of the dog was not removed and the transplanted liver was implanted in an ectopic location.

Although the surgical problem appeared to be one which could probably be solved, the immunological barriers to transplantation were just being defined and the possibility of overcoming this barrier was being approached.[2] The first successful solid organ transplant was reported by the Brigham group from Boston between identical twins.[3]

Meanwhile, Thomas Starzl at Northwestern University, Chicago, was working on techniques of liver transplantation in dogs in the course of his studies on portal blood flow and its effect on the liver.[4] He applied for and won a Markle scholarship. This scholarship was designed to encourage academics in medicine and the scholar was expected to take up a problem which would be a lifetime commitment. Starzl took on the challenge of developing liver transplantation into a clinically viable procedure. He also got a 5-year grant from the National Institute of Health.[5]

While the technical problems of replacing the liver were being solved, the immunological problems of transplantation between a nonidentical donor and a recipient remained problematic. Whole body irradiation remained an extremely dangerous method of preventing rejection and the gap between a dose that is enough to prevent rejection and a dose that would cause lethal toxicity was small. This changed with the introduction into clinical practice of 6-mercaptopurine[6] and then its derivative azathioprine which would produce immunosuppression at doses which were not prohibitively myelotoxic.[7,8] The success of the azathioprine-prednisone cocktail in preventing rejection in kidney transplantation led to the first attempts at liver transplantation.

Liver transplantation, of course, was a much more formidable surgical undertaking than kidney transplantation. The experiments performed on dogs had shown that the liver requires a portal venous inflow without which it shrinks and fails.[4] Removal of the cirrhotic liver was a formidable surgical exercise due to portal hypertension and coagulopathy. The experiments performed on dogs had shown that the vena cava and the portal vein could not be clamped for any sustained duration of time and it was assumed that the situation would be similar in humans. A passive bypass system was used to carry blood from the portal system and from the lower half of the body back into the systemic circulation. It would later become evident that patients with cirrhosis of the liver have porto-systemic collaterals which decompress the splanchnic circulation during portal clamping and this passive bypass system likely did more harm than good. The patients who survived the operation had blood clots in the lung which must have formed partly due to the passive bypass system and partly due to overcorrection of coagulopathy. In any case, none of the seven liver transplants attempted in 1963 was successful with the longest survivor dying 22 days after the operation.[9] A voluntary moratorium on liver transplant activity resulted for the next 3.5 years.

In 1966, antilymphocyte globulin was introduced and its use in canine liver and kidney transplants and in human kidney transplants encouraged the resurrection of human liver transplantation.[10] The first successful human liver transplant was reported by Starzl et al. from the University of Colorado Medical Center, Denver.[11] Roy Calne's clinical program at Cambridge reported its first successful liver transplant soon after.[12]

The initial liver transplants were done using donors after cardiac death. Femoral canulation and perfusion was used to cool the organs after cardiac arrest had taken place. In 1968, the definition of brain death was standardized by a committee constituted for the purpose at the Harvard Medical School and brain death became an acceptable indication for organ procurement.[13] This allowed much safer organ procurement.

Although liver transplantation was now being performed from time to time at a few centers in the United States, France, UK, and Germany, results were poor and long-term survivals were in the minority. Only 20% of the first 170 liver transplants performed at the University of Colorado before 1979 survived for 5 years.[14]

In 1976, Borel et al. described a fungal metabolite called cyclosporine A which had a strong inhibitory effect on cellular immunity without much myelotoxicity.[15] Calne recognized the potential of cyclosporine A in organ transplantation and reported his results with the use of cyclosporine A as the only immunosuppressant in 34 recipients of cadaveric organ transplants: 32 kidney transplants and two liver transplants.[16] Starzl's group (now in Pittsburgh) demonstrated that addition of prednisone to cyclosporine A was more effective than cyclosporine A alone.[17] With this combination, they reported an 80% 1-year liver recipient survival.[18]

A liver transplant was still a somewhat virtuoso performance and the speed of implantation was critical as patients would not tolerate a long period of clamping of the vena cava and the portal vein. There is no doubt that training the next generation of transplant surgeons was difficult as the implantation had to be performed by the fastest surgeon available and there was no room for a learning curve. This situation changed somewhat with the reintroduction of veno-venous bypass. Pump-driven veno-venous bypass allowed a more leisurely and controlled implantation of the liver with less hemodynamic instability while avoiding the problem of clots embolizing to the lungs as in the early passive bypass systems.[19,20] With veno-venous bypass, fellows could be trained to perform all the steps of this operation and both the Pittsburgh and Cambridge groups trained surgeons who established new liver transplant programs all over the world. Liver transplantation became the standard of care for liver failure. Over the next few years, techniques to procure organs safely from deceased donors were standardized.[21,22]

Efforts to improve the preservation of organs to ensure better function or to permit a longer period of preservation in order to allow transport over longer distances resulted in the development of the University of Wisconsin solution (UW solution). Organ preservation is discussed in more detail in another section but extension of the cold ischemia time to 12 hours for liver and 48 hours for kidneys allowed sharing of organs across the country and even between countries.[23,24]

The classical liver transplant operation involved removing the native liver along with the retrohepatic vena cava. The donor liver was procured along with the corresponding segment of cava and the corresponding caval cuffs were anastomosed to restore venous continuity. A modification of this technique was to remove the native liver, leaving the vena cava in place. The donor liver was still procured along with a length of the cava but the lower cava was closed and the upper cava was anastomosed to an opening in the native cava created by joining the orifices of the hepatic veins. This technique had the advantage of avoiding one venous anastomosis, hence reducing the warm ischemia time and also avoiding prolonged cross clamping of the vena cava. This method had been described in pediatric transplants, both at Denver[25] and at Cambridge.[12] However, it was popularized by the Starzl group in Pittsburgh in the late 1980s.[26] In most cases, it obviated the need for venovenous bypass and more and more transplants were done without the bypass.

With excellent results, the shortage of organs and the widening gap between the number of patients who needed liver transplantation and the number of organs available from brain dead donors became a major factor in healthcare policy. One of the approaches to bridge the gap was to use organs which were being discarded at the time. The Pittsburgh group identified the factors which increased the risk of nonfunction or poor function of the transplanted liver and suggested extending the criteria used to select livers.[27] The use of these "marginal" livers helped bridge the gap to some extent at a largely acceptable increase in complications, morbidity and mortality but the waiting list mortality remained high.

Children were particularly disadvantaged while waiting for a liver due to the size mismatch. The number of brain dead donors in the pediatric population was small. One way of improving the availability of livers for children was to reduce the size of an adult liver by performing a partial hepatectomy. This procedure was probably first performed in Denver by Starzl's team but they did not report it until 1990.[28] The operation was first reported by Bismuth's group in Paris[29] and by Broelsch et al. from Hanover.[30]

In view of the organ shortage the idea of splitting the liver and using both sides for different recipients was soon implemented, initially by Pichlmayr in Germany in 1989 and then by Bismuth in Paris and Broelsch in Chicago.[31] By this time, many centers were performing major liver resections with low mortality. Starzl et al.[32] reported 11 right trisegmentectomies, five right hepatectomies, five left hepatectomies, and three left lateral segmentectomies without mortality. In view of the scarcity of organs, particularly for children, the idea of living donor liver transplantation was proposed where a part of a liver of a voluntary donor would be resected and transplanted into a child. The first attempts at this procedure were reported by Raia from Brazil but without long-term survival.[33] The first successful report came from Brisbane, Australia.[34] In view of the ongoing shortage of organs, particularly for pediatric recipients, living donor liver transplantation was very appealing. Broelsch et al.[35] reported the first large series and did much to standardize both the operation and the ethical aspects of the procedure. In view of size restrictions, partial liver transplantation remained restricted to pediatric recipients and was confined to left lateral or left lobe grafts. The first report of the use of the right side of the liver came from Yamaoka et al.[36] The plan was to use the left side of the liver but then was changed intraoperatively due to adverse arterial anatomy. The first adult-to-adult living donor liver transplant (using a left lobe) was reported by Ichida et al. in 1995.[37] The right lobe living donor liver transplant for adults was first reported and then largely standardized by the Queen Mary Hospital team from Hong Kong.[38,39] Living donor liver transplantation has grown to become the predominant form of liver transplantation in much of Asia.[40]

In summary, liver transplantation has become the standard of care for management of end-stage liver failure with excellent results. The next major steps in the field of transplantation are anticipated to be tolerogenic immunosuppression[41] (where a donor-specific tolerance can be achieved and the nonspecific immunosuppression and other side effects of current immunosuppressive regimens can be avoided) and the generation of bioengineered organs from stem cells.[42]

REFERENCES

1. Welch CS. A note on transplantation of the whole liver in dogs. Transplant Bull. 1955;2:54-5.
2. Billingham RE, Brent L, Medawar PB. Actively acquired tolerance of foreign cells. Nature. 1953;172:603.
3. Guild WR, Harrison JH, Merrill JP, et al. Successful homotransplantation of the kidney in an identical twin. Trans Am Clin Climatol Assoc. 1955-56;67:167-73.
4. Starzl TE, Kaupp HA, Brock DR, et al. Reconstructive problems in canine liver homotransplantation with special reference to the postoperative role of hepatic venous flow. Surg Gynecol Obstet. 1960;111:733-43.
5. Hurst J. A modern Cosmas and Damian: Sir Roy Calne and Thomas Starzl receive the 2012 Lasker-Debakey Clinical Medical Research Award. J Clin Invest. 2012;122:3378-82.
6. Schwartz R, Dameshek W. Drug-induced immunologic tolerance. Nature. 1959;183:1682-3.
7. Calne RY. The rejection of renal homografts: inhibition in dogs by 6-mercaptopurine. Lancet. 1960;1:417-8.
8. Starzl TE, Marchioro TL, Wadell WR. The reversal of rejection in human renal allografts with subsequent development of homograft tolerance. Surg Gynecol Obstet. 1963;117:385-95.
9. Starzl TE, Marchioro TL, Von Kaulla KN, et al. Homotransplantation of the liver in humans. Surg Gynecol Obstet. 1963;117:659-76.
10. Starzl TE, Marchioro TL, Porter KA, et al. The use of heterologous antilymphoid agents in canine renal and liver homotransplantation and in human renal homotransplantation. Surg Gynecol Obstet. 1967;124:301-18.
11. Starzl TE, Groth CG, Brettschneider L, et al. Orthotopic homotransplantation of the human liver. Ann Surg. 1968;168:392-415.
12. Calne RY, Williams R. Liver transplantation in man. I. Observations on technique and organization in five cases. Br Med J. 1968:4:535-40.
13. Definition of irreversible coma: report of the ad-hoc committee of the Harvard Medical School to examine the definition of brain death. JAMA. 1968;205:337.
14. Starzl TE, Demetris AJ, Trucco M, et al. Cell migration and chimerism after whole-organ transplantation: the basis of graft acceptance. Hepatology. 1993;17:1127-52.
15. Borel JF. Biological effects of cyclosporine A: a new antilymphocytic agent. Agents Actions. 1976;6:468-75.
16. Calne RY, Rolles K, White DJ, et al. Cyclosporin A initially as the only immunosuppressant in 34 recipients of cadaveric organs: 32 kidneys, 2 pancreases and 2 livers. Lancet. 1979;2:1033-6.
17. Starzl TE, Weil R III, Iwatsuki S, et al. The use of Cyclosporine A and prednisone in cadaver kidney transplantation. Surg Gynecol Obstet. 1980;151:17-26.
18. Starzl TE, Klintmalm GAG, Porter KA, et al. Liver transplantation with use of Cyclosporin A and Prednisone. N Engl J Med. 1981;305:266-9.
19. Denmark SW, Shaw BW Jr, Starzl TE, et al. Veno-venous bypas without systemic anticoagulation in canine and human liver transplantation. Surg Forum. 1983;34:380-2.
20. Shaw BW Jr, Martin DJ, Marquez JM, et al. Venous bypass in clinical liver transplantation. Ann Surg. 1984;200:524-34.
21. Starzl TE, Hakala TR, Shaw BW Jr, et al. A flexible procedure for multiple cadaveric organ procurement. Surg Gynecol Obstet. 1984;158:223-30.
22. Starzl TE, Miller C, Brozniak B, et al. An improved technique for multiple organ harvesting. Surg Gynecol Obstet. 1987;165:343-8.
23. Jamieson NV, Sundberg R, Lindell S, et al. Successful 24-30 hour preservation of the canine liver: a preliminary report. Transplant Proc. 1988;20(Suppl 1):945-7.
24. Kalayoglu M, Sollinger HW, Stratta RJ, et al. Extended preservation of the liver for clinical transplantation. Lancet. 1988;1:617-9.
25. Starzl TE. Experience in hepatic transplantation. Philadelphia: WB Saunders; 1969. pp. 131-5.
26. Tzakis A, Todo S, Starzl TE. Orthotopic liver transplantation with preservation of the inferior vena cava. Ann Surg. 1989;210:649-52.
27. Makowka L, Gordon RD, Todo S, et al. Analysis of donor criteria for the prediction of outcome in clinical liver transplantation. Transplant Proc. 1987;1987:2378-82.
28. Demetris AJ, Starzl TE. Liver transplantation: a 31-year perspective. Chicago: Year Book; 1990. pp. 38-41.
29. Bismuth H, Houssin D. Reduced sized orhtotopic liver graft in hepatic transplantation in children. Surger. 1984;95:367-70.
30. Broelsch CE, Neuhaus P, Burdelski M, et al. Orthotopic transplantation von lebegmenten bei mit gallendangatresien. In: Kolsowski L. Chirurgisches Forum 1984. Berlin: Springer Verlag; 1984. pp. 105-9.
31. Broelsch CE, Emond JC, Whitington PF, et al. Application of reduced size liver transplantation as split grafts, auxiliary orthotopic grafts and living related segmental transplants. Ann Surg. 1990;212: 368-75.
32. Starzl TE, Bell RH, Beart RW, et al. Hepatic trisegmentectomy and other liver resections. Surg Gynecol Obstet. 1975;141:429-37.
33. Raia S, Nery JR, Mies S. Liver transplantation from live donors. Lancet. 1989;2:497.
34. Strong RW, Lynch SV, Ong TH, et al. Successful liver transplantation from a living donor to her son. N Engl J Med. 1990;322:1505-7.
35. Broelsch CE, Whitington PF, Emond JC et al. Liver transplantation in children from living related donors. Surgical techniques and results. Ann Surg. 1991;214:428-37.
36. Yamaoka Y, Washida M, Honda K, et al. Liver transplantation using a right lobe graft from a living related donor. Transplantation. 1994;57:1127-30.
37. Ichida T, Matsunama H, Kawasaki S, et al. Living-related donor liver transplantation from adult to adult for primary biliary cirrhosis. Ann Int Med. 1995;122:275-6.
38. Lo CM, Fan ST, Liu CL et al. Extending the limit on the size of adult recipients in living donor liver transplantation using extended right lobe grafts. Transplantation. 1997;63:1524-8.
39. Fan ST, Lo CM, Liu CL. Transplantation of the right hepatic lobe. N Engl J Med. 2002;63:615-8.
40. Ng KK, Lo CM. Liver transplantation in Asia: past, present and future. Ann Acad Med Singapore. 2009;38:322-31.
41. Starzl TE, Murase N, Abu-Elmagd K, et al. Tolerogenic immunosuppression for organ transplantation. Lancet. 2003;361:1502-10.
42. Takebe T, Sekine K, Enomura M, et al. Vascularized and functional human liver from an iPSC-derived organ bud transplant. Nature. 2013;499:481-4.

CHAPTER 105

Liver Transplantation in India

Vinay Kumaran

BACKGROUND

Liver transplantation is a recent addition to the armamentarium in the battle against liver failure in India. The first attempts at transplanting the liver to save the lives of patients with liver failure or liver cancer were made in 1963 by Thomas Starzl's team in Denver. The initial attempts were not successful.[1] The first successful transplants were performed by the same team in 1967, soon followed by Sir Roy Calne's team in Cambridge.[2,3] By the 1980s, with the introduction of cyclosporine for safer immunosuppression, results had improved dramatically and 1-year survival was over 80%.[4] Liver transplantation had now become the standard of care for management of decompensated liver disease. India, at this time was very much a "third world" country and standards of medical care were not comparable to those at the "developed" countries. The best medical care was being provided by a few elite teaching hospitals run by the government. Private hospitals were, by and large, small and did not provide high-end services. The 1990s saw a change in mind-set. The liberalization of the economy led to many changes. India became increasingly perceived as a growing and healthy economy, somewhat immune to the ailments plaguing the more "developed" economies. The field of healthcare also underwent a revolution of sorts in India. The private sector developed large super-speciality hospitals which provided high-end medical care at a cost that was affordable to a considerable proportion of the population. High-end medical care was now within reach. The growth of liver transplantation in India is a microcosm of the development of healthcare in general.

THINKING ABOUT IT

The first mention of liver transplantation in the Indian literature was a review by Choksi in the Journal of the Association of Physicians of India in 1988.[5] This did not specifically assess the logistics of starting liver transplantation in India but did serve to bring the concept of liver transplantation to the Indian physicians. The magnitude of the problem of end-stage liver disease in India is not easily available. All reviews quote an editorial in Tropical Gastroenterology in 1990[6] which estimated that about 200,000 deaths due to liver failure occur in India every year. Of course, this does not imply that all these patients would have been candidates for liver transplant but it does give some idea that the problem is an important one which needs to be addressed.

In an opinion piece in the Indian Journal of Gastroenterology, Mathur addressed the possibility of starting liver transplantation in India.[7] Since there was no legal recognition for the concept of brain death, he suggested the possibility of procuring organs from nonbeating donors. The poor long-term results of livers obtained from donation after cardiac death were not yet reported. The same issue also contained an article by Saxena and Kaushik looking at the potential cost of establishing liver transplantation in India. Although we now know that their estimate was on the lower side, they did conclude that the cost would not be prohibitive.[8] They calculated that for the cost of each liver transplant on an Indian patient in the United States, one center for liver transplant could be established in India.

FIRST STEPS

The late 1980s and early 1990s were a period when economic reforms and a change in mindset was taking place in India. The then Prime Minister, Rajiv Gandhi returned from a visit abroad and asked the Health Minister why heart and liver transplants were not being done in India.[9] A working group was constituted to look into the question. This group submitted a report identifying four problems:

1. The lack of doctors trained in transplant surgery, medicine, and anesthesia.

2. The poorly regulated kidney transplant sector had been tainted by instances of organ trading.
3. The law did not recognize brain death.
4. The operation and the care of the patient before and after the operation would be very expensive, more so than any other routinely performed medical procedure.

None of these objections seemed insuperable. There were Indian surgeons trained in major liver transplant centers abroad who would be glad to return if given the opportunity. Careful regulation would be required to ensure that the mistakes made with kidney transplantation would not be repeated. Changes to the law would be required to recognize brain death as death. As Saxena and Kaushik[8] had already noted, the cost of a liver transplant in India would likely be a fraction of the cost abroad.

With the support of the Health Ministry and the World Health Organization, a series of meeting were held in the major cities and key opinion leaders were consulted about the acceptability of the concept of brain death. With support from these meetings and after passing through various committees, the Transplantation of Human Organs Bill was passed by the Lok Sabha in 1994 and became law in 1995. The act lays down the laws and rules governing organ donation in India.[10] For living donor transplants it defines who can donate without legal formalities: parents, siblings, children, and spouse. However, in most cases even first-degree relatives are appraised by an internal committee at the transplant center. If the relationship is more distant, the recipient and donor have to seek permission for the transplant from a government appointed authorization committee. For brain death, it laid down the requirement of two certifications, 6 hours apart. For regulation of transplant activities, the composition of authorization committees was laid down. Hospitals would be allowed to perform organ transplants only with the permission of the committee.

The first transplant from a brain-dead donor was a heart transplant at All India Institute of Medical Sciences in 1994.[9] Initial attempts at liver transplantation at Apollo Chennai and All India Institute of Medical Sciences in 1995 and 1996 were unsuccessful. Partial success was obtained at Apollo Chennai when a Malaysian national, transplanted by a surgeon from Singapore (KC Tan), survived for 4 months.[9] The first indigenous success was at Apollo Delhi where a deceased donor liver transplant was successfully performed on November 6, 1998 with long-term survival.[9] The same team, soon after, performed a successful living donor liver transplant on an 18-month-old child with biliary atresia.[9]

The Apollo Delhi team of Rajasekar and Soin remained the only team to perform successful liver transplants on a regular basis for the next few years but early outcomes were certainly not comparable with the major centers abroad. Sibal et al.[11] reported in 2005, that 13 liver transplants had been performed of which eight had been successful.

CATCHING FIRE

By this time two things had become obvious: organ donation by brain dead cadavers was a rare event and likely to remain so for the near future and the government sector was not going to take the lead in liver transplantation. The emphasis shifted to living donor liver transplantation. The first center to take off in a big way was probably Sir Ganga Ram Hospital where Soin and Gupta, under the mentorship of Nundy, established a predominantly living donor liver transplant program. They reported the first 36 cases at the International Liver Transplantation Society meeting in 2006.[12] They described the technical changes which led from a 66% mortality in the first 6 cases to a 90% 1-year survival in the next 30 cases. By May 2007, 318 liver transplants had been performed in 18 centers.[13] In total, 90% of the operations had been performed in the private sector and 73% were living donor transplants.

Since then, several centers have developed established liver transplant programs with excellent outcomes. As of 2011, the centers which had performed more than 50 liver transplants included (in alphabetical order): Amrita Institute of Medical Sciences and Research, Kochi (75), Apollo Hospital, Chennai (70), Apollo Indraprastha, Delhi (401), Global Hospitals, Hyderabad and Chennai (100), Medanta, the Medicity, Gurgaon (56), and Sir Ganga Ram Hospital, Delhi (571).[9] Since then, there are no published figures but according to verbal communications, Apollo Indraprastha, Delhi and Medanta, and Gurgaon are performing close to 300 liver transplants a year. Of the centers on this list, the only predominantly deceased donor program is Apollo Chennai. Organ donation rates in Chennai have been well above the dismal national average. The other center with predominantly deceased donor transplants has been the Army Research and Referral Hospital in Delhi.

INNOVATIONS

With high volumes of living donor liver transplants without the backup of deceased donor options, Indian centers have become innovators, accepting anatomical variations that would be considered contraindications to liver transplant at less experienced centers. The Sir Ganga Ram Hospital team (now divided between Ganga Ram, Medanta, and Kokilaben Hospitals) reported the hilar plate Glissonian sheath approach to the bile duct resulting in a decrease in recipient biliary complications to an unprecedented 5.3%.[14] The group has also described their technique (a modification of that described by the Hong Kong group[15]) for including most or part of the middle hepatic vein with the graft in right lobe transplants.[16] The Apollo Delhi team has described a novel protocol for monitoring and deciding whether to treat CMV infection in liver transplant recipients in a population in which exposure to CMV occurs early in life and nearly all recipients have antibodies to CMV at the time of transplant.[17] Both the Medanta and the Amrita Institute teams have recently reported successful ABO incompatible liver transplants.[18,19]

CONTROVERSIES

With all the advances in the field, it would have been surprising had there been no controversies. There is no liver transplant registry and hence no record of the number of transplants performed at various centers or the outcomes. Certainly each living donor liver transplant passes through an authorization process and hence records exist but these are not compiled, audited or published. What is even more concerning is the lack of transparency concerning donor outcomes. A donor hepatectomy is not without risk and the mortality is not zero. The deaths of at least five living donors have been reported.[20] What is of even more concern is that more donor deaths are known to have occurred but have not been reported. Certainly, a registry of donor outcomes is required.

FUTURE

With a view of making the process of liver transplantation easier, the Transplantation of Human Organs Act was amended in 2011 and the rules are under a process of revision.[21] The new provisions include:

1. The expansion of the definition of "near relative" to include grandparents and grandchildren.
2. To require the doctor in an intensive care unit to inform the relatives of a brain dead patient about the option of organ donation and to ascertain whether they would consent.
3. To allow swapping of organs between a pair of recipients and donors who can donate to each other's recipients but not to their own.
4. To designate centers other than transplant centers where organ procurement may be performed.
5. To enhance the penalty for unauthorized removal of human organs and for receiving or making payment for human organs.

One hopes the government will also put in place systems for implementing these rules and facilitating the process of donation of organs by a brain dead donor. There are many patients dying of organ failure who do not have living donors in the family due to medical or social reasons. The majority of these patients still die waiting for an organ. Even apart from this population, every organ from a deceased donor avoids the requirement of operating on a healthy person. One also hopes that more government hospitals establish liver transplant programs to make the option accessible to those who cannot afford to pay for a liver transplant at a private hospital.

A registry recording not only the number of transplants performed but also the outcomes, including donor outcomes would make the system more transparent and increase public confidence.

REFERENCES

1. Starzl TE, Marchioro TL, Von Kaulla KN, et al. Homotransplantation of the liver in humans. Surg Gynecol Obstet. 1963;117:659-76.
2. Starzl TE, Groth CG, Brettschneider L, et al. Orthotopic homotransplantation of the human liver. Ann Surg. 1968;168:392-415.
3. Calne RY, Williams R. Liver transplantation in man. I. Observations on technique and organization in five cases. Br Med J. 1968;4:535-40.
4. Starzl TE, Klintmalm GAG, Porter KA, et al. Liver transplantation with use of Cyclosporin A and Prednisone. N Engl J Med. 1981;305:266-9.
5. Choksi AP. Liver transplantation: medical aspects. JAPI. 1988;34:263-6.
6. Shenoy S. Liver transplantation in India (editorial). Trop Gastroenterol. 1990;11:53-5.
7. Mathur SK. Liver transplantation in India. Are we ready? Indian J Gastroenterol. 1991;10:142-3.
8. Saxena R, Kaushik SP. Liver transplantation in India. Can we afford it now? Indian J Gastroenterol. 1991;10:140-1.
9. Varma V, Mehta N, Nundy S. Liver transplantation in India: the history. In: Soin AS, Nundy S, editors. Liver transplantation, ECAB clinical update: surgical gastroenterology and liver transplantation. New Delhi: Elsevier; 2011. pp. 8-14.
10. Shroff S. Legal and ethical aspects of organ donation and transplantation. Indian J Urol. 2009;348-56.
11. Sibal A, Pao M, Sharma S, et al. First successful liver transplant in India. Apollo Med. 2005;2:324-7.
12. Soin AS, Gupta S, Saigal S, et al. Evolution of a successful living donor liver transplant program in India: an analysis of 36 consecutive cases. Liver Transpl. 2006;12:C15.
13. Kakodkar R, Soin AS, Nundy S. Liver transplantation in India: its evolution, problems and the way forward. Natl Med J India. 2007;20:53-6.
14. Soin AS, Kumaran V, Rastogi AN, et al. Evolution of a reliable biliary reconstruction technique in 400 consecutive living donor liver transplants. J Am Coll Surg. 2011;211:24-32.
15. Fan ST, Lo CM, Liu CL, et al. Safety and necessity of including the middle hepatic vein in the right lobe graft in adult-to-adult live donor liver transplantation. Ann Surg. 2003;238:137-48.
16. Soin AS, Mohanka R, Singla P, et al. Segment IV preserving middle hepatic vein retrieval in right lobe living donor liver transplantation. J Am Coll Surg. 2011;213(2):e5-16.
17. Wadhawan M, Gupta S, Goyal N, et al. Cytomegalovirus infection: its incidence and management in cytomegalovirus-seropositive living related liver transplant recipients: a single-center experience. Liver Transpl. 2012;18:1448-55.
18. Soin AS, Raut V, Mohanka R, et al. The use of ABO-incompatible grafts in living donor liver transplantation-first report from India. Trop Gastroenterol 2013;34(3)Suppl 1:S38-9.
19. Chacko S. ABO incompatible liver transplant: our experience, outcome and feasibility. Trop Gastroenterol 2013;34(3)Suppl 1:S34.
20. Desai HG. Living donor for an adult-to-adult liver transplantation: need for more regulation? Natl Med J India. 2011;24:243.
21. http://pib.nic.in/newsite/erelease.aspx?relid=52689

CHAPTER 106

Indications and Contraindications for Liver Transplantation

Vibha Varma, Vinay Kumaran

INTRODUCTION

Liver transplantation is a life-saving measure for patients with chronic end-stage liver disease and also some patients with acute liver failure. This requirement is judged on the basis of scoring systems which help in proper allocation of a scarce resource of donor liver, especially in the deceased donor liver transplant (DDLT) programs. Over the years, liver transplantation procedure and the outcome has undergone phenomenal change leading to improved patient and graft survival. This improvement is because of better understanding and refinement of the surgical procedure, better perioperative care and development of effective immunosuppressive drugs. Reported 1- and 3-year survival post primary liver transplant according to the UNOS 2013 is 87.7 and 79.9% respectively.[1] Survival figures for adult patients posttransplant at 1-, 3-, and at 5-years according to the UK liver transplant audit report 2012 for elective transplants was 87.5, 81.2, and 75.1% respectively.[2]

According to one report in 2007, worldwide about 11,000–13,000 liver transplants are performed annually, even then the waiting list of patients for liver transplant in the United States alone is 17,000.[3] Waiting list as on December 31, 2011 in the United States was 15,330 for adult patients with end stage liver disease, and the number of liver transplants in the same year was 5,596 DDLT and 186 living donor liver transplants.[4]

The surgical techniques like transplantation of reduced-size organs, transplantation of "split-livers" and living-related liver transplant are an offshoot of shortage of donor organs. The advantages of living donor liver transplantation (LDLT) is the elective selection of an ideal donor, gives time to optimize the recipient, and is associated with relatively short cold ischemia time. However, while LDLT adds to the donor organ pool, donor safety remains an important concern. Living donor liver transplantation is the predominant form of liver transplant in countries like Japan, Korea, and India, where there is virtually no deceased donor program.

SCORING SYSTEMS AND TIMING OF REFERRAL

Child–Turcotte–Pugh score takes few objective and few subjective parameters to calculate a score which basically stratifies patients according to the severity of liver disease and prognosticates regarding the mortality following surgery. In addition, it is being used to decide about the treatment plan whether it should be medical treatment or there is a need for liver transplant. As there are subjective parameters in this scoring system, it has been superseded by more objective mathematical scoring systems.

It is very important to have an objective scoring system for prioritization of patients for organ allocation. These scoring systems were formulated basically for organ allocation in a DDLT program. However, these mathematical models [model for end-stage liver disease (MELD), and pediatric end-stage liver disease (PELD)], are a useful tool for listing patients even in a LDLT program. These are risk-based prognostic models (based on objective and verifiable medical data) and helps in predicting the mortality in these patients with end-stage liver disease in the absence of liver transplant. The purpose of MELD scores is to help the transplant surgeons in selecting patients who would get greater benefit from transplantation.

Timely referral is very important for these patients with chronic end-stage liver disease or those presenting with acute liver failure for liver transplantation so that there is optimum benefit from the procedure. Patients with a MELD score of >10 and/CTP score of >7 are listed for DDLT.[5] Apart from the above scores, there are other indications for listing these patients - in the form of variant syndromes: intractable ascites, hepatopulmonary syndrome, chronic hepatic encephalopathy, as well as health-related quality of life issues such as persistent and intractable itching, and recurrent cholangitis.

Exceptions to the Model for End-stage Liver Disease Scoring System

There are certain standard exceptions to the MELD scoring system, these conditions are associated with impaired survival, but they are not accounted for in the MELD scores. These exceptions include hepatocellular carcinoma, and other nonhepatocellular carcinoma (HCC) exceptions like hepatopulmonary syndrome, portopulmonary syndrome, familial amyloid polyneuropathy, primary hyperoxaluria, cystic fibrosis, and hilar cholangiocarcinoma.

Extra MELD points are given to HCC patients depending upon the size of the tumor and the 3 months predicted survival in these patients. These extra points are justified because these patients may have a relatively preserved liver function and with the calculated scores they may not get the liver on time leading to drop out due to tumor growth in this period and the associated increased mortality and morbidity. This extra point led to sixfold increase in the proportion of patients being transplanted for HCC.[6] Hepatocellular carcinoma exception policy with Milan criteria originally gave extra 15% mortality risk point for those with tumor <2 cm (MELD 24), and 30% mortality risk for those with solitary tumor >2 cm to <5 cm or 2-3 nodules largest being <3 cm (MELD 29). This prioritization policy has been revised on three occasions and presently there is no extra risk score given for tumors <2 cm and for those with T2 tumor 15% mortality risk point is given (MELD 22). Patients with HCC require recertification every 3 months to confirm that the tumor is still within the criterion for transplantation and if it is, then they receive extra 10% mortality risk points (~5 MELD points) (Table 1).

Other conditions which are included in the standard MELD exception include:

1. Portopulmonary syndrome: These patients have high pulmonary artery pressure and if the mean pulmonary artery pressure is >35 mmHg, the outcomes following liver transplant are poor. In order to receive MELD exception points, the mean pulmonary artery pressure has to be confirmed as below 35 mmHg (might require treatment otherwise it becomes a contraindication for liver transplant).
2. Hepatopulmonary syndrome is another condition where the PaO_2 is <60 mmHg on room air and these patients receive MELD exception points.
3. Familial amyloid polyneuropathy is another condition included in MELD exception.
4. Primary hyperoxaluria requiring combined liver kidney transplantation.

Table 1: Evolution of MELD exception points for HCC

	Original	*April 2003*	*Jan 2004*	*Jan 2005*
Stage I (T1) Single nodule <2 cm	15% risk MELD 24	8% risk MELD 20	Lab MELD	Lab MELD
Stage II (T2) Single nodule ≥2, <5 cm, *or* 2–3 nodules, maximum ≤3 cm	30% risk MELD 29	15% risk MELD 24	15% risk MELD 24	15% risk MELD 22

MELD, model for end-stage liver disease.

Table 2: UNOS status for listing a patient and for organ allocation[7]

Status 1	Fulminant liver failure with life expectancy <7 days • Fulminant hepatic failure as traditionally defined • Primary graft nonfunction <7 days of transplantation • Hepatic artery thrombosis <7 days of transplantation • Acute decompensated Wilson's disease
Status 2a	Hospitalized in ICU for chronic liver failure with life expectancy <7 days, with a Child–Pugh score of ≥10 and one of the following: • Unresponsive active variceal hemorrhage • Hepatorenal syndrome • Refractory ascites/hepatic hydrothorax • Stage 3 or 4 hepatic encephalopathy
Status 2b	Requiring continuous medical care, with a Child–Pugh score of ≥10, or a Child–Pugh score ≥7 and one of the following: • Unresponsive active variceal hemorrhage • Hepatorenal syndrome • Spontaneous bacterial peritonitis • Refractory ascites/hepatic hydrothorax Or, presence of hepatocellular carcinoma
Status 3	Requiring continuous medical care, with a Child–Pugh score of ≥7, but not meeting criteria for status 2b
Status 7	Temporary inactive

ICU, intensive care unit.

5. Cystic fibrosis with FEV1 <40%.
6. Hilar cholangiocarcinoma.

Patients listed with MELD exceptions as mentioned above, are reassessed every 3 months and if they continue to meet the criteria for listing, an additional 10% increase in their MELD score is granted while on the waiting list. Apart from the MELD/PELD score, organ allocation is also according to the UNOS status of patient. Priority is given to patients with status 1, followed by those with MELD/PELD score ≥15, then those having a score of ≤14. UNOS listing status is 2a if the MELD score ≥30, it is 2b if the score is 24–29, and if it is <24, the status is 3 (Table 2). The UNOS status is detailed in Table 2 and this is helpful in organ allocation once the organ is available hence it is applicable in a DDLT program.[7]

Patient Selection and Allocation Policies in the United Kingdom

The National Health Service Blood and Transplant (NHSBT) Organ Donation and Transplantation Directorate monitor the patient selection and organ allocation. This selection and allocation policy is for DDLT. There are two different criteria for selection of adult and pediatric patients requiring elective and emergency transplantation (super-urgent transplantation criteria).[8,9]

Selection Criteria for Adult Elective Transplantation

1. The United Kingdom Model for end-stage liver disease (UKELD—parameters considered serum sodium, creatinine, bilirubin, and international normalized ration) score of ≥49 predicts the projected 1 year liver disease mortality of >9% without transplant and this scoring system is used as a criterion for listing of patients with chronic liver disease for liver transplant.

2. CLD patients with porto-pulmonary hypertension who demonstrate clinically significant response to one of the long acting prostacyclin, sildenafil, or bosentan.
3. Hepatocellular carcinoma—criteria for transplant listing include: single nodule ≤5 cm diameter, or up to 5 lesions all ≤3 cm, or solitary tumor >5 cm and ≤7 cm diameter with stable disease in the last 6 months. While on waiting list locoregional therapy should be administered. Absolute contraindications to transplantation for HCC patients include tumor rupture, AFP >10,000 IU/mL, macroscopic vascular invasion, and extrahepatic spread.
4. Variant syndrome in patients with UKELD score <49 who are considered for transplantation:
   a. Diuretic-resistant ascites
   b. Hepatopulmonary syndrome
   c. Chronic hepatic encephalopathy
   d. Persistent and intractable pruritus
   e. Familial amyloidosis
   f. Primary hyperlipidaemia
   g. Polycystic liver disease
   h. Recurrent cholangitis
   i. Hepatic epithelioid haemangioendothelioma
   j. Sickle cell hepatopathy

Selection Criteria for Pediatric Elective Transplantation

1. Chronic liver disease—any of the mentioned factors due to liver disease
   a. Life expectancy <18 months
   b. Unacceptable quality of life
   c. Growth failure or impairment
   d. Reversible neuro-developmental impairment
2. Rare indications
   a. Organic acidemia requiring liver transplantation
   b. Unresectable hepatic malignancies without extrahepatic spread
   c. Diffuse hepatic hemangioendothelioma unresponsive to alternative treatments
   d. Langerhans cell histiocytosis
   e. Selected mitochondrial respiratory chain disorders with chronic liver disease
   f. Intestinal failure-associated liver disease
   g. Hepatoblastoma

   Rare indications for liver transplantation are audited regularly.

Selection Criteria for Adult Super-urgent Transplantation

The super-urgent liver scheme is available to Group 1 patients in the UK and Republic of Ireland. A requirement to be registered for the super-urgent liver scheme is the presence of at least one of the criteria mentioned in the Table 3.

Selection Criteria for Pediatric Super-urgent Transplantation

1. Acute liver failure in children <2 years with grade 3/4 encephalopathy or INR >4
2. Acute liver failure due to seronegative hepatitis, hepatitis A, or hepatitis B, or an idiosyncratic drug reaction with any grade of encephalopathy and any three from the following:
   a. Unfavorable etiology (seronegative hepatitis, idiosyncratic drug reaction)

Table 3: Selection criteria for adult super-urgent transplantation in the UK

Category 1	Paracetamol poisoning	pH <7.5, > than 24 h after overdose and after fluid resuscitation
Category 2	Paracetamol poisoning	Prothrombin time >100 s or INR >6.5 and serum creatinine >300 µmol/L or anuria, and grade 3–4 encephalopathy
Category 3	Paracetamol poisoning	Serum lactate >24 h after over dose >3.5 mmol/L on admission or >3.0 mmol/L after fluid resuscitation
Category 4	Paracetamol poisoning	Two of the three criteria from category two with clinical evidence of deterioration (e.g. increased ICP, FiO_2 >50%, increased inotrope requirement) in the absence of clinical sepsis
Category 5	Seronegative hepatitis, hepatitis A, hepatitis B, or an idiosyncratic drug reaction	Prothrombin time >100 s or INR >6.5, and any grade of encephalopathy
Category 6	Seronegative hepatitis, hepatitis A, hepatitis B, or an idiosyncratic drug reaction	Any grade of encephalopathy, and any three from the following: unfavorable aetiology, age >40 years, jaundice to encephalopathy time >7 days, serum bilirubin >300 µmol/L, prothrombin time >50 s or INR >3.5
Category 7	Acute presentation of Wilson's disease, or Budd–Chiari syndrome	Combination of coagulopathy, and any grade of encephalopathy
Category 8	Hepatic artery thrombosis on days 0–21 after liver transplantation	
Category 9	Early graft dysfunction on days 0–7 after liver transplantation	At least two of the following: AST >10.000, INR >3.0, Serum lactate >3 mmol/L, absence of bile production
Category 10	Total absence of liver function (e.g. after total hepatectomy)	
Category 11	Live liver donor—develops severe liver failure within 4 weeks of the donor operation	

b. Age <10 years
c. Jaundice to encephalopathy time >7 days
d. Serum bilirubin >300 µmol/L
e. Prothrombin time >50 seconds
f. INR >3.5

3. Acute liver failure due to Budd-Chiari syndrome, Wilson's disease, paracetamol poisoning, or early graft dysfunction

Hepatocellular Carcinoma

This indication needs more detailed explanation for various reasons. One the criteria for listing are different in a DDLT program as against a LDLT program. However, there are certain common contraindications for listing in both situations:

1. Extrahepatic spread
2. Vascular invasion (portal vein or hepatic vein invasion)

For this reason a metastatic work-up is done before listing a patient for liver transplantation which is in the form of bone scan and high resolution computed tomography (CT) scan of the chest or a PET-CT scan. Once it is confirmed that above contraindications are not there then depending upon the kind of program (DDLT vs. LDLT) other criteria are taken into consideration. Initially, there were stringent criteria in the DDLT setting which was widely followed and it is the Milan criteria (solitary nodule ≤5 cm, 2–3 nodules largest ≤3 cm, Child's C cirrhosis with no extrahepatic or vascular spread).[10] This is supposed to provide a 4-year survival of 75% with <15% recurrence rate. Later expanded criteria came up to include some more patients who were being denied a curative option of liver transplant because they were beyond the Milan criteria. This was given by Yao et al. (solitary tumor ≤6.5 cm or ≤3 nodules with largest being <4.5 cm and the total diameter of tumor being ≤8 cm).[11,12] Survival in these patients following transplant was shown to be similar to those within Milan criteria.

Other criterion that is more often considered in the LDLT program is the Asian Medical Center criteria where up to five tumors with maximum diameter being ≤5 cm is considered for transplantation.[13] Another multicenter study by the Metroticket Investigator Study Group which looked into the survival of patients who were transplanted outside the Milan criteria ("up-to-7 rule"—where the sum of the number of lesions and the diameter of the largest tumor in cm is not >than 7), concluded that more patients could be transplanted with a 5-year overall survival of 71.2%.[14] Milan criteria are still the gold standard for listing a patient for transplantation, the MELD exception takes MC into consideration. However, the extended criteria are being followed especially in the LDLT scenario to include more patients who would benefit from liver transplant and have equally good results in terms of survival and recurrence.

INDICATIONS FOR LIVER TRANSPLANTATION

Patients with acute liver failure (fulfilling criteria for emergency liver transplant), chronic liver disease, and malignancy are the broad categories under which the indications could be listed (Table 4).

1. *Acute liver failure:* These patients present with a triad of encephalopathy, coagulopathy, and jaundice, without any evidence of preexisting liver disease. The presentation could be fulminant or subfulminant. The cause for acute liver failure is varied (Table 4). In the West, paracetamol poisoning is the commonest cause for acute liver failure, acute viral hepatitis (A, E, B), seronegative hepatitis, and drug-induced liver failure are other common etiological factors. Acute liver failure, as a cause for liver transplant, occurs in about 5–6% of cases.[15] King's College criteria are most commonly followed for deciding the

Table 4: Indications for liver transplantation
Acute liver failure
Infection—viral (hepatitis A, B, C, D, E)
Seronegative hepatitis
Toxic—acute acetaminophen, mushroom poisoning, and others
Acute fatty liver (pregnancy, tetracyclines, Reye syndrome)
Acute multiorgan (liver) failure following cardiac surgery
Ischemic (ligation of hepatic artery, other surgery)
Vascular cause(acute Budd–Chiari syndrome)
Autoimmune hepatitis
Drugs—idiosyncratic–antituberculous drugs
Wilson's disease, Budd–Chiari syndrome
Neonatal hemochromatosis
Cryptogenic
Cirrhosis from chronic liver disease
Infectious—chronic HBV, HCV, HDV liver disease, coinfection (HBV + HIV)
Alcoholic liver disease
Cryptogenic liver disease
Cholestatic liver diseases
Primary biliary cirrhosis
Primary sclerosing cholangitis
Secondary biliary cirrhosis
Biliary atresia
Alagille syndrome
Byler's disease
Malignant diseases of the liver
Hepatocellular carcinoma
Carcinoid tumor, primary neuroendocrine tumor
Islet cell tumor
Epithelioid hemangioendothelioma
Cholangiocarcinoma*
Metabolic liver disease
Wilson's disease
Hereditary hemochromatosis
Alpha-1 antitrypsin deficiency
Glycogen storage disease
Cystic fibrosis
Glycogen storage disease I and IV
Crigler–Najjar syndrome
Galactosemia
Type 1 hyperoxaluria
Familial homozygous hypercholesterolemia
Hemophilia A and B
Vascular diseases of the liver
Budd–Chiari syndrome
Veno-occlusive disease
Miscellaneous
Nonalcoholic fatty liver disease
Autoimmune hepatitis (PBC—overlap syndrome)
Chronic drug induced—methotrexate, etc.
Adult polycystic liver disease
Nodular regenerative hyperplasia
Caroli's disease
Severe graft-versus-host disease
Amyloidosis
Sarcoidosis
Hepatic trauma

Table 5: Criteria for liver transplantation in acute liver failure

King's College Criteria	
Acetaminophen-induced ALF	*Non-acetaminophen ALF*
1. Arterial pH <7.3 *irrespective* of grade of encephalopathy OR 1. PT >100 s 2. Serum creatinine >3.4 mg/dL 3. Stage 3 or 4 encephalopathy	1. INR >6.5 (PT >100 s), *irrespective* of grade of encephalopathy OR any 3 of the following: 1. INR >3.5 (PT >50 s) 2. Age <10 or >40 years 3. Serum bilirubin >18 mg/dL 4. Jaundice to encephalopathy interval >7 days 5. Non-A, non-B hepatitis, idiosyncratic drug reaction

Revised Wilson Prognostic Index (RWPI)[19]

Score	*Bilirubin (μmol/L)*	*INR*	*AST (IU/L)*	*WCC (10^9/L)*	*Albumin (g/L)*
0	0–100	0–1.29	0–100	0–6.7	>45
1	101–150	1.3–1.6	101–150	6.8–8.3	34–44
2	151–200	1.7–1.9	151–300	8.4–10.3	25–33
3	201–300	2.0–2.4	301–400	10.4–15.3	21–24
4	≥301	>2.5	>401	>15.4	<20

Patients with a RWPI ≥11 needed urgent liver transplantation.

need for emergency liver transplant. Once the patient fulfills the criteria, the chances of survival without liver transplant are <10% (Table 5). These patients give a very short window period and if not transplanted have a very poor chance of survival and this is either due to liver failure per se or due to multiorgan failure and sepsis.[16] Hence, these patients require rapid work-up and transplantation. They are placed in the status 1 in the UNOS or category 1 in the NHSBT categorization and are offered organ on a priority basis. In the LDLT scenario, the living donor is identified, family is counseled, and emergency transplant is carried out after evaluation of both, the donor and the recipient. Apart from the King's College criteria, there are other criteria like the UK blood and transplant criteria, Clichy criteria (acute viral hepatitis), and Wilson's prognostic index (original and the revised) for Wilson's disease with fulminant presentation, these are all followed in the acute liver failure scenario to decide the need for urgent transplantation.[17-19]

2. *Chronic liver disease:* The American Society of Transplant Physicians and the American Association for the Study of the Liver Disease in 1997 proposed the minimum listing criteria for patients with end-stage liver disease and this was based on the risk of mortality at 1-year without transplant. Patients with chronic liver disease who have ≤90% chance of surviving without transplant at 1 year were deemed candidates for listing according to the proposed minimum listing criteria. However, for other indications which were exceptions to the above (cholestatic liver disease with pruritus or repeated cholangitis), there was a need of a method for listing for transplantation. These are included in quality of life indications for transplantation. Patients with cirrhosis of liver without decompensation have a 5-year survival of 91% as compared with 50% in those with decompensated liver disease.[20] Patients who have ascites without spontaneous bacterial peritonitis have a 1-year cumulative probability of survival of 66% versus 38% in those who had spontaneous bacterial peritonitis.[21] Other complication of ascites is hepatorenal syndrome and patients who developed hepatorenal syndrome had a median survival of 1.7 weeks in the Barcelona series.[22,23] Cirrhosis of liver with decompensation which can be in the form of variceal bleeding, intractable ascites, bacterial peritonitis, encephalopathy, hepatorenal syndrome, hepato-pulmonary syndrome, or development of cancer, are all considered for liver transplantation. The cause for end-stage liver disease can be categorized under various heads. Table 4 gives us the list of causes of chronic liver disease which would require liver transplant.
3. *Cholestatic liver disease:* In adults' primary biliary cirrhosis, primary sclerosing cholangitis and overlap syndrome with autoimmune hepatitis form an important indication for liver transplant. The indication was classically defined using the Mayo model which gave a risk score to predict the mortality at 1 year without transplant and if the risk was >10% then these patients were listed for transplant.[5] Other indications in patients with cholestatic liver disease is quality of life indications (fatigue, pruritus, cholangitis). CTP score of ≥7, Mayo risk score, and quality of life indications are hence taken into consideration for listing. In pediatric population, extrahepatic biliary atresia is one of the commonest indications for liver transplantation. These children may present with decompensated liver disease early or they may present after having had a decompressive procedure in the form of Kasai's procedure. Biliary atresia accounts for about 60–70% of pediatric patients undergoing liver transplantation.
4. *Alcoholic liver disease:* This is a major etiological factor for chronic liver disease and these patients are candidates for liver transplant only if they are abstinent and have been seen and cleared by a psychiatrist for listing for transplant. Period of abstinence is arbitrary and a 6-month period of abstinence is generally required.[24] This period of abstinence is helpful in two ways: first it gives adequate time for the liver to recover from the acute insult and some patients might improve to an extent where transplant may not be indicated, second it gives an idea about the compliance of the patient to remain abstinent

so that they remain abstinent after transplant. The psychiatrist assesses the social support system and the compliance of the patient so there is proper allocation of organs to these patients. Acute alcoholic hepatitis is acute presentation of these patients where the patient is actually in active alcohol abuse and presents with decompensation. These patients are sick and the severity of acute alcoholic hepatitis is evaluated using the Maddrey discriminant function (DF) score. Discriminant function score predicts the risk of early death in these patients. If the DF is >32, they are put on medical treatment. Role of liver transplant in these patients is controversial. Presently there are mixed opinions; on one side there is hesitancy to offer transplant due to active alcohol abuse (absence of period of abstinence), ethical issues involved (denial of treatment in the presence high risk of mortality), high chance of recidivism, and due to acute shortage of organs. However, on the other hand there are reports stating that in these patients presenting with acute hepatitis, not responding to medical treatment, with proper selection early transplant will actually provide a better outcome. The requirement of mandatory period of abstinence is questioned as this is considered to be a poor predictor of relapse of alcoholism.[25] The consensus is still awaited and till then indication for transplanting these patients is controversial.

5. *Malignancy:* Hepatocellular carcinoma in a cirrhotic liver as mentioned earlier is an indication for liver transplantation, provided the disease is confined to the liver with no extrahepatic disease. The priority in DDLT scenario with extra MELD exception points is already discussed in the earlier sections. The advantage of transplant is that apart from it being curative and reducing the chance of recurrence, it also takes care of the cirrhotic liver. In LDLT program, the criteria are not restrictive for being candidate for transplantation and if the 3- and 5-year survival is >50% in these patients following transplant, patients should be given this fair chance. Other malignancy in the liver for which transplant is an option is epitheloid hemangioedothelioma, and hepatoblastoma. Amongst the metastatic tumors patients with neuroendocrine tumor, where the primary tumor has been resected and liver is the only site of metastases, transplant is an indication due to the good prognosis. Rest of the metastatic tumors do not merit a transplant due to poor prognosis.
6. *Metabolic syndromes:* Those metabolic diseases causing decompensation and liver failure are indications as in any chronic liver disease; these are Wilson's disease, hereditary hemochromatosis, and α1 antitrypsin deficiency. Other metabolic disorders where the synthetic function is preserved but there is extrahepatic organ involvement like in Type 1 primary hyperoxaluria, where the patient presents with chronic renal failure and combined liver kidney transplant is indicated. In pediatric patients, metabolic syndromes could present as acute liver failure, extrahepatic manifestations (neurological involvement, cerebral, cardiac, or renal failure), or as chronic end-stage liver, kidney, and heart disease, or with quality of life issues (dietary restrictions, etc.). All these form an indication for liver transplant. It is a challenge to diagnose the exact metabolic disorder and evaluate these patients before transplantation.
7. *Vascular disorders of the liver:* Patients with Budd Chiari syndrome would need a transplant if they have a fulminant presentation, once there is established cirrhosis, and if the portal decompression is technically not feasible. These patients generally require lifelong anticoagulation as Budd Chiari syndrome is associated with myeloproliferative disorders in majority (50%), and hypercoagulable state, or malignancy (25%).[26]
8. *Miscellaneous indications:* Complicated polycystic liver disease either alone or with polycystic kidney disease is an indication for liver transplantation or combined liver kidney transplantation. Nonalcoholic steatohepatitis-related cirrhosis is an emerging cause for liver transplantation. Caroli's disease, hepatic trauma, etc. are other rare causes requiring liver transplantation.

CONTRAINDICATIONS

There are few absolute contraindications and some relative contraindications for liver transplantation. Severe cardiopulmonary compromise is an absolute contraindication for transplantation. Patients with severe pulmonary artery hypertension (mean pulmonary arterial pressure ≥50 mmHg) have 100% risk of mortality following transplant, hence are not candidates for transplant.[27] There is 50% risk of mortality in patients with moderate pulmonary hypertension (PAP 35–50 mmHg), hence those with <35–40 mmHg pressure are suitable candidates for transplant. Similarly in patients with HPS, in the presence of arterial hypoxemia (<50 mmHg PaO_2), the risk of mortality following transplant is about 30%.[28] Pulmonary conditions like advanced fibrosis or oxygen dependency in patients with chronic obstructive airway disease are absolute contraindications for transplantation. Relative contraindications are reversible conditions as mentioned in Table 6.

Table 6: Contraindications for liver transplant
Absolute contraindications
• Severe cardiopulmonary disease: – Severe HPS – Severe pulmonary fibrosis – Oxygen dependent COPD – Symptomatic coronary artery disease – Severe ventricular dysfunction – Advanced cardiomyopathy – Severe valvular heart disease and aortic stenosis • Extrahepatic malignancy • Active alcohol/substance abuse • Acute alcoholic hepatitis • Active infection/uncontrolled sepsis • Lack of psychosocial support • Brain death
Relative contraindications
• Reversible pulmonary conditions: – Reactive airway disease – Hepatic hydrothorax – Muscle wasting and infection • Advanced age • Morbid obesity • Acquired immune deficiency syndrome • Cholangiocarcinoma • Diffuse portal vein thrombosis • Previous abdominal surgery • Retransplant for HCV infection

Severe coronary artery diseases which are absolute contraindications for transplant are: severe ventricular dysfunction, advanced cardiomyopathy, severe valvular heart disease, and aortic stenosis. However, if these conditions are resolved following corrective surgery, these candidates could be listed for transplant. At times, patients with end-stage liver disease undergo simultaneous cardiac surgery and liver transplant in that sequence, as none can be done safely without the other.

Patients who have active alcohol abuse as already mentioned are not candidates for liver transplant because of various reasons: both clinical and ethical in the presence of shortage of organs. Similarly, patients who are on active substance abuse or polydrug abuse are not candidates for transplant as the posttransplant period requires psychiatric assessment and treatment and there is high risk of noncompliance in these patients. These above reasons are hence relative contraindications.

Advanced age >65–70 years is a relative contraindication (some centers accept up to 70 years) as the survival following transplant is shown to be low. These patients need extensive evaluation to rule out cardiopulmonary disease contraindicating transplant.[29,30]

Morbid obesity [body mass index (BMI) >40] is associated with high mortality following transplant and this is due to cardiovascular morbidity. Hence, obesity with BMI >35 needs an approach on a case-to-case basis.

Similarly, patients who do not have a psychosocial support system would be relative contraindication for transplant due to issues related to noncompliance and the fear of graft loss.

The absolute contraindication in patients with HIV infection is uncontrolled HIV disease (multidrug resistant), with leukoencephalopathy, advanced malnutrition, requirement of life support, and presence of opportunistic infection. Transplant is selectively offered to patients who have virus control and posttransplant management is done in collaboration with experts managing these patients with HIV.[31]

Presence of ongoing sepsis and active infection of any site (osteomyelitis, pneumonia, bacteremia, fungaemia, etc.) is an absolute contraindication and these need to be treated adequately before listing. These are indications for delisting these patients temporarily.

Other miscellaneous relative contraindications (previous abdominal surgery, portal vein thrombosis, cholangiocarcinoma) and areas of controversy (retransplant for HCV infection, acute alcoholic hepatitis) are listed in Table 6.

DELISTING CRITERIA

Delisting is temporary for patients who develop active infection, or require dialysis, or mechanical ventilation. There is no consensus on the delisting criteria but by the norm of listing if the patients clinical status deteriorates and they are too sick to transplant (have a MELD score of >40, have a predicted survival of <50% at 5 years), or they develop metastatic disease, then these patients are taken off the list.

LIVING DONOR LIVER TRANSPLANT

The advantage in LDLT scenario is the availability of an organ, if the patient presents with the donor. In patients with HCC, the stringent criteria are not necessarily applicable hence those beyond Milan and UCSF criteria, the waiting period is absent and the results are good. Waiting list mortality and drop out due to metastatic disease is not applicable. Patients who have benign liver lesions which are symptomatic (hemangioma, hemangioendothelioma, etc.), or those with metabolic disorder (hyperoxaluria, familial amyloidosis, tyrosinemia, etc.), or cholestatic liver disease, where the MELD score is not very high, get benefitted in the LDLT program as there is no waiting period. The advantage in LDLT over DDLT is the elective situation except in patients with acute liver failure, the short cold ischemia time, both of which accounts for improved graft and patient survival. Donor selection and safety is however of utmost importance in this program. The contraindications in LDLT are the same as in those for DDLT. However, there are certain donor issues that can contraindicate a transplant: presence of a fatty liver with macrosteatosis >20% on liver biopsy, remnant liver volume of <25%, other relative contraindications would be a BMI of >30 in the donor, certain donor anatomical issues like the presence of type E portal vein (multiple sectoral veins draining separately, and >3 bile ducts in the graft.[32,33]

CONCLUSION

With advances in the understanding of transplant immunology and the introduction of better immunosuppressant protocols, along with better surgical techniques, and perioperative management, the outcomes of liver transplantation have improved over the years. The indications and contraindications have been changing but are probably less controversial with better mathematical scoring systems in place and the various clinical scores for acute liver failure. It still has substantial areas which are controversial and which require referral to review board in the DDLT scenario. Introduction of LDLT program has definitely improved the donor organ pool and reduced the waiting period for patients who would not get an organ otherwise. It is definitely the main source of organ pool in countries where deceased organ donation is rare.

REFERENCES

1. http://optn.transplant.hrsa.gov/latestData/rptStrat.asp.
2. http://www.rcseng.ac.uk/surgeons/research/surgical-research/docs/liver-transplant-audit-report-2012.
3. http://www.liver-products.com/liver-therapy/liver-transplantation.html
4. http://srtr.transplant.hrsa.gov/annual_reports/2011/default.aspx
5. Lucey MR, Brown KA, Everson GT, et al. Minimal criteria for placement of adults on the liver transplant waiting list: a report of a national conference organized by the American Society of Transplant Physicians and the American Association for the Study of Liver Diseases. Liver Transpl Surg. 1997;3(6):628-37.
6. Ioannou GN, Perkins JD, Carithers RL Jr. Liver transplantation for hepatocellular carcinoma: impact of the MELD allocation system and predictors of survival. Gastroenterology. 2008 May;134(5):1342-51. doi: 10.1053/j.gastro.2008.02.013.
7. http://www.unos.org/ initially implemented in July 1997 later modified in January 1998 and August 1998.
8. NHS Blood & Transplant and British Transplantation Society. Guidelines for consent for solid organ transplantation in adults. April 2013.
9. NHSBT Liver Advisory Group. Protocols and Guidelines for Children Undergoing Deceased Donor Liver Transplantation in the UK. April 2010.
10. Mazzaferro V, Regalia E, Doci R, et al. Liver transplantation for the treatment of small hepatocellular carcinomas in patients with cirrhosis. N Engl J Med. 1996;334(11):693-9

11. Yao FY, Ferrell L, Bass NM, et al. Liver transplantation for hepatocellular carcinoma: expansion of the tumor size limits does not adversely impact survival. Hepatology. 2001;33:1394-403.
12. Fernández JA, Robles R, Marin C, et al. Can we expand the indications for liver transplantation among hepatocellular carcinoma patients with increased tumor size? Transplant Proc. 2003;35:1818-20.
13. Lee SG, Hwang S, Moon DB, et al. Expanded indication criteria of living donor liver transplantation for hepatocellular carcinoma at one large-volume center. Liver Transpl. 2008;14:935-45. doi: 10.1002/lt.21445.
14. Mazzaferro V, Llovet JM, Miceli R, et al. Metroticket Investigator Study Group. Predicting survival after liver transplantation in patients with hepatocellular carcinoma beyond the Milan criteria: a retrospective, exploratory analysis. Lancet Oncol. 2009;10:35-43. doi: 10.1016/S1470-2045(08)70284-5.
15. Merion RM, Schaubel DE, Dykstra DM, et al. The survival benefit of liver transplantation. Am J Transplant. 2005;5:307-13.
16. Lee WM. Acute liver failure. N Engl J Med. 1993;329:1862-72.
17. Bernuau J, Samuel D, Durand F, et al. Criteria for emergency liver transplantation in patients with acute viral hepatitis and factor V below 50% of normal: a prospective study [abstract]. Hepatology. 1991;14:49A.
18. Nazer H, Ede RJ, Mowat AP, et al. Wilson's disease: clinical presentation and use of prognostic index. Gut. 1986;27:1377-81.
19. Dhawan A, Taylor RM, Cheeseman P, et al. Wilson's disease in children: 37-year experience and revised King's score for liver transplantation. Liver Transpl. 2005;11:441-8.
20. Fattovich G, Giustina G, Degos F, et al. Morbidity and mortality in compensated cirrhosis type C: a retrospective follow-up study of 384 patients. Gastroenterology. 1997;112:463-72.
21. Andreu M, Sola R, Sitges-Serra A, et al. Risk factors for spontaneous bacterial peritonitis in cirrhotic patients with ascites. Gastroenterology. 1993;104:1133-8.
22. Ginès A, Escorsell A, Ginès P, et al. Incidence, predictive factors, and prognosis of the hepatorenal syndrome in cirrhosis with ascites. Gastroenterology. 1993;105:229-36
23. Lucey MR, Brown KA, Everson GT, et al. Minimal criteria for placement of adults on the liver transplant waiting list: a report of a national conference organized by the American Society of Transplant Physicians and the American Association for the Study of Liver Diseases. Transplantation. 1998;66:956-62.
24. Everhart JE, Beresford TP. Liver transplantation for alcoholic liver disease: a survey of transplantation programs in the United States. Liver Transpl Surg. 1997;3:220-6.
25. Mathurin P, Moreno C, Samuel D, et al. Early liver transplantation for severe alcoholic hepatitis. N Engl J Med. 2011;365:1790-800. doi: 10.1056/NEJMoa1105703.
26. Klein AS. Management of Budd-Chiari syndrome. Liver Transpl. 2006;12:S23-8
27. Krowka MJ, Plevak DJ, Findlay JY, et al. Pulmonary hemodynamics and perioperative cardiopulmonary-related mortality in patients with portopulmonary hypertension undergoing liver transplantation. Liver Transpl. 2000;6:443-50.
28. Krowka MJ, Porayko MK, Plevak DJ, et al. Hepatopulmonary syndrome with progressive hypoxemia as an indication for liver transplantation: case reports and literature review. Mayo Clin Proc. 1997;72:44-53.
29. Keswani RN, Ahmed A, Keeffe EB. Older age and liver transplantation: a review. Liver Transpl. 2004;10:957-67.
30. Lipshutz GS, Hiatt J, Ghobrial RM, et al. Outcome of liver transplantation in septuagenarians: a single-center experience. Arch Surg. 2007;142:775-81; discussion 781-4.
31. Fink SA, Brown RS. Current indications, contraindications, delisting criteria, and timing for liver transplantation. In: Busuttil RW, Klintmalm GB, editors. Textbook on liver transplantation. Chap. 7, 2nd ed. New York: Elsevier; 2009. pp. 95-113.
32. Nakamura T, Tanaka K, Kiuchi T, et al. Anatomical variations and surgical strategies in right lobe living donor liver transplantation: lessons from 120 cases. Transplantation. 2002;73:1896-903.
33. Huang TL, Cheng YF, Chen CL, et al. Variants of the bile ducts: clinical application in the potential donor of living-related hepatic transplantation. Transplant Proc. 1996;28:1669-70.

CHAPTER 107

Organ Preservation in Liver Transplant

Raghavendra Raja, Vinay Kumaran

INTRODUCTION

Improvement in organ preservation is responsible for a revolution in organ transplantation, along with improvements in surgical techniques and immunosuppression. Effective organ preservation techniques provide the time leverage for transportation of the organ and identification of the correct recipient in terms of urgency, size, and immunological matching.

WHY ORGAN PRESERVATION?

It is obvious that any organ without nutritional supply is destined to die, but the time for this irreversible damage varies with different organs depending on their metabolism. Organ transplantation entails transport of the organ with reperfusion of the same in another human being before irreversible damage has set in, which at times involve substantial time. At normal temperatures lack of oxygen and perfusion (warm ischemia) leads to rapid decline in cell adenosine triphosphate (ATP) levels, due to which several essential processes, one of which also is to maintain transmembrane ionic concentrations, are disturbed (mainly by transmembrane Na-K ATPase). This further leads to a change in osmotic concentration of intracellular fluid, activation of hydrolytic enzymes, and disruption of intracellular organelles resulting in cell breakdown. As can be seen, ATP loss is a critical factor. Studies have demonstrated the beneficial effect of exposing the stored organ to oxygen for possible aerobic metabolism[1,2] and stimulating anaerobic metabolism for ATP synthesis in explanted organs ex vivo.[3,4] In similar lines, reports of adverse effects of inhibiting ATP synthesis on organ preservation too exist.[5] In organ transplantation ATP loss has to be slowed down at least, if not totally blocked. Whenever possible, provision for ATP synthesis would be ideal for the organ to regain its function upon transplantation into another human being.

History

Initial focus during the years 1940–1960 was basically on preventing rejection of allografts.Once Murray demonstrated successful kidney transplantation between monozygotic twins, efforts started at improving organ preservation.[6] Initially, hypothermia was the cornerstone of preservation with its effect on metabolic inhibition.[7] This included both simple surface cooling with ice slush as used by Moore[8] and core cooling of organ by flushing with cold solution developed by Starzl.[9] The organs were flushed and immersed in cold saline or lactated ringer's solutions. Later came the preservative solutions to overcome the effects of hypothermia (mainly cell swelling), to give a compatible extracellular environment for the cells similar to in vivo scenario, continuous supply of nutrients and removal of metabolites. Initially cold saline, blood, plasma, and cryopreserved plasma were used for this purpose to keep it similar to the extracellular compartment in the body. Later, synthetic preservative solution came into experimental and then for clinical use, the first major one being Collins solution. These were predominantly extracellular type solutions (potassium-rich), and became the standard solutions for organ preservation. Thereafter, various modifications of the Collins solution—mainly *University of Wisconsin* (UW) and histidine-tryptophan-ketoglutarate (HTK) solutions were developed.

Components of Organ Preservation

Hypothermia

This has been the earliest and major component of organ preservation even today. Hypothermia should be maintained at both the internal and external milieu of organ. This involves surrounding or covering the organs with ice (external) and perfusing the organ with cold perfusates through organ inflow, which involves infusion through both aorta (always) and portal vein (sometimes) for liver and abdominal multiorgan transplants. The success of this therapy depends on maintaining the temperature at less than 4°C. It has been demonstrated that decreasing the temperature to 4°C and less slows down enzymatic actions by 10 times.[10] Hypothermia decreases ATP loss rate by decreasing metabolism, but this alone may not explain its beneficiary effect. It also inhibits hydrolytic enzymes, which has been shown to improve the tolerance of tissues to ischemia.[11] Hypothermia only decreases the rate of metabolism, but does not completely stop it; hence end products of metabolism continue to accumulate, although at a slower rate which at some point may damage the tissues irreversibly.

Preservative Solutions

Although hypothermia is a critical factor in organ preservation, there are other considerations too. Hypothermia by its effect on decreasing the metabolic rate and enzymatic reaction and in late stages with loss of ATP inhibits many of the essential cell services maintaining transmembrane ionic concentrations, which would result in high intracellular osmolarity, fluid influx into cell, and cell disruption, although at a rate much slower than that would have ensued under normothermia. This may be prevented to some extent by maintaining effective extracellular osmotic pressure with the use of impermeant molecules.[12,13] Normally, this balance is maintained by Na-K ATPase with high Na concentration outside and high K concentration inside the cell. In preservative solutions, various saccharides (sucrose, mannitol, and glucose), anions (lactobionate, gluconate, phosphate) and colloids (hydroxyl starch, polyethylene glycol, and dextran) are used as impermeants.

Although impermeant is an essential component of the preservative solution, other components are added to prevent storage/reperfusion injury or assist in recovery. The studies regarding their roles and efficacy are controversial.

The cold stored organs are deficient in natural antioxidants, vitamin E and glutathione.[14,15] The formation of oxygen free radicals in ischemic/reperfused tissues has been demonstrated in many previous studies[16-18], and others have demonstrated the protective effects of antioxidants in experiments.[19-21] The major antioxidants used clinically are glutathione and allopurinol (xanthine oxidase inhibitor) in UW solution.

Logically thinking, the need for colloids in preservative solutions exists to counteract the hydrostatic pressure in continuous machine perfusion of organs. However, few reports do exist regarding its beneficial effect in simple cold storage too.[22,23] Hydroxyethyl starch is the colloid predominantly studied for this purpose.

Electrolyte content of the solution is another major issue. Most of the solutions are "intracellular type" with high potassium and low sodium. The reason for this is to prevent hypothermia-induced K-efflux from the cell. But some studies have shown electrolyte composition may not be important for short-term preservation[24,25] and some have even reported-high potassium may be detrimental.[26]

ATP loss is, as seen before, one of the critical factors in organ injury during its storage. One hypothesis was that early regeneration of ATP on reperfusion would be important for successful functioning. ATP is broken down during storage to purine and phosphate. Purine being permeable crosses cell membrane and is flushed out.[27] Adenosine is added to UW solution with this idea to regenerate ATP early on reperfusion.[28]

Main Preservative Solutions (Table 1)

1. Euro-Collins solution: This is a modification of Collins solution and was the earliest liver preservative solution used. It is an isotonic, potassium-rich solution with glucose as impermeant and phosphate as buffer. It is effective in liver preservation only for short period (<6 hours) and is not much in clinical use for liver now.
2. University of Wisconsin solution (UW): The solution was culmination of works of Folkert Belzer and James Southard.[29] This is isotonic, potassium-rich, sodium-rich solution with raffinose and lactobionate as impermeants, phosphate as buffer. Glutathione and allopurinol are added as free radical scavengers, hydroxyethyl starch as colloid, and dexamethasone as a membrane stabilizer.
3. HTK solution (Custodiol)/Bretschneider's solution: It is an isotonic solution with low sodium and potassium. Histidine is used as buffer against acidity, tryptophan as a membrane stabilizer and free radical scavenger, and ketoglutarate as a substrate for anaerobic metabolism.

With so many preservative solutions around, one can be sure that an ideal solution is yet to be discovered. Their usage basically depends on institutional practice. In India, with predominantly living donor liver transplantation (LDLT) setting HTK solution is used by and large in most centers, while in centers with dominant deceased donor liver transplant setting, UW solution is favored. Taking cost factor into consideration and if the duration of preservation is short, Euro-Collins solution may be an option.

With UW solution entering the arena of organ preservation before HTK and rapidly gaining widespread acceptance worldwide, introduction of HTK faced many problems. Several studies compared HTK solution with the then gold standard preservative, UW solution in organ transplantation. Majority of the studies demonstrated almost equal efficacy and safety of HTK solution when compared to UW solution with similar graft and patient survival rates.[30-32]

HTK solution being less viscous is thought to have better penetration in the microcirculation. The same reason was thought to be responsible for lower late biliary complication rate seen with HTK solution in few studies.[33,34] Besides, studies have shown that in LDLT setting with piggyback reconstruction of liver implantation, low potassium content in HTK may obviate the need for in situ flush (cold/warm) before revascularization.[33,35]

The only caution with the use of HTK solution probably appears to be in multiorgan transplants involving pancreas. Few of the studies have documented either increased rates of pancreatitis or acute rejection or graft loss due to vascular thrombosis but many others have also revealed similar graft and patient survival when compared with UW solution.

Table 1: Main preservative solutions

Component	*Euro-Collins*	*UW*	*HTK*
Potassium ion (mmol/L)	115	125	10
Sodium ion (mmol/L)	10	125	15
Magnesium (mmol/L)		5	4
Calcium (mmol/L)			0.015
Chloride (mmol/L)	15		
Bicarbonate (mmol/L)	10		
Sulphate (mmol/L)		5	
Phosphate (mmol/L)	57.5	25	
Glucose (mmol/L)	194		
Raffinose (mmol/L)		30	
Lactobionate (mmol/L)		100	
Adenosine (mmol/L)		5	
Glutathione (mmol/L)		3	
Allopurinol (mmol/L)		1	
Hydroxyethyl starch (Gm/L)		50	
Histidine (mmol/L)			198
Tryptophan (mmol/L)			2
Ketoglutarate (mmol/L)			1
mOsm/L	320	320	310

Methods of Use

1. *Simple cold storage*: This method, explained by Collins, involves flushing out the organ of warm, deoxygenated blood with a suitable solution and cooling it at both internal and external surfaces.[36] The organ is then stored in the preservative solution at temperature less than 4°C.
2. *Continuous machine perfusion*: In this method, developed by Belzer, the organ is perfused with a preservative solution at 4–6°C temperature in a pulsatile manner of about 60 beats/min at 40–50 mm of Hg to simulate the physiological flow.[37] This method appears to be superior at least theoretically, by continuous supply of oxygen, nutrients, and removal of metabolic end products. It is shown to be better than simple storage in clinical studies on kidney preservation with decreased delayed graft function rates. Experimental studies in liver preservation have shown it to be safe.

REFERENCES

1. Pegg DE, Foreman J, Hunt CJ, et al. The mechanism of action of retrograde oxygen persulfflation in renal preservation. Transplantation. 1989;48:210-7.
2. Fujino Y, Kuroda Y, Suzuki Y, et al. Preservation of canine pancreas for 96 hours by a modified two-layer (UW solution/perfluorochemical) cold storage method. Transplantation. 1991;51:1133-5.
3. Anundi I, King J, Owen DA, et al. Fructose prevents hypoxic cell death in liver. Am J Physiol. 1987;253:G390-6.
4. Brass CA, Crawford JM, Narciso J, et al. Hypoxic liver injury and the ameliorating effects of fructose: The glucose paradox revisited. Am J Physiol. 1992;263:G293-300.
5. Stringham JC, Southard JH, Hegge J, et al. Limitations of heart preservation by cold storage. Transplantation. 1992;53:287-93.
6. Merrill JP, Murray JE, Harrison JH, et al. Successful homotransplantation of the human kidney between identical twins. J Am Med Assoc. 1956;160:277-82.
7. Pegg DE, Calne RY, Pryse-Davies J, et al. Canine renal preservation using surface and perfusion cooling techniques. Ann N Y Acad Sci. 1964;120:506-23.
8. Moore FD, Smith LL, Burnap TK, et al. One stage homotransplantations of the liver following total hepatectomy in dogs. Transplant Bull. 1959;6:103-7.
9. Kaupp HA Jr, Starzl TE. The use of an external bypass during experimental total hepatectomy. Surgery. 1960;48:330-1.
10. Fuller BJ. The effects of cooling on mammalian cells. In: Fuller BJ, Grout BWW, editors. Clinical applications of cryobiology. Boca Raton: CRC Press; 1991. pp. 1-22.
11. Imberti R, Nieminen A, Herman B, et al. Mitochondrial and glycolytic dysfunction in lethal injury to hepatopcytes and t-butylhydroxide: protection by fructose, cyclosporin A and trifluoperazine. J Pharmacol Exp Ther. 1993;265:392-400.
12. Sumimoto R, Kamada N. Lactobionate as the most important component in UW solution for liver preservation. Transplant Proc. 1990;22:2198-9.
13. Southard JH, van Gulik TM, Ametani MS, et al. Important components of the UW solution. Transplantation. 1990;49:251-7.
14. Vreugdenhil PK, Belzer FO, Southard JH. Effect of cold storage on tissue and cellular glutathione. Cryobiology. 1991;28:143-9.
15. Marubayashi S, Dohi K, Sumimoto K, et al. Role of free radicals in ischemic rat liver preservation: prevention of damage by vitamin E, CoQ, or reduced glutathione. Transplant Proc. 1988;20:974-5.
16. Bulkley GB, Morris JB. Role of oxygen-derived free radicals as mediators of post-ischemic injury: a clinically oriented overview. In: Proceedings of the fourth international conference superoxide and SOD 1990;1-7.
17. Land W, Messmer K. The impact of ischemia/reperfusion injury on specific and non-specific, early and late chronic events after organ transplantation. Transplant Rev. 1996;10:236-53.
18. Lemasters JJ, Bunzendahl H, Thurman RG. Reperfusion injury to donor livers stored for transplantation. Liver Transplant Surg. 1995;1:124-38.
19. Cosenza CA, Cramer DV, Cunneen SA, et al. Protective effect of the lazaroid U74006F in cold ischemia-reperfusion injury of the liver. Hepatology. 1994;19:418-25.
20. Bromley PN, Cottam SJ, Hilmi I, et al. Effects of intraoperative n-acetylcysteine in orthotopic liver transplantation. Br J Anaesth. 1995;75:352-4.
21. Rabl H, Khoschsorur G, Colombo T, et al. A multivitamin infusion prevents lipid peroxidation and improves transplantation performance. Kidney Int. 1993;43:912-7.
22. Ploeg RJ, Boudjema K, Marsh D, et al. Importance of a colloid in canine pancreas preservation. Transplantation. 1992;53:735-41.
23. Wicomb WN, Collins GM. 24-hour rabbit heart storage with UW solution: effects of low-flow perfusion, colloid, and shelf storage. Transplantation. 1989;48:6-9.
24. Howden BO, Jablonski P, Self G, et al. Effective organ preservation with modified HES-free UW solution with lowered potassium content. Transplant Proc. 1992;24:2274-5.
25. Moen J, Claesson K, Pienaar BH, et al. Preservation of dog liver, kidney, and pancreas using the Belzer-UW solution with a high-sodium and low-potassium content. Transplantation. 1989;47:940-5.
26. Cartier R, Dagenais F, Hollmann C, et al. The role of preservation solutions in coronary endothelial damage during cold storage. Transplantation. 1993;56:997-1000.

27. Osswald H, Schmitz HJ, Kemper R. Tissue content of adenosine, inosine and hypoxanthine in the rat kidney after ischemia and postischemic recirculation. Pflugers Arch. 1977;371:45-9.
28. Southard JH, Belzer FO. The University of Wisconsin organ preservation solution: components, comparisons, and modifications. Transpl Rev. 1993;7:176-90.
29. Belzer FO, Southard JH: Organ preservation and transplantation. Prog Clin Biol Res. 1986;224:291-303.30.
30. Gubernatis G, Pichlmayr R, Lamesch P, et al. HTK-solution (Bretschneider) for human liver transplantation. First clinical experiences. Langenbecks Arch Chir. 1990;375:66-70.
31. Erhard J, Lange R, Schere R, et al. Comparison of histidine-tryptophan-ketoglutarate (HTK) solution versus. University of Wisconsin (UW) solution for organ preservation in human liver transplantation. A prospective, randomized study. Transpl Int. 1994;7:177-81.
32. Eghtesad B, Fontes P, Cacciarelli TV, et al. Comparison of histidine-tryptophan-ketoglutarate (HTK) solution vs. University of Wisconsin (UW) solution for organ preservation in liver transplantation. Hepatology. 2002;36(2):2052.
33. Chan SC, Liu CL, Lo CM, et al. Applicability of histidine-tryptophan-ketoglutarate solution in right lobe adult-to-adult live donor liver transplantation. Liver Transpl. 2004;10:1415-21.
34. Canelo R, Hakim NS, Ringe B. Experience with histidine-tryptophan-ketoglutarate versus University of Wisconsin preservation in transplantation. Int Surg. 2003;88:145-51.
35. Testa G, Malago M, Nadalin S, et al. Histidine-tryptophan-ketoglutarate versus University of Wisconsin solution in living donor liver transplantation: results of a prospective study. Liver Transpl. 2003;9:822-6.
36. Fondevila C, Hessheimer AJ, Maathuis MH, et al. Superior preservation of DCD livers with continuous normothermic perfusion. Ann Surg. 2011;254(6):1000-117.37.
37. op den Dries S, Karimian N, Sutton ME, et al. Ex vivo normothermic machine perfusion and viability testing of discarded human donor livers. Am J Transpl. 2013;13(5):1327-35.

CHAPTER 108

Anesthetic Management in Liver Transplantation

Vijay Vohra

INTRODUCTION

Liver transplantation has become a viable option for patients with advanced liver disease to prolong life with improved quality. Advances in anesthesia and perioperative care, improvement in immunosuppression and surgical techniques have all contributed to this reality. The anesthetic management of these patients still remains complex and challenging. Preoperative evaluation aims to identify patients who need to be optimized before surgery. The results of liver transplant surgery have improved throughout the 1990s but major bleeding, coagulopathy, electrolyte disturbances, and cardiovascular instability still occur more frequently than in any other routine surgical procedure.

The organs from cadaveric donors are limited while the number of the patients on the waiting list for orthotopic liver transplantation continues to grow. This is a major issue in Asian countries where availability of cadaveric organs is limited due to social and cultural reasons. This has led to development of live donor liver transplant (LDLT) program which forms the major share of organs transplanted in India at present.

Although deceased donor liver transplant (DDLT) has less complications and better survival, LDLT also has some advantages. One advantage is that the liver donation from a healthy individual is usually of predictable good quality. The operation can be planned and there is potential good tissue matching. The decreased waiting time reduces the potential deaths from decompensation while waiting for deceased liver. The surgical procedure for LDLT, however, is technically challenging. The main drawback with LDLT is the risk to healthy donor, who is otherwise well. A wide range of complications are reported in the donors after LDLT. This modality may have a potential psychological burden on the donor but can also give satisfaction of having done something noble and fulfilling. Psychological assessment is essential for the donors. The donor is made aware that the liver grows up to 85% of its normal size within a period of weeks.

Donor safety is paramount in living donor transplants and only donors who have no significant comorbid condition are taken up for organ donation. The number of LDLT performed in Asia has continued to increase with cadaveric transplants contributing to the overall numbers in a very small way. On the other hand in the United States, LDLT accounted for less than 5% of liver transplants and cadaveric transplants remain the mainstay of liver transplant program. The number of LDLT procedures performed in Japan, Korea, India, China, and Hong Kong has progressively increased over the years. In India, both live donor and deceased donor programs are operational but well-established transplant centers are practicing more of live donor transplants. At our center at Medanta, The Medicity Hospital in Gurgaon, India it is mainly LDLT with only sporadic cases of cadaveric transplants. The main reason is that the awareness about cadaveric organ donation is lacking apart from the religious beliefs, which form hindrance in the way of organ donation after brain death is pronounced. Cardiac standstill is still practiced as death of an individual, unless there is possibility of organ donation. Cadaveric liver transplant programs have been successfully undertaken in Chennai and in Research and Referral Hospital of army. For DDLT, organ allocation is based on Child–Turcotte–Pugh (CTP) score, which is the widely used method of assessing severity of liver disease. It has a number of fallacies, including subjective nature of assessment of encephalopathy and ascites, besides the score being discontinuous in nature. There is a ceiling for the objective variables as well, that is, if international normalized ratio (INR) is more than 2.3, bilirubin >3 mg%, and albumin<2.5 g%. This has led to change in the allocation policy which is not based on the duration the patient is on the waiting list. The new organ allocation policy uses model for end-stage liver disease (MELD) score as a predictor of mortality and for priority of organ allocation on the waiting list for liver transplantation.[1,2]

Preanesthetic Evaluation

Preoperative evaluation is done in two stages. In the first stage, all the listed transplant candidates are examined and evaluated. The second stage assessment is performed 1 or 2 days before the surgery. The aim of the assessment is firstly to identify prohibitive risks, which must be addressed before attempting transplant, e.g., significant pulmonary hypertension and gross hyponatremia. Neurologic deterioration since the first stage evaluation, any infection, metabolic acidosis, or sepsis should be sought and corrected. Similarly coagulopathy, cardiovascular instability, pulmonary infection, should also be treated to ensure that patient is optimized for surgery. Packed red cells can be infused to build up preoperative hemoglobin, aiming for 10 g% but fresh frozen plasma, cryoprecipitate and platelets, are infused only if there are bleeding tendencies. Relevant investigations—hemoglobin, total counts, arterial blood gases, urea, creatinine, liver function test, and electrolytes including coagulogram are repeated as they serve as a baseline reference.

Assessment of renal function in the perioperative phase is critical for these patients. Poor renal function predicts poor prognosis, higher risk for intraoperative blood loss and postoperative need for dialysis.[3] Creatinine clearance is more sensitive than serum creatinine and is preferred indicator for renal function. Hepatorenal syndrome (HRS) should be suspected as the cause of renal failure and treated aggressively. Vasopressin analogues, terlipressin in the dose of 0.5–2.0 mg upto four times a day along with albumin infusion has been seen to improve renal function with improvement of serum creatinine levels and creatinine clearance. Large volume paracentasis along with albumin infusion has also shown beneficial results in terms of improved renal function.

Cardiovascular assessment is done with electrocardiography and echocardiography. Patients of chronic liver disease can easily develop fluid overload and functional tricuspid regurgitation might be visible on echocardiography. Cardiomyopathy is known to exist in alcoholic liver disease, which is revealed on echocardiography or on stress testing. End-stage liver disease is associated with low systemic vascular resistance and high cardiac output and may precipitate ischemic event in patients with compromised coronary vasculature.

Ascites of portal hypertension is sometimes accompanied with hydrothorax. Hydrothorax is normally left alone unless it causes respiratory compromise in which event therapeutic drainage is done. If there is doubt of underlying pathology, computerized tomography of the chest is done to rule out consolidation underlying the hydrothorax. In the Indian subcontinent, pulmonary tuberculosis should be ruled out in presence of fluid in the chest.

Risk Stratification

The disease severity scoring of these patients is based on two clinical and three laboratory parameters (Table 1), originally based on Child-Pugh classification and later modified to CTP.

Although CTP score gives a fair estimate of severity of the disease, it does not correlate very well with the outcome of the patient following liver transplantation.

Table 1: Child–Turcotte–Pugh score

	1	*2*	*3*
Encephalopathy	None	1 and 2	3 and 4
Ascites	Absent/slight	Moderate	Not controlled by diuretics
Bilirubin mg%	1–2	2–3	>3
Albumin g%	>3.5	2.8–3.5	<2.8
PT (INR)	<1.7	1.7–2.3	>2.3

*Child–Pugh Class A: 5–6, Class B: 7–9, Class C: 10–15.

Modifications in Child–Turcotte–Pugh Score

There have been attempts to modify CTP score as it has a few drawbacks. The major drawback of having parameters which are subjective in nature has been taken care of by MELD score. There have been attempts to incorporate serum creatinine in the CTP score, in the score suggested by Samiullah et al.[4] They found usefulness of creatinine modified CTP score only in patients in CTP class B.

Model for End-stage Liver Disease Score

This was first used in reference to patients of portal hypertension undergoing trans-jugular intrahepatic porto-systemic shunts (TIPS). Since 2002, it has replaced CTP score for allocation of organs in patients awaiting liver transplants in the United States. Using MELD for organ allocation has reduced the mortality of waiting list patient for liver transplant.

Model for end-Stage liver disease is another method of categorizing the patients awaiting liver transplantation. It takes into consideration serum bilirubin, prothrombin time (INR), and serum creatinine. Patient having had hemodialysis pretransplant affects the calculation of MELD score. If patient has had two dialyses in last 1 week creatinine is taken automatically as four in the calculations. It is a mathematical calculation and is calculated by the following formula:

$$\text{MELD score} = 0.957 \times \text{Loge (creatinine mg/dL)} + 0.378 \times \text{Loge (bilirubin mg/dL)} + 1.120 \times \text{Loge (INR)} + 0.6431$$

Multiply the score by 10 and round it to the nearest whole number.

Laboratory values less than 1.0 are set to 1.0 for the purposes of the MELD score calculation

Model for end-stage liver disease is modified in case of hepatocellular carcinoma. Irrespective of other parameters, the minimum score automatically becomes 22.

Extra-MELD points are also given to patients who have developed hepatopulmonary syndrome. Their PaO_2 values are less than 70 mmHg, implying the advanced nature of liver dysfunction and prioritization of such patients.

There have been further modifications of MELD as well. Among those which have been found useful in categorizing disease severity are Na MELD and Delta MELD. Both these MELD variants do need to be validated on a larger scale.

Pediatric End-stage Liver Disease Score

For children under the age of 12 years, different criteria for listing them for liver transplantation, pediatric end-stage liver disease

(PELD) score is used. Besides age, it takes into consideration serum albumin, Prothrombin time (INR), weight, and bilirubin. The mathematical calculation is as follows:

$$\text{PELD score} = 10 \times (0.480 \times (\text{bilirubin}) + 1.857 \times (\text{INR}) - 0.687 \times (\text{albumin}) + 0.436$$

Pediatric end-stage liver disease score calculation takes into account if the child is less than 1 year and if there is growth failure.

There have been developments in incorporating other parameters for assessing disease severity, the most prominent being serum sodium. Hyponatremia indicates severity of chronic liver disease and is associated with poor prognosis. Serum sodium is incorporated in the recently adopted score in United Kingdom and is called United Kingdom end-stage liver disease (UKELD). The validity of this score in organ allocation or outcome after transplant is yet to be established in prospective studies. The calculation is done as follows:

$$\text{UKELD score} = (5.395 \times \text{INR}) + (1.485 \times \text{S. Creatinine}) + (3.13 \times \text{S. Bilirubin}) - (81.565 \times \text{S. Na}) + 435$$

A score of 49 is required before a patient is listed for transplantation and this signifies 9% 1 year mortality risk. A score of 60, on the other hand is associated with 50% mortality in 1 year.[5]

ACUTE LIVER FAILURE

The patients with acute liver disease cannot be rated according to CTP or MELD. The most accepted criteria for Fulminant hepatic failure are the King's College Criteria and Clichy's Criteria.

1. **Criteria of King's College, London**
   This is the criteria accepted for patients to be listed for liver transplantation. The criteria differs for those who develop liver failure from acetaminophen and those from non acetaminophen causes.
   I. Acetaminophen toxicity patients
      a. pH<7.3 or
      b. Prothrombin time >6.5 (INR) and serum creatinine level >3.4 mg/dL
   II. Other patients (non-acetaminophen)
      a. Prothrombin time >6.5(INR) or
      b. Any three of the following variables:
         1. Age <10 years or >40 years
         2. Etiology: non-A, non-B hepatitis, halothane hepatitis, idiosyncratic drug reaction
         3. Duration of jaundice before encephalopathy >7 days
         4. Prothrombin time >3.5 (INR)
         5. Serum bilirubin level >17.6 mg/dL
2. **Clichy's criteria**
   This is based on French data on patients with viral hepatitis. Patients qualifying to undergo emergency liver transplant are:
   1. Age < 30 years - Factor V level <20%
   2. Age > 30 years - Factor V level < 30%

Preoperative Preparation

Preoperative preparation includes reevaluation of the patient, especially if the patient has been admitted from home. All patients must undergo screening process to rule out any infective issues. Culture of blood, urine and ascitic fluid is done. A chest X-ray is done to check if there was hydrothorax or gross ascites, which can affect lung bases. Arterial blood gases analyses are done to rule out metabolic acidosis, which is seen especially if there is development of portal vein thrombosis. Poor oxygenation is seen in hepatopulmonary syndrome for which liver transplant is curative though these patients may have a prolonged intensive care stay. Echocardiography is done to rule out pericardial effusion and any alteration of cardiac function. The need for incentive spirometry is emphasized and patients educated about its use. Premedication with anxiolytics is generally not required except in children or younger patients.

Induction and Intubation

All patients are induced in operating theatre and the patient is placed on a gel mattress which is thermostatically controlled with warm water circulating at 39–41°C. Forced air warmer can also be used to keep upper and lower body warm. An electrocardiogram (ECG) monitor, pulse oximeter and automatic blood pressure monitor are attached to the patient before induction. In sicker patients, it is better to have arterial cannulation done before induction to monitor and to take appropriate action during the induction process. In sicker patients, it is better to have arterial cannulation before induction of anesthesia to monitor hemodynamic responses during the process of induction. Anesthesia is usually induced with midazolam 1–2 mg, fentanyl 1–1.5 mcg/kg and propofol 1–2 mg/kg. Induction dose requirement of propofol may be higher in chronic liver disease due to increased volume of distribution.

This may be followed by suxamethonium if the patient has gross ascites or is likely to be full stomach, otherwise a nondepolarizing relaxant can be used to facilitate endotracheal intubation. Anesthesia is maintained with fentanyl 1–2 mcg/kg/h with air/oxygen/desflurane or isoflurane. Use of nitrous oxide is avoided as it causes distension of intestines on prolonged use by diffusion into the intraluminal space in the bowel.[6] There is always possibility of air embolism in liver transplant surgery, which makes use of nitrous oxide hazardous as it increases the size of embolic air bubbles instead of getting absorbed quickly.

The volatile agent of choice has been isoflurane, which preserves splanchnic blood flow better than other volatile agents.[7] There is evidence that hepatic artery buffer response is better preserved with isoflurane than other inhalational agents.[8] Rocuronium or vecuronium are the preferred muscle relaxants, rocuronium probably has a slight advantage as this relaxant does not have any active metabolite. In a patient where an early extubation is not planned, either of the agents can be used as none of them has any hepato-toxic effects. Atracurium is metabolized by Hoffman's elimination which is pH dependent and is unaffected by liver or kidney function. The breakdown product of atracurium is laudanosine which is excreted by the kidney. This becomes relevant in the event of patients with hepatic encephalopathy in presence of preexisting renal dysfunction as laudanosine has central nervous system effects.

Vascular Access

Venous

Liver transplant surgery is associated with unpredictable blood loss. Losses are expectedly more if there is a history of previous upper abdominal surgery or the patient is highly coagulopathic and has significant portal hypertension. Peripheral venous access

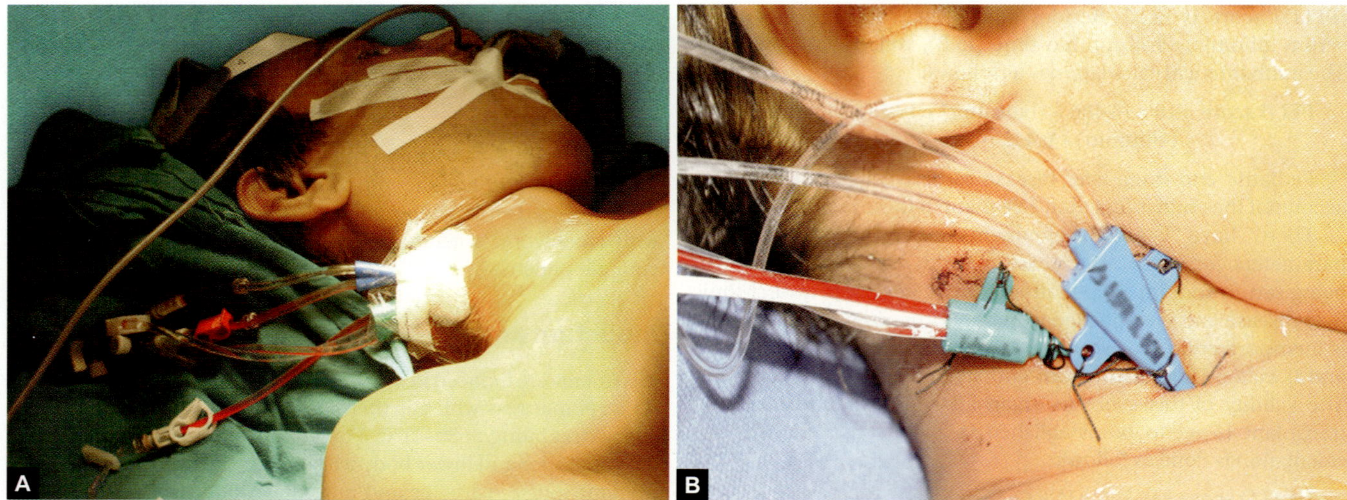

Figure 1 Vascular access in adults (A) and children (B). Preferred site right internal jugular

may be difficult if the patient has had previous hospital admissions before the transplant.

Large-bore intravenous infusions are set up in the arms if peripheral access is available. After induction of anesthesia, central venous cannulation is done. As the patients are generally coagulopathic it is better to use ultrasound guidance for location of internal jugular vein thereby preventing inadvertent arterial puncture and hematoma formation. There is generally no need to correct coagulopathy before obtaining central venous access when ultrasound is being used for guidance. Typically two central venous catheters are inserted, among them one is a large bore for rapid infusion and another triple/four lumen for infusion of drugs and blood products (Fig. 1A). In children also two central venous catheters are inserted and the preferred side is right internal jugular vein (Fig. 1B). Pulmonary artery catheter (PAC) is floated to monitor pulmonary artery pressures. Internal jugular vein, preferably the right side, is the route selected due to the straighter course of the vein. At Medanta, The Medicity Hospital, we use advance venous access catheter 7.5F which has triple lumen and a port for floating PAC. If veno-venous bypass is to be used then either 10F catheter is used or axillary vein is used on the left side. If axillary vein is to be used for inflow, open access is usually obtained surgically. Veno-venous bypass has not been used at our institution for any of the last 500 patients undergoing liver transplantation.

Arterial

Arterial access is required for direct measurement of blood pressure as well as for frequent blood sampling during transplantation. Radial artery is the preferred artery and nondominant side (generally left) is used for this purpose. Other sites that can be used are dorsalis pedis, femoral, or even brachial. Some centers prefer using two arteries—radial and femoral, one each for monitoring and sampling. Our practice is to use one artery and the radial is the preferred one. In small children radial access may be difficult and femoral arterial cannulation may be required. Seldinger technique is used for arterial cannulation using 20G or 22G cannula depending on the age of the recipient.

Intraoperative Monitoring

Special emphasis is on comprehensive monitoring of hemodynamic, coagulation, renal, and respiratory systems. The hemodynamic changes can be sudden and extreme in nature with cardiac output varying drastically during vena caval clamping and reperfusion. Blood loss could be sudden and massive, besides coagulopathy adding to the continuous blood loss and blood product infusion.

A multifunction patient monitored along with cardiac output monitoring is essential for these patients (Fig. 2). Continuous intravascular pressure monitoring is mandatory and there is a case for having two arterial catheters. All patients do have central venous catheters and in selected patients, there is need to have PAC as well. Pulmonary artery catheter can be used for measuring

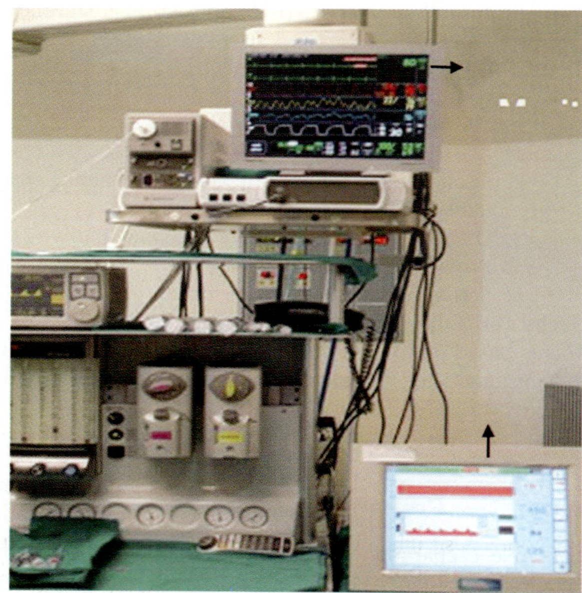

Figure 2 Multifunction patient monitor and lithium dilution cardiac output monitor

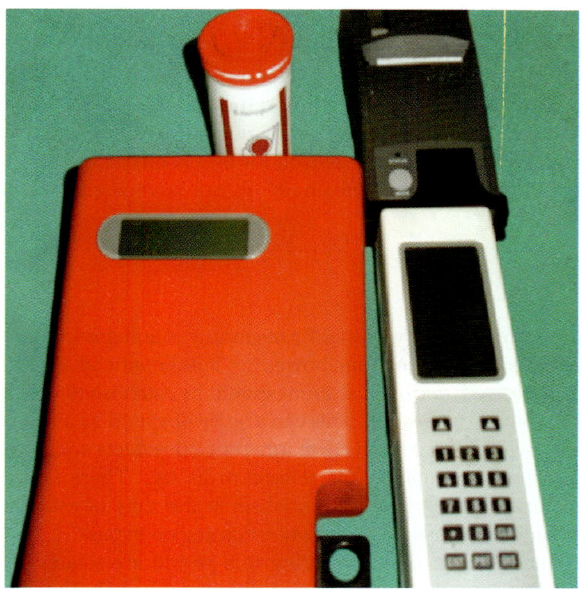

Figure 3 Hemoglobinometer and blood gas analyzer

cardiac output by thermodilution method as well as to monitor pulmonary artery pressures which are increased in patients with porto-pulmonary hypertension. Mean pulmonary artery pressure (MPAP) higher than 35 mmHg is associated with poor prognosis post liver transplant and will require therapeutic measures to keep MPAP well below 35 mmHg. Mixed venous oxygen saturation can act as a good indicator of graft function at the time of reperfusion.

Another monitoring noninvasive tool which can be of use is transesophageal echocardiography (TEE). Discretion for its use is required in patients with large esophageal varices, which could bleed during insertion and manipulation of the TEE probe. It is useful to assess the volume status as well as contractility of the ventricles. It is also useful in diagnosing air embolism as well as thromboembolism, which is always a possibility during this surgery.

Temperature monitoring is essential as hypothermia affects the activity of clotting factors. The maximum temperature drop occurs in the initial induction stage and early in dissection phase. Patient should not be left exposed, except at the time of insertion of lines or during the cleaning and draping procedure. Warming mattress, heating blanket, and fluid warmers are used to keep temperature closer to 37°C.

Arterial blood gases are monitored on a regular basis, starting from induction of anesthesia (Fig. 3). It gives an account of blood oxygenation, sodium, potassium, pH, calcium, glucose, and hemoglobin. These parameters are subject to change during surgery and their regular monitoring is essential for safe conduct of anesthesia. The use of blood and blood products could lead to citrate toxicity as it is not metabolized by the liver which is sub-optimal in function. Citrate binds to calcium and will lead to hypocalcemia and would need correction with calcium chloride on a continuous basis if blood or blood products are infused. Equally important is monitoring of sodium as a significant number of these patients have hyponatremia and rapid correction of sodium can lead to pontine myelinosis, which has a very grave prognosis.

Intraoperative Coagulation

Most patients with end-stage liver disease have coagulopathy along with low platelet count. Low fibrinogen level with dysfibrinogenemia and raised level of fibrinogen degradation products suggest on going fibrinolysis.

Coagulation screen and full blood count along with PT/INR is done in all patients. A full coagulation screen, including platelet count, fibrinogen levels, and thromboelastography (TEG), are routinely done to monitor coagulation.[9]

Intraoperatively the coagulation parameters—PT, APTT, platelet, and TEG are monitored and if required FFP and or platelets are infused accordingly. Absolute number of platelets probably does not reflect state of coagulation in these patients of chronic liver disease with portal hypertension and hypersplenism. Thromboelastography is a better modality to ascertain requirement of platelets in this group of patients. Prolonged reaction time along with maximum amplitude less than 40 mm justifies platelet supplementation.

At Medanta, The Medicity, it is our practice to have onsite coagulation monitoring in operating theatre and TEG is used for assessing coagulation status and administering blood products (Figs 4 and 5). Thromboelastometry is done at the start of the surgery, once or twice during dissection phase, during anhepatic phase, an hour after reperfusion, and at any time there is unexplainable bleeding. Other coagulation monitoring methods are also available which provide global coagulation monitoring. These are rotational thromboelastometry (ROTEM) and sonoclot.

High-risk patients (those with portal hypertension, history of upper abdominal surgery, or bacterial peritonitis) may require prophylactic antifibrinolytic therapy. Subclinical fibrinolysis is present in most patients with chronic liver disease and some centers advocate the use of antifibrinolytic therapy in all patients for liver transplant for chronic liver disease as this is known to reduce overall blood and blood product requirement. There are case reports implicating use of antifibrinolytics with thrombotic events in the recipients.

Antifibrinolytic therapy is used in the form of Tranexamic acid, 1 g bolus followed by 6 g over 24 hours. Other option is aprotinin infusion 50,000 unit test dose, and after 15 minutes, 2 million units

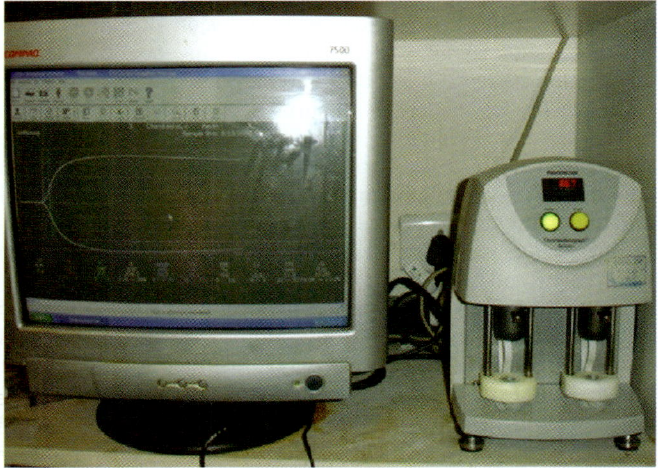

Figure 4 Two-channel TEG machine with active monitoring screen

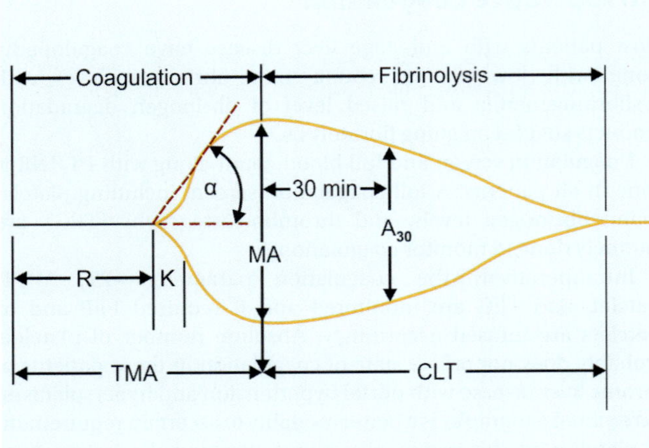

Figure 5 Thromboelastograph showing various components –R, K, R +K time, α angle, MA A 60

over 30 minutes, followed by 500,000 units per hour till the end of surgery. Patients with Budd-Chiari syndrome, hepatocellular carcinoma or those with a history of deep vein thrombosis or other thrombotic tendency are excluded from prophylactic antifibrinolytic therapy.

Phases of Transplantation

Dissection Phase

The beginning of the surgery itself gives a clue to the likely course of the transplant procedure. Coagulopathy, earlier, should be corrected promptly and aggressively, as chasing the abnormal numbers leads to more and more blood loss. On the other hand, abnormal coagulation numbers like increased prothrombin time is not always accompanied with excessive bleeding. The major cardiovascular changes associated with this stage are those related to intravascular volume depletion as a result of blood loss, manipulation of liver, and handling of the inferior vena cava (IVC). During this period, the most important consideration is to maintain intravascular volume by infusion of blood, blood products and colloids, depending on the hematocrit and coagulation status. The blood loss in this phase could be massive, especially in those patients with portal hypertension and previous upper abdominal surgery. Calcium chloride/gluconate must be added in adequate dose to avoid hypotension due to hypocalcemia caused by blood and blood products infusion. Citrate in the blood and blood products binds the calcium forming calcium citrate. As the liver is not functioning adequately, citrate is not metabolized to bicarbonate and calcium is not released.

Once dissection of the liver is done and all the vessels and bile duct have been isolated, trial clamping of IVC is performed to see how well this manoeuvre will be tolerated when new liver is being revascularized. The trial clamping is done for at least 1 minute to see the hemodynamic effects. There is an expected drop in cardiac output and it is to be assessed whether this period of IVC clamping can be managed with vasopressors and volume adjustments. Adequacy of the patient's ability to withstand caval clamping is thereby assessed. If the systolic pressure falls to less than 70% of its previous value, (or SAP<80–90 mmHg, or MAP <60 mmHg), in the presence of adequate blood replacement, or if ECG changes occur, bypass support may be needed. In our center at Medanta, The Medicity we rarely resort to veno-venous bypass during IVC clamping. One reason for that is the patients who are accepted for transplants normally do not have significant heart disease.

Anhepatic Phase

Clamping of portal vein marks the beginning of anhepatic phase and this causes congestion of the bowel.[10,11] If anhepatic phase is likely to be prolonged, porto-caval shunt should be established which will prevent bowel congestion. This can also be obviated by using veno-venous bypass, but it has its own inherent side effects and potential of developing complications related to its use. There is distinct possibility of developing air embolism at the time of establishing veno-venous bypass as well as when coming on bypass.[12]

Hemodynamic changes during this period are related to IVC cross-clamping and to physiological changes caused by the removal of the liver. Some patients, who were unstable during dissection phase start stabilizing during anhepatic phase because the liver which was producing various vasoactive substances is now out of circulation. On the other hand with liver out, some patient would start showing signs of fibrinolysis as tissue plasminogen activator is not being removed from the circulation. Inferior vena cava cross-clamping results in a decrease in cardiac output which is more marked in the absence of extensive collaterals as seen in patients with hepatocellular carcinoma. Inferior vena cava side-clamping is done if the patient does not tolerate cross-clamping or if there is preoperative renal dysfunction. Removal of the native liver leads to reduction in oxygen consumption, which also contributes to the fall in cardiac output. Absence of liver function results in inability to metabolize citrate; citrate intoxication presents with decreased ionized calcium and myocardial depression. Hypocalcemia must be corrected before reperfusion to counter the effects of release of potassium from the ischemic and cold preserved liver graft when it comes into circulation.

Attempts to increase filling pressures by blood and fluid replacement must be cautious at this stage, due to the danger of fluid overload at the time of liver revascularization, when normal venous return and central blood volume is restored. Piggyback technique decreases the need for VVB.[13-17]

Reperfusion Phase

Reperfusion of the new liver is accompanied with changes due to ischemia reperfusion injury. The extent of this injury can be minimized by giving prednisolone before reperfusion in the dose of 10 mg/kg. Still reperfusion can cause dramatic cardiovascular changes, which may or may not last for a long time.[18] There is a sudden increase in serum potassium levels, which may be offset by giving calcium bolus. There could be sudden decrease in heart rate, mean arterial pressure and systemic vascular resistance due to release of vasoactive substances from ischemic liver graft and from static blood from the gut. It is important to ensure that ionized calcium levels are greater than 1.1 mmol/L before reperfusion. Treat hypotension with phenylephrine, or noradrenaline, which should be connected through a syringe pump connected to a running infusion. It is common practice to use one of these prophylactically, along with calcium chloride, at the time of unclamping of the portal vein. Normally there is no more blood loss after this stage but at times anastomotic vascular bleed and fibrinolysis continues and may require continued antifibrinolytic therapy and blood products.

Maintenance of renal function and fluid balance: Renal dysfunction in patients with HRS is due to renal vasoconstriction without any intrinsic damage to the kidneys.[19] Hepatorenal syndrome is seen in up to 10% of patients of chronic liver disease presenting with cirrhosis and ascites.[20] Kidneys are prone to get affected during the transplant with the rapidly altering cardiac output. Effort must be made to maintain urine output during the procedure; although oliguria is usual and even anuria may occur during the period when IVC is clamped. Crystalloid infusion in the form of 5% dextrose is started from the beginning to prevent hypoglycemia. Other crystalloid used is plasmalyte A which is a pH corrected solution having pH of 7.4. Hartman's solution contains lactate which is normally metabolized in the liver and therefore may not be good choice if large volume of fluids is required. Intravascular volume is maintained with Albumin, 6% hydroxyl ethyl starch, blood, and blood products as indicated by measurements of hematocrit and TEG. Mannitol is given as free radical scavenger and as osmotic diuretic in a dose of 0.5–1.0 g/kg before IVC clamping, when an abrupt fall or temporary cessation of urine output is usual. Vena caval clamping is done while the venous anastomosis and portal venous system is being established for the new liver and this period of vena caval clamping lasts for less than 1 hour. Vasopressors may be required at this stage, nor-adrenaline, adrenaline, phenylephrine have all been used. There may be need to give intravenous fluids if there is inadequate response to vasopressors. Dopamine 200 mg in 50 mL, 5% glucose can be used at 0.5–2 mL/h if there is still inadequate urine output with the measures outlined above. Urine output maintenance is desirable although the use of low-dose dopamine for this reason is unproven.[21]

If there is evidence of renal dysfunction preoperatively, one should consider use of veno-venous bypass which maintains renal blood flow during periods of portal vein and vena caval clamping which otherwise produces low flow states.

Option to consider in patients with renal dysfunction is to avoid complete venous clamping and instead use a side clamp whereby a partial vena caval clamp is applied and venous return is not hampered.

Chronic liver disease is often associated with hyponatremia and rapid correction of sodium is accompanied with dire consequences. Sodium level should be maintained closer to the preoperative levels and certainly not increase by more than 10–12 mmol/L in 24 hours which can lead to central pontine myelinosis.[22]

Intraoperative Issues

Major bleeding: This procedure has a potential to have rapid and sudden blood loss and it is essential to transfuse at a rate sufficient to maintain hemodynamic parameters in the near normal range. Some form of rapid infusion device should be available to correct the changing hemodynamic status. It should be remembered that concentrated and washed cells must be supplemented with colloids. Rapid blood replacement causes citrate intoxication leading to hypocalcemia, and even hyperkalemia.

Air/thromboembolism: This is likely to occur during dissection as well as when the graft gets back into circulation. Air embolism is seen at the time of dissection in the area of inferior vena cava. Any hole in the vena cava during dissection entraps air as vena cava is a fixed structure. This is more likely to happen if the venous pressures are low. Thromboembolism happens during re perfusion, as micro thrombi in hepatic circulation or from the veno-venous bypass circuit (if used) get back into the circulation

Metabolic acidosis: There is likelihood of developing metabolic acidosis during dissection and anhepatic phase. Metabolic acidosis develops due to tissue hypoperfusion resulting from shunting of blood from intestines to systemic circulation. Treatment should be aimed at correcting the volume status and by mild hyperventilation. Sodium bicarbonate should be used cautiously as this adds to sodium load. On reperfusion of the liver, metabolic acidosis typically worsens as a result of sudden release into the circulation of acidotic material from the ischemic liver and obstructed splanchnic bed. This is generally self-limiting and resolves over a few hours without specific treatment. It could lead to what is described as postreperfusion syndrome which is seen more in cadaveric donor liver transplant and is rare in LDLT patients.

Hypocalcemia: Ionized calcium measurements are made at regular intervals during the operation. Levels tend to be low even in the early part of the operation in patients with poor liver function, as a result of the citrate in blood products. In spite of calcium administration, these may fall further during anhepatic phase, when citrate metabolism ceases completely. If blood loss is not substantial, values return to normal after reperfusion without the need for further treatment. The aim should be to keep serum calcium within the normal range (1.1–1.3 mmol/L) at all times, especially during the period preceding reperfusion.

Hyperkalemia: This occurs on release of the clamps on portal and hepatic vein but the effect is short lasting and no specific treatment apart from prophylactic calcium chloride is indicated. When hyperkalemia is present or is likely to occur before reperfusion measures to prevent a further marked increase are essential to reduce the risk of hyperkalemic arrest at reperfusion. These include washing of bank blood (if using cell saver), glucose/insulin infusion, and calcium. Other measures used include bleed out of some portal blood and/or bleeding out a predetermined amount of blood from the hepatic veins before establishing reperfusion.

Initial poor graft function: Persistence of metabolic acidosis after reperfusion and continued hemodynamic instability should sound warning bells for poor graft functioning (Table 2). Congested or greyish appearance of the liver, coagulopathy, poor urine output, and hypotension are signs of poor graft function. Poor graft function is seen in poor quality of liver grafts mainly from

Table 2: Signs of poor graft function

1.	Hemodynamic instability
2.	Acid-base imbalance
3.	Poor urine output—renal dysfunction
4.	Persistent hypothermia
5.	Continued coagulopathy
6.	Raised liver enzymes and bilirubin
7.	Failure to regain consciousness

cadaver donors. These marginal donors are being accepted for transplantation due to shortages of donor organs and increasing waiting lists. These are more prone for ischemia reperfusion injury compared to normal grafts. This issue is almost nonexistent in live donor liver transplants. Management includes continued use of N-acetylcysteine 5-10 mg/kg/h, vasopressors, and control of metabolic acidosis. It could take 24 hours or longer before the liver functions start improving. There is continuous requirement for supporting coagulation-fresh frozen plasma, cryoprecipitates, as well as antifibrinolytics.

Hyponatremia: As the liver disease advances, the patient with chronic liver disease is likely to develop low serum sodium levels. In other words, hyponatremia is an indicator of disease severity. This is corrected by fluid restriction, limiting the intake to 800-1000 mL/day. Rapid correction of sodium is not advisable and correction should be in a gradual manner. Generally, a cut off value of sodium 125 mmol/L is taken as the minimum value at which the patient should be undertaken for transplantation. Intra operatively a closed watch should be kept in such patients so as to prevent rise in serum sodium levels. An acceptable limit of serum sodium is 8-10 mmol increase in 24 hours. This becomes relevant if the patient develops metabolic acidosis which needs correction by giving sodium bicarbonate infusion. This will lead to rapid rise in sodium level and makes patient prone to developing central pontine mylenosis, which has very poor outcome.

Postreperfusion syndrome: This is defined as decrease in mean arterial pressure of more than 30%, occurring in the first 5 minutes after reperfusion of the graft and lasting for more than 1minute. The incidence of post reperfusion syndrome (PRS) varies significantly and is seen in up to 50% of the liver transplant recipients.[23,24] There are various known factors which contribute to development of PRS. These could be related to the donor variables as well as surgical factors. Older patients greater than 50 years of age, large dose of inotropes in the deceased donor, prolonged cold ischemia time, fatty liver, long warm ischemia time are some of the factors associated with post reperfusion syndrome. Post reperfusion syndrome would require inotropic support and calcium supplementation. If the metabolic acidosis is pronounced, it will require correction with sodium bicarbonate infusion. The hospital stay as well as the intensive care stay of the patient with PRS could be prolonged.[25]

Blood Conservation Strategies

Blood transfusion during liver transplantation is associated with increased morbidity and mortality.[26] Liver transplantation is at times associated with large blood losses and various conservation strategies are adopted to minimize blood/blood product requirement. Plasma transfusion for correction of coagulation defect may not decrease blood loss during liver transplantation; it can even lead to a hypervolemic state which can even increase blood loss during surgery. Various approaches have been practiced to minimize blood transfusion and each one has its own advantages and drawbacks.

Low central venous pressure: To reduce blood losses during liver dissection before the anhepatic phase, various measures can be employed One of them is lowering of central venous pressure (CVP). Central venous pressure can be lowered by fluid restriction, phlebotomy, and by avoiding plasma transfusion in order and hence diminish the transfusion of blood products. This practice of reducing CVP does not result in any deleterious results.[27] Hepatorenal syndrome is seen in up to 30% of patients of liver transplant for end-stage liver disease and fluid restriction in these patients could be detrimental for the renal outcome. Judicious fluid therapy has to be adopted in this group of patients.

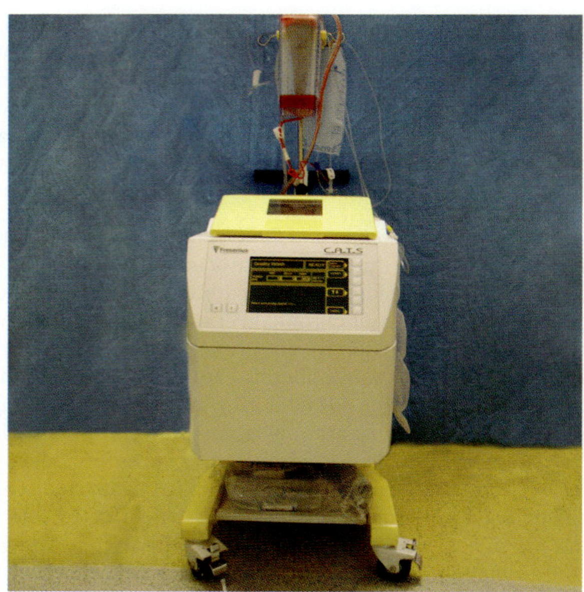

Figure 6 Cell saver

Cell saver: The use of intraoperative cell saver shows a reduction of blood and components transfusion. In a prospective study published recently, the use of cell saver was shown not only to reduce transfusion but also could be cost effective.[28] Cell saver (Fig. 6) use has the potential to reduce the need for heterologous transfusion, thereby reducing the risks of disease transmission and allied cost. One aspect that needs to be kept in mind is that with cell saver, one is using blood which has come out of the abdominal cavity, gone into collection bags, washed, collected into other bags, and then reinfused. During this travel from the abdominal cavity to reinfusion, there is a possibility of contamination and infection.

Thromboelastography: This is method of monitoring whole blood coagulation by measuring viscoelastic changes occuring in the process of clot formation. Thromboelastography is the only test which measures dynamic steps of clot formation. The test starts from initial clot formation and shows the clot lysis, if it occurs after initial clot formation.

Routine use of TEG in the surgical theatre is another means to reduce transfusion of blood components, especially fresh frozen plasma and platelets. Another means of blood loss reduction is the use of recombinant activated factor VII (rFVIIa). Two recent retrospective studies obtained favorable results with reduced transfusion of packed red blood cells and fresh frozen plasma in the patients treated with rFVIIa.[29,30]

Antifibrinolytic: Use of antifibrinolytic can also reduce intra operative bleeding, as there is some amount of fibrinolysis going on in most patients with chronic liver disease. This is due to presence of circulating tissue plasminogen activator during the anhepatic phase and its burst release during reperfusion of the liver graft. Aprotinin has been shown to reduce transfusion requirements in surgeries with significant blood loss.[31] The European multicenter study of aprotinin in liver transplant showed a reduction in the use of red blood cells with high and regular dose of aprotinin in liver transplant recipients.[32] Tranexamic acid is another agent which has been used successfully in preventing fibrinolysis thereby reducing blood loss. Its use was first reported in liver transplant recipient in 1980s. The dose regime has been variable ranging from 2 mg/kg/h to 40 mg/kg/h.[33]

Postoperative Care

Monitoring continues in the postoperative period from where it was left in the operating theater. Pulmonary artery pressure (PAP) monitoring may be discontinued in the intensive care unit, if the pressures are near normal and remain stable. The PAC should be removed after having seen position on chest X-ray. Most patients' posttransplant is ventilated for a variable period depending on their preoperative status and the intraoperative course. Selected patients can be extubated early in the immediate postoperative period on transfer to the intensive care unit. Postoperative routine investigations include hemoglobin, PT, APTT, platelet count, SGOT, SGPT, sodium, potassium, calcium, and creatinine.

There has been an interest to fast track some of these patients from the intensive care unit. To fast track successfully, patients should be chosen carefully and short-acting drugs should be used. Use of benzodiazepine and narcotics is calculated to allow early return of spontaneous breathing and consciousness at the end of surgery. Patients with encephalopathy, large blood and blood product requirement, obesity, high Child-Pugh score are not good candidates for fast tracking. Similarly, patients with obesity and preoperative encephalopathy are poor candidates for immediate extubation. One must be very careful in selecting patients for fast tracking. It is not true that endotracheal extubation at the end of surgery will result in shorter intensive-care-unit stay or in cost saving. All patients postoperatively still require close monitoring.

Keeping a low venous pressure enables a better venous drainage from the newly grafted liver. So if positive end expiratory pressure and intermittent positive pressure can be avoided or minimized in the perioperative period, it may be beneficial for the new liver. Aggressive chest physiotherapy is done post extubation and incentive spirometry. All patients are counseled preoperatively about the need to do incentive spirometry in postoperative phase in the intensive care unit, though it is not possible in patients with encephalopathy.

Vascular Doppler is carried out at least once a day to know the blood flow in portal vein, hepatic vein, and hepatic artery. In children, the Doppler studies are conducted twice a day. The re-exploration rate is much higher in children due to hepatic artery thrombosis or other vascular flows. Some of the children may require heparin infusion postoperatively to prevent thrombotic complications.

Abdominal drain is monitored for the quantity of drainage produced every hour. If required drain hemoglobin is measured and if the value is close to patient's hemoglobin, intra-abdominal bleed, or coagulopathy should be strongly suspected. Thromboelastography at this stage may help in differentiating medical bleed from surgical bleed. In surgical bleed the TEG will be near normal

Postoperative infection is a major hazard in these patients. Over 80% mortality in liver transplant is related to infective issues. Barrier nursing, hand hygiene and appropriate antibiotic therapy should be used in these immunocompromised patients. Immunosuppression in liver transplants can be introduced up to 72 hours posttransplant as liver is much less immunogenic compared with other organs like kidney.

Liver transplantation is at a threshold in this country and is ready to take off and become a routine procedure. The number of liver transplant centers in India has grown significantly in the last 5 years. It requires dedicated multidisciplinary approach with commitment from surgery, anesthesiology, hepatology, blood transfusion services, intensivists, physiotherapist, and intensive care nursing staff.

REFERENCES

1. Kamath PS, Wiesner RH, Malinchoc M, et al. A model to predict survival in patients with end-stage liver disease. Hepatology. 2001;33:464-70.
2. United Network for Organ Sharing Liver Disease Severity Score Committee, Wiesner R, Edwards E, et al. Model for end stage liver disease (MELD) and allocation of donor livers. Gastroenterology. 2003;124:91-6.
3. Pham PT, Pham PC, Wilkinson AH. The kidney in liver transplantation. Clin Liver Dis. 2000;3:567-90.
4. Samiullah S, Qasim R, Khalid S, et al. Evaluation of creatinine modified Child Pugh score for predicting short term prognosis in patients with decompensated cirrhosis of liver as compared to original Child Pugh score. J Ayub Med Coll Abbottabad. 2009;21(2):64-7.
5. Asrani SK, Kim WR. Organ allocation for chronic liver disease: model for end-stage liver disease and beyond. Curr Opin Gastroenterol. 2010;26(3):209-13.
6. Scheinin B, Lindgren L, Scheinin TM. Peroperative nitrous oxide delays bowel function after colonicsurgery. Br J Anaesth. 1990;64:154-8.
7. O'Riordan J, O'Beirne HA, Young Y, et al. Effects of desflurane and isoflurane on splanchnic microcirculation during major surgery. Br J Anaesth. 1997;78:95-6.
8. O'Riordan J, O'Beirne HA, Young Y, et al. Effects of desflurane and isoflurane on splanchnic microcirculation during major surgery. Br J Anaesth. 1997;78:95-6.
9. Ozier Y, Pessione F, Samain E, et al. Institutional variability in transfusion practice for liver transplantation. Anesth Analg. 2003;97:671-9.
10. Haagsma EB, Gips CH, Wesenhagen H, et al. Liver disease and its effect on haemostasis during liver transplantation. Liver. 1985;5:123-8.
11. Bechstein WO, Neuhaus P. Bleeding problems in liver surgery and liver transplantation. Chirurg. 2000;71:363-8.
12. Budd JM, Isaac JL, Bennett J, et al. Morbidity and mortality associated with large-bore percutaneous venovenous bypass cannulation for 312 orthotopic liver transplantations. Liver Transpl. 2001;7:359-62.
13. Tzakis A, Todo S, Starzl TE. Orthotopic liver transplantation with preservation of the inferior vena cava. Ann Surg. 1989;210:649-52.
14. Veroli P, el Hage C, Ecoffey C. Does adult liver transplantation without venovenous bypass result in renal failure? Anesth Analg. 1992;75:489-94.

15. Schwarz B, Pomaroli A, Hoermann C, et al. Liver transplantation without venovenous bypass: morbidity and mortality in patients with greater than 50% reduction in cardiac output after vena cava clamping. J Cardiothorac Vasc Anesth. 2001;15: 460-2.
16. Wall WJ, Grant DR, Duff JH, et al. Liver transplantation without venous bypass. Transplantation. 1987;43:56-61.
17. Wu Y, Oyos TL, Chenhsu RY, et al. Vasopressor agents without volume expansion as a safe alternative to venovenous bypass during cavaplasty liver transplantation. Transplantation. 2003;76:1724-8.
18. Blanot S, Gillon MC, Ecoffey C. Circulating endotoxins during orthotopic liver transplantation and post-reperfusion syndrome [letter]. Lancet. 1993;342:859-60.
19. Moreau R, Lebrec D. Hepatorenal syndrome—definitions and diagnosis. Aliment Pharmacol Ther. 2004;20(Suppl 3):24-8.
20. Gines A, Escorsell A, Gines P, et al. Incidence, predictive factors, and prognosis of hepatorenal syndrome in cirrhosis. Gastroenterology. 1993;105:229-36.
21. Swygert T. Effect of intraoperative low-dose dopamine on renal function in liver transplant recipients. Anesthesiology. 1991;75:571-6.
22. Oh MS, Kim H-J, Carroll HJ. Recommendations for treatment of symptomatic hyponatremia. Nephron. 1995;70:143-50.
23. Ramsay M. The reperfusion syndrome: have we made any progress? Liver Transpl. 2008;14:412-4.
24. Ayanoglu HO, Ulukaya S, Tokat Y. Causes of postreperfusion syndrome in living or cadaveric donor liver transplantation. Transplant Proc. 2003;35:1442-4.
25. Hilmi I, Horton CN, Planinsic RM, et al. The impact of postreperfusion syndrome on short-term patient and liver allograft outcome in patients undergoing orthotopic liver transplantation. Liver Transpl. 2008;14:504-8.
26. Ramos E, Dalmau A, Sabate A, et al. Intra operative red blood cell transfusion in liver transplantation: influence on patient outcome, prediction of requirements, and measures to reduce them. Liver Transpl. 2003;9:1320-7.
27. Massicotte L, Lenis S, Thibeault L, et al. Effect of low central venous pressure and phlebotomy on blood product transfusion requirements during liver transplantations. Liver Transpl. 2006;12:117-23.
28. Phillips SD, Deshpande R, Muiesan P, et al. A prospective study investigating the cost effectiveness of intraoperative blood salvage during liver transplantation. Transplantation. 2006;81:536-40.
29. Kalicinski P, Markiewicz M, Kaminski A, et al. Single pretransplant bolus of recombinant activated factor VII ameliorates influence of risk factors for blood loss during orthotopic liver transplantation. Pediatr Transplant. 2005;9:299-304.
30. Niemann CU, Behrends M, Quan D, et al. Recombinant factor VIIa reduces transfusion requirements in liver transplant patients with high MELD scores. Transfus Med. 2006;16:93-100.
31. Lentschener C, Roche K, Ozier Y. A review of aprotinin in orthotopic liver transplantation: can its harmful effects offset its beneficial effects? Anesth Analg. 2005;100:1248-55.
32. Porte RJ, Molenaar IQ, Begliomini B, et al. Aprotinin and transfusion requirements in orthotopic liver transplantation: a multicentre randomised double-blind study. Lancet. 2000;355:1303-9.
33. Boylan JF, Klinck JR, Sandler AN, et al. Tranexamic acid reduces blood loss, transfusion requirements, and coagulation factor in primary orthotopic liver transplantation. Anesthesiology. 1996;85:1043-8.

CHAPTER 109

Immunology of Liver Transplantation

Manav Wadhawan, John Joseph

INTRODUCTION

Liver transplantation has emerged as an ideal option for treatment of end stage liver disease. The patient survival at one year and five years after liver transplant has been reported to be 90 and 75% respectively.[1] The outcome of the liver transplantation has improved dramatically with newer immunosuppressive regimens that protect allografts from acute rejection. Hyperacute rejection is very uncommon after liver transplant, despite a positive T-cell cross match. Also, the incidence of chronic rejection is very low after liver transplant, unless patients are noncompliant with the immunosuppressive medications. Understanding immune mechanisms in liver transplant is important to identify rejection, make early diagnosis, deliver appropriate treatment, and develop strategies to minimize rejection.

TYPES OF GRAFTS

Four types of liver grafts have been described: autograft, isograft, allograft, and xenograft.[2] Autograft refers to a process where a tissue or organ is transferred from one site of the body to another within the same individual. The autografts have an obvious advantage of spontaneous tolerance, and hence do not need immunosuppressive drugs. Autografts avoid the problem of liver shortage.

An isograft is a tissue or organ transplanted between identical twins, having the same advantages as the autograft.

An allograft or homograft is a tissue or organ transplanted between different members of the same species. Allografts are prone to both acute as well as chronic rejection.

A xenograft refers to a tissue or an organ transplanted between different species. Xenotransplants are till date prone to hyperacute rejection leading to graft dysfunction.

IMMUNE SYSTEM

The immune system consists of the innate and adaptive immunities. Innate or natural immunity refers to the nonspecific response to various antigens. This response is expressed via recruitment of macrophages, neutrophils, other cells as well as cytokines even without prior exposure to these antigens. Adaptive immunity involves recognition of specific antigen as foreign and subsequent mounting immune response against these antigens via T- and B-lymphocytes. The immune response against the transplanted organ is mediated by adaptive immunity via recruitment of lymphocytes against major histocompatibility complex (MHC) molecules expressed on the surface of donor cells.

Transplantation Antigens

Transplantation antigens against which immune response is mounted are MHC molecules, minor histocompatibility antigens, endothelial cell antigens, or ABO blood group antigens.

Human Major Histocompatibility Complex

Human MHC antigens are encoded by MHC genes in short arm of chromosome 6. Human MHC antigens are called HLA (human leukocyte antigen). There are three classes of HLA complex genes: MHC class I and II genes which encode HLA cell surface antigens, and class III genes responsible for the components of the complement system (C2, C4, and factor B).

MHC class I antigens are ubiquitous in human body; these are present on all the cells and encoded by genes of the HLA-A, HLA-B, or HLA-C loci. They present intracellular parasites mainly viruses or cytoplasm derived peptides. The expression of MHC class II antigens is more restricted; they are present only on B-cells, activated T-cells, monocytes, macrophages, dendritic cells, endothelium, and epithelial cells. Class II MHC is encoded by genes of HLA-D locus. Class II MHC proteins (HLA DP, DQ, and DR) bind peptides derived from extracellular proteins. HLA class I molecules are recognized by CD8 T-cells whereas HLA class II molecules are recognized by CD4 T-cells.

Human leukocyte antigens are transmitted in generations in an autosomal dominant pattern. Haplotype are antigens of one HLA region inherited from one parent. HLA-B and DR antigens are generally considered more important than others in impacting the graft loss after transplantation.

Immunological Basis of Allograft Rejection

Allorecognition refers to identification of donor antigens as nonself by the recipient immune system. Allorecognition is largely dependent on MHC incompatibility between the host and the donor. The immune response mounted by the host lymphocytes to the donor alloantigens leads to rejection of the graft. The first step in rejection cascade is allorecognition and activation of the host CD4 and CD8 T-cells and B-cells. This is followed by activation of inflammatory cascade, which leads to destruction of the graft.[3-4] Host T-cells are responsible for the activation and perpetuation of immune response against the alloantigens of the transplanted organ.

Major histocompatibility complex incompatibility between host and donor is more important for rejection; however, recognition of minor histocompatibility (mH) antigens can also cause rejection in MHC matched organs. Further, the importance of mH antigens is evidenced by incidence of graft versus host disease and need of immunosuppression in recipients of HLA identical organs.

Hyperacute Rejection

Hyperacute rejection is seen in patients who have preformed antibodies against the MHC class I antigens of the donor. The preformed antibodies bind to endothelial antigens of the graft, and trigger activation of complement and mononuclear cells of the host causing ischemic damage, intravascular thrombosis, and hemorrhage in the graft. Such preformed antibodies are universal in case of ABO incompatible transplants, but are also seen in sensitized individuals who have received multiple transfusions. Hyperacute rejection is rarely reported in liver transplant, but is more common in kidney and other solid organ transplants. It can be prevented by cross matching donor and recipient sera prior to transplant.[2,4]

Acute Rejection

Acute rejection most commonly occurs after the first week following transplantation, but has been seen at any time after transplant. Most common precipitant is inadequate immunosuppression. Cell-mediated as well as humoral immune responses are involved in the process, and lead to both vascular and parenchymal injury of the graft. It is primarily caused by host T-cell reaction against MHC molecules present on endothelial and parenchymal cells of the graft. The initial step is activation of host CD4+ T-cells which secrete cytokines, subsequently activating cytotoxic CD8+ T-cells which recognize and lyse graft cells.

Alloreactive T-cells are activated by two distinct mechanisms: direct and indirect pathways as depicted in Figure 1.[5,6]

The primary cause of acute rejection is T-cells directly recognizing allogeneic MHC antigens. The donor alloantigens are directly presented to host T-cells by donor antigen presenting cells (APCs). This results in the production of host cytotoxic and helper T-cells. Passenger leukocytes (donor leukocytes present within the graft) migrate from the graft to the host's spleen and lymph nodes activating host T-cells.[4] These activated T-cells then launch an immune attack against the graft/foreign antigens.

The second pathway involves processing of shed allogeneic MHC molecules of donor tissue by recipient antigen presenting cells (Indirect recognition). MHC antigens are internalized by endocytosis, broken down by proteases in endosomes, and further presented to the recipient's T-cells by recipient APCs. The rejection cascade is propagated by memory T-cells due to their rapid immune response upon rechallenge. In the rejection episode, the relative contribution of direct and indirect pathways is 10 and 90%, respectively.[2]

The incidence of acute rejection has declined significantly with triple drug regimens. Rejection rates are highest with young patients with autoimmune disease and lowest with old patients with alcoholic liver disease. Rejection episodes generally start 1 week after the transplantation, and are reported to be highest in the first 42 days after liver transplant.[1] Acute rejection episodes are usually

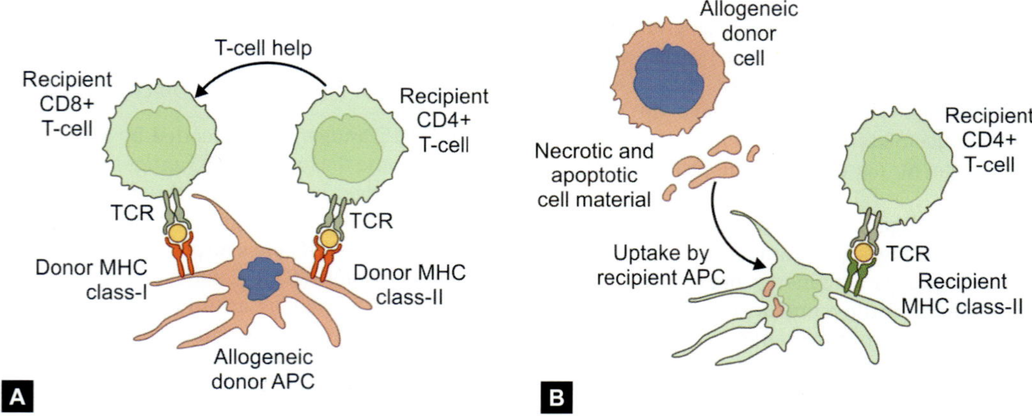

Figure 1 Pathways of alloantigen presentation: (A) Direct; (B) Indirect

mild, and respond to increasing immunosuppression (CNIs and/or steroids). Liver biopsy shows a classical picture of mixed infiltrates with predominance of lymphocytes mixed with eosinophils.

Chronic Rejection

Chronic rejection is the foremost cause of graft rejection late in the course after transplant. It can occur months but generally years after transplantation, and is marked by irreversible fibrosis and loss of graft function.[4] It is characterized by loss of bile ducts on liver biopsy, so called vanishing bile duct syndrome. Risk factors increasing the incidence of chronic rejection are previous acute rejection, ischemic injury, HLA incompatibility, inadequate immunosuppression, and infections. Activated lymphocytes in graft vessel wall induce macrophage recruitment, which initiates fibrosis. Chronic rejection is not prevented with immunosuppressives.

Clinical Human Leukocyte Antigen Testing

Role of HLA testing in liver transplantation is less established than in kidney transplant. Liver allograft is considered less prone to chronic rejection as compared to any other solid organ transplant. HLA testing before transplantation include HLA typing of the donor and recipient, screening of HLA antibodies in the recipient and cross-matching of recipient antibodies with lymphocytes of a prospective donor. This cross matching identifies recipient anti HLA antibodies to antigens on donor cells, which if present can lead to hyperacute rejection. Traditional complement dependent cytotoxicity assays have now been replaced by more sensitive assays like enzyme-linked immunosorbent assay and flow cytometry. DNA-based HLA-typing methods using molecular techniques are also available.[3]

Correlation has been noted with the development of anti-MHC class I antibodies during the posttransplant period, and development of chronic rejection. However, the exact role is still under investigation. Antibody monitoring may be an effective way to predict an impending chronic rejection.

Immunosuppressive Drugs

Immunosuppressives medications act at various sites of lymphocyte activation shown in Figure 2.[5] Donor and recipient dendritic cells activated by foreign antigens migrate to secondary lymphoid organs where they engage naïve T-cells, alloantigen and memory cells activate lymphocyte through T-cell receptor (CD3)—signal 1. CD80 and CD86 markers engage CD28 receptors on T-cells and provide costimulation or signal 2. Both signals activate signal transduction pathways including calcium calcineurine and Ras/mitogen-activated protein kinase pathways. This further triggers transcription of IL-2 and other cytokines, and activate target of rapamycin pathway and cell proliferation—signal 3. The effector T-and B-cells then elicit inflammatory response in the allograft by secretion of TNF alfa and beta, fas ligand expression, and cytotoxins like perforin and granzyme F.[1]

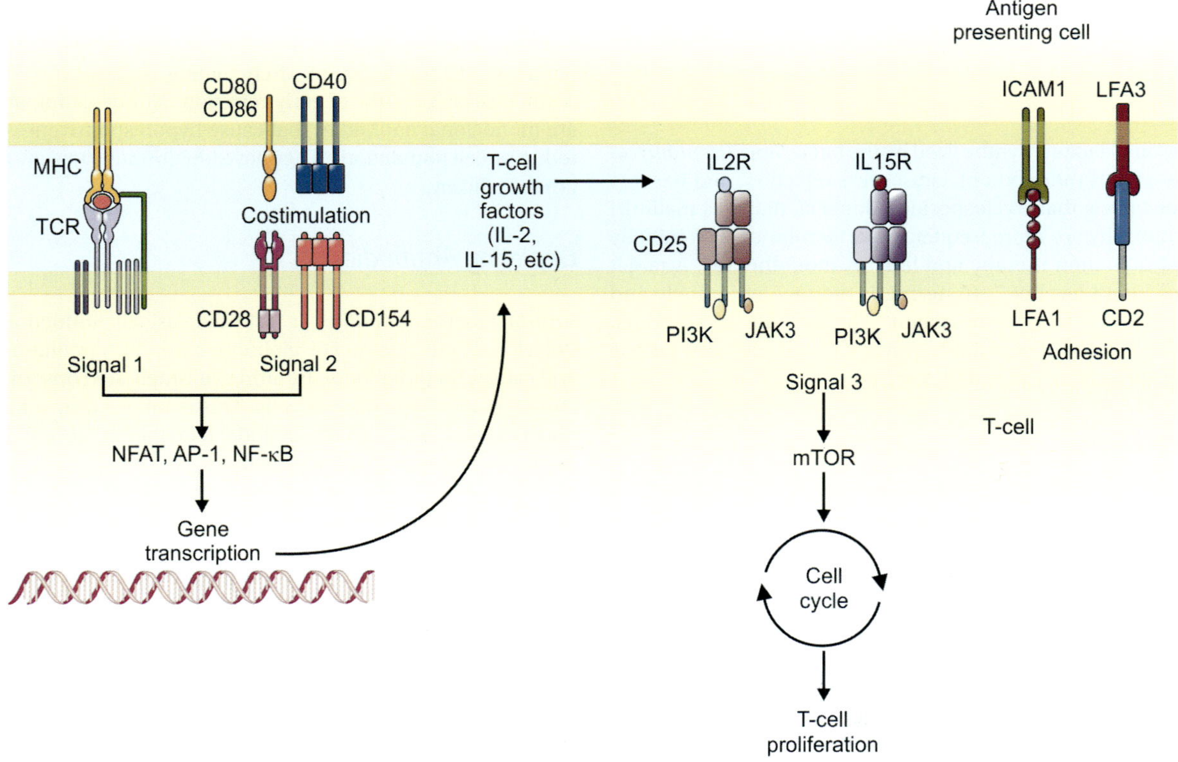

Figure 2 Targets of immunosuppressive drugs

Immunosuppressive drugs can be broadly classified in two categories:

- Pharmacological or small molecule drugs and
- Biological drugs—monoclonal or polyclonal antilymphocyte antibodies which can be lymphocyte depleting or nonlymphocyte depleting agents.[1]

Corticosteroids

Corticosteroids were introduced in late 1950s as an immunosuppressive agent. Currently, they are used at multiple stages after transplant: at the time of liver implantation as intravenous bolus (induction therapy), to prevent rejection, and in treatment of established acute cellular rejection (maintenance therapy).[1]

Steroids are tapered off in 3–6 months in maintenance therapy, except for autoimmune liver diseases. Induction therapy uses high-dose IV methylprednisolone that causes resolution in majority of acute cellular rejection.

Immunophilin Binding Agents

Calcineurin inhibitors (CNI) that suppress T-cell activation are cyclosporine and tacrolimus.

Cyclosporine

It is a cyclic fungal peptide extracted from *Cylindrocarson lucidum*. It enters cells through diffusion and active transport. Its $t_{½}$ is approximately 15 hours. In the first postoperative month, the target trough levels (C0 levels) are 250–400 ng/mL that gradually decreases to 100–200 ng/mL upto 1 year and 100 ng/mL or less later. 10% of patients on cyclosporine develop renal failure by renal vasoconstriction requiring dialysis or renal transplant in 10 years.[7]

Tacrolimus

It is a macrolide lactone synthesized by the bacterium *Streptomyces tsukubaensis*. It is more potent, causes less rejection, and has less severe side effects than cyclosporine. Alopecia, diabetes mellitus, and neurotoxicity are more frequent with tacrolimus. It is initially used in combination therapy and later as monotherapy. A target tacrolimus blood level of 7–10 ng/mL is maintained initially and 5–7 ng/mL at 1-year posttransplant. The half-life is 12 hours. A new oral congener of tacrolimus, Advagraf, with extended release characteristics enables once daily dosing.[2]

Antimetabolites

Antimetabolites like azathioprine and mycophenolate inhibit DNA replication and contain B-and T-cell proliferation. As they act distal in the immunologic cascade, these are weaker immunosuppressants than calcineurin inhibitors. The main role of these drugs is as CNI-sparing agents, hence mitigating renal toxicity by CNIs.

Azathioprine

Azathioprine interferes with salvage pathway of purine synthesis. Its active metabolite 6-mercaptopurine acts as a purine analog. The half-life is 3 hours. Thiopurine methyltransferase genotyping helps to identify patients at increased risk of toxicity. It is used in combination therapy but is now largely replaced by mycophenolate mofetil (MMF).

Mycophenolate Mofetil

It is the prodrug of the natural fermentation product mycophenolic acid (MPA) produced by Penicillium fungus. *Mycophenolate mofetil* is metabolized in liver to MPA. The major advantage of MMF over azathioprine is more selective inhibition of lymphocytes. It lacks renal toxicity and has calcineurin sparing effect. It is useful in patients at high-risk for rejection like young patients transplanted for fulminant liver failure and autoimmune liver disease. Monotherapy causes increased rejection. Side effects respond to dose reduction.[7]

Mammalian Target of Rapamycin (mTOR) Inhibitors

Sirolimus is a macrocyclic antibiotic produced by *Streptomyces hygroscopicus*. An important side-effect of sirolimus is impaired wound healing which precludes its use early after transplant. A black box warning for sirolimus is probable development of hepatic artery thrombosis (HAT) in early posttransplant period. However, newer trials report that HAT may not be more common with sirolimus therapy. The half life is 79 hours. It acts synergistically with cyclosporine. It is used mainly for its renal sparing effect, and has antineoplastic effects in hepatocellular carcinoma. Loading dose has to be given at the initiation of therapy.

Everolimus is a derivative of sirolimus and acts as an mTOR inhibitor. It reduces chronic allograft vasculopathy.[2]

Biologic Agents

These agents interfere with both cell-mediated and humoral immune response. Antibodies interact with lymphocyte surface antigens causing depletion of circulating lymphocytes. Depleting antibodies reduce risk of early rejection. Nondepleting antibodies are monoclonal antibodies that cause hyporesponsiveness without reducing cell populations. They have low-immune toxicity and have limited efficacy.

Depleting Antibodies

Anti-thymocyte globulin: It is used as an induction agent. Polyclonal anti-thymocyte globulin binds all circulating T-cells and causes their depletion by either cell-mediated opsonization or complement-mediated cytolysis. This is followed by macrophage phagocytosis. Side effects include leucopenia, serum sickness, nephritis, and thrombocytopenia.

Muromonab or OKT3

It is used for induction and treating rejection. Prophylaxis against cytomegalovirus, pneumocystis and fungi is required. CD3 counts have to be monitored. Due to very potent immunosuppressive effect, it is rarely used these days.

Alemtuzumab

It is a humanized recombinant monoclonal antibody and is utilized for treating refractory B-cell chronic lymphocytic leukemia.

Nondepleting Antibodies

IL-2 receptor antibodies: Basiliximab and daclizumab are chimeric monoclonal antibodies produced by recombinant DNA technology. They bind to IL-2 receptor on activated T-cells, and are generally well-tolerated. They are used for induction therapy in renal failure.[8]

Costimulation Blockade

Cytotoxic T-lymphocyte-associated antigen 4 competes with CD28 for CD80/86 binding. Belatacept is a soluble recombinant immunoglobulin fusion protein which stimulates CTLA-4 activity, and has a beneficial effect on chronic allograft rejection. It is given as a once monthly injection. The role of costimulation blocking antibodies is still investigational.

The mechanisms of action and adverse effects of commonly used immunosuppressives are enlisted in Table 1

Drug Interactions of Immunosuppressive Drugs

Drug interactions are common in the first 6 months as the number of medicines as well the dosage of immunosuppresants required is high. Drug interactions are grouped into two types:

- Pharmacokinetic interactions—drug interferes with the absorption, distribution, or elimination of another drug.
- Pharmacodynamic interactions—drug potentiates or alter the action or side effects of another.[7]

Common drug interactions are summarized in Table 2

Phases of Immunosuppression

The phases of immunosuppression can be grouped into three time frames:

- Induction phase—This refers to the first month after transplant when high doses of immunosuppressants are required. Triple drug regimen consisting of CNI with antimetabolite and steroids is the most common induction regimen followed all over the world. The use of induction antibodies is decreasing as induction agents, although these are still widely used in some specific subgroups like patients with hepatorenal syndrome.
- Maintenance phase—It refers to immunosuppressive regimen after first month posttransplant. During the maintenance therapy, the number as well as the dose of medicines is decreased. Steroids are generally stopped by the end of 3-6 months. Most patients receive monotherapy with a CNI a few years after liver transplant.

Table 1: Mechanism of action and adverse effects of immunosuppressive drugs

Immunosuppressives	*Mechanisms of action*	*Adverse effects*
Corticosteroids	Bind to intracellular receptors, modulates transcription of genes encoding cytokines, and reduces T-cell proliferation. Reduce B-cell clonal expansion and antibody synthesis. Suppress cell-mediated and humoral immunity. Inhibits epithelial and endothelial cell adhesion, macrophage differentiation, and release of inflammatory mediators	Hyperglycemia, hypertension, hyperlipidemia, neurological impairment, early and severe recurrence of hepatitis C, weight gain, Cushingoid appearance, osteoporosis, cataracts, myopathy, and acute adrenal insufficiency on sudden discontinuation
Cyclosporine	Binds to cyclophilin, a cytoplasmic receptor protein which binds to calcineurin, a calcium-activated serine threonine phosphatase and inhibits IL-2 gene transcription, which limits the activation and proliferation of lymphocytes	Nephrotoxicity, hirsutism, gingival hypertrophy, hypertension, diabetes mellitus, hyperlipidemia, hepatotoxicity, hypomagnesemia, hyperkalemia, and neurotoxicity
Tacrolimus	Blocks the activation of calcineurin, and inhibits T-cell activation gene transcription factors by binding to cytosolic protein FK-506 binding protein (FKBP)	Nephrotoxicity, hirsutism, gingival hypertrophy, hypertension, diabetes mellitus, cardiomyopathy in children, hyperlipidemia, hypomagnesemia, hyperkalemia, and neurotoxicity
Sirolimus	Binds to FKBP-12, inhibits activity of mTOR, which inhibits IL-2-mediated signal transduction, and causes T-and B-cell cycle arrest in the G1-S phase. Prevents plasma cell differentiation and reduces production of IgM, IgG, and IgA antibodies	Anemia, leukopenia, thrombocytopenia, hypercholesterolemia, hypertriglyceridemia, hypokalemia, proteinuria, leg edema, oral ulcers, mucositis, delayed wound healing, lymphocele formation, pneumonitis, and increased recurrence of hepatitis C
Azathioprine	Purine analog that interferes with de novo purine synthesis, and DNA and RNA synthesis. Results in decreased production of T-and B-cells, reduced immunoglobulin and IL-2 secretion	Alopecia, dyspepsia, hypersensitivity reaction, reversible hepatotoxicity, and pancreatitis
Mycophenolatemofetil	Noncompetitive reversible inhibition of inosine monophosphate dehydrogenase which interferes with purine synthesis and blocks lymphocyte proliferation	Nausea, anorexia, gastritis, diarrhea, leukopenia, and thrombocytopenia. Increased incidence of CMV, HSV, Candida, and PML. Increased risk of teratogenicity and abortions
Muromonab/OKT3	Anti-CD3 antibody. Binds and depletes mature T-cells	Cytokine release syndrome, tachyphylaxis, severe HCV recurrence, and pulmonary edema
Alemtuzumab	Anti-CD52 monoclonal antibody. Depletes circulating lymphocytes	Pancytopenia, infections, autoimmunity, and HCV recurrence

Abbreviations: FKBP, FK-506 binding protein; mTOR, mammalian target of rapamycin CMV, cytomegalovirus; HSV, herpes simplex virus; PML, progressive multifocal leukoencephalopathy.

Table 2: Drug interactions of immunosuppressive drugs

Drugs	*Increase IS levels*	*Decrease IS levels*	*Increase toxicity*
Cyclosporine A, Sirolimus, and Tacrolimus	Macrolides, chloramphenicol, ciprofloxacin, chloroquine, HIV protease inhibitors, telaprevir, boceprevir, azoles, calcium channel inhibitors, benzodiazepines, serotonin uptake inhibitors, danazol, OCPs, and allopurinol bind to and inhibit CYP3A4. Vinblastine inhibits the MDR gene p-glycoprotein	Phenytoin, phenobarbital, carbamazepine, rifampicin, and rifabutin induce CYP3A4 metabolism. Ticlopidine reduces bioavailability. Orlistat, octreotide, and metoclopramide reduce absorption	Hyperkalemia increased by ACE inhibitors and potassium-sparing diuretics. Hypomagnesemia increased by amphotericin B. Renal toxicity increased by aminoglycosides, sulphonamides, vancomycin, NSAIDs, acyclovir, ganciclovir, amphotericin B, and melphalan. Statins cause rhabdomyolysis and renal failure. Neurotoxicity enhanced by Imipenem/ cilastatin
Azathioprine		Decreases warfarin levels	Allopurinol, 5-ASA, sulfasalazine, sirolimus and ACE inhibitors increase bone marrow toxicity
Mycophenolatemofetil	Acyclovir and probenecid reduce renal excretion tacrolimus increases levels	Antacids and cholestyramine reduce absorption	
Adrenal steroids	–	Impair hypoglycemic effect of OHA, and natriuretic effect of diuretics	Increases cyclosporine levels
OKT3	–	–	Increases cyclosporine levels

Abbreviations: MDR, multidrug resistance; ACE, angiotensin-converting enzyme; NSAIDs, nonsteroidal anti-inflammatory drugs; 5-ASA, 5-aminosalicylic acid.

- Treatment of acute cellular rejection—After histological diagnosis of acute rejection made, doses of immunosuppressive drugs are increased. Corticosteroid therapy is administered with high-dose intravenous bolus methylprednisolone for three doses. Antilymphocyte antibodies—ATG or Muromonab—are utilized in ~10% of acute rejection episodes which are steroid resistant.[2]

Immunologic Basis of Tolerance

Full immunologic tolerance is a condition where allograft functioning normally does not require any immunosuppression, with the host in a normal immune state and not suffering from any drug-related side effects, infections, or neoplasia. It is a state of donor-specific unresponsiveness.

Tolerance can occur by central and peripheral mechanisms, deletional, and nondeletional mechanisms.

Central Tolerance

Central tolerance destroys naive lymphocytes, encountered in primary lymphoid organs, with reactivity for self-antigens. It occurs by varied mechanisms.[9]

Clonal Deletion

Here, tolerance results from apoptotic deletion of autoreactive T-cells during thymic T-cell development. T-cells specific for self-antigens bound to MHC peptides are eliminated by this method. Antigen presenting cells induce deletion of thymocytes until they reach final maturation. In the thymus, over 95% of T-cells die in situ by apoptosis. Self-reactive B-cells are removed in the bone marrow during the maturation phase from the pre-B to mature B-cell stage.

Clonal Anergy

It is an induction of functionally silent state in B-and T-cells. Anergy occurs if there is B-cell stimulation in the absence of activation of T-cells. These cells lose their ability to proliferate and antibody secretion on antigenic stimulation. Absence of a second costimulatory signal during T-cell activation results in functional unresponsiveness and anergy of T-cells. In the absence of costimulatory signal, T-cells are not able to produce IL-2 and hence cannot proliferate on exposure to the antigen.

Receptor Editing

It is a mechanism where rearrangements of secondary heavy-and light-chain gene occur on exposure to autoantigen that alter the specificity of BCR and eliminate autoreactivity. This mechanism is also responsible for B-cell tolerance.

Peripheral Tolerance

This is required for lymphocytes that have not been silenced in primary organs. It is a dynamic but reversible process which operates through multiple mechanisms.

Immune Deviation

Preferential activation of Th2-type response also leads to induction of tolerance. A shift of the immune response to an antibody-mediated TH2-type from a cell-mediated TH1-type causes tolerance.

Suppression

This is done by both suppressor and cytotoxic T-cells which inhibit lymphocyte activity of T-cells, eliminate APCs- and lyse antigen-specific B-cells.

Immune Privilege

In immune-privileged sites like the liver, tolerance occurs by apoptosis through interactions between T-cells and normal tissue cells.

Coreceptor Modulation

T-cells need two signals for activation. The first signal is the presentation of processed peptide on APC. Interaction of CD28 and CTLA4 receptors on T-cells with costimulatory molecules CD80 and CD86 on APCs is the second signal. T-cells become unresponsive without the costimulatory signal.

Similarly, B-cells also require two signals for activation. The first signal is B-cell receptor ligation and second signal is interactions of costimulatory molecules (class II MHC and B7 and their T-cell binding receptors). B-cells develop tolerance and become refractory to antigenic stimulation without T-cell costimulation.[9]

Role of Dendritic Cells and Regulatory T-cells in Tolerance

Dendritic cells are key mediators of immunological tolerance. They possess the unique ability to stimulate naive T-cells, and serve as a link between the adaptive and innate immunity. There are two classes of DCs: classical DCs (cDCs) and plasmacytoid DCs (pDCs). Classical DCs serve the role of antigen presentation and stimulating T-cells. Plasmacytoid DCs are equipped for cytokine secretion and antigen presentation after pathogen-induced activation. DCs induce central tolerance by two mechanisms: Negative selection of thymocytes by self-antigen presentation and clonal deletion or T-regulatory cell (Treg) generation by recirculating peripheral DCs into the thymus, which present peripheral self-antigen. Antigen presentation by DCs induces T-cell unresponsiveness leading to peripheral tolerance. DCs help in maintaining the homeostasis of regulatory T-cells through costimulatory molecules CD80/CD86. The role of DCs to induce and maintain peripheral Tregs in turn limit DC generation by a negative feedback pathway.[10]

The most promising mediators of tolerance after transplant are regulatory T-cells. ~10–15% of CD4+ T-cells are Tregs and express CD25. They suppress the activity of clonal T-cell. T-regulatory cells are anergic to T-cell antigen-mediated activation and are recognized by FoxP3 expression. They produce suppressive cytokines transforming growth factor -beta and IL-10 to regulate peripheral tolerance.[2]

Induction of Tolerance

Although we are far from achieving induction of tolerance, the aim of current search is to device strategies for inducing tolerance. This includes interference with either costimulatory receptors or the T-cell antigen receptor that in turn inhibit alloreactive T-lymphocytes in an antigen-specific manner.[5] At the time of transplantation, patients who achieve tolerance have been treated mostly with T-cell-depleting antibodies. Major impediments to inducing tolerance are the presence of memory T-cells that react or cross react with histocompatibility antigens and inflammation which promotes cytopathic immune responses.

Tolerogenic Immunosuppression

Tolerogenic or minimal immunosuppression is applied to patients who are able to sustain stable graft function with a very low-dose of calcineurin inhibitors. Till date, operational tolerance or successful withdrawal of immunosuppression has been possible only in a small subgroup of patients. Most of these would have accidentally stopped medications, a small proportion would have been taken off due to posttransplant lymphoproliferative disorder, life-threatening infections or those enrolled in weaning protocols. Those patients, where withdrawal of immunosuppression is attempted should have at least 2-year follow-up on low immunosuppression and a prewithdrawal liver biopsy showing no inflammation. Patients with no prior acute rejection episodes and nonautoimmune primary liver disease, generally do better after withdrawal.[11]

Operationally tolerant recipients might have a signature of tolerance that could be used to identify patients, in whom immunosuppressive therapy could be stopped. Markers of tolerance include increase in natural killer gene signatures, increase in hepcidin genes and increased frequency of regulatory T-cells. A 3 gene signature associated with natural killer cell function predicts tolerance with a positive predictive value of 100% in children.[12] Lower phytohemagglutinin stimulation index also identifies those likely to develop tolerance.[13] If immunosuppression withdrawal is done after careful weaning, 20–40% of adults and up to 60% of children can achieve operational tolerance.

CONCLUSION

The aim of transplant immunology is to build up strategies for preventing transplant rejection. There are paucity of markers of rejection or tolerance, and poor correlation between rejection and drug levels. Rejection leads to graft loss in less than 5% cases. The aim of immunosuppression is to control alloreactivity at the lowest possible dose of immunosuppressants. Alloreactivity and the need for immunosuppression subside with time. Despite advances in immunological knowledge, indefinite graft survival with immune tolerance is rare. The ultimate goal of transplant immunology is to develop therapeutic strategies to support tolerance.

REFERENCES

1. Eugene SR, Willis MC, Michael RS. Schiff's diseases of the liver. 11th ed. John Wiley & Sons Ltd; 2012.
2. Abdeldayem H, Allam N. Liver transplantation—basic issues. Intech;2012.
3. Ayala Garc´ıa MA, Gonz´alezYebra B, L´opez Flores AL, et al. The major histocompatibility complex in transplantation. J Transplant. 2012;2012.
4. Ch. Otto, K. Ulrichs. The immunology of allograft rejection: a survey of current knowledge and a discussion of peptide-specific anti-rejection Transplantationsmedizin. 2004;16. Jahrg:S. 158.
5. Sanchez-Fueyo A, Strom TB. Immunologic basis of graft rejection and tolerance following transplantation of liver or other solid organs. Gastroenterology. 2011;140:51-64.
6. David S. Game, Robert I. Lechler. Pathways of allorecognition: implications for transplantation tolerance. Transpl Immunol. 2002;10:101-8.
7. Killenberg PG and Clavien PA. Medical care of the liver transplant patient. 3rd Ed. John Wiley & Sons Ltd;2006.

8. Fung J, Kelly D, Kadry Z, et al. Immunosuppression in liver transplantation beyond calcineurin inhibitors. Liver Transpl. 2005;11:267-80.
9. Moncef Z. Immunological tolerance: mechanisms. Encyclopedia of life sciences 2001.
10. Kanako LL, Boris R. Dendritic cells: arbiters of immunity and immunological tolerance. Cold Spring Harb Perspect Biol. 2012;4:a007401.
11. Lerut J, Sanchez-Fueyo A. An appraisal of tolerance in liver transplantation. Am JTransplant. 2006;6:1774-80.
12. McCaughan GW, Bowen DG, and Bertolino P. Operational tolerance in liver transplantation: Shall we predict or promote? Liver Transpl. 2013;19:933-6.
13. de la Garza RG, Sarobe P, Merino J et al. Trial of complete weaning from immunosuppression for liver transplant recipients: factors predictive of tolerance. Liver Transpl. 2013;9:937-44.

CHAPTER 110

Pediatric Liver Transplant

Mohammed A Nayeem

INTRODUCTION

The first liver transplantation (LT) was performed on a small child suffering from biliary atresia in 1963, who died of hemorrhage during the operation.[1] The first successful liver transplant was eventually performed by Starzl, on an infant girl with hepatocellular cancer in the year 1967.[2] She lived for 13 months after surgery and died of metastatic disease.

The scarcity of size matched donor organs in children necessitated the development of new techniques like split-liver, reduced liver, and live liver donors to enhance the organ pool. Reduced size donor LT from cadaver livers was first described by Bismuth and Houssin,[3] and later developed by Broelsch.[4] This operation, which is now of historical importance was used to overcome size disparity between small recipients and large donors, potentially allowing the use of a donor more than 10 times larger than the weight of the recipient. It only shifted the use of donor organs from adults to children, while the total pool of available organs remained constant.

The first attempted living-related liver transplantation (LRLT) was performed in 1988 by Silvano Raia et al, at Brazil[5]. Though it resulted in unfortunate death of the child on the sixth postoperative day due to medical complications, Raia's attempt firmly established the technical feasibility of the procedure. Strong et al.[6] (1989) reported from Brisbane, the first successful live donor liver transplant in a pediatric recipient using a left lobe from his mother. The child required retransplantation because of chronic rejection, from a cadaver donor 14 months after the first transplantation.[6] Christopher Broelsch et al performed the first successful series of LRLT in the world on 20 patients.

The surgical innovations along with advances in anesthesia, critical care, and immunosuppression have contributed to remarkable increase in the long-term survival in children undergoing LT. Despite most of the surgical innovations both attempted and successful, were first performed on children, there nonetheless remain substantial issues to be addressed in pediatric LT, even though a high survival rate has been achieved.

According to United Network for Organ Sharing database, Kaplan–Meier graft survivals showed that pediatric patients receiving livers from pediatric aged donors had an 81% 3-year graft survival as compared with 63% if children received livers from donors >18 years.[7] In contrast, adult recipients receiving pediatric livers have poor 3-year graft survivals. Because the outcome of small pediatric donor livers in adult recipients is poor, and small pediatric donors are a precious source of lifesaving organs for the infant recipient, the use of small pediatric donor livers in adults should be avoided.

In 2002, the Model for End-Stage Liver Disease (MELD) score was introduced to allocate cadaver livers based on the severity of recipient liver disease. This allocation model ensured that priority is given to the sickest individuals. The Pediatric End-stage Liver Disease (PELD)[8] score allocation model is used for children up to 12 years of age. It is calculated from a formula based on the following factors namely International Normalized Ratio (INR), total bilirubin, serum albumin, age less than 1-year, and height less than 2 standard deviations from the mean for age and gender. Pediatric recipients (<12 years) get priority to receive cadaver livers from pediatric donors, (<18 years) over adults with the same MELD score.

The need for LT in children for end-stage liver disease has a bimodal age of distribution, the first peak occurring in children less than 2 years of age, and the second peak in those above 10 years.

The **indications** for LT in children can be broadly grouped into (1) decompensated end-stage liver disease, (2) acute liver failure, (3) metabolic liver disease, and (4) unresectable primary liver tumors. There are, however, several indications in which there is a dilemma about decision to transplant. This dilemma is mostly with some of the metabolic syndromes, many of which are very rare and present only in children.

The areas of controversy are as follows:

1. Metabolic diseases that have major extrahepatic manifestations, particularly involving the central nervous system like organic acidemias (e.g., methylmalonic acidemia and propionic acidemia), urea cycle defects, and storage disorders like Gaucher's disease. The most crucial aspect is to determine the degree of central nervous system compromise, and the projected progression of dysfunction over time after LT.

   Children with storage diseases may have progressive central nervous system and cardiac involvement after transplantation, if the abnormal glycogen or lipid reaccumulates. On the contrary, several of the organic acidemias may have benign variants in which minimal central nervous system compromise occurs, and for which LT has been successful. The essence lies in the early identification of children with benign variants, who could be considered as candidates for transplantation. Involvement of the expert pediatric neurologist early in decision making is essential.
2. Diseases for which medical therapy is available, but the debate is how long the LT can be safely delayed, and the overall treatment cost. Examples include the use of 2-(2-nitro-4-trifluoromethylbenzoyl)-1,3 cyclohexanedione (NTBC) to treat tyrosinemia, chelation therapy for Wilson's disease, exchange transfusions and phototherapy to treat Crigler–Najjar syndrome, and antioxidant therapy for neonatal hemochromatosis.

Biliary Atresia

The most common (~70%) indication for LT in children worldwide including India is biliary atresia (BA) Majority of these children require transplant before the age of 2 years. Not surprisingly, there are very few pediatric organ donors who are less than 5 years of age for transplanting these young children.[13]

Biliary artesia may be associated less commonly (10%) with congenital anomalies, some of which are preduodenal portal vein, gut malrotation, Meckel's diverticulum, splenic malformations, and situs inversus. The presence of these malformations per se does not contraindicate liver transplant, and the results of the transplant in this group are not inferior.

Kasai portoenterostomy has been traditionally the primary surgical procedure for all infants with BA who present early on. Primary liver transplant for BA is indicated in kids who present in late infancy (>120 days) or who develop complications from cirrhosis.[7] In India however, most children with extrahepatic biliary atresia either are diagnosed late or have not undergone the Kasai procedure. Nearly half of the infants who undergo Kasai will fail to achieve adequate biliary drainage, and require liver transplant within the first 2 years of life.[9] A majority of children who have successful establishment of biliary drainage with normal postoperative serum bilirubin levels still progress to cirrhosis, though they usually do not require liver transplant until adolescence. Nearly 70% of BA patients may have prolonged transplant-free survival, if the serum bilirubin falls to <2 mg% within 3 months following portoenterostomy.[10,11] Children whose serum bilirubin does not fall below 6 mg% 3 months after the Kasai procedure rarely improve, and should be referred for LT.[12] Though more than 80% of all BA patients who undergo Kasai procedure will eventually need a liver transplant, the sequential use of the Kasai procedure followed by LT is still routinely recommended as it buys time, optimizes overall survival and makes transplant procedure less formidable in an older grown-up child.[14,15]

Hypoplastic portal veins, often measuring only a few millimeters in diameter, are seen in infants with BA and can make LT difficult. The presence of a small portal vein (4 mm or less in diameter) in these infants on preoperative imaging predicts a higher risk of development of portal vein thrombosis in the postoperative period, and requires close monitoring.[16] Parents of these infants should be adequately counseled about this particular risk and the overall outcome. Children who had undergone successful portoenterostomies, but who need transplantation years later due to advanced cirrhosis would have developed near normal size portal veins, justifying the initial Kasai procedure.

Redo portoenterostomies for failed Kasai should not be done as a routine, and be reserved for select patients where there has been a good initial long-term drainage that has abruptly stopped. This usually happens due to concretions or local scarring, which if removed by an experienced surgeon can reestablish the bile flow. Failed portoenterostomy, usually results in only a brief period of bile drainage, and multiple attempts to redo the procedure should be avoided in this group, because repeated surgery can make subsequent LT difficult.

Other cholestatic conditions such as intrahepatic cholestasis syndromes and Alagille syndrome may require LT.

Progressive Familial Intrahepatic Cholestasis

Progressive familial intrahepatic cholestasis (PFIC) also known as Byler's disease, begins in infancy as a cholestatic syndrome, and usually progresses to cirrhosis within the first 2 decades of life.[17] It is inherited in an autosomal recessive pattern and is believed to be due to a defect in transport proteins involved in bile acid secretion resulting in an increase in bile acids in serum. Presenting features include severe pruritus, self-mutilation, jaundice, and growth retardation. Early onset hepatocellular cancer may be a feature of PFIC-2 variant. Low to normal gamma glutamyl transpeptidase (γ-GT) level is characteristic of PFIC (except PFIC-3 which has high γ-GT) and differentiates it from other childhood cholestatic disorders. Ursodeoxycholic acid should be started for all PFIC variants, as soon as the diagnosis is made particularly in PFIC-3 where the response is good.[18] Liver transplantation is usually curative and not known to recur in the graft. Progressive familial intrahepatic cholestasis –1 variants usually have associated extrahepatic manifestations like diarrhea and fatty liver, which may persist after LT and the parents must be adequately counseled. Restoration of biliary bile salt secretion in this variant after LT may sometimes aggravate liver steatosis, or even lead to nonalcoholic steatohepatitis with cirrhosis.[19] Partial biliary diversion procedures provide relief from severe pruritus and improvement in liver function tests. They may be helpful in patients who do not have cirrhosis, or who are not willing for LT. Progressive familial intrahepatic cholestasis-1 must be differentiated from another related disease benign recurrent intrahepatic cholestasis (BRIC-1), both of which are caused by mutations of same gene and have similar clinical presentation, but with asymptomatic periods in the latter. Patients with BRIC must be reassured, that their disease is benign and will not progress to cirrhosis or liver failure.

Biliary Hypoplasia (Alagille's syndrome)

Biliary hypoplasia is a less common cholestatic disorder, but is an important cause of liver disease in children where LT is curative. Biliary hypoplasia may be syndromic or nonsyndromic. Alagille's syndrome is transmitted as autosomal dominant and caused by mutation in the Jagged 1 gene. It presents with chronic cholestasis, posterior embryotoxon, butterfly-like vertebral arch defects, characteristic facies, and hypoplasia of pulmonary artery.[20,21] Most children present with intense pruritus and intact synthetic function. Progression to cirrhosis is uncommon. The prognosis depends on its severity with an overall probability of 75% survival into the third decade. Intense pruritus and/or deforming xanthomas can severely affect the child's quality of life and warrant liver transplant, (in approximately 20–30% children) despite preserved synthetic function. The levels of serum bile acids, γ-GT, and cholesterol are all elevated. The nonsyndromic variant has paucity of interlobular bile ducts on liver biopsy (defined as <0.9 duct per portal tract), without the other components of Alagille's syndrome.[22,23] Related willing donors of inheritable disease Alagille's syndrome should be screened with liver biopsy and cholangiography to rule out the subclinical phenotype (particularly if they share common alleles), which would contraindicate donation.[24]

Fulminant Hepatic Failure

Fulminant hepatic failure (FHF) is the second most common indication among Indian children who require LT. In India, hepatitis A is one of the commonest cause of FHF in children. However, in most other cases the etiology is not clear. Sudden onset jaundice and encephalopathy in previously healthy children with no drug toxicity and negative hepatitis serology is common. There are some unique causes of fulminant liver disease in newborns. Herpes simplex virus is the most common of the viral etiologies leading to acute liver failure (ALF) in neonates. Fatty acid oxidation defects, mitochondrial respiratory chain defects, tyrosinemia type I, and hemophagocytic lymphohistiocytosis also can cause ALF.

Patients who develop sudden onset ALF without known previous liver disease present a challenge both for diagnosis and in assessing their prognosis without liver transplant. Establishment of a primary diagnosis may be impossible before taking up the child for emergency transplant, and precious time should not be wasted in doing so, if the child's condition is deteriorating. Encephalopathy is difficult to assess in children and worsening coagulopathy (INR >2) should be considered as an indication for LT.[25]

Neonatal Hemochromatosis

Neonatal hemochromatosis is an important cause of ALF in the newborn period in the west, though not seen or reported in India. It is distinct from hereditary hemochromatosis seen in adults. The cause is not clear and is believed to be a gestational alloimmune disease process.[26] It is both a diagnostic and therapeutic challenge. Diagnosis is made by demonstrating iron deposition in a lip or minor salivary gland biopsy, or by MRI demonstrating deposition of iron in the extrahepatic reticuloendothelial system.[27] Treatment with an antioxidant cocktail, (N-acetyl cysteine, deferoxamine, or its oral form deferasirox, selenium, and prostaglandin E1) usually is commenced when neonatal hemochromatosis is suspected but a failure to respond within 48–72 hours mandates transplantation.[28] Liver transplantation is life saving, but success rates of approximately 50% are reported.[29]

Hemophagocytic Lymphohistiocytosis

Hemophagocytic lymphohistiocytosis (HLH) is a rare syndrome of pathologic immune activation characterized by clinical signs, and symptoms of severe inflammation. Hemophagocytic lymphohistiocytosis can be congenital or acquired, triggered by infection in an immunocompromised patient. Inappropriate activation of macrophages and natural killer cells causes severe hepatocyte injury. It presents in many forms: pyrexia of unknown origin, hepatitis or acute liver failure, sepsis, Kawasaki disease, and neurologic abnormalities. It should be considered in the differential diagnosis of acute liver failure, especially if lymphocytic infiltrates and macrophages are noted on biopsy. The role of LT in the treatment of patients with HLH is not clearly established and should not be recommended at present, as recurrence in the graft is common. The primary treatment of HLH is bone marrow transplant and immunosuppressive therapies, rather than liver replacement.[30]

Hepatoblastoma

Hepatoblastoma is the most common primary hepatic malignancy found in children followed by hepatocellular carcinoma (HCC).[31] Resection in combination with systemic chemotherapy is the preferred method of treatment for hepatoblastoma and achieves long-term survival.[32] Liver transplantation is indicated for unresectable hepatoblastoma localized to the liver usually after downsizing with chemotherapy.[33] If the tumor is unresectable after appropriate chemotherapy, transplantation may still be offered if there has been a demonstrable response to therapy sometimes even in the presence of isolated pulmonary metastases.[34] When needed, transplantation is best undertaken before completing chemotherapy, so that another two cycles of chemotherapy can be given after transplantation.[35] Hepatocellular carcinoma is rare in children and when present, usually occurs in the setting of another chronic underlying disease such as tyrosinemia or PFIC (type 2).

Hereditary Tyrosinemia

Type I, also known as hepatorenal tyrosinemia, is an autosomal recessive disorder characterized by deficiency of the enzyme fumaryl-acetoacetase, the final enzyme in the tyrosine degradation pathway. The main organs affected are the liver, kidneys, and peripheral nerves. The clinical presentation is variable and includes a peculiar boiled cabbage-like odor, porphyria-like symptoms, neurological crises, rickets, cardiomyopathy, and liver failure or hepatocellular carcinoma. Dysplastic nodules develop in the underlying liver, tyrosinemia being the inborn error with the highest incidence of progression to hepatocellular carcinoma. The affected infants on screening show markedly raised alpa-fetoprotein (AFP) levels, and coagulopathy but with near normal serum transaminases. An elevated blood tyrosine levels are associated with several clinical entities and is not useful for diagnosis. The most useful diagnostic test for tyrosinemia is by measuring succinylacetone in urine. Earlier the presentation in infancy, poorer is the prognosis. Survival, when symptoms develop before 2 months of age is 38% as compared with 96% when child develops symptoms after 6 months.[36] Child should be started on a diet low in tyrosine and phenylalanine (nonanimal protein) and a modified amino acid medical formula (available as Tyrex or Tyros) as soon as the diagnosis is made.

Hereditary tyrosinemia should be distinguished from another disorder transient neonatal hypertyrosinemia, seen primarily in premature infants and a major cause of tyrosine elevation detected on newborn screening. It spontaneously resolves during the first month of life, and usually requires no treatment apart from giving low protein milk formulas or breast milk.

2-(2-nitro-4-trifluoromethylbenzoyl)-1,3 cyclohexanedione a drug with herbicidal activity has become the gold standard for management of these patients, along with the special diet. It (nitisinone/orfadin) prevents the formation of toxic metabolites and produces rapid clinical improvement along with normalization of AFP in most cases.[37] Although all the manifestations of the disease resolve with NTBC, the risk of hepatocellular carcinoma (37% after 2 years of age in untreated children)[38] is reduced to less than 5% but is not eliminated. Surveillance with AFP and liver imaging is recommended at regular intervals.

The treatment of tyrosinemia with NTBC has led to an increase in the mean age of LT by few years. The indications[39,40] for LT now include: (1) fulminant liver failure, (2) rising AFP while on NTBC, (3) increase in the size or number of dysplastic nodules, and (4) inability to afford the expensive NTBC treatment.[41] Liver transplant recipients may still need low-dose NTBC treatment lifelong to prevent ongoing renal tubular dysfunction resulting from the succinylacetone generated in renal tissue.[42]

Though the drug NTBC is well tolerated with negligible side effects, it is not easily available, and is prohibitively expensive. The organization for rare diseases and the drug manufacturer though is delivering the drug free of cost at select centers for the underprivileged.

The adverse effects from lifelong immunosuppression along with potential ongoing renal tubular dysfunction even after liver transplant should be taken into consideration in decision-making against the prohibitive cost of the long-term nitisinone therapy in addition to the potential though small, risk of developing malignancy while still on medical treatment.

Maple Syrup Urine Disease

Maple syrup urine disease (MSUD) is caused by mutations in the gene encoding the branched chain alpa-keto acid dehydrogenase complex resulting in an inability to break down the essential amino acids valine, leucine, and isoleucine.[43] Classic variant MSUD patients manifest as severe leucine intolerance. The resulting metabolites are excreted in sweat and urine giving rise to a sweet odor resembling maple syrup. The treatment consists of a diet restrictive of the above essential amino acids along with the dietary supplements. However, during times of stress or illness children are at risk of cerebral edema resulting from the metabolic decompensation. Recurrent attacks of metabolic decompensation lead to neurological sequelae like spastic paraperesis, dystonia, and mental retardation.[44] Adherence to a restrictive diet, use of MSUD metabolic formulas, and weekly monitoring of plasma amino acids is essential. Seasonal flu vaccines along with the routine scheduled vaccinations are important to prevent recurrent infections. Long-term medical care of such kids is cumbersome with the continuing threat of neurological injury with each intercurrent illness. Liver treatment is essentially curative, immediately allowing removal of dietary restriction and preventing further neurological damage. Maple syrup urine disease is one of the rare ideal settings, wherein domino transplant can be performed.[45] The explanted liver from MSUD patient undergoing liver transplant is transplanted to another recipient without MSUD, thus not adversely affecting the overall organ pool. The domino recipients of the MSUD liver have inexplicably normal branch chain amino acid metabolism with no sequelae.[46]

Crigler–Najjar syndrome type I: It is characterized by unconjugated hyperbilirubinemia persisting in the neonatal period due to complete deficiency of the liver enzyme uridine diphosphate glucuronosyl transferase. Partial deficiency (type 2) of this enzyme is not lethal and treatable with phenobarbital. Type 1 does not respond to phenobarbital and is treated with exchange transfusions, and long duration phototherapy early on to prevent permanent brain damage (kernicterus). Liver transplantation replaces the deficient enzyme, and is curative in these children if done before permanent brain damage occurs.

Auxiliary partial orthotopic liver transplantation (APOLT) has been applied particularly in Crigler–Najjar syndrome, and a few other metabolic syndrome patients where there is a functionally normal liver apart from the particular enzyme defect.[47] Auxiliary LT implies transplantation of a donor liver without removing the entire native liver. Substitution of only a part of the liver (left lateral segment) is sufficient enough to overcome the enzyme deficiency. Studies have shown that only 1–2% of the normal hepatocytes are needed for adequate bilirubin conjugation. Auxiliary partial orthotopic liver transplantation provides the missing enzyme, uridine diphosphate glucuronosyl transferase, while the preserved native liver acts as a safety net in case of graft dysfunction. It also potentially allows withdrawal of immunosuppression should gene therapy become available in future. Auxiliary partial orthotopic liver transplantation is a technically challenging operation though, and the survival rates are less compared with conventional transplantation.

Urea Cycle Disorders

Urea cycle disorders (UCD): Urea cycle is limited to the liver, requires six enzymes and removes nitrogen waste from protein catabolism. The deficiencies of ornithine transcarbamylase (OTC), carbamoylphosphate synthetase, and n-acetylglutamine synthetase, have severe metabolic derangement and worst outcome.[48] Urea cycle disorders are inherited in an autosomal recessive manner except for OTC deficiency, which is X-linked. Typically affected neonates present within hours to days after birth with poor feeding, lethargy, vomiting, and tachypnea progressing rapidly to coma and death. The clinical picture is similar to sepsis and is often missed. Serum ammonia level is usually very high and may be in thousands. In children with UCD, particularly for the above three variants, liver transplant is not only lifesaving but also cures the underlying disease. Liver transplant should be considered before the consequences of the defect result in severe neurologic injury that may contraindicate transplantation, usually within the first year of life, or even as early as 3 months.[49] It is essential to prevent central nervous system injury using dialysis combined with medical therapy in lowering serum ammonia levels until transplantation. Patients with UCD who have repetitive hyperammonemic crisis sustain significant neurologic injury resulting in mental retardation. Early transplantation eliminates episodes of hyperammonemic crisis preserving neurologic function.[50] Related carriers of UCD can donate liver allowing early transplantation.

Organic Acidemias

These are characterized by increased excretion of nonamino organic acids in urine. Different types exist, of which methylmalonic acidemia (MMA) and propionic acidemia (PA) are the commonest and result from defective catabolism of the amino acids isoleucine, valine, methionine, and threonine.[51] Presentation is varied from mild to severe, with severe forms typically presenting with hyperammonemia, ketoacidosis, and neurological problems, including coma very soon after birth. To minimize neurological sequelae, intensive clinical management, including aggressive treatment such as dialysis or hemofiltration, is required. Despite early diagnosis and maximal metabolic control, many patients develop considerable neurological, psychological, cardiac, and renal complications. Liver transplant is indicated in children with organic acidemia, who have significant hyperammonemia, toxic encephalopathy or neurological symptoms such as seizures.[52] Clinical experience with effects of LT on the natural history of PA and MMA is limited due to low prevalence of these diseases. Successful LT achieves metabolic control, growth and development of the child, improvement of cardiac function, and less strict dietary restrictions.[53] However, other consequences of the disease such as stroke and renal dysfunction can still manifest despite successful LT, especially in patients who also have the cobalamin defects.

Differentiation between UCDs and organic acidemias is sometimes difficult as both present with hyperammonemia. The key to distinction is the presence or absence of acidosis, ketosis, or hypoglycemia. Urea cycle defects usually present with respiratory alkalosis due to the hyperpnoea, induced by severe hyperammonemia. In contrast, the initial presentation of many organic acidemias is severe metabolic acidosis with an increased ion gap. The second distinguishing feature of the urea cycle defects is the absence of ketosis. Hypoglycemia can be a feature of organic acidemias but not UCDs. In the absence of acidosis, ketosis, and hypoglycemia, diagnosis of urea cycle defect should be considered vis-à-vis organic acidemia.

Glycogen Storage Disorder

Glycogen storage disorders (GSD) have varied presentation according to the various subtypes and the enzyme deficiency. Glycogen storage disorders can affect the liver, muscle, heart, and brain. Patients typically present with recurrent fasting hypoglycemia. Medical treatment for GSD exists, but is cumbersome and not all individuals are compliant, leading to significant morbidity. Metabolic control in GSD type I requires nocturnal continuous enteral drip feeding to avoid fasting hypoglycemia, and frequent oral uncooked corn starch for prolonged glucose release.[54] For patients with GSD types III, VI, and IX a high-protein diet combined with uncooked cornstarch is the mainstay of therapy. Despite these interventions remarkably improving metabolic control and prolonging survival, long-term complications still do occur.[55] The incidence of hepatic adenomas is high and the risk of hepatocellular cancer increases with age. Liver transplant in GSD is indicated for subtypes I, III, and IV, wherein the patients have poor metabolic control despite medical management, decompensated cirrhosis, or liver tumor. For GSD type IV, LT is particularly indicated and often the first line of treatment as they usually do not have extrahepatic manifestations.[56] In patients with GSD I, kidney disease can progress and hyperuricemia, neutropenia (in GSD Ib) may persist after liver transplant. The child may continue to have neuromuscular and cardiac complications even after LT in GSD type IIIa.

Mitochondrial respiratory chain abnormalities represent disorder in the electron transport proteins due to mitochondrial mutations or deletions and primarily present with neurologic symptoms. Liver can sometimes be affected and present either as fulminant liver failure or as decompensated chronic liver disease. The screening tests include elevated serum and cerebrospinal fluid lactate, elevated serum lactate/pyruvate ratio >20, increased serum ammonia, and hypoglycemia.[57] These disorders are particularly important to recognize during the evaluation process, as they have multisystem involvement and are progressive. In cases of acute liver failure, where there is a suspicion of mitochondrial deficit disorder, tests such as muscle biopsy and magnetic resonance spectroscopy of the brain should be done to look for evidence of systemic disease. Parents should be counseled that although liver transplant replaces the mitochondria in the liver leading to normal liver function, the long-term outcome depends on mitochondrial function in the rest of the body.[58] Liver transplantation for these abnormalities is generally not indicated as the results are dismal (50% survival) even when performed in a highly select group of patients without overt neurologic disease.[59]

Children presenting with nystagmus or secondary mitochondrial defects due to valproate toxicity or Alper's syndrome should never be transplanted. Pediatric neurologist should be involved early in the consultation, as neurologic deficits can be difficult to diagnose in small, critically ill children. Due to the wide spectrum of deficits in mitochondrial disease, it is difficult to predict how neurologic function may evolve in individual patient.

CONTRAINDICATIONS

The absolute contraindications to liver transplant in children include the following:

1. Uncontrolled systemic sepsis
2. Hepatocellular carcinoma with extra hepatic disease
3. Severe multisystem mitochondrial myopathies
4. Alper's disease and valproate-induced liver failure
5. Hemophagocytic lymphohistiocytosis

PERIOPERATIVE CHALLENGES

A pediatric liver transplant recipient is not a miniature adult liver transplant patient. Different spectrum of diseases is seen in pediatric patients like BA, congenital, and metabolic liver disorders. Infants and children have fewer of the comorbidities seen in adult patients and have a greater healing potential, but their reserve is far less. Children have a longer time span to live and the implications of treatment are considerable. Pediatric LDLT is usually done using the left lateral segment or left lobe, which is technically less challenging than the right lobe liver transplant. Pediatric patients may have undergone prior surgeries such as

Kasai portoenterostomy leading to vascularized adhesions. They have smaller vessels and a vascular complication is more likely. A big liver in a small infant or child causes multiple problems, unlike in adults, where a low graft-to-recipient weight ratio (GRWR) graft is more commonly encountered. Roux-en-Y biliary-enteric anastomosis is more commonly performed than the direct choledochocholedochostomy in small children.

The perioperative challenges for LT in children are:

Preoperative Issues

The important aspects of the preparation are optimizing nutrition, immunization, treatment of complications of liver disease, and counseling.

As most of the children with end stage liver disease and metabolic syndromes are malnourished, optimizing nutrition is vital. Children who have chronic cholestasis can be extremely malnourished and have vitamin deficiencies. Calorie-enhanced predigested formula and fat-soluble vitamins are often necessary. Nasogastric feeding tubes may be required in children who have poor appetite or a version to these high-calorie unpalatable diets. Parenteral nutrition should be avoided because it increases the risk of sepsis and liver decompensation.

Administration of age-appropriate immunizations should be done prior to transplantation if time permits, allowing at least 4 weeks between the final live viral immunizations and transplantation. Children who have not completed the necessary vaccine schedule should receive vaccinations at an accelerated schedule. Live vaccines are usually contraindicated in the immunosuppressed child at least for a full year after transplantation. The child should atleast be immunized for diphtheria, pertussis, tetanus, bacillus Calmette–Guerin, hepatitis B, and polio. Measles, mumps, rubella, and varicella vaccines should be brought forward if necessary, and they can be given as early as 6 months of age if the child is scheduled for LT. However, completing the immunization with live vaccines is not possible in children undergoing emergency LT. Vaccination of family members of children scheduled for transplant provides additional protection to the child. The household contacts should be fully immunized using both live and attenuated virus vaccines, except for the oral polio vaccine, which is contraindicated.

Growth and development, especially neurologic development, are areas that need special consideration in pediatrics. Infections are common in children with liver failure and should be evaluated and treated accordingly. Fever without a focus in children who have BA should be treated as cholangitis with appropriate antibiotics.

Cardiac Assessment

Several pediatric liver diseases are associated with congenital heart disease, the most common of which is Alagille syndrome. Although relatively benign forms of pulmonary stenosis are the most common defects, other children may have complex right-heart lesions such as tetralogy of Fallot, which may need surgical correction before LT is undertaken. Biliary atresia may be associated with congenital cardiac disease for example, atrial and ventricular septal defects, which may need to be addressed. Cardiomyopathy may develop secondary to tyrosinemia type I and the organic acidemias. Failure to thrive and stunting are commonly seen in children with genetic disorders particularly Alagille's syndrome.

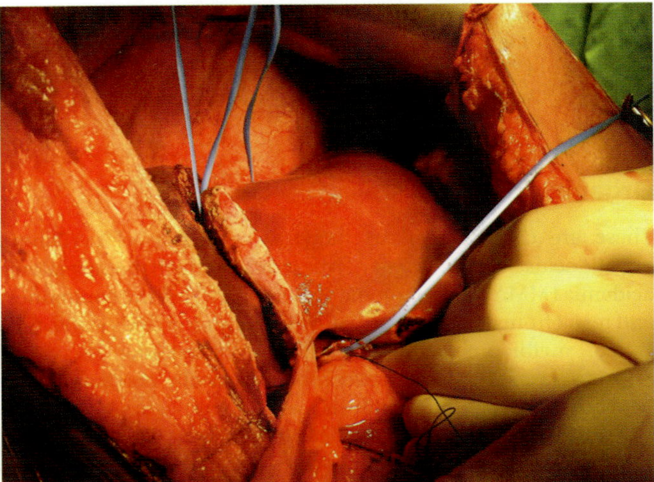

Figure 1 Left lateral segment graft: the line of transection seen about 5 mm to the right of falciform ligament can be seen

The socioeconomic and educational status of the family should be assessed by a multidisciplinary team. It is important to educate and counsel the child's family about lifelong immunosuppressive therapy, its side effects and the need for follow-up at regular intervals.

Intraoperative Issues

The growing discrepancy between the need and the availability of pediatric donor livers has led to newer surgical techniques in LT to expand the donor pool. As a rule of thumb, in infants the left lateral segment is transplanted (Fig. 1); in small children below 12 years of age, the left lobe is adequate; and in adolescents right lobe grafts are used. A GRWR expressed, as percent of body weight between 1.0 and 4.0 is optimal (Fig. 2).[60]

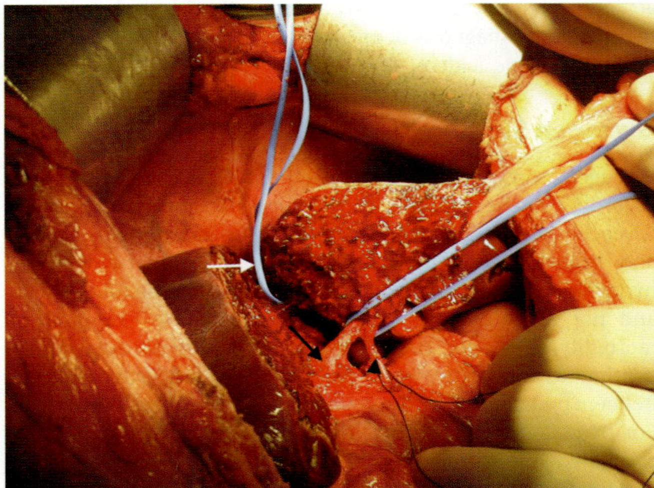

Figure 2 Left lateral segment graft after transection: left portal vein (black arrow), left hepatic artery also supplying segment 4 (arrowhead), and left hepatic vein looped (white arrow) can be seen

Technical complications remain the single most important factor contributing to mortality after pediatric LT. The risk of postoperative complications is higher in children as compared with adults for many reasons:

1. In the virgin abdomen, removal of the native liver in children is usually straightforward. Multiple prior surgeries for BA, or multiple episodes of spontaneous bacterial peritonitis/cholangitis lead to extensive vascularized adhesions, and make it a technically demanding operation increasing the risk of intestinal perforation and bleeding during native hepatectomy. It is advisable to keep ahead of the blood loss, as the reserve in children is less.
2. Blood vessels in children are smaller and so are the vessels of the small left lateral graft increasing the risk of vascular complications. Children are more likely to be hypercoagulable with near normal platelet counts as compared with adults increasing the risk of vascular thrombosis. The incidence of hepatic artery thrombosis in pediatric liver transplant recipients has been reported to be 18%, portal vein thrombosis to be 17%, and hepatic venous outflow obstruction to be 6.6%.[61] The use of partial or split-liver grafts makes biliary reconstruction more difficult, and thus increases the risk of biliary complications.

   In pediatric LRLT, portal vein reconstruction is one of the most crucial elements for success. Recipient portal vein should be anastomosed to the graft left portal vein allowing no twists, kink, rotation, or laxity (Fig. 3). Proper orientation of the graft and recipient portal vein is essential particularly in small children as even a 15° rotation can potentiate thrombosis. Initial marking of one of the surface of the left portal vein with a suture before graft retrieval to guide the orientation is quite helpful.

   Left lateral segment and left-lobe allografts are at great risk for outflow obstruction if the left hepatic vein experiences any rotation. Allograft venous outflow must be unimpeded, and to the confluence of all three hepatic venous orifices to achieve wide and effective outflow (Fig. 4). Impaired outflow leads to allograft swelling, increased vascular resistance, and subsequent inflow (portal) thrombosis. Portal vein Doppler must be done in small babies and children before and after abdominal closure and two to three times a day for the first postoperative week. Small kids should be put on anticoagulants, initially on heparin, and then switched over to antiplatelet agents.

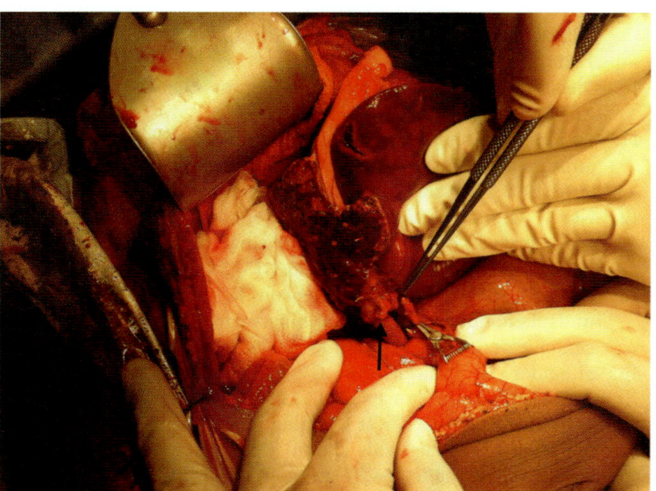

Figure 3 Portal vein reconstruction: recipient portal vein anastomosed to the graft left portal vein allowing no twists, kink, laxity, or tension. Well-perfused left lateral segment graft can be seen

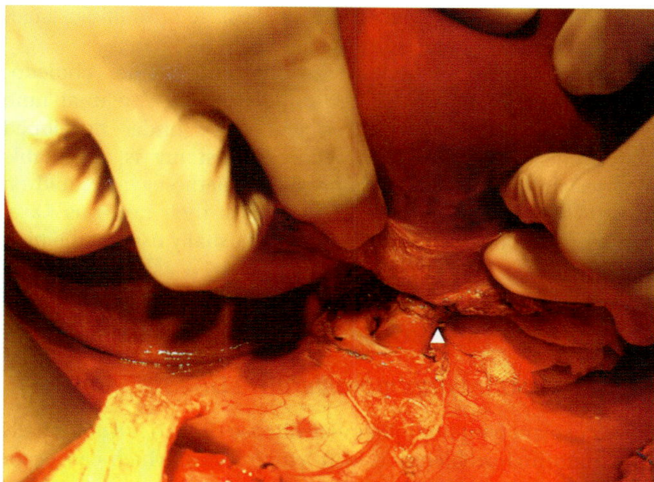

Figure 4 Outflow reconstruction in a left lateral segment graft: left hepatic vein anastomosed to the vena cava at the confluence of three hepatic veins (arrowhead)

3. Large liver graft in a small child (GRWR >4–5%), referred to as big liver syndrome, leads to multiple problems. Small babies may be unable to perfuse a relatively large graft resulting in relative ischemia. Ligation of the coronary vein or ligation of a large portosystemic shunt may help in augmenting the portal blood flow.

Secondly, difficult abdominal wall closure leads to compression and inadequate perfusion of the transplanted liver resulting in surface necrosis adding to the graft dysfunction. Tight abdominal closure further leads to splinting of the diaphragm and delayed extubation contributing to poor outcomes in a small already malnourished child.

In small babies weighing 5–10 kg, even the left lateral segment (LLS) grafts can be too large. Monosegment (usually segment 3) and reduced left lateral segment grafts may be required to overcome the problem of large-for-size grafts.[62] Either bench reduction of the LLS grafts can be done, where the GRWR is high or in situ reduction after the graft is perfused and the measured portal flows are low.

The peripheral nonanatomical reduction of LLS grafts does not address problems related to antero-posterior thickness of segment III which is a major impediment in abdominal closure without tension. Some LLS grafts are short and thick, whereas others are thin and long. The thin long grafts pose less of a problem because a further reduction of part of segment II alone may suffice. However, with short and thick LLS grafts, the removal of segment II alone may not be adequate.

Neonates who have no significant portal hypertension, hepatomegaly, or ascites, the abdominal cavity is usually small. When closing the abdomen, increased intra-abdominal pressure should be avoided. Abdominal closure may be done using a temporary composite mesh, but this is associated with complications like ascitic leak and mesh infection. The use of mobilized skin flaps with running monofilament skin closure while avoiding fascia closure is advisable and is successful in most cases. Musculofascial abdominal wall closure can be completed in a single stage or multiple stages approximately 5–7 days posttransplant.

Bile duct reconstruction as an end-to-side choledochojejunostomy into an isoperistaltic Roux-en-Y jejunal limb is preferred in young children who have under developed native bile duct. Choledocho-choledochostomy is acceptable in older children without primary biliary pathology. In children with BA who have a Roux-en-Y loop from their previous Kasai portoenterostomy the same Roux loop is usually used at the time of transplant.

Specific Complications

Post-transplant Lymphoproliferative Disease

Posttransplant lymphoproliferative disease (PTLD) is a potentially fatal abnormal proliferation of B-lymphocytes, which can occur in any patient who is on immunosuppressive medications. The increased frequency of PTLD in pediatric liver transplant recipients is attributed to the intensity of the immunosuppression required for lifetime duration, and the absence of prior exposure to Epstein–Barr-virus infection in up to 80% of pediatric recipients. Posttransplant lymphoproliferative disease is more likely to follow primary EBV infection, and thus is mostly encountered in pediatric, EBV-naive recipients of allografts from EBV-positive donors.[63] This is a polyclonal or monoclonal lymphoid proliferation of rapid onset. It is more common in children who have received extensive rejection treatment, and is usually extra nodal.

Posttransplant lymphoproliferative disease is the most common tumor in children following transplantation representing almost half of all the tumors compared with 15% among adults. About 80% occur within the first 2 years following transplantation.[64] Posttransplant lymphoproliferative disease is one of the great masqueraders in pediatric transplant medicine and can involve any organ. It may present as a common and usually benign, pediatric complaint such as sinusitis or diarrhea. The index of suspicion is heightened in children with lymphadenopathy, symptoms of airway obstruction caused by enlarged tonsils and adenoids, diarrhea (particularly if associated with protein or blood loss), unexplained fever, weight loss, general malaise, anorexia, headache, new onset of seizures, graft dysfunction, pneumonia, or any new mass lesion.[65] It is essential to make a tissue diagnosis and to evaluate the nature of the lymphocytic proliferation.

Treatment of PTLD is by decreasing or discontinuing immunosuppression and institution of antiviral therapy to allow the immune system to clear EBV. If tumor cells on histopathology express B-cell surface marker CD20, then the anti-CD20 monoclonal antibody rituximab may be used along with cyclophosphamide and prednisone.[66]

Patients with polyclonal PTLD have a better prognosis than monomorphic disease.[67] Serial determination of EBV viral loads is currently the best tool in targeting preemptive therapy, especially in seronegative patients. Monitor for PTLD by EBV PCR 3–6 monthly particularly for the first 2 years, and measure serum albumin, as a decreasing albumin level may be an early sign of gut PTLD.

Tolerance

Complete withdrawal of immunosuppression in children is by serendipity and rarely induced by active treatment. Only a few cases have been reported in literature. Children are more likely to become tolerant after transplantation, as they require less immunosuppression. They are also less likely to develop rejection than older children and adults, perhaps owing to a greater T-helper response than adults.

Immunosuppression

Basic immune suppression protocols in pediatric recipients are similar to those employed in adults. In children, however, early steroid withdrawal to prevent growth retardation is much more widely practiced. Neoral is preferably avoided in young girls to prevent hirsutism. Noncompliance is common particularly among adolescents, and they should be closely monitored. Surveillance of children treated by calcineurin inhibitors for EBV viral infections and appropriate prophylaxis and treatment is essential to prevent the development of posttransplant lymphoproliferative disorder.

REFERENCES

1. Starzl TE, Kaulla KN, Hermann G, et al. Homo transplantation of the liver in humans. Surg Gynecol Obstet. 1963;117:659-76.
2. Starzl TE, Groth CT, Brettschneider L, et al. Orthotopic homotransplantation of the human liver. Ann Surg. 1968;68:392-415.
3. Bismuth H, Houssin D. Reduced-sized orthotopic liver graft in hepatic transplantation in children. Surgery. 1984;95:367-70.
4. Broelsch CE, Emond JC, Whitington PF, et al. Application of reduced-size liver transplants as split grafts, auxiliary orthotopic grafts, and living related segmental transplants. Ann Surg. 1990;212:368-75.
5. Raia S, Nery JR, Mies S, Liver transplantation from live donors. Lancet. 1989;2:497.
6. Strong RW, Lynch SV, Ong TH, et al. Successful liver transplantation from a living donor to her son. N Engl J Med. 1990;322:1505-7.
7. Mc Diarmid SV, Davies DB, Edwards EB. Improved graft survival of paediatric liver recipients transplanted with paediatric-aged liver donors. Transplantation. 2000;70(9):1283-91.
8. Mc Diarmid SV, Anand R, Lindblad AS. Development of a paediatric end-stage liver disease score to predict poor outcome in children awaiting liver transplantation. Transplantation. 2002;74(2):173-81.
9. Kasai M, Mochizuki I, Ohkohchi N, et al. Surgical limitation for biliary atresia: indication for liver transplantation. J Pediatr Surg. 1989;24(9):851-4.
10. Busuttil RW, Seu P, Millis JM, et al. Liver transplantation in children. Ann Surg. 1991;213:4.
11. Ryckman F, Fisher R, Pedersen S, et al. Improved survival in biliary atresia patients in the present era of liver transplantation. J Pediatr Surg. 1993;28(3):382-5 [discussion: 386].
12. Nio M, Ohi R, Hayashi Y, et al. Current status of 21 patients who have survived more than 20 years since undergoing surgery for biliary atresia. J Pediatr Surg. 1996;31(3):381-4.
13. Goss JA, Shackleton CR, Swenson K, et al. Orthotopic liver transplantation for congenital biliary atresia. An 11-year single-center experience. Ann Surg. 1996;224:276-87.
14. Shneider BL, Mazariegos GV. Biliary atresia: a transplant perspective. Liver Transpl. 2007;13:1482-95.
15. Otte JB, de Ville de Goyet J, Reding R, et al. Sequential treatment of biliary atresia with Kasai portoenterostomy and liver transplantation: a review. Hepatology. 1994;20(1 Pt 2):41S-8S.
16. Altman RP, Lilly JR, Greenfeld J, et al. A multivariable risk factor analysis of the portoenterostomy (Kasai) procedure for biliary atresia: twenty-five years of experience from two centers. Ann Surg. 1997;226(3):348-53 [discussion: 353-5].

17. Jacquemin E. Progressive familial intrahepatic cholestasis: genetic basis and treatment. Clin Liver Dis. 2000;4:753-63.
18. Jacquemin E, Hermans D, Myara A, et al. Ursodeoycholic acid therapy in pediatric patients with progressive familial intrahepatic cholestasis. Hepatology. 1997;25:519-23.
19. Lykavieris P, van Mil S, Cresteil D et al. Progressive familial intrahepatic cholestasis type 1 and extrahepatic features: no catch-up of stature growth, exacerbation of diarrhea, and appearance of liver steatosis after liver transplantation. J Hepatol. 2003;39:447-52.
20. Alagille D, Odièvre M, Gautier M, et al. Hepatic ductular hypoplasia associated with characteristic facies, vertebral malformations, retarded physical, mental, and sexual development, and cardiac murmur. J Pediatr. 1975;86:63-71.
21. Cardona J, Houssin D, Gauthier F, et al. Liver transplantation in children with Alagille syndrome—a study of twelve cases. Transplantation. 1995;60(4):339-42.
22. Tzakis AG, Reyes J, Tepetes K, et al. Liver transplantation for Alagille's syndrome. Arch Surg. 1993;128(3):337-9.
23. Hoffenberg EJ, Narkewicz MR, Sondheimer JM, et al. Outcome of syndromic paucity of interlobular bile ducts (Alagille syndrome) with onset of cholestasis in infancy. J Pediatr. 1995;127(2):220-4.
24. Kasahara M, Kiuchi T, Inomata Y, et al. Living-related liver transplantation for Alagille syndrome. Transplantation. 2003;75:2147-50.
25. Bucuvalas J, Yazigi N, Squires RH Jr. Acute liver failure in children. Clin Liver Dis. 2006;10(1):149-68.
26. Whitington PF, Malladi P. Neonatal hemochromatosis: is it an alloimmune disease? J Pediatr Gastroenterol Nutr. 2005;40(5):544-9.
27. Smith SR, Shneider BL, Magid M, et al. Minor salivary gland biopsy in neonatal hemochromatosis. Arch Otolaryngol Head Neck Surg. 2004;130(6):760-3.
28. Flynn DM, Mohan N, McKiernan P, et al. Progress in treatment and outcome for children with neonatal hemochromatosis. Arch Dis Child Fetal Neonatal Ed. 2003;88(2): F124-7.
29. Rodrigues F, Kallas M, Nash R, et al. Neonatal hemochromatosis medical treatment versus. transplantation: the king's experience. Liver Transpl. 2005;11(11):1417-24.
30. McClean P, Davison SM. Neonatal liver failure. Semin Neonatol. 2003;8(5):393-401.
31. Pimpalwar AP, Sharif K, Ramani P, et al. Strategy for hepatoblastoma management: transplant versus non-transplant surgery. J Paediatr Surg. 2002;37(2):240-5.
32. Tiao GM, Bobey N, Allen S, et al. The current management of hepatoblastoma: a combination of chemotherapy, conventional resection and liver transplantation. J Paediatr. 2005;146(2):204-11.
33. Srinivasan P, McCall J, Pritchard J, et al. Orthotopic liver transplantation for unresectable hepatoblastoma. Transplantation. 2002;74(5):652-5.
34. Avila LF, Luis AL, Hernandez F, et al. Liver transplantation for malignant tumors in children. Eur J Paediatr Surg. 2006;16(6):411-4.
35. Faraj W, Dar F, Marangoni G, et al. Liver transplantation for hepatoblastoma. Liver Transpl. 2008;14(11):1614-9.
36. Sherlock S, Dooley J. Nutritional and metabolic liver diseases. In: Sherlock S, Dooley J, editors. Diseases of the liver and biliary System, 11th ed. Oxford: Blackwell Science; 2002. pp. 423-52.
37. Holme E, Lindstedt S. Non-transplant treatment of tyrosinemia. Clin Liver Dis. 2000;4(4):805-14.
38. Weinberg AG, Mize CE, Worthen HG. The occurrence of hepatoma in the chronic form of hereditary tyrosinemia. J Pediatr. 1976;88(3):434-8.
39. Jonas MM, Perez-Atayde AR. Liver disease in infancy and childhood. In: Schiff ER, Sorrell MF, Maddrey WC, editors. Schiff's diseases of the liver, 10th ed. Philadelphia: Lippincott Williams & Wilkins; 2007. pp. 1307-47.
40. Mohan N, McKiernan P, Preece MA, et al. Indications and outcome of liver transplantation in tyrosinaemia type 1. Eur J Pediatr. 1999;158 Suppl 2:S49-54.
41. El-Karaksy H, Fahmy M, El-Raziky M, et al. Hereditary tyrosinemia type 1 from a single center in Egypt: clinical study of 22 cases. World J Pediatr. 2011;7(3):224-231.
42. Pierik LJ, van Spronsen FJ, Bijleveld CM, van Dael CM. Renal function in tyrosinemia type I after liver transplantation: a long-term follow-up. J Inherit Metab Dis. 2005;28(6):871-76.
43. Strauss KA, Wardley B, Robinson D, et al. Classical maple syrup urine disease and brain development: principles of management and formula design. Mol. Genet. Metab. 2010;99(4):333-45.
44. Morton DH, Strauss KA, Robinson DL, et al. Diagnosis and treatment of maple syrup disease: a study of 36 patients. Pediatrics. 2002;109 (6) 999-1008.
45. B.A. Barshop, A. Khanna, Domino hepatic transplantation in maple syrup urine disease, N. Engl. J. Med. 2005;353:2410-11.
46. Badell IR., Hanish SI, Hughes CB, et al. Domino liver transplantation in maple syrup urine disease: a case report and review of the literature. Transplant. Proc. 2013;45:806-9.
47. Rela M, Muiesan P, Vilca-Melendez H, et al. Auxiliary partial orthotopic liver transplantation for Crigler-Najjar syndrome type I. Ann Surg. 1999;229(4):565-9.
48. Seminara J, Tuchman M, Krivitzky L, et al. Establishing a consortium for the study of rare diseases: the urea cycle disorders consortium. Mol. Genet. Metab. 2010;100 (Suppl. 1):S97-105e.
49. Haberle J, Boddaert N, Burlina A, et al. Suggested guidelines for the diagnosis and management of urea cycle disorders. Orphanet J Rare Dis. 2012;7:32.
50. Ah Mew N, Krivitzky L, McCarter R, et al. Urea cycle disorders consortium of the Rare diseases clinical research, clinical outcomes of neonatal onset proximal versus distal urea cycle disorders do not differ. J Pediatr. 2013;162:324-29(e321).
51. Deodato F, Boenzi S, Santorelli FM et al. Methylmalonic and propionic aciduria. Am. J. Med. Genet. C: Semin Med Genet. 2006;142C:104-12.
52. Nagao M, Tanaka T, Morii M, et al. Improved neurologic prognosis for a patient with propionic acidemia who received early living donor liver transplantation. Mol Genet Metab. 2013;108:25-9.
53. Vara R, Turner C, Mundy H, et al. Liver transplantation for propionic acidemia in children, Liver Transpl. 2011;17 661-7.
54. Koeberl DD, Kishnani PS, Chen YT, Glycogen storage disease types I and II: treatment updates. J Inherit Metab. Dis. 2007;30: 159-64.
55. Kishnani PS, Austin SL, Arn P, et al. Glycogen storage disease type III diagnosis and management guidelines. Genet Med. 2010;12:446-63.
56. J. Hicks, E. Wartchow, G. Mierau, Glycogen storage diseases: a brief review and update on clinical features, genetic abnormalities, pathologic features and treatment. Ultrastruct Pathol. 2011;35:183-96.
57. W.S. Lee, R.J. Sokol, Liver disease in mitochondrial disorders. Semin Liver Dis. 2007;27:259-73.
58. E.M. Sokal, R. Sokol, V. Cormier et al. Liver transplantation in mitochondrial respiratory chain disorders, Eur. J Pediatr. 1999;158 (Suppl. 2):S81-4.
59. W.S. Lee, R.J. Sokol, Mitochondrial hepatopathies: advances in genetics, therapeutic approaches, and outcomes, J Pediatr. 2013;163:942-48.
60. Farmer DG, Venick RS, Mc Diarmid SV et al. Predictors of outcomes after paediatric liver transplantation: an analysis of more than 800 cases performed at a single institution. J Am Coll Surg. 2007;204:904-6.
61. Krishna Kumar G, Sharif K, Mayer D et al. Hepatic venous outflow obstruction in paediatric liver transplantation. Paediatr Surg Int. 2010;26:423-425.

62. Higashiyama H, Yamaguchi T, Mori K, et al. Graft size assessment by preoperative computed tomography in living related partial liver transplantation. Br J Surg. 1993; 80:489.
63. Smets F, Sokal EM. Epstein-Barr virus-related lymphoproliferation in children after liver transplant: role of immunity. diagnosis, and management. Paediatr Transplant. 2002;6(4):280-7.
64. Morrison VA, Dunn DL, Manivel JC, et al. Clinical characteristics of post-transplant lymphoproliferative disorders. Am J Med. 1994; 97:14-24.
65. Smets F, Sokal EM. Lymphoproliferation in children after liver transplantation. J Pediatr Gastroenterol Nutr. 2002;34(5):499-505.
66. Orjuela M, Gross TG, Cheung YK, et al. A pilot study of chemo immunotherapy (cyclophosphamide, prednisone, and rituximab) in patients with post-transplant lymphoproliferative disorder following solid organ transplantation. Clin Cancer Res. 2003;9(10 Pt 2):3945S-52.
67. Gross TG. Low-dose chemotherapy for children with post-transplant lymphoproliferative disease. Recent Results Cancer Res. 2002;159:96-103.

CHAPTER 111

Liver Transplantation in Acute Liver Failure

Dronacharya Routh, CS Naidu

INTRODUCTION

Sudden and severe hepatic injury due to varied causes results in a clinical condition called acute liver failure (ALF). Sudden loss of hepatic tissue leads to a deranged coagulation profile, impaired metabolic and immunological function, hepatic encephalopathy (HE), and may progress to multiorgan failure. Acute liver failure, though infrequent in occurrence, is seen mainly in young adults and has been linked to high mortality and financial burden to the society. Diverse etiologies, the relative rarity of the condition along with rapid deterioration make detailed studies difficult. Hence, there are very few evidence-based studies to guide the clinicians. Although orthotopic liver transplantation (OLT) was started initially for treating patients with chronic end-stage liver disease, it is currently being used routinely for the treatment of ALF. The mortality rate in ALF was 80–85% before the use of OLT as a salvage therapy.[1] Over the last decade, there have been technical refinements in the field of liver transplantation and critical care, which have led to improved 1-year survival rates after OLT for ALF from 60 to 80%.[2-5] However, survival rate is still lower following emergency transplantation for ALF than those following elective transplantation. It is also important for clinicians to note that less than 15% of these group of patients have spontaneous recovery,[1] so the decision as to which subset of patients would likely benefit from liver transplantation is critical. The necessity of emergency transplant in ALF has been given due credence world over. The United Network for Organ Sharing (UNOS) in the United States places this group of patients as status 1A (urgent) and similarly in the United Kingdom as "super-urgent" patients, thereby increasing their chances of getting a deceased donor liver at the shortest time. However, till date ALF accounts for less than 11 and 10% of transplants in Europe and the United States, respectively.[6]

DEFINITION

In 1970, Trey C first coined the term fulminant hepatic failure to describe a potentially reversible condition that resulted from severe liver injury in the absence of preexisting liver disease, with encephalopathy within 8 weeks of symptom appearance.[7] Since then a large number of definitions for ALF were given in literature but the key elements of the original definition remained relevant. In 1983, O'Grady et al.[8] classified ALF in adults on the basis of time of presentation. The time for onset of encephalopathy from jaundice classifies ALF into three groups: hyperacute, acute, and subacute. This classification is clinically important, in that it helps to identify the etiology of disease, likely complications, and probable prognosis (Table 1). In 1986, Bernuau et al.[1] categorized ALF into fulminant and subfulminant on the basis of the interval from jaundice to encephalopathy. Importantly, in children, these definitions are clinically irrelevant as clinical encephalopathy is often absent or late in the course of disease. Thus, in 1996, Bhaduri et al. defined ALF in pediatric age group as a systemic disorder with severe impairment of liver function, with or without encephalopathy, occurring with hepatocellular necrosis in a patient with absence of underlying chronic liver disease.[10]

INCIDENCE

The overall incidence of ALF is between one and six cases per million people each year.[11-13] However, data from other regions, including India, are sparse, although different studies have shown that the rates are likely high in areas where infective hepatitis is frequent and there is nonavailability of medical treatment to interrupt hepatic injury progression and involvement of extrahepatic organs.

Table 1: Classification, clinical features, and prognosis of the three subtypes of acute liver failure.

	Hyperacute	*Acute*	*Subacute*
Time from jaundice to encephalopathy	0–1 week	1–4 weeks	4–12 weeks
Severity of coagulopathy	+++	++	+
Severity of jaundice	+	++	+++
Degree of intracranial hypertension	++	++	+/–
Survival rate without emergency liver transplantation	Good	Moderate	Poor
Typical cause	Paracetamol, hepatitis A and E	Hepatitis B	Non-paracetamol drug-induced liver injury

Source: Data from O'Grady et al. (1993)8 and Ichai and Samuel (2008).[9]
+++ = high severity; ++ = medium severity; + = low severity; +/– = present or absent.

ETIOLOGY

The etiology of ALF has wide geographic variations (Table 2).[14] In the West, the most common causes of ALF are acetaminophen overdose, non-A non-E hepatitis, and idiosyncratic drug reactions.[1,15-19] In contrast, in the Indian subcontinent, more than 90% of cases of ALF are due to viral hepatitis. Hepatitis E virus (HEV) followed by hepatitis A virus (HAV) and hepatitis B virus (HBV) are the most common viruses causing ALF as per the incidence.[20-22] Mixed viral infections are not an uncommon cause of ALF. Hepatitis E virus has a high predilection for pregnant women in endemic areas and is a poor prognostic factor in the outcome of ALF.[23] Antitubercular drugs and herbal preparations, which are quite commonly used in our country, are also important etiological factors for ALF. Although uncommon, inherited disorders causing ALF need attention as a differential diagnosis, especially in newborns. This subset of children even before presentation have a variable degree of liver damage and need to be managed with dietary manipulation or other disease-specific therapy that might be life-saving in them and for some cases, liver transplantation might be contraindicated.[24]

Table 2: Etiology of acute liver failure

Common causes		
	Viral	Hepatitis E virus
		Hepatitis A virus
		Hepatitis B virus
	Drugs (idiosyncratic reaction)	Acetaminophen
		Antitubercular drugs
		Herbal preparations
		NSAIDs
	Drug toxicity	Carbamazepine
	Vascular diseases	Ischemic hepatitis in sepsis
		Acute Budd–Chiari syndrome
		Right heart failure
	Toxins	*Bacillus cereus* toxin
		Amanita phalloides toxin
	Metabolic diseases	Acute fatty liver of pregnancy
		Reye syndrome
		Wilson's syndrome
	Autoimmune diseases	Autoimmune hepatitis
Rare causes	Viral	Herpes simplex virus
		Cytomegalovirus
		Epstein–Barr virus
		Adenovirus
		Varicella zoster virus
		Human herpes virus-6
	Toxins	Carbon tetrachloride
		Yellow phosphorus
	Malignant infiltration	Lymphoma
		Metastatic breast cancer

NSAIDs, nonsteroidal anti-inflammatory drugs.

PRINCIPLES OF MANAGEMENT IN ACUTE LIVER FAILURE

Due to rapidly progressing deterioration in liver function, there is severe multiorgan failure with unpredictable complications in ALF. This group of patients is best managed in the liver intensive care units where specialized care is available. The general principle of management is to support the diseased liver and to achieve maximal hepatic regeneration. Intensive care is delivered as per standard protocol to support the failing organs with other measures aimed at recognition and removal of the insult that lead to hepatic injury and prevent development of complications. Etiology-directed interventions, intensive monitoring, and treatment of encephalopathy and intracranial hypertension or cerebral edema remain pivotal during the course of treatment.[25,26] However, the most important decision that needs to be taken by the treating physician is as to which subset of patients of ALF would benefit from emergency liver transplantation. It is necessary to identify patients early in the course who will not achieve adequate regeneration to increase the chance of successful emergency transplantation.

PROGNOSTICATION OF PATIENTS FOR LIVER TRANSPLANTATION

A substantial percentage of patients with ALF have spontaneous recovery with best supportive care. It is essential to recognize the other subset of patients who will benefit from emergent OLT, and at the same time recognize patients who are too sick to benefit from OLT. Orthotopic liver transplantation has its own disadvantages, including operative risk and lifelong immunosuppression. So, to minimize the risk a balance needs to be drawn between delayed transplantation to allow spontaneous recovery against the risk of mortality with the delay and risk of surgery itself. Twenty percent of ALF patients listed for transplantation recover spontaneously without it; however, a significant proportion die awaiting availability of donor organ. Development of complications during the course of the disease, such as hemodynamic abnormalities, sepsis, cerebral edema, and multiorgan system failure, often makes these patients unsuitable for transplantation. In the United Kingdom, 30% of patients initially listed for OLT turn out to be untransplantable after the development of such complications.[26] Moreover, patients have medical or psychosocial conditions, including cardiovascular disease, irreversible brain injury, infection/sepsis, drug or alcohol abuse, lack of family support, and uncontrolled psychiatric disorder, which prohibits transplant.[27]

Therefore, for predicting good postoperative outcome, it is essential to develop a reliable predictive model of survival and need of OLT. These would permit to differentiate those patients who will have a spontaneous recovery and allow a judicious utilization of scarce organs. There are presently no standardized criteria to list patients of ALF for OLT. Although there are several prognostic models for identifying appropriate candidates for transplantation, unfortunately, they have several limitations with varied predictive accuracy.[28,29]

Factors Affecting Prognosis

Etiology

It is one of the most important predictors of outcome in ALF.[30] The outcome following emergency liver transplant in ALF secondary to acetaminophen toxicity is the best with a reported mortality rate of ~30%, while HEV- and HAV-induced hepatitis and pregnancy-related ALF have a very high mortality rate reaching to ~50%.[30-32] Therefore, the knowledge of etiological factors prevalent in a particular region helps in early assessment and listing of patients for OLT. Drug-induced liver injury leading to ALF predominates in North America and Europe, with majority of acetaminophen-induced ALF in the United Kingdom and the United States.[4,30,31,33,34] In developing countries like India, viral hepatitis is the predominant cause and is present in almost 90–100% of cases in the published literature. Over a period of 11 years, the US ALF study group included 1,198 patients with ALF. A total of 133 patients (11.1%) had drug-induced ALF, and with successful transplantation in 42.1%, overall survival was 66.2%; however, the transplant-free (3-week) survival was poor (27.1%).[30]

Clinical and Laboratory Criteria

The criteria to list patients of ALF vary from center to center. The UNOS group stratifies ALF as status 1A based on certain parameters (Table 3). The exclusion criteria for emergency liver transplantation are elderly age group (>70 years); severe infection; uncontrolled septic shock; presence of certain malignancies; severe cardiac, lung, or multiple organ failure; and brain death, as these patients do not tolerate OLT and the outcome is dismal.[35,36] Similarly, patients with sustained elevation in intracranial pressure >50 mmHg, cerebral perfusion pressure <40 mmHg, grade 3–4 encephalopathy with fixed pupils, and history of seizures or brain death are usually not suitable candidates for OLT.[2,36] Biochemical parameters have also been extensively studied to prognosticate ALF. Serum bilirubin level correlates well with the severity of the disease and has been taken into consideration in various prognostic models like the King's College criteria. However, the degree of increase in liver enzymes (aspartate transaminase, alanine transaminase, gamma-glutamyl transferase) does not predict prognosis. In spite of worsening HE, coagulation profile (international normalized ratio), and bilirubin level, there has been improvement of aminotransferase levels. This is an ominous sign and occurs in complete liver failure.

Table 3: UNOS status 1A listing criteria for ALF
Age ≥18 years
Life expectancy <7 days without a liver transplant
Onset of encephalopathy <8 weeks from the first symptom of liver disease
Absence of **preexisting** liver disease (except: Fulminant Wilson's disease)
Residence in the intensive care unit
At least one of the following: ventilator dependence, renal replacement therapy, or INR >2.0

ALF, acute liver failure; INR, international normalized ratio; UNOS, United Network for Organ Sharing.

Multiorgan Failure

The degree of multiorgan failure is also a poor prognostic factor for posttransplant survival. In a multivariate analysis of UNOS data from 1988 to 2003 by Barshes et al., four risk factors were identified for predicting posttransplant survival: recipient age >50 years, pretransplant use of life support, serum creatinine >2 mg/dL, and recipient body mass index ≥30 kg/m^2. The 5-year posttransplant survival with all these risk factors was 44–47%; however, it increased to 82–83% without these features.[37]

Hepatic Encaphalopathy

Mortality rates increase with increase in severity of HE. A study done by Daas et al. showed a mortality rate of 30% for grade 2, 45–50% for grade 3, and 80–90% for grade 4 HE.[36] A similar multicenter study in the United States by Schiødt et al. showed that 39% participants had acetaminophen-induced ALF, with 3-week transplant-free survival being 52% in patients with grade 1–2 HE and 33% with grade 3–4 HE.[32] Interestingly, it has been seen in studies that those with a shorter interval between the development of symptoms and HE (i.e, acetaminophen induced) appear to have a better result than those with longer progression to HE (i.e., other drug-induced liver injury).[1,8,38,39] A characteristic feature of ALF-induced HE is the development of cerebral edema, which by itself is a poor prognostic marker in outcome of ALF. Eighty percent of patients with grade 4 HE develop cerebral edema that leads to intracranial hypertension, subsequently brainstem herniation or ischemic brain damage, accounting for mortality in 50% of patients.[40,41]

Infection

It is often difficult to distinguish ALF-induced hemodynamic changes from superadded infection and sepsis. The most common sites of infection being pulmonary (47%), blood (26%), and urine

(23%) and these account for death in up to 37% of cases.[42] Fungal infections, mainly Candida sp., are seen in around 32% of cases, which occur later in the course of disease, particularly after use of antibiotics or in the background of renal dysfunction.[43,44] Orthotopic liver transplantation is contraindicated in the setting of active infection. The empirical role of antibiotics is controversial and although prophylactic antibiotics decrease the risk of infections, they do not alter the overall outcome.[45-47] Some centers administer antibiotics/antifungals routinely to patients who have clinical evidence of systemic inflammatory response syndrome, have refractory hypotension, progression to stage 3–4 HE, or have significant isolates on surveillance cultures.[47] Early detection of bacterial and fungal infections needs biochemical parameters, periodic surveillance cultures, and frequent chest radiographs.

Psychological Issues

Orthotopic liver transplantation in ALF requires an intensive postoperative follow-up and lifelong immunosuppression, which significantly affects the posttransplant quality of life (QOL). Therefore, before consideration for transplantation in ALF, certain psychosocial factors like substance and/or alcohol abuse, and adequacy of social and financial support need to be looked into. Blei et al. reported death of four patients (12%) in the posttransplant follow-up period from deliberate self-harm.[28]

Prognostic Models

The decision to transplant in ALF is critical and has to be timely for it to be beneficial. While premature transplant will not allow spontaneous recovery in a subset of patients and at the same time, exposing the patient to surgical complications and lifelong immunosuppression, delaying transplant is associated with a high degree of complication and mortality. As stated earlier, multiple prognostic models have been formulated in various studies to determine the benefit of OLT and the likelihood of spontaneous recovery in ALF patients (Table 4).[48-59] However, critical analyses showed that many of these models are subject to bias and are methodologically flawed. In addition, the positive predictive value of these models is falsely elevated as many equate OLT with death.[52]

King's College Criteria

It is the most commonly practiced prognostic model developed from a retrospective cohort of nearly 600 patients.[55,60] The King's College criteria incorporate both etiology of ALF (acetaminophen versus non-acetaminophen-induced ALF) and clinical parameters of disease.[55] A systemic review and meta-analysis of studies using the King's College criteria, by Bailey et al. in 2003, showed the pooled sensitivity and specificity to be 69 and 92%, respectively.[49] These criteria appear to have better positive predictive values (80% in acetaminophen-induced ALF and 70–90% in non-acetaminophen-induced ALF) but inferior negative predictive values (70–90 and 25–50%, respectively). McPhail et al. published a meta-analysis in 2010 which reported that the criteria for non-acetaminophen-induced ALF have a good specificity, particularly for patients with high-grade encephalopathy.[61] It is useful in identifying patients who may require OLT; however, in up to 20% of those fulfilling the criteria may still survive without undergoing OLT and those not meeting the criteria for OLT may still need transplantation. A couple of studies by Bernal et al. in 2002 and

Table 4: Various prognostic scoring systems for acute liver failure

Variable	*Clichy criteria*	*King's criteria : acetaminophen*	*King's criteria: non-acetaminophen*	*APACHE II*	*MELD*
Clinical parameters					
Age	+	–	+	+	–
Etiology	–	–	+	–	–
Presence of hepatic encephalopathy	+	+	–	+	–
Duration of jaundice	–	–	+	–	–
Vital signs	–	–	–	+	–
Laboratory parameters					
INR	–	+	+	–	+
Arterial pH	–	+	–	+	–
Serum creatinine	–	+	–	+	+
Serum bilirubin	–	–	+	–	+
Factor V	+	–	–	–	–
pO_2	–	–	–	+	–
Serum Na and K	–	–	–	+	–
Hematocrit	–	–	–	+	–
Total leukocyte count	–	–	–	+	–

APACHE II, Acute Physiology and Chronic Health Evaluation II; INR, international normalized ratio; MELD, model for end-stage liver disease, pO_2, partial pressure of oxygen.

MacQuillan et al. in 2005 had shown that sensitivity of the above model can be improved by adding arterial blood lactate levels.[60,62]

Clichy Criteria

The Clichy criteria are based on a cohort of French patients with acute HBV infection where a multivariate analysis of factors affecting prognosis in fulminant liver failure was done.[50] These criteria suggest that a serum factor V level of <30% in any patient with grade 3–4 HE or <20% in patients younger than 30 years is a predictor of mortality with a sensitivity and specificity of 86 and 76%, respectively. However, the drawback of these criteria is that factor V level measurements are less commonly available to the clinician than are the parameters in the King's criteria; therefore, this prognostic model is not usually utilized.[63,64] In addition, this model has not been validated in patients with other etiological factors causing ALF.

Acute Physiology and Chronic Health Evaluation II

Although being used commonly in critical care patients, Acute Physiology and Chronic Health Evaluation II (APACHE II) is not routinely used for prognostication of patients with ALF. It is inadequate in predicting the survival of patients without transplantation because many patients who do not fulfill the severity criteria will eventually die of subsequent complications.[65]

Model for End-stage Liver Disease Score

The model for end-stage liver disease (MELD) scoring system is an excellent prognostic model for predicting mortality in chronic liver disease[66-69]; however, it has limited utility in prognostication in ALF patients. Predictors of ALF, such as age, etiology of ALF, and duration of jaundice, are not accounted in the MELD score. It has a sensitivity and specificity of <75% for predicting outcome in all forms of ALF.[70] Whether modification of the MELD with these important factors will improve the MELD as a standard scoring system in prognosis of ALF remains to be seen.

Other Prognostic Models

Dhiman et al. performed a multivariate regression analysis of factors from the Indian subcontinent at a center where liver transplantation was not available. They identified six independent clinical prognostic indicators at admission: age >50 years, jaundice to encephalopathy time greater than 7 days, cerebral edema, grade 3–4 HE, prothrombin time ≥35 seconds, and serum creatinine ≥1.5 mg/dL associated with a poorer prognosis.[71] The presence of three or more of these factors was superior to either King's College criteria or MELD score in predicting an adverse outcome.

A low volume of liver (<1,000 mL) on preoperative computed tomography imaging is also associated with a high mortality rate, a finding that has been validated in studies by Shakil et al. and Yamagishi et al.[72,73] Based upon these findings, a prognostic formula has been proposed, but is not widely utilized. Liver biopsy may also be helpful in determining the cause of the ALF and theoretically, it can also assess the severity and extent of liver damage, but is not done routinely in clinical practice considering the deranged coagulation profile of the patient. In a study by Scotto et al. in 1973, hepatic necrosis of more than 70% was associated with a transplant-free survival of <10%.[74] More recently, studies by Miraglia et al. and Voigt et al. found that the magnitude of necrosis was not predictive of mortality.[75,76] Based upon the available literature, the current prognostic scoring systems based on liver volume or necrosis have not consistently showed reliable accuracy in predicting indications for OLT and outcome from ALF.

The prognostic models that assess the need for liver transplantation in pediatric age group are even more confusing. The Nazer score for Wilson's disease is widely used.[77] A Nazer score of >7 is predictive of the need for liver transplantation in fulminant Wilson's disease. The King's College had modified the Nazer score and showed that a score of >11 predicted mortality with a sensitivity of 93% and specificity of 96% in patients without liver transplantation.[78] The pediatric end-stage liver disease score has also been used to assess the need for transplantation in the pediatric age group. A score >25 was one of the factors that predicted the need for early transplant in children with ALF.[79]

Thus, till date, an ideal prognostic model remains elusive. It should be simple, widely applicable across all age groups and varied etiologies, and multiphasic involving frequently used laboratory and clinical parameters.

WHO WOULD BENEFIT FROM LIVER TRANSPLANTATION?

It remains controversial to identify and select patients who would likely benefit from emergency liver transplantation. Based on the previously discussed prognostic models, patients are listed for OLT. An inaccurate selection will have serious effects—a patient who would otherwise have a spontaneous recovery with medical management and has wrongly received a transplant will be subjected to a needless surgical procedure and lifelong immunosuppression, which is associated with major financial burden and an increased risk of death. Furthermore, a deceased donor graft that could be used in a more suitable candidate will be lost. On the other hand, the consequence of inability to recognize a patient with ALF who would survive only with emergency liver transplantation is of equal magnitude, because a potentially preventable death will ensue. Given the rapid progression of the disease process and clinical deterioration in ALF, patients should be urgently listed for liver transplantation where indicated. Thus, these groups of patients are listed as status 1A or super-urgent for the purpose of early organ allocation in the United States and the United Kingdom.[80,81]

SURGICAL OPTIONS

With the introduction of emergency transplantation for patients with ALF, the 1-year survival rate has risen to 80%.[82,83] However, the outcomes of emergency transplantation are consistently inferior to those for elective conditions, with high mortality rate in early period, mainly as a result of sepsis and multiorgan failure.

Liver transplantation may be performed in various ways depending on the availability of donor organ: deceased heartbeating or a non-heartbeating donor, living donor, auxiliary liver transplants, and variable ABO status. In view of organ shortage, the risk of death waiting for an organ should be balanced against the risk of complications or failure using an alternative graft.

Deceased Donor Liver Transplant

It is the gold standard of treatment if available in patients of ALF with a 1-year survival of as high as 80%. Other surgical options need to be compared against it.[2] Reduced size of graft (split grafts) and marginal grafts lead to reduced survival and are poor prognostic signs. The time to listing and availability of an organ varies from country to country. The wait for an organ often allows natural selection with spontaneous recovery in a small proportion of patients and avoids unnecessary lifelong immunosuppression; however, simultaneously many patients deteriorate and die while waiting. As per the UNOS data in the United States, 50 % of patients of ALF listed as status 1A are expected to receive a deceased donor organ within 15 days.[84] There are often limitations of deceased donor liver transplantation (DDLT) with increased usage of marginal grafts or use of non-heart-beating livers due to urgency of the situation. Longer cold ischemia time can lead to a higher incidence of poor graft function.[85] In a multivariate analysis by Barshes et al., predictors of poor graft function were analyzed. Body mass index >30 kg/m^2, age >50, creatinine >2mg/dL, and a history of use of life support predicted poor function in the recipient.[37] Eighty two percent of patients without any negative factors survived, while only 42% patients with the presence of all factors survived. While waiting for availability of graft, patients often develop "toxic liver syndrome" with extreme hemodynamic instability. Such patients often benefit from a two-staged procedure with a total hepatectomy and porto-caval shunt as an initial procedure followed by liver transplantation when a deceased donor graft is available.[86,87] However, the outcome of this procedure depends on the availability of a donor graft in a reasonable period of time.

Living Donor Liver Transplant

With the increasing shortage of deceased donors, living donor liver transplant (LDLT) in the setting of ALF is being increasingly practiced, especially in the Indian subcontinent.[88-91] There is no consensus on "adequate graft volume." While some researchers have proposed that patients with ALF will require a smaller size graft due to absence of portal hypertension, others believe that the high metabolic demand in ALF mandates a larger volume graft. The study by Lo et al. from Hong Kong reported good survival in an adult with a graft volume (GV) 25% of the standard liver volume (SLV).[92] Despite good survival with smaller grafts, it is generally believed that GV/SLV >40% and preferably >50% is ideal for success in ALF.[93] Results are superior with a graft-to-recipient weight ratio (GRWR) more than 0.8, with 1.0 being ideal.[94,95] In the absence of small-for-size syndrome following LDLT, the graft and donor livers regenerate to full size in a matter of 4 weeks.[95] Despite these risks, right lobe LDLT has an improved survival in ALF possibly because of the increased GRWR, with overall 1-year survival rates between 60 and 90%.[88,91,96-98]

Studies done by Casas et al. and Emre et al. on pediatric age group with ALF had shown a 1-year survival ranging from 67 to 89% and death on the waiting list was decreased to 9% following LDLT.[99,100] It has also been seen that split liver transplantation done in pediatric patients did not influence the outcome of LDLT.[101]

In the United States and Europe, the frequency of LDLT for ALF is 5% compared with more than 90% in Asia, excluding China. Using data from the Intractable Liver Disease Study Group of Japan,[98] the author reported that LDLT was performed in 209 ALF patients. The 1-year, 5-year, and 10-year cumulative survival rates following LDLT were 79, 74, and 73%, respectively. This study showed the benefit of LDLT in ALF in countries where DDLT is rarely done. In this study, it was seen that short- and long-term mortality is affected by patient age; however, donor age impacts only long-term patient mortality. They concluded that the nature of liver disease or treatment offered does not influence long-term patient survival following LDLT.

Certain legal and ethical issues exist in the assessment of donor for LDLT in ALF. Donor evaluation must be expedited due to the urgent need for an organ. The time required for detailed evaluation of donor may often be curtailed by the clinician in the setting of rapid clinical worsening of the planned recipient.[102] However, this carries an increased donor risk due to incomplete evaluation. In areas where cadaveric organs are not readily available, the risk of the recipient's mortality while waiting for a cadaveric organ must be valued against the risk to the living donor, including risk of 0.2% donor mortality.[103,104] In India, the requirement of legal documentation prior to transplantation makes it often difficult to perform LDLT in ALF patients on an urgent basis.

Auxillary Liver Transplant

It has been seen that a few, but significant number of patients with ALF (15%) who fulfill the criteria for transplantation will have total morphological and functional recovery of their liver even if they do not undergo OLT.[105] This fact has led to the concept of auxiliary liver transplantation (ALT). It allows the native liver for potential spontaneous regeneration and possibility of stopping immunosuppressive drugs in the future.[106-109] In ALT, the recipient's liver is left in place while a partial left or right lobe from the donor is transplanted that serves as a temporary liver support to the recipient's injured liver till the native liver regenerates and takes over. Ideally, once the native liver recovers, immunosuppression may be withdrawn and the graft is either allowed to atrophy naturally or removed surgically.[110,111]

Based on the operative procedure, ALT is classified into two types: heterotopic auxiliary transplantation and auxiliary partial liver transplantation. The former is technically easier compared with the latter. In the former, the partial graft is placed below the native liver while in the latter the graft replaces a resected right or left native lobe. Heterotopic graft implantation onto the infrahepatic vena cava may cause venous outflow obstruction that results in slower regeneration of hepatocyte probably due to cytokine release from remnant necrotic liver tissue. As compared with auxiliary partial liver transplantation, heterotopic auxiliary transplantation is associated with an increased incidence of portal vein thrombosis and primary graft nonfunction.[114]

The results of ALT are comparable to conventional OLT; however, unique postoperative complications may develop following ALT, including biliary and neurologic problems.[113] The regeneration of the native liver and graft function may be impaired as portal blood flow is partially diverted from the native liver to the auxiliary graft. Moreover, neurologic dysfunction and cerebral edema may persist or progress due to the smaller size of the transplanted graft.[110] In addition, severe infective complications like multisystem organ failure due to immunosuppression may develop by leaving the necrotic graft in situ.[111,114]

The overall survival for ALT has been reported to be between 60 and 65% in various studies, and 85% of these survivors were able to discontinue immunosuppressive therapy by 1 year following transplantation.[110-112,115] The results of 1-year survival in auxiliary partial transplantation are better than those who underwent heterotopic transplantation.[112] Fifteen percent of the patients who underwent ALT would require retransplantation for various reasons. More recently, Faraj et al. looked at the long-term outcome of 20 children who underwent ALT in the United Kingdom; the 1-, 5-, and 10-year survival rate in this group of children was 85%.[116] Of the 17 survivors, successful regeneration of their native liver was noted in 14 (82%) patients and in 11 children (65% of the survivors), immunosuppressives were withdrawn at a median interval of 23 months (range: 4–106) after transplantation.

Auxiliary liver transplantation is a technically challenging procedure with high rates of complication and retransplantation.[117] Outcomes have improved considerably, in part due to improvements in surgical technique, but also from proper patient selection. Now, many centers consider ALT only for young patients with liver failure due to specific causes, stable extrahepatic organ dysfunction, and optimum availability of graft.[118, 119]

ABO Incompatible Transplant

In emergency situations like ALF, ABO-incompatible (ABO-I) LDLT has become an inevitable option either due to nonavailability of deceased donor or limited living donor. Refusing ABO-I LDLT may lead to expeditious death of the patient. Therefore, in these situations, the use of such grafts from ABO-I donors might be the only option available.[120]

Initial experiences with ABO-I LDLT had shown risk of early mortality in adults, however, relatively safe in infants of <1 year old. The reason for mortality was infection secondary to over-immunosuppression or antibody-mediated rejection, which usually presents as intrahepatic biliary complications or hepatic necrosis.[121] In 2008, Egawa et al. reported similar outcome of transplantation between cases with compatible blood types and cases with identical blood types. The survival rates at 5 years were 81, 76, and 59% in identical, compatible, and incompatible cases, respectively.[122] Todo et al. in 2000 reported first ABO-I liver transplant.[123] They published the overall Japanese experience of ABO-I LDLT in adult patients reporting 2-year survival rate of about 20%. The factors associated with morbidity and poor outcome were older age and pretransplant ABO titer levels. In patients receiving an ABO-I allograft, the incidence of antibody-mediated rejection, biliary complications, and hepatic artery thrombosis is higher.[124-126] In most clinical studies, two methods have been used to decrease antibody-mediated complications. Firstly, plasmapheresis or immunoadsorption before transplantation is used to reduce preformed isoaglutinins in the recipient. Secondly, suppression of isoaglutinins restoration by splenectomy, by specifically interfering activation or maturation of B cells or reinforced immunosuppression is done.[127-135] Splenectomy decreases antibody titers in this subset of patients but it may also cause portal vein thrombosis due to decreased portal flow. Recently, instead of splenectomy, anti-CD20 monoclonal antibody (rituximab) is being used.[136]

OUTCOME

The sudden onset of disease and rapid deterioration of clinical condition with associated complications in ALF results in poor outcome in patients undergoing liver transplantation. Posttransplantation, poorer outcome and high mortality rate reflect the critical condition of these patients. Studies have shown that even with the best pre- and posttransplant supportive care, 30% mortality is observed during the index admission with another 11% of patients succumbing during follow-up.[137,138] The multisystemic impact and the physiological instability of patients with ALF are illustrated by the fact that the main causes for mortality in the perioperative period are sepsis, cardiovascular events, and multiorgan failure. Another important reason for the high mortality in ALF is the quality of donor graft. In multivariate analyses, ABO-I grafts, reduced graft size, and graft steatosis have all been shown to decrease the graft and patient survival.[2,139] Acute liver failure patients are listed on the super-urgent/status 1A transplant candidate and thereby receive the first available (and usable) graft. This graft may not be an ideal graft in every situation. Thus, the combination of a critical recipient and a marginal graft is distant from ideal conditions leading to inferior outcome. In these situations, one could afford to be more careful in the use of marginal grafts. However, the unpredictability of organ availability, the urgency of the patient, and an increased proportion of marginal grafts being retrieved have led to an increased use of such livers for ALF.

In a study of infants with ALF transplanted between 1986 and 2000, spontaneous recovery was noted in only 24%. Nearly half (47%) succumbed to sepsis or multiorgan failure, and 29% underwent OLT, of which half were still alive at a mean follow-up of 5 years. The authors concluded that since the etiology was more commonly an inborn error of metabolism, infants had worse prognosis with ALF.[140] On a multivariate analysis, risk factors for posttransplant mortality included age less than 1 year, grade 4 HE, and use of pretransplant dialysis.[101]

QUALITY OF LIFE

There are many studies related to health-related quality of life (HRQoL) posttransplantation for chronic liver disease; however, there is paucity of data measuring HRQoL following liver transplantation for ALF.[141] In a study conducted by Sargent et al. in 2006, a majority of transplanted ALF recipients have a good QOL posttransplant comparable with their pretransplantation lifestyle. However, the recovery in the early postoperative period is often complex and linked to the physical changes incited by multiorgan failure and intensive care stay, which can cause numerous emotional and physical challenges. Acute liver failure recipients had significant physical inactivity and fatigue due to loss of weight and muscle tone in the initial 3–6 months posttransplantation.[141,142]

FUTURE PERSPECTIVES

Unlike in renal failure, there are few established liver support systems which are of proven efficacy in ALF. Extracorporeal supportive devices like molecular adsorbing recirculating system have been advocated in ALF patients to replace liver function either by buying time for the recovery of native liver or to stabilize the patient and serve as a bridging therapy before liver transplantation, with reduced risk of cerebral complications. Despite individual randomized trials and many uncontrolled case series, no convincing evidence of benefit to ALF patients from liver support systems has been reported.[143,144] Outside a trial situation, there is no published report to prove superiority of either biological or nonbiological systems as a sole treatment when emergency liver transplantation is available.

Hepatocyte transplantation (HT) is a promising alternative to OLT in patients of inborn errors of metabolism where the target is to replace a single deficient enzyme or its product.[145-148] As compared to OLT, this is a less invasive procedure and can be performed repeatedly. More than 30 patients, including 10 children at King's College Hospital,[149, 150] were treated with HT. Hepatocyte transplantation has also been used in ALF patients, where the aim is to maintain liver function until the native liver regenerates or acts as a bridge to OLT.[151] In a review by Storm et al. from six centers in the United States, HT has been used in more than 40 patients, and 18 of them received HT for ALF.[152] Although a fall in the levels of bilirubin and ammonia, as well as improvements in HE, was noticed, HT did not significantly influence the clinical outcome of these patients. In the absence of any randomized controlled trial, it is difficult to draw any conclusions about the efficacy of HT in ALF. However, there is a need to overcome the technical limitations. There is scarcity of unused donor livers to isolate hepatocytes. The grafts are usually steatotic, although addition of N-acetylcysteine improves the quality of the cells harvested. Hepatocytes are cryopreserved for later use; however, thawing leads to harmful effects on metabolic function. There are now better cryopreservation techniques but these require further improvement,[149] and alternative sources of hepatocytes are under investigation. Currently, mesenchymal stem cells are being investigated mainly for their hepatotropic effects. With a better supply of hepatocytes, a wider use of HT can be possible in future. Thus, with more refinements and development of reliable sources providing adequate hepatocyte mass, HT holds promise to reverse or attenuate ALF. This will eliminate the need for emergency transplantation or will maintain the patient till emergency transplantation is feasible.

A substantial advancement has been achieved in the management of ALF over the past few decades; however, much more needs to be done. A simple and reliable marker to identify patients who are unlikely to respond to conservative management is still awaited. Emergency liver transplantation will continue to play a pivotal role till newer management options are explored.

REFERENCES

1. Bernuau J, Rueff B, Benhamou J. Fulminant and subfulminant liver failure: definition and causes. Semin Liver Dis. 1986;6(2):97-106.
2. Bismuth H, Samuel D, Castaing D, et al. Orthotopic liver transplantation in fulminant and subfulminant hepatitis. The Paul Brousse experience. Ann Surg. 1985;222(2):109-19.
3. DeVictor D, Desplanques L, Debray D, et al. Emergency liver transplantation for fulminant liver failure in infants and children. Hepatology. 1992;16(5):1156-62.
4. Hoofnagle J, Carithers RJ, Shapiro C, et al. Fulminant hepatic failure: summary of a workshop. Hepatology. 1995;21(1):240-52.
5. Lee WM. Acute liver failure in the United States. Semin Liver Dis. 2003;23(3):217-26.
6. Freeman RB Jr, Steffick DE, Guidinger MK, et al. Liver and intestine transplantation in the United States, 1997-2006. Am J Transplant. 2008;8(4):958-76.
7. Trey C, Davidson CS. The management of fulminant hepatic failure. Prog Liver Dis. 1970;3:282-98.
8. O'Grady JG, Schalm SW, Williams R. Acute liver failure: redefining the syndromes. Lancet. 1993;342:273-75.
9. Ichai P, Samuel D. Etiology and prognosis of fulminant hepatitis in adults. Liver Transpl. 2008;14 Suppl 2:S67-79.
10. Bhaduri BR, Mieli-Vergani G. Fulminant hepatic failure: pediatric aspects. Semin Liver Dis. 1996;16:349-55.
11. Bower WA, Johns M, Margolis HS, et al. Population-based surveillance for acute liver failure. Am J Gastroenterol. 2007;102:2459-63.
12. Brandsaeter B, Hockerstedt K, Friman S, et al. Fulminant hepatic failure: outcome after listing for highly urgent liver transplantation—12 years experience in the nordic countries. Liver Transpl. 2002;8:1055-62.
13. Escorsell A, Mas A, de la Mata M, et al. Acute liver failure in Spain: analysis of 267 cases. Liver Transpl. 2007;13:1389-95.
14. Lee WM, Sorrell MF. Developing a world view toward acute liver failure. Hepatology. 1996;24:270-1.
15. Lian TJ, Jeffers L, Reddy RK, et al. Fulminant or subfulminantnon-A, non-B viral hepatitis: the role of hepatitis C and E viruses. Gastroenterology. 1993;104:556-62.
16. Vale JA, Proudfoot AT. Paracetamol (acetaminophen) poisoning. Lancet. 1995;346:547-52.
17. Schiodt FV, Rochling FA, Casey DL, et al. Acetaminophen toxicity in an urban county hospital. N Engl J Med. 1997;337:1112-7.
18. Wright TL. Etiology of fulminant hepatic failure: is anothervirus involved? Gastroenterology. 1993;104:640-53.
19. Fagan EA. Acute liver failure of unknown pathogenesis: the hidden agenda. Hepatology. 1994;19:1307-12.
20. Khuroo MS. Acute liver failure in India. Hepatology. 1997;26:244-6.
21. Nanda SK, Yalchinkaya K, Panigrahi AK, et al. Etiological role of hepatitis "E" virus in sporadic fulminant hepatitis. J Med Virol. 1994;42:133-7.
22. Acharya SK, Dasarathy S, Kumer TL, et al. Fulminant hepatitis in a tropical population: clinical course, cause, and early predictors of outcome. Hepatology. 1996;23:1448-55.
23. Khuroo MS, Teli MR, Skidmore S, et al. Incidence and severity of viral hepatitis in pregnancy. Am J Med. 1981;70:252-5.
24. Bhaduri BR, Mieli-Vergani G. Fulminant hepatic failure: pediatric aspects. Semin Liver Dis. 1996;16:349-55.
25. Stravitz RT. Critical management decisions in patients with acute liver failure. Chest. 2008;134:1092-102.
26. Bernal W, Wendon J, Rela M, et al. Use and outcome of liver transplantation in acetaminophen-induced acute liver failure. Hepatology. 1998;27(4):1050-5.
27. Simpson KJ, Bates CM, Henderson NC, et al. The utilization of liver transplantation in the management of acute liver failure: comparison between acetaminophen and non-acetaminophen etiologies. Liver Transpl. 2009;15(6):600-9.
28. Blei A. Selection of acute liver failure: have we got it right? Liver Transpl. 2005;11(2):S30-4.
29. Anand A, Nightingale P, Neuberger J. Early indicators of prognosis in fulminant hepatic failure: an assessment of the King's criteria. J Hepatol. 1997;26(1):62-8.
30. Ostapowicz G, Fontana R, Schiødt F, et al. Results of a prospective study of acute liver failure at 17 tertiary care centers in the United States. Ann Intern Med. 2002;137(12):947-54.
31. Larson AM, Polson J, Fontana RJ, et al. Acetaminophen induced acute liver failure: results of a United States multicenter, prospective study. Hepatology. 2005;42(6):1364-72.
32. Schiødt FV, Davern TJ, Shakil AO, et al. Viral hepatitis related acute liver failure. Am J Gastroenterol. 2003;98(2):448-53.
33. Schiødt FV, Atillasoy E, Shakil A, et al. Etiology and outcome for 295 patients with acute liver failure in the United States. Liver Transpl Surg. 1999;5(1):29-34.
34. Williams R. Classification, etiology, and considerations of outcome in acute liver failure. Semin Liver Dis. 1996;16(4):343-8.
35. Samuel D, Bismuth H. Transplantation in patients with fulminant hepatitis. In: Maddrey W, Schiff E, Sorrell M, editors.

Transplantation of the liver. 3rd ed. Philadelphia: Lippincott Williams & Williams; 2001. p. 361-70.
36. Daas M, Plevak DJ, Wijdicksc EF, et al. Acute liver failure: results of a 5-year clinical protocol. Liver Transpl Surg. 1995;1(4):210-9.
37. Barshes NR, Lee TC, Balkrishnan R, et al. Risk stratification of adult patients undergoing orthotopic liver transplantation for fulminant hepatic failure. Transplantation. 2006;81(2):195-201.
38. Elinav E, Ben-Dov I, Hai-Am E, et al. The predictive value of admission and follow up factor V and VII levels in patients with acute hepatitis and coagulopathy. J Hepatol. 2005;42(1):82-6.
39. O'Grady JG, Alexander GJ, Thick M, et al. Outcome of orthotopic liver transplantation in the aetiological and clinical variants of acute liver failure. Q J Med. 1998;68(258): 817-24.
40. Clemmesen JO, Larsen FS, Kondrup J, et al. Cerebral herniation in patients with acute liver failure is correlated with arterial ammonia concentration. Hepatology. 1999;29(3):648-53.
41. Jalan R, OldeDamink SW, Deutz NE, et al. Moderate hypothermia in patients with acute liver failure and uncontrolled intracranial hypertension. Transplantation. 2003;75(12):2034-9.
42. Bernal W. Changing patterns of causation and the use of transplantation in the United Kingdom. Semin Liver Dis. 2003;23(3): 227-37.
43. Rolando N, Harvey F, Brahm H, et al. Fungal infection: a common, unrecognised complication of acute liver failure. J Hepatol. 1991;12(1):1-9.
44. Vaquero J, Polson J, Chung C, et al. Infection and the progression of hepatic encephalopathy in acute liver failure. Gastroenterology. 2003; 125(3):755-64.
45. Rolando N, Harvey F, Brahm H, et al. Prospective study of bacterial infection in acute liver failure: an analysis of fifty patients. Hepatology. 1990;11(1):49-53.
46. Rolando N, Philpott-Howard J, Williams R. Bacterial and fungal infection in acute liver failure. Semin Liver Dis. 1996;16(4):389-402.
47. Stravitz RT, Kramer AH, Davern T, et al. Intensive care of patients with acute liver failure: recommendations of the US Acute Liver Failure Study Group. Crit Care Med. 2007;35(11):2498-508.
48. Antoniades CG, Berry PA, Bruce M, et al. Actin-free Gc globulin: a rapidly assessed biomarker of organ dysfunction in acute liver failure and cirrhosis. Liver Transpl. 2007;13(9):1254-61.
49. Bailey B, Amre DK, Gaudreault P. Fulminant hepatic failure secondary to acetaminophen poisoning: a systematic review and meta-analysis of prognostic criteria determining the need for liver transplantation. Crit Care Med. 2003;31(1):299-305.
50. Bernuau J, Goudeau A, Poynard T, et al. Multivariate analysis of prognostic factors in fulminant hepatitis B. Hepatology. 1986;6(4):648-651.
51. Bernuau J. Selection for emergency liver transplantation. J Hepatol. 1993;19(3):486-7.
52. Craig DG, Ford AC, Hayes PC, et al. Systematic review: prognostic tests of paracetamol-induced acute liver failure. Aliment Pharmacol Ther. 2010;31(10):1064-76.
53. Harrison PM, O'Grady JG, Keays RT, et al. Serial prothrombin time as prognostic indicator in paracetamol induced fulminant hepatic failure. BMJ. 1990;301(6758):964-6.
54. Itai Y, Sekiyama K, Ahmadi T, et al. Fulminant hepatic failure: observation with serial CT. Radiology. 1997;202(2):379-82.
55. O'Grady JG, Alexander GJ, Hayllar KM, et al. Early indicators of prognosis in fulminant hepatic failure. Gastroenterology. 1989;97(2):439-45.
56. Pereira LM, Langley PG, Hayllar KM, et al. Coagulation factor V and VIII/V ratio as predictors of outcome in paracetamol induced fulminant hepatic failure: relation to other prognostic indicators. Gut. 1992;33(1):98-102.
57. Rolando N, Wade J, Davalos M, et al. The systemic inflammatory response syndrome in acute liver failure. Hepatology. 2000;32(4):734-9.
58. Schiødt FV, Rossaro L, Stravitz RT, et al. Gc-globulin and prognosis in acute liver failure. Liver Transpl. 2005;11(10):1223-7.
59. Van Thiel DH. When should a decision to proceed with transplantation actually be made in cases of fulminant or subfulminant hepatic failure: at admission to hospital or when a donor organ is made available? J Hepatol Vol. 1993;17(1):1-2.
60. Bernal W, Donaldson N, Wyncoll D, et al. Blood lactate as an early predictor of outcome in paracetamol-induced acute liver failure. Lancet. 2002;359(9306):558-63.
61. McPhail MJ, Wendon JA, Bernal W. Meta-analysis of performance of Kings's College Hospital Criteria in prediction of outcome in non-paracetamol-induced acute liver failure. J Hepatol. 2010;53(3):492-9.
62. MacQuillan GC, Seyam MS, Nightingale P, et al. Blood lactate but not serum phosphate levels can predict patient outcome in fulminant hepatic failure. Liver Transpl. 2005;11(9):1073-9.
63. Izumi S, Langley PG, Wendon J, et al. Coagulation factor V levels as a prognostic indicator in fulminant hepatic failure. Hepatology. 1996;23(6):1507-11.
64. Pauwels A, Mostefa-Kara N, Florent C, et al. Emergency liver transplantation for acute liver failure. Evaluation of London and Clichy criteria. J Hepatol. 1993;17(1):124-7.
65. Mitchell I, Bihari D, Chang R, et al. Earlier identification of patients at risk from acetaminophen-induced acute liver failure. Crit Care Med. 1998;26(2):279-84.
66. Schmidt LE, Larsen FS. MELD score as a predictor of liver failure and death in patients with acetaminophen-induced liver injury. Hepatology. 2007;45(3):789-96.
67. Wiesner RH. MELD/PELD and the allocation of deceased donor livers for status 1 recipients with acute fulminant hepatic failure, primary nonfunction, hepatic artery thrombosis and acute Wilson's disease. Liver Transpl. 2004;10(10, Suppl 2):S17-22.
68. Yantorno SE, Trentadue J, Ruf A. The model for end-stage liver disease (MELD): a useful tool to access prognosis in fulminant hepatic failure. Liver Transpl. 2004;10:C36.
69. Zaman MD, Hoti E, Qasim A, et al. MELD score as a prognostic model for listing acute liver failure patients for liver transplantation. Transplant Proc. 2006;38(7):2097-8.
70. Bernal W, Hall C, Karvellas CJ, et al. Arterial ammonia and clinical risk factors for encephalopathy and intracranial hypertension in acute liver failure. Hepatology. 2007;46(5):1844-52.
71. Dhiman RK, Jain S, Maheshwari U, et al. Early indicators of prognosis in fulminant hepatic failure: an assessment of the Model for End-Stage Liver Disease (MELD) and King's College Hospital criteria. Liver Transpl. 2007;13(6):814-21.
72. Shakil AO, Jones BC, Lee RG, et al. Prognostic value of abdominal CT scanning and hepatic histopathology in patients with acute liver failure. Dig Dis Sci. 2000;45(2):334-9.
73. Yamagishi Y, Saito H, Ebinuma H, et al. A new prognostic formula for adult acute liver failure using computer tomography-derived hepatic volumetric analysis. J Gastroenterol. 2009;44(6):615-23.
74. Scotto J, Opolon P, Etévé J, et al. Liver biopsy and prognosis in acute liver failure. Gut. 1973;14(12):927-33.
75. Miraglia R, Luca A, Gruttadauria S, et al. Contribution of transjugular liver biopsy in patients with the clinical presentation of acute liver failure. Cardiovasc Intervent Radiol. 2006;29(6):1008–10.
76. Voigt M, Onwuameze O, LaBrecque D, et al. Liver biopsy to predict mortality in fulminant hepatic failure [abstract]. Hepatology. 2007;46:499A.
77. Nazer H, Ede R, Mowat ARW. Wilson's disease: clinical presentation and use of prognostic index. Gut. 1986;27:1377-81.
78. Dhawan A, Taylor RM, Cheeseman P, et al. Wilson's Disease in children: 37 year experience and revised King's score for liver transplantation. Liver Transpl. 2005;11:441-8.
79. Farmer DG, Venick RS, McDiarmid SV, et al. Fulminant hepatic failure in children: superior and durable outcomes with liver

transplantation over 25 years at a single centre. Ann Surg. 2009;250:484-93.
80. 2009 Annual Report of the U.S. Organ Procurement and Transplantation Network and the Scientific Registry of Transplant Recipients: Transplant Data 1994-2003. Department of Health and Human Services, Health Resources and Services Administration, Healthcare Systems Bureau, Division of Transplantation, Rockville, MD; United Network for Organ Sharing, Richmond, VA; University Renal Research and Education Association, Ann Arbor, MI.
81. Bernal W, Cross TJS, Auzinger G, et al. Outcome after wait-listing for emergency liver transplantation in acute liver failure: a single centre experience. J Hepatol. 2009;50:306-13.
82. Wigg AJ, Gunson BK, Mutimer DJ. Outcomes following liver transplantation for seronegative acute liver failure: experience during a 12-year period with more than 100 patients. Liver Transpl. 2005;11:27-34.
83. Shiffman ML, Saab S, Feng S, et al. Liver and intestine transplantation in the United States, 1995-2004. Am J Transplant. 2006;6:1170-87.
84. Farmer DG, Anselmo DM, Ghobrial RM, et al. Liver transplantation for fulminant hepatic failure: experience with more than 200 patients over a 17-year period. Ann Surg. 2003;237(5):666–675;discussion 675-6.
85. Ringe B, Lubbe N, Kuse E, et al. Total hepatectomy and liver transplantation as a two-stage procedure. Ann Surg. 1993;218(1):3-9.
86. Yanaga K, Eguchi S, Takatsuki M, et al. Two-staged living donor liver transplantation for fulminant hepatic failure. Hepatogastroenterology. 2010;57:146-8.
87. Campsen J, Blei AT, Emond JC, et al. Outcomes of living donor liver transplantation for acute liver failure: the adult-to-adult living donor liver transplantation cohort study. Liver Transpl. 2008; 14(9):1273-80.
88. Liu CL, Fan ST, Lo CM, et al. Right-lobe live donor liver transplantation improves survival of patients with acute liver failure. Br J Surg. 2002;89(3):317-22.
89. Nishizaki T, Hiroshige S, Ikegami T, et al. Living donor liver transplantation for fulminant hepatic failure in adult patients with a left-lobe graft. Surgery. 2002;131(1):S182-9.
90. Uemoto S, Inomata Y, Sukarai T, et al. Living donor liver transplantation for fulminant hepatic failure. Transplantation. 2000;70(1):152-7.
91. Kawasaki S, Makuuchi M, Matsunami H, et al. Living related liver transplantation in adults. Ann Surg. 1998;227(2):269-74.
92. Lo CM, Fan ST, Chan JKFD, et al. Minimum graft volume for successful adult-to-adult living donor liver transplantation in fulminant hepatic failure. Transplantation. 1996;62:696.
93. Marcos A, Fisher RA, Ham JM, et al. Liver regeneration and function in donor and recipient after right lobe adult to adult living donor liver transplantation. Transplantation. 2000;69(7): 1375-79.
94. Kiuchi T, Kasahara M, Uryuhara K, et al. Impact of graft size mismatching on graft prognosis in liver transplantation from living donors. Transplantation. 1999;67:321-4.
95. Man K, Fan ST, Lo CM, et al. Graft injury in relation to graft size in right lobe live donor liver transplantation: a study of hepatic sinusoidal injury in correlation with portal hemodynamics and intragraft gene expression. Ann Surg. 2003;237(2):256-4.
96. Ichida T, Todo S, Fujiwara K, et al. Living related-donor liver transplantation for adult fulminant hepatic failure [abstract]. Hepatology. 2000;32:340A.
97. Lee SG, Ahn CS, Kim KH. Which types of graft to use in patients with acute liver failure? (A) Auxiliary liver transplant (B) Living donor liver transplantation (C) The whole liver. (B) I prefer living donor liver transplantation. J Hepatol. 2007;46(4):574-8.
98. Miwa S, Hashikura, Y, Mita A, et al. Living-related liver transplantation for patients with fulminant and subfulminant hepatic failure. Hepatology. 1999:30(6):1521-26.
99. Casas A, Falkenstein K, Gallagher M, et al. Living donor liver transplantation in critically ill children. Transplant. 1999:3(2):104-8.
100. Emre S, Schwartz ME, Shneider B, et al. Living related liver transplantation for acute liver failure in children. Liver Transplant Surg. 1999;5(3):161-5.
101. Baliga P, Alvarez S, Lindblad A, et al. Posttransplant survival in pediatric fulminant hepatic failure: the SPLIT experience. Liver Transpl. 2004;10(11):1364-71.
102. Abouna G. Emergency adult to adult living donor liver transplantation for fulminanthepatic failure—is it justifiable? Transplantation. 2001;71(10):1498-500.
103. Ghobrial RM, Freise CE, Trotter JF, et al. Donor morbidity after living donation for liver transplantation. Gastroenterology. 2008;135(2):468-76.
104. Yasutomi M, Uemoto S, Inomata Y, et al. Liver failure following living donor liver transplantation for fulminant hepatic failure. Transplant Proc. 2000;32(7):2133-6.
105. Wolf HK, Michalopoulos GK. Hepatocyte regeneration in acute fulminant and nonfulminant hepatitis: a study of proliferating cell nuclear antigen expression. Hepatology. 1992;15:707-13.
106. Moritz MJ, Jarrell BE, Armenti V, et al. Heterotopic liver transplantation for fulminant hepatic failure—a bridge to recovery. Transplantation. 1990;50:524-6.
107. Gubernatis G, Pichlmayr R, Kemnitz J, et al. Auxiliary partial orthotopic liver transplantation (APOLT) for fulminant hepatic failure: first successful case report. World J Surg. 1991;15:660-6.
108. Moritz MJ, Jarrell BE, Munoz SJ, et al. Regeneration of the native liver after heterotopicliver transplantation for fulminant hepatic failure. Transplantation. 1993;55:952-4.
109. Boudjema K, Jaeck D, Siméoni U, et al. Temporary auxiliary liver transplantation for subacute liver failure in a child. Lancet. 1993;342:778-9.
110. Bismuth H, Azoulay D, Samuel D, et al. Auxiliary partial orthotopic liver transplantation for fulminant hepatitis. The Paul Brosse experience. Ann Surg. 1996;224(6):712-26.
111. Chenard-Neu MP, Boudjema K, Bernuau J, et al. Auxiliary liver transplantation: regeneration of the native liver and outcome in 30 patients with fulminant hepatic failure. A multicenter study. Hepatology. 1995;23(5):1119-27.
112. Van Hoek B, De Boer J, Boudjema K, et al. Auxiliary versus orthotopic liver transplantation for acute liver failure: EURALT Study Group, European Auxiliary Liver Transplant Registry. J Hepatol. 1999;30(4):699-705.
113. Azoulay D, Samuel D, Ichai P, et al. Auxiliary partial orthotopic versus standard orthotopic whole liver transplantation for acute liver failure: a reappraisal from a single center by a case-control study. Ann Surg. 2001;234(6):723-31.
114. Pereira SP, McCarthy M, Ellis AJ, et al. Auxiliary partial orthotopic liver transplantation for acute liver failure. J Hepatol. 1997;26(5):1010-7.
115. Boudjema K, Bachellier P, Wolf P, et al. Auxiliary liver transplantation and bioartificial bridging procedures in treatment of acute liver failure. World J Surg. 2002;26(2):264-74.
116. Faraj W, Dar F, Bartlett A, et al. Auxiliary liver transplantation for acute liver failure in children. Ann Surg. 2010;251(2):351-6.
117. Terpstra OT. On behalf of the European Auxiliary Liver Transplant Registry Study Group. Auxiliary versus orthotopic liver transplantation for acute liver failure. J Hepatol. 1999;30:699-705.
118. Quaglia A, Portmann BC, Knisely AS, et al. Auxiliary transplantation for acute liver failure: histopathological study of native liver regeneration. Liver Transpl. 2008;14:1437-48.

120. Hiramatsu A, Takahashi S, Aikata H, et al. Etiology and outcome of acute liver failure: retrospective analysis of 50 patients treated at a single center. J Gastroenterol Hepatol. 2008;23(8):1216-22.
121. Takada Y. Some aspects of adult living donor liver transplantation: small-for-size graft and ABO mismatch. Hepatobiliary Pancreat Dis Int. 2009;8:121-3.
122. Toso C, Al-Qahtani M, Alsaif FA, et al. ABO-incompatible liver transplantation for critically ill adult patients. Transpl Int. 2007;20:675-81.
123. Egawa H, Teramukai S, Haga H, et al. Present status of ABO-incompatible living donor liver transplantation in Japan. Hepatology. 2008;47:143-52.
124. Todo S, Furukawa H, Jin MB, et al. Living donor liver transplattaion in adults: outcome in Japan. Liver Transpl. 2000;6:S66-72.
125. Srinivas Reddy M, Wilson C, Torpey N, et al: ABO incompatible liver transplantation: a case of immediate need (letter). Transpl Int. 2007;20:904-5.
126. Ikegami T, Soejima Y, Taketomi A, et al. Living donor liver transplantation for fulminant hepatic failure from ABO-incompatible donors (letter). Transpl Int. 2008;21:284-5.
127. Egawa H, Oike F, Buhler L, et al. İmpact of recipient age on outcome of ABO-incompatible living donor liver transplantation. Transplantation. 2004;77:403-11.
128. Miyata R, Shimazu M, Tanabe M, et al. Clinical characteristics of thrombotic microangiopathy following ABO incompatible living donor liver transplantation. Liver Transpl. 2007;13:1455-62.
129. Testa G, Vidanovic V, Chejfec G, et al. Adult living-donor liver transplantation with ABO-incompatible grafts. Transplantation. 2008;85:681-6.
130. Kawagishi N, Takeda I, Miyagi S, et al. Management of anti-allogeneic antibody elimination by apheresis in living donor liver transplantation. Ther Apher Dial. 2007;11:319-24.
131. Saliba F, Ichai P, Azoulay D, et al. Successful long-term outcome of ABO-incompatible liver transplantation using antigen-specific immunoadsorption columns. Ther Apher Dial. 2010;14:116-23.
132. Kozaki K, Egawa H, Ueda M, et al. The role of apheresis therapy for ABO incompatible living donor liver transplantation: the Kyoto University experience. Ther Apher Dial. 2006;10:441-8.
133. Song GW, Lee SG, Hwang S, et al. Dual living donor liver transplantation with ABO-incompatible and ABO-compatible grafts to overcome small-for-size graft and ABO blood group barrier. Liver Transpl. 2010;16:491-8.
134. Troisi R, Noens L, Montalti R, et al. ABO-mismatch adult living donor liver transplantation using antigen-specific immunoadsorption and quadruple immunosuppression without splenectomy. Liver Transpl. 2006;12:1412-7.
135. Matsuno N, Nakamura Y, Mejit A, et al. Long-term follow-up ABO-incompatible adult living donor liver transplantation in cirrhotic patients. Clin Transplant. 2007;21:638-42.
136. Goralczyk AD, Obed A, Schnitzbauer A, et al. adult living donor liver transplantation with ABO-incompatible grafts: a german single center experience. J Transplant. 2009; 125(2):1-8.
137. Ikegami T, Taketomi A, Soejima Y, et al. Rituximab, IVIG, and plasma exchange without graft local infusion treatment: a new protocol in ABO incompatible living donor liver transplantation. Transplantation. 2009;88:303-7.
138. Devlin J, Wendon J, Heaton N, et al. Pretransplant clinical status and outcome of emergency transplantation for acute liver failure. Hepatology. 1995;21(4):1018-24.
139. Moore, K, Taylor G, Ward P, et al. Aetiology and management of renal failure in acute liver failure. In: Williams, R, Hughes R, editors. Acute liver failure: improved understanding and better therapy. Welwyn Garden City, UK: Smith Kline Beecham Pharmaceuticals; 1991; p. 47-53.
140. Bernal W, Wendon J, Rela M, et al. Use and outcome of liver transplantation in acetaminophen-induced acute liver failure. Hepatology. 1998;27(4):1050-5.
141. Durand P, Debray D, Mandel R, et al. Acute liver failure in infancy: a 14-year experience of a pediatric liver transplantation center. J Pediatr. 2001;139(6):871-6.
142. Sargent S, Wainwright S. Quality of life following emergency liver transplantation for acute liver failure. NursCrit Care. 2006;11:168-76.
143. Sargent S, Wainwright S. A qualitative study exploring patients' perceived quality of life following an emergency liver transplant for acute liver failure. Intensive Crit Care Nurs. 2007;23:272-80.
144. Lee KH, Lee MK, Sutedja DS, et al. Outcome from molecular adsorbent recycling system (MARS) liver dialysis following drug-induced liver failure. Liver Int. 2005;25:973-7.
145. Koivusalo AM, Kantola T, Arola J, et al. Is it possible to gain extra waiting time to liver transplantation in acute liver failure patients using albumin dialysis? Ther Apher Dial. 2009;13:413-8.
146. Fox IJ, Roy-Chowdhury J. Hepatocyte transplantation. J Hepatol. 2004;40(6):878-86.
147. Dhawan A, Mitry RR, Hughes RD. Hepatocyte transplantation for liver-based metabolic disorders. J Inherit Metab Dis. 2006;29(2-3):431-5.
148. Fisher RA, Strom SC. Human hepatocyte transplantation: worldwide results. Transplantation. 2006;82(4):441-9.
149. Dhawan A, Puppi J, Hughes RD, et al. Human hepatocyte transplantation: current experience and future challenges. Nature Rev Gastroenterol Hepatol. 2010;7:288-98.
150. Dhawan A, Mitry RR, Hughes RD, et al. Hepatocyte transplantation for inherited factor VII deficiency. Transplantation. 2004;78(12):1812-4.
151. Puppi J, Tan N, Mitry RR, et al. Hepatocyte transplantation followed by auxiliary liver transplantation—a novel treatment for ornithine transcarbamylase deficiency. Am J Transpl. 2008;8(2):452-7.
152. Strom SC, Chowdhury JR, Fox IJ. Hepatocyte transplantation for the treatment of human disease. Semin Liver Dis. 1999;19(1):39-48.

CHAPTER 112

Deceased Donor Liver Transplantation

Mohamed Rela, Gomathy Narasimhan

INTRODUCTION

Transplantation is a unique specialty of surgery where the role of a surgeon extends far beyond the operating room and successful outcome relies on multiple factors, including patient selection and evaluation for transplantation, timing of surgery, management of donor factors, multidisciplinary approach in postoperative care, and understanding the immunology of transplantation. The purpose of this chapter is to give the reader an overview on deceased donor liver transplantation (DDLT), which has been in practice for the last 50 years. Liver transplantation involves not only the technique but also, more importantly, the thought process and the aggressive approach to patient management to make it successful.

HISTORY

"The history of medicine is that what was inconceivable yesterday and barely achievable today often becomes routine tomorrow" - Thomas Starzl.

The first human liver transplantation was done in 1963 by Thomas Starzl on a 3-year-old boy with biliary atresia; the child died before completion of the surgery. This attempt was done after several years of experiments on animals and the failure was followed once again by going back and forth to the experiments on animals. The next few were also unsuccessful attempts[1] and the procedure evolved slowly. Technical principles of liver transplantation, which guide us even today, were gradually established in this phase. In 1967, Starzl et al. at the University of Colorado performed the first successful clinical liver transplantation. Over the next decade, although a few centers all over the world were venturing into liver transplantation, it was the perseverant work of Starzl, initially at Colorado, subsequently at Pittsburgh, and simultaneously in the UK, Sir Roy Calne's efforts at Cambridge and King's College program in London that made liver transplantation a success with good long-term outcome. Initial hurdles were in getting the patient alive from the transplant surgery, later it shifted to dealing with the aftermath of what had happened in the operating room (massive blood loss, fluid balance, pulmonary issues, renal failure). The next major hurdle, when patients were carefully managed through the immediate postoperative phase, was to deal with rejection. Knowledge regarding immune suppression was largely derived from experience in renal transplant patients. To start with, liver patients received double drug regimen (azathioprine with steroids) followed by trial with one of the other available options as the third agent—cyclophosphamide, antilymphocyte serum or thoracic duct drainage with not very promising results. The "golden era" of transplantation which started in 1980 was ushered in by the use of cyclosporin. Cyclosporin was isolated from the fungus *Tolypocladium inflatum* and its immunosuppressive activity was discovered by Jean Borrel et al. in 1976. It was then put to clinical use by Sir Roy Calne and shown to have a significant impact in controlling rejection (Fig. 1). With development of standard technique for organ retrieval, liver transplantation, immune suppression, and postoperative care, liver transplantation has become a well-established treatment option for patients with chronic or acute liver failure (ALF). The predominant type of transplant in the world is DDLT and in regions of the world where the concept of deceased donation is not well established (mainly due to cultural reasons), the majority is living donor liver transplantation. Although the overall principles of managing both these types of liver transplants remain the same, there are certain features unique to each of them and we shall deal with DDLT in this chapter.

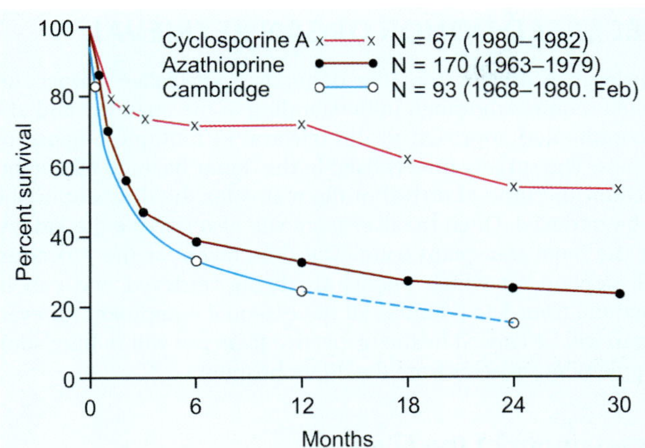

Figure 1 Actuarial survival of patients treated with cyclosporine A and low-dose steroids compared with the actuarial survival obtained under azathioprine and steroids at Pittsburgh and at Cambridge
Source: Adapted from Starzl et al. (1982).

DONOR IN DECEASED DONOR LIVER TRANSPLANTATION

The donor from whom the organs will be retrieved for the purpose of transplantation in DDLT is a deceased person and will be either "donation after brain death (DBD) or donation after cardiac death (DCD)" (previously "non-heartbeating donor"). Brain death is secondary to irreversible damage to the brain stem, first described in 1959 by Mollaret and Goulon as "Le Coma Depasse" a definable condition from which recovery was impossible.[2] This is confirmed by testing for brain stem reflexes and by the apnea test. Once the family has consented to donate the organs, the cascade of events get initiated starting from donor maintenance to optimize the organ function, activating the network for organ allotment, intimation of the recipient hospital of the organ offer for their recipient on the waitlist, logistics for multiorgan retrieval, the retrieval process itself and completion of formalities associated with medico legal documentation and finally culminating in the handing over of the donor to the family for the funeral.

The key to the successful clinical outcome of this whole process is in good donor maintenance and coordination among the donor hospital, the retrieving teams and the recipient hospital. The vitality of the organs is maintained by supporting the circulatory, the respiratory and the endocrine system in a controlled hospital setting in the donor hospital.

Details to be acquired from the donor hospital by the liver recipient team:

1. Admission details—age, sex, diagnosis, days in intensive care unit (ICU)
2. Time of brain death declaration
3. Details of cardiac arrest and resuscitation, if any since admission
4. Current hemodynamics and vasopressor dosages, hourly urine output
5. Details of alcohol intake/smoking/IV drug abuse
6. Past medical and surgical history
7. Labs—liver function and renal function on admission and on the date of brain death declaration with peak sodium values.

Table 1: Extended criteria donor and donor risk index criteria

Extended criteria donor
General criteria
Tumor
Drug abuse
Sepsis
Meningitis
Hepatitis B or C
Liver-specific ECD
Donor >65
ICU stay >7
High BMI
Steatosis
Hypernatremia
High AST, ALT, bilirubin
Donor risk index[4]
Age (<40, 40–49, 50–59, 60–69, >70)
African–American race (vs. white)
Donor height (per 10 cm increase)
Cause of death = cerebrovascular accident
Cause of death = Other
Donation after cardiac death
Split liver transplantation

AST, aspartate aminotransferase, ALT, alanine transaminase

These values help in identifying the risk factors for liver donation. As per the Eurotransplant criteria donor age >65 years, an ICU-stay of more than 7 days, a high body mass index (BMI), steatosis, hypernatremia (>160 mmol) and high levels of aspartate aminotransferase (AST), alanine transaminase (ALT) and bilirubin are being considered as marginal or extended criteria donor (ECD).[3] The more recently introduced donor risk index[4] (Table 1) was validated in Eurotransplant and was found to be the most accurate predictor of transplant outcome.[5] In spite of any number of predictors that are available to assess the outcome, the final decision depends on the clinician to decide between the risk associated with waiting for the next organ for the recipient and the "marginality" of the donor. It is preferable to offer a marginal donor liver to a low-risk patient and liver from a donor with no extended criteria to be offered to a high-risk patient as the low-risk patient may be able to cope better with "stormy" postoperative period that is anticipated with a ECD liver transplantation. Caution is used while offering liver from an elderly donor to a recipient with Hepatitis C as donor age is the strongest predictor of graft loss in patients with HCV cirrhosis.[6] What is definitely important is to know the absolute contraindications on a donor.

Contraindications to organ donation (as per policy statement odt.nhs.uk)

1. Any cancer with evidence of spread outside affected organ (including lymph node) within 3 years of donation (however, localized prostate, thyroid, in situ cervical cancer, and non-melanotic skin cancer are acceptable)
2. Melanoma (except completely excised stage 1 cancers)
3. Choriocarcinoma
4. Active hematological malignancy (myeloma, lymphoma, leukemia)
5. Tuberculosis active and untreated

6. Human immunodeficiency virus infection (exception is when the organs from such donors can be transplanted into HIV infected patients)

DONOR MAINTENANCE

Optimal medical management of the potential organ donor is an important factor in determining the outcome of the transplant on the recipient. The donor should continue to have critical support in intensive care focused on protective strategies to keep donor organs optimized for transplantation. This critical period is important for the maintenance of physiologic homeostasis and allows organs to be procured in best possible condition. The donor care should be a collaborative multidisciplinary effort, including the retrieving units and the critical care team. Hemodynamic instability is commonly seen in the potential donor which is secondary to multiple factors—hypovolemic (therapeutic dehydration for cerebral edema, hemorrhage, diabetes insipidus with massive diuresis, osmotic diuresis due to hyperglycemia), neurogenic [defective vasomotor control and subsequent progressive loss of systemic vascular resistance (SVR)], cardiogenic (hypothermic depression of myocardial contractility and left ventricular dysfunction), and temperature control >35°C (Ref: Fung J, ILTS uploads)

Guidelines for deceased donor maintenance:

Rule of 100s

- Maintain SBP >100
- HR <100 BPM
- UOP >100 mL/h
- PaO_2 >100 mm Hg

Active fluid resuscitation to restore and maintain intravascular volume.

Hormonal Support

Brain death may lead to interruption of hypothalamic pituitary axis leading to hypothyroidism and adrenal insufficiency which causes organ instability due to attenuation of the mitochondrial ability to regenerate adenosine triphosphate.[7] In addition, central diabetes insipidus sets in characterized by excessive diuresis causing hypovolemia and electrolyte instability (hypernatremia). Management of free water loss is by replacement with hypotonic saline or dextrose in water. Electrolytes are added as required. Vasopressin in the dose of 0.5–0.6 units/h helps reduce urine output. Severe cases with urine output >1000 mL/h may respond to 1-desamino-8-D-arginine vasopressin 0.3 mcg/kg. Guidelines for standardized hormonal resuscitation package for deceased donor is given in Table 2.[8] The goal of hormonal management of the brain dead donor is treatment of diabetes insipidus, cardiac arrhythmias, metabolic acidosis, and hypotension.

Table 2: Guidelines for hormonal treatment of deceased donor
1. Methylprednisolone 15 mg/kg bolus
2. Triiodothyronine (T3) 4 mcg bolus, 3 mcg/h
3. Thyroxin (T4) 20 mcg bolus, 10 mcg/h
4. Arginine vasopressin 1 unit bolus, 0.5–4 units/h
5. Insulin Infusion titrate blood glucose to 120–180 mg/dL

DECEASED DONOR ORGAN RETRIEVAL

Retrieval of organs from the donor is a specialized procedure which requires thorough understanding of the anatomy and also a coordinated approach to the retrieval of multiple organs and tissues. The surgery time is fixed in the donor hospital taking into account the time of arrival of the teams for the different organs to be retrieved. Often the liver team will also retrieve the kidneys for the renal transplant team. The time taken for the procedure will depend on which organs are being retrieved and can be anything from 3 to 5 hours. All the essential equipment for every organ will be carried by the respective team but will require some supplementary items from the donor hospital.

Assessment of the Liver

A midline incision from the suprasternal notch to the symphysis pubis allows access to all abdominal and chest organs (Fig. 2). Laparotomy is done to exclude any unsuspected disease and dissection of the organs is commenced. Liver quality assessment is done by inspection and palpation. Biopsy should be obtained in all donors where there is a degree of suspicion. Livers that are yellow in color, have a rubbery to firm consistency, have rounded edges, are too large in size, or have an abnormal appearance should be biopsied. Other indications for biopsy are when the etiology of death is anoxia or hypoxia (like in drowning) to assess for nuclear pyknosis or cellular drop out suggestive of hepatocyte damage and impending cellular death. Steatosis is graded as mild (<30%), moderate (30–60%) and severe (>60%). Acceptance of liver with more than 35–40% steatosis requires experience and should take into account donor age, cold ischemia time, vasopressors used on the donor, severity of illness of the recipient and individual factors that may arise in specific case.

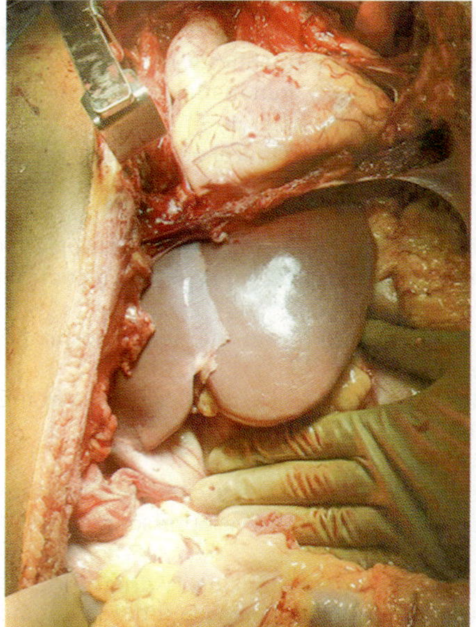

Figure 2 Donor operation: thoracotomy and laparotomy at multiorgan retrieval exposing the heart and the liver

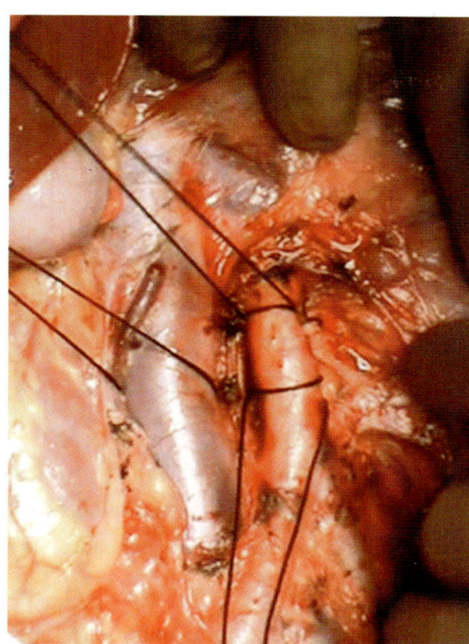

Figure 3 Donor operation: infrarenal aorta and IVC isolated and looped ready for aortic cannulation. Origin of left renal vein is seen
Abbreviation: IVC, inferior vena cava

Steps of Retrieval

The initial mobilization of the liver begins by division of the falciform and the left triangular ligament. The gastrohepatic ligament is incised and the lesser omentum is visually and digitally explored to identify any accessory or replaced left hepatic artery arising from the left gastric artery (occurring in about 15% of patients). If it is present, it has to be dissected to its origin from the left gastric artery and the left gastric artery ligated distal to the origin of the accessory vessel. The right triangular ligament is released and the right lobe mobilized to approach the inferior vena cava (IVC). Next, the structures in the portal triad are palpated by finger encircling the foramen of Winslow to see for accessory or replaced right hepatic artery from superior mesenteric artery (SMA), posterior to the bile duct. Bile duct is hooked and the distal end-ligated and proximal end-transected taking care not to injure the aberrant right artery if it had been palpated posterior to the bile duct. The gall bladder is opened and flushed with saline solution until clear of bile. The hilum dissection is completed by identifying and ligating the gastroduodenal artery. Dissection of the hepatic artery should be done proximal to the gastroduodenal artery (GDA), which involves identifying the left gastric and splenic artery. Further dissection of coeliac artery up to its origin is often done in the cold phase.

Mobilization of the cecum, right colon, and small bowel mesentery reveals the distal IVC and abdominal aorta with exposure of the SMA (Fig. 3). The tissue over the first 2 cm of the SMA is cleared to look for origin of accessory or replaced right hepatic artery. The left and right renal veins are identified, essentially to help with marking the line of transection of the infrahepatic IVC above the renal veins at a later point. Space around left kidney is cleared by mobilizing the left colon down for cooling subsequent to cross-clamp.

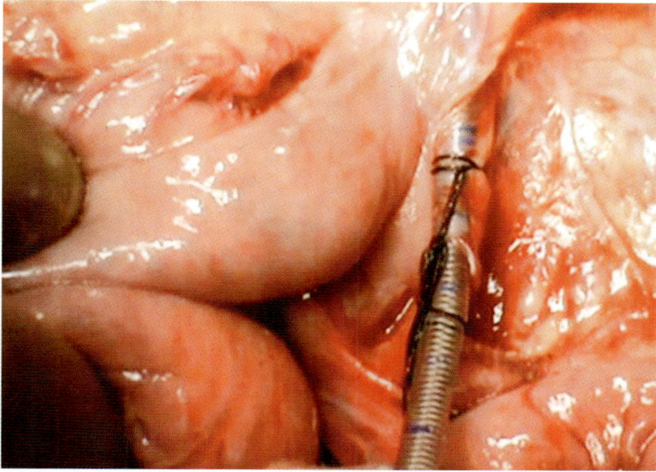

Figure 4 Donor operation: inferior mesenteric vein cannulated for portal vein flush

The distal abdominal aorta is isolated and prepared for cannulation. The superior mesenteric vein (or alternately, the inferior mesenteric vein if pancreas is being retrieved) is isolated for cannulation to perfuse the portal vein (Fig. 4). The supracoeliac aorta is isolated by dividing the crus of the diaphragm and prepared for cross-clamping.

Time is allowed for the cardiac and lung teams to do the dissection prior to cross-clamping and perfusion. Once all the teams are ready, the donor is given 300–500 units/kg of Heparin IV and 3 minutes later, cannulation of the SMV/inferior mesenteric vein (IMV) (for portal vein perfusion) and abdominal aorta (for abdominal organs) follows. The supracoeliac aorta is cross-clamped, blood let out from liver, and abdominal organs by incising the suprahepatic vena cava just below the pericardium and subsequently cold perfusion with University of Wiskonsin solution or histidine-tryptophan-ketoglutarate (HTK) solution started through the aortic and portal cannula. The abdominal cavity is filled with ice slush (which is kept ready prior to cross-clamp) until the perfusion is completed (usually about 3–4 L through the aorta and 2 L through the portal cannula. The cross-clamp time is noted and indicates the start of the "cold ischemia" time (CIT). This is the time from cross-clamp of the donor aorta to reperfusion of the transplanted liver in the recipient after completion of the caval and portal venous anastomoses. The accepted upper limit for CIT is 12 hours and the safe limit may be lower based on the other factors operating in the donor and recipient.

Cold phase dissection involves division of the portal vein at the junction of the splenic vein/SMV, the aorta with the coeliac and SMA origin (taking precaution with the origin of the renal arteries), IVC division at the diaphragm and above the renal veins. The liver is then perfused in the back table once again and then packed in three bags with some cold preservation solution around it and placed in ice box for transport to the recipient hospital. The kidney retrieval proceeds next, followed by retrieval of the iliac arteries and iliac veins. The arteries and veins may be required on the recipient for interposition or jump grafts in specific situations. The donor incision is then closed in a cosmetically acceptable manner with continuous sutures and handed over to the family by the transplant coordinators.

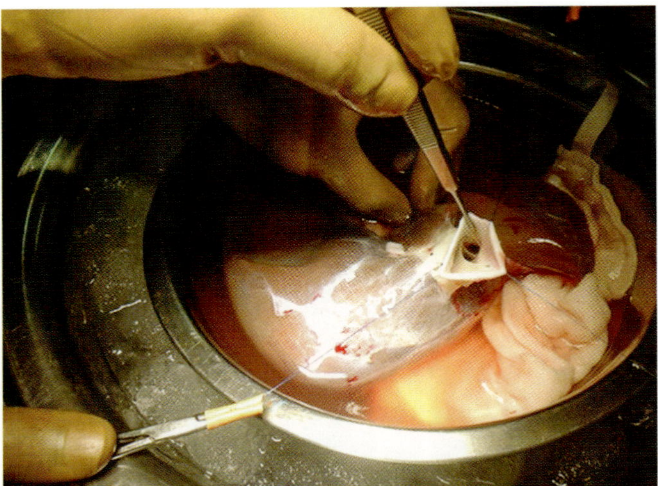

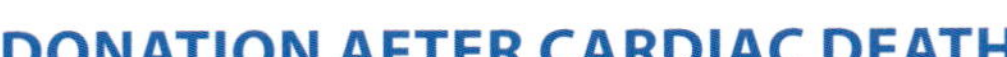

Figure 5 Back table preparation of the inferior vena cava—the hepatic vein orifices seen inside the lumen of the suprahepatic cava

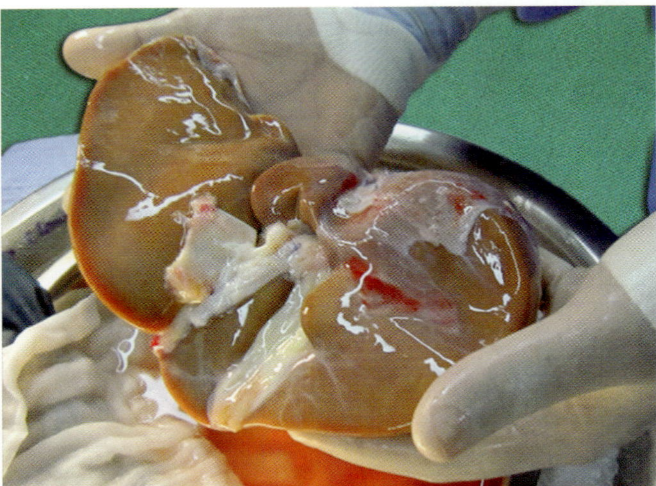

Figure 6 Donor liver ready for implantation after back table preparation

DONATION AFTER CARDIAC DEATH

Donation after cardiac death refers to organ donation after death has been declared on the basis of cardio pulmonary criteria as opposed to neurological criteria in brain death. Donation after cardiac death happens in a gravely ill patient who is expected to die shortly after withdrawal of life support and this is done under controlled situation. There is a fixed time between withdrawal of support, death and organ retrieval, exceeding which the organs will not be viable and hence in that situation, organ donation will not proceed. In order to prevent conflict of interest, no member of the transplant team will be involved in the withdrawal of care from the potential donor. The retrieval starts immediately after declaration of death. Effort is made to cannulate the aorta at the earliest and minimize the elapsed ischemic time between onset of asystole and organ harvest. This is crucial for successful organ donation from deceased donors. These times are organ specific and for the liver it is 30 minutes.[9] The outcome of DCD liver is still considered inferior to liver from DBD and is associated with higher biliary complications.[10]

Back Table Preparation of the Liver Graft

This is done at the recipient hospital to remove diaphragmatic and fibro fatty tissues around blood vessels. Potential bleeding points are repaired on the IVC, portal vein, and hepatic artery (Fig. 5). Reconstruction of the right accessory or left accessory artery, if required is done in the back table by anastomosing it usually to the GDA or the splenic artery stump or at an appropriate location. The liver is once again packed and placed in ice box until the time of implantation into the recipient (Fig. 6)

RECIPIENT SURGERY

Preparation and Anesthesia

All recipients for DDLT would have undergone extensive multiorgan preoperative evaluation before placement on the wait list. Any specific risk factors, if present in the form of hepatorenal syndrome, hepatopulmonary syndrome, porto-pulmonary hypertension, significant portal hypertension, portal vein thrombosis, previous spontaneous bacterial peritonitis (SBP) would have been identified at that stage. As DDLT is always an emergency procedure and the patient is admitted only a few hours before commencement of surgery, a quick check is done to look for any interim change and for evidence of ongoing infection. If infection is detected, the next in the waiting list is called for transplantation. On table monitoring lines include arterial line, central venous line, pulmonary artery catheter sheath (often used as large bore access for rapid infusions) with floatation of Swan Ganz catheter in selected patients and temperature control mechanisms. Infrastructure required in a transplant operation theater include-thromboelastogram machine, continuous renal replacement therapy (CRRT) machine, fluid warmer, rapid infuser, cell saver, bypass pump (occasionally used nowadays), defibrillator with paddles on the table, blood bank with capability to provide blood, and components in a short notice, laboratory to support with stat complete blood count, coagulation and blood gas parameters. It is imperative to have close communication between the surgeons and the anesthetists during the course of the transplant.

Recipient Surgery: The transplantation surgery can be divided into three phases: recipient hepatectomy, anhepatic phase, which comprises implantation of the new liver graft, and reperfusion phase.

Recipient Hepatectomy

This is a crucial step during the orthotopic transplantation of the liver and the key to the ultimate success of operation.[11] It can be quite challenging in presence of severe degree of portal hypertension, adhesions and an unstable patient. A bilateral subcostal incision with midline extension (named Mercedes Benz incision by Sir Roy Calne) or a right subcostal with midline extension is made depending on the access required. The falciform ligament is divided all the way to the suprahepatic cava and all the tissue with the accompanying collaterals are removed up to the xiphoid. A mechanical retractor is used with bilateral subcostal blades. The left and right triangular ligaments are released and the gastrohepatic liagment is opened. The hepatic hilum is addressed next. The dissection is carried down to the hepatic artery, which is divided above its bifurcation. Care should be taken to avoid undue force or traction during artery isolation as it can lead to dissection of the hepatic artery posing a problem for arterial anastomosis during implantation. The bile duct is then divided. In DDLT, it is usually not necessary to divide above the level of cystic duct, however, division above the cystic duct entrance can provide additional length of the bile duct. Accessory right artery, if present, is located posterior to the bile duct in 95% of cases and is ligated. The portal vein is the only structure left at the hilum. The tissues around the portal vein are divided between ligatures and the portal vein is skeletonized.

Subsequent steps that describe caval dissection depend on whether the "classic technique" or the "piggyback technique" is to be adopted for caval reconstruction.

CLASSIC TECHNIQUE

The hepatectomy involves removing the retro hepatic cava along with the cirrhotic liver after achieving control of the supra and infrahepatic cava (Fig. 7). In this technique, use of veno-venous bypass may be required for hemodynamic stability in some patients. The infrahepatic IVC and suprahepatic IVC are circumferentially dissected out, the adrenal vein has to be ligated and divided as it inserts into the part of IVC to be removed. The dissection on the left side of the cava is done up to the insertion of the left hepatic vein. The tissue posterior to the cava is divided and surgeon's finger hooked behind the suprahepatic cava so as to allow enough space for placement of suprahepatic clamp. Dividing right and left phrenic veins helps in further mobilizing suprahepatic IVC if needed. Following this, a trial clamp of the infrahepatic cava is performed and cross-checked with the anesthesia team regarding the patient's hemodynamic stability. If the patient tolerates the trial clamp, the portal vein is clamped proximally and ligated at the bifurcation followed by division of the portal vein. The infra and suprahepatic cava are clamped in that order using vascular clamps and the hepatectomy is completed. This technique avoids the extra time and morbidity involved by going on a veno-venous bypass but in a hemodynamically unstable patient or in situations where there is limited exposure, small recipient or large donor liver, there is a high possibility of having a very edematous bowel by the end of implantation. It is important to anticipate this situation and accordingly plan to go on veno-venous bypass. But, it is to be acknowledged that bypass is very selectively used nowadays, especially with the caval preservation technique along with the use of temporary porto-caval shunts addressing all the concerns mentioned.[12]

PIGGYBACK TECHNIQUE

In this technique, the vena cava is preserved by dissecting the native liver of the IVC completely.[13] No dissection is done posterior to the cava. Dissection is commenced from the infrahepatic cava and the caudate and short hepatic veins are ligated and the liver is mobilized off the anterior surface of the IVC (Fig. 8). This has to be completed before ligation of the portal vein. Alternately, a temporary porto-caval shunt can be performed followed by dissection anterior to the cava. The advantages of a porto-caval shunt is to help reduce mesenteric congestion and allow hemodynamic stability.[14,15] In addition, it reduces bleeding, reduces liver congestion and allows good exposure and mobility of the liver. The use of a shunt is more important in patients who have not developed adequate collateralization as in patients who are transplanted for ALF or in patients transplanted for non-cirrhotic liver disease. Adequate mobilization of the infrahepatic IVC to allow placement of a side clamp and of the portal vein to be swung toward the IVC for shunt is done and an end-to-side portal vein (PV) to IVC anastomosis is done. It is very important to position the portal vein correctly as a kink in the shunt will cause flow restriction and the purpose of the shunt is defeated. If shunt is not performed, the portal vein should be left intact prior to removing the liver for as long as possible.[16] The caval dissection proceeds until the right hepatic vein is reached, followed by isolating the middle hepatic vein (MHV) and left hepatic vein (LHV) trunks. The right hepatic vein is clamped separately and the MHV and

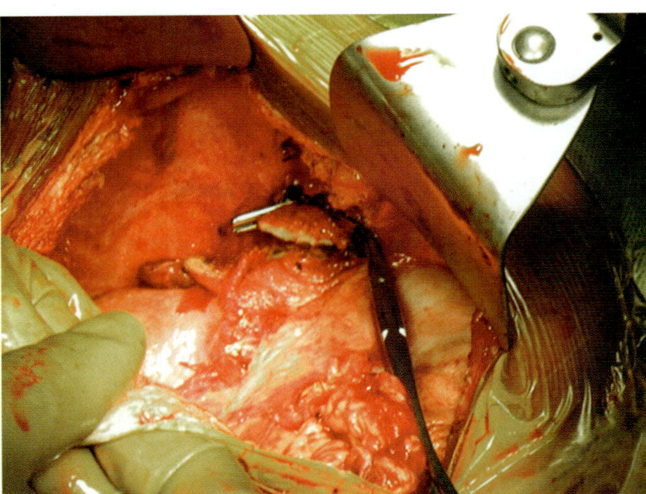

Figure 7 Anhepatic phase in the recipient—planned for cava interposition. Vascular clamp on suprahepatic cava cuff

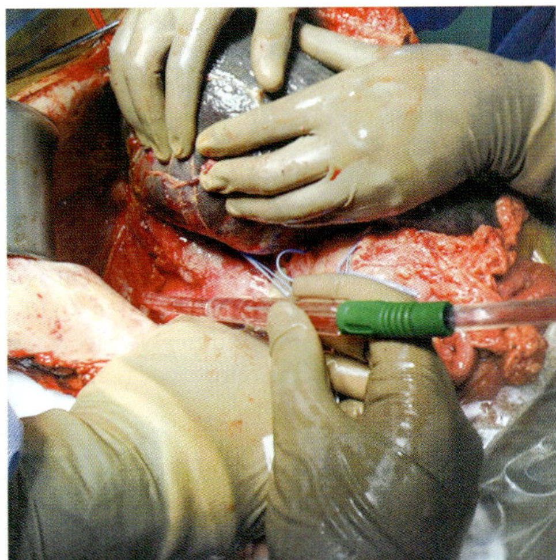

Figure 8 Cava preservation—cholestatic liver in a recipient with primary sclerosing cholangitis—medial rotation of right lobe to enable ligation of short hepatic veins

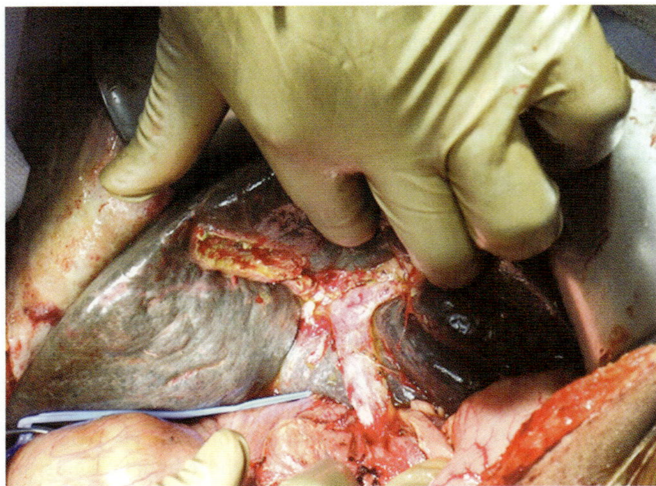

Figure 9 Portal vein at the hilum is intact throughout the dissection of the cava and is clamped just prior to hepatectomy

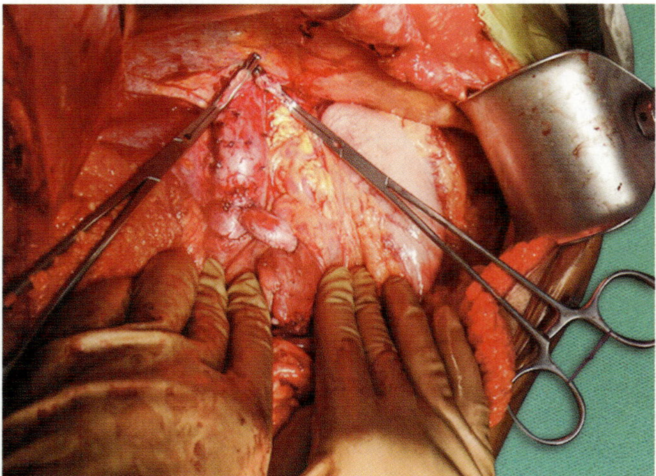

Figure 10 Temporary porto-caval shunt with cava preservation—anhepatic phase. Clamps on the right hepatic vein and the common cuff of the middle and left hepatic veins

LHV are clamped as a common trunk. Intrahepatic transection of veins is done to preserve length and the hepatectomy is completed (Figs 9 and 10).

During the anhepatic phase, the operative field is examined carefully and hemostasis is secured. Areas that require special attention are the right adrenal, retroperitoneal surface corresponding to the bare area of the liver, and the retro-caval region.

IMPLANTATION OF THE LIVER

The implantation of the liver graft into the recipient comprises of four anastomoses and is done in the following order:

1. Vena Cava: Suprahepatic and infrahepatic in the caval interposition technique single caval anastomosis in the piggyback or cavocaval anastomosis.
2. Portal vein anastomosis followed by reperfusion of the liver, which marks the end of the cold ischemia time.
3. Hepatic arterial anastomosis
4. Bile duct anastomosis

Cava Anastomosis

Classic Technique

This comprises two anastomosis—the suprahepatic and the infrahepatic cava. The suprahepatic cava is prepared after explant of the native liver. The openings of the three hepatic veins are opened to create a common ostium. The phrenic opening is sutured. The donor liver is then brought onto the recipient table. The suprahepatic anastomosis is done with 3-0 Prolene continuous sutures after placing two corner stitches. The left corner is first tied and the anastomosis done from left to right, keeping the right corner untied. The posterior (back wall) is intentionally made a little shorter than the anterior (front wall). This allows the sutures to bring the posterior wall closer and the anterior wall to be retracted providing good exposure. The right corner is tied and the anterior wall completed from left to right. The suprahepatic anastomosis is the most difficult when donor liver is large and good exposure and assistance is of paramount importance for accurate anastomosis in addition to good technique. After this, the infrahepatic anastomosis is done. Care should be taken to ensure correct orientation and adequate length (short) of the donor and recipient infrahepatic cava cuffs as an error can lead to kinking after completion of the anastomosis. This anastomosis is done with 4-0 Prolene continuous sutures in a fashion similar to the suprahepatic one. On completion of the posterior wall, the liver graft is perfused with normal saline with 25 g of albumin at room temperature through the portal vein and effluent drained through the infrahepatic vena cava. This is done to remove by-products of metabolism, air, and the preservation solution which is rich in potassium. The anterior wall is then completed.

Piggyback Technique

In this technique, the right hepatic vein opening of the recipient is sutured vertically along its long axis. The openings of the MHV and LHV are converted into one ostium and extended horizontally toward the right vein cuff to allow for a wider cuff. There is only one caval anastomosis in the piggyback technique. In the classic piggyback technique, it is done between the donor IVC and the recipient hepatic vein cuff or if it is a cavocavoplasty modification, it is done by a longitudinal anastomosis between the donor and recipient cava. Side-to-side cavocavoplasty modifications have been evolved to overcome the outflow problems that was encountered in the early days following piggyback anastomosis.[17] But the issue has been overcome with the extension of the opening onto the IVC to create a larger opening.[18] The graft is flushed and drained through the inferior cava or prior to completion of the anterior wall depending on the technique used. The graft infrahepatic IVC is doubly ligated on completion of the flush.

Portal Vein Anastomosis

If the patient has been on a porto-caval shunt, the portal vein is clamped followed by side clamp on the cava and the anastomosis

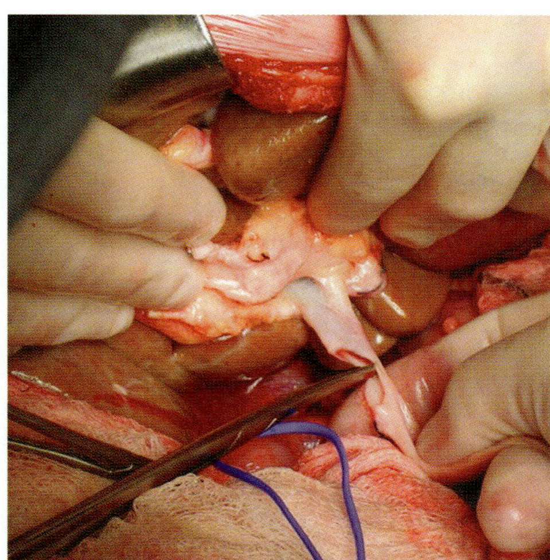

Figure 11 Portal vein of the donor liver trimmed for excess length in preparation for the portal vein anastomosis

is divided. The caval opening is closed with 4-0 Prolene. Prior to starting the anastomosis, the portal vein is flushed to remove any newly formed clots by releasing the clamp and reclamping just above the duodenum. Correct orientation of the portal vein without twists is maintained. The liver is brought down into the abdomen by placing sponges superior and posterior to the liver. Both these maneuvers ensure that the orientation and length are adequate thereby preventing kinks in the anastomosed portal vein. Both the donor and recipient portal veins are trimmed appropriately and the anastomosis is done with 6-0 Prolene continuous sutures from left to right after placing two corner stitches similar to the caval anastomosis (Fig. 11). The running suture is tied in the right corner by allowing a growth factor (an air knot) of about one half the diameter of the portal vein. This is done to avoid narrowing at the suture line.

Reperfusion Phase

In simple terms, reperfusion refers to when the clamps are released from the cava and portal vein on completion of the anastomosis and the donor liver is once again perfused with blood. This marks the end of the CIT (calculated from the time the donor aorta is cross clamped at retrieval). But the relevance to understanding the reperfusion is much more from the physiological sense, more so in a DDLT than in a LDLT. At reperfusion, blood that has been in cold perfusion for the last few hours circulates through the liver and goes to the heart. In the process, the blood takes along with it the metabolic products from the ischemic liver that has been building up with no perfusion and associated with it will be the perfusion solution which has a high content of potassium. This insult to the heart results in the phenomenon called "reperfusion syndrome". Significant reperfusion syndrome is defined as severe hemodynamic instability, persistent hypotension (greater than 30% of the anhepatic level), asystole, or significant arrhythmias.[19] The severity of reperfusion syndrome has been corelated in some studies to the age of the graft, steatosis and the ischemia time.[20] In order to minimize the insult or rather to have a controlled situation in the event of a major reperfusion syndrome, a few techniques are adopted by the surgeon during reperfusion. The anesthetist is intimated about 5 minutes prior to reperfusion (around the start of the portal vein anterior wall anastomosis). The cava clamp/clamps is/are released first. This allows the right heart filling and helps dilute the blood when the portal clamps are released subsequently. After release of the cava-clamps, about 2 minutes is allowed, the caval anastomosis is inspected for hemostasis. The portal clamp is then slowly released over a 2-minute period monitoring the fall in blood pressure, rise in CVP (which is bound to happen with the return of the blood and with the vasopressors used by the anesthetist to counter the reperfusion syndrome), electrocardiogram changes (tall T waves with hyperkalemia). The portal vein release is gradually done and slowed down further if hemodynamic instability is present. It is very important for the surgical team to be prepared to use the paddles in case of a cardiac arrest at reperfusion. An alternate practice for reperfusion is called blood flush where the initial few hundred mL of the blood which reperfuses the liver is let out through the infraheaptic cava and then complete ligation of the infrahepatic cava (in piggyback) or complete the anterior wall of the cava in the caval interposition technique. This prevents the potassium rich blood from reaching the right heart but does not alter the reperfusion syndrome.[21]

Hepatic artery anastomosis: The recipient hepatic artery is carefully mobilized up to the GDA or even proximally depending on the length required to get a tension free, caliber match anastomosis. It is extremely important to avoid undue traction during isolation of the artery as this might leading to dissection of the artery and make it unusable for anastomosis. If a dissection happens inadvertently, we may have to resort to using an interposition graft (deceased donor iliac/SMA or polytetrafluoroethylene graft) as a conduit from the recipient aorta (supracoeliac or infrarenal) to the donor artery. The presence of a coeliac axis stenosis or median arcuate ligament syndrome should be recognized on preop computed tomography and the GDA should be preserved during recipient artery dissection as the GDA will probably be the main inflow from the arcade through the SMA. Once mobilization is complete, the donor and recipient artery are trimmed to an adequate length (without redundancy or too much tension) (Fig. 12). The anastomosis is performed using 7-0 Prolene interrupted sutures starting from the midline in the posterior wall and moving up simultaneously on both sides and then completing the anterior wall. On releasing the clamps on the donor and recipient arteries, the graft is rearterialized. In patients with accessory/replaced right or left artery, arterial reconstruction to one of the branches of the coeliac axis may have been done on the back table itself. But, in some instances, the decision will be taken on table after the arterial anastomosis depending on the back flow.[22] If a good back flow is present from the aberrant artery, it may be decided to not reconstruct the accessory artery. If the back flow is not good, a second anastomosis will be done to an appropriately located and size matched branch of the recipient artery.

Subsequent to total reperfusion of the liver, sufficient time is spent in achieving absolute hemostasis. Once the bile duct anastomosis is complete, it may not be very convenient to rotate the liver to inspect the caval region for hemostasis. At the same time, correction of coagulation if grossly abnormal, is done to assist with hemostasis. Absolute normalization of coagulation is not aimed for as the trend in the international normalized ratio and fibrinogen after reperfusion will serve as a marker of graft function. Presence of bile flow from the donor duct is

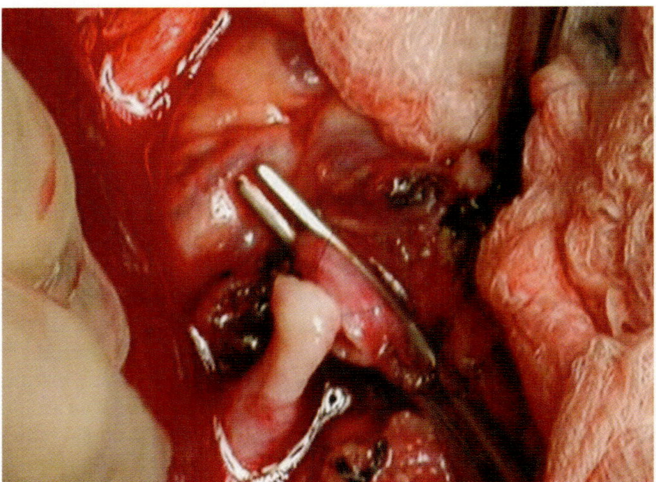

Figure 12 Hepatic artery anastomosis—donor and recipient artery approximated without tension or redundancy

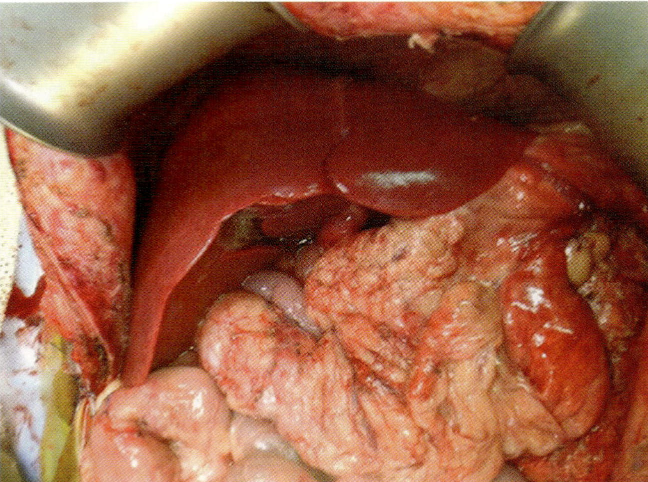

Figure 13 Transplanted liver after completion of all anastomoses and cholecystectomy—abdomen ready for closure with complete hemostasis

an indicator of graft function. Cholecystectomy is performed followed by Doppler ultrasound of the liver and the flow pattern and volume of the portal vein, hepatic artery and the hepatic vein is recorded.

Biliary reconstruction: The last anastomosis is the bile duct reconstruction. In adults, this anastomosis is usually performed between the donor and recipient common hepatic ducts. Alternately, a Roux-en-Y choledochojejunostomy is performed when the recipient duct is unhealthy like in choledocholithiasis, biliary atresia, secondary biliary cirrhosis, and in primary scelrosing cholangitis (PSC). Some recent data do suggest the use of duct to duct in selected patients with PSC with equal outcomes to that of choldochojejunostomy.[23] It is important to remember that the bile duct derives its blood supply by vessels running laterally in the 3 o'clock and 9 o' clock position. Between the donor and the recipient ducts, the blood supply to the donor duct is tenuous and hence it will be prudent to trim the donor duct to adjust for length rather than to trim the recipient duct to prevent ischemic stricture of the anastomosis. Care should also be taken in the event of size discrepancy between the two ducts to adjust during anastomosis. The technique involves interrupted sutures with 6-0 PDS. T tubes are no longer used in DDLT although it was the routine in the early days of transplantation. Roux-en-Y choldochojejunostomy is done with 6-0 PDS interrupted sutures when indicated. (Fig. 13)

SPECIAL SITUATIONS

Portal Vein Thrombosis

Portal vein thrombosis was considered a contraindication for liver transplantation in the early days and Shaw et al. in 1985 reported the first successful liver transplant in patient with portal vein thrombosis.[24] Since then several technical innovations have made it possible to transplant patients with varying degrees of portal vein thrombosis. Portal vein thrombosis may have been identified in the preoperative imaging or may be a finding discovered on table. It may be of help to have a Doppler done at admission to evaluate portal vein status as the initial pretransplant evaluation may have been several months prior to transplant in most patients. Portal vein thrombosis is either partial or total (Yerdel classification 1- and 2-partial, 3- and 4-total). In partial portal vein thrombosis, removal of the thrombus can almost always be accomplished and in total thrombosis removal is possible in 63% of cases and in the rest, jump graft between the superior mesenteric vein and the graft portal vein (donor iliac vein can be used for this purpose) or porto-caval hemi transposition will be the option.[25]

Split Liver Transplantation

Split liver transplantation is an innovative strategy that has been introduced with the aim to increase the number of available organs for transplantation where a whole donor liver is split into two and used on two recipients.[26] Split for a child and an adult has become a routine procedure performed in larger centers with patient and graft survivals equivalent to that after full-size liver transplantation. However, split liver transplantation for two adult recipients is still considered a challenge. The splitting technique involves dividing a whole donor liver in two portions with respective vascular pedicle, venous outflow, and bile duct. Two techniques for liver splitting have been described, ex situ splitting, following liver retrieval as a bench procedure in the recipient hospital and in situ splitting, in the donor before procurement. In situ technique has the advantage of reducing cold ischemia time which enables sharing of the two lobes by two different centers, decreasing incidence of bile leak and for better hemostatic control of the cut surface. However, in situ technique prolongs the retrieval time in the donor hospital, requires coordination between several retrieval teams and requires specialist equipments and considerable surgical expertise. The early results of in situ splitting have demonstrated superior outcome compared to the ex situ technique with better patient and graft survival rates and lower incidence of complications.[27] However, data from King's College showed equivalent short- and long-term transplant outcomes in both techniques.[28] Bench cholangiogram may be useful for the biliary anatomy during ex situ splitting. Similarly, intraoperative cholangiogram can be performed in the in situ technique.

Ex situ Technique

The hilar dissection involves preparation of hepatic artery branches, portal vein, and exploration of the bile ducts with a fine probe. Routinely, the IVC, hepatic artery, main portal vein, and the common bile duct are preserved for the right extended graft. The left hepatic artery is usually divided at its bifurcation. The left portal vein is divided immediately distal to the bifurcation. The small branches to the caudate lobe posteriorly are divided followed by the branches to segment 4 at the umbilical fissure. The bile duct is probed and the left hepatic duct is divided close to the umbilical fissure in order to get a single duct draining segments 2 and 3. It is not uncommon to have two separate ducts draining segments 2 and 3 for subsequent anastomosis in the recipient. The liver parenchyma is transected immediately to the right of the falciform ligament and the various small vessels and bile ducts on the cut surface handled with ligation.

In situ Split Technique

The in situ technique is similar to the living donor left lateral segment donation. The left side of the hepatic triangular ligament is dissected and the left lateral segment is mobilized. The hepatic artery is isolated and the portal vein is dissected at the bifurcation and the left branch is isolated by ligation of the caudate branches. The parenchyma is then transacted to the right of the falciform ligament using cavitron ultrasound aspirator. Toward the end of parenchymal transection the left bile duct is divided. The two hepatic lobes are perfused and retrieved in block. The division of the portal vein, hepatic artery, and hepatic vein is performed ex situ as described above.

Full-left Full-right Split

The disparity in donor supply and demand in adults has motivated interest to supply two adults by extension of split techniques. This technique involves moving the transection plane from the umbilical fissure to the principle plane between the right and left lobes of the liver (Fig. 14). This allows for the left lobe grafts (segments 1–4) to be used for a small adult recipient weighing up to 60 kg or large children weighing over 40 kg.

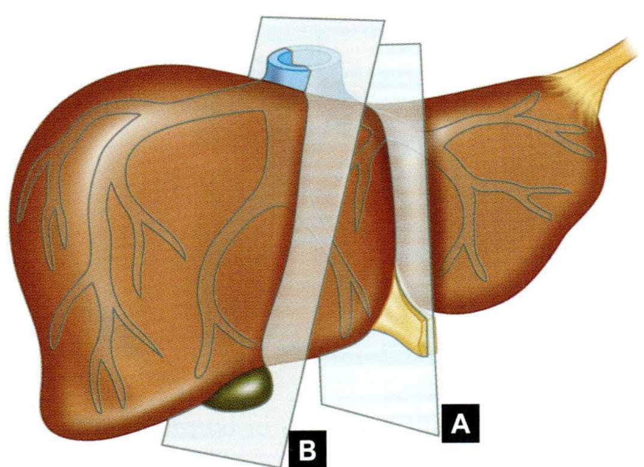

Figure 14 Split liver transplantation splitting plane in (A) standard split and (B) full left and right split

Pediatric Liver Transplantation

Pediatric transplantation in the initial years had a unique problem of size match between the large liver and the small pediatric recipient. Until the 1980s, the only option for children was to wait for an appropriate size matched cadaveric donor. This led to high wait list mortality for pediatric patients. Bismuth et al. described the reduced liver graft where a whole adult liver was reduced in the back table by doing a right or an extended right hepatectomy resulting in a size matched left lobe or left lateral graft for the pediatric recipient.[29]. The disadvantage though was drawing from the adult donor pool. With the development of split liver techniques, the role for reduced grafts no longer exist and pediatric DDLT is only one of the two-size matched whole liver graft from a pediatric donor or split liver graft.

Auxiliary Partial Orthotopic Liver Transplantation

In auxiliary partial orthotopic liver transplantation (APOLT), only a portion of the recipient's liver is replaced by a graft (split or reduced) from a deceased donor. This option is considered in specific situations of the recipient like ALF and metabolic disease without liver damage like Crigler–Najjar syndrome type 1 (CNS 1). In ALF, there is potential for the liver to recover from the acute insult provided there is some liver mass to take the patient through the acute phase.[30] In metabolic syndrome, the requirement is for a small liver mass to help with enzymatic production.[31] Auxiliary liver transplant in ALF allows for the placement of a part of the liver while allowing for the regeneration and recovery of the native liver and this can be followed by withdrawal of immune suppression leading to atrophy of the transplanted liver. In metabolic disease, the hope for future gene therapy and withdrawal of immune suppression is the rationale behind APOLT.

REFERENCES

1. Starzl TE, Iwatsuki S, Van Thiel DH, et al. Evolution of liver transplantation. Hepatology. 1982;2(5):614-36.
2. Machado C, Kerein J, Ferrer Y, et al. The concept of brain death did not evolve to benefit organ transplants. J Med Ethics. 2007;33(4):197-200.
3. Braat AE, Blok JJ, Putter H, et al. The Eurotransplant donor risk index in liver transplantation: ET-DRI. Am J Transplant. 2012;12(10):2789-96.
4. Feng S, Goodrich NP, Bragg-Gresham JL, et al. Characteristics associated with liver graft failure: the concept of a donor risk index. Am J Transplant. 2006;6(4):783-90.
5. Blok JJ, Braat AE, Adam R, et al. Validation of the donor risk index in orthotopic liver transplantation within the Eurotransplant region. Liver Transpl. 2012;18(1):112-9.
6. Lake JR, Shorr JS, Steffen BJ, et al. Differential effects of donor age in liver transplant recipients infected with hepatitis B, hepatitis C and without viral hepatitis. Am J Transplant. 2005;5(3):549-57.
7. Novitzky D, Cooper DK, Morrell D, et al. Change from aerobic to anaerobic metabolism after brain death, and reversal following triiodothyronine therapy. Transplantation. 1988;45(1):32-6.
8. Rosendale JD, Kauffman HM, McBride MA, et al. Hormonal resuscitation yields more transplanted hearts, with improved early function. Transplantation. 2003;75(8):1336-41.
9. Sladen RN, Shonkwiler RJ. Donation after cardiocirculatory death: back to the future? Can J Anaesth. 2011;58(7):591-4,594-8.

10. Callaghan CJ, Charman SC, Muiesan P, et al. Outcomes of transplantation of livers from donation after circulatory death donors in the UK: a cohort study. BMJ Open. 2013;3(9):p. e003287.
11. Stieber AC, Marsh JW Jr, Starzl TE. Preservation of the retrohepatic vena cava during recipient hepatectomy for orthotopic transplantation of the liver. Surg Gynecol Obstet. 1989;168(6):542-4.
12. Reddy K, Mallett S, Peachey T. Venovenous bypass in orthotopic liver transplantation: time for a rethink? Liver Transpl. 2005;11(7):741-9.
13. Tzakis A, Todo S, Starzl TE. Orthotopic liver transplantation with preservation of the inferior vena cava. Ann Surg. 1989;210(5):649-52.
14. Cherqui D, Lauzet JY, Rotman N, et al. Orthotopic liver transplantation with preservation of the caval and portal flows. Technique and results in 62 cases. Transplantation. 1994;58(7):793-6.
15. Llado L, Figueras J. Techniques of orthotopic liver transplantation. HPB (Oxford). 2004;6(2):69-75.
16. Lerut J, Ciccarelli O, Roggen F, et al. Cavocaval adult liver transplantation and retransplantation without venovenous bypass and without portocaval shunting: a prospective feasibility study in adult liver transplantation. Transplantation. 2003;75(10):1740-5.
17. Lerut J, Gertsch P. Side-to-side cavo-cavostomy: a useful aid in "complicated" piggy-back liver transplantation. Transpl Int. 1993;6(5):299-301.
18. Cescon M, Grazi GL, Varotti G, et al, Venous outflow reconstructions with the piggyback technique in liver transplantation: a single-center experience of 431 cases. Transpl Int. 2005;18(3):318-25.
19. Ramsay M. The reperfusion syndrome: have we made any progress? Liver Transpl. 2008;14(4):412-4.
20. Nanashima A, Pillay P, Crawford M, et al. Analysis of postrevascularization syndrome after orthotopic liver transplantation: the experience of an Australian liver transplantation center. J Hepatobiliary Pancreat Surg. 2001;8(6):557-63.
21. Millis JM, Melinek J, Csete M, et al. Randomized controlled trial to evaluate flush and reperfusion techniques in liver transplantation. Transplantation. 1997;63(3):397-403.
22. Kubota K, Makuuchi M, Takayama T, et al. Simple test on the back table for justifying single hepatic-arterial reconstruction in living related liver transplantation. Transplantation. 2000;70(4):696-7.
23. Esfeh JM, Eghtesad B, Hodgkinson P, et al. Duct-to-duct biliary reconstruction in patients with primary sclerosing cholangitis undergoing liver transplantation. HPB (Oxford). 2011;13(9):651-5.
24. Shaw BW Jr, Iwatsuki S, Bron K, et al. Portal vein grafts in hepatic transplantation. Surg Gynecol Obstet. 1985;161(1):66-8.
25. Ravaioli M, Zanello M, Grazi GL, et al. Portal vein thrombosis and liver transplantation: evolution during 10 years of experience at the University of Bologna. Ann Surg. 2011;253(2):378-84.
26. Emond JC, Whitington PF, Thistlethwaite JR, et al. Transplantation of two patients with one liver. Analysis of a preliminary experience with 'split-liver' grafting. Ann Surg. 1990;212(1):14-22.
27. Reyes J, Gerber D, Mazariegos GV, et al. Split-liver transplantation: a comparison of ex vivo and in situ techniques. J Pediatr Surg. 2000;35(2):283-9; discussion 289-90.
28. Rela M, Vougas V, Muiesan P, et al. Split liver transplantation: King's College Hospital experience. Ann Surg. 1998;227(2):282-8.
29. Bismuth H, Houssin D. Reduced-sized orthotopic liver graft in hepatic transplantation in children. Surgery. 1984;95(3):367-70.
30. Belghiti J, Sommacale D, Dondero F, et al. Auxiliary liver transplantation for acute liver failure. HPB (Oxford). 2004;6(2):83-7.
31. Rela M, Muiesan P, Vilca-Melendez H, et al. Auxiliary partial orthotopic liver transplantation for Crigler–Najjar syndrome type I. Ann Surg. 1999;229(4):565-9.

CHAPTER 113

Living Related Liver Transplantation

Subhash Gupta, Neerav Goyal, Shaleen Agarwal

BACKGROUND

Complex operations on the liver have been hindered by its complex anatomy and vascularity. With advances in surgical and anesthesia techniques progressively more complex operations on the liver are being performed. Though kidney donation has become quite common, living donor liver transplantation (LDLT) is still restricted to some specialized centers due to the complexity of this operation. Donor safety being paramount, selection of the donor needs experience, as the anatomy of the liver is highly variable. Due to the shortage of deceased donor livers and the absence of an organized organ-sharing network in India and most other Asian countries, LDLT has emerged as the only viable option for end-stage liver disease. Even in the United States and Europe, where there are established transplant programs, the gap between the demand and the availability of deceased donor grafts continues to grow.

HISTORY

Raia performed the first LDLT in Brazil in 1987. Though the recipient did not survive, this paved the way for modern LDLT. The first successful LDLT was reported from Australia the same year by Strong and the technique was further refined by Dr. Christopher Broelsch at the Chicago Medical Center. His first recipient Alyssa Smith, transplanted in 1989, graduated from college in 2010 and is off immunosuppression. The credit for pioneering adult-to-adult LDLT goes to the Japanese surgeons. The Shinshu group did the first successful adult-to-adult LDLT in 1993. A 53-year-old woman with primary biliary cirrhosis received a left lobe graft from her son. Thus, began a new era in LDLT giving hope to all those adult patients with decompensated chirrhosis who had no hope of getting a deceased donor graft in time.

While increasing the donor pool, the other advantages of living donor transplantation are that these grafts are of extremely good quality and the cold ischemia time is much less as compared with deceased donor grafts. The disadvantages are that this procedure requires a perfectly normal individual to undergo a complex operation with its inherent risks. Today the complications of the procedure have been reduced but not eliminated. However, many large series of donor hepatectomy have been reported without any mortality.

The liver has an amazing regenerative capacity allowing us to resect upto 80% of normal liver volume. However, during donor hepatectomy, the resected graft volume that can be resected should never exceed 70%. The regenerative capacity of the liver has been described in Greek mythology 2,500 years ago. Prometheus was cursed by the Gods to endure eternal pain for revealing the secret of fire to man. He was chained to Mount Caucasus and his liver was eaten daily by the eagle of Zeus. He would not die as his liver regenerated only to be eaten again the next day.

Donor Selection

Donor selection is a complex process involving a full hematological, biochemical, radiological, and cardiopulmonary workup. Further, the donor must also undergo a complete psychological evaluation prior to medical fitness (Table 1). During donor evaluation, the tests must be done to ensure that the graft will work well after implantation and that the donor does not come to harm.

Candidates for donation:

1. Age group 18–55 years
2. Blood group compatible (mostly)
3. Body mass index <30
4. Healthy fit individual with no comorbidity and normal blood workup

5. No active substance abuse
6. Predicted graft volume should be adequate
7. Remnant liver volume should be adequate
8. Favorable vascular and biliary anatomy
9. Approved by the ethics committee of the hospital.

ABO Incompatible Donation

ABO incompatible liver donation is possible and in this the preformed antibody in the recipient needs to be removed by plasmapheresis. Further, rituximab prevents antibody formation. For quick preparation such as in acute liver failure, intravenous immunoglobulin may be used to counter hyperacute rejection from complement activation. Results of ABO incompatible transplant in pediatric age group are sometimes comparable to ABO compatible transplant. At our center, due to the costs involved and somewhat unpredictable results of ABO incompatible transplant, we generally prefer a swap transplant, which is legal.

Radiological Investigations

Plain Computed Tomography Abdomen

Measurement of liver attenuation index is the first step (Fig. 1). This must be greater than + 5. Donor with LAI less than +5 should undergo liver biopsy for estimation of steatosis. Subtracting the splenic density from the liver density on a non-contrast scan gives the attenuation index. Less than + 5 increases the likelihood of steatosis.

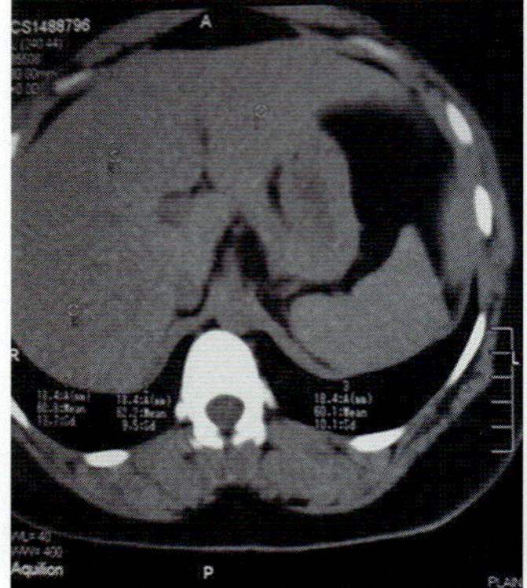
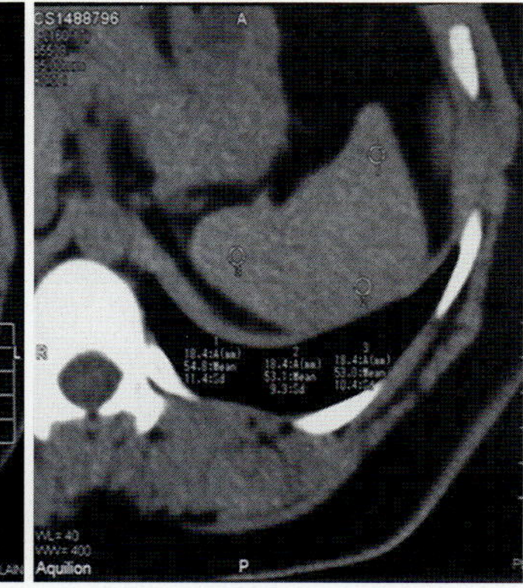

Figure 1 Plain CT—measurement of LAI. CT, computed tomography; LAI, liver attenuation index

Computed Tomography Liver Angiogram

This will delineate the hepatic arterial, portal, and venous anatomy of the liver. In case of a right lobe graft the major area of interest is the

Table 1: Donor evaluation protocol

History	*Age* *Blood group* *Relationship* *Comorbidities/previous illness* *Substance abuse* *Previous surgery and allergies*	
Hematological workup	Complete hemogram	Hemoglobin, platelet count, WBC counts
	Liver function test	Total/Direct bilirubin, SGOT/SGPT, ALP/GGT, total protein and albumin prothrombin time and INR
	Renal function	B. urea, S. creatinine and electrolytes
	Fasting lipid profile	Total cholesterol, triglycerides LDL/VLDL
	Thyroid function tests	T3, T4, TSH
	Fasting blood sugar and HBA1c	
	Serology	HBsAg, anti-HCV, HIV I and II, CMV IgG
Cardiopulmonary evaluation	Pulmonary	Chest radiograph, Pulmonary function test
	Cardiac	ECG 2D echocardiogram Stress echocardiogram (if older than 40 years)
Radiological investigations	USG abdomen/pelvis with Doppler Plain CT abdomen CT liver angiogram MRCP	Routine screen Liver attenuation index Liver volumes Arterial, portal, and hepatic venous anatomy Biliary anatomy and fat estimation
Biopsy (in selected cases)	Fatty change, inflammation	
HLA tissue typing and cross match		

WBC, Whilte blood count; SGOT, Serum glutamic oxaloacetic transaminase; SGPT, serum glutamic-pyruvic transaminase; ALP, Alkaline phosphatase; GGT, gamma-glutamyl transpeptidase; INR, international normalized ratio; LDL, low-density lipoprotein; VLDL, very low-density lipoprotein; TSH, thyroid-stimulating hormone; HBsAg, hepatitis B surface antigen; HCV, hepatitis C virus; HIV, human immunodeficiency virus; ECG, electrocardiogram; USG, ultrasonography; CT, computed tomography; HLA, human leukocyte antigen; MRCP, magnetic resonance cholangiopancreatography; 2D, 2-dimensional.

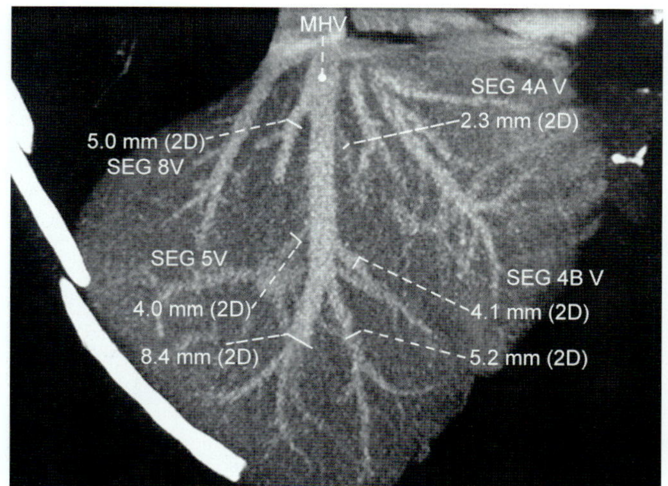

Figure 2 Hepatic venous anatomy—the MHV and its tributaries. Note the drainage of the segment 4 veins. MHV, middle hepatic vein.

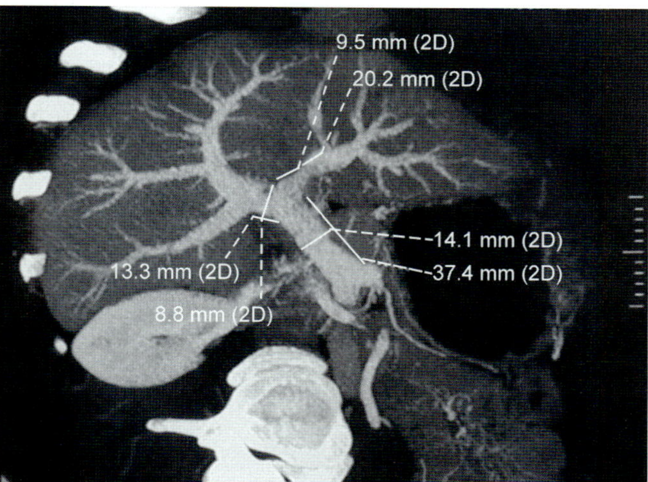

Figure 3 Portal venous anatomy

drainage area of segment IV into middle heaptic vein (MHV). This helps in deciding whether MHV can be taken with the graft or not.

The CT scan images are reconstructed to delineate the vascular structures (Figs 2 and 3). For adults, usually a right lobe graft is procured and this can be either a standard right lobe graft without venous reconstruction of anterior sector drainage, or a modified right lobe with venous reconstruction or an extended right lobe graft where the MHV has been retrieved with the graft. When the MHV is being retrieved with the graft, the draining vein of segment 4a must be preserved. It is believed that segment 4b will drain via tributaries around the falciform ligament.

Controversy surrounds MHV drainage in right lobe grafts. The Hong Kong group routinely retrieves the MHV with the graft. However, they recommend that strict donor selection is essential for a safe outcome. As the same results in recipients can be obtained by reconstructing a new MHV, it seems prudent to use a modified right lobe graft. Unfortunately, the reconstruction would require a venous graft, which is difficult to procure in India, as cadaveric donation is limited. We have developed a technique where the explanted liver provides long venous grafts from either the portal or hepatic vein.

During explanation of the diseased liver, the portal vein is clamped and divided just proximal to the bifurcation. This part of the vein is then stitched with 5-0 Prolene. With careful dissection, the right portal vein is dissected till its bifurcation into anterior and posterior branches. Similarly, the left portal vein is dissected all the way till the umbilical vein. Quite often the umbilical vein can be opened to create a long venous graft. The side branches of the left portal vein can be used to join multiple 5 or 8 tributaries. The patency rates of these grafts are over 70%.

There are many situations where extended right lobe graft is safe such as in young donors, those with less than 5% steatosis, large remnant liver volume or bifid MHV.

Liver Volumetry

The approximate volume of the proposed liver graft and the volume of residual liver are measured on the CT liver angiogram. The remnant liver should be at least 30% of the total liver volume.

Once the volume of the proposed graft is measured, the graft recipient body weight ratio (GRBWR) is calculated. This should preferably be above 0.8 in living donor transplantation. However this continues to be a matter of debate as the original ratio was described by Tanaka when using the right lobe graft without anterior sector drainage. It is possible to have a good results using grafts with GRBWR less than 0.8. In the end, each transplant center must decide what is acceptable for them. From our experience of over 1,400 LDLT, GRBWR has the least impact on recipient outcome. At our center, we would accept a liver graft with GRBWR as low as 0.6.

$$\text{GRBWR} = (\text{Graft weight in grams/Patient weight in grams}) \times 100$$

Magnetic resonance cholangiogram: This modality outlines the biliary anatomy. During scanning for biliary anatomy, inphase/outphase scanning and spectroscopy is done to quantify the fat content. This seems to have a good correlation with liver biopsy results and also has the advantage of looking at fatty change in all segments of the liver (Figs 4 and 5).

Livers with left-sided gall bladder are generally not suitable for donation. Donors with prior history of cholecystectomy pose a special challenge to safe dissection of the porta. Sometimes donors with multiple ducts may be rejected. However, most ducts that have been divided can be joined safely and therefore do not constitute a strict contraindication. The Type IIIa anatomy may pose a problem in bile duct reconstruction if the posterior ducts inserts very high up on the left bile duct (Figs 6 to 8 and Table 2).

Operation: Donor Right Hepatectomy

A self-retaining retracting system such as the Thompson or the Omni-tract retractor should be available. Apart from the routine surgical instruments, a good vascular set with venous clamps and arterial bulldog clamps should be available. The anesthesia team proceeds with induction of the patient and aims for a low central venous pressure (CVP) throughout the transection phase of the surgery. An arterial line and a peripheral long line are usually placed after induction. Deep vein thrombosis prophylaxis is given with graduated compression pumps and stockings. Pressure point protection is essential and a body warmer is used to

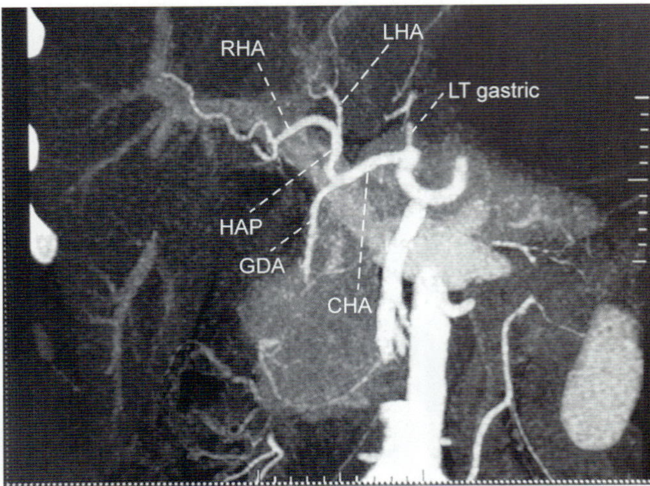

Figure 4 Hepatic arterial anatomy

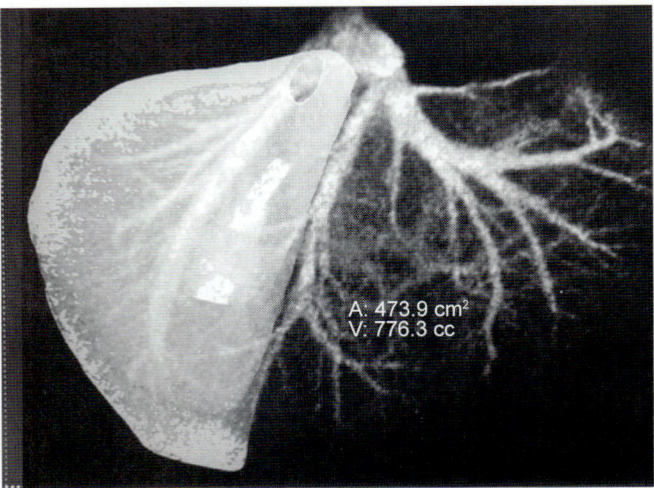

Figure 5 CT volumetry. CT, computed tomography

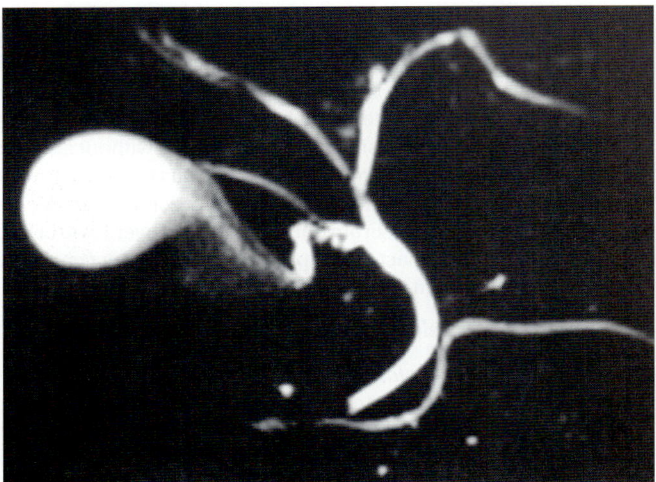

Figure 6 A good quality MRCP helps in defining bile duct anatomy. MRCP, magnetic resonance cholangiopancreatography

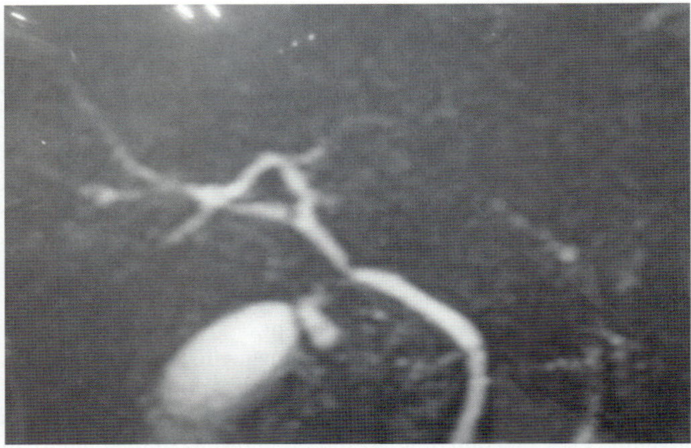

Figure 7 The posterior duct inserts very high in the left duct

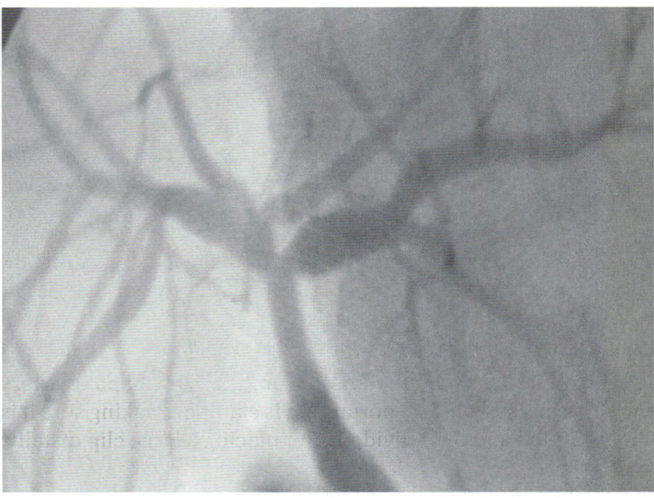

Figure 8 Unsuitable for donation

prevent hypothermia. Vigorous retraction should be avoided and periodically released whenever possible.

The incision used in our unit is a hockey stick incision (reverse L), which is basically a right subcostal incision with an upper midline extension. Midline incisions or laparoscopic-aided hepatectomy are also possible and there are now reports of complete laparoscopic right donor hepatectomy (Fig. 9).

The falciform ligament is divided and the suprahepatic vena cava is exposed. The next step is cholecystectomy and intraoperative cholangiogram. The hilar plate is lowered and a clip is placed over the right hepatic duct just beyond the confluence. The intraoperative cholangiogram is probably the most important step of the operation and no effort should be spared in getting a good cholangiogram. Later in the procedure, the clip will guide the line of division of the bile duct. Abnormal biliary anatomy should be noted. Very rarely abnormal biliary anatomy may result in aborting the donor operation and therefore the recipient operation should only start after the cholangiogram has been done in the donor (Fig. 10).

Next the right lobe is dissected off the IVC and all caudate veins are ligated. The end point of this part of the dissection is the

Table 2: Types of liver grafts

Graft type	*Segments*	*Hepatic vein taken*
Right lobe graft		
1. Extended right lobe graft	4–8	RHV/full MHV taken with graft
2. Modified right lobe graft	4–8	RHV/partial MHV with reconstruction
3. Standard right lobe graft	4–8	RHV/MHV not taken or reconstructed
4. Posterior sector graft	6, 7	RHV based
Left lobe graft	2–4	LHV/MHV
Left lobe with caudate	1–4	LHV/MHV
Left lateral segment	1–3	LHV
Monosegmental graft	2 or 3	LHV

RHV, right hepatic vein; MHV, middle hepatic vein; LHV, left hepatic vein.

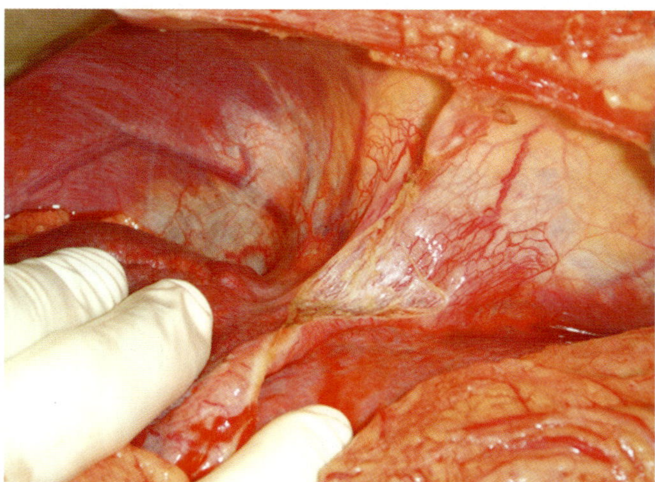

Figure 9 Suprahepatic dissection—IVC exposed. IVC, inferior vena cava

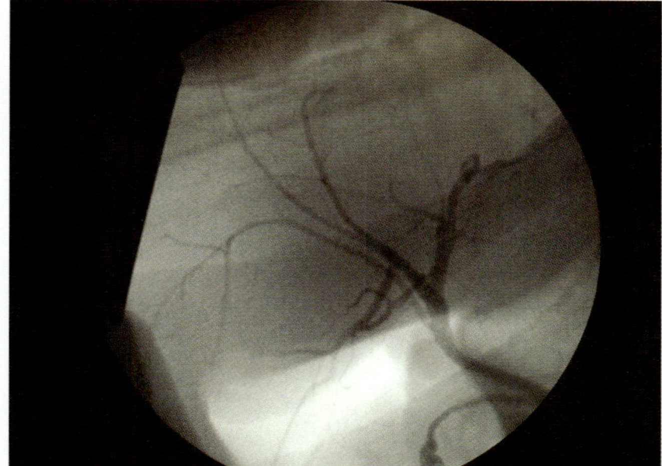

Figure 10 Intraoperative cholangiogram

looping of the right hepatic vein (RHV) (Table 2). If an inferior hepatic vein (IHV) larger than 5 mm is encountered, it is preserved for reconstruction. The RHV is freed from the diaphragm after dividing the inferior phrenic veins. This helps in excluding the diaphragm from the clamp when it will be applied later on. Once the lobe is mobilized, the porta hepatis is dissected. The right hepatic artery to the right of the bile duct and the right portal vein behind the bile duct are dissected and looped. This area is entered by dividing the glissonian capsule lateral to the portal vein. The cystic artery is ligated close to the hepatic artery once again and this allows the artery to fall away from the bile duct. No attempt is made to loop the bile duct at this stage. Bulldog clamps are applied to the artery and portal vein, to delineate the transection plane, which is marked with a diathermy.

Middle Hepatic Vein: Right Hepatic Artery Clamp

In right lobe donation, the area drained by the MHV can be determined by clamping the MHV and LHV and the right hepatic artery. The extent of anterior sector congestion can then be assessed. Usually if the congestion area is less than 20% a standard right lobe graft will suffice. If the area of congestion is more in the segment 8 area, the branches of this area must be reconstructed carefully (Figs 11 and 12).

The parenchyma is divided using either a water jet or an ultrasonic aspirator by staying in the ischemic plane. Small branches are divided till a big branch is seen. This is looped just proximal to the segment 4b branch. Segment 5 vein is dissected by completing the transection till the confluence of bile duct. Similarly a segment 8 vein tributary is used to guide the transection of segment 8 till a sizeable vein is seen and then it is looped.

In case the MHV is planned to be retrieved, the branches to the left of the vein are ligated and divided till the 4a branch is reached and then the vein is looped in preparation for division later on.

Once the segment 8 vein has been looped, the bile duct is divided after a second cholangiogram by staying to the right of the marking clip. The caudate lobe is then divided and the remaining liver slung using a Ryle's tube by placing it superior to the portal structures and to the left of RHV. This maneuver helps in transecting the deeper parts of the liver.

Heparin is given to the donor after transection is completed and hemostasis secured. The hepatic artery is divided after ligating proximally with double ties and also transfixed later. The segment 4 branch if it arises from the right hepatic artery should be preserved. The portal vein is clamped making sure it is not crumpled and then divided after placing a large clip distally. The segment 5 and 8 tributaries are divided using a vascular stapler. The RHV is clamped and then divided (Figs 13 to 15).

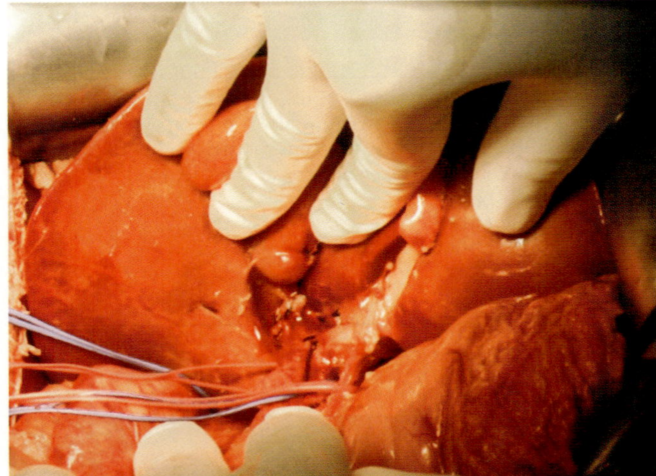

Figure 11 Dissection of the porta hepatis

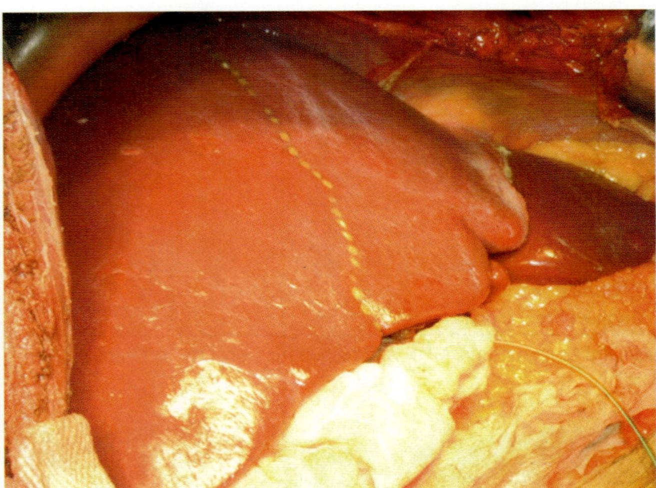

Figure 12 Marking the transection line

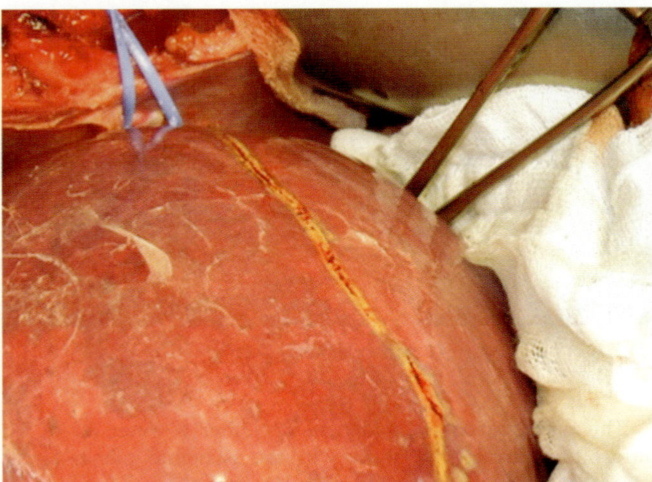

Figure 13 MHV–right hepatic artery clamp test. MHV, middle hepatic vein

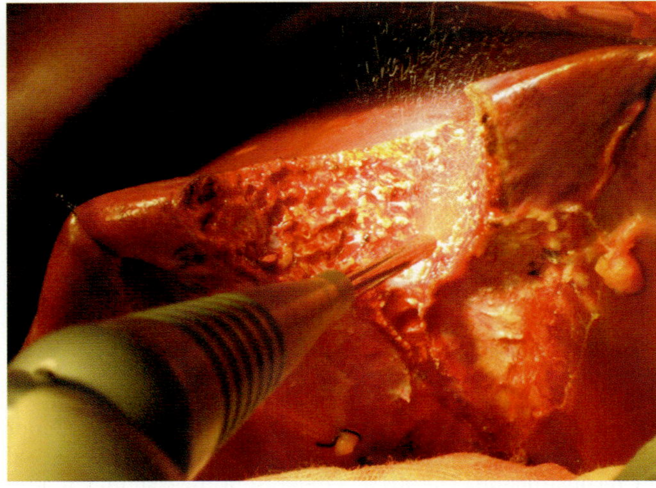

Figure 14 Parenchymal transection with CUSA. CUSA, cavitron ultrasonic surgical aspirator

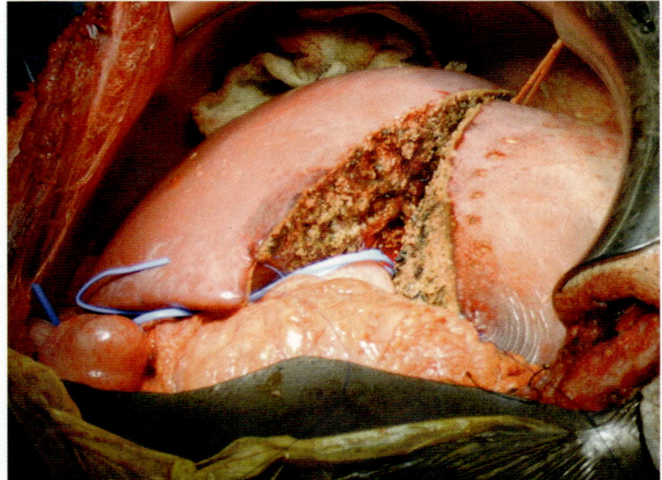

Figure 15 Parenchymal transection complete

The graft is removed and perfusion with cold preservative solution at 4°C is started. The stump of the bile duct is over sewn, the hepatic artery stump transfixed, and the portal and RHV stumps are over sewn.

The ties on the IVC are inspected and the larger branches will need to be transfixed with 5-0 Prolene. The CVP is raised and hemostasis is rechecked prior to closure. A check cholangiogram is done to ensure there is no bile leak and the stump has been closed accurately. A soft drain is placed.

Complications

Most donors have a smooth postoperative recovery and are ambulant by the third postoperative day. The overall mortality reported in literature for right lobe donors is 0.2–0.5%.[1]

While the overall morbidity rates are 12–16%, the incidence of serious morbidity is low.[7] Reported early complications are bleeding, bile leak, intra-abdominal collection, wound sepsis, respiratory complications, and venous thrombosis. Long-term morbidity is usually related to biliary complications.[1] With proper preparation and care the donor complications in major transplant centers are low. Only 0.5% of the donors require a blood transfusion. Biliary complications, which are mainly minor bile leaks, are usually 4–8%. Long-term morbidity in the form of strictures occurs in 0.5–1% of donors. Pain and a feeling of tightness along the incision are common but temporary. Nearly 100% of donors are back to normal activity in 3 months.

Ethical Dilemmas

One of the issues with a donor hepatectomy is that a normal healthy individual is subjected to a major operation. There is intense pressure on the donor when a loved one is unwell. Of concern is the fact that loved ones are willing to donate regardless of the risk to them. In these situations, a simple informed consent is insufficient and a "cooling off" period is necessary. Physicians have a duty to prevent individuals from taking this risk unless the chance of success is proportionately large. Of equal concern is the fact that family members may be under pressure to donate leading to those who are reluctant to do so to feel coerced. This can be eliminated by a private interview with the donor who is then rejected for medical reasons. Also of concern is that this type of donation has the potential for making possible the buying and selling of organs, and hence the strict protocol of ethical committee clearance is followed.

CONCLUSION

Despite all concerns, today donor hepatectomy is a safe procedure in expert hands. In India and most Asian countries, living donor transplantation remains the only hope for most patients with end-stage chronic liver disease. Though it is a major operation our understanding of liver anatomy and the regenerative capacity of liver has advanced to a point where major complications are unheard off.

REFERENCES

1. Florman S, Miller CM. Live donor liver transplantation. Liver Transpl. 2006;12:499-510.

BIBLIOGRAPHY

1. Broelsch CE, Emond JC, Thistlethwaite JR, et al. Liver transplantation with reduced size donor organ. Transplantation. 1988;45:519-24.
2. Chung-Mau Lo. Complications and long-term outcome of living liver donors: a survey of 1,508 cases in five Asian centers. Transplantation. 2003;75:s12-5.
3. Hashikura Y, Makuuchi M, Kawasaki S, et al. Successful living-related partial liver transplantation to an adult patient. Lancet. 1994;343:1233-4.
4. Raia S, Nery J, Mies S. Liver transplantation from live donors. Lancet. 1989;2:497.
5. Strong RW, Lynch SV, Ong TH, et al. Successful liver transplantation from a living donor to her son. N Eng J Med. 1990;322:1505-15.
6. Sugawara Y, Makuuchi M. Advances in adult living donor liver transplantation: a review based on reports from the 10th anniversary of the adult-to-adult living donor liver transplantation meeting in Tokyo. Liver Transpl. 2004;10:715-20.
7. Truog RD. The ethics of organ donation by living donors. N Eng J Med. 2005;353:444-6.

RECIPIENT SURGERY

In the case of cadaveric transplant, once a donor is available, the recipient is called to the hospital. A quick history and examination is done to know the current status and this information is collated with the pretransplant evaluation data. Blood is sent for complete blood count, liver function test, and renal chemistry and cross-matched for blood transfusion. In the case of LDLT, they are admitted 48 hours before the surgery and started on antibiotics, diagnostic ascitic tap is done, and bowel is prepared and oral amphotericin given for prophylaxis against mucormycosis.

TECHNIQUE

The operating room (OR) is prepared with electrocardiogram monitoring, temperature probes, cardiac output measurement, and lines are placed for rapid infusion, two arterial lines and occasionally Swan Ganz catheter. In the OR, real time measurement of arterial blood gas, electrolytes, hemoglobin, prothrombin time, and thromboelastogram (TEG) should be done hourly.

Preoperative Preparation

A. Patient is given preoperative antibiotics half an hour before incision. At our center we give
   1. Piperacillin–Tazobactum
   2. Teicoplanin
   3. Fluconazole.
B. Patient is scrubbed with betadine paint and solution.
C. Intercostal tube drainage is put if patient has significant pleural effusion. This also benefits the operating surgeon in right lobe mobilization as well as during implantation.
D. Special precaution is taken for support of pressure points, deep venous thrombosis prophylaxis (Figs 16 and 17), Shoulder braces, and leg splints to prevent foot drop.
E. A dialysis line may need to be placed in anticipation for need of intraoperative dialysis support.
F. Cell saver may be needed rarely. Instead we aim to control bleeding as we proceed during the operation.
G. Thermal blanket or mattress is used to control the body temperature.
H. Three tiers of liver drapes are put in order to prevent seepage of fluid to the back and this prevents cautery burns (Figs 18 and 19).
I. Apart from retractors, surgical instruments and microsurgery set, argon beam coagulator, harmonic scalpel, two cautery tips, two suction cannulae with a sump drain connection, and a small suction cannula are organized. A headlight is essential.

Incision (Figs 20 to 24)

A bilateral subcostal incision is given with upper midline extension. The incision extends from the left mid-clavicular line to the right side mid-axillary line.[1] The xiphoid process is excised (Fig. 20). The incision is made with a diathermy and all bleeding controlled as and when it happens.

The umbilical ligament is ligated and divided but can be preserved if there is a large shunt till the time of liver explantation.

The falciform ligament is divided till the loose connective tissue surrounding the hepatic veins (Figs 23 and 24). Hooking the left

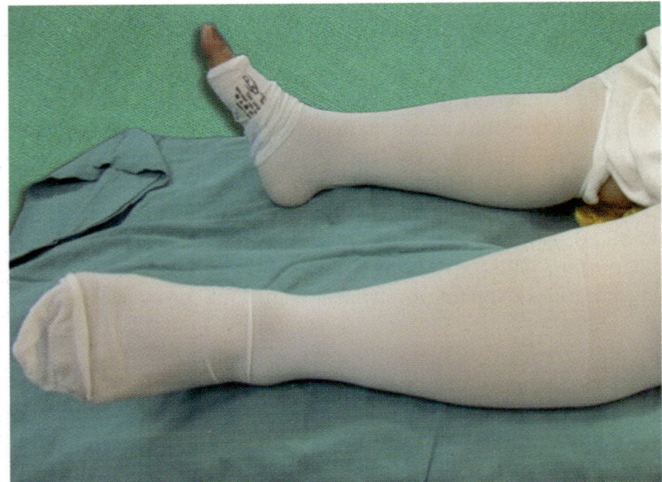

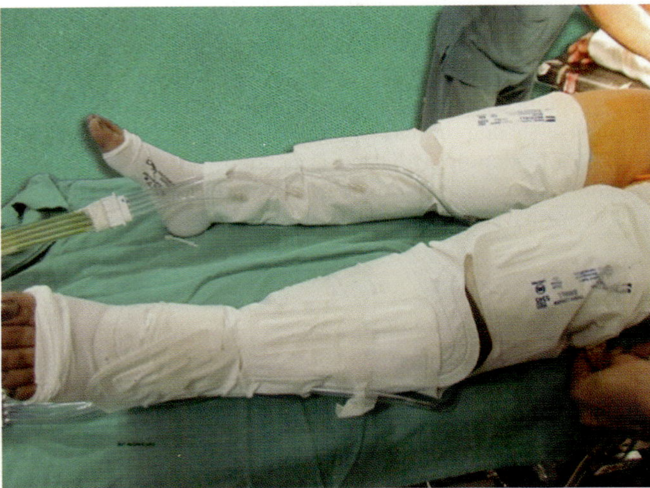

Figures 16 and 17 DVT prophylaxis. DVT, deep venous thrombosis

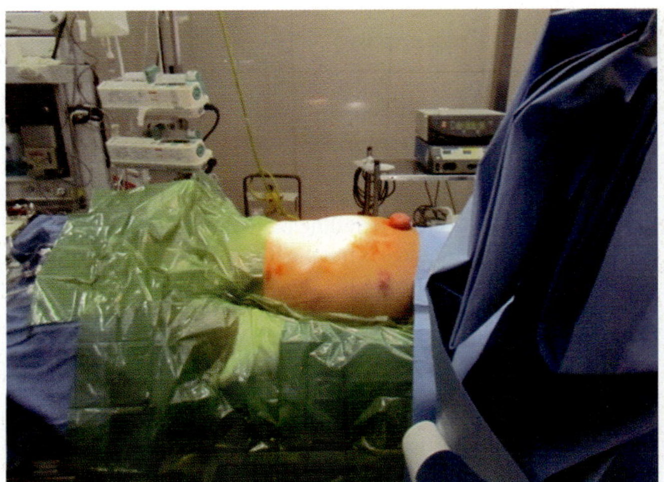

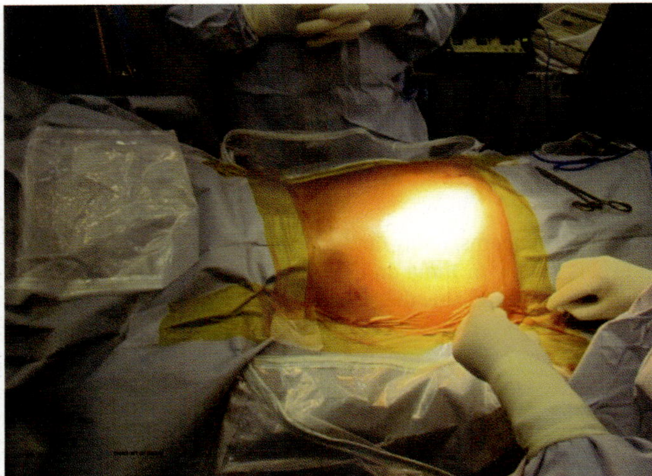

Figures 18 and 19 Three tiers of drapes

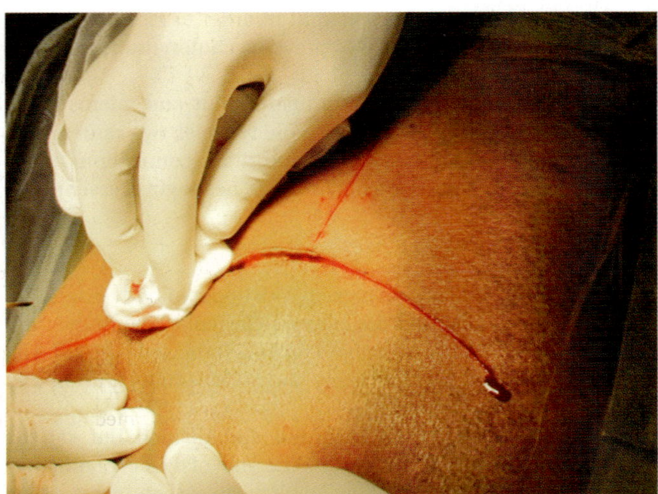

Figure 20 Bilateral subcostal incision extending to xiphisternum in midline

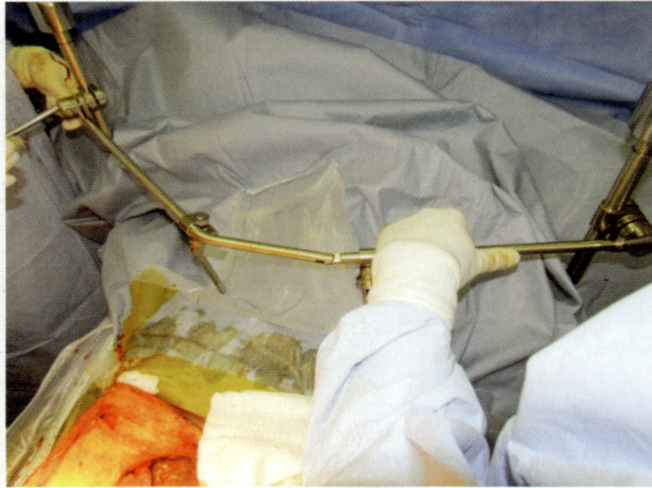

Figure 21 Applying the Omni-tract retractor

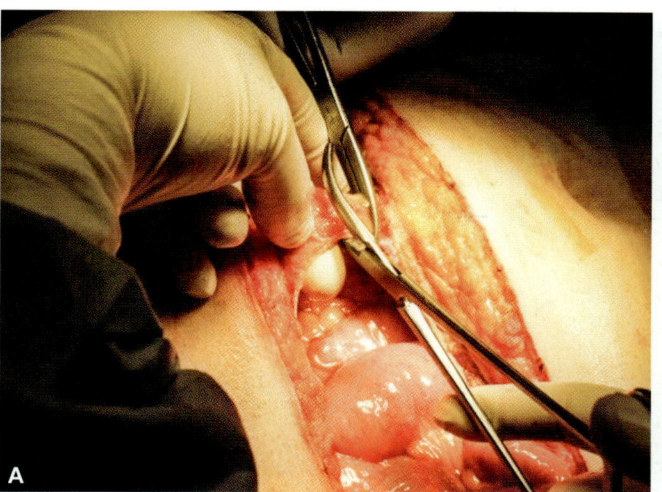

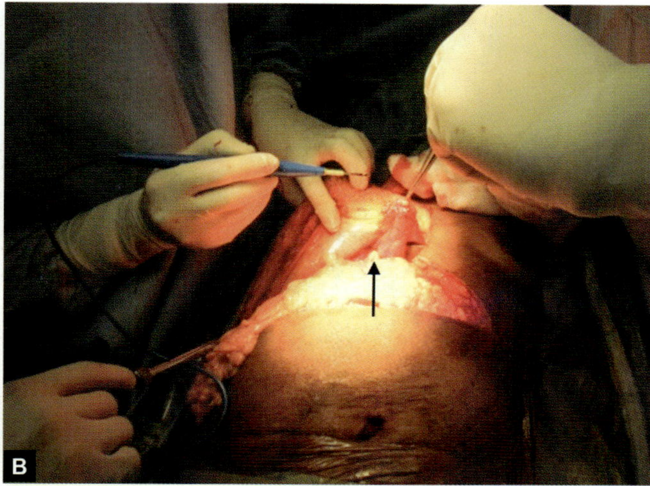

Figure 22A and B Division of falciform ligament

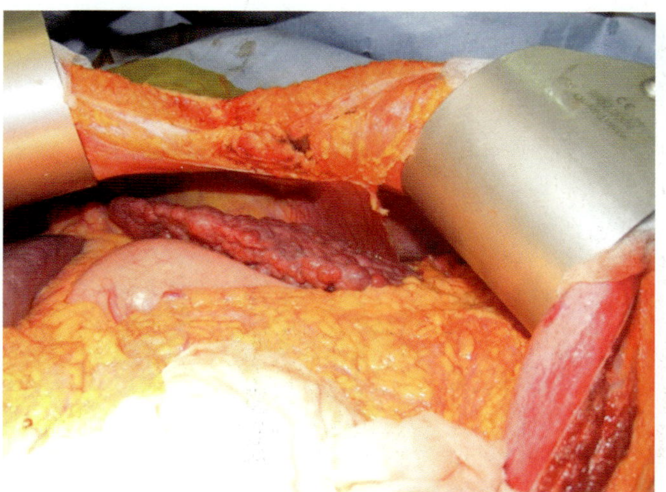

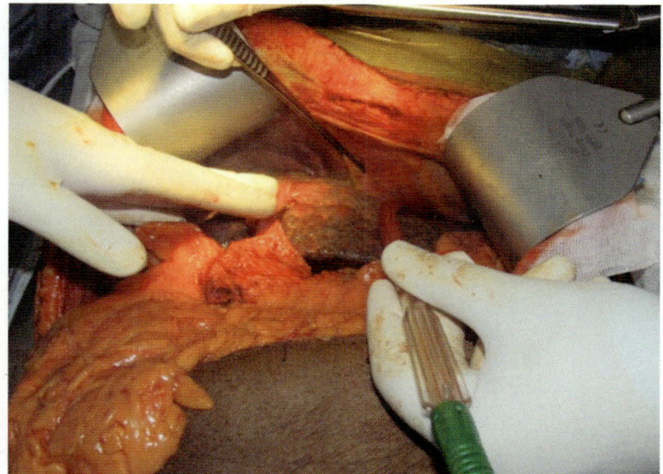

Figures 23 and 24 Division of xiphisternum and left coronary ligament

lobe with the right hand and using the diathermy with the left hand the left coronary ligament is divided. The costal margins are elevated for proper exposure using Thompson or Omni-tract retractor system (Fig. 21).

Assessment

In patients with hepatocellular carcinoma, abdominal survey is done with special attention to the recto-vesical pouch, peritoneum, porta, and liver surface. Any suspicious node in the hepato-duodenal region or along the hepatic artery is sent for frozen section. Usually the recipient surgery is started first, prior to the donor surgery, to rule out any extrahepatic disease in the recipient. However, in an analysis of over 100 cases, no patient was found to have extrahepatic disease after laparotomy.

Left Lobe Mobilization

The lesser omentum is divided taking care to preserve the accessory left hepatic artery (Figs 25 and 26). The left triangular ligament is divided in the following manner. The surgeon lifts the left lobe from beneath while the assistant gives a gentle traction on upper pole of spleen; a mop is placed beneath the left lobe and the triangular ligament overlying the anterior surface of stomach and anterior surface of upper pole of spleen. Then the triangular ligament is divided from lateral end. The whole of ligament is avascular apart from overlying collaterals, which are meticulously cauterized (Fig. 27). The lateral end often carries a vessel, which must be ligated and divided (Fig. 28). After division of the lesser omentum, the ligament of Arantius is divided between ties.

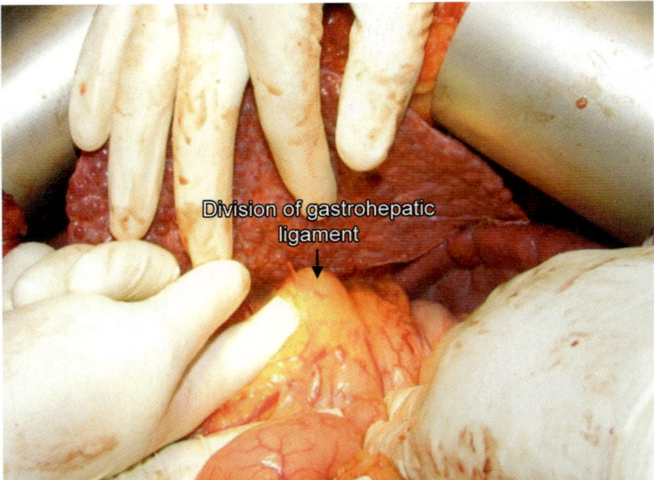

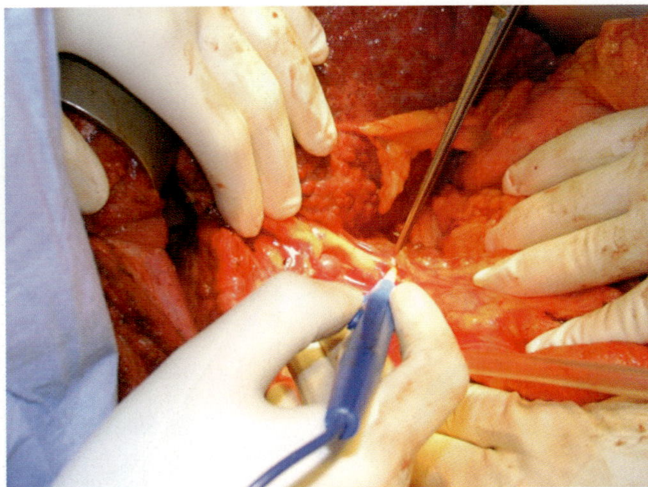

Figures 25 and 26 Division of gastro-hepatic omentum

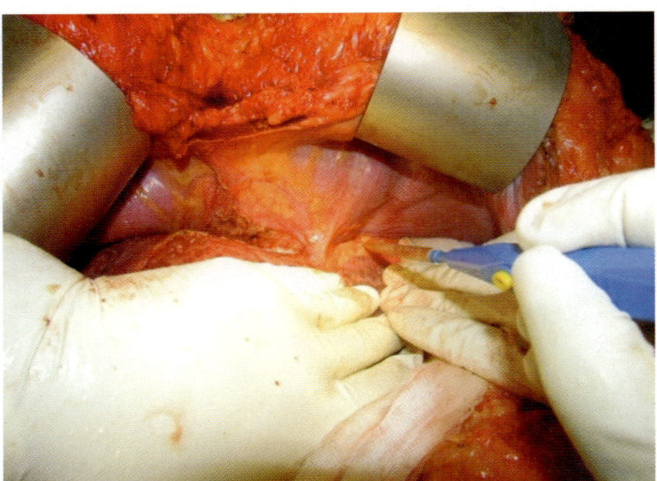

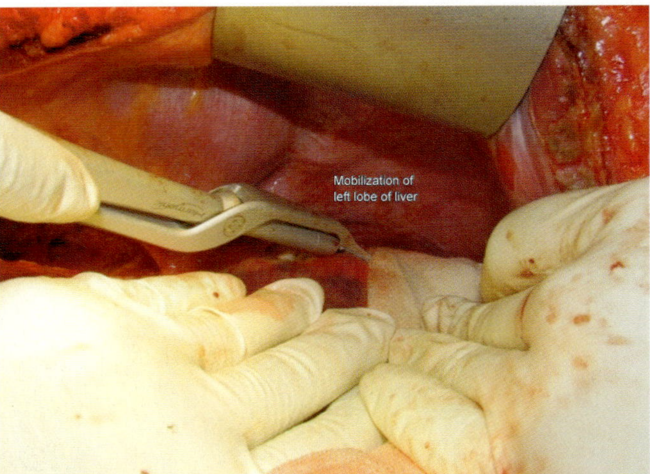

Figures 27 and 28 Division of left triangular ligament

Right Lobe Mobilization

It starts with dividing the right triangular and the coronary ligaments (Fig. 29). Once the right triangular ligament is divided (Fig. 30), the dissection is continued medially dividing superior and inferior coronary ligament with traction from the assistant to rotate the right lobe medially into the surgical field. The bare area of the liver is exposed and the retroperitoneal attachments are divided as the right lobe is further rotated medially.

Right Adrenal Gland Separation

The right adrenal gland must be separated carefully from the right lobe of the liver. Occasionally, this is very adherent to the liver in which case it may need to be kept with the right lobe partially. However, staying close to the liver capsule, one may be able to separate the adrenal gland completely from the liver. By instilling saline on top of the IVC one may be able to open this plane easily. Near the IVC, a vein will often be encountered from the liver to the adrenal vein. This needs to be ligated and divided.

Inferior Vena Cava Clearance

The retrohepatic vena cava is hence exposed. The short-hepatic veins draining the posterior aspect of the right lobe and the caudate are then ligated. The peritoneum over the vena cava inferior to the caudate lobe of the liver is incised and extended circumferentially to loop the cava (Figs 31 and 32). The division of short-hepatic veins is continued up to the level of the RHV such that almost whole of the caval anterior surface is cleared and the RHV is looped after dividing the hepato-caval ligament (Figs 33 and 34).

This is necessary with LDLT where the piggyback technique of caval preservation is necessary. In case of cadaveric transplant with caval replacement, this may not be necessary where once the lower cava is looped, space can be created by blunt dissection so

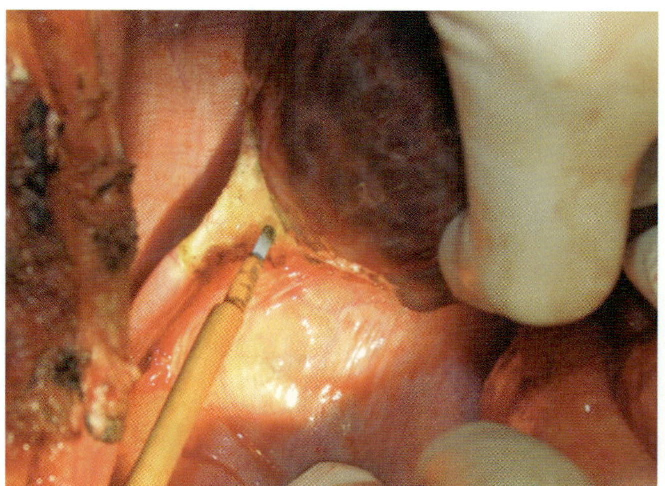

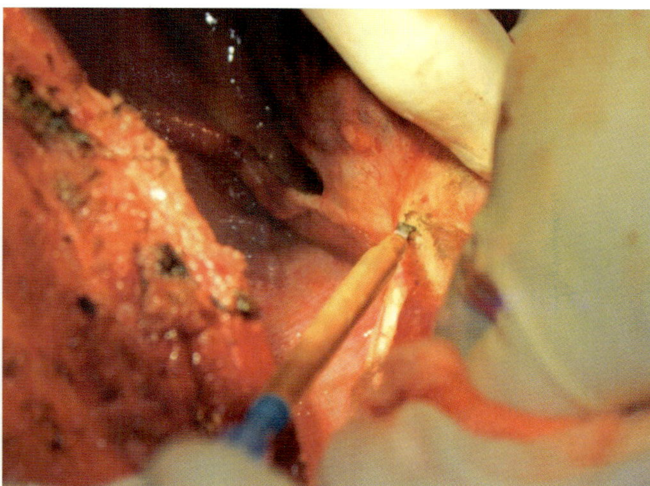

Figures 29 and 30 Division of right triangular ligament

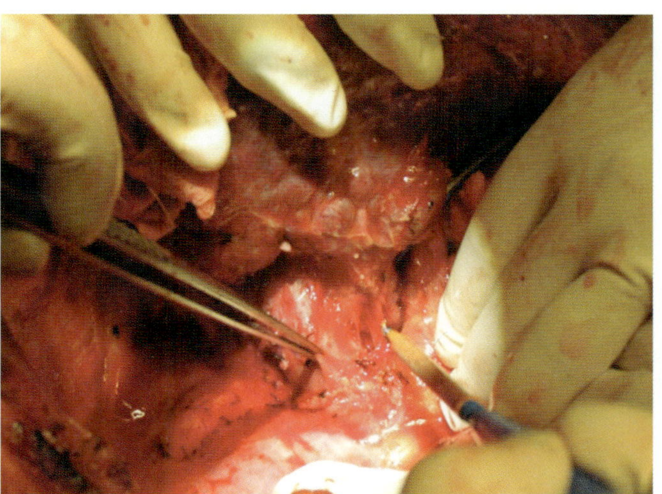

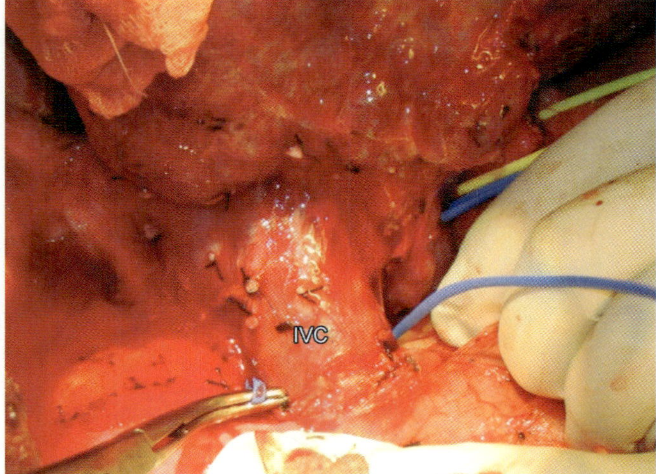

Figures 31 and 32 Division of peritoneum around cava and application of loop

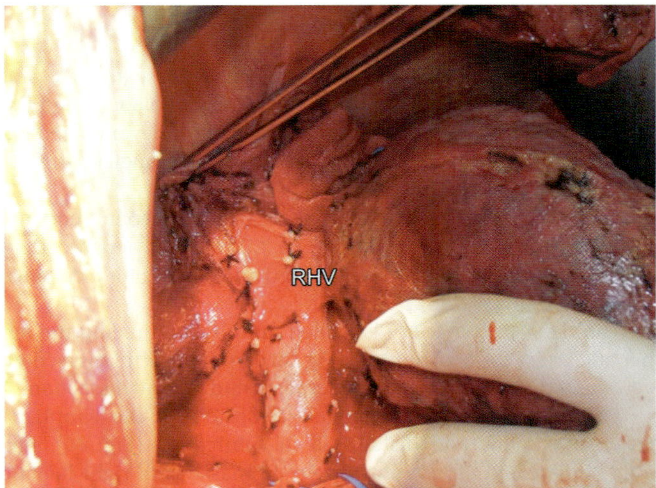

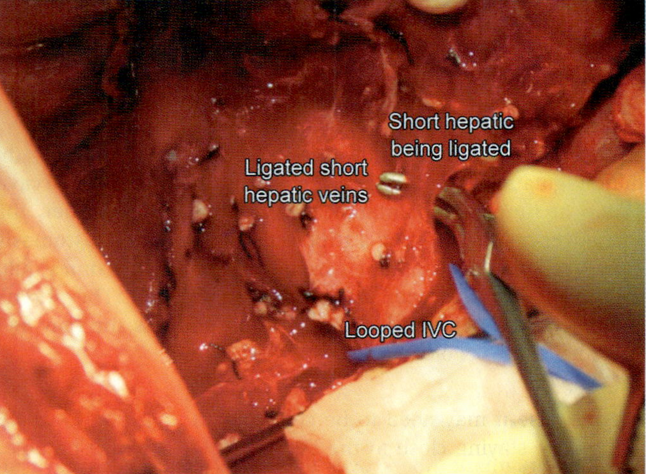

Figures 33 and 34 Division of short hepatic veins with exposure of RHV. RHV, right hepatic vein

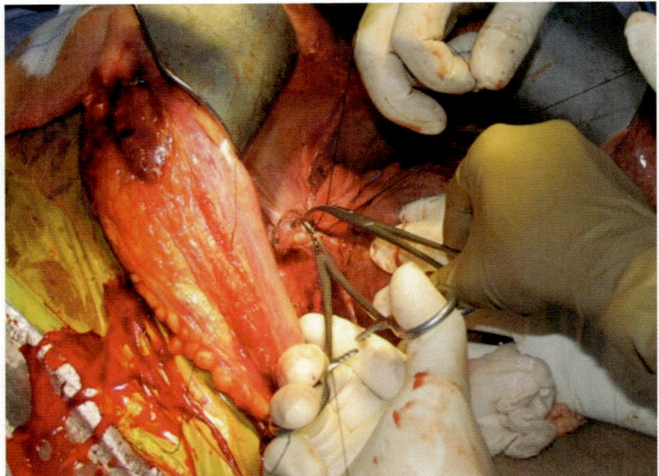

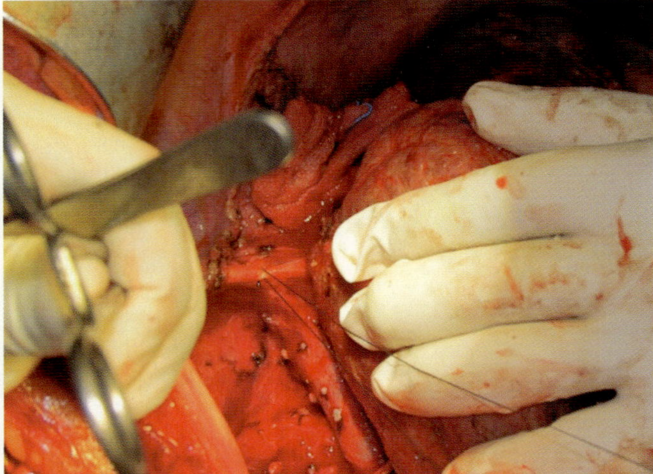

Figures 35 and 36 Division of right phrenic veins

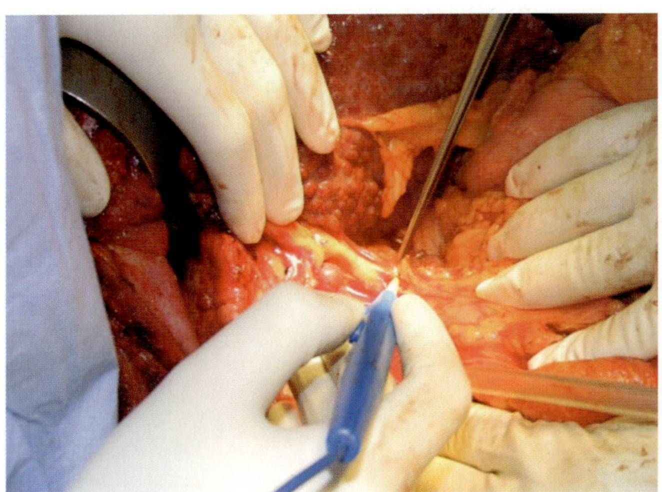

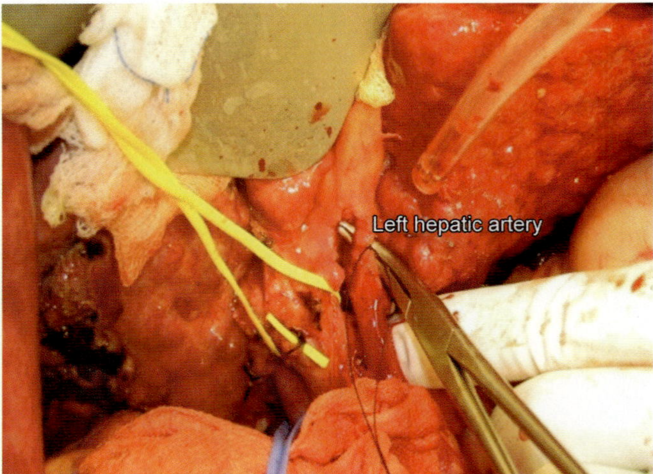

Figures 37 and 38 Division of hepatoduodenal ligament and exposure of left hepatic artery

that the suprahepatic cava with the diaphragm can be clamped with a stout clamp such as the one named after Sir Roy Calne.

Phrenic Veins

Ligating the right phrenic veins frees the IVC from the diaphragmatic attachments and facilitates the application of caval clamp at time of explantation and implantation. Further, this maneuver helps in getting a triphasic outflow after anastomosis. However, this must be done carefully as the IVC becomes quite thin at this level particularly in the posterior part. The phrenic veins are doubly ligated keeping in mind that this site may be a potential source of bleeding (Figs 35 and 36).

Suprahepatic Cava

The diaphragmatic fibers over the suprahepatic vena cava are cleared for a distance of 1.5–2 cm for proper placement of clamps. At this stage attention is turned to portal dissection.

Portal Dissection

There may be vascularized adhesions between segment 6 and rest of the abdomen as well as between the gall bladder and the duodenum. These must be separated in order to prevent bleeding. The cystic artery is ligated and divided in Calot's triangle; the cystic duct stump is kept long.

The anterior layer of the peritoneum over the hepatoduodenal ligament is incised with cautery (Fig. 37). The left hepatic artery and its segment 4 branch are dissected and cleared for a distance of around 2 cm (Fig. 38).

The right gastric artery is ligated and divided freeing the left hepatic artery for anastomosis (Fig. 39). At the time of dissection, care should be taken to avoid vasospasm and intimal dissection.

The portal trunk is completely dissected off the lymphatic tissue proximally and distally till its bifurcation (Fig. 40). Bile duct is dissected off the portal vein en masse with right hepatic artery preserving the soft tissue and ductal branches from the right hepatic artery (Figs 40 and 41). The right hepatic artery

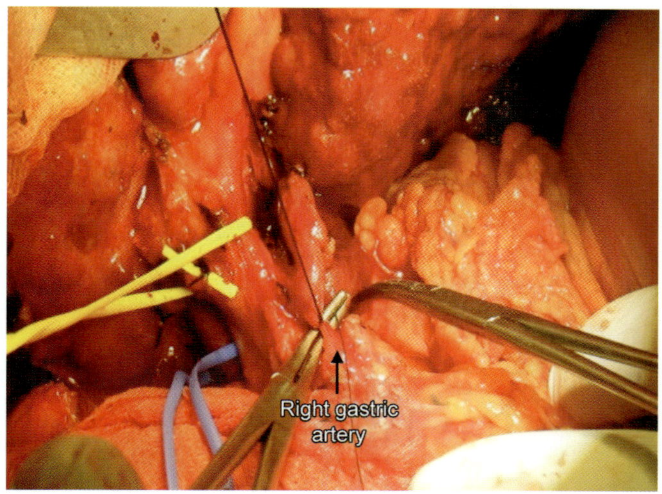

Figure 39 Division of right gastric artery

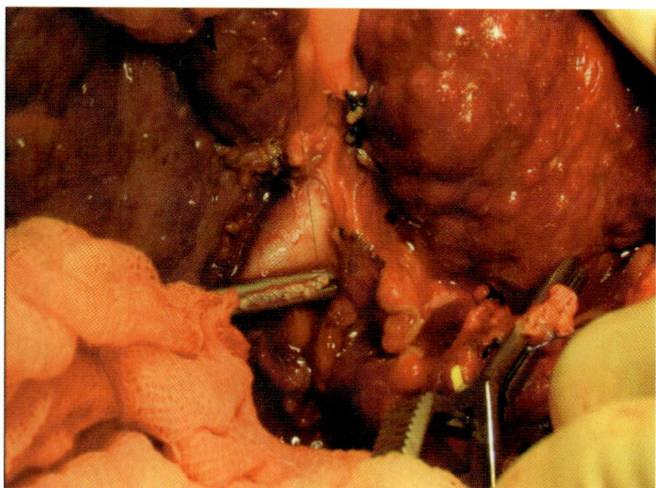

Figure 42 Division of portal vein

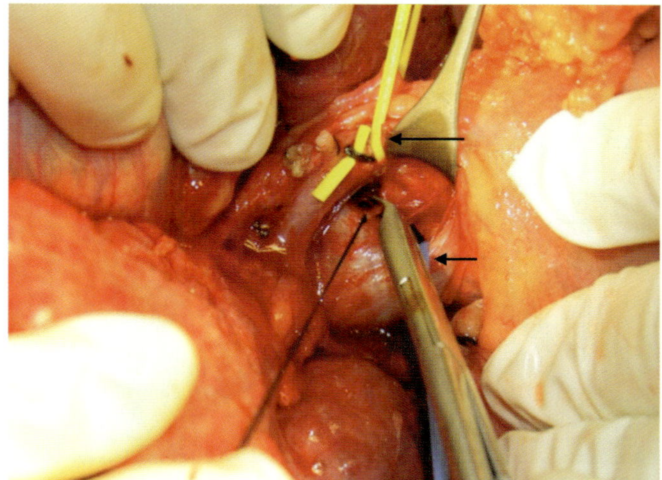

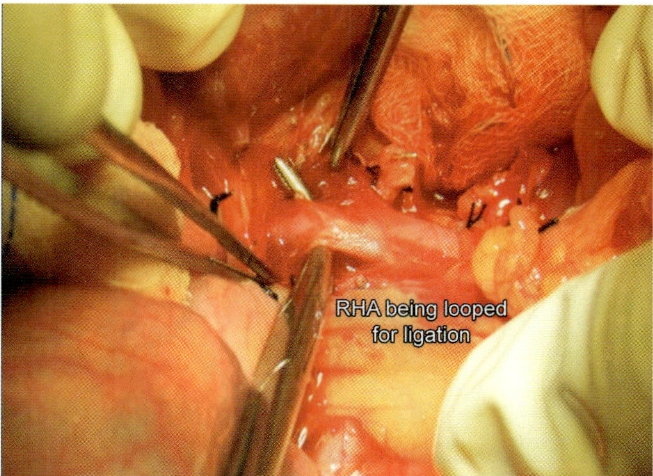

Figures 40 and 41 Portal vein dissection and division of and exposure of right hepatic artery

is ligated and divided high up in the hilum to the right of bile duct (Fig. 41).

Thus the portal structures are freed with loops around the bile duct right hepatic artery complex. The left and the middle hepatic arteries are looped and divided distally. The portal vein is also looped after dividing the lymphatic tissue posterior to the portal vein.

Division of Porta

Once the parenchymal transection has been completed in the donor liver, the diseased liver of the recipient is explanted by clamping/ligating and dividing the hepatic inflow and outflow structures. In this manner, the anhepatic phase can be kept short and both the donor and the recipient liver can be taken out at the same time. In special circumstance like fulminant hepatic failure, hepatocellular carcinoma, portal vein thrombosis, excessive bleeding or when the patient has hepatorenal syndrome, the portal vessels are ligated first to create a portocaval shunt quickly.

The portal vein is temporarily clamped and the bile duct is divided as distally as possible to get both the right and left ducts in a sheath. The portal vein clamp is released and dividing the coronary or the lateral pancreatic branch lengthens the portal vein. The portal vein clamp is reapplied and another clamp is applied anterio-posteriorly just proximal to bifurcation and the portal vein is divided 2 mm distal to it (Fig. 42). The distal end is closed with continuous 5-0 Prolene sutures making sure there is no leak or narrowing.

Explantation

The peritoneal layer reflection over the IVC is divided parallel and close along the length of IVC till the left hepatic vein (LHV). The loose tissue posterior to the cava is gently separated and the lower cava freed till the level of renal veins. A long length of IVC is necessary when there is an IHV to be anastomosed.

At this moment the liver is attached to the IVC only by the hepatic veins. The RHV is divided between clamps and the liver removed after clamping and dividing the middle and LHV (Figs 43 to 46).

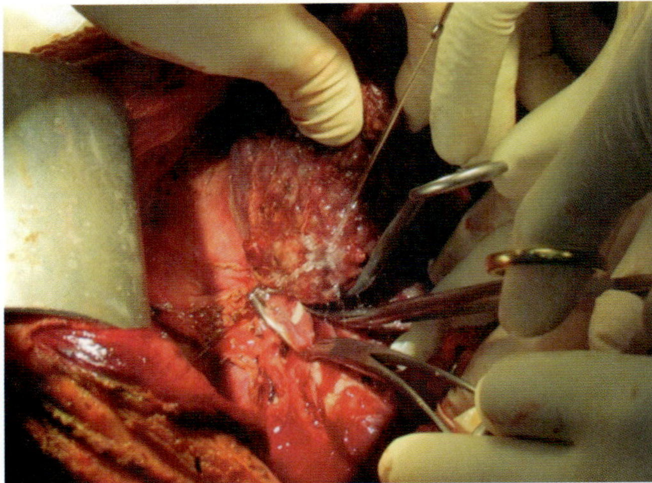

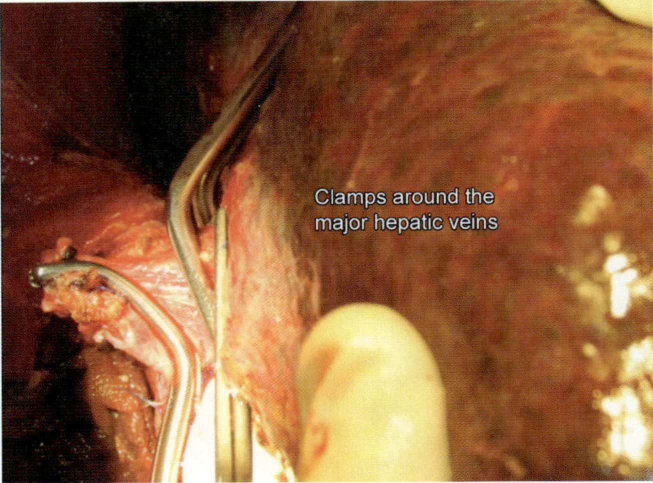

Figures 43 and 44 Clamping and division of RHV. RHV, right hepatic vein

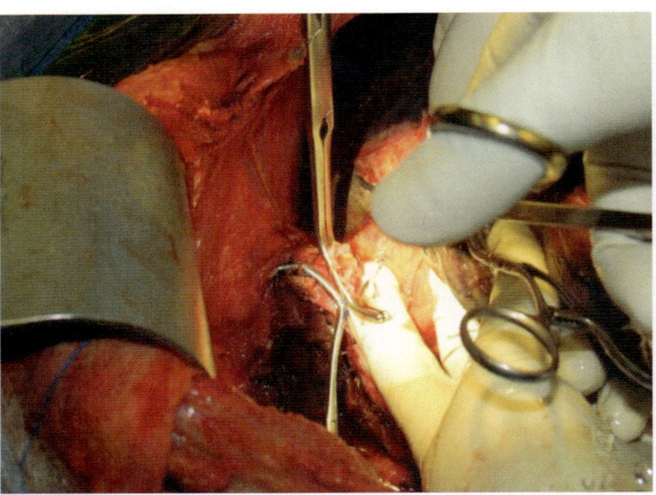

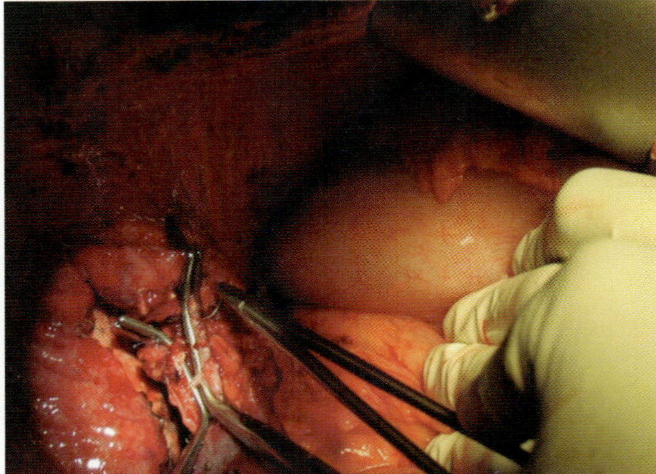

Figures 45 and 46 Clamping and division of middle and LHV and closure of stump. LHV, left hepatic vein

Anhepatic Phase

The common stump of left and MHV opening into the IVC is closed with a double layer of Prolene 5-0 continuous sutures. In case the liver has a tumor, the abdomen is lavaged with a tumoricidal agent. A temporary portocaval shunt is usually performed unless there is significant shunting. In case, there is a large lienorenal shunt, the left renal vein is looped and if necessary ligated in continuity if the portal flow is less. Trial clamping is done to see whether the recipient will tolerate total IVC clamping during the implantation procedure.

Benching

At the back table the donor graft is examined and if necessary veins may be joined or lengthened to facilitate subsequent anastomosis. If a significant segment VII vein is present it is unioned with the main RHV. In case of extended right lobe grafts, the middle vein is lengthened with a portal vein graft. As most of our grafts are modified right lobe grafts, segment 5 and 8 veins are joined to the portal vein graft retrieved from the explanted liver.

We use the recipient portal vein with or without dilating the umbilical vein as a venous conduit for reconstructing the "neo MHV". The obliterated umbilical vein can usually be dilated and opened up in most cases. In case the portal vein is thrombosed, cadaveric vein graft is used if available. Prosthetic graft is used only if venous autograft or allograft is not available.

In case of dual portal vein in the graft, the two veins will need to be joined on the back table prior to implantation and then a cuff is anastomosed to the joined portal vein.

If the right hepatic artery is of short length it can be extended with an arterial graft from the recipient.

Dealing with Portal Vein Thrombosis

Portal vein thrombus if present is dealt with in the following manner.

Patients with chronic organized thrombus which is completely epithelialized and with good portal flow do not require thrombectomy. a good portal vein flow, does not require thrombectomy. However, care must be taken that the thrombus does not get detached from the wall. from the wall. A few tacking stitches may help.

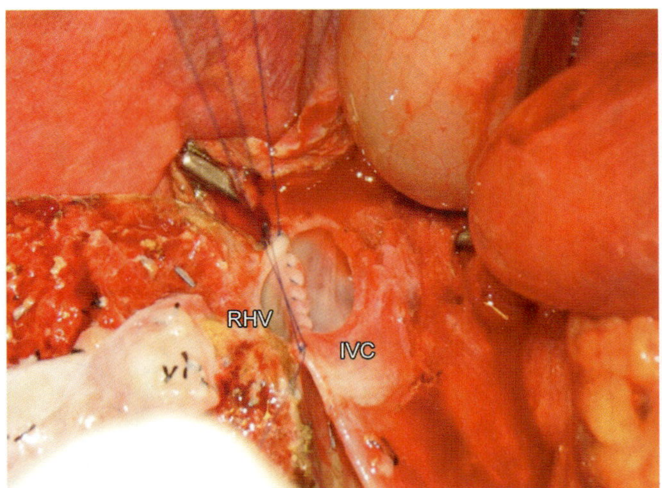

Figure 47 Anastomosis between RHV and IVC. RHV, right hepatic vein; IVC, inferior vena cava

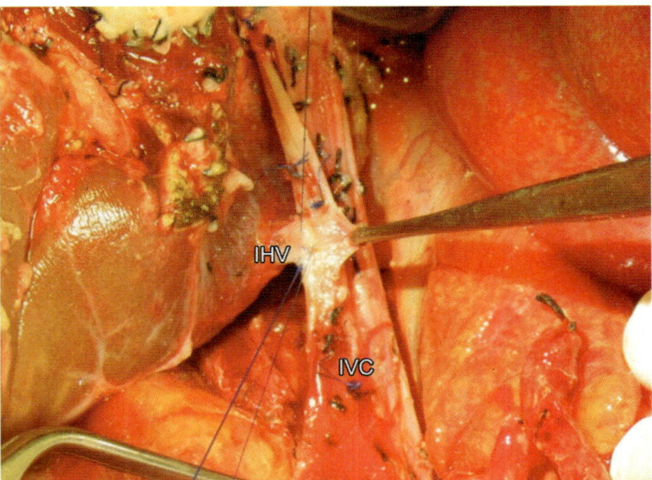

Figure 48 Anastomosis between IHV and IVC. IHV, inferior hepatic veins; IVC, inferior vena cava

A partial thrombus is dissected off the wall and gripped with an artery forceps and then pulled out of the portal vein. Prior to this, one may need to dissect out the portal vein circumferentially right up to the superior border of pancreas, as eversion thrombectomy may also be possible.[2-4] It may also be necessary to display the junction of splenic and superior mesenteric vein for antegrade thrombectomy. When the thrombus cannot be removed, a jump graft may be possible from any part of portal venous system.[5,6]

Implantation

Implantation can be done by either total or partial IVC clamping. For total clamping vascular clamps are applied superiorly above the insertion of hepatic veins and inferiorly above the insertion of renal veins. The hepatic veins are then anastomosed sequentially. During partial IVC clamping each heaptic vein is anastomosed after applying a side biting vascular clamps at venous orifice in the IVC. After the anastomosis is done, a bulldog clamp is applied to prevent backflow from IVC till reperfusion.

The stump of the RHV in the recipient is extended longitudinally and inferiorly to size match the diameter of the donor RHV.

The RHV is anastomosed end to side to the cava with continuous 4-0 Prolene suture (Fig. 47).

In the presence of an IHV, end-to-side anastomosis to the cava is performed by opening the cava longitudinally and anastomosing with 5-0 Prolene continuous sutures (Fig. 48).

The extended MHV or the neo MHV (the portal vein conduit in which the segment 5 and 8 veins have been anastomosed) is anastomosed to either the opening of the middle and LHV or directly to a new opening in the IVC with 5-0 Prolene continuous suture (Fig. 49). The knot is tied loosely with a growth factor. Before knotting, the IVC is flushed with heparinized saline.

In case of a left lobe graft, a common stump of the right, middle and LHV is created for anastomosis to the left and middle vein stump of the graft.

Portal vein is anastomosed in a standard end-to-end fashion with 5-0 Prolene continuous suture allowing a growth factor equivalent to portal vein diameter (Figs 50 and 51).

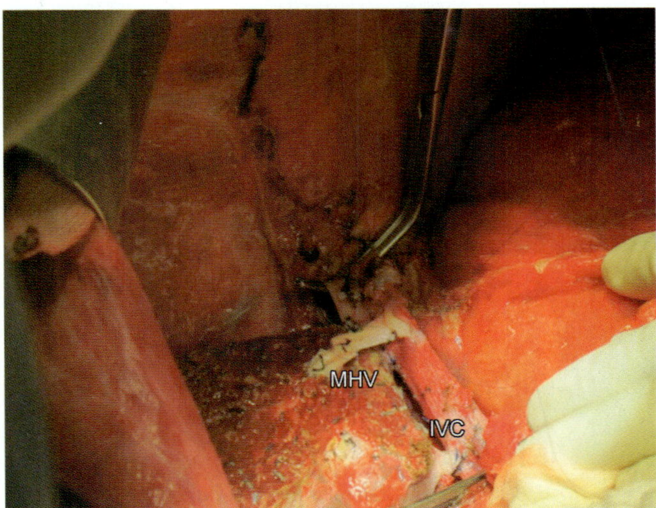

Figure 49 Anastomosis between MHV and IVC. MHV, middle hepatic vein; IVC, inferior vena cava

After this the graft is reperfused by releasing hepatic venous clamps from the IVC and then the portal clamp (Fig. 52). The anesthetist must be on guard as blood pressure does tend to fall on releasing the clamps, the so-called reperfusion syndrome.

Hepatic Artery Anastomosis

Although the use of microscope is popular in many centers, we prefer to do perform the hepatic artery anastomosis using surgical loupes of magnification 3.5 to 4 X with 8-0 Prolene interrupted suture.[7] The right wall is done first and then the left wall is flipped over for the remaining stitches (Figs 53 and 54).

The artery preferred is the left hepatic artery, which usually has a good size match with the donor hepatic artery.

If the hepatic artery is not suitable, then the left gastric artery is dissected for anastomosis.

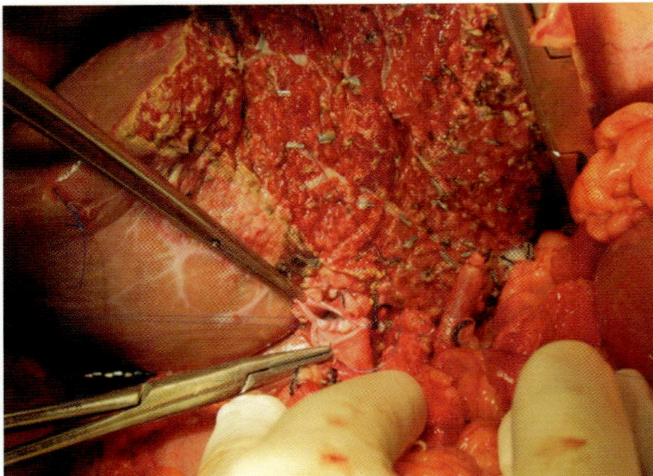

Figure 50 Portal vein reconstruction

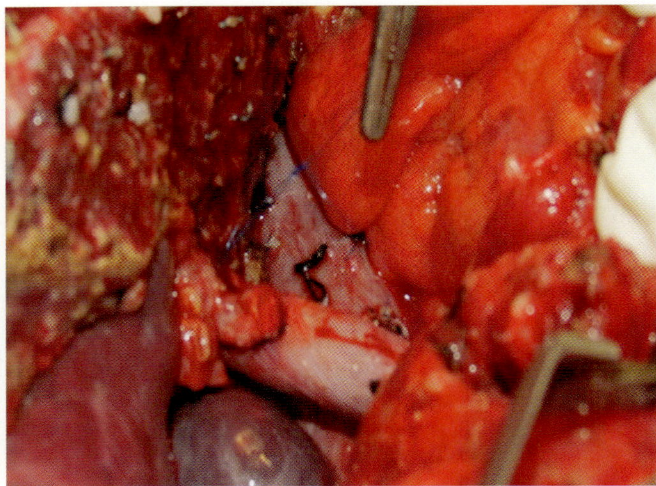

Figure 51 Growth factor left after portal vein anastomosis

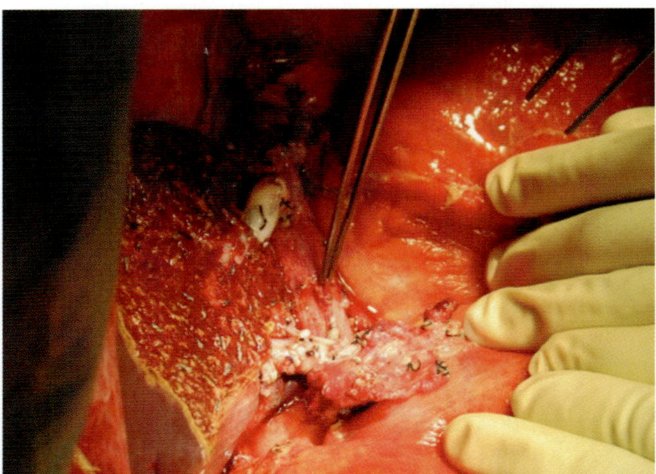

Figure 52 Graft following reperfusion

In case of dual arterial supply to the graft, it is generally preferable to do a size-matched anastomosis of both the arteries to two different arteries of the recipient even if there is a good pulsatile back flow in the second donor artery after the first anastomosis. This reduces the chances of hepatic artery thrombosis.

Intraoperative Doppler is performed to look for drainage from the hepatic vein. This must ideally be triphasic or at least biphasic. The portal vein anastomosis is checked for alignment and the volume flow is measured. The ideal situation would require a portal volume flow of between 150 and 400 mL/100 g of liver tissue. The hepatic artery flow velocity should be greater than 25 mL/min and the resistive index between 0.5 to 0.8.[8-9]

Low portal flow may require "graft inflow modulation", which involves ligation of left renal vein in the presence of a sizeable lieno-renal shunt or ligation of coronary vein or any other large collateral responsible for shunting of blood away from the liver.

High portal flow may require modulation in form of splenic artery ligation. In general, if the graft functioning is good, then we prefer to do inflow modulation postoperatively since a high portal flow sometimes aids in rapid liver regeneration.

The portal venous pressure is measured after the completion of implantation by cannulating a large omental vein. Postoperatively if there is early graft dysfunction and the intra operative portal pressure was high (>15 mm of Hg), then the splenic artery may be ligated postoperatively.

Corrected portal pressure of >15 mmHg is associated with early graft dysfunction with high drain output, delay in normalization of serum bilirubin and INR and a higher rate of re-exploration.

Biliary Reconstruction

Usually this is a single duct-to-duct anastomosis performed under loupe magnification with interrupted 6-0 PDS. In case of multiple ducts, ductoplasty is preferred if the ducts are close to each other. If ductoplasty cannot be done and the recipient duct has two suitable openings, two anastomoses are done. Otherwise one duct is joined to the bile duct and the second one to a Roux loop of jejunum.[10-11]

The anastomosis is assessed by saline instillation through the cystic duct stump followed by an intra-operative cholangiogram. (Figs 55 to 58).

The cystic duct is closed with suture and clips.

Drain Placement

We prefer to use 2 Jackson-Pratt drains, one in the morrisson's pouch and the other in the pelvis. The pelvic drain helps in preventing post operative pelvic collections.

Closure

This is done in two layers with Vicryl 2-0 continuous sutures for the peritoneum and inner muscle layer and 1/0 loop Ethilon for outer muscle layer. Continuous running subcuticular sutures with 3/0 Monocryl suture. This technique of abdominal wound closure prevents the troublesome ascitic fluid seepage from the wound in post-operative period. Wound is covered with aseptic dressing.

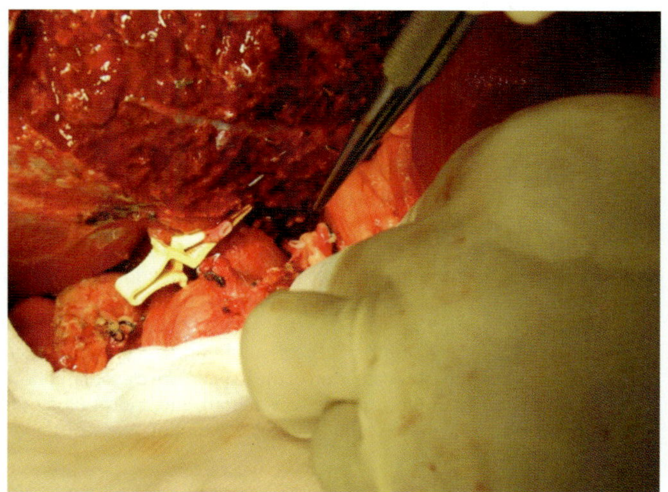

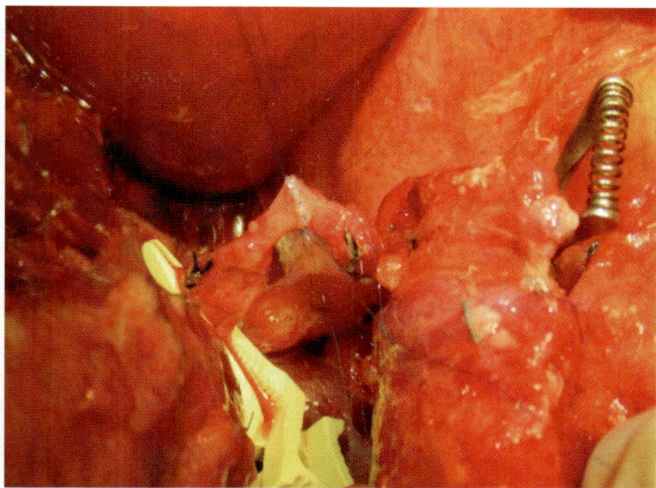

Figures 53 and 54 Anastomosis between donor and recipient hepatic artery

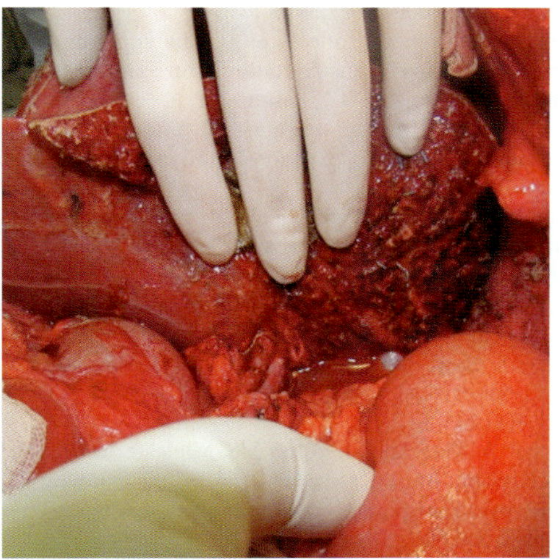

Figure 55 Ductoplasty

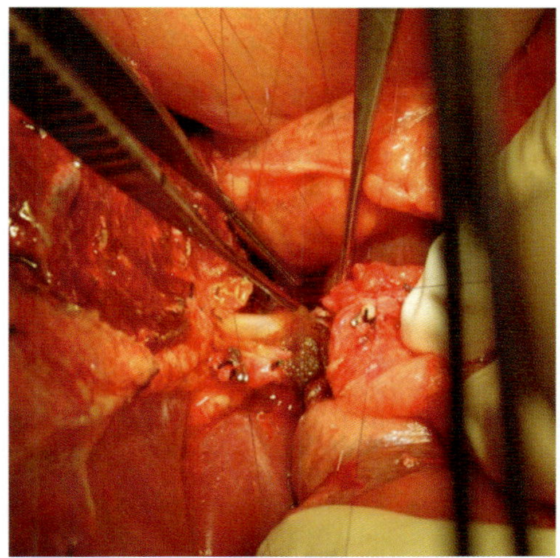

Figure 56 Duct-to-duct anastomosis

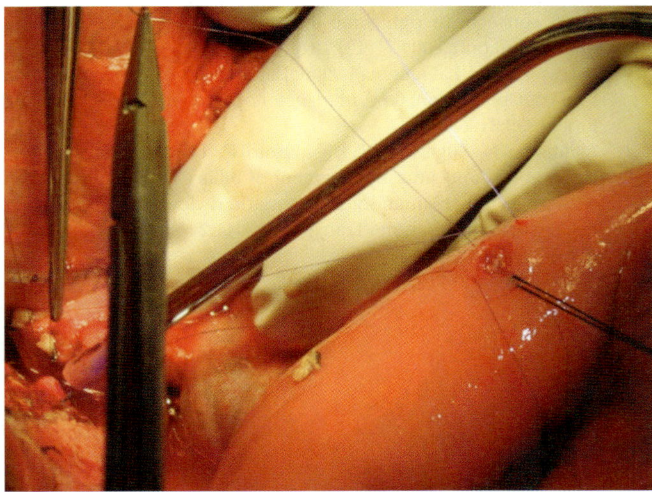

Figure 57 Hepaticojejunostomy

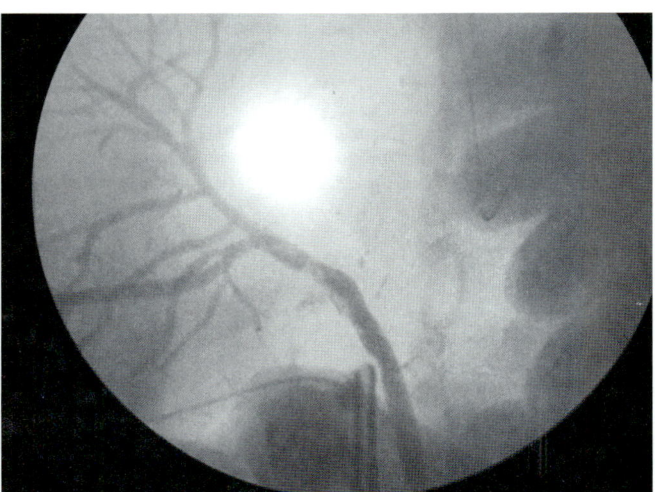

Figure 58 Intraoperative cholangiogram

BIBLIOGRAPHY

1. Murray KF, Carithers RL. AASLD practice guidelines: evaluation of the patient for liver transplantation. Hepatology. 2005;41(6):1407-32.
2. Consensus conference: indications for Liver Transplantation, January 19 and 20, 2005, Lyon-Palais Des Congrès: text of recommendations (long version). Liver Transpl. 2006;12(6):988-1011.
3. Fox AN, Brown RS Jr. Is the patient a candidate for liver transplantation? Clin Liver Dis. 2012;16(2):435-48.
4. Alqahtani SA. Update in liver transplantation. Curr Opin Gastroenterol. 2012;28(3):230-8.
5. Thuluvath PJ. Evaluation of liver transplant recipients. *J Clin Exp Hepatol.* 2011;1(3):199-203.
6. Koffron A, Stein JA. Liver transplantation: indications, pretransplant evaluation, surgery, and posttransplant complications. Med Clin North Am. 2008;92:861-88.
7. Lucey MR, Brown KA, Everson GT, et al. Minimal criteria for placement of adults on the liver transplant waiting list: a report of a national conference organized by the American Society of Transplant Physicians and the American Association for the Study of Liver Diseases. Liver Transpl Surg. 1997;3(6):628-37.
8. Freeman RB. Overview of the MELD/PELD system of liver allocation indications for liver transplantation in the MELD era: evidence-based patient selection. Liver Transpl. 2004;10(10)S2-3.
9. Olthoff KM, Brown RS, Delmonico FL, et al. Summary report of a national conference: evolving concepts in liver allocation in the MELD and PELD Era. Liver Transpl. 2004;10(10):A6-22.
10. Evaluation Alan Koffron, MD, FACS*, Julie A. Stein, MD Med Clin North Am 92 (2008) 861–888.
11. Krowka MJ, Porayko MK, Plevak DJ, et al. Hepatopulmonary syndrome with progressive hypoxemia as an indication for liver transplantation: case reports and literature review. Mayo Clin Proc. 1997;72(1):44-53.
12. O'Grady JG, Alexander GJM, Hayllar KM, Williams R. Early indicators of prognosis in fulminant hepatic failure. Gastroenterology. 1989;97(2):439-45.
13. Mazzaferro V, Regalia E, Doci R, et al. Liver transplantation for the treatment of small hepatocellular carcinomas in patients with cirrhosis. N Engl J Med. 1996;334(11):693-9.
14. Saigal S, Shah SR. Liver transplantation—economics in the less developed world. Indian J Gastroenterol. 2012;31(1):13-4. Epub 2012 Jan 7.
15. Yao FY, Ferrell L, Bass NM, et al. Liver transplantation for hepatocellular carcinoma: expansion of the tumor size limits does not adversely impact survival. Hepatology. 2001;33(6):1394-403.
16. Zhang J, Fallon MB. Hepatopulmonary syndrome: update on pathogenesis and clinical features. Nat Rev Gastroenterol Hepatol. 2012;9(9):539-49.
17. Sussman NL, Kochar R, Fallon MB. Pulmonary complications in cirrhosis. Curr Opin Organ Transplant. 2011;16(3):281-8.
18. Krowka MJ. Management of pulmonary complications in pretransplant patients. Clin Liver Dis. 2011;15(4):765-77. doi: 10.1016/j.cld.2011.08.012.
19. Krowka MJ, Plevak DJ, Findlay JY, et al. Pulmonary hemodynamics and perioperative cardiopulmonary-related mortality in patients with portopulmonary hypertension undergoing liver transplantation. Liver Transpl. 2000;6(4):443-50.
20. Al-Khafaji A, Huang DT. Critical care management of patients with end-stage liver disease. Crit Care Med. 2011;39(5):1157-66.
21. Nadim MK, Davis CL, Sung R, et al. Simultaneous liver-kidney transplantation: a survey of US transplant centers. Am J Transplant. 2012;12(11):3119-27.
22. Angeli P, Sanyal A, Moller S, et al. Current limits and future challenges in the management of renal dysfunction in patients with cirrhosis: report from the International Club of Ascites. Liver Int. 2012;33(1):16-23.
23. Liu YI, Kamaya A, Jeffrey RB, et al. Multidetector computed tomography triphasic evaluation of the liver before transplantation: importance of equilibrium phase washout and morphology for characterizing hypervascular lesions. J Comput Assist Tomogr. 2012;36(2):213-9.

REFERENCES

1. Lladó L, Figueras J. Techniques of orthotopic liver transplantation. HPB (Oxford). 2004;6(2):69-75.
2. Steiber AC, Zetti G, Todo S, et al. The spectrum of portal vein thrombosis in liver transplantation. Ann Surg. 1991;213:199-206.
3. Cherqui D, Duvoux C, Rahmouni A, et al. Orthotopic liver transplantation in the presence of partial or total portal vein thrombosis: problems in diagnosis and management. World J Surg. 1993;17:669-74.
4. Sheil R, Thompson JF, Stephen MS. Mesoportal graft for thrombosed portal vein in liver transplantation. Clin Transplant. 1987;1:18-20
5. Figueras J, Torras J, Rafecas A. Extra-anatomic venous graft for portal vein thrombosis in liver transplantation. Transpl Int.
6. Gupta S, Singhal A, Goyal N, et al. Portal biliopathy treated with living-donor liver transplant: index case. Exp Clin Transplant. 2011;9(2):145-9.
7. Marcos A, Killackey M, Orloff MS, Mieles L, Bozorgzadeh A, Tan HP. Hepatic arterial reconstruction in 95 adult right lobe living donor liver transplants: evolution of anastomotic technique. Liver Transpl. 2003;9(6)570-4.
8. Azzam AZ, Tanaka K. Management of vascular complications after living donor liver transplantation. Hepatogastroenterology. 2012;59(113):182-6.
9. Gondolesi GE, Varotti G, Florman SS, et al. Biliary complications in 96 consecutive right lobe living donor transplant recipients. Transplantation. 2004;77(12):1842-8.
10. Torras J, Lladó L, Figueras J, et al. Biliary tract complications after liver transplantation: type, management, and outcome. Transplant Proc. 1999;31:2406.
11. Akamatsu N, Sugawara Y, Hashimoto D. Biliary reconstruction, its complications and management of biliary complications after adult liver transplantation: a systematic review of the incidence, risk factors and outcome. Transpl Int. 2011;24(4):379-92.

CHAPTER 114

Complications in Living Donor Liver Transplantation

AS Soin, Punit Singla

INTRODUCTION

In Asia, low deceased donor organ donation rates due to religious, cultural, or political obstacles[1] necessitated the rise of living donor liver transplantation (LDLT). Over the past two decades, adult-to-adult LDLT has negotiated a long learning curve of technical difficulties in addition to the continuing ethical concerns[2] about donor safety, and has moved ahead of deceased donor liver transplantation (DDLT)[3-6] to become the standard of care for cirrhotic patients in this part of the world. The success rate with LDLT is now >90% with acceptable mortality and morbidity in high-volume centers.

Post-transplant care involves monitoring of hemodynamic, clinical, and laboratory parameters; timely detection and management of complications; and balanced immunosuppression to prevent graft rejection and avoid infection. It is generally delivered through a multidisciplinary dedicated team of transplant surgeons, physicians, anesthesiologists, intensivists, nurses, technicians, coordinators, and specialists from many allied specialties.

The surgical challenges in LDLT are different from DDLT and include procurement of an adequate size graft, optimal graft and remnant vascular inflow, outflow, and biliary drainage. The reconstruction is tailored to the respective anatomical variations.[7] Inappropriate technique for any of these can lead to devastating complications in the postoperative period. In addition, distressing medical complications may supervene, including infection, rejection, and disease recurrence, which need timely diagnosis and appropriate management.

Early complications, within first 3 months, are generally related to graft quality, technical problems (vascular and biliary complications), rejection, and infections. Complications during the intermediate period, from 3 to 12 months, are due to opportunistic infections and rejection. The late complications, after 12 months, are related to biliary stricture, long-term drug toxicity, recurrent disease, malignancy, metabolic syndrome, cardiovascular complications, and chronic rejection (CR). Complications result in morbidity and increased costs, and may lead to graft loss and mortality.

In this chapter, we shall be discussing the incidence, presentation, diagnosis, and management of such complications.

VASCULAR COMPLICATIONS

Hepatic Artery Thrombosis

This is the commonest vascular complication, often requiring retransplantation.[9,10] hepatic artery thrombosis (HAT) is seen in children (6–8%)[11,12] more than adults (4%)[13] and more so in LDLT than DDLT. Very low rates (1 %) have been reported from high-volume LDLT centers. Hepatic artery thrombosis is commoner in grafts with multiple arterial anastomoses.[14-18]

The occurrence of HAT in LDLT is influenced by the surgeon's experience,[19] type of graft, number of grafts, and the size and number of hepatic arteries (anatomical variations).[20] Various risk factors for HAT include technical factors like small size artery, young recipient (<10 kg),[21] hepatic artery angulation/kink, intimal flaps, multiple anastomotic attempts, and medical reasons such as over use of blood products, high vasopressor requirement, repeated rejection episodes, nonfunction of graft, ABO incompatibility, and cytomegalovirus (CMV) infection.[22] Incidence of late HAT has been found to be lowered with use of antiplatelet prophylaxis,[23] but some studies have shown increased risk of gastrointestinal bleed with equivocal benefit in prevention of HAT.[24] Some centers claim that arterial anastomosis performed using microsurgical technique has less thrombosis rate than using surgical loupe.[25] Continuous sutures have a higher incidence of HAT than interrupted sutures.[26]

Table 1: Post-liver transplant complications

Early (<3 months)	*Intermediate (3–12 months)*	*Late (>12 months)*
• Vascular complications • Primary graft nonfunction • Infections (bacterial) sepsis • Small-for-size syndrome • Biliary leak • Rejection • Surgical site infections	• Biliary strictures • Hepatic vein stenosis • Rejection • CMV infection • EBV infection, PTLD • Hypertension • Poor growth	• Biliary strictures • Renal dysfunction • Hypertension • NODM • Recurrence (HCV, HBV, HCC) • Malignancies (including PTLD) • Growth failure • Osteopenia • Hernia[8]

CMV, cytomegalovirus; PTLD, posttransplant lymphoproliferative disorder; NODM, new onset diabetes mellitus; HCV, hepatitis C virus; HBV, hepatitis B virus; HCC, hepatocellular carcinoma.

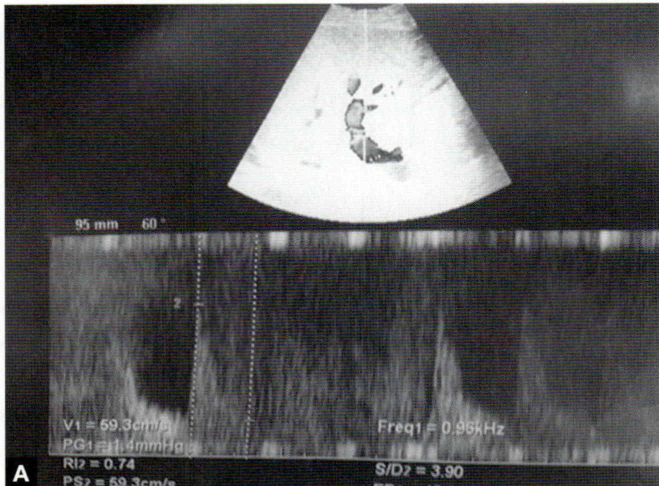

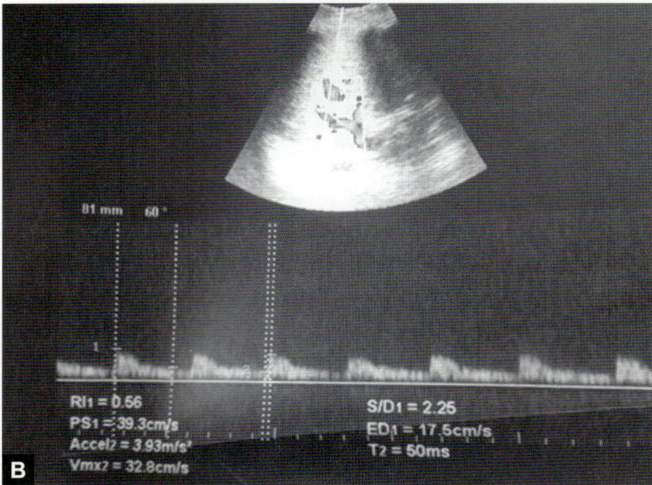

Figure 1 Ultrasound Doppler of hepatic artery. (A) Showing normal waveform pattern; and (B) Decreased hepatic artery velocity

Clinical Presentation and Diagnosis

The clinical presentation of HAT ranges from an asymptomatic patient with minimal deranged liver function to fulminant hepatic failure (Table 1). Hepatic artery thrombosis may be partial or complete. Partial HAT is generally an incidental diagnosis on Doppler ultrasound (DUS).

Complete HAT may present clinically as one of the following ways:

- Mild form/incidental diagnosis: It may present as a dramatic increase in liver enzymes (transaminitis). However, in few cases, it may be incidentally diagnosed on routine DUS even before enzymes or lactate increase. In such a presentation, patients are conscious with minimum/no coagulopathy and encephalopathy.
- Graft failure: Hepatic artery thrombosis may present as severe graft failure in about one-third of cases. These patients have hepatic decompensation in form of hyperbilirubinemia, deranged coagulation profile, encephalopathy, and at times, sepsis due to acute necrosis of the graft.
- Biliary complications may be seen in few patients, where HAT occurs gradually with formation of collaterals, which may prevent necrosis of the graft. Here, the patient may present with transamintis, cholangitis, biliary complications, or rarely sepsis. Usually this type of presentation is late after liver transplantation (LT), may be after few weeks to months.

Doppler ultrasound (Figs 1A and B) is the first line of investigation in patients with suspicion of HAT.[27] Low peak systolic velocity, resistive index <0.5 or >0.8, focal increase in velocity, absent diastolic flow, high systolic acceleration time, and parvus tardus waveform are predictive of HAT.[28] Complete block would be seen as absent flow in hepatic artery. Postoperative routine DUS can detect the HAT in asymptomatic patients but it does not reduce its incidence. It, however, helps in early diagnosis and timely management.[25] Doppler ultrasound can have false positive and false negative findings. Contrast-enhanced ultrasonography (USG) is one of the newer modalities to diagnose HAT; it can be used selectively with reasonable accuracy.[29]

Although selective conventional digital subtraction angiography remains the gold standard investigation for confirmation of diagnosis, computed tomography (CT) angiography (Fig. 2), being

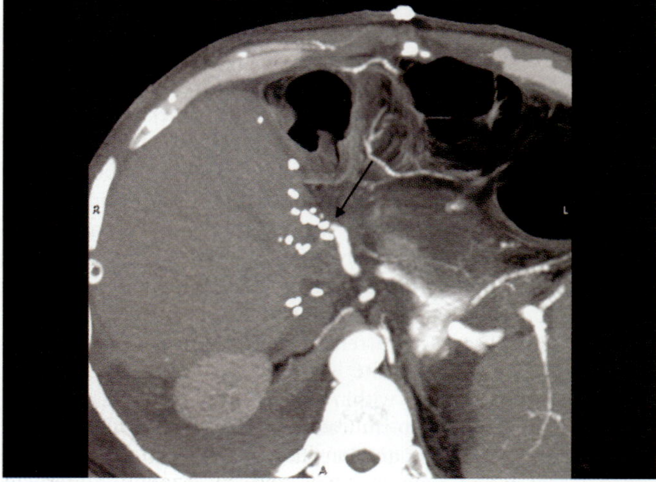

Figure 2 Computed tomography angiography showing no flow in hepatic artery intrahepatically

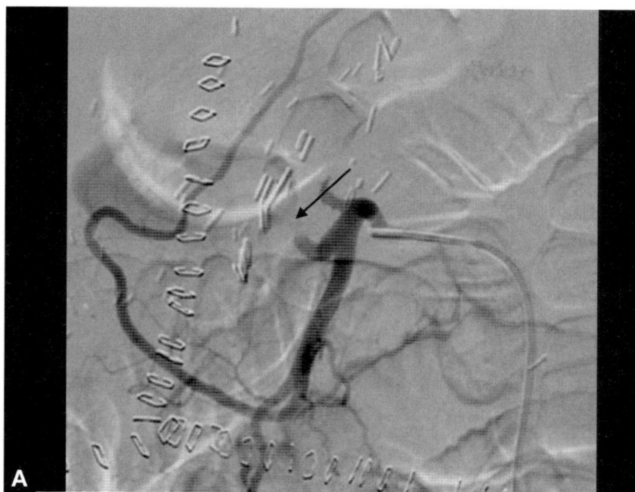

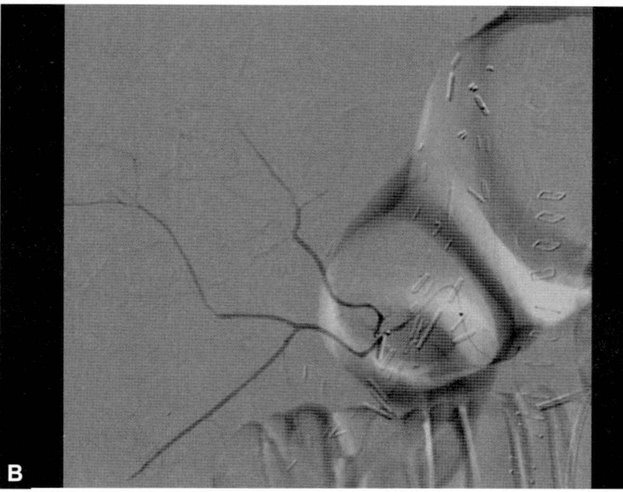

Figure 3 Conventional angiography. (A) Showing hepatic artery thrombosis; and (B) After thrombolysis—completely thrombolysis with good intrahepatic arterial flow

noninvasive, is the next line of investigation after DUS. At present, with faster CT machines and better software, conventional angiography is rarely required just for confirmation of the diagnosis. Digital subtraction angiography (Figs 3A and B) may be preferred over CT angiography in patients with raised creatinine, as less contrast is needed, and in patients who would benefit more with thrombolysis than with surgery.

Treatment

Patients with partial thrombosis, stenosis, spasm, or low flow in the hepatic artery can be treated with low molecular weight heparin (LMWH) and extensive monitoring with frequent DUS.

Treatment of patients with complete HAT depends on the mode of presentation, duration of thrombosis, and day of presentation after LT.[19] Patients with HAT presenting with raised enzymes should undergo surgical revascularization. Complete timely revascularization of the graft is the key to salvage the graft. Generally, in patients with early detection of thrombosis, i.e., within <12 hours of occurrence, the graft may be salvaged.[25] Patients presenting with liver failure need resuscitation, correction of coagulopathy, and urgent retransplantation.

Patients who are at a poor surgical risk, and/or having long duration of thrombosis, can be primarily offered catheter-directed intra-arterial thrombolysis using urokinase/streptokinase and angioplasty by an experienced interventional radiologist.[25,30] Very few cases may require stenting. Both angioplasty and stenting have almost equal success rate with similar complication, patency, and survival rate.[31] Rethrombosis rate is 30%,[30] and 50–70% of successful cases may require another intervention.[32] Acute and intermediate lesions have better response rate than chronic lesions after thrombolysis.[33] If thrombolysis fails, surgical thrombectomy is needed. Retransplantation is indicated if revascularization fails.

Patients presenting with late HAT (2 months after LT) with biliary sepsis can rarely be managed with endobiliary stenting alone, but eventually often require retransplantation due to recurrent sepsis without transplantation.

Role of expectant management in HAT is controversial, but few patients who develop collaterals can be managed with conservative management; however, these patients have high incidence of biliary complications.[34]

Our Protocol for Managing Hepatic Artery Thrombosis

Technique of anastomosis: The most important factor in preventing HAT is appropriate surgical technique. Important points to be kept in mind while doing arterial anastomosis are as follows:

- Appropriate size match, lie, and orientation of arteries
- Avoid intimal injury and flaps on recipient and donor side
- Avoid kinking of vessels
- Gentle handling
- Minimal and judicious use of blood products
- Liberal use of systemic anticoagulation intraoperatively and postoperatively in difficult anastomoses and pediatric patients
- Extension of short stump of artery or two vessels on bench using microscope

We do all anastomoses with 2.5–3.5 × surgical loupes, using Prolene 7-0/8-0 (depending upon size of vessels), inside out, interrupted sutures.

General precautions: The following are the general precautions:

- Routine DUS is performed daily for first week, then biweekly until discharge, and weekly for the first 2 months after LDLT. Doppler ultrasound is performed twice a day for the first week in children <10 kg, difficult arterial anastomosis, multiple anastomoses, and redo anastomosis.
- We prefer to maintain adequate positive fluid balance and tend to keep hemoglobin level around 10 g/dL, and employ venesection if hemoglobin is higher.
- Use blood products judiciously during and after LDLT.
- Use of heparin in children <10 kg and LMWH in small, difficult, or low flow arterial anastomosis, and redo anastomosis.
- Routine use of antiplatelet (low-dose ecosprin) for first 3 months after LDLT.

Patients with partial thrombus are treated with LMWH in form of clexane at doses of 20–40 mg subcutaneously twice a day.

Patients presenting with HAT with raised enzymes require surgical revascularization. We follow the "golden hour" rule to do

DUS, angiography (CT/conventional for confirmation), and shift to operation theatre within an hour of suspicion. During the surgical procedure, we need to look for the condition of the graft, undo the anastomosis, remove the loose thrombus using Fogarty catheter, give thrombolytic agent like urokinase, and ensure graft hepatic artery backflow. Once good inflow is ensured, 5,000 IU of heparin is given and arterial ends are freshened. Anastomosis can be performed with inflow from native hepatic artery (common, right, left), from celiac axis, gastroduodenal artery, splenic artery,[35] or directly from supraceliac aorta using avascular (autologous/homologous, saphenous/venous, or arterial) conduit. We prefer surgical revascularization in cases with HAT occurring within first 10 days after LDLT.

Patients with primary presentation of HAT as liver failure or patients with failure of revascularization are started on supportive medication, broad-spectrum antibiotics. A donor is worked up from the first-degree relatives, and the patient is taken up for retransplantation on an urgent basis.

We prefer to do catheter-directed thrombolysis in the poor surgical candidates, patients with long duration of thrombosis (>6–12 hours), and HAT occurring after 10 days of LT. Availability of an experienced interventional radiologist and appropriate renal function is a must to go ahead with thrombolysis.[33] (Fig. 3B)

We follow our HAT patients closely, especially for long-term biliary complications. We try to manage patients with developing biliary issues (usually stricture or cholangiolar abscess) using endobiliary stenting and drainage of abscess. If the patient requires recurrent admission or frequent stent exchange due to recurrent biliary sepsis, that patient is considered for retransplantation.

We offer expectant management in HAT in highly selected patients. It is offered to those who are discharged from hospital, present after 2–4 weeks post LDLT with no/minimal clinical or biochemical derangement, without any additional biliary complication, infection, or any features of ischemia.[33]

The incidence of HAT in our series is 36/1,482 LDLT (2.4 %).

Portal Vein Thrombosis

Portal vein thrombosis (PVT) is a rare complication with reported incidence of 3–7%[15,36,37] and seen more commonly in children.[15,38] It is generally related to technical issues such as kinking or redundancy of PV, anastomotic stricture, portal vein extension graft, external compression, stenosis,[39] preoperative thrombosis, and rejection.

Preoperatively detected PVT (8% of cirrhotic for LT[40]) once used to be a relative contraindication for LT, is not a contraindication anymore. But, careful intraoperative complete thrombectomy and confirmation of smooth intimal continuity before portal venous anastomosis are a must to decrease postoperative PVT.[41,42] In cases of persistent poor portal flow, inadequate removal of thrombus, or bad intima, revascularization of portal vein using jump graft with inflow from superior mesenteric vein or in some cases from splenic vein can be successful. Complete PVT affects the survival, especially the short term.[43] Postoperatively, drainage of any collection around porta, timely treatment of rejection, and judicious administration of blood products help in preventing PVT.

Clinical Presentation and Management

Early/acute PVT can present as elevated liver enzymes, intestinal congestion, ascites, and variceal hemorrhage. Routine DUS, which is the first investigation[27] of choice, can detect changes in velocity and flow volume in PV, absence of respiratory variation, intraluminal thrombus, and post-stenotic increased velocity or sometimes, poor arterial flow. Computed tomography angiography remains the confirmatory investigation. Surgical thrombectomy, revascularization, correction of technical problem, ligation of large collaterals, and if necessary, reconstruction of portal vein with occasional requirement of bypass grafting from SMV are the mainstays of treatment.[44]

Portal vein thrombosis later than the first week may be amenable to percutaneous transhepatic radiological intervention. PV stenosis is usually diagnosed by DUS by turbulent flow, confirmed by trans-anastomotic PV pressure gradient, and can be treated by PV stenting.[33] Late PVT and portal vein stenosis may not threaten graft survival but can lead to troublesome portal hypertension, variceal hemorrhage,[38] persistent ascites, and splenomegaly. Doppler ultrasound remains the investigation of choice.[27] Computed tomography angiography can show portal vein stenosis and collateral formation (Fig. 4A). Direct repair of portal vein is difficult. Patients with significant varices (gastroesophageal/ectopic) may require transhepatic stent placement,[45] if an experienced interventional radiologist is available. Otherwise, porto-systemic/selective shunt may be required to correct portal hypertension,[38] but preoperatively, adequate liver function should be ensured to prevent encephalopathy.

Our Protocol for Managing Portal Vein Thrombosis

An appropriate technique of anastomosis with appropriate lie, length, orientation of vein, adequate growth factor is the key to avoid portal vein-related problems. Whenever there are two portal veins (Nakamura type C or D[46]) on the graft side (i.e., right anterior and posterior portal vein are separate), we extend the veins using the "Y"-shaped cryopreserved or fresh portal vein from the recipient's explanted liver. Lie and orientation are extremely important in such "Y"-shaped extension grafts. In adults, we use Prolene 6-0/7-0, continuous sutures, and in children 7-0 Prolene posterior wall continuous and anterior wall interrupted sutures with 2.5–3.5× loupes are used. We use anticoagulant in patients with portal vein extension graft and in patients with preoperative PVT.

Our incidence of PVT is <1%.[33] Doppler ultrasound detects portal vein flow velocity and volume across the anastomosis; however, the trend of flow volume is more important than a single value. Computed tomography angiography is used for confirmation. If there is early partial clot, we start the patient on heparin and try to maintain activated partial thromboplastin time ~2.5–3 times the normal and closely monitor for portal vein flow. In case of early complete clot within the first week of transplantation, we prefer to do surgical thrombectomy and reanastomosis. At re-exploration, thrombectomy is performed using a Fogarty catheter; urokinase is used for thrombolysis. Once backflow from the liver and adequate inflow are confirmed, redo anastomosis of portal vein is performed.

Percutaneous transhepatic dilatation and stenting (Figs 4B to 4D) is preferred in patients presenting with portal vein stenosis and PVT after a week of LT with surgery reserved for cases with failed interventional procedure.

Hepatic Venous Outflow Obstruction

Hepatic venous outflow obstruction is a relatively uncommon complication. It can occur because of thrombosis in hyper-

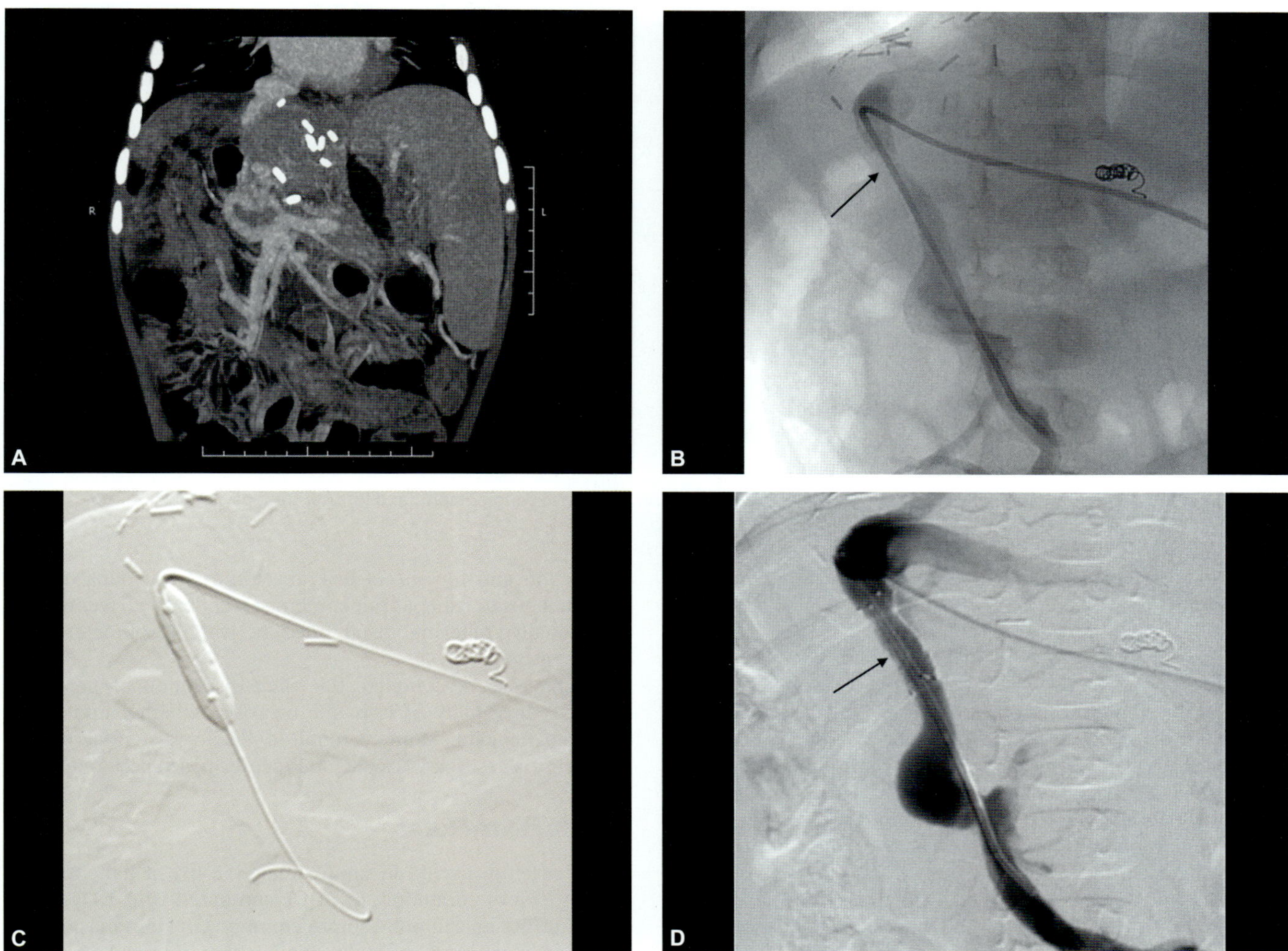

Figures 4A to D (A) CT angiography showing portal vein stenosis, cavernoma formation and preserved SMV–SV junction in left-lobe LDLT; (B) Portal vein stenosis on percutaneous transhepatic angiography; (C) Portal vein stenosis—percutaneous transhepatic portal vein dilatation; (D) Portal vein stenosis—percutaneous transhepatic stent placement. CT, computed tomography; SMV–SV, superior mesenteric vein–splenic vein; LDLT, living donor liver transplantation

coaguable states,[47] twist, or narrowing of HV related to technique. It is common with left compared to right lobe grafts. It can be prevented with a wide anastomosis and use of anticoagulants in patients with hyper-coaguable states.

It can present as deranged liver functions in early posttransplant period, and in severe form can lead to graft rupture,[33] liver surface bleed, which presents as drain bleed, and shock. Such patients need urgent resuscitation and evaluation and high index of suspicion is required to detect the problem. Echogenic contents in the peritoneal cavity on USG abdomen and obvious bleed in the drain help in the diagnosis. Computed tomography scan may not be feasible due to the unstable condition. The patient requires urgent exploration and control of bleeding using various measures like bipolar diathermy and argon laser, but rarely may require perihepatic packing. Operative correction of hepatic venous obstruction is rarely possible except in kinking. Urgent percutaneous/transjugular angioplasty with stent placement[33,48,49] is required after control of bleed. Side-to-side cavocavostomy with an endovascular stapler may be useful for severe hepatic vein and/or inferior vena cava (IVC) outflow obstruction after piggyback implantation.[50]

Late or partial hepatic venous obstruction can present as ascites, gastrointestinal bleed, and sometimes raised enzymes. Doppler ultrasound would show monophasic flow, low velocity, and change of pattern of flow; triphasic CT scan would confirm the diagnosis. Computed tomography is more accurate than DUS for right hepatic vein stenosis after LDLT, with venous pulsatility index as the sole sonographic criterion.[51] Conventional venography can help in diagnosis (Fig. 5A), and pressure gradient across the anastomosis can be measured simultaneously. Operative correction is rarely possible; percutaneous angioplasty with stent placement[52] (Fig. 5B) is the treatment of choice.

BILIARY COMPLICATIONS

Biliary tract complications can occur any time after LT with a duration varying from days to years. Once considered the "Achilles heel" of LDLT, they are the most common technical complications, more often seen with HAT. With technical refinement, their incidence has fallen at high-volume centers.[53] A total of 10–20% of such patients require reoperation. Advances in

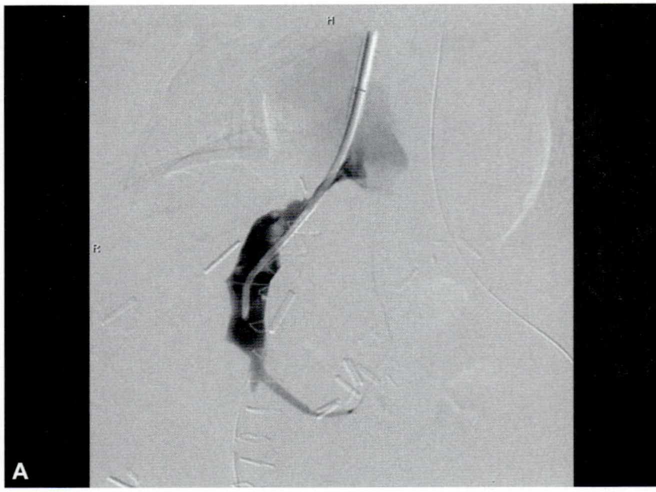

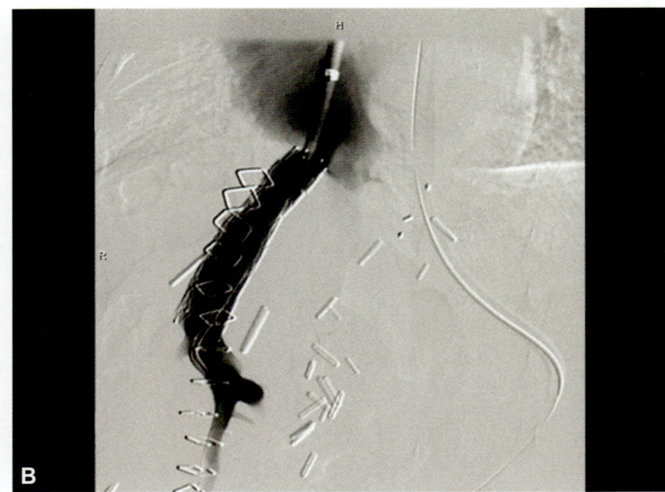

Figures 5A and B Left hepatic vein stenosis. (A) As seen on transjugular angiography; and (B) after stent placement

endoscopic/percutaneous intervention has reduced the need for surgical correction.[54]

Bile Leak

Bile leak can occur from the anastomotic site (most common), cut surface of liver, and from the site of T-tube insertion (uncommon these days). Early bile leak (<4 weeks) is commonly anastomotic or from the cut surface in partial grafts,[55-57] whereas late leak may occur after T-tube removal.[58] Early anastomotic leaks are generally due to poor vascularity and tension at the anastomotic site, or ischemic necrosis due to HAT.

Although LDLT was associated with higher bile leak in the past,[54] currently, with improved techniques and experience, incidence is as low as 5–10%, which is comparable to DDLT.[15,53,55] Bile leak incidence is unrelated to type of biliary anastomosis, i.e., duct-to-duct or Roux-en-Y hepaticojejunostomy.[59,60] However, it is related to the number of anastomosis required with least bile leak incidence in patients with single duct-to-duct anastomosis and higher with double or triple duct anastomoses.[61]

Clinical Presentation and Management

The patient may present with obvious biliary fluid in the drain, abdominal distention/collection, vomiting, abdominal/shoulder pain, fever, raised leukocyte counts, or deranged liver function tests (LFTs).

Ultrasonography of the abdomen, CT scan, or magnetic resonance cholangiopancreatography (MRCP) will detect intra-abdominal collection. Diagnosis of site of leak can be confirmed by cholangiography [through choledochal tube, if placed; MRCP or endoscopic retrograde cholangiopancreatography (ERCP)].

Any intra-abdominal collection should be treated with percutaneous drain placement and appropriate antibiotics. A small leak from the anastomosis or cut surface gradually stops spontaneously, but (unlike in the non-transplant situation), bigger leaks may not close or convert to a stricture owing to the antifibrotic effects of steroids. This is especially so if there is a distal obstruction. In such a situation, a stent may be placed across the obstruction and the site of leak/anastomosis by endoscopic or percutaneous transhepatic or combined (rendezvous) techniques. Occasionally, relieving distal pressure with a sphincterotomy alone may help.[62]

In the case of complete bile duct disruption or persistent bile leak, possibility of ischemic necrosis is higher and Roux-en-Y hepaticojejunostomy is required. Placing a stent across the anastomosis at surgery is a personal/center-based preference.

Bile Duct Strictures

Biliary stricture occurs in approximately 5–9% of patients after LT,[53,55,60] more commonly in LDLT compared with DDLT, and can be at the anastomotic (more common) or non-anastomotic sites. Technical error, multiple, small caliber, thin-walled, poorly vascularized hepatic ducts are the possible causative factors, but previous bile leak and HAT increase the chances of biliary stricture. Other factors associated with development of biliary stricture include acute cellular rejection (ACR), prolonged cold ischemia time,[60] stent use, CR, and CMV infection. Non-anastomotic strictures may occur early (within a year of LT) or late. Early onset strictures are associated with advanced donor age, high model for end-stage liver disease (MELD) score, arterial ischemia, and ABO incompatibility, while the late ones arise in bilio-enteric anastomoses and in patients with recurrent primary sclerosing cholangitis (PSC).[63]

Clinical Presentation and Management

Biliary strictures can present any time after transplantation, usually within weeks to months, but may occur after years. Anastomotic site stricture usually develops within first year of transplant. Patients may present with fever, persistent pruritus, or occasionally with severe cholangitis and sepsis, and deranged liver function (obstructive pattern) with elevated alkaline phosphatase, glutamyl transferase, with or without elevated bilirubin or transaminase levels. Associated undrained bile leak can lead to increased leukocyte counts, peritonitis, sepsis, and ileus. Abdominal USG, MRCP may be required to confirm the diagnosis, site, extent, and severity.[64]

Endoscopic retrograde cholangiopancreatography is the best modality to manage anastomotic strictures, since it confirms the diagnosis and a stent can be placed[65] at the same time. However, it is less efficacious in treating ischemic strictures.[66] Complete resolution and remodeling of anastomotic strictures is possible in 65% of cases, and it does not have a higher complication rate in LT patients.[67,68] Few patients may require percutaneous transhepatic biliary drainage (PTBD). The PTBD drain is initially external, which is internalized later on.[69] Surgical correction is required in a few cases with better results in early surgery (<6 months from diagnosis) and in younger grafts.[70] Few studies have shown a beneficial role of fully covered self-expanding metallic stents in cases with failed standard endoscopic treatment before offering them surgery.[71]

In cases with diffuse intrahepatic strictures, although an extrahepatic dominant stricture can be managed by stenting, a retransplant may eventually be required. After stenting, long-term surveillance and periodic stent exchange are required until stricture remodeling, after which they can be removed.[65]

Our Protocol for Managing Biliary Complications

Biliary complications can be prevented by good anastomotic technique, which is based on the following principles:

- Tension free anastomosis
- Appropriate orientation of hepatic ducts while anastomosis
- Adequate vascularity of the hepatic duct (recipient side)
- Well-vascularized hepatic duct with a sheath of supporting tissue and hilar plate and Glissonian sheath (HPGS) in the donor[53]

We preferably do a duct-to-duct anastomosis using 5-0 or 6-0 polydioxanone sutures, taking preplaced anterior layer, and all interrupted sutures.[53] Use of single or more anastomosis, cystic duct, or Roux loop depends upon number, distance, and lie of the graft ducts. We do not use T-tube but internal stent is used in selected cases with very small duct or with ampullary stenosis. Roux loop hepaticojejunostomy is used in patients with PSC or those within adequate length or doubtful vascularity of biliary duct.

Using "HPGS" technique, our biliary complication rate has decreased from 15.8 to 5.3%.[53]

Bile Leak and Management

In the first week posttransplant, drain bilirubin higher than serum bilirubin should raise a suspicion of bile leak. Clinical and biochemical findings supported by imaging help in the diagnosis. Ultrasonography or preferably plain CT scan is performed to detect intra-abdominal collection.

Conservative management with adequate drainage (from intraoperatively placed drain or percutaneous drain) of the collection is enough in cases with minor anastomotic or cut surface leak with no sepsis, and with normal LFTs. In patients with early large-volume leak, during the first 10 days, we prefer surgical intervention over ERCP before sepsis supervenes. Biliary leak detected in the first 10–30 days is difficult to manage surgically due to inflammatory adhesions intraperitoneally, and hence we prefer to perform ERCP and stenting, for which an experienced interventional gastroenterologist is the key. This endobiliary stent needs to be changed every 3–4 months till the leak site is adequately healed.

In cases with frank biliary peritonitis, undrained or undrainable collections, more than half the circumference disruption or failure of interventional procedures, operation in the form of peritoneal toilet is required with revision of biliary anastomosis or Roux-en-Y hepaticojejunostomy depending upon vascularity of the hepatic ducts.

Biliary Stricture and Management

Patients with obstructive pattern of LFTs undergo USG abdomen and MRCP (Figs 6A to C). Endoscopic retrograde cholangiopancreatography and stent placement are the preferred treatment modalities (Figs 7A to C), and ERCP is difficult but can still be tried in patients with Roux-en-Y hepaticojejunostomy by experienced gastroenterologists.[68] Few patients may require PTBD alone or combined (rendezvous)[69] with ERCP in patients with ERCP failure, and as a primary modality in cases with Roux-en-Y anastomosis. In "rendezvous" technique, PTBD is performed and a catheter is placed across the stricture, which acts as a guide for internal stenting during ERCP. Percutaneous transhepatic biliary drainage placement and placement of guide wire across is itself a challenging procedure (Figs 8A to C) and requires an experienced interventional radiologist. Stent is exchanged 3 monthly or until the stricture is remodeled. The patients with failed attempts at interventional techniques need elective surgical management and biliary "redo." wherein the original anastomosis is taken down and a Roux-en-Y hepaticojejunostomy or "redo" Roux anastomosis is performed.

PRIMARY NONFUNCTION OF GRAFT

There is no uniform definition of primary graft nonfunction but various definitions include progressively increasing transaminases, coagulopathy/worsening of prothrombin time, hepatic coma, increased bilirubin, lactate acidosis, and/or hemodynamic instability.[72]

The incidence of primary nonfunction (PNF) is 4.6–9% in DDLT,[73] and 0.3% in LDLT.[74-76] It is one of the most common reasons for retransplantation. Various donor risk factors, such as advanced age, moderate to severe steatosis, high serum sodium, hemodynamic instability, prolonged intensive care unit (ICU) stay, delay in procurement, and prolonged cold ischemia time,[77] have been implicated as causative factors.[78-80] Recipients with renal failure, high MELD score, and cases of retransplantation have higher incidence of PNF. The pathogenesis for graft dysfunction is generally linked to ischemia/reperfusion injury, damage from reactive oxygen species, and sinusoidal endothelial cell damage.

Postoperative trends in the prothrombin time, hepatic encephalopathy, metabolic acidosis, lactate level trend, and urine output have been reliable predictors of graft function and outcome. Such patients are prone to renal dysfunction or infection, which can adversely affect the patient outcome. Serum cytokine levels, lower preoperative interlukin (IL)-6 and higher IL-2R levels, can predict occurrence of graft dysfunction perioperatively.[81] Transjugular biopsy of the liver may reveal massive zonal necrosis, inflammatory infiltrate, and ballooning hepatocytes.

Various treatment modalities involve use of antioxidants, N-acetylcysteine (NAC), a glutathione precursor, vasoactive mediators [AT II, TXA2, nitric oxide, prostaglandins like prostaglandin E1 (PGE1) and prostacyclin], anti-inflammatory

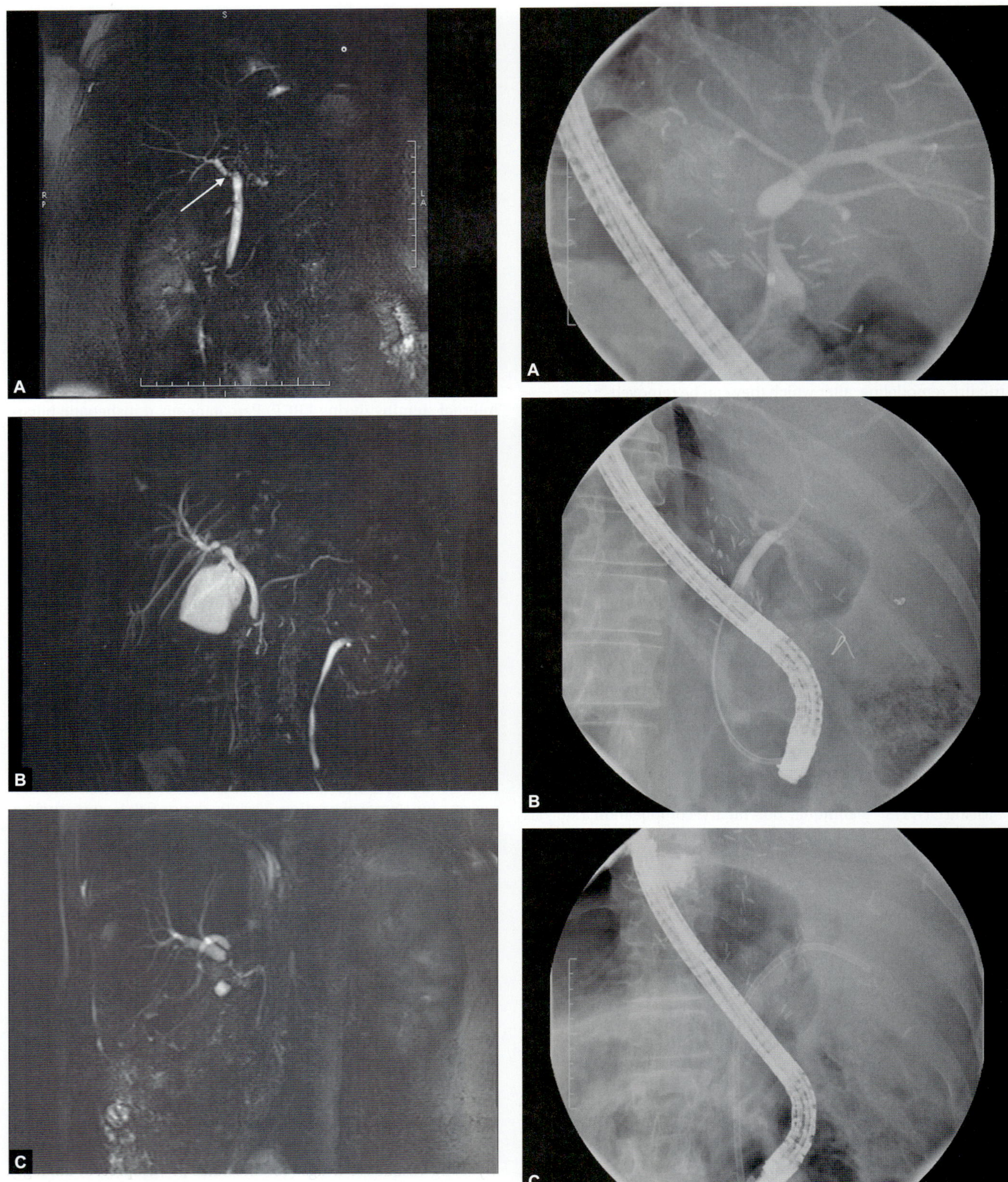

Figures 6A to C (A) MRCP showing biliary stricture in right-lobe LDLT; (B) MRCP showing biliary stricture and bilioma in right-lobe LDLT; (C) MRCP showing two separated ducts with biliary strictures. MRCP, magnetic resonance cholangiopancreatography; LDLT, living donor liver transplantation

Figures 7A to C (A) ERCP showing long biliary stricture; (B) Balloon dilatation during ERCP; (C) Biliary stent placement across the stricture. ERCP, endoscopic retrograde cholangiopancreatography

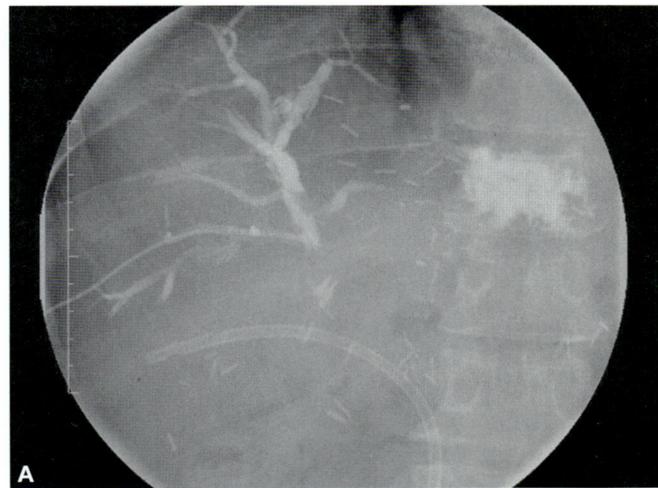

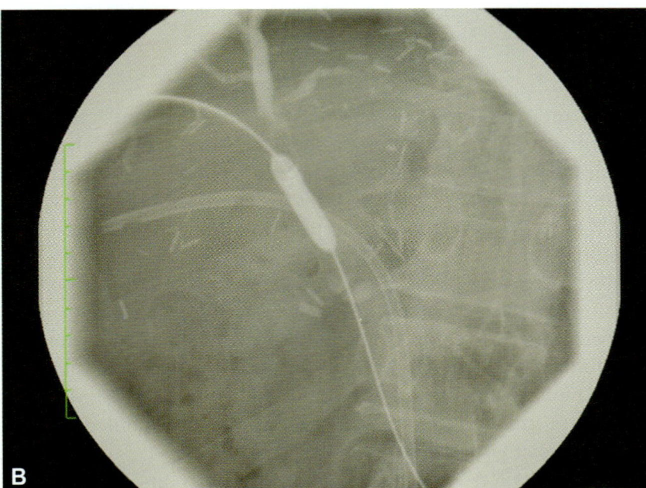

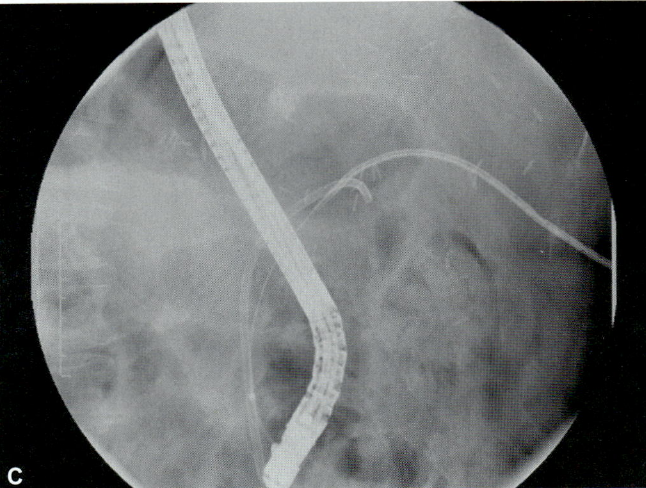

Figures 8A to C (A) Percutaneous transhepatic cholangiogram—showing undrained segment after ERCP; (B) Percutaneous transhepatic biliary dilatation and wire placement; (C) Post-ERCP stenting of one sector, another sector stented using "rendezvous" technique catheter placed by PTBD and stenting by ERCP. ERCP, endoscopic retrograde cholangiopancreatography; PTBD, percutaneous transhepatic biliary drainage

drugs, antiapoptotic strategies (mitochondrial permeability transition inhibitors, anti-Fas or anti-Fas ligand antibodies, antiapoptotic proteins, caspase inhibitors), pharmacological preconditioning, and plasmapharesis. Apart from those discussed below, the remaining are rarely employed, as the data supporting their use are scarce.

Three modalities are often used, with limited evidence of efficacy. First, NAC, a glutathione precursor, which acts by replenishing endogenous glutathione, has been found to improve hemodynamics and oxygen transport, is claimed to decrease ischemia/reperfusion injury, results in lower peak transaminases, improves liver synthetic function, and lowers the incidence of PNF.[82] However, the benefit is not supported by robust data.[83] Second, PGE1 and prostacyclin (PGI2) may be beneficial in resolving or preventing graft dysfunction by vasodilation of small vessels,[84] inhibition of platelet aggregation, and increase in splanchnic flow. Third, plasmapharesis may help by removing preformed antibodies.[85]

Patients need supportive management with broad-spectrum antibiotics, adequate perfusion to maintain renal function, and correction of coagulopathy.

Until more is known about the causes and treatment of PNF, prevention by avoidance of predisposing donor factors and retransplantation of established PNF[73] remain the mainstay of management.

SMALL-FOR-SIZE SYNDROME

"Small-for-size syndrome" (SFSS) is a multifactorial pathophysiological entity seen in partial grafts, which was originally described in patients who received grafts with inadequate hepatocyte mass or functional volume for their metabolic needs. Reported incidence in LDLT varies from 2.9 to 12.5%.[86]

Causes of SFSS, including a small graft size, i.e., graft-to-recipient body weight ratio (GRWR) <0.8 or standard liver volume (SLV) <35%,[87] poor graft quality (moderate steatosis, fibrosis), portal hyperperfusion (leading to sinusoidal congestion, hemorrhagic necrosis of perisinusoidal hepatocytes[88] due to relative hypoxia because of HA buffer response[89], outflow obstruction leading to selective reversal of portal flow in some segments and consequent hyperperfusion injury in remaining segments, are better understood. The following are the four most important factors that play a role in SFSS: the recipient status, the portal pressure and inflow, the venous outflow, and the functional graft volume (determined by the GRWR and graft quality).[90,91]

Small-for-size syndrome currently lacks a consensus definition, but is generally characterized by synthetic dysfunction, coagulopathy, and prolonged cholestasis with or without ascites. Diagnosis of "SFSS" is established after exclusion of graft rejection and vascular, biliary, or primary septic complications.

Strategies to prevent or treat SFSS include prevention of portal hyperperfusion, either by surgically reducing portal flow by splenectomy, splenic artery ligation, splenic artery embolization, or hemiportocaval shunt (aiming to maintain portal flow <400 mL/100 g of graft or portal pressure <20 mm Hg[15,92,93]), or pharmacologically by using vasoactive drugs (somatostatin or vasopressin analogs). We routinely drain the anterior sector either by keeping middle hepatic vein on the graft side or dissecting out the segment V and VIII outflow drainage separately and extending them using cryopreserved or recanalised umbilical veins. With an adequately drained anterior sector, the chances of congestion of posterior sector and thus possibility of functional SFSS decrease.[94-97]

After SFSS is established, a patient needs supportive management with broad-spectrum antibiotics, adequate fluid and electrolyte balance, and correction of coagulopathy. Synthetic function can improve in 3–4 days but cholestasis may take a few weeks to settle. The worsening of acidosis, encephalopathy, and synthetic function beyond 2–3 days decreases the chances of recovery and may necessitate retransplantation. Somatostatin reduces portal vein pressure and downregulates intrahepatic endothelin 1, which reduces formation of microthrombi in liver and improves intrahepatic microcirculation. Role of PGE1 is not clearly defined in SFSS. Various other agents such as endothelin receptor A antagonist, PGE1, thromboxane A_2 synthetase inhibitor, and Pentoxifylline have been tried with variable success rates.[98]

While low graft volume is believed to be the main cause, grafts with GRWR of <0.7 with inflow modulation have been shown to function well in some studies. Few studies have shown successful transplantation in adults with left lobe with modified techniques.[99] Auxiliary partial orthotopic liver transplantation and dual lobe transplantation[100] have also been used to provide adequate volume to the recipients.

ALLOGRAFT REJECTION

Graft rejection results from cell-mediated and humoral immune responses against the donor human leukocyte antigens (HLA) expressed on graft hepatocytes. Liver tends to be relatively resilient to rejection, especially antibody mediated, compared with other organs.[101] This is probably due to the large size of the allograft, minimal class I HLA expression on hepatocytes, production of soluble major histocompatibility complex I molecules, or transfer of passenger donor cells with the graft to the recipient that help in establishing tolerogenic microchimerism.[102] Thus, the need for pharmacological immunosuppression in LT is less compared with other organs. Despite being immunologically privileged, liver grafts may develop acute orCR.

Acute Cellular Rejection

It is histologically characterized by inflammatory infiltrate in the portal triad, predominantly lymphocytes but often mixed infiltrate, that disrupts the biliary epithelium and vascular endothelium (endothelitis) (Fig. 9).[103-106]

Acute cellular rejection occurs in 30–80% of liver grafts, more commonly in children, and can develop anytime after transplantation, with most episodes occurring within the first 3 months.[104] Late ACR (>3 months after LT[107]) is generally seen with low immunosuppression levels,[108] more common in young, females, and patients with autoimmune hepatitis (AIH), primary biliary cirrhosis (PBC), and PSC,[109] and is associated with long-term complications.[110,111] It is becoming increasingly uncommon with the current tacrolimus-based immunosuppression regimens. Late ACR may have atypical histological changes with centrilobular necrosis.

Acute cellular rejection episodes are generally mild, may not cause clinically significant symptoms or histological architectural sequelae and their risk decreases with time. A total of 20% can have a second episode, and fewer still, a third, but generally ACR does not adversely affect graft or patient survival. With current immunosuppression protocols, graft loss secondary to rejection is uncommon.

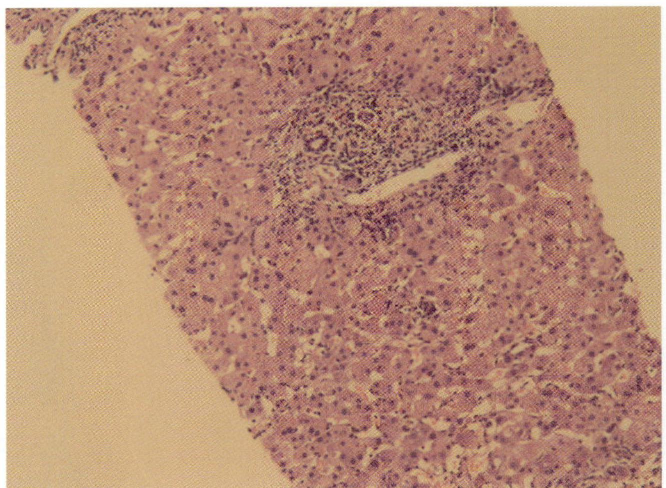

Figure 9 Histopathology showing acute cellular rejection (score 7) showing mixed cellular infiltrates

It is more common in the young, black patients, females, recipients of grafts from elderly donors, patients with fulminant hepatic failure or autoimmune disease, longer cold ischemia times, and in patients with mild liver disease. The most common cause of ACR is inadequate immunosuppression due to lower doses and inadequate absorption or poor compliance.

Most patients are clinically asymptomatic, but sometimes present with nonspecific fever, malaise, fatigue, raised transaminases; none are specific for rejection and patients need histological confirmation. Liver function tests often show raised transaminases and bilirubin levels. Fine-needle aspiration, biliary aspirates, and cytokines profiling or granzyme expression have not been validated and do not have sensitivity or specificity similar to biopsy.

Diagnosis of ACR is based on liver biopsy and histological examination, with no correlation between the serum values and histological abnormalities. The Banff international consensus document criteria for diagnosis are based on grading the severity of portal inflammation, bile duct (cholangiolitis), and venous endothelial injury (endotheliatis).[105] Each category is scored from 0 to 3 and the total score varies from 0 to 9.

Severity of rejection is graded as follows:

- 0–2: no rejection
- 3: borderline
- 4–5: mild rejection
- 6–7: moderate rejection
- 8–9: severe rejection

Once biopsy confirmation of ACR is obtained, high-dose bolus steroid is the initial treatment of choice, which is successful in most of the cases. There is no consensus for optimal dosage, or length of treatment with steroids. However, generally, intravenous methylprednisolone (MP) at 500–1,000 mg daily for 3 days and a rapid taper with increase of the maintenance immunosuppression (tacrolimus, cyclosporine, and mycophenolate) is used to treat ACR. If LFTs do not improve after steroids, a repeat biopsy may be required with another steroid course, if it reveals rejection. If LFTs still do not improve, it is taken as steroid-resistant ACR that may require treatment with thymoglobulin, antilymphocytic antibodies, and other newer agents.

Treatment for late ACR is essentially same as that for ACR.

Our Protocol for Managing Acute Cellular Rejection

We use triple immunosuppression comprising steroid, mycophenolate, and tacrolimus. During the anhepatic phase, intravenous MP at 10 mg/kg is administered, continued postoperatively at 1 mg/kg, and gradually tapered. Tacrolimus/cyclosporine (when tacrolimus is not tolerated) trough levels are monitored on alternate days with a target trough level of 8–12 ng/mL for tacrolimus during the first month and 5–8 ng/mL thereafter, and C0 200–250 ng/mL, C2 800–1,000 in the first month, C0 100–200 ng/mL, C2 800–1,000 up to 3 months, and C0 100–150 ng/mL, C2 600–800 thereafter for cyclosporine.

Steroids are generally withdrawn at 3 months except in patients with hepatitis C virus (HCV) and autoimmune disease. Mycophenolate is withdrawn at 18–24 months and tacrolimus is continued lifelong. However, immunosuppression is individualized for every patient, and tacrolimus and mycophenolate are given/tapered according to renal function, liver function, and complete blood counts. Steroids are continued in small doses for lifelong in patients with autoimmune liver disease, and slowly tapered over 9–12 months in HCV patients. In patients with hepatocellular carcinoma (HCC), we switch over from tacrolimus to sirolimus at 2–3 months.

Acute cellular rejection generally presents as raised liver enzymes, for which infection, vascular, and biliary complications must be ruled out requiring DUS/plain CT scan and MRCP. Percutaneous liver biopsy is performed after correction of coagulation profile, and in selected cases with small vessels and low platelet counts, where adequate coagulation correction may not be possible; a transjugular liver biopsy is performed. We prefer to give high-dose steroids only for biopsy-proven rejection; if biopsy is not possible, then smaller steroid boluses are empirically given and the response is monitored.

In patients with unexplained mildly elevated liver enzymes, maintenance immunosuppression should be increased/optimized. In patients with biopsy-proven rejection with significant increase in enzymes, steroid boluses are given. In adults >40 kg, steroid pulse therapy is given as MP 500 mg intravenous daily for 3 days, and then tapered. In children or adults <40 kg, steroid pulse is given as MP 10–20 mg/kg intravenous daily for 3 days and then tapered. Steroid-resistant ACR is treated with thymoglobulin at dosage of 1.5 mg/kg daily for 7–10 days.

Chronic Rejection

It is also a histological diagnosis characterized by loss of bile ducts (ductopenia) in more than 50% of portal tracts on evaluation of >20 portal tracts (Fig. 10), sometimes along with portal fibrosis, centrilobular degeneration, arteriopathy, and venulitis. Over the years, its incidence has fallen from 5–10% in the 1990s to 3–5% in the present era. It may occur after multiple episodes of refractory acute rejection, or de novo usually due to poor compliance. It generally occurs 2 months or more after transplantation. Although CR can be preceded by episodes of ACR, ACR is not necessarily a risk factor for CR. Patients with autoimmune liver disease and those undergoing retransplantation for CR are predisposed to CR. Low calcineurin inhibitor (CNI) levels early posttransplant may be a risk factor for CR.[110] Chronic rejection more often leads to graft failure and has worse prognosis than ACR. After the introduction of tacrolimus, the incidence of CR has decreased.[111] Retransplantation remains the only effective treatment of CR.

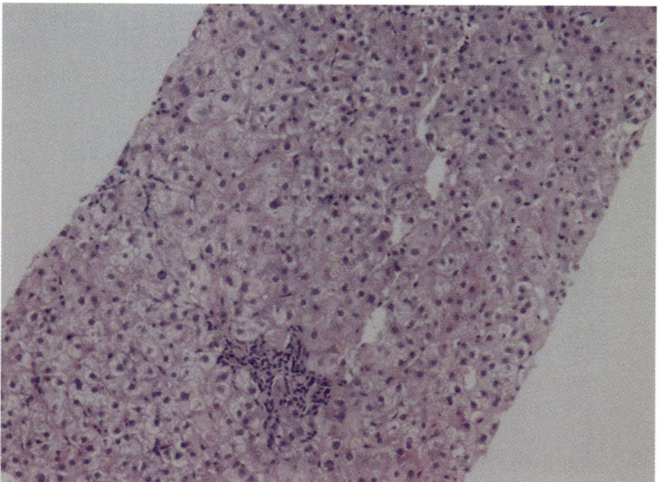

Figure 10 Histopathology showing chronic rejection showing ductopenia

RENAL DYSFUNCTION

Renal dysfunction remains one of the major causes of morbidity and mortality in cirrhotic patients, both before and after LT. Post-transplant survival directly correlates with pretransplant renal function. Hepatorenal syndrome is a major reason for renal dysfunction in cirrhotic patients, which can be temporarily managed with appropriate treatment and should theoretically reverse after LT. Accompanying intrinsic renal disease may require combined liver and kidney transplantation depending on severity of renal failure.

Although postoperative renal dysfunction can occur in any patient after LT, it is more common in patients with preoperative renal dysfunction. The various risk factors include fluid imbalance leading to prerenal type of renal failure, native renal disease, liver graft failure, infection, or drug-induced renal toxicity. Prerenal azotemia due to hypovolemia and hypotension is the most common cause of early renal dysfunction (occurring within the first month) after transplant in patients with normal preoperative renal function and with good graft function. Calcineurin inhibitor-induced renal dysfunction is another common factor, although it is generally seen later.

Mild renal dysfunction is usually associated with oliguria and transient increase in serum creatinine. When severe, it presents as renal failure with anuria requiring dialysis. Postoperative renal dysfunction may lead to requirement of dialysis, prolonged ICU stay, chest-related complications, and increased mortality. In cases with pretransplant renal dysfunction, most liver transplant teams omit the early use of CNIs and use induction agents instead.[112]

Our Protocol for Managing Renal Dysfunction

Renal dysfunction in cirrhotics is defined as serum creatinine >1.5, need for hemodialysis, or creatinine clearance <40 mL/min. Patients having severe renal dysfunction, requiring hemodialysis for more than 6 weeks, or creatinine clearance <30 mL/min are considered for combined liver and kidney transplant with each organ from two different donors.

Patients who do not require combined liver kidney transplant undergo liver transplant alone with "renal protocol"[112] which consists of the following:

- Preoperatively
  - Optimization of the patient: transplant at best renal function (wait till creatinine reaches its nadir, with adequate urine output and not on dialysis)
  - Judicious use of nephrotoxic drugs, including diuretics
  - Optimize fluid and electrolyte balance
- Intraoperatively
  - Proactive intraoperative hemodynamic monitoring and management to avoid hypotension
  - Dialysis machine on standby
  - Side rather than total cross-clamping of IVC to maintain adequate venous return
- Postoperatively
  - Induction with IL-2 receptor antibody
  - Delayed introduction of CNI

All patients with some form of renal dysfunction should be informed about possibility of renal dysfunction postoperatively, requiring more ICU stay, requirement of dialysis, higher incidence of sepsis, and prolonged ventilator requirement.

INFECTION

Infectious complications are seen in up to two thirds of the patients and are the commonest cause of mortality. As immunosuppression may mask common signs of infection, promote rapid progression, and predispose to atypical infections, close surveillance, meticulous evaluation, and aggressive treatment is a must. Bacterial infections are the most common, accounting for nearly 50–60% of infections, 20–40% are viral, 5–15% are fungal, and less than 10% are protozoal. Patients routinely receive prophylactic antibiotics and antifungals, whereas prophylactic antiviral medications are reserved for high-risk patients. Viral infections caused due to human immunodeficiency virus, CMV, hepatitis B virus (HBV), HCV and herpes simplex virus, and various bacterial and atypical organisms can be transmitted with the donor allograft.

Children should receive age-appropriate immunization before transplant as live vaccines are contraindicated after LT.

Various risk factors predisposing to posttransplant/nosocomial infections are as follows:

- Preoperative: underlying medical comorbidity, malnutrition, donor and recipient viral infection status, diabetes, renal failure, ventilation requirement and indwelling catheter, fulminant hepatic failure, high MELD score, and extended use of systemic antibiotics
- Intraoperative: prolonged surgery, prolonged ischemia time, massive blood loss/blood transfusions, and bowel injury
- Postoperative: immunosuppression, indwelling vascular or bladder catheters, prolonged ventilation, re-exploration, vascular complications, poor graft function, biliary obstruction, retransplantation, prolonged antibiotic administration, and renal failure

Early Infections (<1 Month)

Bacterial infections may occur in about 30–60% of patients, mostly in the first 3 months after transplantation.[113,114] Liver transplant recipients are prophylactically covered by antibiotics for Gram-positive, Gram-negative, and anaerobic microorganisms. Common bacterial pathogens include Gram-negative organisms found in the bile and bowel (*Escherichia coli, Enterobacter* species, *Pseudomonas* species, and *Klebsiella*) and Gram-positive organisms (*Staphylococcus aureus,* coagulase-negative staphylococci, and group D streptococci). These microorganisms require antibiotics as per sensitivity.

The cornerstone of treatment for serious infections is temporary reduction or cessation of immunosuppression, along with appropriate antimicrobial therapy and correction of any underlying predisposing factor. Infections associated with operative complications, i.e., bile leak, obstruction, or vascular thrombosis may require radiological intervention or surgical correction in addition to pharmacotherapy. Antibiotics must be changed from empirical to sensitivity-specific and stopped after adequate therapy to avoid super-added infections.

Intermediate Infections (1–6 Months)

While CMV infection is asymptomatic in the general population, it can cause significant morbidity and rarely, mortality in immunosuppressed recipients. It usually occurs after 3–4 weeks of LT. Cytomegalovirus infection may be seen in up to 45% of the post-LT patients, but remains asymptomatic in the majority, manifesting as disease in only 25% of them.[115] The commonest risk factor is a CMV seronegative recipient receiving a graft from a seropositive donor. Patient can present with fever, malaise, hepatitis, bone marrow suppression (leukopenia, thrombocytopenia), chest infection, gastrointestinal bleeding/ulcers, gastroenteritis, and retinitis. Infection to disease conversion rate, severity of disease, graft loss, and mortality are higher in late CMV infection.[115] Antiviral prophylaxis or preemptive therapy[116] is widely used in high-risk patients without any additional risk of opportunistic infections, HCV recurrence, or mortality[117]; both oral and intravenous ganciclovir are effective. Ganciclovir is safe and effective both for prophylaxis and treatment of CMV. Initial intravenous ganciclovir is required in patients with manifested disease or high CMV titers along with reduction of immunosuppression, after which it can be switched to oral medication. Foscarnet is nephrotoxic but can be a useful alternative in cases of ganciclovir resistance. Prolonged subclinical and chronic CMV infection is associated with cholestatic hepatitis, an increased risk of CR, and occasionally, graft failure.[118] Disadvantages of prophylactic treatment are prolonged drug exposure, development of resistance, and development of late-onset CMV disease, and that of preemptive strategy is the need for more frequent laboratory monitoring.[119]

Our Protocol for Cytomegalovirus

Posttransplant prophylaxis is given to seronegative recipients receiving grafts from seropositive donors. Patients undergo quantitative CMV DNA as indicated clinically usually after the first week of transplant, and intravenous ganciclovir is given for CMV DNA >1,000 copies, which is converted to oral valganciclovir after 2 weeks and continued for 6 weeks or until two serial CMV DNA reports are negative, whichever is later. Patients with tissue-invasive CMV disease (detected on tissue biopsy, e.g., gastrointestinal biopsy) are continued on antivirals for 3 months.

Herpes simplex infection: It is usually immunosuppression-induced reactivation of the disease, seen in a few patients after LT. It commonly manifests as mild mucocutaneous, oral or genital disease, and occasionally as hepatitis (diagnosis based on biopsy and DNA positivity). Early diagnosis and treatment are important as it can progress as a systemic disease and can affect the graft as well. It responds well to acyclovir treatment—topical and/or systemic for cutaneous disease and systemic for invasive disease. Reactivation of varicella zoster viral infection (herpes zoster) causes painful blisters in unilateral dermatomal distribution, and responds well to topical and systemic valcyclovir, especially when instituted early.

Epstein-Barr virus: Infection related to this virus is characterized by a mononucleosis-like syndrome. It plays a key role in the pathogenesis of posttransplant lymphoproliferative disorder (PTLD) because of unrestricted proliferation of B cells. This disorder is discussed later in this chapter.

Pneumocystis carinii pneumonia: It is now an uncommon infection because of routine cotrimoxazole (trimethoprim/sulfamethoxazole) prophylaxis.[120,121] We use prophylaxis for 3 months after LT.

Incidence of opportunistic infections with atypical organisms such as *Aspergillus, Nocardia, Listeria, Cryptococcus, Mycobacterium tuberculosis,* respiratory syncytial virus, human herpes virus 6, influenza, and adenovirus infections may be increasing due to universal prophylaxis.

Fungal infections: They are less common but may have serious consequences. Among them candidiasis is the commonest. Disseminated fungal infection has high morbidity and mortality. Culture or histology is required to confirm the diagnosis. Prophylaxis with topical clotrimazole is effective in reducing mucosal infections such as oral candidiasis, esophagitis, or vaginitis, although systemic antifungal prophylaxis with oral fluconazole is commonly used. The role of amphotericin B lipid complex prophylaxis against invasive candida infection is controversial, but a recent study has shown significantly lower infection rate with no extra risk of renal toxicity.[122] Aspergillus is the second most common type of fungal infection. It is acquired by inhalation, affects the lungs, and occasionally the central nervous system. Mucormycosis affecting the cerebrofacial region has almost 100% mortality. We routinely use systemic antifungal medications for the first 2–3 weeks.

Mycobacterial infections: They are commonly seen in patients with preoperative or previously treated mycobacterial infection. Pulmonary disease is the commonest primary/latent/treated site and remains the most common site of posttransplant tuberculosis. We use antitubercular (ATT) medications based on preoperative status of tubercular infection, and graft function postoperatively. Patients with poor graft function postoperatively are given "liver-friendly" ATT drugs, i.e., ethambutol and second-line medications such as levofloxacin, ofloxacin, linezolid, and amikacin; isoniazid is given in patients with good graft function. Patients with a history of previously treated tubercular infection are given prophylactic isoniazid.[123] Prospective recipients with active/inadequately treated tuberculosis are given modified ATT for 4–8 weeks preoperatively, and 9 months posttransplant.[124]

Late Infections (>6 Months)

Community-acquired and opportunistic infections are seen more commonly once prophylaxis is discontinued; patients recover from surgery and go back to the community. Pneumonia, urinary infection, legionella, listeriosis, cryptococcus, histoplasma, coccidioides, and blastomyces are seen occasionally.

IMMUNOSUPPRESSIVE DRUG TOXICITY

The most common agents used for immunosuppression in liver transplant recipients are CNI, i.e., cyclosporine or tacrolimus, in combination with steroids and mycophenolate mofetil. Acute toxicity and infectious complications may be seen in the early posttransplant period.

Chronic immunosuppression is associated with an increased incidence of various malignancies such as PTLD, basal skin cancer, Kaposi's sarcoma, and uterine tumors. Steroid therapy is associated to glucose intolerance (which is generally dose related), hypertension, obesity, bone disease, fluid retention, muscle weakness, pancreatitis, and growth retardation in children. Calcineurin inhibitors (cyclosporine and tacrolimus) are nephrotoxic and may lead to renal dysfunction and electrolyte imbalance such as hyperkalemia, hyperuricemia, hypophosphatemia, and hypomagnesemia. In addition, they may cause seizures, headache, and tremor. Nephrotoxic effects are generally reversible with reduction of the CNI doses but occasionally, irreversible chronic renal disease can develop. Troublesome neurological symptoms such as tremors and seizures with CNI may warrant switching to another CNI agent and antiepileptic drugs. In addition, cyclosporine is more related to gingival hyperplasia and hirsutism. Mycophenolate mofetil can lead to gastrointestinal disturbances and bone marrow depression, which are also dose related and respond to reduction in doses, and sometimes need conversion to the more "gastrointestinal-friendly" mycophenolate sodium.

LONG-TERM COMPLICATIONS

In the long term, metabolic and cardiovascular complications, drug toxicity, and recurrence of disease are the major causes of morbidity and mortality. While patients may have risk factors for some of these conditions, toxicity due to long-term usage of immunosuppression has an additive effect.

Metabolic Syndrome

It includes hypertension, hyperlipidemia, and obesity, and is common after LT, and usually thought to be related to immunosuppression. It increases risks of cardiovascular disease, cardiovascular death, and overall mortality. Hypertension is the most common, seen in up to 70% of the patients, whereas hyperlipidemia is observed in approximately 40%. Hypercholesterolemia is seen in 15–45% and hypertriglyceridemia in 40%. It is due to corticosteroid-induced rise in low-density lipoprotein production, and is common with the use of cyclosporine[125] and sirolimus. Judicious use and selection of steroids, CNIs, and mammalian target of rapamycin inhibitors might help reduce long-term morbidity after LT.[126] Patients should be advised fish oil that contains ω-3 fatty acids to reduce hyperlipidemia, low-fat diet, alcohol avoidance, regular exercise, and lipid lowering and antihypertensive medication as per requirement. Hyperlipidemia is managed with HMG-CoA reductase inhibitors. While some statins are hepatotoxic, gemfibrozil carries a risk of myositis,[127] and bile acid-binding resins like cholestyramine may reduce CNI absorption. Hypertension needs to be managed with weight reduction, salt restriction, regular exercise, calcium channel blockers, steroid taper, and reducing CNI use in addition to dietary modification. New onset coronary artery disease is seen in about 5% of patients.[128-130] Obesity is seen in 17–42% of patients and is mainly attributed to high-dose steroids. Risk modification remains the main preventive strategy. Sibutramine and orlistat reduce CNI absorption and are not recommended.

New onset diabetes mellitus/posttransplant diabetes (NODM, PTD) is seen in 12–20% of recipients,[131] is less common in LDLT, and its overall prevalence in LT decreases with time from 12% at 1 year to 1% at 3 years.[131] Steroid-induced insulin resistance and CNI-related B-cell toxicity seem to be primary mechanisms, and PTD is associated with more infections, renal dysfunction, and accelerated fibrosis progression in HCV patients.

Hyperuricemia is seen in about 40% recipients but clinical gout occurs in about 6–25% of them, especially with cyclosporine use. Allopurinol can be used for prophylaxis, and nonsteroidal anti-inflammatory drugs or steroids are used for acute gout as colchicine is poorly tolerated.

Bone Diseases

Bone diseases like osteopenia and osteoporosis are seen in 10–60% of cases. Osteoporosis affecting the spine and hip is common, especially in patients with cholestatic liver disease.[132] Causes of bone dystrophy are multifactorial, which can include steroid therapy, cholestasis, hepatic osteodystrophy, secondary hyperparathyroidism, hypogonadism, and vitamin D deficiency. Osteoporosis is generally related to steroids, commonly seen after 4–9 months, and gradually recovers as steroids are tapered. Atraumatic bone fractures, avascular necrosis, and vertebral body collapse can occasionally be seen. Management of bone diseases includes vitamin D and calcium supplementation, and antiresorptive agents, including calcitonin, etidronate, calcium, sodium fluoride, and bisphosphonates.

Renal Dysfunction

It occurs in 4–9% of the LT recipients mainly related to use of CNI, presence of pretransplant renal dysfunction, and other renal diseases. Management includes avoiding CNI and strict control of risk factors like hypertension and diabetes.[133-135]

Neuropsychiatric Complications

These complications are generally in the form of anxiety, depression, sometimes as seizures, altered conscious level, cerebral ischemia, and bleed or infection. Encephalopathy may be related to metabolic imbalances, sepsis, poor graft function, and hypoxia. Patients presenting with neurological symptoms should undergo CT/magnetic resonance imaging scan to rule out a cerebrovascular event or infection. Neurologic problems associated with immunosuppression (mostly related to CNI) include seizures, tremors, and headache, can be avoided with dose and drug level monitoring, and managed by change of CNI and reducing the dosage, if possible.

Recurrent Diseases

Hepatitis B recurrence used to have high reinfection and recurrence rate, which significantly reduced (<5%) after introduction of peri-transplant hepatitis B immune-globulin (HBIg) and novel antiviral agents such as lamivudine, adefovir, tenofovir, and entecavir,[136] and even allowed transplantation of hepatitis B core antibody-positive livers into low-risk patients. Hepatitis B patients are taken up for transplant once their viral load is ideally zero, or at least reduced by 2–5 logs with single or combination antiviral drug therapy, given according to response and/or time available prior to transplant. All potential LT recipients should be screened for hepatitis B surface antibody (HBsAb) titers and be vaccinated if inadequate. Prophylaxis for HBV recurrence consists of hyper-immunization of live donors, HBIg during anhepatic phase and postoperatively to keep anti-HBsAb titers >500 IU/L for first month and >100 U/L thereafter,[136,137] and antiviral medications such as entecavir and/ortenofovir. Immunoglobulin is given daily for first week, then weekly for 1 month, and then monthly for 1 year. Few centers do not use immunoglobulin routinely. With effective anti-viral medications, HBV recurrence is rare.

Recurrent hepatitis C infection (Fig. 11) after LT is universal. According to data from centers with DDLT recipients with genotype 1 HCV, acute lobular hepatitis develops in about 75% of HCV recipients with recurrence; half of these would progress to severe disease and 25–30% progress to cirrhosis in 5 years requiring retransplantation.[138] Older donors,[139] prolonged ischemia time, genotype 1B,[140] high pre- and posttransplant viral loads, graft steatosis,[141] CMV infection, use of T-cell-depleting therapies or bolus steroids,[142] and PTD are various risk factors related to HCV recurrence.

Preliminary LDLT data from our center, however, are much more encouraging. We found that only around 30% of HCV recipients (86% genotype 3) need antiviral treatment posttransplant, with more than 70% sustained viral response.[143] Of 368 LDLT recipients (out of a total of 1,482 LDLTs) transplanted for HCV cirrhosis, not a single one has progressed to established cirrhosis over 1–12 months, or needed a retransplant for recurrence [In Press].While there is still some controversy about the effect of steroid withdrawal, majority of studies suggest that steroid-free immunosuppression is well tolerated by patients, and results in lower steroid-related complications without any major difference

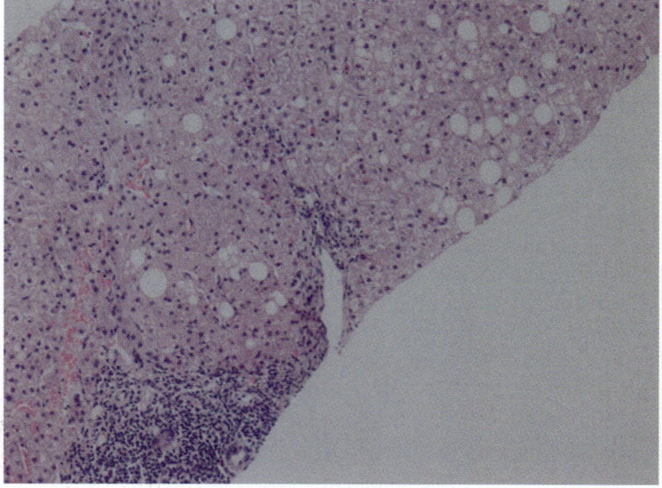

Figure 11 Histopathology showing hepatitis C virus recurrence

in the HCV recurrence pattern.[144-146] Recurrent HCV infection is best diagnosed by high HCV viral load and protocol-based liver biopsy. It, however, may be difficult to differentiate from ACR.[147] Histological changes may be seen as early as the first postoperative week.[148] Treatment of recurrent HCV with pegylated interferon and ribavirin has improved virologic and histologic response,[149] although optimal timing of starting therapy is still unclear.[150,151] Early concern about faster recurrence in LDLT[152,153] has not been seen in recent series.[143,154] We do HCV RNA viral quantitative test biannually, protocol biopsy annually, and treat the recurrence with ribavarin and pegylated interferon.

Recurrence of *autoimmune diseases* such as PSC, PBC, and AIH may be as high as 15% at 3 years to 30% at 10 years. Autoimmune hepatitis patients require lifelong low-dose steroid prophylaxis, and recurrence typically responds to increased immunosuppression.

Active *alcohol abuse,* concerns of recidivism, and compliance are common reasons for denial of transplant listing, especially in DDLT-predominant countries. About 8–20% patients resume drinking after transplant[155] and have poor long-term survival.[156] In our experience with 230 alcoholic liver disease patients who underwent LT, the incidence of recidivism is 10.7%, of which majority are occasional/moderate drinkers [In Press].

In *HCC* patients undergoing LT, tumor-free survival rates of 85–90%, 70–75%, and >60% at 1, 3, and 5 years, respectively, have been reported[157] with no significant influence of DDLT or LDLT. Preoperative treatments, alpha-fetoprotein (AFP) >30 ng/mL, exceeding Milan criteria at final histology, poor tumor differentiation, neutrophil-to-lymphocyte ratio >5, and presence of microvascular invasion predict a lower recurrence-free survival.[158]

Our Experience with Living Donor Liver Transplantation for Hepatocellular Carcinoma

Since live liver donation is a private gift and a "no competition" situation, our policy is to accept HCC for LDLT irrespective of tumor number and size, provided there are no extrahepatic metastases or major vascular invasion. We perform positron emission tomography-CT scan and bone scan in all patients with HCC before LDLT. Of 203 patients undergoing LDLT for HCC, overall survival at 1 and 3 years is 95 and 89% respectively; recurrence-free survival at 1 and 3 years is 83 and 72%, respectively. Pretransplant AFP ≥ 200 ng/mL, HCC beyond UCSF criteria, and presence of microvascular tumor invasion were found to be bad prognostic factors for recurrence free survival [In Press].

SUMMARY

Liver transplantation is lifesaving for patients with end-stage liver disease. It leads to remarkable recovery from symptoms of liver failure or metabolic disease with expectation of long-term survival and a good quality of life. Complications related to preexisting morbidity, graft quality, the complexity of the procedure, and immunosuppression may lead to increased hospital stay, make patients more susceptible to further complications especially infections, increase financial burden, and increase risk of graft loss and mortality. Many technical complications such as vascular and biliary problems can be reduced with experience and expertise, and are seen less frequently in high-volume centers.[33,53] Immunosuppression is a double-edged sword with suboptimal use leading to episodes of rejection and excessive use leading to infections and life-threatening neoplasms. Prevention, anticipation, early diagnosis, and aggressive management of complications help in reducing the associated morbidity and mortality. An evolved multidisciplinary setup and team with expertise in transplant surgery, gastroenterology, hepatology, anesthesia and intensive care, interventional radiology, pathology, and laboratory medicine are essential to ensure good outcomes in these patients.

REFERENCES

1. Todo S, Furukawa H, Jin MB, et al. Living donor liver transplantation in adults: outcome in Japan. Liver Transpl. 2000;6(6 Suppl 2):S66-72.
2. Soin AS. Ethical dilemmas in living donor liver transplantation. Issues Med Ethics. 2003;11(4):104-5.
3. Kakodkar R, Soin A, Nundy S. Liver transplantation in India: its evolution, problems and the way forward. Natl Med J India. 2007;20(2):53-6.
4. Soin AS, Kakodkar R. Living donor liver transplantation in India. Trop Gastroenterol. 2007;28(3):96-8.
5. Soin AS, Vasudevan KR. A successful deceased-donor liver transplant program is not a prerequisite for a living-donor program. Indian J Gastroenterol. 2006;25(6):305-7.
6. Sibal A, Rajasekar MR, Soin AS. Liver transplantation in the developing world. Indian J Pediatr. 1999;66(1 Suppl):S120-3.
7. Renz JF, Yersiz H, Farmer DG, et al. Changing faces of liver transplantation: partial-liver grafts for adults. J Hepatobiliary Pancreat Surg. 2003;10(1):31-44.
8. Perwaiz A, Mehta N, Mohanka R, et al. Right-sided diaphragmatic hernia in an adult after living donor liver transplant: a rare cause of post-transplant recurrent abdominal pain. Hernia. 2010;14(5):547-9.
9. Akun E, Yaprak O, Killi R, et al. Vascular complications in hepatic transplantation: single-center experience in 14 years. Transplant Proc. 2012;44(5):1368-72.
10. Stange BJ, Glanemann M, Nuessler NC, et al. Hepatic artery thrombosis after adult liver transplantation. Liver Transpl. 2003;9(6):612-20.
11. Drazan K, Shaked A, Olthoff KM, et al. Etiology and management of symptomatic adult hepatic artery thrombosis after orthotopic liver transplantation (OLT). Am Surg. 1996;62(3):237-40.
12. Sanada Y, Wakiya T, Hishikawa S, et al. Risk factors and treatments for hepatic arterial complications in pediatric living donor liver transplantation. J Hepatobiliary Pancreat Sci. 2013. doi: 10.1002/jhbp.49. [Epub ahead of print]
13. Silva MA, Jambulingam PS, Gunson BK, et al Hepatic artery thrombosis following orthotopic liver transplantation: a 10-year experience from a single centre in the United Kingdom. Liver Transpl. 2006;12(1):146-51.
14. Hashikura Y, Kawasaki S, Okumura N, et al. Prevention of hepatic artery thrombosis in pediatric liver transplantation. Transplantation. 1995;60(10):1109-12.
15. Duffy JP, Hong JC, Farmer DG, et al. Vascular complications of orthotopic liver transplantation: experience in more than 4,200 patients. J Am Coll Surg. 2009;208(5):896-903.
16. Bekker J, Ploem S, de Jong KP. Early hepatic artery thrombosis after liver transplantation: a systematic review of the incidence, outcome and risk factors. Am J Transplant. 2009;9(4):746-57.
17. Lisman T, Porte RJ. Hepatic artery thrombosis after liver transplantation: more than just a surgical complication? Transpl Int. 2009;22(2):162-4.
18. Soin AS, Friend PJ, Rasmussen A, Saxena R, Tokat Y, Alexander GJ, Jamieson NV, Calne RY. Donor arterial variations in liver transplantation: management and outcome of 527 consecutive grafts. Br J Surg. 1996;83(5):637-41.

19. Pareja E, Cortes M, Navarro R, et al. Vascular complications after orthotopic liver transplantation: hepatic artery thrombosis. Transplant Proc. 2010;42(8):2970-2.
20. Warner P, Fusai G, Glantzounis GK, et al. Risk factors associated with early hepatic artery thrombosis after orthotopic liver transplantation—univariable and multivariable analysis. Transpl Int. 2011;24(4):401-8.
21. Neto JS, Pugliese R, Fonseca EA, et al. Four hundred thirty consecutive pediatric living donor liver transplants: variables associated with posttransplant patient and graft survival. Liver Transpl. 2012;18(5):577-84.
22. Shay R, Taber D, Pilch N, et al. Early aspirin therapy may reduce hepatic artery thrombosis in liver transplantation. Transplant Proc. 2013;45(1):330-4.
23. Vivarelli M, La Barba G, Cucchetti A, et al. Can antiplatelet prophylaxis reduce the incidence of hepatic artery thrombosis after liver transplantation? Liver Transpl. 2007;13(5):651-4.
24. Wolf DC, Freni MA, Boccagni P, et al. Low-dose aspirin therapy is associated with few side effects but does not prevent hepatic artery thrombosis in liver transplant recipients. Liver Transpl Surg. 1997;3(6):598-603.
25. Azzam AZ, Tanaka K. Management of vascular complications after living donor liver transplantation. Hepatogastroenterology. 2012;59(113):182-6.
26. Coelho GR, Leitao AS Jr, Cavalcante FP, et al. Continuous versus interrupted suture for hepatic artery anastomosis in liver transplantation: differences in the incidence of hepatic artery thrombosis. Transplant Proc. 2008;40(10):3545-7.
27. Tamsel S, Demirpolat G, Killi R, et al. Vascular complications after liver transplantation: evaluation with Doppler US. Abdom Imaging. 2007;32(3):339-47.
28. Nolten A, Sproat IA. Hepatic artery thrombosis after liver transplantation: Temporal accuracy of diagnosis with duplex-US and the syndrome of impending thrombosis. Radiology 1996;198:553-9.
29. Lu Q, Zhong XF, Huang ZX, et al. Role of contrast-enhanced ultrasound in decision support for diagnosis and treatment of hepatic artery thrombosis after liver transplantation. Eur J Radiol. 2012;81(3):e338-43.
30. Abdelaziz O, Hosny K, Amin A, et al. Endovascular management of early hepatic artery thrombosis after living donor liver transplantation. Transpl Int. 2012;25(8):847-56.
31. Rostambeigi N, Hunter D, Duval S, et al. Stent placement versus angioplasty for hepatic artery stenosis after liver transplant: a meta-analysis of case series. Eur Radiol. 2013;23(5):1323-34.
32. Singhal A, Stokes K, Sebastian A, et al. Endovascular treatment of hepatic artery thrombosis following liver transplantation. Transpl Int. 2010;23(3):245-56.
33. Singla P, Amit Rastogi, B. Menon, et al. Multidisciplinary management of vascular complications in living donor liver transplantation. Liver Transpl. 2013;19(S1):S307.
34. Fouzas I, Sklavos A, Bismpa K, et al. Hepatic artery thrombosis after orthotopic liver transplantation: 3 patients with collateral formation and conservative treatment. Transplant Proc. 2012;44(9):2741-4.
35. Piskin T, Demirbas T, Yalcin L, et al. Recipient splenic artery utilization for arterial re-anastomosis in living donor liver transplantation:single-center experience. Hepatogastroenterology. 2012;59(116):1263-4.
36. Seu P, Shackleton Seu P, et al. Improved results of liver transplantation in patients with portal vein thrombosis. Arch Surg. 1996;131(8):8404.
37. Kishi Y, Sugawara Y, Matsui Y, et al. Late onset portal vein thrombosis and its risk factors. Hepatogastroenterology. 2008;55(84):1008-9.
38. Jensen MK, Campbell KM, Alonso MH, et al. Management and long-term consequences of portal vein thrombosis after liver transplantation in children. Liver Transpl. 2013;19(3):315-21.
39. Sood D, Kumaran V, Kakodkar R, et al. Portal vein stenosis following living donor liver transplant: manifestations and management. Transpl Int. 2009;22(4):496-9.
40. Suarez Artacho G, Barrera Pulido L, Alamo Martinez JM, et al. Outcomes of liver transplantation in candidates with portal vein thrombosis. Transplant Proc. 2010;42(8):3156-8.
41. Ravaioli M, Zanello M, Grazi GL, et al. Portal vein thrombosis and liver transplantation: evolution during 10 years of experience at the University of Bologna. Ann Surg. 2011;253(2):378-84.
42. Hibi T, Nishida S, Levi DM, et al. When and Why Portal Vein Thrombosis Matters in Liver Transplantation: A Critical Audit of 174 Cases. Ann Surg. 2013. [Epub ahead of print]
43. Rodríguez-Castro KI, Porte RJ, Nadal E, et al. Management of nonneoplastic portal vein thrombosis in the setting of liver transplantation: a systematic review. Transplantation. 2012;94(11):1145-53.
44. Carnevale FC, Santos AC, Seda-Neto J, et al. Portal vein obstruction after liver transplantation in children treated by simultaneous minilaparotomy and transhepatic approaches: initial experience. Pediatr Transplant. 2011;15(1):47-52.
45. Woo DH, Laberge JM, Gordon RL, et al. Management of portal venous complications after liver transplantation. Tech Vasc Interv Radiol. 2007;10(3):233-9.
46. Nakamura T, Tanaka K, Kiuchi T, et al. Anatomical variations and surgical strategies in right lobe living donor liver transplantation: lessons from 120 cases. Transplantation. 2002;73(12):1896-903.
47. Wozney P, Zajko AB, Bron KM, et al. Vascular complications after liver transplantation: a 5-year experience. AJR Am J Roentgenol. 1986;147(4):657-63.
48. Wang SL, Sze DY, Busque S, et al. Treatment of hepatic venous outflow obstruction after piggyback liver transplantation. Radiology. 2005;236(1):352-9.
49. Yamagiwa K, Yokoi H, Isaji S, et al. Intrahepatic hepatic vein stenosis after living-related liver transplantation treated by insertion of an expandable metallic stent. Am J Transplant. 2004;4(6):1006-9.
50. Quintini C, Miller CM, Hashimoto K, et al. Side-to-side cavocavostomy with an endovascular stapler: rescue technique for severe hepatic vein and/or inferior vena cava outflow obstruction after liver transplantation using the piggyback technique. Liver Transpl. 2009;15(1):49-53.
51. Hwang HJ, Kim KW, Jeong WK, et al. Right hepatic vein stenosis at anastomosis in patients after living donor liver transplantation: optimal Doppler US venous pulsatility index and CT criteria—receiver operating characteristic analysis. Radiology. 2009;253(2):543-51.
52. Abouljoud M, Yoshida A, Kim D, et al. Transjugular intrahepatic portosystemic shunts for refractory ascites after liver transplantation. Transplant Proc. 2005;37(2):1248-50.
53. Soin AS, Kumaran V, Rastogi AN, et al. Evolution of a reliable biliary reconstructive technique in 400 consecutive living donor liver transplants. J Am Coll Surg. 2010;211(1):24-32.
54. Kim SH, Lee KW, Kim YK, et al. Tailored telescopic reconstruction of the bile duct in living donor liver transplantation. Liver Transpl 2010;16:1069-74.
55. Soejima Y, Taketomi A, Yoshizumi T, et al. Biliary strictures in living donor liver transplantation: incidence, management, and technical evolution. Liver Transpl. 2006;12:979-86.
56. Gastaca M. Biliary complications after orthotopic liver transplantation: a review of incidence and risk factors. Transplant Proc. 2012;44(6):1545-9.
57. Akamatsu N, Sugawara Y, Hashimoto D. Biliary reconstruction, its complications and management of biliary complications after

adult liver transplantation: a systematic review of the incidence, risk factors and outcome. Transpl Int. 2011;24(4):379-92.

58. Riediger C, Müller MW, Michalski CW, et al. T-Tube or no T-tube in the reconstruction of the biliary tract during orthotopic liver transplantation: systematic review and meta-analysis. Liver Transpl. 2010;16(6):705-17.
59. Shah SA, Grant DR, McGilvray ID, et al. Biliary strictures in 130 consecutive right lobe living donor liver transplant recipients: results of a Western center. Am J Transplant. 2007;7(1):161-7.
60. Chok KS, Chan SC, Cheung TT, et al. Bile duct anastomotic stricture after adult-to-adult right lobe living donor liver transplantation. Liver Transpl. 2011;17(1):47-52.
61. Melcher ML, Pomposelli JJ, Verbesey JE, et al. Comparison of biliary complications in adult living-donor liver transplants performed at two busy transplant centers. Clin Transplant. 2010;24(5):E137-44.
62. Kim JH, Ko GY, Sung KB, et al. Bile leak following living donor liver transplantation: clinical efficacy of percutaneous transhepatic treatment. Liver Transpl. 2008;14(8):1142-9.
63. Howell JA, Gow PJ, Angus PW, et al. Early-onset versus late-onset nonanastomotic biliary strictures post liver transplantation: risk factors reflect different pathogenesis. Transpl Int. 2012;25(7):765-75.
64. Beswick DM, Miraglia R, Caruso S, et al. The role of ultrasound and magnetic resonance cholangiopancreatography for the diagnosis of biliary stricture after liver transplantation. Eur J Radiol. 2012;81(9):2089-92.
65. Hwang S, Lee SG, Sung KB, et al. Long-term incidence, risk factors, and management of biliary complications after adult living donor liver transplantation. Liver Transpl. 2006;12(5):831-8.
66. Buxbaum JL, Biggins SW, Bagatelos KC, et al. Predictors of endoscopic treatment outcomes in the management of biliary problems after liver transplantation at a high-volume academic center. Gastrointest Endosc. 2011;73(1):37-44.
67. Sanna C, Giordanino C, Giono I, et al. Safety and efficacy of endoscopic retrograde cholangiopancreatography in patients with post-liver transplant biliary complications: results of a cohort study with long-term follow-up. Gut Liver. 2011;5(3):328-34.
68. Chahal P, Baron TH, Poterucha JJ, et al. Endoscopic retrograde cholangiography in post-orthotopic liver transplant population with Roux-en-Y biliary reconstruction. Liver Transpl. 2007;13(8):1168-73.
69. Chang JH, Lee IS, Chun HJ, et al. Usefulness of the rendezvous technique for biliary stricture after adult right-lobe living-donor liver transplantation with duct-to-duct anastomosis. Gut Liver. 2010;4(1):68-75.
70. Reichman TW, Sandroussi C, Grant DR, et al. Surgical revision of biliary strictures following adult live donor liver transplantation: patient selection, morbidity, and outcomes. Transpl Int. 2012;25(1):69-77.
71. Traina M, Tarantino I, Barresi L, et al. Efficacy and safety of fully covered self-expandable metallic stents in biliary complications after liver transplantation: a preliminary study. Liver Transpl. 2009;15(11):1493-8.
72. Uemura T, Randall HB, Sanchez EQ, et al. Liver retransplantation for primary nonfunction: analysis of a 20-year single-center experience. Liver Transpl. 2007;13(2):227-33.
73. Varotti G, Grazi GL, Vetrone G, et al. Causes of early acute graft failure after liver transplantation: analysis of a 17-year single-centre experience. Clin Transplant. 2005;19(4):492-500.
74. Busuttil RW, Farmer DG, Yersiz H, et al. Analysis of long-term outcomes of 3200 liver transplantations over two decades: a single-center experience. Ann Surg. 2005;241(6):905-16.
75. Jain A, Reyes J, Kashyap R, et al. Long-term survival after liver transplantation in 4,000 consecutive patients at a single center. Ann Surg. 2000;232(4):490-500.
76. Johnson SR, Alexopoulos S, Curry M, et al. Primary nonfunction (PNF) in the MELD Era: an SRTR database analysis. Am J Transplant. 2007;7(4):1003-9.
77. Stahl JE, Kreke JE, Malek FA, et al. Consequences of cold-ischemia time on primary nonfunction and patient and graft survival in liver transplantation: a meta-analysis. PLoS One. 2008;3(6):e2468.
78. Furukawa H, Todo S, Imventarza O, et al. Effect of cold ischemia time on the early outcome of human hepatic allografts preserved with UW solution. Transplantation. 1991;51(5):1000-4.
79. Abt PL, Desai NM, Crawford MD, et al. Survival following liver transplantation from nonheart-beating donors. Ann Surg. 2004;239(1):87-92.
80. Strasberg SM, Howard TK, Molmenti EP, et al. Selecting the donor liver: risk factors for poor function after orthotopic liver transplantation. Hepatology. 1994;20(4 Pt 1):829-38.
81. Friedman BH, Wolf JH, Wang L, et al. Serum cytokine profiles associated with early allograft dysfunction in patients undergoing liver transplantation. Liver Transpl. 2012;18(2):166-76.
82. Thies JC, Teklote J, Clauer U, et al. The efficacy of N-acetylcysteine as a hepatoprotective agent in liver transplantation. Transpl Int. 1998;11 Suppl 1:S390-2.
83. Hilmi IA, Peng Z, Planinsic RM, et al. N-acetylcysteine does not prevent hepatorenal ischaemia-reperfusion injury in patients undergoing orthotopic liver transplantation. Nephrol Dial Transplant. 2010;25(7):2328-33.
84. Takaya S, Doyle H, Todo S, et al. Reduction of primary nonfunction with prostaglandin E1 after clinical liver transplantation. Transplant Proc. 1995;27(2):1862-7.
85. Mandal AK, King KE, Humphreys SL, et al. Plasmapheresis: an effective therapy for primary allograft nonfunction after liver transplantation. Transplantation. 2000;70(1):216-20.
86. Ben-Haim M, Ernre S, Fishbein TM, et al. Critical graft size in adult-to-adult living donor liver transplantation: Impact of the recipient's disease. Liver Transpl. 2001;7:948-53.
87. Fan ST, Lo CM, Liu CL, et al. Determinants of hospital mortality of adult recipients of right lobe live donor liver transplantation. Ann Surg. 2003;238(6):864-69.
88. Demetris AJ, Kelly DM, Eghtesad B, et al. Pathophysiologic observations and histopathologic recognition of the portal hyperperfusion or small-for-size syndrome. Am J Surg Pathol. 2006;30(8):986-93.
89. Marcos A, Olzinski AT, Ham JM, et al. The interrelationship between portal and arterial blood flow after adult to adult living donor liver transplantation. Transplantation. 2000;70(12):1697-703.
90. Emond JC, Renz JF, Ferrell LD, et al. Functional analysis of grafts from living donors. Implications for the treatment of older recipients. Ann Surg. 1996;224(4):544-52.
91. Soin AS. Smoothing the path: reducing biliary complications, addressing small-for-size syndrome, and making other adaptations to decrease the risk for living donor liver transplant recipients. Liver Transpl. 2012;18 Suppl 2:S20-4.
92. Humar A, Beissel J, Crotteau S, et al. Delayed splenic artery occlusion for treatment of established small-for-size syndrome after partial liver transplantation. Liver Transpl. 2009;15(2):163-8.
93. Troisi R, Ricciardi S, Smeets P, et al. Effects of hemi-portocaval shunts for inflow modulation on the outcome of small-for-size grafts in living donor liver transplantation. Am J Transplant. 2005;5(6):1397-404.
94. Soin AS, Mohanka R, Singla P, et al. Segment IV preserving middle hepatic vein retrieval in right lobe living donor liver transplantation. J Am Coll Surg. 2011;213(2):5-16.
95. Soin AS, Kakodkar R, Saigal S, et al. Recanalized umbilical vein as a conduit for anterior sector venous outflow reconstruction in right lobe grafts. Surgery. 2007;141(6):830.
96. Kakodkar R, Nundy S, Soin AS. Use of banked cryopreserved veins from explanted recipient livers in living donor liver transplantation. Surgery. 2008;144(1):93-5.
97. Kamei H, Fujimoto Y, Nagai S, et al. Impact of non-congestive graft size in living donor liver transplantation: new indicator for

additional vein reconstruction in right liver graft. Liver Transpl. 2007;13:1295-301.
98. Suehiro T, Shimada M, Kishikawa K, et al. Effect of intraportal infusion to improve small for size graft injury in living donor adult liver transplantation. Transpl Int. 2005;18(8):923-8.
99. Botha JF, Langnas AN, Campos BD, et al. Left lobe adult-to-adult living donor liver transplantation: small grafts and hemiportocaval shunts in the prevention of small-for-size syndrome. Liver Transpl. 2010;16(5):649-57.
100. Soejima Y, Taketomi A, Ikegami T, et al. Living donor liver transplantation using dual grafts from two donors: a feasible option to overcome small-for-size graft problems? Am J Transplant. 2008;8(4):887-92.
101. Tippner C, Nashan B, Hoshino K, et al. Clinical and subclinical acute rejection early after liver transplantation: contributing factors and relevance for the long-term course. Transplantation. 2001;72(6):1122-8.
102. Sanchez-Fueyo A, Strom TB. Immunological tolerance and liver transplantation. J Hepatol. 2004;41(5):698-705.
103. Demetris AJ, Ruppert K, Dvorchik I, et al. Real-time monitoring of acute liver-allograft rejection using the Banff schema. Transplantation. 2002;74(9):1290-6.
104. Demetris A, Adams D, Bellamy C, et al. Update of the International Banff Schema for Liver Allograft Rejection: working recommendations for the histopathologic staging and reporting of chronic rejection. An international panel. Hepatology. 2000;31(3):792-9.
105. Demetris A, Batts K, Dhillon A. Banff schema for grading liver allograft rejection: an international consensus document. Hepatology. 1997;25(3):658-63.
106. Fisher LR, Henley KS, Lucey MR. Acute cellular rejection after liver transplantation: variability, morbidity, and mortality. Liver Transpl Surg. 1995;1:10-5.
107. Junge G, Tullius SG, Klitzing V, et al. The influence of late acute rejection episodes on long-term graft outcome after liver transplantation. Transplant Proc. 2005;37(4):1716-7.
108. D'Antiga L, Dhawan A, Portmann B, et al. Late cellular rejection in paediatric liver transplantation: aetiology and outcome. Transplantation. 2002;73(1):80-4.
109. Uemura T, Ikegami T, Sanchez EQ, et al. Late acute rejection after liver transplantation impacts patient survival. Clin Transplant. 2008;22(3):316-23.
110. Soin AS, Rasmussen A, Jamieson NV, et al. CsA levels in the early posttransplant period-predictive of chronic rejection in liver transplantation? Transplantation. 1995;59(8):1119-23.
111. Soin AS, Jamieson NV. Lessons learnt from the multicentre randomized trials of tacrolimus in liver transplantation. Natl Med J India. 1996;9(5):224-6.
112. Singla P, Mohanka R, Tamang TY, et al. Outcome of patients with chronic liver disease and renal dysfunction referred for living donor liver transplant at a high volume centre. Liver Transpl. 2012;18 Suppl 1:S262.
113. Chari RS, Gan TJ, Robertson KM, et al. Venovenous bypass in adult orthotopic liver transplantation: routine or selective use? J Am Coll Surg. 1998;186(6):683-90.
114. Benedetti E, Pirenne J, Troppmann C, et al. A percutaneous technique for venous return cannula insertion for veno-venous bypass in hepatic transplantation. Transplantation. 1995;59(5): 789-91.
115. Kim JM, Kim SJ, Joh JW, et al. Early and delayed onset cytomegalovirus infection of liver transplant recipients in endemic areas. Transplant Proc. 2010;42(3):884-9.
116. Onor IO, Todd SB, Meredith E, et al. Evaluation of clinical outcomes of prophylactic versus preemptive cytomegalovirus strategy in liver transplant recipients. Transpl Int. 2013;26(6):592-600.
117. Bodro M, Sabé N, Lladó L, et al. Prophylaxis versus preemptive therapy for cytomegalovirus disease in high-risk liver transplant recipients. Liver Transpl. 2012;18(9):1093-9.
118. Evans PC, Soin A, Wreghitt TG, et al. An association between cytomegalovirus infection and chronic rejection after liver transplantation. Transplantation. 2000;69(1):30-5.
119. Lautenschlager I. CMV infection, diagnosis and antiviral strategies after liver transplantation. Transpl Int. 2009;22(11):1031-40.
120. Choi YI, Hwang S, Park GC, et al. Clinical outcomes of Pneumocystis carinii pneumonia in adult liver transplant recipients. Transplant Proc. 2013;45(8):3057-60.
121. Trotter JF, Levi M, Steinberg T, et al. Absence of pneumocystis jiroveci pneumonia in liver transplantation recipients receiving short-term (3-month) prophylaxis. Transpl Infect Dis. 2008;10(5):369-71.
122. Saliba F, Delvart V, Ichaï P, et al. Outcomes associated with amphotericin B lipid complex (ABLC) prophylaxis in high-risk liver transplant patients. Med Mycol. 2013;51(2):155-63.
123. Fábrega E, Sampedro B, Cabezas J, et al. Chemoprophylaxis with isoniazid in liver transplant recipients. Liver Transpl. 2012;18(9):1110-7.
124. Yehia BR, Blumberg EA. Mycobacterium tuberculosis infection in liver transplantation. Liver Transpl. 2010;16(10):1129-35.
125. Charco R, Bilbao I, Chavez R, et al. Low incidence of hypercholesterolemia among liver transplant patients under tacrolimus monotherapy immunosuppression. Transplant Proc. 2002;34(5):1555-6.
126. Muller R, Samuel D, Fassati LR, Benhamou JP, Bismuth H, Alexander GJ. 'EUROHEP' consensus report on the management of liver transplantation for hepatitis B virus infection. European Concerted Action on Viral Hepatitis. J Hepatol. 1994;21(6):1140-3.
127. Imagawa DK, Dawson S 3rd, Holt CD, et al. Hyperlipidemia after liver transplantation: natural history and treatment with the hydroxy-methylglutaryl-coenzyme A reductase inhibitor pravastatin. Transplantation. 199615;62(7):934-42.
128. Simo KA, Sereika S, Bitner N, et al. Medical epidemiology of patients surviving ten years after liver transplantation. Clin Transplant. 2011;25(3):360-7.
129. Textor SC, Wiesner R, Wilson DJ, et al. Systemic and renal hemodynamic differences between FK506 and cyclosporine in liver transplant recipients. Transplantation. 1993;55(6):1332-9.
130. Desai S, Hong JC, Saab S. Cardiovascular risk factors following orthotopic liver transplantation: predisposing factors, incidence and management. Liver Int. 2010;30(7):948-57.
131. Yadav AD, Chang YH, Aqel BA, et al. New onset diabetes mellitus in living donor versus deceased donor liver transplant recipients: analysis of the UNOS/OPTN Database. J Transplant. 2013;2013:269096.
132. Guañabens N, Parés A. Management of osteoporosis in liver disease. Clin Res Hepatol Gastroenterol. 2011;35(6-7):438-45.
133. Aucejo F, Rofaiel G, Miller C. Who is at risk for post-transplant lymphoproliferative disorders (PTLD) after liver transplantation? J Hepatol. 2006;44(1):19-23.
134. Evens AM, Roy R, Sterrenberg D, et al. Post-transplantation lymphoproliferative disorders: diagnosis, prognosis, and current approaches to therapy. Curr Oncol Rep. 2010;12(6):383-94.
135. Jain AB, Marcos A, Pokharna R, et al. Rituximab (chimeric anti-CD20 antibody) for posttransplant lymphoproliferative disorder after solid organ transplantation in adults: long-term experience from a single center. Transplantation. 200527;80(12):1692-8.
136. Gane EJ, Angus PW, Strasser S, et al. Lamivudine plus low-dose hepatitis B immunoglobulin to prevent recurrent hepatitis B following liver transplantation. Gastroenterology. 2007;132(3):931-7.
137. Terrault NA, Zhou S, Combs C, et al. Prophylaxis in liver transplant recipients using a fixed dosing schedule of hepatitis B immunoglobulin. Hepatology. 1996;24(6):1327-33.

138. Ponziani FR, Gasbarrini A, Pompili M, et al. Management of hepatitis C virus infection recurrence after liver transplantation: an overview. Transplant Proc. 2011;43(1):291-5.
139. Jain A, Orloff M, Abt P, et al. Transplantation of liver grafts from older donors: impact on recipients with hepatitis C virus infection. Transplant Proc. 2005;37(7):3162-4.
140. Gayowski T, Singh N, Marino IR, et al. Hepatitis C virus genotypes in livertransplant recipients: impact on posttransplant recurrence, infections, response to interferon-alpha therapy and outcome. Transplantation. 1997;64(3):422-6.
141. Subramanian V, Seetharam AB, Vachharajani N, et al. Donor graft steatosis influences immunity to hepatitis C virus and allograft outcome after liver transplantation. Transplantation. 2011;92(11):1259-68.
142. Gane EJ. The natural history of recurrent hepatitis C and what influences this. Liver Transpl. 2008;14 Suppl 2:S36-44.
143. Choudhary NS, Saigal S, Saraf N, et al. Genotype 3 and favorable IL28B polymorphism as predictors of good response for HCV recurrence post liver transplantation. Liver Transpl. 2013;19 (6) Suppl 1:S146-7.
144. Kato T, Gaynor JJ, Yoshida H, et al. Randomized trial of steroid-free induction versus corticosteroid maintenance among orthotopic liver transplant recipients with hepatitis C virus: impact on hepatic fibrosis progression at one year. Transplantation. 200715;84(7):829-35.
145. Krämer BK, Klinger M, Vítko Š, et al. Tacrolimus-based, steroid-free regimens in renal transplantation: 3-year follow-up of the ATLAS trial. Transplantation. 2012;94(5):492-8.
146. Klintmalm GB, Davis GL, Teperman L, et al. A randomized, multicenter study comparing steroid-free immunosuppression and standard immunosuppression for liver transplant recipients with chronic hepatitis C. Liver Transpl. 2011;17(12):1394-403.
147. Jain A, Ryan C, Mohanka R, et al. Characterization of CD4, CD8, CD56 positive lymphocytes and C4d deposits to distinguish acute cellular rejection from recurrent hepatitis C in post-liver transplant biopsies. Clin Transplant. 2006;20(5):624-33.
148. Dickson RC, Caldwell SH, Ishitani MB, et al. Clinical and histologic patterns of early graft failure due to recurrent hepatitis C in four patients after liver transplantation. Transplantation. 1996;61(5):701-5.
149. Lavezzo B, Franchello A, Smedile A, et al. Treatment of recurrent hepatitis C in liver transplants: efficacy of a six versus a twelve month course of interferon alfa 2b with ribavirin. J Hepatol. 2002;37(2):247-52.
150. Terrault NA. Treatment of recurrent hepatitis C in liver transplant recipients. Clin Gastroenterol Hepatol. 2005;3(10 Suppl 2): S125-31.
151. Firpi RJ, Abdelmalek MF, Soldevila-Pico C, et al. Combination of interferon alfa-2b and ribavirin in liver transplant recipients with histological recurrent hepatitis C. Liver Transpl. 2002;8(11): 1000-6.
152. Garcia-Retortillo M, Forns X, Llovet JM, et al. Hepatitis C recurrence is more severe after living donor compared to cadaveric liver transplantation. Hepatology. 2004;40(3):699-707.
153. Gaglio PJ, Malireddy S, Levitt BS, et al. Increased risk of cholestatic hepatitis C in recipients of grafts from living versus cadaveric liver donors. Liver Transpl. 2003;9(10):1028-35.
154. Schmeding M, Neumann UP, Puhl G, et al. Hepatitis C recurrence and fibrosis progression are not increased after living donor liver transplantation: a single-center study of 289 patients. Liver Transpl. 2007;13(5):687-92.
155. Dew MA, DiMartini AF, Steel J, et al. Meta-analysis of risk for relapse to substance use after transplantation of the liver or other solid organs. Liver Transpl. 2008;14(2):159-72.
156. Cuadrado A, Fábrega E, Casafont F, et al. Alcohol recidivism impairs long-term patient survival after orthotopic liver transplantation for alcoholic liver disease. Liver Transpl. 2005;11(4):420-6.
157. Bozorgzadeh A, Orloff M, Abt P, et al. Survival outcomes in liver transplantation for hepatocellular carcinoma, comparing impact of hepatitis C versus other etiology of cirrhosis. Liver Transpl. 2007;13(6):807-13.
158. Bertuzzo VR, Cescon M, Ravaioli M, et al. Analysis of factors affecting recurrence of hepatocellular carcinoma after liver transplantation with a special focus on inflammation markers. Transplantation. 2011;91(11):1279-85.

SECTION 10

Miscellaneous

CHAPTER 115

Variceal Upper Gastrointestinal Bleeding

Patta Radhakrishna, Pavan Addala

INTRODUCTION

Varices are vascular channels connecting the systemic and portal venous circulations and are the consequence of portal hypertension (PHT). They can be associated with both cirrhotic and non-cirrhotic livers. Non-cirrhotic PHT accounts for only 10% of all the cases with PHT. Bleeding from varices account for 10–30% of all cases of upper gastrointestinal (UGI) bleeding.[1] With the presently available knowledge, in addition to liver transplantation, management of cirrhosis is limited to the treatment of its complications like PHT and the entities complicating it like ascites, bleeding, spontaneous bacterial peritonitis, portal hypertensive gastropathy (PHG), enteropathy, colopathy, portopulmonary syndrome, hepatopulmonary syndrome, hepatorenal syndrome, and hepatic encephalopathy. Of all these, PHT-associated variceal bleed is commonly seen in the emergency department requiring emergent care, not only requiring significant man power but also abundant resources in its management. In spite of our better understanding of this condition, mortality rate associated with variceal bleed is still around 10–20%.

DEFINITION

Definition of PHT varies in literature depending on the site at which it is measured. A normal hepatic venous pressure gradient (HVPG) is 3–5 mmHg.[1] However, a HVPG of more than 5 mmHg is universally accepted in defining PHT.[2] An increase in the portosystemic pressure gradient in any portion of the portal venous system is also considered PHT in a broader sense. Portosystemic collateralization is stimulated at pressures of 8–10 mmHg and is clinically significant as it predicts the clinical course of the patients with cirrhosis and also the formation of varices.[3-5] However, varices are commonly found to bleed when the wedged hepatic venous pressure (WHVP) is 12 mmHg or more.

EPIDEMIOLOGY

Though varices can occur at any site in the entire gastrointestinal (GI) system, gastroesophageal junction is the most common site for its formation. At the time of diagnosis, approximately 30–40% of compensated cirrhotic patients and 60% of the decompensated cirrhotic patients have esophageal varices.[1] Of all the cases with UGI bleed, 10–30% have bleeding from the varices.[1] Among those without any varices at the time of diagnosis of cirrhosis, varices develop at the rate of 5–8% per year.[1] Varices are also seen in 90% of cirrhotics at 10 years following the diagnosis of cirrhosis.[1] One-third to one-half of the patients with varices bleeds in life time, of which 40–70% die due to variceal bleed. As the Child's status increases the incidence of varices also increase, with 40% in Child's A and 85% in Child's B patient.[1] Sometimes the diagnosis of cirrhosis is made after the patient presents for the first time with variceal bleed. When untreated, 10–30% of the patients bleed within 2 years. Overall mortality following an acute bleed is about 25–30% overall in patients with cirrhosis and 5–10% in non-cirrhotics and well-compensated cirrhotics), of which half of the deaths are due to uncontrolled bleeding.[1] The primary cause of these deaths is the underlying poor hepatic functional reserve. A 6-week mortality of 12–20% has been observed and two-thirds of them rebleed in 2 years, if no effective treatment is provided.[1] Variceal hemorrhage is the second most common cause of death in cirrhotic patients next to hepatic failure.

ETIOLOGY

Though cirrhosis is the cause of PHT in most of the cases, the causes for cirrhosis of liver are varied. Cirrhosis of the liver makes portal pressure noticeable with the various complications and impending dangers associated with it. Alcoholic liver disease, autoimmune hepatitis and hemochromatosis can all cause PHT even without cirrhosis. However, PHT secondary to

Table 1: Causes of PHT

Common causes	*Less common causes*
• Schistosomiasis • Cirrhosis • Extrahepatic portal vein thrombosis: - Hematologic disorders (polycythemia vera, myeloproliferative disorders) - Prothrombotic conditions (protein C, protein S antithrombin deficiency; antiphospholipid syndrome) - Paroxysmal nocturnal hemoglubinuria - Oral contraceptive use - Intra-abdominal neoplasms (GI adenocarcinomas) - Trauma (including postoperative state) - Intra-abdominal inflammations (pancreatitis, inflammatory bowel disease, diverticulitis) • Idiopathic PHT, Non-cirrhotic portal fibrosis (NCPF)	• Splanchnic arteriovenous fistula • Hereditary hemorrhagic telangiectasia • Sarcoidosis • Nodular regenerative hyperplasia • Fibropolycystic liver disease

PHT, portal hypertension; GI, gastrointestinal.

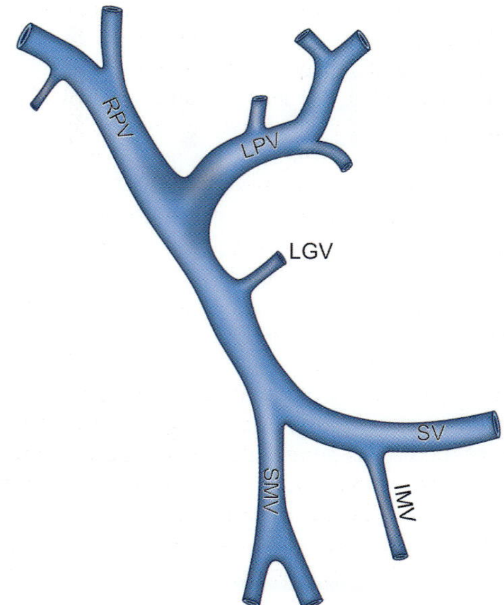

Figure 1 Portal vein
RPV, right portal vein, LPV, left portal vein, LGV, left gastric vein, SV, splenic vein, IMV, inferior mesenteric vein, SMV, superior mesenteric vein.

schistosomiasis probably is the second most common cause globally. It occurs due to the deposition of eggs of *Schistosoma mansoni* and *Schistosoma japonicum* in the presinusoidal portal venules, inducing a granulomatous inflammation around the area resulting in presinusoidal and periportal "clay pipe stem" or "pipe stem" fibrosis. Another commonly seen prehepatic, presinusoidal cause of PHT in the Indian population is extrahepatic portal vein thrombosis. Older studies have shown an incidence of portal vein thrombosis of 25% in patients with cirrhosis, whereas in non-cirrhotics it is confined to 6%. Non-cirrhotic portal Fibrosis, a condition similar to "idiopathic PHT" is diagnosed when the portal pressure is raised without any portal vein obstruction or significant hepatic histological changes like in cirrhosis. This phenomenon is rather commonly seen in the Asiatic countries and particularly in the Indian subcontinent. Other uncommon causes of PHT are mentioned in Table 1.

PORTAL CIRCULATION ANATOMY

Portal circulation is different from systemic venous system in that (a) it is devoid of valves, (b) starts with capillaries and ends with capillaries and (c) it is possible to decompress the system at any point by creating a connection to the systemic circulation. This valve less system allows it to accommodate high flow at low rates because of low resistance. It distributes blood from the spleen, pancreas, and the digestive tract to the liver. Portal vein is formed by the joining superior mesenteric veins (SMV) and splenic vein (SV) posterior to the neck of the pancreas at the level of the second lumbar vertebra in most of the patients. Inferior mesenteric vein (IMV) usually joins the SV (38%) and sometimes SMV (29%). In approximately one-third of the patients, portal vein is formed by SV, SMV, and IMV joining together (Fig. 1). Portal vein is approximately 5–9 cm in length, 0.6–1.2 cm width, with an average diameter of approximately 1 cm. in the hepatoduodenal ligament, it lies posterior to the hepatic artery and common bile duct, usually a little to the left of the duct. It then divides into right and left branches supplying right lobe and left lobe of the liver respectively. The caudate lobe is also supplied by two to three branches arising from the site of bifurcation or the right or left branches. This portal system is connected to the systemic system at various levels by small tributaries which can enlarge to form significant sized collaterals in the event of PHT. Portal vein provides 75% of the total blood flow to the liver and about 50% of its oxygen supply.

The most important of these connections (collaterals) are:
1. The coronary vein (connects esophago-cardiac venous plexus with splenic or portal vein)
2. The short gastric and the left gastro-epiploic (connects esophageal and gastric plexus to the splenic vein)
3. Retroperitoneal portal radicles (connects left renal vein via the left adrenal vein)
4. Umbilical and periumbilical veins connecting to the left portal vein
5. Inferior mesenteric vein connecting via the superior hemorrhoidal vein to the middle and inferior hemorrhoidal vein of the systemic circulation

Variations in portal vein:

1. Portal vein is rarely found anterior to the neck of the pancreas and duodenum.
2. Might directly drain into the vena cava.
3. Rarely, a pulmonary vein may enter the portal vein.
4. There may be a congenital absence of the left portal vein (right portal vein may curve around the liver on the right and supply the left lobe of the liver).
5. Right anterior sectoral vein may arise from the left portal vein.

PATHOPHYSIOLOGY

Varices are a consequence of PHT, which in most of the patients are secondary to the cirrhotic liver. This is attributed to a structural component and a dynamic component in cirrhotic liver. Structural component includes distortion of the liver microcirculation by fibrosis, nodule formation, angiogenesis, and vascular occlusion. Increased hepatic vascular tone owing to the contraction of activated hepatic stellate cells and myofibroblasts around the hepatic sinusoids and in the fibrous septa and of the vascular smooth muscle cells make the dynamic component. In less than 10% of the patients, it occurs due to obstruction of the outflow system like in portal venous thrombosis, non-cirhhotic portal fibrosis (NCPF), extrahepatic portal vein obstruction (EHPVO), Budd–Chiari syndrome, etc. However, in rare situations, idiopathic PHT can be seen in patients with hyperdynamic circulation. As a result, there will be splenomegaly, a hyperdynamic circulatory state and the growth of extensive collateral that shunt portal blood into the systemic circulation.

On an average 1500 mL of blood flows through the liver tissue per minute, which represents about 25% of the cardiac output. Two-thirds of the flow is contributed by the portal vein and one third by the hepatic artery. However, the oxygen supply to the liver is equally contributed by both the portal venous system and the hepatic artery. The portal venous flow is related to the splanchnic arterial flow and the hepatic arterial flow is regulated by the circulating catecholamines and the sympathetic nervous stimulation. The changes in the portal venous system which depend on the splanchnic arterial system are thus compensated by the relative changes in the hepatic arterial flow acting as a buffer. This buffer response of the hepatic artery is responsible in maintaining a constant flow of blood to the hepatic parenchyma.

Depending upon the level of obstruction, PHT can be divided into prehepatic (involves the spleno-portal-mesenteric venous systems), intrahepatic, and the posthepatic. Portal vein thrombosis is the main cause of prehepatic PHT and can present with acute or chronic thrombosis. Intrahepatic PHT can be further divided into presinusoidal, sinusoidal, and postsinusoidal depending on the level of obstruction. However, mixed scenarios are often seen in different conditions affecting the liver. Presinusoidal PHT is characterized by normal or slightly increased HVPG values and normal or slightly increased WHVP and a normal free hepatic venous pressure (FHVP) (Table 2).

The end result of the increasing pressures of the portal system is progressive increase in the size of varix with thinning out of the wall, and tendency to rupture when the pressures increase beyond a certain point. Hence measuring PHT becomes an important part of the evaluation so that management can be directed toward decreasing these pressures. Portal hypertension is best assessed by using the WHVP. It represents the perfusion pressure of the liver with portal blood. The probability of a varix rupturing is directly proportional to the pressure within the portal system and the wall tension. This depends on various factors like the size/diameter of the varix, thickness of the wall of the varix, and the pressure that is mounting within the varix. The three variables that are most predictive of variceal bleed are Child–Turcotte–Pugh (CTP) class, variceal size, and the presence of red wale marking on esophago-gastro-duodeno (EGD) scopy.

Increased splanchnic circulation in the advanced cirrhotic patients plays a major role in maintaining and aggravating PHT. This occurs secondary to marked splanchnic arteriolar vasodilatation and neoangiogenesis in response to an increased release of Vascular Endothelial Growth Factor (VEGF), nitric oxide, and other splanchnic vasodilators. This marked rise in splanchnic circulation results in the formation of ascites, systemic hypotension, renal dysfunction, and increased cardiac index.

HEMODYNAMICS IN PORTAL HYPERTENSION

The factors that influence the pressure in the portal system and the outcomes thereof, can be explained by three basic physical laws:

Ohm's law states that pressure is directly determined by the flow and the resistance to the flow within the blood vessel.

$$D_p = Q \times R$$

(D_p is change in pressure, Q is flow, R is resistance in the vessel)

Resistance itself is determined by other factors like the diameter of the vessel, viscosity of the fluid flowing through the vessel, and the length of the vessel. According to Poiseuille's law:

$$R = 8n\,L/\pi r^4$$

(R = resistance; n = coefficient of viscosity, L = length of the vessel, r = radius of the vessel)

The third law is the Laplace's law. According to Groszmann, the variceal wall tension can be explained by Laplace's law, which states that the tension on the wall is directly related to the transluminal pressure and radius of the vessel and indirectly related to the thickness of the wall.

$$T = \text{TP} \times r/w$$

(T = tension, TP = trans-luminal pressure, r = vessel radius, w = wall thickness).

Table 2: Hepatic venous pressure in various types of PHT

	HVPG	*WHVP*	*FHVP*	*Examples*
Prehepatic	N	N	N	Portal vein thrombosis, EHPVO, NCPF
Presinusoidal	N/↑	N/↑	N	Idiopathic PHT, nodular degenerative hyperplasia, schistosomiasis, sarcoidosis, tuberculosis, early primary biliary cirrhosis
Sinusoidal	↑↑	↑↑	N	Cirrhosis
Postsinusoidal	↑↑	↑↑	N	
Posthepatic	–	–	Hepatic vein cannot be cannulated	Heart failure Budd–Chiari syndrome

PHT, portal hypertension; HVPG, hepatic venous pressure gradient; WHVP, wedged hepatic venous pressure; FHVP, free hepatic venous pressure; EHPVO, extrahepatic portal vein obstruction; NCPF, non-cirhhotic portal fibrosis.

CLINICAL FEATURES

Ascites, which is the most common complication of PHT secondary to cirrhosis is less commonly seen with presinusoidal PHT in both cirrhotic and non-cirrhotic livers. The median survival of patients with ascites in cirrhosis is only 50% over 2 years.[6]

Measurement of Portal Pressure

Indirect and direct means have been described for the measurement of portal pressure. They include direct measurement of the portal vein pressure, splenic pulp pressure, endoscopic variceal pressure, HVPG, ultrasound fibroelastography, and magnetic resonance elastography. The most commonly used and most validated method for predicting the development of complications of PHT is HVPG, which is an indirect method.

Hepatic Vein Pressure Gradient

The HVPG is defined as the difference between the WHVP and free hepatic vein pressure. It represents the gradient between the pressure in the portal vein and the intra-abdominal inferior vena cava (IVC) pressure. Measurement of HVPG is not altered by increase in the intra-abdominal pressure and variations in the zero reference point have no impact on HVPG. Disadvantages are, values may be altered with fibrosis grade in the lobe of the liver which is being drained by the wedged vein and it underestimates sinusoidal pressures in primary biliary cirrhosis and other presinusoidal cause of PHT.

At present, measurement of HVPG is indicated in the following situations:

1. To monitor effectiveness of medical therapy as prophylaxis and as an end point in trials in which they are used for the treatment of PHT
2. To monitor prognosis in patients with cirrhosis and acute alcoholic hepatitis
3. To assess the risk of hepatic resection in patients with cirrhosis. Hepatectomy is contraindicated when HVPG is >10 mmHg due to high risk of irreversible hepatic decompensation within 3 months.[7] To delineate the cause of PHT with a combination of other modalities like venography, right-sided heart pressure measurements, and transjugular liver biopsy
4. Evaluation of progression and regression of chronic liver disease [e.g., in chronic viral hepatitis, HCV recurrence after liver transplantation, evaluation of portal pressure gradient after transjugular intrahepatic portosystemic shunt (TIPS) placement]

Hepatic vein pressure gradient allows the physician in identifying the responders to nonspecific β-blockers (NSBB) prophylaxis, in prognostication and planning the therapeutic intervention, in patients with PHT. Hence, in the centers where adequate expertise and resources are available, HVPG measurements should be routinely done. Target of effective prophylactic medical therapy should be a HVPG of ≤12 mmHg or a drop of at least 20% from the baseline HVPG.[1] Patients with a 10% drop in HVPG or a HVPG of ≤12 mmHg following treatment with NSBB (propranolol) are considered responders (Tables 3 and 4).

Table 3: HVPG and its significance

Value	*Significance*
≤5 mmHg	Normal portal pressure
6–9 mmHg	Subclinical PHT
≥10 mmHg	Clinically significant Varices appear Risk of PHT related complications.[8]
>12 mmHg	Variceal bleeding risk increases
>16 mmHg	Increased mortality risk in patients with previous decompensation.[9]
>20 mmHg	Predicts failure to control bleeding during acute bleeding when measure within 48 h.[10] Low 1-year survival.[11]

HVPG, hepatic vein pressure gradient; PHT, portal hypertension.

Table 4: Methods of measuring portal pressure

	Use	*Remarks*
Splenic pulp pressure	Presinusoidal PHT	Indirect method Rarely used Potential high risk for bleeding
Portal vein pressure	Posthepatic PHT, Intrahepatic presinusoidal PHT	Direct method e.g., Budd–Chiari syndrome, Idiopathic PHT
Endoscopic variceal pressure	Prehepatic, presinusoidal PHT	Direct method It is measurement of the difference between the intravariceal pressure and pressure within the esophageal lumen

PHT, portal hypertension.

METHODS TO DETECT VARICES

Varices are detected commonly with either endoscopy or by imaging in practice. A combination of international normalized ratio (INR) >1.5, a portal vein diameter of >13 mm and thrombocytopenia are proposed to predict the presence of varices in patients with cirrhosis. The success rate of predicting varices has been <10, 20–50, 40–60, and >90% when none, one, two, or all these of these conditions are met.[12] However, it should be noted that 10% of the UGI bleed in patients with known PHT, is due to causes other than varices. Upper gastrointestinal endoscopy is the most commonly used method and is also most effective screening tool in either case. At present radiological investigations cannot be recommended as screening tools for detecting varices in PHT. Capsule endoscopy and computed tomography (CT) are considered alternatives for screening in patients who are not candidates for endoscopy.

Defining the Varices Based on Endoscopic Findings

Grading varices on endoscopy is quite subjective. Various descriptors are used in defining the varices like size, site, form (tortuous, straight, beady, nodular), location (upper, middle, lower third of the esophagus, gastric—diffuse, fundal), red color signs (red wale markings, cherry-red spots, hematocytic spots, diffuse redness), and portal gastropathy. Usually esophageal varices are graded as shown in Table 5.[13]

Varices are considered small when they are <5 mm in diameter and large when they are >5 mm in diameter (Baveno IV classification). Patients with large varices, Child's C status, and red color signs have the highest risk of variceal bleeding at the end of 1 year.

Gastric varices are less common than the esophageal varices with an incidence of 10–20% of varices. Though most commonly seen with esophageal varices, gastric varices can present without esophageal varices and should raise the suspicion of left sided PHT secondary to SV thrombosis. Of note, these gastric bleeds are especially difficult to control, difficult to treat with high recurrence and mortality rates. Most often, gastroesophageal varices (GOV) are just extension of the gastric varices on to the esophagus and are subclassified based on Sarin's classification (Table 6).

As 10% of the bleeds are non-variceal origin, it is suggested that a bleed should be attributed to varices only when a bleeding varix is identified on EGD which is the case in approximately 25% of the cases or when moderate to large size varices are identified on EGD scope with no other lesions in patients who had a recent episode of major UGI bleed which is defined as loss of more than 2 units of blood.

Portal hypertensive gastropathy can present in a mosaic pattern (mild grade) or with red-point lesions, cherry-red spots or black-brown spots (severe grade). It is more often seen in body and fundus of the stomach and is due to increased gastric mucosal perfusion (hyperemia). Though incidence is unknown, its prevalence increases with eradication of esophageal varices. Gastric antral vascular ectasia (GAVE) is characterized by red patches and spots in a diffuse or linear pattern in the gastric antrum, gastric ectasia, and dilatation. Gastric antral vascular ectasia is a nonspecific feature of PHT, with only 30% of the GAVE cases seen in the presence of PHT.

Table 5: Grading of esophageal varices

Grade I	Small and straight, collapse but do not disappear with insufflations
Grade II	Tortuous and occupying less than one-third of the esophageal lumen (>5 mm in diameter)
Grade III	Large and occupying more than one-third of the esophageal lumen

Table 6: Grading of gastric varices

GOV1	Most common Extend along the lesser curvature Can bleed at relatively low HVPG
GOV2	Extend from esophageal varices along the fundus
IGV1	Isolated gastric varices located on the fundus alone Can bleed at relatively low HVPG
IGV2	Isolated gastric varices located in the body, antrum, and along the pylorus Can bleed at relatively low HVPG

HVPG, hepatic venous pressure gradient; GOV1, Gastroesophageal varices Type I; GOV2, Gastroesophageal varices Type II; IGV1, isolated gastric varices Type I; IGV2, isolated gastric varices Type II.

Ultrasonography

When combined with Doppler, the features that are suggestive of PHT are splenomegaly, collateral vessels between the portal and systemic circulation, and reversal of flow direction (hepatofugal) in the portal vein (normal is hepatopetal). Other nonspecific features suggestive of PHT are a portal vein diameter >13 mm and the absence of respiratory variations in the splenic and the mesenteric veins. It is also useful in detecting portal venous thrombosis, SV thrombosis, and the cavernous transformation of the portal vein. Though useful in the initial evaluation of PHT, it is limited by lack of quantitative assessment in follow up after initiating the therapy. Endoscopy combined with ultrasonography (endoultrasound) is the most sensitive method to diagnose esophageal varices, as insufflation during a regular EGD scope may compress small varices resulting in a negative study. Transient elastography may be useful, but cannot be recommended at present.

COMPUTED TOMOGRAPHY

Computed tomography is establishing its role not only in identifying the abnormal configuration of liver and other organs, but also in the identification of ascites, collateral vessels, and early esophageal varices. It is valuable in differentiating submucosal from pergastric fundal varices. Though it is noninvasive and at least as reliable as endoscopic ultrasonography in the detection of varices, it is not recommended as a screening method as it is not cost-effective and does not reach therapeutic requirements.

Magnetic Resonance Imaging

Gadolinium enhanced magnetic resonance imaging (MRI), is increasingly being used for the measurement of azygous and portal blood flow, portal venous thrombosis, spleen stiffness and gives excellent details of the hepatic vasculature. It can also accurately measure the stiffness of fatty liver.

Endoscopic Ultrasonography

Its main uses are in measuring the variceal cross structure to identify patients at increased risk of bleeding, to note the changes after the endoscopic therapy, recurrence after treatment with band ligation and in measuring the size and flow of left gastric vein, azygous vein, and paraesophageal collaterals. When combined with endoscopic measurement of transmural variceal pressure, it allows prediction of bleeding by estimating variceal wall tension.

MANAGEMENT OF VARICES

Preprimary Prophylaxis

As a HVWP ≥10 mmHg is predictive of formation of varices and the clinical course of the patients with cirrhosis,[14] all the patients should undergo a screening EGD at the time of diagnosis of cirrhosis. Presence or absence of varices, in the esophagus, and stomach is then noted. When present, these varices should be graded using any standard classification system American Association for Study of Liver Disease (AASLD suggests small, medium, and large based on the size). However, it is suggested that the character of these varices should be noted down in detail as these classification systems are bound to change with the understanding of this disease. Size, location, number, shape, presence, or absence of red wale markings or red signs should all be noted down in detail.

A preprimary prophylaxis involves the prevention of the formation of the varices. Such a strategy helps us in preventing the development of complications associated with PHT. This group includes patients with cirrhosis and without GOV. Patients with varices at other sites are not included. In case of compensated cirrhosis with no varices, EGD should be repeated every 3 years as the incidence of esophageal varices is 5–10% per year in this patient group, whereas, in decompensated cirrhotic patients with no varices, EGD is recommended every year. If varices are found on surveillance EGD, it should be managed according to the grade of varices. However, in these patients treatment is mainly directed toward the management of the disease liver to prevent further damage to the liver and to delay the onset of complications associated with it. There is no indication at this point of time, with regard to the need to use β-blockers in preventing the formation of varices. Measuring HVPG is only recommended in the context of clinical trials in the Baveno V consensus.

Management of Non-bleeding Varices (Primary Prophylaxis)

The main goals in the management of the incidentally found varices at the time of evaluation of recently diagnosed cirrhotic patients or varices that are identified during surveillance EGD scope of a previously diagnosed cirrhotic on follow up, is prevention of the first episode of bleeding, delay the progression of varices and eradicate them. When these goals can be achieved, associated mortality and morbidity from a bleeding varix can be decreased. Prognosis and management of patients with cirrhotic liver and non-bleeding varices depends on the grade of the varices, level of decompensation of the liver (Child's class) and associated comorbidities. Patients with small varices at the esophago-gastric junction (EGJ) can be arbitrarily divided into low risk (Child's A/B) and increased risk (Child's C, presence of red wale marks on varices) bleed groups.

Low-risk group with small varices at EGJ may be treated with NSBB with intent to prevent the progression of varices and bleeding. Whereas high-risk group of patients have an increased risk of bleeding and hence should be started with NSBB. As all the patients with medium to large size varices at EGJ have a higher risk of bleeding, these patients should receive treatment either with β-blockers of endoscopic variceal ligation (EVL), subject to the availability of resources and expertise, patient's preference and characteristics, tolerability to the medical therapy, and contraindications to the modality of treatment selected. Combination therapy (NSBB, isosorbide-5-mononitrate, spironolactone, EVL) is not supported by enough data to be supported at this moment. Though specific data on gastric varices is not available, NSBB's are recommended in primary prophylaxis.

Management of Bleeding Varices

When the patient presents for the first time with upper GI bleed he should be managed as described below, and once the acute situation is tided over, he should undergo the assessment for the cirrhotic liver and PHT-associated complications.

Resuscitation

On presentation to the emergency room, the standard airway, breathing, circulation of the patient are managed to achieve hemodynamic stability. Two large bore (18G) intravenous cannulas should be placed and resuscitation started after taking the blood for analysis which includes the hemogram, liver function test, coagulation profile, and blood cross matching. Adequate blood (minimum of 6 units) should be reserved for transfusion. A urinary catheter is secured and patient intubated in case of severe hypovolemic shock, encephalopathy, or when other high-risk factors are present. Inotropes and vasopressors are also started as required to maintain adequate mean arterial pressure (MAP) for maintaining adequate perfusion to the vital organs. Patient is then shifted immediately to a high dependency unit or an intensive care unit as required. The main goal of the resuscitation should be to preserve tissue perfusion. Volume resuscitation is initiated with crystalloids and packed red blood cell (PRBC) transfusion is done conservatively at a target hemoglobin level between 7–8 g/dL.[15] Over enthusiastic correction should not be attempted, as higher blood pressure would only result in further increase in blood loss as it can increase the portal pressure.[16] A MAP aimed at 60 mmHg with a systolic pressure above 100 mmHg has been the target in our institute in such patients. Patients with systemic diseases like diabetes and cardiac issues deteriorate fast and fail to mount appropriate response with acute blood loss. Hence, these patients need to be more aggressively resuscitated.

Prophylactic antibiotics should be started in patients with cirrhosis as UGI bleeds precipitate encephalopathy in these patients due to altered NH_3 metabolism. Oral quinolones are recommended in general. However, intravenous ceftriaxone is given in patients with advanced cirrhosis, in patients on previous quinolone prophylaxis and in hospital settings with high prevalence of quinolone-resistant bacterial infections. Vasoactive agents like terlipressin, somatostatin, octreotide, and vapreotide are started in suspected cases of cirrhosis. Prophylactic measures to prevent hepatic encephalopathy are usually started. Measures are taken by adequately hydrating the patient to prevent or precipitate renal failure.

Once the patient is stabilized, prognostication is done by measuring the HVPG, determining the Child's status, calculating the model for end-stage liver disease (MELD) score and by performing an EGD score to identify any active bleeding, and risk factors for recurrent bleeding. Hepatic venous pressure gradient ≥20 mmHg, active hemorrhage at endoscopy and Child–Pugh class C consistently associated with 5-day treatment failure. Whereas a Child–Pugh class C, MELD score ≥18, and failure to control bleeding/early rebleeding in the hospital reliably predict 6-week mortality. This warrants an early EGD scopy with therapeutic intention (preferably within 12 hours) after admission in all the patients with UGI bleeding and any evidence of cirrhosis.

Management of Bleed

An early endoscopy should be planned preferably within 12 hours of admission into the emergency department. Endoscopic variceal ligation is the treatment of choice in any acute variceal bleeding. Sclerotherapy is now only recommended in difficult cases of EVL. For isolated gastric varices (IGV) and gastroesophageal varices Type II (GOV2) type of gastric varices, endoscopic therapy with tissue adhesive is recommended. For gastroesophageal varices Type I (GOV1), both EVL and tissue adhesive can be tried. All patients with high risk for treatment failure should be considered for TIPS within 72 hours after they have received initial treatment with pharmacological agents and endoscopic therapy. These patients include those with CTP C with score of <14 and CTP B with active bleeding. The role of balloon tamponade has faded with the advent of effective pharmacological agents and improving endoscopic techniques. However, it still provides a temporary bridge until definitive treatment can be instituted in certain situations. Self-expanding covered metal stents may be useful in refractory cases.

Management of Treatment Failure

Baveno V definitions and criteria for failure to control bleeding[17]

1. The time frame for the acute bleeding episode should be 120 hours (5 days).
2. Failure is defined as death or need to change therapy defined by one of the following criteria:
   a. Fresh hematemesis or nasogastric (NG) aspiration of ≥100 mL of fresh blood ≥2 h after the start of a specific drug treatment or therapeutic endoscopy.
   b. Development of hypovolemic shock
   c. Drop of 3 g in hemoglobin (9% drop in hematemesis) within any 24-hour period if no transfusion is administered. This time frame need to be further validated.
   d. The potential value of an index of blood transfusion requires prospective validation.

The best timing for the measurement of hematocrit and hemoglobin and the ideal cut off value of adjusted blood requirement index (ABRI) score needs to be further validated. The transfusion target should be a hematocrit of 24% or hemoglobin of 7–8 g/dL. These targets should take into the consideration other comorbidities the patients suffering fr om, age, hemodynamic status and the ongoing bleeding. At present there is no available data to recommend management aspects of coagulability and thrombocytopenia in these patients. Any standard protocol that addresses the correction of coagulability and thrombocytopenia can be followed. A second attempt with endoscopy is warranted in these patients within the first 5 days. When failed, these patients are best managed by TIPS with covered PTFE stents.

Pharmacologic Agents

Pharmacologic agents that are used in PHT act in different mechanisms and hence divided into two groups with the ultimate goal to reduce the portal pressure. The first group includes the drugs that act by decreasing the portal blood flow and include nonselective β-adrenergic blocking agents, vasopressin, and somatostatin and its analogues. The second group act by decreasing the intrahepatic resistance to the blood flow and include α_1-adrenergic blocking agents (e.g., prazocin), angiotensin receptor blocking agents and the nitrates (Table 7).

Endoscopic Therapy

Crawford and Frenckner in 1939 for the first time performed sclerotherapy. For the past many years, endoscopic therapy has been at the center stage in the prevention and control of acute and rebleeding from the varices. Both sclerotherapy and EVL are accepted modalities in the management of varices. However, EVL has been proved to have definite edge over sclerotherapy in many situations. In acute bleeding, both the sclerotherapy and EVL are equally efficacious in controlling the bleed with a success rate of about 80–90% and a rebleed rate of 20–50%. Endoscopic variceal ligation has been established as the endoscopic modality of choice in the control of acute bleeding and eradication of the varices. The incidence of complications associated with sclerotherapy precludes its use as a first line therapy in variceal bleeding (Table 8). Current indications for sclerotherapy include failure of EVL due to poor visualization due to bleeding varices. Though many sclerosants are available in the market no sclerosant is superior to the other. Some of them are sodium tetradecyl sulfate, sodium morrhuate, ethanolamine oleate, and absolute alcohol.

Balloon Tamponade

Balloon tamponade was first introduced by Westphal in 1930. Since then its role in the management of acute variceal bleed has taken noticeable changes. However, at present its role is limited to immediate cessation of the acute bleed and buying time for interventional radiological techniques and surgery, when pharmacological drugs and endoscopy have failed to control the bleed. High recurrent bleed rates (more than 50%) and high complication rates are responsible for this paradigm shift in the usage of balloon. Considerable discomfort, esophageal perforation, ischemic necrosis of the esophagus, airway obstruction, and aspiration are all mentioned following the usage of balloon tamponade. Various types of balloon tubes are available (Table 9).

Transjugular Intrahepatic Portosystemic Shunt

Transjugular intrahepatic portosystemic shunt was first performed by Rosch in 1969 in animals and Colapinto in humans in 1983. Transjugular intrahepatic portosystemic shunt principally acts by deploying a stent between the hepatic vein and the intrahepatic portal vein branch, thus reducing the pressure in the portal system. Technically it is a side-to-side portocaval shunt with a mortality of less than 1–2% with a success rate up to 95% in deploying the stent. However, a stenosis rate of 20–78% has been noted. Decreased stenosis rates have been achieved with the use of coated stents (Viatorr, Gore, Flagstaff, Arizona). Wall stent and the Palmatz stents have been used in the past with higher stenosis rates. Doppler ultrasound has a low negative predictive value and a high positive predictive value in identifying the stenosis. Recurrence of the problem that necessitated TIPS is the predictor for stenosis and can be confirmed with TIPS venogram and measurement of the portocaval pressure gradient. Transjugular intrahepatic portosystemic shunt is associated with considerable complications as shown in Table 10.

Table 7: Pharmacological agents used in lowering portal pressure		
Drug	*Mechanism of action*	*Remarks*
Vasopressin (endogenous peptide hormone)	Splanchnic vasoconstriction	Kenhe in 1956 has first discovered vasopressin Side effects: ischemia and necrosis of the bowel, direct negative inotropic and chronotropic effects on the myocardium decreasing the cardiac output and causing bradycardia, hypertension and coronary vasoconstriction, antidiuresis resulting in hyponatremia
Terlipressin (semisynthetic analogue of vasopressin)	Splanchnic vasoconstriction	Lower systemic side effects compared to vasopressin. Superior safety profile Increases in survival
Somatostatin	Inhibits release of glucagon thus decreasing portal blood flow	Short acting Also decreases postprandial portal blood flow decreasing portal pressure
Octreotide	Inhibits release of glucagon thus decreasing portal blood flow	Analogue of somatostatin Equivalent in effect to somatostatin Longer acting (80–120 min) Does not affect portal pressure despite decreasing postprandial portal blood flow
Vaptreotide		Analogue of somatostatin Improved control of bleeding without reduction in the survival rates
NSBBs (e.g., propranolol, nadolol)	Decreases cardiac output (β_1 blockade) Decreased portal flow (β_2 blockade)	Nadolol—excreted predominantly by kidneys, low lipid solubility, low risk of central nervous system side effects
Nitrates	Decreasing portal flow by causing veno-dilatation	Hypotension is the main side effect. Seldom used in PHTOnly role is in secondary prophylaxis in combination with NSBBs to lower HVPG appropriately
Prazosin	Vasoconstriction	Worsening of systemic hyperdynamic circulation with long term treatment Sodium retention and ascites
Losartan, irbesartan	Angiotensin type II receptor antagonist	
Simvastatin	Liver selective NO release decreasing intrahepatic resistance	

Table 8: Comparison of sclerotherapy and EVL	
Sclerotherapy	*EVL*
Complications: • During injection—retrosternal discomfort, chest pain • Sclerosant-induced esophageal ulcer-related bleeding, stricture and perforation • Mediastinitis • Systemic complications like mesenteric venous thrombosis, pulmonary embolism, sepsis, aspiration pneumonitis, portal vein thrombosis • Worsening of bleed • 1–3% of mortality	Complications: • Esophageal ulcer, strictures, dysmotility
Advantages over EVL: • Useful during active bleeding when visibility is poor • Can be used in fundal varices as a substitute to glue	Advantages over sclerotherapy include: • Fewer complication rates than sclerotherapy • Simpler to perform than injection • EVL during bleeding is not associated with sustained increase in the HVPG

EVL, endoscopic variceal ligation; HVPG, hepatic venous pressure gradient.

The main use of TIPS has been in acute bleeding after failure of endoscopic and medical management and in patients with rebleeding and are refractory to medical therapy and endoscopic therapy. It is also considered as a bridging procedure for the patients waiting for transplant with refractory ascites, hydrothorax, Budd-Chiari syndrome and hepatorenal syndrome as well, particularly in patients with Child's B or C status. Transjugular intrahepatic portosystemic shunt is successful in controlling bleeding in up

Table 9: Types of balloons

Type	*Balloon type*	*Remarks*
Sengstaken–Blakemore tube	Esophageal + gastric balloon	Allows gastric aspiration but not esophagus. A Ryle's tube need to be attached for esophageal aspiration
Minnesota tube	Esophageal + gastric balloon	Provision for esophageal and gastric aspiration
Linton–Nicholas tube	Gastric balloon only	Provision for esophageal and gastric aspiration

Table 10: TIPS-related complications

Local: Hematoma locally at the puncture site Pain Carotid artery puncture **Stent related:** Shunt thrombosis Stent migration Shunt stenosis **Liver related:** Hepatic encephalopathy Progressive hepatic failure Portal vein thrombosis	**Systemic:** Fever Cardiac arrhythmias Hemolytic anemia Pulmonary artery hypertension Reactions to contrast media Cardiopulmonary failure Intraperitoneal hemorrhage Sepsis

TIPS, transjugular intrahepatic portosystemic shunt.

to 90% of the patients with acute esophageal or refractory gastric variceal bleed. However, the rate of encephalopathy is much higher in patients undergoing TIPS, in comparison with endoscopic therapy. Absolute contraindications for performing TIPS are high INR (>1.4), low platelets (<60,000), right-sided heart failure and polycystic liver disease. Other relative contraindications include portal vein thrombosis, hyper-vascular liver tumors and encephalopathy. Table 11 compares TIPS with other therapeutic options in the control of acute variceal bleeding.

Secondary Prophylaxis

Secondary prophylaxis is started in all patients from day 6 of the index variceal bleed. At present, NSBB with EVL with an eradication attitude is the standard of care in these patients. This combination therapy has a lesser rebleeding rates as compared with any one individual therapeutic modality. Hemodynamic response to NSBB provides information about rebleeding risk and the survival at 1 year. In nonresponders to NSBB's, isosorbide mono nitrate can be added, and this has been shown to be efficacious. Combination drug therapy is also recommended in patients who are not fit to undergo EVL and those who are unwilling to undergo EVL. There is also a group of patients who are either intolerant to the medical therapy or medical therapy is contraindicated, and EVL is offered as the sole therapy in this group. Transjugular intrahepatic portosystemic shunt is only offered as a bridging therapy in those patients who are to undergo liver transplantation or in those who fail to respond to a combination of medical therapy and EVL. In the end, transplantation is the only mode of treatment which gives a solution to both the cause and effect of the disease. In patients with IGV1 or GOV2, endoscopic glue therapy or TIPS can be offered. Patients with GOV1 may be treated with endoscopic glue therapy, EVL or NSBB. Portal hypertensive gastropathy is best managed with NSBBs. In patients in whom NSBBs are contraindicated, TIPS or surgical shunts should be considered. Management strategy after the index bleed is shown in Flow chart 1.

Baveno V defines failure of secondary prophylaxis as any single episode of rebleeding which is significant from any of the portal hypertensive sources after day 5 of index bleed. Bleed is considered significant in case of recurrent melena or hematemesis resulting in any of the following:

1. Hospital admission
2. Blood transfusion
3. Drop of 3 g in hemoglobin
4. Death within 6 weeks

Table 11: Comparison between pharmacological, endoscopic, balloon tamponade, and TIPS in the control of acute bleeding

Treatment modality	*Success rates (%)*	*Mortality (%)*	*Recurrence of bleeding (%)*
Pharmacological	80–90	1–3	
Balloon tamponade	80–90	20	50
Endoscopic sclerotherapy + EVL	80–90	1–3	20–50
TIPS	95	1–2	

TIPS, transjugular intrahepatic portosystemic shunt.

PROPHYLACTIC THERAPY IN PATIENTS WITH PORTAL HYPERTENSION

Algorithm for prophylactic therapy in patients with PHT (Flow chart 2).

ROLE OF SURGERY

Even though portosystemic shunts are the most effective means of controlling PHT and preventing portal hypertensive bleed, they are not without any adverse effects. Due to the diversion of hepatotrophic hormones and nutrients either completely or partially, these patients prone for hepatic failure and other adverse events like encephalopathy. In fact, the most common cause of death in patients who undergo a nonselective shunt is hepatic failure. These shunt procedures can be divided into nonselective, selective, and devascularization techniques depending on whether they are going to completely or partially decompress the portal venous system or compartmentalize the system.

Nonselective Shunts

Blakemore is credited with performing portocaval shunts for the first time in a clinical setting for bleeding varices in 1935. Vidal in 1903 first performed a portocaval shunt for ascites. It was Eck in 1877 who performed a portocaval shunt for the first time in dogs, which was an end-to-side nonselective shunt (Fig. 2A). Other nonselective shunts are variants of side-to-side portocaval shunt (Fig. 2B) and are usually more than 10 mm in size. They include

Flow chart 1 Management strategy after the index bleed

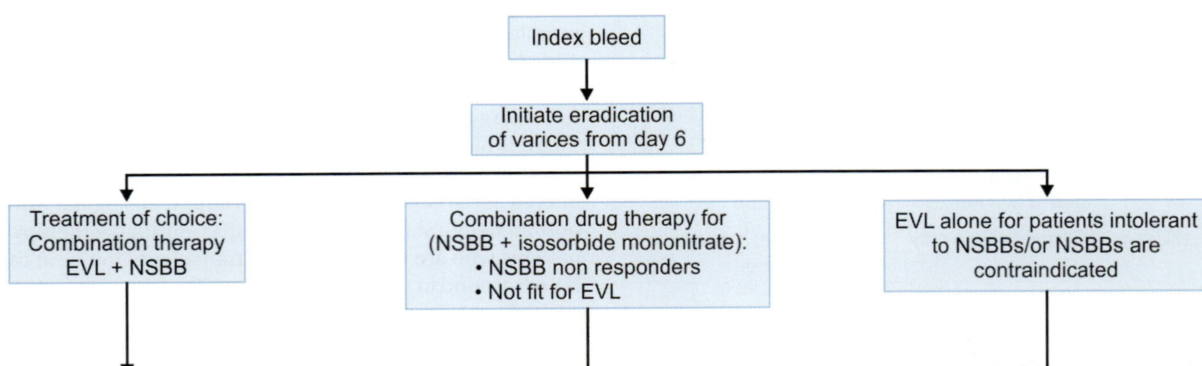

Flow chart 2 Management strategy of prophylactic therapy

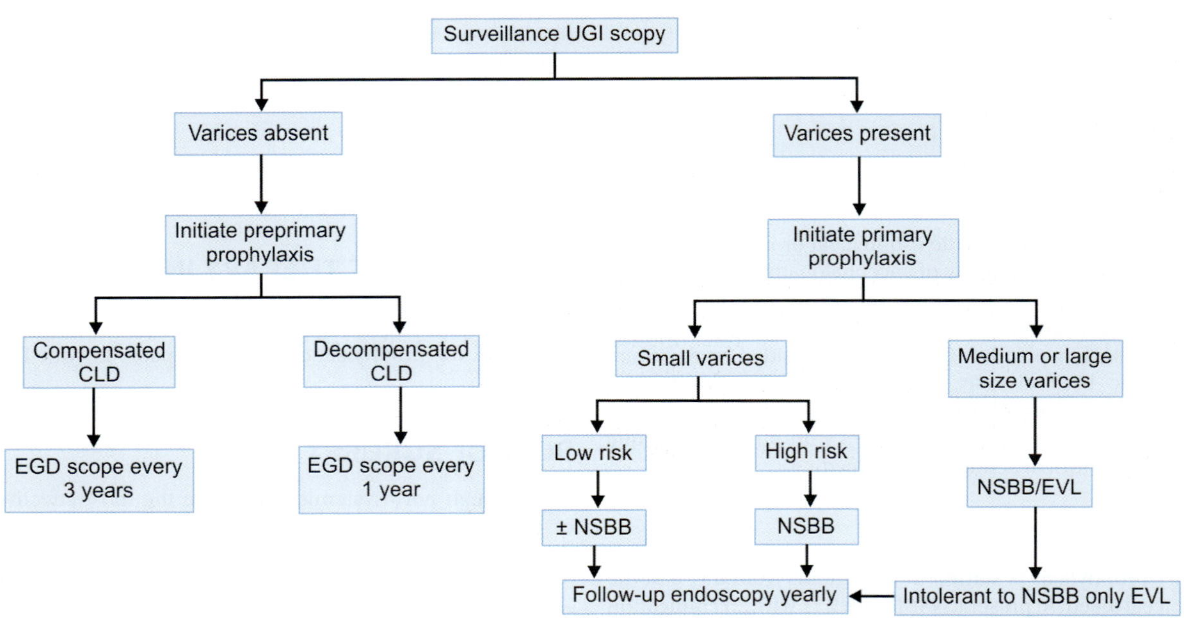

a side-to-side portocaval shunt, large diameter interposition shunt (H - graft shunt), the mesocaval C graft shunt, and the conventional proximal splenorenal shunt (Linton shunt) (Fig. 4). Encephalopathy occurs with a frequency of up to 20–40% in patients undergoing a shunt procedure. By decompressing the portal system and diverting majority of blood from the portal system into the systemic circulation, thus decongesting the intestines, nonselective shunts are very effective in the control of ascites and variceal bleed as well. A major disadvantage of interposition shunts is higher graft thrombosis in the late postoperative period, to the rate of 35%. To overcome this autologous vein grafts have been used. What makes this procedure appealing is the ease at construction, making future transplantation easy by avoiding the porta, and in the event of development of encephalopathy, these shunts can be easily occluded. The small caliber of the proximal SV in proximal splenorenal shunt (PSRS) makes these shunts vulnerable for early shunt thrombosis. The main advantage of this procedure is that hypersplenism is eliminated with splenectomy which is invariable with PSRS (Figs 2A and B).

Indications for nonselective shunts:

1. Failure of medical and endoscopic management for variceal bleed in the acute setting
2. In patients with both variceal bleed and intractable ascites
3. As a bridge to transplantation in patients in whom variceal bleeding is not controlled by either endoscopic management or TIPS.
4. Bleeding from PHG unresponsive to pharmacotherapy
5. Budd–Chiari syndrome with occluded hepatic veins and a patent inferior vena cava (IVC)

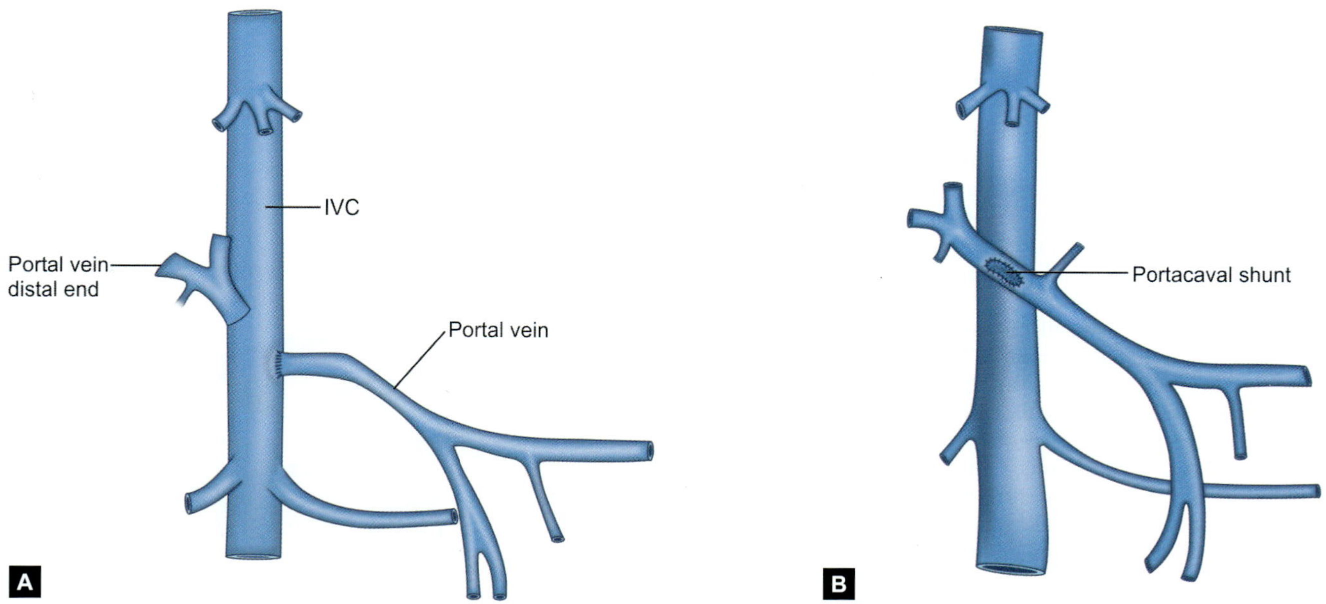

Figures 2A and B (A) End-to-side portocaval shunt; (B) Side-to-side portocaval shunt

Selective Shunts

Selective shunts are devised to counteract the shortcomings of the nonselective shunts. The most popular among these is distal splenorenal shunt (DSRS). Distal splenorenal shunt was introduced by Warren in 1967, followed by left gastric venacaval shunt by Inokuchi in 1968. Other selective shunts are the Rex shunt (mesenterico left portal vein bypass), splenocaval shunt (Basu shunt), and mesenterico caval shunt. As all these result in partial diversion of the portal flow, the incidence of the adverse effects associated with selective shunts due to the diversion of hepatotrophic hormones and the nutrients are less. However, these are not emergency procedures, as portal pressure is not controlled to a level to arrest bleeding immediately after the reconstruction of shunt (Figs 3A and B).

Distal Splenorenal Shunt

Probably DSRS is the most commonly performed selective shunt after it was introduced by Warren in 1967. In this, all the collateral vessels connecting the superior mesenteric component and the gastro-splenic component of the splanchnic circulation are disconnected and the distal end of the SV is anastomosed to the left renal vein. Variations include DSRS with spleno-pancreatic disconnection and the distal splenocaval shunt. As the gastro-splenic component is selectively decompressed, mesenteric system is still under high pressure, and maintains hepatic perfusion at the same time thus decreasing the adverse effects of the nonselective shunts. This will translate to 85% preservation of the hepatic flow from the portal venous system. However, as the patients develop collaterals between the high-pressure mesenteric system to the

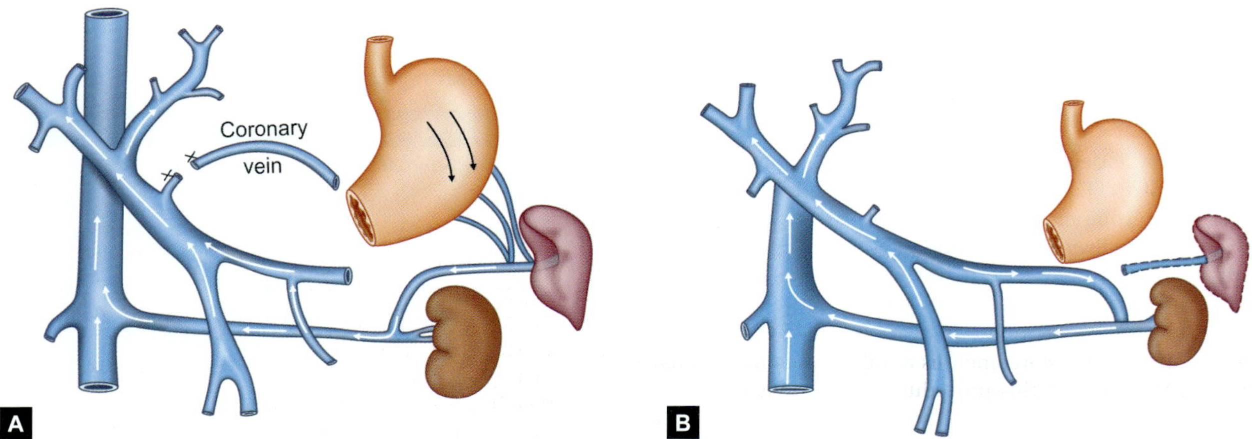

Figures 3A and B (A) Distal spleno-renal shunt; (B) Proximal spleno-renal shunt

shunt, 50% of the DSRS become nonselective by the end of 1 year. So, for DSRS to be effective for a longer duration, extensive devascularization of the collateral connecting the superior mesenteric component to the gastro-splenic component should be carried out during the shunt procedure and should include the coronary vein also. Though technically very demanding, the pancreatic siphon which results in late failure of these cases can be delayed by spleno-pancreatic disconnection. It has also been shown that collateral form rapidly between the portal flow and shunt in patients with ethanol-related cirrhosis when compared to nonalcoholic liver cirrhosis.

As it involves extensive dissection of the area, and an intact high-pressure mesenteric system in cirrhotic patients with high sinusoidal pressure, it might result in the aggravation of ascites. Prior splenectomy and medically intractable ascites are absolute contraindication for this procedure. Small diameter of the SV (<7 mm) is a relative contraindication for DSRS because of higher rates of shunt thrombosis. Patients with transient ascites following an acute insult can still undergo DSRS. However, there is no survival advantage in patients undergoing DSRS in comparison to that of the nonselective shunts in alcoholic cirrhotic patients. The incidence of recurrent bleed is however the same and that of the hepatic encephalopathy has been shown to be less in three randomized controlled trials. Distal splenorenal shunt has been shown to have some survival advantage and low encephalopathy rates, thus increasing the quality of life in patients with nonalcoholic cirrhosis or non-cirrhotic PHT.

Distal splenorenal shunt has definitive advantage over endoscopic therapy in that even though the incidence of encephalopathy in both the groups is same, the rate of recurrent bleed is less in DSRS and thus there is definite survival advantage with improved quality of life. This should probably be offered to all the patients when indicated, particularly is semi-urban and rural population where access to immediate skilled endoscopist is difficult. When compared with TIPS, which acts like a side-to-side nonselective shunt, DSRS has definite advantage with regards to encephalopathy rates, rebleeding rates, and shunt thrombosis rates.

Inokuchi Shunt

As proposed by Inokuchi from Japan, selective decompression of the gastro-esophageal varices by creating a shunt between the coronary vein and the vena cava (left gastric venacaval shunt) is done. An operative mortality of 3% with a rebleeding rate of 8% has been described.

Partial Shunts

As described by Sarfeh, a small 8–10 mm interposition portocaval shunt made of PTFE can achieve the same goal as total shunt, which is the decompression of the varices while preserving the portal flow to the liver unlike in the total shunt. Partial shunt is performed by devascularization of the collaterals followed by anastomosing a PTFE graft of 10 mm or less between the portal venous system and the systemic circulation (IVC). As the hepatic blood flow is preserved in more than 80% with a 8 mm graft and more than 50% with a 10 mm graft, there has been lower frequency of encephalopathy (10–15%) in these patients than that of the patients who underwent nonselective and selective shunts.

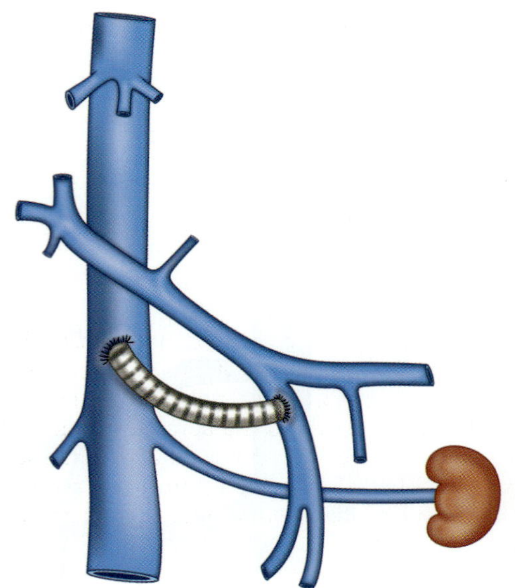

Figure 4 Meso-caval (graft) shunt

However, the survival rates remain the same and the control of the variceal bleeding has been the same. As these shunts are of larger diameter than that of TIPS, they have lower overall failure rates, with stenosis rates approaching 20% (Fig. 4).

Nonshunt Operations

The modalities that are described for nonshunt surgery in PHT, has only one main objective—compartmentalization of the portal flow. This is achieved by either extensive interruption of collateral vessels between high-pressure portal venous components or ablation of the varices. One exception is the left-sided PHT in which case a splenectomy is done (Table 12).

The possible indications for these nonshunt procedures include:

1. Failed medical and endoscopic therapy in patients with ongoing or recurrent variceal bleedingExtensive thrombosis of the splenic and mesenteric veins, precluding shunt procedure
2. Patients with high risk for encephalopathy following a shunt procedure

Table 12: Nonshunt procedures

No shunt surgeries for variceal hemorrhage include:	
Splenectomy Sugiura procedure Mathur's modification of Sugiura procedure Hassab procedure Stapled esophageal transection Splenectomy and coronary vein ligation Tanner's procedure Boerema button	Omentopexy, splenopneumopexy Coronary vein ligation Transthoracic ligation of varices (Boerema–Crile and Milnes–Walker) Total gastrectomy Hepatic and splenic artery ligation

3. Absence of expertise for endoscopic management in the emergency setting
4. Left-sided PHT with mild liver dysfunction and gross splenomegaly

Sugiura Procedure

Classically described as a two-stage approach, is a more radical surgical procedure for the control of variceal bleeding. As a first stage, distal intrathoracic esophagus is devascularized and an esophageal transection performed via a left thoracotomy. After 6 weeks from then, intra-abdominal esophagus and proximal stomach are devascularized by the division of lesser curve and greater curve via an abdominal incision. This procedure always includes a vagotomy and pyloroplasty added to the devascularization. However, this procedure is now performed as a modified single stage procedure through an abdominal incision, providing access to the lower esophagus by dividing the crura. After splenectomy, upper two third stomach and distal 7 cm of oesophagus are devascularized (Fig. 5) by dividing the perforating veins. Left gastric vein is preserved and only the cardiac branches are tied. Oesophageal transection is done 4-5 cm proximal to G E junction using a circular stapler. This is omitted by many surgeons due to its high morbidity. Vagotomy and pyloroplasty is done.

Hassab Procedure

The Hassab procedure commences with the ligation of the splenic artery followed by splenectomy. It is then followed by the devascularization of the proximal stomach and the distal 7–8 cm of the esophagus after mobilization of the vagii. The distal 3 cm of the esophagus and the proximal 5 cm of the stomach are then opened longitudinally, allowing under sewing of each column of the varix within the esophagus. Nasogastric tube is then placed inside the stomach and the esophagogastrostomy is then closed in layers.

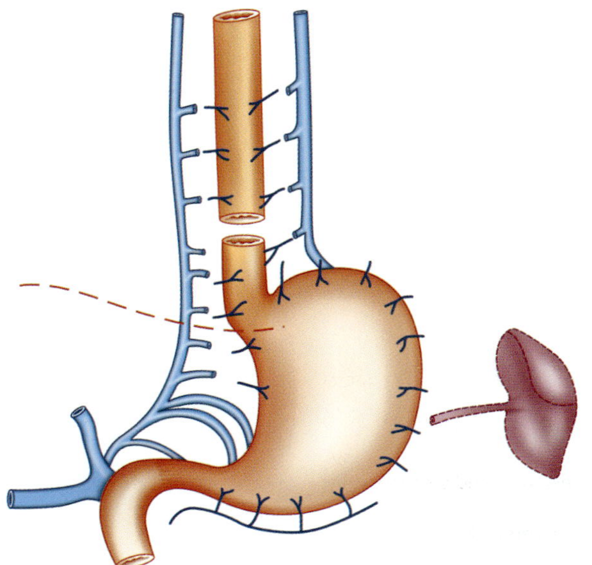

Figure 5 Gastric devascularization

Management of Variceal Bleed in Non-cirrhotic Portal Hypertension

Massive variceal bleeding is a well-documented and life-threatening complication of PHT due to non-cirrhotic PHT. There is very little published data on the management of acute variceal bleed in PHT in a non-cirrhotic setting. The principles of management remain the same as those for patients with cirrhosis which include blood transfusions, intravenous fluids in a standard intensive care setting.[17,18] As compared to non-cirrhotics with acute variceal bleeding (5–7%), bacterial infections are more common in patients with cirrhosis with variceal bleeding (35–66%).[19] Infected cirrhotic patients have a higher rate of variceal rebleeding (43%) than noninfected patients (10%).[20] The role of prophylactic antibiotics in non-cirrhotic patients with variceal bleeding is not known though wherein they seem to improve in survival in patients with cirrhosis and variceal bleeding.[21,22] There is also no data on the efficacy of vasoactive drugs in patients with non-cirrhotic PHT.

Endoscopic Sclero-therapy (EST) and EVL are effective in controlling acute bleeding from esophageal varices and preventing rebleeding in 80–90% of patients. Presently, variceal band ligation with its lower complication rate is preferred. In cirrhotics combination of endoscopic therapy with drugs is more effective than either of them alone for control of acute bleeding (88 vs. 76%) and prevention of rebleeding for 5 days (77 vs. 58%), although there is no difference in mortality.[17,18] However, there is very limited data for non-cirrhotic PHT. Present treatment fails to control or prevent early rebleeding in 8–12% of patients, and these patients should be treated with alternative modes of treatment, like surgery in the form of portosystemic shunts or esophago-gastric devascularization especially in patients with EHPVO. These are shown to be effective[23-25] but carry mortality rates ranging from 10–30%.[26] Indian experience[27,28] has shown that splenectomy and a lieno-renal shunt when performed by experienced surgeons carries a low-operative mortality of 1.9% (elective: 1/140 [0.7%]; emergency 2/20 [10%]), rebleeding rate was 11% and actuarial survival at 15 years by life-table analysis was 95%. It also removes the large spleen, reverses hypersplenism, and is not followed by portosystemic encephalopathy. Importantly, it is a one-time procedure suited to those with little access to blood transfusion and sophisticated medical facilities. Patients with NCPF with acute variceal bleed are also managed in the same way except that a small subset of patients, especially those with a nodular type of NCPF are likely to develop post-shunt encephalopathy. Devascularization is a better choice in these patients. Transjugular intrahepatic portosystemic shunt is also an alternative in select cases.

REFERENCES

1. World Gastroenterology Organization practice guidelines: esophageal varices. June 2008.
2. Groszmann RJ, Bosch J, Grace ND, et al. Hemodynamic events in a prospective randomized trial of propranolol versus placebo in the prevention of a first variceal hemorrhage. Gastroenterology. 1990;99:1401-7.
3. Groszmann RJ, Garcia-Tsao G, Bosch J, et al. β-blockers to prevent gastroesophageal varices in patients with cirrhosis. N Engl J Med. 2005;353:2254-61.
4. Garcia-Tsao G, Groszmann RJ, Fisher RL, et al. Portal pressure, presence of gastroesophageal varices and variceal bleeding. Hepatology. 1985;5:419-24.5.

5. Ripoll C, Groszmann R, Garcia-Tsao G, et al. Hepatic venous pressure gradient predicts clinical decompensation in patients with compensated cirrhosis. Gastroenterology. 2007;133:481-8.
6. D´Amico G, Morabito A, Pagliaro L, et al. Survival and prognostic indicators in compensated and decompensated cirrhosis. Dig Dis Sci. 1986;31(5):468-75.
7. Bruix J, Castells A, Bosch J, et al. Surgical resection of hepatocellular carcinoma in cirrhotic patients: prognostic value of preoperative portal pressure. Gastroenterology. 1996;111(4):1018-22.
8. Ripoll C, Groszmann RJ, Fisher RL, et al. Portal pressure, presence of gastroesophageal varices and variceal bleeding. Hepatology. 1985;5(3):419-24.
9. Merkel C, Bolognesi M, Bellon S, et al. Prognostic usefulness of hepatic vein catheterization in patients with cirrhosis and esophageal varices. Gastroenterology. 1992;102(3):973-9.
10. Moitinho E, Escorsell A, Bandi JC, et al. Prognostic value of early measurements of portal pressure in acute variceal bleeding. Gastroenterology. 1999;117:626-31.
11. Rincon D, Lo Iacono O, Ripoll C, et al. Prognostic value of HVPG for in-hospital mortality of patients with severe acute alcoholic hepatitis. Aliment Pharmacol Ther. 2007;25:841-8.
12. Vinel JP, Cassigneul J, Levade M, et al. Assessment of short-term prognosis after variceal bleeding in patients with alcoholic cirrhosis by early measurement of portohepatic gradient. Hepatology. 1986;6:116-7.
13. The North Italian Endoscoppic Club for the study and treatment of esophageal varices (NIEC). Prediction of the first variceal hemorrhage in patients with cirrhosis of the liver and esophageal varices. A prospective multicenter study. N Engl J Med. 1998;319:983-9.
14. Casado M, Bosch J, Garcia-Pagan JC, et al. Clinical events after transjugular intrahepatic portosystemic shunt: correlation with hemodynamic findings. Gastroenterology. 1998;114(6):1296-303.
15. Colomo A, Hernandez-Gea V, Muniz-Diaz E, et al. Transfusion strategy in patients with cirrhosis and acute gastrointestinal bleeding. Hepatology. 2008;48:413A.
16. Kravetz D, Sikuler E, Groszmann RJ. Splanchanic and systemic hemodynamics in portal hypertensive rats during hemorrhage and blood volume resuscitation. Gastroenterology. 1986;90:1232-40.
17. Franchis R. Evolving consensus in portal hypertension report of the Baveno IV consensus workshop on methodology of diagnosis and therapy in portal hypertension. J Hepatol. 2005;43:167-76.
18. Garcia-Tsao G, Sanyal AJ, Grace ND, et al. Prevention and management of gastroesophageal varices and variceal hemorrhage in cirrhosis. Hepatology. 2007;46(3):922-38.
19. Goulis J, Patch D, Burroughs AK. Bacterial infection in the pathogenesis of variceal hemorrhage. Lancet. 1999;353:139-42.
20. Bernard B, Cardanel JF, Valla D, et al. Prognostic significance of bacterial infection in bleeding cirrhotic patients: a prospective study. Gastroenterology. 1995;108:1828-34.
21. Bernard B, Grange JD, Khac EN, et al. Antibiotic prophylaxis for the prevention of bacterial infections in cirrhotic patients with gastrointestinal bleeding: A meta-analysis. Hepatology. 1999;29:1655-61.
22. Hou MC, Lin HC, Liu TT, et al. Antibiotic prophylaxis after endoscopic therapy prevents rebleeding in acute variceal hemorrhage: a randomized trial. Hepatology. 2004;39:746-53.
23. Mathur SK, Shah SR, Soonawala ZF, et al. Transabdominal extensive oesophagogastric devascularization with gastro-oesophageal stapling in the management of acute variceal bleeding. Br J Surg. 1997;84(3):413-7.
24. Sharma A, Vijayaraghavan P, Lal R, et al. Salvage surgery in variceal bleeding due to portal hypertension. Indian J Gastroenterol. 2007;26(1):14-7.
25. Goyal N, Singhal D, Gupta S, et al. Transabdominal gastroesophageal devascularization without transection for bleeding varices: results and indicators of prognosis. J Gastroenterol Hepatol. 2007;22(1):47-50.
26. Mitra SK, Kumar V, Datta DV, et al. Extrahepatic portal hypertension: a review of 70 cases. J Pediatr Surg. 1978;13(1):51-4.
27. Prasad AS, Gupta S, Kohli V, et al. Proximal splenorenal shunts for extrahepatic portal venous obstruction in children. Ann Surg. 1994;219:193-6.
28. Pande GK, Reddy VM, Kar P, et al. Operations for portal hypertension due to extrahepatic obstruction: results and 10 year follow up. Br Med J (Clin Res Ed). 1987;295:1115-7.

CHAPTER 116

Management of Nonvariceal Hemorrhage

Patta Radhakrishna, Pavan Addala

INTRODUCTION

Upper gastrointestinal (UGI) bleeding constitutes more than 80% of all cases of acute bleeding from the gastrointestinal (GI) tract, and nonvariceal bleeds account for 80% of the UGI bleeding.[1] Nonvariceal upper GI bleeding is amongst the commonest clinical problems presenting in the emergency room. It has diverse manifestations with a varied etiology often requiring emergent care. Peptic ulcer bleeding assumes the most common cause of nonvariceal UGI bleeding. The incidence of acute nonvariceal UGI bleed increases with age, with a slight increased preponderance in the male population. The incidence is of acute nonvariceal UGI is also higher in the hospitalized patients, especially in those undergoing major surgeries. Management essentially includes a multidisciplinary approach, with a great deal of man power and finances involved in this process. Such a team should include an emergency physician, gastroenterologist, intensive care specialist, surgeon, and an interventional radiologist. Surgeons and the gastroenterologists working in tandem from the time the patient arrives in to the hospital can help establish the goals of treatment, such that the best results can be achieved.

The majority of patients with acute UGI bleed stop bleeding spontaneously allowing time for elective evaluation. Approximately, 15% of the patients continue to have a major bleed, requiring treatment either in the form of therapeutic endoscopic intervention or surgery.[2] Eventually, 5–10% of the patients hospitalized for acute UGI bleeding need operative intervention.[3] Improved endoscopic techniques and technology, greater understanding of the disease processes, combined with standardized surgical techniques, and improved critical care management have further decreased the mortality in patients with acute nonvariceal UGI bleeding. Despite all these improvements in its management, the mortality still remains 5% and more.

ETIOLOGY

Incidence of various causes for UGI bleed[4-7]	
Peptic ulcer (Fig. 1)	31–67%
Erosions (Fig. 2)	7–31%
Variceal bleeding	4–20%
Esophagitis	3–12%
Mallory Weiss	4–8%
Neoplasms (Fig. 3)	2–8%
Others (hemobilia, hemosuccus pancreaticus, UGI anastomosis, endoscopic sphincterotomy, PEG insertion, Dieulafoy's lesion (Fig. 4), aortoenteric fistula, pancreatic pseudoaneurysm rupture, portal hypertensive gastropathy)	2–8%

Peptic Ulcer Disease

Peptic ulcer disease (Fig. 1) is the most common cause of nonvariceal UGI bleed. With the advent of proton pump inhibitors and other antiacid secretory drugs the incidence of admission, complications of peptic ulcer disease, mortality, and surgery for peptic disease have significantly decreased in the recent past. This decrease is mainly due to the understanding of ulcer pathogenesis and the role of *H. pylori* and nonsteroidal antinflamatory drugs (NSAIDs). Approximately, 90% of the duodenal ulcer and 75% of the gastric ulcers are associated with *H. pylori* infection. However, a 25% overlap presence is noted in patients with NSAID-induced ulcers. *H. pylori* causes ulcers by the production of toxins that cause local tissue injury (urease, cytotoxins, mucinase, phospholipases, and platelet activating factor), by induction of local mucosal immune response and increasing the gastric levels, and thus increasing acid secretion by reducing the D-cell number

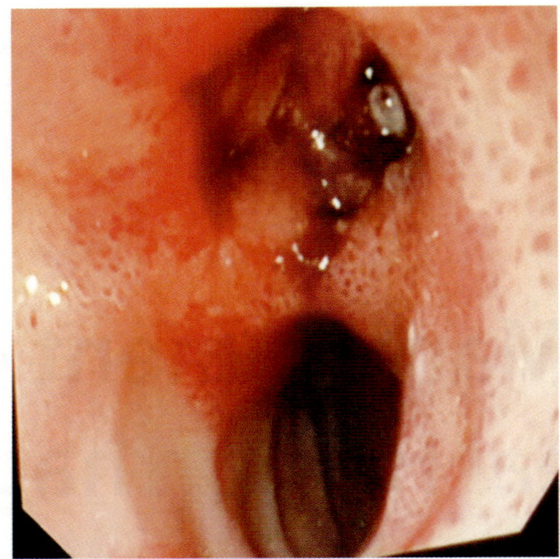

Figure 1 Large duodenal ulcer with stigmata of recent bleed. Visible vessel in the base of ulcer

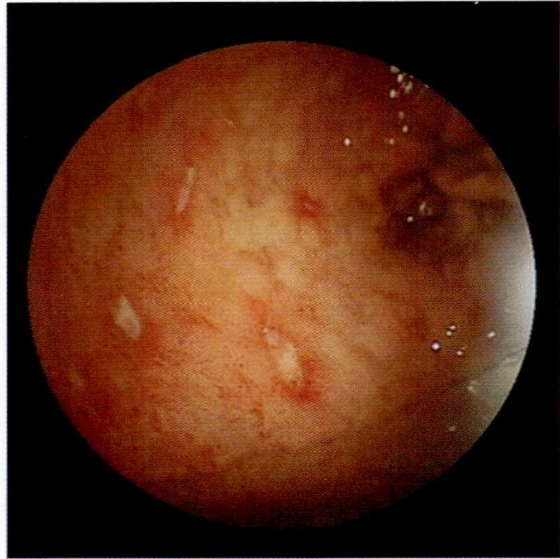

Figure 2 Multiple superficial erosions. History of nonsteroidal anti-inflammatory drug intake was present

in the mucosa. Thus, an ulcer healing rate of 90% can be achieved with eradication of *H. pylori* and a standard proton pump inhibitor (PPI) course of 4 weeks. In contrast to 25% recurrence rates with ulcer healing medications alone, only 2% ulcer recurrence has been noted in patients receiving medication for the eradication of *H. pylori* followed by ulcer healing medications at short term, and 64 and 15% respectively, at long term. In the subset of patients needing long-term NSAIDs intake for medical illnesses, a 2-10-fold increase in the risk for ulcer related complications have been noted. This group is particularly old aged, medically fragile, with prior GI events, and receiving concomitant steroid therapy or anticoagulants. The risk increases in proportion to the potency of the NSAID for the antiinflammatory effect. They act by inhibiting the production of prostaglandins which are responsible for the protective mucous layer secretion over the epithelium.

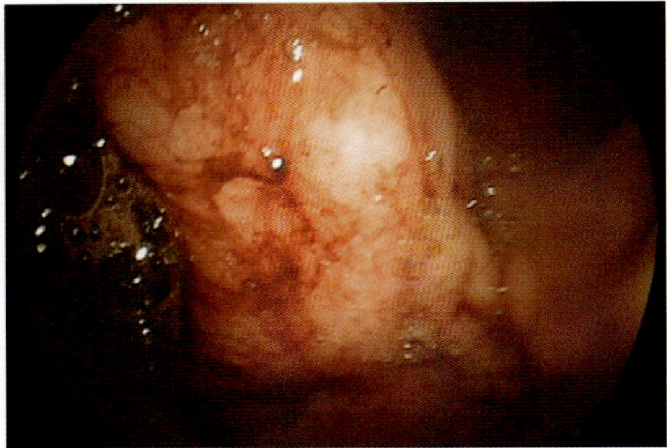

Figure 3 Gastric GIST with bleed

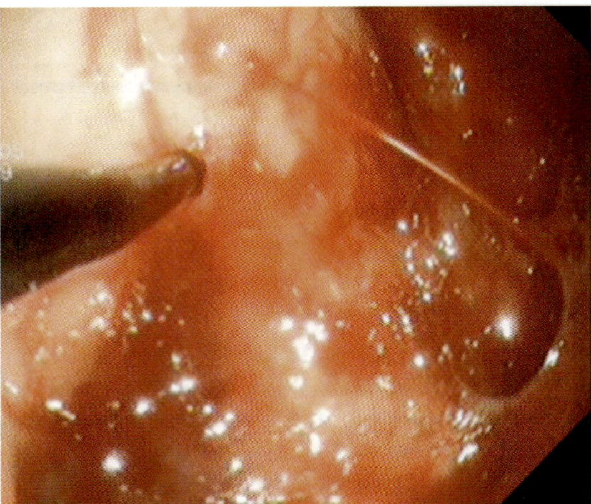

Figure 4 Dieulafoy's lesion with spurting vessel

Stress Gastritis

Acid injury in combination with ischemia due to hypoperfusion states in critically ill patients has been suggested to cause diffuse erosions of the stomach. In patients with head injury, these are called "Cushing's ulcers" and in patients with major burns these are called "Curling's ulcers." With improvement in the overall management of the critically ill patients and with introduction of various acid suppressive drugs, the incidence of stress ulcers has come down.

Mallory–Weiss Tears

These are seen at the gastroesophageal junction more commonly along the lesser curve, and are limited to the mucosa and the submucosal layers. They are typically seen in patients with intense retching and vomiting, following binge alcoholic drinking and hyperemesis gravidarum. The main clue to the diagnosis is typical history and is confirmed on retroflexion maneuver during endoscopy. An increased intragastric pressure due to forceful contraction of the abdominal muscles against an unrelaxed cardia is suggested as the mechanism for these tears.

Dieulafoy's Lesion

These are vascular malformations seen predominantly within the first 6 cm of the esophagogastric junction along the lesser curvature of the stomach. These abnormally enlarged arterioles (1–3 mm) create a constant pressure due to pulsations on the mucosa resulting in a 2–5 mm mucosal defects. As these are not associated with acid peptic disease or infection, surrounding mucosa appears normal, making these lesions difficult to identify. Rupture of the arterioles, usually results in intermittent massive bleeding episodes (Fig. 4). They are diagnosed primarily on endoscopy, and in some instances may need an angiography to determine the site of bleeding.

Aortoenteric Fistula

Aortoenteric fistula follows infection of the aortic graft, and is associated with a massive GI hemorrhage which is devastating with a 50% mortality rate. Its incidence is higher following an end to side proximal anastomosis, as it is more difficult to cover the prosthesis with viable tissue.

Approach to the Patient

1. Initial assessment

   At initial presentation airway and breathing take the priority as in any other case presenting to the emergency. Circulatory system is then assessed, and takes priority and forms the basis for further management. Aggressiveness in the management of patients with acute UGI bleed depends on the magnitude of the bleed, preexisting deficits, and the comorbidities of the patient. This warrants a detailed history including the magnitude and frequency of the bleeding, existing comorbidities, in particular ischemic heart disease, diabetes mellitus, anemia, and drug history (aspirin, clopidogrel, and heparin). Attention is then diverted to stratifying the patients based on the risk factors.
2. History and physical examination: as described in etiology
3. Risk stratification: See Table 1

Table 1: Risk factors for morbidity and mortality in acute upper gastrointestinal bleed

Age	OR for mortality is 3 for age >60 years and 12 for age >75 years
Comorbidity	One comorbidity almost doubles mortality (OR 1.8) e.g., Renal failure, liver disease, respiratory insufficiency, cardiac disease (OR 1.8), malignancy (OR 3.8)
Inpatients	Compared with new patients, inpatients have threefold increased risk of death (comorbidities)
Persistent or recurrent hemorrhage	
Magnitude of hemorrhage	SBP <100 mm Hg on presentation Transfusion requirement Tachycardia Presence of initial hematemesis (2×), hematochezia (2×)
Need for surgery	
Elevated blood urea	

OR, odds rato; SBP, systolic blood pressure.

Nonsteroidal anti-inflammatory drugs (NSAIDs) and anticoagulants do not worsen the prognosis of patients presenting with UGI bleeding. Many scoring systems have been developed to prognosticate patients with UGI bleed. Some are nonspecific (APACHE II), while some are specific (BLEED classification, Rockall score, Blatchford score). BLEED scoring system is a clinical scoring system, and includes four clinical criteria and one laboratory value:

1. Ongoing bleeding
2. SBP <100 mmHg
3. Altered mental status
4. Unstable comorbid condition that require management in intensive care setting
5. Prothrombin time more than 1.2 times the control.

Rockall and Blatchford clinical and endoscopic scoring systems are given in Table 2.

Rockall score predicts death accurately as the score increases. *If a person aged >60 years has a bleed Rockall score becomes minimum 1 and patient should probably be admitted. However, he may be considered for early discharge if otherwise stable* (Table 3). Blatchford risk score predicts mortality and need for treatment (transfusion, endoscopic treatment, and surgery) in patients with UGI bleed. A Blatchford score more than 0 is 99–100% sensitive for identifying a severe bleed, but only 4–44% specific. Clinically, it is far more important to identify all severe UGIB even if it means admitting some patients who prove to have a minor bleed, and could have avoided admission. It should be emphasized that good clinical judgment should guide us in managing these patients, and scoring systems help us but are not the ultimate in deciding the patients' management.[8]

Management: Not all patients with acute UGI bleed present with severe hemorrhage. There is a subset of patients presenting with UGI bleed that can be managed conservatively, and can be

Table 2: Rockall and Blatchford clinical and endoscopic scoring systems

Low-risk patients as per Blatchford risk score
- Urea <6.5 mmol/L
- Hemoglobin ≥13.0 g/dL (men) or ≥12.0 g/dL (women)
- Systolic blood pressure ≥110 mmHg
- Pulse <100/min
- Absent:
  - Melena
  - Syncope

Total Score	*Frequency (% of Total)*	*Rebleeding Rate (%)*	*Mortality Rate (%)*
0	4.9	4.9	0
1	9.5	3.4	0
2	11.4	5.3	0.2
3	15.0	11.2	2.9
4	17.9	14.1	5.3
5	15.3	24.1	10.8
6	10.6	32.9	17.3
7	9.0	43.8	27.0
≥8	6.4	41.8	41.1

Table 3: Rockall scoring for nonvariceal upper GI hemorrhage				
Score				
Variable	0	1	2	3
Age (years)	<60	60–79	>80	
Shock	Non (BP >100; pulse <100)	Tachycardia (pulse >100. BP >100)	Hypotension (BP <100, pulse >100)	
Comorbidity	Nil major		Cardiac failure, ischemic heart disease, major comorbidity	Renal failure, liver failure, disseminated malignancy
Diagnosis	Mallory–Weiss tear, no lesion, no SRH	All other diagnosis	Upper GI malignancy	
Major SRH	None or dark spot		Blood in upper GI tract, adherent clot, visible or spurting vessel	
Maximum total score = 11				
SRH, stigmata of recent hemorrhage; GI, gastroinstestinal; BP, blood pressure.				

discharged without any observation and hospital stay. This group includes those who have Rockall and Blatchford score of 0.

All patients who are aged >70 years (>60 years preferably) should be admitted. Patients with witnessed hematemesis or hematochezia (suspected continued bleeding), hemodynamic instability (systolic blood pressure <100 mm Hg, pulse ≥ 100 beats per minute), patients with comorbidities, patients with known liver disease or varices should be admitted, resuscitated and planned for early endoscopy after stabilization.

Resuscitation

As soon as the patient presents in the emergency room, at least one large-bore (14- or 16-gauge) intravenous cannula should be placed. It is difficult to predict at the initial assessment as to which patients are likely to have further bleeding. Hence, every attempt should be made to secure two cannulae. Ringer's lactate is infused rapidly (2 liters bolus) or as needed to maintain the systolic blood pressure (SBP) >100 mmHg and pulse rate (PR) below 100/min. Please refer to Table 4, for assessment of hypovolemia and fluid resuscitation. Blood should be sent for laboratory investigations, which include hemogram, liver function tests, renal function test, coagulation profile, and cross matching along with viral serology. Foley catheter is inserted to assess renal perfusion. A central line for monitoring perfusion status should be considered. Transfusion with packed red cells and other blood products should be started right away in patients with massive bleeding as per local protocols. Basis for blood transfusion should be full clinical picture, recognizing that over-transfusion may be as damaging as under-transfusion. Platelet transfusion should not be started in patients who are not actively bleeding and are hemodynamically stable. Packed red blood cells transfusion is started when initial Hb <7 g. Platelet transfusions are started in patients who are actively bleeding, and have a platelet count of less than 50,000/mL. Fresh frozen plasma (FFP) is transfused to patients who have either a fibrinogen level of less than 1 g/L, or a prothrombin time (PT) (international normalized ratio-INR) or activated partial thromboplastin time (PTT) greater than 1.5 times normal. Transfusion targets should be:

1. Hematocrit >24%
2. Platelet count >50,000/mm^3
3. PT <15 seconds

Hemoglobin and hematocrit are measured every 6 hours. In patients with active ongoing hematemesis with altered mental status endotracheal intubation should be considered to prevent aspiration pneumonia.[9]

A nasogastric (NG) tube should be introduced, though its role is controversial. It helps in:

Table 4: Assessment of hypovolemia and fluid resuscitation				
Blood loss	<750	750–1500	1500–2000	>2000
Blood loss (%bw)	<15%	15–30%	30–40%	>40%
Pulse	<100	100–120	120–140	>140
BP	>100	>100	<100	<100
Pulse volume	normal	↓	↓	↓
Respiration rate	14–20	20–30	30–35	>35
Hourly urine output	>30	20–30	<20	<20
Mental status	Marked anxiety	Mild anxiety	Anxiety/ confusion	Confusion/ Drowsines
Fluid therapy	Crystalloids	Crystalloids	Ciystalloids/ Colloids/ Blood	Crystalloids/ colloid/Blood

1. Identifying the source of bleed (coffee ground or fresh blood suggests UGI bleed).
2. Assessing the rate of ongoing bleeding.
3. Clearing the stomach of blood, thus allowing visualization during endoscopy.
4. In giving a cold saline lavage, which presumably causes vasoconstriction and clears irritant gastric contents, thus avoiding further bleeding.
5. Clear bilious aspirate minimizes the chance of an ongoing active GI bleed.

It should be emphasized that almost 20% of the patients with a clear NG aspirate still have UGI tract as a source of bleeding.[10] However, UGI scopy should be considered in all the patients with a suspected UGI source of bleed, irrespective of the NG aspirate.

Localization of Bleeding

Endoscopy is crucial in localizing the bleeding site in patients with acute UGI bleed. However, in patients with slow ongoing bleed resulting in anemia and in patients with intermittent bleeding, the role of endoscopy is limited, particularly if there is no identifiable pathology on esophagogastroduodenoscopy (EGD) scope.

Role of Esophagogastroduodenoscopy in Uppergastrointestinal Bleeding

In patients with ongoing UGI bleeding, EGD is highly accurate in identifying the source, and localizing the bleed. Efficacy is further increased by doing EGD scopy within the first 24 hours following the sentinel bleed even in the stable patients.[11] Endoscopy sooner than 24 hours has not been shown to be beneficial.[12,13] Urgent endoscopy (within 24 hours of presentation) is endorsed for patients presenting with hematemesis or hematochezia, hemoglobin less than 8 g/dL, suspected malignant disease or cirrhosis and signs of hypovolemia. However, it should not be generalized, and the Table 5 shown below is just for guidance in deciding the timing of endoscopy.

In an unstable patient urgent EGD scope has been found to decrease the mortality and transfusion requirements. Complications are seen in 1% of the patients undergoing emergency EGD scopy, and include gastrointestinal perforation. Other complications are hypoxia, hypotension, aspiration pneumonia, induced hemorrhage, and adverse medication reaction. Failure to visualize the source of bleeding has been noted in 1-2% of the patients due to profuse bleeding.[14] Aggressive lavage and erythromycin injection at the start of the EGD scope might increase the visualization during the procedure.[15] Erythromycin acts by increasing the gastric emptying time. The initial EGD findings determine the need for subsequent evaluation in the form of lower GI endoscopy, angiography, tagged RBC scan, capsule endoscopy, enteroscopy, and the need for surgery.

Table 5: Timing of endoscopy

Indication	*Remarks*
Super urgent (in operation theatre)	In patients with massive bleeding and refractory hypotension in the operating room with the immediate availability of surgical management
Urgent (immediately in endoscopy suite)	Unstable patients with severe acute upper GI bleeding
Emergent (within 6–12 hours)	Cirrhotic patients, aortoenteric fistula patients and patients who rebleed in the hospital, and hemodynamically stable patients with no evidence of an on-going bleed
Elective (within 24 hours of sentinel bleed)	Stable patients with no ongoing bleed after admission

Angiography: Its main role is in the diagnosis and treatment of severe bleeding, particularly when EGD scopy and colonoscopy have failed to elucidate the cause. It has good specificity and positive predictive value if bleeding is at least 0.5 mL/min but low sensitivity (30–50%). Sensitivity is more for active bleed than for recurrent acute or chronic occult bleeding and a specificity of 100%. Therapeutic intraarterial infusion of vasopressin or transcatheter embolization of actively bleeding vessel can be done at the same time. It does not however, ascertain the precise cause for the bleeding. Complications following angiography include femoral artery thrombosis, hemorrhage and hematomas at the puncture site, contrast reactions, acute renal injury, intestinal ischemia, and transient ischemic attack.

Radionuclide imaging: This can be rapidly performed and helps to localize approximate area of bleeding. It can then be used to guide subsequent investigations like endoscopy and angiography, or surgery. Radionuclide imaging is sensitive for detecting an ongoing bleeding as low as 0.04 mL/min. Two tracers are used for detecting bleeding sites.

- Technetium sulfur colloid (albumin scan): It is used to identify acute, active bleeding. It is rapidly cleared from the circulation.
- Technetium pertechnetate-labeled autologous RBC: -It remains longer in the blood stream (up to 24 hours) and is best utilized for repeated scanning in patients with intermittent bleeding.

Disease-specific Management

Peptic ulcer disease: A spectrum of lesions can be seen in patients with peptic ulcer disease, ranging from erosions in the esophagus, stomach, duodenum, and ulcers in the duodenum (Fig. 1) and stomach, blood clots, bleeding vessels, nonbleeding pulsatile vessels, and even perforation. Each finding is associated with a specific rebleeding risk and with a certain increased risk with stigmata of recent bleeding. Forrest's classification for endoscopic finding and rebleeding risks in peptic ulcer disease has been very useful for considerable time now in prioritizing these patients. (Table 6 and Fig. 5)

Endoscopic therapy is recommended in patients with type Ia and IIa lesions, failing which management should be directed towards surgical therapy. Endoscopic therapy can be in the form of a mechanical method (e.g., clips) with or without adrenaline or thermal coagulation with adrenaline or fibrin, or thrombin with adrenaline.[8] No single modality has been found to be superior to the other.[16] However, a combination therapy, for example, epinephrine injection with cautery or clips, is superior to epinephrine or cautery alone for treatment of high-risk lesions, and significantly reduces the risk of rebleeding, surgery, and mortality.[8,17-20] In the case of peptic ulcer

Table 6: Forrest's classification

Grade	*Description*	*Rebleeding risk (%)*
Ia	Active, pulsatile bleeding	90
Ib	Active, nonpulsatile bleeding	10
IIa	Nonbleeding visible vessel	50
IIb	Adherent clot	33
IIc	Ulcer with black spot	7
III	Clean, nonbleeding ulcer bed	3

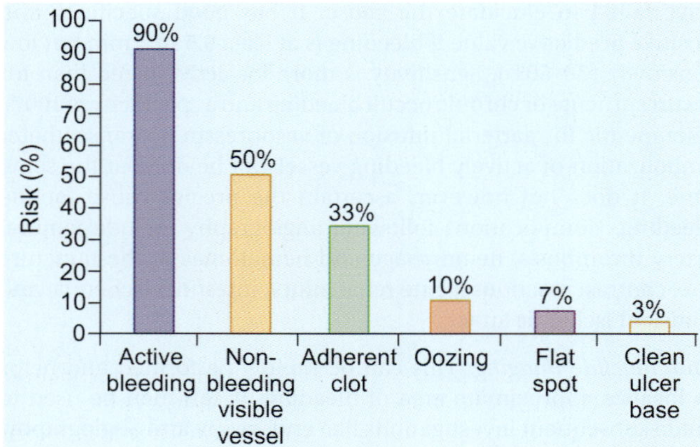

Figure 5 Risk of rebleeding as per Forrest's classification

with adherent clots (Forrest type IIb), no convincing data is there to support endotherapy. A metaanalysis of six RCT (240 patients) for endoscopic versus medical management for adherent clots suggested that endoscopic therapy is superior to medical therapy for preventing recurrent bleeding (pooled relative risk, 0.43; 95% confidence interval, 0.19–0.98). There was however no significant difference in the need for surgery, length of hospital stay, transfusion requirements, or mortality between endoscopic approaches. Another meta-analysis of five RCT (189 patients) with adherent clots showed no significant differences in the risks of rebleeding, need for surgery, or mortality with endoscopic therapy versus no endoscopic therapy.[20] Thus, practice of clot removal followed by endoscopic therapy cannot be recommended for all cases and should be individualized. For Forrest type Ib (with no other stigmata of bleeding), IIc and III endoscopic therapy is not recommended.

After emergency endoscopy, a high dose of intravenous infusion of proton pump inhibitors is recommended for the first 72 hours, followed by eradication of *H. pylori*.[21-24] Surgery for peptic ulcer disease is rarely required in the present era, with its role limited to perforation, suspected malignancy, endoscopically uncontrolled bleeding, and obstruction secondary to chronic fibrosis of the ulcer. Most common vessels involved bleeding in patients with peptic ulcer are gastroduodenal artery in case of duodenal ulcer, and the left gastric artery in case of gastric ulcer. It is probably required to do a wedge resection for hemostasis, and biopsy in the case of gastric ulcer bleed. However, a simple U-stich taken over the bleeding ulcer after a duodenotomy will suffice in case of bleeding from the duodenal ulcer.

Surgery should be followed by infusion of high-dose of PPIs, and eradication of *H. pylori* commenced once the culture and sensitivity of the organism is confirmed. The older notion of combining a vagotomy in emergency do not hold good anymore in the era of PPI domination in ulcer healing over vagotomy. Vagotomy is successful in inhibiting the acid secretion upto 70% less with a morbidity of 20% associated with it. Proton pump inhibitors can decrease up to 98% of the acid secretion when dosaged properly, with an ulcer healing rates of 75% when given alone and 90% when combined with eradication of *H. pylori*. This benefit of PPI with anti-*H. pylori* medication is superior to benefits of vagotomy. Hence, vagotomy as a part of emergency surgery for peptic ulcer complications cannot be recommended and should be obsolete.

Stress gastritis: In the pre-PPI era, significant bleeding from stress ulcers used to be a common phenomenon. Now, with the understanding of its physiology in patients with shock and sepsis, and concomitant use of acid suppressive protocols, significant bleeding is rarely (0.1% as per The Canadian Critical Care Trials Group) encountered nowadays. Hence, the primary goal should always be resuscitation aggressively. High-risk patients for stress gastritis should be identified in the intensive care unit setting, and should be started on local antiulcer protocols. In the event of failure, somatostatin and its analogues, endotherapy, interventional radiological techniques have all been tried with futility. In the rare event of severe bleeding, surgery has been tried and includes gastrotomy with oversewing of the hemorrhage combined with vagotomy and pyloroplasty, and even a near total gastrectomy has been tried. However, it should be remembered that these surgeries are rarely required now and carry high mortality rates.

Esophagitis: Any causative infection, if it is the cause of bleeding should be treated. If erosions are secondary to peptic disease, acid suppression is warranted. Endotherapy is rarely required.

Mallory-Weiss tears: Ninety percent of the times, these mucosal bleeds are self-limiting with approximately 100% mucosal healing rates within the first 72 hours. In rare cases of severe bleeding, endotherpy is warranted in the form of thermal coagulation or injection therapy. Anecdotal cases of successful intervention embolization techniques have been reported, but should be analyzed with caution, as bleeding from other vessels supplying the stomach is real due to rich submucosal plexus. In rare case of failed endotherapy, surgical therapy in the form of high gastrotomy and direct suturing of the mucosal tear should be resorted to.

Dieulafoy's lesion: Endotherapy is the treatment of choice with success rates of 80–100% being reported. When these cannot be controlled endoscopically, lesions should be tattooed to guide the surgeon in the operation theatre. Lesions are identified after a gastrotomy and then are oversewn. In case of inability to locate a lesion, a partial gastrectomy may be performed.

Malignancy: As the rebleeding rates following endotherapy are high, a surgical resection is warranted in patients with bleeding secondary to malignancy after failed endoscopic therapy.

Aortoeneteric fistula: Surgery is the only options in these patients with removal of the prosthesis and doing an extraanatomical bypass. Duodenal rent is then closed primarily.

Others: For both hemobilia and hemosuccus pancreaticus, angiography can be both diagnostic and therapeutic and is the preferred modality. In the event of failure to control bleeding in hemosuccus pancreaticus, a distal pancreatectomy is done in amenable patients. In case of bleeding following an endoscopic sphincteromy, injection therapy is often successful and surgery is rarely required. It occurs in less than 2% of the patients, and majority are self-limiting. Patients with ongoing bleeding are taken up for surgery, a duodenotomy is performed by a lazy S incision, site of bleeding is then oversewn. Three percent of the patients undergoing a percutaneous endoscopic gastrostomy (PEG) present with UGI bleeding. A small percentage of these is from the mucosal side and can be controlled endoscopically. Bleeding from the anastomotic sites is usually of small quantity, and in the majority of patients is self-limiting. In the event of ongoing bleeding from UGI anastomosis, endotherapy can be attempted with minimal insufflation and maximum care.

Recurrent Bleeding Following Endoscopy

A recurrent bleed of 24%, has been noted in high-risk patients following initial endotherapy. Use of PPI therapy in addition to combination endoscopic therapy reduced this recurrence rate to approximately 10%. A routine second-look endoscopy, is defined as a planned event performed within 24 hours of the initial endoscopy, and is not recommended. If there are concerns about inadequacy of therapy delivered and initial endoscopy failed to identify the source of bleeding, a repeat endoscopy is warranted and it is recommended that these patients be adequately resuscitated before repeating the procedure.[8,25-27] Patients with recurrent bleeding generally respond favorably to repeat endoscopic therapy. A second attempt at endoscopic therapy is therefore recommended.

Acknowledgment

Image courtesy Dr Sanjiv Sachdeva, Associate Prof Gastroenterology, G B Pant Institute of Medical Education and Research, Delhi.

REFERENCES

1. Peura DA, Lanza FL, Gostout CJ, et al. The American College of Gastroenterology Bleeding Registry: preliminary findings. Am J Gastroenterol. 1997;92:924-8.
2. Dulai GS, Gralnek IM, Oei TT, et al. Utilization of health care resources for low-risk patients with acute , nonvariceal upper GI haemorrhage: an historical cohort study. Gastrointst Endosc. 2004;60:85-93.
3. Peura DA, Lanza FL, Gostout CJ, et al. The American College of Gastroenterology Bleeding Registry: preliminary findings. Am J Gastroenterol. 1997;92:924-8.
4. Theocharis GJ, Thomopoulos KC, Sakellaropoulos G, et al. Changing trends in the epidemiology and clinical outcome of acute upper gastrointestinal bleeding in a defined geographical area in Greece. J Clin Gastroenterol. 2008;42:128-133.
5. van Leerdam ME, Vreeburg EM, Rauws EA, et al. Acute upper GI bleeding: did anything change? Time trend analysis of incidence and outcome of acute upper GI bleeding between 1993/1994 and 2000. Am J Gastroenterol. 2003;98:1494-9.
6. Paspatis GA, Matrella E, Kapsoritakis A, et al. An epidemiological study of acute upper gastrointestinal bleeding in Crete, Greece. Eur J Gastroenterol Hepatol. 2000;12:1215-20.
7. Czernichow P, Hochain P, Nousbaum JB, et al. Epidemiology and course of acute upper gastro-intestinal hemorrhage in four French geographical areas. Eur J Gastroenterol Hepatol. 2000;12:175-81.
8. ASGE guidelines. The role of endoscopy in the management of acute non-variceal upper GI bleeding. Gastrointest Endosc. 2012;75(6):1132-8.
9. Acute upper gastrointestinal bleeding: management NICE clinical guideline 2012.
10. Rockey DC.Gastrointestinal bleeding. Gastroenterol Clin North Am. 2005;34:581-88.
11. Cooper GS, Chak A, WayLE, et al. Early endoscopy in upper gastrointestinal haemorrhage: associations with recurrent bleeding, surgery, and length of hospital stay. Gastrointest endosc. 1999;49:145-52.
12. Tsoi KK, Ma TK, Sung JJ. Endoscopy for upper gastrointestinal bleeding: how urgent is it? Nat Rev Gastroenterol Hepatol. 2009;6:463-9.
13. Sarin N, Monga N, Adams PC. Time to endoscopy and outcomes in upper gastrointestinal bleeding. Can J Gastroenterol. 2009;23:489-93.
14. Cheng CL, Lee CS, Liu NJ, et al. Overlooked lesions at emergency endoscopy for acute nonvariceal upper gastrointestinal bleeding. Endoscopy. 2002;34:527-30.
15. Frossard JL, Spahr L, Queneau PE, et al. Erythromycin intravenous bolus infusion in acute upper gastrointestinal bleeding: a randomized, controlled, double blinded trial. Gastroenterology. 2002;123:17-23.
16. Laine L, McQuaid KR. Endoscopic therapy for bleeding ulcers: an evidence-based approach based on meta-analyses of randomized controlled trials. Clin Gastroenterol Hepatol. 2009;7:33-47.
17. Vergara M, Calvet X, Gisbert JP. Epinephrine injection versus epinephrine injection and a second endoscopic method in high risk bleeding ulcers. Cochrane Database Syst Rev. 2007;18 CD005584.
18. Barkun AN, Martel M, Toubouti Y, et al. Endoscopic hemostasis in peptic ulcer bleeding for patients with high-risk lesions: a series of metaanalyses. Gastrointest Endosc. 2009;69:786-99.
19. Marmo R, Rotondano G, Piscopo R, et al. Dual therapy versus monotherapy in the endoscopic treatment of high-risk bleeding ulcers: a meta-analysis of controlled trials. Am J Gastroenterol. 2007;102:279-89.
20. Laine L, McQuaid KR. Endoscopic therapy for bleeding ulcers: an evidence-based approach based on meta-analyses of randomized controlled trials. Clin Gastroenterol Hepatol. 2009;7:33-47.
21. Laine L, McQuaid KR. Endoscopic therapy for bleeding ulcers: an evidence-based approach based on meta-analyses of randomized controlled trials. Clin Gastroenterol Hepatol. 2009;7:33-47.
22. Lau JY, Sung JJ, Lee KK, et al. Effect of intravenous omeprazole on recurrent bleeding after endoscopic treatment of bleeding peptic ulcers. N Engl J Med. 2000;343:310-6.
23. Leontiadis GI, Sharma VK, Howden CW. Proton pump inhibitor treatment for acute peptic ulcer bleeding. Cochrane Database Syst Rev. 2006;CD002094.
24. Sung JJ, Barkun A, Kuipers EJ, et al. Intravenous esomeprazole for prevention of recurrent peptic ulcer bleeding: a randomized trial. Ann Intern Med. 2009;150:455-64.
25. Management of acute upper and lower gastrointestinal bleeding. A national clinical guideline. September 2008. Scottish Intercollegiate Guidelines Network.
26. ASGE guidelines. The role of endoscopy in the management of patients with peptic ulcer disease. Gastrointest Endosc. 2010;71(4)663-8.
27. Holster IL, Kuipers EJ. Management of acute nonvariceal upper gastrointestinal bleeding: current policies and future perspectives. World J Gastroenterol. 2012;18:1202-07.

CHAPTER 117

Approach to the Management of Lower Gastrointestinal Hemorrhage

Atul Sharma

INTRODUCTION

Gastrointestinal (GI) hemorrhage is an alarming occurrence, both for the patient and the care providers; however, a structured management approach can effectively treat the majority. Conventionally, the hemorrhage is called *upper gastrointestinal* if it originates above the duodenal-jejunal flexure and *lower gastrointestinal* it occurs below it, although it should correctly be called only intestinal hemorrhage for obvious reasons. However, if the origin cannot be detected by routine investigations, it is considered *obscure,* be it *overt* or *occult.* This chapter is aimed at outlining the epidemiology and the current techniques used to evaluate and treat patients with intestinal hemorrhage for the benefit of the residents and practicing surgeon.

Endoscopy, angiography, and radionuclide scans are used to diagnose and manage lower gastrointestinal hemorrhage (LGIH). Endoscopic procedures include colonoscopy esophagogastroduodenoscopy, wireless capsule endoscopy, push enteroscopy, and double-balloon enteroscopy. How and when each of these is utilized depends on clinical presentation, hemodynamic status, and rate of bleeding.

EPIDEMIOLOGY

The incidence of LGIH in the adult population has been estimated to be 20–30 per 100,000 persons at risk, and is correlated in Western literature with increasing age. The bleed stops spontaneously in 80%, rebleeding occurs in 25%, and in 10% the source of hemorrhage cannot be identified.[1] Data from the United States suggest that LGIH constitutes less than 1% of all hospital admissions. Longstreth estimated the annual incidence to be 20.5 patients per 100,000 (24.2 in males vs. 17.2 in females) and that the incidence increases from the third to the ninth decade by 200 times.[2] Although data from India is scanty, LGIH is considered to be about one tenth as common as upper gastrointestinal hemorrhage (UGIH).[3-5] It has been pointed out that LGIH is under reported even in the United States, because a significant number of patients do not seek medical attention.[6] The experience from All India Institutes of Medical Sciences (AIIMS), New Delhi, shows that the mean age of Indian patients reporting with LGIH to a tertiary care center is 41 years as compared with 70 years in the United States.[5]

Etiology

In a retrospective review from a western urban center of 1,112 medical records with acute LGIH published in 2009, the common etiology of bleeding was reported to be diverticulosis (33.5%), hemorrhoids (22.5%), and malignancy (12.7%),[7] which is similar to the results of a previous review of seven series of patients with LGIH published in 1999.[8]

Bhargava et al. from AIIMS, India, published a study of 244 consecutive patients with recurrent LGIH evaluated by colonoscopic examination. Predominant lesions in adults were nonspecific colitis and ulcers (58%), polyps (19%), cancer (10%), rectal varices (4%), and tuberculosis (3%). Juvenile polyps (77%) and nonspecific colitis and ulcers (23%) were the cause of bleeding in children. A total of 92% lesions involved the left colon.[9]

In another review, which collated data of 91 patients with massive LGIH from three tertiary care hospitals of the Indian Army, the mean age of the patients was 38.9 years; in 45% the hemorrhage originated from the ileo-cecal region and in 34%, it was related to inflammatory bowel disease (IBD). Diverticulosis and colorectal cancer were found to be the cause in only 5.5% each and angiodysplasia or ischemic colitis in only 3.3%.[3]

Current analysis of records of 296 patients who underwent surgery for LGIH at the Department of GI Surgery, AIIMS, from

Table 1: Epidemiology of LGIH in patients operated at GI Surgery, AIIMS, New Delhi from 1985 to 2012 (n = 296). Mean age: 38.1 (range 12–76) M:F = 227:69 = 3.4:1

Etiology	*n*	%
Nonspecific ulcer	96	32.4
Enteric ulcer	40	13.5
Tuberculosis	21	7.1
Vascular	32	10.8
Meckel's diverticulum	12	4.1
IBD	16 (Crohn's disease—2)	5.4
Carcinoma	12 (small bowel—2)	4.1
Ischemic etiology	13	4.4
GIST	19	6.4
Polpys	10	3.4
Diverticulosis	8	2.7
Amebic ulcers	4	1.4
Miscellaneous	13	4.4

AIIMS, All India Institutes of Medical Sciences; LGIH, lower gastrointestinal hemorrhage; IBD, inflammatory bowel disease; GIST, gastrointestinal stromal tumor.

1985 to 2012 (Table 1) reveals that the commonest cause continues to be nonspecific ulcers in 32% and another 20% had either enteric or tubercular ulcers, whereas a vascular cause was found only in 10.8% and diverticulosis in 2.7%. There has been no change in the mean age of these patients (38.1; range 12–76 years) over the past 20 years [Personal Communication].

DIAGNOSIS

Presentation

Lower gastrointestinal hemorrhage has a wide spectrum of presentations, ranging from streaking the side of well-formed stools, splattering of the pan after passage of hard stools, bloody diarrhea, tarry black stools (malena) in 11%, passage of maroon stools in 16.7%, to the recurrent passage of large amounts of fresh blood (hematochezia) in 55.5%.[7]

The clinical presentation differs with the amount, source, and etiology of the hemorrhage. Bleeding from the small intestine presents as malena, right colon as maroon stools, while a left colonic bleed usually reveals itself as bright red blood per rectum. A massive UGIH or a brisk right-sided colonic bleed may also present as hematochezia.[10] On the other hand, cecal hemorrhage may also present sometimes as tarry black stools, which is more typically seen after UGIH. Therefore, the color of stool does not accurately point to the anatomic source of hemorrhage. The presentation of LGIH may also vary depending on the etiology. The hemorrhage may be mild and intermittent from angiodysplasia or moderate to severe if diverticular in origin.

Depending on the nature and severity of bleeding, LGIH has been classified broadly for ease of management, into four overlapping categories[11]:

1. Minor self-limiting
2. Chronic intermittent
3. Massive intermittent
4. Massive ongoing

In the majority (75–90%), the bleeding is minor and self-limiting and mostly responds to conservative therapy. In patients with chronic intermittent bleeding, etiology is often elusive and needs extensive investigation. The third category of patients has episodes of severe bleeding with hemodynamic stability in between the episodes. Urgent colonoscopy has both a diagnostic and therapeutic role in this group. Alternatively, investigating these patients during the episode with ^{99m}Tc-labeled red blood cell scan has also been found to be useful, prior to performing angiography. Patients with massive ongoing hemorrhage, many of whom may be hemodynamically unstable, need urgent therapeutic intervention either by colonoscopy, angiography or surgery.

Traditionally, LGIH is also defined as *acute* when it is of recent onset and leads to hemodynamic instability, and is called *massive* when it is life-threatening and presents with passage of maroon stools or bright red blood from the rectum, a systolic blood pressure of <90 mmHg, and a hemoglobin level <6 g%. It also includes patients in whom the bleeding continues for 3 days or who have rebleeding within a week. Massive hemorrhage is life-threatening and requires substantial blood transfusion. Such patients may be elderly who have multiple comorbidities and 10–20% of them end in mortality.

Clinical Evaluation

Despite advances in investigative modalities, a proper history and physical examination as always are the most essential part of the evaluation of a patient presenting with LGIH and can provide valuable pointers into the etiology and source of hemorrhage. Significant history of acid peptic disease, liver disease, IBD, and the use of nonsteroidal anti-inflammatory drugs (NSAIDs) or anticoagulants is required to be documented. Previous history of malignancy may suggest exposure to radiation and/or chemotherapy.

Symptoms are also important in identifying the source of bleeding. Patients with IBD may present with pain, and frequent stools mixed with blood and mucus. Fever, dehydration, abdominal cramps, and hematochezia in the young point toward infectious or nonspecific colitis; however, older patients presenting with the same symptoms may even have ischemic colitis. An elderly patient with painless bleeding and minimal symptoms may be suffering from diverticulosis or angiodysplasia; on the other hand, a patient with atherosclerotic heart disease may present with syncope following intermittent LGIH due to angiodysplastic lesions.

On physical examination, special attention should be paid to skin rashes, purpuric or ecchymotic spots, and hemangiomata. The oral cavity should be examined for melanosis, and a detailed examination of the abdomen, perineum, and anal canal should be performed. Passage of a nasogastric tube, digital rectal examination, and proctoscopy are part of the routine physical examination in all patients presenting with LGIH.

Up to 15% of patients with suspected LGIH have upper GI bleeding, which highlights the significance of eliminating a gastroduodenal source in patients with hematochezia. The presence of bilious aspirate in the nasogastric tube virtually excludes UGIH but aspiration of clear gastric fluid does not, in which case a gastric lavage with saline may succeed in aspirating some duodenal secretions to clarify the issue. Once hemorrhage is established to be originating from the lower GI tract, the amount of blood loss should be swiftly assessed and a protocol-based approach adopted.

APPROACH TO MANAGEMENT

The essential components of management of LGIH, which should all be done simultaneously, are as follows:

- Clinical assessment and resuscitation
- Localization of bleeding site
- Intervention to stem the bleeding

Clinical Assessment, Resuscitation, and Indications for Blood Transfusion

Massive LGIH is a life-threatening condition and initial resuscitation is most important for its management. These patients should receive intravenous isotonic crystalloids through two wide-bore IV cannulae. A simultaneous rapid assessment of vital parameters is performed, and postural hypotension (a fall of blood pressure >10 mmHg) usually suggests blood loss of >1,000 mL.

Fall of hematocrit of 6% or a level less than 18% is suggestive of substantial blood loss, which needs blood transfusion. The aim should be to maintain a hematocrit of 20–25% in younger and around 30% in high-risk, older patients. An international normalized ratio of >1.5 may indicate coagulopathy, and infusion of fresh frozen plasma is required. Thrombocytopenia should be improved with platelet concentrates.

Indications for admission to an intensive care unit are (a) patients in shock, (b) those needing multiple blood transfusions, (c) those with continuous active bleeding and/or associated comorbidities, or (d) those with an acute abdomen. Extensive evaluation and aggressive resuscitation should be started with early involvement of both a gastroenterologist and GI surgeon. Early identification of high-risk patients and aggressive management are strategic to reducing morbidity and mortality.

Etiopathology

Complete description of the various etiologies is beyond the scope of this chapter and the reader is advised to refer to specific texts for the same; however, a brief pathophysiology of common and some rarer causes of LGIH are outlined below.

Diverticulosis: Diverticulosis has a high prevalence in Western societies mainly because the societies are aging and have a low residue diet. Up to 50% of adults above 60 years of age have evidence of this disease. The prevalence in India is reported to be much lower,[3,4] although no population-based study is available. A sac-like protrusion or diverticulum develops at the point of weakness where the penetrating vessel perforates the circular muscle coat of the colonic wall. This occurs because of constipation and recurrent straining at stools. Etiopathogenesis of diverticular bleeding was studied with histologic data and angiography in the 1970s.[12]

Stercoral trauma and repeated contraction and relaxation of muscularis propria may lead to the thinning of the media. Rupture of the intramural branches of the marginal artery with thinning of the media at or near the bleeding point is usually seen at the dome of the diverticulum or at its antimesenteric margin. Up to 20% of patients with diverticular disease experience bleeding, which stops spontaneously in 80%, but in 5%, the bleeding can be massive. The predicted recurrence rates for bleeding in patients with diverticular hemorrhage who have been managed expectantly are 9, 10, 19, and 25% at 1, 2, 3, and 4 years, respectively.[2] Sixty percent of bleeding is localized to right on arteriogram although diverticula are more commonly seen on the left side.[13-15] In contrast, in about 60% of patients with a colonoscopic diagnosis of diverticular bleeding, the source is left sided.[16] Probably the more serious diverticular bleed is right colonic as 0.5–1 mL/min of bleeding is required for angiography to delineate extravasation.[8] In a reappraisal of the natural history and management of bleeding colonic diverticula, McGuire Jr had reported that the bleeding stopped spontaneously in 75% but continued in most patients who required 4 or more units per day.[17]

Angiodysplasia: Angiodysplasias are ectatic blood vessels in the mucosa and submucosa of the GI tract. Their prevalence was found to be 0.83% in three prospective studies reporting the results of colonoscopic screening of 964 asymptomatic individuals.[18] Colonic angiodysplasias are mostly located in the cecum and ascending colon. They are seen commonly in persons older than 60 years and have been associated with a number of systemic disorders such as atherosclerotic cardiovascular disease, chronic kidney disease, collagen disorders, cirrhosis of the liver, and chronic obstructive pulmonary disease. However, the associations are varied and may only be age-related coincidental occurrences. These degenerative and ectatic blood vessels develop due to chronic, intermittent, low-grade colonic contractions that obstruct the mucosal venous drainage. The mucosal capillaries progressively dilate, become incompetent, and form arterio-venous malformations. At endoscopy, colonic angiodysplasia appear as red, flat lesions, 2–10 mm in diameter, at times with a feeding vessel or a pale mucosal halo (Fig. 1). The shape may be round, oval, or stellate and the margins may be reported as sharp or indistinct.[19]

Hemorrhage from angiodysplasia is veno-capillary in origin and is less torrential than from diverticular disease, but as compared to diverticular bleeding approximately 80% of patients with spontaneously resolved angiodysplasia experience rebleeding.[20] Saperas et al. found that in patients with colonic angiodysplasia, a previous history of brisk bleeding, presence of

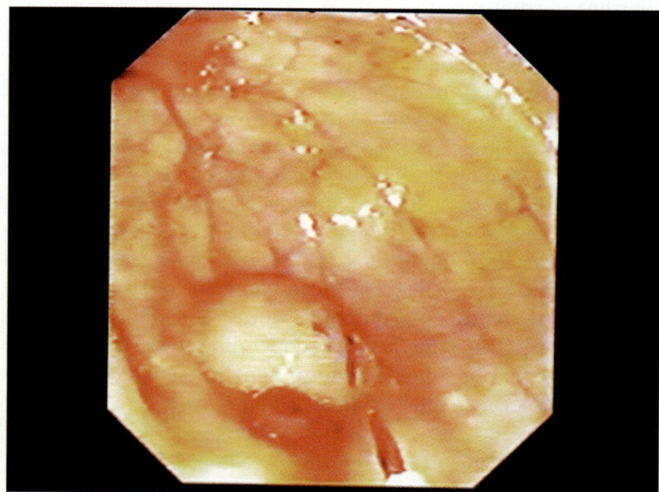

Figure 1 Colonoscopic appearance of angiodysplasia cecum

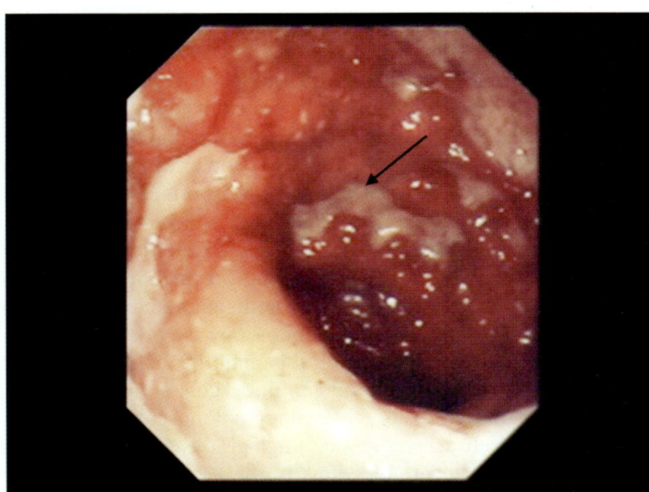

Figure 2 Ulcers in colon

multiple lesions, and aggressive anticoagulation tends to predict recurrent hemorrhage.[21]

Inflammatory diseases: Inflammation and ulcerations due to various causes account for 6–30% of acute LGIH (Fig. 2). This category includes IBD, radiation colitis, infectious colitis, and idiopathic ulcers.[8] Even though IBD causes LGIH, it is seldom massive. Ulcerative colitis can cause mild to moderate bloody diarrhea in about 50% of patients, with up to 7% of patients experiencing massive bleeding.[22,23]

Severe GI bleeding accounts for 6–10% of emergency surgical resections for ulcerative colitis.[24] However, acute life-threatening lower intestinal bleeding has been reported in 0.6–1.3% of patients with Crohn's disease and occurs more frequently in those with colonic involvement than with small bowel involvement alone.[25,26]

Ischemic colitis: Ischemic colitis accounts for 3–9% of patients with acute lower intestinal bleeding.[2,27] It is a disease of the elderly and is frequently associated with comorbidities such as cardiac failure and arrhythmia. It frequently involves watershed areas such as the splenic flexure and the rectosigmoid junction, sparing the rectum. Hypotension and vasoconstriction cause ischemic injury, which leads to mucosal friability leading to mucosal and partial-thickness colonic wall sloughing, edema, and hemorrhage. Precipitating event cannot be identified in most cases. Also ischemic colitis is not usually associated with major blood loss or hematochezia, pain and bloody diarrhea being the main symptoms. Colonoscopic findings often resemble changes of IBD.

Colon carcinoma: Colonic neoplasia may present with bleeding in 2–26% of the cases. Colonic cancers bleed mainly from erosions on the luminal surface, and ulcerated cancers are found to be the cause of acute lower intestinal bleeding in 21%.[8] In a large epidemiologic study looking at the etiology of acute lower intestinal bleeding, nine of 219 patients (4%) had post-polypectomy hemorrhage.[2]

Anorectal disease: Anal fissure is diagnosed with blood streaking of stools, perianal pain, and blood on the toilet paper or splattering the toilet bowl. Hemorrhoidal bleed is in spurts and is fresh and painless. Anorectal disease can cause intermittent rectal bleeding leading to severe anemia and at times even massive rectal bleeding has been reported, especially in patients with human immunodeficiency virus/acquired immune deficiency syndrome-associated thrombocytopenia.[28]

Discovery of benign anorectal disease that is very common should not exclude the possibility of more proximal bleeding from the lower GI tract. The presence of hemorrhoids may just be a red herring, and a source of bleeding higher in the rectum, such as rectal cancer, varices, or a Dieulafoy lesion must be looked for in such situations.[29-31]

Stercoral ulcer and solitary rectal ulcer syndrome: Stercoral ulcers and the solitary rectal ulcer syndrome can also cause LGIH in the elderly. Constipation with hard impacted stool in the rectum causes mucosal damage and stercoral ulcers. Injury may also occur by manipulation or a foreign body such as a rectal tube in the hospitalized patient. The solitary rectal ulcer syndrome is thought to occur due to rectal prolapse and mucosal damage from constipation and straining.[32] Whether acute hemorrhagic rectal ulcer syndrome is a distinct clinical entity remains controversial, it is characterized by sudden onset, painless, and massive hemorrhage from rectal ulcer(s) in patients with serious underlying illnesses and does account for 2.8% of patients with massive LGIH.[33]

Characteristic colonoscopic appearance is a lesion located about 5 cm from the dentate line. There may be solitary or multiple rectal ulcers with round, circumferential, geographical or Dieulafoy like lesions. On histology, the lesions appear as denudation of covering epithelium with hemorrhage, necrosis and multiple thrombi in the vessels of the mucosa and underlying stroma. The histological picture is quite similar to stress-related mucosal injury. In a series from Taiwan, hemostasis was obtained in 14 of 19 patients using therapeutic endoscopy. Prognosis depends on precise diagnosis and management of the underlying conditions and comorbidities.[33]

Radiation-induced colitis and other causes of vasculitis: Radiation therapy induces mucosal telangiectasia and inflammatory changes prone to bleeding. A significant number of patients given pelvic radiotherapy for prostate or uterine cancer develop proctopathy, with 5% reporting hematochezia daily and 9% at least once a week.[34] Preventive treatment with topical rectal beclomethasone dipropionate reduces postradiation risk of bleeding in patients.[35]

Other vasculitic entities include polyarteritis nodosa and Wegener's granulomatosis. These cause sloughing of the mucosa because of vasculitis-induced necrosis.

Lower gastrointestinal hemorrhage may also occur due to thrombocytopenia secondary to immunosuppressive therapy. Aorto-colonic fistulas are a rare cause of LGIH which develops after aortic graft surgery. Importantly, it can cause hemorrhage even 10–20 years after the initial surgery.[8]

Drug-induced lower gastrointestinal hemorrhage: Drug-induced bleeding is common in the elderly, caused mainly by indiscriminate and poorly supervised use of low-dose aspirin and NSAIDs. Low-dose aspirin given for cardiovascular prophylaxis can also produce bleeding, although the risk of bleeding is dose dependent.[36] Anticoagulants and antiplatelet agents can potentiate or exacerbate hemorrhage from preexisting lesions. Oral anticoagulants or corticosteroids should be cautiously used in patients at risk of LGIH, especially in patients already on regular low-dose aspirin or NSAIDs.[37]

Causes of lower gastrointestinal hemorrhage in children: The causes of LGIH in infants, children, and adolescents are at variance from those found in adults and reported in 0.3% of children presenting to the pediatric emergency department of Postgraduate Institute of Medical Education and Research, Chandigarh. Among Indian children the common causes are colitis and polyps. In most of the cases of LGIH, the bleeding is scanty and self-limiting, but conditions like Meckel's diverticulum often presents with life-threatening bleeds.[38]

Uncommon causes of lower gastrointestinal hemorrhage: Other rare causes of lower GI bleeding[29,30,39-41] that may need to be considered are as follows:

- Small bowel diverticulosis/Meckel's diverticulum
- Colonic/rectal varices/portal colopathy
- Diversion colitis
- Dieulafoy lesion of colon or small bowel
- Intussusception
- Endometriosis
- Gastrointestinal bleeding in long-distance runners
- Rupture of arterial pseudoaneurysm following surgery or acute pancreatitis

Localization of Bleeding Site

Clinicians called upon to manage LGIH have a number of diagnostic and therapeutic options such as rigid/flexible sigmoidoscopy, colonoscopy, radionuclide scintigraphy, computed tomography (CT), and angiography. Although no modality has emerged as the gold standard in the management of LGIH, colonoscopy has several advantages, such as the ability to identify the bleeding source regardless of the rate or the presence of active bleeding, the ability to provide a definite histological diagnosis, and multiple therapeutic possibilities. However, there is a need for colonic preparation, endoscopy facilities with experienced staff, and the possibility of the rare but serious complication of perforation.[42] The 2008 Scottish Intercollegiate Guidelines Network (SIGN) guidelines also recommend early colonoscopy in the diagnostic workup of massive LGIH. It may be used along with CT scanning or CT/digital subtraction angiography because when colonoscopy fails to define the site of bleeding in patients with massive LGIH, angiographic transarterial embolization controls the hemorrhage.[37]

Colonoscopy

Diagnostic colonoscopy: The role of urgent colonoscopy in LGIH remains controversial. Few studies advocate colonoscopy within 12–24 hours of admission to improve diagnostic yield and reduce rebleeding and surgery.

Laine and Shah[10] reported the results of a randomized trial of urgent (12 hours from admission) vs. elective (36–60 hours from admission) colonoscopy in 72 patients with LGIH. Commenting on this study, Strate in a recent editorial stated that majority of patients stopped bleeding spontaneously and there was no difference in rebleeding, blood transfusions, diagnostic or therapeutic interventions, length of hospital stay, or hospital charges in patients undergoing urgent vs. elective colonoscopy. However, the limited number of patients in this study and the fact that patients in the urgent colonoscopy arm appeared to have more severe bleeding than those undergoing elective examinations make it difficult to draw conclusions regarding the utility of urgent vs. elective colonoscopy in LGIH.[43]

Bhargava et al. describing their experience of 240 consecutive patients at AIIMS, New Delhi with recurrent lower GI bleeding studied by colonoscopic examination reported that the procedure was successful either in identifying the lesion or in excluding it up to the cecum in 90%. A total of 92% of these lesions involved the left colon mainly involving the rectum and sigmoid colon.[4]

Also, colonoscopy is almost invariably required following the outcome of imaging modalities, whether positive or negative, to confirm the source of bleeding or exclude colorectal malignancy or diverticulosis, which is why colonoscopy is considered to be the most efficient initial test for the majority of patients with LGIH who can be stabilized and can undergo colon preparation. In a study by Jensen et al., emergency colonoscopy and upper endoscopy as well as emergency angiography were performed in 22 patients with severe bleeding. In the 17 patients with lower intestinal sources of bleeding, the diagnostic yield of colonoscopy was 82 vs. 12% for angiography.[44] Similarly, in a retrospective study by Strate et al., initial colonoscopy within 24 hours of admission offered a diagnostic yield of 85 vs. 45% for initial scintigraphy and angiography.[45]

In hemodynamically stable patients with moderate to severe bleeding, diagnostic colonoscopy is the investigation of choice. Compared with angiography, colonoscopy has a higher yield and lower complication rate.[44-46] The 2009 American Association of Family Physicians (AAFP) recommendations also emphasize that urgent colonoscopy in the context of lower GI bleeding is a safe procedure and tends to improve outcomes.[47]

Therapeutic colonoscopy: Once diagnosis is made, colonoscopic hemostasis can be achieved by epinephrine or saline injection, thermal contact, argon plasma coagulation, clipping, or band ligation. A review of published series by Strate et al.[48] revealed that endoscopic therapy was applied to 10–40% of patients undergoing colonoscopy for LGIH, and the commonest intervention used was thermal contact plus injection. Their review of 71 cases of diverticular bleeding treated with endoscopically placed hemoclips had a 100% success rate for homeostasis with no complications. Colonoscopy with or without intervention for LGIH is considered a safe procedure. In a review of four studies with 664 patients, there were two perforations with an overall complication rate of 0.3% for colonoscopy and 0.6% if colonoscopy was performed urgently.[48]

Best results of colonoscopy are seen in patients who are hemodynamically stable and bleeding slowly or who have stopped bleeding. Those who have brisk bleeding have a lower diagnostic yield. Unstable patients may deteriorate with colonoscopy. Therefore, patients of LGIH should be carefully screened before colonoscopy. The bowel needs to be prepared well, with a rapid oral or nasogastric tube purge, as performing colonoscopy on an unprepared bowel is difficult, time consuming, and may not yield useful information. Both colonoscopy and bowel preparation should not be done in suspected perforation. In cases of suspected perforation or obstruction, plain abdominal radiography should be performed before colonoscopy to rule out this complication. Bowel preparation otherwise does not initiate or aggravate bleeding.

Colonoscopy in an unstable patient may be undertaken in operating room with full preparation for anesthesia and surgery.

If patients become unstable during colonoscopy in the endoscopy suite, the procedure should be abandoned. If colonoscopy reveals an active fulminant inflammation, the procedure should be again aborted. Incidentally discovered lesions should ideally be left alone.

Nuclear Scintigraphy

Radionuclide scanning, also known as nuclear scintigraphic imaging, has been used in the diagnosis of patients with LGIH but its role remains controversial. The modalities include Technetium-99 (^{99}Tc) sulfur colloid scan, the ^{99m}Tc pertechnetate-labeled autologous red blood cell scan (TRBC scan), and the indium-111 (^{111}In)-labeled RBC scintigraphy. Nuclear scintigraphy has a sensitively of 86% and can detect hemorrhage at rates as low as 0.1–0.5 mL/min, as opposed to angiography, which detects bleeding at rates of 1–1.5 mL/min. This technique is reported to be 10 times as sensitive than mesenteric angiography in detecting ongoing bleeding, but has a specificity of only 50% when compared with endoscopy or angiography due to its limited resolution, which is why scintigraphic imaging is used primarily as a screening method to select patients for angiography because a negative scan can eliminate the requirement for an unnecessary and invasive angiography.[49]

^{99m}Tc Pertechnetate-labeled Autologous Red Blood Cell Scans: Ng et al. recommend TRBC scintigraphy as a pre-screening test for selective mesenteric angiography after a retrospective review of records of 86 patients with positive TRBC scintigraphy. On TRBC scintigraphy, immediate (within 2 minutes) or delayed blush was seen. Immediate blush had a positive predictive value of 75% for angiography, while a delayed blush had a negative predictive value of 93% for angiography.[50] They concluded that patients with immediate blush should undergo mesenteric angiography, while those with delayed blush are better off with colonoscopic evaluation instead of angiography. The 2009 AAFP recommendations state that TRBC or arteriography may be used in patients with continued bleeding when endoscopy has not aided in diagnosis.[47]

The TRBC scan is preferred, because its half-life is longer and abdominal scans can be obtained for up to 24 hours. This is advantageous in patients with intermittent bleeding. These scans have a high sensitivity ranging from about 80 to 98% and can detect slow bleeding. The bleeding spot can be correctly recognized when intraluminal accumulation of TRBC is observed during the dynamic phase of scanning.

^{99m}Tc Sulfur Colloid Scans: ^{99m}Tc sulfur colloid scan can be done without any preparation. Imaging is to be done quickly as this agent has a very short half-life (2.5–3.5 minutes). Colloid is rapidly cleared by the reticuloendothelial system. Due to short half-life, these scans are not useful in patients with intermittent bleeding. While interpreting scans it should be borne in mind that bleeding from hepatic flexures and the splenic flexures may be concealed as ^{99m}Tc sulfur colloid enhances the liver and spleen.

^{111}Indium-labeled Red Blood Cell Scintigraphy: There is paucity of literature in the use of ^{111}In labeled-RBC scintigraphy. It has the advantage of prolonged half-life (67 hours) and can therefore be useful for detection of intermittent bleeding. However, it is expensive, labor intensive, and gives poor localization of bleed. Because of intestinal motility, images could also be poor. It is useful especially when conventional methods have failed. Schmidt et al. published a study where ^{99m}Tc scanning was initially futile,[51] but later scintigraphy with ^{111}In-labeled RBCs detected the bleeding site in six patients. In another report in a 70-year-old patient with intermittent bleeding and severe anemia, Mole et al. detected synchronous, small and large intestinal adenocarcinomas with ^{111}In-labeled RBC scintigraphy.[52]

The difficulty of localization using nuclear scintigraphy was demonstrated in a study by Hunter et al. In this study, eight patients had an unnecessary procedure and the results of TRBC scanning were incorrect in about one fourth of patients.[53] Poor localization in radionuclide scans of the bleeding site is perhaps due to the rapid passage of tagged RBCs in the large bowel as also overlapping bowel segments. Recurrent lower GI bleeding after negative TRBC scintigraphy has been reported to be as high as 27%.[54]

Computed Tomographic Scanning

Although the clinical features of intestinal ischemia are very typical and intramural hemorrhage rarely causes continuous pain in the abdomen associated with rigidity of the anterior abdominal wall, the ability of CT scanning to differentiate between intestinal ischemia and intramural hemorrhage has been studied by Macari et al. who found that ischemia typically involves a long segment with wall thickening of less than 1 cm, whereas intramural hemorrhage usually involves a shorter segment and is associated with a bowel wall thickness of 1 cm or more.[55]

Ernst et al. from France reported a study on 24 patients with LGIH. Three-phase helical CT of the abdomen was done for diagnosis. The diagnosis of the bleeding site was shown by at least one of the following: enhanced bowel wall; spontaneous hyperdensity of the peri-bowel fat; extravasation of the contrast into lumen, polyp, or tumor; or vascular ectasia. Presence of diverticula alone did not establish the bleeding site.[56] However, pooling of contrast medium has been found to be a useful sign.[57]

The results of CT were compared with the diagnosis obtained by colonoscopy, enteroscopy, or surgery. A definite diagnosis was made in 19 patients. The bleeding site was located in the small bowel in five patients and the colon in 14 patients. The CT correctly located four small bowel hemorrhages and 11 colonic hemorrhages. Diagnosis of the primary lesion responsible for the bleeding was made in 10 patients. These results suggest helical CT to be a good diagnostic tool in acute lower GI bleeding to help the physician to diagnose the bleeding site.[57]

Computes tomography scanning was compared with colonoscopy and conventional angiography (CA) for locating the bleeding site in patients of LGIH in a pilot study.[58] It suggested CT to be a convenient, safe, and accurate diagnostic tool for acute LGIH. The sensitivity of CA was questionable. The authors proposed a management algorithm for such patients, using CT as the pre-CA screening tool, where a positive CT should be followed by therapeutic angiography, while patients with a negative CT may be triaged to alternative management pathways.

Lee et al. from Fremantle, Western Australia, after a review of 15 studies found that CT diagnosed a potential causative pathology or the presumed bleeding site in 80% of patients. They proposed that multidetector computed tomography (MDCT) should be used as the preliminary swift investigation to triage patients presenting with LGIH for supplementary investigation and management.[59] Frattaroli et al. comparing the sensitivity of MDCT scanning with endoscopy in identifying the site and etiology of acute LGIH reported that the sensitivity in identifying the site and etiology of bleeding was 100 and 88.2%, respectively, for MDCT scan, compared with 52.9 and 52.9% for endoscopy.[60] The overall sensitivity, specificity, positive and negative predictive values (PPV and NPV), and accuracy of MDCT angiography have recently been reported to be 86.0, 100, 100, 60.6, and 88.5%, respectively.[61]

Computes tomography angiography is thus a valuable investigation for LGIH. In an animal model of colonic hemorrhage, Kuhle et al.[62] reported that a single detector helical CT angiography could detect active hemorrhage at rate of 0.3 mL/min, which was better than the sensitivity of mesenteric angiography of 0.5 mL/min and approaching values of RBC scintigraphy of 0.2 mL/min. In a meta-analysis, Wu et al.[63] found numerous studies that gave evidence to the role of CT relative to CA for the diagnostic workup of patients suffering from acute GI bleeding. Several studies besides this analysis have shown that CT can diagnose bleeding where angiography failed to locate the source.[58,64,65]

Advantages of MDCT for the diagnostic workup of LGIH patients are its minimal invasiveness, speed, and reproducibility. Multidetector computed tomography scanning can easily delineate small bowel which is difficult to access with endoscopy.[63] When a bleeding site is identified on CT then angiography even when initially negative, can be pursued for repeat assessment and embolization.[66]

Recently, in an effort to assess the utility of dual-source dual-energy computed tomography angiography (DSDECTA) in the diagnosis of active GI bleeding, 58 consecutive patients underwent the procedure. An active bleeding source was identified in 67.2%, all of which were confirmed by one or more reference standards. In the negative group, 15/19 patients went home without any episode. The overall sensitivity, specificity, PPV, NPV, and accuracy of DSDECTA were 88.6, 100, 100, 73.7, and 91.4%, respectively. The AUC was 0.935 ± 0.063. The dose reduction of a dual-phase DSDECTA protocol was approximately 30%, compared with that of a triple-phase protocol used in a previous study.[67]

Intervention to Stem the Bleeding

Besides therapeutic colonoscopy, the other options are angiographic embolization or surgery, both of which are considered below:

Emergency Angiography

The utility of mesenteric angiography in the diagnosis and management of LGIH has been well established and is done when colonoscopy is either inconclusive or precluded by active bleeding. Bleeding at a rate of more than 0.5 mL/min can be detected by selective mesenteric angiography (Fig. 3).

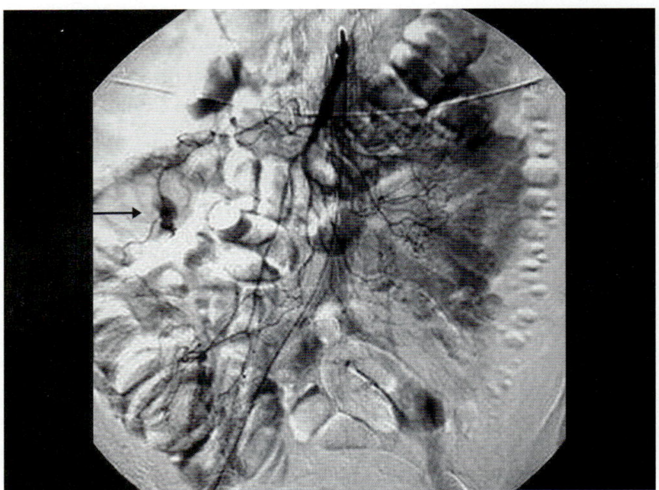

Figure 3 Angiographic appearance of angiodysplasia

Emergency angiography is indicated when after 4 units of blood transfusion in the first 2 hours following hospital admission, the systolic blood pressure remains <100 mmHg. Browder et al. reported the outcome of 50 such patients initially managed with emergency angiography. The average age was 67.2; mean hematocrit, 23.7; and average transfusion, 7.6 units. Bleeding site could by located in 72%; however, the etiologies of bleeding were mostly colonic in origin from diverticular disease ($n = 19$) and arteriovenous malformations ($n = 15$), which is at variance from the epidemiology seen in our population. Twenty of 22 (91%) patients receiving selective intra-arterial vasopressin stopped bleeding but 50% rebled on cessation of vasopressin. Thirty-five of 50 (70%) patients underwent surgery, with 57% operated on electively after vasopressin therapy. A total of 17 patients had segmental colectomy, with no rebleeding. Operative morbidity in these 35 patients was significantly improved when compared with previously reported patients undergoing emergency subtotal colectomy without angiography (8.6 vs. 37%; $P<0.02$). The authors claim that angiography successfully locates the bleeding site, allowing for segmental colectomy. Vasopressin infusion transiently halts bleeding, permitting elective surgery in many instances.[68] Details of the techniques used, outcomes, and complications have been reviewed by Cherian et al. from the Kovai Medical Center and Hospital, Coimbatore.[69]

The disadvantages of angiography are that it has a sensitivity of approximately 30–47%, can only be performed during active bleeding, and has a complication rate of about 9%. The risk of bowel ischemia and cardiac arrhythmia seen with vasopressin infusions have been reduced with newer super-selective embolization techniques. However, in a review of 20 studies utilizing super-selective embolization for control of LGIH, major complications requiring surgery or resulting in death were seen in as many as 17%.[48] Another significant concern for both angiography and MDCT is renal compromise secondary to infusion of contrast.[70]

Provocative Mesenteric Angiography

Acute LGIH usually stops spontaneously. In patients with recurrent bleed, when the source cannot be identified on angiography, provocative visceral arteriography has been advocated for diagnosis. Prior studies using streptokinase, urokinase, or tissue plasminogen activator have reported a 33–37.5% rate of identifying the site of hemorrhage. Widlus and Salis reported a retrospective analysis of nine patients with recurrent massive bleed and unidentified source in whom provocative visceral arteriography was performed using reteplase as the fibrinolytic agent. Colonic hemorrhage was induced in 89% of patients with no procedure-related complications. These patients subsequently underwent micro-embolization, segmental resection, or were treated conservatively. The authors concluded that reteplase is a safe and effective provocative agent, to allow localization in patients with occult, recurrent, and massive LGIH, but no further studies have been reported as yet.[71]

More recently provocative mesenteric angiography was performed using a protocol of systemic anticoagulation with heparin followed by selective transcatheter injection of vasodilator and tissue plasminogen activator into the arterial distribution of highest suspicion on 34 patients with obscure and recurrent LGIH. The authors also concluded that patients with melena and patients admitted for reasons other than acute LGIH were significantly less likely to benefit from provocative mesenteric angiography.[72]

Table 2: Outcome of management in lower gastrointestinal hemorrhage ($n = 91$)[3]

	n	%
Bleed stopped on conservative therapy	18	20
(including five where no diagnosis could be made)		
Diagnosis made on colonoscopy	36	40
Remaining subjected to emergency laparotomy	**37**	
Diagnosis obvious on exploratory laparoscopy	25/37	67
Diagnosis by intraoperative endoscopic	12/37	33
Overall mortality	4	(4)*

* One due to rebleed after surgery from an additional lesion.

Surgical Options and Outcome

Emergency Surgery

Emergency surgery is required in about 10–25% of patients with LGIH in whom nonoperative management is unsuccessful or unavailable. Following are the indications for emergency surgery suggested by the AAFP[49]:

1. Persistent hemodynamic instability with active bleeding
2. Persistent or recurrent bleeding
3. Transfusion of more than 4 units packed RBCs in a 24-hour period, with active or recurrent bleeding

It is also suggested that comorbid disease and local expertise available must be considered before deciding to take the patient for emergency surgery.

Surgical Options

Surgical options depend on whether the bleeding source has been accurately identified preoperatively. Segmental bowel resection after accurate localization of the bleeding point gives the best results with low recurrence rates and morbidity and mortality. However, if the diagnosis is still not clear, the abdomen is invariably explored through a midline vertical incision. The intraoperative strategy to use multiple non-crushing intestinal clamps to identify the segment that fills up with blood has largely been given up. Transillumination of bowel may sometimes reveal abnormal vessels or ulcers. Intraoperative enteroscopy (IOE) is done with the help of a gastroenterologist in case the site/cause of bleeding is not obvious on laparotomy. A colonoscope is usually introduced by the surgeon through an enterotomy and he/she then assists its passage. Enteroscopy is performed while advancing the scope as manipulation of the small bowel with the colonoscope itself may cause iatrogenic mucosal tears and hematomas, which may be mistakenly identified as a source of bleeding. If the bleeding point cannot still be diagnosed through intraoperative pan-intestinal endoscopy, options available for a surgeon are a closure or to perform a right hemicolectomy or a subtotal colectomy.

"Blind" Right Hemicolectomy

"Blind" right hemicolectomy has been advised and followed in a number of GI surgical centers in India, before the expertise for performing a full-length colonoscopy/angiography in a hemodynamically unstable patient was available even in tertiary care centers, leave aside the facility of intraoperative endoscopy. The procedure is still relevant in India if left-sided colonoscopy/sigmoidoscopy is negative, as in most of our patients the causative lesion lies in the terminal ileum/right colon.[3,73] If on exploratory laparotomy, the causative lesion is not obvious, a blind right-sided hemicolectomy may reveal the cause on examining the specimen in the operation theatre. Whether or not to perform a primary anastomosis depends upon the hemodynamic stability and whether the cause has been located. Performing an ileostomy and mucous fistula has the advantage of safety and being able to localize the site of bleed to small/large bowel if the bleed recurs, the attendant morbidity notwithstanding. On the other hand, in Western literature, subtotal colectomy is considered the procedure of choice in patients who are actively bleeding from an unknown source.

Outcome

The outcome of evaluation and treatment of 91 patients with massive LGIH in tertiary care hospitals of the Indian Army[3] are detailed in Table 2. Analysis of recently collated data of 296 patients with LGIH who underwent surgery from 1985 to 2012 at the Department of GI Surgery, AIIMS, intraoperative endoscopy was required in 84, 129 (44%) patients underwent a right hemicolectomy (45 with a stoma), and 104 (35%) segmental resection of the small bowel (22 with a stoma). Subtotal colectomy was undertaken in only 26 (9%). Twenty three (8%) patients had recurrence of LGIH, 12 of who required reoperation. The overall 30-day operative mortality was 46/296 (15.5%). [Personal communication].

OBSCURE GASTROINTESTINAL BLEED

Definition

Obscure gastrointestinal bleeding (OGIB), be it overt or occult, represents about 5% of all GI hemorrhage,[74,75] and is defined as bleeding from the GI tract that persists or recurs without an obvious etiology after an initial evaluation using bidirectional endoscopy and imaging with a small bowel radiograph.[76]

Etiology

The hemorrhage originates most commonly from the small bowel and the common cause, as in LGIH, is very different in Indians as compared with the reports from Western literature. In the West, the most common cause of OGIB is a vascular lesion, typically found in the small bowel which at times may be associated with renal failure, scleroderma, CREST syndrome (The acronym "CREST" refers to the five main features: calcinosis, Raynaud's phenomenon, esophageal dysmotility, sclerodactyly, and telangiectasia.), radiation injury, collagen vascular disease, or Von Willebrand disease. Other vascular causes include Dieulafoy lesions, ectopic varices, and hemorrhoids.[77,78]

Hayashi et al. demonstrated that only 12% of patients with OGIB were found to have NSAID-induced ulcers or erosions in the small bowel among 61 patients who had undergone double-balloon endoscopy (DBE) for GI bleeding or anemia, at Jichi Medical School Hospital, Japan.[79] On the other hand, in a large study from Kolkata of 222 patients with definite lesions at capsule endoscopy (CE), 156 (70%) had ulcers/erosions. Tumors of the small bowel were found in 48 and angiodysplasia only in 18. The authors found it difficult to characterize ulcers/erosions, but at least 12 were considered to be tubercular (based on abdominal CT scan ± fine-needle aspiration cytology and follow-up), 42 patients were considered to have Crohn's disease (based on fissuring serpiginous ulcers with cobblestone appearance, or histology from tissue obtained at enteroscopy or surgery), and only 12 ulcers were NSAID induced.[73]

Neoplasms of the small intestine are an important cause of OGIB and benign tumors tend to bleed more than malignant tumors. Gastrointestinal stromal tumor (GIST) (Fig. 4) is the most common neoplasm causing OGIH. Other neoplastic causes include carcinoids, adenocarcinoma, ampullary adenoma, and metastatic lesions such as melanoma.[78]

The authors justifiably concluded that DBE is a useful diagnostic tool with high clinical practice value and should be considered the gold standard for the investigation of small bowel tumors.

Evaluation of Obscure Gastrointestinal Bleeding

For the ease of evaluation, patients with OGIB have been further classified into three categories by Goenka et al.[73] as follows:

1. Persistent overt bleeding (bleeding documented within 48 hours at the time of first evaluation)
2. Recent overt bleeding (last episode of bleeding > 48 hours prior to the first evaluation)
3. Obscure occult bleeding (anemia associated with positive fecal occult blood without overt bleeding)

Capsule Endoscopy

The ability of CE to identify a definite bleeding source (Figs 5 to 8) was found to be significantly higher for category I than category II and III patients ($p < 0.05$), but there was no significant difference in the diagnostic yield when comparing category II and III patients.[73]

In the status report by the Technology Assessment Committee of the American Society for Gastrointestinal Endoscopy evaluating a series of 260 patients with OGIB, the yield of CE was 87% in patients with ongoing overt OGIB and 46% in those with occult OGIB,[80] whereas workers from Shanghai suggest that the optimum timing of CE in OGIB is within the first few days, with an acceptable maximum duration of 2 weeks.[81]

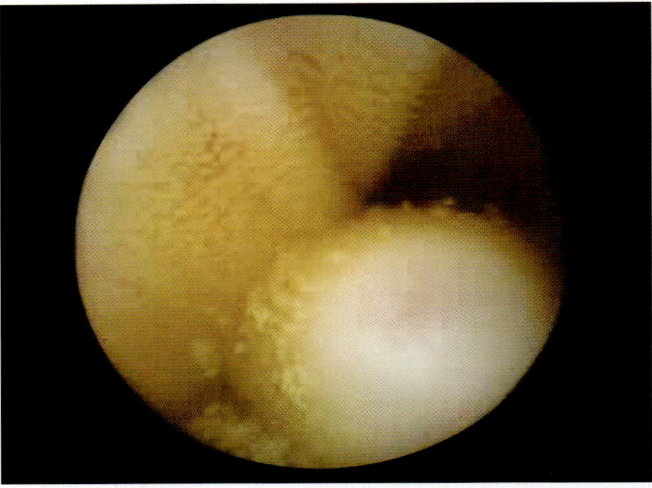

Figure 5 Capsule enteroscopy showing a globular mass in jejunum with loss of villous pattern and shining overlying mucosa

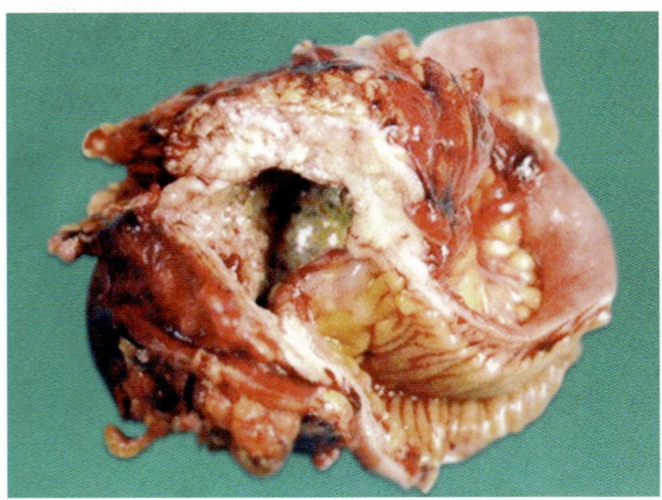

Figure 4 Resected specimen of gastrointestinal stromal tumor (GIST) of the ileum

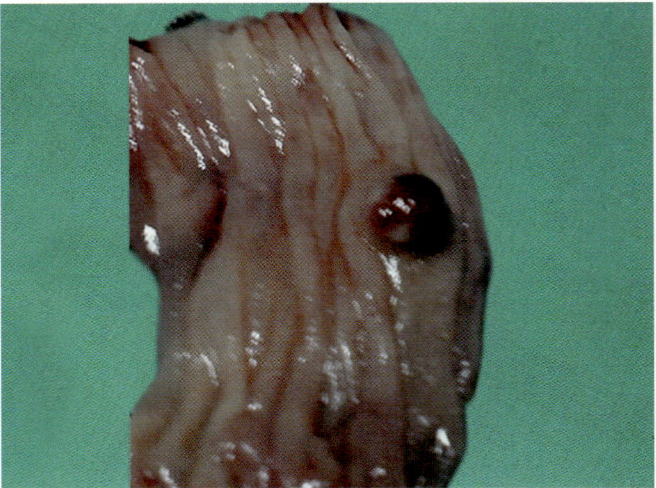

Figure 6 Resected segment of the jejunum showing a small polypoidal lesion with an adherent clot on its surface

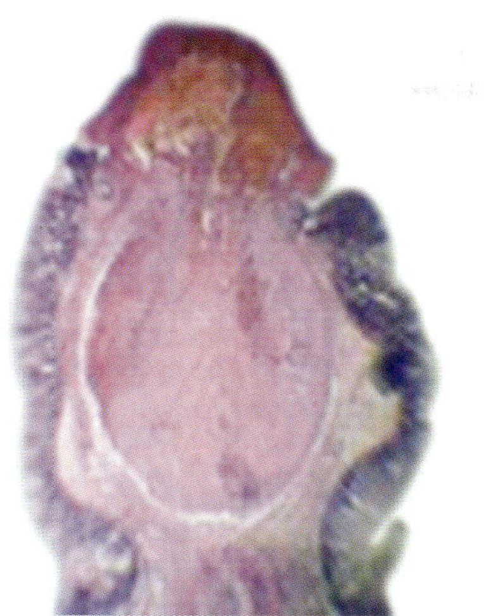

Figure 7 Whole mount view of the jejunal submucosal polyp showing bleed from the mucosal surface (H&E stain ×4)

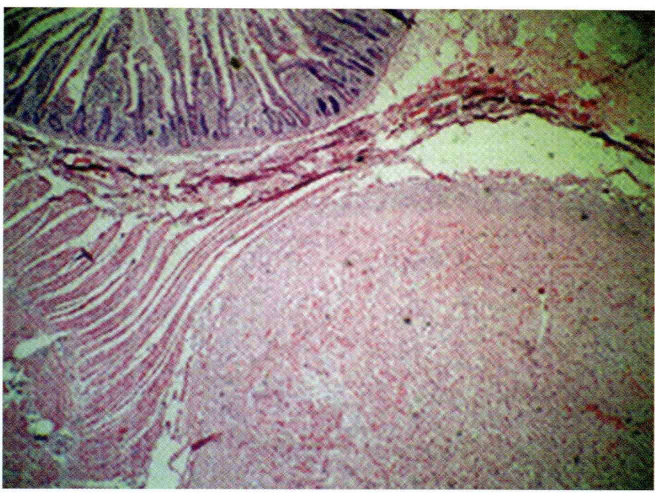

Figure 8 Microphotograph of the jejunal polyp showing myxoid areas with stellate cells and blood vessels (H&E ×100)

Capsule endoscopy, balloon-assisted enteroscopy, spiral enteroscopy, and CT enterography have overcome the limitations of older diagnostic tests. Capsule endoscopy is presently endorsed for the evaluation of patients with OGIB after a negative bidirectional endoscopy. However, balloon-assisted enteroscopy is useful for both the diagnosis and endoscopic management of OGIB.[82] Computed tomographic enterography on the other hand is superior to small bowel radiography for luminal and extraluminal lesions. Such advances in small bowel imaging and the therapeutic ability have resulted in a trend toward noninvasive evaluation and endoscopic management of OGIB.[73,76,83,84]

Use of CE in diagnosis of OGIB is hampered by the lack of control on the capsule, inability to biopsy the lesion or attempt endoscopic treatment, and the possibility of retaining the capsule proximal to a stenotic lesion in the bowel.[85] The contraindications to CE are dementia leading to inability to swallow the capsule, strictures in the esophagus, or subacute small bowel obstruction.

Double-balloon Endoscopy

The diagnosis of OGIB has been markedly improved with the development of total enteroscopy with a nonsurgical steerable double-balloon method by Yamamoto et al. in 2001.[86] Double-balloon endoscopy may be performed either through the mouth or anus and is able to explore a large part of the small bowel. It also has the advantage of image clarity, manual control, option of performing a biopsy, and endoscopic treatment,[87] and has been demonstrated to be a safe and useful procedure for the diagnosis of OGIB.[88] In a recent single-center study from the Zhejiang Province, China, 440 consecutive DBE examinations were performed in 400 patients between January 2007 and April 2012. Small bowel tumors were diagnosed in 78 patients, of whom 67 were diagnosed using DBE, resulting in a diagnostic yield of 16.8% (67/400). Adenocarcinoma (29.5%, 23/78), GIST (24.4%, 19/78), and lymphoma (15.4%, 12/78) were the most common tumors. Among the 78 tumors, 60.3% (47/78) were located in the jejunum, and the overall number of malignant tumors was 74.4% (58/78). Double-balloon endoscopy examinations were frequently performed in patients with OGIB (47.4%) and abdominal pain (24.4%). The positive detection rate for DBE in the 78 patients with small bowel tumors was 85.9% (67/78), which was higher than that of a CT scan (72.9%, 51/70). Based on the operation results, the accuracy rates of DBE for locating small bowel neoplasms, such as adenocarcinoma, GIST, and lymphoma, were 94.4, 100, and 100%, respectively. The positive biopsy rates for adenocarcinoma and lymphoma were 71.4 and 60%, respectively.[82]

However, diagnostic yield of CE has been found to be significantly higher compared with a single DBE examination done via the oral or anal route (137/219 vs. 110/219, odds ratio: 1.67, 95% confidence interval: 1.14–2.44, $p < 0.01$).[89]

Capsule endoscopy has also been found to have higher diagnostic yield and comparable long-term outcomes when compared with angiography. In a recent study from Hong Kong, 60 consecutive patients presenting OGIH were randomized to receive small bowel CE or angiography and followed up for a mean duration of 48.5 months. The diagnostic yield of immediate CE was significantly higher than angiography (53.3 vs. 20.0%, $p = 0.016$). The cumulative risk of rebleeding in the angiography and CE group was 33.3 and 16.7%, respectively ($p = 0.10$, log-rank test). There was no significant difference in the long-term outcomes between the two groups, including further transfusion, hospitalization for rebleeding, and mortality.[90]

Liu and Kaffes after a recent review of all full original articles in English-languaged journals in the PubMed database from 1985 to 2010 relevant to the investigation of OGIH recommend CE and DBE to be both first-line investigations as they are complimentary procedures, with comparable high diagnostic yields and DBE also provides the opportunity for therapeutic intervention. Imaging modalities such as CT enterography and CT enteroclysis may be considered when CE or DBE are contraindicated. Repeating the gastroscopy and/or colonoscopy may be fruitful in some situations. Older diagnostic modalities such as enteroclysis, CT, angiography, and TRBC scintigraphy still play a complementary but increasingly selective role.[91]

Intraoperative Enteroscopy

It involves the endoscopic evaluation of the small bowel by surgical assistance usually via laparotomy. The diagnostic yield of this procedure ranges between 58 and 88%.[92] However, rebleeding has been reported to occur in up to 60% of patients after IOE,[93] as pathology may not be noticed due to limited visibility and the evanescent nature of vascular ectasias. Other complications of IOE include serosal tears, perforation, avulsion of mesenteric vessels, and prolonged post-procedure ileus.[94] At present, this procedure is reserved for patients with negative diagnostic yield on other modalities, including CE and DBE and requiring multiple transfusions.[77]

SUMMARY

Although the epidemiology of LGIH in India is very different from the West, a full-length colonoscopy is the initial diagnostic method of choice as in addition to its diagnostic utility, colonoscopy offers the opportunity for therapeutic intervention.

Advances in diagnostic and therapeutic endoscopy, CT, and interventional angiography have resulted in a shift away from the need for surgical treatment in the elderly with multiple comorbidities suffering from diverticulosis or angiodysplasia. This has also reduced healthcare costs and, more importantly, patient morbidity and mortality in developed countries. If surgery is required, precise localization and segmental resection give better outcome than the subtotal colectomy.

However, for Indian patients, if the left-sided colonoscopy is negative and facilities for IOE/CE/DBE/MDCT/selective angiography are not available and the patient has already been transfused 6 units of blood, an exploratory laparotomy should be performed. If the diagnosis is not obvious on laparotomy, performing a "blind" right hemicolectomy may be a life-saving procedure. Effort should normally be made to locate the site of bleed by utilizing modern modalities such as CT angiography, DBE, CE, and angiography. Per-operative enteroscopy can be used if the facilities exist and the site of bleeding is still elusive.

Despite improvements in diagnostic imaging and procedures, 10–20% of patients with OGIB have no demonstrable bleeding source, and 5–10% of patients may present with recurrent episodes of massive hemorrhage. Such patients undergo repeated transfusions and multiple invasive investigations repeatedly. This unresolved problem requires systematic and orderly evaluation at a tertiary care center by a multidisciplinary team.

REFERENCES

1. Imdahl A. Genesis and pathophysiology of lower gastrointestinal bleeding. Langenbeck's Arch Surg. 2001;386:1-7.
2. Longstreth GF. Epidemiology and outcome of patients hospitalized with acute lower gastrointestinal haemorrhage: a population-based study. Am J Gastroenterol. 1997;92:419-24.
3. Anand AC, Patnaik PK, Bhalla VP, et al. Massive lower intestinal bleeding—a decade of experience. Trop Gastroenterol. 2001;22:131-4.
4. Bhargava DK, Rai RR, Dasarathy S, et al. Colonoscopy for unexplained lower gastrointestinal bleeding in a tropical country. Trop Gastroenterol. 1995;16:59-63.
5. Govil D, Sahni P. Lower gastrointestinal haemorrhage. GI Surg Ann. 1994;93-103.
6. Talley NJ, Jones M. Self-reported rectal bleeding in a United States community: prevalence, risk factors, and health care seeking. Am J Gastroenterol. 1998;93:2179-83.
7. Gayer C, Chino A, Lucas C, et al. Acute lower gastrointestinal bleeding in 1,112 patients admitted to an urban emergency medical center. Surgery. 2009;146:600.
8. Zuckerman GR, Prakash C. Acute lower intestinal bleeding. Part II: etiology, therapy, and outcomes. Gastrointest Endosc. 1999;49:228-38.
9. Bhargava DK, Rai RR, Dasarathy S, et al. Colonoscopy for unexplained lower gastrointestinal bleeding in a tropical country. Trop Gastroenterol. 1995;16:59-63.
10. Laine L, Shah A. Randomized trial of urgent vs. elective colonoscopy in patients hospitalized with lower GI bleeding. Am J Gastroenterol. 2010;105:2636-41.
11. Sahni P, Nundy S. Lower gastrointestinal hemorrhage In: Srivastava SK, editor. Modern concepts in surgery. New Delhi: Tata McGraw Hill; 1992. pp. 129-34.
12. Meyers MA, Alonso DR, Gray GF, et al. Pathogenesis of bleeding colonic diverticulosis. Gastroenterology. 1976;71:577-83.
13. Koval G, Benner KG, Rosch J, et al. Aggressive angiographic diagnosis in acute lower gastrointestinal haemorrhage. Dig Dis Sci. 1987;32:248-53.
14. Casarella WJ, Galloway SJ, Taxin RN, et al. "Lower" gastrointestinal tract haemorrhage: new concepts based on arteriography. AJR Am J Roentgenol. 1974;121:357-68.
15. DeMarkles MP, Murphy JR. Acute lower gastrointestinal bleeding. Med Clin North Am. 1993;77:1085-100.
16. McGuire HH, Haynes BW. Massive haemorrhage from diverticulosis of the colon: guidelines for therapy based on bleeding patterns observed in fifty cases. Ann Surg. 1972;175:847-53.
17. McGuire HH Jr. Bleeding colonic diverticula: a reappraisal of natural history and management. Ann Surg. 1994;220:653-6.
18. Foutch PG, Rex DK, Lieberman DA. Prevalence and natural history of colonic angiodysplasia among healthy asymptomatic people. Am J Gastroenterol. 1995;90:564.
19. Krevsky B. Detection and treatment of angiodysplasia. Gastrointest Endosc Clin N Am. 1997;7:509.
20. Gupta N, Longo WE, Vernava AM 3rd. Angiodysplasia of the lower gastrointestinal tract: an entity readily diagnosed by colonoscopy and primarily managed non-operatively. Dis Colon Rectum. 1995;38:979-82.
21. Saperas E, Videla S, Dot J, et al. Risk factors for recurrence of acute gastrointestinal bleeding from angiodysplasia. Eur J Gastroenterol Hepatol. 2009;21:1333-9.
22. GK Pande, S Nundy. Ulcerative colitis. In: Srivastava SK, editor. Modern concepts on surgery. New Delhi: Tata McGraw Hill; 1992. pp. 221-6.
23. Pal S, Sahni P, Pande GK, et al. Outcome following emergency surgery for refractory severe ulcerative colitis in a tertiary care centre in India. BMC Gastroenterol. 2005;5:39.
24. Robert JH, Sachar DB, Aufses AH, et al. Management of severe haemorrhage in ulcerative colitis. Am J Surg. 1990;19:550-5.
25. Robert JR, Sachar DB, Greenstein AJ. Severe gastrointestinal bleeding in Crohn's disease. Ann Surg. 1991;213:207-11.
26. Cirocco WC, Reilly JC, Rusin LC. Life-threatening haemorrhage and exsanguination from Crohn's disease: report of four cases. Dis Colon Rectum. 1995;38:85-95.
27. Peura DA, Lanza FL, Gostout CJ, et al. The American College of Gastroenterology bleeding registry: preliminary findings. Am J Gastroenterol. 1997;92:924-8.
28. Chalasani N, Wilcox CM. Etiology and outcome of lower gastrointestinal bleeding in patients with AIDS. Am J Gastroenterol. 1998;93:175-8.
29. Krishna RP, Singh RK, Ghoshal UC. Recurrent lower gastrointestinal bleeding from idiopathic ileocolonic varices: a case report. J Med Case Reports. 2010;4:257.
30. Enns R. Dieulafoy's lesions of the rectum: a rare cause of lower gastrointestinal bleeding. Can J Gastroenterol. 2001;15:541-5.
31. Nishimuta Y, Tsurumaru D, Komori M, et al. A case of rectal Dieulafoy's lesion successfully treated by transcatheter arterial embolization. Jpn J Radiol. 2012;30:176-9.

32. Chait MM. Lower gastrointestinal bleeding in the elderly. World J Gastrointest Endosc. 2010;2(5):147-54.
33. Tseng CA, Chen LT, Tsai KB, et al. Acute hemorrhagic rectal ulcer syndrome: a new clinical entity? Report of 19 cases and review of the literature. Dis Colon Rectum. 2004;47:895-903; discussion 9035.
34. Crook J, Esche B, Futter N. Effect of pelvic radiotherapy for prostate cancer on bowel, bladder, and sexual function: the patient's perspective. Urology. 1996;47:387-94.
35. Fuccio L, Guido A, Laterza L, et al. Randomised clinical trial: preventive treatment with topical rectal beclomethasone dipropionate reduces post-radiation risk of bleeding in patients irradiated for prostate cancer. Aliment Pharmacol Ther. 2011;34:628-37.
36. Huang ES, Strate LL, Ho WW, et al. Long-term use of aspirin and the risk of gastrointestinal bleeding. Am J Med. 2011;124:426-33.
37. Scottish Intercollegiate Guidelines Network (SIGN). Management of acute upper and lower gastrointestinal bleeding. A national clinical guideline. SIGN publication no 105. Edinburgh (Scotland): Scottish Intercollegiate Guidelines Network (SIGN); 2008. pp. 34-6.
38. Balachandran B, Singhi S. Emergency management of lower gastrointestinal bleed in children. Indian J Pediatr. 2013;80:219-25.
39. Miller LS, Barbarevech C, Friedman LS. Less frequent causes of lower gastrointestinal bleeding. Gastroenterol Clin North Am. 1994;23:21-52.
40. Mate AD, Surnare KR, Deolekar SS, et al. Lower gastrointestinal bleeding due to hepatic artery pseudoaneurysm following laparoscopic cholecystectomy. J Minim Access Surg. 2013;9:31-3.
41. Sanchez LD, Tracy JA, Berkoff D, et al. Ischemic colitis in marathon runners: a case-based review. J Emerg Med. 2006;30:321-6.
42. Lhewa DY, Strate LL. Pros and cons of colonoscopy in management of acute lower gastrointestinal bleeding World J Gastroenterol. 2012;18:1185-90.
43. Strate LL. Editorial: Urgent colonoscopy in lower GI bleeding: not so fast. Am J Gastroenterol. 2010;105,2643-5.
44. Jensen DM, Machicado GA. Diagnosis and treatment of severe hematochezia. The role of urgent colonoscopy after purge. Gastroenterology. 1988;95:1569-74.
45. Strate LL, Syngal S. Predictors of utilization of early colonoscopy vs. radiography for severe lower intestinal bleeding. Gastrointest Endosc. 2005;61:46-52.
46. Cohn SM, Moller BA, Zieg PM, et al. Angiography for preoperative evaluation in patients with lower gastrointestinal bleeding: are the benefits worth the risk? Arch Surg. 1998;133:50-5.
47. Wilkins T, Baird C, Pearson AN, et al. Diverticular bleeding. Am Fam Physician. 2009;80:977-83.
48. Strate LL, Naumann CR. The role of colonoscopy and radiological procedures in the management of acute lower intestinal bleeding. Clin Gastroenterol Hepatol. 2010;8:333-43.
49. Emslie JT, Zarnegar K, Siegel ME, et al. Technetium-99m-labeled red blood cell scans in the investigation of gastrointestinal bleeding. Dis Colon Rectum. 1996;39:750-4.
50. Ng DA, Opelka FG, Beck DE, et al. Predictive value of technetium Tc 99m-labeled red blood cell scintigraphy for positive angiogram in massive lower gastrointestinal hemorrhage. Dis Colon Rectum. 1997;40:471-7.
51. Schmidt KG, Rasmussen JW, Grove O, et al. The use of indium-111-labelled platelets for scintigraphic localization of gastrointestinal bleeding, with special reference to occult bleeding. Scand J Gastroenterol. 1986;21:407-14.
52. Mole DJ, Hughes SJ, Khosraviani K. ^{111}Indium-labelled red-cell scintigraphy to detect intermittent gastrointestinal bleeding from synchronous small- and large-bowel adenocarcinomas. Eur J Gastroenterol Hepatol. 2004;16:795-9.
53. Hunter JM, Pezim ME. Limited value of technetium 99m-labeled red cell scintigraphy in localization of lower gastrointestinal bleeding. Am J Surg. 1990;159:504-6.
54. Hammond KL, Beck DE, Hicks TC, et al. Implications of negative technetium 99m-labeled red blood cell scintigraphy in patients presenting with lower gastrointestinal bleeding. Am J Surg. 2007;193:404-7; discussion 407-8.
55. Macari M, Chandarana H, Balthazar E, et al. Intestinal ischemia versus intramural hemorrhage: CT evaluation. AJR Am J Roentgenol. 2003;180:177-84.
56. Ernst O, Bulois P, Saint-Drenant S, et al. Helical CT in acute lower gastrointestinal bleeding. Eur Radiol. 2003;13:114-7.
57. Yamaguchi T, Yoshikawa K. Enhanced CT for initial localization of active lower gastrointestinal bleeding. Abdom Imaging. 2003;28:634-6.
58. Sabharwal R, Vladica P, Chou R, et al. Helical CT in the diagnosis of acute lower gastrointestinal hemorrhage. Eur J Radiol. 2006;58:273-9.
59. Lee S, Welman CJ, Ramsay D. Investigation of acute lower gastrointestinal bleeding with 16- and 64-slice multidetector CT. J Med Imaging Radiat Oncol. 2009;53:56-63.
60. Frattaroli FM, Casciani E, Spoletini D, et al. Prospective study comparing multi-detector row CT and endoscopy in acute gastrointestinal bleeding. World J Surg. 2009;33:2209-17.
61. Sun H, Jin Z, Li X, et al. Detection and localization of active gastrointestinal bleeding with multi-detector row computed tomography angiography: a 5-year prospective study in one medical center. J Clin Gastroenterol. 2012;46:31-41.
62. Kuhle WG, Sheiman RG. Detection of active colonic hemorrhage with use of helical CT: findings in a swine model. Radiology. 2003;228:743-52.
63. Wu LM, Xu JR, Yin Y, et al. Usefulness of CT angiography in diagnosing acute gastrointestinal bleeding: a meta-analysis. World J Gastroenterol. 2010;16: 3957-63.
64. Kennedy DW, Laing CJ, Tseng LH, et al. Detection of active gastrointestinal hemorrhage with CT angiography: a 4(1/2)-year retrospective review. J Vasc Interv Radiol. 2010;21:848-55.
65. Jaeckle T, Stuber G, Hoffmann MH, et al. Detection and localization of acute upper and lower gastrointestinal (GI) bleeding with arterial phase multi-detector row helical CT. Eur Radiol. 2008;18:1406-13.
66. Lin S, Rockey DC. Obscure gastrointestinal bleeding. Gastroenterol Clin North Am. 2005;34:679-98.
67. Sun H, Xue HD, Wang YN, et al. Dual-source dual-energy computed tomography angiography for active gastrointestinal bleeding: a preliminary study. Clin Radiol. 2013;68:139-47.
68. Browder W, Cerise EJ, Litwin MS. Impact of emergency angiography in massive lower gastrointestinal bleeding. Ann Surg. 1986;204:530-6.
69. Cherian MP, Mehta P, Kalyanpur TM, et al. Arterial interventions in gastrointestinal bleeding. Semin Intervent Radiol. 2009;26:184-96.
70. Yoon W, Jeong YY, Shin SS, et al. Acute massive gastrointestinal bleeding: detection and localization with arterial phase multi-detector row helical CT. Radiology. 2006;239:160-7.
71. Widlus DM, Salis AI. Reteplase provocative visceral arteriography. J Clin Gastroenterol. 2007;41:830-3.
72. Kim CY, Suhocki PV, Miller MJ Jr, et al. Provocative mesenteric angiography for lower gastrointestinal hemorrhage: results from a single-institution study. J Vasc Interv Radiol. 2010;21:477-83.
73. Goenka MK, Majumder S, Kumar S, et al. Single center experience of capsule endoscopy in patients with obscure gastrointestinal bleeding. World J Gastroenterol. 2011;17:774-8.
74. Raju GS, Gerson L, Das A, et al . American Gastroenterological Association (AGA) Institute technical review on obscure gastrointestinal bleeding. Gastroenterology. 2007;133:1697-717.
75. Cellier C. Obscure gastrointestinal bleeding: role of videocapsule and double-balloon enteroscopy. Best Pract Res Clin Gastroenterol. 2008;22:329-40.
76. Pasha SF, Hara AK, Leighton JA. Diagnostic evaluation and management of obscure gastrointestinal bleeding: a changing paradigm. Gastroenterol Hepatol (NY). 2009;5:839-50.

77. Kochhar GS, Sanaka MR, Vargo JJ. Therapeutic management options for patients with obscure gastrointestinal bleeding. Therap Adv Gastroenterol. 2012;5:71-81.
78. Rockey DC. Occult and obscure gastrointestinal bleeding: causes and clinical management. Nat Rev Gastroenterol Hepatol. 2010;7:265-79.
79. Hayashi Y, Yamamoto H, Kita H, et al. Non-steroidal anti-inflammatory drug-induced small bowel injuries identified by double-balloon endoscopy. World J Gastroenterol. 2005;11:4861-64.
80. Mishkin DS, Chuttani R, Croffie J, et al. ASGE Technology Status Evaluation Report: wireless capsule endoscopy. Gastrointest Endosc. 2006;63:539-45.
81. Ge ZZ, Chen HY, Gao YJ, et al. Best candidates for capsule endoscopy for obscure gastrointestinal bleeding. J Gastroenterol Hepatol. 2007;22:2076-80.
82. Chen WG, Shan GD, Zhang H et al. Double-balloon enteroscopy in small bowel tumors: a Chinese single-center study. World J Gastroenterol. 2013;19:3665-71.
83. Koh SJ, Im JP, Kim JW, et al. Long-term outcome in patients with obscure gastrointestinal bleeding after negative capsule endoscopy. World J Gastroenterol. 2013;19:1632-8.
84. Pasha SF, Leighton JA. Endoscopic techniques for small bowel imaging. Radiol Clin North Am. 2013;51:177-87.
85. Rondonotti E, Villa F, Mulder CJ, et al. Small bowel capsule endoscopy in 2007: indications, risks and limitations. World J Gastroenterol. 2007;13:6140-49.
86. Yamamoto H, Sekine Y, Sato Y, et al. Total enteroscopy with a nonsurgical steerable double-balloon method. Gastrointest Endosc. 2001;53:216-20.
87. Matsumoto T, Esaki M, Moriyama T, et al. Comparison of capsule endoscopy and enteroscopy with the double-balloon method in patients with obscure bleeding and polyposis. Endoscopy. 2005;37:827-32.
88. Wu CR, Huang LY, Song B, et al. Application of double-balloon enteroscopy in the diagnosis and therapy of small intestinal diseases. Chin Med J (Engl). 2007;120:2075-80.
89. Ran ZH, Tong JL. A meta-analysis of the yield of capsule endoscopy compared to double-balloon enteroscopy in patients with small bowel diseases. World J Gastroenterol. 2007;13:4372-78.
90. Leung WK, Ho Simon SM, Suen BY, et al. Capsule endoscopy or angiography in patients with acute overt obscure gastrointestinal bleeding: a prospective randomized study with long-term follow-up. Am J Gastroenterol. 2102;107:1370-6.
91. Liu K, Kaffes AJ. Review article: the diagnosis and investigation of obscure gastrointestinal bleeding. Aliment Pharmacol Ther. 2011;34:416-23.
92. Douard R, Wind P, Panis Y, et al. Intraoperative enteroscopy for diagnosis and management of unexplained gastrointestinal bleeding. Am J Surg. 2000;180:181-4.
93. Zaman A, Sheppard B, Katon RM. Total peroral intraoperative enteroscopy for obscure GI bleeding using a dedicated push enteroscope: diagnostic yield and patient outcome. Gastrointest Endosc. 1999;50:506-10.
94. Lopez MJ, Cooley JS, Petros JG, et al. Complete intraoperative small-bowel endoscopy in the evaluation of occult gastrointestinal bleeding using the sonde enteroscope. Arch Surg. 1996;131:272-7.

CHAPTER 118

Bariatric and Metabolic Surgery

Mahendra Narwaria, Ahmad Jan

INTRODUCTION

There has been a dramatic increase in the number of obese population worldwide. In the last three decades alone, its incidence has doubled with an estimated over half a billion obese individuals globally.[1] Apart from being a debilitating condition with variable medical illnesses[2] (Table 1), obesity is also associated with physiopsychological disorder like social isolation, depression, and other somatic abnormalities. Thus, long-term obesity is detrimental to a patient's health and well-being.[3]

The pathophysiology of obesity is complex and remains poorly understood. Its etiology is multifactorial, involving genetic, behavioral, psychological, and other causes. Among theses, it is postulated that the abnormal habit in dietary intake and reduced physical activity has pivotal role in increasing the incidence of obesity.[4]

Obesity is defined as abnormal or excessive fat accumulation that may impair health and it is classification mainly based on measuring the body mass index (BMI). For those in the Asia-Pacific region, the BMI was modified from internationally accepted guidelines, the latter based mainly on data from Europe and the United States. This modification is justified, given that Asians have a higher percentage of body fat for a given body weight, and are more highly predisposed to central abdominal adiposity than are other ethnicities. Thus, the proportional high body fat composition ultimately poses a high risk for developing obesity-related complications even with decreased BMI.[5-6] World health organization has established modified cutoff values for Asians[7] (Table 2). Furthermore, the International Diabetes Federation (IDF) endorsed waist circumference measurement as a parameter in detecting early incidence of metabolic syndrome in obese Asians because of their high propensity of central (abdominal) adiposity. It has been endorsed that Waist circumference of more than 90 cm in men and 80 cm in women is a marked point for the risk of developing metabolic syndrome.[12]

Modalities of Weight Management

Methods of weight management are generally divided in to two main categories, conservative and surgical. The former is further subdivided into: nutritional modification, physical exercises, and weight reducing medication. The Surgical options are ranging between either pure restrictive, malabsorbative or mixed procedures. When considering a successful weight managing tool, surgical intervention has been already supported by robust studies which proved its superiority compared to any other alternatives. Besides its long lasting effect on reducing excess weight, bariatric surgery also declared itself effective in preventing and controlling other co-morbidites attributed to the obesity.[8,9]

Modalities other than bariatric surgery are beyond the scope of this chapter and the discussion will be only limited to different surgical approaches commonly used in overweight management.

Indications for Bariatric Surgery

The Asian Pacific Metabolic and Bariatric Surgery Society has endorsed certain criteria for surgical intervention in Asian population (Table 3).[10]

These guidelines were further modified at the 2nd International Federation for the Surgery of Obesity-Asia-Pacific Chapter (IFSO-APC) Congress[11] as following:

- Surgery should be considered in the treatment of obesity among acceptable Asian candidates with BMI ≥35 with or without comorbidities.

Table 1: Comorbidities associated with obesity

GERD	Malignancies (Breast, endometrial, colorectal)	Venous stasis
Cardiovascular dysfunction (CAD, CHF)	Sexual hormone dysfunction	Degenerative arthritis (chronic joint pain)
Respiratory insufficiency (sleep apnea, asthma)	Infections	*Pseudotumor cerebri*
Metabolic syndrome (hyperlipidemia, HTN, T2DM)	Skin disorder	Psychosocial illness

GERD, gastroesophageal reflux disease; CAD, coronary artery disease; CHF, congestive heart failure; HTN, hypertension; T2DM, type 2 diabetes mellitus.

- Bariatric/gastrointestinal (GI) metabolic surgery should be considered in the treatment of type 2 diabetes mellitus (T2DM) or metabolic syndrome in patients who are inadequately controlled by lifestyle alterations or medical treatment for candidates with BMI = 30.
- The surgical approach may be considered a nonprimary alternative to treat inadequately controlled T2DM or metabolic syndrome among suitable Asian candidates with BMI ≥27.5.

Metabolic syndrome is considered an adjunct to obesity; thus, the criteria to define this syndrome must be clarified.

A patient is said to manifest metabolic syndrome if he or she has the following:

Central obesity with any two of the following four factors: raised triglyceride, reduced high density lipoprotine, DM and HTN (Table 4).

Contraindication for Bariatric Surgery

- Lack of social support
- Mental impairment that interferes with a patient's ability to weigh the risks against the benefits of surgery
- Active neoplastic disease
- Decompensated liver cirrhosis (Child Class C) with signs of portal hypertension.
- Life-threatening unstable or incurable preexisting comorbidities, including unstable coronary artery disease and uncontrolled severe obstructive sleep apnea with pulmonary hypertension
- Pregnancy

Table 2: World Health Organization proposed classification of body mass index in adult Asians

Classification	*Europids*	*Asians*	*Risk of comorbidities*
Underweight	<18.5	<18.5	Low
Normal range	18.8–24.9	18.5–22.9	Average
Overweight	>25	>23	Increased
Obese I	30–34.9	>25	Moderate
Obese II	35–39.9	>30	Severe
Obese III	>40	–	–

Note: No Obese III classification (morbid obesity) in Asians.

Table 3: Indications for bariatric surgery per Asian Pacific Metabolic and Bariatric Surgery Society consensus meeting, 2005

Patients with BMI >37 kg/m
Patients with BMI >32 kg/m and presence of diabetes or two significant obesity-related comorbidities
Patients unable to lose or maintain weight loss by dietary or medical measures
Patients >18 years but <65 years
Bariatric surgery may be performed on children <18 years after proper consultation with a pediatrician

- Immobility (e.g., wheelchair or scooter dependence)
- Inability to follow-up and lack of willingness to comply with postoperative regimens, including vitamin and mineral supplementation, and dietary changes
- Active substance abuse

Bariatric Surgery

Surgical procedures can be categorized into restrictive and combined restrictive-malabsorbtive procedures. International Federation for the Surgery of Obesity-Asia-Pacific Chapter Congress recommends the following procedures for bariatric and metabolic surgery for Asians: sleeve gastrectomy, gastric banding, gastric bypass, and biliopancreatic diversion with duodenal switch (BPD-DS). Laparoscopy-based bariatric surgery has become widely used because of advancements in laparoscopic instrumentation and training. This resulted in improved surgical outcomes, namely reduced pain, faster recovery, and fewer wound-related complications.

Rarely Performed Procedures

Procedures that were commonly performed in the past have to be mentioned because patients who have undergone these procedures are still encountered in practice.

Table 4: The new International Diabetes Federation definition

Elevated triglycerides	≥150 mg/dL (1.7 mmol/L) or specific treatment for this lipid abnormality
Reduced HDL cholesterol	<40 mg/dL (1.03 mmol/L) in males <50 mg/dL (1.29 mmol/L) in females or specific treatment for this lipid abnormality
Elevated blood pressure	Systolic BP ≥ 130 or diastolic BP ≥ 85 mm Hg or treatment of previously diagnosed hypertension
Elevated fasting plasma glucose	FPG ≥100 mg/dL (5.6 mmol/L), or previously diagnosed type 2 diabetes If above 5.6 mmol/L or 100 mg/dL, OGTT is strongly recommended but not necessary to define the presence of the syndrome

Note: If BMI is >30 kg/m^2, central obesity may be assumed and waist circumference need not be measured.
BMI, body mass index; HDL, high-density lipoprotein; FPG, fasting plasma glucose; OGTT, oral glucose tolerance test.

Intestinal Bypass

A purely malabsorbative procedure called jejunoileal bypass (JIB), performed in the 1960s and the 1970s, was abandoned in the early 1980s because of the significant risk of severe nutritional deficiency associated with intestinal bypass.

Vertical Gastroplasty

Vertical gastroplasty was introduced in 1980 as a purely restrictive bariatric procedure. The original (horizontal) gastroplasty involved stapling the stomach into a small partition, leaving only a small opening for food to pass from the upper stomach pouch into the lower stomach pouch. Inappropriate attempts to increase weight loss by narrowing the outlet led to pouch obstruction, staple line disruption, and high rate of reoperation, resulting in an extremely poor long-term weight loss. Thus, vertical gastroplasty is no longer performed.

Commonly Performed Procedure

Restrictive

Sleeve gastrectomy (SG): It was introduced by Hess in 1988[13] and Marceau in 1990[14] as part of biliopancreatic diversion surgery. In 2000, Regan et al. described the isolated sleeve gastrectomy as a first-stage surgery part of two-stage laparoscopic BPD-DS[15].

Technical approach: The surgical technique used in creating sleeve gastrectomy has often been a subject of debate. These controversies include the size of the bougie used in stomach remnant calibration, the distance between first stapler firing and the pylorus and plication of the stapler line. The following steps are recommended to achieve a desired tight sleeve:

a) Calibration of the stomach on the bougie size between 32 and 36 F.
b) Complete posterior dissection-resection of the thin layer of the posterior fundus from the left crus, and the crus should be visualized.
c) First antrum firing (5- 6 cm) from the pylorus.

SG can be conducted by two different approaches: the classical approach and the transomental approach. In the classical type, dissection commences by freeing the stomach from the greater omentum before creating the sleeved stomach. While in the transomental approach, dissection usually starts with creating a large greater trans-omental window followed by complete dissection of the posterior stomach wall from the structures in the lesser sac before embarking on sequential stapler firing to create the sleeve. In comparing the two approaches, in our experience, we found that, though, the operative time can be equal between the classical and transomental approach, however, the later technique can secure an extra safety measures in reducing the incidence of bleeding from the inadvertently teared short gastric or the gastroepiploic vessels. This is achieved by the lower pulling force that is exerted while separating the greater omentum off the specimen in the last stage of procedure after creating the sleeve (Figs 1 and 2).[16]

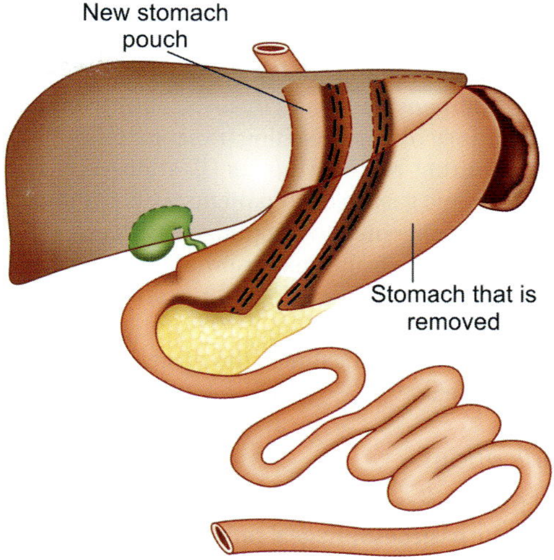

Figure 1 Sleeve gastrectomy

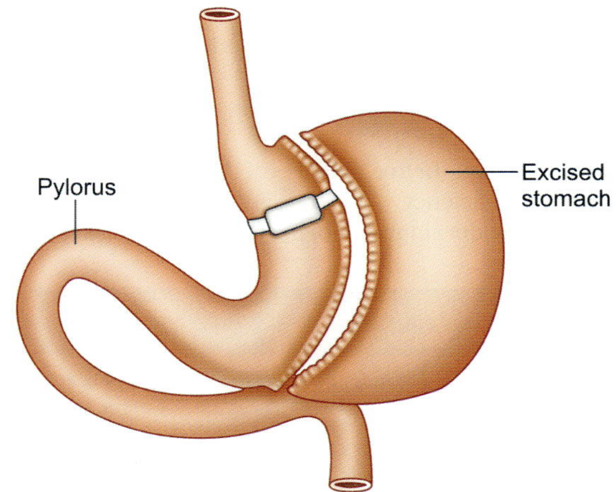

Figure 2 Banded sleeve gastrectomy

Mechanism of Action

- Food restriction: The newly created stomach remnant is 10% of its original size; thus, the amount of ingestion will be restricted.
- The level of ghrelin (also known as the hunger hormone), which is mainly secreted from cells located in the fundus, is markedly reduced after SG.[17]
- Enterohormonal changes: Accelerated emptying of gastric content into the duodenum and the intestine leads to changes in enterohormone secretion.[18]
- Although limited, SG can influence the secretion of the incretin hormones glucagon-like peptide-1 (GLP-1) and peptide tyrosine tyrosine. Thus, this type of surgery can be effective in diabetes mellitus management.[19]

Indications

- Stand-alone procedure in BMI <50
- Staged procedure in BMI >50 with severe metabolic syndrome

- Obesity with short history of well-managed metabolic syndrome (less than 5 years)
- Obesity in the elderly and adolescents
- Obesity in compensated liver cirrhosis, obesity in patient with end-stage kidney disease awaiting transplantation[20]
- Patients requiring periodic upper GI endoscopy for chronic ulcer and chronic gastritis and patients with cirrhotic liver who may require management of esophageal varices
- Patients precluded from malabsorbative procedure due to inflammatory bowel disease, chronic anemia, and chronic medication
- Surgery is not contraindicated in the presence of less than 5 cm hiatal hernia defect[16]

Contraindications

- Ulcer in the lesser curvature[21]
- Symptomatic gastroesophageal reflux disease (GERD)
- Barret's esophagus[21]

Advantages

- Technically simpler and less demanding than other types of bariatric surgery
- Can be a stand-alone procedure that needs no further adjustments
- Associated with better quality of life as it has no major nutritional deficiency
- Precludes the development of post-diet dumping syndrome

Table 5: Management of commonly encountered laparoscopic sleeve gastrectomy complications

Problem	*Possible cause*	*Suggested management*
Sleeve Leak	Tissular causes Ischemic—mechanical causes	Salvageable RYGB (Thal Patch) Gastric stent
GERD	Incomplete fundal resection Narrowing at incisura angularis Improper hiatal hernia defect closure De novo reflux disease	Endoscopy, esophageal manometery for diagnosis PPI for 3 months Conversion to GB in refractory condition
Early failure of weight loss	Technical cause (large bougie/extra fundus)	Revision surgery
Late food intolerance	Gastric stricture	Endoscopic dilation Seromyotomy Revision surgery
Early nausea and vomiting	Dehydration	Strict rehydration
Late persistent vomiting ± gait ataxia, blurred vision, amnesia	Wernicke's syndrome	Thiamine replacement

RYGB, Roux-en-Y gastric bypass; PPI, proton pump inhibitor; GERD, gastroesophageal reflux disease; GB, gastric bypass.

Disadvantages/Complications (Table 5)

- Presence of a long stapler line that can contribute to perioperative mortality and morbidity
- Irreversibility of the procedure
- Overall morbidity and mortality rates of 0–24% and 0.39%, respectively[22]
- Sleeve leakage
- Staple line bleeding
- Gastric stricture
- Weight regain

Outcomes

- Excessive body weight loss 5 years postsurgery reached 57% in some series.[23]
- Sucandy et al., indicated in their study of 131 patients 1 year post laparoscopic sleeve gastrectomy, the highest resolution of comorbidities was seen with DM (72%), followed by hypertension (55.5%), and hyperlipidemia (50%). All diabetic patients who participated in the study gained control of their hyperglycemia (either complete resolution or less severe disease) 18 months postsurgery.[24]
- Vidal et al. showed that the short-term outcomes of SG can be comparable to those of gastric bypass in terms of T2DM remission.[25]

Adjustable Gastric Band

The adjustable gastric band (AGB) has rapidly gained popularity globally, particularly in the United States and Australia because of its safety and effectiveness. Silicon gastric banding has been used since 1983, and its modification called stoma adjustable silicon gastric band has been used since 1986. Dr. Kuzmak is credited for the use of AGB, and the introduction of the stoma calibration device.[26] Many types of gastric bands are available: Bioenteric lap band system, realize band, midband and holigast. Gastric bands have an inflatable silicone device (which creates a small gastric pouch) connected by Silastic tubing to an injection (access) port. Access port is placed subcutaneously in the anterior abdominal wall through which saline can be injected or withdrawn using a fine needle to adjust the band and thereby the stoma (outlet) of the gastric pouch. Good weight loss and its maintenance, combined

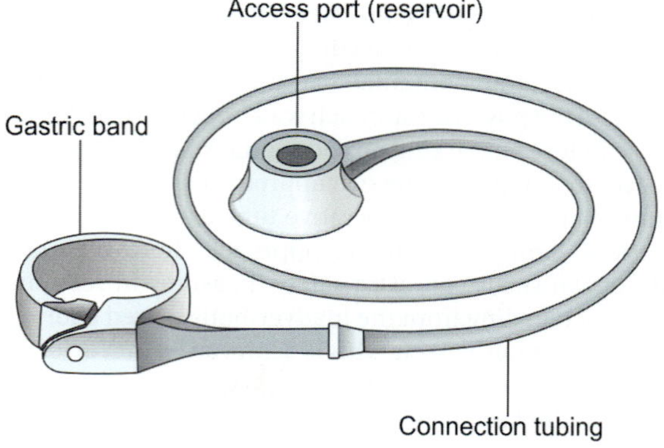

Figure 3 The LAP-BAND adjustable gastric banding system

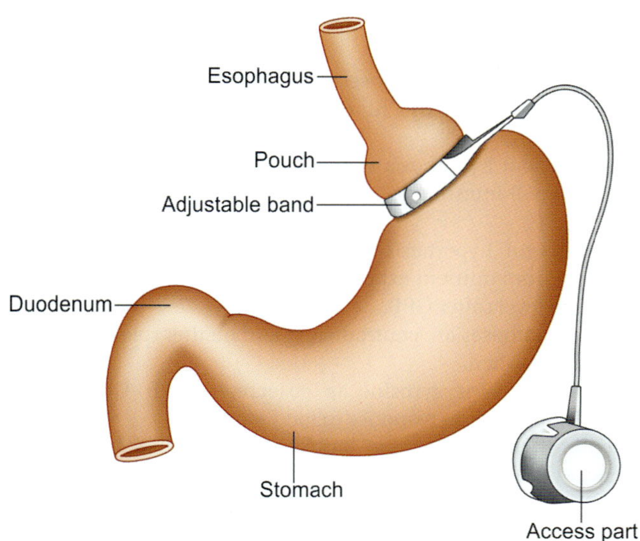

Figure 4 Lap adjustable gastric banding

with the ability to nonsurgically adjust the stoma size led to the wide adoption of the procedure in treating bariatric patients (Figs 3 and 4). However, band erosion/herniation and band slippage became a major long-term concern in the long run.

The AGB used to be a preferred bariatric procedure because it was perceived as less invasive completely reversible. However, this perception changed when long-term observation of the procedure showed a high failure rate of up to 40% in some series, and a complication rate of 33%.[27,28]

Mixed Malabsorbative and Restrictive Procedures

Roux-en-Y Gastric Bypass

History: After a remarkable weight loss and satiety in a patient who had undergone subtotal gastrectomy and Billroth II reconstruction for peptic ulcer management, Mason introduced gastric bypass surgery in 1966 as a restrictive method. [29] The procedure initially

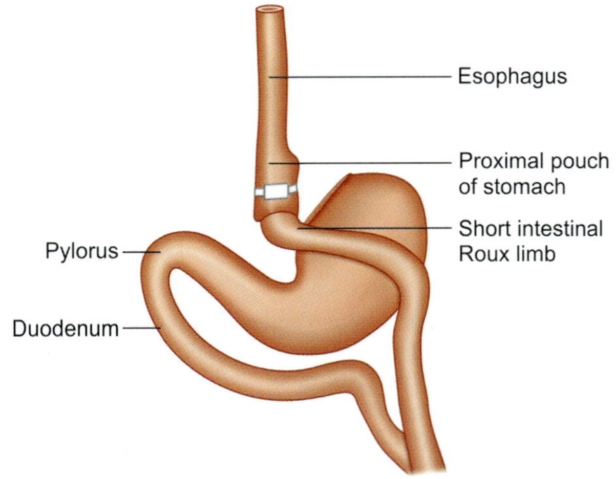

Figure 5 Banded gastric bypass

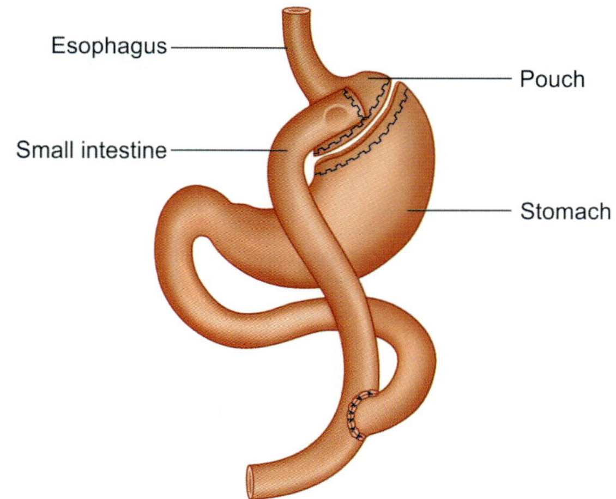

Figure 6 Gastric bypass Roux-en-Y

involved horizontal proximal gastric division with the creation of a 100–150 mL gastric pouch. The pouch was drained by an alimentary passage with a short afferent biliopancreatic limb (Fig. 5). The size of the gastrojejunal stoma was 12 mm. Mason modified the technique by reducing the pouch size to 50 ml to improve postoperative weight loss. Since then, the technique of constructing Roux-en-Y gastric bypass (RYGB) underwent multiple modifications by different surgeons (Fig. 6). Torres and Oca introduced an advanced gastric bypass procedure by creating a 35 ml gastric pouch on the lesser curvature almost 4 cm distal to the cardia, and then detaching the gastric pouch from the stomach remnant. The jejunum was divided at 45 cm from the ligament of Treitz, and the gastrojejunal anastomosis was performed with a 21 mm circular stapler. The biliopancreatic and alimentary anastomosis was created at 90 cm. This type of surgery was further promoted by Wittgrove in 1994,[30] when he performed the first minimally invasive gastric bypass surgery.

Technical approach: The RYGB is the most commonly performed bariatric operation worldwide and remains to be the gold standard surgery for obesity management and associated metabolic syndrome. The method combines excellent restriction with mild malabsorption. The procedure consists of, the creation of a proximal pouch about 30 cc in size by dividing the pouch from the remaining stomach with the use of a 35 mm stapler. The newly created pouch is connected with a Roux limb of bowel that is created by dividing the proximal jejunum about 70 cm below the ligament of Treitz. The divided distal segment, also known as the alimentary limb, is brought up to form a gastroenterostomy 2.5 cm in diameter. The created proximal segment (biliopancreatic limb) is anastamosed back to the distal limb at about 150 cm below the point of division to create a common channel. Although, the procedure is becoming increasingly standardized in certain facilities worldwide, debates related to the technique arise.

The arguments lie in the differences in the size of the gastric pouches, construction of the gastrojejunostomies, use of a constrictive ring at the gastroenterostomy to limit outflow, length of the Roux-en-Y limbs, and placement of the small bowel in front or behind the colon.[31]

Table 6: Debates related to different techniques in Roux-en-Y gastric bypass

Problem	*Possible effect*	*Recommendation*
Gastric pouch size	Can lead to weight loss failure, if pouch is too large	Use a 36 Fr bougie, use the 2nd vessel as a rough landmark for the first stapler firing
Gastrojejunostomy size	Narrow opening can lead to obstruction Wide opening can lead to failure of weight loss	Liner stapler versus circular Stoma size of 2.5 cm
Length of the RYGB limb	Long limb, severe malabsorption Short limb, failure of the procedure	Based on DM history <5 years, 150 cm >5–0 years, 180 cm 10 years, 200 cm Based on BMI BMI <50, 150 cm BMI >50, 200 cm
Placement of pouch ring	--------	Indicated for BMI >50

Lists of problems related to the procedure and recommendations to address them in Table 6.

Mechanism of Action

The overall mechanism of gastric bypass action in obesity is not fully understood. However, consideration of multiple factors can improve the benefits of the bariatric procedure.

- Food restriction: The postoperative weight loss acts inversely with the size of the pouch. Because of pouch dilation, weight regain may occur after an initial period of efficient weight loss. Thus, the application of a restrictive band on the pouch is recommended to avoid similar problems in the future, particularly for extremely obese patients (BMI >50).[32]
- Adjustment of eating behavior: This can occur when the patient avoids having a high-calorie diet and eat small quantities of food to avoid postprandial dumping symptoms (sweating, flushing, weakness, tachycardia, nausea, abdominal cramping, bloating, and diarrhea). Postgastric bypass patients also experience less hunger and have better compliance with the postoperative diet, which can be explained by the lower levels of ghrelin hormone found mainly in the excluded fundus and the duodenum.[33]
- Endocrine effect:
  - Bariatric surgery acts mainly on two major gut hormones known as incretins. The two hormones are gastric inhibitory peptide (GIP) and (GLP-1). The GIP is mainly secreted in the duodenum from the K-cells, whereas GLP-1 is secreted from the L-cells found mainly in the ileum. [34-35]
  - Incretins mainly stimulate glucose-dependent insulin secretion.
  - Apart from its insulinotropic effect on the β-cells, GLP-1 also assists in lowering blood glucose by inhibition of gastric emptying, enhancement of insulin sensitivity and inhibition of glucagon secretion from the liver. [36,37]
  - The GLP-1 effect may persist from 6 months to 1 year postsurgery.[38]

Two hypotheses proposed on the increase in incretin levels after GBP are the hindgut hypothesis and the foregut hypothesis.

- The hindgut hypothesis states that the rapid exposure of the lower small intestine to nutrients leads to increased incretins after GBP.
- The foregut hypothesis proposes that the exclusion of the foregut from nutrient exposure is responsible for the increased incretin levels after GBP.
- Both hypotheses are contradictory and neither roles have been well established.
- Peptide tyrosine tyrosine is cosecreted with GLP-1 from intestinal L cells in response to food intake.
- Peptide tyrosine tyrosine has been responsible in reducing caloric intake post-GB.[39]

Indications

- Sweet eaters
- Any BMI with DM >5 years or presence of metabolic syndrome >5 years
- Severe obesity or BMI >50
- Obesity associated with symptomatic GERD

Contraindications for Gastric Bypass

- Presence of endocrine diseases causing obesity (hypothyroidism, Cushing's disease)
- Presence of psychotic diseases (depression, schizophrenia)
- Eating disorders (binge eating, anorexia)
- Patients not committed to lifelong postoperative follow-up

Perioperative Complications

Early complications

- Anastomotic leakage, which occurs in about 1.3–4% of patients[40-41]
- Pulmonary embolism, which occurs in about 0.6–1.1 % of patients[41]
- Hemorrhage, which occurs in about 0–3% of patients[42]

Late postoperative complications

- Stoma stenosis, which occurs in about 0.8–34.5% of the patients[41-42]
- Stoma ulceration, which occurs in about 4–12% of the patients[43]
- Intestinal obstructions caused mainly by internal herniation
- Nutritional deficiency

Expected Outcomes

- Weight loss: The reported percentage of excessive weight loss (EWL) 2–5 years postsurgery ranges from 65–75%.[43,44]
- Resolution of metabolic syndrome
  - DM: up to 97% resolution rate[45]
  - HTN: up to 62% resolution rate[43]
  - Hyperlipidemia: up to 75% resolution rate[46]

Biliopancreatic Bypass with Duodenal Switch

Biliopancreatic diversion (BPD) was initially developed in 1976 by Scopinaro as an alternative procedure to jejunoileal bypass surgery.[47] Hess modified the procedure in 1998 to BPD with duodenal switch (BPD-DS). The first laparoscopic BPDS was performed in 1999 by Michel Gagner.

The surgery requires a restrictive component and a malabsorptive component. The method can be conducted as a single-step surgery or a two-step procedure. Because of a high chance of complication or mortality incidence in extremely obese patients, some surgeons have favored conducting the surgery in two steps. The first step consists of sleeve resection. After a significant weight loss, the second step, which is the duodenal switch, is then performed.

Eligibility for this surgery should be highly restrictive in certain patient categories. As mentioned previously, this procedure should not be performed on patients needing permanent oral medication, patients who cannot commit to long-term follow-up, patients with a history of chronic bowel disease, patients with a severe psychiatric disorder, and patients who are pure vegetarians.

The procedure is ideally recommended to severely obese patients (BMI >60) presenting with related metabolic syndrome.

Apart from some modifications, the newly introduced BPDS technique applies techniques similar to those used in the classical BPD described by Scopinaro. In the modified surgery, the pylorus is preserved, the stomach is vertically resected (instead of horizontally resected) with the use of a 32–34 Fr gastric tube and the length of the common channel is elongated from 50–70 or 100 cm. The stomach remnant is drained with end-to-side duodeno-jejunal anastomosis.

As previously mentioned, this procedure can be performed as a single- or a two-step surgery. Some super obese patient did not need the second step for sufficient weight reduction 2 years after primary sleeve gastrectomy. Thus, it may be rarely needed to perform a one-step duodenal switch surgery initially except for selected patients with severe metabolic syndrome (Fig. 7).

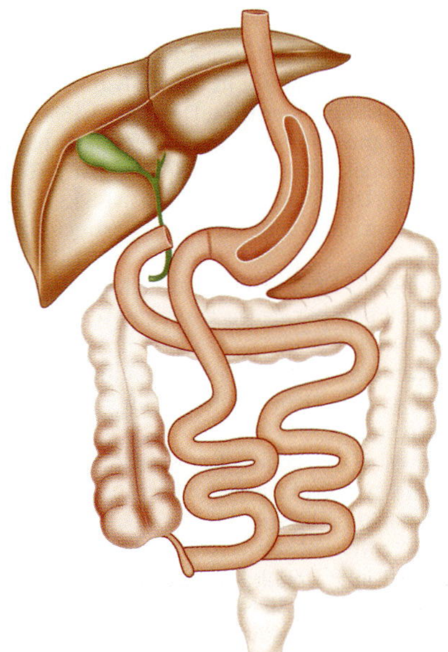

Figure 7 Biliopancreatic diversion with duodenal switch

Outcomes

- Compared with conventional RYGB, biliopancreatic diversion with or without duodenal switch shows greater excessive weight loss at 5 years postoperative. An EWL of about 75% compared with 58% after RYGB is indicated.[48]
- In a meta-analysis of multiple control studies, Buchwald et al. showed complete remission of DM in 98.9% of patients operated by BPD compared with that in 83.7% of postgastric bypass surgery patients.[49]
- Lemmens et al. reported variable types of late complications in a series of 1,040 patients after conventional BPD. These complications included iron deficiency anemia in 40% of the patients and protein malnutrition in 12.4% of the patients. Total parenteral nutrition was needed in 7% of the patients. Chronic diarrhea/steatorrhea and flatulence/odor problem were reported in 30 and 10% of the patients, respectively.

Despite the superiority of BPD over RYGB in long-term weight management and resolution of obesity-related metabolic syndrome, such an extensive surgery must be recommended only to carefully selected patients who are fully aware of the surgical consequences and committed to long-term postoperative follow-up.

Revision Surgery

Indications

- Early sleeve leak
- Weight regain >2 kg per month for longer than 6 months
- Failure of restriction: Dilation of pouch or sleeve, band slippage or migration, symptomatic GERD with dysfunction of lower esophageal sphincter
- Insufficient weight control 2 years postsurgery
- Poor quality of life: recurrent emesis, abdominal pain, diarrhea, dumping syndrome (early and late), and severe nutritional deficiency
- Procedural complications: Recurrent ulcerations of stomas, stoma stenosis (not responding to other endoscopic treatment)

Workup

- Detailed eating habits of the patient and the patient's psychological status
- Assessment of the patient's physical activity

Flow chart 1 Revision surgery in a failed procedure due to not intact anatomy

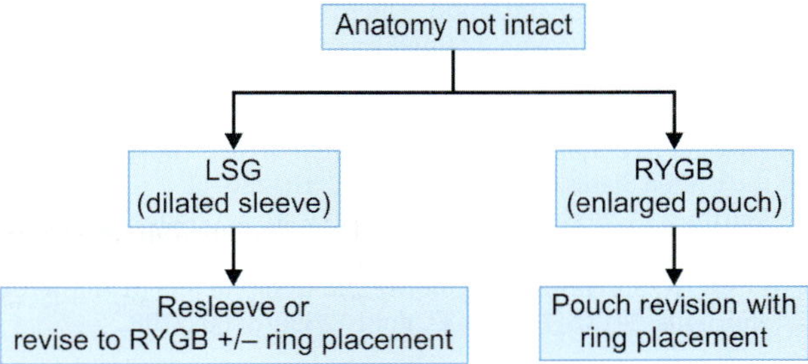

- Detailed information regarding the stomach pouch volume, either by contrast abdominal X-ray or by a more sophisticated technique such as computed tomography with 3D reconstruction [50]
- Upper GI endoscopy inspection of the esophagus and stomach pouch. *Helicobacter. pylori* test is recommended prior to any revision surgery in the stomach[51]
- Esophageal manometry and 24 hr Ph

Revision Surgery Algorithms (Flow charts 1 to 3)

Flow chart 2 Revision surgery in a failed procedure with intact anatomy

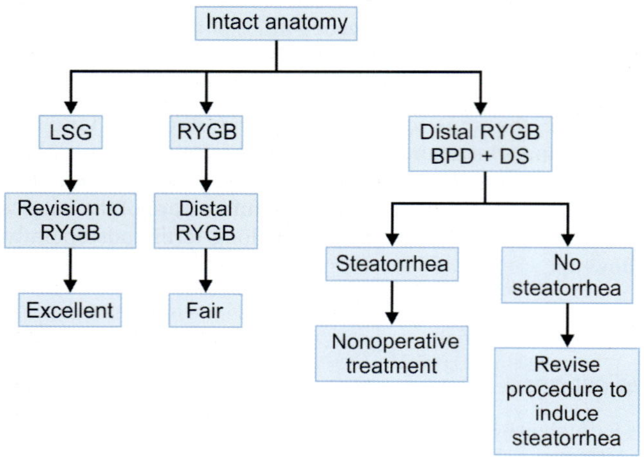

Flow chart 3 Revision surgery in failed gastric bypass

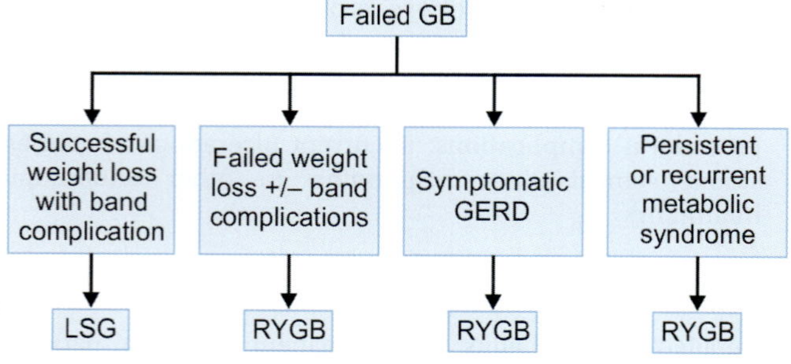

REFERENCES

1. World Health Organization. Obesity and overweight: factsheet. 2014. http://www.who.int/mediacentre/factsheets/fs311/en/
2. Malnick SD1, Knobler H. The medical complications of obesity. QJM. 2006;99(9):565-79.
3. Mokdad AH, Marks JS, Stroup DF, et al. Actual causes of death in the United States, 2000. JAMA. 2004;291:1238-45.
4. Martinez JA, Body-weight regulation: causes of obesity. Proc Nutr Soc. 2000;59(3):337-45.
5. Misra A1, Shrivastava U. Obesity and dyslipidemia in South Asian Nutrients. 2013;5(7):2708-33. doi:10.3390/nu5072708.
6. Huxley R, James WP, Barzi F, et al. Obesity in Asia Collaboration. Ethnic comparisons of the cross-sectional relationships between measures of body size with diabetes and hypertension. Obes Rev. 2008;9 Suppl 1:53-61.
7. WHO Expert Consultation. Appropriate body-mass index for Asian populations and its implications for policy and intervention strategies. Lancet. 2004;363:157-63.
8. Christou NV, Sampalis JS, Liberman M, et al. Surgery decreases long-term mortality, morbidity, and health care use in morbidly obese patients. Ann Surg. 2004;240:416-24.
9. Batsis JA, Romero-Corral A, Collazo-Clavell M. Effect of bariatric surgery on the metabolic syndrome: a population-based, long-term controlled study. Mayo Clin Proc. 2008;83(8):897-907. doi:10.4065/83.8.897
10. Asia-Pacific Perspective: Redefining Obesity and its Treatment http://www.wpro.who.int/nutrition/documents/docs/Redefiningobesity.pdf.
11. IFSO-APC Consensus Statements 2011, Obes Surg. 2012;22:677-84. doi 10.1007/s11695-012-0610-7.
12. Alberti KG, Zimmet P, Shaw J, et al. Metabolic syndrome—a new world-wide definition. A consensus statement from the International Diabetes Federation. Diabet Med. 2006;23(5):469-80.
13. Hess DS, Hess DW. Biliopancreatic diversion with duodenalswitch. Obes Surg. 1998;8:267-82.
14. Lagace M, Marceau P, Marceau S, et al. Biliopancreatic diversion with a new type of gastrectomy: some previous conclusions revisited. Obes Surg. 1995;5:411-18.
15. Ren C, Patterson E, Gagner M. Early results of laparoscopic biliopancreatic diversion with duodenal switch: a case series of 40 consecutive patients. Obes Surg. 2000;10:514-23.
16. Dapri G, Vaz C, Cadière GB, et al. A prospective randomized study comparing two different techniques for laparoscopic sleeve gastrectomy. Obes Surg. 2007;17:1435-41.
17. Langer FB, Hoda R, Bohdjalian A, et al. Sleeve gastrectomy and gastric banding: effects on plasma ghrelin levels. Obes Surg. 2005;15:1024-29.
18. Melissas J, Koukouraki S, Askoxylakis J, et al. Sleeve gastrectomy—a restrictive procedure? Obes Surg. 2007;17:57-62.
19. Karamanakos SN, Vagenas K, Kalfarentzos F, et al. Weight loss, appetite suppression, and changes in fasting and postprandial ghrelin and peptide-YY levels after Roux-en-Y gastric bypass and sleeve gastrectomy: a prospective, double blind study. Ann Surg. 2008;247:408-10.
20. Takata MC, Campos GM, Ciovica R, et al. Laparoscopic bariatric surgery improves candidacy in morbidly obese patients awaiting transplantation. Surg Obes Relat Dis. 2008;4:159-64.
21. Parikh M, Gagner M, Heacock L, et al. Laparoscopic sleeve gastrectomy: does bougie size affect mean% EWL? Short-term outcomes. Surg Obes Relat Dis. 2008;4:528-33.
22. ASMBS position statement on sleeve gastrectomy as a bariatric procedure.
23. Patricia Siebere , Markus Gass, Beatrice Kern, et al. Five-year results of laparoscopic sleeve gastrectomy. Surg Obes Relat Dis. 2014;10(2); 243-9.
24. Iswanto S, Gintaras A, Fernando B. Resolution of Diabetes Mellitus, Hypertension, and Hyperlipidemia after Laparoscopic Vertical Sleeve Gastrectomy.
25. Vidal J, Ibarzabal A, Nicolau J et al. Short-term effects of sleeve astrectomy on type 2 diabetes mellitus in severely obese subjects. Obes Surg. 2007;17:1069-74.
26. Kuzmak LI, A review of seven years experience with silicon gastric banding. Obes Surg. 1991;1:403-8.
27. DeMaria EJ, Sugerman HJ, Meador JG, et al. High failure rate after laparoscopic adjustable silicone gastric banding for treatment of morbid obesity. Ann Surg. 2001;233:809-18.

28. Weiner R, Blanco-Engert R, Weiner S, et al. Outcome after laparoscopic adjustable gastric banding—8 years experience. Obes Surg. 2003;13:427-34.
29. Mason EE, I to C. Gastric bypass in obesity. Surg Clin N Am. 1967;47:1345-51.
30. Wittgrove AC, Clark GW, Tremblay LJ. Laparoscopic gastric bypass, Roux-en-y preliminary reports of five cases. Obes Surg. 1994;4:353-7.
31. Shauer P, Ikramuddin S, Gourash W, et al. Outcomes after laparoscopic Roux-en-Y gastric bypass for morbid obesity. Ann Surg. 2000;232:515-29.
32. Ernst B, Thurnheer M, Wilms B, et al. Differential changes in dietary habits after gastric bypass versus gastric banding operations. Obes Surg. 2009;19:274-80.
33. Cummings DE, Weigle DS, Frayo RS, et al. Plasma ghrelin levels after diet induced weight loss or gastric bypass surgery. N Engl J Med. 2002;346:1623-30.
34. Holst JJ The physiology of glucagon-like peptide 1. Physiol Rev. 2007;87:1409-39.
35. Kreymann B, Williams G, Ghatei MA et al. Glucagon peptide-1: a physiological incretin in man. Lancet. 1987;2:1300-04.
36. Zander M, Madsbad S, Madsen JL et al. Effect of 6-weekcourse of glucagon like peptide-1 on glycaemic control, insulin sensitivity, and beta cell function in type 2 diabetes: a parallel group study. Lancet. 2002;359:824-30.
37. Meier JJ, Gallwitz B, Salmen S, et al. Normalization of glucose concentrations and deceleration of gastric emptying after solid meals during intravenous glucagons like peptide-1 in patients with type 2 diabetes. J Clin Endocrinol Metab. 2003;88:2719-25.
38. Laferrere B, Tran , Egger JR, et al. The increase in GLP-1levels and incretin effect after Roux-en-Y gastric bypass surgery persists up to 1 year in patients with type 2 diabetes mellitus. The Obesity Society Annual Meeting. New Orleans: Nature Publishing Group; 2007. p. A7.
39. Batterham RL, Cowley MA, Small CJ, et al. Inhibition of food intake in obese subjects by peptide YY3-36. N Engl J Med. 2003;349:941-48.
40. Lujan JA, Hernandez Q, Frutos MD, et al. Laparoscopic gastric bypass in the treatment of morbid obesity. Surg Endosc. 2002;16:1658-62.
41. Nguyen NT, Goldman C, Rosenquist J, et al. Laparoscopic versus open gastric bypass :a randomized study of outcomes, quality of life, and costs. Ann Surg. 2001;234:279-91.
42. Nguyen NT, Tivers R, Wolfe BM. Early gastrointestinal hemorrhage after laparoscopic gastric bypass. Obes Surg. 2003;13:62-65.
43. White S, Brooks E, Jurikova L et al. Long-term outcomes after gastric bypass. Obes Surg. 2005;15:155-63.
44. Dhabuwala A, Cannan RJ, Stubbs RS. Improvement inco-morbidities following weight loss from gastric bypass surgery. Obes Surg. 2000;10:428-35.
45. Mottin CC, Padoin AV, Schroer CE et al. Behavior of type 2 diabetes mellitus in morbid obese patients submitted to gastric bypass. Obes Surg. 2008;18:179-81.
46. Alexandrides TK, Skroubis G, Kalfarentzos F. Resolution of diabetes mellitus and metabolic syndrome following Roux-en-Y gastric bypass and variant of biliopancreatic diversion in patients with morbid obesity. Obes Surg. 2007;17:176-84.
47. Scopinaro N, Gianetta E, Civalleri D, et al. Biliopancreatic bypass for obesity: II. Initial experience in man. Br J Surg. 1979;66(9):618-20.
48. Maggard MA, Shugarman LR, Suttorp M, et al. Meta-analysis: surgical treatment of obesity. Ann Intern Med. 2005;142(7):547-59.
49. Buchwald H, Avidor Y, Braunwald E, et al. Bariatric surgery: a systematic review and metaanalysis. JAMA. 2004 13;292(14):1724-37.
50. Karcz WK, Kuesters S, Marjanovic G, et al. 3D-MSCT gastric pouch volumetry in bariatric surgery—preliminary clinical results. Obes Surg. 2009;19(4):508-16.
51. Hartin CW, Jr., Remine DS, Lucktong TA. Preoperative bariatric screening and treatment of Helicobacter pylori. Surg Endosc. 2009;23(11):2531-4.

CHAPTER 119

Robotics in Gastrointestinal Surgery

Arvind Kumar, Belal Bin Asaf

INTRODUCTION

It is over a decade now since robotic-assisted laparoscopic technology was used for abdominal surgery. Nearly every gastrointestinal (GI) surgery has been done and demonstrated as safe, feasible, and reproducible.

Laparoscopic surgery has few limitations—such as two-dimensional vision of the surgical field, limited instrument dexterity and reduced degree of motion, and counterintuitive movements—that encouraged even experienced laparoscopic surgeons to test the potential of surgical robotics. The da Vinci Surgical System with its magnified high-definition (HD) three-dimensional (3D) view of the operative field and articulating instruments with intuitive movement and seven degrees of freedom of movement enhances the surgical skills to allow complex surgeries by minimally invasive approach in otherwise difficult to reach areas (accessing the inaccessible) .

DA VINCI SURGICAL SYSTEM AND ITS COMPONENTS

Technically speaking, the word robot is actually a misnomer. As per the widely accepted definition, *the word "robot" refers to a machine competent enough to carry out a complex series of actions automatically, particularly one programmable by a computer."* The emphasis is on the word "automatically." In reality, the surgical robot works on the master–slave concept and there is no automation involved. Every move by the surgical system is controlled by the surgeon. Therefore, in true sense of it, the da Vinci Surgical System is actually a surgical tele-manipulator, wherein the surgeon is able to perform the surgery sitting at the surgical console at a distance from the patient.

The latest generation robot is the da Vinci Si Surgical System, manufactured by Intuitive Surgical (Sunnyvale, CA, USA) and is made up of three integrated components:

1. *Surgeon console:* It is an ergonomically designed unit, which is typically placed in the same operating room (OR) as the patient. The surgeon operates while seated comfortably at the surgeon console (Fig. 1), viewing a binocular 3D image of the operative site (Fig. 2). As the surgeon moves the master controllers at the console, the instruments inserted into patient through ports attached to interactive robotic arms perform the exact same movements inside the patient's body, albeit the movements are scaled down and any tremors are filtered. The master controller at the console (Fig. 3) consists of two multijoint fingertip joystick-like controllers, one for each hand. The surgeon moves the controller using the thumb and index fingers, and makes movement that he/she would be doing if he/she was doing an open surgery using his/her hands and these movements at master control are replicated exactly at the instrument tip. The console also has a footswitch panel that enables the surgeon to execute multiple tasks such as swapping between different arms and using energy instruments.
2. *The patient (robotic) cart:* The patient cart in da Vinci Si model consists of four arms, mounted on a moveable wheel base which is motorized for easy navigation (Fig. 4). The cart is connected to the master console by means of cables. Each of the robotic arms has multiple joints, resembling the human arm with a shoulder (setup joint), an elbow, and a wrist (effector instrument). The instruments are attached to a carriage on the robotic arm, which moves the instrument in and out of the port. This acts as the elbow of the robotic arm and pivots at the entry point into the specific body cavity. Out of the four arms, the middle arm is for the camera. The robotic arms are compatible with specially designed metallic ports, which come in 5, 8,

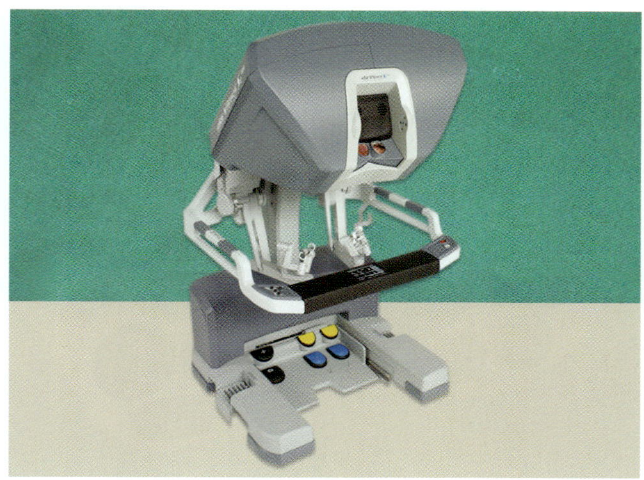

Figure 1 Surgeon console
Source: Intuitive Surgicals, *http://www.intuitivesurgical.com/company/media/images/#sthash.omV63fwL.dpuf*

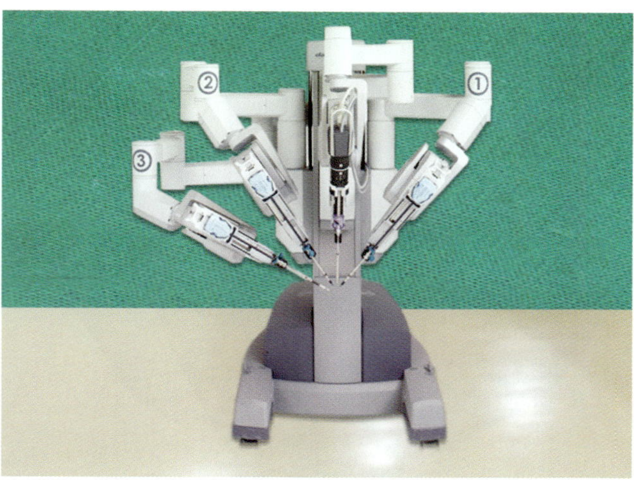

Figure 4 Patient cart
Source: Intuitive Surgicals, *http://www.intuitivesurgical.com/company/media/images/#sthash.omV63fwL.dpuf*

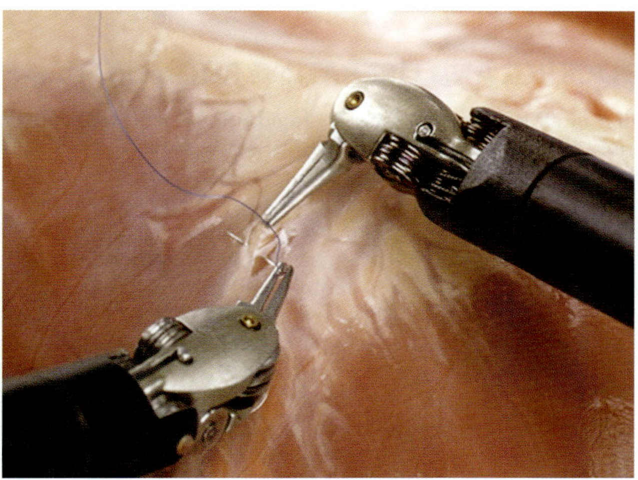

Figure 2 Stereoscopic high-definition (1080i HD) surgical vision
Source: Intuitive Surgicals, *http://www.intuitivesurgical.com/company/media/images/#sthash.omV63fwL.dpuf*

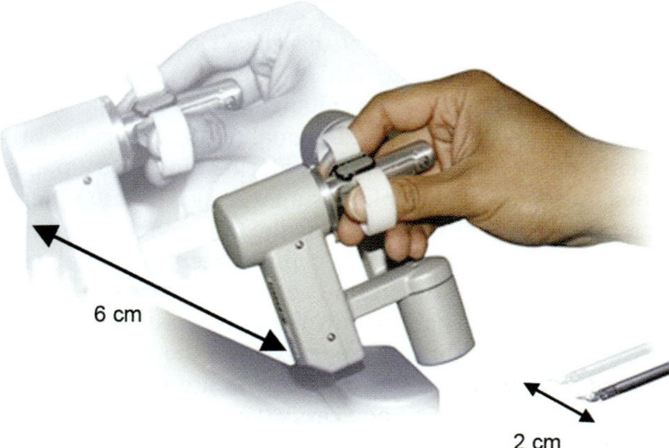

Figure 3 Master controller (movements are scaled and tremors filtered)
Source: Intuitive Surgicals, *http://www.intuitivesurgical.com/company/media/images/#sthash.omV63fwL.dpuf*

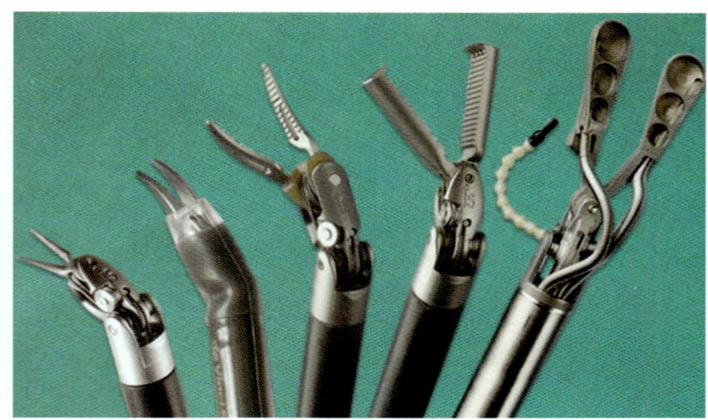

Figure 5 Robotic instruments with EndoWrist technology. (EndoWrist® Technology, Intuitive Surgical Inc.)
Source: Intuitive Surgicals, *http://www.intuitivesurgical.com/company media/images/#sthash.omV63fwL.dpuf*

and 12 mm dimensions. During use in surgery, the robotic arms need to be draped using disposable custom-made sterile plastic drapes for the arms to ensure a sterile operating field. The robotic system is provided with a wide range of specially designed instruments (Fig. 5) provided with a wrist (EndoWrist® technology, Intuitive Surgical Inc.). A cable system connected to four wheels on the instrument's head controls the endowristed movements. The robot can move them simultaneously to make complex movements mimicking the motion of the human wrist. The wrist in the instrument provides seven degrees of freedom of movement (Fig. 6). This count is maintained by the system. The instruments can be sterilized and reused for 10 sessions only after which they have to be discarded. This is what leads to a recurring cost of robotic system usage.

3. *The vision cart* (Fig. 7): It is a trolley that houses the endovision system and the central processing unit that integrates the two key components of the system, namely, the console and the patient cart. To facilitate team communication, it has a wide touch screen with telestration capability. The magnified view helps assistants in improved visualization of anatomy and incoming instruments from the periphery.

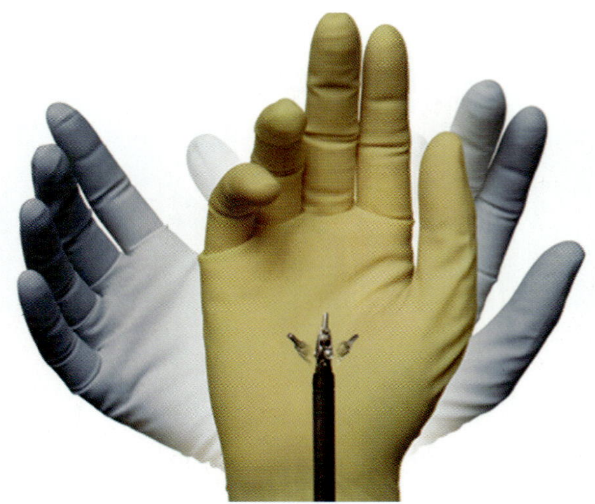

Figure 6 Freedom of movement
Source: Intuitive Surgicals, *http://www.intuitivesurgical.com/company/media/images/#sthash.omV63fwL.dpuf*

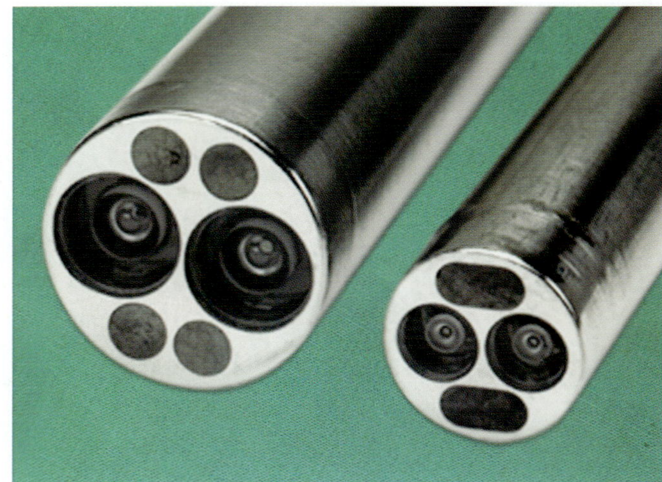

Figure 8 12 mm and 8.5 mm da Vinci telescopes with dual viewing channels
Source: Intuitive Surgicals, *http://www.intuitivesurgical.com/company/media/images/#sthash.omV63fwL.dpuf*

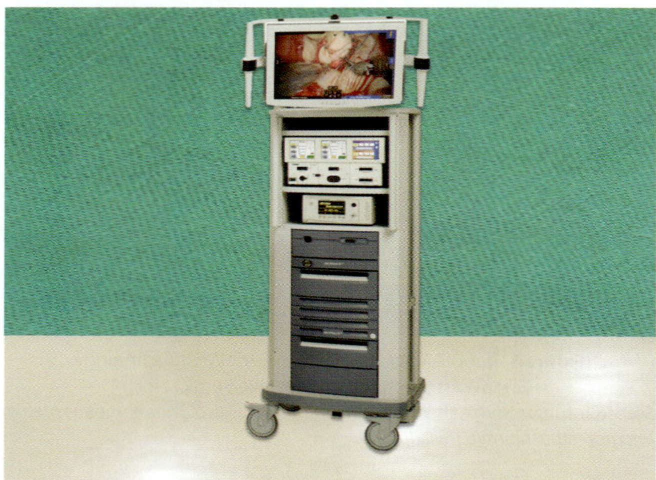

Figure 7 The vision cart
Source: Intuitive Surgicals, *http://www.intuitivesurgical.com/company/media/images/#sthash.omV63fwL.dpuf*

The endovision system has a unique three-chip camera, which is mounted on a telescope (12 and 8.5 mm) (Fig. 8). These telescopes have dual viewing channels (each connected to a camera) providing two independent optical systems representing the surgeon's right and left eye. These optical systems project a HD 3D binocular view to the surgeon at the console. The level of magnification can be controlled by adjusting the depth of camera inserted in the operating field.

Following are the key components of the vision cart:

- Core (central processing point for the system)
- Illuminator (light source for endoscope view)
- Camera assembly (provides the HD 3D view)
- Camera control unit (carries out image processing)
- Touch screen (which provides audio and video control patient side)
- Tank holders (support insufflation tanks)

DOCKING AND OPERATING ROOM SETUP

First of all the patient to be operated upon is anesthetized and subsequently positioned on the operating table as desired for the specific surgery. Painting and draping of the patient is done in an aseptic manner. The patient cart with robotic arm draped by the sterile drapes is then positioned close to the operating table in a configuration that ensures that the camera, the target anatomy, and the central column of the patient cart are aligned in a straight line with the target anatomy in center. The arms are then moved manually by using the clutch button provided near each joint in the arm and the arms of the robot are appropriately positioned. The cannula mounts on the robotic arms are then connected to the appropriately placed ports on the patient. This process is known as *docking*. Once the arms are connected to the patient, further movement of the patient cart is not allowed. The telescope attached to the camera is inserted into the camera port through the camera arm. Instruments are then inserted into the ports and connected to the instrument arms and under direct vision, the assisting surgeon parks the instrument tip inside the appropriate patient cavity at a convenient and safe place. The surgeon takes his place at the master console, placing his head in the binocular view finder and elbows on the padded rest bars. The surgery is then initiated by the console surgeon. Any bedside assistance with additional ports is provided by the assistant surgeon who also helps in changing instruments as needed during the course of the surgery. The OR setup diagram below (Fig. 9) depicts schematically the OR configuration during a robotic-assisted surgery. When the surgery is completed or when conversion is needed, the surgeon presses the stand by button on the control panels provided in the master console. This causes the robotic arms to disengage from the master controls. The instruments placed within the ports are removed and the arms are separated from the ports at the cannula mounts and the patient cart is moved aside. This is known as *undocking*. If necessary, the patient can be repositioned and the surgery can be continued in the desired way.

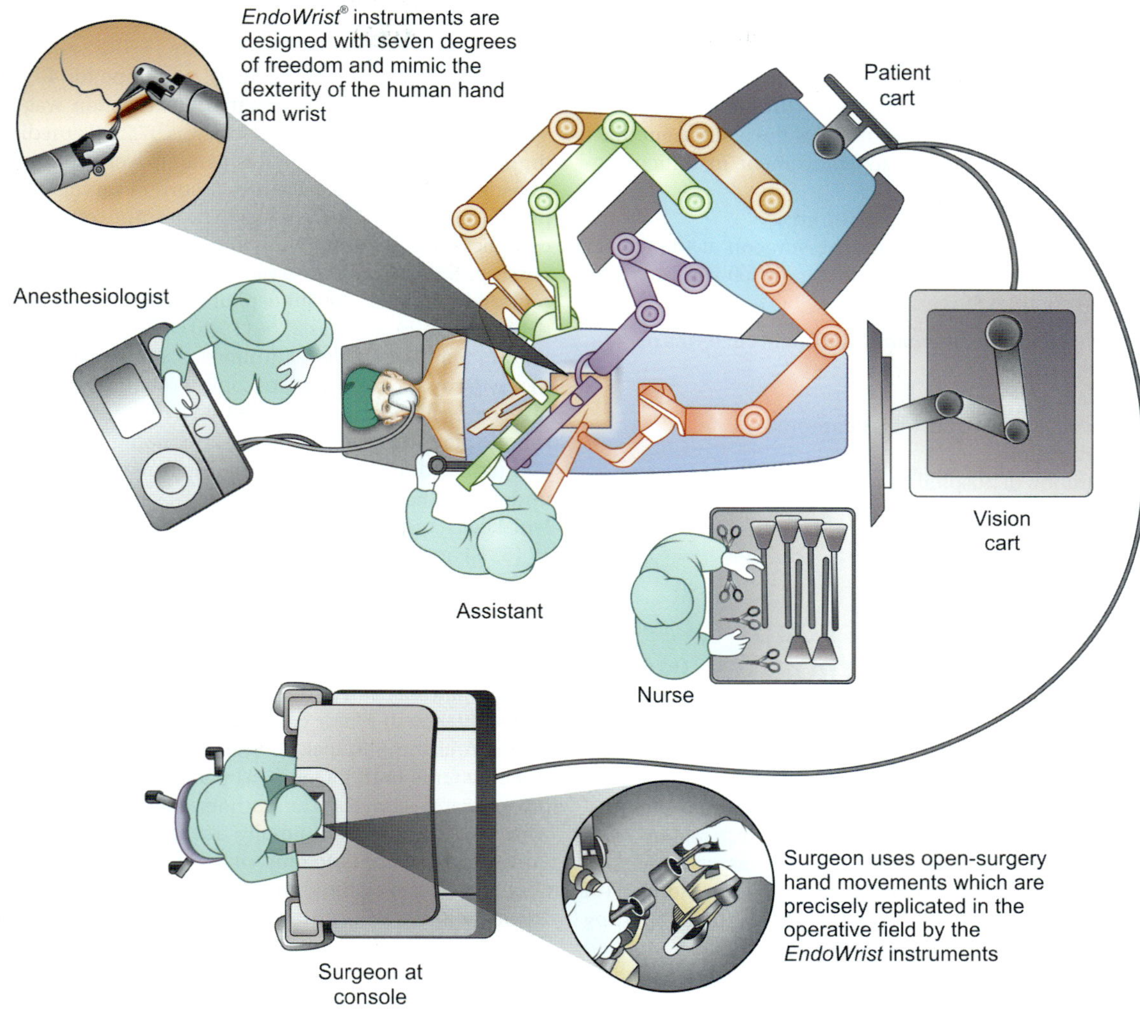

Figure 9 Operating room (OR) configuration
Source: Intuitive Surgicals, *http://www.intuitivesurgical.com/company/media/images/#sthash.omV63fwL.dpuf*

ADVANTAGES OF ROBOTIC SURGERY OVER CONVENTIONAL LAPAROSCOPIC SURGERY

The large incisions required in open conventional surgeries provided excellent unhindered access to the desired organ. However, one should bear in mind that patients requiring such major surgeries are usually nutritionally deprived and with less than optimum general condition. They have a hard time recovering from these large incisions. Therefore, after having undergone these surgeries, patients' lives are saved but their quality of life does not necessarily improve. Minimal access surgery (MAS) helps improve the quality of life after a major abdominal surgery by reducing the trauma of access to the diseased organ. However, on the other hand, the MAS has made otherwise simple procedures into technically complex and skill-demanding procedures due to:

- Loss of stereoscopic depth perception
- Loss of natural hand-eye coordination
- Loss of dexterity due to long, rigid instruments that operate on a fixed fulcrum at the point of entry of the trocars
- Counterintuitive movements

All these together with loss of the degrees of freedom from six degrees to two degrees further compromise on the dexterity during the laparoscopic procedure. Intracorporeal suturing and knot-tying are particularly difficult. Furthermore, the long rigid instruments compromise the ergonomics and thereby contribute significantly to surgeon fatigue and longer learning curves.

The da Vinci surgical system addresses the shortcomings of MAS. The surgical robot restores the faculties lost when using MAS techniques while maintaining the advantages of MAS:

- High-definition stereoscopic 10× magnified 3D visualization provides vision which is even more detailed than in open surgery.
- Improved hand-eye coordination due to both visual and spatial alignment of the surgeon's hand motions to the motion of the surgical tool.

- The EndoWrist® technology provides increased dexterity and intuitive movements and restores the degrees of freedom lost in conventional laparoscopy
- Motion scaling, another novel feature of the system, scales down large movements made by the surgeon on the master console to smaller more precise micromovements of the instrument tip.
- Tremor filtering allows for steady movement in difficult-to-access areas.
- There is no fatigue factor in the robotic arms.
- The ergonomic sitting position for the surgeon at the master console further reduces the fatigue factor, which is vital in long duration and complex surgeries.

These benefits translate into patients' benefits in terms of

- Much less blood loss
- Much less pain after surgery
- Much lower incidence of postop pneumonia
- Quicker healing time
- Reduced duration of hospital stay
- Reduced use of pain medication
- Faster return to work.
- Small incisions

CURRENT APPLICATION OF ROBOTIC SURGICAL SYSTEM IN GASTROINTESTINAL SURGERY

Esophagus

The first robotic-assisted esophagectomy was reported in 2003.[1] The distal esophagus was resected using the transhiatal route with the da Vinci robot. Foregut continuity was reestablished by a gastric pull-up with cervical esophagogastrostomy. Till date, there are 26 articles in the literature on this topic reporting experience with approximately 295 robotic esophagectomies in the management of malignant and benign esophageal diseases, including transthoracic esophagectomy with lymphadenectomy and transhiatal esophagectomy. Most reports have described transthoracic esophagectomy and have demonstrated the feasibility and safety of esophagectomy using the surgical robot. Few of the largest reported series are described below.

The first report of completely robotic esophagectomy was by Kernstine et al.[2] in 2007, who reported the use of surgical robot in 14 patients undergoing esophagectomy. Eight of the 14 patients underwent complete robotic esophagectomy with OR time of 11.1 ± 0.8 hours and estimated blood loss was 400 ± 300 mL.

Boone et al.[3] reported their experience of 47 transthoracic robotic esophagectomy (TRE). They reported a 14.9% conversion rate. The median blood loss was 625 mL, median operating time was 450 minutes, and the mean hospital stay was 18 days. Pulmonary complications were noted in 21 out of 47 patients with three inpatient mortalities. R0 resection was achieved in 76.6% patients and a median of 29 (range 8–68) lymph nodes were dissected.

From India, Puntambekar et al.[4] have reported a series of 32 cases. The average blood loss was 80 mL and mean operative time was 210 minutes. They reported no conversions and concluded that TRE is a better alternative than thoracoscopic esophagectomy in view of the reduced stress to the surgeon. Cerfolio et al.[5] reported successful Robotic Ivor Lewis with chest anastomosis in 22 patients. Dunn et al.[6] presented their 3-year single-center experience about dissection of thoracic esophagus by transhiatal robotic esophagectomy (THRE) and its associated morbidity. In their institute, THRE was done for 40 patients with resectable esophageal carcinoma. R0 resection was achieved in 94.7% of patients. Mean blood loss was 97.2 mL, median operative time was 311 minutes, and five patients were converted to open. Anastomotic leak and stricture, recurrent laryngeal nerve palsy, pneumonia, and pleural effusion were noticed as postoperative complications. Twenty five percent leak rate and 35% laryngeal nerve paresis rate were somewhat higher as compared with the reported literature. No inhospital mortality was noted; however, the 30-day mortality was 2.5% (1/40).

An early, single-institution experience of combined thoracoscopic and laparoscopic robotic-assisted minimally invasive esophagectomy was shared by Sarkaria[7] using a four-arm robotic platform, with particular attention given to complications and pitfalls during procedure development. Twenty one patients underwent the procedure with a four-arm robotic platform (17 by Ivor Lewis and four by McKeown). R0 resection was achieved in 17 (81%) and induction treatment was given to 16 (76%) patients; the majority [14/21 (67%)] received chemoradiation. The median estimated blood loss was 307 mL, median operative time was 556 minutes, which reduced to 414 minutes in last five cases of the series and median length of hospital stay was 10 days. Conversion rate to open was 24% (5) and 20 was the median number of lymph nodes dissected. Major complications was noted in five patients (24%). Anastomotic leak as well as airway fistula was noted in three patients (14%). One (5%) patient died of complications on postoperative day 70. The authors concluded that as compared with the standard minimally invasive esophagectomy, four-arm robotic esophagectomy may offer advantages; however, its adoption in a structured program needs critical evaluation of its adverse effects and subsequent alteration of technique which is paramount to reduce complications, increase patient safety, and improve the conduct of operation early in the learning curve.

Kim et al. reported the safety and feasibility of robot-assisted thoracoscopic esophagectomy for esophageal cancer in the prone position.[8] Robot-assisted thoracoscopic esophagectomy was performed in 21 patients in the prone position by a surgical oncologist who was inexperienced with thoracoscopic esophagectomy. The prime result of this study was the potential role of a robotic system to achieve an adequate learning curve by an inexperienced surgeon with thoracoscopic esophagectomy.

Most of these studies have showed the feasibility and safety of robotic-assisted esophagectomy. However, further trials are required to establish its superiority as compared with open and thoracoscopic procedures.

Apart from esophagectomy, the robotic surgical system has been used for Heller's myotomy. Robotic Heller's myotomy also gained popularity and has emerged as a safe and effective option. Reports suggest that the robotic technique allows more precise dissection, especially during the myotomy itself, owing to better maneuverability of instruments and improved visualization. In comparison with conventional laparoscopy, mucosal perforations during the procedure seem to occur less often with robotic assistance, but the actual clinical benefits need to be established further. Melvin et al.,[9] in a prospective, multi-institution study, reported the outcomes of 104 patients of achalasia who underwent robotic Heller's myotomy with partial fundoplication using the da

Vinci system. No mucosal perforations were noted in the study group and the average duration of hospital stay was 1.5 days. In a postoperative symptom survey, 76% of all patients reported a significant improvement of symptoms. During the average follow-up of 16 months, none of the patient required reoperation; however, one needed endoscopic esophageal balloon dilation.

In a retrospective study by Horgan et al.,[10] comparing laparoscopic Heller myotomy with robot-assisted Heller myotomy, a total of 121 patients underwent operative intervention with 62 cases done by laparoscopic approach and 59 cases robotically. The average operative time for the laparoscopic approach was 122 minutes compared with 141 minutes for the robotic-assisted approach. The rate of mucosal perforation was found to be less in the robot-assisted group compared with the laparoscopic group with the incidence of postoperative reflux and symptom improvement being comparable between the two groups. Huffmanm et al.[11] reported that patients who underwent Heller's myotomy through robotic approach had better quality of life compared with those who had laparoscopically. Though the operative time was longer in robotic group, no mucosal perforation was noted as opposed to 8% perforation rate in the laparoscopic myotomy group. Shaligram et al.[12] reported a retrospective study using 2,683 patients with achalasia to compare perioperative outcomes for open, laparoscopic, and robotic Heller myotomy. Both laparoscopic and robotic approach had better results compared with the open approach. Compared with open group, only the robotic surgery group had statistically significant reductions in need for intensive care unit (ICU) admission, postoperative morbidity, and length of hospital stay. No statistical differences were noted in mortality and morbidity needing ICU admission, length of stay, or 30-day readmissions between the robotic and the laparoscopic group. The cost of laparoscopic Heller's Myotomy was obviously lower than the robotic approach. But surprisingly, laparoscopic surgery was cheaper than the open procedure.

On the basis of available data, robotic Heller's myotomy appears as safe and efficacious as laparoscopic Heller myotomy. Mucosal perforation rates during myotomy may be lower with robotic intervention; however, the actual clinical significance of this finding is uncertain.

Robotic-assisted esophageal surgery is a developing field, and level 1 evidence to support this approach when compared with other is lacking. The benefits are uncertain when compared with a conventional laparoscopic approach. High cost of treatment and prolonged operative times are obstacles to accept these techniques. Further research in the field of robotic esophageal surgery may provide better technology and reduced costs that will generate more interest and acceptance in the near future.

Stomach

The major advantage of robotic gastric surgery is the ease and reproducibility of D2 lymphadenectomy. Even the intracorporeal digestive restoration is facilitated by the use of the robotic approach, particularly following total gastrectomy has been reported. Robotic dissection is associated with lesser blood loss, compared with robot-assisted with laparoscopic gastrectomy (LG). The learning curve and reproducibility also appear to be shorter with robotic surgery. The potential to reproduce D2 lymphadenectomy, extended resections, and ability to perform complex reconstructions, combined with advantages of minimal access, provides robotic surgery with an important role in delineating the therapeutic strategy for advanced gastric cancer.

No significant differences in adequacy of oncological resection, morbidity, or mortality were noted when robot-assisted and conventional LG were compared. However, indications and effectiveness of robotic surgery in gastric carcinoma need to be explored with more studies.

INDICATIONS FOR ROBOTIC GASTRECTOMY

The indications for robotic gastrectomy (RG) are the same as those for laparoscopic ones: Minimally invasive surgery (MIS) for early gastric cancer is based on the recommendations of the Japanese gastric cancer treatment guidelines and classification[13,14] as well as the fact that the oncological safety of MIS for advanced gastric cancer remains controversial.

Accepted indications for a RG can be summarized as:

- Indications for RG with limited lymphadenectomy: stage IA.
- Indications for RG requiring D2 lymphadenectomy: stage IB-IIA

Endoscopic resection should be considered first for strictly mucosal and submucosal tumor, if eligible. In case of failed attempts or for patients not suitable to this approach, RG with limited lymphadenectomy can be considered.

Contraindications for robotic surgery, similar to laparoscopic surgery, include intolerance to pneumoperitoneum and oncologically contraindicated preoperative findings of T4b cancers or distant metastases.

The robotic surgical system facilitates the procedure of performing laparoscopic surgery by providing a 10 times magnified and HD 3D image. The surgical robot's spontaneous transformation of the instrument handle to the tip movement eliminates the mirror image effect. This computer-operated surgical system allows surgeons to overcome various difficulties during laparoscopic gastric surgery, particularly dissection of splenic vessels, isolation of diaphragmatic crura, and in performing more extensive lymphadenectomy, including LN #14v, #8a, #9, #11p, #11d, and #12a.[15] The robotic surgical system helps in lymphadenectomy in obese and bleeding control. The surgeon can define the bleeding vessels more clearly and control them using robotic system more easily than in conventional laparoscopic surgery.

The first report of RG was published by Hashizume et al. in 2003.[16] Since then multiple case series of RGs for gastric cancer involving over 700 patients have been published in literature. A brief review of the important studies in English literature is presented herein.

Marano et al.[17] conducted a comprehensive review of the database up to July 2012 on PubMed, EMBASE, and the Cochrane Library.[17] Studies comparing RG versus laparoscopic gastrectomy or open gastrectomy were included in the study.

In this meta-analysis, 1,967 patients included from seven studies compared robotic (n = 404) with open (n = 718) or laparoscopic (n = 845) gastrectomy. The author concluded that in RG, there was a shorter hospital stay compared with the open group and reduced blood loss compared with the laparoscopic group. However, operative time was significantly prolonged. No significant difference was noted when the number of lymph nodes were retrieved and overall complication rates were analyzed between the groups. The authors concluded that reduced intraoperative blood loss and short length of hospital stay were noted in RG for gastric cancer when compared with laparoscopic gastrectomy and open gastrectomy at a cost of a longer operating time. Robotic gastrectomy also provides an oncologically adequate lymphadenectomy. However, to evaluate both short- and long-term outcomes, high-quality prospective studies were recommended.

Song et al.[20] published their experience of 100 consecutive RGs with lymph node dissection in 2009 wherein they analyzed clinic-pathological characteristics and surgical outcomes. Most of these reports prove the safety and feasibility of RG with D2 lymphadenectomy (Table 1). An optimal R0 resection and adequate lymph node retrieval were achieved with low postoperative morbidity and shorter hospital stays.

Some common limitations were reported like longer duration of surgery, loss of tactile feedback, and the extra cost involved. However, randomized trials and longer follow-up period are needed to provide long-term outcome and clinical advantages.

Robot-assisted gastrectomy (RAG) was compared with laparoscopic or open approach in some retrospective studies. Most of these reports prove the safety and feasibility of RAG with D2 lymph node dissection by experienced laparoscopic surgeons. They have found RAG to be oncologically as effective as open surgery[30] with lesser blood loss and short duration of hospital stay compared with laparoscopic and open gastrectomy (OG).[31] Pernazza et al.[32] for the first time compared RAG and OG in terms of the survival after a mean follow-up of 26 months. The study reported that robotic surgery may have some long-term benefits which were more evident in patients with advanced disease. At the end of learning curve for RAG, no statistically significant difference was noted in operative time between the two groups. The postoperative mortality rates were higher in the conventional group. They concluded that robotic D2 lymphadenectomy is convincingly as accurate as open surgery and easier than laparoscopic surgery.

Caruso et al.[30] published a case control study that showed no significant difference between the number of lymph nodes retrieved during the laparoscopic and open procedures. In the robotic group, all the resected margins were free of tumor as opposed to presence of tumor in two resected specimens in the open group. Despite longer operative time, the RAG group was favored due to lesser blood loss and a shorter length of hospital stay. However, no difference in survival rate was noted in short-term follow-up between the two approaches. The study concludes that compared with open approach, RAG with D2 lymph node dissection is technically feasible, safe, and oncologically effective.

Some authors reported their results about the comparison of RAG versus LG. Demographic features, intraoperative factors, postoperative complications, and oncologic parameters were evaluated in these trials. The robotic approach showed a favorable trend due to less blood loss in two studies[33,34] and shorter hospital stay than the laparoscopic group. One of the studies reported a lower morbidity in the robotic group. In most of the other studies, the morbidity between RAG and LG was comparable.

Some studies described sound oncologic operative outcomes.[34,35] Unlike the laparoscopic group, positive resection margins (tumor involvement in the resection line) were not noted in any of the specimens in the robotic group. Lymph node retrieval was sufficient and comparable between the two techniques.

The limitation of these studies is the lack of answer to the question of long-term oncological outcomes. Only one group reported intermediate survival after RAG. The operative time in RAG also appears to be too long. Robot-assisted gastrectomy was compared with both open and laparoscopic group by Kim et al.[36] in a small subset of patients and reported better short-term surgical outcomes in terms of blood loss and hospital stay with RAG group. Improved survival may be linked to the precise dissection by robotic technique that helped to decrease the blood loss and transfusion rate. By overcoming the technical limitations of conventional laparoscopy, RAG has the potential to reduce the conversion rates and reduce the stress experienced by surgeons during advanced laparoscopy.

Table 1: Major series of robotic gastrectomies[18-29]

Authors	*Year*	*Country*	*Number of patients*	*Number of nodes*	*Surgery*	*Level of invasion*	*R0 resection*	*Mean operative time (min)*	*Hospital stay in days*	*Blood loss (mL)*
Anderson et al.	2007	United States	7	24	RSTG	EGC, AGC	Yes	420	4	
Patriti	2008	Italy	13	28.1 ± 8.3		EGC, AGC	Yes	286 ± 32.6	11.2 ± 4.3	103 ± 87.5
Song et al.	2009	Korea	100	36.7	RTG/RSTG	EGC	Yes	231	7.8 ± 17.1	
Hur et al.	2010	Korea	7	–	RTG/RTSG	EGC	Yes	205	9	–
Liu et al.	2010	China	9	19–24	RTG/STG	–	–	150–440	–	10–100
Isogaki et al.	2011	Japan	61	43 ± 14	RTG/STG	–		520 ± 177	13.3	
D'Annibale	2011	Italy	24	28 (23–34)	RTG/STG	EGC/AGC	Yes	267.50 (255–305)	6	30
Lee et al.	2011	Korea	12	(46921–115)	RADG	EGC	Yes	253	6.6 ± 1.6	135
Uyama I et al	2012	Japan	25	44.3 ± 18.4	RADG	EGC	Yes	361 ± 58.1	12.1 ± 3.2	51.8 ± 38.2
Kang et al.	2012	Korea	100	–	RTG					93.25 ± 84.59
Liu et al.	2013	China	104	23.1 ± 5.3.	RTG	EGC/AGC	Yes	272.52 ± 53.91	6.2	81
Hyun	2013	Korea	38	23.4 ± 7.0	–	–	–	234.4 ± 48.0		

RSTG, robotic subtotal gastrectomy; RTG, robotic total gastrectomy; RADG, robotic-assisted distal gastrectomy; EGC, early gastric cancer; AGC, advanced gastric cancer.

Similar results were noted with other authors[37] when investigated on the same aspects in a larger group, except longer hospital stay. The advantage of robotic system in dissecting lymph nodes are due to the stability of the camera, the 3D magnified view and seven degrees of freedom of movement has been exemplified especially in the infrapyloric and suprapancreatic area. The disadvantages of robotic surgery in comparison with laparoscopic or open surgery include higher cost, longer operation time, and loss of tactile feedback.

In RAG, operating times and cost are at present certainly higher than in laparoscopic and open gastric surgery. The operative time can be lowered after achievement of the learning curve of both surgical and nursing staff; this has been published in many trials. To establish the oncological and long-term adequacy of RAG, multicenter, randomized, controlled trials are still in need.

BARIATRIC SURGERY

Laparoscopic bariatric surgery can be quite demanding. Bariatric operations are complex and carry a potential risk of hemorrhage or leakage in view of long staple lines or GI anastomosis. Due to the body habitus of these patients, substantial difficulty is added to the procedures. During surgery, movements of long, narrow laparoscopic instruments may become difficult due to less compliant thick abdominal wall and may make the operation tiresome for the surgeon. Dissection is also difficult due to enlarged left lobe of liver that hampers the view of gastroesophageal junction and the angle of His. These problems can be overcome with the help of robotic surgical system, which has stiff instruments with consistent mechanical power of its arm. Laparoscopic Roux-en-Y Gastric Bypass (LRYGBP) is the most extensively studied robotic bariatric surgery.[38-40] It involves fashioning of a gastrojejunal and a jejunojejunal anastomosis with the help of staplers or manually. Laparoscopic RYGBP requires the surgeon to possess advanced suturing skills. However, in robotic surgery, the surgeon enjoys the seven degrees of freedom and 3D magnified view over the conventional laparoscopic ones, filtering of the otherwise normal tremor, and the ability to be effectively ambidextrous, transform technically challenging and arduous task to a straightforward manual task thereby making the learning curve for this procedure rather easier.

On the other hand, laparoscopic sleeve gastrectomy (LSG) is a relatively simpler operation that requires division of the gastrosplenic and gastrocolic ligaments till the angle of His, and the longitudinal division of the stomach by an endoscopic stapler. Some say that the use of robotic techniques may not be cost effective or worthwhile for an operation that requires less laparoscopic skills. However, proponents of the use of robotic sleeve gastrectomy (RSG) object to this consideration. Laparoscopic sleeve gastrectomy is easier than RYGBP but it is not always true. Dissection and mobilization of greater curvature of stomach is usually tricky, especially in the uppermost part of the gastrosplenic ligament, and can become more difficult in the presence of sliding hernia. The main reason for poor postoperative weight loss may be secondary to retention of part of gastric fundus due to difficulty in mobilization of herniated part of the stomach from the left crus. Leakage from staple line may occur due to imprecise application of stapler causing partial esophageal resection.[41] These technical difficulties are more commonly encountered during an operation on super obese patients. Robotic surgical system application can help the surgeon to tackle all these possible problems. However, the application of robotics to LSG might increase the cost of treatment but gives a sense of safety to the surgeon, which results in short operative time.

Romero et al.[42] from South Miami Hospital, Florida, published a study that compared their preliminary experience with RSG versus the descriptive results of a systematic review of the laparoscopic approach. Data from their RSG experience were retrospectively collected. Information was compared with a systematic review of 22 selected studies that included 3,148 LSG cases. This study included 134 RSG versus 3,148 LSG. Leaks were found in 0 RSG versus 1.97% LSG, strictures in 0 versus 0.43%, bleeding in 0.7 versus 1.21%, and mortality in 0 versus 0.1%, respectively; mean surgical time was calculated to be 106.6 ± 48.8 versus 94.5 ± 39.9 minutes; and mean hospital length of stay was 2.2 ± 0.6 versus 3.3 ± 1.7 days, respectively. Four (2.9%) complications were found in robotic series. This series shows that RSG is a safe alternative when used in bariatric surgery, showing similar results as the laparoscopic approach. Surgical time was longer in the robotic approach, while hospital length of stay was lower. No leaks or strictures were found in the robotic cases.

In a systematic review of robotic bariatric surgery by Cirocchi et al.[43], 22 studies were reviewed. In biliopancreatic diversion, anastomotic leak rate was 8.51% and 30-day reoperation rate was 1.14% in Roux-en-Y gastric bypass and 1.16% in sleeve gastrectomy. Major complication rate in Roux-en-Y gastric bypass is 4.26% compared with sleeve gastrectomy (1.2%). Similarly, mean hospital stay was longer in Roux-en-Y gastric bypass (range 2.6–7.4 days). Small sample size, heterogeneity of the enrolled patients, and the lack of data from metabolic and bariatric outcomes were the major limitations of these studies. Majority of these cases were completed with stapled anastomosis despite the use of robot. The authors concluded that the present evidence does not support the hypothesis that robotic surgery is better in complex cases. Robotic surgery is mainly useful at some of the surgical steps (vertical gastric resection in the RSG or gastrojejunostomy and jejunojejunostomy in the robotic Roux-en-Y gastric bypass). Further trials will be required to establish with certainty the long-term benefits and absolute advantages.

Colon and Rectum

The first robotic-assisted procedure on large bowel was done by Weber et al. in 2001[44] for diverticulitis. The greatest advantage with robotic colorectal surgeries is better approach and maneuverability in the depth of pelvis, where traditional laparoscopic instrumentation may be particularly difficult. A more detailed review of robotic colorectal surgery is dealt in another chapter in the book.

PANCREATIC SURGERY

Pancreatic surgery is challenging for both surgeon and patients alike. Even a decade after adoption of robotic technology for abdominal surgery, robotic pancreatic surgery has had a relatively slower start, because these surgeries are technically demanding and require not only robotic expertise but also an absolute knowledge of the various anatomical variations which are fairly common in this area. In the last few years, many authors have approached the pancreas laparoscopically using the assistance of the surgical robot, some with very promising results in terms of surgical and oncological outcomes. However, parameters like meticulous dissection, hemostasis, and oncologic results must be matched as established principles of open pancreatic surgery. This approach needs thorough assessment before adopting as a new technique. We present a brief review of the techniques and outcomes of robotic-assisted pancreatic resections.

Robotic abdominal operation including first pancreatic transaction was presented by Giulianotti et al. in 2003,[45] and robotic excision of neuroendocrine tumor was reported by Melvin et al.[46] (Table 2). Most pancreatic surgeries performed until recently were for pancreatic adenocarcinoma, and most often required a Whipple's operation. Whipple's procedure is technically challenging, lengthy, and carries with it significant morbidity.[47,48] Small, asymptomatic, and incidental pancreatic lesions are frequently diagnosed due to increase in body imaging.[49,50] These include cystic and neuroendocrine tumors, which have a much better prognosis than adenocarcinoma.[49,50] These lesions favor laparoscopic or robotic approach due to their small size and lesser chances of vascular involvement. Most robotic pancreatic procedures reported in literature (60–70%) are performed for benign lesions less than 3 cm.[51-54] This may be due to sound clinical judgment but it leads to selection bias.

Robotic-assisted surgery for various pancreatic pathologies was reported by Giulianotti et al. in 134 patients and this is the biggest series of robotic pancreatic surgery reported to date.[55] Mean operating time was 331 minutes and mean hospital stay was 9.3 days. Fourteen cases converted to open; morbidity rate was 26% and mortality rate was 2.23% (three patients). Various operations performed were 60 pancreaticoduodenectomies, 23 splenopancreatectomies, 23 spleen-preserving distal pancreatectomies, 3 enucleations, three middle pancreatectomies, and one total pancreatectomy. A total of 21 patients underwent different surgical procedures for treatment of acute and chronic pancreatitis.

Kang et al.[56] compared the laparoscopic and robot-assisted spleen-preserving pancreatectomy in 45 patients (20 robotic and 25 laparoscopic). However, mean operation time was shorter in the laparoscopic group; the spleen-preserving rate was superior in the robotic group with no difference in the oncologic outcome.

Boggi et al.[57] first reported the feasibility of robot-assisted pancreatic transplantation. Till date they have performed three pancreatic transplants, and their preliminary data have been encouraging.

In most high-volume centers, open distal resections take less than 1 hour and pancreaticoduodenal resections 2.5–3 hours,[58] both performed with minimal blood loss (<150 cm^3), short hospital stay (5–8 days), and few pancreatic fistulas (0–6%).[59,60] In a study by Wayne et al.,[58] their first robotic resection took 3 hours, and the latest one 1 hour and 30 minutes. Two hours and 22 minutes was the mean operative time reported. Table 2 summarizes four published case series of robotic distal pancreatectomy (RP).

The safety and feasibility of robotic pancreatic surgery with few conversions to open surgery and a greater splenic preservation rate compared with laparoscopic surgery were reported.[56,62] Despite being done by surgeons with large experience in laparoscopic pancreatic surgeries, reported robotic operating times were long. The extra treatment cost is a well-founded concern with the robotic surgery. The cost of open pancreatectomy (OP), RP, and laparoscopic distal pancreatectomy (LP) in 77 cases was compared by Waters et al.[51] The mean operating time and hospital stay were

Table 2: Reported series on robotic pancreatectomy[51-53,61]

Authors	*Number of patients*	*Operative time (h min)*	*Hospital stay (days)*	*Blood loss (mL)*	*Fistula*
Giulianotti et al.	46	5 h and 31 min	9.3	323	9
Daoudi et al.	30	4 h and 53 min	6.1	212	14
Kang et al.	20	4 h and 58 min	7.18	372	-
Waters et al.	17	4 h and 58 min	4	279	0

Reports of robotic central resection include three, five, and nine patients with mean operating times from 5 hours and 20 minutes to 8 hours.[62-64] Their fistula rates were one in three,[64] one in five,[65] and seven in nine,[62] respectively, and the hospital stay ranged from 9 to 28 days.

3 hours, 42 minutes and 8 days for OP; 4 hours, 5 minutes and 6 days for LP; and 4 hours, 58 minutes and 4 days for RP. The total cost for RP was US$16,059, which was higher than for OP (US$10,588) and LP (US$12,986).

Robotic surgery facilitates pancreatic MIS as it enables difficult technical maneuvers to be performed with ease. Therefore, robotic pancreatic surgery is safe and feasibly advantageous in appropriately selected cases.

ROBOTIC GALLBLADDER SURGERY

The first robotic surgery ever to be performed on human was a robotic-assisted cholecystectomy in March 1997, performed by Cadiere and Himpens in Brussels, Belgium, using a da Vinci robot. Numerous groups have reported their experience. Vidovszky et al.[66] reported that the time of robotic surgery is dependent on the surgical experience. Their mean setup time for robotics was 24 ± 8.8 minutes. However, the setup time decreased after the first 16 cases: from 30.6 ± 10.7 minutes (first 16 cases) to 18.3 ± 4.0 minutes (cases 33–48). Technical advancement has made it possible for decreasing the number of incisions in robotic surgery and now single-site surgery has also been reported. Wren et al.[67] reported their experience of nine robotic single-site cholecystectomies. Average OR time was 105.3 minutes as compared to standard laparoscopic group (106.1 minutes). After an average follow-up of 3 months, no serious adverse events were noted in the robotic surgery group.

Vidovszky[68] described their early experience about single-site robotic cholecystectomy (SSRC) and its applicability to patients. A total of 95 patients underwent SSRC and were prospectively evaluated. Procedural times, postoperative complications, hospital stay, and readmissions were evaluated. In the study population, 71.6% were female and had a mean body mass index (BMI) of 30.1 ± 7.1 kg/m. Mean total operative time (TOT) was 88.63 ± 32.0, ranging from 49 to 220 minutes and six cases converted to laparoscopy, one to open, and one aborted. At total of 11.6% of patients required hospital admission, 6.3% readmission, or 1.1% reoperation. Conversion rate or TOTs is not affected significantly by patient factors like obesity. During the study interval, no bile duct injury or death was encountered. The authors concluded that SSRC is a safe, promising technique, has a manageable learning curve, and can be offered to a wide array of patients.

Morel et al.[69] from Geneva collected prospective data on all consecutive SSRC. Demographic, intra- and postoperative data of

82 patients who underwent SSRC were analyzed at their institution. Cholelithiasis was the main disease encountered. Mean operative time was 91 minutes and intraoperative complications occurred in 2.4% of cases. Two patients needed an additional laparoscopic trocar and one converted to open surgery in view of gallbladder carcinoma intraoperatively. Mean length of hospital stay was 2.4 days, and the rate of postoperative complications was 4.9%. When compared with patients' normal BMI, longer operative time but similar conversion rate and complications was noted in patients with higher BMI.

Robot has also been used in radical resections of gallbladders, though the experience has been anecdotal. Robot-assisted radical resection of gallbladder was reported in five patients by Shen et al in 2012.[70] The mean operative time was 200 minutes (12–300 minutes), mean hospital course was 7.4 days (range = 7–8 days), and mean number of lymph nodes dissected was 9 (range = 3–11). No complications were reported at the time of discharge. The author concluded that dissection in narrow, deep space like skeletonization of hepatoduodenal ligament, hepatic artery and the celiac axis and lymph node retrieval from peripancreatic and hepatoduodenal ligament is better with robotic surgery.

In the field of MIS, robotics and single-incision techniques are the latest additions. Due to better cosmetic results, enthusiasm has increased for single-incision techniques, but these are also associated with several technical disadvantages. The robotic platform may provide a solution to these issues. Pros and cons of robotic system for cholecystectomy and its comparison with single-site technique was reported by Romero-Talamás and Kroh.[71] After reviewing available literature, they concluded that although this technique is still not extensively tested, it is at least comparable to laparoscopic cholecystectomy in selected patients. However, to further evaluate and to add this technique in a surgeon's armamentarium, a larger well-controlled study is required in future.

ROBOTIC LIVER SURGERY

In the beginning of the twentieth century, liver resection was done infrequently because of the inherent friability of liver and high tendency for bleeding. However, by the end of last century, due to advanced imaging techniques, improved anesthesia, critical care, transfusion medicine, and postoperative care, liver surgery was performed routinely with reduced morbidity and mortality. Furthermore, laparoscopic liver surgery is possible now due to the technological advancements in the liver parenchymal transection techniques.

An international consensus conference was convened to assess the status of laparoscopic liver surgery.[72] According to this consensus report, the best indications for laparoscopic liver resection were solitary lesions less than 5 cm, located in the peripheral liver segments, whereas lesions adjacent to major vessels or near the liver hilum were not considered suitable for laparoscopic liver resection because of the potential risk of massive bleeding and the potential need for biliary reconstruction. Malignant tumors [colorectal liver metastases and hepatocellular carcinoma (HCC)] are not a contraindication to minimally invasive resection as demonstrated in various comparative studies, as long as there is no compromise in the oncologic integrity of the procedure. Although robotic liver surgery was not discussed in the consensus conference manuscript, the same rules can be applied to the technique as long as patient safety and oncologic results are not compromised.

One of the major concerns of laparoscopic liver resection is major bleeding from vascular structures within the parenchyma pushing hepatobiliary surgeons away from performing major liver resections using a minimally invasive technique. The da Vinci robot may prove useful in managing bleeding without conversion to an open surgery. The surgical robot has provided advantage to surgeons in controlling major bleeding with the help of robotic arms where endowrist instruments work as vascular clamps and perform intracorporeal suturing and tying in difficult locations.

With rising incidence of HCC, more patients will benefit from minimally invasive surgical resection because of limited availability of liver allografts (Table 3). Less postoperative adhesions after minimal invasive surgery make subsequent dissection relatively easy, is especially useful in patients with HCC who may require repetitive surgery or future transplantation.

Ho et al.[73] reported a systematic review of robotic liver resection where 19 series describing 217 patients were reviewed. In this review, patients of colorectal liver metastasis and HCC were analyzed in terms of demographics, perioperative outcomes, and oncological results. Wedge liver resections and

Table 3: Major reports on robotic liver resections[74-91]

Year	*Authors*	*Journal*	*Number of patients*	*Malignant*	*Benign*
2011	Giulianotti et al.	Surgery	70	42	28
2012	Choi et al.	Surg Endosc	30	21	9
2011	Chan et al.	J Hepatobiliary Pancreat Sci	27	21	6
2011	Giulianotti et al.	Arch Surg	24	17	7
2011	Casciola et al.	Surg Endosc	23	19	4
2011	Ji et al.	Ann Surg	13	8	5
2012	Lai et al.	Int J Surg	10	9	1
2010	Berber et al.	HPB	9	9	0
2009	Patriti et al.	J Hepatobiliary Pancreat Surg	6	6	0
2011	Wakabayashi et al.	J Hepatobiliary Pancreat Sci	4	3	1
2008	Choi et al.	Yonsei Med J	3	2	1
2008	Vasile et al.	Chirurgia (Bucur)	3	1	2
2011	Panaro et al.	JSLS	1	1	0
2011	Holloway et al.	Gynecol Oncol	1	1	0
2010	Giulianotti et al.	J Laparoendosc Adv Surg Tech A	1	1	0
2009	Machado et al.	Arq Gastroenterol	1	1	0
2011	Giulianotti et al.[b]	J Hepatobiliary Pancreat Sci	1	0	1
2012	Giulianotti et al.	Transplant Int	1	0	1

segmentectomy were the most commonly performed procedures. The overall complication rate is 20.3% and conversion rate is 4.6%, and the most common reason for conversion was unclear tumor margin and not bleeding. Intra-abdominal collection is the most common cause of morbidity. Mean operative blood loss was 50–660 mL, with main blood loss occurring with major hepatectomies. Mean operation time was 200–507 minutes and mean postoperative hospital stay was 5.5–11.7 days. Twenty five months is the mean follow-up for HCC and 36 months follow-up for colorectal liver metastasis. However, overall survival was not reported; disease-free survival was comparable with that after laparoscopic procedure for mixed malignancies. Short-term results are comparable to conventional laparoscopic liver resection; however, long-term oncologic results are unclear. The author concluded that for surgeons with advanced laparoscopic skills, robotic liver resection is safe and feasible.

As surgeons' experience with robotics improves, major hepatectomies will be more commonplace at busy liver centers. The delicate dissection that can be performed with the robotic platform to achieve inflow and outflow control and safe parenchymal transection will be recognized as a distinct advantage over laparoscopic instruments for major liver resections. Although robotic liver surgery is in its infancy, the advantages offered by surgical robots will undoubtedly expand its use for this purpose in the future.

ROBOTIC BILIARY-ENTERIC RECONSTRUCTION

Bilio-enteric anastomoses have to be performed meticulously so as to not compromise the anastomotic integrity and to avoid any technical errors that result in anastomotic stricture formation from improper suturing or vascular compromise. These complex biliary procedures can be performed with conventional laparoscopic technique albeit with extremely high laparoscopic skills. The difficulty arises secondary to the restrictive movement of laparoscopic instruments, combined with the fulcrum effect of laparoscopy, poor ergonomics, and compromised dexterity.

The surgical robot is ideally suited for biliary dissection and biliary-enteric anastomosis, thereby expanding its usage to a multitude of benign conditions, including choledochal cyst excision, benign common bile duct strictures, and biliary atresia. Woo et al. in 2006 reported the use of da Vinci surgical system for the minimally invasive treatment of a type I choledochal cyst.[92] Robotic surgical system was used in a 5-year-old girl for complete resection of the choledochal cyst and a Roux-en-Y hepaticojejunostomy. In current available literature, multiple series of robotic resection of choledochal cysts and hepaticojejunostomy have been reported.[92-99]

Chang et al.[98] reported their experience with da Vinci robotic surgical system for resections of choledochal cysts in 14 children. Data were analyzed retrospectively. Patient's demographics, operative methods, and postoperative outcomes, including operative time, hospital days, and complications, were reported. In 11 consecutive cases, complete resection of the choledochal cyst and Roux-en-Y hepaticojejunostomy were performed without any complication.

Dawrant et al.[99] reported their experience in robotic choledochal cyst excision in children weighing less than 10 kg. The da Vinci surgical system was used for resection of choledochal cysts and hepaticojejunostomy in five children. Type 1C cyst was present in all cases and three were very large. The Roux loop was fashioned extracorporeally. One year was the mean age (range: 0.5–1.4), and mean weight was 8.5 kg (range: 7.6–9.5). They reported no conversions. After a median of 4 days, feeding was established and after a median of 6 days, patients were discharged without postoperative complications. The authors found that for this complex minimal access procedure, robotic surgery has the advantage due to its ergonomics, and these are feasible even in children less than 10 kg.

Meehan et al.[95] performed four complex hepatobiliary procedures with the da Vinci surgical robot in children (Intuitive Surgical, Sunnyvale, CA): two Kasai portoenterostomies and two choledochal cyst resections. Roux-en-Y jejunojejunostomy was done extracorporeally in both Kasais through the 12 mm umbilical port site; however, it was done intracorporeally in both choledochal cysts. All bilio-enteric anastomosis were performed intracorporeally. For the Kasai procedure, total average time was 6 hours and 12 minutes and for the choledochal cysts, it was 7 hours and 38 minutes. Average duration of hospital stay was 4 days, and no intraoperative or perioperative complications were encountered.

The surgeon sits comfortably at the console that made the ergonomics better. Robotic arm has features that help not only dextrous but also ambidextrous operators, and also help in tremor filtration and motion scaling (large movements by the operator are translated into small movements of the instruments). All these help in making dissection, suturing, and knot tying easier, so that hepaticojejunostomy anastomosis become far easier than with conventional laparoscopic surgery. The major disadvantage with robotic surgery is loss of haptic feedback compared with conventional laparoscopic surgery, but improved vision allowing visual feedback may compensate for this. Surgery of the hepatobiliary system has progressed tremendously. Improved techniques to achieve vascular control and technological advancements have facilitated parenchymal transection, resulting in decreased mortality and morbidity from liver surgery. In addition to the advantages offered by minimally invasive hepatobiliary surgery, robotic surgery offers improved visualization and enhanced functionality and maneuverability, and increases surgeon comfort that helps in expanding the horizon of minimally invasive liver surgery.

CONCLUSION

As of today, there is lack of conclusive evidence regarding the long-term benefits of robotic abdominal surgery, particularly in terms of long-term oncological equivalence. However, enough studies have demonstrated the safety, feasibility, and reproducibility of robotic surgery. With its improved 3D vision along with excellent range of movements due to endowrist, robotic surgery has definitely expanded the horizon of conventional laparoscopic surgery allowing safe performance of even complex procedures that were earlier thought to be unapproachable by conventional laparoscopy. With more and more centers adopting this technology, the coming years are bound to take "robotics in gastrointestinal disorders" from the realm of curiosity to an established reality.

REFERENCES

1. Horgan S, Berger RA, Elli EF, et al. Robotic-assisted minimally invasive transhiatal esophagectomy. Am Surg. 2003;69(7):624-6.
2. Kernstine KH, DeArmond DT, Shamoun DM, et al. The first series of completely robotic esophagectomies with three-field lymphadenectomy: initial experience. Surg Endosc. 2007;21(12):2285-92.
3. Boone J, Schipper ME, Moojen WA, et al. Robot-assisted thoracoscopicoesophagectomy for cancer. Br J Surg. 2009;96(8):878-86.
4. Puntambekar SP, Rayate N, Joshi S, et al. Robotic transthoracic esophagectomy in the prone position: experience with 32 patients with esophageal cancer. J Thorac Cardiovasc Surg. 2011;142(5):1283-4.
5. Cerfolio RJ, Bryant AS, Hawn MT. Technical aspects and early results of robotic esophagectomy with chest anastomosis. J Thorac Cardiovasc Surg. 2012. [Epub ahead of print]
6. Dunn DH, Johnson EM, Morphew JA, et al. Robot-assisted transhiatal esophagectomy: a 3-year single-center experience. Dis Esophagus. 2012. doi: 10.1111/j.1442-2050.2012.01325.x.
7. Sarkaria IS, Rizk NP, Finley DJ, et al. Combined thoracoscopic and laparoscopic robotic-assisted minimally invasive esophagectomy using a four-arm platform: experience, technique and cautions during early procedure development. Eur J Cardiothorac Surg. 2013;43(5):e107-15. doi: 10.1093/ejcts/ezt013.
8. Kim DJ, Hyung WJ, Lee CY, et al. Thoracoscopic esophagectomy for esophageal cancer: feasibility and safety of robotic assistance in the prone position. J Thorac Cardiovasc Surg. 2010;139(1):53-59.e1.
9. Melvin WS, Dundon JM, Talamini M, et al. Computer-enhanced robotic telesurgery minimizes esophageal perforation during Heller myotomy. Surgery. 2005;138(4):553-8; discussion 558-9.
10. Horgan S, Galvani C, Gorodner MV, et al. Robotic-assisted Heller myotomy versus laparoscopic Heller myotomy for the treatment of esophageal achalasia: multicenter study. J Gastrointest Surg. 2005;9(8):1020-9; discussion 1029-30.
11. Huffmanm LC, Pandalai PK, Boulton BJ, et al. Robotic Heller myotomy: a safe operation with higher postoperative quality-of-life indices. Surgery. 2007;142(4):613-8; discussion 618-20.
12. Shaligram A, Unnirevi J, Simorov A, et al. How does the robot affect outcomes? A retrospective review of open, laparoscopic, and robotic Heller myotomy for achalasia. Surg Endosc. 2012;26(4):1047-50.
12. Baek SJ, Lee DW, Park SS, et al. Current status of robot-assisted gastric surgery. World J Gastrointest Oncol. 2011 Oct;3(10):137-43.
13. Japanese Gastric Cancer Association. Japanese classification of gastric carcinoma: 3rd English edition. Gastric Cancer. 2011;14:101-12.
14. Japanese Gastric Cancer Association. Japanese gastric cancer treatment guidelines 2010 (ver. 3) Gastric Cancer. 2011;14:113-23.
15. Kim MC, Heo GU, Jung GJ. Robotic gastrectomy for gastric cancer: surgical techniques and clinical merits. Surg Endosc. 2010;24:610-15.
16. Hashizume M, Sugimachi K. Robot-assisted gastric surgery. Surg Clin North Am. 2003;83:1429-44.
17. Marano A, Choi YY, Hyung WJ, et al. Robotic versus laparoscopic versus open gastrectomy: a meta-analysis. J Gastric Cancer. 2013;13(3):136-48. doi: 10.5230/jgc.2013.13.3.136.
18. Anderson C, Ellenhorn J, Hellan M, et al. Pilot series of robot-assisted laparoscopic subtotal gastrectomy with extended lymphadenectomy for gastric cancer. Surg Endosc. 2007;21(9):1662-6.
19. Patriti A, Ceccarelli G, Bellochi R, et al. Robot-assisted laparoscopic total and partial gastric resection with D2 lymph node dissection for adenocarcinoma. Surg Endosc. 2008;22(12):2753-60.
20. Song J, Oh SJ, Kang WH, et al. Robot-assisted gastrectomy with lymph node dissection for gastric cancer: lessons learned from an initial 100 consecutive procedures. Ann Surg. 2009;249(6):927-32.
21. Hur H, Kim JY, Cho YK, et al. Technical feasibility of robot-sewn anastomosis in robotic surgery for gastric cancer. J Laparoendosc Adv Surg Tech A. 2010;20:693-97.
22. Liu FL, Lv CT, Qin J, et al. [Da Vinci robot-assisted gastrectomy with lymph node dissection for gastric cancer: a case series of 9 patients]. Zhonghua Wei Chang Wai Ke Za Zhi. 2010;13(5):327-9.
23. Isogaki J, Haruta S, Man-I M, et al. Robot-assisted surgery for gastric cancer: experience at our institute. Pathobiology. 2011;78(6):328-33.
24. D'Annibale A, Pende V, Pernazza G, et al. Full robotic gastrectomy with extended (D2) lymphadenectomy for gastric cancer:surgical technique and preliminary results. J Surg Res. 2011;166(2).
25. Lee HH, Hur H, Jung H, et al. Robot-assisted distal gastrectomy for gastric cancer: initial experience. Am J Surg. 2011;201(6):841-5.
26. Uyama I, Kanaya S, Ishida Y, et al. Novel integrated robotic approach for suprapancreatic D2 nodal dissection for treating gastric cancer: technique and initial experience. World J Surg. 2012;36(2):331-7.
27. Kang BH, Xuan Y, Hur H, et al. Comparison of surgical outcomes between robotic and laparoscopic gastrectomy for gastric cancer: the learning curve of robotic surgery. J Gastric Cancer. 2012;12(3):156-63. doi: 10.5230/jgc.2012.12.3.156.
28. Liu XX, Jiang ZW, Chen P, et al. Full robot-assisted gastrectomy with intracorporeal robot-sewn anastomosis produces satisfying outcomes. World J Gastroenterol. 2013;19(38):6427-37.
29. Hyun MH, Lee CH, Kwon YJ, et al. Robot versus laparoscopic gastrectomy for cancer by an experienced surgeon: comparisons of surgery, complications, and surgical stress. Ann Surg Oncol. 2013;20(4):1258-65. doi: 10.1245/s10434-012-2679-6.
30. Caruso S, Patriti A, Marrelli D, et al. Open vs robot-assisted laparoscopic gastric resection with D2 lymph node dissection for adenocarcinoma: a case-control study. Int J Med Robot. 2011;7(4):452-8. doi: 10.1002/rcs.416.
31. Glantzounis G, Ziogas D, Baltogiannis G. Open versus laparoscopic versus robotic gastrectomy for cancer: need for comparative-effectiveness quality. Surg Endosc. 2010;24:1510–12.
32. Pernazza G, Gentile E, Felicioni L, et al. Improved early survival after robotic gastrectomy in advanced gastric cancer. Surg Laparosc Endosc Percutan Tech. 2006;16:286.
33. Pugliese R, Maggioni D, Sansonna F, et al. Subtotal gastrectomy with D2 dissection by minimally invasive surgery for distal adenocarcinoma of the stomach: results and 5-year survival. Surg Endosc. 2010;24:2594-02.
34. Woo Y, Hyung WJ, Pak KH, et al. Robotic gastrectomy as an oncologically sound alternative to laparoscopic resections for the treatment of early-stage gastric cancers. Arch Surg. 2011;146:1086-92.
35. Yoon HM, Kim YW, Lee JH, et al. Robot-assisted total gastrectomy is comparable with laparoscopically assisted total gastrectomy for early gastric cancer. Surg Endosc. 2012;26:1377-81.
36. Kim MC, Heo GU, Jung GJ. Robotic gastrectomy for gastric cancer: surgical techniques and clinical merits. Surg Endosc. 2010;24:610-15.
37. Huang KH, Lan YT, Fang WL, et al. Initial experience of robotic gastrectomy and comparison with open and laparoscopic gastrectomy for gastric cancer. J Gastrointest Surg. 2012;16(7):1303-10.
38. Hubens G, Balliu L, Ruppert M, et al. Roux-en-Y gastric bypass procedure performed with the Da Vinci robot system: is it worth it? Surg Endosc. 2008;22:1690-6.
39. Mohr CJ, Nadzam GS, Curet MJ. Totally robotic Roux-en-Y gastric bypass. Arch Surg. 2005;140:779-86.

40. Yu SC, Clapp BL, Lee MJ, et al. Robotic assistance provides excellent outcomes during the learning curve for laparoscopic Roux-en-Y gastric bypass: results from 100 robotic-assisted gastric bypasses. Am J Surg. 2006;192:746-9.
41. Diamantis T, Alexandrou A, Nikiteas N, et al. Initial experience with robotic sleeve gastrectomy for morbid obesity. Obes Surg. 2011;21(8):1172-9.
42. Romero RJ, Kosanovic R, Rabaza JR, et al. Robotic sleeve gastrectomy: experience of 134 cases and comparison with a systematic review of the laparoscopic approach. Obes Surg. 2013;23(11):1743-52.
43. Cirocchi R, Boselli C, Santoro A, et al.Current status of robotic bariatric surgery: a systematic review. BMC Surg. 2013;13(1):53.
44. Weber PA, Merola S, Wasielewski A, et al. Telerobotic-assisted laparoscopic right and sigmoid colectomies for benign disease. Dis Colon Rectum. 2002;45(12):1689-94; discussion 1695-6.
45. Giulianotti PC, Coratti A, Angelini M, et al. Robotics in general surgery: personal experience in a large community hospital. Arch Surg. 2003;138(7):777-84.
46. Melvin WS, Needleman BJ, Krause KR, et al. Robotic resection of pancreatic neuroendocrine tumor. J Laparoendosc Adv Surg Tech A. 2003;11:33-6.
47. Cooperman AM. Pancreatic cancer: the bigger picture. Surg Clin North Am. 2001;11:557-74.
48. Cooperman AM, Fader A, Cushin B, et al. Surgery and cancer of the pancreas: will common sense become common practice? Hematol Oncol Clin North Am. 2002;11:81-94.
49. Tanaka S, Nakao M, Ioka T, et al. Slight dilatation of the main pancreatic duct and presence of pancreatic cysts as predictive signs of pancreatic cancer: a prospective study. Radiol. 2010;11:965-72.
50. Sahani DV, Saokar A, Hahn PF, et al. Pancreatic cysts 3 cm or smaller: how aggressive should treatment be? Radiol. 2006;11:912-9.
51. Waters JA, Canal DF, Wiebke EA, et al. Robotic distal pancreatectomy: cost effective? Surgery. 2010;148(4):814-23.
52. Kang CM, Kim DH, Lee WJ, et al. Conventional laparoscopic and robot-assisted spleen-preserving pancreatectomy: does da Vinci have clinical advantages? Surg Endosc. 2011;11:2004–9.
53. Daouadi M, Zureikat AH, Zenati MS, et al. Robot-assisted minimally invasive distal pancreatectomy is superior to the laparoscopic technique. Ann Surg. 2013;11:128-32.
54. Giulianotti PC, Sbrana F, Bianco FM, et al. Robot-assisted laparoscopic pancreatic surgery: single-surgeon experience. Surg Endosc. 2010;11:1646-57.
55. Giulianotti PC, Sbrana F, Bianco FM, et al. Robot-assisted laparoscopic pancreatic surgery: single-surgeon experience. Surg Endosc. 2010;24(7):1646-57.
56. Kang CM, Kim DH, Lee WJ, et al. Conventional laparoscopic and robot-assisted spleen-preserving pancreatectomy: does da Vinci have clinical advantages? Surg Endosc. 2011;25(6):2004-9.
57. Boggi U, Signori S, Vistoli F, et al. Laparoscopic robot-assisted pancreas transplantation: first world experience. Transplantation. 2012;93(2):201-6.
58. Wayne M, Steele J, Iskandar M, et al. Robotic pancreatic surgery—no substitute for experience and clinical judgment: an initial experience and literature review. World J Surg Oncol. 2013;11(1):160.
59. Cooperman AM, Schwartz ET, Fader A, et al. Safety, efficacy, and cost of pancreaticoduodenal resection in a specialized center based at a community hospital. Arch Surg. 1997;11:744-47.
60. Coopermann AM. Pancreaticoduodenal resection: pearls, perils, and pitfalls. Surg Clin North Am. 2001;11:579-93.
61. Giulianotti PC, Sbrana F, Bianco FM, et al. Robot-assisted laparoscopic pancreatic surgery: single-surgeon experience. Surg Endosc. 2010;11:1646-57. doi: 10.1007/s00464-009-0825-4.
62. Winer J, Can MF, Bartlett DL, et al. The current state of robotic-assisted pancreatic surgery. Nat Rev Gastroenterol Hepatol. 2012;11:468-76.
63. Coopermann AM. Pancreaticoduodenal resection: pearls, perils, and pitfalls. Surg Clin North Am. 2001;11:579-93.
64. Giulianotti PC, Sbrana F, Bianco FM, et al. Robot-assisted laparoscopic middle pancreatectomy. J Laparoendosc Adv Surg Tech A. 2010;11:135-39.
65. Kang CM, Kim DH, Lee WJ, et al. Initial experiences using robot-assisted central pancreatectomy with pancreaticogastrostomy: a potential way to advanced laparoscopic pancreatectomy. Surg Endosc. 2011;11:1101-06.
66. Vidovszky TJ, Smith W, Ghosh J, et al. Robotic cholecystectomy: learning curve, advantages, and limitations. J Surg Res. 2006;136(2):172-8.
67. Wren SM, Curet MJ. Single-port robotic cholecystectomy: results from a first human use clinical study of the new da Vinci single-site surgical platform, Arch Surg. 2011;146(10):1122-7.
68. Vidovszky TJ, Carr AD, Farinholt GN, et al. Single-site robotic cholecystectomy in a broadly inclusive patient population: a prospective study. Ann Surg. 2013. [Epub ahead of print]
69. Morel P, Buchs NC, Iranmanesh P, et al. Robotic single-site cholecystectomy. J Hepatobiliary Pancreat Sci. 2014;21(1):18-25.
70. Shen BY, Zhan Q, Deng XX, et al. Radical resection of gallbladder cancer: could it be robotic? Surg Endosc. 2012. [Epub ahead of print]
71. Romero-Talamás H, Kroh M. Cholecystectomy by using a surgical robotic system. J Hepatobiliary Pancreat Sci. 2014;21(1):11-7.
72. Buell JF, Cherqui D, Geller DA, et al. The international position on laparoscopic liver surgery: the Louisville statement, 2008. Ann Surg. 2009;250(5):825-30.
73. Ho CM, Wakabayashi G, Nitta H, et al. Systematic review of robotic liver resection. Surg Endosc. 2013;27(3):732-39.
74. Giulianotti PC, Coratti A, Sbrana F, et al. Robotic liver surgery: results for 70 resections. Surgery. 2011;149(1):29-39.
75. Choi GH, Choi SH, Kim SH, et al. Robotic liver resection: technique and results of 30 consecutive procedures. Surg Endosc. 2012;26(8):2247-58.
76. Chan OC, Tang CN, Lai EC, et al. Robotic hepatobiliary and pancreatic surgery: a cohort study. J Hepatobiliary Pancreat Sci. 2011;18(4):471-80. doi: 10.1007/s00534-011-0389-2.
77. Giulianotti PC, Sbrana F, Coratti A, et al. Totally robotic right hepatectomy: surgical technique and outcomes. Arch Surg. 2011;146(7):844-50.
78. Casciola L, Patriti A, Ceccarelli G, et al. Robot-assisted parenchymal-sparing liver surgery including lesions located in the posterosuperior segments. Surg Endosc. 2011;25(12):3815-24.
79. Ji WB, Wang HG, Zhao ZM, et al. Robotic-assisted laparoscopic anatomic hepatectomy in China: initial experience. Ann Surg. 2011;253(2):342-8.
80. Lai EC, Tang CN, Li MK. Robot-assisted laparoscopic hemi-hepatectomy: technique and surgical outcomes. Int J Surg. 2012;10(1):11-5.
81. Berber E, Akyildiz HY, Aucejo F, et al. Robotic versus laparoscopic resection of liver tumours. HPB (Oxford). 2010;12(8):583-6.
82. Patriti A, Ceccarelli G, Bartoli A, et al. Laparoscopic and robot-assisted one-stage resection of colorectal cancer with synchronous liver metastases: a pilot study. J Hepatobiliary Pancreat Surg. 2009;16(4):450-7.
83. Wakabayashi G, Sasaki A, Nishizuka S, et al. Our initial experience with robotic hepato-biliary-pancreatic surgery. J Hepatobiliary Pancreat Sci. 2011;18(4):481-7.
84. Choi SB, Park JS, Kim JK, Hyung WJ, Kim KS, Yoon DS, Lee WJ, Kim BR. Early experiences of robotic-assisted laparoscopic liver resection.Yonsei Med J. 2008 Aug 30;49(4):632-8.

85. Vasile S, Sgarbură O, Tomulescu V, et al. The robotic-assisted left lateral hepatic segmentectomy: the next step. Chirurgia (Bucur). 2008;103(4):401-5.
86. Panaro F, Piardi T, Cag M, et al. Robotic liver resection as a bridge to liver transplantation. JSLS. 2011;15(1):86-9.
87. Holloway RW, Brudie LA, Rakowski JA, et al. Robotic-assisted resection of liver and diaphragm recurrent ovarian carcinoma: description of technique. Gynecol Oncol. 2011;120(3):419-22.
88. Giulianotti PC, Sbrana F, Bianco FM, et al. Robot-assisted laparoscopic extended right hepatectomy with biliary reconstruction. J Laparoendosc Adv Surg Tech A. 2010;20(2):159-63.
89. Machado MA, Makdissi FF, Surjan RC, et al. [First robotic-assisted laparoscopic liver resection in Latin America].ArqGastroenterol. 2009;46(1):78-80.
90. Giulianotti PC, Addeo P, Bianco FM. Robotic right hepatectomy for giant hemangioma in a Jehovah's Witness. J Hepatobiliary Pancreat Sci. 2011;18(1):112-8.
91. Giulianotti PC, Tzvetanov I, Jeon H, et al. Robot-assisted right lobe donor hepatectomy. Transpl Int. 2012;25(1):e5-9.
92. Woo R, Le D, Albanese CT, et al. Robot-assisted laparoscopic resection of a type I choledochal cyst in a child. J Laparoendosc Adv Surg Tech A. 2006;16(2):179-83.
93. Klein MD, Langenburg SE, Lelli JL, et al. Pediatric robotic surgery: lessons learned from a clinical experience. J Laparoendosc Adv Surg Tech A. 2007;17:265-71.
94. Kang CM, Chi HS, Kim JY, et al. A case of robot-assisted excision of choledochal cyst, hepaticojejunostomy, and extracorporeal Roux-en-y anastomosis using the da Vinci surgical system. Surg Laparosc Endosc Percutan Tech. 2007;17(6):538-41.
95. Meehan JJ, Elliott S, Sandler A. The robotic approach to complex hepatobiliary anomalies in children: preliminary report. J Pediatr Surg. 2007;42(12):2110-4.
96. Geiger JD. Robotic excision of choledochalcyst. In: Holcomb GW, Georgeson KE, Rothenberg SS, editors. Atlas of pediatric laparoscopy and thoracoscopy. Philadelphia, PA: Saunders Elsevier; 2008. pp. 211-5.
97. Alqahtani A, Albassam A, Zamakhshary M, et al. Robot-assisted pediatric surgery: how far can we go? World J Surg. 2010;34:975-78.
98. Chang EY, Hong YJ, Chang HK, et al. Lessons and tips from the experience of pediatric robotic choledochal cyst resection. J Laparoendosc Adv Surg Tech A. 2012;22(6):609-14.
99. Dawrant MJ, Najmaldin AS, Alizai NK. Robot-assisted resection of choledochal cysts and hepaticojejunostomy in children less than 10 kg. J Pediatr Surg. 2010;45(12):2364-8.

CHAPTER 120

Tumor Markers in Gastrointestinal Malignancy

Nilesh Patil, Kunal Parasar, Sundeep Singh Saluja

INTRODUCTION

The National Institute of Health Biomarker Working Group has defined tumor marker as "a characteristic that is objectively measured and evaluated as an indicator of normal biological processes, pathogenic processes, or pharmacologic responses to a therapeutic intervention."[1] An ideal tumor marker should have the following characteristics:

A. It is produced only by the tumor cells and is detected in all patients with the specific tumor.
B. Tumor load correlates well with the blood levels of the marker.
C. Patients with stable disease should have a consistent concentration of the tumor marker.
D. The half-life of the marker needs to be short enough so that when production drops, the level of the marker falls off rapidly.
E. The assay for the marker should be analytically sensitive, specific, easy to perform, inexpensive, rapid, and reproducible.

At present there is no single tumor marker fulfilling all above criteria. The tumor markers may be protein or nonprotein. In addition, nonprotein markers are further categorized into ribonucleic acid (RNA)-based markers (such as altered expression of transcripts or micro RNAs) and deoxyribonucleic acid (DNA)-based markers such as single nucleotide polymorphism, chromosomal translocations, changes in DNA copy number, microsatellite instability, or epigenetic changes.[2] These tumor markers may be found either in body fluids, especially blood and urine or in the tumor tissue itself. The markers detected in body fluids have the highest potential for clinical use due to the ease of access and repeated sampling, besides being cost-effective. The important clinical applications of tumor markers are diagnostic, prognostic, and predictive. Generally immunoassay methods are employed to detect these markers. The newer techniques for measuring tumor markers are focusing on gene expression microarray, proteomics, and detection of circulating tumor cells. The common tumor markers and their uses are summarized in Table 1.

Tumor Markers in Specific Gastrointestinal Malignancies

Colorectal Cancer

Carcinoembryonic antigen: It is a glycoprotein with a molecular weight of 200 kd, normally found in embryonic entodermal epithelium. It belongs to a group of tumor markers referred to as oncofetal proteins. The molecule itself is released into the blood circulation and is also detected in the secretions of stomach, small intestine, and biliary tree. It plays important role in cell adhesion, besides being antiapoptotic. Its normal level in serum is <2.5 ng/mL and is raised if level exceeds 5 ng/mL. The borderline levels of 2.5–5 ng/mL may be found in smokers and benign conditions such as chronic obstructive pulmonary disease, cirrhosis, inflammatory bowel disease, and pancreatitis. The half-life of carcinoembryonic antigen (CEA) is 7–14 days. It is the most thoroughly investigated serological marker in colorectal cancer (CRC).

Screening: Most expert panels including American Society of Clinical Oncology[3] and European Group on Tumor Markers (EGTM)[4] do not recommend CEA as a screening modality due to its low sensitivity in detecting early stage disease.[3] Only 5–40% of patients with localized disease have elevated levels of CEA. Carcinoembryonic antigen has high specificity for detecting occult metastatic disease; therefore, raised CEA levels in a patient with colorectal cancer warrant further evaluation for distant metastasis, and thereby helps in treatment planning.

Table 1: Common tumor markers and their use

Tumor marker	*Normal value*	*Tumor type*	*Utility*
CEA	2.5–5 ng/mL	Colorectal cancer	Prognosis Response to neoadjuvant therapy Postoperative surveillance
MSI	–	Suspected lynch syndrome	Diagnosis Screening siblings
AFP	0–10 ng/mL	Hepatocellular carcinoma	Adjunct in screening
CA19-9	0–37 IU/mL	Pancreatic cancer	May help in Diagnosis Prognosis Follow-up to detect recurrence
Chromogranin A	2–15 ng/mL	Neuroendocrine tumor	Diagnosis Postoperative surveillance

CEA, carcinoembryonic antigen; MSI, microsatellite instability; AFP, alfa-fetoprotein; CA19-9, carbohydrate antigen 19-9.

Prognosis: The increased CEA level reflects the tumor burden and the degree of elevation in CEA levels correlates well with higher stage. Also, 5-year survival is significantly poor in patients with elevated preoperative levels than in those with normal levels. So, CEA is measured routinely preoperatively in newly diagnosed patients of CRC, as it has prognostic value and is an independent predictor of survival, especially in stage-2 patients. However, there is insufficient data in the literature to support the application of CEA to select CRC patients who could get benefit from adjuvant treatment.[4]

Monitoring: There is level I evidence supporting CEA for postoperative surveillance, especially in the situation of elevated preoperative levels. A meta-analysis comparing outcomes in patients with intensive versus minimal or no follow-up using CEA revealed that patients on intensive follow-up had 20–30% reduction in hazard rate for all causes of mortality. Since different follow-up regimen were used in various studies, it is difficult to conclude about the best combination of tests and its frequency. However, EGTM panel recommend that CEA should be measured at baseline and then every 3 months for at least 3 years in all stage 2/3 patients. Subsequently, it may be measured every 6 months for 5 years. The raised CEA levels are found in approximately 75% of patients with recurrent CRC before the development of clinical symptoms. Most expert panels recommend serial CEA determinations during the follow-up after curative resection for CRC, because it is more sensitive in detection of early recurrent disease as compared with other diagnostic modalities.[4] However, CEA is more sensitive for hepatic or retroperitoneal metastasis compared with pulmonary, local, or peritoneal metastasis. As the elevation of CEA could be transient, repeat measurement should be done by the same laboratory assay in order to confirm the trend.

In advanced CRC patients, CEA is used for monitoring response to systemic therapy. Studies have showed favorable agreement between radiological and CEA-defined responses.[5,6] There was more than 90% agreement between imaging and CEA response for both stable and disease progression after systemic therapy. However, it is important to remember that a transient or spurious rise in CEA level can occur immediately after initiation of specific chemotherapy. This is due to necrosis and/or apoptosis of cancer cells.

Fecal and genetic markers in colorectal cancer: As randomized clinical trials have demonstrated reduction in the mortality from CRC due to screening with fecal occult blood test (FOBT), (EGTM) has recommended the use of FOBT for screening of CRC and advanced colorectal adenomas. Fecal occult blood test is slowly being replaced by newer fecal immunochemical tests (FIT) because of its lack of specificity for human hemoglobin (Hb), and relatively low sensitivity and specificity for colorectal neoplasia. Recently, tests for fecal DNA markers such as mutant ras, mutant p53, mutant APC, and specific methylated genes are becoming popular due to their superiority over FOBT. However, these tests are expensive and technically demanding.

Lynch syndrome (LS), an autosomal dominant disorder constitutes about 3% of all CRCs. Besides CRC, it predisposes an individual to other malignancies such as endometrium, stomach, and small bowel cancer. Many observational studies have reported reduced cancer rates and mortality due to the close surveillance of subjects with LS, although there are no randomized clinical trials addressing this issue. The mutations in mismatch repair (MMR) genes like MLH1, MSH2, PMS2, and MSH6 result in microsatellite instability (MSI). Microsatellite instability/mismatch repair is present in >90% of patients with LS. Therefore patients suspected to have LS are subjected to MSI testing. If they test positive then one should look for specific gene mutations. Previously, MSI/MMR protein determination in CRC was confined to the individuals fulfilling the Amsterdam and Bethesda criteria. It is important to remember that 12–17% of sporadic CRC can also have MSI/MMR due to loss of MLH1 or MSH2. More recently, several organizations including EGTM, recommended such testing in all CRC patients due to advantages of cost effectiveness, and improved sensitivity for detecting mutation carriers. However, such a universal testing may not be possible in developing countries due to limited resources. In the presence of MSI or defective MMR activity, a subject should undergo genetic counseling and germ line gene testing for LS. Many randomized trials have now reported a favorable outcome in colon cancer patients (especially stag II and III) carrying MSI or defective MMR. This provides a strong evidence for utility of MSI/MMR status as a prognostic biomarker. It may also be a predictive biomarker for response to adjuvant 5-fluorouracil-based chemotherapy. Presence of MSI is associated with lack of benefit from adjuvant treatment. This finding along with better prognosis of patients with positive MSI suggest, that one may subject Stage II CRC patients to MSI testing while deciding upon adjuvant treatment.

Recently, monoclonal antibodies to epidermal growth factor regulator such as cetuximab and panitumumab are being used either alone or in combination with cytotoxic chemotherapy to treat advanced CRC patients. The response rate of such a treatment was found to be only 10–15%. Subsequently, it was seen that the positive results was not found in patients carrying mutations especially in codon 12 of the K-ras gene. So, various expert panels now recommend testing for K-ras gene mutations before initiation of such therapy in advanced CRC cases. It has clinical and cost benefit bearing for the use of monoclonal antibodies.

Pancreatic Cancer

Carbohydrate antigen 19-9: It is a sialyated Lewis blood group antigen, which is widely used serum marker for pancreatic malignancy. It is an oligosaccharide and is normally absorbed on the surface of erythrocyctes. This epitope is normally present in the biliary tree and is also expressed by pancreatic cancer cells.

Screening: For a healthy adult, the upper limit of normal is 37 U/mL. It is not an effective screening test for pancreatic ductal adenocarcinoma, (PDA) due to its low sensitivity in early stage disease.[7] But with increasing the cutoff values, CA 19-9 diagnoses the PDA more accurately. The reported sensitivities and specificities of CA 19-9 in diagnosis of PDA varies from 67 to 92%, and 68 to 92%, respectively. However, its utility as a diagnostic marker is limited due to following reasons: (a) it cannot be used in cases with negative Lewis blood group antigen which constitutes 5–10% of general population; (b) serum CA 19-9 levels can be elevated up to the hundreds or thousands (U/mL) in patients with benign biliary tract disease; (c) raised CA 19-9 may be also found in patients with acute or chronic pancreatitis; and (d) besides PDA, CA 19-9 levels are also increased in other malignancies such as those of biliary tree, stomach, colon, liver, and lung. Thus, when used for diagnostic purpose, assessment of CA19-9 levels should be done in conjunction with other modalities (imaging and/or biopsy).

Prognosis: Preoperative CA 19-9 has *limited prognostic value* both in localized and advanced PDA because of the variable expression of Lewis antigen in many patients and falsely increased CA 19-9 levels due to biliary obstruction, which is found in majority cases of PDA and different benign pancreatobiliary conditions.[7] However, persistently raised CA 19-9 levels even after biliary drainage may suggest underlying malignant pathology more accurately.[8] The hazard ratio using CA 19-9 is 2.0 or less, which is similar to that predicted by pathological characteristics such as lymph nodes and resection margins. This shows that preoperative value does not have much prognostic significance.

Some ability of preoperative CA 19-9 levels to determine the *resectability* of pancreatic cancer has been shown by a recent study. The study reported unresectable disease in one third of patients with levels above 300 U/mL.[9] In patients with early stage or locally advanced PDA, the postoperative CA 19-9 values following curative resection provides better prognostic information than the preoperative ones.[7] Studies have reported poor survival in patients whose CA 19-9 levels failed to normalize after resection. However, 3 to 6 months may be required for normalization of CA 19-9 levels after surgery.[10]

Monitoring: Rise in CA 19-9 levels following curative resection can predict the recurrence 2 to 9 months before any clinical or radiological evidence. But, the confirmation should be done by imaging and/or biopsy before initiating any therapy. Serial determination of CA 19-9 plays an important role in monitoring response to the therapy (either radiotherapy or chemotherapy). Improved survival has been reported in patients with a biochemical response after therapy in patients with locally advanced or metastatic PDA.[11,12] A fall in CA 19-9 levels by >75% was associated with median survival of more than 1 year.

Other markers like CEA and CA-125 are not very useful therefore not recommended in routine use while diagnosing or managing carcinoma pancreas.

Markers in pancreatic secretions: Since, invasive pancreatic cancer is associated with shedding of the tumor cells, pancreatic juice can serve as a potential rich source of tumor markers. But the assessment of both conventional (CA 19-9, CEA, and many others) and molecular (mutant K-ras and P53) markers are associated with several limitations such as modest sensitivity, false positive elevations in benign pancreatobiliary disorders, low yield in case of pancreatic duct obstruction, and requirement of invasive procedure for collection of specimen.

Recently, several other tumor markers either serum [CA-242, CEA, Detection of a pancreatic cancer-associated antigen-2, tissue polypeptide-specific antigen, tumor M2-pyruvate kinase, insulin-like growth factor binding protein-1, (IGF-1), and macrophage inhibitory cytokine] or tissue based (k-ras, p53, specific mucins, microRNAs, p21, SMAD4, and BCL-2) have been investigated for pancreatic cancer. None of them have demonstrated superiority over CA19-9. So, they are not widely used in clinical practice.

Hepatocellular Carcinoma

Alfa-fetoprotein: It is an oncofetal antigen with a molecular weight of 70 kd. This glycoprotein is produced by fetal hepatocytes and yolk sac during pregnancy.

Screening: The cutoff level for a healthy nonpregnant adult is <25 ng/mL. The estimated sensitivity and specificity of alfa-fetoprotein (AFP) for diagnosing hepatocellular carcinoma (HCC) is 25–75% and 76–94%, respectively. But it is important to note that both sensitivity and specificity varies with the chosen cutoff value. Also, the sensitivity of AFP declines with decrease in the size of tumor (52% for >3 cm versus 25% for <3 cm). Screening for HCC is indicated in high risk group which include all patients with cirrhosis, and some hepatitis B virus and hepatitis C virus infected patients. Alfa-fetoprotein is the most widely used tumor marker along with ultrasonography (USG) (every 6–12 months) for *surveillance* of HCC in high risk patients, and as a diagnostic tool in patients with focal liver lesions and suspected HCC. Combining USG with AFP increases the efficacy of screening. In general, consistently increased serum AFP levels of >200 ng/mL are diagnostic of HCC; but, such high values are seen in less than one third cases of HCC. AFP has several limitations as a diagnostic marker: (a) the positive yield of AFP in HCC is only 60–80%[13] with low sensitivity in early stage disease; (b) serum AFP levels are not always elevated in HCC and values may fluctuate during natural history of the disease; (c) the normal levels of AFP are found in majority patients with fibrolamellar and sarcomatoid variants of HCC; (d) false positive results may occur in pregnancy, hepatitis, cirrhosis; and IBD and

(e) besides HCC, significant elevation in serum AFP levels may occur in other gastrointestinal malignancies (such as gastric, pancreatic, or colorectal), lung cancer, and embryonal carcinoma.

Prognosis: Alfa-fetoprotein *correlates well with stage and prognosis* in patients with AFP-producing HCCs. Its level reflects the tumor size. Values >400 ng/mL are usually associated with large-sized tumors and multinodular disease. Also, the doubling time of preoperative AFP levels can predict early post operative recurrence and prognosis.[14] Alfa-fetoprotein concentration (<or >400 ng/mL) is one of the four independent factors of Cancer of the Liver Italian Program staging system which establishes prognosis for HCC patients. In a review of patients from the Scientific Registry of Transplant Recipients database, Toso et al.[15] reported AFP as an independent risk factor for poor survival (<50% survival at 3 years. in patients with an AFP level >400 ng/mL). Thus, incorporating AFP level in selection criteria may further improve posttransplant outcome.

Monitoring: Along with computed tomography or magnetic resonance imaging, serial measurements of AFP levels after resection or ablation are useful for monitoring the response and early detection of recurrence. With effective treatment AFP levels *drop to <10 ng/mL within a month,*[16] and rising trend in AFP values over the course reflects the recurrence. In case of advanced HCC, the reduction in AFP values following palliative therapy such as transarterial chemoembolization or chemotherapy suggest a favorable response. But, the monitoring of AFP levels becomes clinically significant only when AFP is raised before any treatment.

Other Commonly Used Markers in Hepatocellular Carcinoma

Alfa-fetoprotein-L3: AFP has three different isoforms. The AFP-L1 is the most common type. It has minimal affinity for lens culinaris agglutinin (LCA). It is increased in conditions like cirrhosis and hepatitis. Alfa-fetoprotein-L2 has an intermediate affinity for LCA. It is increased in patients with yolk sac tumors and pregnancy. Alfa-fetoprotein-L3 (lens culinaris agglutinin-reactive) glycoform of AFP is produced only by malignant cells. Studies [13,17] have reported >95% specificity for HCC with a cutoff value >10% of total serum AFP. So, it may be used for early diagnosis when tumor size is <2 cm.[13] In addition, AFP-L3 is a marker of biologically aggressive tumor and indicates poor prognosis. Such patients develop early vascular invasion and intrahepatic metastasis.

Des-γ-carboxy-prothrombin: It is abnormal prothrombin produced by malignant hepatocytes due to acquired defect in vitamin K-dependent posttranslation carboxylation. *Des-γ-carboxy-prothrombin* is involved in angiogenesis of HCC with potential mitogenic and migratory activities. It has been recognized as an excellent tumor marker for diagnosis of HCC and the commonly used cutoff level is 40 mAU/mL. Several studies have reported sensitivity of 48–62% and specificity of 81–98%.[18,19] Recently, Baek et al. reported superior diagnostic accuracy than that of AFP irrespective of the HCC size.[20] In addition, Volk et al. showed that DCP is significantly better than AFP and AFP-L3 in differentiating HCC from cirrhosis.[21] The sensitivity of diagnosing HCC increases to >85% with combined AFP and DCP assay. Its serum levels correlates well with vascular invasion or intrahepatic metastasis. Recently, more attention is given to DCP as it has been found to be an independent prognostic factor for recurrence, and survival irrespective of the treatment (resection, transplant, ablation, or transarterial chemoembolization) received.

Glypican-3: It belongs to the family of heparin sulfate proteoglycans. It regulates cell adhesion, migration, and cytoskeleton organization in tumor cells. As glypican-3 is exclusively expressed by HCC tumor cells, it can be considered as a potential tumor marker for diagnosis of early HCC. Although, some studies have reported sensitivity and specificity of 77 and 96%, respectively for glypican-3,[22] there is *no consensus regarding its diagnostic role.* Simultaneous measurement of AFP and glypican-3 could increase the diagnostic sensitivity significantly. Recently, few studies have reported glypican-3 as an independent prognostic marker and it can detect recurrence early in HCC patients after surgery.[23,24]

Neuroendocrine Tumors (Table 2)

General Markers

Chromogranin (Cg): Chromogranin (Cg) belongs to family of glycoproteins. They are the most important general tumor markers for neuroendocrine tumors (NETs). They are present

Table 2: Various serum and urinary biomarkers used in neuroendocrine tumors

	Tumor marker	*Gastrointestinal NET*	*Pancreatic NET*
	Plasma		
	General Markers		
1	Chromogranin A	+	+
2	Chromogranin B	+	+
3	Neuron-specific enolase	+	+
4	Pancreatic polypeptide	+	+
	Specific		
1	Ghrelin	+	–
2	Neuropeptide K	+	–
3	Gastrin	–	Gastrinoma
4	Insulin	–	Insulinoma
5	Vasoactive intestinal peptide	–	Vipoma
6	Calcitonin	–	+
7	Somatostatin	–	Somatostatinoma
8	Substance P	+	+
	Urinary		
1	5-Hydroxy indolacetic acid	+	–
2	Tele methylimidazoleacetic acid	–	+

NET, neuroendocrine tumors.

in the secretory vesicles of NET cells throughout the body. The clinically relevant markers among them are Cg A and Cg B. Adrenal contains equal amount of Cg A and Cg B, while stomach and parathyroid contains mainly Cg A. Chromogranin A is a better tumor marker than Cg B as it is found more abundantly than Cg B in most NETs. For various types of NETs, the reported sensitivity and specificity of Cg A are 60–100% and 70–100%, respectively.[25,26] However, false positive results for Cg A are seen in conditions such as type A chronic atrophic gastritis, impaired kidney function and in patients on proton pump inhibitors. Chromogranin B is more specific for NETs as its levels are not affected by above conditions, but there is no commercially available assay for its measurement.[25] The circulating Cg A levels correlate with *both tumor burden and biological activity*. Chromogranin A is an independent prognostic marker for small intestinal NET, as it determines both tumor burden and biologic activity. In patients with NETs, raised Cg A levels reflect poor overall prognosis and early decline in the values following treatment may indicate a favorable outcome.[27] It is important to note that circulating Cg A levels does not correlate well with tumor mass in patients treated with somatostatin analogues as they block synthesis, and release of Cg A. The North American Neuroendocrine Tumor Society, 2013 guidelines[28] recommend *monitoring of Cg A levels* in advanced disease with raised Cg A levels at the *time of diagnosis*. In addition, it also suggests *following its levels* in patients undergoing resection.

Pancreatic polypeptide: Pancreatic polypeptide (PP) is another general tumor marker, elevated in NETs of both GI tract and pancreas. Its sensitivity varies from 50 to 80%.[26] However, a lot of clinical conditions such as chronic kidney diseases, advanced age, inflammatory diseases of gut, diarrhea, and laxative abuse can cause falsely elevated levels of pancreatic polypeptide. With *simultaneous measurement of Cg A and PP*, particularly in patients with nonfunctional pancreatic endocrine tumors, a *sensitivity of almost 95%* can be achieved.[26,29] Its secretion is stimulated by protein meal, therefore a mixed meal stimulation is useful in diagnosing patients with MEN 1 and PETs.

Neuron-specific enolase (NSE): Neuron-specific enolase (NSE), present in the cytoplasm of neuroendocrine cells, serves as a potential tumor marker for NETs. Its level has been found to be increased in pancreatic endocrine tumors and 30–50% of cases with intestinal NETs. Sometimes NSE could be of value, particularly in patients with poorly differentiated NETs, as they have elevated levels of NSE despite the normal Cg A values. In addition, some authors have reported higher sensitivity with the combined NSE and Cg A assay compared with either marker alone.[30]

Specific Markers

The choice of the specific tumor marker to be tested for NETs can be predicted by the anatomic site of primary tumor (if this is known) and clinical presentation such as: urinary 5-hydroxyindolacetic acid level in patients with mid- or foregut tumors producing symptoms of carcinoid syndrome. All three types of gastric NETs have raised Cg A levels. They vary in serum gastrin levels where type I and II have raised gastrin level unlike type III. Duodenal NET are mainly gastrinoma that present as Zollinger-Ellison syndrome. They have elevated serum gastrin level which aids in diagnosis whenever clinically suspected. Duodenal somatostatinoma are diagnosed histologically by presence of characteristic psammoma bodies.

Pancreatic NETs are either functional or nonfunctional types. Functional NET have specific clinical presentation due to specific substance release. Identification of elevated levels of specific substance in serum helps in diagnosing tumors like insulin and pro-insulin levels during a 48–72 hour fast in cases with insulinoma, serum gastrin levels in cases of gastrinoma, serum vasoactive intestinal polypeptide, and glucagon levels in patients with VIPoma and glucagonoma syndrome, respectively. Nonfunctional PNET are either truly nonfunctional or PPoma. They are diagnosed using general markers such as Cg A, NSE, or PP. Among these Cg A is most commonly used and recommended as described above.

Carcinoma Gallbladder

At present there are no effective tumor markers available for carcinoma gall bladder (Ca GB) with good sensitivity and specificity.[31] The commonly used tumor makers in clinical practice for Ca GB are CA19-9, CEA, CA-125, and CA-242. CA 19-9 and CEA are most widely studied. However, there is no strong evidence to support isolated use of either CA19-9 or CEA for diagnostic purpose due to poor sensitivity in early stage disease and low specificity.[31] CA-125 is increased in 58% of cases with Ca GB and can differentiate Ca GB from GSD.[32] Low specificity limits its use as a diagnostic marker as serum levels are raised in other GI or gynecological malignancies. CA-242 is associated with high specificity (83%) for Ca GB, and its levels are rarely affected by stone disease.[33,34] But its sensitivity is low (64%) and it cannot differentiate Ca GB from pancreatic cancer, as CA-242 is also highly expressed by pancreatic cancer.[33,34] Recently, combined measurement of these markers has been reported to be associated with increased diagnostic accuracy.[34] At present tumors markers in diagnosis of gall bladder cancer are having little significance as compared with high index of clinical suspicion and good quality imaging. Among these markers CA 19-9 is a better predictor of malignant pathology and its pretreatment levels has been validated as an independent prognostic factor for Ca GB patients.[34] It must be taken into account that these tumor markers can be useful in monitoring a patient of Ca GB for recurrence if their levels are raised at the time of diagnosis, and normalize after treatment.

Cholangiocarcinoma

Cholangiocarcinomas are relatively uncommon malignancies with characteristic slow growth and majority of patients presents in advanced stage. The major hurdle in the diagnosis of cholangiocarcinoma is limited availability of tissue samples. So, there are need of tumor markers for better early diagnosis and therapeutic approach. There is no single diagnostic and/or prognostic marker for cholangiocarcinoma.[36] The most extensively studied tumor marker is CA 19-9. Studies evaluating CA 19-9 have failed to provide a sufficient evidence for its use as a diagnostic marker because of previously mentioned limitations. But its level can be assessed in conjunction with other imaging tests to diagnose cholangiocarcinoma. In addition, there is no conclusive evidence in the literature regarding the ability of CA 19-9 to detect cholangiocarcinoma early in patients with primary sclerosing cholangitis.[36]However, consistent rise in its level on periodic testing should raise the suspicion of possible development of cholangiocarcinoma in PSC patients. Many studies including a meta-analysis on its prognostic role have shown pretreatment raised serum levels of CA 19-9 predictive of survival. But most of the studies were either observational or retrospective and were not well defined.[36,37] Carcinoembryonic antigen is not a useful marker for diagnosing cholangiocarcinomas as it cannot differentiate bile duct cancers from benign biliary diseases. It does not have any prognostic value also.[36] In spite of low specificity, CA 125 is better than CA19-9 in detecting cholangiocarcinoma and differentiating benign, and malignant biliary obstruction as its levels are not influenced by cholangitis or stones.[35] Few authors have reported specific mucins (MUC1 and MUC5AC) in the serum as promising prognostic markers in cholangiocarcinomas. Their elevated levels are associated with worse prognosis. Recently, several other potential diagnostic (interleukin-6, trypsinogen-2, and matrix metalloproteinases) and prognostic(C-reactive protein) markers have been investigated in single studies. But all these studies do not provide a good level of evidence and their results have not been validated in other cohorts.

Some groups have also evaluated the strength of combined assay using two or more different markers which may increase diagnostic accuracy. Ramage et al.[38] reported 100% specificity and positive predictive value with an index defined as CA 19-9 + (CEA × 40). But sensitivity obtained was only 67%. Recently, by simultaneous measurement of transthyretin and CA 19-9 levels in a formula, Liu et al.[39] were able to differentiate cholangiocarcinoma from other benign biliary diseases with 98% sensitivity and 100% specificity. The important drawbacks of these studies are limited number of patients studied, and need for verification of their results in other study populations. Studies evaluating significance of levels CA 19-9 and CEA in the bile showed variable sensitivity and specificity. But, the new bile markers such as IGF-1, pancreatic elastase/amylase, MCM-5, and Mac-2BP have shown some promising results in single studies on small group of patients.

Carcinoma Esophagus

The only curative modality available at present is surgery with or without neoadjuvant chemo radiotherapy. But the patients undergoing potentially curative resection still have poor long-term prognosis. The prediction of tumor biology based on tumor markers in serum or tissue biopsy specimens may help the practicing surgeon to guide surgery and adjuvant therapy. At present, tumor markers for diagnostic purpose are of minimal clinical value compared to endoscopy and biopsy. Recently, Scarpa et al.[40] (reported that preoperative serum CA19-9 and CEA levels can be used for the prediction of resectability in esophageal carcinoma, particularly in esophageal adenocarcinoma. Regarding prognosis, Chen et al.[41] in his systematic review and meta-analysis found some potential tumor biomarkers predicting outcome in esophageal cancer patients such as vascular endothelial growth factor, cyclin D1, Ki-67, and squamous cell carcinoma antigen in esophageal squamous cell carcinoma; cyclooxygenase-2 and human epidermal growth factor receptor-2 in esophageal adenocarcinoma; and p21, p53, C-reactive protein, and hemoglobin level in esophageal carcinoma. But most of the studies analyzed had heterogeneity with respect to assessment of marker expression and cutoff point selection.

Carcinoma Stomach

Most commonly evaluated markers in carcinoma stomach are CEA, CA 19-9, and CA 72-4, which may be elevated at various stages in patients with gastric cancer. Other useful markers in gastric cancer are AFP, CA-125 and serum sialyl-Tn antigen. Although there are no prospective trials, several studies have shown clinical significance of the each of these markers. But low sensitivity and specificity prevent their use as diagnostic markers in early detection of gastric cancer. Also, National Comprehensive Cancer Network guidelines for gastric cancer do not recommend measurement of serum markers for preoperative evaluation and staging. Recently, in a systematic review of literature, the Task Force of the Japanese Gastric Cancer Association[42] reported that the combinations of CEA, CA 19-9, and CA 72-4 has improved positive rates for gastric cancer and CA 72-4 is the most useful marker for detecting advanced disease, besides being an independent prognostic factor. Also, the monitoring during posttreatment follow-up is important in patients with positive markers to detect early recurrence. Alfa-fetoprotein is helpful in detecting and predicting hepatic metastasis, while CA 125 and STN are useful for detecting peritoneal deposits.[41]

In addition, overexpression of HER2 is seen in 10–25% of cases with gastric or gastroesophageal junction (GOJ) carcinomas [4] As seen in breast cancer, these HER-2 positive tumor cells are highly sensitive to the anti-HER2 antibody. In a randomized, prospective, multicenter, phase III trial (Trastuzumab for Gastric Cancer study), Bang et al.[43] demonstrated benefit from trastuzumab in combination with chemotherapy in HER2 positive advanced gastric or GOJ cancers. So, NCCN and EGTM[40] 2014 guidelines recommend determination of HER2 status before initiation of anti-HER2 antibody therapy in patients with metastatic gastric or GOJ cancers.

REFERENCES

1. Biomedical, F.A.S.T. "NIH Definition of Biomarker." Clin Pharmacol Ther. 69(2001):89-95.
2. Ludwig JA, Weinstein JN. Biomarkers in cancer staging, prognosis and treatment selection. Nat Rev Cancer. 2006;5:845-56.
3. Locker GY, Hamilton S, Harris J, et al. ASCO 2006 update of recommendations for the use of tumor markers in gastrointestinal cancer. J Clin Oncol. 2006;24(33):5313-27.
4. Duffy MJ, Lamerz R, Haglund C, et al.. Tumor markers in colorectal cancer, gastric cancer and gastrointestinal stromal cancers: European group on tumor markers 2014 guidelines update. Int. J. Cancer. 2014;134:2513-22.
5. de Haas RJ, Wicherts DA, Flores E, et al. Tumor marker evolution: comparison with imaging for assessment of response to chemotherapy in patients with colorectal liver metastases. Ann Surg Oncol. 2010;17:1010-23.
6. Iwanicki-Caron I, Di Fiore F, Roque I, et al. Usefulness of the serum carcinoembryonic antigen kinetic for chemotherapy monitoring in patients with unresectable metastasis of colorectal cancer. J Clin Oncol. 2008;26:3681-6.
7. Winter JM, Yeo CJ, Brody JR. Diagnostic, Prognostic, and Predictive Biomarkers in Pancreatic Cancer. J Surg Oncol. 2013;107:15-22.
8. Marrelli D, Caruso S, Pedrazzani C, et al. CA 19-9 serum levels in obstructive jaundice: clinical value in benign and malignant conditions. Am J Surg. 2009;198:333-9.
9. Maithel SK, Maloney S, Winston C, et al. Preoperative CA 19-9 and the yield of staging laparoscopy in patients with radiographically

resectable pancreatic adenocarcinoma. Ann Surg Oncol. 2008;15:3512-20.

10. Montgomery RC, Hoffman JP, Riley LB, et al. Prediction of recurrence and survival by post-resection CA 19-9 values in patients with adenocarcinoma of the pancreas. Ann Surg Oncol. 1997;4:551-6.
11. Ziske C, Schlie C, Gorschluter M, et al. Prognostic value of CA 19-9 levels in patients with inoperable adenocarcinoma of the pancreas treated with gemcitabine. Br J Cancer. 2003;89:1413-17.
12. Hammad N, Heilbrun LK, Philip PA, et al. CA 19-9 as a predictor of tumor response and survival in patients with advanced pancreatic cancer treated with gemcitabine based chemotherapy. Asia Pac J Clin Oncol. 2010;6:98-105.
13. Yan-JieZhao, QiangJu Guan-Cheng Li. Tumor markers for hepatocellular carcinoma (Review). Mol Clin Oncol. 2013;1:593-8.
14. Masuda T, Beppu T, Horino K, et.al. Preoperative tumor marker doubling time is a useful predictor of recurrence and prognosis after hepatic resection of hepatocellular carcinoma. J Surg Oncol. 2010;102(5):490-6.
15. Toso C, Asthana S, Bigam DL, et al. Reassessing selection criteria prior to liver transplantation for hepatocellular carcinoma utilizing the Scientific Registry of Transplant Recipients database. Hepatology. 2009;49(3):832-8.
16. Han SJ, Yoo S, Choi SH, et al. Actual half-life of alphafetoprotein as a prognostic tool in pediatric malignant tumors. Pediatr Surg Int. 1997;12:599-602.
17. Aoyagi Y, Suzuki Y, Isemura M, et al. The fucosylation index of alpha-fetoprotein and its usefulness in the early diagnosis of hepatocellular carcinoma. Cancer. 1988;61:769-74.
18. Murata K, Sakamoto A. Impairment of clathrin-mediated endocytosis via cytoskeletal change by epithelial to fibroblastoid conversion in HepG2 cells: a possible mechanism of des gamma-carboxyprothrombin production in hepatocellular carcinoma. Int J Oncol. 2008;33:1149-55.
19. Grizzi F, Franceschini B, Hamrick C, et al. Usefulness of cancer-testis antigens as biomarkers for the diagnosis and treatment of hepatocellular carcinoma. J Transl Med. 2007;5:3.
20. Baek YH, Lee JH, Jang JS, et al. Diagnostic role and correlation with staging systems of PIVKA-II compared with AFP. Hepatogastroenterology. 2009;56:763-7.
21. Volk ML, Hernandez JC, Su GL, et al. Risk factors for hepatocellular carcinoma may impair the performance of biomarkers: a comparison of AFP, DCP, and AFPL3. Cancer Biomark. 2007;3:79-87.
22. Shirakawa H, Kumnuma T, Nishimura Y, et al. Glypican-3 is a useful diagnostic marker for a component of hepatocellular carcinoma in human liver cancer. Int J Oncol. 2009;34:649-56.
23. H. Shirakawa, H. Suzuki, M. Shimomura, et al. "Glypican-3expression is correlated with poor prognosis in hepatocellular carcinoma." Cancer Sci. 2009;100:1403-07.
24. Ning S, Bin C, Na H, et al. Glypican-3, a novel prognostic marker of hepatocellular cancer, is related with postoperative metastasis and recurrence in hepatocellular cancer patients. Mol Biol Rep. 2012;39:351-7.
25. O'Toole D, Grossman A, Gross D, et al. ENETS Consensus guidelines for the standards of care in neuroendocrine Tumors: biochemical markers. Neuroendocrinology. 2009;90:194-202.
26. Vinik AI, Silva MP, Woltering EA, et.al. Biochemical testing for neuroendocrine tumors. Pancreas. 2009;38:876-89.
27. Yao JC, Pavel M, Phan AT, et al. Chromogranin A and neuron-specific enolase as prognostic markers in patients with advanced pNET treated with everolimus. J Clin Endocrinol Metab. 2011;96(12):3741-49.
28. Kunz PL, Reidy-Lagunes D, Anthony LB, et al. North American Neuroendocrine Tumor Society. Consensus guidelines for the management and treatment of neuroendocrine tumors. Pancreas. 2013;42(4):557-77.
29. Metz DC, Jensen RT. Gastrointestinal neuroendocrine tumors: pancreatic endocrine tumors. Gastroenterology. 2008;135:1469-92.
30. Oberg K, Stridsberg M. Neuroendocrine tumors. in tumor markers. Physiology, pathobiology, technology, and clinical applications. 2002;339-49.
31. Srivastava K, Srivastava A, Mittal B. Potential biomarkers in gall bladder cancer: present status and future directions (Review article). Biomarkers. 2013;18(1):1-9.
32. Chaube A, Tewari M, Singh U, et al. CA 125: a potential tumor marker for gall bladder cancer. J Surg Oncol. 2006;93:665-9.
33. Rana S, Dutta U, Kochhar R, et al. Evaluation of CA 242 as a tumor marker in gall bladder cancer. J Gastrointest Cancer. 2012;43(2):267-71.
34. Wang YF, Feng FL, Zhao XH, et al. Combined detection tumor markers for diagnosis and prognosis of gall bladder cancer. World J Gastroenterol. 2014;20(14):4085-9.
35. Malaguarnera G, Giordano M, Paladina I, et al. Markers of bile duct tumors. World J Gastrointest Oncol. 2011;3(4):49-59.
36. Grunnet M., Mau-Sørensen M. Serum tumor markers in bile duct cancer—a review. Biomarkers. 2014;19(6):437-43.
37. Shang-Long L, Zi-Fang S, Qing-Gang H, et al. Serum carbohydrate antigen (CA) 19-9 as a prognostic factor in cholangiocarcinoma: a meta-analysis. Front Med China. 2010, 4(4):457-62.
38. Ramage JK, Donaghy A, Farrant JM, et al. Serum tumor markers for the diagnosis of cholangiocarcinoma in primary sclerosing cholangitis. Gastroenterology. 1995;108:865-9.
39. Liu L, Wang J, Liu B, et al. Serum levels of variants of transthyretin down-regulation in cholangiocarcinoma. J Cell Biochem. 2004;104:745-55.
40. Scarpa M, Noaro G, Saadeh L, et al. "Esophageal Cancer Management: Preoperative CA19. 9 and CEA Serum Levels May Identify Occult Advanced Adenocarcinoma." World journal of surgery 39.2 (2015): 424-432.
41. Meilan Chen, Jizheng Huang, Zhenli Zhu, et al. Systematic review and meta-analysis of tumor biomarkers in predicting prognosis in esophageal cancer. BMC Cancer. 2013;13:539.
42. Shimada H, Noie T, Ohashi M, et al. Clinical significance of serum tumor markers for gastric cancer: a systematic review of literature by the Task Force of the Japanese Gastric Cancer Association. Gastric Cancer. 2014;(1):26-33.
43. Bang YJ, Van Cutsem E, Feyereislova A, et al. ToGA Trial Investigators. Trastuzumab in combination with chemotherapy versus chemotherapy alone for treatment of HER2-positive advanced gastric or gastro-esophageal junction cancer (ToGA): a phase 3, open-label, randomized controlled trial. Lancet. 2010;376:687-97.

CHAPTER 121

Chylous Ascites

Vageesh BG, PK Mishra

The human body is a tube and tank machine with an electrical system that is made up of trillions of cells and two fluids, which are designed to create and react to chemistry. While this machine can malfunction, malfunctions can be fixed.

—*Kevin W. Reese*

INTRODUCTION

Accumulation of lipid-rich lymph in the peritoneal cavity due to disruption of the lymphatic system secondary to traumatic injury or obstruction is called chylous ascites (CA) or milky ascites. In children congenital abnormalities of lymphatic system and trauma are the most common causes. Abdominal malignancy, cirrhosis, and infections are common causes in adults. The presence of a milky, creamy appearing ascitic fluid with triglyceride content above 200 mg/dL is diagnostic, and, in the majority of cases, unless there is a strong suspicion of malignancy, further investigations are not required in patients with cirrhosis. If an underlying cause is identified, targeted therapy is possible, but most cases will be treated conservatively, with dietary support including high-protein and low-fat diets supplemented with medium-chain triglycerides, therapeutic paracentesis, total parenteral nutrition, and somatostatins. Rarely, resistant cases have been treated by transjugular intrahepatic portosystemic shunt, surgical exploration, or peritoneovenous shunt.

HISTORY

Lympha from Latin denotes water Goddess.[1] Although lymphatic system was described in the seventh century B.C. Hippocrates was one of the first to allude to the lymphatic system in fifth century B.C. The lymphatic system consists of a network of vessels containing tissue fluid or lymph and it is an integral part of the circulatory system. Olaus Rudbeck and Thomas Bartholin independently described the lymphatic system in the seventh century. Jean Pecquet in 1651 described the cisterna chyli in dogs. He traced the flow to return to the heart via thoracic duct which after reaching the neck emptied into the venous system.

ANATOMY AND PHYSIOLOGY OF LYMPH

Circulatory system filters about 20 L of plasma daily from the blood capillaries. Out of these 20 L, 17 L get reabsorbed into the circulation directly. Rest of the 3 L move via the interstitial spaces to the lymphatic channels which provides an alternate route of their return. Lymphatic channels are present in all body tissues and have one way valve to direct the excess unabsorbed fluid.[2] Lymphatic channels from abdomen and lower part of the body converge to empty into the cisterna chyli. Cisterna chyli lies between inferior vena cava (IVC) and aorta in the retroperitoneum at the level of first and second lumbar vertebra. Cisterna chyli which receives lymphatics from small intestines has lymph rich in lymphocytes triglycerides and fatty acids. Lymph from the cisterna chyli goes upward via the thoracic duct. Thoracic duct enters thoracic cavity through the aortic hiatus and travels along the right side of esophagus between the aorta and azygous till the fifth thoracic vertebra. At this point, it crosses behind the esophagus to lie to the left of the esophagus. It enters the superior mediastinum behind the aortic arch and then goes into the neck. It empties into the circulatory system at the junction of internal jugular and subclavian vein (Fig. 1).

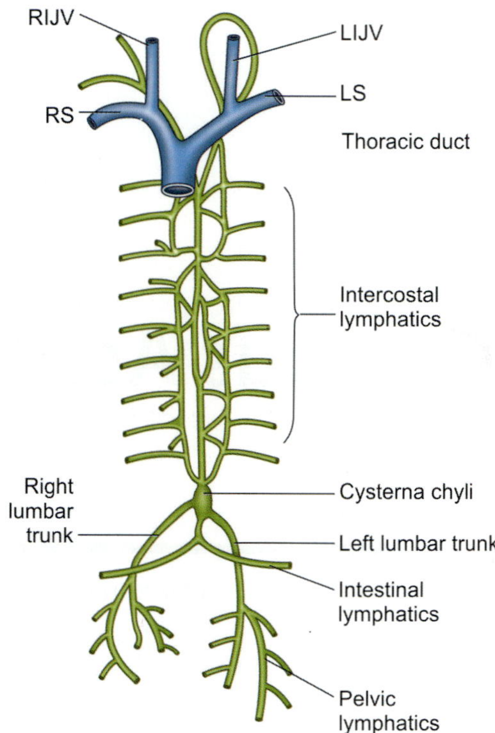

Figure 1 The lymphatic system

PATHOPHYSIOLOGY

Flow chart 1 Pathophysiology of Chylous Ascites

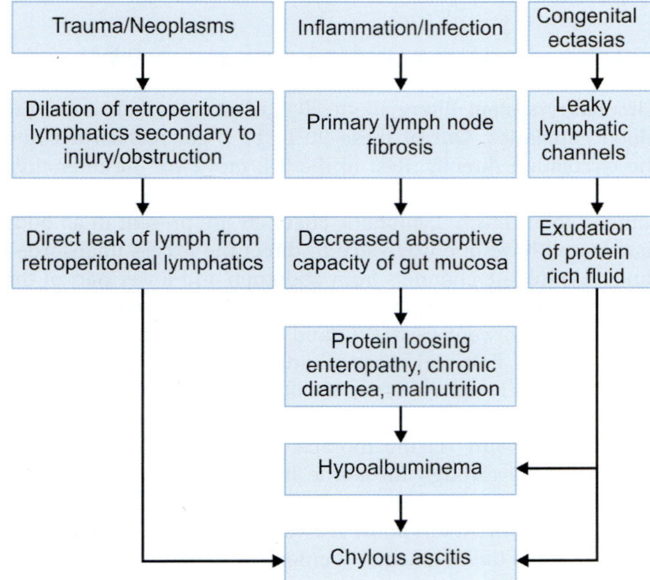

ETIOLOGY

Chylous ascites may be divided into traumatic and atraumatic causes (Table 1, Flow chart 1), in which the underlying etiology determines the long-term management. In India, *Mycobacterial, Filarial* infections form the majority of cases while malignancy and liver cirrhosis form >60% of cases in the Western countries.

Traumatic

Blunt or penetrating abdominal trauma may cause serious injury to main abdominal lymph vessels causing lymph leak and CA. Chylous ascites can occur weeks to months after surgical procedures depending on type of surgery and area of surgical dissection.[3] In most of the studies the incidence of postoperative CA is around 1%. Patients undergoing gastric, esophageal, retroperitoneal, or cytoreductive surgeries are found to have high incidence of CA. Whipples procedure, IVC resection, distal splenorenal shunts are the other surgeries which may lead to CA. Radiotherapy to abdomen or pelvis can cause lymphatic vessel fibrosis with in small intestine and mesentery leading to CA.[4]

Atraumatic

Most common cause of CA in children is congenital lymphatic abnormalities. Chylous ascites may be secondary to hyperplastic or hypoplasia of lymphatics. Primary lymphatic hyperplasia can present in two types. Bilateral hyperplasia is a type with undilated lymphatics having valves. In lymphangiectasia there is a gross dilation of lymphatics without any valves. Latter is the most common variety. Klippel–Trenaunay syndrome and yellow nail syndrome are types of hypoplastic lymphatic disorders causing CA.

Mycobacterial infections can cause CA. Multidrug-resistant tuberculosis (TB), atypical mycobacterial infections are of challenge in managing modern day TB. Filariasis is a helminthic infection commonly found in eastern belts of India. *Wuchereria bancrofti* is the parasite responsible organism, which can cause severe inflammatory changes in lymphatics leading to CA.

Neoplasms are the most common cause of CA in adults. Lymphomas account for >30% of cases. Tumors from esophagus, stomach, pancreas, kidney, and uterus can cause extrinsic compression or direct invasion of lymphatics leading to CA.

Liver cirrhosis causes rupture of serosal lymphatics leading to CA.[5] Nephrotic syndrome and right heart failure are some of the other important causes of CA.

CLINICAL FEATURES

Patient presenting with isolated ascitic features is rare in CA. Manifestation of an underlying etiology is common. Symptoms include heaviness of abdomen, dragging pain, fever, and vomiting.

Cancer cachexia is a classical picture in cases of neoplasms. Signs include progressive increase in abdominal girth, features of liver cell failure in cases of cirrhosis, and palpable lymph nodes.

COMPLICATIONS OF CHYLOUS ASCITIS

Loss of protein rich fluid in to peritoneal cavity leads to most of the complications. Malnutrition and serious electrolyte imbalances are the most common complications. Secondary infections can lead to fatal complications like septic shock and multiple organ dysfunction syndrome. Neurological complications like demyelination syndromes are known to occur in long standing CA. Mortality perse due to CA is rare but most commonly due to underlying cause.

Table 1: Causes of chylous ascites

Traumatic:
- Trauma
  - Blunt abdominal trauma
  - Battered baby syndrome
- Postoperative
  - Abdominal aneurysm repair
  - Retroperitoneal node dissection
  - Catheter placement for peritoneal dialysis
  - Inferior vena cava resection

Radiotherapy

Atraumatic:
- Congenital (more common in pediatric population)
  - Primary lymphatic hypoplasia
  - Klippel–Trenaunay syndrome
  - Yellow nail syndrome
  - Bilateral hyperplasia
  - Primary lymphatic hyperplasia
  - Intestinal lymphangiectasia

Infectious:
- Tuberculosis
  - Filariasis (*Wuchereria bancrofti*)
  - *Mycobacterium avium* intracellulare
- Inflammatory
  - Pancreatitis
  - Retroperitoneal fibrosis
  - Constrictive pericarditis
  - Coeliac sprue
  - Sarcoidosis
  - Whipple's disease
  - Retractile mesenteritis

Neoplastic (common in adult population):
- Lymphoma
  - Lymphangiomyomatosis
  - Carcinoid tumors
  - Kaposi's sarcoma

Other Causes:
- Cirrhosis
- Right heart failure
- Dilated cardiomyopathy
- Nephrotic syndrome

MANAGEMENT

Diagnosis

Laboratory Findings

On routine blood tests, lymphocytic leucocytosis may be one of the important findings. Ascitic fluid analysis establishes the diagnosis.[4] Classically the fluid is milky in appearance, lymphocytosis on cell count, increased total protein levels, serum ascites-albumin gradient <1.1 mg/dL, negative for bilirubin, amylase, and lactic dehydrogenase. Gram stain and culture are also negative. Ascitic fluid triglyceride is typically >200 mg/dL. Depending on underlying etiology adenosine deaminase may be positive in abdominal TB, cytology may be positive for malignant cells in selected cases. Table 2 shows the differential diagnosis and important laboratory features in these conditions.

IMAGING

Ultrasonography abdomen may show fluid collection and may help in approximate quantification. It is also useful in guided aspiration or drainage procedures. Liver condition and other solid organ malignancies can be ruled out. Contrast enhanced computed tomography abdomen (Fig. 2) is helpful in finding the primary cause, demonstrating intra-abdominal lymphadenopathy, and site of lymph leak. Appearance of fat-fluid level on recumbent position is a pathognomonic feature of CA.

Intraoperative localization can be done by using methylene blue dye test. In this, methylene blue is given through the Ryle's tube (RT) placed in to jejunum and retroperitoneal area is cautiously visualized for any extravasation of dye from lymphatic vessels (Fig. 3).

TREATMENT

Medical

Diet Therapy

Goal of nutrition therapy is to decrease production of chyle, replace fluid and electrolytes, and maintain or improve nutrition

Table 2: Characterization of different types of ascites

Feature	*Cirrhotic ascites*	*Tubercular ascites*	*Chylous ascites (Non-tubercular)*	*Malignant ascites*
Etiology	Cirrhosis	Mycobacteria	Multifactor	Neoplasms
Color	Transluscent	Straw Yellow	Milky	Bloody
Cell count	High (If SBP) (PMN Predominent)	High (Lympocyte Predominent)	High (Lympocyte Predominent)	High (RBC Predominent)
Cytology	Benign cells	Benign cells	Benign cells	Malignant cells
Glucose	Normal	Normal/Low	High	High
Protein	Low	High	High	Low
SAAG	>1.1 g/dL	<1.1 g/dL	<1.1 g/dL	<1.1 g/dL
Triglyceride	Normal	Normal	High	Normal
ADA	Negative	Positive	Negative	Negative

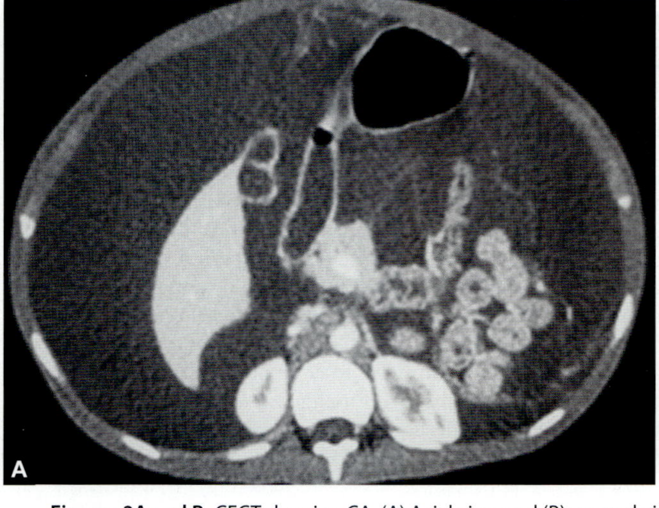

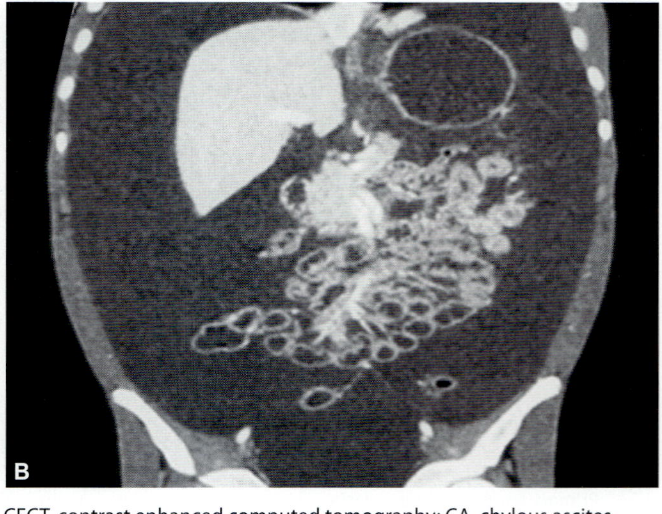

Figures 2A and B CECT showing CA. (A) Axial view and (B) coronal view. CECT, contrast enhanced computed tomography; CA, chylous ascites

status. This can be best achieved with high-protein, low-fat diet with medium chain triglycerides (MCT). These MCTs are directly absorbed into intestinal cells and transported as free fatty acids and glycerol directly to liver via portal vein.[7] In patients with advanced cirrhosis, MCT oil should not be used as narcosis and coma may occur. Such patients should be managed with a low-sodium diet and diuretics such as spironolactone. In resistant cases, total parenteral nutrition (TPN) is a good option as it bypasses the gut lumen. Total parenteral nutrition in combination with somatostatin or octreotide has shown better results in management.

Drugs

In cases of cirrhotic ascites, potassium sparing diuretics like spironolactone is used along with salt and fluid restriction. Orlistat, a reversible inhibitor of gastric and pancreatic lipases, was reported to minimize ascites and triglyceride levels in ascitic fluid in a patient with CA due to cirrhosis. Anti-tuberculosis treatment is used if TB is found to be the cause. Diethylcarbamazine can be used in filarial CA. Etilefrine is a sympathomimetic drug which was used to cause resolution of post-esophagectomy CA.

Abdominal Paracentesis

In most of the patients, treating the underlying cause will cure CA. This is especially true with infectious diseases. In refractory cases with dyspnea therapeutic tap will relieve symptoms. USG/CT-guided diagnostic tap is done to establish the diagnosis. Use of albumin in precentesis period is still under investigation. Large volume paracentesis are performed in end-stage disease with refractory ascites.

Tranjugular Intrahepatic Portosystemic Shunt

Tranjugular intrahepatic portosystemic shunt is an established modality of treatment in resistant CA. But in cases of cirrhotic patients it should be used with caution. Shunt blockage is a common complication.

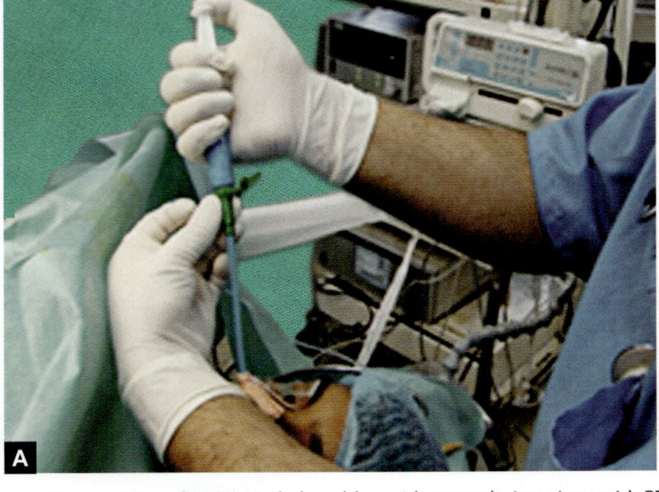

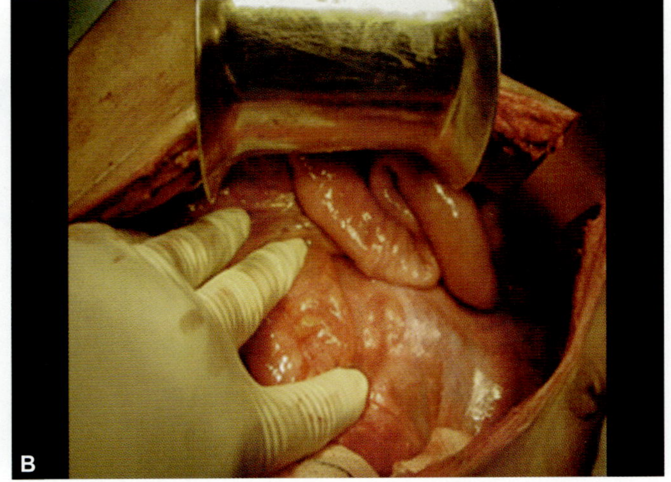

Figures 3A and B (A) Methylene blue with cream being given with RT placed in jejunum, (B) bluish-stained lymphatics in the retroperitoneum

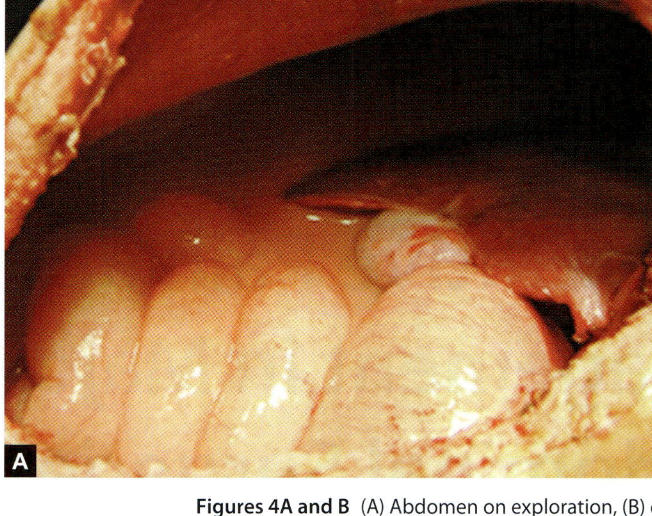

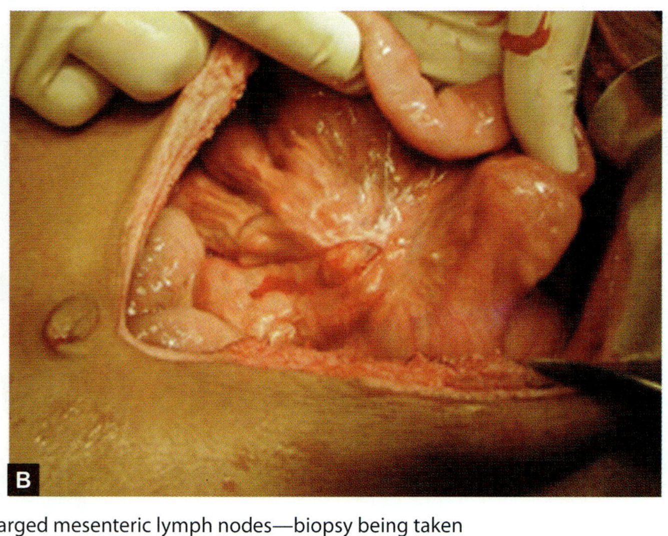

Figures 4A and B (A) Abdomen on exploration, (B) enlarged mesenteric lymph nodes—biopsy being taken

Peritoneovenous Shunting

LeVeen and Denver shunts are types of peritoneovenous shunts used in refractory ascites.[8] These are outdated modality at present due to serious complications associated with it like sepsis, disseminated intravascular coagulation, and air embolism. Viscous chyle causes frequent blockage of these shunts.

Angiography

It is a very useful modality in managing postoperative chyle leaks in terms of localization and embolization. Technical expertise and cost are the limiting factors.

Surgical (Figs 4A and B)

Indications
1. Chylous ascites refractory to medical management
2. Congenital lymphangiectasia
3. Neoplasms
4. Postoperative causes

In most of the cases, primary diagnosis is established preoperatively and hence there is less scope for diagnostic laparoscopy. On laparotomy milky fluid, peritoneal nodules, enlarged mesenteric, and retroperitoneal lymph nodes are classical findings.

Neoplasms of solid organs mainly carcinoma stomach, pancreas, and kidney may cause extrinsic compression on lymphatics. Studies have shown even in advanced disease tumor debulking may give symptomatic relief in CA. Congenital intestinal lymphangiectasia (Waldmanns disease) needs segmental small bowel resection.[9] In postoperative CA, localization of leak site is the key. For this fat challenge test with fresh cream through RT, or methylene blue dye test is conducted. If the site is localized, ligation is the treatment of choice. Fibrin glue application is tried in some cases.[10]

PROGNOSIS

Prognosis mainly depends on underlying cause. Best prognosis is seen in CA due to infectious etiology and some inflammatory pathology. Bad prognosis is seen with advanced malignancy, cirrhosis of liver, and congenital ectatic diseases. Morbidity associated with postoperative ascites is high. Mortality in CA is mainly due to underlying advanced malignancy or liver cirrhosis.

REFERENCES

1. Lymph - Definition and More from the Free Merriam-Webster Dictionary.
2. Uriz J, Cárdenas A, Arroyo V. Pathophysiology, diagnosis and treatment of ascites in cirrhosis. Baillières Best Pract Res Clin Gastroenterol. 2000;14(6):927-43.
3. Cárdenas A, Chopra S. Chylous ascites. Am J Gastroenterol. 2002;97(8):1896-900.
4. Aalami O, Allen DB, Organ CH. Chylous ascites: a collective review. Surgery. 2000;128:761-78.
5. Sultan S, Pauwels A, Poupon R, et al. Chylous ascites in cirrhosis. Retrospective study of 20 cases. Gastroenterol Clin Biol. 1990;14:842-7.
6. Runyon BA, Montano AA, Akriviadis EA, et al. The serum ascites albumin gradient is superior to the exudate-transudate concept in the differential diagnosis of ascites. Ann Intern Med. 1992;117:215-20.
7. Aoki H, Takakura N, Shiozaki S, et al. Milk-based test as a preventive method for chylous ascites following pancreatic resection. Dig Surg. 2010;27(5):427-32.
8. Rubinstein D, McInnes I, Dudley F. Morbidity and mortality after peritoneovenous shunt surgery for refractory ascites. Gut. 1985;26(10):1070-3.
9. Zeidan S, Delarue A, Rome A, et al. Fibrin glue application in the management of refractory chylous ascites in children. J Pediatr Gastroenterol Nutr. 2008;46(4):478-81.
10. Antao B, Croaker D, Squire R. Successful management of congenital chyloperitoneum with fibrin glue. J Pediatr Surg. 2003;38(11):E7-8.

CHAPTER 122

Acute Postoperative Pain and its Management in Major Abdominal Surgeries

Baljit Singh, Indira Malik

INTRODUCTION

Pain is an inevitable accompaniment of surgery anywhere in the body but its significance is more in the upper abdominal region. Tissue injury due to surgery results in release of histamine and inflammatory mediators like serotonin, bradykinin, prostaglandins, and nerve growth factor.[1] These mediators cause activation of peripheral nociceptors which further relays the information to the central nervous system (CNS) and initiate neurogenic inflammation. This is followed by release of neurotransmitters like substance P and calcitonin gene-related peptide which induces peripheral vasodilation and plasma extravasation. All these changes are responsible for the pain. Apart from the patient's suffering, its effect on the respiratory system can be severe. Pain leads to splinting of the diaphragm as the patient cannot breathe deeply. This promotes pooling up of the secretions in the basal regions of the lungs and collapse of the alveoli. In a patient who has some preexisting respiratory disorder, the likelihood of developing pneumonia is much higher if the pain is treated inadequately. The pain following major upper abdominal surgery, therefore, deserves special attention. Apart from the avoidable suffering, there are certain acute and chronic effects that can alter the postoperative course of the patient.

EFFECTS OF POSTOPERATIVE PAIN

Acute Effects

Uncontrolled perioperative pain may potentiate postoperative pain. Transmission of nociceptive stimuli from the periphery to the CNS results in a neuroendocrine stress response. The dominant response involves the hypothalamic-pituitary-adrenocortical and sympathoadrenal interactions. Suprasegmental reflex response to pain causes increased sympathetic tone which results in increased catecholamine release along with catabolic hormones while the secretion of anabolic hormones is decreased. Oxygen consumption and metabolism are increased and more substrates are mobilized from storage depots. Levels of blood glucose, ketone bodies, free fatty acids, and lactate are raised and sodium water retention occurs.[2]

The stress response may be an important element in the development of hypercoagulability,[3] immunosuppression,[4] and hyperglycemia[5] postoperatively. Sympathetic hyperactivity increases myocardial oxygen consumption and decrease coronary blood flow which may lead to myocardial ischemia and infarction. Over activity of the sympathetic system and increased inhibitory inputs from central and local factors may result in delayed return of gastrointestinal motility and aggravate paralytic ileus triggered by handling of the gut during surgery.

Postoperative respiratory function is markedly reduced, especially following major upper abdominal surgery and the spinal reflex inhibition of phrenic nerve activity is an important component of this phenomenon. Control of pain enables the patient to breathe deeply, cough out secretions, and mobilize early which reduces not only the incidence of developing postoperative pulmonary complications but the deep vein thrombosis also.

Chronic Effects

Postoperative pain which is poorly controlled, may predict the development of chronic persistent pain after surgery.[6] It is more common after breast and gall bladder surgery, sternotomy, thoracotomy, and limb amputation. Continued peripheral nociceptive input from the surgical site maintains central sensitization and causes chronic pain. Therefore, prevention of central sensitization and control of acute postoperative pain assumes more significance.

PRE-EMPTIVE ANALGESIA

Amplification of postoperative pain results from central sensitization and hyper excitability after the surgical incision. Preemptive analgesia is administration of analgesics before the surgical incision. It prevents the establishment of central sensitization due to the incisional injury occurring during surgery as well as inflammatory injury due to the release of neurotransmitters.[7] Thus, preemptive analgesia along with multimodal analgesic interventions may reduce acute postoperative pain and prevent chronic pain after surgery. Its use in the last decade has decreased as the results from various studies have been equivocal.

MULTIMODAL PERIOPERATIVE PAIN MANAGEMENT

The principle of multimodal strategy includes control of postoperative pain to allow early mobilization, early enteral nutrition, and education and attenuation of perioperative stress response through the use of regional anesthetic techniques and a combination of analgesic agents. It involves a combination of different techniques and different drugs to achieve the desired effect and keeping the side effects to the minimum. Epidural anesthesia and analgesia is an integral part of this strategy because it confers superior analgesic and physiological benefits.[2]

METHODS TO TREAT ACUTE POSTOPERATIVE PAIN

Regional Analgesic Techniques

Regional techniques are commonly used for effective postoperative pain management. They provide better analgesia compared to systemic opioids and also reduce the overall morbidity and mortality associated with surgery. However, these procedures are associated with certain risks and a careful assessment of the risk-benefit ratio for every patient should be performed. The neuraxial block may be single dose, intermittent boluses by the clock or continuous infusion of low-dose local anesthetic with or without narcotics.

Single-Dose Neuraxial Opioid

Administration of a single dose of opioid as the sole or an adjuvant analgesic agent, epidurally or intrathecally, is a useful mode of treating pain. Highly lipophilic opioids like fentanyl and sufentanil offer rapid onset of analgesia with rapid clearance from the cerebrospinal fluid (CSF). The development of adverse effects like the delayed respiratory depression is attributed to the delayed cephalic spread. Hydrophilic opioids like morphine have greater cephalic spread and remain in the CSF for a longer period thereby increasing the incidence of delayed respiratory depression. A single bolus of epidural fentanyl, 50–100 µg diluted in 10 mL normal saline provides rapid postoperative analgesia. A single-dose epidural opioid is very useful when the catheter location is incongruent with the surgical incision. More often, opioids are used in conjunction with low concentration local anesthetic drugs, bupivacaine or ropivacaine.

Intermittent Bolus Administration

In this mode, the drugs are delivered by the clock in the postoperative period every 2 hours or as per the protocol of the institution. In the author's institution, the local anesthetic drug, bupivacaine 0.125%, (1–1.5 mL per dermatome) is given every 2 hours and in combination with fentanyl 1 µg every 4 hours. This is a fairly useful method in centers where there is facility for close monitoring in the postoperative area.

Continuous Epidural Analgesia

Drugs can be administered as infusion through an indwelling epidural catheter. It is a safe and an effective method for management of acute pain. It is labor saving arrangement too, as it saves the nursing or the medical staff from administering frequent top ups. It is important to keep in mind that intraoperative use of general–epidural anesthetic technique using the epidural catheter results in less pain and early recovery after surgery compared with general anesthesia followed by systemic opioids.[2]

ANALGESIC DRUGS

Local Anesthetics

The precise site of action in the epidural space is unclear but the potential sites are the spinal nerve roots, dorsal root ganglion or the spinal cord. However, the use of local anesthetic as the sole analgesic agent is less common due to quick regression of sensory block leading to poor analgesia and high motor block resulting in hypotension.[8]

Opioids

These are beneficial in that they do not cause hypotension and motor block. Also, the duration of action is longer than the local anesthetics alone. Respiratory depression, early and late besides pruritus is the side effects that are of major concern.

Local Anesthetic-Opioid Combination

It has several advantages over using either opioids or local anesthetic agents alone. There is better postoperative analgesia, regression of sensory block is limited and also the dose of local anesthetic is reduced. However, the overall incidence of side effects may not be diminished.[2] Interaction between local anesthetics and opioids may be both synergistic and additive. Bupivacaine, ropivacaine, or levobupivacaine are preferred because these produce differential sensory blockade with minimal impairment of motor function. The concentration of local anesthetics used for analgesia is typically less than that used for regional anesthesia. Bupivacaine or levobupivacaine in a concentration ≤ 0.125% or ropivacaine ≤ 0.2% are sufficient. Lipophilic opioids like fentanyl, 2–5 µg/mL or sufentanil, 0.5–1 µg/mL combined with local anesthetics allow for rapid titration of analgesia.

Adjuvant Drugs

Clonidine and epinephrine are the most commonly used adjuvants. Clonidine mediates analgesia primarily through the descending noradrenergic pathway and its epidural dosing is 5–20 µg/h.[9]

However, it has undesirable side effects like hypotension, sedation, and bradycardia limiting its use. Epinephrine may improve epidural analgesia, increase sensory block, and is administered in a dose of 2–5 μg/mL. N-methyl D-aspartate antagonists like ketamine can theoretically diminish central sensitization and increase the analgesic effects of epidural opioids.

Dosing of Neuraxial Opioids[2] (Table 1)

Table 1: Dosing of neuraxial opioids

Drug	*Intrathecal single dose*	*Epidural single dose*	*Epidural continuous infusion*
Fentanyl	5–25 μg	50–100 μg	25–100 μg/h
Sufentanil	2–10 μg	10–50 μg	10–20 μg/h
Alfentanil		0.5–1 mg	0.2 mg/h
Morphine	0.1–0.3 mg	1–5 mg	0.1–1 mg/h
Diamorphine	1–2 mg	4–6 mg	
Hydromorphone		0.5–1 mg	0.1–0.2 mg/h
Meperidine	10–30 mg	20–60 mg	10–60 mg/h
Methadone		4–8 mg	0.3–0.5 mg/h

LOCATION OF CATHETER INSERTION

Optimal postoperative analgesia is a function of insertion of the epidural catheter congruent to the incisional dermatome. This ensures superior analgesia as well as minimal side effects. Lumbar epidural catheters more commonly result in lower extremity blocks and urinary retention along with earlier termination of epidural analgesia. Thoracic epidural blocks for abdominal surgeries do not cause sympathetic inhibition in the lower extremities and avoid urinary retention. Placement of epidural catheter in the thoracic region though technically difficult, appears to be as safe as those in the lumbar region.[2]

RECOMMENDED LOCATION OF CATHETER INSERTION FOR VARIOUS ABDOMINAL SURGICAL PROCEDURES[2] (TABLE 2)

Table 2: Recommended location of catheter insertion for various abdominal surgical procedures

Location of incision	*Surgical procedure*	*Congruent epidural catheter placement*
Upper abdominal	Cholecystectomy, esophagectomy, gastrectomy, hepatic resection, Whipple's procedure	T6–8
Mid abdominal	Cystoprostatectomy, nephrectomy	T7–10
Lower abdominal	Abdominal aortic aneurysm repair, colectomy, radical prostatectomy, total abdominal hysterectomy	T8–11

SIDE EFFECTS OF NEURAXIAL ANALGESIC DRUGS

1. Hypotension: Blockade of sympathetic fibers by local anesthetics may contribute to postoperative hypotension. It may be treated by decreasing the dose of local anesthetic administered.
2. Motor block: Approximately 2–3% patients may experience lower extremity motor block which may contribute to pressure sores on the back of heels. This usually resolves within 2 hours of discontinuing the infusion. A lower concentration of local anesthetic or an incision-congruent placement of epidural catheter may avoid motor block. However, if the weakness does not resolve after discontinuation of the infusion, the patient must be evaluated promptly and spinal hematoma, spinal abscess, or intrathecal migration of catheter should be ruled out.
3. Nausea and vomiting: Neuraxial administration of opioids in a single dose may cause nausea and vomiting in approximately 20–50% patients while those receiving infusions may have an incidence up to 45–80%. This phenomenon is related to the cephalic migration of opioids within the CSF to the area postrema in the medulla.[10] This explains the reason why nausea and vomiting is more common with infusions of morphine than with those of fentanyl. Droperidol, metoclopramide, dexamethasone, naloxone, and transdermal scopolamine have been successfully used to treat this complication.
4. Pruritus: It is seen in 60% patients of epidural or intrathecal administration of opioids. It does not have any serious consequences but can be very distressing for the patient. This may be related to central activation of an "itch center" in the medulla or opioid receptors in the trigeminal nucleus or nerve roots due to cephalad migration of opioids. Intravenous administration of naltrexone, nalbuphine, naltrexone, naloxone, and droperidol may be effective in controlling opioid-induced pruritus.
5. Respiratory depression: Respiratory depression with neuraxial opioids is dose dependent and incidence ranges from 0.1–0.9%. Lipophilic opioids cause less delayed respiratory depression than hydrophilic opioids. Risk factors associated with respiratory depression due to neuraxial opioids include, increasing age, higher dose, concomitant systemic opioids or sedative use, comorbid conditions, prolonged or extensive surgery, and thoracic surgeries. It can be successfully treated with naloxone in 0.1–0.4 mg increments.
6. Urinary retention: Urinary retention results from the interaction of neuraxial opioids with the opioid receptors in the spinal cord which decreases the strength of detrusor muscle contraction.[10] The incidence with neuraxial opioid administration may be as high as 70–80%. Epidural local anesthetics may also cause urinary retention with an incidence of 10–30%.

PATIENT-CONTROLLED EPIDURAL ANALGESIA

Patient-controlled epidural analgesia (PCEA) allows for individualization of postoperative analgesic requirements and has several advantages over continuous epidural infusions. Lipophilic opioids hasten the onset of analgesia and have a shorter duration of action besides having a lower incidence of respiratory depression. Thus these are preferred for use with PCEA. The commonly used regimens are listed in Table 3[2]:

Table 3: Commonly used regimens

General regimens	*Continuous rate (mL/h)*	*Demand dose (mL)*	*Lockout interval (min)*
0.05% bupivacaine + 4 µg/mL fentanyl	4	2	10
0.0625% bupivacaine + 5 µg/mL fentanyl	4–6	3–4	10–15
0.1% bupivacaine + 5 µg/mL fentanyl	6	2	10–15
0.2% ropivacaine + 5 µg/mL fentanyl	5	2	20
Abdominal surgery			
0.0625% bupivacaine + 5 µg/mL fentanyl	4–6	3–4	10–15
0.125% bupivacaine + 0.5 µg/mL sufentanil	3–5	2–3	12
0.1–0.2% ropivacaine + 2 µg/mL fentanyl	3–5	2–5	10–20

Benefits of Epidural Analgesia

Epidural analgesia can decrease the incidence of postoperative gastrointestinal, pulmonary and cardiac complications following major abdominal surgeries.

Gastrointestinal

- Early return of gastrointestinal motility
- Less incidence of anastomotic dehiscence

Pulmonary

- Decreased incidence of pulmonary infections and atelectasis

Cardiac

- Decreased in postoperative myocardial infarction by attenuation of sympathetically mediated coronary vasoconstriction and improved coronary blood flow to areas at risk for ischemia.
- Attenuation of stress response and hypercoagulability.

Use of epidural technique for analgesia is associated with an overall improvement in pain relief and other outcomes such as patient satisfaction and health-related quality of life.[11]

Risks of Epidural Analgesia

As mentioned earlier, the risk-benefit ratio must be weighed carefully for every individual patient. Complications are related to the placement of epidural catheters as well as indwelling catheters. The concurrent use of anticoagulants in patients receiving neuraxial anesthesia and analgesia has been highlighted due to the increased incidence of spinal hematomas, especially after the introduction of low molecular weight heparin (LMWH). The American Society of Regional Anesthesia and Pain Medicine (ASRA) has listed a series of consensus statements based on available literature for the insertion and removal of epidural catheters and administration of neuraxial blocks in the presence of various anticoagulants, like warfarin, antiplatelets, fibrinolytics-thrombolytics, standard unfractionated heparin, and LMWH.[12]

Infections associated with epidural analgesia may result from both exogenous and endogenous sources. Meningitis and spinal abscesses are rare but superficial inflammation and cellulitis (4–14%) is common with a high incidence of catheter colonization (20–35%).

Migration of epidural catheters into the intrathecal, intravascular, or subcutaneous spaces increases the failure rate and decreases analgesic efficacy. Use of an epinephrine containing local anesthetic test dose, administration of fractionated doses of local anesthetic and aspiration of the catheter before administration of the bolus dose are recommended to avoid the complications associated with intrathecal or intravascular placement.

SYSTEMIC ANALGESICS (TABLE 4)

Beyond the immediate postoperative period where epidural or parenteral analgesics have a major stake, systemic analgesics is the mainstay of postoperative pain management.[13] These analgesics may be opioids or non-opioids

a. Non-opioid analgesics: Aspirin, acetaminophen, nonsteroidal anti-inflammatory drugs, and selective cyclooxygenase-2 inhibitors are the principal drugs in this category, used for treating mild to moderate postoperative pain. Routes of administration are mostly oral or intramuscular but acetaminophen (paracetamol) is also available in intravenous preparations.

Table 4: Systemic analgesics

Drug	*Route of administration*	*Maximum recommended dose (mg)*
Aspirin	PO	3600
Ibuprofen	PO	3200
Ketorolac	IM/PO	120
Mefenamic acid	PO	1000
Diclofenac sodium	IM/PO	200
Acetaminophen	IV/IM/PO	1200

b. Opioid analgesics: Morphine and its related compounds exert their analgesic effects by acting on a group of receptors known as opioid receptors. The major sites of action of systemically administered opioids are periaqueductal and periventricular gray mater, nucleus reticularis gigantocellularis, medial thalamus, mesencephalic reticular formation, lateral hypothalamus, raphe nucleus, and spinal cord. However, systemic opioids are responsible for some unpleasant and undesirable side effects which include sedation, respiratory depression, euphoria, miosis, constipation, and dependence.

Tramadol, a synthetic cyclohexanol, is a centrally acting analgesic and has a weak affinity for the µ-opioid receptor. It is one tenth as potent as morphine, causes less respiratory depression, and has less abuse potential.

Another group of drugs is constituted by the opioid agonist-antagonists which include pentazocine, nalbuphine, and butorphanol.

PATIENT-CONTROLLED ANALGESIA (TABLE 5)

This technique combines the advantages of a continuous infusion with the flexibility of administering small bolus doses and patient-initiated doses as analgesic requirements may vary from patient to patient. Lockout interval is the minimum time that must elapse between two subsequent patient-activated doses. Morphine and fentanyl are the drugs used most commonly by this route.[13]

Table 5: Patient-controlled analgesia

Drug	*Bolus (mg)*	*Lockout interval (min)*	*Infusion (mg/h)*
Fentanyl	0.015–0.05	3–10	0.02–0.1
Morphine	0.5–3	5–20	0.1–1
Buprenorphine	0.03–0.2	10–20	1–8

LOCAL INFILTRATION

The instillation of local analgesic in the vicinity of the surgical incision is a simple method of providing postoperative analgesia. Before injection, needle aspiration must always be carried out to avoid intravascular injection. However, analgesia is short-lived and it corresponds to the duration of action of the local anesthetic. Bupivacaine and ropivacaine are the most commonly used local anesthetic drugs due to their longer duration of action.

NEUROLYTIC NERVE BLOCKS

Neurolytic nerve blocks are preferable in terminally ill cancer patients. The extent and duration of analgesia is limited by regrowth of axons and development of denervation dysesthesia. The principal disadvantage associated with these blocks is that it is not possible to precisely control the spread of the neurolytic agent. Alcohol and phenol are the most commonly used agents for prolonged interruption of neural function. Phenol injection is painless and takes about 15 minutes to exert its effect while alcohol injections though painful are prompt in creating neurolysis.[15,16]

Celiac Plexus Block

Celiac plexus block is the most effective neurolytic block for chronic pain associated with upper abdominal malignancy. Injection of 25 mL 50% alcohol is given on either side of the celiac plexus. This block should be performed with radiological assistance, endo-ultrasound, fluoroscopy, or CT guidance as the needle traverses very close to vital structures on its way to the plexus. The classical technique for percutaneous injection involves bilateral placement of the block needles anterior to the body of the L1 vertebra and anterolateral to the aorta at the level of celiac trunk. It is preferable to put in the needle on the left side first because if the needle enters the aorta inadvertently, it can be pushed further to go across the anterior wall (transaortic technique). The injection in this approach is given as one single bolus of 40–50 mL of 50% alcohol after aspiration and confirming that the needle tip is not in the aorta. Computer tomography-guided injections are more precise as the needle can be accurately placed in relation to the celiac trunk.[14] There is less risk of the injected solution spreading more posteriorly to the paravertebral nerve roots or the sympathetic chain thus minimizing the risk of paresis or orthostatic hypotension. Fluoroscopy can also be used to guide needle placement. In patients with chronic pancreatitis, or any chronic pain of pancreatic pain, an injection of 80 mg depomedrol mixed with low-dose local anesthetic (bupivacaine 0.125%) in a total volume of 40 mL can be given for a long-lasting relief. For those patients who cannot lie prone for the standard posterior approach, anterior approach under ultrasound guidance has shown good results. The patient should be admitted overnight for observation after the block as some have loose motions due to unopposed parasympathetic activity. Also, it is recommended that the patient should be given a fluid preload of 15–20 mL/kg lactated ringer before the injection to minimize the incidence of hypotension that occurs due to the sympathetic block leading to vasodilatation.

SUPERIOR HYPOGASTRIC PLEXUS BLOCK

Patients with pelvic pain associated with gynecological, rectal, or genitourinary malignancies may benefit from the interruption of pelvic innervations at the level of the superior hypogastric plexus. The block is performed by introducing needles medially and caudally through the space between the L5 spinous process and the upper border of the sacrum bilaterally under fluoroscopic control. The needles are positioned anterior to the sacral promontory and neurolytic or steroid solution is injected as required.[14]

IONTOPHORESIS

Although, patient controlled analgesia has demonstrated efficacy and patient satisfaction, the current techniques of IV infusions has certain limitations like programming errors and restricted patient mobility due to syringes, tubing and pumps. The patient controlled fentanyl hydrochloride iontophoretic transdermal system (fentanyl ITS) is designed to address these issues. It is a very novel technique where a small device, approximately of the size of a credit card, is attached to the skin anywhere on the body, usually the forearm and is activated by the patient himself. The drug is delivered with the noninvasive iontophoretic technology by application of an external electrical field, based on the principle that like charges repel each other.[14] Fentanyl is most suitable for this technique because it requires that the drug should be lipid soluble, have a low molecular mass, and ionizable. It allows patients to maintain an acceptable level of pain control following titration to comfort with a loading dose of opioid. Patient satisfaction is demonstrated by the low number of withdrawals due to inadequate analgesia and the high percentage of patients rating pain control with this technique as good or excellent. Further, the patient mobility is not restricted as there is no tubing or lines attached to the system that confine the patient to the bed. Early mobilization reduces venous stasis and minimizes the incidence of deep vein thrombosis.

RELATIONSHIP BETWEEN ACUTE PAIN AND CHRONIC PAIN

Development of a chronic pain syndrome may be an extension of inadequately treated acute pain postoperatively. Pain persisting for more than 30 days following surgery can be considered as chronic.

This involves altered mechanisms of nociceptive modulation, centralization and amplification of neural responses that account for differences in clinical presentation, and therapeutic modality.

SUMMARY

The traditional belief that pain has to be endured after surgery is now undergoing a sea change. The belief that it is one way of natural justice has probably contributed to its neglect over the years. With the World Health Organization declaring pain as the fifth vital sign, it is now beginning to get the recognition that it deserves. Untreated postoperative pain is associated with undesirable physiological changes that are detrimental to the recovery of the patient. Besides, it entails a very traumatic experience that the patients often do not forget all their life. Chronic persistent postsurgical pain is now increasingly being realized as due to inadequately treated acute pain. The patient suffering apart, persistent postsurgical pain can lead to long-term psychological effects that can affect the quality of life and robs the patient of his right to well- being. Effective pain management entails a comprehensive team work—surgeon to realize that pain is harmful to the patient, anesthesiologist to assess and prescribe analgesics, and the nursing staff to effectively implement the strategies to treat pain.

REFERENCES

1. Julius D, Basbaum AI. Molecular mechanisms of nociception. Nature. 2001;413:203.
2. Hurley RW, Wu CL. Acute postoperative pain. In: Miller RD, editor. Miller's anesthesia, 7th ed. vol. 2, Philadelphia, Pennsylvania: Churchill Livingstone; 2010. pp. 2757-81.
3. Rosenfield BA. Benefits of regional anesthesia on thromboembolic complications following surgery. Reg Anesth. 1996;21(suppl):9-12.
4. Desborough JP. The stress response to trauma and surgery. Br J Anaesth. 2000;85:109.
5. Pomposelli JJ, Baxter JK 3rd, Babineau TJ, et al. Early postoperative glucose control predicts nosocomial infection rate in diabetic patients. JPEN J Parenter Enteral Nutr. 1998;22:77.
6. Macrae WA. Chronic pain after surgery. Br J Anaesth. 2001;87:88.
7. Kissin I. Preemptive analgesia. Anesthesiology. 2000;93:1138.
8. Wheatley RG, Schug SA, Watson D. Safety and efficacy of postoperative epidural analgesia. Br J Anaesth. 2001;87:47.
9. Curatolo M, Schnider TW, Petersen-Felix S, et al. A direct search procedure to optimize combinations of epidural bupivacaine, fentanyl, and clonidine for postoperative analgesia. Anesthesiology. 2000;92:325.
10. Chaney MA. Side effects of intrathecal and epidural opioids. Can J Anesth. 1995;42:891.
11. Carli F, Mayo N, Klubien K, et al: Epidural analgesia enhances functional exercise capacity and health-related quality of life after colonic surgery: results of a randomized trial. Anesthesiology. 2002;97:540.
12. Horlocker TT, Wedel DJ, Rowlingson JC, et al. Regional anesthesia in the patient receiving antithrombotic or thrombolytic therapy. Reg Anesth Pain Med. 2010;35:64-101.
13. Lubenow TR, Ivankovich AD, Barkin RL. Management of acute postoperative pain. In: Barash PG, Cullen BF, Stoelting RK, editors. Clinical anesthesia. 5th ed. Philadelphia: Lippincott Williams & Wilkins; 2006. pp. 1405-41.
14. Abram SE. Chronic pain management. In: Barash PG, Cullen BF, Stoelting RK, editors. Clinical anesthesia. 5th ed. Philadelphia: Lippincott Williams & Wilkins; 2006. pp. 1441-72.
15. Singler RC. An improved technique for alcohol neurolysis of the celiac plexus. Anesthesiology. 1982;56:137.
16. Mattia C, Coluzzi F. Acute postoperative pain management: Focus on iontophoretic transdermal fentanyl. Ther Clin Risk Manag. 2007;3:19-27.

CHAPTER 123

Telemedicine: Principles and the Future

Shuzi Shimizu, Ho-Seong Han, Kuriko Kudo, Yoshiko Houkabe, Yasuaki Antoku, Naoki Nakashima

WHY TELEMEDICINE NOW?

Telemedicine has various meanings and can be classified into two major categories. The first is telemedicine between doctor and patient, and the second is between doctors. The former category can be further divided in two: remote consultation, where doctors see patients remotely through monitors, and telesurgery, where doctors operate remotely using consoles to manipulate a robot in a remote operating theater.[1,2] Telemedicine between doctors can also be divided into two categories: remote consultation with specialists, for example, in the fields of telepathology or teleradiology, and remote education, in which doctors discuss cases by teleconference or demonstrate live surgeries for remote audiences.[3-5] This chapter focuses on the very last category, remote medical education.

One can imagine the convenience of remote education in saving time and travel expenses, especially when communicating with colleagues abroad. In addition, remote education is highly efficient because it is easily repeatable and allows a large audience at once. Imagine a situation in which you want to visit a hospital to watch a skilled surgeon perform an advanced operation. Only a few doctors could spare the time and most would be able to visit only once, not many times. However, with telemedicine, you can watch the operation frequently with many of your colleagues and without any travel expenses.

When the Internet became available in the 1990s, many groups attempted to use it for remote education in surgery and other medical fields. Remote education was quite successful in the fields of telepathology, teleradiology, and teledermatology, because the contents were fixed images.[6] Even large image files could reach remote sites and start discussion within a few seconds. Surgery, however, requires entirely different conditions, because we need video rather than still images. We know that to some extent fixed images can help us understand the key points of surgery as described in textbooks or journals, but for full understanding we really need whole streaming to see live surgery or recorded videos.

Transmission of video has been a big technical challenge because as many as 30 frames must be transmitted continuously to have satisfactory video quality at remote sites. Technology in the early stages of the Internet age had serious problems with insufficient bandwidth. Hence, the main target of engineering research at that time was optimizing compression algorithms to preserve video quality for transmission in limited bandwidth. As a result, video quality was inevitably degraded and often sluggish, leaving surgeons unsatisfied with image quality and resulting in loss of interest in remote education. Satellite was another available technology, but its extremely high cost did not successfully attract surgeons, either.

In 2002, there was a dramatic change in these circumstances: Japan and Korea were connected by a huge internet. Bandwidth drastically increased from 8 Mbps to 2 Gbps, a growth of three orders of magnitude resulting in more than 200 times more bandwidth. The FIFA World Cup was hosted between Japan and Korea in 2002 as well, and various technological advancements occurred in both countries around that time. With the development of this huge bandwidth, concerns about limiting transmission volume disappeared, and original quality surgical steaming without compression could be sent to remote sites through sufficient network space. The quality of surgical streaming was well preserved, and today we believe that improvements in both quality and cost allow the practical use of telemedicine in surgery. Here we present new technologies needed, activities we have performed, and new trends to keep in mind.

WHAT YOU NEED TO START

Two basic components are required to begin remote surgical education with satisfactory quality and low cost. The first is a research education network (REN) and the second is a digital video transport system (DVTS).

Research education network is an internet, but is totally different from the normal commercial Internet that you use at home. It is usually government funded or nonprofit, and its use is limited to research and education purposes. Therefore, regular companies cannot connect to REN for their business, and access is privilege restricted to universities and research institutions. Available bandwidth is much larger with REN than with the commercial Internet. Other details for comparison are shown in Table 1. Domestic RENs are present in many advanced countries, and international RENs also exist to connect these domestic lines. The list of major RENs is summarized in Table 2. Science Information Network is a Japanese REN, for example, connecting approximately 700 institutions, which are listed on its homepage. Internet2 is a REN in the United States, with a membership of approximately 250 universities. The Asia-Pacific Advanced Network (APAN) in Asia, GEANT2 in Europe, and RedClara in Latin America are international RENs. The first step in starting remote surgical education is to see if your hospital is a member of a domestic REN so that you can take advantage of the advanced internet.

Digital video transport system is a tool developed in Japan in 1999 that converts digital video signals directly to Internet protocols.[7] It is authorized by the International Communications Union and is freely downloadable from the Internet (http://www.sfc.wide.ad.jp/DVTS/). This software must be installed on a personal computer and connected to a video camera or surgical equipment via IEEE 1394 interface. In contrast to conventional systems that require an initial investment in costly videoconferencing equipment, DVTS allows you to try the system

Table 1: Basics of research and education network compared with commercial network

	Research and education network	*Commercial network*
Funding	Governments	Telecommunications Companies
Profits	Nonprofit	Profit-oriented
Benefits for	Public	Private
Cost paid by	Universities/institutions	Companies or individuals
Bandwidth	~500 Gbps	~1 Gbps
Network	Dedicated	Best effort in many cases
Stability	Stable	Not stable
Support	24 × 7	Depends on contract
Transmission style	Large-scale data	Millions of small data

Table 2: Major research and education networks

Country and region	*Name*	*Website*
Asia		
Australia	AARNet	www.aarnet.edu.au
China	CERNET	www.cernet.edu.cn
Hong Kong	HARNET	www.jucc.edu.hk/harnet/
India	NKN	www.nkn.in
Indonesia	INHERENT	www.itb.ac.id
Japan	SINET	www.sinet.ad.jp
Kazakhstan	KazRena	www.kazrena.kz
Kyrgyzstan	KRENA	www.krena.kg
South Korea	KOREN	www.korennetwork.com
Malaysia	MYREN	www.myren.net.my
Nepal	NREN	www.nren.net.np
New Zealand	REANNZ	www.reannz.co.nz
Pakistan	PERN	www.pern.edu.pk
Philippines	PREGINET	www.pregi.net
Sri Lanka	LEARN	www.learn.ac.lk
Taiwan	NCHC	www.nchc.org.tw/en
Thailand	ThaiREN	www.thairen.net.th
United Arab Emirates	ANKABUT	www.ankabut.ae
Vietnam	VinaREN	www.vinaren.vn
North America		
United States	Internet2	www.internet2.edu
Canada	Canarie	www.canarie.ca
Latin America		
Argentina	INNOVA RED	www.innova-red.net
Brazil	RNP	www.rnp.br
Colombia	RENATA	www.renata.edu.co
Costa Rica	RedCONARE	www.conare.ac.cr
Chile	REUNA	www.reuna.cl
Mexico	CUDI	www.cudi.edu.mx
Peru	RAAP	www.raap.org.pe
Uruguay	RAU2	www.rau.edu.uy/redavanzada
Europe		
Belgium	BELNET	www.belnet.be
Czech Republic	CESNET	www.cesnet.cz
France	RENATER	www.renater.fr
Italy	GARR	www.garr.it
Lithuania	LITNET	www.litnet.lt
Netherlands	SURFnet	www.surfnet.nl
Norway	UNINETT	www.uninett.no

Contd...

Contd...

Country and region	*Name*	*Website*
Spain	RedIRIS	www.rediris.es and www.red.es
Sweden	SUNET	www.sunet.se
Turkey	ULAKBIM	www.ulakbim.gov.tr
UK	JANET	www.ja.net
Africa		
Egypt	EUN	www.eun.eg
Morocco	MARWAN	www.marwan.ma
South Africa	TENET	www.tenet.ac.za
International		
Africa	UbuntuNet	www.ubuntunet.net
Asia Pacific	APAN	www.apan.net
Asia Pacific	TEIN	www.teincc.org/teincc
Central Asia	CAREN	caren.dante.net
Europe	GÉANT	www.geant.net
Global	GRORIAD	www.gloriad.org/gloriaddrupal
Latin America	RedCLARA	www.redclara.net
Mediterranean	EUMEDCONNECT	www.eumedconnect3.net

with common, easily located equipment. You can set up the system without much difficulty, and if you are not satisfied, little has been lost. However, it is important to note that DVTS does not work well on commercial networks and so DVTS and REN must be paired to work efficiently.

WHAT YOU CAN DO

Telemedicine activity began between Japan and Korea. The first international transmission of recorded surgical videos with DVTS occurred in February 2003, and the first live surgery, laparoscopic gastrectomy for early gastric cancer, was transmitted in August 2003. Regular teleconferencing between Seoul National University Bundang Hospital in Korea and Kyushu University Hospital in Japan began in 2005 for pre- and postoperative cases. These teleconferences were highly educational, especially for young staff, not only as a means of gaining academic knowledge but also for easy exposure to an international atmosphere in English, which is the second language for both countries.[8] The same system was used at a large, formal Congress of Urology in 2006, where the surgical image quality was very highly rated by participants.[9]

As many surgeons found this combined system very useful, telemedicine rapidly expanded in the Asia-Pacific region.[10] China, Taiwan, Australia, and the United States joined in 2004, and many others followed.[11-13] As of November 2013, we have connected 44 countries and regions, and have organized 405 programs with 272 institutions. In Japan, we performed many advanced endoscopy surgeries and transmitted them abroad, but at the same time, we learned a lot from others. One good example is bariatric surgery. Because bariatric surgery was rare in Japan, we asked Flinder's University Hospital in Australia to transmit live video of this surgery to our country. Expansion beyond Asia has not been difficult, either. Laparoscopic surgery was transmitted to Norway in 2009 and to South Africa in 2011, with very satisfactory results.[14,15] Because REN is rapidly expanding in Latin America, we have been working to establish good links to Mexico, Colombia, Chile, Brazil, and other countries.[16] In India, we connected via NKN (previously called ERNET) first to Tata Memorial Hospital in 2007, followed by the Asian Institute of Gastroenterology and the Institute of Liver Biliary Sciences in 2011, GB Pant Hospital in 2012, and more institutions await connection. We shared a total of 37 programs with these Indian hospitals.

In addition to surgery, we have organized many programs in gastrointestinal endoscopy, where moving images are prerequisite to learning new procedures and skills such as endoscopic submucosal dissection, endoscopic ultrasonography (EUS), EUS-guided punctures, per-oral endoscopic myotomy, and stenting for stenosis or pancreato-biliary stone extraction.[17,18] Other programs have included robotic surgery, transplantation, cardiology, prenatal ultrasonography, and programs for medical students and nurses as well (Figs 1 and 2). Statistics show that three-quarters of our activities have been teleconferences where slides and recorded

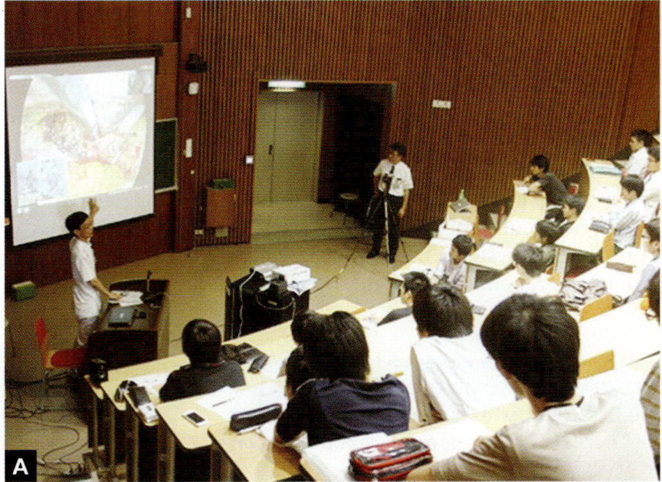

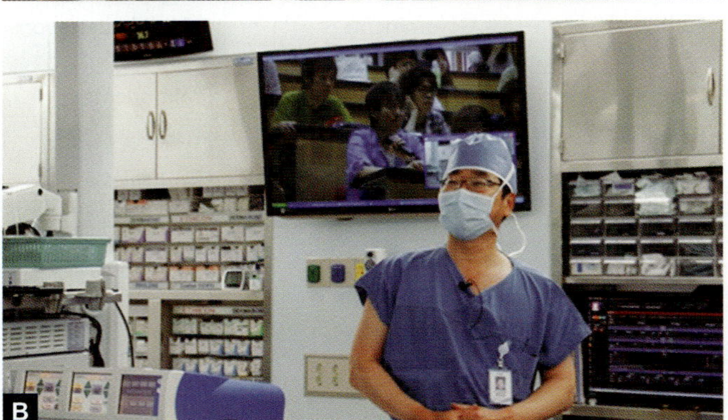

Figure 1 Live surgery transmitted from Korea to Japan using digital video transport system. (A) Medical students in Japan, watching live surgery transmitted from Korea. (B) Operating theater in Korea, with a doctor talking to a Japanese class

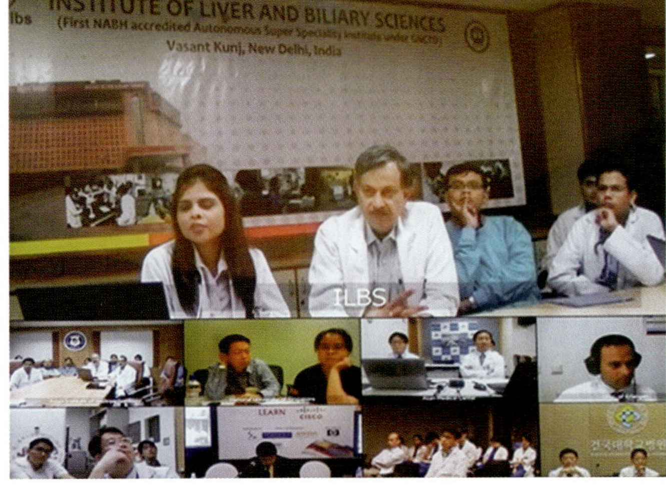

Figure 2 Endoscopic case conference in Asia and beyond. Two Indian hospitals join with those from Korea, Taiwan, Hong Kong, Malaysia, Singapore, Sri Lanka, and Germany. Endoscopic videos and slides were shown during the conference using Vidyo

videos are used with active discussion and one-quarter have been live demonstrations with patients. For multiple DVTS connections, we have used the QualImage/Quatre system (Information Services International-Dentsu, Ltd., Tokyo, Japan), which came into use in 2005.[14] The ratio of multiple connections has increased year by year to over 70% in 2012 for multisite discussion. As far as security issues are concerned, no patient data are included in transmissions and patient privacy is strictly preserved.

NEW TRENDS AND THE FUTURE

Combining DVTS and REN was a novel invention that allowed the progress of telemedicine in the early 2000s and it has been very useful in improving image quality and cost. However, it is not surprising that changing needs have led to further demands from medical staff as new medical devices have been introduced and technology has developed.

The first challenge is that many hospitals without REN have become interested in telemedicine and want to join with narrower bandwidth on the regular commercial network. The second is the need for high-definition (HD) images. Standard-definition video quality was satisfactory until HD images became available several years ago and have prevailed in the medical community. The third is the possibility of using mobile devices, which have become so common and handy in daily life. All of these requests were quite understandable, and they have been fulfilled accordingly.

Thanks to the emergence of new technologies and improvements in commercial networks, we can now provide good solutions to all three challenges. Because so many new systems exist in various countries, our team has selected three technologies as standard tools for remote medical education.[19] The selection criteria are as follows: (1) global availability and support, (2) satisfactory image quality for medical videos, and (3) cost as inexpensive as possible. In addition to DVTS, we now use the HD type of H.323, and Vidyo® (Hackensack, NJ, USA). Some representative companies for H.323 include Polycom (San Jose, CA, USA), Cisco (San Jose, CA, USA), Lifesize (Austin, TX, USA), and Sony (Tokyo, Japan). The key differences among these three technologies are summarized in Table 3. Limitations persist in all three systems and a perfect system is not yet available. We need to choose systems depending on availability at each participating site and the contents to be used in the program.

Table 3: Comparison of teleconference systems in use

	DVTS	*HD-H.323*	*Vidyo*
Resolution	Standard definition	High definition	High definition
Compression	Minimal	Yes	Yes
Bandwidth	30 Mbps	~12 Mbps	~6 Mbps
Global IP	Necessary	Necessary	Not necessary for client
Equipment	Software	Hardware	Hardware and software
Price	Free	US$6,000–US$30,000	US$25,000–US$60,000
Mobile compatibility	No	Yes	Easy
Multiple connection	Usually 4, up to 16	20 or more	20 or more
Multicontrol unit	Quatre	MCU for H.323	Vidyo Portal
Setup	Time-consuming	Easy	Easy
Availability	Download from homepage	Various vendors	Vidyo Co.
Limitations	Big network	Expensive equipment, MCU quality	Poor sending image, expensive server

Abbreviations: DVTS, digital video transport system; IP, Internet protocol; MCU, multipoint control unit.

From our experience of more than 10 years, we can point out some current problems with telemedicine. The first and fundamental issue is the relationship between doctors and engineers. With very limited exceptions, doctors alone cannot establish and run the systems because they lack familiarity with the technology and have busy routine clinics. Therefore, doctors require a good engineering team to help them. The reality we have found, however, is that there is little communication between doctors and engineers, even within the same hospital, and it can be very challenging to find or newly hire enough engineers to support this activity. However, once doctors and engineers collaborate, the result is a win–win situation to promote these attractive programs. The second challenge is the diversity of technological availability at different hospitals in various countries. Some are well equipped with sufficient network and audiovisual equipment, but others lack these tools, especially in Asia, where many countries are still developing. Differences in cultures, customs, and ideas can cause misunderstandings and minor frictions as well. Time differences are another big problem that cannot be easily overcome, especially when connecting across continents.

We have better future prospects than when we started this project, because the technological situation is much better now than previously. We are sure to encounter fewer technical problems ahead than we have experienced in the past. However, to efficiently facilitate telemedicine activities, domestic and international organizations are needed through which doctors and engineers can share their attractive programs and technological troubleshooting. With the final goal of globally standardized medicine for patients, the fusion of medical needs and technological support is essential.

ACKNOWLEDGMENTS

The authors are appreciative of the kind cooperation and great expertise of the entire medical and engineering staff in program organization and network preparations at all involved hospitals and institutions. We give special thanks to the APAN- and TEIN-NOC teams for intensive network preparations. This project was funded in part by Grant-in-Aid No. 23256005 for Scientific Research from the Japan Society for the Promotion of Science.

REFERENCES

1. Edirippulige S, Martin-Khan M, Beattie E, et al. A systematic review of telemedicine services for residents in long term care facilities. J Telemed Telecare. 2013;19(3):127-32.
2. Marescaux J, Leroy J, Gagner M, et al. Transatlantic robot-assisted telesurgery. Nature. 2001;413(6854):379-80.
3. Weinstein RS, Graham AR, Lian F, et al. Reconciliation of diverse telepathology system designs. Historic issues and implications for emerging markets and new applications. APMIS: Acta Pathol Microbiol Immunol Scand. 2012;120(4):256-75.
4. Bradley WG Jr. Teleradiology. Neuroimaging Clin N Am. 2012;22(3):511-7.
5. Li X, Liu J, Huang J, et al. An analysis of the current educational status and future training needs of China's rural doctors in 2011. Postgrad Med J. 2013;89(1050):202-8.
6. Senel E. History of teledermatology: a technique of the future in dermatology. Skinmed. 2010;8(3):167-70.
7. Ogawa A, Kobayashi K, Sugiura K, et al. Design and implementation of DV stream over Internet. Proceedings of the Internet Workshop IWS 99. 1999:255-60.
8. Shimizu S, Nakashima N, Okamura K, et al. International transmission of uncompressed endoscopic surgery images via super-fast broadband Internet connections. Surg Endosc. 2006;20:167-70.
9. Eto M, Lee TY, Gill IS, et al. Broadcast of live endoscopic surgery from Korea to Japan using the digital video transport system. J Endourol. 2007;21(12):1517-20.
10. Shimizu S, Han HS, Okamura K, et al. Technologic developments in telemedicine: state-of-the-art academic interactions. Surgery. 2010;147(5):597-601.
11. Huang KJ, Qiu ZJ, Fu CY, et al. Uncompressed video image transmission of laparoscopic or endoscopic surgery for telemedicine. Telemed J E Health. 2008;14(5):479-85.
12. Huang KJ, Cen G, Qiu ZJ, et al. Application of International Videoconferences for Continuing Medical Education Programs Related to Laparoscopic Surgery. Telemed J E Health. 2014; 20(2):157-60.
13. Colin K, Shimizu S, Okamura K, et al. High definition digital video links for surgical training. J Telemed Telecare. 2006;12 Suppl 3:S26-8.
14. Shimizu S, Okamura K, Nakashima N, et al. High-quality telemedicine using digital video transport system over global research and education network. In: Graschew G, Roelofs TA, editors. Advances in telemedicine: technologies, enabling factors and scenarios. Rijeka, Croatia: Intech; 2011. pp. 87-110.
15. Shimizu S, Thomson S, Doyle G, et al. Live surgery broadcast from Japan to South Africa: high-quality image transmission over a high-speed academic network. J Int Soc Telemed eHealth. 2013;1(3):80-5.
16. Shimizu S, Kudo K, Antoku Y, et al. Telemedicine in the Asia-Pacific region transmitted over a research and education network. In: Mathias I, Monteiro A, editors. Gold book [digital book]: technological innovation in education and health. Rio de Janeiro: EdUERJ; 2012. pp. 552-72.
17. Kaltenbach T, Muto M, Soetikno R, et al. Teleteaching endoscopy: the feasibility of real-time, uncompressed video transmission by using advanced-network technologies. Gastrointest Endosc. 2009;70(5):1013-7.
18. Shimizu S, Itaba S, Yada S, et al. Significance of telemedicine for video image transmission of endoscopic retrograde cholangiopancreatography and endoscopic ultrasonography procedures. J Hepatobiliary Pancreat Sci. 2011;18(3):366-74.
19. Cao MD, Shimizu S, Antoku Y, et al. Emerging technologies for telemedicine. Korean J Radiol. 2012;13 Suppl 1:S21-30.

CHAPTER 124

Surgery for Portal Hypertension

Joseph George, Rajesh Panwar, Sundeep Singh Saluja, Peush Sahni

INTRODUCTION

In 1945, on the basis of an idea that Eck proposed 68 years before, Whipple reported the first series of patients with portal hypertension who had been treated successfully for variceal bleeding by means of a portacaval shunt.[1] Since then, the role of surgery in the management of portal hypertension has seen a lot of changes. For over 25 years, surgical intervention was the only way of treating this problem till Grace et al[2] and Resnick et al[3] assessed the long-term results of patients with a portacaval shunt. They showed no difference in the survival rates between patients who had undergone surgery and those who had not. Those who had undergone portacaval shunts were dying from liver failure.

New surgical techniques such as selective or partial portosystemic shunts and devascularization procedures that could preserve the portal blood flow to the liver and at the same time decrease variceal bleeding rates were done more frequently during the 1970s.[4,5] The advent of endoscopic sclerotherapy (EST) and systemic vasopressors in the 1980s, the establishment of orthotopic liver transplantation as a curative procedure, and the development of transjugular intrahepatic portosystemic shunt (TIPS) changed the management of portal hypertension. It relegated to the background portosystemic shunts in the management of patients with portal hypertension due to cirrhosis.

HEMODYNAMICS WITH RESPECT TO SURGERY

The portal vein carries about 1500 mL/minute of blood from the intestine and spleen to the liver. Obstruction of the portal venous flow results in a rise in portal venous pressure. This obstruction can occur at three levels in relation to the liver, that is, prehepatic, intrahepatic, or posthepatic. However, the classification of obstruction is understood better in relation to the hepatic sinusoids (Fig. 1).

1. Presinusoidal obstruction: This could be either prehepatic as in extrahepatic portal venous obstruction (EHPVO) or intrahepatic as in noncirrhotic portal fibrosis (NCPF) or schistosomiasis.
2. Postsinusoidal obstruction: This could be either intrahepatic as in veno-occlusive disease or posthepatic as in right-sided heart failure, hepatic venous outflow tract obstruction or inferior vena caval obstruction.
3. Sinusoidal obstruction: This occurs in cirrhosis.

A pressure difference between the systemic and portal circulations can cause the formation of portosystemic collaterals by the opening and dilatation of pre-existing vascular channels connecting the portal venous system and the superior and inferior vena cava. These vessels are commonly located at the gastroesophageal junction below the mucosa and present as gastric and esophageal varices.

The hepatic venous pressure gradient (HVPG) is a surrogate marker of portal pressure and is the difference between the wedged and free hepatic venous pressures. Hepatic venous pressure gradient >5 mmHg is defined as portal hypertension, regardless of clinical evidence. Varices form when the HVPG is >10 mmHg and HVPG >12 mmHg is considered the threshold pressure for variceal rupture.[6]

PORTOSYSTEMIC SHUNTS

As the name suggests, these shunts create a connection between the portal and systemic circulations. The vascular channels on the portal side include mainly the portal vein, the splenic vein, and the superior mesenteric vein, while those on the systemic side include the inferior vena cava and the left renal vein. These shunts decompress the high-pressure portal system into the low-pressure

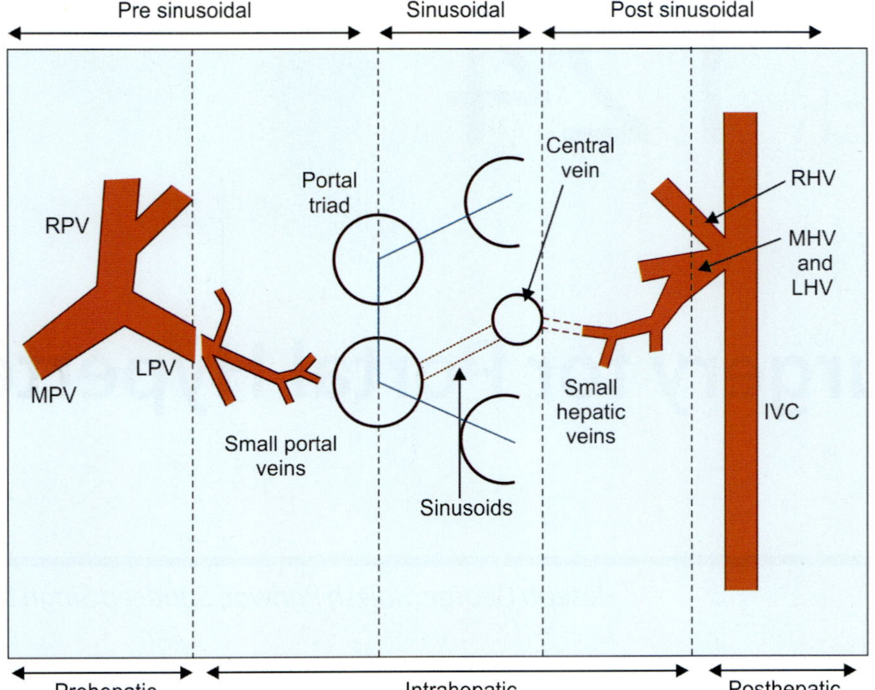

Figure 1 Schematic representation of various sites of obstruction to portal blood flow in portal hypertension
Abbreviations: RPV, right portal vein; MPV, main portal vein; LPV, left portal vein; RHV, right hepatic vein; MHV, middle hepatic vein; LHV, left hepatic vein; IVC, inferior vena cava

systemic circulation, thereby decreasing the portal pressure. Owing to their large size, these shunts decrease the blood flow through the smaller natural portosystemic connections such as esophageal varices. This decrease in portal pressure and diversion of blood flow away from the varices decreases the risk of variceal bleeding. However, in patients with cirrhosis, there is increased resistance to blood flow in the liver itself, so portosystemic shunts divert the blood away from the liver resulting in an increased risk of hepatic encephalopathy. These shunts may be classified as nonselective, selective, or partial depending on how much portal blood flow to the liver is preserved.

Nonselective shunts divert the large portal flow completely (Fig. 2) into systemic circulation. These are as follows:

1. Portacaval
   a. End-to-side
   b. Side-to-side
   c. Interposition graft [autologous: internal jugular; synthetic: dacron, polytetrafluoroethylene (PTFE)]
2. Proximal lienorenal
3. Side-to-side lienorenal[7]
4. Mesocaval

A transjugular intrahepatic portosystemic shunt (Fig. 3) behaves like a nonselective side-to-side portacaval shunt.

Selective shunts attempt to decompress only the varices-bearing compartment of the portal venous system while preserving some portal flow to the liver. The typical example is Warren's distal lienorenal shunt[4] (Fig. 4) that allows selective decompression of the stomach and gastroesophageal junction through gastric venous collaterals into the spleen through carefully preserved short gastric veins into the splenic vein. The blood drains into the lower pressure left renal circulation through the end-to-side distal lienorenal shunt. Blood from the inferior and superior mesenteric veins continues to perfuse the liver through the intact portal vein. Failure to ligate the coronary vein leads to rapid collateralization between the gastric and mesenteric venous systems. Collaterals may also form through the pancreatic venous drainage (pancreatic siphon) that can be prevented by dissecting the full length of the splenic vein from the pancreas (splenopancreatic disconnection). Inokuchi's coronary caval shunt is another example of a selective shunt.[8,9]

Partial shunts incompletely decompress the portal system because they have a small diameter (<1 cm) and thus maintain some blood flow to the liver. Sarfeh's small diameter (8 mm) interposition graft portacaval shunt[10] is an example of a partial shunt. Most small diameter partial shunts either thrombose or dilate and become nonselective over time. A small diameter PTFE shunt, when combined with coronary vein ligation and division of collaterals, provides a fixed resistance and is more likely to maintain hepatopetal portal flow. Compared with larger, nonselective portacaval interposition shunts, the smaller (8 mm) PTFE shunt is followed by improved survival and less encephalopathy in some studies.

The general principles that guide the selection of a shunt procedure are as follows:

1. The incidence of encephalopathy depends not only on the type of shunt but also on the functional status of the liver. Thus, patients with preserved liver function (e.g., EHPVO) do not develop hepatic encephalopathy even with nonselective

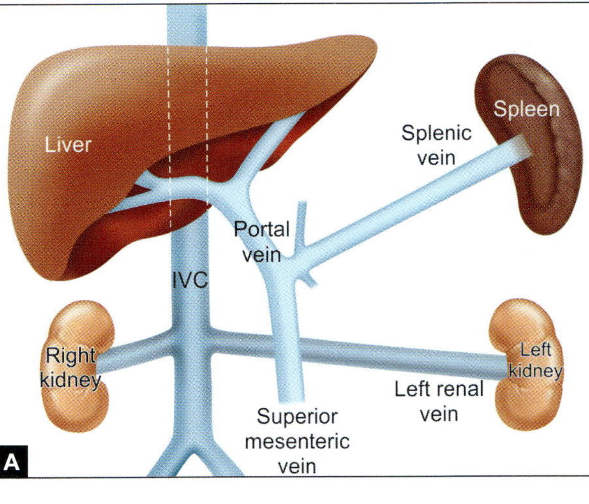

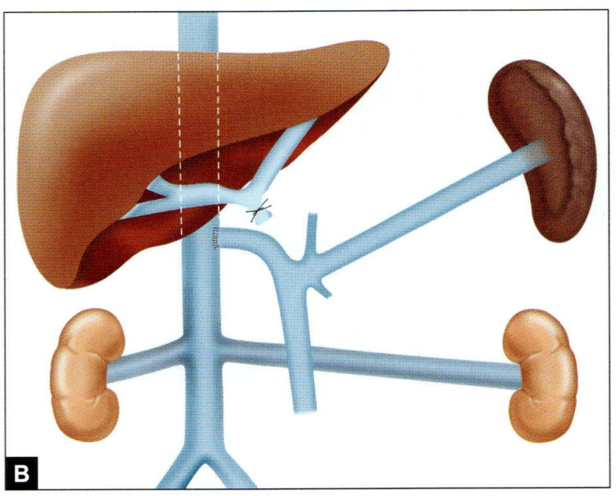

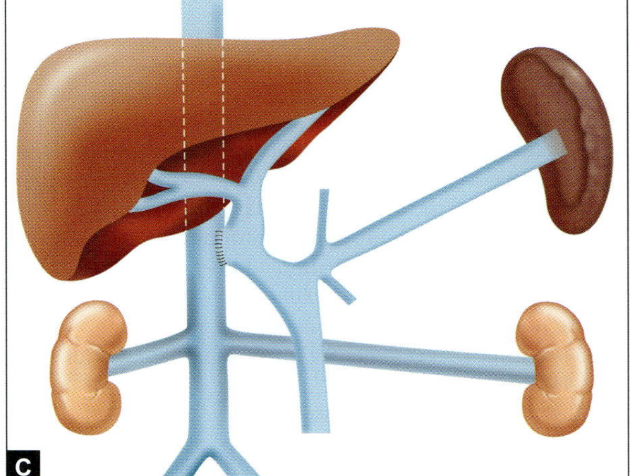

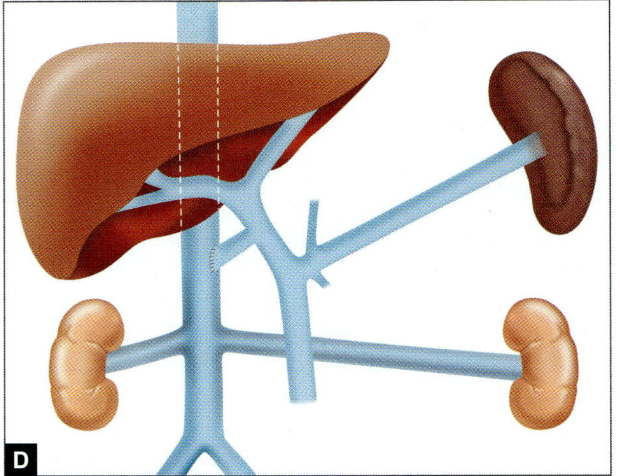

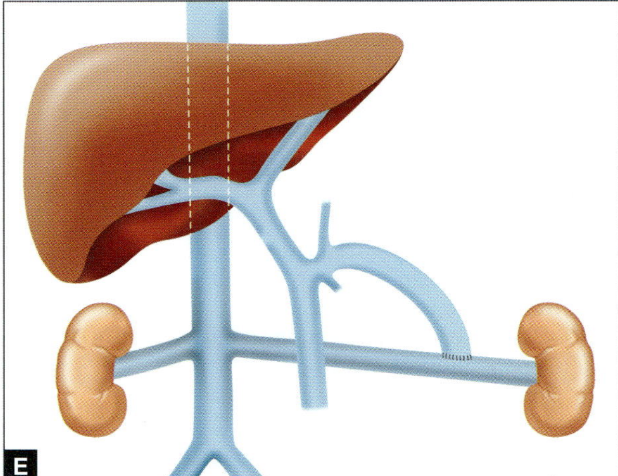

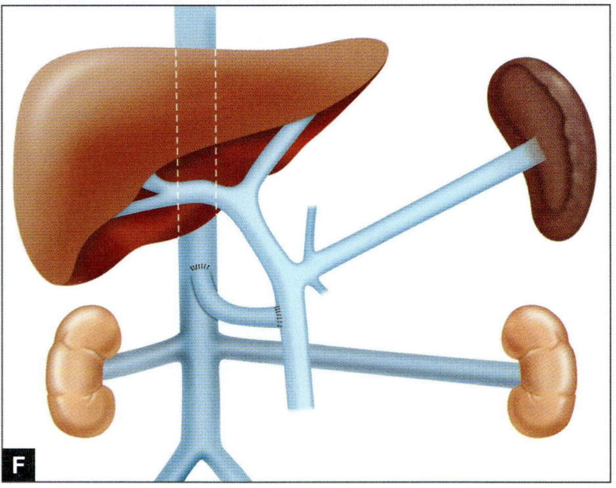

Figures 2A to F Schematic representation of nonselective portosystemic shunts: (A) Normal anatomy with labels, (B) end-to-side portacaval shunt, (C) side-to-side portacaval shunt, (D) portacaval shunt with interposition graft, (E) proximal lienorenal shunt, and (F) mesocaval shunt.
Abbreviation: IVC, inferior vena cava

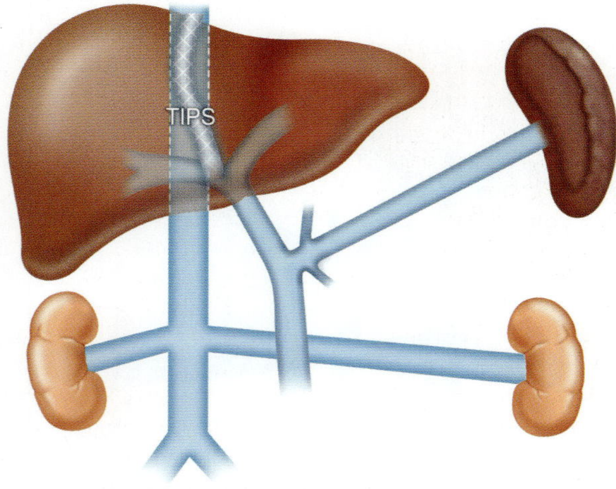

Figure 3 Schematic representation of transjugular intrahepatic portosystemic shunt

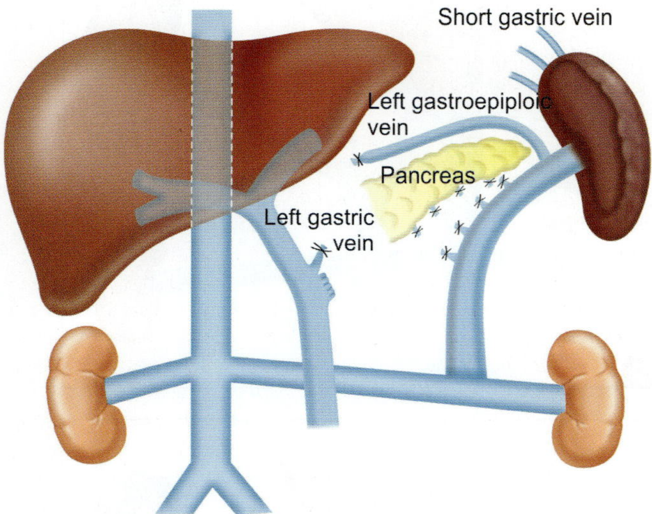

Figure 4 Schematic representation of Warren's (distal lienorenal) shunt

shunts, while patients with severe liver dysfunction may develop encephalopathy even after partial or selective shunts.

2. The risk of shunt thrombosis increases with decreasing diameter of the afferent vascular channel.
3. Patients with liver dysfunction may become candidates for liver transplantation in the future. This should be kept in mind before offering shunt surgery to these patients as any dissection around the porta hepatis would make future liver transplant surgery more difficult.
4. The relief of ascites requires decompression of the splanchnic circulation as well as the hepatic sinusoids. An end-to-side portacaval shunt does not decompress the hepatic sinusoids, while partial shunts only do so partially and thus are not effective in relieving ascites. Selective shunts do not decompress the splanchnic circulation or the sinusoids and in addition disrupt the retroperitoneal collaterals (distal lienorenal shunt) and thus may worsen the ascites.
5. A portacaval shunt may be technically difficult or impossible in patients with very large caudate lobes.
6. Lack of patency of portal or splenic veins may limit the options for shunt surgery.

INDICATIONS FOR SHUNT SURGERY

Elective:

1. Secondary prophylaxis for variceal bleeding in patients with noncirrhotic portal hypertension, for example, EHPVO and NCPF and cirrhosis with preserved liver function (Child's score: 5–7).
2. Primary prophylaxis for variceal bleeding in patients with EHPVO.

Emergency:

1. Uncontrolled acute variceal bleeding where endotherapy has failed or is not available.
2. Exsanguinating variceal bleeding not amenable to endotherapy.

PREOPERATIVE EVALUATION

The preoperative evaluation of a patient with portal hypertension being considered for surgery includes:

1. Detailed history: History of upper gastrointestinal (GI) bleeding, symptoms suggestive of liver decompensation such as jaundice, encephalopathy, ascites, spontaneous bacterial peritonitis, hepatorenal syndrome, and hepatopulmonary syndrome.
2. Physical examination: Stigmata of liver disease, icterus, dilated abdominal veins, ascites, splenomegaly, etc.
3. Diagnosis of portal hypertension:
   a. Presence of esophageal varices on upper GI endoscopy
   b. HVPG (if required)
4. Diagnosis of hypersplenism
   a. History of gum bleeding, epistaxis, menorrhagia, etc.
   b. Hemoglobin, total leukocyte count, platelet count
5. Differentiation between cirrhotic and noncirrhotic portal hypertension
   a. Liver function tests: bilirubin, albumin, transaminases, prothrombin time
   b. Ultrasound abdomen
   c. Fibroscan
   d. Liver biopsy (if required)
6. Etiology of liver disease
   a. History of alcohol intake
   b. Viral markers
   c. Autoimmune markers
   d. Iron and copper studies
7. Assessment of vascular anatomy for feasibility of shunt surgery
   a. Doppler ultrasound
   b. Computed tomography portography

OUTCOME OF SHUNT SURGERY IN PATIENTS WITH CIRRHOSIS

The outcome of shunt surgery varies according to the indication for which it was done. In general, shunt surgery is most beneficial in patients with a preserved liver function (Child's A/early B status), those with refractory variceal bleed, or in those who do not have easy access to tertiary healthcare with the availability of endoscopy or interventional radiology techniques (TIPS).

Role in Primary Prophylaxis

Controlled trials have shown that prophylactic shunt surgery in patients with cirrhosis is associated with a higher rate of liver failure despite protection from variceal bleeding.[11,12] Hence, surgery has no role in the primary prophylaxis of variceal bleeding in portal hypertension due to cirrhosis.[13,14]

Surgery for Acute Variceal Bleeding

A surgical shunt may be considered in patients with cirrhosis who are Child's A/B functional status when other modalities have failed to control the variceal bleeding, and if expertise is available.[15] In a randomized controlled trial by Orloff et al,[16] 211 patients with cirrhosis and acute variceal bleeding who required at least two units of blood transfusion were randomized to endoscopic sclerotherapy (EST; $n = 106$) or emergency portacaval shunt (EPCS; $n = 105$) within 8 hours of initial presentation. Endoscopic sclerotherapy achieved permanent control of bleeding in only 20% of patients, whereas EPCS controlled bleeding in all patients ($P \leq 0.001$). Survival after EPCS was also significantly higher at all time intervals and in all Child's classes ($P \leq 0.001$).

In case of inadequate control of variceal bleeding with pharmacotherapy and endotherapy, a Sengstaken–Blakemore tube can be used and the gastric balloon inflated for 12–24 hours. The early use of TIPS (within 72 hours) has been associated with significant reduction in treatment failure and mortality as compared with continuation of vasoactive drug therapy followed by long-term endoscopic band ligation (EBL) in patients with cirrhosis and Child's B/C functional status who were at high risk of endoscopic treatment failure for active bleeding. During a median follow-up of 16 months, rebleeding or failure to control bleeding occurred in 14 patients in the pharmacotherapy–EBL group as compared with 1 patient in the early-TIPS group ($P = 0.001$). The 1-year actuarial survival was 61% in the pharmacotherapy–EBL group versus 86% in the early-TIPS group ($P < 0.001$).[17] Since TIPS is a less invasive radiological intervention that can be performed under local anesthesia, it is generally accepted that TIPS should be preferred in patients with an acute variceal bleed refractory to endoscopic intervention. However, a surgical shunt can be life saving if TIPS fails or is not available.

Emergency shunt surgery has a higher mortality in both patients with and without cirrhosis.[15,18] Under-running of the esophagogastric varices helps in resuscitation and allows semielective shunt surgery to be done.[19,20] Patients with portal venous anatomy unsuitable for surgical shunts, those with shunt failures, and Child's B/C status with uncontrolled bleeding can be considered for devascularization procedures. Patients treated with devascularization have a lower incidence of postoperative encephalopathy compared with patients treated with a shunt but at the expense of higher rebleed rates.[21]

Role in Secondary Prophylaxis

The current recommendations for the prevention of variceal rebleeding suggest that all patients receive secondary therapy namely beta-blockers and endoscopic variceal ligation to prevent recurrent variceal bleeding.[22] Transjugular intrahepatic portosystemic shunt has been shown to give better long-term control of variceal bleeding in a number of randomized trials. A meta-analysis showed that TIPS was associated with significantly reduced risk of variceal bleeding and death due to bleeding but significantly increased risk of encephalopathy. However, EST was the modality for endoscopic treatment in the majority of studies included. Despite the improved control of bleeding, TIPS did not lead to a survival benefit.[23]

Henderson et al[24] showed excellent outcomes in patients with cirrhosis and Child's A/B status with refractory bleeding who received surgical shunts. In their series, the overall survival and rebleeding rates were 86% and 6.3%, respectively, with a median follow-up of 36 months. In a meta-analysis of all randomized clinical trials, shunt therapy had significantly less rebleeding (odds ratio, OR, 0.24, 95% confidence interval, CI, 0.18–0.30), but significantly more acute hepatic encephalopathy (OR 2.07, 95% CI 1.59–2.69) than endoscopic therapy.[25] There were no significant differences in mortality and duration of hospital stay. No survival advantage over endotherapy was demonstrated with any shunt.

The role of TIPS versus a surgical shunt for the prevention of rebleeding has been studied in a randomized clinical trial comparing the two treatments in patients who did not respond to medical therapy. No significant difference was found in rebleeding rates (5.5% for distal splenorenal shunt versus 10.5% for TIPS), encephalopathy, or survival. Patients undergoing TIPS required more interventions, although the study used uncovered stents and concluded that the two treatments were of equal efficacy in preventing recurrent variceal bleeding.[26] In a subsequent cost analysis study of the same patients, TIPS was also found to be cost-effective especially with the use of coated stents.[27]

The choice between TIPS and surgical shunts depends on the patient's hepatic reserve and timing of possible transplantation. If transplantation is expected within 1–2 years, TIPS is likely to bridge the patient to transplantation without the need for surgical intervention. However, if transplantation is unlikely to occur within 1–2 years, a surgical shunt may be needed; more than 50% of patients undergoing TIPS require reintervention within this time period.

Endoscopic treatment of varices alone will not be enough in patients with cirrhosis as they have other complications such as infections including spontaneous bacterial peritonitis, hepatorenal syndrome, and worsening liver failure, which lead to death. Reducing the portal pressure by portosystemic shunts may worsen the hepatocellular function because of the diverted portal blood flow. Hence, liver transplantation remains the only curative option in them.

OUTCOME OF SHUNT SURGERY IN PATIENTS WITH NONCIRRHOTIC PORTAL HYPERTENSION

Patients with EHPVO and NCPF, who account for 40–50% of acute variceal bleeds in India, have preserved hepatocellular function.[20] These patients are young and have moderate/massive splenomegaly. They may also have growth retardation, symptomatic hypersplenism, and may develop symptomatic portal biliopathy in the long term due to compression of the bile duct by the periportal cavernoma. Lowering the portal pressure by portosystemic shunts in these patients provides good control of variceal bleeding without the adverse effects of hepatocellular decompensation. Unlike endoscopic treatment of varices, portosystemic shunts have been shown to lead to a growth spurt and cure of symptomatic hypersplenism. These are also one-time treatment options.[28] Endoscopic eradication of esophageal varices may also lead to formation of duodenal or colorectal ectopic varices that are less accessible sites.[29]

Several studies have shown that shunts can be successfully used in children of any age with a rebleed rate <10%.[30,31] There is no evidence of altered liver function or hepatic encephalopathy after shunt surgery for EHPVO, even on long-term follow-up in a large series of patients.[19,32] Portacaval shunts cannot be done in patients with EHPVO because the portal vein is replaced by a cavernoma. A selective shunt does not provide any additional benefit as (i) post-shunt encephalopathy does not occur in EHPVO unlike in patients with cirrhosis, (ii) hypersplenism may persist in up to 40% of patients, and (iii) the distal splenorenal shunt is technically more difficult in patients with large spleens. Prasad et al.[32] in a study with 15-year follow-up after a proximal lienorenal shunt in EHPVO showed a rebleeding rate of 11%. Mortality after elective surgery was 0.7% and the 15-year survival was 95%.

Thus, although shunt surgery has gone out of favor in patients with cirrhosis, it still has an important place in the management of patients with noncirrhotic portal hypertension. Many of these patients have symptomatic splenomegaly and hypersplenism. A proximal lienorenal shunt removes the spleen in addition to effectively preventing variceal bleeding and is the most common portosystemic shunt procedure in India.

TECHNIQUE OF PROXIMAL LIENORENAL SHUNT

Position: Semiprone 30–45° left side up with the patient's right loin at the kidney bridge. A rolled towel is placed over the kidney bridge.

Incision: Left oblique, thoracoabdominal over the eighth intercostal space, crossing the midline of the abdomen at the midpoint between the umbilicus and the tip of the xiphoid.

Procedure:

1. The diaphragm is incised radially after cutting a small segment of the cartilage of the costal margin. While cutting the diaphragm, the bleeding points are caught by Allis' forceps on either side and secured later with figure-of-eight 1/0 silk stitches. They are held as stays.
2. A self-retaining chest retractor is inserted and its blades are stitched to the margins of the opening.
3. The lesser sac is opened by dividing the gastrocolic omentum from its middle toward the upper pole of the spleen.
4. The splenic artery is identified along the upper border of the pancreas and doubly ligated in continuity. The tails of the proximal tie are kept long to identify the artery easily.
5. The splenocolic ligament is incised and the retroperitoneal space entered between the layers of the lienorenal ligament and the splenic flexure. The space behind the posterior layer of the lienorenal ligament and the spleen is opened by sharp dissection and the lienorenal ligament is divided between the ligatures.
6. The spleen along with the tail of pancreas is turned to the right and the splenic vein is dissected from behind the pancreas. The small tributaries coming from the pancreas are ligated with 4/0 silk and divided. After it is mobilized all around, the vein is divided close to the hilum between 4/0 ligatures.
7. The tail of pancreas is mobilized from the splenic hilum and the rest of the structures at the hilum are divided between clips and the spleen is removed. The splenic vein is dissected for a length that is necessary for it to reach the renal vein without tension.
8. The left renal vein is identified at the renal hilum and looped with a no 1 silk held by straight clips at either end. A 2.5–3 cm length of the renal vein is dissected in order to allow safe application of a vascular clamp.
9. Lienorenal shunt: The splenic vein is held as far distally as possible with a curved vascular forceps. The anesthetist is asked to heparinise the patient. The opening in the renal vein is slightly larger than the diameter of the splenic vein by excising an elliptical piece of its wall. Two 6/0 double ended Prolene sutures are used for the anastomosis. First an outside in stitch is taken from the posterior lip of the right corner of the opening in the splenic vein and then an inside out stitch is taken on the corresponding corner of the renal vein using the other end of the Prolene suture. The next stitch is from outside in on the anterior lip of the renal vein and the final stitch is from inside out on the anterior wall of the splenic vein and the suture is tied. A similar stitch is taken on the other corner using the other Prolene suture. The posterior wall anastomosis is started from the right side with one of the strands of Prolene. The anastomosis is done using a continuous stitch taking uniform bites 1 mm apart and 1 mm from the margin. When the suture reaches the left corner, the needle is brought out on the renal vein side anteriorly and tied with one of the strands of the Prolene suture at that corner. Now one of the strands of Prolene at the left corner is used to complete the anterior wall of the anastomosis till the center. The suture on the right corner is used to reach the middle of the anterior wall from the other end. The splenic vein clamp is opened to allow clots and air to escape before a loose knot (with "growth factor") is tied in the middle of the anterior wall. The vascular clamps are taken out and a dry sponge is placed on the anastomosis till the blood stops leaking.
10. Hemostasis: The cut edges of the lienorenal ligament are oversewn and any other bleeding point in the splenic bed is suture ligated.
11. Tube drains are placed in the chest and splenic bed. The diaphragm is closed with interrupted, transverse mattress stitches taken with 2/0 Prolene. The ribs are apposed with two, interrupted, Ethibond sutures. The incision is closed using a loop nylon suture for the sheath and staples or 3/0 nylon for the skin.

COMPLICATIONS OF SHUNT SURGERY (PROXIMAL LIENORENAL SHUNT)

A shunt surgery is relatively safe in experienced hands with low complication rates in patients without liver dysfunction. However, some of the complications can be life threatening or may be associated with significant morbidity.

1. Intraoperative complications: These occur rarely and include:
   a. Life-threatening hemorrhage that can occur during mobilization of the spleen because of the presence of large collaterals or dense vascular adhesions between the spleen and the diaphragm. This complication is best avoided by meticulous hemostasis and careful dissection.
   b. Injury can occur to adjacent organs such as the stomach and colon. There may be dense adhesions between the upper pole of the spleen and fundus of the stomach especially in patients who have had glue injection for gastric varices.
2. Early postoperative:
   a. Hemorrhage that may require reoperation.

   b. Basal atelectasis and respiratory tract infection may occur as the pain associated with a thoracoabdominal incision may restrict respiratory movements. Placing an epidural catheter can provide effective pain relief but may be contraindicated if the platelet counts are low or the coagulation deranged.
   c. Ascites may occur transiently possibly due to disruption of retroperitoneal collaterals.
   d. Pancreatic, gastric, or colonic fistulae may occur due to injury to the pancreatic tail, fundus of the stomach, or splenic flexure of the colon, respectively.
3. Late postoperative
   a. Shunt-related
      i. Post-shunt encephalopathy occurs in patients with cirrhosis and may also occur in patients with NCPF but in a smaller proportion (7%). This is usually easily treated with a change in diet, good bowel movements, and the use of oral sodium benzoate. Patients with EHPVO do not develop shunt-related encephalopathy.
      ii. Rebleeding occurs in around 10% of patients. These patients may be treated with endoscopic variceal ligation. Shunt thrombosis occurs in a larger number of patients. However, all patients with shunt thrombosis do not rebleed.
      iii. Shunt nephropathy and myelopathy are rare complications that occur more commonly in patients with NCPF as compared to patients with EHPVO.
   b. Splenectomy related
      i. Overwhelming postsplenectomy infection (OPSI) is a dreaded complication and routine polyvalent vaccination has been recommended 2 weeks before splenectomy. However, in our experience, the risk of OPSI was negligible despite a policy of no vaccination.
      ii. Postsplenectomy thrombocytosis is another complication that may lead to shunt thrombosis. Patients with platelet counts>1,000,000/cmm should be treated with antiplatelet agents such as aspirin; those with counts >1,200,000/cmm should receive anticoagulants till the platelet count decreases to <1,000,000/cmm.

MESENTERICOPORTAL (REX) SHUNT

While portosystemic shunts provide only palliation of portal hypertension, a Rex shunt is considered to be a curative option. A Rex shunt is a porto-portal shunt between the superior mesenteric vein and the left branch of the portal vein (Fig. 5). It bypasses the obstruction in the portal vein and directs the blood to its normal path toward the liver. The shunt is useful only in a selected group of patients with prehepatic portal hypertension and patent portal vein branches and is used for the treatment of EHPVO in children. A retrospective study by Guerin et al.[33] found the success rate of Rex shunt to be 60% compared with 100% of a portosystemic shunt. Thus, the Rex shunt is a good option but can be offered to only some patients with EHPVO.

DEVASCULARIZATION AND OTHER NONSHUNT PROCEDURES

These procedures are more akin to endoscopic therapy in that they do not reduce the portal pressure. While the incidence of postoperative encephalopathy and hepatocellular dysfunction is

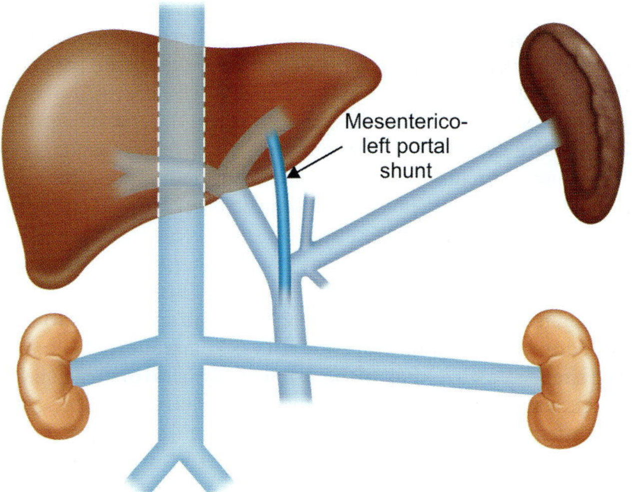

Figure 5 Schematic representation of a Rex shunt

Table 1: Nonshunt procedures for variceal bleeding

Category	*Procedure*
Direct ligation of varices	Crile's procedure Boerema's procedure
Resection procedures	Transthoracic esophagogastric resection Total gastrectomy Partial esophagogastrectomy with jejunal interposition Partial esophagogastrectomy with colonic interposition
Transection procedures	Esophageal transection Milnes Walker Johnston Gastric transection Tanner
Devascularization	Hassab's procedure Modified Hassab's procedure Sugiura and Futagawa procedure Modified Sugiura's procedure Ginsberg Hidalgo Huerta Johnson Orozco Mathur

lower, the rebleeding rates are higher than those with shunts.[21] These procedures can be broadly classified into direct ligation of varices, resection procedures, transection procedures, and devascularization procedures (Table 1). A number of nonshunt procedures have been described, but except for devascularization procedures most of the others have gone out of favor because of a high rebleed rate, high morbidity rate, or both.

DEVASCULARIZATION PROCEDURES

The gastroesophageal junction, the lower esophagus, and the upper part of the stomach are the sites responsible for most bleeding episodes in patients with portal hypertension. This is because of the presence of superficial dilated veins in these locations that act as natural portosystemic shunts and drain a significant part of the portal blood into the systemic circulation. These veins have very thin walls and thus are prone to rupture and the risk of rupture is directly proportional to the portal pressure. The devascularization procedures aim at disconnecting these veins from the portal circulation that would block the transmission of high pressure to them and thus prevent bleeding.

The devascularization procedures done presently have evolved from the procedures initially described by Hassab[34] in 1964 and by Sugiura and Futagawa[5] in 1973. Hassab's devascularization procedure included splenectomy, devascularization of the lower esophagus, the upper half of the stomach, division of the left gastric vessels, and separation of the stomach from its bed.

Sugiura and Futagawa described a two-stage (initial thoracic followed by abdominal procedure 4–6 weeks later) esophagogastric devascularization with splenectomy, sutured esophageal anastomosis as well as truncal vagotomy and pyloroplasty. They reported a very low rebleed rate of 1.5% that could not be reproduced by other centers. The thoracic part was done through the 6th or 7th intercostal space, and 30–50 perforating veins were carefully ligated along 12–18 cm of the lower esophagus. The esophageal transection was done at the level of the diaphragm where the anterior muscular and mucosal layers were divided, while the posterior layer was left intact. In the second stage, 4–6 weeks later, the abdominal part of the procedure was done starting with splenectomy, followed by devascularization along the greater curvature and cardia and then along the lesser curvature. As both vagi were divided to facilitate devascularization, a pyloroplasty was always added. Devascularization of at least 7 cm of the stomach from the cardia was considered adequate.

Various modifications of Sugiura's procedure have been reported to decrease the morbidity and achieve similar outcomes. Ginsberg et al[35] modified the procedure and did it in one stage, through the abdomen and using a subcostal incision. The esophageal transection was done using a 29 mm circular stapler unless previous sclerotherapy or thickness of the esophagus precluded its use when a 25 mm stapler was used. The pyloroplasty was done without opening the mucosa, while Nissen fundoplication was done to prevent reflux after surgery.

Another modification was described by Mathur et al[36] This entailed devascularization of the upper two-thirds of the greater and lesser curvature of the stomach, ligation of the retrogastric collaterals, transhiatal devascularization of 7–10 cm of the lower esophagus and fundoplication. Besides these essential compulsory steps, esophageal transection, subcardiac gastric stapling, under-running of gastric varices, vagal preservation or pyloroplasty/pyloromyotomy, and splenectomy or splenic artery ligation were optional steps.

INDICATIONS FOR DEVASCULARIZATION PROCEDURES

Elective:

1. EHPVO with failure of endoscopic therapy and nonshuntable anatomy
2. NCPF with symptomatic hypersplenism but a nonbleeder

Emergency:

1. Cirrhosis with active variceal bleeding and failed endoscopic management
2. EHPVO/NCPF with active variceal bleeding, failed endoscopic management, and nonshuntable anatomy

COMPLICATIONS

Procedure-related:

1. Leaks and strictures are related to esophageal transection (2–28%).
2. Postvagotomy gastric disturbances.
3. Postsplenectomy: Portal vein thrombosis could be secondary to decrease in flow or thrombocytosis with a reported rate of 1–6%.

Disease-related:

1. In patients with cirrhosis, the occurrence of decompensation depends on the Child's status.
2. Ascites occurs in 3–28% of patients and is treated with diuretics.
3. Encephalopathy does not occur in EHPVO and NCPF but may occur in patients with cirrhosis.

TECHNIQUE OF SPLENECTOMY AND DEVASCULARIZATION (MODIFIED HASSAB)

Position: Same as for proximal lienorenal shunt

Incision: Left oblique thoracoabdominal, left subcostal or midline. The operation can also be done through a Mercedes-Benz incision if the patient is old, sick, or obese.

Procedure:

1. The spleen is mobilized as described earlier in the technique of proximal lienorenal shunt and removed first. In an emergency, where the patient is actively bleeding from varices, a gastrotomy and suture ligation of bleeding varices is the first step of the procedure (Figs 6 and 7).
2. The upper half of the greater curvature gets devascularized as the short gastric vessels are divided for splenectomy. The devascularization is extended by ligating the branches of the gastroepiploic arcade near the gastric wall till the upper two-thirds of the greater curvature are devascularized.
3. The upper half of the lesser curvature of the stomach is devascularized next by ligating the vessels close to gastric wall as described for the procedure of highly selective vagotomy.
4. The left gastric vessels are ligated and divided and the stomach is separated from the pancreas. An accessory or replaced left hepatic artery if present should be preserved.
5. The gastroesophageal junction and the abdominal esophagus are mobilized next and the abdominal esophagus is looped, if possible. Usually, there are multiple collaterals around the gastroesophageal junction that should be dissected and ligated carefully. Continuous oozing from these vessels can spoil the surgical field making the subsequent steps very difficult.
6. The esophagus is then mobilized from the hiatus by dividing the phrenoesophageal membrane and the thoracic cavity is entered.
7. The lower thoracic esophagus is mobilized all around for a distance of 5 cm to complete the devascularization. An energy source such as a harmonic scalpel makes this step easier.

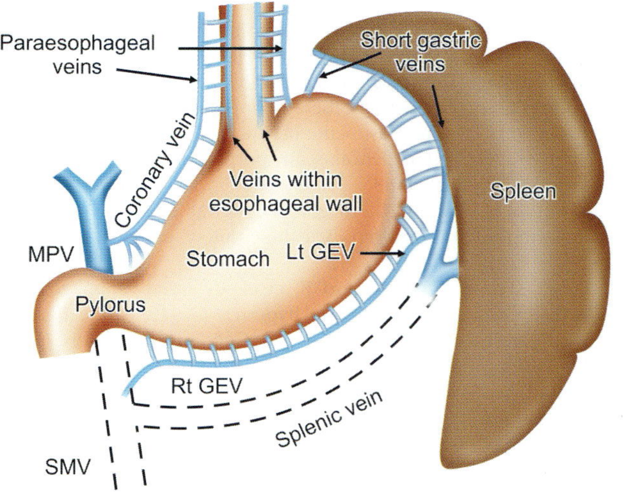

Figure 6 Schematic representation of anatomy related to esophagogastric devascularization procedures.
Abbreviations: Lt GEV, left gastroepiploic vein; MPV, main portal vein; Rt GEV, right gastroepiploic vein; SMV, superior mesenteric vein

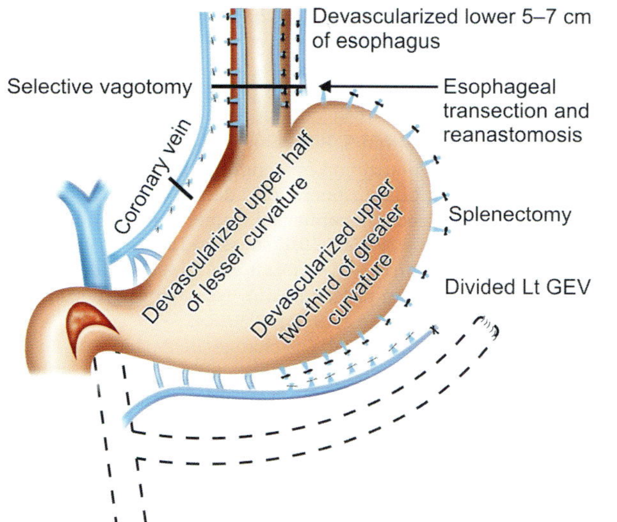

Figure 7 Schematic representation of esophagogastric devascularization procedures
Abbreviation: Lt GEV, left gastroepiploic vein

8. A pyloric stretching may be done if there is doubt regarding the integrity of the vagi.
9. Hemostasis is achieved and the incision is closed after placing tube drains in the chest and the splenic bed.

Studies have shown that esophagogastric devascularization without esophageal stapled transection was a safe and effective procedure for adequate control of variceal bleeding with similar results and lesser morbidity when compared with devascularization with esophageal transection.[37]

Orozco et al[38] showed that the no-splenectomy group had fewer blood transfusions and less postoperative portal vein thrombosis, and similar rebleeding and encephalopathy rates compared with the splenectomy group.

Contrary to other studies, Zhang et al[39] found improved hyperdynamic circulation, decreased portal venous flow, and increased hepatic artery flow after splenectomy with periesophagogastric devascularization, which resulted in short-term improvement in hepatic functional reserve.

SUMMARY

Surgery for portal hypertension has undergone a sea change over the past 3–4 decades. From a disease condition treated primarily by surgical intervention, it is presently treated with a selective approach. The liver function and cause of portal hypertension are important determinants of the best modality for the treatment of a particular patient. Patients with acute variceal bleeding are managed primarily with endoscopic therapy and pharmacotherapy with surgery being used as a salvage procedure. In patients with cirrhosis, a nonshunt procedure is a better choice, while in those with a noncirrhotic cause, a portosystemic shunt is a better procedure. Similarly, for secondary prophylaxis, noncirrhotic patients are most suitable for a portosystemic procedure, while patients with cirrhosis are better managed by nonsurgical methods.

REFERENCES

1. Whipple AO. The problem of portal hypertension in relation to the hepatosplenopathies. Ann Surg. 1945;122:449-75.
2. Grace ND, Muench H, Chalmers TC. The present status of shunts for portal hypertension in cirrhosis. Gastroenterology. 1966;50:684-91.
3. Resnick RH, Iber FL, Ishihara AM, et al. A controlled study of the therapeutic portacaval shunt. Gastroenterology. 1974;67:843-57.
4. Warren WD, Zeppa R, Fomon JJ. Selective trans-splenic decompression of gastroesophageal varices by distal splenorenal shunt. Ann Surg. 1967;166:437-55.
5. Sugiura M, Futagawa S. A new technique for treating esophageal varices. J Thorac Cardiovasc Surg. 1973;66:677-85.
6. Kumar A, Sharma P, Sarin SK. Hepatic venous pressure gradient measurement: time to learn! Indian J Gastroenterol. 2008;27:74-80.
7. Mitra SK, Rao KL, Narasimhan KL, et al. Side-to-side lienorenal shunt without splenectomy in noncirrhotic portal hypertension in children. J Pediatr Surg. 1993;28:398-401.
8. Inokuchi K. A selective portacaval shunt. Lancet. 1968;2:51-2.
9. Inokuchi K, Beppu K, Koyanagi N, et al. Fifteen years' experience with left gastric venous caval shunt for esophageal varices. World J Surg. 1984;8:716-21.
10. Sarfeh IJ, Rypins EB. Partial versus total portacaval shunt in alcoholic cirrhosis. Results of a prospective, randomized clinical trial. Ann Surg. 1994;219:353-61.
11. Burroughs AK, D'Heygere F, McIntyre N. Pitfalls in studies of prophylactic therapy for variceal bleeding in cirrhotics. Hepatology. 1986;6:1407-13.
12. Jackson FC, Perrin EB, Smith AG, et al. A clinical investigation of the portacaval shunt. II. Survival analysis of the prophylactic operation. Am J Surg. 1968;115:22-42.
13. Sarin SK, Kumar A, Angus PW, et al. Primary prophylaxis of gastroesophageal variceal bleeding: Consensus recommendations of the Asian Pacific Association for the Study of the Liver. Hepatol Int. 2008;2:429-39.

14. The Veterans Affairs Cooperative Variceal Sclerotherapy Group. Prophylactic sclerotherapy for esophageal varices in men with alcoholic liver disease. A randomized, single-blind, multicenter clinical trial. N Engl J Med. 1991;324:1779-84.
15. de Franchis R, Baveno VF. Revising consensus in portal hypertension: Report of the Baveno V consensus workshop on methodology of diagnosis and therapy in portal hypertension. J Hepatol. 2010;53:762-8.
16. Orloff MJ, Isenberg JI, Wheeler HO, et al. Randomized trial of emergency endoscopic sclerotherapy versus emergency portacaval shunt for acutely bleeding esophageal varices in cirrhosis. J Am Coll Surg. 2009;209:25-40.
17. Garcia-Pagan JC, Caca K, Bureau C, et al. Early use of TIPS in patients with cirrhosis and variceal bleeding. N Engl J Med. 2010;362:2370-9.
18. Bosch J, Berzigotti A, Garcia-Pagan JC, et al. The management of portal hypertension: Rational basis, available treatments and future options. J Hepatol. 2008;48 Suppl 1:S68-92.
19. Pande GK, Reddy VM, Kar P, et al. Operations for portal hypertension due to extrahepatic obstruction: results and 10 year follow up. Br Med J. 1987;295:1115-17.
20. Rao TH, Pande GK, Sahni P, et al. The management of upper gastrointestinal haemorrhage in a tropical country. Arch Emerg Med. 1991;8:169-76.
21. Ezzat FA, Abu-Elmagd KM, Aly MA, et al. Selective shunt versus nonshunt surgery for management of both schistosomal and nonschistosomal variceal bleeders. Ann Surg. 1990;212:97-108.
22. Garcia-Tsao G, Sanyal AJ, Grace ND, et al. Prevention and management of gastroesophageal varices and variceal hemorrhage in cirrhosis. Hepatology. 2007;46:922-38.
23. Zheng M, Chen Y, Bai J, et al. Transjugular intrahepatic portosystemic shunt versus endoscopic therapy in the secondary prophylaxis of variceal rebleeding in cirrhotic patients: Meta-analysis update. J Clin Gastroenterol. 2008;42:507-16.
24. Henderson JM, Nagle A, Curtas S, et al. Surgical shunts and TIPS for variceal decompression in the 1990s. Surgery. 2000;128:540-7.
25. Khan S, Tudur Smith C, Williamson P, et al. Portosystemic shunts versus endoscopic therapy for variceal rebleeding in patients with cirrhosis. Cochrane Database Syst Rev. 2006;4:CD000553.
26. Henderson JM, Boyer TD, Kutner MH, et al. Distal splenorenal shunt versus transjugular intrahepatic portal systematic shunt for variceal bleeding: a randomized trial. Gastroenterology. 2006;130:1643-51.
27. Boyer TD, Henderson JM, Heerey AM, et al. Cost of preventing variceal rebleeding with transjugular intrahepatic portal systemic shunt and distal splenorenal shunt. J Hepatol. 2008;48:407-14.
28. Kato T, Romero R, Koutouby R, et al. Portosystemic shunting in children during the era of endoscopic therapy: Improved postoperative growth parameters. J Pediatr Gastroenterol Nutr. 2000;30:419-25.
29. Sarin SK, Agarwal SR. Extrahepatic portal vein obstruction. Semin Liver Dis. 2002;22:43-58.
30. Bismuth H, Franco D, Alagille D. Portal diversion for portal hypertension in children. The first ninety patients. Ann Surg. 1980;192:18-24.
31. Orloff MJ, Orloff MS, Girard B, et al. Bleeding esophagogastric varices from extrahepatic portal hypertension: 40 years' experience with portal-systemic shunt. J Am Coll Surg. 2002;194:717-28; discussion 728-30.
32. Prasad AS, Gupta S, Kohli V, et al. Proximal splenorenal shunts for extrahepatic portal venous obstruction in children. Ann Surg. 1994;219:193-6.
33. Guerin F, Bidault V, Gonzales E, et al. Meso-Rex bypass for extrahepatic portal vein obstruction in children. Br J Surg. 2013;100:1606-13.
34. Hassab MA. Gastroesophageal decongestion and splenectomy. A method of prevention and treatment of bleeding from esophageal varices associated with bilharzial hepatic fibrosis: Preliminary report. J Int Coll Surg. 1964;41:232-48.
35. Ginsberg RJ, Waters PF, Zeldin RA, et al. A modified Sugiura procedure. Ann Thorac Surg. 1982;34:258-64.
36. Mathur SK, Shah SR, Nagral SS, et al. Transabdominal extensive esophagogastric devascularization with gastroesophageal stapling for management of noncirrhotic portal hypertension: long-term results. World J Surg. 1999;23:1168-74.
37. Johnson M, Rajendran S, Balachandar TG, et al. Transabdominal modified devascularization procedure with or without esophageal stapler transection—an operation adequate for effective control of a variceal bleed. Is esophageal stapler transection necessary? World J Surg. 2006;30:1507-18; discussion 1519.
38. Orozco H, Mercado MA, Martinez R, et al. Is splenectomy necessary in devascularization procedures for treatment of bleeding portal hypertension? Arch Surg. 1998;133:36-8.
39. Zhang Y, Wen T, Yan L, et al. The changes of hepatic hemodynamics and functional hepatic reserve after splenectomy with periesophagogastric devascularization. Hepatogastroenterol. 2009;56:835-9.

CHAPTER 125

Ethics in Surgery

Sanjay Nagral

INTRODUCTION

The field of medical ethics (Greek *ethos*, behavior) broadly deals with moral values as they apply to medicine. As an academic discipline, it covers its practical application to clinical settings as well as the relevant history, philosophy, and sociology. On a practical level, knowledge of the accepted ethical framework in a particular social context can help in dealing with day-to-day dilemmas that medical practitioners face. From this perspective, it is useful for practitioners of the surgical science to be aware of the relevant ethical concerns and consensus.

The idea of an ethical code for practitioners of medicine is perhaps as old as the profession itself. Western medical ethics may be traced back to historical guidelines stipulated by Hippocrates and early Christian teachings. By the 18th century, medical ethics has crystallized into a definite subject. In England, Thomas Percival, a physician wrote the first modern code of medical ethics in 1803 in which he coined the expressions "medical ethics" and "medical jurisprudence."[1] In 1847, the American Medical Association adopted its first code of ethics based mainly on Percival's work.[2] Various bodies in countries across the world later came up with their own versions of ethical codes.

The wide acceptance of these ethical codes was a tacit understanding with the society, wherein medicine obtained social recognition as a profession and in turn it agreed to regulate its practice within certain ethical tenets. Historically, what is rather unique to this profession, the idea of self-regulation was largely accepted by the society and the state. The British model of medical councils largely controlled by the profession itself was also inherited by us in India.

A common and widely acceptable framework used in contemporary medical ethics is based on the "four principles" stipulated by Beauchamp and Childress in their textbook "Principles of Biomedical Ethics."[3] It identifies four basic principles, namely:

- Beneficence—a practitioner should primarily act in the best interest of the patient.
- Non-maleficence—"first, do no harm."
- Autonomy—the patient has the right to refuse or choose their treatment.
- Justice—fair distribution of scarce health resources including ensuring equality.

Another concept that emerged very early as a cardinal principle was "informed consent." This refers to the notion that a person (in this case a patient) must be explicitly informed about and made to appreciate potential benefits and risks in the treatment, that the patient is offered or opts for. Informed consent, it does not only mean the process of obtaining consent or the legal requirements for eligibility or capability to consent which vary from place to place. Patients can make their own medical decisions, or can authorize another person to make decisions. Informed consent is closely related to the value of autonomy and is also a continuous process in the doctor patient interaction.

Another term called bioethics was first coined in 1926 by Fritz Jahr, in an article about the "bioethical imperative," as he called it, regarding the scientific use of animals and plants.[4] The field of bioethics is now much broader than medical ethics. Issues such as palliative care, abortion, euthanasia which talk about end of life, allocation of scarce health care resources, and individual's right to refuse any treatment for any reason including religious or cultural, have been discussed more often in bioethics than medical ethics. The two fields often overlap and the distinction is in a sense superfluous. Whatever the terminology, there is no doubt however that the scope of current ethical debate has moved well beyond the confines of the doctor patient relationship to include areas like human rights and health care policy.

The growing influence of ethics in contemporary medicine has influenced institutional review boards (IRB) to evaluate experiments on human subjects critically and also has led to increasing role of clinician ethicists and the integration of ethics into medical school curricula.

DISTINCTION BETWEEN ETHICS AND LAW

A fundamental distinction needs to be made between the ideas of "medical ethics" and "medical law" or the more commonly used term "medico legal". Although there is a significant overlap between the two areas, legality refers to the narrow field of the laws of the land, whereas ethics goes much beyond that. What is deemed legal by the state may not be considered ethical by the profession and *vice versa*. For example, the participation of medical professionals in torture and execution of prisoners maybe perfectly "legal" in many countries, but many large professional bodies have called upon its members not to participate in such activities as they have deemed it "unethical". A more contemporary example familiar to Indian readers would be the phenomenon of "commissions" or "fee splitting." While this has not yet been declared illegal, it is certainly considered unethical partly by consensus as also by the ethics guidelines of the Medical Council of India (MCI).

INDIAN SCENARIO

Medicine in India is marked by a wide variety of practitioners as well as systems of medicine. Also, there are huge geographical, cultural, and socioeconomic disparities. Although the situation is slowly changing, the practice of medicine in India is still largely unregulated. Although India's access to scientific ideas and technology has vastly improved, there is a deficit in structures, processes, and protocols. The major issue in healthcare in India has been its paradigm shift from public health provider to private healthcare industry.[5] In the last decade, the private healthcare sector has grown greatly in all dimensions. Medical education, until a few decades back entirely in the public sector, has also slowly moved into the hands of the private sector, both at the undergraduate and postgraduate levels. The pharmaceutical and medical equipment industries also have grown and now exert significant influence over the medical profession and on the public too.

In the last decade, we have also witnessed the entry of a new group of market players generating their own dynamics in what is now perhaps more aptly termed the "healthcare industry."[5]

This includes corporate hospitals, especially hospital chains, international tie-ups, the medical tourism sector, clinical research organizations, and insurance companies. These new forces are especially relevant to a high-end super speciality discipline like surgical gastroenterology. The economic liberation has led to the availability of the latest technology that has helped both the equipment industry and the Pharmaceutical industry. Pharmaceutical companies are in a position to dictate medical opinion with money and power. This has led to the emergence of new ideas, special emphasis on areas of specialization, new developments driven by an alliance of industry, media and sections of the profession are spring up periodically. A classic example of this is the emergence of bariatric surgery as a niche speciality, as well as a market for obesity control as a quick fix for what is really a lifestyle disease.

The changing paradigm of healthcare is affecting healthcare workers and their outlook.[5] Private healthcare industry is in the practice of setting income targets for its employees, pay employees in the same organization differently as per income generated, and even terminate its employees including doctors at short notice. Turf wars between corporate hospitals and between big corporate hospitals and small hospitals have become open, and there is poaching of "salable doctors." There is a "no holds barred" advertising by the industry. On the other hand, there is growing discontent in civil society about what are perceived as "unethical" practices, which has manifested in increasing litigation in courts.

In many countries of the world, self-regulation is performed by quasi-judicial medical councils and professional associations acting as peer groups in maintaining the profession's credibility. Unfortunately, both these forms have been less than active in India, and have partly lost their credibility both in the public eye as well as amongst medical professionals. It may be pertinent to note that as a result of this inaction and also as a response to media and public anger, we have seen increasing judicial intervention in areas, which should have been internally regulated. The Pre-Natal Diagnostic Techniques Act and the Human Organs Transplant Act are examples of such interventions.[5]

There are some aspects of contemporary health care practice in India, which need urgent ethical debate and action. For example, it would be reasonable to say that today a large majority of referrals from family physicians to specialists, cross referrals between specialists, and from doctors to diagnostic centers, etc. involve some kind of a kickback. If cash transactions without due receipts or transparency constitute corruption in any trade, then this aspect demands either self-regulation or state intervention. But beyond that it is also a matter of ethics, which the profession needs to debate and act upon.

The MCI has a set of ethics guidelines for its members.[6] The MCI is a qausi-judicial body, and its code, though not law, is ethically binding on all practitioners of modern medicine in India. The code has been periodically amended and now covers a wide range of areas. It also has an ethics committee, which looks at specific complaints. State medical councils are also active in most states. Professional medical associations in India have, however, been found wanting in developing guidelines concerning important ethical areas in their speciality. For example, the Association of Surgeons of India has not gone beyond token discussion on issues of significant ethical dilemmas for practising surgeons. The Indian Association of Surgical Gastroenterology, which is, now recognized as the leading body in this discipline made a small beginning by debating ethical case scenarios in its annual conferences, a few years back. However, it also has still to formally address and evolve guidelines on pertinent issues like live donor liver transplantation an area that is an ethical quagmire.

WHY SHOULD SURGICAL ETHICS BE ADDRESSED SEPARATELY?

Surgery is intrinsically an invasive intervention with significant potential for grievous injury and harm. It involves the almost total submission by an individual to a surgeon's control during the perioperative period. It is potentially intimidating and often sudden. In this sense, it makes special demands on the surgeon to recognize and respect ethical principles at every stage. Also, there are new complex situations, which have emerged with the evolution of the scope of surgery in the last few decades. Thus, although the basic overarching principles remain applicable to surgery, there are several specific areas which deserve special discussion. The following part of this chapter attempts to highlight some of these areas.

INFORMED CONSENT IN THE CONTEXT OF SURGERY

The extent, detail, and methodology of informed consent for surgical intervention have naturally been the subjects of intense discussion. For example, the extent of disclosure of complications during the consent process is an area needing clarity. For example, should all patients undergoing cholecystectomy be informed about the small but definite risk of bile duct injury? Should this disclosure vary based on the patients' cultural background? Should the figures for complication rates that are quoted be from international data or local data? Is bile duct injury negligence or an acceptable complication? Is there a case for compensation? While some of these questions are complex and border on the medico legal, the nature of consent and extent of disclosure are in the realm of good ethical practice and can be standardized.

In the context of a surgical training program, is it ethically necessary to inform the patient that the surgery would be performed by a junior or a trainee? If so does the patient have a right to insist that the senior surgeon does the procedure? Should the same parameters be applied to a patient in the public sector and the private sector? If not, is this a case of discrimination, an issue being increasingly recognized as an ethical imperative?

There can be no rigid standardization of informed consent. But if contested in law, the basic principles of complete, documented disclosure in a language the patient understands would be tested.

For example, in the performance of major procedure like a pancreatoduodenectomy the possibility of postoperative mortality, morbidity as well the fact that tumor has a significant chance of recurrence would constitute an acceptable genuine informed consent.

INNOVATIVE SURGERY

Surgery is inherently a field which lends itself to innovation often for the advancement of science, and in the interest of the patient. Thus the use of a new surgical technique, a new technology, or even a new protocol is often necessary, but raises questions of special consent and experimentation. The extent of disclosure (you are the first patient we are going to try this technique on!) is important. The reuse of disposables, a common practice in the Indian scenario also raises ethical concerns.[7] By and large, the guiding principles include respect for the other person, due consideration of a risk-benefit ratio in favor of the patient, and clear intention to do only what appears to be justifiable in a given situation.[8]

END OF LIFE AND WITHDRAWAL OF CARE

Although this area is relevant to the entire field of medical care, our ability to treat and prolong life with complex interventions and intensive care now regularly brings up serious ethical dilemmas in this area, in the practice of surgical gastroenterology. Thus, for example, what should be the approach to a very elderly patient with advanced colorectal malignancy who presents with a perforation, and is likely to be on one hand at very high risk for the procedure and on the other need the creation of a stoma? Is there a case for withholding care and letting the patient die? Should it be dictated by the patients' wishes or of the family members? Can the patients' views in this situation be considered acceptable?

Or in another example, how should we approach a young patient who presents with extensive gangrene of almost the entire small bowel as a result of mesenteric vascular disease? When we understand that resection of the entire small bowel is almost certainly going to lead to a slow and miserable death which may also lead to financial devastation are we justified in withholding the resection, and in turn hasten death? In other words, what are the ethical parameters under which a form of passive euthanasia is acceptable?

There is a vast amount of literature in the ethics discourse, which deals with these issues. The ethical principles of autonomy and justice are invoked in this context, and well-structured protocols for withdrawal or withholding of care have evolved. In fact some countries have gone on to extend the scope of active euthanasia.

However, the confounding factors of treatment costs, cultural beliefs and, multiple players in the family make the situation more complicated in India. The case for national or institutional guidelines in the Indian scenario is therefore very strong. The issue of euthanasia was extensively debated in India in the context of the Aruna Shanbaug case. The debate in India is confounded by the issue of cost of healthcare. No definite policy seems to have emerged from the churning.[9] Till then, all of us will have to use personal judgment keeping in mind sound ethical principles to deal with individual cases.

ORGAN TRANSPLANTATION AND LIVER TRANSPLANTATION

The field of organ transplantation is an ethical minefield. The success of transplantation as a lifesaving procedure in a strange way has also led to some of the fiercest ethical challenges in modern medicine. The number of patients desperately needing a transplant far outnumbers the available organs. This inevitably leads to a competition for organs, which in turn severely tests the principles of transparency and distributive justice.

In the field of surgical gastroenterology in India, liver transplantation has seen tremendous strides in the last few years. While this is a good development from the viewpoint of those suffering and dying from end-stage liver disease, it has led to the inevitable ethical questions. Although the activity in the field of deceased donation in India is still minimal, questions about fair distribution of the organs have already come up. Ensuring distributive justice in a scenario where only the rich can afford a transplant mainly in the private sector is in itself an ethical challenge.

In addition, the eternal question of whether the organ should go to the sickest patient, (who is likely to have a bad result but needs it the most) or the fittest patient (who is likely to have the best result but can wait) is also relevant. Organ sharing protocols in some of the active states are currently varied, but do not go by the justice-based principle of the most deserving first.

In response to the shortage of deceased-donor organs, living donor liver transplantation has grown exponentially and is now the predominant form of liver transplantation in India. While this has significantly increased the number of procedures, it has thrown up a different set of ethical challenges.[10] The foremost among these is the potential threat to the life of the living donor, which is inherent in what is an extremely major surgical procedure. The nature of the informed consent, the inherent pressures of being asked to save the life of a close relative sometimes in an emergency scenario, and familial or social pressures to donate have all been the subject of intense debate across the world.

The nature and power relations in the Indian family often result in a disproportionately high number of female donors. There have been some reported donor deaths in India,[11] but an unknown number of donor deaths have not been reported. The lack of a national registry to record donor mortality and morbidity further compounds the problem. There have been calls both in the deceased and living donor settings to legalize some form of incentives to the donor. This is of course in stark contradiction to the various international consensus ethical guidelines in transplantation, which have unequivocally opposed the idea of incentivization and paid donation.

A detailed discussion of the ethical dilemmas confronting liver transplantation is beyond the scope of this chapter, but it needs to be mentioned that this is one area of surgery where our ethical foundations and clarity will continue to be severely tested.

CLINICAL TRIALS

There has been a tremendous growth in the number of clinical trials being conducted in India. Although some of this is a result of increased interest in scientific documentation and research, a large number of these trials are a result of the outsourcing industry, and its recent interest in India as a fertile ground for human subjects. A growing number of clinical research organizations now act as the link between the pharmaceutical industry and clinicians.

The very basis for this sudden arrival of the clinical trial industry to India has been questioned for its sociopolitical bias,[12] wherein the use of Indian patients as guinea pigs has been questioned. In the actual performance of these trials questions about the nature of the consent, violation of safety protocols, and compensation in case of severe injury have already come up for discussion both in legal cases as well as media exposes. The functioning of institutional review boards has also been under scrutiny.

A recent amendment of the MCI addresses industry-sponsored research.[13] It recommends that researchers ensure that the particular research proposal has due permission from the competent concerned authorities including clearance of national, state or institutional ethics committees. It also recommends that the researcher ensures that the source and amount of funding is publicly disclosed at the beginning of the project, and that proper care and facilities are provided to human volunteers, if they are necessary for the research. Finally, the guidelines state that, while accepting such an assignment a medical practitioner shall have the freedom to publish the results of the research in the greater interest of society by inserting such a clause in the document for the assignment. Although all these areas (and their violations) have been highlighted by health activists, these guidelines coming from the MCI will have added weight.

RELATIONSHIP WITH PHARMACEUTICAL AND EQUIPMENT INDUSTRY

Throughout the world, the relationship between the pharmaceutical industry and the medical profession has come under the ethical scanner. Both in the context of marketing tactics as well as sponsored research, there have been numerous well-documented attempts at inappropriate influencing of physician behavior.[14] Attempts by the industry at changing physician prescription habits by influencing content in conferences, journals, and medical association guidelines are well known. However, it is direct bribing by sponsorship of activities such as paid holidays that have exploded onto the public domain. The response of the medical profession to such controversy has been variable, but in some countries national medical organizations have come out with codes of conduct for their members. The American Medical Association in its code of ethics has a separate section dealing with gifts to physicians from the industry, which explicitly details what is acceptable and what is not.[14] In the UK, both the General Medical Council in its "good medical practice'" document as well as the British Medical Association have laid down guidelines on the issue. From the industry side, the International Federation of Pharmaceutical Manufacturers and Associations has a detailed code in place which was modified in 2007. The Organization of Pharmaceutical Producers of India has also adopted a modified version of this code. The medical profession and its associations in India have, unfortunately, been largely silent on the subject.

There is good evidence to suggest that gifting and hospitality by the pharma industry does influence prescription habits. A large review of published articles from 1994 onwards concluded that meetings with pharmaceutical representatives were associated with requests by physicians for adding the drugs to the hospital formulary and changes in prescribing practice. Attending sponsored continuing medical education events and accepting funding for travel or lodging for educational symposia were associated with increased prescription rates of the sponsor's medication.[14]

The MCI in another amendment to its existing code of conduct, the Indian Medical Council (professional conduct, etiquette, and ethics) regulations 2002, has proposed sweeping guidelines on the relationship between the pharmaceutical industry and the medical profession in India.[15] This is an attempt at a code of ethical conduct for doctors and professional associations in their relationship with the pharmaceutical and allied health sector industry. The impact of these guidelines on ground reality remains to be seen, but if recent news items are to be believed, by doing so the MCI has at the least succeeded in breaking the conspiracy of silence that surrounded this issue in India. The guidelines also cover clinical trials sponsored by the industry, an area of current relevance. Following the initial guidelines, the MCI has now gone a step further by announcing a list of punishments which are graded based on the financial quantum of the gift received.

The MCI code now specifically prohibits practitioners from accepting gifts, travel facilities, hospitality, and monetary grants from the healthcare industry either in their name or in the names of their family members. It also bars doctors and their family members from accepting rail or air travel facilities, cruise tickets, hospitality, and paid vacations from the industry. The guidelines are much more specific on these issues than on many others because they actually do not leave room for interpretation of what is often termed "reasonable hospitality."[15]

SURGICAL WORKSHOPS

"Live surgical workshops," where operative procedures are beamed "live" to an audience from the operating room, has arrived on the scene with a bang in the past few years. Many surgical conferences in India and abroad are now dominated by such sessions. There have been several ethical concerns raised about the conduct of such workshops.[16]

The main concern is about the patient's involvement and consent for the process. Is the patient clearly told that she/he will be the subject of a "live" demonstration by a visiting faculty in front of a large audience? And that the operating surgeon is unlikely to be available to deal with postoperative complications, if they arise? How often does the person performing the procedure himself explain the procedure to the patient and family? Are the principles of a proper informed consent respected in the setting of such workshops? There is, therefore, a larger ethical issue that this debate raises. What ground rules should govern the use of patients in the learning process? To quote from an editorial in the journal gastrointestinal endoscopy by the well-known endoscopist, Peter Cotton[17] "How detailed is the informed consent process? How many experts have declined to do a procedure because they cannot see a good indication when confronted with the patient on the table, and an expectant audience? How many experts check on key environmental factors that they take for granted at home—such as local practices for disinfection, antibiotic prophylaxis, sedation, and monitoring. If it appears that the local practices are different, should you insist on your own standards or bend them for the benefit of 'the show'? If you compromise at all, how does this square with being an expert teacher? The pressure to do what the organizer wants and to 'succeed' can be substantial. It takes real courage to 'fail' on camera or to desist when the benefit–risk ratio appears inadequate—indeed to behave totally responsibly, especially when jetlagged and well entertained." In a letter to a leading national journal a few years ago a senior surgical gastroenterologist from India listed some shocking examples of what he thought were gross ethical transgressions in the conduct of such workshops in India. This is one area of ethical debate where there is still complete deficit of opinion/guidelines from any organization or association in India.

Thus, the scope and nature of the discourse of medical ethics is rapidly changing. It has a special relevance to the surgical discipline not only to the surgical procedure, but a wide gamut of related fields. Although the Indian healthcare scenario is culturally different from that of the West, in some areas it is beginning to resemble the developed world. Should the current parameters and consensus on ethics, which largely originate in the Western world, be applied *in toto* to medical practice in India? This is a complex question with no easy answers. A vibrant Indian ethics movement which derives relevant ideas from the global movement and modifies them to suit local conditions is urgently needed. One positive sign in this direction is the increasing amount of writing on the subject in India. Worthy of mention in this regard is the Indian Journal of Medical Ethics which started as a small publication in 1993 has now evolved into a full-fledged indexed and reputed journal. Senior members of the surgical fraternity in India are regularly writing on issues related to ethics in professional journals.[8] That a book like this chooses to include a chapter on ethics is also welcome evidence of this phenomenon.

REFERENCES

1. Percival T. Medical ethics. John Henry Parker; 1849. pp. 49-57.
2. Berlant J. Profession and Monopoly: a study of medicine in the United States and Great Britain. University of California Press; 1975. ISBN 0-520-02734-5.
3. Gillon R. "Medical ethics: four principles plus attention to scope". BMJ. 1994;309:184-8. doi:10.1136/bmj.309.6948.184.
4. Goldim JR. Revisiting the beginning of bioethics: the contributions of Fritz Jahr (1927). Perspect Biol Med. 2009;52:377-80.
5. Nagral S. Ethics, equity and justice: a view from the belly of the beast. Indian J Med Ethics. 2011;8(1):9-12.
6. http://www.mciindia.org/RulesandRegulations/Code of Medical EthicsRegulations2002.aspx. Accessed on June 6, 2014.
7. Hussain M, Balsara KP, Nagral S. Reuse of single-use devices: looking back, looking forward. Natl Med J India. 2012;25(3):151-5.
8. Kaushik SP. Ethics in surgical practice: an Indian viewpoint. Natl Med J India. 2002;15(1):34-6.
9. Nagral S. Euthanasia cost factor is a worry. http://timesofindia.indiatimes.com/home/sunday-toi/all-that-matters/Euthanasia-cost-factor-is worry/articleshow/7690155.cms
10. Nagral S. A deceased-donor liver transplant program must precede a living-donor program. Indian J Gastroenterol. 2006;25(6):302-4.
11. Reddy MS, Narasimhan G, Cherian PT, et al. Death of a living liver donor: opening Pandora's box. Liver Transpl. 2013;19(11):1279-84.
12. Kietinun S, Gupte MD, Sengupta A. A clinical trial in a developing country: many questions, few answers. Issues Med Ethics. 2003;11(3):89-90.
13. Code of Ethics Regulations, 2002. Medical Council of India, amendment Notification, New Delhi, the 10th December, 2009. http://mciindia.org/know/rules/ethics.htm. Accessed on February 2, 2010.
14. Nagral S, Roy N. The Medical Council of India guidelines on industry-physician relationship: breaking the conspiracy of silence. Natl Med J India. 2010;23(2):69-71.
15. Available from: http://www.mciindia.org/Rules-and Regulation/Gazette%20Notifications%20-%20Amendments/Ethics%20-%20 10.12.2009.pdf. Accessed on June 6, 2014.
16. Nagral S. Live operative workshops: a critique. Natl Med J India. 2004;17(2):100-2.
17. Cotton PB. Live endoscopy demonstrations are great, but... Gastrointest Endosc. 2000;51(5):627-9.

Appendix

GENERAL

1. *Cockcroft and Gault creatinine clearance (CrCl):*

   $$\text{CrCl (mL/min)} = \frac{N \times [\text{140-age (years)}] \times \text{weight}^* \text{(kg)}}{\text{Serum creatinine (micromol/L)}}$$

   Where N = 1.23 males, 1.04 females

   IBW (kg) = (no of inches over 5 ft × 2.3) + 50 (male) or 45.5 (female)

   The formula given is for GFR which is not same as creatinine clearence
2. Fractional excretion of Na^+ = Urine Na^+ × serum Cr/urine Cr × serum Na^+ × 100%
3. Anion gap = Na^+ to (Cl^- + HCO_3^-) normal value 8-12 mEq/L
4. Sodium deficit = TBW (total body water) × (140 – serum sodium)

   TBW = Male, 0.6 × lean body weight
   Female, 0.5 × lean body weight
5. Water deficit = ([Plasma Na concentration – 140]/140) × total body water
6. HCO_3^- deficit (mmol/L) = Body weight × 0.4 × (desired HCO_3^- measured HCO_3^-)
7. Postoperative replacement calculation
   - *Carbohydrate:* 2.75 gm/kg/day
   - *Sodium:* 1-2 mmol/kg
   - *Potassium:* 0.5-1 mmol/kg/day
   - *Calcium:* 0.2-0.3 mEq/kg
   - *Magnesium:* 0.35-0.45 mEq/kg
8. Plasma osmolarity (mOsm/kg) = 2[Na^+] + [Glucose]/18 + [BUN]/2.8

   Intracellular fluid = 2/3 TBW

   Extracellular fluid (ECF) = 1/3 TBW
   ECF = Intravascular (1/3) + interstitial (2/3)
   Interstitial fluid = 3/4 ECF
   Plasma = 1/4 ECF
   Whole blood = 75 mL/kg
   Intracellular fluid = 2/3 TBW

   Maintenance fluid calculations
   100 mL/kg for the first 10 kg
   50 mL/kg for the second 10 kg
   20 mL/kg for each subsequent 10 kg
9. Body fluid composition (mEq/L)

Fluid	*Na^+*	*Cl^-*	*K^+*	*HCO_3^-*	*H^+*	*Volume (L/day)*
Saliva	30–60	15–40	20	15–50	–	0.5–1.5
Gastric	60–100	90–140	10	–	30–100	1–4
Duodenum	140	80	5	50	–	1–3
Bile	140	100	5	50	–	0.5–1.5
Pancreas	140	75	5	90	–	1
Jejunum	100	100	5	10		1–2
Ileum	130	110	10	30		1–2
Colon	60	40	30	20	–	–

10. Composition of commonly used intravenous fluids (mEq/L)

Fluid	*Na*	*Cl*	*K*	*Ca*	*Base*	*Glucose*	*pH*	*mOsm/L*
Ringer's lactate (Hartmann's)	130	109	5	2	28	0	6.5	277
Normal saline (0.9% NaCl)	154	154	0	0	0	0	5.0	292
5% Dextrose	0	0	0	0	0	50	4.0	274

Contd...

*Use ideal body weight (IBW) if actual weight is greater than 120% IBW

Contd...

Fluid	*Na*	*Cl*	*K*	*Ca*	*Base*	*Glucose*	*pH*	*mOsm/L*
5% Dextrose and Normal saline (DNS)	154	154	0	0	0	50	5.0	565
5% Albumin	154	154	0	0	0	0	7.0	310
Hetastarch	154	154	0	0	0	60	5.5	300
Plasmalyte	140	98	5	0	27	0	5.0	294

11. Grades of abdominal hypertension

Degree of hypertension	Mesenteric pressure
Normal pressure	5–7 mm Hg
Grade 1 hypertension	12–15 mm Hg
Grade 2 hypertension	16–20 mm Hg
Grade 3 hypertension	21–25 mm Hg
Grade 4 hypertension	>25 mm Hg

12. Clavien-Dindo grading system for the classification of surgical complications

Definition	
Grade I:	Any deviation from the normal postoperative course without the need for pharmacological treatment or surgical, endoscopic and radiological interventions. Allowed therapeutic regimens are: drugs as antiemetics, antipyretics, analgetics, diuretics and electrolytes and physiotherapy. This grade also includes wound infections opened at the bedside.
Grade II:	Requiring pharmacological treatment with drugs other than such allowed for grade I complications. Blood transfusions and total parenteral nutrition are also included.
Grade III:	Requiring surgical, endoscopic or radiological intervention
Grade IIIa:	Intervention not under general anesthesia
Grade IIIb:	Intervention under general anesthesia
Grade IV:	Life-threatening complication (including CNS complications: brain hemorrhage, ischemic stroke, subarachnoid bleeding, but excluding transient ischemic attacks) requiring IC/ICU management.
Grade IVa:	Single organ dysfunction (including dialysis)
Grade IVb:	Multiorgan dysfunction
Grade V:	Death of a patient
Suffix 'd':	If the patients suffers from a complication at the time of discharge, the suffix "d" (for 'disability') is added to the respective grade of complication. This label indicates the need for a follow-up to fully evaluate the complication.

13. Unit conversions
    Pressure: 1 mm Hg = 0.735 cm H_2O
    1 cm H_2O = 1.36 mm Hg
    Serum bilirubin: 1 mg/dL = 17.1 μmol/L
    Blood sugar: 1 mmol/L = 18 mg/dL

BILIARY SYSTEM

1. Milwaukee classification system of Sphincter of Oddi dysfunction
   Type 1:
   - Pancreatobiliary pain *and*
   - Elevated liver or pancreatic biochemistries *and*
   - Dilated bile or pancreatic duct *and*
   - [Delayed drainage of contrast on endoscopic retrograde cholangiopancreatography (ERCP)]

   Type 2:
   - Pancreatobiliary pain and
   - Elevated liver or pancreatic biochemistries or
   - Dilated bile or pancreatic duct or
   - [Delayed drainage of contrast on ERCP]

   Type 3:
   - Pancreatobiliary pain *only*
2. Modified Alonso-Lej classification of choledochal cyst
   Type 1: Solitary fusiform extrahepatic cyst
   Type 2: Extrahepatic supraduodenal diverticulum
   Type 3: Intraduodenaldiverticulum; choledochocele
   Type 4a: Fusiform extra- and intrahepatic cysts
   Type 4b: Multiple intrahepatic cysts
   Type 5: Multiple intrahepatic cysts; Caroli disease
3. Bismuth classification of biliary stricture
   1. *Low common hepatic duct stricture:* hepatic duct stump >2 cm
   2. *Proximal common hepatic duct stricture:* hepatic duct stump <2 cm
   3. *Hilar stricture with no residual common hepatic duct:* hepatic duct confluence intact
   4. *Destruction of hepatic duct confluence:* right and left hepatic ducts separated
   5. Involvement of aberrant right sectoral hepatic duct alone or with concomitant stricture of the common hepatic duct.
4. Hinchey's classification of left colonic diverticulitis
   Stage I: Pericolic or mesenteric abscess
   Stage II: Walled-off pelvic abscess
   Stage III: Generalized purulent peritonitis
   Stage IV: Generalized fecal peritonitis

LIVER

1. Model for end-stage liver disease (MELD) score: $0.957 \times \log_e(\text{serum creatinine}) + 0.378 \times \log_e(\text{serum bilirubin}) + 1.12 \times \log_e(\text{INR}) + 0.643$
2. Pediatric end-stage liver disease (PELD) score = $0.480 \log(\text{bilirubin mg/dL}) + 1.857 \log(\text{INR}) + 0.687 \times \log(\text{albumin g/dL})$
   Stage liver disease (PELD) score =

$$\frac{0.436, \text{ if patient} <1 \text{ year of age}}{0.667, \text{ if growth failure } (\leq 2 \text{ standard deviations})}$$

Multiply the score by 10 and round to the nearest whole number. Lab values less than 1 are set to 1 for the purpose of MELD calculation.

3. Stages of encephalopathy
   I Irritability, altered sleep cycles
   II Disorientation, asterixis
   III Confusion, somnolence
   IV Coma
4. Modified Barcelona Clinic Liver Cancer staging system.
   Very early stage: Single hepatocellular carcinoma (HCC) mass <2 cm, carcinoma *in situ*
   Early stage: 1 HCC or 3 nodules ≤3 cm,
   Intermediate stage: No portal vein thrombosis, multinodular
   Advanced stage: Portal invasion, metastases
   Terminal stage
5. Milan criteria
   Offer transplantation to patients with
   1 lesion <5 cm
   2 to 3, none >3 cm
   Absence of macroscopic vascular invasion
   Absence of extrahepatic spread
6. University of California San Francisco (UCSF) criteria
   Offer transplantation to patients with
   Single tumor less than 6.5 cm
   Fewer than three tumors, the total diameter of all being less than 8 cm and the largest tumor less is than 4.5 cm
   Absence of macroscopic vascular invasion
   Absence of extrahepatic spread
7. American Association for the Surgery of Trauma (AAST) liver injury scale
   I. Hematoma Subcapsular, nonexpanding <10 cm surface area
   Laceration Capsule tear, nonbleeding <1 cm depth
   II. Hematoma Subcapsular, nonexpanding 10–50% surface area
   Intraparenchymal nonexpanding <10 cm diameter
   III. Hematoma Subcapsular, >50% surface area or expanding, ruptured
   Laceration <3 cm depth (parenchyma)
   IV. Hematoma Ruptured intraparenchymal hematoma with active bleeding
   Laceration Parenchymal disruption 25–75% of lobe
   V. Laceration <75% parenchymal disruption
   Vascular Juxtahepatic venous injury
   VI. Vascular Hepatic avulsion
8. Child–Pugh classification

	Score		
Parameter	1	2	3
Bilirubin (mg/dL)	<2	2–3	>3
Albumin (g/dL)	>3.5	2.8–3.5	<2.8
Ascites	Absent	Moderate	Severe
Encephalopathy	Absent	Moderate	Severe
Prothrombin time			
Seconds prolonged	<4	4–6	>6
International normalized ratio (INR)	<1.7	1.7–2.3	>2.3

Grade A: 5–6 points
Grade B: 7–9 points
Grade C: 10–15 points

In primary, sclerosing cholangitis and primary biliary cirrhosis, the bilirubin level upper limit for class 1 is 4 mg/dL and upper limit for class 2 is 10 mg/dL reflecting the fact that these diseases feature high conjugated bilirubin levels.

PANCREAS

1. *Classification of postpancreatectomy hemorrhage:* International Study Group of Pancreatic Surgery

Grade	*Time of onset, location, severity, clinical impact*	*Clinical condition*	*Diagnostic consequence*	*Therapeutic consequence*
A	Early, intra- or extraluminal, mild	Well	Observation, blood count, ultrasonography, computed tomography (CT)	No
B	Early,intra or extraluminal, severe Late, intra or extraluminal, mild	Often well/ intermediate; very rarely life-threatening	Observation, blood count, ultrasonography (USG), CT, angiography, endoscopy	Transfusion, intensive care unit (ICU), Therapeutic endoscopy, embolization, relaparotomy for early postpancreatectomy hemorrhage (PPH)
C	Late, intra or extraluminal, severe	Severely impaired, life-threatening	Angiography, CT, endoscopy	Localization of bleeding, angiography, and embolization, endoscopy, Relaparotomy

2. Criteria for grading pancreatic fistula – International study group definition

Criteria	*No fistula*	*Grade A fistula*	*Grade B fistula*	*Grade C fistula*
Drain amylase	<3 times normal serum amylase	>3 times normal serum amylase	>3 times normal serum amylase	>3 times normal serum amylase
Clinical condition	Well	Well	Often well	Ill/bad
Specific treatment	No	No	Yes/no	Yes
USG/CT	Negative	Negative	Negative/positive	Positive
Persistent drainage >3 weeks	No	No	Usually yes	Yes

Contd...

Contd...

Criteria	*No fistula*	*Grade A fistula*	*Grade B fistula*	*Grade C fistula*
Signs of infection	No	No	Yes	Yes
Readmission	No	No	Yes/no	Yes/no
Sepsis	No	No	No	Yes
Reoperation	No	No	No (percutaneous intervention)	Yes
Death	No	No	No	Yes

3. *Classification of delayed gastric emptying (DGE):* International Study Group definition

Grade	*Nasogastric tube (NGT) required*	*Unable to take solid oral intake by postoperative day (POD)*	*Vomiting/ gastric distension*	*Use of prokinetics*
A	4–7 days, reinsertion >POD3	7	+−	+−
B	7–14 days, reinsertion >POD7	14	+	+
C	>14 days, reinsertion >POD14	21	+	+

4. Ranson's prognostic criteria for non-gallstone pancreatitis

At presentation:
- Age >55 years
- Blood glucose level >200 mg/dL
- WBC >16,000 cells/mm^3
- Lactate dehydrogenase level >350 IU/L
- Aspartate aminotransferase >250 IU/L

After 48 hours of admission
- Hematocrit: Decrease >10%
- Serum calcium level <8 mg/dL
- Base deficit >4 mEq/L
- Blood urea nitrogen level[†]: Increase >5 mg/dL
- Fluid requirement >6 L
- PaO_2 <60 mm Hg

Ranson score ≥3 defines severe pancreatitis.

Ranson's prognostic criteria for gallstone pancreatitis

At presentation
- Age >70 years
- Blood glucose level >220 mg/dL
- WBC >18,000 cells/mm^3
- Lactate dehydrogenase level >400 IU/L
- Aspartate aminotransferase level >250 IU/L

After 48 hours of admission
- Hematocrit: Decrease >10%
- Serum calcium level <8 mg/dL
- Base deficit >5 mEq/L
- Blood urea nitrogen level[†]: Increase >2 mg/dL

* As compared with admission value.
† As compared with admission value.

- Fluid requirement >4 L
- PaO_2: Not available

Ranson score ≥3 defines severe pancreatitis.

5. Computed tomography severity index (CTSI) for acute pancreatitis

Feature	*Points*
Pancreatic inflammation	
Normal pancreas	0
Focal or diffuse pancreatic enlargement	1
Intrinsic pancreatic alterations with peripancreatic fat inflammatory changes	2
Single fluid collection/or phlegmon	3
Two or more fluid collections or gas, in or adjacent to the pancreas	4
Pancreatic necrosis	
None	0
≤30%	2
30–50%	4
>50%	6

CTSI, 0–3, mortality 3%, morbidity 8%; CTSI, 4–6, mortality 6%, morbidity 35%; CTSI, 7–10, mortality 17%, morbidity 92%.

6. Revised Atlanta classification of fluid collections in acute pancreatitis

The revised Atlanta classification distinguishes an early phase (1st week) in which clinical parameters determine treatment from a later phase (after the 1st week) in which treatment is determined on the basis of clinical parameters and morphologic criteria defined by CT.

Severe acute pancreatitis is defined in the first phase as organ failure lasting more than 48 hours or death; and during the second phase, as persistent organ failure, death, or complications resulting from acute pancreatitis.

Fluid collections are defined by presence or absence of necrosis and infection:

acute peripancreatic fluid collections (in the first 4 weeks without necrosis),

pseudocysts (encapsulated fluid collections after 4 weeks, without necrosis),

acute necrotic collections (ANCs; in first 4 weeks, with necrosis),

walled-off necrosis (WON; encapsulated collections after 4 weeks, with necrosis).

Intraparenchymal fluid collections due to pancreatitis are referred to as ANCs or WONs, not as pseudocysts.

ANC, acute necrotic collection; APFC, acute peripancreatic fluid collection; WON, walled-off necrosis.

7. Rosemont consensus-based endoscopic ultrasound features for diagnosis of chronic pancreatitis

Parenchymal features

Major A criteria
- Hyperechoic foci with postacoustic shadowing

Major B criteria
- Honeycombing lobularity*

Minor criteria

- Hyperechoic, nonshadowing foci ≥3 mm in length and width
- Lobularity including three or more noncontiguous lobules in the body or tail
- Pancreatic cysts ≥2 mm in short axis
- At least three strands*

Ductal features

Major A criteria

- Main pancreatic duct calculi†

Minor criteria

- Irregular main pancreatic duct contour
- Dilated side branches‡
- Main pancreatic duct dilation (≥3.5 mm in the body or ≥1.5 mm in the tail)
- Hyperechoic main pancreatic duct margin >50% of the main pancreatic duct in the body and tail*

Diagnosis of chronic pancreatitis

Consistent chronic pancreatitis

- One major A criteria + three or more minor criteria
- One major A criteria + major B criteria
- Two major A criteria

Suggestive of chronic pancreatitis¶

- One major A criteria + less than three minor
- Major B criteria + three or more minor criteria
- Five or more minor criteria

Indeterminate chronic pancreatitis¶

- 3–4 minor criteria in the absence of major
- Major B criteria + less than three minor criteria

Normal

- Fewer than three minor criteria

8. American Association for the Surgery of Trauma Pancreatic Injury Grading

Grade		*Description*
I	Hematoma	Minor contusion without ductal injury
	Laceration	Superficial laceration without ductal injury
II	Hematoma	Major contusion without ductal injury or tissue loss
	Laceration	Major laceration without ductal injury or tissue loss
III	Laceration	Distal transaction or pancreatic parenchymal injury without ductal injury
IV	Laceration	Proximal transection or pancreatic parenchymal injury involving the ampulla
V	Laceration	Massive disruption of the pancreatic head

‡The presence of calculi in the main pancreatic duct, regardless of its the location, is the most predictive finding of chronic pancreatitis.

§Defined as at least three tubular anechoic structures, each one ≥1 mm in width, budding from the main pancreatic duct.

¶With suggestive and indeterminate chronic pancreatitis, the diagnosis needs to be confirmed with another imaging modality.

ESOPHAGUS AND STOMACH

1. Savary–Miller scoring of esophageal injury in gastroesophageal reflux disease (GERD)
   1. Indicates erythema
   2. Linear ulceration
   3. Confluent ulceration
   4. Stricture
2. Three phases of tissue injury from alkali ingestion

Phase	*Tissue injury*	*Onset*	*Duration*	*Inflammatory response*
1.	Acute necrosis	1–4 days	1–4 days	Coagulation of intracellular proteins Inflammation
2.	Ulceration and granulation	3–5 days	3–12 days	Tissue sloughing Granulation of ulcerated tissue bed
3.	Cicatrization and scarring	3 weeks	1–6 months	Adhesion formation Scarring

3. Endoscopic grading and treatment of corrosive esophageal and gastric burns

Degree of burn	*Endoscopic evaluation*	*Treatment*
First degree	• Mucosal hyperemia • Edema	• 48-hour observation • Acid suppression
Second degree	• Limited hemorrhage • Exudates • Ulceration • Pseudomembrane formation	• Aggressive IV resuscitation • IV antibiotics • Acid suppression
Third degree	• Mucosal sloughing • Deep ulcerations • Massive hemorrhage • Complete luminal obstruction • Charring • Perforation	• Inhaled steroids • Fiberoptic intubation (if needed)

4. Gastric ulcer types

Type	*Location*	*Acid level*
I	Lesser curve at incisura	Low to normal
II	Gastric body with duodenal ulcer	Increased
III	Prepyloric	Increased
IV	High on lesser curve	Normal
V	Anywhere	Normal, Nonsteroidal anti-inflammatory drug (NSAID-induced)

5. Forrest classification for endoscopic findings and rebleeding risks in peptic ulcer disease

Grade	*Description*	*Rebleeding risk*
Ia	Active, pulsatile bleeding	High
Ib	Active, nonpulsatile bleeding	High
IIa	Nonbleeding visible vessel	High
IIb	Adherent clot	Intermediate
IIc	Ulcer with black spot	Low
III	Clean, nonbleeding ulcer bed	Low

6. Grouping of regional lymph nodes (Groups 1–3) by location of primary tumor in stomach

Lymph node		*Location of primary tumor in stomach*		
Station (no.)	*Description*	*Upper third*	*Middle third*	*Lower third*
1	Right paracardial	1	1	2
2	Left paracardial	1	3	M
3	Lesser curvature	1	1	1
4sa	Short gastric	1	3	M
4sb	Left gastroepiploic	1	1	3
4d	Right gastroepiploic	2	1	1
5	Suprapyloric	3	1	1
6	Infrapyloric	3	1	1
7	Left gastric artery	2	2	2
8a	Anterior comm. hepatic	2	2	2
8p	Posterior comm. hepatic	3	3	3
9	Celiac artery	2	2	2
10	Splenic hilum	2	3	M
11p	Proximal splenic	2	2	2
11d	Distal splenic	2	3	M
12a	Left hepatoduodenal	3	2	2
12b, p	Posterior hepatoduodenal	3	3	3
13	Retropancreatic	M	3	3
14v	Superior mesenteric vein	M	3	2
14a	Superior mesenteric artery	M	M	M
15	Middle colic	M	M	M
16a1	Aortic hiatus	3	M	M
16a2, b1	Para-aortic, middle	M	3	3
16b2	Para-aortic, caudal	M	M	M

COLON

1. Clinical criteria for hereditary nonpolyposis colorectal cancer (HNPCC)

Amsterdam criteria

At least three relatives with colon cancer and all of the following:
- One affected person is a first-degree relative of the other two affected persons
- Two successive generations affected
- At least one case of colon cancer diagnosed before age 50 years
- FAP excluded

Modified Amsterdam criteria

Same as the Amsterdam criteria, except that cancer must be associated with HNPCC (colon, endometrium, small bowel, ureter, renal pelvis) instead of specifically colon cancer

Bethesda criteria

The Amsterdam criteria or one of the following:
- Two cases of HNPCC-associated cancer in one patient, including synchronous or metachronous cancer
- Colon cancer and a first-degree relative with HNPCC-associated cancer and/or colonic adenoma (one case of cancer diagnosed before age 45 years and adenoma diagnosed before age 40 years)
- Colon or endometrial cancer diagnosed before age 45 years
- Right-sided colon cancer that has an undifferentiated pattern (solid, cribriform) or signet-cell histopathologic characteristics diagnosed before age 45 years
- Adenomas diagnosed before age 40 years

2. Modified Spigelman classification for staging duodenal polyposis in FAP patients

Variable/points	*1*	*2*	*3*
Polyp number	1–4	5–20	>20
Polyp size (mm)	1–4	5–10	>10
Histology	Tubular	Tubulovillous	Villous
Dysplasia	Low		High grade

3. Vienna classification of Crohn's disease

Age at diagnosis (year) A1: <40
A2: >40
Behavior B1: Nonstricturing, nonpenetrating
B2: Stricturing
B3: Penetrating
Location L1: Terminal ileum
L2: Colon
L3: Ileocolon
L4: Upper gastrointestinal tract

Index

Page numbers followed by *f* refer to figure, *fc* to flow chart and *t* refer to table

A

B

D

E

H

I

J

K

L

M

P

Q

R

S

T

U

V

W

X

Z